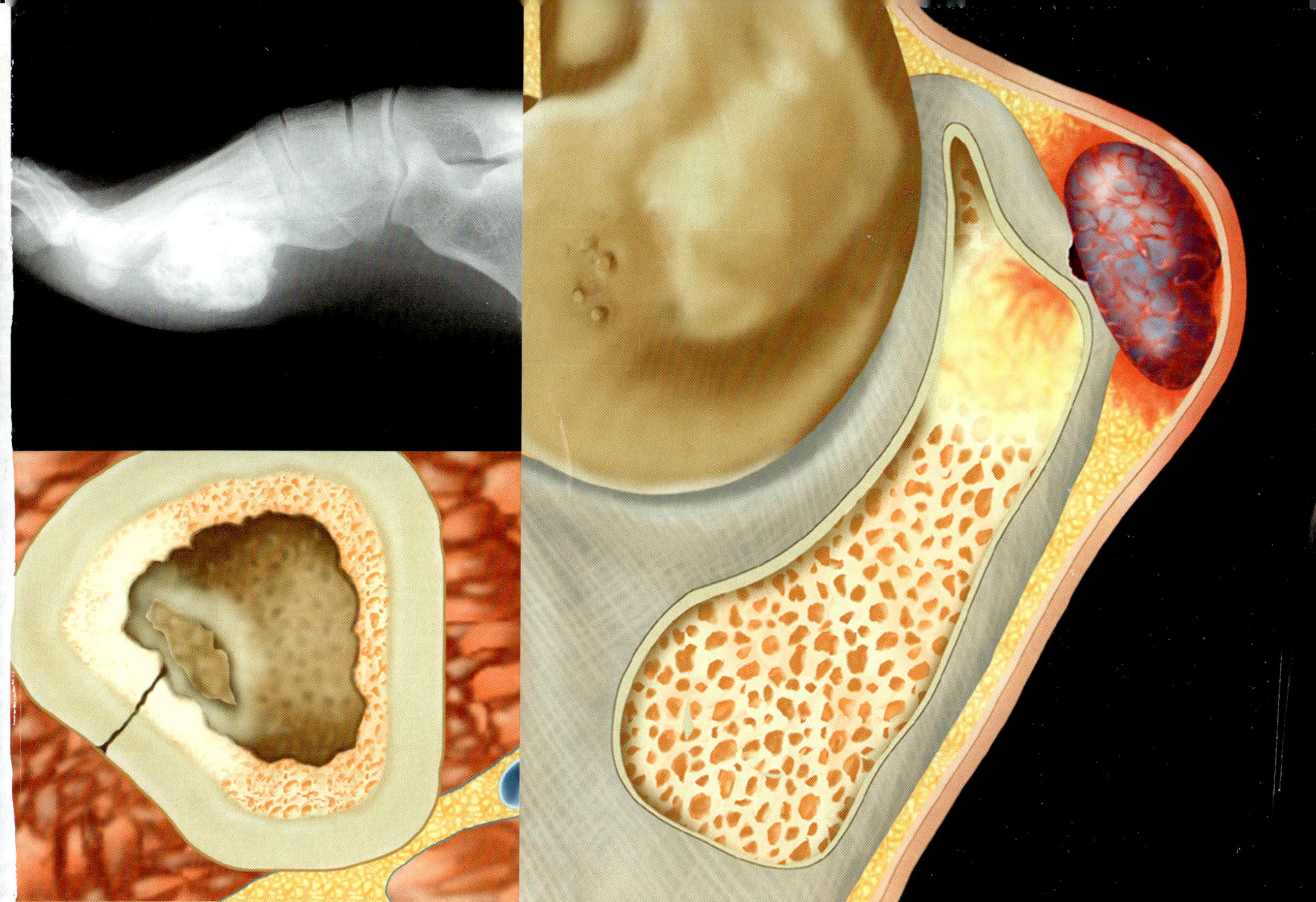

Diagnostic Imaging

Musculoskeletal Non-Traumatic Disease

SECOND EDITION

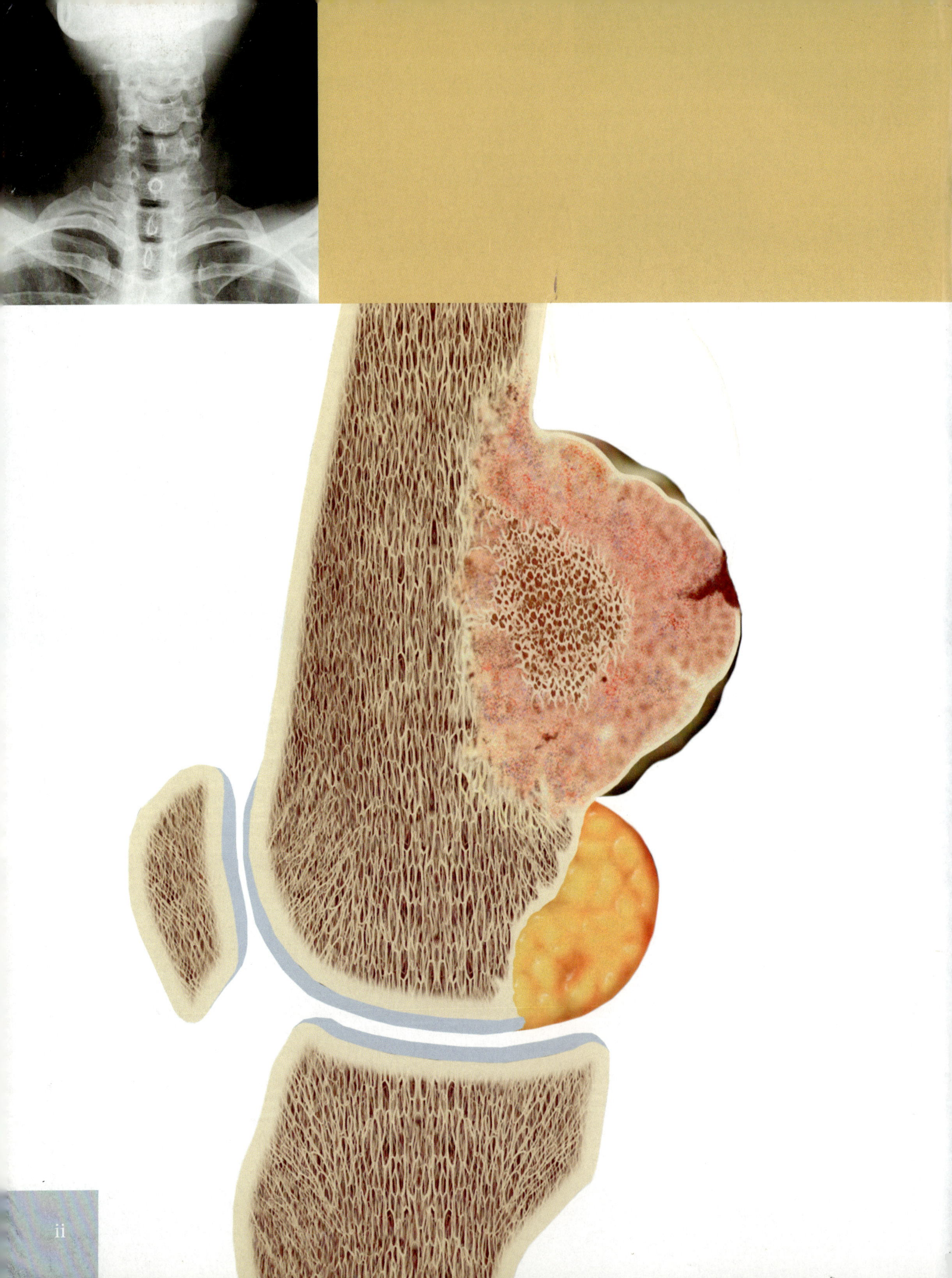

Diagnostic Imaging

Musculoskeletal Non-Traumatic Disease

SECOND EDITION

B.J. Manaster, MD, PhD, FACR

Emeritus Professor
Department of Radiology
University of Utah School of Medicine
Salt Lake City, Utah

ELSEVIER

1600 John F. Kennedy Blvd.
Ste 1800
Philadelphia, PA 19103-2899

DIAGNOSTIC IMAGING: MUSCULOSKELETAL: NON-TRAUMATIC DISEASE, SECOND EDITION ISBN: 978-0-323-39252-5

Notices

Knowledge and best practice in this field are constantly changing. As new research and experience broaden our understanding, changes in research methods, professional practices, or medical treatment may become necessary.

Practitioners and researchers must always rely on their own experience and knowledge in evaluating and using any information, methods, compounds, or experiments described herein. In using such information or methods they should be mindful of their own safety and the safety of others, including parties for whom they have a professional responsibility.

With respect to any drug or pharmaceutical products identified, readers are advised to check the most current information provided (i) on procedures featured or (ii) by the manufacturer of each product to be administered, to verify the recommended dose or formula, the method and duration of administration, and contraindications. It is the responsibility of practitioners, relying on their own experience and knowledge of their patients, to make diagnoses, to determine dosages and the best treatment for each individual patient, and to take all appropriate safety precautions.

To the fullest extent of the law, neither the Publisher nor the authors, contributors, or editors, assume any liability for any injury and/or damage to persons or property as a matter of products liability, negligence or otherwise, or from any use or operation of any methods, products, instructions, or ideas contained in the material herein.

Publisher Cataloging-in-Publication Data

Names: Manaster, B. J.
Title: Diagnostic imaging. Musculoskeletal : non-traumatic disease / [edited by] B.J. Manaster.
Other titles: Musculoskeletal : non-traumatic disease.
Description: Second edition. | Salt Lake City, UT : Elsevier, Inc., [2016] | Includes bibliographical references and index.
Identifiers: ISBN 978-0-323-39252-5
Subjects: LCSH: Musculoskeletal system--Imaging--Handbooks, manuals, etc. | MESH: Musculoskeletal Diseases--diagnosis--Atlases. | Musculoskeletal System--radiography--Atlases. | Diagnostic Imaging--methods--Atlases.
Classification: LCC RC925.5.D537 2016 | NLM WE 39 | DDC 616.7'0754--dc23

International Standard Book Number: 978-0-323-39252-5

Cover Designer: Tom M. Olson, BA
Cover Art: Laura C. Sesto, MA

Printed in Canada by Friesens, Altona, Manitoba, Canada

Last digit is the print number: 9 8 7 6 5 4 3 2 1

Dedication

This book is dedicated to all my family members, colleagues, and students. I have learned much from each of you and treasure the association.

BJM

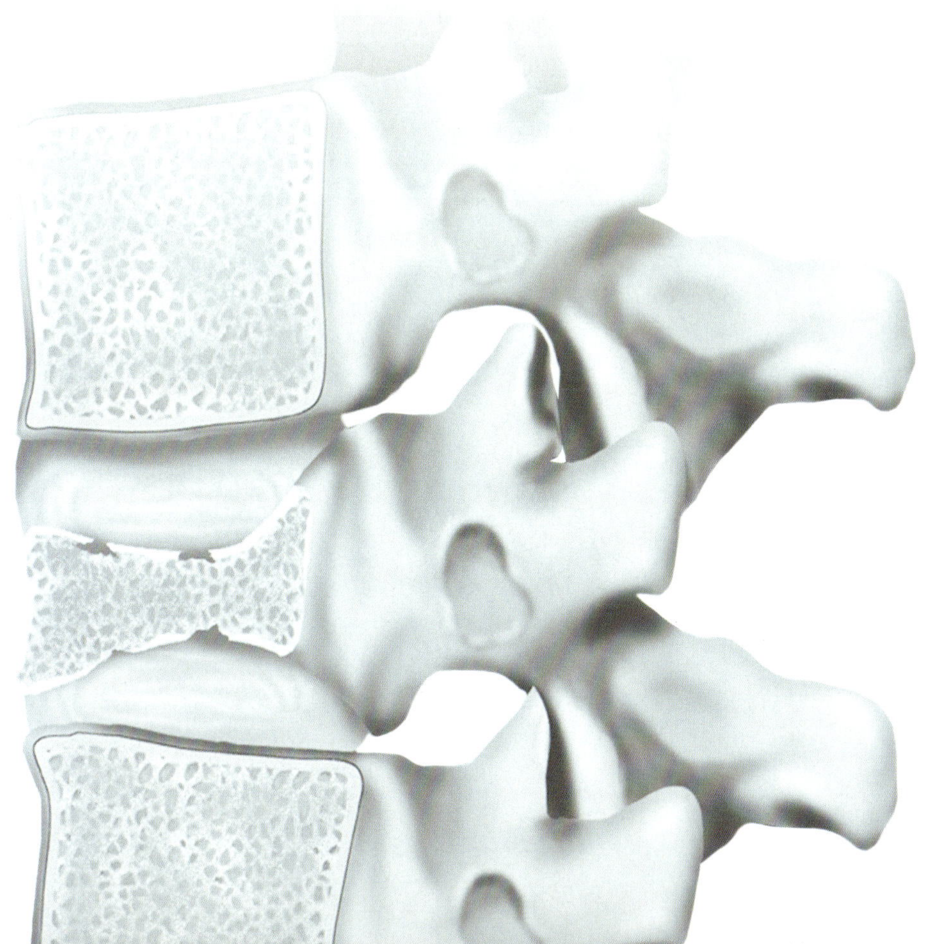

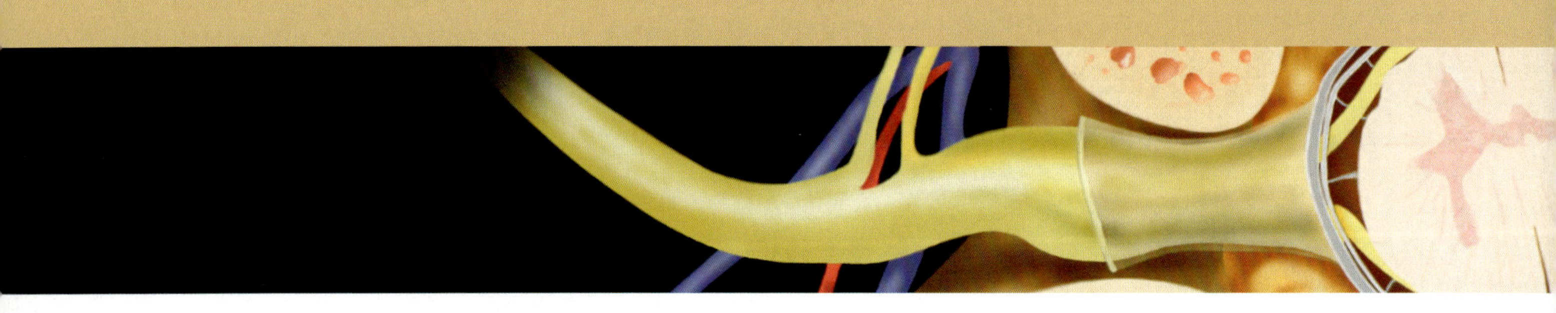

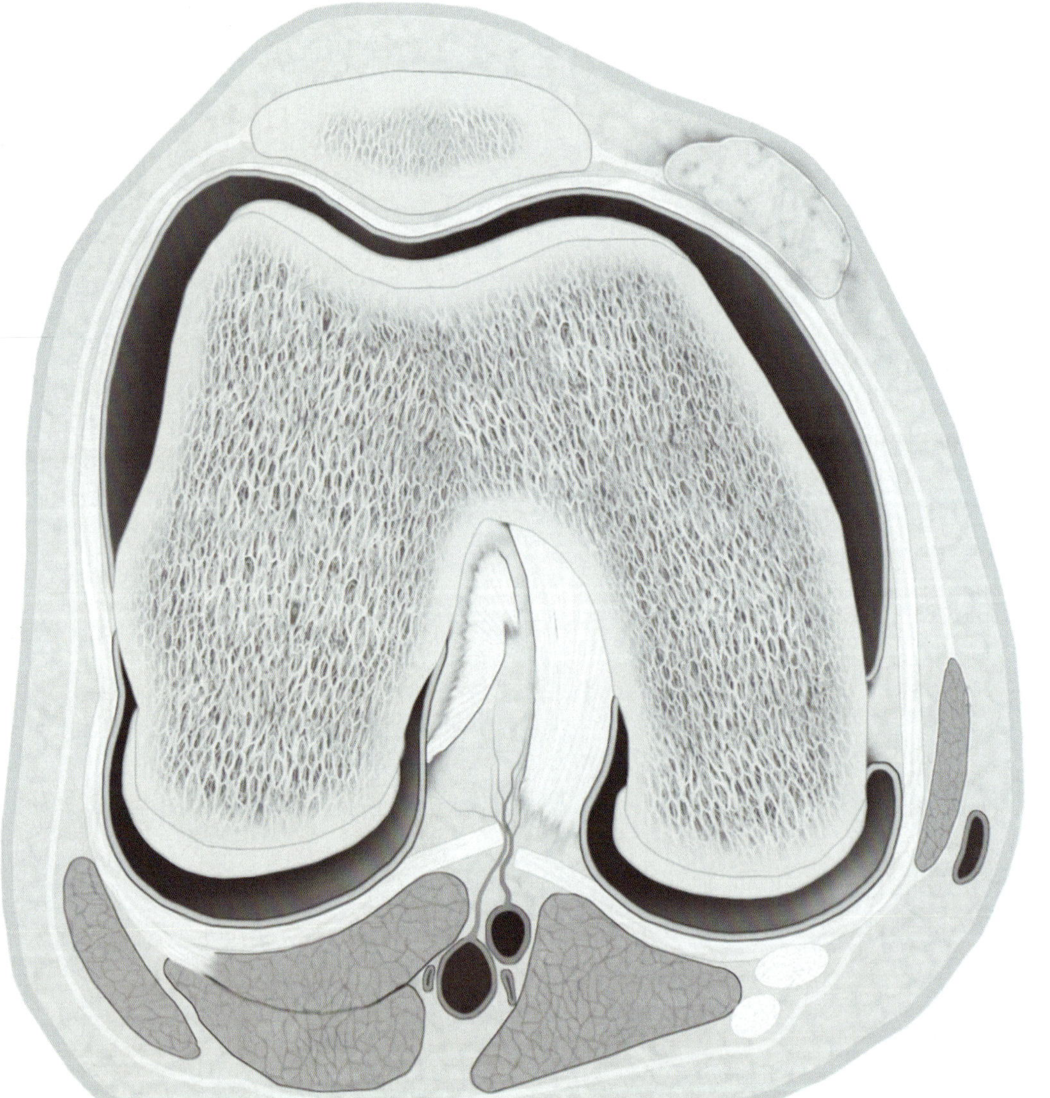

Contributing Authors

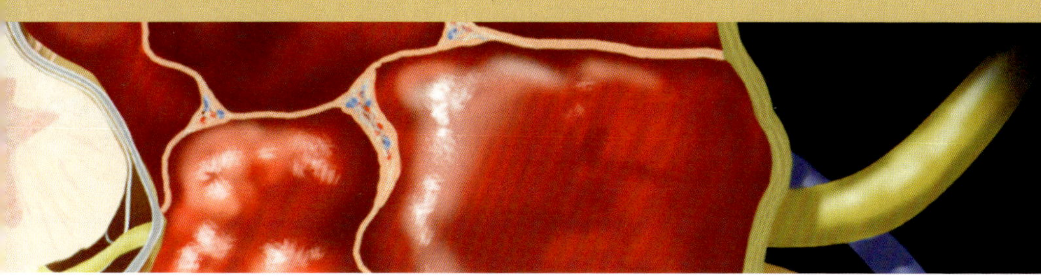

Catherine C. Roberts, MD
Professor of Radiology
Mayo Clinic
Scottsdale, Arizona

Cheryl A. Petersilge, MD, MBA
Clinical Professor of Radiology
Cleveland Clinic Lerner College of Medicine
Case Western Reserve University
Cleveland, Ohio

Julia R. Crim, MD
Chief of Musculoskeletal Radiology
Professor of Radiology
University of Missouri at Columbia
Columbia, Missouri

Sandra Moore, MD
Assistant Clinical Professor
New York University Medical Center
Hospital for Joint Diseases
New York, New York

Christopher J. Hanrahan, MD, PhD
Associate Professor
Musculoskeletal Division Section Chief
Department of Radiology and Imaging Sciences
University of Utah School of Medicine
Salt Lake City, Utah

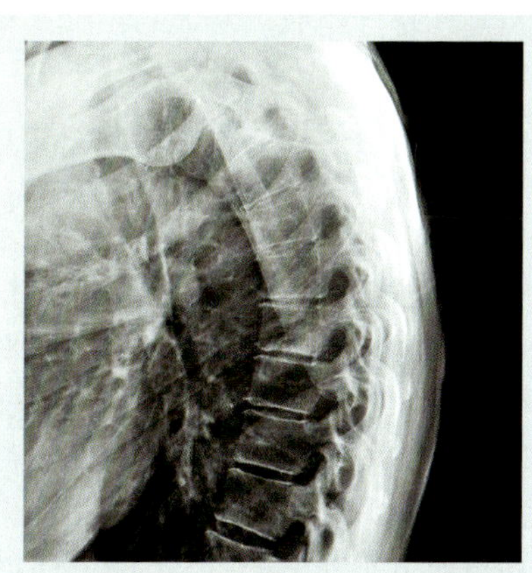

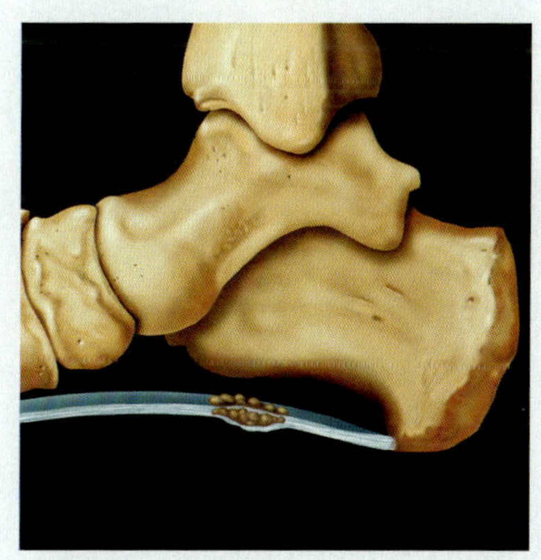

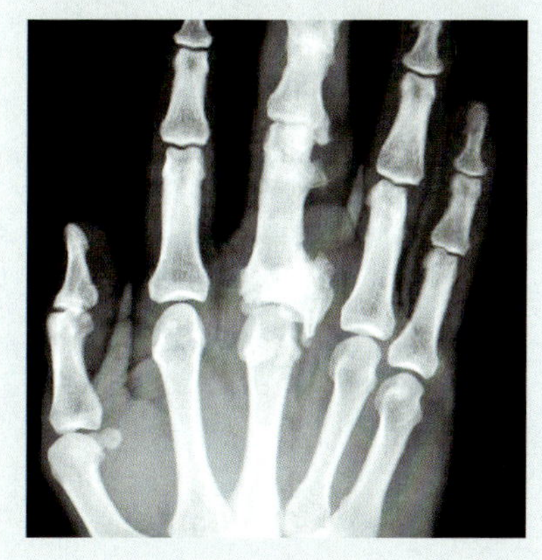

Preface

We are delighted to present the second edition of *Diagnostic Imaging: Musculoskeletal: Non-Traumatic Disease.* Along with its companion book, *Diagnostic Imaging: Musculoskeletal: Trauma*, we offer complete coverage of the extensive topic of musculoskeletal imaging in the standard *Diagnostic Imaging* text format. More than 1,000 pages and thousands of images provide a detailed understanding of arthritis, osseous tumors, soft tissue tumors, metabolic bone disease, infectious processes, systemic diseases contributing to osseous abnormalities, drug and nutritional abnormalities contributing to bone disease, and congenital/developmental musculoskeletal abnormalities. One might expect to find the topics of orthopedic implants and "hardware" in either the traumatic or non-traumatic disease books; we have chosen to include these topics in the present book.

As with the initial edition, we have kept the authoring team small. This maintains the advantage of consistent quality throughout the book and ensures that there is no duplication of topics or information, while being certain of complete coverage of topics.

We have maintained the signature *Diagnostic Imaging* format of bulleted text and Key Facts boxes. Prose introductions to major sections offer the author's approach to difficult topics and are worth an initial perusal. Tabular offerings as well as graphics enhance understanding of some topics and may serve as quick references.

The clinical images have been updated for this edition and, as with the initial edition, are seen in far larger numbers than can be accommodated in most textbooks. Since many, if not most, musculoskeletal diseases rarely have a single imaging presentation, we have included the variations in appearance

and have not wasted space showing similar-appearing cases. We have also enlarged the ebook gallery for many of the topics, showing additional cases that will help the reader appreciate the variability of these disease processes.

Text and references have been updated for this edition. Some new topics have been added, particularly in the section of Drug-Induced and Nutritional MSK Conditions. The authors hope and expect that you will find our offering valuable in your practice.

B.J. Manaster, MD, PhD, FACR

Emeritus Professor
Department of Radiology
University of Utah School of Medicine
Salt Lake City, Utah

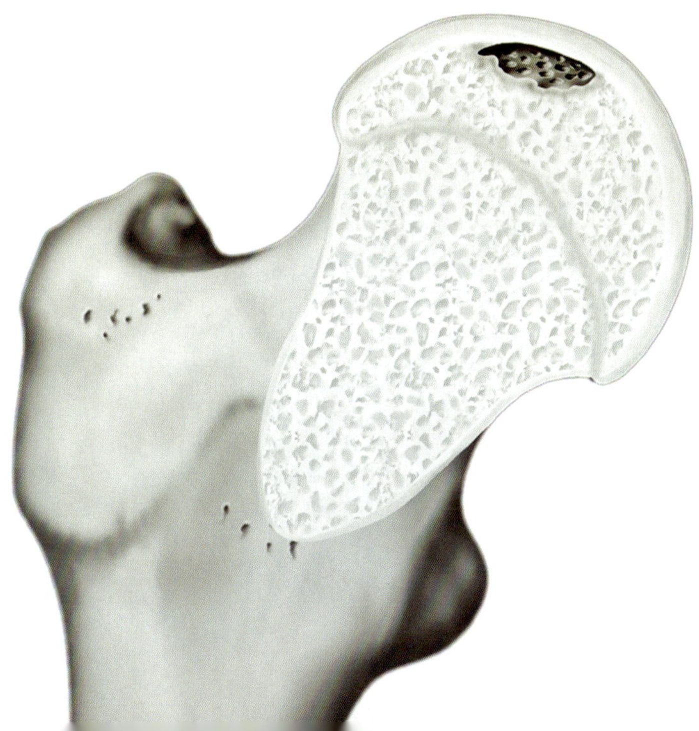

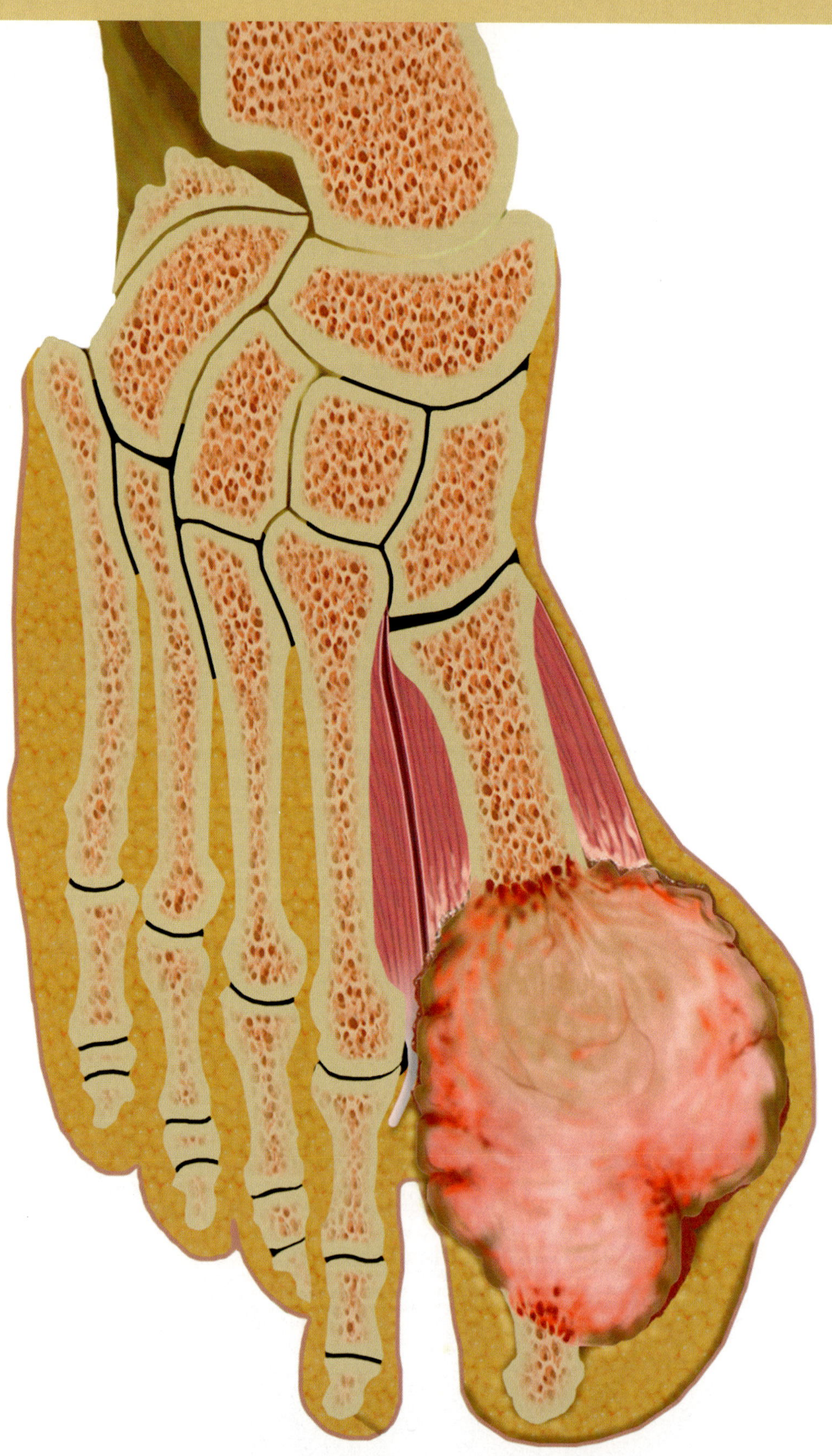

Acknowledgments

Text Editors

Arthur G. Gelsinger, MA
Nina I. Bennett, BA
Terry W. Ferrell, MS
Karen E. Concannon, MA, PhD
Emily C. Fassett, BA
Matt Hoecherl, BS
Tricia L. Cannon, BA

Image Editors

Jeffrey J. Marmorstone, BS
Lisa A. M. Steadman, BS

Medical Editor

Megan K. Mills, MD

Illustrations

Richard Coombs, MS
Lane R. Bennion, MS
Laura C. Sesto, MA

Art Direction and Design

Tom M. Olson, BA
Laura C. Sesto, MA

Lead Editor

Lisa A. Gervais, BS

Production Coordinators

Angela M. G. Terry, BA
Rebecca L. Hutchinson, BA

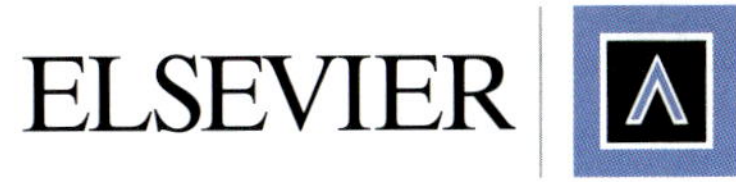

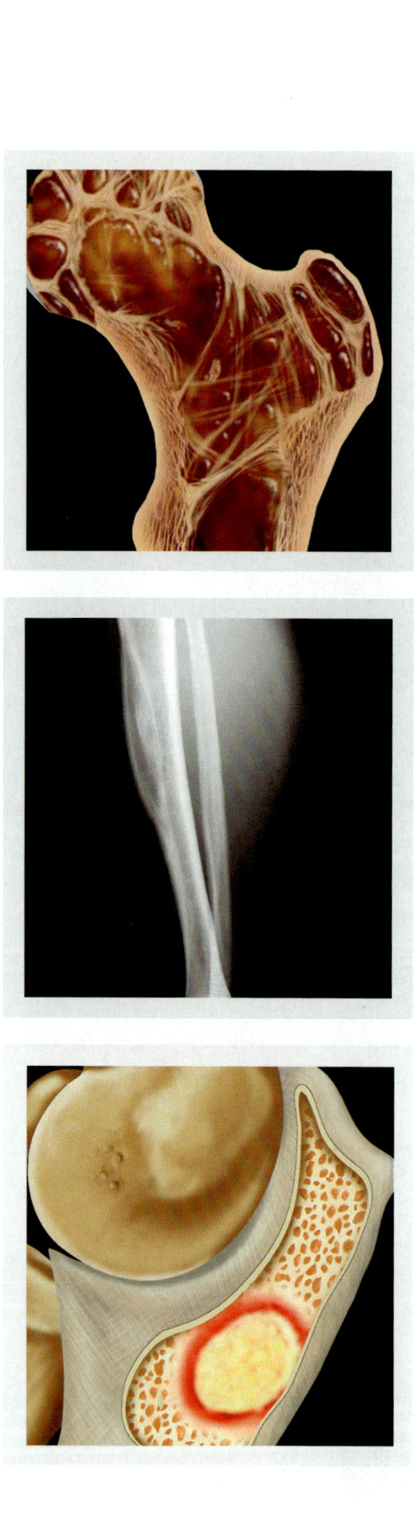

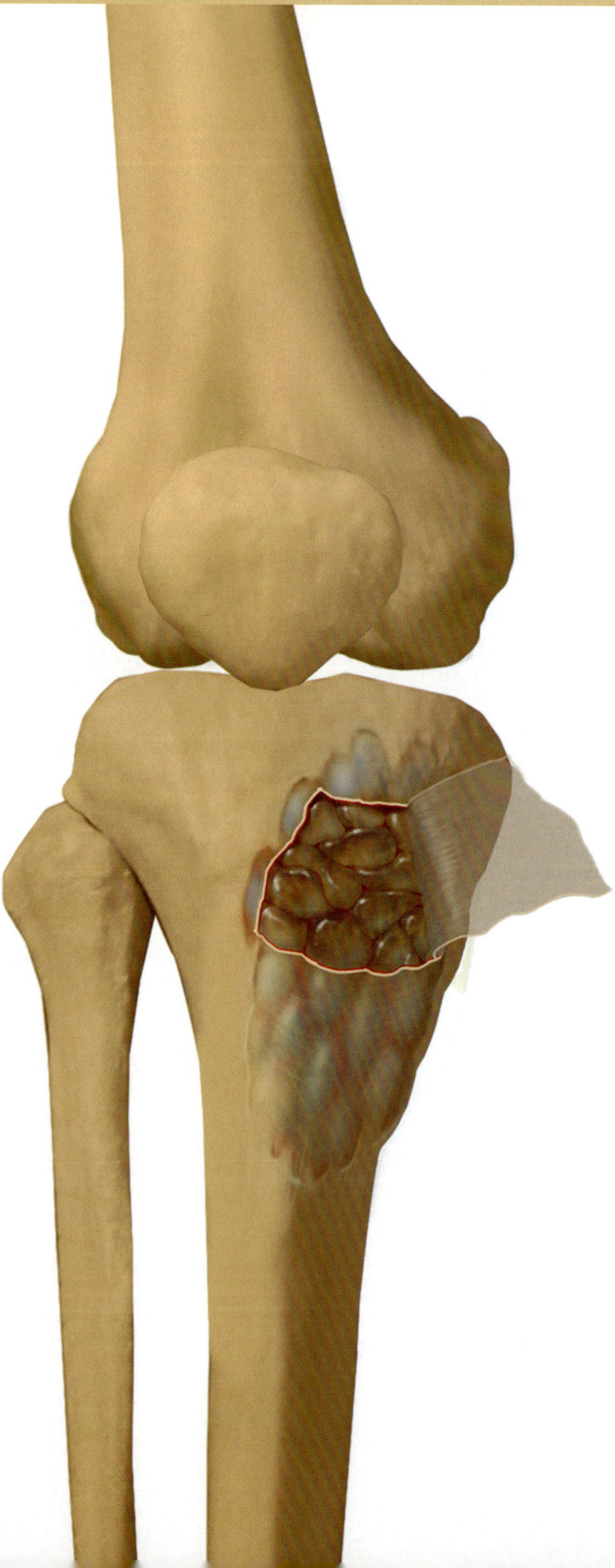

Sections

TABLE OF CONTENTS

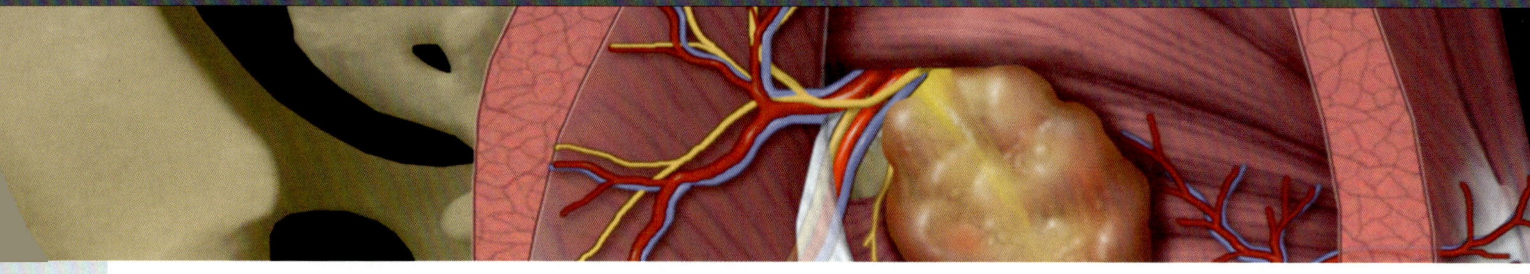

SECTION 1: ARTHRITIS

INTRODUCTION AND OVERVIEW

EROSIVE

PRODUCTIVE

MIXED EROSIVE AND PRODUCTIVE

DUE TO BIOCHEMICAL DISORDERS OR DEPOSITIONAL DISEASE

MISCELLANEOUS JOINT DISORDERS

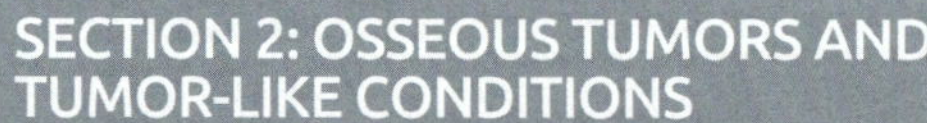

SECTION 2: OSSEOUS TUMORS AND TUMOR-LIKE CONDITIONS

INTRODUCTION AND OVERVIEW

TABLE OF CONTENTS

TABLE OF CONTENTS

TABLE OF CONTENTS

TABLE OF CONTENTS

TABLE OF CONTENTS

SECTION 6: SYSTEMIC DISEASES WITH MSK INVOLVEMENT

GENERAL

STORAGE DISORDERS

CONNECTIVE TISSUE DISORDERS

CONNECTIVE TISSUE DISORDER WITH ARACHNODACTYLY

SOFT TISSUE DISORDERS

VASCULAR

SECTION 7: ORTHOPEDIC IMPLANTS OR ARTHRODESIS

ARTHROPLASTIES AND ARTHRODESIS

INTERNAL FIXATION

TABLE OF CONTENTS

TABLE OF CONTENTS

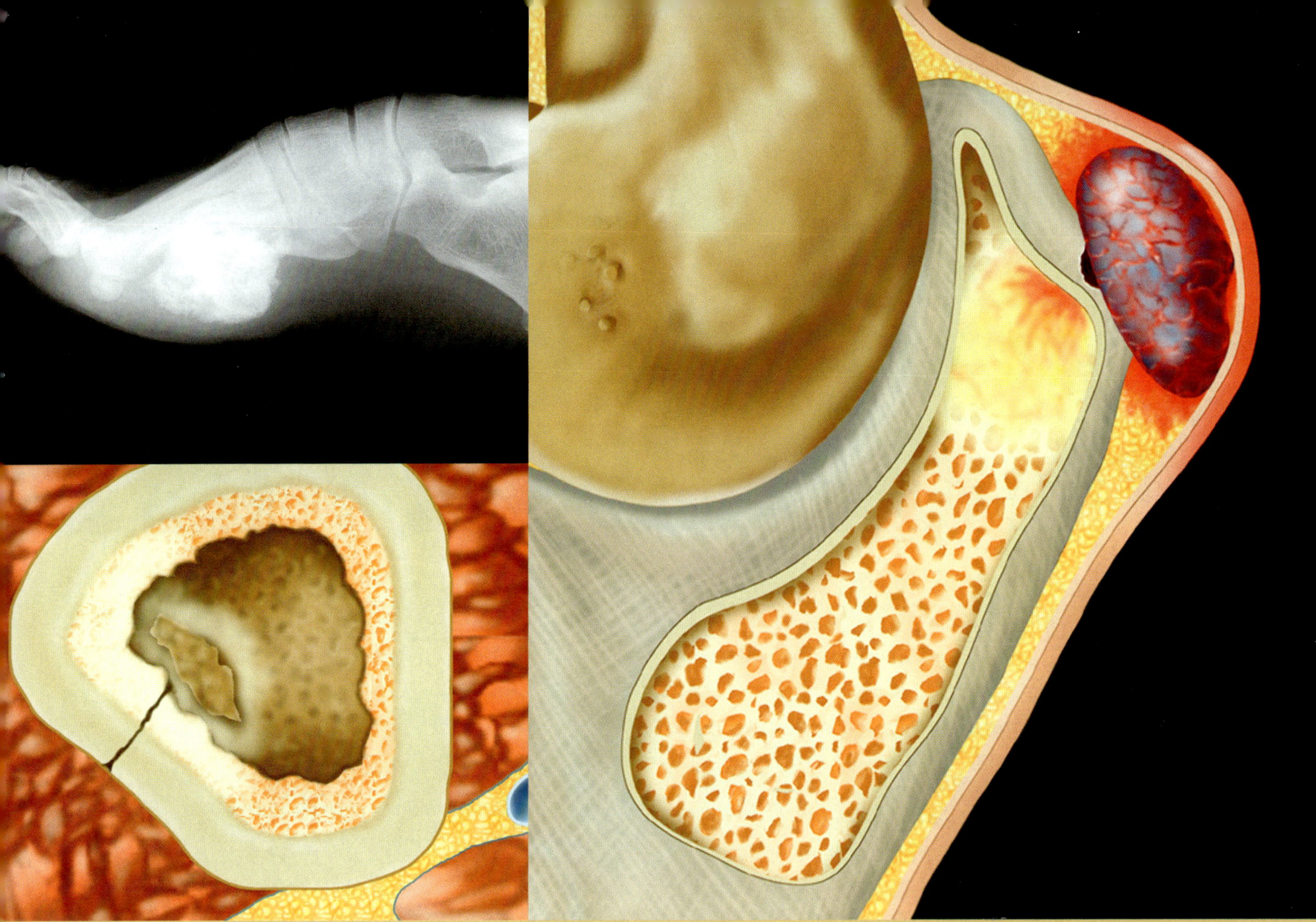

Diagnostic Imaging

Musculoskeletal Non-Traumatic Disease

SECOND EDITION

SECTION 1
Arthritis

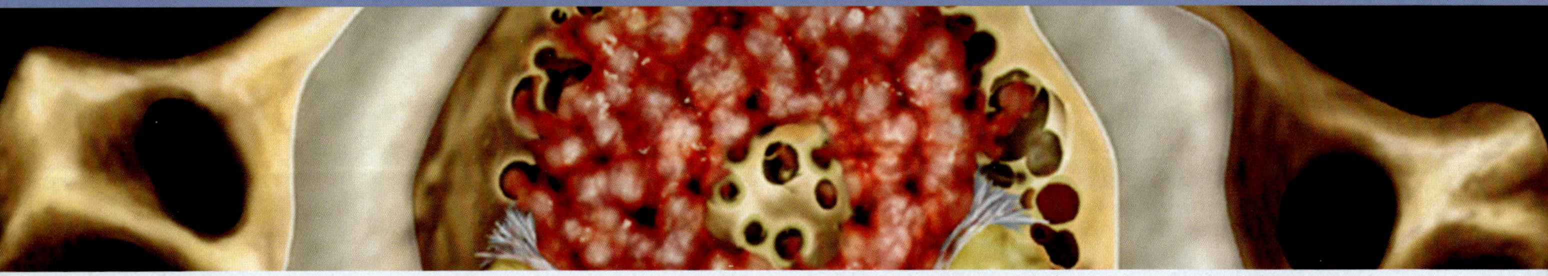

Introduction and Overview

Erosive

Productive

Mixed Erosive and Productive

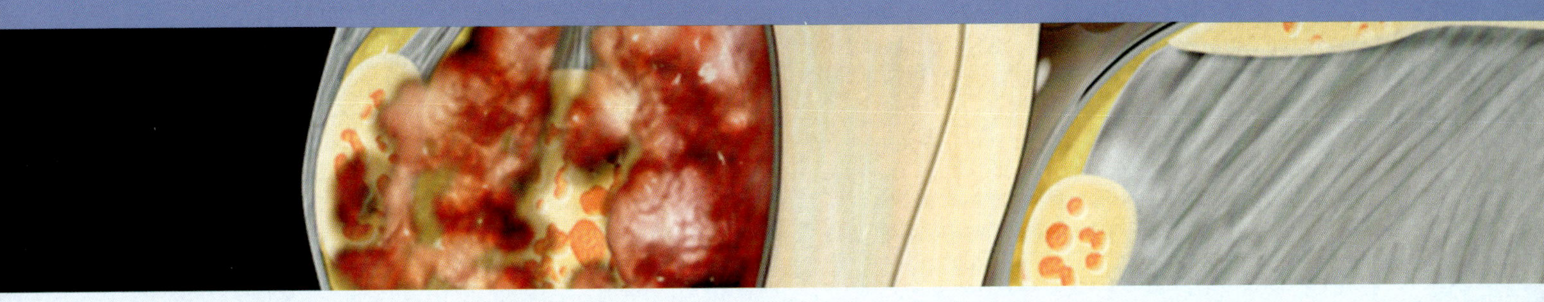

Due to Biochemical Disorders or Depositional Disease

Miscellaneous Joint Disorders

Classic Appearance of Arthritic Processes

When an arthritic process is well established in a particular patient, it will usually achieve a typical appearance, which allows diagnosis by means of imaging. At such a moderately early or mid stage of disease, radiographs are usually sufficient to make the correct diagnosis. The diagnosis usually depends on the location of the joint abnormalities and a host of other radiographic characteristics.

Location of involved joints can often eliminate some diagnoses and raise the probability of others. For example, distal interphalangeal joint disease is commonly seen in psoriatic arthritis, osteoarthritis, and erosive osteoarthritis. However, it is not seen in rheumatoid arthritis until extremely late in the disease; thus RA should not be considered in an early arthritis. Similarly, a disease involving the sacroiliac joints would raise the possibility of ankylosing spondylitis, inflammatory bowel disease arthritis, psoriatic spondyloarthropathy, chronic reactive arthritis, osteoarthritis, and DISH. Common locations of joint involvement are illustrated in diagrammatic fashion in this section. Note the joints that are involved earliest and most commonly are distinguished from those involved less frequently or in end-stage disease.

While the location of the joints involved certainly contributes to establishing a list of reasonable diagnoses, the lists can be relatively long, as in the examples above. There are several other parameters that are useful in honing that list to a single diagnosis that are outlined in the tables that follow. Further explanation regarding some of these parameters may be helpful, as follows.

Age and gender may be the easiest parameters to apply. There are a minimal number of arthritic processes that affect children (juvenile inflammatory arthritis, hemophilic arthropathy, inflammatory bowel disease arthropathy, and septic joint) and teenagers (in addition to those affecting children, early onset adult rheumatoid arthritis and ankylosing spondylitis). Some diseases are gender specific (hemophilic arthropathy and hemochromatosis), while others are found in one gender far more frequently (gout, ankylosing spondylitis, chronic reactive arthritis in males, and rheumatoid arthritis in females).

One of the most important parameters is the **character of the process**. Some arthritides are **purely erosive**; rheumatoid arthritis is the hallmark for this group. Others are **purely bone-forming** (also termed "productive"). This bone formation may appear in the form of osteophytes (as in osteoarthritis), enthesopathy or ligamentous ossification (as in ankylosing spondylitis, DISH, and OPLL), or periositis (as in psoriatic arthritis, chronic reactive arthritis, and juvenile idiopathic arthritis). Other processes may be **mixed**, sometimes starting with erosions but progressing to osteophytes (as in pyrophosphate arthropathy or gout) or starting with periostitis and progressing to mixed erosions and osteophytes (as in psoriatic arthritis or chronic reactive arthritis). These processes tend to be distinctive for each type of arthritis by the time they are well established; between evaluating the character of the process and its primary location in an individual, the diagnosis can usually be secured.

Bilateral symmetry of an arthritic process can be a useful characteristic. Rheumatoid arthritis is especially well known for appearing bilaterally symmetric. Note that rheumatologists do not require specific joints of specific digits to qualify the arthritis as symmetric. For example, 5th PIP left hand and 3rd PIP right hand would be considered symmetric disease simply because of PIP involvement of each hand. Note also that bilateral symmetry may not be present in early stages of arthritic disease, even in rheumatoid arthritis. Similarly, while we usually think of the sacroiliitis of ankylosing spondylitis as being bilaterally symmetric, in its early stages the symmetry is often strikingly absent. Therefore, useful generalizations regarding bilateral symmetry are most often made in the mature stages of the disease process. However, rigid application of "rules" of symmetry should be avoided when evaluating early arthritis.

Soft tissue swelling can be the key to finding the earliest changes of arthritis on a radiograph. The sausage digit may lead to the discovery of subtle periostitis, even in the absence of joint space narrowing or erosions. Swelling around a metacarpophalangeal joint may lead to closer examination of a metacarpal head showing cortical indistinctness or the dot-dash pattern of early inflammatory disease. Be sure to window every image to evaluate the soft tissues, as these abnormalities can lead to closer examination of adjacent joints.

Soft tissue masses are not frequently seen in conjunction with arthritic processes. However, they may lead to specificity in diagnosis. Gouty tophi, seen as a mass containing a variable degree of dense tissue, can be diagnostic. As another example, soft tissue nodules, combined with acroosteolysis and interphalangeal joint erosions, leads to the rare diagnosis of multicentric reticulohistiocytosis.

In differentiating between the ligamentous ossification of DISH/OPLL, osteophytes of spondylosis deformans, syndesmophytes of ankylosing spondylitis, and paravertebral ossification of psoriatic arthritis and chronic reactive arthritis, the **character of paravertebral ossification** can often suggest the correct diagnosis. However, as with other parameters, it is important to note that mature paravertebral ossification in each of these entities may all have a similar appearance. True osteophytes may bridge across the disc space and give the appearance of the flowing ligamentous ossification of DISH. Mature ankylosing spondylitis has much bulkier syndesmophytes than the thin vertical ones depicted in early disease.

Subchondral cysts are seen in virtually all arthritic processes and therefore are rarely useful in differentiating among them. However, occasionally the subchondral cysts are so large that this characteristic becomes useful in diagnosis. Particularly large subchondral cysts in a setting that otherwise resembles rheumatoid arthritis lead to the diagnosis of robust rheumatoid arthritis. Very large cysts are also noted in pyrophosphate arthropathy and pigmented villonodular synovitis. Osteoarthritis and gout may also produce very large subchondral cysts.

Bone density must always be interpreted within the context of patient age and gender. An elderly female will usually have diffuse osteoporosis, with or without superimposed rheumatoid arthritis (classically described as causing juxtaarticular, followed by diffuse osteoporosis). Thus, though we state that normal bone density is a characteristic of osteoarthritis and gout, in an older patient those arthritic processes may be seen in the presence of diffuse osteoporosis. Another example that may cause confusion is the young adult with end-stage renal disease and a renal transplant. Erosive disease in these patients is likely to be gout or amyloid. However, the bone density will be decreased due to both their renal osteodystrophy and likely use of steroids for their transplant. In this case, gout should be suggested to explain erosive disease, despite the bone appearing osteoporotic. Focal osteoporosis can also be helpful in identifying joints with active inflammation, as the hyperemia from the inflammatory process leaches the calcium from the bone.

The **pattern and timing of cartilage destruction** may be another useful parameter. Some arthritides, such as gout, classically cause prominent erosions before significant cartilage destruction, while most inflammatory arthritides, such as rheumatoid arthritis, result in early marginal erosions but also relatively early cartilage destruction. The pattern of cartilage destruction also distinguishes the inflammatory arthropathies, where it is uniform throughout the joint as opposed to the more focal cartilage destruction seen in the weight-bearing portions of the joint in osteoarthritis.

Adjacent calcific or ossific densities may be particularly helpful in diagnosis. Chondrocalcinosis is not unique to pyrophosphate arthropathy but is most frequently seen in that disease. The presence of chondrocalcinosis should also raise the question of traumatic osteoarthritis and hemochromatosis. Calcifications in gouty tophi are usually unique in their appearance. Calcific or ossific bodies in synovial chondromatosis are different from the osseous debris seen with a Charcot joint. Therefore, the character of adjacent calcific or osseous densities may be useful in the diagnostic process.

Ankylosis of the peripheral joints is most commonly seen in psoriatic arthritis and juvenile idiopathic arthritis. It is commonly found in the spine of patients suffering from spondyloarthropathies (most frequently ankylosing spondylitis), DISH, and juvenile idiopathic arthritis. Other more rare arthritic processes may show ankylosis as well. On the other hand, ankylosis in cases of rheumatoid arthritis is exceedingly rare. Do not be fooled by a surgical arthrodesis in a patient with severe rheumatoid arthritis. Arthrodesis is often attempted to stabilize the digits in this disease, and may mimic ankylosis.

Early Appearance of Arthritic Processes

We are now diagnosing arthritic processes at an earlier stage, prior to any radiographic change. This ability is essential, since early application of disease-modifying drug therapy may halt joint destruction. The benefit of early diagnosis is obvious, yielding longer patient productivity and decreasing the need for arthroplasty. However, the diagnosis may be difficult with subtle or absent radiographic findings and relies on MR or ultrasound. Early tenosynovitis and joint effusions may be identified on ultrasound, and MR may demonstrate tenosynovitis, effusion, and bone marrow edema long before actual erosions are seen in rheumatoid arthritis. Inflammatory change at vertebral body corners may be identified on MR, indicating early spondyloarthropathy. Even more subtle may be the enthesitis and adjacent marrow edema found in early ankylosing spondylitis, which are often found at the "corners" of the image (interspinous ligaments, iliac spine, greater trochanter) and are easily overlooked. Close attention should be paid to these locations, even when evaluating a "routine lower back pain" spine MR exam.

Late Appearance of Arthritic Processes

End-stage arthritic processes may have a classic appearance. Classic changes are often seen in the deformities and erosive change in rheumatoid patients or in the postural changes with vertebral column fusion in ankylosing spondylitis patients. However, at times an arthritic process, particularly when ineffectively treated, may attain a potentially confusing nonstandard appearance. An example of this is the rheumatoid patient who has failed drug therapy, resulting in an arthritis mutilans appearance of the hands (remember that pencil-in-cup and arthritis mutilans are not exclusively seen in psoriatic arthritis). Another example is the Native American ankylosing spondylitis patient who is treated without the use of Western medications and may present not only with the spondyloarthropathy expected in ankylosing spondylitis, but also with erosive disease involving all the peripheral joints, including hands and feet. Finally, the classic disease process that may be confusing is end-stage gout, which, if misdiagnosed or undertreated, may result in spectacular erosive disease at unexpected locations. It is important to remember that gout can look like anything and can be located at any joint!

Coexistence of Arthritic Processes

It is not unusual for two of the more common arthritic processes to coexist, particularly in the elderly patient. This may be confusing initially but can be worked out through understanding the prevalence of the diseases in the patient population, as well as by paying attention to the appearance and location of the abnormalities present. The most common combination is a new onset of rheumatoid arthritis superimposed on osteoarthritis. In this case, the osteoarthritis is usually well-established, involving the 1st carpometacarpal and interphalangeal joints in classic fashion, but there is new inflammatory change seen in the metacarpophalangeal joints. The elderly patient may also develop pyrophosphate arthropathy, superimposed over osteoarthritis or rheumatoid arthritis. The patient with a diabetic Charcot joint may develop superimposed septic arthritis. Keeping these possibilities in mind is useful to the interpreter, as the pattern of disease may not be classic.

Conclusion

There are many subtleties involved at specific joint locations in specific diseases, which cannot be discussed in such a broad introduction. These will be covered in proper detail in the individual sections that follow.

Selected References

1. Navallas M et al: Sacroiliitis associated with axial spondyloarthropathy: new concepts and latest trends. Radiographics. 33(4):933-56, 2013
2. Rowbotham EL et al: Rheumatoid arthritis: ultrasound versus MRI. AJR Am J Roentgenol. 197(3):541-6, 2011
3. Narváez JA et al: MR imaging of early rheumatoid arthritis. Radiographics. 30(1):143-63; discussion 163-5, 2010
4. Emad Y et al: Can magnetic resonance imaging differentiate undifferentiated arthritis based on knee imaging? J Rheumatol. 36(9):1963-70, 2009
5. Haavardsholm EA et al: Magnetic resonance imaging findings in 84 patients with early rheumatoid arthritis: bone marrow oedema predicts erosive progression. Ann Rheum Dis. 67(6):794-800, 2008
6. Kim NR et al: "MR corner sign": value for predicting presence of ankylosing spondylitis. AJR Am J Roentgenol. 191(1):124-8, 2008

Characteristics of Arthritic Processes

Arthritis Type	Gender	# of Joints	Symmetry	Bone Density	Character	Cartilage Destruction
RA	M < F (1:3)	Polyarticular	Yes, by end stage	Density ↓	Erosive	Early, diffuse
Robust RA	M > F	Polyarticular	Yes, by end stage	End stage ↓	Erosive	Early, diffuse
JIA	M < F (1:4-5)	Pauci- or polyarticular	Generally no	End stage ↓	Erosive	Early, diffuse
Hemophilia	M only	Pauciarticular	No	Normal	Erosive	Early, diffuse
Adult Still disease	M = F	Polyarticular	Generally no	End stage ↓	Erosive	Early, diffuse
MCRH	M < F	Polyarticular	Yes	Related to age	Erosive	Early, diffuse
Osteoarthritis	M < F	Polyarticular	Often	Normal	Produces bone	Early, focal
DISH/OPLL	M > F (2:1)	Nonarticular	Nonarticular	Normal	Produces bone	None
AS/IBD arthritis	AS: M > F (2.5-5:1); IBD: M = F	Polyarticular	Yes, by end stage	Mid to end stage ↓	Mixed	Mid stage, diffuse
PSA/CRA/HIV	PSA: M = F; CRA/HIV: M > F (5-6:1)	Polyarticular	Generally no	Normal	Mixed	Mid stage, diffuse
Gout	M > F (9:1)	Polyarticular	No	Normal	Mixed	Late disease
Pyrophosphate	M < F (1:2-7)	Polyarticular	Generally no	Related to age	Mixed	Mid stage, diffuse
Hemochromatosis	M only	Polyarticular	Generally no	Normal	Produces bone	Late disease
Amyloid	M > F	Pauciarticular	No	Density ↓	Erosive	Early, focal
PVNS	M < F (1:2)	Monoarticular	No (single joint)	Normal	Erosive	Late, focal
PSC	M > F	Monoarticular	No (single joint)	Normal	Erosive	Late, focal
Charcot	M = F, relates to etiology	Mono- or pauciarticular	No	Not unless diabetic	Destructive	Early, diffuse
Septic arthritis	M = F	Monoarticular	No (single joint)	Normal	Erosive	Early, diffuse

Characteristics of Arthritic Processes (Continued)

Arthritis Type	Subchondral Cysts	Enthesopathy	Periostitis	Adjacent Density	Ankylosis	Soft Tissue Masses
RA	Yes	No	No	No	No	Rheumatoid nodules
Robust RA	Yes, large	No	No	No	No	Rheumatoid nodules
JIA	Yes	No	Yes, early	No	Yes	No
Hemophilia	Yes	No	No	No	No	No
Adult Still disease	Yes	No	No	No	Yes	No
MCRH	Yes	No	No	No	No	Nodules
Osteoarthritis	Yes	Yes	No	Rare chondrocalcinosis	No	Heberden nodes
DISH/OPLL	No	Yes, prominent	No	No	Yes	No
AS/IBD arthritis	Yes	Yes, prominent	No	No	Yes	No
PSA/CRA/HIV	Yes	Yes	Yes, prominent	No	Yes	No
Gout	Yes	No	No	Yes, tophus	No	Tophi
Pyrophosphate	Yes, large	No	No	Chondrocalcinosis	No	No
Hemochromatosis	Yes	No	No	Chondrocalcinosis	No	No
Amyloid	Yes, large	No	No	No	No	Amyloid nodules
PVNS	Yes, large	No	No	No	No	No
PSC	Yes	No	No	Calcified bodies	no	Rare extraarticular
Charcot	Yes	No	Occasionally	Osseous debris	No	Large fluid collections
Septic arthritis	If chronic	No	Yes	No	Rare	No

Rheumatoid arthritis = RA, juvenile idiopathic arthritis = JIA, multicentric reticulohistiocytosis = MCRH, diffuse idiopathic skeletal hyperostosis = DISH, ossification posterior longitudinal ligament = OPLL, ankylosing spondylitis = AS, inflammatory bowel disease = IBD, psoriatic arthritis = PSA, chronic reactive arthritis = CRA, pigmented villonodular synovitis = PVNS, and primary synovial chondromatosis = PSC.

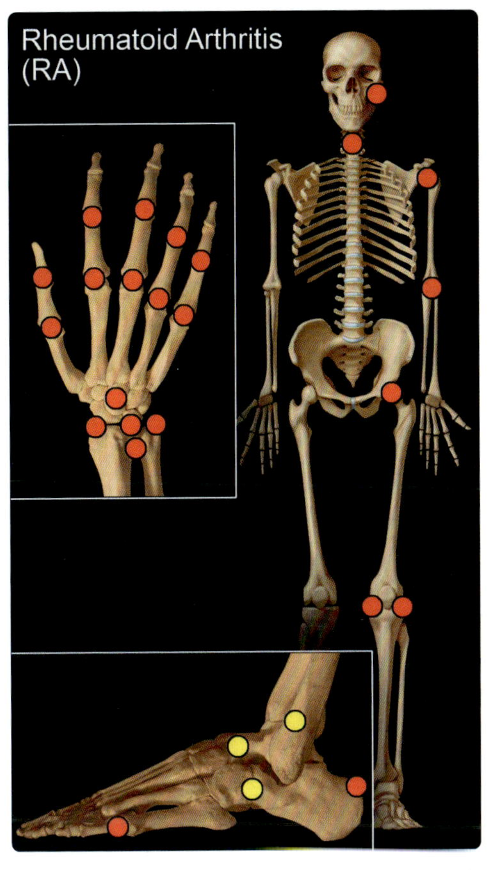

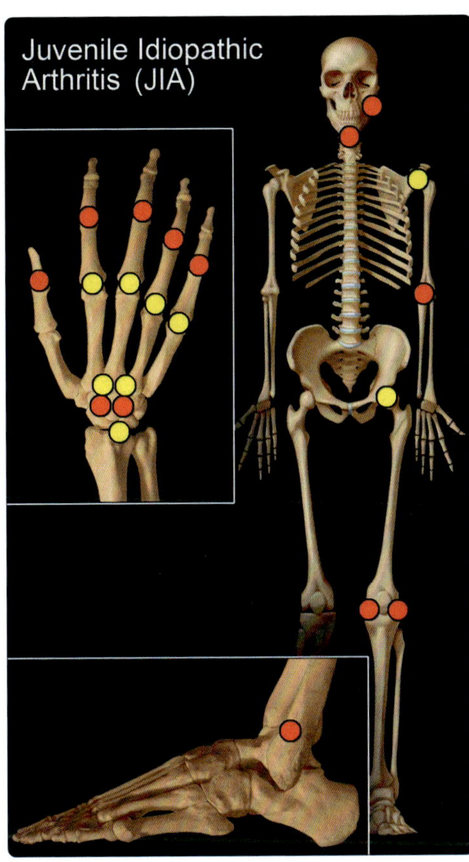

(Left) *RA distribution (common: Red; less common: Yellow) is shown. The hand is the hallmark of the disease, with distal radioulnar joint, radiocarpal joint, intercarpal joint, MCP & PIP joint involvement. Retrocalcaneal and 5th MTP involvement is most common in the foot, with other ankle/hindfoot joints involved less commonly. Hip, knee, shoulder, elbow, temporomandibular, and cervical involvement are common as well.* **(Right)** *JIA distribution is shown. The knee, ankle, and elbow are most frequently involved. In the hand, pericapitate and proximal interphalangeal joints are most frequent, followed by radiocarpal, carpometacarpal, and metacarpophalangeal joints. Cervical spine and temporomandibular involvement are common, while the shoulder and hip are less so.*

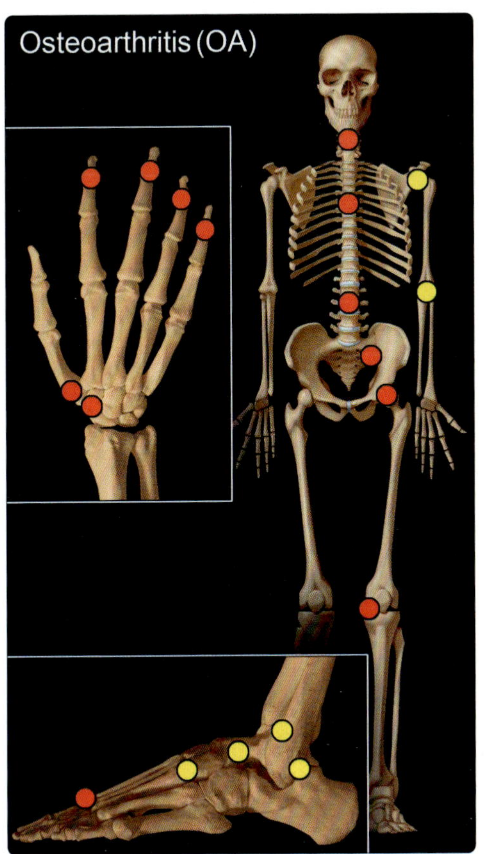

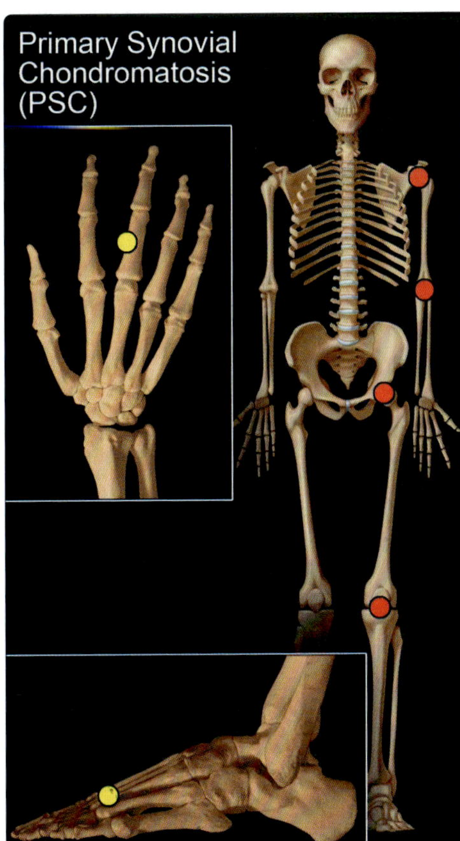

(Left) *OA distribution (common: Red; less common: Yellow) is shown. Hands show common involvement of the 1st carpometacarpal and scapho-trapezio-trapezoid joints, as well as the distal interphalangeal joints. Foot involvement is most frequent at the 1st metatarsophalangeal joint, with the ankle, subtalar, talonavicular, and tarsometatarsal joints less frequently involved. Hip and knee OA are common, while shoulder and elbow are less common. All elements of the spine are commonly affected.* **(Right)** *PSC distribution is shown. Knee involvement is most common, followed by elbow, shoulder, and hip. Axial involvement is virtually never seen. The rare process tenosynovial chondromatosis affects the hands and feet.*

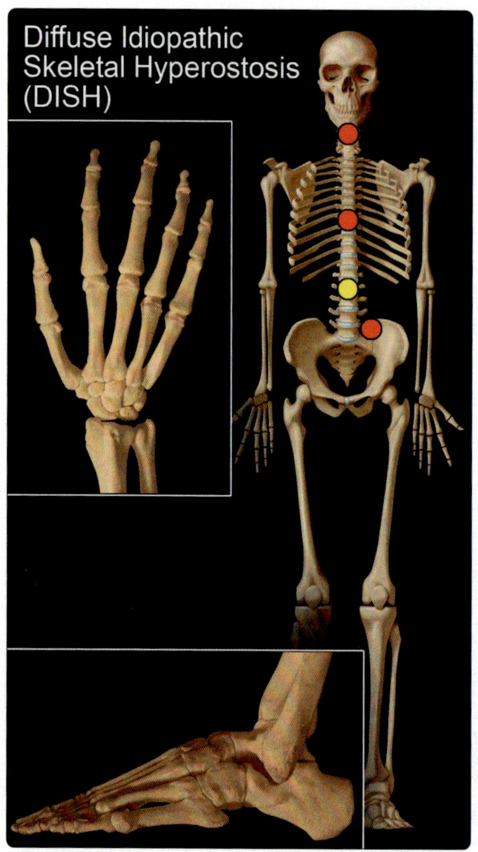

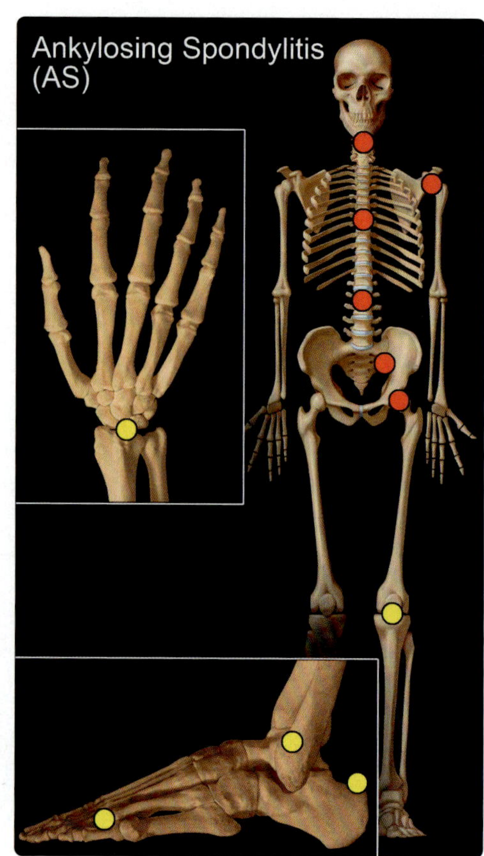

(Left) *DISH and ossification of posterior longitudinal ligament (OPLL) distribution (common: Red; less common: Yellow) are shown. These processes are shown together since they have considerable overlap in distribution, with OPLL predominating in the cervical spine and DISH predominating in the thoracic spine. The nonsynovial portions of the sacroiliac joints (upper 1/2 to 2/3) are affected in DISH.* **(Right)** *AS & inflammatory bowel disease spondyloarthropathy (IBD) distribution are shown. These are shown together; their distribution is identical. All elements of the spine may be involved, along with the sacroiliac joints and large proximal joints (hips, shoulders, and less commonly, knees). With advanced disease, the wrist and ankles may be affected.*

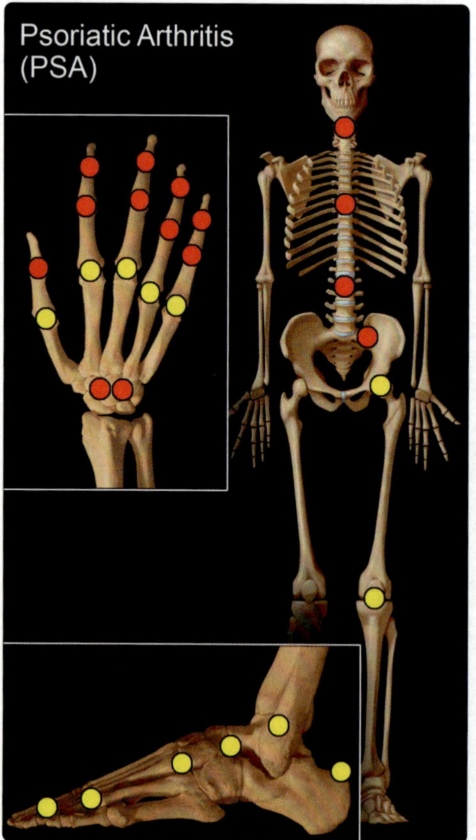

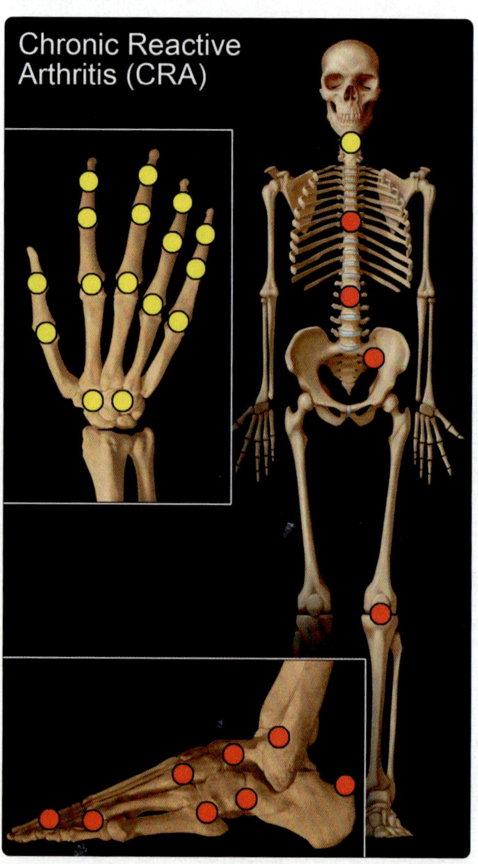

(Left) *PSA distribution (common: Red; less common: Yellow) is shown. The spondyloarthropathy involves all the elements of the spine as well as the sacroiliac joints. The hands show the most frequent peripheral joint involvement, especially in the pericapitate and IP joints. Less frequently, the lower extremities may be involved (foot, ankle, knee, hip).* **(Right)** *CRA distribution is shown. The spondyloarthropathy involves all the elements of the spine as well as the sacroiliac joints. This axial distribution is identical to that of psoriatic arthritis. The feet show the most frequent peripheral joint involvement, with the retrocalcaneal, hindfoot, midfoot, and forefoot all at risk. Knee involvement is also seen. Hand and wrist involvement is considerably less frequent, seen either in advanced disease or sporadically.*

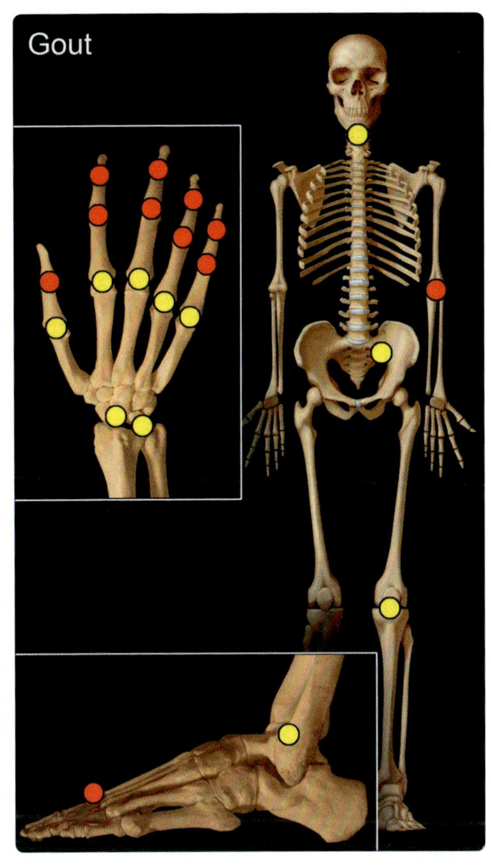

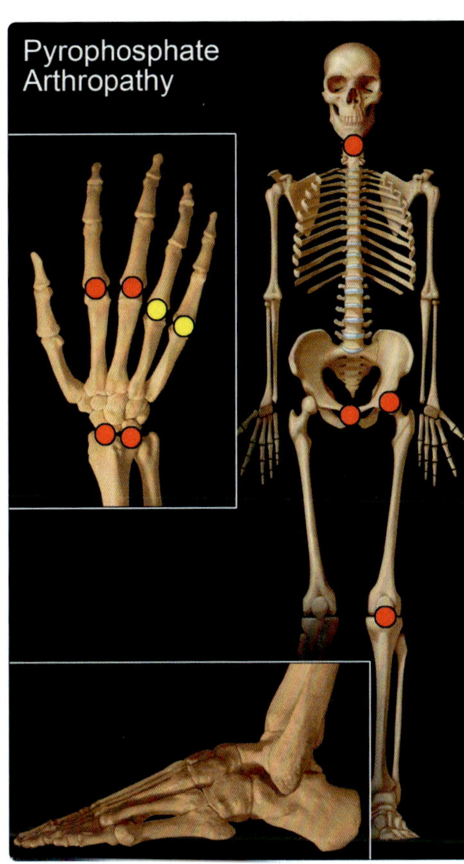

(Left) *Gout distribution (common: Red; less common: Yellow) is shown. Involvement of the 1st MTP joint is the hallmark of the disease, though other foot & ankle joints may be affected. In the hand, the IP joints are much more frequently affected than the MCP or carpals. Of the more proximal joints, the elbow is more frequently involved than the knee. Axial involvement of the C spine & SI joints is uncommonly seen.* **(Right)** *Pyrophosphate arthropathy distribution is shown. The wrist shows a specific predilection for radiocarpal involvement, often leading to SLAC deformity, while the MCP joints are affected in the hand (2nd & 3rd earlier and more frequently than 4th & 5th). The knee is commonly involved, as are the hips & symphysis pubis. The upper elements of the C spine are often affected as well.*

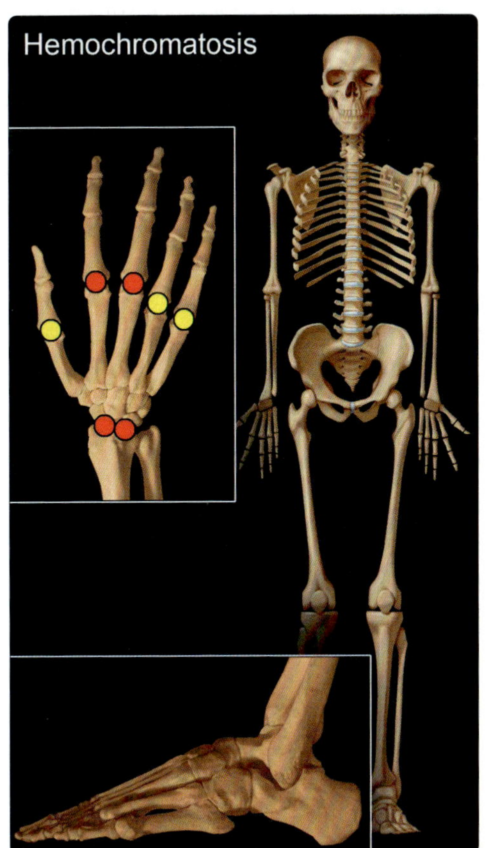

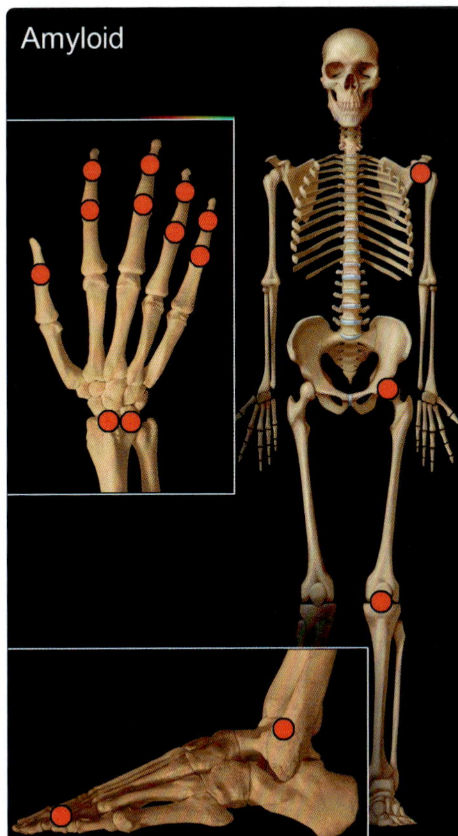

(Left) *Hemochromatosis distribution (common: Red; less common: Yellow). Disease affecting the wrist shows a distinct predilection for the radiocarpal joint. In the hand, the metacarpophalangeal joints are distinctively involved; the 2nd and 3rd are found to be abnormal both earlier and more severely than the 1st, 4th, and 5th. Note that this distribution is similar to that of pyrophosphate arthropathy in the wrist and hand. The remainder of the skeleton is only rarely affected.* **(Right)** *Amyloid distribution. The large proximal joints (shoulder, hip, and knee) are particularly prone to involvement. In the hand, any joint may be involved, but the interphalangeal joints and radiocarpal joints are more frequently abnormal. Ankle and foot interphalangeal joints may be affected as well.*

Rheumatoid Arthritis of Axial Skeleton

KEY FACTS

TERMINOLOGY

- Chronic progressive systemic inflammatory disease in which joints are primary target

IMAGING

- Purely erosive disease, most frequently involving C1-C2
- Radiographic findings
  - Dens erosions
  - Atlantoaxial subluxation
  - Atlantoaxial impaction: May be unilateral or bilateral
    - If unilateral, collapse results in torticollis
  - Subaxial subluxation
  - Sternoclavicular joints involved in 30% of patients with RA but difficult to visualize on radiograph
  - Osteoporosis
- Radiographs must include lateral flexion-extension
- CT: Additive to radiographs
  - Extent of erosive disease more apparent
  - Atlantoaxial (AA) impaction well shown
- MR: Additive to radiographs
  - Pannus, usually around odontoid, distinctly seen
  - Cord compression and damage directly visualized

CLINICAL ISSUES

- Patients with axial disease rarely show associated symptoms until very late
  - Cord symptoms with AA impaction
  - Cord symptoms with > 9 mm AA subluxation
  - Unilateral C1-C2 facet disease → painful torticollis
- Patients with axial disease virtually always have significant peripheral disease (hands/feet) as well

DIAGNOSTIC CHECKLIST

- Watch location of anterior arch of atlas relative to odontoid to evaluate for AA impaction
  - Anterior arch should align with upper portion of dens
- Remember AA subluxation may be underestimated on neutral lateral radiograph and CT

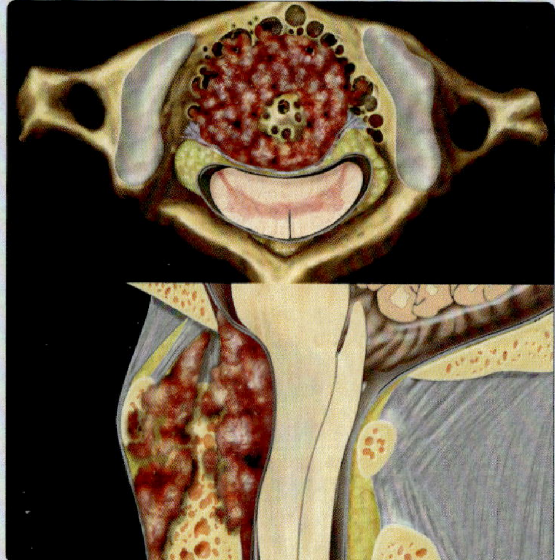

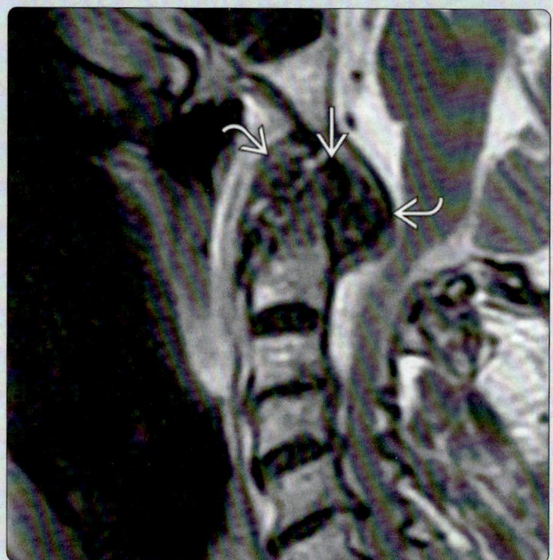

(Left) *Graphic in axial and sagittal planes through the atlantoaxial level of the cervical spine demonstrates the inflammatory pannus surrounding the odontoid process that frequently occurs in patients with rheumatoid arthritis (RA). Note the erosion of the odontoid, as well as focal compression of the spinal cord.* **(Right)** *Sagittal T2WI MR shows extensive erosive changes of the odontoid process ➡, as well as a large amount of pannus ➡ with effacement of the thecal sac and posterior displacement of cord.*

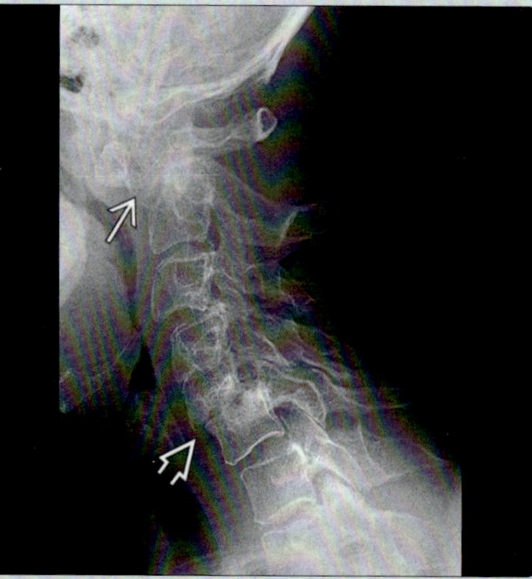

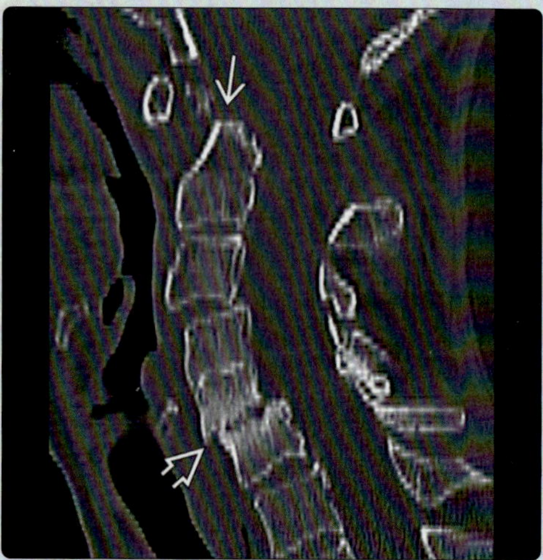

(Left) *Lateral x-ray shows severe (> 9 mm) atlantoaxial (AA) subluxation ➡ and impaction. Note the disruption of the spinolaminar line at C1-C2. Many of the facets are eroded, and abnormal motion of osteoporotic bone results in endplate destruction and subluxation at the C5-C6 level ➡.* **(Right)** *Sagittal CT in the same patient emphasizes the severe odontoid erosion ➡ and AA subluxation with impaction. There is no soft tissue swelling at C5-C6 ➡, indicating that the disc space loss is mechanical rather than infectious.*

TERMINOLOGY

Abbreviations

- Rheumatoid arthritis (RA)

Definitions

- Chronic progressive systemic inflammatory disease in which joints are primary target
  - Atlantoaxial subluxation = C1-C2 subluxation = atlantoaxial (AA) subluxation
  - Atlantoaxial impaction = cranial settling = C1-C2 impaction = AA impaction

IMAGING

General Features

- Best diagnostic clue
  - Purely erosive disease, most frequently involving C1-C2 articulation
- Location
  - C1 and C2 facets, uncovertebral joints, dens, peridens bursa
  - Subaxial (below C2) involvement of cervical facets and uncovertebral joints
  - Sternoclavicular joints involved in 30% of patients with RA but difficult to visualize on radiograph
  - Thoracolumbar spine and sacroiliac joints may have microscopic involvement not manifested on radiographs
- Size
  - Ranges from mild pannus formation to significant instability with cord involvement

Radiographic Findings

- Dens erosions
  - Due to inflammatory pannus in surrounding bursa
  - Seen on lateral or open mouth odontoid views
- AA subluxation
  - Due to disruption of transverse ligament by inflammatory pannus
  - Normal distance between inferior margin of anterior arch of atlas and dens < 4 mm
    - AA subluxation generally not symptomatic until distance reaches 9 mm
  - Evaluated on lateral radiograph
    - May not be apparent without flexion-extension views
      - Flexion generally shows maximal subluxation
      - Extension may indicate pannus preventing full reduction
- AA impaction
  - Due to erosions and collapse of facet joints at C1-C2
    - With bilateral facet collapse, dens may protrude through foramen magnum and cause cord symptoms
  - Evaluated on lateral radiograph
    - Anterior arch of atlas should normally be adjacent to upper portion of dens
      - Anterior arch location adjacent to body of dens or body of C2 indicates AA impaction
    - Impaction of dens through foramen magnum may not be easily seen due to overlying mastoids on lateral radiograph
      - If impaction suggested by position of anterior arch of atlas relative to C2, CT will show extent of process
- Unilateral AA impaction
  - Due to erosions and collapse of single facet joint at C1-C2
    - Unilateral collapse results in acute torticollis
- Subaxial subluxation
  - Due to combination of ligament instability, facet and uncovertebral joint erosive disease, and osteoporosis
    - Erosions and ligament disruption allow abnormal motion across vertebral body endplates → subluxation
    - Uncovertebral joint pannus, combined with underlying osteoporosis and abnormal motion → endplate destruction
  - Seen on lateral radiograph as stair-step deformity
    - Associated endplate destruction may suggest infection
  - Fusion in adult RA extremely uncommon but may occur following endplate destruction
- Osteoporosis

CT Findings

- Extent of erosive disease more apparent
- May see pannus around dens
- Coronal and sagittal reformats show extent of facet and uncovertebral erosions
- AA impaction may be much more evident
  - Projection of dens > 5 mm above Chamberlain line (extends from hard palate to opisthion on sagittal)
  - Intersection of dens with Wackenheim line (extends along clivus on sagittal)
- Note that AA subluxation may be reduced (and therefore underestimated) on CT since patient is supine in scanner

MR Findings

- T1WI
  - Pannus is mass-like low signal
- T2WI
  - Pannus has heterogeneous low and high signal
  - High signal synovial fluid in facets and uncovertebral joints
  - High signal erosions and marrow edema
- STIR
  - Same as T2WI, but abnormal cord signal may be more apparent
    - Contusion or syrinx
- T1WI C+ FS
  - Increased sensitivity in diagnosis of early RA
  - Pannus shows avid enhancement
  - Early erosions enhance

Imaging Recommendations

- Best imaging tool
  - Radiographs, with lateral flexion-extension
  - CT: Additive to radiographs
    - Erosion extent better visualized
    - AA impaction well shown
  - MR: Additive to radiographs
    - Pannus distinctly seen, usually around odontoid
    - Cord compression and damage directly visualized

DIFFERENTIAL DIAGNOSIS

DDx of Atlantoaxial Subluxation

- Seronegative spondyloarthropathies
  - Subluxation may be seen in ankylosing spondylitis, enteropathic spondylitis, psoriatic spondylitis, or chronic reactive spondylitis
  - Syndesmophytes indicate spondyloarthropathy
  - Vertebral body or facet fusion indicate spondyloarthropathy; fusion occurs extremely rarely in adult RA
- Juvenile idiopathic arthritis
  - Often have fused levels, with waisting of hypoplastic bodies

DDx of Endplate Abnormalities

- Disc space infection
  - Single level more suggestive of infection
  - Normal bone density at adjacent levels suggests infection
- Spondyloarthropathy of hemodialysis
  - Endplate destruction, often with listhesis
  - May be multilevel
  - Generally does not involve C1-C2

PATHOLOGY

General Features

- Etiology
  - Unknown etiology for RA
  - Pathophysiology presumed to relate to persistent immunologic response of genetically susceptible host to some unknown antigen
- Genetics
  - Genetic predisposition
    - Concordance in monozygotic twins (25%)
    - 1st-degree relatives develop RA at rate 4x that of general population
  - Still, individual not likely to have affected family member

Gross Pathologic & Surgical Features

- Synovial lining is hypertrophic, edematous
- Joint distension, bone erosion, cartilage destruction

Microscopic Features

- Organized accumulations of CD4 helper T cells, antigen presenting cells, lymphoid follicles
- Large amounts of immunoglobulin produced, including rheumatoid factor
- Angiogenesis in synovium

CLINICAL ISSUES

Presentation

- Most common signs/symptoms
  - Patients with axial disease rarely show associated symptoms until very late
    - Cord symptoms with AA impaction
    - Cord symptoms with significant AA subluxation (> 9 mm)
    - Painful torticollis with unilateral C1-C2 facet collapse
  - Patients with axial disease virtually always have significant peripheral disease (hands/feet) as well

Demographics

- Age
  - Peak age of onset: 4th-5th decades
- Gender
  - M:F = 1:3
- Epidemiology
  - RA in 1% of worldwide population
    - 5% in some Native American populations
  - 50% of RA patients have cervical spine involvement

Natural History & Prognosis

- With severe disease, may develop radiculopathy or cervical myelopathy
- ↑ morbidity and mortality if patient has craniocervical junction instability

Treatment

- Treatment of RA: Generally combination, aimed at pain relief while escalating therapy rapidly to suppress disease prior to joint destruction
  - Nonsteroidal antiinflammatory drugs
    - Symptomatic relief; do not alter disease process
  - Glucocorticoids (oral or intraarticular)
    - Controls inflammation rapidly; allows time for slower-acting drugs to take effect
  - Disease-modifying antirheumatic drugs
    - Suppresses joint destruction (e.g., methotrexate, sulfasalazine, antimalarials, gold)
  - Biologics: Anti-TNF-α drugs, antiinterleukin-1
    - Role of cytokines (especially tumor necrosis factor-α and interleukin-1) in pathophysiology of RA now recognized
- Treatment of symptomatic cervical spine instability
  - Transoral odontoidectomy
  - Posterior fusion occiput-C1-C2
  - Laminectomy and facet fusion/stabilization
- Some believe liberal surgical treatment of C1-C2 instability may improve morbidity and mortality

DIAGNOSTIC CHECKLIST

Image Interpretation Pearls

- Watch location of anterior arch of atlas relative to odontoid to evaluate for AA impaction
- Remember AA subluxation may be underestimated on neutral lateral radiograph and CT

SELECTED REFERENCES

1. Wallis D et al: Tumour necrosis factor inhibitor therapy and infection risk in axial spondyloarthritis: results from a longitudinal observational cohort. Rheumatology (Oxford). 54(1):152-6, 2015
2. Del Grande M et al: Cervical spine involvement early in the course of rheumatoid arthritis. Semin Arthritis Rheum. 43(6):738-44, 2014
3. Kaito T et al: Predictors for the progression of cervical lesion in rheumatoid arthritis under the treatment of biological agents. Spine (Phila Pa 1976). 38(26):2258-63, 2013
4. Narváez JA et al: Bone marrow edema in the cervical spine of symptomatic rheumatoid arthritis patients. Semin Arthritis Rheum. 38(4):281-8, 2009
5. Restrepo CS et al: Imaging appearances of the sternum and sternoclavicular joints. Radiographics. 29(3):839-59, 2009

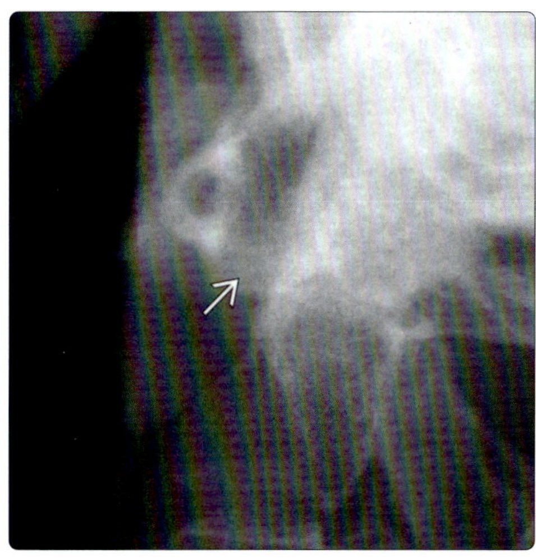

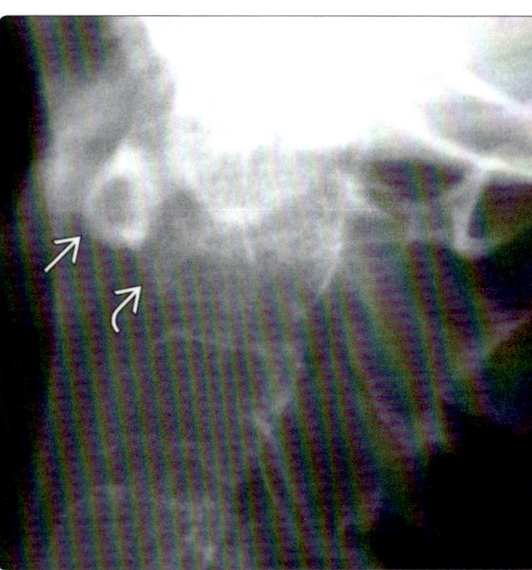

(Left) *Lateral radiograph shows AA subluxation ➡. Even more importantly, the anterior arch of the atlas is in a low position relative to the odontoid. This indicates AA impaction. The actual impaction is difficult to visualize radiographically because of superimposed mastoid processes.* **(Right)** *Lateral radiograph of the same patient 1 year later shows the anterior arch of the atlas ➡ located at the level of the body of the odontoid ➡. The AA impaction is severe.*

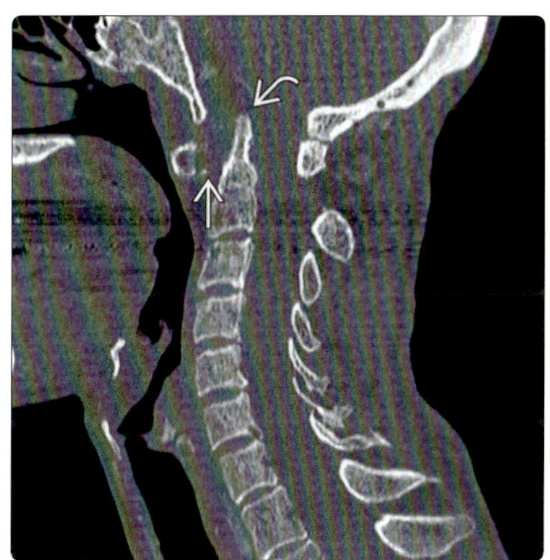

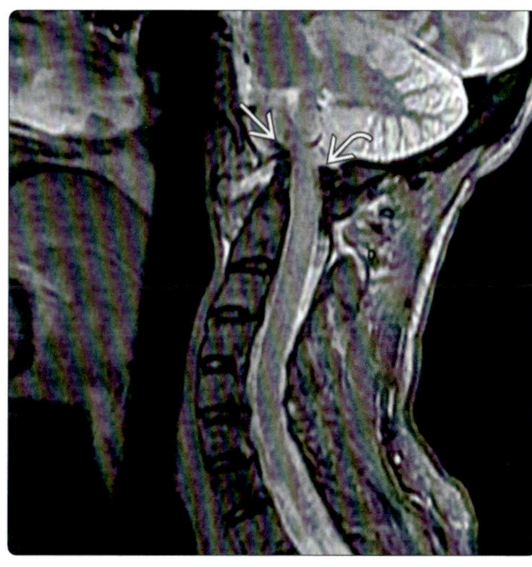

(Left) *Sagittal CT shows a typical pattern of cranial settling in RA due to AA impaction. There is upward translocation of the dens with respect to the foramen magnum ➡; Wackenheim clival line is abnormal. Dens erosion and AA subluxation ➡ are noted as well.* **(Right)** *Sagittal STIR MR of the same patient shows the impacted dens position ➡ and narrowing of the subarachnoid space at the foramen magnum with cord compression between the odontoid and opisthion ➡.*

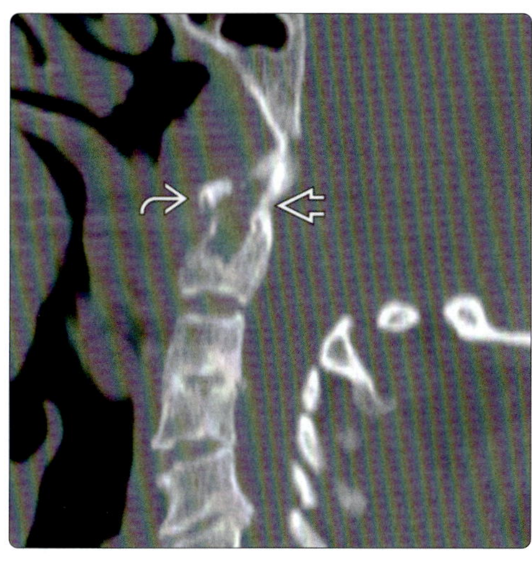

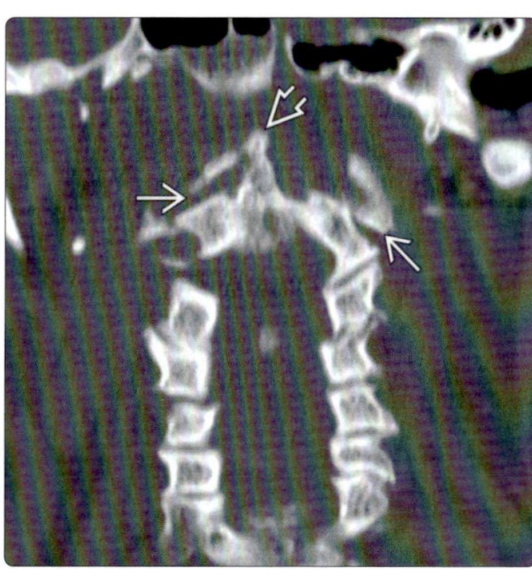

(Left) *Sagittal NECT shows severe erosive changes of C1 and odontoid process ➡. The location of the remnant of anterior arch of C1 ➡ opposite the body of C2 indicates AA impaction.* **(Right)** *Coronal NECT shows the impacted tip of the eroded odontoid ➡. It also demonstrates the erosions and collapse of the lateral masses (facets) at C1-C2 ➡. Compare this to the facets of the subaxial spine, which are normal. It is the collapse of the lateral masses that results in AA impaction.*

(Left) *Sagittal bone CT in a patient with RA shows erosions at multiple levels in the cervical spine, causing instability at occiput-C1, AA subluxation ➡, AA impaction (cranial settling) ➡, as well as endplate erosions and uncovertebral erosions at lower levels ➡. Such diffuse involvement is common.* **(Right)** *AP radiograph in a patient with RA shows angulation of the mandible ➡. The cervical spine is straight; this mandibular tilt should suggest unilateral AA impaction.*

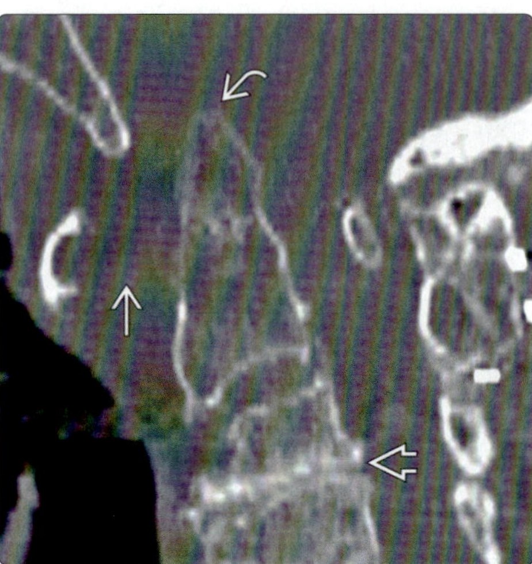

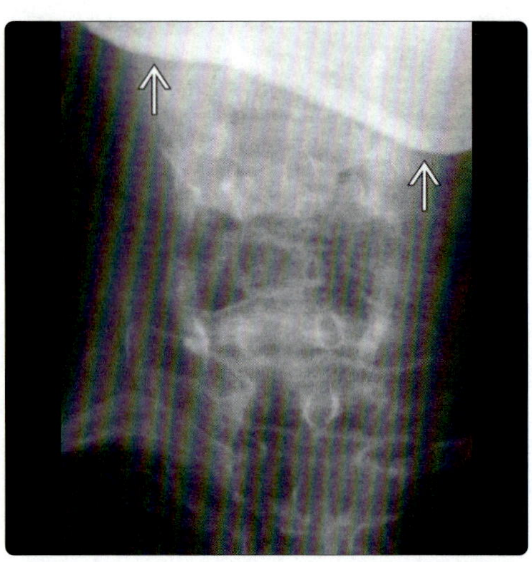

(Left) *Open mouth odontoid radiograph in an RA patient with acute torticollis shows a normal right C1-C2 facet ➡ but eroded left C1-C2 facet ➡. This discrepancy may result in unilateral collapse of this joint and associated painful torticollis.* **(Right)** *Coronal bone CT of the same patient confirms the erosions and collapse of the left C1-C2 facet ➡ compared with the normal right C1-C2 facet ➡. Note that the occiput-C1 facets ➡ are normal as well.*

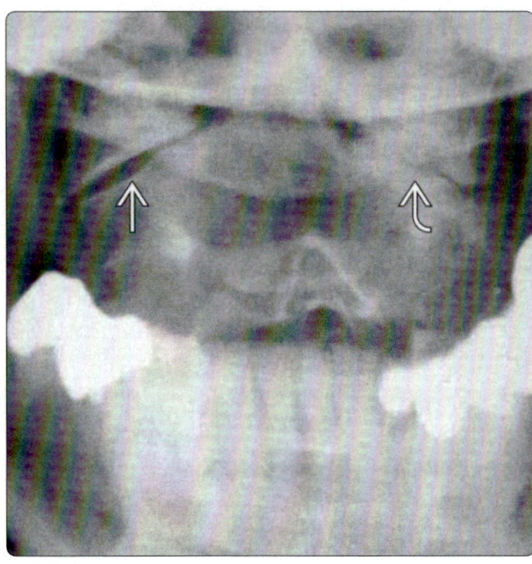

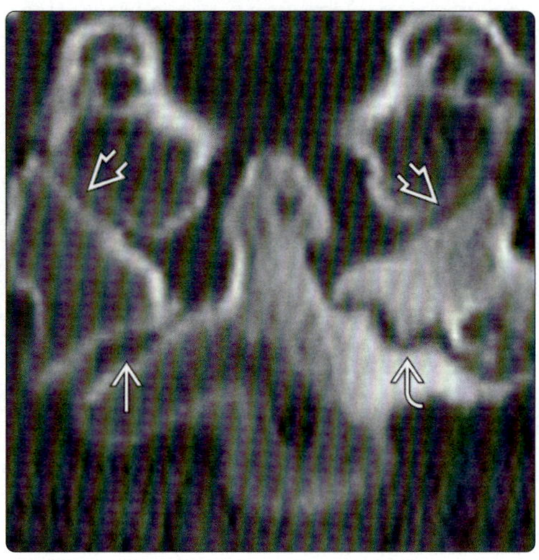

(Left) *Sagittal bone CT in this same RA patient shows the erosions and collapse of the left C1-C2 facet ➡.* **(Right)** *The normal right C1-C2 facet joint ➡ in this same patient is shown for comparison. Facet joints are at risk for erosive disease at any location of the spine. However, C1-C2 facets seem particularly at risk. If both C1-C2 facets erode and collapse, the patient may develop AA impaction. With unilateral collapse, the patient develops a painful torticollis.*

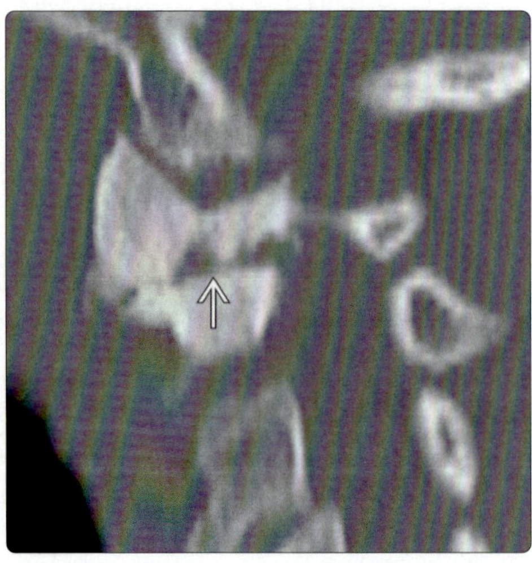

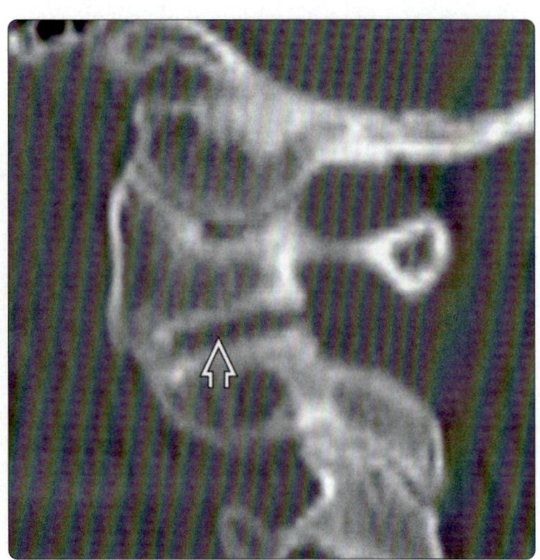

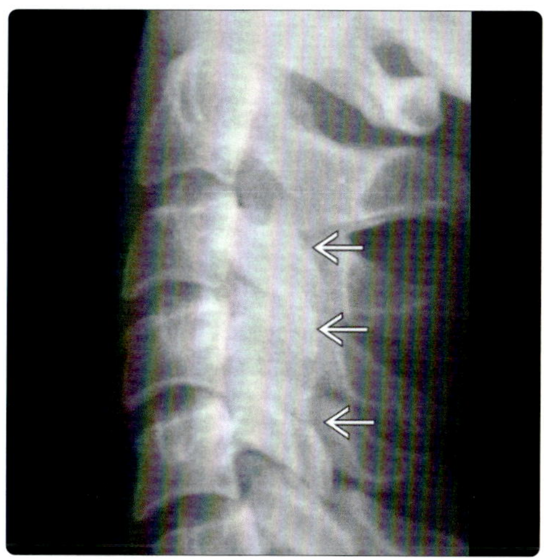

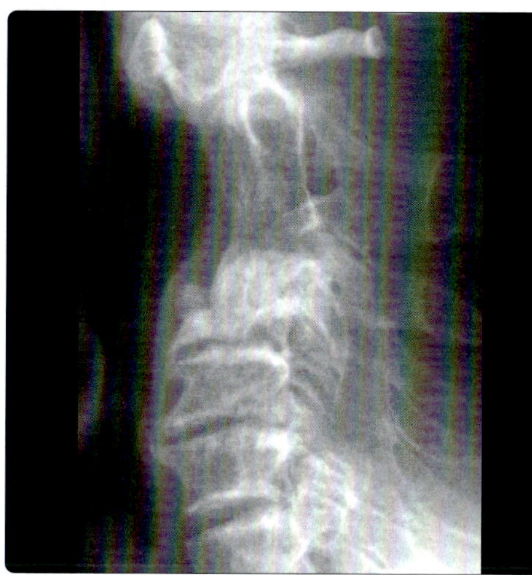

(Left) *Lateral radiograph in an RA patient with normal AA structures shows erosive change of multiple facet joints ➡. This has not yet resulted in abnormal alignment or endplate destruction.* **(Right)** *Lateral radiograph in a patient with RA shows severe erosive disease, resulting in AA subluxation, facet erosions, and presumed ligamentous disruption. The combination leads to malalignment and subsequent endplate mechanical erosions and disc destruction.*

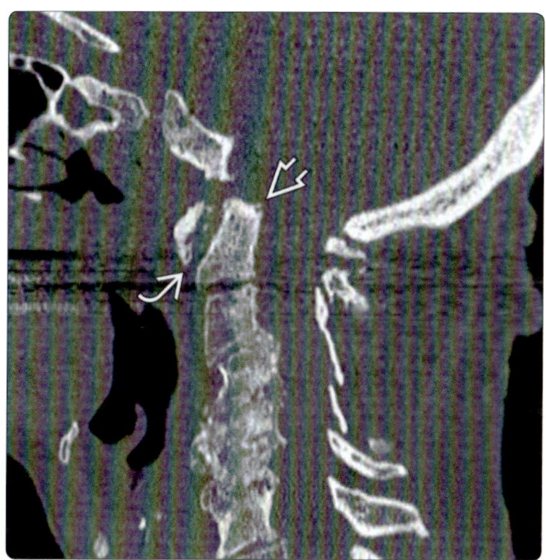

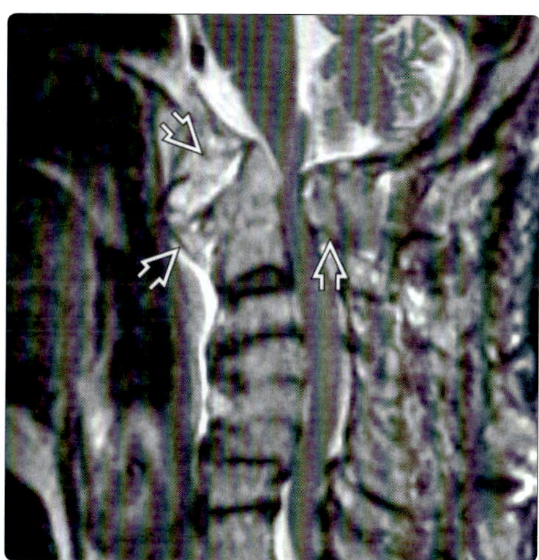

(Left) *Sagittal NECT shows C1-C2 impaction ➡. The odontoid process is eroded ➡. The subaxial spine shows marked diffuse disc and endplate degeneration due to a combination of ligamentous disruption and facet/uncovertebral joint erosions.* **(Right)** *Sagittal STIR MR shows pannus formation ➡ causing severe cord compression. C1-C2 subluxation and impaction are prominent. Multilevel subluxations of the subaxial cervical spine reflect facet and uncovertebral involvement.*

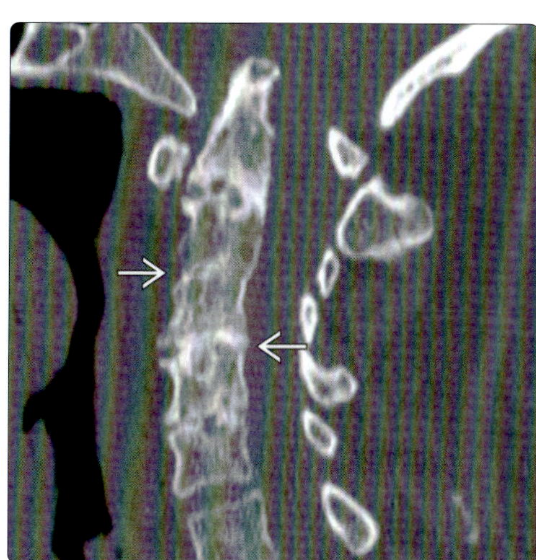

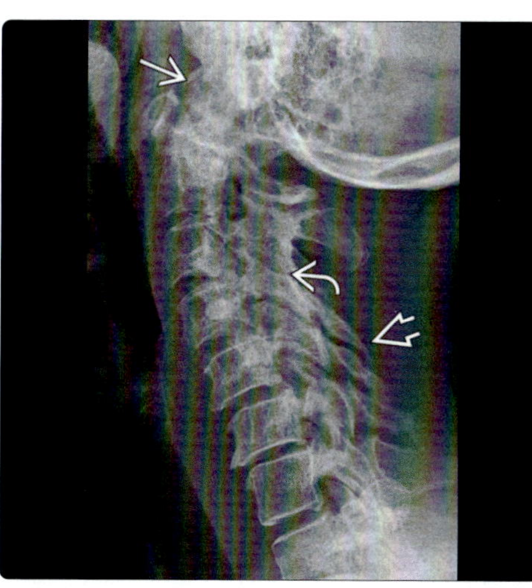

(Left) *Sagittal CT shows RA C1-C2 impaction. Note the fusion at several vertebral bodies ➡. Fusion in RA is uncommon but may occur at the site of these mechanical erosions and disc degeneration.* **(Right)** *Lateral x-ray shows mild AA subluxation and severe AA impaction ➡. Note also the eroded facets at multiple levels ➡ as well as the thinned spinous processes ➡, typical of RA. The patient has mild stair-step subluxations of the vertebral bodies secondary to a combination of abnormal motion and osteoporosis.*

Rheumatoid Arthritis of Shoulder and Elbow

KEY FACTS

TERMINOLOGY

- Chronic progressive systemic inflammatory disease in which joints are primary target

IMAGING

- Purely erosive arthropathy
- Uniform cartilage narrowing
- Osteoporosis
- Glenohumeral joint
  - Largest and earliest erosions at margin
  - Eventually, erosions uniformly involve humeral head and glenoid
  - Subchondral cysts may be large, but underlying osteoporosis may mask their size
  - Elevation of humeral head due to rotator cuff tear
  - Hatchet-like mechanical erosion at medial surgical neck of humerus
  - Swelling of joint may be prominent due to decompression of synovial fluid through rotator cuff tear (RCT) into subacromial/subdeltoid bursa
- Elbow joint
  - Effusion (elevated anterior and posterior fat pads)
  - Olecranon bursitis common in rheumatoid arthritis (RA)
  - Erosions uniform throughout joint
- MR in RA
  - Thickened, low signal, avidly enhancing pannus and synovium
  - Low signal rice bodies within effusion
  - Subchondral marrow edema
  - RCT, partial or complete
  - Decompression of synovial effusion well seen

DIAGNOSTIC CHECKLIST

- Other causes of synovitis, especially infection if monoarticular

(Left) *AP radiograph shows erosions of the distal end of the clavicle ➡ as well as at the coracoclavicular ligament insertion site of the clavicle ➡, typical sites of erosions in rheumatoid arthritis (RA).* **(Right)** *Coronal graphic shows advanced RA of the shoulder. Thickened synovium lining the capsule is distended by effusion. Cartilage is thinned uniformly. Large marginal erosions are seen where bone is not covered by cartilage, and smaller subchondral erosions are present. Marrow edema and rotator cuff tear complete the picture.*

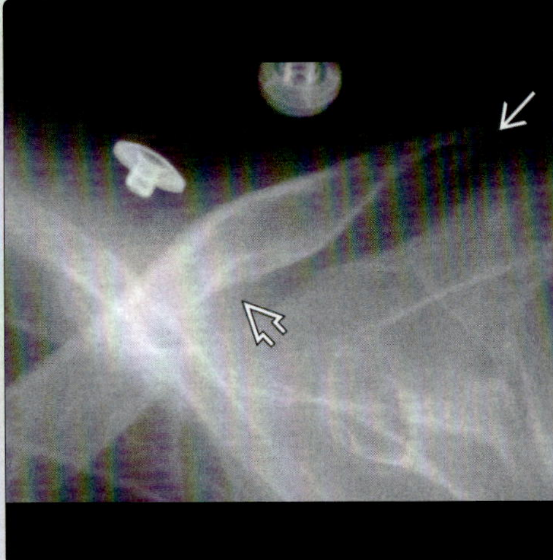

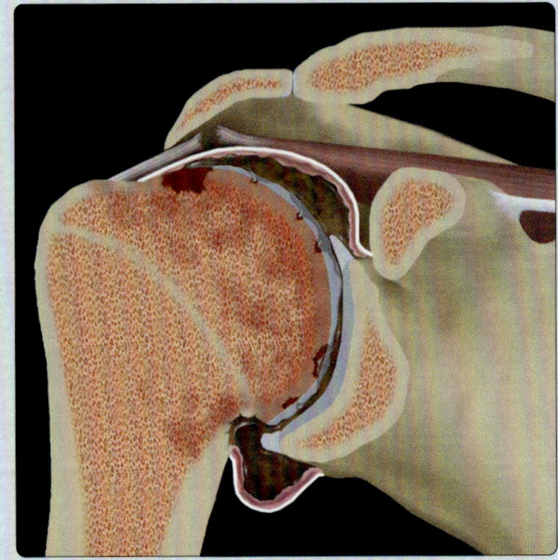

(Left) *Axial bone CT demonstrates the typical uniform glenohumeral cartilage loss ➡ that is seen in RA, along with humeral head erosions and subchondral cysts ➡.* **(Right)** *Coronal bone CT shows marginal erosion at the humeral head ➡. The head is subluxated superiorly secondary to chronic rotator cuff tear. This results in a mechanical erosion of the osteoporotic bone at the surgical neck of the humerus ➡; this puts the patient at additional risk of fracture.*

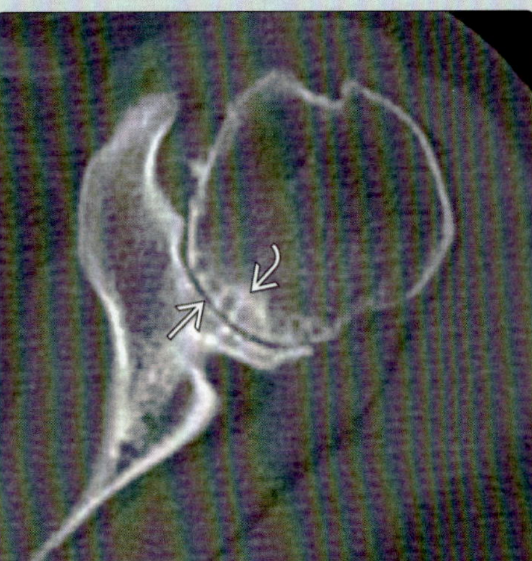

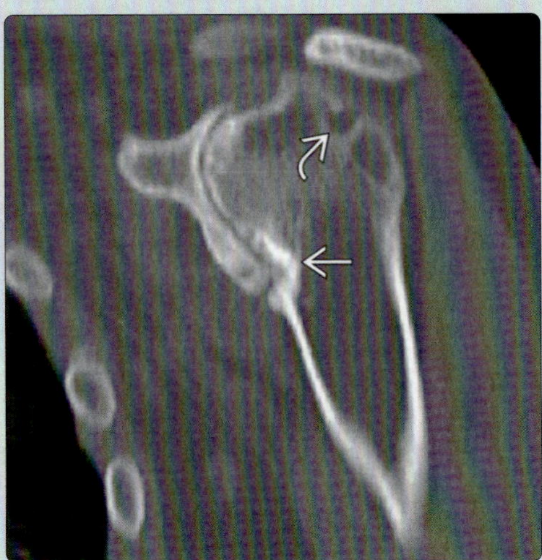

TERMINOLOGY

Abbreviations

- Rheumatoid arthritis (RA)
- Rotator cuff tear (RCT)

Definitions

- Chronic progressive systemic inflammatory disease in which joints are primary target

IMAGING

General Features

- Best diagnostic clue
  - Purely erosive arthropathy
  - Uniform cartilage narrowing
  - Osteoporosis
- Location
  - Earliest changes are in synovium, followed by cartilage and bone

Radiographic Findings

- Acromioclavicular (AC) joint
  - Erosions on both sides of joint
  - End-stage penciling of clavicle into thin point
  - May resorb clavicle at insertion of coracoclavicular ligaments
- Glenohumeral joint
  - Uniform cartilage narrowing
  - Erosions
    - Largest and earliest at margin (junction of cartilage-covered humeral head and greater tuberosity)
    - Eventually, erosions uniformly involve humeral head and glenoid
    - End-stage destruction of entire head and glenoid
  - Subchondral cysts may be large, but underlying osteoporosis may mask their size
  - Elevation of humeral head due to RCT
    - With chronicity, head seems to articulate with underside of acromion, molding acromion into concavity
  - Hatchet-like mechanical erosion at medial surgical neck of humerus
    - Due to chronic elevation of humeral head and consequent rubbing of osteoporotic humeral neck against inferior glenoid
    - Increases risk of insufficiency fracture across surgical neck
  - Swelling of joint may be prominent due to decompression of synovial fluid through RCT into subacromial/subdeltoid bursa
- Elbow joint
  - Effusion (elevated anterior and posterior fat pads)
  - Swelling about joint
    - Over olecranon: Olecranon bursitis common in RA
    - Elsewhere due to decompression of synovial fluid through capsule or into bicipital radial bursa
  - Erosions uniform throughout joint
    - Equally involving capitellum, trochlea, ulna, radial head/neck
    - End-stage uniform destruction of osseous structures

CT Findings

- Same osseous findings as noted on radiograph
  - Erosions and subchondral cysts more apparent
- Inflamed synovium enhances

MR Findings

- T1WI
  - Thickened low signal pannus
  - Low signal effusion, erosions, and subchondral cysts
  - If superimposed amyloid, deposits are low signal
    - Intraarticular or within thickened tendons
- Fluid-sensitive sequences
  - Effusion is high signal
  - Thickened low signal pannus lines synovium
  - Low signal rice bodies within effusion
  - Erosions and subchondral cysts high signal
  - Subchondral marrow edema
  - RCT, partial or complete
  - Decompression of synovial effusion well seen
    - Shoulder: Generally through RCT into subacromial/subdeltoid bursa
    - Elbow: Into bicipital radial bursa or into adjacent soft tissues
  - If amyloid deposits present, they remain low signal
  - ↑ signal ulnar nerve from elbow impingement
- T1WI FS + contrast
  - Avid enhancement of thick pannus along synovium
  - Subchondral cysts and erosions have high signal surrounding low signal fluid contents

Imaging Recommendations

- Best imaging tool
  - Radiographs generally make diagnosis
  - MR often adds information
    - Integrity of rotator cuff
    - Early (preradiographic) diagnosis: Synovitis
    - Early osseous destructive phase: More accurate evaluation of erosions and subchondral cysts

DIFFERENTIAL DIAGNOSIS

Septic Arthritis

- In differential of early RA
- Enhancing synovitis, effusion
- Marrow edema or early erosions

Charcot, Neuropathic

- In differential of late shoulder RA
- Destruction of humeral head and glenoid
- Large effusion, decompressing into subdeltoid via RCT
- Presence of osseous debris and lack of pannus helps to differentiate
- Generally unilateral; etiology is syringomyelia

Spondyloarthropathies

- Ankylosing spondylitis and enteric spondylitis often involve large proximal joints (shoulder, hip)
- Early in disease, may appear purely inflammatory, with synovitis and erosions
- Later in disease, generally mixed erosive/productive
- Spine/SI joint involvement differentiates from RA

PATHOLOGY

General Features

- Etiology
  - Unknown etiology
  - Pathophysiology presumed to relate to persistent immunologic response of a genetically susceptible host to some unknown antigen
- Genetics
  - Genetic predisposition
    - Concordance in monozygotic twins: 25%
    - 1st-degree relatives develop RA at rate 4x that of general population
  - Individual not likely to have affected family member
- Associated abnormalities
  - Subcutaneous rheumatoid nodules in 30%
    - Extensor surfaces (ulna, Achilles) and digits
  - Amyloid deposition
  - Thoracic: Pleural effusions, rheumatoid nodules, rarely interstitial fibrosis
  - Vasculitis
  - Felty syndrome: RA + splenomegaly + leukopenia
  - Sjögren syndrome: RA + keratoconjunctivitis + xerostomia
  - ↑ risk of lymphoma
  - Lifetime of systemic inflammation may contribute to ↑ risk of cardiovascular disease, renal disease, and infection
  - ↑ mortality rate, reduced survival by 10-18 years

Gross Pathologic & Surgical Features

- Synovial lining is hypertrophic, edematous
- Joint distension, osseous erosion, cartilage destruction
- Rice bodies: Detached synovial villi

Microscopic Features

- Organized accumulations of CD4 helper T cells, antigen presenting cells, lymphoid follicles
- Large amounts of immunoglobulin produced, including rheumatoid factor
- Angiogenesis in synovium

CLINICAL ISSUES

Presentation

- Most common signs/symptoms
  - Symmetric polyarthritis, especially small joints
  - Constitutional symptoms of fatigue, low-grade fever
  - Usually presents over course of weeks or months; occasionally fulminant disease
- Other signs/symptoms
  - Shoulder/elbow
    - Pain, swelling, ↓ range of motion
    - RCT symptoms

Demographics

- Age
  - Peak age at onset: 3rd-5th decades
- Gender
  - M:F = 1:3
- Epidemiology
  - RA in 1% of worldwide population
    - 5% in some Native American populations
  - Shoulder involved in 60% of patients with RA
  - Acromioclavicular involved in 50% of patients with RA
  - Elbow involved in 50% of patients with RA

Natural History & Prognosis

- Up to 60% go into remission
  - With aggressive multidrug Rx, most improve
- With severe erosions and RCT, poor prognosis for shoulder function

Treatment

- Treatment of RA: Generally combination of drugs, aimed at pain relief while escalating therapy rapidly to suppress disease prior to joint destruction
  - Nonsteroidal antiinflammatory drugs
    - Symptomatic relief; do not alter disease progress
  - Glucocorticoids (oral or intraarticular)
    - Controls inflammation rapidly; allows slower acting drugs to take effect
  - Disease-modifying antirheumatic drugs
    - Suppresses joint destruction (e.g., methotrexate, sulfasalazine, antimalarials, gold)
  - Biologics: Anti-TNF-α drugs, antiinterleukin-1
    - Role of cytokines (especially tumor necrosis factor-α and interleukin-1) now recognized
- Surgical treatment
  - Synovectomy may arrest/delay progression
  - Shoulder
    - Poor prognosis for RCT repairs
    - Arthroplasty: Often reverse shoulder device is chosen because of rotator cuff tear
      - RA patients at particular risk for periprosthetic fracture, especially of acromion
  - Elbow
    - Radial head resection → symptomatic relief
    - Arthroplasty often fails (loosening, periprosthetic fracture) due to thin osteoporotic bone

DIAGNOSTIC CHECKLIST

Consider

- Other etiologies of synovitis, especially infection if monoarticular

SELECTED REFERENCES

1. Levy O et al: Surface replacement arthroplasty for glenohumeral arthropathy in patients aged younger than fifty years: results after a minimum ten-year follow-up. J Shoulder Elbow Surg. 24(7):1049-60, 2015
2. Morris BJ et al: Risk factors for periprosthetic infection after reverse shoulder arthroplasty. J Shoulder Elbow Surg. 24(2):161-6, 2015
3. Cross MB et al: Results of custom-fit, noncemented, semiconstrained total elbow arthroplasty for inflammatory arthritis at an average of eighteen years of follow-up. J Shoulder Elbow Surg. 23(9):1368-73, 2014
4. van der Zwaal P et al: The natural history of the rheumatoid shoulder: a prospective long-term follow-up study. Bone Joint J. 96-B(11):1520-4, 2014
5. Jämsen E et al: The decline in joint replacement surgery in rheumatoid arthritis is associated with a concomitant increase in the intensity of anti-rheumatic therapy: a nationwide register-based study from 1995 through 2010. Acta Orthop. 84(4):331-7, 2013
6. Bøyesen P et al: Prediction of MRI erosive progression: a comparison of modern imaging modalities in early rheumatoid arthritis patients. Ann Rheum Dis. 70(1):176-9, 2011
7. Narváez JA et al: MR imaging of early rheumatoid arthritis. Radiographics. 30(1):143-63; discussion 163-5, 2010

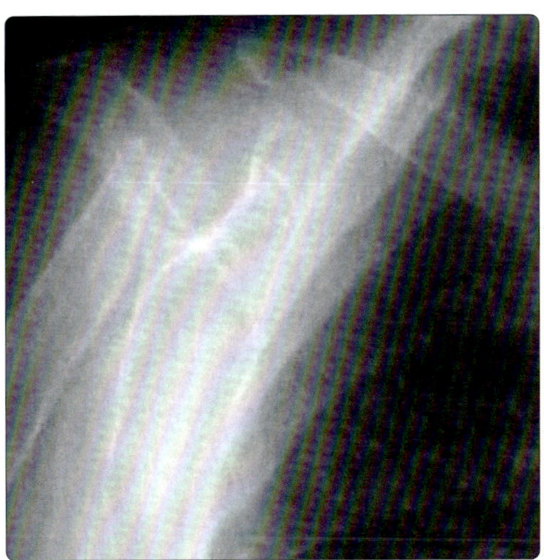

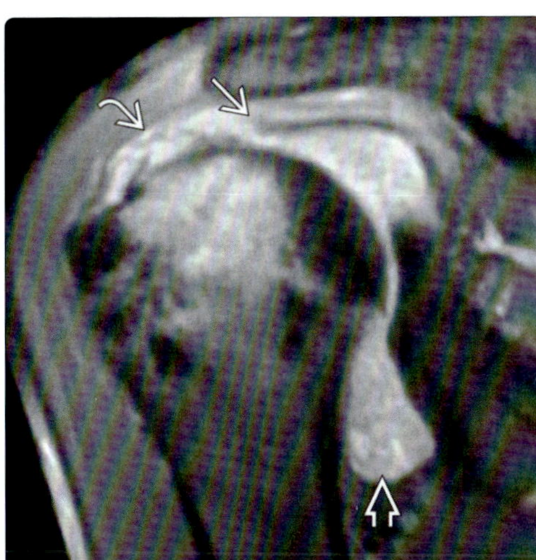

(Left) *AP radiograph shows a case of severe, long-term RA, with erosions of the clavicle, glenoid, and humeral head.* **(Right)** *Coronal PD FS MR shows the retracted infraspinatus tendon ➡, part of the chronic rotator cuff tear that is usually seen with advanced RA. There is mild edema in the humeral head. The glenohumeral joint is distended, and low signal synovitis fills the axillary bursa ➡ and extends across the rotator cuff tear into the subacromial bursa ➡. Note the humeral head elevation.*

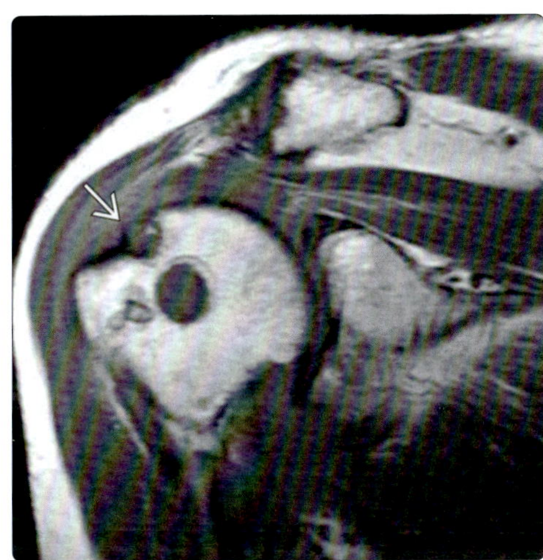

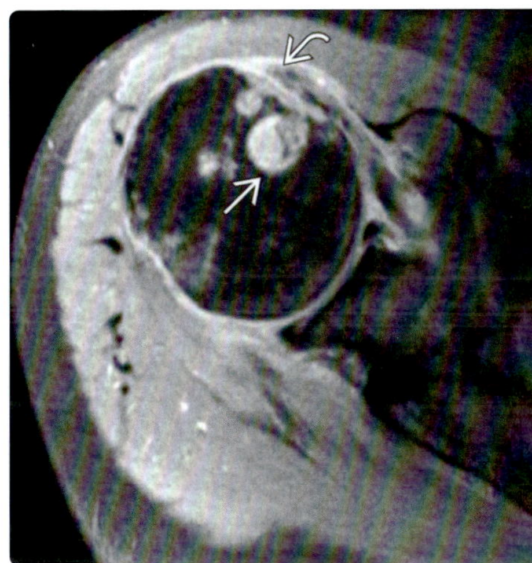

(Left) *Coronal T1WI MR shows typical findings of RA in the shoulder. There are low signal subchondral cysts, as well as a marginal erosion of the humeral head ➡.* **(Right)** *Axial PD FSE FS MR in the same patient shows subchondral cysts as well as a marginal erosion ➡. Note the thin and disrupted subscapularis tendon ➡, with fluid seen both in the glenohumeral joint and subdeltoid bursa. It seems remarkable that the radiograph in this case appeared normal.*

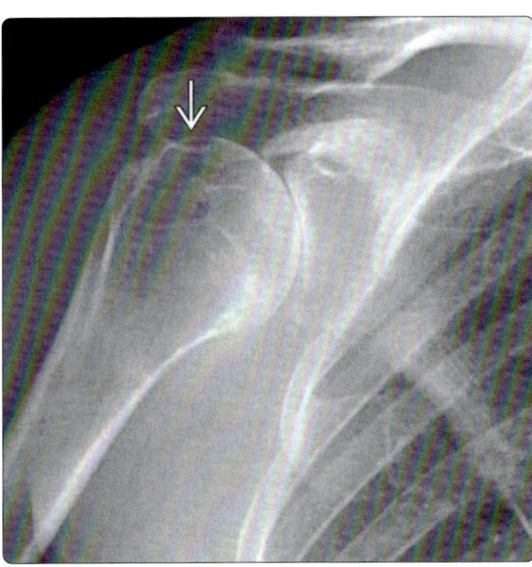

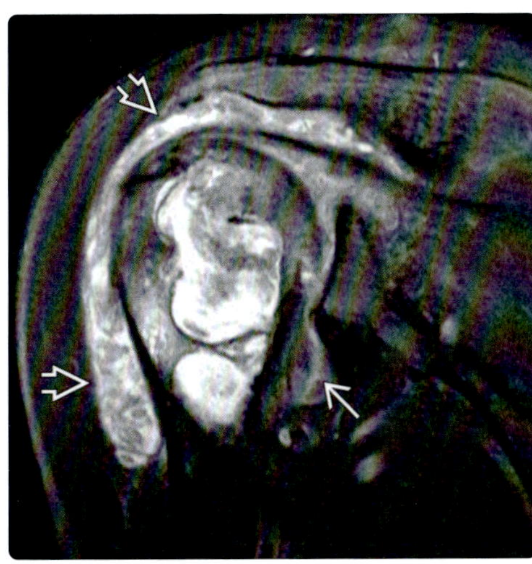

(Left) *AP radiograph in a patient with RA shows only osteopenia and a small marginal erosion ➡. The osteopenia seen on radiographs in patients with RA often disguises the full extent of erosive disease and subchondral cysts.* **(Right)** *Coronal T2WI FS MR in the same patient shows tremendous synovitis in both the glenohumeral joint ➡ and subacromial/subdeltoid bursa ➡. The diffuse nodular low signal masses within the fluid are synovitis.*

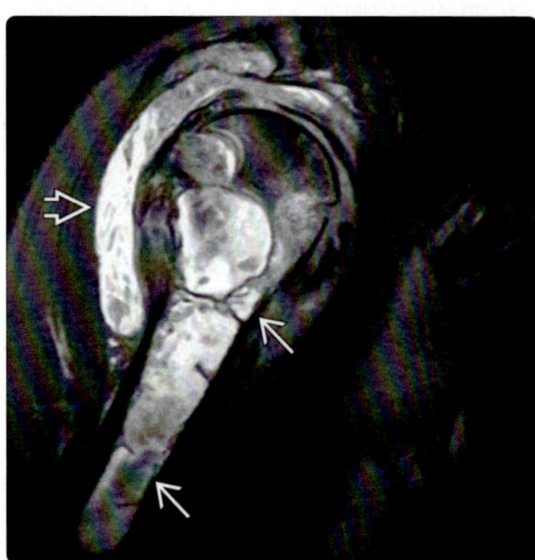

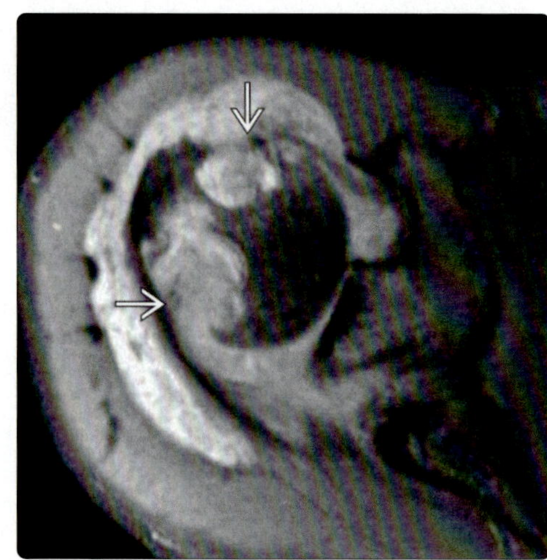

(Left) *Sagittal T2WI FS MR in the same patient emphasizes the tremendous synovitis in both the glenohumeral joint and subacromial/subdeltoid bursa ➡. Both the synovitis and extent of subchondral cysts extending down the marrow ➡ are well depicted.* **(Right)** *Axial PD FS MR in the same patient shows the size of the erosions ➡. It is quite remarkable that the radiographs showed only osteopenia and a small erosion, even in retrospect. This humeral metadiaphysis is at risk for fracture.*

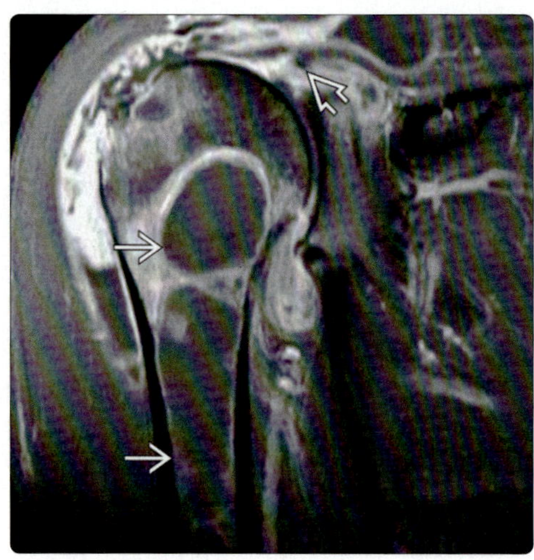

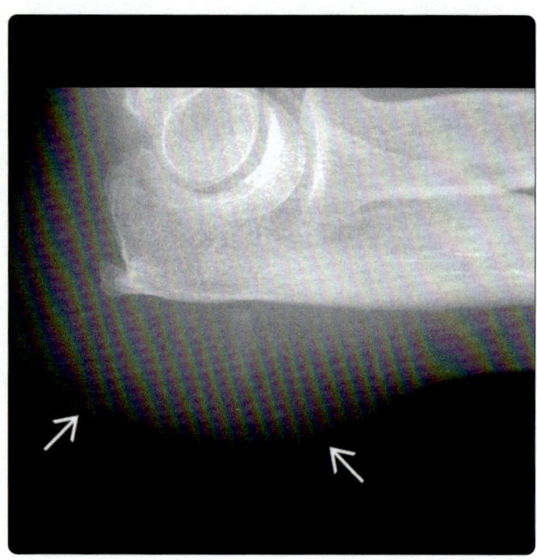

(Left) *Coronal T1 FS postcontrast MR in the same patient confirms that the marrow abnormality represents erosions and subchondral cysts, with low signal fluid surrounded by enhancing synovitis ➡. A rotator cuff tear is seen as well, with retraction of supraspinatus ➡.* **(Right)** *Lateral radiograph of the elbow shows diffuse osteopenia and soft tissue swelling over the olecranon ➡. The location is typical for olecranon bursitis, secondary to RA in this case.*

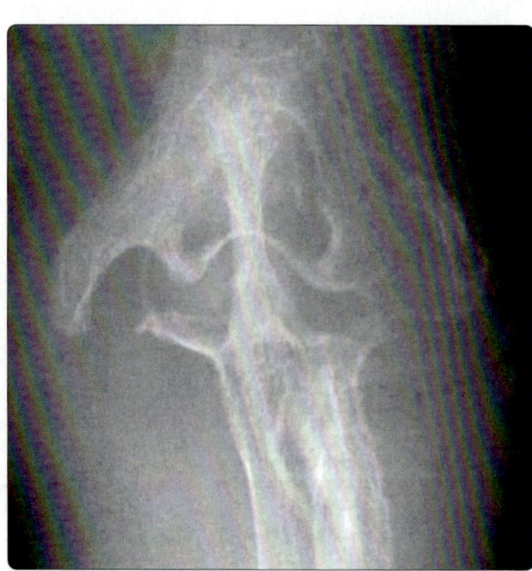

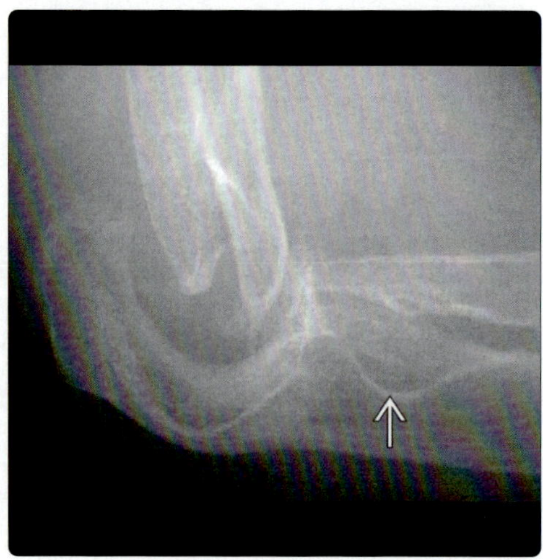

(Left) *Anteroposterior radiograph shows a classic case of severe and long-term RA. There is symmetric erosive disease of the distal humerus, proximal radius, and proximal ulna, along with osteopenia.* **(Right)** *Lateral radiograph confirms the erosions, as well as a mechanical erosion at the proximal shaft of the ulna ➡ where the remnant of radial head has been rubbing. The symmetry of the process and purely erosive nature make the diagnosis RA.*

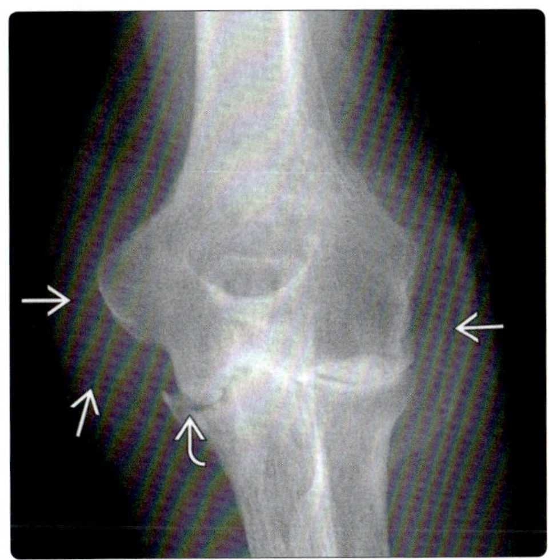

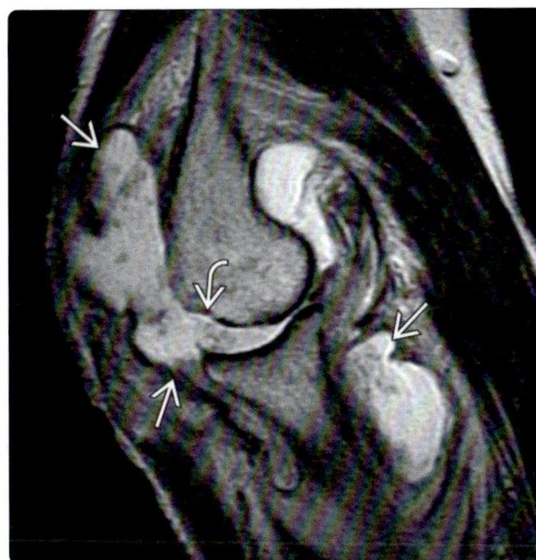

(Left) *AP radiograph shows extensive uniform thinning of cartilage throughout the elbow and subchondral erosions at the coronoid. There is extensive soft tissue swelling and diffuse osteopenia. No productive change is seen; the findings are typical of RA.* **(Right)** *Sagittal T2FS MR in the same case of RA shows complete loss of cartilage and thinning of cortex at the capitellum. The fluid is all contained within an extremely distended joint and contains low signal material that has been termed rice bodies.*

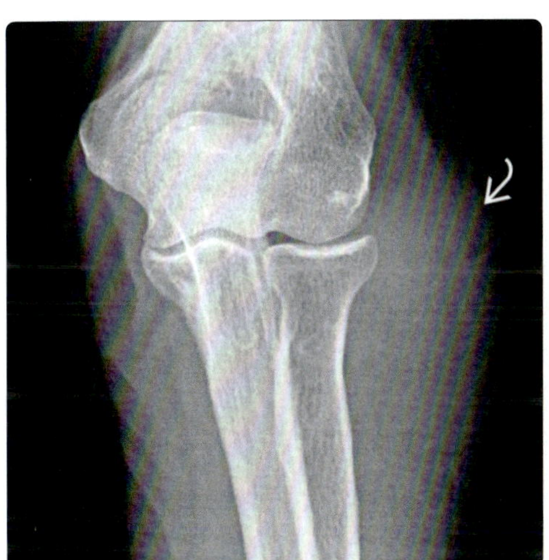

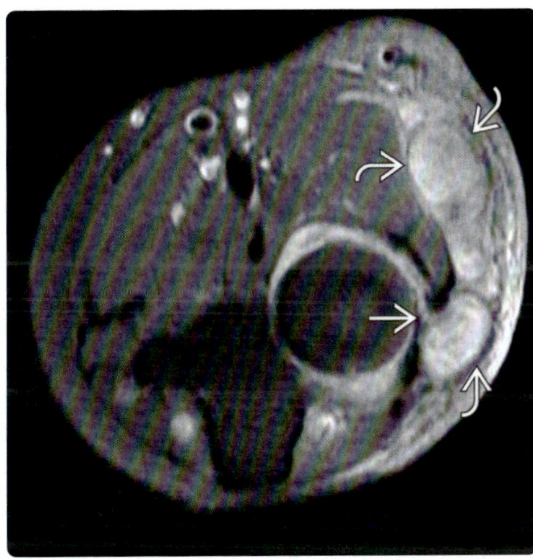

(Left) *AP radiograph shows a lateral soft tissue mass but no other abnormalities in a patient with RA.* **(Right)** *Axial PD FS MR performed to evaluate the soft tissue mass in the same patient shows synovitis and fluid surrounding the radial neck. There is a thin neck of fluid extending from the joint effusion to the mass. This proves that the mass is simply fluid from the joint, which has decompressed into the soft tissues laterally, as happens in restricted joints with active synovitis.*

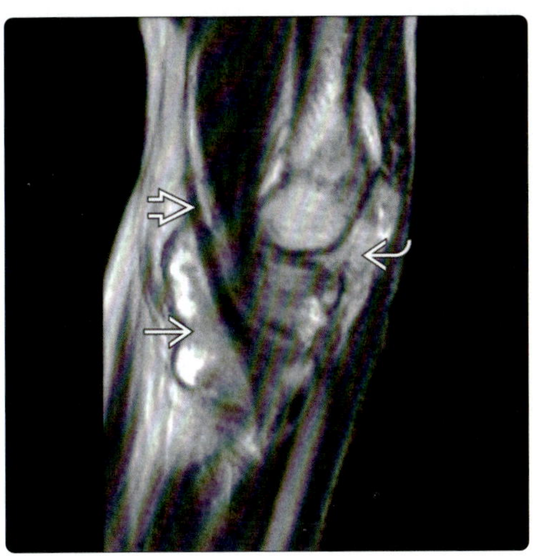

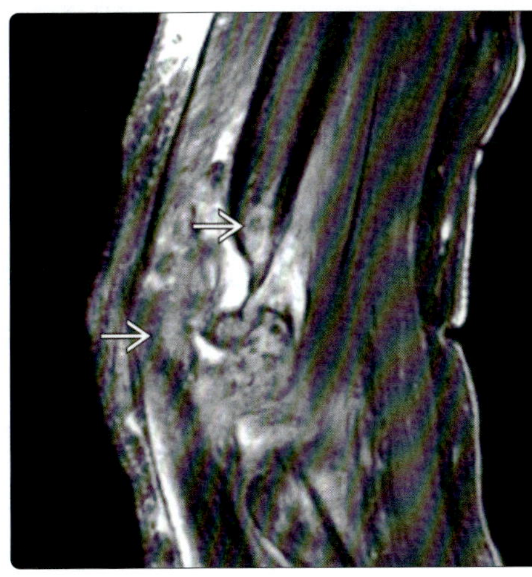

(Left) *Sagittal T2WI MR shows bicipital radial bursitis related to RA. Lobular-enhancing synovitis is seen in the bicipital radial bursa around the biceps tendon. Fluid and synovitis are also seen in the elbow joint.* **(Right)** *Sagittal T2WI MR in a patient with RA shows joint destruction, large effusion, and abnormal bone marrow signal. These findings could be due simply to advanced RA, but infection must be considered and was proved surgically.*

KEY FACTS

IMAGING

- Erosions
  - Earliest osseous pattern is loss of cortical distinctness, followed by dot-dash pattern of cortical loss
  - Marginal erosions tend to occur early in portion of bone which is within capsule but not covered by cartilage
  - Direct subchondral erosions
  - Late aggressive disease: Pencil-in-cup appearance in phalanges
- Ulnar styloid may show capping: Only site of productive change in RA
- Malalignment due to ligament/tendon disruption
- MR: Pannus: Thick, nodular low signal synovium outlined by effusion
  - Marrow edema: Subchondral high signal
  - Thickened, avidly enhancing synovium outlines low signal effusion and erosions
  - Tenosynovitis may be earliest soft tissue abnormality, though nonspecific
- US: Excellent for early effusions in small joints
  - Tenosynovitis and tendon rupture seen directly

CLINICAL ISSUES

- RA in 1% of worldwide population
  - 5% in some Native American populations
- Female > male (3:1)
- Carpus involved in 80% patients with RA
- MCPs involved in 85% patients with RA
- Hand PIP involved in 75% patients with RA

DIAGNOSTIC CHECKLIST

- Earliest RA may be monostotic or asymmetric
  - Must differentiate from septic joint
- Use sites of focal soft tissue swelling to guide you to subtle osseous findings on radiograph
- Watch for cortical indistinctness and dot-dash pattern for earliest radiographic signs of erosion

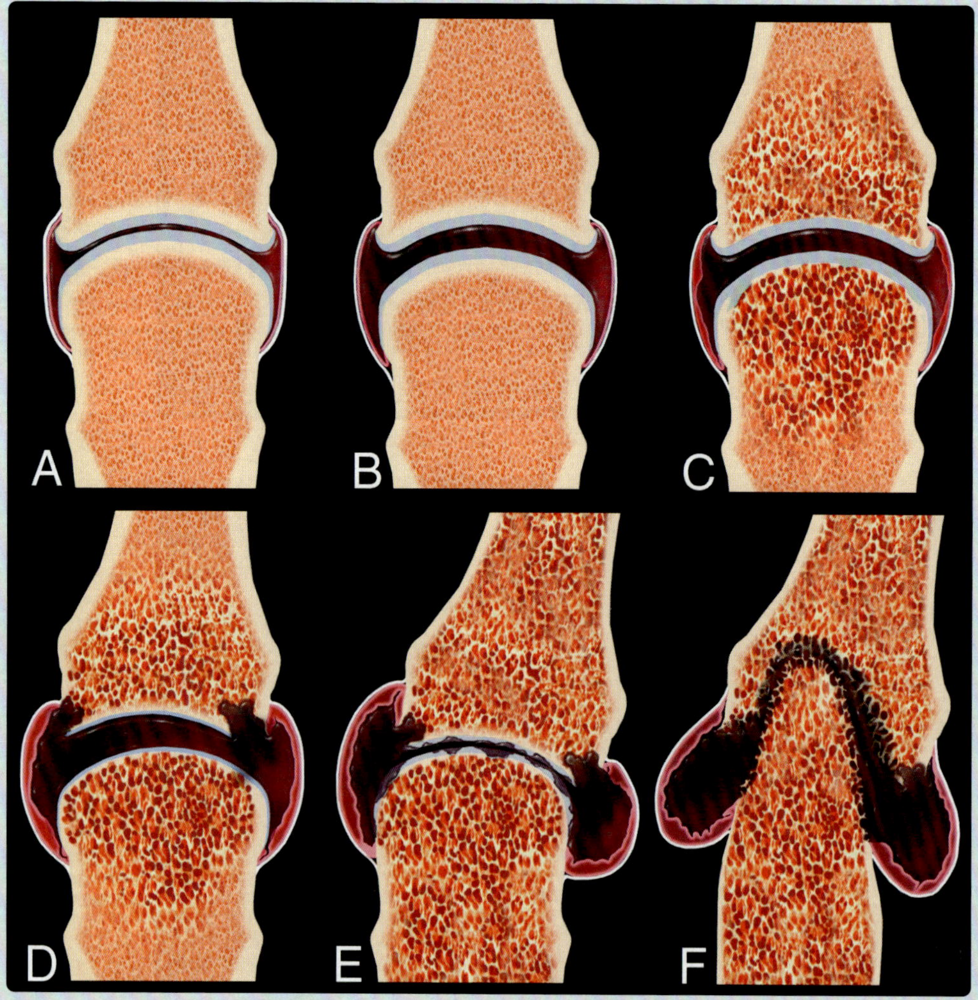

PA graphic of a PIP joint shows progressive destruction of the joint. (A) is normal, with intact cortex, cartilage, bone density, and capsule. (B) shows early disease, with only synovitis and effusion. (C) shows juxtaarticular osteopenia, with cortex becoming indistinct, the dot-dash pattern. (D) shows thinning of cartilage and marginal erosions in the portion of bone which is intracapsular but not protected by cartilage. (E) shows progression of osteopenia and subchondral erosions extending through cartilage defects. (F) shows arthritis mutilans, with pencil-in-cup deformity, seen in end-stage disease.

TERMINOLOGY

Abbreviations

- Rheumatoid arthritis (RA)

Definitions

- Chronic progressive systemic inflammatory disease in which joints are primary target

IMAGING

General Features

- Best diagnostic clue
  - Purely erosive disease
  - Osteoporotic
  - Malalignment
- Location
  - Symmetry of disease is classic
    - Early in disease, may be unilateral
  - Early involvement of disease
    - Metacarpophalangeal (MCP) or proximal interphalangeal joint (PIP)
    - Distal radioulnar joint (DRUJ)
    - Radiocarpal joint (RC)
  - Later involvement
    - Intercarpal joints
  - Distal interphalangeal joints (DIP) and 1st carpometacarpal (CMC) joints not involved until end stage

Radiographic Findings

- Hand and foot have earliest involvement; watch for subtle changes
- Focal soft tissue swelling may be clue to underlying bone involvement
  - Especially about MCP, PIP, ulnar styloid
- Osteoporosis
  - Early: Juxtaarticular
  - Later: Diffuse
- Erosions
  - Earliest pattern is loss of cortical distinctness, followed by dot-dash pattern of cortical loss
  - Marginal erosions tend to be early in portion of bone, which is within capsule but not covered by cartilage
    - Mouse ears appearance at base of phalanges
    - Ulnar and radial styloid processes
  - Direct subchondral erosions
  - Late severe destruction of osseous structures
    - May give pencil-in-cup appearance in phalanges
    - May destroy distal ulna or proximal carpal row
- Cartilage destruction
  - Initial radiographs may make joint space appear wide due to distension from effusion
  - Cartilage thinning and narrowing of joint are uniform
- Subchondral cysts frequent finding in RA but nonspecific
- Ulnar styloid may show capping: Only site of productive change in RA
- Malalignment due to ligament/tendon disruption
  - Carpus
    - Ulnar translocation (carpals subluxate ulnarly such that lunate mostly articulates with ulna)
    - Volar subluxation of carpus on radius
    - Scapholunate dissociation
    - Volar or dorsal intercalated segmental instability (VISI or DISI)
  - Digits
    - Ulnar drift at MCPs
    - Volar subluxation of MCPs
    - Hitchhiker's thumb
    - "Boutonnière" (hyperflexion PIP, hyperextension DIP) and "swan neck" (hyperextension PIP, hyperflexion DIP) deformities

CT Findings

- Mirror radiographic findings; rarely used except in postoperative evaluation

MR Findings

- T1WI
  - Low signal effusion, erosions
- Fluid-sensitive sequences
  - High signal effusion, erosions, subchondral cysts
  - High signal tenosynovitis
  - Pannus: Thick, nodular, low signal synovium outlined by effusion
  - Marrow edema: Subchondral high signal
- T1WI C+ FS
  - Thickened, avidly enhancing synovium outlines low signal effusion and erosions
  - Tenosynovitis: Enhancement of involved tendons
  - Median nerve may enhance if impinged by tenosynovitis in carpal tunnel

Ultrasonographic Findings

- Excellent for early effusions in small joints
- Tenosynovitis: Hyperechoic
- Tendon rupture: Direct visualization
- Color Doppler evaluates hypervascularity
- Rheumatoid nodule: Homogeneous hypoechoic mass

Imaging Recommendations

- Best imaging tool
  - Initial imaging is radiograph
  - If negative, US or MR useful to detect early disease
    - Excellent for detection, but not prognostic for individual
  - Following therapy (generally drug studies)
    - US with Doppler good for effusions, inflammation
    - MR best for following early erosions
- Protocol advice
  - Radiographs: PA and open-book view (Norgard)
    - Open-book view helpful to identify early MCP, triquetral, and pisiform erosions
    - If carpal alignment evaluation is required, true lateral view should be added
  - Half dose contrast at 3T MR sufficient for assessing synovitis/tenosynovitis in early RA

DIFFERENTIAL DIAGNOSIS

Systemic Lupus Erythematosus

- Deformities in similar pattern but reducible
- Nonerosive until late in disease; prominent tenosynovitis

Erosive Osteoarthritis

- Erosive, but distribution is that of OA
  - DIP > PIP; 1st carpometacarpal joint, scapho-trapezoid-trapezium joint

Psoriatic Arthritis

- May initially be purely erosive
- Distribution favors DIP joints but may involve others
- Distribution in carpus unpredictable
- May have evidence of periostitis (fluffy periosteal reaction along shafts or at bases of digits)
- Dynamic enhancement pattern may differentiate psoriatic arthritis from RA at 15 minutes

Hyperparathyroidism

- Subchondral resorption at ends of digits or carpal bones may collapse, simulating erosion
- Other signs of hyperparathyroidism: Subchondral resorption, tuft resorption, vascular calcification

PATHOLOGY

General Features

- Etiology
  - Unknown etiology
  - Pathophysiology presumed to relate to persistent immunologic response of genetically susceptible host to some unknown antigen
- Genetics
  - Genetic predisposition
    - Concordance in monozygotic twins: 25%
    - 1st-degree relatives develop RA at rate 4x that of general population
  - Individual not likely to have affected family member

Gross Pathologic & Surgical Features

- Synovial lining is hypertrophic, edematous
- Joint distension, osseous erosion, cartilage destruction

CLINICAL ISSUES

Presentation

- Most common signs/symptoms
  - Symmetric polyarthritis, especially involving small joints of hand and foot
    - May be asymmetric or monoarticular initially
  - Constitutional symptoms of fatigue, low-grade fever
  - Usually presents over course of weeks or months; occasionally fulminant disease
- Other signs/symptoms
  - Wrist and hand deformities
    - Ulnar translocation of carpus
    - Scapholunate dissociation; carpal instability
    - Volar subluxation and ulnar drift MCPs
    - "Boutonnière," "swan neck," "hitchhiker" deformities

Demographics

- Age
  - Peak onset: 3rd-5th decades
- Gender
  - Female > male (3:1)
- Epidemiology
  - RA in 1% of worldwide population
    - 5% in some Native American populations
  - Carpus involved in 80% patients with RA
  - MCPs involved in 85% patients with RA
  - Hand PIP involved in 75% patients with RA

Natural History & Prognosis

- May have remission with aggressive multidrug Rx
- Those resistant to therapy show continued worsening of erosions, ligament, and tendon disease
  - Progressive pain and loss of function

Treatment

- Generally combination of drugs, aimed at pain relief while escalating therapy rapidly to suppress disease prior to joint destruction
  - Biologics: Anti-TNF-α drugs, anti-interleukin-1
    - Role of cytokines (especially tumor necrosis factor-α and interleukin-1) in pathophysiology of RA now recognized
- Surgical treatment
  - Synovectomy, tenosynovectomy
  - Carpus
    - Resection of distal ulna
    - Proximal carpectomy
    - Arthrodesis (generally dorsal plating of radius, through scaphoid, lunate, capitate, to 3rd MC)
    - Carpal arthroplasty; may fail and be complicated by massive osteolysis
  - MCPs, PIPs
    - Arthrodesis, often IP of thumb and digits
    - Arthroplasty: Complications common
      - Fracture of devise or digit
      - Massive osteolysis and synovitis

DIAGNOSTIC CHECKLIST

Consider

- Early on, RA may be monostotic or asymmetric
  - Must differentiate from septic joint

Image Interpretation Pearls

- Use soft tissue swelling around hand to guide you to subtle osseous findings on radiograph
- Watch for cortical indistinctness and dot-dash pattern for earliest radiographic signs of erosion

SELECTED REFERENCES

1. Navalho M et al: Bilateral MR imaging of the hand and wrist in early and very early inflammatory arthritis: tenosynovitis is associated with progression to rheumatoid arthritis. Radiology. 264(3):823-33, 2012
2. Bøyesen P et al: Prediction of MRI erosive progression: a comparison of modern imaging modalities in early rheumatoid arthritis patients. Ann Rheum Dis. 70(1):176-9, 2011
3. Rowbotham EL et al: Rheumatoid arthritis: ultrasound versus MRI. AJR Am J Roentgenol. 197(3):541-6, 2011

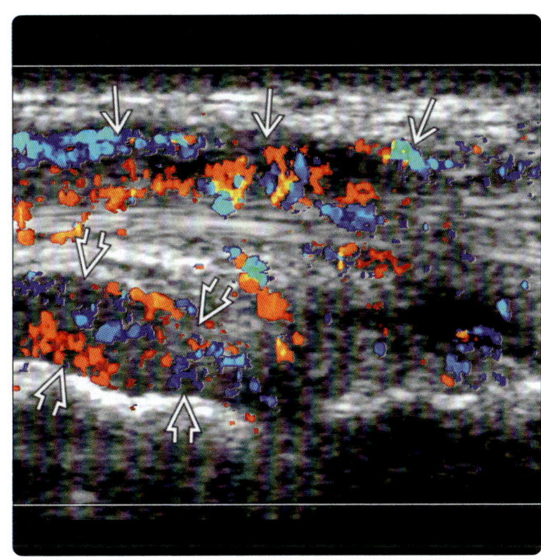

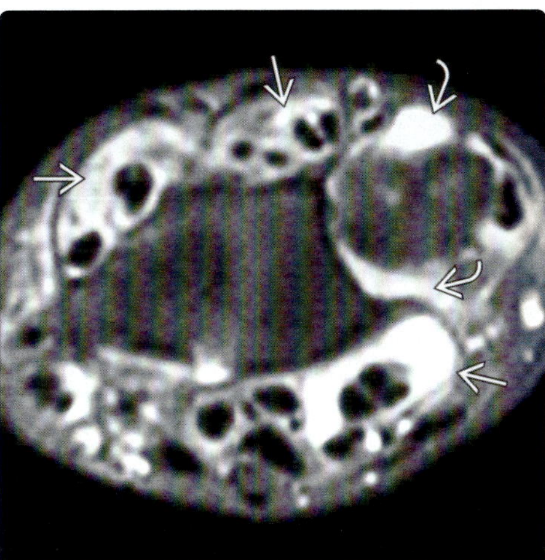

(Left) *Longitudinal color Doppler ultrasound shows typical tenosynovitis with marked increase in vascularity, indicating hyperemia ➡. There is also synovial thickening and hyperemia of the palmar aspect of the joint capsule ➡, indicating joint synovitis. This proved to be early RA, normal on radiograph.* **(Right)** *Axial T2WI FS MR shows high signal tenosynovitis ➡ surrounding normal extensor and flexor tendons and synovitis in the DRUJ ➡. There are no erosions; radiograph was normal.*

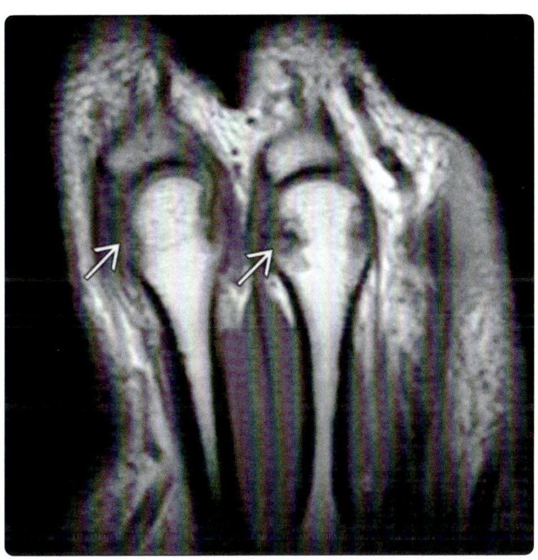

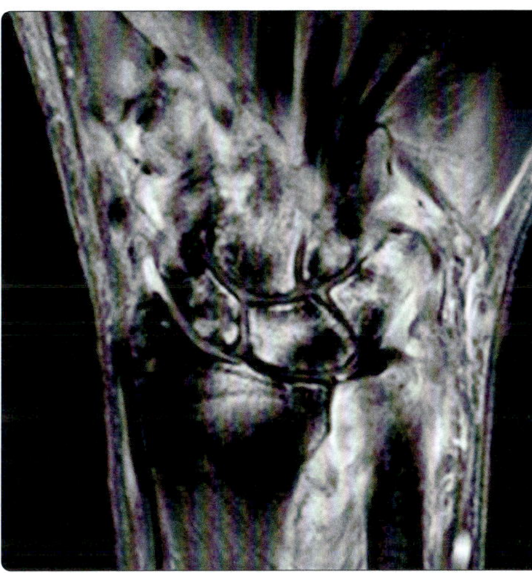

(Left) *Coronal T1WI MR, obtained in a patient with a new onset of unilateral joint pain and swelling, shows the MC heads with marginal erosions ➡. These erosions were not visible on radiograph.* **(Right)** *Coronal T2WI FS MR in the same patient shows involvement beyond the MCPs. The carpal bones, radiocarpal joint, and DRUJ show similar findings of effusion and both marginal and subchondral erosions. The distribution and pattern of erosive disease is typical of RA.*

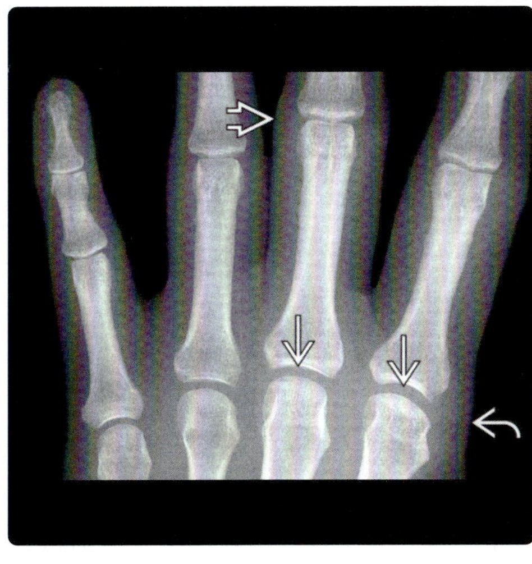

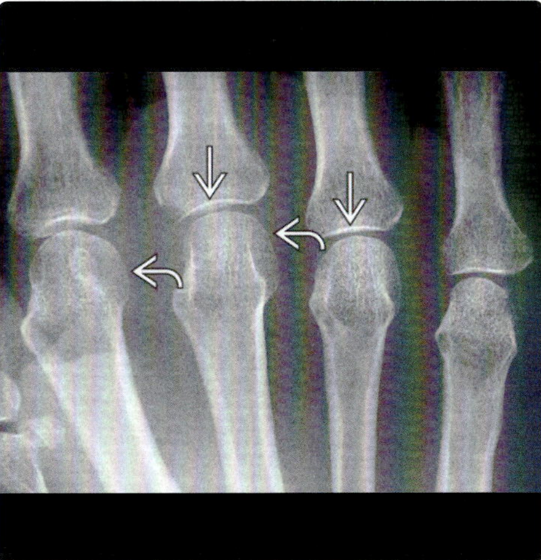

(Left) *PA radiograph in a patient with new-onset hand pain and swelling shows swelling at the MCPs ➡ and PIPs ➡. There is no focal osteoporosis or erosion, but distension of MCPs 2 and 3 is seen ➡. This is due to synovitis and effusion, very early radiographic signs of RA.* **(Right)** *PA radiograph shows juxtaarticular osteopenia and cartilage narrowing at the MCPs ➡. Cortical indistinctness on the MC heads ➡ is the dot-dash pattern, indicating early erosive change.*

(Left) *PA radiograph shows a typical case of marginal erosions in RA ➲. These are seen early in the erosive process, occurring in bone that is intracapsular but not protected by cartilage. This is the region of bone that is most vulnerable to the inflammatory process.* **(Right)** *PA radiograph in a patient with early RA shows that the bone density is normal. The only involved joint is a PIP ➲, showing erosion and severe cartilage damage. Remember that early erosions in RA are as likely to involve the PIP as the MCP.*

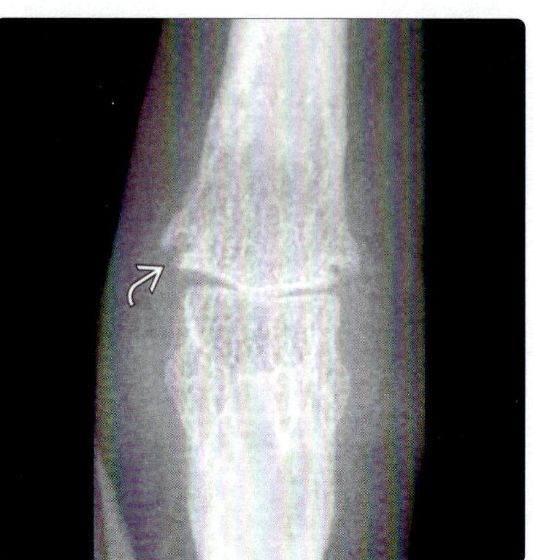

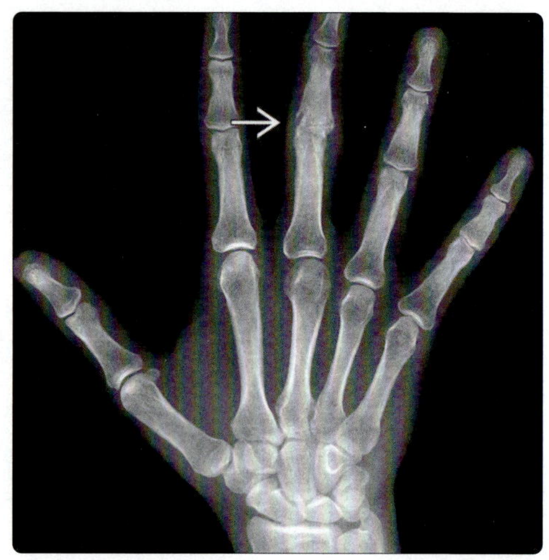

(Left) *PA radiograph shows a nodule ➲, which causes scalloping of underlying bone ➲. Note the decreased cartilage width at the 2nd MCP, along with the marginal erosion of the MC head ➲. The appearance and distribution is typical for RA with a rheumatoid nodule.* **(Right)** *PA radiograph in a 48-year-old man shows severe rapid-onset osteopenia in a band-like pattern of the distal radius ➲ as well as soft tissue swelling and likely erosion at the ulnar styloid ➲.*

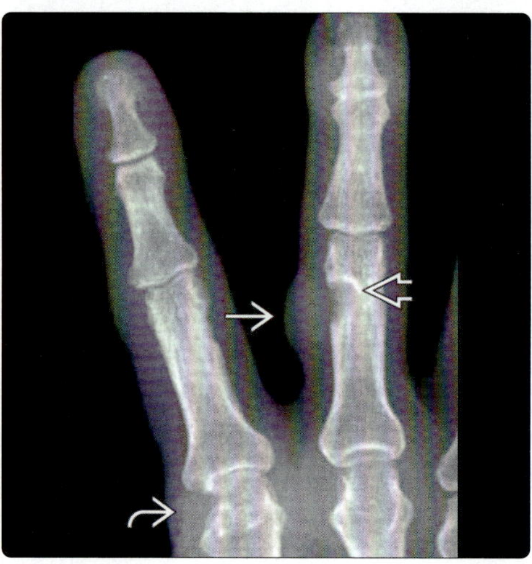

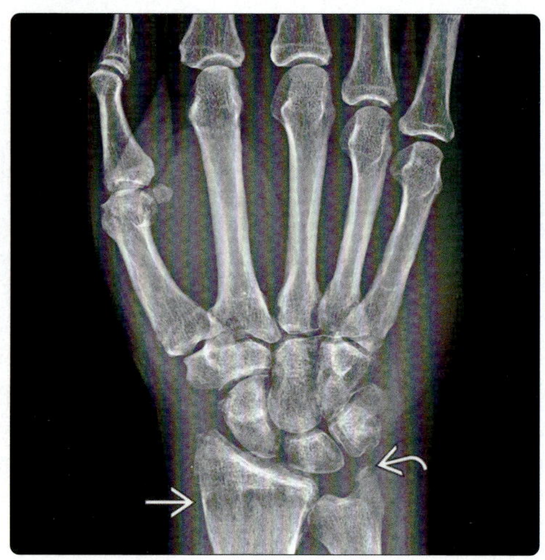

(Left) *Coronal T1 MR arthrogram of the same patient shows edema and erosions of the ulnar styloid and triquetrum ➲. In addition, there is disruption of the scapholunate ligament ➲.* **(Right)** *Coronal T2 FS MR in the same patient confirms the erosions in the ulnar styloid, triquetrum, and demonstrates another in the scaphoid ➲. Note the mild thinning of cartilage at the radioscaphoid joint ➲, with other cartilage appearing normal. This patient's erosions are more extensive than suspected on radiograph.*

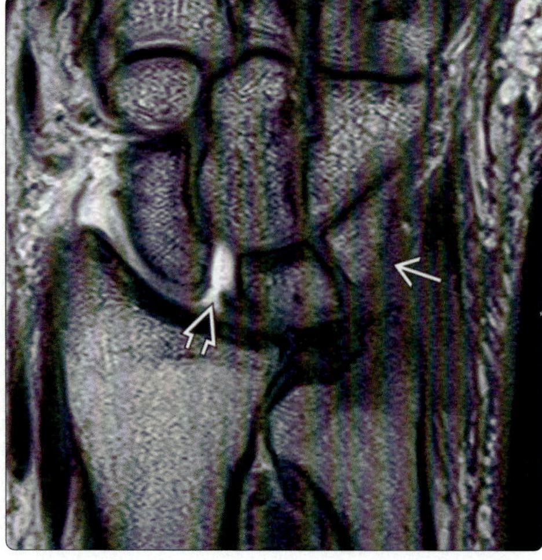

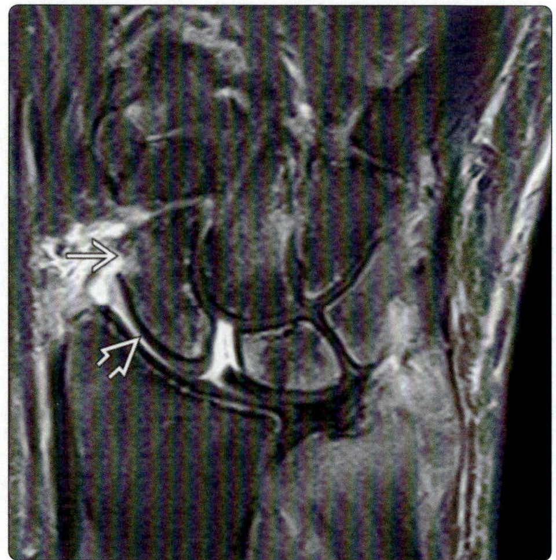

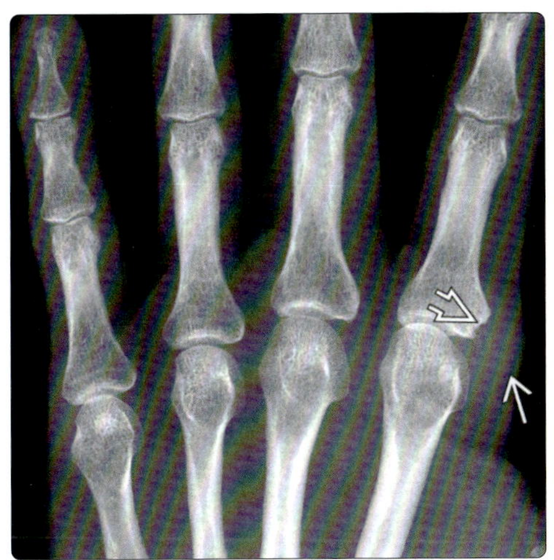

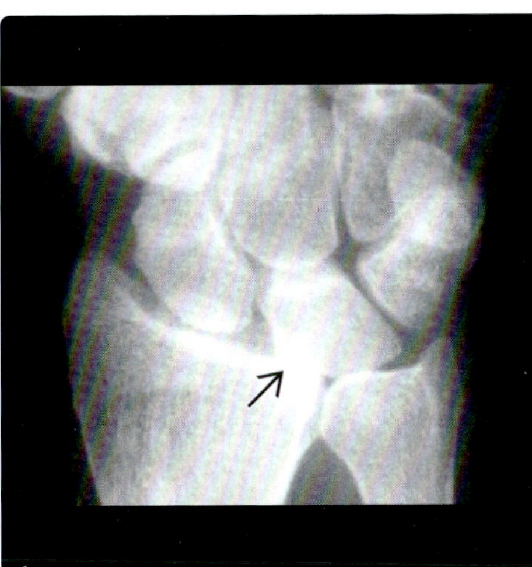

(Left) *PA radiograph shows normal bone density and only a single MCP with soft tissue swelling ➡ and single associated erosion ➡. This is the only radiographic sign of RA in this young woman.* **(Right)** *PA radiograph in a patient with early RA shows radiocarpal joint narrowing, as well as ulnar translation of the entire carpus ➡. Note that the majority of the lunate overlies the ulna, confirming that translation.*

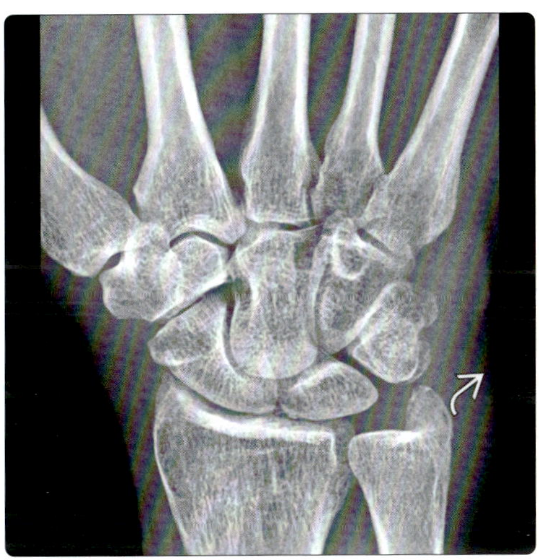

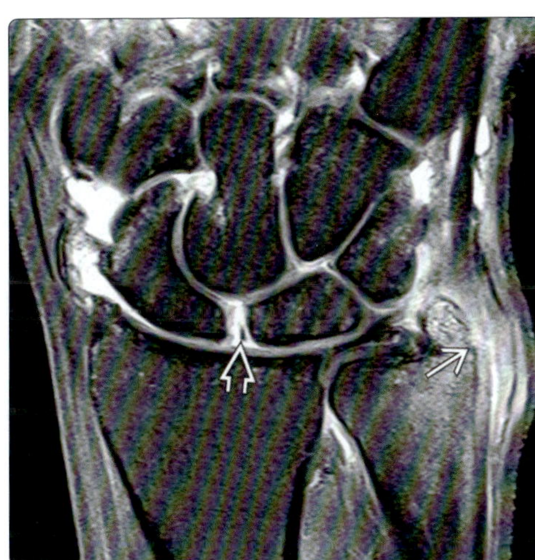

(Left) *PA radiograph in a middle-aged man with joint pain shows only soft tissue swelling ➡ near the ulnar styloid. This should suggest early RA.* **(Right)** *In the same patient, an indirect T2 C+ FS MR arthrogram shows ulnar-sided tenosynovitis and small ulnar styloid erosion ➡ with extensive edema. There is also scapholunate ligament disruption ➡.*

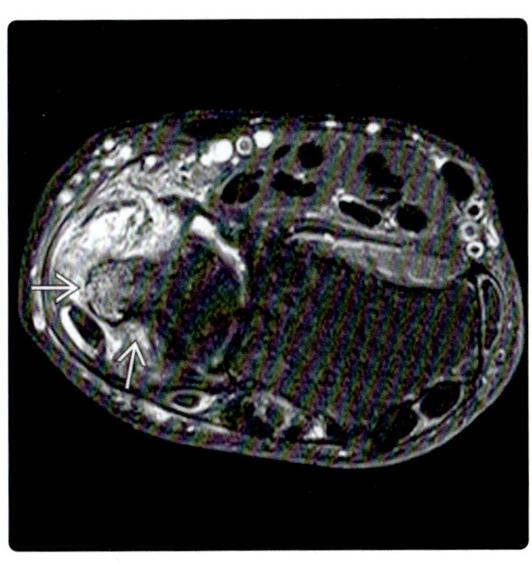

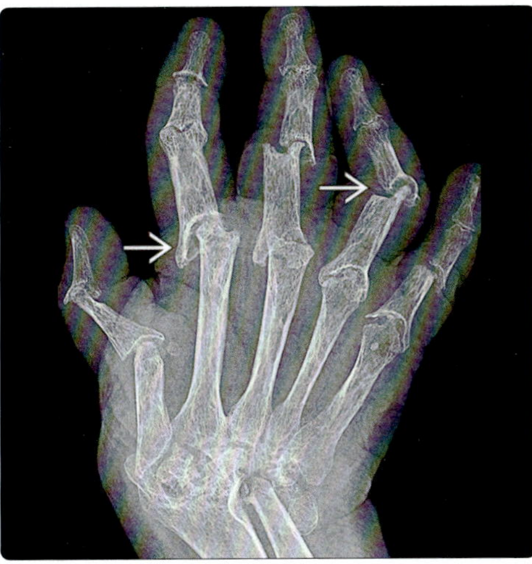

(Left) *Axial PD C+ FS MR in the same patient, through the distal carpus, shows more extensive erosion of the distal ulna ➡ than was suspected on the coronal.* **(Right)** *PA radiograph demonstrates severe osteopenia with arthritis mutilans. The erosions are so severe that "pencil-in-cup" morphology is seen in multiple joints ➡. Although arthritis mutilans is a hallmark for psoriatic arthritis, it is also seen in any severe inflammatory arthropathy, including RA.*

Rheumatoid Arthritis of Hip

KEY FACTS

IMAGING

- Radiographs often diagnostic
  - Bilaterally symmetric uniform cartilage narrowing
  - Protrusio
  - Osteoporosis
  - Insufficiency fractures
    - Femoral neck: Medial basicervical and midcervical
    - Femoral head and weight-bearing acetabulum
  - Pathologic fracture subtrochanteric region in patients taking bisphosphonates for osteoporosis
    - Visualized as linear sclerosis adjacent to bump on lateral cortex in subtrochanteric region
- MR T1WI: Soft tissue complications
  - Ruptured and retracted gluteus tendon surrounded by high-signal fat
  - Gluteal fatty atrophy if tendon chronically torn
  - Linear low-signal insufficiency fracture
- MR fluid-sensitive sequences
  - High-signal marrow edema
  - Thick low-signal synovial thickening and pannus with high-signal effusion
  - Decompressed effusion shows high-fluid signal in iliopsoas bursa
  - With effusion, labral tear and cartilage thinning may be directly seen
  - High-signal tenosynovitis and tendon rupture
- MR: Osteonecrosis secondary to steroid use

DIAGNOSTIC CHECKLIST

- Bilateral protrusio is seen in other processes as well but most frequently in rheumatoid arthritis (RA)
- Soft tissue mass in iliopsoas bursa showing fluid characteristics is most likely decompressed synovial fluid in patient with RA; hip capsule is weakest anteriorly
- Watch for insufficiency fractures, both in medial cervical region and femoral head/acetabulum

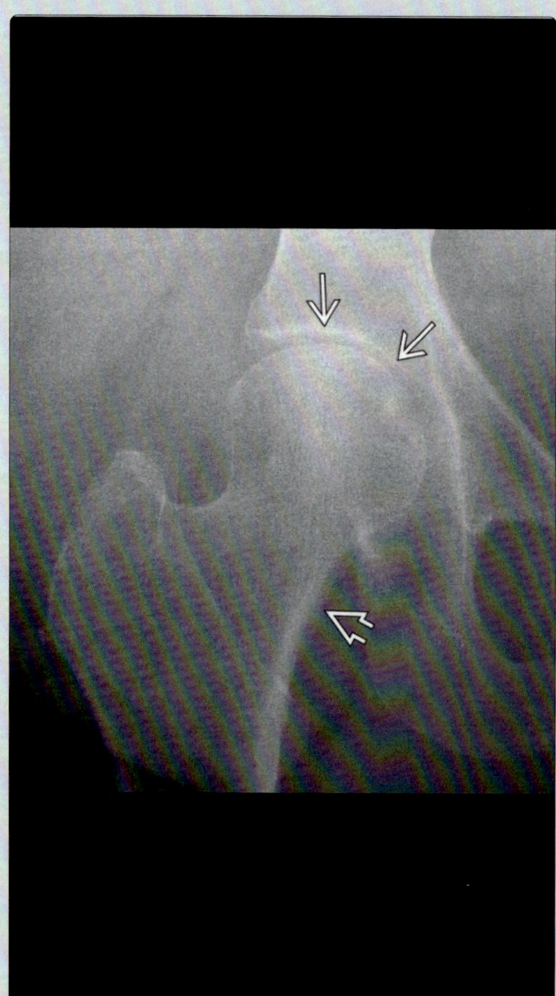

AP radiograph shows diffuse osteopenia, definitely abnormal for this 52-year-old woman. In addition, there is uniform cartilage thinning in the hip joint ➡. The patient has not yet developed protrusio, erosions, or subchondral cysts, but there is calcar buttressing ➡.

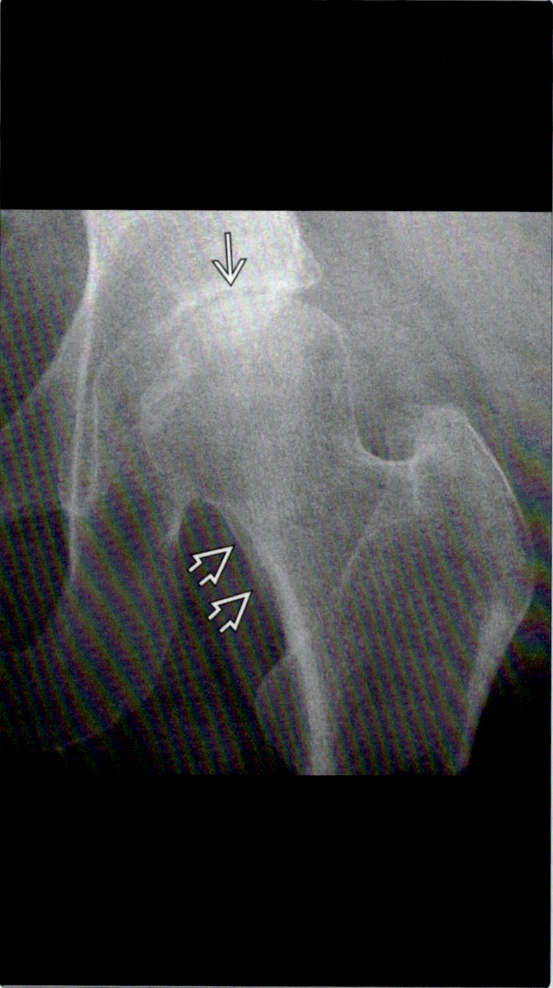

AP radiograph of the contralateral hip in the same patient also shows diffuse symmetric cartilage thinning ➡ and more prominent calcar buttressing ➡. The primary disease process is RA, but the patient is developing secondary osteoarthritis, as indicated by the buttressing.

TERMINOLOGY

Abbreviations

- Rheumatoid arthritis (RA)

Definitions

- Chronic progressive systemic inflammatory disease in which joints are primary target

IMAGING

General Features

- Best diagnostic clue
  - Bilaterally symmetric uniform cartilage narrowing
  - Protrusio
  - Osteoporosis

Radiographic Findings

- Diffuse osteopenia
  - Hip involvement occurs after peripheral involvement, so patient has usually developed moderate to severe osteoporosis
- Effusion
  - Distended fat pads
    - Iliopsoas, gluteal, obturator
- Uniform cartilage narrowing
  - Cartilage covers all of femoral head
  - Acetabular cartilage is horseshoe-shaped
    - Medial portion of acetabulum is not covered with cartilage
- Erosions
  - Initially, marginal erosions
    - Noted at cutback of femoral head and neck, region of bone that is within capsule but not protected by cartilage
  - Later, diffuse subchondral erosions around femoral head and acetabulum
  - With osteopenia and diffuse erosions, femoral head migrates medially (protrusio)
- Subchondral cyst formation common
- Insufficiency fractures
  - Femoral neck: Medial basicervical and midcervical
    - Visualized as linear sclerosis; fracture line rarely seen on radiograph
  - Weight-bearing portion is femoral head and acetabulum
  - Subtrochanteric region in patients taking bisphosphonates for osteoporosis
    - Initially seen as focal sclerotic bone production along lateral cortex, 5-8 cm below trochanters
    - Represents region of disordered bone at site of maximal stress
      - Bisphosphonates inhibit osteoclasts, so bone formed in reaction to stress cannot remodel
      - Disordered bone at this site is weak
    - Visualized as linear sclerosis adjacent to bump on lateral cortex in subtrochanteric region
      - May complete fracture
- Osteonecrosis secondary to steroid use
  - Central sclerosis in femoral head
  - With progression, subchondral fracture and collapse

CT Findings

- CT mirrors radiographic findings of erosions, cysts, altered morphology
- Insufficiency fractures may be more easily visualized
- Enhancement of synovitis
- Synovial fluid decompresses into iliopsoas bursa

MR Findings

- T1WI
  - Low-signal pannus and effusion
  - Low-signal bone marrow edema, erosions, and subchondral cysts
  - Linear low-signal insufficiency fracture lines
  - Subchondral low-signal indicating osteonecrosis (secondary to steroid use)
  - Soft tissue complications
    - Ruptured and retracted gluteus tendon surrounded by high-signal fat
    - Fatty atrophy of gluteus muscle if tendon chronically torn
- Fluid-sensitive sequences
  - High-signal marrow edema
  - Thick low-signal synovium and pannus surrounded by high-signal effusion
  - High-signal erosions and subchondral cysts
  - Hip effusion decompresses into iliopsoas bursa → high-signal anterior mass
  - With effusion, labral tear and cartilage thinning may be directly seen
  - High-signal tenosynovitis and tendon rupture
  - Insufficiency fracture may show linear high signal, or edema may obscure fracture line
  - Double line sign of osteonecrosis
- T1WI C+ FS
  - Avid enhancement of thick synovium surrounding low-signal effusion
  - Proves fluid characteristics of decompressed fluid in iliopsoas bursa

Ultrasonographic Findings

- Effusion and bursal fluid well seen

Imaging Recommendations

- Best imaging tool
  - Radiograph is diagnostic for mid to late disease
  - MR often more useful
    - Proves early disease
    - Diagnoses insufficiency fractures
    - Diagnoses soft tissue complications

DIFFERENTIAL DIAGNOSIS

Septic Arthritis

- Unilateral process
- Effusion, erosions, synovial reaction may not be distinguishable from RA

Paget Disease

- Softened bone results in protrusio, similar to morphology in RA
- Early Paget disease may show diffuse osteoporosis (or due to disuse if patient is bedridden)

- Disordered trabecular pattern and cortical thickening of hip/pelvis should help differentiate
- No erosions

Osteomalacia/Hyperparathyroidism

- Softened bone results in protrusio, similar to RA morphology
- Diffuse osteopenia
- Subperiosteal resorption, vascular calcification may differentiate
- No true erosions

PATHOLOGY

General Features

- Etiology
  - RA: Unknown etiology
  - Pathophysiology presumed to relate to persistent immunologic response of genetically susceptible host to some unknown antigen
- Genetics
  - Genetic predisposition
    - Concordance in monozygotic twins: 25%
    - 1st-degree relatives develop RA at rate 4x that of general population
  - Individual not likely to have affected family member
- Associated abnormalities
  - Subcutaneous rheumatoid nodules in 30%
    - Extensor surfaces (ulna, Achilles) and digits
  - Amyloid deposition
  - Thoracic: Pleural effusions, rheumatoid nodules, rarely interstitial fibrosis
  - Vasculitis
  - Felty syndrome: RA + splenomegaly + leukopenia
  - Sjögren syndrome: RA + keratoconjunctivitis + xerostomia
  - ↑ risk of lymphoma
  - ↑ mortality rate, reduced survival by 10-18 years
    - Lifetime of systemic inflammation may contribute to ↑ risk of CV disease, renal disease, and infection

Gross Pathologic & Surgical Features

- Synovial lining is hypertrophic, edematous
- Joint distension, osseous erosion, cartilage destruction

Microscopic Features

- Organized accumulations of CD4 helper T-cells, antigen-presenting cells, lymphoid follicles
- Large amounts of immunoglobulin produced, including rheumatoid factor
- Angiogenesis in synovium

CLINICAL ISSUES

Presentation

- Most common signs/symptoms
  - Symmetric polyarthritis, especially of small joints of hand and foot
  - Constitutional symptoms of fatigue, low-grade fever
  - Usually presents over course of weeks or months; occasionally fulminant disease
- Other signs/symptoms
  - Soft tissue mass anterior to hip, secondary to synovial fluid decompression into iliopsoas bursa

Demographics

- Age
  - Peak onset: 3rd-5th decades
- Gender
  - M:F = 1:3
- Epidemiology
  - 1% of worldwide population
    - 5% in some Native American populations
  - Hip involved in 50% of patients with RA

Natural History & Prognosis

- If remission not accomplished by drug therapy, progresses to painful decreased range of motion
- Insufficiency fracture risk is high

Treatment

- Generally combination, aimed at pain relief while escalating therapy rapidly to suppress disease prior to joint destruction
  - NSAIDs
    - Symptomatic relief; do not alter disease progress
  - Glucocorticoids (oral or intraarticular)
    - Controls inflammation rapidly; allows slower-acting drugs to take effect
  - Disease-modifying antirheumatic drugs
    - Suppresses joint destruction (e.g., methotrexate, sulfasalazine, antimalarials, gold)
  - Biologics: Antitumor necrosis factor (TNF)-α drugs, anti-interleukin-1
    - Role of cytokines (especially TNF-α and interleukin-1) in pathophysiology of RA now recognized
- Surgical treatment
  - Synovectomy
  - Arthroplasty
    - At greater risk for periprosthetic fracture, early loosening, infection
    - Larger number of revisions than arthroplasties placed for osteoarthritis
    - Comorbidity of RA → extended hospital stay
  - Intramedullary rodding of fracture

DIAGNOSTIC CHECKLIST

Consider

- Bilateral protrusio is seen in other processes as well but most frequently in RA
- Soft tissue mass in iliopsoas bursa showing fluid characteristics in patient with RA is most likely decompressed synovial fluid

Image Interpretation Pearls

- Watch for insufficiency fractures, both in medial cervical region and lateral subtrochanteric region

SELECTED REFERENCES

1. Bause L: Short stem total hip arthroplasty in patients with rheumatoid arthritis. Orthopedics. 38(3 Suppl):S46-50, 2015
2. Nikiphorou E et al: The effect of disease severity and comorbidity on length of stay for orthopedic surgery in rheumatoid arthritis: results from 2 UK Inception Cohorts, 1986-2012. J Rheumatol. 42(5):778-85, 2015

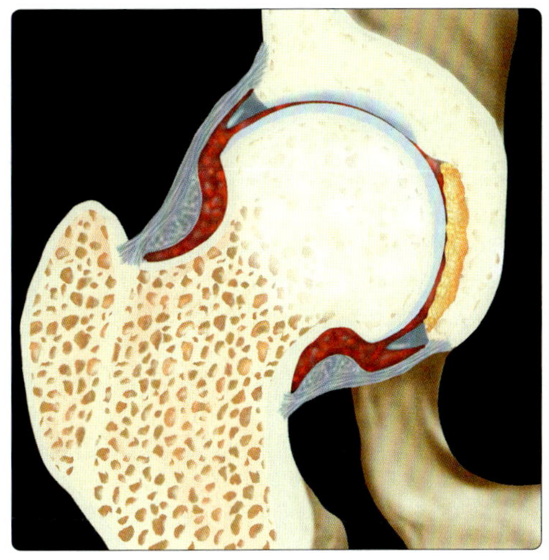

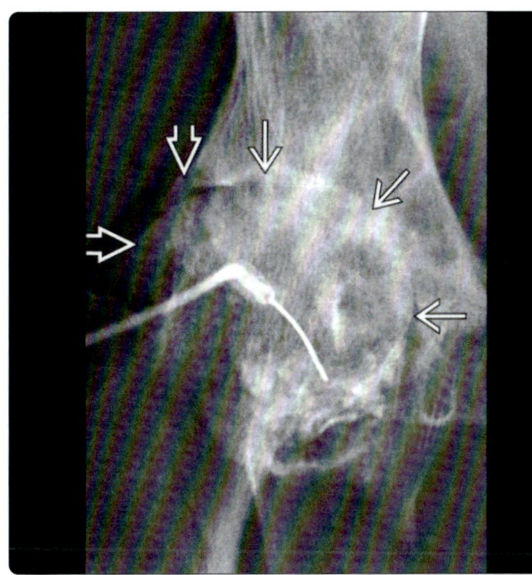

(Left) *Coronal graphic shows an early, preerosive phase of rheumatoid arthritis, with hypertrophic synovium (red), diffuse cartilage thinning (yielding concentric joint space narrowing), and reactive marrow edema in the femoral head and acetabulum.* **(Right)** *AP radiograph obtained during the arthrographic portion of a therapeutic injection in a known rheumatoid arthritis (RA) patient shows uniform cartilage loss ➡ with large accompanying erosions. There are osteophytes ⇨; secondary osteoarthritis has developed.*

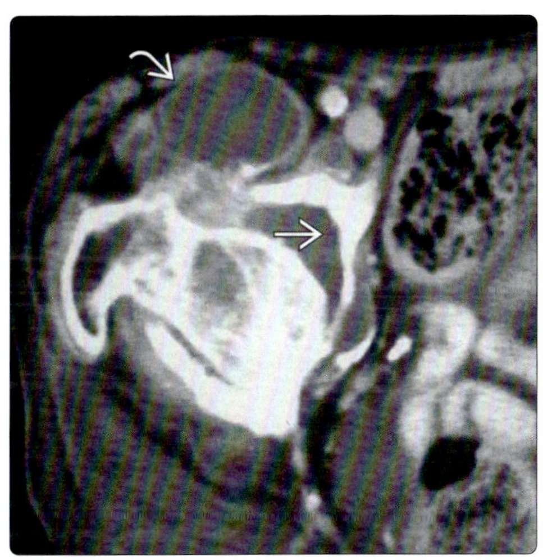

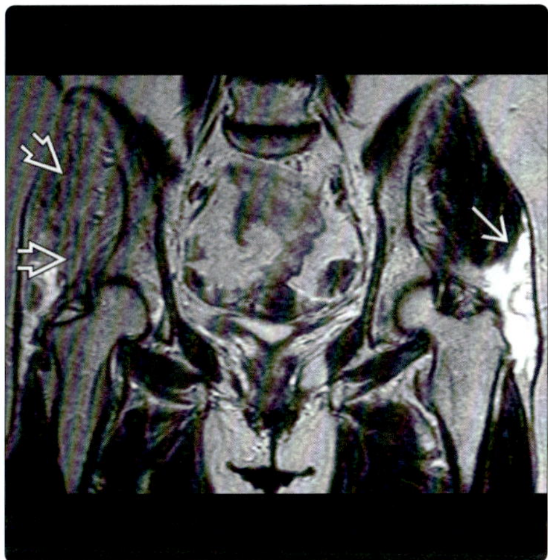

(Left) *Axial CECT shows erosions of the left hip ➡ in a patient with RA. There is also a fluid collection in the iliopsoas bursa ↷. The hip joint is not capacious, and synovial fluid decompresses through the weak anterior capsule.* **(Right)** *Coronal T2WI MR shows soft tissue complications of RA, with acute rupture of the left gluteal muscle insertion at the greater tuberosity ➡. There is chronic disruption on the right side, with fatty atrophy of the muscle ⇨.*

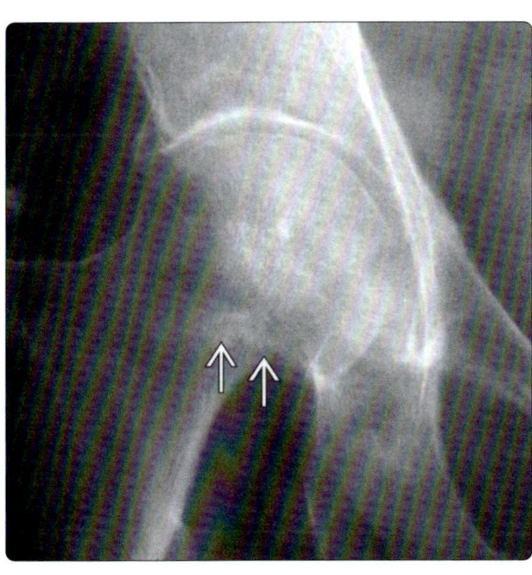

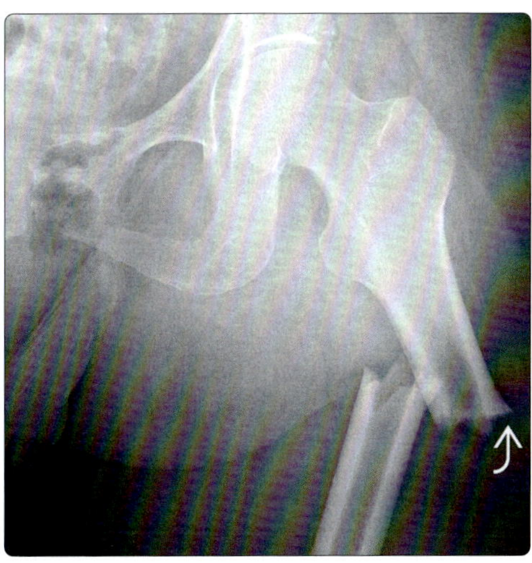

(Left) *AP radiograph shows severe osteopenia and uniform joint space loss, typical of RA. This patient had recent worsening of pain; the linear sclerosis at the medial femoral neck ➡ represents an insufficiency fracture, a frequent risk in these patients.* **(Right)** *AP radiograph in a patient treated with bisphosphonates for osteoporosis related to RA and steroid use is shown. The transverse fracture in the subtrochanteric femoral diaphysis with lateral beak ↷ is a typical complication of bisphosphonate use.*

Rheumatoid Arthritis of Knee

KEY FACTS

IMAGING

- Radiographs: Osteopenia
  - Effusion distorts suprapatellar recess, Hoffa fat pad
  - Common decompression into popliteal cyst
  - Uniform cartilage thinning, visualized as joint space narrowing, involving all 3 compartments
  - Erosions initially marginal (tibial plateau, patella)
  - Deformity, related to ligament and capsular laxity
- T1WI MR
  - Low signal marrow edema, early erosions
  - Low signal linear insufficiency fracture lines
- Fluid-sensitive MR sequences
  - High signal effusion surrounded by low signal thickened synovium
  - Cartilage seen directly, especially in fat-saturated sequences, which show different signal in cartilage relative to effusion
  - High signal marrow edema
  - Ligamentous injury well seen
  - PD sequences show associated meniscal tears
- T1WI C+ FS MR
  - Avid synovial enhancement, surrounding low signal effusion and popliteal cyst

CLINICAL ISSUES

- RA in 1% of worldwide population
- 5% in some Native American populations
- Knee involved in 75% patients with RA

DIAGNOSTIC CHECKLIST

- Popliteal (Baker) cysts may dissect proximally and distally so far as to be confusing
- Ruptured popliteal cyst may be confusing clinically as well as by imaging; may be mistaken for tumor
- Watch for linear sclerosis, indicating insufficiency fracture, both pre- and postarthroplasty
  - Prearthroplasty: In femoral condyles, tibial metaphysis

(Left) *AP radiograph in a 43-year-old woman shows findings of early RA. There is slight uniform cartilage thinning and a single erosion ➔ is seen on this image. Osteopenia might be suspected but is difficult to evaluate early in the process.* **(Right)** *Lateral radiograph in the same patient again shows mild uniform cartilage thinning. There is a large suprapatellar effusion ➔ and a suggestion of deossification at the inferior patellar margin ➔. At this point, the process appears to be purely erosive but undifferentiated.*

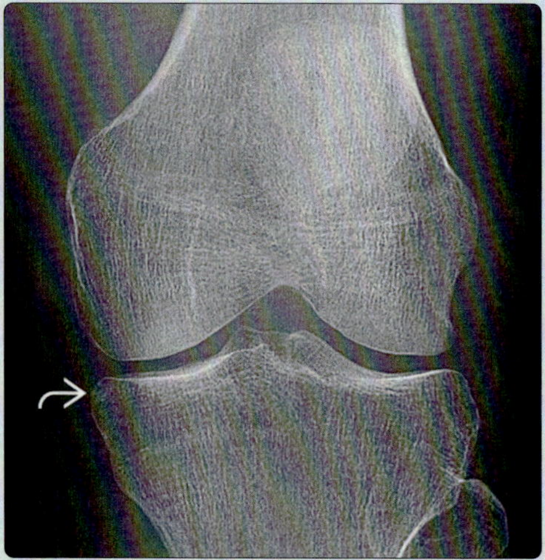

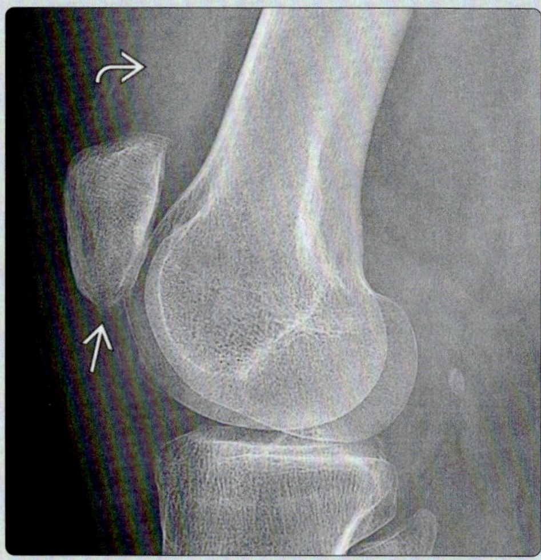

(Left) *Coronal T1 MR in the same patient confirms the single erosion ➔. Note also that both meniscal bodies are torn. PD is more accurate than T1, but the information is present on this image.* **(Right)** *Axial T2 FS MR shows rice bodies ➔ within the large effusion, typical of RA. In addition, the patellar cartilage is virtually absent ➔ and there is prominent subchondral cyst formation ➔. Findings are typical of RA, and the diagnosis was confirmed on serology.*

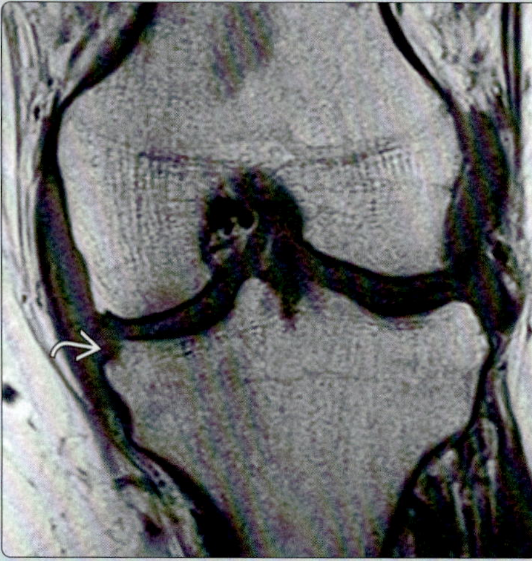

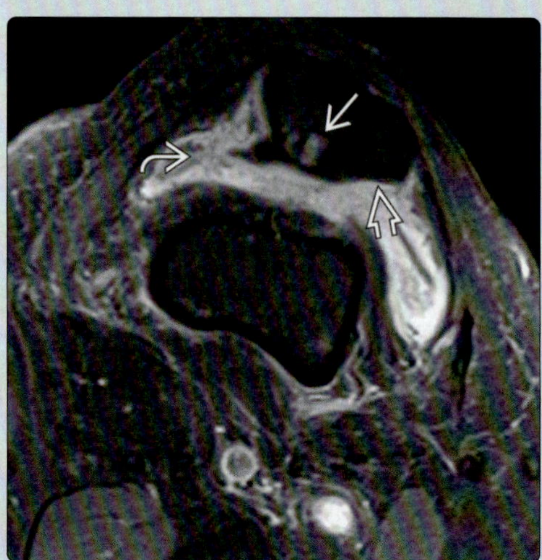

TERMINOLOGY

Abbreviations

- Rheumatoid arthritis (RA)

Definitions

- Chronic progressive systemic inflammatory disease in which joints are primary target

IMAGING

General Features

- Best diagnostic clue
  - Symmetric, uniform joint space narrowing
  - Purely erosive disease
  - Osteoporosis
  - Valgus deformity

Radiographic Findings

- Osteopenia
  - Initially: Juxtaarticular
  - Later: Diffuse
  - Watch for associated linear sclerosis, indicating insufficiency fracture (particularly medial tibia)
- Large effusion
  - Distorts suprapatellar recess, Hoffa fat pad
  - Common decompression into popliteal (Baker) cyst
    - May be large, dissecting proximally or distally
- Uniform cartilage thinning, visualized as joint space narrowing, involving all 3 compartments
- Erosions
  - Initially marginal
    - Tibial plateau, immediately below joint line
    - Femoral condyles, 1-2 cm above joint line
    - Patella, nonarticular edges
  - With advanced disease, subchondral and uniform
- Subchondral cysts prominent
- Deformity, related to ligament and capsular laxity
  - Valgus angulation (collateral ligament)
  - Medial or lateral translation of tibia relative to femur (capsule, collateral ligament)
  - Anterior or posterior translation of tibia (cruciates)

MR Findings

- T1WI
  - Low signal effusion, popliteal cyst
  - Low signal erosions, subchondral cysts, marrow edema
  - Low signal linear insufficiency fracture lines
- Fluid-sensitive sequences
  - High signal effusion, surrounded by low signal thickened synovium
  - High signal popliteal cyst
    - Identify in gastrocnemius-semimembranosus bursa, dissecting proximally or distally
    - Ruptured cyst shows less defined high signal, with surrounding soft tissue edema; often has neck showing original location/anatomy
  - Cartilage seen directly, especially in fat-saturated sequences, which show different signal in cartilage relative to effusion
  - High signal marrow edema
  - High signal erosions, subchondral cysts
  - High signal along linear fracture lines
  - Ligamentous and tendinous injury well seen
    - Quadriceps at risk in RA
  - PD sequences show associated meniscal tears
- T1WI C+ FS
  - Avid synovial enhancement, surrounding low signal effusion and popliteal cyst
  - Enhancing edges of bone around low signal fluid in erosions and subchondral cysts
- One study showed MR to help differentiate RA from undifferentiated arthritis &/or spondyloarthropathy involving knee
  - RA showed more destructive changes (synovial thickening, bone marrow edema, erosions)
  - Spondyloarthropathy showed enthesitis (absent in RA)

Ultrasonographic Findings

- Confirms popliteal cyst

Imaging Recommendations

- Best imaging tool
  - Diagnosis made on radiograph when disease has progressed to joint space narrowing
  - MR makes earlier diagnosis and adds information about internal derangement

DIFFERENTIAL DIAGNOSIS

Septic Arthritis

- Similar appearance of thickened reactive synovium, cartilage destruction, osseous erosions
- Monostotic process should differentiate; extremely rare for RA to be monostotic involving only knee

Ankylosing Spondylitis

- Osteopenia is similar
- Early disease may be purely erosive, like RA
- Knee involved late in disease; should have axial involvement & enthesitis, allowing differentiation

Psoriatic Arthritis/Chronic Reactive Arthritis

- May involve knee, though relatively late in disease
- Involvement may be initially purely erosive, then becoming mixed erosive/productive
- Axial involvement, if present, allows differentiation from RA

Juvenile Idiopathic Arthritis

- Knee commonly involved, with effusion, cartilage destruction, and erosions
- Enlarged metaphyses and epiphyses (related to hyperemia and overgrowth while skeletally immature) differentiates from adult RA

Hemophilic Arthritis

- Knee commonly involved, with effusion, cartilage destruction, and erosions
- Enlarged metaphyses and epiphyses (related to hyperemia and overgrowth while skeletally immature) differentiates from adult RA
- Generally unilateral, always male gender

PATHOLOGY

General Features

- Etiology
  - RA: Unknown etiology
  - Pathophysiology presumed to relate to persistent immunologic response of genetically susceptible host to some unknown antigen
- Genetics
  - Genetic predisposition
    - Concordance in monozygotic twins: 25%
    - 1st-degree relatives develop RA at rate 4x that of general population
  - Individual not likely to have affected family member
- Associated abnormalities
  - Subcutaneous rheumatoid nodules in 30%
    - Extensor surfaces (ulna, Achilles) and digits
  - Amyloid deposition
  - Thoracic: Pleural effusions, rheumatoid nodules, rarely interstitial fibrosis
  - Vasculitis
  - Felty syndrome: RA + splenomegaly + leukopenia
  - Sjögren syndrome: RA + keratoconjunctivitis + xerostomia
  - ↑ risk of lymphoma
  - Lifetime of systemic inflammation may contribute to ↑ risk of CV disease, renal disease, and infection
  - ↑ mortality rate, reduced survival by 10-18 years

Staging, Grading, & Classification

- Criteria for clinical diagnosis of RA (2010 American College of Rheumatology/European League Against Rheumatism)
  - Score-based algorithm: Add score of categories A-D; score of ≥ 6/10 is needed for classification of patient as having definite RA
    - (A) Joint involvement
      - 1 large joint scores 0
      - 2-10 large joints scores 1
      - 1-3 small joints scores 2
      - 4-10 small joints scores 3
      - > 10 joints (at least 1 small joint) scores 5
    - (B) Serology (at least 1 test result is needed for classification)
      - Negative rheumatoid factor (RF) **and** negative anti-citrullinated protein antibody (ACPA) scores 0
      - Low-positive RF or low-positive ACPA scores 2
      - High-positive RF or high-positive ACPA scores 3
    - (C) Acute-phase reactants (at least 1 test result is needed for classification)
      - Normal CRP (C-reactive protein) **and** normal ESR scores 0
      - Abnormal CRP or abnormal ESR scores 1
    - (D) Duration of symptoms
      - < 6 weeks scores 0
      - ≥ 6 weeks scores 1

CLINICAL ISSUES

Presentation

- Most common signs/symptoms
  - Constitutional symptoms of fatigue, low-grade fever
  - Pain, development of valgus deformity of knees
  - Posterior mass (popliteal cyst); painful if ruptures
  - Usually presents over course of weeks or months; occasionally fulminant disease

Demographics

- Age
  - Peak onset at 3rd-5th decades
- Gender
  - M:F = 1:3
- Epidemiology
  - 1% of worldwide population
    - 5% in some Native American populations
  - Knee involved in 75% patients with RA

Natural History & Prognosis

- Process is often arrested by aggressive drug therapy
- Those who do not develop remission progress to significant joint destruction, pain, and functional disability

Treatment

- Generally combination, aimed at pain relief while escalating therapy rapidly to suppress disease prior to joint destruction
  - Nonsteroidal antiinflammatory drugs (NSAIDs)
    - Symptomatic relief; do not alter disease progress
  - Glucocorticoids (oral or intraarticular)
    - Controls inflammation rapidly; allows slower acting drugs to take effect
  - Disease-modifying antirheumatic drugs (DMARDs)
    - Suppresses joint destruction (e.g., methotrexate, sulfasalazine, antimalarials, gold)
  - Biologics: Anti-TNF-α drugs, anti-interleukin-1
    - Role of cytokines (especially tumor necrosis factor-α and interleukin-1) in pathophysiology of RA now recognized
- Surgical treatment
  - Arthroscopy for repair of associated meniscal injury
  - Arthroplasty; watch for complications of infection, loosening, periprosthetic fractures

DIAGNOSTIC CHECKLIST

Consider

- Popliteal cysts may dissect proximally and distally so far as to be confusing
- Ruptured popliteal cyst may be confusing clinically as well as by imaging; may be mistaken for tumor

Image Interpretation Pearls

- Watch for linear periarticular sclerosis, indicating insufficiency fracture, both pre- and postarthroplasty

SELECTED REFERENCES

1. Nikiphorou E et al: The effect of disease severity and comorbidity on length of stay for orthopedic surgery in rheumatoid arthritis: results from 2 UK inception cohorts, 1986-2012. J Rheumatol. 42(5):778-85, 2015
2. Flemming DJ et al: MR imaging assessment of arthritis of the knee. Magn Reson Imaging Clin N Am. 22(4):703-24, 2014
3. Bøyesen P et al: Prediction of MRI erosive progression: a comparison of modern imaging modalities in early rheumatoid arthritis patients. Ann Rheum Dis. 70(1):176-9, 2011

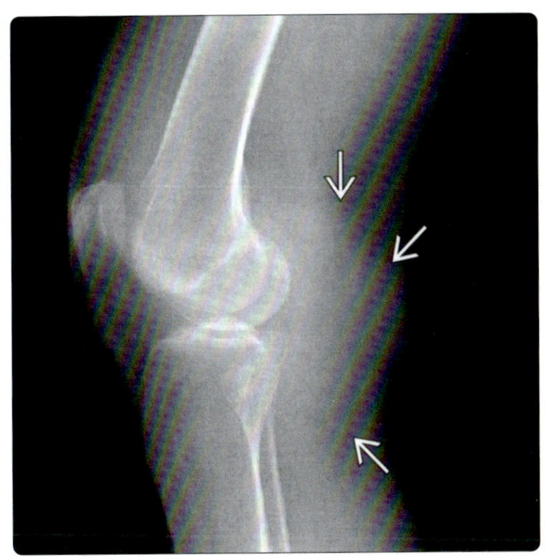

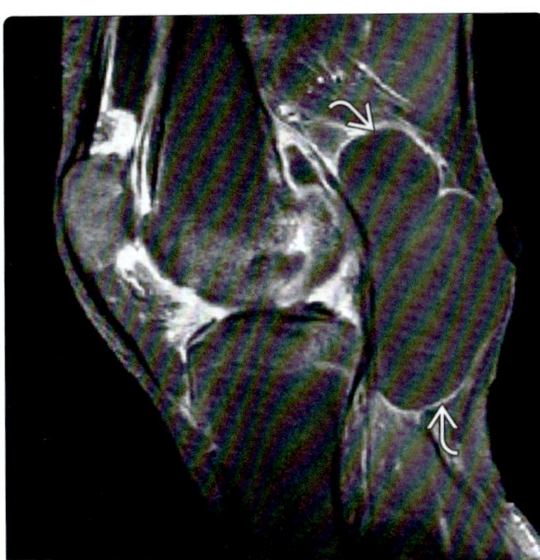

(Left) *Lateral radiograph shows osteopenia, joint effusion, and a posterior soft tissue mass ➡ without definite osseous destruction. This appearance is nonspecific.* **(Right)** *Sagittal T1WI C+ FS MR in the same patient shows the mass ➡ to be a fluid collection; axial images proved it to be a popliteal cyst. Note the thick, enhancing wall of the cyst, indicating synovitis, similar to that seen in the joint proper. There is severe cartilage thinning, small erosions, and bone marrow edema, all typical of RA.*

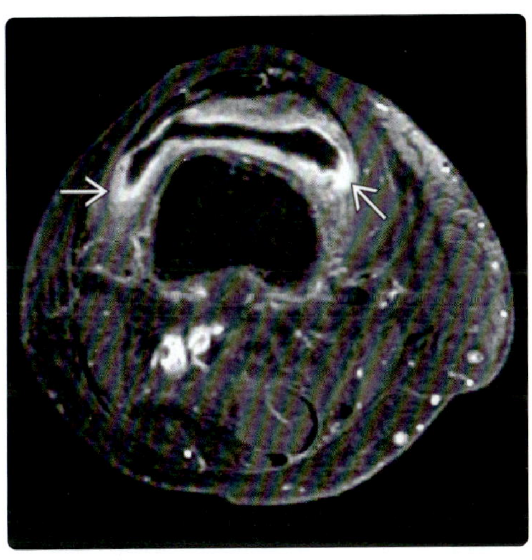

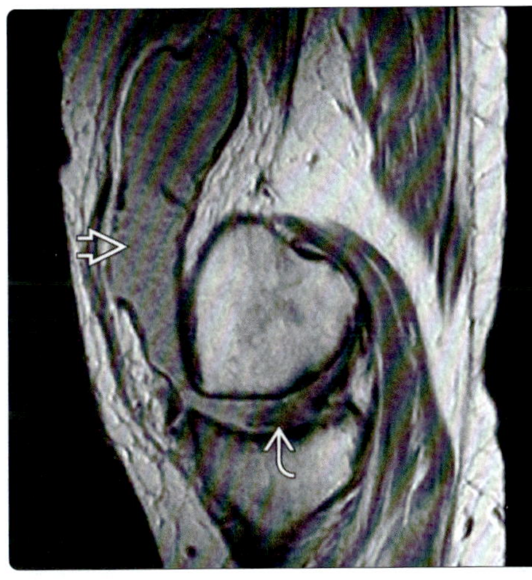

(Left) *Axial T1WI C+ FS MR demonstrates enhancing thickened synovial lining ➡ confirming synovitis, but this is nonspecific and certainly could be from a septic joint. Aspiration revealed no organisms or crystals. Patient was treated for a flare of RA and the pain subsided.* **(Right)** *Sagittal PD MR shows a huge effusion, containing innumerable tiny bodies ➡, consistent with rice bodies seen in inflammatory joint disorders. Complete cartilage loss is seen, along with meniscal destruction ➡.*

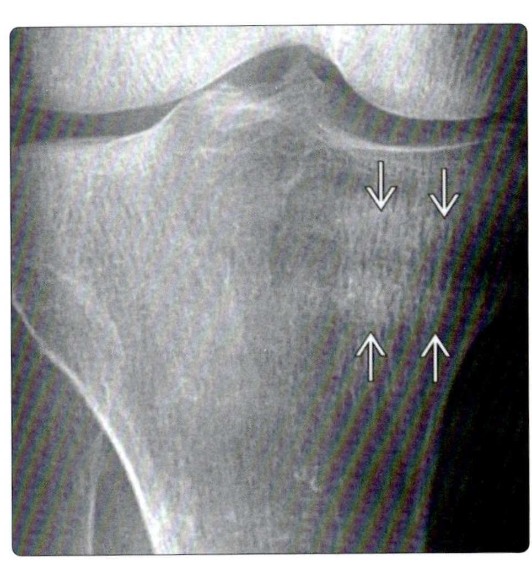

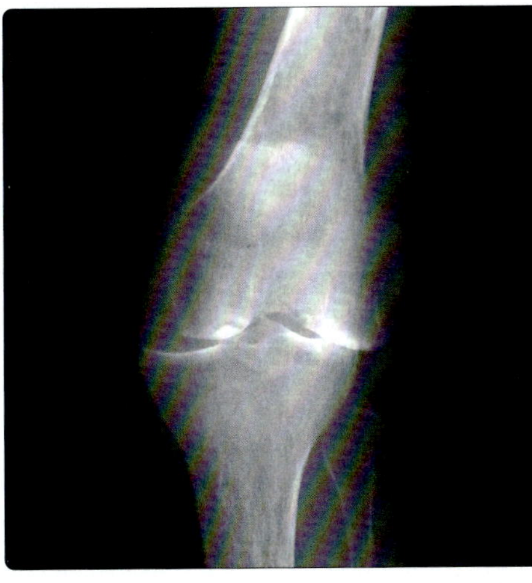

(Left) *AP radiograph shows osteopenia and modest medial compartment narrowing in a patient with RA and new onset of pain. Note also the 2 sclerotic lines in the medial tibial condyle ➡. These features are diagnostic of insufficiency fracture.* **(Right)** *AP radiograph is classic for the diagnosis of RA. There is uniform loss of joint width. The bones are severely osteopenic. There is also ligamentous laxity, as seen with the medial displacement of the tibia relative to the femur. Note also the typical valgus alignment of the knee.*

KEY FACTS

IMAGING

- Radiograph
  - Effusions, especially tibiotalar and metatarsophalangeal (MTP)
  - Pre-Achilles bursitis
  - Location of earliest erosion in foot is MTP (especially 5th)
  - Erosions posterior calcaneal tubercle
  - Osteoporosis, increasing risk of insufficiency fracture (seen as linear sclerosis)
- MR T1WI
  - Low signal bone marrow edema, erosions, subchondral cysts
  - Linear low signal insufficiency fractures
- MR fluid-sensitive sequences
  - Thick, low signal synovium bathed in high signal synovial fluid
  - High signal marrow edema and erosions
  - High signal bursitis (especially pre-Achilles)
  - High signal tenosynovitis and abnormal morphology partial tendon tears
- Avid enhancement of synovium, with adjacent low signal fluid
- US: Confirm fluid collections and effusions
  - Direct visualization of tendon ruptures

CLINICAL ISSUES

- Tibiotalar joint involved in 75% patients with RA
- Midfoot involved in 60% patients with RA
- MTP involved in 75% patients with RA
- Malalignment of ankle and toes; painful posterior calcaneus

DIAGNOSTIC CHECKLIST

- Posterior calcaneal tubercle erosions seen in RA; chronic reactive arthritis is not only diagnosis to consider
- On radiographs, focal soft tissue swelling should direct careful examination of adjacent joint space and bones
- Watch for insufficiency fractures

(Left) *AP radiograph shows a soft tissue mass ➡ separating the 1st and 2nd metatarsophalangeal (MTPs). The mass was painful in this 45-year-old woman. There is a tiny marginal erosion at the base of the 1st proximal phalanx ➡. This, along with the patient's age and gender, should suggest RA, but the mass needs further evaluation.* **(Right)** *Sagittal T1 MR in the same patient shows the mass ➡ to be rather featureless and intermediate intensity. The portion of the 1st metatarsal that is in plane ➡ is unremarkable.*

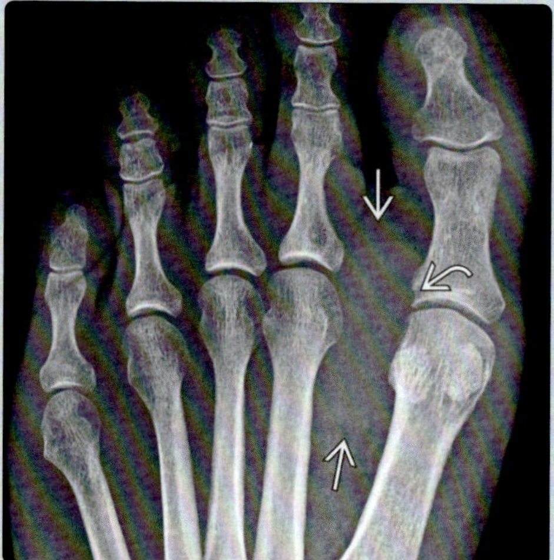

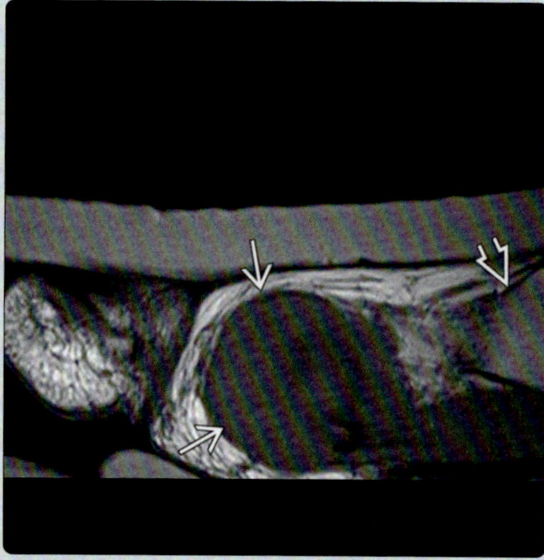

(Left) *Short axis T2FS MR, same patient, shows marrow edema within the entire 1st metatarsal head ➡. A joint effusion ➡ at the 1st MTP displaces the extensor tendon. There is a mixed signal mass ➡ separating metatarsals 1 and 2.* **(Right)** *Short axis postcontrast T1FS shows enhancing synovium encasing the effusion at the 1st MTP ➡. More importantly, the mass is shown to be low-signal fluid with a thick enhancing rim ➡. Given the constellation of findings, the mass is intermetatarsal inflammatory bursitis in a patient with RA.*

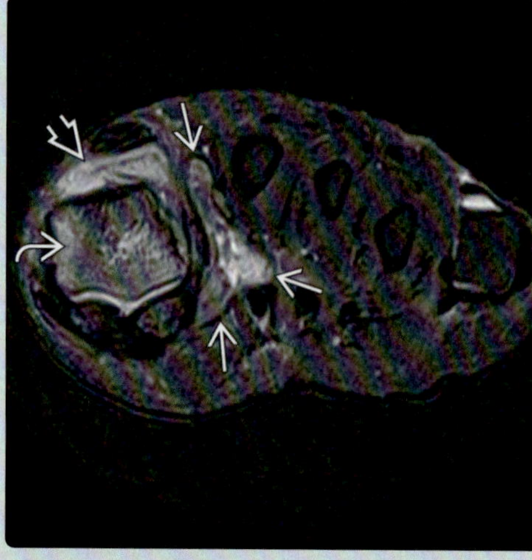

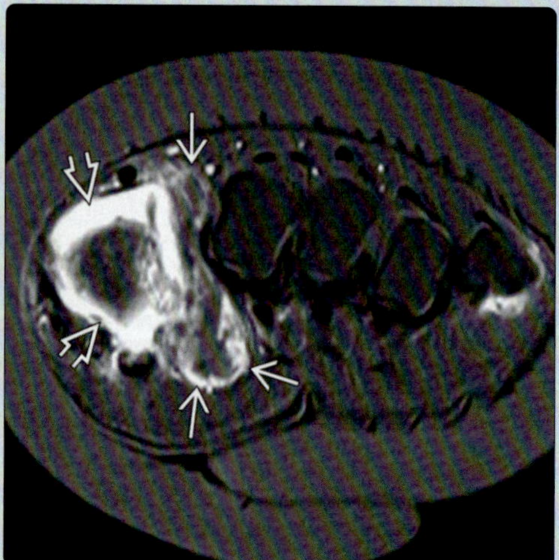

TERMINOLOGY

Abbreviations

- Rheumatoid arthritis (RA)

Definitions

- Chronic progressive systemic inflammatory disease in which joints are primary target

IMAGING

General Features

- Best diagnostic clue
  - Diffuse osteoporosis
  - Bilaterally symmetric uniform joint space narrowing, hindfoot and midfoot joints
  - Bilaterally symmetric erosions, especially at 5th metatarsophalangeal (MTP) joints

Imaging Recommendations

- Best imaging tool
  - Radiographs are utilized 1st; useful once erosions and joint space narrowing have occurred
  - MR shows earlier disease

Radiographic Findings

- Osteopenia
  - Initially juxtaarticular
  - Eventually diffuse
  - Sclerotic insufficiency fracture line, related to osteopenia
    - Distal fibula and tibia, posterior calcaneus, metatarsal neck
- Soft tissue swelling
  - Effusions, especially tibiotalar and MTP
  - Pre-Achilles and other sites of bursitis
- Cartilage destruction
  - Uniform, seen on radiograph as joint space narrowing
- Erosions
  - Early cortical indistinctness and dot-dash pattern
  - Location of earliest erosion is MTPs, particularly 5th
  - Erosions of posterior calcaneal tubercle
  - Later erosions may be severe, with subchondral destruction
    - Pencil-in-cup deformity may be seen in RA (not specific for psoriatic arthritis)
- Deformity
  - Metatarsus primus varus, hallux valgus
  - Hammer toe
  - Valgus hindfoot, collapse midfoot

CT Findings

- Mirrors osseous radiograph findings
- Erosions more clearly delineated
- Enhancement of synovium

MR Findings

- T1WI
  - Low signal synovium, effusions
  - Low signal edema, erosions, subchondral cysts
  - Linear low signal insufficiency fractures
- Fluid-sensitive sequences
  - Thick, low signal synovium bathed in high signal synovium
  - High signal bursitis (especially pre-Achilles)
  - High signal erosions, subchondral cysts
  - High signal marrow edema
  - High signal edema around insufficiency fracture; may obscure actual fracture line
  - Tendon damage
    - High signal tenosynovitis
    - High signal, abnormal morphology partial tendon ruptures (particularly posterior tibial tendon and Achilles tendon)
- T1WI FS + contrast
  - Avid enhancement synovium; adjacent low signal fluid

Ultrasonographic Findings

- Confirm fluid collections and effusions
- Semiquantitative evaluation articular cartilage
- Doppler evaluation of synovitis monitors therapy
- Direct visualization of tendon ruptures

DIFFERENTIAL DIAGNOSIS

Chronic Reactive Arthritis

- Abnormalities prominent in foot and calcaneus, as in RA
  - Posterior tubercle of calcaneus generally shows mixed erosive and productive change in chronic reactive arthritis (CRA)
  - With active inflammation, osteoporosis and erosions predominate, mimicking RA
- Look for other findings of CRA
  - Spondyloarthropathy; enthesitis on MR
  - Urethritis, conjunctivitis

Psoriatic Arthritis

- Abnormalities most prominent in hand but often involve foot as well, psoriatic arthritis (PSA) similar to RA in this respect
  - Posterior tubercle of calcaneus and MTPs generally show mixed erosive and productive change in PSA
    - Occasionally purely erosive in PSA, mimicking RA
- Look for other findings of PSA
  - Spondyloarthropathy
  - Periostitis

Septic Arthritis

- Monoarticular; RA almost always polyarticular
- Synovitis, cartilage damage, erosions may be indistinguishable from RA by imaging
- Septic arthritis is also risk in RA; if concerned, joint should be aspirated

PATHOLOGY

General Features

- Etiology
  - RA: Unknown etiology
  - Pathophysiology presumed to relate to persistent immunologic response of genetically susceptible host to some unknown antigen
- Genetics
  - Genetic predisposition

- Concordance in monozygotic twins: 25%
- 1st-degree relatives develop RA at rate 4x that of general population
  - Still, individual not likely to have affected family member
- Associated abnormalities
  - Subcutaneous rheumatoid nodules in 30%
    - Extensor surfaces (ulna, Achilles) and digits
  - Amyloid deposition
  - Thoracic: Pleural effusions, rheumatoid nodules, rarely interstitial fibrosis
  - Vasculitis
  - Felty syndrome: RA + splenomegaly + leukopenia
  - Sjögren syndrome: RA + keratoconjunctivitis + xerostomia
  - ↑ risk of lymphoma
  - Lifetime of systemic inflammation may contribute to ↑ risk of cardiovascular disease, renal disease, and infection
  - ↑ mortality rate, reduced survival by 10-18 years

Staging, Grading, & Classification

- Criteria for clinical diagnosis of RA (2010 American College of Rheumatology/European League Against Rheumatism)
  - Score-based algorithm: Add score of categories A-D; score of ≥ 6/10 is needed for classification of patient as having definite RA
    - (A) Joint involvement
      - 1 large joint scores 0
      - 2-10 large joints scores 1
      - 1-3 small joints scores 2
      - 4-10 small joints scores 3
      - > 10 joints (at least 1 small joint) scores 5
    - (B) Serology (at least 1 test result is needed for classification)
      - Negative rheumatoid factor (RF) **and** negative anticitrullinated protein antibody (ACPA) scores 0
      - Low-positive RF or low-positive ACPA scores 2
      - High-positive RF or high-positive ACPA scores 3
    - (C) Acute-phase reactants (at least 1 test result is needed for classification)
      - Normal C-reactive protein (CRP) **and** normal erythrocyte sedimentation rate (ESR) scores 0
      - Abnormal CRP or abnormal ESR scores 1
    - (D) Duration of symptoms
      - < 6 weeks scores 0
      - ≥ 6 weeks scores 1

CLINICAL ISSUES

Presentation

- Most common signs/symptoms
  - Symmetric polyarthritis, especially small joints
  - Constitutional symptoms: Fatigue, low-grade fever
  - Usually presents over course of weeks or months; occasionally fulminant disease
- Other signs/symptoms
  - Malalignment of ankle and toes; painful heel

Demographics

- Age
  - Development peaks at 3rd-5th decades
- Gender
  - M:F = 1:3
- Epidemiology
  - RA in 1% of worldwide population
    - 5% in some Native American populations
  - Tibiotalar joint involved in 75% patients with RA
  - Midfoot involved in 60% patients with RA
  - MTP involved in 75% patients with RA

Natural History & Prognosis

- Remission may occur with aggressive multidrug therapy
- Those who do not have remission progress to painful, deformed foot

Treatment

- Treatment of RA: Generally combination; aimed at pain relief while escalating therapy rapidly to suppress disease prior to joint destruction
  - NSAIDs
    - Symptomatic relief; do not alter disease progression
  - Glucocorticoids (oral or intraarticular)
    - Controls inflammation rapidly; allows slower acting drugs to take effect
  - DMARDs
    - Methotrexate, sulfasalazine, antimalarials, gold
    - Suppresses joint destruction
  - Biologics: Anti-TNF-α drugs, antiinterleukin-1
    - Role of cytokines (especially tumor necrosis factor-α and interleukin-1) in pathophysiology of RA now recognized
- Surgical treatment of RA
  - Resection heads/bases phalanges
  - Synovectomy
  - Tenodesis
  - Arthrodesis (difficult to accomplish due to osteoporosis but often improves function)
  - Arthroplasty
    - Ankle: May have good result; watch for loosening, infection, periprosthetic fracture
    - Digits: Silastic arthroplasties may fail
      - Ligament abnormality causes malalignment
      - Abnormal motion on osteoporotic bone causes osseous debris and device failures
      - May result in massive osteolysis

DIAGNOSTIC CHECKLIST

Consider

- Posterior calcaneal tubercle erosions seen in RA; CRA and PSA not only diagnoses to consider

Image Interpretation Pearls

- On radiographs, focal soft tissue swelling should direct careful examination of joint space and bones
- Watch for insufficiency fractures

SELECTED REFERENCES

1. Naredo E et al: Predictive value of Doppler ultrasound-detected synovitis in relation to failed tapering of biologic therapy in patients with rheumatoid arthritis. Rheumatology (Oxford). 54(8):1408-14, 2015
2. Onodera T et al: A comparative study with in vitro ultrasonographic and histologic grading of metatarsal head cartilage in rheumatoid arthritis. Foot Ankle Int. 36(7):774-9, 2015

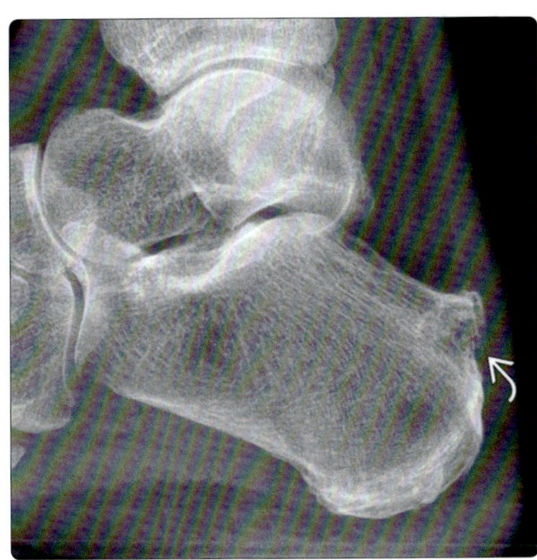

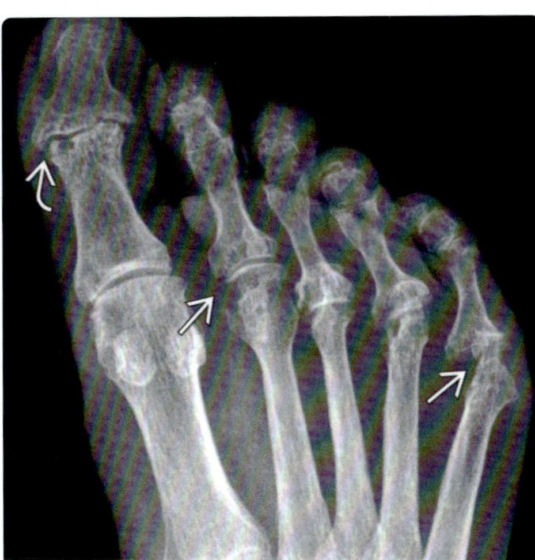

(Left) *Lateral radiograph shows erosion* ➡ *at the posterior calcaneal tubercle. This is a nonspecific finding of inflammatory arthropathy; RA is just as likely a diagnosis as psoriatic or chronic reactive arthritis.* **(Right)** *AP radiograph in the same patient shows significant erosive disease involving MTP 2-5* ➡ *as well as the 1st IP joint* ➡*. There is no periostitis to suggest psoriatic or chronic reactive arthritis. The distribution is typical for RA and confirms the diagnosis.*

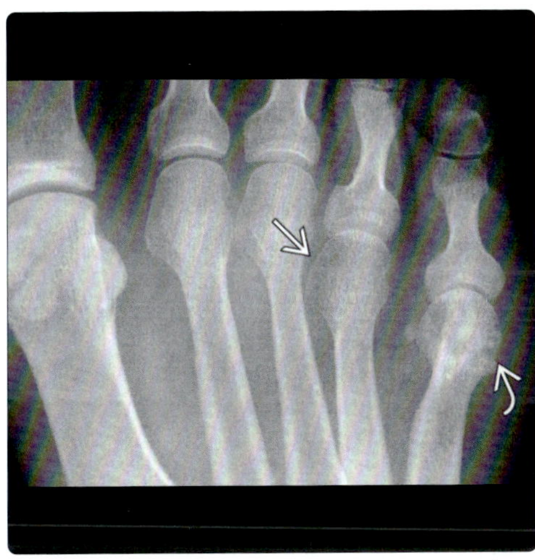

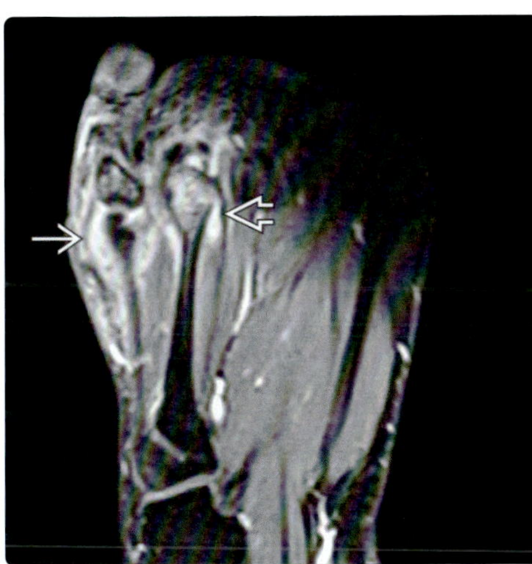

(Left) *AP x-ray shows focal osteopenia at the 4th and 5th MTPs, with cortical indistinctness at the 4th MT head* ➡*. True erosions and subchondral cysts are seen at the 5th MT head* ➡*, the most frequent location for RA in the foot. MR would show further disease.* **(Right)** *Axial STIR MR in a patient with normal x-rays shows erosive disease of the 5th MTP, along with effusion and synovitis* ➡*. Though there is no erosion at the 4th MTP, there is edema in the 4th metatarsal head as well as effusion* ➡*. The findings are of early RA.*

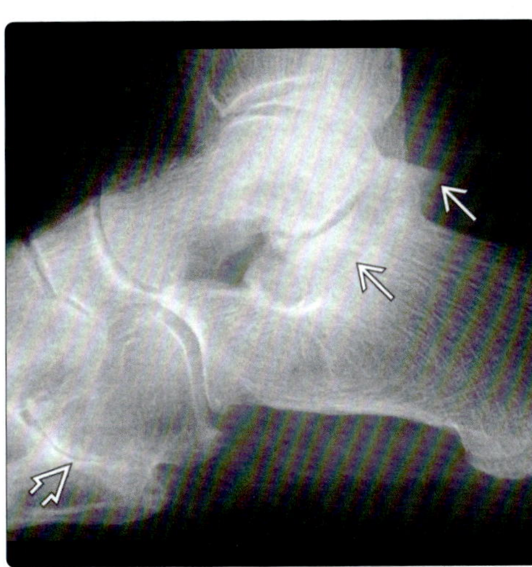

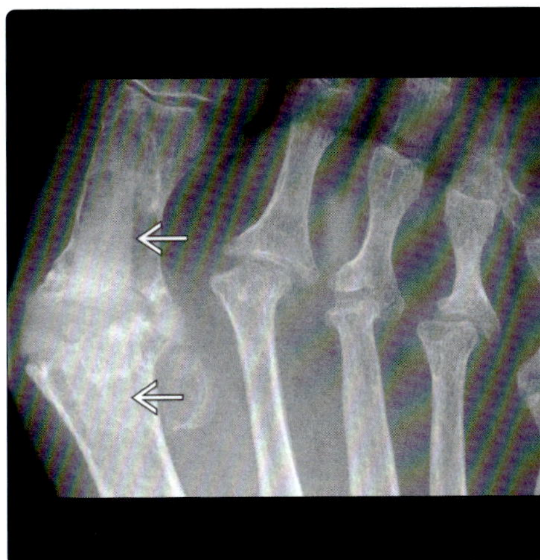

(Left) *Lateral radiograph shows erosive disease of the midfoot* ➡*, typical of RA. Note also the sclerotic linear offset in the calcaneus* ➡*. This insufficiency fracture might easily be overlooked, as are others in these patients.* **(Right)** *AP radiograph shows resection of the heads of MT 2-4, a frequent treatment of the painful deformities of MTPs in patients with RA. The 1st MTP has been replaced with a Swanson arthroplasty* ➡*, which has failed; the particles result in massive osteolysis.*

KEY FACTS

TERMINOLOGY

- Robust rheumatoid arthritis: Variant of RA in which subchondral cyst formation is particularly prominent and normal bone density is often maintained

IMAGING

- Findings are most prominent in wrist and hand
  - Other locations, particularly feet, may be involved
- Generally, location is typical of RA
  - Distribution in wrist: Distal radioulnar, radiocarpal joints
  - Distribution in hand: MCP and IP joints
- Generally, appearance is typical of RA
  - Bilaterally symmetric disease
  - Uniform cartilage loss and resultant narrowing
  - Erosions, both marginal and subchondral
  - Deformities: Ulnar translocation of carpus, carpal instability, MCP volar subluxation, and ulnar deviation
  - Synovial proliferation
  - Rheumatoid nodules
- Bone density may be variable
  - If not fully advanced and hand does not suffer from disuse, may retain normal bone density
  - If advanced, osteopenia is diffuse
- Large subchondral cyst formation
  - Major differentiating factor from conventional RA
  - Cyst formation is disproportionate to erosive disease

CLINICAL ISSUES

- Usually occurs in males
- Patients generally active and pursue physical labor
- Pain & stiffness limited compared with routine RA patients
- Etiology thought to relate to continued use of hands, particularly with manual labor
  - Continued use helps maintain bone density
  - Continued use forces effusions and pannus through cartilage and articular surface defects into subchondral cysts, elevating pressure, and causing gradual enlargement of cysts

(Left) *PA radiograph shows cartilage narrowing predominantly in the MCPs ➡ and small marginal erosions at the MCPs ➡ typical of RA. However, these are not nearly as impressive as the large subchondral cysts seen at several sites ➡. Note also the bone density is normal. This 52-year-old man is a manual laborer and has robust RA.* **(Right)** *PA of contralateral hand shows soft tissue swelling (presumed synovitis) ➡ and large subchondral cysts ➡ in a symmetric distribution, confirming the diagnosis.*

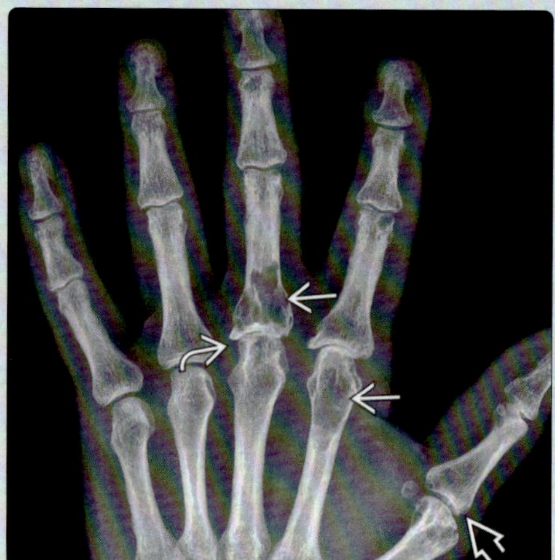

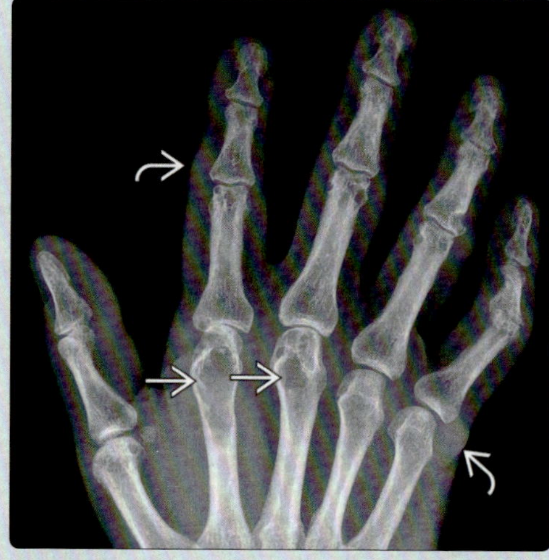

(Left) *AP radiograph shows cartilage narrowing at the 1st MTP and multiple small marginal erosions ➡ in a typical distribution of RA. However, the foot shows normal density and an extremely large subchondral cyst ➡, making this atypical for routine RA. The constellation is in fact that of robust RA in this active man who does not have significant complaints of pain.* **(Right)** *Contralateral foot shows erosions and normal bone density but fewer cysts. Rheumatoid factor levels were high, confirming the diagnosis.*

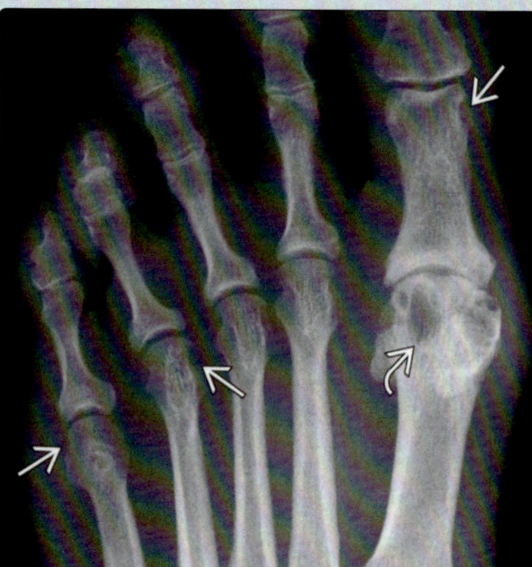

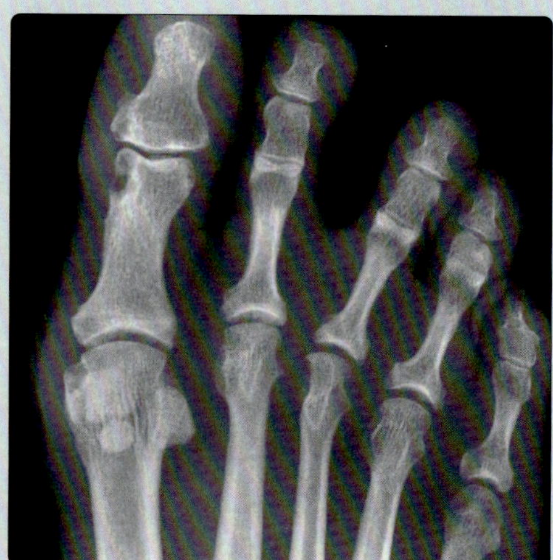

KEY FACTS

TERMINOLOGY

- Felty syndrome: Triad of
  - Rheumatoid arthritis (RA)
  - Splenomegaly
  - Neutropenia

IMAGING

- Usually severely deforming RA
  - Erosions
  - Cartilage destruction
  - Joint deformities
- May have other extraarticular manifestations of RA
  - Rheumatoid nodules
  - Vasculitis
  - Sjögren syndrome
  - Pericarditis

CLINICAL ISSUES

- Rare process
- Usually Caucasian female
- High titer rheumatoid factor (RF)
- Often have HLA-DR4 and other alleles associated with disease severity in RA
- Etiology unknown
  - Neutropenia may result from splenic sequestration of granulocytes
- Treatment parallels that of RA
  - Disease-modifying drug therapy; rituximab (monoclonal anti CD20 antibody) reported effective
  - Arthroplasty, arthrodesis as needed to regain function
- Consider splenectomy if
  - Splenomegaly is massive
  - Patient suffers recurrent infections
- Associated large granular lymphocytic leukemia in 40% of cases
- Most cases of neutropenia in RA are acquired, not Felty syndrome
  - Related to medications used for RA

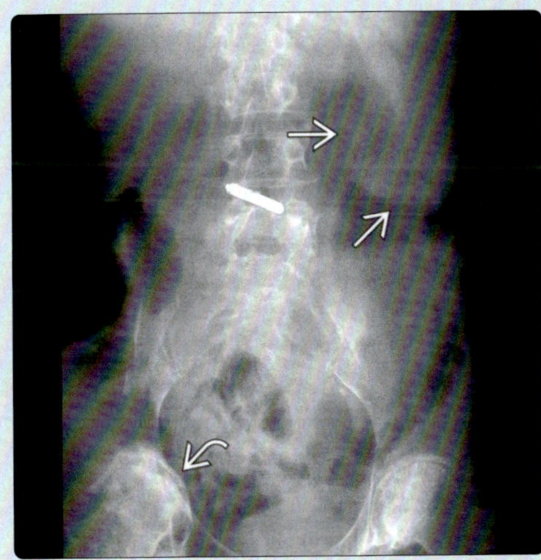

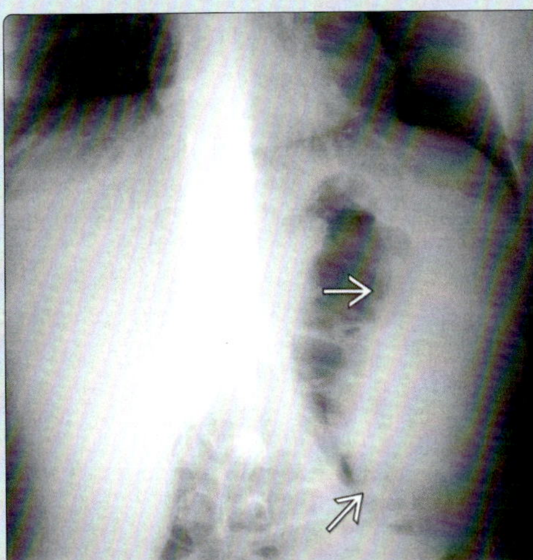

(Left) *Anteroposterior radiograph shows splenomegaly ➡, along with severe erosive disease of the hips, resulting in protrusio ➡. This is a typical case of Felty syndrome; the patient also had neutropenia. In this rare syndrome, the arthritic process is usually severe, as in this case.* **(Right)** *Anteroposterior radiograph shows severe splenomegaly ➡ as outlined by the bowel gas in the splenic flexure. No other abnormality is present, and there is a wide differential based on this image alone.*

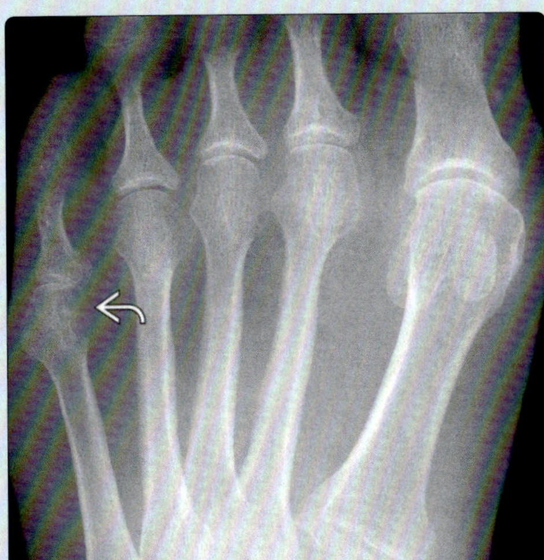

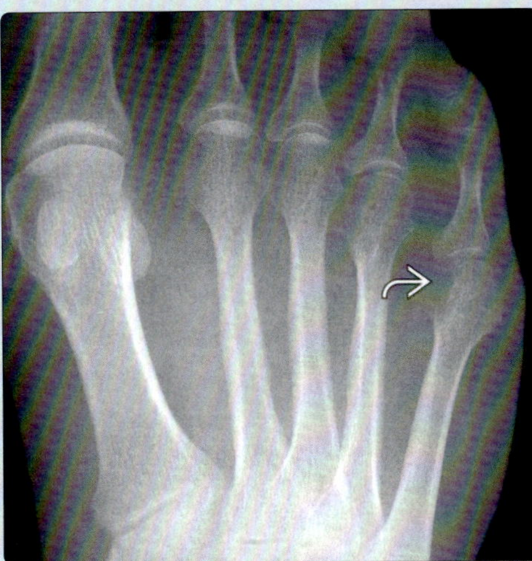

(Left) *AP radiograph of the forefoot in the same patient shows joint space narrowing and erosive change of the 5th metatarsal head ➡.* **(Right)** *AP radiograph of the contralateral foot shows a symmetric pattern of cartilage narrowing and erosive change at the 5th metatarsophalangeal joint ➡. The patient proved to have rheumatoid arthritis and neutropenia, as well as the noted splenomegaly, completing the triad of Felty syndrome. It is unusual for the RA to appear so mild in a patient with Felty syndrome.*

KEY FACTS

TERMINOLOGY

- Group of inflammatory arthropathies affecting children < 16 years old

IMAGING

- 4 subtypes differ in clinical presentation and prognosis
- Any affected joint has similar attributes
  - Bilateral but not always symmetric
  - Large effusions, erosions, cartilage destruction
  - End-stage ankylosis
- Growth abnormalities common
  - Gracile long bones (narrow diameter, thin cortex)
  - Short stature, hypoplastic iliac wings
  - Hypoplastic cervical vertebral bodies
  - Ballooned (enlarged) epiphyses
  - Enlarged intercondylar and trochlear notches
  - Micrognathia: Hypoplastic angle of mandible with temporomandibular joint erosions
- Earliest radiographic signs
  - Periostitis: Seen only at earliest stages, in young child
  - Differential growth of epiphysis
    - Focal hyperemia results in focal advanced growth of epiphyses
    - Often need contralateral side for comparison to make diagnosis
- MR generally not utilized but may provide information at early stage, prior to radiographic changes
  - Effusions, tenosynovitis: High T2WI signal
  - Marrow edema: Low T1WI, high T2WI signal
  - Erosions: Low T1WI, high T2WI signal
  - Pannus: Thickened synovium, low signal on T1 and T2, enhances

TOP DIFFERENTIAL DIAGNOSES

- Hemophilic arthropathy
- Toxic synovitis of hip
- Chronic septic joint

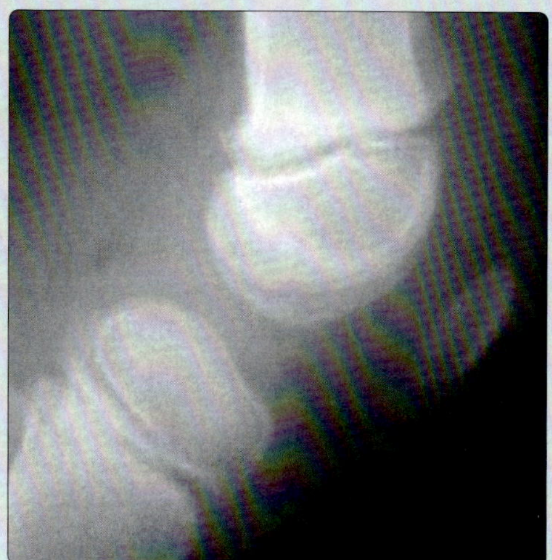

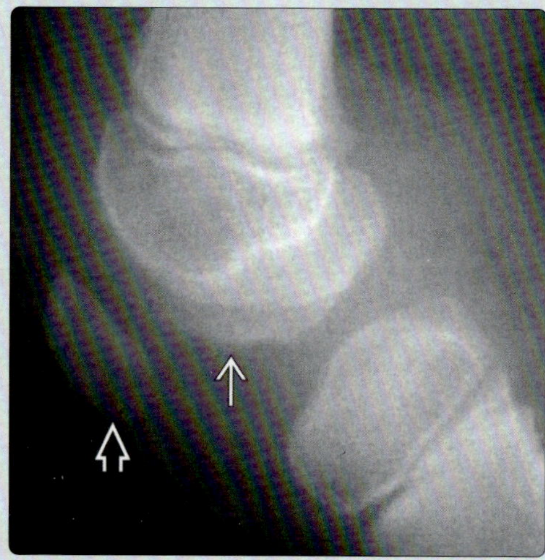

(Left) *Lateral radiograph shows the unaffected knee in a child with oligoarticular juvenile idiopathic arthritis (JIA). This is shown for comparison.* **(Right)** *Lateral radiograph shows the contralateral affected knee in the same patient. Although at 1st glance this radiograph appears normal, there is significant overgrowth of the epiphyses of this knee. Note the femoral condyles, proximal tibial epiphysis, and in particular the patella ➲. There is also crenulation or irregularity along the femoral condyles ➲.*

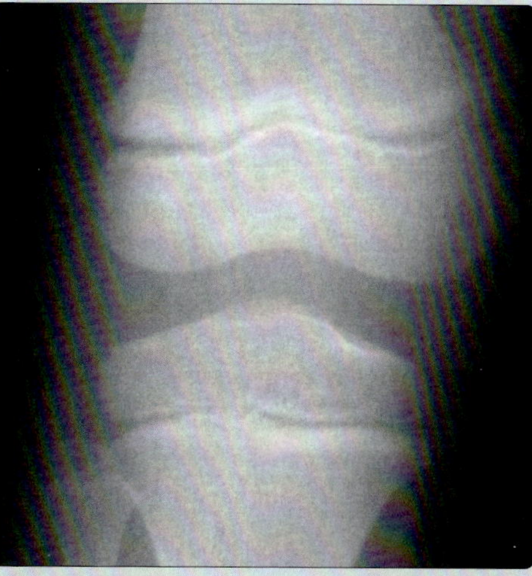

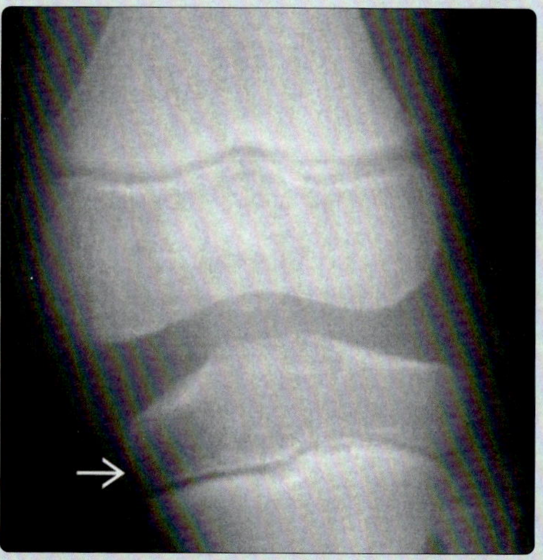

(Left) *AP radiograph shows the normal knee in the same child.* **(Right)** *AP radiograph of the affected knee was taken at the same distance and time. Note the enlargement of the femoral condylar and proximal tibial epiphyses. This occurs due to the hyperemia of the joint secondary to inflammation and synovitis. Such overgrowth, or ballooning, is often the 1st radiographic sign of JIA. Note also the more mature morphology of the medial tibial epiphysis ➲. Without comparison radiographs, it may easily be missed.*

TERMINOLOGY

Abbreviations

- Juvenile idiopathic arthritis (JIA)

Synonyms

- Juvenile chronic arthritis
- Juvenile rheumatoid arthritis
- Systemic JIA: Still disease

Definitions

- Group of inflammatory arthropathies affecting children < 16 years old; 4 subsets generally recognized

IMAGING

General Features

- Best diagnostic clue
  - 4 subtypes differ in clinical presentation and prognosis
  - Any affected joint has similar attributes
    - Large effusions
    - Osseous erosions
    - Cartilage destruction
    - Often bilateral but usually not symmetric
    - End-stage ankylosis
      - Carpus most frequent site of fusion
      - If cervical spine involved, fusion of bodies and posterior elements frequently occurs
    - Osteoporosis
- Location
  - Subsets differ in joints most likely to be affected
    - Oligoarticular (> 50% of cases)
      - Generally only 2-4 joints
      - Knee most frequent, followed by ankle and elbow
    - Psoriatic arthritis/enthesitis-related arthritis (10% of cases)
      - Sacroiliac joints, knee, ankle, hip
    - Polyarticular [RF(+) or RF(-)] (30% of cases)
      - 5+ joints
      - Hands/feet; may involve all joints as in adult RA
    - Systemic (10% of cases)
      - Polyarticular, following pattern of adult RA
  - Location in hand/wrist different from adult RA
    - Pericapitate erosions predominate in carpus
    - Metacarpophalangeal involvement does not dominate interphalangeal involvement
- Morphology
  - Growth abnormalities common
    - Gracile long bones (narrow diameter, thin cortex)
      - Due to chronic illness
    - Short stature, hypoplastic iliac wings
      - Due to chronic illness, lack of weight bearing
      - Early epiphyseal closure due to hyperemia
    - Hypoplastic cervical vertebral bodies
      - Due to body fusion prior to skeletal maturity
      - Morphology is normal, but fused bodies are uniformly small relative to unfused bodies
    - Micrognathia: Hypoplastic angle of mandible with temporomandibular joint erosions
    - Ballooned (enlarged) epiphyses
      - Overgrowth of epiphysis due to hyperemia from inflammatory synovitis
      - Results in prominent, enlarged epiphyses relative to diaphyses
      - Clinically, knobby enlarged joints
      - Especially prominent in knee, ankle, elbow
    - Enlarged notches
      - Due to pressure erosion from pannus
      - Noted in intercondylar notch of knee and trochlear notch in elbow

Radiographic Findings

- Uniform osteopenia
- Earliest radiographic signs
  - Periostitis: Seen only at earliest stages, in young child
  - Differential growth of epiphysis; often need contralateral side for comparison
- Purely erosive disease
- Uniform cartilage narrowing
- Large effusions
- Progressive destruction, with ankylosis at end-stage
- Growth abnormalities
  - Short stature
  - Gracile long bones
  - Overgrown epiphyses with enlarged notches

MR Findings

- MR provides information at early stage, prior to radiographic change
  - Effusions, tenosynovitis: High T2WI
  - Marrow edema: Low T1WI, high T2WI signal
  - Erosions: Low T1WI, high T2WI signal
  - Pannus: Thickened synovium
    - Low signal on T1WI
    - Low signal on T2WI, may be nodular, outlined by high signal effusion
    - Enhances with contrast administration
  - Menisci may appear small or compressed due to effusion
  - Contrast essential to distinguish active synovial inflammation from nonenhancing effusion or fibrotic pannus
- May be used to evaluate for early physeal fusion when evaluating for growth potential

DIFFERENTIAL DIAGNOSIS

Hemophilic Arthropathy

- Restricted to male population
- Most commonly affects knee, ankle, elbow
- Chronic intraarticular bleeding → identical to JIA
  - Purely erosive, destructive disease
  - Epiphyseal overgrowth due to hyperemia
  - Enlarged notches due to pannus
  - MR low signal synovial deposition of hemosiderin from chronic intraarticular bleeds

Chronic Septic Joint

- Tuberculous or fungal infection
- Chronicity allows slow destruction of joint
  - → erosives and cartilage/bone destruction
  - Long-term hyperemia → epiphyseal overgrowth

Characteristics of Juvenile Idiopathic Arthritis Subsets

Subsets of JIA	Oligoarticular	Psoriatic Arthritis/ERA	Polyarticular [RF(+) or RF(-)]	Systemic
Frequency	50%	10%	30%	10%
Age of onset (years)	1-10	9-16	3-16	3-16
Gender predominance	M:F = 1:5	M:F = 4:1	M:F = 1:4	M = F
Arthritis pattern	Mono- or pauciarticular (1-4 joints)	Sacroiliitis or asymmetric oligoarthritis	Polyarticular (> 5 joints), symmetric	Polyarticular; 1 or more
Extraarticular features	Rare	Psoriasis, enthesitis, inflammatory bowel disease	Rheumatoid nodules, weight loss	Fever, rash, lymphadenopathy, serositis
Uveitis	10-50%	10%	Rare	Rare
Laboratory findings	RF(-), 85% ANA(+)	50% HLA-B27(+)	80% RF(-), 40% ANA(+)	Leukocytosis, ESR > 50 mm/h, anemia, ↑ LFTs; RF(-), ANA(-)
Prognosis	Joints: Excellent; eyes: Guarded	Risk of spondylitis (20-50%)	Severe erosive arthritis (50%)	Chronic arthritis (50%), severe erosive arthritis (20%)

Undifferentiated JIA: Those cases that fit into none or at least 2 of the other categories.
ERA = enthesitis-related arthritis.

PATHOLOGY

General Features

- Etiology
  - Cause unknown
    - Disordered immunoregulation reported
    - Possible latent viral infection (rubella suggested)
    - Likely not common cause among subsets
- Genetics
  - Associated with *IL2RA* (CD25) gene (IL-2 receptor α)
    - General susceptibility gene for autoimmune diseases; likely represents JIA susceptibility locus
  - JIA patients carrying TNF-α -308 GA/AA and -238 GA genotypes → worse prognosis and lower response to anti-TNF-α drugs
- Associated abnormalities
  - Oligoarticular: Serious risk of uveitis
    - May be complicated by blindness
  - Psoriatic arthritis/enthesitis-related arthritis
    - 50% HLA-B27(+)
  - Polyarticular: Constitutional symptoms
    - Low-grade fever, weight loss
    - Lymphadenopathy
    - Rheumatoid factor positive in 20-30%
    - ANA(+) in 40%
  - Systemic
    - Quotidian (daily spiking) fever, rash
    - Lymphadenopathy
    - Hepatosplenomegaly
    - Weight loss, myalgia
    - Neutrophilic leukocytosis, anemia
    - Rheumatoid factor and ANA (-); ↑ ESR

CLINICAL ISSUES

Demographics

- Age
  - Onset usually before 9 years of age
    - Younger onset in oligoarticular (< 6 years)
    - Older onset in psoriatic arthritis/ERA (9-16 years)
- Gender
  - M:F = 1:4-5 for oligoarticular and polyarticular
  - M:F = 4:1 for psoriatic arthritis/ERA
  - M = F for systemic JIA
- Epidemiology
  - Relatively rare; 2 different studies quote 12-20/100,000 and 57-113/100,000

Natural History & Prognosis

- Oligoarticular
  - If treated, joint function usually remains excellent
  - Ophthalmic prognosis guarded: All patients should have routine ophthalmologic exam every 3-6 months
- Psoriatic arthritis/ERA
  - 20-50% go on to chronic spondyloarthropathy
- Polyarticular
  - 20-50% develop severe erosions, similar to adult RA
- Systemic onset
  - 50% chronic arthritis
  - 20% develop severe erosive arthritis

Treatment

- Aggressive combined drug therapy, as in adult RA

DIAGNOSTIC CHECKLIST

Image Interpretation Pearls

- Watch for morphologic changes: Growth delay or overgrown epiphyses

Reporting Tips

- If possible, evaluate enough of skeleton to help place patient in appropriate subset
  - Affects prognosis; ophthalmic implications

SELECTED REFERENCES

1. Hinze C et al: Management of juvenile idiopathic arthritis: hitting the target. Nat Rev Rheumatol. 11(5):290-300, 2015
2. Sheybani EF et al: Imaging of juvenile idiopathic arthritis: a multimodality approach. Radiographics. 33(5):1253-73, 2013

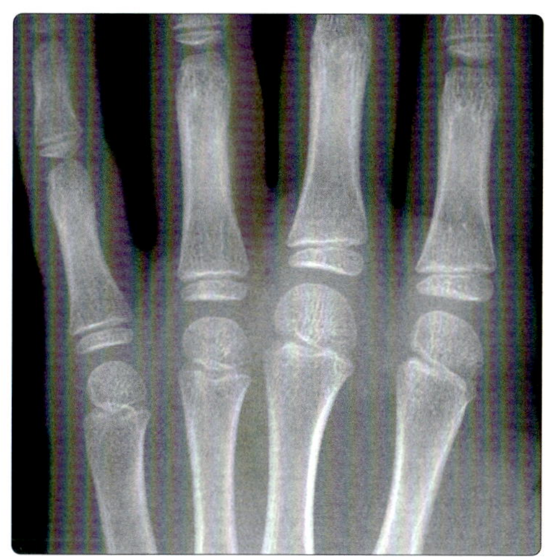

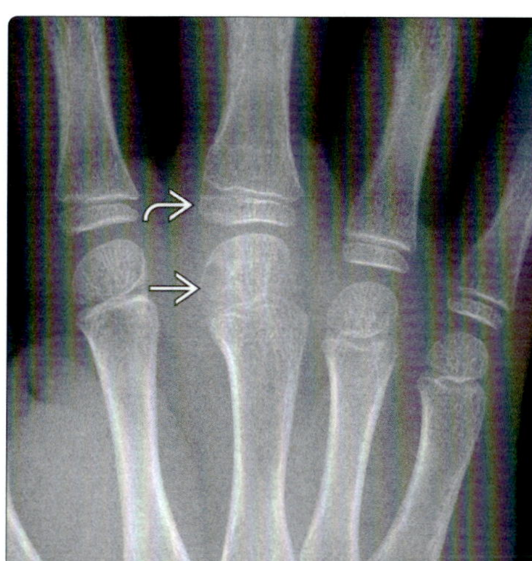

(Left) *PA radiograph shows the hand in a child with new onset of metacarpophalangeal pain and swelling (the right worse than the left). This left hand appears normal.* **(Right)** *PA radiograph of the right hand in the same patient is shown. Compare the 3rd metacarpal head ➡; it is enlarged and eroded. Additionally, there is relative overgrowth of the base of the proximal phalanx ➡. Note the soft tissue swelling. This focally advanced skeletal maturation is secondary to hyperemia from the inflammatory process.*

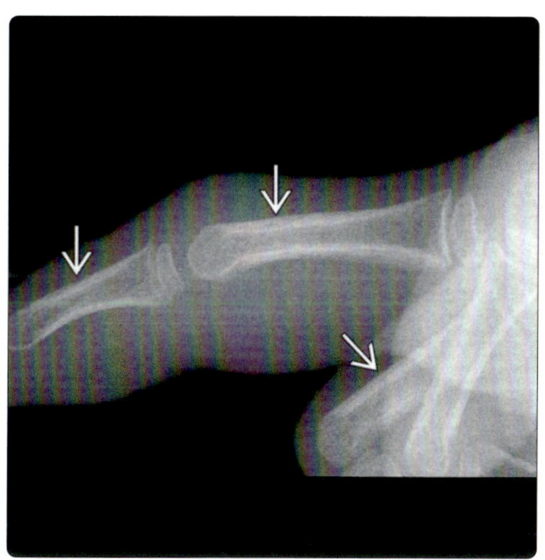

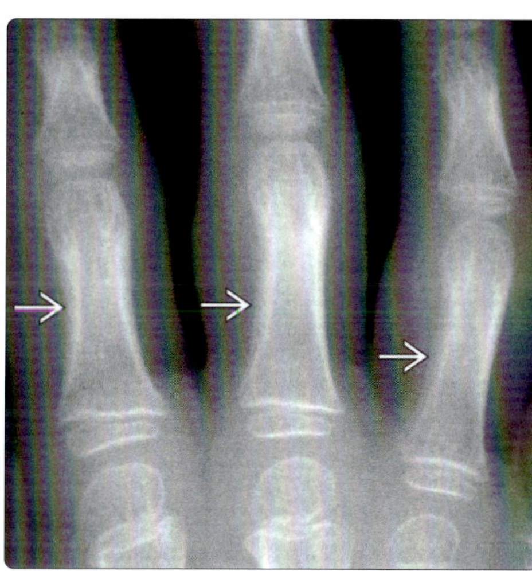

(Left) *Lateral radiograph in a young child shows regular periosteal reaction extending along the phalanges ➡. There is soft tissue swelling but no articular abnormality.* **(Right)** *PA radiograph in the same child shows the same subtle but regular periosteal reaction ➡. The differential diagnoses for this appearance include JIA, sickle cell dactylitis, and tuberculosis dactylitis. This proved to be an early manifestation of JIA.*

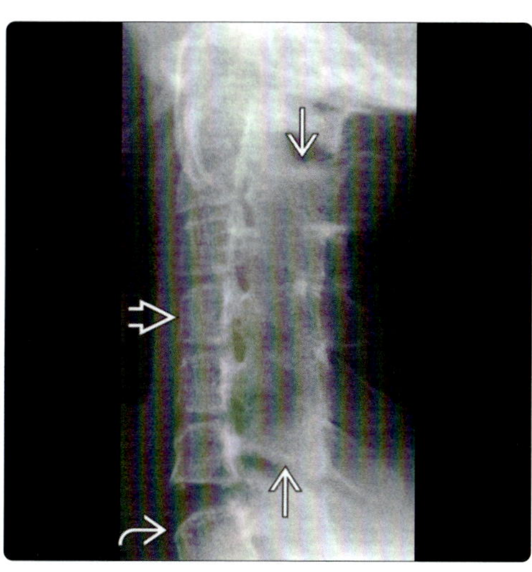

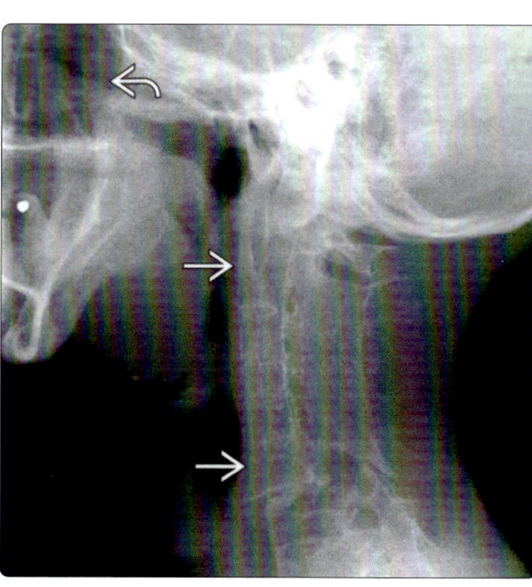

(Left) *Lateral radiograph of the cervical spine in JIA shows the typical ankylosis of posterior elements as well as vertebral bodies, extending from C2-C6 ➡. With fusion at a young age, growth is arrested, leaving hypoplasia of the involved bodies ➡ compared with uninvolved ones ➡.* **(Right)** *Lateral radiograph in a JIA patient with C2-C6 fusion ➡ and hypoplasia over that interval is shown. There is micrognathia, with hypoplastic angles of the mandible and eroded temporomandibular joints ➡.*

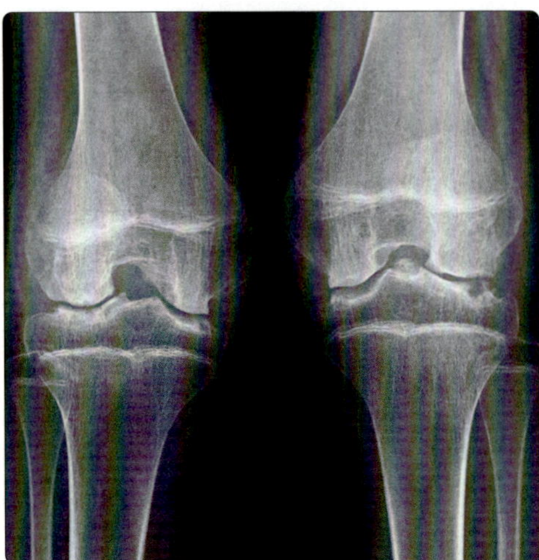

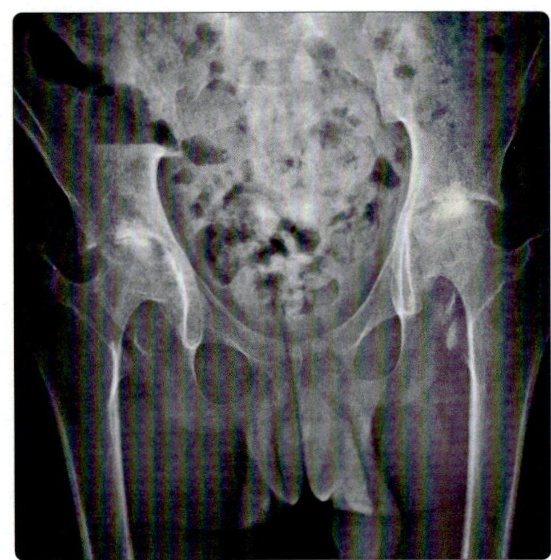

(Left) *AP radiograph of the knees in a patient with longstanding JIA shows ballooned overgrowth of the femoral condyles and widening of the intercondylar notch. Additionally, there is uniform cartilage thinning and prominent subchondral erosions.* **(Right)** *AP radiograph in the same patient shows destruction of the hip joints with associated protrusio, typical of JIA.*

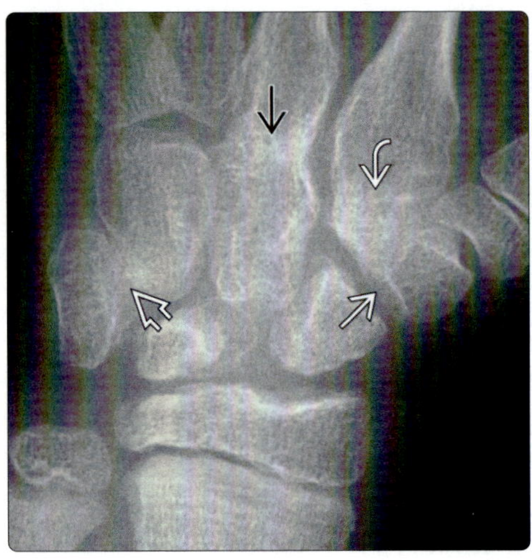

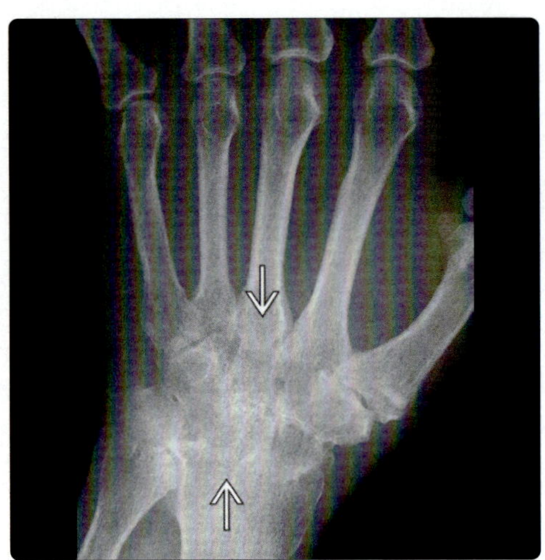

(Left) *PA radiograph of the carpus in a child with JIA shows early fusion at several sites, including capitate-metacarpal ➙, trapezoid-metacarpal ➙, trapezium-trapezoid ➙, and hamate-triquetrum ➙. The cortex appears slightly irregular or crenulated. Carpal ankylosis is typical of JIA.* **(Right)** *PA radiograph in a young adult who developed JIA as a teenager shows near-complete carpal ankylosis ➙. This is common in JIA but is not expected in adult rheumatoid arthritis.*

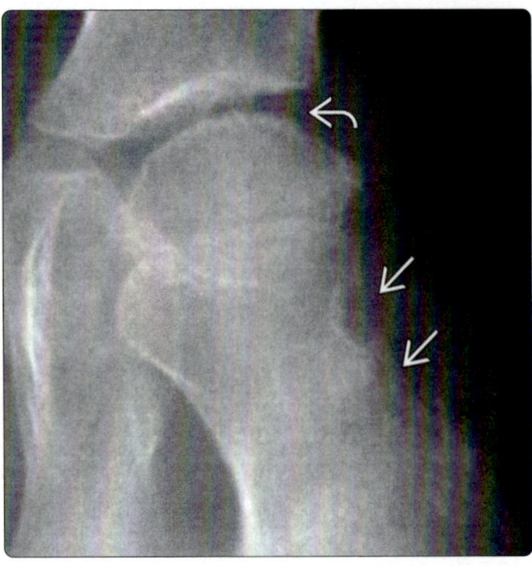

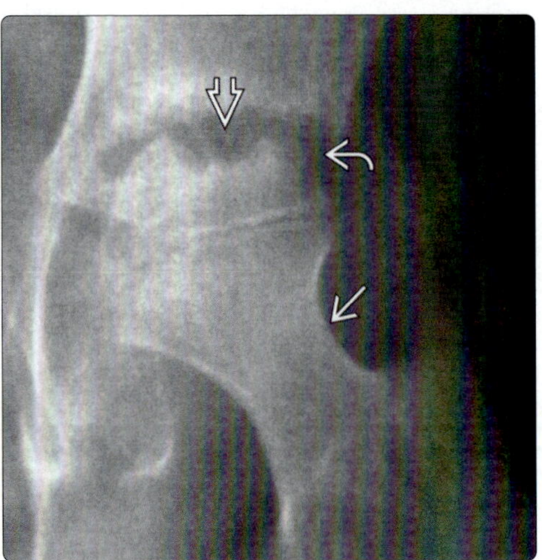

(Left) *AP radiograph in a child with JIA shows erosions along the lateral femoral neck ➙. This portion of the hip is within the capsule and constitutes a bare area of bone, which is not protected by cartilage. It is at risk for early erosion. There is also cartilage narrowing ➙.* **(Right)** *AP radiograph in the same child, 1 year later, shows the neck erosions have smoothed ➙, leaving a thin neck at risk for fracture. There is complete cartilage loss ➙ as well as subchondral erosions ➙.*

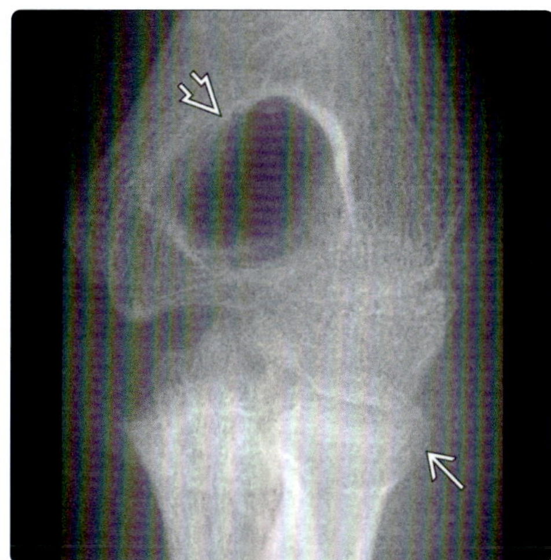

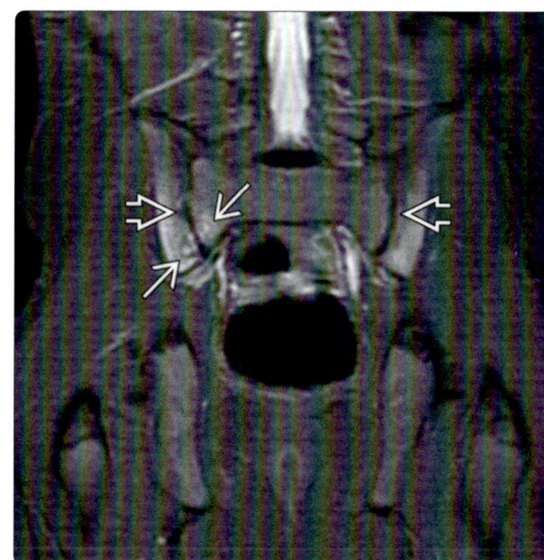

(Left) *AP radiograph shows JIA, with widening of the trochlear notch ➡ due to pressure erosion from pannus over a long period of time. The radial head is relatively enlarged ➡ due to continual hyperemia in the joint. All growth centers may enlarge, but in the elbow, the radial head shows disproportionate overgrowth.* **(Right)** *Coronal STIR MR of the sacroiliac joints in an 8 year old shows bilateral asymmetric sacroiliitis ➡, with erosions and cysts ➡. This is the enthesitis-related arthritis subtype of JIA.*

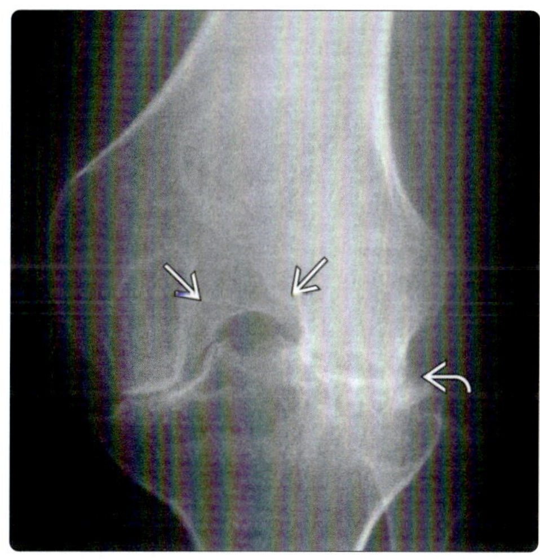

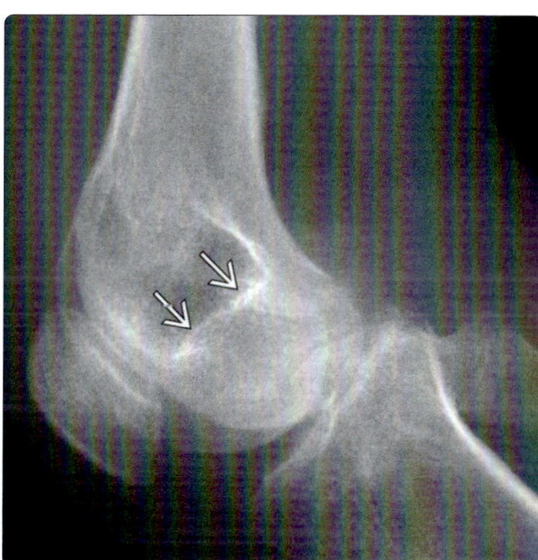

(Left) *AP radiograph shows classic severe JIA in a patient who is now an adult. There is overgrowth of the femoral condyles and a widened intercondylar notch ➡ superimposed on the erosive destructive inflammatory changes ➡.* **(Right)** *Lateral radiograph shows overgrowth of the femoral condyles and patella, developed secondary to chronic hyperemia prior to skeletal maturation. The widened intercondylar notch can be diagnosed on the lateral view by bowing of the Blumensaat line ➡.*

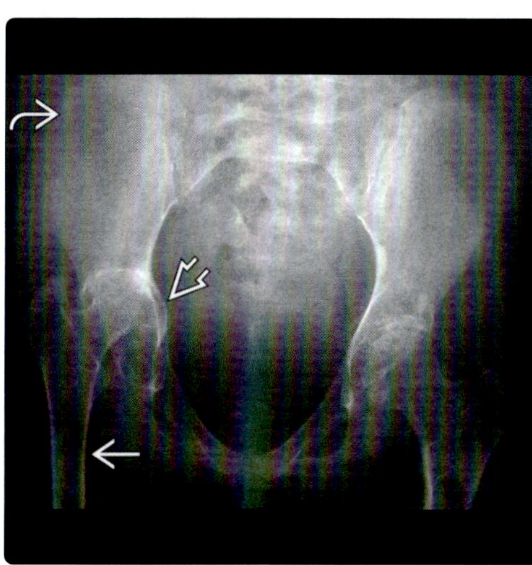

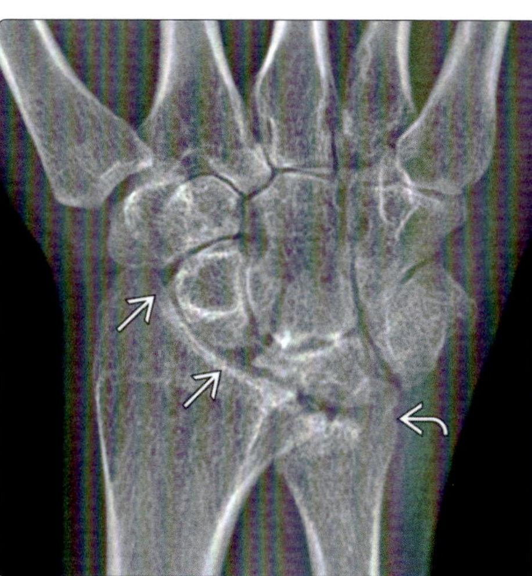

(Left) *AP radiograph shows the adult sequela of JIA, with iliac wing hypoplasia ➡ and gracile femur ➡, which are the results of chronic illness and infrequent weight bearing. There is protrusio of the hip, with severe destruction ➡.* **(Right)** *PA radiograph shows ulnar tilt due to overgrowth of the radial styloid ➡ during the hyperemic growing stage of JIA. Note the matching overgrowth of the ulnar styloid ➡. The collapsed radial aspect of the lunate likely resulted from erosions & impaction from mild trauma.*

Adult Still Disease

KEY FACTS

TERMINOLOGY

- Systemic inflammatory disease, featuring triad
  - Quotidian fevers (spiking, daily)
  - Evanescent rash
  - Chronic polyarthritis
- Considered adult continuum of juvenile idiopathic arthritis (JIA)

IMAGING

- Hand: Interphalangeal (IP) joints more commonly affected than metacarpophalangeal (MCP) joints
  - Proximal interphalangeal (PIP) joints (50%)
  - Distal interphalangeal (DIP) joints (20%)
  - MCP joints (33%)
- Wrist: Involved in 74% of cases
  - Pericapitate (midcarpal and carpometacarpal) disease is classic, but any pattern of carpal involvement may be seen
- Uniform cartilage loss
- Erosions, similar to RA
- Carpus may be remarkable for joint space narrowing, without significant erosive change
- Ankylosis, especially at carpus

TOP DIFFERENTIAL DIAGNOSES

- Psoriatic arthritis (PSA)
  - IP > MCP joint involvement is similar
  - Ankylosis is similar
  - Rash and constitutional symptoms differentiate adult Still disease from PSA
- Chronic reactive arthritis
  - Constitutional symptoms may be suggestive
  - Location of arthritic changes is likely different in adult Still, with hand/wrist predominating
  - Foot/ankle may be involved, similar to CRA

CLINICAL ISSUES

- 75% have onset between 16 and 35 years; M = F

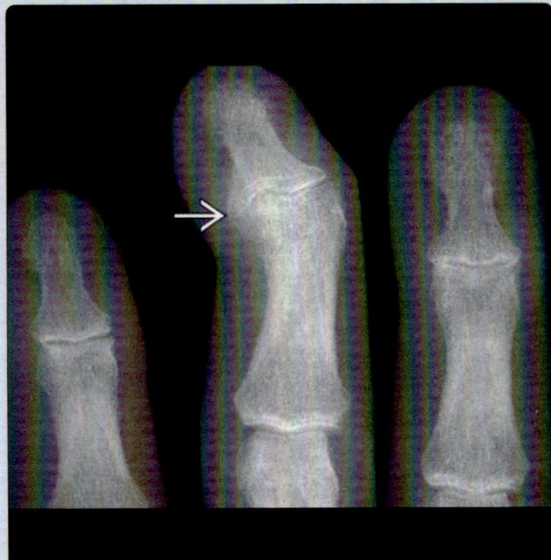

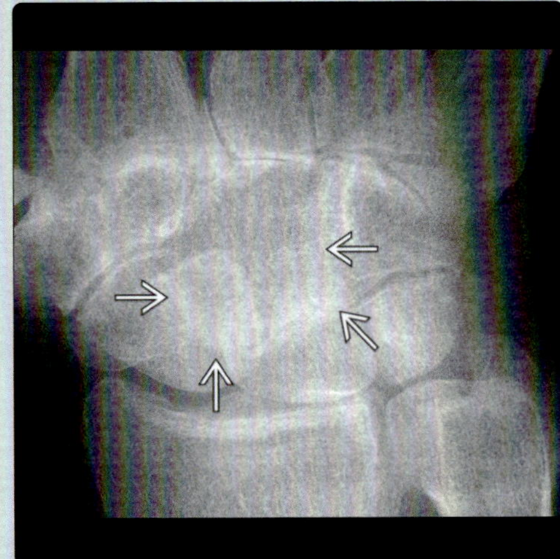

(Left) *PA radiograph of the fingers in a patient with constitutional symptoms suggests adult Still disease. There is joint space narrowing and erosive change of a distal interphalangeal (IP) joint* ➡*. The other IP joints showed narrowing but no erosions. The MCP joints were normal.* **(Right)** *PA radiograph of the carpus in the same patient is shown. While there is diffuse joint space narrowing, it is most prominent in the pericapitate distribution* ➡*. No erosions are seen, but there may be ankylosis. This is classic adult Still disease.*

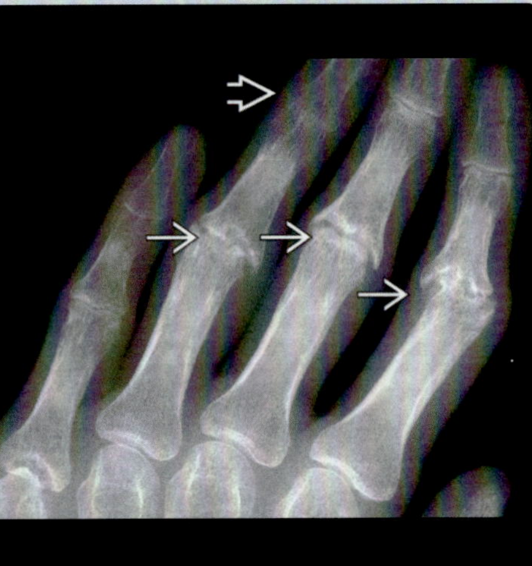

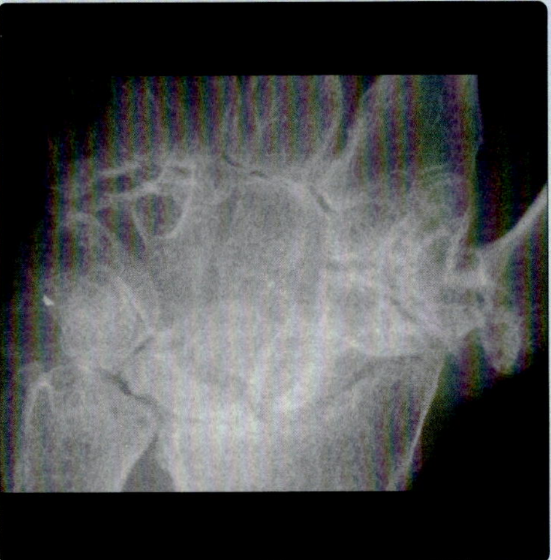

(Left) *PA radiograph of the hand in a patient with rash and daily fevers is shown. There are significant IP joint erosions* ➡ *and ankylosis of a single distal interphalangeal joint* ➡*. The appearance may suggest psoriatic arthritis, but the constitutional symptoms help make the diagnosis of adult Still disease.* **(Right)** *PA radiograph of the carpus in the same patient is shown. There is diffuse cartilage loss and erosive change. This is a nonspecific appearance and does not serve to differentiate psoriatic from adult Still disease.*

TERMINOLOGY

Synonyms

- Wissler-Fanconi syndrome, subsepsis hyperallergica

Definitions

- Systemic inflammatory disease, featuring triad
  - Quotidian fevers (spiking, daily)
  - Evanescent rash
  - Chronic polyarthritis
- Considered adult continuum of juvenile idiopathic arthritis (JIA)

IMAGING

General Features

- Best diagnostic clue
  - Diagnosis of exclusion
  - 25% develop destructive polyarthritis, behaving like rheumatoid arthritis (RA)
- Location
  - Hand
    - Interphalangeal (IP) joints more commonly affected than metacarpophalangeal (MCP) joints
      - Proximal interphalangeal (PIP) joint (50%)
      - Distal interphalangeal (DIP) joint (20%)
      - MCP joint (33%)
  - Wrist
    - Involved in 74% of cases
    - Pericapitate (midcarpal and carpometacarpal) disease is classic, but any pattern of carpal involvement may be seen
  - Foot: Midtarsal and tarsal-metatarsal joints
  - Knee: 84% involvement, at least with arthralgias

Radiographic Findings

- Uniform cartilage loss
- Erosions similar to RA
- Carpus may be remarkable for joint space narrowing, without significant erosive change
- Ankylosis, especially at carpus
- Distribution of involved joints differentiates from RA
- No periostitis; may differentiate from psoriatic

DIFFERENTIAL DIAGNOSIS

Psoriatic Arthritis

- IP > MCP joint involvement is similar
- Ankylosis is similar
- Rash and constitutional symptoms differentiate adult Still disease from psoriatic arthritis

Chronic Reactive Arthritis

- Constitutional symptoms may be suggestive
- Location of arthritic changes is likely different in adult Still, with hand/wrist predominating
  - Foot/ankle may be involved, similar to chronic reactive arthritis

Inflammatory Bowel Disease

- Constitutional symptoms may be suggestive
- Distribution of destructive arthralgias usually different; axial and proximal joints predominate in inflammatory bowel disease

PATHOLOGY

General Features

- Etiology
  - Unknown; adult continuum of JIA
    - Same manifestations and clinical course
  - Prodromal sore throat common (70%)
  - Associated with variety of viral infections

CLINICAL ISSUES

Presentation

- Most common signs/symptoms
  - Triad of daily spiking fever, evanescent rash, and chronic polyarthritis (usually hands, feet)
- Other signs/symptoms
  - Myalgia
  - Weight loss
  - Lymphadenopathy
  - Hepatosplenomegaly
  - Pleuritis, pericarditis
  - May have abrupt onset myocardial injury
- No specific diagnostic test
  - Seronegative for rheumatoid factor and ANA

Demographics

- Age
  - 75% have onset between 16 and 35 years
    - 10% onset after 50 years of age
- Gender
  - M = F
- Ethnicity
  - No predilection for race or ethnic origin
- Epidemiology
  - Rare (0.16/100,000)

Natural History & Prognosis

- If chronic, 50% develop carpal ankylosis
- Intermittent flares throughout life
- Systemic manifestations do not ↑ mortality

Treatment

- Arthritis managed with same drug therapy as RA
- Steroids for severe systemic manifestations

DIAGNOSTIC CHECKLIST

Image Interpretation Pearls

- Pericapitate predominance in carpal disease and IP predominance in hand disease, with ankylosis, is highly suggestive
  - Primary differential with these findings is psoriatic arthritis; constitutional symptoms differentiates

SELECTED REFERENCES

1. Dong MJ et al: 18F-FDG PET/CT in patients with adult-onset Still's disease. Clin Rheumatol. 34(12):2047-56, 2015
2. Kadavath S et al: Adult-onset Still's disease-pathogenesis, clinical manifestations, and new treatment options. Ann Med. 47(1):6-14, 2015

KEY FACTS

TERMINOLOGY

- Noninflammatory arthropathy, progressive cartilage loss leading to hypertrophic change in bone

IMAGING

- Diagnosis of osseous productive change made on radiographs
  - Anterior and lateral vertebral body osteophyte formation (spondylosis deformans)
  - Facet joint narrowing and hypertrophy
  - Uncovertebral (apophyseal) joint osteophytes
    - Restricted to cervical spine
  - Baastrup disease
    - Shaggy bony production at spinous processes
    - Apposing surfaces hypertrophied and flattened
    - Most prevalent in lumbar spine
- Severity of canal/foraminal stenosis evaluated on MR
  - Oblique sagittal MR images useful to evaluate foraminal stenosis
- SI joints: Generally 2 appearances
  - Sclerosis along cortex of synovial portion
  - Marginal osteophytes

TOP DIFFERENTIAL DIAGNOSES

- Diffuse idiopathic skeletal hyperostosis
- Ankylosing spondylitis
- Retinoid-associated spondylosis
- Spondyloarthropathy of psoriatic of chronic reactive arthritis

PATHOLOGY

- Mechanical
- Inflammatory arthritis (usually inactive rheumatoid arthritis in cervical spine)
- Metabolic
- Biochemical changes in cartilage

CLINICAL ISSUES

- 12% prevalence in USA (20 million people)

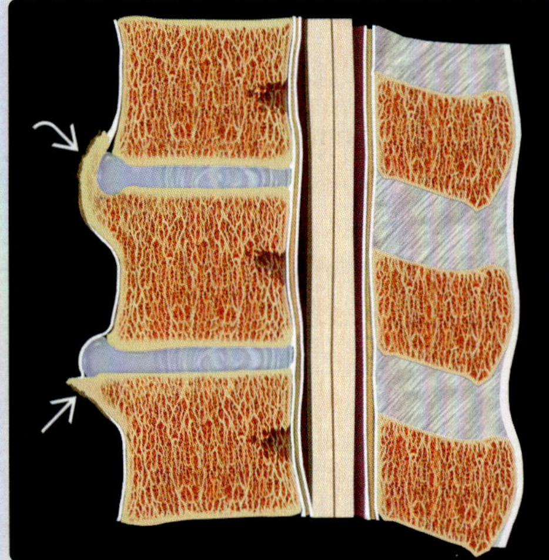

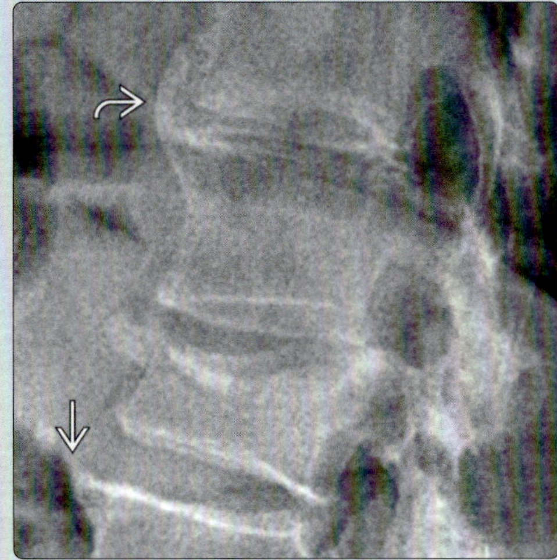

(Left) *Graphic shows the initial horizontal osteophyte ➡, which forms upon stretching of Sharpey fibers by a bulging annulus fibrosus. Thus, spondylosis deformans or vertebral body osteophytes are related to degenerative disc disease. With continued growth, the osteophyte is directed more vertically and may eventually bridge the disc space ➡.* **(Right)** *Lateral radiograph demonstrates the horizontal osteophyte ➡ arising from the cortex of the body as well as a larger bridging osteophyte ➡.*

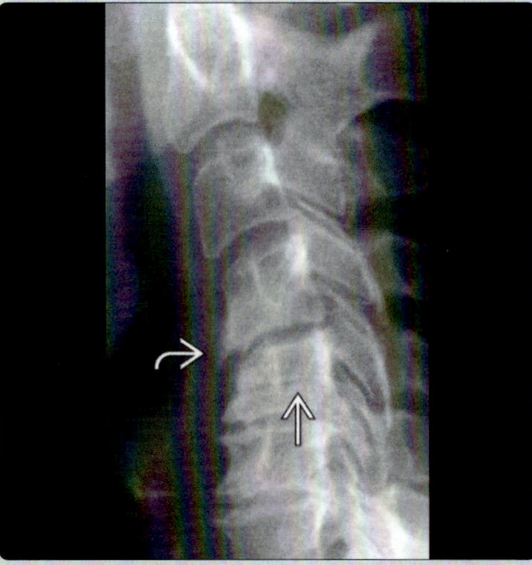

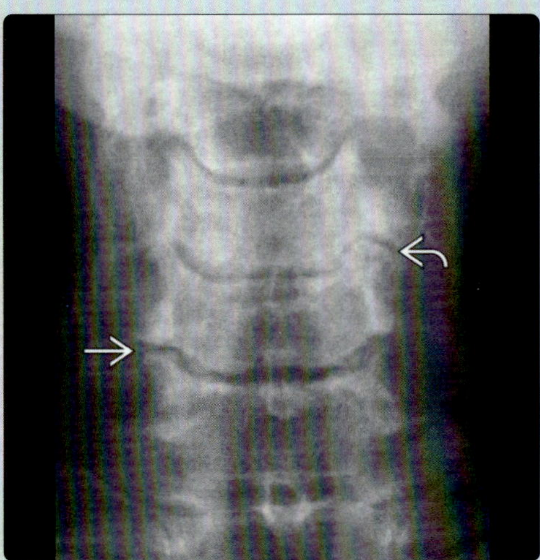

(Left) *Lateral radiograph shows typical osteoarthritis (OA) of the cervical spine, with anterior spondylosis ➡ at a level of disc degeneration. The osteophytes formed at apophyseal joints often appear as a lucency crossing the vertebral body ➡. This lucency extends surprisingly far anteriorly.* **(Right)** *AP radiograph in the same patient shows OA of the apophyseal joints, most prominent on the right at C5-6 ➡ and the left at C4-5 ➡. These, along with C6-7, are the most frequent levels involved.*

TERMINOLOGY

Abbreviations

- Osteoarthritis (OA)

Synonyms

- Degenerative joint disease
- Facet arthropathy
- Uncovertebral OA
- Osteophytosis, spondylosis deformans

Definitions

- Noninflammatory arthropathy, with progressive cartilage loss and resultant hypertrophic change in bone
- For ease of discussion, nonarthritic axial osseous hypertrophic change is included in this section
  - Spondylosis deformans: Osteophyte production at anterior and lateral vertebral body, adjacent to endplate, arising from osseous cortex
  - Baastrup disease: Bony proliferation between spinous processes

IMAGING

General Features

- Best diagnostic clue
  - Bone production at vertebral bodies, facet joints, uncovertebral joints
  - Generally has associated degenerative disc disease
- Location
  - Spondylosis deformans: Osteophytes at vertebral body anteriorly and laterally
  - Facet joints
  - Uncovertebral (apophyseal) joints (posterolateral vertebral bodies, cervical spine)
  - Baastrup disease: Most commonly lumbar spine
- Size
  - Ranges from subtle to large osseous formation
- Morphology
  - Normal bone formation; if large enough, hypertrophic bone contains marrow

Imaging Recommendations

- Best imaging tool
  - Diagnosis made on radiographs
  - Severity of canal or foraminal stenosis evaluated on MR
- Protocol advice
  - Oblique sagittal images useful on MR to evaluate foraminal stenosis

Radiographic Findings

- Normal bone density
- Eburnation of vertebral body endplates
- Spondylosis deformans (spinal osteophytosis)
  - Bony projection arising from cortex of vertebral body endplate, adjacent to disc
  - Not associated with synovial joint
  - Usually associated with disc space narrowing
- Uncovertebral (apophyseal) OA
  - Posterolateral vertebral body joints located only in cervical spine
  - Osseous projection seen in 3 views
    - Posterior bony projection on lateral view, with transverse lucency projected over posterior 1/2 of vertebral body
    - AP: Superior bony projection at lateral edge of vertebral body
    - Oblique: Osseous projection from body into neural foramen
- Facet OA
  - Increased density of facets on AP and lateral views
  - Osseous projection into neural foramen on cervical oblique view
- Hypertrophic bone formation around odontoid and anterior arch of atlas
- Ossification of posterior longitudinal ligament
- Baastrup disease
  - Shaggy bony production around spinous processes
  - Processes become hypertrophied and flattened
  - May result in neoarthrosis and formation of adventitious bursa
- SI joints: Generally 2 appearances
  - Sclerosis along cortex of synovial portion of joints
    - No erosion or ankylosis
  - Marginal osteophytes
    - Either at bottom of SI joint or at junction of synovial and nonsynovial portion (1/2 to 1/3 of distance from top of SI joint)
    - Appears as round density; occasionally mistaken for bone island or metastatic disease

CT Findings

- Hypertrophy of bone at all sites described above easily seen
- Additional findings of
  - Disc herniation
  - Spinal stenosis
  - Foraminal stenosis
  - Ligamentum flavum hypertrophy
- Baastrup disease
  - Shaggy bone formation surrounding spinous processes, with eburnation of bone
  - Osseous cystic formation in spinous processes
- SI joint marginal osteophytes: Anterior bridging easily seen

MR Findings

- Osseous hypertrophy
  - If small, osteophytes appear as low signal on T1WI as well as fluid-sensitive sequences
  - If large, osteophytes contain marrow, which follows normal marrow signal intensity on MR
- Disc herniation, annular tears
- Ligamentum flavum hypertrophy (low signal on all sequences) contributes to stenosis
- Synovial cysts arising from facets may cause impingement/stenosis
- Assess degree of spinal and foraminal narrowing
- Baastrup disease
  - Low signal hypertrophied bone surrounding spinous process
  - High signal cysts on fluid-sensitive sequences
  - Hypertrophied interspinous ligament (low signal all sequences) may contribute to spinal stenosis

DIFFERENTIAL DIAGNOSIS

Ankylosing Spondylitis

- Character of syndesmophytes is different than that of osteophytes
- Osteoporosis in ankylosing spondylitis; normal density on OA
- Sacroiliitis, erosions, &/or ankylosis

Diffuse Idiopathic Skeletal Hyperostosis

- Ossification of anterior longitudinal ligament generally differs in appearance from osteophytes
- Occasionally bone formation in diffuse idiopathic skeletal hyperostosis (DISH) will be indistinguishable from spondylosis deformans
- Disc degeneration generally absent in DISH
- Facet arthrosis generally absent in DISH

Retinoid-Associated Spondylosis

- Spondylosis indistinguishable from that in degenerative spine disease
- Younger patient; no disc or facet disease

Spondyloarthropathy of Psoriatic or Chronic Reactive Arthritis

- Bulky paravertebral ossification tends to arise slightly distant from endplate/disc junction
- Paravertebral ossification extends farther from vertebral body than most osteophytes
- Ossification better seen on AP than lateral view
- Sacroiliitis

PATHOLOGY

General Features

- Etiology
  - Mechanical
    - Trauma
    - Stress/repetitive microtrauma
    - Obesity
    - Abnormal morphology or connective disease
      - Dysplasia
      - Marfan disease
      - Ehlers-Danlos disease
  - Inflammatory arthritis
    - Usually inactive rheumatoid arthritis (especially cervical spine)
    - Ligamentous abnormality from prior injury → abnormal stress on abnormal bone
  - Metabolic
    - Wilson disease
    - Ochronosis
    - Hemochromatosis
  - Biochemical changes in aging cartilage
    - ↓ water content, ↓ proteoglycans and collagen, ↓ number of chondrocytes → softened cartilage and ↑ risk of damage from any source of trauma
- Genetics
  - Multigenic trait, based on twin and familial studies
  - Genetic predisposition for females with OA of distal interphalangeal joints (may be as high as 65%)
- Associated abnormalities
  - Diagnostic laboratory tests normal
  - Synovial fluid normal

Gross Pathologic & Surgical Features

- Relevant anatomy
  - Sharpey fibers attach outer fibers of annulus fibrosus to vertebral body cortex
  - With protrusion of annulus fibrosis, Sharpey fiber attachment on vertebral body is elevated
  - Osteophytes form at Sharpey fiber attachment
    - Extend horizontally
    - With growth, start to extend vertically
    - May eventually bridge disc space
- Gross pathology
  - Fissuring, pitting, ulceration of cartilage
  - Adjacent reactive bone (osteophyte, subchondral sclerosis)
  - Synovium normal or mildly inflamed

CLINICAL ISSUES

Presentation

- Most common signs/symptoms
  - Pain related to use (no pain at rest)
  - Self-limited morning stiffness
  - Crepitus
  - Decreased range of motion
  - Subchondral cysts in odontoid may predispose to fracture from low velocity fall
  - Baastrup disease universally associated with other degenerative spine disease
    - Caution should be used in diagnosing it as cause of back pain
- Other signs/symptoms
  - No swelling/warmth
  - No constitutional symptoms

Demographics

- Age
  - Usually > 65 years old
    - Seen in 80% of people > 75 years old
- Gender
  - M < F
- Epidemiology
  - 12% prevalence in USA (20 million people)

Natural History & Prognosis

- May progress to spinal canal and foraminal stenosis

Treatment

- Analgesics for pain relief and maintenance of function
- Physical therapy, weight loss
- Intraarticular corticosteroid injection
- Surgical decompression of canal or foraminal stenosis
- Fusion for instability

SELECTED REFERENCES

1. Raastad J et al: The association between lumbar spine radiographic features and low back pain: a systematic review and meta-analysis. Semin Arthritis Rheum. 44(5):571-85, 2015
2. Maataoui A et al: Association between facet joint osteoarthritis and the Oswestry Disability Index. World J Radiol. 6(11):881-5, 2014

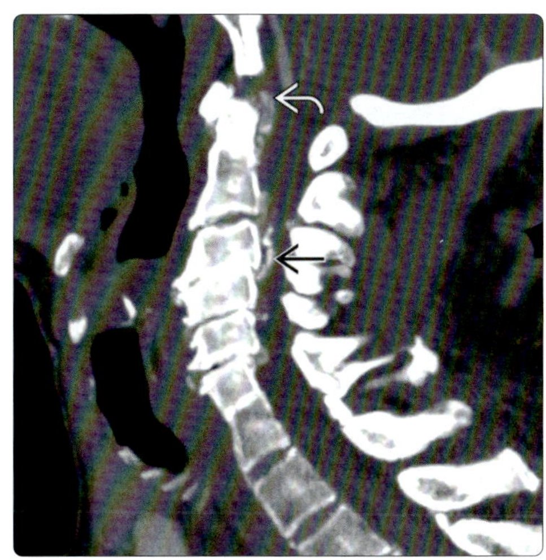

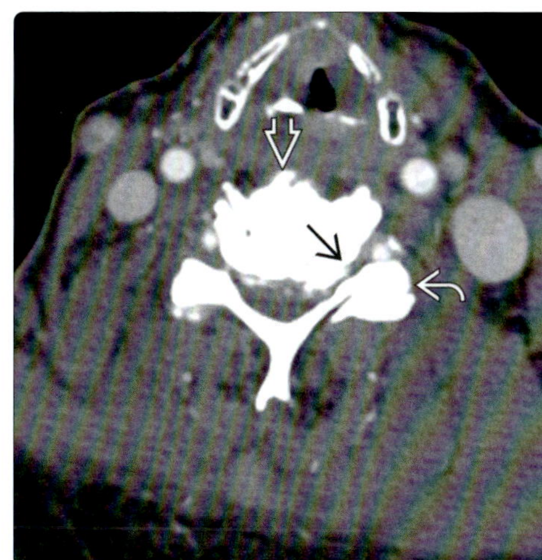

(Left) *Sagittal CECT shows multilevel cervical spondylosis with severe central canal stenosis. Multilevel disc disease is seen with bony sclerosis at the endplates. Bony hypertrophy around C1-2* ➡ *is common. Ossification of posterior longitudinal ligament* ➡ *contributes to stenosis.* **(Right)** *Axial CECT in the same patient shows severe bilateral foraminal stenosis with uncovertebral joint hypertrophy* ➡*. Spondylosis deformans* ➡ *and facet hypertrophy* ➡ *are seen as well.*

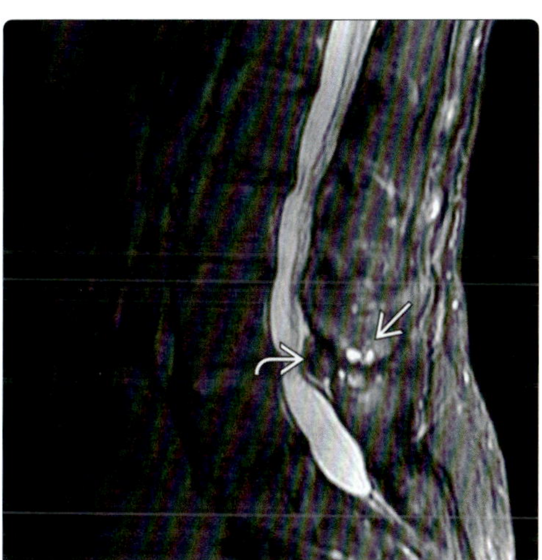

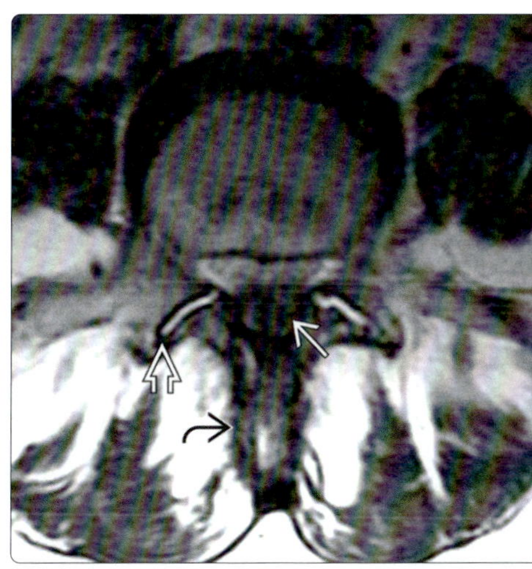

(Left) *Sagittal STIR MR shows typical interspinous process degeneration (Baastrup disease). There is cystic degeneration of the L4-5 ligament with areas of rounded T2 hyperintensity* ➡ *amid low signal hypertrophied ligament* ➡*.* **(Right)** *Axial T2WI MR in the same patient shows degenerative changes of the adjacent cortical margins of the posterior spinous processes* ➡*. The redundant ligamentum flavum* ➡ *and facet hypertrophy* ➡ *contribute to canal stenosis.*

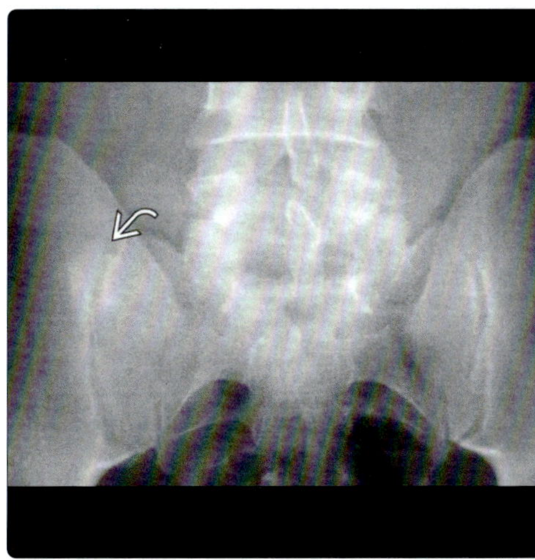

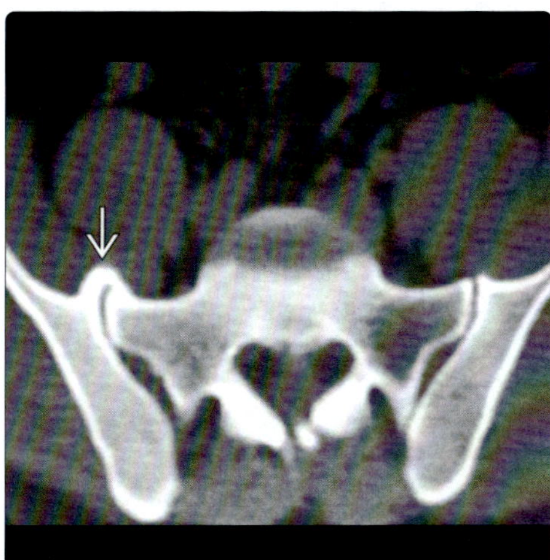

(Left) *AP radiograph shows a sclerotic "lesion" at the level of the upper right SI joint* ➡*. It is important to remember that OA of the SI joints may either present as diffuse sclerosis of the cortex, or as a rounded sclerosis, either at the superior or inferior edge of the synovial portion of the joint.* **(Right)** *Axial bone CT in the same patient proves the sclerotic focus represents a typical marginal osteophyte bridging the SI joint* ➡*.*

DISH

KEY FACTS

TERMINOLOGY

- **D**iffuse **i**diopathic **s**keletal **h**yperostosis (DISH)
- Bone-forming diathesis primarily affecting spine, with ossification of tendons and ligaments

IMAGING

- Radiographs make diagnosis
- Spine
  - Flowing anterior ossification
  - No significant facet arthropathy or ankylosis, minimal degenerative disc disease
  - Normal bone density
  - If bulky enough, marrow is seen within ossification
  - Adjacent ligament ossification around cervical spine may result in pain &/or dysphagia
  - May have associated ossification of posterior longitudinal ligament
- Sacroiliac (SI) joints
  - Involves superior, nonsynovial portions
  - Synovial portions of SI joints remain normal
  - Often see nearby ligament ossification
- Extensive fluffy enthesopathy at tendon, ligament, or joint capsule insertions
- CT for evaluation of complications
  - Transverse fractures following minor trauma
  - Seen with long column fusion and osteoporosis (relatively rare in DISH compared with AS)
- MR: Evaluate cord following transverse fracture
  - Displacement of critical structures in neck

CLINICAL ISSUES

- Usually incidental finding
  - Appearance generally worse than clinical findings
- DISH becoming much more prevalent
  - Associated with aging population, obesity, and type 2 diabetes
- Rare carrot stick fracture of vertebral column may result in severe cord damage

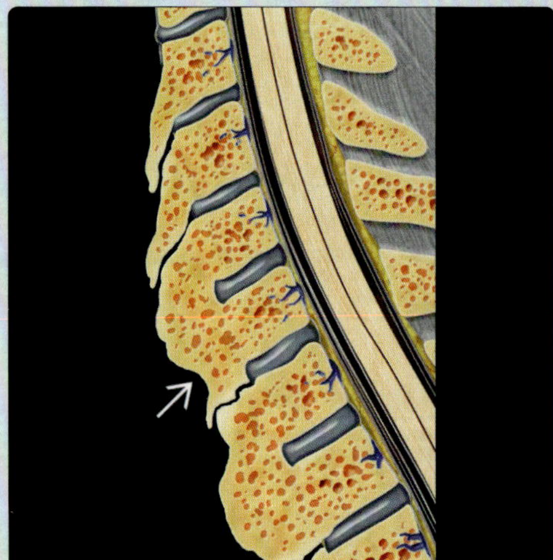

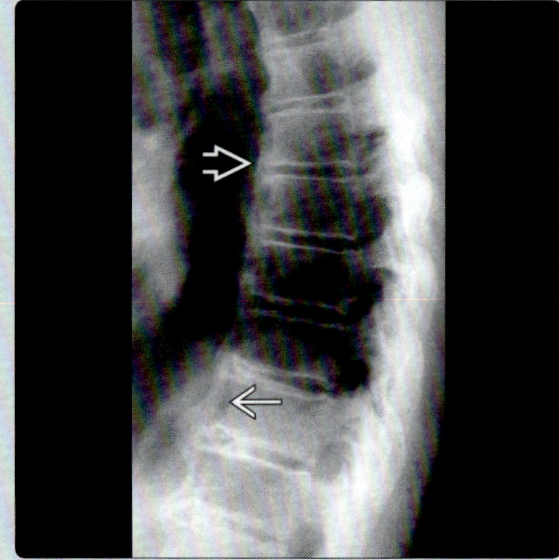

(Left) *Sagittal graphic depicts diffuse idiopathic skeletal hyperostosis (DISH) of the cervical spine. The essential parameters contributing to the diagnosis include anterior flowing ossification ➡ often bridging vertebral bodies along with normal discs and normal facet joints.* **(Right)** *Lateral radiograph of the thoracic spine shows classic flowing ossification. Though the majority of the vertebral bodies have the ossification applied anteriorly along the full extent of the body ➡, at least 1 shows lucency at the concavity ➡.*

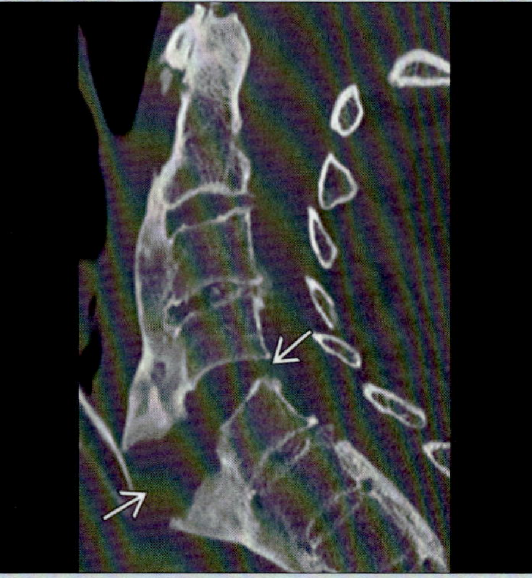

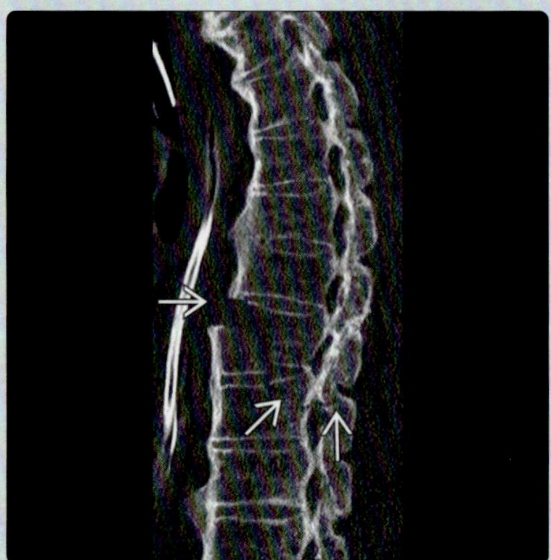

(Left) *Sagittal CT shows flowing anterior ossification typical of DISH. This 81 YO fell out of bed; the combination of long column fusion and osteoporosis made him vulnerable for the fracture ➡. 40% of these patients admitted with fracture will have neurologic deficits; there is a 20% mortality rate within 3 months.* **(Right)** *Sagittal CT in a 75 YO shows a transverse fracture ➡ through a T spine with long column fusion and osteoporosis related to DISH. This patient was an obese type-2 diabetic, at particular risk for DISH.*

TERMINOLOGY

Abbreviations

- **D**iffuse **i**diopathic **s**keletal **h**yperostosis (DISH)

Synonyms

- Forestier disease, ankylosing hyperostosis

Definitions

- Bone-forming diathesis primarily affecting spine, with ossification of tendons and ligaments

IMAGING

General Features

- Best diagnostic clue
  - Anterior flowing ossification involving anterior longitudinal ligament (ALL), adherent to anterior and right-lateral vertebral bodies
    - No significant facet arthropathy or ankylosis, minimal degenerative disc disease
- Location
  - Thoracic spine: 100%
    - R > L (attributed to effect of repetitive aortic pulsations inhibiting bone proliferation on left)
  - Lumbar spine: > 90%
  - Cervical spine: 75%
  - Sacroiliac joints: Nonsynovial portions involved
- Size
  - Small (early stages) to bulky, large ossification
- Morphology
  - Ossification rather than calcification

Imaging Recommendations

- Best imaging tool
  - Radiographs for diagnosis
  - CT for complications
    - Transverse fractures following minor trauma
      - Cervicothoracic or thoracolumbar junction
      - Seen with long column fusion and osteoporosis [relatively rare in DISH compared with ankylosing spondylitis (AS)]
  - MR for complications
    - Evaluate cord following transverse fracture
    - Displacement of critical structures in neck

Radiographic Findings

- Spine
  - Flowing anterior ossification
    - Earliest formation is adjacent to anterior midvertebral body
    - May also have early bone formation with appearance of spondylosis
    - If bulky, ossification contains marrow
    - May have hyperostosis of odontoid and anterior arch of atlas
  - Bone density usually normal
    - Will become osteoporotic if extensive long column fusion
  - Adjacent ligament ossification around cervical spine may result in pain &/or dysphagia
    - Stylohyoid ligament ossification
  - Often have associated ossification of posterior longitudinal ligament (OPLL)
- Sacroiliac (SI) joints
  - Involves superior, nonsynovial portions
    - Bony production and bridging may occur
  - Synovial portions of SI joints remain normal
  - Often see nearby ligament ossification
    - Iliolumbar
    - Sacrospinous
    - Sacrotuberous
- Entheses
  - Extensive fluffy enthesopathy at tendon, ligament, and joint capsule insertions
    - Iliac crest: 66%
    - Ischial tuberosities: 53%
    - Femoral trochanters: 40%
    - Nonarticular portion of patella: 29%

CT Findings

- Confirms location of ossification and presence of marrow
- Confirms nonsynovial SI joint involvement
- Often required to show subtle transverse fractures following minor trauma

MR Findings

- T1WI of ossification
  - Low signal in early ossification
  - Develops high marrow signal with progressively bulkier ossification
- Fluid-sensitive sequences
  - ALL ossification may be hypointense unless so large that fatty marrow is prominent
  - High signal spinal cord injury after trauma
- Minimal enhancement in absence of fracture

DIFFERENTIAL DIAGNOSIS

Degenerative Spine Disease

- Spondylosis, if advanced, may appear identical to ossification of DISH
- Also shows degenerative change in facet and apophyseal joints
- Degenerative disc disease helps differentiate

Ankylosing Spondylitis

- Osteoporosis in AS is prominent differentiating feature
- AS syndesmophytes: Thin, vertical, forming in annulus
- Severe late AS may extend to ossify ALL
- Long column fusion may have similar appearance
- Sacroiliac joint involvement is synovial portion

Retinoid-Related Degenerative Change

- Long use of retinoids results in prominent osteophyte formation, which may bridge disc space
- Not true ALL ossification
- Generally in younger population than seen with DISH

Fluorosis

- Bony proliferation in spine
- Enthesitis
- Osteoporotic, with fragile bones

PATHOLOGY

General Features

- Etiology
  - Unknown
- Associated abnormalities
  - 50% have associated ossification of posterior longitudinal ligament (OPLL)
    - Conversely, 44% of patients with OPLL have concomitant anterior vertebral hyperostosis
    - If disease with both features is more prominent in thoracic spine, it is called DISH
    - If disease with both features is more prominent in cervical spine, it is called OPLL
  - Minor trauma may cause transverse (carrot stick) fracture, analogous to that seen with AS
    - Much less common complication than in AS
    - Seen in cases with long column fusion and some degree of osteoporosis

Gross Pathologic & Surgical Features

- Anatomy: ALL attaches to anterior surface of body
  - ALL less adherent to intervertebral disc than bodies; may relate to different appearance of ossification in DISH
- 3 distinct types of pathologic development of DISH are recognized
  - Type 1: Purely limited to ALL
  - Type 2: Identical to spondylosis deformans
  - Type 3: New bone formation seen in midanterior portion of vertebral body
- It is not important to distinguish these pathologic types

Microscopic Features

- Normal-appearing bone and marrow within ossifications

Diagnostic Criteria, Radiographic Only

- Strict criteria
  - Flowing ossification along anterolateral aspect of at least 4 contiguous bodies
    - Arbitrary, but differentiates DISH from spondylosis deformans
  - Relative preservation of intervertebral disc height, without vacuum sign or vertebral body sclerosis
    - Differentiates DISH from degenerative spine with spondylosis deformans
  - No apophyseal bony ankylosis
    - Differentiates from spondyloarthropathies
  - No sacroiliac joint erosion or fusion
    - Meant to differentiate from AS and other spondyloarthropathies
    - Remember: DISH may have sacroiliac joint abnormalities, which are distinct from those of AS
- These strict criteria likely underestimate DISH population by ignoring patients with both DISH and degenerative spine disease

CLINICAL ISSUES

Presentation

- Most common signs/symptoms
  - Spine stiffness and decreased mobility
    - Spine pain generally not as prominent as extent of ossification may suggest
  - Dysphagia in up to 25% due to prominent anterior cervical bone production
    - Combination of direct mechanical compression and inflammation/fibrosis of esophageal wall

Demographics

- Age
  - Generally > 50 years old
- Gender
  - M:F = 2:1
- Epidemiology
  - 12% of individuals over age 65
    - Another study based on chest radiograph: 25% males and 15% females over age 50
  - Increasing prevalence of DISH in USA due to its association with aging population, obesity, and type-2 diabetes
  - Prevalence likely underestimated if strict criteria of DISH are used to eliminate those individuals with concomitant degenerative spine disease
  - Prevalence decreased in African Americans, Native Americans, and Asians relative to Caucasians

Natural History & Prognosis

- Usually incidental finding; no significant morbidity
- Appearance by imaging generally is worse than clinical findings
- Rare carrot stick fracture of vertebral column may result in severe cord injury
  - 40% have neurologic deficits if admitted with fracture
  - 20% mortality within 3 months if admitted with fracture

Treatment

- Analgesics, NSAIDS for pain and stiffness
- Osteophyte resection if severe symptoms due to mass effect (particularly in neck; rare)

DIAGNOSTIC CHECKLIST

Consider

- In uncommon DISH patient with long column fusion and osteoporosis, watch for carrot stick fracture following minor trauma
  - CT often required to make this diagnosis since fracture may be nondisplaced

Image Interpretation Pearls

- Watch for concomitant OPLL and possible myelopathy
- Watch for rare anterior cervical ossification, which may impinge on critical structures

SELECTED REFERENCES

1. Carmona R et al: MR imaging of the spine and sacroiliac joints for spondyloarthritis: influence on clinical diagnostic confidence and patient management. Radiology. 269(1):208-15, 2013
2. Campagna R et al: Fractures of the ankylosed spine: MDCT and MRI with emphasis on individual anatomic spinal structures. AJR Am J Roentgenol. 192(4):987-95, 2009
3. Westerveld LA et al: Spinal fractures in patients with ankylosing spinal disorders: a systematic review of the literature on treatment, neurological status and complications. Eur Spine J. 18(2):145-56, 2009

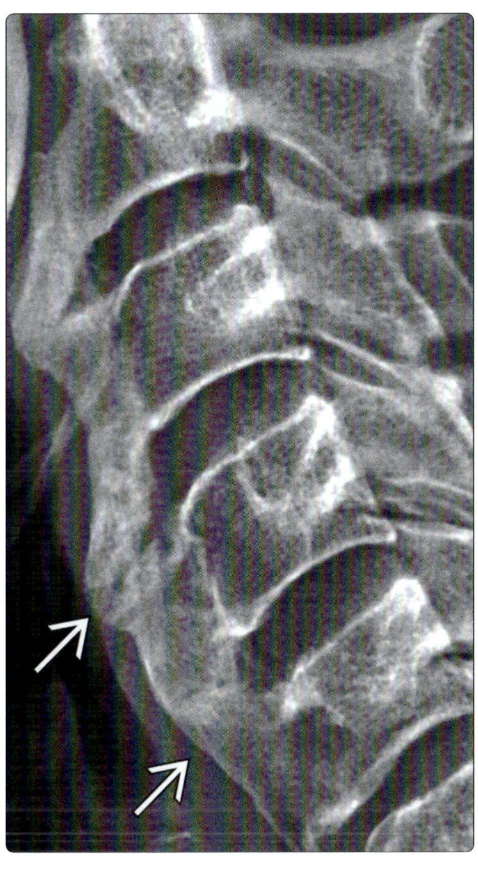

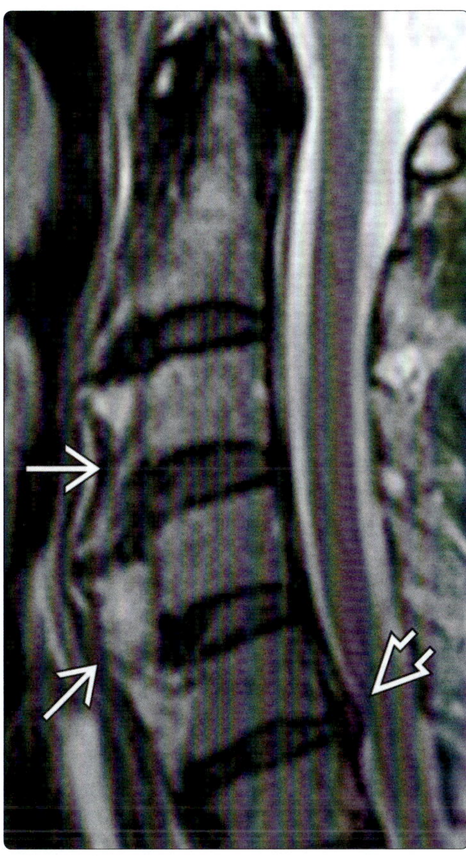

(Left) *Sagittal radiograph shows a typical anterior-flowing bone formation ➔ diagnostic of DISH. Note that the disc spaces are relatively normally maintained, though there is mild narrowing at C5-C6. The facets do not show significant arthritic change. This patient has significant neck pain.* **(Right)** *Sagittal T2WI FSE MR in the same patient confirms the marrow-containing anterior bone formation ➔. However, the MR adds significant information; there is a disc herniation at C5-C6 ⇨, the cause of the patient's pain. It is unusual for DISH to be the etiology of significant new pain, and other reasons should be sought. Disc disease and fracture with pseudarthrosis may be etiologies of radiculopathy or myelopathy; dysphagia results from the anterior bone formation.*

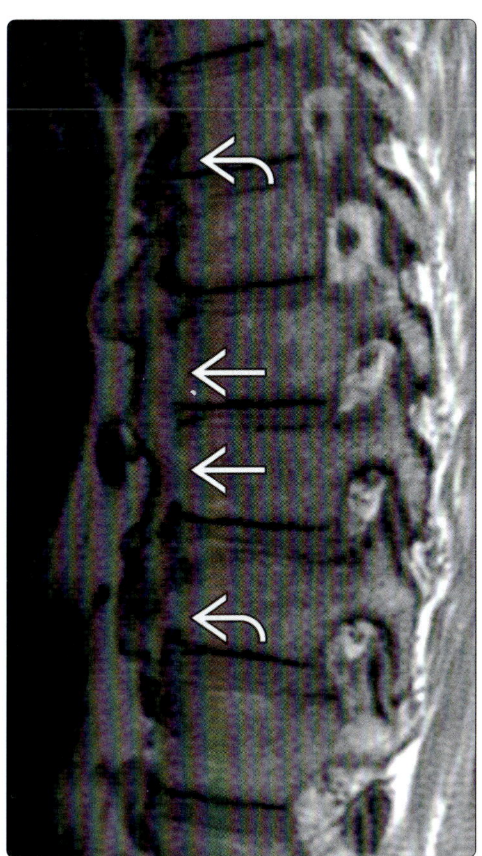

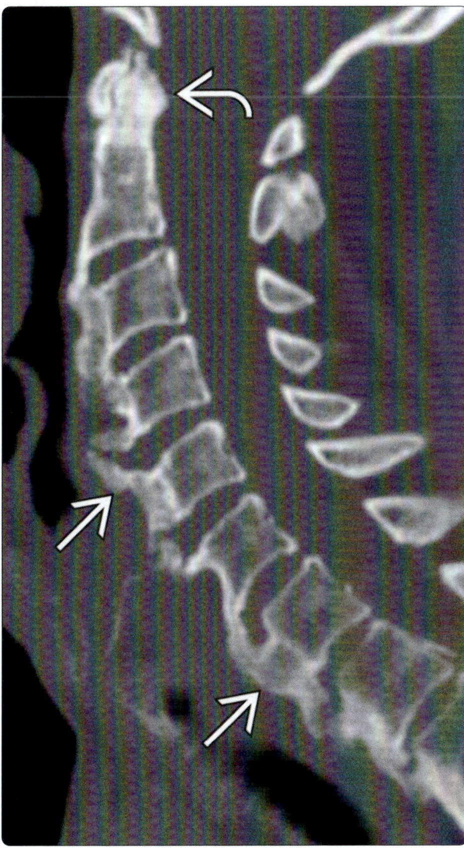

(Left) *Sagittal T1 MR shows a patient with DISH. The image is right parasagittal; the anterior-flowing bone formation is far more prominent here than on the left (not shown). The anterior bone production arises directly from the center of the vertebral body in some locations ➔ but from the inferior or superior vertebral body in others ↶. Either is typical of this disease. The discs remain normal as do the facet joints. DISH is not a true arthropathy, although in some cases there is overlap with degenerative spine disease.* **(Right)** *Sagittal CT shows the anterior-flowing bone formation of DISH ➔. Alignment is normal as is disc space. There is no suggestion of apophyseal joint osteoarthritis. Note the bone formation around the odontoid process ↶ as well as the anterior arch of the atlas; this is typical but not unique to DISH.*

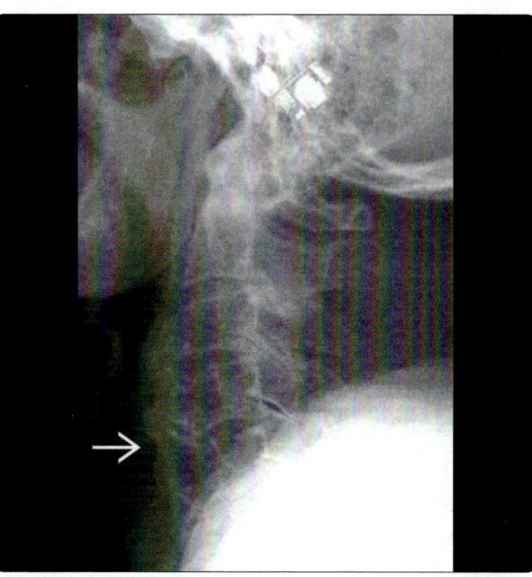

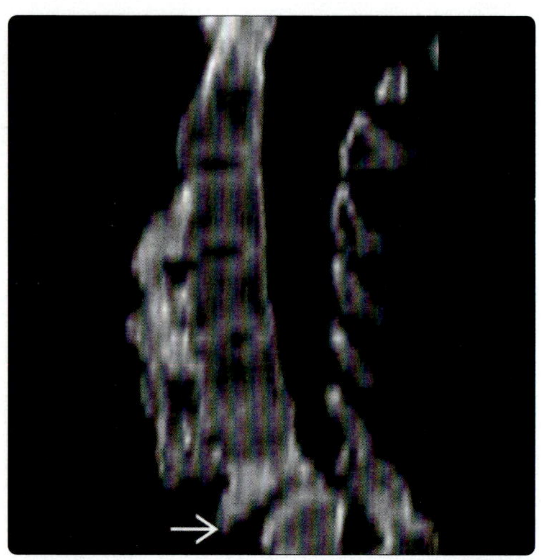

(Left) *Lateral radiograph obtained in the emergency department following a motor vehicle accident (MVA) shows bulky anterior flowing osteophyte formation ➡, typical of DISH. There is no prevertebral soft tissue swelling. However, given the degree of osteoporosis and effective cervical spine fusion, fracture must be considered.* **(Right)** *Sagittal bone CT confirms a carrot stick fracture at the C6-C7 level ➡. This was a devastating injury to this patient who sustained massive cord injury from this relatively minor trauma.*

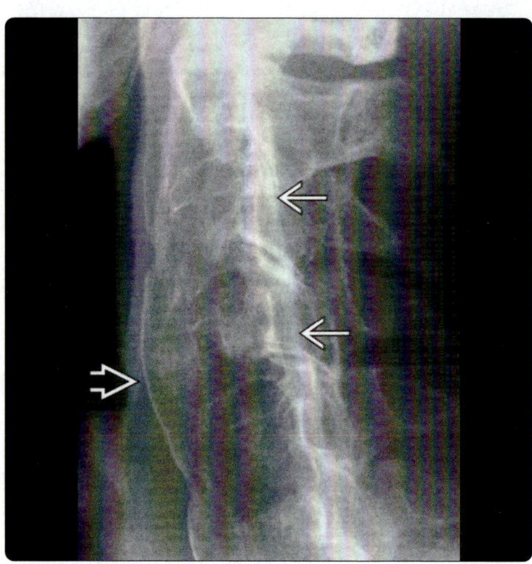

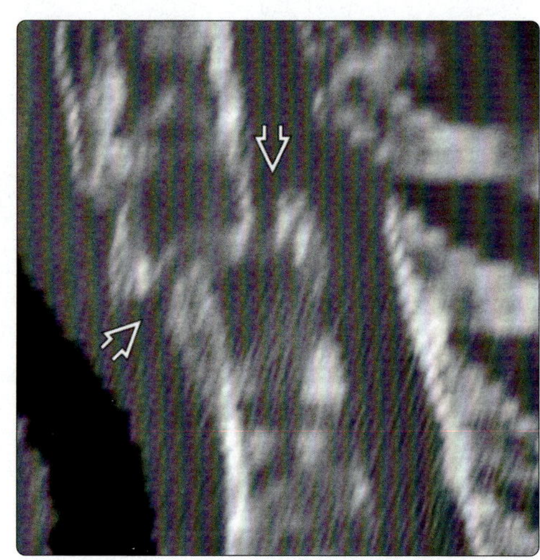

(Left) *Lateral radiograph obtained after a minor MVA shows ossification of the posterior longitudinal ligament ➡, a finding typically seen in OPLL but also seen in DISH. The anterior osteophytes have merged, leaving a solid column of osteoporotic bone ➡. This finding should raise the possibility of a hidden fracture near the cervicothoracic junction, as it does in patients with ankylosing spondylosis.* **(Right)** *CT is confirmatory ➡ with a displaced carrot stick type of fracture.*

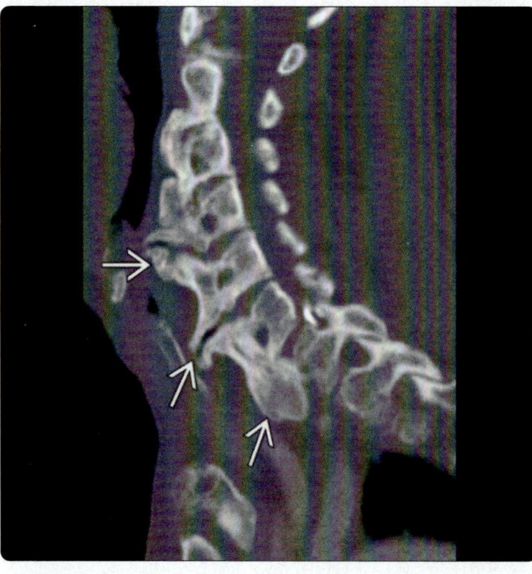

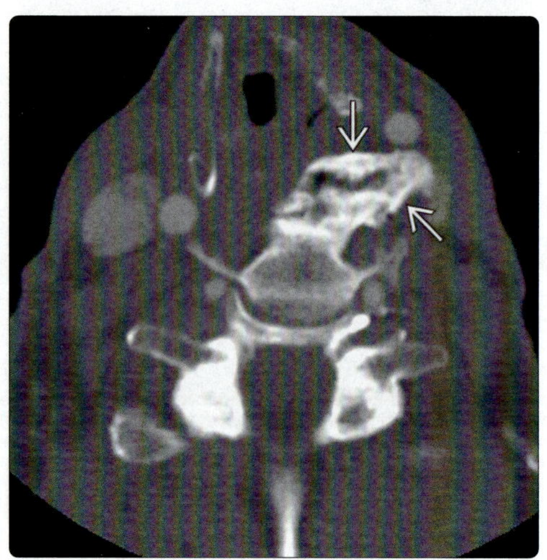

(Left) *Sagittal NECT shows exuberant anterior osteophyte formation ➡ throughout the cervical and upper thoracic spine, typical of DISH.* **(Right)** *Axial NECT in the same patient shows a huge osteophyte displacing the left carotid artery and effacing the left hypopharynx ➡. Large anterior or anterolateral osteophytes may cause significant dysphagia and occasionally involve other adjacent structures, as in this case.*

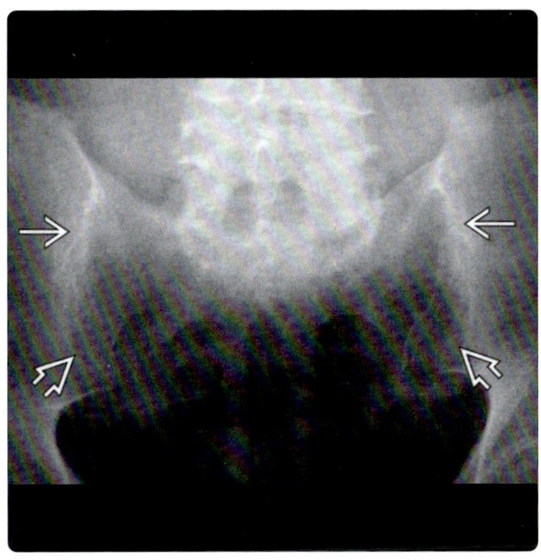

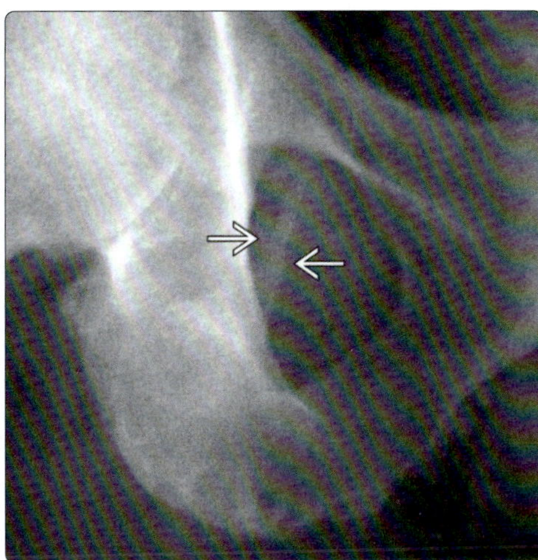

(Left) *Anteroposterior radiograph of the sacroiliac joints in DISH shows the superior nonsynovial portion of the joint to be fused ➡, while the anteroinferior synovial portion of the SI joint remains normal ➡.* **(Right)** *Anteroposterior radiograph of the lower pelvis in the same patient shows linear calcification superimposed on the obturator foramen. This represents sacrotuberous ligament ossification ➡. Both the pattern of SI joint involvement and the ligament ossification are typical of DISH.*

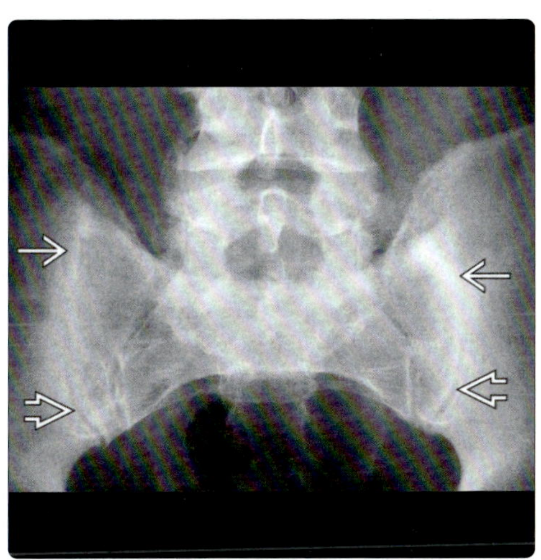

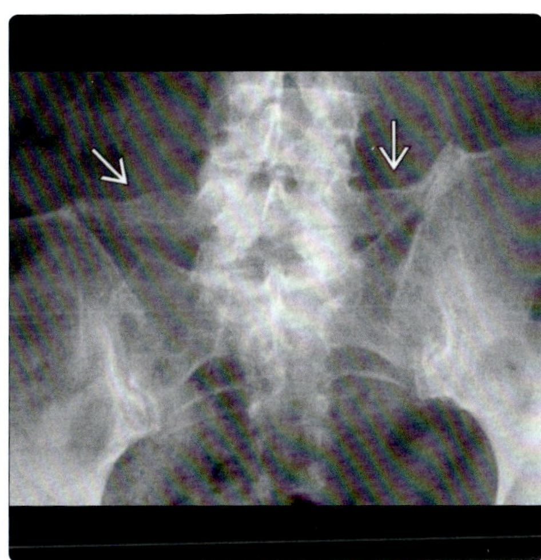

(Left) *Anteroposterior radiograph of the sacroiliac joints shows the typical and specific appearance of DISH. There typically is fusion across the superior nonsynovial portions ➡, while the inferior, synovial portions of the joints remain normal ➡. Note the normal bone density as well.* **(Right)** *AP radiograph in a patient with a classic spine appearance of DISH shows prominent iliolumbar ossification ➡. The upper portions of the SI joints show sclerosis but are not yet fused.*

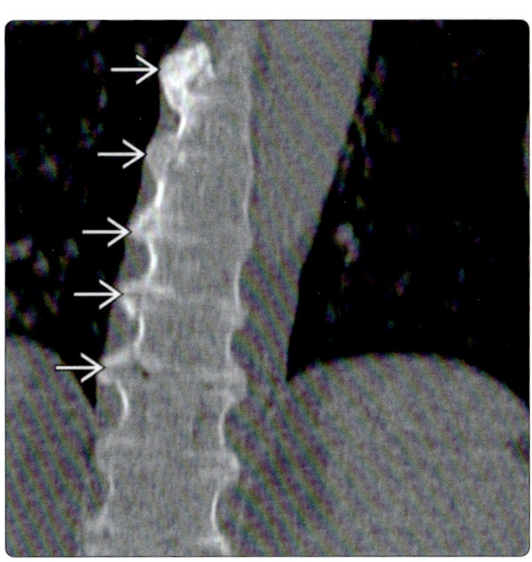

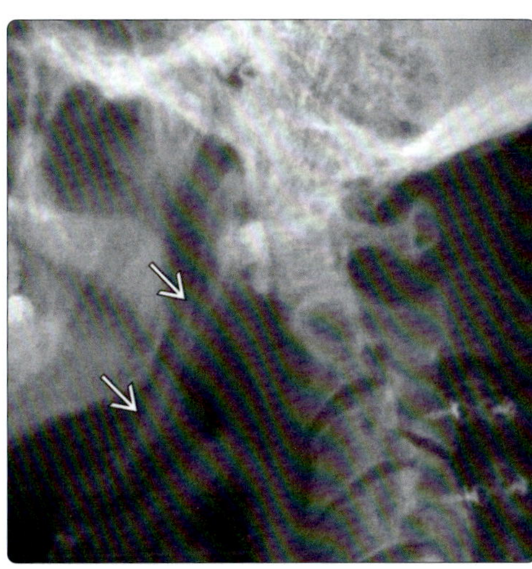

(Left) *Coronal bone CT shows a typical case of thoracic DISH. The preferential right-sided localization of the bone formation is noted ➡, with sparing of the spine along the left next to the aorta.* **(Right)** *Lateral radiograph in a patient with thoracic DISH shows dense ossification of the stylohyoid ligaments ➡. This may cause neck pain; the constellation has been termed Eagle syndrome. This patient had superimposed degenerative disease of the cervical spine and has had an open-door laminectomy.*

KEY FACTS

TERMINOLOGY

- Ossification posterior longitudinal ligament (OPLL)
- Definition: Replacement of posterior longitudinal ligamentous tissue by ectopic new bone

IMAGING

- Radiograph: Most frequent at 4th and 5th cervical levels
  - May involve thoracic or lumbar spine (20%)
  - May be seen at C1 level, posterior to dens
- CT to fully evaluate extent of ossification
- In patient with clinical signs of myelopathy, MR to evaluate spinal cord
  - Linear sclerosis of OPLL may be easily overlooked on MR
- 44% of patients with OPLL have concomitant anterior hyperostosis
- If significant concomitant diffuse idiopathic skeletal hyperostosis (DISH) and OPLL, may develop long column fusion

CLINICAL ISSUES

- If canal diameter < 6 mm, symptomatic myelopathy nearly universal
- If canal diameter > 14 mm, symptomatic myelopathy rare
- Spastic paresis progressing to paralysis: 17-22%
- If OPLL has prominent DISH and ankylosis, minor trauma may result in transverse fracture
- Mild cases asymptomatic; incidentally discovered

DIAGNOSTIC CHECKLIST

- Evaluate carefully for extension to level of C1
  - Extension to C1 often not expected or sought
  - If considering decompression surgery, must cover full extent of lesion
- In presence of anterior longitudinal ligament ossification, consider possibility of long column fusion
  - Puts patient at risk for transverse fracture with minor trauma; may have devastating effect

(Left) *Cut sagittal graphic of the cervical spine shows mature bone formation flowing along the course of the posterior longitudinal ligament, OPLL. It attaches firmly to the posterior vertebral bodies as well as annulus fibrosus fibers of the discs.* **(Right)** *Lateral radiograph shows subtle linear ossification in the path of the posterior longitudinal ligament ➡, representing OPLL. The process may be this thin or may be considerably more thick and dense. However, either may easily be missed on x-ray.*

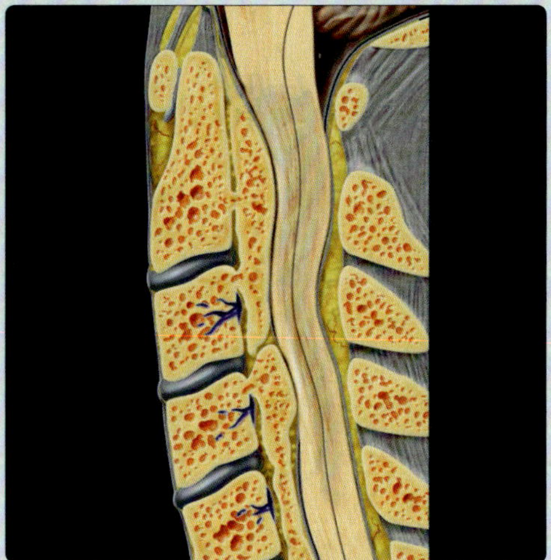

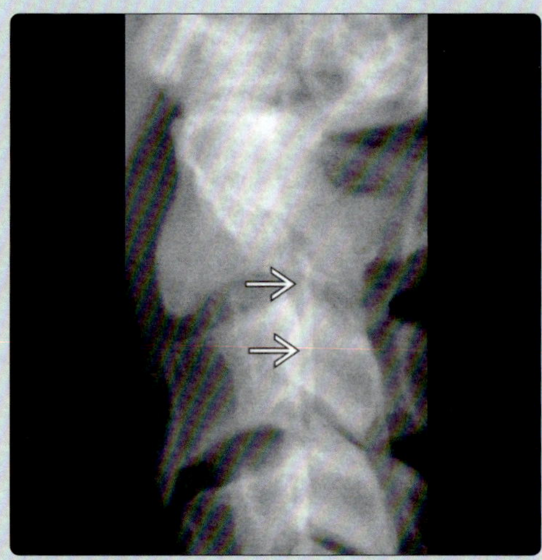

(Left) *Sagittal CT in a 30-year-old man shows productive change at the anterior bodies & ligamentum flavum but even more prominent linear bone formation posterior to the vertebral bodies ➡. This case of OPLL extends along the entire cervical spine.* **(Right)** *Axial bone CT shows OPLL ➡ that demonstrates a significant degree of stenosis produced in this patient. (Previously published in Musculoskeletal Imaging: The Requisites. 2nd ed. Philadelphia, PA: Mosby, Elsevier; 2002.)*

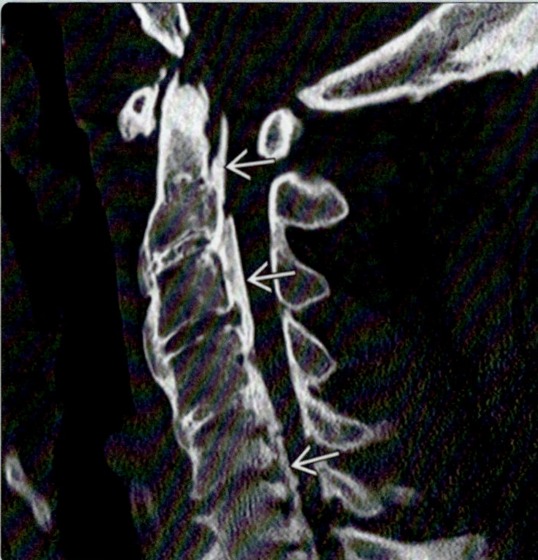

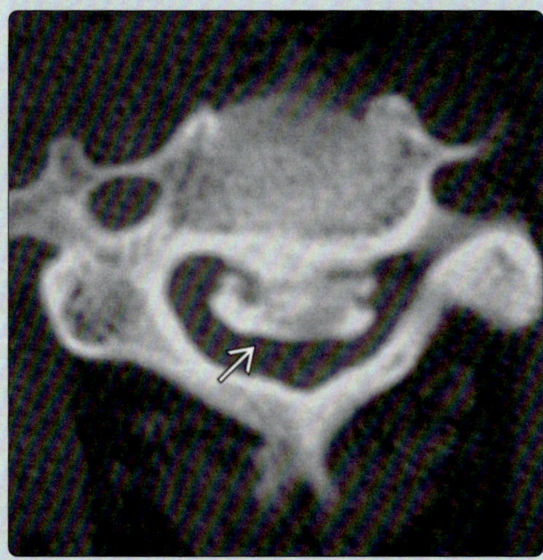

TERMINOLOGY

Synonyms

- Ossification posterior longitudinal ligament (OPLL)

Definitions

- Replacement of posterior longitudinal ligamentous tissue by ectopic new bone

IMAGING

General Features

- Best diagnostic clue
  - Flowing ossification posterior to vertebral bodies
- Location
  - Posterior longitudinal ligament (PLL)
  - Most frequent at 4th and 5th cervical levels
  - May involve thoracic or lumbar spine (20%)
    - Generally not continuous, typically more focal
  - May be seen at C1 level, posterior to dens
    - May result in cervical myelopathy
    - Extremely subtle on radiograph
      - Superimposed C1 lateral masses obscure ossification at this site
    - Likely underdiagnosed; recent survey showed its presence in 25% of patients with OPLL at C4-5
    - Usually have thoracolumbar involvement, often segmental rather than continuous
    - Often have ossification of anterior longitudinal ligament (ALL) as well
- Size
  - Ranges from thin to thick and bulky
    - Associated range of spinal canal stenosis
- Morphology
  - Mature linear ossification
  - Location in anterior spinal canal puts patient at risk for spinal stenosis

Imaging Recommendations

- Best imaging tool
  - CT to fully evaluate extent of ossification
    - Carefully evaluate for involvement posterior to C1
    - Spinal canal stenosis
  - In patient with clinical signs of myelopathy, MR to evaluate spinal cord

Radiographic Findings

- Linear ossification along path of PLL
- Attachment to posterior aspect of vertebral bodies and annulus fibrosus
  - Continuous or discontinuous
- Generally linear rather than undulating
- May have involvement beyond subaxial C spine
  - May be discontinuous
  - Upper cervical spine difficult to evaluate secondary to overlying tissue: Mastoids, C1 facets, ear lobe
- No associated disc disease or facet/apophyseal joint osteoarthritis
- No associated sacroiliac joint or peripheral arthritis
- May have associated ossification of anterior longitudinal ligament [diffuse idiopathic skeletal hyperostosis (DISH)]
  - 44% of patients with OPLL have concomitant anterior hyperostosis
  - Conversely, 50% of patients with DISH also have ossification of PLL
- Bone density usually normal
  - If significant concomitant DISH and OPLL, may develop long column fusion
  - If fused chronically, may develop osteoporosis
    - Combination of fusion and osteoporosis puts patient at risk for transverse fracture from minor trauma, similar to ankylosing spondylitis

CT Findings

- Essential to find all sites of PLL ossification for complete evaluation and surgical planning
- Ossification following path of PLL
  - Generally smooth
  - Rarely, with advanced disease, may see marrow
- May be contiguous with vertebral body or separate
- Axial: Upside-down T formation (termed bow tie)
- Narrowed spinal canal
- Generally normal disc spaces, facet, and apophyseal joints
- If post trauma with significant component of DISH, watch for transverse fracture through fused column
  - May be subtle since usually nondisplaced

MR Findings

- T1WI
  - Ossification is low signal; if thin, may be difficult to differentiate from normal PLL
  - If thick and chronic enough to develop marrow, ossification may have high T1 marrow signal; this appearance is unusual
  - Best seen on sagittal images
  - Axial: Upside-down T configuration
- Fluid-sensitive sequences
  - Ligament ossification usually low signal on all sequences
  - Evaluate degree of spinal stenosis
    - Possible cord hyperintensity secondary to myelomalacia
- If concomitant DISH and OPLL, evaluate for fracture across fused segment and associated cord injury
- MR may underestimate all sites of PLL ossification; may also need CT

DIFFERENTIAL DIAGNOSIS

Diffuse Idiopathic Skeletal Hyperostosis

- DISH and OPLL are frequently seen together
  - 44% of OPLL patients have flowing ALL ossification
  - 50% of DISH patients have PLL ossification
- Rule of thumb: Name by predominant location
  - If anterior flowing ossification predominates in thoracic spine, name it DISH, despite presence of OPLL
  - If ALL ossification is predominant in cervical spine with dense OPLL, name it OPLL

Osteoarthritis With Spondylosis Deformans

- Osteophytes, especially from apophyseal joints, may give appearance of posterior ossification
- Does not show contiguity across > 1 body
- Facet and disc degenerative change

Progressive Systemic Sclerosis

- Deposition, generally around C1-C2 vertebrae
- Pyrophosphate and hydroxyapatite
- Most frequently cloud-like rather than linear

Pyrophosphate Arthropathy

- Calcium pyrophosphate deposition usually occurs around C1-C2 level in cervical spine
- May be very dense
- Crowned dens syndrome
- Much less likely to involve subaxial levels

Spondyloarthropathy of Hemodialysis

- Curvilinear dural calcification; may be circumferential
- Patients on chronic hemodialysis
- Often have concurrent disc destruction and endplate irregularity with resorption

Meningioma

- Avidly enhancing dural-based mass + dural tail, smooth margins
- Often T2 hypointense secondary to calcification
- Lack characteristic T-shaped PLL ossification on axial imaging

Calcified Herniated Disc

- Focal calcified mass centered at single disc space
- Lacks characteristic T-shaped PLL ossification

PATHOLOGY

General Features

- Etiology
  - Not known
  - May be part of spectrum, with early-stage OPLL in evolution noted
    - Hypertrophied PLL with punctate calcification rather than smooth flowing ossification
    - Difficult to distinguish from spondylosis
  - Possible etiologies include autoimmune disorders, trauma, or infection
- Genetics
  - Chromosome 6 *COL11A2* gene related to OPLL
- Associated abnormalities
  - DISH seen in 50% of cases of OPLL
  - Enthesopathy if concomitant DISH

Staging, Grading, & Classification

- Stenosis
  - If canal diameter < 6 mm, symptomatic myelopathy is nearly universal
  - If canal diameter > 14 mm, symptomatic myelopathy is rare
  - Variable symptoms if canal diameter 6-14 mm
    - More likely symptomatic if spine is highly mobile

CLINICAL ISSUES

Presentation

- Most common signs/symptoms
  - Frequently is incidental finding
  - Myelopathy referable to stenotic level
  - Classic: Japanese patient with progressive quadriparesis or paraparesis

Demographics

- Age
  - Usually > 50 years
  - Rare if < 30 years
- Gender
  - M:F = 2:1
- Epidemiology
  - 2-4% prevalence in Japan (originally described in this population)
  - Prevalence in Caucasians is less, but disease seen more frequently with increased use of CT and MR

Natural History & Prognosis

- Mild cases asymptomatic; incidentally discovered
- Parameters correlated with progressive myelopathy
  - > 60% canal stenosis
  - Highly mobile cervical spine
- Spastic paresis progressing to paralysis: 17-22%
  - If patient presents with myelopathy, progression is likely
- If OPLL has prominent DISH and ankylosis, minor trauma may result in transverse fracture
  - Cord damage may be significant

Treatment

- If asymptomatic → observation, nonsurgical management
- Symptomatic or high-grade stenosis → choice of
  - Posterior decompression (laminectomy or laminoplasty)
  - Anterior corpectomy and fusion

DIAGNOSTIC CHECKLIST

Consider

- Evaluate carefully for extension to level of C1
  - Extension to C1 often not expected or sought
  - If considering decompression surgery, must cover full extent of lesion

Image Interpretation Pearls

- In presence of ALL ossification, consider possibility of long column fusion
  - If chronic long fusion, may become osteoporotic
  - Puts patient at risk for transverse fracture with minor trauma; may have devastating effect
- Segmental ossification of PLL may be found at multiple levels
  - Evaluate for stenosis &/or spinal cord damage at each of these levels

SELECTED REFERENCES

1. Fujimori T et al: Ossification of the posterior longitudinal ligament of the cervical spine in 3161 patients: A CT-based study. Spine (Phila Pa 1976). 40(7):E394-403, 2015

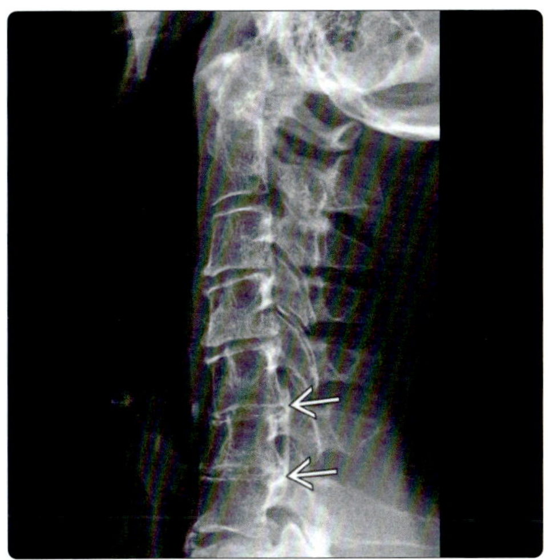

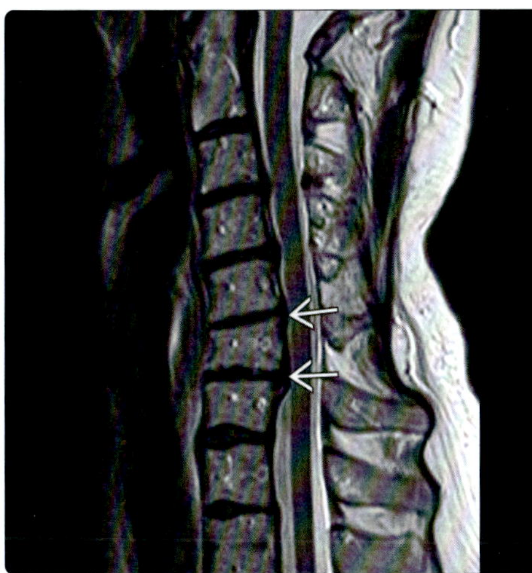

(Left) *Lateral radiograph in a patient with widespread degenerative disc disease also shows OPLL as a linear density posterior to vertebral bodies C5-C7 ➡. With careful observation, this finding is easily seen on radiograph.* **(Right)** *Sagittal T2WI MR in the same patient shows disc disease at multiple levels. The low-signal-intensity OPLL is present ➡ but is easy to overlook on MR. It is interesting that OPLL is one of the few spinal findings that is more visible on radiograph and CT than MR.*

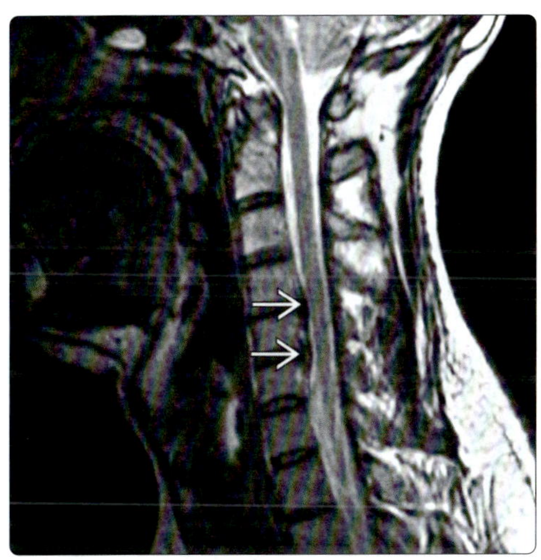

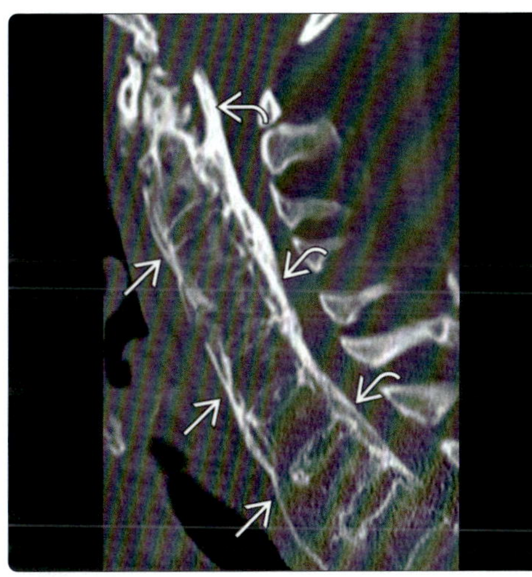

(Left) *Sagittal T2WI MR shows a typical case of mild cervical OPLL. There is flowing posterior longitudinal ligament ossification at C4 through C6 ➡. Signal intensity is similar to adjacent vertebral marrow, indicating the ossific nature of the lesion.* **(Right)** *Sagittal bone CT shows OPLL extending along the length of the cervical spine ➡. Its thickness at the C2-C4 level is concerning for spinal stenosis. There is also flowing anterior ossification, suggesting diffuse idiopathic skeletal hyperostosis (DISH) ➡; the 2 may coincide.*

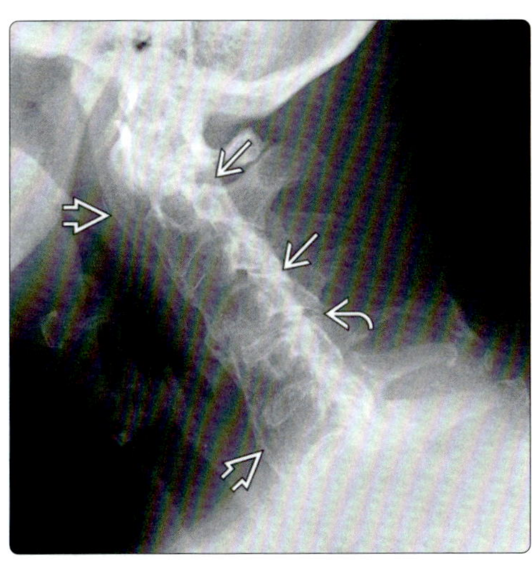

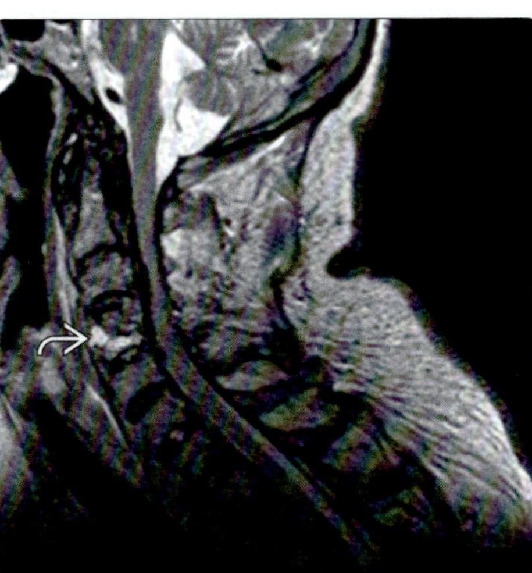

(Left) *Lateral radiograph shows an unusual case of OPLL with superimposed DISH, which over time has resulted in long column fusion. The thick and densely ossified posterior longitudinal ligament is seen ➡, along with anterior flowing osteophytes ➡. The patient had minor trauma, and a fracture of the column can be seen ➡.* **(Right)** *Sagittal T2WI MR in the same patient confirms OPLL, DISH, and superimposed fracture ➡, analogous to the carrot stick fracture seen in AS.*

Osteoarthritis of Shoulder and Elbow

KEY FACTS

TERMINOLOGY

- Noninflammatory arthritis characterized by progressive loss of cartilage
  - Resultant hypertrophic change in bone

IMAGING

- Shoulder radiograph
  - Osteophyte rings anatomic neck of humeral head
  - Osteophyte rings glenoid; often best seen on axillary lateral
  - Subchondral sclerosis
  - Normal bone density
  - Subchondral cysts
  - Intraarticular loose bodies
- Subluxation of glenohumeral joint may occur, based on underlying abnormality
  - Superior subluxation humeral head if chronic rotator cuff tear (RCT)
  - Posterior subluxation of humeral head if chronic
- Elbow radiograph
  - Osteophyte formation: Olecranon, coronoid, ringing radial head/neck
  - Intraarticular loose bodies
- CT or CT arthrography to search for loose bodies
- MR or MR arthrography to search for early cartilage damage prior to osteophyte formation
  - Osteochondral defect
  - Loose bodies
  - Shoulder: Enhancement axillary nerve in quadrilateral space if huge osteophyte (rare)
  - Elbow: Enhancement ulnar nerve in cubital tunnel (uncommon)

PATHOLOGY

- Etiology
  - Primary: Chronic microtrauma and aging
  - Secondary: Chronic RCT, trauma, calcium pyrophosphate or hydroxyapatite deposition disease

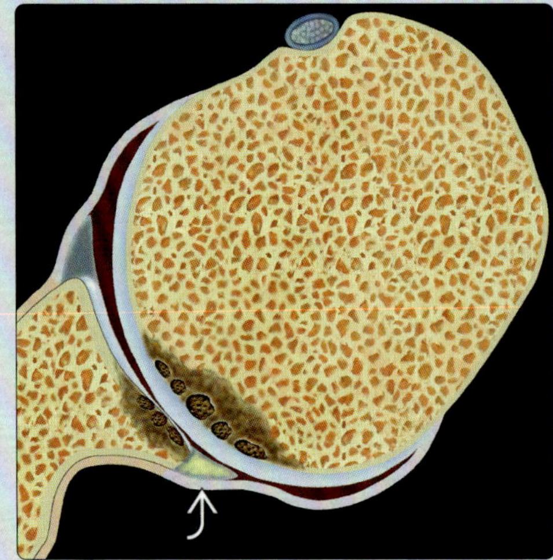

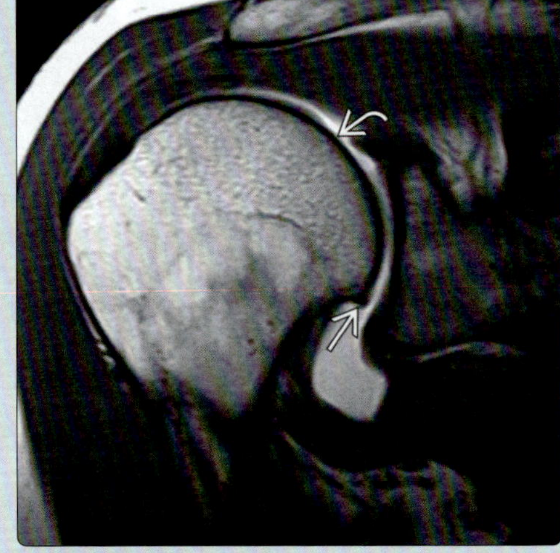

(Left) *Graphic in axial plane shows osteoarthritis (OA) of the glenohumeral (GH) joint, with posterior subluxation of the humerus, cartilage thinning on the glenoid, subchondral cyst formation, and labral degeneration ➔.* **(Right)** *Coronal T2 MR shows early signs of OA of the GH joint. There is a small inferior osteophyte ➔, but, more importantly, there is a 1-cm focal site of severe cartilage damage on the weight-bearing portion of the humeral head ➔, outlined by effusion. The labrum and rotator cuff are intact.*

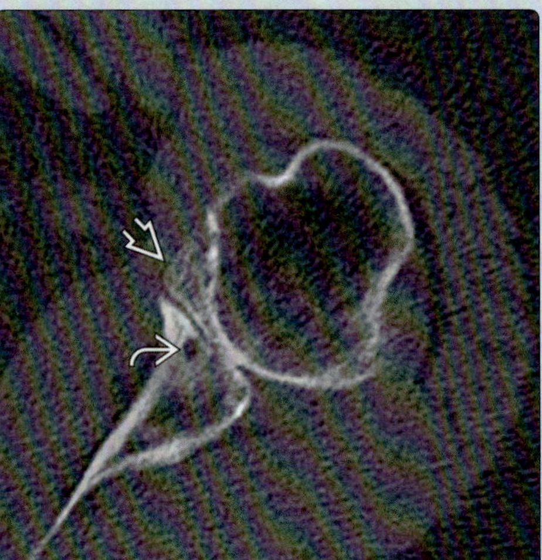

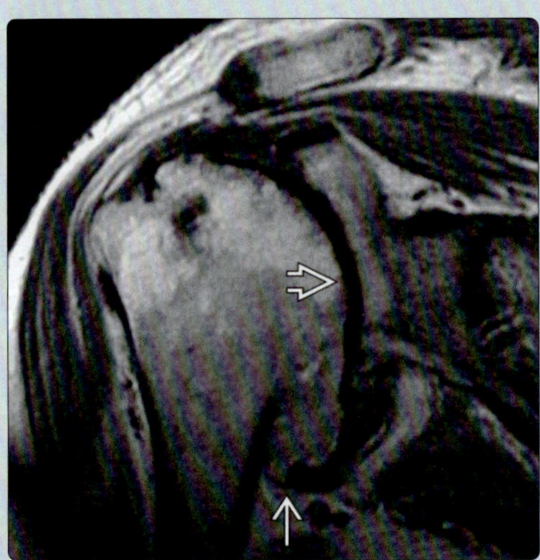

(Left) *Axial NECT of the GH joint demonstrates severe osteophyte formation ➔, as well as joint space narrowing and subchondral cyst formation ➔. The osteophyte is in the typical inferomedial marginal position.* **(Right)** *Coronal T1WI MR shows marked inferomedial humeral head osteophyte formation ➔ and GH joint space narrowing ➔, consistent with severe OA. This large osteophyte extended posteriorly, compressing the neurovascular bundle of the quadrilateral space.*

TERMINOLOGY

Abbreviations

- Osteoarthritis (OA)

Synonyms

- Osteoarthrosis, degenerative joint disease (DJD)

Definitions

- Noninflammatory arthritis characterized by progressive loss of cartilage
  - Resultant hypertrophic change in bone
- Often specified as primary vs. secondary OA
  - Primary OA: DJD resulting from chronic microtrauma and aging
    - Shoulder and elbow not as predisposed to primary OA as hip, knee, interphalangeal joints, and 1st carpometacarpal joint
  - Secondary OA: DJD resulting from specific traumatic event, abnormal underlying morphology, infection, or metabolic abnormality

IMAGING

General Features

- Best diagnostic clue
  - Cartilage loss in weight-bearing portions of joint
  - Osteophyte formation
  - Normal bone density, subchondral sclerosis
- Location
  - Shoulder
    - Superomedial humeral head earliest site of cartilage loss
  - Elbow
    - Radiocapitellar, ulnotrochlear, or both
- Size
  - Ranges from subtle to large osteophyte formation
    - Shoulder particularly may develop huge inferomedial marginal osteophytes on head
- Morphology
  - Bone production: Sclerosis, osteophytes

Radiographic Findings

- Shoulder
  - Normal bone density
  - Subchondral sclerosis
  - Osteophyte formation
    - Rings glenoid; often best seen on axillary lateral
    - Rings anatomic neck of humeral head (marginal)
      - Most prominent growth is inferomedial, into axillary pouch
  - Subchondral cysts
  - Joint space narrowing
  - Subluxation of glenohumeral joint may occur, based on underlying abnormality
    - Superior subluxation of humeral head if chronic rotator cuff tear
    - Posterior subluxation of humeral head if chronic instability (seen on axillary lateral view)
  - Intraarticular loose bodies
    - May be difficult to visualize on radiograph unless joint is distended by effusion
    - Watch for ossified bodies in axillary and subcoracoid recesses
- Elbow
  - Normal bone density
  - Subchondral sclerosis
  - Osteophyte formation
    - Olecranon process
    - Coronoid process
    - Ringing radial head/neck
  - Subchondral cyst formation
  - Joint space narrowing
  - Subluxation
  - Intraarticular loose bodies
    - Difficult to see on radiograph in absence of effusion
    - Watch for ossified bodies in anterior and posterior joint recesses, outlined by fat pads

CT Findings

- Elbow
  - CT used to search for loose bodies
    - If loose bodies are not ossified, CT arthrography may be necessary

MR Findings

- T1WI
  - Low signal: Subchondral cysts, subchondral sclerosis
  - Marrow signal within large mature osteophytes
  - If inferomedial humeral head osteophyte is large, use T1WI sagittal and axial to evaluate its proximity to axillary nerve in quadrilateral space
- Fluid-sensitive sequences
  - Low signal: Subchondral sclerosis
  - High signal: Bone marrow edema, subchondral cysts
  - Synovitis seen as thickening, low-signal, adjacent to high-signal effusion
  - If effusion present, watch for focal cartilage defects or diffuse thinning
  - Loose bodies within effusion
  - Associated tendon tear or tendinopathy
  - High-signal neuropathy
    - Shoulder OA: Axillary nerve in quadrilateral space
    - Elbow OA: Ulnar nerve in cubital tunnel

Imaging Recommendations

- Best imaging tool
  - Radiograph diagnoses mild to moderate OA
  - CT or CT arthrography to search for loose bodies
  - MR or MR arthrography to search for early cartilage damage prior to osteophyte formation

DIFFERENTIAL DIAGNOSIS

Shoulder Osteoarthritis

- Osteonecrosis
  - Occurs at same superomedial site on humeral head as early OA
  - Double line sign might simulate subchondral sclerosis
- Septic arthritis
  - Cartilage thinning (joint space narrowing)
  - Effusion

- Loss of cortical distinctness or cortical bone plate; distinguishes septic joint from bone-forming OA
- If suspected, must aspirate joint

- Chronic rotator cuff tear
  - Results in secondary OA
- "Milwaukee" shoulder
  - Hydroxyapatite crystal deposition
  - May result in severe degenerative changes, with cartilage destruction followed by osteophyte formation

Elbow Osteoarthritis

- Juvenile idiopathic arthritis (JIA)
  - Overgrowth of epiphyses, particularly radial head
  - When JIA active, synovitis much more prominent than in OA
  - Loose bodies, erosions, cartilage destruction
- Hemophilic arthropathy
  - Overgrowth of epiphyses, particularly radial head
  - When active joint bleeding, synovitis much more prominent than in OA
  - Loose bodies, erosions, cartilage destruction
  - Blooms on gradient echo imaging secondary to hemosiderin deposition in synovium
- Primary synovial chondromatosis (PSC)
  - Loose bodies tend to be of similar size in PSC
  - May result in OA

PATHOLOGY

General Features

- Etiology
  - Primary OA of shoulder or elbow
    - Biochemical changes in cartilage
      - ↓ water content, ↓ proteoglycans, ↓ number of chondrocytes → abnormal cartilage, ↑ risk of damage with microtrauma
    - Low levels of estrogen have been associated with increased risk of OA
  - Secondary OA of shoulder
    - Trauma
      - Prior fracture or dislocation
      - Occupational overload
    - Prior untreated complete rotator cuff tear
      - Elevation of head → abnormal articulation
    - Prior inflammatory arthropathy
      - Cartilage destruction
      - Ligamentous/tendinous laxity → instability
    - Crystal deposition disease
      - Usually hydroxyapatite deposition
    - Abnormal morphology
      - Hypoplastic glenoid
      - Metaphyseal and epiphyseal morphologic abnormalities in various dysplasias
      - Ligamentous laxity in collagen vascular diseases
  - Secondary OA of elbow
    - Trauma (prior fracture with malunion)
    - Valgus extension overload injury
    - Joint destruction from prior inflammatory arthropathy
    - Joint destruction from bodies in synovial chondromatosis
- Genetics
  - Certain genes are markedly upregulated in osteoarthritic compared with nonosteoarthritic shoulders
    - *GJA1, COX2, VCAN, COL1A1, ADAMTS5, MMP3*, and *TNF* expression significantly ↑
    - May serve as biomarkers

CLINICAL ISSUES

Presentation

- Most common signs/symptoms
  - Shoulder
    - Progressive pain with motion; no pain at rest
    - Often antecedent or occupational trauma
    - Decreased range of motion, crepitus
  - Elbow
    - Progressive pain with use of joint
    - Limited flexion and extension
    - Clicking, locking secondary to loose bodies
    - Subluxation, deformity
- Other signs/symptoms
  - Axillary neuropathy secondary to shoulder OA (rare)
  - Ulnar neuropathy secondary to elbow OA (rare)

Demographics

- Age
  - Primary OA: Elderly patient
  - Secondary OA: Younger patient
- Gender
  - M > F for both shoulder and elbow
    - Opposite of gender ratio in knee and interphalangeal hand OA
    - Relates to traumatic and occupational etiology in shoulder and elbow
- Epidemiology
  - Shoulder
    - 1 in 6 adults suffers from chronic shoulder pain
    - > 1/2 of those adults with current shoulder symptoms still have symptoms 5 years later
    - Populations with occupational stress on shoulder are at greater risk for long-term shoulder OA
    - In 2004, shoulder disorders caused longest absences from work compared with other occupational musculoskeletal injuries in USA
  - Elbow: Affected less frequently than weight-bearing joints, such as hip and knee

Natural History & Prognosis

- Progressively debilitating disease without intervention

Treatment

- Usually conservative
  - Physical therapy, NSAIDs
  - Intraarticular steroid injection
- Surgery: Arthroplasty if OA is severe

SELECTED REFERENCES

1. Kawanishi Y et al: The association between cubital tunnel morphology and ulnar neuropathy in patients with elbow osteoarthritis. J Shoulder Elbow Surg. 23(7):938-45, 2014

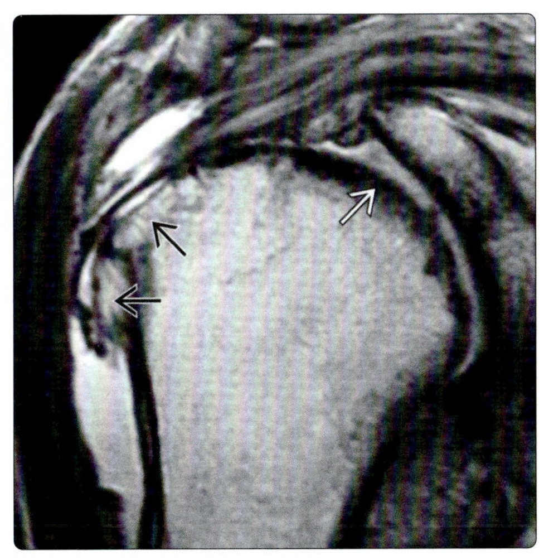

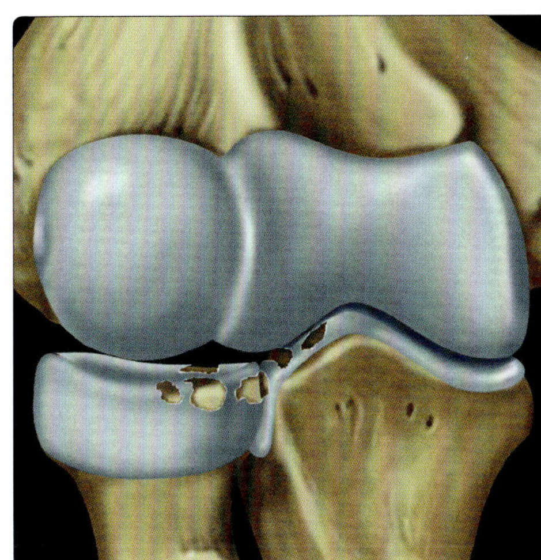

(Left) *Coronal PD MR demonstrates OA, including complete cartilage loss, subcortical sclerosis ➡, and superior marginal osteophyte formation ➡. There is severe thinning of the supraspinatus tendon; other cuts showed a full-thickness rotator cuff tear. Effusion is seen in both the GH joint and the subacromial-subdeltoid bursa.* **(Right)** *Graphic shows OA in the elbow, with several focal cartilage defects. Elbow OA often results from prior trauma &/or loose bodies.*

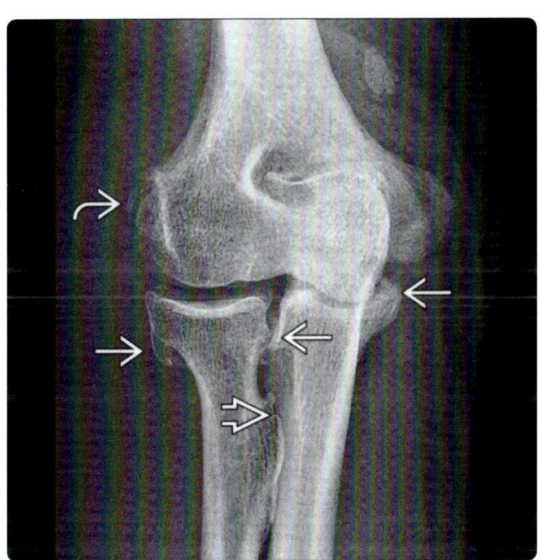

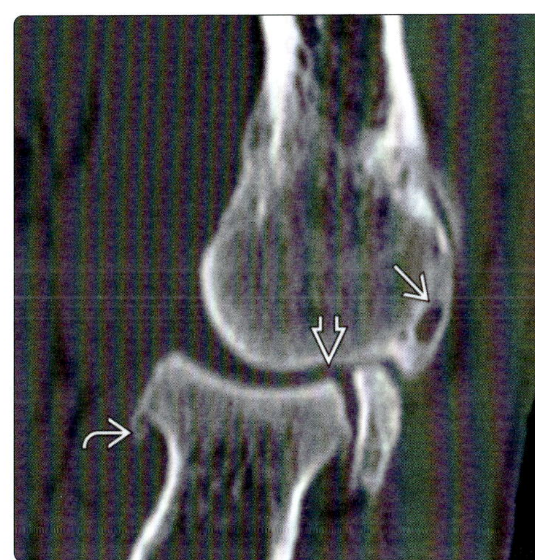

(Left) *AP radiograph shows moderate elbow OA with osteophytes ➡ and hypertrophic bone at the radial tuberosity ➡. A corticated ossicle in the proximal extensor tendon ➡ is consistent with chronic tendinopathy or prior tear.* **(Right)** *Sagittal NECT shows chronic elbow OA with subchondral cysts ➡, osteophytes ➡, and joint space narrowing ➡. The extent of osseous disease is sometimes better demonstrated on CT than radiograph.*

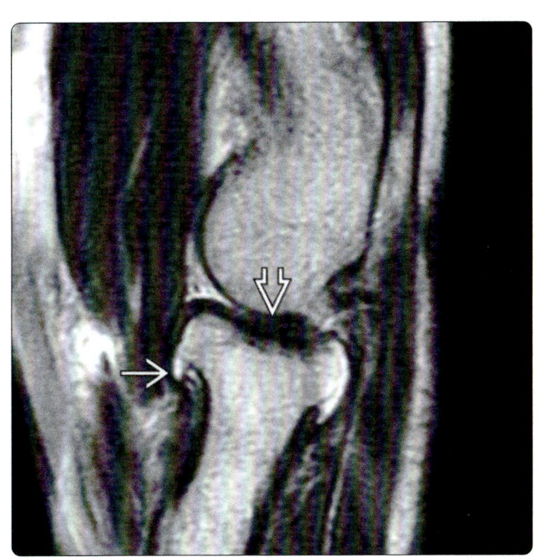

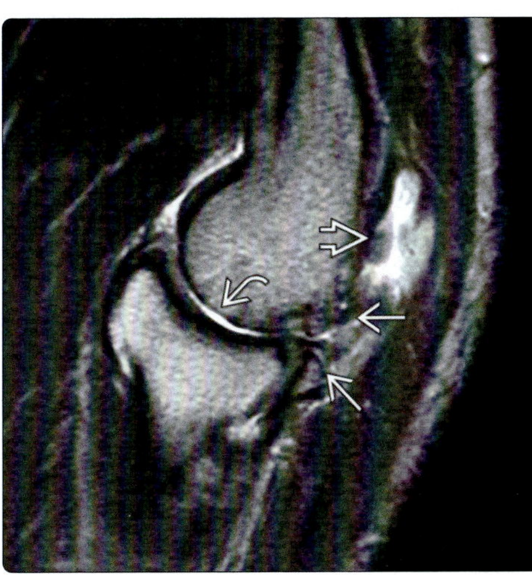

(Left) *Sagittal T2WI MR shows mild to moderate OA of the elbow, with osteophytes ➡ and mild chondral thinning ➡.* **(Right)** *Sagittal T2WI MR shows OA of the radiocapitellar joint with loose bodies within the distended posterior recess ➡. Osteophytosis is noted posteriorly ➡, and there are subchondral sclerosis and cartilage loss ➡. Loose bodies can be difficult to identify on MR or radiograph unless they are large.*

Osteoarthritis of Wrist and Hand

KEY FACTS

TERMINOLOGY

- Osteoarthritis (OA): Noninflammatory arthritis due to progressive loss of cartilage
  - Resultant hypertrophic change in bone
- Erosive osteoarthritis (EOA): Inflammatory variant of OA

IMAGING

- Both OA and EOA are highly location specific
  - IP joints (particularly DIP)
  - 1st CMC and STT joints in carpus
- OA: Cartilage narrowing + osteophytes
- EOA: Cartilage narrowing + erosions, ± osteophytes
- MR fluid-sensitive sequences
  - ↑ signal inflammatory sites, early erosions
  - ↑ signal marrow edema

TOP DIFFERENTIAL DIAGNOSES

- EOA DDx
  - Psoriatic arthritis
  - Adult Still disease
  - Multicentric reticulohistiocytosis
  - Hyperparathyroidism

CLINICAL ISSUES

- M < < F for IP joints of hand
- M < < < F for EOA (M:F = 1:12)
- Symptoms of EOA
  - Acute articular attacks, generally interphalangeal joints
- Symptoms of OA
  - Joint pain related to use
  - Self-limited morning stiffness

DIAGNOSTIC CHECKLIST

- To differentiate EOA from other erosive inflammatory arthropathies, use carpal distribution
  - EOA virtually always also has changes in 1st CMC &/or STT joints due to either EOA or standard OA

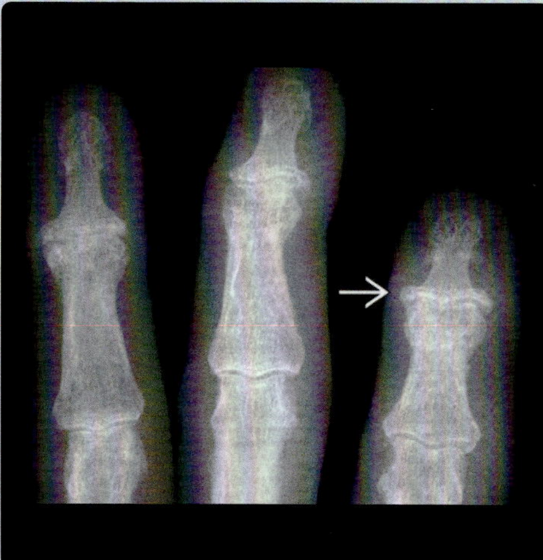

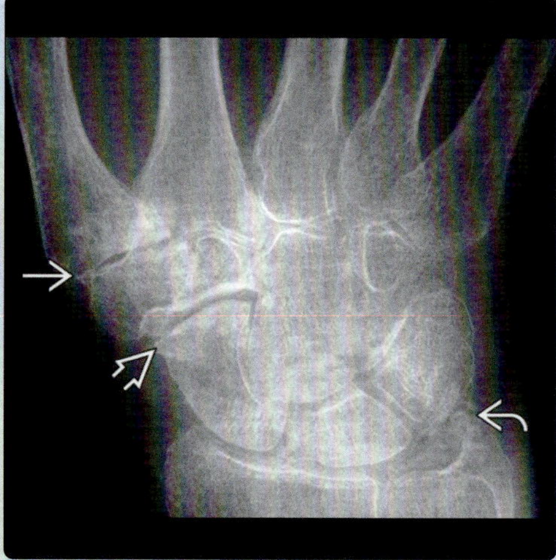

(Left) *PA radiograph shows joint space narrowing at all of the distal interphalangeal (DIP) joints; less severe narrowing is present at the proximal interphalangeal (PIP) joints. There are osteophytes at all of the DIPs ➡, without erosive change. This is typical osteoarthritis (OA).* **(Right)** *PA radiograph of the same hand shows sclerosis and narrowing at the 1st carpometacarpal (CMC) ➡ as well as scapho-trapezium-trapezoid (STT) ⇨ joints, typical of OA. There is trauma-related chondrocalcinosis ⮌.*

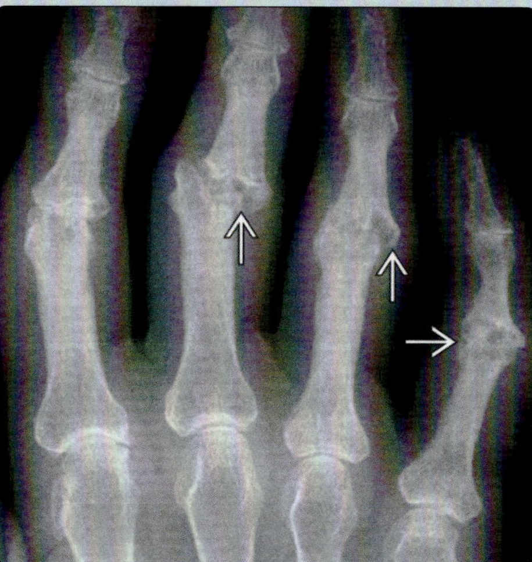

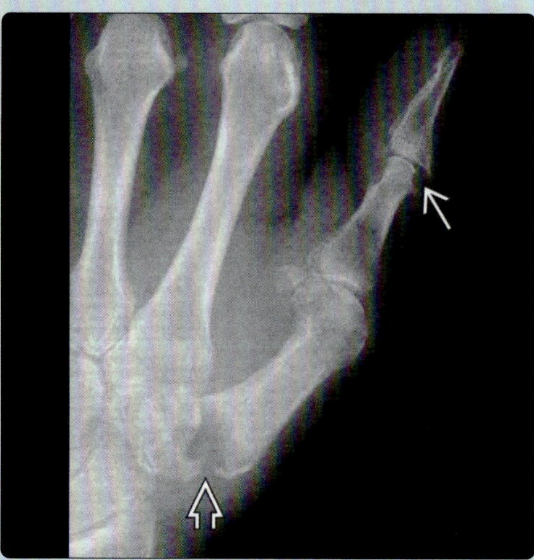

(Left) *PA radiograph shows a classic case of erosive osteoarthritis (EOA). The DIP joints show nonspecific narrowing. The PIP joints show significant erosive disease ➡. Bone density is normal. Either EOA or psoriatic arthropathy might be considered.* **(Right)** *PA radiograph, same patient, shows significant erosive disease of the interphalangeal joint of the thumb ➡ as well as large erosions at the 1st CMC ⇨. The location of erosive change at the 1st CMC joint secures the diagnosis of EOA; psoriatic arthritis does not involve this joint.*

TERMINOLOGY

Abbreviations

- Osteoarthritis (OA)

Synonyms

- Degenerative joint disease (DJD), osteoarthrosis
- Variant: Erosive osteoarthritis (EOA)
  - Inflammatory osteoarthritis

Definitions

- OA: Noninflammatory arthritis due to progressive loss of cartilage
  - Resultant hypertrophic change in bone
- EOA: Inflammatory variant of OA

IMAGING

General Features

- Best diagnostic clue
  - Both OA and EOA are highly location-specific
    - In hand/wrist, interphalangeal (IP) joints and 1st carpometacarpal joint &/or scaphotrapeziotrapezoid joints
  - OA: Cartilage narrowing + osteophytes
  - EOA: Cartilage narrowing + erosions, ± osteophytes
- Location
  - OA locations in hand
    - Distal interphalangeal joints (DIP)
    - Proximal interphalangeal joints (PIP)
    - Metacarpophalangeal (MCP) joints only if other predisposing factors
      - e.g., trauma, hemochromatosis
  - OA locations in wrist
    - 1st carpometacarpal (1st CMC) joint
    - Scapho-trapezium-trapezoid (STT) joint
    - Other involved carpal joints may have secondary OA, related to trauma
      - Ulno-lunate or ulno-triquetrum, secondary to ulnar-positive variance
      - 4 corners (lunate-triquetrum-capitate-hamate) related to lunate morphology
      - Radial styloid-scaphoid related to scapholunate dissociation or radial fracture
  - EOA location
    - Same hand locations as OA: DIP, PIP
    - Same carpal locations as OA: 1st CMC, STT
    - Seen in IP joints of foot
    - Described, but rarely seen in MCP, knee, hip
- Morphology
  - OA: Purely productive arthritis, osteophyte formation
  - EOA: Erosive or mixed erosive-productive arthritis

Radiographic Findings

- Normal bone density
  - Caveat: Elderly women may have osteoporosis related to age and gender; may still have OA
- Joint space narrowing
  - Symmetric in small joints of hand and wrist
- Osteophytosis
  - IP joints: Often dorsal, best seen on lateral view
  - 1st CMC: Osteophytes may be extremely large, especially on radial aspect of joint
- Subchondral bone cysts
- Malalignment
  - At 1st CMC, metacarpal often subluxated in radial direction
  - Otherwise, malalignment is not significant part of process
- Erosions
  - Do not occur in OA
  - EOA: Erosions are, by definition, part of process
    - In IP joints, erosions located centrally at head, slightly lateral from center at adjacent base
      - Location of these erosions, with sclerosis along subchondral bone, results in gull wing pattern
      - Gull wing pattern typical of EOA, though not pathognomonic
    - Carpal location of disease is same as OA: 1st CMC and STT
      - Carpal disease may be erosive
      - More frequently, carpal disease is either mixed erosive-productive or purely productive, with cartilage narrowing and osteophytes
- Chondrocalcinosis
  - Generally not thought of, but is often seen as manifestation of OA
    - Does not necessarily imply pyrophosphate arthropathy
  - Chronic trauma at triangular fibrocartilaginous complex (TFCC) may result in chondrocalcinosis
    - Chronically torn TFCC
    - Ulnar-positive variance
- Ankylosis
  - Not common in OA; may be seen in EOA
- Symmetry: Generally present
  - Disease progression may be more rapid in dominant hand

CT Findings

- Higher detection rate for carpal OA than radiographs

MR Findings

- MR generally not utilized for OA of hand/wrist
  - Large osteophytes follow marrow signal
  - Bone marrow edema, subchondral sclerosis
- MR in EOA
  - Fluid-sensitive sequences
    - High signal marrow edema
    - High signal inflammatory sites, early erosions
    - High signal effusions
- Chondrocalcinosis may be either high or low signal

Ultrasonographic Findings

- US evaluation for synovitis correlates with progression of disease at 5 years

Imaging Recommendations

- Best imaging tool
  - Diagnosed by radiograph

DIFFERENTIAL DIAGNOSIS

DDx of Erosive Osteoarthritis

- Psoriatic arthritis (PSA)
  - IP joint disease predominates in PSA
  - PSA is erosive disease but may have superimposed osteophytes
  - Character of soft tissue swelling (sausage digit) may differentiate from EOA
  - Periostitis in PSA, not in EOA
- Adult Still disease
  - IP erosive disease often predominates over MCP
  - Pericapitate carpal disease may differentiate it from EOA
  - Ankylosis more frequent in Adult Still disease
- Multicentric reticulohistiocytosis
  - DIP and PIP erosions
  - Soft tissue nodules
  - Tuft resorption (acroosteolysis)

PATHOLOGY

General Features

- Etiology
  - Mechanical: Trauma, stress, abnormal morphology
  - Biochemical change in cartilage
    - Accumulation of glycation end products in cartilage → increased brittleness of collagen matrix
    - With age, ↓ water content, ↓ # chondrocytes, ↓ production of proteoglycans
      - Leads to softened cartilage, ↑ risk damage
    - ↑ tumor necrosis factor and interleukin-1 found in OA; ↑ in degradative enzymes
  - Postulated association with decreased estrogen in elderly
- Genetics
  - Twin and familial studies: OA is multigenic trait
  - Genetic predisposition for women with OA of DIP joints; may be as high as 65%

Gross Pathologic & Surgical Features

- Fissuring, pitting, ulceration cartilage
- Reactive bone: Osteophytes, subchondral sclerosis
- Synovium
  - OA: Normal to mild synovial inflammation
  - EOA: Mild to severe synovial inflammation

CLINICAL ISSUES

Presentation

- Most common signs/symptoms
  - Symptoms of OA
    - Joint pain related to use
      - No pain at rest
    - Self-limited morning stiffness
    - Crepitus
    - ↓ range of motion
    - No swelling or warmth
    - No constitutional symptoms
  - Symptoms of EOA
    - Acute articular attacks, generally IP joints
      - Rheumatoid-like

Demographics

- Age
  - Most common in patients > 65 years
  - OA in > 80% of individuals > 75 years
- Gender
  - M < F for all forms of OA
  - M < < F for IP joints of hand
  - M < < < F for EOA; (M:F = 1:12)
- Ethnicity
  - More common in Caucasians than African Americans
  - More prevalent in Native Americans than general population
- Epidemiology
  - Most common arthropathy; 20 million in USA
  - 12% prevalence in USA

Natural History & Prognosis

- OA: Progressive pain and debility
- EOA
  - May be self-limited with conservative therapy
  - Some cases progress to clinical manifestations like rheumatoid arthritis

Treatment

- Objective: Relieve pain, maintain function
  - Physical therapy
  - Nonnarcotic analgesics
  - Intraarticular corticosteroid
- Arthrodesis
- Arthroplasty
  - Current arthroplasties have high failure rate
    - Loosening, osteolysis
- Other carpal surgical options
  - Ligament reconstruction/tendon interposition (LRTI)/suspensionplasty
    - For 1st CMC OA
    - Resection of trapezium, forearm ligament rolled and placed in defect, threaded through base of 1st metacarpal
  - Radial column fusion (scaphoid-trapezoid-trapezium)
  - Ulnar (4-corner) fusion: Lunate-trapezoid-hamate-capitate
  - Proximal row carpectomy

DIAGNOSTIC CHECKLIST

Image Interpretation Pearls

- In differentiating EOA from other erosive inflammatory arthropathies, use carpal distribution
  - EOA virtually always also has changes in 1st CMC &/or STT joints due to either EOA or standard OA
  - Other arthropathies do not localize to these sites

SELECTED REFERENCES

1. Haugen IK et al: Increasing synovitis and bone marrow lesions are associated with incident joint tenderness in hand osteoarthritis. Ann Rheum Dis. ePub, 2015
2. Mathiessen A et al: Ultrasound-detected inflammation predicts radiographic progression in hand osteoarthritis after 5years. Ann Rheum Dis. ePub, 2015
3. Saltzherr MS et al: Computed tomography for the detection of thumb base osteoarthritis: comparison with digital radiography. Skeletal Radiol. 42(5):715-21, 2013

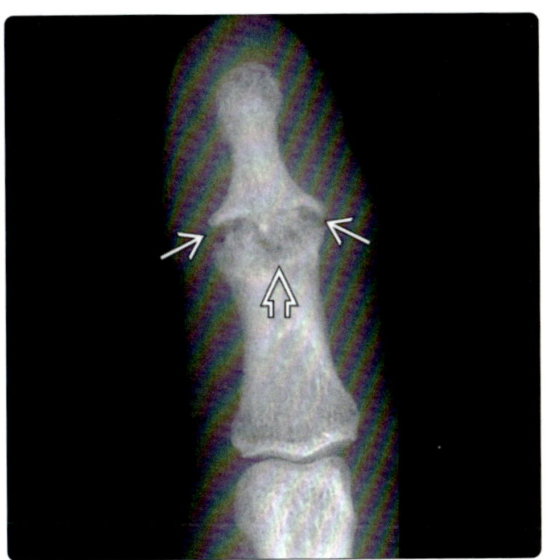

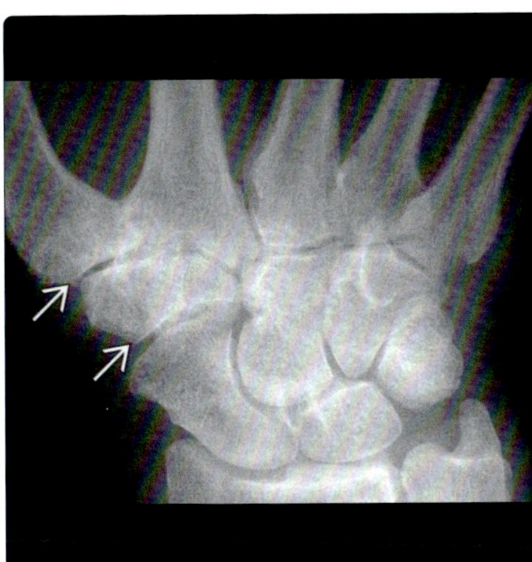

(Left) *PA radiograph shows the classic "gull wing" deformity of EOA. The "gull" body is formed by a direct central subchondral erosion of the middle phalanx ➡, and the "gull wings" are formed by more lateral erosions at the base of the distal phalanx ➡.* **(Right)** *PA radiograph of the same hand shows narrowing of both the 1st CMC and STT joints ➡, without either osteophytes or erosions. This distribution of carpal disease confirms the diagnosis of EOA given the appearance of the DIP.*

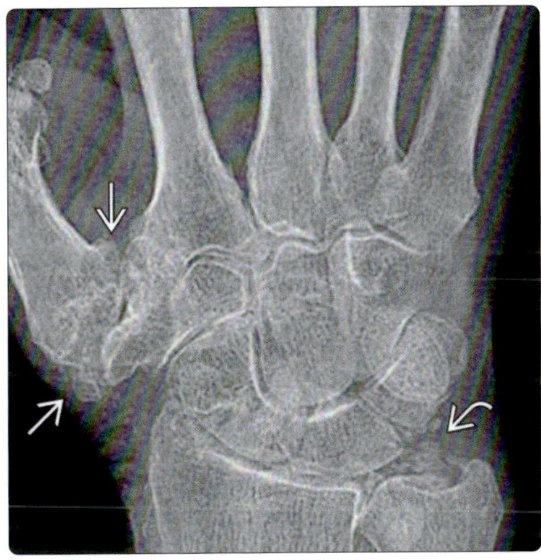

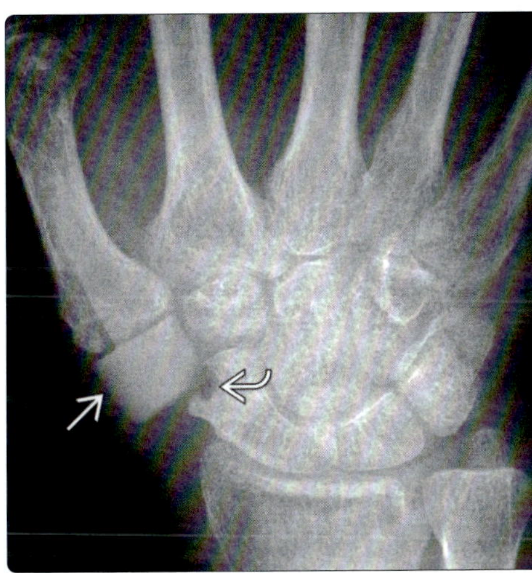

(Left) *PA radiograph of the wrist shows tremendous osteophyte formation at the 1st CMC ➡. This is a common and painful manifestation of OA. Note the chondrocalcinosis ➡. This may be present due to OA or else due to trauma from the ulnar-positive variance; it need not imply CPPD.* **(Right)** *PA radiograph shows resection of trapezium for OA and placement of a Silastic prosthesis ➡. These arthroplasties often fail, resulting in osteolysis. A mechanical erosion is seen in the scaphoid ➡.*

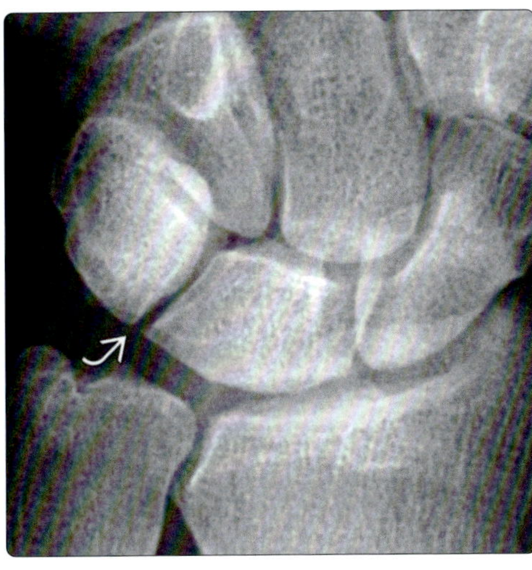

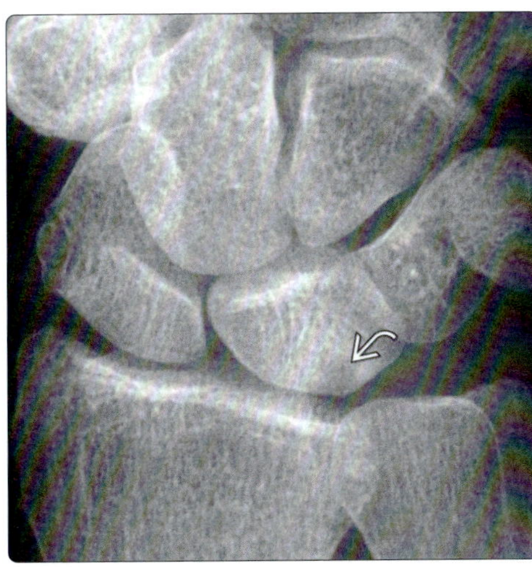

(Left) *PA radiograph shows secondary OA of the lunate and triquetrum ➡ related to ulnar-positive variance. If OA involves carpal articulations other than the 1st CMC or STT, a secondary cause such as this should be sought.* **(Right)** *PA radiograph shows subchondral cyst and osteophyte formation on the lunate ➡. This results from ulnar abutment due to positive ulnar variance. It is a secondary, rather than primary, form of osteoarthritis.*

Osteoarthritis of Hip

KEY FACTS

TERMINOLOGY

- Noninflammatory arthritis resulting from progressive cartilage degeneration
  - Resultant hypertrophic change in bone

IMAGING

- Radiograph
  - Normal bone density, narrowed joint space
  - Osseous productive change
    - Osteophytes
    - Femoral neck (calcar and lateral) buttressing
      - Most specific finding for osteoarthritis (OA) (92%)
  - Subchondral cyst formation (Egger cyst in acetabulum)
    - Solitary acetabular cyst termed Egger cyst
      - May mimic tumor
  - Subluxation femoral head
    - 80% superolateral, 20% medial (protrusio)
  - Often associated with underlying morphologic abnormality in young adults
    - Femoroacetabular impingement (FAI)
    - Developmental dysplasia of hip (DDH)
- MR: Bone marrow edema
  - Volume of edema correlates with severity of hip pain, severity of radiographic OA, and number of microfractures in subchondral bone
  - Cartilage defects are seen if outlined by fluid
  - Cartilage in hip is thin, and capsule is tight, making cartilage more difficult to evaluate than in knee
  - Labral tear or degeneration

DIAGNOSTIC CHECKLIST

- When evaluating OA in young adult, consider etiology other than primary OA
  - FAI or DDH (may be subtle)
  - Spondyloarthropathy, such as ankylosing spondylitis (look at sacroiliac joints)
- Protrusio occurs in 20% of hip OA; do not assume rheumatoid arthritis with this appearance

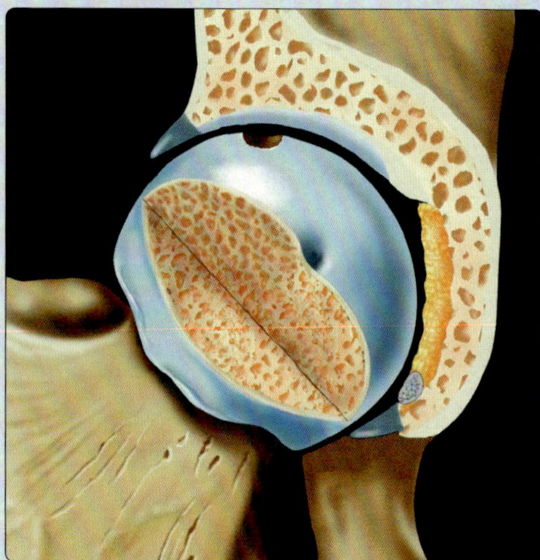

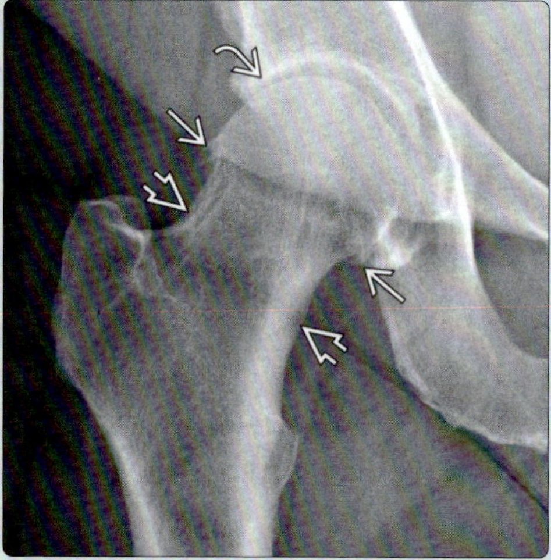

(Left) *Graphic of early osteoarthritis (OA) of the hip shows a focal cartilage defect in the weight-bearing portion of the femoral head. The bone density is normal, and the patient has not yet developed subchondral cysts or osteophytes. The labra are normal as well.* **(Right)** *AP radiograph shows classic hip OA. There is mild superolateral subluxation, and cartilage narrowing is seen superolaterally ➙. A ring osteophyte is seen ➙, as is extensive buttressing ➙ of the calcar (medial femoral neck) & lateral femoral neck.*

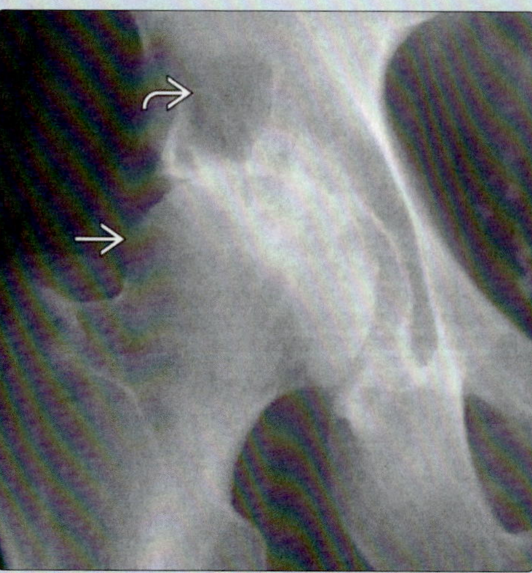

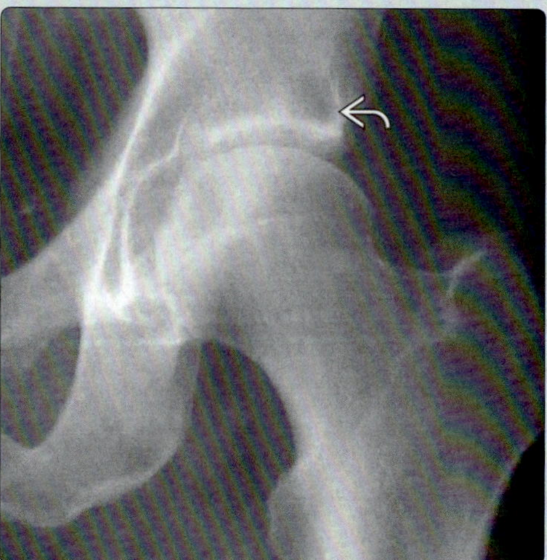

(Left) *AP radiograph shows OA, with ↓ cartilage in the superior weight-bearing portion of the joint, mild superolateral subluxation of the femoral head, ring osteophytes around the femoral head ➙, and a large acetabular subchondral cyst ➙.* **(Right)** *AP radiograph of the left hip in the same patient shows more subtle abnormality but with normal cartilage. There is a single small acetabular subchondral cyst ➙ so typical of OA that it has been termed an Egger cyst and is the early hallmark of the disease.*

TERMINOLOGY

Abbreviations

- Osteoarthritis (OA)

Synonyms

- Degenerative joint disease

Definitions

- Noninflammatory arthritis resulting from progressive cartilage degeneration
  - Resultant hypertrophic change in bone

IMAGING

General Features

- Best diagnostic clue
  - Radiograph: Joint-space narrowing in weight-bearing portion, osteophytes, subchondral cysts
  - MR: Cartilage defect or thinning, labral damage, subchondral cysts
- Location
  - Weight-bearing (anterosuperior) portion of joint

Radiographic Findings

- Normal bone density
- Joint-space narrowing (sensitivity 91%, specificity 60%)
  - Focal, weight-bearing portion of joint
- Osseous productive change
  - Osteophytosis (sensitivity 89%, specificity 90%)
    - Ring osteophytes at femoral head; largest inferomedially
    - Acetabular rim
  - Buttressing: Calcar and lateral femoral neck (92% specificity)
- Subchondral cyst formation
  - Most prominent in acetabulum (termed Egger cyst)
    - May be early isolated finding; may mimic tumor
- Subluxation femoral head
  - 80% superolateral, 20% medial (protrusio)
- Look for underlying morphologies that lead to hip OA
  - Lateral femoral head/neck junction bump → cam-type femoral acetabular impingement (FAI)
  - Coxa magna deformity (Legg-Calvé-Perthes or slipped capital femoral epiphysis) → cam-type FAI
  - Acetabular rim overgrowth → pincer-type FAI
  - Retroverted acetabulum (crossover sign) → pincer-type FAI
  - Otto disease (failure of triradiate cartilage fusion) → protrusio → pincer-type FAI
  - Developmental dysplasia (DDH) → often combined cam- and pincer-type FAI
    - Usually decreased acetabular coverage of femoral head laterally or anteriorly
    - Coxa valga deformity of femoral neck
- Findings often associated with FAI and subsequent OA
  - Os acetabulum
  - Pits located at anterolateral femoral neck
- Insufficiency fracture of femoral head
  - Rarely noted on radiograph initially
  - Progresses rapidly to OA
  - May progress to destruction of entire femoral head → "hatchet" deformity
  - Constellation termed rapidly progressive OA

CT Findings

- CT rarely used for hip evaluation
  - As part of "gunsight" exam to evaluate for torsion, may see retroversion of acetabulum or femoral neck
  - CT arthrography to evaluate for loose bodies, labral tear, cartilage damage

MR Findings

- T1WI
  - Osteophytes contain marrow if large enough
  - Low-signal sclerosis, buttressing, subchondral cysts
- Fluid-sensitive sequences
  - Bone marrow edema
    - Volume of edema correlates with severity of hip pain, severity of radiographic OA, and number of microfractures in subchondral bone
  - Cartilage defects seen if outlined by fluid
    - Cartilage in hip is thin, and capsule is tight, making cartilage more difficult to evaluate than in knee
  - Labral tear or degeneration
  - Subchondral or paralabral cysts
- MR arthrography
  - Labral tear or detachment
  - Cartilage: Focal defect, diffuse thinning, or delamination
  - Osteophytes
  - Subchondral or paralabral cysts
  - Morphology associated with DDH or FAI

Imaging Recommendations

- Best imaging tool
  - Radiograph for mild to advanced OA
  - MR arthrography for early cartilage or labral injury
- Protocol advice
  - MR or CT arthrography: Tight joint limits amount of contrast outlining cartilage
    - Traction during injection helps move contrast around femoral head
    - Traction during MR has been advocated for, with contrast outlining cartilage well
  - Oblique axial sequence has highest yield for labral tears; need several sequences to see subtle cartilage damage

DIFFERENTIAL DIAGNOSIS

Osteonecrosis

- Early to fairly late osteonecrosis (ON) results in femoral head flattening without articular abnormalities
- OA only seen in late-stage ON

Femoral Acetabular Impingement

- Impingement anterolateral head/neck junction (cam)
- Impingement anterolateral acetabulum (pincer)
- Morphology must be recognized as risk for early OA

Developmental Dysplasia

- Shallow acetabulum laterally, possibly anteriorly
- Morphology must be recognized due to risk of developing early OA

Pyrophosphate Arthropathy (CPPD)

- CPPD in cartilage and labrum
- Degenerative changes in hip, with osteophytes; erosions difficult to visualize; mimics OA
- Subchondral cysts may be large

PATHOLOGY

General Features

- Etiology
  - OA pathogenesis not fully understood; heterogeneous risk factors
  - Microtrauma applied to cartilage with biochemical changes of aging
    - ↓ water content, ↓ proteoglycans, ↓ number of chondrocytes
      - Leads to brittle or soft cartilage, at risk for fissuring, ulceration, and delamination
  - Trauma
    - Acetabular or femoral head fracture, generally related to hip dislocation
    - Abnormal weight bearing due to trauma or degenerative change in other joints
      - Limb-length discrepancy with pelvic tilt
      - Scoliosis with pelvic tilt
      - Knee arthritis with malalignment and relative limb shortening
  - Developmental abnormalities
    - Legg-Calvé-Perthes (ON in childhood)
    - Slipped capital femoral epiphysis
  - Abnormal morphology (developmental)
    - DDH
      - Acetabular dysplasia (most common)
      - Rotational malalignment of femoral neck
    - Femoral acetabular impingement morphology
      - Cam type: Anterolateral femoral neck bump
      - Pincer type: Overcoverage of head by acetabulum
      - Cam and pincer types often coexist
      - Several etiologies for each of these types
  - Abnormal morphology (congenital)
    - Epiphyseal abnormalities, such as spondyloepiphyseal dysplasia
  - Low levels of estrogen have been associated with ↑ risk of OA
- Genetics
  - Twin and familial studies suggest OA is multigenic trait

Gross Pathologic & Surgical Features

- Fissuring, pitting, ulceration of cartilage
- Adjacent reactive bone
- Synovium: Normal to mild inflammatory changes

Microscopic Features

- Bone marrow edema pattern on MR correlates with several histopathologic findings
  - Subchondral sclerosis
  - Bone marrow fat necrosis
  - Subchondral pseudocysts
  - Bone marrow fibrosis
  - Microfractures in various stages of healing
  - Normal bone marrow elements
  - Only small amount of true bone marrow edema is seen histopathologically

CLINICAL ISSUES

Presentation

- Most common signs/symptoms
  - Joint pain related to use (no pain at rest); pain may localize to groin
  - Self-limited morning stiffness
  - Crepitus, decreased range of motion
  - No swelling or warmth
  - No constitutional symptoms

Demographics

- Age
  - Most common > 65 years old
  - Seen in 80% of those > 75 years old
- Gender
  - M > F for hip OA
- Epidemiology
  - OA has 12% prevalence in USA
  - Framingham study: Symptomatic OA in 0.7-4.4% of American adults
  - Results in placement of several hundred thousand hip arthroplasties per year

Natural History & Prognosis

- May stabilize with conservative therapy
- May lead to debilitating hip pain, limiting function

Treatment

- Physical therapy, NSAIDs
- For early OA in FAI
  - Labral repair, osteochondroplasty
- For early OA in DDH
  - Labral repair, periacetabular or femoral neck rotational osteotomy
- Arthroplasty

DIAGNOSTIC CHECKLIST

Consider

- When evaluating OA in young adult, consider etiology other than primary OA
  - FAI or DDH (may be subtle)
  - Spondyloarthropathy, such as ankylosing spondylitis (look at sacroiliac joints)
- Protrusio occurs in 20% of hip OA; do not assume rheumatoid arthritis with this appearance

Image Interpretation Pearls

- With FAI or DDH morphology, evaluate for both cam and pincer mechanisms

SELECTED REFERENCES

1. Xu L et al: The diagnostic performance of radiography for detection of osteoarthritis-associated features compared with MRI in hip joints with chronic pain. Skeletal Radiol. 42(10):1421-8, 2013
2. Taljanovic MS et al: Bone marrow edema pattern in advanced hip osteoarthritis: quantitative assessment with magnetic resonance imaging and correlation with clinical examination, radiographic findings, and histopathology. Skeletal Radiol. 37(5):423-31, 2008

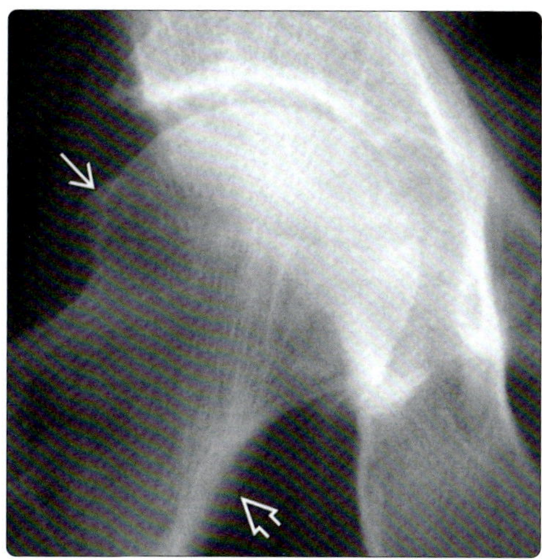

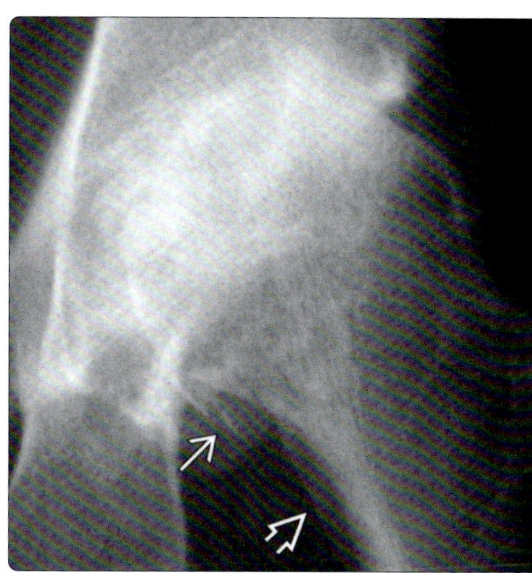

(Left) *AP radiograph shows OA with ring osteophyte ➡ and calcar buttressing ➡. There is medial rather than superior joint narrowing, but this OA is still typical.* **(Right)** *AP radiograph of the left hip in the same patient shows more severe OA, with a large inferior marginal osteophyte ➡ and complete cartilage loss. There is superolateral subluxation of the head relative to the acetabulum. Buttressing along the calcar (medial weight-bearing portion of the femoral neck) is prominent as well ➡.*

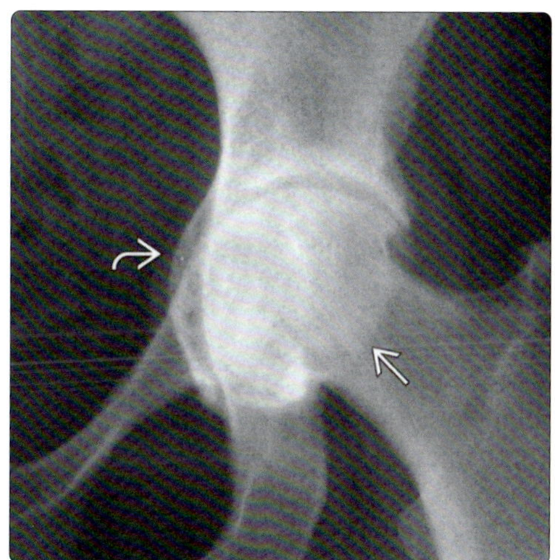

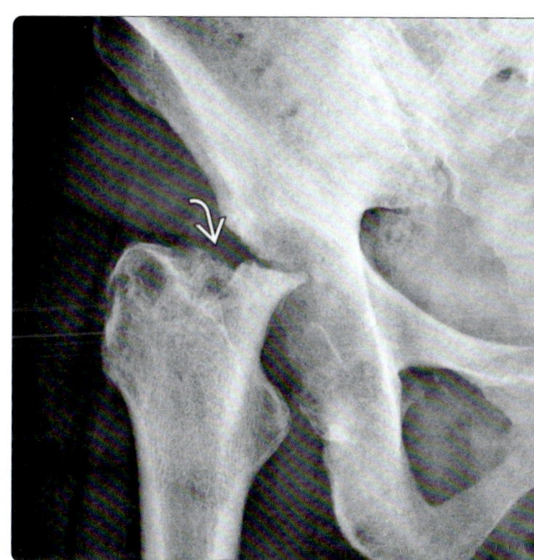

(Left) *AP radiograph shows OA with ring femoral head osteophyte ➡, cartilage narrowing, and protrusio ➡. Protrusio occurs in up to 20% of cases of hip OA.* **(Right)** *AP radiograph shows a "hatchet" deformity, with complete destruction of the femoral head ➡. This destruction often progresses over a matter of weeks and has been termed rapidly destructive OA of the hip or Postel OA. The distinguishing features are the straight margin at the femoral neck and the rapidity of the process.*

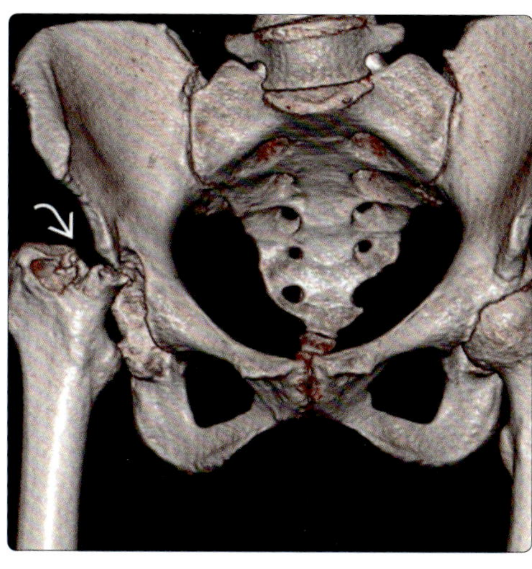

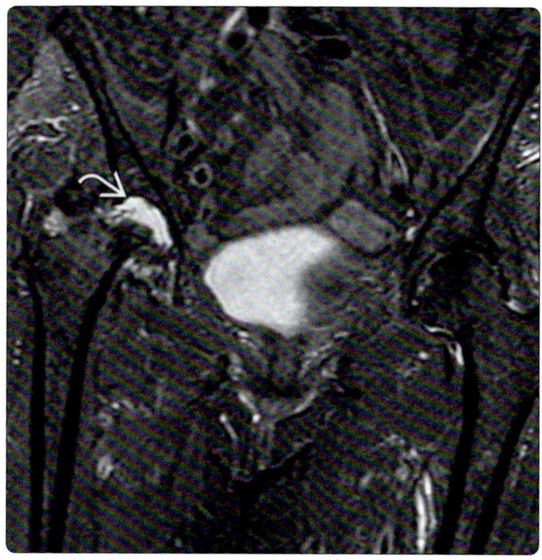

(Left) *Anterior 3D CT of same patient obtained 3 weeks later shows further destruction of the acetabulum and femoral head/neck ➡. Rapidly destructive OA of the hip is thought to occur secondary to subchondral insufficiency fracture, but the original fracture is rarely seen. Both septic hip and Charcot hip must be ruled out.* **(Right)** *Coronal STIR MR of the same patient shows there is a relatively small amount of fluid in the destroyed hip joint ➡. This, plus aspiration, effectively rules out both septic and Charcot hip.*

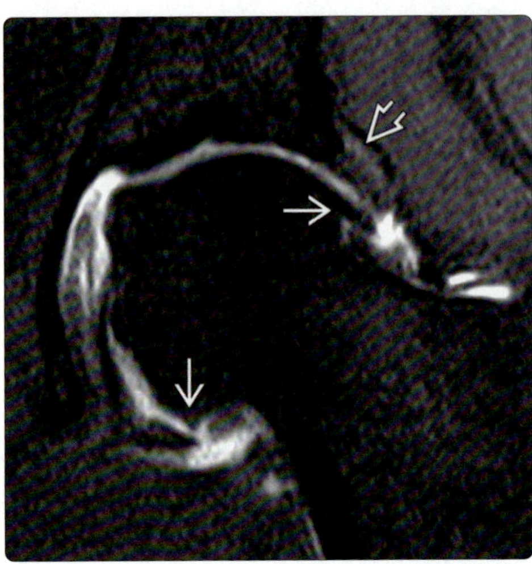

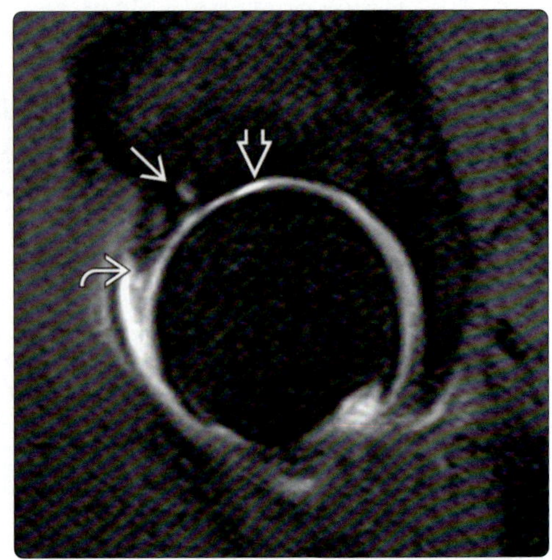

(Left) *Coronal T1WI FS MR arthrogram shows a typical MR appearance of OA, with diffuse irregularity of all articular cartilage. Osteophyte formation is present at the margins of the articular surface ➡. Focal degeneration is present within the labrum ➡.* **(Right)** *Sagittal T1WI FS MR arthrogram in the same patient shows severe thinning of weight-bearing cartilage ➡. Foci of subchondral signal change are seen in the acetabulum ➡, and there is labral degeneration with detachment ➡.*

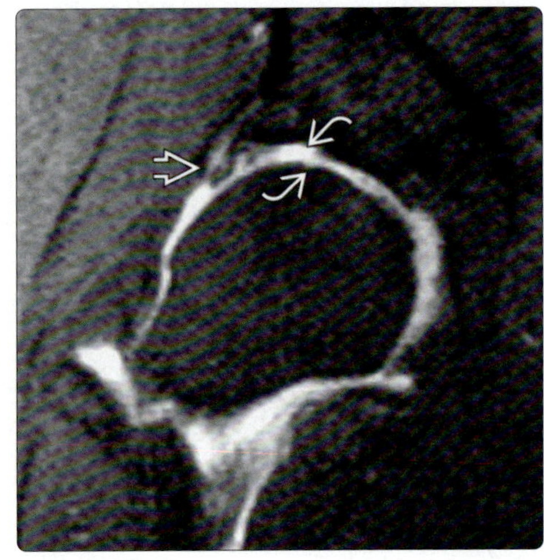

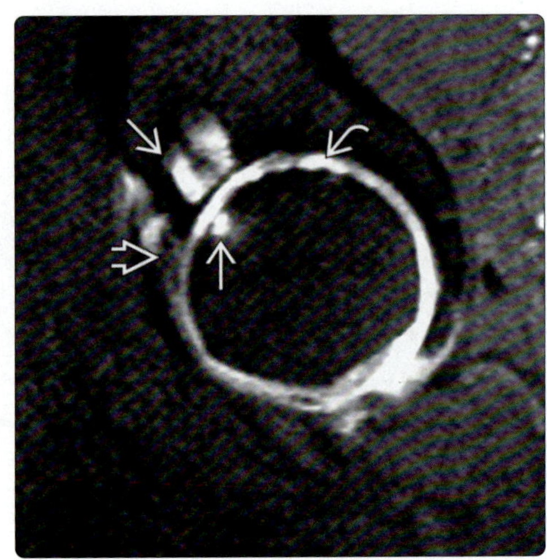

(Left) *Coronal T1WI FS MR arthrogram is shown. Although it is uncommon to perform an MR arthrogram in a patient with OA, this has classic findings. Cartilage thinning is greatest in the weight-bearing portion ➡, and labral damage is severe ➡.* **(Right)** *Sagittal T1WI FS MR arthrogram in the same patient shows large subchondral cysts located in both the acetabulum and femoral head ➡. As on the coronal image, the complete cartilage loss is apparent ➡, and labral signal and morphology are abnormal ➡.*

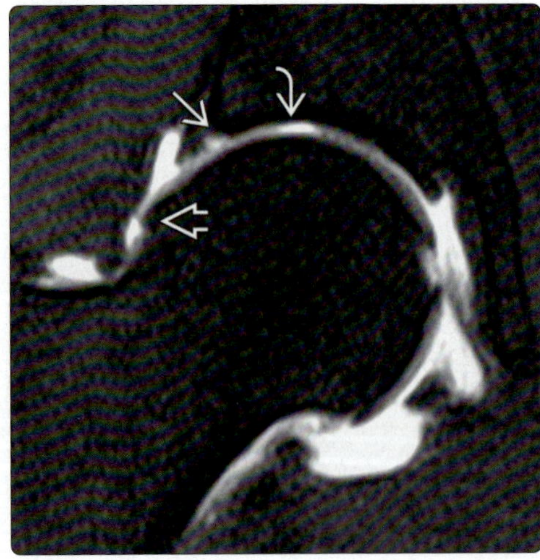

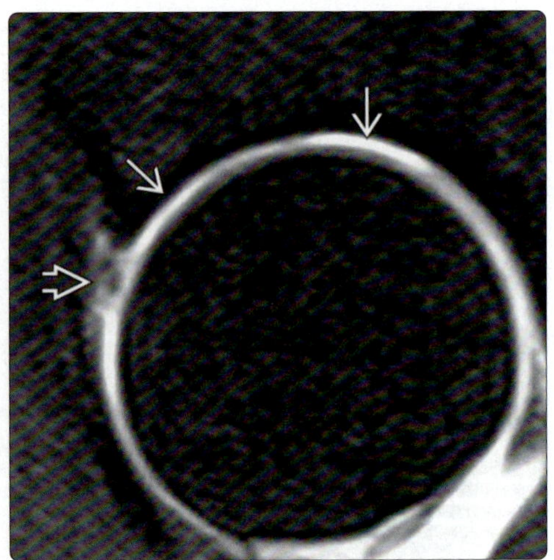

(Left) *Coronal T1WI FS MR arthrogram shows typical femoral acetabular impingement, resulting in OA. This young patient has a lateral femoral neck bump ➡ as well as a focal cartilage defect ➡ and detached labrum ➡.* **(Right)** *Sagittal T1WI FS MR arthrogram in the same patient shows 2 distinct sites of cartilage loss ➡ as well as the detached labrum ➡. It is notable that the radiographs in this case showed only the femoral bump; the extent of early OA was not recognized prior to the MR arthrogram.*

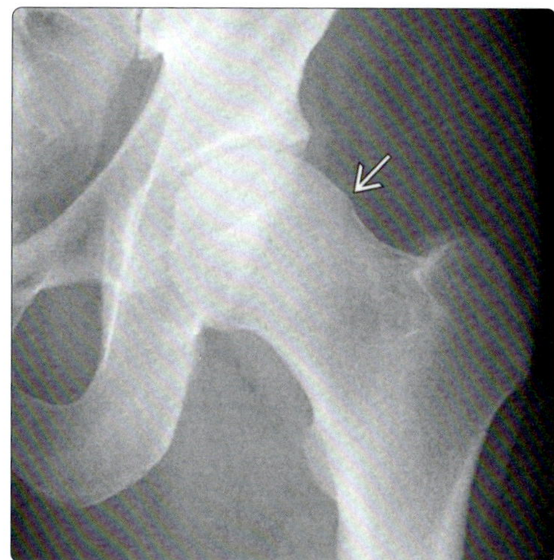

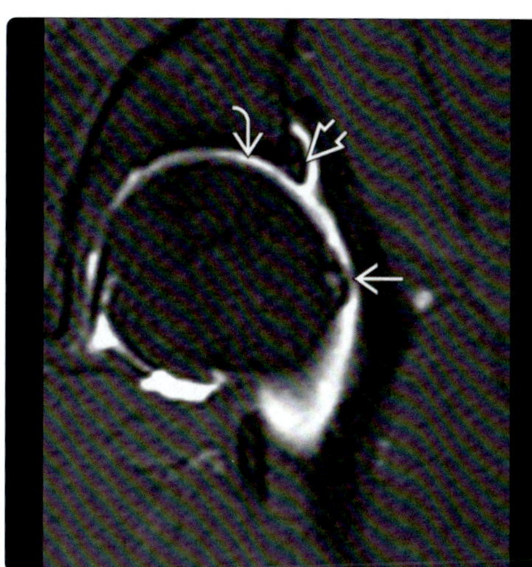

(Left) *AP radiograph shows a lateral bump ➡ at the junction of the femoral head and neck; this appearance has been associated with cam-type femoral acetabular impingement (FAI). There are no other signs of OA.* **(Right)** *Coronal T2WI FS MR arthrogram in the same patient shows that this is a typical case of FAI. The bump is present ➡, along with thinning of the superior cartilage ➡, indicating early OA. The labrum does not appear torn or detached but has signal suggesting degeneration ➡.*

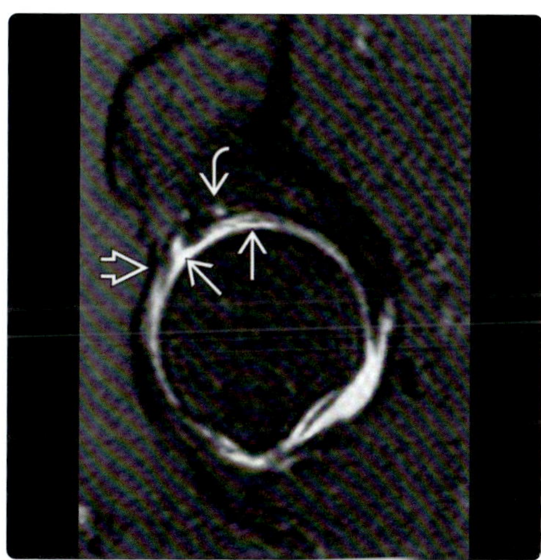

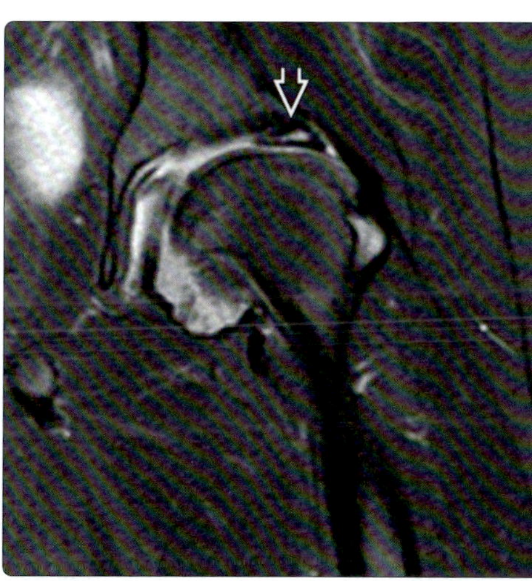

(Left) *Sagittal MR arthrogram in the same patient shows cyst formation ➡ as well as thinning of cartilage ➡. A complex tear is seen in the labrum ➡. The findings are of significant FAI.* **(Right)** *Coronal T2WI FS MR shows a coxa magna deformity. Because the acetabulum shows normal width, the deformity is due to Legg-Calvé-Perthes disease. This results in abnormal articulation and secondary hypertrophy of the labrum. The morphology results in a cam-type FAI; labral tear ➡ is seen.*

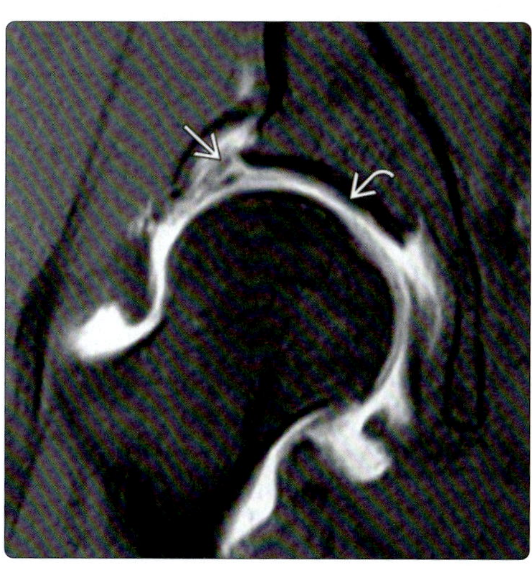

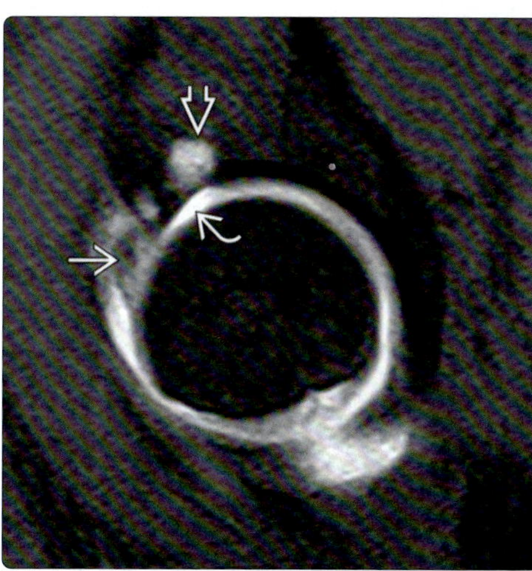

(Left) *Coronal T1WI FS MR shows mild developmental dysplasia of the hip (DDH, note the abnormally low center-edge angle) with a labral tear and detachment ➡. Cartilage irregularity is present throughout the joint ➡.* **(Right)** *Sagittal T1WI FS MR in the same patient shows the full extent of the tear as well appreciated ➡. Focal full-thickness cartilage loss is seen ➡; at this site, a cyst is present within the subchondral bone ➡. Remember the association of DDH with labral tears and early OA; DDH may be subtle.*

KEY FACTS

TERMINOLOGY

- Arthritis developing secondary to cartilage degeneration
  - Results from imbalance between biosynthesis and degradation of cartilage constituents; degradative processes outpace repair
  - Presently defined as productive radiographic changes in combination with joint pain
  - Cartilage loss occurs for several years before there are changes of OA on radiographs; definition may be refined in future

IMAGING

- Radiographic findings for OA
  - Joint space narrowing, commonly medial
  - Osteophytosis, marginal and subchondral
  - Subchondral cysts
  - Malalignment, varus > valgus
- MR findings predictive of early OA
  - Cartilage defects or thinning
  - Bone marrow edema: Thought to correlate with pain in many individuals
  - Meniscal tears or degeneration
  - Cruciate or medial/lateral supporting structure insufficiency
  - High correlation of meniscal tears with adjacent cartilage damage, either focal or diffuse thinning
  - Meniscal extrusion common in advanced OA and correlates with radiographic joint space narrowing

DIAGNOSTIC CHECKLIST

- Early cartilage damage must be sought on all MR exams
  - If there is meniscal tear, search for adjacent cartilage damage
  - Bone marrow edema without traumatic event often signals overlying cartilage damage
- Characterize type of cartilage damage
  - Diffuse, focal, delamination
- Look for subchondral osteophytes

(Left) *Graphic shows moderately advanced osteoarthritis (OA) of the knee. Marginal osteophytes and sclerosis of the subchondral bone show the productive nature of the disease. Cartilaginous defects and loose bodies are present as well.* **(Right)** *AP radiograph shows near-complete cartilage loss in the medial compartment ➡ resulting in varus abnormality. There is slight subchondral sclerosis, but no significant osteophyte formation is seen. This is a typical appearance of moderate OA.*

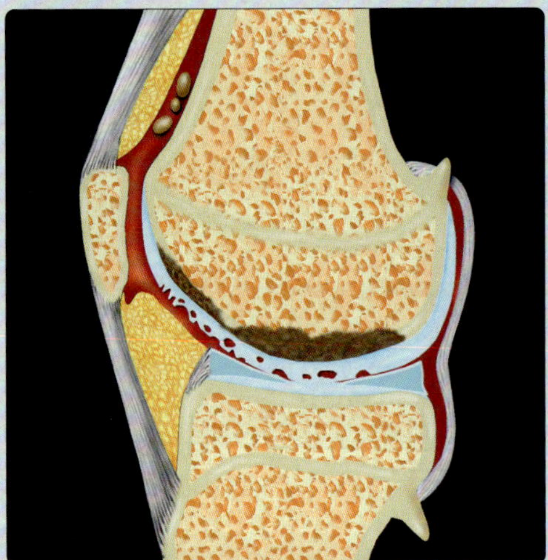

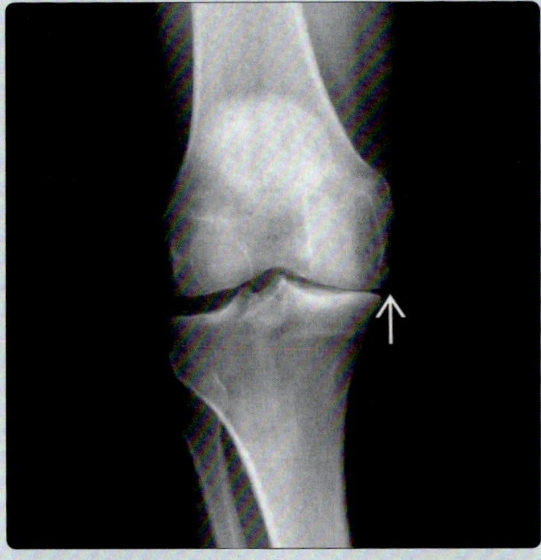

(Left) *AP radiograph shows tiny osteophytes in both the lateral and medial compartments, along with medial cartilage narrowing ➡. In isolation, this might be interpreted as mild osteoarthritis.* **(Right)** *Coronal T2 FS MR in the same patient demonstrates extrusion of the medial meniscus ➡; note that extrusion may be seen with simple OA and does not necessarily imply posterior root tear. There is also complete loss of cartilage on both the medial femoral and tibial condyles ➡.*

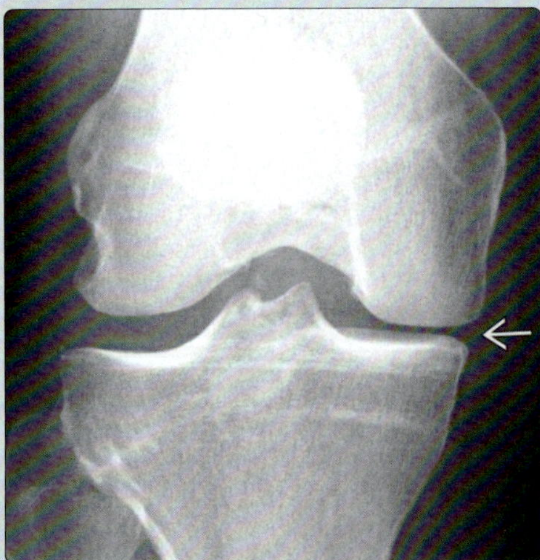

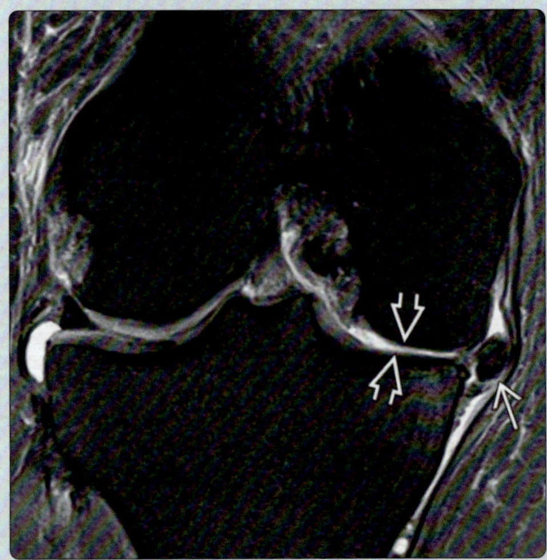

TERMINOLOGY

Abbreviations

- Osteoarthritis (OA)

Synonyms

- Degenerative joint disease (DJD)

Definitions

- Arthritis developing secondary to cartilage degeneration
  - Results from imbalance between biosynthesis and degradation of cartilage constituents; degradative processes outpace repair
  - Presently defined as productive radiographic changes in combination with joint pain
  - Cartilage loss occurs for several years before OA seen on radiograph; definition may be refined in future

IMAGING

General Features

- Best diagnostic clue
  - Radiograph: Joint space narrowing + osteophytes
  - MR: Focal or diffuse cartilage defects ± osteophytes

Radiographic Findings

- Joint space narrowing
  - Frequently evaluated on AP and PA with 15° flexion (notch view), both weight-bearing
    - Medial compartment often 1st or more severely involved
      - Primary lateral involvement is not rare, so should not dissuade one from diagnosis
    - Patellofemoral compartment more severely involved if patient has tracking disorder
- Osteophytosis
  - Marginal and tibial spine is most frequent
  - Subchondral (weight-bearing surface) osteophytes less common but more symptomatic and associated with cartilage damage
- Subchondral cysts
- Malalignment
  - Varus (lateral angulation of joint) is most common; relates to medial compartment cartilage loss
  - Valgus (medial angulation of joint) is less common, relates to lateral compartment cartilage loss
  - Patellar subluxation, usually lateral, relates to tracking disorder
- Normal bone density
- Chondrocalcinosis, especially in hyaline cartilage, may be seen in end-stage OA

MR Findings

- T1WI
  - Particularly useful for identifying osteophytosis
    - Watch for subchondral osteophytes; these result in greater cartilage damage than marginal ones
- Fluid-sensitive sequences
  - Cartilage: Multiple specialized imaging sequences
    - Cartilage usually assessed adequately in clinical setting with routine PDWI FS and T2WI FS
  - Bone marrow edema (hyperintense): Thought to correlate with pain in many individuals
    - Watch for increasing number and size of lesions, but correlation with pain is not strict
    - Progressive marrow edema associated with high risk of cartilage loss in same region
  - Menisci
    - Meniscal tear or degeneration is seen best on PD
      - High correlation with adjacent cartilage damage, either focal or diffuse thinning
    - Meniscal extrusion common in advanced OA and correlates with radiographic joint space narrowing
  - Ligamentous injury
    - Watch for cruciate or medial/lateral supporting structure insufficiency
    - Instability → mechanical trauma to cartilage
  - Thickened plica associated with cartilage injury
  - Subchondral cysts: 45% prevalence in OA
    - Communicating cysts adjacent to cartilage defect
      - 33% prevalence in severe OA
    - Noncommunicating interspinous tibial cysts
      - 38.5% prevalence in severe OA
      - Likely secondary to repetitive cruciate stress

Imaging Recommendations

- Best imaging tool
  - Radiograph for mild to moderate OA
  - MR for early cartilage degradation, prior to development of osteophytes

DIFFERENTIAL DIAGNOSIS

Pyrophosphate Arthropathy

- Chondrocalcinosis (may be present in OA as well)
- Predominant patellofemoral disease (in absence of tracking abnormality)

PATHOLOGY

General Features

- Etiology
  - Trauma
    - Unclear whether repetitive trauma (e.g., long distance running) contributes to OA of knee
      - Study shows tendency toward rapid recovery of cartilaginous and meniscal volumes 1 hour post 20 km run (menisci lag cartilage recovery)
      - One 10-year study shows long distance runners to not incur permanent damage without significant preexisting damage
    - Direct trauma may lead to focal cartilage defect or delamination
    - Ligamentous instability or meniscal tears
      - Chronic instability from cruciate disruption or medial/lateral supporting structures → mechanical trauma → OA
      - OA occurs frequently 10-20 years after anterior cruciate or meniscal tear
      - Isolated medial posterior meniscal root tear associated with incident & progressive medial tibiofemoral cartilage loss
  - Normal aging of cartilage

Cartilage Damage Classification Systems

Gross Description	MR (Modified Outerbridge)	Surgical Evaluation (Outerbridge)	Arthroscopic Evaluation (Noyes)
Normal	Grade 0	Grade 0	Grade 0
Cartilage swelling, softening; intact surface	Grade I: T2 signal alteration with intact surface	Grade I: Softening and swelling	Grade IA: Moderate softening
			Grade IB: Extensive softening and swelling of articular surface
Superficial fragmentation and fissuring	Grade II: Surface irregularity extending < 50% of depth	Fragmentation and fissuring ≤ 0.5 inch diameter	Grade IIA: Surface irregularity < 1/2 cartilage thickness
Deep fragmentation and fissuring	Grade III: Defect extends to deep 50% of cartilage thickness	Fragmentation and fissuring > 0.5 inch diameter	Grade IIB: Surface irregularity > 1/2 cartilage thickness
Exposed bone	Grade IV: Exposed bone	Grade IV: Exposed bone	Grade IIIA: Exposed bone
			Grade IIIB: Cavitation or erosion of exposed bone

Adapted from Mosher TJ et al: Degenerative Disease. In Pope et al: Imaging of the Musculoskeletal System. Philadelphia: Saunders, 2008.

  - Chondrocytes ↓ in number, ↓ production of proteoglycans → ↑ brittleness of collagen matrix
  - ↑ tumor necrosis factor and interleukin in OA
    - Increases degradative enzymes
- Abnormal morphology
  - Patellar tracking abnormality → patellofemoral OA
  - Metaphyseal or epiphyseal dysplasia → early OA
- Genetic mutations of type II cartilage collagen gene
  - Syndromes that show premature onset of OA
- Low levels of estrogen have been associated with ↑ risk of OA

Gross Pathologic & Surgical Features

- Bone is richly innervated and may be source of knee pain in many patients

CLINICAL ISSUES

Presentation

- Most common signs/symptoms
  - Pain with activity, not at rest
  - Crepitus, locking
  - Varus or valgus deformity

Demographics

- Epidemiology
  - 25% of adults age > 55 experience frequent knee pain
    - 1/2 of these have radiographic OA; others may only have early signs, visible only on MR
  - Framingham study: Symptomatic knee OA in 6.1% of adults age > 30
    - Incidental meniscal findings on MR are common in general population & ↑ with age

Natural History & Prognosis

- Knee pain is common; identifying which patients will progress to functional debilitating OA is not easy
  - Generic factors show reasonable correlation with outcome: Body mass index, severity of pain at presentation, mood disturbance
  - Clinical history, physical examination, and severity of radiographic OA are all of limited predictive value

Treatment

- NSAIDs and physical therapy
- Intraarticular glucocorticoid injection
- Intraarticular hyaluronic acid injection
  - Several studies show good clinical response relative to placebo in knee (but not other joints)
- Focal cartilage repair options
  - Microfracture: Drilling of cartilage, hoping to induce fibrocartilage formation
  - Autologous chondrocyte graft: Chondrocytes grown in lab, injected under periosteal sleeve into defect
  - Autologous osteochondral transplant: Transplanted plugs of cartilage and bone, usually from trochlea
  - Cadaver osteochondral transplant
- Altered weight-bearing
  - High tibial osteotomy introduces varus or valgus to change weight-bearing to lateral or medial compartment, respectively
- Total knee arthroplasty

DIAGNOSTIC CHECKLIST

Image Interpretation Pearls

- Early cartilage damage must be sought on all MRs
  - If meniscal tear, search for adjacent cartilage damage
  - Bone marrow edema without traumatic event often signals underlying cartilage damage

Reporting Tips

- Characterize type of cartilage damage
  - Diffuse, focal, delamination
- Look for subchondral osteophytes

SELECTED REFERENCES

1. Alizai H et al: Cartilage lesion score: comparison of a quantitative assessment score with established semiquantitative MR scoring systems. Radiology. 271(2):479-87, 2014
2. Guermazi A et al: Medial posterior meniscal root tears are associated with development or worsening of medial tibiofemoral cartilage damage: the multicenter osteoarthritis study. Radiology. 268(3):814-21, 2013
3. Kijowski R et al: Evaluation of the articular cartilage of the knee joint: value of adding a T2 mapping sequence to a routine MR imaging protocol. Radiology. 267(2):503-13, 2013

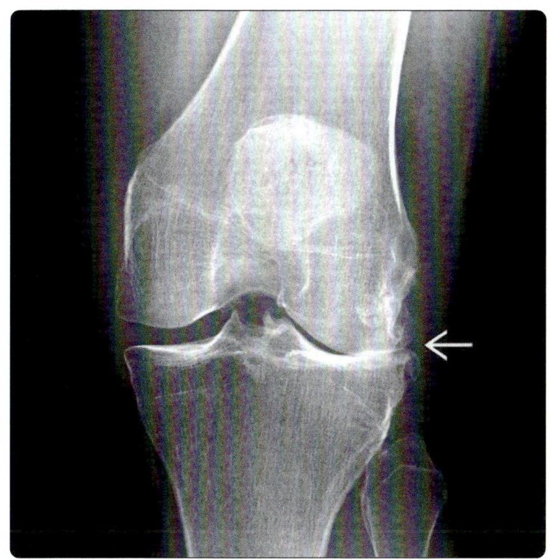

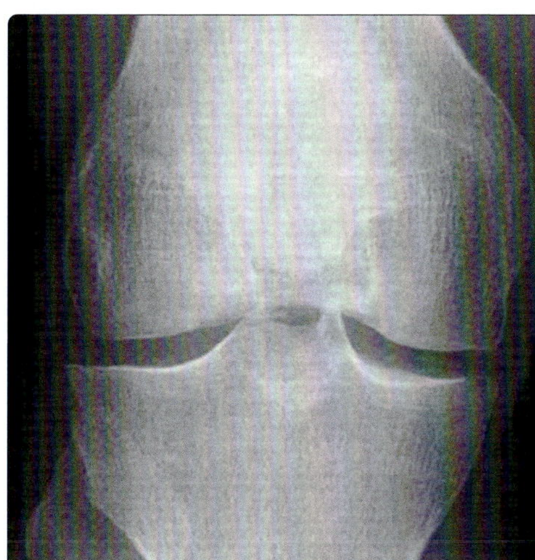

(Left) *AP radiograph shows lateral compartment OA ➡. Osteophytes and complete cartilage loss are seen with valgus deformity. Although medial compartment involvement is considered typical of OA, lateral compartment predominance may be seen.* **(Right)** *AP radiograph shows a case of early OA related purely to osteophyte formation. The radiograph is weight-bearing and shows no malalignment or significant cartilage loss. There are osteophytes seen on the tibial spines but not elsewhere.*

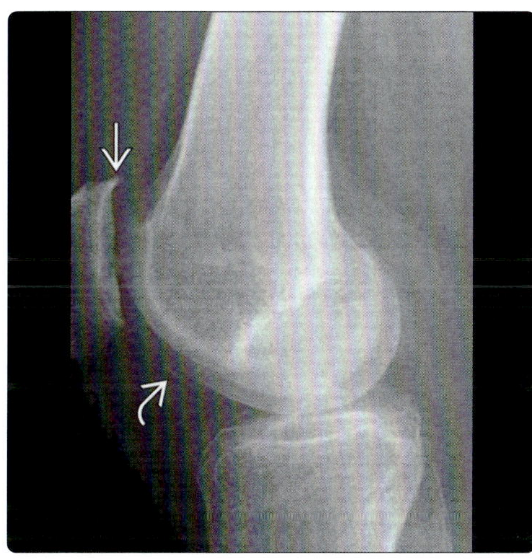

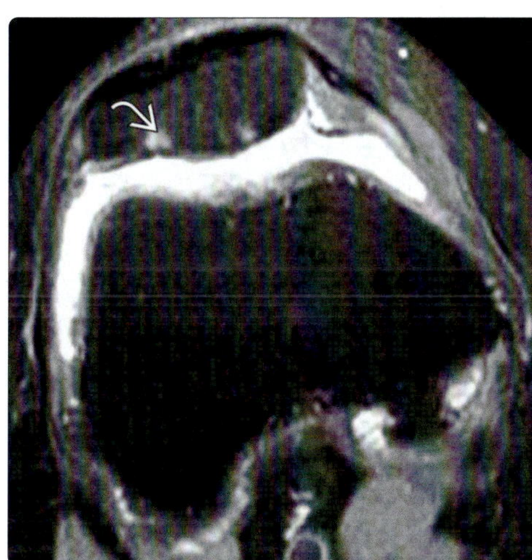

(Left) *Lateral radiograph in the same patient shows patellar osteophytes ➡. There is also a subchondral osteophyte on the femoral condylar surface ➡. Subchondral osteophytes often have an associated focal cartilage defect, as was proven on MR in this case. Note that no loose bodies are seen.* **(Right)** *Axial PD MR in the same patient shows complete cartilage loss involving both patellar facets ➡. This severe disease may be surprising, juxtaposed with the less impressive radiographs.*

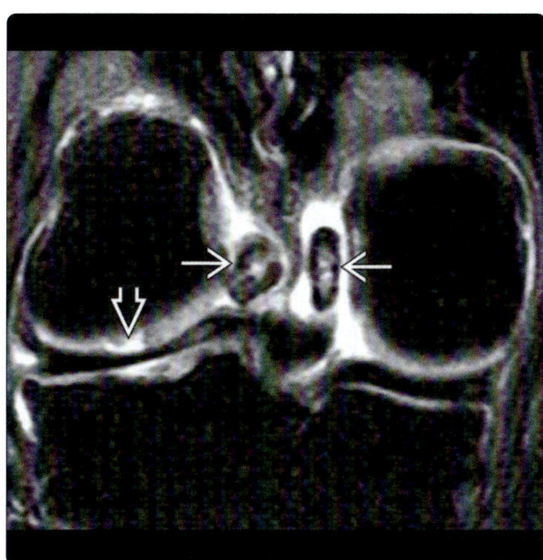

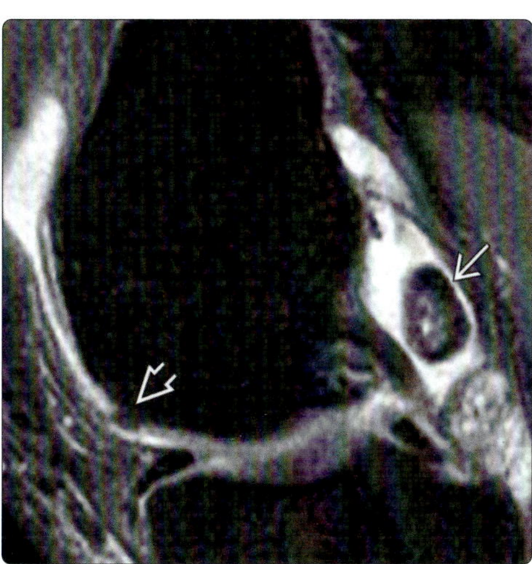

(Left) *Coronal PD FS MR in the same patient shows loose bodies ➡ not seen on radiograph. There is a deep focal cartilage defect ➡.* **(Right)** *Sagittal PD FS MR in the same patient demonstrates another loose body ➡. There is a subchondral osteophyte with cartilage defect ➡. The stabilizing structures were intact. The early OA relates to the loose bodies and subchondral osteophytes with their associated cartilage defects. These findings are not seen on radiograph so MR is valuable in this case.*

(Left) *AP radiograph shows medial cartilage narrowing and a sizable subchondral osteophyte ➡, with only minimal marginal osteophytes.* **(Right)** *Sagittal T2WI FS MR in the same patient is located slightly medial to the subchondral osteophyte, but shows the extensive loss of cartilage along the weight-bearing portion of the medial femoral condyle ➡, along with signs of delamination. Subchondral osteophytes signal significant associated cartilage damage.*

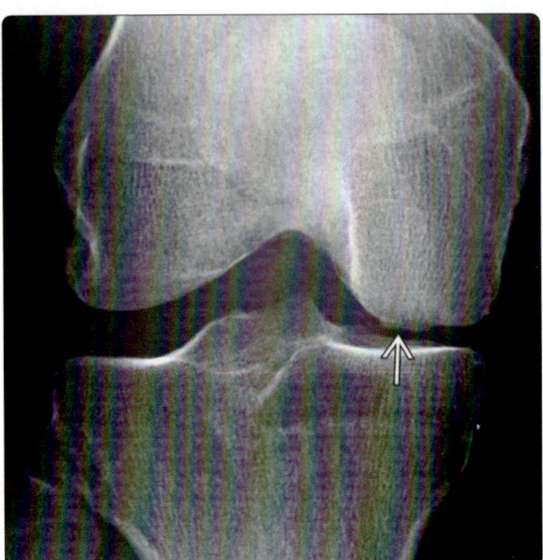

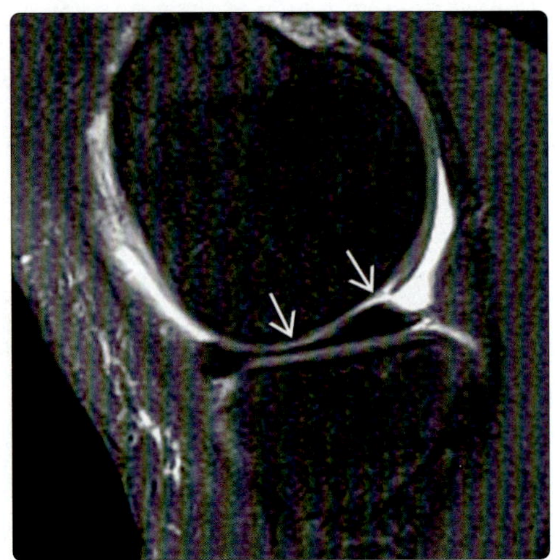

(Left) *Sagittal T2WI FS MR shows a large trochlear cartilage defect ➡ along with marrow edema. It is important to inspect the trochlear regions carefully, and it can be difficult to evaluate the extent of trochlear damage since the surface is usually not orthogonal to the plane of imaging.* **(Right)** *Arthroscopic photograph shows the large, full-thickness defect at the trochlea of the same patient, prior to attempted cartilage repair procedure.*

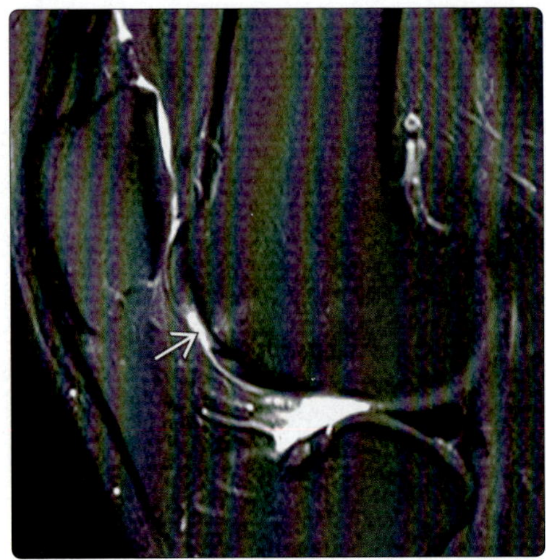

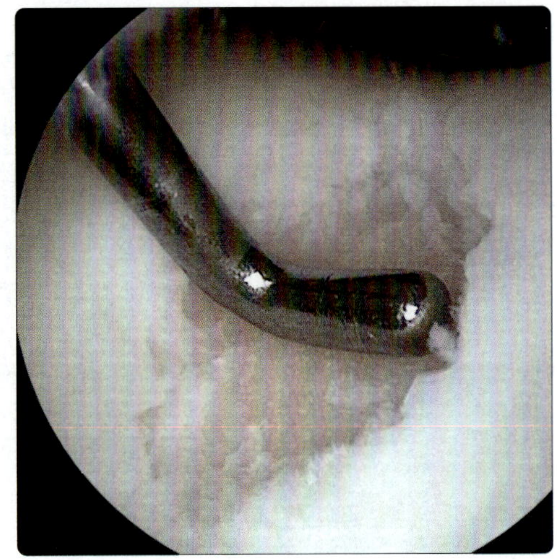

(Left) *Axial T2WI FS MR shows a focal fissure of the patellar cartilage at the apex ➡, reaching the subchondral bone. Note the defect extends laterally at the bone plate ➡; delamination should be a concern here.* **(Right)** *Axial T2WI FS MR demonstrates increased signal intensity and partial thickness cartilage loss, predominantly on the lateral facet of the patella, particularly well seen due to the effusion. There is also underlying bone edema ➡. The cartilage abnormality is grade II to III.*

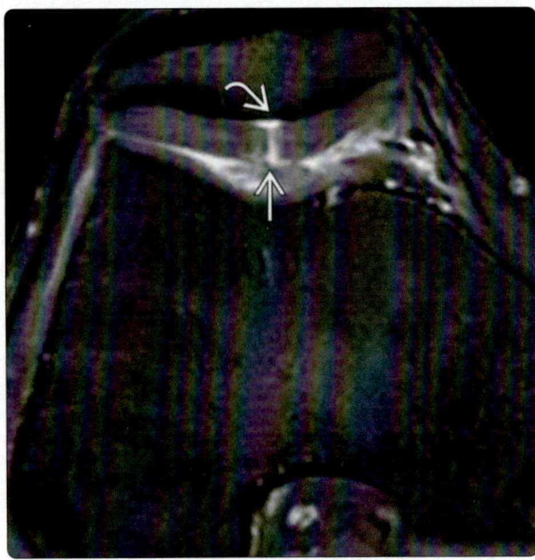

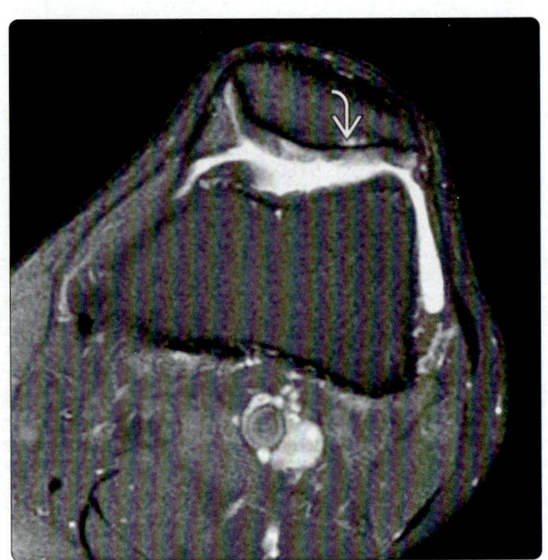

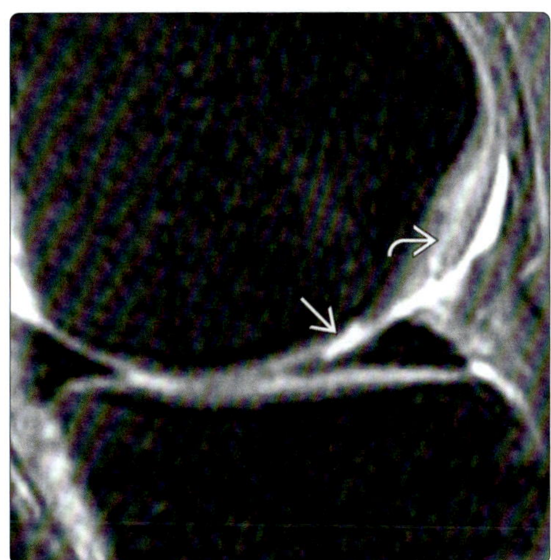

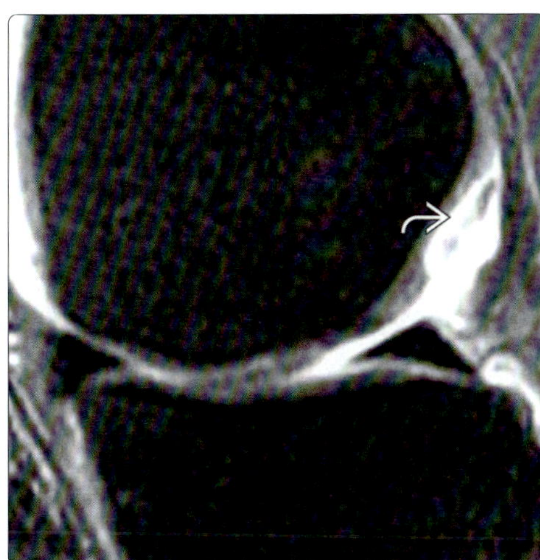

(Left) *Sagittal T2WI FS demonstrates a focal cartilage defect* ➔*. It is important to not overlook the linear high signal in the more posterior portion of the femoral condyle* ↪*; this heralds delamination.* **(Right)** *Sagittal T2WI FS in the same patient shows the delamination of a large portion of femoral condylar cartilage to much better advantage* ↪*. This patient had normal radiographs but most certainly has osteoarthritis.*

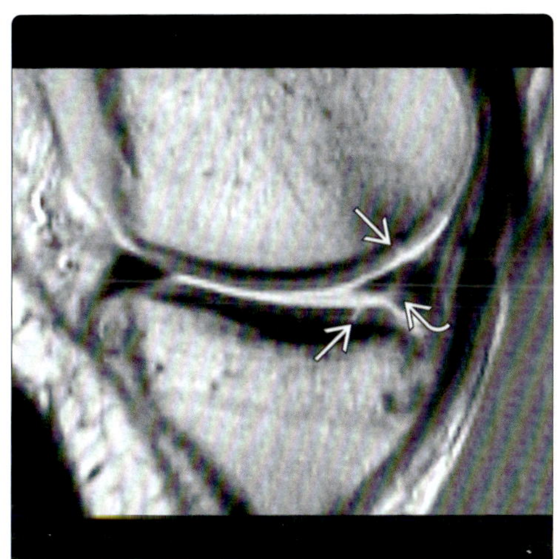

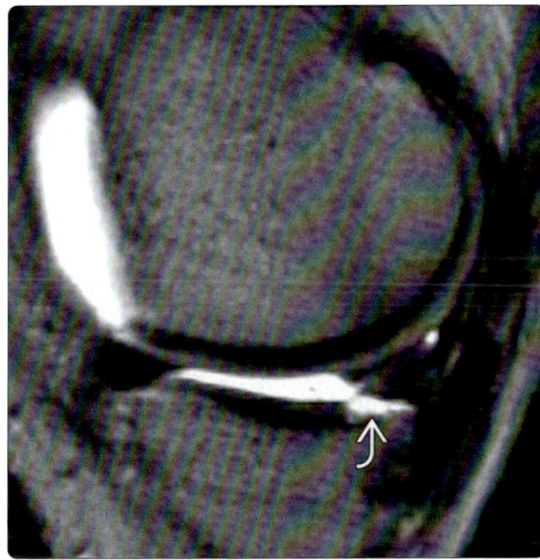

(Left) *Sagittal PD MR shows a tear of the posterior horn, medial meniscus* ↪*, and the blunt posterior horn suggests chronicity. Cartilaginous defects and thinning are seen* ➔*.* **(Right)** *Sagittal T2WI MR in the same patient shows the tibial osteochondral defect even more prominently because it is outlined by fluid* ↪*. This large defect puts this young patient at risk for early OA. Remember that meniscal tears are often associated with adjacent chondral defects, which should be actively sought.*

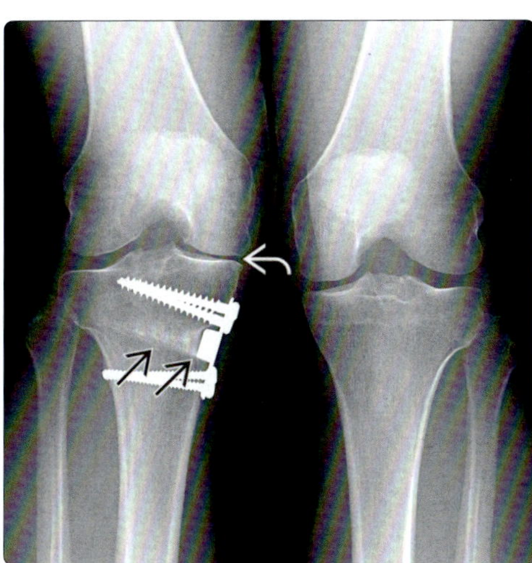

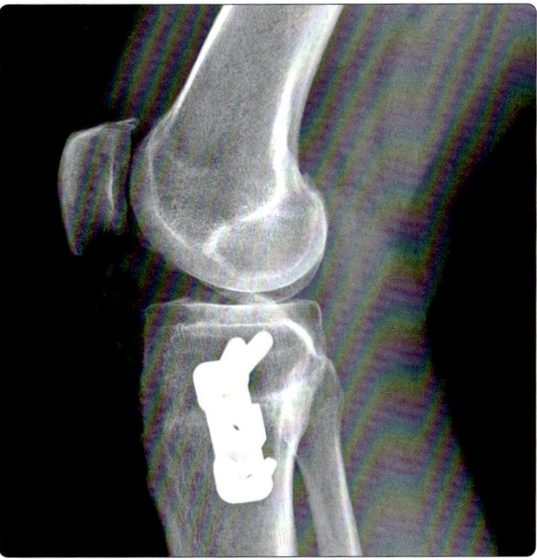

(Left) *AP radiograph shows medial compartment OA* ↪*. The patient has undergone tibial opening wedge osteotomy, with the wedge placed medially* ⇨ *to promote increased lateral compartment weight-bearing.* **(Right)** *Lateral radiograph in the same patient shows the wedge osteotomy and plate/screws. This procedure is employed in relatively young patients with single compartment OA, with the hope that reducing weight-bearing in that compartment yet retaining motion may induce fibrocartilage repair.*

Ankylosing Spondylitis

KEY FACTS

IMAGING

- Radiographs show more advanced disease
  - Spine
    - Osteopenia: Diffuse, especially with fusion
    - Sacroiliitis: Usually bilaterally symmetric
    - Osteitis at anterior corners of vertebral bodies
    - Eventual long column fusion of bodies and facets
      - "Bamboo spine" with dagger sign
  - Remainder of axial skeleton
    - Erosions and eventual fusion: Sternoclavicular, costochondral, costovertebral, pubis
  - Peripheral disease: Usually hip and shoulder
- MR shows earliest changes
  - High signal enthesopathy may be earliest sign
  - Romanus lesions: Inflammatory change (high signal) at vertebral body corners
- CT most useful in evaluating for subtle transverse fracture following trauma

CLINICAL ISSUES

- 0.1% prevalence
- ↑ prevalence in some Native American populations
- Less prevalent in African Americans than Caucasians
- M > F (M:F = 2.5-5:1)
- Peak age of onset: 15-30 years

DIAGNOSTIC CHECKLIST

- Earliest signs on MR easily overlooked
  - Thin syndesmophytes more easily recognized on radiograph than CT/MR
  - Must watch for other sites of abnormality to suggest diagnosis: Enthesopathy, Romanus lesions
- Be suspicious for AS in young males with low back pain
- Following even minor trauma in patient with AS, must perform CT to evaluate for fracture
  - If fractured, MR to evaluate spinal cord
  - High morbidity/mortality rate for these patients when admitted to ER with fracture

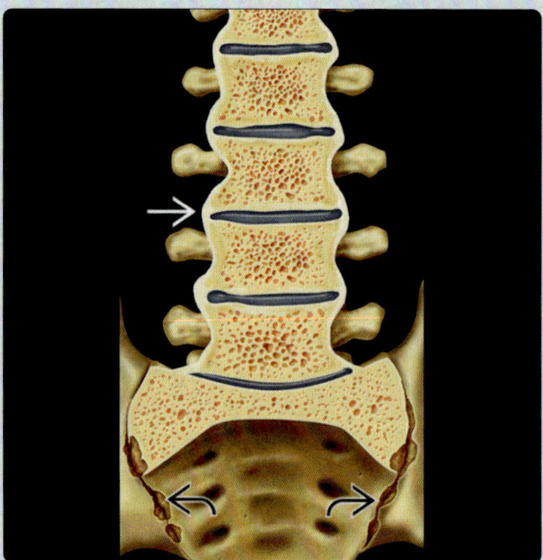

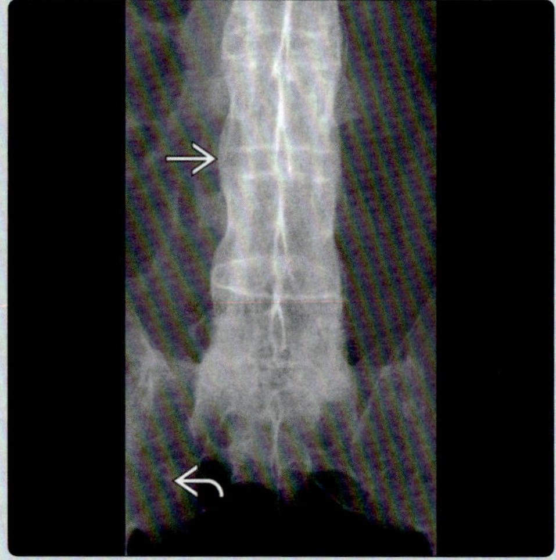

(Left) *Coronal graphic illustrates the findings of advanced ankylosing spondylitis. The vertical syndesmophytes appear to undulate ➡, and there is a solid column fusion ("bamboo spine"). The sacroiliac (SI) joints show symmetric erosive disease ↩.* **(Right)** *AP radiograph is immediately recognizable as a case of AS. The bridging vertical syndesmophytes ➡ show column fusion and associated diffuse osteoporosis. The inferior SI joints are eroded ↩ and undergoing early fusion.*

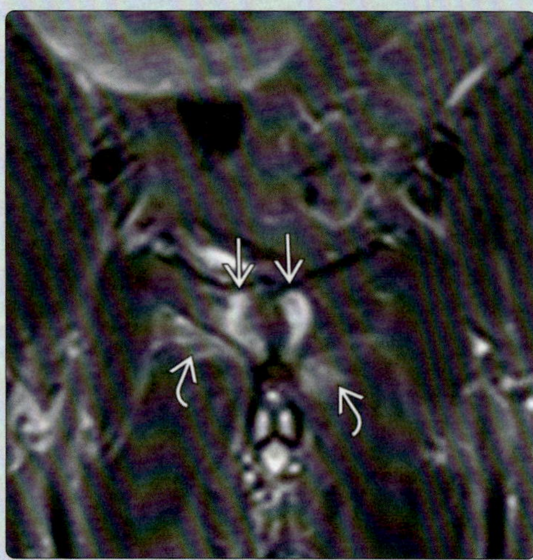

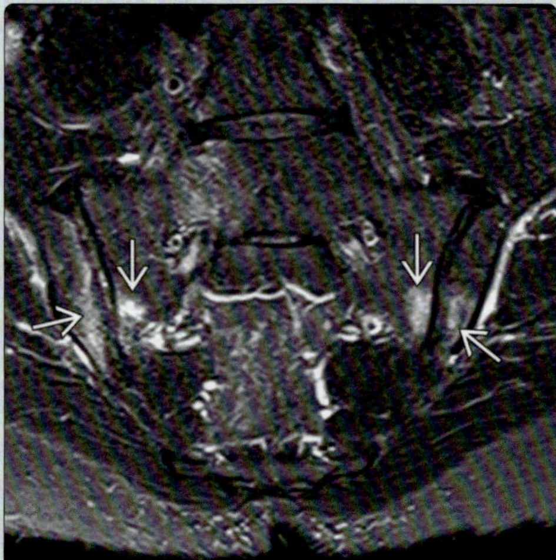

(Left) *Coronal T2 FS MR in a 45-year-old man with known AS shows hyperintense SI at the pubic symphysis ➡ as well as at the adductors bilaterally ↩. This appearance suggests an athletic pubalgia from sports injury; however, he did not exercise more vigorously than using an elliptical machine. Remember that AS may demonstrate enthesitis and periostitis, as seen here.* **(Right)** *Oblique coronal T2 FS MR, same patient, shows abnormal SI on both sides of the SI joints ➡, typical of active inflammation in AS or other spondyloarthropathies.*

TERMINOLOGY

Abbreviations

- Ankylosing spondylitis (AS)

Definitions

- Inflammatory arthropathy and enthesopathy with predilection for axial skeleton

IMAGING

General Features

- Best diagnostic clue
  - Thin vertical syndesmophytes with concomitant bilateral sacroiliitis
- Location
  - Sacroiliac joints (SIJ): Synovial portion (lower 1/2-1/3)
  - Vertebral column
    - Anterior corners vertebral bodies
    - Anterior fibers annulus fibrosus; eventually anterior longitudinal ligament involved
    - Lumbar predominance in 1st 20 years of disease
      - Post 20 years, cervical spine equally involved
    - Conventional wisdom: Spondylosis starts at lumbosacral or thoracolumbar junction and progresses, without skipping segments
      - Do not use this to eliminate diagnosis, especially early in disease
      - MR shows by location of Romanus lesions that this is not invariable; much more diffuse involvement, with skips, early in disease
  - Peripheral: Proximal large joints (hips, shoulders)
  - Entheses: Axial and proximal appendicular location

Imaging Recommendations

- Best imaging tool
  - Moderate to advanced disease: Radiograph
  - Early disease: MR
  - Complications of trauma: CT, perhaps with MR
- Protocol advice
  - MR SIJs: Oblique coronal STIR and with contrast

Radiographic Findings

- Osteopenia: Diffuse, especially with fusion
- Axial disease
  - Sacroiliitis
    - Bilateral symmetric most common (86%)
      - Early in disease may be asymmetric
    - Erosions and widening; eventual fusion
  - Spine
    - Thin vertical syndesmophytes form in outer fibers of annulus fibrosus
    - Osteitis at anterior corners of vertebral bodies
      - Fluffy amorphous bone → "shiny corners"
      - Resorption of corners → squaring of body
    - Eventual long column fusion of bodies and facets
      - "Bamboo spine" with dagger sign
      - Complete fusion in 28% with AS > 30 years, 43% with AS > 40 years
    - Fusion + osteoporosis puts spine at risk for transverse fracture from mild trauma
      - "Carrot stick" fracture; often nondisplaced
      - Difficult to visualize on radiograph
      - Often at C-T or T-L junctions
      - Usually involves 3 columns; injury to posterior osteoligamentous component is hallmark
    - May have atlantoaxial subluxation
  - Other axial joints: Erosions and eventual fusion
    - Sternoclavicular, costochondral, costovertebral
- Peripheral disease
  - Usually large joints (hip > shoulder)
  - Often asymmetric side-to-side
  - Cartilage loss
  - May have either erosive or bony productive change
    - Osteophytes on hip may suggest lateral femoral head/neck bumps
    - Do not mistake for cam-type morphology of femoral acetabular impingement
  - More distal peripheral disease less common or seen with inadequate treatment
- Enthesopathy: Interspinous ligaments & around pelvis

CT Findings

- CT most useful in evaluating for subtle transverse fracture following trauma; sagittal/coronal reformats required

MR Findings

- T1WI
  - Romanus lesions: Low signal triangular edema at corners of vertebral bodies
  - SI joint marrow edema (low signal)
  - More chronic Romanus and SI joint lesions develop fatty marrow changes (high signal)
  - Once anterior syndesmophytes are mature and thick, high signal marrow is seen within them
- Fluid-sensitive sequences
  - Early high signal enthesopathy may be earliest sign
    - Watch interspinous ligaments, iliac spines, greater and lesser trochanters, pubic rami
  - Romanus lesions: Inflammatory change (high signal) at vertebral body corners
    - Often seen prior to syndesmophyte formation and heralds their formation
    - Easily overlooked or presumed to be degenerative
    - Chronic lesions replaced by fat
  - Anderson lesions: Same as Romanus but located more centrally at discovertebral junction
  - Low signal syndesmophytes themselves are difficult to see on MR until thickened significantly
  - Watch for transverse fracture in fused column
    - High signal ligament and cord damage
  - Synovial portions of SIJs show high signal
    - Coronal oblique sequences most useful
- T1 FS post contrast shows enhancement of
  - Active Romanus and Anderson lesions
  - Active enthesopathy
  - Early SIJ synovitis best seen post contrast

DIFFERENTIAL DIAGNOSIS

Inflammatory Bowel Disease Arthritis

- Identical appearance of sacroiliitis and spondylitis
- Identical peripheral joint disease and distribution

Psoriatic Spondyloarthropathy

- Generally, bilateral asymmetric sacroiliitis
- Bulky asymmetric paravertebral ossification
- Normal bone density
- Peripheral joint distribution: Hands > other sites

Chronic Reactive Arthritis

- Generally, bilateral asymmetric sacroiliitis
- Bulky asymmetric paravertebral ossification
- Normal bone density
- Peripheral joint distribution: Feet > other sites

Osteoarthritis

- Vertebral body osteophytes arise slightly further from disc and are directed more horizontally than syndesmophytes
- Degenerative endplate changes may mimic Romanus lesions on MR; generally more broad in shape and associated with degenerative disc disease
- Associated disc disease and facet osteoarthritis
- Sclerosis and marginal osteophytes at SI joints
- Normal bone density

Diffuse Idiopathic Skeletal Hyperostosis

- Anterior flowing ossification of ligament rather than formation of syndesmophytes
- Generally, no involvement of facet joints
- No true sacroiliitis; ossification of nonsynovial superior portion of SI joint
- Normal bone density

Femoral Acetabular Impingement

- Lateral femoral neck bumps in cam-type morphology resemble osteophytes in AS but no sacroiliitis in FAI

PATHOLOGY

General Features

- Genetics
  - Strong multigenic inherited component
  - HLA-B27 is strongest association
    - HLA(+) in > 90% of Caucasians with AS
    - HLA(+) in only 50% of African Americans with AS
    - AS develops in 1-2% of HLA(+) individuals
    - 20% risk of AS if HLA(+) & 1st-degree relative with AS

CLINICAL ISSUES

Presentation

- Most common signs/symptoms
  - Insidious onset low back pain and stiffness
  - Asymmetric oligoarticular peripheral disease
  - ↓ chest expansion (< 4 cm)

Demographics

- Age
  - Peak onset: 15-30 years
- Gender
  - M > F (M:F = 2.5-5:1)
    - Females likely underdiagnosed
      - Less axial and hip disease in females
      - More peripheral joint involvement, osteitis pubis, and isolated cervical spine disease
- Ethnicity
  - ↑ prevalence in Native American populations (5%)
  - Less prevalent in African Americans than Caucasians
- Epidemiology
  - 0.1% prevalence

Natural History & Prognosis

- With therapy, majority maintain spinal mobility
- Often require hip or knee arthroplasty
- Romanus lesions on MR are predictive of formation of syndesmophytes
  - Treatment with anti-TNF-α may resolve MR evidence of inflammation but does not seem to affect likelihood of syndesmophyte formation at those sites
- Postural change (severe thoracic kyphosis and decreased lumbar lordosis) if untreated
- Untreated uveitis → loss of vision
- Overall survival comparable to general population
- Juvenile-onset AS has minor differences compared with adult-onset AS
  - Less severe axial involvement by radiograph
  - ↑ hip involvement with ↑ need for arthroplasty
  - Slightly higher proportion of women
  - Similar functional outcomes
- At risk for spine fracture with minor trauma; must CT
  - Spinal cord at risk; even if fx nondisplaced, must MR
  - On admission, 67% of AS patients with spine fracture have neurologic deficits
    - Secondary deterioration occurs frequently
  - Mortality rate within 3 months after injury = 17.7%

Treatment

- Aimed at decreasing pain and stiffness, maintaining posture and mobility
- Anti-TNF-α: Promising but only short follow-up in studies thus far
  - Dramatic improvement in symptoms and spinal mobility
  - Not clear if it modifies disease progression

DIAGNOSTIC CHECKLIST

Consider

- Syndesmophytes more easily recognized on radiograph than CT/MR
  - Must look carefully for these on CT/MR
  - Must watch for other sites of abnormality to suggest diagnosis: Enthesopathy, Romanus lesions
  - Be suspicious for AS in young males with back pain
- Following even minor trauma in patient with AS, must perform CT or MR to evaluate for fracture

Image Interpretation Pearls

- Earliest signs on MR easily overlooked
  - High signal enthesopathy
  - Romanus lesions: High signal, enhancing vertebral corner lesions when active

SELECTED REFERENCES

1. Canella C et al: MRI in seronegative spondyloarthritis: imaging features and differential diagnosis in the spine and sacroiliac joints. AJR Am J Roentgenol. 200(1):149-57, 2013

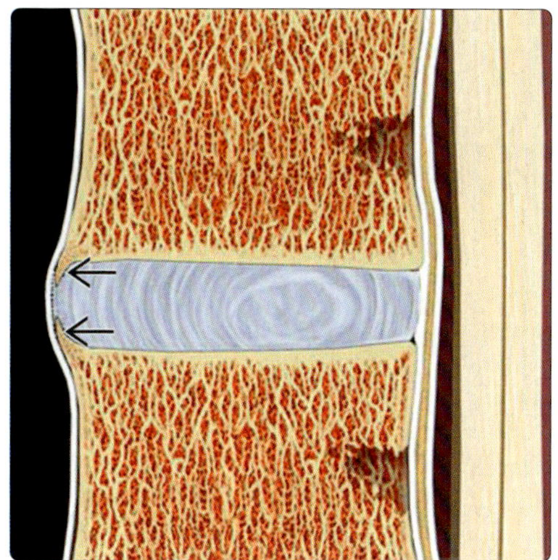

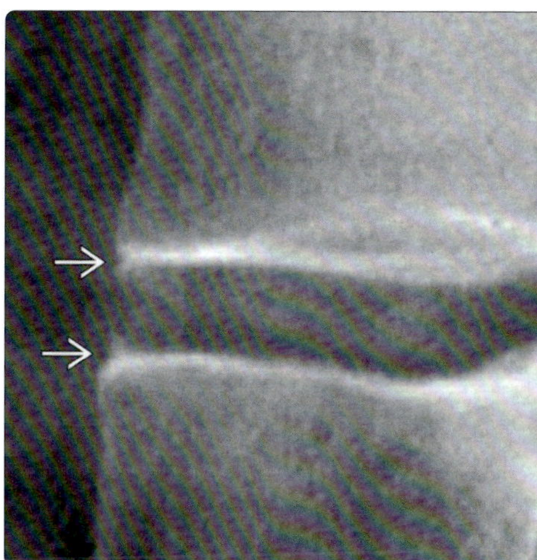

(Left) *Sagittal cut graphic through vertebral bodies demonstrates thin vertical syndesmophytes forming in the annulus fibrosus of adjacent bodies ➡. It is these syndesmophytes that eventually fuse, resulting in body ankylosis.* **(Right)** *Lateral radiograph matches the graphic, showing the earliest radiographic signs of actual syndesmophyte formation ➡. These bony projections generally are better seen on lateral than AP view. Note that there is no squaring or sclerosis of the bodies.*

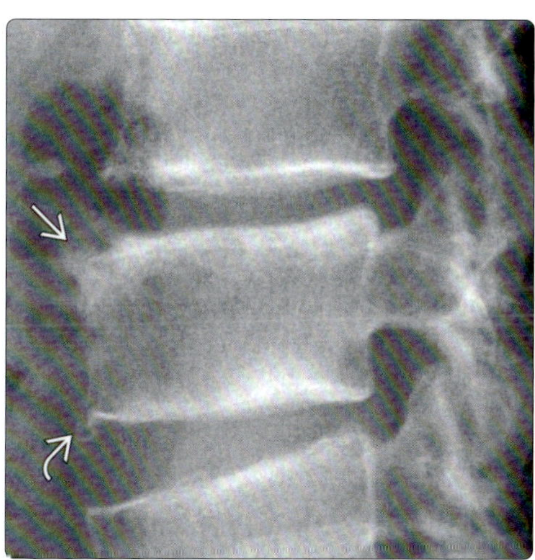

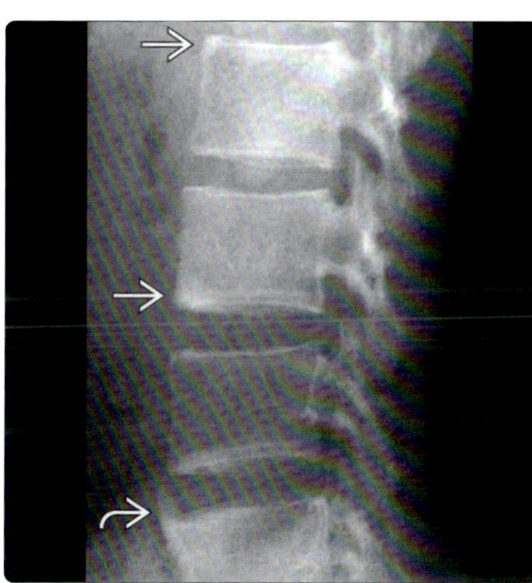

(Left) *Lateral radiograph shows 2 sites of syndesmophyte formation. The 1st shows amorphous bone production that has not yet formed a syndesmophyte ➡, while the 2nd shows a well-defined, more mature syndesmophyte containing marrow ➡.* **(Right)** *Lateral radiograph shows osteitis, or "shiny corners," at 2 vertebral bodies ➡. Note the squaring of the bodies. There is a vertical syndesmophyte seen at a lower lever ➡; all are typical findings of ankylosing spondylitis.*

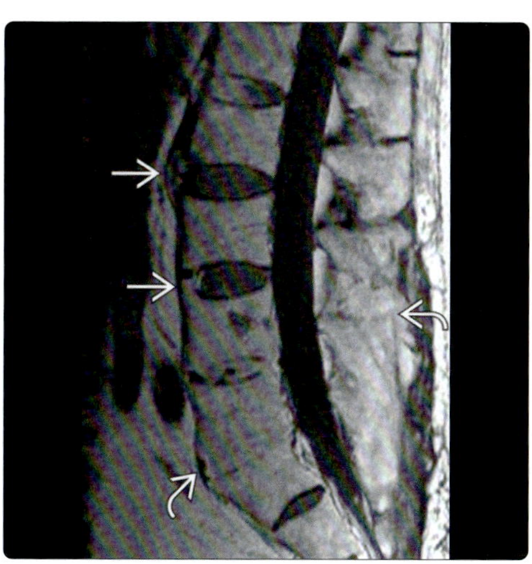

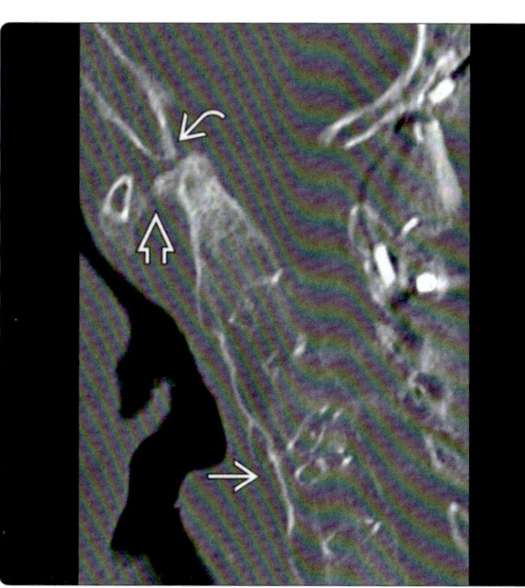

(Left) *Sagittal T1WI MR shows advanced AS, with ossification of the ALL as well as syndesmophyte formation ➡. Several levels of posterior element as well as body ankylosis are seen ➡. These advanced findings might be overlooked if only disc disease is evaluated.* **(Right)** *Sagittal bone CT shows AS, with osteoporosis and long column fusion ➡. Hyperostosis at the odontoid and anterior arch of C1 ➡ as well as atlantoaxial subluxation ➡, as seen here, are not unusual findings in AS.*

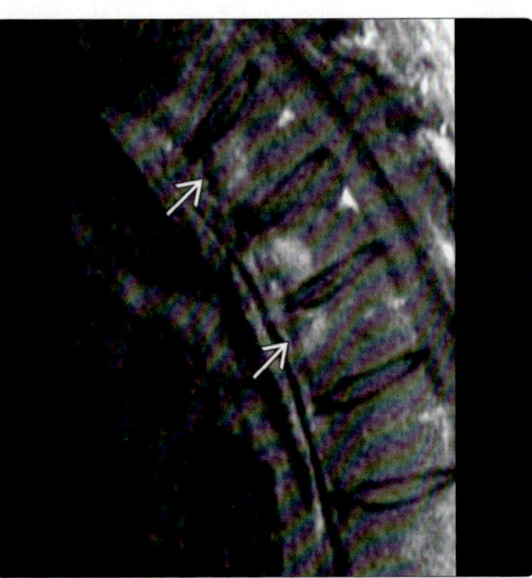

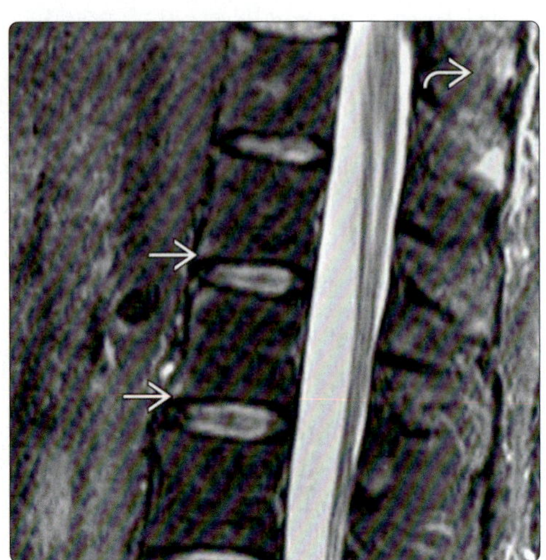

(Left) *Sagittal STIR MR shows advanced Romanus lesions ➡. The anterior corner sites of osteitis are prominently seen; the patient does not yet have syndesmophytes.* **(Right)** *Sagittal T2WI FS MR in a different patient shows more subtle Romanus lesions at the anterior corners ➡. The radiographs were normal, and it may be easy to overlook these early abnormalities on MR. However, other hints may be present. In this case, there is edema within the intraspinous ligaments ➡, another early abnormality indicating enthesitis in AS.*

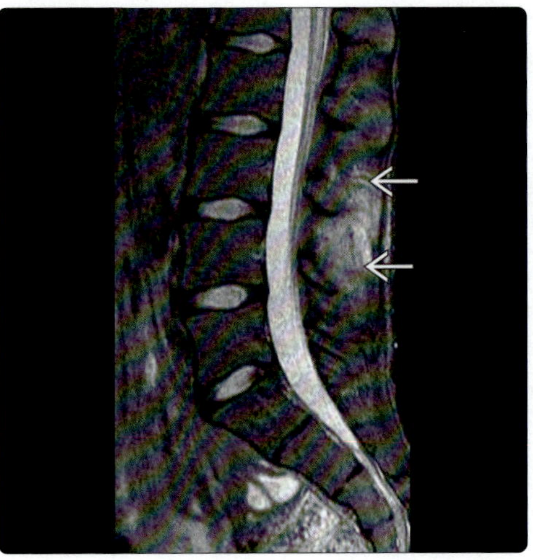

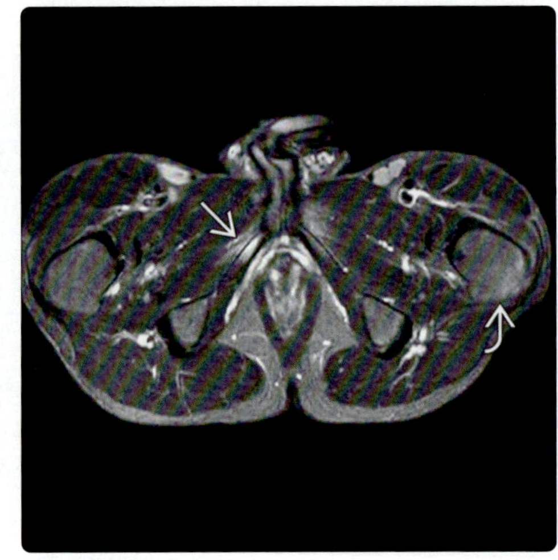

(Left) *Sagittal T2WI FS MR in a young adult male athlete shows no evidence of syndesmophytes, osteitis, or other vertebral signal abnormality. Nevertheless, there is enthesitis at the interspinous ligaments ➡. This should raise the question of spondyloarthropathy.* **(Right)** *Axial T2WI FS MR in the same patient shows marrow edema and enthesitis at the pubic ramus site of origin of the adductors ➡ as well as the greater trochanter ➡. Enthesitis is an early sign of AS and may be present as the earliest finding.*

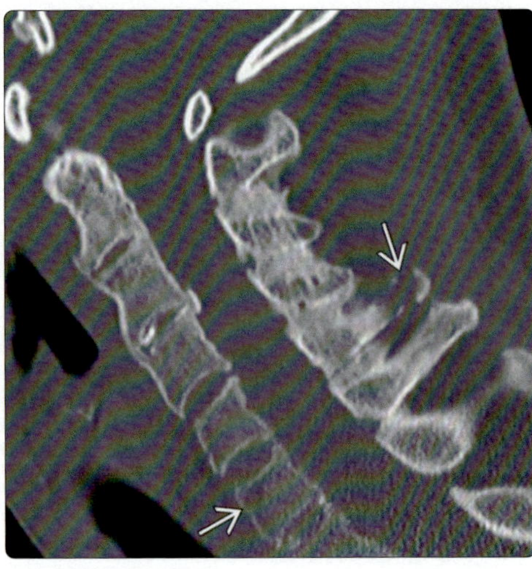

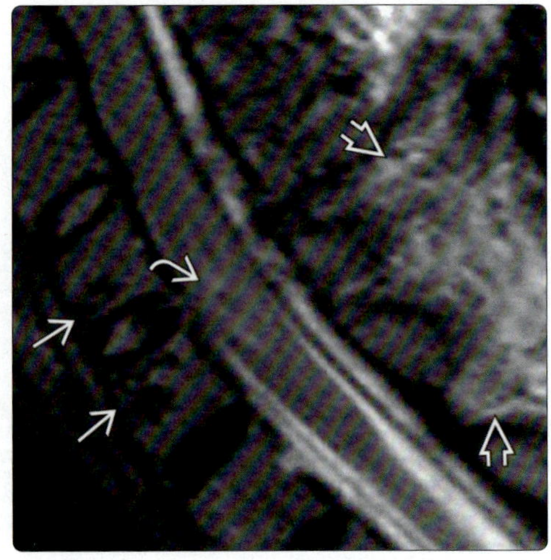

(Left) *Sagittal CT in a 40-year-old man shows ankylosis and osteoporosis typical of AS. The patient had a minor MVA; small nondisplaced fractures were seen at several sites ➡. Because morbidity is significant in these patients who present with fractures, MR must be obtained to evaluate the spinal cord, despite the fact that the fractures are nondisplaced.* **(Right)** *Sagittal T2 FS MR, same patient, shows cord hemorrhage ➡ along with 2 nondisplaced fractures ➡. There is significant ligament injury ➡ as well.*

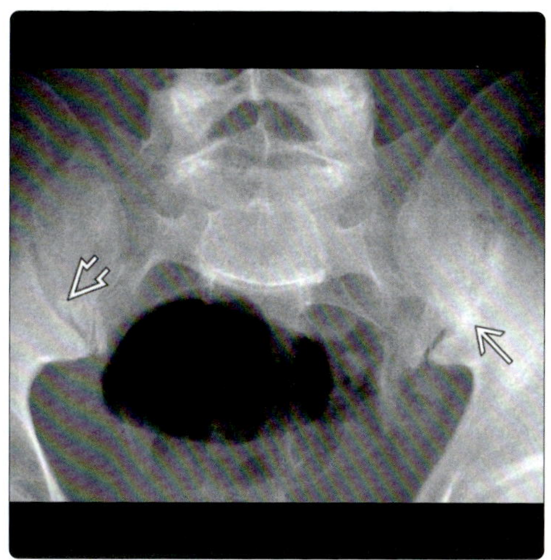

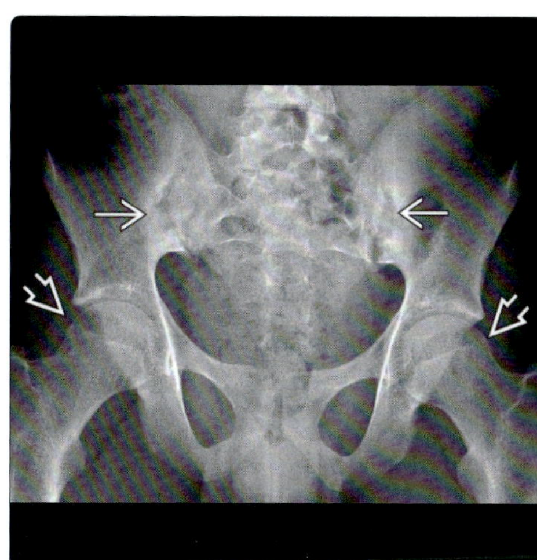

(Left) *AP radiograph shows bilateral but highly asymmetric SI joint disease. The left SI joint shows erosions and sclerosis ➡, while the right shows only subtle loss of cortical distinctness ➡. Early AS may present with asymmetric SI joint disease, as in this case.* **(Right)** *AP radiograph shows bilateral lateral femoral head/neck junction bumps ➡. These might mistakenly be considered the morphology of cam-type femoral acetabular impingement. However, the bilateral sacroiliitis ➡ confirms the diagnosis of AS.*

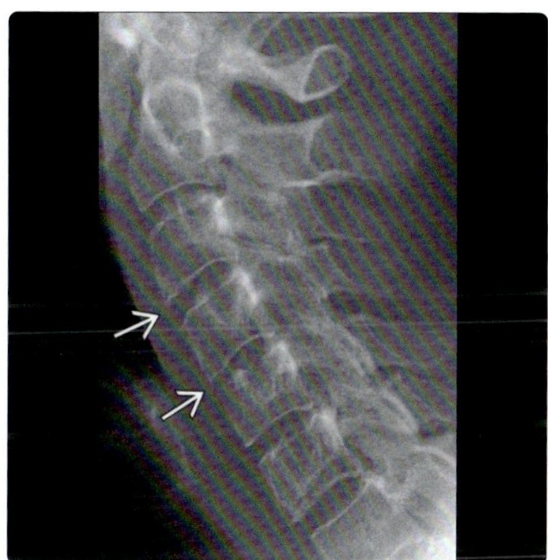

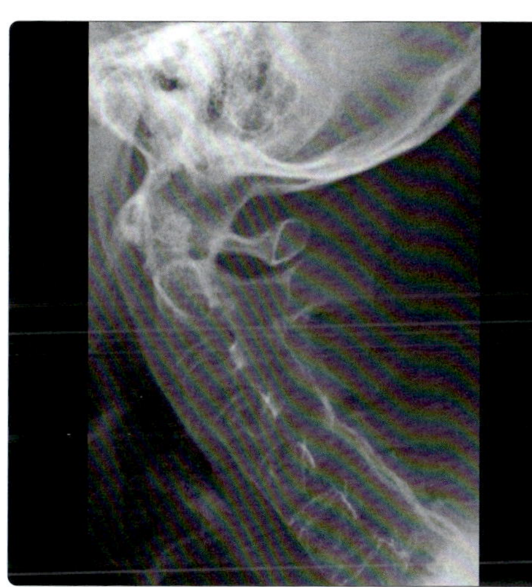

(Left) *Lateral radiograph in a 21-year-old man shows early syndesmophyte formation ➡ as well as some indistinctness (though not fusion) at the facet joints. The bones are osteoporotic for a man of this age.* **(Right)** *Lateral radiograph in the same patient obtained 10 years later, shows significant progression of the disease, with fusion of all the bodies and facets as well as some of the spinous processes. This degree of progression is, unfortunately, typical of AS.*

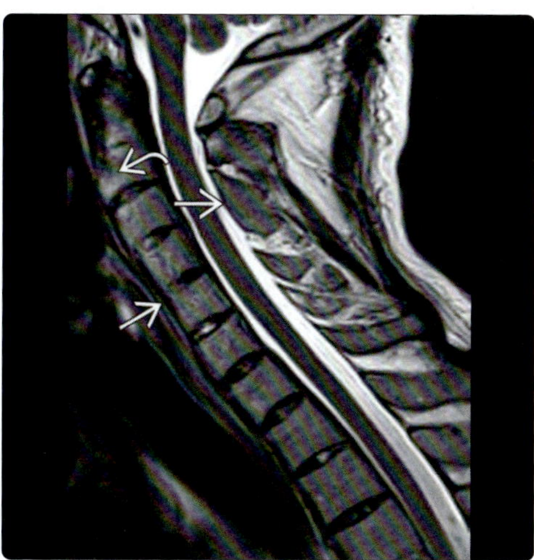

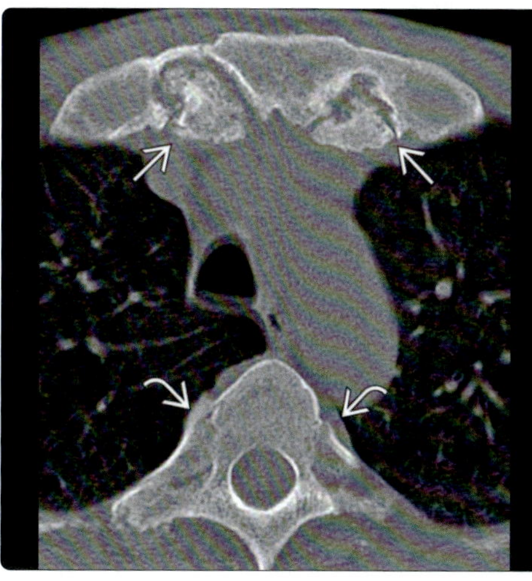

(Left) *Sagittal T2 MR, same patient, obtained at the same time as the 2nd x-ray, shows how subtle the signs of advanced AS may be on MR. Osseous fusion is present ➡ but not obvious. There is some inflammatory change at vertebral body corners ➡. MR can appear deceptively benign in these patients.* **(Right)** *Axial CT shows abnormalities of the axial skeleton in a patient with AS, with erosive change in the sternoclavicular joints ➡ and ankylosis of the costovertebral joints ➡. These findings may alert the reader to the likelihood of AS.*

KEY FACTS

TERMINOLOGY

- Inflammatory bowel disease with associated peripheral arthritis &/or spondyloarthropathy

IMAGING

- Radiographs: Spondyloarthropathy similar to that of ankylosing spondylitis (AS)
  - Bilateral sacroiliitis
  - Syndesmophytes, often → vertebral body fusion
  - Peripheral arthropathy, generally proximal joints
  - Signs of surgery for IBD
- Peripheral small joints affected by polyarthropathy
  - Generally no osseous changes
- Steroid use for IBD puts skeleton at risk for osteonecrosis, particularly femoral heads
- MR fluid-sensitive sequences
  - Soft tissue edema at sites of enthesitis, including vertebral body corners (Romanus lesions)
  - High signal early inflammatory signs in SI joints and peripheral joints

TOP DIFFERENTIAL DIAGNOSES

- Ankylosing spondylitis
- Osteoarthritis (OA), femoral acetabular impingement (FAI) if pronounced hip disease

DIAGNOSTIC CHECKLIST

- When considering diagnosis of OA or FAI in young adult, always look at SI joints to be certain that IBD or AS arthritis has not been missed
- CT for abdominal pain in patients with IBD
  - Do not forget to look at axial skeleton with bone algorithm for osseous abnormalities
- Consider diagnosis of IBD arthropathy in patient with skeletal appearance of AS plus bowel surgery
- On MR, watch for enthesitis on fluid-sensitive imaging as hint of early disease

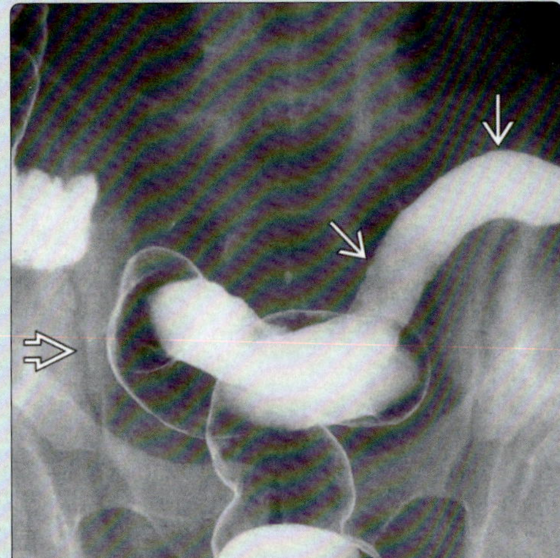

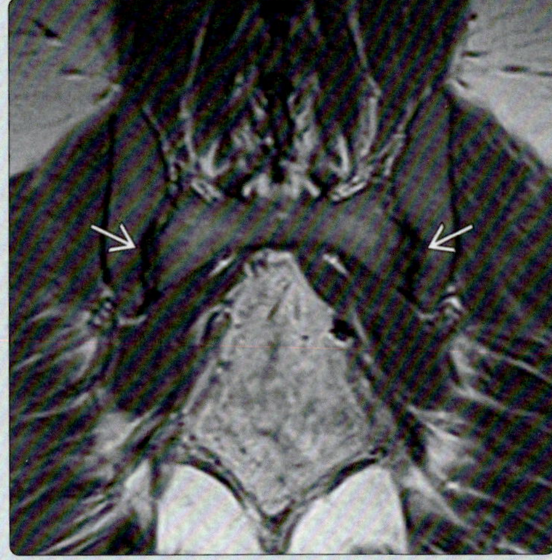

(Left) *AP radiograph in a 30-year-old man undergoing barium enema shows tubular ulcerated bowel ➡ typical of ulcerative colitis. Loss of haustral folds has been termed lead pipe appearance. Sacroiliac joints show bilateral widening & erosions ➡. Sclerosis is greater on the left than the right, but the findings are reasonably symmetric. The appearance is classic for inflammatory bowel disease (IBD) spondyloarthropathy.* **(Right)** *Coronal T1 MR in a 29-year-old man with low back pain shows sclerosis of the sacroiliac joints bilaterally ➡.*

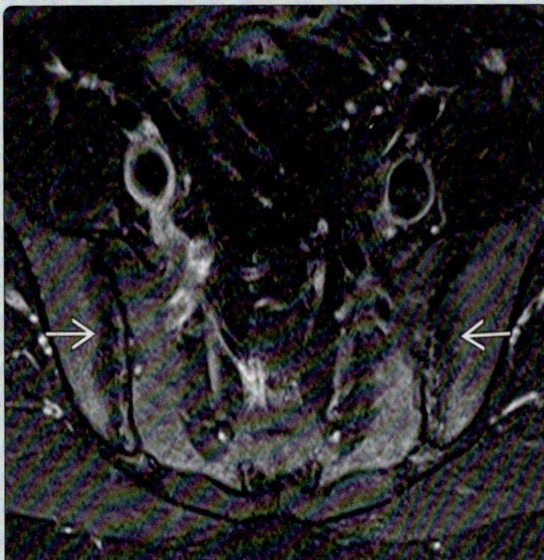

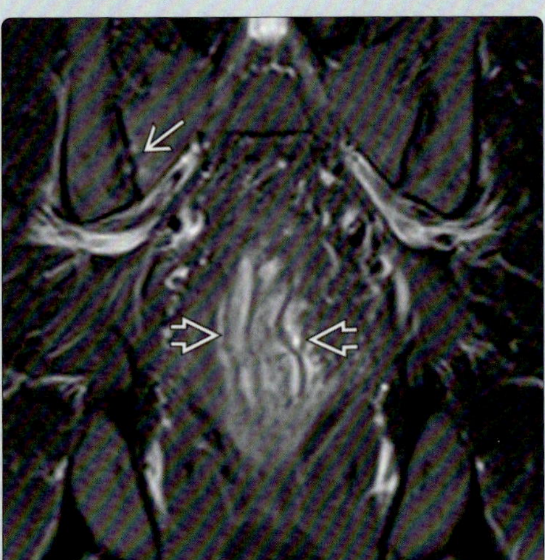

(Left) *Axial oblique T2 FS MR in the same patient confirms bilateral sacroiliac joint sclerosis ➡ and small erosions but no fusion; the radiograph (not shown) confirmed this density.* **(Right)** *Coronal T2 FS MR in the same patient confirms sacroiliitis ➡. There is also thickening of the rectal folds with associated edema ➡. The rectal findings are typical of Crohn disease; the patient has IBD spondyloarthropathy.*

TERMINOLOGY

Abbreviations

- Inflammatory bowel disease (IBD)

Synonyms

- Enteropathic arthritis

Definitions

- Inflammatory bowel disease with associated peripheral arthritis &/or spondyloarthropathy

IMAGING

General Features

- Best diagnostic clue
  - Spondyloarthropathy similar to that of ankylosing spondylitis (AS)
    - Bilateral sacroiliitis
    - Syndesmophytes, often → vertebral body fusion
  - Peripheral arthropathy, generally proximal joints
  - Signs of surgery for IBD
- Location
  - Sacroiliac (SI) joints
  - Spine, thoracolumbar > cervical
  - Large proximal joints: Hip > shoulder

Imaging Recommendations

- Best imaging tool
  - Diagnosis made on radiograph when disease is moderately advanced
  - Early, preradiographic diagnosis made on MR

Radiographic Findings

- Sacroiliac joints
  - Bilaterally symmetric inflammatory disease, identical to findings of AS
    - Early erosions and widening
    - Later sclerosis and fibrous ankylosis
    - Usually bilaterally symmetric
      - May be asymmetric at any time in disease process of any individual patient
      - Even if asymmetric, it is almost always bilateral
      - Do not use asymmetry of sacroiliitis to eliminate IBD arthropathy as diagnosis
- Spine
  - Thin, vertical syndesmophytes form in outer fibers of annulus fibrosus
    - Early disease best seen on lateral images
    - Early disease may show amorphous bone rather than organized syndesmophyte
  - Shiny corners → squaring of vertebral bodies
  - May extend to involve anterior longitudinal ligament and bridge vertebral bodies
  - Long column fusion of spine may result
    - Bamboo spine with dagger appearance along spinous processes on AP radiograph
    - Chronic fusion results in osteoporosis
    - At risk for transverse, 3-column fracture from relatively minor trauma, as in AS
- Other axial joints
  - Costovertebral, costochondral, sternoclavicular
    - Erosions, eventually resulting in ankylosis
- Peripheral joints
  - Proximal joints predominate (hips > shoulders, knees)
    - Erosions or osteophyte formation
    - Do not mistake osteophytes in young patient for morphology of femoral acetabular dysplasia
  - Peripheral small joints affected by polyarthropathy
    - Generally no osseous changes
    - If active, see subtle transient abnormalities
      - Soft tissue swelling
      - Osteopenia, focal loss of cortical distinctness
- Osteonecrosis (ON)
  - Steroid use for IBD puts skeleton at risk for ON, particularly femoral heads
  - Subchondral fracture
  - Flattening in weight-bearing anterosuperior portion
- Eventual osteoporosis
- Signs of bowel surgery
  - Colostomy
  - Staple lines in pelvis suggesting resection
  - Ileo-anal pull-through staple pattern

CT Findings

- CT generally not utilized for osseous evaluation in IBD arthropathy
  - Exception: Posttrauma evaluation for fracture if long column fusion
- CT often performed for abdominal pain in patients with IBD
  - Diagnosis of IBD should alert one to search for skeletal abnormalities in axial skeleton

MR Findings

- T1WI
  - Low signal edema at sites of early inflammation
  - Low signal syndesmophytes
    - Easily overlooked on MR
- Fluid-sensitive sequences
  - High signal early inflammatory signs
    - Soft tissue edema at sites of enthesitis
      - Interspinous ligaments
      - Entheses around pelvis: Pubic rami, ischium, iliac spines, trochanters
    - Sacroiliac joints
    - Romanus lesions at vertebral body corners
    - Osseous edema in peripheral joints
      - Hip most frequent: Edema, early erosions
      - Hands, feet may show edema and effusions, which usually resolve without osseous damage
  - Osteonecrosis: Double line sign femoral head
- T1WI C+ FS
  - Enhancement at active soft tissue or bone lesions

DIFFERENTIAL DIAGNOSIS

Ankylosing Spondylitis

- Spine, SI joints, peripheral arthritis identical to IBD

Osteoarthritis

- Hip osteophytes in IBD arthritis often suggest osteoarthritis (OA)
- OA patients generally older

- Sacroiliac and spine disease distinguish the two

Psoriatic Arthritis

- Mixed erosions and osteophytes may appear similar
- Sacroiliitis may appear similar if symmetric in psoriatic arthritis (PSA)
- Bulky paravertebral ossification usually distinguishes PSA from IBD or AS

Chronic Reactive Arthritis

- Same appearance as PSA; occasionally similar to IBD if sacroiliitis is symmetric or spinal ossification not as bulky as expected in chronic reactive arthritis (CRA) or PSA

Femoral Acetabular Impingement

- Lateral femoral head/neck "bump" may mimic osteophyte in IBD or AS
  - Always check SI joints when considering diagnosis of OA or femoral acetabular impingement (FAI) in young patient

PATHOLOGY

General Features

- Etiology
  - Evidence of predisposing genes, which modulate host-pathogen interaction at mucosal surfaces
    - Links between joint and gut inflammation suggested in several studies
- Associated abnormalities
  - Activity of peripheral arthritis parallels gut inflammation
    - Axial arthritis does not have this association
  - Close association with ankylosing spondylitis
    - 60% of patients with AS have subclinical change in large or small bowel
  - HLA-B27(+) in 50% of patients with IBD arthritis

Microscopic Features

- Synovial fluid: Sterile inflammatory changes

CLINICAL ISSUES

Presentation

- Most common signs/symptoms
  - Abdominal pain, weight loss, diarrhea
  - GI symptoms usually antedate or coincide with onset of arthritis
  - Arthritis clinically indistinguishable from that of AS
    - Low back pain, stiffness
    - ↓ chest expansion (< 4 cm)
    - Hip pain and stiffness
    - Peripheral joint swelling and pain

Demographics

- Gender
  - M = F for IBD-associated peripheral arthritis
  - M > F for IBD-associated axial arthritis
- Epidemiology
  - Arthritis is most common extraintestinal abnormality in IBD
  - 10-25% of IBD patients develop arthritis
    - Axial arthritis develops in 10-15% of IBD patients
    - Peripheral arthritis develops in 20% of IBD patients (may not have osseous damage)

Natural History & Prognosis

- *Salmonella, Yersinia, Shigella*
  - Self-limited polyarthritis; rare radiographic changes
  - Only rare sacroiliac changes
- Ulcerative colitis, Crohn disease, Whipple disease
  - 10-15% develop arthropathy
    - Most mild and peripheral with few osseous changes
    - 20-30% develop spondyloarthropathy like AS
- With adequate treatment, mobility and function generally maintained
  - Hip or knee arthroplasty may be necessary
- Without adequate treatment, may have severe postural changes
  - Thoracic hyperkyphosis and flattening of lumbar spine, similar to AS
- Long column fusion + osteoporosis puts patient at risk for 3-column fracture from minor trauma
- If treated with steroids for bowel disease, at risk for osteonecrosis

Treatment

- Similar to treatment for AS
- NSAIDs, DMARDs
  - Improve inflammatory symptoms, control pain
  - No effect on disease progression
- Corticosteroids
  - Often used to control bowel disease; puts skeleton at risk for osteonecrosis
  - Intraarticular steroids may be used for monoarthritis
- Anti-TNF-α for refractory axial disease
  - Improves function and ↓ inflammatory changes on MR
  - Long-term control of disease progression not yet proven
- Colectomy
  - Peripheral joint disease may improve, but in minority of cases

DIAGNOSTIC CHECKLIST

Consider

- When considering diagnosis of OA or FAI in young adult, always look at SI joints to be certain IBD or AS arthritis are not being missed

Image Interpretation Pearls

- CT often performed for abdominal pain in IBD
  - Do not forget to look at axial skeleton with bone algorithm for osseous abnormalities
- Consider diagnosis of IBD arthropathy in patient with skeletal appearance of AS plus bowel surgery
- On MR, watch for enthesitis on fluid-sensitive imaging as hint of early disease

SELECTED REFERENCES

1. Bazsó A et al: Importance of intestinal microenvironment in development of arthritis. A systematic review. Immunol Res. 61(1-2):172-6, 2015
2. Gamsjaeger S et al: Altered bone material properties in HLA-B27 rats include reduced mineral to matrix ratio and altered collagen cross-links. J Bone Miner Res. 29(11):2382-91, 2014
3. Paparo F et al: Seronegative spondyloarthropathies: what radiologists should know. Radiol Med. 119(3):156-63, 2014

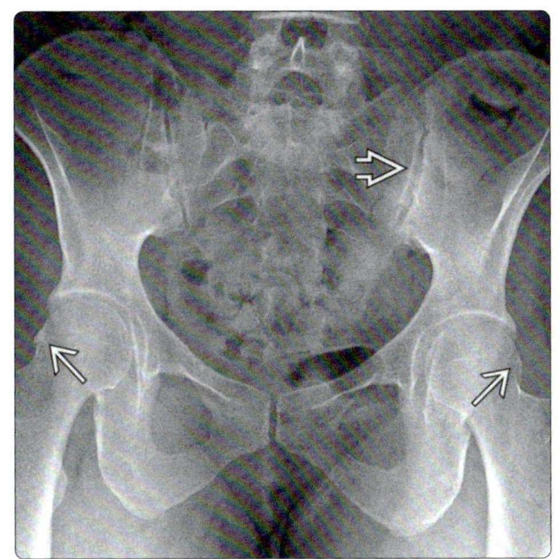

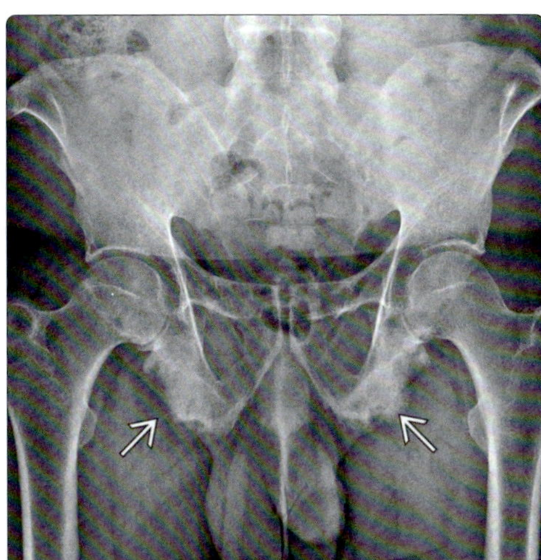

(Left) *AP radiograph shows bilateral bumps at the femoral head/neck junction ➡. These are in a position to cause femoral acetabular impingement, and indeed the patient had symptoms of that process. However, there are also asymmetric SI joint erosions ➡. The patient had IBD; the bumps as well as sacroiliitis result from the associated spondyloarthropathy.* **(Right)** *AP radiograph shows fusion of both SI joints and enthesopathy ➡, typical of either AS or IBD advanced spondyloarthropathy.*

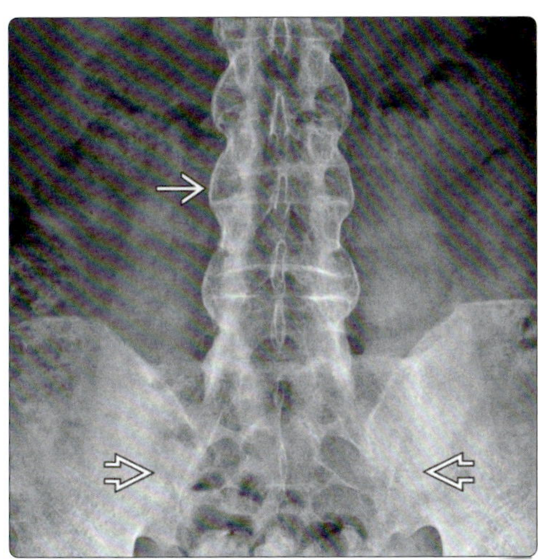

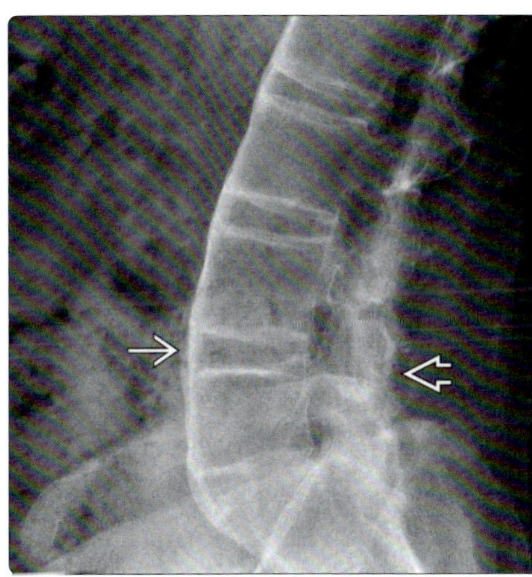

(Left) *AP radiograph in the same patient shows bamboo lumbar spine ➡ (complete ankylosis) and symmetric near-complete SI joint fusion ➡.* **(Right)** *Lateral radiograph of the same patient shows vertical syndesmophytes and complete fusion of the bodies of the lumbar spine ➡. Note the fusion of the lumbar facets as well ➡. This severe osseous disease was, amazingly, previously unsuspected prior to the patient's visit to the clinic for low back pain. He carried a diagnosis of IBD.*

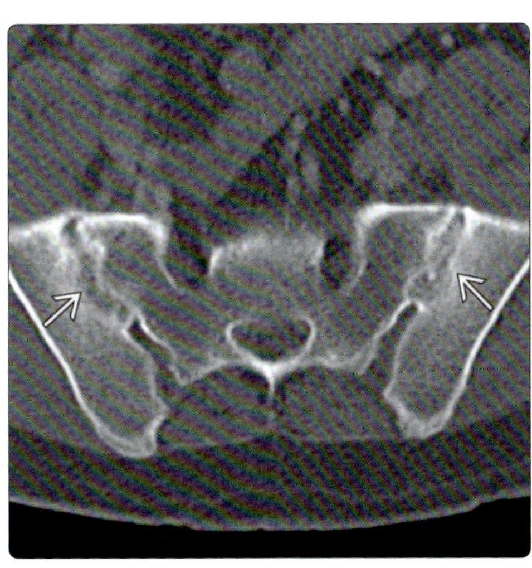

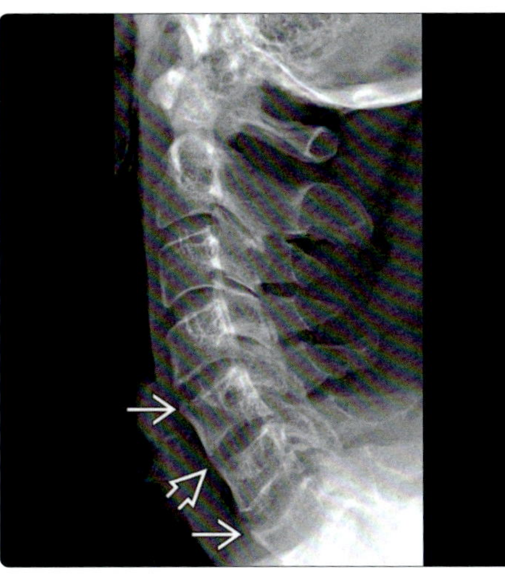

(Left) *Axial CT in the same patient 5 years earlier shows severe, bilaterally symmetric SI disease ➡, which was not noted. The diagnosis could easily have been established at time of this CT and therapy instituted.* **(Right)** *Lateral radiograph in a patient with IBD shows 1 typical vertical syndesmophyte ➡ and 2 other sites of less well-organized, earlier syndesmophyte formation ➡. L-spine was completely ankylosed; C-spine is generally less severely involved than the thoracolumbar spine in these patients.*

(Left) *Coronal CT in a patient with known ulcerative colitis (UC) shows thickened bowel wall & submucosal ulcerations along the transverse colon ➡, the lead pipe appearance. There is prominent mesenteric fat, typical in UC patients.* **(Right)** *Coronal CT in the same patient shows classic findings of IBD spondyloarthropathy. Syndesmophytes have merged ➡, resulting in ankylosis and bamboo appearance. The SI joints have symmetric fibrous ankylosis ➡. This is not distinguishable from AS, but the bowel disease secures the diagnosis.*

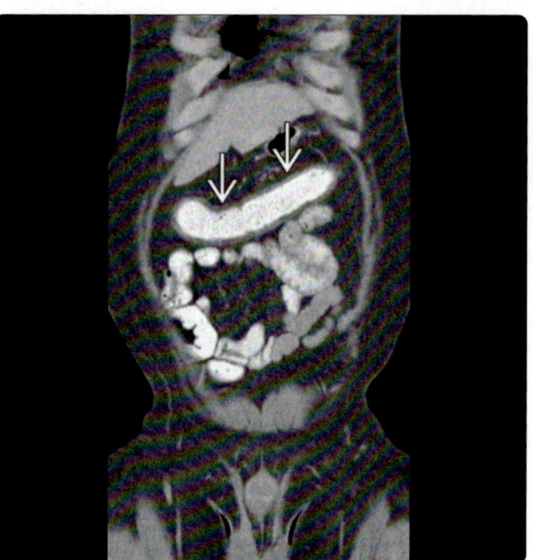

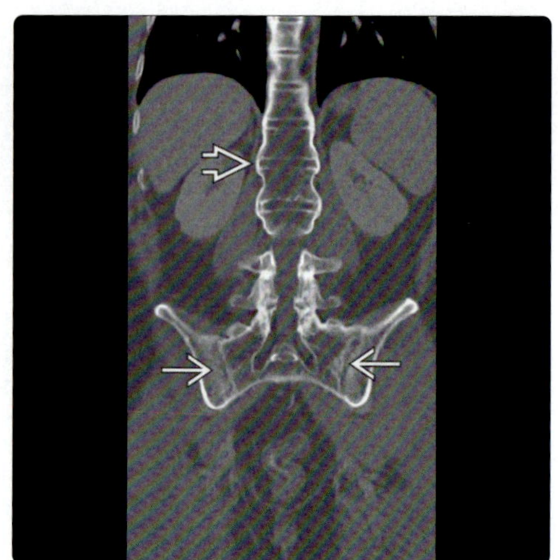

(Left) *Coronal CT in the same patient, located more posteriorly, shows notable mesenteric fat within the pelvis. The osseous findings are classic, with symmetric thin vertical syndesmophytes ➡. The sclerosis and enthesopathy along the ischium ➡ is remarkable and typical.* **(Right)** *AP radiograph shows bilateral sacroiliitis ➡. The staple row indicates ileo-anal pull-through ➡ and a diagnosis of IBD spondyloarthropathy. There is also osteonecrosis ➡ of the left femoral head, resulting from steroid use.*

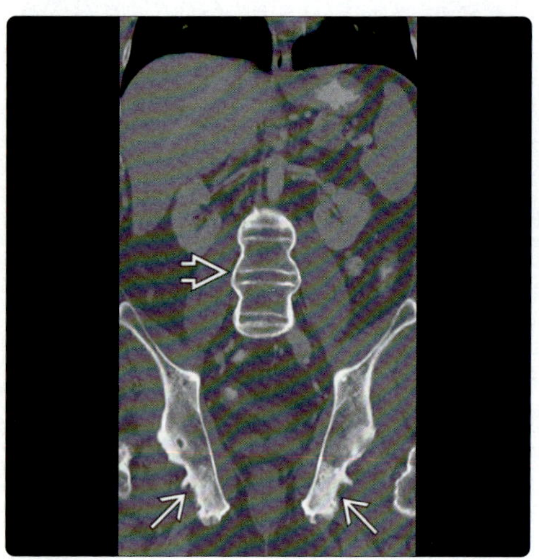

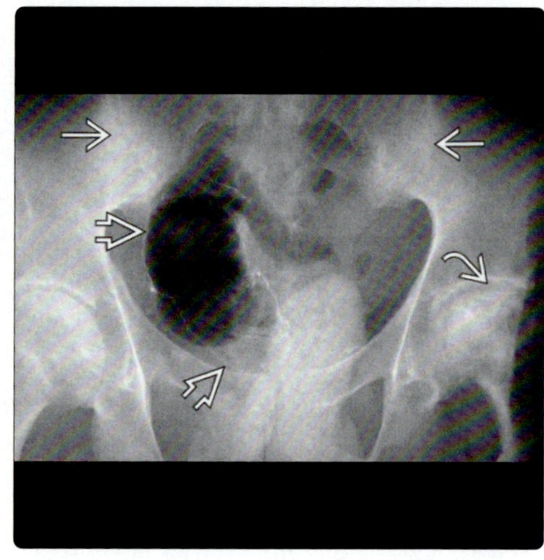

(Left) *Axial abdominal CT shows thickening of the bowel wall in a patient with IBD arthritis. There is linear fatty deposition within the bowel wall ➡, typical of inflammatory bowel disease. Note the fibrofatty mesenteric proliferation and prominent lymph nodes, also typical of this disease.* **(Right)** *Lateral radiograph of the knee in the same patient shows longstanding enthesopathy at the infrapatellar tendon ➡. As in ankylosing spondylitis, enthesopathy is prominent in IBD arthritis.*

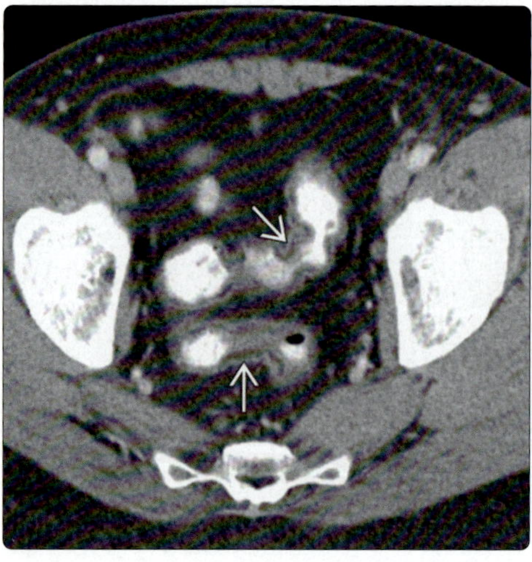

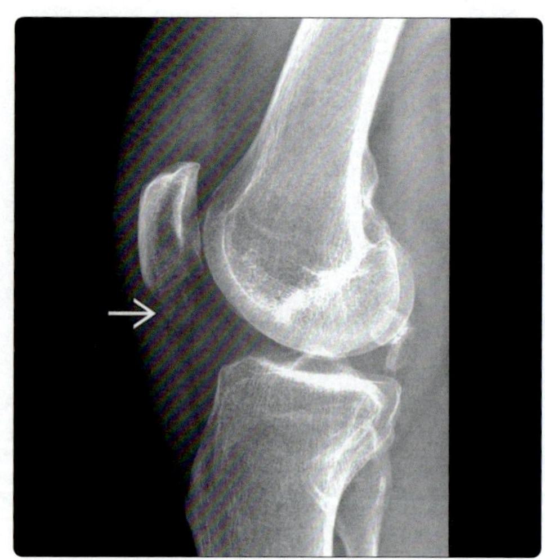

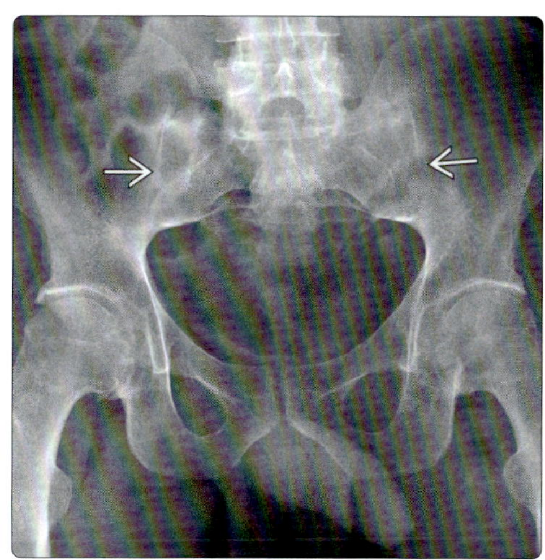

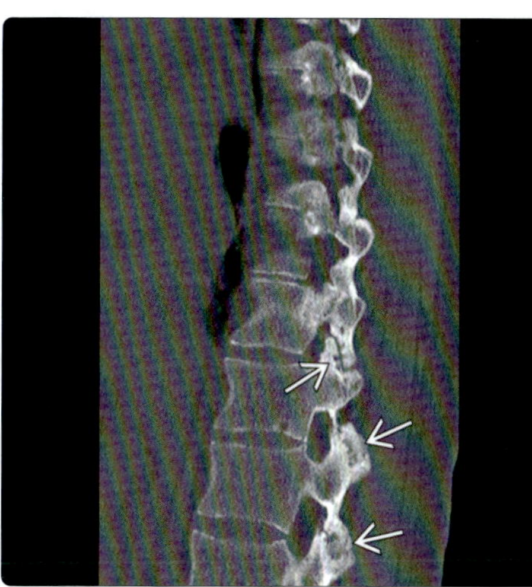

(Left) *AP radiograph in a young man with known IBD shows bilateral fusion of the SI joints ➡. There is also mild productive change at the hips, typical of IBD spondyloarthropathy.* **(Right)** *Sagittal CT in the same patient shows both sclerosis and erosions at the facet joints of the thoracolumbar spine ➡. IBD spondyloarthropathy, like AS, is a mixed erosive/productive process.*

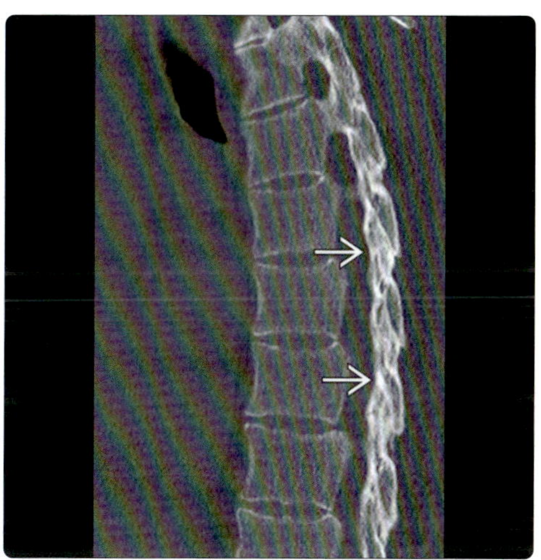

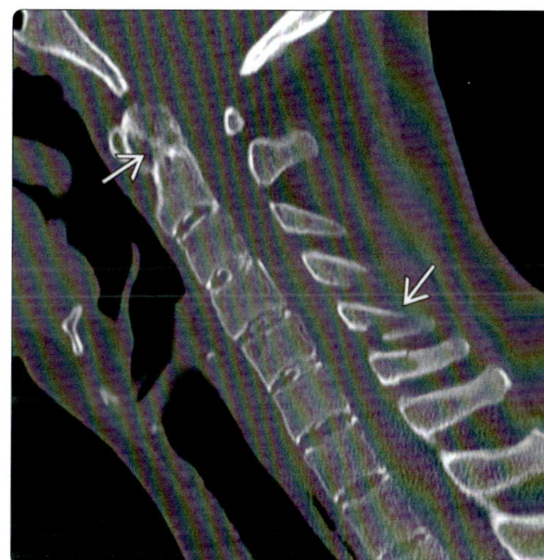

(Left) *Sagittal CT, more centrally in the same patient, shows complete fusion of the spinous processes ➡, though the bodies are not yet fused.* **(Right)** *Sagittal CT of the C-spine in the same patient was obtained following minor trauma. Multiple nondisplaced fractures are seen ➡. However, in patients like this with long-column fusion, such fractures may not be innocuous. MR is required to evaluate for cord damage.*

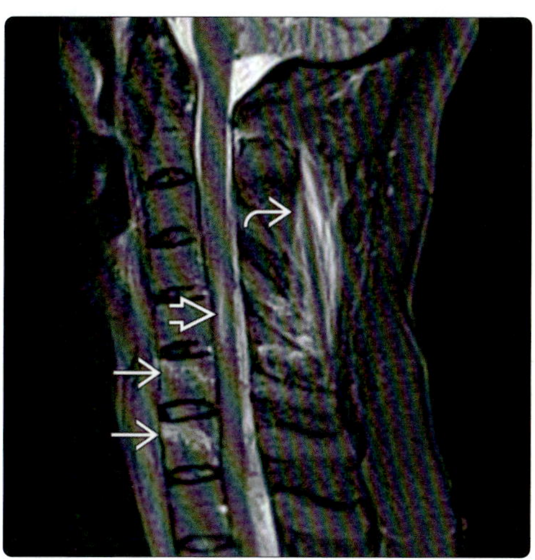

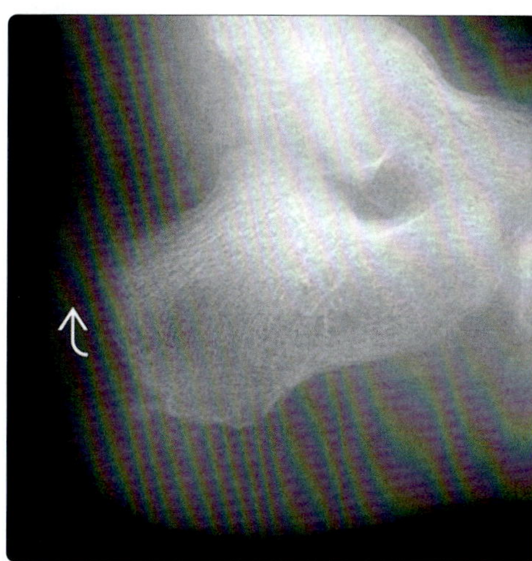

(Left) *Sagittal T2 FS MR in the same patient shows previously undetected fractures of 2 bodies ➡, ligamentous injury ➡, and evidence of cord trauma ➡. There is high morbidity associated with even minor spine fractures in patients such as this with long-column fusion.* **(Right)** *Lateral radiograph shows a subtle abnormality of the calcaneus. There is swelling of the soft tissues posterior to the Achilles tendon ➡ and obliteration of the pre-Achilles fat pad, indicating inflammatory change in a child with IBD.*

Psoriatic Arthritis

KEY FACTS

TERMINOLOGY

- Inflammatory arthritis, usually developing after or coincident with skin changes of psoriasis
  - Arthritis precedes skin changes by 2 years in 15%

IMAGING

- Diagnosis most frequently made on radiographs
- Peripheral arthropathy in hands/feet
  - Row pattern
    - Interphalangeal (IP) joints predominate
    - Erosive; may progress to arthritis mutilans
    - "Pencil-in-cup" deformities, "telescoping" fingers
  - Ray pattern
    - Productive, with enthesopathy, periostitis
    - Soft tissue swelling, sausage digit
- Sacroiliitis: 35% of patients
  - Usually begins asymmetrically, but bilaterally
  - At any time in course, may appear symmetric
- Spondylitis: 30% of patients
  - Bulky paravertebral ossifications
  - More prominently seen on AP than lateral view
  - Asymmetric with skipped levels
- Ankylosis is common feature
- Normal bone density
- Bilaterality and symmetry less frequent than in rheumatoid arthritis
- In early disease, MR shows abnormalities, though usually nonspecific
  - Edema, synovitis in peripheral joints nonspecific
  - Marrow edema
  - Enthesopathy, periostitis

DIAGNOSTIC CHECKLIST

- Watch for periostitis along metaphyses and shafts of digits; may be subtle
  - May be seen on either radiograph or MR
  - Differentiates from rheumatoid arthritis and erosive osteoarthritis

(Left) *PA radiograph in a young adult shows cartilage loss and mild erosive change at the 2nd PIP ➔ but more severe erosive change along with soft tissue swelling and enthesopathy ➔ at the 3rd PIP. Note the normal MCP joints and normal bone density. This is typical psoriatic arthritis.* **(Right)** *PA radiograph in the same patient, 9 years later, shows advanced mixed erosive and productive disease of the DIP ➔ and PIP ➔ joints. This is now more convincingly a typical row pattern of psoriatic arthritis.*

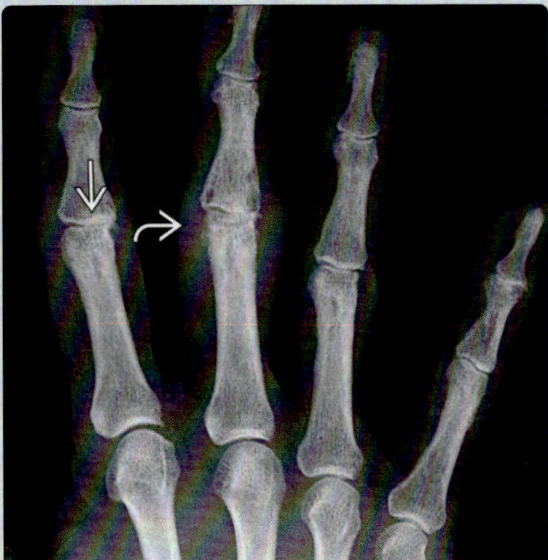

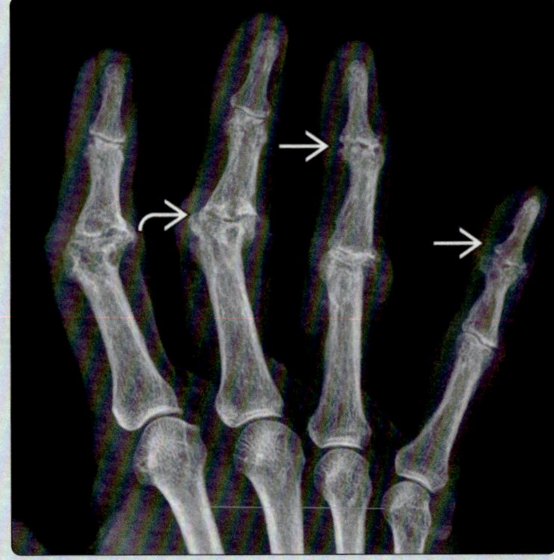

(Left) *AP radiograph of the foot shows disease involving only the great toe. There is diffuse soft tissue edema ➔, mild acroosteolysis ➔, and distinct periostitis ➔. The remaining joints imaged are normal. This appearance is classic for the ray pattern of psoriatic arthritis.* **(Right)** *Oblique radiograph in the same patient, 9 years later, shows the disease remains monoarticular but that periostitis has resolved while the IP joint has developed severe erosive change ➔. The character may have changed, but the disease remains PSA.*

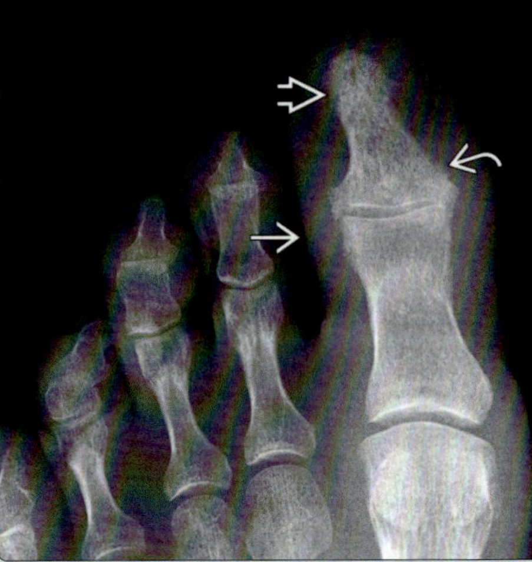

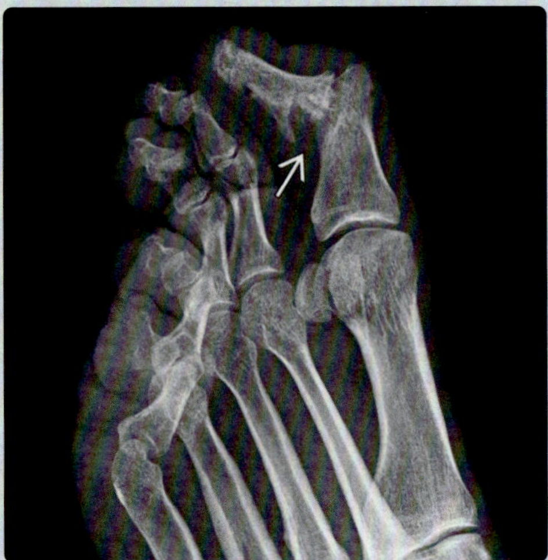

TERMINOLOGY

Abbreviations

- Psoriatic arthritis (PSA)

Synonyms

- Psoriatic spondyloarthropathy
  - Not true synonym; spine and sacroiliac disease found in subset of patients with PSA

Definitions

- Inflammatory arthritis, usually developing after or coincident with skin changes of psoriasis
  - Arthritis precedes skin change up to 2 years in 15%

IMAGING

General Features

- Best diagnostic clue
  - Spondyloarthropathy
    - Bulky paravertebral ossification
      - Better seen on AP than lateral radiograph
      - Asymmetric with skips
    - Bilateral but asymmetric sacroiliitis
  - Peripheral arthropathy
    - Row pattern
      - Interphalangeal (IP) joints predominate
      - Erosive; may progress to arthritis mutilans
      - Productive, with ankylosis, periostitis
    - Ray pattern
      - Sausage digit, enthesopathy
- Location
  - Spondyloarthropathy
    - Thoracolumbar > cervical; skips segments
    - Bilateral sacroiliac (SI) joints, asymmetric
  - Peripheral arthropathy: Hand > foot > other joints
    - IP joints > metacarpophalangeal (MCP) or metatarsophalangeal (MTP) joints
  - 2/3 asymmetric and mono- or oligoarticular
  - 1/3 polyarticular; may mimic rheumatoid arthritis (RA)

Imaging Recommendations

- Best imaging tool
  - Diagnosis most frequently made on radiographs
  - For early disease, MR shows abnormalities
    - Edema, synovitis in peripheral joints: Nonspecific
    - Ray pattern more specific on MR
      - Marrow and periosteal edema
      - Enthesopathy, periostitis
    - One study showed frequent foot involvement by MR criteria in psoriatic patients without joint symptoms
      - Achilles tendinitis (57%), retrocalcaneal bursitis (50%), joint effusion/synovitis (46%)
- Protocol advice
  - SI joints: Angled coronal, thin-section, T2WI FS or STIR MR

Radiographic Findings

- Normal bone density
- Bilaterality and symmetry less frequent than in RA
- Hand
  - Involved in 25%
  - Row pattern: DIP prevalence
    - Begins as marginal erosions
    - Progresses to aggressive erosions
      - "Pencil-in-cup" deformity: Pencil-like thinning of proximal portion, cup-like erosion of distal portion of joint
      - Typical, but not specific to PSA
    - 5% develop arthritis mutilans
      - Destruction so significant that much of phalanx is resorbed
      - Clinical "telescoping" fingers, where finger can be pulled out to normal length
    - May resorb bone at tufts (acroosteolysis)
    - MCPs eventually involved if poorly controlled
    - Ankylosis is common in moderately advanced PSA
  - Ray pattern: Soft tissue edema of entire ray termed sausage digit
    - Productive change is important feature
      - Periostitis along shafts of digits
      - Enthesitis at sites of ligament/tendon insertion
- Wrist
  - Any compartment may be involved; fairly nonspecific
  - Pericapitate disease is slightly more prominent but may not help diagnose individual case
  - Erosive disease
  - Enthesopathy may be subtle but often present
- Foot
  - Not as frequently involved as hand but common
  - IP disease predominates
  - MTP disease not uncommon
  - Same features as in hand: Row pattern of erosive disease, ray pattern of edema and periostitis
  - Rare sclerosis in distal phalanges: Ivory phalanx
- Ankle
  - Enthesitis
    - Achilles and plantar aponeurosis insertion
  - Hindfoot more frequently involved in early PSA changes than forefoot
  - Erosions, especially posterior tubercle calcaneus
- Proximal joints
  - Hip is uncommonly involved relative to more acral joints, but may show erosions
- Sacroiliitis: 35% of patients with PSA; 20-40% of PSA patients with peripheral arthritis
  - Usually begins asymmetrically, but bilaterally
  - At any time in course, may appear symmetric
  - End stage: Bilateral ankylosis
- Spondylitis: 30% of patients
  - Thoracolumbar spine predominates
  - Bulky paravertebral ossifications
    - Arise from vertebral body, extend vertically around disc to eventually bridge
    - In early stage, appear as amorphous ossification
    - Later develop mature bone marrow
    - More prominently seen on AP than lateral view
    - Asymmetric with skipped bodies
  - Ankylosis of facets less common than in ankylosing spondylitis (AS)

MR Findings

- T1WI
  - Low signal edema at sites of early erosions
  - Low signal effusions
  - Late in spondylitis, marrow signal within paravertebral ossifications
- Fluid-sensitive sequences and T1 C+ FS sequence
  - Entheseal inflammatory change: High signal
    - Achilles insertion and plantar fasciitis
    - Around pelvis
    - Interspinous ligaments
    - Vertebral body corners
  - Row pattern of IP joints
    - High signal erosions and subchondral cysts
    - High signal effusion containing lower signal synovitis
    - Nonspecific synovial membrane enhancement
    - PSA not distinguishable from RA based on joint and synovial MR characteristics
      - Early reports show PSA may show more abrupt drop (washout) in synovial contrast enhancement 15 minutes postinjection
  - Ray pattern of hands/feet more specific for PSA
    - High signal periosteal edema along diaphysis
    - Bone marrow edema begins at capsular insertion of phalanx and spreads to involve entire bone
    - Soft tissue edema may spread to subcutis
    - Muscular fascial thickening may be seen

Ultrasonographic Findings

- Joint effusions, tenosynovitis; nonspecific

DIFFERENTIAL DIAGNOSIS

DDx of Spondyloarthropathy in Psoriatic Arthritis

- Chronic reactive arthritis (CRA)
  - Same appearance of bilateral but asymmetric sacroiliitis
  - Same bulky paravertebral ossification

DDx of Peripheral Arthritis in Psoriatic Arthritis

- Chronic reactive arthritis (CRA)
  - Same IP distribution of erosive disease
  - Same sausage digits with periostitis
  - Lower extremity predominates in CRA; upper in PSA
- Erosive osteoarthritis (EOA)
  - Interphalangeal erosions may appear identical, though EOA erosions central rather than marginal
  - IP > MCP involvement
  - Carpal distribution different: 1st carpometacarpal and scapho-trapezium-trapezoid in EOA
- Rheumatoid arthritis (RA)
  - MCP > IP involvement (DIP disease unusual except in advanced cases)
  - No periostitis
  - May give similar appearance of arthritis mutilans in advanced disease
  - Carpal distribution does not always differentiate, but distal radioulnar joint and radiocarpal joints predominate in RA

PATHOLOGY

General Features

- Etiology
  - Unknown: Likely combination of environmental and hereditary factors
- Associated abnormalities
  - Skin changes of psoriasis
  - Nail changes: Pitting, ridging, onycholysis

CLINICAL ISSUES

Presentation

- Most common signs/symptoms
  - Often family history of psoriasis
  - Dactylitis
  - Usually oligoarticular; occasionally polyarticular
  - Occasionally back pain
  - Pain from enthesitis, especially Achilles or plantar

Demographics

- Age
  - Peak onset of psoriatic arthritis 30-35 years
- Gender
  - M = F for psoriatic arthritis
  - M > F (M:F = 2-3:1) for psoriatic spondylitis
- Epidemiology
  - 0.1% prevalence in USA
  - Arthritis in 5-20% of patients with psoriasis

Natural History & Prognosis

- Morbidity can be substantial
  - Worse with
    - Positive family history
    - Positive HLA-B27
    - Onset before age 20
    - Polyarticular disease

Treatment

- Same as other spondyloarthropathies
  - Anti TNF-α: Promising, but only small studies with short follow-up thus far

DIAGNOSTIC CHECKLIST

Consider

- Because both psoriasis and PSA may be presenting features of HIV, this disease should be ruled out

Image Interpretation Pearls

- Watch for periostitis along metaphyses and shafts of digits; may be subtle
  - Differentiates PSA from RA and erosive osteoarthritis

SELECTED REFERENCES

1. Lew PP et al: Imaging of disorders affecting the bone and skin. Radiographics. 34(1):197-216, 2014
2. Braum LS et al: Characterisation of hand small joints arthropathy using high-resolution MRI–limited discrimination between osteoarthritis and psoriatic arthritis. Eur Radiol. 23(6):1686-93, 2013
3. Spira D et al: MRI findings in psoriatic arthritis of the hands. AJR Am J Roentgenol. 195(5):1187-93, 2010

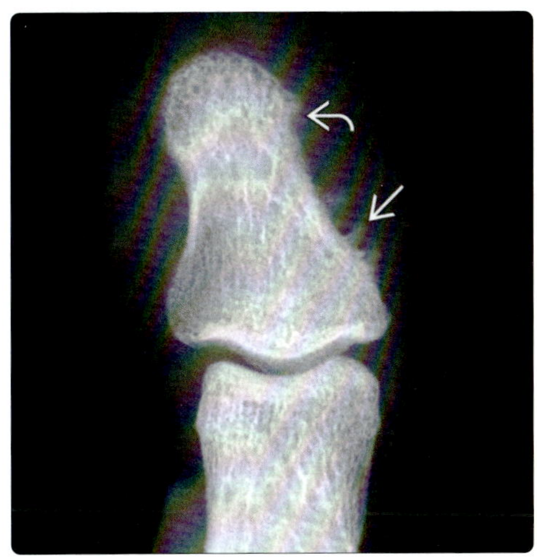

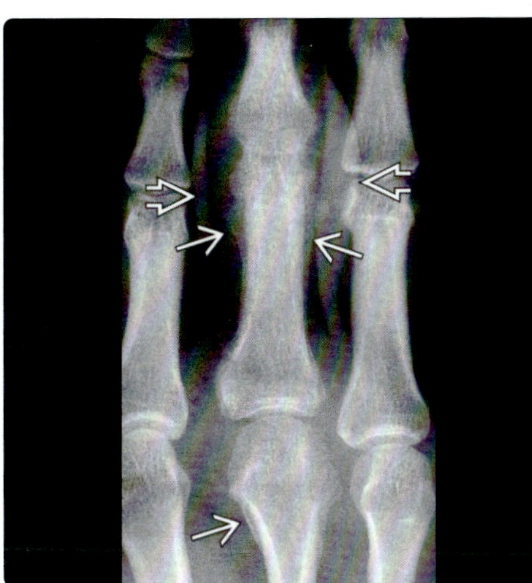

(Left) *AP radiograph of the great toe shows both periostitis ➡ and a hint of acroosteolysis ➡. The combination strongly suggests psoriatic arthritis, although chronic reactive arthritis is also considered. The patient had psoriasis.* **(Right)** *PA radiograph shows an outstanding example of the single ray pattern of involvement in a patient with PSA. There is tremendous soft tissue swelling ➡ overlapping the other digits. Cartilage narrowing is seen, and the periostitis along the shafts is prominent ➡.*

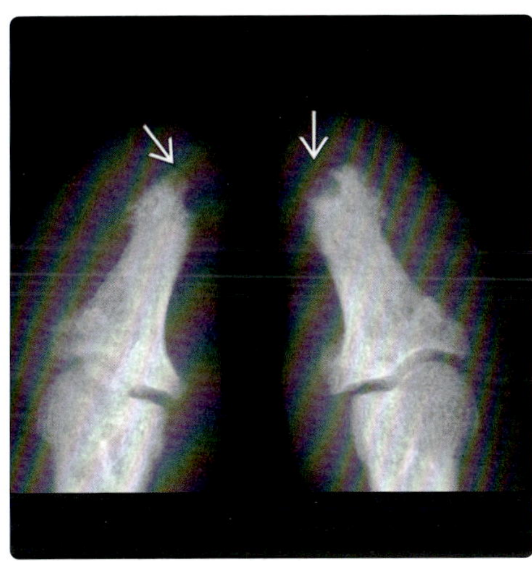

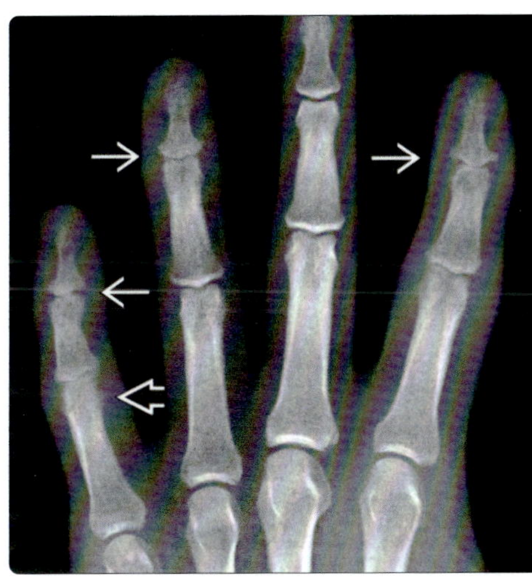

(Left) *Oblique radiograph of both thumbs shows acroosteolysis ➡ at the tufts. This is a somewhat unusual finding in patients with PSA, but it is much more frequently seen in PSA than in the other common arthritides.* **(Right)** *PA radiograph shows early PSA. The carpus and MCP joints were normal (not shown). The fingers show diffuse IP joint disease, with juxtaarticular osteopenia, swelling, joint narrowing, and marginal erosions ➡. Subtle periostitis is best seen at the 5th proximal phalanx ➡.*

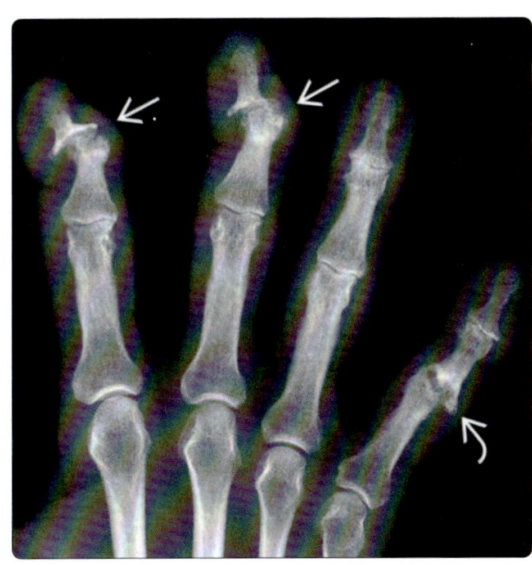

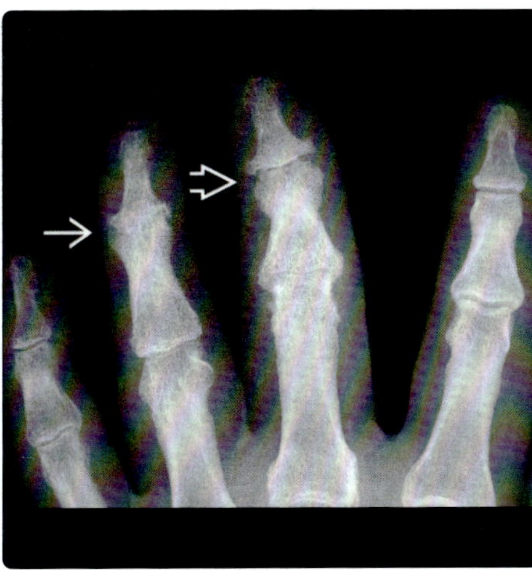

(Left) *PA radiograph shows mixed erosive and productive changes in a row pattern involving the DIP ➡ and PIP ➡ joints. Note that the MCP joints are normal as is the bone density. This is typical psoriatic arthritis.* **(Right)** *PA radiograph shows erosive disease and developing ankylosis in 1 DIP joint ➡ and purely erosive disease in another ➡, typical of psoriatic arthritis. The bone density is normal, and the digits are diffusely swollen.*

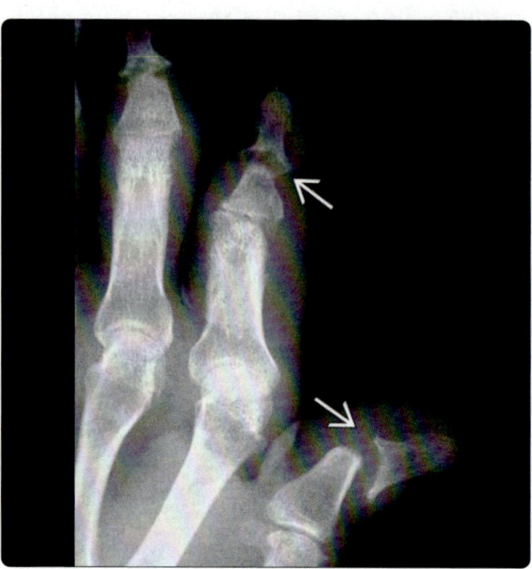

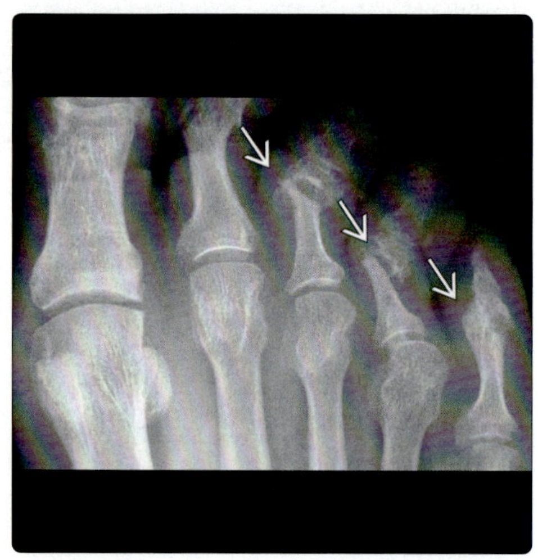

(Left) *PA radiograph shows normal bone density, but there is such severe erosive interphalangeal disease ➡ that it qualifies for the term "arthritis mutilans," which is sometimes used in these cases and most typically seen in psoriatic arthritis. Clinically, these digits are "telescoping," as they can be pulled out to length.* **(Right)** *AP radiograph in a patient with PSA shows arthritis mutilans at the IP joints ➡. The MTP joints are less severely involved. This is a typical appearance, but it may be seen in either PSA or CRA.*

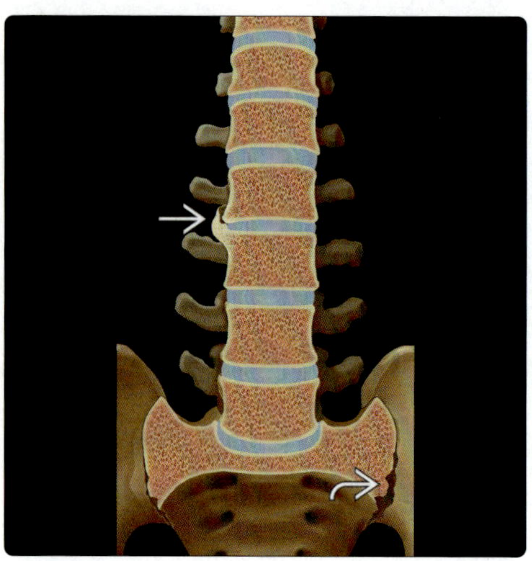

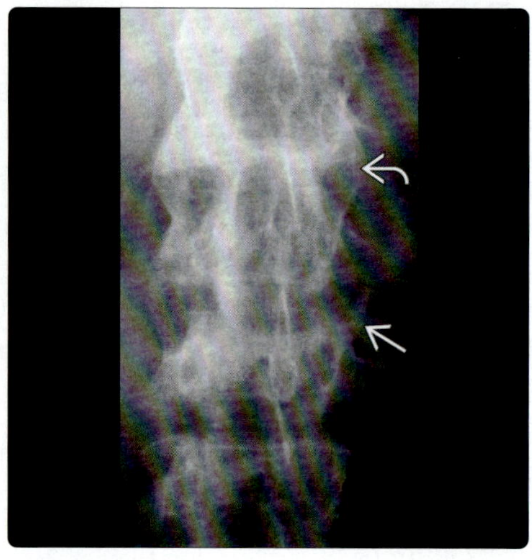

(Left) *Graphic depicts the appearance of early PSA. The paravertebral ossification, best seen on the AP view, is bulky ➡ and may eventually bridge the disc space. Erosive sacroiliitis is bilateral but usually asymmetric ➡ early in the disease.* **(Right)** *AP radiograph of a patient with PSA shows an early osteophyte extending initially away from the vertebral body, then vertically around the disc space ➡. At another level, a bulky paravertebral osteophyte fully bridges the disc space ➡.*

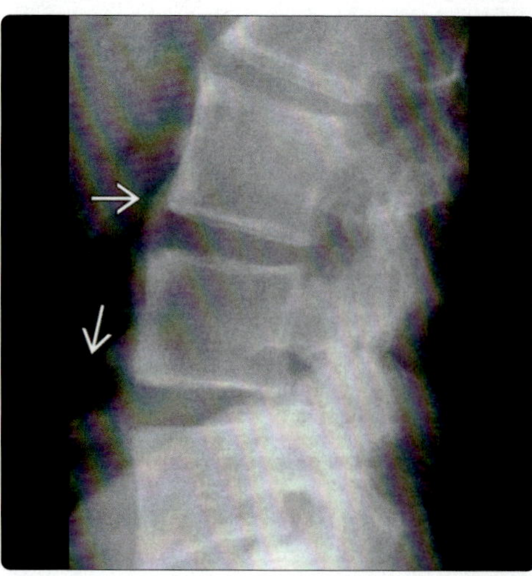

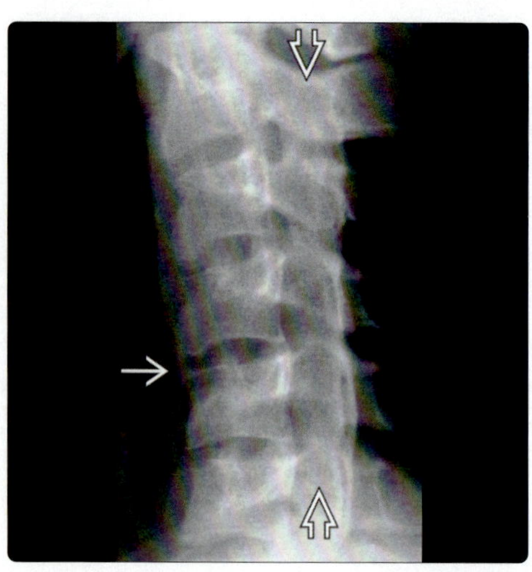

(Left) *Lateral radiograph of the lumbar spine in a patient with psoriatic spondyloarthropathy shows early paravertebral ossification ➡. At this early stage, the ossification appears fluffy and rather amorphous; later it attains a mature bony appearance.* **(Right)** *Lateral radiograph shows a single vertical osteophyte ➡, along with complete ankylosis of the cervical spine facets ➡. It is uncommon but not unheard of to have such a long segment of ankylosis in psoriatic arthritis.*

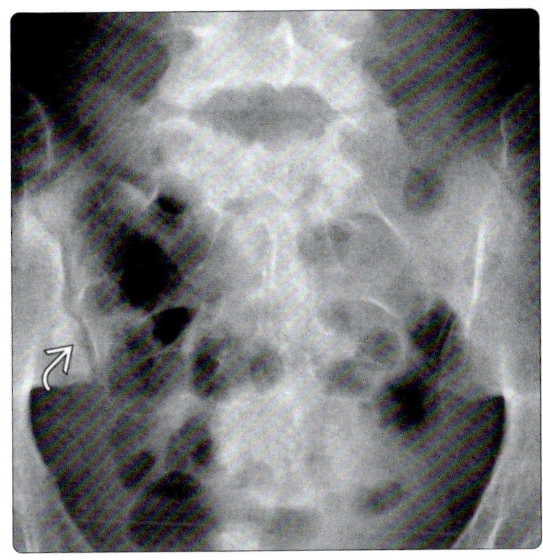

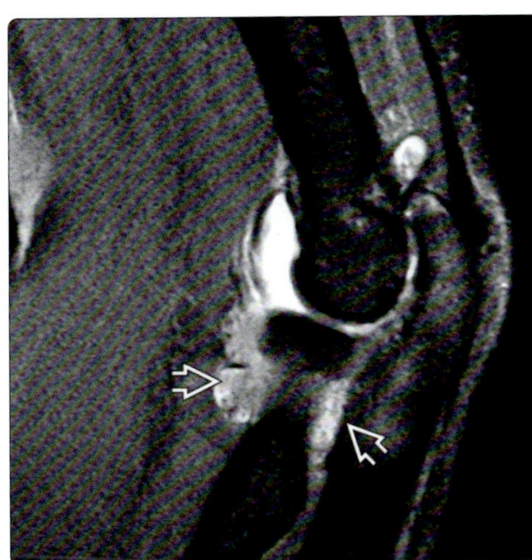

(Left) *AP radiograph shows a nearly normal left SI joint, but the right shows mild widening and sclerosis ➙. This bilateral asymmetry is typical of either psoriatic or chronic reactive spondyloarthropathy. The patient developed typical skin changes of psoriasis within a year.* **(Right)** *Sagittal MR arthrogram shows synovial proliferation surrounding the proximal radius ➙. MR findings are nonspecific; diagnosis was made based on radiographs, serology, culture, and synovial pathology.*

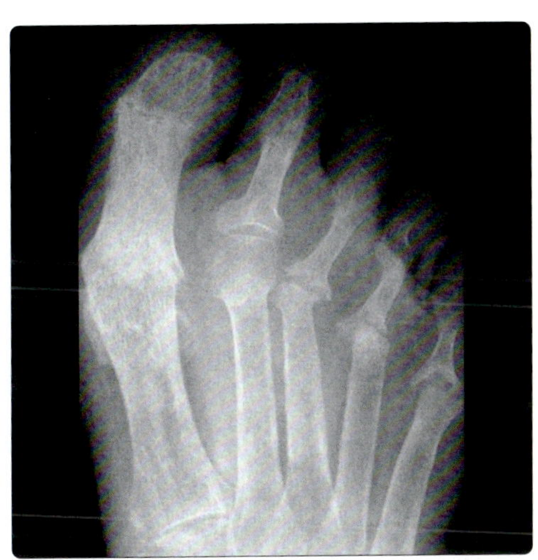

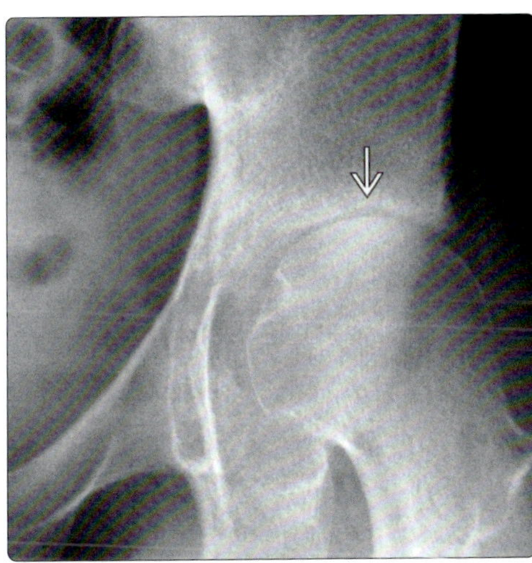

(Left) *AP radiograph shows long-term psoriatic arthritis with ankylosis of the great toe and severe erosive disease involving not only the IP joints but also the MTP joints. The diagnosis based on this radiograph alone is either PSA or chronic reactive arthritis.* **(Right)** *AP radiograph of the hip in a young woman shows cartilage loss ➙ without erosive or osteophyte change. She had asymmetric but bilateral sacroiliitis. While the proximal joint disease most suggests ankylosing spondylitis or IBD, she proved to have PSA.*

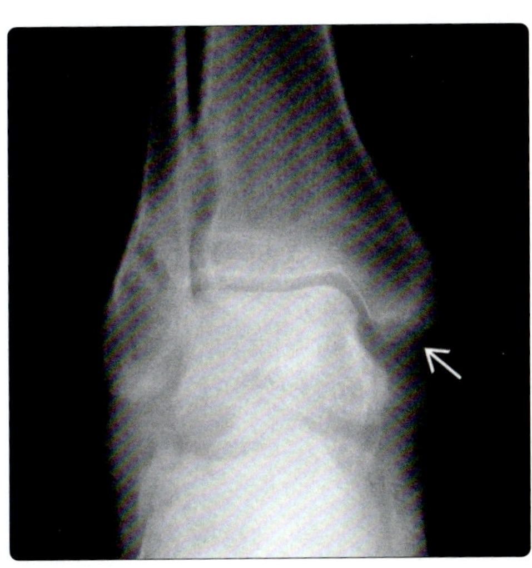

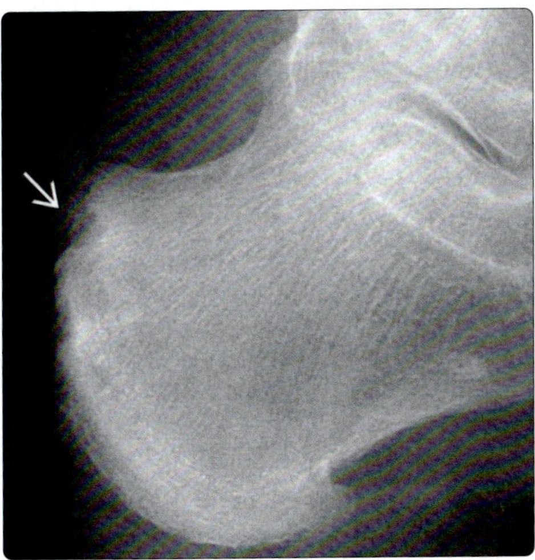

(Left) *AP radiograph demonstrates extensive enthesopathy at the malleoli ➙. There was a large effusion seen as well. This productive change may be seen in PSA, chronic reactive arthritis, advanced ankylosing spondylitis, or inflammatory bowel disease.* **(Right)** *Lateral radiograph of the calcaneus in the same patient shows advanced erosive disease at the posterior tubercle ➙. As with the enthesopathy, this is a nonspecific finding among the spondyloarthropathies; the patient proved to have PSA.*

KEY FACTS

TERMINOLOGY

- Arthritis seen as part of triad of arthritis, urethritis (cervicitis), and conjunctivitis
- < 33% manifest full triad at presentation

IMAGING

- Radiographs usually make diagnosis
  - Calcaneus: Classical location of abnormality
    - Early: Posterior tubercle deossification
    - Later: Posterior tubercle erosions, enthesitis
  - Sausage digit, periostitis, especially toes
- Axial disease
  - Bilateral sacroiliitis, often but not invariably asymmetric
  - Bulky paravertebral ossification
    - Asymmetric: Skips bodies; does not always involve right and left sides; best seen on AP view
- Early disease requires MR to establish inflammatory change, which has not yet resulted in radiographic findings

CLINICAL ISSUES

- Heel pain in 61%
  - One of most disabling features
- M:F = 5-6:1
- Caucasians affected more commonly than African Americans or other racial groups (4:1)
- Small joints of feet (64%)
- Sausage digits (52%)
- Low back pain in 61% (radiograph changes in 20%)

DIAGNOSTIC CHECKLIST

- Axial disease in CRA is identical to that of PSA
- Look carefully at soft tissues; sausage digit is highly directive finding for either CRA or PSA
- Posterior calcaneal erosions not unique to CRA
  - Consider also RA, PSA, AS/IBD arthritis
- CRA may present with severe symptoms in HIV patients; consider this underlying disease

(Left) *Coronal cut graphic of the lumbosacral spine depicts the axial abnormalities commonly found in chronic reactive arthritis (CRA). There is bilateral though asymmetric sacroiliitis ➡. There is also bulky paravertebral ossification bridging the vertebral bodies ➡.* **(Right)** *AP radiograph in a patient with CRA shows bulky paravertebral ossification ➡. This need not be as symmetric, and there are often skip areas. The sacroiliac joints both show widening and sclerosis, left more advanced than right ➡.*

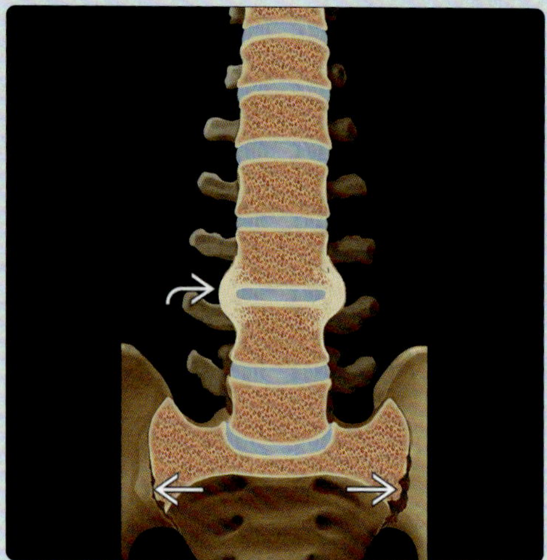

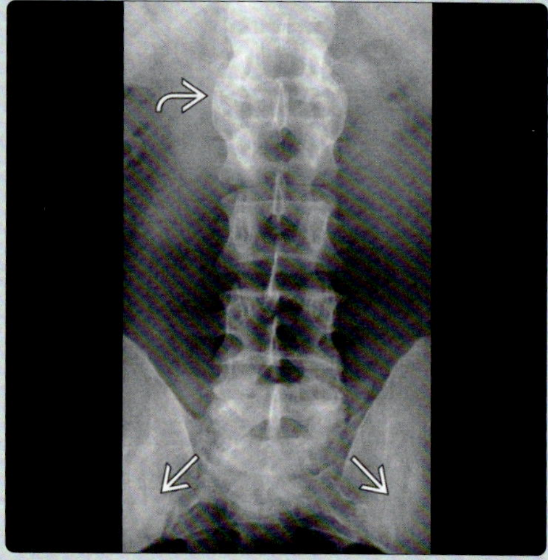

(Left) *Lateral radiograph in patient with CRA shows bridging syndesmophytes ➡ at two levels of C spine. Patient had more advanced and bulky syndesmophytes involving thoracolumbar spine (not shown). Note the normal bone density. Given advanced disease, normal bone density makes CRA or psoriatic spondyloarthropathy (PSA) more likely than ankylosing spondylitis (AS)/inflammatory bowel disease arthritis.* **(Right)** *AP radiograph, same patient, shows bilateral asymmetric sclerosis of the SI joints (right more narrow than left).*

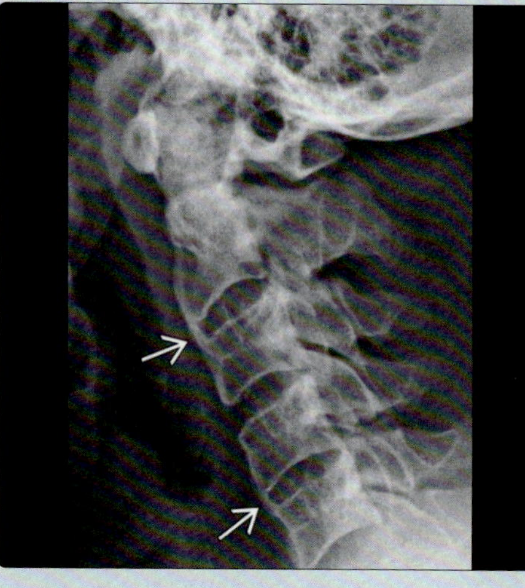

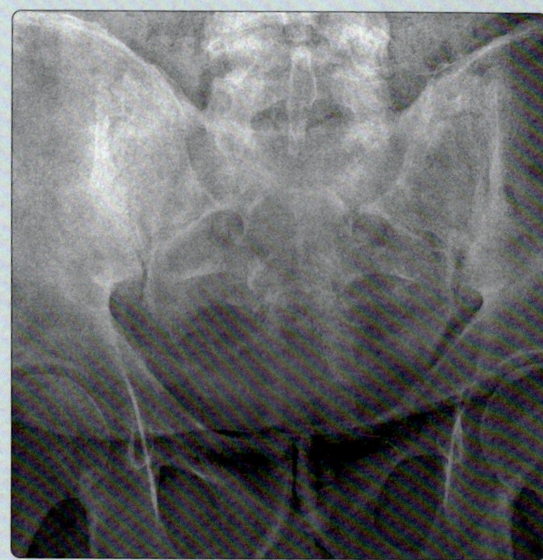

TERMINOLOGY

Abbreviations

- Chronic reactive arthritis (CRA)

Synonyms

- Reactive arthritis, sexually acquired reactive arthritis, HIV-related arthritis, Reiter disease
  - Term "Reiter" no longer in use due to recent discovery of his criminal mistreatment of prisoners

Definitions

- Arthritis seen as part of triad of arthritis, urethritis (cervicitis), and conjunctivitis
  - < 33% manifest full triad at presentation

IMAGING

General Features

- Best diagnostic clue
  - Calcaneus: Erosions and enthesitis at posterior tubercle
  - "Sausage digit," periostitis, especially toes
    - Digits of hands occasionally involved
  - Axial disease
    - Bilateral sacroiliitis
    - Bulky, asymmetric paravertebral ossification
- Location
  - Calcaneus > toes > other lower extremity joints
  - Sacroiliac joints
  - Thoracolumbar > cervical spine
- Morphology
  - Erosions, periostitis, ankylosis

Imaging Recommendations

- Best imaging tool
  - Radiographs usually make diagnosis
  - Early disease requires MR to establish inflammatory change, which has not yet resulted in radiographic findings

Radiographic Findings

- Bone density: Generally normal
  - Juxtaarticular osteopenia at active site, later normalizes
- Symmetry: Less frequent than in rheumatoid arthritis (RA) or ankylosing spondylitis (AS)
- Enthesopathy is prominent finding
  - Ossification at tendinous insertion
    - Achilles insertion on calcaneus
    - Patella
    - Pelvis: Iliac spines, ischial tuberosities, pubis
- Peripheral joints
  - Calcaneus
    - Early: Posterior tubercle deossification
    - Later: Posterior tubercle erosions
    - Posterior tubercle enthesitis, reactive bone
  - Digits
    - Sausage digit: Soft tissue swelling along entire ray, rather than about single joint
    - Periostitis: Osseous reaction along shafts of phalanges, at tendinous insertions
    - Erosions: Late osteophytes
- Axial skeleton
  - Sacroiliac joints
    - Bilateral sacroiliitis
      - Involves synovial portion of joint (inferior 1/2 to 2/3)
      - Usually asymmetric early in disease
      - Early: Erosions, widening
      - May become symmetric at any point in disease; do not use symmetry to rule out CRA
      - Late: Sclerosis, fibrous or bony ankylosis
  - Spine
    - Thoracolumbar > cervical involvement
    - Bulky paravertebral ossification
      - Seen best on AP view; extends around disc space, rather than adjacent to annulus fibrosis
      - Asymmetric: Skips bodies; does not always involve right and left sides
    - Usually can be differentiated from both spondylosis of osteoarthritis and syndesmophytes of AS
      - Early bone formation is fluffy and amorphous in all these processes, and less easily differentiated
    - Cervical spine less frequently or severely involved
      - May show atlantoaxial subluxation
    - Facet fusion may be seen
      - Less frequent and severe than in AS
      - Presence should not be used to rule out CRA
  - Other axial joints may show inflammatory change
    - Costovertebral, sternoclavicular

CT Findings

- Generally not utilized in CRA; mirrors radiographic findings
- Watch for sacroiliac changes in spine CT obtained for low back pain

MR Findings

- Advanced findings mirror radiographic appearance
  - Erosions, inflammatory change
  - Marrow in bulky paravertebral ossification
  - High signal sacroiliitis on fluid sequences, or low signal ankylosis
- Early MR findings similar to those in other arthritis processes
  - On fluid-sensitive sequences
    - Enthesopathy
      - Especially at Achilles, plantar aponeurosis, interspinous ligaments, around pelvis
    - Bone marrow edema at early sites of osseous inflammation
      - Posterior calcaneus, toes
      - Sacroiliac joints, vertebral bodies

Ultrasonographic Findings

- Synovitis, tenosynovitis

DIFFERENTIAL DIAGNOSIS

Psoriatic Spondyloarthropathy

- Axial disease identical
  - Bilateral sacroiliitis, often asymmetric
  - Bulky paravertebral ossification
- Peripheral disease: Hands predominate in psoriatic spondyloarthropathy (PSA) (feet in CRA), but toes and heel often involved in both

Rheumatoid Arthritis

- MTP and posterior calcaneal tubercle erosive disease appear similar
- No productive change (periostitis, enthesitis, osteophyte formation) in RA

Ankylosing Spondylitis/Inflammatory Bowel Disease Arthritis

- Axial disease usually different
  - Bilateral sacroiliitis more symmetric
  - Thin vertical syndesmophytes rather than bulky paravertebral ossifications
- Peripheral disease: Usually hips, knees, shoulders in AS/ inflammatory bowel disease (IBD)
  - Advanced disease may involve toes and calcaneus
- Osteoporosis in advanced AS or IBD, not in CRA

PATHOLOGY

General Features

- Etiology
  - Unknown, but strong HLA-B27 association
    - HLA(+) in 65-75% Caucasians with CRA
    - HLA(+) in 30-50% African Americans with CRA
  - May be triggered by GU (*Chlamydia*) or GI infections (*Shigella, Salmonella, Yersinia, Campylobacter*)
    - Arthritis generally lags infection by 1-4 weeks
    - Cultures of synovium and joint fluid are sterile (hence term "reactive")
    - Often no history of antecedent infection, which may be subclinical
- Genetics
  - + HLA-B27 association
- Associated abnormalities
  - Indirect association with HIV
    - Prevalence and severity of CRA ↑ in persons with HIV
    - Etiology may be sexually transmitted disease caused by microorganisms common to both CRA and HIV

Gross Pathologic & Surgical Features

- Reactive bone formation

Microscopic Features

- Sterile but inflammatory synovium and effusions

CLINICAL ISSUES

Presentation

- Most common signs/symptoms
  - Heel pain (61%)
    - Radiographic changes on calcaneus in 16%
    - One of most disabling features
  - Knee pain (68%)
  - Ankle pain (49%)
  - Small joints of feet (64%)
    - Small joints of hands (42%)
    - Sausage digits (52%)
  - Low back pain
    - Pain in 61%
    - Only 20% have axial radiographic changes (likely greater if imaging with MR)
      - Sacroiliitis by radiograph (17%)
      - Spondylitis by radiograph (7%)
  - Urethritis/cervicitis: Mucocutaneous ulcerations
  - Conjunctivitis in 33%; usually mild
  - Urethritis/conjunctivitis may predate articular symptoms
- Other signs/symptoms
  - 25% have keratoderma blennorrhagicum
    - Rash on soles/palms; clinically resembles pustular psoriasis
  - Fever relatively common
  - Weight loss may be striking
  - Aortitis in 1-2%; patients with longstanding disease
  - Amyloidosis (rare)

Demographics

- Age
  - Onset: 16-60 years old
  - Mean: 26 years old
- Gender
  - M:F = 5-6:1
- Ethnicity
  - Caucasians affected more commonly than African Americans or other racial groups (4:1)
    - Non-Caucasians have lower frequency of positive HLA-B27
- Epidemiology
  - 3.5 cases/100,000 males < 50 years old

Natural History & Prognosis

- Majority spontaneously resolve over months
- Substantial minority (15%): Relapsing course with persistent and disabling arthritis/enthesitis
  - 70% of these develop axial arthritic changes

Treatment

- Same as for AS and psoriatic arthritis
- NSAIDs, DMARDs for symptomatic relief
- Injection of glucocorticosteroid for monoarticular
- Anti-TNF-α is promising, affording symptomatic relief and ↓ inflammation
  - Not yet proven to delay progression of disease

DIAGNOSTIC CHECKLIST

Consider

- CRA may present with severe symptoms in HIV patients; consider this underlying disease

Image Interpretation Pearls

- Axial disease in CRA is identical to that of PSA
- Posterior calcaneal erosions not unique to CRA
  - Consider also RA, PSA, AS, IBD arthritis
- Look carefully at soft tissues; sausage digit is highly directive finding for either CRA or PSA
  - Usually will see periostitis and early articular disease

SELECTED REFERENCES

1. Keithlin J et al: Systematic review and meta-analysis of the proportion of non-typhoidal Salmonella cases that develop chronic sequelae. Epidemiol Infect. 143(7):1333-51, 2015
2. Lew PP et al: Imaging of disorders affecting the bone and skin. Radiographics. 34(1):197-216, 2014
3. Hannu T: Reactive arthritis. Best Pract Res Clin Rheumatol. 25(3):347-57, 2011

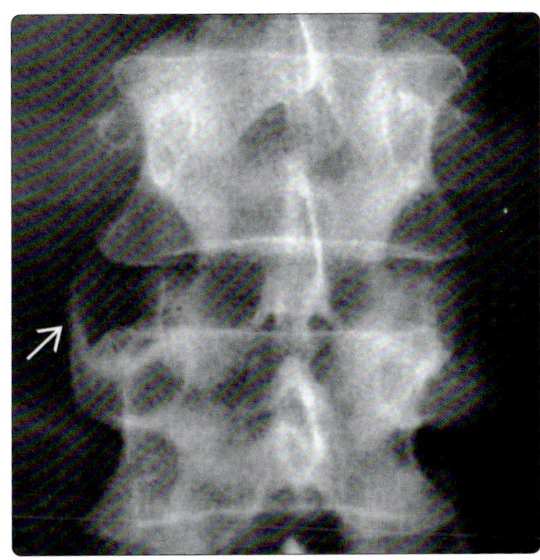

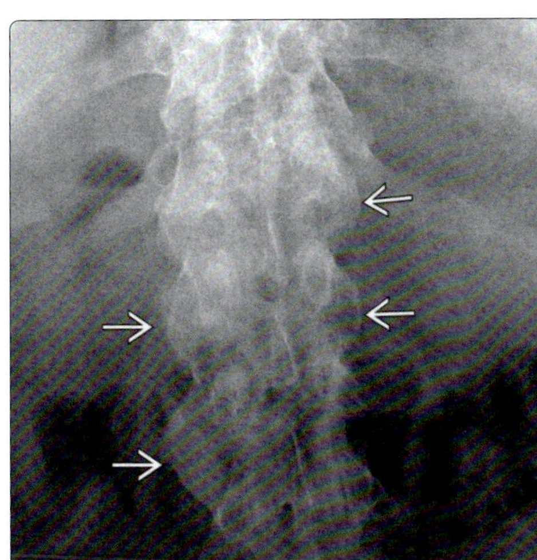

(Left) *AP radiograph shows the spine in a patient with CRA. The character of an early paravertebral ossification is seen ➡ arising from the vertebral body at some distance from the endplate and bridging toward the adjacent vertebral body, differentiating it from a syndesmophyte.* **(Right)** *AP radiograph of the thoracolumbar junction in a 48-year-old man with CRA shows advanced bulky and somewhat asymmetric syndesmophyte formation ➡, typical of the disease process.*

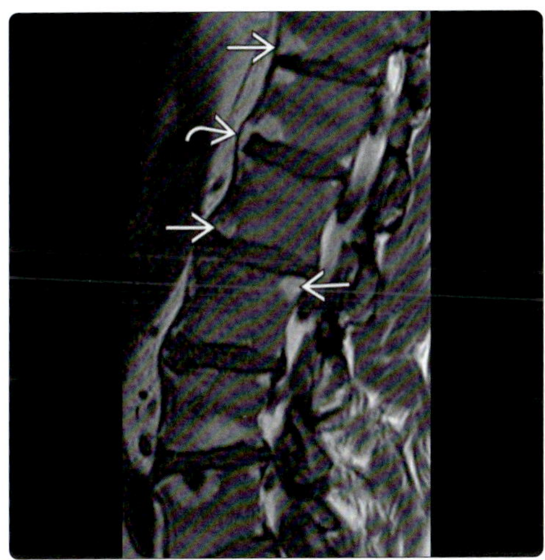

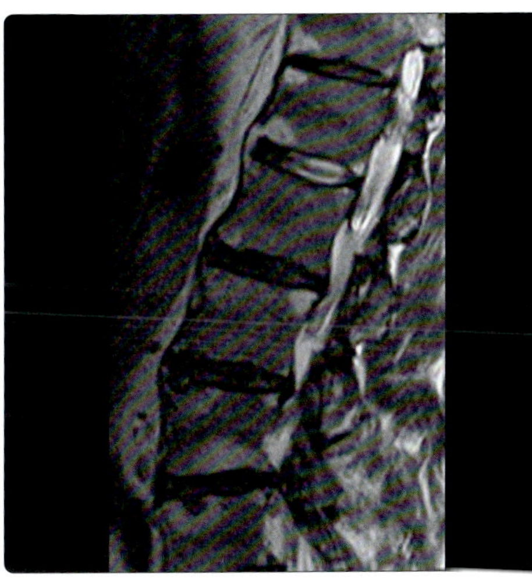

(Left) *Sagittal T1 MR, same patient, shows bridging syndesmophytes, some containing fatty marrow ➡. Note also the high-signal corner Romanus lesions ➡. The fact that these lesions are high signal on T1 indicates chronicity of the process, with fat replacing the site of previous inflammation. If the inflammation were active, it would be low SI on T1, but hyperintense on T2.* **(Right)** *Sagittal T2 MR also shows the Romanus lesions and fatty marrow in the syndesmophyte since the sequence was not fat saturated.*

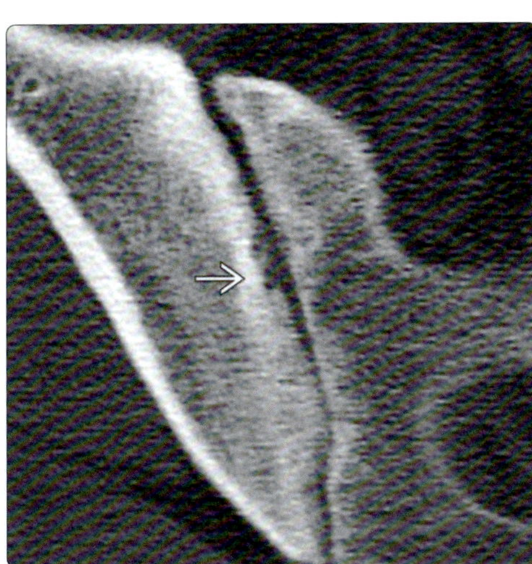

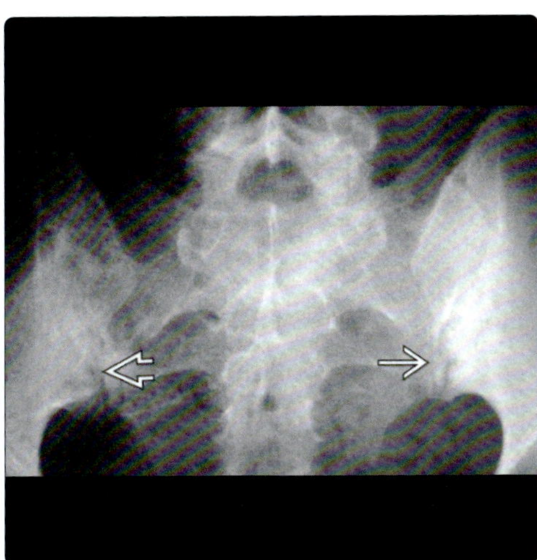

(Left) *Axial bone CT shows early, somewhat subtle axial abnormalities, with early erosive change ➡ of the sacroiliac joint, and mild associated sclerosis. This was more prominent on the right than the left side; the patient proved to have CRA.* **(Right)** *AP radiograph is classic for CRA. The sacroiliac joints show bilateral but asymmetric erosive change with sclerosis, the left ➡ worse than the right ➡.*

(Left) *AP radiograph shows SI joints that are both abnormal, with sclerosis and erosions. The abnormality is bilateral but asymmetric, the left ➔ worse than the right ➔. Remember, however, that any CRA patient may demonstrate symmetric disease at some point in the process.* **(Right)** *AP radiograph shows advanced changes of CRA with bilateral SI joint fusion. There is unilateral erosion of the hip ➔; when the disease is longstanding, proximal joints may become involved.*

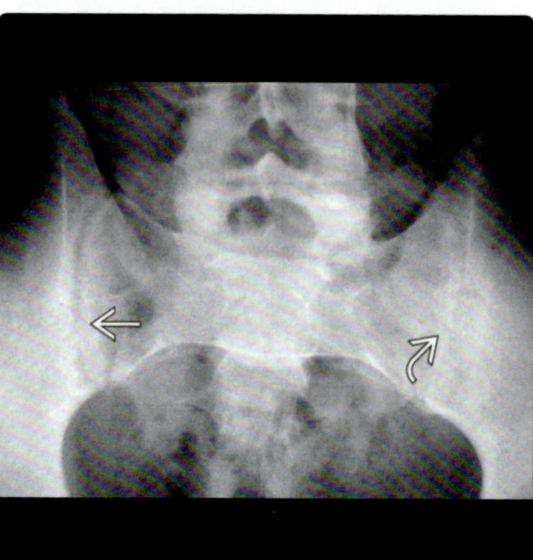

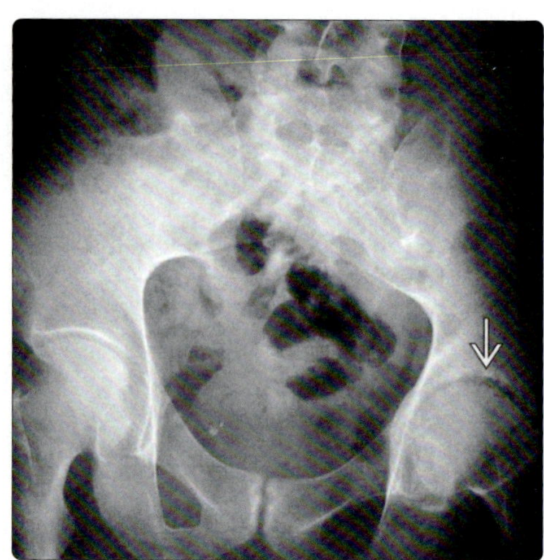

(Left) *Lateral radiograph demonstrates prominent erosions of the posterior calcaneus ➔. The bone density is normal. Findings are typical, though not pathognomonic, for CRA. Other erosive arthritides, such as RA, PSA, and AS, are possible, though less likely.* **(Right)** *Lateral radiograph shows a classic presentation of CRA, with dense reactive change and enthesopathy at the Achilles insertion ➔ as well as the plantar aponeurosis ➔. Such reactive change should not be seen in RA or AS.*

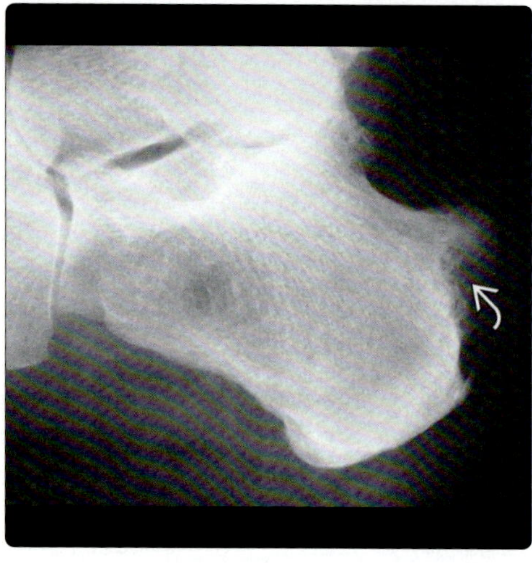

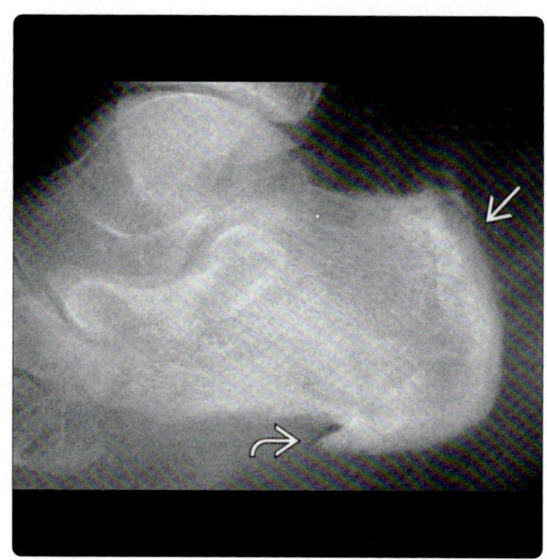

(Left) *Lateral radiograph of the left calcaneus in a patient with CRA is normal, showing distinct cortex ➔ and a clear pre-Achilles fat pad. It is presented for comparison.* **(Right)** *Lateral radiograph of the contralateral heel in the same patient is abnormal with indistinctness of the cortex ➔ and early erosive change. The pre-Achilles fat pad is replaced by inflammatory tissue. This is early disease, which may be subtle on radiograph and must be actively sought.*

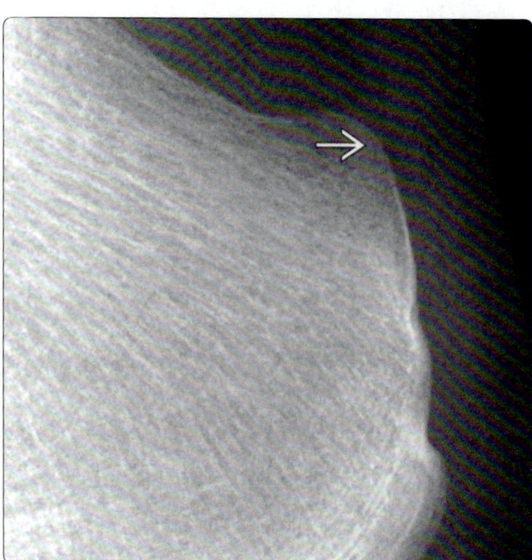

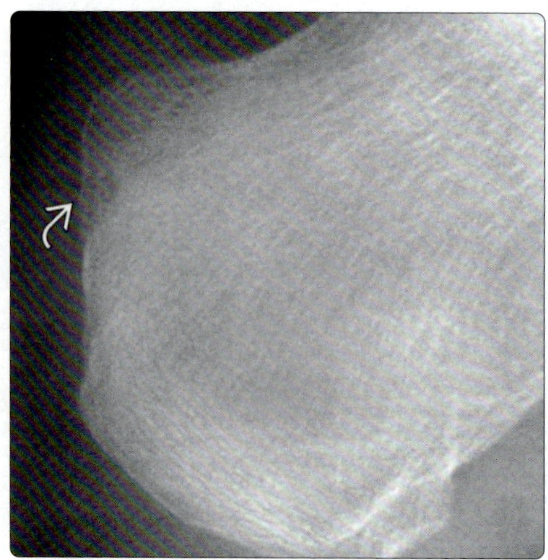

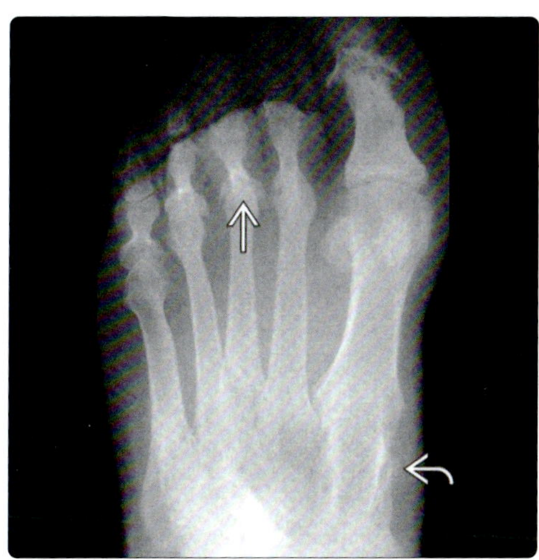

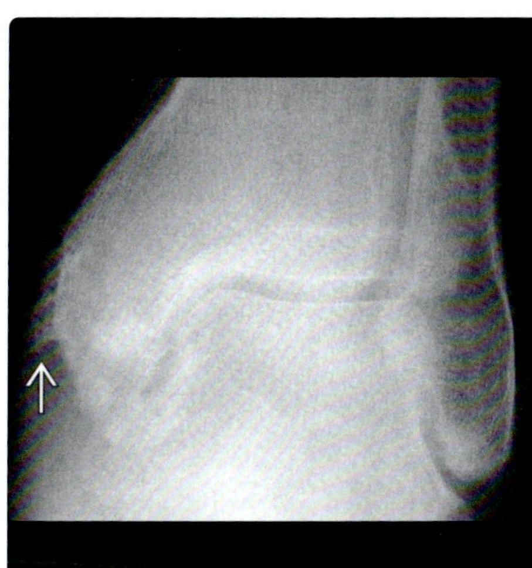

(Left) *AP radiograph of the forefoot in a patient with CRA shows predominantly erosive change at the MTP and IP joints. There is a suggestion of enthesopathy at the medial cuneiform. Remember that all of the spondyloarthropathies may, at any time in their process, exhibit erosive, productive, or mixed patterns of arthritic disease.* **(Right)** *AP radiograph in the same patient shows productive change with enthesopathy at the malleoli. The location and appearance is typical of CRA.*

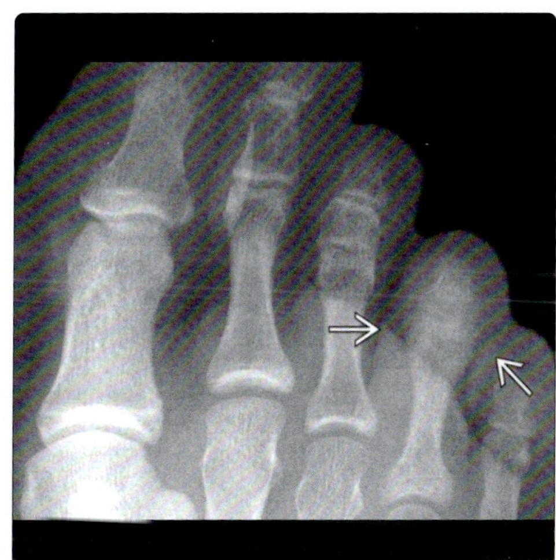

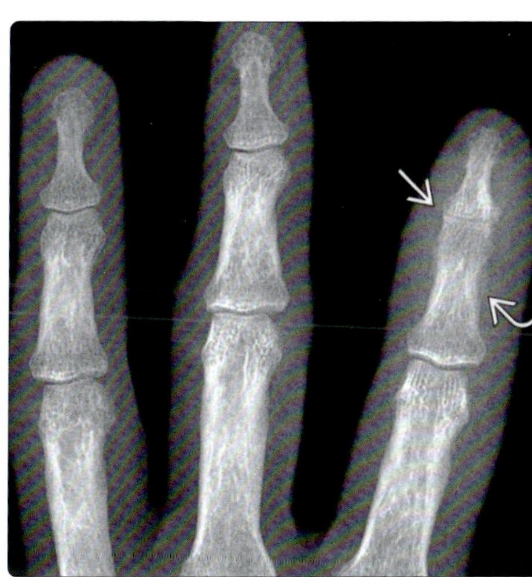

(Left) *AP radiograph in a patient with CRA and toe pain shows a "sausage digit" with swelling of the entire ray. There is no periostitis or erosive change at this time (the toe is flexed, obliterating the IP joint space). Sausage digits are seen in CRA and PSA.* **(Right)** *PA radiograph shows sausage digit with periostitis, as well as cartilage narrowing in the DIP. This sausage digit may be seen in PSA or CRA. The latter diagnosis is associated with HIV patients, as in this case.*

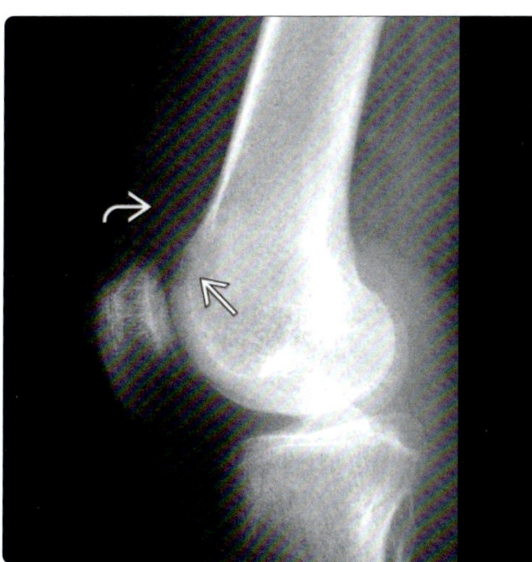

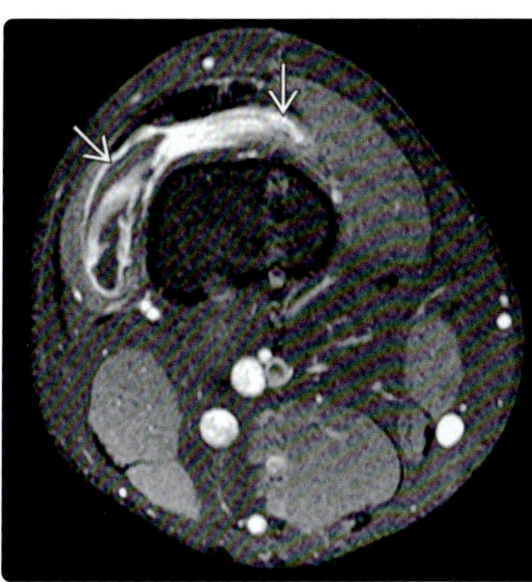

(Left) *Lateral radiograph of the knee shows an effusion with juxtaarticular osteoporosis and early erosive change. This patient has CRA; the joints of the lower extremity are most at risk for involvement.* **(Right)** *Axial T1WI C+ FS MR shows typical synovitis with irregular, mildly thickened and enhancing synovium. The appearance is nonspecific. Aspirate to exclude infection showed no organisms or culture growth. Further work-up led to the diagnosis of CRA.*

Gout

KEY FACTS

TERMINOLOGY

- Hyperuricemia, resulting in sodium urate crystal deposition in soft tissues and joints
  - Primary gout: Results from abnormalities in purine metabolism or from idiopathic ↓ renal excretion of urate
  - Secondary gout: Results from increased serum uric acid levels resulting from associated disorder
    - Neoplasm, lymphoproliferative disease
    - End-stage renal disease (ESRD)
    - Drugs (diuretics, ethanol, cytotoxics)

IMAGING

- Best clue: Dense tophi, juxtaarticular erosions with overhanging edges
- Location: 1st metatarsal phalangeal (MTP) most frequent site
  - 50% of patients have this as initial site
  - 80-90% involve this site at some point in disease
- Radiographs usually normal 1st 7-10 years of disease
- Normal bone density maintained
- Cartilage damage occurs only late in disease
- Erosions are well circumscribed with sclerotic margins
- Erosions may have overhanging edge
- Tophi: Dense nodules
- MR: Synovial pannus: Thickened, low T1 & T2 signal with peripheral enhancement
  - Adjacent soft tissue &/or bone marrow edema: Low signal T1, high signal T2
  - Gouty tophus has constant T1WI MR appearance: Intermediate homogeneous signal intensity
  - Gouty tophus appears variably on T2 & other fluid-sensitive sequences: Mixed low and high signal
  - Gouty tophus enhances with contrast

DIAGNOSTIC CHECKLIST

- Gout can look like anything and present anywhere in musculoskeletal system
- Gout is common; maintain high index of suspicion

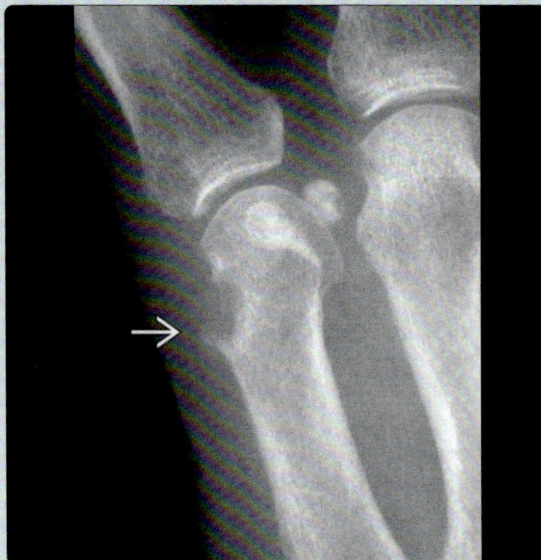

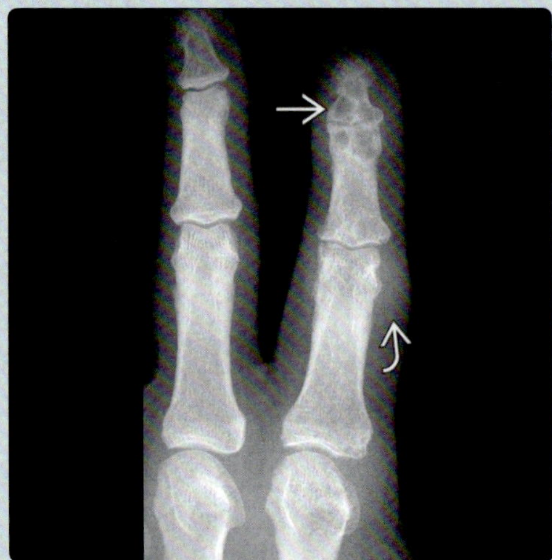

(Left) *PA radiograph shows a classic appearance of gout with soft tissue swelling at the 5th MCP. A juxtaarticular erosion has an overhanging edge ➡, extending perpendicularly from the metaphysis. Note that the cartilage width is normal.* **(Right)** *PA radiograph shows particularly well-marginated erosions at the DIP ➡; this type of margination is typical of gout. Other less well-marginated erosions are seen at the PIP, along with juxtaarticular swelling containing density typical of tophus ⮳.*

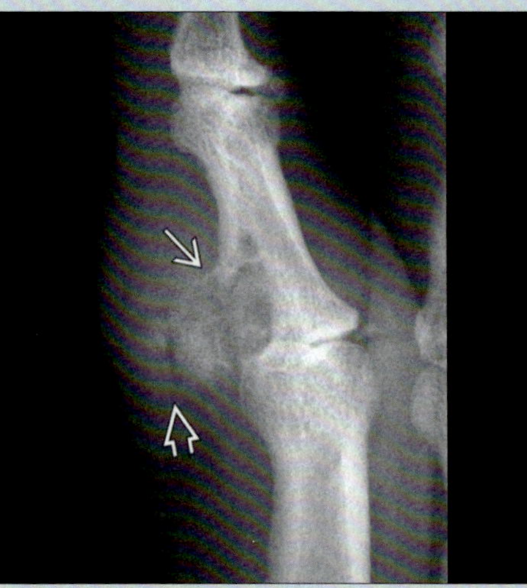

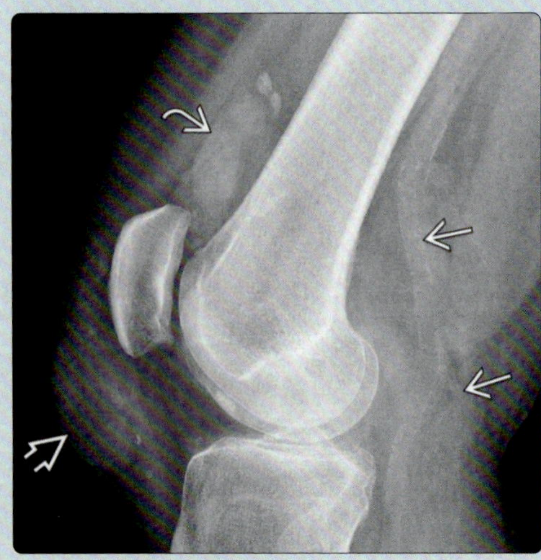

(Left) *Oblique radiograph shows an impressive soft tissue tophus containing density typical of sodium urate deposition ⇨. A large erosion at the PIP has resulted in a classic overhanging edge ➡. Gout is the only possible diagnosis.* **(Right)** *Lateral radiograph in a 55 year old with end-stage renal disease shows an unusually dense effusion ⇨ as well as a prepatellar dense tophus ➡. Prominent large and small vessel calcification ⮳ is noted as well, typical of ESRD. Gouty deposits are not uncommon in these patients.*

TERMINOLOGY

Synonyms

- Gouty arthritis, tophaceous gout

Definitions

- Hyperuricemia, resulting in sodium urate crystal deposition in soft tissues and joints
  - Primary gout: Results from abnormalities in purine metabolism or from idiopathic ↓ renal excretion of urate
  - Secondary gout: Results from increased serum uric acid levels resulting from associated disorder
    - Neoplasms, lymphoproliferative disease
    - Chronic renal failure
    - Drug therapy (diuretics, ethanol, cytotoxics)
  - Saturnine gout: Results from chronic lead intoxication from either occult or occupational exposure or ingestion of moonshine

IMAGING

General Features

- Best diagnostic clue
  - Tophi, juxtaarticular erosions, overhanging edges
- Location
  - 1st metatarsal phalangeal (MTP) most frequent site
    - 50% of patients have this as initial site
    - 80-90% involve this site at some point in disease
  - Lower extremity > upper extremity
  - Axial disease in 14% gout patients; L > T or C-spine
  - Small joints > large joints
  - Any musculoskeletal site can be involved
  - Usually oligoarticular but may be polyarticular
  - Generally not symmetric
- Size
  - Tophi and erosive disease may be small and discrete (few millimeters) or several centimeters in size
- Morphology
  - Overhanging edge said to be characteristic: Excrescence of juxtaarticular erosion extending perpendicularly from underlying bone

Radiographic Findings

- Radiographs usually normal 1st 7-10 years of disease
- Classic radiographic features
  - Normal bone density maintained
  - Cartilage damage occurs only late in disease
  - Erosions are well circumscribed with sclerotic margins
    - Erosions may have overhanging edge
    - Erosions often intraarticular but classically are juxtaarticular as well
  - Tophi: Dense nodules
    - Density is usually cloudy, amorphous
    - Tophi occasionally contain distinct calcifications
    - Eccentric, not necessarily associated with joint
- Unusual, late radiographic features
  - Rare intraosseous calcifications
    - Simulate appearance of enchondroma or infarct
    - Related to intraosseous penetration of crystals
    - Usually longstanding gout with severe renal disease
    - Distal aspect of 1st metatarsal most frequent site; may have adjacent soft tissue calcification
  - Tophus may be so large and osseous destruction so severe that tumor is suspected
    - Look for any sign that process may be articular; destructive articular tumors are rare

Ultrasonographic Findings

- Combination of effusion, tophus, erosion, & double contour sign (hyperechoic line of crystals with underlying hyperechoic line of subchondral bone) diagnostic in 97%

CT Findings

- Dual-energy CT useful in challenging cases
  - Differentiates urate crystals from calcium using specific attenuation coefficients

MR Findings

- Effusion: Low T1 and high T2 signal; seen in 50%
- Synovial pannus: Thickened, low T1 and T2 signal with peripheral enhancement
- Erosion (intraarticular or juxtaarticular)
- Adjacent soft tissue &/or bone marrow edema: Low signal T1, high signal T2
- Characteristics of gouty tophi
  - Gouty tophus has constant T1WI MR appearance: Intermediate homogeneous signal intensity
  - Gouty tophus has variable appearance on T2 & other fluid-sensitive sequences: Mixed low and high signal
    - Variable whether tophus is soft tissue or intraosseous
    - Variability related to amount of calcium present
    - Most common appearance on fluid-sensitive sequences: Intermediate to low signal, heterogeneous
  - Gouty tophus enhances with contrast

DIFFERENTIAL DIAGNOSIS

Inflammatory Arthritides (RA, CPPD)

- Any single erosive site may have similar appearance
- Thickened hypervascular pannus/synovium

Amyloid Deposition

- Intraarticular and extraarticular deposition has similar MR signal characteristics to gout
- May cause erosions

PVNS and Giant Cell Tumor of Tendon Sheath

- Nodular mass has similar MR signal characteristics to gout but may bloom with GRE
- Erosions/subchondral cysts may be prominent

Synovial Osteochondromatosis

- May form conglomerate, nodular-appearing mass, which may have similar MR signal characteristics
- May cause erosions

Brown Tumor of Hyperparathyroidism

- Subchondral location may simulate erosion
- Low signal intensity on both T1 & T2 MR imaging simulates that of intraosseous gout
- With treatment, brown tumor may hyperossify over time, differentiating it from deposition diseases
- Patients with end-stage renal disease are at risk for brown tumor formation, gout, and amyloid

PATHOLOGY

General Features

- Etiology
  - Biochemical derangement: Hyperuricemia → deposition of urate crystals in soft tissue, cartilage, and bone → inflammatory response and destruction
    - Minority of patients with elevated serum urate level develop acute attacks of gouty arthritis
    - Tophaceous gout: Chronic phase of disease (rarely, tophi noted at time of 1st attack)
  - Majority of cases are idiopathic; may be familial
  - Minority of cases seen in patients with chronic disease (end-stage renal disease, psoriasis) or high rate of cellular turnover (treated widespread tumor)
- Associated abnormalities
  - May cause gouty nephropathy: Crystals impair renal function (pyelonephritis, urinary obstruction)

Microscopic Features

- Sodium urate deposition in cartilage, bone (usually epiphyseal), periarticular structures, kidney
- Tophus: Mass of urates
  - Either crystalline or amorphous
  - Surrounded by vascular inflammatory reaction (macrophages, lymphocytes, fibroblasts)
- Synovial fluid
  - Negative birefringent needle-shaped crystals under polarized light microscopy
  - White blood cell count: 7,000-10,000

CLINICAL ISSUES

Presentation

- Most common signs/symptoms
  - Patients usually have had gout 10-12 years before tophi are seen radiographically or on physical exam
  - Classic presentation is sudden onset of pain at 1st MTP, often at night (podagra)
  - Clinical presentation of soft tissue tophus may be atypical of gout
    - Occasionally presents with swelling and erythema, without erosive or articular process
    - Clinical consideration of painful mass may be infection or neoplasm
    - Rarely presents with nerve compression by tophus
- Other signs/symptoms
  - Up to 40% may have normal serum uric acid levels at time of initial attack

Demographics

- Age
  - 30-60 years at onset, unless predisposing factor
- Gender
  - M:F = 20:1
  - Rare in premenopausal females but incidence increases after menopause
- Ethnicity
  - Pacific Islanders > Caucasians > African Americans
- Epidemiology
  - < 5% of patients with hyperuricemia develop gout
  - Prevalence of asymptomatic hyperuricemia: 5-8% in USA
  - < 0.5% of USA population has symptomatic gout
  - 5% of all patients with arthritis have gout
  - In families affected by gout, incidence range: 6-80%
- Other predisposing factors
  - Metabolic syndrome patients (obesity, hypertension, hyperlipidemia, diabetes, prothrombotic state, proinflammatory state): Remarkably high prevalence of gout
  - Use of thiazide diuretics
  - Lead toxicity (particularly from home-made stills)
  - Heavy alcohol consumption
  - End-stage renal disease
  - Tumor lysis syndrome (rapid increase in uric acid with rapid response to oncologic therapy)
  - Innate immune system may relate to response to hyperuricemia

Natural History & Prognosis

- If untreated, causes significant episodic pain
- Over time, progressively destructive arthritic disease

Treatment

- Acute attacks: Nonsteroidal antiinflammatory medications, particularly indomethacin
- Long-term control
  - Probenecid: Enhances uric acid excretion
  - Allopurinol: Inhibits uric acid production
  - Various forms of uricase: Catalyzes conversion of uric acid to more readily excreted allantoin
    - Difficulty with antigenicity; new forms being produced; may be used as induction agent
- Dietary and alcohol consumption modifications
- Consider strong association of metabolic syndrome and gout; recognize and treat comorbidities
- Studies are currently underway to show efficacy of MR, CT, and US to monitor pharmacological treatment

DIAGNOSTIC CHECKLIST

Consider

- Radiograph usually diagnostic; obviates need for MR
- MR of mass should not be interpreted without corresponding radiograph (or gout may not be considered)
- Septic arthritis & crystal-induced arthropathy can occur simultaneously; aspirated fluid must be evaluated for both

Image Interpretation Pearls

- Gout can look like anything and present anywhere in musculoskeletal system
  - Location of disease may be atypical
  - Soft tissue tophus may mimic infection or tumor
  - Gout is common; maintain high index of suspicion

SELECTED REFERENCES

1. Girish G et al: Advanced imaging in gout. AJR Am J Roentgenol. 201(3):515-25, 2013
2. Lumezanu E et al: Axial (spinal) gout. Curr Rheumatol Rep. 14(2):161-4, 2012
3. Desai MA et al: Clinical utility of dual-energy CT for evaluation of tophaceous gout. Radiographics. 31(5):1365-75; discussion 1376-7, 2011
4. Glazebrook KN et al: Identification of intraarticular and periarticular uric acid crystals with dual-energy CT: initial evaluation. Radiology. 261(2):516-24, 2011
5. Konatalapalli RM et al: Gout in the axial skeleton. J Rheumatol. 36(3):609-13, 2009

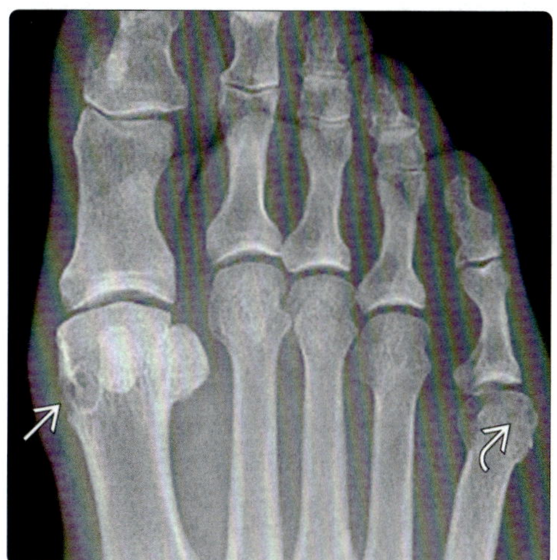

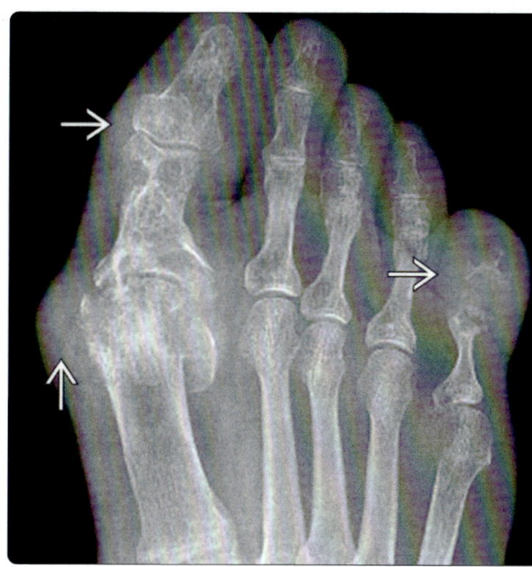

(Left) *AP radiograph shows early gout with a well-marginated erosion in a juxtaarticular position near the 1st MTP ➡. Joint space and bone density are normal. No intraarticular erosions are seen at this joint, though there is one at the 5th MTP ➡.* **(Right)** *AP radiograph shows much more advanced gout. Tophi are seen at several sites ➡ along with highly destructive erosive disease. By this point in the process, cartilage destruction is seen as well. Given the tophi, gout is the only possible diagnosis.*

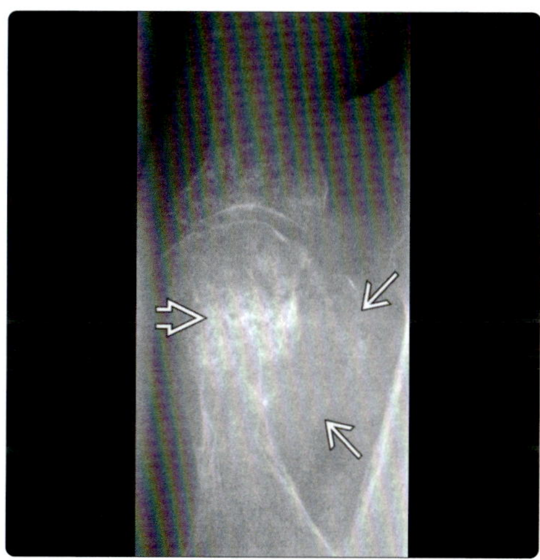

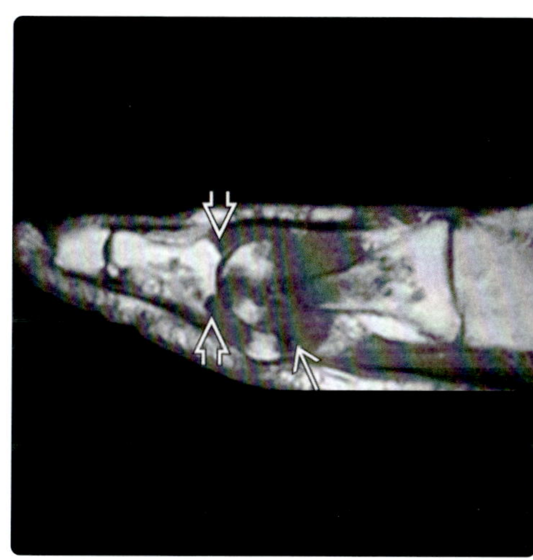

(Left) *AP radiograph shows a destructive process at the neck of the 1st MT. The metatarsal itself contains calcifications ➡. The soft tissue mass also contains faint calcifications ➡. Either matrix-containing tumor or advanced gout can show such soft tissue and intraosseous calcifications.* **(Right)** *Sagittal T1 MR, same patient, suggests the articular nature of the process. Besides the severe circumferential destruction of the neck of the 1st metatarsal, there are erosions involving the plantar base of the proximal phalanx ➡ as well as the sesamoid ➡.*

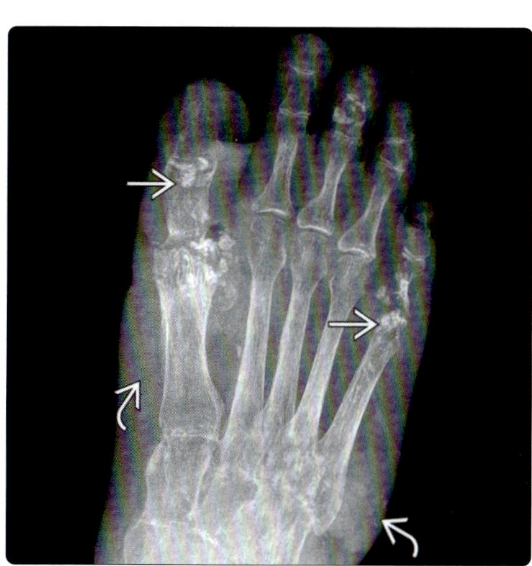

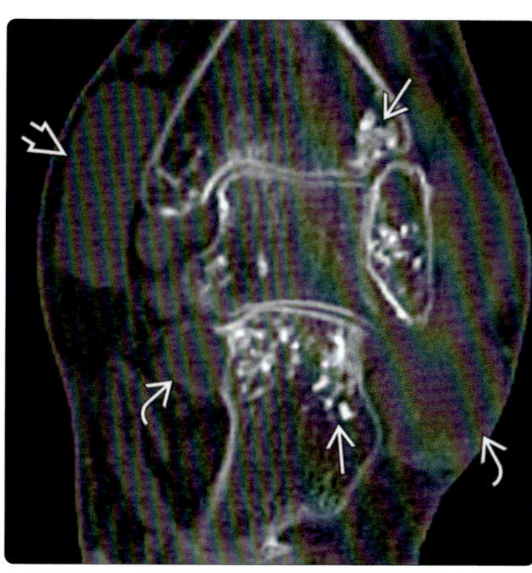

(Left) *AP radiograph in a 65-year-old woman allergic to colchicine shows advanced gout, with tophaceous deposits throughout the soft tissues ➡ as well as unusual intraosseous dense deposits ➡. Erosions are prominent in the 1st and 5th MTPs.* **(Right)** *Coronal CT, same patient, shows the intraosseous deposits ➡ even better than on radiograph. In addition, there are soft tissue masses, some of which are tophi ➡ and some of which are abscesses ➡ in this patient with chronic insufficiently treated gout.*

(Left) *Axial PD MR of the elbow in a 60-year-old man shows an intermediate intensity mass ➡ within the olecranon bursa, extending through the triceps tendon ➡ to directly erode the olecranon ➡.* **(Right)** *Sagittal PD FS MR, same patient, shows inhomogeneously hyperintense tophus within the olecranon bursa ➡. Bone marrow edema and erosion ➡ are noted, as is disruption and infiltration of much of the triceps tendon ➡. The process is entirely extraarticular; there is no actual joint involvement in this patient with gout.*

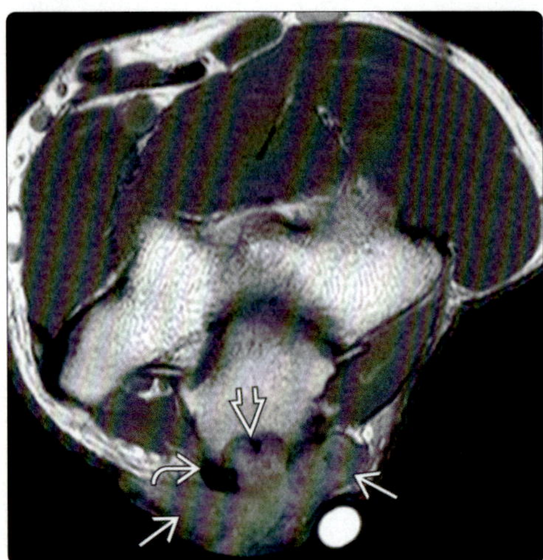

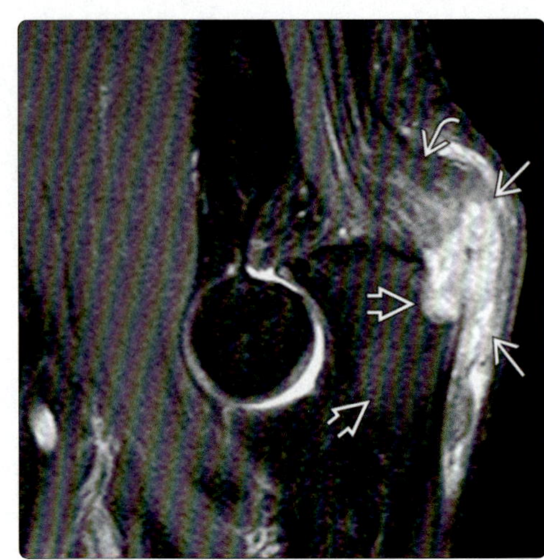

(Left) *Lateral radiograph shows an enlarged olecranon bursae containing relatively dense calcifications ➡. Gouty tophi usually have more amorphous density, but rarely the calcification will be as prominent as seen in this case.* **(Right)** *Coronal T1 MR in a 52-year-old man shows a single site of marrow edema ➡ and associated erosion ➡. The radiographs were normal; this finding is nonspecific.*

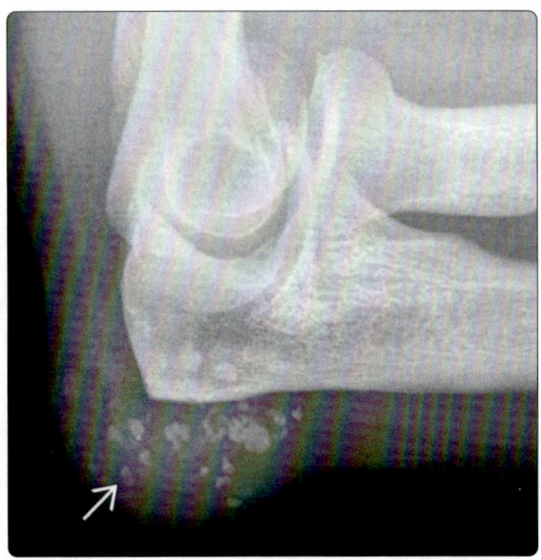

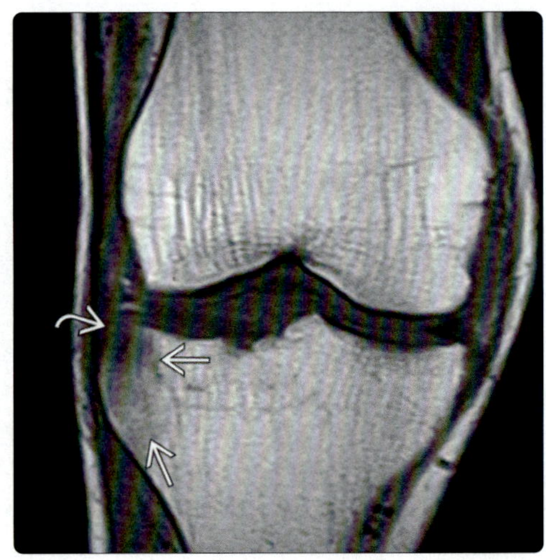

(Left) *Axial T2 FS MR, same patient, through the tibial plateau shows multiple sites of marrow edema ➡ in a juxtaarticular position. Small effusion is present.* **(Right)** *Sagittal T1 C+ FS MR in same patient shows marrow edema ➡, small erosion ➡, and mild synovial thickening with surrounding enhancement ➡. These findings remain nonspecific, and could represent any inflammatory arthropathy; aspiration proved gout.*

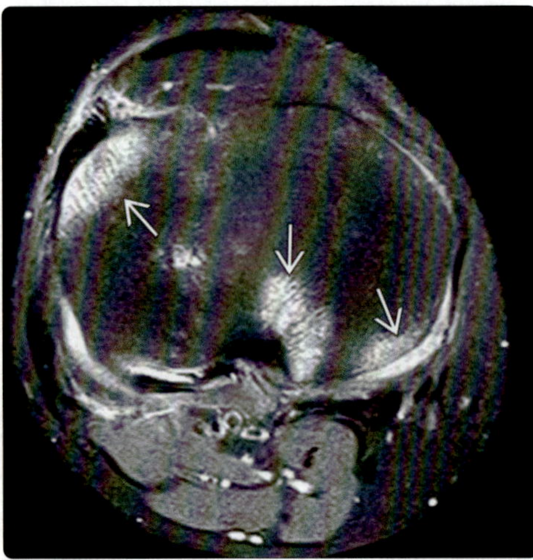

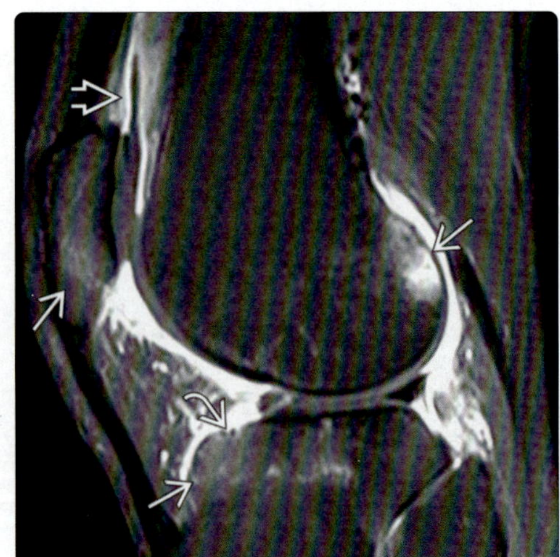

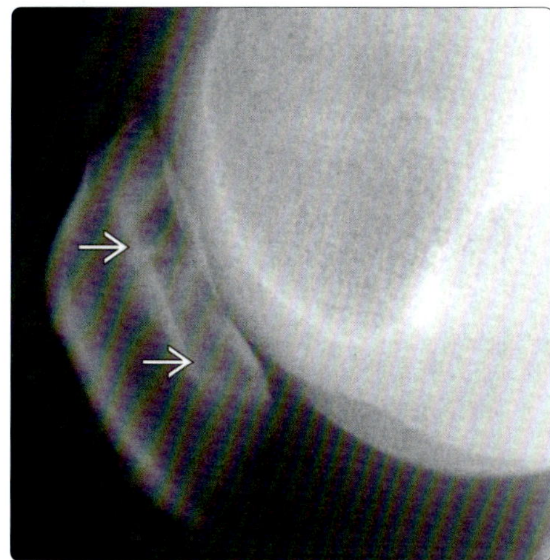

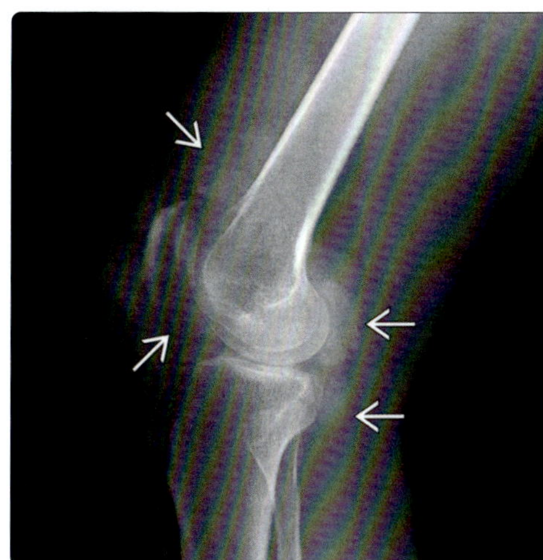

(Left) *Lateral radiograph shows a lytic lesion within the articular portion of the patella ➡, without other abnormalities. This proved to be gout; remember that the patella is a commonly involved bone in this process.* **(Right)** *Lateral radiograph demonstrates dense nodules ➡ centered within and around the knee. Bone density is normal, and there are no erosions. Gout can be extremely painful, usually from the associated synovitis/inflammation. The joint was aspirated, revealing urate crystals.*

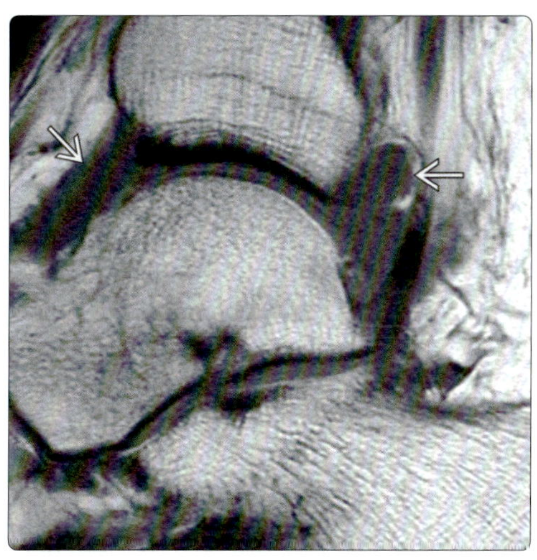

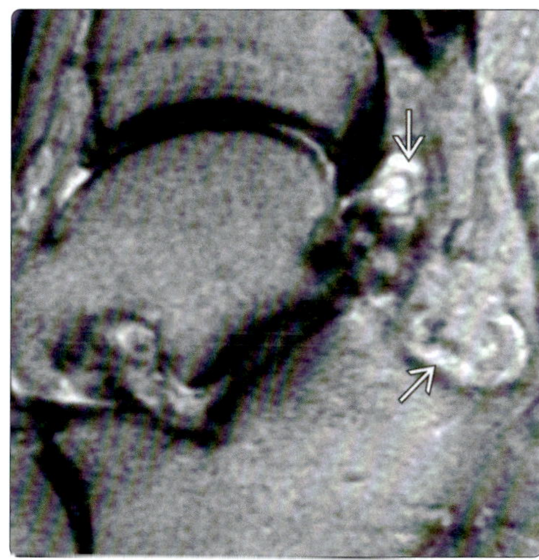

(Left) *Sagittal T1WI MR shows findings that result in a differential diagnosis of gout vs. pigmented villonodular synovitis (PVNS). Both disease entities can be monoarticular; either could have the low signal density within the tibiotalar joint seen in this case ➡.* **(Right)** *Sagittal T2WI MR in the same patient shows heterogeneity but largely low signal ➡. The patient is middle-aged, which slightly favors the diagnosis of PVNS over gout. At aspiration, this proved to be gout.*

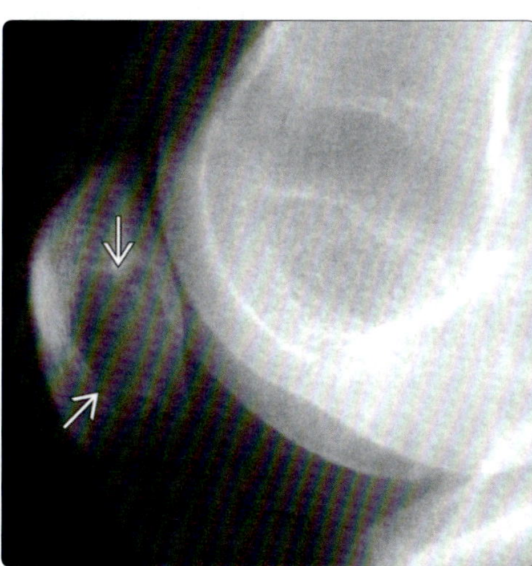

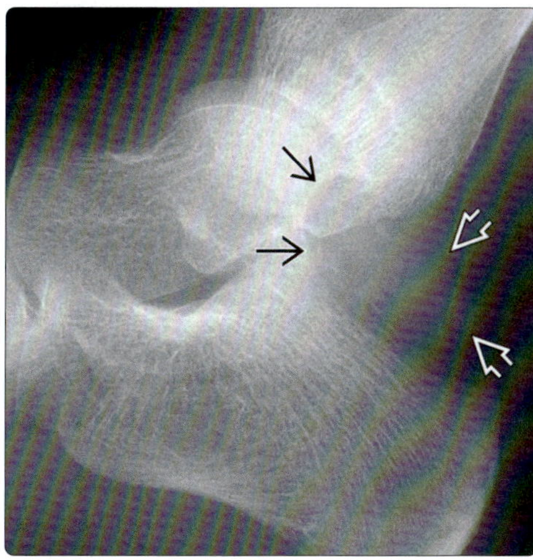

(Left) *Lateral radiograph shows a large erosion or lytic lesion within the patella ➡. Nothing else characterizes the lesion.* **(Right)** *Lateral radiograph in the same patient shows a large soft tissue mass at the posterior talus ➡ eroding the bones ➡. The extrinsic nature of the talar lesion suggests an erosive process. This young patient has end-stage renal disease and is at risk for deposition disease, such as gout or amyloid. Biopsy proved gout at each of these sites.*

Pyrophosphate Arthropathy

KEY FACTS

TERMINOLOGY

- Terminology has been confusing since terms have been used interchangeably
  - Chondrocalcinosis: General term for cartilage calcification (seen by pathology or imaging)
  - Pyrophosphate arthropathy: Specific pattern of structural joint damage that occurs from CPPD crystal deposition, intra- and paraarticular
  - Pseudogout: Gout-like clinical syndrome produced by CPPD crystal deposition; **not** radiologic diagnosis

IMAGING

- Location is distinctive
  - Chondrocalcinosis: Knee > symphysis pubis > wrist > hip (acetabular labrum) > shoulder > elbow
  - Arthropathy: Knee > wrist > hand > shoulder, hip
    - Knee: Patellofemoral shows isolated or greater involvement than medial or lateral compartments
    - Wrist: Radiocarpal + 2nd and 3rd MCP
  - Spine: Particularly at dens ("crowned dens")
- Radiographic appearance
  - Chondrocalcinosis (not invariably present)
  - Early arthropathy may be mixed or even purely erosive (1/8 will show erosion)
  - Hook-like or "drooping" osteophytes metacarpal heads
  - Subchondral cysts common
  - Scapholunate advanced collapse wrist
- CT: Calcific densities may be more conspicuous than on radiograph or MR
- MR of chondrocalcinosis
  - Chondrocalcinosis may be low or high signal on either T1WI or fluid-sensitive sequences
    - May not be conspicuous
  - Meniscus may appear enlarged
    - Chondrocalcinosis signal mimics meniscal tear
  - Calcifications surrounding dens are low signal; can suggest pannus of rheumatoid arthritis
    - At risk for fracture or myelopathy

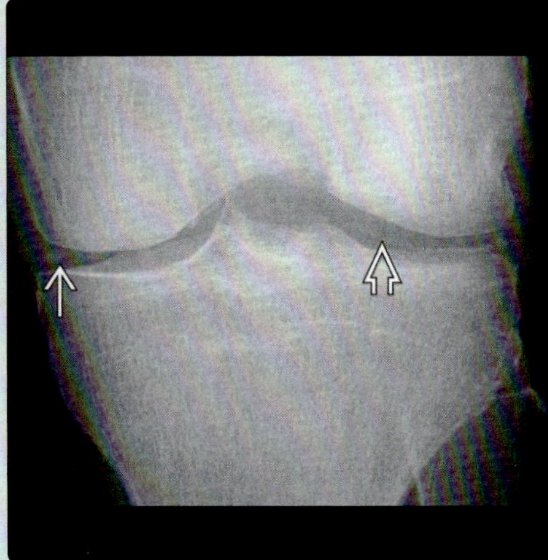

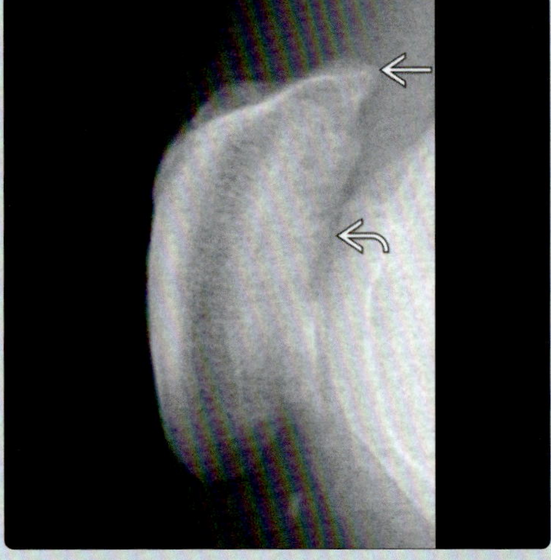

(Left) *AP radiograph in a 63-year-old patient shows dense chondrocalcinosis in both the meniscus (fibrocartilage) ➡ and hyaline cartilage ➡. There is mild osteophyte formation, but based on this image alone, one can diagnose only chondrocalcinosis, not pyrophosphate arthropathy.* **(Right)** *Lateral radiograph in the same patient shows mixed arthritic changes with large central erosion ➡ as well as osteophyte formation ➡. The predominance of patellofemoral arthritic change leads to the diagnosis of pyrophosphate arthropathy.*

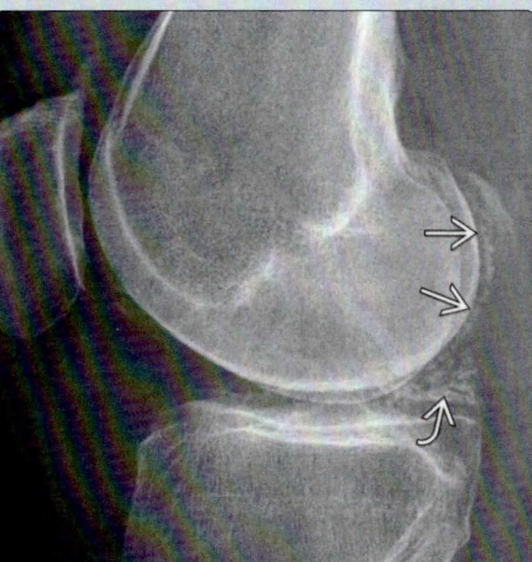

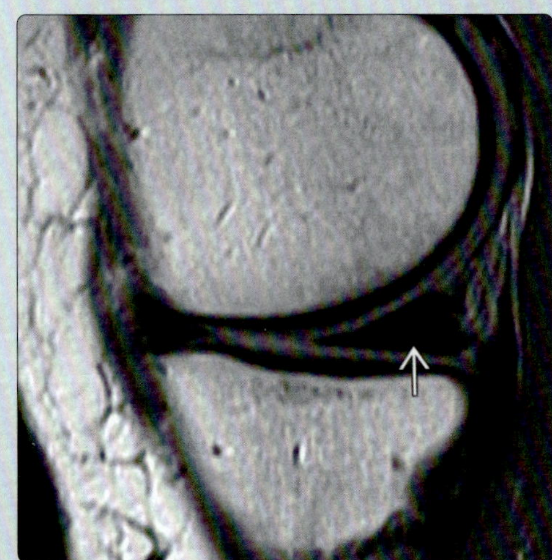

(Left) *Lateral radiograph in a 55-year-old patient shows preferential arthritis in the patellofemoral compartment; also shows chondrocalcinosis in both hyaline ➡ and fibrocartilage (meniscus) ➡.* **(Right)** *Sagittal PD MR in the same patient shows mild, somewhat linear, signal within the posterior horn of medial meniscus ➡. When interpreted without benefit of radiograph, this might be considered degenerative, but it is in fact due to crystal deposition in this case of pyrophosphate arthropathy.*

Pyrophosphate Arthropathy

TERMINOLOGY

Abbreviations

- Calcium pyrophosphate dihydrate (CPPD)

Synonyms

- CPPD crystal deposition disease, pseudogout, chondrocalcinosis
  - Not true synonyms, but often incorrectly used interchangeably

Definitions

- Chondrocalcinosis: General term for cartilage calcification (seen by pathology or imaging)
  - May or may not result in arthropathy
  - Calcification may be within hyaline or fibrocartilage
  - Calcification may be deposition of pyrophosphate, calcium hydroxyapatite, or dicalcium phosphate dihydrate crystals (or combinations thereof)
- Pyrophosphate arthropathy: Specific pattern of structural joint damage that occurs from CPPD crystal deposition in intraarticular and paraarticular locations
- Pseudogout: Gout-like clinical syndrome produced by CPPD crystal deposition; **not** radiologic diagnosis

IMAGING

General Features

- Best diagnostic clue
  - Knee or hand with chondrocalcinosis + radiocarpal, MCP, or patellofemoral arthropathy
- Location
  - Usually polyarticular and symmetric (2/3)
  - Chondrocalcinosis: Knee > symphysis pubis > wrist > hip (acetabular labrum) > shoulder > elbow
  - Arthropathy: Knee > wrist > hand > shoulder, hip
    - Knee: Patellofemoral shows isolated or greater involvement than medial or lateral compartments
    - Wrist: Radiocarpal joint
    - Hand: Metacarpals, particularly 2nd and 3rd
  - Rare pseudorheumatoid location, involving interphalangeal as well as MCPs
  - Spine: Particularly surrounding dens ("crowned dens")
- Morphology
  - Scapholunate advanced collapse (SLAC) is common associated wrist deformity

Imaging Recommendations

- Best imaging tool
  - Radiograph

Radiographic Findings

- Chondrocalcinosis (usually, not invariably, present)
  - Need not be present radiographically for arthropathy to develop
  - May line hyaline cartilage
    - In knee, particularly along femoral condyles
    - In wrist, particularly at lunatotriquetral or scapholunate articulation
  - May be easiest to see in fibrocartilage
    - Triangular shape in menisci
    - Triangular or amorphous shape in triangular fibrocartilage complex
  - Less frequently seen in synovium and joint capsule
    - Linear or, less commonly, globular
- Arthropathy
  - Appearance
    - Arthropathy is generally productive
      - Hook-like or "drooping" osteophytes are distinctive at metacarpal heads
    - Early arthropathy may be mixed or even purely erosive (1/8 will show erosion)
    - Rare pseudoneuropathic appearance with fragmentation and severe destruction
  - Location: Quite specific
    - Hand and wrist: Radiocarpal and MCP (2nd and 3rd)
    - Knee: Patellofemoral compartment significantly more affected than medial or lateral
- Cartilage narrowing
- Normal bone density maintained
- Subchondral cysts common
  - Well delineated with sclerotic margin
  - May be large, simulating neoplasm
- Malalignment
  - Radial deviation MCPs is common
  - SLAC is common
    - Separation of scaphoid and lunate, with capitate migrating proximally, forcing itself between them
    - Scaphoid erodes into distal radial articular surface
- Cervical spine
  - Calcification surrounding dens (crowned dens)
  - Erosions and remodeling of dens; at risk for fracture
  - Calcification of ligamentum flavum
  - Calcification of intervertebral disks with narrowing

CT Findings

- Mirrors findings on radiographs
  - Calcific densities may be more conspicuous than on radiograph or MR
- Particularly noted in spine
  - Lobulated calcified mass in ligamentum flavum or facet joint capsule
  - Disc calcifications
  - Pressure erosions, subchondral cysts around dens
  - Occasional fracture (usually odontoid)

MR Findings

- ± chondrocalcinosis
  - May not be conspicuous on MR
  - Meniscus may appear enlarged
  - May be low or high signal on either T1WI or fluid-sensitive sequences
    - Signal alterations from chondrocalcinosis significantly decreases sensitivity and specificity for diagnosis of meniscal tears
    - Interpretation in conjunction with radiograph helps prevent false-positive diagnosis of tear
- Arthropathy: Findings nonspecific except by distinctive location
  - Inflammatory changes, granulation tissue, fibrosis
- Calcifications surrounding dens are low signal; can suggest pannus of rheumatoid arthritis (RA)

DIFFERENTIAL DIAGNOSIS

Septic Arthritis

- Clinical presentation very similar (red, swollen)
- Septic arthritis may show deossification
- Aspirate should be analyzed for crystals and infection

Hemochromatosis

- Younger males may develop arthropathy identical to pyrophosphate arthropathy
  - Arthropathy develops in up to 50% of those with hemochromatosis
- Hook-like character of MCP osteophytes is said to be more prominent in hemochromatosis but time dependent

Giant Cell Tumor

- Subchondral cysts of pyrophosphate arthropathy can be so large as to simulate subchondral giant cell tumor
- Differentiate by presence of chondrocalcinosis and multiplicity of cysts in pyrophosphate arthropathy

Chondrosarcoma

- Amorphous chondrocalcinosis mimics chondroid matrix in temporomandibular joint and spine
- Lobulated calcified mass of chondrocalcinosis causes adjacent erosion, not as likely seen in chondrosarcoma

Rheumatoid Arthritis

- CPPD mass around dens mimics pannus of RA on MR
- Erosions and remodeling of dens similar in RA and CPPD
- Calcification seen on CT or radiograph serves to differentiate; RA does not calcify

PATHOLOGY

General Features

- Etiology
  - Enzyme or saturation abnormalities allow formation of excess pyrophosphate
  - Pyrophosphate deposits in cartilage, resulting in inflammatory cascade
  - Amplification loop hypothesis: Aging cartilage may predispose to crystal deposition because of changes in concentration of proteoglycan
- Associated abnormalities
  - CPPD crystal deposition can be seen in association with several metabolic abnormalities
    - Hemochromatosis, Wilson disease, hyperparathyroidism
  - CPPD crystal deposition can be associated with osteoarthritis (OA)
    - May be synchronous and unrelated to OA, or may be due to repetitive microtrauma

CLINICAL ISSUES

Presentation

- Most common signs/symptoms
  - May be asymptomatic (10-20%)
  - Pseudogout: Acute self-limited attacks simulating gout or septic arthritis (10-20%)
  - Pseudo-OA: Chronic degenerative joint changes without acute exacerbations (35-60%)
  - Pseudo-RA: More continuous acute attacks simulating RA clinically and in distribution (2-6%)
  - Pseudoneuropathic arthropathy: Rapidly destructive form of arthritis (< 2%)
  - Diagnosis proven by joint aspiration
- Other signs/symptoms
  - Pain, swelling, fever, ↑ ESR
    - May accompany pseudogout attacks
    - Simulates infection
  - Crowned dens syndrome
    - Acute presentation of pyrophosphate arthropathy involving dens
    - Pain, elevated C-reactive protein
    - Occasional instability

Demographics

- Age
  - Rare before age 30 then increases significantly in elderly (27-50% occur in patients aged 85-90 years)
- Gender
  - M < F (M:F = 1:2-7)
- Epidemiology
  - Appendicular location: 5% of adults
  - Atlantoaxial location: 12.5% of adults
    - Prevalence increases with age
      - □ 34% if ≥ 60 years, 49% if ≥ 80 years

Natural History & Prognosis

- Progressive pain and disability with chronic CPPD

Treatment

- Based on prevention of crystal formation, dissolution of crystals, and decreasing biologic consequences
- Joint lavage, intraarticular injection of hyaluronan
- NSAIDs, corticosteroids, low doses of colchicine

DIAGNOSTIC CHECKLIST

Consider

- Remember that chondrocalcinosis need not be present to diagnose pyrophosphate arthropathy
- Distribution of arthropathy suggests diagnosis
  - Very specific joint distribution within wrist/hand
  - Specific compartment distribution within knee (patellofemoral > medial or lateral)
- If septic joint is suspected clinically in joint showing chondrocalcinosis
  - Remember that pyrophosphate arthropathy often has similar clinical presentation (pseudogout)
  - Send aspirate for crystal analysis as well as culture

Image Interpretation Pearls

- MR of chondrocalcinosis can be confusing
  - Chondrocalcinosis on MR may be invisible, subtle, high or low SI on either T1WI or fluid-sensitive sequences
  - Sensitivity and specificity for diagnosis of meniscal tear is adversely affected by chondrocalcinosis

SELECTED REFERENCES

1. Chang EY et al: Frequency of atlantoaxial calcium pyrophosphate dihydrate deposition at CT. Radiology. 269(2):519-24, 2013

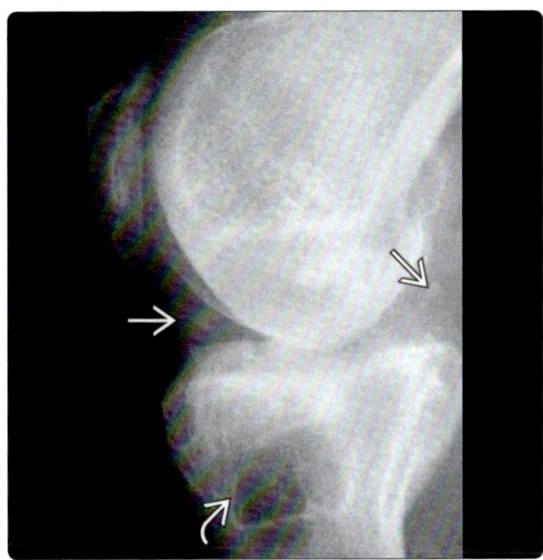

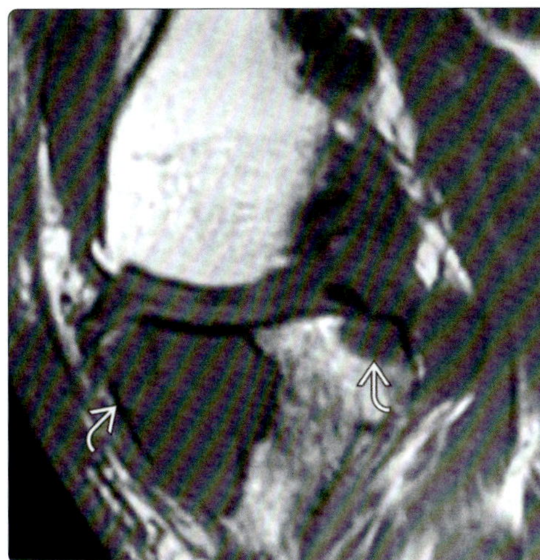

(Left) *Lateral radiograph shows a large lytic lesion in the proximal tibia ➡. This could possibly be misinterpreted as a tumor. However, careful observation also shows chondrocalcinosis ➡, which should lead to consideration of the diagnosis of pyrophosphate arthropathy.* **(Right)** *Sagittal T1WI MR in the same patient shows multiple subchondral cysts ➡. This secures the diagnosis of pyrophosphate arthropathy. Note that the chondrocalcinosis itself is not visualized on MR in this case.*

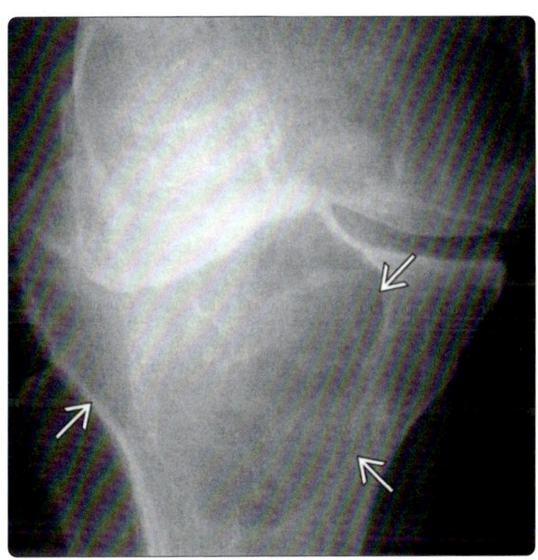

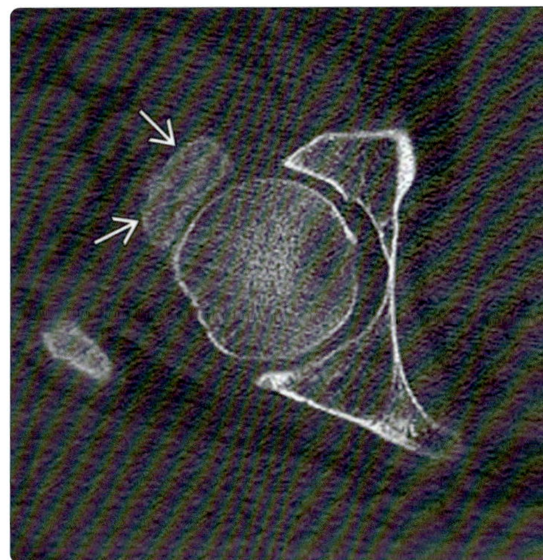

(Left) *AP radiograph shows a pathologic fracture into a large lytic lesion occupying the tibial subchondral region ➡. While one might consider diagnosis of tumor, note that there is also joint disease. This proved to be pyrophosphate arthropathy.* **(Right)** *Axial CT shows a mineralized mass within the hip joint ➡. This could represent a loose body, intraarticular chondroma, conglomerate synovial chondromatosis, or an unusually nodular form of chondrocalcinosis deposition within the synovium.*

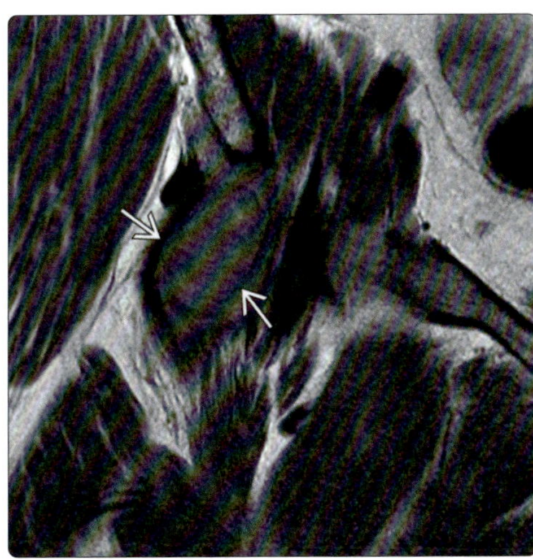

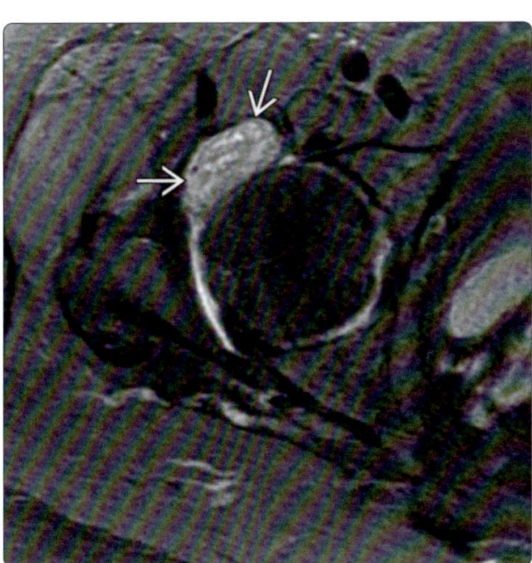

(Left) *Coronal T1 MR, same patient, shows the mass ➡ to be mildly inhomogeneous and of SI similar to skeletal muscle.* **(Right)** *Axial T2FS MR shows the mass to have mildly ↑ SI but contains foci of lower SI ➡. Without the radiograph, one might consider pigmented villonodular synovitis, nodular synovitis, gout, amyloid, or hemophilia. However, none of these diagnoses should show the mineralization seen on CT. This proved to be a nodular deposit of chondrocalcinosis, and the diagnosis was calcium pyrophosphate dihydrate (CPPD).*

(Left) *PA radiograph shows pyrophosphate arthropathy with chondrocalcinosis in the triangular fibrocartilage complex (TFCC) ➡ as well as advanced radiocarpal arthropathy. Scapholunate advanced collapse SLAC wrist deformity ⇨ seen, and large subchondral cysts inside carpal bones.* **(Right)** *PA radiograph shows chondrocalcinosis in the TFCC ➡, as well as within the scapholunate joint ↪. There is radiocarpal arthropathy typical of pyrophosphate arthropathy with SLAC wrist deformity ⇨ and subchondral cyst formation.*

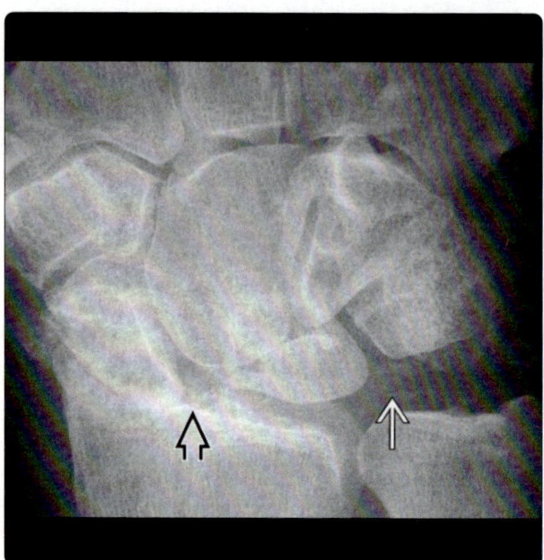

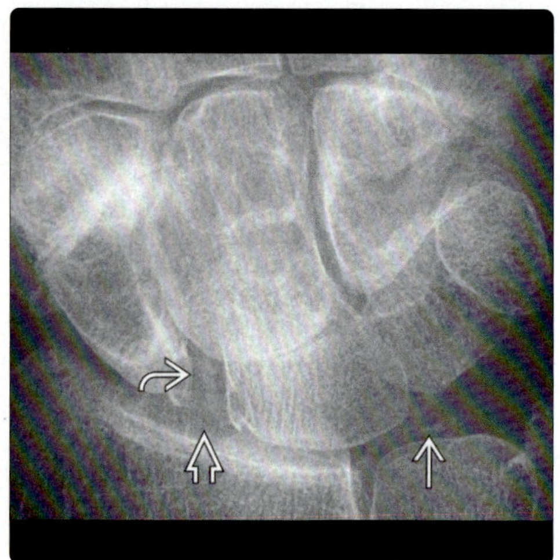

(Left) *PA radiograph shows tremendous subchondral cyst formation as well as dense chondrocalcinosis within the TFCC and other portions of the joint ➡. There is a SLAC wrist deformity with scapholunate widening and with excavation of the radius by the scaphoid ⇨.* **(Right)** *Lateral radiograph in the same patient shows dorsal and volar chondrocalcinosis ➡, as well as soft tissue swelling. The diagnosis of pyrophosphate arthropathy is straightforward with these findings.*

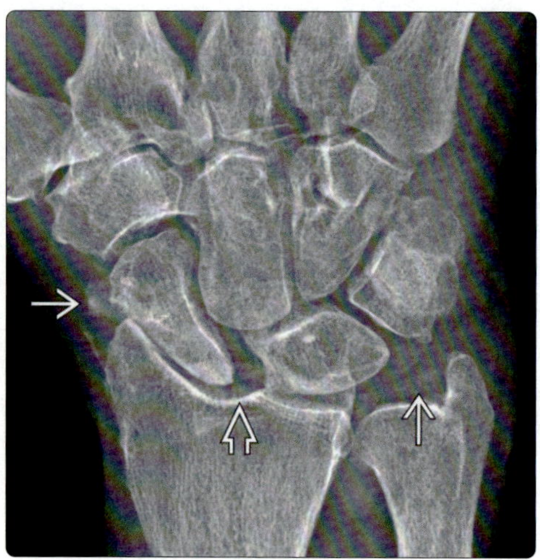

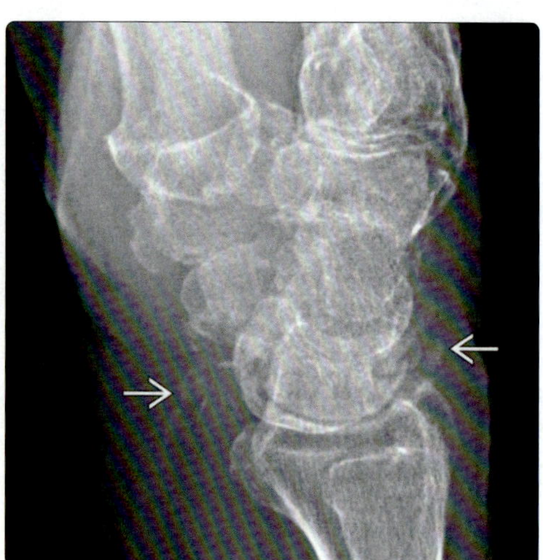

(Left) *Coronal T2WI FS MR in the same patient shows a large effusion extending throughout the radiocarpal ➡, midcarpal, and distal radiocarpal joints. Large cysts are seen within the carpal bones ↩, which contain both high and low signal material; this is joint fluid with crystal deposits.* **(Right)** *Coronal T2WI FS MR shows effusion, decompressed along the volar tendon sheaths ➡. Globular heterogeneous lower signal material ⇨ represents nodular collections of crystals within the joint.*

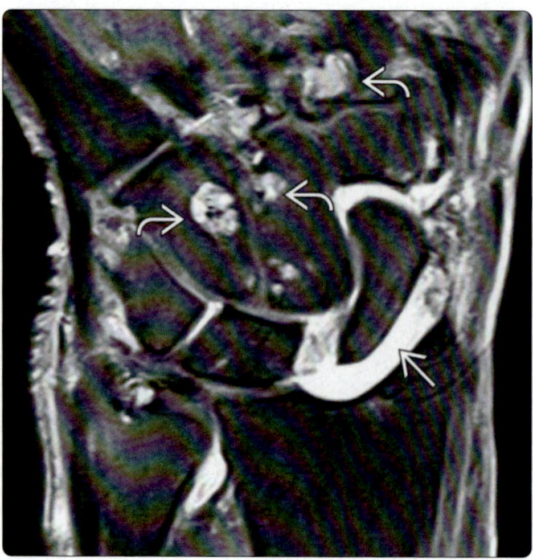

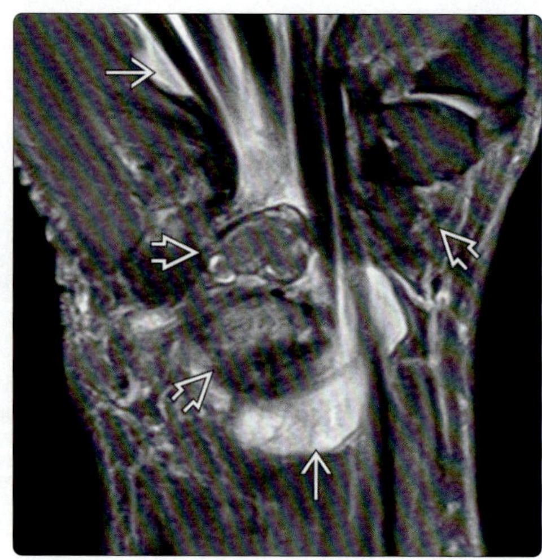

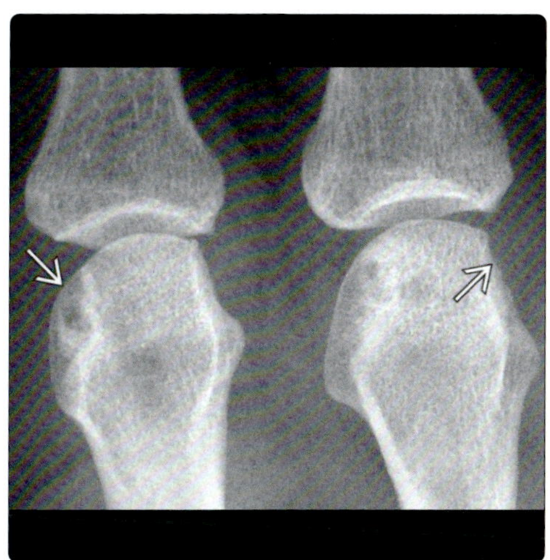

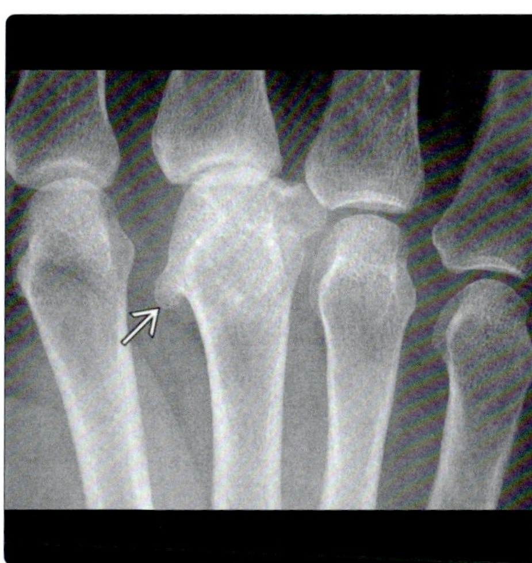

(Left) *PA radiograph shows classic pyrophosphate arthropathy. The 2nd and 3rd MCPs show early erosive change ➡. Although osteophytes at the MCPs are typical, it should be remembered that pyrophosphate arthropathy may present as primarily erosive disease.* **(Right)** *PA radiograph shows large hook-like osteophytes at the 3rd MCP ➡. This distribution of productive disease suggests the diagnosis of pyrophosphate arthropathy; this patient had confirmatory wrist findings.*

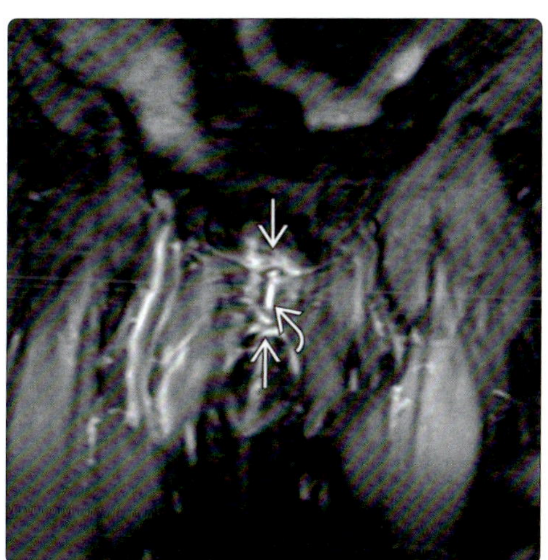

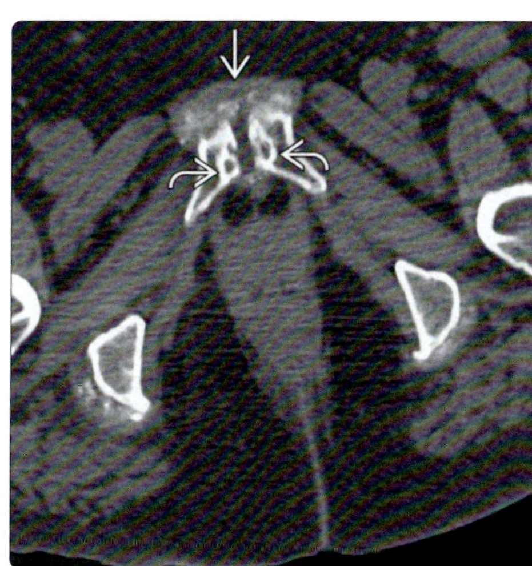

(Left) *Coronal STIR MR shows edema around the symphysis pubis ➡ and fluid within the symphysis ➡. Findings are nonspecific; they may be related to osteoarthritis, crystal deposition disease, microinstability, or previous injury.* **(Right)** *Axial NECT in the same patient shows soft tissue fullness ➡ with accompanying mineralization. There are subchondral cysts ➡ but no bone destruction. Aspiration and biopsy appeared normal, but crystal analysis confirmed CPPD.*

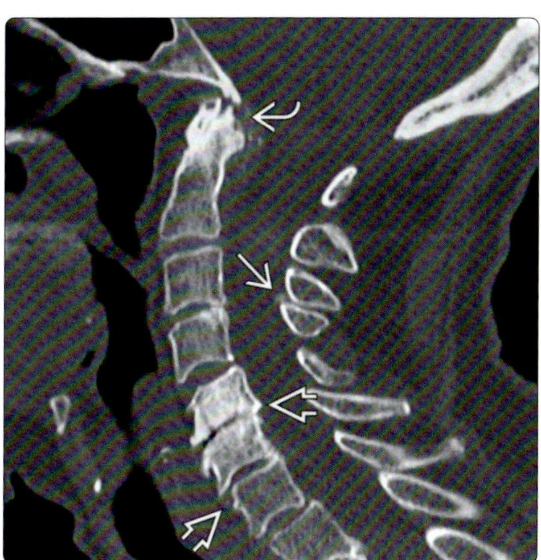

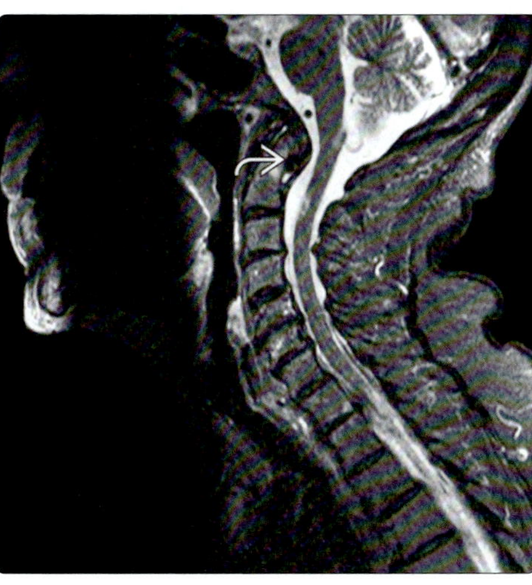

(Left) *Sagittal bone CT shows calcifications posterior to the dens ➡ as well as cysts in the dens and anterior arch of C1. Calcifications are also seen in the ligamentum flavum ➡ and intervertebral discs ➡. These findings are characteristic of CPPD arthropathy.* **(Right)** *Sagittal STIR MR in the same patient shows mass surrounding the dens ➡, which is a nonspecific appearance. On MR, CPPD surrounding the dens often mimics the pannus of rheumatoid arthritis. CT differentiates the 2 disease processes.*

Hydroxyapatite Deposition Disease

KEY FACTS

TERMINOLOGY

- Broad spectrum of musculoskeletal pathology due to hydroxyapatite crystal deposition
  - Primary HADD includes calcific tendonitis and bursitis

IMAGING

- Homogeneous calcification located at tendon or bursa
- Generally monoarticular
- Shoulder most frequent (69%)
  - External rotators of hip next most common
  - Spine, elbow, knee, wrist, ankle
- Character of calcification changes over time
  - Inhomogeneous, faintly seen initially
  - Becomes more well defined and dense
  - Eventually may disappear
- Rare cortical erosions
  - Tail of calcifications extends from eroded surface
- MR: Globular focus of low signal on all sequences
  - May have hyperintensity in adjacent soft tissues
  - Bone marrow edema due to HA deposition
  - Gradient-echo imaging: Blooming of deposit
  - Fusiform enlargement of affected tendon
- US: Hyperechoic foci within tendon showing other signs of tendinopathy

CLINICAL ISSUES

- Treatment: Generally conservative
- Deposits may be needled and aspirated
  - 13% of these develop painful bursitis within 3 months

DIAGNOSTIC CHECKLIST

- Cortical invasion by low signal material
  - Watch for continuity with tendinous insertion
- With reactive-appearing hyperintensity on MR at site of tendon insertion, consider HADD
  - Use radiograph to make diagnosis easily
  - Small calcifications frequently overlooked on both MR and radiograph

(Left) *Sagittal STIR MR shows tremendous fusiform enlargement of the peroneus longus tendon ➡ along its middle 1/3, with fairly homogeneous low signal throughout. Without a radiograph, differential includes entities with extensive fibrous tissue.* **(Right)** *AP radiograph in the same patient demonstrates homogeneous calcification extending over much of the length of the tendon ➡. The radiograph makes it easy to diagnose surprisingly extensive hydroxyapatite deposition (HADD).*

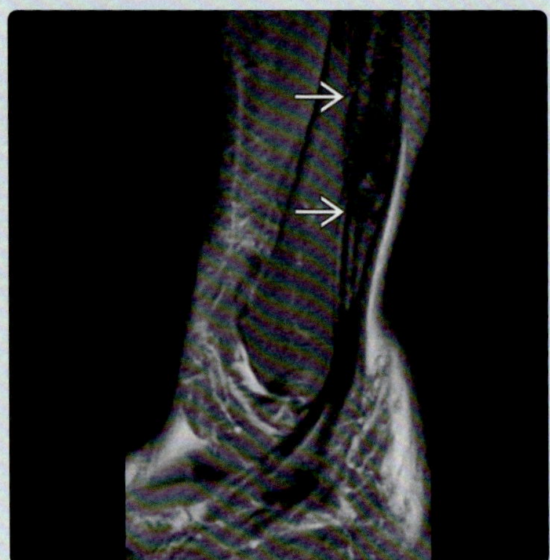

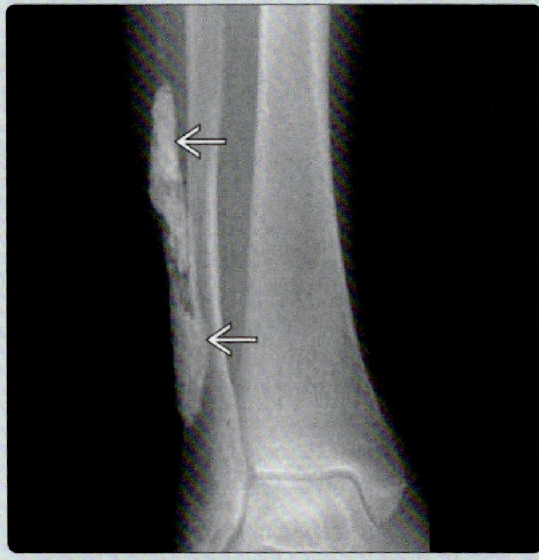

(Left) *AP radiograph shows a patchy sclerotic density superimposed on the humeral head ➡. Another view is required to determine whether the density is in soft tissues or bone.* **(Right)** *Axillary lateral radiograph provides the orthogonal view to secure the diagnosis. The calcific density is now seen to be entirely within the soft tissues posterior to the humeral head, in the position of the infraspinatus tendon ➡. This is calcific tendinitis; remember that the supraspinatus is not the only site affected in the shoulder.*

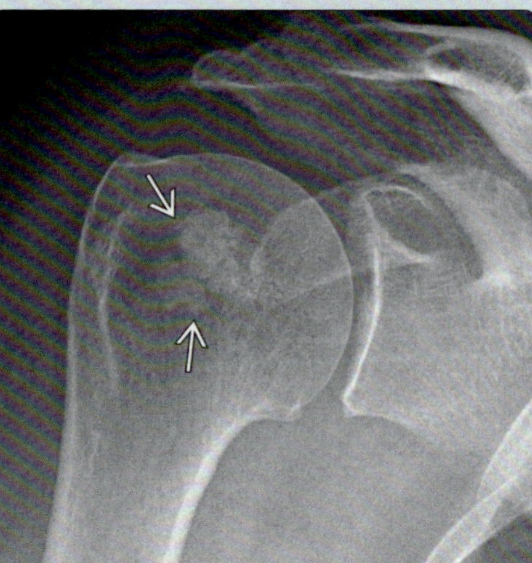

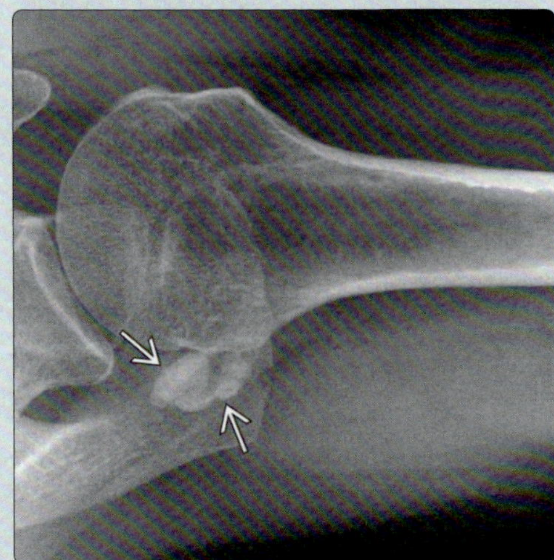

TERMINOLOGY

Abbreviations

- Hydroxyapatite deposition disease (HADD)

Synonyms

- Milwaukee shoulder, calcific tendinitis, calcific bursitis

Definitions

- Broad spectrum of musculoskeletal pathology due to hydroxyapatite crystal deposition
  - Primary HADD includes calcific tendonitis and bursitis
  - Secondary hydroxyapatite related to underlying disease; not further discussed in this section
    - End-stage renal disease
    - Collagen vascular disease
    - Vitamin D intoxication
    - Tumoral calcinosis

IMAGING

General Features

- Best diagnostic clue
  - Homogeneous calcification located at site of tendon or bursa
- Location
  - Generally monoarticular
  - Shoulder most frequent (69%)
  - External rotators of hip next most common
  - Spine: Likely more common than generally recognized
    - Longus coli
    - Ligamentum flavum
  - Elbow: Triceps, forearm flexor, and extensor insertions
  - Knee: Quadriceps tendon, inferior patellar tendon insertions
  - Wrist: Especially flexor carpi ulnaris at pisiform
  - Hand: Periarticular (metacarpophalangeal, interphalangeal)
  - Ankle
- Size
  - Ranges from tiny to large
    - Large deposits extend along path of tendon
- Morphology
  - Homogeneous without internal characteristics

Imaging Recommendations

- Best imaging tool
  - Calcifications seen on radiograph
    - May need tangential or oblique view so that small calcification is not superimposed on bone
  - MR frequently obtained secondary to unexplained pain
    - Reactive high signal may be much more apparent than tiny calcifications that incite it
    - Obtaining radiograph may be extremely useful in interpreting MR

Radiographic Findings

- Globular homogeneous calcific density
  - May be ovoid, linear, even triangular
  - No internal characteristics, such as trabeculation
  - No well-defined cortication
- In distribution of tendon or bursa
- Character of calcification changes over time
  - Initially, inhomogeneous, faintly seen
  - Becomes more well defined and dense
  - Eventually may disappear
- Rare cortical erosions
  - Usually at pectoralis or gluteal insertions
  - Tail of calcifications extends from eroded surface

CT Findings

- Follows radiographic characteristics
- If osseous erosion present, may see comet tail of calcific crystal deposition
  - Extends from erosion into adjacent soft tissues
  - Extension is along path of tendinous insertion

MR Findings

- Globular focus of low signal on all sequences
  - Unless deposit is large, easily overlooked on MR
- Fusiform enlargement of affected tendon
  - Signal of tendinopathy: Often higher signal than expected on fluid-sensitive sequences
- May have hyperintensity in adjacent soft tissues
  - Reactive inflammation: Myositis or bursitis
  - Ovoid or elongated region of abnormality
  - Usually not round or tumor-like
- Bone marrow edema due to HA deposition in adjacent bone
- Gradient-echo imaging: Blooming of deposit
- Postcontrast imaging
  - HA deposition itself does not enhance
  - Surrounding inflamed soft tissues enhance intensely

Ultrasonographic Findings

- Hyperechoic foci within tendon showing other signs of tendinopathy
  - US sensitive for calcific foci as small as 2 mm
  - Calcific foci may or may not shadow

DIFFERENTIAL DIAGNOSIS

Tendinopathy or Tenosynovitis

- Must differentiate low signal normal tendon from globular low signal HA deposits on MR
- HADD may have associated tendinopathy

Tumor

- Large soft tissue deposits with surrounding edema may mimic tumor
- Soft tissue deposits with local osseous invasion may mimic tumor
  - Consideration of parosteal or periosteal osteosarcoma is of particular concern
  - Proximal humerus (pectoralis insertion) or proximal femur (trochanters or adductor insertion) are sites where one must be vigilant
  - Watch for comet tail shape of associated calcification extending from ossific erosion

Dystrophic Calcification

- If tendinous calcification is extensive, may mimic other soft tissue deposition
  - Progressive systemic sclerosis

- Polymyositis/dermatomyositis
- Hyperparathyroidism
- Dialysis-related disease, metastatic calcification
- Tumoral calcinosis
- Location within tendon serves to differentiate HADD from these entities
- Many of these dystrophic deposits are more amorphous or cloud-like than deposits of HADD

PATHOLOGY

General Features

- Etiology
  - Pathogenesis unknown
  - Hypothesis: Microtrauma or stress within tendon → hypovascular region → degenerative tear → necrosis and calcification
  - Hypothesis: Focal intratendinous hypoxia due to mechanical or metabolic factors → fibrocartilaginous transformation of tendon → calcification
- Associated abnormalities
  - Osteoarthritis (OA)
    - Prevalence of HA crystals in synovial fluid of OA not known
      - 1 study showed HA crystals in 44/100 synovial aspirates of patients with OA
      - Pyrophosphate crystals also found in some samples of synovial fluid from OA patients
      - HA crystals have also been detected in cartilage of patients with OA
    - Milwaukee shoulder epitomizes association
      - Generally elderly women
      - Destructive arthropathy of glenohumeral joint with HA in synovial fluid
      - High incidence of rotator cuff tear
      - High levels of activated collagenase and neutral protease enzymes

Gross Pathologic & Surgical Features

- Calcific tendinitis itself may be indolent
  - HA deposition may cause painful inflammatory response in adjacent soft tissues

Microscopic Features

- HA crystals very small compared with sodium urate or pyrophosphate crystals
- No birefringence
- Phagocytosis of crystals by neutrophils →
  - Release of chemotactic factors →
  - Attracts additional neutrophils →
  - Activation and enhancement of acute inflammation

CLINICAL ISSUES

Presentation

- Most common signs/symptoms
  - Range of symptoms
    - May be asymptomatic
      - HADD is frequently incidental finding
    - Acute onset of pain
      - Decreased range of motion
      - Erythema, periarticular edema
      - Tenderness to palpation
- Other signs/symptoms
  - Low-grade fever
  - Leukocytosis
  - Elevated ESR
  - Elevated C-reactive protein
- Clinical profile
  - Affects sedentary individuals more frequently than manual laborers
    - May be associated with repetitive activity or microtrauma typical for degenerative tendinopathy

Demographics

- Age
  - Peak incidence: 4th-6th decades
- Gender
  - Slight ↑ prevalence in men overall
  - M < F in shoulder
- Epidemiology
  - 3% general population estimated

Natural History & Prognosis

- Tends to be self-limiting with resolution of both clinical and imaging findings

Treatment

- Generally conservative
- Steroid injection if intensely painful
- Deposits may be needled, lavaged, and aspirated
  - 50% improvement; 10% minor complications
  - 13% develop painful bursitis within 3 months following treatment

DIAGNOSTIC CHECKLIST

Consider

- With reactive-appearing hyperintensity on MR at site of tendon insertion, consider HADD
  - Use radiograph to make diagnosis easily
  - Small calcifications frequently overlooked on both MR and radiograph

Image Interpretation Pearls

- Cortical invasion by low signal material
  - Watch for continuity with tendinous insertion

SELECTED REFERENCES

1. Greis AC et al: Evaluation and Nonsurgical Management of Rotator Cuff Calcific Tendinopathy. Orthop Clin North Am. 46(2):293-302, 2015
2. Lanza E et al: Ultrasound-guided percutaneous irrigation in rotator cuff calcific tendinopathy: what is the evidence? A systematic review with proposals for future reporting. Eur Radiol. ePub, 2015
3. Del Castillo-González F et al: Treatment of the calcific tendinopathy of the rotator cuff by ultrasound-guided percutaneous needle lavage. Two years prospective study. Muscles Ligaments Tendons J. 4(4):407-12, 2014
4. Gabra N et al: Retropharyngeal calcific tendinitis mimicking a retropharyngeal phlegmon. Case Rep Otolaryngol. 2013:912628, 2013
5. Torbati SS et al: Acute calcific tendinitis of the wrist. J Emerg Med. 44(2):352-4, 2013
6. Ogon P et al: Prognostic factors in nonoperative therapy for chronic symptomatic calcific tendinitis of the shoulder. Arthritis Rheum. 60(10):2978-84, 2009
7. Serafini G et al: Rotator cuff calcific tendonitis: short-term and 10-year outcomes after two-needle us-guided percutaneous treatment–nonrandomized controlled trial. Radiology. 252(1):157-64, 2009

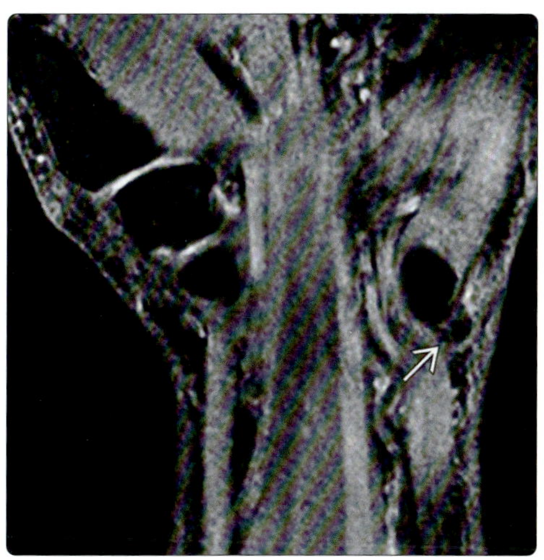

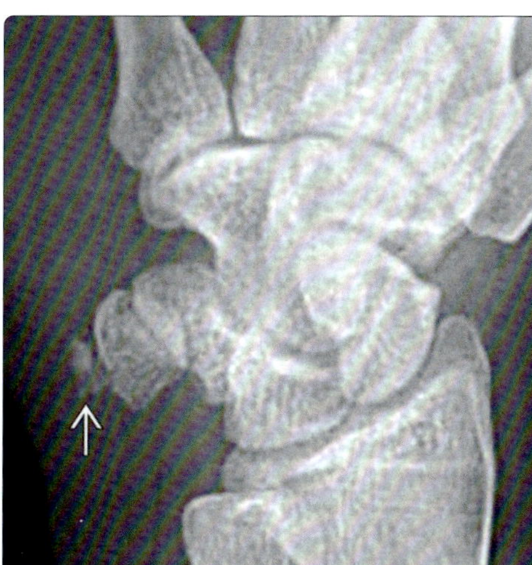

(Left) *Coronal STIR MR demonstrates a low signal focus adjacent to the pisiform at the insertion of the flexor carpi ulnaris* ➡*. This patient had chronic pain at this location on the volar and ulnar aspect of the wrist; there was no history of trauma.* **(Right)** *Oblique radiograph in the same patient confirms globular calcification adjacent to the pisiform* ➡*. This is a typical appearance as well as the location of HADD in the carpus. It may be difficult to visualize on routine views of the wrist.*

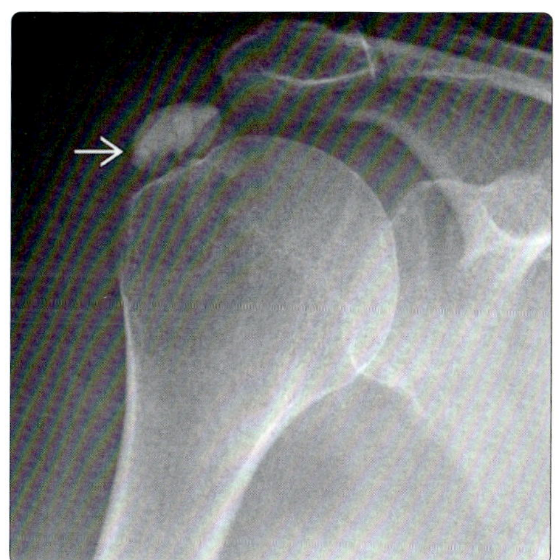

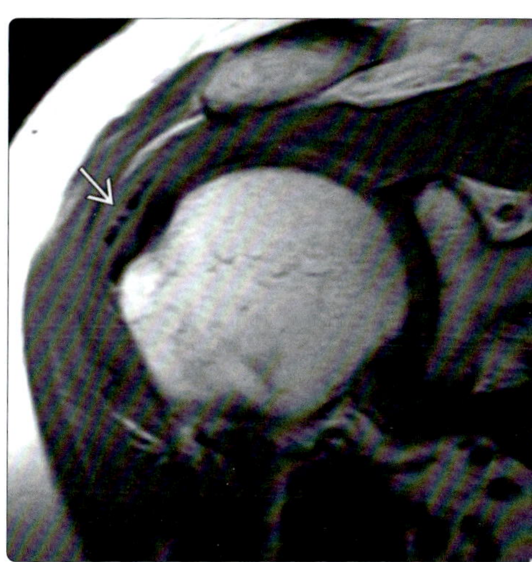

(Left) *AP radiograph of a painful shoulder demonstrates a large globule of calcification* ➡ *within the supraspinatus tendon, typical of calcific tendinitis.* **(Right)** *Coronal T1 MR confirms the position of the calcification* ➡ *within the supraspinatus tendon. The tendon appears swollen; fluid-sensitive sequence (not shown) would likely show inflammatory change surrounding the calcific body. It was determined that the patient should be treated with needling and aspiration of the calcific focus.*

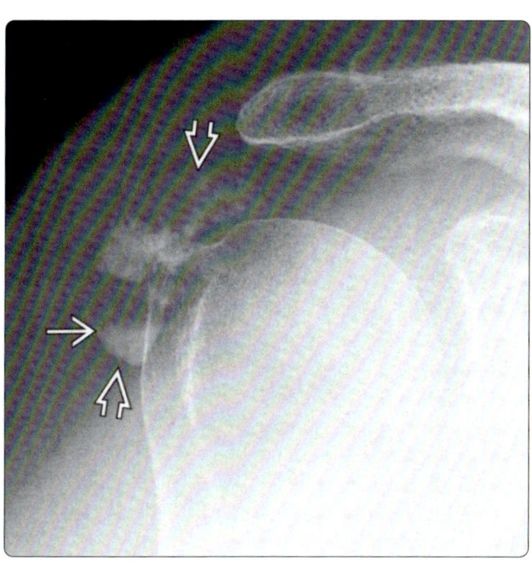

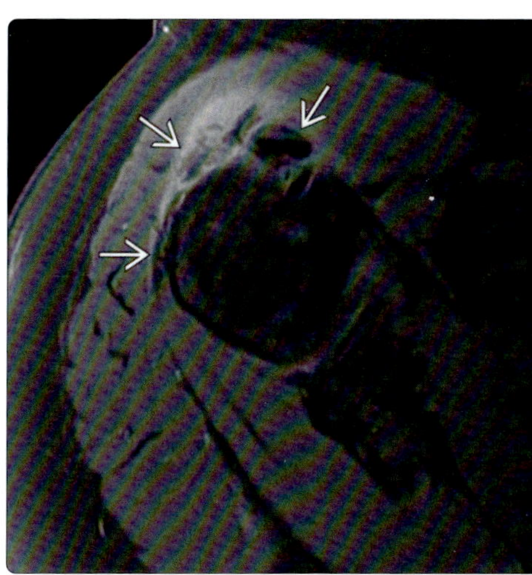

(Left) *AP radiograph in the same patient was obtained 2 weeks following needling and aspiration of the calcific focus. At this time, much of the calcification has dispersed into and outlines the subdeltoid bursa* ➡*. There is a fluid-calcification level* ➡ *seen in this upright image.* **(Right)** *Axial T2 FS MR confirms the calcification is within the subdeltoid bursa* ➡*. One study shows 13% of patients develop painful bursitis within 3 months of needling and aspiration of calcific tendinitis.*

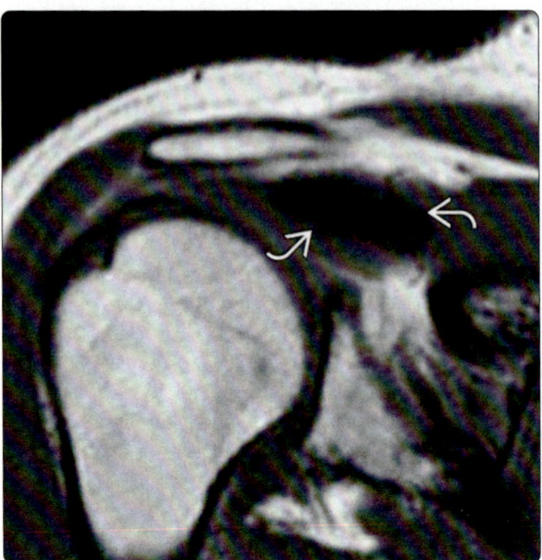

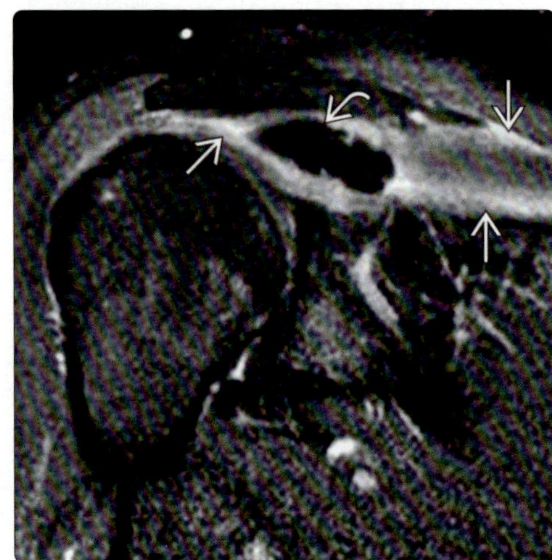

(Left) *Coronal T1WI MR appears very nearly normal. However, a large region of differential low signal is faintly seen within the supraspinatus muscle* ➢. **(Right)** *Coronal T2WI C+ FS MR in the same patient better shows the globular low signal material* ➢. *This is a huge focus of HA calcification. There is surrounding inflammation in the muscle and tendon, which enhances intensely* ➔; *this inflammatory reaction likely causes any acute symptoms the patient may be experiencing.*

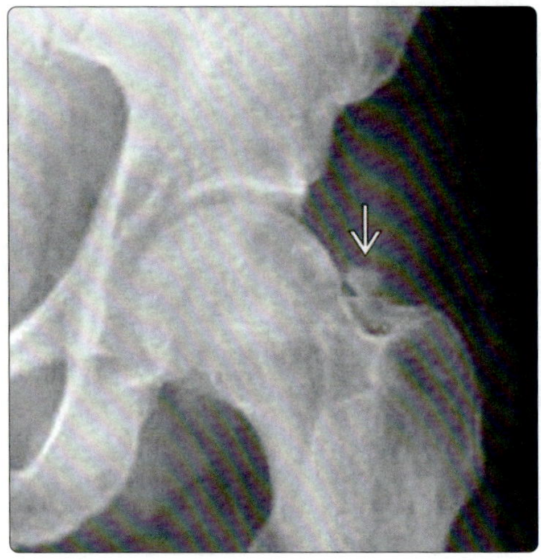

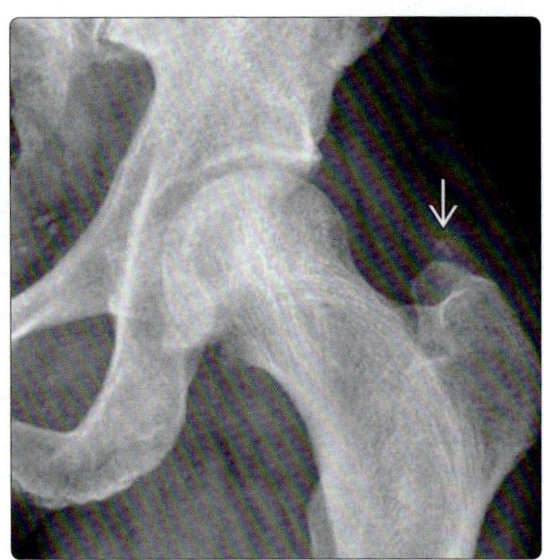

(Left) *Series of 2 images demonstrates the evolution of HADD. This AP radiograph shows a large globular focus adjacent to the greater trochanter* ➔. *However, this was an incidental finding; the image was obtained following trauma and the patient had no associated symptoms.* **(Right)** *AP radiograph obtained 7 months later in the same patient shows the calcification to have changed character. It is less well defined and much smaller* ➔. *Despite this apparent resolution, the patient has become quite symptomatic.*

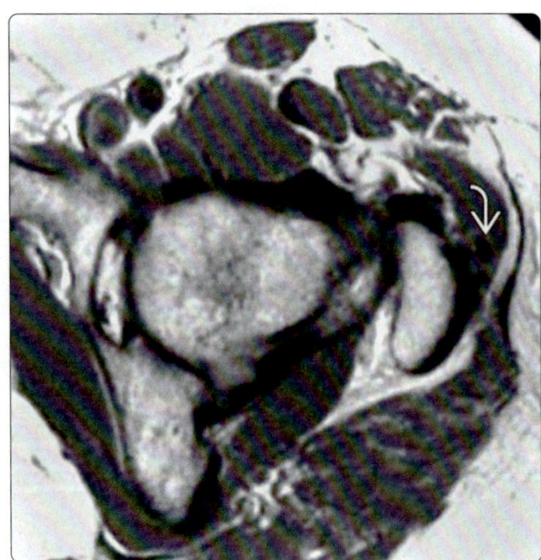

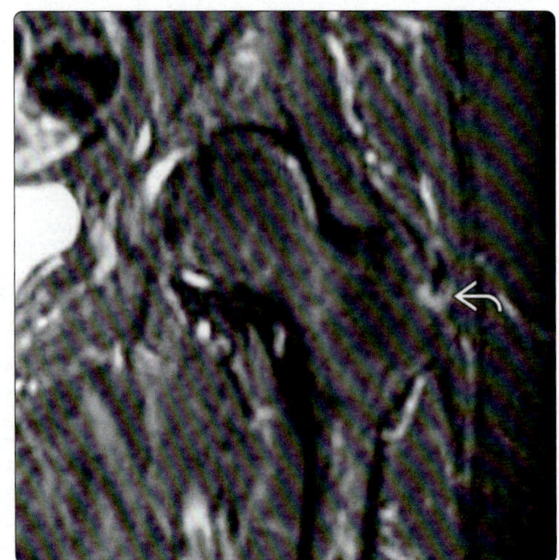

(Left) *Axial T1WI MR in the same patient, obtained at the time he had intense hip pain, shows the small focus of HA deposition within the gluteus medius tendon* ➢ *corresponding to the radiograph.* **(Right)** *Coronal STIR MR obtained at the same time shows surrounding soft tissue hyperintensity, indicating inflammation* ➢. *It is worthwhile to remember that the calcification in HADD undergoes an evolution in its appearance. It is often more symptomatic as it appears to be resolving.*

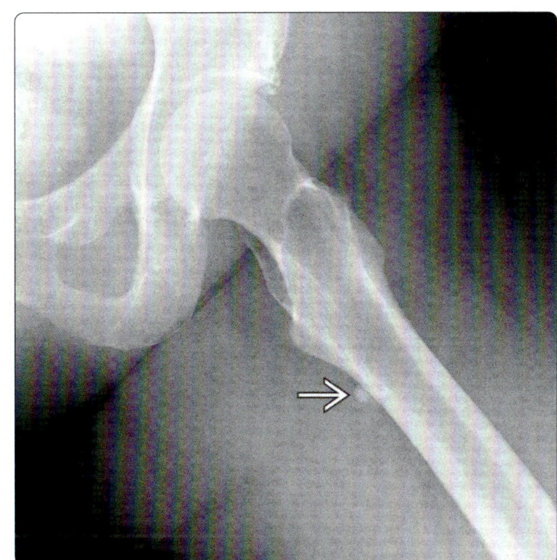

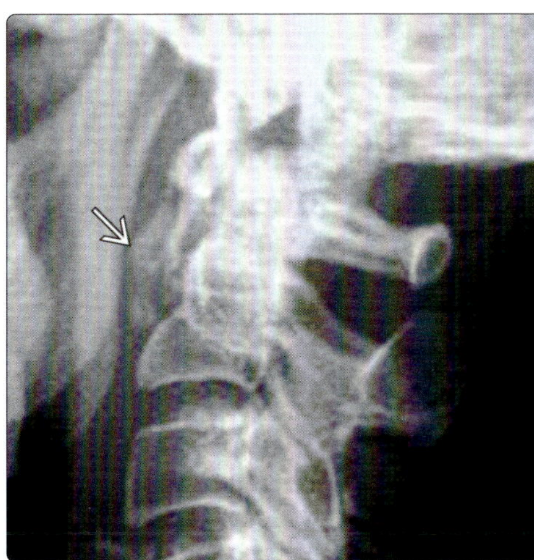

(Left) *Lateral radiograph demonstrates an amorphous calcific deposit at the insertion of the gluteus maximus tendon ➡. It is worthwhile to remember the distal extent of gluteal insertion. These calcific deposits can produce severe pain. In rare cases, these deposits may produce erosion of the bone adjacent to the deposit.* **(Right)** *Lateral radiograph shows globular calcification anterior to the cervical spine ➡. This represents hydroxyapatite deposition within the longus coli.*

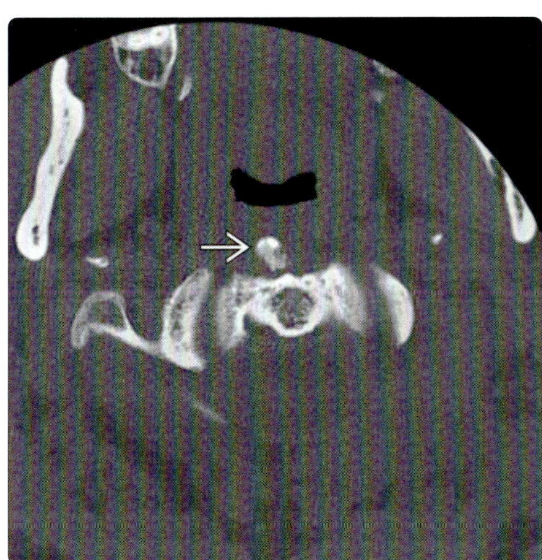

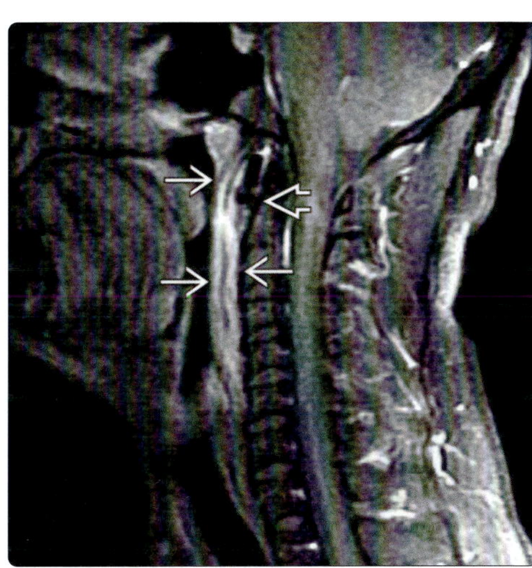

(Left) *Axial bone CT shows globular calcification located anterior to C2 ➡. This is the location of longus coli and is a relatively common site of HADD in the spine.* **(Right)** *Sagittal T1WI C+ FS MR in the same patient demonstrates the typical elongated and tapering configuration of longus coli tendonitis. The enhancing inflammatory process ➡ forms a thick rim around a narrow fluid collection. The calcific deposit is seen ➡ corresponding to the abnormality seen on CT.*

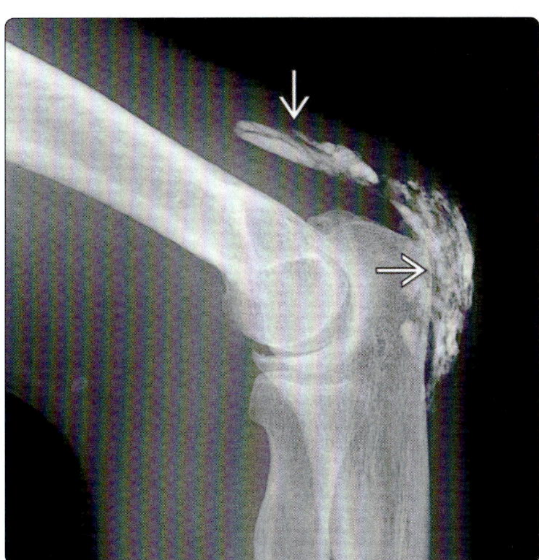

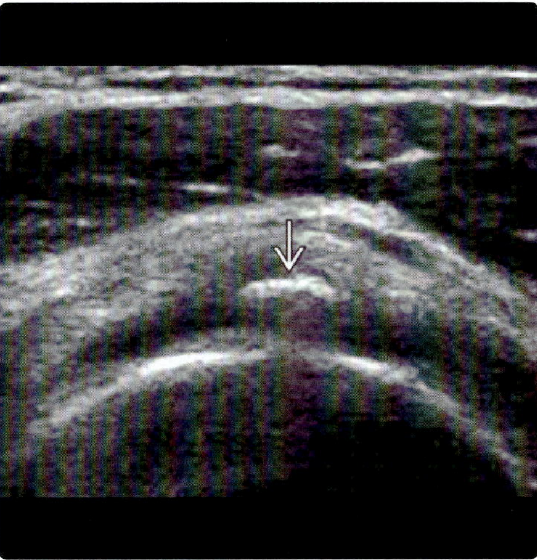

(Left) *Lateral radiograph of the elbow demonstrates extensive dense mineralization in the region of the olecranon bursa ➡, indicative of HADD. The dense and well-defined nature indicates longstanding involvement of the bursa.* **(Right)** *Longitudinal US through the shoulder shows a small hyperechoic focus with acoustic shadowing ➡. This represents a calcification within the supraspinatus tendon, diagnostic for HADD. The tendon itself is thickened and tendinotic.*

Amyloid Deposition

KEY FACTS

TERMINOLOGY

- Multisystem disorder caused by deposition of fibrillar protein aggregates

IMAGING

- MR much more definitive than radiograph
- Periarticular tendinous thickening
  - Low signal infiltration of tendons on all sequences
  - Tendon enlargement particularly notable at shoulder & wrist (flexor tendons of carpal tunnel)
- Large effusions and bursitis, low signal on T1 and high signal on fluid-sensitive sequences
- Low signal capsular thickening, all sequences
- Nodular or thick synovitis (low signal on all sequences) outlined by effusion
- Large erosions filled with low signal material
  - Fluid-sensitive sequences may show mixed low and high SI within erosions

PATHOLOGY

- Primary (AL) amyloidosis
  - Monoclonal population of plasma cells produces amyloidogenic immunoglobulin light-chain protein (λ more often than κ)
- Dialysis-related amyloid arthropathy
  - Glomerular filtration failure → ↑ β2 microglobulin → amyloid fibril deposition

CLINICAL ISSUES

- Only 10-15% of patients with multiple myeloma have amyloidosis
- Nearly 100% of patients treated with dialysis 15-20 years develop amyloidosis

DIAGNOSTIC CHECKLIST

- Thickened tendons and joint capsule + low signal erosions on all sequences suggest amyloidosis

(Left) *Sagittal T1WI MR shows extreme thickening with uniform low signal intensity of the quadriceps tendon ⮳. There is an effusion.* **(Right)** *Sagittal T2WI MR, matching the site in the same patient, shows the thickened quadriceps tendon to remain low signal ⮳. The effusion contains nodular soft tissue masses. This patient has chronic renal failure and has been treated with dialysis for 18 years. The deposition, thickening the tendons, is a classic presentation of dialysis-related amyloidosis.*

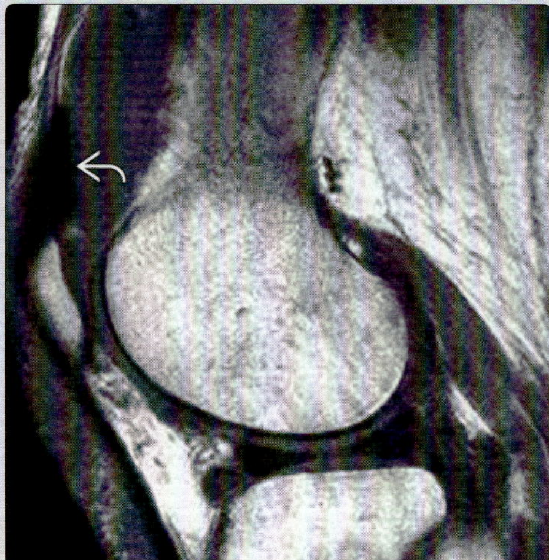

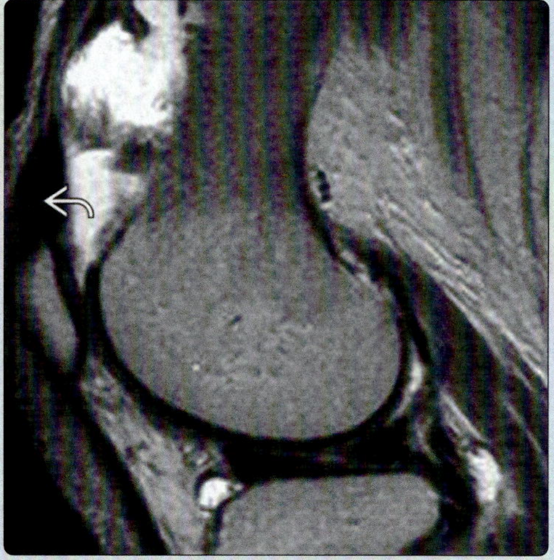

(Left) *Sagittal T1WI MR shows low signal material within the entire intercondylar notch ➘, surrounding the cruciate ligaments and thickening the posterior capsule ⮳. There is an erosion as well ➡.* **(Right)** *Sagittal T2WI MR in the same patient shows that the tissue occupying the intercondylar notch and thickening the posterior capsule remains low signal ➘. Though the low signal material within a joint may not be specific, the thickening of the capsule helps confirm the diagnosis of amyloidosis.*

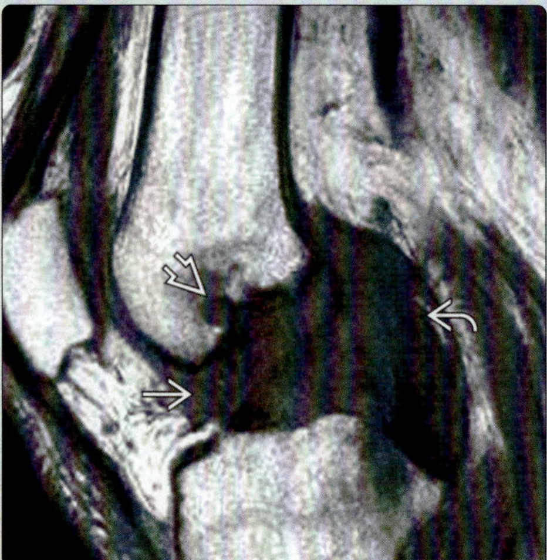

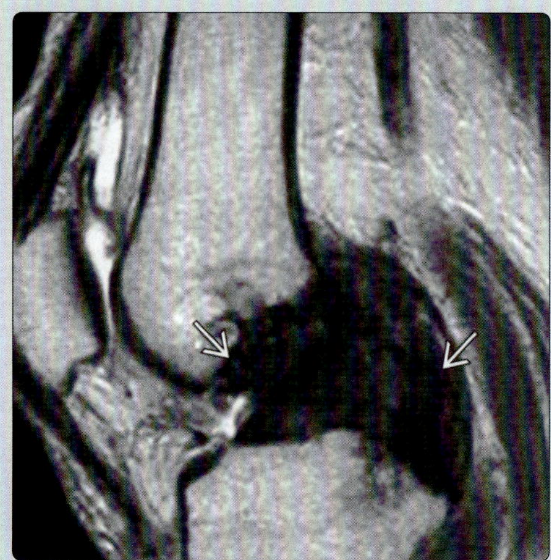

TERMINOLOGY

Definitions

- Multisystem disorder caused by deposition of fibrillar protein aggregates
  - Interfere with structural integrity and function of involved organs and tissues
- 4 main types, distinguished by deposited proteins and clinical associations

IMAGING

General Features

- Best diagnostic clue
  - Prominent soft tissue swelling, effusion, large cysts, with low signal on all MR sequences
- Location
  - Shoulder, hip, wrist, knee, spine
- Size
  - Tendon infiltration and osseous erosion may be large, especially in shoulder (shoulder pad sign)

Imaging Recommendations

- Best imaging tool
  - MR much more definitive than radiograph

Radiographic Findings

- Peripheral joints
  - Nondescript soft tissue swelling
  - Large effusion
  - Large subchondral "cysts" (actually erosions)
    - Well defined; may have fine sclerotic margin
  - Cartilage narrowing
  - Pathologic fracture
- Spine: Irregular destruction of endplates

MR Findings

- Periarticular tendinous thickening
  - Low signal infiltration of tendons on all sequences
  - Tendon enlargement, particularly notable at shoulder and wrist (flexor tendons of carpal tunnel)
- Large effusions and bursitis, low signal on T1 and high signal on fluid-sensitive sequences
- Low signal capsular thickening on all sequences
- Nodular or thick synovitis (low signal on all sequences) outlined by effusion
- Large erosions filled with low signal material
  - Fluid-sensitive sequences may show mixed low and high signal intensity
- No paramagnetic effect on gradient imaging
- Contrast: Synovitis and material within erosions shows moderate enhancement
- Carpal tunnel abnormalities
  - Tendon thickening, median nerve enlargement or enhancement, volar bowing of retinaculum
- Pathologic fracture, complete or incomplete
  - Linear low SI on T1, surrounding high SI edema on T2
- Spine abnormalities
  - Endplate irregularity with increased signal on fluid-sensitive sequences; disc space narrowing
  - May progress rapidly and involve multiple levels
- Amyloidoma: Rare discrete mass mimicking tumor

Ultrasonographic Findings

- Erosions filled with echogenic material
- Tendon thickening
- Echogenic "pads" of material between muscle layers
- Abnormal fluid collections

DIFFERENTIAL DIAGNOSIS

Gout

- Similar low T1 and mixed T2 MR signal in deposits
- Similar well-marginated erosions
- Does not tend to have as prominent tendinous infiltration but more focal tophi

Brown Tumors

- Low T1 and T2 signal (or inhomogeneous)
- If adjacent to cortex, may give appearance of erosion, as in amyloid
- Tendon ruptures occur with both amyloid and hyperparathyroidism

Hemophilic Arthropathy

- Low T1, fairly low T2 (inhomogeneous) signal deposits
- Erosions likely to be filled with high signal fluid
- "Blooming" of iron depositions on GRE

Pigmented Villonodular Synovitis

- Low T1, fairly low T2 (inhomogeneous) signal deposits
- Erosions likely to be filled with high signal effusion
- "Blooming" of nodular hemosiderin deposits on GRE

Rheumatoid Arthritis

- Primary amyloid may appear similar, with symmetric erosions, subchondral cysts, nodularity
- Erosions in rheumatoid arthritis contain high signal material

PATHOLOGY

General Features

- Etiology
  - Primary (AL) amyloidosis
    - Monoclonal population of plasma cells produces amyloidogenic immunoglobulin light-chain protein (λ more often than κ)
  - Secondary (inflammatory-related or AA) amyloidosis
    - Inflammatory stimuli → liver production of serum amyloid A protein → amyloid fibril production
  - Hereditary amyloidosis
    - Group of autosomal dominant diseases
    - Gene mutations → amyloidogenic proteins → amyloid fibrils
    - No associated monoclonal gammopathy
  - Dialysis-related amyloid arthropathy
    - Glomerular filtration failure → ↑ β2 microglobulin → amyloid fibril deposition

Microscopic Features

- Electron microscopy: Characteristic fibrillary array
  - Low signal intensity on both T1 and T2 may be due to fibrous nature of amyloid-containing tissues
- Light microscopy: Stains with Congo red
- Polarized light microscopy: Apple-green birefringence
- Amyloid deposits seen in synovium & synovial fluid

Types of Amyloid

Amyloid Type	Clinical Syndrome	Protein	Associated Disease	MSK Involvement
Immunoglobulin (AL)	Primary amyloidosis	Ig light chains	Plasma cell dyscrasias	Yes, often rheumatoid-like
Reactive (AA)	2° (inflammatory disease)	Amyloid A	RA, FMF	Rare
Hereditary	Familial	Various non-Ig proteins	Genetic, none	Rare
β-2-microglobulin	Dialysis-related amyloid	β-2-microglobulin	End-stage renal disease	Common, joints & tendons

CLINICAL ISSUES

Presentation

- Most common signs/symptoms
  - Primary (AL) amyloid
    - Fatigue, involuntary weight loss
    - Reflects organ systems involved
      - Nephrotic syndrome (30-50%), congestive heart failure (40%), hepatomegaly (25%), carpal tunnel syndrome (25%), peripheral neuropathy (20%)
    - Systemic polyarthritis with pain and swelling
      - Joint disease resembling RA, with pain, stiffness, swelling, nodules, and symmetry
  - Secondary (inflammatory or AA) amyloid
    - 99% have renal insufficiency
    - 20% have nausea, diarrhea
  - Hereditary amyloidosis
    - Peripheral neuropathy
    - Cardiac and kidney involvement less common
  - Dialysis-associated amyloidosis
    - 1st symptom may be at carpal tunnel (CTS)
      - Direct relationship between prevalence of CTS & dialysis: Prevalence after 10 years (20%), after 15 years (30-50%), after 20 years (80-100%)
    - Joint pain in 50% after 10 years of dialysis
    - Spondyloarthropathy of hemodialysis

Demographics

- Age
  - Any, depending on underlying cause
- Primary (myeloma-related or AL) amyloidosis
  - Rare: 8 cases per 1 million
  - Affects older population (usually > 65 years)
  - Males (65%) > females
  - Only 10-15% of patients with multiple myeloma (MM) have amyloidosis
    - Unusual for MM to develop in patients with amyloidosis
- Secondary (inflammatory or AA) amyloidosis
  - Seen with RA > familial Mediterranean fever (FMF) > psoriatic arthritis, ankylosing spondylitis, reactive arthritis, adult Still disease, juvenile idiopathic arthritis, systemic lupus erythematosus, chronic infection (tuberculosis), decubitus ulcers
    - 75% of cases occur with RA
    - Amyloid does not develop in most RA patients
  - Time from diagnosis of underlying inflammatory disease to development of amyloid: 10-20 years
- Dialysis-associated amyloidosis
  - Nearly 100% of patients treated with dialysis for 15-20 years develop amyloid deposits
  - Occurs with either hemo- or peritoneal dialysis
  - May also develop in chronic renal insufficiency not treated by dialysis

Natural History & Prognosis

- Diagnosis made by tissue biopsy
- Cardiomyopathy resistant to medical therapy
- Primary amyloidosis: 20% survival 5 years after diagnosis
  - Multisystem involvement, rapid progression
- Secondary amyloidosis has slower course and longer median survival: > 10 years after diagnosis
- Hereditary amyloidosis: Prolonged survival if liver transplant prior to organ failure
- Dialysis-associated amyloidosis
  - Most patients on long-term dialysis develop amyloidosis
  - Prognosis determined by underlying kidney disease
  - Joint and tendon destruction may significantly impair quality of life

Treatment

- Primary amyloidosis
  - Chemotherapy with melphalan and prednisone
    - Not clear that this prolongs survival
  - Autologous stem cell bone marrow transplant
  - Support of involved organs
- Secondary amyloidosis
  - Treatment: Control underlying inflammatory process
  - Colchicine in patients with FMF
- Anti-TNF-α may benefit both 1° and 2° forms
  - Small, uncontrolled studies at this time
- Hereditary amyloidosis
  - Liver transplantation, supportive measures
- Dialysis-associated amyloidosis
  - Symptomatic: NSAIDs, local steroid injection
  - Surgery for CTS, tendon rupture
  - Kidney transplantation halts progression

DIAGNOSTIC CHECKLIST

Consider

- Thickened tendons, joint capsule suggest amyloidosis
- Predominantly low signal within erosions suggestive, but not specific, for amyloid

SELECTED REFERENCES

1. Loizos S et al: Amyloidosis: review and imaging findings. Semin Ultrasound CT MR. 35(3):225-39, 2014
2. Beggs SA et al: A chronic thigh mass in a 69-year-old man. Amyloidoma presenting as a chronic soft tissue mass. Skeletal Radiol. 39(12):1237, 1259-61, 2010

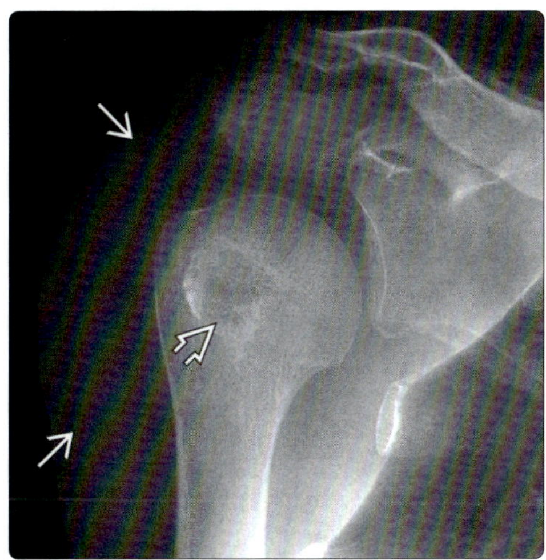

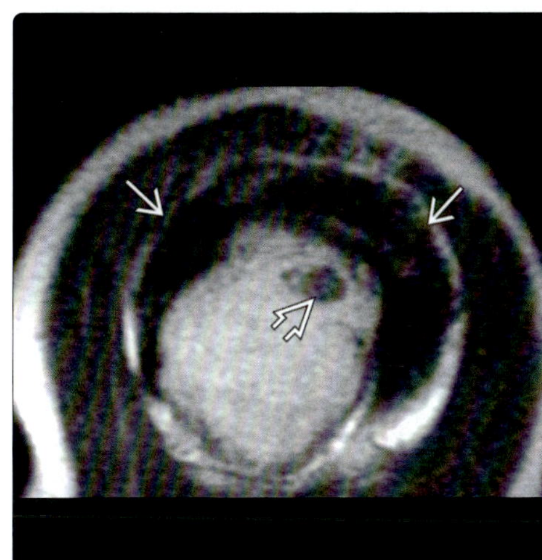

(Left) *AP radiograph shows diffuse osteoporosis. There is a large soft tissue mass, which has obliterated all fat planes, surrounding the glenohumeral joint ➡ and a large erosion within the humeral head ➡. This is chronic hemodialysis-related amyloid.* **(Right)** *Sagittal T2WI MR in the same patient shows tremendous low signal thickening of the rotator cuff tendons ➡ as well as an erosion containing low signal material ➡. It should not be surprising that clinically the shoulder pad sign applies.*

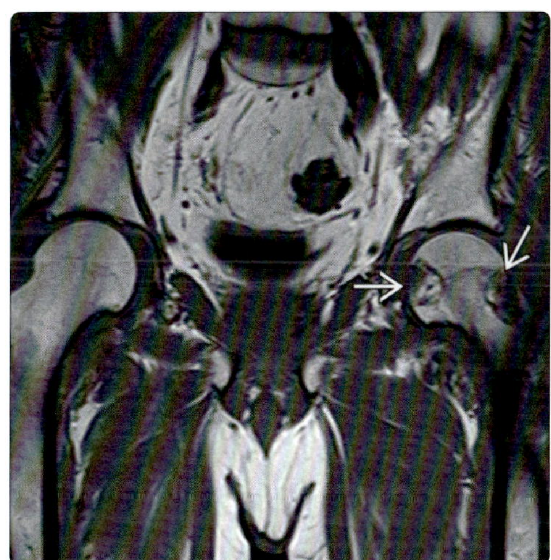

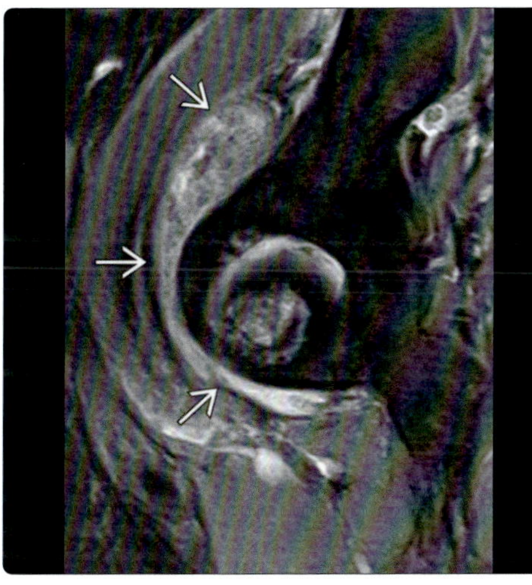

(Left) *Coronal T1WI MR in a 68-year-old man shows large erosions involving the left femoral head and neck ➡. The erosions contain mostly low signal nodular material. The right hip shows minimal osteoarthritis but otherwise is normal. Considerations for diagnosis of the left hip include PVNS, gout, hemophilic arthropathy, and amyloid deposition.* **(Right)** *Sagittal PD FS MR in the same patient shows extension from the anterior capsule into the iliopsoas bursa ➡. The contents remain mostly low SI, bathed in high SI fluid.*

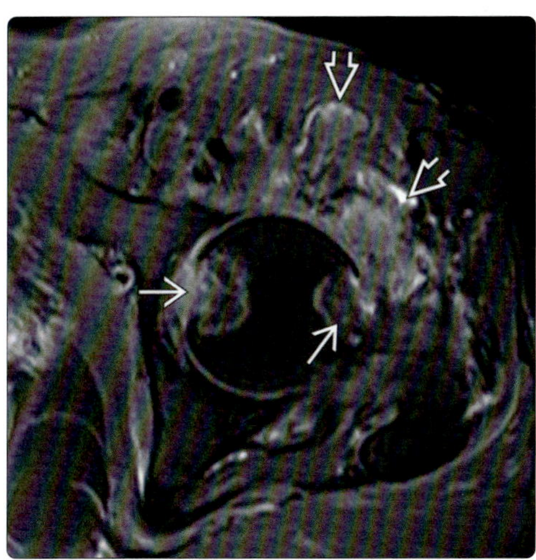

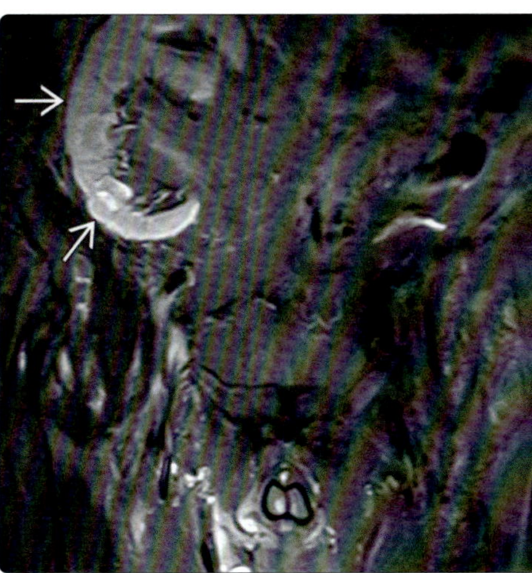

(Left) *Axial T2 FS MR, same patient, shows the large femoral erosions ➡ containing mostly low signal material, with similar material in the distended capsule and iliopsoas bursa ➡. The differential diagnosis remains unchanged.* **(Right)** *Coronal T2 FS MR, cut more anteriorly in the patient, shows a functioning kidney transplant ➡. This patient with end-stage renal disease had been on dialysis for many years prior to his transplant; biopsy of the hip proved amyloid deposition.*

(Left) *AP radiograph shows erosions of the capitellum ➡ as well as the trochlea and ulna ➡. There is osteopenia and diffuse soft tissue swelling. Based on the radiograph alone, this could represent rheumatoid arthritis but proved to be amyloid deposition.* **(Right)** *AP radiograph shows diffuse osteoporosis as well as large masses within the hip joints ➡. There is also a suggestion of femoral neck erosion ➡. The history of chronic hemodialysis leads to the diagnosis of dialysis arthropathy.*

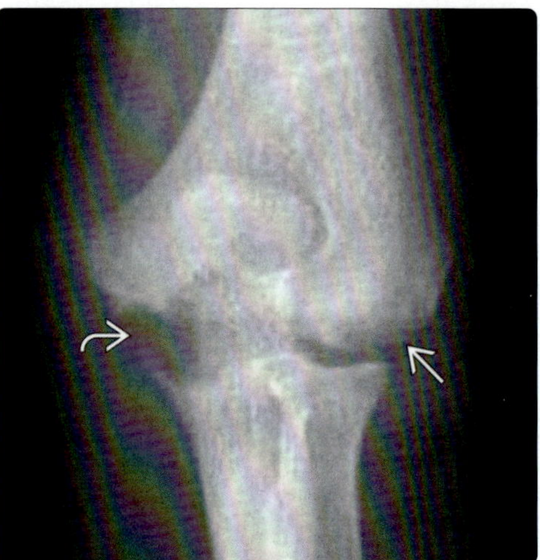

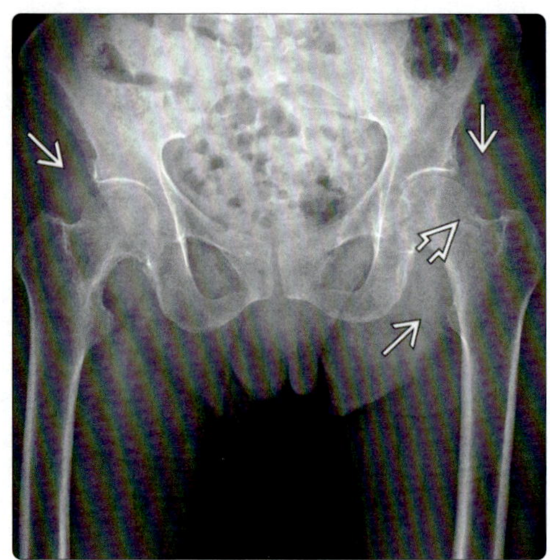

(Left) *Coronal T1WI MR in the same patient located anteriorly in the joint shows large, low-signal collections within distended joints ➡.* **(Right)** *Coronal T1WI MR located slightly posteriorly in the same patient confirms femoral head/neck erosion on the left ➡. The low signal intraarticular material may consist of a mixture of pyrophosphate and sodium urate crystals, along with amyloid deposition. Amyloid is proven by tissue biopsy; gout proven by synovial fluid evaluation.*

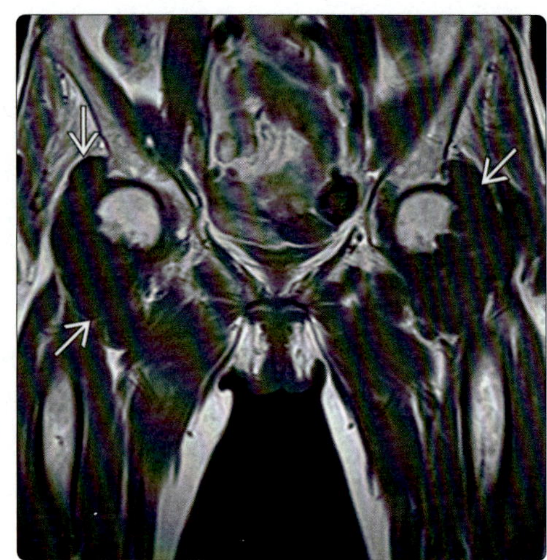

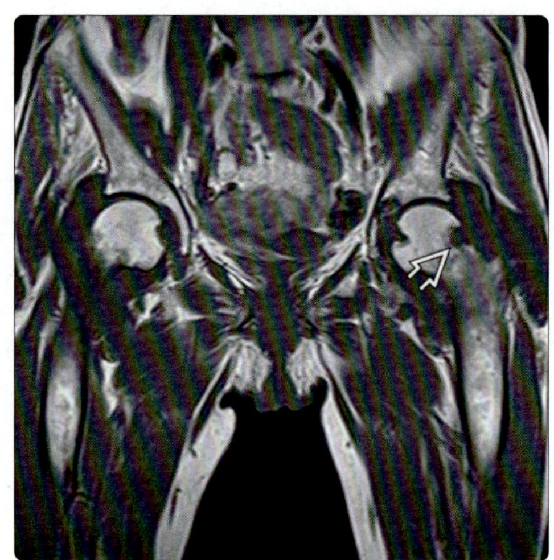

(Left) *Sagittal T2WI FS MR of the left hip in the same patient shows the intraarticular material to be predominantly low signal with regions of high signal intermixed ➡. It distends the joint anteriorly.* **(Right)** *Axial PD FS MR of the same hip shows acetabular erosion containing the mixed signal ➡ and the anterior joint distension containing the same material ➡. This is extensive dialysis-related amyloid deposition involving the capsule, bones, and synovium.*

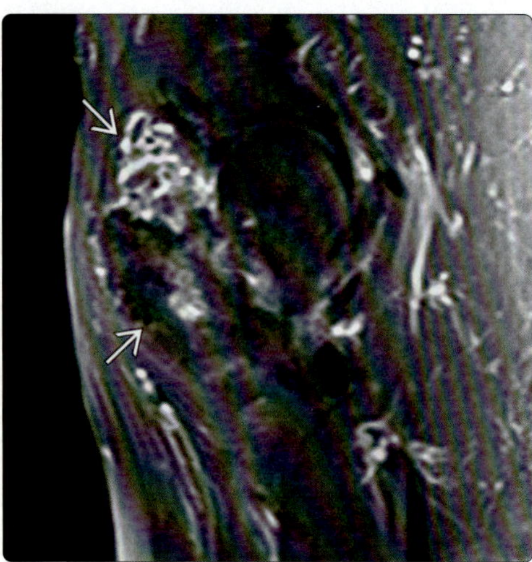

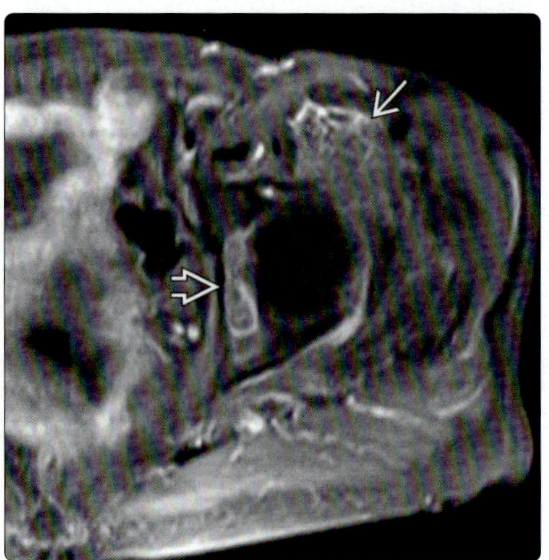

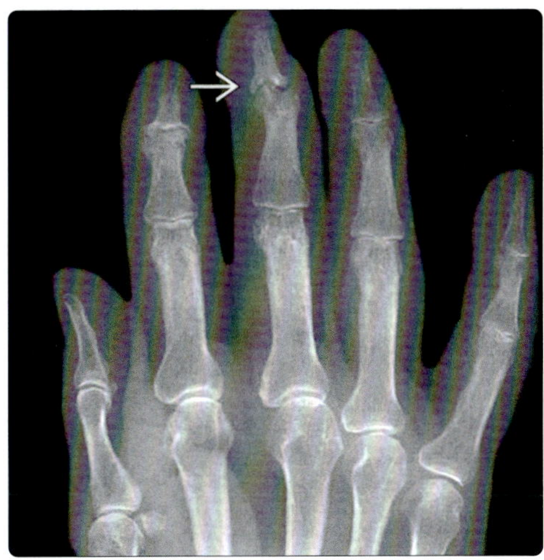

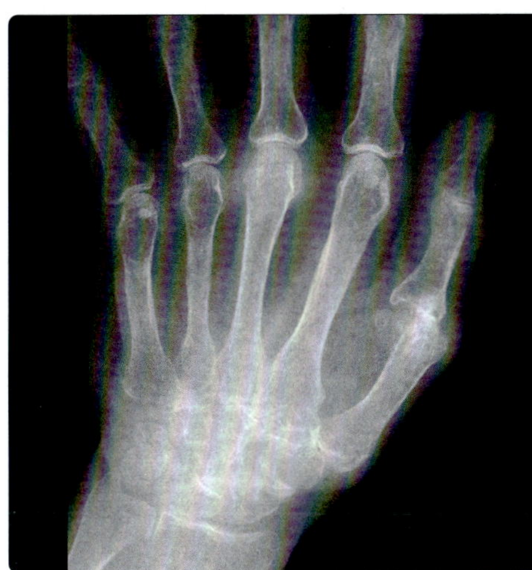

(Left) *PA radiograph demonstrates erosive change at the DIP joints →. Amyloid deposition within a joint can result in erosions, which itself is nonspecific, but in the company of large soft tissue masses is highly suggestive.* **(Right)** *PA radiograph suggests rheumatoid arthritis with MCP soft tissue swelling, erosions, and osteoporosis. The patient history of multiple myeloma and a negative rheumatoid factor should make one consider the diagnosis of amyloid deposition, which was proven at biopsy.*

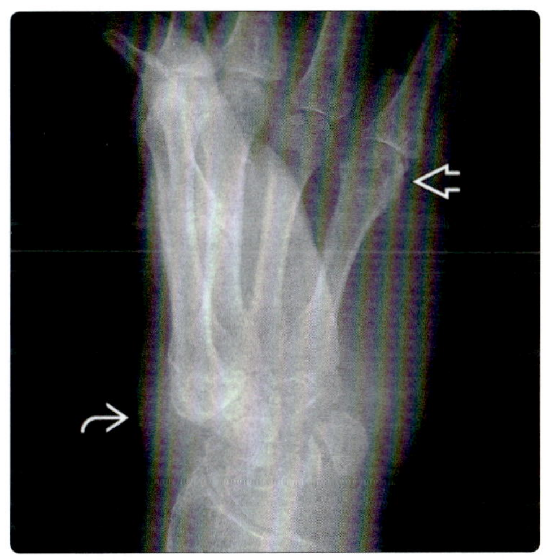

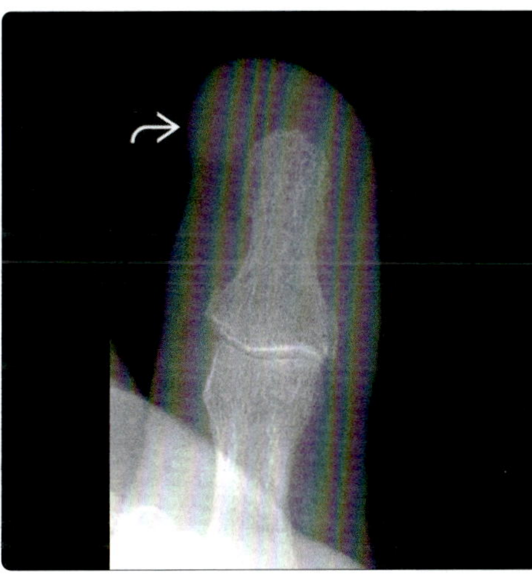

(Left) *Oblique radiograph shows dorsal soft tissue nodular swelling → as well as erosions at the 5th MCP joint →.* **(Right)** *PA radiograph in the same patient shows a soft tissue nodule →. This collection of findings most frequently yields the diagnosis of rheumatoid arthritis, but the patient was rheumatoid factor negative. Biopsy of the carpal erosions demonstrated amyloid. This patient did not have renal failure; the diagnosis of primary amyloidosis from multiple myeloma might be considered.*

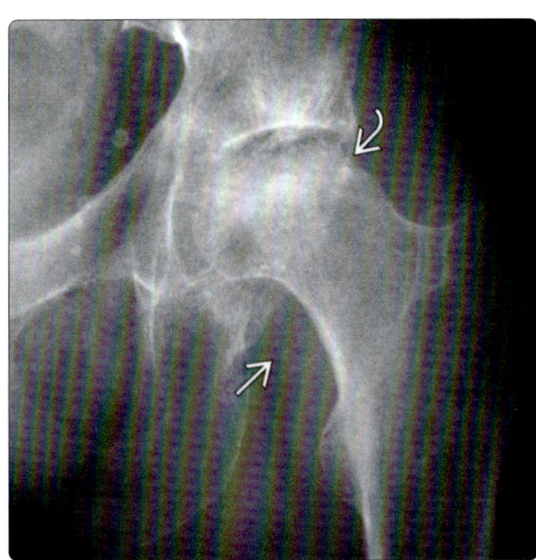

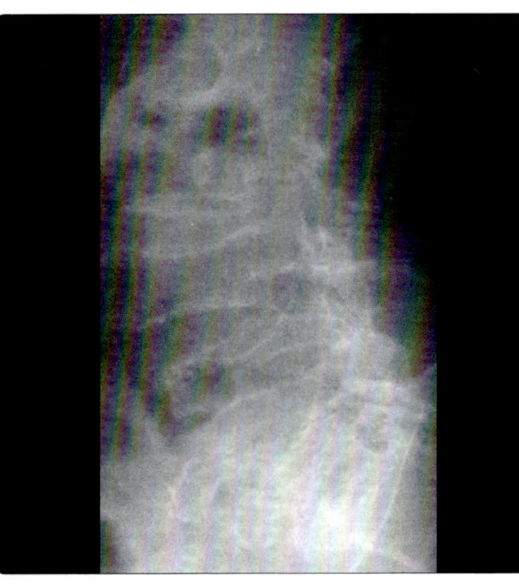

(Left) *AP radiograph in the same patient shows distension of the joint → and severe erosive disease → with collapse of the femoral head.* **(Right)** *Lateral radiograph in the same patient shows diffuse osteoporosis and compression fractures of all the lumbar vertebrae. No focal lesions are seen. Biopsy showed multiple myeloma. Amyloid may be seen secondary to multiple myeloma and should be considered when lumpy soft tissue swelling is seen with erosions that are not typical of rheumatoid arthritis.*

KEY FACTS

TERMINOLOGY

- Arthritis associated with hemochromatosis
  - Hemochromatosis: Progressive ↑ in total body iron stores; abnormal iron deposition in multiple organs

IMAGING

- Best diagnostic clue: Large hook-like osteophytes involving 2nd and 3rd metacarpophalangeal (MCP) joints
- Location: Preferentially involves MCP joints
  - Initially 2nd and 3rd; eventually involves all MCPs
  - Radiocarpal joint
  - Rarely involves shoulder, elbow, hip, knee
- Radiologic abnormalities
  - Cartilage thinning (joint space narrowing)
  - Subchondral sclerosis and cysts
  - Osteophytes on MC heads eventually become large and hook-like, curving away from MCP joint
  - Normal bone density
  - Symmetric in that both hands usually involved
  - Chondrocalcinosis (fibro- and hyaline cartilage)

TOP DIFFERENTIAL DIAGNOSES

- Pyrophosphate arthropathy (CPPD)
  - Chondrocalcinosis
  - Preferential involvement 2nd and 3rd MCP joints
  - Osteophytes generally not as large as in hemochromatosis
  - Generally older patient population for CPPD

PATHOLOGY

- Primary hemochromatosis: Genetic disorder
  - Autosomal recessive disorder
  - Single site mutation on *HFE* gene
  - Allows cellular uptake of iron-based transferrin
  - Patients also have ↑ in intestinal iron absorption
- Secondary hemochromatosis: Variety of etiologies but usually results from chronic hemolytic anemia
  - Hemosiderosis from multiple blood transfusions
- Arthropathy develops in 25-50% of patients with primary hemochromatosis, usually relatively early in disease
- Liver is main organ of deposition
  - Initially involves periportal hepatocytes
  - Progresses to perilobular fibrosis and cirrhosis
- Pancreas also commonly involved
  - Results in insulin resistance and type 1 diabetes
- Cardiomyopathy and arrhythmias
- Hyperpigmentation of skin
- Iron present in joint fluid, synovium, and cartilage

CLINICAL ISSUES

- Clinical symptoms
  - Swelling at MCP joints
  - Decreased range of motion
  - Pain with use, not at rest
- Onset in adults: Young to middle-aged
- M:F = 1.8:1
- 0.4-1% in Caucasians (less in other ethnic groups)
- No ↑ in mortality unless cirrhosis develops
  - 1/3 of patients who die from hemochromatosis with cirrhosis develop hepatocellular carcinoma
- Presence of arthropathy does not affect overall prognosis of hemochromatosis

DIAGNOSTIC CHECKLIST

- Consider: Radiographic signs of hemochromatosis arthropathy may occur prior to other signs of primary hemochromatosis
- Consider: Hook-like osteophytes need not be present to make diagnosis
  - Size and morphology of osteophytes relates to longevity of disease
- If arthritic pattern suggestive of pyrophosphate arthropathy develops in young adult (particularly male), consider diagnosis of hemochromatosis
  - Pyrophosphate arthropathy rare in patients < 30 years old; generally in elderly patients

(Left) *PA radiograph shows cartilage narrowing at the metacarpophalangeal (MCP) joints with subchondral cysts ➡. The osteophytes formed at the metacarpal heads are large and have acquired a hook-like appearance ➡, typical of hemochromatosis.* **(Right)** *PA radiograph in a young adult man with MCP arthritis, shows cartilage narrowing ➡ and osteophytes ➡. This is relatively early disease compared with others showing the typically described large hook-like osteophytes, but distribution is typical.*

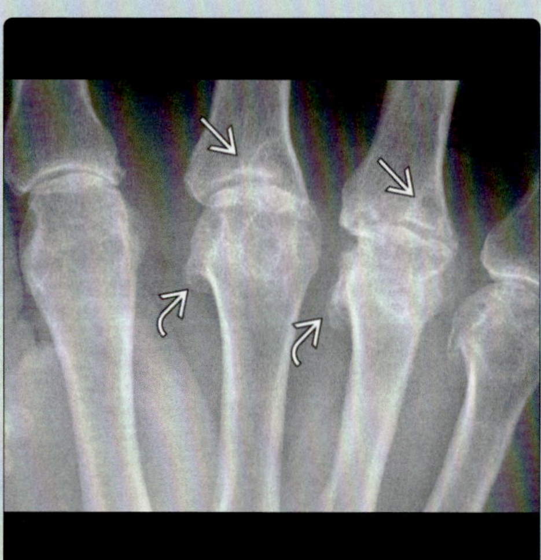

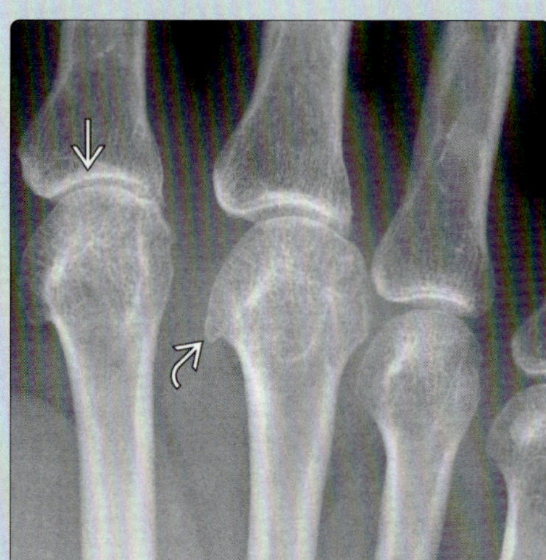

KEY FACTS

TERMINOLOGY

- Pathologic pigmentation of connective tissues in patients with alkaptonuria
  - Enzymatic defect: Deficiency of homogentisic acid oxidase

TOP DIFFERENTIAL DIAGNOSES

- Ankylosing spondylitis: Severe ochronosis may result in bony bridging and osteoporosis, similar to ankylosing spondylitis
- Rheumatoid arthritis: Peripheral joint osteoporosis, cartilage loss, osseous fragmentation may simulate rheumatoid arthritis

CLINICAL ISSUES

- Generally not noted prior to age 20-30
- Blue-gray: Pigmentation of ears or sclerae
- Young adults develop low back pain and arthritis of large proximal joints
- Spinal abnormalities
  - Osteoporosis
  - Calcification/ossification of discs
  - Disc space narrowing and vacuum phenomena
  - Few osteophytes
  - With longstanding disease, ossification may bridge vertebral bodies
- Other axial abnormalities
  - Calcification/ossification at sacroiliac joints and symphysis pubis
- Large peripheral joints (shoulder, hip, knee)
  - Joint space narrowing
  - Osseous collapse and fragmentation
  - Intraarticular loose bodies
  - Few, small osteophytes
  - Tendinous calcification/ossification
  - Small joint involvement rare
  - MR: Nonspecific marrow edema, effusion, subchondral cysts

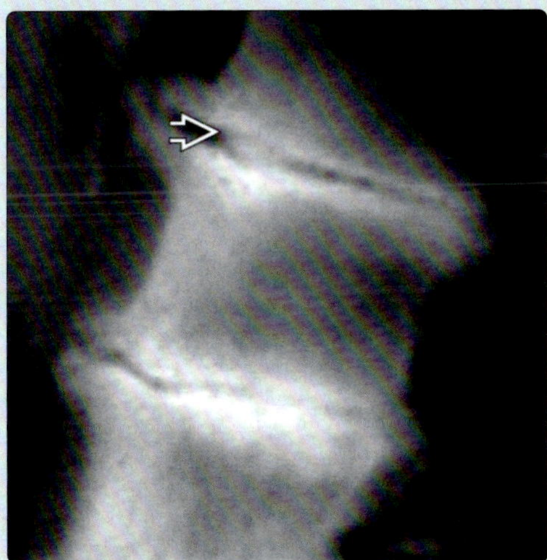

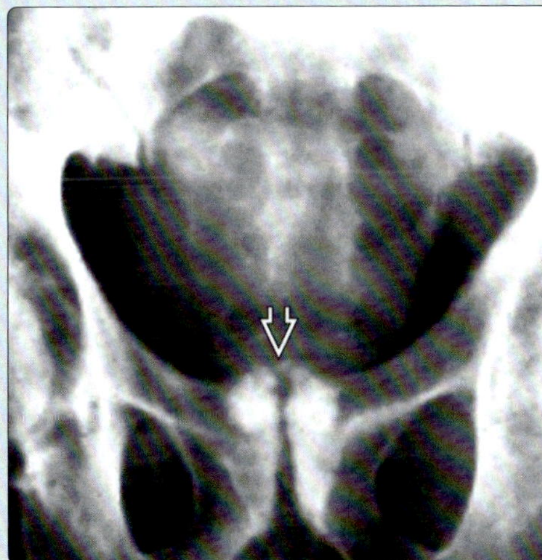

(Left) *Lateral radiograph shows the classic appearance of ochronosis (alkaptonuria). There is calcification in the intervertebral discs ➡ and severe disc space narrowing. The endplates show sclerosis, but the underlying bone density is osteoporotic.* **(Right)** *AP radiograph of the pelvis in the same patient shows calcification of the pubic symphysis ➡. Ochronosis is an extremely rare cause of calcification at these sites. CPPD is a much more common cause of calcification in both regions.*

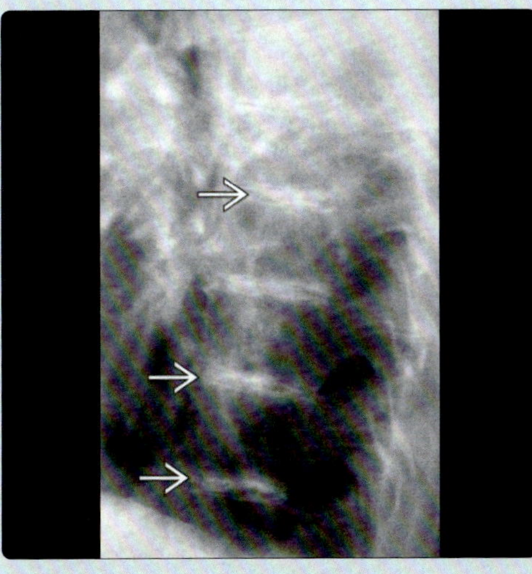

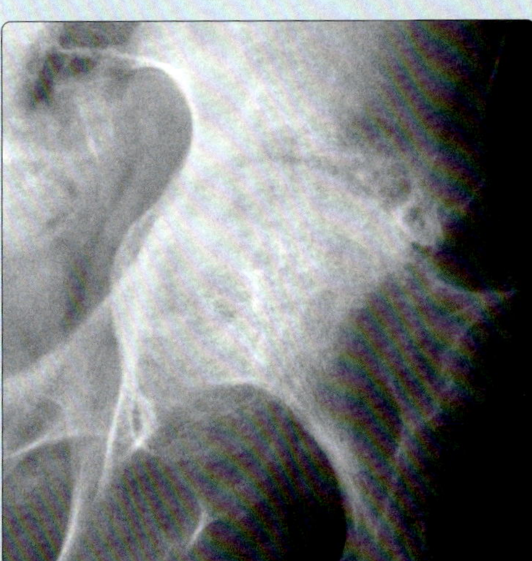

(Left) *Lateral radiograph of the spine shows diffuse osteoporosis plus dense calcification of most of the discs ➡. Though one may see disc calcification from degenerative change, the combination of osteoporosis and extensive disc calcification is seen with ochronosis.* **(Right)** *AP radiograph of the hip shows diffuse osteoporosis, protrusio, and complete loss of cartilage. Occasionally long-term ochronosis results in cartilage fragmentation and secondary degenerative disease, as in this case.*

Wilson Disease

KEY FACTS

TERMINOLOGY

- Synonym: Hepatolenticular degeneration
- Definition: Inherited disorder characterized by accumulation of copper in tissues

IMAGING

- Best diagnostic clue: Osteopenia + ossicles or osseous excrescences
- Location: Knee, hand, wrist, elbow, shoulder, hip
  - Patellofemoral joint predominates in knee
  - Metacarpophalangeal and radiocarpal joints
- Osteopenia in 50%
  - May be associated with pathologic fractures
- Chondrocalcinosis has been reported
  - Some believe most cases are ossicles rather than true chondrocalcinosis
- Cartilage narrowing
- Subchondral bone irregular and indistinct ("paintbrush")
  - Excrescences arising from subchondral bone contribute to this appearance
- Focal areas of fragmentation of articular surface
  - May result in presence of well-corticated ossicles
  - If larger, gives appearance of osteochondral defect
- Subchondral cysts
- Periostitis at trochanters and inferior calcaneus
- Spine
  - Irregularities in endplate contour: Schmorl nodes, may resemble Scheuermann disease
  - Anterior wedging in midthoracic vertebral bodies

TOP DIFFERENTIAL DIAGNOSES

- Osteoarthritis
  - Subchondral cyst and cartilage narrowing
  - Fragmentation of osteophyte may suggest Wilson
  - Excrescences in Wilson disease are distinctly different from osteophytes
- Pyrophosphate arthropathy and hemochromatosis
  - Chondrocalcinosis appears similar
  - Similar distribution, particularly patellofemoral, radiocarpal, and metacarpophalangeal joints
  - Small ossicles and excrescences in Wilson disease should differentiate it

PATHOLOGY

- Autosomal recessive inheritance
  - Mutation in *ATP7B* gene → dysfunction of ATP7B protein and ↓ copper excretion by hepatocytes
- Associated findings
  - Degenerative changes in basal ganglia
  - Cirrhosis of liver
  - Kayser-Fleischer rings in cornea
  - Renal tubular disease
- Articular cartilage may have copper deposition
- Source of fragmentation within joints uncertain
  - Minor injury from patient tremors and spasticity may result in damage to cartilage and bone
  - Renal tubular dysfunction may cause osteomalacia resulting in bone fragility
  - Copper in articular cartilage may cause degradation of collagen and proteoglycans

CLINICAL ISSUES

- 1st manifestations generally hepatic and neurologic
  - Tremor, rigidity, dysarthria, personality change
  - Abnormal liver function tests, eventual cirrhosis
- Articular symptoms
  - Seen in 50% of adults; may be asymptomatic
  - Pain and swelling may occur
- Fever, hemolytic anemia
- Proteinuria, aminoaciduria, phosphaturia
- Mean age of diagnosis 9.5 years; many asymptomatic; discovered by abnormal liver function tests, screening
- Age of onset: 50% symptomatic by 15 years of age
- Gender: Male slightly more common than female
- Symptoms improve with treatment: D-penicillamine, copper chelating drugs, liver transplant

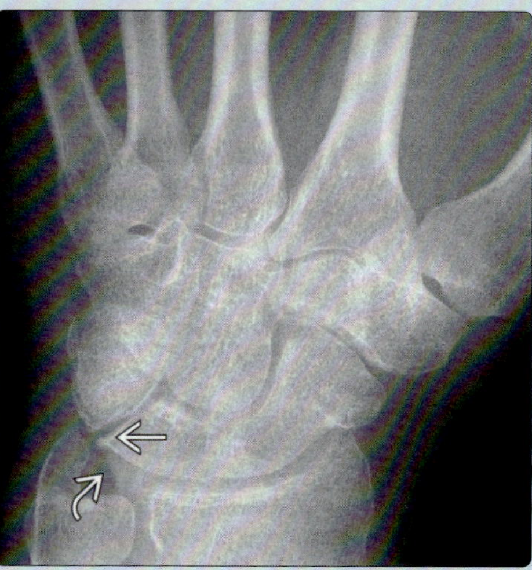

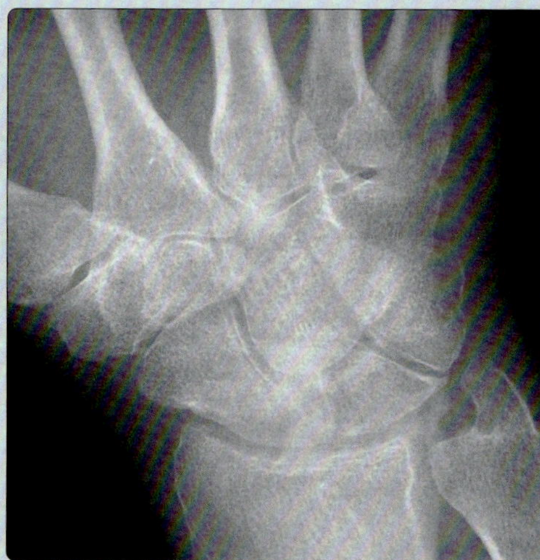

(Left) *PA radiograph of a patient with Wilson disease demonstrates bones that are diffusely osteoporotic for a young woman. The wrists show fairly prominent osseous excrescences arising from the lunate ➡ and radius ↷.* **(Right)** *PA radiograph of the contralateral hand in the same patient shows symmetric carpal excrescences. These osseous excrescences are often seen in Wilson disease, but they may also have the appearance of small ossicles. There may be chondrocalcinosis, but it is not seen in this case.*

KEY FACTS

TERMINOLOGY

- Deposition of calcium oxalate in tissues, including bone

IMAGING

- Best diagnostic clue: Sclerotic bones associated with nephrocalcinosis
- Location
  - Spine: Vertebral bodies &/or endplates
  - Metaphyses of long bones
- Radiographic findings: Varied patterns of sclerosis
  - Generalized osseous sclerosis
  - Patchy sclerosis
  - Metaphyseal dense bands: All long bones
  - Subchondral sclerosis of proximal humerus and femur (may mimic osteonecrosis)
  - Bone-within-bone appearance: Ilium, sternum, vertebral bodies
  - Drumstick configuration of metacarpals (widening of bone at metacarpal head and neck)
  - Endplate sclerosis vertebral bodies (simulates rugger jersey spine)
- Transverse pathologic fracture
- Resorptive patterns secondary to renal failure
- Chondrocalcinosis
- Calcification of adjacent ligaments and tendons
- Vascular and soft tissue calcifications
- CT: Small, contracted kidneys
  - May have dense calcification in cortex and medullary portions
  - Sclerotic bones

TOP DIFFERENTIAL DIAGNOSES

- Renal osteodystrophy
- Hyperparathyroidism
  - Nephrocalcinosis, but kidneys generally not as severely contracted
- Sclerosing dysplasias
  - No kidney abnormality; should differentiate

PATHOLOGY

- Gross pathology in bone: Oxalate crystals surrounded by granulomatous reaction
- Calcium deposition in kidneys, small arteries, eyes, soft tissues, bone
- Kidneys
  - Nephrolithiasis
  - Nephrocalcinosis: Cortical and medullary involvement
  - Glomeruli unaffected
  - Small, contracted kidneys
  - Eventually, kidneys replaced by fibrous septa and crystal deposits
- Osseous structures
  - Density due to direct crystal deposition
  - Foreign body giant cell reaction superimposed and stimulates new bone formation
- Joints
  - Crystal deposition in synovium and articular cartilage are rare
  - Crystals rarely found in synovial fluid
  - Generally not true arthropathy
- Primary etiology: Rare hereditary process
  - Autosomal recessive, 2 types
  - Overproduction of oxalate related to enzymatic defects
- Secondary etiology
  - Related to chronic renal disease
  - Hyperoxaluria related to small bowel resections

CLINICAL ISSUES

- Primary oxalosis usually apparent by 5 years of age
- M = F
- Progressive renal failure and uremia
- Prolonged survival of primary oxalosis now possible
  - Dialysis
  - 2-step renal transplantation
  - Prominent crystal deposition still occurs

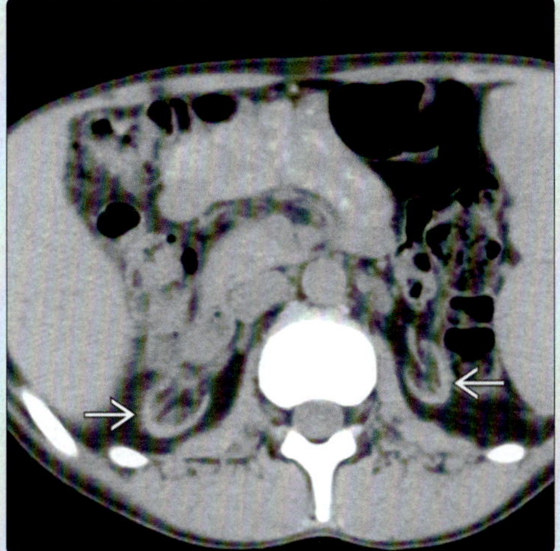

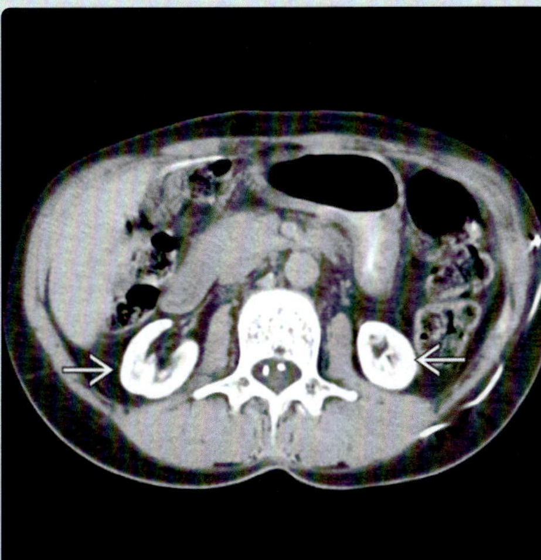

(Left) *Axial NECT shows small end-stage kidneys ➡ with high density throughout the cortex and medulla (global nephrocalcinosis). Also evident are very dense bones, another typical feature of oxalosis.* **(Right)** *Axial NECT shows extremely dense and small kidneys ➡, a characteristic feature of some patients with oxalosis. The nephrocalcinosis in this patient is global, both cortical and medullary. The density of the bones is also increased due to deposition of calcium oxalate crystals.*

KEY FACTS

IMAGING

- Location
  - Single focus; joints, bursae, tendon sheaths
  - Intraarticular PVNS: 80% occur in knee
- Morphology
  - May be focal nodular mass
  - May be diffuse, with villonodular proliferation of entire synovium and in all potential joint recesses
- MR demonstrates extent; characteristic but not pathognomonic (diagnostic in 95%)
  - Gradient-echo imaging usually shows blooming phenomenon of hemosiderin-laden nodules
- Large effusion on radiograph or MR
  - Rarely, after repeated bleeding, effusion appears dense on radiograph
- ± erosion; occurs in 50%
- ± large, well-marginated subchondral cyst

TOP DIFFERENTIAL DIAGNOSES

- Nodular synovitis
- Gout
- Amyloid
- Hemophilic arthropathy
- Synovial chondromatosis

CLINICAL ISSUES

- 5% of all primary soft tissue "tumors"
- Treatment
  - Resection with synovectomy
  - Incomplete resection has high recurrence rate

DIAGNOSTIC CHECKLIST

- If suspicious of PVNS, use gradient-echo sequence to elicit blooming
- Search carefully for all regions of involvement, including all recesses, to achieve complete resection

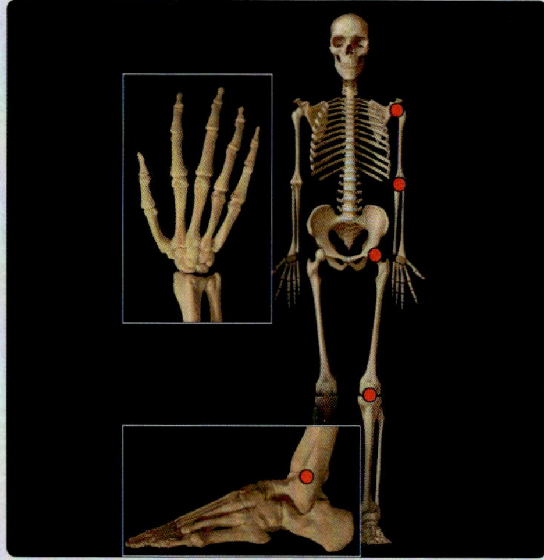

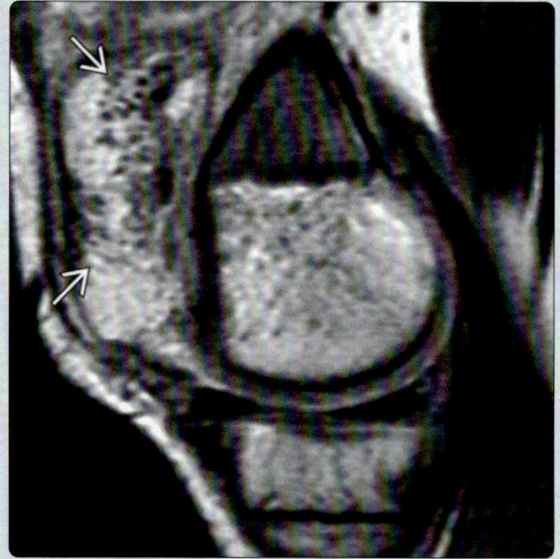

(Left) *Graphic depicting the most common locations for pigmented villonodular synovitis (PVNS). The knee joint is by far the most common location of those shown.* **(Right)** *Sagittal PD MR shows a classic case of PVNS. There is a large suprapatellar effusion which contains low signal nodularity ➡. PVNS may present either with diffuse nodularity, as in this case, or as a focal nodular mass. Large effusions are almost invariable. The patient is a teenager, which can be quite typical.*

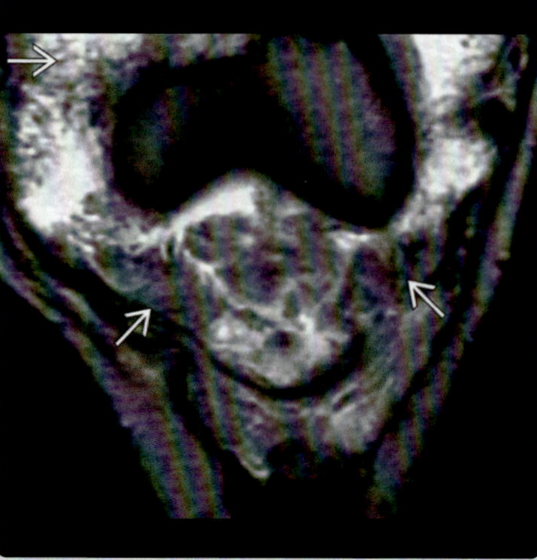

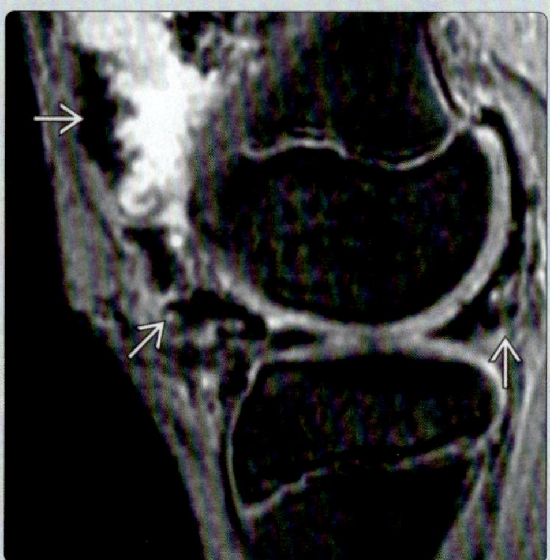

(Left) *Coronal T2WI MR in the same patient shows the high signal effusion containing innumerable low signal nodules ➡. The synovium is thickened and the Hoffa fat pad is flattened and displaced by the extensive fluid collection.* **(Right)** *Sagittal T2* GRE MR shows blooming of the low signal nodules ➡. The nodules appear larger and even lower in signal intensity than they did on T2 imaging. Blooming occurs when these nodules contain hemosiderin, as they usually do. This feature confirms the diagnosis.*

TERMINOLOGY

Synonyms

- Pigmented villonodular synovitis (PVNS); benign synovioma; nodular tenosynovitis
- Giant cell tumor of tendon sheath: Pathologically identical but fully discussed in separate section

Definitions

- Monoarticular proliferation of hemorrhagic synovium
- Occurs in joint, bursa, tendon sheath
  - PVNS: Diffuse, articular form
  - Giant cell tumor of tendon sheath: Localized, extraarticular form

IMAGING

General Features

- Best diagnostic clue
  - Radiograph: Large effusion ± associated erosions and subchondral cysts
  - MR: Effusion with synovial proliferation, low signal on all sequences, and usually blooms on gradient-echo
- Location
  - Single focus; joints, bursae, tendon sheaths
    - Rare reports of multifocal occurrence
  - PVNS (intraarticular): 80% occur in knee
    - Knee > ankle > hip > shoulder > elbow
  - Giant cell tumor of tendon sheath
    - Hand and wrist (65-89%): Volar aspect of digits
    - Foot and ankle
- Size
  - Begins as small focal mass attached to synovium
  - May enlarge to involve entire joint, lining entire synovial surface
- Morphology
  - May be focal nodular mass
  - May be diffuse, with villonodular proliferation of entire synovium and in all potential joint recesses
    - In knee, can extend down popliteus tendon sheath and into posterolateral compartment, coronary recess, meniscofemoral recess, popliteal cyst, intercondylar notch, and even along collateral ligaments

Imaging Recommendations

- Best imaging tool
  - MR demonstrates extent of process; appearance characteristic but not pathognomonic (diagnostic in 95%)
- Protocol advice
  - Gradient-echo imaging shows blooming phenomenon of hemosiderin-laden nodules in most cases

Radiographic Findings

- Intraarticular PVNS
  - Large effusion
    - Rarely, after repeated bleeding, may appear dense
  - Normal bone density
  - Cartilage preserved until late in process
    - Cartilage narrowing only with secondary degenerative change
      - □ Osteophytes generally present at this late stage
  - ± erosion; occurs in 50%
  - ± large, well-marginated subchondral cyst
  - Very rarely and late, may show dystrophic calcification
- Giant cell tumor of tendon sheath
  - Soft tissue mass, generally on volar side of finger
  - Pressure erosions of underlying bone (15%)
  - Rare dystrophic calcifications

CT Findings

- Nonspecific, but may be suggestive if subchondral cysts are large
- Effusion, soft tissue mass
  - May have increased attenuation related to hemosiderin deposits
  - Synovium enhances post contrast
- Well-defined erosions with sclerotic margins

MR Findings

- Effusion, generally large
- Erosions (may be subtle)
- Synovial-based masses
  - May be solitary nodular mass or multiple nodules
  - May result in thickening and nodularity of synovium throughout most of joint
  - May extend through capsular defects along juxtaarticular ligaments
  - T1WI MR: Low signal, homogeneous
    - Rare foci of high signal: Lipid-laden macrophages
  - T2 and other fluid-sensitive sequences: Variably low signal and inhomogeneous
    - Majority of mass is usually low signal on fluid-sensitive sequences
    - Variability relates to variable amounts of fat, fibrous tissue, blood products, and edema present
  - GRE sequence: Blooms, relating to presence of hemosiderin
  - Postcontrast imaging: Moderate to intense inhomogeneous enhancement
    - May increase conspicuity for evaluation of extent of lesion, but not required for diagnosis

DIFFERENTIAL DIAGNOSIS

Intraarticular Nodular Synovitis

- Most frequently in knee, especially infrapatellar fat pad
- MR signal intensity may be identical to PVNS
- Lesion is nodular, similar to nodular form of PVNS
- Generally less hemosiderin present than PVNS
- Generally smaller effusion than PVNS

Gout

- T1: Low signal intensity nodular lesions
- T2: Low/inhomogeneously mixed signal intensity
- Juxtaarticular location (if present) makes gout more likely than PVNS

Amyloid

- Similar to gout, with low signal intensity T1 and T2 articular and juxtaarticular mass
- Enhances with contrast, but no blooming with GRE
- Generally due to underlying disease process

Hemophilic Arthropathy

- Effusion with low signal synovial proliferation on T1 and T2, same as PVNS
- Proliferative synovium enhances with contrast
- Blooms on GRE, same as PVNS
- Erosions of adjacent bone, same as PVNS
- Morphology, with overgrowth of epiphyses/metaphyses should differentiate hemophilic arthropathy from PVNS
- Familial (X-linked, so found only in males)

Synovial Chondromatosis

- Generally bodies are seen as separate entities, often following signal of bone or cartilage
- Usually bodies are seen on radiograph, making differentiation of diagnoses simple
- Occasional conglomerate low signal mass in synovial chondromatosis, not seen on radiograph, may be confused with PVNS
  - Does not bloom with GRE imaging

PATHOLOGY

General Features

- Etiology
  - Unknown etiology; likely reactive inflammatory process
  - Treated as low-grade, locally aggressive neoplasm
  - Abnormal synovium is prone to hemorrhage with minor trauma
    - Repeated hemorrhagic effusions result in iron deposition in synovium and nodules
  - With proliferation of abnormal synovium, focal erosions and subchondral cysts develop
- Genetics
  - Clonal chromosomal aberrations, aneuploidy
  - Gene and protein expression patterns suggest ongoing proliferation is sustained by apoptosis resistance

Gross Pathologic & Surgical Features

- Intraarticular PVNS
  - Joint filled with unclotted dark brown blood
  - Villonodular frond-like proliferation of synovial membrane
    - Cut surface: Yellow-brown (iron deposition)

Microscopic Features

- Synovial proliferation
  - Multinucleated giant cells, hemosiderin-laden macrophages
  - Intra- and extracellular hemosiderin; uncommonly, may contain little hemosiderin

CLINICAL ISSUES

Presentation

- Most common signs/symptoms
  - Painful swollen joint; insidious onset
  - Limited, painful range of motion
  - Sharp, sudden ↑ of pain if nodule is torsed
  - Nearly always monoarticular
  - Effusion is often grossly chocolate brown color
  - Rapid reaccumulation of effusion
  - Rare pathologic fracture through large subchondral cyst

Demographics

- Age
  - Intraarticular PVNS
    - Wide range; adolescents to elderly
    - Most frequent: 30-40 years
  - Giant cell tumor of tendon sheath: 30-50 years
- Gender
  - Intraarticular PVNS: M:F = 1:2
  - Giant cell tumor of tendon sheath: M = F
- Epidemiology
  - 5% of all primary soft tissue "tumors"
  - Giant cell tumor of tendon sheath: 2nd most common soft tissue mass of hand

Natural History & Prognosis

- Benign, locally aggressive lesion
- If untreated, repeated bleeding and proliferation leads to joint destruction

Treatment

- Resection with synovectomy
- Incomplete resection has high recurrence rate
  - Overall recurrence of intraarticular PVNS: 20-50% (higher rate related to incomplete synovectomy)
- Open procedure may be required as arthroscopic synovectomy unlikely to have complete access to some lesion locations
  - Posterior to cruciate ligaments
  - Superior to femoral condyles
  - Inferior to tibial plateau
- Radiation synovectomy is occasionally used following recurrence or as adjuvant in initial extensive disease
- Refractory cases with severe osteoarthritis require arthroplasty or arthrodesis

DIAGNOSTIC CHECKLIST

Consider

- If suspicious of PVNS, use gradient-echo sequence to elicit blooming

Image Interpretation Pearls

- Blooming on GRE is not pathognomonic for PVNS; hemophilia is other major consideration
  - Conversely, lack of blooming on GRE does not rule out PVNS since there may be little hemosiderin present
- Search carefully for all regions of involvement, including all recesses, to achieve complete resection

SELECTED REFERENCES

1. Mollon B et al: Combined arthroscopic and open synovectomy for diffuse pigmented villonodular synovitis of the knee. Knee Surg Sports Traumatol Arthrosc. 24(1):260-6, 2014
2. Manaster BJ et al: Musculoskeletal Imaging: The Requisites. 2nd ed. Philadelphia: Mosby, Elsevier, 2002

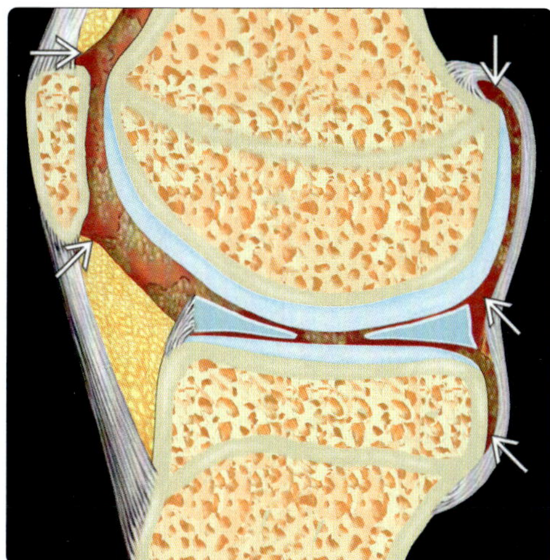

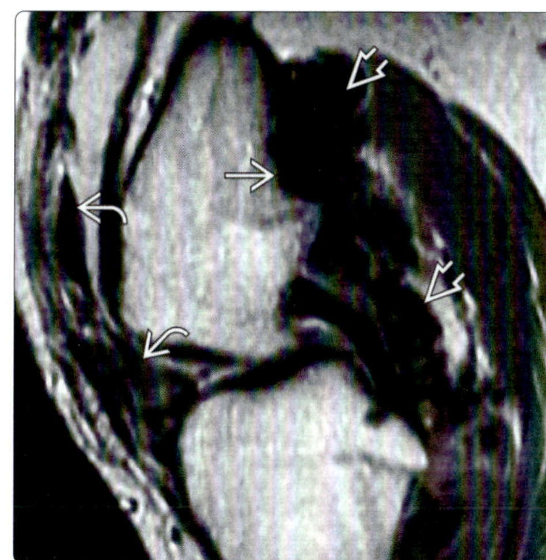

(Left) *Sagittal graphic shows the diffuse form of PVNS, with innumerable small nodules lining the synovium and filling all possible recesses of the joint* ➡. **(Right)** *Sagittal PD MR shows an extensive case of PVNS. Note the nodularity lining the synovium within the anterior part of the joint, as well as the Hoffa fat pad* ➡. *There are even more extensive low signal nodular deposits outlining the posterior cruciate ligament and posterior capsule* ➡. *An erosion of the posterior femur is seen* ➡.

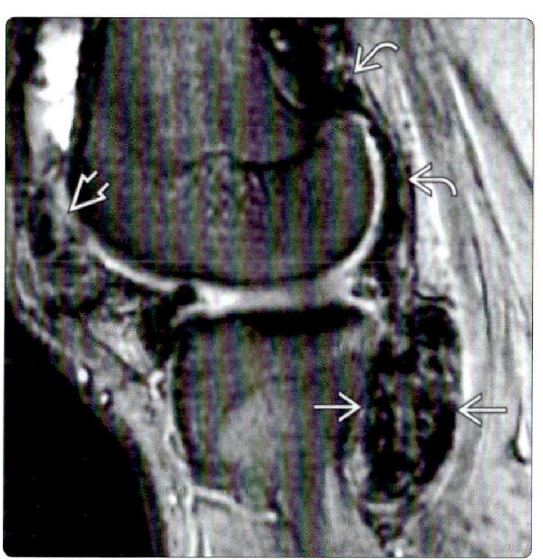

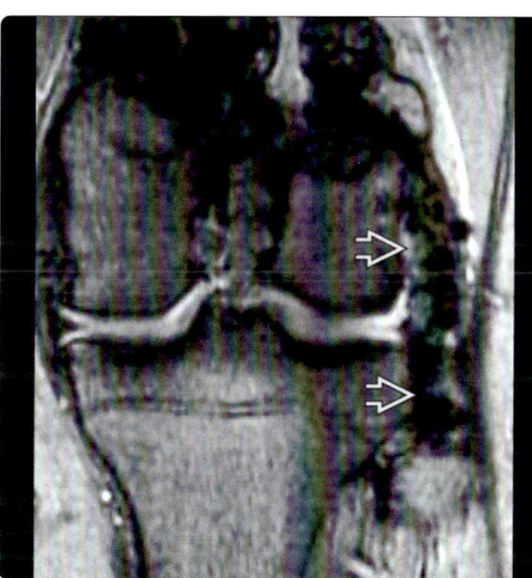

(Left) *Sagittal T2* GRE MR in the same patient shows the expected blooming of the nodular densities due to their retained hemosiderin. The same blooming is seen along the anterior synovium* ➡ *and along the posterior capsule* ➡. *Deposits of PVNS have extended through the popliteal hiatus to surround the popliteus muscle, extraarticularly* ➡. **(Right)** *Coronal T2* GRE MR in the same patient shows that the nodular deposits line the fibular collateral ligament* ➡. *PVNS in this case is both intra- and extraarticular.*

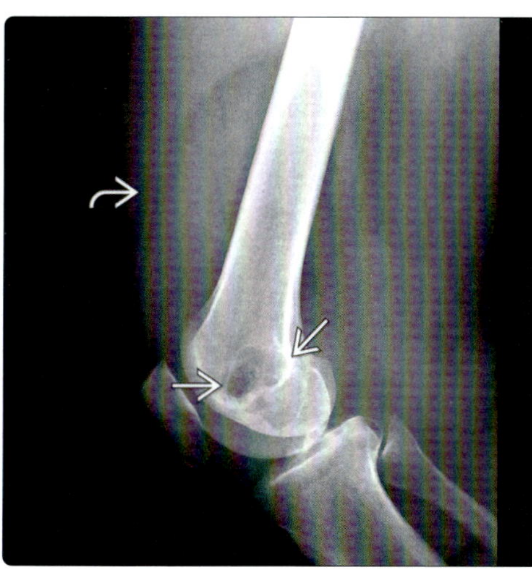

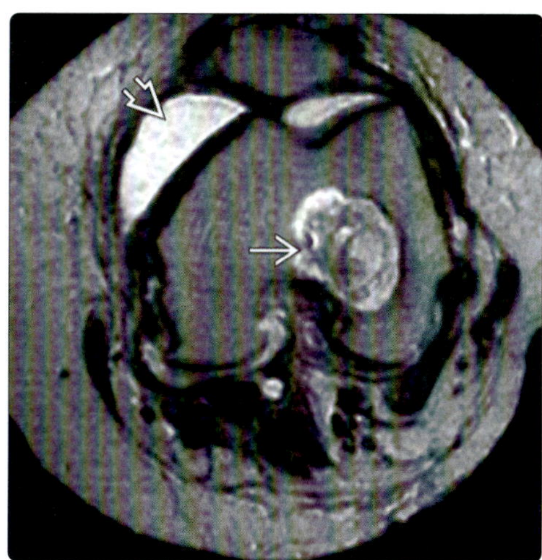

(Left) *Lateral radiograph shows an enormous effusion* ➡ *in a patient with PVNS. A large lytic lesion is seen within the femoral metaphysis* ➡. **(Right)** *Axial T2WI FS MR in the same patient shows the contents of the lesion with a largely heterogeneous low signal* ➡; *note also that there are innumerable tiny nodular low signal densities within the effusion* ➡, *typical of PVNS. A single huge erosion is a bit uncommon, but remember that erosions are not uncommonly seen in PVNS.*

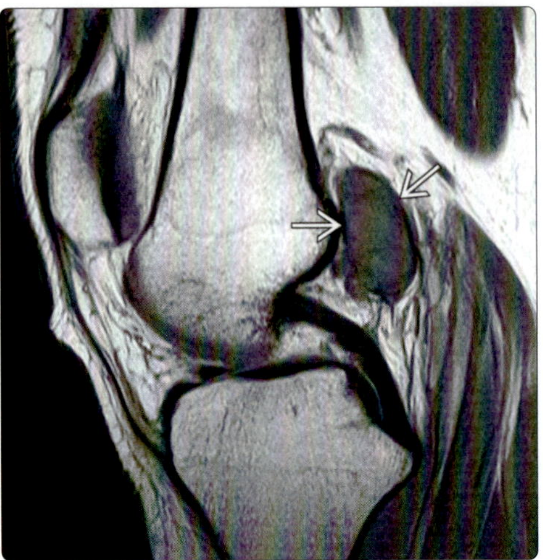

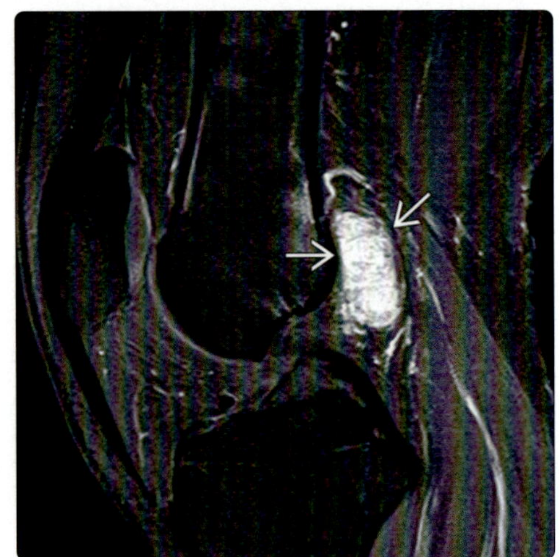

(Left) *Sagittal PD MR in a young woman complaining of fullness posterior to her knee shows a single fairly homogeneous intraarticular mass → with signal similar to muscle. The mass remained somewhat heterogeneously low signal on T2WI FS imaging (not shown).* **(Right)** *Sagittal post-contrast T1WI C+ FS MR in the same patient shows intense enhancement →. Although there is a differential diagnosis, the location and signal characteristics are typical of PVNS in this young adult patient.*

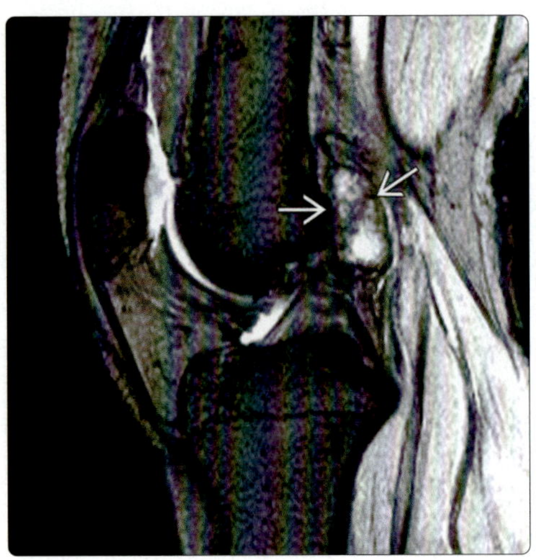

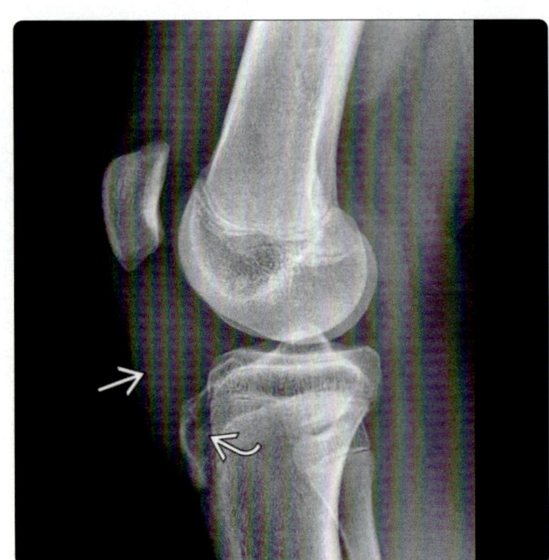

(Left) *Sagittal GRE MR in the same patient shows no blooming within the inhomogeneous mass →. Lack of blooming does not rule out the diagnosis of PVNS; at pathology, PVNS was proven and there was very little hemosiderin present.* **(Right)** *Lateral radiograph shows a mass → occupying the Hoffa fat pad region, displacing the inferior patellar tendon and replacing normal fat. The mass has eroded the adjacent tibial apophysis, resulting in an apparent lytic lesion ↪. The most likely diagnosis in this teenager is PVNS.*

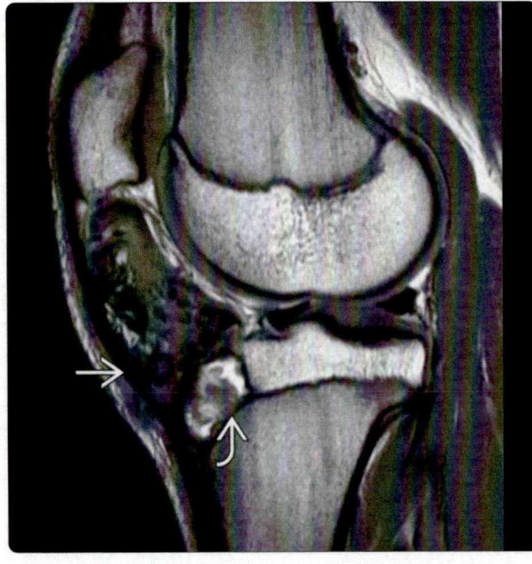

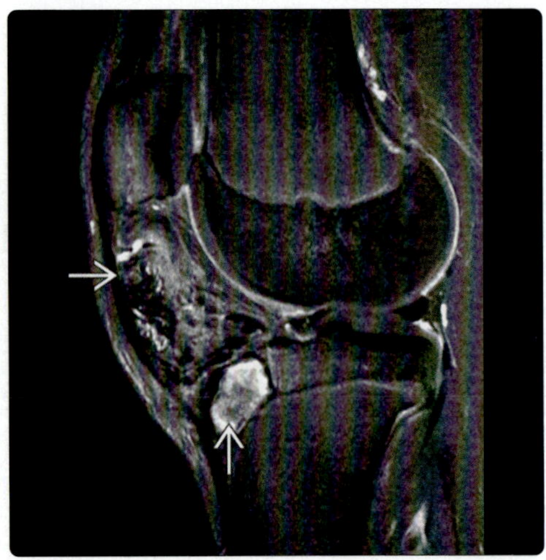

(Left) *Sagittal T1WI MR in the same patient shows that the mass completely replaces the fat pad. The mass is inhomogeneously low signal, both within the Hoffa fat pad region → and the bony erosion ↪. There is some residual fat in both regions. Much of the lesion remained low signal on T2 (not shown).* **(Right)** *Sagittal T1WI C+ FS MR shows mild enhancement of the mass and material within the tibial erosion →. The patient's age and signal characteristics make PVNS the most likely diagnosis, proven at surgery.*

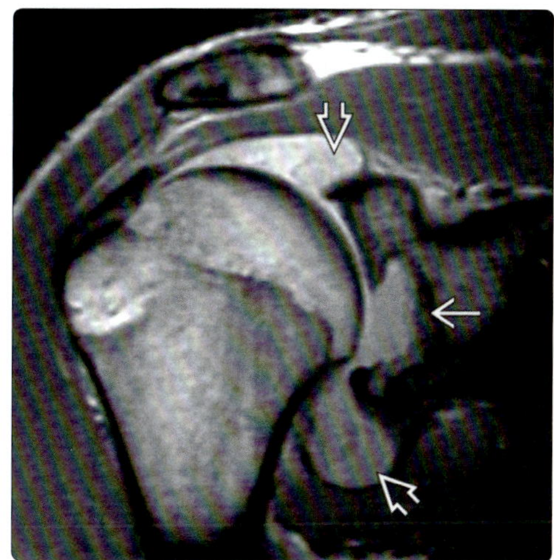

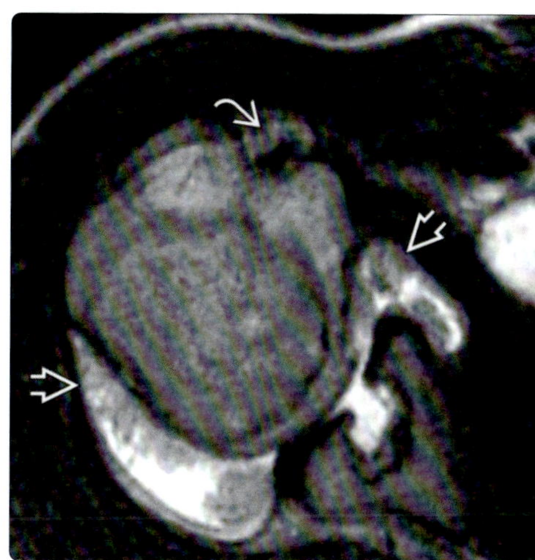

(Left) *Coronal PD MR shows a classic case of PVNS with large glenoid erosion ➡, as well as low signal nodularity lining the synovium surrounding a huge effusion ➡.* **(Right)** *Axial T2WI MR shows more prominently the nodular low signal material lining the synovium ➡ as well as extending down the bicipital tendon sheath ➡. This monoarticular process was proven to be PVNS. (Previously published in Musculoskeletal Imaging: The Requisites. 2nd ed. Philadelphia, PA: Mosby, Elsevier; 2002.)*

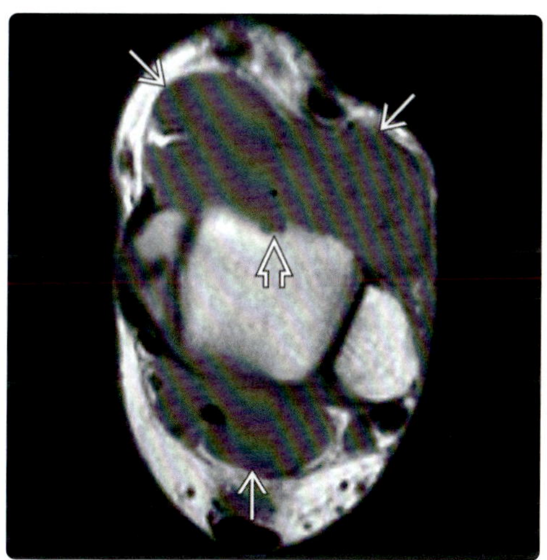

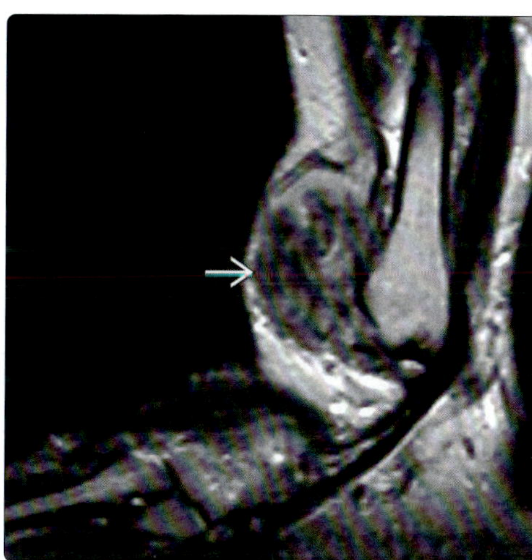

(Left) *Axial T1WI MR in a patient who presented with a large soft tissue mass at the tibiotalar joint shows an intraarticular process, with low signal intensity in the soft tissue mass ➡ and an erosion in the anterosuperior aspect of the talus ➡.* **(Right)** *Sagittal T2WI MR in the same patient shows inhomogeneous but mostly low signal intensity within the mass ➡. Overall, the findings in this monoarticular process are diagnostic of PVNS, which was proven at biopsy.*

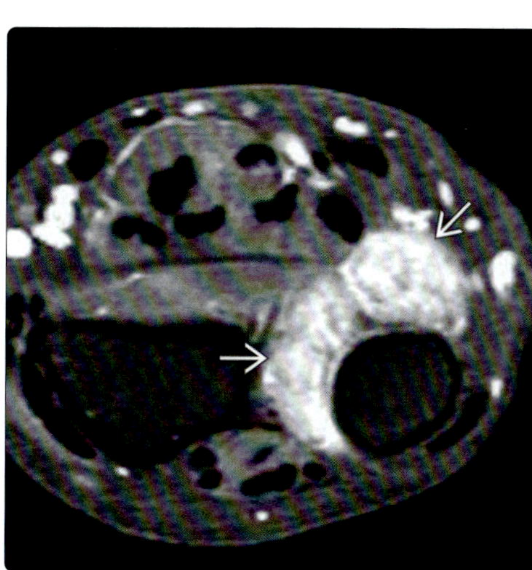

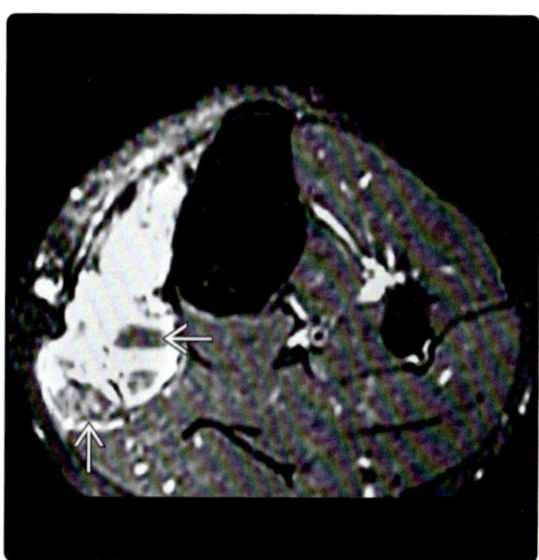

(Left) *Axial T1WI C+ FS MR of a wrist mass involving the distal radioulnar joint shows distension and enhancement with low signal nodularity ➡. The wrist is an uncommon location for PVNS; gout might also be considered, but PVNS was proven.* **(Right)** *Axial T1WI C+ FS MR shows a highly unusual case of PVNS in the pes anserinus. Normally, a pes anserinus bursitis would simply show fluid surrounding the tendons of the pes. In this case, biopsy showed the low signal nodularity ➡ within the bursa to be PVNS.*

KEY FACTS

TERMINOLOGY

- Soft tissue mass containing cartilage, generally arising in infrapatellar fat pad of knee

IMAGING

- Location
  - Intraarticular
  - Knee > > any other joints
  - Hoffa fat pad > > any other location within knee joint
- Lateral radiograph of knee
  - Soft tissue mass obliterates fat density of Hoffa fat pad
  - Chondroid matrix (rings, arcs, or punctate calcifications) often present
  - May have adjacent mechanical erosion of bone
- T1WI MR
  - Rounded mass, not infiltrative, in Hoffa fat pad
  - Inhomogeneously low signal, slightly hyperintense to muscle
  - Contains low signal matrix
- Fluid-sensitive MR sequences
  - Inhomogeneous high signal, containing low signal matrix
  - If matrix is sparse, may see high signal lobules typical of benign cartilage tumor
  - ± adjacent high signal osseous erosion
  - Generally no effusion
- Postcontrast MR
  - Lesion enhances, variably bright

TOP DIFFERENTIAL DIAGNOSES

- Nodular synovitis
  - Rounded mass containing ↓ SI on most sequences; may (rarely) contain calcification
- Pigmented villonodular synovitis
  - Areas of ↓ SI all sequences 2° to hemosiderin deposit; blooms on GRE; does not calcify
- Intraarticular chondrosarcoma
  - Extremely rare; most often arises from degeneration of synovial chondromatosis

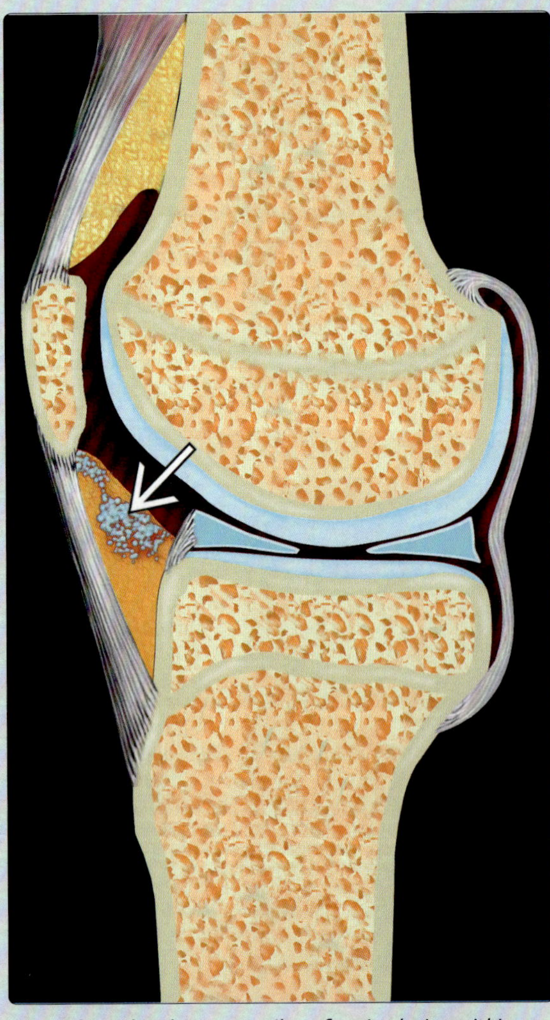

Sagittal graphic shows a cartilage-forming lesion within Hoffa fat pad ➡. The lesion often forms a typical chondroid matrix, making it recognizable on radiograph. The knee is the most common site of intraarticular chondroma.

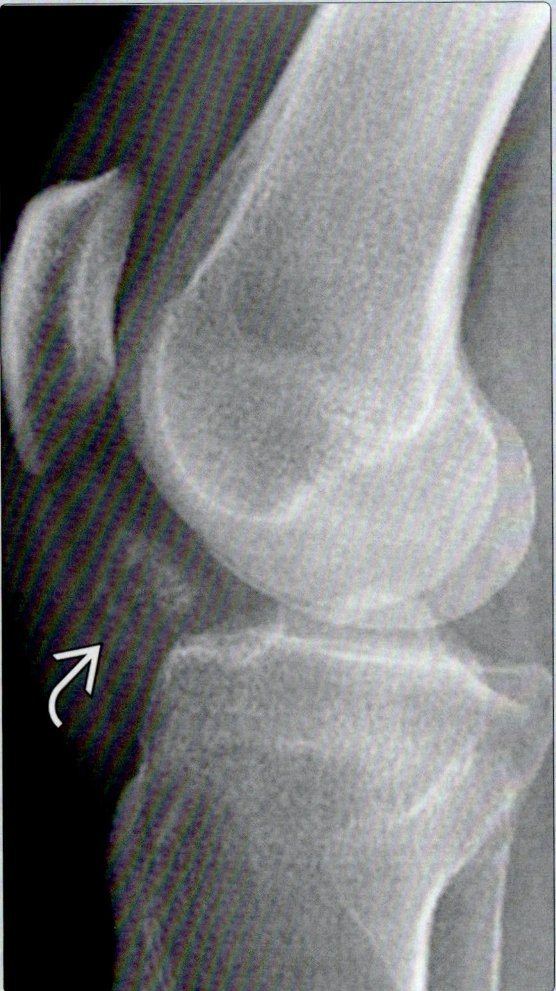

Lateral radiograph shows a large intraarticular lesion located within Hoffa fat pad ➡. The lesion produces a chondroid matrix, seen as punctate and curvilinear densities. This is a typical appearance of intraarticular chondroma.

TERMINOLOGY

Synonyms

- Giant ossifying chondroma
- Giant intraarticular synovial osteochondroma
- Intracapsular chondroma
- Chondroma of infrapatellar fat pad
- Osteochondroma of infrapatellar fat pad

Definitions

- Soft tissue mass containing cartilage, generally arising in infrapatellar fat pad of knee

IMAGING

General Features

- Best diagnostic clue
  - Chondroid matrix within soft tissue mass occupying Hoffa fat pad
- Location
  - Intraarticular
  - Knee > > any other joints
  - Hoffa fat pad > > any other location within knee joint
- Size
  - Greatest diameter generally < 5 cm
- Morphology
  - Ovoid to round mass

Imaging Recommendations

- Best imaging tool
  - Radiograph: Lateral required to evaluate for calcified chondroid matrix
  - MR: Required to evaluate for full extent of lesion and to define cartilage content

Radiographic Findings

- Lateral radiograph of knee
  - Soft tissue mass obliterates fat density of Hoffa fat pad
  - Chondroid matrix (rings, arcs, or punctate calcifications) often present
  - May have adjacent mechanical erosion of bone

CT Findings

- Same as radiograph

MR Findings

- T1WI
  - Rounded mass, not infiltrative, generally in Hoffa fat pad
  - Inhomogeneously low signal, slightly hyperintense to muscle
  - Contains low signal matrix
  - ± adjacent low signal erosion
- Fluid-sensitive sequences
  - Inhomogeneous higher signal, containing low signal matrix
  - If matrix is sparse, may see high signal lobules typical of benign cartilage tumor
  - ± adjacent high signal osseous erosion
  - Generally no effusion
- T1WI FS + contrast: Lesion enhances, variably bright

DIFFERENTIAL DIAGNOSIS

Nodular Synovitis, Intraarticular

- Rounded mass containing low signal on most sequences is typical and similar to intraarticular chondroma
- May (rarely) contain calcification
- Knee is most common articular location
- Location within knee is usually (though not invariably) Hoffa fat pad

Pigmented Villonodular Synovitis

- May appear as nodular mass
- Contains areas of low signal on all sequences due to hemosiderin deposit; these bloom on gradient-echo
- Does not calcify
- Large effusion
- Knee is most common articular location
- Location within knee is variable; may be within Hoffa fat pad

Synovial Chondrosarcoma

- Most often arises from degeneration of synovial chondromatosis
- Contains chondroid matrix
- Knee is most common articular location
- Location within knee is variable; Hoffa fat pad location is possible but not invariable

PATHOLOGY

General Features

- Etiology
  - Unknown; hypothesized to be end-stage Hoffa disease, related to chronic inflammation, fibrosis, and impingement

Gross Pathologic & Surgical Features

- Hyaline cartilage nodules
- ± enchondral calcification

CLINICAL ISSUES

Presentation

- Most common signs/symptoms
  - Anterior knee pain and swelling
  - Locking, clicking

Demographics

- Epidemiology
  - Rare lesion

Treatment

- Surgical resection

SELECTED REFERENCES

1. Malinowski K et al: Selected cases of arthroscopic treatment of popliteal cyst with associated intra-articular knee disorders primary report. Ortop Traumatol Rehabil. 13(6):573-82, 2011
2. Ozkur A et al: Hoffa's recess in the infrapatellar fat pad of the knee on MR imaging. Surg Radiol Anat. 27(1):61-3, 2005
3. Helpert C et al: Differential diagnosis of tumours and tumour-like lesions of the infrapatellar (Hoffa's) fat pad: pictorial review with an emphasis on MR imaging. Eur Radiol. 14(12):2337-46, 2004
4. Jacobson JA et al: MR imaging of the infrapatellar fat pad of Hoffa. Radiographics. 17(3):675-91, 1997

(Left) *Anteroposterior radiograph shows a small erosion involving the anterior tibial plateau ➭. This is a nonspecific erosion and may be either based on an inflammatory arthritis or a mechanical process. No other abnormality is seen.* **(Right)** *Sagittal PDWI FS MR in the same patient shows a relatively large mass located in the Hoffa fat pad. The mass has heterogeneous signal in this proton density sequence, with portions slightly hyperintense to muscle. It contains multiple punctate and rounded regions of lower signal ➭ scattered throughout. These correspond to the chondroid matrix seen on the initial lateral radiograph. The appearance is typical of intraarticular chondroma. If no calcified matrix had been present, diagnosis of pigmented villonodular synovitis might be considered.*

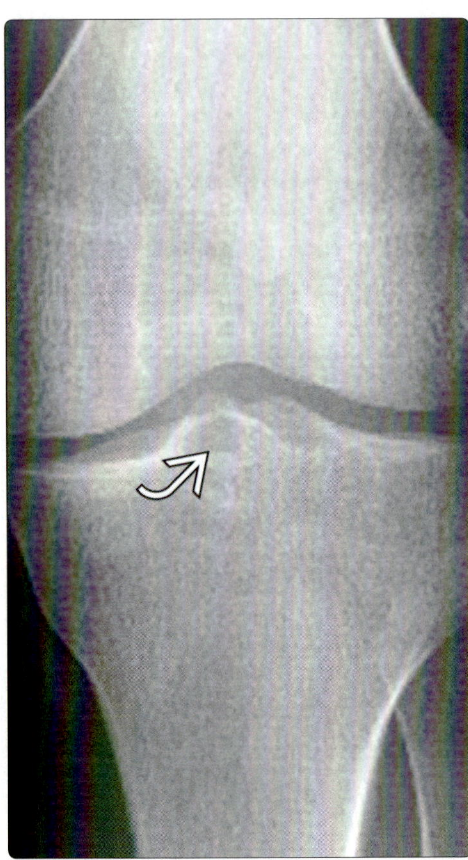

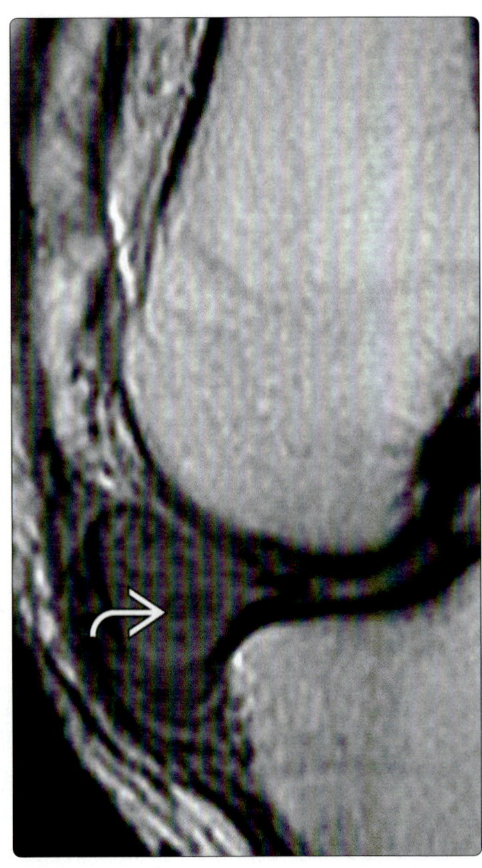

(Left) *Sagittal T2 MR in the same patient shows the mechanical erosion of the anterior tibial plateau ➭. There is no effusion, signaling that the process is not an inflammatory arthritis. Similarly, PVNS usually has a large accompanying effusion, so it is an unlikely diagnosis. The lesion contains a few regions of high SI with T2 weighting but mostly consists of rounded, low signal material ➭. While the low SI is suspicious for matrix, radiograph is necessary to confirm the chondroid nature of the lesion.* **(Right)** *Axial T2 MR, same patient, shows the large extent of the lesion ➭, contained entirely within Hoffa fat pad. In addition to the low signal chondroid matrix, there are a few regions of lobulated high signal ➭; this appearance is typical of a benign cartilage lesion. The entire picture is that of intraarticular chondroma.*

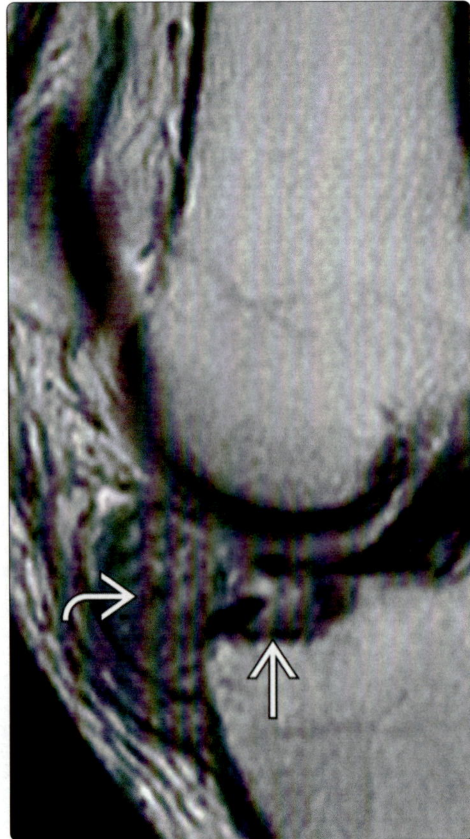

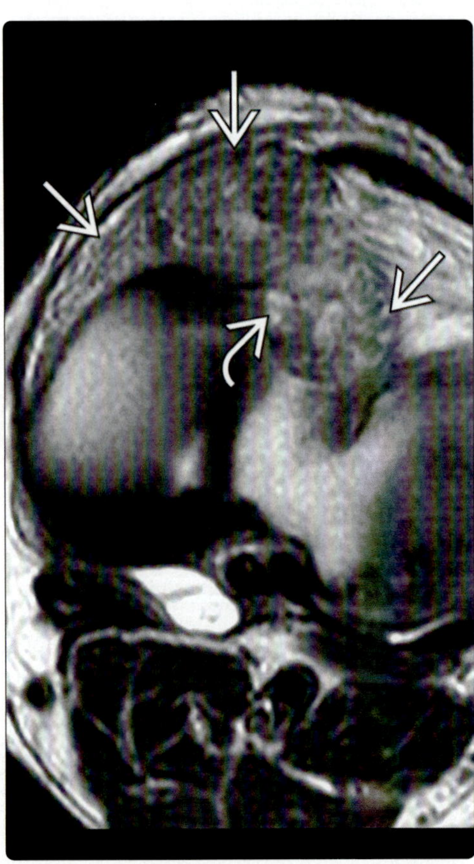

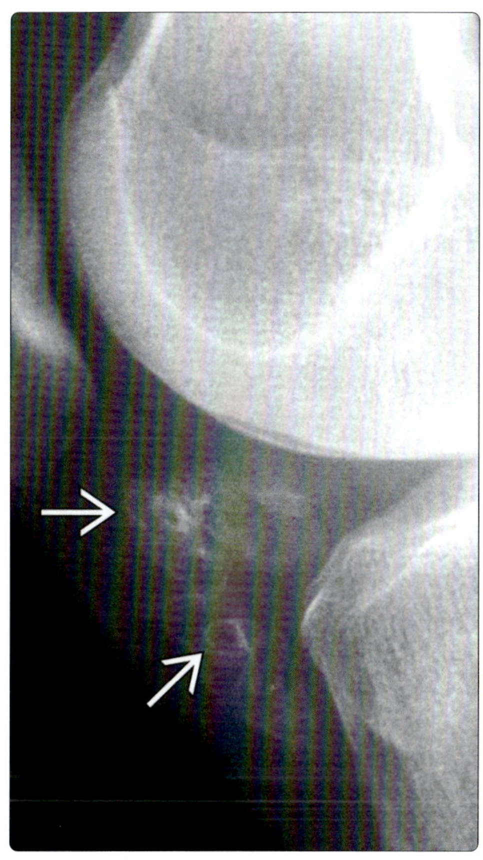

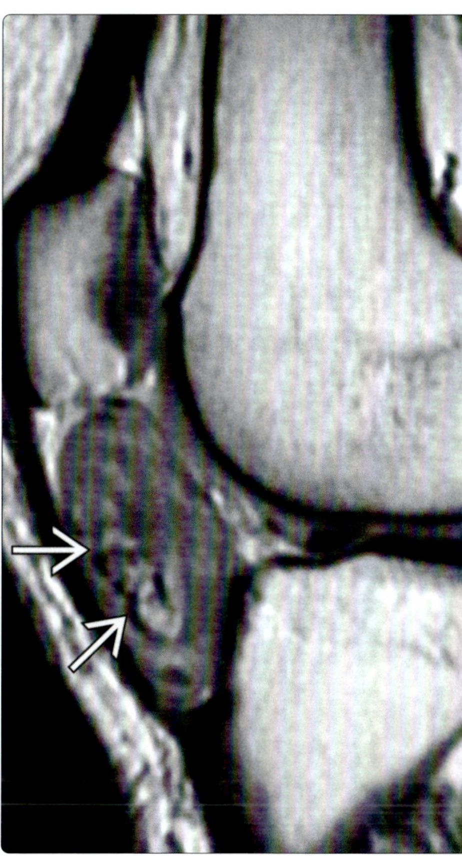

(Left) *Lateral radiograph shows a large mass involving the entire extent of Hoffa fat pad. The lesion contains faint calcification* ➔ *that is curvilinear, suggestive of a cartilage lesion. The most frequent cartilage lesion occurring in this location is intraarticular chondroma, the most likely diagnosis in this case.* **(Right)** *Sagittal PDFS MR in the same patient shows the lesion to occupy the entire extent of Hoffa fat pad. Curvilinear low signal sites are present throughout the lesion* ➔. *The lesion is heterogeneous, with the majority of signal being slightly hyperintense to muscle. Scattered regions of higher signal are contained within the lesion. Without the radiographic confirmation of cartilage matrix, this appearance might be suggestive of pigmented villonodular synovitis; however, PVNS does not develop calcification.*

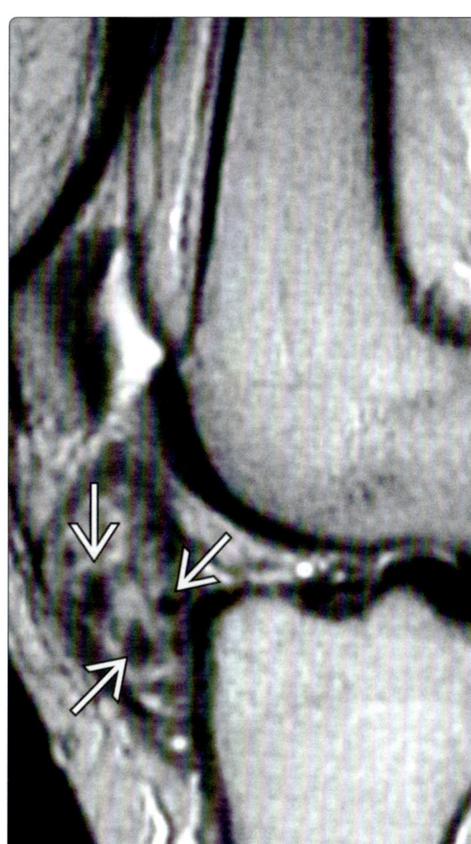

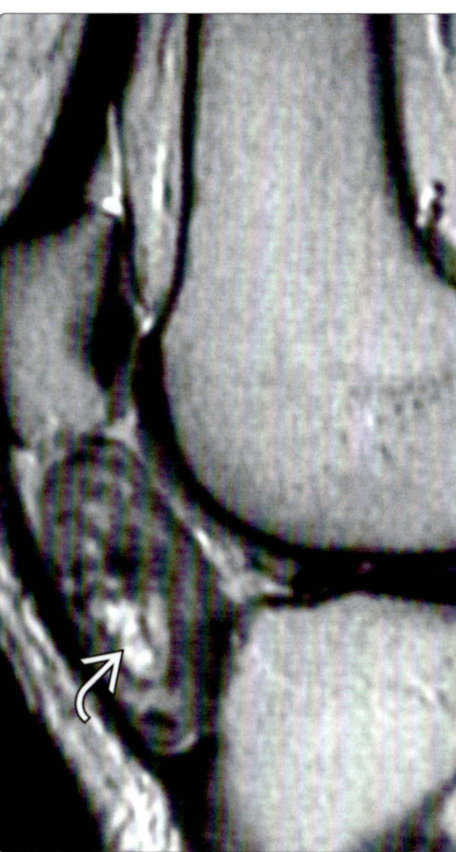

(Left) *Sagittal T2WI MR in the same patient shows the scattered rounded low signal sites of calcification* ➔, *matching those seen on the radiograph. The tissue surrounding the calcification is heterogeneous.* **(Right)** *Sagittal T2WI MR in the same patient and adjacent cut shows scattered low signal calcification. This section also shows a few areas of lobulated high signal* ➔, *which is typically seen in benign cartilage lesions. However, this is only a small region and is not specific. There is no effusion. Both the lack of effusion and the presence of matrix makes the diagnosis of pigmented villonodular synovitis unlikely. Nodular synovitis may rarely contain calcification, but this rarity, as well as the lack of effusion, makes nodular synovitis far less likely than intraarticular chondroma.*

Nodular Synovitis (Intraarticular)

KEY FACTS

TERMINOLOGY

- Localized synovial proliferation

IMAGING

- Location: Within knee, infrapatellar (Hoffa) fat pad > > suprapatellar recess > posterior intercondylar notch
- Lateral radiograph: Soft tissue nodule may be outlined by fat if lesion is within fat pad
- T1WI MR
  - Intermediate to slightly higher signal intensity relative to skeletal muscle
  - May be mildly inhomogeneous
- Fluid-sensitive sequences
  - Inhomogeneous, relatively high signal intensity
  - Variable circular regions of low signal intensity (hemosiderin)
- Small effusion may be present
- Moderate to prominent enhancement; inhomogeneous

TOP DIFFERENTIAL DIAGNOSES

- Pigmented villonodular synovitis (PVNS)
- Intraarticular chondroma
- Hoffa disease
- Gout

CLINICAL ISSUES

- Adults; wide age range
- Presents with pain, swelling
  - Rarely acute pain, related to torsion
- Slow growth, not infiltrative
- Surgical excision
  - Synovectomy not required
  - Recurrence with this treatment is rare

DIAGNOSTIC CHECKLIST

- Remember to consider this diagnosis since behavior and treatment are different than for PVNS

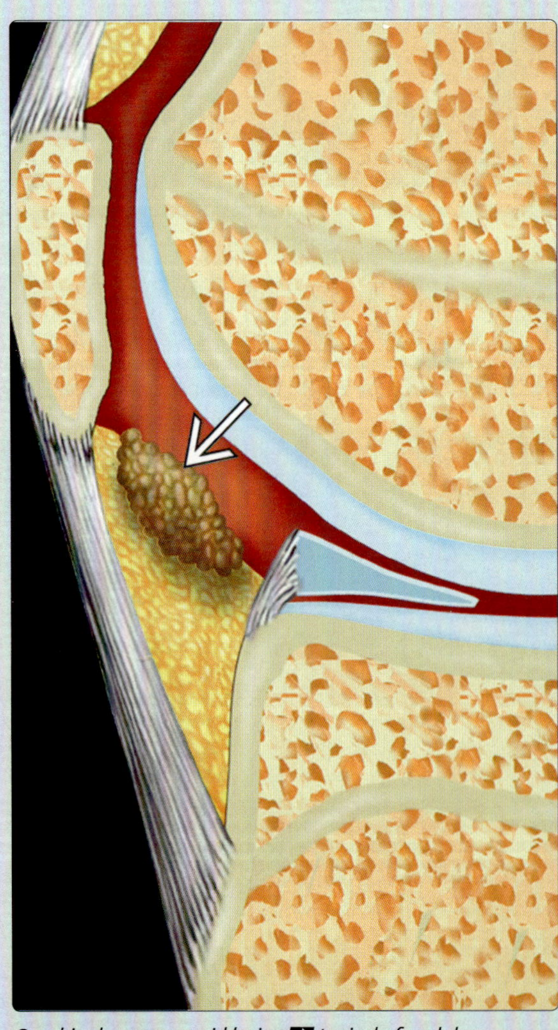

Graphic shows an ovoid lesion ➔ typical of nodular synovitis displacing a portion of Hoffa fat pad. There is no cartilage (as would be seen with intraarticular chondroma) or hemosiderin (as would be seen in the focal nodular form of PVNS) within the lesion.

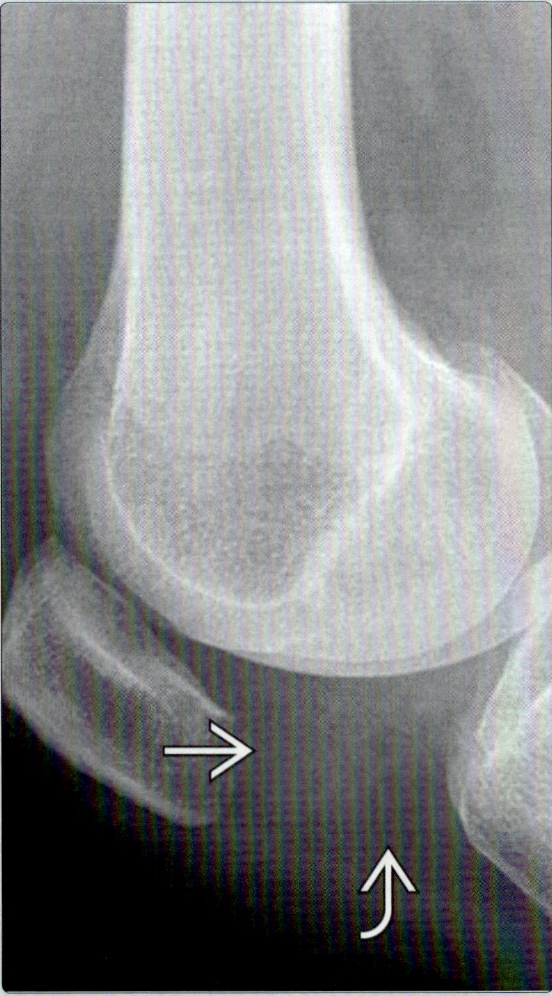

Lateral radiograph shows a rounded soft tissue mass ➔ located within and displacing the fat density of Hoffa fat pad ⮣. There is no calcification, which makes intraarticular chondroma less likely. The most likely diagnoses are nodular synovitis or a focal form of PVNS.

TERMINOLOGY

Synonyms

- Synovial giant cell tumor
- Intraarticular giant cell tumor
- Localized nodular synovitis

Definitions

- Localized synovial proliferation

IMAGING

General Features

- Best diagnostic clue
  - Soft tissue mass, particularly within Hoffa fat pad
- Location
  - When process is intraarticular, knee > ankle
    - Within knee, infrapatellar (Hoffa) fat pad > > suprapatellar recess > posterior intercondylar notch, adjacent to posterior cruciate ligament

Imaging Recommendations

- Best imaging tool
  - MR
- Protocol advice
  - Add gradient echo sequence to demonstrate extent of hemosiderin deposition (generally less than in PVNS)

Radiographic Findings

- Soft tissue nodule may be outlined by fat if lesion is within fat pad
  - If not outlined by fat, mass likely is not visible on radiograph
- Should not contain calcification

CT Findings

- Similar to radiograph: Intraarticular rounded soft tissue mass

MR Findings

- T1WI: Intermediate to slightly higher signal intensity relative to skeletal muscle
  - May be mildly inhomogeneous
- Fluid-sensitive sequences
  - Inhomogeneous, relatively high signal intensity
  - Variable circular regions of low signal intensity (hemosiderin)
  - Linear or cleft-like high signal internal regions reported
  - Small effusion may be present
  - May have associated chondromalacia
- Gradient echo sequence: Small amounts of hemosiderin may bloom
- Postcontrast imaging
  - Moderate to prominent enhancement; inhomogeneous
  - If effusion is present, may show mild synovitis

DIFFERENTIAL DIAGNOSIS

Pigmented Villonodular Synovitis

- May be nodular and occur in Hoffa fat pad as well as elsewhere in joint
- Statistically far more common than nodular synovitis
- MR features may be identical, with mass containing inhomogeneous areas of low signal
- Gradient echo imaging usually shows blooming of low signal areas, due to hemosiderin deposition
  - Amount of hemosiderin deposit generally much greater in pigmented villonodular synovitis (PVNS) than in nodular synovitis
- Large hemorrhagic effusion generally present
- Requires more extensive surgery (synovectomy)
- High incidence of recurrence

Intraarticular Chondroma

- Located in Hoffa fat pad
- Often contains calcified matrix visible on radiograph
- Lobulated ↑ SI cartilage on fluid-sensitive MR

Hoffa Disease

- Inflammation and fibrosis within fat pad
- Ill-defined margin

Gout

- Areas of ↓ SI on fluid-sensitive sequences similar
- Intense enhancement
- Associated erosions if longstanding

PATHOLOGY

Gross Pathologic & Surgical Features

- Yellow to brown well-defined mass
- May have pedicle extending to synovium

Microscopic Features

- Variable amounts of hemosiderin deposits
- Features which differentiate it from PVNS
  - No villous fronds
  - No hemorrhage
  - Fewer deposits of hemosiderin

CLINICAL ISSUES

Presentation

- Most common signs/symptoms
  - Pain, swelling
    - Rarely acute pain, related to torsion
  - Locking, limited range of motion

Natural History & Prognosis

- Slow growth, not infiltrative

Treatment

- Surgical excision; synovectomy not required
  - Recurrence with this treatment is rare

DIAGNOSTIC CHECKLIST

Consider

- Remember to consider this diagnosis since behavior and treatment differ from PVNS

SELECTED REFERENCES

1. Park JH et al: Localized nodular synovitis of the infrapatellar fat pad. Indian J Orthop. 47(3):313-6, 2013
2. Walker EA et al: Magnetic resonance imaging of benign soft tissue neoplasms in adults. Radiol Clin North Am. 49(6):1197-217, vi, 2011

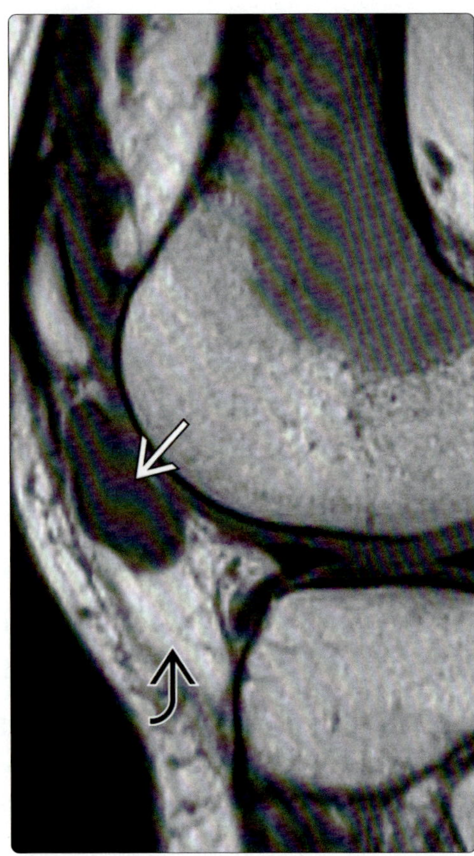

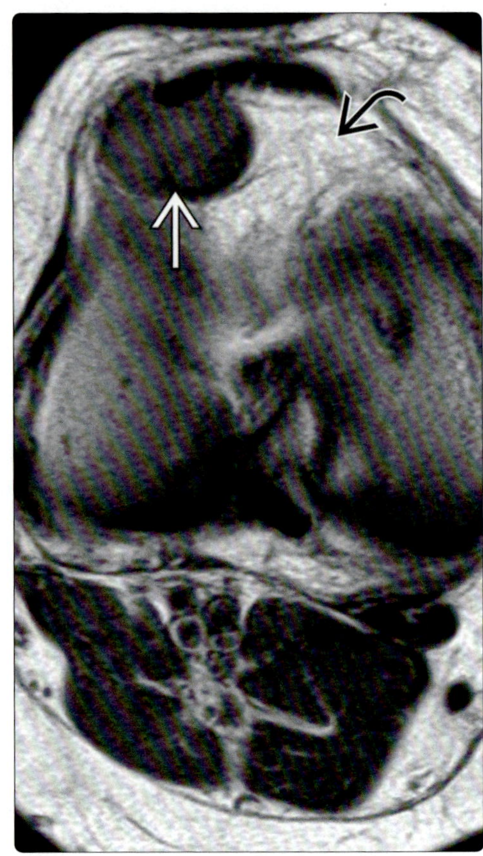

(Left) *Sagittal PDWI MR in the same patient shows a rounded mass ➡ located within (and displacing) the Hoffa fat pad ➩. The mass is not infiltrative and does not affect the adjacent bone or cartilage. It is homogeneous and fairly isointense to muscle. There is no low signal focus within the mass to suggest either calcification or hemosiderin deposition.* **(Right)** *Axial T1WI MR in the same patient shows the lesion ➡ to be slightly inhomogeneous, with lower signal areas in a portion of the periphery. The location within the fat pad ➩ is noted, as is the lack of surrounding tissue disturbance. This sequence does not serve to further narrow the differential of nodular synovitis, intraarticular chondroma, and pigmented villonodular synovitis (PVNS).*

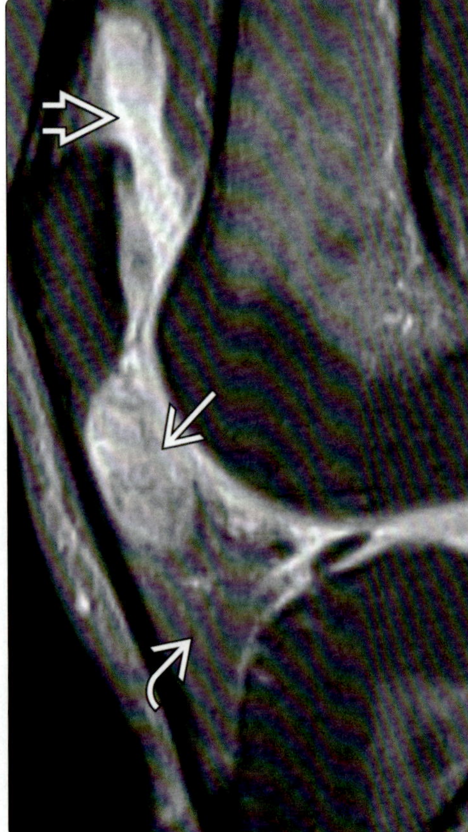

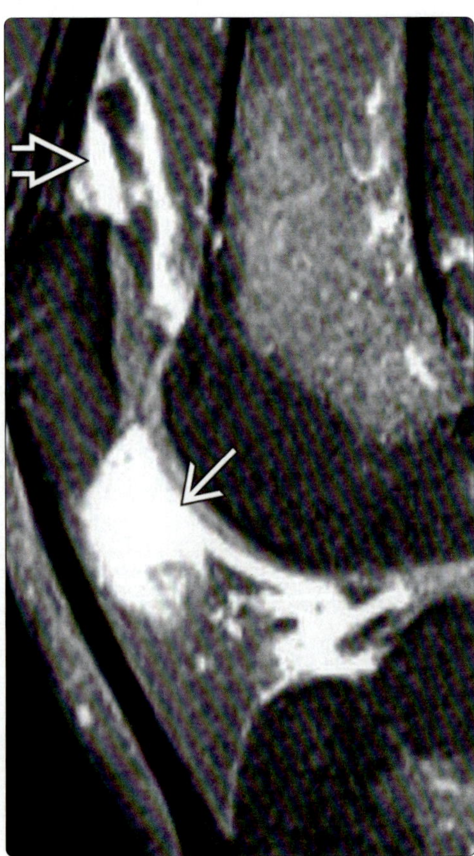

(Left) *On sagittal T2 WI FS MR, the lesion ➡ is mildly inhomogeneous with high SI. There is no low signal to suggest hemosiderin or calcific deposition. Adjacent Hoffa fat pad ➩ is undisturbed, without edema or fibrosis. There is a small effusion ➡ that has a mildly complicated appearance, suggesting synovitis. This is helpful in differentiating the possible diagnoses. While intraarticular chondroma generally does not elicit an effusion, PVNS usually has a much larger effusion than is seen here.* **(Right)** *Sagittal T1 WI C+ FS MR in the same location shows the mass to enhance intensely ➡. The suprapatellar recess shows intense enhancement of the thickened synovium ➡, with relatively little effusion. Although the other lesions under consideration also are expected to enhance, the overall appearance is most typical of nodular synovitis.*

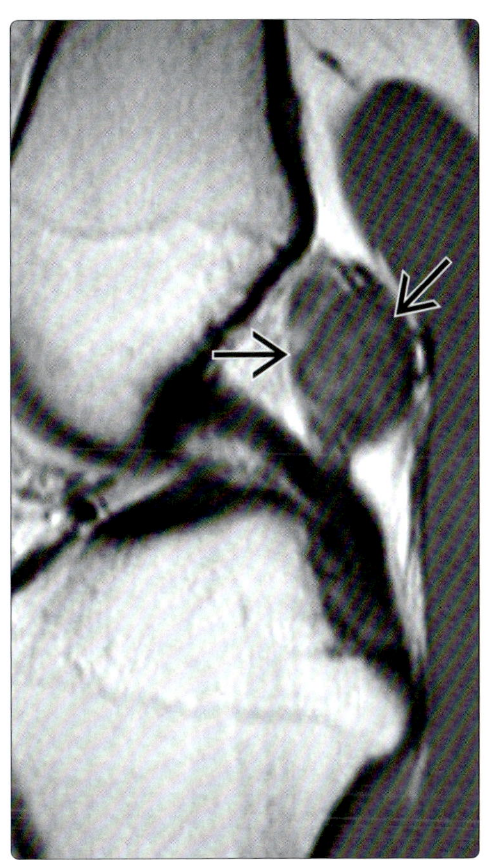

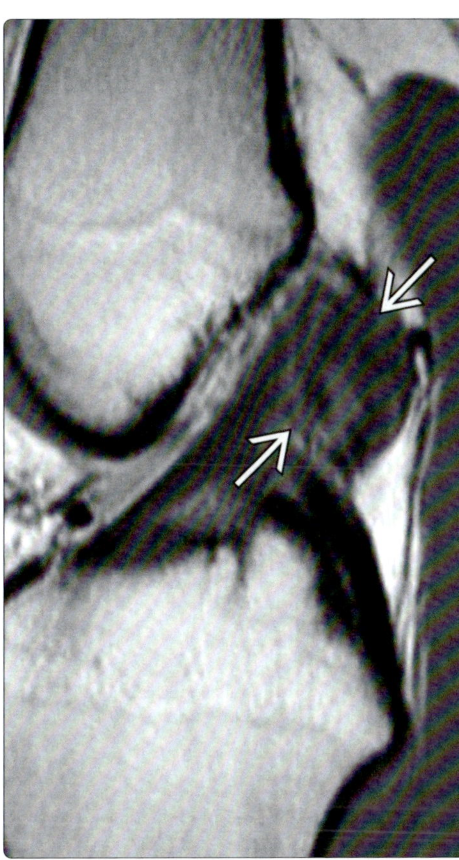

(Left) *Sagittal PDWI MR shows a large, rounded mass located in the posterior knee joint ⇒, adjacent to the posterior cruciate ligament and Wrisberg ligament. The lesion is slightly inhomogeneous but is mostly isointense to skeletal muscle.* **(Right)** *Sagittal PDWI MR, adjacent cut, shows the lesion ⇒ to be in close association with the proximal fibers of the anterior cruciate ligament, and to slightly bow the posterior capsule. There is no focus of low signal to suggest either calcification or hemosiderin deposition. The most likely diagnosis in this teenager is pigmented villonodular synovitis (PVNS), but nodular synovitis in an unusual location should be considered as well. Though this latter process most frequently is located within Hoffa fat pad, it occasionally occurs elsewhere within the knee joint.*

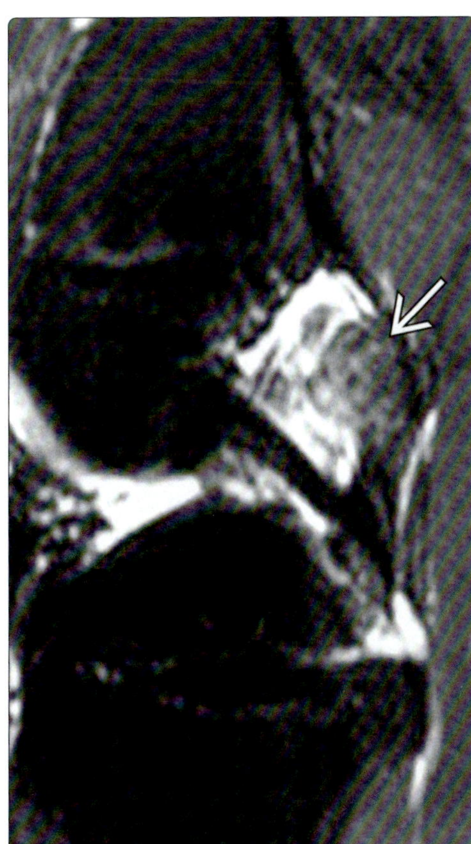

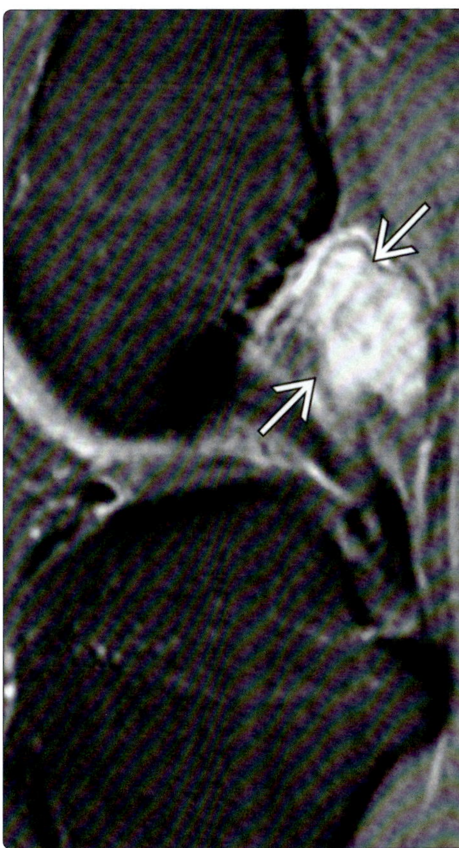

(Left) *Sagittal T2 FS MR in the same patient shows the mass ⇒ is heterogeneous, containing high signal regions but also abundant low signal areas. This may be seen in either nodular synovitis or PVNS. GRE imaging might differentiate the two if the hemosiderin of PVNS were to bloom, but it was not done in this case. Nodular synovitis may contain small amounts of hemosiderin, but generally less than is found in PVNS. Note the lack of effusion; this makes nodular synovitis more likely than PVNS, which usually has a large effusion.* **(Right)** *Sagittal T1 C+ FS MR shows intense enhancement ⇒. This does not serve to differentiate PVNS from nodular synovitis. Biopsy showed the lesion to be nodular synovitis, with no hemosiderin present. Remember that nodular synovitis is not restricted in location to Hoffa fat pad. (Courtesy K. Suh, MD.)*

KEY FACTS

TERMINOLOGY

- a.k.a. lipoid dermatoarthritis
- Infiltration of lipid-laden histiocytes into various tissues: Skin, bone, cartilage, synovium
  - Results in triad of soft tissue nodules, acro-osteolysis, and chronic destructive polyarthritis

IMAGING

- Focal skin nodules without calcification
- Symmetric interphalangeal (IP) joint destruction, with well-defined erosions; MCP less frequent
- Less frequent erosive involvement in wrist, shoulder, hip, knee
- Acro-osteolysis

TOP DIFFERENTIAL DIAGNOSES

- Psoriatic arthritis (PSA)
  - Acro-osteolysis
  - IP erosions are mimic of PSA
  - Nodules are small and distinct, very different from "sausage digit" of PSA
- Rheumatoid arthritis (RA)
  - Nodules similar to rheumatoid nodules
  - Erosions more distinct than those in RA
  - IP joints more commonly involved than MCPs; this is opposite of distribution of RA
  - Acro-osteolysis not seen in RA

CLINICAL ISSUES

- Nodules resemble rheumatoid nodules
  - Most prominent on hands and wrist
  - Also seen on ears, chest, face, mucosal surfaces
  - May present as granuloma annulare
- Progressive disease; etiology unknown (infectious agents such as *Mycobacterium* suspected)
- Seronegative for rheumatoid factor
- Diagnosis made by biopsy
- Treated with corticosteroids and cytotoxic drugs

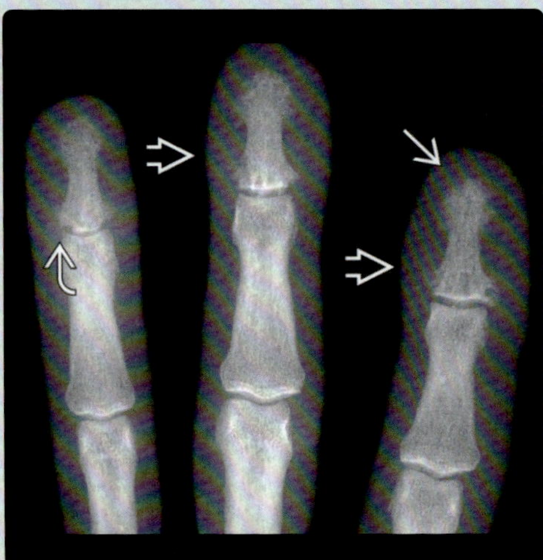

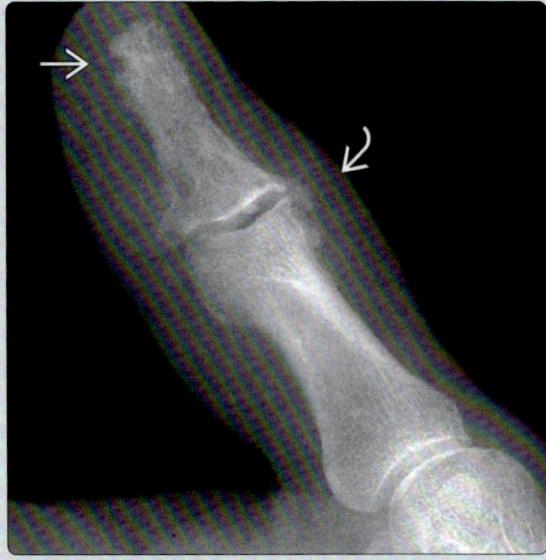

(Left) *PA radiograph demonstrates acro-osteolysis ➔ as well as nodularity of the fingers ➔. There are erosions at the DIP joints ➔. The hands were otherwise completely normal.* **(Right)** *PA radiograph in the same patient shows acro-osteolysis ➔ as well as nodularity of the fingers ➔ and subtle IP erosions. The acro-osteolysis and DIP joint disease is suggestive of psoriatic arthritis, but the nodularity is unusual for that disease. Multicentric reticulohistiocytosis was proven at biopsy.*

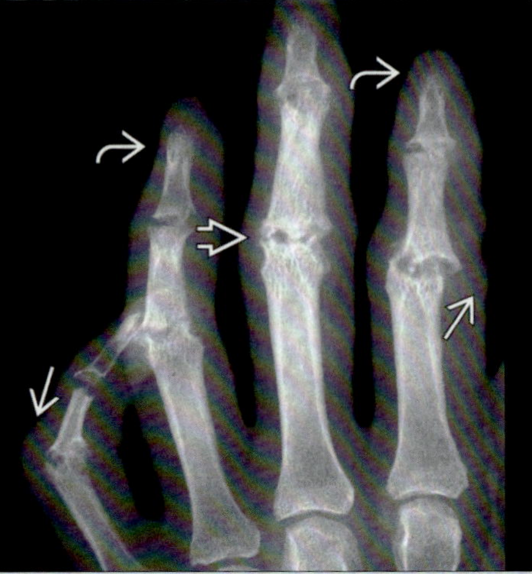

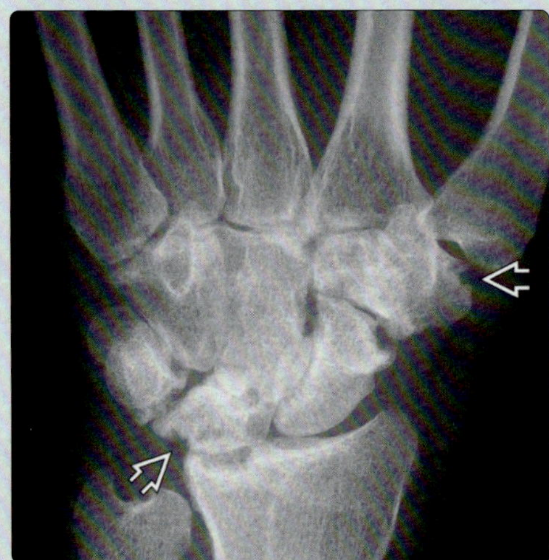

(Left) *PA radiograph in a different patient shows nodularity ➔ as well as acro-osteolysis ➔. Additionally, there are well-defined erosions, particularly involving the IP joints ➔.* **(Right)** *PA radiograph in the same patient shows prominent well-defined erosions within the carpus ➔. The combination of findings is typical of multicentric reticulohistiocytosis (lipodermatoarthritis). The soft tissue nodules help to differentiate this disease from psoriatic arthritis.*

KEY FACTS

TERMINOLOGY

- Vascular malformation arising in intraarticular location
- Synonym: Synovial hemangioma

IMAGING

- Knee > elbow and ankle > other joints
- Effusion, soft tissue mass
- Well-marginated pressure erosions
  - Related to repeated episodes of bleeding
  - Not inflammatory; may mimic hemophilic arthropathy
- Rare appearance of phleboliths
- MR or CT may show crucial information
  - Intraarticular dilated, tortuous vessels
  - Classify as juxtaarticular, intraarticular, or intermediate (features of both)
  - May appear localized or diffuse within joint
  - Isointense to muscle on T1; inhomogeneous hyperintensity on fluid-sensitive sequences
  - Variable enhancement of mass and vessels following contrast administration

TOP DIFFERENTIAL DIAGNOSES

- Hemophilic arthropathy (has prominent low SI)
- Pigmented villonodular synovitis (prominent low SI, blooms on GRE)

CLINICAL ISSUES

- Clinical presentation
  - History of slowly growing mass
  - Recurrent effusions and pain
  - Mechanical symptoms
  - May relate to minimal trauma causing bleeding
  - Palpable, spongy mass may be present
  - May decrease in size with elevation of extremity; increases in size when in dependent position
- Age: Generally young patients (child, teenager)
- Treatment: Surgical excision + synovectomy

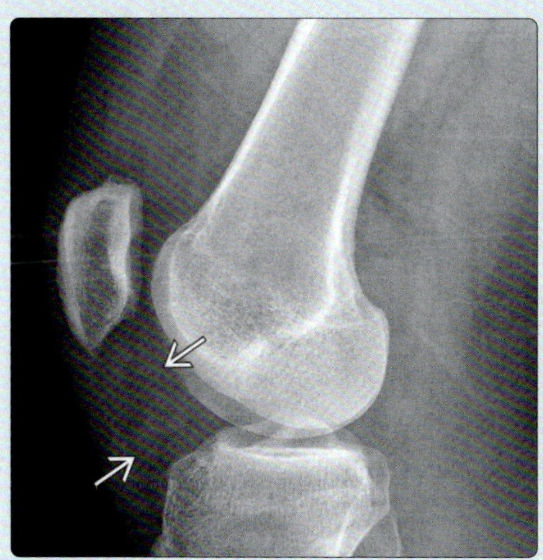

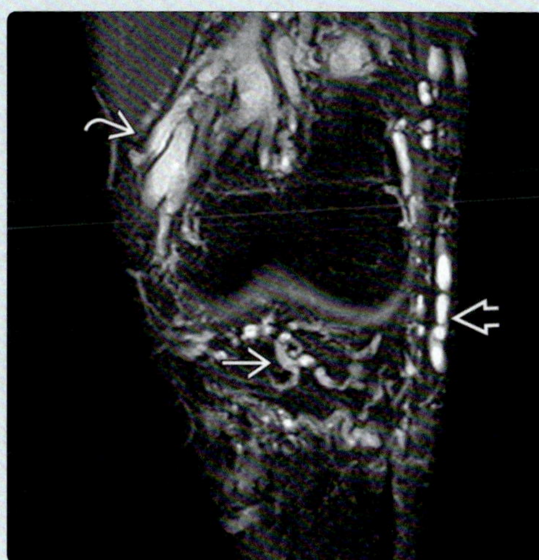

(Left) *Lateral radiograph of the knee in a young adult who reported a spongy painful mass that varied in size shows an effusion. Careful examination also shows rounded and elongated soft tissue masses ➡ coursing through Hoffa fat pad.* **(Right)** *Coronal T2 MR in the same patient, anteriorly in the joint, shows large vessels ➡ contributing flow to smaller vessels, both within Hoffa fat pad ➡ and in an extraarticular position ➡.*

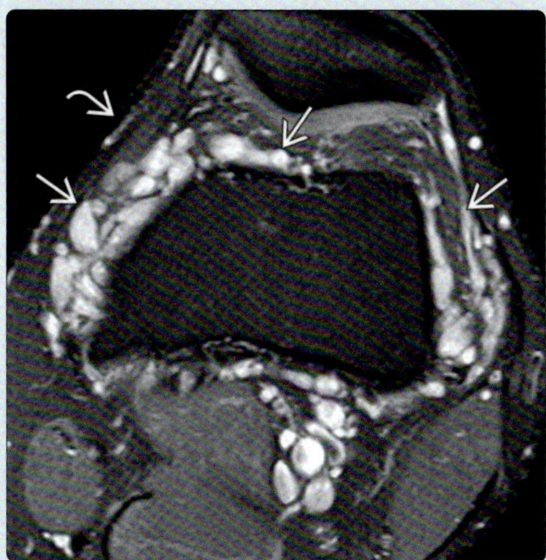

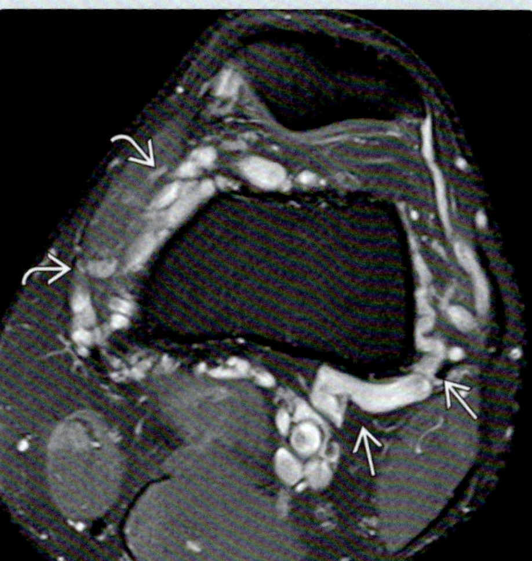

(Left) *Axial T2 FS MR in the same patient shows the tortuous vessels surrounding the femoral metaphysis ➡ with smaller extraarticular vessels ➡ as part of the same process.* **(Right)** *Axial T2 FS MR, located slightly more proximally, shows the large feeding vessels ➡ leading to this vascular malformation. This malformation is predominantly intraarticular with a small extraarticular component (seen here within vastus medialis ➡). This lesion was formerly known as synovial hemangioma.*

KEY FACTS

TERMINOLOGY

- Benign neoplasm with synovial membrane proliferation and formation of cartilaginous or osseous bodies
- May be within joint, bursa, or tenosynovial structures

IMAGING

- Multiple round bodies of similar size and variable calcification
- Range from tiny speckled calcifications to large round, lamellated cartilage or ossified bodies
- Bodies may form in conglomerate mass rather than free-floating
- Degree of calcification highly variable
- Associated erosions not uncommon
- Occasionally, bodies not calcified and only soft tissue mass ± osseous erosion is seen radiographically
- Bodies are of variable MR signal, depending on proportion of calcium, chondroid, and mature ossific tissue
    - Ranges from low signal bodies on all sequences to marrow signal bodies on all sequences
    - Majority (77%) have low to intermediate T1 signal, with hyperintense T2 signal intensity
    - Those with marrow signal may contain hypointense calcifications
- Malignant transformation: Extremely rare and no reliable distinguishing feature

DIAGNOSTIC CHECKLIST

- Consider diagnosis if radiograph shows monoarticular osteopenia and erosions
    - Calcification/ossification of bodies absent in 15%; MR makes diagnosis
- Consider diagnosis in extraarticular locations
    - Bursae or tendon sheaths, especially hands and feet
- With multiple recurrences and aggressive osseous destruction beyond surface erosions, consider degeneration to chondrosarcoma

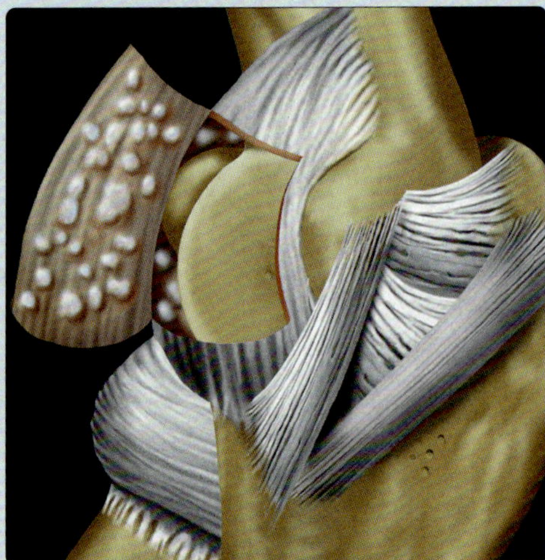

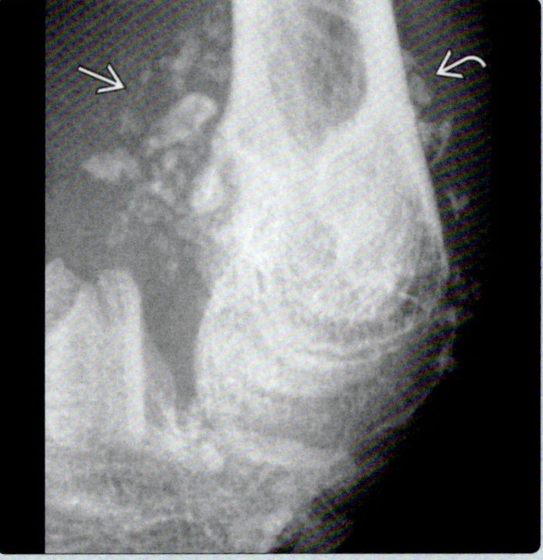

(Left) *Graphic of the lateral elbow with reflected anterior capsule shows multiple rounded bodies, some attached to the synovium and others loose within the joint space. This is a depiction of the gross appearance of synovial chondromatosis.* **(Right)** *Lateral radiograph shows a classic case of synovial chondromatosis. This adolescent patient has innumerable tiny ossified bodies, all of similar size, seen on this view to be distending both the anterior ➡ and posterior ➡ joint space.*

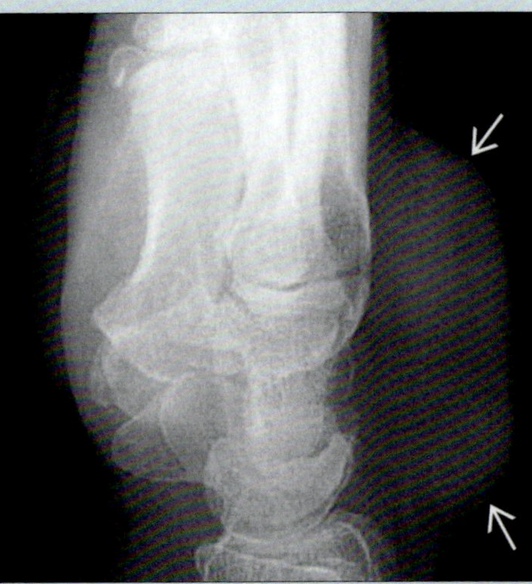

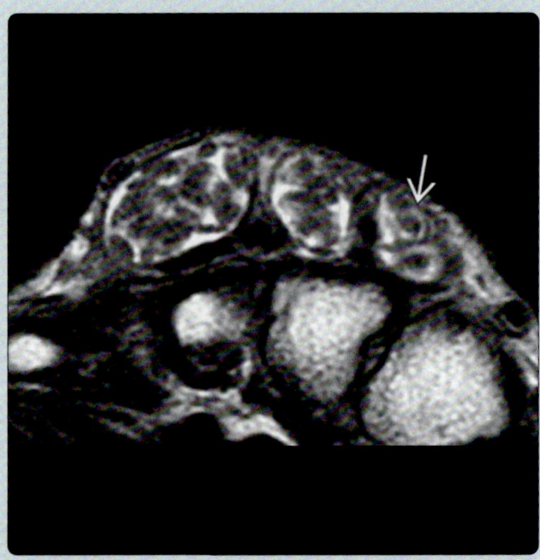

(Left) *Lateral radiograph shows a soft tissue mass ➡ known to be chronic. There is no calcification within the mass or any other characterizing feature.* **(Right)** *Axial T1 MR shows multiple distended dorsal tendon sheaths ➡. Each contains multiple low signal round lesions. This represents tenosynovial chondromatosis. It is worthwhile to remember that synovial chondromatosis may arise within any closed space lined by synovium.*

TERMINOLOGY

Abbreviations

- Primary synovial chondromatosis (PSC)

Synonyms

- Synovial osteochondromatosis (if there has been enchondral ossification of cartilage)

Definitions

- Benign neoplasm with synovial membrane proliferation and formation of cartilaginous or osseous bodies
  - Within joint, bursa, or tenosynovial structures

IMAGING

General Features

- Best diagnostic clue
  - Multiple, round, similar-sized calcified bodies seen on radiograph
    - 85% of cases are calcified sufficiently for detection by radiograph
  - Detection and evaluation by MR for those that are not calcified
- Location
  - Generally monoarticular (not invariably)
  - Intraarticular, particularly in large joints
    - Knee (50-65%) > hip > shoulder > elbow
  - Bursal locations: Subdeltoid, popliteal are most common
  - Tenosynovial chondromatosis: Hands and feet are most common
  - Extracapsular spread through usual sites of joint decompression
    - Across rotator cuff tear into subacromial/subdeltoid bursa
    - From hip into iliopsoas bursa
  - Rare extension into adjacent muscle and fascial tissue
- Size
  - Ranges from mm to > 2-cm bodies
- Morphology
  - Rounded bodies, generally of similar size
  - Bodies may appear lamellated, with concentric rings of calcification
  - Occasionally will form conglomerate mass within joint or extend into extracapsular tissues

Imaging Recommendations

- Best imaging tool
  - Radiograph, MR

Radiographic Findings

- Multiple round bodies of similar size and variable calcification
  - Range from tiny speckled calcifications to large round, lamellated cartilage or ossified bodies
  - Bodies may be formed in conglomerate mass rather than free-floating
  - Degree of calcification highly variable
- Associated osseous erosions not uncommon
  - Caused by saucerization; well marginated
  - May be difficult to visualize on radiograph (20-50%), though occur more frequently
- Occasionally, bodies not calcified and only a mass with occasional erosion is seen radiographically
- Extraarticular form: Generally hands or feet
  - Calcifications in tendon sheaths or bursae
  - May cause saucerization (pressure erosion) of adjacent bone

MR Findings

- 80% have erosions detectable by MR
- Large effusion (hyperintense on fluid-sensitive sequences, low signal on T1)
- Bodies are of variable MR signal, depending on proportion of calcium, chondroid, and mature ossific tissue
  - May follow signal of either mature bone or cartilage throughout all sequences or may be less determinate
    - Ranges from low signal bodies on all sequences to marrow signal bodies on all sequences
      - Majority (77%) have low to intermediate T1 signal, with hyperintense T2 signal intensity
      - Those with marrow signal may contain hypointense calcifications
  - Bodies are round, multifaceted
  - Bodies may be loose and dependent in joint
  - Bodies may be conglomerate, appearing as "mass" within and extending from joint
- Contrast with T1WI FS imaging shows hyperplastic synovium as enhancing, surrounding low signal effusion and bodies (often obscured)
- Malignant transformation: Extremely rare and no reliable distinguishing feature
  - Watch for snowstorm appearance of calcification, which has different appearance from that of chondromatosis
  - Watch for associated soft tissue mass or osseous destruction, especially following multiple resections

DIFFERENTIAL DIAGNOSIS

Synovial Chondrosarcoma

- Significantly more rare than PSC
- PSC that has transformed to chondrosarcoma may not be differentiated by imaging
  - Snowstorm appearance of calcified cartilage, with different overall appearance from other PSC bodies may be suggestive

Intraarticular Chondroma

- Most frequently located in Hoffa fat pad
- Calcification can mimic nodular mass-like presentation of PSC

Pigmented Villonodular Synovitis

- May be confusing if only MR is available or if bodies of PSC are not calcified
- Intraarticular nodularity that causes extrinsic erosions, similar to PSC
- Low signal on both T1 and T2, with blooming on gradient-echo sequences, demonstrates hemosiderin in pigmented villonodular synovitis

Secondary Synovial Osteochondromatosis

- Coexistent osteoarthritis
- Generally, bodies are of different size and shape as well as fewer in number

- Concentric rings of growth seen pathologically and occasionally radiographically

PATHOLOGY

General Features

- Etiology
  - Genetic features suggest benign neoplastic etiology
  - Once formed, nodules grow
    - If remain attached to synovium, develop blood supply and may become osseous
    - If loose within joint, nourished by synovial fluid and become cartilaginous
  - Articular cartilage destruction is likely of mechanical origin; not inflammatory
- Genetics
  - Chromosome 6 abnormalities common in PSC
    - Suggests neoplastic rather than metaplastic origin
  - Bone morphogenic proteins (BMP: Multifunctional growth factors) likely involved in pathobiology of cartilaginous and osteogenic metaplasia
    - High levels of BMP present in bodies and synovium isolated from these patients
  - Dysregulation of hedgehog signaling seems to play important role in PSC
    - Feature of several other benign cartilage tumors

Gross Pathologic & Surgical Features

- Hyperplastic synovium covering bluish-white nodular projections of hyaline cartilage
- Bodies may fuse together, forming conglomerate

Microscopic Features

- Hyaline cartilage, surrounding synovial lining
- Often hypercellular with atypical features
  - Correlation with imaging features required to distinguish PSC from rare differentiation into chondrosarcoma
- Cell cultures from PSC are enriched with osteoprogenitors
  - Differentiate along osteogenic and chondrogenic lineages
  - Distinct from cell cultures established from osteoarthritis or normal synovium

CLINICAL ISSUES

Presentation

- Most common signs/symptoms
  - Mass, generally centered on joint
  - Generally painful, but may be asymptomatic
    - Pain often of several years duration
  - Clicking, locking, restricted range of motion
- Other signs/symptoms
  - Occasionally present with monoarticular osteopenia and restrictive capsulitis

Demographics

- Age
  - 3rd-5th decades most frequent
  - Wide range, with less frequent cases seen in adolescents and elderly
- Gender
  - M > F

Natural History & Prognosis

- Generally slow enlargement
- Progresses to osteoarthritis when intraarticular
- Rare progression to synovial chondrosarcoma (5-6%)
  - In longstanding disease
    - Mean time from diagnosis to malignant transformation 20 years, with wide range
  - Generally following multiple attempts at resection
  - Rapidity of recurrence and extent of destruction may help differentiate from simple recurrence
  - Represents most frequent etiology of synovial chondrosarcoma

Treatment

- Resection of bodies, along with synovectomy, shown in some studies to reduce recurrence rate
  - Controversial; some advocate arthroscopic removal of bodies without synovectomy
- Extensive disease has high recurrence rate, even with synovectomy (range of 3-23%)
- Tenosynovial chondromatosis has particularly high recurrence rate
- After multiple recurrences, radiation therapy has been successfully used

DIAGNOSTIC CHECKLIST

Image Interpretation Pearls

- Consider diagnosis if radiograph shows monoarticular osteopenia and erosions
  - Calcification/ossification of bodies absent in 15%; MR makes diagnosis
- Consider diagnosis in extraarticular locations
  - Bursae or tendon sheaths, especially hands and feet
- With multiple recurrences and aggressive osseous destruction beyond surface erosions, consider degeneration to chondrosarcoma

SELECTED REFERENCES

1. de Sa D et al: Arthroscopic surgery for synovial chondromatosis of the hip: a systematic review of rates and predisposing factors for recurrence. Arthroscopy. ;30(11):1499-1504, 2014
2. Evans S et al: Synovial chondrosarcoma arising in synovial chondromatosis. Sarcoma. 2014:647939, 2014
3. Yao MS et al: Synovial chondrosarcoma arising from synovial chondromatosis of the knee. JBR-BTR. 95(6):360-2, 2012
4. Nakanishi S et al: Bone morphogenetic proteins are involved in the pathobiology of synovial chondromatosis. Biochem Biophys Res Commun. 379(4):914-9, 2009
5. Zamora EE et al: Synovial chondrosarcoma: report of two cases and literature review. Eur J Radiol. 72(1):38-43, 2009
6. Bui-Mansfield LT et al: Magnetic resonance appearance of intra-articular synovial sarcoma: case reports and review of the literature. J Comput Assist Tomogr. 32(4):640-4, 2008
7. Murphey MD et al: Imaging of synovial chondromatosis with radiologic-pathologic correlation. Radiographics. 27(5):1465-88, 2007

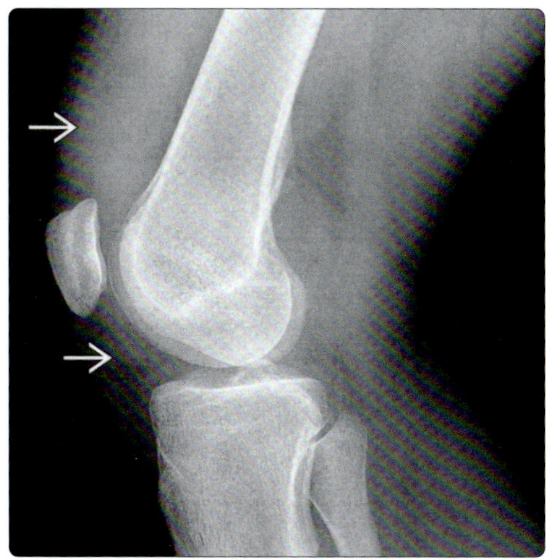

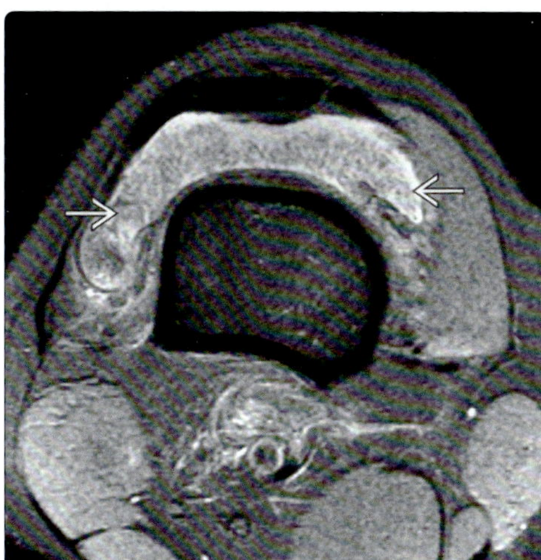

(Left) *Lateral radiograph shows joint effusion ➡ and no calcifications, an entirely nonspecific finding.* **(Right)** *Axial PD FS MR in the same patient shows innumerable filling defects, characteristic of primary synovial chondromatosis ➡. At arthroscopy, a snowstorm of these tiny bodies was seen. It must be remembered that, in a minority of cases, the bodies in synovial chondromatosis are not calcified enough to be visible on radiograph.*

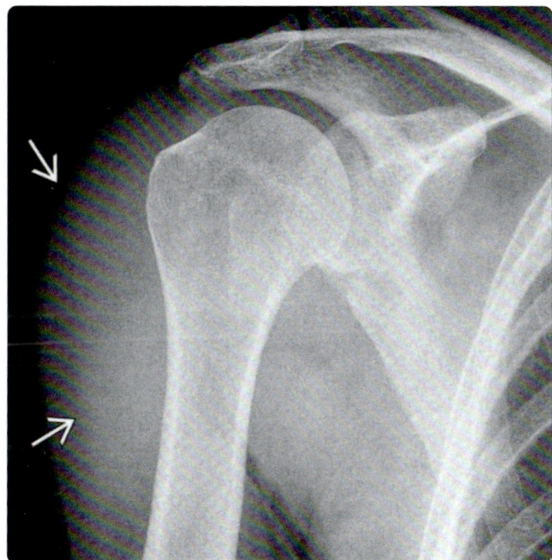

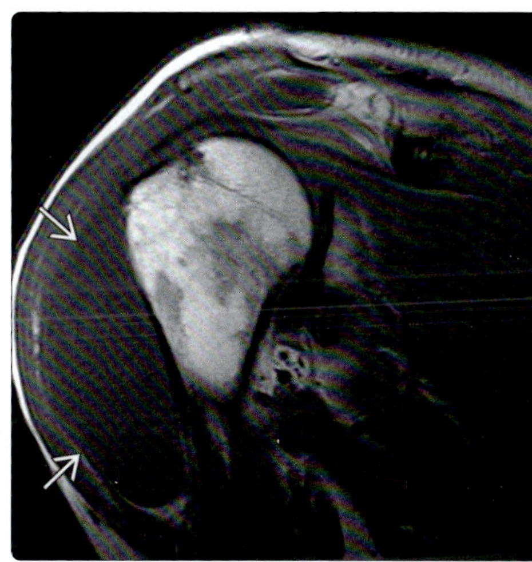

(Left) *AP radiograph demonstrates a soft tissue mass ➡ in the region of the deltoid in this 57-year-old woman. There is no calcification or other finding to further characterize the lesion.* **(Right)** *Coronal T1 MR in the same patient shows homogeneous low signal distending the subdeltoid bursa ➡. There is no evidence on this sequence of anything other than fluid within the bursa.*

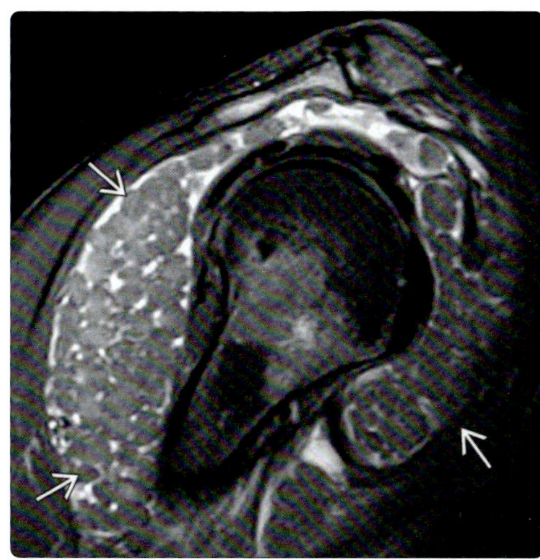

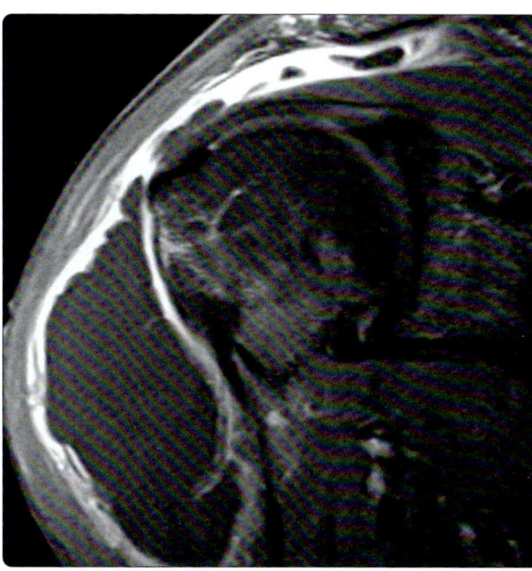

(Left) *Sagittal T2 FS MR shows the subdeltoid bursa to be packed with multiple round bodies ➡, surrounded by synovial fluid. The bodies in synovial chondromatosis may show different signal intensities in different cases, depending on their composition (predominantly cartilage versus bone).* **(Right)** *Coronal T1 C+ FS MR shows enhancing synovium; again, the bodies are not seen.*

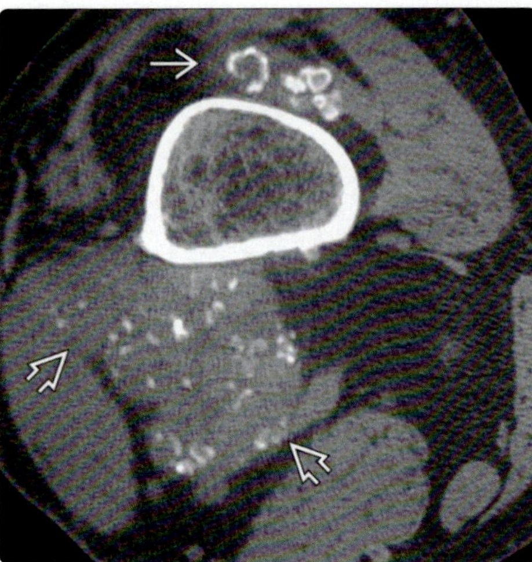

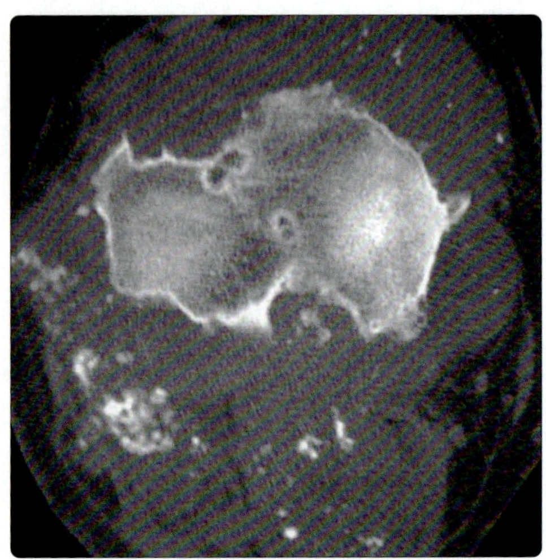

(Left) *Axial bone CT shows multiple round calcifications of similar but not identical sizes located both intraarticularly ➡ and extraarticularly, appearing to form a mass that invades the biceps femoris muscle ➡.* **(Right)** *Axial bone CT in the same patient shows rounder calcified bodies scattered throughout the extraarticular soft tissues of the leg. There is also significant erosive disease involving the tibia. This is an example of extraarticular extension of synovial chondromatosis.*

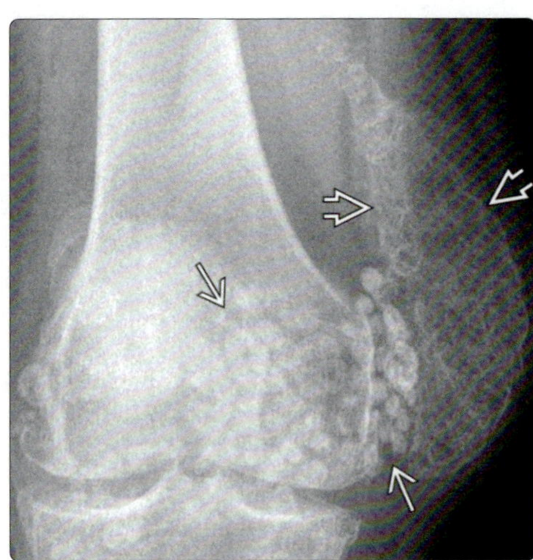

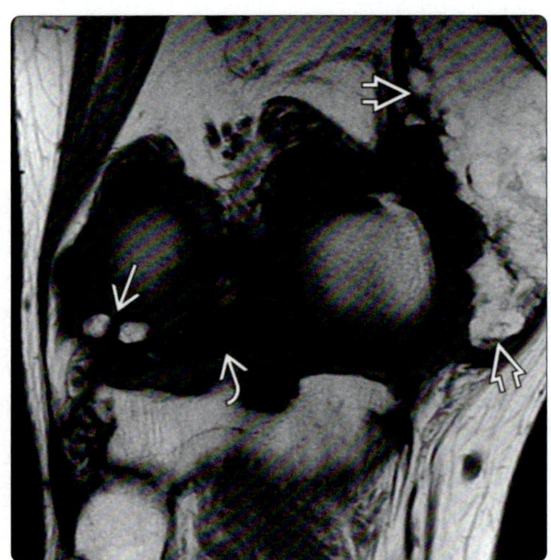

(Left) *AP radiograph shows multiple round bodies ➡ proven to be within the knee joint. In addition, there is a mass that appears more conglomerate ➡ located medial to the joint.* **(Right)** *Coronal T1 MR in the same patient shows some of the rounded bodies to have marrow signal ➡ and others ➡ are low signal, typical of synovial chondromatosis. In addition, the conglomerate mass ➡ is marrow signal, suggesting that it is bone.*

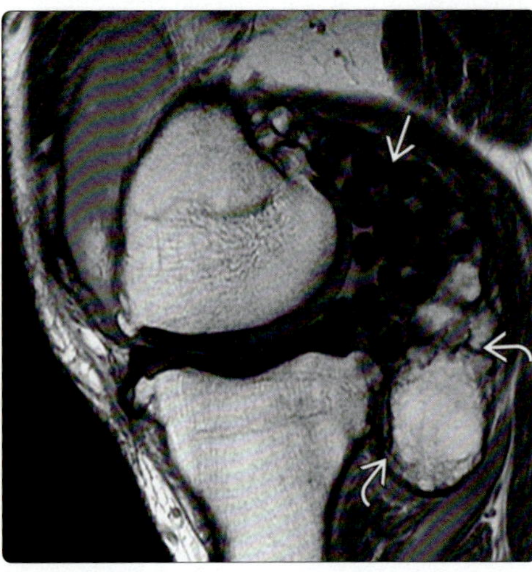

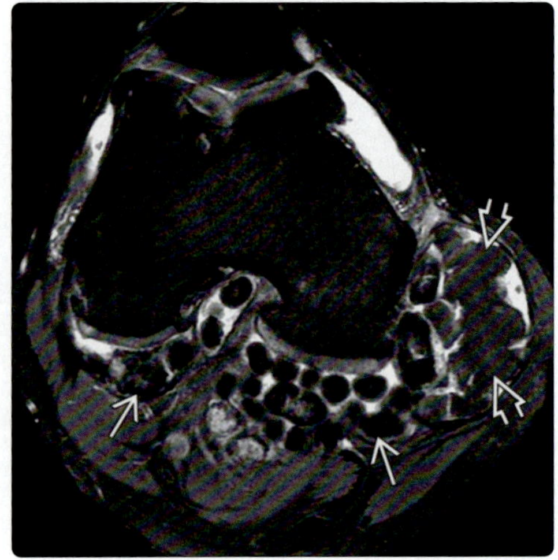

(Left) *Sagittal PD MR in the same patient confirms the multiple intraarticular bodies of synovial chondromatosis ➡. The conglomerate mass ➡ is partially seen and continues to show signal matching bone marrow.* **(Right)** *Axial T2 FS MR confirms the regular appearance of synovial chondromatosis ➡. The medial mass ➡ saturates out, as does bone marrow. This patient has an unusual combination of both multiple bodies and conglomerate mass, both representing synovial chondromatosis.*

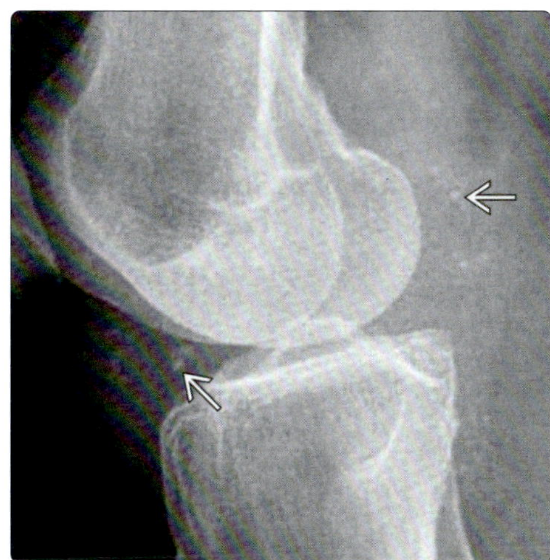

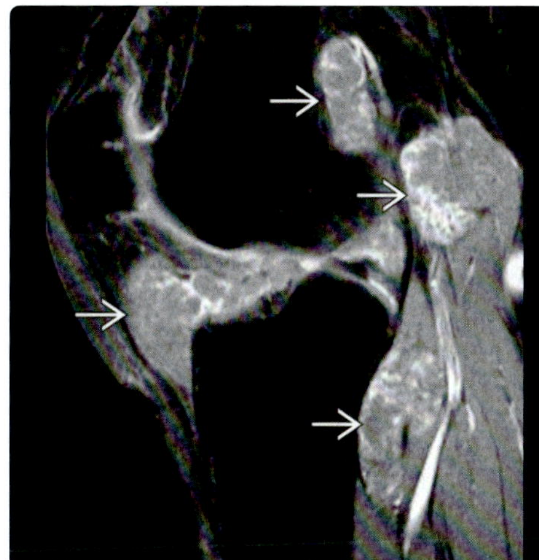

(Left) *Lateral radiograph shows multiple punctate bodies located within the knee joint ➡. These had been observed on prior radiographs and had not changed over 1 year. The diagnosis was presumed to be stable PSC.* **(Right)** *Sagittal T1WI C+ FS MR in the same patient shows that the extent of disease was underestimated by radiograph. Enhancement in and around several masses ➡ is seen, both intra- and extraarticularly, typical of PSC. At excision, there was no area of sarcomatous degeneration.*

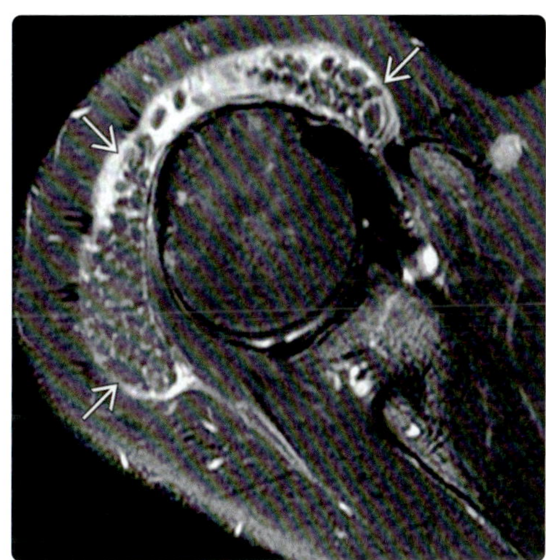

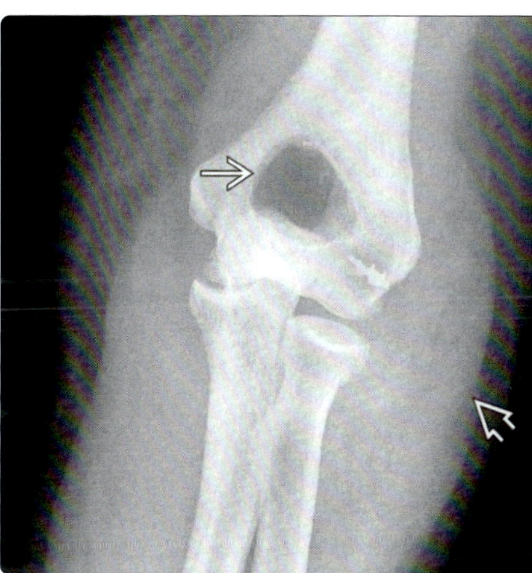

(Left) *Axial T2WI FS MR shows a distended deltoid bursa containing multiple low signal round bodies ➡. The rotator cuff was intact, and no intraarticular bodies were seen. This is bursal PSC.* **(Right)** *AP radiograph in a patient status post multiple previous resections shows erosion of the notch ➡ and a large mass within the brachioradialis muscle ⇨. Note that there is no calcification, though pathology showed synovial chondromatosis at each of the prior resections.*

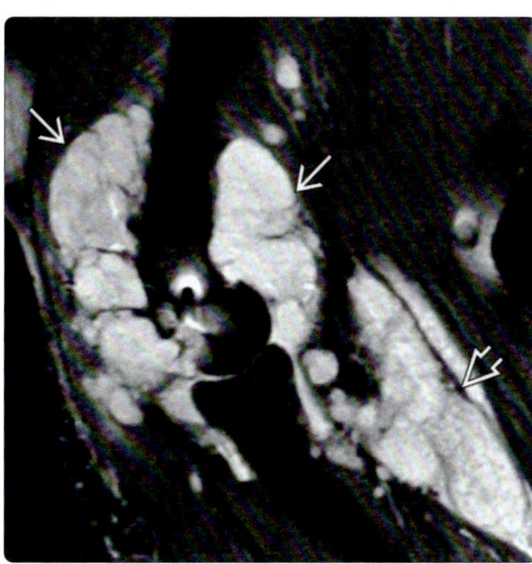

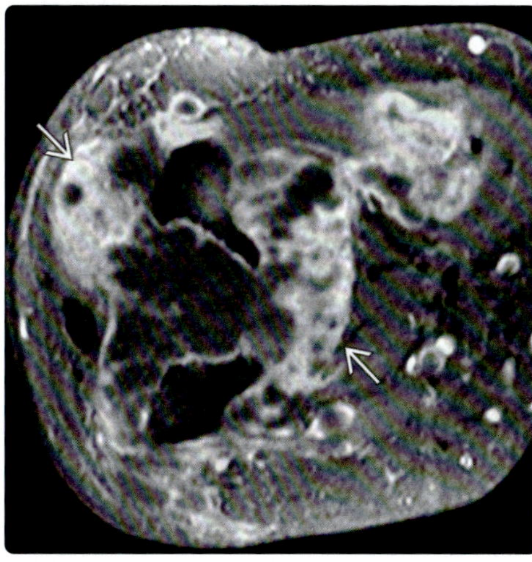

(Left) *Sagittal T2WI FS MR in the same patient details the extent of the recurrent lesion, both intra- ➡ and extraarticularly ⇨.* **(Right)** *Axial T1WI C+ FS MR shows the synovium enhances significantly, while much of the mass remains low signal with some foci of enhancement ➡. Pathology revealed enough cellular atypia to alter the diagnosis to synovial chondrosarcoma. This represents one of the rare cases of PSC that degenerated to synovial chondrosarcoma.*

KEY FACTS

TERMINOLOGY

- Severely and rapidly destructive joint process, with etiology often suggested by location

IMAGING

- Best imaging clue: **5 Ds**
  - Normal bone **density** for patient
  - Joint **distension**
  - Bony **debris**
  - Cartilage **destruction**
  - Joint **disorganization** (or **dislocation** or **deformity**)
- Location is strongly suggestive of etiology
  - Shoulder: Syringomyelia
  - Wrist: Diabetes, syringomyelia
  - Spine: Spinal cord injury, tabes, diabetes
  - Hip: Alcohol, tabes
  - Knee: Tabes, congenital indifference or insensitivity to pain, steroid injection
  - Ankle/foot: Diabetes
- Rate of destruction can be extremely fast
- MR of joint is used for problem solving
  - May help in differentiation of Charcot foot from osteomyelitis developing in Charcot foot
    - T1 and postcontrast MR imaging far more useful than fluid-sensitive sequences in attempting to differentiate infection from neuropathic changes
    - Significant overlap exists

CLINICAL ISSUES

- Up to 30% have near normal proprioception
- 15% of diabetics develop Charcot joints
- 20% of syringomyelia patients develop Charcot joints

DIAGNOSTIC CHECKLIST

- Debris and other findings may be distant from joint
  - Establish that primary process is articular, which helps make diagnosis

(Left) *Graphic shows common (red) and less common (yellow) sites of Charcot joints. Etiology is suggested by location.* **(Right)** *Sagittal T1WI MR, part of a series in a patient with diabetic Charcot foot, shows numerous abnormalities. Charcot joints are noted at navicular cuneiforms ➔. There is ↓ signal in the plantar soft tissues, with confluent ↓ signal in the adjacent cuboid ➔, concerning for osteomyelitis. It also shows diffuse ↓ signals throughout the talus ➔, an unexpected finding.*

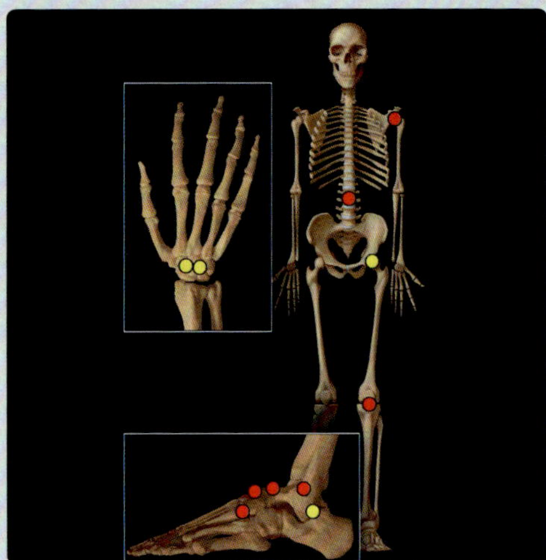

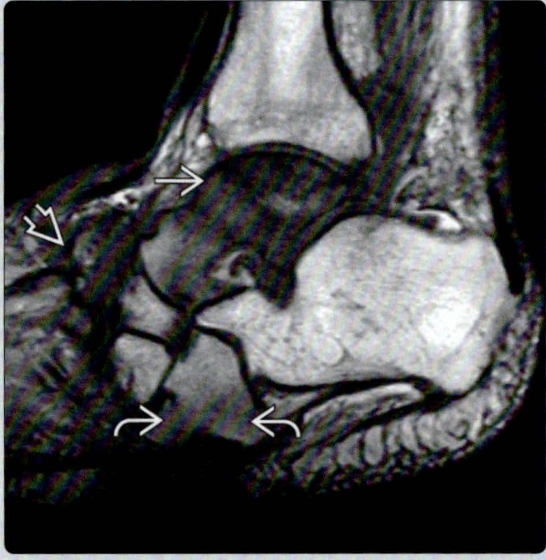

(Left) *Sagittal STIR MR in the same patient further defines the talar abnormality as an insufficiency fracture of the dome ➔.* **(Right)** *Sagittal T1WI C+ FS MR, adjacent slice, shows a wedge-shaped region of hypointensity ➔, representing a segment of osteonecrosis (ON) in the body of the talus. Remember that the talus is prone to ON and that the tarsal bones are prone to insufficiency fracture in diabetic feet. Sinus track ➔ led to the cuboid, confirming osteomyelitis, which was suspected based on both T1 and STIR.*

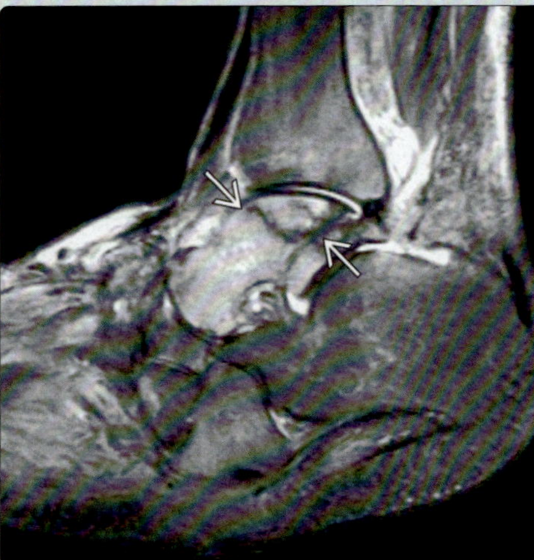

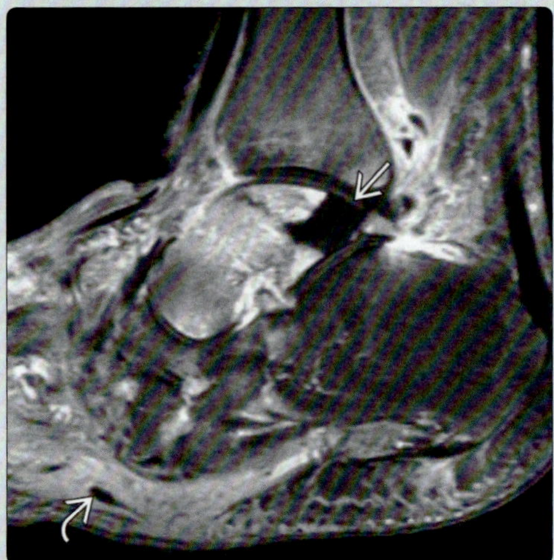

TERMINOLOGY

Synonyms

- Charcot = neuropathic joint

Definitions

- Severely and rapidly destructive joint process, with etiology often suggested by location

IMAGING

General Features

- Best diagnostic clue
  - **5 Ds**
    - Normal bone **density** for patient
    - Joint **distension**
    - Bony **debris**
    - Cartilage **destruction**
    - Joint **disorganization** (or **dislocation** or **deformity**)
- Location
  - **Location is strongly suggestive of etiology**
  - Shoulder: Syringomyelia
  - Wrist: Diabetes, syringomyelia
  - Spine: Spinal cord injury, tabes, diabetes
    - Mobile segments caudad to stabilized segment of spine in paraplegic are at risk
  - Hip: Alcohol, tabes
  - Knee: Tabes, congenital indifference or insensitivity to pain, steroid injection
  - Ankle/foot: Diabetes
    - Lisfranc (tarsal-metatarsal) > talonavicular > intertarsal > Chopart (hindfoot-midfoot), tibiotalar, subtalar
- Morphology
  - Hypertrophic (prominent bony debris): 20%, particularly seen in knees
  - Atrophic (bony debris mostly resorbed): 40%, particularly seen in diabetic ankle/foot
  - Combined hypertrophic and atrophic: 40%

Radiographic Findings

- Rate of destruction can be extremely fast, rivaling that of septic joint
- All Charcot joints have large effusions
  - Effusions can be so tense that they may present as "mass"
    - Massive effusions in shoulder often extend from glenohumeral joint across rotator cuff tear to subacromial/subdeltoid bursa
  - Large effusions can decompress, carrying osseous debris away from joint
    - Seen particularly in knee with debris dissecting down fascial planes of leg
  - Large fluid collections around Charcot joint in foot or ankle may be mistaken for abscess
  - Paraspinous fluid collections in Charcot spine
- Bony debris (whether prominent in hypertrophic form or minimal in atrophic form)
  - Density is osseous, not chondroid or calcific
  - Debris floats within large effusions, so may be placed several centimeters away from joint
  - Debris may decompress along with effusions and dissect away from joint
- Density of bone is typically normal, unless underlying density is decreased as in elderly or diabetic patient
- Early cartilage destruction
- Mixed erosive and productive osseous changes
  - Shoulder Charcot can be significantly atrophic, resorbing nearly entire humeral head and neck; may have appearance of surgical resection
- Ligamentous laxity, with joint subluxation/dislocation
  - Judge subluxation at Lisfranc joint on AP for 1st and 2nd TMT joints, on oblique for 3rd-5th TMT joints

CT Findings

- Generally not utilized for this diagnosis
- Shows articular destruction
- Shows distended joint space containing osseous debris
  - Because of tremendous distension, this debris within apparent mass may appear several centimeters distant from joint
  - Be careful not to misinterpret this appearance as mass containing matrix (i.e., chondrosarcoma)
- Reformats show disorganization of joint

MR Findings

- MR can be used to problem solve, establishes articular nature of process
- T1
  - Osseous destruction of both sides of joint
  - Adjacent bone may show reactive low signal
    - If low signal is hazy and reticulated, it is likely to be reactive
    - If low signal is confluent and prominent, it is more likely osteomyelitis
  - Surrounding low signal effusion
- Fluid-sensitive sequences
  - Shows huge effusion distending joint
  - May show effusion decompressed into adjacent bursa or fascial planes
  - Debris located within fluid collection
  - Osseous destruction on both sides of joint, outlined by effusion
  - Adjacent bone may show reactive hyperintense signal; difficult to differentiate from osteomyelitis
- Contrast-enhanced sequences
  - High signal rim surrounds fluid collections, either effusions or decompressed pockets of fluid
  - Osseous enhancement adjacent to destroyed articular bone
    - This enhancement may be seen in simply reactive bone and need not imply osteomyelitis

Imaging Recommendations

- Best imaging tool
  - Diagnosis usually made by radiograph
  - If shoulder arthropathy is determined to be neuropathic, MR of cervical spine should be obtained to evaluate for syrinx
  - MR of joint is used for problem solving
    - May help in differentiation of Charcot foot from osteomyelitis developing in Charcot foot, but significant overlap exists

DIFFERENTIAL DIAGNOSIS

Osteomyelitis or Septic Joint, Ankle/Foot

- Neuropathic and septic joint may coexist
- Both can have large effusions/fluid collections
- Both diagnoses can have enhancement of bone
- There are a few factors that may favor infection
  - Abnormal T1 signal in infected bone is confluent; hazy/reticular pattern is reactive
    - Fat replacement rather than infiltration
  - Fluid collections have less bony debris in cases of infection
  - Air in sinus tract leading to abnormal bone diagnoses infection

Chondrosarcoma, Shoulder

- Surprisingly, even though the 2 lesions are distinctive, Charcot joint is often misdiagnosed on radiograph as chondrosarcoma
  - Matrix in chondrosarcoma is chondroid, rather than bony debris seen in Charcot shoulder
  - Mass in chondrosarcoma is not intraarticular

Osteoarthritis or Inflammatory Arthritis

- Early stage osteoarthritis resembles early Charcot
- Osseous debris generally less prominent
- Joint dislocation should not be seen in arthritis
- Effusions generally smaller in arthritis

Discitis, Spine

- Both discitis and Charcot spine may have paraspinal soft tissue mass/fluid collections
- Both show disc and endplate destruction with debris
- Both may show subluxation
- Patients with spinal cord injury or diabetes are at risk for both discitis and Charcot spine
- Presence of prominent debris, subluxation, vacuum disc, and facet involvement makes Charcot more likely
- Many cases will require aspiration to prove diagnosis

PATHOLOGY

General Features

- Etiology
  - Primary pathogenesis uncertain
  - Likely initial alteration in sympathetic nerve control of osseous blood flow →
    - Hyperemia and active bone resorption
  - **Secondary neurotraumatic mechanism resulting in destructive cycle**
    - Blunted pain sensation and proprioception →
    - Relaxation of skeletal supporting structures →
    - Chronic instability →
    - Recurrent injury by normal biomechanical stresses, but abnormal joint loading →
    - Osseous fragmentation and joint disorganization
  - Diabetes: Mostly peripheral joints (foot, hand)
  - Tabes dorsalis: Affects spine, knee > hip, ankle/foot
  - Syringomyelia: Shoulder, wrist
  - Spinal cord injury: Spine, more caudad than site of injury (unprotected motion)
    - Active paraplegic patients (weightlifting, wheelchair athletics) put nonstabilized portion of their spinal column at risk
  - Congenital insensitivity/indifference to pain: Lower extremity (knee, ankle)
  - Intraarticular steroid use: Knee is most common
  - Alcoholism: Hip, metatarsophalangeal, IP joints
  - Amyloidosis: Knee and ankle
  - Leprosy: IP joints of hand, MTP joints of foot
  - Multiple sclerosis
  - Meningomyelocele: Ankle and intertarsal joints
  - Neurologic conditions: Charcot-Marie-Tooth, Riley-Day syndrome (dysautonomia)
  - Navajo neuropathy: Sensorimotor neuropathy; progressive CNS white matter lesions

Gross Pathologic & Surgical Features

- Significant amount of cartilaginous and osseous debris within synovial membrane

CLINICAL ISSUES

Presentation

- Most common signs/symptoms
  - Swollen, unstable joint
  - Up to 30% have near normal proprioception
    - Careful exam elicits neurological abnormality
    - Response to deep pain and proprioception may be ↓

Demographics

- Age
  - Relates to underlying etiology
    - Depends on age of onset of diabetes
    - Congenital pain insensitivity/indifference: Teens
- Epidemiology
  - 15% of diabetics develop Charcot joints
  - 20% of syringomyelia patients develop Charcot joints
  - Worldwide, 10-20% of patients with tabes dorsalis develop Charcot joints

Natural History & Prognosis

- Rapidly progressive destruction
- With worsening alignment, at risk for skin ulceration, and eventual osteomyelitis

Treatment

- If conservative treatment fails, needs reconstruction
- Arthrodesis difficult to achieve; 25% recur or have significant complications

DIAGNOSTIC CHECKLIST

Image Interpretation Pearls

- Even though debris and other findings may be distant from joint, establish that primary process is articular; this makes diagnosis

SELECTED REFERENCES

1. Peters EJ et al: Diagnosis and management of infection in the diabetic foot. Med Clin North Am. 97(5):911-46, 2013
2. Johnson PW et al: Diagnostic utility of T1-weighted MRI characteristics in evaluation of osteomyelitis of the foot. AJR Am J Roentgenol. 192(1):96-100, 2009

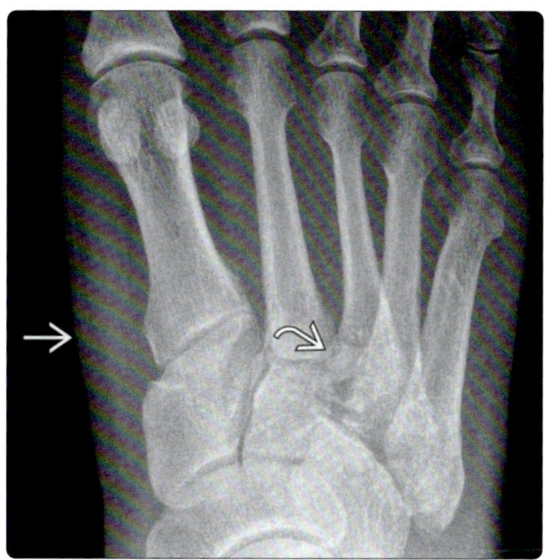

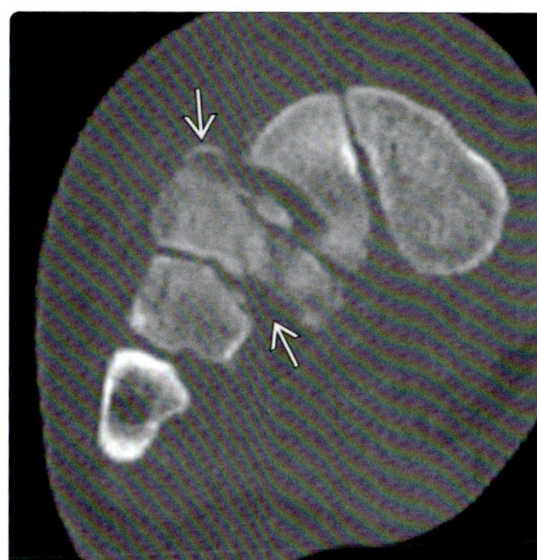

(Left) *AP radiograph shows swelling about the tarsometatarsal joints ➡. Careful observation reveals fragmentation ➡ at the base of the 3rd metatarsal, with likely fragmentation of the bases of the 4th and 5th as well. There was no history of trauma; this is a Charcot foot.* **(Right)** *Short-axis CT, same patient, proves the fragmentation and mild subluxation of the metatarsal bases ➡; it is often far more severe than suspected on the basis of radiographs. As one would expect, the patient is diabetic.*

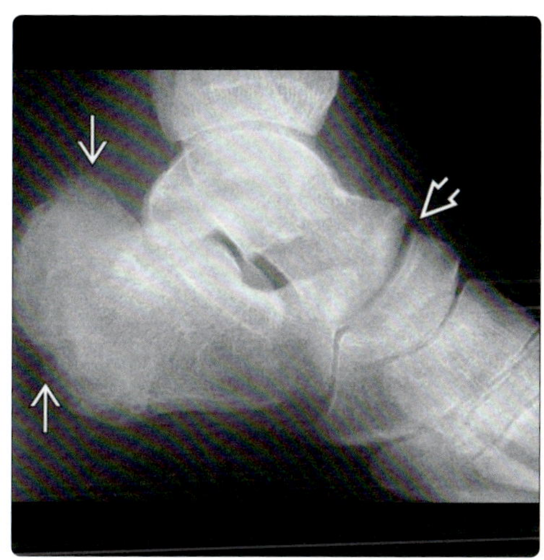

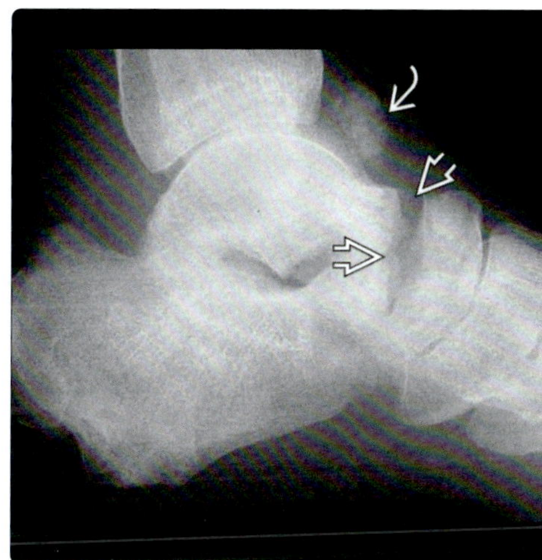

(Left) *Lateral radiograph shows an old and healed calcaneal insufficiency avulsion fracture ➡, typical in diabetics. The talonavicular joint shows concavity of the articular surface of the talus, along with some sclerosis ➡, suspicious for early Charcot joint.* **(Right)** *Lateral radiograph of the same foot 2 months later shows ongoing destruction at the talonavicular joint ➡. Debris has migrated dorsal to the talus, contained within a distended joint capsule ➡. This is a classic Charcot joint.*

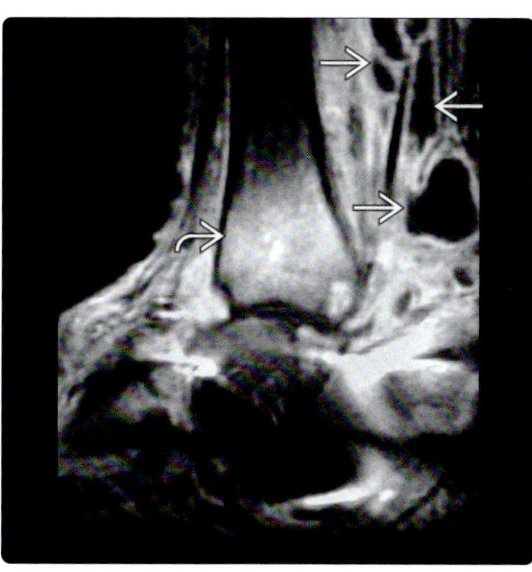

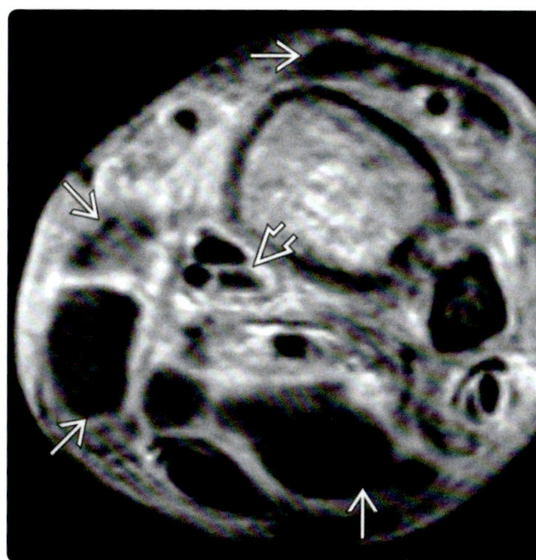

(Left) *Sagittal T1WI C+ FS MR in a Charcot foot shows fluid collections (some containing debris) surrounding the ankle ➡ and abnormal signal within the distal tibia ➡. Metallic artifact obscures the subtalar, talonavicular, and calcaneocuboid joints.* **(Right)** *Axial T1WI C+ FS MR in the same patient shows fluid collections in the soft tissues ➡ and tendon sheaths ➡. These are neuropathic fluid collections. Bones enhance, related to reactive change. There was no infection at biopsy.*

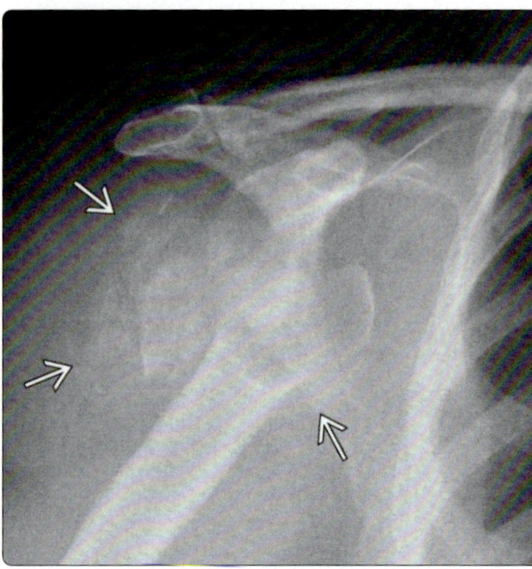

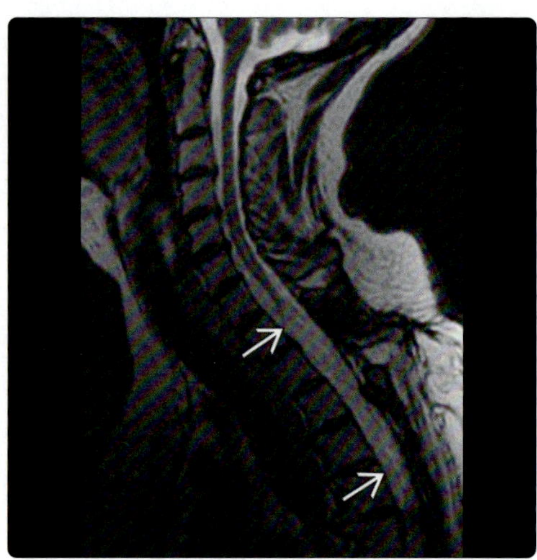

(Left) *AP radiograph shows a dislocated shoulder with severe fragmentation and bony debris. The placement of the debris suggests massive distension of the glenohumeral joint and subacromial/subdeltoid bursa ➡. The combination of findings is typical of Charcot (neuropathic) shoulder.* **(Right)** *Sagittal T2 MR, same patient, shows a large cervicothoracic syrinx ➡. Syringomyelia is the most common etiology of Charcot changes in the glenohumeral joint.*

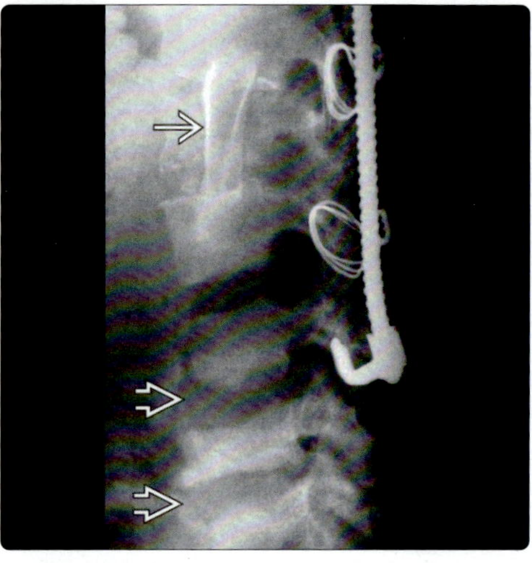

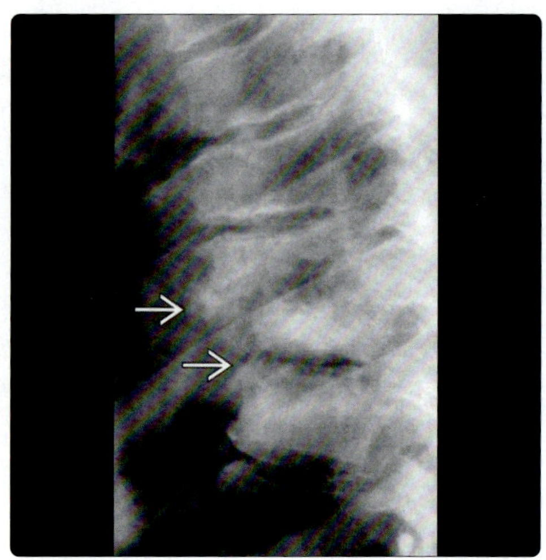

(Left) *Lateral radiograph of a paraplegic shows a burst fracture of L1 treated with partial corpectomy, strut graft ➡, and posterior rods. Note the osseous destruction and instability at the next 2 levels ➡. These Charcot vertebrae are typically located immediately caudad to the stabilized spine.* **(Right)** *Lateral radiograph shows significant subluxation and destruction of endplates with osseous debris at 2 adjacent levels ➡. This paraplegic patient developed instability and Charcot spine.*

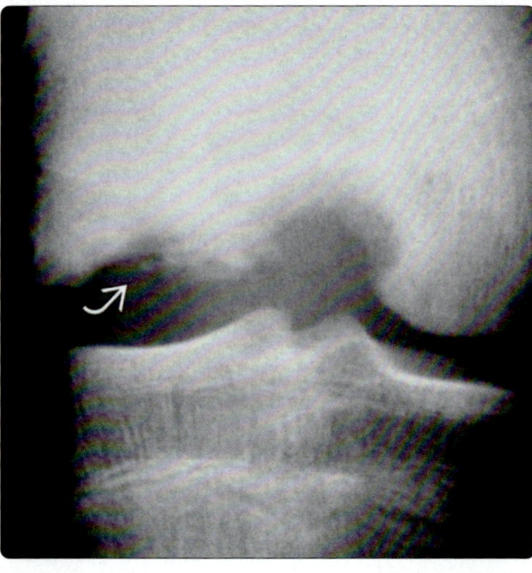

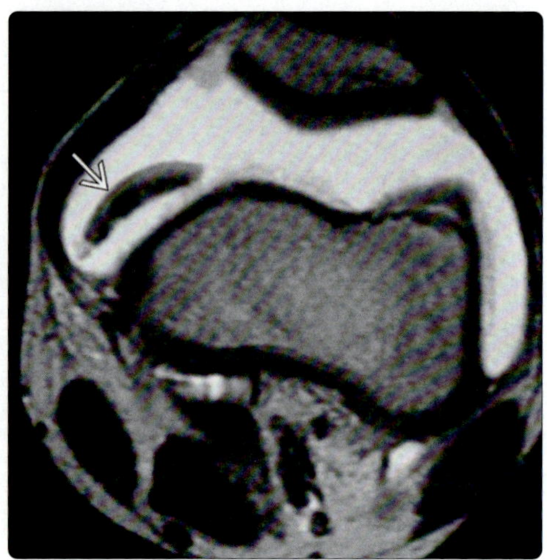

(Left) *AP radiograph shows ragged destructive changes of the femoral condyle and osseous debris ➡ in a young patient. His contralateral AP knee had similar abnormalities.* **(Right)** *Axial T2WI MR in the same patient shows a large effusion and 1 of multiple pieces of osteocartilaginous debris ➡. This patient's knees show the debris, distension, and destruction typical of neuropathic joints. The etiology in this case is congenital insensitivity to pain.*

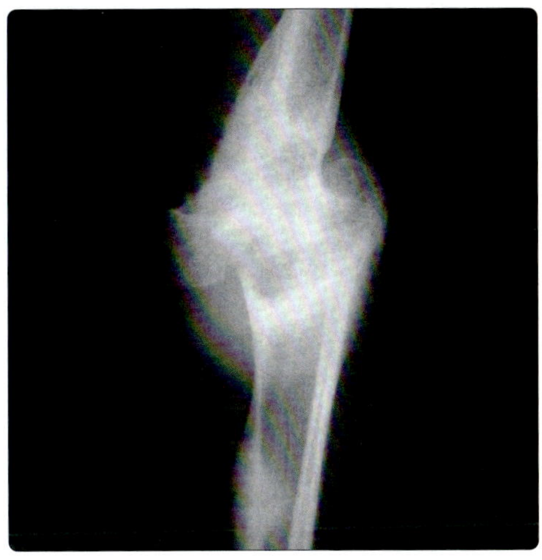

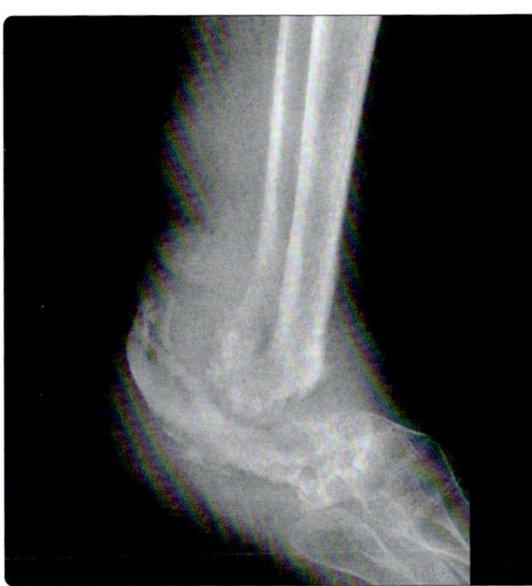

(Left) *AP radiograph shows an unusual case of neuropathic joint, resulting from congenital indifference to pain. The left knee shows severe disruption with subluxation, fragmentation, attempted repair, and complete destruction of the joint.* **(Right)** *Lateral radiograph of contralateral limb in same patient shows just as severe disruption with destruction of the tibiotalar, subtalar, and midfoot joints. Congenital indifference to pain is an unusual cause of Charcot joint and is often polyarticular.*

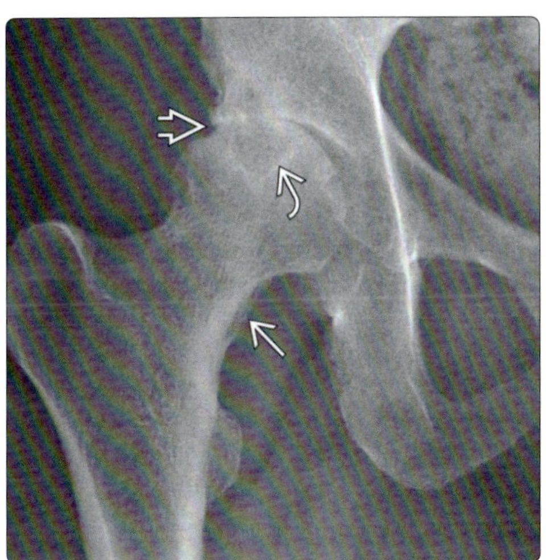

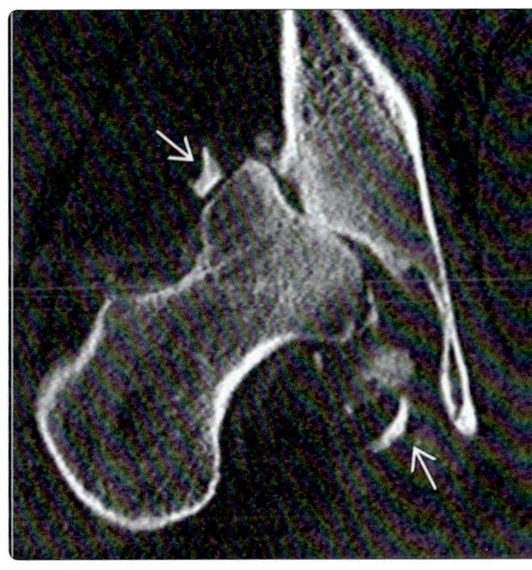

(Left) *AP radiograph in a middle-aged patient gives the initial impression of uncomplicated osteoarthritis, with cartilage loss ➡, large subchondral cyst formation ➡, superolateral subluxation of the hip, and calcar buttressing ➡.* **(Right)** *Coronal CT, obtained 2 months later in the same patient, shows severe and rapid progression of destruction of the femoral head and acetabulum. Abundant debris ➡ is seen within the joint.*

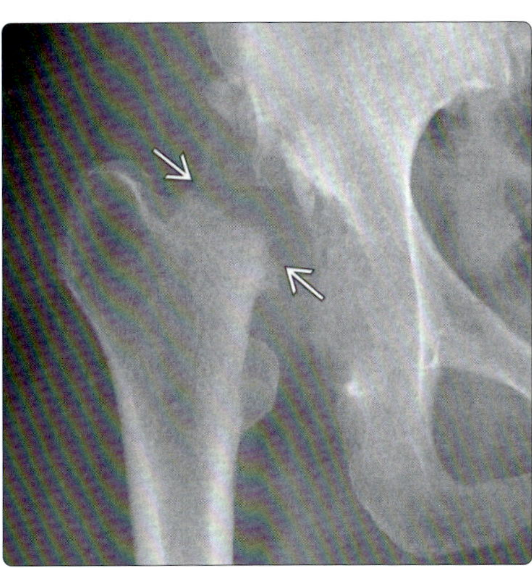

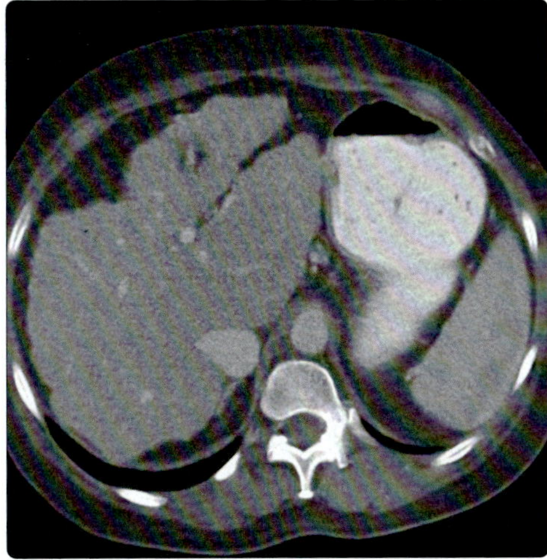

(Left) *AP radiograph in the same patient 7 months later shows the classic hatchet sign ➡ of rapid destruction of the hip. The rapidity of the destruction and the appearance suggest a diagnosis of rapidly destructive osteoarthritis of the hip. However, one must also consider Charcot arthropathy as an etiology.* **(Right)** *Axial CT from the same patient shows a small, nodular liver, typical of cirrhosis. The most common etiology of Charcot hip is alcoholism; the cirrhosis proves the etiology in this case.*

Hypertrophic Osteoarthropathy

KEY FACTS

TERMINOLOGY

- Syndrome characterized by proliferation of skin (1°) and bone (1° and 2°) in distal extremities

IMAGING

- Radiograph/CT
  - Periosteal reaction without underlying osseous lesion or injury
  - Tibia, fibula, radius, ulna are most frequent
  - Less common in phalanges
  - Degree of bone production, width, and extent along cortex relates to duration of disease
  - No underlying marrow or soft tissue abnormality
  - Clubbing of digits
- Joints
  - Soft tissue swelling
  - No joint space narrowing
  - No erosions or other arthritic changes
- Bone scan: Dense, fairly linear and symmetric uptake along long bones
  - Digits may be more apparent on bone scan secondary to clubbing

PATHOLOGY

- 1° hypertrophic osteoarthropathy (HOA) familial (autosomal dominant): Pachydermoperiostosis
- 2° HOA: Mechanisms uncertain
  - Pulmonary: Cancer, cystic fibrosis, pulmonary fibrosis, chronic infection
  - Pleural: Mesothelioma, pleural fibroma
  - Cardiac: Cyanotic congenital heart disease, patent ductus arteriosus, bacterial endocarditis
  - Gastrointestinal: Inflammatory bowel disease, cancer, cirrhosis

CLINICAL ISSUES

- 95-97% of HOA is 2° form
- 90% of 2° HOA cases associated with malignancy

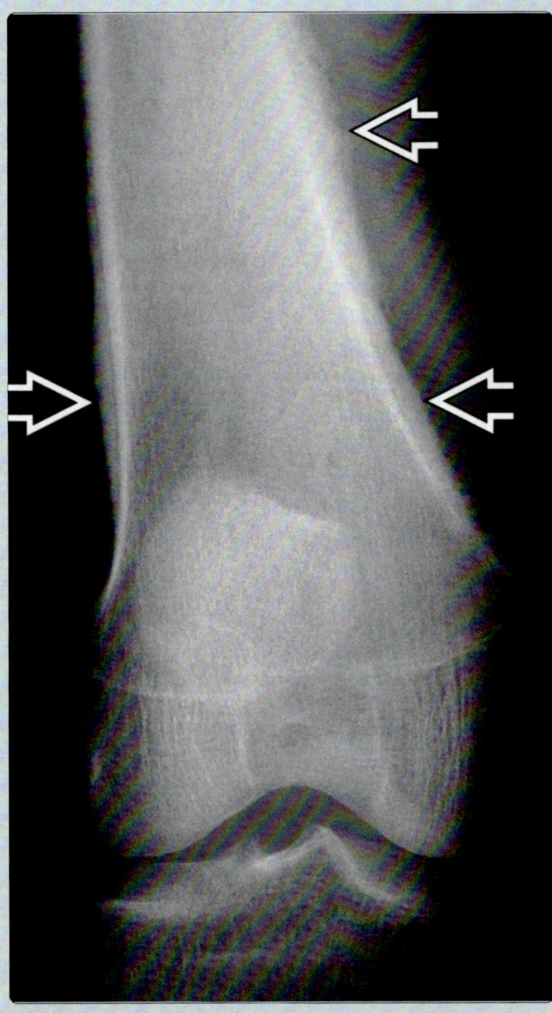

Anteroposterior radiograph shows dense, linear periosteal reaction along the diaphysis of the femur ➾. The underlying marrow is normal. The patient complained of knee pain and swelling, but the joint appears completely normal.

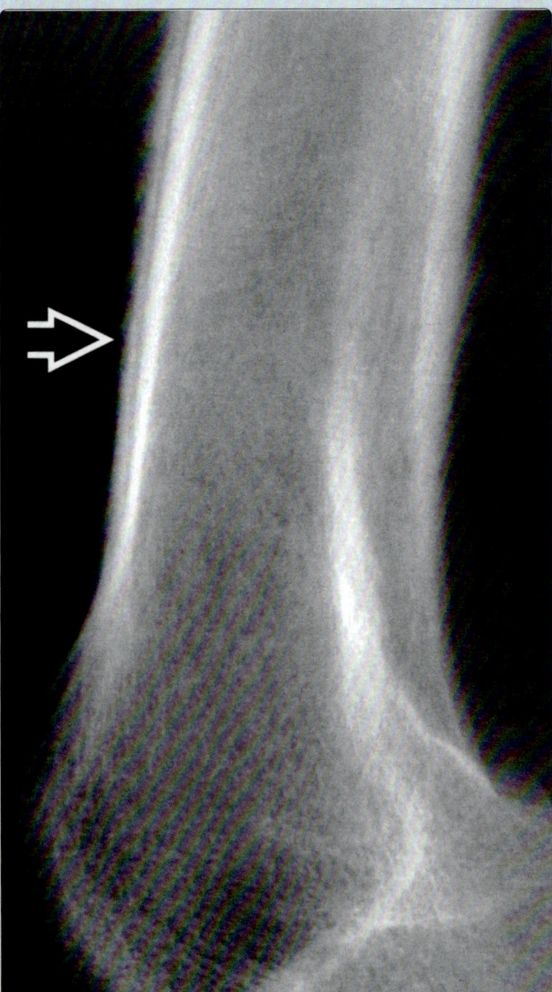

Lateral radiograph of the same knee confirms very regular periosteal reaction ➾. In this patient with complaints of severe arthritic pain, a secondary cause must be sought. This patient proved to have lung cancer, unsuspected prior to this exam.

TERMINOLOGY

Abbreviations

- Hypertrophic osteoarthropathy (HOA)

Synonyms

- Hypertrophic pulmonary osteoarthropathy; acropachy; secondary HOA; Marie-Bamberger syndrome
- Primary HOA = pachydermoperiostosis

Definitions

- Syndrome characterized by proliferation of skin (1°) and bone (1° and 2°) in distal extremities

IMAGING

General Features

- Best diagnostic clue
  - Periosteal reaction without underlying osseous lesion or injury
- Location
  - Tibia, fibula, radius, ulna are most frequent
    - Less common in phalanges
- Size
  - Degree of bone production, width, and extent along cortex relates to duration of disease
- Morphology
  - Periosteal reaction varies from dense and linear to fluffy and exuberant

Radiographic Findings

- Usually symmetric periosteal reaction
  - May be thick, linear, dense, layered
  - May be fluffy, exuberant
  - Thickness/extent dependent on disease duration
    - Shorter duration of disease → diaphyseal; later extends to metaphyses and epiphyses
- No underlying marrow or soft tissue abnormality
- Clubbing of digits
- Tuft hypertrophy or acroosteolysis (uncommon)
  - Acroosteolysis more commonly seen in patients with primary HOA and cyanotic heart disease
  - Hypertrophy at tufts more commonly seen in patients with malignancy
  - May be evolutionary, dependent on underlying disease duration
- Joints
  - Soft tissue swelling
  - No joint space narrowing
  - No erosions or other arthritic changes

CT Findings

- Same as radiographic findings
- Shows underlying chest or abdominal abnormalities

MR Findings

- T1: Low signal periosteal reaction; normal marrow
- Fluid-sensitive sequences: Linear high signal may be seen on either side of low signal periosteal reaction

Nuclear Medicine Findings

- Bone scan: Dense, fairly linear and symmetric uptake along long bones
  - Occasionally not symmetric
  - Digits on bone scan may be more apparent secondary to clubbing

DIFFERENTIAL DIAGNOSIS

Multifocal Osteomyelitis

- Associated marrow abnormality with infection

Neoplasm

- Associated marrow, soft tissue abnormality with tumor

Stress Reaction, Especially of Tibiae

- May be bilateral, symmetric, and indistinguishable from HOA

Venous Stasis: Lower Extremities

- May elicit periosteal reaction; look for varicosities

Multifocal Periosteal Reaction in Child

- Caffey disease
- Hypervitaminosis A: Younger than expected for primary HOA
- Progressive diaphyseal dysplasia (Camurati-Engelmann disease): Endosteal as well as periosteal thickening
- Leukemia: Osteoporosis, marrow infiltration

PATHOLOGY

General Features

- Etiology
  - Primary HOA: Genetic
  - Secondary HOA: Mechanisms uncertain
    - Pulmonary: Cancer, cystic fibrosis, pulmonary fibrosis, chronic infection
    - Pleural: Mesothelioma, pleural fibroma
    - Cardiac: Cyanotic congenital heart disease, patent ductus arteriosus, bacterial endocarditis
    - Gastrointestinal: Inflammatory bowel disease, cancer, cirrhosis
    - Systemic malignant disorders: Lymphoma, POEMS
    - Reported in HIV-AIDS patients who have coexistent pulmonary infections
  - Unilateral secondary HOA reported in infected aortic or axillary-axillary graft
  - Final common pathway thought to involve release of PDGF by megakaryocytes
    - Deposited in peripheral tissues secondary to lung's inability to filter
  - Reports of tumor containing GHRH → high serum GH
    - Resolution of HOA after resection of tumor and simultaneous ↓ serum GH also reported
  - Clubbing: Platelet precursors fail to fragment within pulmonary circulation
    - → fragments entrapped in peripheral vasculature
    - → PDGF and VEGF
    - → promotion of vascularity → clubbing
- Genetics
  - Primary HOA familial (autosomal dominant)
  - Mutations in *HPGD* identified (encoding 15-hydroxyprostaglandin dehydrogenase, main enzyme of prostaglandin degradation)
- Associated abnormalities

- Reported association of primary HOA with myelofibrosis

Gross Pathologic & Surgical Features

- New bone formation on cortical surfaces
  - Gradual conversion of newly formed cancellous bone into compact outer sheath
  - Progressive rarefaction of compact outer layers of original cortex
- Clubbed digits: Increased numbers of fibroblasts
- Synovial membranes may have proliferative features

CLINICAL ISSUES

Presentation

- Most common signs/symptoms
  - Arthritis: Patients claim arthritis (joint pain) though only radiographic finding is periostitis
    - Arthritis is often presenting symptom
      - Pain worse at night, aggravated by motion
    - Arthritis clinically manifests as swelling, stiffness, decreased range of motion
    - Articular symptoms in 30-40% of secondary HOA
  - Clubbing of digits
    - Skin thickening
    - Hyperhidrosis
- Other signs/symptoms
  - Primary HOA
    - Thickening of skin (pachydermia), forehead, dorsum of hand
    - Skin also coarse with furrowing and oiliness
    - Excessive sweating
    - Bone and joint pain
    - Endocrine abnormalities
    - May develop myelofibrosis
  - Thyroid acropachy
    - Clubbing
    - Periostitis of digits said to be fluffy rather than linear
    - Exophthalmos
    - Pretibial myxedema

Demographics

- Age
  - Primary HOA: Child or young adult presentation
  - Secondary forms present in later adulthood, associated with underlying abnormality
- Gender
  - Male > > female (7:1) in 1° HOA
  - 2° HOA: No gender predominance
- Ethnicity
  - 1° HOA is more common in African Americans than in Caucasians
- Epidemiology
  - 95-97% of HOA is secondary form
  - 90% of secondary HOA cases associated with malignancy
    - Non-small cell lung cancer is most common
    - Secondary HOA occurs in 4-17% patients with lung carcinoma
    - Secondary HOA occurs in 20-35% of patients with pleural mesothelioma

Natural History & Prognosis

- Primary HOA is usually self-limited; pain decreases or resolves in adulthood
  - Average time from onset to resolution of symptoms: 10 years (range: 5-20)
  - Does not affect lifespan
  - Morbidity may be significant, with kyphosis and neurologic symptoms
- Secondary HOA pain and imaging abnormalities may resolve with treatment of underlying abnormality
  - Mortality related to underlying disease rather than HOA

Treatment

- NSAIDs for symptoms
- Bisphosphonates may relieve symptoms
- Treat underlying disease for secondary forms

DIAGNOSTIC CHECKLIST

Consider

- If symmetric periosteal reaction is seen, or there is periosteal reaction without underlying osseous abnormality, consider secondary HOA
  - Search for chest abnormality, particularly tumor
  - If chest is normal, consider abdominal abnormality

Image Interpretation Pearls

- Radiographs will often be centered on joint since patient complains of arthritis
  - Watch for periosteal reaction on long bones adjacent to joints (edge of radiograph finding)

SELECTED REFERENCES

1. Li S et al: Primary hypertrophic osteoarthropathy with myelofibrosis and anemia: a case report and review of literature. Int J Clin Exp Med. 8(1):1467-71, 2015
2. Tüysüz B et al: Primary hypertrophic osteoarthropathy caused by homozygous deletion in HPGD gene in a family: changing clinical and radiological findings with long-term follow-up. Rheumatol Int. 34(11):1539-44, 2014
3. Booth TC et al: Update on imaging of non-infectious musculoskeletal complications of HIV infection. Skeletal Radiol. 41(11):1349-63, 2012
4. Drakonaki EE et al: Ten-year-old boy with finger and toe swelling. Skeletal Radiol. 41(8):1003, 2012
5. Drakonaki EE et al: Hypertrophic osteoarthropathy in a child due to thoracic Hodgkin's disease. Skeletal Radiol. 41(8):1027-8, 2012
6. Ede K et al: Hypertrophic osteoarthropathy in the hepatopulmonary syndrome. J Clin Rheumatol. 14(4):230-3, 2008
7. Martinez-Lavin M et al: Hypertrophic osteoarthropathy: a palindrome with a pathogenic connotation. Curr Opin Rheumatol. 20(1):88-91, 2008
8. Narla VV et al: Atypical presentation of hypertrophic pulmonary osteoarthropathy on Tc-99m MDP bone scintigraphy. Clin Nucl Med. 33(10):702-4, 2008
9. Armstrong DJ et al: Hypertrophic pulmonary osteoarthropathy (HPOA) (Pierre Marie-Bamberger syndrome): two cases presenting as acute inflammatory arthritis. Description and review of the literature. Rheumatol Int. 27(4):399-402, 2007
10. McNaughton DA et al: AJR teaching file: Cavitated mass with hypertrophic osteoarthropathy. AJR Am J Roentgenol. 188(3 Suppl):S7-9, 2007
11. Bachmeyer C et al: Myelofibrosis in a patient with pachydermoperiostosis. Clin Exp Dermatol. 30(6):646-8, 2005
12. Castori M et al: Pachydermoperiostosis: an update. Clin Genet. 68(6):477-86, 2005

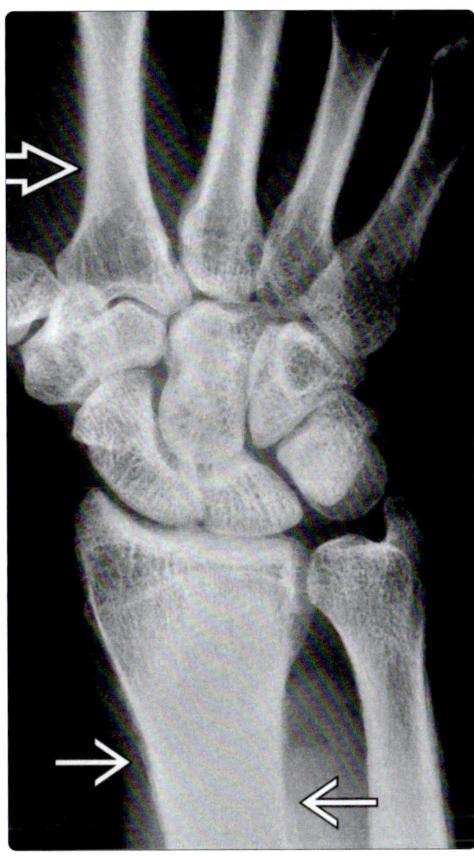

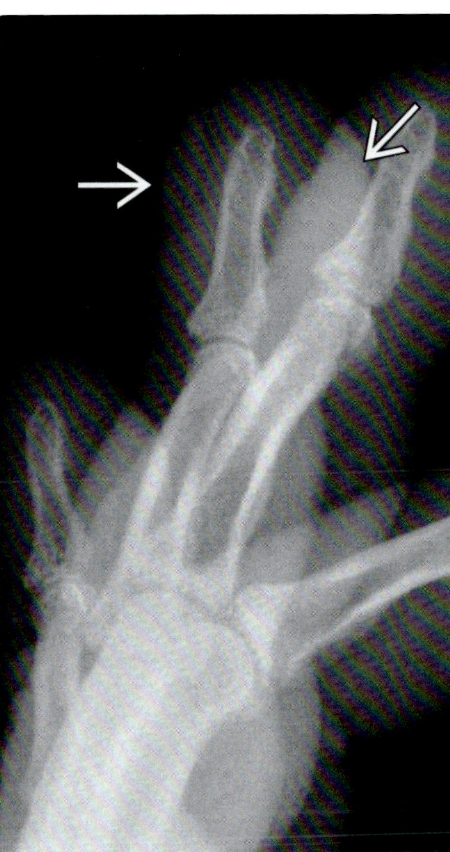

(Left) *PA radiograph obtained for wrist pain and swelling shows a completely normal carpus. However, there is dense, somewhat fluffy periosteal reaction along the diaphysis of the radius ➡. Much more subtle periosteal reaction is seen along the 2nd metacarpal ➡. There is no underlying osseous abnormality seen. The periosteal abnormalities may easily be missed in these cases, since the interpreter tends to focus on the joints.* **(Right)** *Lateral radiograph from the same hand demonstrates no periosteal reaction but clubbing at the terminal digits. Note the soft tissues of the 4th digit ➡. The tuft does not show either acroosteolysis or hyperostosis, as may sometimes be seen in cases of secondary hypertrophic osteoarthropathy (HOA). The combination of clubbing and periosteal reaction strongly suggest the diagnosis of HOA.*

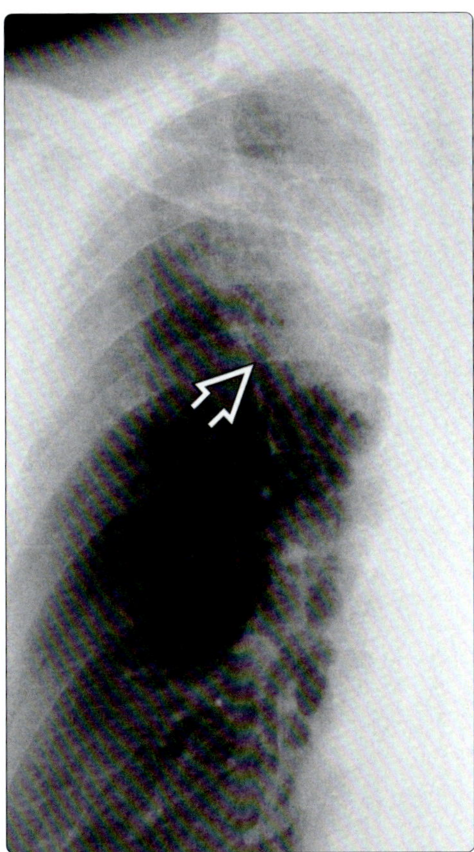

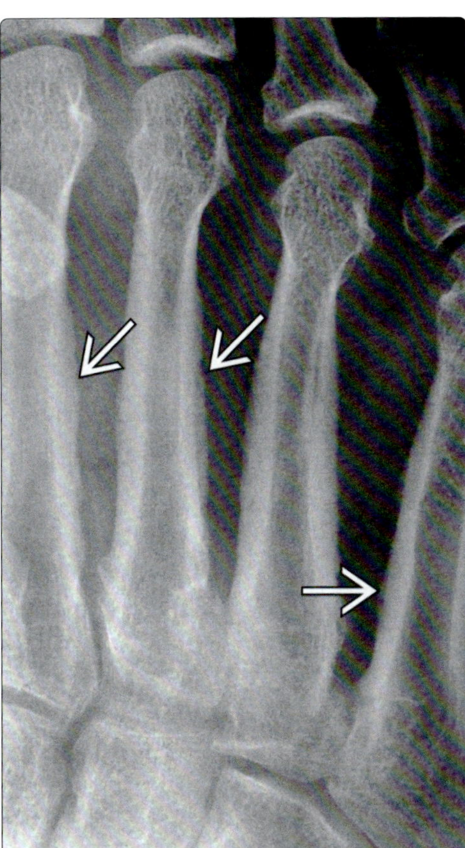

(Left) *Coned PA radiograph of the chest in the same patient is shown. The wrist and hand radiographs showed periosteal reaction and clubbing suggesting secondary HOA. Accordingly, a chest examination was suggested. This confirms an upper lobe mass ➡. The most frequent association with secondary HOA is malignancy, most frequently non-small cell lung cancer.* **(Right)** *AP radiograph of the foot, obtained for arthritis pain, demonstrates dense periosteal reactive bone formation ➡. The patient had similar findings along the diaphysis of the tibia, and the findings were bilateral. At the suggestion of the radiologist, a chest radiograph was obtained. It confirmed the presence of lung carcinoma (not shown). It is not rare for unsuspected lung tumors to be discovered by the association with HOA.*

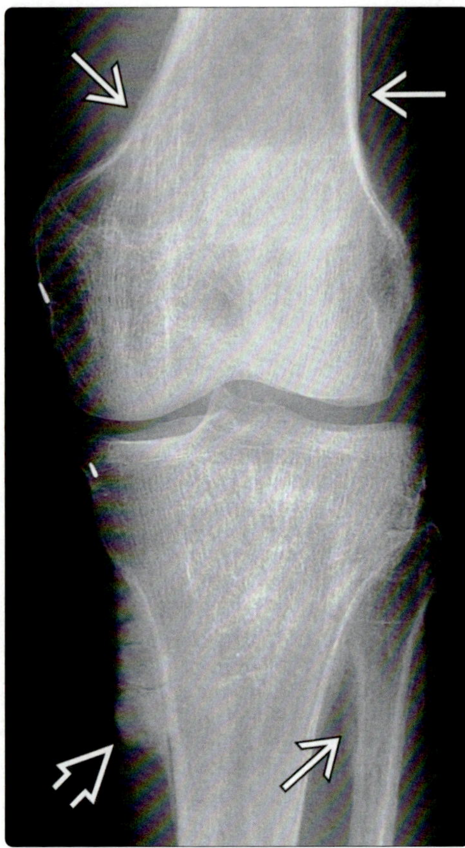

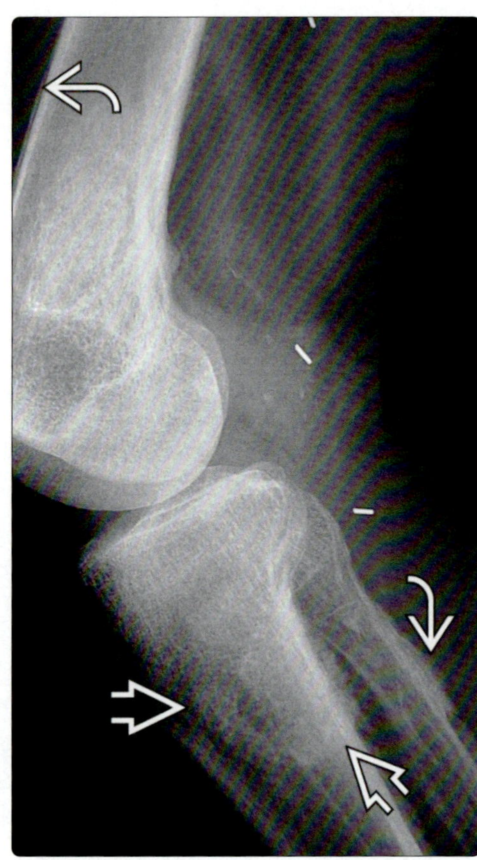

(Left) *AP radiograph obtained for joint pain is shown. The joint is normal, but there is exuberant bone formation adjacent to the medial tibial metadiaphysis ➩. This is a highly unusual appearance; the morphology might initially be concerning for a tumor or exostosis. Note also other sites of periosteal reaction, more regular and linear, at the femur and fibula ➩. This is typical of HOA. The exuberant bone formation on the tibia is an extreme example of HOA. (From: DI Musculoskeletal Imaging.)* **(Right)** *Lateral radiograph of the same knee shows exuberant periosteal bone superimposed on the tibial metaphysis ➩, but the fibular and femoral regular reaction is more easily seen ➩. The underlying abnormality was lung cancer.*

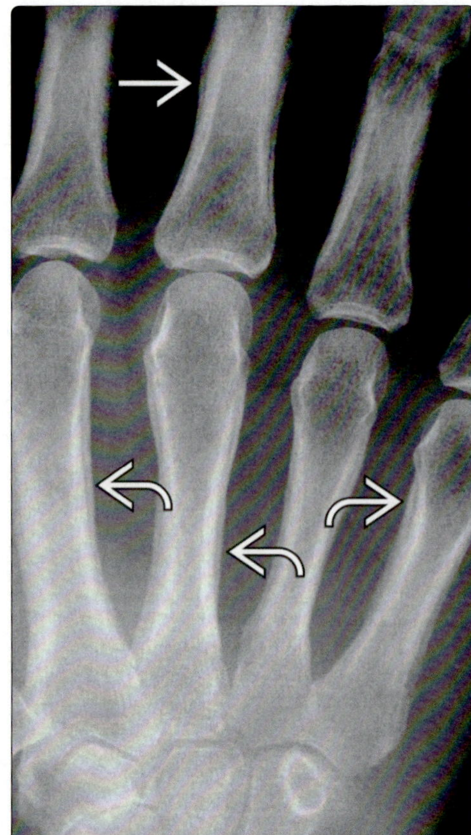

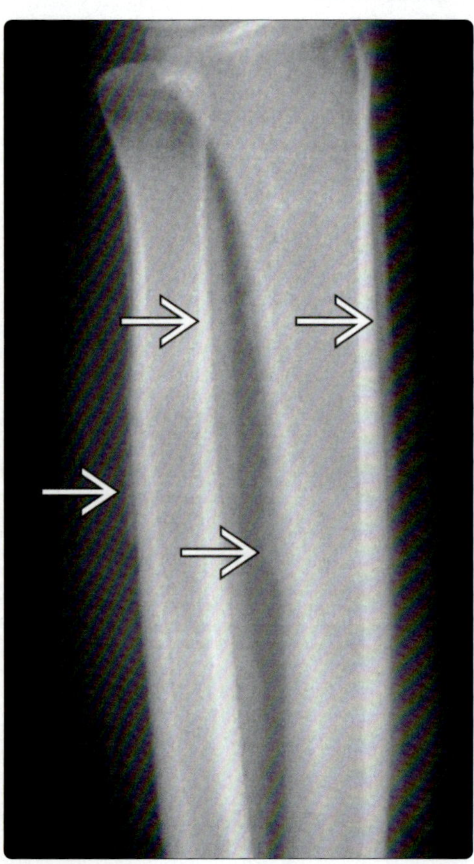

(Left) *PA radiograph of a hand demonstrates regular periosteal reaction in the metacarpals ➩ and, more subtly, the phalanges ➩. The bone formation is far too regular and symmetric from bone to bone to represent a periostitis as might be seen in psoriatic arthritis. Despite the fact that the patient presented with arthritis, the joints are normal and secondary HOA must be strongly considered. In this case, the lungs were normal. The etiology was found to be intraabdominal: Cirrhosis.* **(Right)** *AP radiograph of the forearm of a young adult male shows dense, thick, slightly fluffy periosteal reaction involving both the radius and ulna ➩. The abnormality is predominantly diaphyseal and extends to the metaphyses. The contralateral forearm showed similar findings; HOA must be considered.*

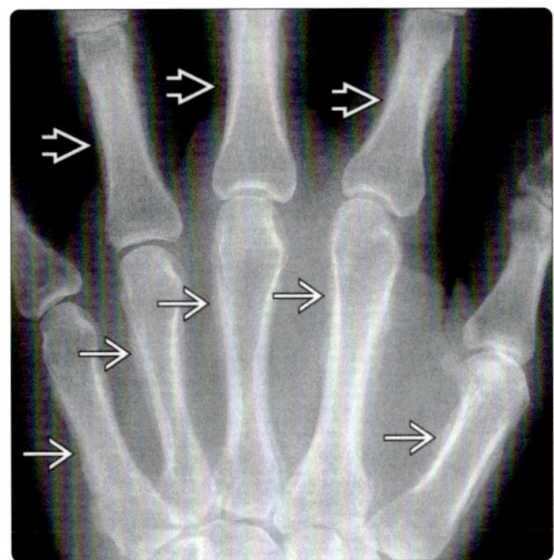

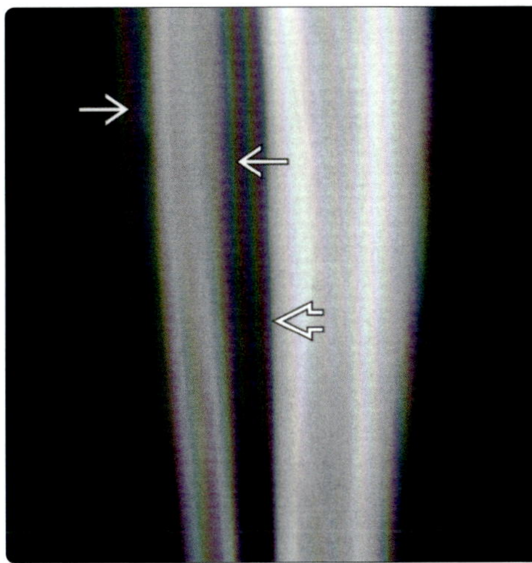

(Left) *PA radiograph in the same patient shows similarly dense periosteal reaction involving the metacarpals ➡ as well as proximal phalanges ➡. The pattern is identical.* **(Right)** *AP radiograph in the same patient shows the same rather fluffy periosteal bone formation along the fibula ➡ and more subtle tibial reaction ➡. With normal marrow and endosteal bone, hypertrophic osteoarthropathy is the diagnosis of choice.*

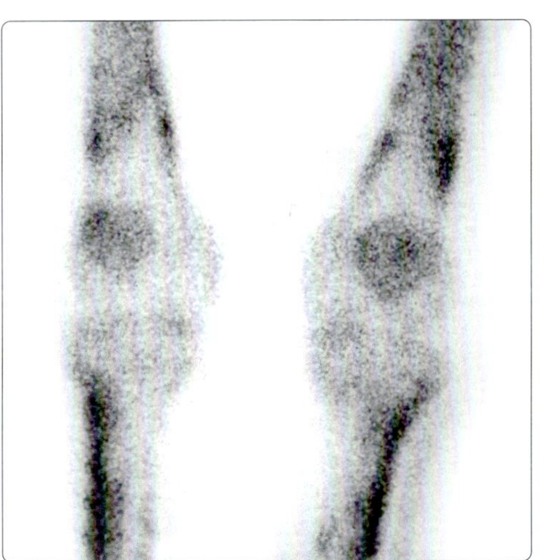

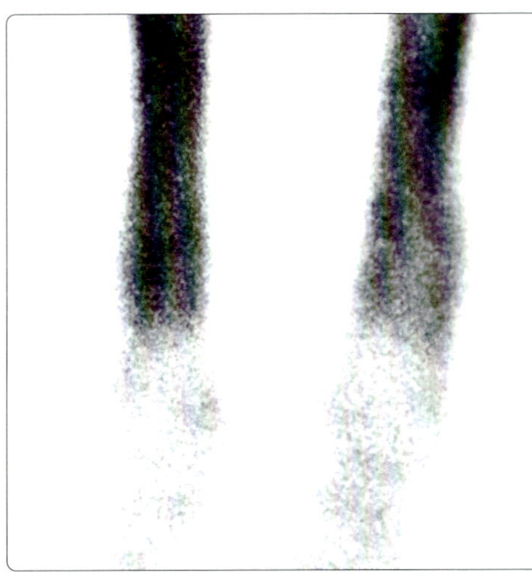

(Left) *Frontal Tc-99m bone scan of the knees in the same patient shows patchy, abnormal uptake along the diaphyses of the femora and tibiae.* **(Right)** *Frontal Tc-99m bone scan in the same patient shows more dense uptake in the distal tibia and fibula. The scan is typical of HOA. This patient had thickening of the skin over the dorsum of his hands as well as his forehead. The imaging and clinical appearance is typical of primary HOA or pachydermoperiostosis.*

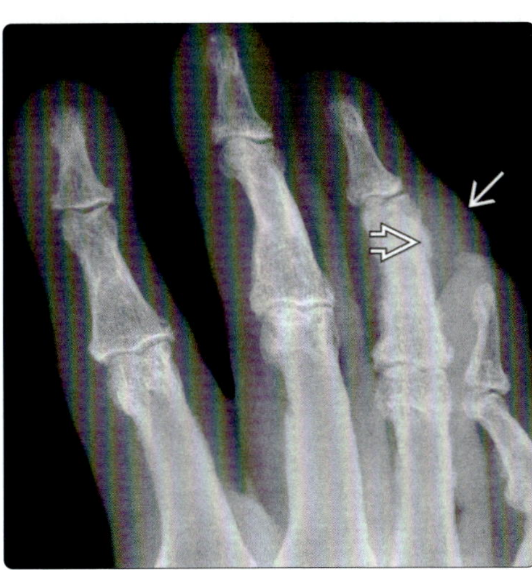

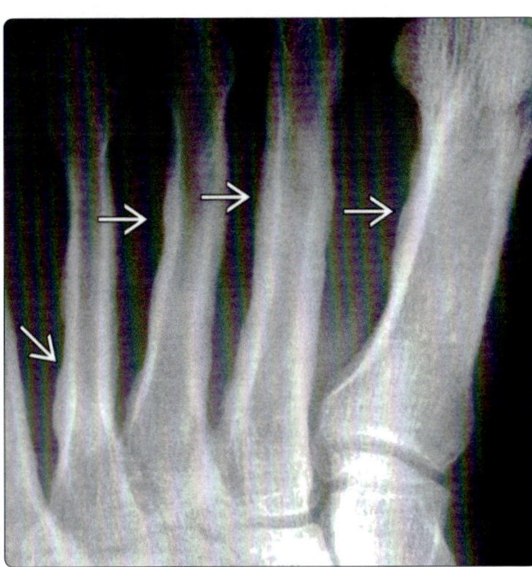

(Left) *Oblique radiograph of the hand demonstrates soft tissue swelling of the fingers ➡ as well as fluffy periostitis ➡. This patient has thyroid acropachy.* **(Right)** *Anteroposterior radiograph shows dense periosteal reaction along all the metatarsals ➡. This is typical of HOA. One most frequently follows this finding with a chest radiograph, since the most common etiology is lung cancer. However, tuberous sclerosis is a rare cause, as is seen in this case.*

Complex Regional Pain Syndrome

KEY FACTS

TERMINOLOGY

- Diffuse persistent pain, usually in extremity, often associated with
  - Vasomotor disturbances
  - Trophic changes
  - Limited range of motion or immobility of joints
- CRPS type 1: No detectable nerve lesion
  - Replaces term reflex sympathetic dystrophy (RSD)
- CRPS type 2: Detectable nerve lesion with resultant pain along distribution of nerve
  - Replaces term causalgia

IMAGING

- Radiographs may show diffuse regional osteoporosis
  - Subcortical changes may predominate
  - Trophic changes in soft tissues may be seen
  - In hand, may be osteoporotic along either ulnar or radial nerve distribution
- T1WI MR: Foci of low signal bone marrow edema
- Fluid-sensitive MR sequences
  - Patchy hyperintense bone marrow edema
  - Watch particularly for subcortical abnormalities
  - Skin thickening, soft tissue edema
- 3-phase bone scan
  - Generally ↑ uptake in blood flow, blood pool, and uptake phases

CLINICAL ISSUES

- 50% still have pain after 2 years
- High intensity on bone scan suggests better prognosis and response to treatment

DIAGNOSTIC CHECKLIST

- Consider: Early bone scan to make early diagnosis, which may respond to therapy
- MR is generally regional examination; be certain abnormality is focal before diagnosing it as CRPS
  - Do not miss diffuse infiltrating disease process

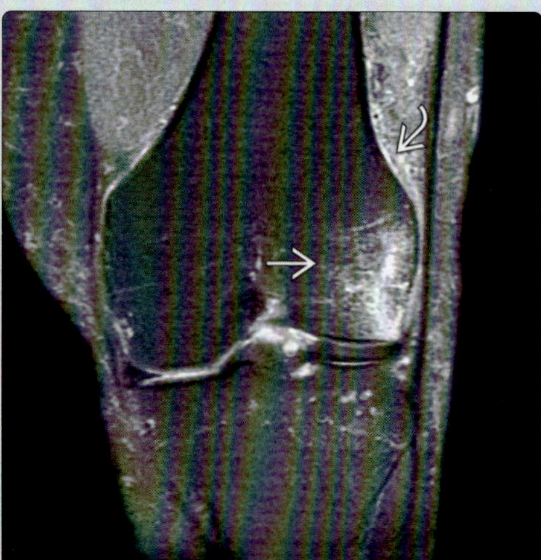

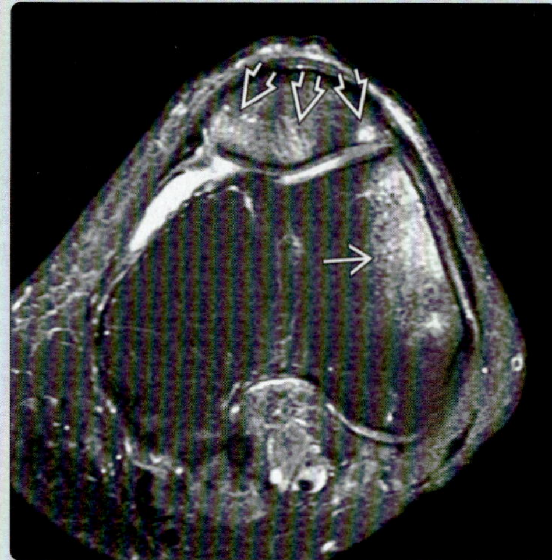

(Left) *Coronal T2WI FS MR demonstrates complex regional pain syndrome (CRPS). Initial presentation shows edema in the lateral femoral condyle ➡. There is also mild edema in the soft tissues adjacent to the femoral condyle ➡.* **(Right)** *Axial T2WI FS MR in the same patient, also obtained at the time of presentation, confirms edema in the lateral condyle ➡. The patella also shows patchy high signal edema ➡. Note that the edema is located predominantly in a subchondral position.*

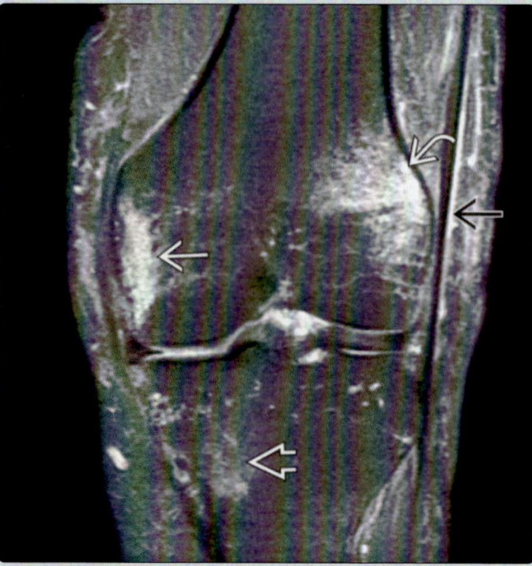

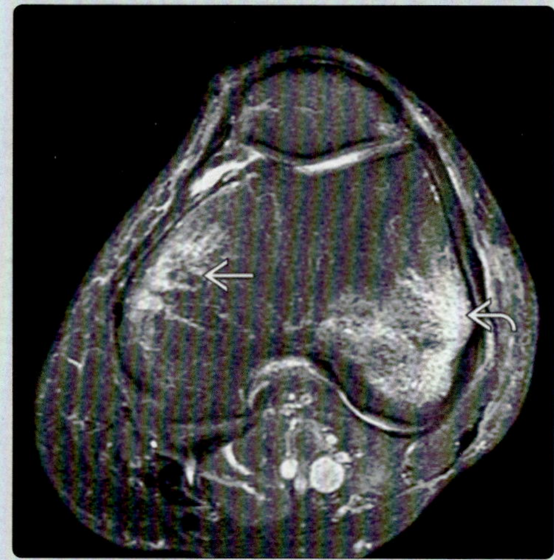

(Left) *Coronal T2WI FS MR shows the same patient approximately 3.5 months later. The knee was still painful, but the edema pattern has changed: The lateral femoral condyle shows a different pattern of edema ➡, and there is new edema in the medial femoral condyle ➡ and tibia ➡. Soft tissue edema is noted along the iliotibial band ➡.* **(Right)** *Axial T2WI FS MR in the same patient at the same time shows the medial ➡ and lateral ➡ femoral condylar marrow edema; edema in the patella has cleared.*

TERMINOLOGY

Abbreviations

- Complex regional pain syndrome (CRPS)

Synonyms

- Reflex sympathetic dystrophy (RSD); shoulder-hand syndrome; Sudeck atrophy, algodystrophy, causalgia

Definitions

- Diffuse persistent pain, usually in extremity; often associated with
  - Vasomotor disturbances
  - Trophic changes
  - Limited range of motion or immobility of joints
- Likely neurologic disorder affecting vascular system and pain receptors
  - CRPS type 1: No detectable nerve lesion
    - Replaces term reflex sympathetic dystrophy (RSD)
  - CRPS type 2: Detectable nerve lesion with resultant pain along distribution of nerve
    - Replaces term causalgia

IMAGING

General Features

- Best diagnostic clue
  - Bone scan: ↑ periarticular activity, particularly distally
  - MR: Patchy marrow edema, soft tissue edema
- Location
  - Usually unilateral (25% bilateral)
  - Upper extremity > lower extremity
    - Exception: In children, lower extremity predominates (5:1)
  - Entire hand/foot, or follows ulnar or radial nerve distribution in hand

Imaging Recommendations

- Best imaging tool
  - Bone scan 80% sensitive and specific overall
    - Sensitivity: 25% stage 1, 85% stage 2, 95% stage 3
  - MR may show soft tissue edema in stage 1; nonspecific
    - Marrow abnormalities seen in stage 2 may be more specific
      - Must identify as regional to increase specificity
  - Comparison study shows poor sensitivity and specificity of both bone scan & MR for early disease
- Protocol advice
  - Compare contralateral side
  - If injecting radionuclide or contrast, inject lower extremity if evaluating upper extremities and vice versa

Radiographic Findings

- Most frequently normal in early disease
- May show diffuse regional osteoporosis
  - Subcortical changes may predominate
  - If severe, cortical tunneling
- In hand, may be osteoporotic along either ulnar or radial nerve distribution
- Trophic changes in soft tissues may be seen (swelling or thinning)

CT Findings

- Bone CT
  - Osteopenia; nonspecific

MR Findings

- T1WI: Foci of low signal bone marrow edema
  - May be diffuse, but watch for subcortical foci
- Fluid-sensitive sequences
  - Patchy hyperintense bone marrow edema
    - Watch particularly for subcortical abnormalities
  - Skin changes
    - Skin thickening, soft tissue edema
    - Skin thinning is late change
  - End stage: Muscle atrophy

Nuclear Medicine Findings

- 3-phase bone scan shows asymmetry in all 3 phases
  - Generally ↑ uptake in blood flow, blood pool, and uptake phases
    - Blood flow may rarely be ↓ due to vasoconstriction; generally in children
  - ↑ periarticular activity distally

DIFFERENTIAL DIAGNOSIS

Senile Osteoporosis

- Generally more diffuse than CRPS
- Regional migratory osteoporosis may be focal; large joints predominate

Disuse Osteoporosis

- Posttraumatic, stroke
- Bone scan early in process shows more prominent ↑ in uptake proximally rather than distally
- Bone scan shows ↓ uptake in chronic disease

Diffuse Marrow Infiltration

- No focal MR abnormality
- May initially present as patchy marrow abnormality without focal lesions
- Patchy marrow is particularly common following treatment of diffuse process, such as multiple myeloma

Normal Patchy Marrow

- Red marrow is replaced in specific order of osseous structures, but may appear patchy in any instance
- Anemia, smoking, various medications may affect distribution and amount of red marrow
- Appears as generalized process

PATHOLOGY

General Features

- Etiology
  - Pathogenesis is obscure
    - Idiopathic in 25-35%
    - Altered morphology noted in prefrontal cortex that may be related to CRPS
    - Antineuronal antibodies may be implicated in a subset of patients
  - Associated processes
    - Trauma
      - Soft tissue injury caused 40% of CRPS in 1 study

- ◻ Fracture (especially Colles) caused of 25% of CRPS in 1 study
  - Hemiplegia (prevalence of CRPS: 12-21%)
  - Arterial thrombosis
  - Peripheral nerve injury
  - Acute coronary artery disease (5-20% develop CRPS)
  - Painful rotator cuff lesions
  - Arthroscopy may predispose to CRPS in knee
  - Herpes zoster with postherpetic neuralgia
  - Spinal cord disorders
- May be disorder of pain signaling & regulation, & persisting neural injury generating pain signals
- Central mechanisms of neuronal hyperresponsivity may be factor
- Regional cortical brain atrophy with altered connectivity is being investigated as etiology

- Genetics
  - HLA-A3, HLA-B7, HLA-DR2(15) implicated
  - HLA-DR2(15) associated with poor treatment response
- Associated abnormalities
  - Emotional disturbances
  - Fibromyalgia
  - Sleep disorders

Staging, Grading, & Classification

- Stage 1: Aching, throbbing, burning pain; cold and touch intolerance; swelling
  - Bone scan usually normal
- Stage 2: Muscle wasting, ↑ pain, vasomotor disturbances, soft tissue edema
- Stage 3: Contracture, ↓ range of motion, waxy skin, ridged nails, ↓ pain

Gross Pathologic & Surgical Features

- Affected bone is hyperemic with patchy osteoporosis
- Synovial proliferation and inflammation
- Thickened, waxy skin
- Hair loss
- Muscle atrophy

Microscopic Features

- Mast cells, neutrophils, macrophages
- Inflammatory cytokines

CLINICAL ISSUES

Presentation

- Most common signs/symptoms
  - Constant, burning, severe pain
  - Swelling, trophic skin changes
  - Signs of vasomotor instability (Raynaud phenomenon, temperature, sweating variation)
  - Pitting or nonpitting edema
  - Exquisite tenderness to light touch
- Other signs/symptoms
  - Tremor, incoordination, weakness, sensory changes

Demographics

- Age
  - 40-60 years most common
  - In children, peripuberty is most common age
- Gender
  - Slight female preponderance
- Ethnicity
  - May be more common in Caucasians

Natural History & Prognosis

- 3 overlapping stages of CRPS
  - Acute stage (3-6 months)
    - Intense limb pain, tenderness, swelling, vasomotor disturbances
  - Subacute stage (6-12 months)
    - Acute symptoms at least partially resolve, while atrophic changes in skin evolve; chronic aching or burning pain
    - Skin dry, may be edematous or develop brawny thickening
  - Atrophic stage
    - Skin and subcutaneous atrophy
    - Contractures
- 50% still have pain after 2 years
- High intensity on bone scan suggests better prognosis and response to treatment

Treatment

- Adults
  - Treat underlying abnormality
  - Analgesia, local heat, ice
  - Physical therapy
  - Stress loading and desensitization programs
  - Prednisone may be useful early in disease
  - Nerve manipulation
    - Sympathetic nerve blocks
    - Transcutaneous electrical nerve stimulation (TENS)
    - Spinal cord stimulation
- Children
  - Good initial response to physical therapy (90% cure rate without medications)
  - Recurrence rate of 30-50% suggests significantly lower long-term cure rate

DIAGNOSTIC CHECKLIST

Consider

- Early bone scan to make early diagnosis, which may respond to therapy
- High intensity on bone scan predictive of good response to early therapy

Image Interpretation Pearls

- MR is generally regional examination; be certain abnormality is focal before diagnosing as CRPS
  - Do not miss diffuse infiltrating disease process

SELECTED REFERENCES

1. Birklein F et al: Complex regional pain syndrome-significant progress in understanding. Pain. 156 Suppl 1:S94-S103, 2015
2. Dirckx M et al: The prevalence of autoantibodies in complex regional pain syndrome type I. Mediators Inflamm. 2015:718201, 2015
3. Lee DH et al: Brain alterations and neurocognitive dysfunction in patients with complex regional pain syndrome. J Pain. ePub, 2015
4. Bove GM: Focal nerve inflammation induces neuronal signs consistent with symptoms of early complex regional pain syndromes. Exp Neurol. 219(1):223-7, 2009
5. Nishida Y et al: Skeletal muscle MRI in complex regional pain syndrome. Intern Med. 48(4):209-12, 2009

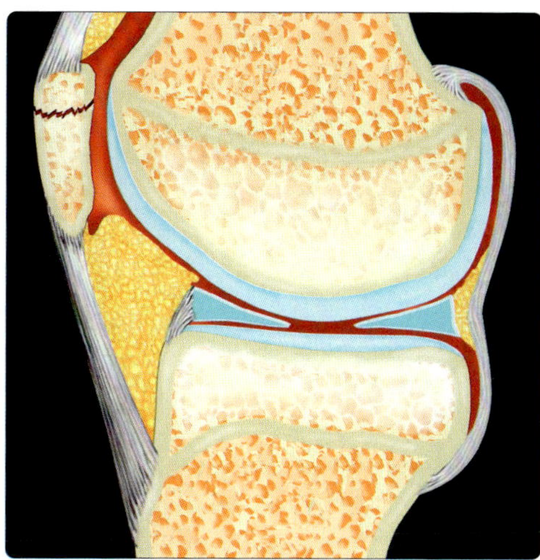

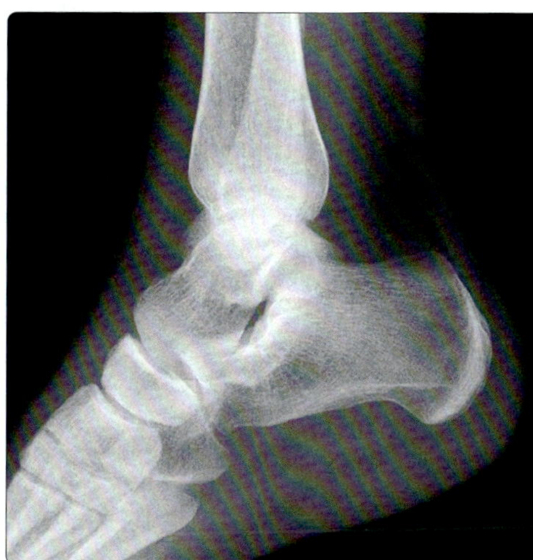

(Left) *Sagittal graphic shows a patellar fracture depicted as the etiology of CRPS. The edema is shown as an ivory-colored subchondral abnormality obscuring the normal trabeculation in the subchondral region of the patella, femoral condyle, and tibial plateau.* **(Right)** *Lateral radiograph of the ankle, obtained at the time of minor twisting injury, shows the osseous structures to be normal. The bone density is also normal in this young individual.*

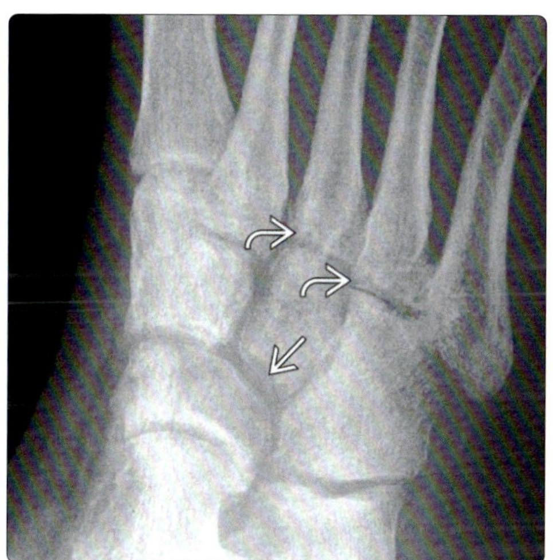

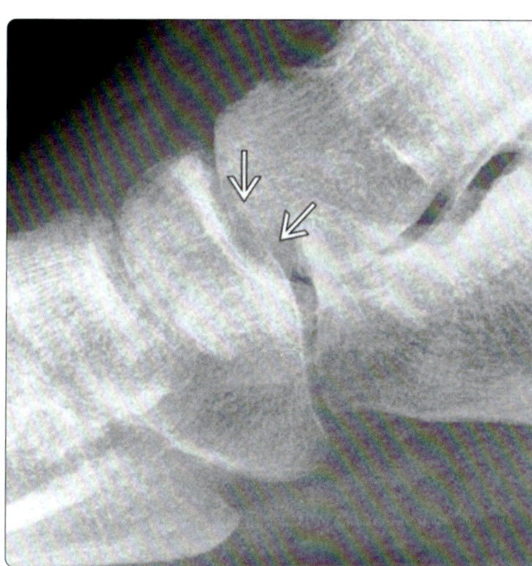

(Left) *Oblique radiograph in the same patient 3 months later, after pain had worsened significantly, reveals a subtle pattern of osteoporosis. Note the subchondral lucency at the metatarsal bases in a spotted pattern ➡ as well as in the lateral cuneiform ➡.* **(Right)** *Lateral radiograph in the same patient shows a similar subchondral spotty appearance in the talar head ➡ This patchy subchondral osteoporosis is one of the earliest radiographic changes that can be identified in patients with CRPS.*

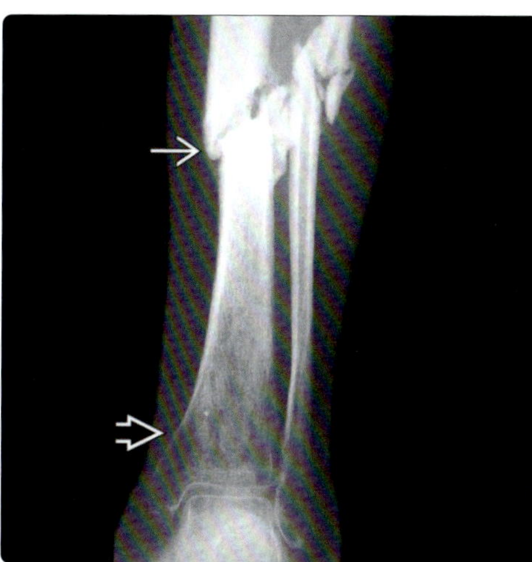

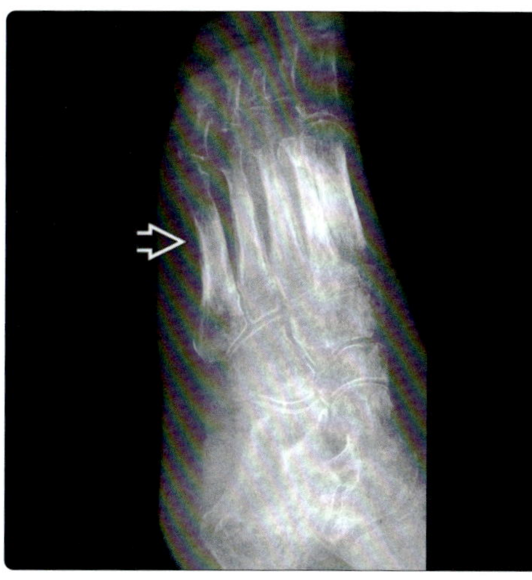

(Left) *Anteroposterior radiograph shows atrophic nonunion of both leg bones ➡. Note that there is no bridging bone, no significant callus, & sclerotic rounding of the edges at the fracture site. The bone density is normal at the site of the fracture. However, distal to the fracture there is severe osteoporosis seen as a moth-eaten permeative pattern of bone with cortical tunneling ➡.* **(Right)** *Oblique radiograph of the same extremity shows osteoporosis with cortical tunneling ➡ representing CRPS.*

(Left) *Anteroposterior radiograph shows an inferior shoulder dislocation known as luxatio erecta ➡. The shoulder was reduced.* **(Right)** *Posteroanterior radiograph of the wrist in the same patient taken 4 weeks later, despite normal and painless function of the shoulder, shows severe osteopenia, not typical of a patient of her age. Patient had complained of worsening pain of the forearm and hand. The diagnosis of complex regional pain syndrome (CRPS) must be considered related to the trauma.*

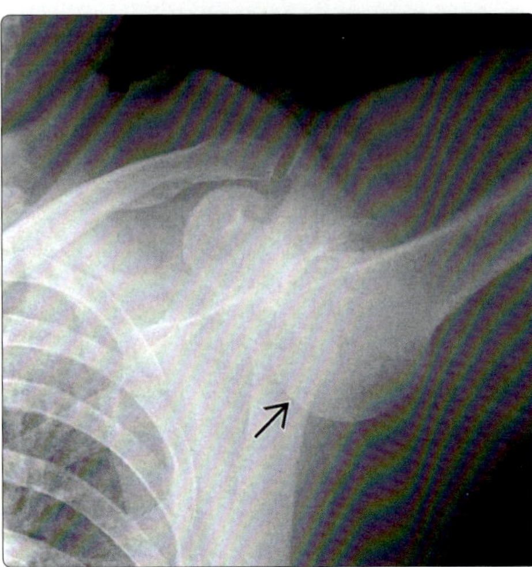

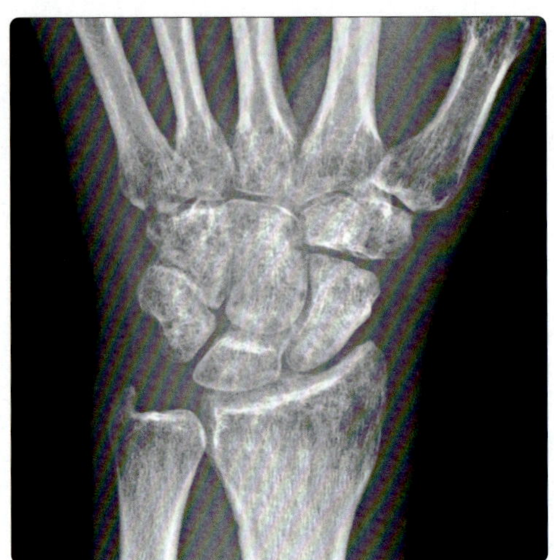

(Left) *Coronal STIR MR in the same patient shows thickening of the posterior cord of the brachial plexus ➡. This, in combination with the history of luxatio erecta, indicates a stretch injury of the nerve. In a patient with documented nerve injury, this represents a case of type 2 CRPS, previously termed "causalgia."* **(Right)** *PA radiograph obtained 2 months following trauma shows an unusual pattern of CRPS following the distribution of the ulnar nerve ➡; the remaining bones are not osteoporotic.*

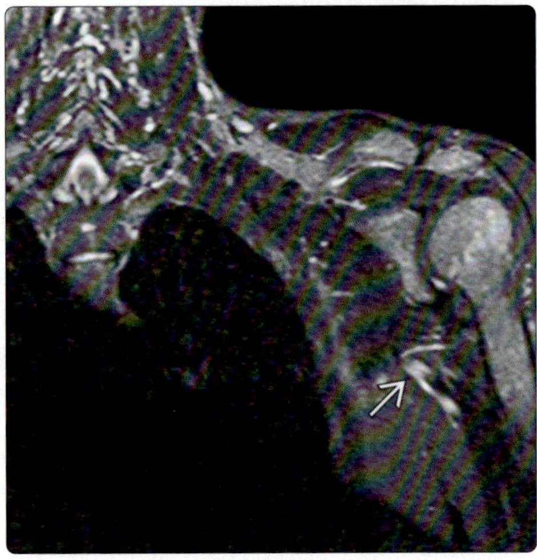

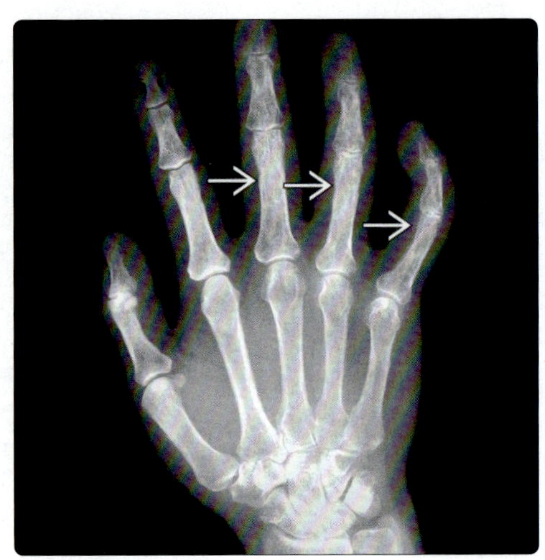

(Left) *Coronal T2WI FS MR in a patient with severe knee pain shows patchy areas of marrow edema ➡. Additionally, there is soft tissue edema along the metaphyseal periosteum ➡.* **(Right)** *Coronal T2WI FS MR in the same patient, slightly more posteriorly, again shows the patchy marrow edema ➡ and mild adjacent soft tissue edema ➡. There was no internal derangement; the patient had a history of mild knee trauma 3 months earlier. The patchy edema and history are diagnostic of CRPS.*

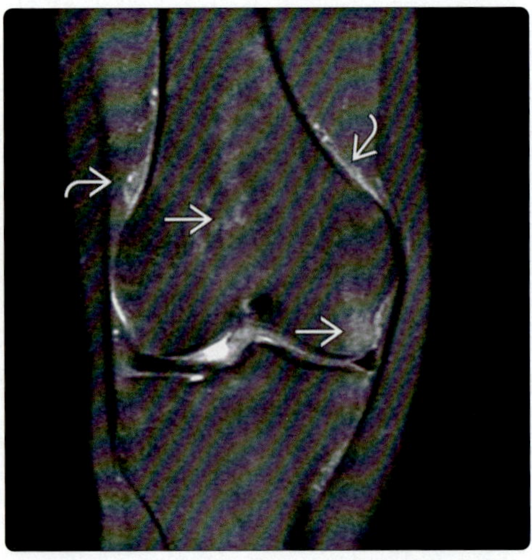

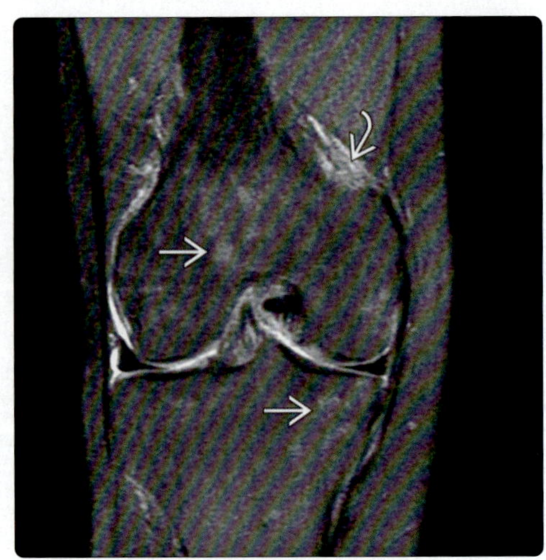

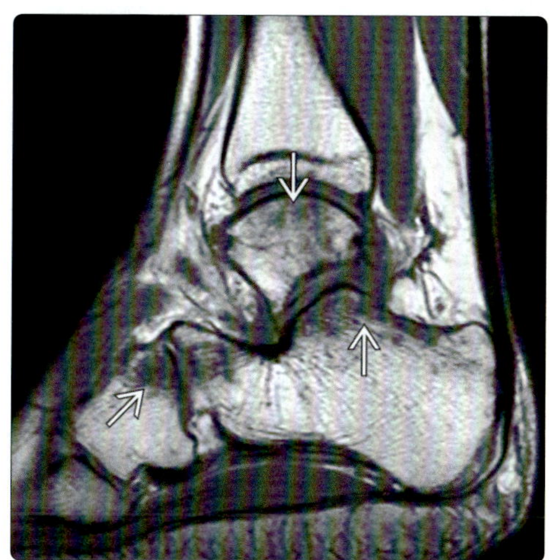

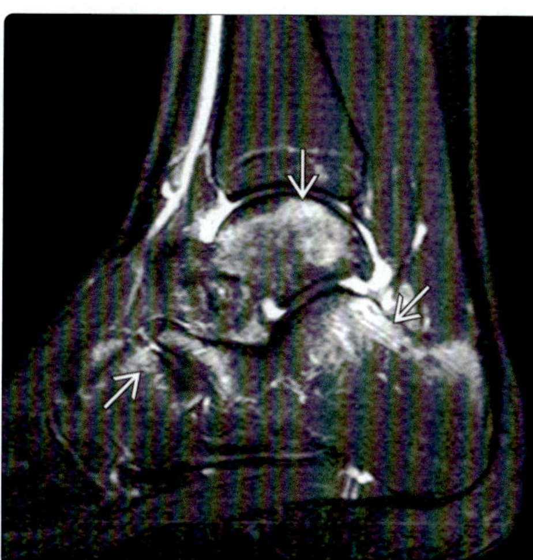

(Left) *Sagittal T1WI MR in a teenager with painful hindfoot several months following surgery for lateral instability shows multiple sites of low signal in the subcortical regions of multiple bones* ➔. *There is no linear low signal to suggest a fracture.* **(Right)** *Sagittal STIR MR in the same patient shows patchy high signal in the same subcortical regions* ➔. *This appearance, combined with the clinical scenario of painful foot in an athletic child following surgery, is typical of complex regional pain syndrome (CRPS).*

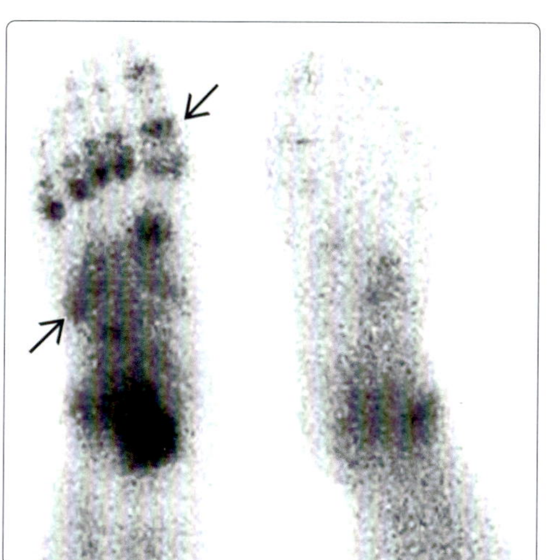

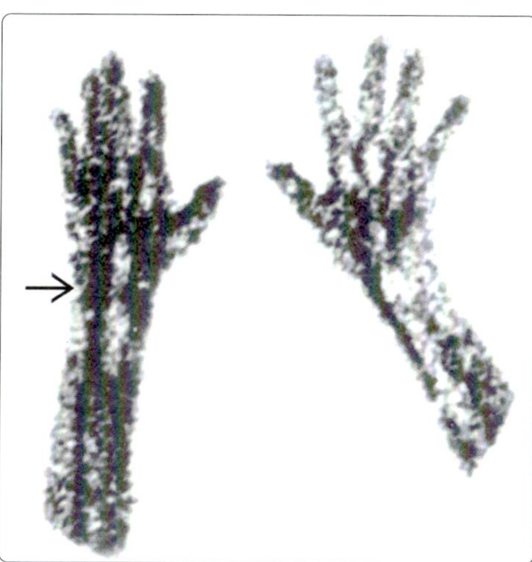

(Left) *Plantar bone scan of the feet in a patient with burning lower extremity pain after minor injury shows increased activity* → *in a periarticular distribution in the right foot, classic findings of CRPS. Note that the plantar image shows distal joints exceptionally well; attention to scanning technique is important when considering this diagnosis.* **(Right)** *Palmar angiographic phase bone scan in a patient with severe right hand pain shows increased blood flow* → *in the painful right upper extremity.*

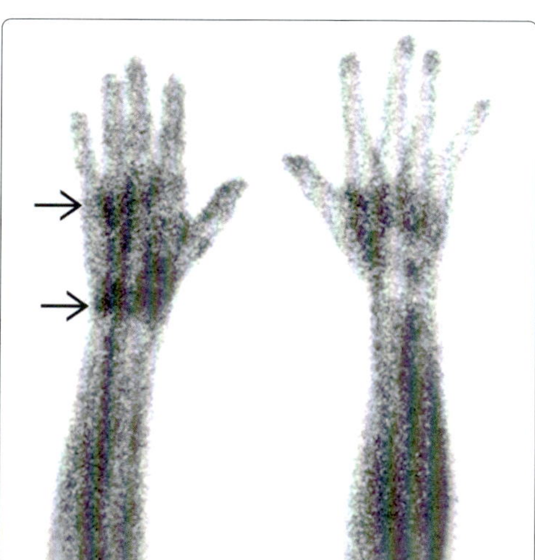

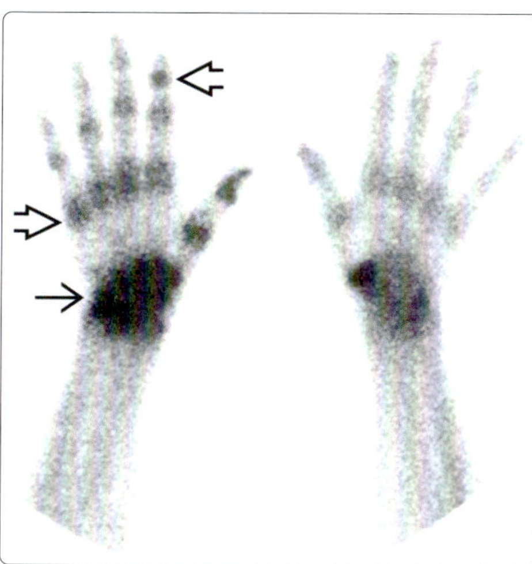

(Left) *Palmar blood pool phase bone scan in the same patient shows increased activity throughout the right upper extremity* → *compared to the left.* **(Right)** *Palmar delayed phase bone scan in the same patient shows increased activity in and around the joints of the right wrist* → *and hand* ⇨*, classic findings of CRPS. Such distinct periarticular activity, asymmetric in side-to-side comparison, is distinctive for this diagnosis. All 3 phases of bone scan are important.*

SECTION 2

Osseous Tumors and Tumor-Like Conditions

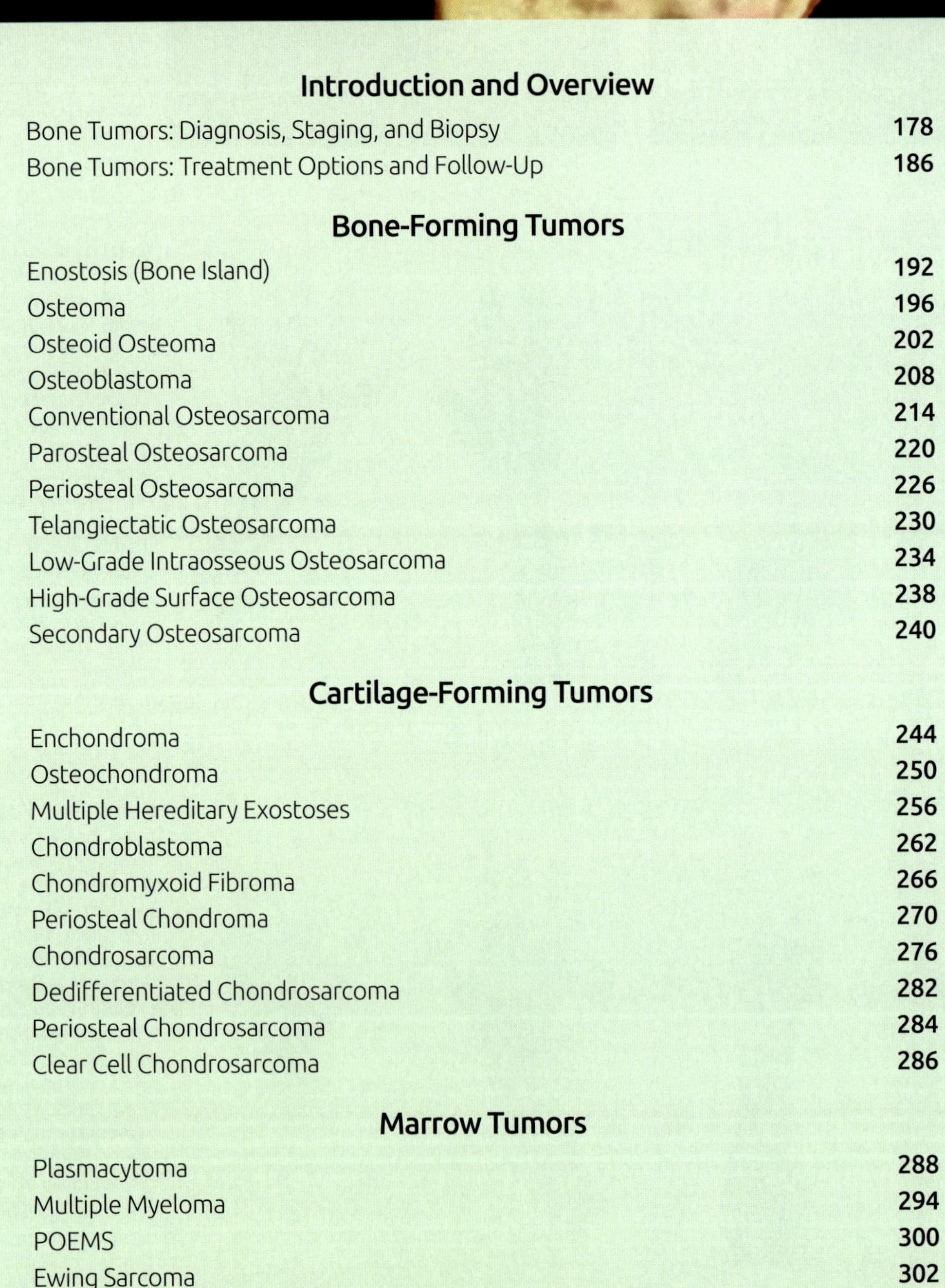

Introduction and Overview

Bone-Forming Tumors

Cartilage-Forming Tumors

Marrow Tumors

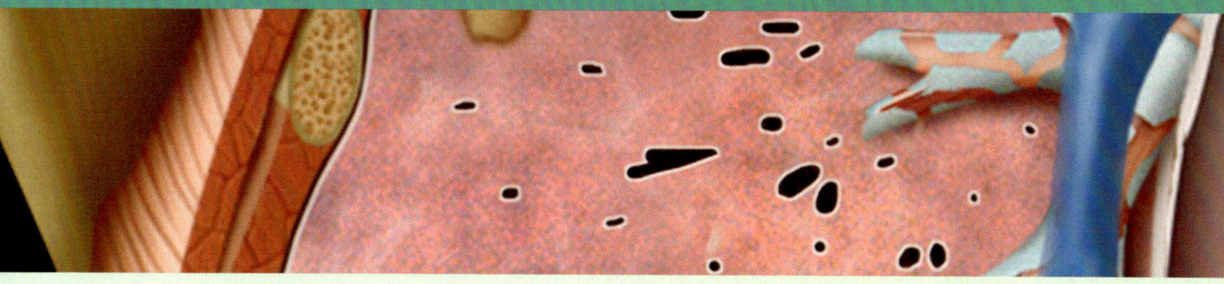

Other Osseous Tumors

Tumor-Like Conditions

Radiation-Induced Abnormalities

Introduction

Primary bone tumors are relatively uncommon, and malignant bone tumors are far less common than benign. The true incidence of benign bone tumors is difficult to estimate since the majority are asymptomatic and therefore are likely never discovered. The incidence of bone sarcoma is estimated to be 0.8/100,000 individuals; bone sarcomas occur 10x less frequently than soft tissue sarcomas. While some bone tumors or tumor-like lesions may be easily identified by radiographic characteristics, many require further imaging. Diagnosis, staging, and biopsy can be challenging and usually depend heavily on imaging.

When evaluating bone tumors, it is important to consider the relative incidence of the lesion. Enchondroma and nonossifying fibroma/benign fibrous cortical defect are the most frequent benign lesions, while metastatic tumor and multiple myeloma are the most common malignant lesions, followed by osteosarcoma, chondrosarcoma, and Ewing sarcoma.

There are also diseases associated with development of bone tumors; these underlying diseases may be known by clinical history or may be apparent on imaging studies. High-risk associations for development of sarcomas include enchondroma (particularly in Ollier and Mafucci disease, degenerating to chondrosarcoma), familial retinoblastoma syndrome (osteosarcoma), and Rothmund-Thompson syndrome (osteosarcoma). Moderate-risk associations include osteochondroma (chondrosarcoma), Paget disease (osteosarcoma and other sarcomas), and previous irradiation (osteosarcoma and other sarcomas). Low-risk associations include bone infarct (malignant fibrous histiocytoma), fibrous dysplasia (fibrosarcoma), chronic osteomyelitis, metallic and polyethylene implants, osteoblastoma, giant cell tumor, and chondroblastoma.

Differentiating Benign From Malignant Bone Tumors

There are a number of radiographic parameters that predict malignancy. These include

- Permeative (nongeographic) pattern
- Wide zone of transition from normal to abnormal
- Absence (or interruption) of sclerotic margin
- Aggressive periosteal reaction
- Cortical breakthrough with soft tissue mass

It must be remembered, however, that some malignant lesions may have a benign or a nonaggressive appearance on radiograph. Telangiectatic osteosarcoma often appears geographic, with a largely sclerotic margin. Chondrosarcoma usually is low grade in its initial presentation, often with a narrow zone of transition and sclerotic margin, and even endosteal thickening. This common lesion may be underdiagnosed, with disastrous results for the patient.

Conversely, some benign lesions may have a highly aggressive or malignant appearance. These include Langerhans cell histiocytosis, giant cell tumor, osteoblastoma, aneurysmal bone cyst, and osteomyelitis. Overdiagnosis of these lesions as malignant may result in unnecessary patient distress and even overtreatment.

MR has a high predictive value for malignancy. It has been observed that the presence of focal normal marrow signal within a tumor is highly suggestive of a benign tumor. Conversely, parameters to look for that suggest malignancy include necrosis and soft tissue mass with prominent enhancement. However, MR is not uniformly reliable in every case in differentiating benign and malignant lesions. For example, as with radiographs, differentiating benign enchondroma from low-grade chondrosarcoma remains challenging, as does recognizing an early aggressive case of Langerhans cell histiocytosis, which may present with soft tissue mass. The techniques of 3-T proton MR spectroscopy and diffusion-weighted MR imaging hold promise as noninvasive tools for characterizing lesions as malignant or benign but are not currently in general use.

Predicting Grade or Prognosis by Imaging

Radiographs or CT often provide the best assessment of biologic activity of an osseous lesion. The permeative nature of a lesion within bone is better appreciated on radiograph/CT than MR, as are a wide zone of transition and the nature of periosteal reaction (aggressive vs. nonaggressive). On the other hand, MR best demonstrates the soft tissue mass, with any necrosis and extension to various compartments, which may also be predictive of grade. Fluorine 18 FDG PET/CT predictive results are encouraging, particularly in FDG-avid lesions, such as Ewing sarcoma or osteosarcoma. There is a suggestion that both high lesion standard uptake value (SUV) and spatial heterogeneity may predict worse patient outcome. However, it must be remembered that many benign lesions show increased FDG uptake.

Predicting Histologic Type of Bone Tumors

Many parameters are used to assist in predicting histologic type of bone tumors. These include

- Tumor matrix: Production of osteoid, chondroid, &/or dystrophic calcification
- Location in flat or tubular bone, axial or appendicular skeleton, or particular bone (such as tibia, mandible)
- Location in epiphysis, metaphysis, or diaphysis
- Location in transverse plane (central, eccentric, cortical, or surface)
- Monostotic vs. polyostotic lesion
- Age of patient
- MR signal characteristics

Once it has been established whether the lesion is aggressive or nonaggressive, utilization of these parameters often results in the correct histologic diagnosis, or at least a limited list of differential considerations.

Staging of Bone Tumors

The AJCC system is the most frequently used for staging malignant bone tumors. Tumor size (T), which is moderately related to prognosis, differentiates the A and B subsets of stages I and II. MR is required for evaluation of tumor size, which may be underestimated by radiograph if the lesion is permeative. Histologic grade (G) of lesion defines the difference between stage I and stage II. Obtaining the correct histologic grade of the lesion is strongly associated with imaging; contrast-enhanced MR demonstrates areas where the lesion is most active and from which the biopsy should be obtained in order to be certain that one is evaluating representative tissue.

"Skip metastases" (2nd lesion within the same bone or immediately adjacent bone) elevate a high-grade lesion to stage III. Evaluation for skip metastases is made by MR; osteosarcoma is particularly at risk for such lesions, and at least one MR sequence of the entire length of bone must be obtained when evaluating such a tumor.

Regional lymph node involvement (N) elevates the lesion to stage IV; it is evaluated by MR or CT. The presence of metastases (M) also elevates the lesion to stage IV. Metastases from bone tumors most frequently involve the lung, with the 2nd most common site being other bones. Lung metastases are evaluated by CT. Osseous metastases may not be actively sought unless there are clinical signs of pain in another bone. However, for lesions that most frequently metastasize to other bones (Ewing sarcoma, osteosarcoma, chondrosarcoma, fibrosarcoma), bone scan or FDG PET/CT may be utilized. It should be noted that, for at least some histologic types of bone sarcomas, the combination of PET/CT and conventional imaging increases accuracy in preoperative tumor staging.

The Musculoskeletal Tumor Society (MSTS) surgical staging system may be preferred by some orthopedic oncologists. The largest difference between this and the AJCC system is in the primary tumor (T) definition. Rather than tumor size, this system emphasizes tumor encapsulation (the reactive tissue that rims tumor tissue) and whether it extends beyond its compartment of origin. The compartments are strictly defined. Additionally, the MSTS system addresses adjacency or involvement of tumor with the neurovascular bundle. Cross-sectional imaging, usually MR, is used for this site evaluation. Whether or not this system is officially utilized by the orthopedic oncologist, all elements of this system (neurovascular bundle and specific muscle/compartment involvement) must be included in any imaging report. These elements help reflect the prognosis for the patient and are used to plan the surgical resection.

Restaging of Bone Tumors

Conventional osteosarcomas, as well as several other high-grade sarcomas, are treated with preoperative chemotherapy. The objectives of this therapy include shrinkage of the tumor from the surrounding soft tissues, making limb salvage more feasible, and control of micrometastases in other tissues. Additionally, preoperative chemotherapy allows evaluation of the effectiveness of the chemotherapy regimen by assessing the degree of tumor necrosis.

Restaging is required in these patients prior to definitive surgery. The restaging includes chest CT to evaluate for lung metastases. It also includes MR in all 3 planes, with contrast administration. The size of the lesion in all dimensions must be evaluated. Description must include soft tissue involvement, including specific muscle and fascial plane violations, as well as compartment involvement. Neurovascular and joint involvement must be evaluated. Finally, it is mandatory to compare key images with the initial staging MR to evaluate the effectiveness of chemotherapy. This comparison must include evaluation of any change in size of the lesion, change in degree of necrosis, and mention of any tissues previously involved that now appear to be free of tumor.

It is important to recognize that osteosarcoma may paradoxically appear to enlarge on posttherapy imaging. As the tumor is treated, previously deposited tumor osteoid may begin to mature; as it does so, the new bone formation may appear both larger and more dense. However, it also appears better organized, which serves as the best hint that the bone is maturing rather than simply increasing in size and not responding to therapy. In these cases, watch for other signs of improvement, such as increased necrosis; size alone is not a dependable criterion.

In many instances, FDG PET/CT is included in restaging to evaluate for nodal, osseous, and other sites of distant metastasis. The comparative standardized uptake value may also correlate with chemotherapeutic response and prognosis.

Biopsy Considerations

Biopsy is performed both to make or confirm the histologic diagnosis and to establish the grade of the lesion if it is malignant. Biopsy may be performed percutaneously or open at surgery. In either case, cross-sectional imaging should be used to determine both the approach for the needle or open procedure and to determine the site of most representative tissue for sampling.

Several requirements must be taken into account when planning a needle biopsy. First, only a single soft tissue compartment should be crossed by the needle. This requires a full understanding of the compartmental anatomy of the limb in question. Second, major neurovascular bundles must be avoided. Third, it is imperative to avoid contaminating an adjacent joint. The most frequent error regarding an adjacent joint is made in biopsies around the knee. An anterior or lateral approach to a distal femoral lesion can easily pass through the suprapatellar recess. Remember that this recess is quite large, whether or not it is distended.

It is important to consult with the oncologic surgeon regarding the location he or she wants for the biopsy track, as the track must be resected at the time of definitive surgery. As a general rule, it is important to not track through tissue that will be needed for a functional limb salvage or through tissue that may be needed to cover a large resection. The most frequent error of this type is in approaching a lesion arising in the iliac wing. If a posterior (gluteal) approach is chosen, that tissue must be resected, which is undesirable in most cases. The preferred approach is anterior, either through the anterolateral iliac crest or, if necessary, through the iliacus.

Please note that these are general guidelines for biopsy planning. For a more comprehensive guide, outlined by site, please reference the tables in the excellent article authored by Liu et al.

Biopsy must include representative tissue in order to allow accurate histologic diagnosis and appropriate grading. The grading in turn affects the staging of the lesion. It is important to avoid biopsying necrotic tissue. MR with contrast demonstrates these nonenhancing regions; avoid them when biopsying a lesion. Conversely, do not biopsy dense tumor matrix or dense reactive bone. These lesions often do not contain enough active tissue to determine the grade of the lesion from a core biopsy. The most frequent error in this regard is aiming for sclerotic matrix in osteosarcoma or chondrosarcoma.

Primary bone tumors often require more tissue than is provided by fine-needle aspiration for evaluating both diagnosis and grade of lesion. It is important to have the pathologist in the room during a biopsy to evaluate the presence of tumor in the sample, as well as to determine whether there is enough tissue quantity for diagnosis. Generally, if the tumor is determined to be nonmetastatic, core needle biopsies should be obtained.

T, N, M, G Definitions for Staging of Primary Malignant Bone Tumor

TNM	Definitions
Primary Tumor (T)	
TX	Primary tumor cannot be assessed
T0	No evidence of primary tumor
T1	Tumor ≤ 8 cm in greatest dimension
T2	Tumor > 8 cm in greatest dimension
T3	Discontinuous tumors in primary bone site
Regional Lymph Nodes (N)	
NX	Regional lymph nodes cannot be assessed
N0	No regional lymph node metastasis
N1	Regional lymph node metastasis
Distant Metastasis (M)	
MX	Distant metastasis cannot be assessed
M0	No distant metastasis
M1	Distant metastasis
M1a	Lung metastasis
M1b	Distant site metastasis other than lung
Histologic Grade (G)	
GX	Grade cannot be assessed
G1	Well differentiated
G2	Moderately differentiated
G3	Poorly differentiated
G4	Undifferentiated; note that Ewing sarcoma is considered G4

AJCC Stage Grouping, Primary Malignant Bone Tumor

Stage	T	N	M	G
IA	T1	N0	M0	G1, 2 (low grade)
IB	T2	N0	M0	G1, 2 (low grade)
	T3	N0	M0	G1, 2 (low grade)
IIA	T1	N0	M0	G3, 4 (high grade)
IIB	T2	N0	M0	G3, 4 (high grade)
III	T3	N0	M0	G3, 4 (high grade)
IVA	Any T	N0	M1a	Any G
IVB	Any T	N1	Any M	Any G
	Any T	Any N	M1b	Any G

All stage I tumors are low grade and have not spread to regional lymph nodes or to other distant sites. All stage II tumors are high grade and have not spread to another site within the bone, to regional lymph nodes, or to other distant sites. Stage III tumors are high grade and have spread to another site within the bone of origin, or to the immediately adjacent bone, but have not spread to regional lymph nodes or to other distant sites. Stage IVA tumors have metastasized to the lung. They may be of any size and grade and have not spread to regional lymph nodes. Stage IVB tumors have spread to regional lymph nodes &/or metastasized to sites other than the lung. They may be of any size and grade. (Tables adapted from 7th edition AJCC Cancer Staging Forms.)

Selected References

1. Subhawong TK et al: Diffusion-weighted MR imaging for characterizing musculoskeletal lesions. Radiographics. 34(5):1163-77, 2014
2. Rakheja R et al: Necrosis on FDG PET/CT correlates with prognosis and mortality in sarcomas. AJR Am J Roentgenol. 201(1):170-7, 2013
3. Subhawong TK et al: Proton MR spectroscopy in metabolic assessment of musculoskeletal lesions. AJR Am J Roentgenol. 198(1):162-72, 2012
4. Omura MC et al: Revisiting CT-guided percutaneous core needle biopsy of musculoskeletal lesions: contributors to biopsy success. AJR Am J Roentgenol. 197(2):457-61, 2011
5. Costelloe CM et al: 18F-FDG PET/CT as an indicator of progression-free and overall survival in osteosarcoma. J Nucl Med. 50(3):340-7, 2009
6. Liu PT et al: Anatomically based guidelines for core needle biopsy of bone tumors: implications for limb-sparing surgery. Radiographics. 27(1):189-205; discussion 206, 2007

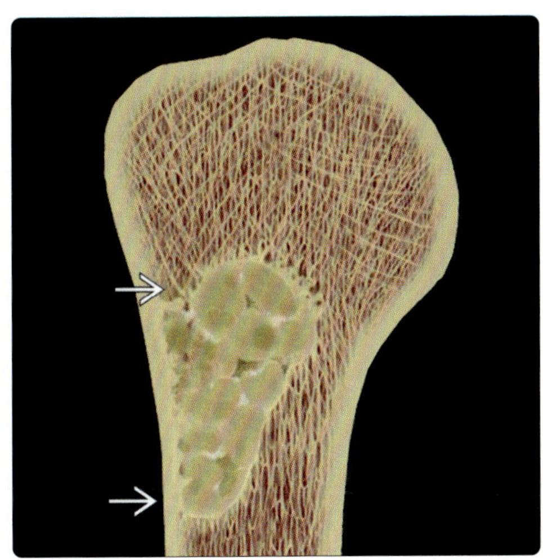

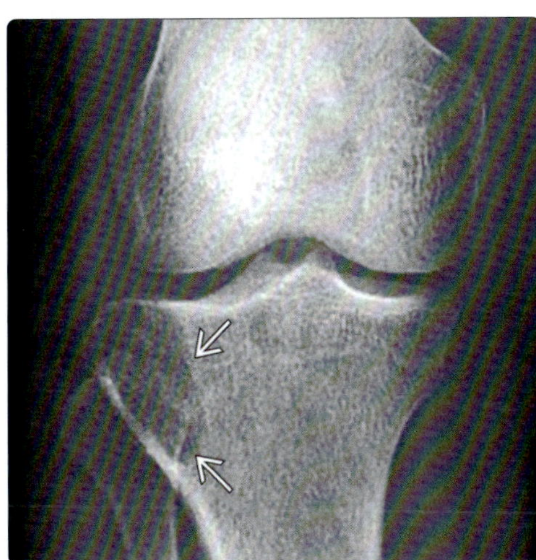

(Left) *Graphic depicts stage IA primary malignant bone tumor. For stage IA, the lesion is T1 (≤ 8 cm in greatest dimension)* ➡*, low grade (G1, 2), and has no nodal or other metastases (N0, M0).* **(Right)** *AP radiograph shows a lytic eccentric lesion with a narrow zone of transition* ➡ *measuring < 8 cm in greatest diameter (T1). There was no nodal involvement (N0) or metastatic disease (M0). The lesion proved to be G2 chondrosarcoma, which is considered low grade. Thus the stage is IA.*

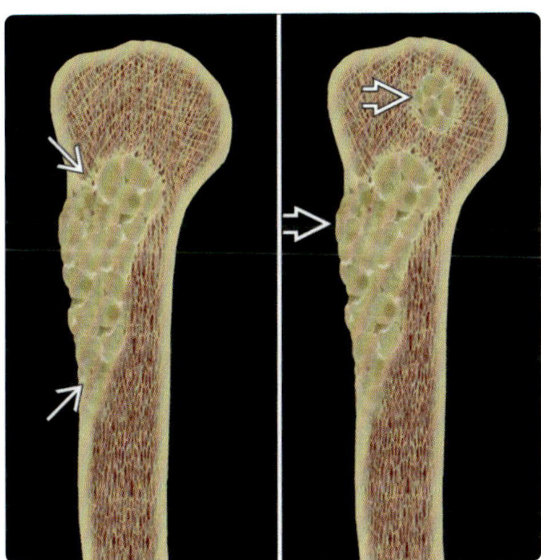

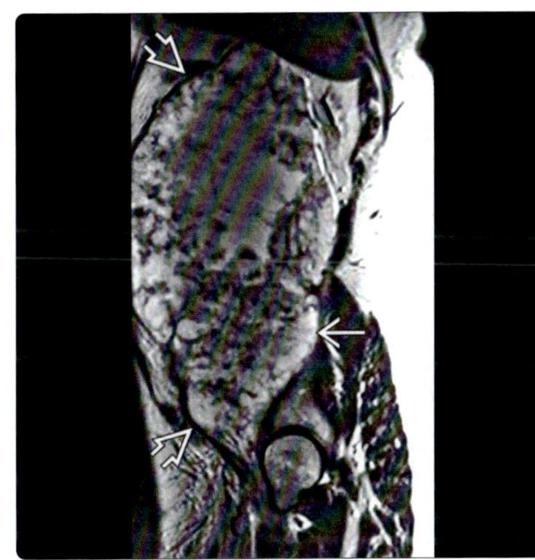

(Left) *Graphic depicts stage IB bone tumor. For stage IB, the lesion is either T2 (> 8 cm in greatest dimension)* ➡ *or T3 (discontinuous tumors in primary site)* ➡*. All are low grade (G1, 2) and N0, M0.* **(Right)** *Sagittal T2WI MR shows a huge lesion (T2)* ➡ *arising from the iliac wing* ➡*. This chondrosarcoma is low grade (G1) and had no nodal or metastatic involvement (N0, M0). Because of size and location, prognosis for wide resection is poor. Nonetheless, the AJCC classification is stage IB.*

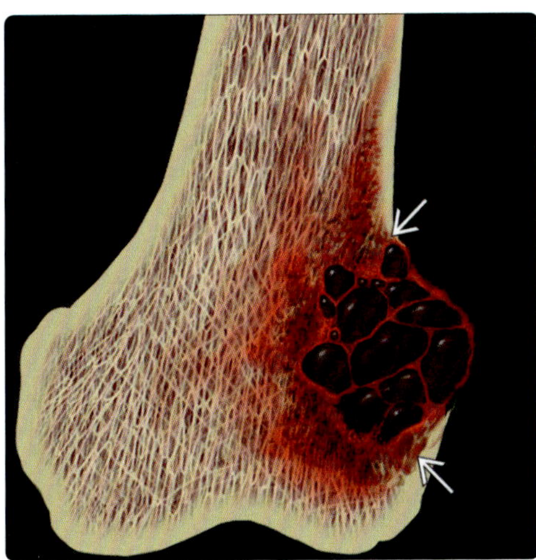

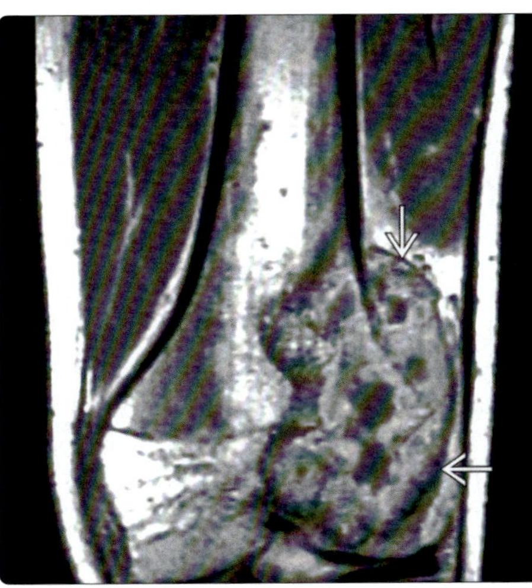

(Left) *Graphic depicts stage IIA primary malignant bone tumor. For stage IIA, the lesion is T1 (≤ 8 cm in greatest dimension)* ➡ *and high grade (G3, 4). No nodal or other metastases can be present (N0, M0).* **(Right)** *Coronal T1WI C+ MR shows a high-grade (G3) telangiectatic osteosarcoma with cortical breakthrough* ➡*. Since it is < 8 cm in greatest diameter (T1) and presented without nodal or metastatic involvement (N0, M0), it is stage IIA.*

(Left) *Graphic depicts stage IIB primary malignant bone tumor. For stage IIB, the lesion is T2 (> 8 cm) → and high grade (G3, 4). No nodal or other metastases can be present (N0, M0).* **(Right)** *Y view radiograph shows a radiation-induced osteosarcoma arising from the scapula →. The very large lesion (T2) was high grade (G4) at biopsy but had no nodes or metastases (N0, M0), making it stage IIB.*

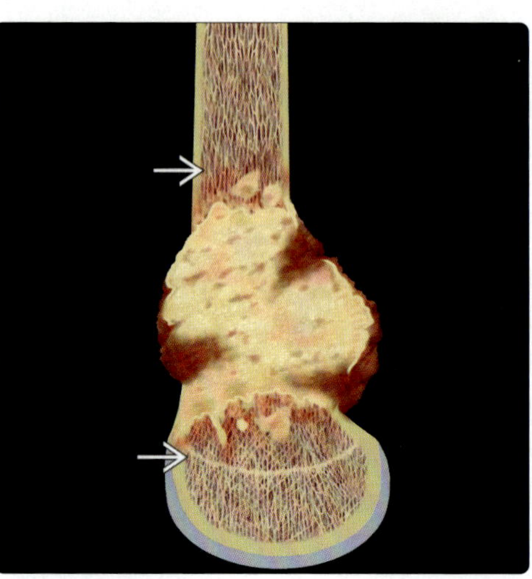

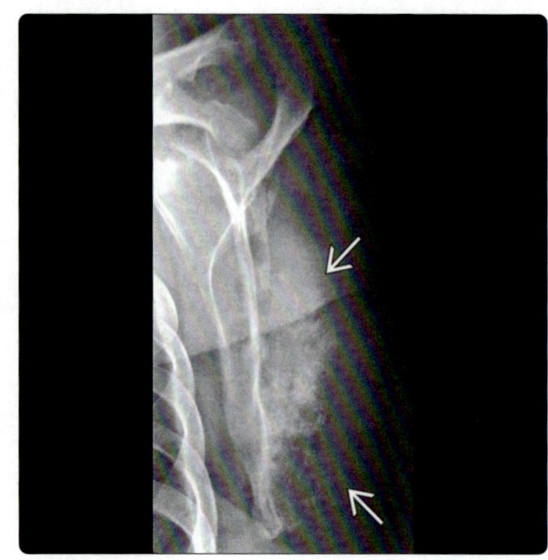

(Left) *Graphic depicts stage III primary malignant bone tumor. Stage III requires a T3 designation, defined as discontinuous tumors within the 1° site. These present as a larger 1° tumor ⇨ with nearby 2° tumor →, shown in this case within the same bone.* **(Right)** *Graphic depicts the 2nd type of stage III primary malignant bone tumor. The discontinuous tumors in this case present as a larger 1° tumor ⇨ with nearby 2° tumor →, in this case, in an immediately adjacent bone.*

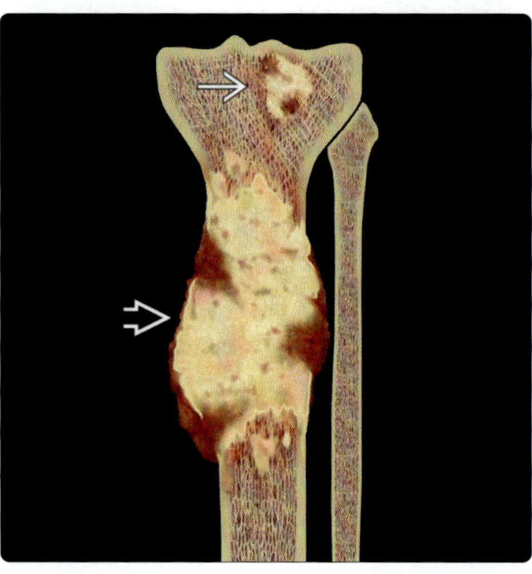

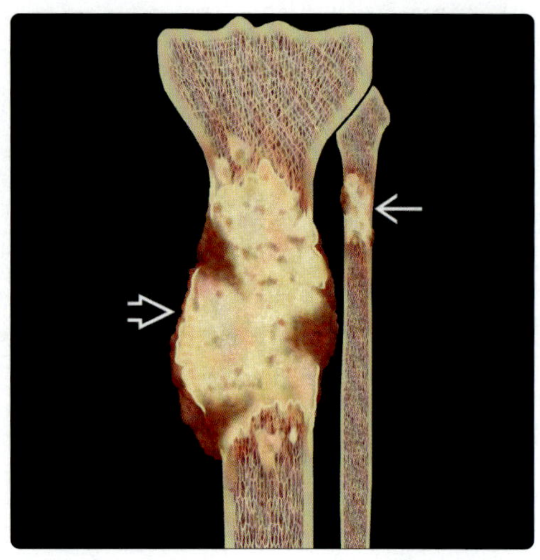

(Left) *Lateral radiograph shows an aggressive osteosarcoma of the fibula →, which proved to be high grade (G3). There were no nodal or distant metastases (N0, M0). By size, it might qualify as T1, and therefore be stage IIA. However, MR resulted in upgrading the staging.* **(Right)** *Coronal T1WI C+ FS MR in the same patient shows a large fibular lesion →. There is a small lesion in the tibia as well ↪, which had the same histology. This is a "skip metastasis," upgrading the lesion (T3, G3, N0, M0) to stage III.*

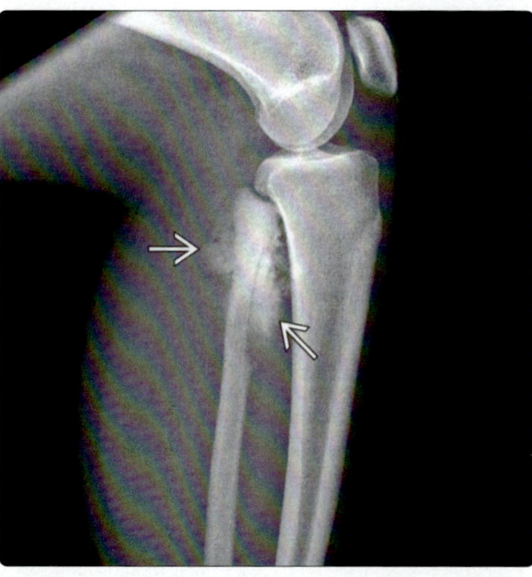

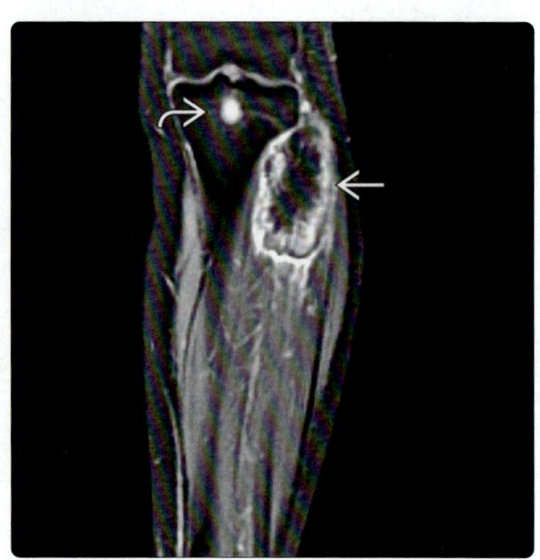

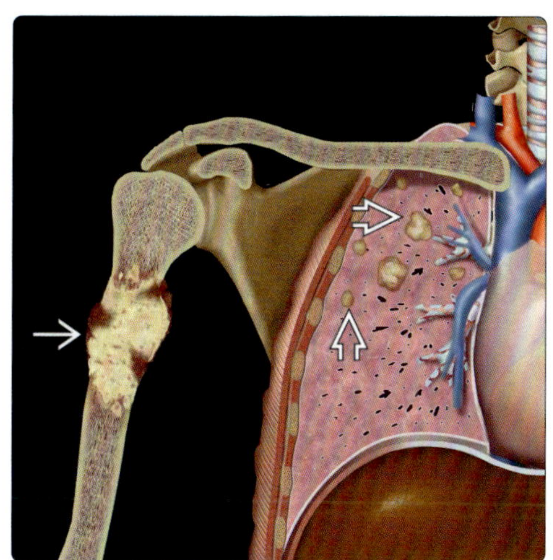

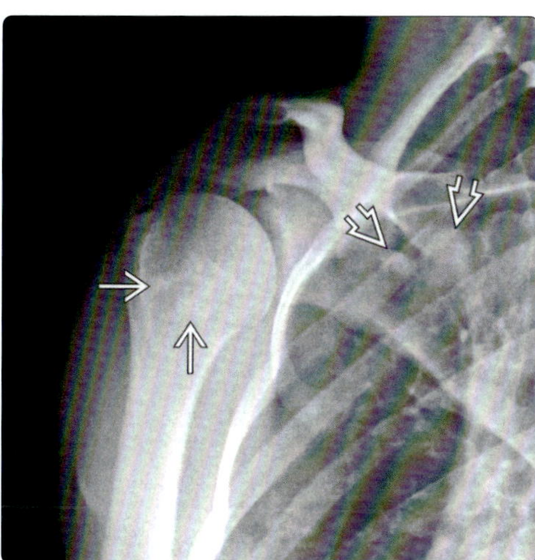

(Left) *Graphic depicts a stage IVA 1° malignant bone tumor. The 1° lesion is within the humerus ➡. It may be of any grade or size (G or T) but does not have regional lymph node involvement (N0). There are metastases within the lung (M1a) ➡ but not at other distant sites.* **(Right)** *AP radiograph shows a subtle sclerotic lesion ➡. This is a small lesion (T1) but proved to be a high-grade (G3) osteosarcoma. There were no involved nodes (N0), but the presence of lung metastases ➡ (M1a) increases the stage to IVA.*

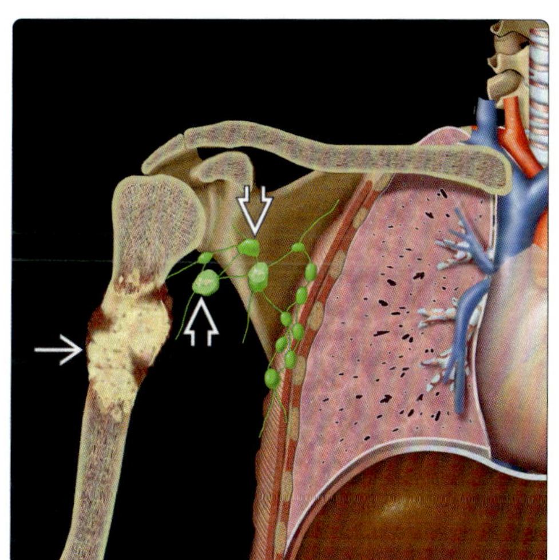

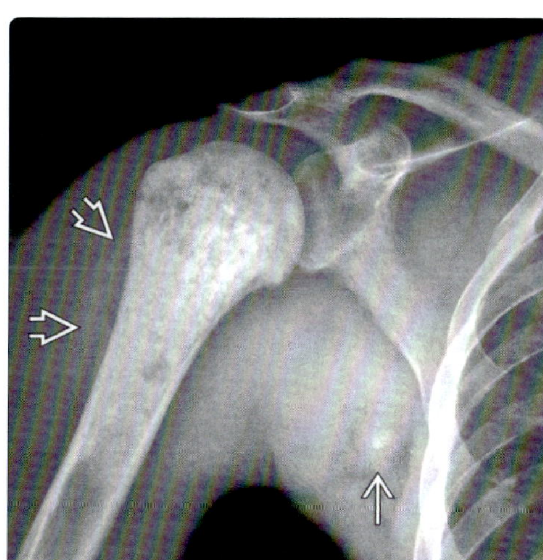

(Left) *Graphic depicts 1 type of stage IVB 1° malignant bone tumor. This 1° lesion is in the humerus ➡. It may be any size (T) or grade (G). There are regional axillary lymph nodes involved (N1) ➡. There may or may not be distant metastases at any site.* **(Right)** *AP radiograph shows a permeative sclerotic lesion (T2), with a faintly seen soft tissue mass ➡. This is diagnostic of osteosarcoma (G4). Note also the faint ossification of an axillary lymph node ➡ (N1). There were no other metastases; the lesion is stage IVB.*

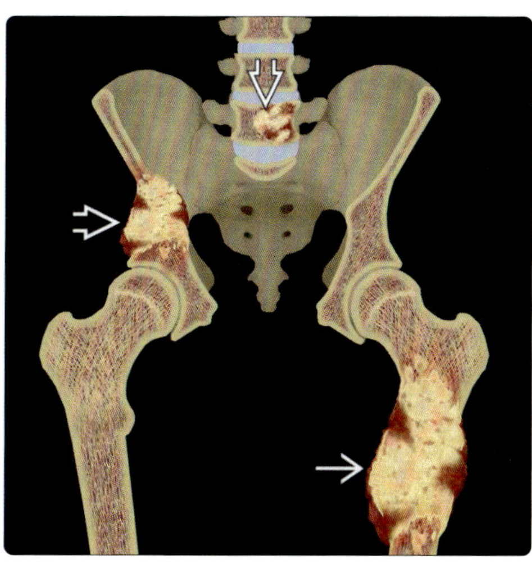

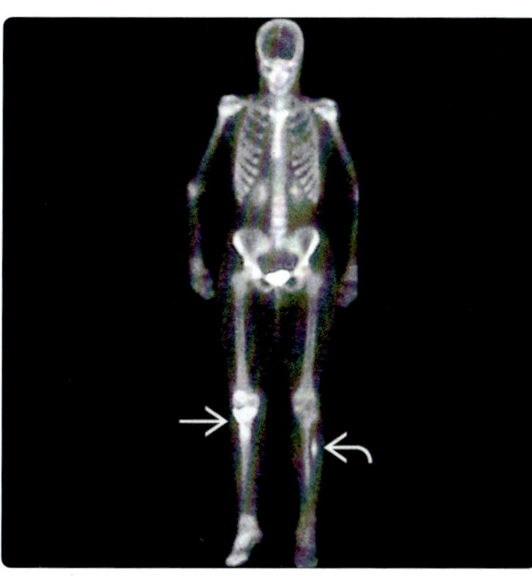

(Left) *Graphic depicts another type of stage IVB 1° malignant bone tumor. Here, the 1° tumor is in the left femur ➡. Lymph nodes may be N0 or N1. There is metastatic disease that involves any organ other than the lung; bone metastases are shown ➡.* **(Right)** *AP bone scan shows uptake at a 1° lesion known to be a small Ewing sarcoma (T1, G4) ➡. Lymph nodes are negative. Uptake is also present in the contralateral fibula ➡, which proved to be an osseous metastasis (M1b). This makes the lesion stage IVB.*

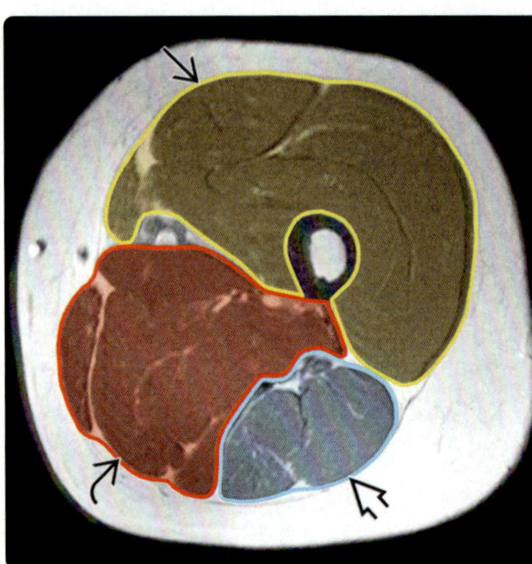

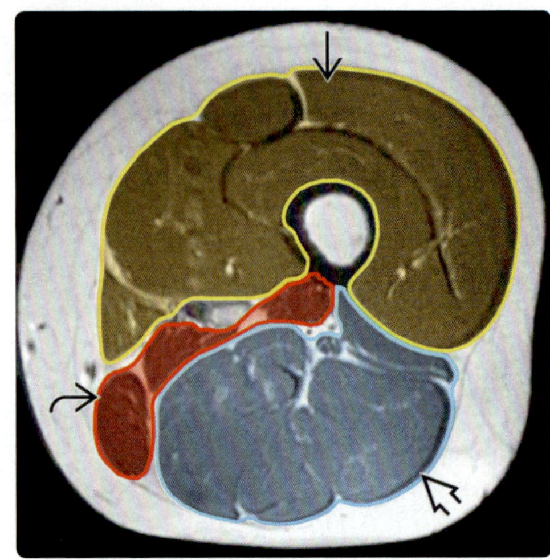

(Left) *Compartmental anatomy of thigh, for biopsy planning, is shown. T1WI MR shows proximal midthigh compartments for biopsy consideration: Anterior, posterior, and medial. Avoid rectus femoris and vastus intermedius; don't violate lateral intermuscular septum (between vastus and lateralis long head of biceps), sciatic nerve, or profunda femoris artery (posteromedial to lateral intermuscular septum).* **(Right)** *Image shows distal midthigh compartments: Anterior, posterior, and medial.*

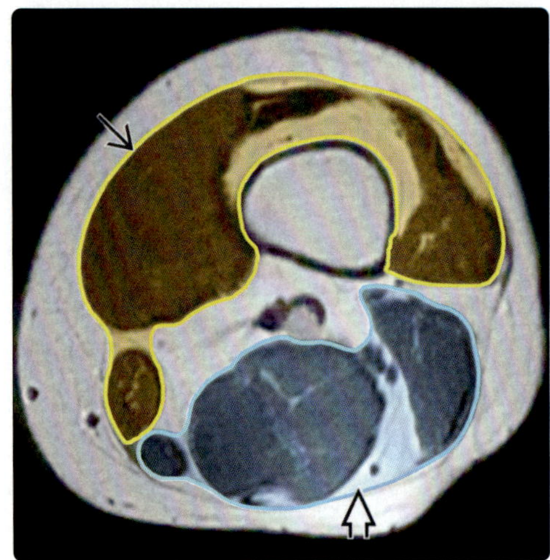

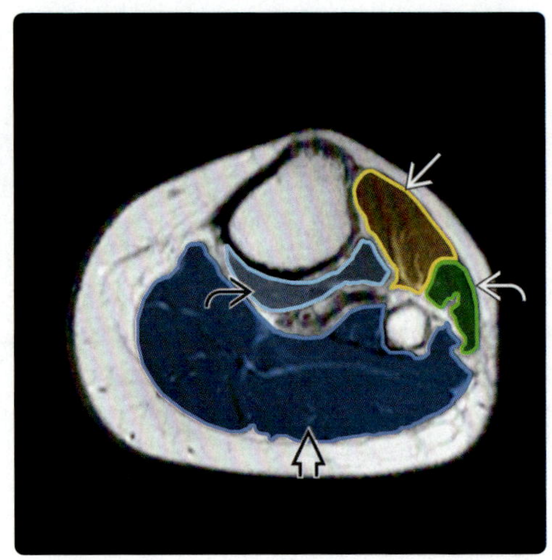

(Left) *Image maps distal thigh compartments: Anterior and posterior. Avoid superficial femoral neurovascular bundle-adductor canal, popliteal neurovascular bundle, and knee joint capsule (suprapatellar recess extends far proximal to femoral condyles).* **(Right)** *Image shows proximal leg compartments: Anterior, lateral, superficial posterior, and deep posterior. Avoid tibial tubercle, anterior, posterior tibial, and peroneal neurovascular bundles.*

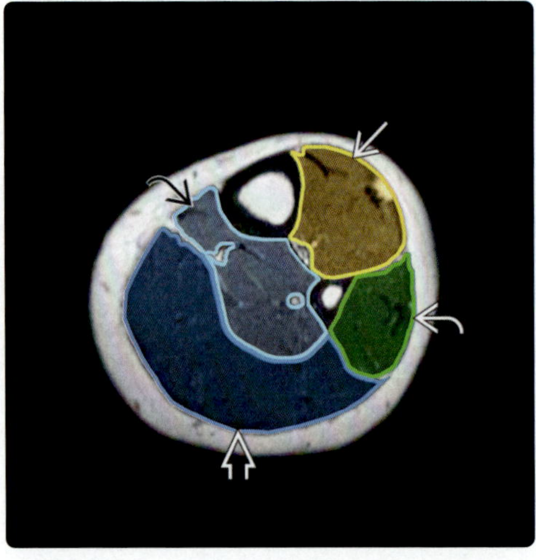

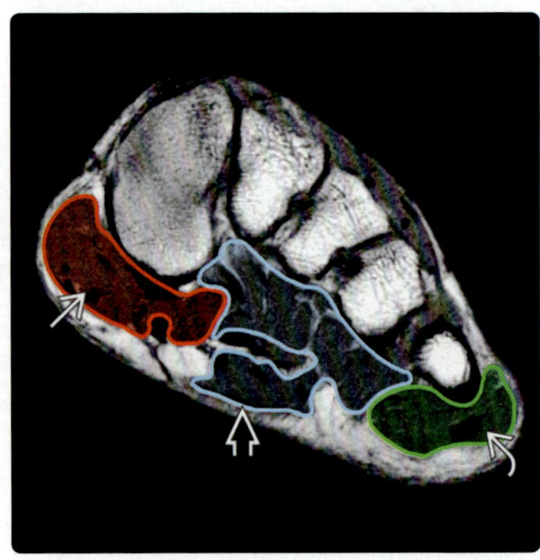

(Left) *Distal leg compartments are depicted: Anterior, lateral, superficial posterior, and deep posterior. Avoid anterior and posterior tibial and peroneal neurovascular bundles, deep peroneal nerve, and distally the peroneus brevis and longus tendons.* **(Right)** *Foot: Plantar aspect of the foot is divided into 3 compartments, the medial, lateral, and central. The dorsum of the foot and ankle are considered extracompartmental.*

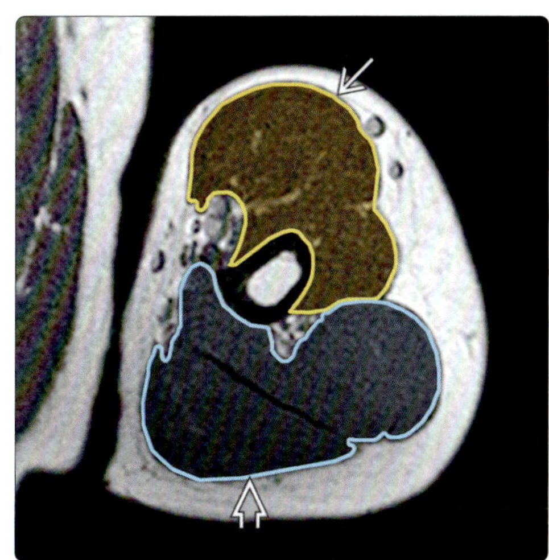

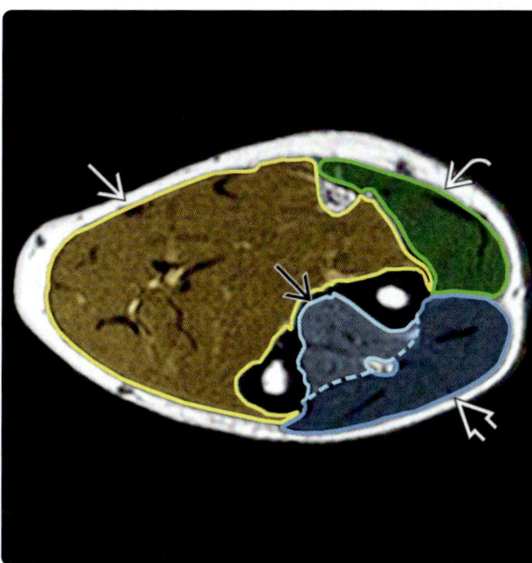

(Left) *Arm compartments are displayed: Anterior ➡ and posterior ➡. Avoid the cephalic vein near the deltopectoral interval proximally, anterolateral aspect of the middle upper arm, and radial nerve posterior to the proximal humeral metaphysis and diaphysis.* **(Right)** *Graphic displays forearm compartments: Volar ➡, superficial dorsal ➡, deep dorsal ➡, and "mobile wad" ➡. Avoid radial nerve/radial artery, medial nerve, and extensor pollicis brevis and abductor pollicis longus distally.*

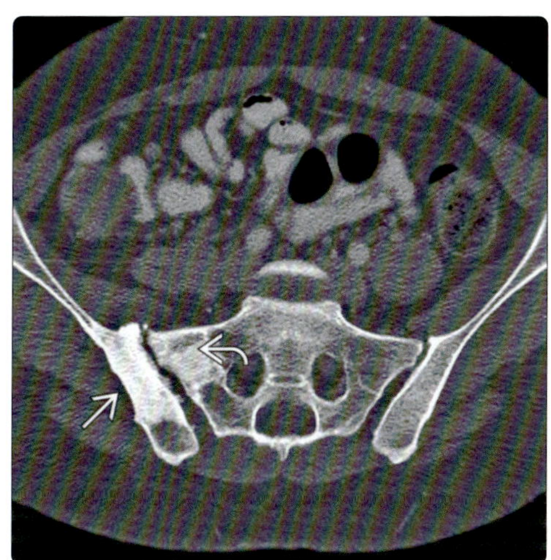

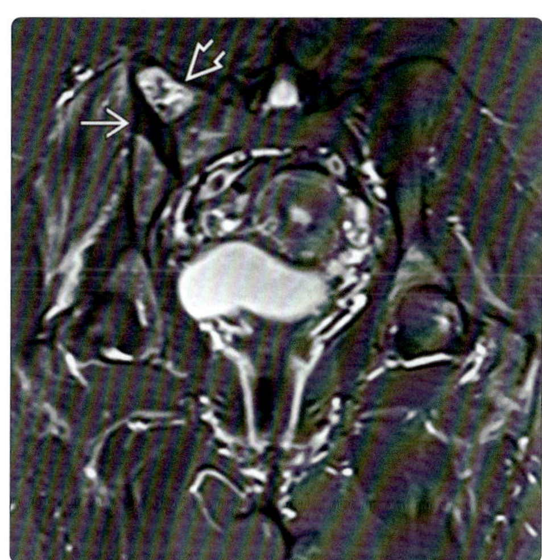

(Left) *This case shows important biopsy considerations. Dense bone formation is seen on axial CT, originating in the iliac wing ➡ and crossing to involve the sacrum ➡. Unfortunately, biopsy of this osteosarcoma was attempted from a posterior approach, into the sclerotic bone, obtaining nondiagnostic tissue.* **(Right)** *Coronal STIR MR in the same patient shows sclerotic bone ➡ at the site of unsuccessful biopsy. The more active high signal soft tissue portion ➡ has a higher probability of yielding diagnostic tissue.*

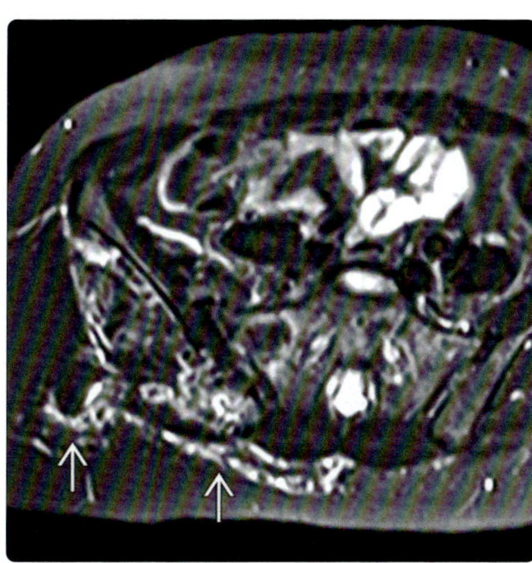

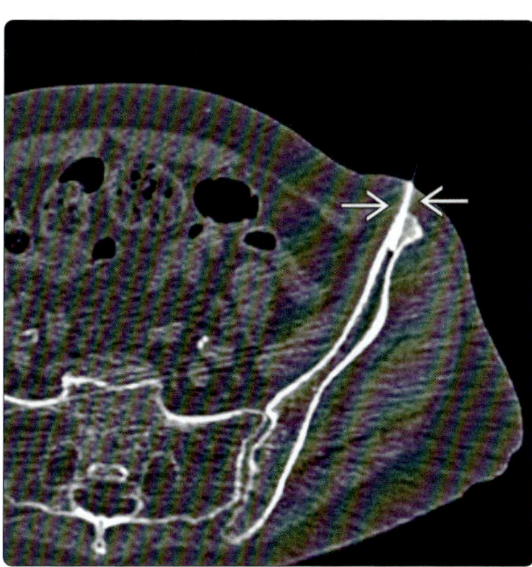

(Left) *Axial T2WI FS MR in the same patient obtained several weeks after posterior biopsy attempt shows tracking of hematoma and tumor cells ➡ through the glutei. This tissue must be resected and is therefore unavailable for coverage of the planned large surgical bed.* **(Right)** *Axial CT shows a biopsy needle entering the anterolateral iliac crest ➡ on a path traversing the long axis of the bone. This is a preferred biopsy approach for an osseous lesion of the iliac crest.*

Treatment Options for Primary Bone Tumors

Intralesional injection may be considered for treatment of simple bone cysts, and rarely other benign lesions, such as Langerhans cell histiocytosis. For simple bone cysts, large bore needles are used (often under imaging guidance), contrast is injected to demonstrate continuity throughout the lesion, the lesion is vigorously flushed, and then steroids are injected.

Radiofrequency ablation (RFA), under general anesthesia and CT guidance, is the treatment of choice for most cases of osteoid osteoma. RFA has also been described as a successful treatment for osteoblastoma. Bone metastases, which are painful and unresponsive to other treatment, may be treated with RFA as well.

Surgery is the primary treatment for the majority of symptomatic or malignant bone tumors. The surgical treatment options are defined as follows.

- Intralesional excision (curettage): Tumor is incompletely resected; procedure usually not appropriate for malignant tumors or tumors with high recurrence rate
- Marginal excision (excisional biopsy): Plane of dissection passes through reactive tissue of lesion; satellites of residual tumor are left behind; generally inadequate for malignant lesions
- Wide excision: Entire lesion is removed, along with reactive tissue, surrounded by intact cuff of normal tissue; this is considered adequate resection for most bone sarcomas
- Radical excision: Lesion is removed along with entire muscle, bone, or other involved tissues in compartment; not commonly required for treatment of bone tumors

Chemotherapy is the first-line therapy for Ewing sarcoma and lymphoma. It serves as adjuvant therapy for most other malignant bone tumors. The exceptions to this are those lesions that are usually low grade and unresponsive to chemotherapy. Such lesions include low-grade chondrosarcoma, periosteal osteosarcoma, and parosteal osteosarcoma. Chemotherapy may be used initially (following biopsy and histologic confirmation of high-grade tumor) for conventional osteosarcoma and many other high-grade sarcomas, prior to definitive surgical treatment. The goal of this therapy is to shrink the soft tissue mass, allowing for easier tumor resection, particularly around neurovascular bundles. It is also hoped that the chemotherapy will control systemic micrometastases. Finally, chemotherapy given preoperatively is used to evaluate tumor responsiveness to the regimen (extent of tumor necrosis is measured), which can help direct postoperative treatment.

Radiation therapy (RT), along with chemotherapy, may be considered first-line therapy for Ewing sarcoma and primary bone lymphoma, depending on the institution. RT may be used preoperatively to help shrink and control tumor mass in high-grade lesions. It is also used postoperatively for lesions with a marginal resection. It may be utilized to treat local tumor recurrence. The exceptions to this are low-grade chondrosarcoma and low-grade osteosarcomas (periosteal, parosteal), which are not responsive to radiation.

Limb Salvage Considerations

Limb salvage operations are defined as those that offer tumor control without sacrifice of the limb. The vast majority of musculoskeletal surgical treatments result in limb salvage; these of course include intralesional excision and marginal excision but also include the majority of wide excisions.

Limb salvage should be attempted only if a functional result is likely. This means that not only the musculoskeletal structures, but also the neurovascular structures must be viable or restored. Growing children present a special difficulty in that limb salvage surgery may not be sensibly attempted if the growth plate cannot be maintained. Because of all these considerations for limb salvage, specific information is required from preoperative tumor imaging. This includes

- Proximal, distal, and transverse extent of osseous and soft tissue involvement
- Location of either the proximal or distal end of the lesion relative to a palpable anatomic landmark (for example, knee joint line or greater trochanter)
- Specific muscles and compartments involved by tumor must be identified
- Major neurovascular involvement must be noted
- Joint involvement
- Tumor extension relative to epiphyseal plate; generally need ~ 2 cm of tumor-free bone adjacent to metaphyseal side of growth plate for adequate limb salvage surgery seeking to retain the physis

Following resection of tumor, the reconstructive choice depends on the location and extent of the lesion, the anticipated functional result and functional demands of the patient, and the likelihood of associated complications. Following removal of all or part of a major joint, either an arthroplasty, osteochondral bone graft, or arthrodesis might be chosen. If the tumor is located in the shaft of a long bone and the resection can spare the joints, reconstruction of the segmental bone defect may be performed with cadaver graft (intercalary graft), perhaps supplemented with vascularized fibular graft. Composite arthroplasties can be constructed by using a large-fragment bone allograft for the skeletal defect and a conventional prosthesis for the articulation. The most predictably good results and early return to function follow endoprosthetic replacements. Modular designs allow different lengths of prostheses. Familiarity with the limb salvage techniques aids the diagnostician in evaluating postoperative imaging. Findings will include expected postoperative change in adjacent tissue, as well as mechanical failure of an endoprosthesis or complications of infection or local tumor recurrence.

Major Treatment Roadblocks

Biopsy tracks that contaminate joints or tissue required for reconstruction may make limb salvage impossible; consult with the orthopedic oncologist as part of planning a biopsy and avoiding such contamination.

Inadequate tumor-free regions for specific limb salvage procedures may be problematic. It is useful for the imager to be aware that for limb salvage in a child, 2 cm of normal metaphyseal bone adjacent to an epiphyseal plate is required. For an internal hemipelvectomy, the surgeon usually needs 2 cm of tumor-free superior acetabulum, and tumor should not extend into zone 2 of the sacrum. Finally, it should be noted that major surgical resections with cadaver bone graft heal poorly and require long periods of protection from bearing weight. Healing is by "creeping substitution" of host bone over the scaffolding provided by cadaver bone. Healing may be further delayed by large muscle resections resulting in poor blood supply and the addition of chemotherapy and local radiation therapy.

Residual Tumor (Postoperative) Grading

Residual tumor is always graded following resection, based on gross surgical as well as microscopic pathologic assessment. Depending on grade of tumor and residual tissue, chemotherapy &/or radiation therapy may be required to adequately or optimally treat the patient. The residual tumor grading system is as follows.

- RX: Residual tumor cannot be assessed
- R0: No residual tumor
- R1: Microscopic residual tumor
- R2: Macroscopic residual tumor

Follow-Up of Primary Bone Tumors

Baseline imaging of the tumor site should be obtained within 3-6 months of the definitive resection. Radiographs are mandatory. MR must be obtained if metallic artifact is not prohibitive; if MR is not diagnostic, CT with reformats &/or US should be considered.

Imaging of massive allografts and articular reconstructions can be difficult. The graft is mated with the residual host bone and stabilized with extensive plates and screws. Nonstructural bone graft as well as structural bone graft (allograft or autograft, the latter often a vascularized fibular segment) may be used as supplements. These elements may obscure the host bone-allograft interface and make it difficult to evaluate for bony bridging.

Osteoarticular allografts require a long period of protected weight-bearing (up to 1-2 years) and complications occur in approximately 50% of these patients. These complications include infection, joint instability, nonunion, and fracture. After approximately three years, articular collapse occurs in a significant proportion of patients, even when the graft has incorporated with the host bone.

Long stem endoprostheses or total arthroplasties placed for limb salvage are often associated with extensive resection of supporting soft tissues. This puts the prosthesis at risk for instability, which in turn may lead to prosthetic loosening (25% reported at 5 years), dislocation, or periprosthetic fracture. Evaluation for these complications is generally made with radiographs, though CT with longitudinal reformats may be useful in discovering subtle fractures.

Besides following the limb salvage constructs for complications of infection, fracture, and nonunion, one must be vigilant for tumor recurrence. The search pattern must include evaluation for osseous destruction, tumor matrix formation, soft tissue mass, and lymph node enlargement. Extensive metallic implants may seem to limit evaluation to radiographs. However, CT with longitudinal reformats may be surprisingly revealing.

If the metallic implants are titanium, MR may yield useful information in all but the most densely metallic regions. Interpretation of MR of massive allografts is not straightforward, however. Progressive revascularization of the implanted grafts occurs in a patchy focal manner. It appears to begin in intertrabecular areas adjacent to cortex, giving an MR appearance of a diffuse granular marrow pattern with focal geographic abnormalities. This may mimic the MR pattern of recurrent tumor or infection. Additionally, radiation or chemotherapy may alter the host bone appearance. Given the variability of expected appearance, biopsy might be utilized liberally if there is suspicion of recurrence based on imaging. On the other hand, if there is intact cortex within the graft and no soft tissue mass, it may be elected to follow these MR abnormalities closely rather than immediately proceeding to biopsy, of course subject to clinical circumstances.

US may also provide useful surveillance for recurrent soft tissue mass as long as the lesion is not excessively deep.

Determining the interval for follow-up for asymptomatic patients is a complicated process, which is based on the patient's likelihood of developing either local recurrence or distant metastases. These, in turn, correlate with the following variables.

- Tumor type
- Tumor stage: Size, grade, and presence of metastases
- Completeness of resection (residual tumor grading)
- Percentage of necrosis found at surgery, which relates to the success of chemotherapy

Follow-up for the asymptomatic patient with malignant disease but low risk may vary by local preference, but usually entails the following evaluations.

- Regional evaluation (radiograph + MR, CT, or US) plus chest CT q6 months for first two years
- Regional evaluation (radiograph + MR, CT, or US) plus chest CT annually thereafter

Follow-up for the asymptomatic patient with high-risk malignancy may vary by local preference, but usually entails the following.

- Regional evaluation (radiograph + MR, CT, or US) plus chest CT q3 months for first two years
- Regional evaluation (radiograph + MR, CT, or US) plus chest CT q6 months for next three years
- Regional evaluation (radiograph + MR, CT, or US) plus chest CT annually thereafter
- Some institutions utilize PET/CT in follow-up, particularly for lesions demonstrated to be FDG avid (for example, Ewing sarcoma and osteosarcoma)
- Generally recurrence and new metastatic disease are unlikely after a 10-year disease-free interval

Follow-up after recurrence

- Regional evaluation (radiograph + MR, CT, or US)
- Chest CT
- Tissue biopsy or resection for documentation prior to treatment with chemotherapy or radiation

Selected References

1. Zbojniewicz AM et al: Posttreatment imaging of pediatric musculoskeletal tumors. Radiographics. 34(3):724-40, 2014
2. Fritz J et al: Imaging of limb salvage surgery. AJR Am J Roentgenol. 198(3):647-60, 2012
3. Chen BB et al: Dynamic contrast-enhanced MR imaging measurement of vertebral bone marrow perfusion may be indicator of outcome of acute myeloid leukemia patients in remission. Radiology. 258(3):821-31, 2011
4. Kotnis NA et al: Magnetic resonance imaging appearances following hindquarter amputation for pelvic musculoskeletal malignancy. Skeletal Radiol. 38(12):1137-46, 2009
5. Motamedi D et al: Thermal ablation of osteoid osteoma: overview and step-by-step Guide. Radiographics. 29(7):2127-2141, 2009
6. Watts AC et al: MRI surveillance after resection for primary musculoskeletal sarcoma. J Bone Joint Surg Br. 90(4):484-7, 2008
7. Davies AM et al: Follow-up of musculoskeletal tumors. I. Local recurrence. Eur Radiol. 8(5):791-9, 1998

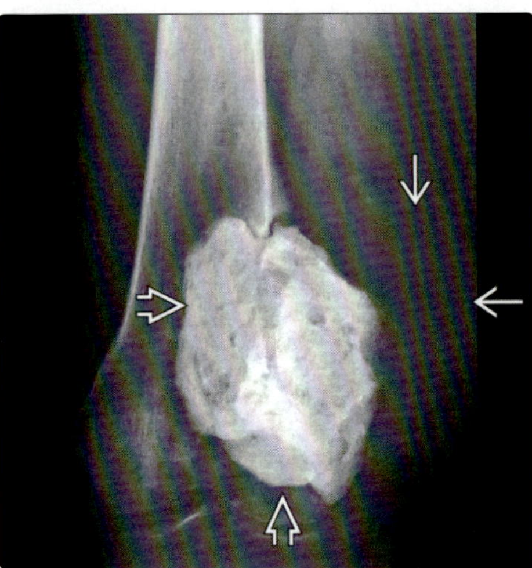

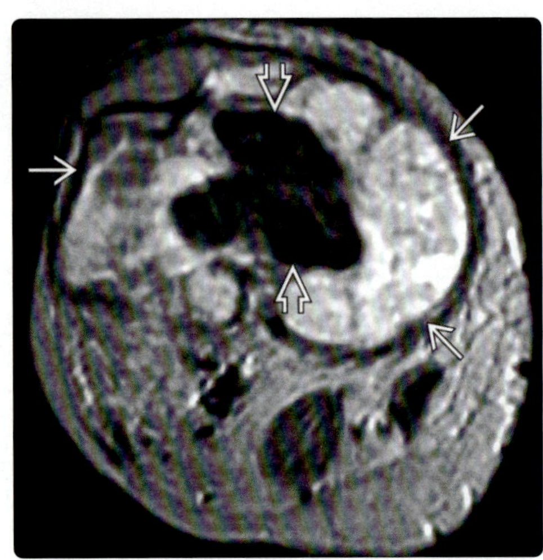

(Left) *AP radiograph shows a surgical site where a lesion was treated with curettage and cement ➡. There is also a large soft tissue mass ➡.* **(Right)** *Axial T2WI MR in same patient shows the cement ➡ with a circumferential soft tissue mass ➡. The treatment was curettage (marginal excision) for a lesion mistakenly presumed to be a giant cell tumor. This is inadequate treatment for proven chondrosarcoma, now recurrent. Adequate biopsy and surgical planning is a common theme in tumor recurrences.*

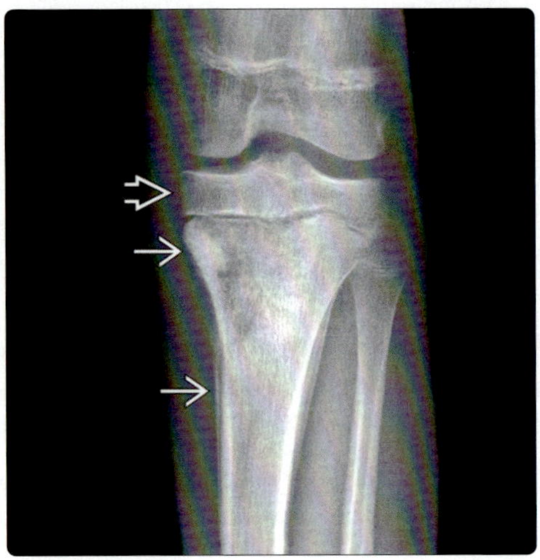

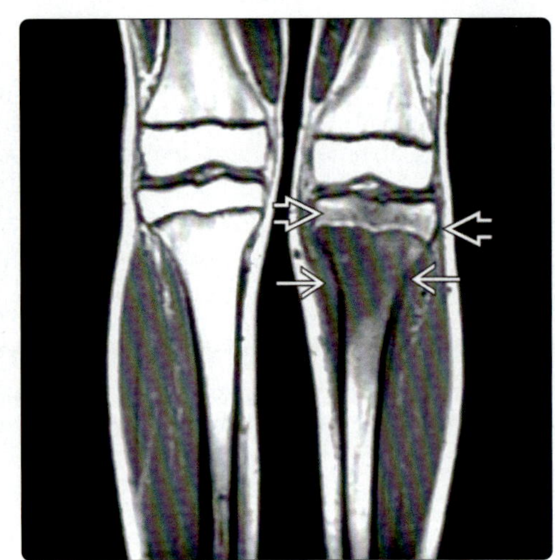

(Left) *AP x-ray shows a permeative eccentric metaphyseal lesion that elicits periosteal reaction ➡, proven at biopsy to be osteosarcoma. The epiphysis appears to be spared ➡.* **(Right)** *Coronal T1WI MR in the same patient shows the tumor ➡ involves the epiphysis ➡, which must be resected; limb length considerations must be a part of the surgical plan. (Previously published in Manaster BJ et al: Musculoskeletal Imaging: The Requisites. 2nd ed. Philadelphia: Mosby, Elsevier; 2002.)*

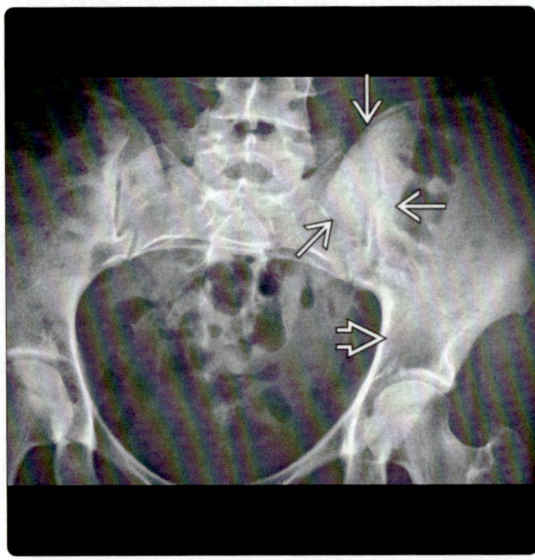

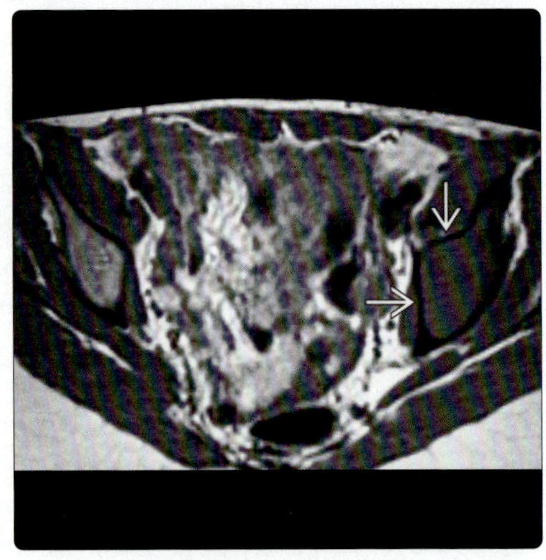

(Left) *AP radiograph shows an osteosarcoma of the posterior iliac wing ➡. In order for an internal hemipelvectomy to be performed (rather than a larger operation resulting in a less functional result), at least 2 cm of superior acetabulum ➡ must be tumor-free.* **(Right)** *T1WI MR of the same lesion at the level of the left superior acetabulum shows low signal tumor involvement ➡. Because there are not 2 cm of tumor-free superior acetabulum, the surgeon recommended against internal hemipelvectomy.*

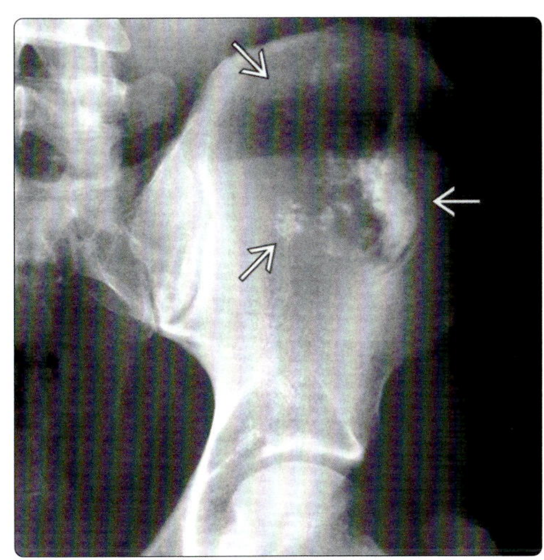

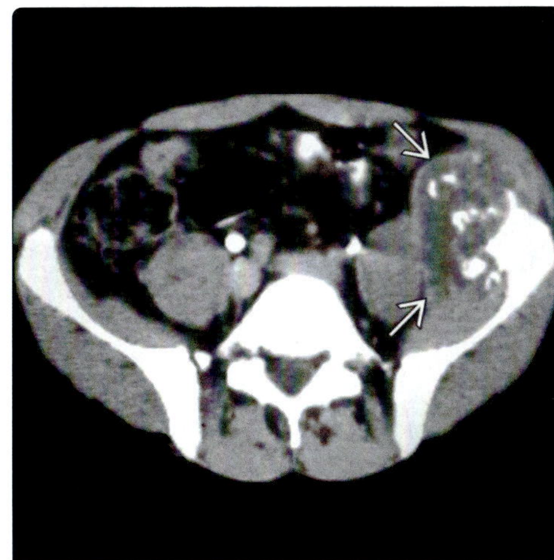

(Left) *AP radiograph shows iliac wing chondrosarcoma ➔ that appears to be in a position amenable to internal hemipelvectomy, with adequate tumor-free superior acetabular bone.* **(Right)** *Axial NECT in the same patient confirms the large soft tissue mass, which contains chondroid matrix and necrotic areas as well as tumor ➔. Even though wide resection is the treatment of choice, care must be taken not to track any tumor. Chondrosarcoma is particularly at risk for local recurrence.*

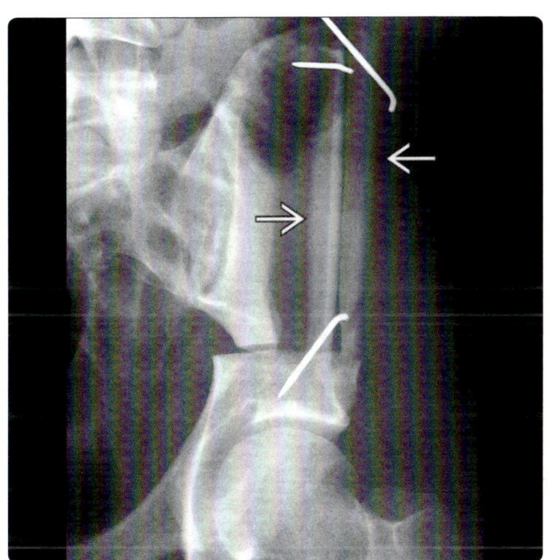

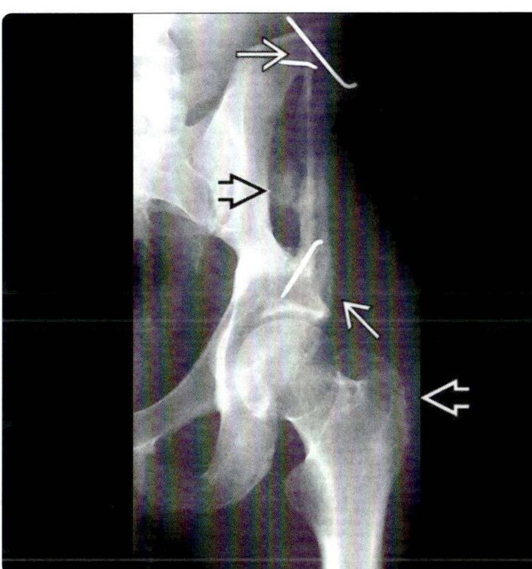

(Left) *AP radiograph in the same patient shows he was treated with an internal hemipelvectomy with stabilizing fibular strut grafts ➔. Pathology showed the margins to be tumor-free (R0).* **(Right)** *AP surveillance radiograph in the same patient 12 months later shows the fibular graft to have incorporated ➔. However, there is new matrix seen within the tumor bed ⇨, as well as adjacent to the greater trochanter ➔, indicating tumor recurrence, likely spread by surgical hematoma. Likelihood of cure is low.*

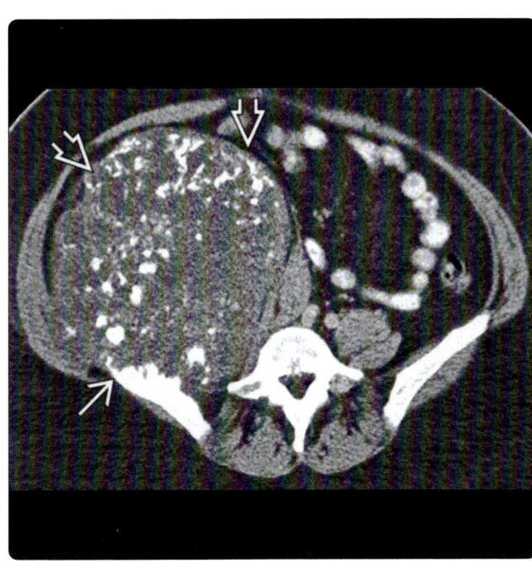

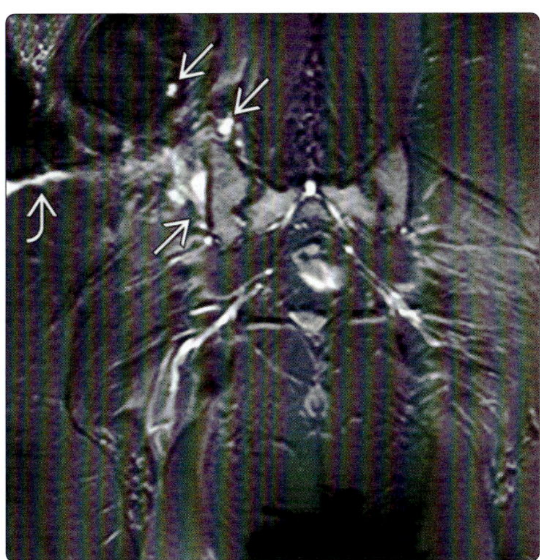

(Left) *Axial bone CT shows a huge chondrosarcoma ➔ arising from the iliac wing ➔. Despite low histologic grade, its size and position make it nearly impossible to achieve a wide en bloc resection. Prognosis is guarded, despite the low grade of the lesion. This proved to be the case; resection grade was R1.* **(Right)** *Coronal STIR MR in the same patient 6 months postoperatively shows multiple nodules of recurrent tumor ➔ and recurrence along the surgical track ➔. The prognosis is poor.*

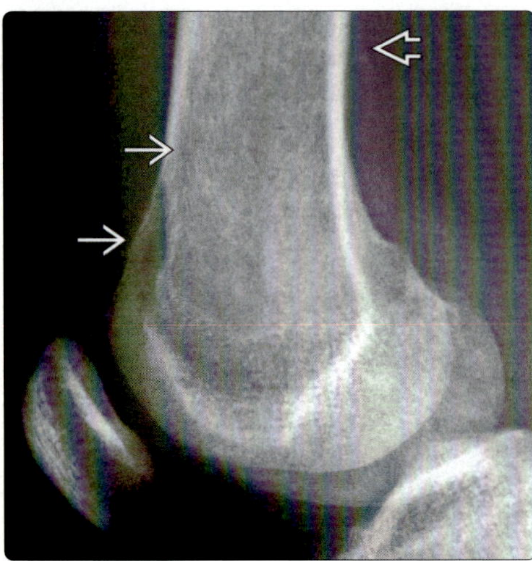

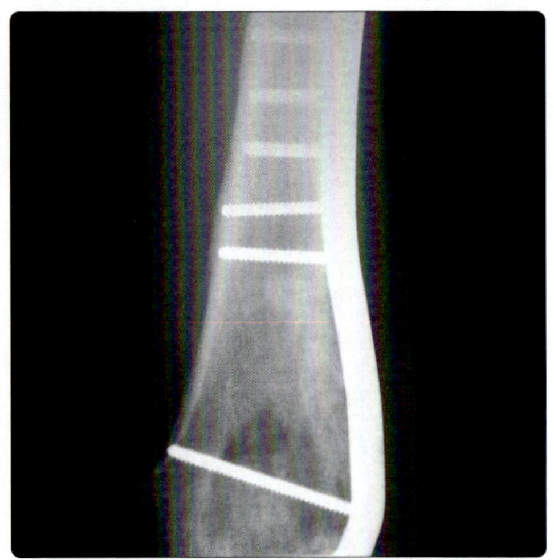

(Left) *Lateral radiograph shows a highly permeative lesion ➡ with periosteal reaction ⇨. However, preoperative histology suggested cyst. The discrepancy between radiographic appearance and pathology report should have been addressed and repeat biopsy considered. However, the lesion was considered by the surgeon to be a cyst, and curettage (marginal excision) was performed.* **(Right)** *Postoperative AP x-ray in the same patient shows curettage of the lesion with bone graft and plating.*

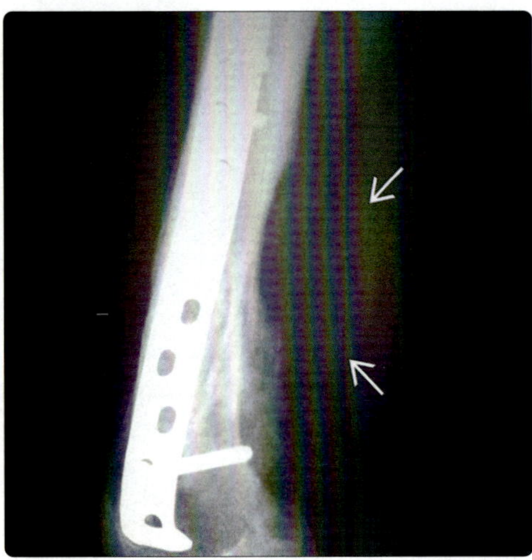

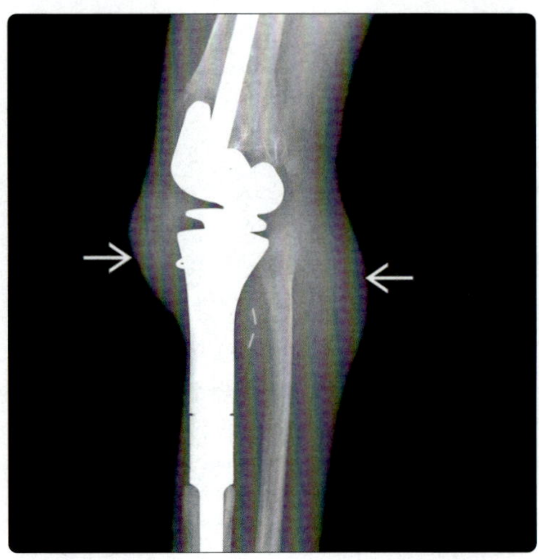

(Left) *Lateral radiograph in the same patient shows osseous destruction and a large recurrent soft tissue mass ➡. The "cyst" was an inadequately treated telangiectatic osteosarcoma. Beware of mismatch of histology and imaging. This patient's chance of survival is now poor.* **(Right)** *Lateral radiograph several months following limb salvage procedure (long stem modular arthroplasty) for osteosarcoma shows a soft tissue mass ➡. US showed the mass to be solid; biopsy proved recurrence.*

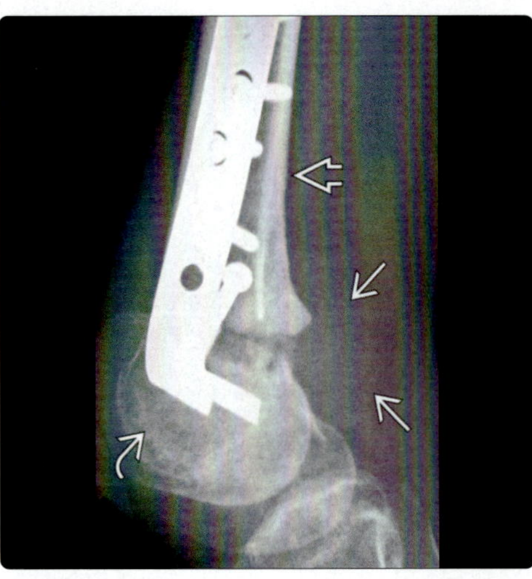

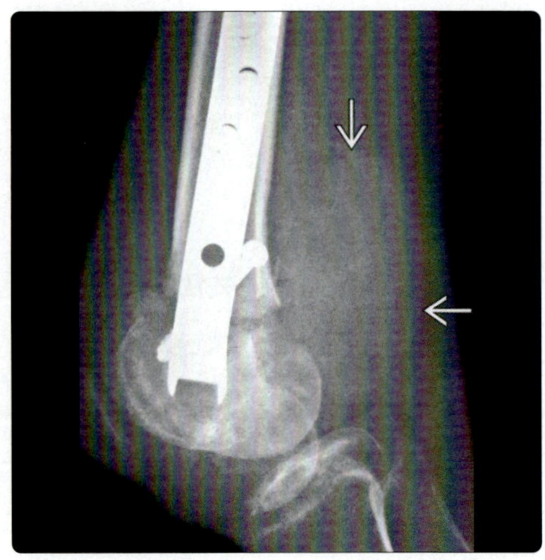

(Left) *Lateral radiograph obtained 6 months after resection of osteosarcoma shows allograft ⇨. The distal metaphysis ↪ and native joint were retained. There is no bone bridging at the host bone/graft interface. However, there is a posterior soft tissue mass ➡; recurrence must be suspected. US showed the mass to be solid; tumor recurrence is confirmed.* **(Right)** *Lateral radiograph 4 months later shows mass enlargement ➡. Lung metastases had also developed.*

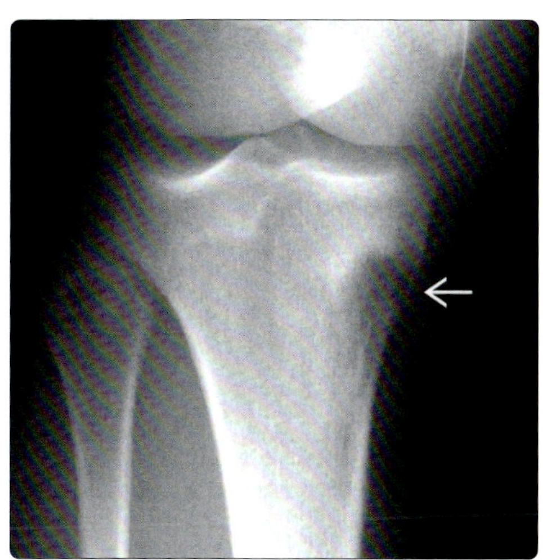

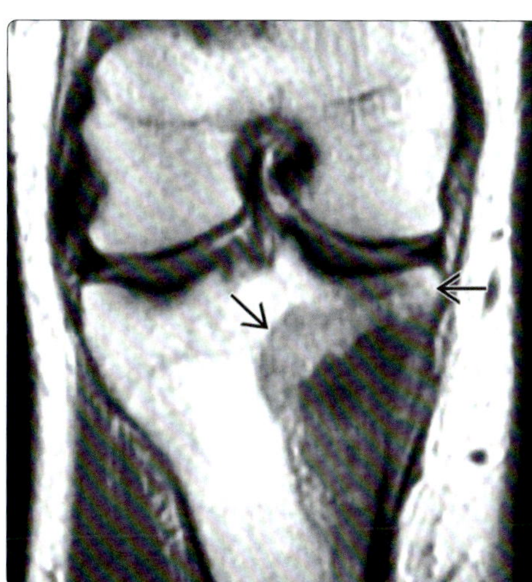

(Left) *Oblique x-ray shows a lytic moderately aggressive lesion* ➡*; biopsy showed osteosarcoma. The size suggests that limb salvage may be successful, but adjacent subchondral bone is a concern.* **(Right)** *Coronal PDWI MR, same patient, shows the mass to be subarticular* ➡*. Therefore, at least part of the patient's knee joint must be resected, making limb salvage more complicated. (Previously published in Musculoskeletal Imaging: The Requisites. 2nd ed. Philadelphia, PA: Mosby, Elsevier; 2002.)*

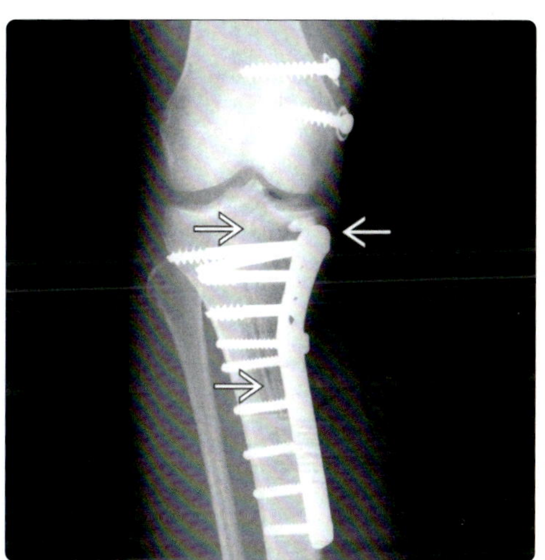

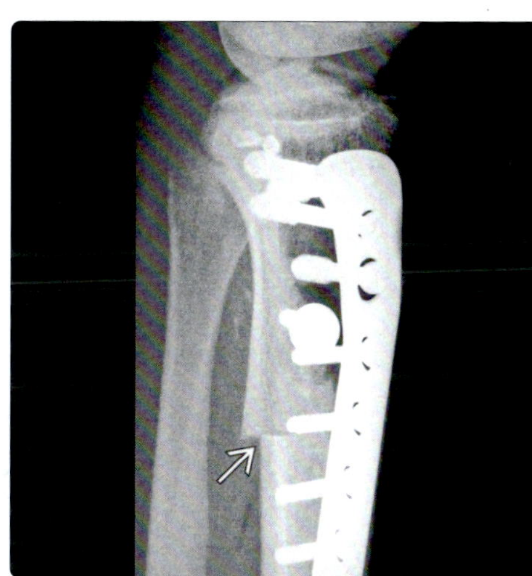

(Left) *AP radiograph in the same patient shows that the lesion was resected and a hemiosteoarticular graft was placed* ➡*.* **(Right)** *Lateral radiograph shows the osteoarticular graft* ➡ *at its junction with the host bone. This is an aggressive limb salvage procedure. The graft may take 2-3 years to incorporate, and there is substantial risk of articular collapse after this time. However, even if there is articular collapse, there will be enough bone stock present to support a routine arthroplasty.*

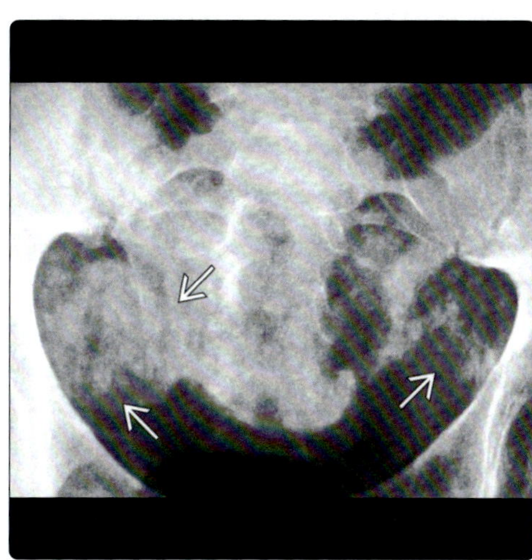

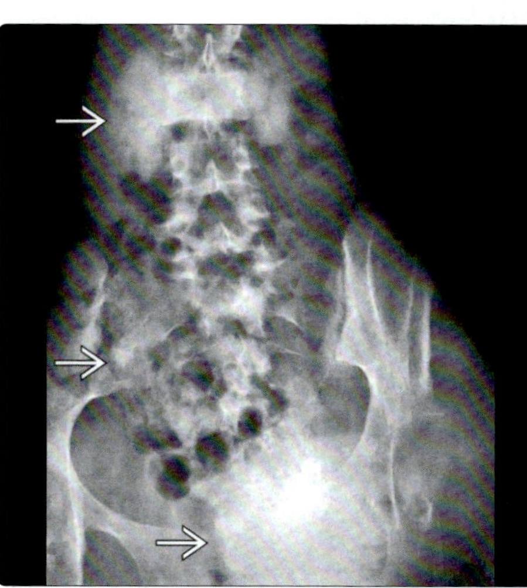

(Left) *AP radiograph obtained in a patient several months following resection of leg osteosarcoma demonstrates amorphous tumor osteoid forming within the iliac lymph nodes* ➡*. Of all the primary malignant bone tumors, osteosarcoma most frequently involves nodes.* **(Right)** *AP radiograph 10 months after left hip disarticulation for osteosarcoma shows multiple sites of osseous metastases* ➡*. The patient had lung metastases as well; bone metastases in osteosarcoma generally develop later than lung metastases.*

Enostosis (Bone Island)

KEY FACTS

TERMINOLOGY

- Benign focus of compact (cortical) bone located within cancellous bone (medullary cavity)

IMAGING

- Generally radiographic diagnosis
  - Homogeneously dense, fading at periphery, and merging into normal trabeculae
  - Periphery described as brush-like; may appear somewhat stellate
  - No associated marrow edema or cortical destruction
  - May be polyostotic
- CT may show peripheral features more distinctly
  - Periphery fades into adjacent trabeculae
- MR: Low signal on all sequences
  - Faintly higher signal than surrounding normal bone on fat-saturated images
  - No enhancement with contrast
- Bone scan may be normal, but often positive
  - Depends on lesion size; generally some ↑ uptake seen if lesion > 1 cm in diameter
  - Does not reliably differentiate bone island from metastasis
- Pelvis, long bones, ribs, spine are most frequent locations
  - May be found in any bone

DIAGNOSTIC CHECKLIST

- Only difficulty in diagnosis occurs in elderly, who are at risk for sclerotic metastases
  - Polyostotic feature slightly favors metastatic disease, but not invariably
  - Bone scan may show ↑ uptake in both enostosis and sclerotic metastasis
  - T1 and T2WI MR may be identical; metastases usually show some contrast enhancement, at least peripherally
  - Rarely, biopsy is required to differentiate
- Peripheral edge of lesion is distinctive, fading into normal bone with subtle finger-like extensions

(Left) *AP radiograph shows a typical large bone island ➡. The sclerosis is regular and shows brush-like edges, fading into normal bone rather than a distinct sclerotic edge.* **(Right)** *Coronal T1 MR in the same patient shows low signal intensity throughout the lesion, similar to that of cortical bone. Particularly at the superior edge of the lesion, one sees the brush-like border of the bone island ➡ melding into normal bone, a typical feature of bone island.*

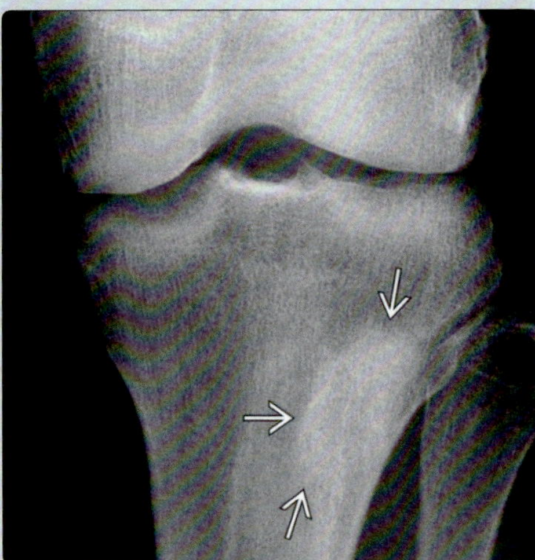

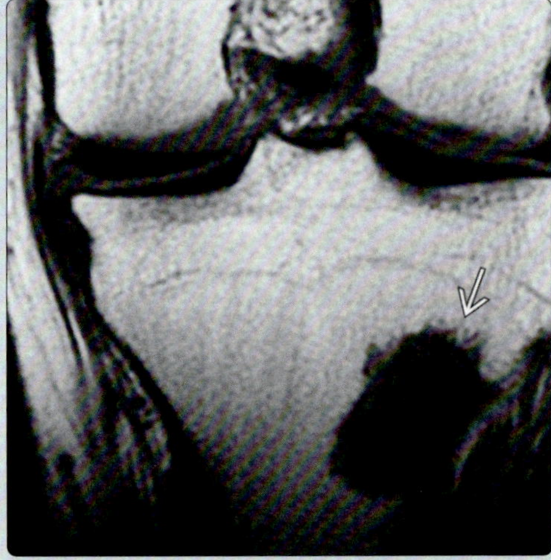

(Left) *Sagittal T2 MR, same patient, shows the homogeneous low signal intensity of the lesion ➡ to be identical to that of cortical bone. This signal intensity feature is typical, and maintains without contrast enhancement.* **(Right)** *Sagittal T2 FS MR, in the same site as the prior T2 image, shows that there is minimally higher signal intensity in the bone island ➡ than in the intensely low signal fat-saturated surrounding bone. This is typical of bone island and should not be misinterpreted as representing a metastasis.*

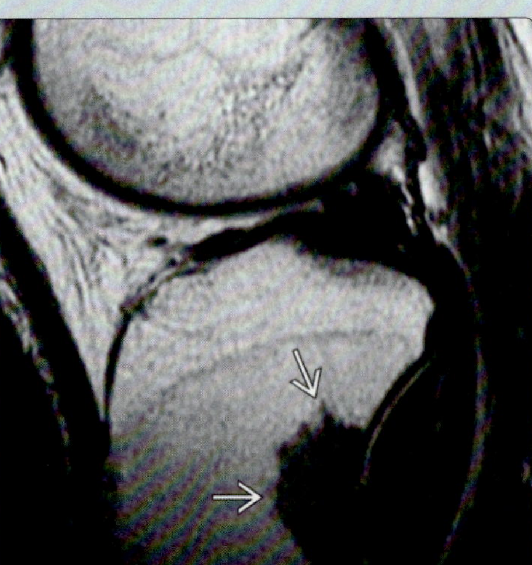

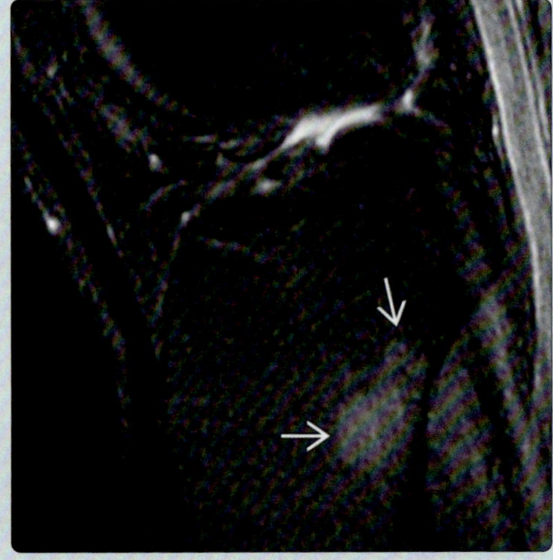

TERMINOLOGY

Definitions

- Benign focus of compact (cortical) bone located within cancellous bone (medullary cavity)

IMAGING

General Features

- Best diagnostic clue
  - Homogeneous lesion with characteristics of cortical bone, occurring within marrow space
- Location
  - Pelvis, long bones, ribs, spine are most frequent
- Size
  - Usually small (< 1 cm); may be giant (several cm)
  - Size may change over time: May enlarge, remain stable, or decrease/disappear
- Morphology
  - Round or oval, oriented along long axis of bone

Radiographic Findings

- Homogeneously dense, fading at periphery, and merging into normal marrow
  - Periphery described as brush-like; may appear somewhat stellate
- No associated cortical destruction
- May be multiple in same bone or polyostotic
  - If multiple and concentrated in metaphyseal region, termed osteopoikilosis

CT Findings

- Sclerotic lesion follows radiographic appearance
- Peripheral extensions into normal adjacent bone (brush border) best seen on CT

MR Findings

- Low signal on all sequences; faintly higher signal than surrounding bone with fat saturation
- Periphery fades into adjacent marrow, as on radiograph and CT
- No enhancement with contrast

Nuclear Medicine Findings

- Bone scan may be either positive or normal
  - Depends in part on lesion size; often some ↑ uptake seen if lesion > 1 cm in diameter

DIFFERENTIAL DIAGNOSIS

Metastatic Disease (Sclerotic)

- May have nearly identical appearance
  - Metastatic focus may not be as homogeneous throughout, allowing differentiation
- Metastases generally show some enhancement on MR

Fibroxanthoma (Nonossifying Fibroma)

- Generally heal during teenage years, with slightly sclerotic bone forming from periphery → center of lesion
- Eventually replaced by normal bone or leave faint trace of homogeneous sclerosis
- Cortically based rather than central

Osteoma

- Dense focus; usual location is paranasal sinus or skull
  - If located peripherally, arises on outer cortex of bone, not within marrow
- Generally homogeneously sclerotic, though may have regions of inhomogeneity

Osteoid Osteoma

- Usually have lytic nidus ± central sclerotic focus
- Nidus may be obscured on radiograph by homogeneous sclerotic bone reaction: Only appearance that could be confused with bone island
  - Lytic nidus always seen either with CT or MR

Cement & Bone Fillers

- Cement usually has peripheral lucent halo
- Bone graft seen as multiple sclerotic foci, which gradually merge as healing occurs

PATHOLOGY

General Features

- Etiology
  - Likely developmental
    - Normal cortical bone, which fails to resorb during growth process of endochondral ossification

CLINICAL ISSUES

Presentation

- Most common signs/symptoms
  - None; incidental finding

Demographics

- Age
  - Seen in adults far more frequently than children
- Epidemiology
  - Incidence reported at 14%; may be higher

Natural History & Prognosis

- No associated morbidity or mortality

DIAGNOSTIC CHECKLIST

Consider

- Only difficulty in diagnosis occurs in elderly, who are at risk for sclerotic metastases
  - Polyostotic feature slightly favors metastatic disease
  - Bone scan usually shows ↑ uptake in both enostosis and sclerotic metastasis
  - T1 and T2WI MR may be identical; metastases usually enhance, at least peripherally
  - Spectral CT may be helpful differentiating sclerotic metastasis from bone island, particularly using standard deviation of CT value on high-energy, virtual monochromatic spectral images
  - Rarely, biopsy is required to differentiate

SELECTED REFERENCES

1. Dong Y et al: Differential diagnosis of osteoblastic metastases from bone islands in patients with lung cancer by single-source dual-energy CT: Advantages of spectral CT imaging. Eur J Radiol. 84(5):901-7, 2015
2. Gould CF et al: Bone tumor mimics: avoiding misdiagnosis. Curr Probl Diagn Radiol. 36(3):124-41, 2007

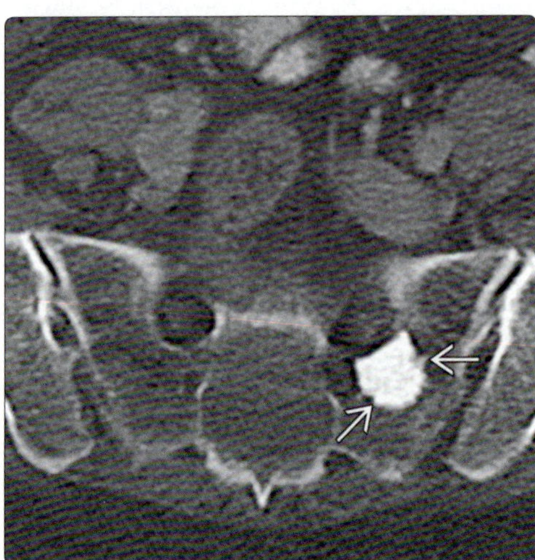

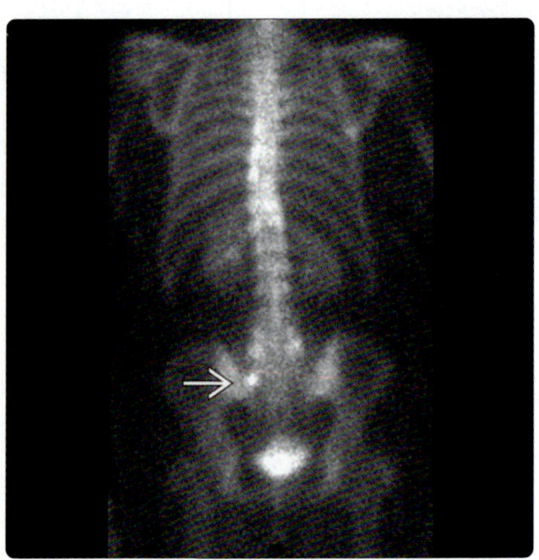

(Left) *Axial bone CT shows an incidentally discovered bone island within the sacrum. The homogeneously sclerotic lesion has the typical appearance of fading into the adjacent bone at its periphery ➡. This may give a brush-like, slightly infiltrative, or stellate appearance, but is typical for the lesion.* **(Right)** *Posterior projection of a bone scan in the same patient shows focal round uptake matching the bone island ➡. If the lesion is large enough, its sclerotic features lead to a positive bone scan.*

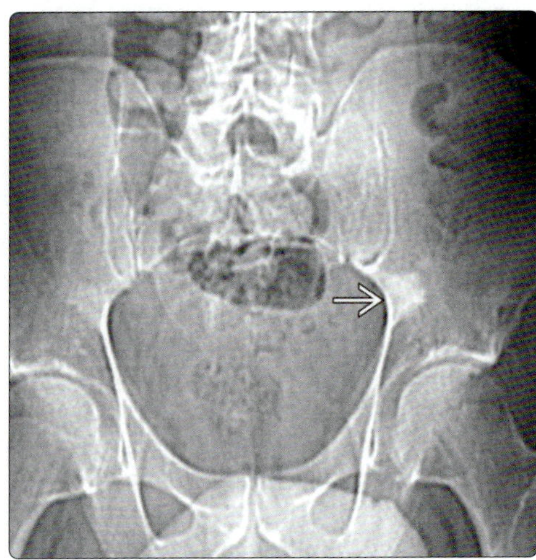

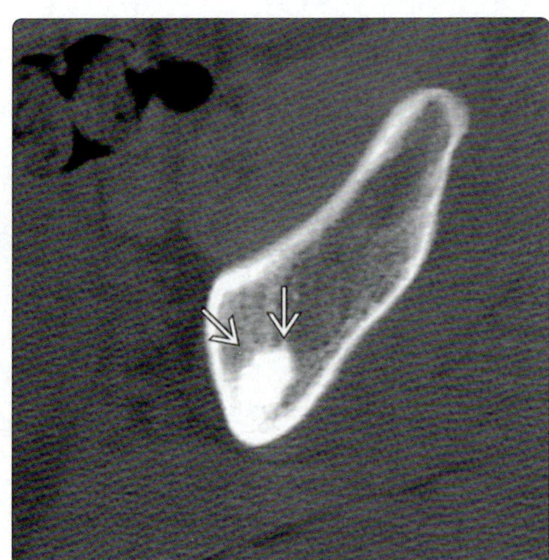

(Left) *CT scanogram demonstrates a rather large bone island ➡. It is homogeneously dense and located in the medullary space. In a middle-aged man such as this, there could be concern for metastatic prostate cancer.* **(Right)** *Axial NECT shows that the lesion blends into the surrounding normal bone with spicules at the periphery ➡, typical of bone island. Do not be surprised to find that this lesion is hot on bone scan. Enostoses, if they are large enough, can show ↑ bone scan uptake.*

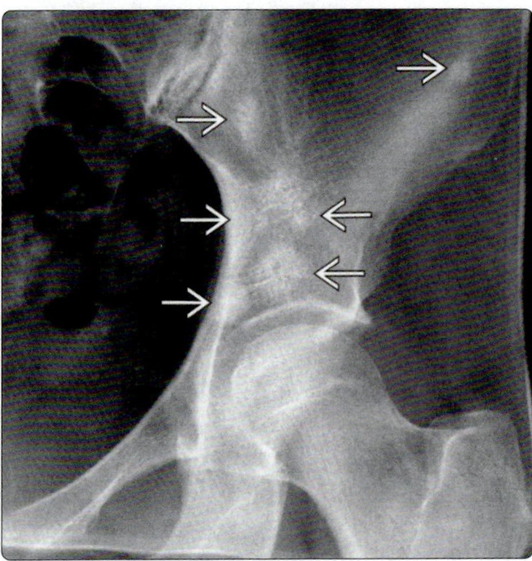

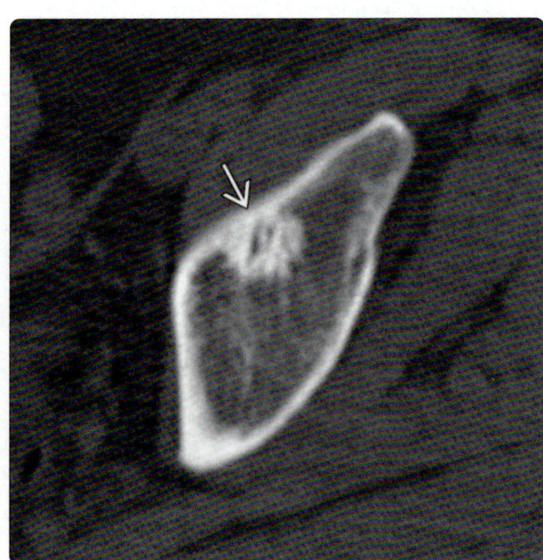

(Left) *AP radiograph performed for contralateral hip pain incidentally noted multiple sclerotic lesions ➡ limited to the left ilium. A bone scan (not shown) had no abnormal tracer uptake. Nonetheless, this unusual cluster of sclerotic lesions is concerning for metastatic disease.* **(Right)** *Axial CT in the same patient shows these lesions to be as dense as cortical bone with spiculated margins ➡. These lesions were stable 4 years later, so no further follow-up is needed; they represent an unusual cluster of enostoses.*

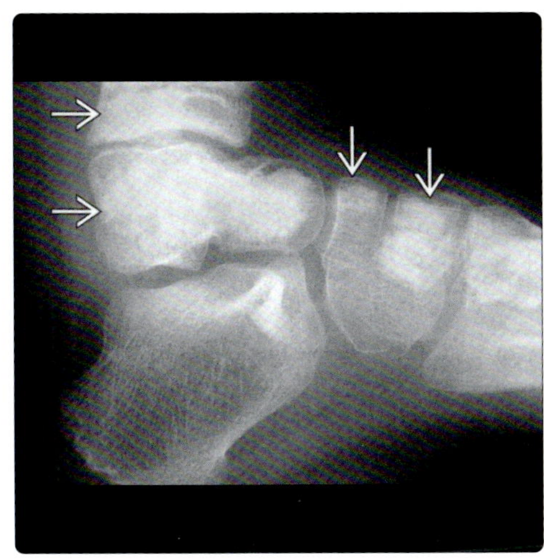

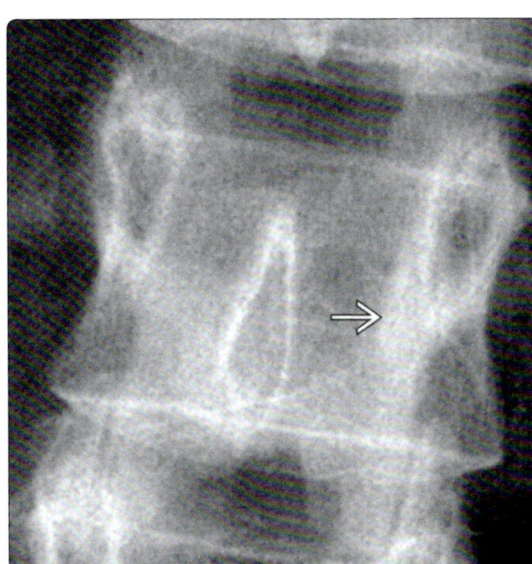

(Left) *Lateral radiograph demonstrates multiple bone islands ➡; they were present at other sites as well. This appearance is termed osteopoikilosis and does not require further work-up.* **(Right)** *AP radiograph shows a typical case of vertebral bone island. The lesion ➡ appears adjacent to the pedicle on this projection but is not otherwise well characterized.*

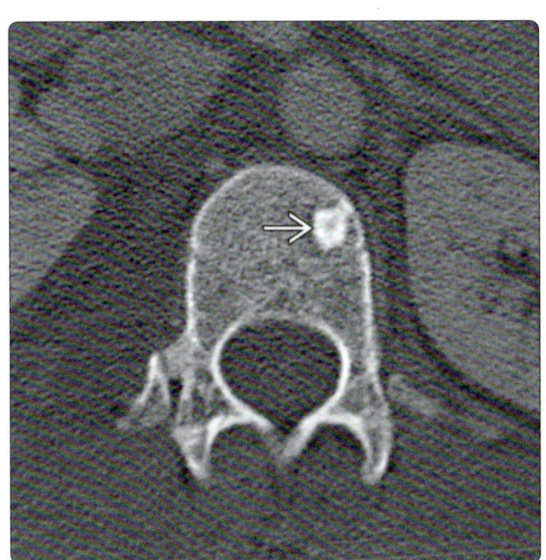

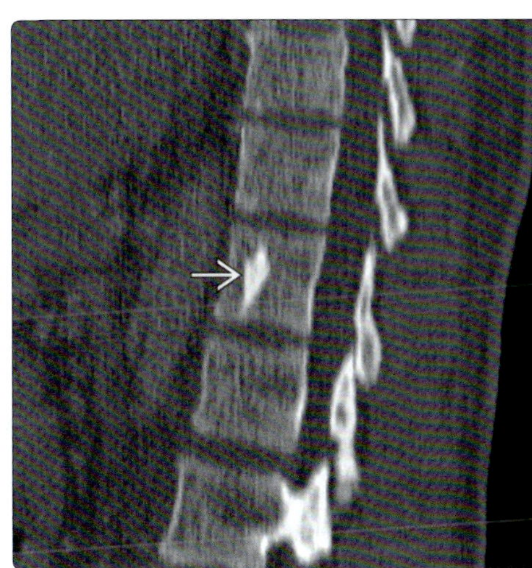

(Left) *Axial bone CT in the same patient was performed to better characterize the lesion seen on radiograph. The lesion is densely sclerotic ➡, with mild spiculation extending from its periphery.* **(Right)** *Sagittal reformatted bone CT confirms dense sclerosis with irregular brush-like margins of a bone island. Note also that the lesion is oriented along the long axis of the vertebral body ➡. Morphology of bone island tends to be either round or oval; there is no other reasonable diagnosis in this case.*

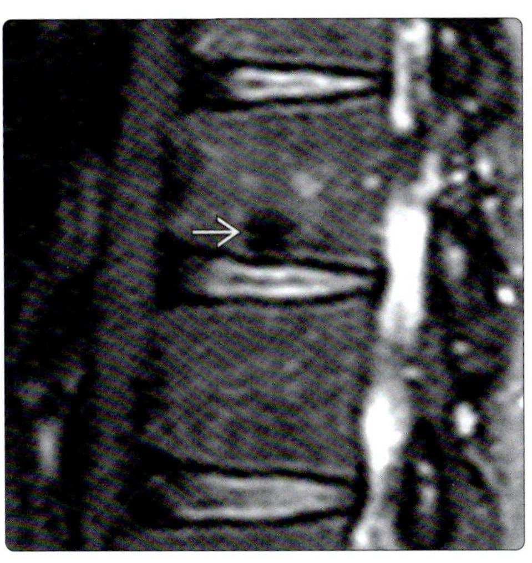

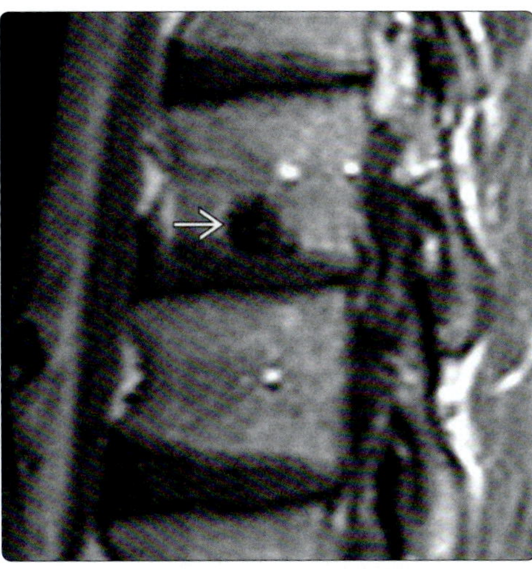

(Left) *Sagittal STIR MR shows a small focal area of markedly diminished signal within a vertebral body ➡. It remained low signal on all sequences. Note that there is no surrounding edema or reactive change on this STIR image.* **(Right)** *Sagittal T1WI C+ MR in the same patient shows no contrast enhancement of the lesion ➡, confirming the diagnosis of bone island. If initial imaging leaves a question regarding bone island vs. metastasis, administration of contrast may provide the answer.*

Osteoma

KEY FACTS

TERMINOLOGY

- Benign tumor that forms mature, well-differentiated bone

IMAGING

- Location: Paranasal sinuses: 75% overall
  - Frontal (80%) > ethmoid (20%) > maxillary
  - Cranium: Outer table
  - Mandible: Surface
  - Tubular bones: Femur > short tubular bones
  - Arises from surface of bone
- Intramedullary extension and expansion rare in long bones; may be seen in sinuses
- Radiograph/CT: Homogeneous bone density is most frequent appearance (well-differentiated lamellar bone production)
  - May have less homogeneously dense regions, but matrix is still clearly osteoid
- MR of dense lamellar osseous portions of lesion
  - Low SI on all sequences without enhancement
- MR of less dense osseous portions of lesion
  - Low SI on T1, similar to other cancellous bone
  - Mildly inhomogeneous SI on fluid-sensitive sequences, similar to other cancellous bone

TOP DIFFERENTIAL DIAGNOSES

- In long bone
  - Sessile osteochondroma
  - Parosteal osteosarcoma
  - Melorheostosis
- In paranasal sinus
  - Fibrous dysplasia
  - Osteoblastoma
  - Osteosarcoma

PATHOLOGY

- Associations: Gardner syndrome & tuberous sclerosis

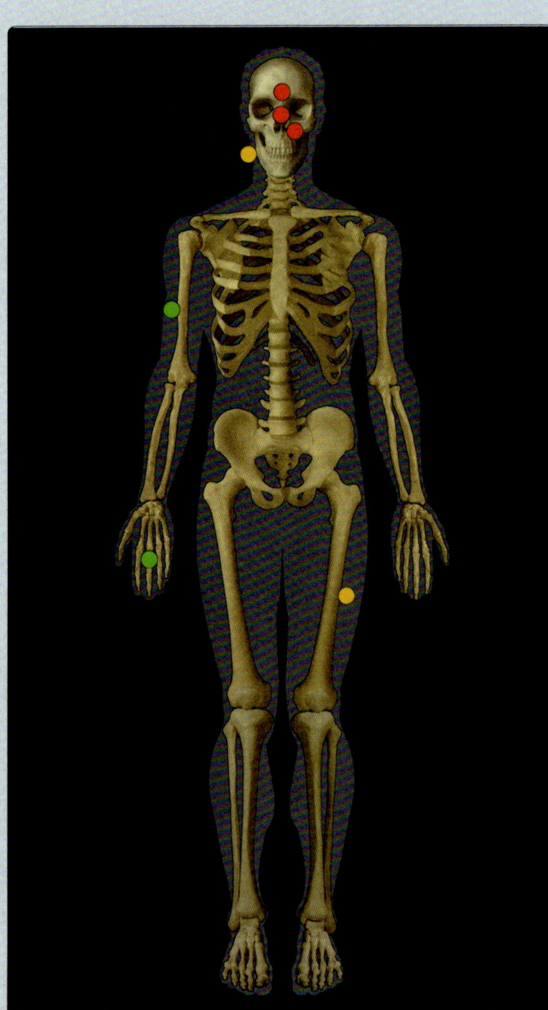

Graphic depicts the most frequent locations of osteoma. The paranasal sinuses are by far the most frequent (red: Frontal > ethmoid > maxillary > sphenoid). Mandibular and tubular bone osteomas are seen less frequently (yellow). Least frequent locations are shown by green.

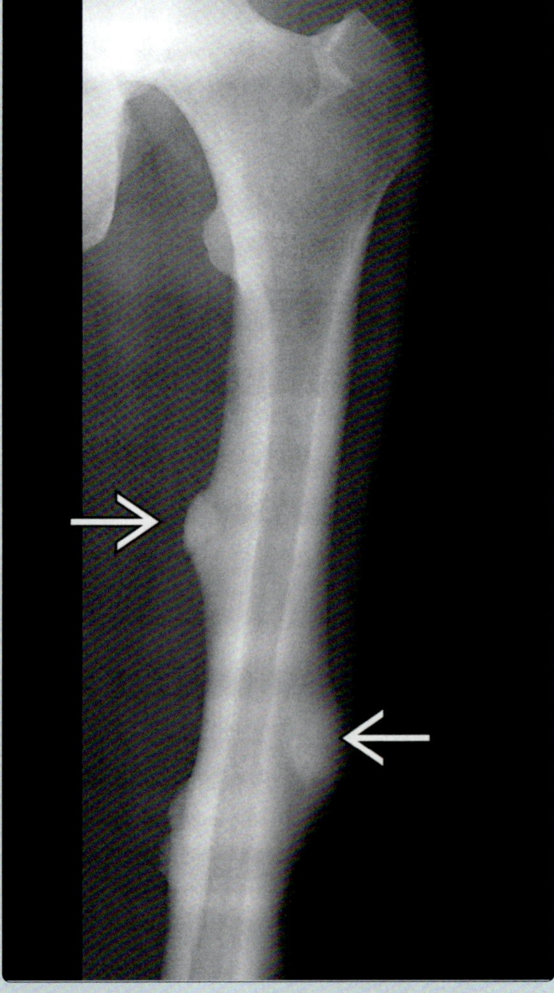

Anteroposterior radiograph shows multiple homogeneously dense osteomas ➡ arising along the surface of the femur. Note that the bone marrow is undisturbed, there is no periosteal reaction, and the lesions produce mature bone matrix.

TERMINOLOGY

Synonyms

- Surface osteoma, parosteal osteoma, ivory osteoma, ivory exostosis, hamartoma of bone

Definitions

- Benign tumor that forms mature, well-differentiated bone

IMAGING

General Features

- Best diagnostic clue
  - Well-differentiated bone formation, without aggressive features
- Location
  - Paranasal sinuses: 75% overall
    - Frontal (80%) > ethmoid (20%) > maxillary > sphenoid
      - Traditionally named for sinus lumen invaded by osteoma, not sinus of origin
    - May extend intraorbitally or intracranially
  - Cranium: Outer table
  - Mandible: Surface; rarely arises centrally
  - Long bones
    - Femur > humerus > short tubular bones
    - Arises from surface of bone
- Size
  - Generally 1-4 cm; range is wider
- Morphology
  - Round to oval, smooth borders
  - Sessile or pedunculated in sinus
  - Sessile in long bone

Radiographic Findings

- Matrix: Osteoid
  - Homogeneous bone density is most frequent appearance (well-differentiated lamellar bone production)
  - May have less homogeneously dense regions, but matrix is still clearly osteoid (woven or cancellous bone production)
    - Mixed lamellar and cancellous bone may be seen in paranasal sinus lesions, giving mixed density, more frequently than long bones
    - One case report of inhomogeneity in osteoma of long bone due to fatty regions within lesion
- Arises from surface of bone
  - Intramedullary extension rare in long bones
  - Intramedullary extension and expansion more frequently seen in sinuses
- No soft tissue mass
  - If ostium is occluded, paranasal sinuses may have mucocele or sinusitis
  - One case report of separate, entirely osseous nodule in adjacent soft tissues
- Periosteal reaction: None, or extremely rare
- Borders sharply demarcated

CT Findings

- Similar to radiograph: Surface bone-producing lesion
- Best defines matrix
  - Smooth, homogeneous, dense bone may comprise entire (or at least majority of) lesion
  - May have adjacent regions of less dense cancellous bone formation
  - Rarely contains regions of fat density
- CT demonstrates any expansion of involved bone (generally in paranasal sinus lesions, not long bones)
- Associated soft tissue abnormalities
  - Mucocele, sinus opacification from blocked ostium

MR Findings

- Dense lamellar osseous portions of lesion
  - Low signal intensity on all sequences
  - Rarely contains regions with fatty signal intensity
  - No enhancement with contrast
- Less dense cancellous osseous portions of lesion
  - Low signal intensity on T1, similar to other cancellous bone
  - Mildly inhomogeneous signal intensity on fluid-sensitive sequences, similar to other cancellous bone
  - None or else very mild enhancement with contrast
- Desmoid tumor may be found nearby if patient has Gardner syndrome
  - Low T1 signal, homogeneous low to heterogeneous high T2 signal, ± enhancement

Imaging Recommendations

- Best imaging tool
  - Diagnosis generally made on radiograph
  - If there is concern for involvement of adjacent structures, MR is most useful
- Protocol advice
  - Enhanced MR or CT best for evaluation of complications
    - Mucocele, pneumatocele
    - Abscess

DIFFERENTIAL DIAGNOSIS

In Long Bone

- Sessile osteochondroma
  - Normal continuum of marrow and cortex from underlying bone differentiates from osteoma
- Parosteal osteosarcoma (OS)
  - If mature, matrix in parosteal OS may appear as dense as in osteoma, with rounding of edges
  - Lesion in parosteal OS is organized with distinctive zoning; mature bone centrally and less mature bone and soft tissue peripherally; zoning differentiates from osteoma
  - Surface origin of parosteal OS is similar to osteoma
  - Parosteal OS often involves adjacent marrow, unlike osteoma
  - One case report of osteoma containing inhomogeneous regions plus adjacent soft tissue osseous nodular focus, leading to misdiagnosis as parosteal OS
- Melorheostosis
  - Endosteal and cortical bone formation, generally more linear
    - Occasionally will appear heaped up on cortex, mimicking osteoma
  - Pathologically, indistinguishable from osteoma

In Paranasal Sinus

- Fibrous dysplasia
  - Mixed sclerotic lesions with ground-glass appearance may mimic osteoma with both cancellous and lamellar bone
  - Predilection for skull base rather than sinuses
- Osteoblastoma
  - Rare lesion; skull is uncommon location, paranasal sinuses even less so
  - May have mixed sclerotic and lytic regions of bone formation, similar to inhomogeneous osteoma
- OS
  - Tumor bone formation may initially appear similar
  - Generally more aggressive: Amorphous bone matrix, osseous destruction
  - Soft tissue mass is usually present

PATHOLOGY

General Features

- Genetics
  - Gardner syndrome: Autosomal dominant
- Associated abnormalities
  - Gardner syndrome
    - Osteomas in tubular bones and mandible
    - Multiple cutaneous and subcutaneous lesions (cysts, fibromas)
    - Desmoid tumors: May be superficial or deep
    - Multiple colonic polyps: Marked propensity to develop adenocarcinoma
  - Tuberous sclerosis has association with osteoma formation
  - Soft tissue osteoma (choristoma): Rare, described in thigh and intraoral locations

Gross Pathologic & Surgical Features

- Gross appearance of hard, white, dense cortical bone

Microscopic Features

- May demonstrate mixture of bone types
  - Many believe cancellous is precursor of compact bone in osteomas with mixed density appearance
  - Cancellous (trabecular, spongy) regions: Thin trabecular architecture, with fatty marrow
    - Contains woven bone
    - Often shows active bone formation with transformation to lamellar bone
  - Woven bone: Fairly mature matrix with prominent collagen fibers
    - High numbers of rounded osteocyte lacunae
  - Lamellar (compact) regions: Narrow parallel layers of mature bone matrix
    - Densely packed collagen fibers with smaller and fewer lacunae
    - No Haversian systems in marrow spaces

CLINICAL ISSUES

Presentation

- Most common signs/symptoms
  - Usually incidental finding; < 5% of osteomas are symptomatic
  - Asymmetric mass; pain is uncommon
  - Uncommonly, abnormalities associated with adjacent soft tissue structures
    - Exophthalmos, diplopia
    - Sinusitis, mucocele
    - Abscess, as complication of sinus blockage

Demographics

- Age
  - > 50% in 50-70 age bracket; range: 10-80 years
- Gender
  - Male > female; ratio 2:1
- Epidemiology
  - 3% incidence in general population
  - Most common benign tumor of paranasal sinuses

Natural History & Prognosis

- Grows slowly; maximal growth occurs as patient approaches skeletal maturation
- Generally remains asymptomatic
- No reported cases of malignant degeneration

Treatment

- Treatment rarely is required
- Treatment recommended for
  - Intracranial or intraorbital extension
  - Location near frontal sinus ostium
  - > 50% of frontal sinus filled by osteoma
  - Unrelenting symptoms
  - Evidence of significant growth occurring in skeletally mature patient
- Marginal surgical resection is curative

DIAGNOSTIC CHECKLIST

Consider

- Be sure to evaluate affect of paranasal sinus osteoma on adjacent structures
- Multiple osteomas should raise the possibility of Gardner syndrome
  - Patient must be evaluated for intestinal polyposis & advised of potential for developing adenocarcinoma

SELECTED REFERENCES

1. Agrawal D et al: External manifestations of Gardner's syndrome as the presenting clinical entity. BMJ Case Rep. 2014, 2014
2. Hansford BG et al: Osteoma of long bone: an expanding spectrum of imaging findings. Skeletal Radiol. 44(5):755-61, 2014
3. de Oliveira Ribas M et al: Oral and maxillofacial manifestations of familial adenomatous polyposis (Gardner's syndrome): a report of two cases. J Contemp Dent Pract. 10(1):82-90, 2009
4. Jack LS et al: Frontal sinus osteoma presenting with orbital emphysema. Ophthal Plast Reconstr Surg. 25(2):155-7, 2009
5. Lee BD et al: A case report of Gardner syndrome with hereditary widespread osteomatous jaw lesions. Oral Surg Oral Med Oral Pathol Oral Radiol Endod. 107(3):e68-72, 2009
6. Chen CY et al: Sphenoid sinus osteoma at the sella turcica associated with empty sella: CT and MR imaging findings. AJNR Am J Neuroradiol. 29(3):550-1, 2008
7. Larrea-Oyarbide N et al: Osteomas of the craniofacial region. Review of 106 cases. J Oral Pathol Med. 37(1):38-42, 2008
8. Sundaram M et al: Surface osteomas of the appendicular skeleton. AJR Am J Roentgenol. 167(6):1529-33, 1996

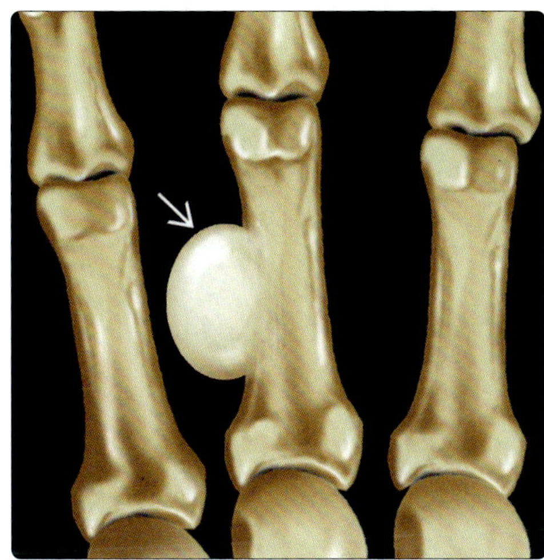

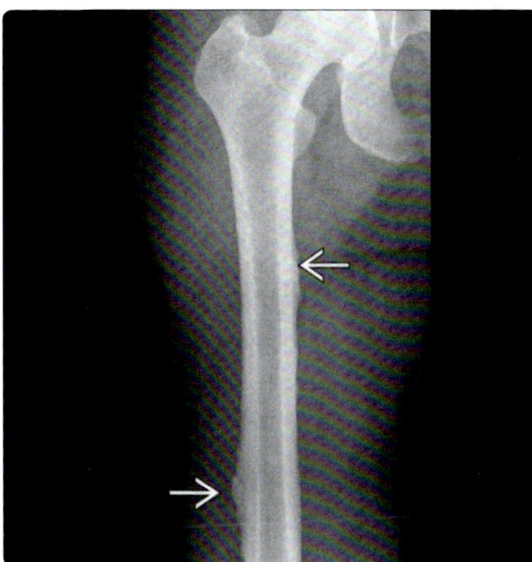

(Left) *Volarly oriented graphic shows an osteoma arising from the surface of a phalanx ➡. The round, white lesion is typical of the gross pathologic appearance of these lesions. The lesions consist of dense lamellar bone, which has no aggressive appearance or behavior.* **(Right)** *AP radiograph, 1st of 5 images in 1 patient, shows lobulated sclerotic cortical masses ➡, typical of osteomas. Since the lesions are multiple, Gardner syndrome should be considered, and associated intestinal polyposis sought.*

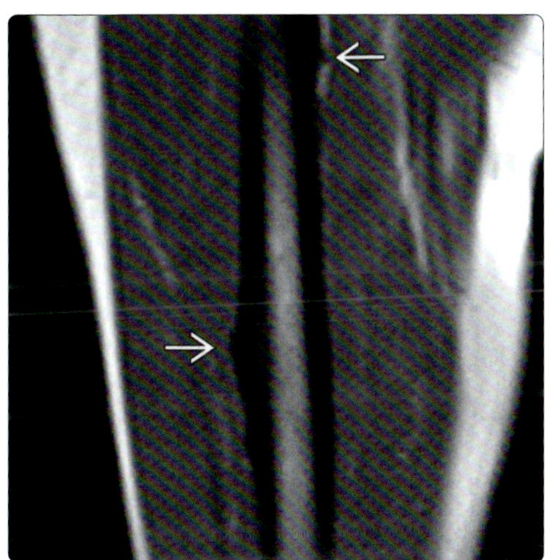

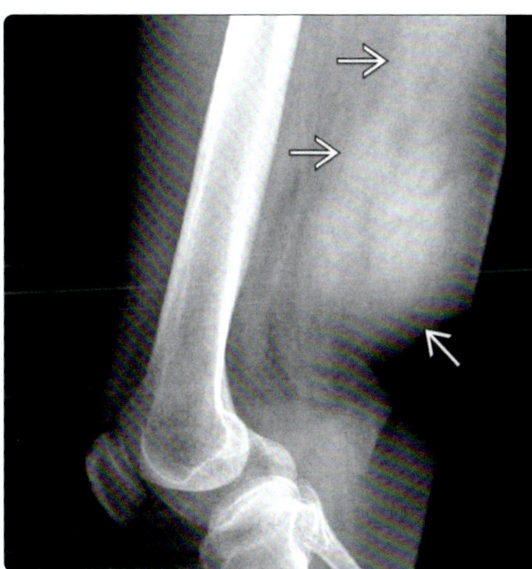

(Left) *Coronal T1WI MR in the same patient confirms the lobulated masses are low signal and restricted to the cortex ➡. Involvement of both medial and lateral cortices makes osteoma a more likely diagnosis than a dysplasia such as melorheostosis.* **(Right)** *Lateral radiograph of the same thigh shows a large soft tissue mass in the posterior thigh ➡, without other characterizing features. Given the multiple osteomas and confirmation of polyposis, the mass most likely represents a desmoid tumor.*

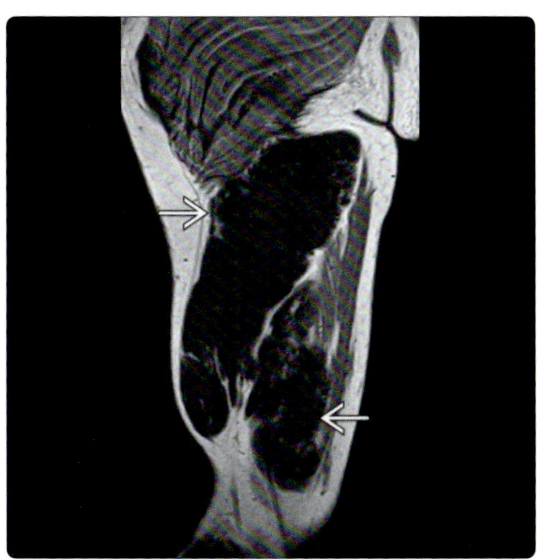

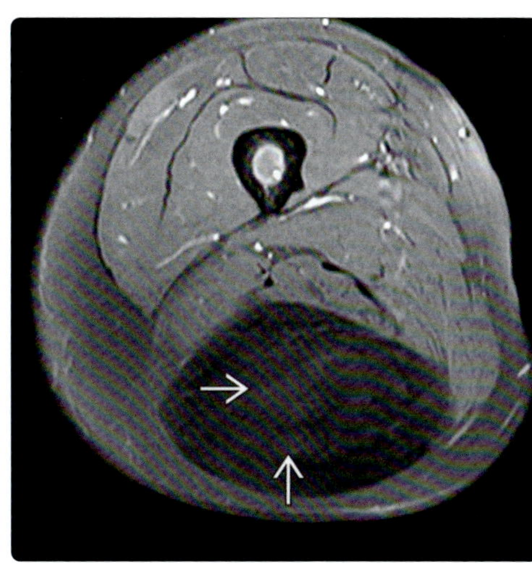

(Left) *Coronal T1WI MR through the posterior thigh shows a large, highly infiltrative mass. The mass is homogeneous and low signal on T1 ➡ as well as fluid-sensitive sequences (not shown).* **(Right)** *Axial T1WI C+ FS MR shows the dense low signal remains prominent post contrast administration; only a hint of contrast enhancement is seen centrally ➡. Desmoid need not be quite this densely low signal and homogeneous, and it generally enhances slightly more than is seen here, but no other diagnosis is possible.*

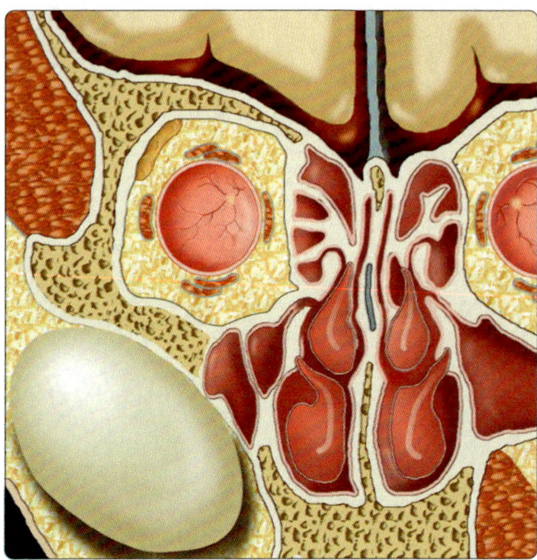

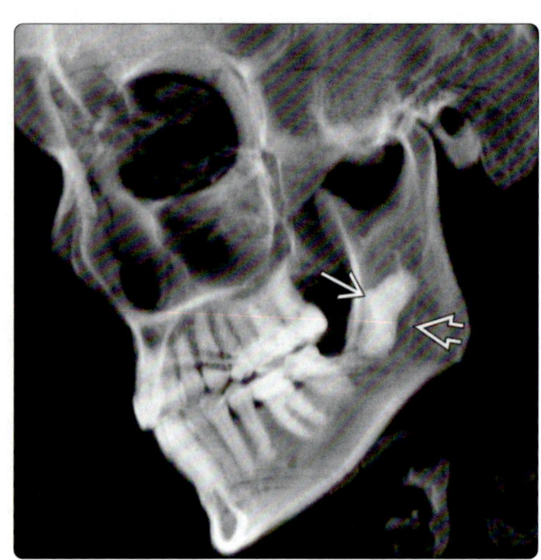

(Left) *Coronal graphic depicts a large, oval, ivory osteoma arising within the mandible. This is a "central" lesion rather than a more common surface osteoma. Although the lesion and expanded mandible are shown abutting the maxilla, there is no invasion or suggestion of aggressive behavior.* **(Right)** *Lateral 3D CT shows a case of a "central" mandibular osteoma. This sharply marginated, homogeneously hyperdense lesion ➡ arises in the left mandible anterior and superior to the inferior alveolar nerve canal ⇨.*

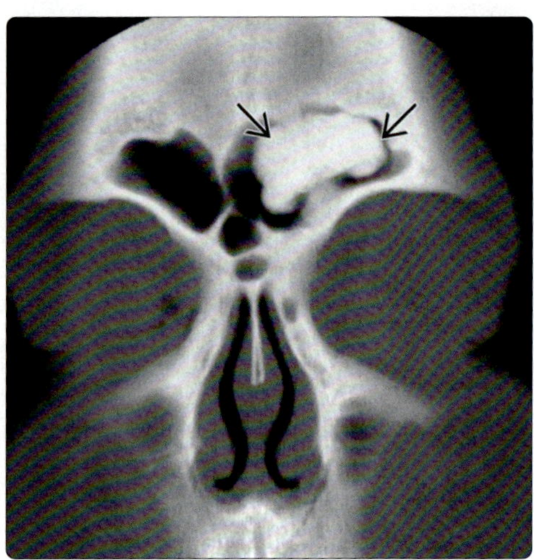

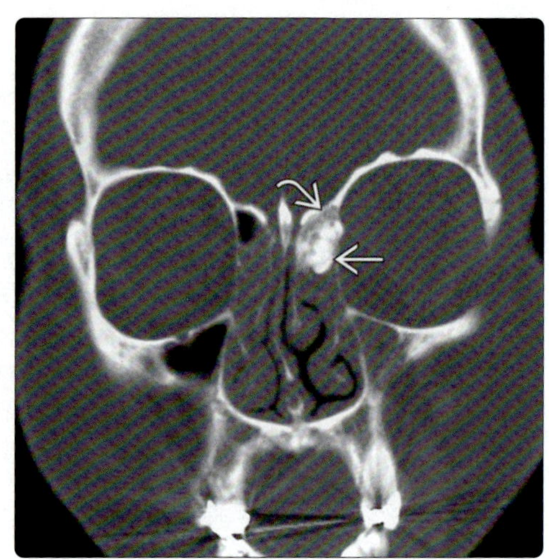

(Left) *Coronal CT shows a uniformly densely ossified mass ➡ in the left frontal sinus typical of an osteoma. The connection to the sinus wall is not seen on these images. There is no surrounding mucosal disease within the sinus. The mass does not obstruct the frontal sinus drainage pathway.* **(Right)** *Coronal CT demonstrates a mixed density osteoma within the left ethmoid sinus ➡, with regions of densely ossified matrix and other areas with a more ground-glass appearance ↷.*

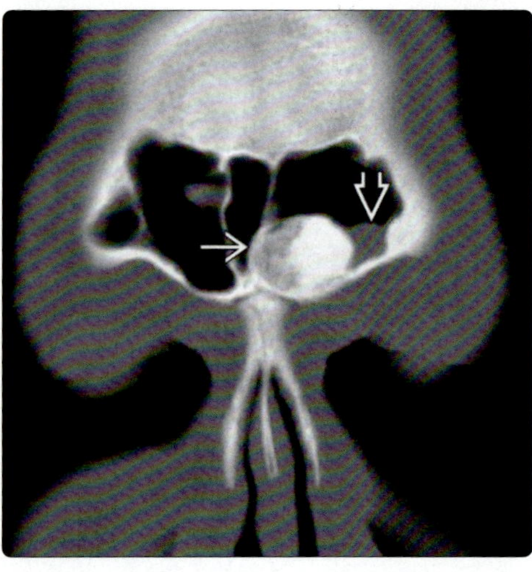

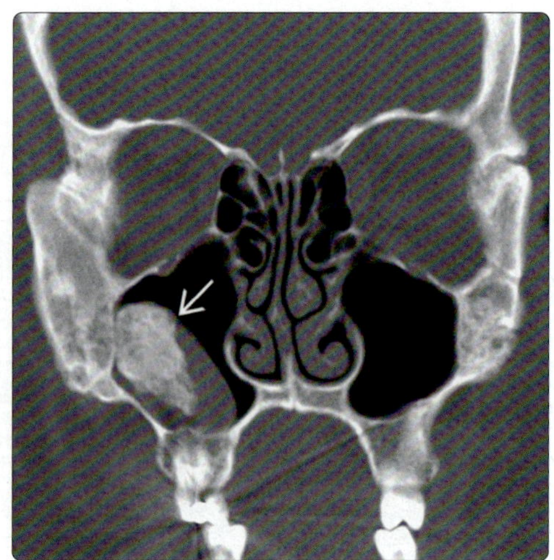

(Left) *Coronal CT demonstrates a well-circumscribed mixed density osteoma ➡ within the left frontal sinus obstructing the frontal sinus drainage pathway. Postobstructive secretions ⇨ are noted lateral to the lesion.* **(Right)** *Coronal CT demonstrates a mixed ossified and soft tissue density mass ➡ arising from the lateral wall of the right maxillary sinus. This "mixed" type of osteoma is composed of varying amount of bone and fibrous tissue. Both the location and appearance are unusual.*

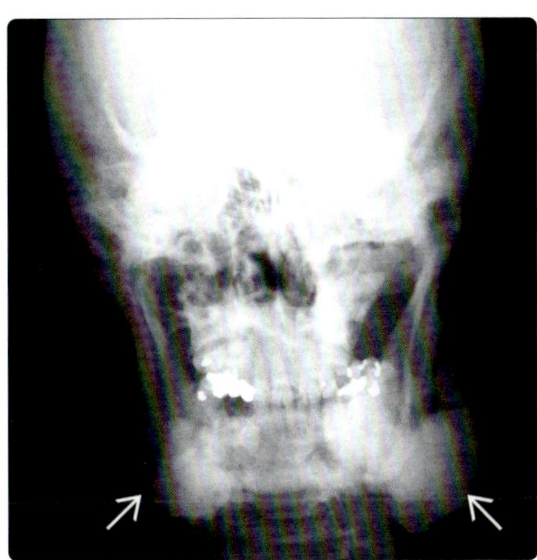

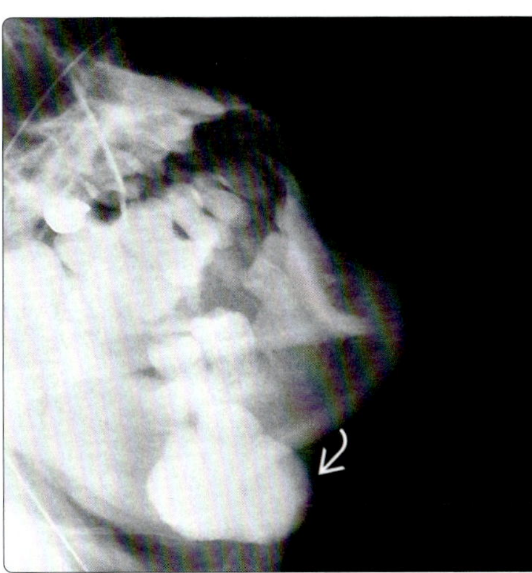

(Left) *AP x-ray shows multiple nodular ossific densities along both mandibular bodies ➡. The large, well-differentiated ossifications represent osteomas and, in this case, are part of Gardner syndrome.* **(Right)** *Lateral radiograph in the same patient shows multiple osteomas. There is a very large, homogeneous, dense bone formation seen at the angle of the mandible on the left side ➡. This patient had a long history of polyposis of the colon. Care must be taken to monitor for adenocarcinoma.*

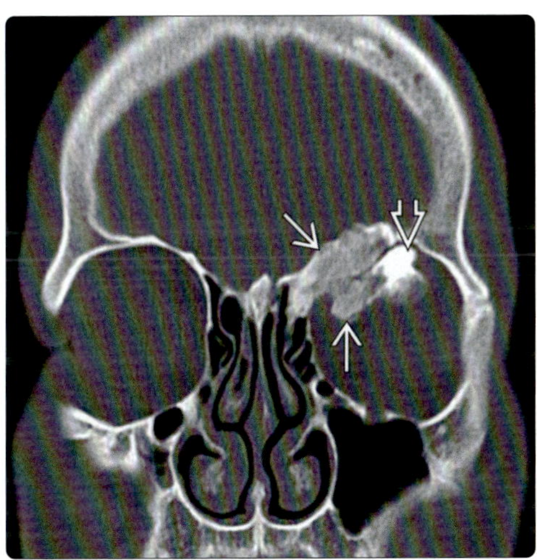

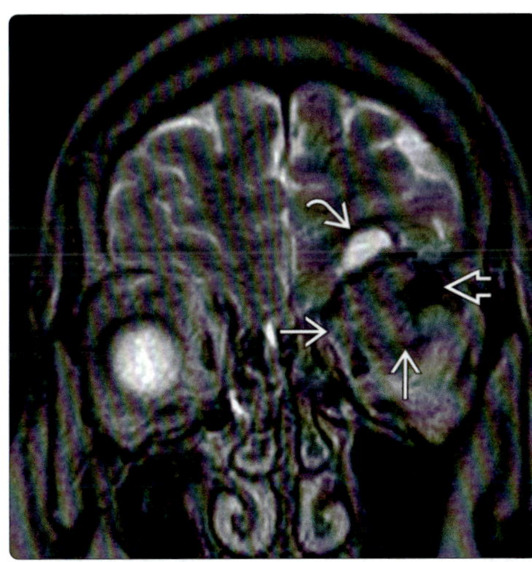

(Left) *Coronal bone CT, 1st of 4 images, shows a mixed density osteoma arising from the frontal sinus. The dense, classic osteoma-like portion is seen coronally ➡ but the majority of the lesion has a less dense appearance ➡, corresponding to cancellous bone.* **(Right)** *Coronal T2WI FS MR in the same lesion shows the low signal of the dense portion ➡ and slightly higher inhomogeneous signal of the cancellous ➡ portion of the lesion. A high signal fluid collection is seen ➡ displacing intracranial contents.*

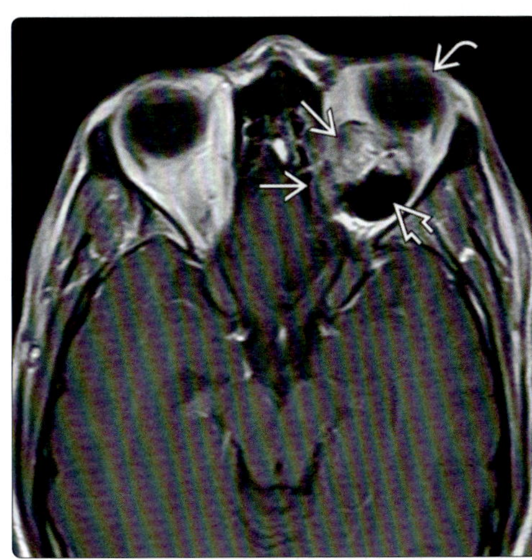

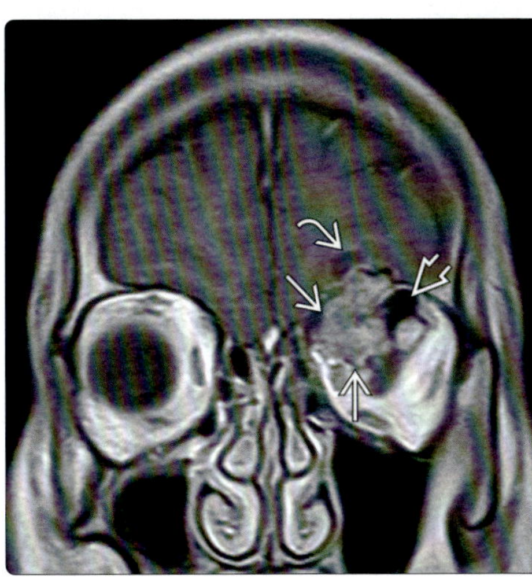

(Left) *Axial T1WI C+ FS MR in the same patient shows the dense lamellar osseous portion to remain low signal ➡, while the less dense cancellous bone ➡ shows slight enhancement. Note the proptosis of the left eye ➡.* **(Right)** *Coronal T1WI C+ FS MR confirms the displacement of orbital contents by this mixed signal osteoma. A low-signal dense portion ➡ and mildly enhancing less dense portion ➡ are noted, with minimal surrounding enhancement. The fluid collection ➡ represents a mucocele.*

KEY FACTS

TERMINOLOGY

- Benign bone-forming tumor characterized by extensive reaction and pain disproportionate to size

IMAGING

- Location
  - Cortical diaphyseal location: 65-70%
  - Femur > tibia; together account for 60% of all OO
  - Intracapsular (most commonly femoral neck)
  - Spine: 10%; usually posterior elements
- Radiographic and CT appearance
  - Oval lytic lesion located within dense cortical bone
  - Sclerosis may obscure underlying lytic nidus on radiograph
  - ± central sclerotic focus within nidus
  - If lesion is intracapsular, sclerotic reactive bone often seen distant from lesion
  - Intracapsular lesions may result in premature osteoarthritis and growth abnormalities
  - Subperiosteal lesion elevates periosteum but does not arise within cortex
  - Spine lesions may develop nonrotatory scoliosis, concave on side of lesion
- MR appearance
  - Reactive periosteal, soft tissue, and marrow edema may mimic more aggressive lesions
- Nidus on MR
  - T2WI: Greater hyperintensity than on T1
  - May have lower intensity nidus, depending on vascularity and whether it is calcified
  - Nidus generally well seen but may be relatively inconspicuous on MR due to volume averaging

CLINICAL ISSUES

- Relatively common; 4-10% of primary bone tumors
- Most common age range: 10-25 years; M:F = 3:1
- Pain becomes unremitting in most untreated cases
- CT or MR-guided ablation is treatment of choice

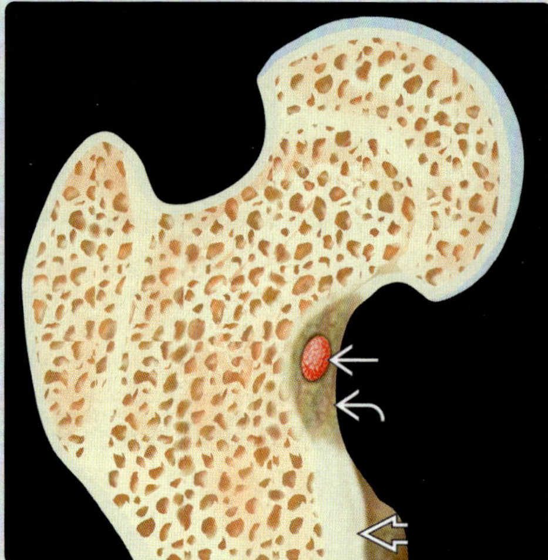

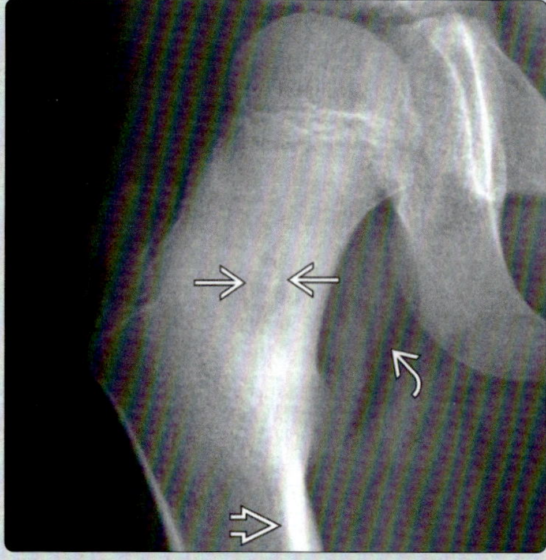

(Left) *Graphic depicts a intracapsular osteoid osteoma (OO). The lesion is located intracortically. It is small ➡ and, in fact, may be obscured by surrounding reactive sclerosis ➡. The reactive bone formation often extends distally far from the lesion ➡.* **(Right)** *AP radiograph of a intracapsular OO, with an oval lytic lesion and central sclerosis ➡ is shown. There is surrounding sclerosis, as well as sclerotic reaction extending down the calcar ➡. Effusion is demonstrated by the distended fat pad ➡.*

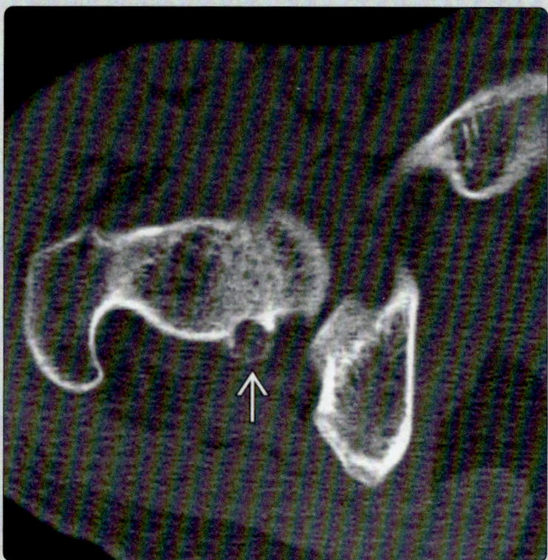

(Left) *Anteroposterior bone scan in a different patient with intracapsular OO shows a focal round region of uptake in the right femoral head and neck region. The lesion shows intense uptake, with surrounding less intense uptake ➡, which has been termed the double density sign.* **(Right)** *Axial NECT of the same lesion demonstrates that it is located on the posterior aspect of the proximal femoral neck ➡. Although adjacent sclerotic reaction is mild, there was more prominent reaction distally.*

TERMINOLOGY

Abbreviations

- Osteoid osteoma (OO)

Definitions

- Benign bone-forming tumor characterized by extensive reaction and pain disproportionate to size

IMAGING

General Features

- Location
  - Has been reported in nearly all bones
  - Cortical diaphyseal location: 65-70%
    - Most common site
    - Femur > tibia: Together account for 60% of all OO
    - Hands and feet: ~ 20% (scaphoid, talus, calcaneus)
  - Intramedullary location is rare
    - Usually carpal and tarsal bones
    - Rarely epiphyses
  - Intracapsular location
    - Most common is femoral neck, often along calcar
    - Reported in elbow, foot, wrist, knee, and facet joints
  - Subperiosteal location
    - Usually intracapsular; hip, talus most common
  - Spine: 10%
    - Posterior elements
    - Lumbar (59%) > cervical > thoracic > sacral
  - Rare multifocal synchronous lesions reported

Radiographic Findings

- Cortical diaphyseal location
  - Oval lytic lesion located within dense cortical bone
  - Surrounding cortical bone thickened and sclerotic
    - Sclerosis may obscure underlying lytic nidus
  - ± central sclerotic focus within lucent nidus
- Intracapsular (intraarticular) location
  - Oval lytic lesion located within cortex
  - ± surrounding sclerotic reactive bone
  - Sclerotic reactive bone often seen distant from lesion, in extracapsular location
  - Joint effusion
  - May result in early osteoarthritis with osteophytes
  - Growth abnormalities if chronic
    - Hyperemia → either overgrowth or early fusion of physis, depending on skeletal age
- Subperiosteal location
  - Round sclerotic focus elevates periosteum but does not arise within cortex
  - ± associated sclerotic reaction; reaction tends to be more limited than OO in other locations
  - Usually intracapsular, associated with effusion
- Intramedullary location
  - Well-circumscribed lesion
  - Partially or completely calcified nidus
  - May have surrounding radiolucent zone
  - Reactive sclerosis minimal or absent
- Spine
  - Posterior elements; difficult to discern on radiograph
    - Uncommon to see lytic nidus
    - May see sclerotic reaction surrounding nidus
  - Nonrotatory scoliosis, concave on side of lesion

CT Findings

- CT useful for diagnosis and specifying location of lesion
  - Cortical vs. subperiosteal or medullary
- Adjacent &/or distant sclerotic reaction
- Lytic nidus, ± central sclerotic focus
- Nidus often adjacent to nutrient vessel
- Associated pathologic fracture (rare)
- CT guidance for percutaneous radiofrequency ablation

MR Findings

- Nidus on MR
  - T1WI: Round lesion, slightly hyperintense to muscle
  - T2WI: Greater hyperintensity
    - May have lower intensity nidus, depending on vascularity and whether it is calcified
  - Nidus enhances avidly
    - Dynamic enhancement: Lesion to marrow differential is greatest in arterial phase
  - Nidus generally well seen but may be relatively inconspicuous on MR due to volume averaging
- Reactive response on MR
  - Cortical thickening and reaction: Low SI on all sequences
  - Reactive change within marrow shows edema in 63%
  - Periosteal elevation or adjacent soft tissue reactive changes in 50%; high SI on fluid-sensitive sequences
  - Intracapsular lesions induce effusion
  - **Caution**: If nidus is not visualized, reactive changes may be misinterpreted as primary tumor
- MR guidance may be used for laser ablation

Nuclear Medicine Findings

- Bone scan shows very intense, round activity at nidus
  - Highly sensitive
  - Double density sign: Very intense central activity at nidus, surrounded by less intensity of reactive bone
  - Round focus helps distinguish from stress fracture, which has more linear activity
- Intensity at nidus may be less in intracapsular than cortical lesions

Imaging Recommendations

- Best imaging tool
  - Often diagnosed on radiograph
  - CT confirms and specifically localizes nidus
- Protocol advice
  - Thin-section CT with reformats required
  - Greatest enhancement in arterial phase
    - Postcontrast MR should either be dynamic study or done 30 seconds following injection

DIFFERENTIAL DIAGNOSIS

DDx of Diaphyseal Cortical Lesion

- Stress fracture
  - Healing elicits sclerotic reaction, similar to OO
  - Reaction is linear, crossing bone; secures diagnosis
  - CT or MR should confirm linearity of fracture
- Chronic cortical osteomyelitis

- Round or oval lytic lesion surrounded by dense sclerotic reaction
- May have serpiginous sinus track, seen by CT or MR
- May contain dense sequestrum

DDx of Intracapsular Lesion

- Arthritis
  - Effusion
  - Reactive osteophyte formation
- Osteosarcoma or Ewing sarcoma
  - Reactive sclerosis &/or marrow edema may mimic these malignant tumors
  - Lack of permeative bone destruction or soft tissue mass in OO should differentiate

PATHOLOGY

Gross Pathologic & Surgical Features

- Round, red, gritty, or granular lesion surrounded by ivory white sclerotic bone

Microscopic Features

- Central region of vascularized connective tissue
  - Contains osteoblasts, which produce osteoid
  - Microtrabecular arrays lined by plump appositional osteoblasts may distinguish OO from osteoblastoma
- Hypervascular sclerotic bone surrounds central lesion
  - Abrupt interface between central lesion and surrounding sclerosis

CLINICAL ISSUES

Presentation

- Most common signs/symptoms
  - Pain, worse at night
    - Initially intermittent, later relentless
      - Early mild symptoms may delay seeking treatment
    - 80% report pain relief by salicylates or nonsteroidal antiinflammatory drugs
  - Intracapsular lesions present with signs of synovitis, joint pain, decreased range of motion
  - Physical exam: Very localized extreme tenderness
    - Possible associated redness and swelling
  - In spine, painful nonrotatory scoliosis, concave to side of lesion
- Other signs/symptoms
  - Premature osteoarthritic change if intracapsular and chronic (occurs in up to 50% of intracapsular femoral neck lesions)
  - Growth abnormalities if intracapsular, depending on skeletal age
  - Rare muscle atrophy
  - Rare neurologic signs

Demographics

- Age
  - Usual range: 10-25 years
    - Children and adolescents most frequently
- Gender
  - M > F (ratio 3:1)
- Epidemiology
  - Relatively common; 4-10% of primary bone tumors (excluding myeloma)

Natural History & Prognosis

- Pain becomes unremitting in most untreated cases
- Reports of involution of lesion and resolution of pain without intervention
  - Varying times, but generally many months to years
- If entire lesion is ablated or excised, recurrence extremely rare
  - Recurrence likely related to incomplete treatment and residual nidus
- No reported cases of malignant degeneration

Treatment

- CT-guided radiofrequency thermal ablation
  - 75-90% initial success rate reported
    - Large or nonspherical lesions may require 2nd ablative procedure
  - Requires careful planning of approach to avoid complications
  - Skin burn must be avoided, especially with superficial lesions
- MR-guided laser ablation and US ablation may be used
- Surgical resection is alternative
  - Resection is usually larger than with thermal ablation, leaving bone weakened
  - Lesion may be missed and sclerotic reaction resected

DIAGNOSTIC CHECKLIST

Consider

- Intracapsular OO diagnosis is often delayed
  - Lesion itself often missed due to small size
  - Distant sclerotic reaction and edema not recognized as reaction but worked-up as lesion of interest
  - Growth abnormalities and arthritis may overshadow lesion itself
- OO should be considered as possible cause of scoliosis in young patients
- Do not be distracted by reactive sclerosis or edema in adjacent bone or soft tissues
- Dynamic MR makes lesion more conspicuous, may aid in diagnosis of lesion in unusual location
- Prior to percutaneous ablation of OO, be certain lesion is not chronic cortical abscess
  - Biopsy for pathologic confirmation of OO in conjunction with ablation
  - Postablation infection may in fact be activation and spreading of preablative focus of infection

SELECTED REFERENCES

1. Aiba H et al: Conservative treatment for patients with osteoid osteoma: a case series. Anticancer Res. 34(7):3721-5, 2014
2. Bourgault C et al: Percutaneous CT-guided radiofrequency thermocoagulation in the treatment of osteoid osteoma: a 87 patient series. Orthop Traumatol Surg Res. 100(3):323-7, 2014
3. Fuchs S et al: Postinterventional MRI findings following MRI-guided laser ablation of osteoid osteoma. Eur J Radiol. 83(4):696-702, 2014
4. Ciftdemir M et al: Atypical osteoid osteomas. Eur J Orthop Surg Traumatol. 25(1):17-27, 2013

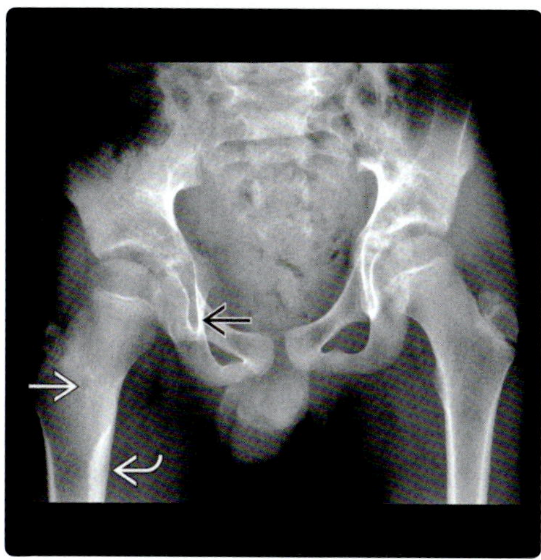
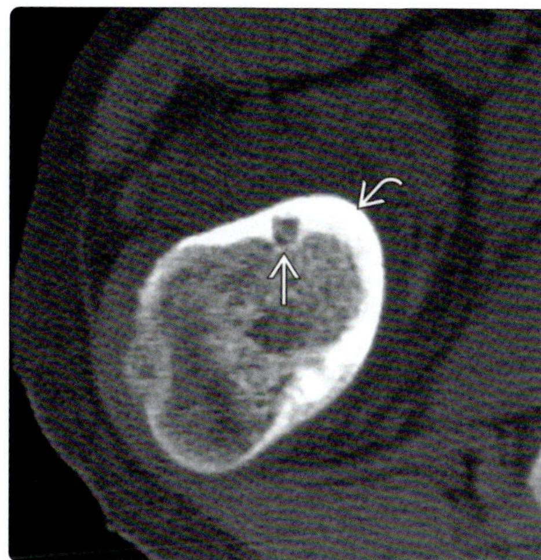

(Left) *AP radiograph shows altered morphology due to a intracapsular OO in a child. There is a subtle lytic lesion in the intertrochanteric region ➡, with calcar buttressing distally ➡. The femoral head is laterally subluxated, due to chronic effusion, which allows the teardrop to overgrow ➡. Finally, there is hip valgus due to chronic subluxation and altered weight bearing.* **(Right)** *Axial NECT in the same patient shows the OO to be located in the anterior cortex ➡, along with calcar reaction ➡.*

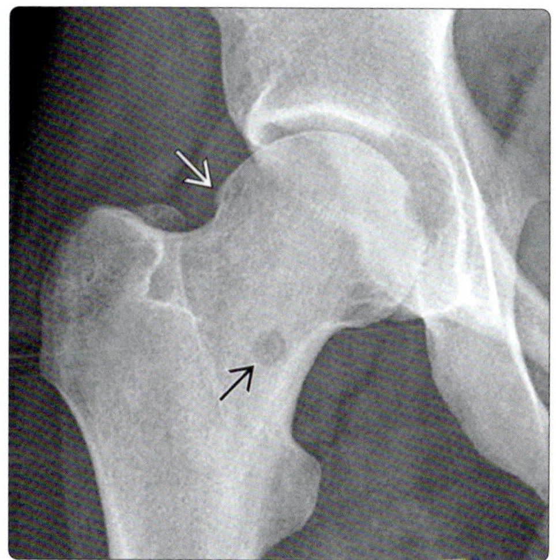
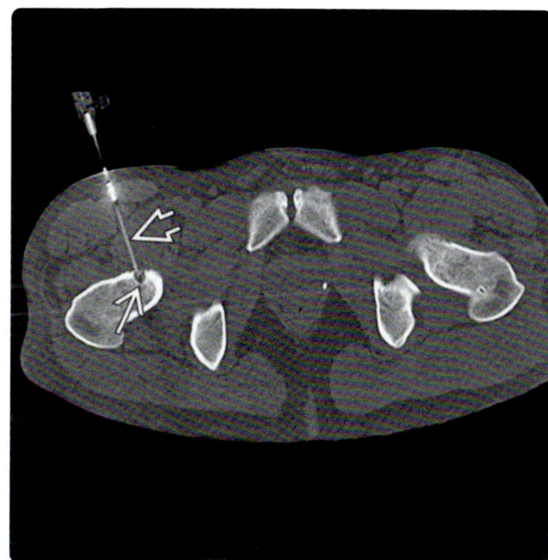

(Left) *AP radiograph demonstrates a typical femoral neck OO in a young adult. The lytic nidus is within the femoral neck ➡ and has elicited prominent reaction, with calcar buttressing and osteophyte formation ➡. There is little sclerosis surrounding the nidus itself; such sclerosis may be less prominent in intracapsular than cortical diaphyseal OO.* **(Right)** *Axial NECT shows the needle ➡ in position for percutaneous thermal ablation of this OO, located in the anterior cortex ➡.*

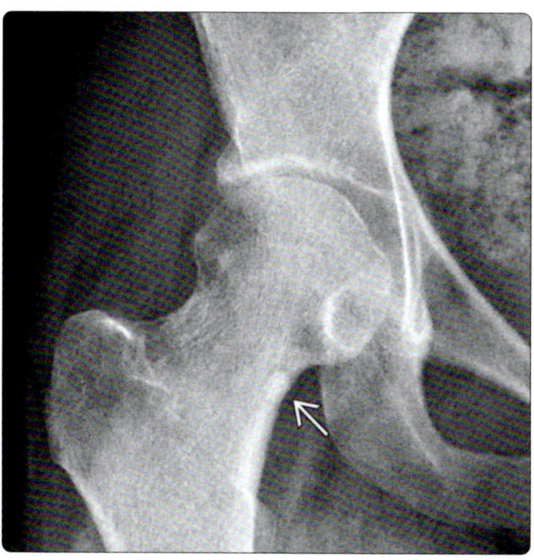
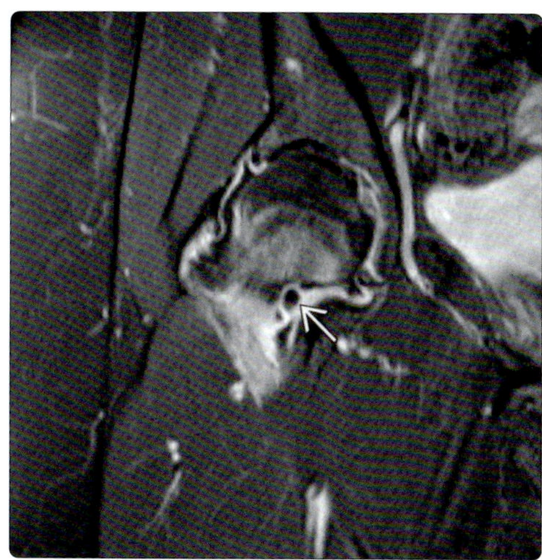

(Left) *AP radiograph of a subperiosteal OO shows a round sclerotic lesion located in or adjacent to the medial cortex of the hip ➡ in a patient whose history suggested OO. Note that there is minimal sclerotic reaction and no periosteal reaction to this lesion, which differentiates it from the usual cortical OO.* **(Right)** *Coronal T1WI C+ FS MR in the same patient shows the lesion to be low signal ➡ and located adjacent to, but not within, the cortex. There is mild surrounding marrow edema.*

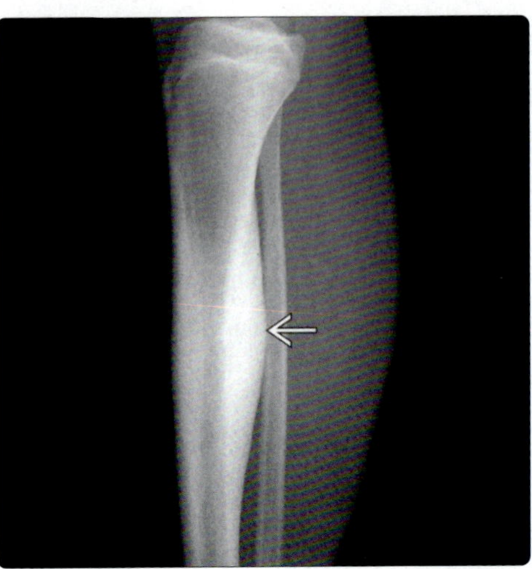

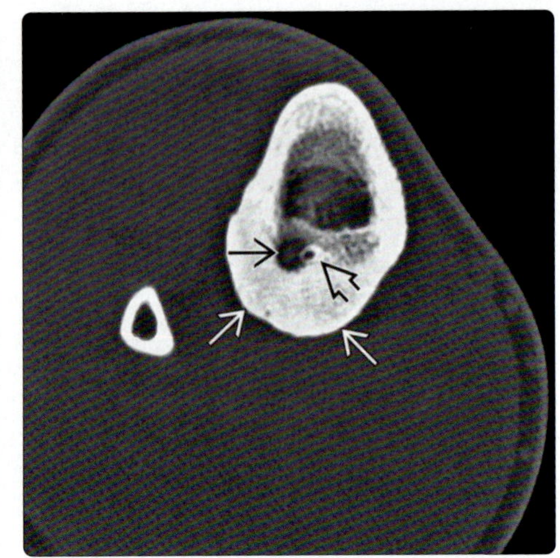

(Left) *Lateral radiograph shows a cortical diaphyseal OO, with prominent thickening of the posterior cortex of the tibia ➡. The thickened reactive bone obscures the nidus itself.* **(Right)** *Axial NECT in the same patient shows the heaped-up posterior periosteal reaction ➡ surrounding a round lytic lesion buried in the deep cortex, almost within the marrow itself ➡. This OO is located immediately adjacent to a nutrient vessel ➡, a relationship that is commonly seen.*

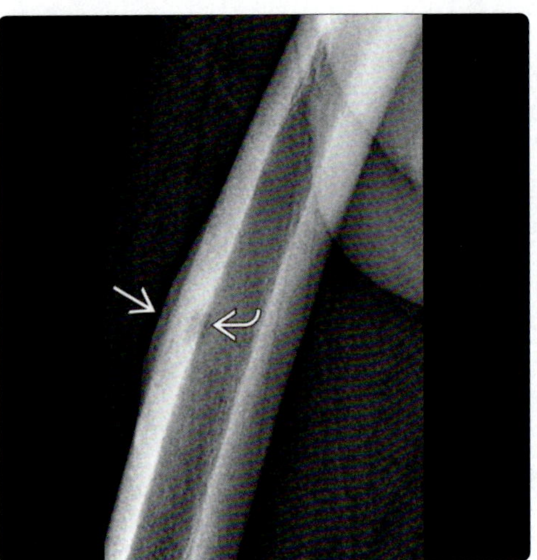

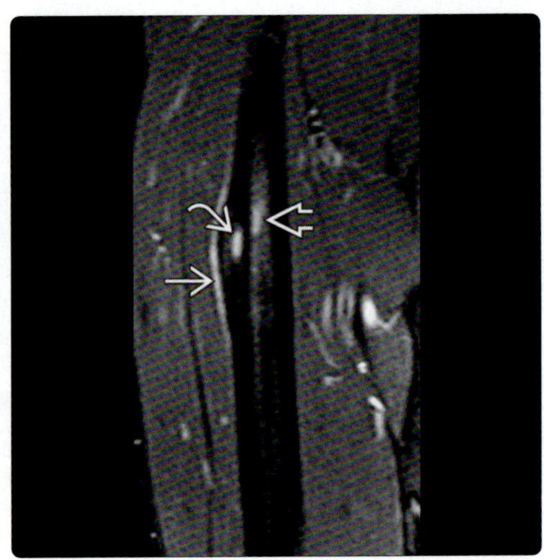

(Left) *Lateral radiograph allows the diagnosis of OO, with an oval lytic lesion ➡ and surrounding dense sclerotic reactive bone formation ➡.* **(Right)** *Coronal STIR MR in the same patient shows the nidus to have typical high signal on STIR ➡. Note that there is also high signal in the adjacent periosteum ➡, as well as within the adjacent marrow ➡. These reactive changes can make the benign lesion seem more aggressive on MR than on radiograph but must be expected with OO.*

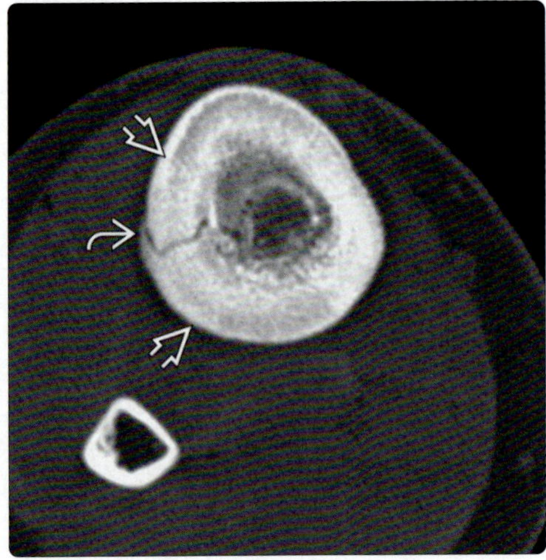

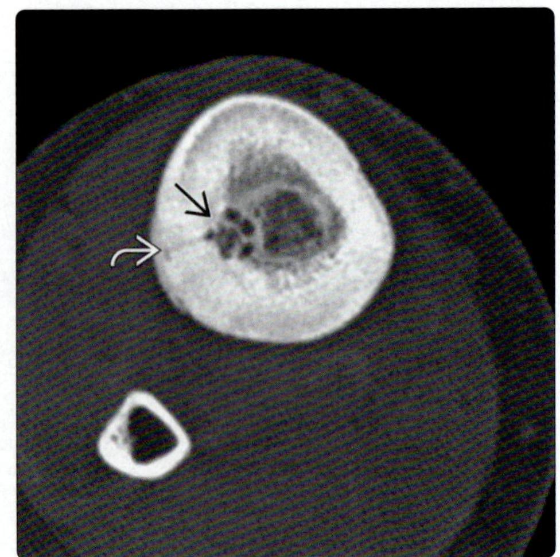

(Left) *Axial NECT shows an interesting case of OO. At this level, there is densely sclerotic cortical bone ➡ surrounding a fracture ➡. It is tempting to simply diagnose the lesion as a stress fracture.* **(Right)** *Axial NECT cut obtained slightly distal to the prior image shows the fracture line ➡ leading to the rather unusual appearing bubbly nidus located deep to the cortex, in the medullary space ➡. This OO has resulted in a pathologic fracture. The cortical reaction is due to both of these processes.*

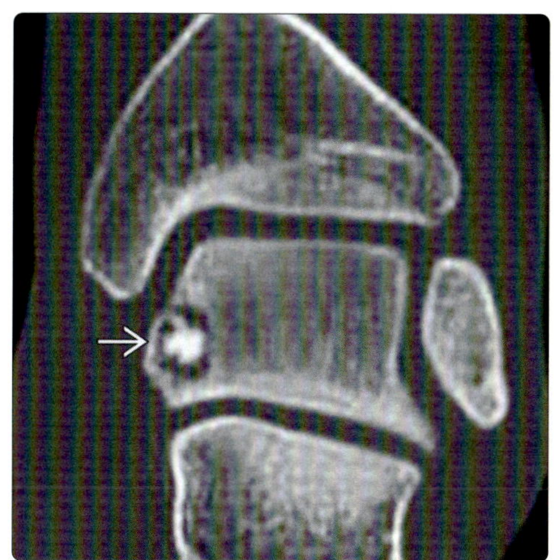

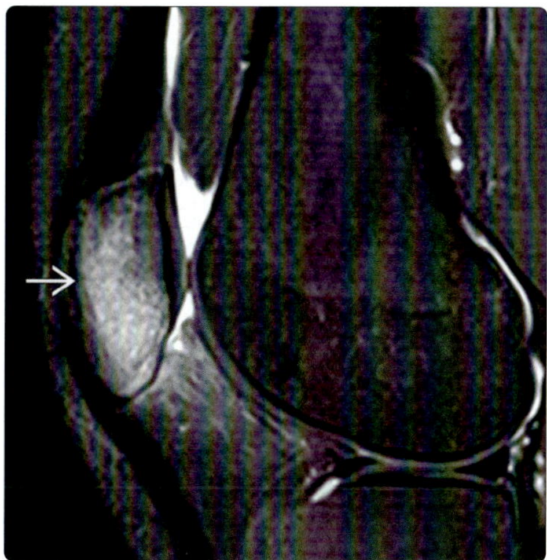

(Left) *Coronal bone CT shows an intramedullary OO within the talus ➡. Note the sclerotic nidus surrounded by a lucent halo, typical of this type of OO. There is no surrounding sclerosis. The hand/foot location is typical.* **(Right)** *Sagittal T2FS MR in a young patient with anterior knee pain shows intense edema within the entire patella ➡ but no focal lesion in this cut. With no nidus seen, the edema may lead to misdiagnosis of a more aggressive lesion.*

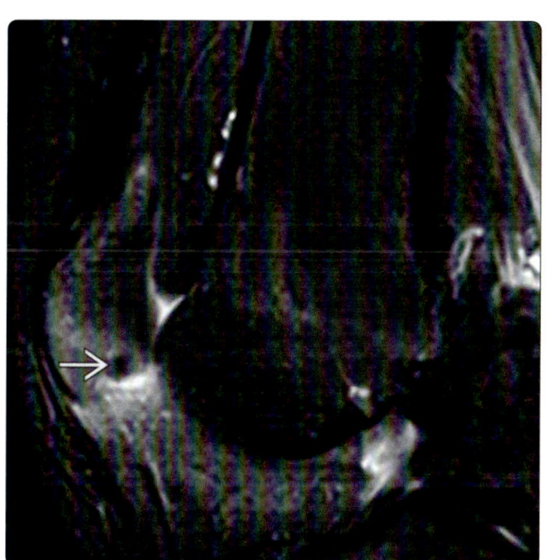

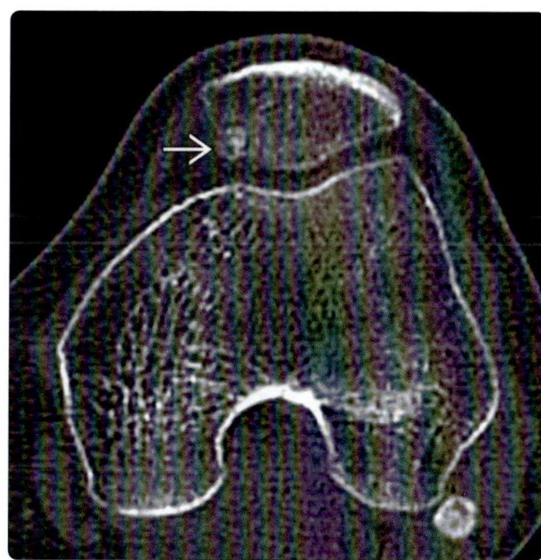

(Left) *Far medial sagittal T2 FS MR cut in the same patient shows a small focal low signal round lesion ➡. With the edema appearing so generalized in the patella, this low signal focus is not specific. While OO must be considered, it could also represent a small bone island with unrelated patellar marrow edema.* **(Right)** *Axial bone CT in the same patient shows the bubbly cortically based lytic lesion ➡ with mild surrounding reaction. With this image, the diagnosis of OO is secure.*

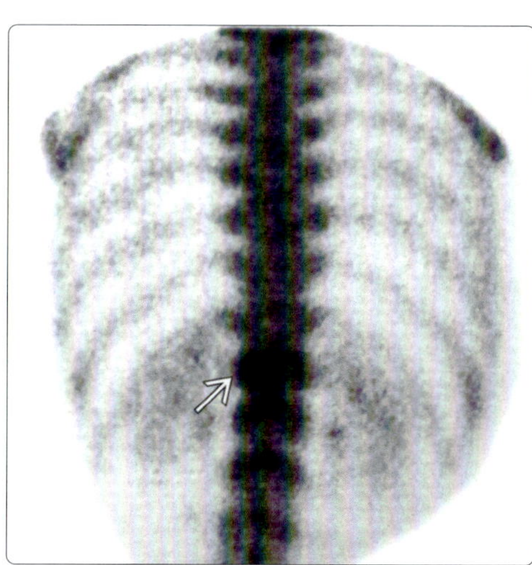

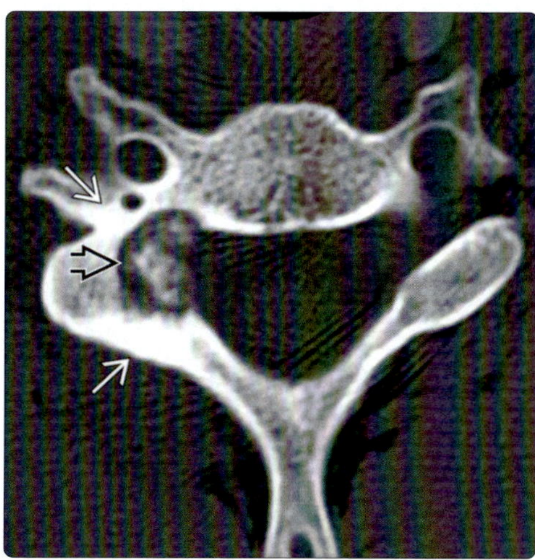

(Left) *Anteroposterior bone scan demonstrates increased uptake within the posterior elements of T12 ➡. The round uptake is at the apex, on the concave side of a scoliosis. CT proved OO at this site. Nonrotatory scoliosis in an adolescent should stimulate a search for OO.* **(Right)** *Axial bone CT shows a classic appearance of OO. There is a sharply demarcated lytic lesion in the neural arch ⇨; the lesion contains bone matrix. Reactive sclerosis is present around the lesion ➡.*

KEY FACTS

TERMINOLOGY

- Rare, benign bone-forming tumor

IMAGING

- Location
  - 40-55% occur in spine or flat bones
  - In spine, most frequently originates in posterior elements (94%) rather than body
  - 26% occur in long tubular bones
- Usually expanded, may be bubbly with thinned cortex
- May be entirely lytic (25-65%); may contain variable degrees of mineralized matrix
- Geographic, nonaggressive (92%)
  - Occasionally will act more aggressively
- MR fluid-sensitive sequences: Ranges from low to high signal intensity with variable degrees of inhomogeneity
  - May have extensive peripheral marrow edema and associated soft tissue edema (flare phenomenon)
  - Most are contained within bone; aggressive varieties have soft tissue mass

CLINICAL ISSUES

- 1st through 3rd decades; 2nd decade is most common
- Male > female, 2:1
- May progress either slowly or fairly aggressively
- Treatment: Surgical excision

DIAGNOSTIC CHECKLIST

- Considerations for cases of bone-forming lesions in typical location for osteoblastoma, but appearing aggressive
  - Atypical or aggressive osteoblastoma may be difficult to differentiate from osteosarcoma
  - Prominent marrow and soft tissue edema seen on MR of osteoblastoma may mimic more aggressive lesion (flare)
  - Aggressive (epithelioid-type) osteoblastomas may develop, without degeneration to osteosarcoma
  - Very rare cases of osteoblastoma degenerating to osteosarcoma have been reported

(Left) *Graphic depicts an osteoblastoma. The location within a posterior element of the spine is typical ➡, as is the expanded nature of the lesion, with a thin intact rim.* **(Right)** *AP radiograph shows a relatively small and lytic osteoblastoma arising in a transverse process ➡. The nonaggressive nature of the lesion, as well as its location, is typical for this diagnosis. A small amount of ossific matrix is present, which secures the diagnosis.*

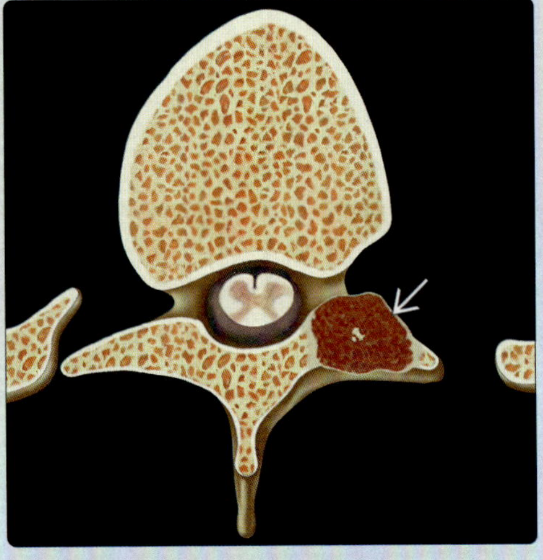

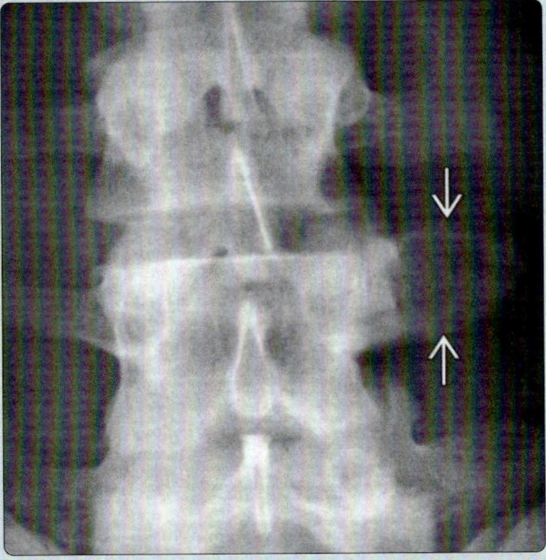

(Left) *Lateral radiograph shows a widely expanded lesion occupying the spinous process ➡. The degree of ossific matrix is remarkable and the lesion appears nonaggressive, allowing the diagnosis of osteoblastoma to be made with certainty. If the lesion was completely lytic, the diagnosis of aneurysmal bone cyst would have to be considered.* **(Right)** *AP radiograph shows a dense but irregularly ossified mass arising at the T3 level ➡. This is another appearance in the spectrum of ossification of osteoblastoma.*

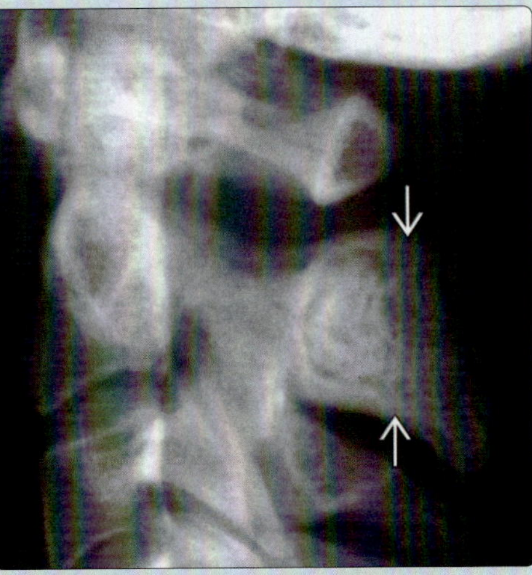

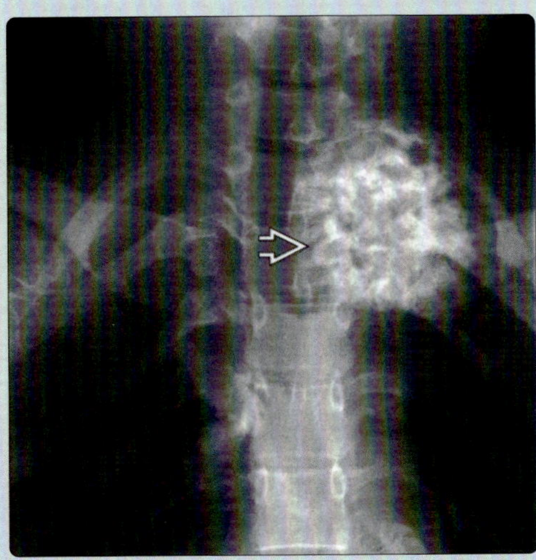

TERMINOLOGY

Abbreviations

- Osteoblastoma (OB)

Synonyms

- Giant osteoid osteoma
  - Incorrect term, but emphasizes its histologic similarity to osteoid osteoma
- Ossifying giant cell tumor
- Osteogenic fibroma (outdated term)

Definitions

- Rare, benign bone-forming tumor

IMAGING

General Features

- Best diagnostic clue
  - Expanded lesion, ± matrix, generally nonaggressive, involving posterior spinal elements or long bones
    - Degree of aggressiveness may truly vary
    - Imaging appearance of aggressiveness may vary, with MR appearing more aggressive than radiograph/CT or clinical behavior of lesion
- Location
  - 40-55% occur in spine or flat bones
    - In spine, most frequently originates in posterior elements (94%) rather than body
      - Lesion may extend from posterior elements to involve vertebral body, especially if aggressive
      - Equal distribution in cervical, thoracic, lumbar, sacral regions
    - Flat bones: Pelvis, scapula
  - 26% occur in long tubular bones
    - Femur is most frequent long bone location
    - Metadiaphyseal
    - Eccentric (46%) or cortically based (42%)
  - 26% in hands and feet
    - Majority in talus, usually at dorsal neck
  - Skull and mandible: Some consider cementoblastoma to be OB (attached to root of tooth)
  - Subperiosteal location is rare, generally confined to facial and cranial locations; may be seen in long bones
  - Soft tissue location is extremely rare
  - Multifocal OB is extremely rare
- Size
  - Generally > 2 cm; may be quite large
- Morphology
  - Generally round to oval

Radiographic Findings

- Usually expanded, with thinned cortex; may be bubbly
- May be entirely lytic (25-65%) or may contain variable degrees of mineralized matrix
- Geographic, nonaggressive (92%)
  - Sclerotic margin in majority of lesions
  - Occasionally will act more aggressively
    - May develop less well-defined, moth-eaten, or permeative perimeter
    - May have cortical breakthrough and soft tissue mass
- Periosteal reaction in 86%; usually linear, lamellated
  - Rarely spiculated reaction
- Scoliosis, concave to side of lesion in spine or rib

CT Findings

- Matches radiographic findings of geographic lesion with occasional aggressive characteristics
  - Matrix ossification may be better visualized on CT
  - Thin cortical rim more apparent on CT than x-ray

MR Findings

- T1WI: Low to intermediate signal, fairly homogeneous
  - Lower signal foci if matrix present
- Fluid-sensitive sequences: Ranges from low to high SI with variable degrees of inhomogeneity
  - Depends on degree of matrix ossification present
- Enhancement ranges from mild to intense, depending on amount of matrix ossification
  - With near complete ossification of lesion, peripheral enhancement is usually seen
- May have extensive peripheral marrow edema and associated soft tissue edema (flare phenomenon)
  - Reactive edema may be so intense and extensive as to make lesion appear more aggressive on MR than on CT
- Most are contained within bone; aggressive varieties have associated soft tissue mass
  - Soft tissue mass characteristics mimic those of bone, depending at least in part on degree of mineralization
- Aneurysmal bone cyst may arise within lesion
  - Fluid-fluid levels seen in portion of lesion

Nuclear Medicine Findings

- Intense focal uptake on bone scan
- All reported cases metabolically active on FDG-PET

DIFFERENTIAL DIAGNOSIS

Aneurysmal Bone Cyst

- In spine, arises in posterior elements, similar to OB
- In long bones, metadiaphyseal and eccentric
- Often has fluid-fluid levels; OB may have them as well
- No calcific matrix

Giant Cell Tumor

- In spine, generally arises in body rather than posterior elements (location of OB)
- Entirely lytic
- No sclerotic margin

Langerhans Cell Histiocytosis

- Lytic lesion, which may have variable degrees of aggressive behavior
- No matrix, but may mimic entirely lytic OB, particularly in pelvic lesion of child

Fibrous Dysplasia

- Variable degree of density (lytic to ground-glass to sclerotic) may mimic OB
- Often polyostotic, which would distinguish it from OB
- In tubular bones is usually central rather than eccentric
- Less frequently in spine than OB unless polyostotic

Osteoid Osteoma

- Generally, distinctly different clinical history and imaging appearance
- Histopathology may be confusing
  - Historically, some authors suggest OB and osteoid osteoma (OO) are different clinical expressions or stages of same pathologic process
  - Subtle pathologic differences do exist; should be evaluated in conjunction with imaging

Osteosarcoma

- Uncommon in spine
- Osteoid production in osteosarcoma (OS) may be difficult to distinguish from matrix in aggressive OB
- May be difficult to distinguish from aggressive OB
  - Generally, OS has more pronounced permeative osseous destruction than OB
  - Generally, OS has larger soft tissue mass than OB
  - Generally, OS has more aggressive periosteal reaction than OB

PATHOLOGY

Gross Pathologic & Surgical Features

- Hemorrhagic, red and brown
- Gritty or granular consistency; may have cystic regions

Microscopic Features

- Osteoid production: Very active formation of osteoid and immature bone trabeculae
  - Compact masses of large osteoblasts
  - Well vascularized
  - Diffusely scattered osteoclast-type multinucleated giant cells
  - Hyaline cartilage may be present
- Aggressive osteoblastoma characterized by epithelioid osteoblasts
  - Significantly larger than normal osteoblasts
  - More prominent nucleoli with abundant cytoplasm
- Histologic differentiation between OB and OO may be difficult
  - Should be interpreted in context of imaging and clinical findings
  - Osteoid production in OB greater than in OO
  - Less organized pattern of trabecular bone than in nidus of OO

CLINICAL ISSUES

Presentation

- Most common signs/symptoms
  - Dull, localized, gradually increasing pain
  - Neurologic symptoms if cord or nerve root compression
    - Reported in 38% of spinal lesions
  - Tenderness to palpation at lesion site
- Other signs/symptoms
  - Scoliosis, concave to side of rib or spine lesion
    - Not as frequent association as in OO
  - Tumor-associated osteomalacia (rare)
  - Preoperative alkaline phosphatase levels may distinguish between conventional and aggressive OB

Demographics

- Age
  - 1st through 3rd decades; 2nd decade is most common
    - Aggressive OB subgroup generally seen in older age group
- Gender
  - Male > female, 2:1
- Epidemiology
  - 1-2% of all bone tumors
  - 3-6% of all benign bone tumors

Natural History & Prognosis

- Progression
  - May progress either slowly or fairly aggressively
  - Rare reports of malignant degeneration to OS
    - Generally following multiple recurrences of aggressive OB
    - Possibility of misdiagnosis of initial lesion should be considered

Treatment

- Surgical excision
  - Wide resection is curative but may not be necessary
  - Marginal excision (curettage) is most frequently chosen if wide resection would result in functional impairment
    - Incomplete excision may result in recurrence (14-24% reported in different series)
    - Progression-free survival 74% at 10 years in 1 study
    - Recurrence may be up to 50% in aggressive OB
- Percutaneous thermal ablation is reported

DIAGNOSTIC CHECKLIST

Consider

- Considerations for cases of bone-forming lesion in typical location for OB, but appearing aggressive
  - Atypical or aggressive OB may be difficult to differentiate from OS
  - Prominent marrow and soft tissue edema seen on MR of OB may mimic more aggressive lesion (flare)
    - May have discordant appearance relative to radiograph or CT
    - Differentiate this flare phenomenon from truly aggressive OB
  - Aggressive (epithelioid-type) OBs may develop, without degeneration to OS
  - Very rare cases of OB degenerating to OS have been reported

SELECTED REFERENCES

1. Orguc S et al: Primary tumors of the spine. Semin Musculoskelet Radiol. 18(3):280-99, 2014
2. Ruggieri P et al: Osteoblastoma of the sacrum: report of 18 cases and analysis of the literature. Spine (Phila Pa 1976). 39(2):E97-E103, 2014
3. Yalcinkaya U et al: Clinical and morphological characteristics of osteoid osteoma and osteoblastoma: a retrospective single-center analysis of 204 patients. Ann Diagn Pathol. 18(6):319-25, 2014
4. Yin H et al: Clinical characteristics and treatment options for two types of osteoblastoma in the mobile spine: a retrospective study of 32 cases and outcomes. Eur Spine J. 23(2):411-6, 2014
5. Al-Muqbel KM et al: Osteoblastoma is a metabolically active benign bone tumor on 18F-FDG PET imaging. J Nucl Med Technol. 41(4):308-10, 2013

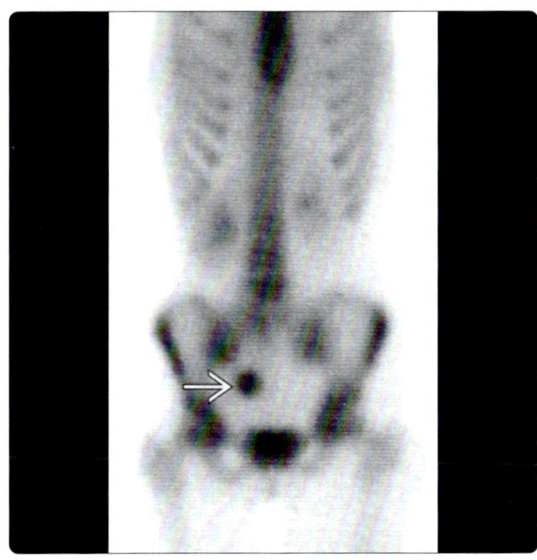

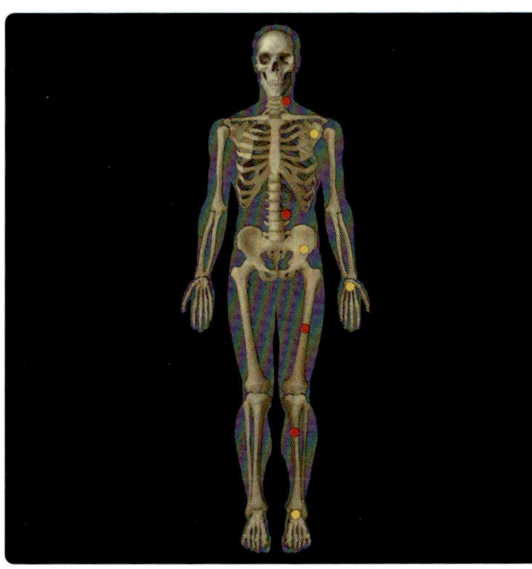

(Left) *AP bone scan shows a focus of uptake superimposed over the right sacrum ➡, corresponding to a site of dull aching pain. The lesion proved to be OB, which invariably shows increased uptake on bone scan and is metabolically active on FDG-PET.* **(Right)** *Graphic depicts the distribution of osteoblastoma. The lesion is seen most frequently in the posterior elements of the spine (red). The femur and tibia are the most frequently involved tubular bones (red). Flat bones and hand/foot bones are less commonly involved (yellow).*

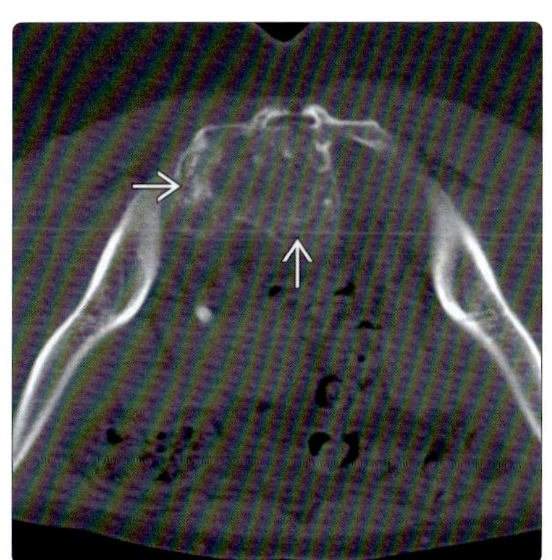

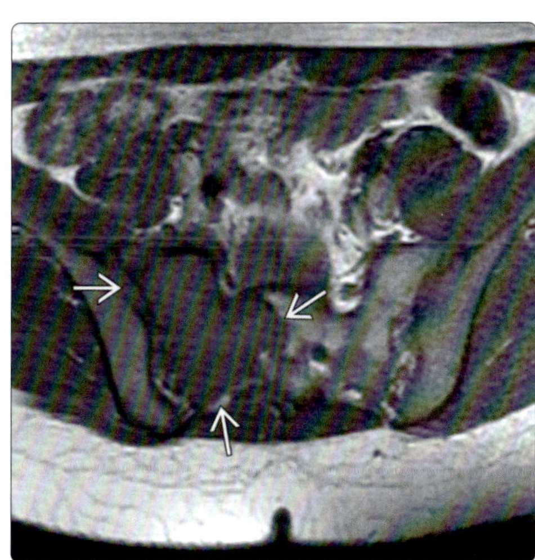

(Left) *Axial bone CT in prone position shows an expanded lesion arising from the sacrum in a 19-year-old woman. There are foci of matrix ➡ within the lesion. No cortical break is seen. Differential diagnoses include osteoblastoma, chordoma, and less likely, chondrosarcoma.* **(Right)** *Axial T1 MR in the same patient shows the lesion ➡ involves both the body and posterior elements of the sacrum. It is fairly homogeneously hypointense, similar to skeletal muscle.*

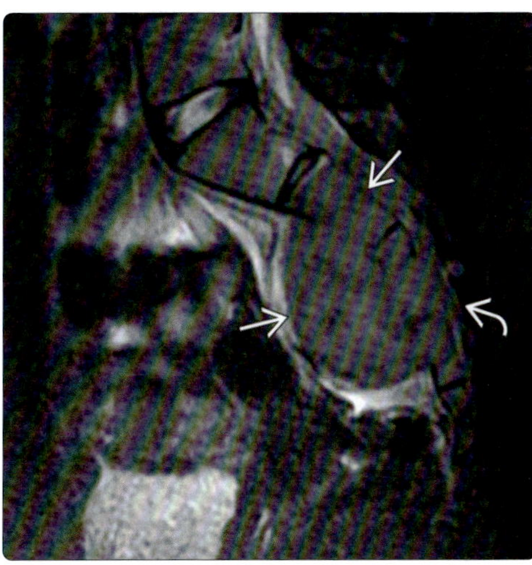

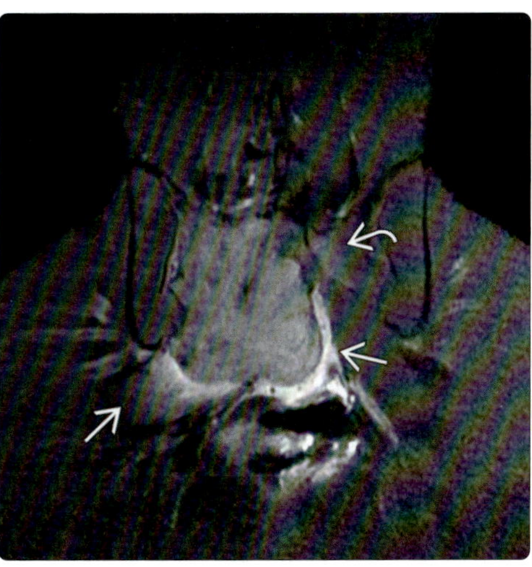

(Left) *Sagittal T2 FS MR shows the large expanded lesion ➡ involve multiple sacral elements and extend into the canal ➡. The signal is inhomogeneous and relatively low, related to the osteoid matrix formation seen on CT.* **(Right)** *Coronal postcontrast T1FS MR shows the inhomogeneously enhancing lesion, but also regions of flare enhancement involving the adjacent sacrum ➡ and soft tissues ➡. This flare is not expected in chordoma or chondrosarcoma, but is seen in OB; this diagnosis was confirmed at biopsy.*

(Left) *Axial T2WI MR shows a typical osteoblastoma of the right L2 lamina. There is a heterogeneous mass that expands the lamina very significantly ➡. The lesion showed moderate, much more homogeneous enhancement with contrast.* **(Right)** *Coronal T2WI MR in the same patient again demonstrates the heterogeneous expanding mass ➡. Note the scoliosis, concave on the side of the lesion. Osteoblastoma should always be considered in the differential diagnosis of painful scoliosis.*

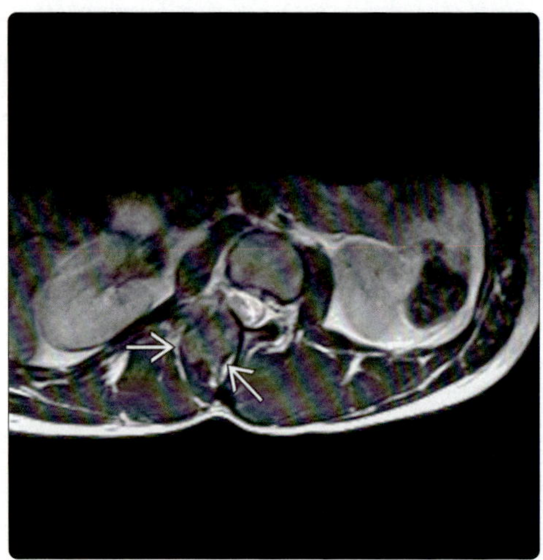

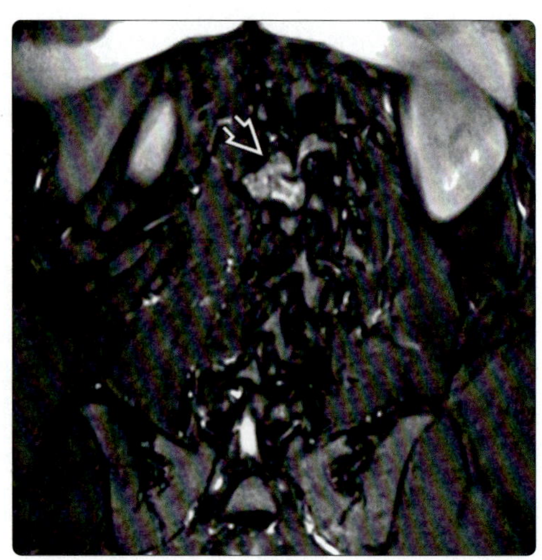

(Left) *Axial bone CT shows a typical osteoblastoma ➡, which is completely lytic, with mild expansion of the lamina. There is no cortical breakthrough, and no hint of aggressive behavior.* **(Right)** *Axial T1WI C+ FS MR of the same lesion shows tremendous enhancement of the epidural tissues ➡, paraspinous muscles ➡, and spinous process ➡, giving a highly aggressive appearance. This MR description is discordant with the nonaggressive CT appearance. This has been termed the flare phenomenon.*

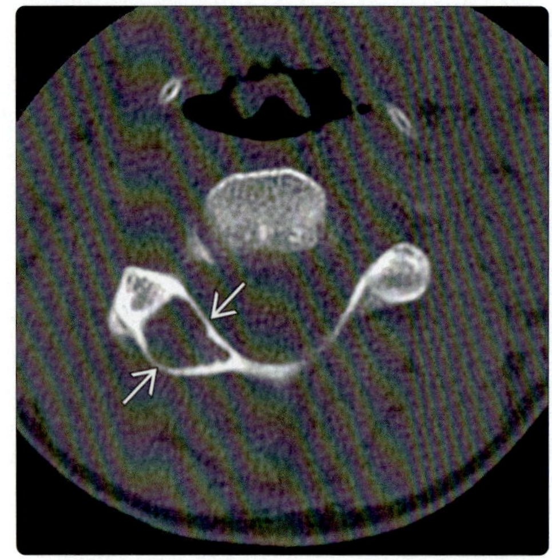

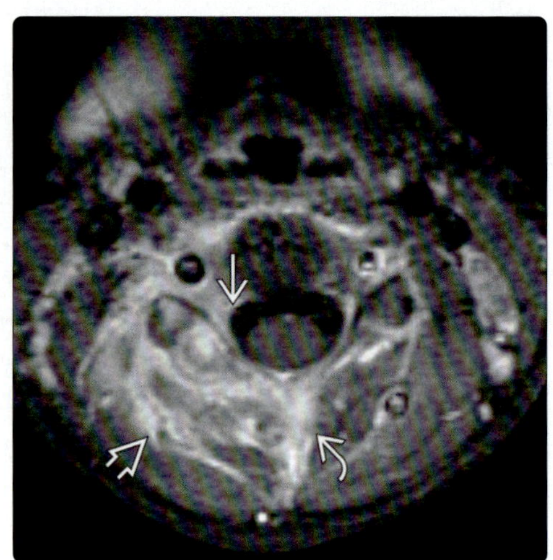

(Left) *AP radiograph shows an eccentric sclerotic metadiaphyseal lesion ➡. The density and central rounded lucencies are unusual for a diagnosis of healing nonossifying fibroma (NOF). Giant bone island is unlikely, given the sharp border.* **(Right)** *Coronal T1WI C+ is mostly low signal, matching the precontrast T1. However, there are regions of contrast enhancement centrally ➡, not expected in either healing NOF or giant bone island. However, a mildly active OB might feature this characteristic. Biopsy proved this diagnosis.*

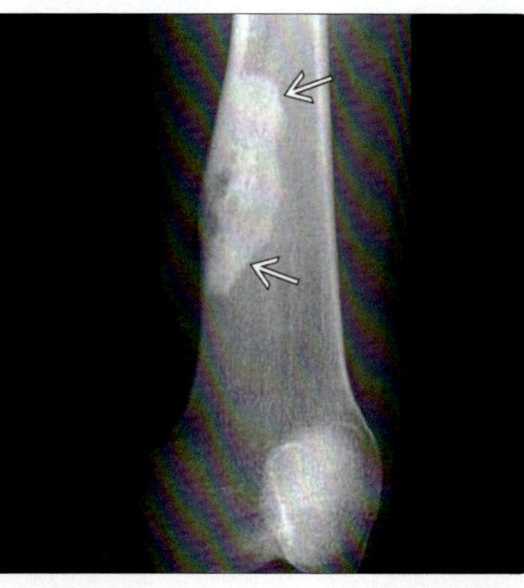

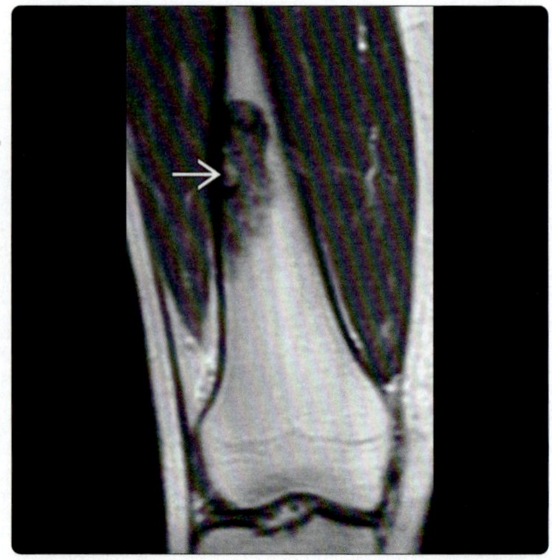

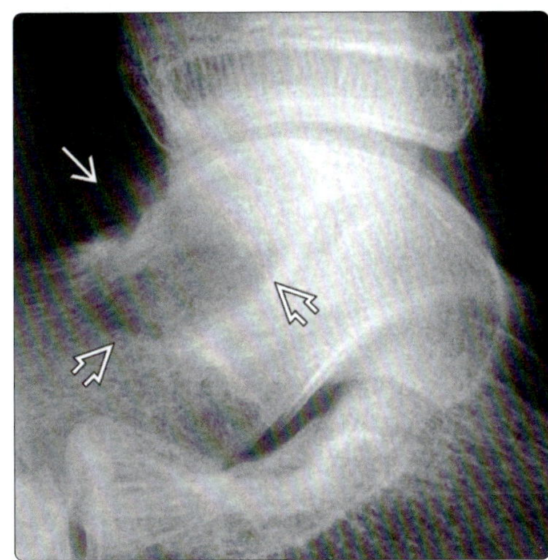

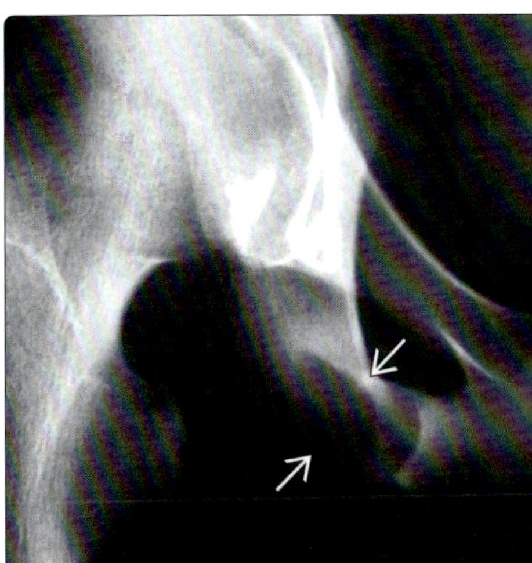

(Left) *Lateral radiograph of the talus shows a lytic "blistering" lesion arising at the dorsal neck of the talus ➡. This is the typical appearance and location of osteoblastoma when it arises in this bone. This patient has developed a secondary aneurysmal bone cyst ⇨.* **(Right)** *AP radiograph shows a lytic lesion, well circumscribed and nonaggressive, arising in the ischium ➡. Without matrix, several other diagnoses are statistically more likely than osteoblastoma, but the latter was proven at biopsy.*

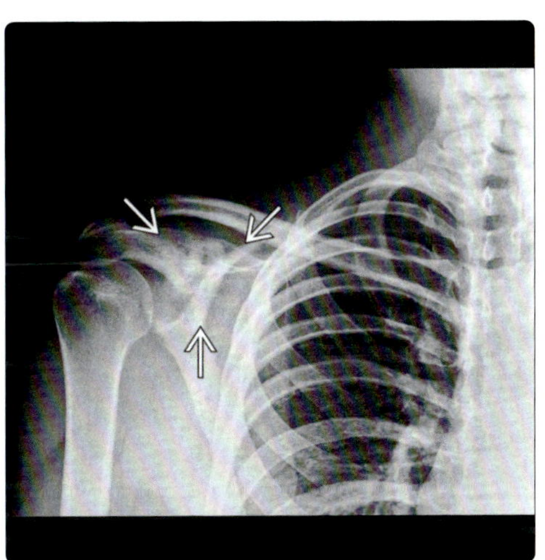

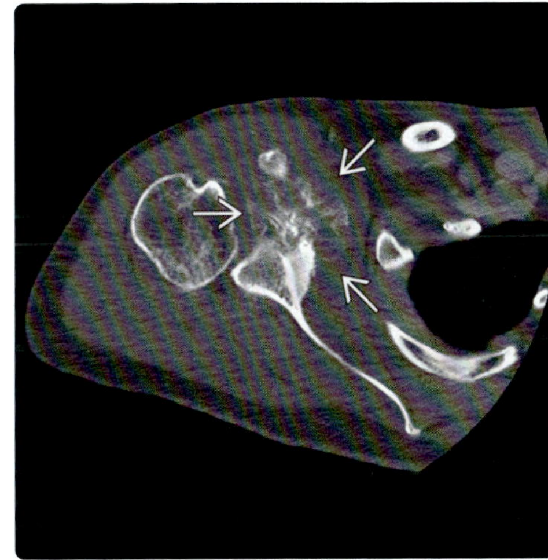

(Left) *AP radiograph reveals an expansile, lytic lesion involving the scapula ➡. This is a nonspecific appearance. By radiograph, no matrix is seen, and the lesion does not appear aggressive.* **(Right)** *Axial NECT in the same patient adds significant information, better demonstrating the lesion to be expanded, arising exophytically from the anterior glenoid. There is internal bony matrix ➡ that was not seen on the initial radiograph. This lesion arises in a periosteal location. Note the subluxated humeral head.*

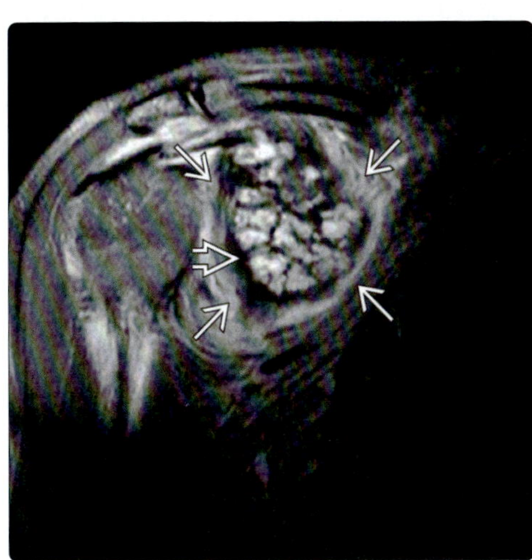

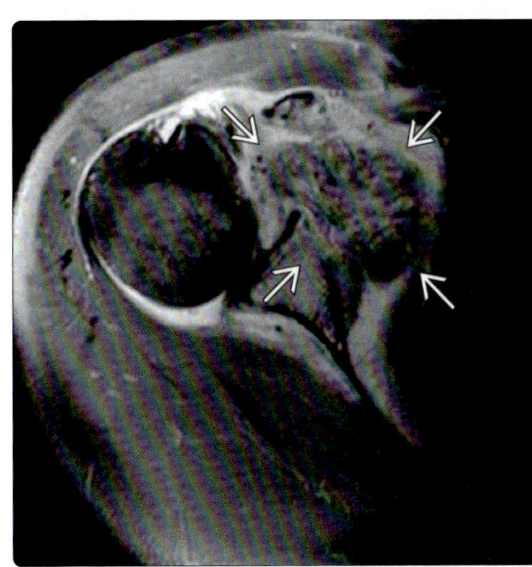

(Left) *Coronal STIR MR in the same patient shows the lesion contains lobulated inhomogeneous high signal tissue ➡. A few fluid levels are present ⇨.* **(Right)** *Axial T1WI C+ FS MR in the same patient emphasizes the lesion arising from a periosteal location on the glenoid ➡. It enhances inhomogeneously. Given the bony matrix, the lesion must be considered either an aggressive periosteal osteoblastoma or a telangiectatic osteosarcoma. Histology revealed epithelioid osteoblastoma, a rare aggressive variant of OB.*

Conventional Osteosarcoma

KEY FACTS

TERMINOLOGY

- Malignant osteoid-producing tumor originating in intramedullary space

IMAGING

- 91% in metaphysis, 9% in diaphysis
  - Note: Epiphyseal involvement should be sought; physis is not effective barrier
    - 75-88% extension to epiphysis in children
- Permeative, destructive lesion, eccentrically located
  - Wide zone of transition, no sclerotic margin
- Density ranges from lytic to intensely sclerotic
  - Visible matrix present in majority (90%)
  - Adjacent nodal metastases may contain osteoid
  - Lung metastases may be ossified
- Cortical destruction, soft tissue mass (90%)
- Rare skip metastases: Noncontiguous lesions in same or adjacent bone
- MR: Fluid-sensitive sequences
  - Peritumoral edema, both in bone and soft tissue, may exaggerate size of mass
- Intense enhancement of marrow and soft tissue mass
  - Differentiates viable regions from areas of necrosis

CLINICAL ISSUES

- Most commonly occur in 2nd decade (75% occur in patients < 25 years of age)
- Male > female, 3:2 ratio (less dramatic gender difference in older population)
- Most common malignant bone tumor in children/adolescents
- 5-10% have pulmonary metastases at presentation
  - Pulmonary > osseous and nodal metastases
- Multidisciplinary therapy results in disease-free survival of 60-80% if patients are good responders to chemotherapy (> 90% tumor necrosis)
- Local recurrence or systemic metastases generally occur within 2 years but long-term surveillance required

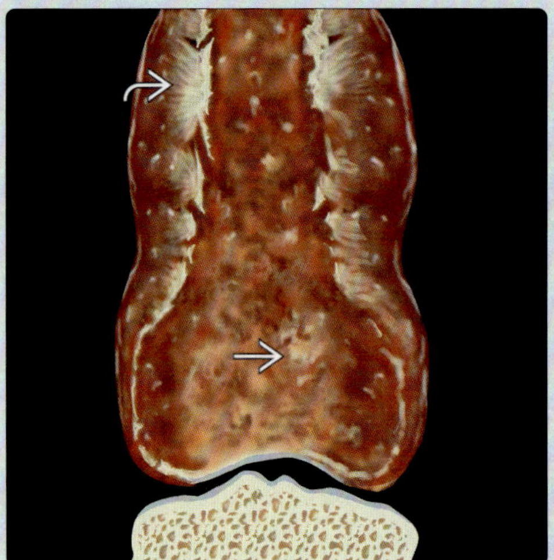

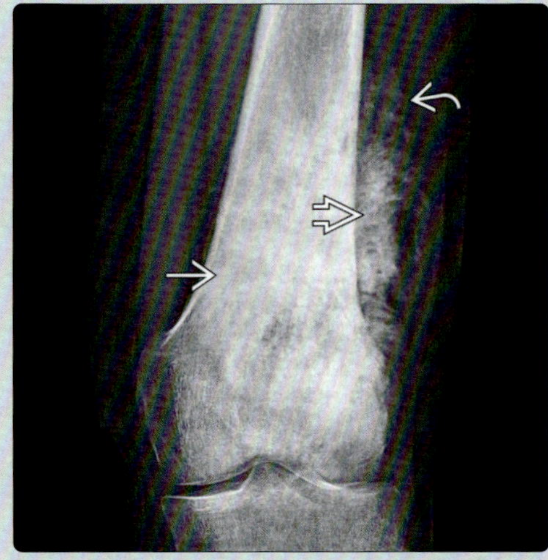

(Left) *Graphic depicts a cut section through osteosarcoma (OS). The permeative lesion destroys osseous architecture and breaks through the cortex, with a circumferential soft tissue mass. Amorphous osteoid is depicted, both within the bone → and in the soft tissues →.* **(Right)** *AP radiograph in a 25-year-old woman shows dense sclerotic tumor osteoid replacing metadiaphyseal marrow → and a soft tissue mass containing both dense → and amorphous → tumor osteoid. Conventional OS is the only possible diagnosis.*

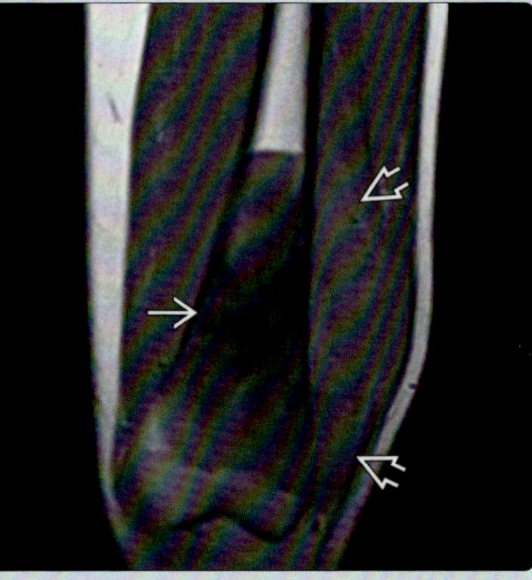

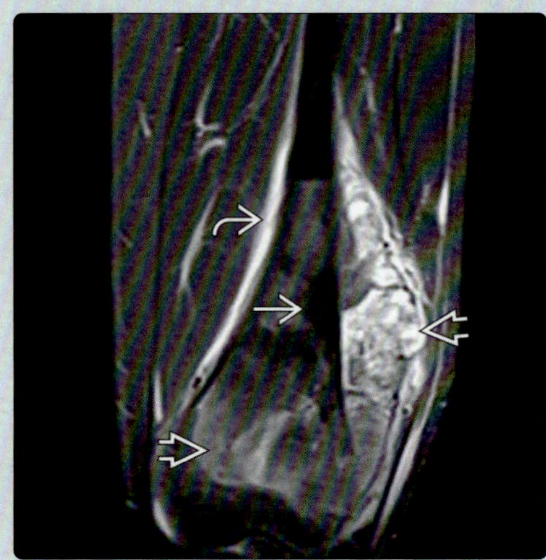

(Left) *Coronal T1 MR in the same patient shows hypointense marrow replacement; the lowest signal represents tumor osteoid →. There is a soft tissue mass → displacing soft tissues.* **(Right)** *Coronal T1 C+ FS MR shows enhancing tissue → along with hypointense tumor osteoid →. Periosteal reaction hyperintensity → and tumor extending through the cortex is noted. This is an extremely aggressive lesion.*

TERMINOLOGY

Abbreviations

- Osteosarcoma (OS)

Synonyms

- Osteogenic sarcoma, central OS, medullary OS, sclerosing osteosarcoma, subtypes osteoblastic sarcoma, chondroblastic OS, fibroblastic OS

Definitions

- Malignant osteoid-producing tumor originating in intramedullary space

IMAGING

General Features

- Location
  - 91% in metaphysis, 9% in diaphysis
    - Note: Epiphyseal involvement should be sought; physis is not effective barrier
      - 75-88% extension to epiphysis in children
      - Primary site of OS in epiphysis is extremely rare
  - Long bones 70-80%
    - 50% around knee
    - Femur (40-45%) > tibia (16-20%) > humerus
  - Other bones involved more frequently in older patients
- Size
  - Rapid growth, often > 6 cm at time of diagnosis

Radiographic Findings

- Permeative, destructive lesion, eccentrically located in metaphysis or metadiaphysis
  - Wide zone of transition, no sclerotic margin
  - Contour of bone usually not expanded; reflects rapid destructive process
- Density ranges from lytic to intensely sclerotic
  - Visible matrix present in majority (90%)
  - Most are mixed lytic/sclerotic
  - Osteoid matrix: Usually less dense than bone, amorphous, and unorganized
- Cortical destruction, soft tissue mass (90%)
  - Soft tissue mass may contain tumor osteoid
- Periosteal reaction: Aggressive
  - Codman triangle, interrupted, "sunburst" types
- Rare skip metastases: Noncontiguous lesions in same or adjacent bone
- Adjacent nodal metastases may contain osteoid matrix
- Lung metastases may be ossified
  - Rarely complicated by spontaneous pneumothorax
- Restaging radiographs, after chemotherapy, often show tumor to have enlarged
  - Tumor osteoid matures as chemotherapy shrinks soft tissue mass; volume of osteoid enlarges as it matures

CT Findings

- May better define osteoid matrix, but rarely necessary
  - Unusual forms (intracortical OS) better defined on CT
- Soft tissue mass seen, with low-attenuation necrosis
- Required for staging of lung metastases

MR Findings

- Osteoid low signal on all sequences
  - MR may demonstrate more regions of low signal osteoid than are evident by calcified matrix on radiograph or CT
- T1: Nonosteoid portions near isointense to muscle
- Fluid-sensitive sequences (generally fat saturated)
  - Heterogeneous ↑ signal soft tissue and osseous mass
  - Peritumoral edema, both in bone and soft tissue, may exaggerate size of mass
- Intense enhancement of marrow and soft tissue mass
  - Differentiates viable regions from ↓ signal necrosis

Nuclear Medicine Findings

- Bone scan demonstrates
  - Skip lesions in same or adjacent bone
    - Assumes lesion at least 1 cm diameter
  - Osseous metastases at other sites
  - May show ossified lymph node or lung metastases
- PET/CT: May be useful as prognostic indicator
  - High standardized uptake value (SUV) before and after chemotherapy suggests worse disease-free survival
  - ↑ total lesion glycolysis (TLG) following chemotherapy associated with worse prognosis
  - > 90% tumor necrosis associated with ↓ SUV
  - 1 study showed PET/CT useful at least once during treatment of 9 of 20 OS patients

Image-Guided Biopsy

- Plan in conjunction with oncologic surgeon
  - Cross only single compartment
  - Needle track will be resected, so do not contaminate tissue needed for reconstructive surgery
- Obtain both fine-needle aspirate and core samples
  - Be certain biopsy is of representative viable tissue
    - Avoid mature bone matrix/necrotic regions

Imaging Recommendations

- Best imaging tool
  - Generally diagnosed on radiograph
  - CT required to evaluate for lung metastases and often used for image-guided biopsy
  - MR with contrast required for site evaluation and biopsy/surgical planning
  - MR used for restaging after initial chemotherapy
  - Bone scan or PET/CT may be used to evaluate for other metastatic sites, generally requested if physical exam suggests additional systemic disease

DIFFERENTIAL DIAGNOSIS

Ewing Sarcoma

- Highly aggressive lesion, generally diaphyseal but may be metadiaphyseal
- May elicit prominent reactive bone formation, mimicking sclerosis of OS
  - Sclerosis in Ewing sarcoma found **only** in bone, not soft tissue mass; differentiating it from OS

Osteoblastoma

- Bone-forming tumor most frequently arising in posterior elements of spine

- Occasionally highly aggressive and even malignant, mimicking OS

PATHOLOGY

General Features

- Etiology
  - Genetic susceptibility in patients with hereditary retinoblastoma and Li-Fraumeni syndrome
- Genetics
  - No specific translocation or other structural alteration; recurrent involvement of certain chromosomal regions

Microscopic Features

- Highly anaplastic, pleomorphic, containing mixtures of several cell types
  - Epithelioid, plasmacytoid, small round cells, giant cells, spindle cells
- Osteoid must be identified for diagnosis
- Varying amounts of cartilage &/or fibrous tissue
  - Histological subdivision of OS into osteoblastic (50%), chondroblastic (25%), and fibroblastic (25%)
  - Imaging appearance and prognosis do not directly correlate with these histologic subtypes

CLINICAL ISSUES

Presentation

- Most common signs/symptoms
  - Nonspecific deep pain, becomes unremitting
  - Tender mass, limitation in function
  - Pathologic fracture in 5-10%

Demographics

- Age
  - Most commonly occurs in 2nd decade (75% occur in patients < 25 years of age)
    - Older patient population often has predisposing lesion with secondary OS
- Gender
  - Male > female, 3:2 ratio (less dramatic gender difference in older population)
- Epidemiology
  - Most common nonhematologic primary bone tumor (4-5/1,000,000 population), 2nd only to myeloma
  - Most common malignant bone tumor in children/adolescents
  - 15% of all biopsied primary bone tumors
  - 85% of all types of OS

Natural History & Prognosis

- Universally fatal if untreated (rapid hematogenous dissemination)
- 5-10% have pulmonary metastases at presentation
- Pulmonary > osseous and nodal metastases
- Prognosis relates to
  - Initial tumor stage (size, grade, metastases)
  - Response to initial chemotherapy
  - Completeness of resection
- 80-90% mortality if treated with wide resection alone
  - Strongly implies frequent presence of subclinical pulmonary micrometastases in majority of cases
- Multidisciplinary therapy results in disease-free survival of 60-80% if patients are good responders to chemotherapy (> 90% tumor necrosis)
  - Nonresponders to chemotherapy (< 90% tumor necrosis) have < 15% survival rate if postoperative therapy not changed
    - If appropriate change in chemotherapy is made, survival may improve
- Local recurrence or systemic metastases generally occur within 2 years; long-term surveillance required

Treatment

- Presume systemic disease at time of presentation, even if not visualized by imaging
  - Initial treatment with chemotherapy ± radiation
  - Wide resection; limb salvage if practicable
  - Postoperative chemotherapy
  - Postoperative radiation therapy if resected tumor margins are not clear
- If there is systemic disease at presentation
  - Pulmonary metastases resected if limited in number
  - More intensive preoperative chemotherapy
  - Suboptimal histologic response (< 90% necrosis) → alteration of and increased intensity of postoperative chemotherapy
  - If metastases progress on chemotherapy, may leave primary tumor in situ
- Pretreatment dual-phase FDG-PET may be useful in predicting histologic response to therapy

DIAGNOSTIC CHECKLIST

Consider

- Lytic permeative lesions may be overlooked initially
- Tumor osteoid within soft tissue mass is pathognomonic for OS
  - May help differentiate OS from Ewing sarcoma, which may have dense reactive bone formation, but it is limited in location to bone, not soft tissue
  - Myositis ossificans has similar disorganized amorphous bone formation 3-8 weeks post injury
- Following initial chemotherapy, OS may appear on radiograph to have enlarged

Reporting Tips

- MR evaluation must include
  - Measurement of tumor location relative to palpable landmark (for surgical planning)
  - Measurement of lesion in all dimensions and identification of violated muscles/compartments
  - Neurovascular involvement
  - Physeal involvement
  - Intraarticular involvement (19-24%)
  - Any known measurements required for limb salvage
  - Skip metastases in same or adjacent bone (< 5%)

SELECTED REFERENCES

1. Byun BH et al: Prediction of response to neoadjuvant chemotherapy in osteosarcoma using dual-phase 18F-FDG PET/CT. Eur Radiol. 25(7):2015-24, 2015

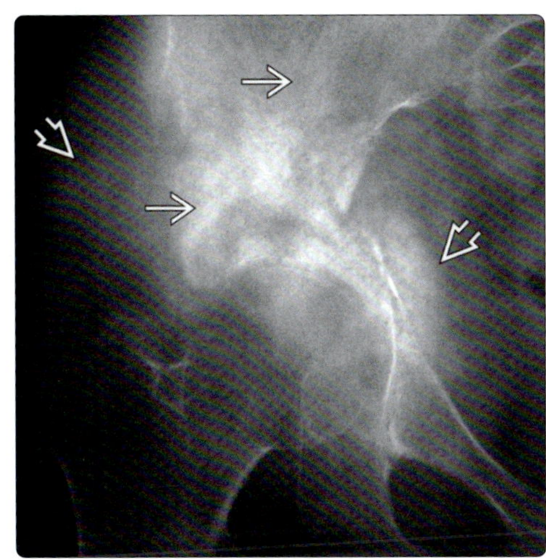

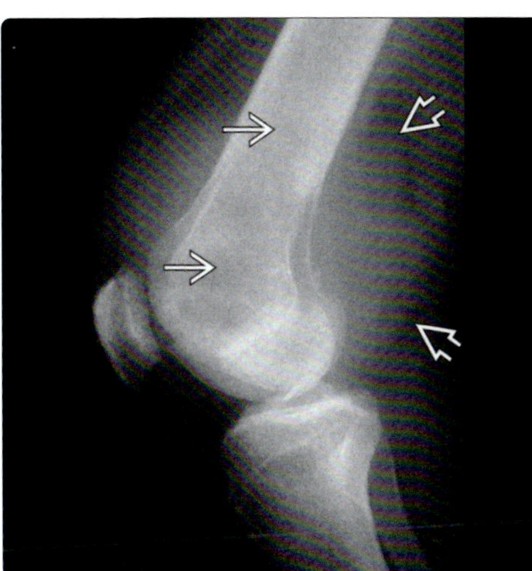

(Left) *AP radiograph of a blastic OS shows easily seen osteoid matrix within both the bone ➡ and soft tissue mass ➡. The permeative change in the bone is easily seen; there is no possible diagnosis other than conventional OS.* **(Right)** *Lateral radiograph of OS in a teenage girl shows a lytic permeative process with only cloudy amorphous matrix ➡. There is a large dense soft tissue mass that should not be mistaken for effusion ➡. This case was misdiagnosed in the emergency department as trauma.*

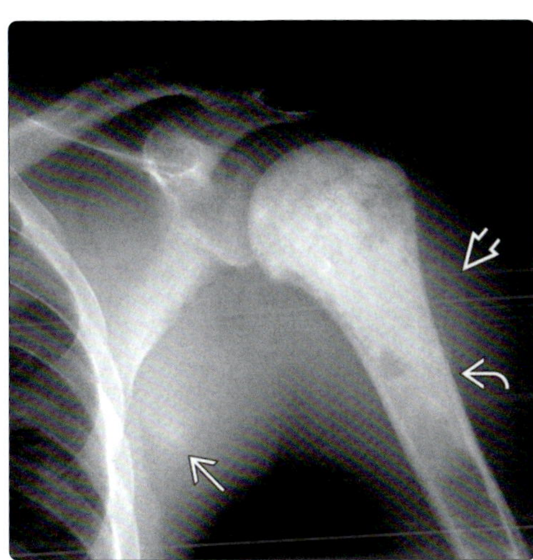

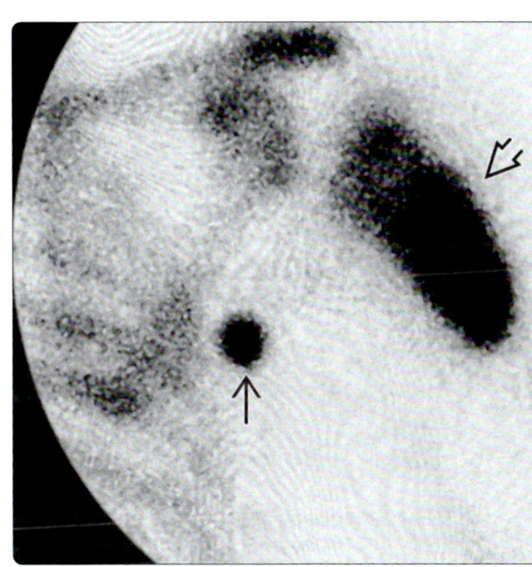

(Left) *AP radiograph shows a classic OS, highly aggressive and forming tumor bone in the proximal humerus. Periosteal reaction is seen ➡, as is a soft tissue mass ➡. Note also the faint matrix within a mass in the axilla ➡. (Previously published in Musculoskeletal Imaging: The Requisites. 2nd ed. Philadelphia, PA: Mosby, Elsevier; 2002.)* **(Right)** *AP bone scan shows uptake in the original lesion ➡ and a hot focus in axilla ➡. This uptake corresponds to the ossification seen on radiograph and represents a nodal metastasis.*

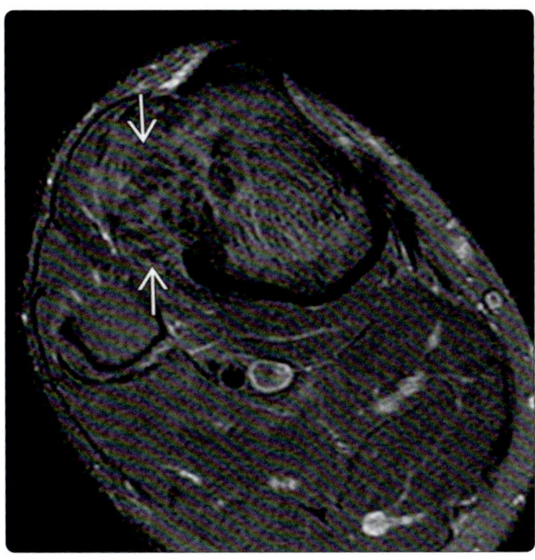

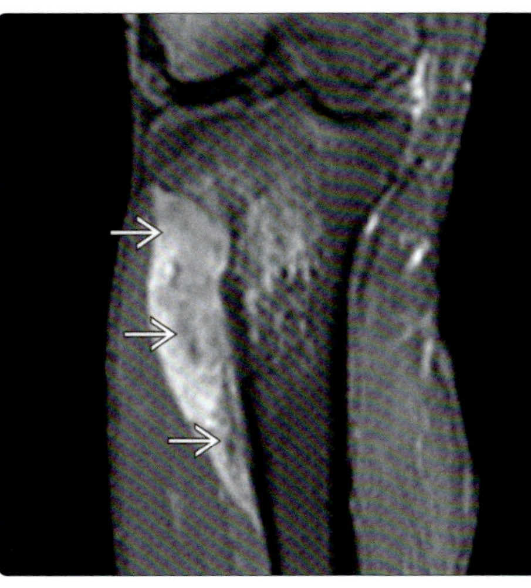

(Left) *Axial T2 FS MR in a 40-year-old man shows a metaphyseal lesion that has almost no hyperintensity. The lesion contains low signal regions ➡ in a sunburst pattern, extending through a cortical breech into a soft tissue mass.* **(Right)** *Coronal T1 C+ FS MR in the same patient confirms the extent of the osseous and soft tissue mass. Note the hypointense regions ➡ within the soft tissue mass, corresponding to tumor osteoid in this conventional OS.*

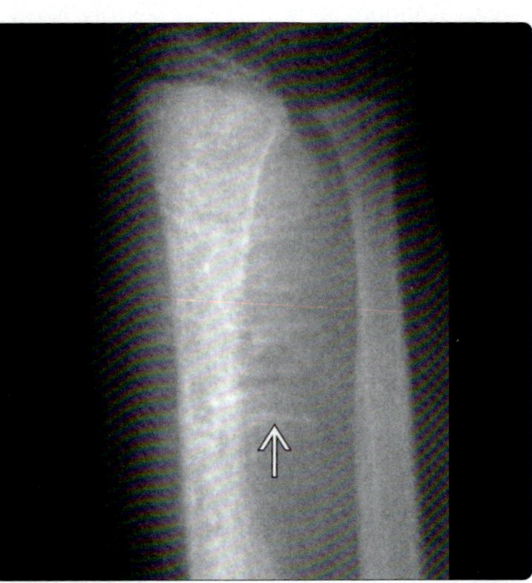

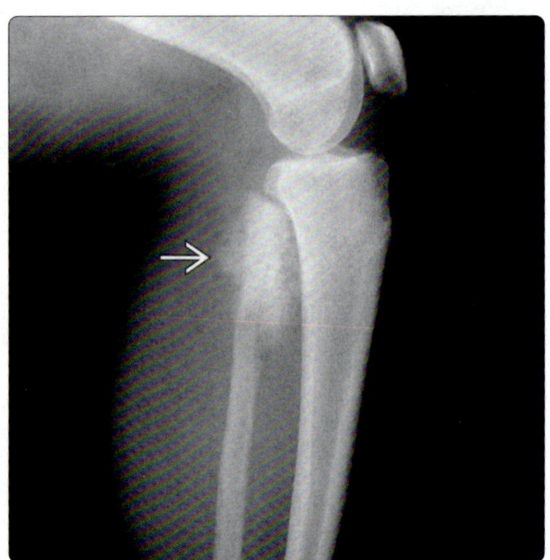

(Left) *AP radiograph shows horizontal periosteal reaction ➔, termed "sunburst." It indicates an aggressive process. Note that there is permeative destruction of the radius, with tumor osteoid formed in both the bone and soft tissue mass. The only possible diagnosis is OS.* **(Right)** *Lateral radiograph shows a typical case of an OS in the proximal fibula. The mass contains osteoid matrix, and has a prominent "sunburst" periosteal reaction ➔ as well as matrix formation in the soft tissue mass. The tibia appears normal.*

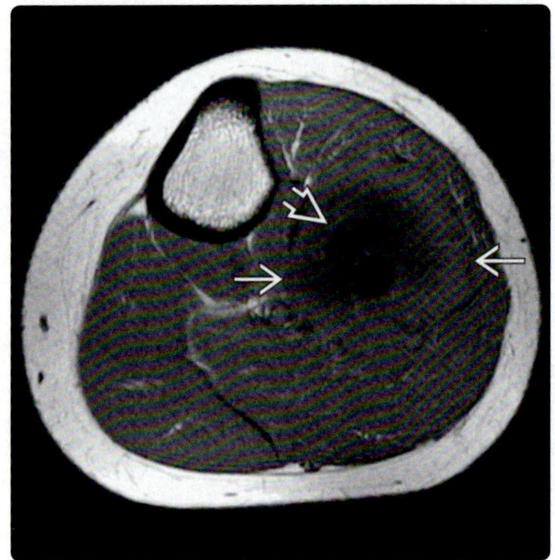

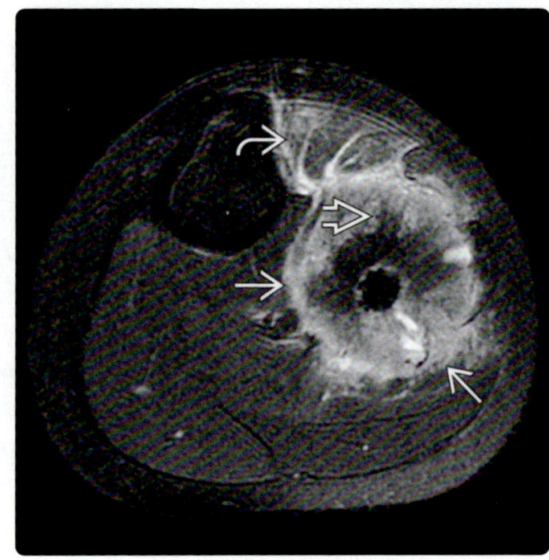

(Left) *Axial T1WI MR in the same patient shows the OS to be isointense to muscle ➔, with the regions of low signal intensity corresponding to the "sunburst" periosteal reaction ➔.* **(Right)** *Axial T2WI FS MR shows the low signal soft tissue bone formation and periosteal reaction to better advantage ➔. The remainder of the OS ➔ is hyperintense to muscle. There is edema involving many of the adjacent muscles, without a definite mass ➔. It may be impossible to be certain that these regions are tumor-free.*

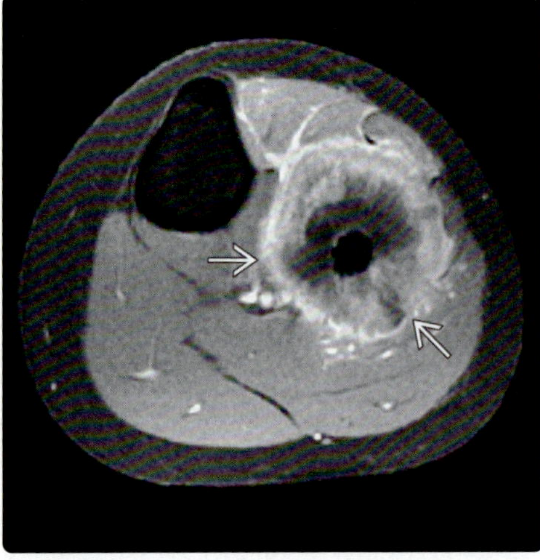

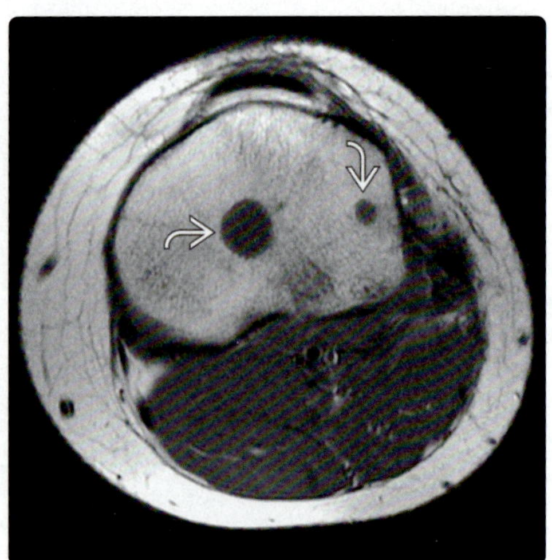

(Left) *Axial T1WI C+ FS MR shows intense, heterogeneous enhancement of the soft tissue mass ➔. The osseous tumor mass remains low signal because of the dense bone formation. The fact that the anterior soft tissues, which showed hyperintensity on the T2W FS image, do not enhance makes it more likely that they are tumor-free.* **(Right)** *Axial T1WI MR more proximal in the same leg shows a critical finding: 2 tibial lesions ➔. Skip metastases are rare and may occur in the parent bone or develop across joints.*

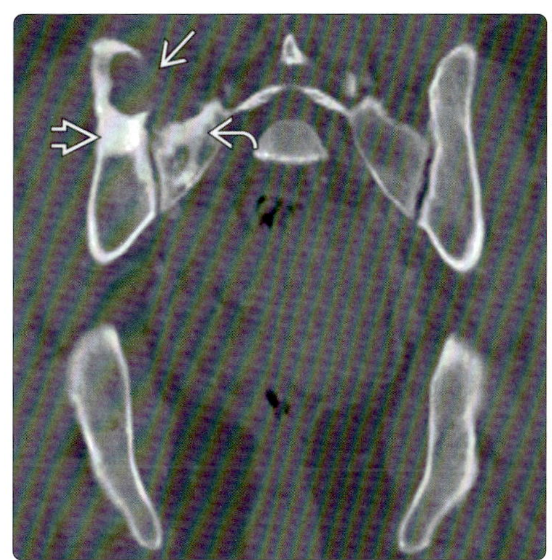

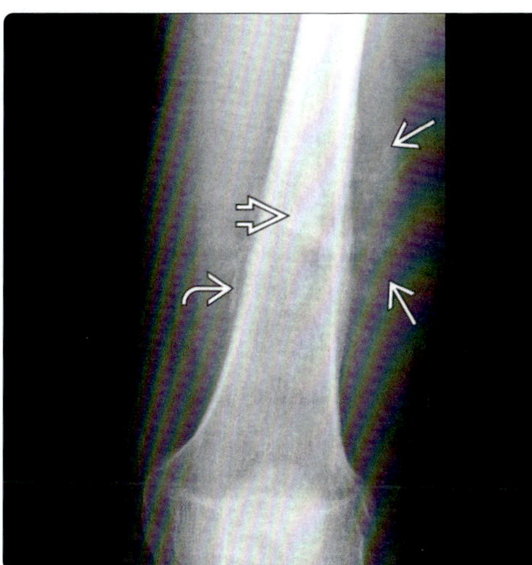

(Left) *Coronal bone CT shows mixed features of an OS with dense sclerosis in a portion ➡ and adjacent completely lytic mass ➡. The latter is the optimal site for biopsy since it is more active. Note that the sacroiliac joint is easily crossed by tumor ➡.* **(Right)** *AP radiograph in a 24-year-old man with a metadiaphyseal lesion shows somewhat amorphous but still definitive tumor osteoid within a soft tissue mass ➡. There is dense intramedullary sclerosis ➡ and prominent periosteal reaction ➡. Diagnosis must be conventional OS.*

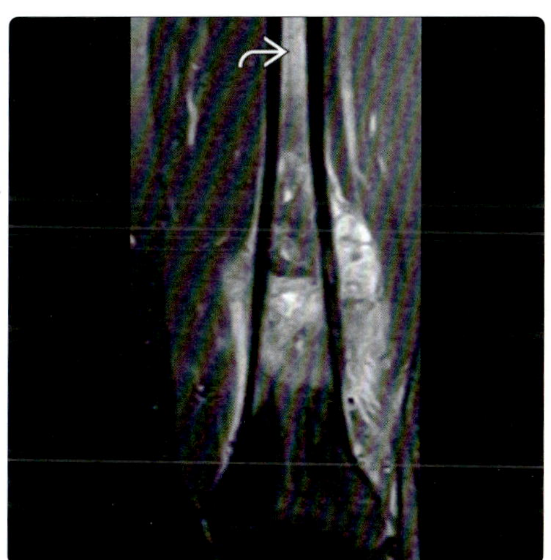

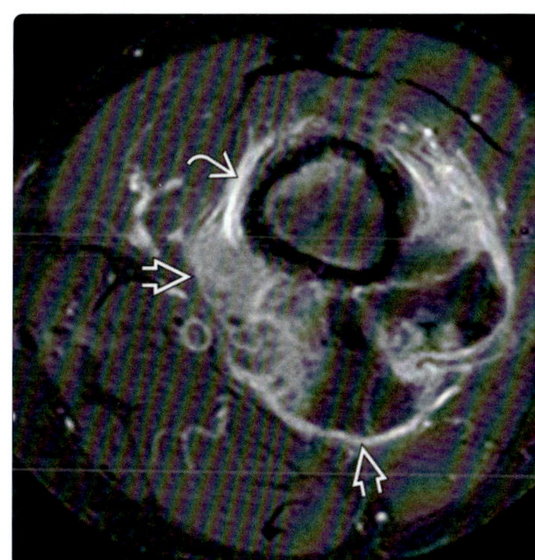

(Left) *Coronal T2 FS MR in the same patient shows mixed sclerosis and hyperintensity in the marrow as well as a soft tissue mass. Periosteal reaction is hyperintense and prominent. Note that marrow involvement extends proximal to the imaged portion of the lesion ➡.* **(Right)** *Axial T1 C+ FS MR in the same patient shows the nearly circumferential soft tissue mass ➡ and hyperintense periosteal reaction ➡. Note the variable sclerosis and hyperintensity within both the marrow and soft tissue mass.*

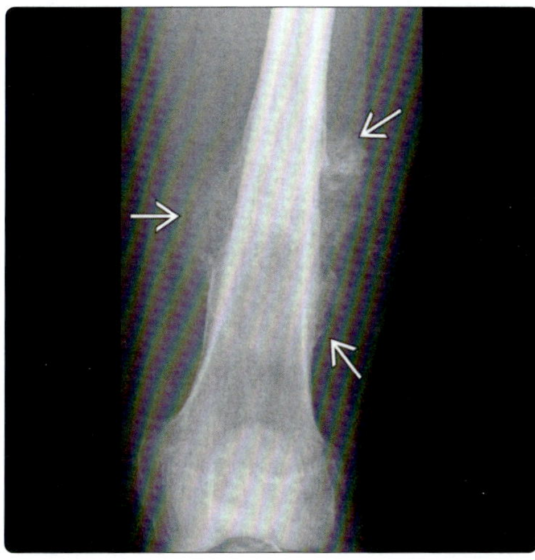

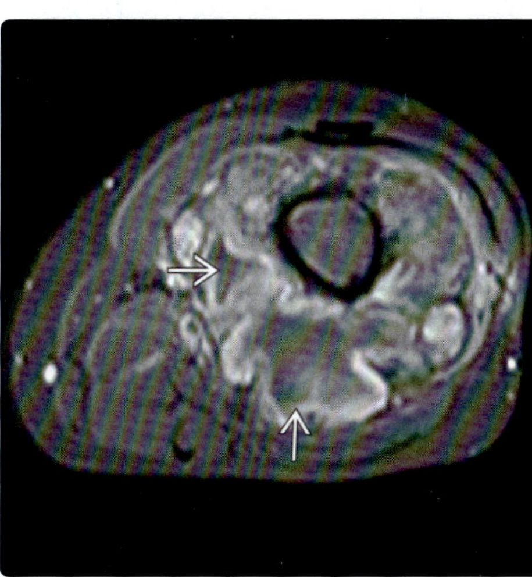

(Left) *AP radiograph obtained 4 months after the previous images and following chemotherapy shows the tumor osteoid has become more dense and appears more organized. The extent of tumor osteoid appears greater ➡ than pretherapy, which is typical in responding OS.* **(Right)** *Axial T1 C+ FS MR, 4 months post therapy, shows extensive areas of tumor necrosis ➡. Note that the lesion may appear to have enlarged, even though there is significant response.*

Parosteal Osteosarcoma

KEY FACTS

TERMINOLOGY

- Low-grade osteosarcoma (OS) arising on surface of bone

IMAGING

- Metaphyseal in 90%
  - Strong site preference for distal femoral metadiaphysis, posterior cortex (65% of all lesions)
- Fusiform along length of bone, with tendency to "wrap around" circumference as it enlarges
  - Intimately associated (contiguous) with surface
  - Initially, may appear as cortical thickening and be misinterpreted as healing stress fracture
  - As lesion enlarges, parts of it may be adjacent to cortex without attaching to it, giving appearance of cleft
- Bone is mature at site of origin, less mature at periphery
  - Opposite zoning pattern of myositis ossificans
- MR fluid-sensitive sequences
  - Heterogeneous high signal, with low signal tumor bone
  - High signal soft tissue seen at periphery of lesion
  - High signal involvement of cortex and marrow
- Enhancement of soft tissue and involved marrow
- Marrow involvement in 40-50%, best seen on MR
  - Intramedullary extension does not alter prognosis as long as resection is complete
- Any regions of differentially prominent nonnecrotic soft tissue mass should be biopsied
  - May represent higher grade region of dedifferentiation to high-grade disease
  - Dedifferentiation to high-grade disease 16-43%

CLINICAL ISSUES

- 3rd and 4th decades most common; generally slightly older than conventional OS
- 4-5% of all OSs
- Most common surface OS (65%)
- 90-95% survival at 5 years
- If foci of dedifferentiation present (either initially or at recurrence), prognosis is similar to conventional OS

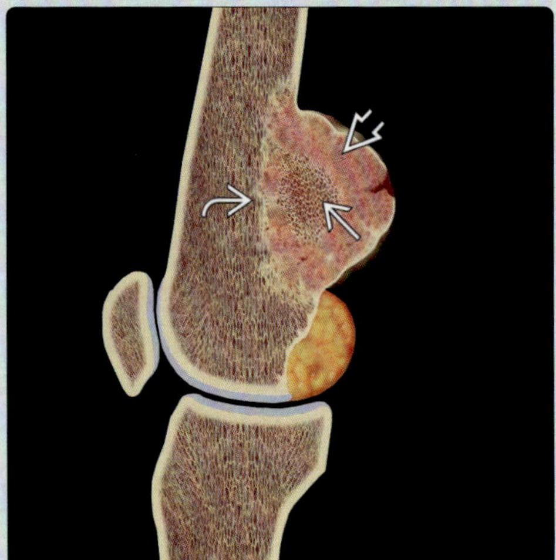

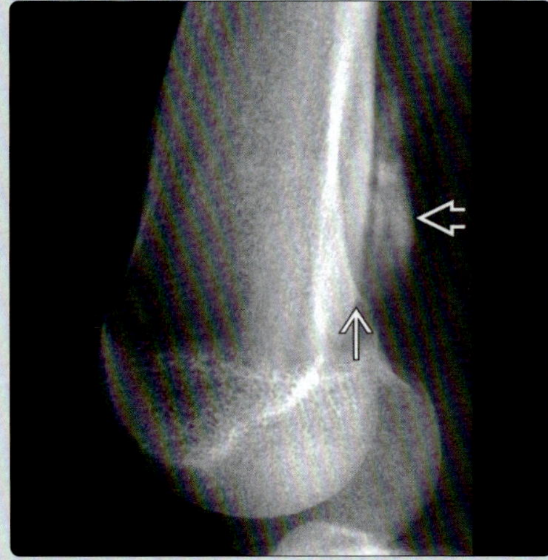

(Left) *Graphic depicts parosteal OS. Note that there is relatively mature bone located centrally within the lesion ➡, surrounded by less mature osteoid ➡ and soft tissue. This zoning pattern is typical of low-grade OS. Additionally, there is intramedullary extension of the lesion ➡; this is a frequent feature of the lesion and must be considered when planning resection.* **(Right)** *Lateral x-ray shows mature bone ➡ in a parosteal OS with apparent cleft at the cortical interface ➡. Clefts are infrequently seen and are not complete.*

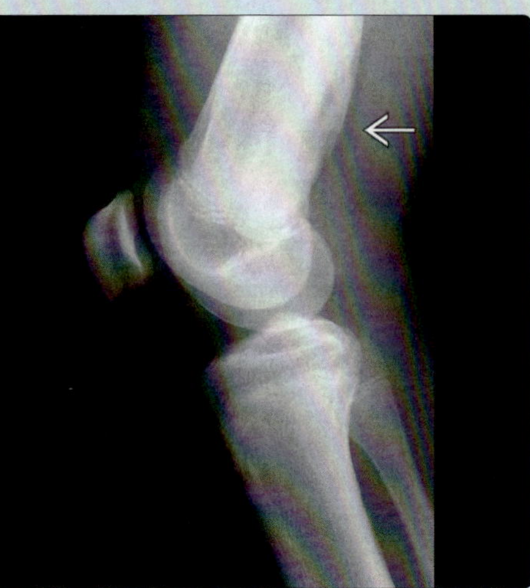

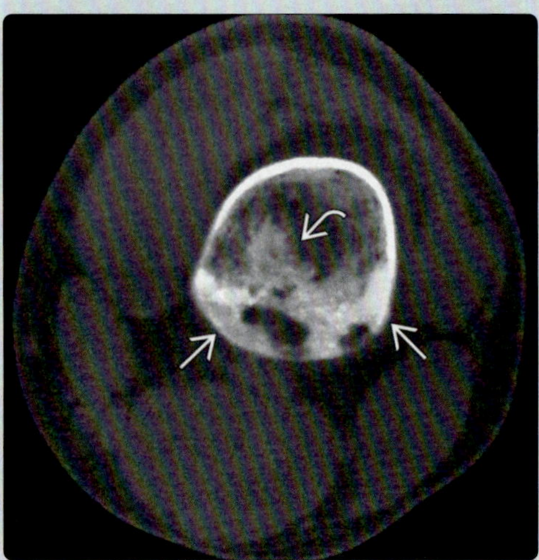

(Left) *Lateral radiograph shows a typical parosteal OS. There is thickening and almost layered appearance of the posterior cortex of the distal femur ➡. The bone formation is quite mature.* **(Right)** *Axial NECT in the same patient confirms thickened cortex at the posterior femur ➡. However, there are lytic regions as well, showing some inhomogeneity. Although there is no soft tissue mass, there is intramedullary involvement, with sclerosis ➡ and lytic lesions. The marrow is usually not completely spared in parosteal OS.*

TERMINOLOGY

Abbreviations

- Osteosarcoma (OS)

Synonyms

- Juxtacortical OS, juxtacortical low-grade OS

Definitions

- Low-grade osteosarcoma arising on surface of bone

IMAGING

General Features

- Best diagnostic clue
  - Mature bone intimately associated with cortex
- Location
  - Metaphyseal in 90%
  - Strong site preference for distal femoral metadiaphysis, posterior cortex (65% of all lesions)
  - Other common sites: Proximal tibia, proximal femur, proximal humerus
  - Flat bones: Rare
- Size
  - Range: 2 cm to very large (> 10 cm) at time of diagnosis
- Morphology
  - Fusiform along length of bone, with tendency to "wrap around" circumference as it enlarges

Imaging Recommendations

- Best imaging tool
  - Radiograph for diagnosis
  - MR for full evaluation of extent and soft tissue/marrow involvement

Radiographic Findings

- Lesion arises from cortical surface
  - Intimately associated (contiguous) with surface
    - Initially, may appear as cortical thickening and be misinterpreted as healing stress fracture
    - As lesion enlarges, parts of it may be adjacent to cortex without attaching to it, giving appearance of cleft (seen on radiograph in 30%)
  - May develop as cortical thickening, partially circumferential
    - Widened cortex contains mixture of disorganized dense bone formation and lytic regions
  - May develop as globular or oval bone formations arising from cortex, but otherwise largely separate from it
    - As these enlarge, may appear to "wrap around" bone
- Bone is mature at site of origin, less mature at periphery
  - Early lesion may contain only immature bone, appearing amorphous
  - With time, bone matures, from center of lesion to periphery
    - Opposite zoning pattern to that of myositis ossificans
  - Long-term lesion may even contain trabeculae
- Cortex is involved but difficult to evaluate by radiograph
  - Endosteal cortex may show sclerotic thickening, mimicking marrow involvement
- Marrow nearly always involved; difficult to evaluate by radiograph
- Soft tissue mass at periphery of bone mass: Inferred on radiograph by displacement of fat planes

CT Findings

- Mimics those of radiograph; cleft seen in 65%
- May be easier to evaluate maturity and zoning of osseous matrix
- Intramedullary involvement demonstrated but extent better evaluated on MR
- Soft tissue mass is more apparent

MR Findings

- T1: Low signal osseous mass; heterogeneous signal fairly isointense to skeletal muscle in soft tissue mass
  - Shows marrow involvement (41% of low-grade lesions, 50% of high-grade lesions)
- Fluid-sensitive sequences
  - Heterogeneous high signal, containing low signal tumor bone
  - High signal soft tissue seen at periphery of lesion
  - High signal involvement of cortex and marrow
    - Intramedullary extension does not alter prognosis as long as resection is complete
- Enhancement of soft tissue and involved marrow
- Watch for any portions of lesion that have more aggressive or different appearance (e.g., fluid levels)
  - May represent higher grade of osteosarcoma within lesion
  - May represent dedifferentiation of lesion into high-grade surface sarcoma, spindle cell sarcoma, or (rarely) telangiectatic OS

Image-Guided Biopsy

- Biopsy should be directed to nonnecrotic soft tissue
- Any regions of differentially prominent soft tissue mass should be biopsied
  - May represent higher grade region of dedifferentiation to high-grade disease
    - Dedifferentiation to high-grade disease 16-43%
    - Seen either initially or at recurrence

DIFFERENTIAL DIAGNOSIS

Osteochondroma

- Continuity of cortex and marrow into stalk of osteochondroma should be feature of differentiation
  - Cross-sectional imaging occasionally required to demonstrate this

Myositis Ossificans

- Mature myositis has opposite zoning pattern from parosteal OS: More mature peripherally, less centrally
- Mature myositis generally not intimately associated with adjacent cortex
- Immature myositis may mimic immature parosteal OS
  - Amorphous bone formation
  - Cortical and periosteal reaction
  - Marrow edema
  - High signal, enhancing mass on MR (larger on immature myositis ossificans than immature parosteal OS)

Periosteal Osteosarcoma

- Surface OS, generally more diaphyseal in location

- Osteoid matrix generally less mature than in parosteal OS
  - Immature parosteal OS may mimic mature periosteal OS
  - Zoning pattern is identical, as is cortical involvement; marrow infrequently involved

Periosteal Chondroma

- Surface cartilage lesion may have similar appearance to early parosteal OS
  - Matrix may appear identical to early amorphous bone; later mature bone in parosteal OS is distinctive
  - Cortical involvement (frequent scalloping) more similar to periosteal OS than parosteal OS

High-Grade Surface Osteosarcoma

- Early parosteal OS may mimic immature osteoid formation of this lesion
- Generally more diaphyseal in location than parosteal OS
- Generally larger soft tissue mass, more rapid growth than parosteal OS
- Much more rare lesion

PATHOLOGY

General Features

- Genetics
  - 1 or more supernumerary ring chromosomes
  - Different than alterations seen in conventional OS
  - Distinctive cytogenetic abnormality resulting in amplification of *CDK4* and *MDM2* genes

Gross Pathologic & Surgical Features

- Hard lobulated mass attached to cortex
- Contains nodules of cartilage, some on surface, mimicking incomplete cartilage cap
- 40-50% invade marrow
- Softer periphery may invade adjacent skeletal muscle
- Fleshy areas must be evaluated for dedifferentiation, particularly in recurrent lesion

Microscopic Features

- Well-formed bony trabeculae, simulating normal bone
  - May or may not show osteoblastic rimming
- Hypocellular stroma; spindle cells show minimal atypia
- 50% show cartilaginous differentiation
  - No columnar arrangement as in osteochondroma
  - May lead to misdiagnosis as fibrous dysplasia
- May have large areas devoid of bone and rich in collagen, similar to desmoplastic fibroma
- 15-43% have areas of high-grade spindle cell dedifferentiation
  - May be present initially or at recurrence
  - Dedifferentiates to OS, fibrosarcoma, or malignant fibrous histiocytoma

CLINICAL ISSUES

Presentation

- Most common signs/symptoms
  - Mass, generally painless or with low-grade pain
  - Lack of full knee flexion (65% in posterior distal femur)

Demographics

- Age
  - 3rd and 4th decades most common; generally older than conventional OS
- Gender
  - Slight female predominance
- Epidemiology
  - 4-5% of all osteosarcomas
  - Most common surface OS (65%)

Natural History & Prognosis

- Slow continued growth
- Late lung metastases
- 90-95% survival at 5 years
- If foci of dedifferentiation present (either initially or at recurrence), prognosis is similar to conventional OS
- If incompletely treated initially, high recurrence rate
  - Recurrence may be of higher grade or dedifferentiation with greater metastatic potential

Treatment

- Wide surgical resection if parosteal OS
- If dedifferentiated, treated as conventional OS

DIAGNOSTIC CHECKLIST

Consider

- Full MR presurgical evaluation required
  - Soft tissue, and particularly marrow, involvement must be outlined to allow for wide resection
  - If resection is marginal, high rate of recurrence
- Potentially dangerous lesion since it may be underestimated
  - Histologic pattern is often misdiagnosed as fibrous dysplasia, leading to incomplete resection
    - Discrepancy between radiologic and pathologic interpretation **must** be rectified
    - Misdiagnosis and related undertreatment may result in low-grade, treatable lesion transforming to high-grade, metastatic
  - Lesion may contain higher grade regions (either primarily or at recurrence)
    - Case series: Wide range of this finding (22-64%)
    - Watch carefully for nonmineralized foci of soft tissue mass

SELECTED REFERENCES

1. Hang JF et al: Parosteal osteosarcoma. Arch Pathol Lab Med. 138(5):694-9, 2014
2. Yarmish G et al: Imaging characteristics of primary osteosarcoma: nonconventional subtypes. Radiographics. 30(6):1653-72, 2010
3. Azura M et al: Parosteal osteosarcoma dedifferentiating into telangiectatic osteosarcoma: importance of lytic changes and fluid cavities at imaging. Skeletal Radiol. 38(7):685-90, 2009

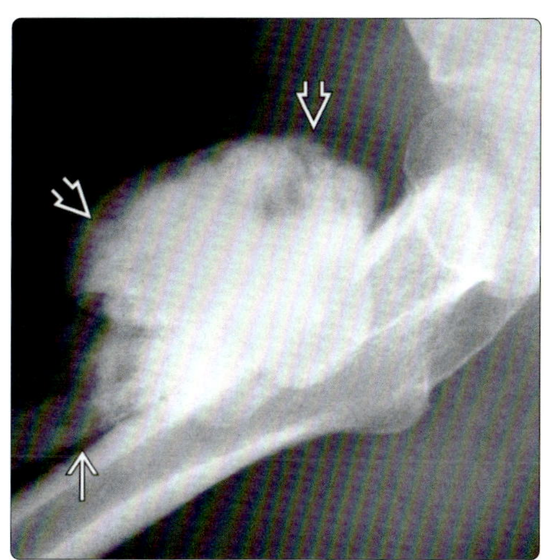

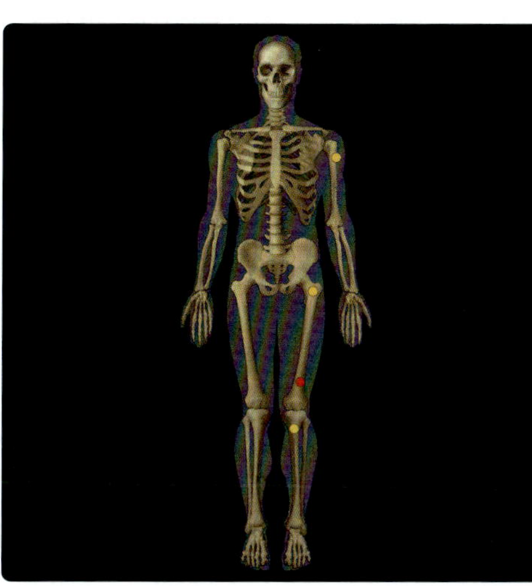

(Left) *Lateral radiograph of the proximal femur in a patient who reports slow growth of this mass for over a year. Note the "pasted on" appearance of mature bone ➡ in a parosteal OS as it wraps around the cortex. A partial cleft is seen ➡.* **(Right)** *Graphic depicts the most likely location of parosteal OS (red; 65% occur in the posterior femoral cortex) and less common locations (yellow: Proximal tibia, proximal femur, proximal humerus). The lesions are metaphyseal.*

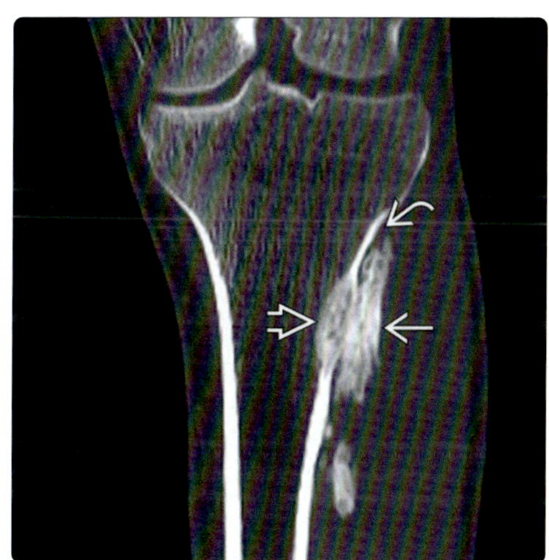

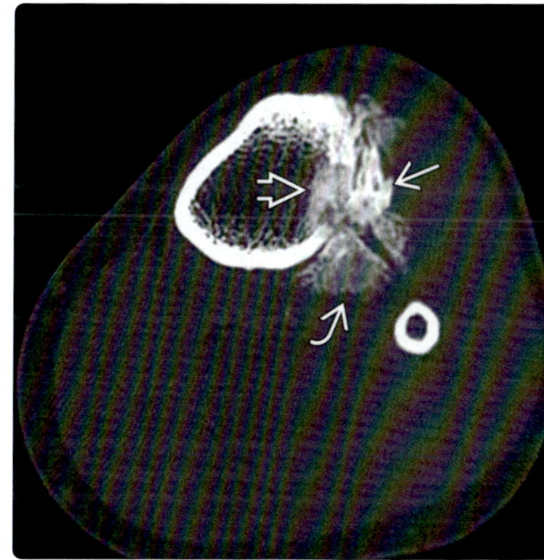

(Left) *Coronal reconstruction CT in a 24-year-old man shows mature osteoid formation ➡ in a surface tumor. There is a partial cleft ➡ at the surface. Marrow involvement is seen ➡; the findings and location are typical of parosteal OS.* **(Right)** *Axial CT, same case, redemonstrates the cortical destruction and intramedullary involvement ➡ in this parosteal OS. Defining the extent of marrow involvement is crucial for surgical planning. Central mature bone formation ➡ with less mature bone peripherally ➡ is typical.*

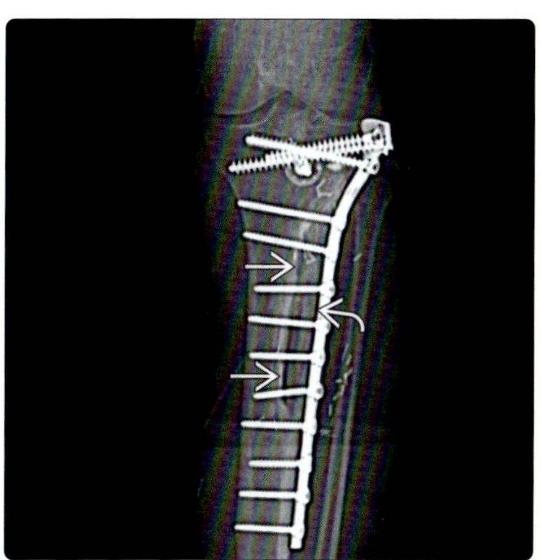

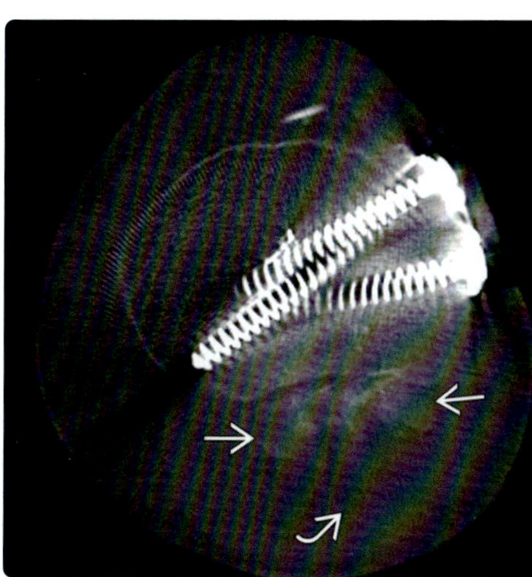

(Left) *Coronal CT scanogram of same patient obtained 5 years later shows treatment by saucerization of the cortex ➡ and adjacent marrow, with support by fibular graft ➡ and plate.* **(Right)** *Axial CT at the proximal end of the plate shows tumor recurrence, with tumor osteoid formed posteriorly ➡, as well as a soft tissue mass ➡ displacing surrounding tissues. A recurrence of parosteal OS is likely to show either a higher grade of tumor or tumor dedifferentiation to conventional OS. Careful tissue sampling is crucial.*

(Left) *AP x-ray gives a bizarre appearance to a parosteal OS. The entire distal femur appears to be expanded ➡. However, note that the bone formation is quite regular, containing trabeculae and not appearing aggressive.* **(Right)** *Lateral x-ray in the same patient shows the fairly regular trabecular pattern of bone formation in parosteal OS ➡. Furthermore, the origin of the lesion appears concentrated in the posterior cortex of the distal femur, extending around the medial and lateral sides, the most common location.*

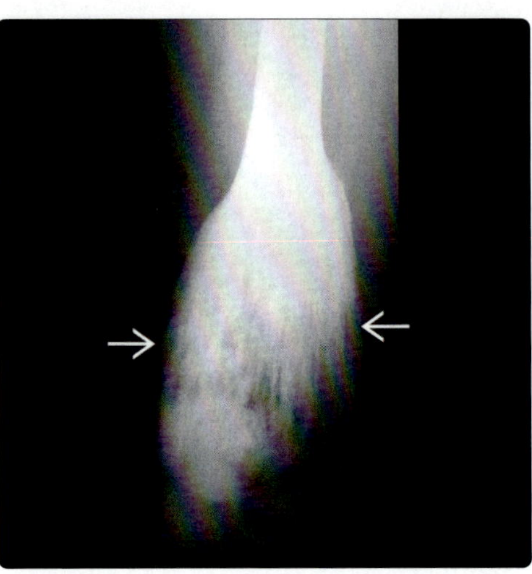

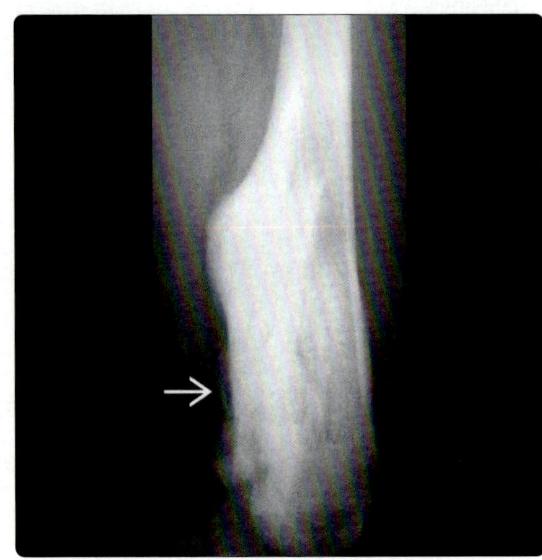

(Left) *Axial CT in the same patient shows the tremendous bone formation surrounding 3/4 of the femoral cortex ➡. There is marrow involvement; there is no doubt of the diagnosis of parosteal OS. However, MR is necessary to adequately assess for soft tissue mass external to the osseous tumor.* **(Right)** *Lateral x-ray, different patient, shows apparent cure of parosteal OS, with saucerization of the posterior femoral cortex and incorporation of bone graft ➡. If the margins were clear of tumor, the cure rate should be > 90%.*

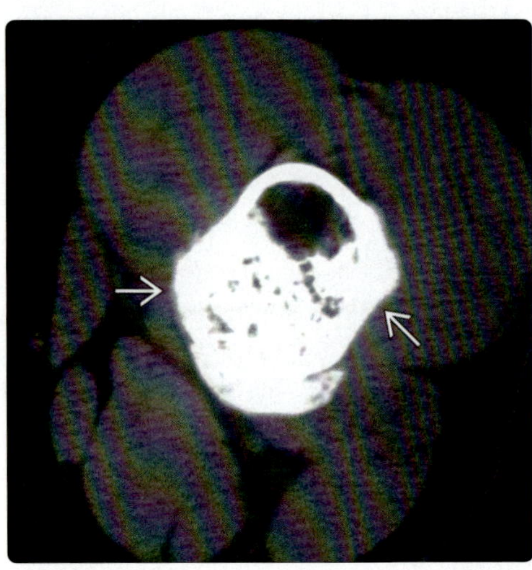

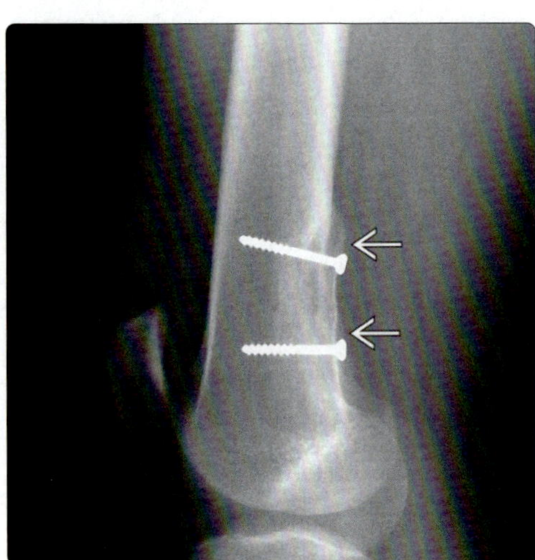

(Left) *Axial NECT in the same patient 8 years later shows tumor recurrence. Note the mature tumor bone formation in the center of the soft tissue mass ➡, with surrounding less mature bone and soft tissue ➡. This is the expected zoning pattern of parosteal OS.* **(Right)** *Axial NECT, more distally in the same patient, shows less mature bone matrix and a sizable soft tissue mass ➡. Recurrence may occur late, as in this case, and is often of higher grade than the original lesion or dedifferentiated to conventional OS.*

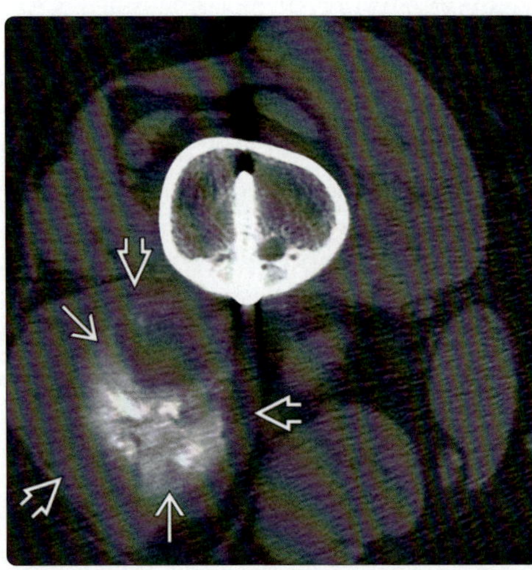

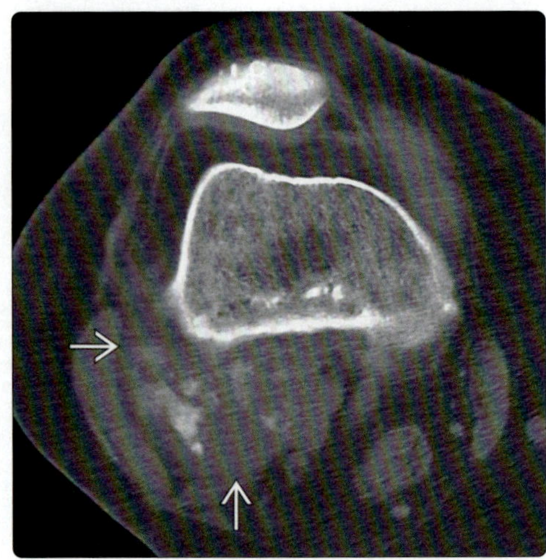

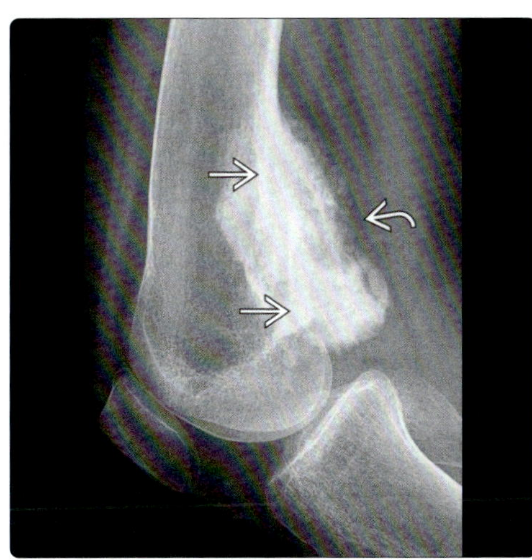

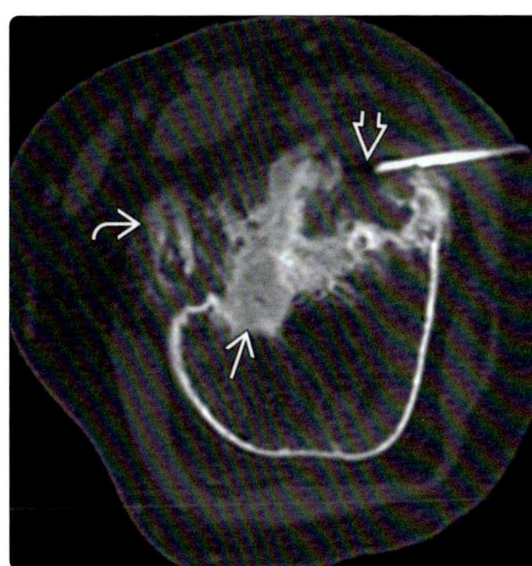

(Left) *Lateral x-ray shows dense osseous matrix that appears to be "pasted on" the posterior femoral metaphysis. The matrix is more mature centrally ➡ than peripherally ↪. The appearance and location are typical of parosteal OS.* **(Right)** *Axial NECT in a prone position during biopsy shows that there is marrow involvement. The central matrix is mature ➡, with less mature matrix peripherally ↪, the typical zoning pattern of parosteal OS. A biopsy needle placed in the soft tissue mass ⇨ showed dedifferentiation.*

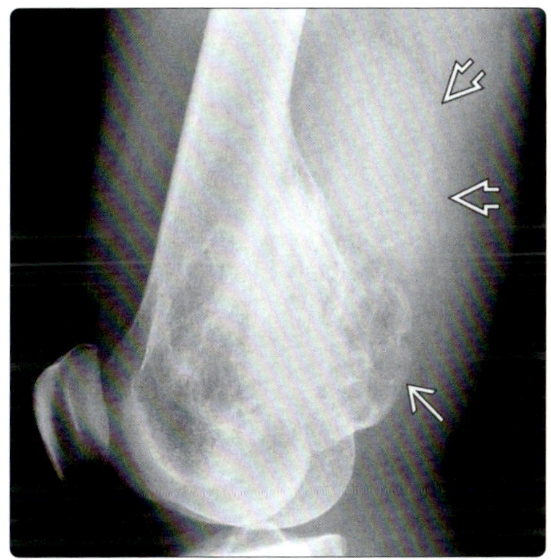

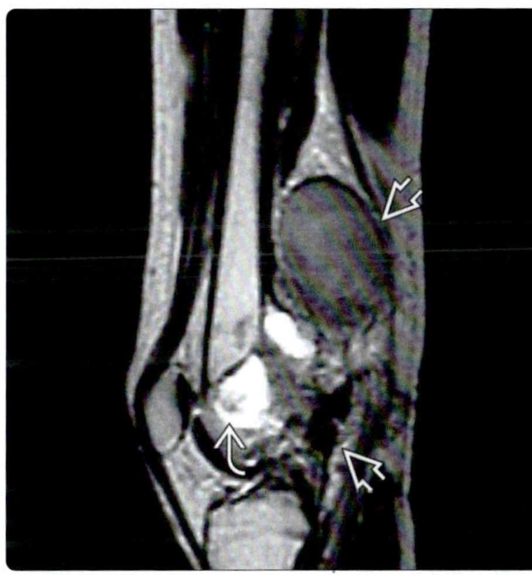

(Left) *Lateral x-ray in a patient who reports having a lump removed 13 years earlier, said to be benign, shows an exophytic bone-producing lesion ➡ with a proximal soft tissue mass ⇨. Recurrent parosteal OS (previously misdiagnosed) must be assumed.* **(Right)** *Sagittal T2WI MR of the lesion shows osseous invasion ↪ and a large mass ⇨. The different character of the tumor at different sites suggests that portions of the recurrent tumor are higher grade than the original. Correct diagnosis at the onset is crucial.*

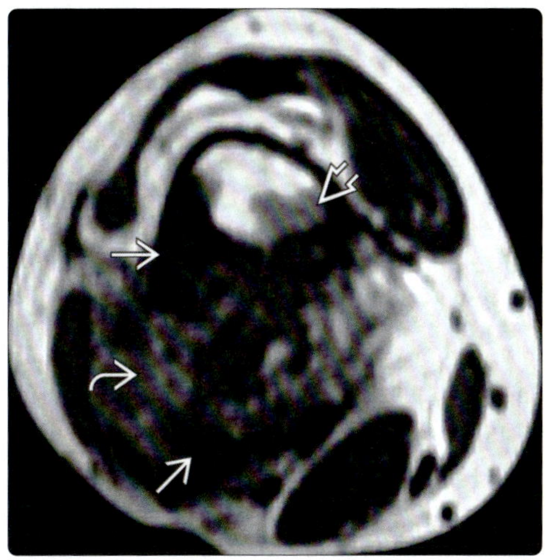

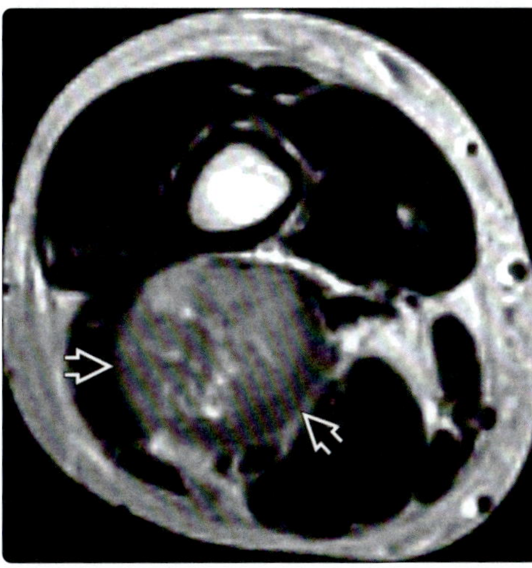

(Left) *Axial T1WI MR in the same patient shows intraosseous invasion by the recurrent lesion ⇨. The large soft tissue mass contains low signal tumor bone ➡, corresponding to that seen on the radiograph, as well as regions of soft tissue tumor isointense to muscle. Note that the neurovascular bundle ↪ is surrounded.* **(Right)** *Axial T2WI MR, at a higher level, shows heterogeneous high signal ⇨ mass without bone. This is the region of higher grade tumor; it should also be evaluated carefully for regions of dedifferentiation.*

Periosteal Osteosarcoma

KEY FACTS

TERMINOLOGY

- Intermediate-grade surface osteosarcoma (OS), usually chondroblastic

IMAGING

- Location: Diaphysis or metadiaphysis of long bones
  - Tibia & femur (85-95%) > ulna & humerus (5-10%)
- Radiograph: Calcified spicules of bone in 68%
  - Arranged perpendicular to cortex; sunburst appearance
  - Bone formation may not be typical; may appear more dense, flocculated
- Bone more organized and dense near cortical surface, less organized and dense along outer edge
  - Zoning pattern of maturation typical of surface osteosarcomas
- Cortex has variable appearance
  - Usually visible cortical involvement: Thickening (82%), which is scalloped (68%)
- Periosteum may be elevated at proximal and distal ends of lesion, mimicking but less aggressive than Codman triangles
- MR: Low signal osteoid matrix displayed as rays perpendicular to cortex (75%)
  - Heterogeneous high signal soft tissue mass, extending from periphery of tumor osteoid
  - Enhancement of soft tissue mass, plus any marrow and cortical involvement
  - Marrow involvement is rare

CLINICAL ISSUES

- 2nd and 3rd decades: Generally slightly later than conventional OS but younger than parosteal OS
- Rare; < 2% of all osteosarcomas
- 25% of all surface osteosarcomas
- Treatment: Wide surgical excision
- Prognosis: 85% 5-year survival with adequate treatment
  - Better than conventional osteosarcoma
  - Poorer than parosteal osteosarcoma

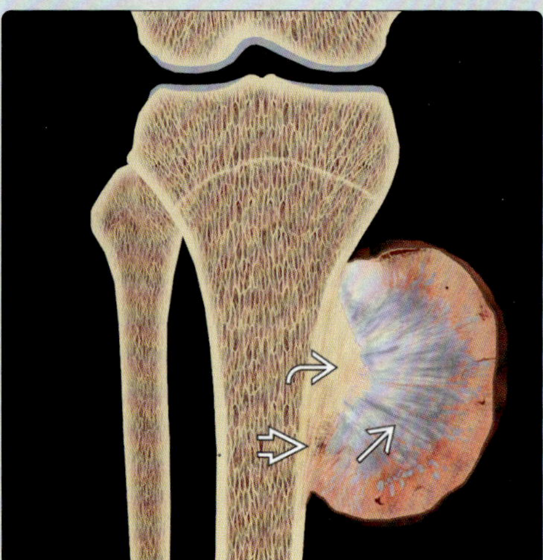

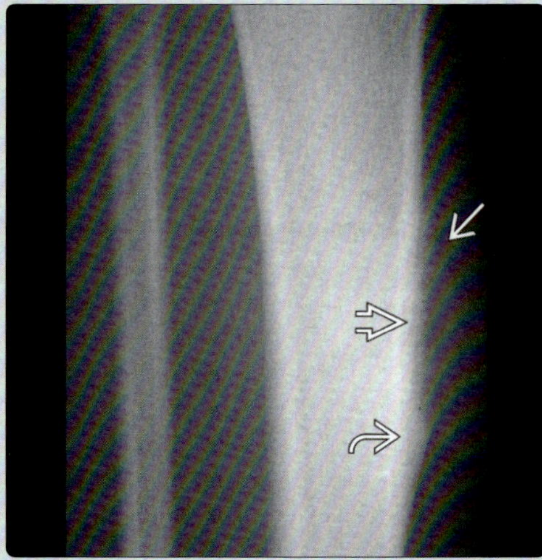

(Left) *Graphic of periosteal OS shows the broad-based lesion arises from the thickened cortex ➡, with some ossified regions blending into the tumor ➡. The soft tissue component contains rays of cartilage or osseous matrix ➡ and regions of spindle cells.* **(Right)** *AP radiograph shows a typical periosteal OS. There is thickening ➡ as well as scalloping ➡ of the cortex related to this surface lesion. The lesion contains faint amorphous osteoid matrix and perpendicular periosteal reaction seen within the soft tissue mass ➡.*

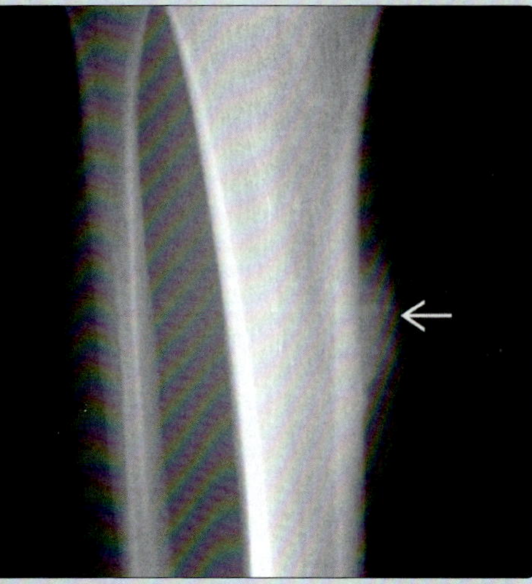

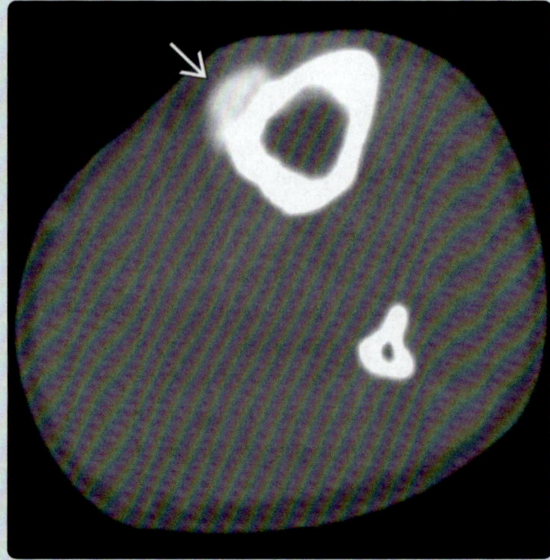

(Left) *AP radiograph (different patient) shows another appearance of periosteal OS. This surface lesion produces more mature-appearing and less spiculated bone ➡. There is no cortical thickening or scalloping.* **(Right)** *Axial NECT (same patient) allows better evaluation of the matrix located completely on the surface ➡. These features are within the range of the expected appearance of parosteal OS but not as classic as cases showing spicules and cortical scalloping. Marrow involvement must be sought by MR.*

TERMINOLOGY

Abbreviations

- Osteosarcoma (OS)

Synonyms

- Juxtacortical chondroblastic OS

Definitions

- Intermediate-grade surface OS, usually chondroblastic; ± marrow involvement

IMAGING

General Features

- Location
  - Diaphysis or metadiaphysis of long bones
  - Tibia & femur (85-95%) > ulna & humerus (5-10%)
  - Rare reports of mandible, clavicle, pelvis, rib, cranium involvement
  - 1 case report of bilateral metachronous lesions & 1 of bilateral synchronous lesions
- Size
  - Generally < 5 cm in length
- Morphology
  - Fusiform along cortical surface

Imaging Recommendations

- Best imaging tool
  - Diagnosis on radiograph, full evaluation on MR

Radiographic Findings

- Calcified spicules of bone in 68%
  - Arranged perpendicular to cortex; sunburst appearance
  - Bone formation may not be typical; may appear more dense, flocculated
  - May have little bone formation visible on radiograph
- Bone more organized and dense near cortical surface, less organized and dense along outer edge
  - Zoning pattern of maturation typical of surface osteosarcomas
- Cortex has variable appearance
  - Usually visible cortical involvement: Thickening (82%), which is scalloped (68%)
  - Cortex may appear irregular and permeated
- Periosteum may be elevated at proximal and distal ends of lesion
  - Thickening may mimic appearance of Codman triangle but not as aggressive in appearance
  - No truly aggressive periosteal reaction

CT Findings

- Mimics findings on radiography
- Character of osteoid matrix, low in attenuation, more clearly delineated than on radiograph
  - Rays perpendicular to cortex seen in 91%
  - Zoning, with more organized bone near cortical surface and less organized bone peripherally should be seen
- True involvement of cortex may be determined
  - May circumferentially involve up to 75% of cortex but usually 25-50%
- May demonstrate small amount of marrow involvement
- Soft tissue mass demonstrated beyond osteoid, but full extent difficult to evaluate on CT

MR Findings

- Necessary to evaluate true extent of involvement
- T1WI shows low signal of cortex and osteoid
  - Soft tissue mass tends to be nearly isointense to skeletal muscle
- Fluid-sensitive sequences: Fat-saturated most helpful
  - Low signal osteoid matrix may be displayed as rays perpendicular to cortex (75%)
  - Heterogeneous high signal soft tissue mass, extending from periphery of tumor osteoid
    - Signal may be so high as to obscure matrix
    - Generally mass extending beyond matrix is not very large
  - High signal within cortex (generally low signal) indicates cortical involvement
  - High signal within fat-saturated marrow, contiguous with tumor indicates marrow extension (uncommon: 2%)
    - Marrow involvement affects choice of surgical resection
    - Marrow involvement is generally sparse but should not preclude diagnosis
    - Abnormal marrow signal not contiguous with tumor is more likely edema than tumor
- Enhancement of soft tissue mass, plus any marrow and cortical involvement

DIFFERENTIAL DIAGNOSIS

Periosteal Chondroma or Chondrosarcoma

- May appear identical to periosteal OS
  - May not be possible to differentiate calcified chondroid from calcified osteoid, respectively
  - Both lesions tend to scallop underlying cortex
  - Both lesions tend to involve metadiaphysis of long bones
- Periosteal chondroma much more common than periosteal OS; periosteal chondrosarcoma is rare

Myositis Ossificans

- Mature myositis has distinct pattern of ossification, more mature peripherally than centrally
- Immature myositis (4-12 weeks post trauma) may mimic periosteal OS
  - Amorphous bone formation
  - Periosteal reaction, edema in marrow and cortex
  - High signal enhancing mass seen on MR
  - Faint halo of peripheral bone may be seen on MR or CT to help distinguish myositis ossificans from periosteal OS

High-Grade Surface Osteosarcoma

- More rare than periosteal OS
- Pattern of tumor osteoid calcification more variable, but may look similar
- Scalloping or destruction of adjacent cortex may have similar appearance
- Metadiaphyseal location, and particular bones involved (femur, tibia, humerus) identical to periosteal OS
- Higher grade lesion, so destruction may occur more rapidly
  - Soft tissue mass tends to be larger

Parosteal Osteosarcoma

- Generally has distinct appearance with mature lesion
  - More organized bone production sometimes containing trabeculae
  - Tumor osteoid is more dense
  - Same zoning pattern, with more organized and mature bone at cortical site of origin, less mature bone and soft tissue mass peripherally
  - May appear to wrap around bone, and may have cleft between at least part of tumor bone and cortex
  - Generally involves cortex and adjacent marrow
- May be difficult to differentiate from periosteal OS in 2 circumstances
  - Early parosteal OS may have small amounts of immature bone in juxtacortical position, mimicking periosteal OS
  - Recurrent parosteal OS may be of higher grade, with less mature osteoid

PATHOLOGY

General Features

- Genetics
  - Little information; complex karyotypic changes reported in 3 of 4 cases
  - Familial incidence described in 1 report

Staging, Grading, & Classification

- AJCC: Incorporates tumor size, grade, and metastases

Gross Pathologic & Surgical Features

- Fusiform, attached to surface
- Spicules of bone arising perpendicular to surface
  - More dense near center of origin; taper to edge
  - Periphery may be uncalcified
- May have glistening, grayish appearance of cartilage in parts of tumor

Microscopic Features

- Ossified mass intimately attached to cortex
  - Mature bone with endochondral ossification
- Chondroblastic: Cartilaginous component predominates
  - Varying degrees of cellular atypia; intermediate grade overall
- Spicules: Elongated vascular cores surrounded by calcified, osseous, or chondro-osseous matrix
  - Entire spicule may be surrounded by noncalcified cartilage
- Periphery: Generally no calcification
  - Fascicles of spindle cells, often with significant mitotic activity

CLINICAL ISSUES

Presentation

- Most common signs/symptoms
  - Painless or low-grade painful mass

Demographics

- Age
  - 2nd and 3rd decades: Generally slightly later than conventional OS but younger than parosteal OS
- Gender
  - Slight male predominance
- Epidemiology
  - Rare; < 2% of all osteosarcomas
  - 25% of all surface osteosarcomas
    - More common than high-grade surface OS
    - Less common than parosteal OS (2:1 ratio parosteal to periosteal)

Natural History & Prognosis

- Slow progression in size
- Prognosis better than conventional OS, not as good as parosteal OS
  - 83% disease-free survival in study (15-year follow-up)
  - Another study showed 5-year survival better if no marrow involvement (90% vs. 75%)
- If inadequately treated (marginal resection), high recurrence rate
  - 70% if margins not clear
- 15% rate of metastasis, generally to lung
- Does not have propensity to dedifferentiation

Treatment

- Wide surgical excision
  - Limb salvage usually feasible since lesion is usually diaphyseal
- Chemotherapy has been used in European study; does not appear to affect survival
  - Chemotherapy and radiation variably used, according to local preferences

DIAGNOSTIC CHECKLIST

Consider

- Pay close attention to soft tissue and intramedullary extent
  - Excisions without clear margins result in significant recurrence rate

Image Interpretation Pearls

- Determining intramedullary involvement by MR may be difficult
  - Uncommonly occurs but affects surgical planning
  - 1 study, based on fairly small numbers, suggests
    - Marrow signal abnormality that is in contiguity with soft tissue mass should be interpreted as marrow involvement by tumor
    - Marrow signal abnormality that is not in contiguity with soft tissue mass should be interpreted as edema

SELECTED REFERENCES

1. Gulia A et al: Oncological and functional outcome of periosteal osteosarcoma. Indian J Orthop. 48(3):279-84, 2014
2. Cesari M et al: Periosteal osteosarcoma: a single-institution experience. Cancer. 117(8):1731-5, 2011
3. Yarmish G et al: Imaging characteristics of primary osteosarcoma: nonconventional subtypes. Radiographics. 30(6):1653-72, 2010
4. Murphey MD et al: Imaging of periosteal osteosarcoma: radiologic-pathologic comparison. Radiology. 233(1):129-38, 2004

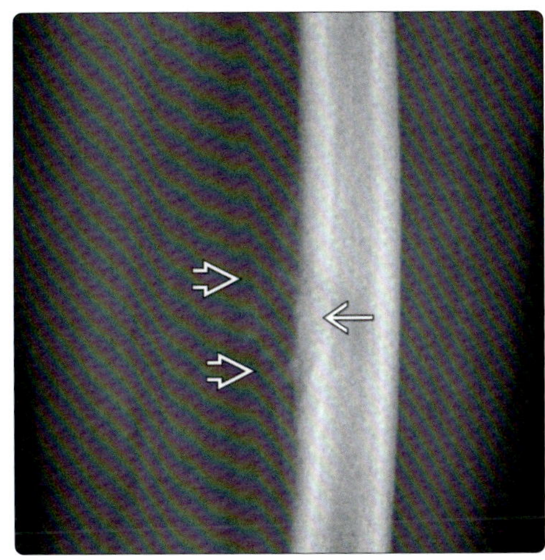

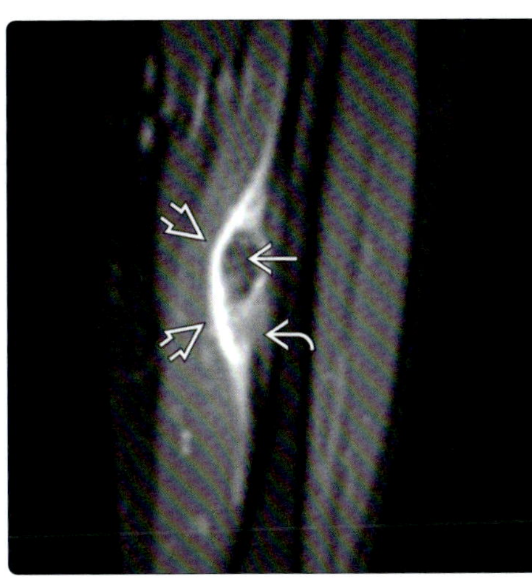

(Left) *Lateral radiograph shows the spiculated matrix extending into a soft tissue mass ➩. The lesion arises from the cortical surface, with irregularity suggesting cortical involvement ➩ & scalloping. No marrow involvement is seen on radiograph.* **(Right)** *Coronal T1WI C+ FS MR shows the low signal of the surface tumor bone ➩, with high signal in the surrounding mass ➩. This is the zoning pattern expected for a surface OS. Faint signal is seen within the cortex ➩, but the medullary cavity is uninvolved. (Courtesy K. Wright, MD.)*

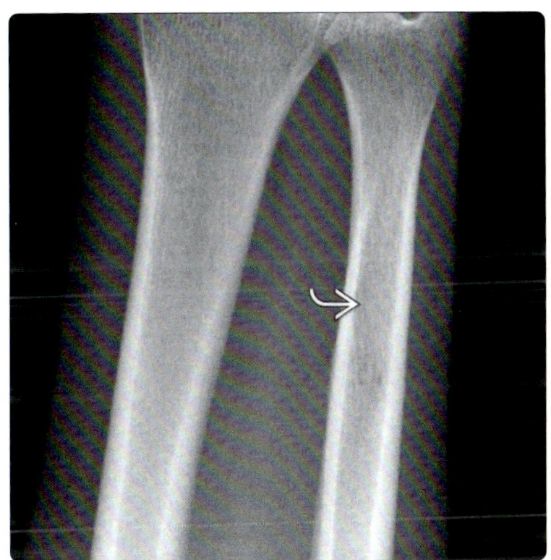

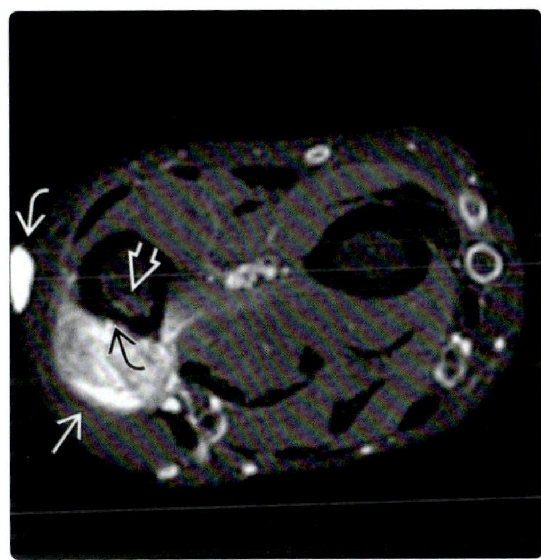

(Left) *AP radiograph in a 31-year-old man with distal forearm pain shows only a faint lucency ➩ to indicate a lesion involving the distal ulna.* **(Right)** *Axial T2 FS MR shows a large inhomogeneous soft tissue mass ➩ that causes cortical scalloping ➩. There is a focus of hyperintensity involving the marrow, suggesting intramedullary extension ➩. An external marker ➩ denotes the site of pain. The surface lesion with cortical scalloping is typical of periosteal OS.*

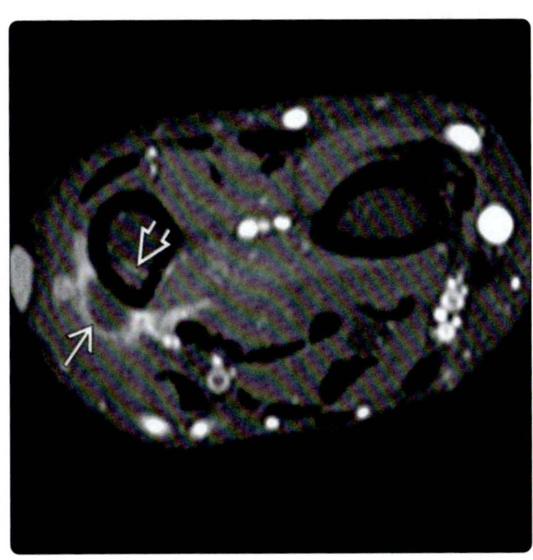

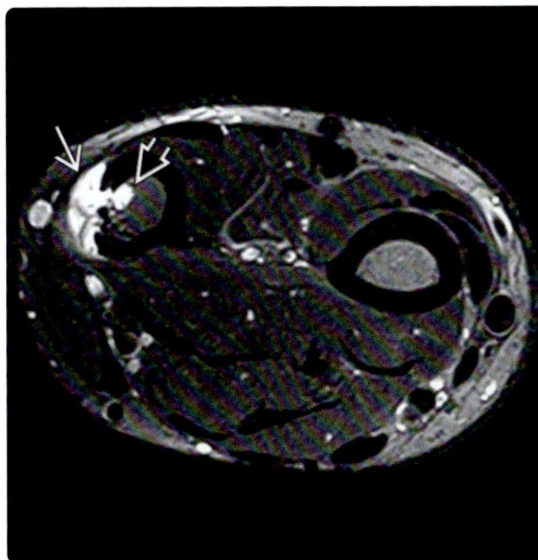

(Left) *Axial T1 C+ FS MR shows the lesion to enhance, surrounding a necrotic region ➩. Most importantly, it also demonstrates enhancement of the suspected focus within the marrow ➩. Marrow involvement must be diagnosed, and wide resection including the marrow is recommended. Unfortunately, the patient received only marginal resection of the soft tissue portion of the lesion.* **(Right)** *Axial T2 FS MR 6 months following marginal resection demonstrates recurrence both in the soft tissues ➩ and marrow ➩.*

KEY FACTS

TERMINOLOGY

- Malignant bone-forming tumor containing or largely consisting of large blood-filled spaces

IMAGING

- Location: 90% tubular bone metaphysis; other locations rare
  - Distal femur (48%) > proximal tibia (14%), proximal humerus, proximal femur
- Lytic; partially geographic lesion
  - Narrow zone of transition may be seen in part, wide zone in other parts
  - Watch for red flag zone where transition from normal to abnormal bone is indistinct
  - Aneurysmal expansion of cortex in 75%, though prominent expansion in fewer cases (19%)
  - Generally matrix only subtly visible as small foci in periphery of lesion (58%)
- T1WI MR: Inhomogeneous signal similar to or slightly higher than muscle intensity
  - May contain ↑ signal due to methemoglobin
  - Focal small ↓ signal in periphery secondary to calcifications
- Fluid-sensitive sequences: Inhomogeneous high signal
  - Fluid-fluid levels in 90%
  - Nodular solid portions of lesions seen within mass, often at periphery
- Enhancement peripherally and in any nodular tissue

CLINICAL ISSUES

- Rare; 4-12% of all cases of osteosarcoma
- 2nd decade most common; wide age range
- 5-year survival rate 68%, similar to conventional osteosarcoma
- Treatment: Same as conventional osteosarcoma

(Left) *Axial bone CT in a 27-year-old woman shows destruction of the fibular head and neck, with little remaining recognizable bone, but with osteoid matrix* ⮳*. The mass* ➔ *is very large and shows attenuation lower than that of muscle.* **(Right)** *Axial T1 MR in the same patient shows the mass to contain regions of fluid levels* ➔ *as well as areas of high signal intensity* ⮳*, indicating hemorrhage. Both findings are typical of telangiectatic osteosarcoma (OS).*

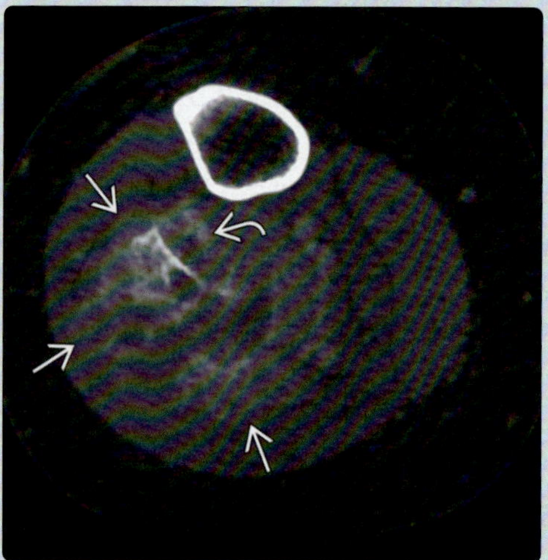

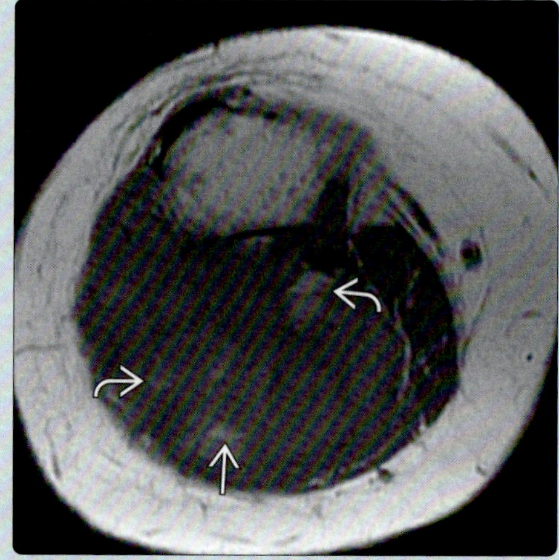

(Left) *Axial STIR MR shows the multiple fluid levels* ➔ *throughout much of the mass to better advantage.* **(Right)** *Axial T1 C+ FS MR obscures the fluid levels but shows intense enhancement of the mass* ➔ *as well as more peripheral edema. There are multiple regions of tumor necrosis* ⮳*, typical of the aggressive nature of telangiectatic OS. With appropriate treatment, this lesion has survival rates similar to those of conventional OS.*

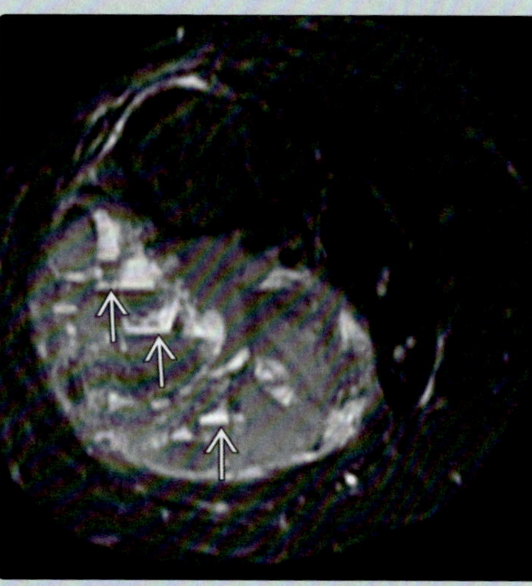

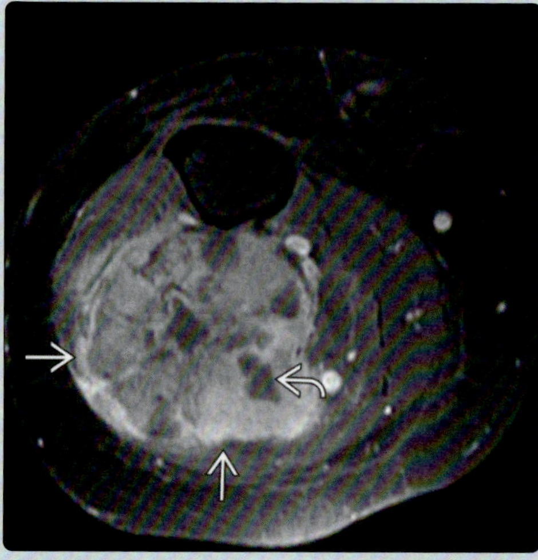

TERMINOLOGY

Synonyms

- Rare malignant bone aneurysm, hemorrhagic osteosarcoma (OS), aneurysmal bone cyst-like OS

Definitions

- Malignant bone-forming tumor containing or largely consisting of large blood-filled spaces

IMAGING

General Features

- Location
  - 90% tubular bone metaphysis; other locations rare
    - Distal femur (48%) > proximal tibia (14%), proximal humerus, proximal femur
  - Metaphyseal lesion extends into epiphysis in 83%

Radiographic Findings

- Lytic; may appear partially geographic
  - Narrow zone of transition may be seen in part, wide zone in other parts
  - May have at least partial sclerotic margin
  - Uncommonly, true permeative pattern is seen
  - Watch for red flag region where zone of transition is indistinct
- Aneurysmal expansion of cortex in 75%, though prominent expansion in fewer cases (19%)
- Generally matrix only subtly visible as small foci in periphery of lesion (58%)
  - In osseous &/or soft tissue portion of lesion
- Cortical interruption (78%) with soft tissue mass in majority, though may be subtle on radiograph
- Aggressive periosteal reaction is common (72%)
- High incidence of pathologic fracture (43-61%)
- Highly aggressive appearance may also occur

CT Findings

- Heterogeneous ↓ attenuation in center of lesion
- Small calcific foci in periphery, generally better seen on CT (85%) than on radiograph (58%)
- Fluid-fluid levels present but only visible in 48%
- Cortical destruction and soft tissue mass
- Enhancement of tumor at periphery and in septa

MR Findings

- T1WI: Inhomogeneous signal similar to or slightly higher than muscle intensity
  - Contain ↑ signal due to methemoglobin (96%)
  - May demonstrate fluid-fluid levels
- Focal small ↓ signal in periphery 2° to calcifications
- Fluid-sensitive sequences: Inhomogeneous high signal
  - Fluid-fluid levels in 90%
  - Nodular solid portions of lesions seen within mass, often at periphery
- Enhancement peripherally and in any nodular tissue

Nuclear Medicine Findings

- Peripheral uptake with central photopenic region (donut) in majority

DIFFERENTIAL DIAGNOSIS

Aneurysmal Bone Cyst

- Expanded lytic lesion arising in metaphysis
- Generally more geographic than telangiectatic OS
- Fluid-fluid levels (rarely solid lesion)
- No enhancing nodularity or tumor osteoid

PATHOLOGY

General Features

- Genetics
  - Few reports show complex chromosomal changes

Gross Pathologic & Surgical Features

- Cystic, filled incompletely with blood clot ("bag of blood")
  - Occupies > 90% of lesion; only small amount is solid

Microscopic Features

- Blood-filled or empty spaces separated by thin septa
  - Septa and periphery contain highly malignant spindle tumor cells
  - Fine osteoid seen in minimal amounts

CLINICAL ISSUES

Presentation

- Most common signs/symptoms
  - Deep bone pain
  - Pathologic fracture in 60%

Demographics

- Age
  - 2nd decade most common; wide age range
- Gender
  - M:F = 1.5-2:1
- Epidemiology
  - Rare; 4-12% of all cases of OS

Natural History & Prognosis

- 5-year survival rate 68%, similar to conventional OS
  - Highly sensitive to chemotherapy, though survival rates not different than OS

Treatment

- Presurgical chemotherapy
- Wide surgical resection, limb salvage if feasible
- Postoperative chemotherapy

DIAGNOSTIC CHECKLIST

Consider

- Watch for red flags to avoid underdiagnosis
  - Lack of geographic border in any part of lesion
  - Cortical breakthrough
  - Soft tissue mass in septa or at edge of lesion

SELECTED REFERENCES

1. Yarmish G et al: Imaging characteristics of primary osteosarcoma: nonconventional subtypes. Radiographics. 30(6):1653-72, 2010
2. Discepola F et al: Telangiectatic osteosarcoma: radiologic and pathologic findings. Radiographics. 29(2):380-3, 2009

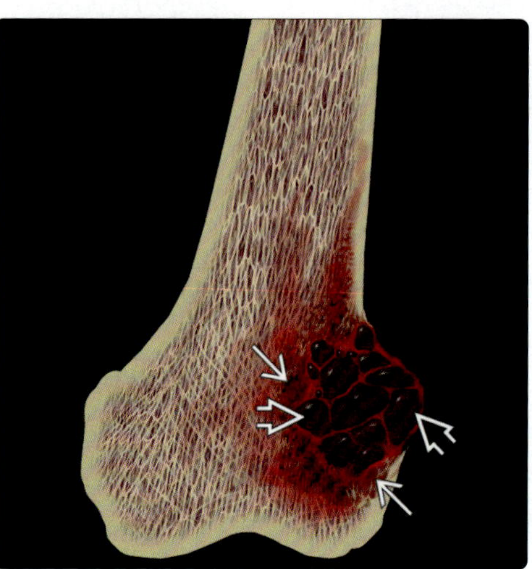

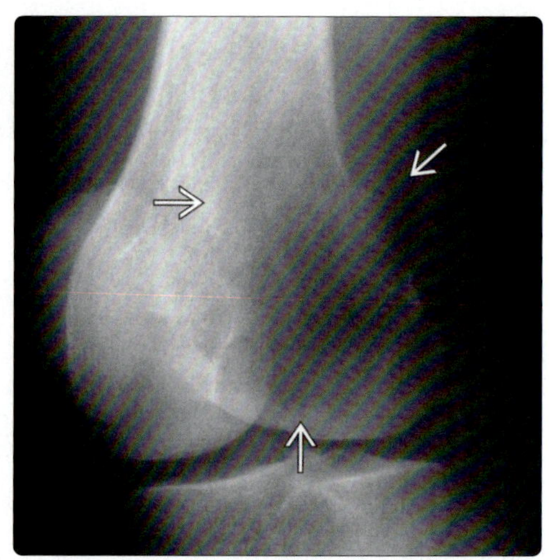

(Left) *Graphic shows telangiectatic OS. Note the extremely hemorrhagic appearance, with blood clots ➡ and also small nodules of tumor ➡.* **(Right)** *Oblique radiograph demonstrates a moderately aggressive lesion with cortical breakthrough and a soft tissue mass ➡. It is located in the distal end of the femur and extends to the subarticular surface. Although there is no matrix present, both chondrosarcoma and OS should be considered, along with aggressive giant cell tumor.*

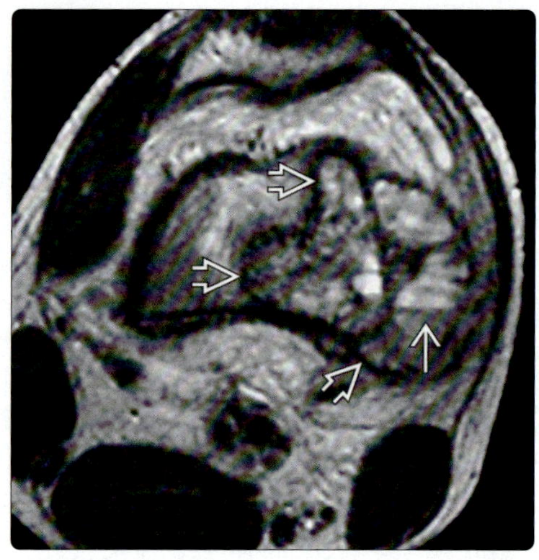

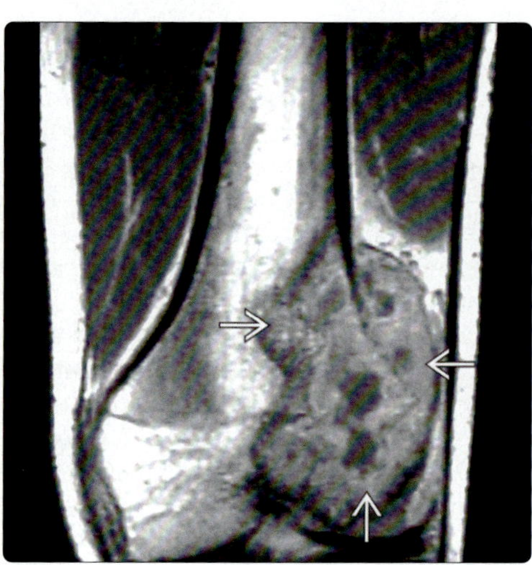

(Left) *Axial T2 MR in the same patient shows a few fluid levels ➡ with a surrounding inhomogeneous solid mass ➡.* **(Right)** *Coronal T1 C+ MR shows enhancement of the lesion ➡ and some cystic or necrotic regions. Biopsy showed telangiectatic OS. This lesion often does not appear as permeative as a conventional OS; they rarely contain matrix and fluid levels are common. The correct diagnosis is crucial since prognosis and treatment are the same as conventional OS; underdiagnosis may prove disastrous.*

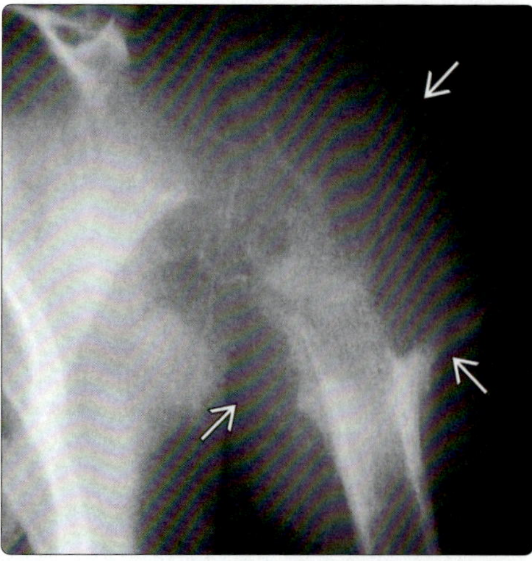

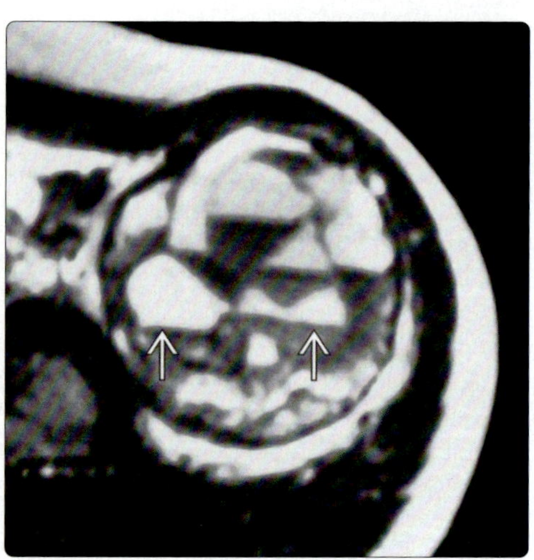

(Left) *AP x-ray shows an unusual case of a severely destructive telangiectatic sarcoma. There is a lytic lesion ➡ that contains amorphous osteoid matrix. There is periosteal reaction and a large soft tissue mass. The picture is that of an aggressive conventional OS.* **(Right)** *Axial T2WI MR in the same patient shows that the majority of the lesion contains fluid levels ➡, more typical of a telangiectatic OS. This is a surprising disparity in the appearance of the radiograph and MR, but the diagnosis was confirmed at surgery.*

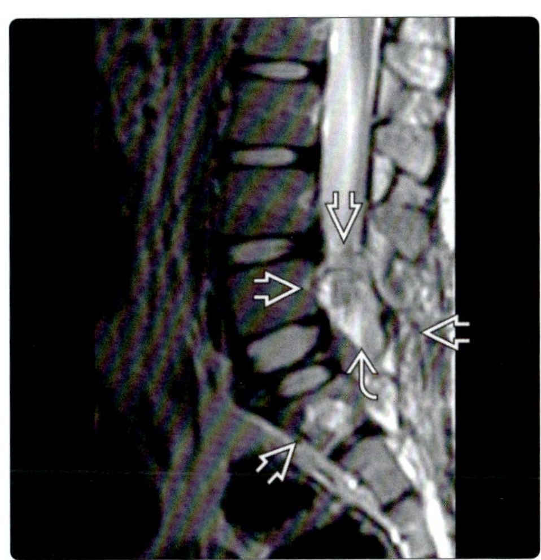

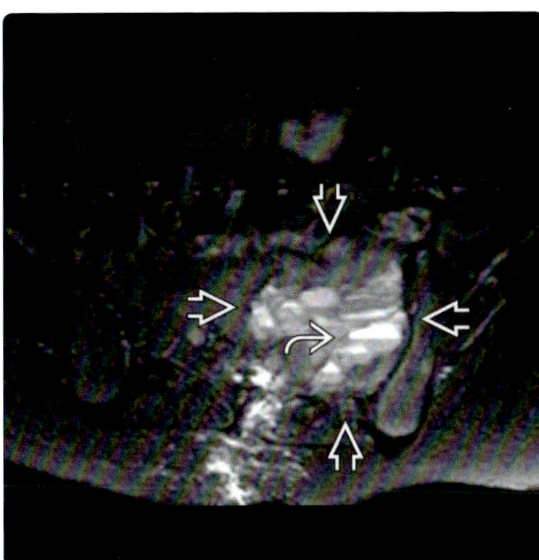

(Left) *Sagittal T2WI MR of telangiectatic OS shows an aggressive mass originating in the (now collapsed) L5 vertebral body. The mass* ➡ *extends into the posterior elements, spinal canal, paraspinous soft tissues, and into the sacrum. Multiple fluid-fluid levels are seen* ➡*.* **(Right)** *Axial T2WI FS MR in the same patient shows the mass* ➡ *along with fluid-fluid levels* ➡*. The latter finding may suggest aneurysmal bone cyst; however, the mass is more extensive than expected for that diagnosis and contains solid portions.*

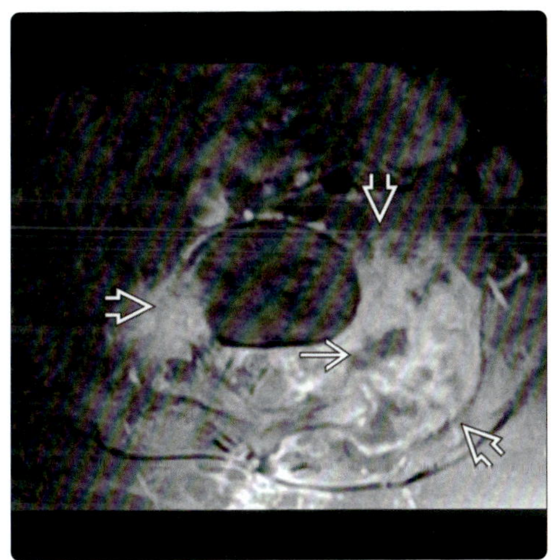

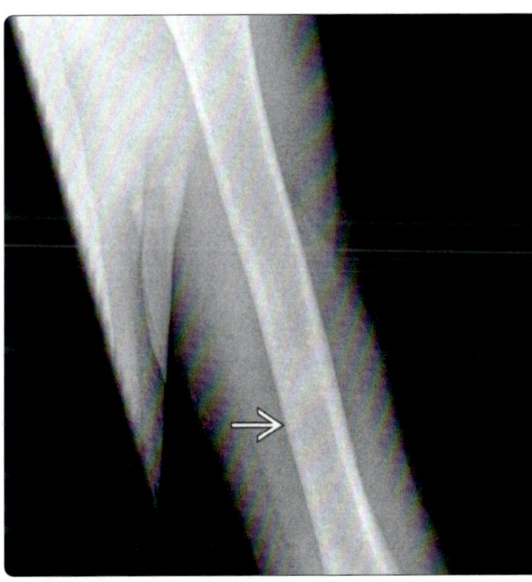

(Left) *Axial T1WI C+ MR obtained more proximally shows enhancement of solid components* ➡ *surrounding nonenhancing, low signal cystic areas* ➡*. The combination of extensive destruction and fluid levels lead to the diagnosis of telangiectatic OS, proven at biopsy.* **(Right)** *AP radiograph shows a subtle lesion of the humerus* ➡ *in a child who complained of pain at this site. This appearance might be most suggestive of Langerhans cell histiocytosis in this child. MR was performed.*

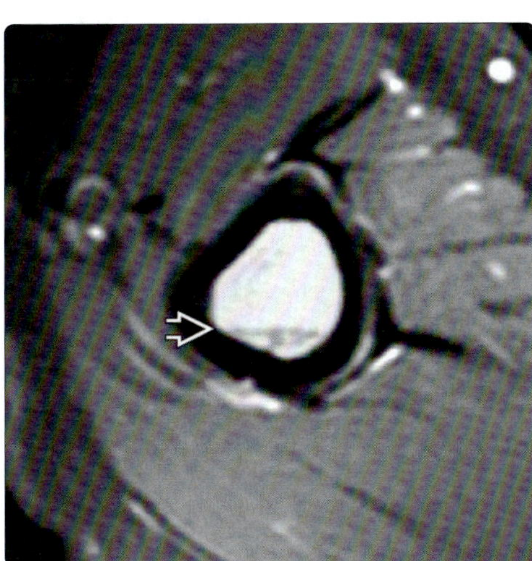

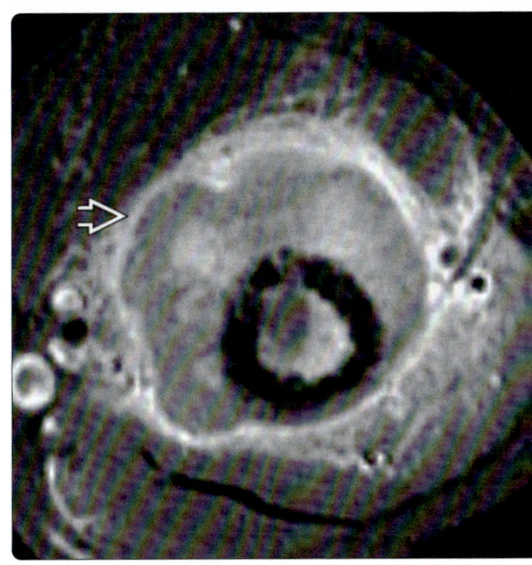

(Left) *Axial T2WI MR shows a fluid level* ➡ *within the humerus, thought at an outside institution to be an aneurysmal bone cyst (ABC).* **(Right)** *Axial T1WI C+ MR obtained 2 months later shows a large soft tissue mass* ➡ *with extensive necrosis and permeative bone destruction. This case demonstrates the aggressive nature of telangiectatic OS, as well as the deceptively nonaggressive appearance it may have initially. The red flag is the disparity between the initial radiograph and MR; this must be addressed.*

KEY FACTS

TERMINOLOGY

- Low-grade osteosarcoma arising within osseous medullary cavity

IMAGING

- Location: Metadiaphyseal, usually long bones, particularly femur and tibia
- Permeative; may be quite subtle
- Poorly marginated
- Up to 1/3 may show well-defined margins
- May contain trabeculation, sclerosis
- Matrix: Variable
- Most will have some degree of cortical destruction
- ± periosteal reaction
- ± relatively small soft tissue mass
- MR often necessary to delineate cortical destruction or soft tissue mass that may be present

CLINICAL ISSUES

- Present with low-grade pain, swelling
  - May be months to years before medical attention sought
- Peak incidence 2nd & 3rd decades (average: 28 years)
- Much more indolent behavior than conventional osteosarcoma
- High incidence of recurrence following inadequate resection

DIAGNOSTIC CHECKLIST

- More aggressive lesions fall within "small round blue cell" list of permeative diaphyseal lesions
- Less aggressive lesions often initially misdiagnosed on pathology as fibrous dysplasia and not recognized until recurrence
  - Local excision with recurrence may result in more aggressive malignancy: Dedifferentiation or metastatic spread

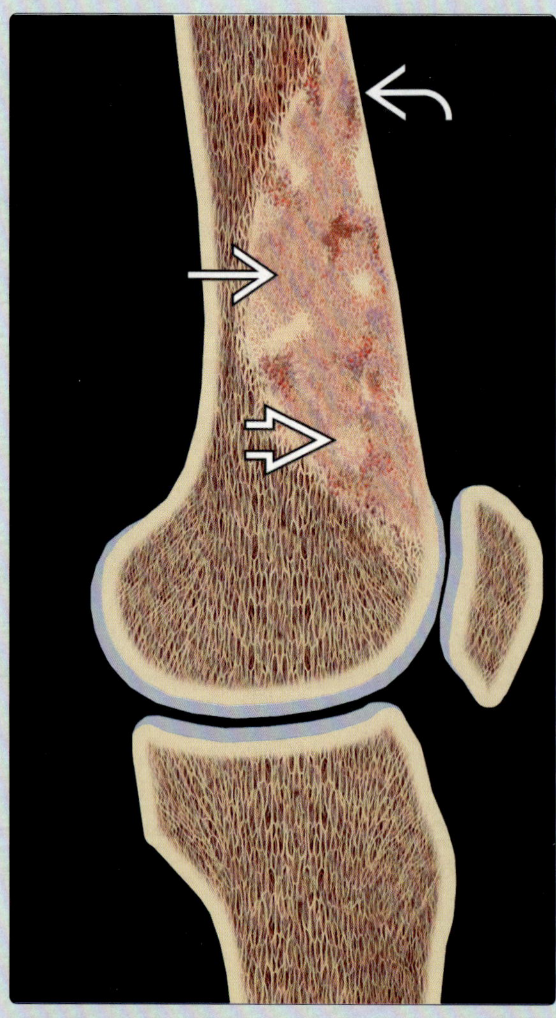

Sagittal graphic depicts a low-grade intraosseous osteosarcoma. There is a mixture of immature osteoid ➡ and mature regions of bone formation ➡. There is no sclerotic or defined margin; the lesion is permeative. The cortex is severely thinned ➡.

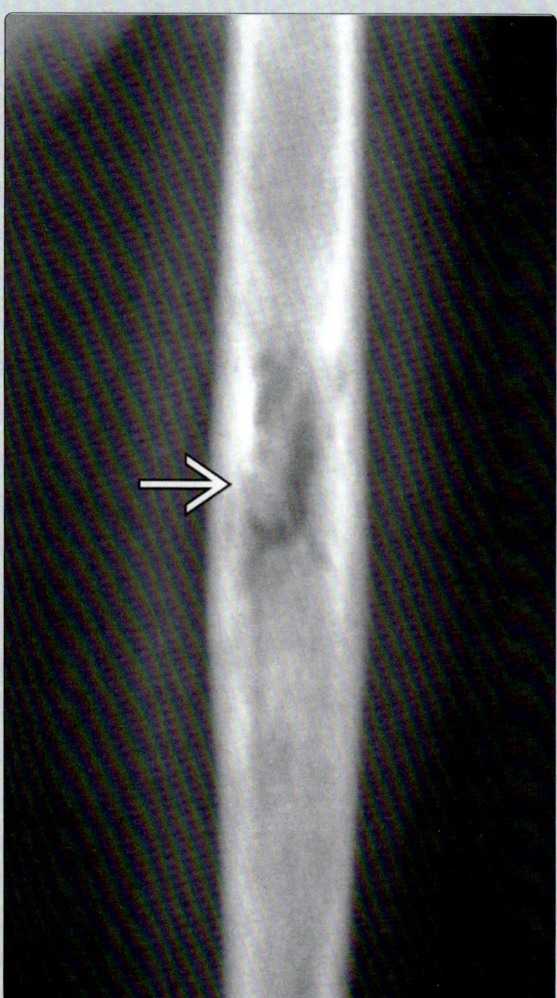

AP radiograph of low-grade intraosseous osteosarcoma demonstrates a permeative lesion within the diaphysis of the humerus ➡. There is no matrix, cortical breakthrough, soft tissue mass, or periosteal reaction.

Low-Grade Intraosseous Osteosarcoma

TERMINOLOGY

Synonyms

- Low-grade central osteosarcoma, well-differentiated intramedullary osteosarcoma, sclerosing osteosarcoma

Definitions

- Low-grade osteosarcoma arising within medullary cavity

IMAGING

General Features

- Best diagnostic clue
  - Permeative metadiaphyseal lesion with moderate appearance of aggressiveness
- Location
  - Usually long bones, particularly femur and tibia
  - Metadiaphyseal
- Size
  - Tend to be large by time of discovery

Radiographic Findings

- Permeative; may be quite subtle
- Poorly marginated
  - Up to 1/3 may show well-defined margins
- May contain trabeculation, sclerosis
- Matrix: Variable
  - May be lytic but often densely mineralized
  - Regions of amorphous mineralization as well
- Most will have some degree of cortical destruction
  - Expansion, thinning of cortex, or permeative
- ± periosteal reaction (22-50% reported)
- ± relatively small soft tissue mass

CT Findings

- Mimics radiographic findings; may show matrix, cortical breakthrough, and periosteal reaction better

MR Findings

- Variability in presence of matrix affects homogeneity and persistent low signal on all sequences
- Generally inhomogeneous low signal on T1 and inhomogeneous high signal on fluid-sensitive sequences, with enhancement
  - Best shows involvement of cortex & soft tissue mass

DIFFERENTIAL DIAGNOSIS

Ewing Sarcoma

- No matrix but may elicit sclerotic bone reaction
- Diaphyseal and permeative
- Most cases have very large soft tissue mass, but minority may appear less aggressive initially

Langerhans Cell Histiocytosis

- Permeative, ranging from nonaggressive to highly aggressive in appearance
- May have soft tissue mass

Fibrous Dysplasia

- Expanded lesion with variable density, thinned cortex
- Initial diagnosis of low-grade intraosseous osteosarcoma is often fibrous dysplasia (FD) on both imaging and histology

PATHOLOGY

General Features

- Genetics
  - Low number of chromosomal imbalances contrasts with complex aberrations in high-grade osteosarcomas

Microscopic Features

- Very difficult to diagnose: May resemble FD, desmoplastic fibroma, osteoblastoma, chondromyxoid fibroma, low-grade parosteal osteosarcoma
- Hypo- to moderately cellular fibroblastic stroma
- Variable amounts of collagen and osteoid production

CLINICAL ISSUES

Presentation

- Most common signs/symptoms
  - Low-grade pain, swelling
  - May be months to years before medical attention sought

Demographics

- Age
  - Peak incidence 2nd & 3rd decades (average: 28 years)
- Gender
  - M = F
- Epidemiology
  - 1-2% of all osteosarcomas

Natural History & Prognosis

- Much more indolent behavior than conventional osteosarcoma
- High recurrence rate following inadequate resection
  - Recurrence may exhibit higher histological grade or dedifferentiation with potential for metastases
- 15-20% progress to high-grade spindle cell sarcoma

Treatment

- Initial wide excision must be definitive to avoid recurrence and possible dedifferentiation

DIAGNOSTIC CHECKLIST

Consider

- More aggressive lesions fall within "small round blue cell" list of permeative diaphyseal lesions
- Less aggressive lesions often initially misdiagnosed on pathology as FD and not recognized as osteosarcoma until recurrence
  - Local excision with recurrence may result in more aggressive malignancy
  - Watch for focal red flags: Cortical destruction, soft tissue mass, periosteal reaction

SELECTED REFERENCES

1. Gilg MM et al: Central low-grade osteosarcoma with an unusual localization in the diaphysis of a 12-year old patient. Radiol Oncol. 47(2):192-6, 2013
2. Yarmish G et al: Imaging characteristics of primary osteosarcoma: nonconventional subtypes. Radiographics. 30(6):1653-72, 2010
3. Andresen KJ et al: Imaging features of low-grade central osteosarcoma of the long bones and pelvis. Skeletal Radiol. 33(7):373-9, 2004

(Left) *AP radiograph shows a typical case of low-grade intraosseous osteosarcoma. A moderately aggressive lytic lesion is seen occupying the marrow space of the proximal tibial metadiaphysis. Much of the lesion appears permeative ➡, but more circumscribed regions are also seen. There is a small region of cortical breakthrough, which shows some amorphous osteoid matrix ➡.* **(Right)** *Lateral radiograph in the same patient shows much of the lesion to appear only moderately aggressive, with geographic regions ➡. The overall radiographic picture is of only moderate aggressiveness, but the single site of cortical breakthrough should alert the diagnostician that something more aggressive than fibrous dysplasia must be considered. MR should be considered mandatory in such a case.*

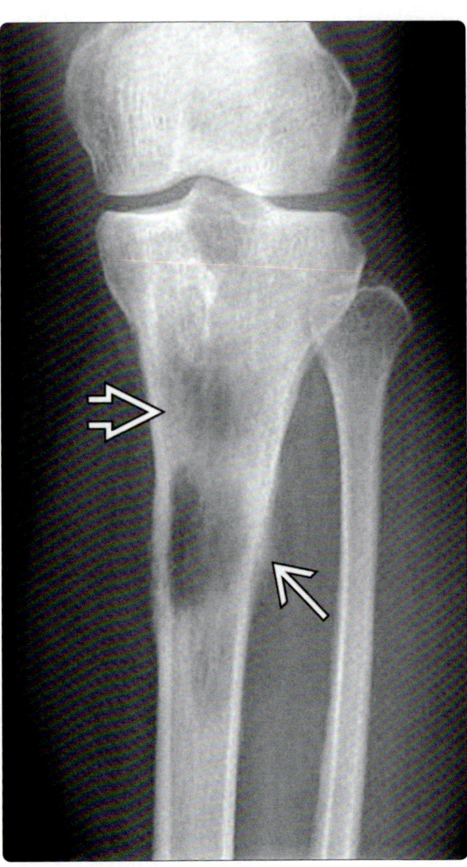

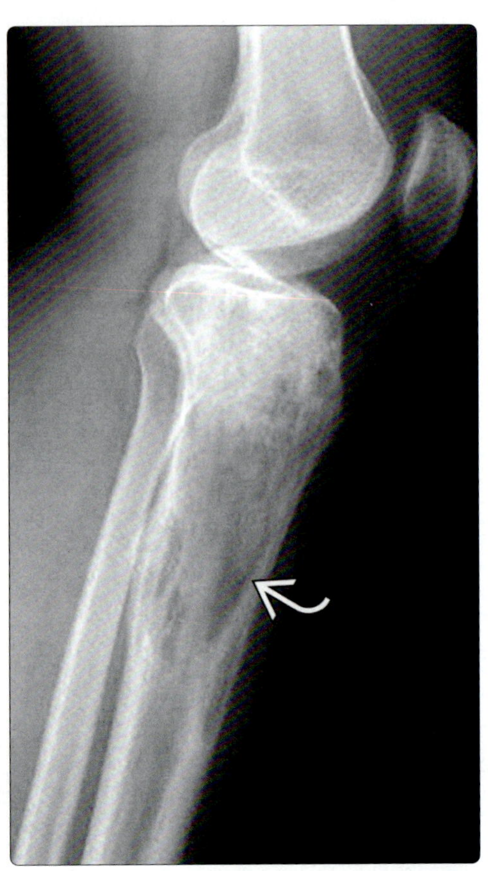

(Left) *Coronal T1WI MR in the same patient shows a permeative lesion arising within the marrow ➡. The cortical breakthrough and soft tissue mass ➡ is larger than was suggested by radiograph.* **(Right)** *Axial T2 FS MR shows inhomogeneous high marrow signal. There is high signal within much of the cortex ➡, indicating permeation and cortical breakthrough ➡. A soft tissue mass is seen circumferentially about the tibia, which could be a conventional osteosarcoma (OS) by imaging criteria. However, there are portions that appear less aggressive on radiograph than most OS, and the soft tissue mass is relatively smaller than is often seen in conventional OS. Therefore one might consider the diagnosis of low-grade intraosseous osteosarcoma, which was confirmed by histology. (Courtesy KJ Suh, MD.)*

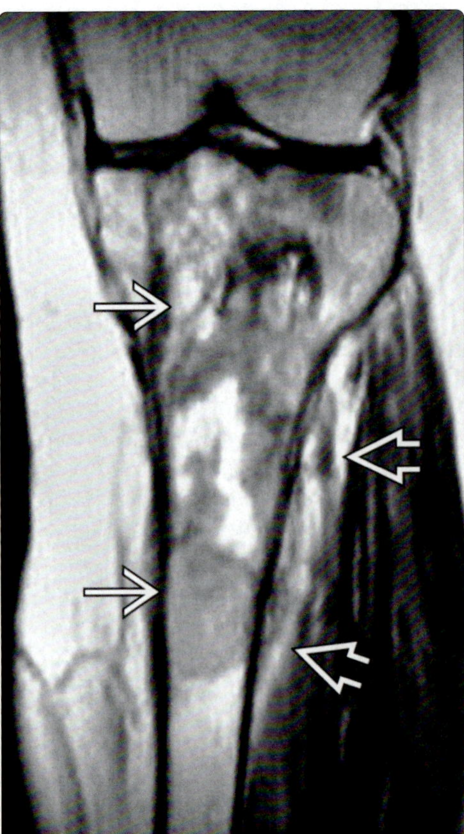

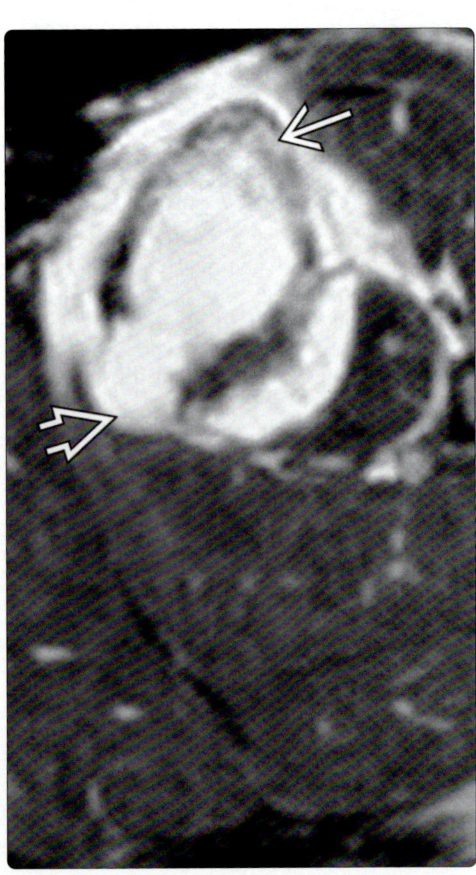

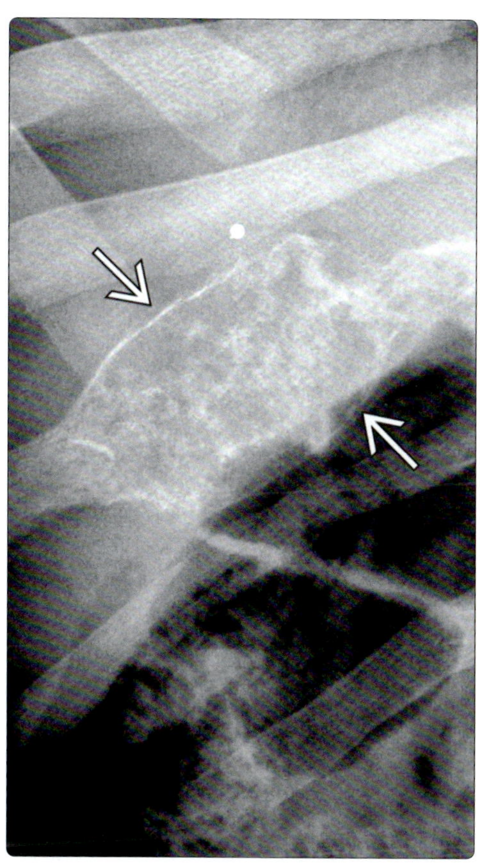

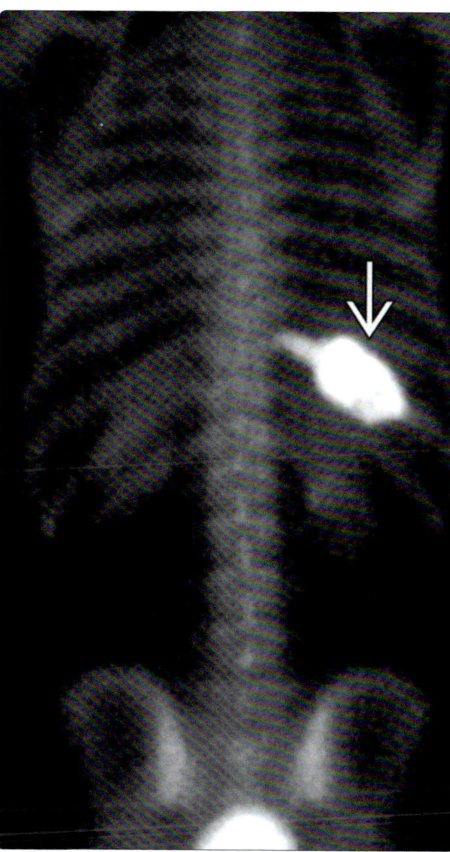

(Left) *AP radiograph shows a solitary rib lesion ➡, which is expanded, well-marginated, and contains matrix. The most frequent matrix-containing lesion in ribs is enchondroma. However, enchondromas of the ribs rarely attain this size. Fibrous dysplasia is common in the rib, but the matrix should not be this distinct. This patient stated that the mass had been present for several years but was now more bothersome.* **(Right)** *Posteroanterior bone scan in the same patient shows the solitary lesion to have intense uptake ➡. Although enchondroma or fibrous dysplasia may show mild uptake, it is rarely this intense; this degree of uptake and the patient's indication of recent increase in discomfort warrants further work-up.*

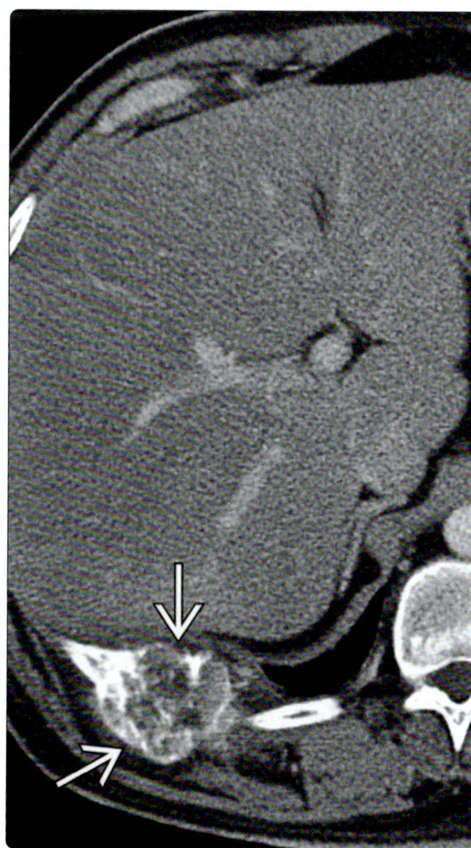

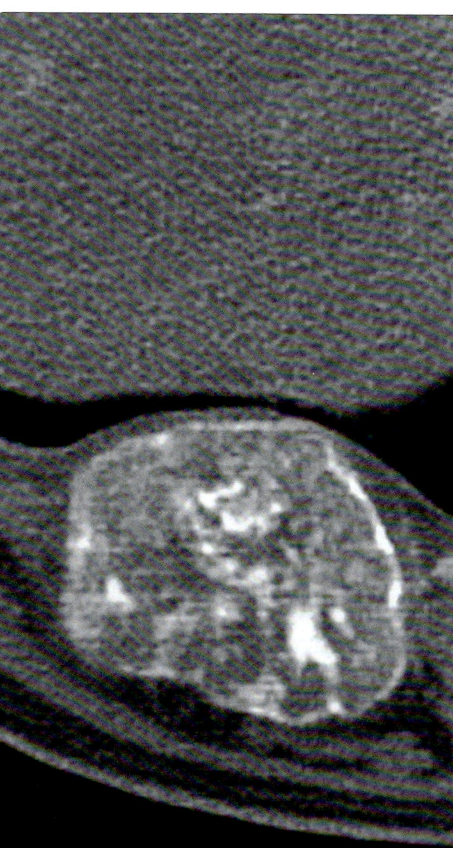

(Left) *Axial CT adds important information, showing no cortical breakthrough or soft tissue mass related to this lesion ➡. The matrix is not identifiable as distinctly osteoid or chondroid.* **(Right)** *Axial CT in a different section confirms that one cannot distinguish between osteoid and chondroid matrix. However, the lesion appears nonaggressive. Statistically, this lesion was expected to be a low-grade chondrosarcoma arising from an underlying enchondroma. The rarity of osteosarcoma relative to cartilage-forming tumors in the ribs led to this diagnosis. However, at surgery, it proved to be a low-grade intraosseous osteosarcoma. Luckily, the treatment of wide resection would be adequate for either.*

High-Grade Surface Osteosarcoma

KEY FACTS

TERMINOLOGY

- High-grade, bone-forming tumor arising from osseous surface

IMAGING

- Location: Diaphyseal, surface
  - Femur (46%) > humerus (16%) > tibia/fibula
- Osteoid matrix usually present in soft tissue mass
- Underlying cortex may be partially destroyed
- Periosteal reaction common; tends to be perpendicular and aggressive
- MR: Soft tissue mass contains variable amounts of low signal tumor osteoid
  - Affects homogeneity and overall signal of mass
  - Generally, fluid-sensitive sequences show inhomogeneous high signal
  - Adjacent soft tissue invasion beyond apparent confines of matrix
  - Minimal medullary involvement may be seen and must be sought
  - Avid enhancement with contrast

TOP DIFFERENTIAL DIAGNOSES

- Imaging appearance may be nearly identical to the following lesions (histology differentiates it)
  - Parosteal osteosarcoma
  - Periosteal osteosarcoma
  - Periosteal chondroma

CLINICAL ISSUES

- Peak incidence in 2nd decade; age distribution similar to conventional osteosarcoma
- < 1% of all osteosarcomas; 10% of all juxtacortical osteosarcomas
- Somewhat better prognosis compared with conventional osteosarcoma
- Same treatment as conventional osteosarcoma

(Left) *Anteroposterior radiograph shows a high-grade surface osteosarcoma with osteoid matrix on the diaphyseal surface ➡, appearing somewhat aggressive in that it is not organized. There is not obvious periosteal reaction or involvement of the underlying cortex or marrow.* **(Right)** *Coronal T1WI MR confirms the lesion to be confined to the surface ➡. It is inhomogeneously low signal, related to the known osseous matrix. Both the marrow ↩ and adjacent cortex appear to be undisturbed by the lesion.*

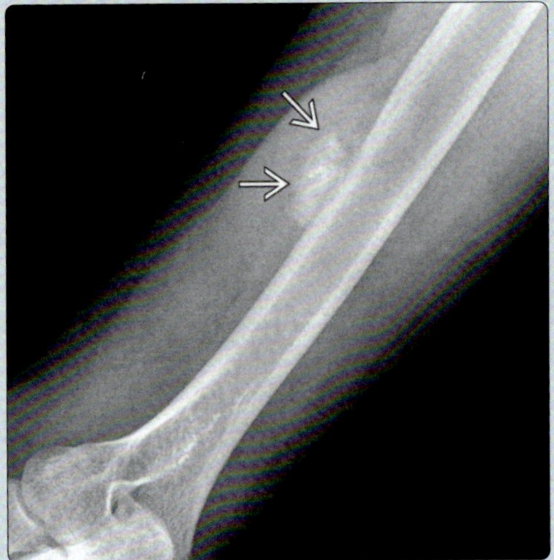

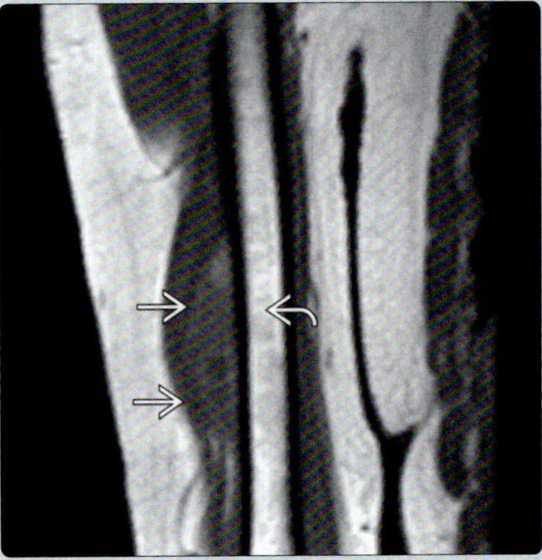

(Left) *Axial T2 FS MR, same patient, shows heterogeneous high signal ➡, with the low signal of the matrix seen more centrally. Note that the lesion extends beyond the confines of the matrix into the soft tissue. There is subtle high signal within the marrow adjacent to the lesion ↩, indicating intramedullary extension.* **(Right)** *Coronal T1WI C+ FS MR shows avid enhancement of the lesion ➡ with extension proximally and distally along the periosteum. There is no cortical signal, but subtle marrow signal ↩ raises concern for involvement.*

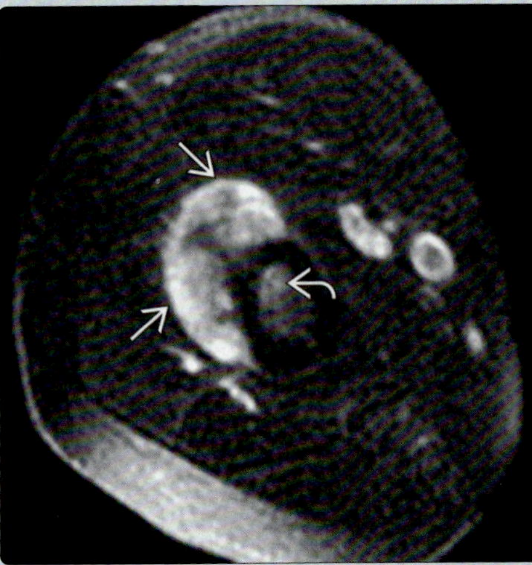

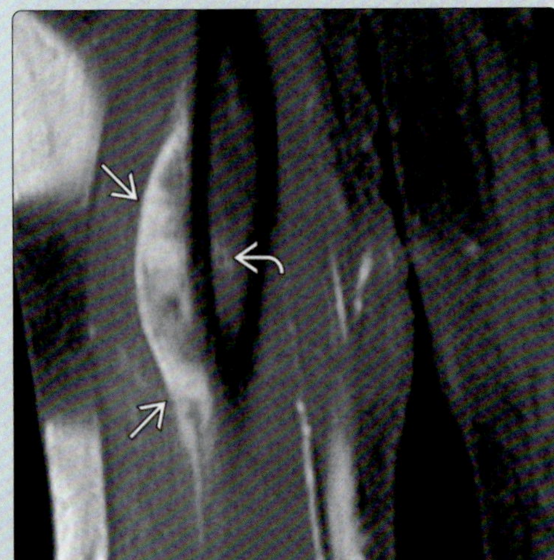

TERMINOLOGY

Synonyms

- Juxtacortical osteosarcoma, surface osteosarcoma

Definitions

- High-grade bone-forming tumor arising from bone surface

IMAGING

General Features

- Best diagnostic clue
  - Osteoid matrix-producing lesion in soft tissues adjacent to and involving surface of long bone
- Location
  - Femur (46%) > humerus (16%) > tibia/fibula
  - Surface lesion, diaphyseal

Radiographic Findings

- Osteoid matrix usually present in soft tissue mass
  - Without matrix, may only see distortion of fat planes around soft tissue mass
- Underlying cortex may be partially destroyed
  - Scalloping of cortex or permeative change
- Periosteal reaction common; tends to be aggressive

CT Findings

- Mimics those of radiograph
- Faint osteoid matrix may be best seen on CT

MR Findings

- Soft tissue mass containing variable amounts of low signal tumor osteoid
  - Affects homogeneity and overall signal of mass
  - Generally, fluid-sensitive sequences show inhomogeneous high signal
  - Adjacent soft tissue invasion beyond matrix
- Periosteal reaction with edema in adjacent cortex
- Minimal medullary involvement may be seen and must be sought (reported in 8-48% of cases)
- Avid contrast enhancement

DIFFERENTIAL DIAGNOSIS

Periosteal Osteosarcoma

- Similar scalloping and involvement of cortex
- Osteoid matrix production in soft tissue surface mass may appear identically amorphous to high-grade surface OS
- May involve lesser circumference of bone than high-grade surface OS, but not a differentiating factor

Parosteal Osteosarcoma

- Routine parosteal osteosarcoma has more mature bone production and appears more organized
- Dedifferentiated parosteal osteosarcoma may have similar amorphous bone production

Periosteal Chondroma

- Benign surface cartilage tumor
  - Matrix is chondroid, though not always easy to differentiate from immature osteoid
- May develop similar scalloping of underlying cortex

PATHOLOGY

Gross Pathologic & Surgical Features

- Multilobulated surface
- Color varies depending on amount of chondroid matrix, osteoid matrix, hemorrhage, and necrosis
- "Soft" spots on surface help to differentiate from parosteal osteosarcoma

Microscopic Features

- Same histology as conventional osteosarcoma
- High-grade cytologic atypia and high mitotic activity

CLINICAL ISSUES

Presentation

- Most common signs/symptoms
  - Painful mass
  - Rarely present with pathologic fracture

Demographics

- Age
  - Peak incidence in 2nd decade; age distribution similar to conventional osteosarcoma
- Gender
  - Slight male predominance (1.6:1)
- Epidemiology
  - < 1% of all osteosarcomas; 10% of all juxtacortical osteosarcomas

Natural History & Prognosis

- Prognosis somewhat better than conventional osteosarcoma
  - 82% 5-year survival rate in 1 series
- Major prognostic factor is response to chemotherapy

Treatment

- Same treatment as conventional osteosarcoma
  - Preoperative chemotherapy, followed by restaging
  - Wide resection
  - Adjuvant postoperative chemotherapy
  - ± radiation therapy, often related to adequacy of tumor margins from surgery

DIAGNOSTIC CHECKLIST

Consider

- May be impossible to differentiate from other surface osteosarcomas by imaging
  - Prognosis and treatment are significantly different
  - Greater aggressiveness in surface osteosarcoma should suggest this diagnosis

SELECTED REFERENCES

1. Yarmish G et al: Imaging characteristics of primary osteosarcoma: nonconventional subtypes. Radiographics. 30(6):1653-72, 2010
2. Staals EL et al: High-grade surface osteosarcoma: a review of 25 cases from the Rizzoli Institute. Cancer. 112(7):1592-9, 2008
3. Murphey MD et al: Imaging of periosteal osteosarcoma: radiologic-pathologic comparison. Radiology. 233(1):129-38, 2004
4. Vanel D et al: Radiological study of 12 high-grade surface osteosarcomas. Skeletal Radiol. 30(12):667-71, 2001

Secondary Osteosarcoma

KEY FACTS

TERMINOLOGY

- Bone-forming sarcoma arising in bone affected by underlying condition making it susceptible to sarcomatous degeneration
  - Paget disease
  - Previously radiated bone
  - Dedifferentiated chondrosarcoma

IMAGING

- Aggressive change in character within underlying lesion
- Paget sarcoma: Underlying changes of Paget disease
  - Either lytic or mixed lytic/sclerotic highly destructive pattern
  - Occurs in any bone affected by Paget disease
  - Similar distribution as Paget disease, except ↓ incidence in vertebrae and ↑ incidence in humerus
- Radiation sarcoma: Underlying changes of prior radiation
  - Short (hypoplastic) bone if radiated as child
  - Mixed lytic & sclerotic changes of radiation osteonecrosis in 50%
  - Superimposed changes of new bone destruction, osteoid matrix, and soft tissue mass
  - Location: Sites of frequent radiation, particularly including shoulder girdle, iliac wing, long bones
- Dedifferentiated chondrosarcoma: Underlying findings of chondrosarcoma
  - Chondroid matrix present, absent, or subtle
  - Superimposed destructive change, often in 1 part of lesion

CLINICAL ISSUES

- Age at presentation variable; tends to be older population
  - Paget sarcoma: Median is 64 years
  - Radiation sarcoma: Median latency period of 11 years following radiation but wide range
  - Dedifferentiated chondrosarcoma: 50-60 years
- Natural history: Extremely poor prognosis

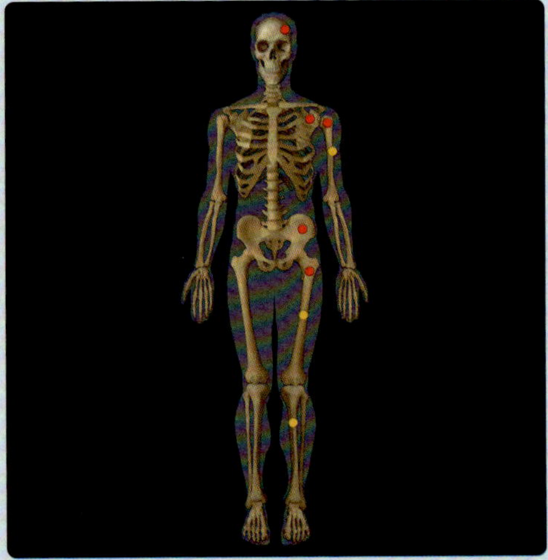

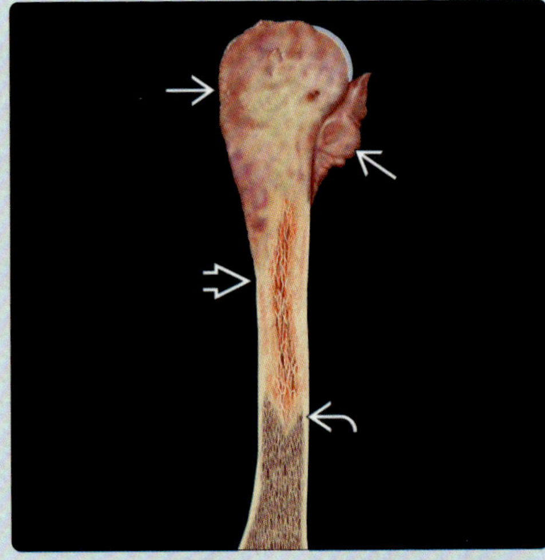

(Left) *Graphic shows the sites typical for development of secondary OS. These are sites that are frequently radiated, or frequent locations for chondrosarcoma or Paget disease.* **(Right)** *Graphic depicts OS arising in Paget disease. There is a large destructive tumor located proximally ➡, with extension into soft tissue. The tumor blends imperceptibly into the Paget disease, showing typical thickened cortex and disordered trabeculae ➡. There is sharp margination between the Paget disease and adjacent normal bone ➡.*

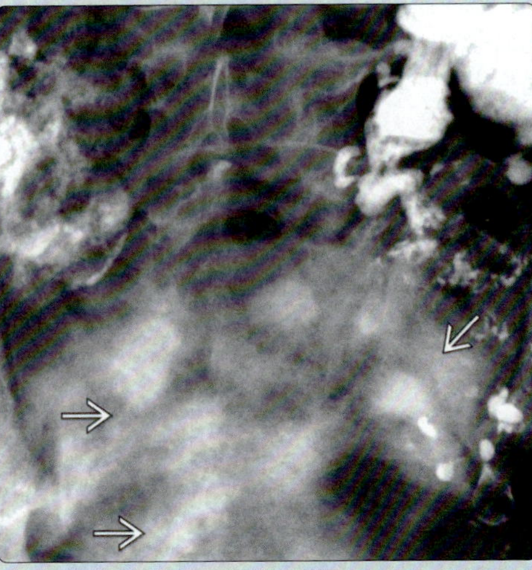

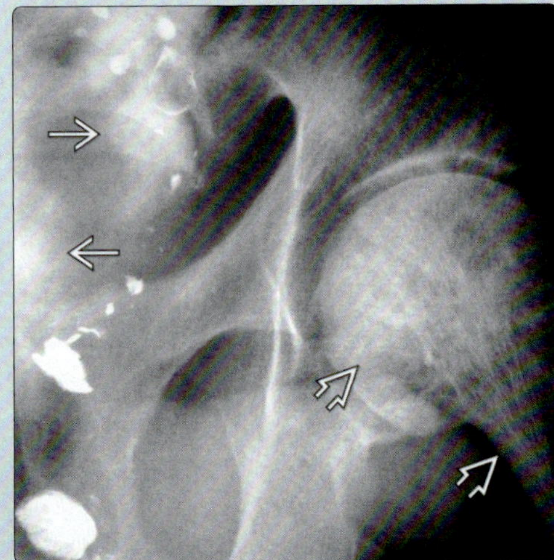

(Left) *AP radiograph shows Paget sarcoma. The sacrum is replaced by fluffy amorphous bone density ➡. The bone is expanded, without normal trabeculae. This appearance can only represent osteosarcoma; patients of this age with osteosarcoma often have an underlying etiology.* **(Right)** *AP radiograph in the same patient shows tumor osteoid replacing the sacrum ➡. The hip has a distinctly different appearance, with thick coarsened trabeculae ➡. This is typical Paget disease, and the sacral lesion is secondary OS.*

TERMINOLOGY

Definitions

- Bone-forming sarcoma arising in bone affected by underlying condition making it susceptible to sarcomatous degeneration
  - Paget disease
  - Previously radiated bone
  - Dedifferentiated chondrosarcoma
  - Other rare disorders, including dedifferentiation of surface osteosarcomas (OS) to high-grade OS

IMAGING

General Features

- Best diagnostic clue
  - Aggressive change within underlying lesion

Radiographic Findings

- Paget sarcoma
  - Underlying Paget disease
    - Coarsened trabeculae, mixed lytic/sclerotic disease, thickened cortex
  - Either lytic or mixed lytic/sclerotic highly destructive pattern
  - Cortical breakthrough, soft tissue mass
- Radiation sarcoma
  - Underlying changes of prior radiation
    - Short (hypoplastic) bone if radiated as child
    - Mixed lytic & sclerotic changes of radiation osteonecrosis in 50%
      - May be whole bone if radiated for Ewing sarcoma or lymphoma
      - May be in port-like configuration; part of bone may be involved if included in therapy field, with other portions normal
  - Superimposed changes of new bone destruction, osteoid matrix, and soft tissue mass
- Dedifferentiated chondrosarcoma
  - Underlying findings of chondrosarcoma
    - Thickened or thin cortex but not aggressive
    - Chondroid matrix present, absent, or subtle
  - Superimposed destruction in 1 portion of lesion
    - New cortical breakthrough, soft tissue mass, osteoid

PATHOLOGY

General Features

- Etiology
  - Paget sarcoma
    - Generally patients have widespread and long-term Paget disease (at least 70%)
    - Uncommonly occurs with monostotic disease
  - Radiation sarcoma
    - Glenoid or proximal humerus: Axillary radiation for breast cancer
    - Proximal shoulder girdle: Mantle radiation for Hodgkin disease
    - Iliac wing: Radiation for Wilms tumor
    - Long bones: Whole bone radiation for Ewing sarcoma or primary bone lymphoma
  - Dedifferentiated chondrosarcoma
    - 10% of chondrosarcomas dedifferentiate
  - Other dedifferentiated sarcomas
    - Parosteal osteosarcoma
      - Incomplete resection → high recurrence rate
      - Recurrence frequently is of higher grade
      - Less commonly, recurrence contains regions of dedifferentiation to conventional OS
    - Bone infarct: Transforms to malignant fibrous histiocytoma (MFH) more commonly than OS
    - Fibrous dysplasia: Rare dedifferentiation to OS, associated with Albright syndrome
    - Metallic implants: Rare development of tumor; usually MFH, few reports of OS

CLINICAL ISSUES

Demographics

- Age
  - Paget sarcoma: Median is 64 years
  - Radiation sarcoma: Median latency period of 11 years following radiation but wide range
  - Dedifferentiated chondrosarcoma: 50-60 years
- Epidemiology
  - 5-7% of all osteosarcomas
  - Paget sarcoma
    - 67-97% of cases of secondary OS
    - Sarcomatous change occurs in 0.7-0.95% of patients with Paget disease
  - Radiation sarcoma
    - 6-22% of secondary osteosarcomas
    - Risk of developing OS in radiated bone 0.03-0.8%
      - Prevalence may be increasing due to longer survival of children treated with radiation
    - Latent period, median: 11 years; range: 2-35 years
  - Dedifferentiated chondrosarcoma
    - 10% of chondrosarcomas dedifferentiate
    - Dedifferentiated portion usually MFH, but may be OS, fibrosarcoma, or rhabdomyosarcoma

Natural History & Prognosis

- Paget sarcoma prognosis
  - Poor prognosis; 11% 5-year survival
  - Metastases present in 25% at initial presentation
- Radiation sarcoma prognosis
  - 68.2% 5-year survival for extremity lesions
  - 27.3% 5-year survival for axial lesions (pelvic, vertebral, shoulder girdle)
- Dedifferentiated chondrosarcoma
  - Dismal prognosis: 10% survival at 2 years

SELECTED REFERENCES

1. Yagishita S et al: Secondary osteosarcoma developing 10 years after chemoradiotherapy for non-small-cell lung cancer. Jpn J Clin Oncol. 44(2):191-4, 2014
2. Murphey MD et al: The many faces of osteosarcoma. Radiographics. 17(5):1205-31, 1997

(Left) *AP radiograph obtained during a venogram shows the normal vein superimposed over an abnormal femur, with cortical thickening along the diaphysis ➡ and sclerosis of the lateral femoral condyle ➡. This is typical Paget disease. The contrast is unusually well seen in the venogram, indicating proximal obstruction.* **(Right)** *Axial NECT in the same patient shows a large OS in the iliac wing ➡, arising in Paget disease and causing vascular obstruction. This is a case of Paget degeneration to OS.*

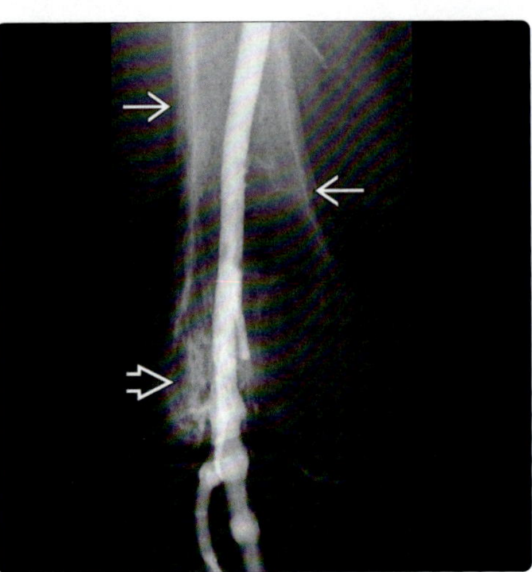

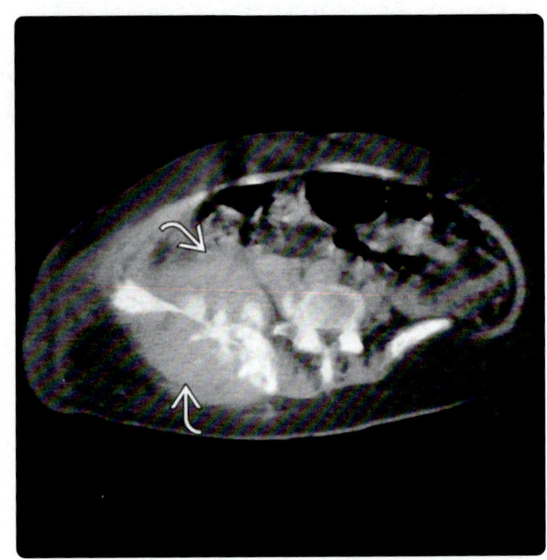

(Left) *Lateral radiograph shows an intramedullary chondrosarcoma, with central matrix ➡ and cortical thickening ➡. Superimposed on this is a focal soft tissue mass, which contains faint amorphous osteoid ➡. This is a case of chondrosarcoma that has dedifferentiated into a highly aggressive OS.* **(Right)** *Axial NECT, the 1st of 3 images, shows the course of a sternal chondrosarcoma. This image was obtained at presentation and shows a mass with scattered chondroid matrix ➡, typical of chondrosarcoma.*

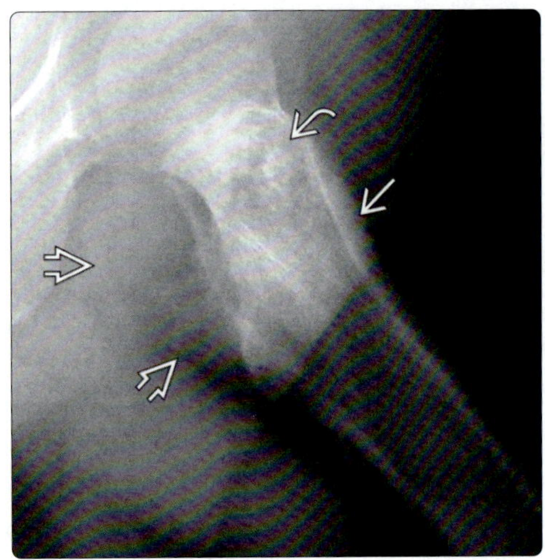

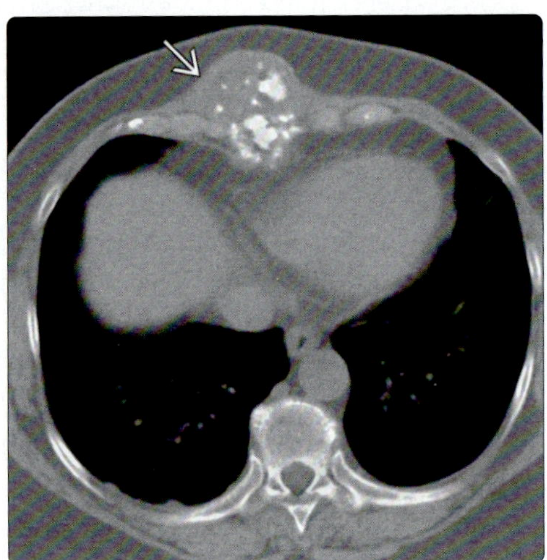

(Left) *Axial NECT shows the patient underwent standard treatment of wide resection, with no suggestion of complication ➡.* **(Right)** *Axial NECT obtained 20 months post resection showed a small mass or thickening at the site of resection. Only 3 months following that scan, this CT was obtained, showing that the mass has enlarged significantly in a very short time. There is no matrix within the mass ➡. At surgery, it was proven to be a chondrosarcoma, dedifferentiated to OS.*

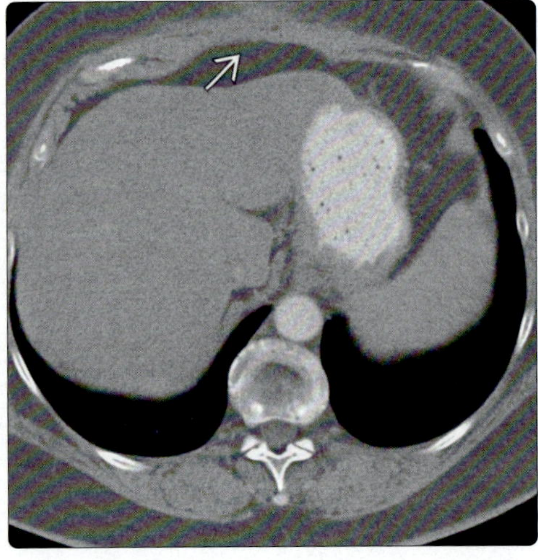

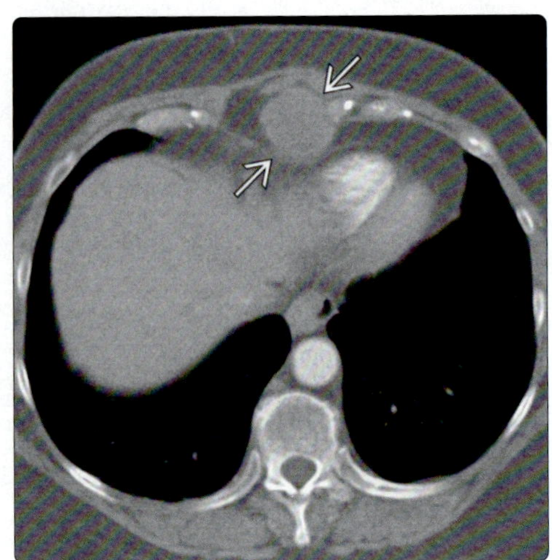

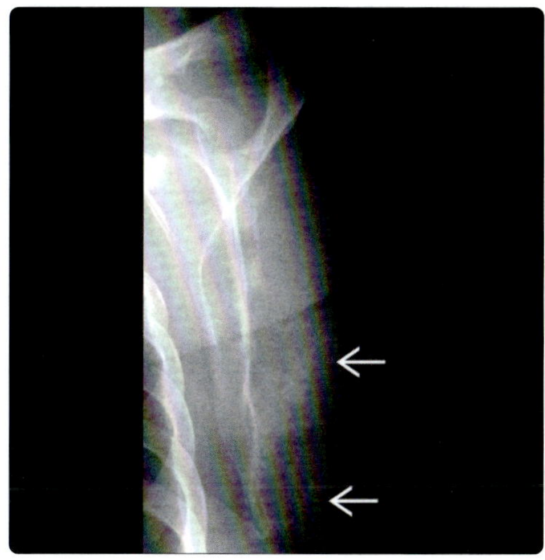

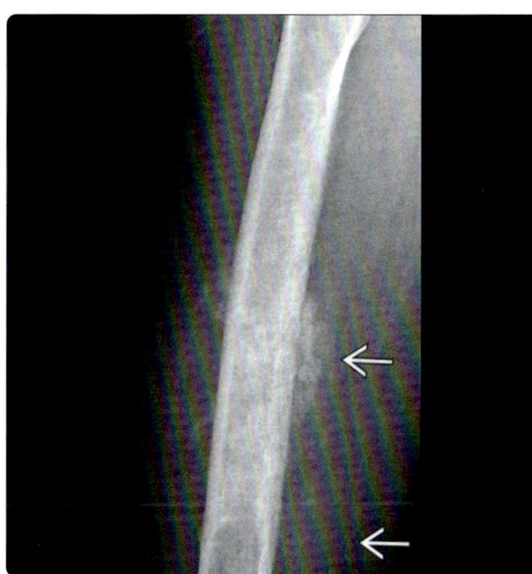

(Left) *Y view radiograph shows a radiation-induced OS. There is a severely destructive lesion of the scapula, with a large soft tissue mass containing osteoid matrix ➡. This region had been radiated 11 years earlier.* **(Right)** *Lateral radiograph in a middle-aged man shows lack of normal trabeculation within the diaphysis of the femur, as well as osteoid matrix both within the bone and a large soft tissue mass ➡. This region had been radiated as treatment of malignant fibrous histiocytoma 31 years earlier.*

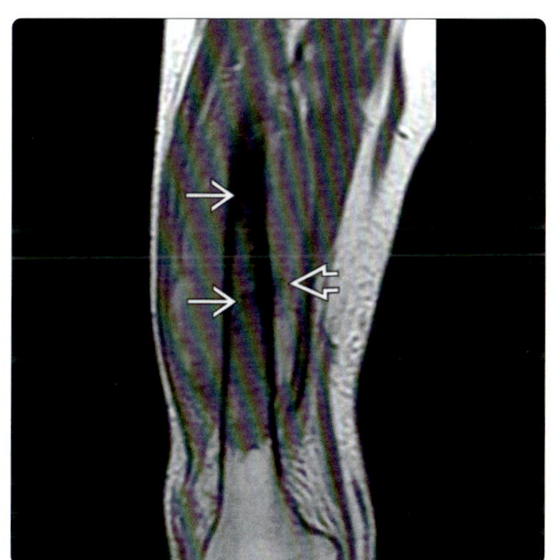

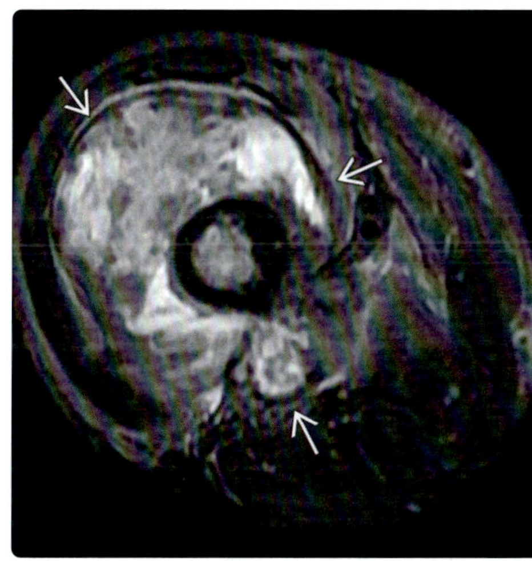

(Left) *Coronal T1 MR in the same patient shows the replacement of fatty marrow by inhomogeneous low signal material, some of which is quite hypointense ➡. There is a large circumferential soft tissue mass containing some low signal foci ➡ as well. This is the amorphous tumor osteoid seen in this patient's secondary OS.* **(Right)** *Axial T2 FS MR, same patient, shows an invasive heterogeneous soft tissue mass ➡ that violates more than 1 compartment. Marrow signal is inhomogeneous as well.*

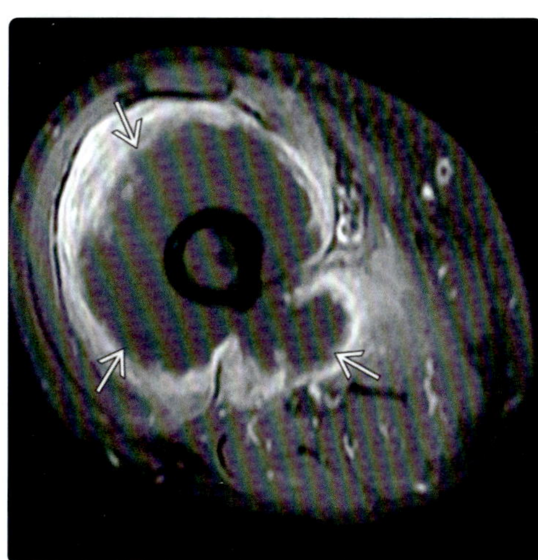

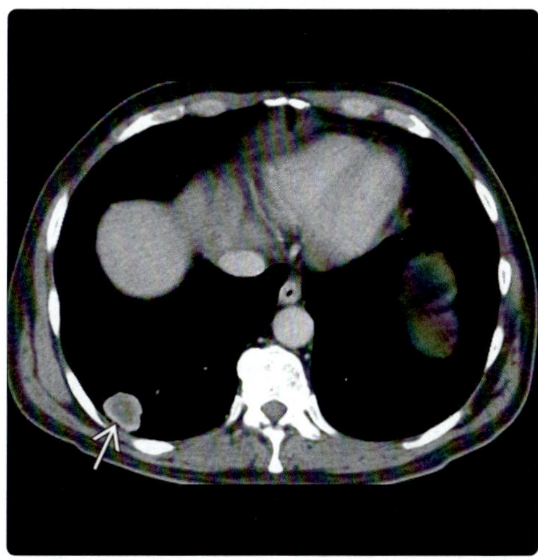

(Left) *Axial postcontrast T1 FS MR of the same region shows that the majority of the soft tissue mass is necrotic ➡. This extensive necrosis indicates the degree of aggressiveness of the lesion.* **(Right)** *Axial CT in the same patient shows metastatic lung disease ➡. The nodule likely contains a small amount of tumor osteoid. Secondary osteosarcomas related to prior radiation, as in this case, may occur several decades following the radiation. They have a dismal prognosis.*

Enchondroma

KEY FACTS

TERMINOLOGY

- Benign tumor of hyaline cartilage originating in medullary bone

IMAGING

- Location: 50% occur in hands and feet
- Long bones: Proximal humerus > proximal and distal femur > proximal tibia
- Geographic central lesion
- No complete cortical destruction or soft tissue mass in absence of pathologic fracture
  - In small tubular bones, may be expanded and bubbly
  - May cause mild scalloping of endosteal cortex over short distances
  - If scalloping > 2/3 cortical thickness or > 2/3 length of lesion, consider transformation to chondrosarcoma (CS)
- Chondroid matrix: May be subtle or absent
- Enchondroma protuberans: Exophytic enchondroma
  - May show cortical defect, appearing aggressive
- MR fluid-sensitive sequences: Lobulated high signal typical of benign cartilage lesions
  - Enhancement: Peripheral and septal, accentuating lobules

CLINICAL ISSUES

- Generally discovered incidentally on x-ray or MR
- Usually asymptomatic

DIAGNOSTIC CHECKLIST

- Differentiation between enchondroma and low-grade CS may be extremely difficult
  - Clinical tumor-like pain (not joint-related) is suggestive of transformation to CS but not diagnostic
- In detecting transformation of enchondroma to low-grade CS, note the following
  - Extensive endosteal scalloping is concerning
  - Change in character of lesion (seen on any modality) is strongly suggestive of transformation, but not diagnostic

(Left) *AP radiograph shows a proximal metaphyseal lesion ➡ containing chondroid matrix. Although the lesion appears geographic, there is no sclerotic margin surrounding it. There is no endosteal scalloping; this is a typical enchondroma.* **(Right)** *Coronal T1 MR in the same patient shows that the lesion is much larger than it appeared on radiograph. There is an intensely low signal at the site of the chondroid matrix ➡ and a more intermediate signal in a lobulated pattern ➡ more peripherally.*

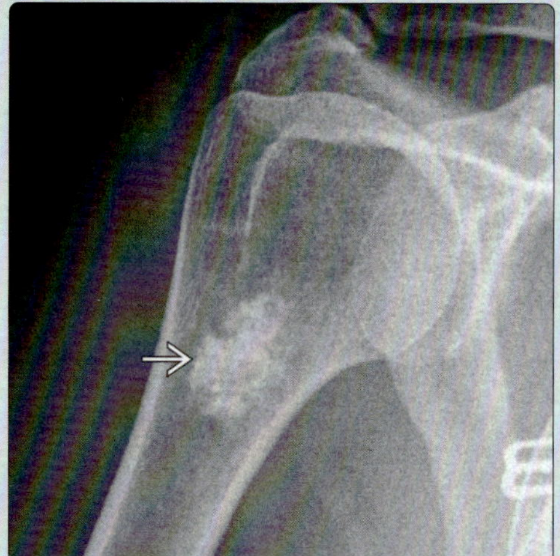

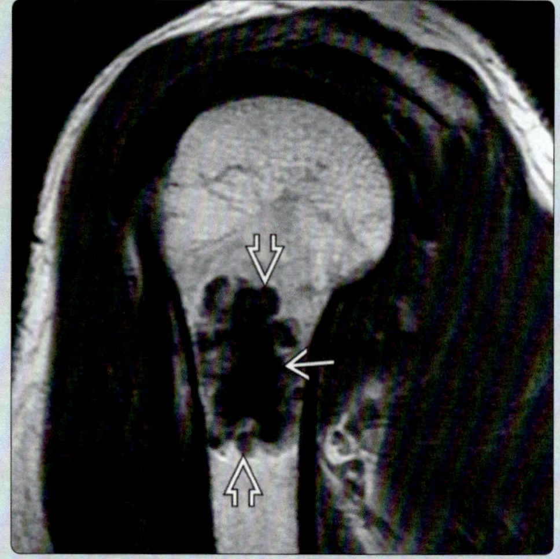

(Left) *Coronal T2 FS MR in the same patient shows the hypointense matrix ➡ with hyperintense lobules ➡. This lobulation is typical of benign cartilage and the combination is that expected in a benign enchondroma.* **(Right)** *Postcontrast T1 C+ FS MR, in the same location, shows the expected peripheral and septal enhancement of the cartilage nodules ➡. This is the expected enhancement pattern of enchondroma. At times, one may also see mild confluent enhancement ➡ that is not as strictly related to the lobules.*

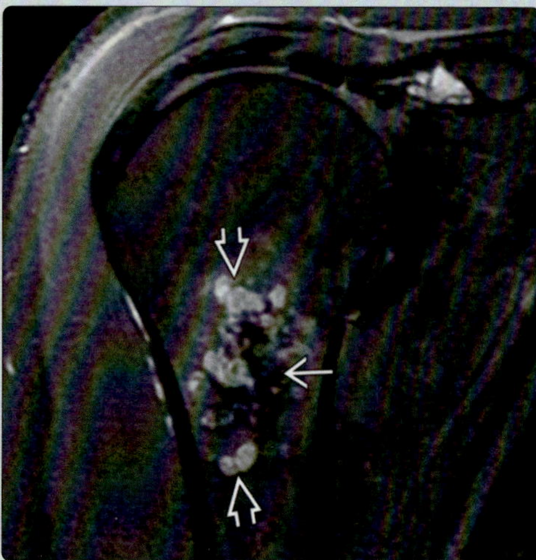

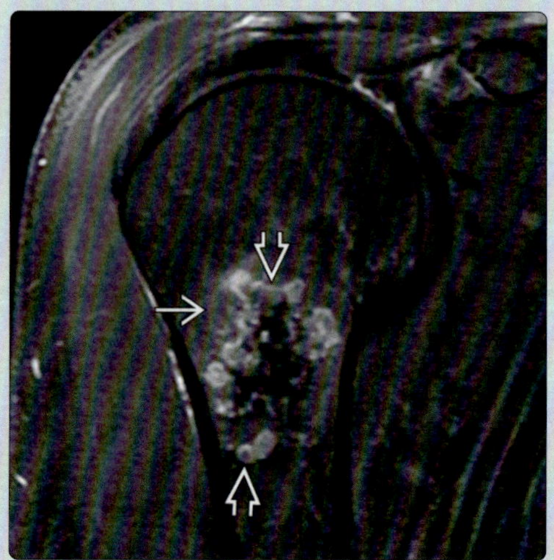

TERMINOLOGY

Synonyms

- Solitary enchondroma, central chondroma

Definitions

- Benign hyaline cartilage tumor originating in bone

IMAGING

General Features

- Location
  - Usually metaphyseal or metadiaphyseal
    - Epiphyseal location is so rare that one must consider chondrosarcoma (CS) in such cases
  - Generally solitary
    - Multiple enchondromas occur, particularly in hands
      - Need not represent multiple enchondromatosis (Ollier disease) in absence of other findings
  - Surgical series: 50% occur in hands and feet
    - Most common tumor of small tubular bones
  - Long bones: Proximal humerus > proximal and distal femur > proximal tibia

Radiographic Findings

- Geographic central lesion; may be eccentric
  - Although geographic, sclerotic rim is rare
  - Metaphyseal is most common location
    - Diaphyseal is less frequent, but not rare
- No complete cortical destruction or soft tissue mass in absence of pathologic fracture
  - In small tubular bones, may be expanded and bubbly
    - Expansion may be so prominent that there is cortical breakthrough
    - May appear quite aggressive in small bones without being malignant
  - In larger bones, enchondroma usually not large enough to cause expansion of bone
    - May cause mild scalloping of endosteal cortex over short distance
      - If scalloping > 2/3 cortical thickness or > 2/3 length of central lesion, consider transformation to CS
      - Eccentric enchondroma arising adjacent to cortex expected to cause endosteal scalloping and even minor cortical disruption
- Chondroid matrix
  - May be flocculent, punctate, or show rings and arcs
  - May be dense and extensive
  - May be extremely subtle or entirely absent
- Enchondroma may change over time
  - May enlarge, increase matrix calcification
  - Watch for change in character of lesion
    - New region of lytic destruction at edge of lesion without matrix suggests transformation to CS
    - Destruction of established chondroid matrix suggests transformation to CS
- Enchondroma protuberans: Exophytic enchondroma
  - Arises in medullary cavity but forms exophytic mass on surface of bone
  - Seen most frequently in ribs and small tubular bones
  - May show cortical defect, appearing aggressive

MR Findings

- T1WI: Low to intermediate signal intensity
  - May contain small regions of normal fatty marrow
  - 1 study suggests predominant intermediate signal intensity suggests transformation to low-grade CS
- Fluid-sensitive sequences: Lobulated high signal typical of benign cartilage lesions
- Matrix seen as low signal or signal void
- Enhancement: Peripheral and septal, accentuating lobules
  - Dynamic contrast and subtraction MR imaging may be useful in differentiating benign from malignant
- Enchondroma protuberans
  - Lesion arises in marrow and extends into exophytic mass; continuity is shown on MR
  - Cortical defect + well-defined rounded soft tissue mass are well seen

Imaging Recommendations

- Best imaging tool
  - Most are incidentally noted on radiograph
  - With routine sports MR, many are incidentally noted
    - 2.1% incidence in routine shoulder MR
  - If concerned with differentiating enchondroma from low-grade CS, MR may be useful but often not diagnostic
- Protocol advice
  - Dynamic contrast enhancement may improve chances of differentiating enchondroma from low-grade CS

Nuclear Medicine Findings

- Unless very small, enchondromas show increased uptake on bone scan (in at least 30%)
- Degree of uptake does not have prognostic implications regarding degeneration

Image-Guided Biopsy

- Biopsy of lesion considered enchondroma vs. low-grade CS is controversial
  - Tracking of tumor cells (via needle track or hematoma) can be devastating if lesion proves to be CS; focal seeding readily occurs
  - Because sarcomatous portion of lesion may be small, tissue sampling errors are likely with needle biopsy
- Many orthopedic oncologists prefer to surgically address lesion as if it were low-grade CS (often with marginal excision)
  - May adjust treatment appropriately if histology of surgically resected tumor shows sarcoma

DIFFERENTIAL DIAGNOSIS

Small Tubular Bone Enchondroma

- Giant cell tumor
  - Inhomogeneous T2 MR signal different from lobulated cartilage signal of enchondroma
- Aneurysmal bone cyst
  - Fluid levels seen on MR
- Simple bone cyst
  - Entirely cystic on MR

Large Bone Enchondroma

- Low-grade CS
  - Alterations in cortex

- Fairly extensive region of endosteal scalloping
- Alternatively, may have endosteal thickening, which is not seen in enchondroma
- Change in character of enchondroma suggestive, though enchondroma itself may change without true transformation to CS
- Giant cell tumor
  - Margin similar to enchondroma (not sclerotic)
  - Location originating in metaphysis but extending toward subchondral bone distinguishes it from enchondroma
  - T2WI MR signal: High, inhomogeneous, often with extensive confluent areas of low signal different from high lobular signal of enchondroma
- Medullary bone infarct
  - Should be distinguishable on radiographs
    - Infarct usually has more prominent sclerotic margin, thicker and denser dystrophic calcification
  - Distinguishable on MR; does not contain high T2 signal lobulated cartilage signal

PATHOLOGY

General Features

- Etiology
  - Uncertain: Hypothesized that foci of dysplastic chondrocytes in physis fail to undergo normal endochondral ossification
    - With growth of bone, foci displaced into metaphysis and eventually diaphysis
    - Theory challenged in studies that showed virtually no such cartilage "rests" in 248 knee MRs

Microscopic Features

- Hypocellular, avascular
- Abundant hyaline cartilage matrix
- Small bone enchondromas may be much more cellular, with greater cytological atypia

CLINICAL ISSUES

Presentation

- Most common signs/symptoms
  - Generally discovered incidentally on x-ray or MR
  - Usually are asymptomatic, but presence or absence of pain is not a reliable parameter for differentiating malignant from benign lesion
    - Enchondroma may be painful
    - Pathologic fracture in enchondroma may be painful
    - Malignant degeneration usually painful

Demographics

- Age
  - 5-80 years old; majority: 3rd-5th decades
- Gender
  - M = F
- Epidemiology
  - 2nd most common benign tumor of bone
  - 10-25% of all benign bone tumors
    - Actual incidence greater since large numbers are discovered incidentally
      - □ MR study shows incidental enchondroma found in knee in 2.9% of routine MR exams; much higher than autopsy series (0.2%)

Natural History & Prognosis

- Generally painless and unchanging throughout life
- Pathologic fracture may occur
- Malignant transformation to CS (rarely other sarcomas)
  - Usually proximal large tubular bones or flat bones
  - Rarely occurs in phalanges
- Rare reports of spontaneous resolution

Treatment

- Incidentally noted small enchondromas
  - Patient may be made aware of them, but decision may be made with patient not to work-up or follow-up as long as there is no associated pain
- Large enchondromas, ± clinical symptoms
  - Work-up with MR of lesion and chest CT
  - If work-up suggests enchondroma rather than CS, marginal or wide resection, depending on expected functionality of limb
  - If work-up suggests low-grade CS, wide resection should be curative
    - If histology proves low-grade CS, appropriate sarcoma follow-up is required

DIAGNOSTIC CHECKLIST

Consider

- Differentiation between enchondroma and low-grade CS may be extremely difficult
  - Tumor-like pain (not joint-related) is suggestive of degeneration but not diagnostic

Image Interpretation Pearls

- In detecting degeneration of enchondroma to low-grade CS, note the following
  - Extensive endosteal scalloping is concerning
    - Endosteal scalloping is normal in enchondroma arising adjacent to cortex
  - Change in character of lesion (seen on any modality) must be considered suggestive of transformation to CS
    - Note that enchondroma may normally enlarge or show change in matrix; does not necessarily indicate transformation to CS, but full work-up and surgery likely required in such circumstances

SELECTED REFERENCES

1. Herget GW et al: Insights into Enchondroma, Enchondromatosis and the risk of secondary Chondrosarcoma. Review of the literature with an emphasis on the clinical behaviour, radiology, malignant transformation and the follow up. Neoplasma. 61(4):365-78, 2014
2. Choi BB et al: MR differentiation of low-grade chondrosarcoma from enchondroma. Clin Imaging. 37(3):542-7, 2013
3. De Coninck T et al: Dynamic contrast-enhanced MR imaging for differentiation between enchondroma and chondrosarcoma. Eur Radiol. 23(11):3140-52, 2013
4. Logie CI et al: Chondrosarcoma: a diagnostic imager's guide to decision making and patient management. Semin Musculoskelet Radiol. 17(2):101-15, 2013

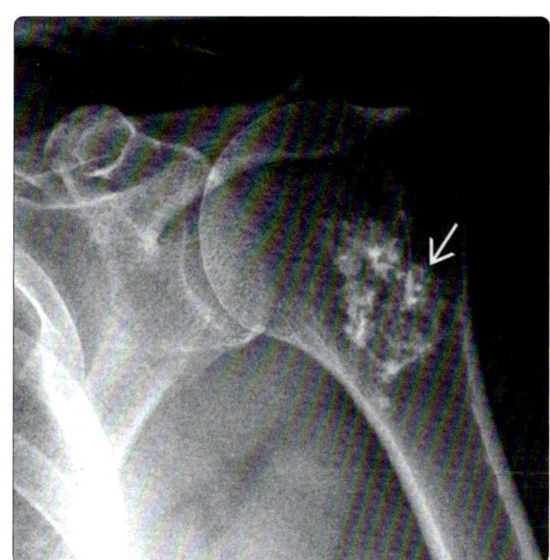

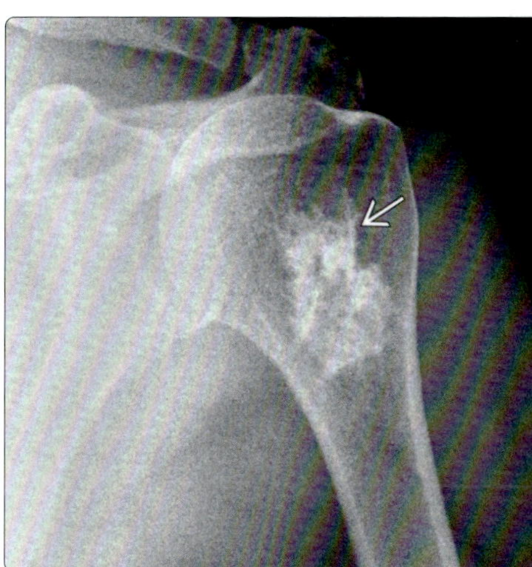

(Left) *AP radiograph of a typical-appearing enchondroma in a 46-year-old woman shows a central metaphyseal lesion containing punctate chondroid matrix ➡ and no aggressive features.* **(Right)** *AP radiograph of the same patient obtained 16 months later shows that the matrix in the lesion has expanded and appears more confluent ➡. This changing pattern over a relatively short time should make one consider the possibility of malignant transformation of the lesion.*

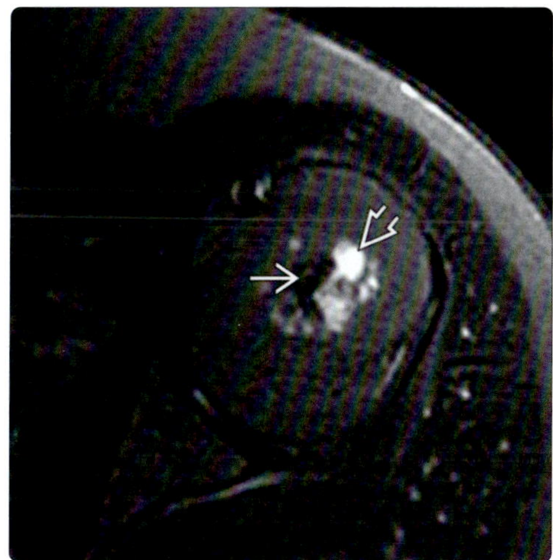

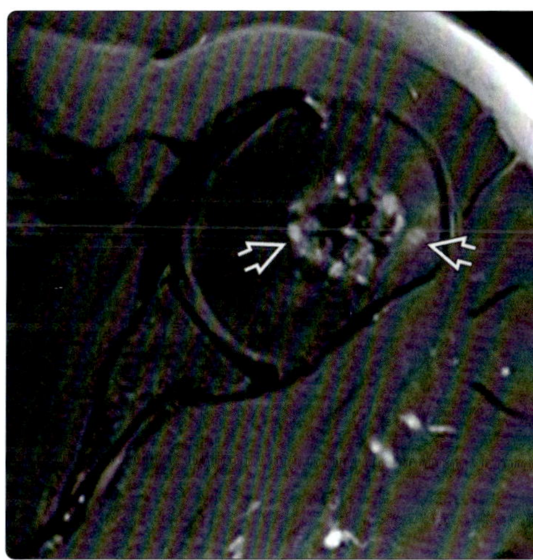

(Left) *Axial T2 FS MR in the same patient, obtained at the time of the initial evaluation, shows both low signal matrix ➡ and high signal lobulation ➡ of the benign cartilage in the enchondroma.* **(Right)** *Matched axial T2 FS MR in the same patient, 16 months later, shows that the lesion has changed significantly. It is larger, with greater central calcification, and has more peripheral hyperintense lobulation ➡. Although it is difficult to perfectly match the images, the entire study convincingly showed change in the lesion.*

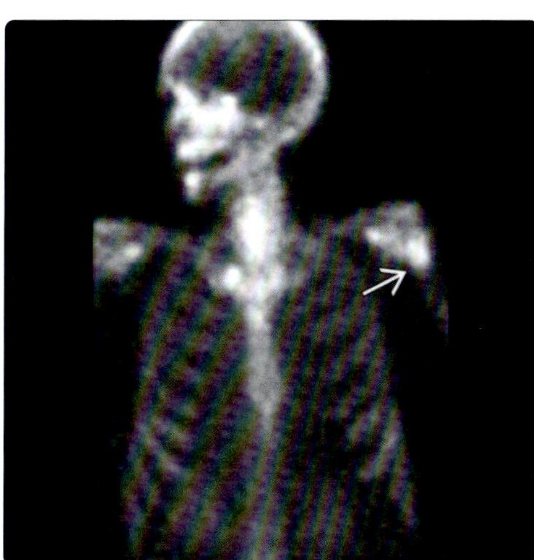

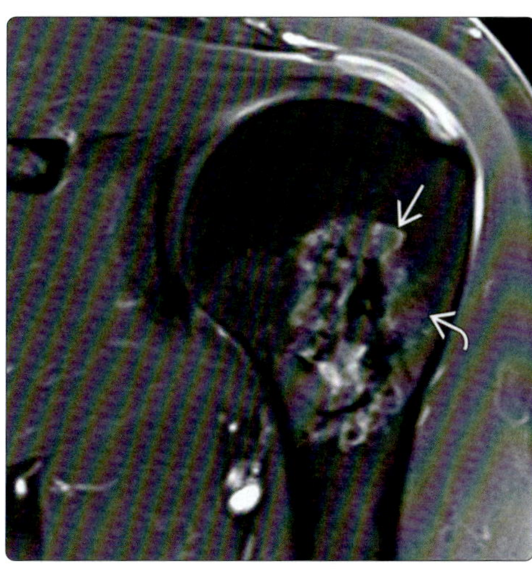

(Left) *AP bone scan shows the lesion to have abnormal uptake ➡. However, this is expected in enchondroma.* **(Right)** *Coronal postcontrast T1 FS MR, same patient, shows peripheral enhancement of the lobulations ➡ as well as nonspecific mild confluent enhancement of bone ➡. In this case, the overall change was concerning for malignant transformation, although, no single imaging factor otherwise pointed to such. The lesion was curetted and pathology showed enchondroma without evidence of chondrosarcoma.*

(Left) *AP radiograph demonstrates the typical chondroid matrix of an enchondroma, with rings and arcs* ➡*. The metaphyseal location is typical for this diagnosis, and there is no aggressive characteristic to the lesion.* **(Right)** *AP follow-up radiograph 4 years later shows a subtle change in the lesion. There is still no suggestion of aggressiveness, but new lobules of matrix are present* ➡*. An enchondroma may show change over time, but any change must be considered to potentially represent transformation.*

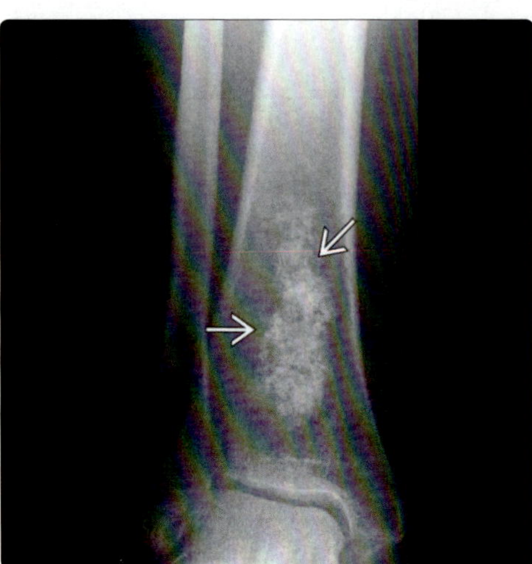

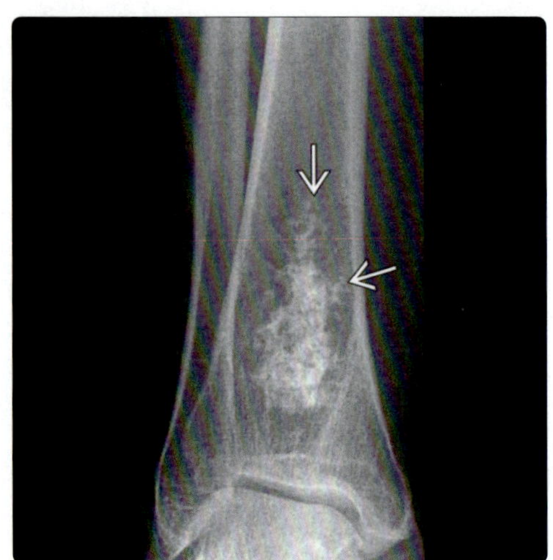

(Left) *Coronal STIR MR in the same patient following the prior radiograph shows the lesion to have high signal lobulations, with low signal matrix, typical of enchondroma.* **(Right)** *Coronal T1WI C+ FS MR shows areas of contrast puddling outside the margin of the lesion seen on the STIR image* ➡*. However, this cannot be considered diagnostic of malignant transformation. Analysis of the curetting demonstrated a few areas of grade 1 chondrosarcoma, with the majority of the lesion representing enchondroma.*

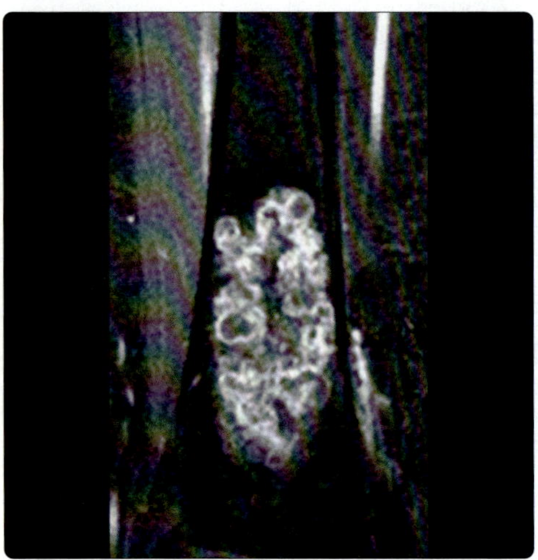

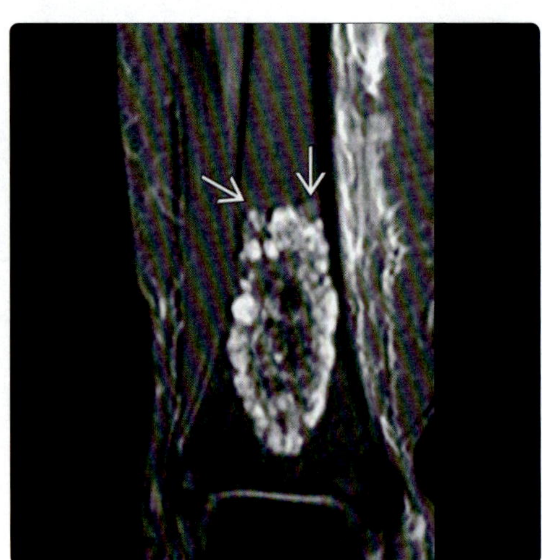

(Left) *Lateral radiograph shows a large but stable enchondroma. The diaphyseal lesion contains prominent chondroid matrix. The lesion is geographic, without sclerotic margin, and causes mild scalloping of the endosteum* ➡*.* **(Right)** *AP radiograph shows central metadiaphyseal humeral lesion. Lesion is large but appears to have a narrow zone of transition. It's completely lytic & scallops the endosteum* ➡ *with no host reaction. All these cases of proven enchondroma show the variable appearance of this lesion.*

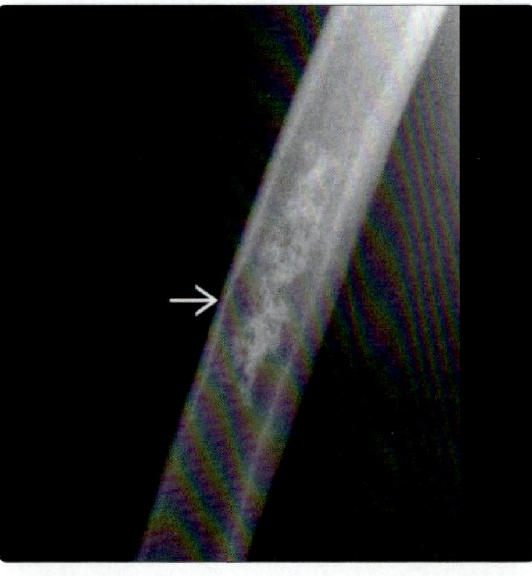

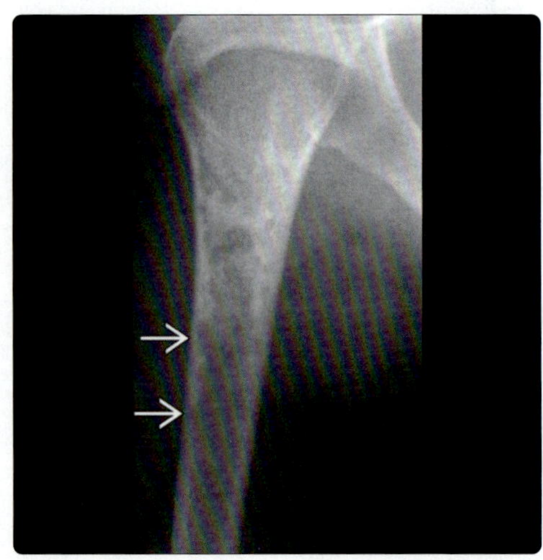

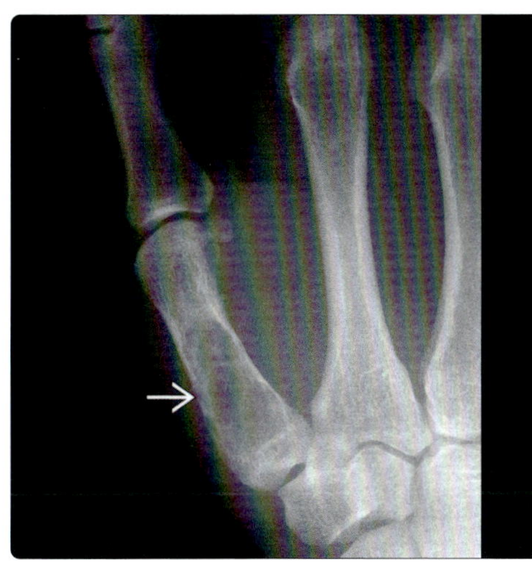

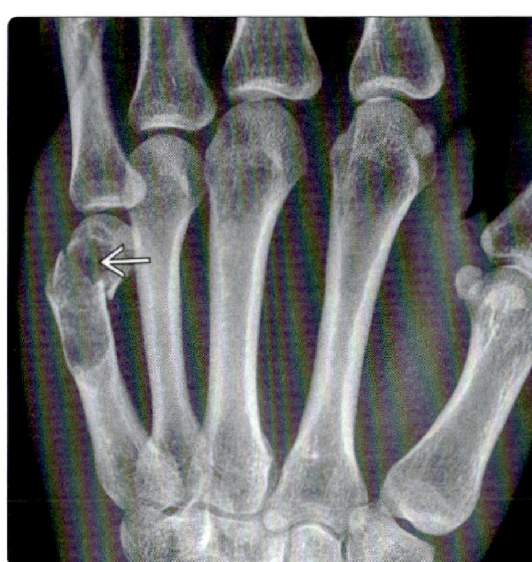

(Left) *AP radiograph shows a slightly expanded lytic lesion involving the diaphysis. Lesion is geographic → and has a narrow zone of transition. The most common lytic lesion of the hand is enchondroma, even in the absence of chondroid matrix, and was proven in this case.* **(Right)** *PA radiograph shows a lytic lesion that mildly expands the bone and significantly scallops the cortex. There is a faint punctate chondroid matrix → seen within the lesion. This typical enchondroma was asymptomatic prior to its pathologic fracture.*

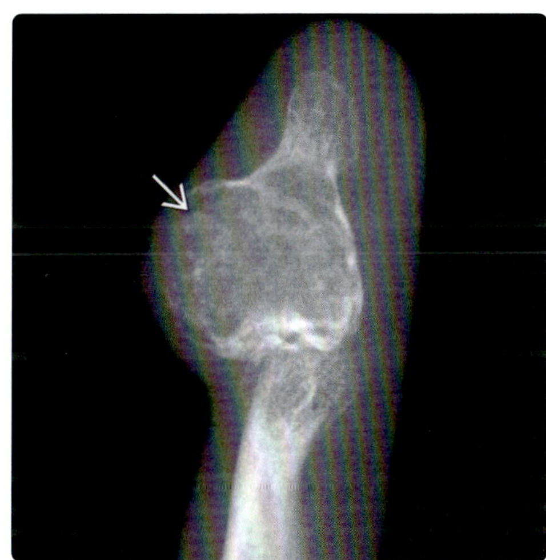

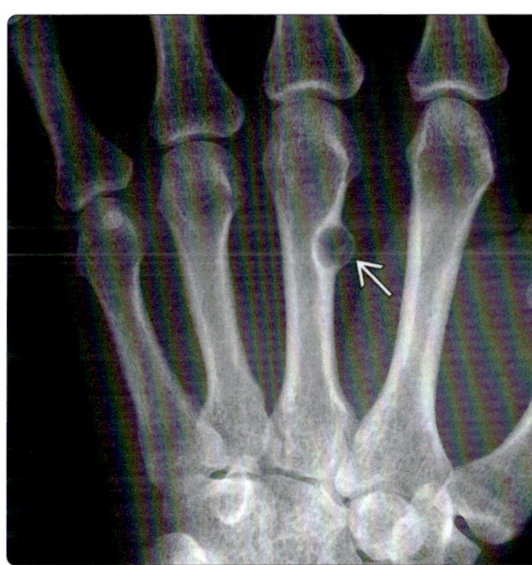

(Left) *Lateral radiograph shows a highly expanded phalangeal lesion, which contains extensive chondroid matrix →. The overlying cortex is severely thinned and, in places, even destroyed. Despite the aggressive appearance, which some phalangeal enchondromas may obtain, transformation to chondrosarcoma is rare in this location. This is a proven enchondroma.* **(Right)** *AP radiograph gives an unusual appearance of enchondroma protuberans, arising within and expanding the cortex but containing typical matrix →.*

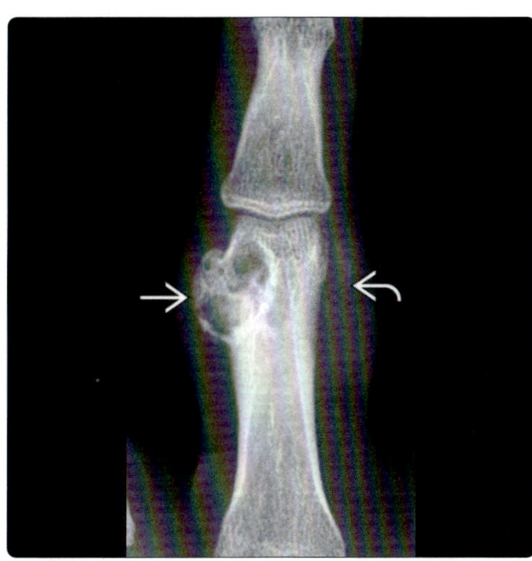

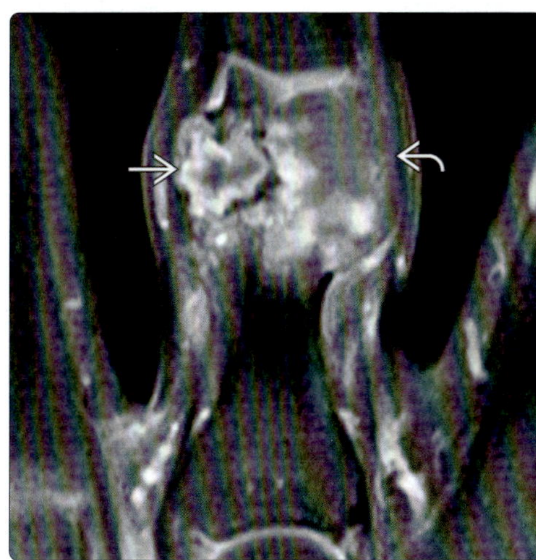

(Left) *PA radiograph shows enchondroma protuberans arising within the medullary cavity but expanding the cortex significantly →. A soft tissue mass is seen ↷.* **(Right)** *Coronal T1WI C+ FS MR in the same patient shows the typical peripheral enhancement of that portion of the lesion, which appeared classic on radiograph → but had less typical enhancement of the portion showing cortical breakthrough ↷. The aggressive appearance is typical of enchondroma protuberans. (Courtesy A. Kingzett-Taylor, MD.)*

Osteochondroma

KEY FACTS

TERMINOLOGY

- Cartilage-capped osseous excrescence with continuous cortex and marrow extending from underlying bone

IMAGING

- Metaphysis or metaphyseal equivalents
  - Femur (30%) > tibia (20%) > humerus (10-20%)
- Composed of stalk, marrow, and cortex; all continuous with normal underlying bone
- Lesion may be sessile (broad-based), mimicking undertubulation of metaphysis
- Calcifications in chondroosseous portion common
- MR: Orderly hyaline cartilage cap, mildly undulating and not exceeding 1 cm in width in adults
  - Cap has lobulated high signal of hyaline cartilage on fluid-sensitive sequences
  - Cap covered by thin perichondrium, low signal on T1 and T2 sequences
  - Enhancement limited to thin fibrovascular tissue covering (nonenhancing) cartilage cap and thin septa within cap

CLINICAL ISSUES

- Knobby mass, long duration
- Mechanical pain from trauma or impingement
- Limited range of motion and snapping tendons from impingement
- Nerve impingement
- Rapid painful "enlargement" from overlying bursa
- Vascular complications
- Fracture of stalk of osteochondroma
- Increasing pain &/or mass enlargement following skeletal maturation suggest degeneration to chondrosarcoma

DIAGNOSTIC CHECKLIST

- Recommendation: Use thickness of > 1 cm as threshold for surgical resection of exostosis

(Left) *Graphic depicts a transected section through a solitary osteochondroma. Note the normal marrow and cortex extending from the underlying bone, along the stalk ➔. The cartilaginous cap is uniformly thin ➔. The exostosis typically grows away from the adjacent joint, as shown.* **(Right)** *Lateral radiograph of a large complex-appearing pedunculated exostosis ➔ shows ossification within the stalk, which may obscure the underlying trabecular pattern. A smaller exostosis, matching the graphic, is also seen ➔.*

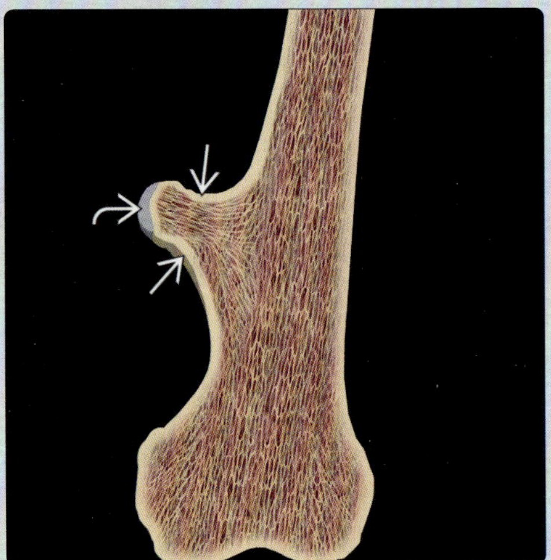

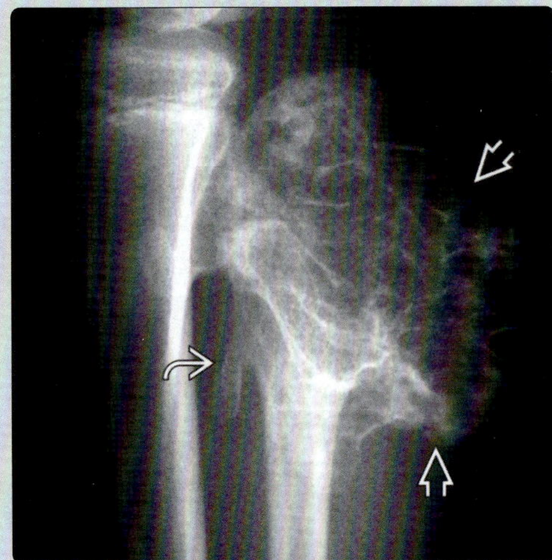

(Left) *AP radiograph shows an exophytic type of exostosis. The stalk is well seen ➔ and the underlying bone is normal. No other destructive pattern is seen to suggest sarcomatous change. This patient had pain related to mechanical impingement.* **(Right)** *Lateral radiograph shows the undulating cortical pattern seen with sessile exostoses ➔. Note that except for the outline the cortex and marrow appear completely normal. The apparent widening may be misdiagnosed as a marrow infiltration process or metaphyseal dysplasia.*

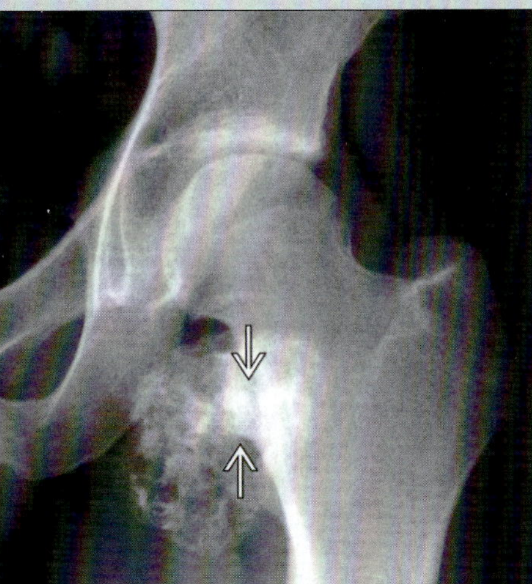

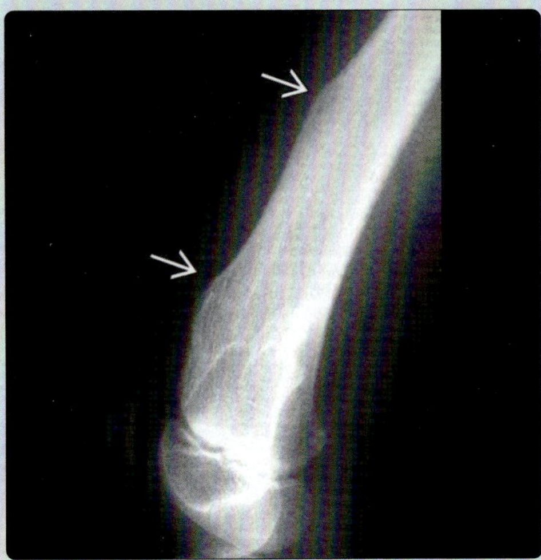

TERMINOLOGY

Synonyms

- Exostosis, solitary osteochondroma, osteocartilaginous exostosis

Definitions

- Cartilage-capped osseous excrescence with continuous cortex and marrow extending from underlying bone

IMAGING

General Features

- Location
  - Metaphysis/metaphyseal equivalents (rarely diaphysis)
  - 95% located in extremities
    - Femur (30%) > tibia (20%) > humerus (10-20%)
    - Lower extremity > upper extremity (2:1)
    - 40% around knee
    - 10% small bones hands/feet
    - Flat bones less frequently involved than long bones: Pelvis (5%) and scapula (4%)
    - Spine (2%)

Radiographic Findings

- Radiography
  - Composed of stalk, marrow, and cortex; all continuous with normal underlying bone
    - If near joint, tends to project away from joint line, growing along forces generated by location of tendons and ligaments
    - Lesions arising in pelvis may become very large before discovery
    - Lesions in ribs most often arise from costochondral junction; may give appearance of pulmonary nodule
    - May have associated deformity of adjacent (otherwise normal) bones
      - Rib deformity from scapular exostosis
      - Pelvic deformity from proximal femoral exostosis
      - Deformity at proximal or distal tibia/fibula
  - Lesion may be sessile (broad-based), mimicking undertubulation of metaphysis
  - Endochondral calcification may be seen within cartilage cap and medullary bone
    - Rings and arcs, punctate, or flocculent calcification
  - Overlying cartilage cap is thin, generally not evaluated by radiograph
    - Size may be inferred by distorted fat planes or contained calcifications
  - Degeneration of lesion to chondrosarcoma suggested by
    - Osseous destruction
    - Change in calcifications (scattered or "snowstorm")
    - Enlargement of cartilage cap, inferred by distorted fat planes

CT Findings

- Mimics those of radiograph; may show relationship of lesion to cortex and marrow better
- Cartilage cap thickness may be evaluated if mineralized or if overlying soft tissues are thin; otherwise may be difficult

MR Findings

- Normal bone marrow extending into exostoses
- Cortex continuous with that of underlying bone
- Orderly hyaline cartilage cap, mildly undulating and not exceeding 1 cm width
  - Cap has lobulated high signal of hyaline cartilage on fluid-sensitive sequences (low to intermediate signal on T1)
  - Cap covered by thin perichondrium, low signal on T1 and T2 sequences
  - In young patients with active growth, cartilage has different normal appearance
    - May be up to 3 cm thick
    - Shows marked heterogeneity on all sequences
- Mineralized areas within cap and exostosis remain low signal on all sequences
- Enhancement limited to thin fibrovascular tissue covering cartilage cap (nonenhancing) and thin septa within cap
- No soft tissue mass
- Fluid in overlying bursa may be seen: High T2 signal, nonenhancing
  - Signal may be altered if bursa complicated by inflammation, infection, or hemorrhage
  - Bursal lining may develop metaplasia, → synovial chondromatosis
- Secondary mechanical changes in exostosis
  - Marrow edema from impingement or trauma
  - Stalk fracture: Linear fracture with adjacent edema
- Neurovascular compromise
  - Pseudoaneurysm (especially in popliteal fossa)
  - Stretched/deviated nerve over osteochondroma
    - Associated denervation signal with hypertrophy or atrophy of muscle

Ultrasonographic Findings

- Thickness and regularity of cartilage cap may be determined by US if lesion is not deep
- Cap is hypoechoic if nonmineralized and differentiated from surrounding hyperechoic fat and muscle
- Mineralization within cap → acoustic shadowing

Nuclear Medicine Findings

- Benign osteochondromas show uptake on bone scan, related to additional bone as well as endochondral calcification within cap
- Chondrosarcoma may show more intense uptake, but this is not a reliable feature for differentiating benign from malignant

Imaging Recommendations

- Best imaging tool
  - Radiograph for diagnosis
  - MR to evaluate for complication
- Protocol advice
  - Contrast administration important
    - Differentiates bursa from thick cartilage cap
    - Helps differentiate chondrosarcomatous change

DIFFERENTIAL DIAGNOSIS

Chondrosarcoma

- Consider if

- Lesion continues to grow following skeletal maturation
- There is new pain, not related to other exostosis complication
- There is change in character of calcified matrix, osseous destruction, or soft tissue mass
- Cartilage cap > 1 cm in thickness

Parosteal Osteosarcoma

- Arises from cortical surface but does not have continuous marrow with underlying bone
- Only with very large lesions might differentiation be difficult; solved by axial imaging

Juxtacortical Myositis Ossificans

- Mature myositis may have similar well-ordered trabeculae to exostosis
- Myositis may elicit periosteal reaction but is not connected to underlying cortex and marrow

PATHOLOGY

General Features

- Etiology
  - Developmental lesion
    - Unknown; possible aberrant growth of physeal plate or herniation of plate into metaphysis
    - Associated with radiation, arising at median of 8-11 years after radiation therapy
- Genetics
  - Cytogenetic aberrations involving 8q22-24.1 (location of *EXT1* gene) found in 10/30 solitary osteochondroma cases
  - Suggests osteochondromas are true neoplasms rather than dysplasia

CLINICAL ISSUES

Presentation

- Most common signs/symptoms
  - Knobby mass, long duration
  - Mechanical pain from trauma or impingement
  - Limited range of motion and snapping tendons from impingement
- Other signs/symptoms
  - Nerve impingement
    - Usually peripheral, around knee
    - Occasional spinal cord impingement from vertebral or rib exostosis
  - Rapid painful "enlargement" from overlying bursa
    - May become inflamed, infected, or hemorrhagic
  - Vascular complications
    - Pseudoaneurysm formation
    - Arterial or venous stenosis/thrombosis
  - Fracture of stalk of exostosis
  - Increasing pain &/or mass enlargement following skeletal maturation suggest degeneration to chondrosarcoma
    - Note: Rare cases reported of continued growth of benign exostosis in adult
    - Degeneration tends to occur in or after 4th decade
    - Malignant transformation occurs in < 1% of solitary lesions
    - Accounts for 8% of all chondrosarcomas
    - Generally low grade (67-85% of cases)

Demographics

- Age
  - Generally discovered in first 3 decades
- Gender
  - M = F
- Epidemiology
  - Found in 3% of population
  - Most common bone tumor: 35-45% of benign bone tumors, 8-12% of all bone tumors
    - May be underestimate, since most lesions are asymptomatic and discovered incidentally
  - 90% are solitary lesions

Natural History & Prognosis

- Exostoses stop growing after skeletal maturation
- Complications of exostosis related to adjacent tissues may occur
- < 1% incidence of degeneration of solitary lesion to chondrosarcoma

Treatment

- Watchful waiting
  - Patient education regarding risk for degeneration
  - Generally no requirement of routine imaging follow-up of lesions; varies on individual basis
- Mechanical complications (bursa formation, nerve irritation, impingement, etc.) treated by simple resection of offending lesion
  - Resection of entire perichondrium required to avoid recurrence (rate: < 2%)
- Concern for degeneration of osteochondroma should lead to full work-up for chondrosarcoma
  - Chondrosarcoma treated by wide surgical resection

DIAGNOSTIC CHECKLIST

Consider

- Question of normal cartilage cap thickness is debated; 1 series shows
  - Cartilage caps < 1.5 cm correlate with benign exostosis
  - Cartilage caps > 2.5 cm correlate with chondrosarcoma
  - Recommendation: Use thickness of > 1 cm as threshold for surgical resection of exostosis

SELECTED REFERENCES

1. Gould ES et al: Osteochondroma of the hip with adjacent bursal chondromatosis. Skeletal Radiol. 43(12):1743-8, 2014
2. Zhang Y et al: Solitary C1 spinal osteochondroma causing vertebral artery compression and acute cerebellar infarct. Skeletal Radiol. 44(2):299-302, 2014
3. Bernard SA et al: Improved differentiation of benign osteochondromas from secondary chondrosarcomas with standardized measurement of cartilage cap at CT and MR imaging. Radiology. 255(3):857-65, 2010
4. Bernard SA et al: Cartilage cap thickness measurement on T2-weighted MRI imaging and the risk of secondary chondrosarcoma in osteochondromas. Presented at Society of Skeletal Radiologists. March, 2008
5. Murphey MD et al: Imaging of osteochondroma: variants and complications with radiologic-pathologic correlation. Radiographics. 20(5):1407-34, 2000

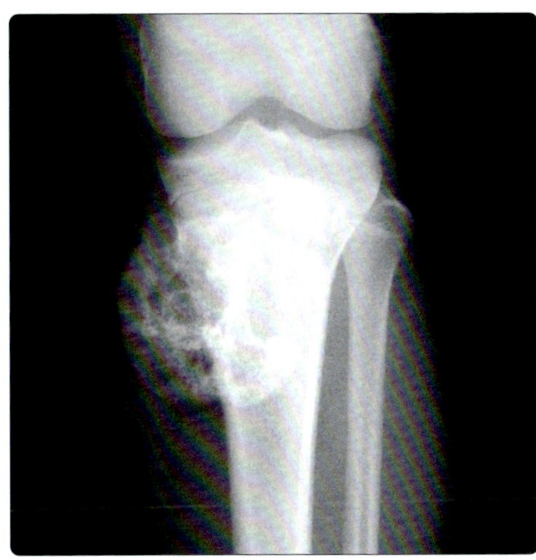

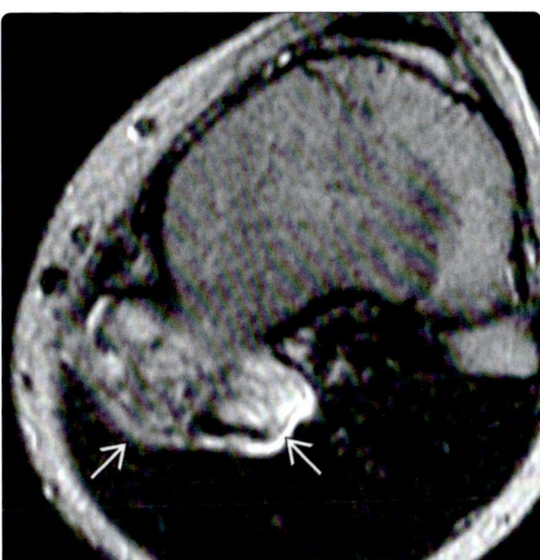

(Left) *AP radiograph shows a typical exostosis arising from a stalk at the metaphysis, with normal underlying bone, though both stalk and bone are obscured by a calcified matrix located within the lesion, largely peripherally. The cartilage cap size cannot be assessed on this radiograph.* **(Right)** *Axial T2WI MR in the same patient demonstrates normal cortex and medullary bone extending from the underlying normal tibia. The cartilage cap is high signal ➡ and thin and regular, confirming benign osteochondroma.*

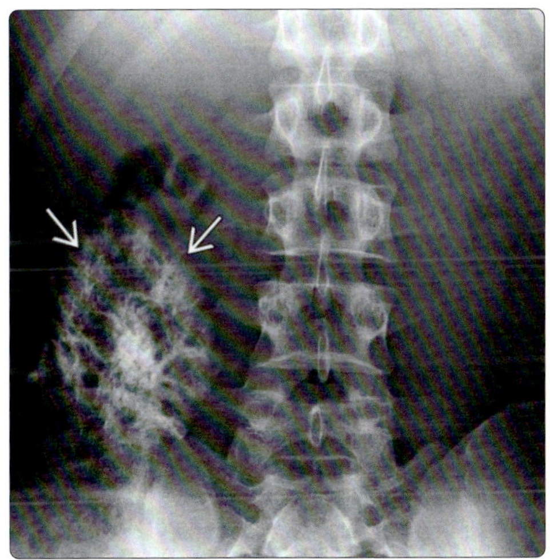

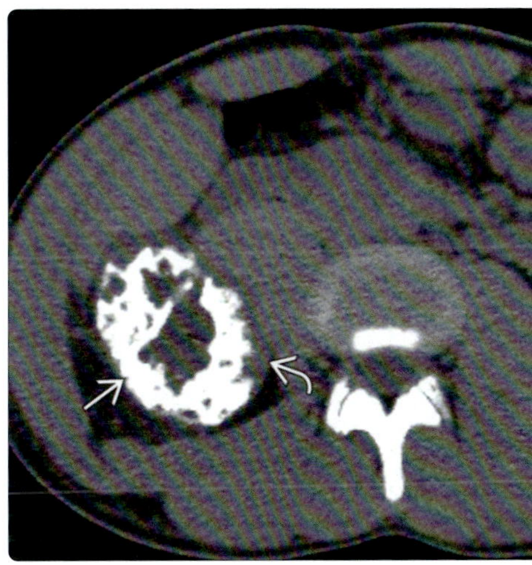

(Left) *AP radiograph shows a large exostosis ➡ arising from the iliac crest. Aside from its impressive size, there is nothing to suggest malignant change.* **(Right)** *Axial CT in the same patient shows the exostosis ➡. There is a suggestion of a somewhat thick cartilage cap in places ↩. However, this is a 19-year-old man who is just becoming skeletally mature, and this cap thickness falls within the expected range.*

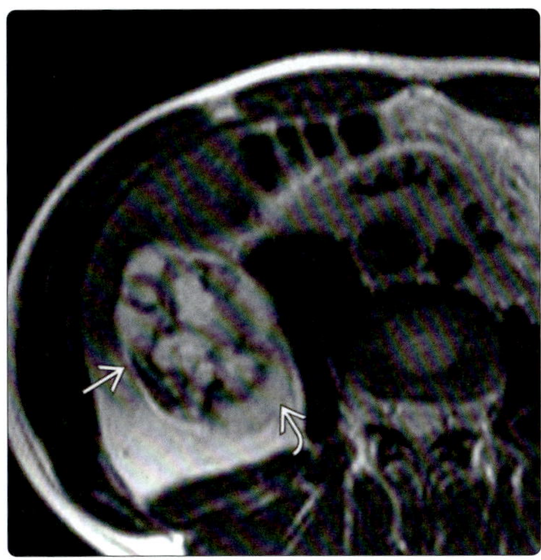

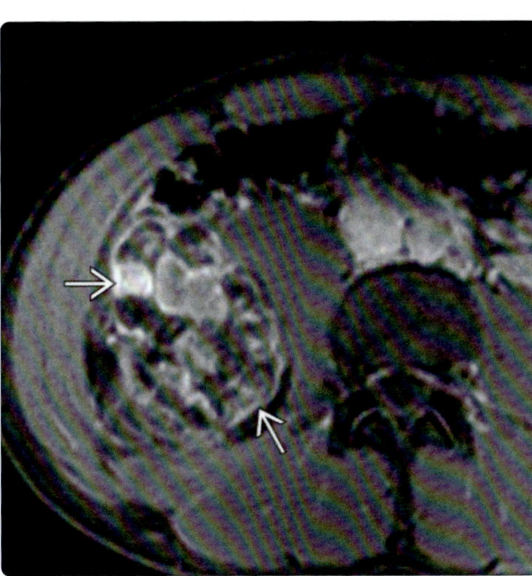

(Left) *Axial T1 MR shows the exostosis ➡ within a bed of fat. There is normal marrow and cortex; the cartilage cap ↩ size is not overly concerning given the patient's age.* **(Right)** *Axial T2 FS MR, in the same patient, does not add specificity to the question of whether there is malignant degeneration of the exostosis ➡. Unfortunately, the findings on MR are not always definitive. Because of its large size, the lesion was excised and there were no malignant features seen at pathology.*

(Left) *Axial cross-sectional graphic depicts osteochondroma arising from the vertebral body ➡, compressing the contents of the spinal canal.* **(Right)** *Axial bone CT shows a vertebral body exostosis extending into the spinal canal ➡. There is marrow and cortical continuity with parent vertebral body, typical for osteochondroma. Note that the cartilaginous cap is not seen. Though axial location is uncommon for a solitary osteochondroma, it may be surprisingly common in patients with multiple hereditary exostoses.*

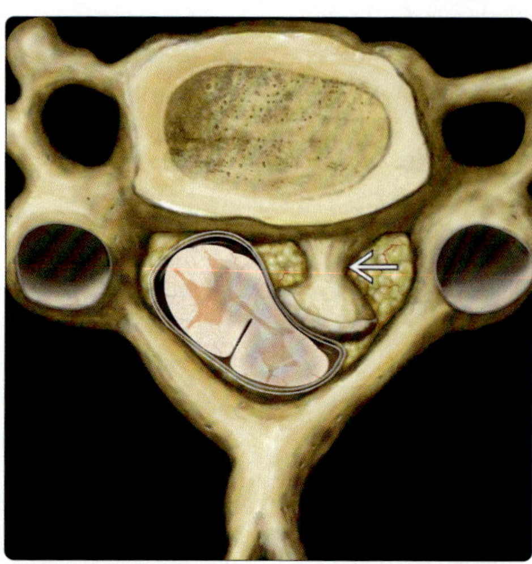

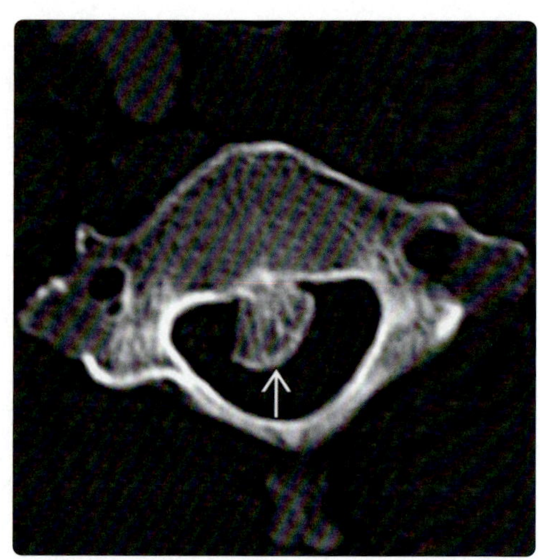

(Left) *AP radiograph shows a large soft tissue mass ➡ centered over a faintly seen osteochondroma ➡. The exostosis, though difficult to see, exhibits standard characteristics of a stalk of normal bone arising from the metaphysis. This growing mass in an adult must generate suspicion of degeneration to chondrosarcoma.* **(Right)** *Coronal T1WI MR in the same patient shows the large mass to be higher signal intensity than muscle ➡, with small associated exostosis ➡.*

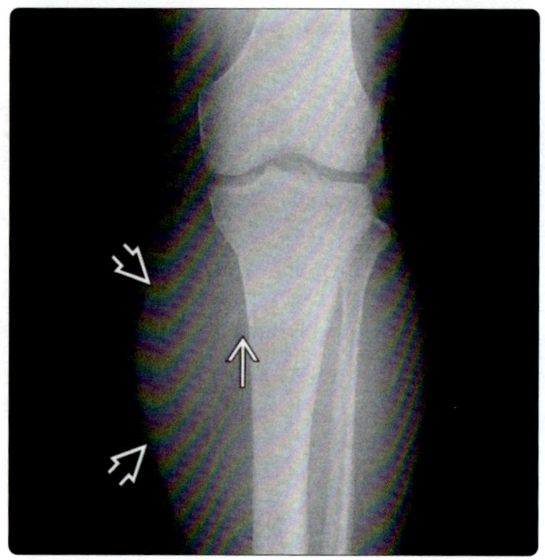

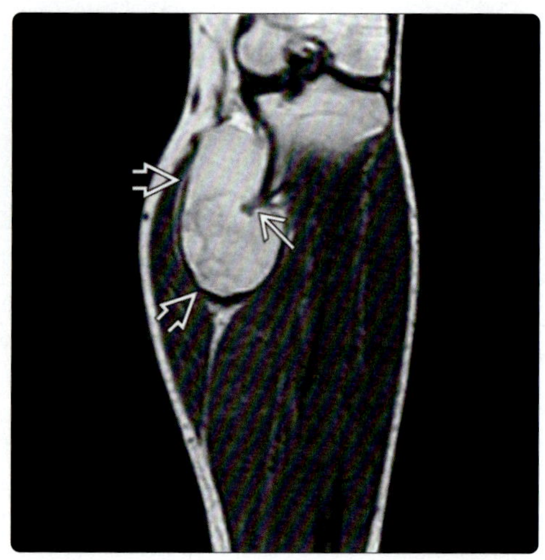

(Left) *Axial T1WI C+ FS MR in the same patient shows the exostosis well ➡. The enhancing mass surrounding it suggests that the fluid content is not simple, but it is not typical of an enlarged cartilage cap. Diagnosis of bursal formation over the exostosis was proven by ultrasound and aspiration of 300 cc of extremely thick gelatinous fluid.* **(Right)** *Sagittal PD FS MR shows a neurologic complication of osteochondroma. The large, classic-appearing exostosis is located such that the sciatic nerve is stretched over it ➡.*

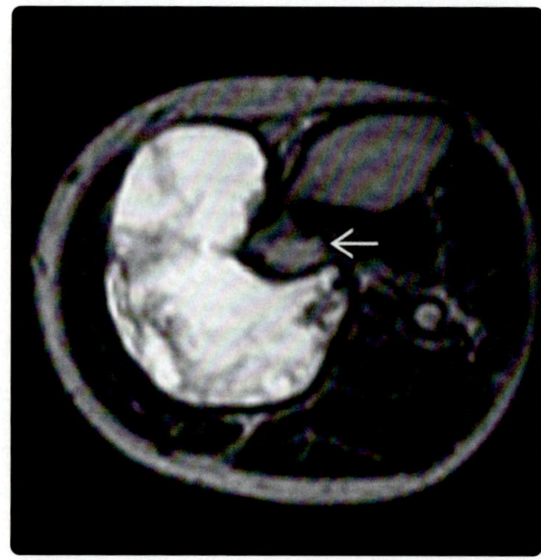

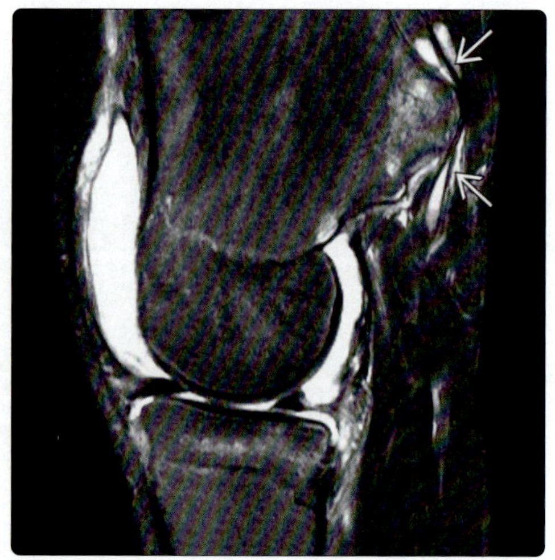

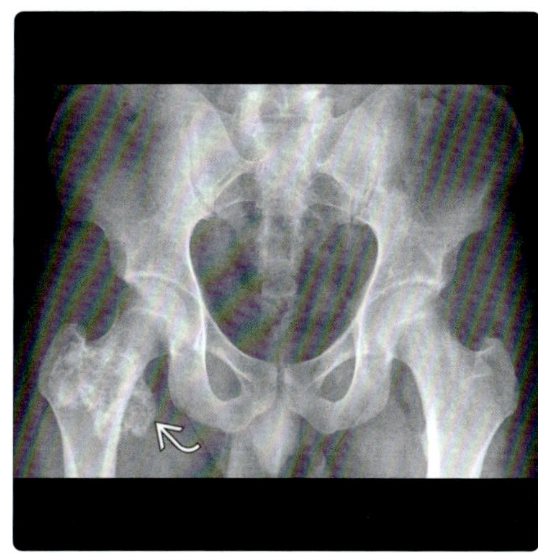

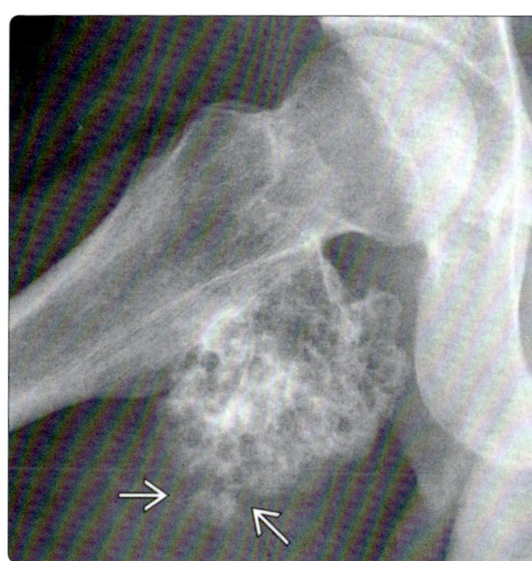

(Left) *AP radiograph shows complications of exostosis. This image was obtained when the patient complained of acute onset of pain. It shows a large femoral metaphyseal osteochondroma ➡. Concerns about complications led to further imaging.* **(Right)** *Frog leg lateral radiograph in the same patient shows the classic osteochondroma arising from normal underlying bone and containing calcific matrix. Note the fracture of the exostosis ➡ due to trauma, likely accounting for the acute symptoms.*

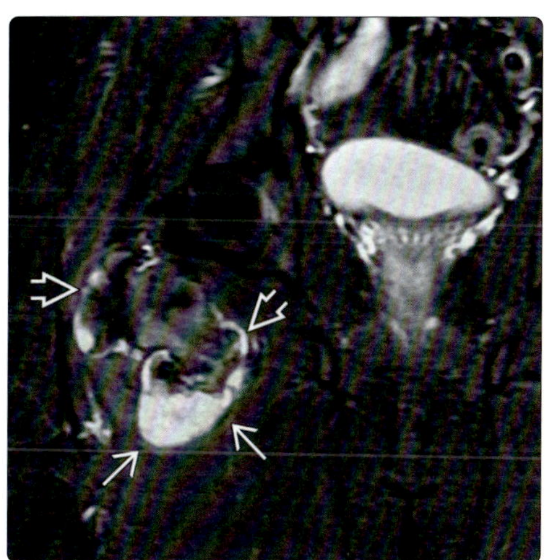

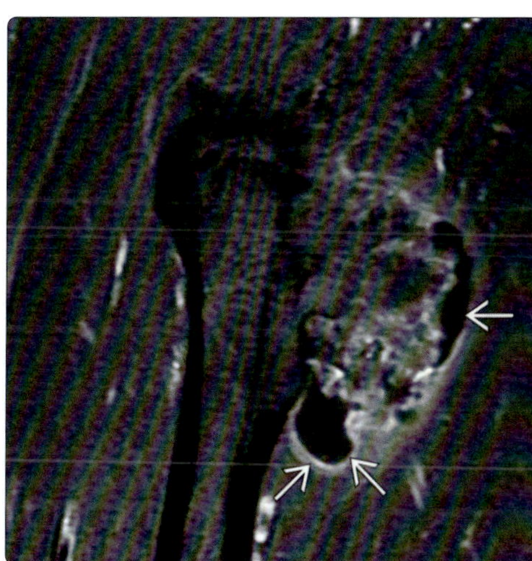

(Left) *Coronal STIR MR in the same patient shows typical exostosis proximally ➡ but more confluent high signal that might initially be concerning for a pathologically thick cartilage cap ➡ more distally.* **(Right)** *Sagittal T1WI C+ FS MR in the same patient shows that the high signal "cap" is in fact a fluid collection ➡. A bursa can form over an exostosis, particularly in the context of trauma, as in this case. Therefore, interval "growth" after skeletal maturation does not always imply malignant transformation.*

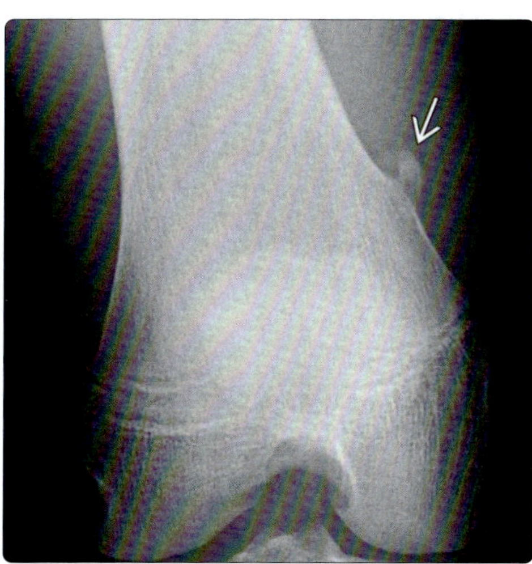

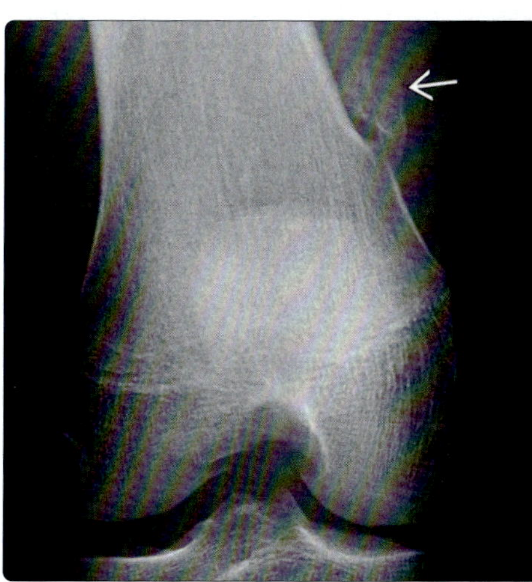

(Left) *AP radiograph shows a single metaphyseal lesion ➡ that shows continuity with normal marrow and cortex. The diagnosis of exostosis is confidently made.* **(Right)** *AP radiograph in the same patient 1 year later shows growth of the lesion ➡. However, it still has the appearance of an uncomplicated exostosis. Interval growth of an exostosis in a skeletally immature patient is expected, analogous to physeal growth. Therefore the "rule" that exostoses should not grow does not apply to children.*

Multiple Hereditary Exostoses

KEY FACTS

TERMINOLOGY

- Multiple osteochondromas, either sessile or pedunculated

IMAGING

- Usually symmetric widening of metaphyses with small exostoses at apex, or cauliflower-like exostoses; normal underlying bone
- Metaphyseal region of tubular bones + metaphyseal equivalents
- Sessile form
  - More common than pedunculated form in MHE
  - Normal underlying bone
  - Metaphyses undertubulated, broad, but with normal marrow and cortex
  - May mimic infiltrative storage disorder or dysplasia
- Pedunculated form
  - Stalk arises from normal underlying bone, with continuous normal marrow and cortex
  - Overlying cartilage cap is thin
  - More likely than sessile form to show endochondral calcification within cartilage cap
- MR: Orderly hyaline cartilage cap, not irregular and not exceeding 1 cm in width
  - Cap has high signal of hyaline cartilage on fluid-sensitive sequences (low to intermediate signal on T1)
  - Enhancement limited to thin fibrovascular tissue covering cartilage cap (nonenhancing) and thin septa within cap
- Thickness and regularity of cartilage cap may be determined by US if lesion is not deep

PATHOLOGY

- Autosomal dominant; 90% familial history MHE

CLINICAL ISSUES

- Knobby masses, especially around knees
- Defective metaphyseal remodeling → deformities
- Short stature from early physeal closure (40%)
- 1-3% incidence of degeneration to chondrosarcoma

(Left) *Graphic depicts transection of iliac wings in patient with multiple hereditary exostoses (MHE). Both wings show a proliferation of broad-based exostoses ➔ containing normal bone. Exophytic lesion with a thick cartilage cap is seen ⇨, representing degeneration to CS.* **(Right)** *Axial NECT shows a large sacral exostosis with typical pattern of a central stalk & normal underlying bone. Note no enlarged cartilage cap, indicated by a thin layer of muscle overlying the cortex of the exostosis ➔.*

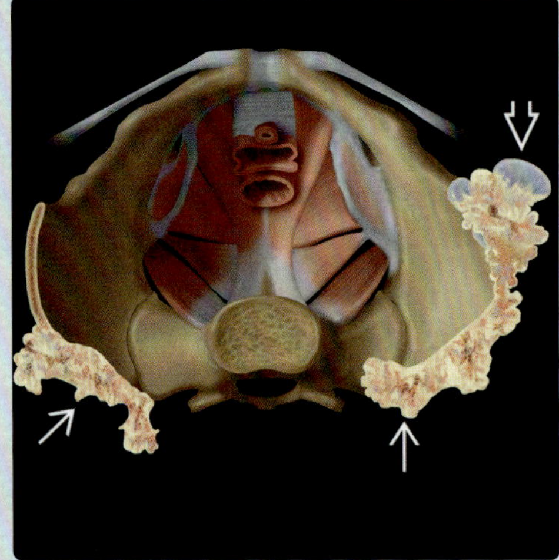

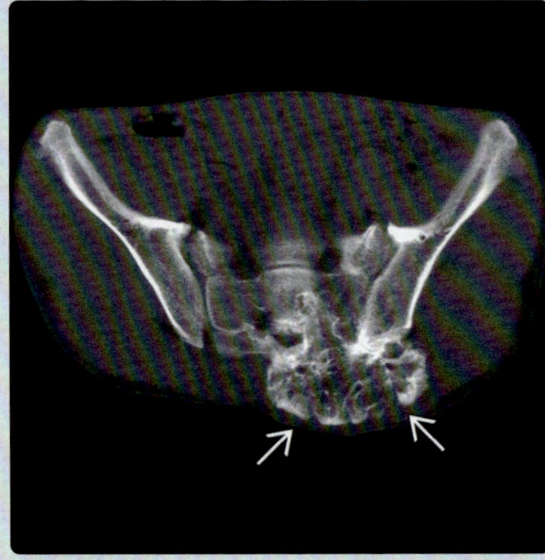

(Left) *Axial NECT in the same patient, proximal to prior image, shows a portion of the large exophytic exostosis ⇨ and broad sessile exostoses occupying both the anterior and posterior aspects of the iliac wings ➔.* **(Right)** *Axial NECT in the same patient more distally shows sessile exostoses involving nearly every bone ⇨. These are not as large and exophytic as the sacral lesion, but represent hundreds of exostoses. This is a very typical pattern for MHE.*

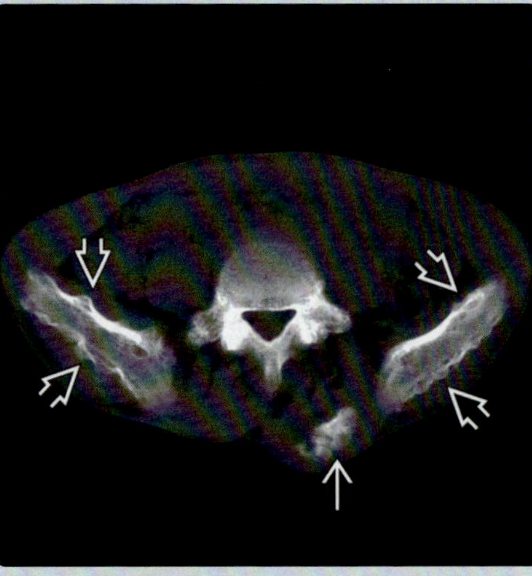

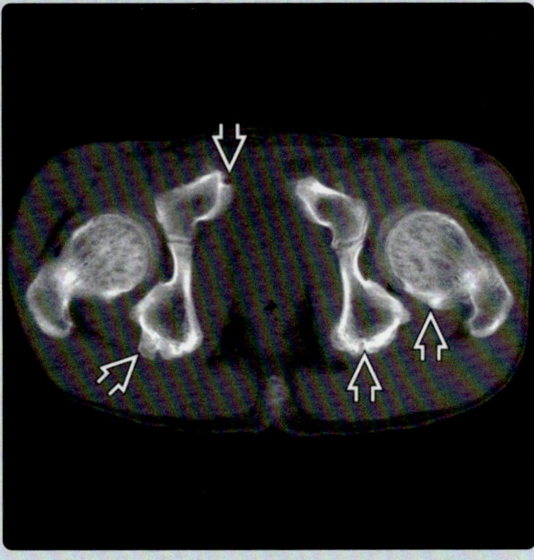

TERMINOLOGY

Abbreviations

- Multiple hereditary exostoses (MHE)

Synonyms

- Hereditary osteochondromatosis, hereditary deforming osteochondromatosis, hereditary chondrodysplasia, diaphyseal aclasis, metaphyseal aclasis, hereditary multiple exostoses, hereditary multiple osteochondromas, familial osteochondromatosis

Definitions

- Multiple osteochondromas, either sessile or pedunculated

IMAGING

General Features

- Best diagnostic clue
  - Usually symmetric widening of metaphyses with small exostoses at apex or cauliflower-like exostoses; normal underlying bone
- Location
  - Metaphyseal region of tubular bones + metaphyseal equivalents
  - Proximal and distal femur, proximal and distal tibia-fibula, proximal humerus, forearm bones
  - Ilium, pubis, ischium
  - Ribs: Costovertebral and costochondral junctions
  - 27% of MHE have involvement of spine
  - Often, but not invariably bilaterally symmetric (depends on phenotype)
- Size
  - Wide range
- Morphology
  - Either sessile (flat, broad-based along cortex) or pedunculated (cauliflower-like, on stalk)

Imaging Recommendations

- Best imaging tool
  - Diagnosed by radiograph
  - MR to evaluate individual lesion complication

Radiographic Findings

- Sessile form
  - More common than pedunculated form in MHE
  - Normal underlying bone
  - Metaphyses undertubulated and broad but with otherwise normal marrow and cortex
  - Apex of sessile lesion may show irregular outline along cortex (especially in pelvic lesions)
  - Thin overlying cartilage usually not seen on radiograph (generally does not contain calcification)
  - Tend to be symmetric, though need not be
    - Rare unilateral forms exist; related to specific genetic type of MHE
  - Associated deformities
    - Bilateral coxa valga
    - Short ulnae, dislocated radial heads
    - Bowing of either or both forearm bones
    - Synostosis of tibia and fibula or radius and ulna
    - Valgus alignment of distal tibia (2%)
    - Limb length inequality (10%)
- Pedunculated form
  - Stalk arises from normal underlying bone, with continuous and normal marrow and cortex
    - If near joint, tends to project away from joint line, growing along direction of tendons
    - Lesions arising in pelvis may become very large before discovery
    - Lesions in ribs most often arise from costochondral junction; may give appearance of pulmonary nodule on chest x-ray
  - Overlying cartilage cap is thin
    - Size may be inferred by distorted fat planes or contained calcifications
  - More likely than sessile form to show endochondral calcification within cartilage cap
    - Rings and arcs, punctate, or flocculent calcification
- Suggestions of lesion degeneration to CS
  - Osseous destruction
  - Scattered (or change in) calcifications (snowstorm appearance)
  - ↑ in size of cartilage cap is inferred by distorted fat planes

CT Findings

- Same findings as those in radiographs

MR Findings

- Normal bone marrow extending into exostoses
- Exostosis cortex continuous with that of underlying bone
- Orderly hyaline cartilage cap, not irregular and not exceeding 1 cm in width
  - Cap has high signal of hyaline cartilage on fluid-sensitive sequences (low to intermediate SI on T1)
  - Cap covered by thin perichondrium, low signal on T1 and T2 sequences
  - Mineralized areas within cap remain low signal
  - In young patients with active growth, cartilage may be up to 3-cm thick and show marked heterogeneity
- Enhancement limited to thin fibrovascular tissue covering cartilage cap (nonenhancing) and thin septa within cap
- No soft tissue mass
- Fluid in overlying bursa may be seen: High T2 signal, low signal following contrast injection
- Secondary mechanical changes in exostosis
  - Marrow edema from impingement or trauma
  - Fracture of stalk

Ultrasonographic Findings

- Thickness and regularity of cartilage cap may be determined by US if lesion is not deep
- Cap is hypoechoic if nonmineralized, differentiating it from surrounding hyperechoic fat and muscle
- Areas of mineralization within cap show acoustic shadowing

Nuclear Medicine Findings

- Benign osteochondromas show uptake on bone scan, related to additional bone and endochondral calcification within cap
- CS may show more intense uptake, but this feature is not reliable for differentiating benign from malignant lesions

DIFFERENTIAL DIAGNOSIS

Chondrosarcoma

- Most important differential for individual lesion
- Consider if lesion continues to grow following skeletal maturation
- Consider if lesion is newly painful, not related to complication of adjacent nerve, bursa, or fracture
- Consider if there is change in character of calcified matrix, thick cartilage cap, or evidence of osseous destruction or soft tissue mass

Metaphyseal Dysplasia

- Widening, undertubulation of metaphyses may be mistaken for dysplasia
  - Mimics Gaucher or Pyle disease
- Misdiagnosis may occur when interpreting chest radiographs and only portion of abnormal proximal humeri are visualized

PATHOLOGY

General Features

- Genetics
  - Autosomal dominant inheritance
    - 90% have positive family history for MHE
    - 96% penetrance
  - *EXT* (likely tumor suppressor) genes show mutations
    - Hypothesized that inactivation of *EXT* gene in cartilaginous cell in growth plate allows formation of exostosis
  - Abnormalities shown at 3 distinct loci
    - Chromosomes 8, 11, and 19
  - 3 phenotypic patterns correlate with 3 genotypes
  - Possible incomplete penetrance in females

Microscopic Features

- Inner layer: Normal bone
- Middle layer: Cartilage cap with superficial clusters of chondrocytes
  - Close to transition to bone, organization of cartilage cells resembles physis undergoing endochondral ossification
- Outer layer: Perichondrium, continuous with periosteum of underlying bone

CLINICAL ISSUES

Presentation

- Most common signs/symptoms
  - Knobby masses, especially around knees
    - Defective metaphyseal remodeling → deformities
      - Madelung-type deformity at wrist and associated radial head dislocation at elbow
      - Bowing of other bones occurs though less consistently
    - Short stature from early physeal closure (40%)
      - Asymmetric early physeal closure → limb length discrepancy
  - Mechanical pain
    - Nerve impingement
    - Rapid painful "enlargement" from overlying bursa
    - Pseudoaneurysm
    - Fracture of stalk of exostosis
  - Increasing pain &/or mass enlargement following skeletal maturation suggests degeneration to CS
    - Note: Rare cases reported of continued growth of benign exostosis in adult

Demographics

- Age
  - Often discovered by age 2
- Gender
  - Male > female, 2:1 ratio
- Epidemiology
  - 1 in 50,000 individuals
  - Of all patients with osteochondromas, 15% have MHE

Natural History & Prognosis

- Exostoses stop growing after skeletal maturation
- Mechanical symptoms (pain, bursa formation, nerve or vessel impingement, fracture of stalk) may require surgery
  - Average of 2 surgical procedures per patient in 1 cohort of MHE
- 1-3% incidence of transformation to CS
  - Relates to greater number of osteochondromas present as well as greater propensity of each to transform
  - Larger incidence reported (up to 20% in 1 series), but case selection presents bias in these reports
  - Lesions around shoulder girdle and pelvis are at most risk for transformation
  - Less common transformation to osteosarcoma, malignant fibrous histiocytoma, dedifferentiated CS

Treatment

- Watchful waiting
  - Patient education regarding risk for degeneration to CS
  - Routine imaging follow-up of lesions generally not advocated; may vary on individual basis
- Mechanical complications (bursa formation, nerve irritation, impingement, etc.) treated by simple resection of offending lesion
- Concern for transformation of osteochondroma should lead to full work-up for CS
  - CS treated by wide surgical resection

DIAGNOSTIC CHECKLIST

Consider

- Question of normal cartilage cap thickness is debated; 1 series shows
  - Caps < 1.5 cm correlate with benign exostosis
  - Caps > 2.5 cm correlate with CS
  - Recommendation: Use thickness of > 1 cm as threshold for surgical resection of exostosis

SELECTED REFERENCES

1. Czajka CM et al: What is the proportion of patients with multiple hereditary exostoses who undergo malignant degeneration? Clin Orthop Relat Res. 473(7):2355-61, 2015

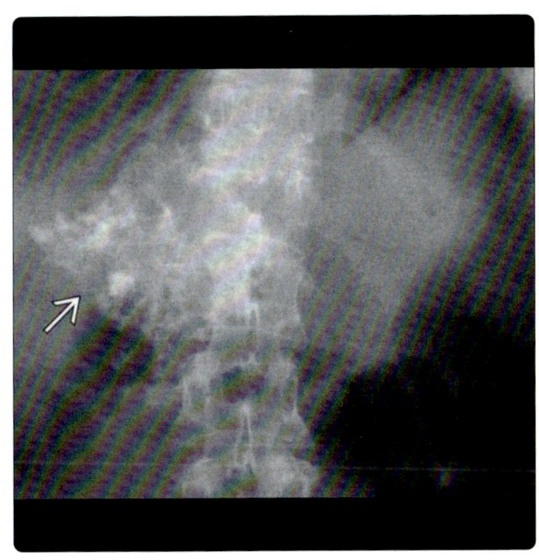

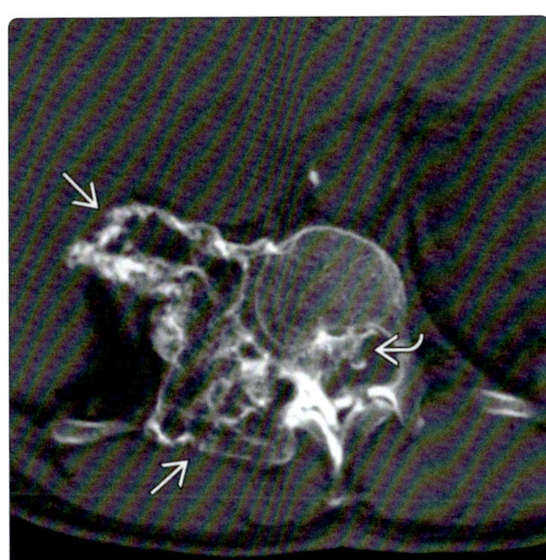

(Left) *AP radiograph, part of a skeletal survey in a patient with MHE, shows destructive changes in the body of T12/L1. Note the very disorganized appearance in a large cartilaginous mass ➡, concerning for degeneration to chondrosarcoma.* **(Right)** *Axial NECT, same patient, shows the lesion to actually be a well-organized exostosis ➡. Given the appearance of deformity without destruction, one can assume the lesion has been present for a long period of time. Note the spinal canal involvement with cord compression ➡.*

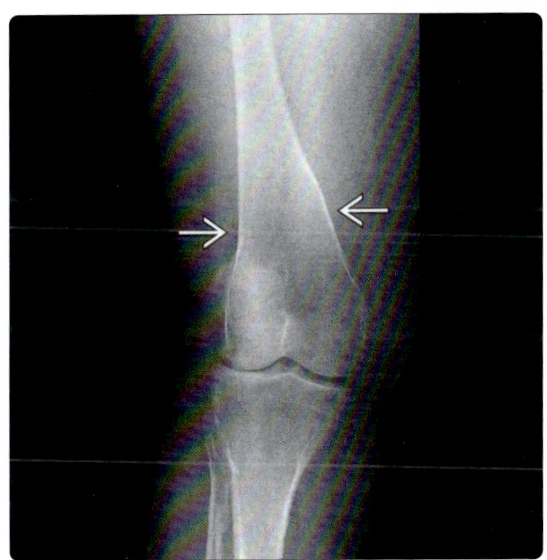

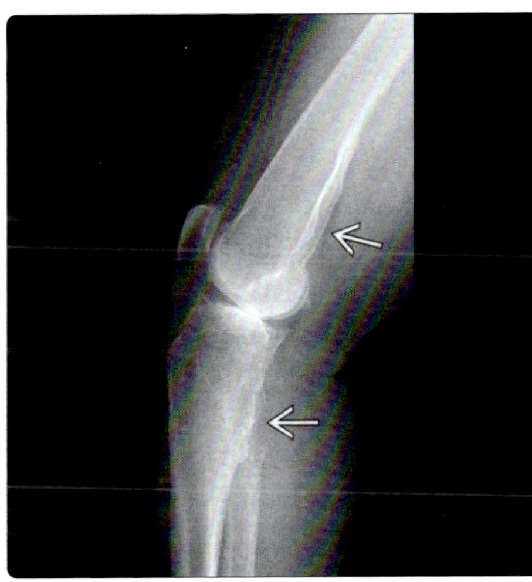

(Left) *AP radiograph shows prominent undertubulation of the distal femoral metadiaphyses ➡ that is bilaterally symmetric. If one is not careful, this might be misdiagnosed as either a marrow infiltration process, such as Gaucher disease, or a dysplasia, such as Pyle disease.* **(Right)** *Lateral radiograph in the same patient allows better appreciation of the sessile osteochondromas of the tibia and femur ➡. Exostoses seen in MHE may be sessile rather than exophytic, frequently resulting in misdiagnosis.*

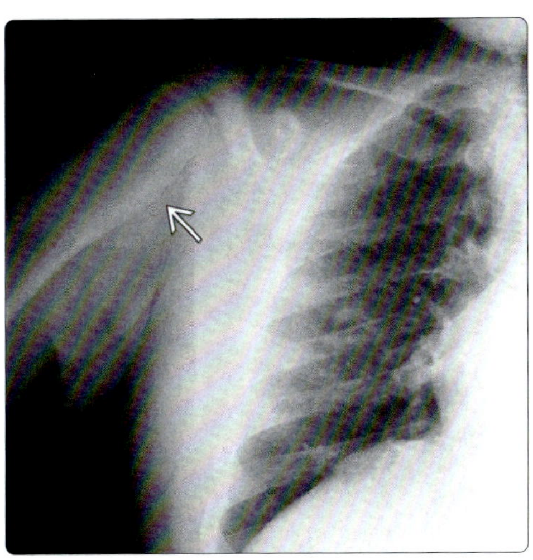

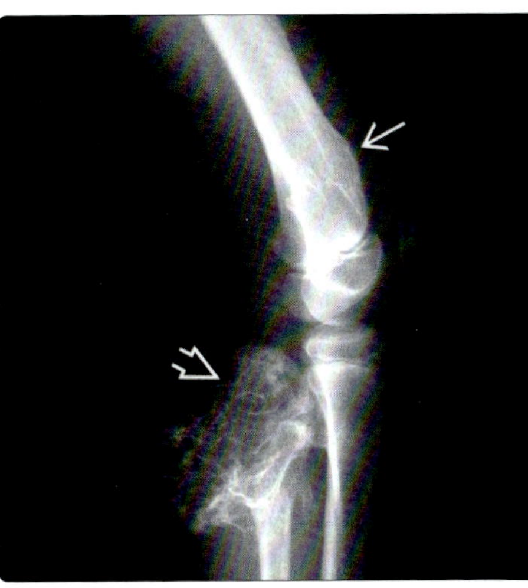

(Left) *AP radiograph shows the broad, rather featureless appearance of sessile exostoses in the humerus ➡ of a patient with MHE. It is not surprising that the diagnosis is often missed or misinterpreted on chest x-ray.* **(Right)** *Lateral radiograph of the knee in a child complaining of a mass and mechanical pain shows an obvious case of MHE. There is a combination of sessile ➡ and pedunculated ➡ exostoses, both of which may normally continue to enlarge until skeletal maturation.*

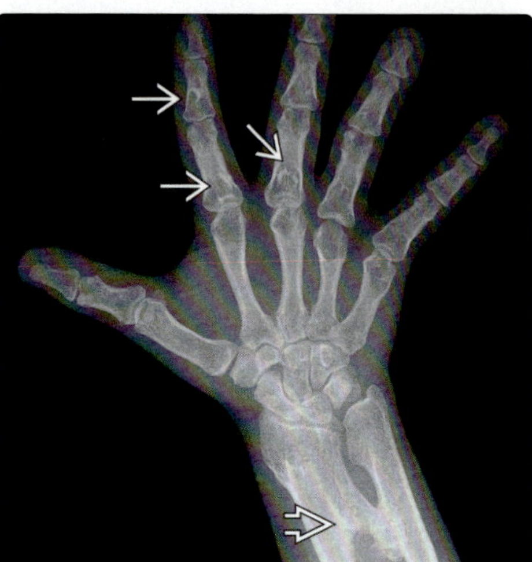

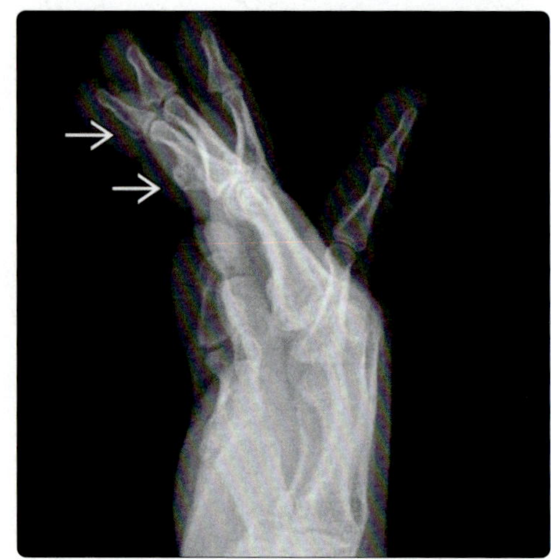

(Left) *PA radiograph demonstrates sessile exostosis bridging between the forearm bones ➩, resulting in synostosis and decreased carpal angle. The patient complained of "lumps" on the fingers, which correspond to the rounded densities seen on the phalanges ➔.* **(Right)** *Lateral radiograph in the same patient shows the phalangeal densities in profile to be exostoses ➔. This patient has MHE. It is not uncommon for forearm deformity to be part of the clinical picture.*

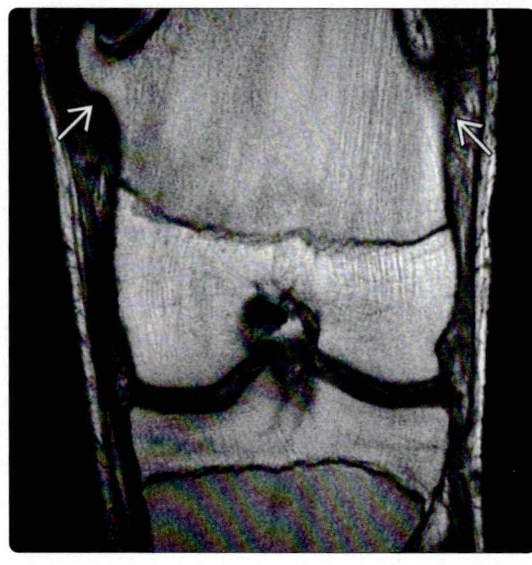

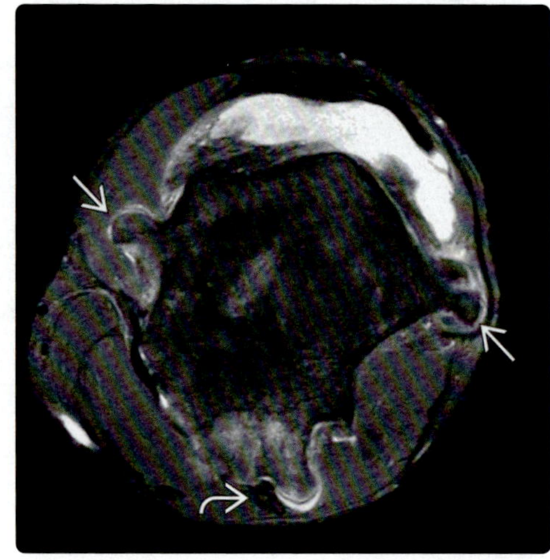

(Left) *Coronal T1WI MR in a patient with MHE shows failure of modeling of the femur and multiple discrete osteochondromas ➔. Note the normal marrow extending into the lesions.* **(Right)** *Axial PD FSE FS MR in the same patient shows the cartilage caps well as thin crescents of high signal intensity, with no thickening to suggest malignant degeneration ➔. Note the marked displacement of the sciatic nerve ➔ by a large posterior osteochondroma. Related symptoms may require surgical excision of the lesion.*

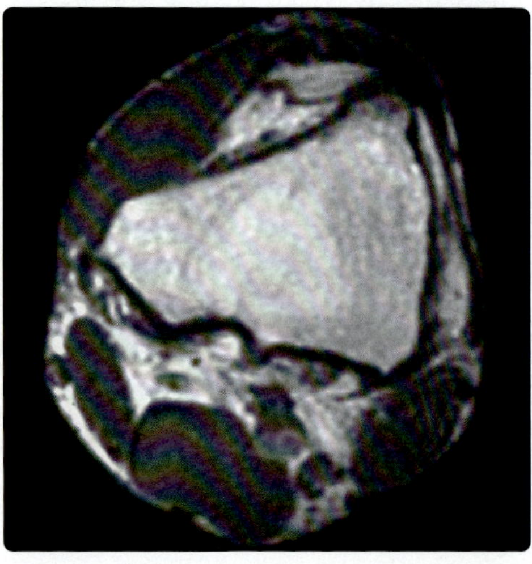

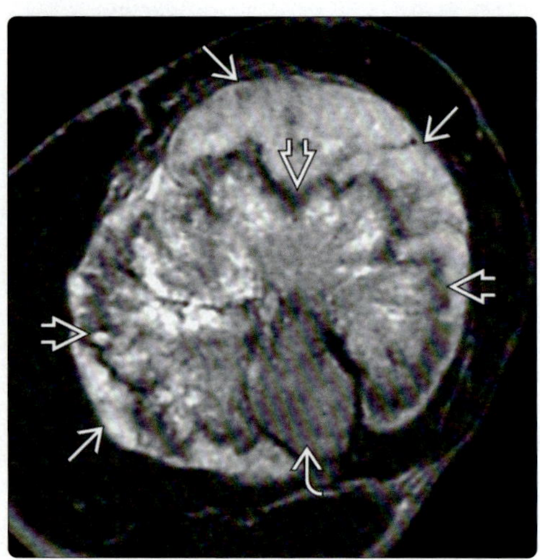

(Left) *Axial T1WI MR shows a distal femoral metaphysis in a patient with MHE. The morphology is very abnormal but typical for MHE with several sessile exostoses.* **(Right)** *Axial T2WI MR in the same patient shows a classic chondrosarcoma arising in a degenerating cartilage cap in the proximal femur. The femoral shaft is seen ➔, with its marrow extending into a large, cauliflower-like exostosis ➩, which is in turn surrounded by an inhomogeneous cartilage cap of variable thickness ➔, > 1 cm at several sites.*

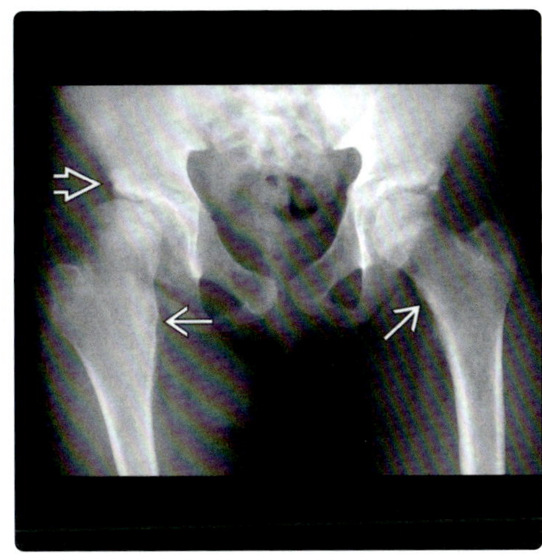
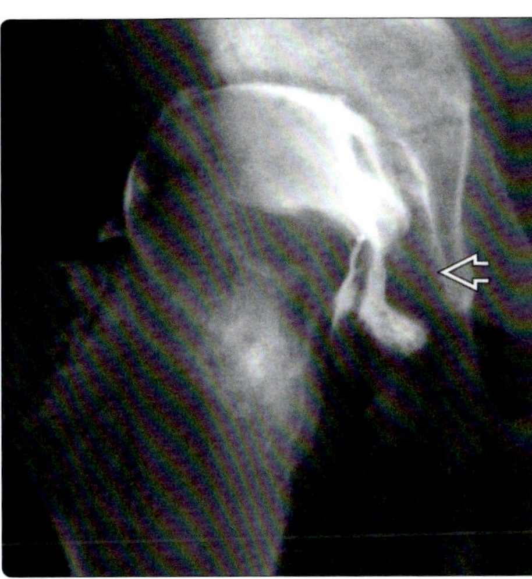

(Left) *AP radiograph of MHE shows sessile exostoses at both femoral necks ➡, along with broadening of the superior pubic ramus bilaterally. Note the valgus configuration of the right femoral neck and the associated acetabular dysplasia ➡, resulting from longstanding subluxation of the femoral head.* **(Right)** *AP arthrogram shows contrast outlining a lucent exostosis ➡, which caused the longstanding subluxation. The deformity must be addressed surgically to prevent osteoarthritis.*

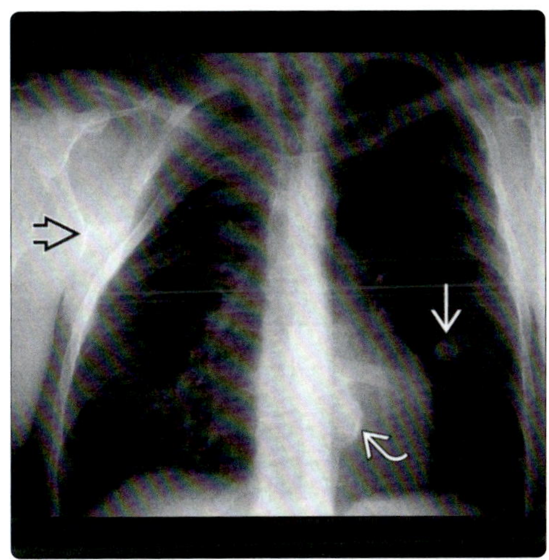
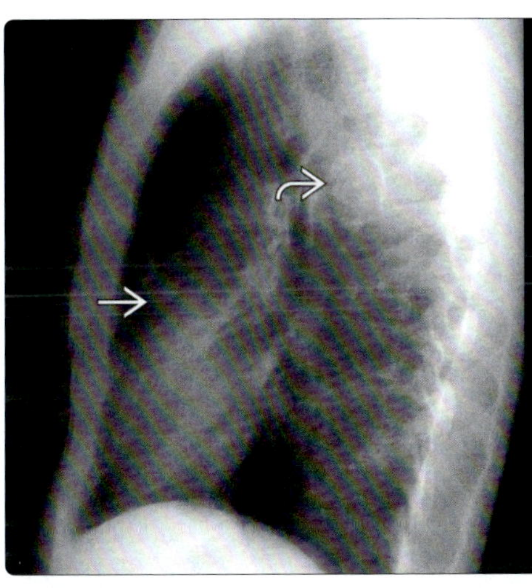

(Left) *AP radiograph shows a typical thorax in a patient with MHE. Note the excrescence arising from a rib ➡, the thoracic spine ➡, and right scapula ➡. The scapular lesion is particularly large, though not radiodense, causing rib cage deformity that at first looks like an old thoracoplasty; however a discrete scapular mass can be seen. Note that rib lesions can give the appearance of lung nodules.* **(Right)** *Lateral radiograph in the same patient confirms the rib ➡ and spine ➡ exostoses.*

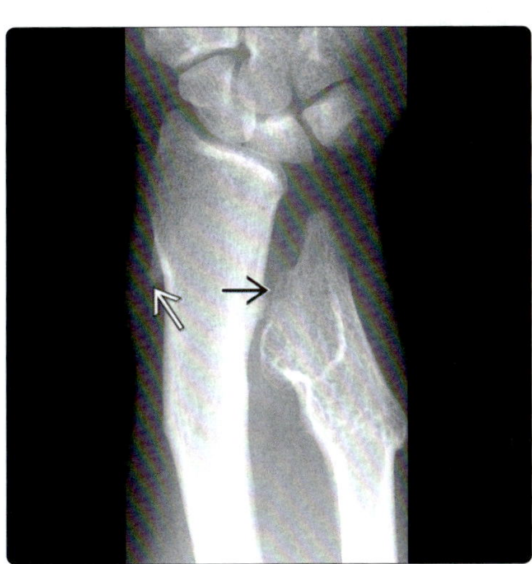
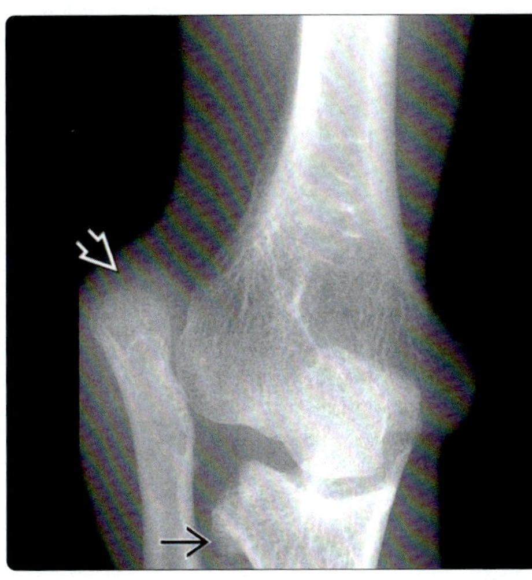

(Left) *AP radiograph shows a typical wrist deformity due to MHE. Multiple exostoses, exophytic ➡ and sessile ➡, are seen. These result in bowing deformity and, in this case, reverse Madelung deformity.* **(Right)** *AP radiograph of the elbow in the same patient shows an exostosis at the proximal ulna ➡. Note also the longstanding radial head dislocation ➡, which can be typically seen in patients with MHE. Not surprisingly, the findings were bilateral, though they need not be.*

KEY FACTS

TERMINOLOGY

- Benign cartilage tumor arising in epiphysis of skeletally immature individuals

IMAGING

- Location
  - > 75% in long bones
  - Epiphyseal origin, often extends into metaphysis
  - Proximal humerus > proximal tibia > proximal and distal femur
- Geographic lytic lesion
- 1/3-1/2 contain chondroid matrix
- Sclerotic margin in majority
- Eccentrically located within epiphysis
- Larger and more longstanding lesions develop smooth thick periosteal reaction (50%)
- Lesion occasionally contains fluid levels (occasionally represents 2° aneurysmal bone cyst)
- MR: Inhomogeneously low signal on T1; inhomogeneously high signal intensity on fluid-sensitive sequences
  - High signal on fluid-sensitive sequences in adjacent cortex, marrow, and soft tissue in majority of cases

CLINICAL ISSUES

- Most frequently affects those 10-25 years old
- M > F (nearly 2:1)
- Surgical treatment: Curettage and bone graft
- Radiofrequency ablation may be considered in small lesions (mean diameter of 1.4 cm in 1 report)

DIAGNOSTIC CHECKLIST

- Though lesion arises in epiphysis, it may extend into metaphysis with growth
- Metaphyseal periosteal reaction and adjacent edema may mimic more aggressive lesion
- Watch for lobulations or serpiginous extension beyond rounded geographic border

(Left) *Graphic shows a transected proximal humerus containing typical chondroblastoma. It depicts a geographic, eccentrically located lesion within the epiphysis. There is a sclerotic margin ⇨ and a few calcifications present within the lesion ➡.* **(Right)** *Radiograph of a classic chondroblastoma seen in a nearly skeletally mature patient is shown. Lytic lesion arises within the epiphysis and extends into the metaphysis ➡. It has no calcific matrix, is geographic, and has a slightly sclerotic margin.*

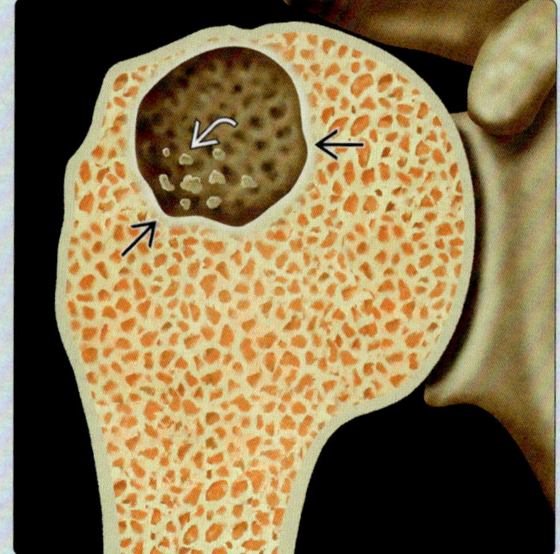

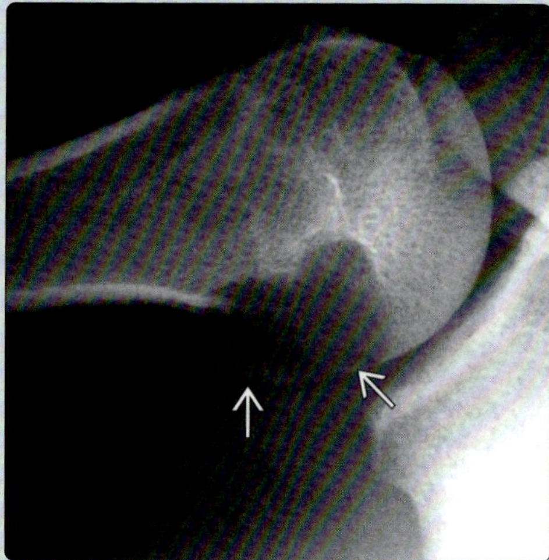

(Left) *Coronal T1WI MR shows a homogeneous epiphyseal lesion arising eccentrically ⇨, typical for chondroblastoma. Dense periosteal reaction is seen along the metaphysis ➡, a typical finding in 50% of these lesions.* **(Right)** *Axial NECT shows a highly eccentric chondroblastoma within the humeral epiphysis ⇨. It contains a small fleck of calcific matrix ➡ and slightly expands the cortex. This patient complained of pain & popping with rotation of the shoulder and originally was unnecessarily arthroscoped rather than imaged.*

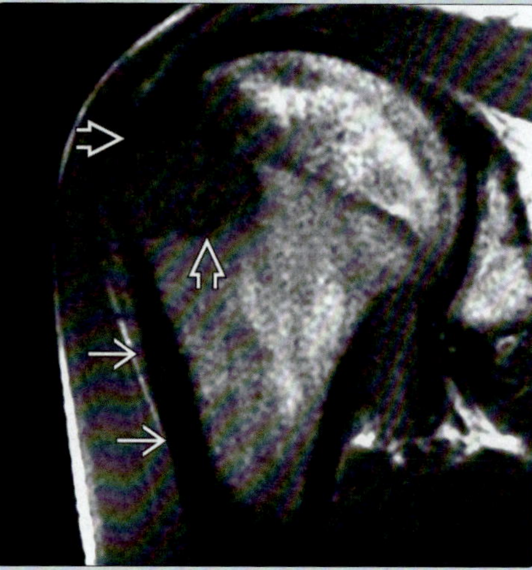

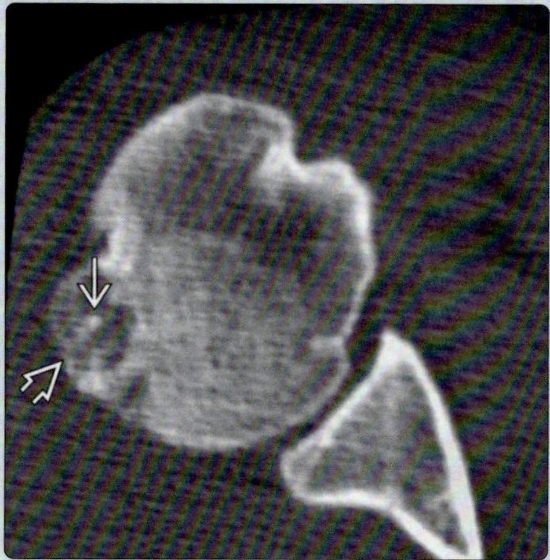

TERMINOLOGY

Synonyms

- Calcifying giant cell tumor, epiphyseal chondromatous giant cell tumor, Codman tumor, chondroblastoma (CB)

IMAGING

General Features

- Best diagnostic clue
  - Lytic geographic lesion arising in epiphysis of skeletally immature patient
- Location
  - > 75% in long bones
  - Epiphyseal origin; often extends into metaphysis
    - Proximal humerus > proximal tibia > femur
  - Metaphyseal/epiphyseal equivalent sites in ilium, acetabulum, patella, and hindfoot/midfoot bones
  - Skull/temporal bone rare and found in older adults

Radiographic Findings

- Geographic lytic lesion
  - 1/3-1/2 contain chondroid matrix
  - Sclerotic margin in majority
- Eccentrically located within epiphysis
  - Extends into metaphysis as it enlarges (25-50%)
- No cortical breakthrough or soft tissue mass
  - Mild cortical expansion or thinning may occur
- Larger and more longstanding lesions develop smooth thick periosteal reaction (50%)
  - Reaction occurs along adjacent metaphysis

CT Findings

- Mirrors radiographic appearance: Geographic lytic lesion
- Chondroid matrix more easily seen than on x-ray
- May show lobulated or serpiginous pattern at edge of lesion in up to 10%; irregular margination → recurrence

MR Findings

- Inhomogeneously low signal on T1; inhomogeneously high signal intensity on fluid-sensitive sequences
  - Inhomogeneity relates to chondroid matrix, calcification, and fluid within lesion
  - Generally, high signal lobulated nodules typical of benign cartilage lesions are **not** present
- Lesion occasionally contains fluid levels (occasionally representing secondary aneurysmal bone cyst)
- Joint effusion in minority of cases (1/3)
- Periosteal reaction in adjacent metaphysis
  - Low SI all sequences; along metaphyseal cortex
- High signal on fluid-sensitive sequences in adjacent cortex, marrow, and soft tissue in majority of cases
  - No distinct soft tissue mass
  - Correlates with degree of periosteal reaction

DIFFERENTIAL DIAGNOSIS

Clear Cell Chondrosarcoma

- Rare lesion; arises in epiphysis
- May be indistinguishable by imaging criteria

Giant Cell Tumor

- Originates in metaphysis, extends to epiphysis; mature CB and mature giant cell tumor (GCT) may occupy similar positions
- Generally has no (or little) sclerosis at margin

PATHOLOGY

Microscopic Features

- Nodules of relatively mature cartilage surrounded by highly cellular tissue
- Giant cells almost always present
- May have fine network of pericellular calcification ("chicken wire" calcification)
- Aneurysmal bone cyst (ABC)-like changes in up to 1/3

CLINICAL ISSUES

Presentation

- Most common signs/symptoms
  - Mild localized pain; may refer to joint

Demographics

- Age
  - Most frequently 10-25 years old
    - Arises prior to skeletal maturation but may not present clinically until after physeal fusion
- Gender
  - M > F (nearly 2:1)
- Epidemiology
  - < 1% of all bone tumors; 9% of benign bone tumors

Natural History & Prognosis

- Curettage and bone grafting successfully cure in 80-90%
- Local recurrence in 14-18%, usually within 2 years
- May have associated ABC, especially in patella
- Rare reports of pulmonary metastases in patients with histologically benign chondroblastomas

Treatment

- Surgical: Curettage and bone graft
  - Addition of cryosurgery reported to ↓ rate of recurrence to 7% but had 14% physeal growth arrest
- Radiofrequency ablation may be considered in small lesions (mean diameter of 1.4 cm in 1 report, 2.5 cm in another)
  - Caution required in subchondral lesions at weight-bearing surface, which are subject to collapse

DIAGNOSTIC CHECKLIST

Consider

- Though lesion arises in epiphysis, it may extend into metaphysis with growth
- Metaphyseal periosteal reaction and adjacent edema may mimic more aggressive lesion

SELECTED REFERENCES

1. Lalam RK et al: Image guided radiofrequency thermo-ablation therapy of chondroblastomas: should it replace surgery? Skeletal Radiol. 43(4):513-22, 2014
2. Tan H et al: Chondroblastoma of the patella with aneurysmal bone cyst. Orthopedics. 37(1):e87-91, 2014

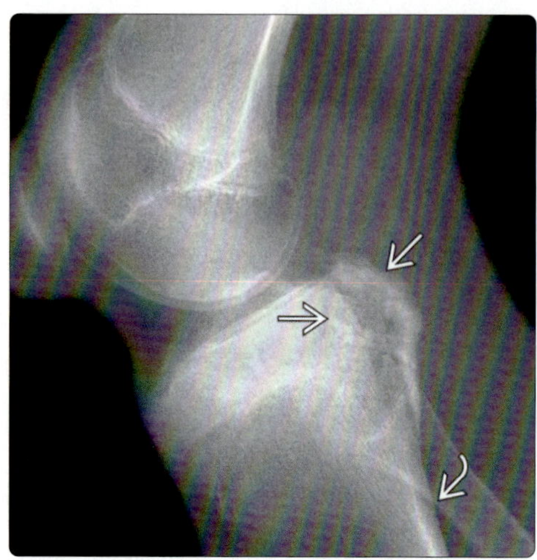

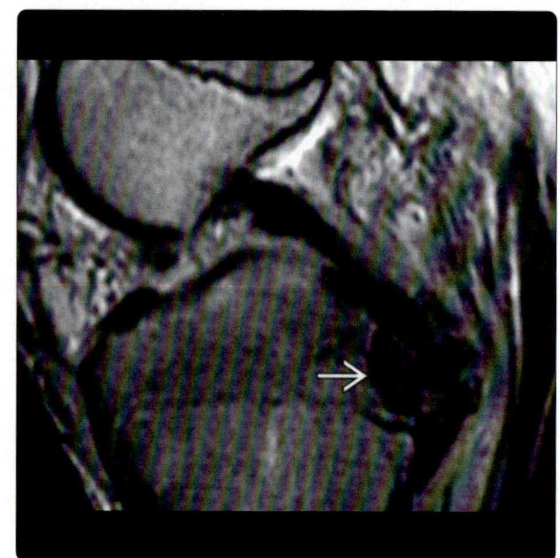

(Left) *Lateral radiograph demonstrates a matrix-forming tumor ➡ located eccentrically in the tibial epiphysis. There is dense linear periosteal reaction extending along the posterior metaphyseal cortex ➡. Though the sclerosis within the lesion is unusual for chondroblastoma, the other features make the diagnosis.* **(Right)** *Sagittal T2WI FS MR in the same patient shows inhomogeneous but largely low signal epiphyseal lesion ➡, related to sclerosis seen on radiograph. This signal is unusual for chondroblastoma.*

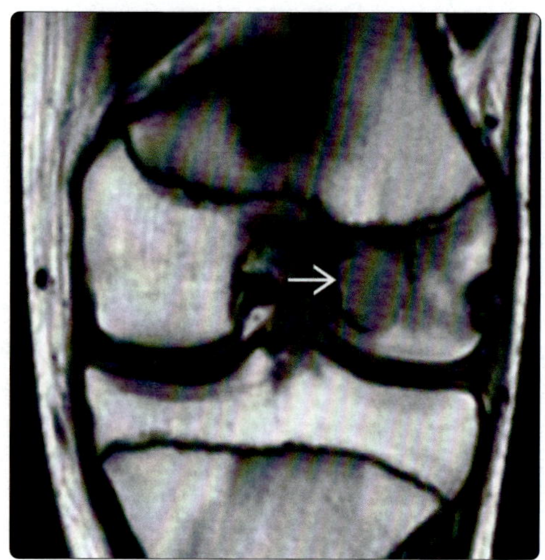

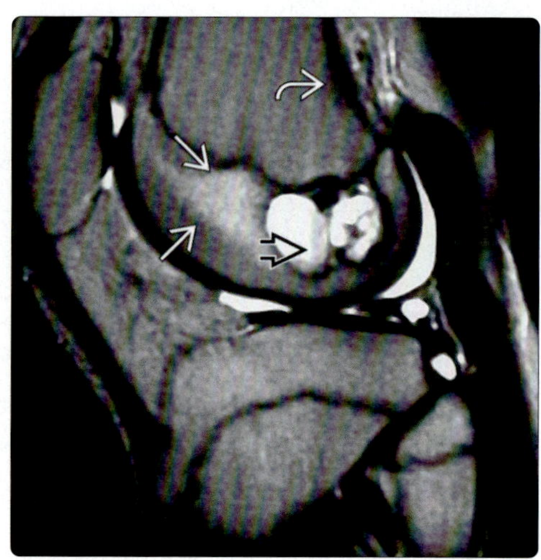

(Left) *Coronal T1WI MR shows a homogeneous moderately low signal lesion eccentrically located within an epiphysis ➡, classic for a chondroblastoma.* **(Right)** *Sagittal T2WI FS MR in the same patient shows the lobulated high signal of this lesion. There is a cystic component that contains a fluid level ➡; this appearance is not uncommon in chondroblastoma. Note also that there is edema in the adjacent marrow ➡ and periosteal reaction in the nearby posterior femoral metaphysis ➡.*

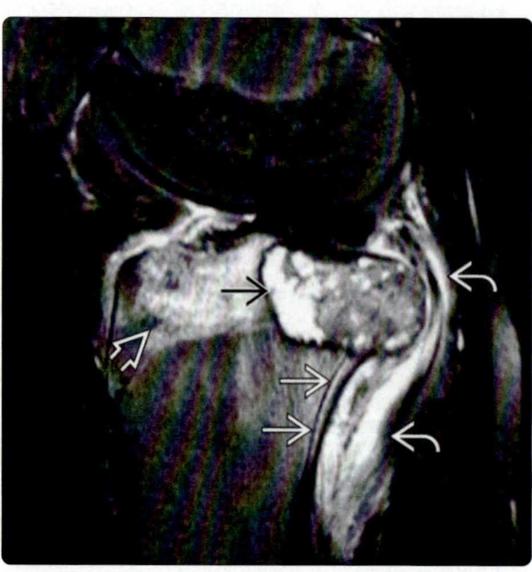

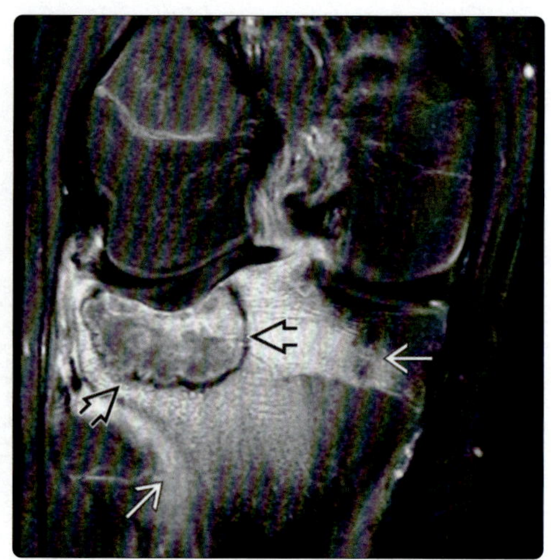

(Left) *Sagittal T2WI FS MR of tibial chondroblastoma is shown. Note the mixed signal intensity lesion with lobular high signal portions ➡ and inhomogeneous lower signal posteriorly. Adjacent marrow edema ➡ and periosteal reaction with cortical edema ➡. Edema within adjacent popliteus muscle is prominent ➡.* **(Right)** *Coronal T1WI C+ FS MR in the same patient shows moderate enhancement within the lesion, surrounding lower signal regions of calcification ➡. Marrow edema enhances intensely ➡.*

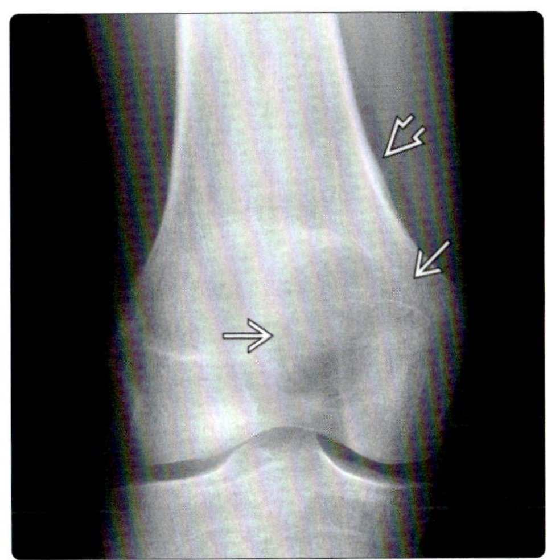

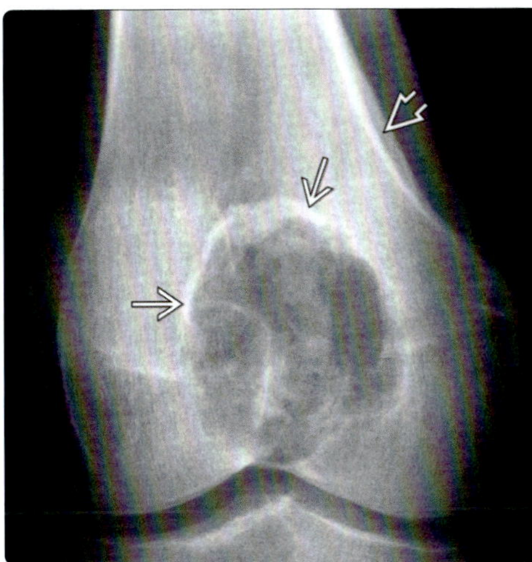

(Left) *AP radiograph series shows a lytic lesion located eccentrically in the metaphysis of the distal femur ➡ in a 27 year old. There is a slightly sclerotic margin, and subtle periosteal reaction is seen ➡. Except for the reaction, the appearance and patient age are suggestive of giant cell tumor.* **(Right)** *AP radiograph obtained 1 year later, without intervening treatment, shows evolution of the findings to those typical of chondroblastoma (proven at biopsy), with greater density of the reaction ➡ and margin ➡.*

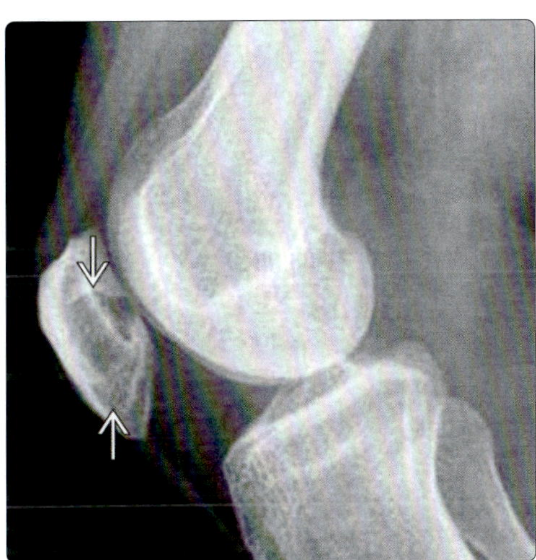

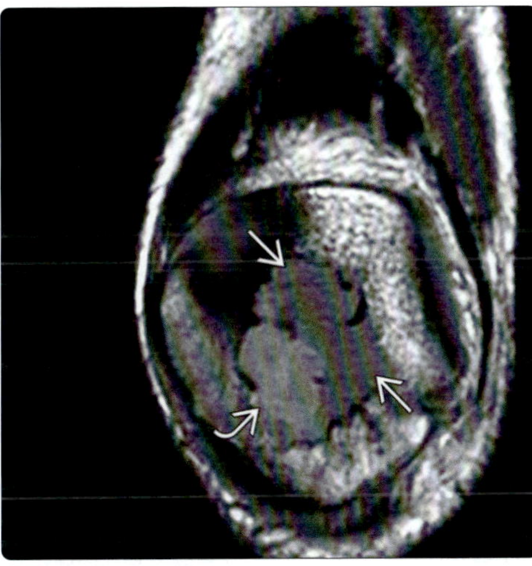

(Left) *Lateral radiograph shows a lytic lesion with a thin sclerotic geographic margin ➡. The lesion has no aggressive features. In this teenager, one might consider diagnoses of giant cell tumor, aneurysmal bone cyst, and chondroblastoma.* **(Right)** *Coronal T1WI MR in the same patient shows a mixed lesion with low homogeneous signal in the superomedial portion ➡ and a more inhomogeneous higher signal inferolateral portion ➡. This suggests 2 distinct regions within the lesion.*

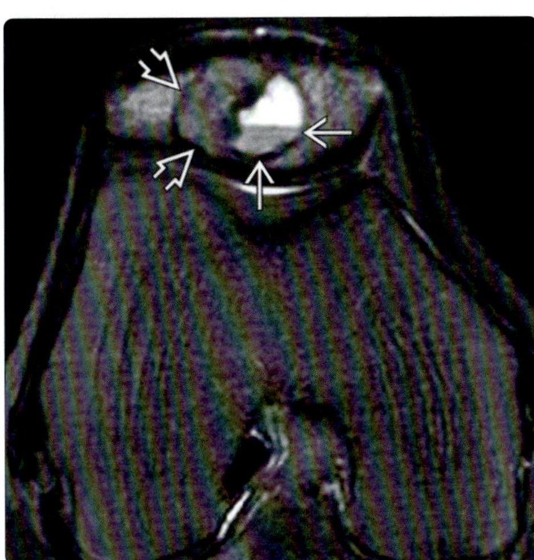

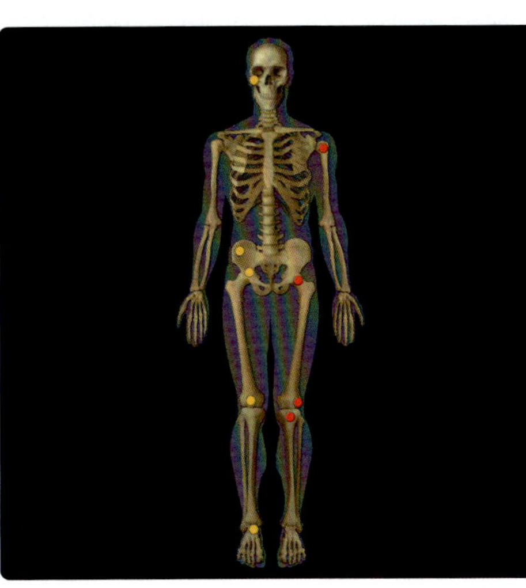

(Left) *Axial PDWI FS MR in the same patient shows the medial portion contains fluid levels ➡, while the lateral portion of the lesion appears more solid with mild inhomogeneity ➡. Chondroblastoma may serve as an underlying lesion for development of aneurysmal bone cyst. Both lesions were proven at biopsy. (Courtesy K. Jin Suh, MD.)* **(Right)** *Graphic depicts common sites of chondroblastoma in red (proximal humerus, proximal tibia, both femoral epiphyses) and less common sites in yellow.*

KEY FACTS

TERMINOLOGY

- Benign lobulated cartilage tumor

IMAGING

- Location: 61% in long bones
  - ~ 50% occur around knee
    - Proximal tibia is single most frequent site
  - 24% in bones of hand/foot
  - 25% in flat bones
    - Of flat bones, iliac wing is most common
- Site of origin: Metaphyseal (53%) or diaphyseal (43%)
- Geographic, with sclerotic margin
- Eccentric (58%), lobulated, with thinning of cortex
- Often expanded (89%)
- Chondroid matrix rare (< 10%)

TOP DIFFERENTIAL DIAGNOSES

- Giant cell tumor (GCT)
  - Similar location (eccentric, originates in metaphysis, extends to subarticular region)
  - GCT also geographic but rarely has sclerotic margin
- Aneurysmal bone cyst
  - Eccentric, metadiaphyseal lesion
  - Geographic, expanded
  - Generally fluid-fluid levels seen on MR; rarely solid

CLINICAL ISSUES

- Wide age range; mean: 23 years, median: 18 years
  - 50% in 2nd decade at presentation
- Slight male predominance
- Rare lesion (< 1% of bone tumors)
  - 2.3% of cartilage tumors (least common benign cartilage tumor)
- Excellent prognosis
- Treatment: Marginal excision (curettage and bone grafting)
  - Recurrence rate of 15-25%

(Left) *Graphic depicts the gross pathologic appearance of chondromyxoid fibroma (CMF). The lesion is well demarcated and has a glistening fleshy appearance. It is eccentrically located and results in mild expansion of the cortex* ➡. **(Right)** *AP radiograph of a typical CMF. The lesion is most frequently found in the tibia, is metaphyseal and eccentric in location, slightly bubbly, and has a sclerotic margin* ➡. *As seen here, CMF need not contain chondroid matrix.*

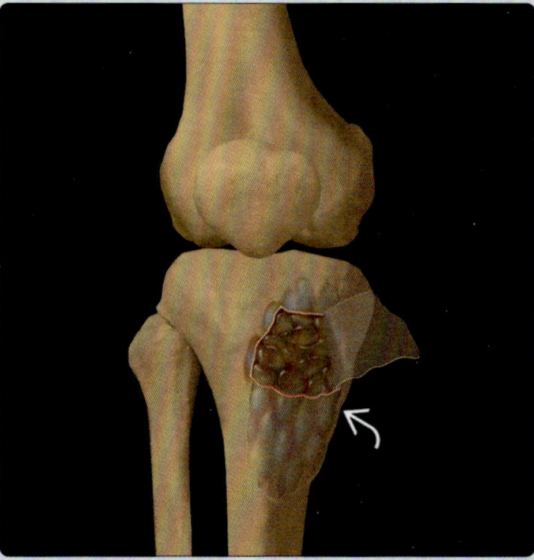

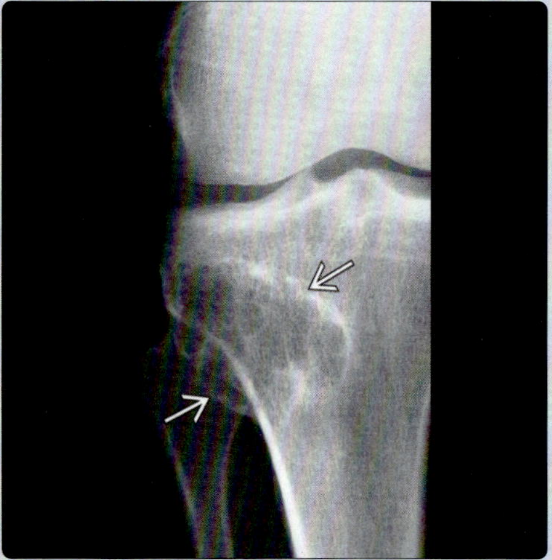

(Left) *AP radiograph shows an unusual CMF in a very young child. This central radial metadiaphyseal lesion is more suggestive of aneurysmal bone cyst, but CMF was proven at biopsy. Note the pseudotrabeculations, which make the lesion appear septated* ➡. **(Right)** *Axial NECT shows a mildly expanded lytic lesion occupying subchondral bone* ➡. *Aneurysmal bone cyst and chondroblastoma would most likely be considered in this teenager. CMF is a relatively rare lesion but was proven at biopsy.*

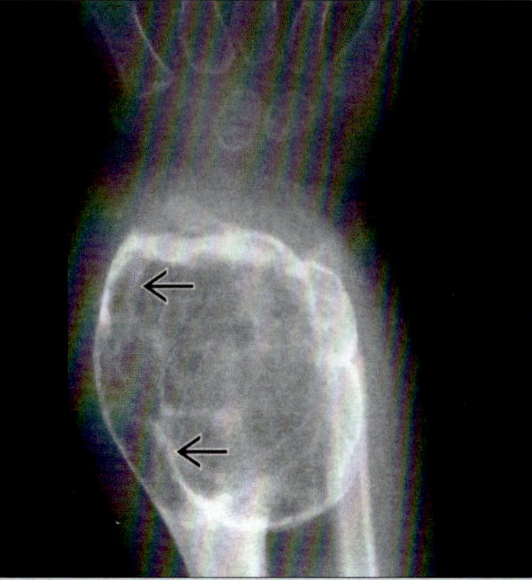

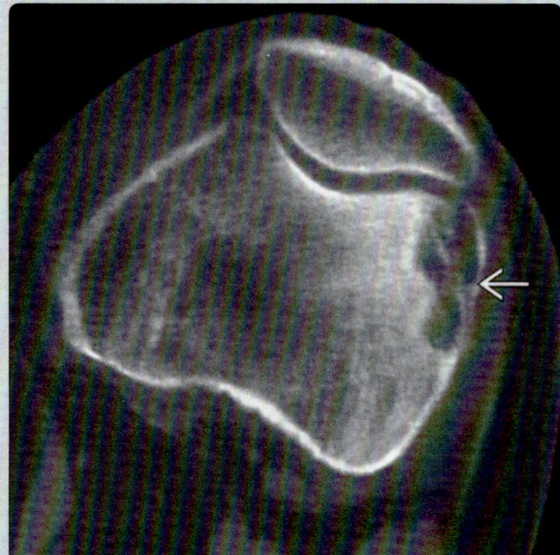

TERMINOLOGY

Abbreviations

- Chondromyxoid fibroma (CMF)

Definitions

- Benign lobulated cartilage tumor

IMAGING

General Features

- Location
  - 61% in long bones
  - ~ 50% occur around knee (proximal tibia is single most frequent site)
  - 25% in flat bones, most frequently ilium
  - 24% in bones of hand/foot
  - Multiple other bones described, but rare (spinal, craniofacial, clavicular, calcaneal locations)

Radiographic Findings

- Geographic, with sclerotic margin
- Metaphyseal (53%) or diaphyseal (43%) site of origin
  - Those centered in metaphysis may extend across physis to subarticular bone
  - Oriented along longitudinal axis of bone
  - Apophyseal origin is reported but rare
- Eccentric (58%), lobulated with thinning of cortex
  - Pseudotrabeculations give appearance of septation
  - Often expanded (89%)
  - May erode bone and rarely results in soft tissue mass
  - Though most are intramedullary, other locations have been described
    - Rare cases of juxtacortical CMF, simulating other surface lesions of bone; rarely intracortical
- No periosteal reaction in absence of pathologic fracture
- Chondroid matrix rare (< 10%)

CT Findings

- Mimics radiographic findings
- Shows matrix and osseous erosion more convincingly

MR Findings

- T1: Isointense to skeletal muscle; internal hyperintense foci in 37%
- Fluid-sensitive sequences: 2 patterns
  - May have peripheral band of intermediate signal, with central hyperintensity (58% in 1 study)
  - Diffusely & homogeneously hyperintense (42%)
  - May be multilobulated
- Postcontrast T1 FS: Peripheral nodular enhancement (69%) or diffuse enhancement (31%)
  - Peripheral nodular enhancement corresponds to peripheral band of intermediate signal on T2 MR

DIFFERENTIAL DIAGNOSIS

Giant Cell Tumor

- Similar location (eccentric, originates in metaphysis, extends to subarticular region)
- Giant cell tumor (GCT) also geographic but rarely has sclerotic margin

Aneurysmal Bone Cyst

- Eccentric, metadiaphyseal lesion
- Geographic, expanded
- Generally fluid-fluid levels seen on MR; rarely solid

PATHOLOGY

General Features

- Genetics
  - Clonal abnormalities of chromosome 6
  - Pronounced expression of type II collagen (marker of chondrocytic cell differentiation and hydrated proteoglycans)

Gross Pathologic & Surgical Features

- Expanded bluish, gray, or white tumor
- No necrosis or cystic change
- Typical hyaline cartilage not usually present

Microscopic Features

- Lobular, with stellate cells in myxoid background
- Hyaline cartilage in 19%
- May contain regions of aneurysmal bone cyst (ABC)

CLINICAL ISSUES

Presentation

- Most common signs/symptoms
  - Mild pain, often present for several years

Demographics

- Age
  - Wide range; mean: 23 years, median: 18 years
    - 50% in 2nd decade at presentation
- Epidemiology
  - < 1% of bone tumors < 2% of benign bone tumors
  - 2.3% of cartilage tumors (least common benign cartilage tumor)

Natural History & Prognosis

- Excellent prognosis

Treatment

- Marginal excision (curettage and bone grafting)
  - Recurrence rate of 15-25%

DIAGNOSTIC CHECKLIST

Consider

- CMF is generally straightforward diagnosis, except
  - When in unusual location, especially when origin is not intramedullary
  - When in unusual bone; locations other than tibia or iliac wing often not suggestive of diagnosis
  - Nuclear atypia may suggest more aggressive lesion, but is common histologic finding

SELECTED REFERENCES

1. Bhamra JS et al: Chondromyxoid fibroma management: a single institution experience of 22 cases. World J Surg Oncol. 12:283, 2014
2. Kim HS et al: MRI of chondromyxoid fibroma. Acta Radiol. 52(8):875-80, 2011

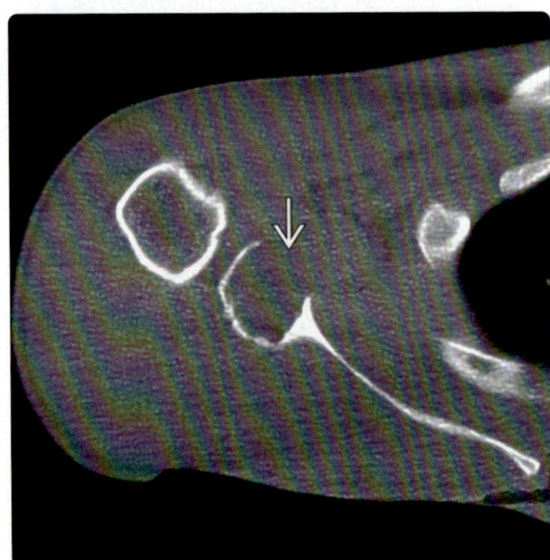

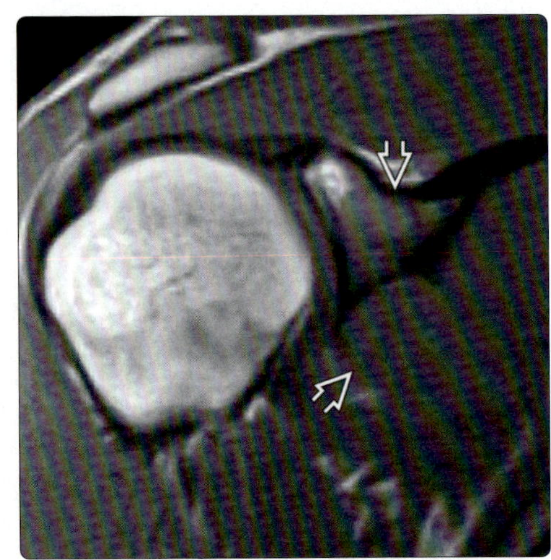

(Left) *Axial NECT shows a CMF in the glenoid; an unusual lesion in an unusual location. The lesion is lytic, expanded, and arises in the glenoid of the scapula ➡. There is cortical breakthrough and an anterior soft tissue mass. There is no matrix present. Because it arises in a flat bone, cartilage lesions should be considered, including chondroblastoma and CMF.* **(Right)** *Coronal T1WI MR in the same patient shows the mass to replace most of the glenoid ➡. The signal is low and isointense to skeletal muscle.*

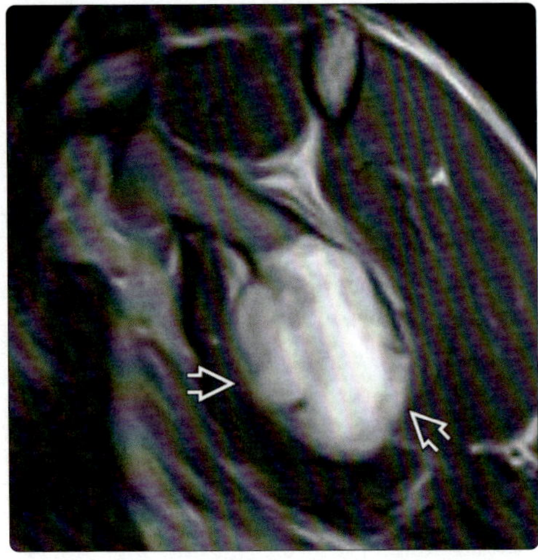

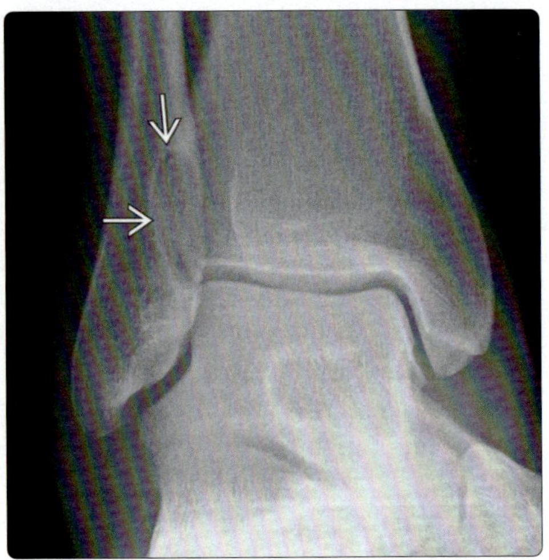

(Left) *Sagittal T2WI MR in the same patient shows inhomogeneous high signal in the lesion ➡. Note that the lesion does not have the usual high signal lobular appearance of benign cartilage; this should not be surprising, as little hyaline cartilage is found in CMF. This diagnosis may be difficult to prospectively suggest because of its rarity and location.* **(Right)** *AP radiograph in a 33-year-old woman shows an eccentrically located lytic lesion ➡ in the distal fibular metaphysis. Part of the lesion has a sclerotic margin. No matrix is seen.*

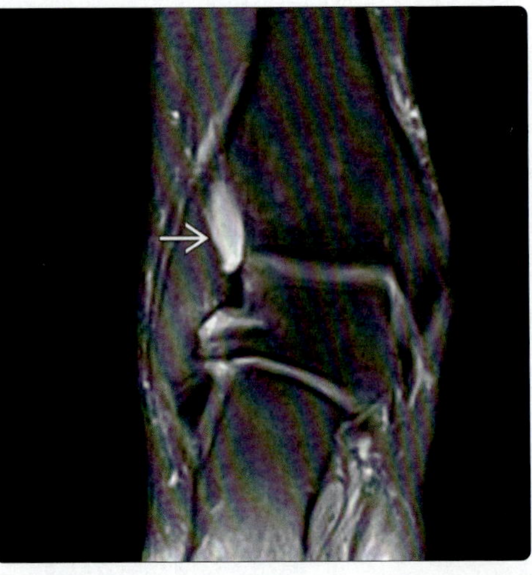

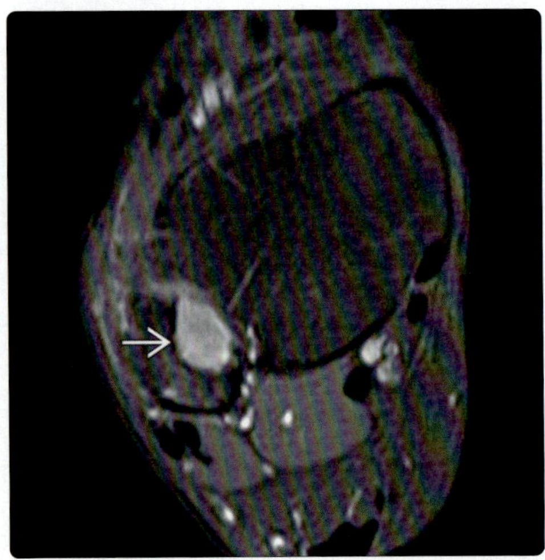

(Left) *Coronal T2 FS MR shows the lesion ➡ to be hyperintense, with only minor inhomogeneity. On T1 MR (not shown), the lesion was homogeneously hypointense, similar in signal to muscle.* **(Right)** *Axial T1 C+ FS MR shows the lesion ➡ to enhance with mild inhomogeneity. There is no marrow edema or soft tissue mass. The imaging findings are not specific for any particular lesion, but CMF was diagnosed at biopsy.*

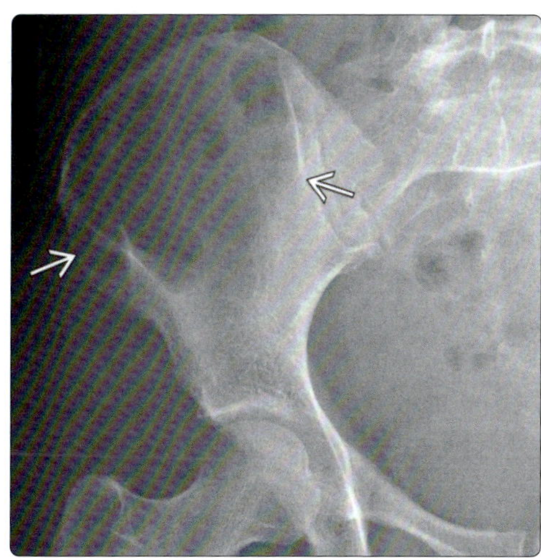

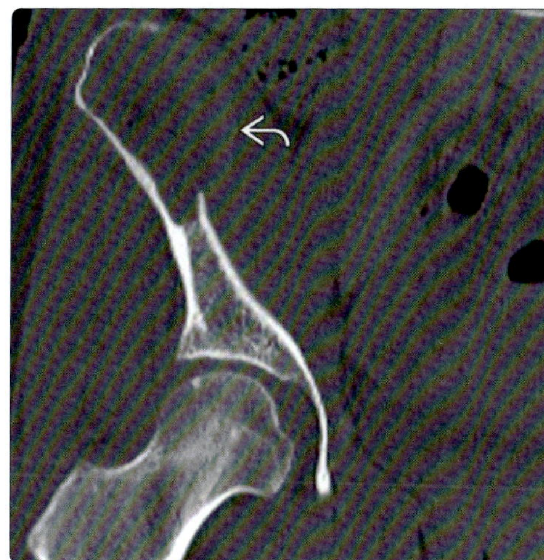

(Left) *AP radiograph in a 35-year-old woman shows a completely lytic lesion involving a large portion of the iliac wing. The lesion appears geographic* ➡ *although only a portion of it shows significant sclerosis at its margin. Aside from the large size, there is no sign of aggressiveness.* **(Right)** *Coronal CT demonstrates the lytic lesion to have the thinnest possible cortex at its medially expanded portion* ➡. *However, the lesion does appear to be contained relative to the adjacent iliacus muscle.*

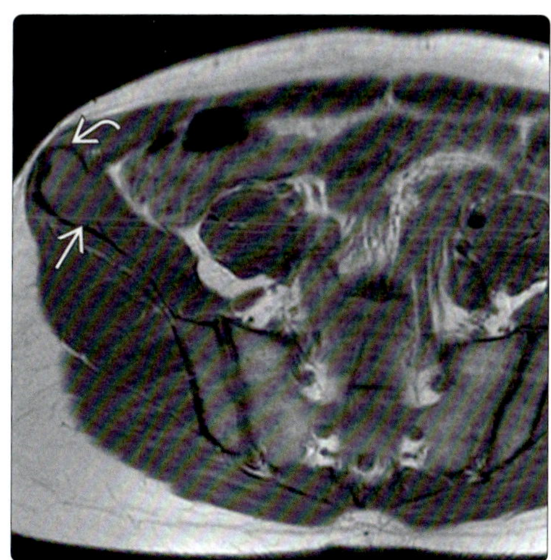

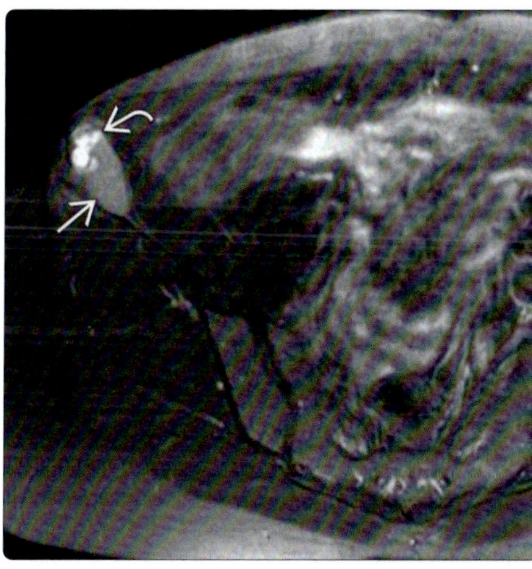

(Left) *Axial T1 MR in the same patient shows the lesion to be largely of similar hypointense signal* ➡ *to skeletal muscle. However, one peripheral portion* ➡ *is less hypointense.* **(Right)** *Axial T2 FS MR shows the majority of the lesion to be mildly hyperintense* ➡, *while the peripheral portion shows more lobular hyperintensity* ➡ *that is suggestive of benign cartilage. Although such cartilage lobulation is not expected in CMF, its presence should not disqualify CMF as a possible diagnosis.*

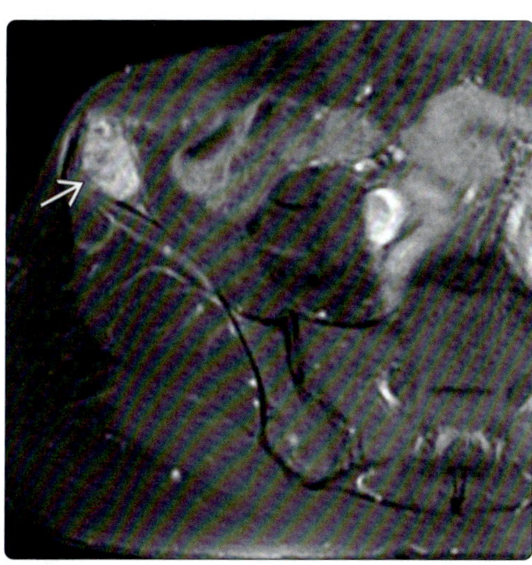

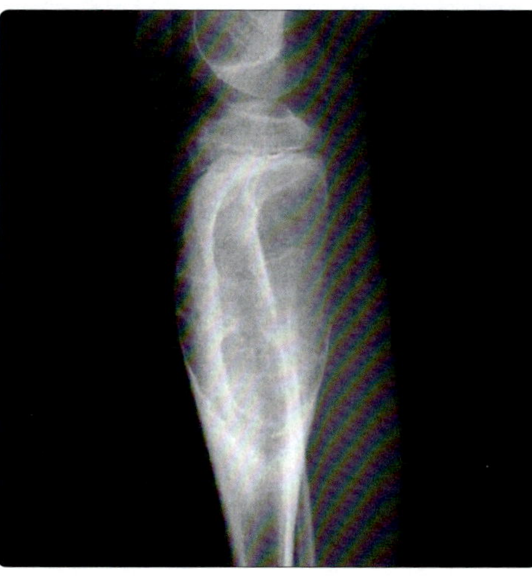

(Left) *Axial T1 C+ FS MR shows mildly inhomogeneous enhancement throughout the lesion* ➡. *In this case, the imaging features are most suggestive of a benign lesion. The T2 sequence suggests cartilage, and the location therefore should raise the possibility of CMF.* **(Right)** *Lateral radiograph shows a large, pathologically proven CMF located in the tibial metaphysis that is eccentric and expansile. It is entirely lytic and shows no cortical breakthrough. Aneurysmal bone cyst should be considered as well.*

Periosteal Chondroma

KEY FACTS

TERMINOLOGY

- Chondroid tumor arising in periosteal layer of tubular bones

IMAGING

- Best diagnostic clue
  - Surface lesion arising from metaphysis of tubular bone, producing chondroid matrix
- Location: Metaphyseal, arising on surface of bone
  - Proximal humerus and femur (70%)
  - Phalanges (25%) (hands > feet)
- Radiographic findings
  - Saucerization of cortex
  - Sclerotic margination
  - Buttressing of cortex at proximal and distal ends of lesion
  - Matrix calcification (75%)
  - Soft tissue mass
- MR findings
  - Lobulated configuration of mass: Important diagnostic finding when present
  - Isointense or low T1 signal intensity
  - Hyperintense T2 signal
  - Heterogeneous enhancement, generally at periphery of lesion
- Intramedullary involvement in 20%

CLINICAL ISSUES

- Age: 2nd-4th decades most frequent; may occur in children
  - Slightly younger age group than periosteal chondrosarcomas
- Epidemiology: Rare: < 2% of all chondromas (majority are enchondroma)
  - Periosteal chondroma > > periosteal chondrosarcoma (3-4:1 ratio)
- Natural History: Slow local progression
- Treatment: Wide excision if practicable

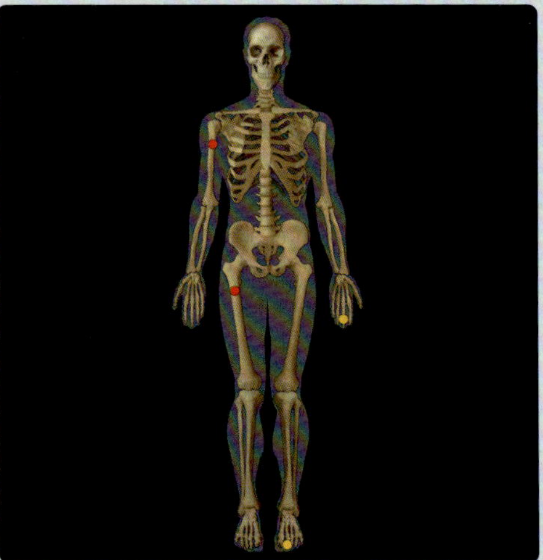

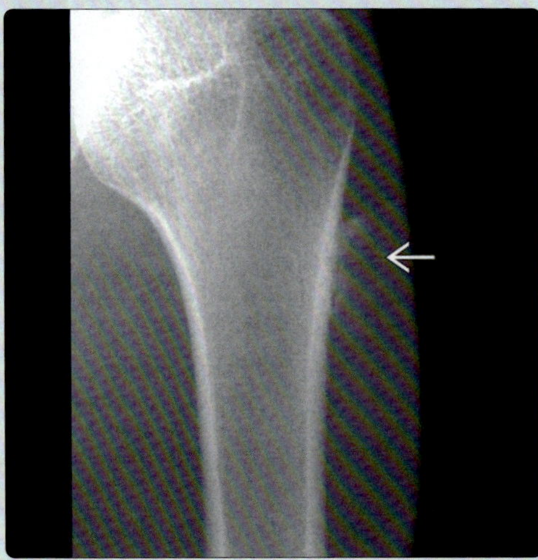

(Left) *Graphic depicts common locations of periosteal chondroma. The most common locations are the proximal metadiaphysis of the humerus and femur (red). Phalanges of the hands and feet are less common locations (yellow).* **(Right)** *AP radiograph shows a typical periosteal (juxtacortical) chondroma. There is a matrix-forming surface lesion of the proximal humeral metaphysis ➡. The cortex appears normal. Differential includes periosteal chondroma, periosteal osteosarcoma, and early parosteal osteosarcoma.*

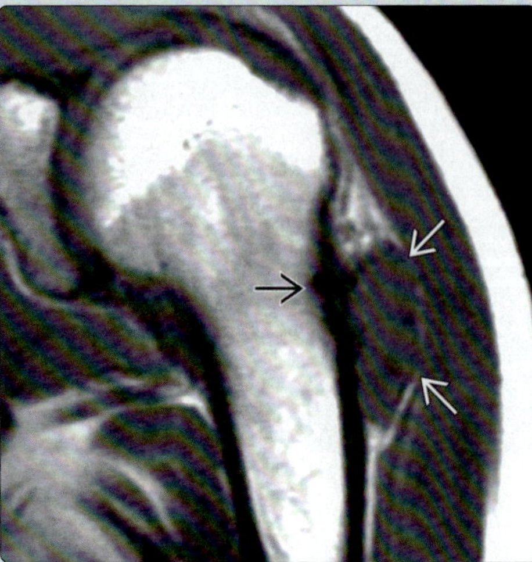

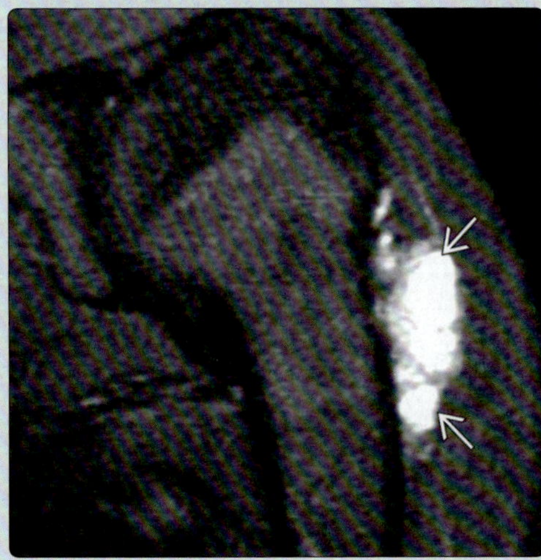

(Left) *Coronal T1WI MR in the same patient shows a low signal lesion containing some spicules of even lower signal ➡. Minimal intramedullary involvement is seen ➡.* **(Right)** *Coronal T2WI MR in the same patient shows the lesion to be lobulated ➡. Compared to the radiograph, the high signal mass extends slightly beyond the matrix. The lobulations are more suggestive of benign cartilage than of a surface osteosarcoma. The lesion is smaller and the patient younger than is usually seen in periosteal chondrosarcoma.*

TERMINOLOGY

Synonyms

- Juxtacortical chondroma, parosteal chondroma

Definitions

- Chondroid tumor arising in periosteal layer of tubular bones

IMAGING

General Features

- Best diagnostic clue
  - Surface lesion arising from metaphysis of tubular bone, producing chondroid matrix
- Location
  - Metaphyseal, arising on surface of bone
  - Proximal humerus and femur (70%)
  - Phalanges (25%) (hands > feet)
  - Rarely multiple
- Size
  - Median: 2.5 cm greatest diameter (mean: 2.2 cm) in 1 study (range: 1-6.5 cm)
    - Tends to be smaller than periosteal chondrosarcoma
      - Size may be one of the more important differentiating factors
- Morphology
  - Extends along long axis of surface of bone

Nuclear Medicine Findings

- Case report: PET/CT reported to be useful in distinguishing periosteal chondroma from periosteal chondrosarcoma using standard uptake value (SUV) max cutoff of 2.0 or 2.3

Imaging Recommendations

- Best imaging tool
  - Radiograph suggests diagnosis and differential
  - MR required to evaluate involvement of soft tissues &/or marrow

Radiographic Findings

- Saucerization of cortex
- Sclerotic margination
- Dense periosteal reaction, especially at proximal and distal ends of lesion
- Buttressing of cortex at proximal and distal ends of lesion
- Matrix calcification (75%)
- Soft tissue mass

CT Findings

- Mimics radiographic findings
- Matrix and saucerization of cortex may be better defined

MR Findings

- Lobulated configuration of mass
- Isointense or low T1 signal intensity
- Hyperintense T2 signal
- Heterogeneous enhancement, generally at periphery of lesion
- Intramedullary involvement (20%)
- Intramedullary edema (20%)
- Irregular soft tissue margins (30%)

DIFFERENTIAL DIAGNOSIS

Periosteal Chondrosarcoma

- Rare surface chondrosarcoma
- Same location as periosteal chondroma
- Usually low grade, so may not appear terribly aggressive
- Nearly identical imaging characteristics as periosteal chondroma
  - Surface lesion
  - Cortical scalloping
  - Matrix calcification
  - Similar MR characteristics
    - Lobulations of low-grade cartilage, high signal on fluid-sensitive sequences
    - Peripheral enhancement; small soft tissue mass
- No reliable differentiating factors from periosteal chondroma, but
  - May be larger than most periosteal chondromas
  - Arise in slightly older patient age group than periosteal chondromas

Periosteal Osteosarcoma

- Intermediate-grade surface osteosarcoma
- Same location as periosteal chondroma
- Nearly identical radiographic characteristics as periosteal chondroma
  - Similar propensity to scallop underlying cortex
  - Matrix calcification usually seen
    - Osteoid characteristics not always easily differentiated from chondroid
  - Soft tissue mass extending from osseous surface
    - MR does not show cartilage lobulation
    - Low signal osteoid central in lesion, with peripheral soft tissue mass

High-Grade Surface Osteosarcoma

- Rare high-grade osteosarcoma
- Same location as periosteal chondroma
- Faster growth pattern than periosteal chondroma
- Osteoid matrix located centrally in soft tissue mass
- Cortical scalloping but may also show invasion

Parosteal Osteosarcoma

- Mature parosteal osteosarcoma should not be confused with periosteal chondroma
  - Mature bone with "pasted on" appearance relative to underlying cortex
  - Common involvement of marrow
  - Location of common lesions is different: Distal femur, proximal tibia
- Immature parosteal osteosarcoma may be more difficult to distinguish from periosteal chondroma
  - Amorphous osteoid may simulate chondroid matrix at surface of bone
  - May be no marrow involvement early in process

PATHOLOGY

General Features

- Associated abnormalities
  - Rarely, associated enchondroma has been reported

- Confusing imaging may suggest chondrosarcoma arising from enchondroma

Gross Pathologic & Surgical Features

- Well marginated; thickened cortex, solid periosteal buttressing

Microscopic Features

- Similar histologic appearance to enchondroma
- Differentiation from periosteal chondrosarcoma may be difficult
  - Both sarcoma and chondroma show cellular atypia

CLINICAL ISSUES

Presentation

- Most common signs/symptoms
  - Pain, swelling
    - Phalangeal lesion: Painful subcutaneous lump
  - May be asymptomatic

Demographics

- Age
  - 2nd-4th decades most frequent; may occur in children
  - Slightly younger age group than periosteal chondrosarcomas
- Gender
  - Male = female
- Epidemiology
  - Rare: < 2% of all chondromas (majority are enchondroma)
  - Periosteal chondroma + periosteal chondrosarcoma account for 1% of bone tumors
    - Periosteal chondroma > > periosteal chondrosarcoma (3-4:1 ratio)

Natural History & Prognosis

- Slow local progression

Treatment

- Wide excision if practicable
  - Local excision sufficient if entire lesion proves to be periosteal chondroma
  - If part of lesion proves to be higher grade, suggesting periosteal chondrosarcoma, local (marginal) excision has high recurrence rate
- Local (marginal) excision if required for functional reasons

DIAGNOSTIC CHECKLIST

Consider

- Surface lesions may be difficult to differentiate from one another
  - Early chondroid and osteoid matrix may not be differentiated on radiographs
  - Parosteal osteosarcoma usually differentiated by maturity of matrix; may be difficult with immature lesion
  - High-grade surface osteosarcoma usually differentiated by rapidity of growth
  - Periosteal osteosarcoma and periosteal chondroma may be particularly difficult to differentiate on radiographs
    - If high signal lobulations are present on T2 MR, more suggestive of periosteal chondroma
- Imaging criteria for differentiating between periosteal chondrosarcoma and periosteal chondroma are sparse
  - Only moderate agreement exists between imaging and pathology in 1 study
  - Considered reasonable to be more concerned for chondrosarcoma if greatest diameter > 3 cm
  - Might consider wide excision of either lesion if practical

SELECTED REFERENCES

1. Kosaka H et al: Imaging features of periosteal chondroma manifesting as a subcutaneous mass in the index finger. Case Rep Orthop. 2014:763480, 2014
2. Morimoto S et al: Usefulness of PET/CT for diagnosis of periosteal chondrosarcoma of the femur: A case report. Oncol Lett. 7(6):1826-1828, 2014
3. Rabarin F et al: Focal periosteal chondroma of the hand: a review of 24 cases. Orthop Traumatol Surg Res. 100(6):617-20, 2014
4. Douis H et al: The imaging of cartilaginous bone tumours. I. Benign lesions. Skeletal Radiol. 41(10):1195-212, 2012
5. Yamamoto Y et al: Concurrent periosteal chondroma and enchondroma of the fibula mimicking chondrosarcoma. Skeletal Radiol. 35(5):302-5, 2006
6. Karabakhtsian R et al: Periosteal chondroma of the rib–report of a case and literature review. J Pediatr Surg. 40(9):1505-7, 2005
7. Hagiwara Y et al: Periosteal chondroma of the fifth toe–a case report. Ups J Med Sci. 109(1):65-70, 2004
8. Kahn S et al: Kissing periosteal chondroma and osteochondroma. Skeletal Radiol. 31(4):235-9, 2002
9. Lucas DR et al: Chondromas: enchondroma, periosteal chondroma, and enchondromatosis. In Fletcher CDM et al: World Health Organization Classification of Tumours: Tumours of Soft Tissue and Bone. Lyon: IARC Press. 237-40, 2002
10. Robinson P et al: Periosteal chondroid tumors: radiologic evaluation with pathologic correlation. AJR Am J Roentgenol. 177(5):1183-8, 2001
11. Woertler K et al: Periosteal chondroma: MR characteristics. J Comput Assist Tomogr. 25(3):425-30, 2001
12. Ishida T et al: Concurrent enchondroma and periosteal chondroma of the humerus mimicking chondrosarcoma. Skeletal Radiol. 27(6):337-40, 1998

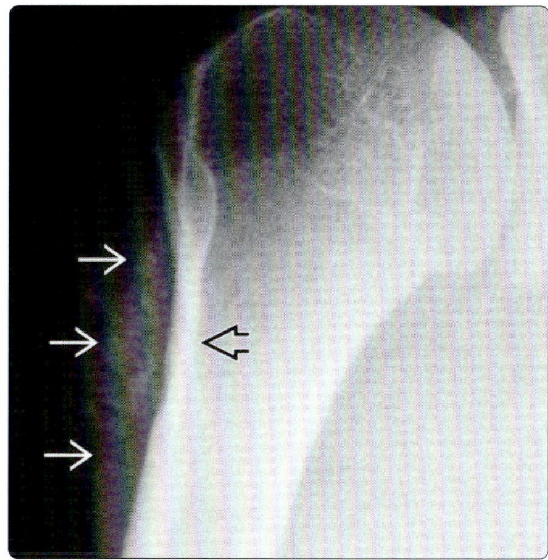

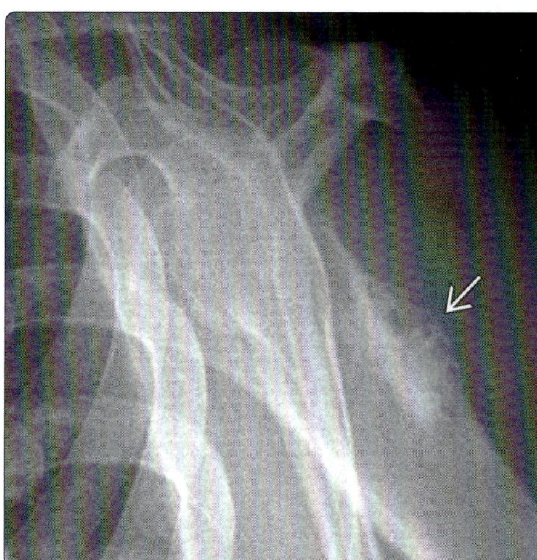

(Left) *AP radiograph shows fairly extensive but nonspecific matrix ➡ within a surface lesion of bone. The lesion has caused mild scalloping of the underlying cortex, which in turn shows some thickening ⇨. The lesion is typical, but not pathognomonic, of periosteal chondroma.* **(Right)** *Scapular Y radiograph shows an incidental finding, typical of periosteal chondroma. The surface lesion arises on the posterior cortex of the humeral metadiaphysis ➡. The lesion scallops the cortex, resulting in cortical sclerosis.*

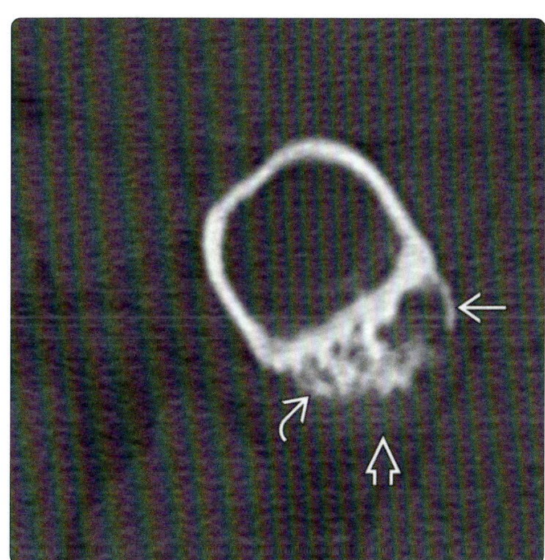

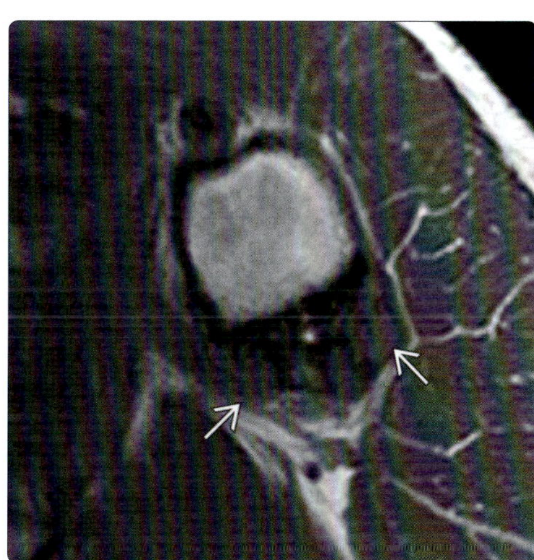

(Left) *Axial CT in the same patient confirms the cortical scalloping. There is a partial periosteal shell ➡ as well as calcified matrix within the lesion ➡. Soft tissue mass extends beyond the matrix ➡. This could represent periosteal chondroma, periosteal chondrosarcoma, periosteal osteosarcoma, or early parosteal osteosarcoma.* **(Right)** *Axial T1WI MR in the same patient shows the surface lesion to be of fairly homogeneous low signal intensity on T1 ➡, without underlying marrow involvement.*

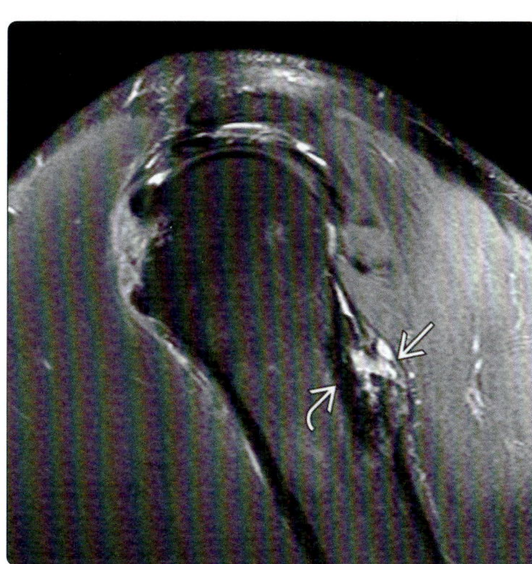

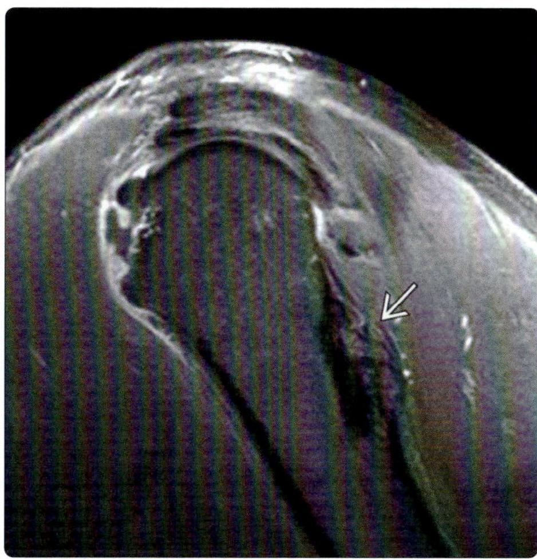

(Left) *Sagittal T2WI FS MR in the same case shows the dense sclerosis of the cortical reaction ➡. More peripherally in the lesion, there is a suggestion of high signal lobulation ➡. This is suggestive, but not diagnostic, of a cartilaginous lesion.* **(Right)** *Sagittal T1WI C+ FS MR shows only minimal enhancement of the chondroid portions of the lesion ➡. No intramedullary extension or edema is seen. The relatively small size and nonaggressive appearance favors periosteal chondroma as the diagnosis.*

(Left) *AP radiograph demonstrates a lesion that is either surface or cortically based ➡ in the metadiaphysis of a skeletally immature patient. If it is a cortically based lesion, this could represent an ossifying fibroma, or possibly even a cortically based fibrous dysplasia or sessile osteochondroma. However, surface lesion must be considered as well.* **(Right)** *AP bone scan shows abnormal uptake in the lesion ➡. It is solitary. The bone scan does not differentiate among the lesions under consideration.*

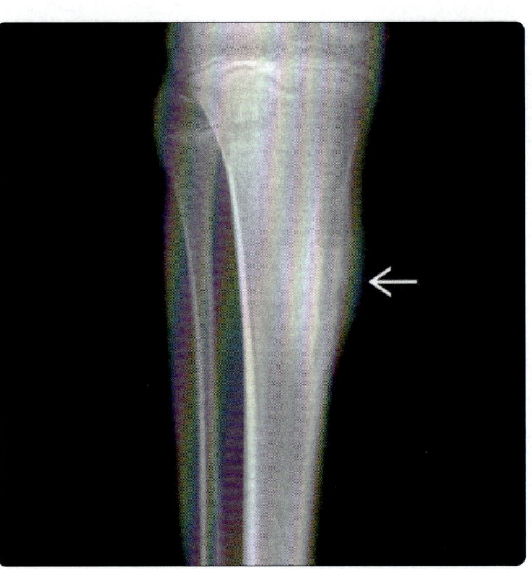

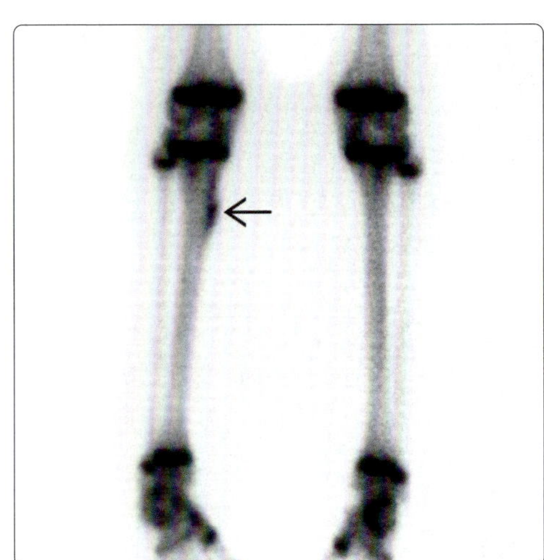

(Left) *Coronal T1WI MR in the same patient shows that there is no evidence of a soft tissue mass but simply matrix formation arising from the cortex ➡ of otherwise normal bone.* **(Right)** *Coronal T2WI MR shows that the lesion is higher signal intensity on T2 ➡. The underlying bone is normal. This removes the possibility of a cortically based lesion and places it as a surface lesion. Given that this is a surface lesion without soft tissue mass, periosteal chondroma is by far the best choice. This was proven at biopsy.*

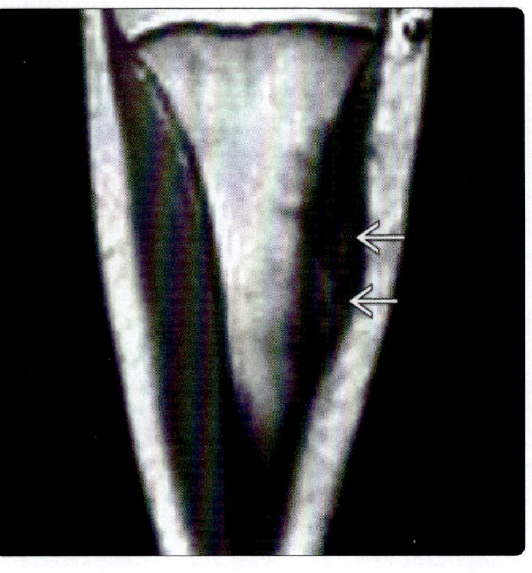

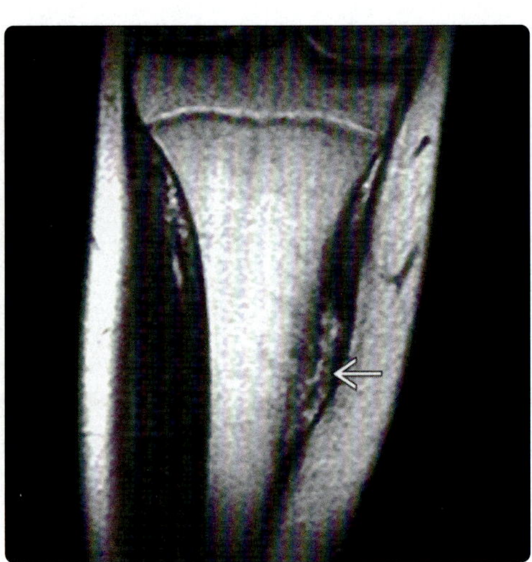

(Left) *Lateral radiograph shows scalloping of the cortex ➡ with cortical buttressing ➡ at the proximal and distal aspects of the lesion. There is no discernible matrix in this surface lesion.* **(Right)** *Axial CT confirms the cortical buttressing ➡ and scalloping ➡. The surface lesion in fact expands into the anterior soft tissues ➡ and contains fine matrix. This appearance may be seen with periosteal osteosarcoma, periosteal chondrosarcoma, or periosteal chondroma. The latter lesion is the most common and was proven.*

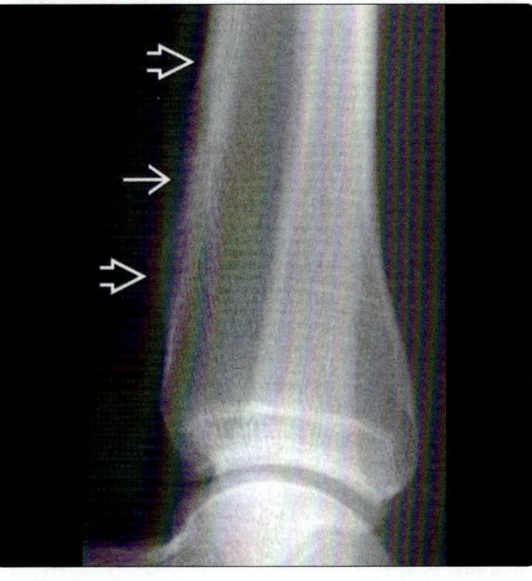

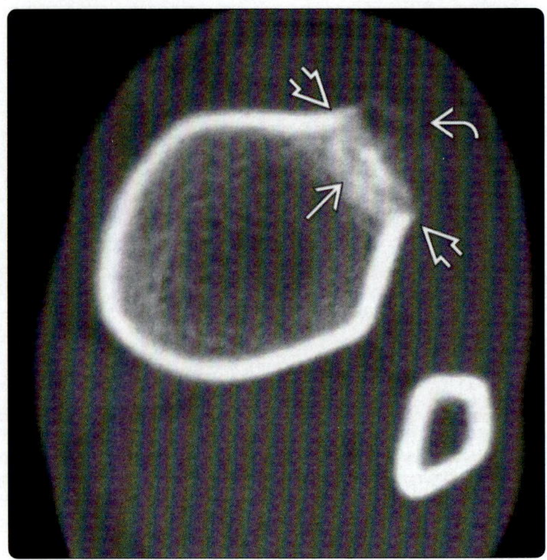

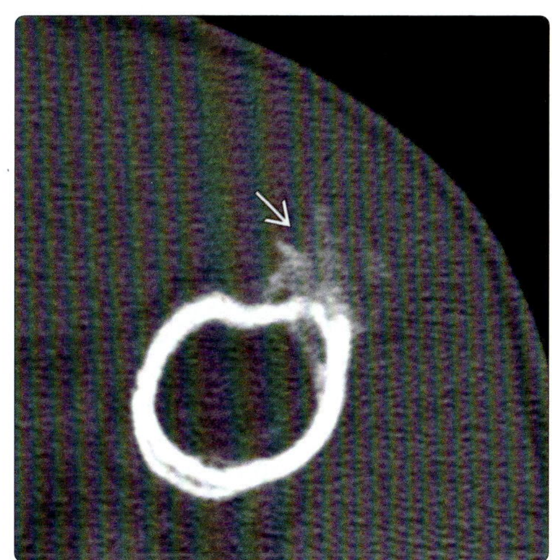

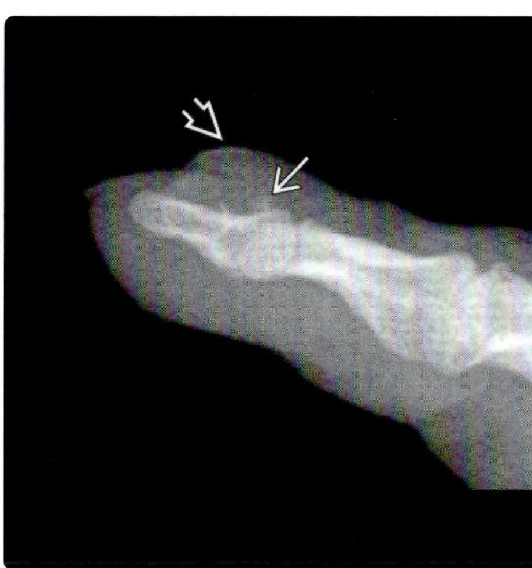

(Left) *Axial CT demonstrates a surface lesion in the metaphyseal region of bone. There is matrix within the soft tissue mass ➡. The lesion slightly scallops the cortex. This appearance is not specific for any of the surface bone lesions. Biopsy proved the most common lesion for this appearance, periosteal chondroma.* **(Right)** *Lateral radiograph demonstrates a soft tissue mass on the dorsum of the distal phalanx ⇨ as well as fairly mature matrix on the surface of the bone ➡. The underlying bone is undisturbed.*

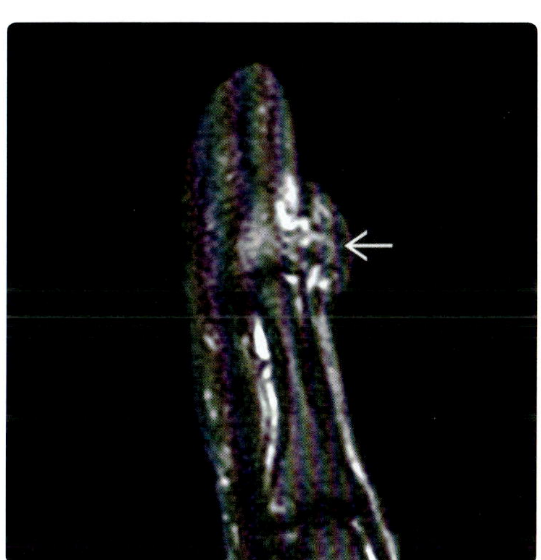

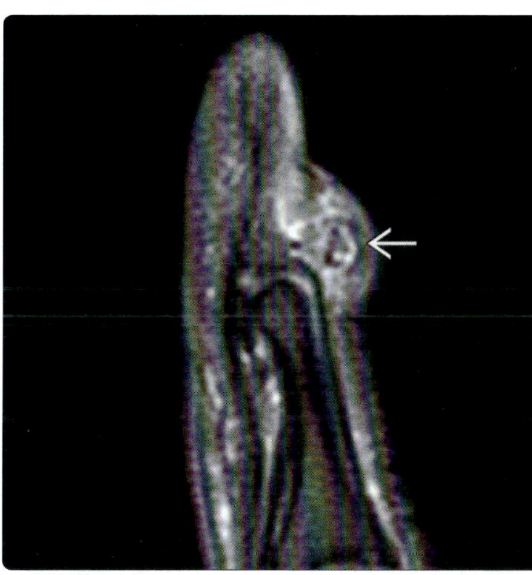

(Left) *Sagittal T2WI FSE MR in the same patient shows low signal matrix and high signal surrounding mass ➡.* **(Right)** *Sagittal T1WI C+ FS MR in the same patient shows enhancement of the mass ➡ surrounding the matrix. Of the surface lesions of bone, periosteal chondroma is the one that most frequently involves the phalanges. Biopsy proved the diagnosis of periosteal chondroma.*

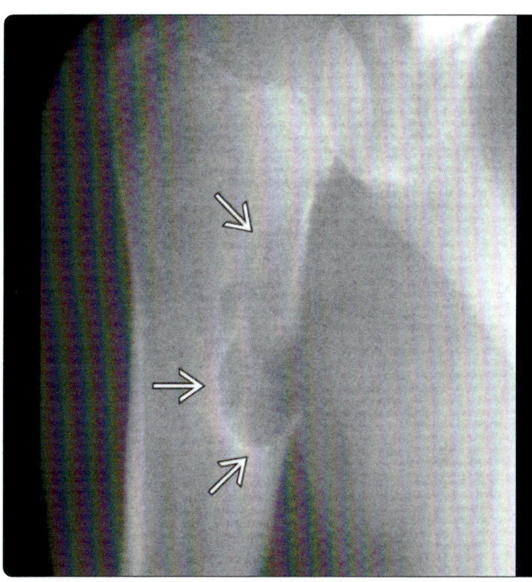

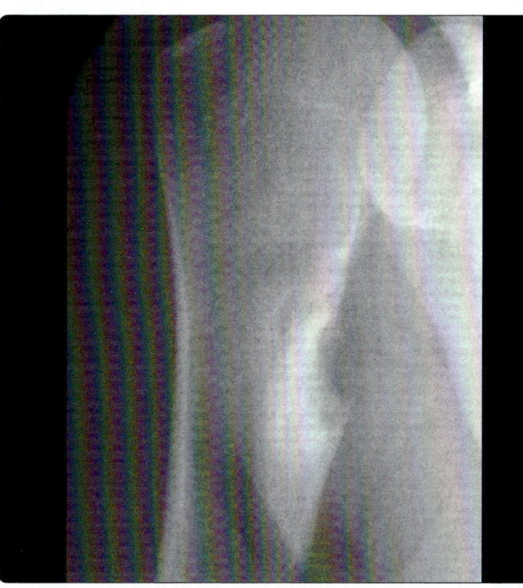

(Left) *AP x-ray shows a surface lesion, proven to be periosteal chondroma. It has scalloped out the underlying bone ➡. It is located in the metaphyseal region, with no obvious matrix or soft tissue mass. Differential diagnosis includes periosteal chondroma, periosteal osteosarcoma, and a cortically based lesion with a very thin rim, such as fibrous dysplasia or aneurysmal bone cyst. Periosteal chondroma was proven at biopsy.* **(Right)** *AP x-ray obtained 5 years later shows spontaneous regression of the lesion.*

Chondrosarcoma

KEY FACTS

TERMINOLOGY

- Malignant hyaline cartilage tumor
    - Primary chondrosarcoma (CS): Originates centrally in previously normal bone
    - Secondary CS: Originates in cartilaginous precursor (enchondroma or exostosis)

IMAGING

- Common locations: Iliac wing > proximal femur > proximal humerus > distal femur
- Chondroid matrix variably present (78%): Punctate, rings and arcs
    - Be aware of entirely lytic lesions that may appear deceptively nonaggressive
- Generally low-grade lesion, with limited appearance of aggressiveness on radiograph
- Scalloping 2/3 width of cortex (75% of CS) or 2/3 length of lesion suggests CS
- Often has endosteal cortical thickening
- Exophytic chondrosarcoma (arising from exostosis): Cartilage cap > 1 cm thick
- MR, T1WI: Lesion fairly isointense to skeletal muscle
    - Entrapped foci of yellow marrow much less frequently seen than in enchondromas
- MR, fluid-sensitive sequences: Variable inhomogeneity and organization of high signal
    - Low-grade lesion: Lobulated high signal appearance of benign or low-grade malignant cartilage (seen in 72% of chondrosarcomas)
    - High-grade lesion: Greater inhomogeneity and less organization of high signal; may not detect lobulation
- MR, postcontrast imaging: Varies with lesion grade
    - Low-grade lesion: Peripheral and septal enhancement around lobulated cartilage, with a few areas of "puddling," generally peripherally located
    - High-grade lesion: More generalized enhancement, surrounding low signal regions of necrosis

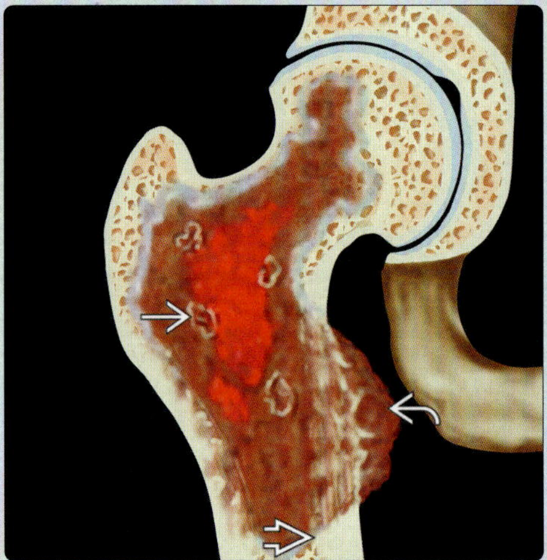

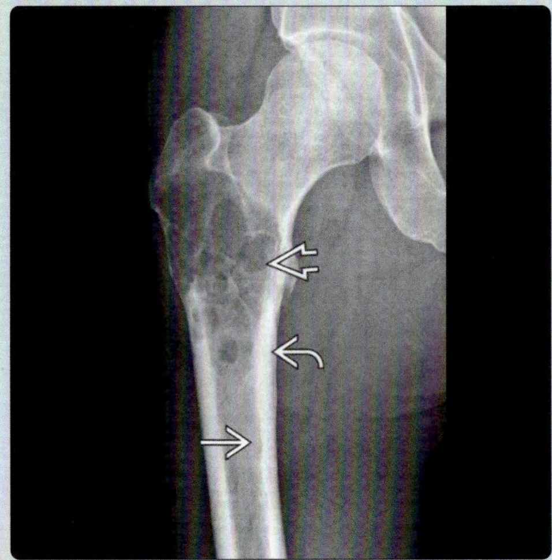

(Left) *Graphic displays intramedullary chondrosarcoma (CS) with islands of chondroid ➡, mild cortical breakthrough and a soft tissue mass ➡, and endosteal thickening ➡. These lesions tend to appear only moderately aggressive.* **(Right)** *AP radiograph shows a slightly bubbly lytic lesion in the metadiaphysis ➡. More distally the lesion changes character; it is more permeative and causes both endosteal scalloping ➡ and thickening ➡. This appearance is typical of low-grade CS.*

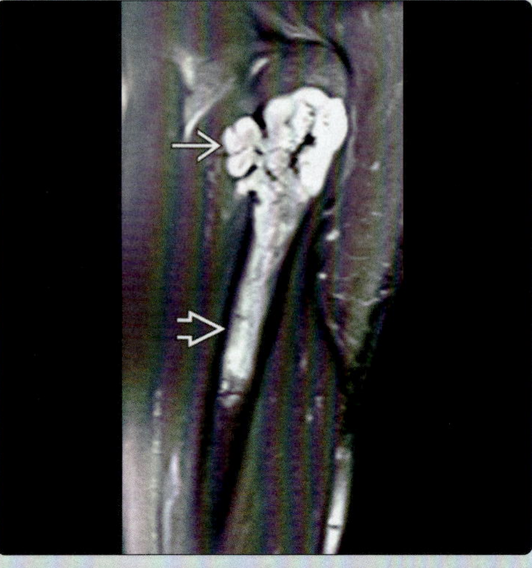

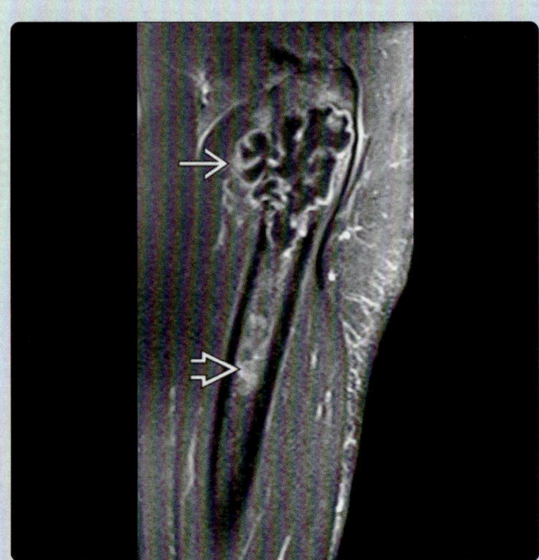

(Left) *Sagittal T2WI FS MR in the same patient shows the lesion to be high signal; proximally it is lobulated, which is typical of a low-grade cartilaginous lesion. There is cortical breakthrough anteriorly ➡. The proximal lobulations are in a region that is lower grade than the distal nonlobulated tumor ➡.* **(Right)** *Sagittal T1WI C+ FS MR at the same site shows peripheral enhancement surrounding lobules ➡. More importantly, there are regions of more confluent enhancement in the distal portion of the lesion ➡.*

TERMINOLOGY

Synonyms

- Primary chondrosarcoma (CS), conventional CS, secondary CS

Definitions

- Malignant hyaline cartilage tumor
  - Primary CS: Originates centrally in previously normal bone
  - Secondary CS: Originates in cartilaginous precursor (enchondroma or osteochondroma)

IMAGING

General Features

- Location
  - Iliac wing > proximal femur > proximal humerus > distal femur
  - Other bones (axial skeleton, craniofacial bones, distal appendicular skeleton) infrequently involved
  - Metaphyseal or metadiaphyseal
    - Epiphyseal lesion is uncommon but should raise a red flag
      - Enchondromas do not arise in epiphysis;a chondroid lesion that is not chondroblastoma at this site should raise suspicion for CS

Radiographic Findings

- Intramedullary CS (primary or secondary)
  - Lytic lesion arising centrally in metaphysis (most frequent) or diaphysis
  - Chondroid matrix variably present (78%): Punctate, rings and arcs (but lesion may be entirely lytic)
  - Generally low-grade lesion, with limited appearance of aggressiveness on radiograph
    - May appear fairly geographic
    - Cortical thinning or scalloping, with mild expansion
      - Scalloping 2/3 width of cortex (75% of CS) or 2/3 length of lesion suggests CS (rather than enchondroma)
      - Note: Enchondroma arising eccentrically adjacent to cortex normally shows similar scalloping
    - Often has endosteal cortical thickening as well
    - No periosteal reaction
    - Little or no cortical breakthrough/soft tissue mass
  - Higher grade intramedullary lesion uncommon; more aggressive appearance
    - Wide zone of transition without sclerotic margin
    - Cortical breakthrough (57% on radiography), soft tissue mass (46%)
  - Secondary CS may show transition from enchondroma to more aggressive chondrosarcoma
- CS in small tubular bones
  - Uncommon (enchondroma in this location may appear aggressive yet not be malignant)
  - Cortical expansion, bubbly appearance
  - Cortical breakthrough, soft tissue mass
  - Periosteal reaction
  - ± chondroid matrix
- Exophytic CS (secondary)
  - Underlying osteochondroma (stalk with normal marrow and cortex arising from normal bone)
  - Evidence of cartilage cap > 1 cm thick
    - Distorted fat planes
  - Snowstorm appearance or evidence of change in character and location of matrix
  - Osseous destruction, soft tissue mass

CT Findings

- Mimics radiographic findings
  - Distance and depth of scalloping better seen on CT
  - Length of scalloping seen well on longitudinal reformatted images
- May better define matrix (seen in 94%)
- May infer size of cartilage cap in exophytic CS, but measurement is usually not reliable

MR Findings

- Matrix (seen in 79%): Low signal on all sequences
- Scalloping of endosteal cortex and extent well seen
  - Scalloping 2/3 depth of cortex seen on MR in 85% of CS
- Soft tissue mass seen on MR in 76% of CS
- T1WI: Lesion fairly isointense to skeletal muscle
  - Entrapped foci of yellow marrow much less frequently seen than in enchondromas
- Fluid-sensitive sequences: Variable inhomogeneity and organization of high signal
  - Low-grade lesion: Lobulated high signal appearance of benign or low-grade malignant cartilage (seen in 72% of CS)
  - High-grade lesion: Greater inhomogeneity and less organization of the high signal; may not detect lobulation
- Postcontrast T1 FS imaging: Varies with lesion grade
  - Low-grade lesion: Peripheral and septal enhancement around lobulated cartilage, with few areas of confluence, generally peripherally located
  - Fast contrast-enhanced gradient-echo MR may help differentiate enchondroma from low-grade CS
    - Earlier enhancement in CS but significant overlap
  - High-grade lesion: More generalized enhancement, surrounding low signal regions of necrosis
- Dynamic contrast-enhanced MR may differentiate enchondroma from low-grade CS
  - Threshold values of relative enhancement = 2 and slope = 4.5 said to diagnose 100% CS but with 37% false-positive diagnosis in enchondromas
- Exophytic CS (secondary)
  - Cartilage cap seen as high signal on fluid-sensitive images, > 1 cm in thickness
  - Soft tissue mass, osseous destruction better defined

Image-Guided Biopsy

- Oncologic centers differ in whether they pursue percutaneous biopsy of cartilage tumors
  - Concern for tissue sampling error
    - Cartilage lesions often require large portions of lesion for correct diagnosis, far larger than obtained with percutaneous biopsy
  - Concern about tracking tumor cells by hematoma or needle, contaminating tissue needed for reconstruction

DIFFERENTIAL DIAGNOSIS

Enchondroma

- Central metaphyseal, usually with chondroid matrix
- Difficult to differentiate from low-grade CS
  - Eccentric enchondroma arising adjacent to cortex is expected to cause endosteal scalloping and even minor cortical disruption

PATHOLOGY

General Features

- Genetics
  - Multistep genetic model for secondary CS
- Associated abnormalities
  - Secondary CS
    - Enchondroma: Rate of degeneration of solitary enchondroma unknown
      - Rate of degeneration in Ollier (multiple enchondromatosis) ~ 25%
      - Rate of degeneration in Maffucci ~ 25%
    - Osteochondroma: Rate of degeneration of solitary lesion < 1%
      - Multiple hereditary exostosis: Rate of degeneration ~ 3%

Staging, Grading, & Classification

- Lesion graded histologically on scale of 1-3
  - Based on nuclear size, hyperchromasia, and cellularity
  - Grade 1 very similar to enchondroma
  - Majority (61%) are grade 1, 36% grade 2, 3% grade 3

Microscopic Features

- Blue-gray cartilage, irregularly shaped lobules separated by fibrous bands
- More cellular than enchondroma, varying by field, with atypical chondrocytes

CLINICAL ISSUES

Presentation

- Most common signs/symptoms
  - Pain and swelling
    - Anecdotally, enchondroma is painless and CS is painful
      - In fact, enchondromas are often reported as painful; pain alone is not enough to differentiate enchondroma from CS
    - Skillful evaluation should differentiate tumor pain from adjacent joint mechanical pain
  - Often of long duration prior to medical attention
    - Particularly so with iliac wing lesions, which are often very large by time of detection

Demographics

- Age
  - Peak incidence 50-70 years of age
  - Wide range; do not use age to eliminate diagnosis of CS in teenager or young adult
- Gender
  - Male predominance (M:F = 1.5:1)
- Epidemiology
  - 3rd most common malignant bone neoplasm
  - Conventional CS accounts for 90% of CS (including less common extraskeletal, periosteal, dedifferentiated)

Natural History & Prognosis

- Prognosis relates to several factors
  - Histologic grade is most important predictor
    - Grade 1: 89% 5-year survival
    - Grade 2 and 3 combined: 53% 5-year survival
  - Tumor necrosis, mitotic count, myxoid matrix
  - Outcome of advanced unresectable central CS: Survival 48% at 1 year, 24% at 2 years, 12% at 3 years
- Late metastases: Lung, bone

Treatment

- Wide resection
- Recurrence related to contamination of surgical bed or to margins that are not tumor-free
  - Any contamination puts patient at risk for recurrence; cartilage tumors do not need to establish significant blood supply to grow
  - 10% of recurrences have higher grade
- Surveillance for recurrence/metastases for 10 years

DIAGNOSTIC CHECKLIST

Consider

- **Caution**: Intramedullary CS of femur or humerus is usually low grade and appears nonaggressive
  - Significant numbers of these lesions are underdiagnosed, either as enchondroma or another lesion if no chondroid matrix is present
  - Large "enchondroma" in either femur or humerus should be viewed with suspicion
  - Any thickening or significant scalloping of cortex should heighten suspicion for CS
- May be extremely difficult to differentiate low-grade CS from enchondroma
  - Scalloping of endosteal cortex over significant length of lesion is suggestive on radiograph/CT
    - Exception: Eccentric enchondroma arising adjacent to cortex expected to cause endosteal scalloping and even minor cortical disruption
  - Increased matrix or enlargement of enchondroma need not imply chondrosarcomatous change; enchondromas may show such alterations normally
  - Cartilage cap thickness > 1 cm suggestive of transformation in exostosis

SELECTED REFERENCES

1. Brown MT et al: How safe is curettage of low-grade cartilaginous neoplasms diagnosed by imaging with or without pre-operative needle biopsy? Bone Joint J. 96-B(8):1098-105, 2014
2. Douis H et al: MRI differentiation of low-grade from high-grade appendicular chondrosarcoma. Eur Radiol. 24(1):232-40, 2014
3. De Coninck T et al: Dynamic contrast-enhanced MR imaging for differentiation between enchondroma and chondrosarcoma. Eur Radiol. 23(11):3140-52, 2013
4. Meftah M et al: Long-term results of intralesional curettage and cryosurgery for treatment of low-grade chondrosarcoma. J Bone Joint Surg Am. 95(15):1358-64, 2013

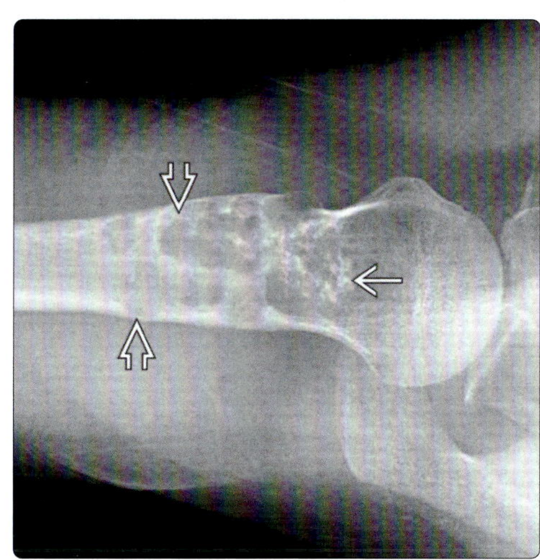

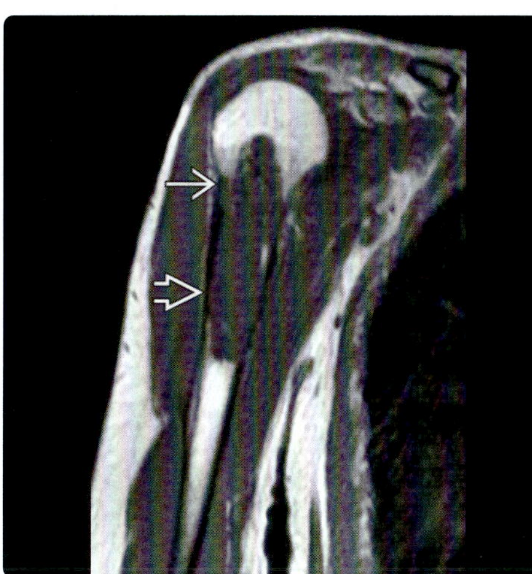

(Left) *Lateral radiograph shows evidence of enchondroma containing chondroid matrix in the proximal humeral metaphysis →. Distal to the enchondroma, there is a lytic lesion that results in mild expansion and cortical scalloping →; this change in character of the lesion represents low-grade CS.* **(Right)** *Coronal T1 MR in the same patient shows the expected hypointensity in both the enchondromatous → and chondrosarcomatous → portions of the lesion.*

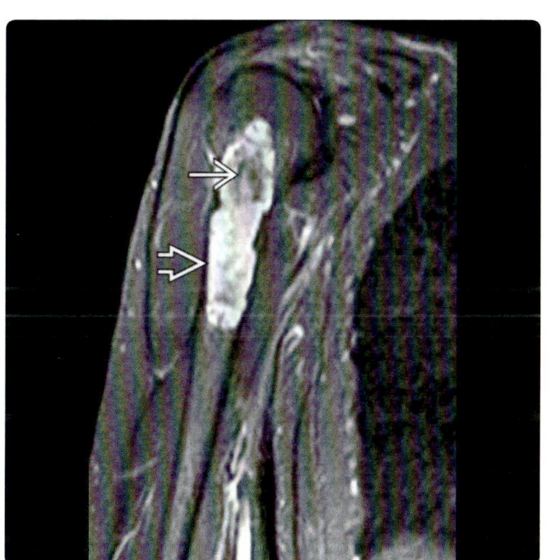

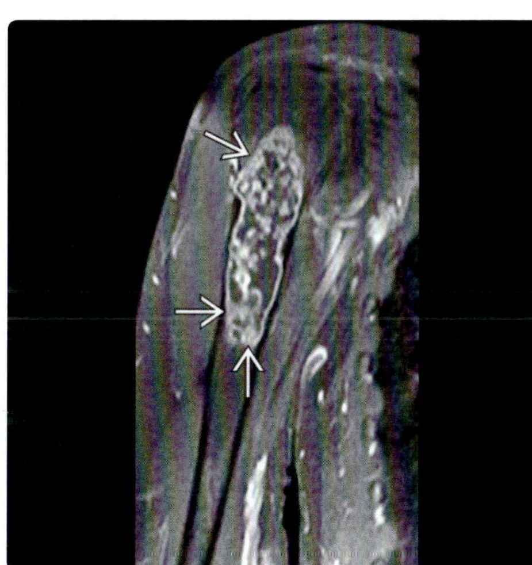

(Left) *Coronal T2WI FS MR in the same site shows low signal located proximally within the lesion, that of the chondroid matrix →. Nonspecific high signal extends distally within the lesion →; there is no cortical breakthrough. Note the lack of distinct cartilage lobulation.* **(Right)** *Coronal postcontrast T1FS MR in the same site shows the expected peripheral enhancement. There is also puddling of contrast at several sites that are not septal →. This may be suggestive, but not diagnostic, of CS; low-grade CS was proven at biopsy.*

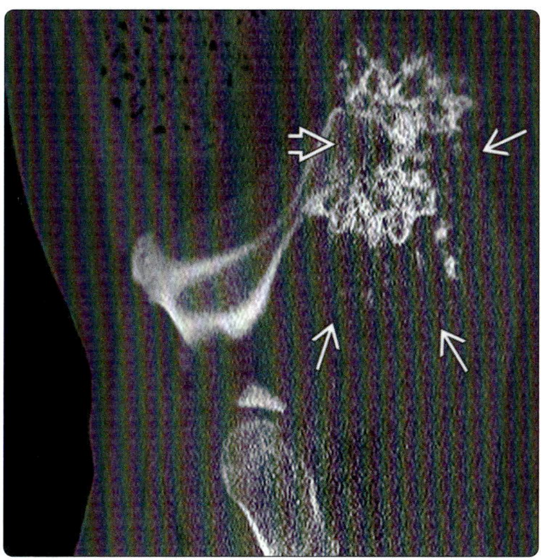

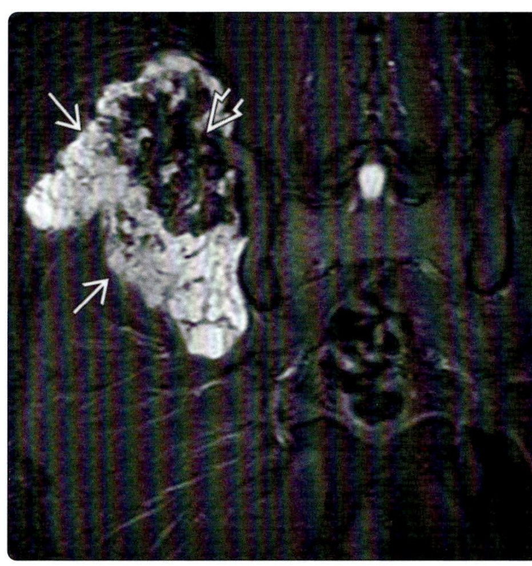

(Left) *Sagittal bone CT reconstruction shows an exostosis arising from the iliac wing →. The regular portion of the exostosis is surrounded by a soft tissue mass that contains a snowstorm appearance of chondroid matrix →. This appearance is classic for transformation of exostosis to CS.* **(Right)** *Coronal STIR MR in the same patient shows the underlying exostosis → with the thick hyperintense cartilage cap → surrounding it, representing chondrosarcomatous transformation.*

(Left) *AP radiograph shows a lytic eccentric lesion with a narrow zone of transition but no sclerotic margin ➔ extending to the subchondral bone. The diagnosis based on the radiograph should be giant cell tumor.* **(Right)** *Coronal T2WI MR in the same patient shows lobulated high signal throughout the lesion ➔, which is more typical of a chondroid lesion than giant cell tumor (high signal, not lobulated, with some central low signal). The MR may suggest enchondroma, but location does not. One must suspect CS.*

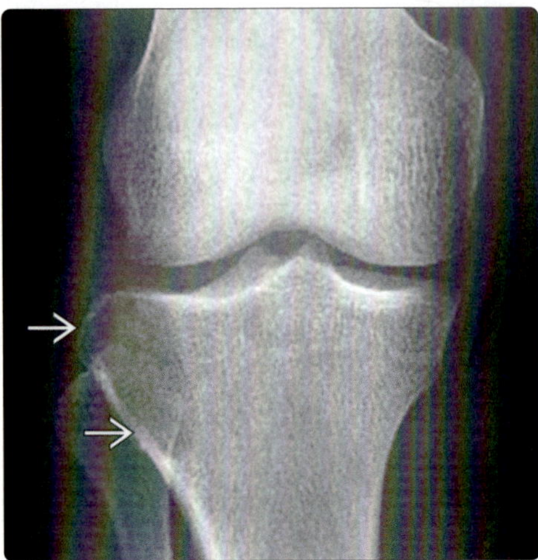

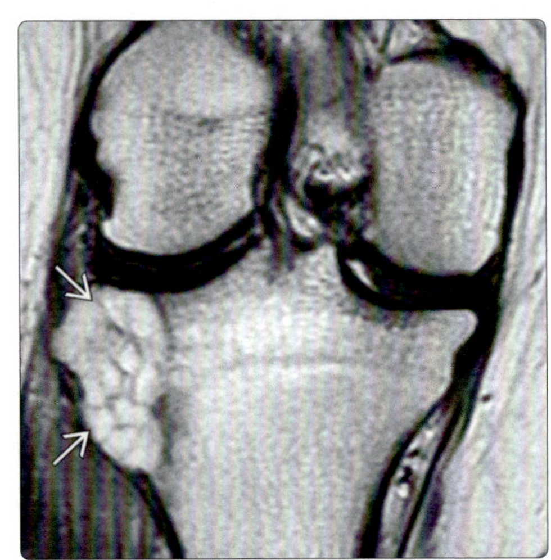

(Left) *Coronal T1 C+ FS MR in the same slice shows peripheral and septal enhancement ➔ as well as a region of more confluent enhancement ⇨. There is marrow edema. At biopsy, this was grade 2 CS.* **(Right)** *AP radiograph shows a completely lytic CS. The lesion is moderately aggressive, with sclerotic margin but cortical breakthrough ⇨ and pathologic fracture. Although this certainly could represent either a metastatic lesion or myeloma, CS should be a consideration. CS may be completely lytic.*

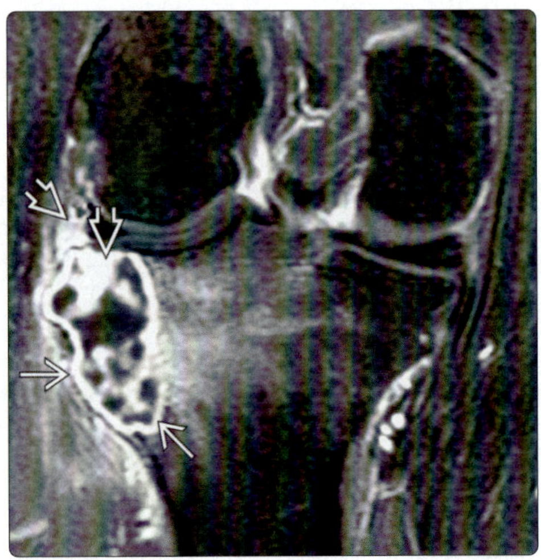

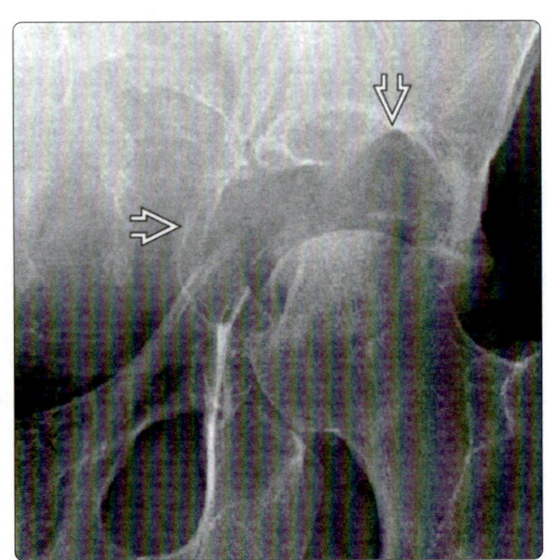

(Left) *Coronal PD FS MR in the same patient shows inhomogeneous ↑ SI ➔. This is diagnostically nonspecific. More important, note the high signal extending along the pelvic wall ⇨, likely representing hematoma due to pathologic fracture.* **(Right)** *Coronal T1WI C+ FS MR in the same slice shows peripheral enhancement with some other regions of high signal outside the original lesion ➔. Biopsy showed low-grade CS, but there was also tumor studding the structures of the left hemipelvis, a serious consequence of fracture.*

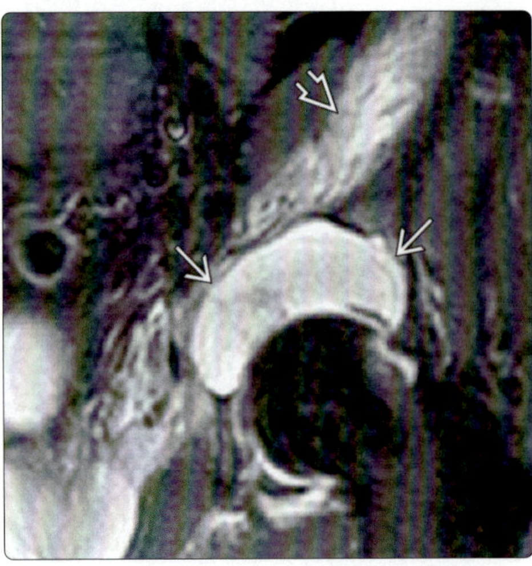

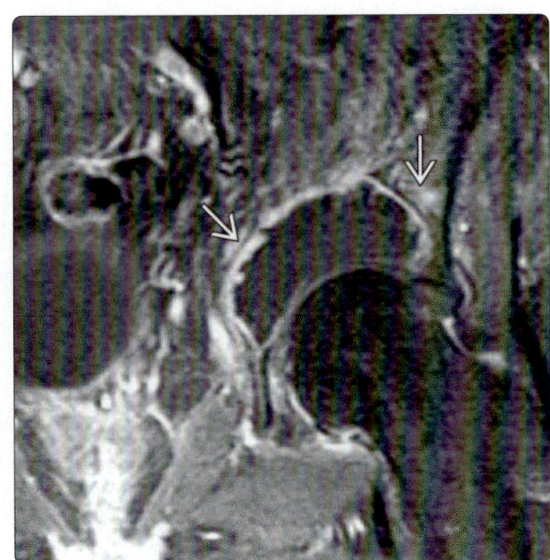

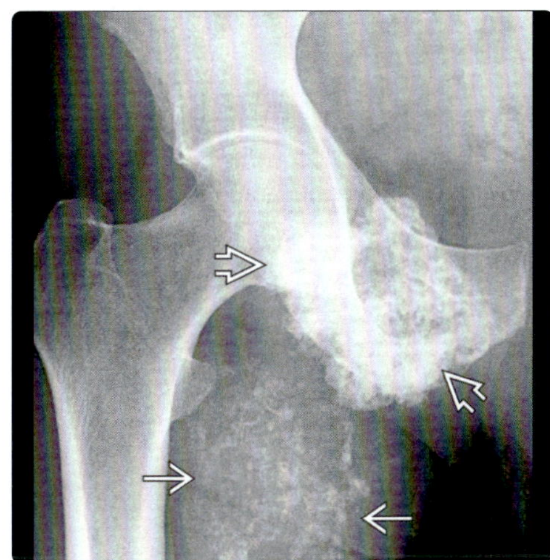

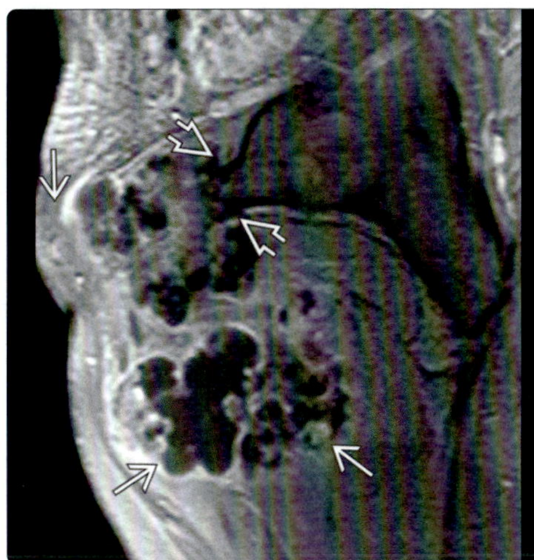

(Left) *AP radiograph shows an exophytic CS. There is a very large soft tissue mass containing chondroid matrix* ➡ *that has a snowstorm appearance. The mass has a different character proximally, where the exostosis arises from the pubic ramus; the chondroid matrix is quite mature and organized* ➡. **(Right)** *Sagittal T1WI C+ FS MR in the same patient shows the exostosis stalk* ➡. *Peripherally, there is a disorganized mass* ➡ *consisting of a thickened cartilage cap and necrotic chondrosarcomatous tissue.*

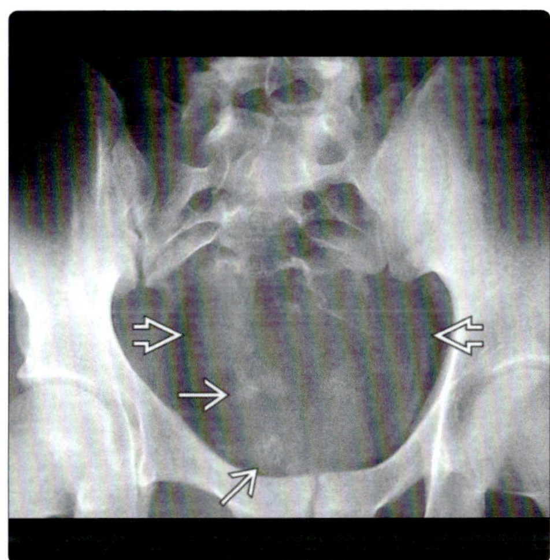

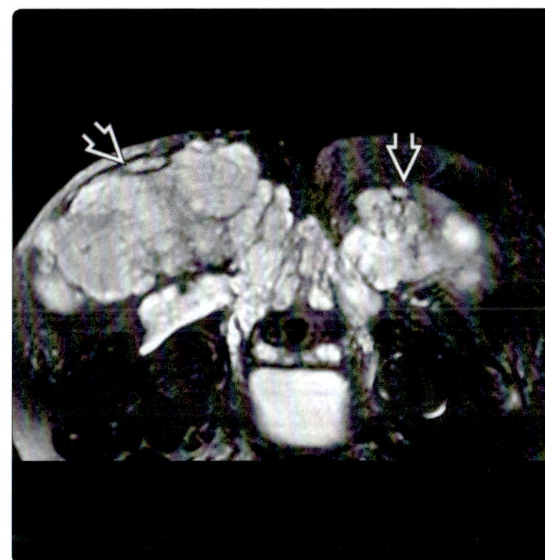

(Left) *AP radiograph shows destruction of the distal elements of the sacrum, with a large soft tissue mass* ➡. *Matrix is seen within the mass* ➡ *that, on radiograph, may either be chondroid or fragments of bone left within a mass, such as a chordoma.* **(Right)** *Axial T2WI MR in the prone position shows the soft tissue mass to be even larger than expected, extending into both buttocks* ➡ *as well as anteriorly. There is extensive high signal lobulation, typical of low-grade CS. CS is a common sacral tumor.*

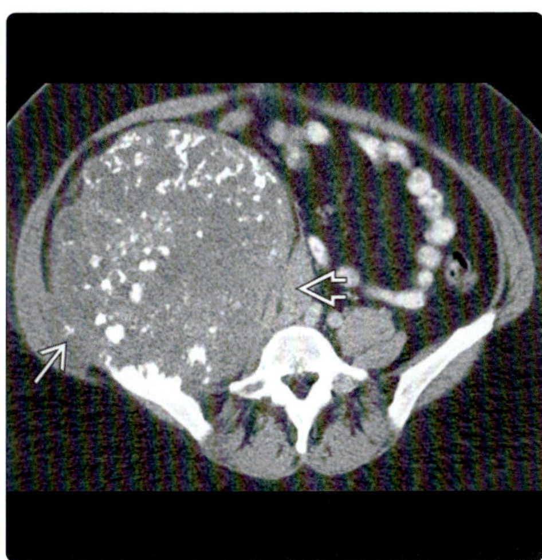

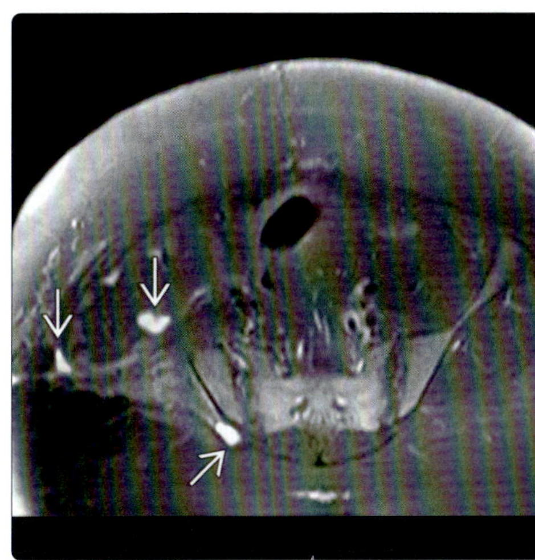

(Left) *Axial CT demonstrates a large, chondroid, matrix-containing mass arising from the right iliac wing* ➡. *It extends anteriorly, displacing the iliopsoas* ➡; *this explains how iliac wing CS may be so large prior to detection. The diagnosis must be CS; treatment is wide resection.* **(Right)** *Axial T2WI FS MR in the same patient obtained 6 months following resection shows multiple sites of recurrence as high signal nodules* ➡. *It is important to recognize that postoperative recurrence of CS is a significant risk.*

Dedifferentiated Chondrosarcoma

KEY FACTS

TERMINOLOGY

- Chondrosarcoma containing 2 distinct components
  - Well-differentiated cartilage tumor (usually low-grade chondrosarcoma, rarely enchondroma or osteochondroma)
  - High-grade noncartilaginous sarcoma (most commonly osteosarcoma or MFH but other sarcomas may occur)

IMAGING

- Location: Femur > pelvis > humerus
- Bimorphic: Low-grade or benign cartilaginous portion and high-grade sarcomatous portion
  - Evident on radiograph in 53% (some patients have findings more typical of conventional chondrosarcoma)
- MR: Bimorphic pattern of high- and low-grade portions of lesion not identified in all cases
  - MR more likely to demonstrate dominant high-grade portion than radiograph or CT
- MR of underlying cartilaginous portion of lesion
  - May be intramedullary or have typical appearance of enchondroma or low-grade chondrosarcoma
  - Low signal chondroid matrix, all sequences (66%)
  - High signal lobulations typical of cartilage
  - May have typical appearance of osteochondroma or exophytic chondrosarcoma
- MR of noncartilaginous high-grade sarcoma
  - Osseous invasion, soft tissue mass
  - Not as much (or as organized) matrix

TOP DIFFERENTIAL DIAGNOSES

- Chondrosarcoma
  - Initial impression of dedifferentiated chondrosarcoma is of conventional chondrosarcoma on radiographs in 85% of cases and CT in 89% of cases
  - If focal region of dedifferentiation is missed, lesion will be undertreated
  - Thorough evaluation of full extent of any cartilage lesion is crucial

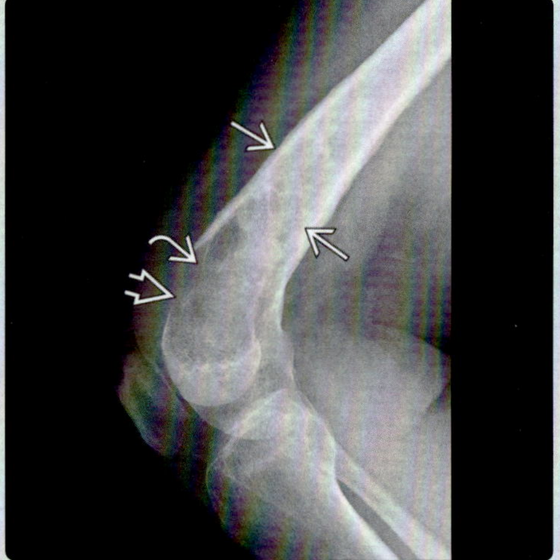

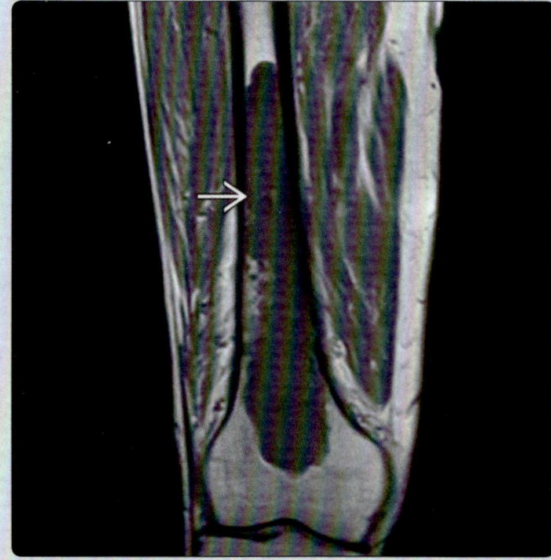

(Left) *Lateral radiograph shows chondroid matrix with mild endosteal scalloping ➡ within a metadiaphyseal lesion. This is typical of chondrosarcoma. However, there is a red flag here: There is a change in character in the distal-most aspect, where the lesion becomes entirely lytic ➡, with anterior cortical breakthrough ➡. One must be concerned for dedifferentiation of this chondrosarcoma.* **(Right)** *Coronal T1 MR shows mostly homogeneous intermediate signal, with some low signal chondroid ➡.*

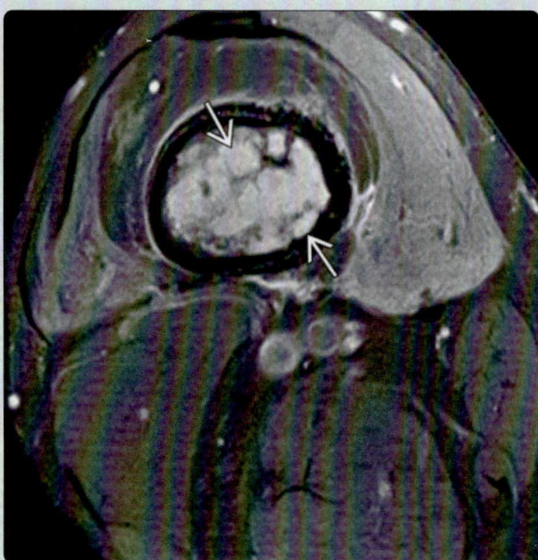

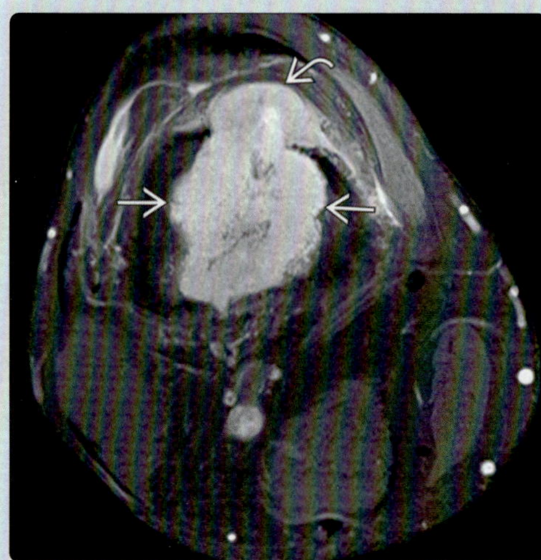

(Left) *Axial T2 FS MR through the metadiaphysis shows typical low-grade chondrosarcoma, with multiple hyperintense lobules ➡ and only mild endosteal scalloping.* **(Right)** *Axial T2 FS MR obtained slightly more distally in the metaphysis shows confluence of the high signal lesion ➡ with anterior cortical breakthrough/soft tissue mass ➡. This is the region of dedifferentiation into high-grade spindle cell sarcoma. Biopsy must be obtained from this more aggressive portion of the lesion.*

TERMINOLOGY

Definitions

- Distinct variety of chondrosarcoma containing 2 distinct components
  - Well-differentiated cartilage tumor (usually low-grade chondrosarcoma, rarely enchondroma or osteochondroma)
  - High-grade noncartilaginous sarcoma (most commonly osteosarcoma or malignant fibrous histiocytoma)

IMAGING

General Features

- Location
  - Femur > pelvis > humerus

Radiographic Findings

- Bimorphic: Low-grade or benign cartilaginous portion and high-grade sarcomatous portion
  - Evident on radiograph in 53%
  - Some patients have findings more typical of conventional chondrosarcoma
- Cartilaginous portion
  - Lytic, often containing chondroid matrix
  - Fairly geographic, but usually no sclerotic margin
  - Cortex: Thinned, scalloped, and expanded (67%)
    - Low-grade chondrosarcoma cortex often shows endosteal thickening (32%)
  - Generally no (or minimal) cortical breakthrough and no soft tissue mass in cartilaginous portion
  - Uncommon: Osteochondroma (sometimes in setting of multiple hereditary osteochondromas)
- Noncartilaginous high-grade sarcomatous portion
  - Distinctly destructive, permeative osseous process
  - More likely lytic, without (or with less) matrix
    - If dedifferentiated portion is osteosarcoma, may contain amorphous osteoid matrix (6% of cases)
  - Cortical breakthrough
  - Soft tissue mass (seen on radiograph in 25-87% in 2 separate series)
  - Aggressive periosteal reaction
  - If arising from osteochondroma, soft tissue mass and destruction of adjacent cortex & exostosis may be seen

MR Findings

- Bimorphic pattern of high- and low-grade portions of lesion **not** identified in all cases
  - MR more likely to demonstrate dominant high-grade portion than radiograph or CT
- Underlying cartilaginous portion of lesion
  - May have typical appearance of enchondroma or low-grade chondrosarcoma
    - ↓ signal chondroid matrix, all sequences, in 66%
    - High signal lobulations typical of cartilage
    - Peripheral nodular enhancement with contrast
  - May have typical appearance of osteochondroma or exophytic chondrosarcoma
    - Cortex and marrow extending from bone
    - High T2 cartilage cap; thin if osteochondroma, > 1-cm thick if chondrosarcoma
- Noncartilaginous high-grade sarcomatous portion
  - Osseous invasion, soft tissue mass
  - Not likely to have as much (or as organized) matrix
  - Inhomogeneous T1 signal isointense with muscle
  - Fluid-sensitive sequences: Heterogeneously ↑ signal
  - Intense enhancement post contrast, with low signal regions of necrosis

DIFFERENTIAL DIAGNOSIS

Chondrosarcoma, Conventional

- Underlying chondroid matrix
- Cortical scalloping, often with other regions of endosteal cortical thickening
- Initial impression of dedifferentiated chondrosarcoma is of conventional chondrosarcoma on radiographs in 85% of cases and CT in 89% of cases
  - Dedifferentiated areas may not be readily visible

PATHOLOGY

General Features

- Genetics
  - No specific chromosomal aberrations
    - Structural and numerical aberrations frequently seen in chromosomes 1 and 9, but not specific
  - Both tumor components appear to share common origin
    - Likely early division of 2 cell clones

CLINICAL ISSUES

Demographics

- Age
  - Typically 50-60 years (range: 29-85 years)
- Gender
  - Slight male preponderance (53%)
- Epidemiology
  - 10% of chondrosarcomas

Natural History & Prognosis

- Overall 24% survival at 5 years (median survival: 13 months)
- Distant metastases present at time of diagnosis in 21%
  - 5-month median survival in these patients
- Patients presenting with no sign of metastases are treated aggressively: 28% survival at 10 years

Treatment

- Wide resection
- Radiation, chemotherapy (not proven to be efficacious)

DIAGNOSTIC CHECKLIST

Consider

- Bimorphic pattern not easily seen in ~ 50% of cases
  - Watch carefully for low-grade cartilage lesions with adjacent high-grade aggressive abnormalities
  - Thorough evaluation of entire lesion in any cartilage tumor is critical

SELECTED REFERENCES

1. Bindiganavile S et al: Long-term outcome of chondrosarcoma: a single institutional experience. Cancer Res Treat. 47(4):897-903, 2015

Periosteal Chondrosarcoma

KEY FACTS

TERMINOLOGY

- Rare variety of chondrosarcoma arising in periosteal layer of tubular bones

IMAGING

- Metadiaphyseal surface lesion, often femur
- Majority contain chondroid matrix (75%)
- May extend slightly into medullary space (25%)
- Rarely elicit intramedullary & soft tissue edema
- Soft tissue extension may have irregular margins

TOP DIFFERENTIAL DIAGNOSES

- Periosteal chondroma
  - 4x more frequent than periosteal chondrosarcoma
  - May appear identical by imaging
  - Tendency toward younger age, smaller lesions (< 3 cm) compared to chondrosarcoma (> 3 cm)
- Periosteal osteosarcoma
  - Surface lesion with similar characteristics of cortical scalloping, minimal osseous invasion
  - Soft tissue mass contains osteoid matrix, which may be differentiated from chondroid

PATHOLOGY

- Histologic differentiation from periosteal chondroma may be difficult
  - Greater cellular atypia in chondrosarcoma
  - Greater osseous & soft tissue invasion than chondroma

CLINICAL ISSUES

- Asymptomatic or mildly painful mass
- Most are well-differentiated, low-grade lesions
  - Wide excision is usually sufficient treatment
  - Metastases rare when adequately treated
  - High recurrence rate with marginal excision

(Left) *Lateral radiograph demonstrates a lobulated, mixed sclerotic and lytic lesion > 3 cm in length arising from the distal femoral metadiaphyseal surface ➡. This was an incidental finding. Differential includes all of the surface lesions (parosteal & periosteal osteosarcoma, periosteal chondroma, & periosteal chondrosarcoma).* **(Right)** *Axial NECT confirms that the lobulated lesion is cortically located, extending into the posterior soft tissues ➡. Along the majority of the lesion, the bone cortex is undulating but intact.*

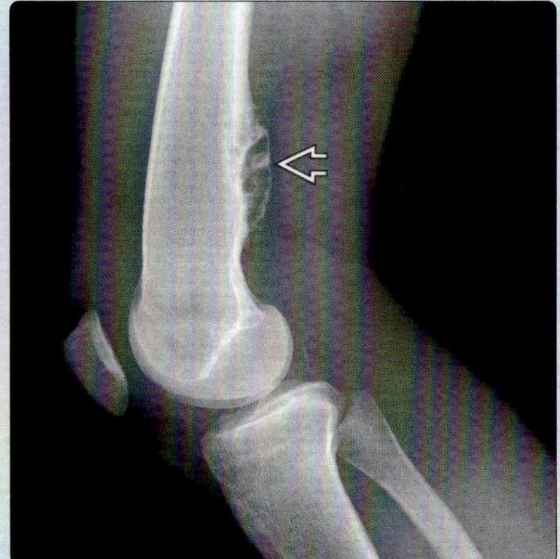

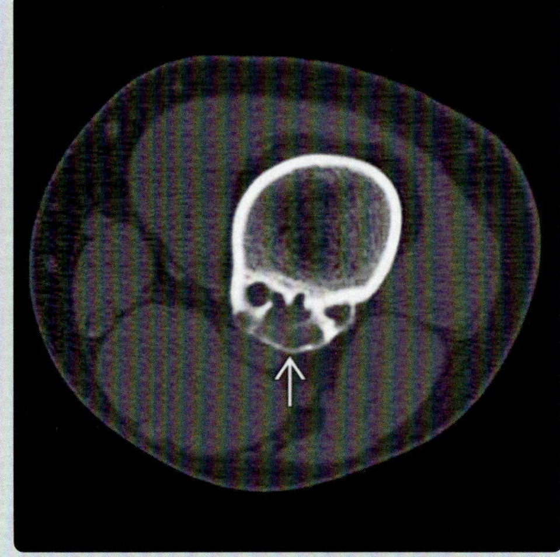

(Left) *Sagittal T2WI FS MR in the same patient reveals that the lobulated contents are markedly hyperintense, a typical pattern for benign or low-grade cartilage lesions. Note the mild invasion of the posterior cortex & marrow ➡. There is no marrow or soft tissue edema.* **(Right)** *Axial T1WI C+ FS MR shows peripheral enhancement of the lobulated portions of the lesion ➡. Imaging therefore confirms a periosteal cartilage lesion but does not differentiate between benign & malignant; histology showed chondrosarcoma.*

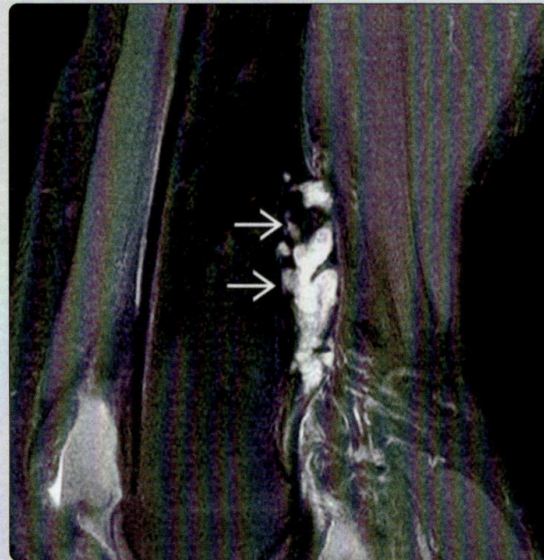

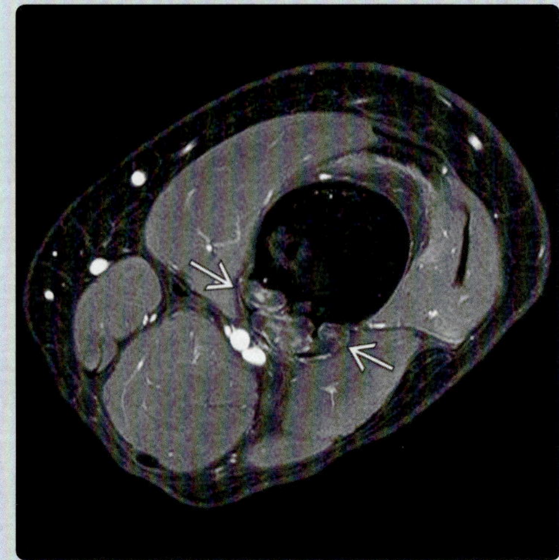

TERMINOLOGY

Synonyms

- Juxtacortical chondrosarcoma

Definitions

- Chondrosarcoma arising in periosteal layer of tubular bones

IMAGING

General Features

- Best diagnostic clue
  - Metadiaphyseal surface lesion
- Location
  - Distal femur (33%) and proximal humerus (33%) most common location
  - Metaphyseal (47%)
- Size
  - Median 4 cm greatest diameter in 1 study (mean 5.3 cm; range: 3-14 cm)

Radiographic Findings

- Cortical scalloping
- Matrix calcification (75%)

MR Findings

- Isointense or low T1 signal
- Hyperintense T2 signal
- Intramedullary involvement (26%)
- Intramedullary edema (30%)
- Irregular soft tissue margins (30%)

Nuclear Medicine Findings

- PET/CT may differentiate periosteal chondrosarcoma from periosteal chondroma
  - Recommend using standard uptake value (SUV) max of 2.0-2.3
  - Very small number of cases

DIFFERENTIAL DIAGNOSIS

Periosteal Chondroma

- 4x more frequent than periosteal chondrosarcoma
- May appear identical by imaging
- Tendency toward younger age group, smaller lesions

Periosteal Osteosarcoma

- Surface lesion with similar characteristics of cortical scalloping, minimal osseous invasion
- Soft tissue mass contains osteoid matrix, which may be differentiated from chondroid

PATHOLOGY

Gross Pathologic & Surgical Features

- Histologic differentiation from periosteal chondroma may be difficult
  - Greater cellular atypia
  - Greater osseous invasion

Microscopic Features

- Generally low histologic grade (53% grade 1, 45% grade 2)

CLINICAL ISSUES

Presentation

- Most common signs/symptoms
  - Asymptomatic or mildly painful mass (44%)

Demographics

- Age
  - 3rd through 6th decades
  - Slightly older age group than periosteal chondroma
- Gender
  - 61% male in 1 study

Natural History & Prognosis

- High recurrence rate if treated with marginal excision
- Most are well-differentiated, low-grade lesions
  - Wide excision is usually sufficient treatment
  - Metastases rare when adequately treated
- Histopathological findings and molecular aberrations not predictive of prognosis

Treatment

- Wide excision

DIAGNOSTIC CHECKLIST

Consider

- Imaging criteria for differentiating between periosteal chondrosarcoma and periosteal chondroma are sparse
  - Only moderate agreement exists between imaging and pathology in 1 study
  - Considered reasonable to be more concerned for chondrosarcoma if greatest diameter > 3 cm
  - Might consider wide excision of either lesion if practical

SELECTED REFERENCES

1. Cleven AH et al: Periosteal chondrosarcoma: a histopathological and molecular analysis of a rare chondrosarcoma subtype. Histopathology. 67(4):483-90, 2015
2. Goedhart LM et al: The presentation, treatment and outcome of periosteal chondrosarcoma in the Netherlands. Bone Joint J. 96-B(6):823-8, 2014
3. Morimoto S et al: Usefulness of PET/CT for diagnosis of periosteal chondrosarcoma of the femur: A case report. Oncol Lett. 7(6):1826-1828, 2014
4. Bertoni F et al: Chondrosarcoma. In Fletcher CDM et al: World Health Organization Classification of Tumours: Tumours of Soft Tissue and Bone. 249-50. Lyon: IARC Press, 2002
5. Chaabane S et al: Periosteal chondrosarcoma. AJR Am J Roentgenol. 192(1):W1-6, 2009
6. Robinson P et al: Periosteal chondroid tumors: radiologic evaluation with pathologic correlation. AJR Am J Roentgenol. 177(5):1183-8, 2001

Clear Cell Chondrosarcoma

KEY FACTS

TERMINOLOGY

- Rare low-grade variant of chondrosarcoma, usually originating in epiphysis

IMAGING

- May contain stippled chondroid matrix
- Well-defined lytic lesion
- Occasional sclerotic margin
- 2/3 occur in humeral or femoral heads
  - Reported in most other bones

TOP DIFFERENTIAL DIAGNOSES

- Chondroblastoma (CB)
  - CB generally occurs in younger age group
  - Strikingly similar imaging appearance

CLINICAL ISSUES

- Clinical presentation
  - Joint pain, limited range of motion
  - Effusion
- 2% of all chondrosarcomas
- M > F; ratio 3:1
- Most patients 25-50 years old
- Natural history
  - Marginal excision or curettage → 86% recurrence rate
  - Mortality 15%, metastases to lung and bone
  - Rare reports of dedifferentiation to high-grade sarcoma
- Treatment
  - Wide excision is curative

DIAGNOSTIC CHECKLIST

- Strong characteristic of this lesion is its epiphyseal location
- Because major differential diagnoses (chondroblastoma, degenerative cyst, giant cell tumor) are benign lesions, misdiagnosis results in inappropriate undertreatment of malignant lesion
- Watch for any red flags in epiphyseal lesions to suggest they may be this unusual sarcoma

(Left) *Axial NECT in a typical patient with clear cell chondrosarcoma is shown. The well-defined epiphyseal lesion has a sclerotic rim ➡ and contains faint internal cartilaginous matrix ➡. These findings cannot be differentiated from chondroblastoma, which is statistically much more likely.* **(Right)** *Axial T1WI C+ FS MR in (same patient) shows a thick, irregular rim of enhancement ➡. Differential diagnosis for this lesion remains chondroblastoma and, as was pathologically proven, clear cell chondrosarcoma.*

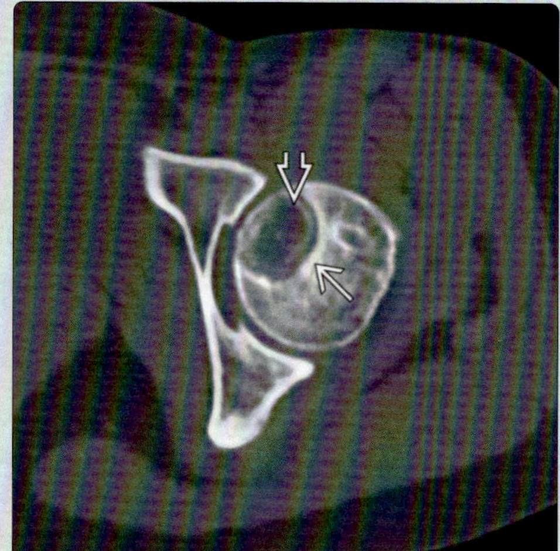

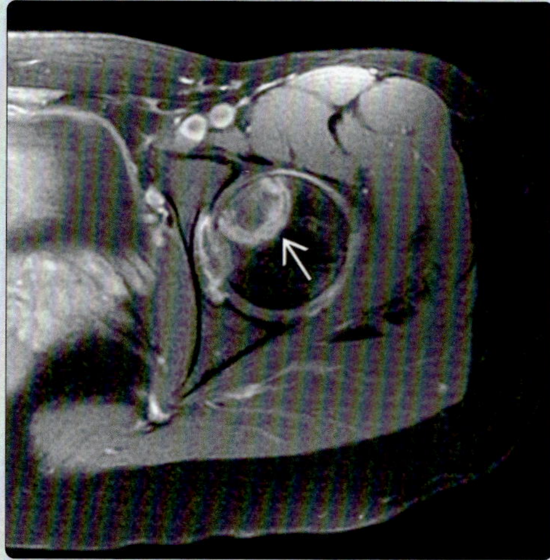

(Left) *AP radiograph of clear cell chondrosarcoma shows a mixed lytic and sclerotic lesion ➡ extending from the humeral head into the metadiaphysis. Chondroid matrix is faintly visible proximally ➡.* **(Right)** *Sagittal T2WI FS MR shows that the large intramedullary lesion ➡ involving the head & proximal humeral shaft is hyperintense relative to skeletal muscle. Low signal chondroid matrix is confirmed ➡, diagnostic of chondrosarcoma. The epiphyseal origin suggests clear cell variant, confirmed at surgery.*

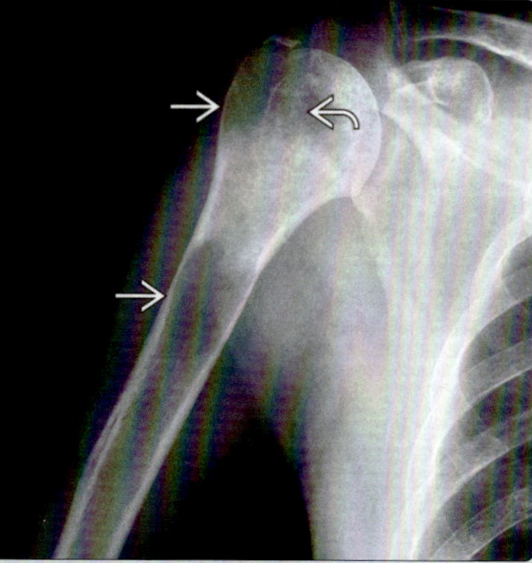

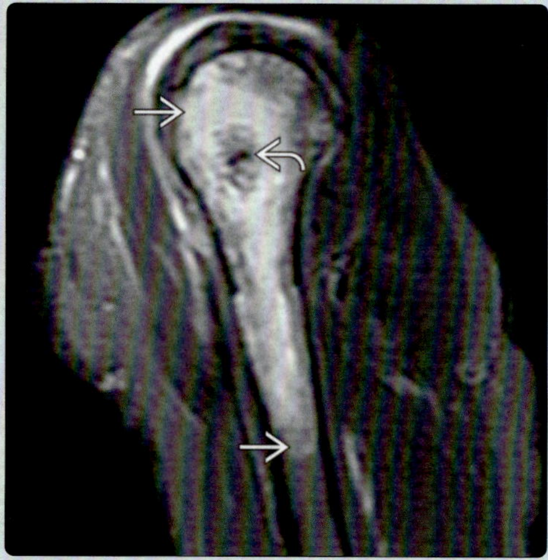

TERMINOLOGY

Definitions

- Rare low-grade variant of chondrosarcoma, usually originating in epiphysis

IMAGING

General Features

- Location
  - 2/3 occur in humeral or femoral heads
    - Scattered reports of lesion occurring in most other bones
  - Multiple synchronous lesions have been reported

Radiographic Findings

- Classic appearance is well-defined lytic epiphyseal lesion
  - Margin may be sclerotic
  - Generally no cortical breakthrough or soft tissue mass
  - Generally no periosteal reaction
- May appear more aggressive, without distinct margination
  - Origin in epiphysis may suggest diagnosis in this case
- May contain stippled chondroid matrix

MR Findings

- T1: Homogeneous intermediate signal
- Fluid-sensitive sequences: Heterogeneous hyperintense signal
- Cystic regions reported as unusual finding but may be confounding, mimicking aneurysmal bone cyst

DIFFERENTIAL DIAGNOSIS

Chondroblastoma

- Strikingly similar imaging appearance
  - Epiphyseal location may be identical
  - May contain chondroid matrix
  - Mild or moderate degree of aggressiveness appears similar
- Chondroblastoma (CB) generally occurs in younger age group
- CB histology distinctly different than clear cell chondrosarcoma
  - With discrepancy between imaging appearance of CB and pathology that does not have CB characteristics, consider diagnosis of clear cell chondrosarcoma

Langerhans Cell Histiocytosis

- May arise in epiphysis, so similar by location
- Entirely lytic lesion
- Mild or moderate degree of aggressiveness appears similar
- Langerhans cell histiocytosis (LCH) generally occurs in younger population than clear cell chondrosarcoma

Epiphyseal Osteomyelitis

- Unusual location of osteomyelitis except in children
- Lytic destructive lesion may appear similar on radiograph
- MR should distinguish by demonstrating abscess formation

Degenerative Cyst in Osteoarthritis

- May be large with sclerotic rim
- May mimic epiphyseal tumor and conversely epiphyseal tumor may mimic degenerative cyst

Giant Cell Tumor

- Arises in metaphysis but often extend to subchondral bone by time of discovery
  - May mimic epiphyseal lesion
- Entirely lytic; usually geographic but without sclerotic rim

PATHOLOGY

Microscopic Features

- Lobulated groups of round cells containing clear cytoplasm seen on cell block material
- Large plasmacytoid cells with foamy cytoplasm, as well as extracellular chondroid-type matrix material
- Contain some regions of conventional low-grade chondrosarcoma in 50% of cases

CLINICAL ISSUES

Presentation

- Most common signs/symptoms
  - Joint pain, effusion, limited range of motion

Demographics

- Age
  - Most patients 25-50 years old
- Gender
  - M:F = 3:1
- Epidemiology
  - 2% of all chondrosarcomas

Natural History & Prognosis

- Wide excision is curative
- Marginal excision or curettage → 86% recurrence rate
  - Mortality 15%, metastases to lung and bone
  - Metastases may be late (reported after 20 years)
- Rare reports of dedifferentiation to high-grade sarcoma

DIAGNOSTIC CHECKLIST

Consider

- 1/2 cases in 1 study were underdiagnoses
  - Results in undertreatment and recurrence of lesion

Image Interpretation Pearls

- Strong characteristic of this lesion is its epiphyseal location
  - Relatively few other lesions primarily reside in epiphysis
- Because major differential diagnoses (CB, degenerative cyst, giant cell tumor) are benign lesions, misdiagnosis results in inappropriate undertreatment of malignant lesion
  - Watch for any red flags in epiphyseal lesions to suggest they may be this unusual sarcoma

SELECTED REFERENCES

1. Jiang XS et al: Clear cell chondrosarcoma: Cytologic findings in six cases. Diagn Cytopathol. 42(9):784-91, 2014
2. Douis H et al: The imaging of cartilaginous bone tumours. II. Chondrosarcoma. Skeletal Radiol. 42(5):611-26, 2013

Plasmacytoma

KEY FACTS

TERMINOLOGY

- Localized clonal proliferation of plasma cells
- Solitary bone plasmacytoma (SBP)
  - Mass of plasma cells centered in bone marrow
- Solitary extramedullary plasmacytoma (EMP)
  - Mass of plasma cells in extramedullary location
- Extramedullary plasmacytoma in presence of multiple myeloma (MM)
  - Mass of plasma cells with known MM

IMAGING

- CT or MR
  - Nonspecific soft tissue mass that enhances with contrast
  - Diagnosis made on biopsy
- SBP
  - Almost always occur in sites of red marrow: Skull, spine, pelvis, or proximal humerus/femur
  - Most common sites: Pelvis and spine (thoracic > lumbar > cervical)
- EMP: 78-85% occur in upper aerodigestive tract
- Extramedullary plasmacytoma in presence of MM
  - 72-85% in soft tissues surrounding axial skeleton

CLINICAL ISSUES

- SBP
  - Majority progress to MM
- EMP
  - < 30% progression to MM
- Extramedullary plasmacytoma with MM
  - Occurs in 10-15% of patients at diagnosis
  - Poor prognosis

DIAGNOSTIC CHECKLIST

- All patients with solitary lesion should undergo whole-body MR to evaluate for MM
  - 30% of suspected SBP have MM at presentation
  - If additional lesions found, will be reclassified and prognosis/treatment altered

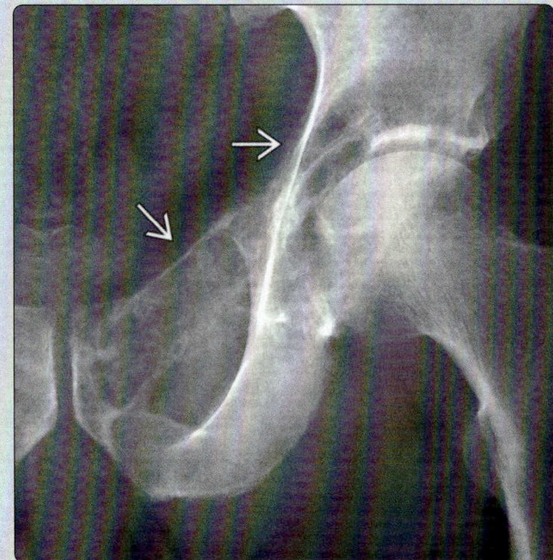

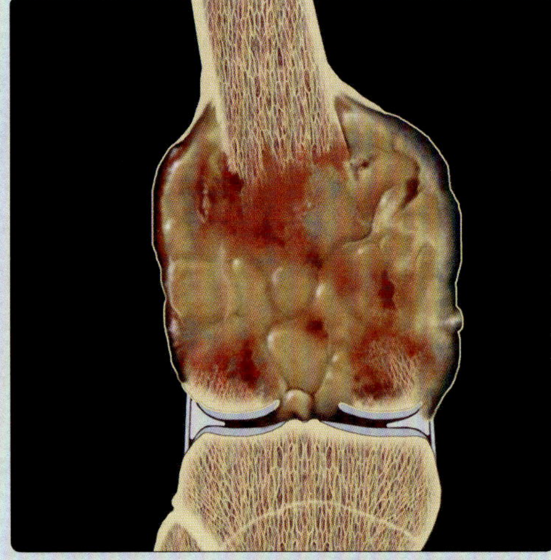

(Left) *AP radiograph of the left innominate bone demonstrates a bubbly lesion occupying the superior pubic ramus ➡ and extending into the acetabulum. There is cortical breakthrough involving the inferior cortex of the ramus.* **(Right)** *Coronal graphic of plasmacytoma demonstrates a mass centered in the metaphyseal bone marrow of the distal femur expanding into the adjacent soft tissues. A thin cortical rim is present about the majority of the lesion.*

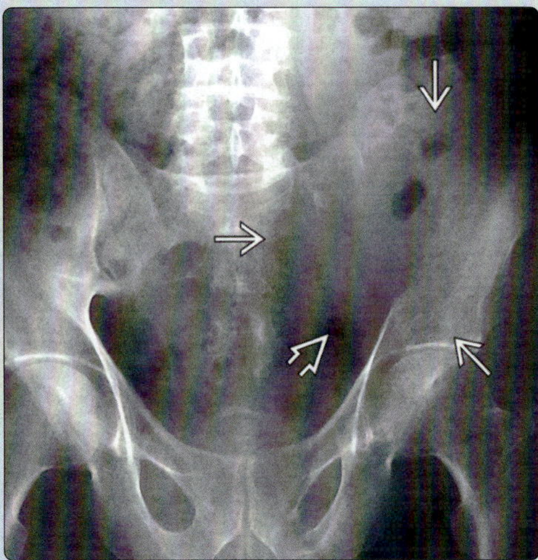

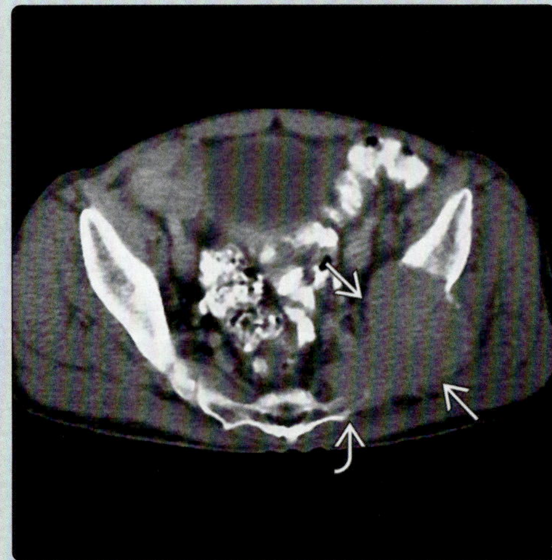

(Left) *AP pelvic radiograph demonstrates a large lytic lesion occupying the entire left iliac wing ➡, extending to the left acetabulum, and crossing the sacroiliac joint (SIJ) to involve the left sacral ala. Note that the SIJ does not serve as an effective barrier. There is no matrix or host response, though cortical breakthrough has occurred along the sciatic notch ➡.* **(Right)** *Axial CT shows the suspected soft tissue mass centered in the left iliac wing ➡ and extending into the left sacral ala ➡. Biopsy proved plasmacytoma.*

TERMINOLOGY

Abbreviations

- Solitary bone plasmacytoma (SBP)
- Extramedullary plasmacytoma (EMP)

Definitions

- Localized clonal proliferation of plasma cells
- Solitary bone plasmacytoma
  - Clonal proliferation of plasma cells centered in bone marrow
- Solitary extramedullary plasmacytoma
  - Clonal proliferation of plasma cells in extramedullary location
- Extramedullary plasmacytoma in presence of multiple myeloma (MM)
  - MM with localized extramedullary clonal proliferation of plasma cells

IMAGING

General Features

- Best diagnostic clue
  - Mass within soft tissues or bone marrow
- Location
  - Variable
  - SBP
    - Almost always occur in sites of red marrow: Skull, spine, pelvis, or proximal humerus/femur
    - Most common sites: Spine (thoracic > lumbar > cervical) and pelvis
  - EMP
    - 78-85% occur in upper aerodigestive tract
    - 2nd most common site: Gastrointestinal tract
    - Can occur anywhere
  - Extramedullary plasmacytoma in presence of MM
    - 72-85% occur in soft tissues around axial skeleton
    - Also occur in lymph nodes, spleen, and liver
    - Rarely occur in lung or CNS
    - Can occur anywhere
- Size
  - Varies
  - > 5 cm more likely to progress to systemic disease

Imaging Recommendations

- Best imaging tool
  - SBP
    - MR to define extent of disease
  - EMP
    - MR most sensitive to evaluate extent of local disease and adjacent lymph node involvement
  - Whole-body MR to exclude systemic disease that would indicate diagnosis of MM

Radiographic Findings

- SBP
  - Geographic lytic lesion centered in bone marrow
  - 44% show multiloculated appearance
  - No identifiable matrix
- EMP
  - Radiographs not useful

CT Findings

- Soft tissue mass that enhances with contrast
- No identifiable matrix
- SBP
  - Usually breaks through thinned cortex
- EMP
  - Most in upper aerodigestive tract

MR Findings

- T1WI
  - Low signal soft tissue mass
- T1WI C+
  - Enhancement of soft tissue mass
- Fluid-sensitive sequences
  - Intermediate signal soft tissue lesion
- Whole-body MR
  - Remainder of bone marrow appears normal
  - No evidence of systemic multiple myeloma

DIFFERENTIAL DIAGNOSIS

Lymphoma

- Usually has intact cortex around bone, unlike SBP
- Usually multiple bilateral lymph nodes involved, unlike EMP

Metastases, Bone Marrow

- Solitary expanded thyroid or renal cell metastasis is most common mimic
- MR or CT will usually demonstrate multiple lesions
- Often known history of malignancy

Chondrosarcoma

- Solitary lesion, often nonaggressive
  - Distinct margins, may not have cortical breakthrough
- Subtle chondroid matrix may be present

Brown Tumor

- Lytic lesion, mildly expanded
- Generally without sclerotic margin
- Abnormal bone density, other findings of resorption

Giant Cell Tumor

- Lytic expanded lesion without sclerotic margin

PATHOLOGY

General Features

- Etiology
  - Unknown
  - Exposure to herbicides, insecticides, benzene, and ionizing radiation may contribute
- Genetics
  - SBP
    - Similar to MM
  - EMP
    - Polysomy common
    - 37% with break at 14q32 (heavy chain locus; 50-70% in MM)
    - Translocation t(4;14) in 16%
    - Lower proliferation indices than MM
  - Extramedullary plasmacytoma in presence of MM
    - Poor prognosis

- Higher association with IgD MM
- Higher prevalence in patients ≤ 55 years of age

- Associated abnormalities
  - SBP
    - 30-50% of suspected SBP have MM at presentation
      - Reclassified and prognosis/treatment altered
      - Whole-body MR used to search for additional foci
      - Multiplanar flow cytometry used to predict likelihood of developing MM; 71% with positive flow evolve to MM, while 8% with negative flow evolve to MM

Staging, Grading, & Classification

- SBP
  - Durie and Salmon PLUS staging of MM
  - In absence of bone marrow disease, SBP is considered stage IA
- EMP
  - No formal staging
  - Smaller lesions have better prognosis
  - Careful analysis needed to differentiate from reactive plasmacytosis, poorly differentiated neoplasms, lymphoma, or plasma cell granuloma

Microscopic Features

- Uniform plasma cells: Cells with eccentric nuclei and basophilic cytoplasm

CLINICAL ISSUES

Presentation

- Most common signs/symptoms
  - SBP
    - Pain at site of lesion
    - Occasionally symptoms and signs of spinal cord or nerve root compression
  - EMP
    - Nasal discharge, epistaxis, nasal obstruction, sore throat, hoarseness, or hemoptysis
  - Extramedullary plasmacytoma with known MM
    - Pain and fever unrelated to infection

Demographics

- Age
  - SBP
    - Median: 50-54 years
  - EMP
    - 70% 51-70 years
- Gender
  - M > F (2.3-3:1)
- Epidemiology
  - < 2% of monoclonal gammopathies
  - 5% of plasma cell neoplasms

Natural History & Prognosis

- SBP
  - Majority progress to MM
  - Median time to progression: 2-4 years
  - High-grade angiogenesis associated with earlier progression to MM
- EMP
  - < 30% progression to MM
  - Local recurrence in ~ 30%
  - Disseminated soft tissue disease in 35-39%
- Extramedullary plasmacytoma with known MM
  - Occurs in 10-15% of patients at diagnosis
  - Arises in 5-10% of patients after treatment (median time: 19 months after treatment initiation)
  - Often associated with fever, elevated serum lactate dehydrogenase, pancytopenia, and decreased serum level of paraprotein

Treatment

- SBP
  - If MR reveals other bone marrow lesions, treat as MM
  - If no other lesions, radiotherapy with 40-50 Gy in 20 fractions
  - If SBP > 5 cm, consider higher dose of radiation therapy (i.e., 50 Gy) and chemotherapy
- EMP
  - If no systemic disease, radiotherapy with 40-50 Gy in 20 fractions
    - Lymph nodes should be included in field
  - Radiotherapy &/or surgery
    - Majority cured by radiotherapy alone

DIAGNOSTIC CHECKLIST

Consider

- All patients with suspected solitary lesion should undergo whole-body MR to evaluate for MM

Image Interpretation Pearls

- Soft tissue mass is nonspecific
- Diagnosis made on biopsy

Reporting Tips

- SBP
  - With vertebral body involvement, posterior cortex or epidural involvement should be documented, as these often cause cord or nerve root compression
- EMP
  - Evaluation of regional lymph node involvement is important
    - Indicates higher rate of progression
    - Lymph node involvement should be specified, as it should be included in radiation therapy field

SELECTED REFERENCES

1. Wang Y et al: Pelvic solitary plasmacytoma: computed tomography and magnetic resonance imaging findings with histopathologic correlation. Korean J Radiol. 16(1):146-53, 2015
2. Katodritou E et al: Clinical features, outcome, and prognostic factors for survival and evolution to multiple myeloma of solitary plasmacytomas: a report of the Greek myeloma study group in 97 patients. Am J Hematol. 89(8):803-8, 2014
3. Paiva B et al: Multiparameter flow cytometry for staging of solitary bone plasmacytoma: new criteria for risk of progression to myeloma. Blood. 124(8):1300-3, 2014
4. Guo SQ et al: Prognostic factors associated with solitary plasmacytoma. Onco Targets Ther. 6:1659-66, 2013

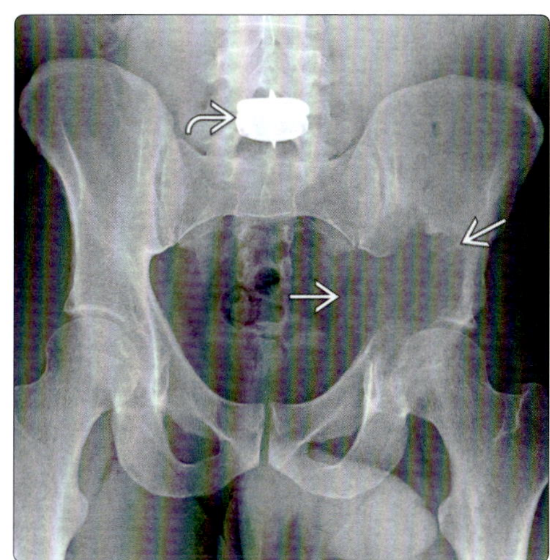

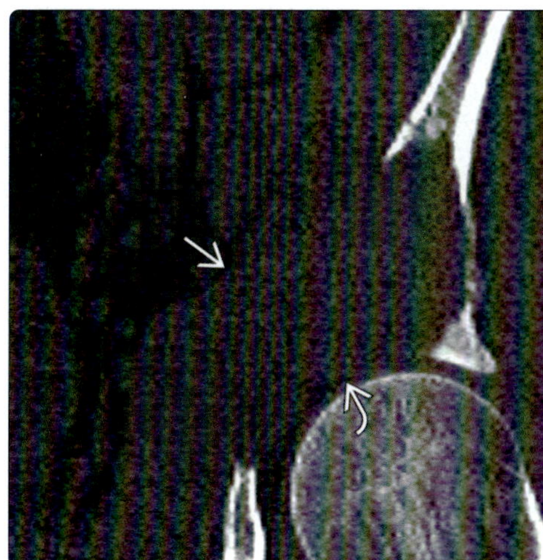

(Left) *AP radiograph from a 35-year-old man who has complained of sciatica for 5 years is shown. There is a large lytic lesion involving the iliac wing and acetabulum ➡ showing cortical breakthrough and soft tissue mass. Note also the disc prosthesis ↪ placed for his sciatic symptoms. His symptoms did not improve since they were due to the pelvic lesion that occupies the sciatic notch. Not all sciatica is spine related.* **(Right)** *Coronal CT proves the lesion to be completely lytic with cortical disruption both medially ➡ and at the acetabular roof ↪.*

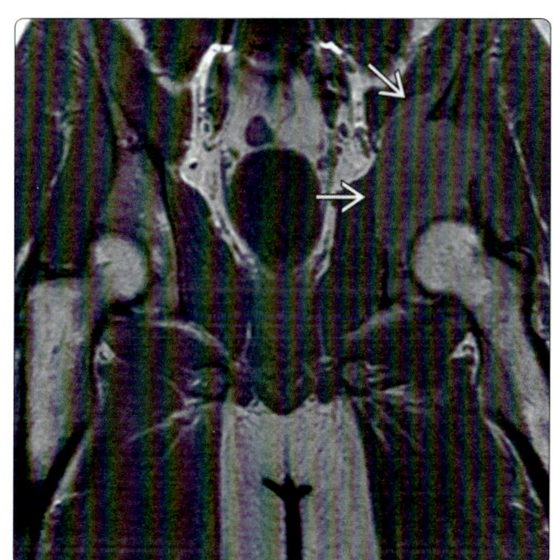

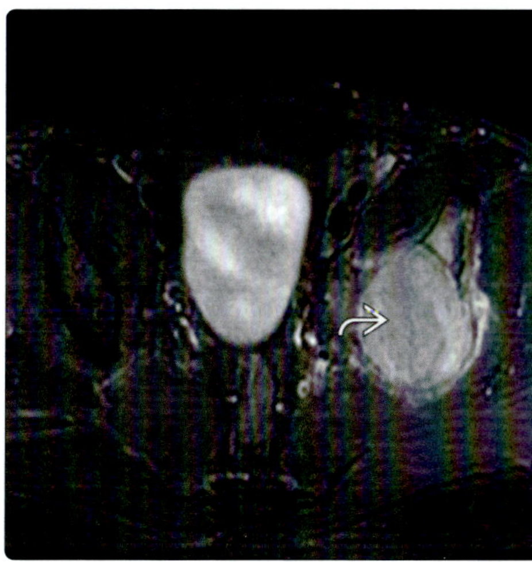

(Left) *Coronal T1 MR shows the lesion ➡ to have intermediate/low signal intensity with slightly lower signal centrally.* **(Right)** *Axial STIR MR shows hyperintensity within the lesion, again with slightly lower signal centrally ↪. Prior to biopsy, differentials include giant cell tumor, lytic chondrosarcoma, malignant fibrous histiocytoma, and lymphoma. The patient's young age should not preclude consideration of plasmacytoma.*

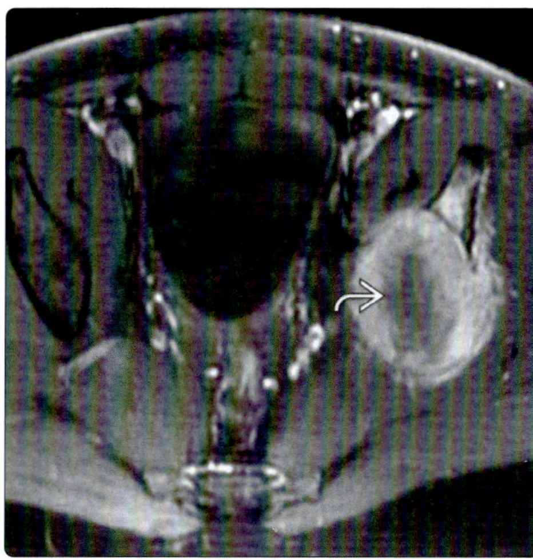

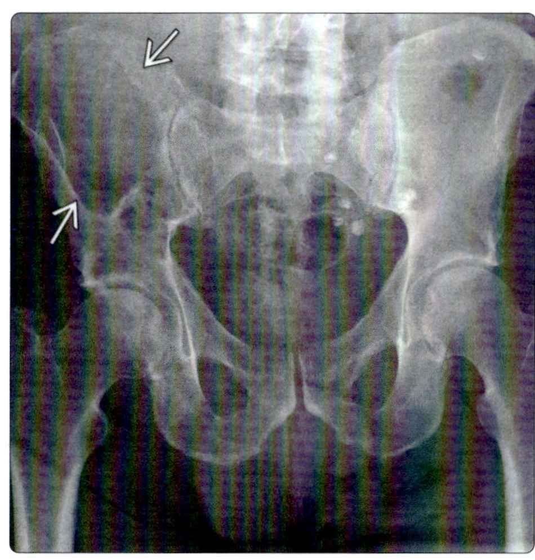

(Left) *Axial postcontrast T1FS MR shows avid enhancement with necrosis centrally ↪. The MR characteristics are nonspecific. Biopsy proved plasmacytoma.* **(Right)** *AP radiograph in a middle-aged man shows a large, lytic, moderately aggressive lesion occupying the iliac wing ➡. Biopsy proved plasmacytoma. The iliac wing is such a common location for this lesion that, in virtually any aged adult, plasmacytoma should be considered a diagnostic possibility in any mildly or moderately aggressive lytic lesion here.*

(Left) *Sagittal T1 MR shows a mildly expanded plasmacytoma involving S1 and S2 vertebral bodies ➡ surrounding the intervening disc.* **(Right)** *Sagittal STIR MR shows the lesion ➡ to be homogeneously hyperintense. The MR is nonspecific and could represent any of the common lesions found in the sacrum, including chordoma and plasmacytoma. GCT is less likely since there is no hypointense signal on STIR. Chondrosarcoma often shows a characteristic nodularity, but higher grade lesions could have this appearance.*

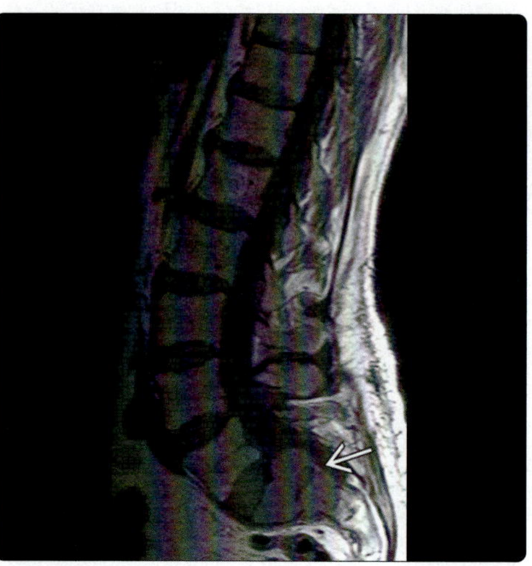

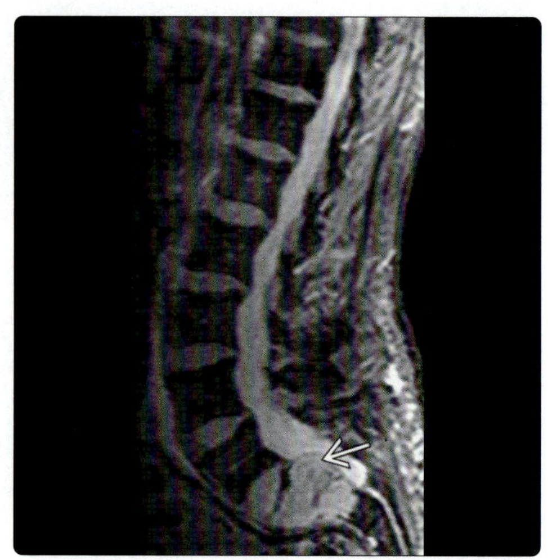

(Left) *Coronal CT shows lytic destruction of the sacrum ➡. No matrix is seen.* **(Right)** *Axial CT in the same patient shows the lesion to have broken through cortex anteriorly and to invade the iliac wings ➡ bilaterally. Though we usually expect a joint to be a barrier to tumor extension, the sacroiliac joint is an exception where there is routine direct extension of tumor. By CT, this lesion could equally represent plasmacytoma, chordoma, giant cell tumor, or lytic chondrosarcoma. Plasmacytoma was biopsy proven.*

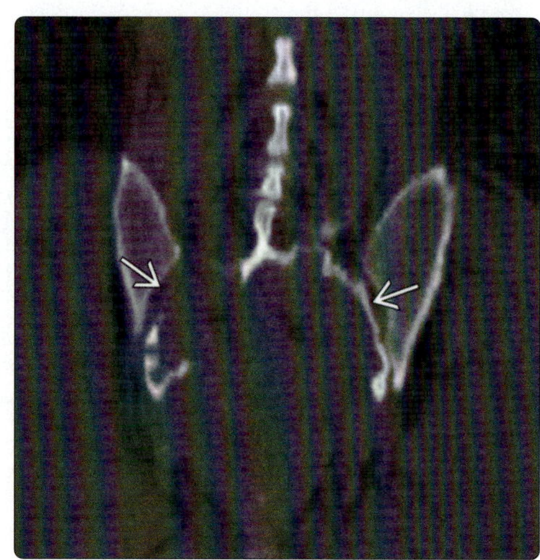

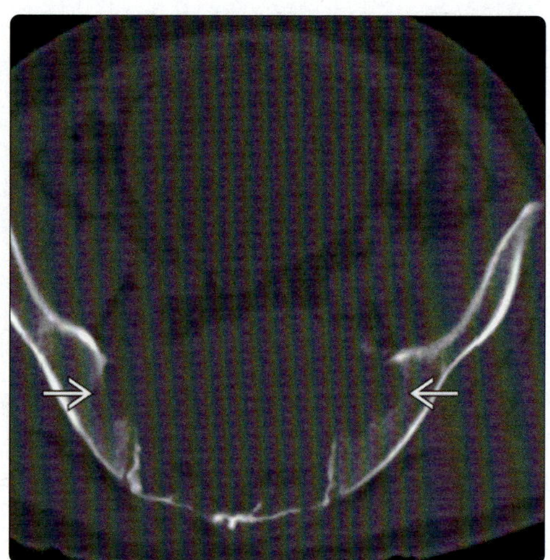

(Left) *Coronal STIR in the same patient shows the sacral lesion to be of nonspecific hyperintensity ➡. However, in addition there is a focal lesion in the right acetabulum ➡.* **(Right)** *Adjacent STIR coronal image again shows the large sacral lesion ➡, as well as a 2nd small focus ➡. The very great size discrepancy between the sacral lesion and the small foci suggests that these smaller lesions represent early lesions of multiple myeloma in a patient with plasmacytoma converting to myeloma. This was proven to be the case at biopsy.*

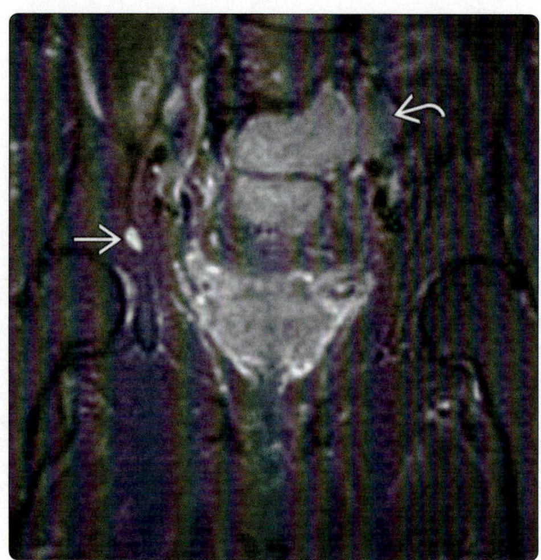

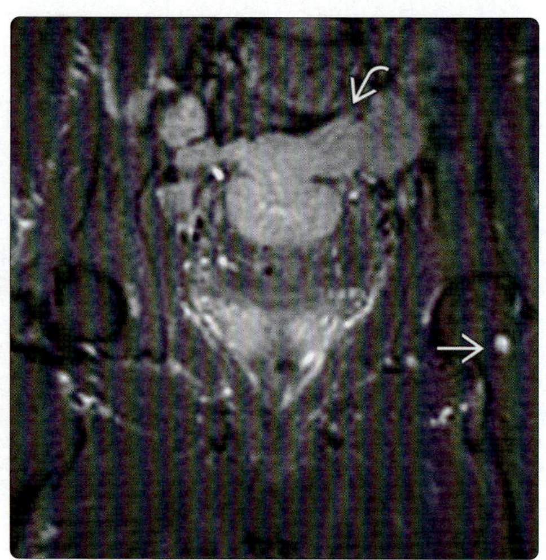

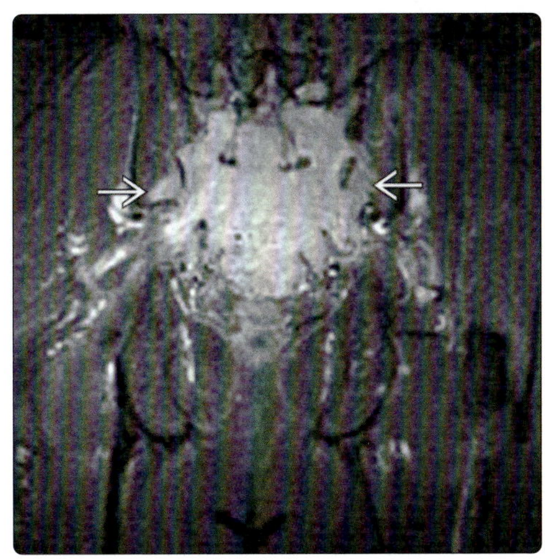

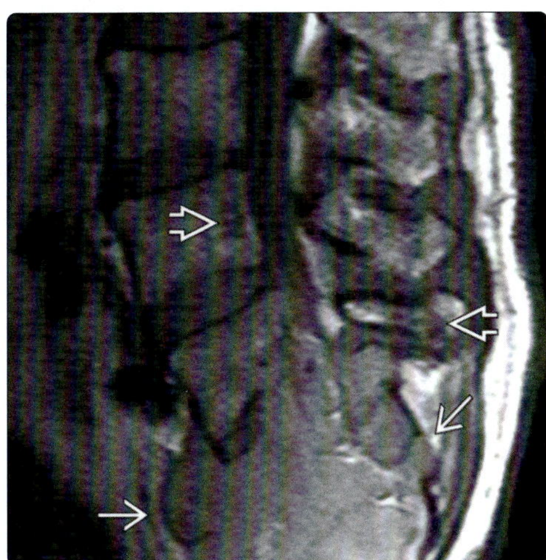

(Left) *Coronal STIR MR demonstrates a very large mass occupying and destroying the majority of the sacrum and extending into the iliac wings ➡. The plasmacytoma has nonspecific low signal on T1 and high signal on STIR MR imaging.* **(Right)** *Sagittal T1WI MR in the same patient shows the sacral mass extending beyond the sacral margins both anteriorly and posteriorly ➡. Low signal T1 areas within the bone marrow fat ➡ correspond to myeloma infiltration. This is SBP that progressed to MM.*

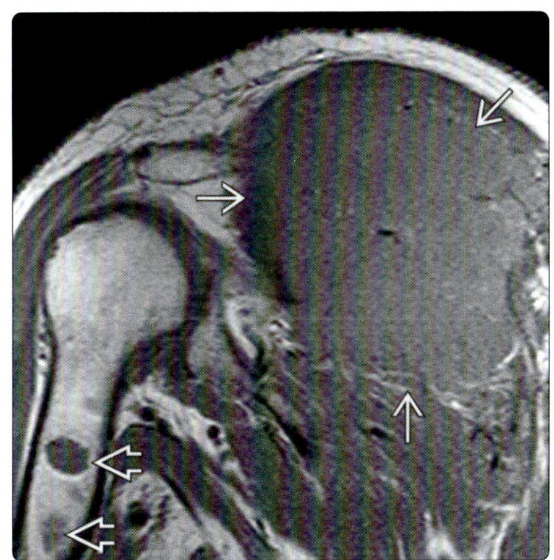

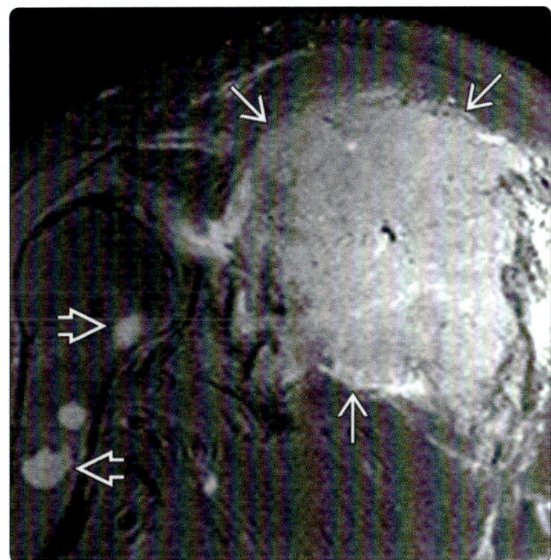

(Left) *Coronal T1WI MR demonstrates a large low T1 signal mass ➡ that arose in the acromion and extended into the adjacent soft tissues. It was present at the time of multiple myeloma diagnosis. The proximal humerus shows multifocal myeloma lesions in the bone marrow ➡.* **(Right)** *Coronal T1WI C+ FS MR in the same patient demonstrates diffuse enhancement of the plasmacytoma ➡ and multifocal medullary lesions ➡, emphasizing the fact that multiple myeloma (MM) should be sought in patients presenting with SBP.*

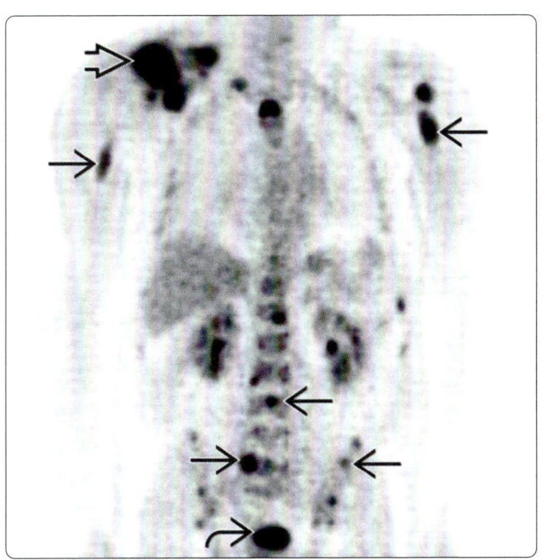

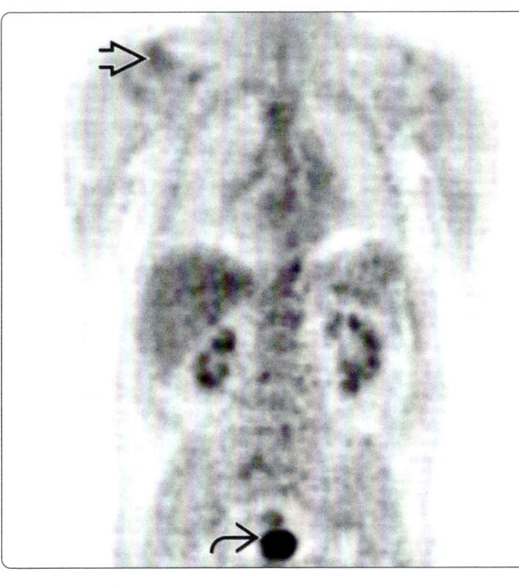

(Left) *Coronal PET in the same patient shows markedly increased uptake within the mass ➡ and extensive medullary disease within the humeri, vertebrae, and iliac wings ➡. Normal bladder activity is noted ➡.* **(Right)** *Coronal PET following treatment, including high-dose chemotherapy with stem cell transplantation and maintenance chemotherapy, shows response with decreased uptake in both the plasmacytoma ➡ and MM lesions. Normal bladder activity is seen ➡.*

KEY FACTS

TERMINOLOGY

- Most common primary malignancy of bone
- Plasma cell disorder → primarily in bone marrow

IMAGING

- Radiographs
  - Intramedullary lytic "punched out" lesions
  - Diffuse osteopenia
- MR or PET/CT
  - Multifocal or diffuse infiltration of bone marrow
- Location
  - Axial > appendicular
  - Proximal > > distal extremities
- Best imaging tool
  - Whole-body-MR (WB-MR)
  - T1 and STIR images most sensitive
- Epidural spread of disease common
  - ± cord compression → oncologic emergency

CLINICAL ISSUES

- Compression fractures
- Steroid complications
  - Osteonecrosis
- Bisphosphonate complications
  - Mandible osteonecrosis
  - Subtrochanteric insufficiency fractures
- Other treatment-related complications
  - Deep vein thrombosis and pulmonary embolism

DIAGNOSTIC CHECKLIST

- Any patient with monoclonal gammopathy of undetermined significance, smoldering multiple myeloma, or solitary bone plasmacytoma
  - Must exclude MM by radiologic skeletal survey → if negative, MR
- Important for staging
  - Number of lesions (< 5, 5-20, > 20)
  - Degree of diffuse disease by MR

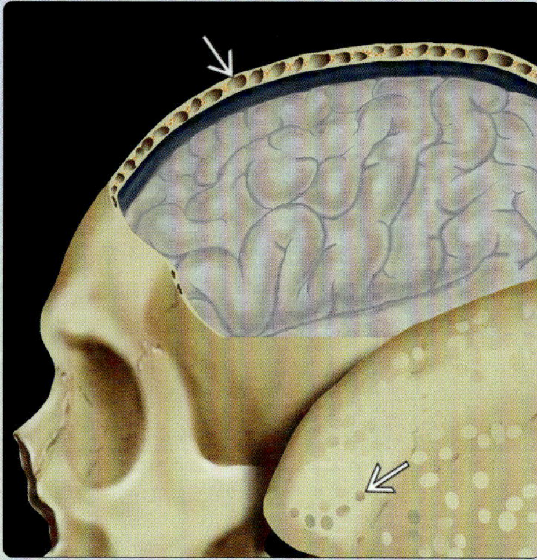
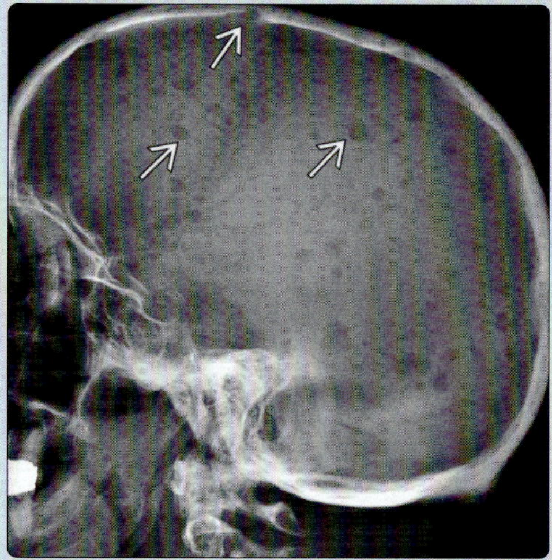

(Left) *Sagittal graphic through the calvaria demonstrates focal well-circumscribed multiple myeloma (MM) lesions within the diploic space ➔. These appear as lytic lesions by radiograph and can be seen as STIR bright lesions by MR.* **(Right)** *Lateral skull from a skeletal radiograph demonstrates numerous lytic multiple myeloma lesions ➔ in this patient with stage IIIA disease.*

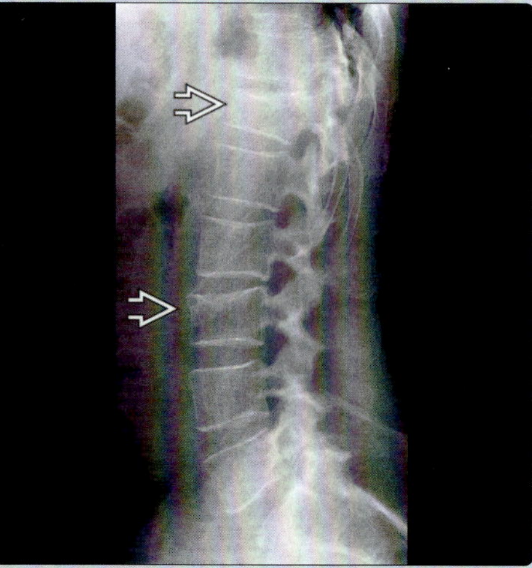
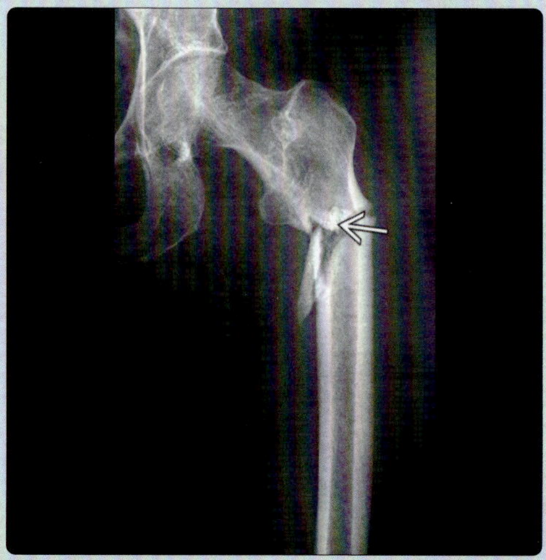

(Left) *Diffuse osteopenia and compression fractures ➔ are seen in this case of MM in a young adult male. Osteopenia out of proportion to that expected for a patient's age should raise suspicion of an underlying cause, such as myeloma, even without focal lesions.* **(Right)** *AP radiograph in a patient being treated for MM shows diffuse osteopenia and a subtrochanteric fracture. The lateral femoral cortex is slightly heaped up ➔. This is a bisphosphonate fracture; remember that treatment of MM often includes bisphosphonates.*

TERMINOLOGY

Abbreviations

- Multiple myeloma (MM)
- Monoclonal gammopathy (MG)
- MG of undetermined significance (MGUS)
- MG of borderline significance (MGBS)
- Smoldering multiple myeloma (SMM)
- Solitary bone plasmacytoma (SBP)

Definitions

- Most common primary malignancy of bone
- Plasma cell disorder → primarily in bone marrow (BM)

IMAGING

General Features

- Best diagnostic clue
  - Radiographs
    - Intramedullary lytic "punched out" lesions
  - MR or PET/CT
    - Multifocal or diffuse infiltration of bone marrow
- Location
  - Intramedullary (virtually always)
    - Axial > appendicular (proximal > > distal)
    - Vertebral bodies as well as posterior elements
  - Extramedullary (uncommon)
- Size
  - Varies: Diffuse infiltration or focal lesions (any size)

Radiographic Findings

- Radiographic skeletal survey
  - Lytic lesions
  - Diffuse osteopenia ± compression fractures
  - Rare manifestation: Sclerotic lesions [POEMS (polyneuropathy, organomegaly, endocrinopathy, M-protein, skin lesions) syndrome]
  - False-negative rate high
    - Underestimates number of lesions and therefore tumor burden

CT Findings

- Intramedullary soft tissue mass producing lytic lesions
- ± endosteal scalloping
- ± cortical breakthrough and soft tissue mass

MR Findings

- Patterns by MR (some may coexist)
  - No visualized disease
  - Micronodular ("variegated" or "salt and pepper")
  - Multifocal (usually ≥ 5 mm)
  - Diffuse marrow infiltration
- T1WI
  - Diffuse or focal: Signal ≤ muscle/disc
- STIR
  - Untreated disease has ↑ signal intensity
- T1WI C+ FS
  - Untreated disease enhances with contrast

PET/CT Findings

- Active lesions: Activity above background
- ↑ detection of nonosseous lesions, rib, and scapular lesions when compared with nonwhole-body MR
- Valuable in nonsecretory multiple myeloma

Response to Therapy

- MR: Replacement of previously infiltrated marrow 1st by red marrow, then by fat
  - Dynamic whole-body contrast may assess Rx
  - Whole-body diffusion-weighted MR may assess Rx
- Decreased FDG uptake
- Prolonged and intense regimen often required before lesions appear to normalize
  - Lytic lesions seen on CT almost always persist even after successful treatment

Imaging Recommendations

- Best imaging tool
  - Whole-body MR (WB-MR) or near-whole-body MR
  - If unable to perform whole-body MR, PET/CT
    - Defines extent of medullary/extramedullary disease
- Protocol advice
  - T1 and STIR images most sensitive
  - T1 post-gadolinium → no ↑ detection of disease
  - Near whole-body MR (facilities without WB-MR)
    - Coronal STIR of skull, sternum, shoulder girdles (to include proximal 2/3 humeri), pelvis (to include proximal 2/3 femur)
    - Sagittal T1 and STIR of entire spine

Nuclear Medicine Findings

- Bone scan not useful in evaluating MM
  - High false-negative rate for individual lesions

DIFFERENTIAL DIAGNOSIS

Differential of Multiple Myeloma Presentation With Multiple Focal Lesions

- Metastases
  - Often less well-defined destruction on radiograph
  - ↑ activity on bone scan
- Leukemia
  - Permeative bone destruction
  - May present with diffuse osteopenia
  - ↑ activity on bone scan

Differential of Multiple Myeloma Presentation as Diffuse Osteopenia

- Leukemia
- Primary osteoporosis

PATHOLOGY

General Features

- Etiology
  - Unknown
  - Cited associations: Herbicides, insecticides, benzene, radiation
- Genetics
  - Plasma cell disorder with genetic alterations
    - Multiple possible; may ↑ during course of disease
  - Rarely hereditary
- Associated abnormalities

Durie and Salmon PLUS Staging*

Disease	STAGE[1]	Bone Marrow	Radiographic Findings[2]	MR Findings[3]	PET/CT Findings
MGUS	None	< 10% plasma cells	No lytic lesions	Normal marrow	Normal marrow
SMM	IA	≥ 10% plasma cells	No lytic lesions	Limited disease or plasmacytoma	Limited marrow disease or plasmacytoma
MM		≥ 10% plasma cells &/or plasmacytoma + EOD[4]	Varies: No lytic lesions → multiple lesions → osteopenia	Varies: Normal marrow to diffuse infiltration	Increased FDG uptake in marrow: Diffuse vs. multifocal
	IIA/B			5-20 FLs[5]; moderate DD	5-20 FLs
	IIIA/B		> 20 lytic lesions	> 20 FLs; severe DD	> 20 FLs

*Lab values not shown. [1]A - Serum creatinine (SCr) < 2.0 mg/dl & no extramedullary disease (EMD); B- SCr > 2.0 mg/dl &/or EMD. [2]Lytic lesions are seldom used as MR & PET/CT are more sensitive. [3]BM appearance is variable. Stage III MM by clinical criteria can have a normal MR appearance of BM → associated with more favorable prognosis. [4]EOD, end organ damage: Includes calcium elevation, renal insufficiency, anemia, or bone abnormalities. [5]FL, focal lesions ≥ 5 mm; DD, diffuse disease. DD is evaluated on T1 images: Mild = micronodular; moderate = diffuse T1 signal < normal marrow but with contrast between vertebral BM disc; severe = low T1 signal of vertebral BM with signal ≤ the adjacent disc.

- Epidural spread of disease

Staging, Grading, & Classification

- Classification
  - MGUS
    - Can be precursor to MM (1% per year)
    - Also → Waldenström, lymphoma, primary amyloidosis, or chronic lymphocytic leukemia
  - MM
    - Sclerotic MM
      - Rare; most often associated with POEMS syndrome
      - Better survival than symptomatic MM
    - SBP
      - Must exclude disseminated disease
      - Usually centered in bone marrow
    - SMM
      - ↑ risk → MM (10% per year for first 5 years)
    - Nonsecretory
      - No M-protein found in blood or serum
      - Best followed by FDG PET/CT
    - Plasma cell leukemia: More aggressive form
      - Presence of > 20% circulating plasma cells
      - Can occur at diagnosis or with progression
- Staging
  - Durie and Salmon PLUS system
  - International staging system (no imaging parameters)

CLINICAL ISSUES

Presentation

- Most common signs/symptoms
  - Bone pain; excessive protein in urine or blood

Demographics

- Age
  - Primarily 40-80 years old
- Gender
  - M > F
- Ethnicity
  - African American > Caucasian American

Natural History & Prognosis

- Eventually uniformly fatal
- Median survival → increase from 2.5-8.5 years with newer Rx

Treatment

- Chemotherapy
  - Dexamethasone
    - ± melphalan
    - ± antiangiogenesis (e.g., thalidomide)
    - ± protease inhibitor (e.g., bortezomib)
- Autologous peripheral stem cell transplantation
  - May be tandem (2nd transplant post recovery from 1st)
- Allogeneic; rarely → unacceptably high mortality rate
- Usual progression of treatment
  - Induction chemo → peripheral stem cell (PSC) harvest → high-dose chemo → PSC transplant → maintenance chemo
  - High-dose chemo → PSC transplant: May be performed more than once
- Treatment complications
  - Compression fractures (pathologic or insufficiency)
  - Osteonecrosis
  - Bisphosphonate complications
    - Mandible osteonecrosis
    - Subtrochanteric insufficiency fractures
  - Deep vein thrombosis and pulmonary embolism

DIAGNOSTIC CHECKLIST

Consider

- Any patient with MGUS, SMM, or SBP
  - Must exclude MM by RSS → if negative, MR

Reporting Tips

- Important for staging
  - Number of lesions (< 5, 5-20, > 20)
  - Degree of diffuse disease by MR

SELECTED REFERENCES

1. Giles SL et al: Whole-body diffusion-weighted MR imaging for assessment of treatment response in myeloma. Radiology. 271(3):785-94, 2014
2. Padhani AR et al: Assessing the relation between bone marrow signal intensity and apparent diffusion coefficient in diffusion-weighted MRI. AJR Am J Roentgenol. 200(1):163-70, 2013

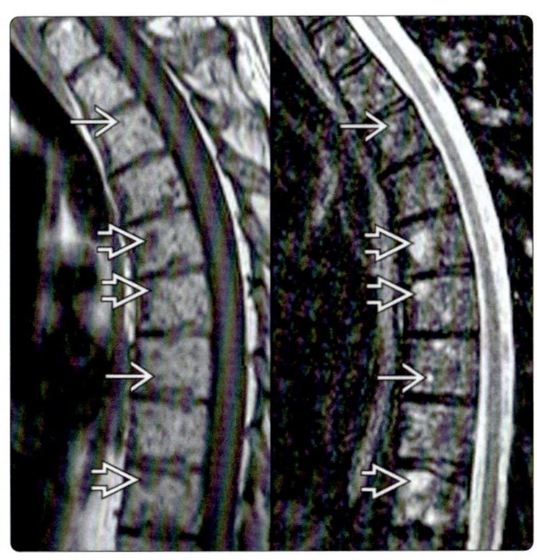

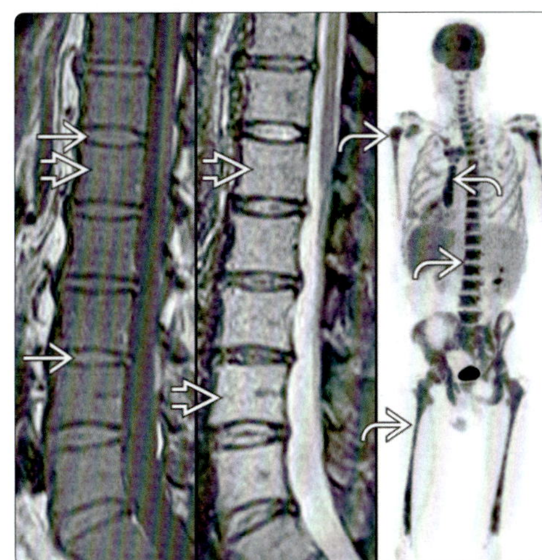

(Left) *Sagittal T1 STIR MR images through the thoracic spine show low T1/high STIR in a multifocal pattern ➡ with micronodular background ➡. An isolated micronodular pattern can be seen with stage I disease, while multifocal is usually associated with stage II/III disease.* **(Right)** *Sagittal T1 STIR and PET MIP images depict diffuse myeloma. Marrow signal ➡ is < disc ➡ on T1, high signal on STIR, and shows diffuse uptake on PET ➡. This pattern can be mistaken for marrow stimulation.*

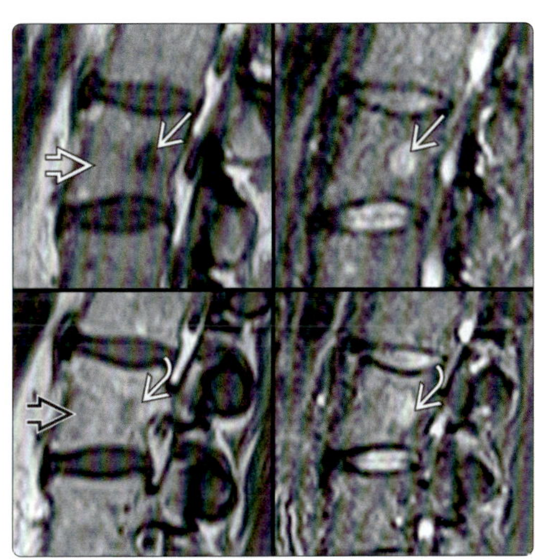

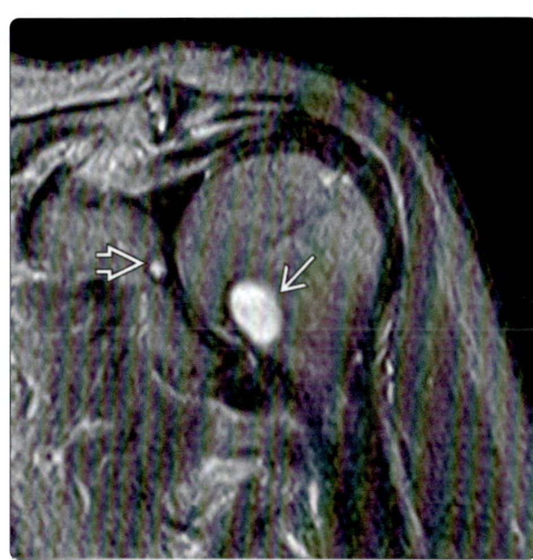

(Left) *Sagittal T1 MR (left) and STIR (right) images prior to therapy (upper) and after 2 transplants (in complete clinical remission) (bottom images) are shown. Focal low T1/high STIR signal lesion ➡ could be mistaken for an atypical hemangioma; however, it shows ↓ size after therapy ➡. Note ↓ fat on T1 ➡ due to myeloma. Increased fat is visible after treatment ➡.* **(Right)** *Coronal STIR MR early in remission shows myeloma lesions (↑ STIR signal) in the humeral metaphysis ➡ and scapula ➡.*

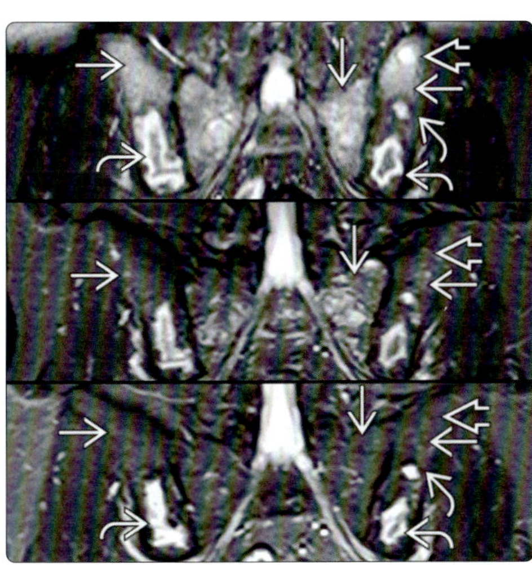

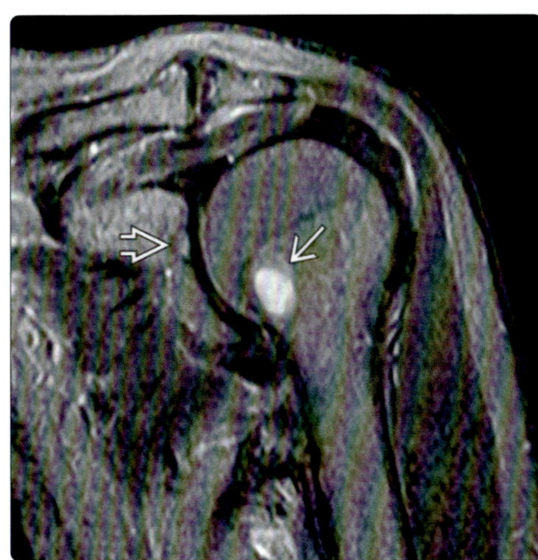

(Left) *Coronal STIR MR of parasacral marrow in the same patient after 5 weeks of therapy (upper), 1st transplant (middle), and 2nd transplant (lower) is shown. Serpentine border lesions ➡ improve minimally, consistent with bone infarcts. Diffuse ↑ marrow signal ➡ and focal lesion ➡ improve after treatment.* **(Right)** *Coronal STIR MR in the same patient in clinical remission on maintenance therapy shows periphery of lesion filling with fat or marrow elements ➡. Scapular lesion is also decreasing in size ➡.*

(Left) *Coronal STIR MR of shoulder depicts myeloma in the distal clavicle → and proximal humerus ⇨ during relapse (upper) that has ↓ signal intensity in complete remission after 3 transplantations (lower).* **(Right)** *Axial CT from PET/CT depicts a lytic lesion within the spinous process prior to initiation of therapy (upper) →. After therapy, the lytic lesion persists ↪. Prior wisdom that spinous process lesions were rare is false. Lytic lesions persist after treatment due to inhibition of osteoblast function.*

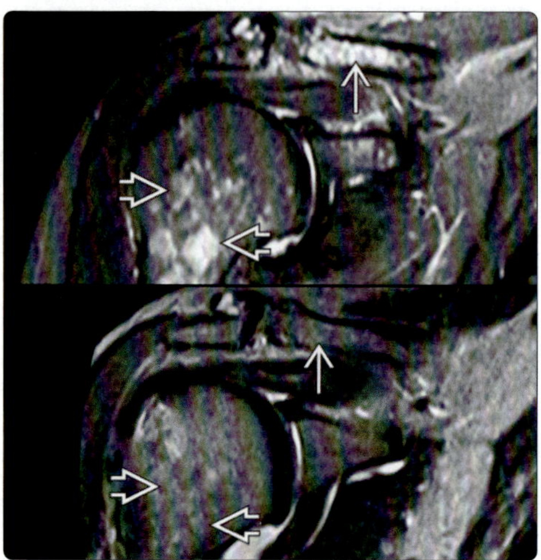

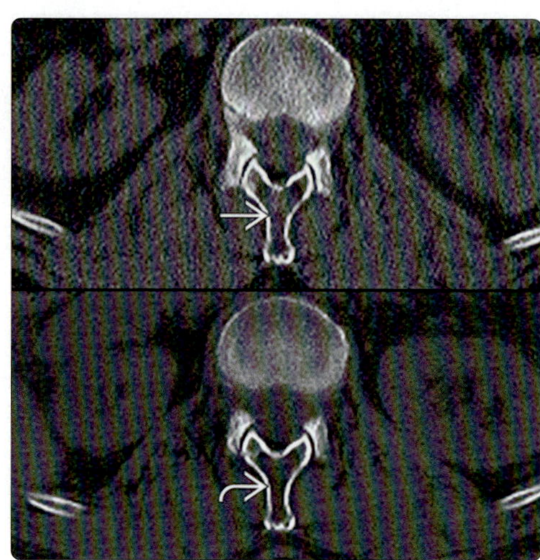

(Left) *Sagittal T1 STIR MR images of the lower spine depict > 10 focal lesions → with background heterogeneously ↓ signal on T1 ⇨ and ↑ STIR signal ↪ indicating extensive multiple myeloma infiltration. Also note pathologic compression fracture at T9.* **(Right)** *Sagittal CT, PET/CT, and PET in the same patient, after 35 days of treatment with lenalidomide and dexamethasone with minimal response, depict heterogeneous diffuse uptake of FDG → with focal uptake in the spinous process of L4 with lytic lesion ⇨.*

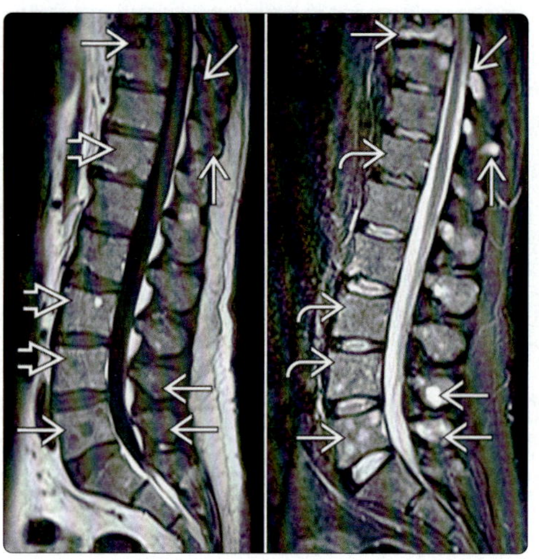

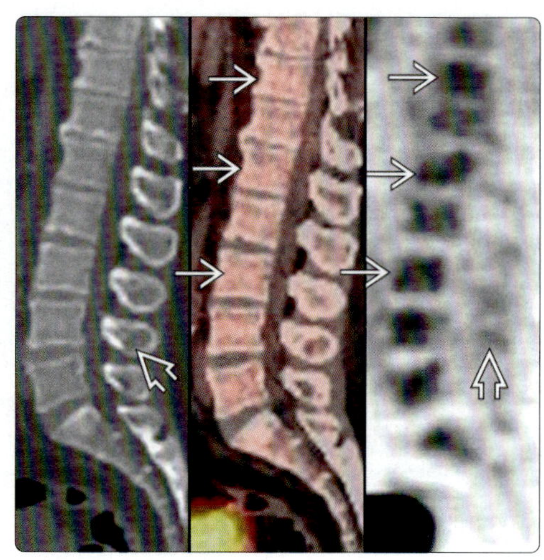

(Left) *Sagittal STIR MR images in the same patient show response to treatment by ↑ marrow fat ⇨ and ↓ STIR signal ↪ in previous areas of marrow infiltration and focal lesions → after tandem autologous transplantation + maintenance therapy. Kyphoplasty of T9 is low on T1/STIR.* **(Right)** *Sagittal CT, PET/CT, and PET depict response to treatment (tandem transplantation + maintenance) showing ↓ uptake of FDG →. Note the persistent L4 lytic lesion ⇨. T9 kyphoplasty shows artifactual ↑ FDG uptake ↪.*

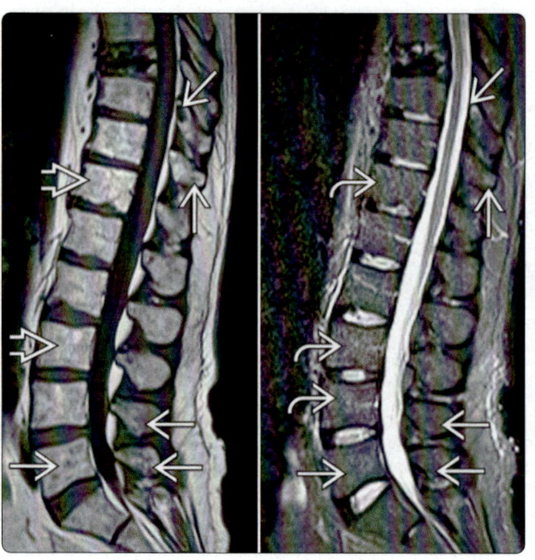

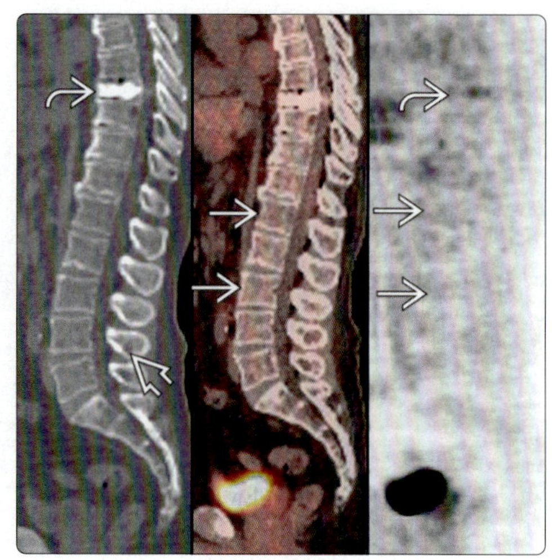

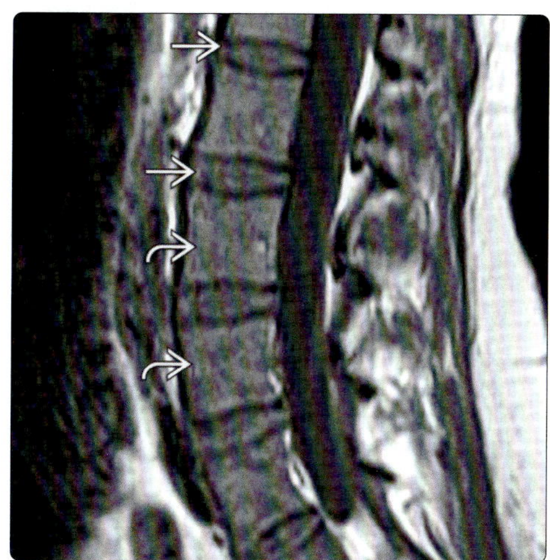

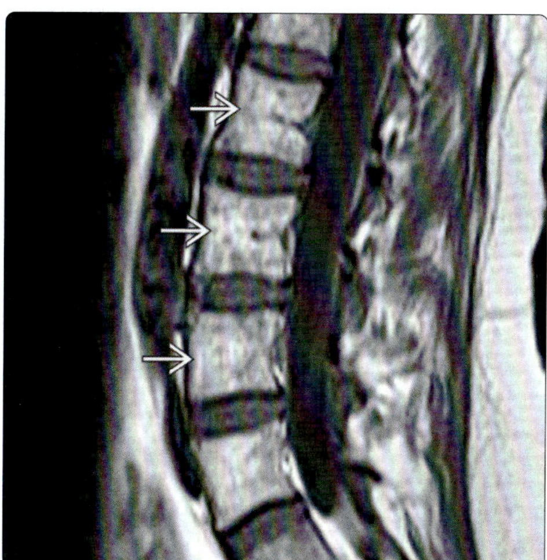

(Left) *Sagittal T1WI MR depicts moderate diffuse marrow infiltration by myeloma. The discs* ➡ *are similar in intensity to the bone marrow* ➡ *throughout the spine. On routine bone marrow biopsy, 90% plasma cells were present.* **(Right)** *Sagittal T1WI MR in the same patient, after induction chemotherapy, high-dose chemotherapy, and 2 stem cell transplantations, shows striking change in appearance with marked increase in fat within the marrow* ➡ *in this patient with complete remission.*

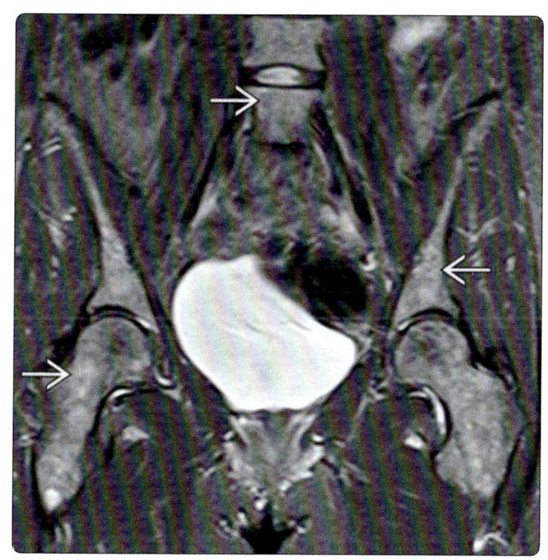

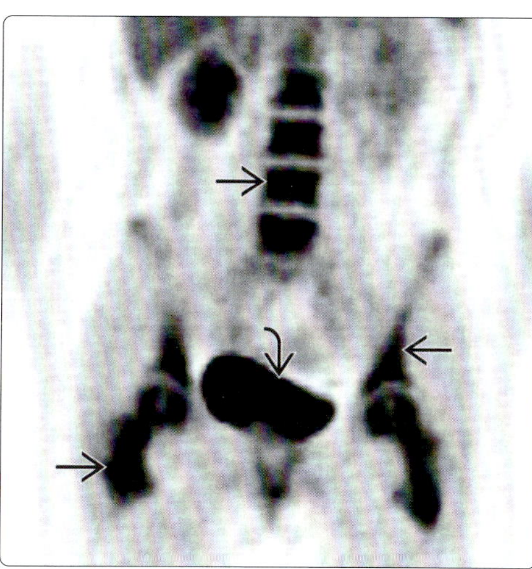

(Left) *Coronal STIR MR through the pelvis prior to treatment demonstrates diffuse relatively homogeneous increased STIR signal within the vertebral bodies, iliac bones, and proximal femora* ➡ *in this patient with diffuse myeloma infiltration.* **(Right)** *Coronal PET before treatment demonstrates marked ↑ FDG activity in the bone marrow* ⇨ *similar to the bladder* ⇨*, which has high activity due to excretion.*

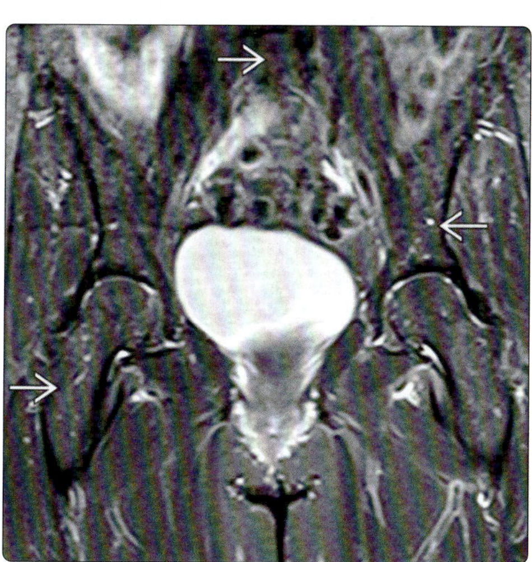

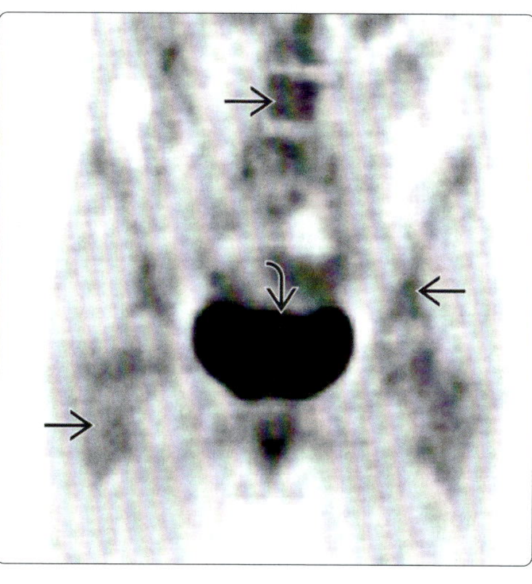

(Left) *Coronal STIR MR in the same patient, after induction chemotherapy followed by high-dose chemotherapy and 2 stem cell transplantations, demonstrates decreased STIR signal* ➡ *consistent with complete remission. Bone marrow biopsy showed no detectable plasma cell dyscrasia.* **(Right)** *Coronal PET after treatment demonstrates marked ↓ FDG activity in the bone marrow* ⇨ *compared to the bladder* ⇨*, which has high activity due to excretion of the tracer.*

POEMS

KEY FACTS

TERMINOLOGY

- **P**olyneuropathy, **o**rganomegaly, **e**ndocrinopathy, **M** protein (monoclonal plasma cell proliferative disorder), **s**kin changes (**POEMS**)
  - Acronym does not include several other important features, among them sclerotic bone lesions

IMAGING

- Location: Osseous lesions found in typical distribution of multiple myeloma
  - Axial skeleton (spine, ribs, sternum)
  - Flat bones (cranium, pelvis, shoulder girdle)
  - Proximal large tubular bones
- Solitary lesion 42%, 2-3 lesions 29%, > 3 lesions 29%
- 47% sclerotic only; 51% mixed lytic & sclerotic
  - Round, completely sclerotic lesions
  - Round, lytic lesions with dense sclerotic rim
  - Diffuse sclerosis; no focal lesions
- MR: Fully sclerotic lesions ↓ SI on all sequences
  - May have peripheral ↑ SI on STIR, post contrast
  - Lytic lesions with sclerotic rim on radiograph show ↓ SI on T1, ↑ SI on fluid sequences with ↓ signal rim, + enhancement

PATHOLOGY

- Ambiguity regarding number of features required for diagnosis
- Association of plasma cell dyscrasia and peripheral neuropathy is strong in POEMS
  - 34-50% of patients with osteosclerotic myeloma have neuropathy
  - 50% of patients with myeloma and peripheral neuropathy have sclerotic bone lesions

CLINICAL ISSUES

- Treated POEMS appears to have slightly longer survival than multiple myeloma: 165 months

(Left) *AP radiograph demonstrates lesions, too numerous to count, which are round and generally about a centimeter in diameter. They are variably fully sclerotic → or lytic with sclerotic rings ⇨. This sclerotic ring pattern is a variant form of the purely sclerotic lesions seen in POEMS.* **(Right)** *AP radiograph shows diffuse pelvic sclerosis, also with smudgy rounded lesions within the femoral necks. This is a variant of the sclerotic bone lesions in POEMS, in which the sclerosis is more diffuse than focal.*

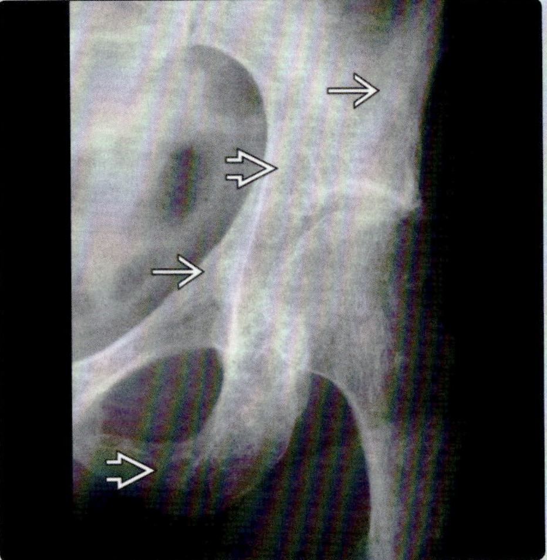

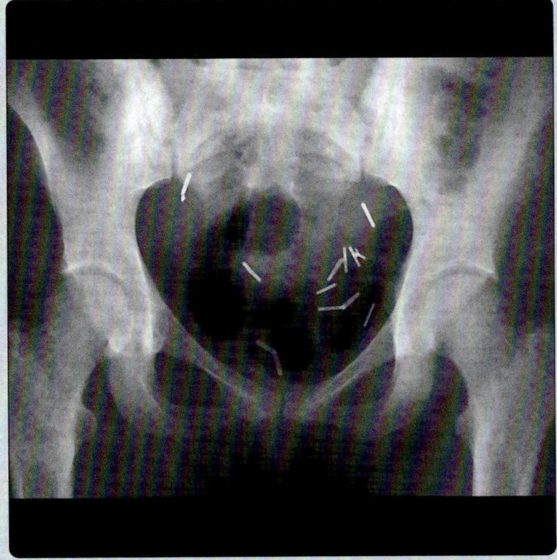

(Left) *Sagittal STIR MR, in a patient with known monoclonal plasma cell proliferation, shows multiple ↓ SI lesions →. There is slight surrounding high signal ↪ at some of the lesions. Ordinarily an active (not POEMS) myeloma lesion would be entirely hyperintense.* **(Right)** *Coronal STIR MR in the same patient shows multiple sternal lesions that are low SI →. They were similarly low signal on T1 imaging. Radiographs showed matching sclerotic foci. The patient has the sclerosing osseous lesions seen in POEMS syndrome.*

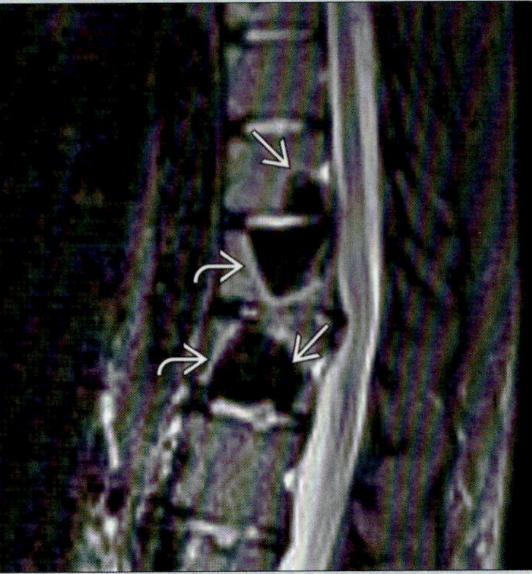

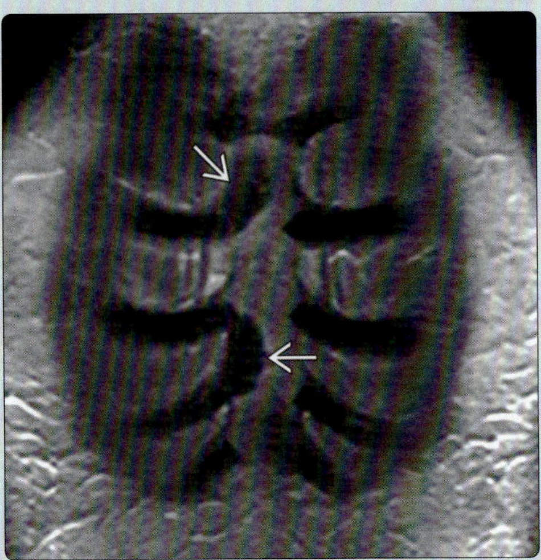

TERMINOLOGY

Definitions

- **P**olyneuropathy, **o**rganomegaly, **e**ndocrinopathy, **M** protein (monoclonal plasma cell proliferative disorder), **s**kin changes (**POEMS**)
  - Acronym does not include several other important features; among them, sclerotic bone lesions

IMAGING

General Features

- Location
  - Osseous lesions: Typical distribution of multiple myeloma
    - Axial skeleton (spine, ribs, sternum)
    - Flat bones (cranium, pelvis, shoulder girdle)
    - Proximal large tubular bones

Radiographic Findings

- Osseous lesions
  - Solitary lesion in 42%; 2-3 lesions in 29%; > 3 lesions 29%
  - 47% sclerotic only; 51% mixed lytic & sclerotic; range of appearance
  - Range of appearance
    - Round, completely sclerotic lesions
    - Round, lytic lesions with dense sclerotic rim
    - Diffuse sclerosis in affected regions; no focal lesions
- Chest radiographs
  - Pleural effusions, ↑ diaphragm, cardiomegaly (23%)

MR Findings

- Osseous lesions with expected signal, according to radiographic findings
  - Fully sclerotic lesions low signal on all sequences
    - May have peripheral ↑ SI on STIR, post contrast
  - Lytic lesions with sclerotic rim on radiograph show low SI on T1, high SI on fluid sequences with low signal rim, + enhancement
  - Often mixed pattern of lesions

DIFFERENTIAL DIAGNOSIS

Sclerotic Bone Metastases

- Breast, prostate most common

Multiple Bone Islands

- Differentiated by feature in bone island of dense lesion blending into normal bone at periphery

Osteopoikilosis

- Clustered bone islands around metaphyses

PATHOLOGY

General Features

- Etiology
  - Etiology unknown
    - Imbalance of proinflammatory cytokines has been implicated
      - ↑ interleukin-1β, IL-6, and tumor necrosis factor-α
      - Vascular endothelial growth factor increased and may be associated with syndrome
  - Establishing diagnosis
    - No single test to confirm diagnosis
    - Linking disparate signs and symptoms used
      - Interconnections between POEMS, sclerotic lesions, and Castleman disease not understood
    - Ambiguity persists about the number of features necessary for diagnosis
      - Makes it difficult to establish therapeutic regimens and understand prognosis
  - Association of plasma cell dyscrasia and peripheral neuropathy is strong in POEMS
    - 34-50% of patients with osteosclerotic myeloma have neuropathy
    - 50% of patients with myeloma and peripheral neuropathy have sclerotic bone lesions
      - Compare with only 1-8% of patients with classic multiple myeloma who have neuropathy
  - Largest retrospective series (Mayo Clinic) used the following criteria to diagnose POEMS syndrome (listed incidences based on this series)
    - Major criteria (100% required for inclusion)
      - Polyneuropathy: Demyelinating, axonal loss
      - Monoclonal plasma cell proliferative disorder
    - Minor criteria (at least 1 required for inclusion)
      - Sclerotic bone lesions (usually present: 95%)
      - Castleman disease (11%)
      - Organomegaly (splenomegaly, hepatomegaly, or lymphadenopathy): 50%
      - Edema (edema, pleural effusion, or ascites): 29%
      - Endocrinopathy (adrenal, thyroid, pituitary, gonadal, parathyroid, pancreatic): 67% have at least 1 manifestation
      - Skin changes (hyperpigmentation most common, hypertrichosis, plethora, hemangiomata): 68%

CLINICAL ISSUES

Presentation

- Most common symptom: Peripheral neuropathy

Natural History & Prognosis

- Treated POEMS appears to have slightly longer survival than multiple myeloma: 165 months
  - Number of features of POEMS present at diagnosis not prognostic of survival
  - May accumulate additional features over time
  - Even patients with multiple bone lesions or with > 10% plasma cells may not progress to overt myeloma
    - Patients tend not to have usual complications of multiple myeloma, such as renal failure

Treatment

- Multisystem disease, so no standardized target therapy
  - Radiation for solitary bone lesion
  - High-dose chemotherapy with autologous stem cell support may be utilized
- Treatment response ranges from ↑ sclerosis to resolution

SELECTED REFERENCES

1. Glazebrook K et al: Computed tomography assessment of bone lesions in patients with POEMS syndrome. Eur Radiol. 25(2):497-504, 2015

KEY FACTS

TERMINOLOGY

- Ewing sarcoma family of tumors: Cytogenetically closely related if not identical lesions on morphologic continuum
  - Ewing sarcoma: Bone and rare soft tissue location
  - Primitive neuroectodermal tumor: Bone & soft tissue tumors with microscopic features indistinguishable from Ewing sarcoma but with histologic rosette formation
  - Askin: Similar lesion, but involving chest wall

IMAGING

- Location: Diaphysis or metadiaphysis of long bones (70%)
  - Tubular bone involvement usually in younger patient age group (1st and early 2nd decades)
- Location: Flat bones (25%): Ilium, scapula, chest wall
  - Usually in older patient age group (late 2nd and 3rd decades)
- Imaging appearance: Permeative osseous destruction
  - No sclerotic margin; wide zone of transition
  - Permeative nature may be so subtle as to appear normal on radiograph
- Aggressive periosteal reaction, often lamellated ("onion skin"), rarely sunburst pattern
- Cortical destruction always present but variable in appearance
  - May be focal & obvious
  - May present as subtle linear canals connecting intramedullary tumor to soft tissue mass
- Soft tissue mass variable
  - May be very large
  - May be small & circumferential
- No true matrix
  - Reactive bone formation often appears as sclerosis within osseous portion of tumor (40%)

CLINICAL ISSUES

- 2nd most common bone sarcoma in children and adolescents (following osteosarcoma)

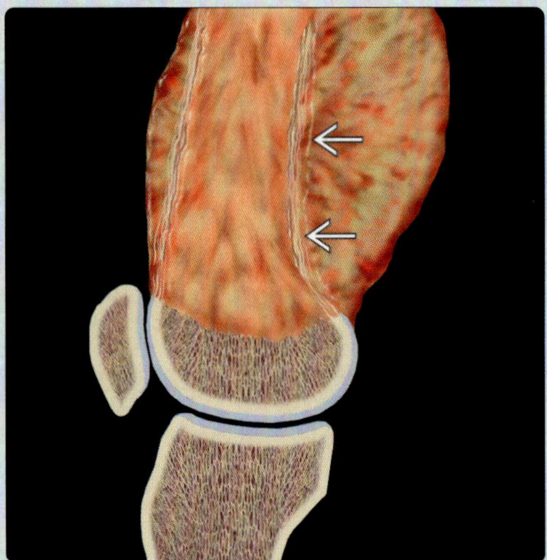

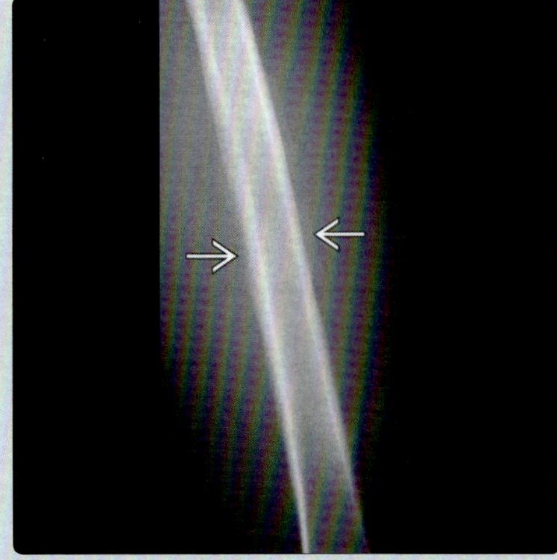

(Left) *Sagittal graphic shows a tumor mass typical of Ewing sarcoma destroying the metadiaphysis, with extension through the cortex to form a large soft tissue mass. Note the interrupted lamellated periosteal reaction* ➡*.* **(Right)** *Lateral radiograph shows typical diaphyseal Ewing sarcoma. The permeative osseous destruction can be difficult to visualize on radiograph. There is aggressive-appearing periosteal reaction* ➡ *and a large soft tissue mass, which is not well seen due to the lack of fat planes in this child.*

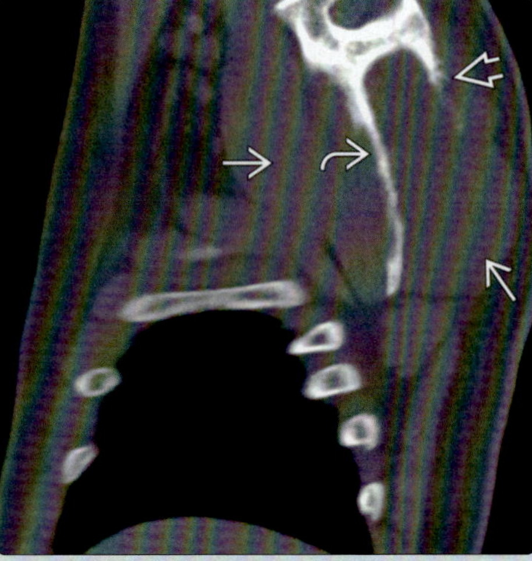

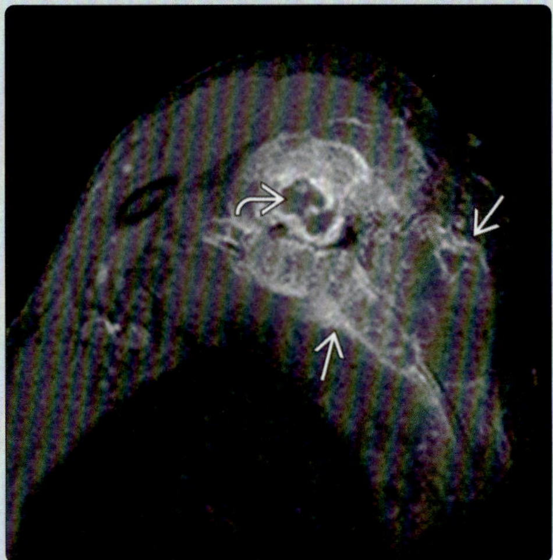

(Left) *Sagittal bone CT in a young adult shows cortical destruction of the body of the scapula* ➡ *and acromion* ➡ *with large soft tissue mass* ➡*.* **(Right)** *Sagittal postcontrast T1FS MR shows predominantly peripheral enhancement of this large Ewing sarcoma* ➡ *that contains necrotic tissue* ➡*. It is interesting that Ewing sarcoma may present either with a huge soft tissue mass and cortical destruction, as in this case, or with a discrete circumferential mass and subtle channels leading to it through the otherwise intact cortex.*

TERMINOLOGY

Abbreviations

- Ewing sarcoma (ES)

Definitions

- ES family of tumors: Cytogenetically closely related if not identical lesions on morphologic continuum
  - ES: Bone and rare soft tissue location
  - Primitive neuroectodermal tumor: Bone & soft tissue tumors with microscopic features indistinguishable from ES but with histologic rosette formation
  - Askin: Similar lesion, but involving chest wall

IMAGING

General Features

- Best diagnostic clue
  - Aggressive permeative osseous lesion with cortical breakthrough and soft tissue mass
- Location
  - Diaphysis (33-35%) or metadiaphysis (44-59%) of long bones
    - Tubular bone involvement usually in younger patient age group (1st and early 2nd decades)
    - Femur (20%), tibia-fibula (18%), upper extremity
  - Flat bones (25%): Ilium, scapula, chest wall
    - Usually in older patient age group (late 2nd and 3rd decades)
  - Axial skeleton: Usually sacrum (6% ES cases)
  - Rare extraskeletal or periosteal location of lesions
  - Location Askin tumor: Thoracic cage

Radiographic Findings

- Permeative osseous destruction (76-82%)
  - No sclerotic margin; wide zone of transition (96%)
  - Permeative nature may be so subtle as to appear normal on radiograph
- No true matrix
  - Reactive bone formation often appears as sclerosis within osseous portion of tumor (40%)
  - Reactive bone formation does **not** appear in soft tissue mass
- Periosteal reaction usually aggressive (95%), often lamellated ("onion skin"), may show sunburst pattern
- Soft tissue mass may be small & circumferential or massive
  - Often shows little overt cortical destruction; small channels through cortex may be seen
- Occasionally has slower course early in process, resulting in less aggressive appearance
  - No cortical breakthrough or soft tissue mass
  - Endosteal reaction results in cortical thickening (21%)

CT Findings

- Required for staging for lung metastases
- Mimic radiographic findings
  - Focal cortical destruction seen well
  - Subtle linear cortical channels extending to soft tissue mass common (66%)
    - May require viewing at wide window settings
    - Only evidence of cortical destruction in 30% of cases

MR Findings

- T1WI: Low to intermediate signal mass
- Fluid-sensitive sequences: Homogeneous (86%) low to intermediate (68%) signal mass; high signal intensity in 32%
  - Reactive bone may produce significant regions of low signal within marrow
  - High signal periosteal reaction
  - Marrow and soft tissue edema; exaggerated by STIR
  - Linear canals connecting marrow to soft tissue mass (only evidence of cortical destruction in 30-40%)
    - Highly suggestive of round cell tumor (ES, lymphoma, leukemia)
- Postcontrast imaging: Inhomogeneous but avid enhancement
  - Often contains regions of ↓ SI tumor necrosis
- Extraskeletal ES: Nonspecific MR appearance
  - Low to intermediate SI on T1, inhomogeneous intermediate to high SI on fluid-sensitive sequences, avid enhancement with necrotic regions
  - Normal adjacent bone marrow and cortex
  - Serpentine high flow vascular channels (low SI on all sequences) in 90%

Nuclear Medicine Findings

- Bone scan: Intense uptake at primary tumor and any osseous metastases
- PET/CT: Particularly useful in ES
  - ES has highest standard uptake value (SUV) of malignant primary bone tumors (mean: 5.3)
  - Used to stage ES
    - Osseous metastasis detection superior to bone scan (sensitivity 88% on PET/CT vs. 37% on bone scan)
  - Used to restage and assess response to therapy
    - SUV < 2.5 following chemotherapy: 79% + predictive value for favorable response (< 10% viable tumor)
  - Used to evaluate for tumor recurrence
    - Sensitivity (96%), specificity (81%), accuracy (90%)
    - Whole-body exam useful in detecting distant mets

DIFFERENTIAL DIAGNOSIS

Osteomyelitis

- Permeative, lytic osseous destruction similar to ES
- Periosteal reaction tends to be linear, more thick than in ES but may not be distinguishable
- Reactive osseous sclerosis may be similar to ES
- Fever, leukocytosis, elevated ESR present in both ES and osteomyelitis
- MR with contrast usually differentiates the 2 due to thick-walled soft tissue abscesses and intramedullary abscess in osteomyelitis

Osteosarcoma

- Usually metaphyseal, but metadiaphyseal location overlaps in osteosarcoma (OS) and ES
- Permeative, aggressive lesion
- Periosteal reaction more likely to be interrupted, sunburst variety than in ES
- Most OS have some degree of osteoid matrix; may be mimicked by reactive bone formation in ES

Langerhans Cell Histiocytosis

- May be highly aggressive, with lytic, permeative bone destruction, mimicking ES
- Periosteal reaction is prominent feature
- May show cortical breakthrough and soft tissue mass, though usually smaller than in ES
- Aggressive Langerhans cell histiocytosis (LCH) may show much faster osseous destruction than ES

Metastasis

- Neuroblastoma metastasis in young patient mimics ES
- Generally more metaphyseal than ES

Lymphoma

- Permeative, lytic, destructive
- Diaphyseal or metadiaphyseal, central, as in ES
- Large soft tissue mass, as in ES
- Occasionally elicits endosteal bone reaction and cortical thickening, as in ES
- May be multifocal, especially when arising in children, mimicking ES with osseous metastases

PATHOLOGY

General Features

- Genetics
  - Ewing family of tumors have recurrent t(11;22) (q24;q12) chromosomal translocation (in 90%)
    - 50% have secondary chromosomal aberrations
  - Nearly all cases of Ewing family of tumors show some type of *EWS/ETS* gene fusion (85%)

Microscopic Features

- Uniform small round cells with round nuclei and scant cytoplasm
- Often PAS-positive glycogen (70-100%)
- Necrosis common, but not extensive, with viable cells in perivascular distribution

CLINICAL ISSUES

Presentation

- Most common signs/symptoms
  - Painful (82-88%) mass (60%)
- Other signs/symptoms
  - Fever (20-49%), anemia, leukocytosis, ↑ ESR (43%)
    - May elevate clinical suspicion of infection
  - Pathologic fracture uncommon (5-15%)

Demographics

- Age
  - Range: 5-30 years (median: 13 years)
  - 80-90% < 20 years
- Gender
  - Male > female (1.5:1)
- Ethnicity
  - Extremely rare in African Americans (0.5-2% of cases)
- Epidemiology
  - 6-12% of primary malignant bone tumors
  - 3% of all childhood malignancies
  - 2nd most common bone sarcoma in children and adolescents (following OS)

Natural History & Prognosis

- 5-year survival rate: 65-82% with wide surgical resection (40% if resection marginal)
- Recurrence rate: 30%; generally occurs within 5 years (85-90%)
- 5-year survival for those with metastatic or recurrent disease: 25-39%
  - Metastatic disease at presentation: 30%
- Prognostic features
  - Stage
  - Anatomic location (proximal lesions, particularly in pelvis, have worse prognosis than distal lesions)
  - *EWS/ETS* fusion status: Type 1 gene fusion associated with better prognosis
  - PET/CT maximum SUV < 2.5 following chemotherapy correlates with improved survival
  - < 90% necrosis with neoadjuvant chemotherapy
- Mets: Hematogenous spread to lung, bone marrow, liver
- Treatment-related secondary malignancies
  - ↑ incidence with recent aggressive chemotherapy
    - 2% develop leukemia or myelodysplastic syndrome, median: 2.6 years following treatment
    - 1.5% develop other solid tumors, median: 8 years following treatment
    - Cumulative risk of 20% at 20 years for developing 2nd bone sarcoma
- Long-term complications of radiation may occur
  - Growth cessation → limb length discrepancy
  - Radiation osteonecrosis
  - Radiation-induced sarcoma

Treatment

- Initial chemotherapy to mitigate micrometastases and augment local control methods
- Initial radiation therapy considered, particularly when marginal resection may be required for functionality
- Wide resection if possible with goal of maximizing local control if limb salvage is possible
- Consolidation therapy ± radiation

DIAGNOSTIC CHECKLIST

Consider

- Ewing sarcoma is so rare in African Americans that another diagnosis (such as lymphoma) should be suggested for lesion appearing to be typical ES
- "Small round cell tumor" differential is interesting; it includes benign and high-grade malignant entities
  - Osteomyelitis, LCH, lymphoma, ES
  - Any of these may be monostotic or polyostotic
  - May not be able to differentiate by imaging

SELECTED REFERENCES

1. Murphey MD et al: From the radiologic pathology archives: ewing sarcoma family of tumors: radiologic-pathologic correlation. Radiographics. 33(3):803-31, 2013
2. Maheshwari AV et al: Ewing sarcoma family of tumors. J Am Acad Orthop Surg. 18(2):94-107, 2010
3. Bestic JM et al: Use of FDG PET in staging, restaging, and assessment of therapy response in Ewing sarcoma. Radiographics. 29(5):1487-500, 2009

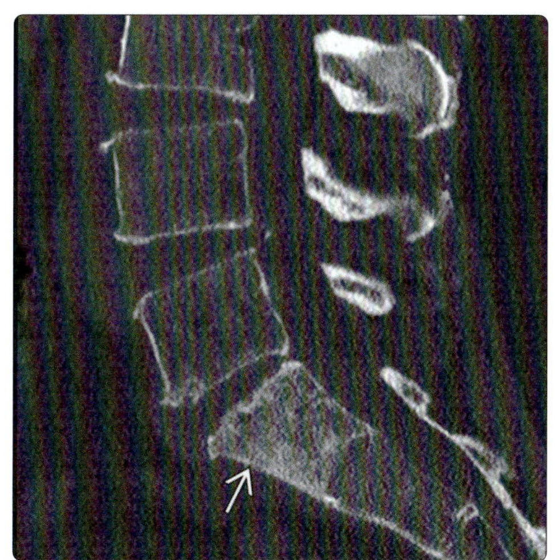

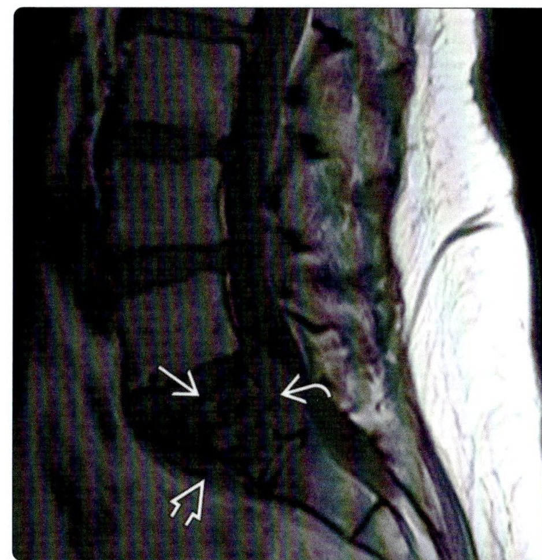

(Left) *Sagittal CT in a 63 year old shows mild sclerosis of S1 ➡. No overt cortical or intramedullary destruction is seen.* **(Right)** *Sagittal T1 MR, same patient, shows inhomogeneous hypointense signal and complete marrow replacement ➡. There is cortical breakthrough, though subtle cortical destruction ➡, and a small circumferential soft tissue mass ➡ is seen. The combination of reactive bone formation and this discrete cortical breakthrough and mass is typical of Ewing sarcoma, biopsy-proven in this case.*

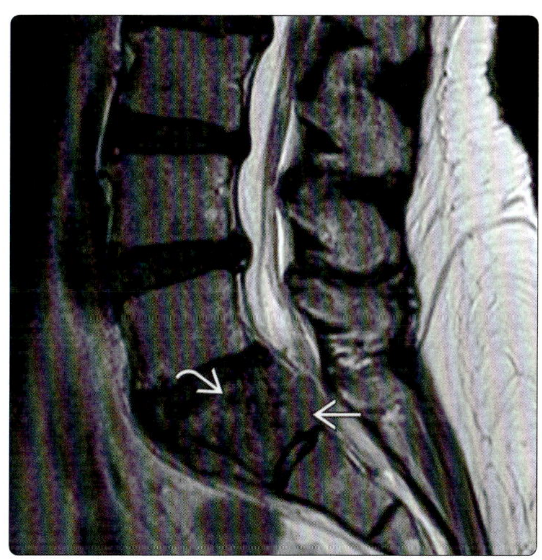

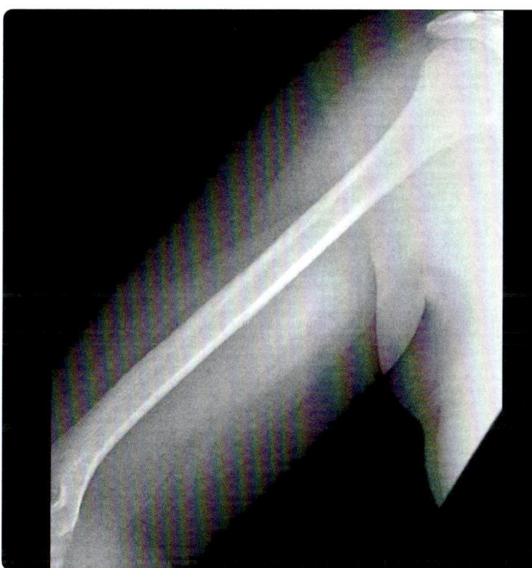

(Left) *Sagittal T2 MR in the same patient shows the low signal sclerotic bone ➡ within S1 and intermediate signal in the remaining tissue ➡, a typical appearance in Ewing sarcoma.* **(Right)** *Lateral radiograph appears completely normal in this unusually slow-growing Ewing sarcoma. There is neither osseous destructive change nor periosteal reaction. The fat planes are undisturbed. However, the arm was painful and deserved further work-up.*

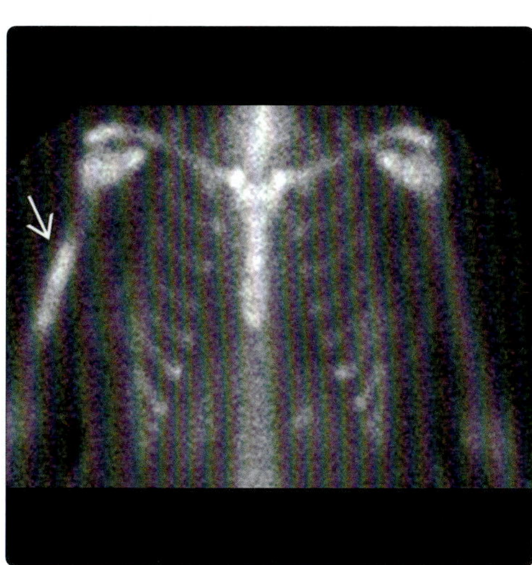

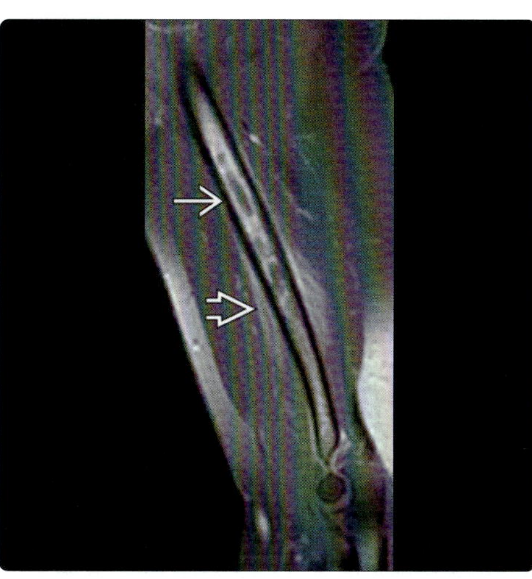

(Left) *AP bone scan in the same patient shows abnormal uptake in the midshaft of the humerus ➡. It is concerning that the abnormality is so highly permeative that it cannot be seen on radiograph, since this may indicate a highly aggressive lesion. Since it involves the midshaft of the humerus in a teenager, Ewing sarcoma must be considered.* **(Right)** *Sagittal T1WI C+ FS MR shows diffuse enhancement within the diaphysis ➡ with some areas of necrosis and mild edema external to it ➡. Ewing sarcoma was proven at biopsy.*

(Left) *Axial bone CT shows subtle osseous destruction along the body of the scapula ➡, giving a permeative appearance. This case of Ewing sarcoma demonstrates how subtle the primary osseous destruction may be in a flat bone, even when the accompanying soft tissue mass is large.* **(Right)** *Coronal T1WI MR in the same patient shows the size and extent of the mass to good advantage ➡; it is minimally hypointense to skeletal muscle and extends superior and inferior to the acromion process.*

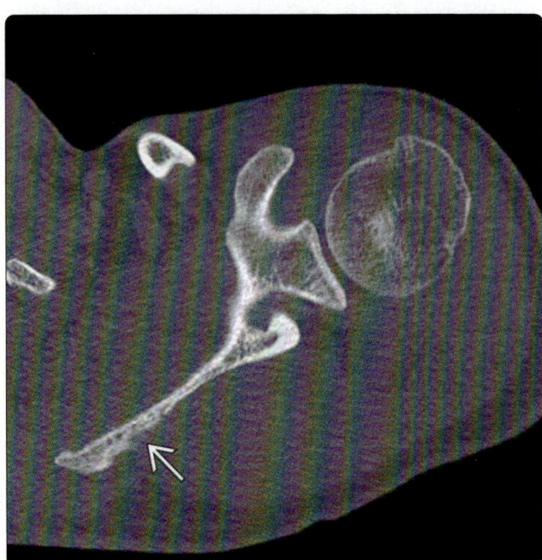

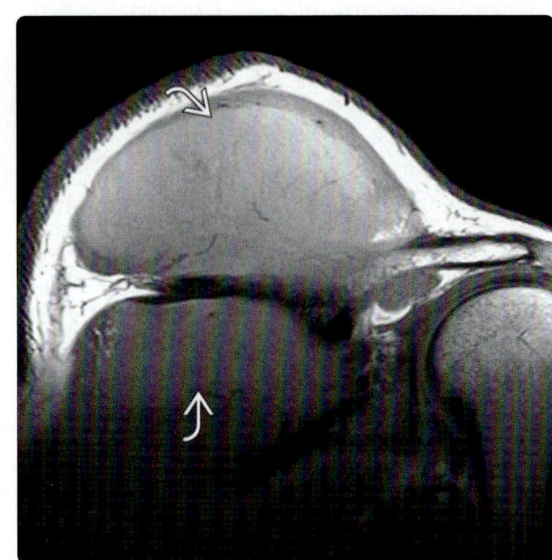

(Left) *Axial PDWI FS MR shows subscapularis and infraspinatus involvement. Soft tissue lesion ➡ is hyperintense, but note how subtle osseous high signal is, seen on MR only in wider portions of bone.* **(Right)** *Coronal T1WI C+ FS MR shows the lesion to enhance significantly and heterogeneously ➡. Note large areas of low signal indicating central tumor necrosis and surrounding edema within the muscle. Subtle abnormality of bone with large soft tissue mass may be seen in ES.*

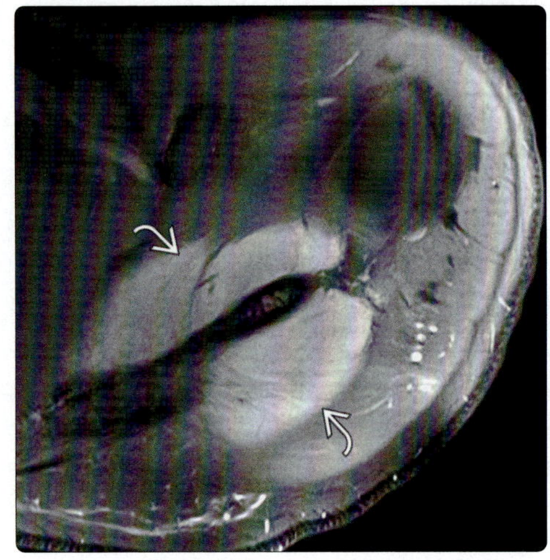

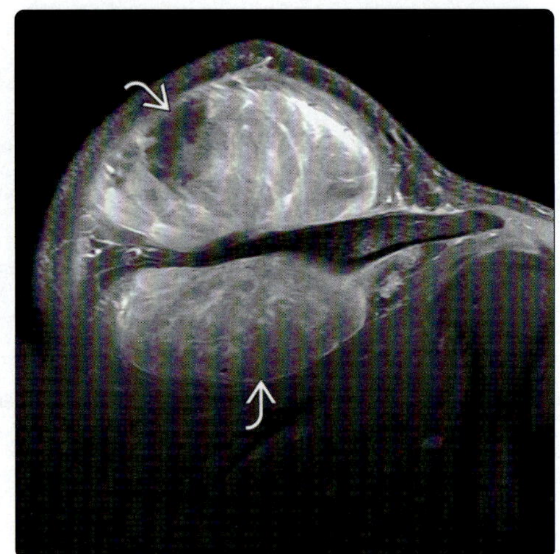

(Left) *Lateral radiograph shows a very dense lesion involving the entire proximal epiphysis of the tibia ➡. The epiphyseal plate appears intact, and no osseous destruction or soft tissue mass is seen.* **(Right)** *Axial T1 C+ FS MR in the same patient shows inhomogeneous hyperintensity in the bone, with low signal sclerosis less diffusely distributed than suggested on the radiograph. There is a relatively small circumferential mass. This case of ES is a reminder of the reactive sclerosis that may develop in these lesions.*

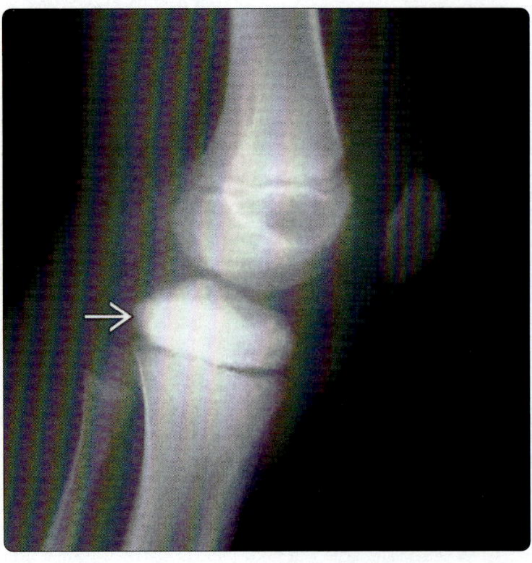

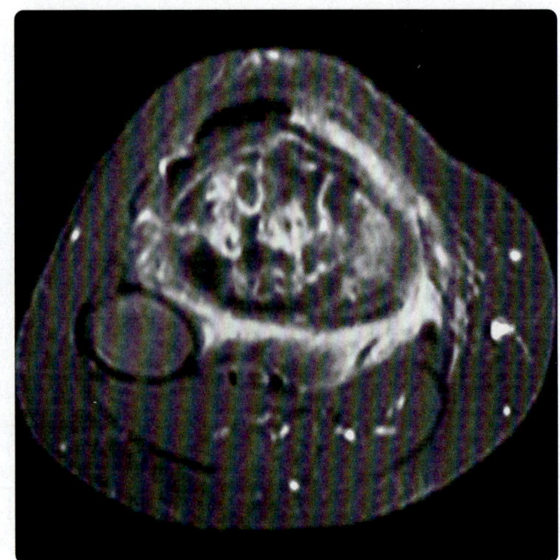

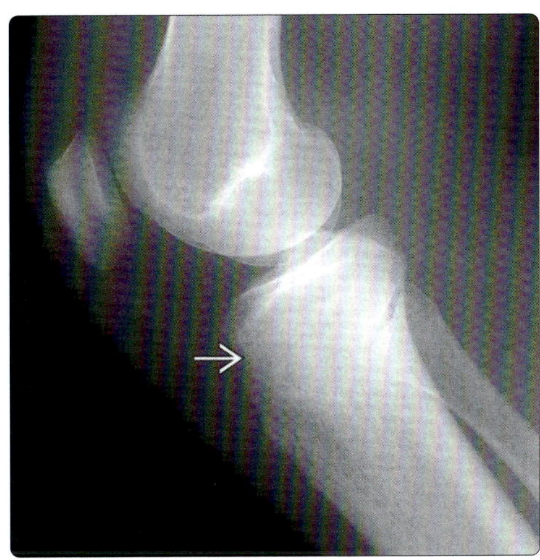

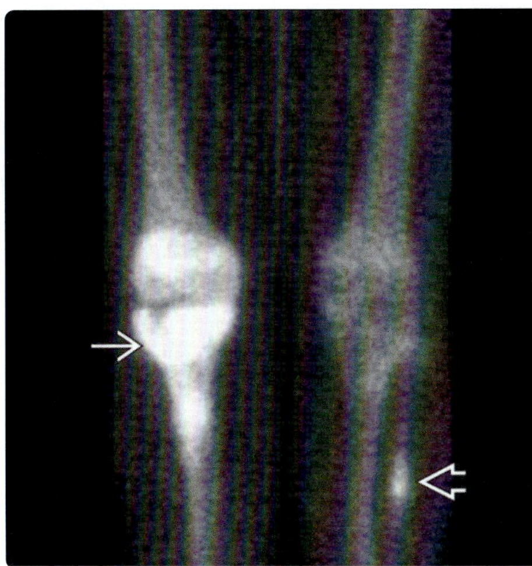

(Left) *Lateral radiograph shows only a suggestion of increased density in the proximal tibia ➡. There is absolutely no periosteal reaction or destruction change seen by radiograph. This is a very difficult radiographic diagnosis of Ewing sarcoma. AP radiograph (not shown) was normal.* **(Right)** *AP bone scan in the same patient shows uptake not only in the right proximal tibia ➡ but also in the diaphysis of the left fibula ⇨. This fibular uptake is nonspecific, but metastatic disease must be considered.*

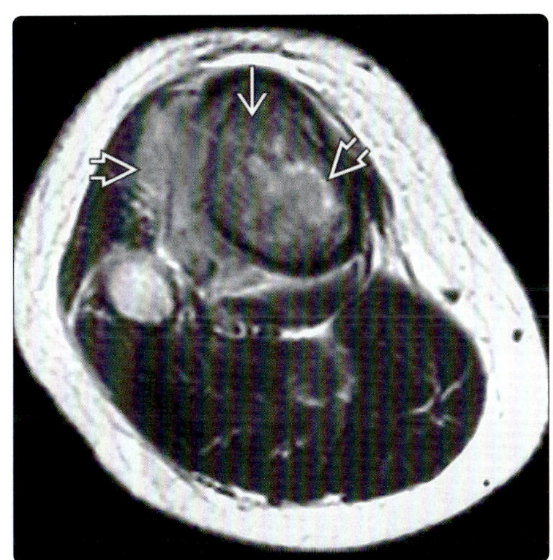

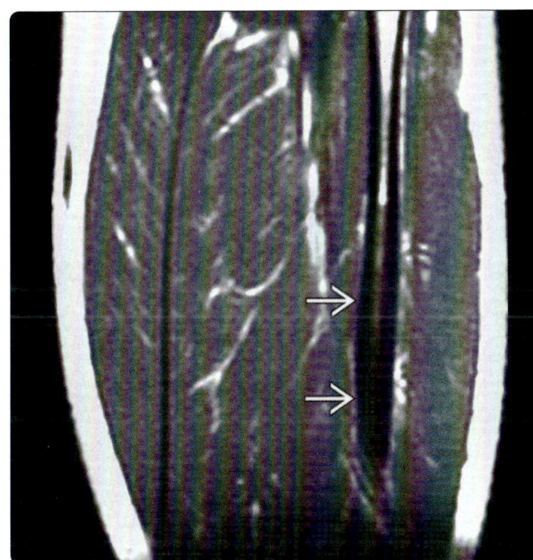

(Left) *Axial T2WI MR shows the lesion to be inhomogeneous, containing relatively low signal ➡ along with inhomogeneous high signal and soft tissue mass ⇨. This low signal suggests either reactive bone formation in Ewing sarcoma or subtle tumor osteoid in osteosarcoma.* **(Right)** *Coronal T1WI MR of the left fibula shows a surprisingly long region of diaphyseal marrow replacement ➡, corresponding to the bone scan abnormality. This represents an osseous metastasis in this case of ES.*

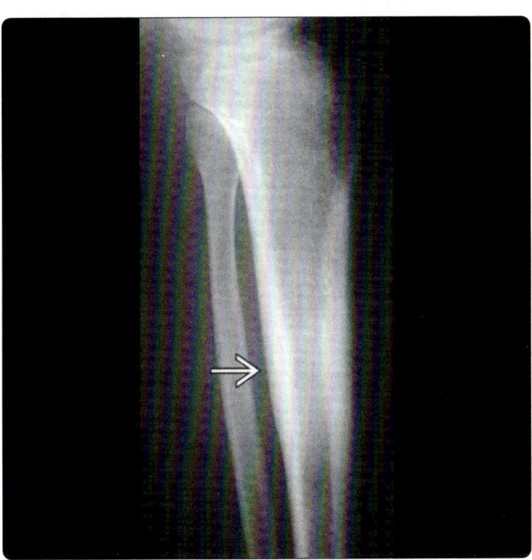

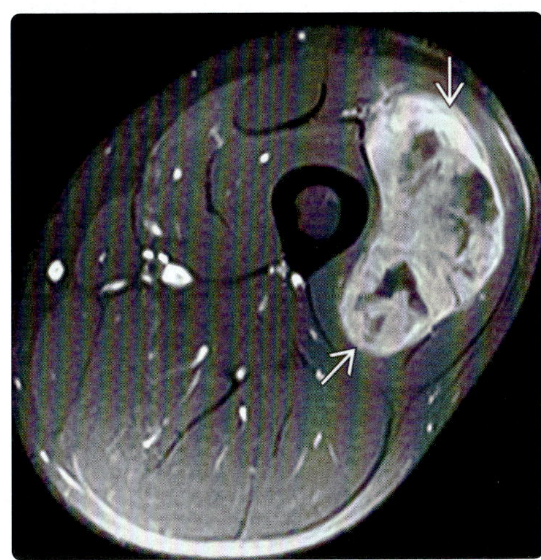

(Left) *Lateral radiograph in a young man complaining of leg pain shows the only abnormality is endosteal thickening and periosteal reaction ➡. Reactive bone masks the permeative bone destruction in this Ewing sarcoma. Occasionally this aggressive lesion presents on radiograph only as cortical thickening.* **(Right)** *Axial T1WI C+ FS MR shows a rare soft tissue Ewing sarcoma lesion. The appearance is nonspecific, with inhomogeneous high signal ➡; femur is normal.*

KEY FACTS

TERMINOLOGY

- Leukemia: Neoplastic disorder of white blood cells
  - May be myeloid or lymphoid in origin
  - May be acute or chronic

IMAGING

- Best diagnostic clue on radiograph
  - Permeative multifocal osseous destruction
  - Child: Radiolucent transverse metaphyseal bands
  - Adult: Diffuse osteopenia without underlying etiology for osteoporosis
- Location in childhood leukemia
  - Femur (24%), humerus (11%), ilium (17%), spine (14%), tibia (9%), scapula (4%)
- Location in adult leukemia: Axial skeleton predominates
- MR, T1WI: Low signal leukemic infiltrate
  - Permeative or patchy
- MR, T2WI: Hypointense or mildly to significantly hyperintense
  - Fat-saturated T2WI or STIR shows hyperintensity

CLINICAL ISSUES

- Most common signs/symptoms
  - Localized or diffuse bone pain
  - Paraarticular arthralgias (75%)
- ALL: Peak 2-10 years (most common childhood leukemia)
- AML: Peak > 65 years (but constitutes 15-20% of childhood leukemia)
- CML: Peak > 40 years (rare in childhood)
- CLL: 50-70 years
- Most common malignancy of childhood
- # 20 cause of cancer death in all age groups
- 5-year survival of combined leukemias: 25-30%
- Children with ALL: Complete remission in 90%
- Treatment
  - Chemotherapy: Induction, consolidation, maintenance
  - Bone marrow transplant
  - Radiation therapy

(Left) *Lateral radiograph in a child with no significant trauma shows diffuse osteopenia and a compression fracture ➡.* **(Right)** *AP radiograph in the same patient shows diffuse osteopenia and metaphyseal linear lucencies ➡. The differential diagnosis of severe osteopenia in a child includes osteogenesis imperfecta and renal osteodystrophy. However, the lucent metaphyseal lines are strongly suggestive of rapid development of osteopenia, making leukemia the most likely diagnosis.*

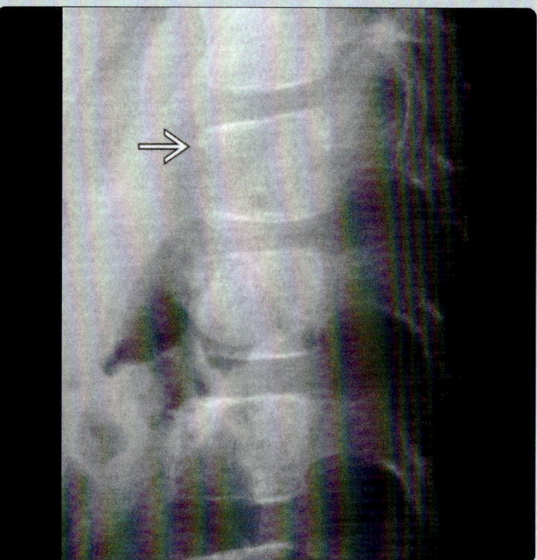

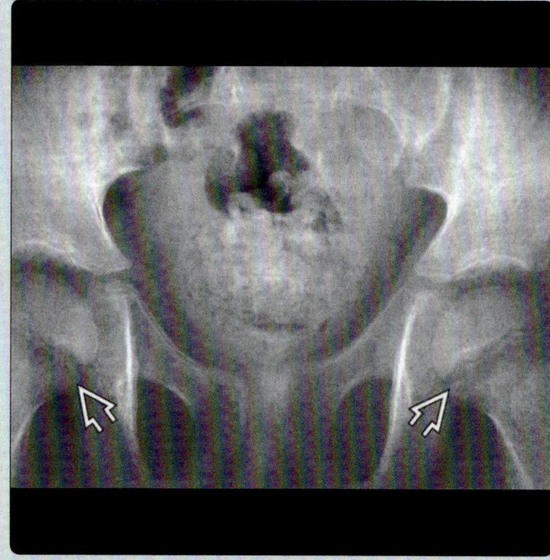

(Left) *Coronal T1WI MR shows an abnormal low signal intensity lesion at the medial aspect of the femur ➡, which is surrounded by multiple satellite lesions ➡. There is no cortical disruption.* **(Right)** *Coronal T2WI FS MR shows the lesions to be heterogeneously hyperintense ➡. Although normal erythropoietic marrow may have a nodular appearance in the distal femur, the leukemic infiltrates in this case can be recognized because they are of lower SI on T1WI and higher SI on T2WI than expected for erythropoietic marrow.*

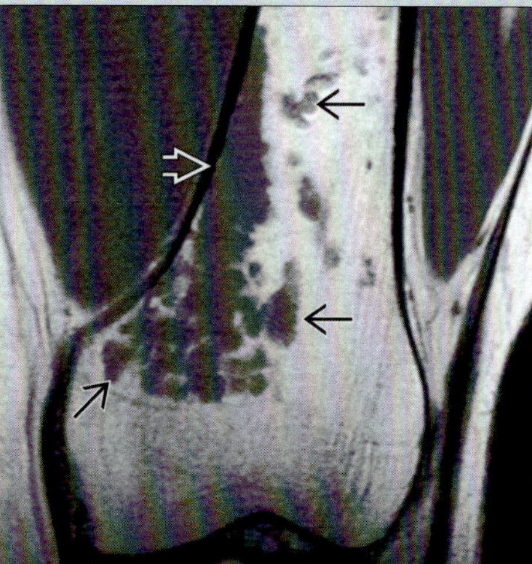

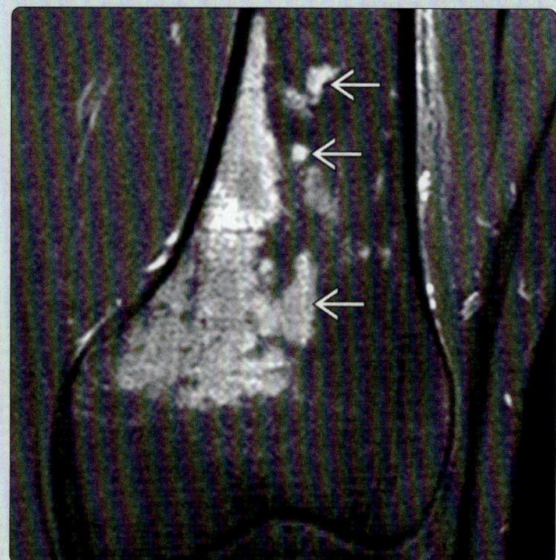

TERMINOLOGY

Abbreviations

- Acute lymphocytic leukemia (ALL)
- Chronic lymphocytic leukemia (CLL)
- Acute myelogenous leukemia (AML)
- Chronic myelogenous leukemia (CML)

Synonyms

- Granulocytic sarcoma, chloroma

Definitions

- Leukemia: Neoplastic disorder of white blood cells
  - May be myeloid or lymphoid in origin
  - May be acute or chronic

IMAGING

General Features

- Best diagnostic clue
  - Permeative multifocal osseous destruction
  - Child: Radiolucent transverse metaphyseal bands
  - Adult: Diffuse osteopenia without underlying etiology for osteoporosis
- Location
  - Childhood leukemia
    - Femur (24%), humerus (11%), ilium (17%), spine (14%), tibia (9%), scapula (4%)
  - Adult leukemia
    - Axial skeleton predominates

Radiographic Findings

- Lesions may be subtle & not recognizable on radiograph
  - Diffuse osteopenia not appropriate for patient age and gender may be best clue
  - Compression fracture without significant trauma should raise suspicion
- Lesions that are visible on radiograph
  - More common in children than adults with leukemia
  - Lucent metaphyseal lines ("leukemic lines") seen in 40-53% of ALL patients
    - Transverse lucent bands in metaphysis
    - Most frequent around knee and in proximal humerus
    - Following therapy, bands become focally dense
    - Not pathognomonic
  - Other lesions may be focally lytic
    - Blastic or mixed lytic/sclerotic lesions are rare
    - Range from permeative to geographic
  - Suture widening in skull with convolutional markings
  - Periostitis in long bones: 12-25%
    - Smooth, lamellated, or sunburst pattern
  - Pathologic fracture
    - Generally through metaphysis/physis
    - Physeal fracture results in slipped epiphysis

CT Findings

- Permeative bone destruction, lucent metaphyseal bands

MR Findings

- T1WI: Low signal leukemic infiltrate
  - Permeative or patchy
  - Iso- or hypointense to skeletal muscle or disc (internal spine standard)
- T2WI: Ranges from hypointense, mildly hyperintense, to significantly hyperintense
  - Fat-saturated T2WI or STIR shows hyperintensity
- Avid enhancement with contrast
- Dynamic contrast-enhanced MR may be predictive of degree of angiogenesis
  - Studies suggest relation to prognosis
- Opposed-phase imaging shows no signal dropout of leukemic foci on out-of-phase sequence

DIFFERENTIAL DIAGNOSIS

DDx of Diffuse Infiltrates Seen as Osteopenia (or Foci Seen Only on MR)

- Multiple myeloma
  - May present only as inappropriate osteopenia (for age and gender) on radiograph
  - Generally lower T1 signal than adjacent disc in spine and adjacent muscle elsewhere
  - T2 signal increase not impressive but generally high STIR signal and contrast enhancement
- Primary multifocal osseous lymphoma
  - Most frequently seen in childhood
  - Lesions may not be discernible on radiograph, or there may only be osteopenia
  - MR makes diagnosis: Low signal T1, high signal STIR, often with serpiginous pattern
- Chronic recurrent multifocal osteomyelitis
  - Occurs in childhood
  - Bone pain but no systemic symptoms
  - Usually not visible on radiograph
  - MR shows abnormality: Low signal T1, high signal STIR, enhancement post contrast
  - Biopsy required for diagnosis
- Systemic nonneoplastic processes leading to (nonsenile) osteoporosis
  - Steroids, alcohol, smoking
  - Malnutrition and anorexia
  - Renal osteodystrophy
  - Rheumatoid arthritis, ankylosing spondylitis
  - Osteogenesis tarda, hypophosphatasia tarda
- Red marrow reconversion
  - Due to hypoxic stress related to high altitude stress, athletic demands, obesity, smoking
  - Patchy, may appear permeative on MR
  - Generally not as low SI on T1 or high SI on T2WI FS as leukemia; distribution may help differentiate
- Marrow repopulation or stimulation
  - Red marrow repopulation with sickle cell anemia and stimulation with various treatments (including bone marrow stimulating drugs)
  - Patchy low T1WI SI, may appear permeative on MR
  - T2 and STIR signal hyperintense; difficult to differentiate from infiltration
  - Opposed-phase imaging useful for differentiation from leukemia

DDx of Child With Radiolucent Metaphyseal Lines

- One of classic presentations of leukemia

- Metastases, bone marrow
  - Especially neuroblastoma; usually 2-5 years
- Chronic illness
  - Includes sickle cell anemia, rickets, juvenile idiopathic arthritis, hemophilia
  - Malnutrition or prolonged hyperalimentation
  - Chemotherapy
- Normal variant of rapid growth
- Trauma, non-weight-bearing

DDx of Multifocal Permeative Lytic Lesions

- One of classic presentations of leukemia
- Metastases, bone marrow
  - Especially neuroblastoma in young child
  - In adult, breast & lung are most common primaries
- Ewing sarcoma
  - Polyostotic when metastasizes to bones (common)
  - Generally, obvious larger primary lesion present
  - Osseous destruction and soft tissue mass are usually more prominent than with leukemia
- Langerhans cell histiocytosis
  - Childhood lesion, often polyostotic
  - Lytic lesion; pattern varies from geographic to highly aggressive with periosteal reaction, cortical breakthrough, soft tissue mass
- Primary multifocal osseous lymphoma
  - Usually lesion of childhood
  - When visible on radiograph, pattern is lytic & destructive

PATHOLOGY

General Features

- Etiology
  - Arises from primitive stem cell either de novo or from preexisting preleukemic state
- Genetics
  - Patients with trisomy 21 and chromosomal translocations are at high risk of developing ALL
  - Trisomy 12 association with CLL
  - 90% of patients with CML have acquired chromosomal abnormality
    - Philadelphia chromosome, translocation between chromosomes 9 and 22
- Associated abnormalities
  - External factors highly associated with leukemia
    - Alkylating drugs
    - Ionizing radiation
    - Chemicals (benzene)
  - Predisposing hematological disorders
    - Aplastic anemia
    - Chronic myeloproliferative disorders

Microscopic Features

- Diffuse infiltration of bone marrow by poorly differentiated blast cells
- ALL: Infiltrates of small blue cells
- AML: Auer rods diagnostic
- CLL: Mature lymphocytes, 55% atypical cells
- CML: Leukocytosis, ↑ in basophils, eosinophils, neutrophils

CLINICAL ISSUES

Presentation

- Most common signs/symptoms
  - Localized or diffuse bone pain
  - Paraarticular arthralgias (75%)
- Other signs/symptoms
  - Fever, elevated ESR
    - May be confused with acute rheumatic fever, rheumatoid arthritis, osteomyelitis
  - Hepatosplenomegaly, lymphadenopathy
  - Joint effusions
  - Petechial hemorrhage, retinal hemorrhage
  - Anemia, frequent infections

Demographics

- Age
  - ALL: Peak 2-10 years (most common childhood leukemia)
  - AML: Peak > 65 years (but constitutes 15-20% of childhood leukemia)
  - CML: Peak > 40 years (rare in childhood)
  - CLL: 50-70 years
- Gender
  - M > F (2:1)
- Epidemiology
  - Most common malignancy of childhood
    - ALL: 75%, AML: 15-20%, CML: 5%
  - # 20 cause of cancer death in all age groups

Natural History & Prognosis

- 5-year survival of combined leukemias: 25-30%
- Children with ALL: Complete remission in 90%
  - 80% disease-free 5 years following treatment
- Adults with ALL: Remission in 60-80%
  - 20-30% disease-free 5 years following treatment
- AML: 5-year survival 45%
- CLL: Median survival is 6 years
- CML: Median survival is 5 years

Treatment

- Chemotherapy: Induction, consolidation, maintenance
- Radiation therapy
- Bone marrow transplant

DIAGNOSTIC CHECKLIST

Consider

- Watch for signs of diffuse osteopenia
  - When present in young adult (especially male) or child, look for underlying etiology
    - If patient has no underlying reason for osteoporosis (steroids, alcoholism, renal osteodystrophy, etc.), report should suggest infiltrative process

SELECTED REFERENCES

1. Fiz F et al: Adult advanced chronic lymphocytic leukemia: computational analysis of whole-body CT documents a bone structure alteration. Radiology. 271(3):805-13, 2014

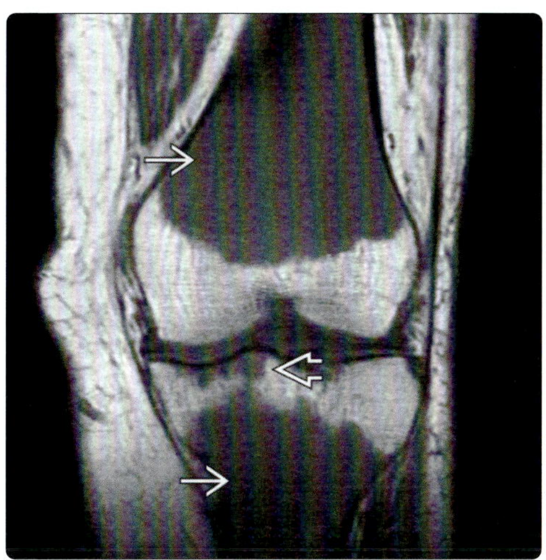

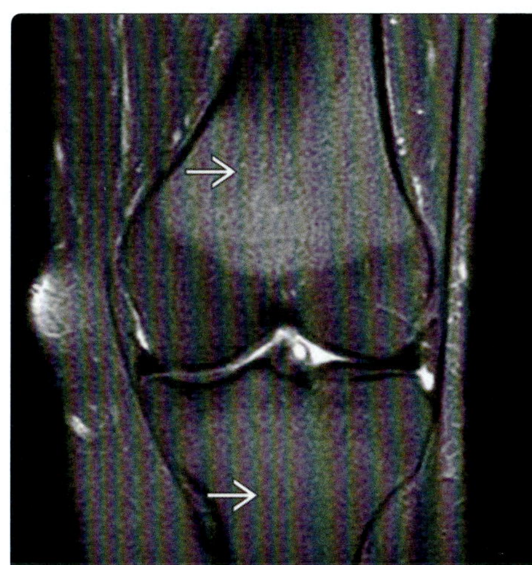

(Left) *Coronal T1WI MR shows abnormal marrow signal in bones around the knee ➡ and patchy involvement of the epiphyseal remnants ⇨.* **(Right)** *Coronal T2 FS MR shows the abnormal marrow signal to be only mildly hyperintense ➡, typical of hematopoietic marrow. However, the distribution, particularly involving the epiphyseal remnants, is highly suggestive of a diffuse marrow infiltrating process and should suggest that further work-up is necessary. Marrow aspiration revealed acute leukemia.*

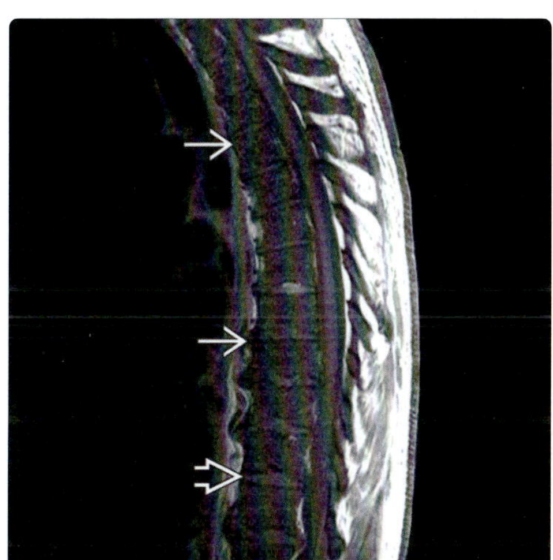

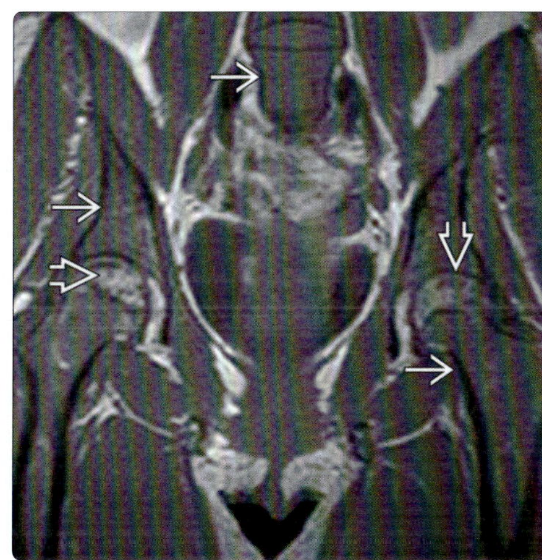

(Left) *Sagittal T1WI MR shows the bone marrow to have diffuse, markedly abnormal low signal ➡. Vertebral body bone marrow should not be lower signal than the intervening disc spaces ⇨ on T1WI MR. Aspiration showed diffuse leukemic infiltration.* **(Right)** *Coronal T1WI MR shows marrow that is diffusely too low signal for a 30 year old ➡. The marrow should have greater fatty conversion than is seen here. Low signal lesions are seen within the epiphyses ⇨ as well, suggesting marrow infiltration.*

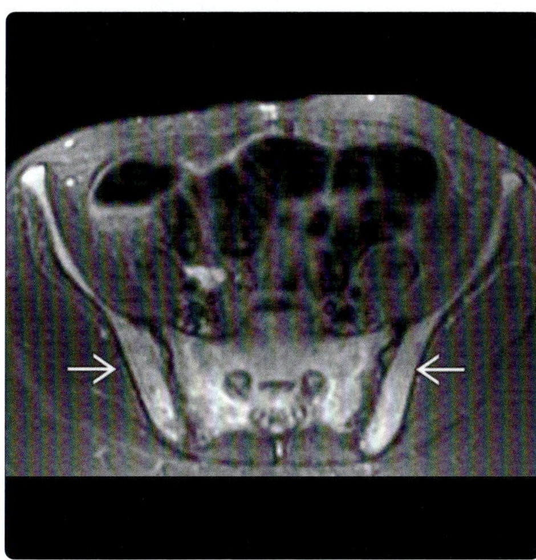

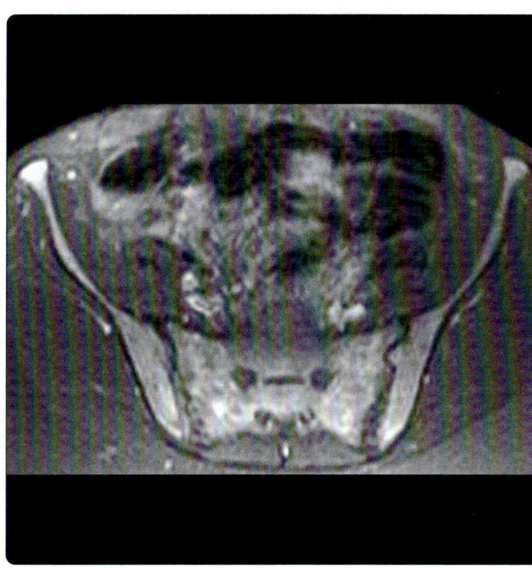

(Left) *Axial STIR MR in the same patient shows diffuse high signal within the pelvis and sacral osseous structures ➡.* **(Right)** *Axial T1WI C+ FS MR, same cut, shows diffuse enhancement of these same structures. The distribution in the proximal femora (including epiphyses) and pelvis, as well as signal abnormality, raises the likelihood of marrow infiltrative disease; biopsy proved leukemia. The radiographs were normal in this patient who complained of diffuse bone pain, a typical scenario. MR diagnosed leukemia.*

Lymphoma of Bone

KEY FACTS

TERMINOLOGY

- Primary lymphoma of bone: Neoplasm composed of malignant lymphoid cells
  - May occur as single skeletal site, ± regional lymph node involvement
  - May present with multiple bone involvement, without visceral or lymph node involvement

IMAGING

- Location: Regions of persistent red marrow in adults
  - Long bones in 71%
  - Flat bones in 25%
- Often extensive involvement of bone with permeative bone destruction (70%)
- Lytic lesion; no true matrix
  - May contain sclerotic reactive bone (30%)
  - Sequestra may be present (16%)
- Cortical (endosteal) thickening may occur
- Periosteal reaction in 60%; tends to be lamellated
- Cortical destruction is more often subtle, not observable on radiograph
- Soft tissue mass may be small and circumferential or disproportionately large
- MR shows permeative pattern of lesion well
  - Tumor serpiginously located between areas of normal marrow and medullary bone

DIAGNOSTIC CHECKLIST

- Image interpretation pearls
  - Radiograph may appear normal or only show endosteal thickening
  - Permeative pattern, leaving normal elements surrounded by tumor, is highly suggestive of primary lymphoma of bone
  - Tumor extension through small cortical channels, without overt cortical destruction, is characteristic
  - Radiographs underestimate prevalence of primary multifocal osseous lymphoma

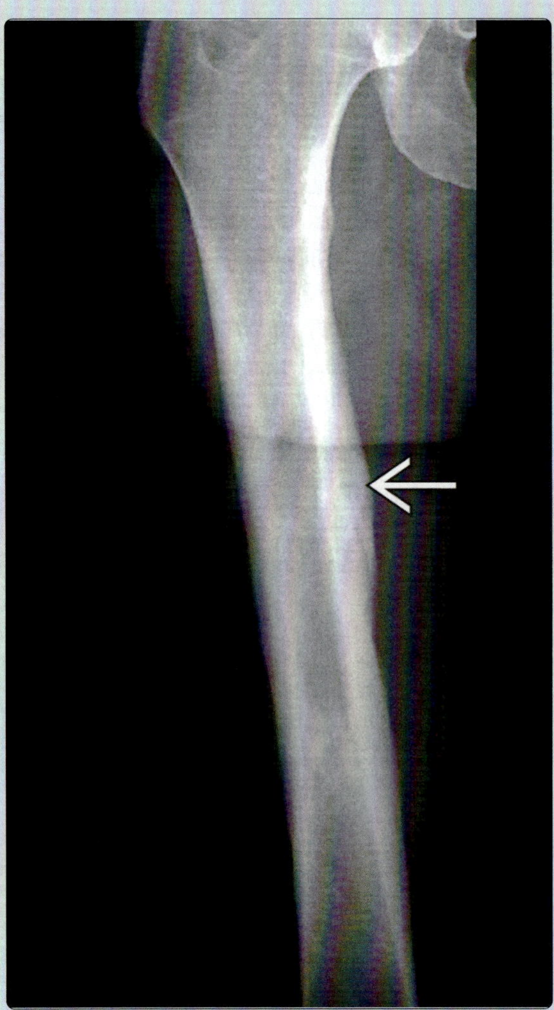

AP radiograph shows a large, highly permeative lesion involving the diaphysis of the femur. The lesion has evoked cortical and endosteal thickening medially ➡. This case of primary bone lymphoma has typical radiographic features.

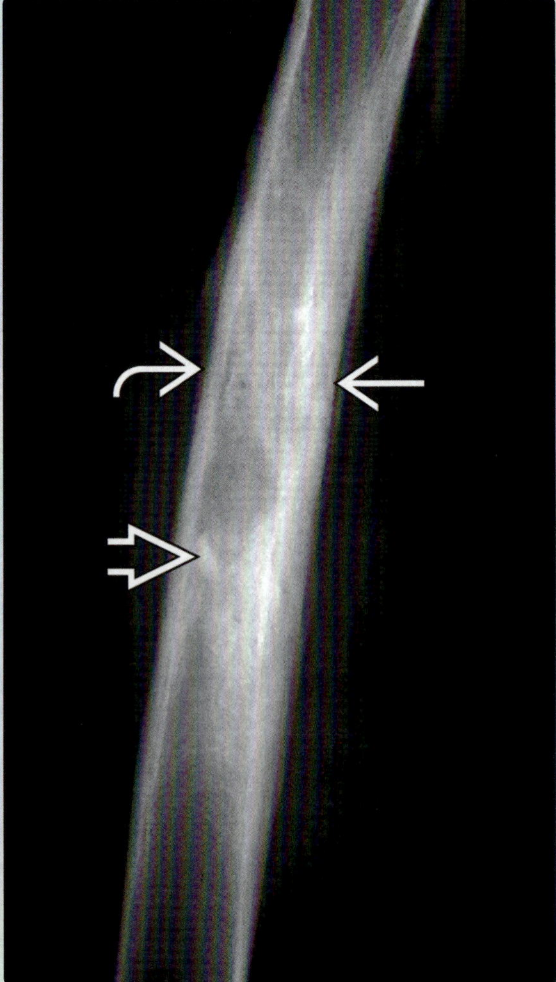

Lateral radiograph in the same patient shows the lesion has anterior periosteal reaction. There is a sequestrum present ➡ and endosteal scalloping anteriorly ↪, despite endosteal thickening posteriorly ➡. This combination is typical of lymphoma.

TERMINOLOGY

Abbreviations

- Primary lymphoma of bone (PLB)

Synonyms

- Reticulum cell sarcoma, primary non-Hodgkin lymphoma of bone, primary lymphoma of bone, osteolymphoma, lymphosarcoma

Definitions

- Neoplasm composed of malignant lymphoid cells
- Divided into 1° or 2° lymphoma of bone
  - PLB
    - Single skeletal site, ± regional lymph node involvement
    - Multiple bone involvement, without visceral or lymph node involvement
      - Termed primary multifocal osseous lymphoma
      - Diagnosis requires absence of involvement of distant lymph nodes or viscera for 6 months following diagnosis
      - More frequent in children than adults
  - Secondary lymphoma of bone
    - Presentation with bone tumor, but work-up shows involvement of viscera or lymph nodes in multiple regions
    - Known soft tissue lymphoma, with bone biopsy demonstrating involvement of bone

IMAGING

General Features

- Best diagnostic clue
  - Permeative osseous destruction with apparently intact cortex but soft tissue mass
- Location
  - Regions of persistent red marrow in adults
    - Long bones in 71%
      - Proximal metadiaphysis femur (25%), humerus (10%), tibia (10%)
    - Flat bones in 25%
      - Pelvis (20%), scapula (5%), clavicle, skull, spine
  - Usually presents as solitary lesion
    - Primary multifocal osseous lymphoma (PMOL) considered subset of PLB
      - Multiple bones affected but no nodal or visceral involvement
      - 10-31% of lymphomas present as PMOL
      - PMOL in metaphysis, diaphysis, and epiphysis
      - Most lesions occur around knee and in skull

Radiographic Findings

- Often extensive involvement of bone with permeative bone destruction (70%)
- Wide zone of transition
- Sclerotic margination is rare
- Lytic lesion; no true matrix
  - May contain sclerotic reactive bone (30%)
  - Sequestra may be present (16%)
- Cortical destruction, may have large soft tissue mass
  - Cortical destruction more often is subtle channels, not observable on radiograph
  - Soft tissue mass may be disproportionately large
- Cortical (endosteal) thickening may occur
- Periosteal reaction in 60%; tends to be lamellated
- PMOL
  - Lesions may be extremely subtle, not visible on radiograph
  - Lytic, permeative, serpiginous when visualized (similar to other small round cell tumors)

CT Findings

- May demonstrate sequestra better than radiograph
- Subtle cortical involvement well demonstrated
- CT used to evaluate chest, abdomen, and pelvis for lymphadenopathy and visceral involvement
  - Differentiates 1° and 2° lymphoma of bone

MR Findings

- Intramedullary involvement on MR
  - Shows permeative pattern of lesion well, with tumor serpiginously located between areas of normal marrow and medullary bone
    - Tumor regions: Low SI T1, high SI T2, enhancing
    - Residual marrow elements show normal bone T1 and T2 signal, without enhancement
      - Heterogeneous combination of low signal tumor and high signal residual marrow on T1WI termed salt and pepper
      - Heterogeneous pattern makes it difficult to differentiate diffuse marrow infiltration from hypercellular marrow on T1
- Cortical destruction may be subtle, even on MR
  - Only 28% show complete cortical disruption
  - Often associated with little overt cortical destruction; small channels through cortex may be seen (52%)
    - Circumferential soft tissue mass permeates cortex and periosteum in 66% of these
- Soft tissue mass on MR
  - May be disproportionately large relative to osseous destruction or small and circumferential
  - Low SI on T1 (isointense to skeletal muscle)
  - Fluid-sensitive sequences: Inhomogeneous ↑ SI
  - Inhomogeneously enhancing; regions of necrosis
- Dynamic contrast enhancement may better demonstrate marrow involvement
  - Likely due to angiogenesis of tumor cells in PLB; especially effective in higher grade lesions
- PMOL
  - Usually serpiginous pattern
  - Heterogeneous mixed high and low signal on fluid-sensitive sequences
  - Soft tissue mass absent in > 60% cases
  - MR detects more pelvic lesions than bone scan

Nuclear Medicine Findings

- Bone scan shows polyostotic lesions
- 16% false-negative rate for lesions on bone scan

DIFFERENTIAL DIAGNOSIS

Solitary Primary Lymphoma of Bone

- Ewing sarcoma (ES)
  - Generally more overtly permeative and destructive than PLB
  - Occasionally, ES shows very subtle destruction, no periosteal reaction but endosteal thickening, similar to some cases of PLB
  - ES generally occurs in younger adults than PLB; overlap exists
- Osteomyelitis
  - Sequestrum, permeative destruction, reactive bone formation similar to PLB
  - MR shows intramedullary &/or soft tissue abscess, which is generally characteristic
  - Systemic symptoms may help differentiate
- Malignant fibrous histiocytoma of bone
  - Generally more destructive than PLB, but lower grade lesions may have similar appearance

Multifocal (Primary Multifocal Osseous Lymphoma)

- ES with osseous metastases
  - Multiplicity of lesions may appear similar
  - Generally has distinctly different primary lesion with smaller secondary lesions
- Langerhans cell histiocytosis (LCH)
  - Like PMOL, LCH may be aggressive and multifocal
  - Both LCH and PMOL may show sequestra
  - Same age group as majority of PMOL cases
- Chronic recurrent multifocal osteomyelitis
  - Radiographs usually normal; MR shows nonspecific polyostotic abnormality
  - Chronic pain, cultures negative, diagnosis by biopsy
- Metastases, bone marrow
  - Metastatic neuroblastoma has similar appearance
  - Same age group as PMOL cases (generally children)
  - Lesions below knee more suggestive of PMOL

PATHOLOGY

General Features

- Genetics
  - Translocation of chromosomes 14 and 18 and chromosomes 8 and 14
- Associated abnormalities
  - May occur as posttransplant lymphoproliferative disease in immunocompromised patients
  - Associated with HIV/AIDS

Microscopic Features

- Generally diffuse large cell types
  - Large B-cell type (92%)
  - Diffuse follicle center cell type (3%), anaplastic large cell type (3%), immunocytoma (2%)
- Tend to show permeation around tissues, leaving behind normal medullary bone and marrow fat cells
  - Residual trabeculae may be normal or thickened

CLINICAL ISSUES

Presentation

- Most common signs/symptoms
  - Bone pain, sometimes mass
    - Insidious; may persist intermittently for months
  - Neurologic symptoms if lesion is in spine
  - Pathologic fractures (22%)

Demographics

- Age
  - Wide range: 1-86 years
  - Rare: < 10 years
  - Incidence increases with age throughout life
  - Peak incidence in 6th to 7th decades
- Gender
  - M > F (1.5:1)
    - Among affected children, M:F ratio is 6:1
- Epidemiology
  - 5-25% of non-Hodgkin lymphoma is extranodal in origin; of these, 5% arise in bone marrow
  - PLB: 3-7% of all osseous malignant tumors
  - 16% of patients with lymphoma eventually have bone involvement
  - 11-31% are multifocal at presentation (2 series)
    - 50% of children present with PMOL
    - Adults rarely present with PMOL

Natural History & Prognosis

- 83-90% 5-year survival
- 46% progression-free at 5 years
- Poor prognostic factors: Older age group (> 60 years of age), higher stage lesions, recurrent tumor

Treatment

- PLB: Chemotherapy is primary treatment
  - Adjuvant radiation therapy
- PMOL in child
  - Chemotherapy only

DIAGNOSTIC CHECKLIST

Image Interpretation Pearls

- Radiograph may appear normal or only show endosteal thickening
  - PLB should be considered and MR performed in such patients who complain of persistent pain
  - ES may rarely have similar presentation
- Permeative pattern, leaving normal elements surrounded by tumor, is highly suggestive of PLB
  - Radiograph: Seen as sequestrum
  - MR: Seen as serpiginous tumor surrounding normal marrow elements + small cortical channels
- Radiographs underestimate prevalence of PMOL
  - MR survey detects more lesions than bone scan

SELECTED REFERENCES

1. Messina C et al: Primary and secondary bone lymphomas. Cancer Treat Rev. 41(3):235-246, 2015

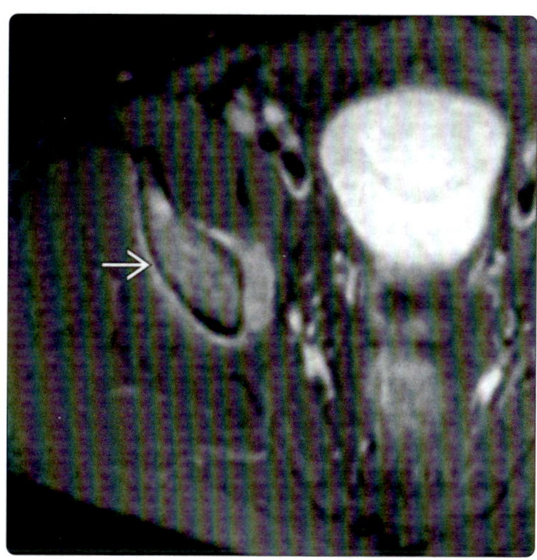

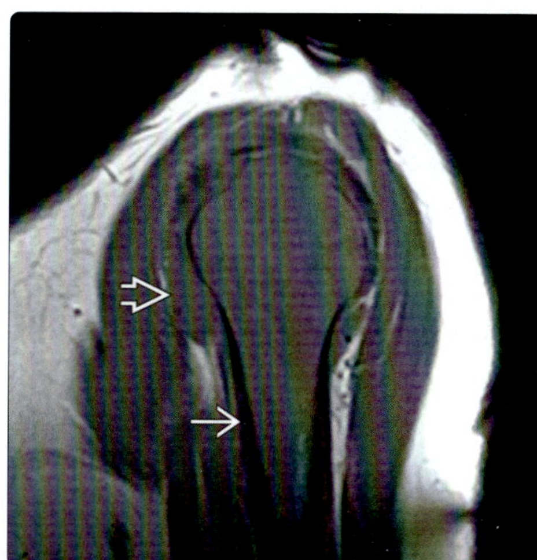

(Left) *Axial T2WI FS MR shows hyperintense bone marrow ➔. The cortex appears intact; tiny channels through the cortex allow a circumferential soft tissue mass to develop. The mass may be small, as in this case, or may be very large. This patient had HIV/AIDS, which may predispose to development of lymphoma.* **(Right)** *Sagittal T1WI MR shows low signal involving the marrow of the proximal humerus ➔. There is a small anterior soft tissue mass extending through apparently intact cortex ⇨.*

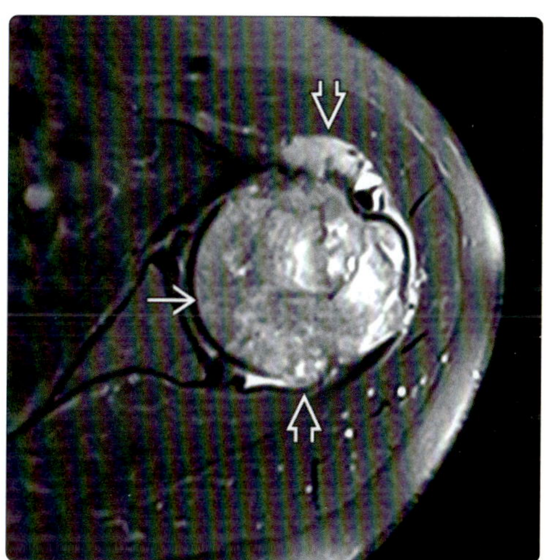

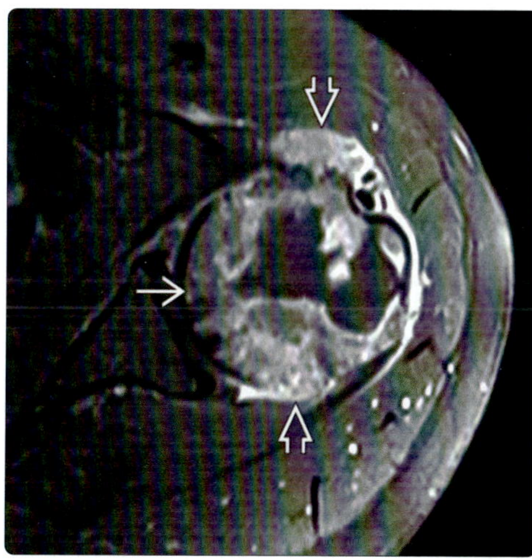

(Left) *Axial T2WI FS MR in the same patient shows inhomogeneous high signal within the marrow ➔. Note also the multiple focal regions of tumor extension through the cortex to form small soft tissue masses ⇨. Only minimal cortical disruption is seen.* **(Right)** *This axial T1WI C+ FS MR shows serpiginous regions of ↓ SI necrotic tissue within the marrow with surrounding inhomogeneous enhancement of bone ➔ and soft tissue masses ⇨. This appearance of mass with minimal cortical disruption is typical of lymphoma.*

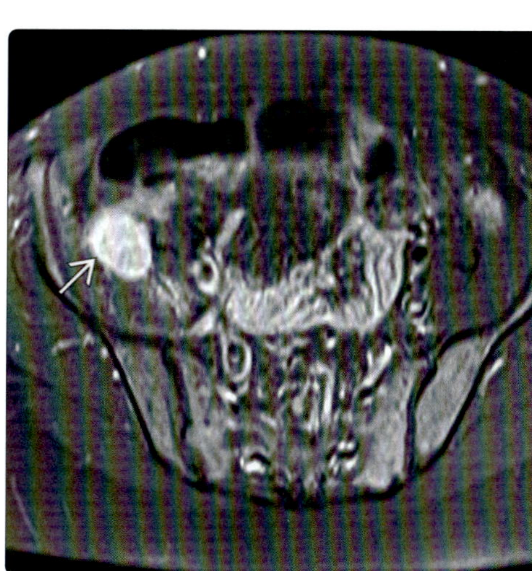

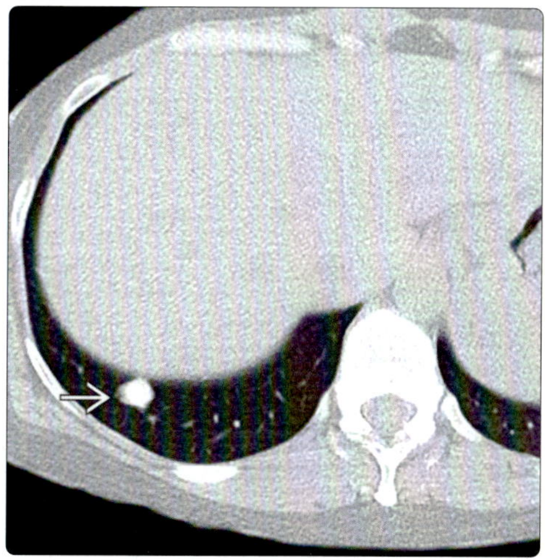

(Left) *Axial T1WI C+ MR of the pelvis in the same patient shows an enhancing lesion ➔; other images showed the lesion to extend from the L2 and L3 nerve roots along the course of the femoral nerve. This proved to be metastatic extension along the epineurium.* **(Right)** *Axial NECT of the lung in the same patient shows pulmonary metastatic disease ➔. Though the patient's major symptoms related to femoral nerve radiculopathy, primary lymphoma developed in her humerus, resulting in distant metastases.*

(Left) *Axial PET/CT in a patient with treated primary bone lymphoma shows a new region of tracer accumulation in the anterior left iliac spine (left ➡, right ➡). **(Right)** Axial bone CT in the same patient demonstrates vague sclerosis ➡ in this region without bone destruction. Since the bone marrow was considered the "organ" involved in this patient's primary disease, return of the disease in a different bone is more accurately termed a recurrence than a metastasis.*

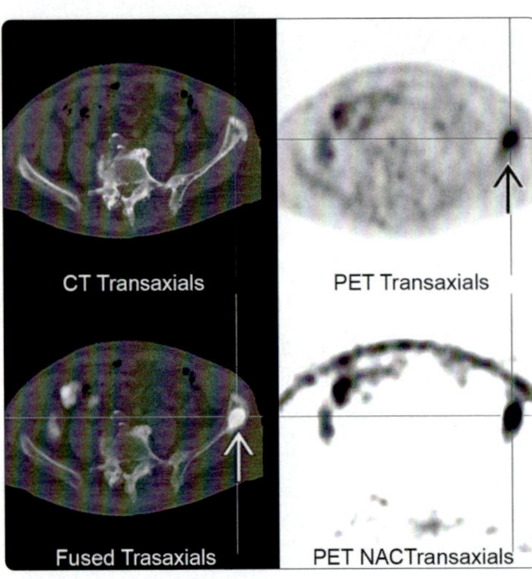

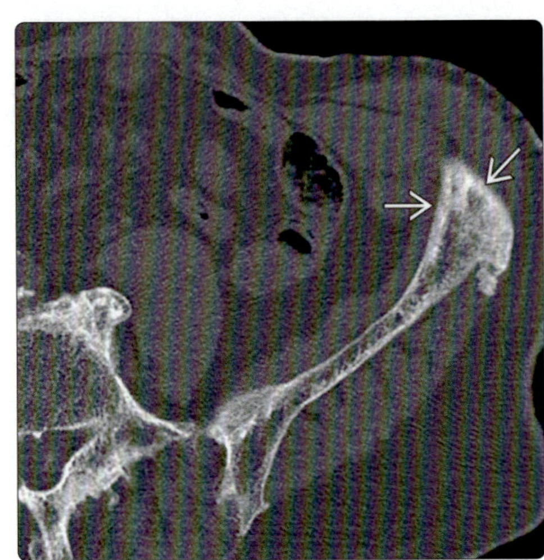

(Left) *This case illustrates the classic small round cell lesion differential diagnosis. There are multiple lytic destructive lesions within the pelvis ➡, as well as mixed lytic and sclerotic lesion in the femur ➡. **(Right)** AP radiograph in the same patient shows a similar lesion in the humeral epiphysis ➡. Differential includes multifocal osteomyelitis, Ewing sarcoma with osseous metastases, Langerhans cell histiocytosis, metastatic neuroblastoma, and polyostotic lymphoma. Biopsy proved lymphoma.*

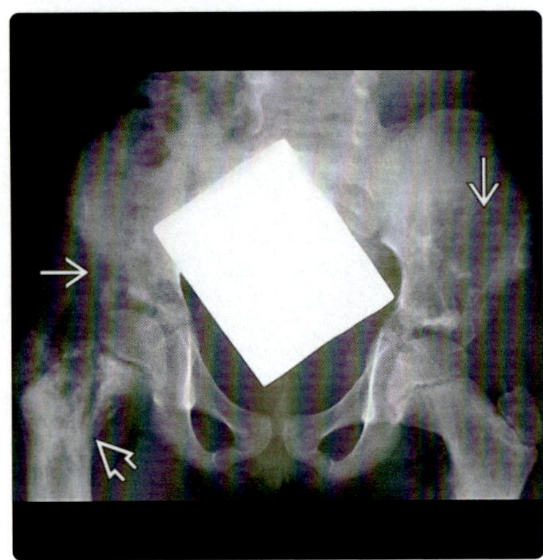

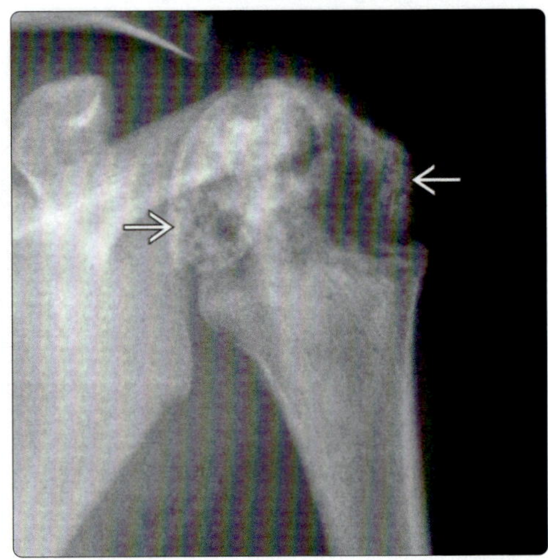

(Left) *Coronal T2WI FS MR shows diffuse but patchy abnormal signal in multiple bones, including the spine, pelvis, and proximal femora ➡. **(Right)** Axial STIR MR in the same patient shows a serpiginous pattern of abnormal signal ➡. Note the high signal in the adjacent muscle and fascia ➡ but no soft tissue mass. Findings are typical of multifocal lymphoma, which usually occurs in children. Of children with lymphoma, 50% present with polyostotic disease. Chemotherapy is the sole treatment.*

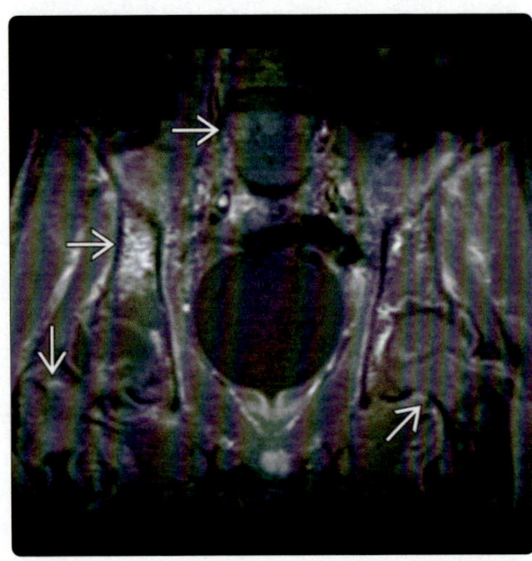

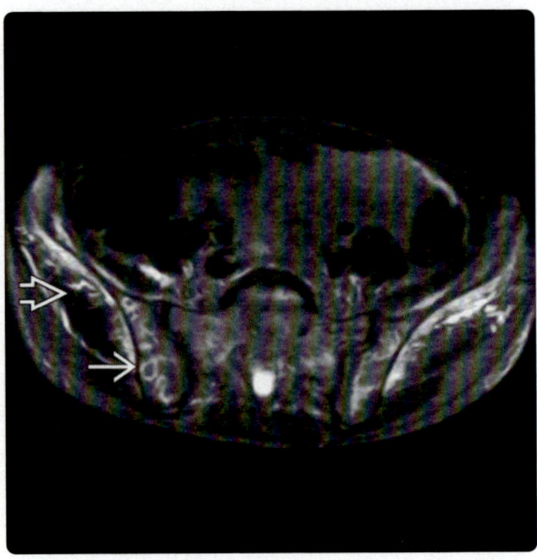

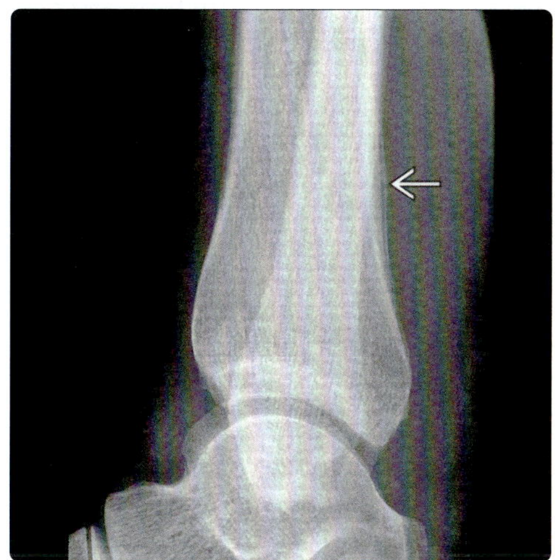

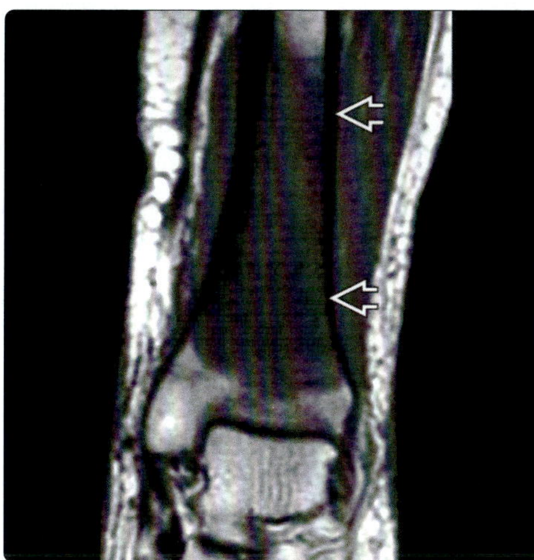

(Left) *Lateral radiograph shows thick, dense periosteal reaction ➡ at the distal tibia but no apparent marrow abnormality. This appearance might prompt consideration of diagnoses such as hypertrophic osteoarthropathy or osteomyelitis.* **(Right)** *Coronal T1WI MR in the same patient shows a very large area of low signal marrow ➡. A lesion that is so permeative that it cannot be seen on radiograph plus thick periosteal reaction suggests aggressive diagnosis such as Ewing sarcoma or primary lymphoma of bone.*

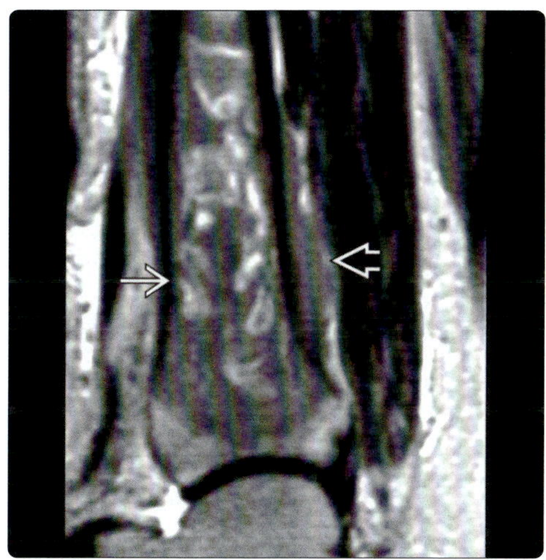

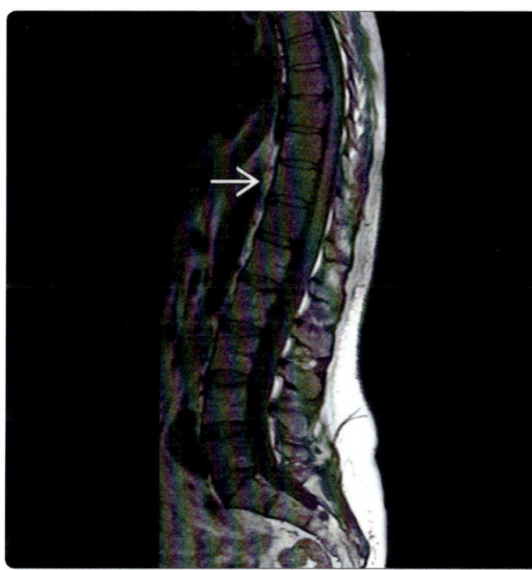

(Left) *Sagittal T2WI MR in the same patient shows inhomogeneous mixed ↓ and ↑ SI that is mostly contained within the marrow ➡ with only a small posterior soft tissue mass ➡. This serpiginous pattern with tumor permeating through an apparently intact cortex is typical of primary lymphoma of bone.* **(Right)** *Sagittal T1WI bone survey MR shows an infiltrative process with diffuse ↓ SI within the vertebrae ➡. This is abnormal; a 60-year-old woman should have nearly all white (fatty) marrow.*

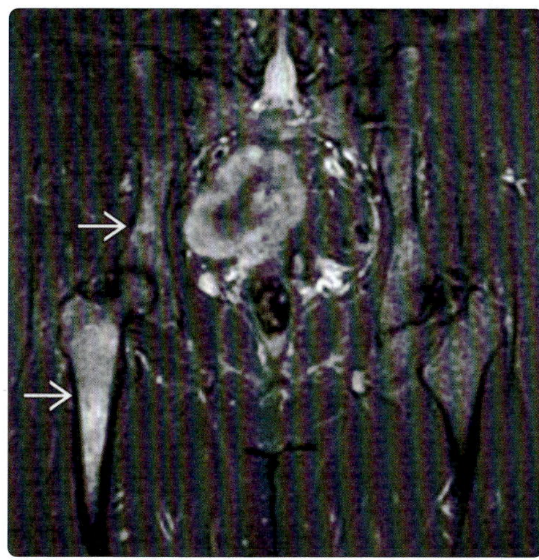

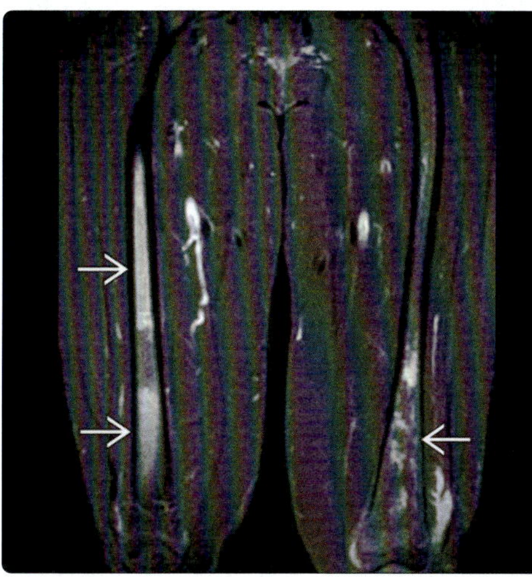

(Left) *Coronal STIR MR (same patient) shows diffuse inhomogeneous high signal within multiple bones ➡, matching regions that were abnormally low signal on T1 imaging.* **(Right)** *Coronal STIR MR of the femora (same patient) shows patchy abnormal hyperintense signal ➡. In a patient of this age, the most likely infiltrative process would be either multiple myeloma or leukemia. However, diagnosis is multifocal lymphoma. This is unusual; adults with PLB most frequently have a single osseous focus.*

KEY FACTS

TERMINOLOGY

- Tumor involving bone which originated from another (distant) site

IMAGING

- Location: Generally bones with persistent red marrow
- Radiograph: Relatively poor sensitivity: 50% of bone mass must be destroyed before lytic lesion visualized
- Breast: 34% lytic, 23% sclerotic, 43% mixed at baseline
- Prostate: Usually sclerotic, but may be lytic or mixed
- Lung: Usually lytic; uncommonly sclerotic
- Thyroid and renal cell: Lytic, often solitary, bubbly
- Adenocarcinomas: Usually lytic; rarely sclerotic or with sunburst reaction mimicking osteosarcoma
- PET/CT: Positive predictive value (PPV) of 98% when PET and CT findings are concordant
  - PET and CT are frequently discordant (58%)

CLINICAL ISSUES

- Skeletal system is 3rd most common site involved by metastatic tumor, following lung and liver
- Prolonged clinical course in several cancers today (for example, 20% of patients with breast metastases to bone survive > 5 years)
- Metastases from uncommon sites now seen more frequently
  - Treatment of painful or unstable bone lesions required in these patients
- Treatment of lesions requires imaging or metabolic measures of response
- Predictors of response to treatment of breast metastases
  - Increasing sclerosis of lesions, decrease in SUV by 8.5% on PET predicts long response duration

DIAGNOSTIC CHECKLIST

- Fracture through lesser trochanter in adult should be considered pathologic until proven otherwise

(Left) *Sagittal graphic depicts a metastasis involving a vertebral body. Previously it was believed that metastases involve the posterior elements preferentially. However, MR series show that the body is more likely to be involved by hematogenous metastases. Such lesions may be difficult to visualize on x-ray prior to destruction of pedicles or development of compression fracture.* **(Right)** *Sagittal T2WI MR shows low signal osteosarcoma metastasis involving the vertebral body ➡, extending into the anterior epidural space ➡.*

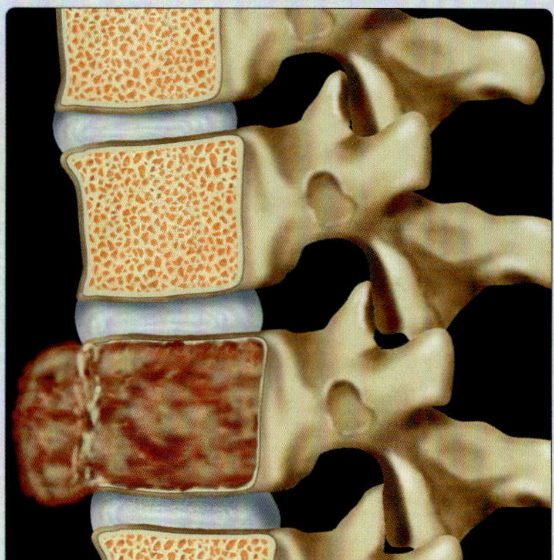

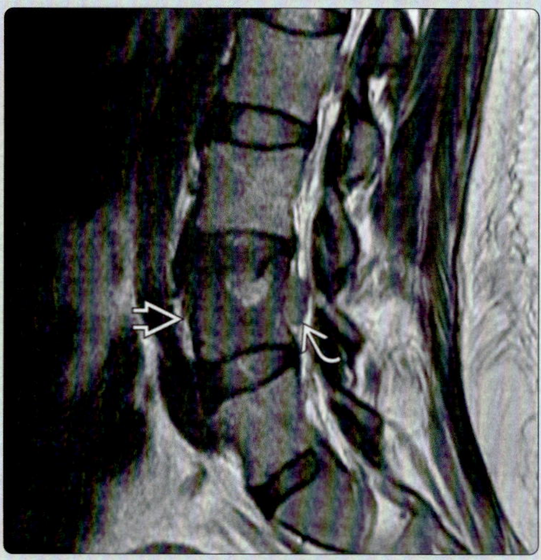

(Left) *AP radiograph shows a lytic acetabular lesion ➡. This geographic lesion proved to be a breast metastasis. While one expects breast metastases to be sclerotic and multifocal, even a solitary lytic lesion in a woman should always lead to consideration of metastatic breast cancer.* **(Right)** *Coronal bone CT shows a typical case of metastatic prostate carcinoma, with multiple sclerotic lesions ➡. Though sclerotic metastases appear more dense than cortical bone, these lesions are not as structurally sound and are at increased risk for fracture.*

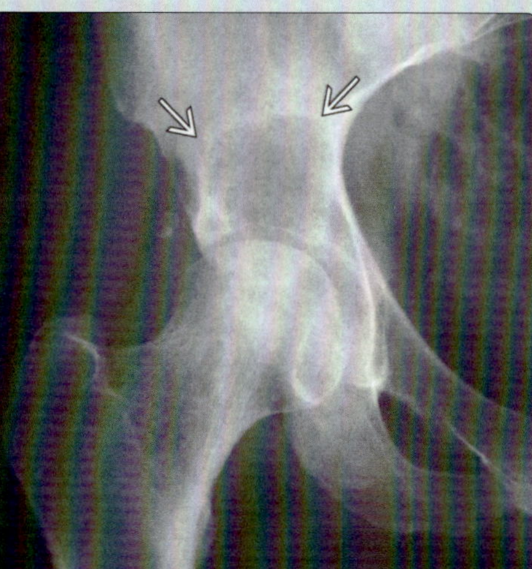

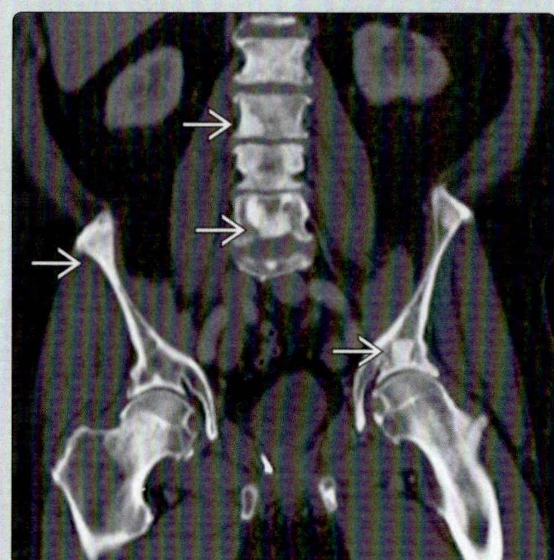

TERMINOLOGY

Synonyms

- Metastatic carcinoma, skeletal deposits, osseous metastasis, secondaries in bone, bony implants

Definitions

- Tumor involving bone which originated from another (distant) site

IMAGING

General Features

- Location
  - Generally bones with persistent red marrow
    - Vertebrae, proximal femur, ribs, sternum, pelvis, skull, shoulder girdle
  - Series of 114 histologically proven cases
    - 44% in axial skeleton
    - 29% in appendicular skeleton
      - Proximal femur most common
    - 27% in mixed location
    - Lesions in small tubular bones: Rare, but consider lung for primary site
  - Generally central in bone
    - If cortically based, consider breast or lung as primary

Radiographic Findings

- Relatively poor sensitivity: 50% of bone mass must be destroyed before lytic lesion is visualized
- Breast
  - Pretreatment: 34% lytic, 23% sclerotic, 43% mixed
  - Pattern may change following therapy
    - Many treated lesions become more sclerotic (48%)
- Prostate
  - Usually sclerotic, but may be lytic or mixed
- Lung
  - Usually lytic; uncommonly sclerotic
- Thyroid and renal cell
  - Lytic, often solitary, bubbly
- Adenocarcinomas
  - Usually lytic; rarely sclerotic or with sunburst reaction mimicking osteosarcoma

MR Findings

- T1WI: SI generally low to intermediate
- Fluid-sensitive sequences: SI generally high; low to mixed if sclerotic lesion
- Enhancement with contrast; may be peripheral
- Tubular signal void may be seen centrally in renal cell met
  - Indicates highly vascular lesion, suggests diagnosis and that embolization may be useful
- Differentiation of vertebral metastasis from insufficiency fracture is difficult
  - Positive findings suggesting metastasis
    - Convex posterior border of vertebral body
    - Abnormal SI of pedicle or posterior element
    - Epidural mass or focal paraspinal mass
    - Presence of other spinal metastases
  - Positive findings suggesting insufficiency fracture
    - Low SI band on T1 and T2 MR
    - Regions of normal bone marrow (fat) signal intensity
    - Retropulsion of posterior bone fragment
    - Multiple other compression fractures
  - Diffusion-weighted MR may be useful
  - Opposed-phase imaging shows no significant signal dropout of metastases on out-of-phase sequence

Nuclear Medicine Findings

- PET
  - False-positives for metastatic disease
    - Fracture: Wide range of SUV values likely relates to acuity of fracture and patient age
      - No SUV cut-off level established to reliably distinguish insufficiency fractures from malignancy
    - Many benign osseous lesions, including fibroxanthoma and fibrous dysplasia
  - Contributes to detection of lytic bone metastasis in breast and other cancers
    - Less efficacious in other tumors, such as prostate
  - Large study shows NaF PET to have high impact on following patients with progressive osseous metastases, resulting in frequent alteration of therapy
- PET/CT
  - CT helps to obviate further imaging or false-positive PET diagnosis of benign entities
  - Positive predictive value (PPV) of 98% when PET and CT findings are concordant
    - PET and CT are frequently discordant (58%)
      - PPV with positive PET and negative CT: 61% (increases if multiple lesions present)
      - PPV of **solitary** lesion with positive PET and negative CT: 43%; these lesions need further corroboration by MR or biopsy
      - PPV with negative PET and positive CT: 17%
  - SUV ↓ by 8.5% following therapy is strong predictor (2.4x) of metastatic bone response
    - Particularly when used in conjunction with change in density of lesion
  - Total lesion glycolysis change is not predictive of metastatic bone response in patients with breast cancer

DIFFERENTIAL DIAGNOSIS

Sclerotic Metastases

- Sclerosing dysplasias: Bone island, osteopoikilosis
- Paget disease
- Healing rib or insufficiency fractures
- Treated hyperparathyroidism/healing Brown tumor
- Mastocytosis
- Sarcoidosis of bone

Lytic Metastases

- Multiple myeloma
- Brown tumor of hyperparathyroidism
- Langerhans cell histiocytosis
- Vascular tumors
- Multifocal primary osseous lymphoma
- Chronic recurrent multifocal osteomyelitis

PATHOLOGY

General Features

- Etiology
  - Local blood flow contributes to pattern
    - Batson plexus: Vertebral venous plexus is high volume, low pressure, valveless
      - Communicates directly with veins of pelvis, proximal half of lower extremity, proximal half of upper extremity: Most likely sites of metastasis

CLINICAL ISSUES

Presentation

- Most common signs/symptoms
  - Pain, swelling
  - Pathologic fracture
    - Particularly spine and proximal femur
  - Neurologic symptoms
- Other signs/symptoms
  - Hypercalcemia (paraneoplastic syndrome) may accompany osteolysis

Demographics

- Age
  - 2/3 are 40-60 years old
- Epidemiology
  - Skeletal system is 3rd most common site involved by metastatic tumor
    - Follows lung and liver metastases in frequency
    - 70% of patients with metastases from known primary tumor have bone lesions
  - Metastatic carcinomas are most common
    - 93% are concentrated in 5 primary tumor types
      - Breast: Bone is most common site of distant metastases; 30% at time of diagnosis, 73% at autopsy
      - Prostate: 30% at time of diagnosis, 80% at autopsy
      - Lung: 33% at autopsy
      - Kidney: 25% at autopsy
      - Thyroid: 50% at autopsy
  - In children, most common are neuroblastoma, rhabdomyosarcoma, clear cell sarcoma of kidney

Natural History & Prognosis

- Metastatic breast cancer
  - Lytic metastases → poorer prognosis than sclerotic
- Bone metastases generally herald incurability
  - Prolonged clinical course in several cancers today (for example, 20% of patients with breast metastases to bone survive > 5 years)
    - Treatment of painful or unstable bone lesions required in these patients
- Metastases from uncommon sites now seen
  - New therapies prolong life, allowing systemic metastases in bones to occur
- Treatment of lesions requires imaging or metabolic measures of response
  - Predictors of response to treatment of breast metastases
    - Increasing sclerosis of lesions predicts good response
    - Decrease in SUV by 8.5% on PET predicts long response duration

Treatment

- Generally palliative
  - Designed to provide pain relief
  - Restore patient mobility to improve quality of life
- Stabilization of fracture or weight-bearing sites at risk of fracture
  - Kypho- or vertebroplasty of collapsing spinal lesion
  - Femur at particular risk for fracture due to combined sheer and bending forces during normal gait
    - Watch for endosteal scalloping, large-sized lesion
    - Combination of intramedullary (IM) rod, plate and screw systems, methylmethacrylate
      - IM rod may further disseminate tumor
    - Arthroplasty may be more suitable, depending on location of lesion
      - High rate of hip dislocations with tumor endoprosthesis
- Radiation therapy
- Percutaneous cryoablation useful for palliation of pain

DIAGNOSTIC CHECKLIST

Consider

- Metastases to vertebrae involve bodies more frequently than posterior elements
  - Hematogenous spread through veins of Batson
- Renal cell or thyroid metastases often present as solitary highly expanded lesions
  - Often mistaken for primary bone sarcoma
  - Often seen in patients younger than normally expected for metastatic disease
- Renal cell carcinoma is highly vascular
  - Biopsy may cause severe bleeding
  - Consider embolization of feeding vessels prior to biopsy &/or surgery
- Osseous metastases are not always shown by PET FDG
  - Some primary tumors have poor likelihood of PET FDG uptake (particularly prostate)
  - PET not routine part of work-up, but if patient pain is not explained by other imaging, consider PET/CT

Image Interpretation Pearls

- Fracture through lesser trochanter in adult
  - Consider pathologic until proven otherwise
- Insufficiency fractures may mimic metastatic disease
  - Subcapital fractures: With rotation and varus malalignment, lytic lesion is mimicked
  - Sacral and pubic ramus insufficiency fracture: Motion and delayed healing → irregularity and lucency
  - Iliac insufficiency fracture (supraacetabular, oblique, superomedial ilium) may mimic metastasis
    - Prior pelvic radiation puts patients at risk

SELECTED REFERENCES

1. Hillner BE et al: 18F-fluoride PET used for treatment monitoring of systemic cancer therapy: Results from the National Oncologic PET Registry. J Nucl Med. 56(2):222-8, 2015

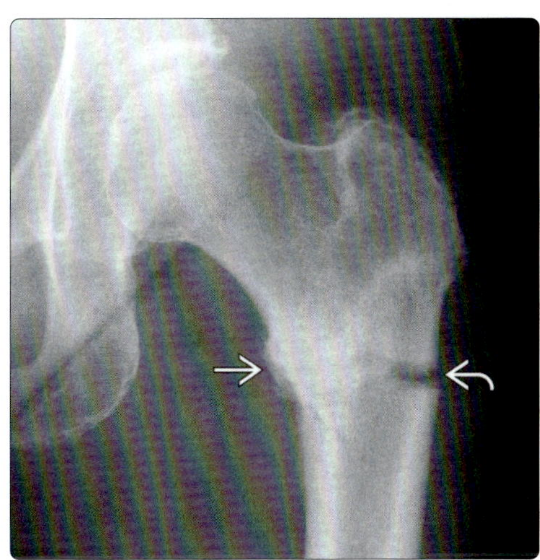

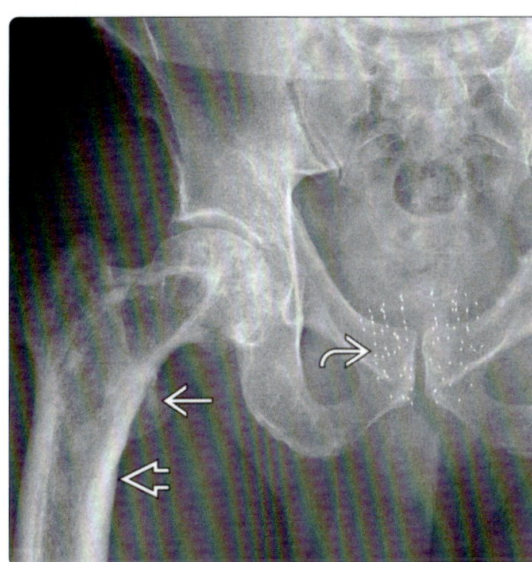

(Left) *AP radiograph shows a sclerotic lesser trochanter ➡ and a pathologic fracture ↪. A transverse fracture either occurs from significant trauma or is pathologic. A sclerotic metastatic lesion in an older woman most frequently is a result of breast cancer, as in this case.* **(Right)** *AP radiograph shows sclerotic metastases ➡ arising in Paget disease ➡. Note the seed implants ↪, indicating treatment for prostate cancer. Hyperemia in Paget bone may lead to preferential deposition of metastases.*

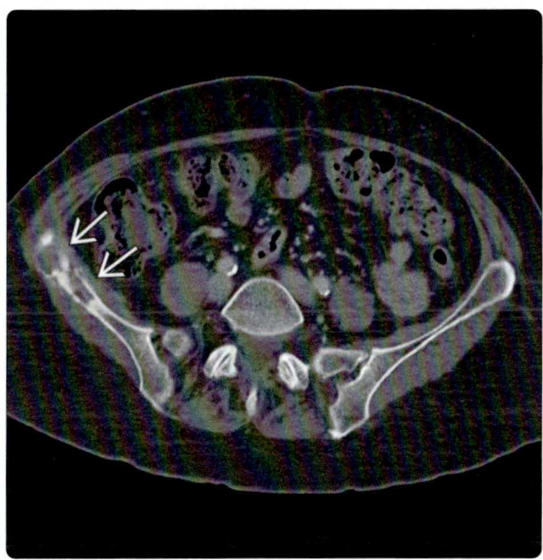

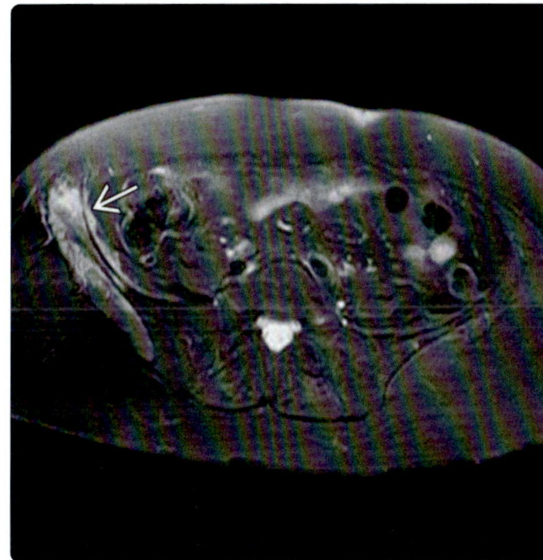

(Left) *Axial CECT shows a typical case of metastatic breast carcinoma, with a mixed lytic and sclerotic destructive lesion ➡. Even if this is a solitary lesion, metastasis should be strongly considered.* **(Right)** *Axial T2WI FS MR in the same case shows high signal in the lesion ➡ and surrounding soft tissues. If there is any question of malignancy T1WI SPGR acquired in- and out-of-phase may be used to prove that the process obliterates normal bone marrow fat, thus favoring malignancy.*

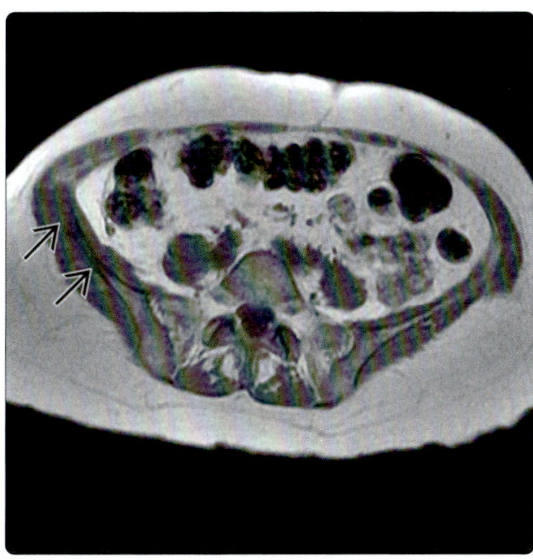

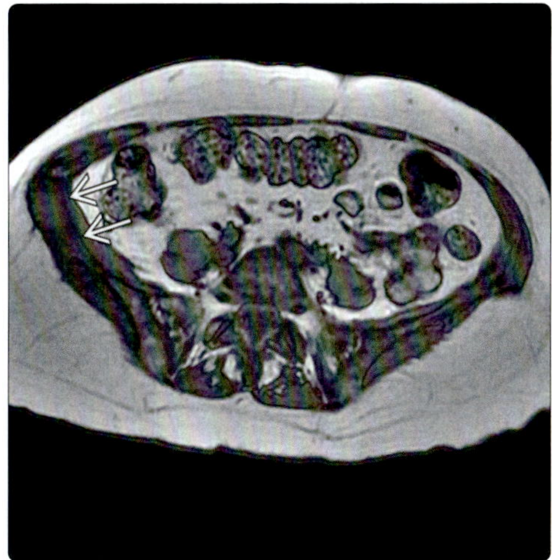

(Left) *In- and out-of-phase imaging was performed in the same case. Axial T1WI SPGR acquired in-phase shows that the lesion ➡ has lower signal than muscle, which is a suspicious finding.* **(Right)** *Axial T1WI SPGR acquired out-of-phase shows that the abnormal region ➡ fails to have drop out of signal, indicating that there is no residual marrow fat to cause signal cancellation. This helps to confirm the impression of marrow infiltration.*

(Left) *AP radiograph demonstrates an avulsion fracture of the lesser trochanter. Note that there is also lytic trabecular disruption. This proved to be pathologic fracture through a metastasis. In an adult patient, avulsion of the lesser trochanter should be considered pathologic until proven otherwise.* **(Right)** *Axial CECT shows multiple sclerotic lesions. Although lung carcinoma metastases are usually lytic, nonsmall-cell lung metastases are occasionally sclerotic, as in this case.*

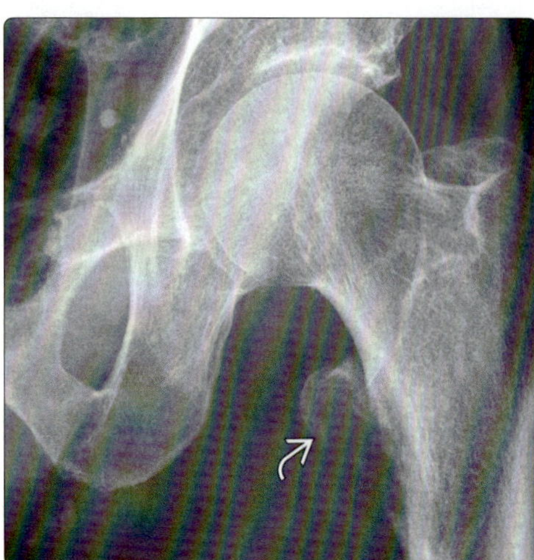

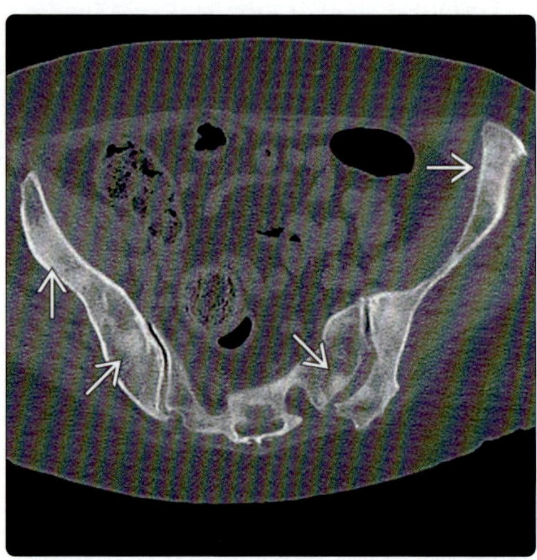

(Left) *Frog leg lateral radiograph of the femur in a young woman shows a cortically based lytic lesion. This proved to be a solitary breast metastasis. Cortically based metastases tend to be either lung or breast in origin. This lesion is at high risk for pathologic fracture; it needs prophylactic rodding.* **(Right)** *Coronal T1WI MR shows an enormous mass involving the scapula and adjacent soft tissues. The mass proved to be metastatic renal cell carcinoma. Kidney or thyroid metastases may present as expanded and solitary lesions.*

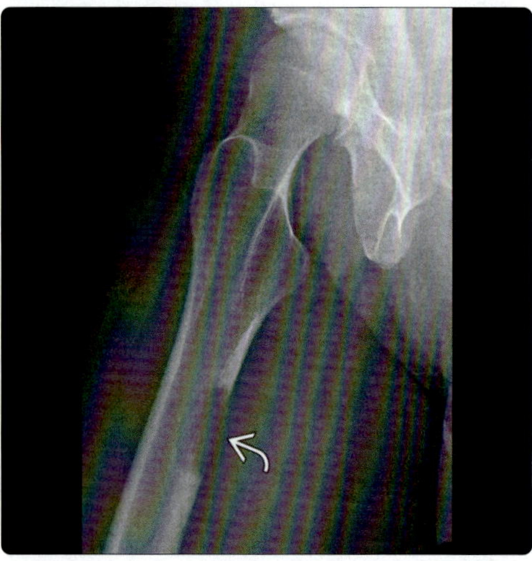

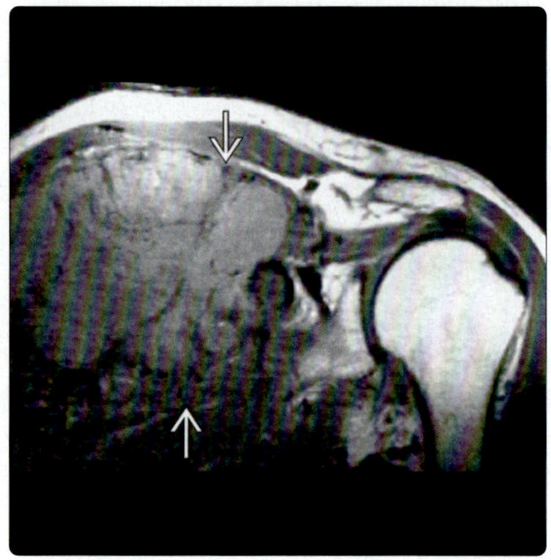

(Left) *Coronal NECT shows a sunburst appearance of metastatic adenocarcinoma from the pancreas. The hemipelvis is occupied by an expanded lesion with sunburst reaction. Though it is unusual to have a single osseous metastasis be clearly dominant relative to others, and even more unusual for a metastasis to have a sunburst type of bone production, it is worth remembering that this pattern may be seen with adenocarcinoma.* **(Right)** *Lateral radiograph shows a medulloblastoma metastasis with sunburst reaction.*

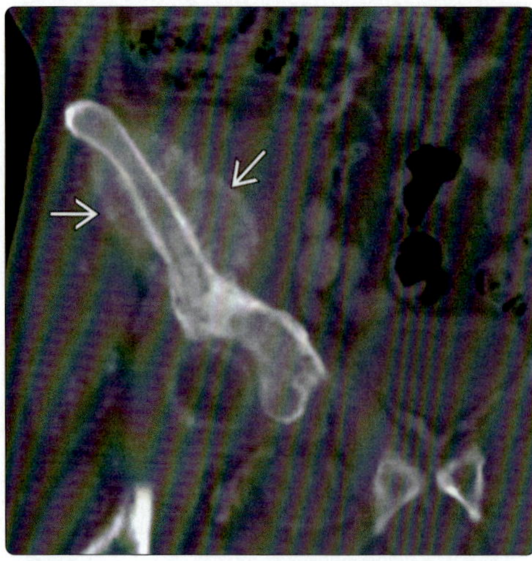

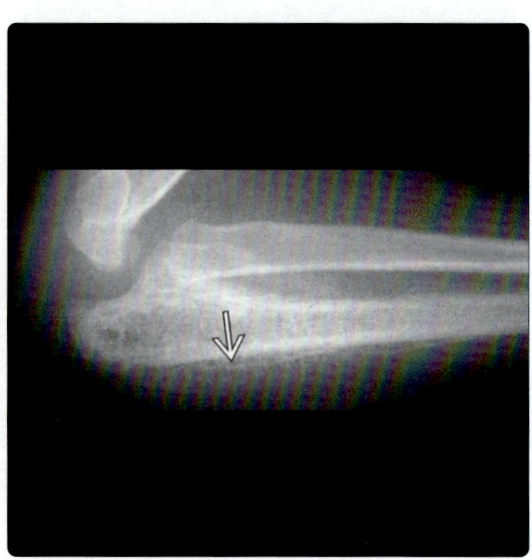

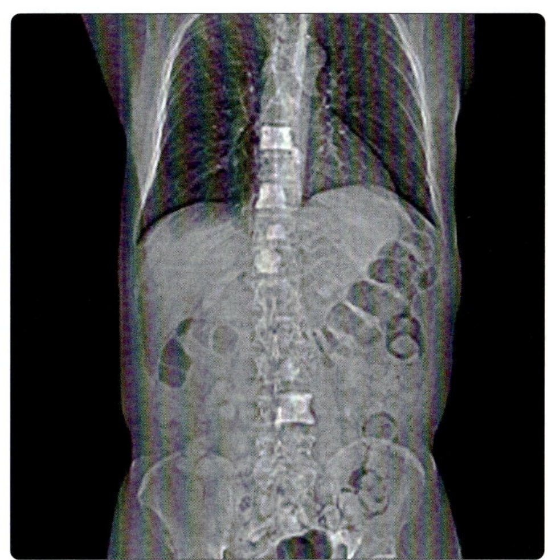

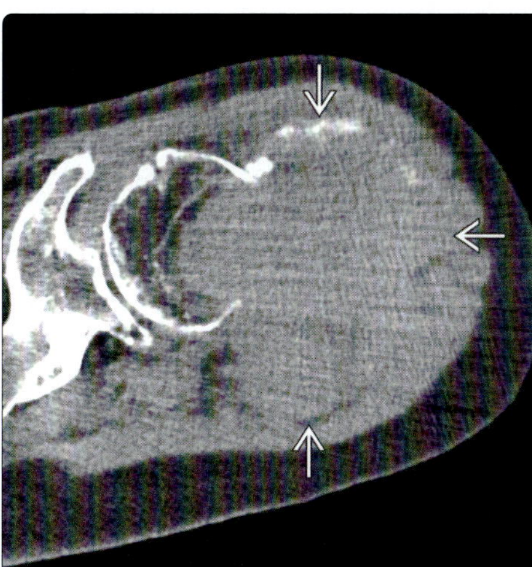

(Left) *Coronal CT scanogram shows extensive osseous abnormalities with sclerotic bone densities throughout the skeleton. There is a wide differential (mostly metastases), but in this case the lesion is metastatic carcinoid, 1 of the less common etiologies.* **(Right)** *Axial NECT shows a large destructive mass ➔, which proved to be hepatocellular metastasis. Most patients have nonosseous metastatic sites (usually lung) identified before skeletal metastases develop, which is not the case here.*

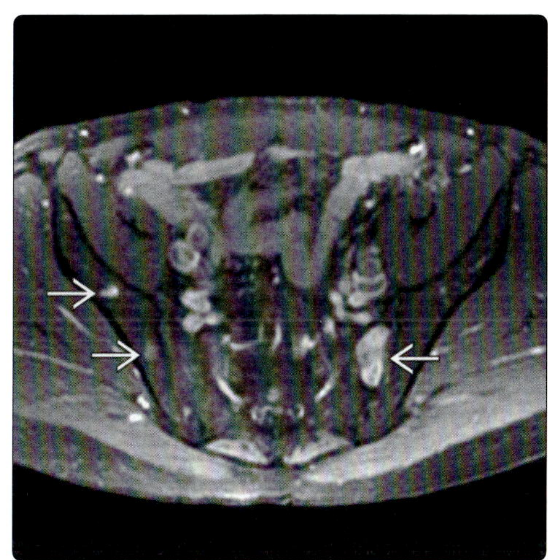

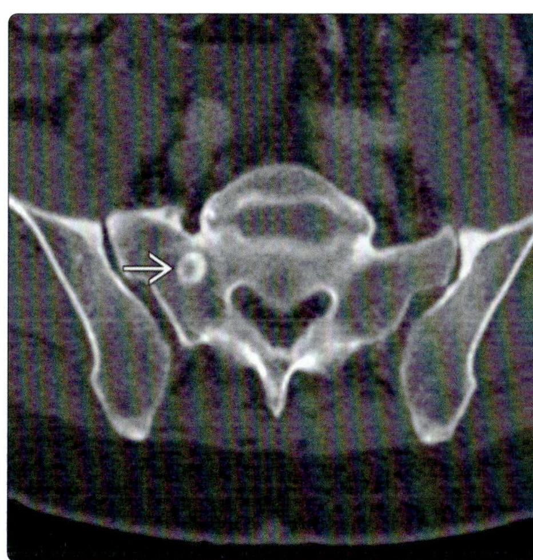

(Left) *Axial T1WI C+ FS MR demonstrates bone metastases from synovial sarcoma ➔. This tumor does not normally metastasize to bone, but it is important to remember that late in the metastatic process, even unusual bone metastases may occur. This patient already had been treated for lung and brain metastases. As patients live longer with malignant tumors, we should expect to see unusual bone metastases.* **(Right)** *Axial CECT shows melanoma metastasis ➔, which may occur anywhere in the body.*

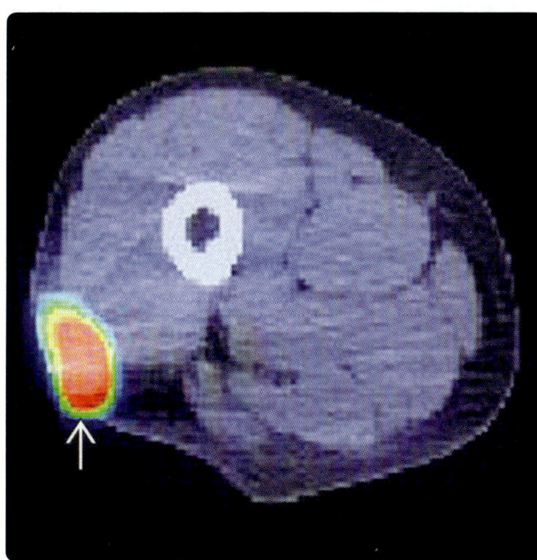

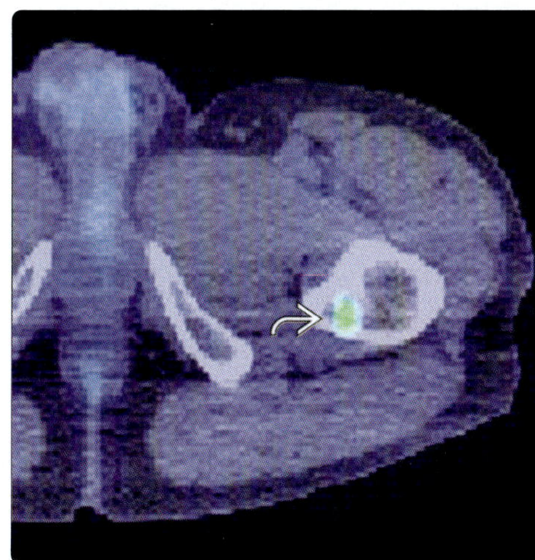

(Left) *Axial PET/CT shows intense FDG uptake of a mass ➔, which proved to be high-grade undifferentiated pleomorphic sarcoma.* **(Right)** *Axial PET/CT in the same patient shows a lesion involving the lesser trochanter ➔, which proved to be metastatic. Osseous metastases may occur from soft tissue malignant lesions, though generally not as frequently as lung metastases, and can also occur from primary bone tumors, most frequently Ewing sarcoma, osteosarcoma, and chondrosarcoma.*

KEY FACTS

TERMINOLOGY

- Rare benign bone tumor consisting of spindle cells with minimal cellular atypia

IMAGING

- Location: Any bone possible; mandible most frequently involved
  - Tubular bones: Metadiaphyseal or diaphyseal
- Best imaging tool: MR is diagnostic; used for evaluation of site
- Predominantly nonaggressive in appearance, with some mildly aggressive features
- Radiograph: Lytic lesion (may contain minimal sclerosis in 13%)
  - Pseudotrabeculation in 63%
  - Geographic or partially geographic in 95%
  - Mild cortical breakthrough in 53% and associated soft tissue mass
- CT: Lytic in 65%
  - Mixed lytic and mildly sclerotic in 35%
  - Cortical breakthrough in 88%; soft tissue mass in 41%
- MR: T1 shows low signal intensity (iso- to hypointense to muscle)
  - Fluid-sensitive sequences (whether or not fat saturated): Iso- to hypointense to muscle
  - Low T2 signal involves at least 50% of lesion
  - Low T2 signal intensity of lesion is most prominent differentiating feature
  - May be confounded by edema and hemorrhage in pathologic fracture
  - Post contrast: Heterogeneous enhancement
- Diagnosis should be strongly considered in nonaggressive, nonsclerotic osseous lesion with low T2 signal

CLINICAL ISSUES

- Most common in adolescents and young adults (range is much wider)
- Rare: 0.1% of all primary bone tumors

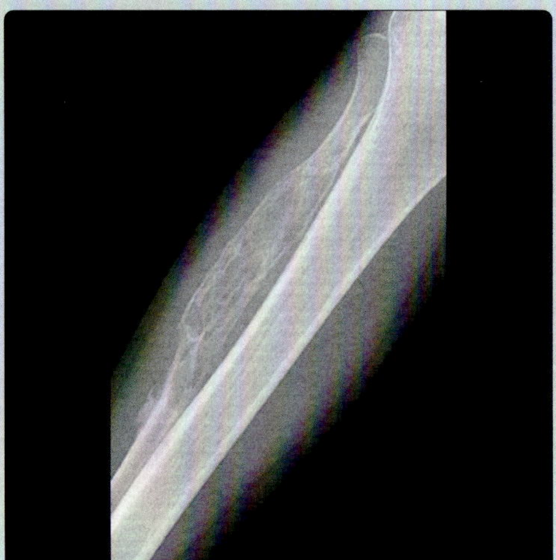

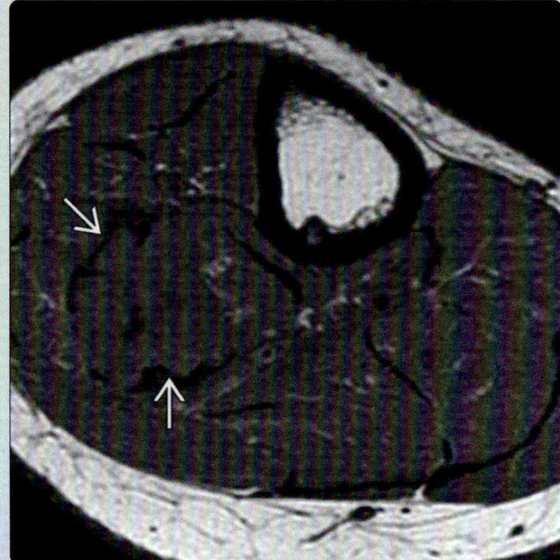

(Left) *AP radiograph shows a moderately aggressive diaphyseal lesion, which is lytic, expanded, contains pseudotrabeculation, and has a distal pathologic fracture. This is nonspecific; nonossifying fibroma and desmoplastic fibroma are 2 of the more likely diagnoses.* **(Right)** *Axial T1WI MR in the same case shows the intraosseous lesion ➡ to be low signal, slightly lower than adjacent muscle. The fibula is significantly expanded. The appearance is nonspecific, though the very low signal suggests a fibrous lesion.*

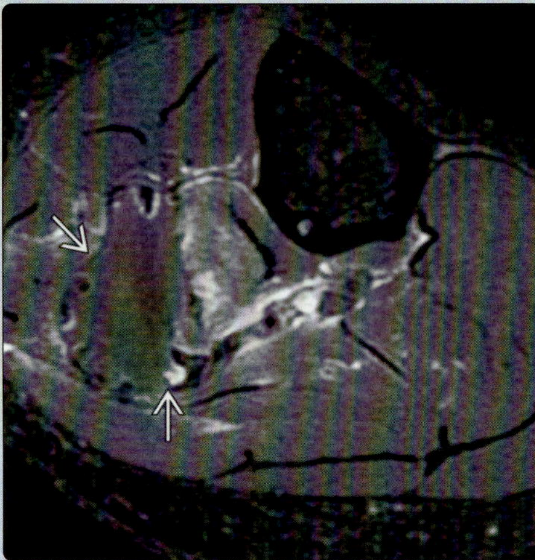

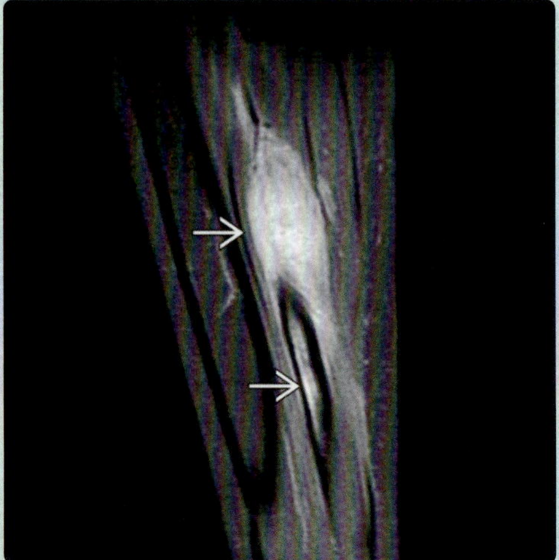

(Left) *Axial T2WI FS MR in the same case shows predominantly low signal ➡ with surrounding mild edema. This low signal occupies the majority of the lesion. Desmoplastic fibroma is the intraosseous form of fibromatosis, or soft tissue desmoid. It is a rare lesion, but can be suggested in a moderately aggressive osseous lesion in which the majority shows low signal on T2 imaging, as in this case.* **(Right)** *Sagittal T1WI C+ FS MR in the same case shows enhancement of the lesion ➡.*

TERMINOLOGY

Synonyms

- Desmoid tumor of bone, intraosseous counterpart of soft tissue fibromatosis

Definitions

- Rare benign bone tumor consisting of spindle cells with minimal cellular atypia

IMAGING

General Features

- Location
  - Any bone possible; mandible most frequently involved
  - Tubular bones: Metadiaphyseal or diaphyseal
- Size
  - Average: 8 cm in longitudinal length

Imaging Recommendations

- Best imaging tool
  - MR is diagnostic; useful for evaluation of tumor site

Radiographic Findings

- Generally nonaggressive appearance, with superimposed mildly aggressive features
- Lytic lesion (may contain minimal sclerosis in 13%)
- Pseudotrabeculation in 63%
- Geographic or partially geographic in 95%
- Central (61%) or eccentric
- Sclerotic margin (46%)
- Mild expansion; cortical thinning
- Mild cortical breakthrough (53%) and associated soft tissue mass

CT Findings

- Lytic in 65%
  - Mixed lytic and mildly sclerotic in 35%
- Cortical breakthrough in 88%; soft tissue mass in 41%

MR Findings

- T1: Low signal intensity (iso- to hypointense to muscle)
- Fluid-sensitive sequences (whether or not fat saturated): Iso- to hypointense to muscle
  - Low T2 signal involves at least 50% of lesion
  - Low T2 signal intensity of lesion is most prominent differentiating feature
  - May be confounded by edema and hemorrhage in pathologic fracture
  - Cystic foci reported in 1 case
- Post contrast: Heterogeneous enhancement

DIFFERENTIAL DIAGNOSIS

Nonossifying Fibroma (Fibroxanthoma, NOF)

- If lesion is in thin tubular bone (fibula, ulna), NOF appears centrally located and may simulate desmoplastic fibroma

Fibrosarcoma or Malignant Fibrous Histiocytoma

- Low-grade spindle cell tumors may appear only moderately aggressive and mimic desmoplastic fibroma
- MR differentiates lesions on basis of T2 signal

PATHOLOGY

General Features

- Genetics
  - Trisomies 8 and 20 appear to be nonrandom
    - Analogous to soft tissue desmoid tumors

Gross Pathologic & Surgical Features

- Creamy white cut surface with whorled pattern
- Well-defined scalloping of adjacent bone

Microscopic Features

- Spindle cells in abundant collagen
- Rarely contains extensive chondroid metaplasia; may lead to mistaken diagnosis of chondrosarcoma
- Cellular atypia & pleomorphism minimal; mitoses rare

CLINICAL ISSUES

Presentation

- Most common signs/symptoms
  - Pain or deformity
  - Pathologic fracture in 13%

Demographics

- Age
  - Adolescents and young adults (range is much wider)
- Gender
  - Slight male predominance
- Epidemiology
  - Rare: 0.1% of all primary bone tumors

Natural History & Prognosis

- Locally progressive/aggressive
- Rare case reports of sarcomatous degeneration, often many years following resection

Treatment

- Wide resection favored
  - Recurrence of 17%
- Marginal resection if required for functional reasons
  - 72% recurrence; may occur several years following resection

DIAGNOSTIC CHECKLIST

Consider

- Diagnosis should be considered in nonaggressive, nonsclerotic osseous lesion with low T2 signal
  - Foci of low T2 signal seen in giant cell tumor and fibrous dysplasia, but do not occupy full extent of lesion as seen in desmoplastic fibroma

SELECTED REFERENCES

1. Okubo T et al: Desmoplastic fibroma of the rib with cystic change: a case report and literature review. Skeletal Radiol. 43(5):703-8, 2014
2. Yin H et al: Desmoplastic fibroma of the spine: a series of 12 cases and outcomes. Spine J. 14(8):1622-8, 2014
3. Wadhwa V et al: Incidental lesion in the femoral metaphysis. Desmoplastic fibroma of the bone. Skeletal Radiol. 42(12):1739-40, 1775-6, 2013
4. Apaydin M et al: Desmoplastic fibroma in humerus. J Med Imaging Radiat Oncol. 52(5):489-90, 2008
5. Rastogi S et al: Desmoplastic fibroma: a report of three cases at unusual locations. Joint Bone Spine. 75(2):222-5, 2008

KEY FACTS

TERMINOLOGY

- Liposclerosing myxofibrous tumor (LSMFT)
  - Benign fibroosseous lesion, typified by propensity to occur in intertrochanteric region

IMAGING

- Location: 85% occur in femur
  - Strong predilection for intertrochanteric region (over 90% of femoral lesions in this location)
- Consists of mixture of tissues, any of which may predominate on imaging
  - Dense sclerosis
  - Matrix calcification
  - Lytic or cystic regions
  - Fat density (uncommon)
- Geographic with sclerotic margin
- Matrix in 72% (range of globular, linear, ring-like)
- MR: Low signal sclerotic rim & matrix
  - Otherwise isointense to muscle on T1
  - Fat signal rarely seen
  - Fluid-sensitive sequences: Inhomogeneous ↑ SI
  - Same regions of myxofibrous tissue showing ↓ attenuation on CT show ↑ signal on MR

TOP DIFFERENTIAL DIAGNOSES

- Fibrous dysplasia
  - Mixture of sclerosis, ground-glass, lytic regions is similar in appearance to LSMFT
- Intraosseous lipoma (involuting stage)
  - Differentiated from LSMFT on imaging studies by ↑ lipomatous tissue in intraosseous lipoma

CLINICAL ISSUES

- Pain in ~ 50%, generally moderate, long in duration
  - Otherwise, usually incidental finding
- Rate of malignant degeneration: 10-16%
  - Likely related to extensive ischemic change
  - Reports of degeneration to osteosarcoma, MFH

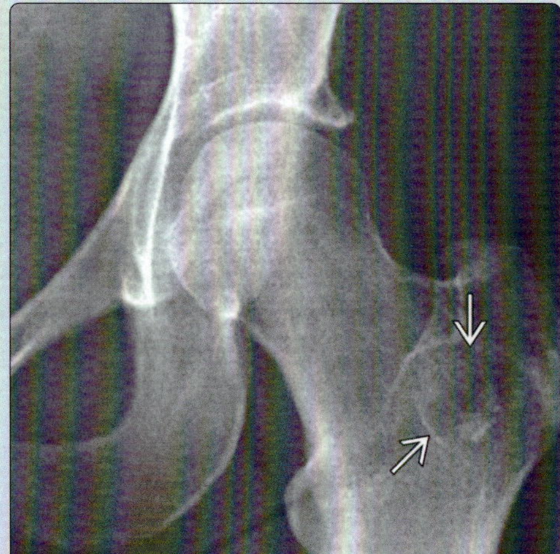

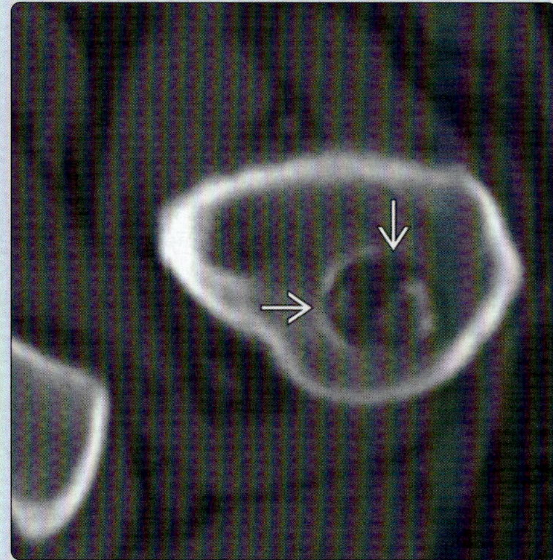

***(Left)** AP radiograph shows a liposclerosing myxofibrous tumor (LSMFT) in the intertrochanteric region of the femoral neck, geographic with a sclerotic margin ➡ and a small amount of central sclerotic matrix. **(Right)** Axial NECT in the same patient mirrors the sclerotic rim ➡ and inner matrix. Regions of lower attenuation in the lesion likely represent a focus of myxofibrous tissue, which would be high signal on MR. Despite the nonaggressive appearance, a small percentage of these lesions may become malignant.*

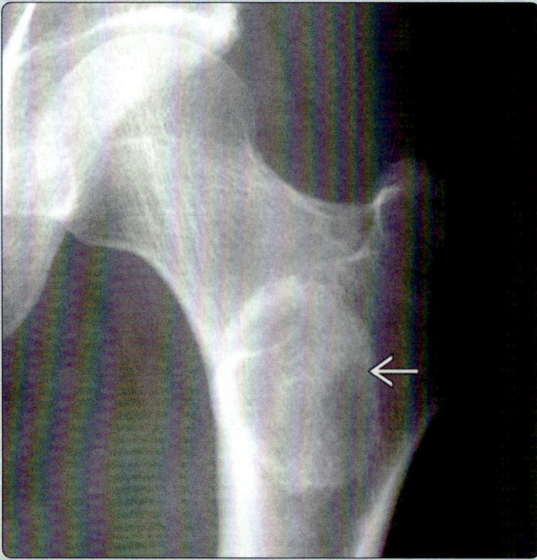

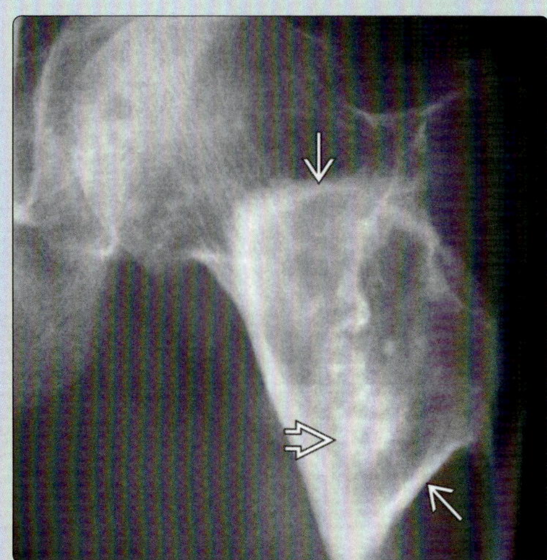

***(Left)** AP radiograph shows a lesion typical of LSMFT, with a sclerotic rim ➡ and mixed lytic and blastic center, geographic and nonaggressive in appearance. The most important feature is its central location within the intertrochanteric region of the proximal femur. Of LSMFTs, 85% occur in the femur, and of those, > 90% arise in this location. **(Right)** AP radiograph shows a large LSMFT within the intertrochanteric region of the femur, with a typical sclerotic rim ➡ and central matrix ⇨.*

TERMINOLOGY

Abbreviations

- Liposclerosing myxofibrous tumor (LSMFT)

Definitions

- Benign fibroosseous lesion, typified by propensity to occur in intertrochanteric region

IMAGING

General Features

- Location
  - 85% occur in femur
    - Strong predilection for intertrochanteric region (more than 90% of femoral lesions in this location)
  - Other bones rarely reported (ilium, humerus, rib)

Radiographic Findings

- Consists of mixture of tissues, any of which may predominate on imaging
  - Dense sclerosis
  - Matrix calcification
  - Lytic or cystic regions
  - Fat density (uncommon)
- Geographic with sclerotic margin
- May be expansile, but generally not significantly
- Matrix in 72% (range of globular, linear, ring-like)

CT Findings

- Mimic radiographic findings
- May demonstrate matrix more conclusively
- Low attenuation of fat rarely seen
  - ↓ attenuation may be seen on CT due to myxofibrous tissue

MR Findings

- Low signal sclerotic rim and matrix
- Otherwise isointense to muscle on T1
  - Fat signal rarely seen
- Fluid-sensitive sequences: Inhomogeneous high signal
  - Same regions of myxofibrous tissue showing ↓ attenuation on CT show ↑ signal on MR

Nuclear Medicine Findings

- Bone scan: Mild to marked uptake

DIFFERENTIAL DIAGNOSIS

Fibrous Dysplasia

- Mixture of sclerosis, ground-glass, lytic regions is similar to appearance in LSMFT
- Fibrous dysplasia (FD) rarely has sclerotic rim
- When FD occurs in femoral neck, there is often a varus deformity (shepherd's crook)

Intraosseous Lipoma (Involuting Stage)

- Intraosseous lipomas may undergo involution
  - Fat necrosis, calcification, cysts, reactive bone
- Differentiated from LSMFT on imaging studies by greater presence of lipomatous tissue in intraosseous lipoma

PATHOLOGY

General Features

- Etiology
  - Possibly derived from involuting intraosseous lipoma: Histologic and imaging similarities

Gross Pathologic & Surgical Features

- Mixture of histologic elements, seen in varying proportions
  - Myxoma, myxofibroma, fibroxanthoma
  - Fibrous dysplasia-like features
  - Cysts
  - Fat necrosis, lipoma
  - Ischemic ossification, cartilage

Microscopic Features

- Proliferating myxofibrous and fibroosseous tissue
- 1 study showed underlying FD, suggesting LSMFT is not distinct lesion

CLINICAL ISSUES

Presentation

- Most common signs/symptoms
  - Pain in ~ 50%, generally moderate and of long duration
    - Otherwise, usually incidental finding
  - Rare pathologic fracture

Demographics

- Age
  - Mean: 42 years; range: 15-69 years (in series of 39 cases)
- Gender
  - Slight male predilection

Natural History & Prognosis

- Rate of malignant degeneration: 10-16%
  - Likely related to extensive ischemic change
  - Reports of degeneration to osteosarcoma, malignant fibrous histiocytoma

Treatment

- Propensity for malignant degeneration should in part direct treatment
  - Painful LSMFT should be resected
  - Lesions that have no pain may be watched
    - MR may be most useful for noting early changes of degeneration

DIAGNOSTIC CHECKLIST

Consider

- LSMFT has greater predilection for malignant transformation than other fibroosseous lesions
  - Watch for evidence of aggressiveness within preexisting benign process: Focal osseous destruction + soft tissue mass

SELECTED REFERENCES

1. Dattilo J et al: Liposclerosing myxofibrous tumor (LSMFT), a study of 33 patients: should it be a distinct entity? Iowa Orthop J. 32:35-9, 2012
2. Campbell K et al: Case report: two-step malignant transformation of a liposclerosing myxofibrous tumor of bone. Clin Orthop Relat Res. 466(11):2873-7, 2008

Malignant Fibrous Histiocytoma of Bone

KEY FACTS

TERMINOLOGY

- Malignant osseous neoplasm composed of fibroblasts and pleomorphic cells exhibiting storiform pattern

IMAGING

- Location: Long bones, central metaphysis or diaphysis (75%)
  - Often extends from metaphysis to epiphysis or diaphysis
  - Femur (30-45%) > tibia, fibula, humerus
- Most high grade, with lytic destructive pattern
  - Permeative, wide zone of transition
  - Cortical breakthrough and soft tissue mass
  - Periosteal reaction often absent; if present, aggressive
- Lower grade lesions may appear at least partially geographic
- May have signs of prior lesion
  - Serpiginous pattern of bone infarct
  - Mixed lytic sclerotic pattern of Paget disease
  - Mixed lytic sclerotic pattern of radiation necrosis
- MR nonspecific unless there are signs of prior lesion
  - T1WI: Isointense to skeletal muscle
  - Fluid sensitive: Heterogeneous high signal
  - Postcontrast: Avid enhancement

CLINICAL ISSUES

- Wide age range; higher incidence in patients > 40 years
  - 10-15% occur in 2nd decade, so do not discount diagnosis in adolescents/young adults
- Usually high grade at presentation
  - Metastases in lung at presentation in 45-50% in 1 series
- Overall survival: 34-50% at 5 years

DIAGNOSTIC CHECKLIST

- Search for subtle calcification in aggressive bone lesion to discover 2° malignant fibrous histiocytoma (MFH)
  - 28% of MFH is secondary
  - Unfavorable prognostic factor: MFH arising in preexisting lesion

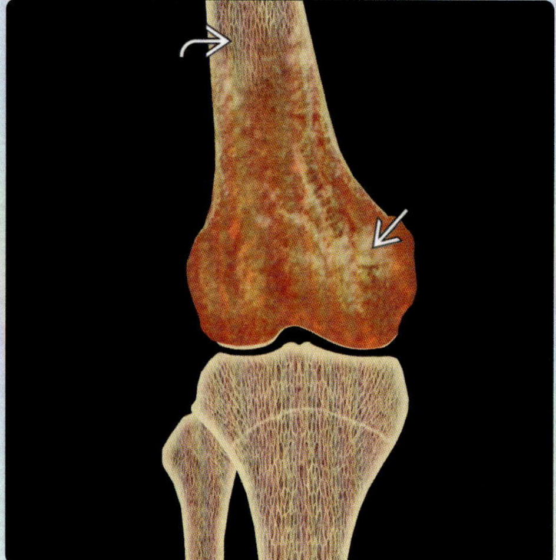

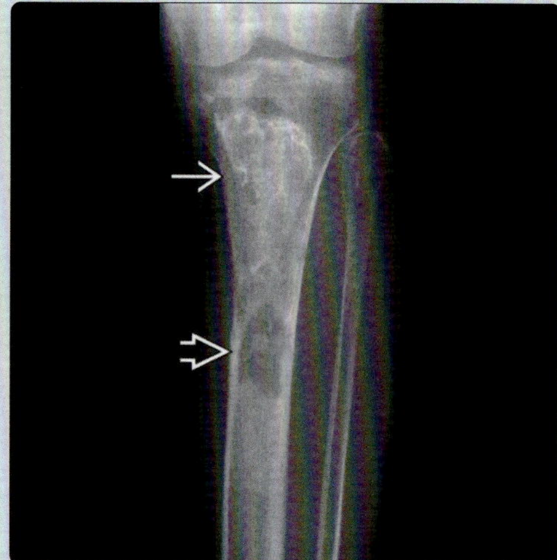

(Left) *Graphic shows transected specimen of MFH of bone arising in a bone infarct. The infarcted bone is seen as opaque yellow tissue ➔ surrounded and infiltrated by fleshy soft tissue, which is the malignant tumor. The lesion is permeative, having no sharp demarcation relative to normal bone ➔.* **(Right)** *AP radiograph of a secondary MFH shows a typical infarct in the proximal tibia ➔ but a change in character of the lesion more distally, where more prominent lysis is seen ➔. This implies an aggressive lesion.*

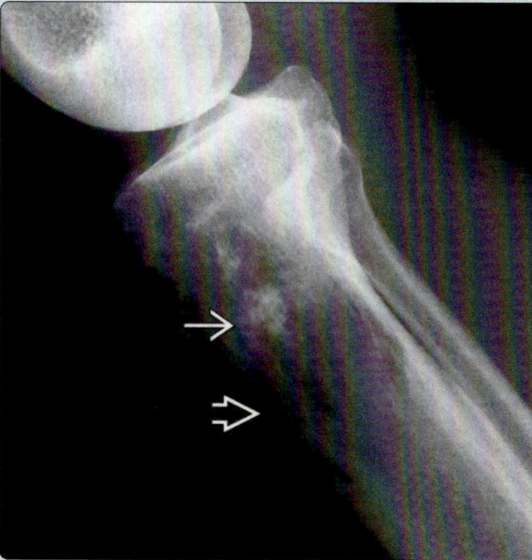

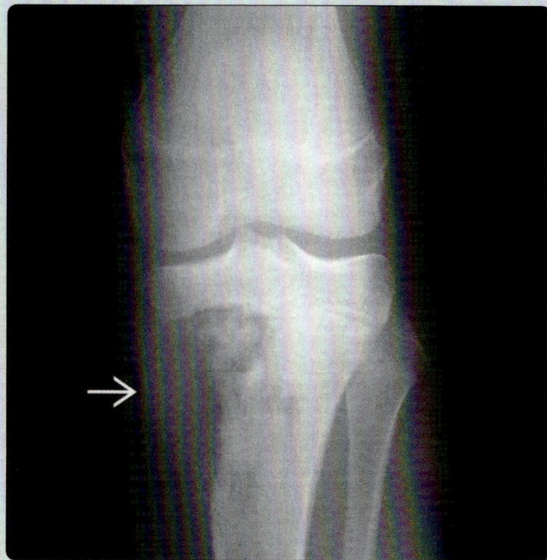

(Left) *Lateral radiograph, different patient, shows calcification in proximal tibia ➔, typical of bone infarct. There is a change in the character of the lesion, with the distal portion becoming lytic with a wide zone of transition ➔, indicating secondary MFH.* **(Right)** *AP x-ray shows a lytic destructive lesion with cortical breakthrough medially and a sizable soft tissue mass ➔. The location and appearance in a patient of this age is most typical of osteosarcoma. However, biopsy proved MFH secondary to bone infarct.*

TERMINOLOGY

Abbreviations

- Malignant fibrous histiocytoma (MFH)

Synonyms

- Malignant histiocytoma, xanthosarcoma, malignant fibrous xanthoma, fibroxanthosarcoma

Definitions

- Malignant osseous neoplasm composed of fibroblasts and pleomorphic cells exhibiting storiform pattern

IMAGING

General Features

- Best diagnostic clue
  - Aggressive osseous lesion, nonspecific unless associated with findings of bone infarct or other preexisting lesion
- Location
  - Long bones, central metaphysis or diaphysis (75%)
    - Often extends from metaphysis to epiphysis or diaphysis
    - Femur (30-45%) > tibia, fibula, humerus
    - 37% occur around knee
    - Flat bones: Pelvis most common
  - Usually solitary; rare multifocal tumors reported

Radiographic Findings

- Most high grade at presentation, with lytic destructive pattern
  - Permeative with wide zone of transition
    - Generally no sclerotic margin, but if present is incomplete
  - Cortical breakthrough and soft tissue mass
    - Cortex generally not expanded
  - Periosteal reaction often absent; if present, aggressive
- Lower grade lesion may appear at least partially geographic
  - Incomplete sclerotic margin
  - Some permeative change and aggressive regions should be present
- May have signs of prior lesion
  - Serpiginous pattern of bone infarct
  - Mixed lytic sclerotic pattern of Paget disease
  - Mixed lytic sclerotic pattern of radiation osteonecrosis
  - Chondroid matrix in dedifferentiated chondrosarcoma or enchondroma
  - Multiple ground-glass lesions in fibrous dysplasia
    - New lucency in sites of previous surgery suggest transformation to sarcoma
  - Cortically based geographic lesion of nonossifying fibroma
  - Thick reactive bone, serpiginous tracking in chronic osteomyelitis

CT Findings

- Mimics radiographic findings

MR Findings

- T1WI: Isointense to skeletal muscle
- Fluid sensitive: Heterogeneous high signal
- Postcontrast: Avid enhancement
- May show preexisting lesion in adjacent bone
  - Double line sign of bone infarct
  - Abnormal trabeculation of Paget disease
  - Cartilage in chondrosarcoma/enchondroma
  - Replacement of marrow by fat in radiation necrosis
  - Multiple lesions, abnormal marrow in fibrous dysplasia
  - Cortically based low signal nonossifying fibroma
  - Chronic osteomyelitis: Thick low signal reactive bone, high signal, enhancing serpiginous tracking, enhancing rim about abscess

Imaging Recommendations

- Best imaging tool
  - Usually picked up on radiograph
  - MR for evaluation of site and biopsy/surgical planning

DIFFERENTIAL DIAGNOSIS

Fibrosarcoma

- Lytic aggressive lesion
- Same locations as MFH
- No difference in imaging appearance from primary MFH

Primary Lymphoma of Bone

- Lytic aggressive lesion
- May have very similar appearance to MFH
- May have endosteal thickening of part of cortex
  - If present, differentiates from MFH

Chondrosarcoma

- If high-grade lytic chondrosarcoma, may not be differentiated from primary MFH by radiograph
- If high-grade chondrosarcoma with chondroid matrix, may be confused with secondary MFH with calcified bone infarct
  - Generally can differentiate chondroid matrix from serpiginous calcified infarct
  - MR allows differentiation of these 2 patterns
- Generally, chondrosarcoma is low grade
  - Less aggressive in appearance than MFH
  - MR shows lobulated high signal cartilage on T2WI sequences

Vascular Sarcoma

- May be highly aggressive; no matrix
- Often multifocal

PATHOLOGY

General Features

- Etiology
  - Primary MFH: Unknown
  - Secondary MFH: 28-43% of cases
    - Prior osseous abnormality or treatment
      - Bone infarct
      - Radiation
      - Paget disease
      - Chondrosarcoma may transform to MFH
      - Fibrous dysplasia (extremely rare complication, < 1% of cases; most of these transform to osteosarcoma)
      - Fibroxanthoma (nonossifying fibroma) (rare)
      - Chronic osteomyelitis (rare)

- Metallic implant reported as association (rare)
- Liposclerosing myxofibrous tumor (rare)

- Genetics
  - Diaphyseal medullary stenosis with MFH: Rare, autosomal dominant bone dysplasia/cancer syndrome
    - Diffuse diaphyseal medullary stenosis with endosteal cortical thickening, metaphyseal striations, and scattered infarctions
    - High rate of malignant transformation
- Associated abnormalities
  - Intramedullary bone infarct may have associated sarcoma
    - Rare development
    - Mean age at development: 53 years
    - African Americans disproportionately represented (36% in 1 study)
    - Most infarcts associated with sarcoma have no known etiology or risk factor
    - 75% of cases have multiple bone infarcts
    - Femur and tibia most common locations
    - Type of sarcoma associated with bone infarcts (1 series of 40 patients)
      - MFH: 73%
      - Osteosarcoma: 18%
    - Poor survival rate: 2-30% at 5 years

Staging, Grading, & Classification

- AJCC staging, including evaluation of lesion size, grade, and presence of metastases

Gross Pathologic & Surgical Features

- Varies in color and firmness
- Areas of necrosis and hemorrhage
- Irregular margins, cortical destruction

Microscopic Features

- Mixed population of spindle, histiocytoid, and pleomorphic cells
- Varying amounts of multinucleated giant cells
- Chronic inflammatory cells
- Characteristic storiform (pinwheel) pattern in fibroblastic areas
- Most are high-grade lesions

CLINICAL ISSUES

Presentation

- Most common signs/symptoms
  - Pain and swelling, occasionally for several months
  - Pathologic fracture (20%)

Demographics

- Age
  - Wide range; higher incidence in patients > 40 years
    - 10-15% occur in 2nd decade, so do not discount diagnosis in adolescents/young adults
  - Note this is a younger age of peak occurrence than pleomorphic sarcoma (soft tissue MFH)
- Gender
  - Male predominance (1.5:1)
- Epidemiology
  - Osseous MFH significantly less common than soft tissue MFH (pleomorphic sarcoma)
  - Rare; 2-5% of all primary malignant bone tumors
  - 28-43% of MFH is secondary

Natural History & Prognosis

- Usually high grade at presentation
- Metastases in lung at presentation in 45-50% in 1 series
  - Other less common sites of metastases: Bone, soft tissue
- Overall survival: 34-53% at 5 years
- In patients with localized disease at presentation, 5-year survival of ~ 50%
- Favorable prognostic factors
  - Young age (< 40 years) at presentation
  - Low histologic grade
  - Adequate wide surgical resection
- Unfavorable prognostic factors
  - MFH arising in preexisting lesion
    - Recent study disputes this, suggesting 1° and 2° MFH have similar prognoses
  - Surrounding inflammatory cells and desmoplasia

Treatment

- Wide resection
- Pre- and postoperative chemotherapy
- ± radiation therapy

DIAGNOSTIC CHECKLIST

Image Interpretation Pearls

- Search for subtle calcification in aggressive bone lesion to discover 2° MFH

SELECTED REFERENCES

1. Qu N et al: Malignant transformation in monostotic fibrous dysplasia: clinical features, imaging features, outcomes in 10 patients, and review. Medicine (Baltimore). 94(3):e369, 2015
2. Romeo S et al: Malignant fibrous histiocytoma and fibrosarcoma of bone: a re-assessment in the light of currently employed morphological, immunohistochemical and molecular approaches. Virchows Arch. 461(5):561-70, 2012
3. Koplas MC et al: Imaging findings, prevalence and outcome of de novo and secondary malignant fibrous histiocytoma of bone. Skeletal Radiol. 39(8):791-8, 2010
4. Domson GF et al: Infarct-associated bone sarcomas. Clin Orthop Relat Res. 467(7):1820-5, 2009
5. Min WK et al: Malignant fibrous histiocytoma arising in the area of total hip replacement. Joint Bone Spine. 75(3):319-21, 2008
6. Hoshi M et al: Malignant change secondary to fibrous dysplasia. Int J Clin Oncol. 11(3):229-35, 2006
7. Richter H et al: Malignant fibrous histiocytoma associated with remote internal fixation of an ankle fracture. Foot Ankle Int. 27(5):375-9, 2006
8. Scottish Bone Tumor Registry et al: Paget sarcoma of the spine: Scottish Bone Tumor Registry experience. Spine (Phila Pa 1976). 31(12):1344-50, 2006
9. Staals EL et al: Dedifferentiated central chondrosarcoma. Cancer. 106(12):2682-91, 2006
10. Tarkkanen M et al: Malignant fibrous histiocytoma of bone: analysis of genomic imbalances by comparative genomic hybridisation and C-MYC expression by immunohistochemistry. Eur J Cancer. 42(8):1172-80, 2006
11. Zlowodzki M et al: CASE REPORTS: malignant fibrous histiocytoma of bone arising in chronic osteomyelitis. Clin Orthop Relat Res. 439:269-73, 2005
12. Murphey MD et al: From the archives of the AFIP. Musculoskeletal malignant fibrous histiocytoma: radiologic-pathologic correlation. Radiographics. 14(4):807-26; quiz 827-8, 1994

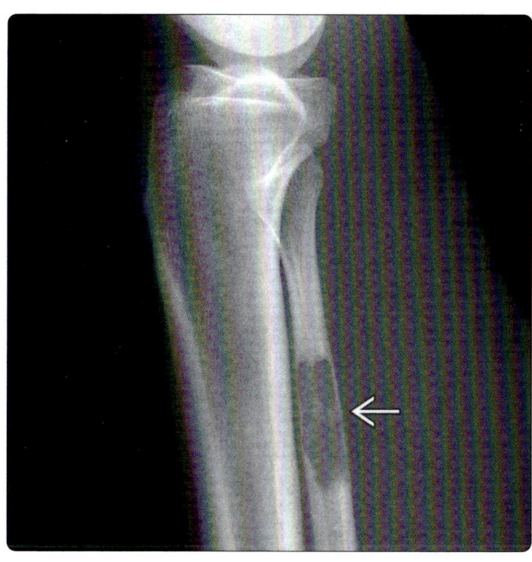

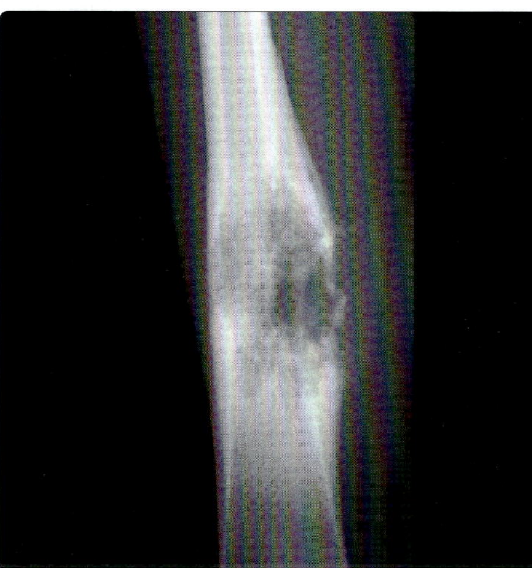

(Left) *Lateral radiograph shows a lytic lesion that has only a mildly aggressive appearance* ➙*. At biopsy, however, this proved to be MFH. Furthermore, it was a high-grade lesion, which is particularly surprising given the radiographic appearance.* **(Right)** *AP radiograph shows a case of primary MFH, a highly aggressive lytic lesion arising in the central diaphysis. There is a wide zone of transition, cortical breakthrough, host reaction, and a soft tissue mass. There is no evidence of underlying lesion.*

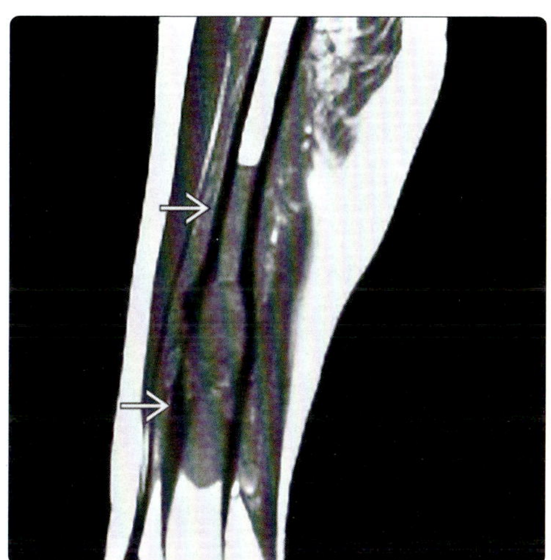

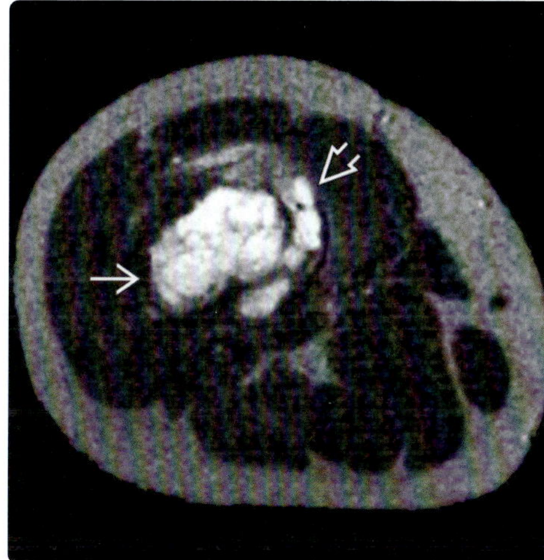

(Left) *Sagittal T1WI MR in the same patient shows the diaphyseal extent of the lesion* ➙*, which is intermediate signal intensity on this sequence. The lesion involves more bone than might have been expected from the radiograph.* **(Right)** *Axial T2WI MR in the same patient shows a rather lobulated high signal lesion* ➙ *occupying the marrow, with medial cortical breakthrough and a modest soft tissue mass* ➙*. The MR does not add specificity to the diagnosis of MFH in this case but allows excellent site evaluation.*

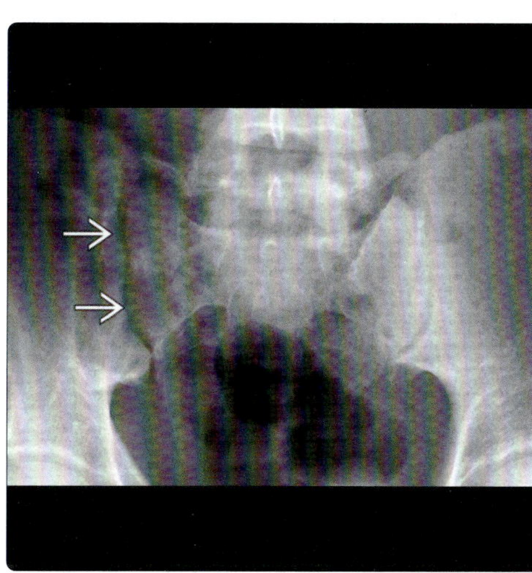

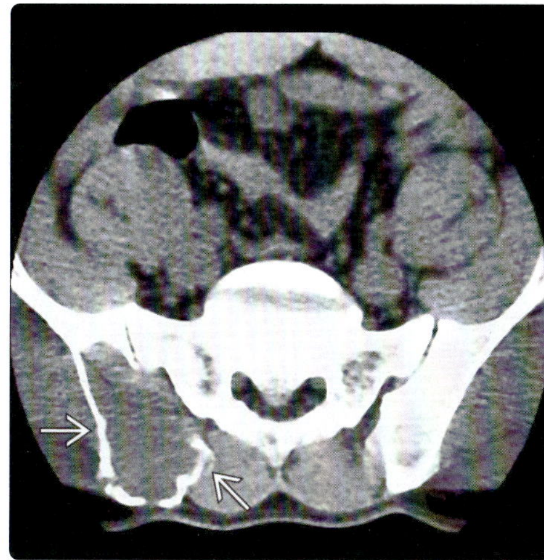

(Left) *AP radiograph shows an easily overlooked MFH. The right sacroiliac joint appears completely lucent* ➙ *(compared to left). This appearance has been termed the "naked" SI joint, indicating that the posterior iliac wing is absent.* **(Right)** *Axial NECT in the same patient shows the expanded lytic lesion* ➙ *replacing the marrow of the posterior right iliac wing. This is a moderately aggressive lesion; MFH is just 1 of several diagnostic possibilities but was proven at surgery.*

Fibrosarcoma

KEY FACTS

TERMINOLOGY

- Malignant spindle cell tumor of bone in which tumor cells are oriented in fascicular or herringbone pattern

IMAGING

- Long tubular bones in 70%
  - Metaphyses of long bones; distal femur most frequent
- Pelvis: 9%
- Aggressive destructive lesion
  - Permeative, wide zone of transition
  - Periosteal reaction need not be present; variable appearance when it is
- Lytic, may contain sequestered bone fragments
- Central or eccentric
- Cortical breakthrough with soft tissue mass

TOP DIFFERENTIAL DIAGNOSES

- Malignant fibrous histiocytoma (MFH)
  - Primary MFH has identical aggressive imaging appearance to fibrosarcoma
- Osteosarcoma (osteolytic)
  - If no matrix, may appear identical, with permeative destructive character
- Primary lymphoma of bone
  - Lytic lesion that may appear as aggressive as fibrosarcoma
  - May induce endosteal bone thickening; if present, differentiates it from fibrosarcoma

CLINICAL ISSUES

- 2nd to 6th decades; rarely reported as early as infancy
- ~ 5% of all primary malignant bone tumors
  - Prevalence difficult to determine due to inconsistency in use of terminology of fibrosarcoma vs. MFH
- Overall 5-year survival: 34%

(Left) *Lateral radiograph shows an aggressive lytic lesion ➡ in a 22-year-old man. The lesion is eccentric, shows periosteal reaction ↶, and has cortical breakthrough with a soft tissue mass ⇨. The lesion is aggressive but nonspecific, with a wide differential.* **(Right)** *Sagittal T1 C+ FS MR shows the lesion with wide associated marrow edema ➡. The soft tissue mass enhances avidly and has a region of central necrosis ↶. Biopsy showed fibrosarcoma. Imaging is nonspecific beyond indicating an aggressive lesion.*

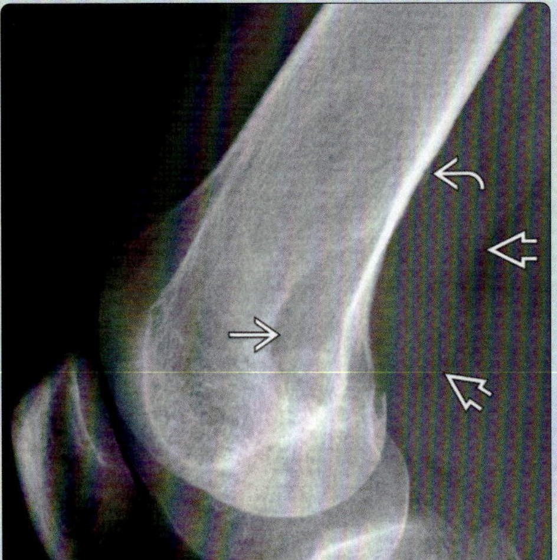

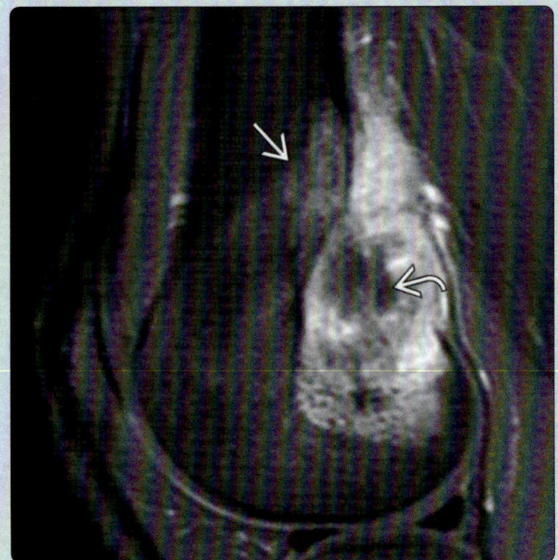

(Left) *Lateral radiograph shows the classic appearance of fibrous dysplasia (FD). The trabeculae are replaced by ground-glass matrix, the bone is expanded, and the cortex is scalloped. There is severe anterior bowing ➡, which was subsequently treated by osteotomy and rodding.* **(Right)** *Lateral radiograph in the same patient several years later shows the osteotomy has healed. However, there is a new destructive lytic lesion replacing the proximal tibia ➡, proven to be a rare degeneration of FD to fibrosarcoma.*

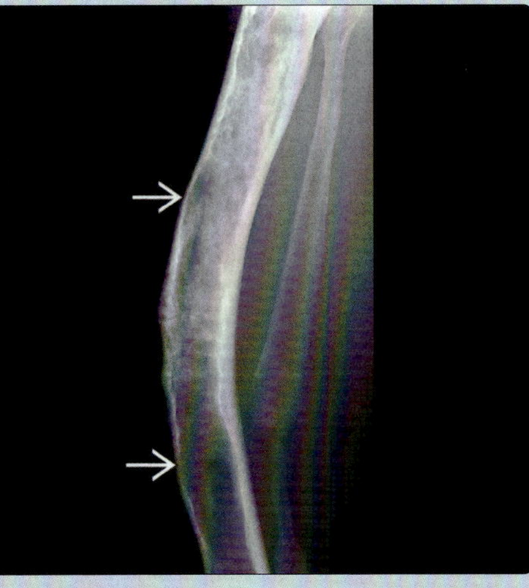

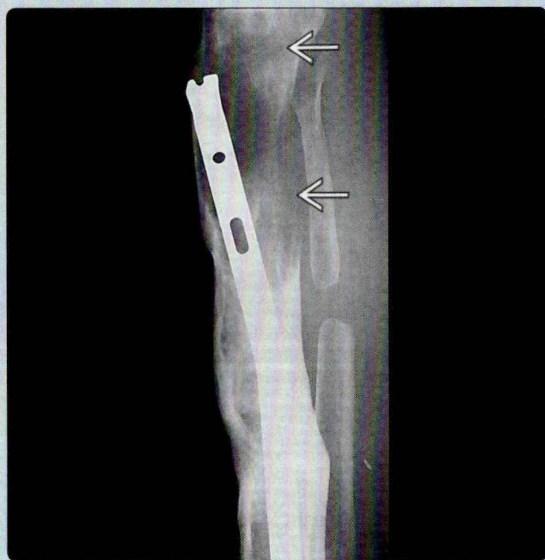

TERMINOLOGY

Definitions

- Malignant spindle cell tumor of bone in which tumor cells are oriented in fascicular or herringbone pattern

IMAGING

General Features

- Best diagnostic clue
  - Lytic aggressive lesion of bone; nonspecific
- Location
  - Long tubular bones: 70%
    - Metaphyses of long bones; distal femur most frequent
    - Other sites: Proximal femur, proximal tibia, distal humerus
  - Pelvis: 9%

Radiographic Findings

- Aggressive destructive lesion
  - Permeative, wide zone of transition
- Periosteal reaction need not be present; variable appearance when it is
- Lytic, may contain sequestered bone fragments
- Central or eccentric
- Cortical breakthrough with soft tissue mass

MR Findings

- Nonspecific aggressive lesion
  - T1 mass isointense to skeletal muscle
  - Fluid-sensitive sequences: Inhomogeneously hyperintense
  - Avid contrast enhancement

DIFFERENTIAL DIAGNOSIS

Malignant Fibrous Histiocytoma

- Primary malignant fibrous histiocytoma (MFH) has identical aggressive imaging appearance compared to fibrosarcoma
- MFH more common than fibrosarcoma
- Differentiated histologically

Osteosarcoma (Osteolytic)

- Generally younger age group
- If no matrix, may appear identical, with permeative destructive character

Chondrosarcoma (Lytic)

- Same age group and locations
- Chondroid matrix need not be present; may mimic other lesions
- Generally lower grade, with thickened endosteal cortex, scalloping of cortex, expansion but not significant cortical breakthrough and mass
- Endosteal thickening may differentiate chondrosarcoma from fibrosarcoma

Primary Lymphoma of Bone

- Lytic, may appear as aggressive as fibrosarcoma
- May induce endosteal bone thickening; if present, differentiates it from fibrosarcoma

PATHOLOGY

General Features

- Etiology
  - Unknown in majority of cases
  - Some cases associated with prior conditions
    - Radiation
    - Paget disease
    - Chondrosarcoma (dedifferentiated)
    - Giant cell tumor
    - Bone infarct
    - Chronic osteomyelitis
    - Fibrous dysplasia
    - Ameloblastic fibroma

Gross Pathologic & Surgical Features

- Firm white lesion on cut section
- Trabeculated
- If poorly differentiated, consistency is softer and more fleshy, with necrosis

Microscopic Features

- Uniform spindle cells arranged in fascicular or herringbone pattern
- Higher grade lesions more cellular, with less collagen and greater nuclear atypia
- Difficult diagnosis; upon review, many are reclassified as other sarcomas

CLINICAL ISSUES

Presentation

- Most common signs/symptoms
  - Pain and swelling
  - Pathologic fracture in 1/3

Demographics

- Age
  - 2nd to 6th decades; rarely reported as early as infancy
- Gender
  - M = F
- Epidemiology
  - Prevalence difficult to determine due to inconsistency in use of terminology of fibrosarcoma vs. MFH
  - ~ 5% of all primary malignant bone tumors

Natural History & Prognosis

- Overall 5-year survival: 34%
- Prognosis strongly related to grade of lesion
  - Low-grade 10-year survival: 83%
  - High-grade 10-year survival: 34%
- Metastases to lung, less frequently to bone

Treatment

- Wide surgical resection
- Chemotherapy, radiation therapy

SELECTED REFERENCES

1. Qu N et al: Malignant transformation in monostotic fibrous dysplasia: clinical features, imaging features, outcomes in 10 patients, and review. Medicine (Baltimore). 94(3):e369, 2015

KEY FACTS

TERMINOLOGY

- Benign intraosseous tumor consisting of adipocytes

IMAGING

- Best diagnostic clue: Fat density lesion on all imaging modalities
  - Other components present during lesional involution
- 71% intramedullary in lower limb
  - Proximal femur > proximal tibia > calcaneus
- Lucent intramedullary lesion
- May be expanded
- Thin sclerotic rim (most)
- May contain central calcification (stage 2 lesions) or less distinct but more extensive calcification (stage 3)
  - 62% in calcaneal lesions; 30% at other sites
- MR in stage 1
  - T1 and T2: ↑ signal, isointense to subcutaneous fat
  - Shows fat-suppression characteristics
- MR in stage 2 or 3 (67% of lesions)
  - Contains regions of typical adipose signal
  - Fat necrosis: Low signal T1, high signal T2
  - Cyst formation: Low signal T1, high signal T2, peripheral enhancement
  - Signal void in regions of calcification

PATHOLOGY

- Milgram staging: Relating to degree of involution present histologically
  - Stage 1: Viable fat cells
  - Stage 2: Transitional, composed partly of viable fat cells plus fat necrosis and calcification
  - Stage 3: Necrotic fat, calcification, variable degrees of cyst formation, reactive bone

CLINICAL ISSUES

- May undergo spontaneous involution
- Reports of extremely rare cases of transformation to liposarcoma or malignant fibrous histiocytoma

(Left) *Lateral radiograph shows a typical intraosseous lipoma showing early involutional changes. The location in the mid to anterior calcaneus is typical. The lesion is geographic and triangular-shaped ➡. It is lucent but contains some punctate calcifications.* **(Right)** *Sagittal bone CT confirms the geographic nature of the lesion, which appears septate. Note small calcific densities ➡ surrounded by fat density (compare to subcutaneous fat). The diagnosis can confidently be made on either CT or radiograph.*

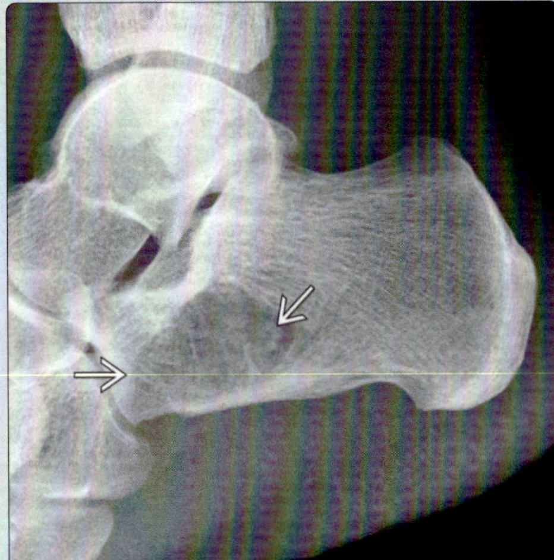

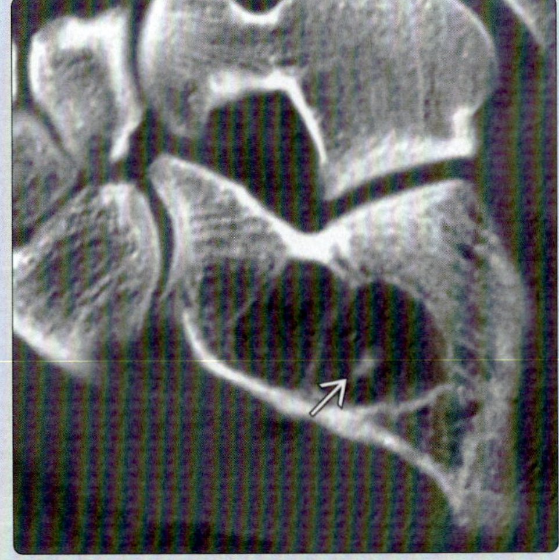

(Left) *Sagittal T1WI MR in the same patient shows the lesion to have high fat signal with small, calcific, low signal densities ➡. Note the low signal round focus ➡.* **(Right)** *Sagittal T2WI FS MR, same slice, shows signal dropout of the majority of the lesion, which consists of fat. A small amount of signal is seen around the calcifications ➡, and the round focus is clearly cystic ➡. With age, as intraosseous lipomas begin to involute, areas of calcification and cystic necrosis may develop.*

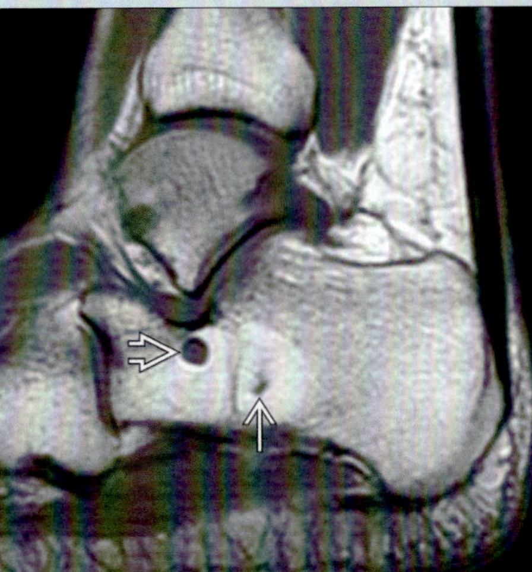

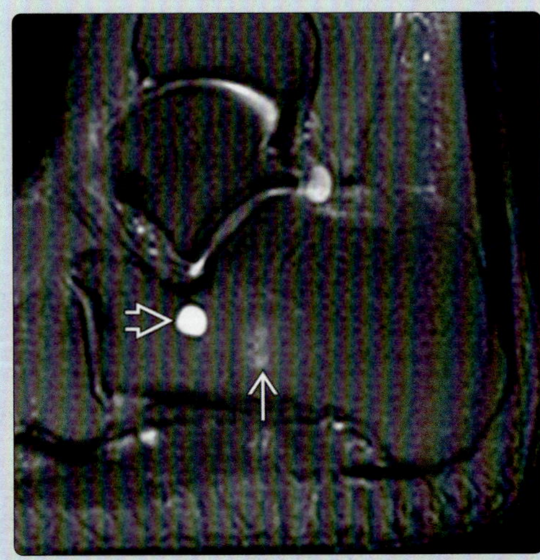

TERMINOLOGY

Synonyms

- Intramedullary lipoma, intracortical lipoma, ossifying lipoma

Definitions

- Benign intraosseous tumor consisting of adipocytes

IMAGING

General Features

- Best diagnostic clue
  - Fat density lesion on all imaging modalities
    - Other components present during involution
- Location
  - 71% intramedullary in lower limb
    - Proximal femur > proximal tibia > calcaneus
  - Intracortical and other locations rare

Radiographic Findings

- Lucent intramedullary lesion
- Thin sclerotic rim (most)
  - Occasionally lesions do not appear geographic with defined margin
  - Stage 3 lesions may have thicker rims than 1 or 2
    - Sclerotic rim most common in calcaneal lesions
- May contain central calcification (stage 2 lesions) or less distinct but more extensive calcification (stage 3)
  - 62% calcaneal lesions; 30% other sites
- Occasional mild cortical expansion

CT Findings

- Fat-attenuation intraosseous lesion; appearance dictated by stage
  - May have expansile remodeling, thin sclerotic rim

MR Findings

- Stage 1
  - T1 and T2: High signal, isointense to subcutaneous fat
  - Signal void with fat suppression
  - Thin rim of low signal sclerosis
- Stage 2 or 3: 67% of lesions
  - Fat necrosis: Low signal T1, high signal T2
  - Cyst formation: Low signal T1, high signal T2, peripheral enhancement
  - Signal void in regions of calcification
  - Portions contain routine fat signal intensity as well

DIFFERENTIAL DIAGNOSIS

Calcaneal Lesions in Same Location as Lipoma

- Simple bone cyst: Thin sclerotic rim, no calcification unless floating fragment
- Physiologic trabecular pattern may mimic lucent lesion

Involutional Lesion, Stage 3 (Any Site)

- May be confused with bone infarct 2° to extensive calcification
- Ground-glass density may suggest fibrous dysplasia
- Liposclerosing myxofibrous tumor has similar sclerosis but little fat

PATHOLOGY

Staging, Grading, & Classification

- Milgram staging: Relating to degree of involution present histologically
  - Stage 1: Viable fat cells organized into lobules
  - Stage 2: Transitional, composed partly of viable fat cells plus fat necrosis and calcification
  - Stage 3: Necrotic fat, calcification of necrotic fat, variable degrees of cyst formation, + reactive bone formation

Gross Pathologic & Surgical Features

- Well-defined, soft, yellow
- Involutional components depend on stage

Microscopic Features

- Lobules of mature adipocytes, may encase trabeculae
- May have fat necrosis

CLINICAL ISSUES

Presentation

- Most common signs/symptoms
  - Usually asymptomatic, though up to 66% may report pain
  - Mild aching pain may occur

Demographics

- Age
  - Wide range; most diagnosed in 4th decade
- Gender
  - Males > females (1.6:1)
- Epidemiology
  - Rare: < 0.1% of primary tumors of bone
  - Likely more prevalent but underdiagnosed

Natural History & Prognosis

- Nonprogressive
- May undergo spontaneous involution
- Possible intralesional ischemic damage
- Reports of extremely rare cases of malignant transformation to liposarcoma or malignant fibrous histiocytoma

Treatment

- If symptomatic, curettage and bone grafting
  - Marginal resection yields rare recurrence
- If asymptomatic, conservative treatment

DIAGNOSTIC CHECKLIST

Consider

- Generally straightforward diagnosis, but involutional changes may confuse appearance

SELECTED REFERENCES

1. Mannem RR et al: AIRP best cases in radiologic-pathologic correlation: intraosseous lipoma. Radiographics. 32(5):1523-8, 2012
2. Eyzaguirre E et al: Intraosseous lipoma. A clinical, radiologic, and pathologic study of 5 cases. Ann Diagn Pathol. 11(5):320-5, 2007
3. Kapukaya A et al: Osseous lipoma: eleven new cases and review of the literature. Acta Orthop Belg. 72(5):603-14, 2006
4. Kwak HS et al: On the AJR viewbox. MR findings of calcaneal intraosseous lipoma with hemorrhage. AJR Am J Roentgenol. 185(5):1378-9, 2005

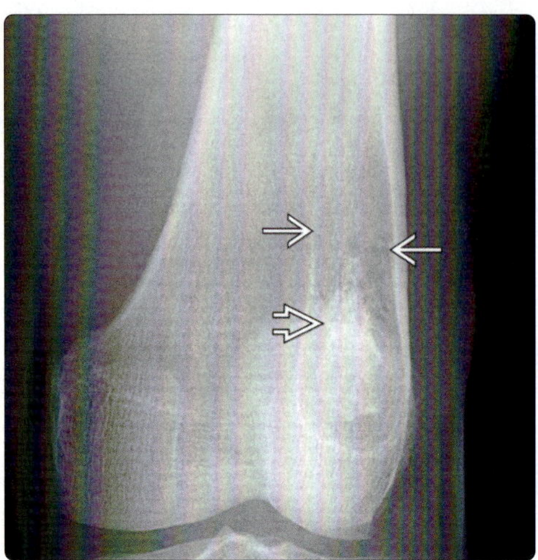

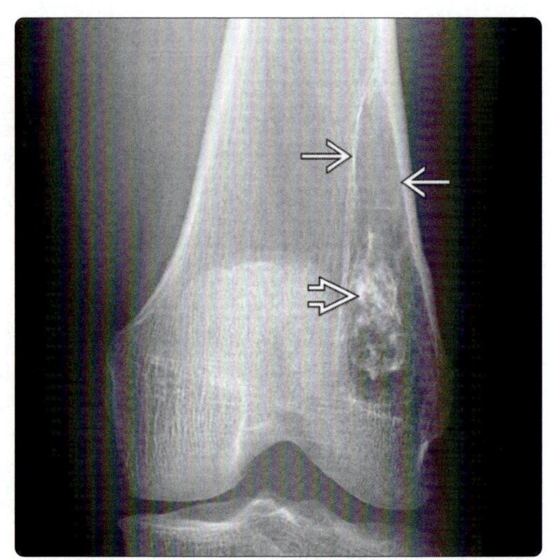

(Left) *AP radiograph shows developing senescence in an intraosseous lipoma. A large, elongated lesion is located eccentrically within the metadiaphysis. The lesion has a thin sclerotic border, with fat density seen inside* ➡*. More centrally, there is dystrophic calcification* ➡*. This is the typical appearance of a stage 2 lipoma.* **(Right)** *AP radiograph in the same patient 5 years later shows the sclerotic margin to be thicker and more distinct* ➡*. The central calcification has matured* ➡*.*

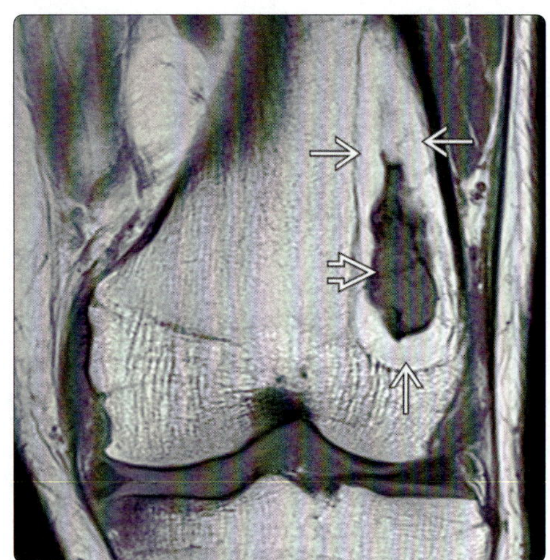

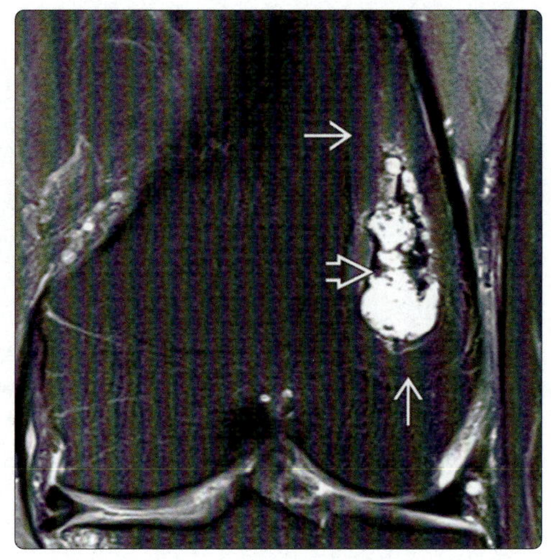

(Left) *Coronal T1WI MR in the same patient shows fat signal inside the lesion's thin sclerotic border* ➡*. Central low signal shows different degrees of low signal intensity, related to both fluid and calcification* ➡*.* **(Right)** *Coronal PDWI FS MR in the same patient shows signal dropout in the lipomatous portion of the lesion* ➡*. There is high signal centrally, indicating cystic necrotic portions* ➡*, interspersed with low signal calcifications. The majority of the lesion shows involutional change.*

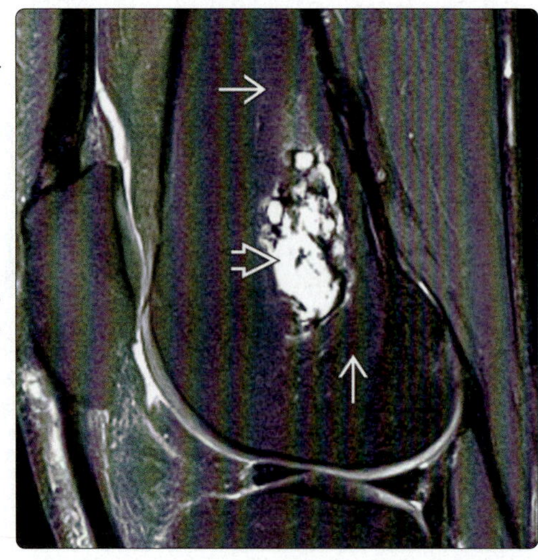

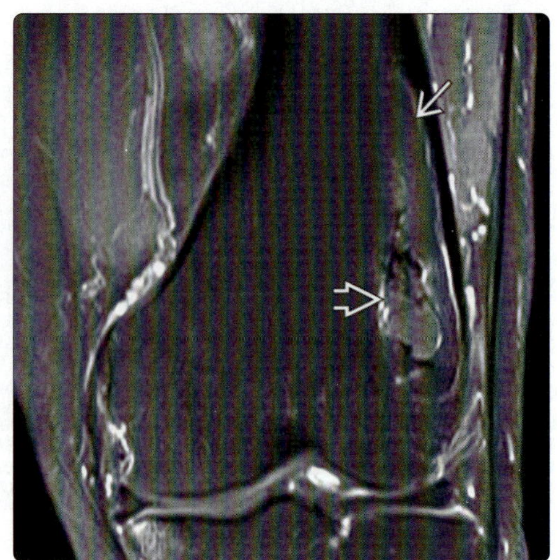

(Left) *Sagittal T2WI FS MR in the same patient shows that the original sclerotic margin of the lesion is no longer visible, and the fat adjacent to the rim shows complete signal dropout with fat saturation* ➡*. High signal central necrosis is again seen* ➡*, along with calcification.* **(Right)** *Coronal T1WI C+ FS MR in the same patient shows only faint, thin rim enhancement around the lesion* ➡ *and cystic degeneration* ➡*. The overall appearance is of a stage 3 intraosseous lipoma, which is undergoing senescence.*

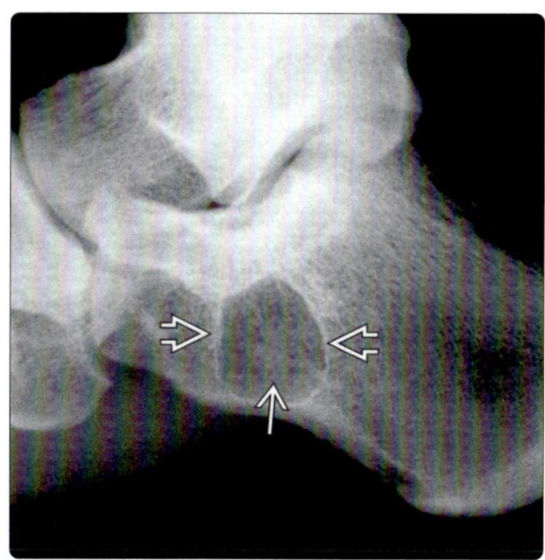

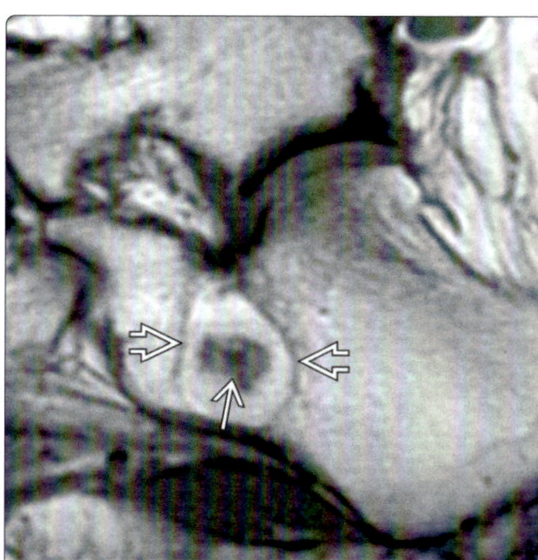

(Left) *Lateral radiograph shows a well-circumscribed lucent lesion* ➡ *with a thin sclerotic rim and faint internal mineralization* ➡. **(Right)** *Sagittal T2WI MR in the same patient shows well-defined fat signal intensity* ➡ *with a central area of low signal intensity* ➡ *due to mineralization. Calcification on radiograph was diagnostic, eliminating diagnosis of either unicameral bone cyst or physiologic pseudotumor due to trabecular arrangement. MR is confirmatory, showing stage 2 intraosseous lipoma.*

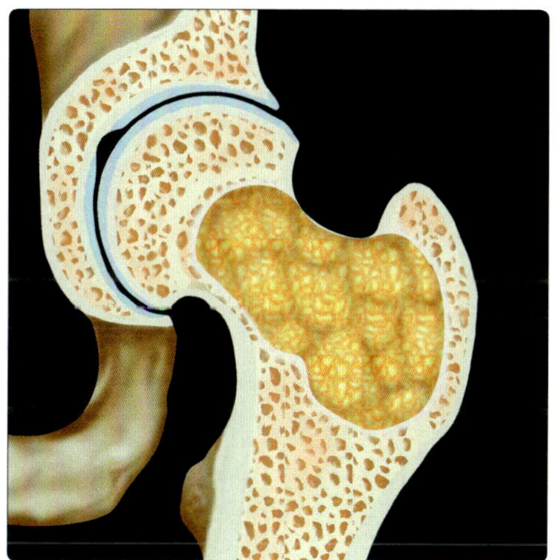

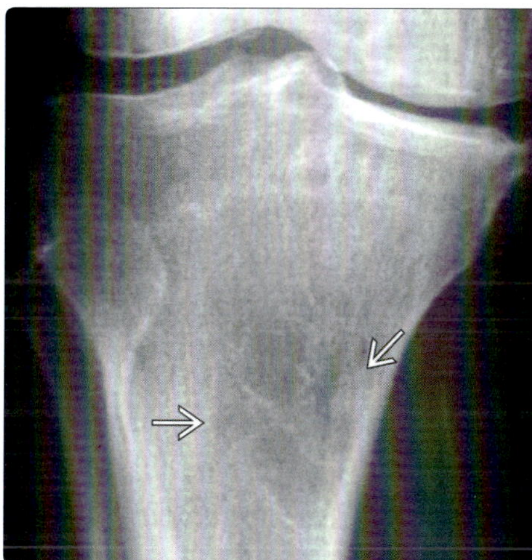

(Left) *Graphic shows a cut section of femur containing a lipoma, appearing lobulated, depicted as stage 1, without necrosis or calcification.* **(Right)** *Radiograph of a lytic lesion within the tibia* ➡ *shows there is no sclerotic rim; one might consider enchondroma or bone infarct. However, there is also fat density, which suggests the diagnosis of an intraosseous lipoma. (Previously published in Musculoskeletal Imaging: The Requisites. 2nd ed. Philadelphia, PA: Mosby, Elsevier; 2002.)*

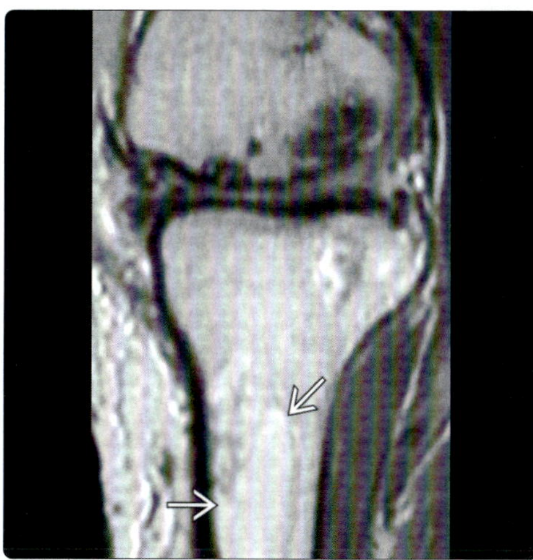

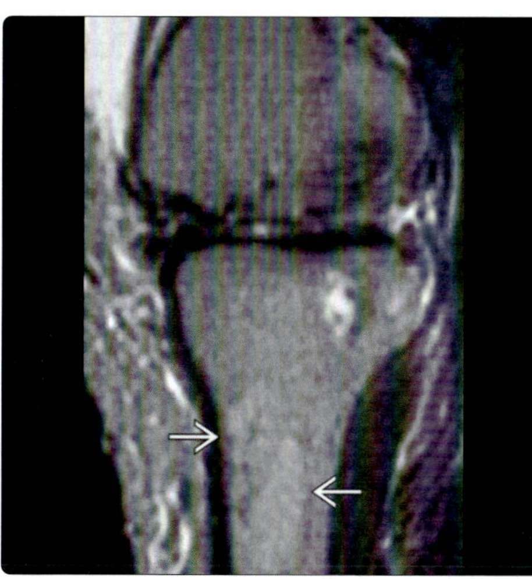

(Left) *Sagittal PDWI MR in the same patient shows the lesion to consist of lobulated fat* ➡ *with the same signal as the subcutaneous fat. There is no other tissue type seen within the lesion.* **(Right)** *Sagittal T2WI FS MR shows the faintest outline of the lesion* ➡, *with complete fat suppression, similar to the marrow, diagnostic of intraosseous stage 1 lipoma. Without any changes of involution, the lesion may be difficult to identify correctly on radiograph. Note also the osteoarthritis, the cause of this patient's pain.*

KEY FACTS

TERMINOLOGY

- Generally benign bone tumor composed of sheets of neoplastic ovoid mononuclear cells interspersed with uniformly distributed large osteoclast-like giant cells
- Rare malignant giant cell tumor (GCT) (5% of all GCT)
  - 1° malignant GCT: Arises in conjunction with benign GCT
  - 2° malignant GCT: Either arises in recurrence of previously benign GCT or arises 2° to treatment of benign GCT with radiation

IMAGING

- Location: Originates in metaphysis, extends into epiphysis, often to subarticular end of bone
  - Distal femur > proximal tibia > distal radius
  - Axial skeleton: Sacrum > other vertebrae
  - Vertebral body > > posterior elements
- Radiographic appearance usually unique
  - Completely lytic lesion in majority of cases
  - ± cortical breakthrough/soft tissue mass (33-50%)
  - Combination of narrow transition zone and nonsclerotic margin suggestive of GCT; unusual in other lesions
  - Generally no periosteal reaction
- Uncommon aggressive or malignant GCT shows increased degree of aggressiveness
- MR T1: Low to intermediate SI, inhomogeneous
- MR fluid-sensitive series: Inhomogeneous high signal intensity with areas of
  - ↓ signal within lesion (63%)
  - Aneurysmal bone cyst components: Loculations with fluid-fluid levels on T2 (14%)

CLINICAL ISSUES

- Peak incidence at age 20-50 (80%)
- Incidence: 20% of all benign primary bone tumors
- High recurrence rate with marginal resection (curettage): 25%
- Rx with denosumab promising; distinctive peripheral calcification in healing lesion

(Left) *Graphic depicting transected specimen of a giant cell tumor (GCT). Soft tissue of this tumor is typically pinkish-tan. Note: The lesion is sharply demarcated from normal bone ➔, but the margin is very thin. Hemorrhagic cystic (ABC) regions are present ➔.* **(Right)** *Coronal CT demonstrates a completely lytic lesion that originates in the metaphysis and extends nearly to the subchondral bone. The margin ➔ is distinct but nonsclerotic. CT shows cortical breakthrough at the medial margin ➔. This is a classic appearance of GTC.*

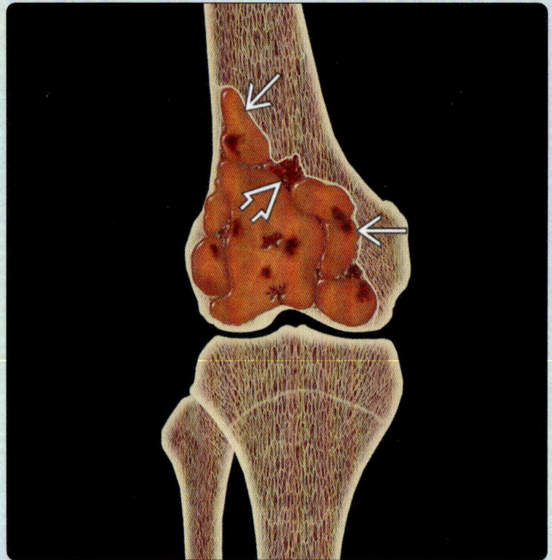

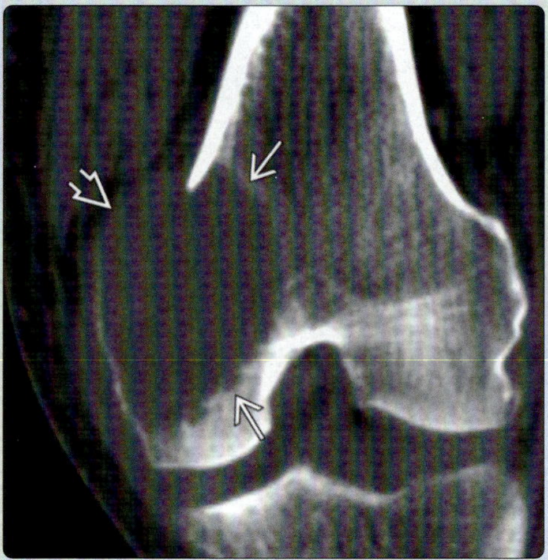

(Left) *Sagittal T2 FS MR (same patient) shows only moderate hyperintensity of the lesion, with regions of distinctly lower signal intensity ➔. These low signal foci are typically seen in GCT, although they may have different morphologies (nodular, zonal, whorled, diffuse). There is mild associated marrow edema.* **(Right)** *Axial postcontrast T1 C+ FS MR in the same patient shows the inhomogeneous mildly enhancing lesion ➔, with a significant region of necrosis. Degrees of necrosis may differ, depending on aggressiveness of the lesion.*

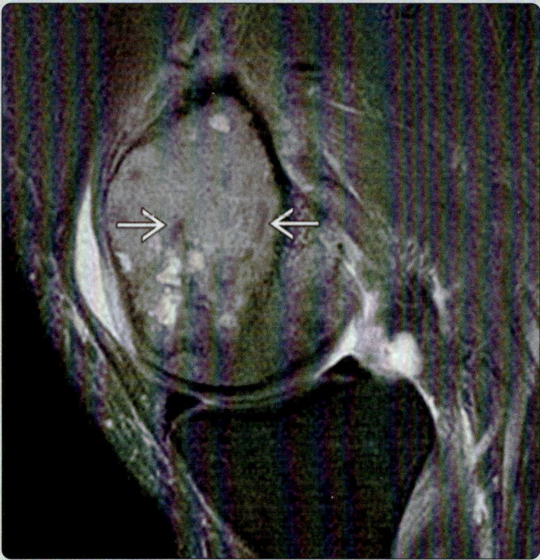

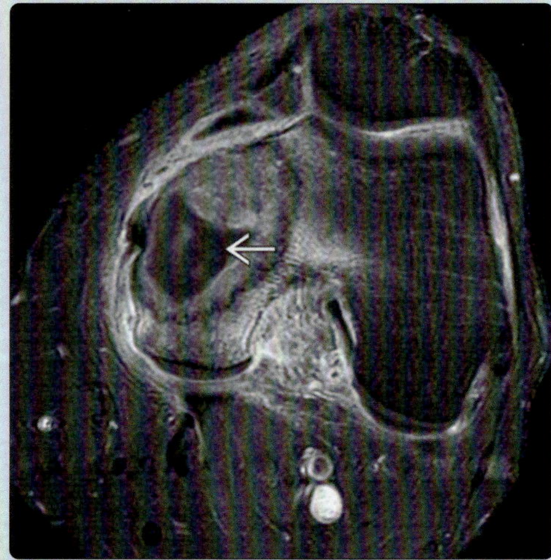

TERMINOLOGY

Abbreviations

- Giant cell tumor (GCT)

Definitions

- Generally benign bone tumor composed of sheets of neoplastic ovoid mononuclear cells interspersed with uniformly distributed large osteoclast-like giant cells
- Rare malignant GCT (5% of all GCT)
  - Primary malignant GCT: Arises within benign GCT
  - Secondary malignant GCT: 2 varieties
    - Majority: Secondary to treatment of initially benign GCT with radiation
    - Minority: Arise in recurrence of once benign GCT

IMAGING

General Features

- Best diagnostic clue
  - Lytic lesion with narrow zone of transition but no sclerotic margin, extending to subchondral bone
- Location
  - Originates in metaphysis, extends into epiphysis, often to subarticular end of bone
    - 84-99% within 1 cm of subarticular bone
    - Since origin is in metaphysis, extension to epiphysis relates to size and duration of tumor
  - 75-90% in long bones: Distal femur > proximal tibia > distal radius
    - 50-65% occur around knee
  - 5% involve flat bones, especially pelvis
  - < 5% involve small tubular bones of hand/foot
  - Axial skeleton: Sacrum > other vertebrae
    - Vertebral body > > posterior elements
  - Very rarely multicentric
    - Tend to be found around knee or in hand/foot
    - Multicentric GCT also related to Paget disease
      - Skull, facial bones, pelvis, spine
  - Very rarely arise in soft tissues

Radiographic Findings

- Completely lytic lesion in majority of cases
  - Rare matrix production
- Eccentric, arising in metaphysis but extending towards subchondral bone plate
- Majority are geographic with narrow transition zone
  - Usually no sclerotic margin (80-85%)
  - Combination of narrow zone of transition and nonsclerotic margin highly suggestive of GCT; unusual in other lesions
- Thinning of cortex; ranges from mildly to significantly expanded
  - Occasional bubbly appearance
- May show pseudotrabeculation (33-57%)
- ± cortical breakthrough/soft tissue mass (33-50%)
- Generally no periosteal reaction
- Uncommon aggressive or malignant GCT shows increased degree of aggressiveness
  - Permeative, cortical breakthrough, soft tissue mass, periosteal reaction

CT Findings

- More accurate assessment of cortical thinning and breakthrough
- Lung metastases, soft tissue implants may show peripheral ossification

MR Findings

- T1: Low to intermediate SI, inhomogeneous
  - Areas of lower SI throughout portions of lesion
- Fluid-sensitive series: Inhomogeneous high SI
  - Inhomogeneous low signal within lesion (63%)
    - May be nodular, zonal, whorled, or diffuse
    - Occupies at least 1/5 of lesion
    - May bloom on gradient-echo imaging
    - May be due to extravasated hemosiderin-containing erythrocytes and phagocytic function of tumor cells or ↑ collagen content
- Postcontrast imaging: Inhomogeneous enhancement
- Aneurysmal bone cyst (ABC) components: Loculations with fluid-fluid levels on T2WI (14%)
  - Peripheral enhancement of cystic portions

DIFFERENTIAL DIAGNOSIS

Chondroblastoma

- Originates in epiphysis rather than metaphysis
- May contain chondroid matrix (generally not)
- Sclerotic margin common, + periosteal reaction
- Generally skeletally immature patients

Chondrosarcoma

- Lytic conventional chondrosarcoma may extend to subchondral bone and mimic GCT
- Clear cell chondrosarcoma originates in epiphysis, mimicking subchondral extension of GCT
- Generally low-grade, fairly narrow zone of transition
- Lobulated high T2 signal differentiates it on MR

Aneurysmal Bone Cyst

- May be present in portion of GCT
- Usually younger when not associated with GCT
- Generally located eccentrically in metadiaphysis
- Fluid levels seen throughout lesion on MR

PATHOLOGY

General Features

- Etiology
  - Most malignant GCT are secondary, related to previous radiation
- Genetics
  - Telomeric association is most frequent chromosomal abnormality
- Associated abnormalities
  - ABC components in 14%
    - Conversely, GCT is most common lesion associated with 2° ABC (39%)
  - Rarely, arise in bone affected by Paget disease

Staging, Grading, & Classification

- 3 similar systems: Enneking, Campanacci, and Bertoni

- Stage 1: Indolent radiographic and histologic appearance (10-15% of GCTs)
- Stage 2: More aggressive radiographic appearance (expanded but intact periosteum) and benign histologic pattern (70-80% of GCTs)
- Stage 3: Aggressive growth with soft tissue mass but histologically benign; distant metastases may occur (benign metastasizing GCT) (10-15% of GCTs)
- MR likely more reliable for predicting clinical behavior

Microscopic Features

- Round to elongated mononuclear cells (neoplastic component) mixed with osteoclast-like giant cells
  - Giant cells may have 50-100 nuclei
  - Mononuclear cells express RANKL → stimulation of formation and maturation of osteoclasts
- Small foci of bone may be found
- Soft tissue or lung metastases have same tissue, often surrounded by thin shell of reactive bone
- Intravascular plugs of tumor are frequent

CLINICAL ISSUES

Presentation

- Most common signs/symptoms
  - Pain, swelling
  - Limited range of motion of adjacent joint
  - Pathologic fracture (5-10%)

Demographics

- Age
  - Peak incidence: 20-50 (80%)
  - Rarely seen in skeletally immature patients
    - Distribution and behavior same as in adults
  - Malignant GCT patients average 10 years older
- Gender
  - Slight female predominance (1.1-1.5:1)
  - Malignant GCT shows male predominance (3:1)
- Ethnicity
  - High prevalence in parts of Asia
- Epidemiology
  - 4-5% of all primary bone tumors
  - 20% of all benign primary bone tumors
  - Malignant transformation of GCT (5% of all GCT)
    - Majority: GCT previously treated with radiation
    - Some are in recurrence of resected GCT
    - Very few GCT are primarily malignant

Natural History & Prognosis

- High recurrence rate with marginal resection (curettage): 25%
  - Recurrent GCT has ↑ likelihood of pulmonary metastases (10%) despite benign local lesion
- Unusual lesional behavior
  - Locally aggressive behavior may occur without lesion being malignant
  - Metastases may occur with primary tumor remaining benign (benign metastasizing GCT) (1.8-5% of GCT)
    - 48% occur following recurrence
    - Pulmonary metastases generally seen within 3 years following diagnosis
      - Some grow very slowly and may even regress spontaneously; some progress more rapidly
- Prognosis in secondary malignant GCT similar to that of other high-grade spindle cell tumors (average 5-year survival: 35-50%)
- Prognosis in primary malignant GCT may be better than secondary; very few patients reported

Treatment

- Wide resection is preferred in order to limit recurrence
  - Often not practicable due to location of lesion
    - Wide resection of subchondral lesion often requires joint arthroplasty or osteochondral graft
      - Neither of these procedures is optimal in young patient being treated for benign lesion
- Because of considerations of functionality, marginal resection is often offered initially
  - Curettage, supplemented by ablative therapy (thermal, phenol, hydrogen peroxide, methylmethacrylate, burring)
    - Adjuvants to curettage appear to decrease recurrence rate significantly
  - Curetted lesion filled with bone graft
    - If greater support is needed, either structural bone graft or methylmethacrylate cement is placed
  - Intravenous bisphosphonates reduced recurrence in 1 trial (4.2% compared to 30% control)
- If in unresectable location, denosumab (antibody to RANKL) shown to be efficacious
  - Healing lesions (and resolving metastases) show distinctive peripheral calcification, followed by progressive central mineralization
  - Slows proliferation and destroys osteoclasts, but stromal cells remain
    - May only partially address treatment of lesion but make subsequent surgical resection possible

DIAGNOSTIC CHECKLIST

Consider

- Recurrence rate following curettage is high; close surveillance and high index of suspicion needed
  - Likelihood of pulmonary metastases increases with recurrence, despite benign histology

Image Interpretation Pearls

- Pattern of low signal intensity on fluid-sensitive sequences suggests diagnosis, even when lesion is in unusual location

SELECTED REFERENCES

1. Hakozaki M et al: Radiological and pathological characteristics of giant cell tumor of bone treated with denosumab. Diagn Pathol. 9:111, 2014
2. Mak IW et al: A translational study of the neoplastic cells of giant cell tumor of bone following neoadjuvant denosumab. J Bone Joint Surg Am. 96(15):e127, 2014
3. Chakarun CJ et al: Giant cell tumor of bone: review, mimics, and new developments in treatment. Radiographics. 33(1):197-211, 2013
4. Raskin KA et al: Giant cell tumor of bone. J Am Acad Orthop Surg. 21(2):118-26, 2013
5. Murphey MD et al: From the archives of AFIP. Imaging of giant cell tumor and giant cell reparative granuloma of bone: radiologic-pathologic correlation. Radiographics. 21(5):1283-309, 2001

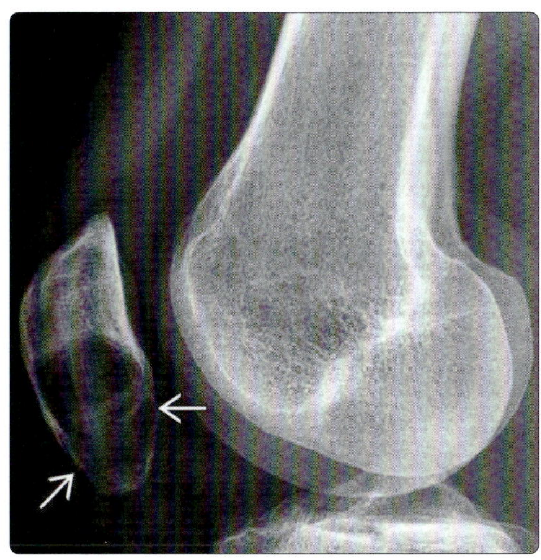

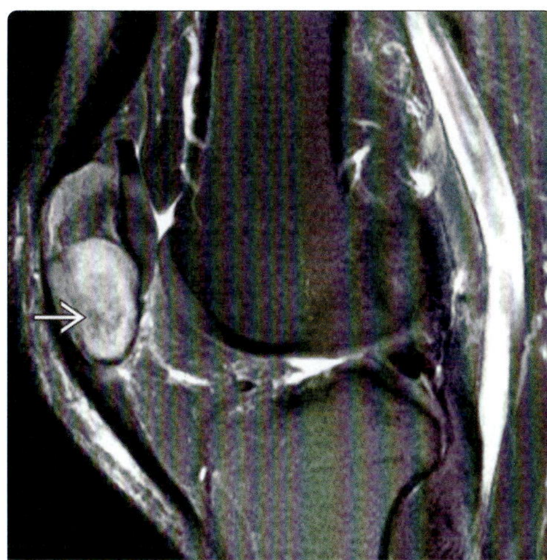

(Left) *Lateral radiograph demonstrates a slightly expanded completely lytic lesion of the patella ➡. The lesion is quite typical in appearance for chondroblastoma; however, the patient is older than most with chondroblastoma. Therefore, giant cell tumor should also be considered.* **(Right)** *Sagittal T2WI FS MR in the same patient shows inhomogeneous low signal ➡ within the surrounding high signal of the lesion. This ↓ SI within the lesion is typical of a giant cell tumor and helps confirm the diagnosis.*

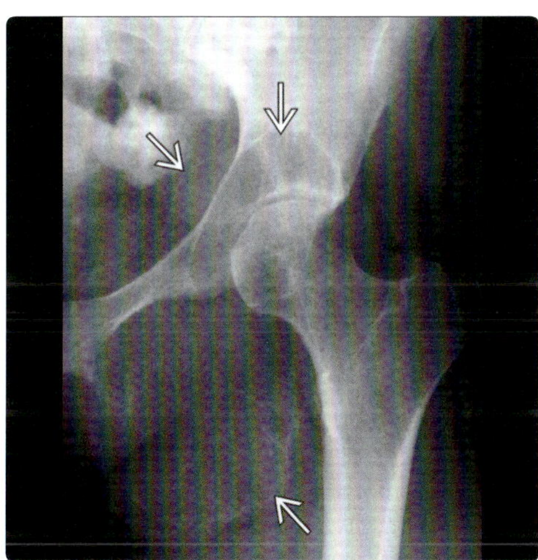

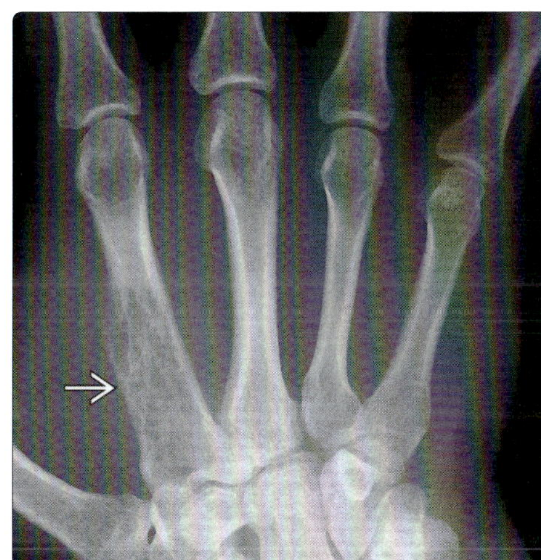

(Left) *AP radiograph demonstrates a lesion involving much of the hemipelvis ➡. It is extremely expansile but has a narrow transition zone and does not appear to have a soft tissue mass. The lesion proved to be a giant cell tumor, which may be significantly expanded and bubbly.* **(Right)** *AP radiograph shows a moderately aggressive lesion that extends from the subarticular surface of the metacarpal distally ➡ and has broken through the cortex and developed periosteal reaction. Consider GCT and enchondroma.*

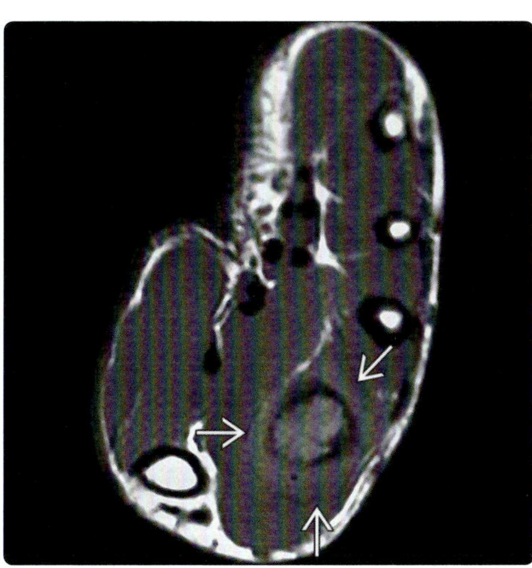

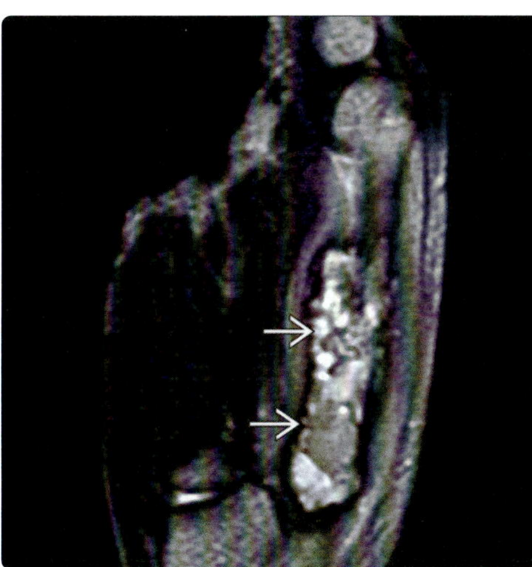

(Left) *Axial T1WI MR in the same patient demonstrates a low signal intensity lesion, which has broken through the cortex; there is a circumferential soft tissue mass ➡.* **(Right)** *Sagittal T2 FS MR of the same lesion shows the moderately aggressive lesion to have mixed high and low signal intensity ➡. This inhomogeneous signal, with prominent low signal regions, is typical of GCT, which was proven at biopsy. Enchondroma would have shown high signal lobulation typical of cartilage.*

(Left) *Sagittal T1WI MR shows complete collapse of the L3 vertebral body with preservation of intervertebral disc space. The lesion is slightly hyperintense to skeletal muscle and shows epidural extension* ➡ *and a large anterior paraspinal soft tissue mass* ➦. **(Right)** *Sagittal T2WI MR in the same patient shows the epidural mass* ➡ *and paraspinous mass* ➦ *to be predominantly low signal intensity. A GCT arises preferentially in the vertebral body rather than posterior elements and has these signal characteristics.*

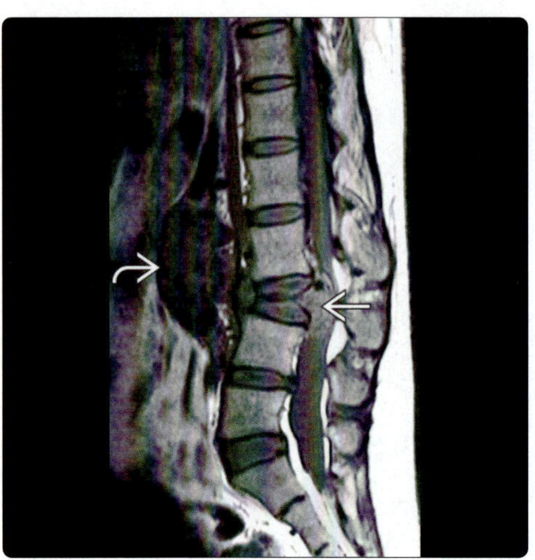

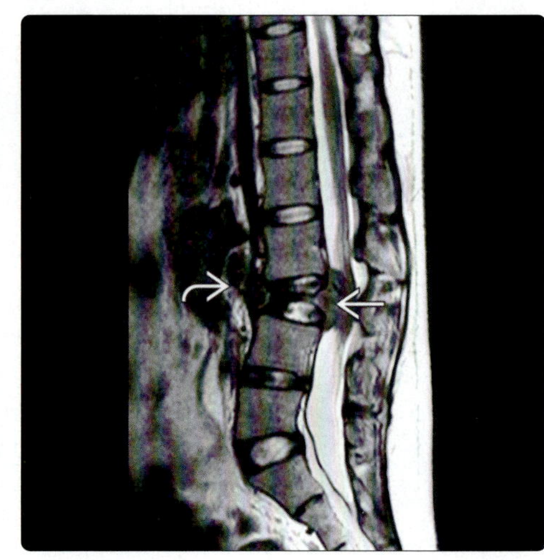

(Left) *Axial T1WI C+ FS MR in the same patient shows diffuse enhancement of the paraspinal mass* ➡. *Note also the invasion of the vena cava by a large intracaval mass displaying the same signal characteristics* ➦. *This proved to be a highly aggressive but benign GCT.* **(Right)** *AP radiograph shows a moderately aggressive tumor, entirely lytic, which is largely geographic* ⇨ *but appears more permeative distally* ➡ *with a wider zone of transition. The location and appearance is typical of an aggressive GCT.*

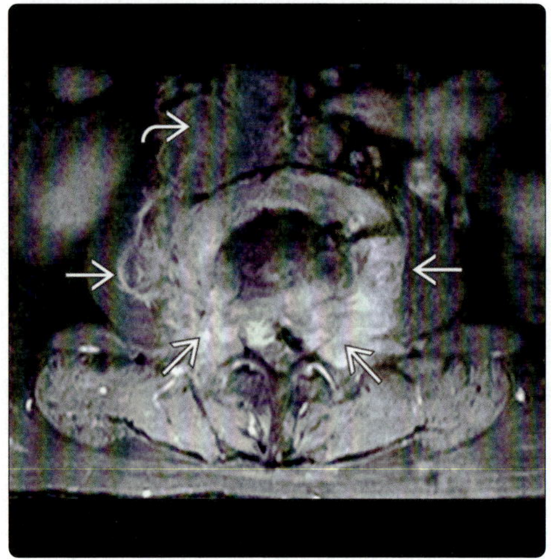

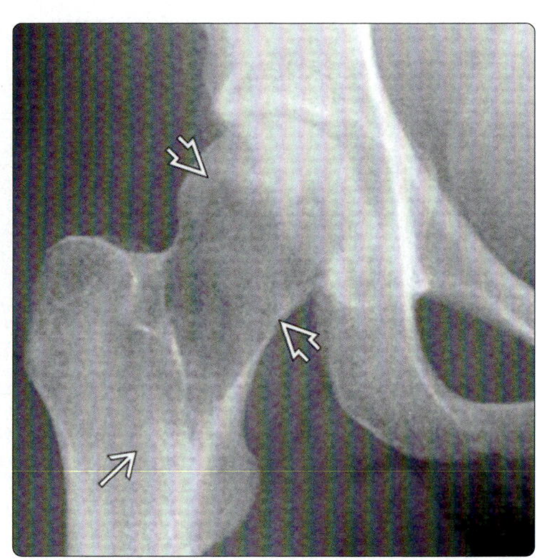

(Left) *Axial NECT in the same patient confirms aggressive features. There is cortical breakthrough anteriorly, with a small soft tissue mass* ➡. *This may still represent a GCT, but more aggressive lesions must be considered.* **(Right)** *Axial T2WI MR in the same patient shows mostly septated-appearing areas of high signal intensity. Note the fluid levels* ➡. *Findings are not typical of a GCT, so telangiectatic osteosarcoma must be considered. At surgery, this proved to be a cystic GCT with regions of aneurysmal bone cyst.*

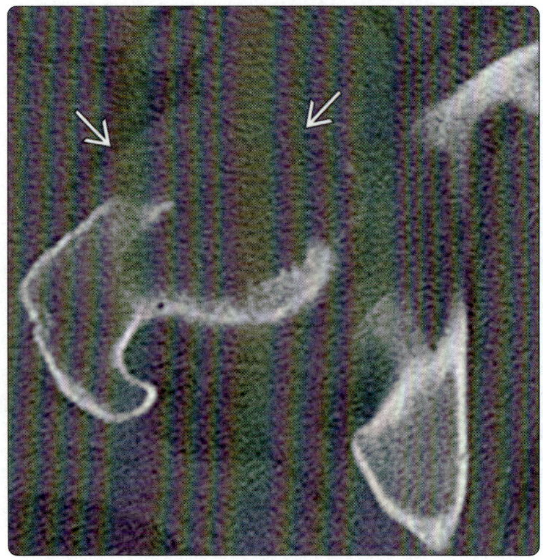

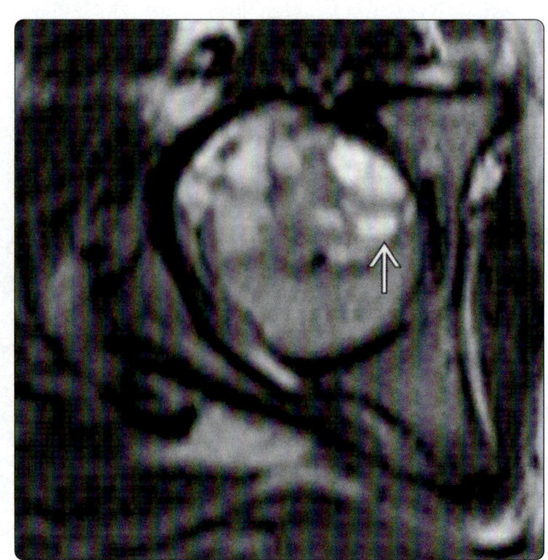

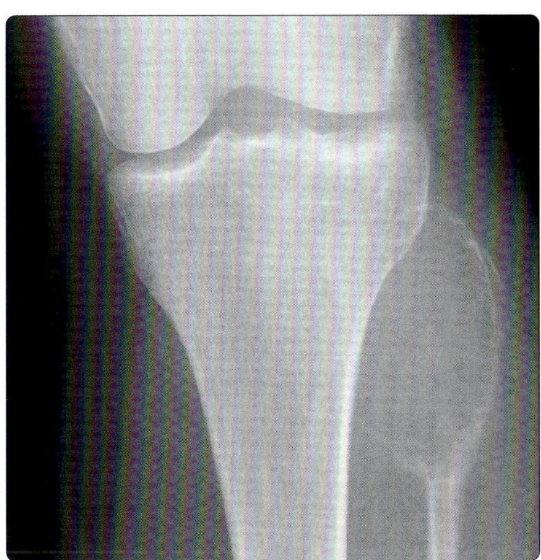

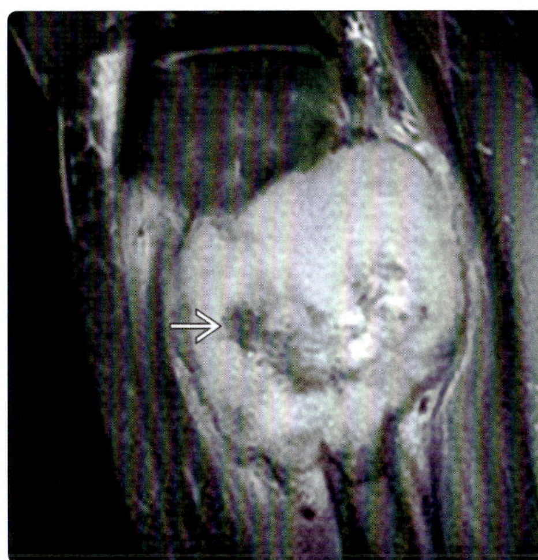

(Left) *AP radiograph shows a large lytic expanded lesion of the fibular metaphysis that extends to the subchondral bone. In a young adult, this appearance is typical of a GCT.* **(Right)** *Sagittal T2FS MR of the fibular lesion shows it to have small regions of cortical breakthrough. The lesion is inhomogeneously hyperintense. There is a central region of hypointensity ➡ that is typically seen on T2 imaging in a GCT.*

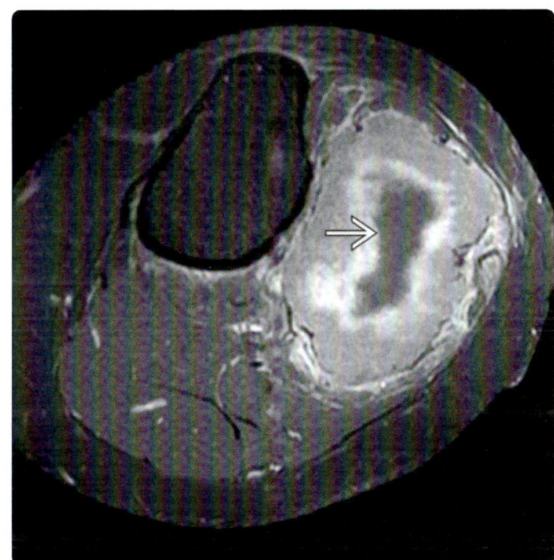

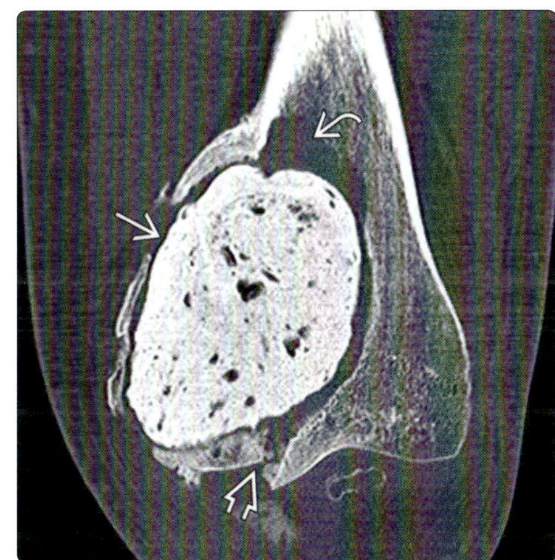

(Left) *Axial postcontrast T1 C+ FS MR of the same fibular lesion shows enhancement as well as a large area of central necrosis ➡, as is often seen in an aggressive GCT.* **(Right)** *Coronal CT in a 25-year-old man who was treated for a GCT 3 months earlier is shown. Treatment consisted of curettage with placement of methylmethacrylate ➡. There is a pathologic fracture ➡ at the subchondral bone, which is the reason for the patient's acute onset of pain. However, there is also a region of osseous destruction ➡, highly suspicious for GCT recurrence.*

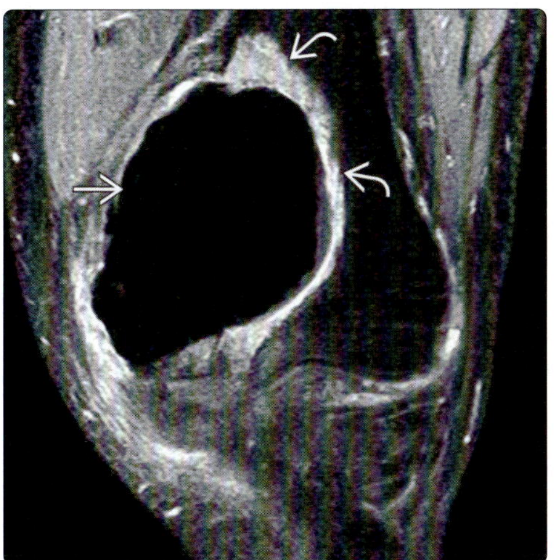

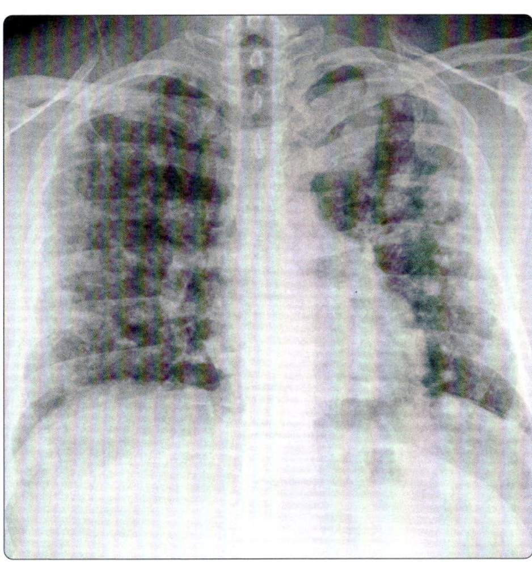

(Left) *Coronal T2 FS MR obtained in the same patient shows the low signal of the cement ➡, with surrounding hyperintense tissue that proved to be recurrent tumor ➡.* **(Right)** *PA chest radiograph of the same patient shows lung metastases, too numerous to count, proven to be a GCT. Although metastatic disease in a GCT is relatively rare, it is more common in patients with recurrence of the initial tumor, as in this case.*

Adamantinoma

KEY FACTS

TERMINOLOGY

- Low-grade malignant lesion most frequently arising in tibial cortex

IMAGING

- Multifocal within same bone (27%)
- Ipsilateral fibula may be involved as well (10%)
- Lytic lesion, often multilobulated and expansile
- Geographic, with sclerotic margin in at least a portion; much or all of lesion appears nonaggressive
- 15% cortical breakthrough seen by radiograph, though breakthrough actually occurs ~ 50%
- MR or CT: Origin of lesion seen in cortex; may extend circumferentially around cortex
- MR: Marrow involvement, as extension of cortical lesion (60%)
  - Fluid-sensitive sequences: Hyperintense, generally homogeneous; inhomogeneous in 40%
- Tissue sampling error may result in incorrect diagnosis of osteofibrous dysplasia (OFD)
  - Should obtain sample from lytic center of lesion

CLINICAL ISSUES

- Median age: 25-35 (range: 3-86 years)
  - Only 3% < 10 years of age; overlap but generally significant difference in age group from OFD
- Treatment: Wide resection
  - Marginal excision often results in recurrence (90%) &/or metastases (12-29%)
  - Recurrence associated with ↑ in epithelium to stroma ratio and more aggressive behavior
- Long-term follow-up to screen for late metastases
- Adamantinoma, OFD-like adamantinoma, and OFD thought by some to represent spectrum of similar disease

(Left) *Lateral radiograph of early adamantinoma shows a thickened cortex with a small, lytic, cortically based lesion ➡, otherwise nonspecific.* **(Right)** *Axial CECT in the same patient confirms that the lesion is cortically based; it has elicited prominent reactive change ➡. The differential diagnosis is in the spectrum of osteofibrous dysplasia, cortically based fibrous dysplasia, and adamantinoma. The imaging findings are not sufficient to differentiate among these. At biopsy, this case proved to be adamantinoma.*

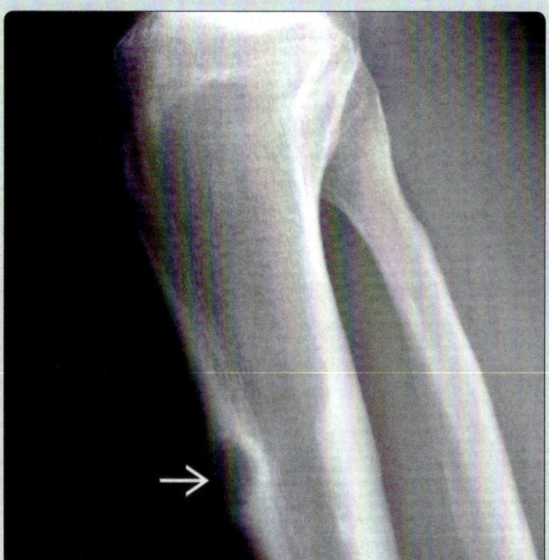

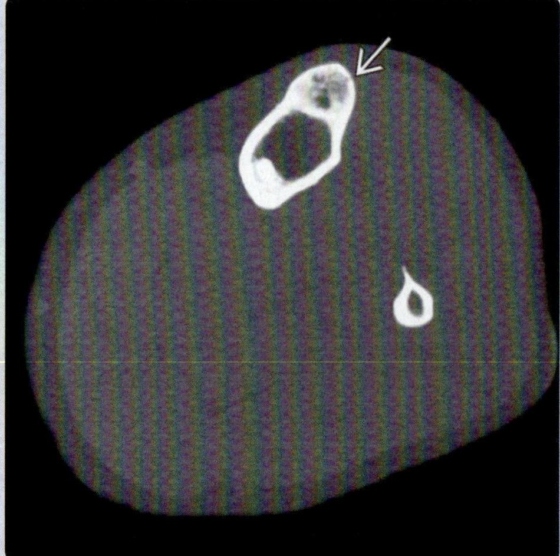

(Left) *AP radiograph shows a corticaly based lytic lesion with expansion but sclerotic margins ➡. There is a suggestion of cortical breakthrough; this lesion had enlarged over a 2-year period.* **(Right)** *Axial CECT in the same patient demonstrates the true behavior of the lesion. It has destroyed the anterior tibial cortex and has developed a soft tissue mass ➡. The location, appearance, and slow growth is typical of adamantinoma. With progressive enlargement, behavior may become aggressive.*

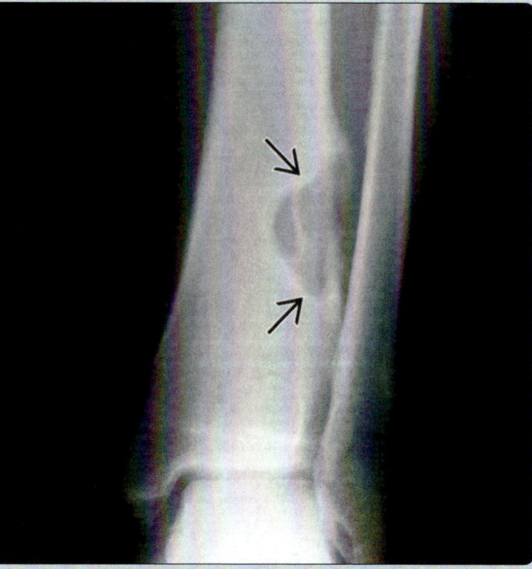

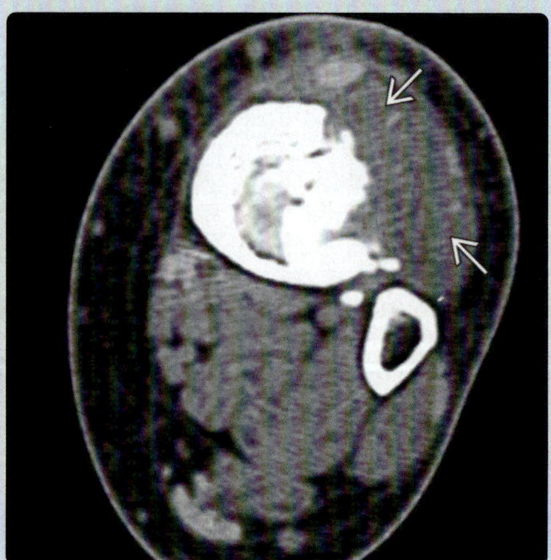

TERMINOLOGY

Synonyms

- Extragnathic adamantinoma, differentiated adamantinoma, juvenile intracortical adamantinoma

Definitions

- Low-grade malignant lesion usually arising in tibial cortex

IMAGING

General Features

- Best diagnostic clue
  - Cortically based lesion in anterior tibia
- Location
  - Tibia (85-90%)
    - Particularly anterior cortex of metadiaphysis (distal more frequent than proximal)
    - Intracortical origin
    - Multifocal within same bone (27%)
    - Ipsilateral fibula may be involved as well (10%)
  - Other bones rarely involved
- Size
  - Large by time of diagnosis (average: 10 cm)

Radiographic Findings

- Cortically based (usually anterior tibia)
  - Expands to involve medullary canal
  - Extends along length of bone; may be large by time of diagnosis
- Lytic lesion, often multilobulated and expansile
  - Cortical thinning; expansion generally not excessive
- Geographic, with sclerotic margin in at least a portion; much or all of lesion appears nonaggressive
- May develop more aggressive appearance with less distinct border, cortical breakthrough, and soft tissue mass
  - 15% cortical breakthrough seen by radiograph, though breakthrough actually occurs ~ 50%
  - Solid periosteal reaction associated with cortical break
- Tibial lesion may be multifocal within same bone or involve ipsilateral fibula

CT Findings

- Mimic of radiographic findings
  - Shows cortical breakthrough & soft tissue mass clearly
  - May show circumferential cortical involvement

MR Findings

- Multiloculated, often with daughter lesions in same bone or ipsilateral fibula
- Origin of lesion seen in cortex; may extend circumferentially around cortex
- Marrow involvement, extension of cortical lesion (60%)
  - Ranges from mild to complete; more complete involvement may help distinguish lesion from osteofibrous dysplasia (OFD)
- MR demonstrates cortical breakthrough (32-50%)
  - Soft tissue mass beyond cortical breakthrough (9%)
- T1: Iso- or slightly hyperintense to skeletal muscle
- Fluid-sensitive images: Hyperintense, different patterns
  - Generally homogeneous ↑ SI; inhomogeneous in 40%
  - Pattern of multiple nodules within lesion (45%)
  - Lobulated pattern in solitary focus (41%)
- Diffuse homogeneous intense contrast enhancement
- MR does not differentiate adamantinoma from OFD-like adamantinoma

Imaging Recommendations

- Best imaging tool
  - Diagnosis by radiograph; MR required for full evaluation

Image-Guided Biopsy

- Tissue sampling error may result in incorrect diagnosis of OFD
  - Epithelial cells tend to be located centrally in adamantinoma and may be missed by fine-needle aspiration
  - Peripheral biopsy may show only findings of OFD or OFD-like adamantinoma
  - Should obtain sample from lytic center of lesion
- Study reports upgrading of needle biopsy diagnosis from OFD or OFD-like adamantinoma to adamantinoma in 21% of 24 cases once surgical tissue available
  - Highlights need for adequate tissue sampling

DIFFERENTIAL DIAGNOSIS

Intracortical Fibrous Dysplasia

- Fibrous dysplasia usually central lesion; may be cortically based in tibia
  - Density ranges from lytic to ground-glass
  - May have cortical breakthrough and soft tissue mass
    - Differentiation from adamantinoma not always possible by means of imaging
  - May have other lesions in same bone; does not serve to differentiate from adamantinoma
    - Lesions in multiple other bones makes diagnosis

Osteofibrous Dysplasia

- Generally younger age group (virtually never seen in adults)
- Similar appearance: Lytic, geographic, cortically based
- Tibia most commonly involved bone
- Lesion tends to have less circumferential involvement of cortex than adamantinoma

Osteofibrous Dysplasia-Like Adamantinoma

- Also termed differentiated adamantinoma or juvenile adamantinoma
- Same appearance on imaging
- Occur in skeletally immature patients
- Osteofibrous dysplasia-like tissue but with small nests of epithelial cells compared with abundant epithelial cells in adamantinoma
- Benign course; in middle of histologic and behavioral spectrum of OFD → adamantinoma

PATHOLOGY

General Features

- Genetics
  - Recurrent numerical chromosomal abnormalities (usually #7, 8, 12, 19)
  - Genetic aberrations restricted to epithelial component

Staging, Grading, & Classification

- AJCC staging, including lesion size, grade, and presence of metastases

Gross Pathologic & Surgical Features

- Yellow-gray firm lobulated tumor
- Peripheral sclerosis
- May be multilobulated, with normal bone between lobules
- Cystic spaces containing blood or straw-colored fluid

Microscopic Features

- Biphasic tumor; variety of patterns in adamantinoma
  - Most commonly epithelial cells surrounded by bland spindle cell osteofibrous component
    - Presence of epithelial cells differentiates adamantinoma from OFD
  - Trabeculae, surrounded by osteoblasts
  - Mitotic activity generally low
- OFD-like adamantinoma
  - Significantly fewer epithelial cells than adamantinoma

CLINICAL ISSUES

Presentation

- Most common signs/symptoms
  - Swelling, mass
  - Often present for multiple years before medical attention sought

Demographics

- Age
  - Median age: 25-35 years (range: 3-86 years; 75% occur in 2nd and 3rd decades)
    - Only 3% < 10 years of age; overlap but generally significant difference in age group from OFD
- Gender
  - Slight male predominance in some series, female in others; not definitive
- Epidemiology
  - 0.4% of all primary bone tumors

Natural History & Prognosis

- Slow, continuous expansion of most lesions
- Extracompartmental growth (soft tissue mass) is poor prognostic factor
- Other poor prognostic factors
  - Male gender
  - Female presenting at young age (< 20 years)
  - Pain at presentation
  - Short duration of symptoms
  - Recurrence
- Marginal excision often results in recurrence (90%) &/or metastases (12-29%)
  - Recurrence associated with ↑ in epithelium to stroma ratio and more aggressive behavior
- With wide resection, cure not always definitive
  - Local recurrence: 19%
  - Mortality: 13%
- Metastases to lungs, regional lymph nodes
  - Less frequently to skeleton, liver, brain

Treatment

- Wide resection
- Radiation and chemotherapy of limited use
- Long-term follow-up required to screen for late metastases
  - Recurrence reported as late as 7 years, metastases 27 years following surgery

DIAGNOSTIC CHECKLIST

Consider

- Adamantinoma, OFD-like adamantinoma, and OFD thought by some to represent spectrum of similar disease
  - Frequent reports of marginal excision of lesions initially reported to be OFD or OFD-like adamantinoma resulting in aggressive recurrence and being reclassified as adamantinoma
  - Histopathology, ultrastructure, and cytopathology suggest they are closely related
    - Progressive complexity of chromosomal aberrations, increasing from OFD to adamantinoma
    - Of these, only adamantinoma develops metastases
    - Suggests multistep neoplastic transformation

Reporting Tips

- Since OFD and adamantinoma cannot reliably be differentiated by imaging, report possibility of both lesions
  - Tissue should be carefully examined to determine where individual case lies along this spectrum

SELECTED REFERENCES

1. Bethapudi S et al: Imaging in osteofibrous dysplasia, osteofibrous dysplasia-like adamantinoma, and classic adamantinoma. Clin Radiol. 69(2):200-8, 2014
2. Giannoulis DK et al: Multiple recurrences and late metastasis of adamantinoma in the tibia: a case report. J Orthop Surg (Hong Kong). 22(3):420-2, 2014
3. Ramanoudjame M et al: Is there a link between osteofibrous dysplasia and adamantinoma? Orthop Traumatol Surg Res. 97(8):877-80, 2011
4. Most MJ et al: Osteofibrous dysplasia and adamantinoma. J Am Acad Orthop Surg. 18(6):358-66, 2010
5. Szendroi M et al: Adamantinoma of long bones: a long-term follow-up study of 11 cases. Pathol Oncol Res. 15(2):209-16, 2009
6. Camp MD et al: Best cases from the AFIP: Adamantinoma of the tibia and fibula with cytogenetic analysis. Radiographics. 28(4):1215-20, 2008
7. Gleason BC et al: Osteofibrous dysplasia and adamantinoma in children and adolescents: a clinicopathologic reappraisal. Am J Surg Pathol. 32(3):363-76, 2008
8. Khanna M et al: Osteofibrous dysplasia, osteofibrous dysplasia-like adamantinoma and adamantinoma: correlation of radiological imaging features with surgical histology and assessment of the use of radiology in contributing to needle biopsy diagnosis. Skeletal Radiol. 37(12):1077-84, 2008
9. Papagelopoulos PJ et al: Clinicopathological features, diagnosis, and treatment of adamantinoma of the long bones. Orthopedics. 30(3):211-5; quiz 216-7, 2007
10. Lee RS et al: Osteofibrous dysplasia of the tibia. Is there a need for a radical surgical approach? J Bone Joint Surg Br. 88(5):658-64, 2006
11. Van Rijn R et al: Adamantinoma in childhood: report of six cases and review of the literature. Pediatr Radiol. 36(10):1068-74, 2006
12. Van der Woude HJ et al: MRI of adamantinoma of long bones in correlation with histopathology. AJR Am J Roentgenol. 183(6):1737-44, 2004
13. Kahn LB: Adamantinoma, osteofibrous dysplasia and differentiated adamantinoma. Skeletal Radiol. 32(5):245-58, 2003
14. Hogendoorn PC et al: Adamantinoma. In Fletcher CDM et al: World Health Organization Classification of Tumours: Tumours of soft tissue and bone. Lyon: IARC Press. 332-4, 2002
15. Springfield DS et al: Relationship between osteofibrous dysplasia and adamantinoma. Clin Orthop Relat Res. (309):234-44, 1994

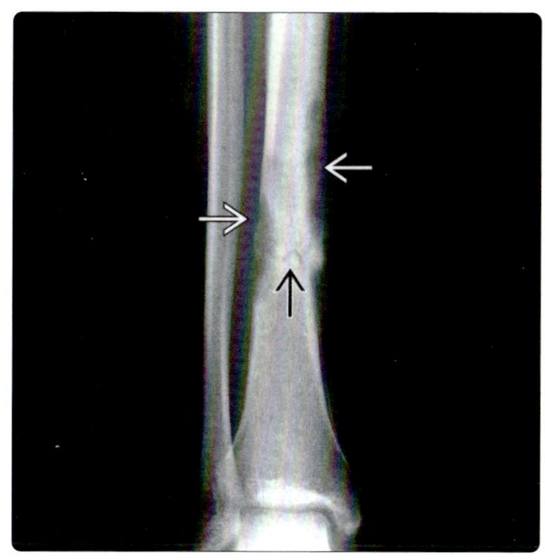

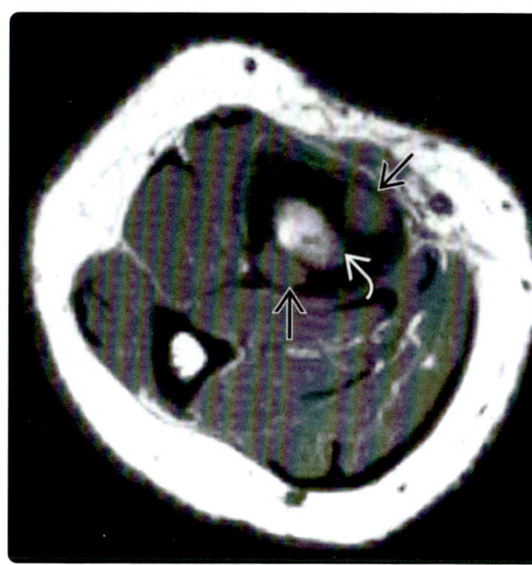

(Left) *AP radiograph shows a cortically based lytic lesion in the distal tibia ➡ with a pathologic fracture extending across its distal aspect ➡. The cortical location in the tibia is typical of adamantinoma.* **(Right)** *Axial T1WI MR in the same patient shows what appears to be 2 lesions, both located within the cortex ➡. More proximal sections showed them to be part of a continuous nearly circumferential cortical lesion. The signal is isointense to skeletal muscle, and there appears to be some marrow involvement ➡.*

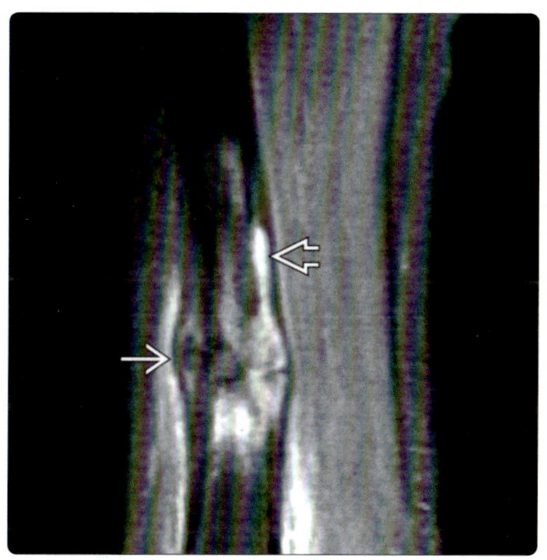

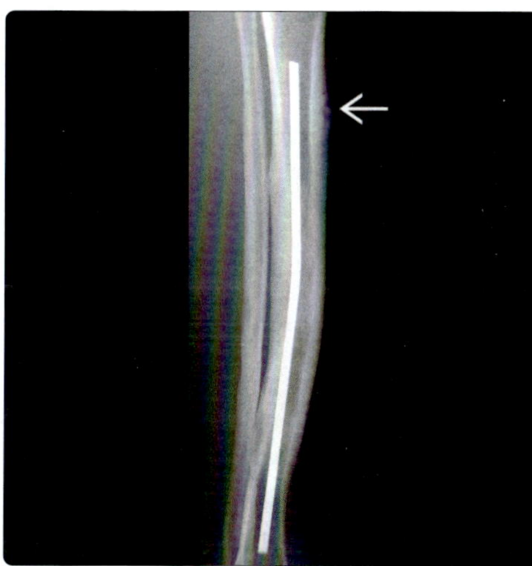

(Left) *Sagittal T2WI MR in the same patient shows the lesion to be high signal ➡ with a healing fracture ➡. Marrow signal may result from tumor involvement or edema. Biopsy proved adamantinoma.* **(Right)** *Lateral radiograph shows recurrent adamantinoma. Previous surgery, with rodding for stabilization, was a marginal resection of adamantinoma. There is now a new cortically based lytic lesion in the proximal anterior tibia ➡. Inadequately treated adamantinoma has a high recurrence rate.*

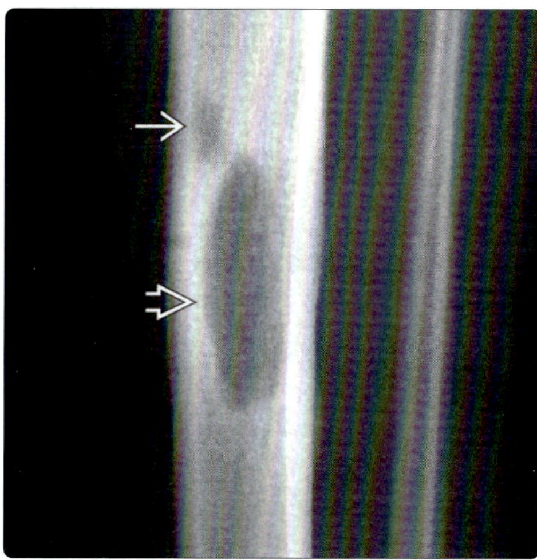

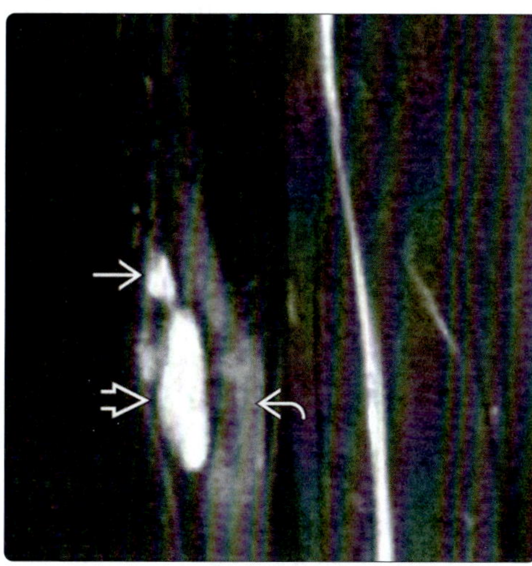

(Left) *AP radiograph shows a moderately aggressive lesion without sclerotic margin ➡. A smaller, similar lesion is seen proximally ➡.* **(Right)** *Sagittal T2WI FS MR in the same patient proves the lesion to be based in the cortex ➡, as is the daughter lesion ➡. There is cortical breakthrough and a soft tissue mass, as well as intramedullary extension ➡. With this degree of aggressiveness, adamantinoma is the favored diagnosis and was proven at biopsy. Treatment is work-up for metastatic disease, then wide resection.*

Hemangioma: Intraosseous

KEY FACTS

TERMINOLOGY

- Hemangioma: Benign lesion composed of blood vessels
- Lymphangioma: Sequestered, noncommunicating lymphoid tissue lined by lymphatic endothelium
- Angiomatosis: Diffuse infiltration of bone or soft tissue by hemangiomas or lymphangiomas
  - Cystic angiomatosis: Extensive involvement of bone by angiomatosis

IMAGING

- Vertebral bodies most common site of hemangioma
  - May extend from body to posterior elements or uncommonly originate in posterior elements
  - 33% of vertebral hemangiomas are multifocal
- Calvaria: Usually frontal and parietal bones
- Long bones: Most frequently in metaphyses of tibia, femur, humerus
- Radiographic findings
  - Vertebral lesions may contain coarse (corduroy) trabeculations, presenting as dense striations
  - Flat bones: Lytic, with sunburst pattern
  - Cranial lesions involve outer table more significantly than inner table
  - Tubular bones: Lytic/may contain trabeculations
- MR: Classic vertebral hemangioma ↑ SI on both T1 and T2, low signal striations on all sequences
  - Not all lesions are classic

CLINICAL ISSUES

- Presentation: Usually incidental finding, particularly in spine
  - Cord compression, pain, neurological symptoms: Uncommon complications of vertebral lesions
  - Angiomatosis: 65% extensive visceral involvement
- Hemangioma: Excellent prognosis
- Cystic angiomatosis: Slow progression

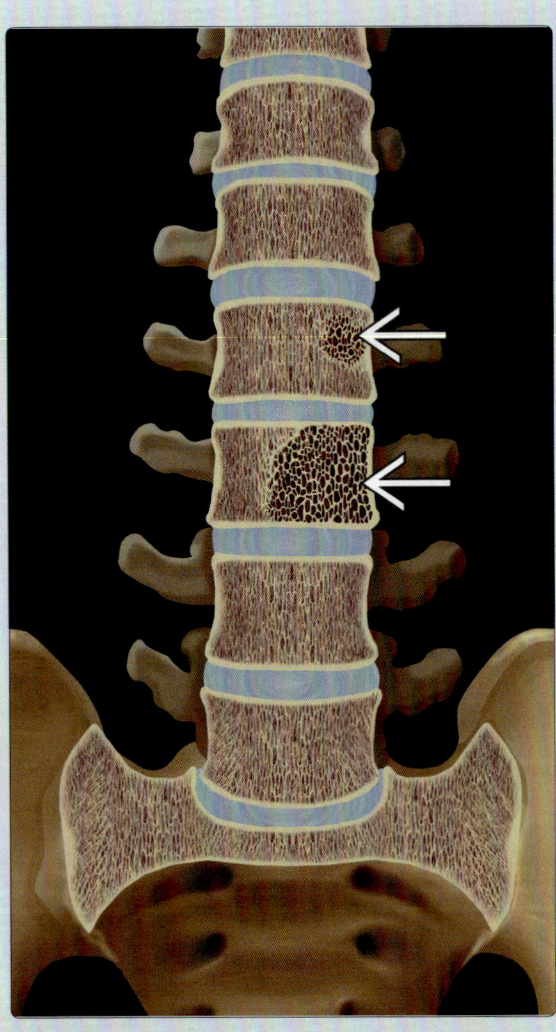

Graphic depicts a transected spine containing intraosseous hemangiomas ➡. These lesions may be large or small; gross appearance is of a well-demarcated, coarsely trabeculated red lesion, clearly distinct from normal cancellous bone.

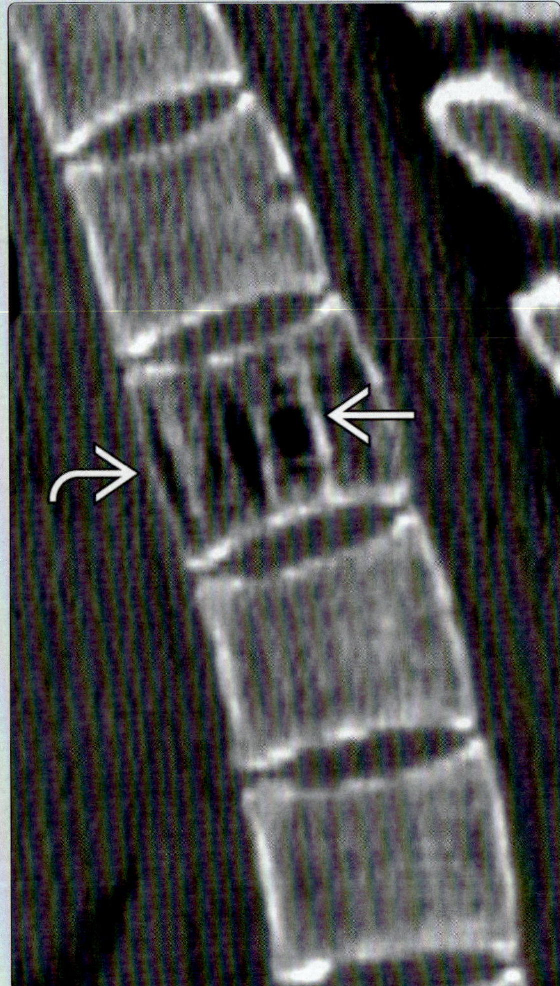

Sagittal reformatted CT shows a typical hemangioma occupying the entire vertebral body. The coarsened vertical trabeculae form a corduroy pattern ➡. Note that the bone is minimally expanded ➡.

TERMINOLOGY

Synonyms

- Capillary hemangioma, cavernous hemangioma, venous hemangioma, angioma, histiocytoid hemangioma, angiomatosis, cystic angiomatosis, skeletal hemangiomatosis, cystic lymphangiectasia, hemolymphangiomatosis
- Gorham disease: Disappearing bone disease, phantom bone disease, massive osteolysis

Definitions

- Hemangioma: Benign lesion composed of blood vessels
  - Capillary hemangioma: Usually in vertebral body
  - Cavernous hemangioma: Usually in flat bone (calvaria, ilium)
  - Venous and arteriovenous hemangiomas involve bone in extremely rare cases; usually soft tissue
- Lymphangioma: Sequestered, noncommunicating lymphoid tissue lined by lymphatic endothelium
- Angiomatosis: Diffuse infiltration of bone or soft tissue by hemangiomatous or lymphangiomatous lesions
  - Cystic angiomatosis: Extensive involvement of bone by angiomatosis
- Massive osteolysis (Gorham or disappearing bone disease) considered to be within spectrum of benign vascular lesions

IMAGING

General Features

- Location
  - Osseous hemangiomas
    - Majority of osseous hemangiomas are central or eccentric
      - Other rare sites of involvement: Intracortical, periosteal, intraarticular
    - Most common site: Vertebral bodies
      - May extend from body to posterior elements or, uncommonly, originate in posterior elements
      - 33% of vertebral hemangiomas are multifocal
    - Craniofacial bones
      - Calvaria, usually frontal or parietal bones
    - Long bones, most frequently in metaphyses of tibia, femur, humerus
      - Rare periosteal or intracortical hemangioma located in anterior tibia
  - Angiomatosis
    - Femur > rib > spine > pelvis > humerus > scapula, and other long bones
  - Gorham disease: Upper arm, shoulder > mandible

Radiographic Findings

- Spine
  - Lytic lesion
  - May contain coarse trabeculations, presenting as dense striations (corduroy pattern)
  - May be multiloculated (honeycomb)
  - May be mildly expanded
  - Pathologic fracture related to hemangioma uncommon
  - Cortical breakthrough and soft tissue mass rare
- Flat bones may have different appearance
  - Significant expansion
  - Lytic, with sunburst pattern of reactive bone
  - Honeycomb pattern: Curvilinear reactive bone
  - Cranial lesions involve outer table more significantly than inner table
- Tubular bones
  - Lytic or may contain coarse striations
    - Occasional honeycomb or lattice-like pattern
  - Mildly expanded
- Angiomatosis: Large localized region or widespread lesions throughout skeleton (cystic angiomatosis)
  - Lytic, expanded, geographic with sclerotic margin
  - Honeycomb or lattice-like appearance, cystic
- Gorham disease
  - Lytic, progressive bone destruction
    - Cortical and cancellous; may result in sharp cut-off or sucked candy appearance
  - With progression, entire bone may disappear
    - May extend across joint

CT Findings

- Spine: Polka dot pattern of coarsened trabeculae
  - Emphasized by low-attenuation fatty stroma
  - CT demonstrates any extension into posterior elements or epidural mass effect
- Calvaria: Shows differential involvement of outer table compared with inner table
  - Widened diploic space
  - Radiating or sunburst pattern of thickened trabeculae (bone adjacent to vascular channels)
- Tubular bones: Linear and circular thickened trabeculae better recognized than on radiograph
  - Periosteal or cortical hemangiomas in anterior tibia identified by serpiginous vascular channels

MR Findings

- Hemangioma
  - Coarsened trabeculae low signal on all sequences
  - T1WI: High signal is classic
    - Variable signal, depending on amount of fat tissue
  - T2WI: High signal, related both to fat tissue and vascular channels
  - STIR: Usually low signal, suppressing fatty stroma
  - Most lesions enhance, though variably
- Angiomatosis
  - Low to intermediate T1 signal
  - Fluid-sensitive sequence: Mixture of low, intermediate, and high signal intensities

Nuclear Medicine Findings

- Bone scan: Ranges from photopenic through normal to moderate increased uptake
  - Requires size > 2 cm to be seen on bone scan

DIFFERENTIAL DIAGNOSIS

Tubular Bone Lesion

- If lesion in small tubular bone lacks trabecular thickening, may mimic aneurysmal bone cyst
- Long tubular bone lesion may mimic fibrous dysplasia with mild expansion and thinning of cortex
- Multifocal lytic lesions mimic other processes
  - Metastases, bone marrow

- Multiple myeloma
- Other multifocal vascular tumors

Vertebral Body Lesion

- Striations, mild expansion may mimic Paget disease
  - Circumferential thickening in Paget may be distinctive
  - Internal coarsened trabeculae in Paget disease is less orderly than in hemangioma
- Lesions with atypical MR signal (low T1, STIR bright) and lacking prominent trabeculae mimic other lesions common to vertebral bodies
  - Metastases, bone marrow
  - Multiple myeloma
  - Langerhans cell histiocytosis, especially if compression fracture in young patient

Cystic Angiomatosis

- Polyostotic fibrous dysplasia (FD)
  - Honeycombing and cystic change less common in FD
- Mastocytosis
  - Generally more evenly sclerotic
- Early purely lytic cystic angiomatosis without thickened trabeculae; may mimic other lytic polyostotic disease
  - Metastases, bone marrow
  - Multiple myeloma
  - Other vascular osseous lesions, including angiosarcoma

PATHOLOGY

General Features

- Associated abnormalities
  - Cystic angiomatosis may have visceral involvement by cavernous hemangiomas (60-70% of cases)
  - Gorham disease: 50% have history of trauma
  - Oncogenic osteomalacia has high association with vascular lesions; most frequently hemangiopericytoma

Gross Pathologic & Surgical Features

- Hemangioma
  - Soft, well-demarcated red mass
  - Honeycomb appearance with sclerotic bone trabeculae, scattered blood-filled cavities
- Cystic angiomatosis
  - Large cavities lined by gray membrane
  - Communicating cysts, separated by thick trabeculae

Microscopic Features

- Capillary and cavernous hemangioma: Thin-walled, blood-filled vessels lined by a single layer of fat
  - Vessels permeate marrow and surround trabeculae
  - Capillary hemangioma: Small vessels consisting of flat endothelium surrounded by basal membrane
  - Cavernous hemangioma: Dilated, blood-filled spaces lined by flat endothelium surrounded by basal membrane
- Epithelioid hemangioma: Large polyhedral neoplastic endothelial cells
  - Vesicular nuclei and abundant eosinophilic cytoplasm
  - Stroma: Loose connective tissue; may contain mixed inflammatory infiltrate
- Angiomatosis
  - Blood or lymphatic vessel origin; occasionally mixture
  - Same histology as capillary hemangioma

CLINICAL ISSUES

Presentation

- Most common signs/symptoms
  - Usually incidental finding, particularly in spine
- Other signs/symptoms
  - Cord compression, pain, neurological symptoms: Uncommon complication
  - Pain from compression fracture and associated hematoma: Uncommon complication
  - Palpable mass lesion, particularly in skull
  - Angiomatosis: 65% extensive visceral involvement
    - May present with pathologic fracture

Demographics

- Age
  - Hemangioma: Peak diagnosis in 5th decade
  - Angiomatosis: First 3 decades
  - Gorham disease: Generally present < 4th decade
- Gender
  - F > M (3:2) in one study; M > F (2:1) in another
- Epidemiology
  - Both osseous and soft tissue hemangiomas common
    - Autopsy series: In vertebrae in 10% of adults
      - Larger numbers seen with MR; one study shows incidence in 27% of individuals
    - Clinically significant lesions are rare
  - Lymphangioma is rare; soft tissue much more common than osseous
  - Angiomatosis: 30-40% of cases are osseous

Natural History & Prognosis

- Hemangioma
  - Excellent prognosis; rarely symptomatic
  - Behavior: Usually as a vascular malformation
  - Progression to angiosarcoma extremely rare
- Cystic angiomatosis: Slow progression and enlargement
- Gorham disease: Rapid dissolution of bone
  - May stabilize, but usually little reparative bone

Treatment

- Asymptomatic lesions not treated
- Symptomatic lesions
  - Embolization and resection
    - Low recurrence rate
  - Vertebroplasty for support
  - ± radiation therapy

SELECTED REFERENCES

1. Rigopoulou A et al: Intraosseous hemangioma of the appendicular skeleton: imaging features of 15 cases, and a review of the literature. Skeletal Radiol. 41(12):1525-36, 2012
2. Murphey MD et al: From the archives of the AFIP. Musculoskeletal angiomatous lesions: radiologic-pathologic correlation. Radiographics. 15(4):893-917, 1995

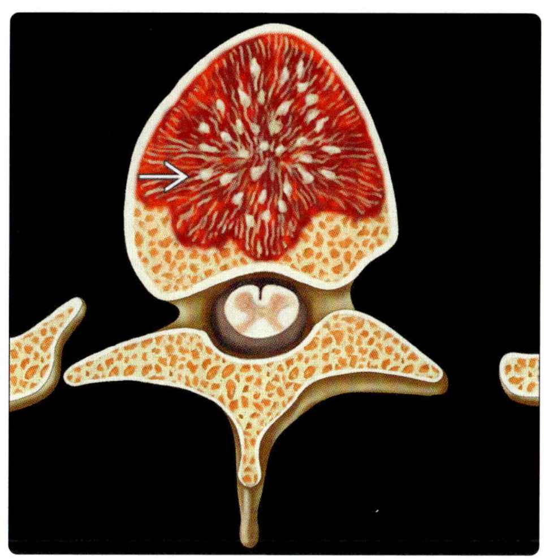

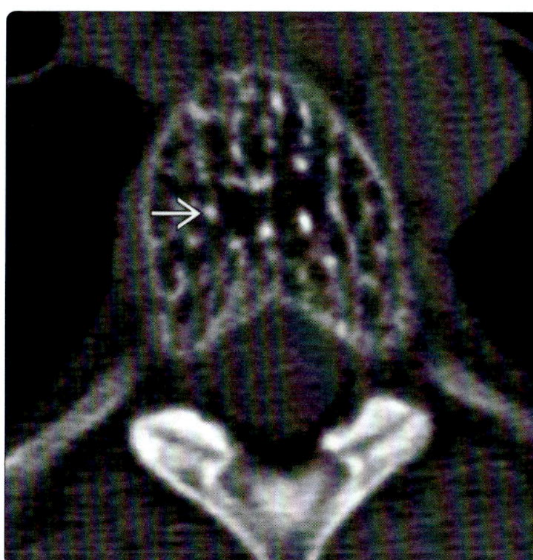

(Left) *Axial graphic shows a vertebral body hemangioma, with central coarsened trabeculae ➡. In the axial plane, these trabeculae form a polka dot pattern, which is quite typical of the lesion. Though this graphic shows the lesion to be completely contained within the body, hemangioma may extend into posterior elements.* **(Right)** *Axial CT through a vertebral hemangioma shows the polka dot pattern of the coarsened trabeculae ➡, typical of the process. This hemangioma occupies the entire body.*

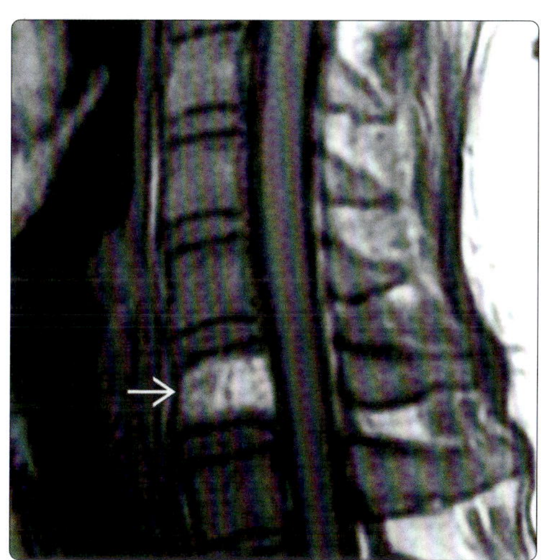

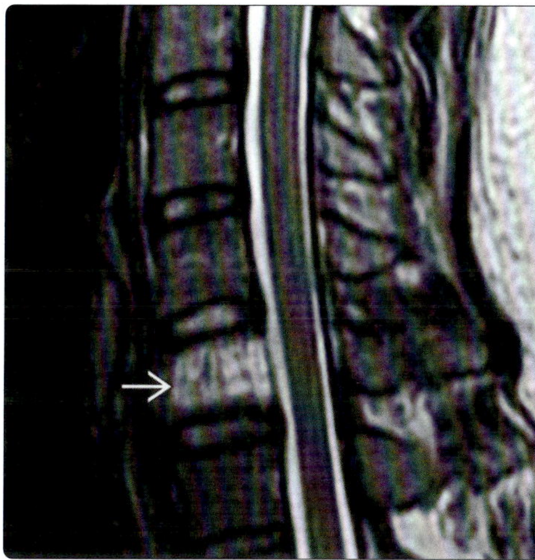

(Left) *Sagittal T1WI MR shows a classical hemangioma of a cervical vertebral body. The body shows some low signal coarse trabeculation within the hyperintense fatty stroma ➡.* **(Right)** *Sagittal T2WI MR in the same patient shows both the corduroy pattern of vertical coarse trabeculation and high signal of the body ➡. The pattern of high T1 and T2 signal is typical of hemangioma. The STIR image is not shown, but it showed signal dropout of fat, leaving this body lower signal than the adjacent vertebrae.*

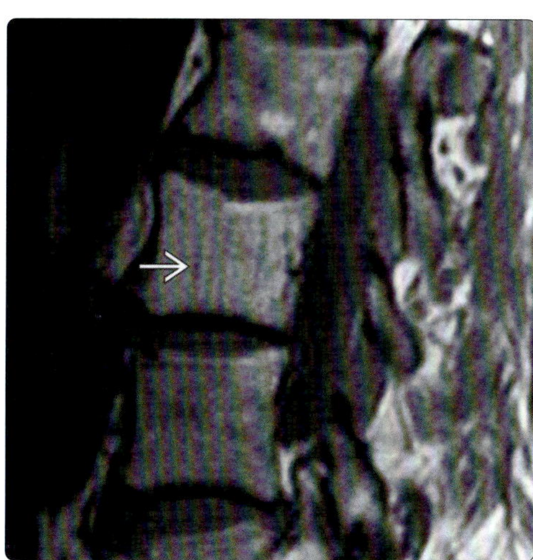

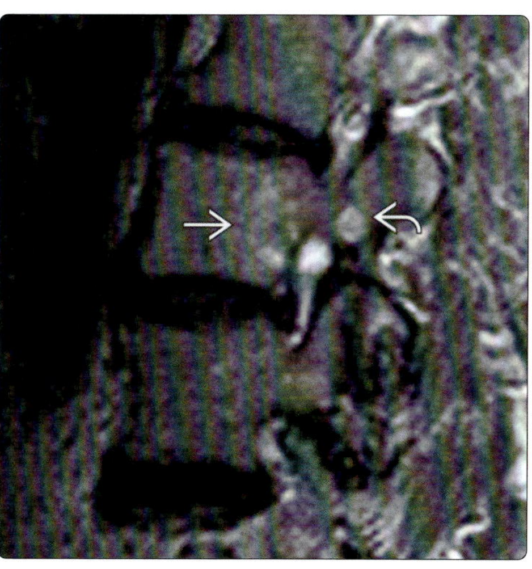

(Left) *Sagittal T1WI MR shows a vertebral hemangioma that occupies the entire body. The low signal coarse trabeculations are evident ➡, but the lesion is not as conspicuous as many hemangiomas because it contains little fat.* **(Right)** *Sagittal T2WI MR in the same patient shows how difficult it can be to see an atypical lesion that contains little fat. The trabecular pattern is faintly seen ➡, with a small amount of nearby fat. A more typical hemangioma is seen in the region of the pars ➡.*

(Left) *Oblique radiograph shows a lesion arising from the iliac wing, which elicits a sunburst pattern of periosteal reaction →. This sunburst pattern of reaction has been described most frequently in hemangiomas of the skull but may be seen elsewhere.* **(Right)** *Axial NECT in the same patient shows the sunburst pattern in the portion of the hemangioma that is expanding on the anterior surface of the iliac wing →. There is a honeycomb pattern in the iliac wing →, the site of origin of the lesion.*

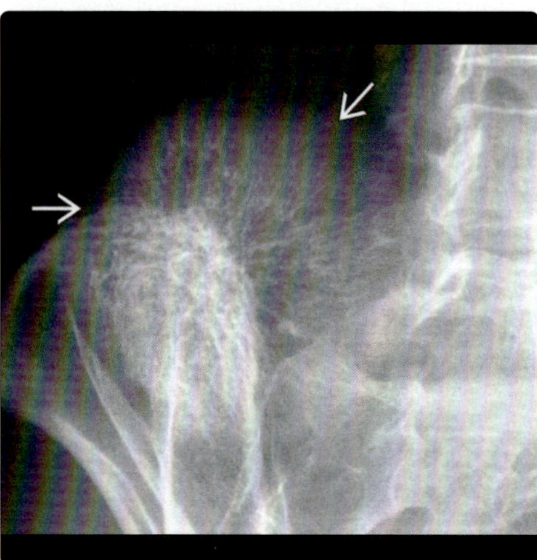

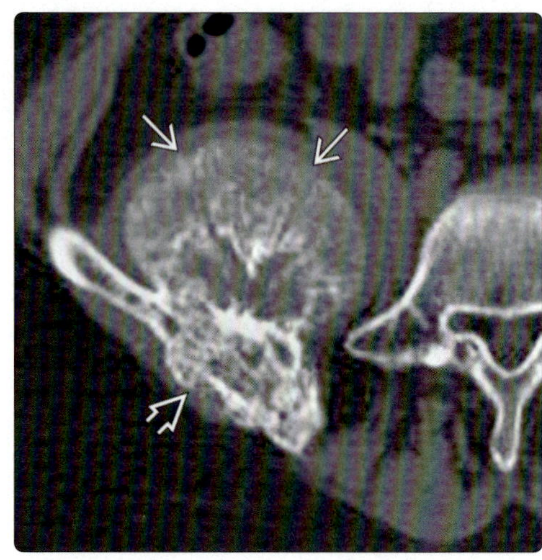

(Left) *Axial T2WI MR in the same patient shows the lesion and its anterior extension to be higher in signal intensity →, but low signal bone reaction is seen within the lesion →.* **(Right)** *Axial T1WI C+ MR shows the lesion to enhance →, with low signal in the honeycomb and sunburst reactive bone →. The expanded lesion is contained within the cortex and there is no soft tissue mass. The iliopsoas is displaced anteromedially and distorted →.*

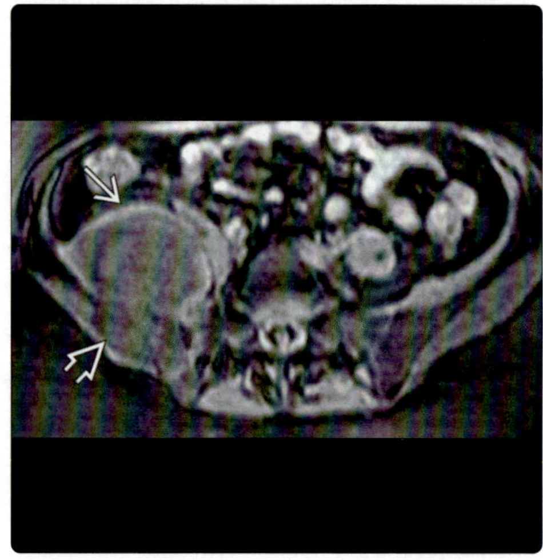

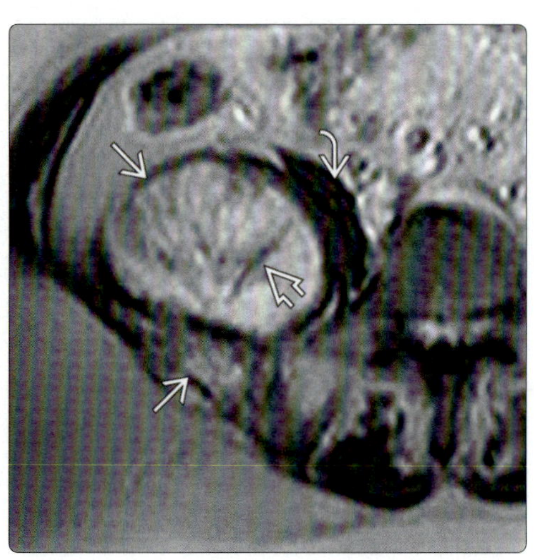

(Left) *Lateral radiograph shows a well-demarcated lesion with a honeycomb appearance →. Note that the outer table is more involved than the inner table. Though the sunburst pattern is described often in the literature, this honeycomb pattern may be more frequently seen.* **(Right)** *Axial T2WI MR reveals a sharply marginated expansile hemangioma with a honeycomb appearance from intradiploic trabecular thickening →; the outer table shows more involvement than the inner table.*

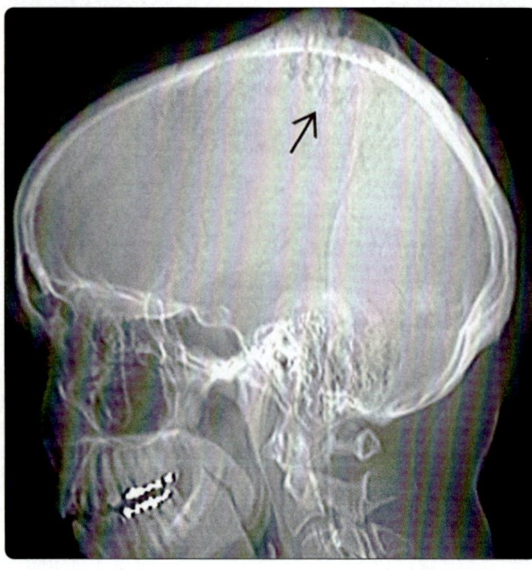

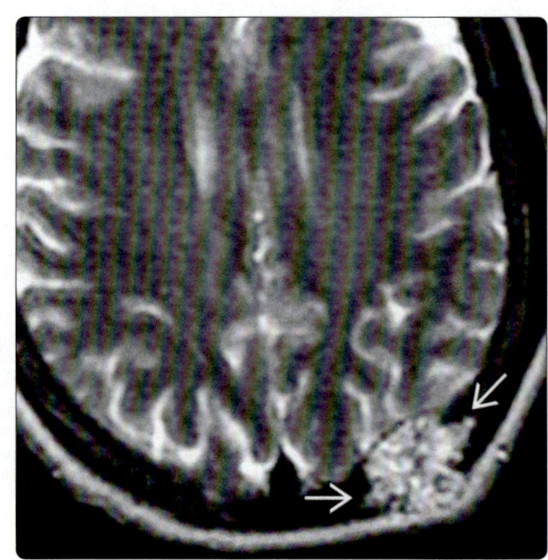

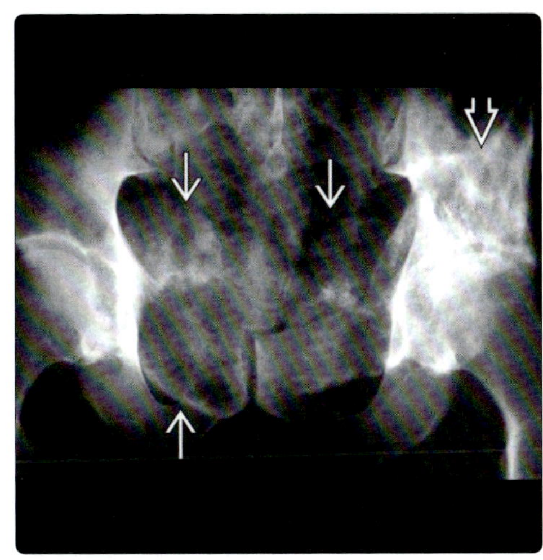

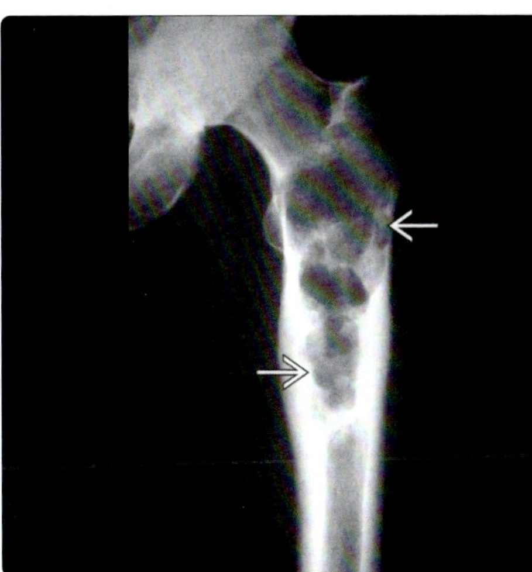

(Left) *AP radiograph shows multiple osseous lesions, which have been present and slowly growing for over 20 years. There is prominent enlargement of the pubic rami* ➡ *and left acetabulum* ➡*. Though large, the lesions do not appear aggressive.* **(Right)** *AP radiograph in the same patient shows an expanded lytic lesion with a honeycomb appearance of reactive bone formation* ➡*. The diagnosis is cystic angiomatosis, a rare benign multicentric manifestation of hemangiomatosis &/or lymphangiomatosis.*

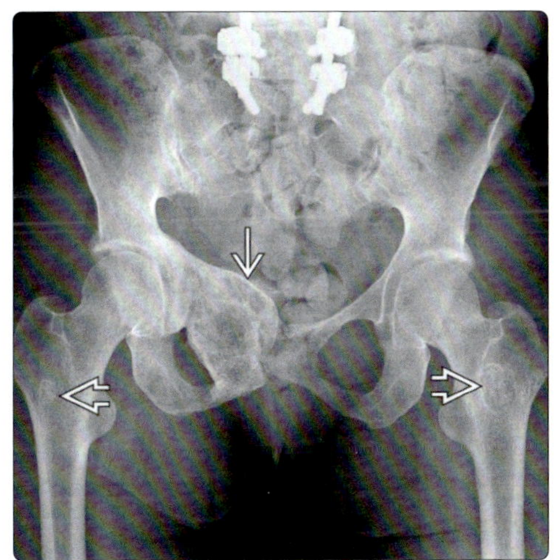

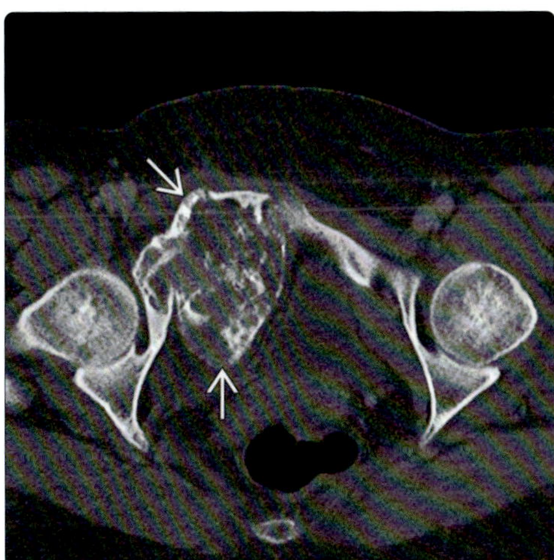

(Left) *AP radiograph shows a longstanding expanded lesion of the pubic ramus* ➡*. Other lesions are noted in the intertrochanteric regions* ➡*, which are variably lytic or sclerotic. The lesions have progressed over a period of several years. This patient has hemangiomatosis involving the bones, skin, and viscera.* **(Right)** *Axial CT in the same patient shows an expanded hemangioma, which displays a honeycomb pattern of reactive bone* ➡*. The lesions of hemangiomatosis display the same findings as those of a solitary lesion.*

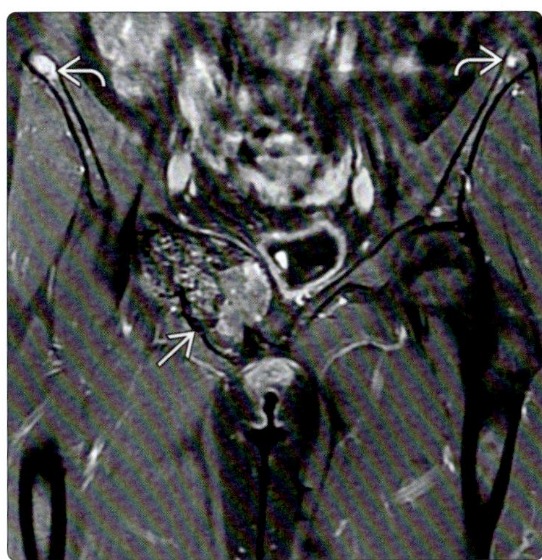

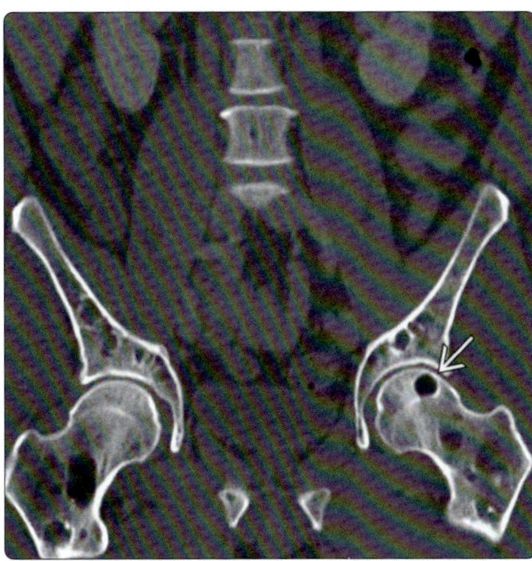

(Left) *T1WI C+ FS MR in the same patient shows enhancement of the large lesion* ➡*, along with low-signal central bone formation. There is enhancement of several other lesions* ➡ *without any other characteristics. None of the lesions appear aggressive in this patient with hemangiomatosis.* **(Right)** *Coronal CT shows multiple lytic lesions that appear nonaggressive* ➡ *in a young man with long-term lymphangiomatosis. The lesions are indistinguishable from multiple hemangiomas.*

Hemangiopericytoma: Osseous

KEY FACTS

TERMINOLOGY

- Intraosseous vascular tumor of pericytic origin, of intermediate or indeterminate malignancy
- Unlike hemangioma, considered true neoplasm

IMAGING

- Location: Osseous hemangiopericytoma much less common than soft tissue lesion
  - 35% of osseous lesions occur in lower extremities
  - Often multicentric; may occur in contiguous anatomic sites, such as bones of ankle/foot
- Radiographic appearance: Lytic in 70%; varying degrees of sclerosis in 30%
  - With sclerosis, may see prominent trabeculae or honeycombing
  - Ranges from non- to moderately aggressive
- MR appearance: Nonspecific
  - Generally ↓ SI on T1, ↑ SI on T2, enhancing
  - May have prominent peripheral vessels

PATHOLOGY

- Arises from cells of Zimmerman located around vessels

CLINICAL ISSUES

- Rare associated hypophosphatemic (oncogenic) osteomalacia
  - Reported more frequently with hemangiopericytoma than other vascular bone lesions
- Age range: 15-48 years
  - If multifocal, average age is 10 years younger
- Rare; < < 1% of primary malignant bone tumors
- Unpredictable behavior
  - Ranges from benign to low-grade malignant

DIAGNOSTIC CHECKLIST

- Pearl: Multiple lesions in contiguous bones (particularly foot/ankle) suggests vascular origin
- Generally cannot differentiate between malignant & benign hemangiopericytoma or among vascular lesions by imaging

(Left) *AP radiograph shows a nonaggressive lytic lesion with a sclerotic rim ➡ in the iliac wing in a 46 year old. The lesion is nonspecific but may suggest plasmacytoma or other lesions in a patient of this age.* **(Right)** *AP radiograph in the same patient shows a more aggressive lesion in the calcar of the contralateral hip. The lesion is lytic and at least part of it has a wide zone of transition ➡. Statistically, the most likely diagnoses are metastases and myeloma, but vascular tumors must also be considered.*

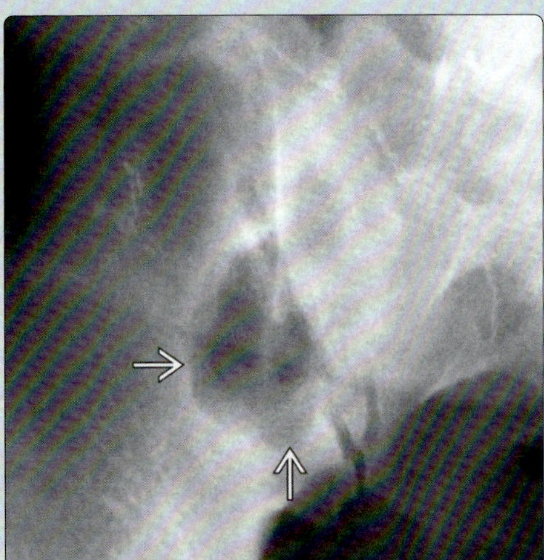

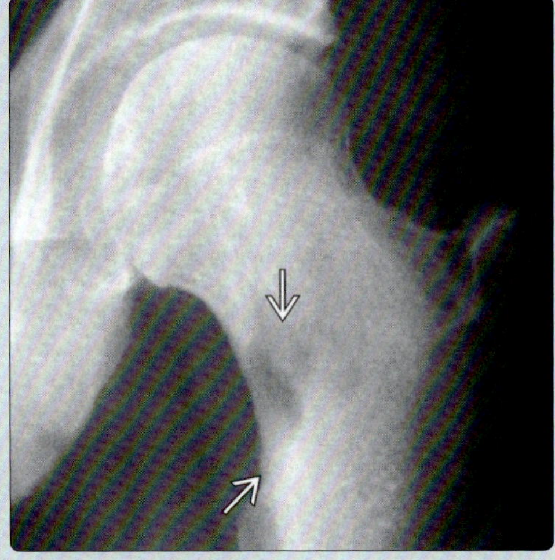

(Left) *Lateral radiograph, same patient, shows a moderately aggressive lesion with a fairly wide transition zone ➡ and significant cortical scalloping ➡. The appearance of holes has been termed honeycomb pattern.* **(Right)** *AP radiograph confirms moderately aggressive features. The constellation of 3 lesions in this case, from nonaggressive to moderately aggressive, is typical of polyostotic vascular tumors, but not specific for any particular one. Malignant hemangiopericytoma was proven at biopsy.*

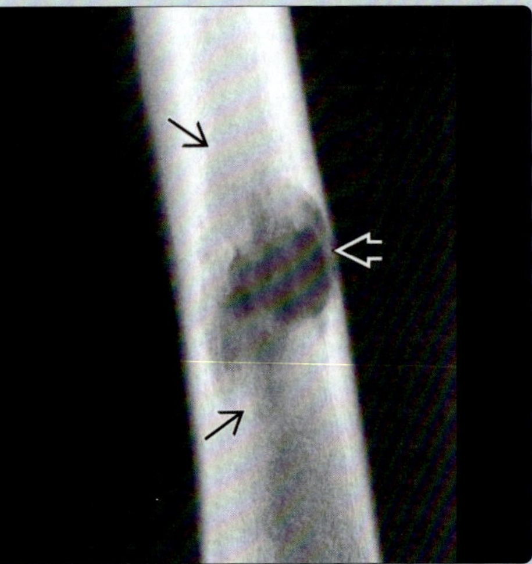

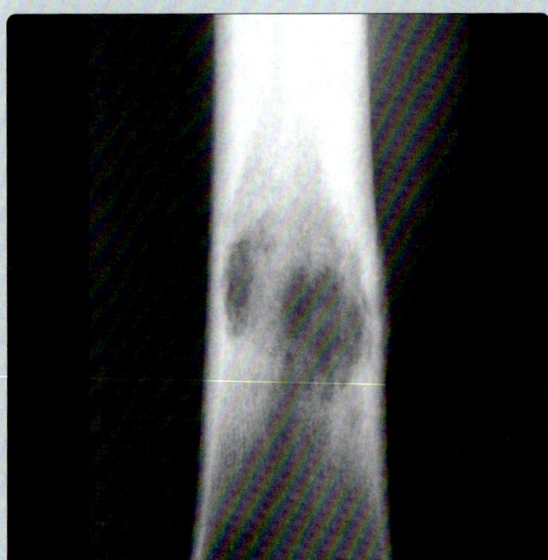

KEY FACTS

TERMINOLOGY

- Intraosseous vascular tumor of endothelial origin, of intermediate or indeterminate malignancy
  - Unlike hemangioma, considered true neoplasm (independent growth potential, nuclear atypia)

IMAGING

- Location: Osseous hemangioendothelioma less common than soft tissue
- Osseous hemangioendothelioma locations
  - Calvaria, spine
  - Tubular bones, usually lower extremities
- May be solitary or multicentric
  - Pearl: Consider diagnosis with multicentric lesions grouped regionally (foot/ankle > wrist/hand)
- MR nonspecific: ↓ SI on T1, ↑ SI on T2, enhancing lesion; variably aggressive appearance
- Radiographic appearance: Lytic lesion, with occasional honeycomb appearance
  - Variable appearance of aggressiveness, from nonaggressive to aggressive with cortical breakthrough and soft tissue mass

PATHOLOGY

- Vascular channels densely arranged, with multiple communications (antler-like pattern)
- Pleomorphic endothelial cells, with hyperchromatic nuclei

CLINICAL ISSUES

- Wide age range: 10-75 years
  - Most commonly presents in 2nd or 3rd decades
  - If multifocal, average age is 10 years younger
- Rare; < < 1% of primary malignant bone tumors
- Unpredictable behavior
  - Ranges from benign to low-grade malignant
- Treatment: Embolization, wide resection
  - ± chemotherapy, radiation, depending on grade
  - Thermal ablation has also been advocated

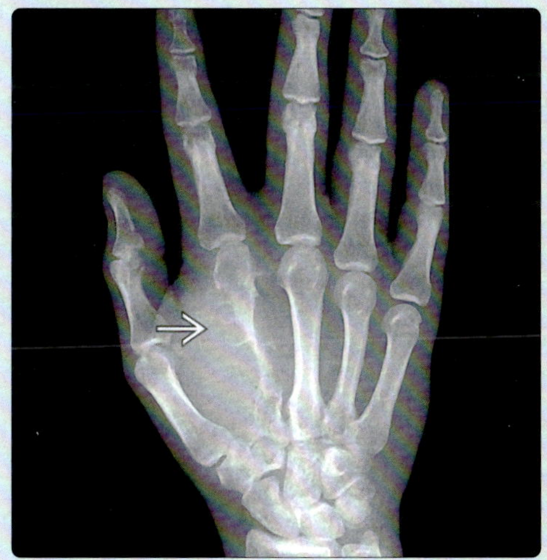
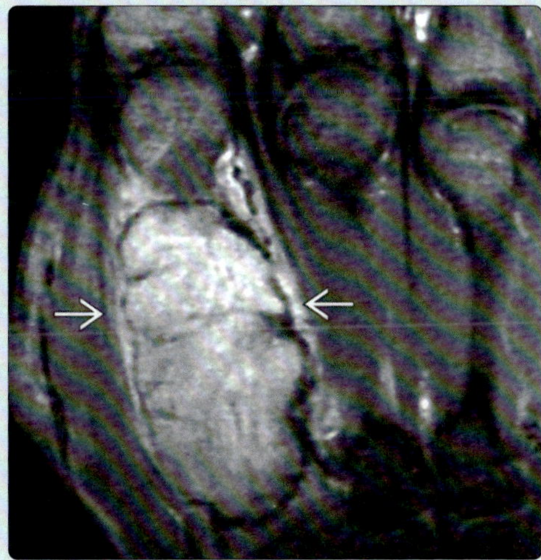

(Left) *AP radiograph shows a highly destructive, nonspecific osseous lesion, proven to be a vascular tumor, arising in the metacarpal and growing rapidly, leaving only wisps of residual bone ➡. No matrix is present.* **(Right)** *Coronal T1WI C+ FS MR, same patient, shows an enhancing soft tissue mass ➡ with a nonspecific pattern, proven to be a hemangioendothelioma at biopsy. This lesion is intermediate within the spectrum of vascular tumors, which ranges from hemangioma to angiosarcoma.*

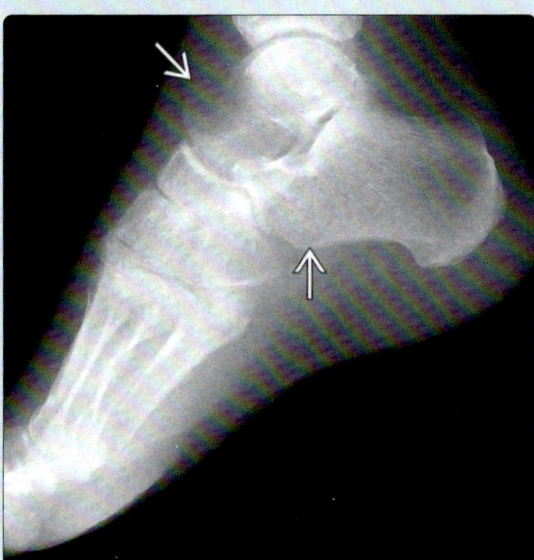
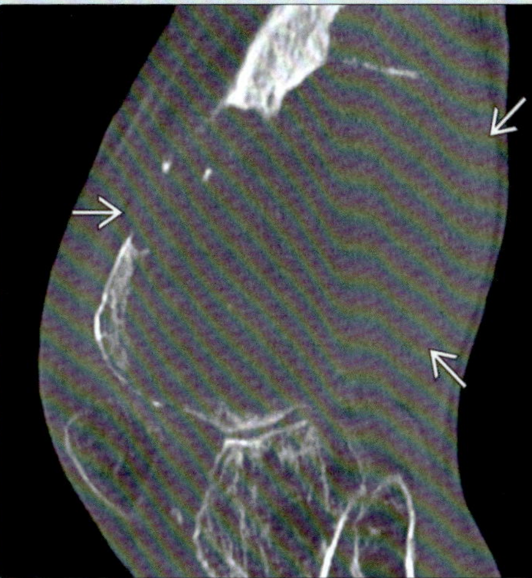

(Left) *Lateral radiograph shows multiple lytic lesions involving the foot ➡, including lesions of the talus, anterior calcaneus, and cuboid. Polyostotic lesions in the lower extremity, particularly when grouped closely in a young adult, should prompt consideration of vascular lesion spectrum. In this case, pathology shows hemangioendothelioma.* **(Right)** *Sagittal bone CT demonstrates a large mass ➡ in a hemophilic pseudotumor, which has degenerated into a malignant epithelioid hemangioendothelioma.*

Angiosarcoma: Osseous

KEY FACTS

TERMINOLOGY

- Aggressive malignant vascular tumor
  - Cells show endothelial differentiation

IMAGING

- Location of osseous angiosarcoma
  - 60% in long bones
  - 7% in pelvis
  - Majority in femur & pelvis in 1 study of 60 patients
- Most are solitary, but may be multifocal (33%)
  - If multifocal, often in lower extremities
  - Multifocal may cluster in adjacent bones
- Imaging appearance
  - Lytic, destructive
  - No (or incomplete) sclerotic margin
  - Bone often expanded if low grade
  - Cortical breakthrough, soft tissue mass if high grade
  - MR is nonspecific

CLINICAL ISSUES

- Peak: 3rd to 5th decades
- M > F = 2:1
- < 1% of malignant bone tumors
- Prognosis poor: 66% of cases developed metastases to lung and other organs in 1 study
- Studies suggest that patients with multifocal lesions may have higher survival rates (not supported in another study)
- < 1% of malignant bone tumors
- Only 6% of angiosarcomas are osseous

DIAGNOSTIC CHECKLIST

- Image interpretation pearl: Clustering of multifocal lesions in single anatomic region
  - Highly suggestive of osseous vascular tumors
  - Usually cannot distinguish between angiosarcoma, hemangioendothelioma, hemangiopericytoma; multifocality may be seen in all 3 lesions
  - Angiosarcoma may be more destructive

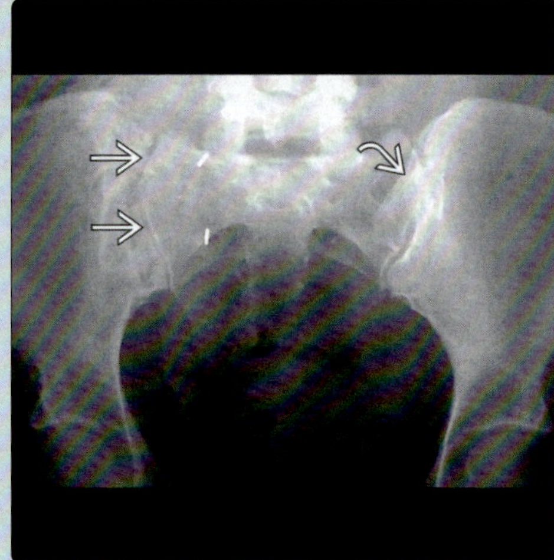

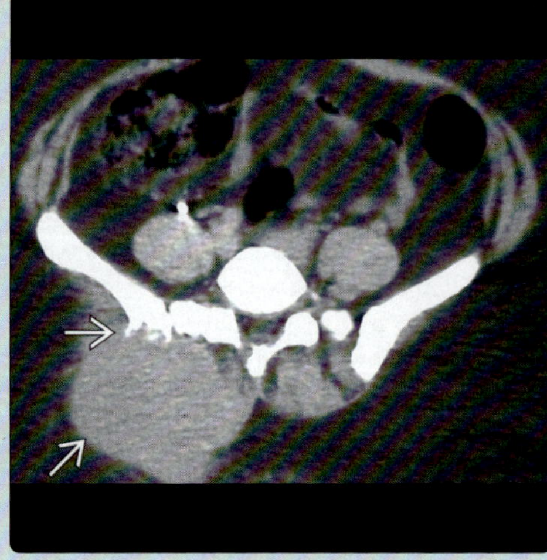

(Left) *AP radiograph shows a "naked" sacroiliac joint. Note the clearly visible right sacroiliac joint ➡. This indicates that the posterior iliac wing is missing. The posterior iliac wing is easily seen superimposed over the SI joint on the normal left side ➡. This naked SI joint is an important diagnostic finding, indicating a large posterior destructive iliac lesion, but can be easily overlooked.* **(Right)** *Axial NECT confirms destruction of the posterior iliac wing ➡ and adjacent sacral ala by proven angiosarcoma.*

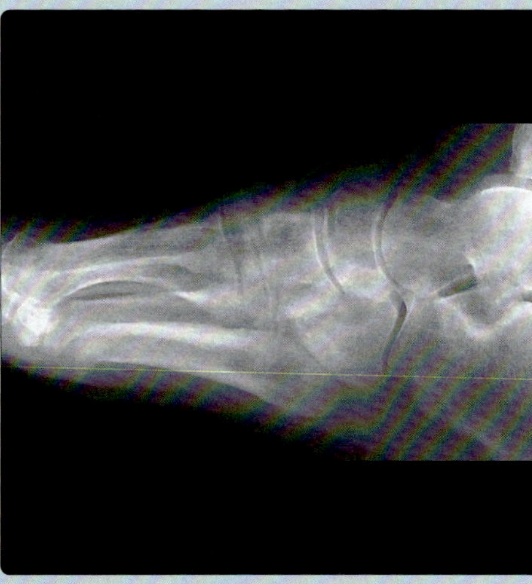

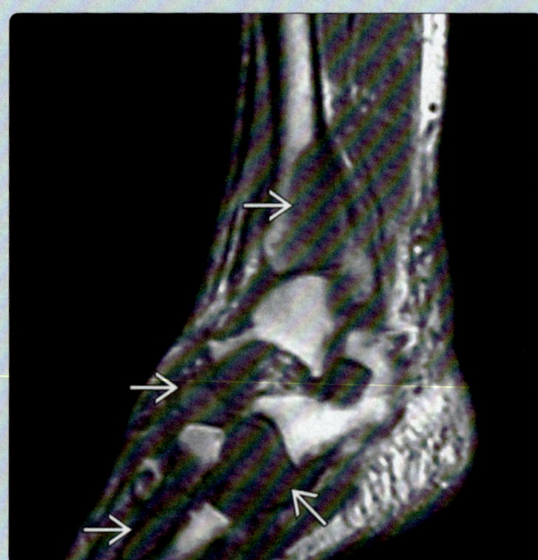

(Left) *Lateral radiograph shows what appears to be diffuse osteopenia, involving multiple bones of the ankle and foot, but no focal lesion.* **(Right)** *Sagittal T1WI MR in the same case shows multiple focal lesions involving, to some extent, nearly every bone of the foot and ankle ➡. The marrow replacement is seen as low signal intensity on T1WI MR. Polyostotic lesions, especially isolated to the lower extremities, should lead to consideration of vascular osseous tumors. In this case, angiosarcoma was proven.*

TERMINOLOGY

Synonyms

- Hemangiosarcoma
- Hemangioendothelial sarcoma
- Epithelioid angiosarcoma

Definitions

- Aggressive malignant vascular tumor
  - Cells show endothelial differentiation

IMAGING

General Features

- Best diagnostic clue
  - When multifocal, 2 findings suggest diagnosis of vascular tumor
    - Lesions predominantly in lower extremity
    - Many lesions clustered in single anatomic region (ankle/foot most common)
    - Not specific for angiosarcoma; also seen in hemangioendothelioma or hemangiopericytoma
- Location
  - Involves skin and soft tissues far more frequently than bone (6%)
  - Location of osseous angiosarcoma
    - Majority in femur & pelvis in 1 study of 60 patients
    - 60% in long bones
      - Tibia > femur > humerus
    - 7% in pelvis
    - Spinal involvement relatively frequent
  - Most solitary, but may be multifocal (33%) primary lesions
    - If multifocal, often in lower extremities
    - Multifocal lesions may cluster in adjacent bones
      - Often foot and ankle
    - Multifocality may in some cases represent metastatic disease from undiagnosed soft tissue angiosarcoma
- Size
  - May be large by time of diagnosis, especially in pelvis

Imaging Recommendations

- Best imaging tool
  - Detected on radiograph
  - More fully evaluated with MR
  - No imaging is specific for diagnosis
  - Evaluate for multifocal lesions: Bone scan may be useful

Radiographic Findings

- Lytic, destructive
  - Wide zone of transition
  - No (or incomplete) sclerotic margin
    - May have honeycomb or hole-within-hole appearance if lesion is of lower grade
  - Bone often expanded if low grade
  - Cortical breakthrough, soft tissue mass if high grade

CT Findings

- Mimics radiographic findings
  - Variable degrees of aggressiveness, depending on grade of lesion

MR Findings

- Nonspecific T1 hypointensity
- Nonspecific T2 hyperintensity, inhomogeneous
- Nonspecific contrast enhancement
  - Central low signal of necrosis is common
- May have prominent peripheral vessels
- 1 case report of fluid-fluid levels within lesion

Nuclear Medicine Findings

- Bone scan: Significantly increased uptake

DIFFERENTIAL DIAGNOSIS

Multifocal

- Metastases, bone marrow
- Multiple myeloma
- Disuse osteoporosis (by radiograph; MR distinguishes)
  - Complex regional pain syndrome would have similar appearance
  - Severe osteoporosis may appear moth-eaten, similar to multifocal lesions, which can be seen in adjacent bones of foot in angiosarcoma
- Other multifocal vascular lesions
  - Hemangioendothelioma, osseous
  - Hemangiopericytoma, osseous

Solitary Lesion

- Plasmacytoma
  - Moderately aggressive
  - Lytic, expanded
- Lymphoma
  - Lytic, aggressive
  - Large soft tissue mass
  - May have thickened endosteum, differentiating it from angiosarcoma
- Fibrosarcoma, malignant fibrous histiocytoma of bone
  - Lytic, aggressive, may have identical appearance

PATHOLOGY

General Features

- Etiology
  - Unknown
  - May be associated with prior radiation
  - Possible association with
    - Long-term metal implants
    - Paget disease
    - Osseous infarction
- Genetics
  - 2 subgroups of angiosarcoma
    - 1 with few or no genetic aberrations
    - 1 with multiple genetic aberrations
      - Most common: Amplification of both 2q and 17q
      - Found in angiosarcoma originating in either bone or soft tissue
    - No difference in 2 groups related to either location of tumor or survival

Staging, Grading, & Classification

- AJCC staging, including consideration of
  - Tumor size

- Tumor grade
- Presence of metastases

Gross Pathologic & Surgical Features

- Bloody and firm in consistency
- Abnormal blood vessels exhibiting complicated infolding and irregular anastomoses

Microscopic Features

- Epithelial cells lining blood vessels show malignant characteristics
  - Small tissue samples may be misdiagnosed as metastatic lesion because of epithelioid cells
- Spindle and epithelioid cells within solid portion of tumor
- Range from well- to poorly differentiated

CLINICAL ISSUES

Presentation

- Most common signs/symptoms
  - Pain and swelling
  - Pathologic fracture

Demographics

- Age
  - 2nd to 7th decade
  - Peak: 3rd to 5th decades
  - Mean age: 54 (in 1 study of 60 patients)
- Gender
  - M > F = 2:1
- Epidemiology
  - < 1% of malignant bone tumors
  - Only 6% of angiosarcomas are osseous

Natural History & Prognosis

- 66% of cases developed metastases to lung and other organs in 1 study
- 40% presented with metastases in 1 study of 60 patients
- Overall 67% 5-year survival in 1 study (included soft tissue and osseous lesions)
- Another study of 60 patients showed 5-year survival of 20%
  - 33% for those presenting with localized disease
    - 46% survival for those with surgical complete remission
  - 0% for those presenting with metastatic disease
- Prognosis also relates to grade of lesion
- Studies suggest that patients with multifocal lesions may have higher survival rates
  - Other studies suggest no difference in survival between solitary & multicentric presentations

Treatment

- Wide resection
  - Complete surgical resection appears to be requirement for any potential of cure
- Chemotherapy
- ± radiation therapy

DIAGNOSTIC CHECKLIST

Image Interpretation Pearls

- Clustering of multifocal lesions in single anatomic region
  - Highly suggestive of osseous vascular tumors
  - Usually cannot distinguish between angiosarcoma, hemangioendothelioma, hemangiopericytoma
    - Angiosarcoma may be more destructive, but differentiation not reliable

SELECTED REFERENCES

1. Verbeke SL et al: Array CGH analysis identifies two distinct subgroups of primary angiosarcoma of bone. Genes Chromosomes Cancer. 54(2):72-81, 2015
2. Balaji GG et al: Primary epithelioid angiosarcoma of the calcaneum: a diagnostic dilemma. J Foot Ankle Surg. 53(2):239-42, 2014
3. Palmerini E et al: Primary angiosarcoma of bone: a retrospective analysis of 60 patients from 2 institutions. Am J Clin Oncol. 37(6):528-34, 2014
4. Sakamoto A et al: Aggressive clinical course of epithelioid angiosarcoma in the femur: a case report. World J Surg Oncol. 12:281, 2014
5. Griffith B et al: Angiosarcoma of the humerus presenting with fluid-fluid levels on MRI: a unique imaging presentation. Skeletal Radiol. 42(11):1611-6, 2013
6. Thariat J et al: Primary multicentric angiosarcoma of bone: true entity or metastases from an unknown primary? Value of comparative genomic hybridization on paraffin embedded tissues. Rare Tumors. 5(3):e53, 2013
7. Errani C et al: Vascular bone tumors: a proposal of a classification based on clinicopathological, radiographic and genetic features. Skeletal Radiol. 41(12):1495-507, 2012
8. Dunlap JB et al: Cytogenetic analysis of a primary bone angiosarcoma. Cancer Genet Cytogenet. 194(1):1-3, 2009
9. Asmane I et al: Adriamycin, cisplatin, ifosfamide and paclitaxel combination as front-line chemotherapy for locally advanced and metastatic angiosarcoma. Analysis of three case reports and review of the literature. Anticancer Res. 28(5B):3041-5, 2008
10. Abraham JA et al: Treatment and outcome of 82 patients with angiosarcoma. Ann Surg Oncol. 14(6):1953-67, 2007
11. Marthya A et al: Multicentric epithelioid angiosarcoma of the spine: a case report of a rare bone tumor. Spine J. 7(6):716-9, 2007
12. Mittal S et al: Post-irradiation angiosarcoma of bone. J Cancer Res Ther. 3(2):96-9, 2007
13. Deshpande V et al: Epithelioid angiosarcoma of the bone: a series of 10 cases. Am J Surg Pathol. 27(6):709-16, 2003
14. Santeusanio G et al: Multifocal epithelioid angiosarcoma of bone: a potential pitfall in the differential diagnosis with metastatic carcinoma. Appl Immunohistochem Mol Morphol. 11(4):359-63, 2003
15. McDonald DJ et al: Metal-associated angiosarcoma of bone: report of two cases and review of the literature. Clin Orthop Relat Res. (396):206-14, 2002
16. Roessner A et al: Angiosarcoma. In Fletcher CDM et al: World Health Organization classification of Tumours: Tumours of soft tissue and bone. Lyon: IARC Press, 2002
17. Choi JJ et al: Angiomatous skeletal lesions. Semin Musculoskelet Radiol. 4(1):103-12, 2000
18. Wenger DE et al: Malignant vascular lesions of bone: radiologic and pathologic features. Skeletal Radiol. 29(11):619-31, 2000
19. Abdelwahab IF et al: Angiosarcomas associated with bone infarcts. Skeletal Radiol. 27(10):546-51, 1998
20. Boulanger V et al: Primary angiosarcoma of bone in Paget's disease. Eur J Surg Oncol. 24(6):611-3, 1998
21. Greenspan A et al: Differential diagnosis of tumors and tumor-like lesions of bones and joints. Philadelphia: Lippincott-Raven, 1998
22. Lomasney LM et al: Multifocal vascular lesions of bone: imaging characteristics. Skeletal Radiol. 25(3):255-61, 1996
23. Murphey MD et al: From the archives of the AFIP. Musculoskeletal angiomatous lesions: radiologic-pathologic correlation. Radiographics. 15(4):893-917, 1995

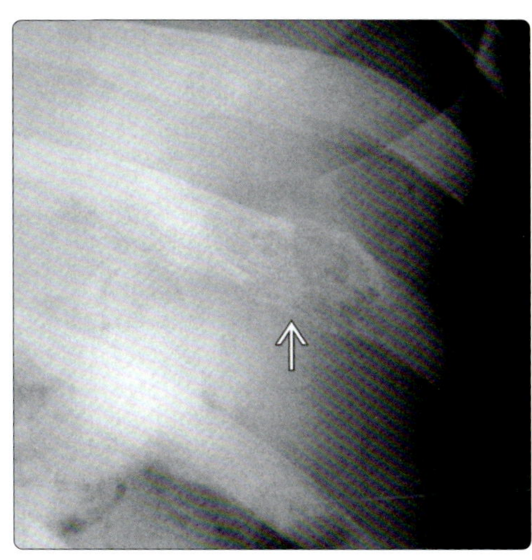

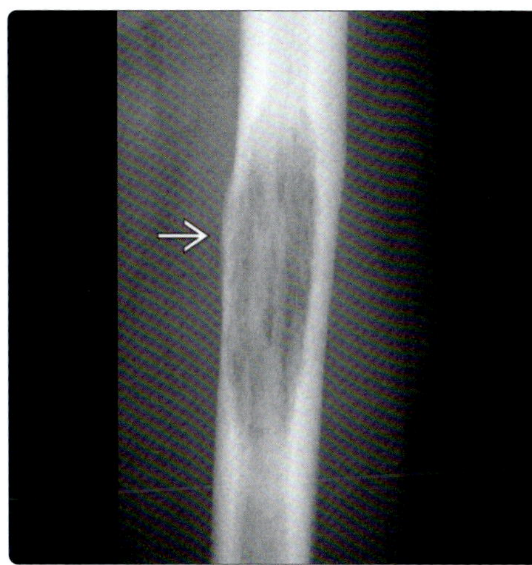

(Left) *AP radiograph in a patient with polyostotic angiosarcoma shows a rib lesion that is lytic and mildly expanded ➡ with cortical breakthrough and appears moderately aggressive.* **(Right)** *AP radiograph in the same case shows a femoral lesion with a fairly wide zone of transition and thinning of the endosteal cortex ➡. Like the rib lesion, this appears moderately aggressive. These 2 lesions should prompt consideration of metastasis or multiple myeloma, though the patient is only in their 30s.*

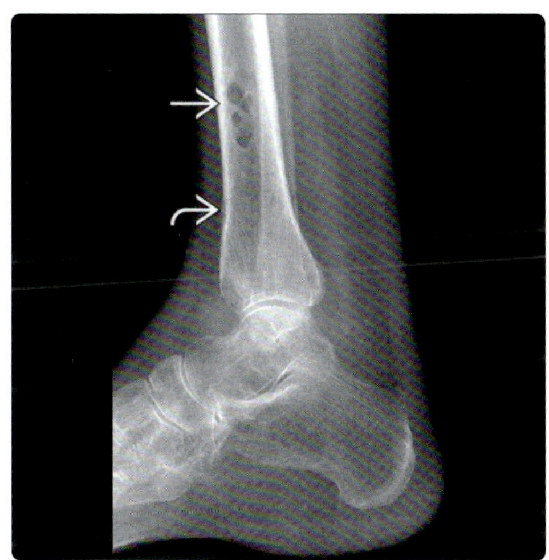

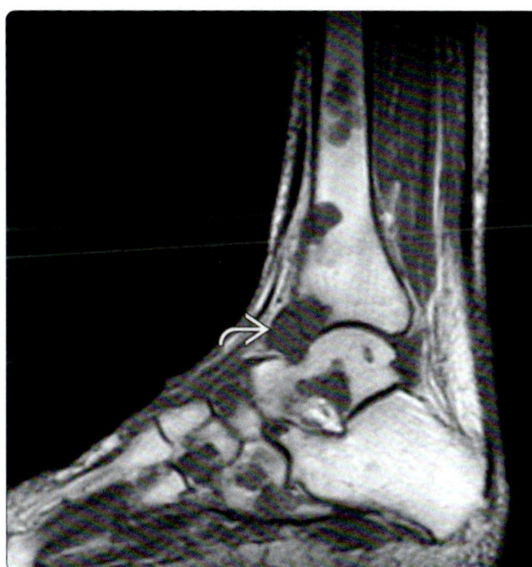

(Left) *Lateral radiograph in a 69-year-old woman with ankle pain shows multiple lytic lesions, the most obvious in the distal tibia. One is lytic and appears to be septated ➡. Another is cortically based ➡. Other lesions throughout the ankle are easily misinterpreted as the moth-eaten pattern of osteoporosis.* **(Right)** *Sagittal T1 MR in the same patient shows far more lesions than were noted on the radiograph. One extends into the ankle joint ➡; this had appeared as an effusion on the x-ray. The lesions are of uniform intermediate intensity.*

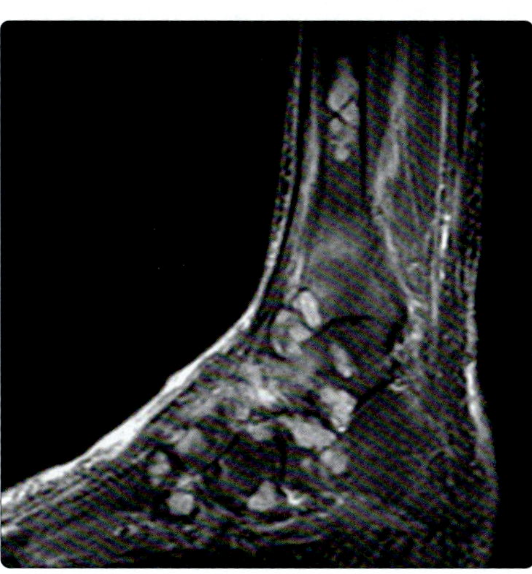

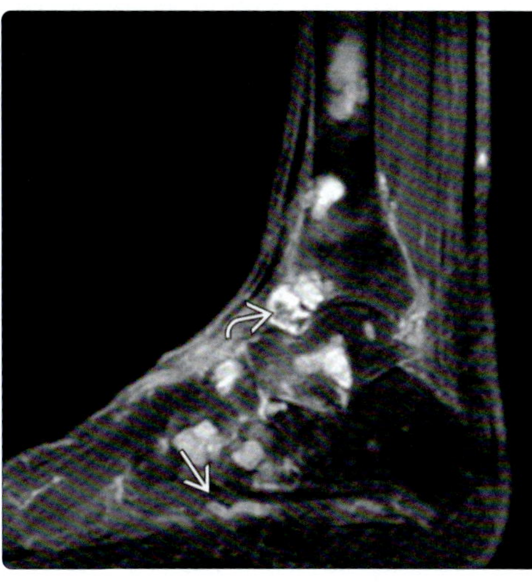

(Left) *Sagittal STIR MR in the same patient shows heterogeneity in the high intensity lesions.* **(Right)** *Sagittal T1 C+ FS MR shows the lesions to enhance avidly with a central area of necrosis in one ➡. There is prominent vascularity ➡. This has been noted to be a feature of vascular tumors, but is not specific. The more specific feature is the cluster of multiple lesions in the lower extremity; there were no other lesions at presentation. This distribution makes metastatic disease highly unlikely.*

KEY FACTS

TERMINOLOGY

- Low- to intermediate-grade malignant tumor that recapitulates notochord

IMAGING

- Location: Sacrum (60%)
  - Sphenooccipital/nasal (25%)
  - Cervical spine (10%)
  - Thoracolumbar spine (5%)
- Radiographic appearance: Lytic destructive lesion
  - Internal calcification may be present (50-70%)
  - Calcification prominent in chondroid chordoma (located virtually only in clivus)
  - Bony debris often carried into soft tissue mass; may mimic matrix
- CT: 90% show calcification
  - Though lesion is locally aggressive, time course is slow enough that it may not appear aggressive
- MR T1WI: Isointense to hypointense; inhomogeneous if dense calcification present
- MR fluid-sensitive sequences: Inhomogeneous but generally very high signal
  - May appear lobulated
  - Significant regions of low signal if dense calcification present

CLINICAL ISSUES

- Slowly growing, often with nonspecific symptoms
  - Eventually develops symptoms related to location of spread into adjacent soft tissues
- 1-4% of primary malignant bone tumors
- Of sacral tumors, 40% are chordomas
- High recurrence rate (80%) with marginal resection
- 5-year survival rate: 50-84% in different studies
- Recent study shows that lesion is highly malignant over long term
- May contain dedifferentiated foci; poorer prognosis

(Left) *AP radiograph of the pelvis in a 44-year-old man shows destruction of the caudal portion of the sacrum ➡. Note there is also faintly seen calcification ⮫. This appearance is typical of either sacral chordoma or chondrosarcoma.* **(Right)** *Axial CT in the same patient shows the large size of the sacral mass. Note that calcification ➡ does not have a chondroid appearance. The calcification is mostly distributed peripherally; this appearance is typical of chordoma. Such calcification is seen in 90% of chordomas by CT.*

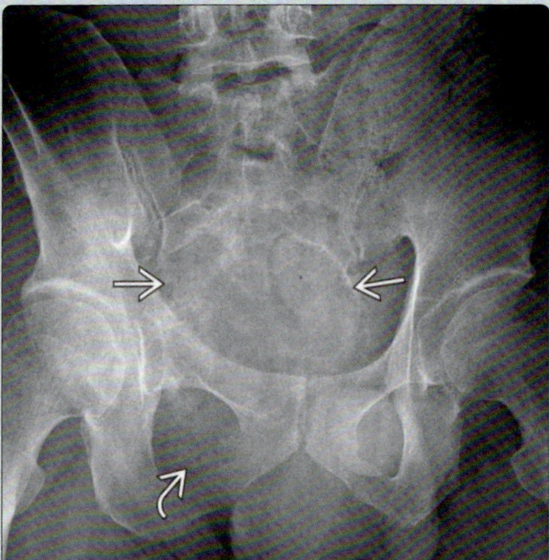

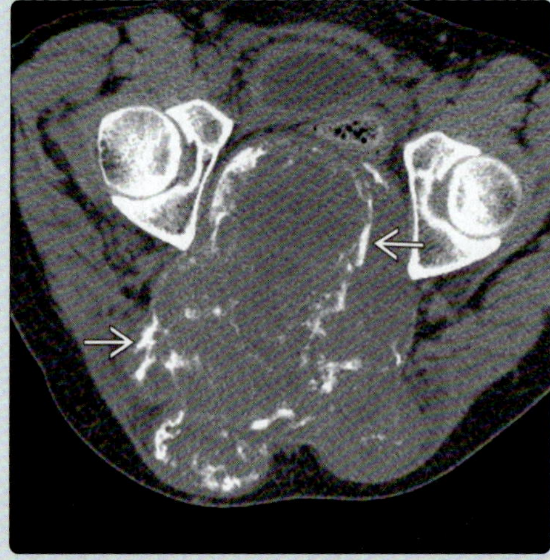

(Left) *Axial T1 MR, same case, shows intermediate to low signal in the mass posteriorly ➡ but higher signal anteriorly ⮫. This combination is typical of chordoma, with the higher signal representing either blood or highly proteinaceous material.* **(Right)** *Axial T2 FS MR shows heterogeneous hyperintensity throughout the mass ➡, with some areas of hypointensity representing the calcifications. Note the anterior displacement of the rectum ⮫ and bladder, typical of chordoma.*

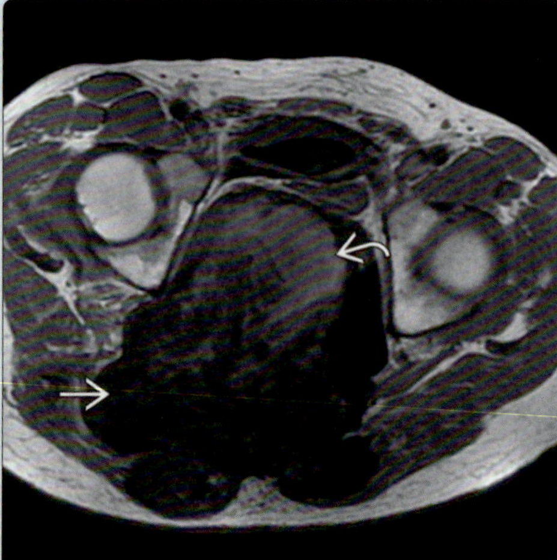

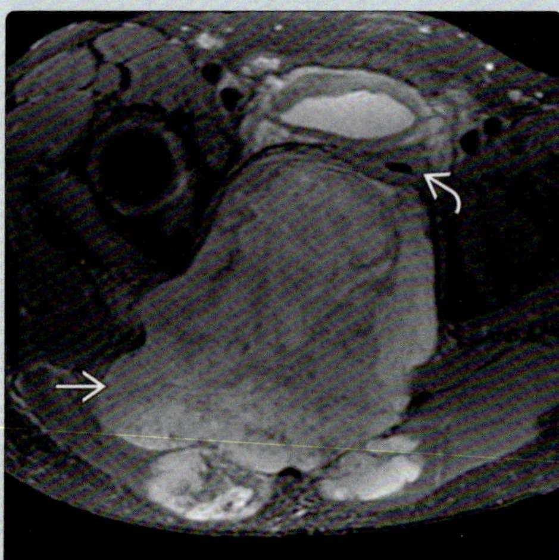

TERMINOLOGY

Definitions

- Low- to intermediate-grade malignant tumor that recapitulates notochord

IMAGING

General Features

- Location
  - Sacrum (60%); predominantly in lower sacral elements
  - Sphenooccipital/nasal (25%)
    - 33% are of chondroid chordoma variety
  - Cervical spine (10%)
  - Thoracolumbar spine (5%)
  - Usually midline in origin

Radiographic Findings

- Lytic destructive lesion
  - No true matrix produced, but internal calcification often present (50-70% by radiograph)
  - Calcification prominent in chondroid chordoma (located virtually only in clivus)
- Though lesion is locally aggressive, time course is slow enough that it may not appear aggressive
  - Narrow zone of transition
  - Margin is often at least partially sclerotic
  - No periosteal reaction
  - Expansion of bone without cortical breakthrough early in process
- Monostotic with rare exceptions
- Soft tissue mass, often prevertebral but may extend into epidural space
  - Sacral lesion displaces bowel/bladder

MR Findings

- Sphenooccipital chordomas usually begin in clivus
  - Rarely occur in nasopharynx, maxilla, paranasal sinuses
  - Rarely multicentric
  - Nodular or scattered calcifications in 20-70%
  - Sagittal images show tumor indenting pons
  - Calcification, hemorrhage, and mucoid areas contribute to heterogeneity
  - MRA required: Tumoral encasement/displacement of vessels in ~ 80%
- Vertebral chordomas begin in vertebral body
  - May extend to posterior elements
  - Displace spinal cord &/or nerve roots
  - Rarely arise in epidural or intradural space
  - Rarely develop posterior mediastinal mass, which is discontinuous with osseous lesion
  - Late in process may involve intervertebral disc and contiguous vertebral bodies
  - Mass hyperintense to disc on T2, often with septations
- Sacral chordomas: Begin in retrorectal location
  - May enlarge so much as to involve buttocks
- MR signal characteristics
  - T1WI: Isointense to hypointense; inhomogeneous if dense calcification present
    - Areas of high intensity due to hemorrhage & high protein content
  - Fluid-sensitive sequences: Inhomogeneous but generally very high signal
    - May appear lobulated
    - Significant regions of low signal if calcification present
    - May have myxoid regions & areas of hemorrhage
  - Moderate inhomogeneous enhancement

DIFFERENTIAL DIAGNOSIS

DDx of Chordoma in Sacrum

- Giant cell tumor (GCT)
  - Arises in body of sacrum, usually upper levels (S1 or S2), expands anteriorly
  - 2nd most common 1° sacral tumor (after chordoma)
  - Lytic lesion; no matrix
  - May appear moderately to highly aggressive
  - MR shows central or swirling low signal on T2/STIR
    - Chordoma may appear similar 2° to calcification
- Chondrosarcoma, conventional
  - Sacrum is most common vertebral site for this lesion
  - Chondroid matrix may mimic peripheral calcification or bony debris in chordoma
  - Low-grade lesion contains high signal lobulations on T2
- Neurofibroma
  - Soft tissue lesion arising in sacral foramen may destroy bone to point of simulating lesion of sacral origin
  - Large presacral mass plus epidural mass
  - T2 often has central low signal; not significantly different from chordoma appearance
- Osteoblastoma
  - Arises in body of sacrum
  - Often produces osteoid matrix; may mimic chordoma
  - May be aggressive or even malignant
- Plasmacytoma
  - Lytic lesion without sclerosis or reactive bone
  - Moderately aggressive

DDx of Chordoma in Vertebral Body

- Multiple myeloma
  - Lesions commonly arise in vertebral body
  - Lytic, moderately aggressive
  - Epidural mass may occur, though not commonly
  - Usually multiple in vertebrae
- Metastases, bone marrow
  - May arise in either body or posterior elements
  - May have epidural mass, similar to chordoma
  - Usually multiple lesions
- Osteoblastoma
  - Arises in vertebral body, similar to chordoma
  - Often produces osteoid matrix; may mimic chordoma
  - May be aggressive or even malignant
- GCT
  - Arises in vertebral body, similar to chordoma
  - Entirely lytic; may extend to epidural space or posterior elements
  - More common in vertebral body than chordoma
- Lymphoma
  - Involvement of disc and contiguous vertebral bodies is similar to late vertebral chordoma

DDx of Chordoma in Clivus

- Chondrosarcoma, conventional
  - Dense calcification in chondroid chordoma mimics chondroid matrix in chondrosarcoma
  - Histologic differentiation is difficult: Cartilaginous foci in chondroid chordoma resembles that in chondroma or chondrosarcoma
    - Immunohistochemical stains demonstrate tumor cells to be reactive for epithelial markers
- Giant invasive pituitary macroadenoma
  - Origin in sella helps to differentiate from chordoma
- Metastases, bone marrow
  - Lytic or mixed lytic-sclerotic, with local extension

PATHOLOGY

General Features

- Etiology
  - Vestigial remnants of notochordal tissue
- Genetics
  - Clonal chromosome aberrations detected in some
  - Familial cases have been described

Microscopic Features

- Individual lobules separated by fibrous bands
- Tumor cells arranged in sheets, cords, or float singly within abundant myxoid stroma
- Pale vacuolated cytoplasm (termed physaliphorous)
- Mild to moderate nuclear atypia
- Chondroid chordoma: Portions of lesion look like low-grade chondrosarcoma

CLINICAL ISSUES

Presentation

- Most common signs/symptoms
  - Slowly growing, often with nonspecific symptoms
    - Eventually develops symptoms related to location of spread into adjacent soft tissues
  - Sacrum
    - Constipation: Rectal displacement/obstruction
    - Presacral mass detected on rectal examination
    - Anesthesia/paresthesia late and uncommon
    - Eventual perineal pain and numbness
  - Sphenooccipital
    - Headache
    - Cranial nerve compression (especially ocular)
      - Blurred vision, diplopia, weakness
    - Endocrine disturbance if pituitary is compressed
    - Inferior spread → nasal obstruction, bleeding
    - Lateral spread: Cerebellopontine angle symptoms
  - Cervical or thoracolumbar spine
    - Symptoms of nerve root/cord compression
      - Pain, numbness, motor weakness, paralysis

Demographics

- Age
  - Generally > 30 years; extremely rare < 20 years
    - Younger patients tend to have sphenooccipital involvement more frequently than other regions
  - Most commonly presents in 6th decade (30%)
  - Skull and spine lesions tend to present 10 years earlier than sacral lesions
- Gender
  - Male > female (1.8:1)
- Epidemiology
  - 1-4% of primary malignant bone tumors
  - Of all sacral tumors, benign or malignant, 40% are chordomas

Natural History & Prognosis

- Initial slow progression; local soft tissue displacement
- Prognosis variable, depending on location and involvement of local tissues
- High recurrence rate (80%) with marginal resection
- Previous surgery & large size of lesion related to ↑ local recurrence
- 5-year survival rate: 50-84% in different studies
  - 10-year survival rate: 30-64%
- Recent study shows that lesion is highly malignant over long term
  - Metastasizes to lung, bone, soft tissue, lymph node
    - Metastasis eventually occurs in up to 40%
- Dedifferentiated chordoma contains malignant spindle cell component
  - May be primary chordoma or recurrent tumors that have been irradiated
  - Very poor prognosis
    - Prognosis worse if lesion is large, marginally resected, or crosses sacroiliac joint
    - Prognosis better if dedifferentiation is small (< 1 cm)
- Chondroid chordoma: Significantly better prognosis
  - 15-year survival: > 50%

Treatment

- Long-term malignant nature of lesion suggests aggressive treatment if possible
  - Wide resection is optimal but often not compatible with acceptable functionality
- Adjuvant radiation appears to ↑ disease-free intervals
- Photon radiation therapy may be useful
- Percutaneous radiofrequency ablation considered in recurrent lesions
- Molecular targeted therapy under development (imatinib)
  - Some assert it may slow disease, but naturally slow progression makes this difficult to prove in short term

DIAGNOSTIC CHECKLIST

Consider

- Sacral lesion difficult to visualize on AP radiograph due to overlying bowel
  - Watch on lateral radiograph for displacement of rectum by presacral mass

SELECTED REFERENCES

1. Si MJ et al: Differentiation of primary chordoma, giant cell tumor and schwannoma of the sacrum by CT and MRI. Eur J Radiol. 82(12):2309-15, 2013

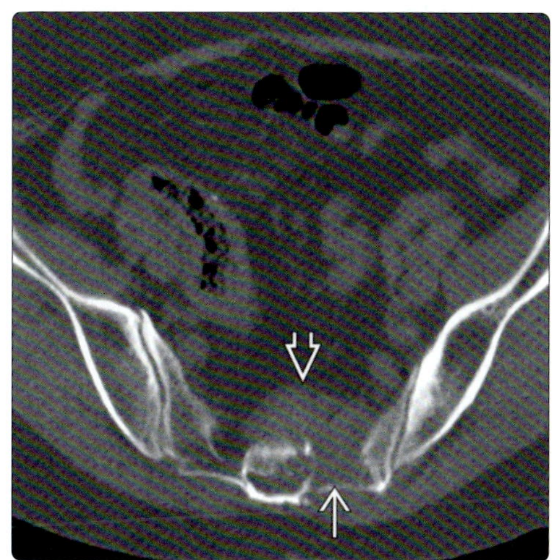

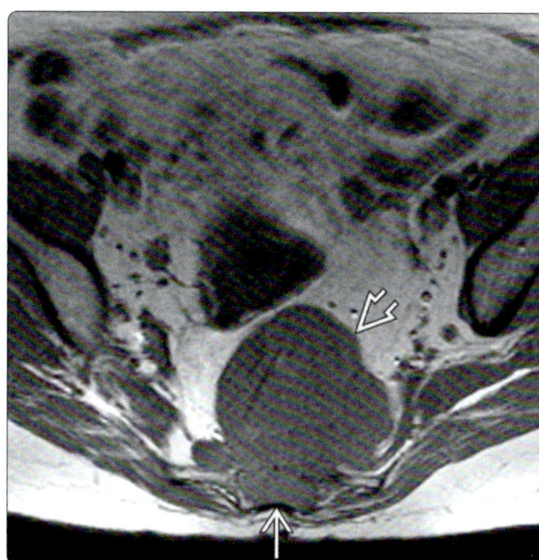

(Left) *Axial NECT shows a lytic bone lesion occupying the left sacral ala ➡ and a prevertebral soft tissue mass extending from the osseous lesion ➡. The location and appearance are typical of chordoma. Other lesions, such as neurofibroma, chondrosarcoma, and giant cell tumor, may have a similar appearance.* **(Right)** *Axial T1WI MR in the same patient shows the osseous lesion ➡ and soft tissue mass ➡ to be homogeneously low signal, isointense to skeletal muscle. The mass displaces bowel contents anteriorly.*

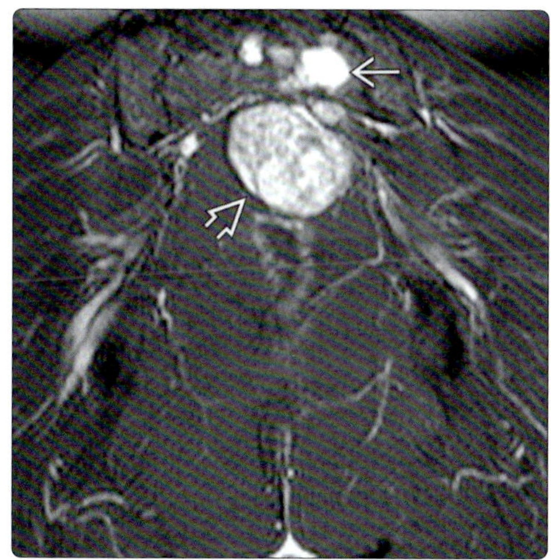

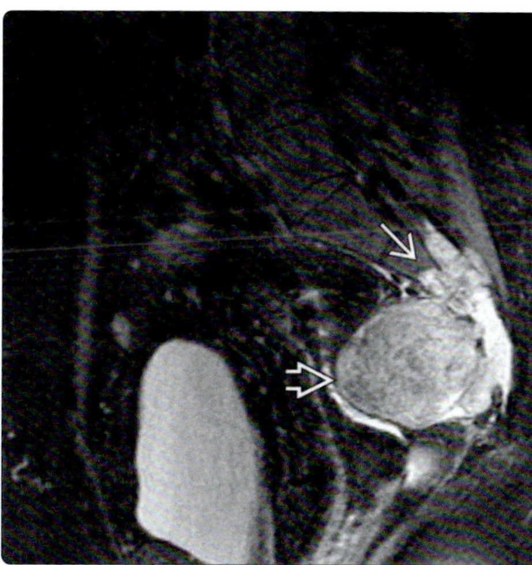

(Left) *Coronal STIR MR in the same patient shows an inhomogeneously hyperintense osseous lesion ➡ and soft tissue mass showing similar characteristics ➡.* **(Right)** *Sagittal T1WI C+ FS MR in the same patient shows significant enhancement of both the bone ➡ and soft tissue masses ➡. Note that the rectum and uterus have been previously resected; if they had been present, they would have been displaced anteriorly. The location and appearance are typical of chordoma.*

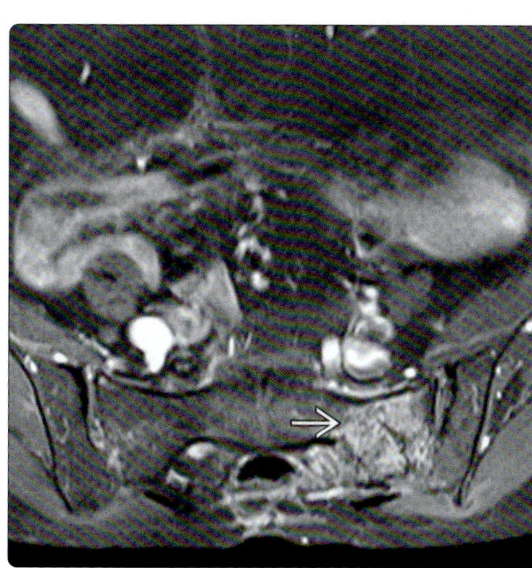

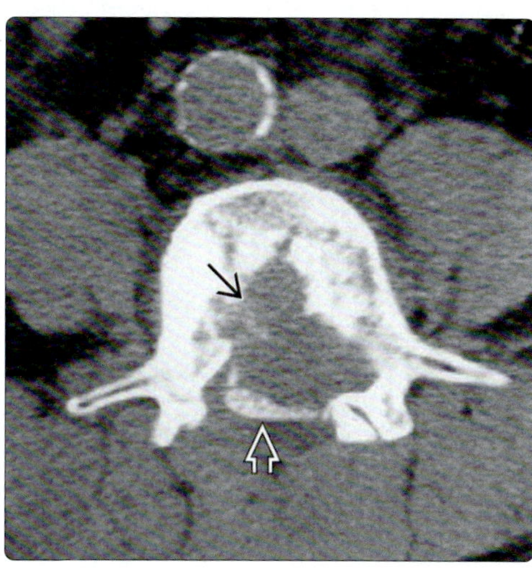

(Left) *Axial T1WI C+ FS MR obtained 1 year following treatment by marginal resection (required to maintain function), shows tumor recurrence within the left sacral ala ➡. Chordoma is a locally aggressive lesion, which has a high rate of recurrence, particularly with a marginal resection. Over time, metastatic disease often develops.* **(Right)** *Axial CT with myelogram shows a chordoma developing in the body of a lumbar vertebra ➡, extending into the epidural space and compressing the thecal sac ➡.*

KEY FACTS

TERMINOLOGY

- Increased and disordered bone turnover and remodeling

IMAGING

- Distribution of Paget disease
  - Monostotic (10-35%) or polyostotic (65-90%)
  - Skull: 25-65% of patients
  - Spine: 30-75% of patients
  - Pelvis: 30-75% of patients
  - Proximal long bones: 25-30% of patients
- Radiographic or CT appearance
  - Early lesions: Lytic, thinned cortex
  - Later lesions: Mixed lytic/sclerotic
  - Disordered, thickened trabeculae
  - Cortical thickening
  - Deformity: Protrusio, varus hips, anterior bowing tibia, basilar invagination
  - Enlargement of involved bone in all dimensions
- Lesion in long bone begins at subchondral region, progresses toward diaphysis
  - Exception: Lesion may rarely begin in diaphysis; usually tibia
- Sharp oblique delineation at lesional border with normal bone
  - Termed blade of grass or flame-shaped
- MR appearance: Variable, depending on phase
  - Histologic composition of marrow space changes from lytic through blastic disease
  - Often contains more marrow fat than adjacent normal bone
- Bone scan: ↑ ↑ uptake when lesions are active

DIAGNOSTIC CHECKLIST

- Preservation of regions of marrow fat in Paget disease
  - May help differentiate regions of early sarcomatous degeneration, where fat is destroyed
- Fat also not seen in presence of fracture

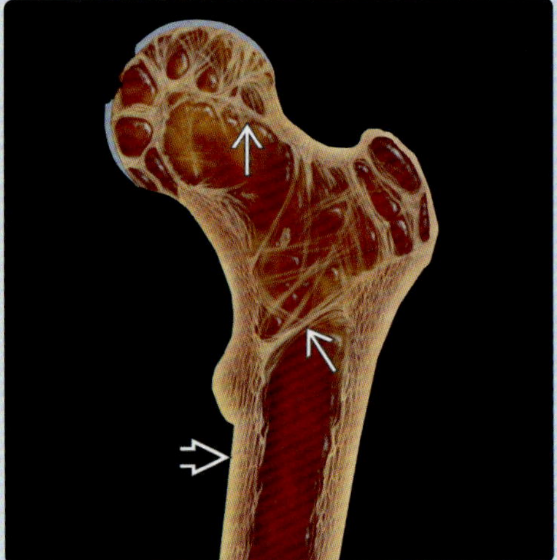

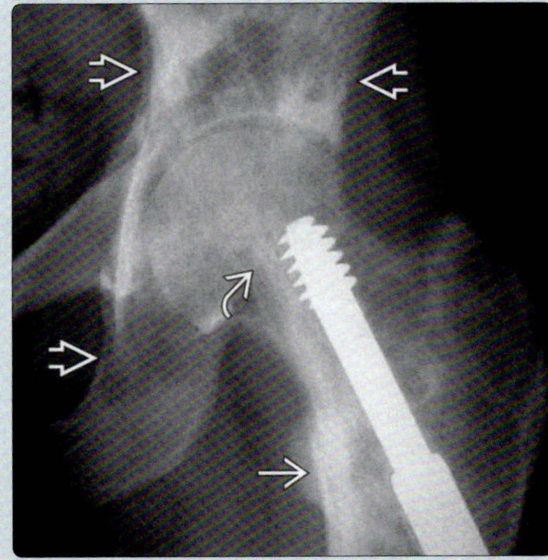

(Left) *Graphic depicts transected femur in advanced Paget disease. There is loss of normal cancellous architecture and replacement by coarse, thick bundles of trabecular bone ➡. The cortex is irregularly thickened and has a coarse granular appearance ➡ in contrast to the smooth ivory appearance of normal cortical bone.* **(Right)** *AP radiograph shows the mixed pattern of Paget disease involving the acetabulum ➡ and femur. Note the coarsened medial femoral cortex ➡ and weight-bearing trabeculae ➡.*

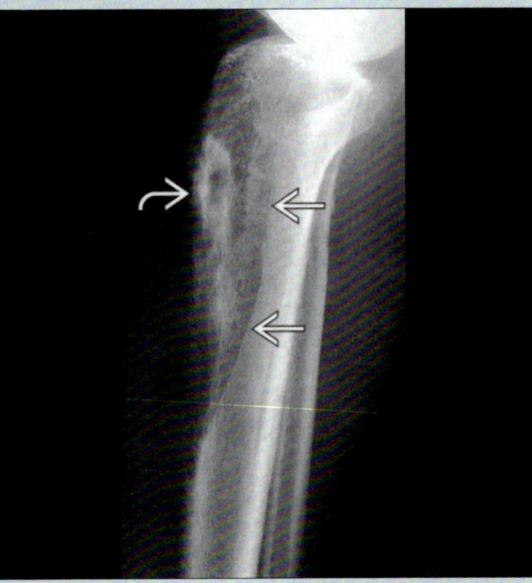

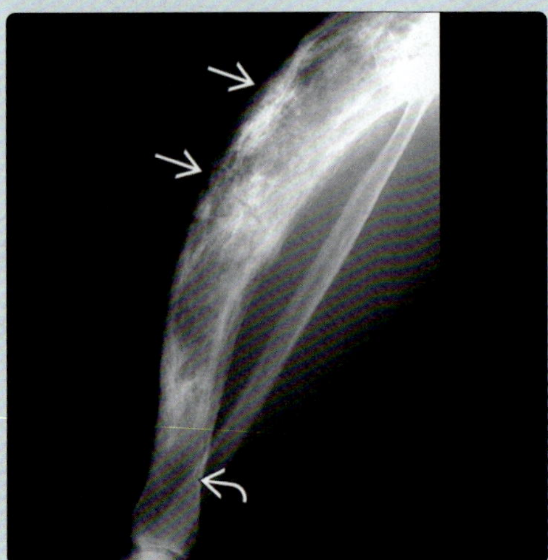

(Left) *Lateral radiograph of Paget disease demonstrates a lytic lesion with small sclerotic areas within it ➡. The lesion extends from the subarticular region distally in a blade of grass or flame-shaped pattern ➡. Early mild enlargement of the bone is seen.* **(Right)** *Lateral radiograph in a contrasting, advanced case of Paget disease shows diffuse involvement; only a small distal region of tibia remains normal ➡. Note the enlargement of bone and anterior bowing, with small "banana" fractures ➡.*

TERMINOLOGY

Definitions

- Increased and disordered bone turnover and remodeling

IMAGING

General Features

- Best diagnostic clue
  - Enlarged bone with coarsened trabeculae
- Location
  - Monostotic (10-35%) or polyostotic (65-90%)
  - Distribution of uncomplicated Paget disease
    - Skull: 25-65% of patients
    - Spine: 30-75% of patients
    - Pelvis: 30-75% of patients
    - Proximal long bones: 25-30% of patients
  - Distribution of Paget sarcoma
    - 2/3 in large limb bones (femur, humerus, tibia)
    - 1/3 in flat bones (pelvis, skull, scapula)
    - Fairly similar to normal distribution of Paget disease, except
      - Increased incidence in humerus
      - Decreased incidence in spine
    - Multifocal Paget sarcoma: 17%
      - Usually femur and skull

Radiographic Findings

- Generalizations
  - Early lesions: Lytic, thinned cortex
  - Later lesions: Mixed lytic/sclerotic
    - Disordered, thickened trabeculae
    - Cortical thickening
    - Enlargement of involved bone in all dimensions
    - Deformity related to softening of bone: Protrusio, varus hips, anterior bowing tibia, basilar invagination
- Skull
  - Lytic phase: Lysis, usually frontal or occipital bones
    - Termed osteoporosis circumscripta
  - Enlargement of skull: Widening of diploic space
    - Both inner and outer tables of calvaria involved
  - Late phase: Focal regions of sclerosis within thickened calvaria
    - Termed cotton wool
  - Basilar invagination
- Long bones
  - Lesion begins at proximal or distal subchondral region, progresses towards diaphysis
    - Exception: Lesion rarely begins in diaphysis; usually tibia
  - Sharp oblique delineation at lesional border with normal bone
    - Termed blade of grass or flame-shaped
  - Incomplete horizontal insufficiency fractures
    - On convex side of bone
    - Progress to "banana" fractures
    - Contribute to abnormal lateral bowing of femur, anterior bowing of tibia
- Pelvis
  - Early cortical thickening and sclerosis of iliopectineal and ischiopubic lines
  - Enlargement, involvement of iliac wing
  - Protrusio acetabulae
- Spine
  - Enlarged vertebrae, thickened sclerotic borders → picture frame appearance
    - Center often radiolucent
  - Ivory vertebra in late blastic phase
- Watch for superimposed neoplasm
  - Sarcomatous degeneration
  - Giant cell tumor

MR Findings

- Variable, depending on phase of disease
  - Histologic composition of marrow space changes from lytic through blastic disease
  - Often contains more marrow fat than adjacent normal bone
  - Often heterogeneous "speckled" on both T1 and T2
  - Inhomogeneous enhancement
- Giant cell tumor or Paget sarcoma
  - Typical findings of these lesions, superimposed on Paget disease
  - Often marrow fat is obliterated by superimposed tumor
    - Absent fat may help differentiate tumor from Paget bone
- Dynamic contrast imaging shows regions of excessive hypervascularity
  - Located in advancing active zone
  - May be useful in evaluating therapeutic effect of medications

Nuclear Medicine Findings

- Bone scan: ↑ ↑ uptake when lesions are active
- Used to assess distribution and skeletal disease extent

DIFFERENTIAL DIAGNOSIS

Sclerotic Metastases

- Blastic lesions in same distribution as Paget disease
- No trabecular coarsening or enlargement of bone

Fibrous Dysplasia

- Calvarial and base of skull distribution identical
  - Appearance may not be distinguishable from Paget disease
- If homogeneous ground-glass appearance is present, diagnostic of fibrous dysplasia (FD)
- FD may enlarge bone but generally without trabecular coarsening or cortical thickening

Multiple Myeloma

- Early lytic lesions of Paget disease may be similar
- Myeloma does not enlarge bone or trabeculae

Myelofibrosis

- Sclerosis but without bone enlargement

PATHOLOGY

General Features

- Etiology
  - Environmental influence (viral etiology) postulated due to regional difference in disease prevalence

- Chronic measles infection may be related
- Intranuclear inclusion bodies resembling those of paramyxovirus found in osteoclasts
- Genetics
  - Predisposition to Paget disease may have genetic component linked to chromosome arm 18q
  - Mutations in gene encoding sequestosome 1 (*SQSTM1*) in familial (25-50%) and sporadic Paget disease

Microscopic Features

- Lytic phase
  - Fibrovascular tissue replaces yellow marrow when active
  - Aggressive bone resorption
  - Increased vascular channels
  - Osteoblastic rimming
- Inactive phase
  - Return to diffuse yellow marrow gradually occurs
  - Decreased bone turnover, coarsened trabeculae
  - Irregular cement lines
  - Loss of excessive vascularity

CLINICAL ISSUES

Presentation

- Most common signs/symptoms
  - May be asymptomatic initially for many years
  - Bone pain: Deep, constant, worse at night
  - Deformity: Protrusio, femoral or tibial bowing
  - Spinal stenosis and related neurologic abnormalities
  - Increased skull size
  - Hearing loss (impingement on cranial nerve VIII)
    - Other cranial nerves affected less frequently
  - Pathologic fracture (12-20%, most often femur)
  - Paget sarcoma: Change in pain pattern
- Other signs/symptoms
  - Elevated alkaline phosphatase and urinary hydroxyproline
  - High-output heart failure (rare)

Demographics

- Age
  - Generally 55-85 years of age
    - Median age of Paget sarcoma: 64 years
  - Only 4% of Paget cases occur < 40 years of age
    - Nonetheless, prevalence is so great that diagnosis must be considered even in young adults
- Gender
  - Male slightly > female
  - Paget sarcoma more common in men (2:1)
- Ethnicity
  - Caucasian predominance, especially in Great Britain, Australia, New Zealand, USA, and Western Europe
- Epidemiology
  - 3% of individuals > 40 years of age
  - 10-11% of individuals > 80 years of age
  - Some suggestions that pattern of disease is changing
    - May be less prevalent and developed later in life
    - May involve fewer bones

Natural History & Prognosis

- Osseous weakening → deformity, fracture
  - Fractures often begin as incomplete fractures on convex side of long bone; progress to "banana" fracture
- Secondary osteoarthritis
- Neurologic symptoms
- Hyperemia may predispose metastases to lodge in bone with underlying Paget disease
- Rare development of giant cell tumor, occasionally multiple
  - Higher prevalence in patients who develop disease early, with polyostotic disease and with + family history
- Rare development of pseudosarcoma
  - Soft tissue mass with aggressive MR appearance, rapid growth, but no malignant cells
- Rare degeneration to sarcoma
  - Of precursors to osseous malignancy, considered in moderate risk category
    - Incidence of sarcomatous change: 0.7-0.95%
  - Generally occurs in patients with widespread Paget disease (70% of sarcoma cases)
  - Most commonly degenerates to osteosarcoma (50-60%) or malignant fibrous histiocytoma, chondrosarcoma
    - Look for underlying Paget disease in population of older patients with osteosarcoma
  - Prognosis for Paget sarcoma poor
    - 11% overall 5-year survival
    - Shorter for multifocal disease
    - Metastases present in 25% at initial presentation

Treatment

- If asymptomatic, no treatment
- Bisphosphonates reduce bone turnover; relatively long-lasting effect
- Calcitonin, Mithramycin
- Surgery: Correction of deformities; arthroplasty
- Paget sarcoma: Depends on whether there are metastases at presentation
  - Aggressive treatment: Systemic chemotherapy, wide resection, radiation
  - Palliative treatment: Stabilization of involved bone as necessary, systemic chemotherapy as indicated

DIAGNOSTIC CHECKLIST

Image Interpretation Pearls

- Preservation of regions of marrow fat in Paget disease
  - May help differentiate regions of early sarcomatous degeneration, where fat is destroyed
  - Fat also not seen in presence of fracture

SELECTED REFERENCES

1. Galson DL et al: Pathobiology of Paget's Disease of Bone. J Bone Metab. 21(2):85-98, 2014
2. Bolland MJ et al: Paget's disease of bone: clinical review and update. J Clin Pathol. 66(11):924-7, 2013

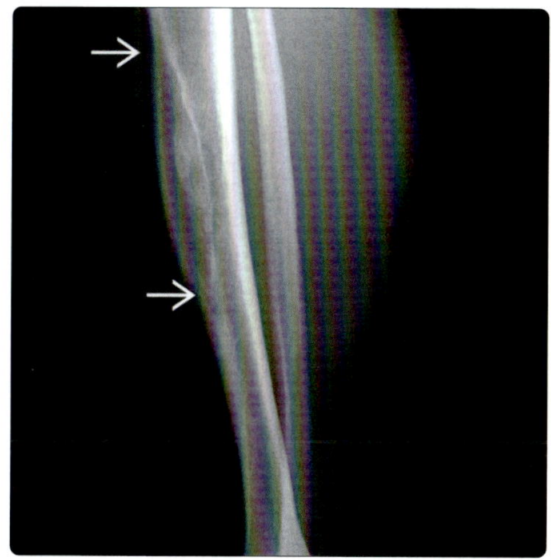

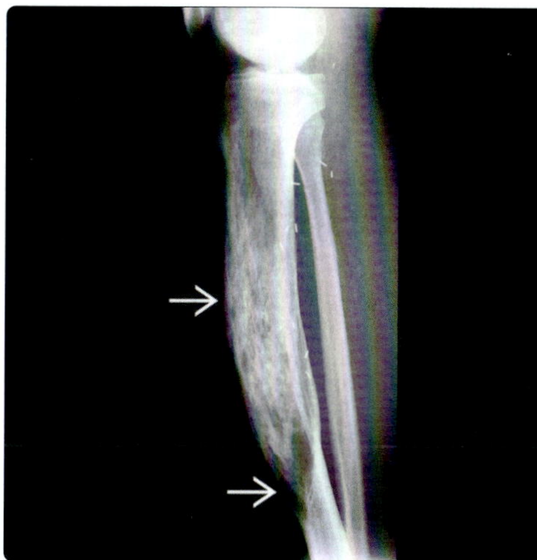

(Left) *Lateral radiograph shows a very well-demarcated mixed lytic/sclerotic lesion arising in the anterior midtibia ➡. Although the early lytic lesion in Paget disease is said to originate at the subchondral cortex of a long bone, it is good to remember that the tibia is the common exception to this rule.* **(Right)** *Lateral radiograph in the same patient 8 years later demonstrates relentless progression of Paget disease. The tibia is significantly expanded, bowed anteriorly, and has a larger and still active lesion ➡.*

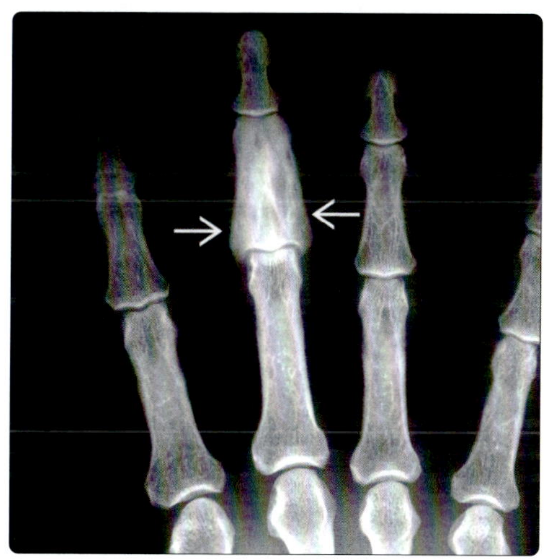

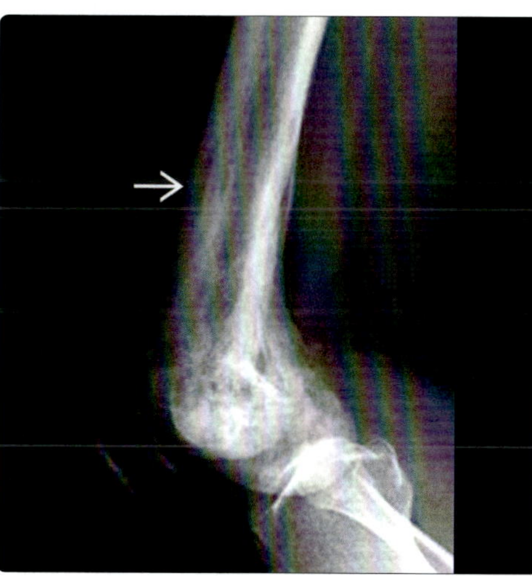

(Left) *AP radiograph shows a solitary focus of Paget disease, with a single densely sclerotic and significantly enlarged phalanx ➡. Though the site is unusual, the appearance allows almost no consideration other than Paget disease.* **(Right)** *Lateral radiograph in a 50-year-old woman shows mature Paget disease, with dense cortical thickening of the femoral cortex ➡. No significantly active lytic process is seen.*

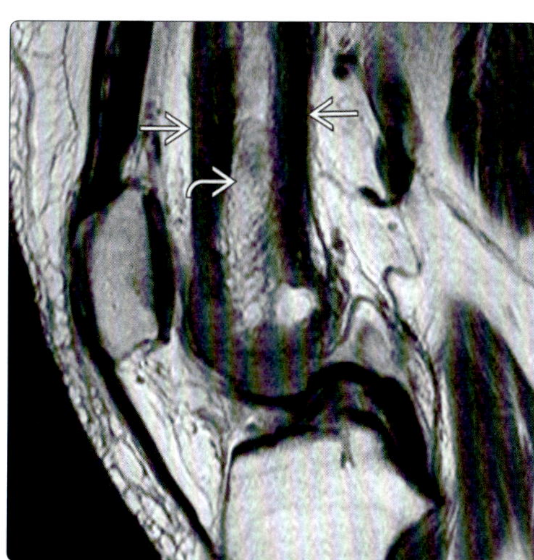

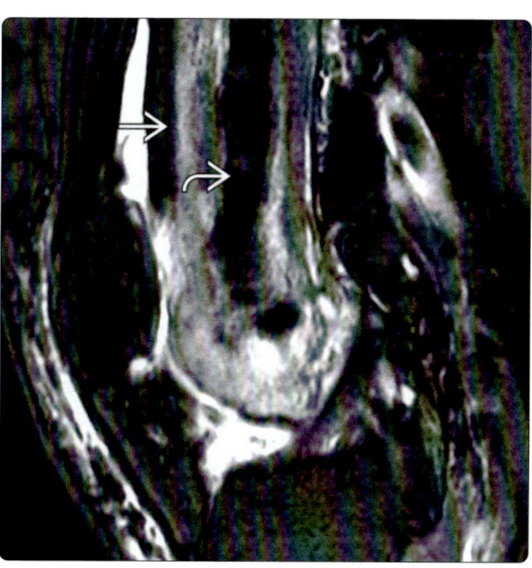

(Left) *Sagittal T1 MR in the same patient confirms the maturity of the process. The thick cortex is fairly uniformly hypointense ➡ and the central marrow ↪ shows fat replacement.* **(Right)** *Sagittal T2 FS MR in the same patient shows mild hyperintensity of the thick cortex ➡, suppression of the fatty marrow ↪, and no focal hyperintense active lesion. This is the expected appearance of a mature site of Paget disease.*

(Left) *Lateral radiograph shows the body and posterior elements of C2 to be enlarged and contain coarsened trabeculae ➡. This pattern is typical and in fact diagnostic of Paget disease. This pattern is not seen in metastatic disease or multiple myeloma.* **(Right)** *Lateral radiograph presents a classic picture frame appearance of a vertebral body ➡. The mixed lytic and dense lesion of this body is seen, along with the overall enlargement of the body. There is no reasonable diagnosis but Paget disease.*

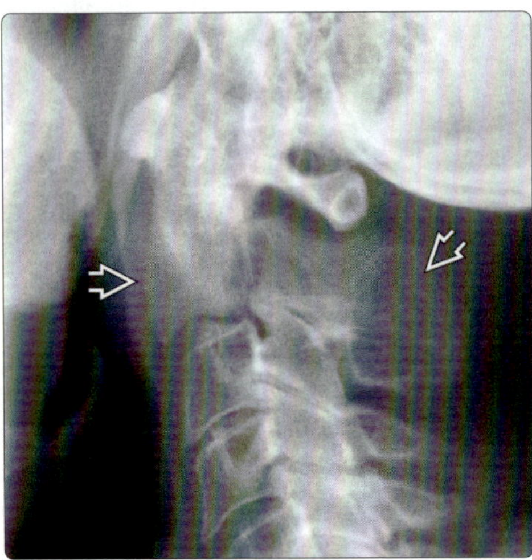

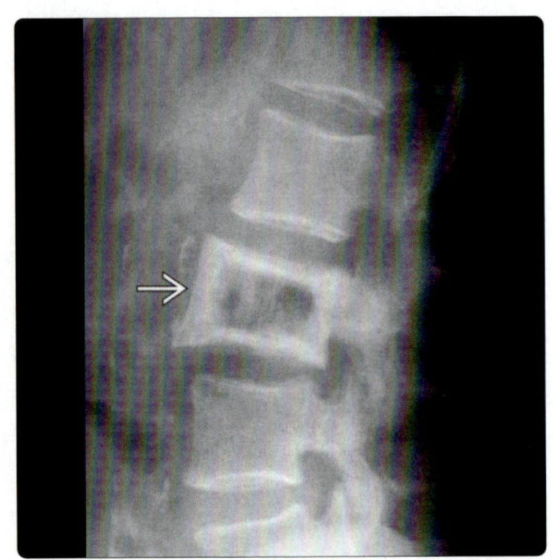

(Left) *Lateral radiograph shows a mild compression fracture but abnormal density in the L5 vertebral body, with coarse trabeculation and expansion of the body ➡. In an elderly patient, this is a typical description for Paget disease. However, there might be concern regarding destructive change anteriorly.* **(Right)** *Sagittal T2WI MR in the same patient shows the expanded vertebral body without evidence of a soft tissue mass ➡. Note the regions of residual fat within the body ➦, typical of uncomplicated Paget disease.*

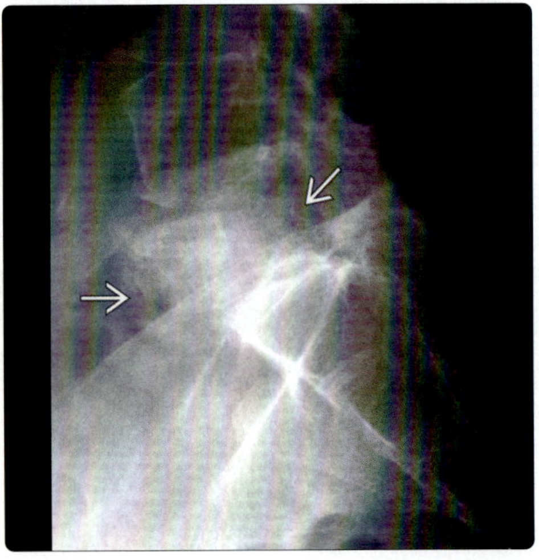

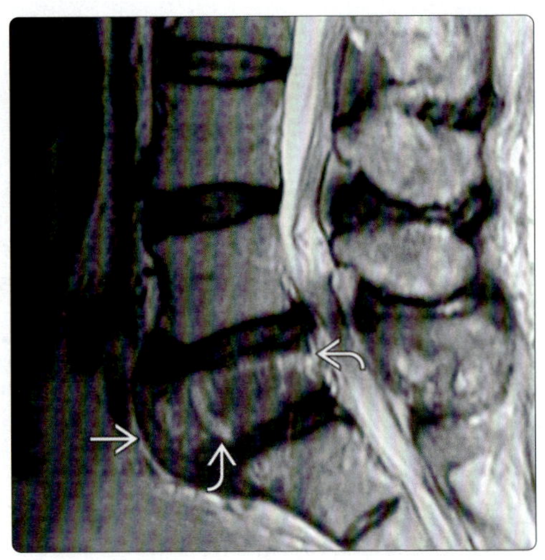

(Left) *Lateral radiograph shows osteoporosis circumscripta. This is early Paget disease involving the skull. Note the confluent lytic region of the occipital bone ➡. There is, in addition, widening of the diploic space ➦, which will progress along with disease progression.* **(Right)** *Axial T2WI MR shows Paget disease with diffuse thickening of the calvaria ➡, with diploic widening and coarsened trabeculae. Marrow exhibits an increased quantity of hyperintense fat ("atrophic marrow").*

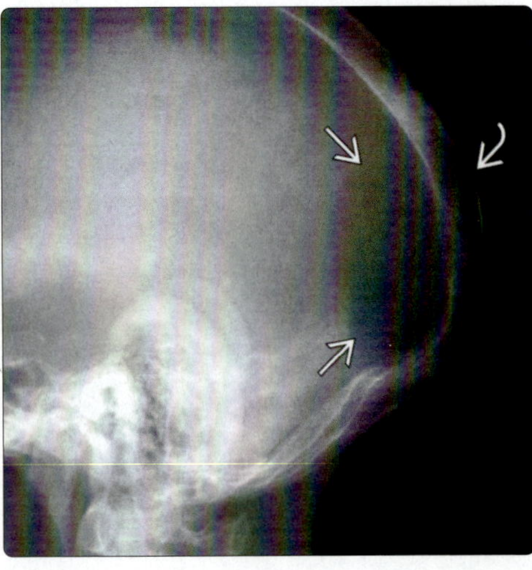

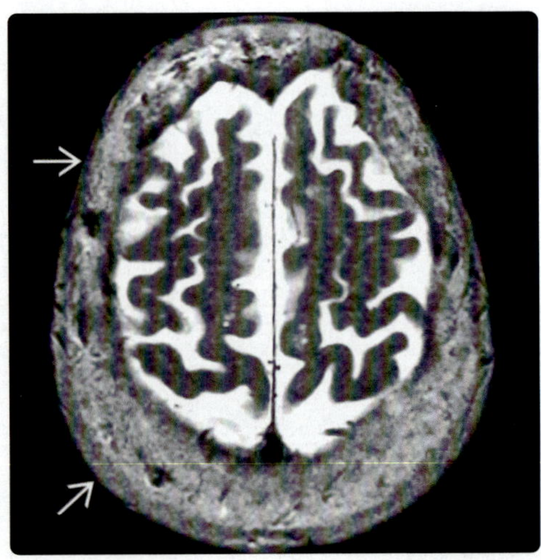

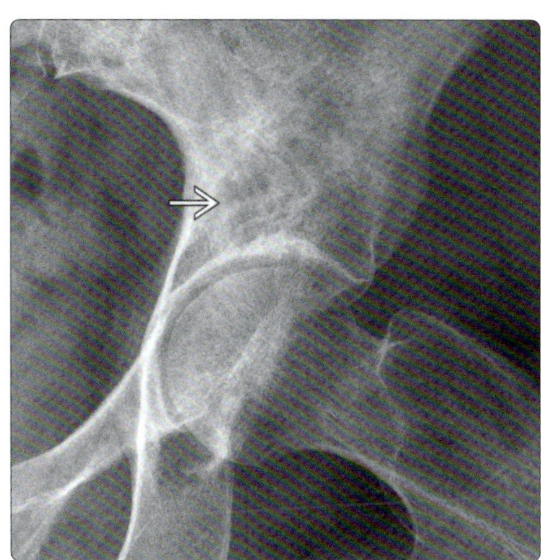

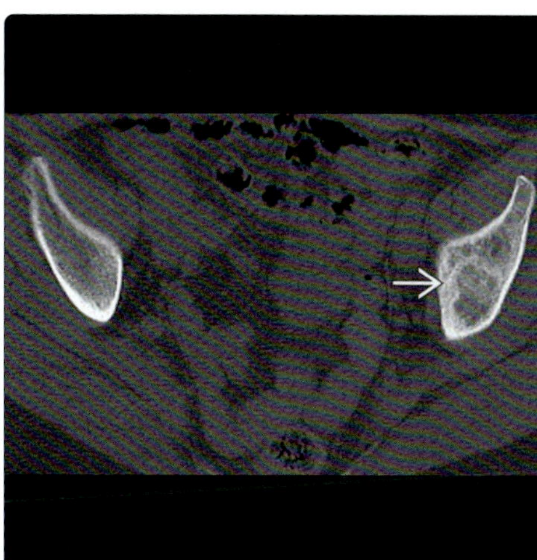

(Left) *Frog leg lateral radiograph in a 67-year-old woman with hip pain shows the trabeculae in the acetabulum ➡ to have a disordered appearance. Normally, the acetabulum shows a triangular-shaped relative lucency at this site.* **(Right)** *Axial bone CT confirms the abnormal trabecular pattern in the left acetabulum ➡. Compared with the normal right side, the left shows a mixed lytic and sclerotic pattern. Although there is only minimal medial cortical thickening, the pattern is still typical of early Paget disease.*

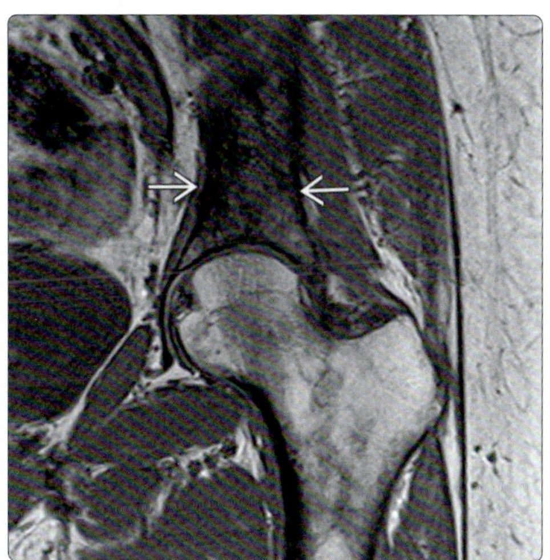

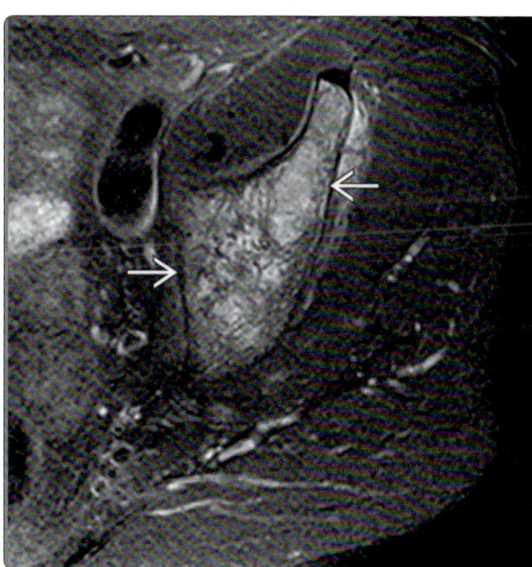

(Left) *Coronal T1 MR in the same patient shows inhomogeneous hypointense signal within the acetabulum ➡. There is no fatty marrow, as would normally be expected in a patient of this age.* **(Right)** *Axial T2 FS MR in the same patient shows inhomogeneous and disordered hyperintensity of the acetabulum ➡. There is no marrow suppression to suggest the presence of fatty marrow. This appearance, in conjunction with the radiograph, is typical of active early Paget disease.*

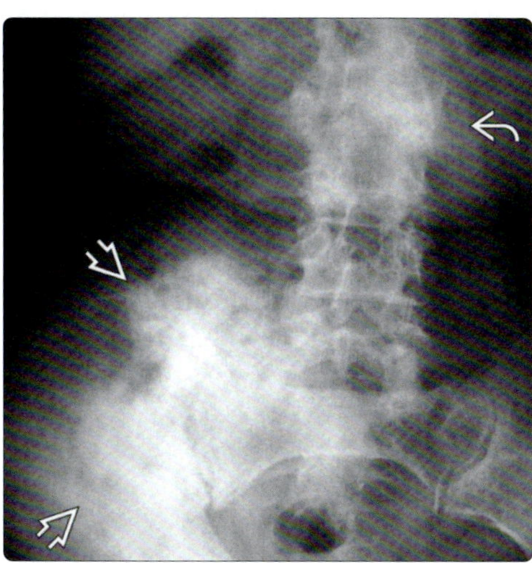

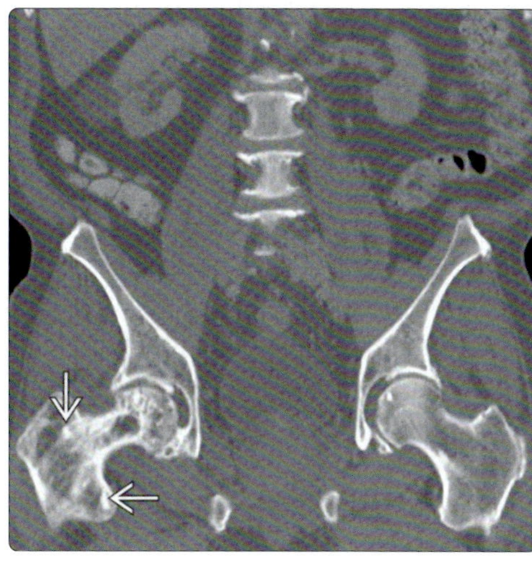

(Left) *AP radiograph shows a large Paget sarcoma arising in the iliac wing ➡ crossing into the sacrum. There is dense osteoid matrix; osteosarcoma is the most frequent type of Paget sarcoma. A 2nd site is found at L2 ➡; this may be metastatic or multifocal.* **(Right)** *Coronal bone CT demonstrates both Paget disease of the right hip and superimposed smudgy sclerotic prostate metastases ➡. It is possible that metastases preferentially are deposited in Paget bone 2° to increased blood flow.*

Langerhans Cell Histiocytosis

KEY FACTS

TERMINOLOGY

- Neoplastic proliferation of Langerhans cells

IMAGING

- Location
  - Flat bones: 65-70%
  - Long bones: 25-30%
  - Spine: 9%
- Monostotic (66-75%) more frequent than polyostotic (25-34%)
- Early lesions at any site may appear highly aggressive
  - Destructive change may be extremely rapid
- More mature lesions: Geographic, less aggressive
- Skull lesions
  - Beveled edge: Differential involvement of inner and outer tables of skull
  - May contain sequestra
- Vertebral lesions
  - Collapse results in vertebra plana; on AP radiograph, thin plate of vertebra plana, intact pedicles
- Fluid-sensitive MR sequences: Heterogeneous, high signal
  - Intense contrast enhancement of marrow abnormality and any soft tissue mass
  - Soft tissue, marrow, and fascial edema prominent, especially in aggressive lesions with cortical breakthrough, mimicking malignant tumor

CLINICAL ISSUES

- Wide age range: A few months to 8th decade
  - Mean age at diagnosis: 5-10 years
  - Disseminated form in younger patients
- Male > female (2:1)
- Generally benign course for LCH with healing following treatment
- Death associated with acute Letterer-Siwe disease
- Imaging work-up may be confusing since initial lesion presentation can be deceptively aggressive

(Left) *Lateral graphic depicts multiple lytic skull lesions, as can be seen in Langerhans cell histiocytosis (LCH). The edge of the lesions is beveled, indicating differential destruction of the inner and outer tables of the skull.* **(Right)** *AP skull radiograph shows some typical beveled edges of classic LCH ➡. The beveled edge is not pathognomonic for LCH, but it is typical and an extremely useful finding when present. In addition, sequestra ➡ are present, a finding which has also been described as typical in this disease.*

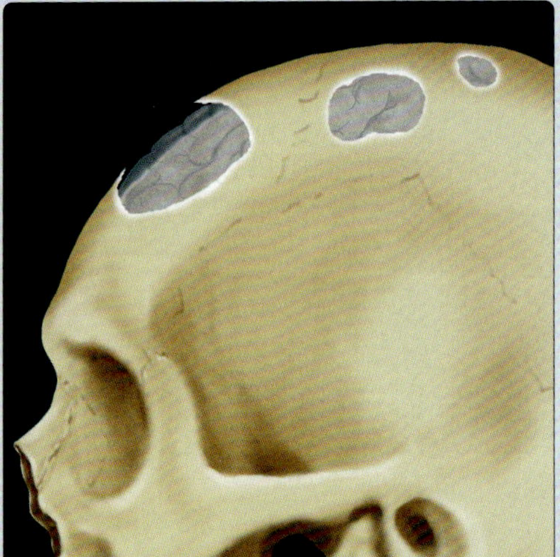

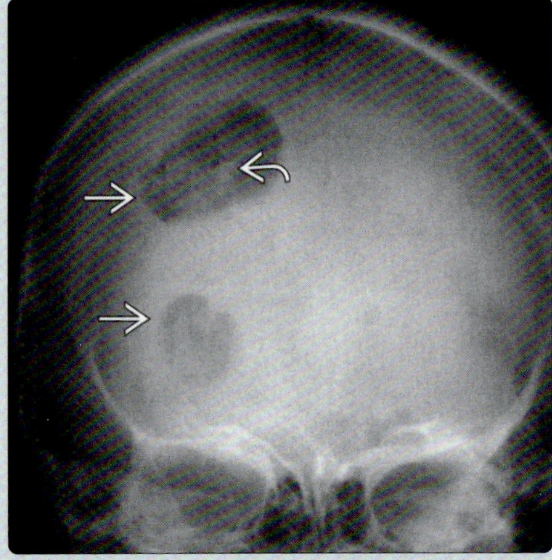

(Left) *Oblique radiograph obtained tangential to a bump on the skull shows there is a lytic lesion occupying the diploic space, which shows a beveled edge ➡. This appearance, especially in a child, is typical of LCH.* **(Right)** *Oblique T1 C+ FS MR shows the lesion to be heterogeneous, with enhancement surrounding lower signal portions of the lesion ➡. Note the differential destruction of the inner and outer tables, confirming the etiology of the beveled edge. (Courtesy K. Suh, MD.)*

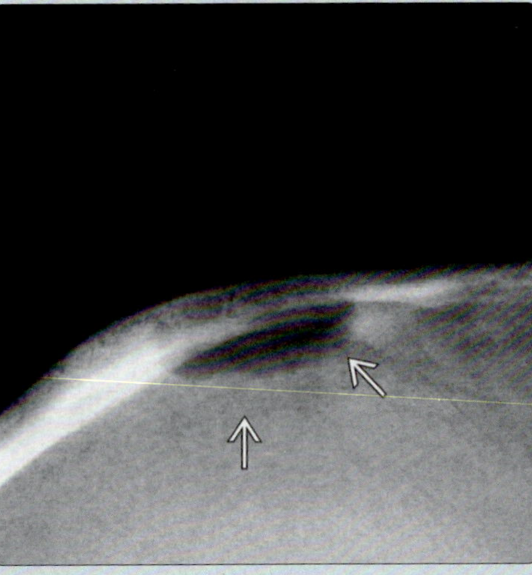

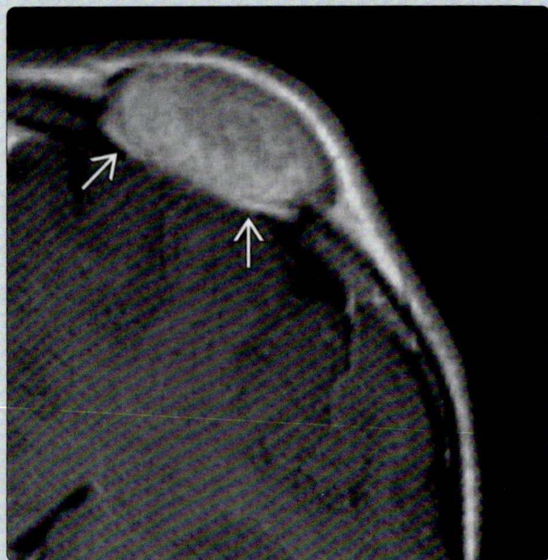

TERMINOLOGY

Abbreviations

- Langerhans cell histiocytosis (LCH)

Synonyms

- Eosinophilic granuloma (EG), Langerhans cell granulomatosis, histiocytosis X
- Clinical variants: Hand-Schüller-Christian disease, Letterer-Siwe (LS) disease

Definitions

- Neoplastic proliferation of Langerhans cells

IMAGING

General Features

- Location
  - Flat bones: 65-70%
    - Calvaria
    - Pelvis
    - Rib (most frequent site in adults)
  - Long bones: 25-30%
    - Femur, tibia, humerus
    - May arise anywhere along length of bone: Diaphysis (majority), metaphysis, epiphysis (relatively rare)
  - Spine: 9%
  - Monostotic (66-75%) > polyostotic (25-34%)
    - Polyostotic lesions appear within 1-2 years of one another
  - Rare occurrence of focal soft tissue LCH
- Size
  - Mean: 4-6 cm, range: 1-15 cm

Radiographic Findings

- Early lesions at any site may appear highly aggressive
  - Permeative, nongeographic
  - No sclerotic margin
  - Periosteal reaction
  - Cortical breakthrough, soft tissue mass
  - Destructive change may be extremely rapid
    - Faster destruction than sarcoma or osteomyelitis
- More mature lesions: Geographic, less aggressive
  - Periosteal reaction is linear if present
  - Endosteal scalloping, minimal expansion of bone
  - No soft tissue mass
- Skull lesions
  - Well-defined lytic lesion
  - Thin or no sclerotic margin
    - Thick sclerotic margin during healing phase
  - Beveled edge: Differential involvement of inner and outer tables of skull
  - May contain sequestra
  - Small lesions may coalesce → large geographic lesion
  - With cortical destruction, may → soft tissue mass
  - Floating tooth with maxillary or mandibular lesion
- Vertebral lesions
  - Affects body preferentially
    - Discs, endplates, posterior elements spared
    - Collapse results in vertebra plana; on AP x-ray, thin plate of vertebra plana, intact pedicles
  - Early in process may see paraspinal or epidural mass
  - With treatment, may reconstitute part of body height

CT Findings

- Beveled edge and sequestra more easily identified
- CT for lung involvement once diagnosis established

MR Findings

- T1WI: Homogeneous low signal
- Fluid-sensitive sequences: Heterogeneous, high signal
- Intense contrast enhancement of marrow abnormality and any soft tissue mass; may be heterogeneous
- Budding appearance of lesion described as helping to differentiate from more aggressive tumors
- Periosteal reaction outlined by high signal on fluid-sensitive and postcontrast imaging
- Marrow edema, especially in early active lesions
- Soft tissue and fascial edema prominent, especially in aggressive lesions with cortical breakthrough

Nuclear Medicine Findings

- Majority show increased uptake on bone scan
  - Normal appearance in 35% of lesions
- PET shows 35% ↑ new or recurrent lesions than x-ray

Imaging Recommendations

- Best imaging tool
  - Often diagnosed on radiograph
  - Aggressive lesion requires further work-up since malignant lesions are in differential
    - MR for site evaluation
    - Percutaneous biopsy
  - Whole-body PET/CT or MR survey to evaluate for polyostotic disease

DIFFERENTIAL DIAGNOSIS

Ewing Sarcoma

- Lytic, aggressive, permeative lesion
- Aggressive periosteal reaction, soft tissue mass
- Systemic symptoms of fever, ↑ ESR, leukocytosis like LCH
- May even mimic polyostotic LCH since Ewing may metastasize to other osseous sites
  - Ewing sarcoma generally has 1 obvious primary site, with metastases appearing smaller
- No imaging definitively differentiates Ewing sarcoma from active LCH; requires biopsy

Osteomyelitis

- Destructive change nearly as rapid as early LCH
- Lytic, permeative, aggressive lesion
- Periosteal reaction
- May have sclerotic reactive bone formation
- Systemic symptoms of fever, ↑ ESR, leukocytosis like LCH
- May not be able to differentiate by radiograph
- MR shows abscesses in bone &/or soft tissue

Metastases, Bone Marrow

- In patient age group matching that of polyostotic LCH, neuroblastoma metastases are most common
- Lytic, aggressive, permeative
- Located most frequently in metaphyses

Primary Multifocal Osseous Lymphoma

- 50% of lymphoma cases in children present multifocally
- Serpiginous, lytic, permeative lesions
- Same distribution as LCH

PATHOLOGY

General Features

- Etiology
  - Group of disorders involving abnormal proliferation of histiocytes in reticuloendothelial system
- Genetics
  - Some LCH cases demonstrated to be clonal
    - Others polyclonal, suggesting it may be reactive
- Associated abnormalities
  - 3 forms of histiocytosis
    - LS disease (acute disseminated form): 10%
      - Acute onset hepatosplenomegaly
      - Rash
      - Lymphadenopathy
      - Skeleton may not be involved in LS
    - Hand-Schüller-Christian disease (chronic disseminated): 20%
      - Exophthalmos
      - Lymphadenopathy (may be massive)
      - Hepatosplenomegaly
      - Pulmonary fibrosis
    - LCH (bone &/or lung): 70%

Gross Pathologic & Surgical Features

- Soft red mass

Microscopic Features

- Langerhans cells: Intermediate in size with indistinct cytoplasmic borders
  - Eosinophilic to clear cytoplasm with oval nuclei
- Langerhans cells found in clusters
- Admixed with inflammatory cells: Eosinophils, lymphocytes, neutrophils, plasma cells
- Necrosis common: Does not portend aggressive course
- Langerhans cells contain unique intracytoplasmic "tennis racket" inclusions (Birbeck granules)

CLINICAL ISSUES

Presentation

- Most common signs/symptoms
  - Pain and swelling
  - Vertebra plana: Back pain &/or neurologic symptoms
  - Fever, elevated ESR, leukocytosis, peripheral eosinophilia
    - Systemic symptoms plus aggressive appearance suggest other aggressive lesions as well as LCH
      - Osteomyelitis or Ewing sarcoma
  - Lung, lymph node involvement common
- Other signs/symptoms
  - Loosening of teeth with mandibular involvement
  - Mucocutaneous involvement in 50-55% of LCH
    - Skin 2nd most common site after bone

Demographics

- Age
  - Wide age range: A few months to 8th decade
    - Mean age at diagnosis: 5-10 years
  - 80-85% in patients under age 30
  - 60% in patients under age 10
  - Disseminated form at younger age (< 2 years)
- Gender
  - Male > female (2:1)
- Ethnicity
  - More common in Caucasian population
- Epidemiology
  - 1% of all osseous tumor and tumor-like lesions

Natural History & Prognosis

- Spontaneous remission of some lesions reported over 3-month to 2-year period
- Generally benign course for LCH with healing following treatment
- Death associated with acute LS disease
- Variable prognosis for Hand-Schüller-Christian disease

Treatment

- Observation if stable and no risk of fracture
- Resolution of LCH observed over period of 11-14 months, regardless of treatment modality
  - Curettage and bone grafting/stabilization if painful or at risk of fracture
  - Steroid injection
  - Chemotherapy if multisystem disease
  - Radiation therapy if surgically inaccessible
    - Risk of radiation-induced sarcoma
    - Avoided if possible; reserve for specific indications
- Spine lesions may require decompression/stabilization

DIAGNOSTIC CHECKLIST

Consider

- Aggressive early phase of LCH may mimic other aggressive "small round blue cell" lesions
  - Ewing sarcoma, osteomyelitis, neuroblastoma metastasis, lymphoma
- Late phase suggests nonaggressive or benign process

Image Interpretation Pearls

- Extremely rapid growth may occur in LCH
  - Lesions may appear over 2-week period
  - Much faster than tumor; slightly faster than infection
  - Sequential radiographs or history (if reliable) showing this rapid evolution may suggest LCH

SELECTED REFERENCES

1. Amini B et al: Soft tissue Langerhans cell histiocytosis with secondary bone involvement in extremities: evolution of lesions in two patients. Skeletal Radiol. 42(9):1301-9, 2013
2. Song YS et al: Radiologic findings of adult pelvis and appendicular skeletal Langerhans cell histiocytosis in nine patients. Skeletal Radiol. 40(11):1421-6, 2011
3. Arkader A et al: Primary musculoskeletal Langerhans cell histiocytosis in children: an analysis for a 3-decade period. J Pediatr Orthop. 29(2):201-7, 2009

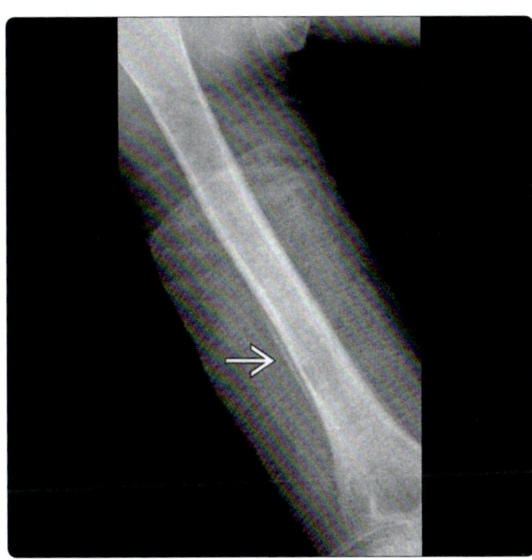

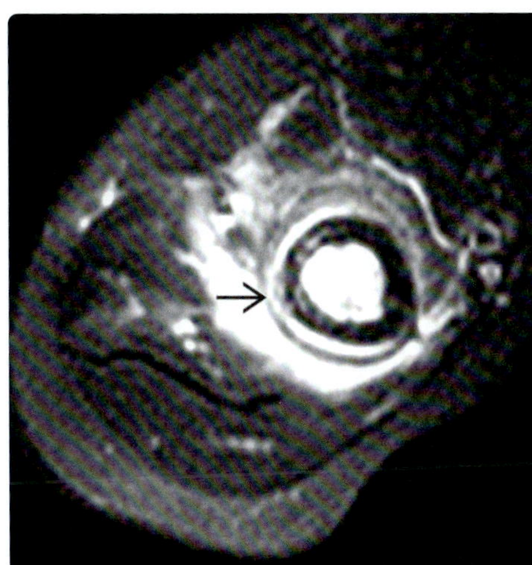

(Left) *AP radiograph obtained immediately following trauma shows an aggressive permeative lesion within the mid diaphysis of the humerus. There is prominent periosteal reaction* ➡. **(Right)** *Axial T2WI FS MR in the same patient shows a hyperintense soft tissue mass surrounding the osseous abnormality. Periosteal reaction is prominent* ➡. *These findings of an aggressive diaphyseal lesion are typical of Ewing sarcoma but either osteomyelitis or LCH may have a similar appearance.*

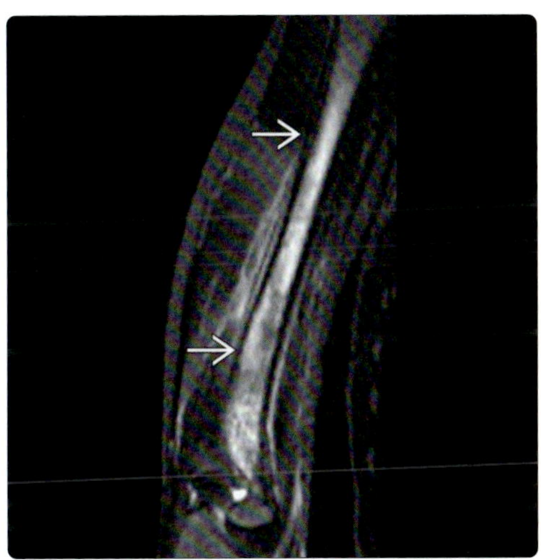

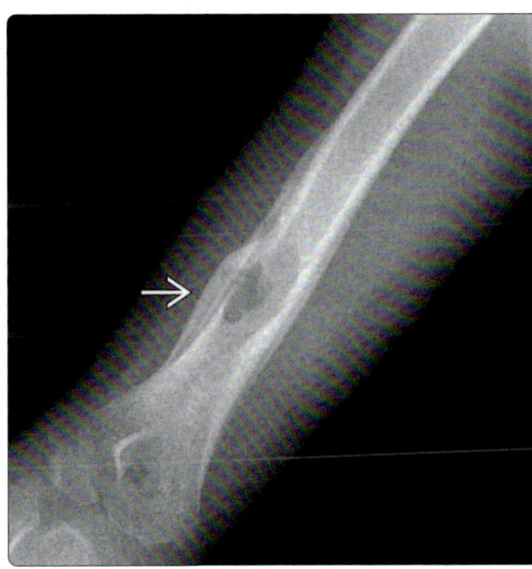

(Left) *Sagittal T1WI C+ FS MR in the same patient shows the osseous abnormality to be even more extensive than suspected* ➡. *No abscess formation is demonstrated, which reduces the differential to Ewing sarcoma vs. LCH. Biopsy proved LCH.* **(Right)** *AP radiograph obtained 1 year later in the same patient shows the lesion is beginning to heal, with thick nonaggressive-appearing periosteal reaction* ➡. *While the early appearance of LCH may be alarming, over time it acts and also appears less aggressive.*

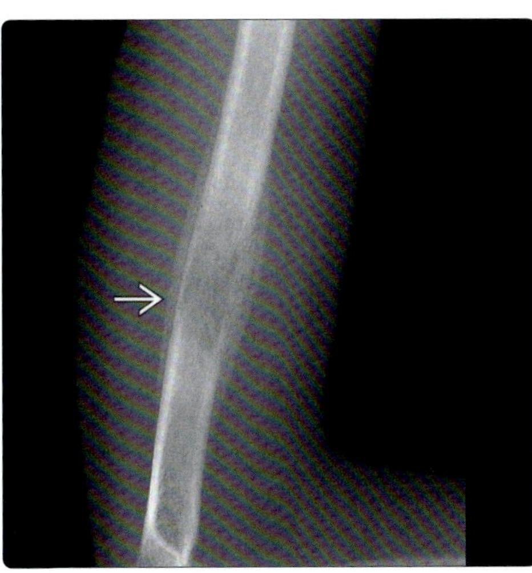

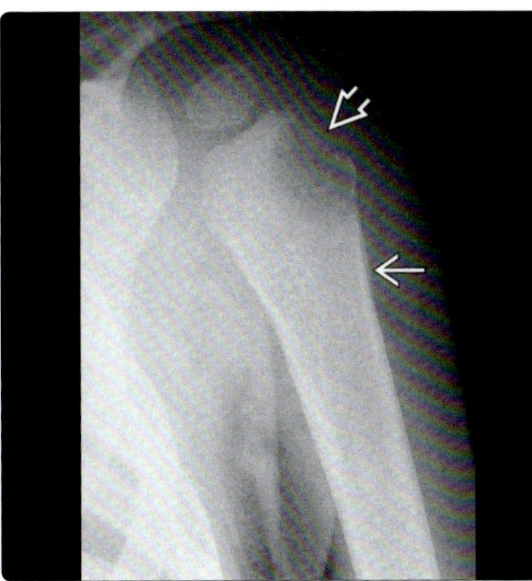

(Left) *Lateral radiograph in a young patient shows a highly permeative diaphyseal lesion, which has engendered prominent periosteal reaction* ➡. *The most likely, and most feared diagnosis for this appearance, is Ewing sarcoma. Biopsy showed LCH.* **(Right)** *AP radiograph shows a lytic, ill-defined lesion* ➡, *which had elicited periosteal reaction* ➡. *Given the young age of the patient (18 months), LCH, osteomyelitis, or neuroblastoma metastasis are more likely than Ewing sarcoma. Biopsy proved LCH.*

(Left) *Lateral radiograph demonstrates a lytic permeative lesion within the distal humeral metaphysis ➡, which has elicited dense periosteal reaction ➡. The most likely differential diagnosis in this patient age group includes Ewing sarcoma, LCH, osteomyelitis, metastases, and leukemia.* **(Right)** *Coronal T2WI FS MR shows the lesion to be heterogeneous but high signal. Periosteal reaction is well demonstrated ➡. Cortical breakthrough with soft tissue mass is confirmed ➡.*

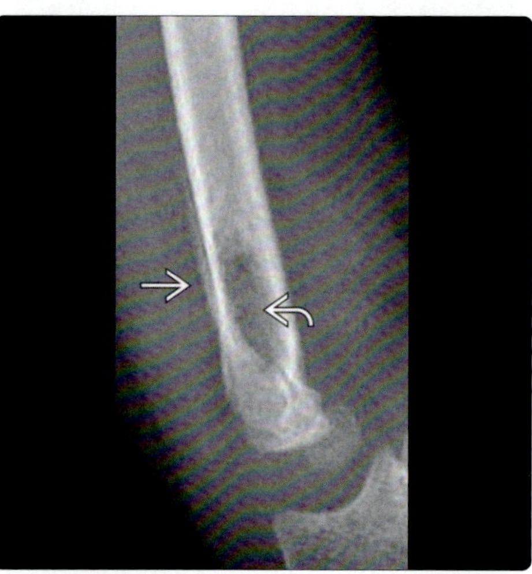

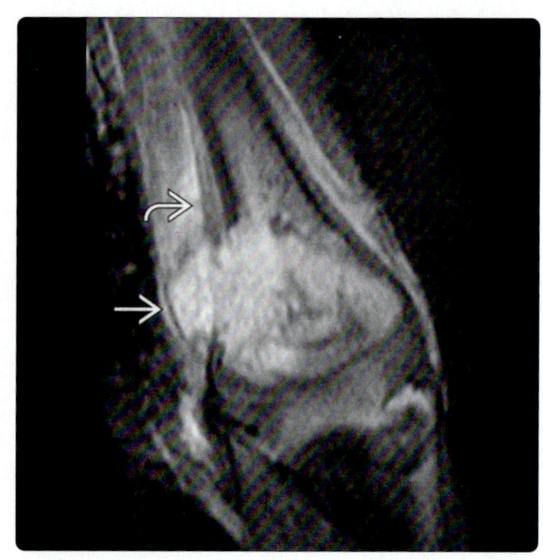

(Left) *Coronal T1WI C+ FS MR shows differential enhancement of the lesion ➡. The MR serves to more fully describe site involvement but does not help differentiate histology. Biopsy showed LCH. It is important to remember that LCH may behave aggressively and cortical breakthrough is not uncommon early in the process. (Courtesy K. Suh, MD.)* **(Right)** *AP radiograph shows polyostotic LCH with multiple lytic osseous lesions in the pelvis ➡, all with a nonaggressive pattern.*

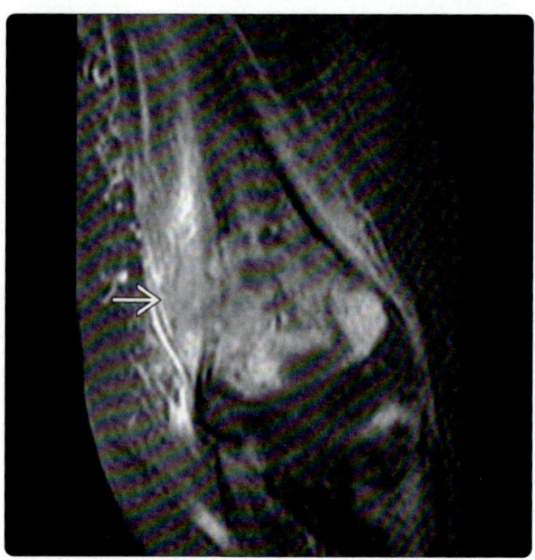

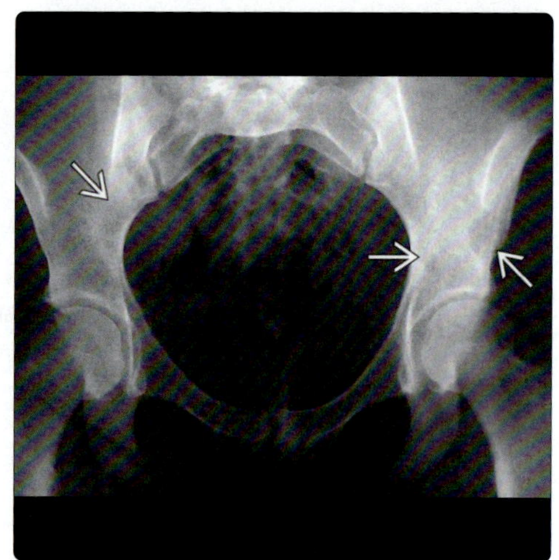

(Left) *AP radiograph shows a well-circumscribed lytic lesion within the left femoral head epiphysis ➡. Differential diagnoses includes LCH, chondroblastoma, and Brodie abscess.* **(Right)** *Coronal T2WI FS MR in the same patient shows a heterogeneously high signal epiphyseal lesion ➡. No joint effusion or physeal involvement is seen. Biopsy revealed LCH. Epiphyseal lesions are uncommon, but in children, LCH should always be considered. Presentation may be either aggressive or nonaggressive, as in this case.*

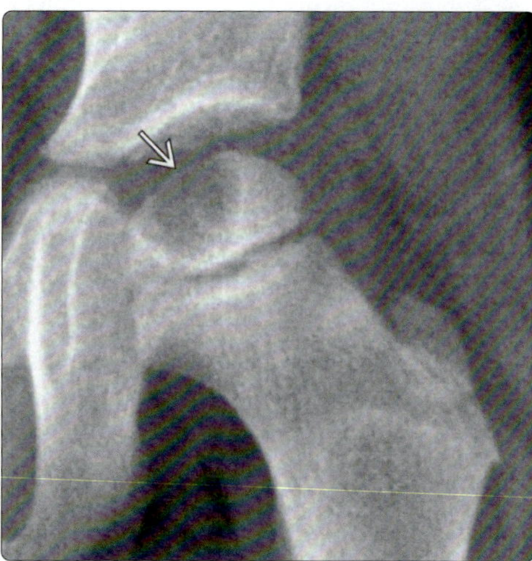

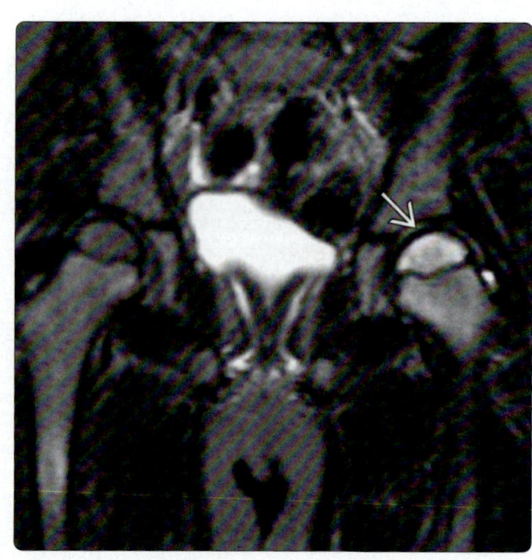

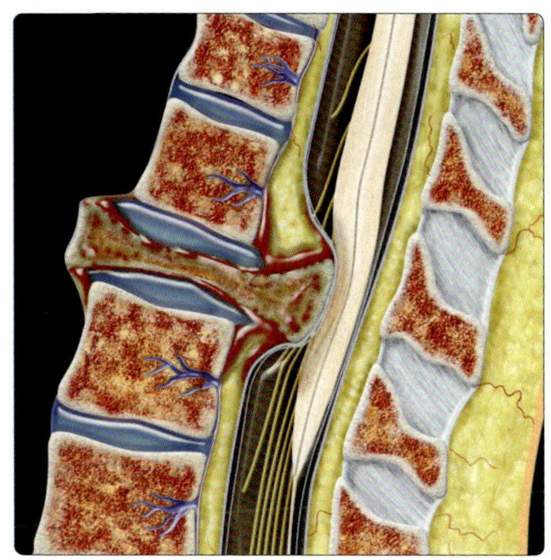

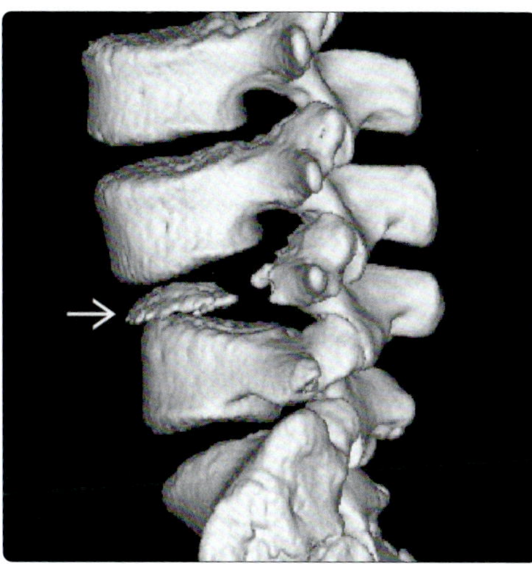

(Left) *Sagittal graphic depicts LCH of the vertebral body. The discs and endplates are usually spared, as are the posterior elements. Involvement of the entire body may result in vertebra plana.* **(Right)** *3D reconstructed NECT shows severe vertebral plana ➡. Despite the severity of body involvement, the posterior elements appear to be intact. Vertebra plana may be seen in children with Ewing sarcoma or neuroblastoma metastases, but LCH should be strongly considered, as was proven by biopsy in this case.*

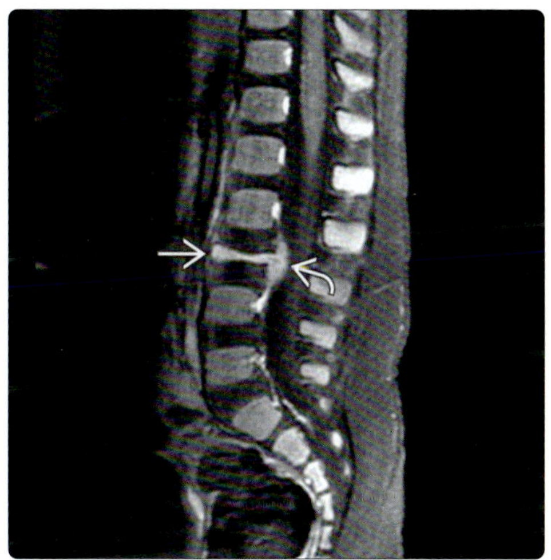

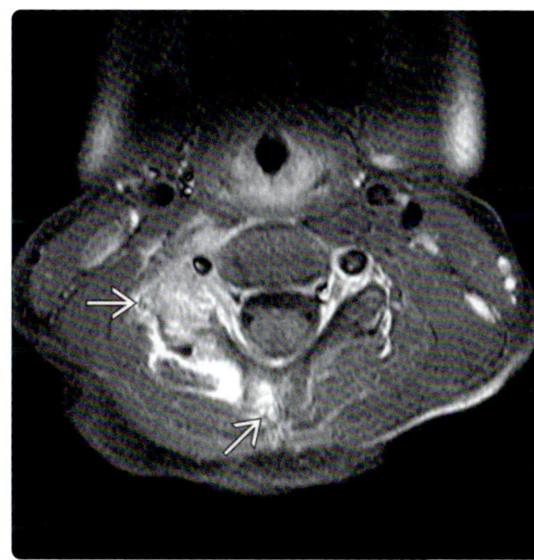

(Left) *Sagittal T1WI C+ FS MR shows a typical case of vertebral plana secondary to LCH ➡. There is posterior epidural extension ↪, which is often present; it lifts and extends under the posterior longitudinal ligament.* **(Right)** *Axial T1WI C+ FS MR shows an unusual case of LCH involving the posterior elements, with marked enhancement of an associated soft tissue mass ➡. Lymphadenopathy is present. Soft tissue masses are common during the early phase of LCH but regress with evolution of lesions.*

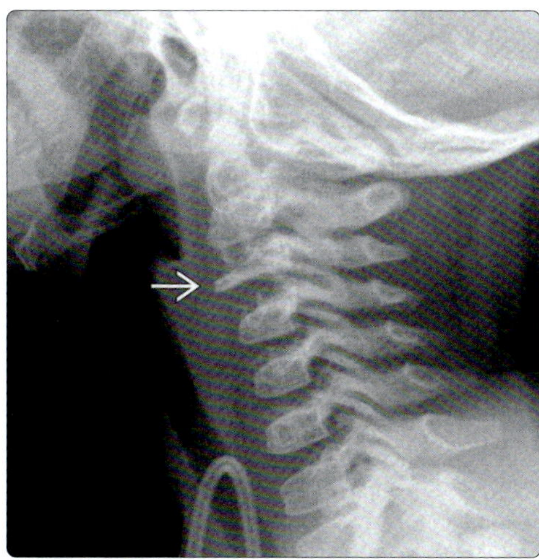

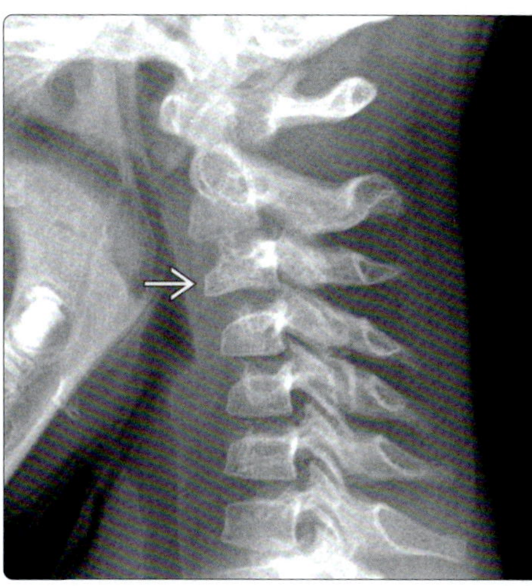

(Left) *Lateral radiograph shows typical C3 vertebral plana ➡ in a child with multiple other skeletal lesions (not visible here). With intact disc spaces and posterior elements, LCH is the most likely diagnosis and was proven by biopsy.* **(Right)** *Lateral radiograph in the same patient 3 years later shows the lesion has resolved and the vertebral height is nearly completely reconstituted ➡. Such reconstitution of height may occur following treatment of LCH since the vertebral endplates generally remain intact.*

Fibrous Dysplasia

KEY FACTS

TERMINOLOGY

- Benign fibroosseous lesion

IMAGING

- Polyostotic in 15-20%
  - Tends to be unilateral, though not reliably
- Location
  - Diaphyseal; often extends to metaphysis and occasionally to epiphysis
  - Lesion usually central within bone, causing varying degrees of expansion
- Radiographic appearance
  - Density varies from lytic to densely sclerotic
    - Lytic bubbly appearance often seen in pelvic lesions
    - Densely sclerotic lesions may be seen in base of skull
    - Most lesions are mildly sclerotic ground glass, relating to amount of woven bone within lesion
  - Bowing deformities of long bones
    - Varus femoral neck ("shepherd's crook")
  - Polyostotic form → limb length discrepancy (70%)
- MR appearance
  - T1WI MR: Homogeneous low signal intensity
  - Fluid-sensitive MR sequences: Range from very high signal to mildly high signal superimposed on low signal
  - Avid heterogeneous enhancement of active lesions; inactive lesions show more mild enhancement
  - May have associated aneurysmal bone cyst with fluid-fluid levels
- FDG PET shows variable metabolic activity

CLINICAL ISSUES

- May be asymptomatic if monostotic
- Polyostotic form: 2/3 symptomatic by age 10
  - McCune-Albright syndrome
  - Mazabraud syndrome
- Extremely rare malignant transformation (0.5%)
- Treatment: Only complications are treated
  - May treat with bisphosphonates

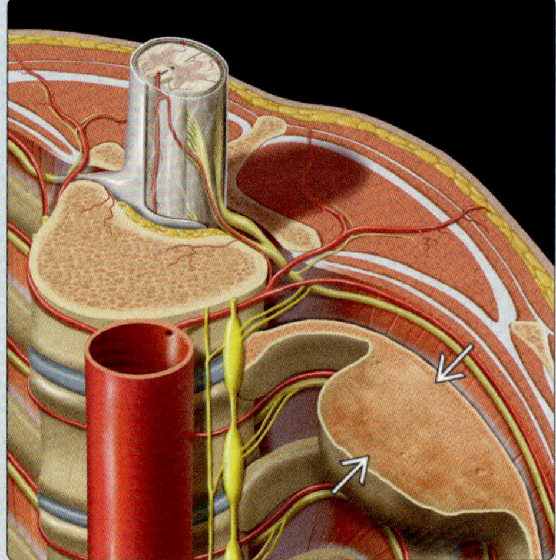

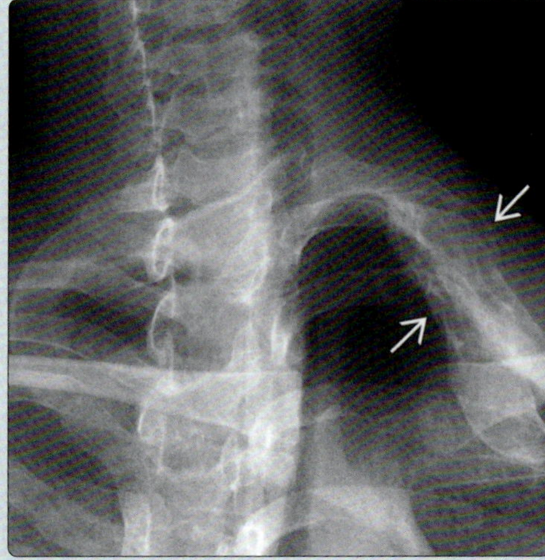

(Left) *Graphic depicts a transected rib containing a focus of fibrous dysplasia (FD). The expanded lesion contains solid white and tan tissue ➡; the cut surface has a gritty consistency due to the irregular foci of woven bone trabeculae. The adjacent rib contains normal cancellous and cortical bone.* **(Right)** *Oblique radiograph in a patient with left brachial plexus symptoms shows a bubbly lytic lesion of the 1st rib ➡, which does not appear aggressive. FD should be strongly considered.*

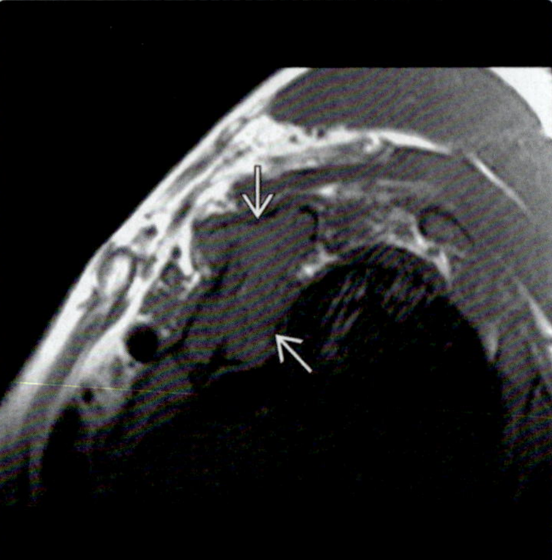

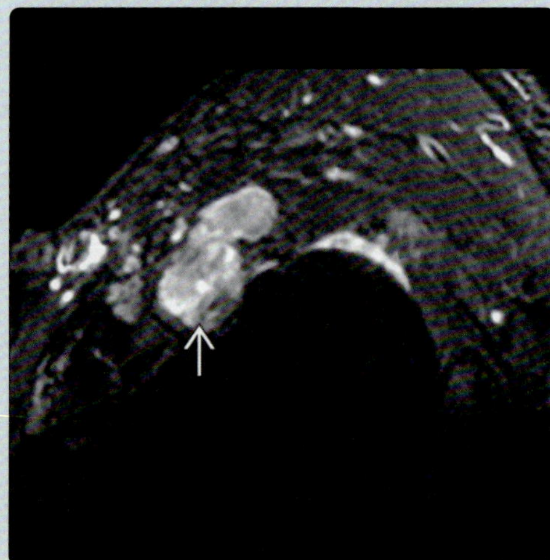

(Left) *Sagittal T1WI MR shows the rib lesion to be relatively homogeneous ➡ and isointense to skeletal muscle. It appears to be contained by thin but intact cortex.* **(Right)** *Sagittal STIR MR shows the expanded lesion to be heterogeneously hyperintense ➡; areas of low signal correspond to regions of ground-glass matrix. The brachial plexus is deviated and compressed. The rib lesion is typical of FD, the most common benign expanded rib lesion found in the adult population.*

TERMINOLOGY

Abbreviations

- Fibrous dysplasia (FD)

Synonyms

- Fibrocartilaginous dysplasia, generalized fibrocystic disease of bone, osteitis fibrosa

Definitions

- Benign fibroosseous lesion

IMAGING

General Features

- Best diagnostic clue
  - Mild to moderate expansion of marrow with range of sclerosis, most commonly ground glass
- Location
  - Polyostotic in 15-20%
    - Pelvis, femur, tibia, virtually any bone
    - Tends to be unilateral, though not reliably
  - Monostotic lesions (80-85%)
    - Long bones
      - Femur (35-40%)
      - Tibia (20%)
    - Skull (cranium, base of skull) (20-34%)
    - Ribs (10-28%)
  - Lesions usually arise centrally within bone
    - Uncommonly based in cortex; tibia is most common site for cortically based FD
  - Diaphyseal; often extend to metaphysis and occasionally to epiphysis
- Size
  - 1 cm to involvement of entire bone

Radiographic Findings

- Geographic lesion
- Density varies from lytic to densely sclerotic
  - Lytic bubbly appearance often seen in pelvic lesions
  - Densely sclerotic lesions may be seen in base of skull
  - Most lesions are mildly sclerotic
    - Termed ground glass, relating to amount of woven bone within lesion
- Lesion usually central within bone, causing varying degrees of expansion
  - Expansion greatest in pelvic lesions
  - Skull and mandible lesions may be so expanded as to give appearance of cherubism
    - Tends to involve only 1 side of skull
  - Long bones tend to have more mild expansion
    - Smooth endosteal thinning
- No periosteal reaction
- No cortical breakthrough or soft tissue mass
- Bowing deformities of long bones
  - Due to microfractures of abnormal bone along primary weight-bearing portion of bone
  - Varus deformity of femoral neck ("shepherd's crook")
  - Anterior tibial bowing
  - Protrusio acetabulum
- Polyostotic form → limb length discrepancy (70%)
  - Due to bowing deformities + hyperemia with early fusion

MR Findings

- T1WI: Homogeneous low signal intensity
- Fluid-sensitive sequences: Lesions range from very high signal to mildly high signal superimposed on low signal
  - Depends on amount of woven bone within lesion
  - Cysts appear rounded, high signal
- Avid heterogeneous enhancement of active lesions; inactive lesions show more mild enhancement
  - Hypointense cysts on T1WI C+ FS
- May have associated aneurysmal bone cyst (ABC)
  - ABC portion of lesion shows loculated cysts with fluid-fluid levels

Nuclear Medicine Findings

- Increased uptake in majority of lesions
- FDG PET shows variable metabolic activity; SUV in late stage may either ↑ or ↓

Image-Guided Biopsy

- Fine-needle aspiration (FNA) generally yields inadequate tissue for biopsy

DIFFERENTIAL DIAGNOSIS

DDx of Skull Fibrous Dysplasia

- Paget disease
  - Focal to diffuse widening of diploic space
  - Density ranges from osteoporosis (osteoporosis circumscripta) to dense (cotton wool appearance)
  - Tends to involve both sides of skull; FD usually involves only 1
- Metastases, bone marrow

DDx of Pelvic Fibrous Dysplasia (Bubbly)

- Giant cell tumor
  - Entirely lytic
  - Narrow zone of transition; no sclerotic margin
- SBC
  - When SBC occurs in adults, it is often in pelvis
  - Nonspecific lytic lesion with mildly sclerotic margin on radiograph
  - MR confirms cystic nature of lesion

DDx of Tubular Bone Fibrous Dysplasia

- Simple bone cyst
  - Central lytic, mildly expanded, thinning of cortex
  - Metaphyseal or metadiaphyseal, depending on age
  - Fallen fragment sign on radiograph
  - MR confirms cystic nature of lesion
- Ollier disease
  - May be polyostotic, often unilateral, as is polyostotic FD
  - Lesions usually metaphyseal, leaving normal diaphysis; FD more often involves diaphysis
  - Striated appearance of lesions; ± chondroid matrix
  - Limb length discrepancy in both Ollier and FD
- In tibia, when originates in cortex, FD is indistinguishable from either of the following
  - Adamantinoma
  - Osteofibrous dysplasia

PATHOLOGY

General Features

- Etiology
  - Developmental dysplasia
    - Abnormal differentiation of osteoblasts → replacement of normal marrow and cancellous bone by immature bone and fibrous stroma
- Genetics
  - Predisposition to somatic mutations of skeleton-forming mesenchymal tissue
    - Activating mutations of *GNAS* gene, encoding α-subunit of stimulatory G protein seen in both mono- and polyostotic forms
    - Clonal chromosome aberrations (3, 8, 10, 12, 15) suggest lesion is neoplastic
    - Increased levels of c-fos oncoprotein

Gross Pathologic & Surgical Features

- Tan-gray tissue
- Firm to gritty texture
- Cysts may be present, containing yellowish fluid
- Blue-tinged, translucent foci of cartilage

Microscopic Features

- Fibrous and osseous tissues in varying proportions
  - Proportions vary from lesion to lesion
  - Proportions vary within lesion
- Fibrous portion: Cytologically bland spindle cells
- Osseous: Irregular curvilinear trabeculae of woven bone
- 10% contain foci of cartilage

CLINICAL ISSUES

Presentation

- Most common signs/symptoms
  - May be asymptomatic if monostotic
  - Polyostotic form: 2/3 symptomatic by age 10
  - Painful if associated with microfractures (particularly femoral neck or tibia)
- Other signs/symptoms
  - May be associated with oncogenic osteomalacia
    - Present with fractures
  - May have abnormal cranio-facial appearance
    - Cherubism: Symmetric involvement of mandible and maxilla
      - Autosomal dominant or sporadic
      - May be considered variant of FD; actually form of giant cell reparative granuloma
      - Variable progression until puberty; may regress in adulthood
    - Leontiasis ossea: Involvement of facial and frontal bones with lion-like physiognomy caused by severe craniofacial osseous thickening
    - Cranial nerve palsies
  - McCune-Albright syndrome
    - Polyostotic unilateral FD
    - Endocrine abnormalities
      - Sexual precocity: Presents with abnormal vaginal bleeding
      - Hyperthyroidism
      - Diabetes mellitus
      - Hyperparathyroidism (presents with rickets)
      - Acromegaly
    - Café au lait spots, coast of Maine appearance
      - May correspond to sites of skeletal involvement
    - Female predominance
  - Mazabraud syndrome
    - Polyostotic FD
    - Multiple fibrous & myxomatous soft tissue tumors
    - Greater incidence of malignant transformation to osteosarcoma

Demographics

- Age
  - May present at any age (usually 5-50 years)
    - 75% present by age 30
  - Polyostotic form tends to present earlier (mean age of 8 years) than monostotic
- Gender
  - M = F (except in McCune-Albright syndrome, in which female patients predominate)
- Epidemiology
  - 1% of biopsied primary bone tumors
  - Most common benign lesion of rib

Natural History & Prognosis

- Monostotic form does not progress to polyostotic FD
- Monostotic: Growth usually stabilizes at puberty
  - Lesion remains; does not involute or heal
  - Lesions may ↑ in size during pregnancy
- Polyostotic form: Lesions tend to become less active after puberty
  - Generally, new lesions do not develop
  - Deformities may progress
- Complications: Microfractures and bowing deformities
- Pathologic fracture heals poorly with dysplastic callus
- Extremely rare malignant transformation (0.5%)
  - May occur in either polyostotic or monostotic FD
  - Osteosarcoma > fibrosarcoma > chondrosarcoma
  - Most frequently involve craniofacial bones or femur
  - 33-50% of those reported had prior radiation and are considered radiation-induced sarcoma
  - Poor prognosis

Treatment

- Only complications are treated
  - Deformities may be treated with osteotomy and bone graft/stabilization
- Attempted curettage and bone grafting results in high rate of recurrence (approaches 100%)
- May treat with bisphosphonates
- Treat associated endocrine abnormalities

DIAGNOSTIC CHECKLIST

Consider

- If percutaneous biopsy of FD requested, FNA generally not adequate; plan on core biopsy

SELECTED REFERENCES

1. Su MG et al: Recognition of fibrous dysplasia of bone mimicking skeletal metastasis on 18F-FDG PET/CT imaging. Skeletal Radiol. 40(3):295-302, 2011

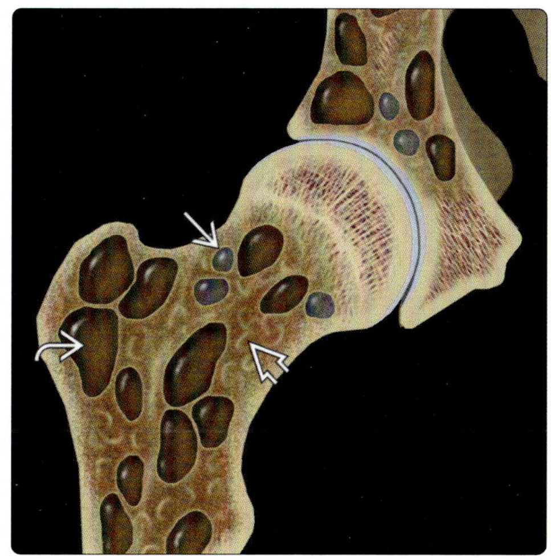

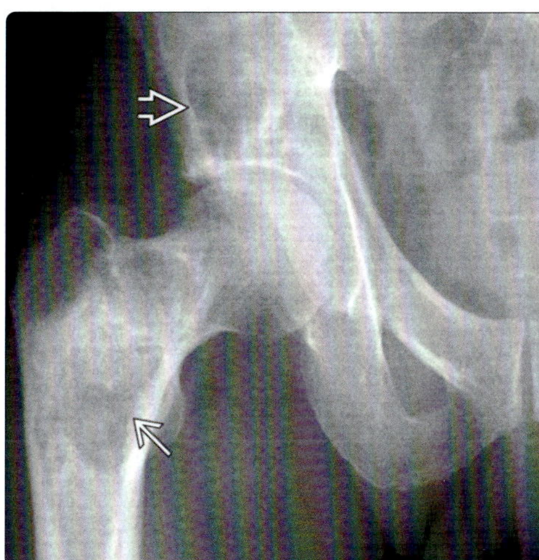

(Left) *Coronal graphic depicts FD. Cystic regions contain yellowish fluid; focal regions of cartilage are seen as well. The tan gritty material consists of spindle cells containing curvilinear woven bone fragments. Note the acetabular involvement, commonly seen associated with femoral neck FD.* **(Right)** *AP radiograph shows mixed lytic sclerotic lesions of the femoral neck typical of FD, with varus deformity of the femoral neck. Note that there is acetabular involvement as well.*

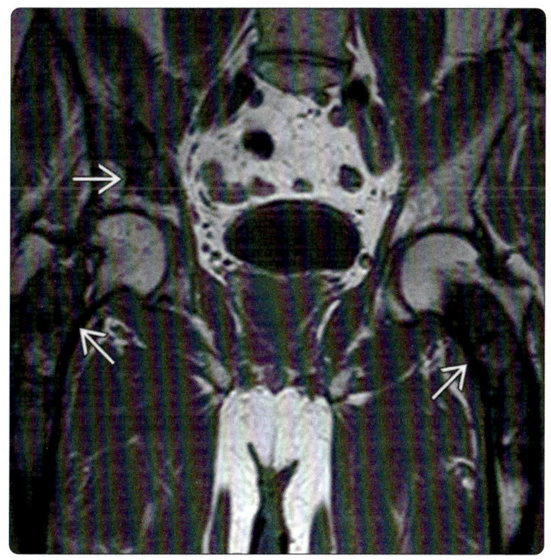

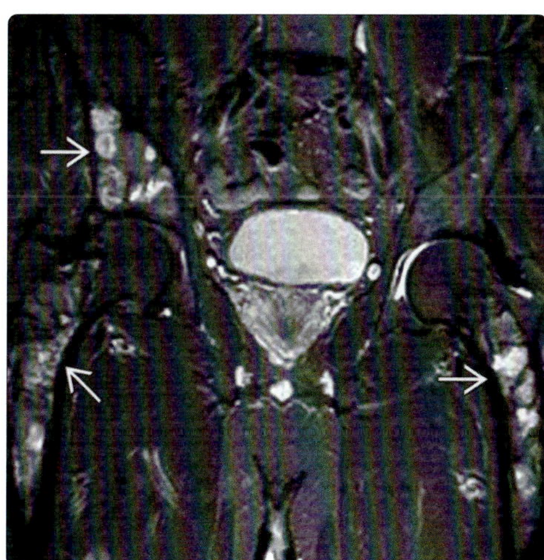

(Left) *Coronal T1WI MR in a patient with polyostotic FD shows fairly uniform hypointensity, similar in signal to skeletal muscle, in all involved areas. Regions of residual bone show normal marrow signal.* **(Right)** *Coronal STIR MR in the same patient shows mixed high and low signal in all regions involved with FD, corresponding to the presence of ground-glass osteoid. There is more involvement of the right femoral neck than the left, resulting in right varus deformity.*

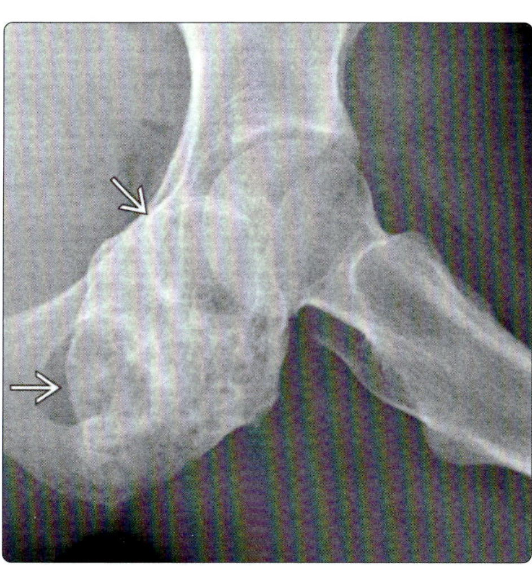

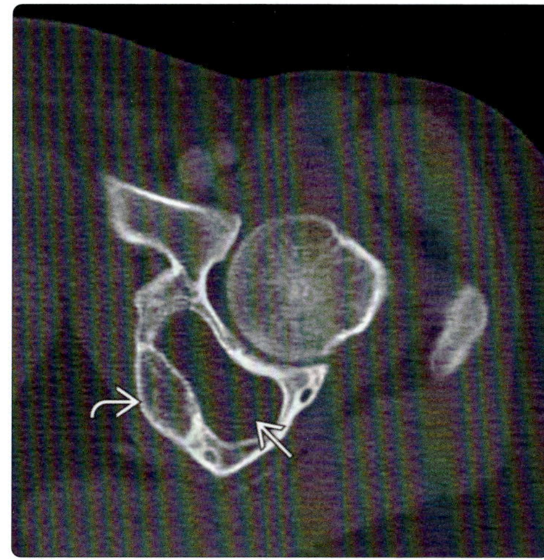

(Left) *AP radiograph demonstrates an expanded, bubbly lesion arising in the left ischium. The lesion is not aggressive; it has mixed lytic and ground-glass sclerotic regions, diagnostic of FD. Without demonstration of a stalk extending to normal bone, exophytic exostosis should not be considered.* **(Right)** *Axial bone CT in the same patient shows the mixed lytic and ground-glass sclerotic regions, which are typical and diagnostic of FD. No further work-up is required.*

(Left) *AP radiograph shows classic FD in the shaft of the tibia, with its mild widening of the bone, thinning of the cortex, and ground-glass dysplasia ➔. There are also round lytic lesions in the distal tibial epiphysis and talus, which represent cystic FD ➯.* **(Right)** *Sagittal T1WI MR in the same patient shows uniform low signal in both the ground-glass tibial shaft lesion ➔ and the cystic talar lesions ➯. The unaffected bone retains normal high-signal marrow.*

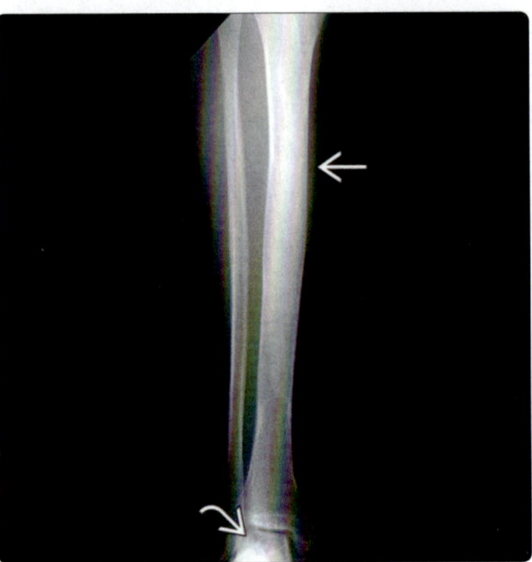

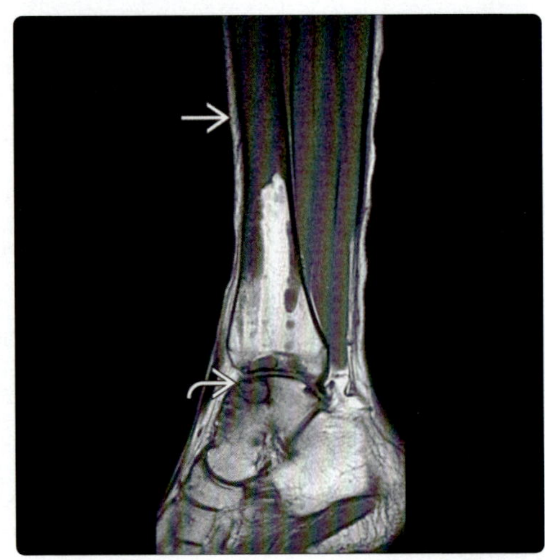

(Left) *Coronal T2WI FS MR shows uniformly high signal in the cystic tibial epiphyseal regions of involvement ➯ and mixed high and low signal in the tibial shaft and talar lesions ➔, which was moderately sclerotic on radiograph. Signal intensity on T2 can be variable in FD, depending on how much woven bone is present.* **(Right)** *AP radiograph shows a cortically based lytic lesion wrapping around the tibia ➔, representing cortically based FD, osteofibrous dysplasia, or adamantinoma.*

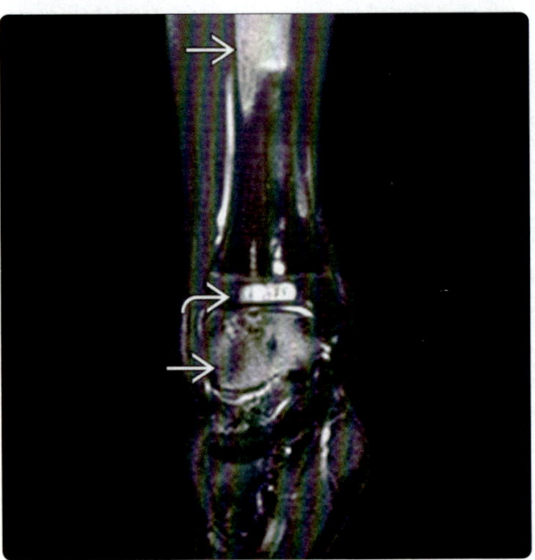

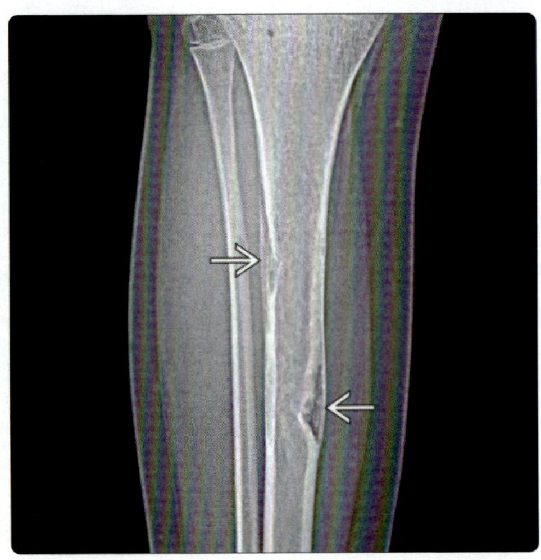

(Left) *Axial NECT in the same patient shows this to be an expanded large cortically based lesion ➔. No cortical breakthrough is seen.* **(Right)** *Axial T2WI MR confirms that the lesion is confined to the cortex ➔; the marrow and surrounding soft tissues are normal. There is no differentiating feature for the 3 possible diagnoses. Of these, cortically based FD is more commonly seen than either osteofibrous dysplasia or adamantinoma. Biopsy was required to establish the suspected diagnosis of FD.*

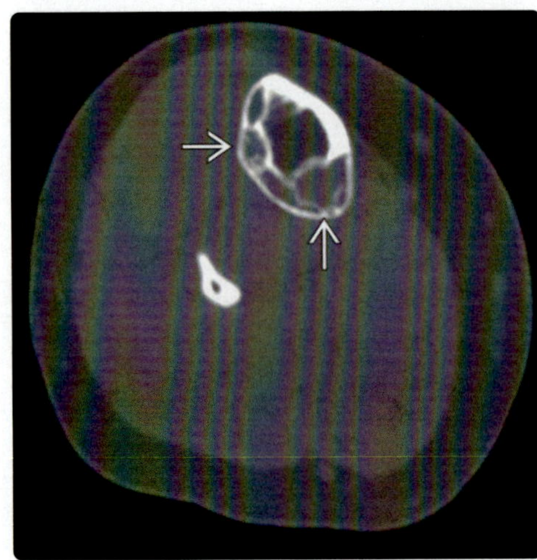

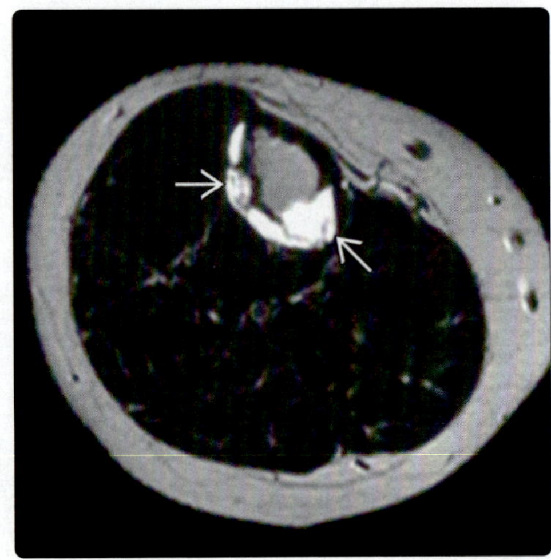

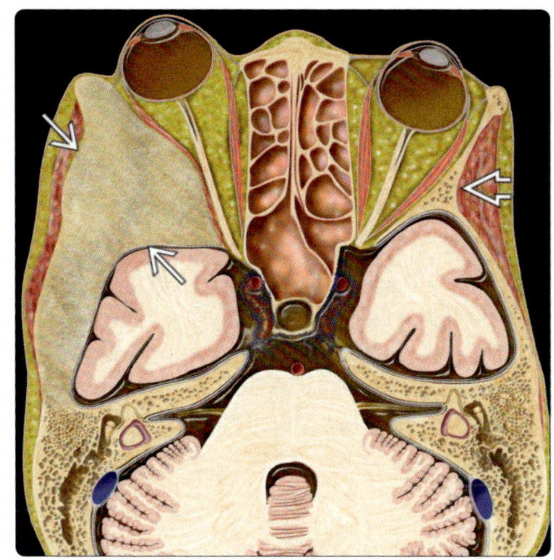

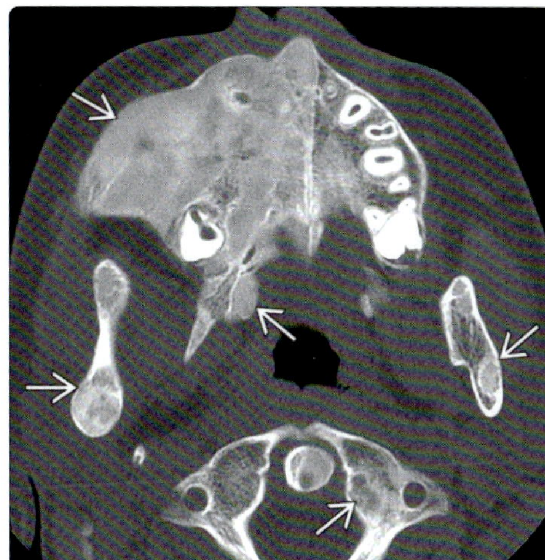

(Left) *Axial graphic shows the expanded base of skull focus of FD ➡, compared to normal marrow on the contralateral side ➡. The tan, gritty-appearing lesion corresponds to the spindle cell stroma containing fragments of woven bone and bits of cartilage.* **(Right)** *Axial NECT of the mandible and maxilla demonstrates extensive multifocal bone expansion with a ground-glass appearance ➡, corresponding to the previous graphic showing the gross appearance of FD.*

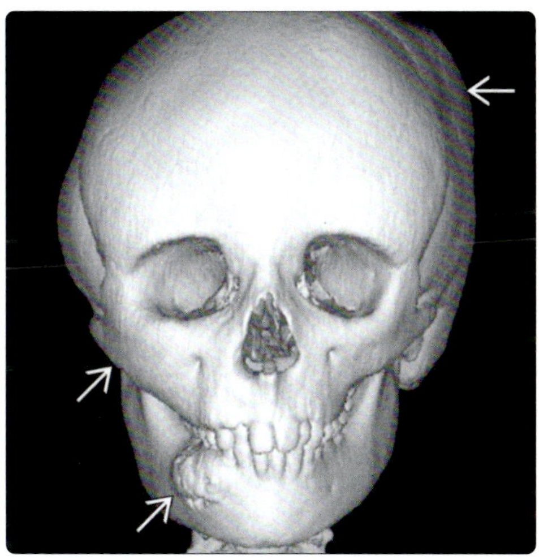

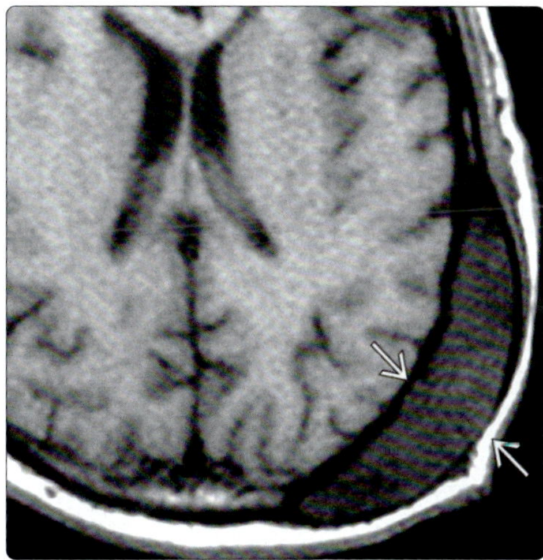

(Left) *3D CT surface reconstruction demonstrates marked asymmetric calvarial, facial bone, and mandibular thickening ➡. Leontiasis ossea, named for the lion-like physiognomy caused by severe craniofacial osseous thickening, is the final outcome in several disorders, including FD, Paget disease, craniodiaphysial dysplasia, and renal osteodystrophy.* **(Right)** *Axial T1WI MR shows focal expansion and inhomogeneously low signal intensity in a focus of cranial FD ➡.*

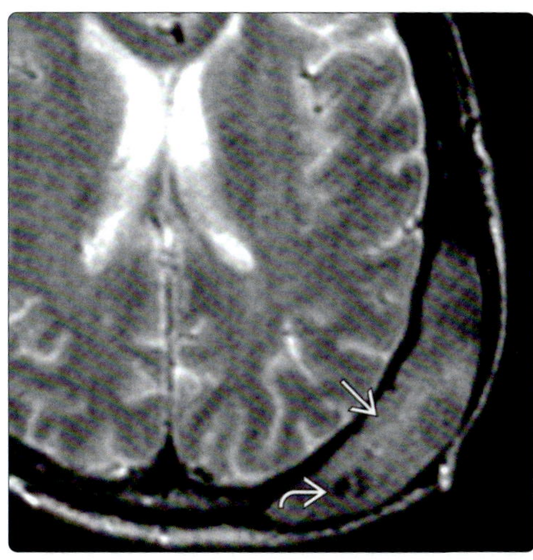

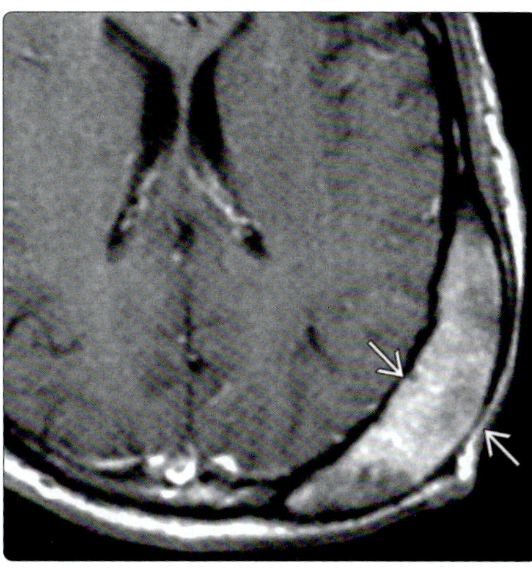

(Left) *Axial T2WI MR of the same region shows mixed signal, with some regions of mild hyperintensity ➡ but others of low signal ➡, corresponding to the ground-glass appearance seen on CT (not shown).* **(Right)** *Axial T1WI C+ MR shows inhomogeneous enhancement ➡. At least mild enhancement is usually seen in FD, and a heterogeneous pattern is typical. Note that both the inner and outer tables of the skull remain intact and only 1 side of the skull is involved.*

Osteofibrous Dysplasia

KEY FACTS

TERMINOLOGY

- Fibroosseous lesion primarily affecting tibia and fibula of children

IMAGING

- Location: Diaphysis (usually proximal) of tibia or fibula
  - Arises in cortex; may extend to medullary canal
- Multifocal or long confluent lesion common
- Lytic (60%) or ground-glass (40%)
- Geographic, sclerotic margin
- Bowing deformity, usually anterior
- Tissue sampling error may result in incorrect diagnosis of OFD when lesion is in fact adamantinoma
  - Upgrading of needle biopsy diagnosis from OFD to adamantinoma once surgical tissue available reported in 21% of 24 cases

TOP DIFFERENTIAL DIAGNOSES

- Intracortical fibrous dysplasia
- Osteofibrous dysplasia-like adamantinoma
- Adamantinoma

CLINICAL ISSUES

- Lesion of childhood; 50% occur < 5 years of age
  - Age thought by many to be distinctive indicator; extremely rare after skeletal maturation
- High recurrence rate if treated with curettage and bone grafting (> 60%)
  - If aggressive behavior warrants surgery, wide resection should reduce recurrence rate to acceptable levels
- No tendency to progress; stabilization and spontaneous regression reported in patients > 10 years of age
- Malignant changes not reported

DIAGNOSTIC CHECKLIST

- Reporting tip: Since OFD and adamantinoma cannot reliably be differentiated by imaging, report possibility of both lesions

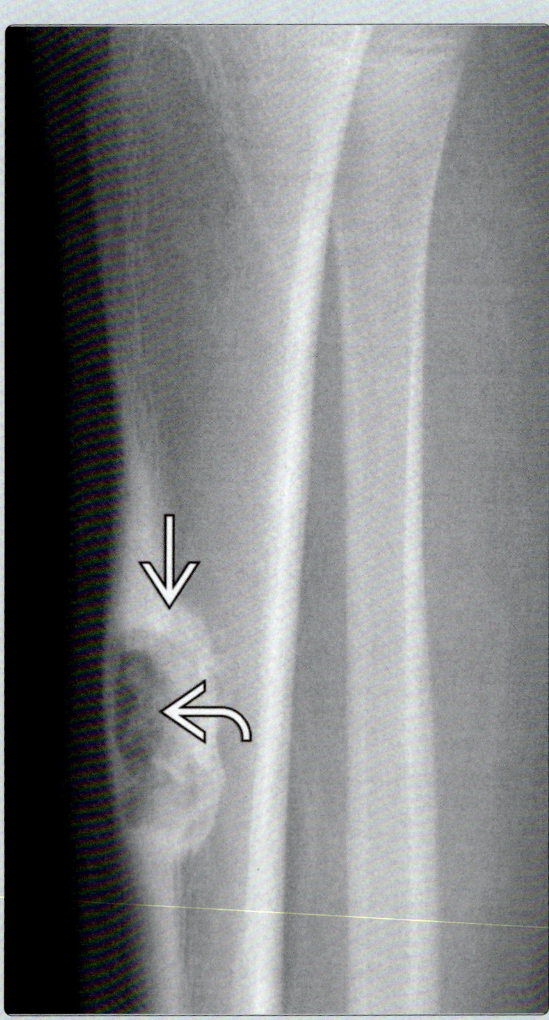

Oblique radiograph shows a typical case of osteofibrous dysplasia (OFD), arising in the cortex in the upper 1/3 of the tibial diaphysis and thinning the anterior cortex. It has a densely sclerotic margin ➡ and contains osteoid matrix ⮐, though the majority of such lesions do not.

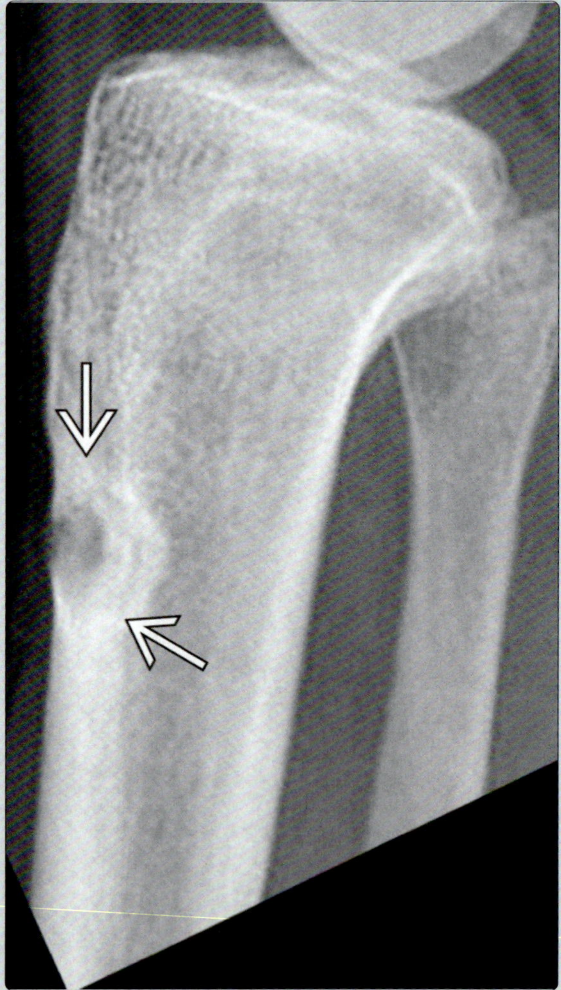

Lateral radiograph demonstrates a geographic lytic lesion located within the anterior cortex of the proximal tibia ➡. The lytic lesion has a dense sclerotic margin with slight anterior expansion. This is a typical OFD except for the patient age of 25 years.

TERMINOLOGY

Abbreviations

- Osteofibrous dysplasia (OFD)

Synonyms

- Ossifying fibroma, osteitis fibrosa cystica
- Congenital fibrous defect of tibia, extragnathic ossifying fibroma, Kempson-Campanacci

Definitions

- Fibroosseous lesion primarily affecting tibia and fibula of children

IMAGING

General Features

- Location
  - Diaphysis (usually proximal) of tibia or fibula, almost exclusively
    - Series of 14 cases showed 13 in tibia, 1 in fibula
      - 2 cases showed 2 lesions in different bones, 1 ipsilateral, 1 bilateral
      - 3 cases showed multiple lesions in same bone
    - Series of 24 cases showed 22 in tibia, 2 in fibula
    - Series of 24 showed 4 were multiple
      - 3 had satellite lesions in same bone
      - 1 showed bilateral tibial involvement
- Size
  - Average: 6 cm in length (smaller than average reported adamantinoma, though overlap exists)

Radiographic Findings

- Lytic (60%) or ground-glass (40%)
- Geographic, sclerotic margin
- Arises in cortex
  - Thinned, expanded cortex
  - May extend from cortex into medullary canal
  - Multifocal or long confluent lesion common
- Pseudotrabeculation; may appear multiloculated
- No periosteal reaction
- Bowing deformity, usually anterior
  - May develop pseudarthrosis after pathologic fracture

CT Findings

- Mimics radiographic findings
- May better demonstrate any ground-glass matrix
- Improved distinction of multiple lesion with normal intervening bone vs. pseudotrabeculated lesion compared with radiograph

MR Findings

- Cortical expansion in 58%
  - Cortical destruction and soft tissue mass rare
- Cortical lesion may extend to medullary canal, well shown on MR
  - 1 study of 24 patients showed intramedullary extension in 100%
- T1 signal intensity: Homogeneous or heterogeneous (50%) intermediate
- Fluid-sensitive sequences: Heterogeneous intermediate to high signal intensity
  - Most frequently heterogeneous but intermediate signal intensity
- 1 study showed intralesional fat in 12%
- Internal low signal bands and multilocular appearance in 91%
- Rare cystic regions
- Mild (if any) adjacent soft tissue edema in absence of pathologic fracture
- Intense contrast enhancement, usually heterogeneous
- No differentiating features from adamantinoma

Image-Guided Biopsy

- Tissue sampling error may result in incorrect diagnosis of OFD when lesion is in fact adamantinoma
  - Epithelial cells located centrally in adamantinoma; may be missed by fine-needle aspiration
  - Peripheral biopsy may show only findings of OFD or OFD-like adamantinoma
    - Should obtain sample from lytic center of lesion
    - Tissue samples should be generous to avoid sampling error
- Upgrading of needle biopsy diagnosis from OFD to adamantinoma once surgical tissue available reported in 21% of 24 cases
- Suggests that needle biopsy diagnosis of OFD should be treated with some skepticism with regard to patient management

DIFFERENTIAL DIAGNOSIS

Intracortical Fibrous Dysplasia (FD)

- In tibia, FD not infrequently originates in cortex
  - May be indistinguishable radiographically from OFD
- Slightly older median age
- Histologic differentiation

Osteofibrous Dysplasia-Like Adamantinoma

- Also termed differentiated adamantinoma or juvenile adamantinoma
- Same appearance on imaging
- Occurs in skeletally immature patients
- OFD-like tissue, but with small nests of epithelial cells
- Benign course; in histologic and behavioral spectrum of OFD to adamantinoma

Adamantinoma

- Imaging appearance may be identical
  - May demonstrate more aggressive appearance, with cortical breakthrough and soft tissue mass
- Occurs in either children or adults
- Histologically, more abundant epithelial cells
- Behaviorally more aggressive
  - High recurrence rates with inadequate resection
  - Significant metastatic potential

PATHOLOGY

General Features

- Etiology
  - Unknown; not certain if neoplastic or dysplasia

Gross Pathologic & Surgical Features

- Pale or yellowish white, gritty

- Softer, more fragile than normal bone
- No cysts seen

Microscopic Features

- Variably cellular fibroblastic proliferation, storiform
- Osteoid or bony trabeculae with variation in shape and orientation, rimmed by osteoblasts
  - Degree of calcification varies
  - No long bony spicules typical of FD
- Collagen fibers in stroma

CLINICAL ISSUES

Presentation

- Most common signs/symptoms
  - Mass, ± pain
  - Pathologic fracture, may result in pseudarthrosis

Demographics

- Age
  - Lesion of childhood; 50% occur < 5 years of age
    - Age thought by many to be distinctive indicator; extremely rare after skeletal maturation
    - 1 report of 5 cases with mean age of 19 years likely skewed by single 63-year-old patient
- Gender
  - M > F

Natural History & Prognosis

- High recurrence rate if treated with curettage and bone grafting (> 60%)
  - Especially if treatment occurs prior to age 5
  - Recurrence may progress to pseudarthrosis
- No tendency to progress; stabilization & spontaneous regression reported in patients > 10 years of age
- Malignant changes not reported

Treatment

- Surgery following needle biopsy diagnosis avoided by some experienced surgeons until after puberty, and then only performed on large lesions
- If aggressive behavior warrants surgery, wide resection should reduce recurrence rate to acceptable levels
- If surgery is suggested due to concern for theoretical progression to adamantinoma, wide resection is preferred method
  - Mitigates concern for unrepresentative needle biopsy sample and for recurrence

DIAGNOSTIC CHECKLIST

Consider

- Adamantinoma, OFD-like adamantinoma, and OFD thought by some to represent spectrum of similar disease
  - Frequent reports of marginal excision of lesions initially reported to be OFD or OFD-like adamantinoma, resulting in aggressive recurrence and reclassification as adamantinoma
  - Histopathology, ultrastructure, and cytopathology suggest these are closely related
    - Progressive complexity of chromosomal aberrations, increasing from OFD to adamantinoma
    - Only adamantinoma develops metastatic disease
    - Suggests multistep neoplastic transformation

Reporting Tips

- Since OFD and adamantinoma cannot reliably be differentiated by imaging, report possibility of both lesions
  - Tissue should be carefully examined to determine where along this spectrum individual case lies

SELECTED REFERENCES

1. Jung JY et al: MR findings of the osteofibrous dysplasia. Korean J Radiol. 15(1):114-22, 2014
2. Wick MR et al: Proliferative, reparative, and reactive benign bone lesions that may be confused diagnostically with true osseous neoplasms. Semin Diagn Pathol. 31(1):66-88, 2014
3. Gleason BC et al: Osteofibrous dysplasia and adamantinoma in children and adolescents: a clinicopathologic reappraisal. Am J Surg Pathol. 32(3):363-76, 2008
4. Khanna M et al: Osteofibrous dysplasia, osteofibrous dysplasia-like adamantinoma and adamantinoma: correlation of radiological imaging features with surgical histology and assessment of the use of radiology in contributing to needle biopsy diagnosis. Skeletal Radiol. 37(12):1077-84, 2008
5. Lee RS et al: Osteofibrous dysplasia of the tibia. Is there a need for a radical surgical approach? J Bone Joint Surg Br. 88(5):658-64, 2006
6. Van der Woude HJ et al: MRI of adamantinoma of long bones in correlation with histopathology. AJR Am J Roentgenol. 183(6):1737-44, 2004
7. Kahn LB: Adamantinoma, osteofibrous dysplasia and differentiated adamantinoma. Skeletal Radiol. 32(5):245-58, 2003
8. Seeger LL et al: Surface lesions of bone. Radiology. 206(1):17-33, 1998
9. Nakashima Y et al: Osteofibrous dysplasia (ossifying fibroma of long bones). A study of 12 cases. Cancer. 52(5):909-14, 1983

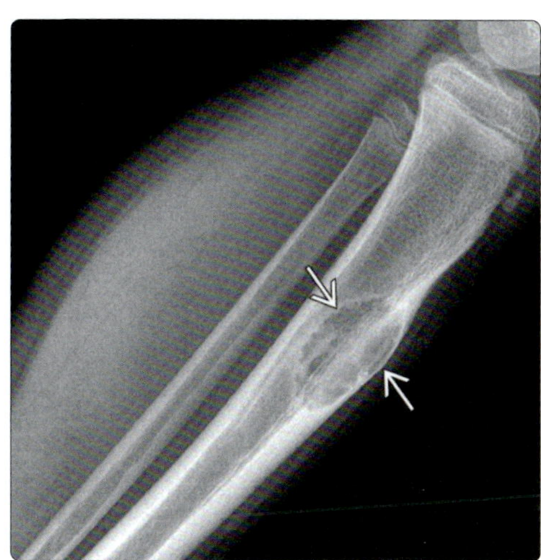

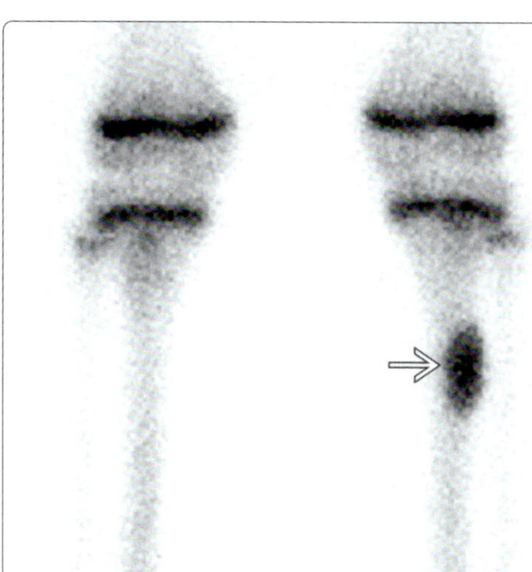

(Left) *Lateral radiograph of a metadiaphyseal lesion in an 8-year-old girl demonstrates mild expansion and a sclerotic rim surrounding a lytic lesion ➡ that originated in the cortex. The lesion contains regions of ground-glass matrix. There is thinning of the endosteal cortex, but no evidence of cortical breakthrough. No satellite lesion is seen. Given the patient age, OFD is a likely diagnosis.* **(Right)** *AP bone scan shows the lesion to have significant increased uptake ➡.*

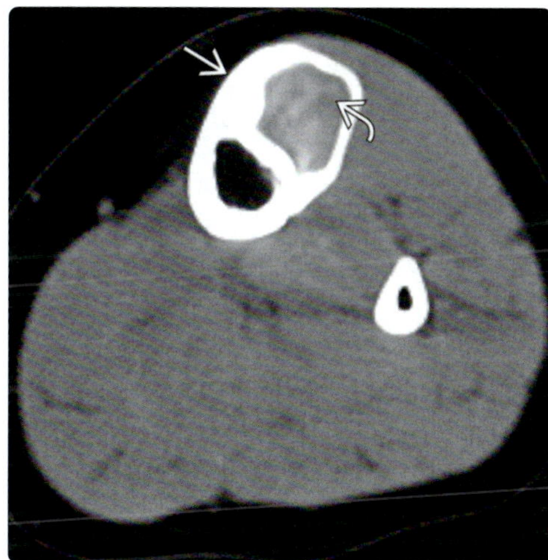

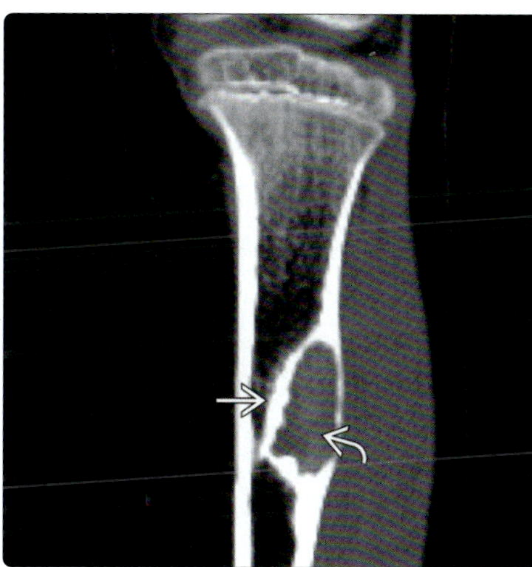

(Left) *Axial CT shows the cortically based tibial lesion ➡ that has a complete sclerotic rim. The center of the lesion has variable ground-glass density ↪.* **(Right)** *Coronal CT reconstruction in the same patient shows the lesion to be contained by a dense sclerotic rim ➡. The matrix is again noted to be of ground-glass density ↪.*

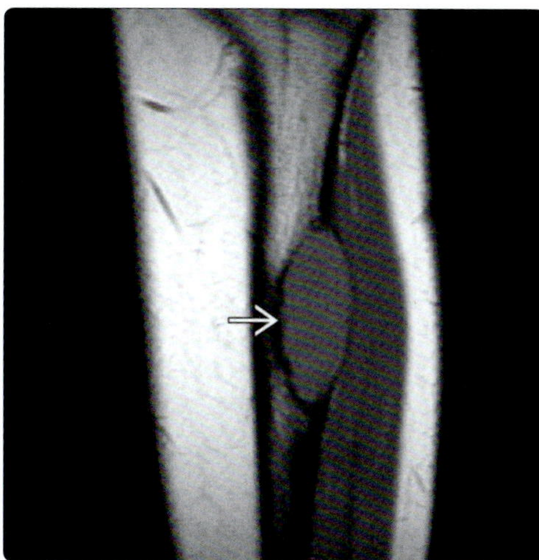

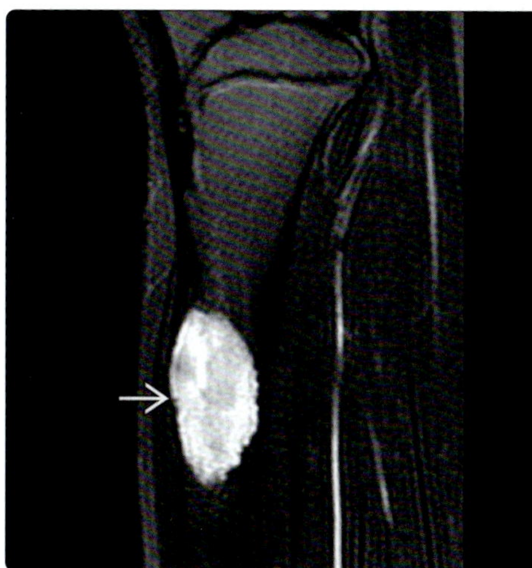

(Left) *Coronal T1 MR shows the lesion contents to be homogeneous ➡, with nonspecific signal intensity similar to that of skeletal muscle.* **(Right)** *Sagittal T2 FS MR shows heterogeneity of the lesion, with predominant signal hyperintensity ➡. None of these studies definitively differentiates this biopsy-proven OFD from OFD-like adamantinoma or adamantinoma.*

(Left) *Oblique radiograph in a 10 month old shows a large lytic lesion occupying the majority of the tibial diaphysis. The radiograph gives the impression of the lesion occupying the marrow centrally, causing expansion* ➡*.* **(Right)** *Sagittal NECT in the same case shows that the well-marginated lesion is in fact based within the cortex of the bone* ➡*. The cortex is expanded and the lesion extends circumferentially. The combination of a well-defined expanded cortical lesion in the tibia and the patient's young age suggests OFD.*

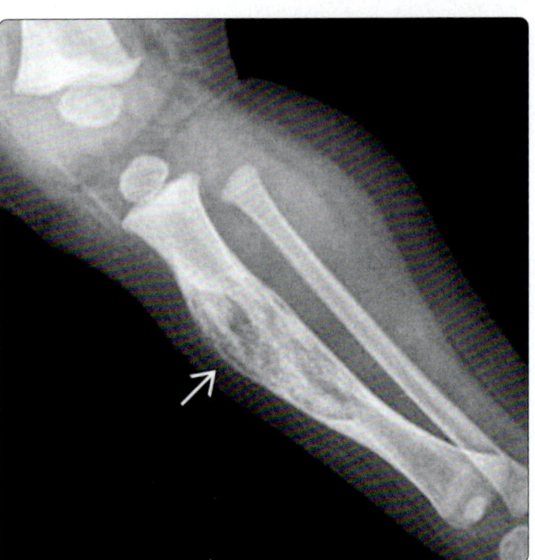

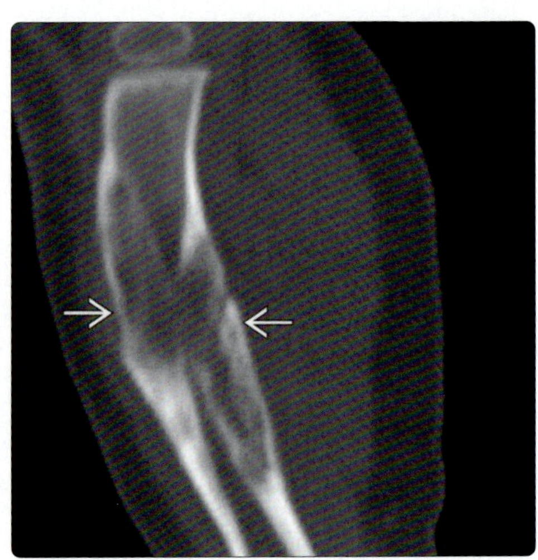

(Left) *Oblique sagittal STIR MR through the medial cortex in the same case shows nonspecific high signal within the lesion and no cortical breakthrough* ➡*. Biopsy proved OFD.* **(Right)** *AP radiograph demonstrates a cortically based lytic lesion within the distal fibular metaphysis* ➡ *in a child. The sclerotic margin is dense. The most common lesion at this site is fibroxanthoma (nonossifying fibroma), but other cortical lesions, such as OFD or adamantinoma, should be considered due to the location in the leg.*

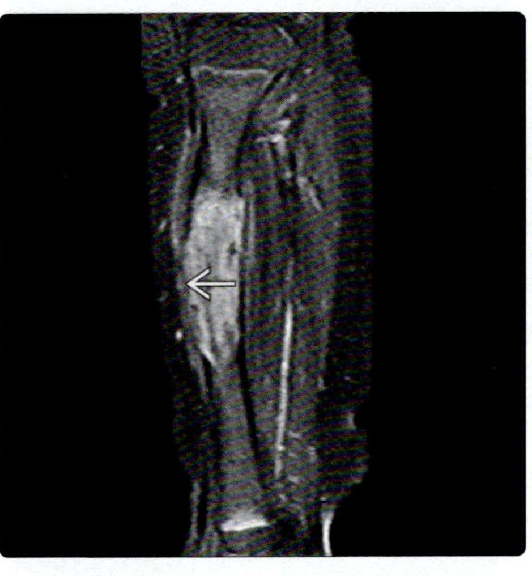

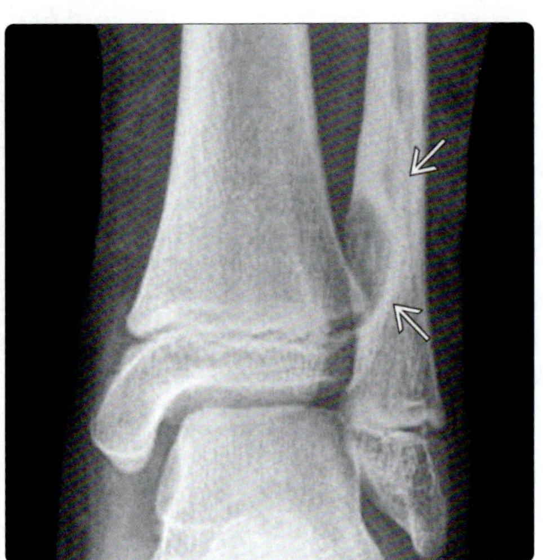

(Left) *Coronal PDWI FS MR shows the same lesion to be fairly homogeneously high signal* ➡ *and suggests that the lesion may be central in location.* **(Right)** *Axial STIR MR in the same case shows that the lesion is in fact eccentric and cortically based* ➡*, leaving a portion of the normal marrow seen laterally* ➡*. This occurs in a cortical lesion within a gracile bone. There is surrounding soft tissue edema, but no true cortical breakthrough. Imaging suggests either OFD or adamantinoma; OFD was proven at biopsy.*

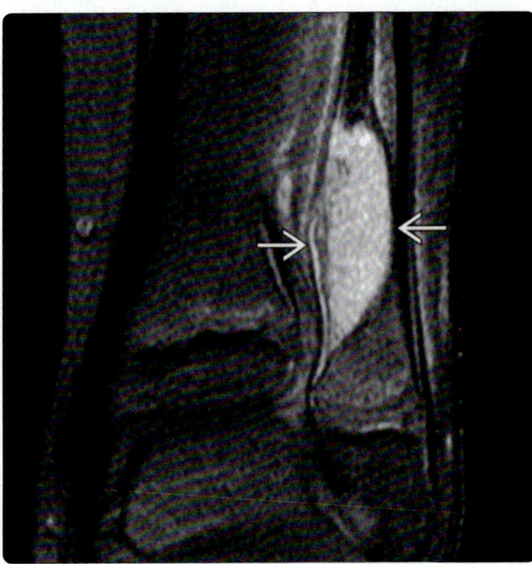

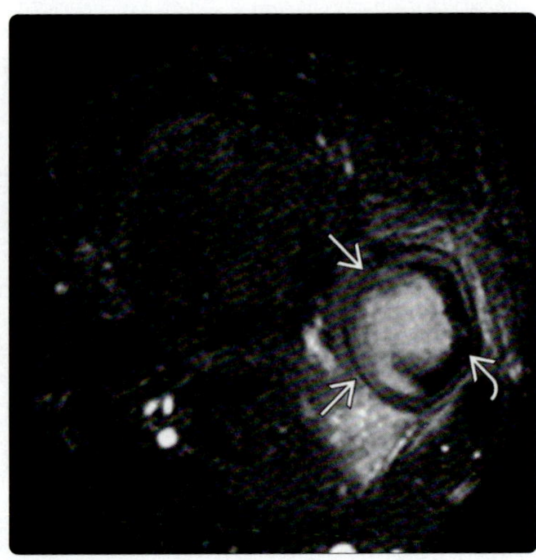

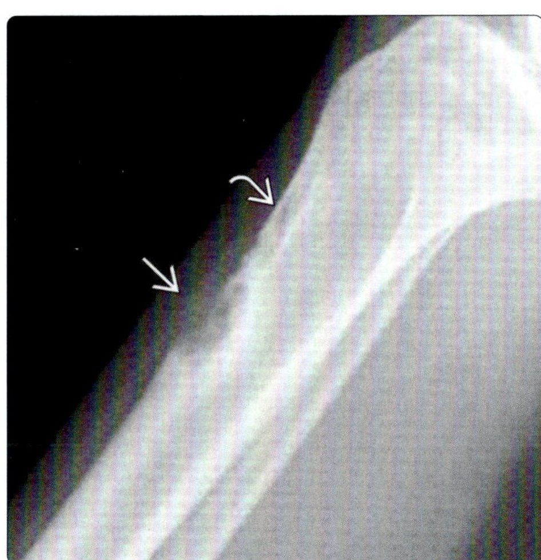

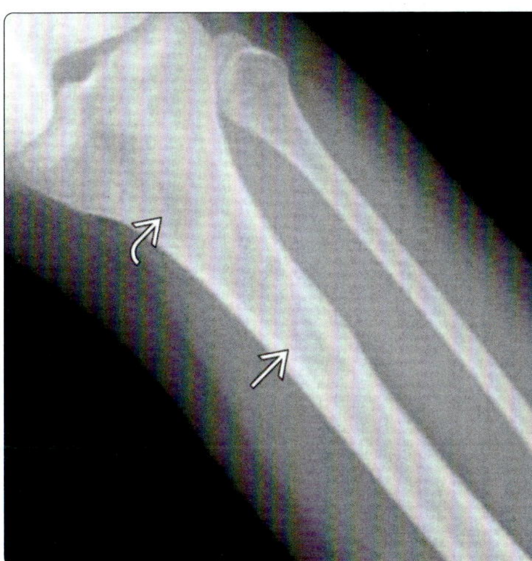

(Left) *Lateral radiograph shows a lytic lesion in the proximal tibial diaphysis, based in the cortex ➡. There appears to be cortical breakthrough anteriorly, but the lesion seems relatively geographic. There is either proximal extension of the lesion or a 2nd focus ↗.* **(Right)** *AP radiograph in the same patient shows the slightly expanded lytic lesion ➡, with the proximal lesion only faintly seen ↗. The differential diagnosis includes the spectrum of cortically based tibial lesions.*

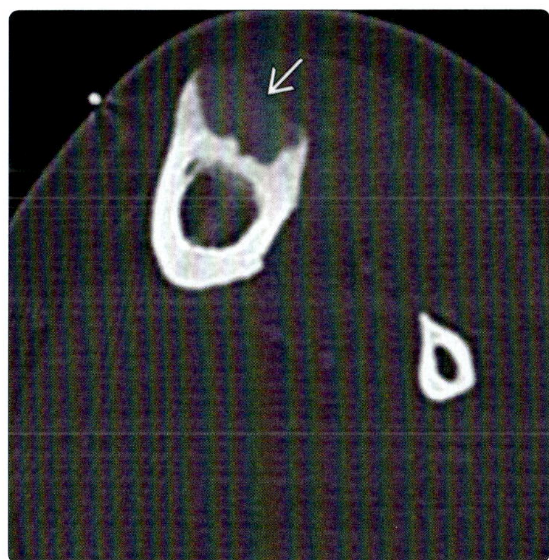

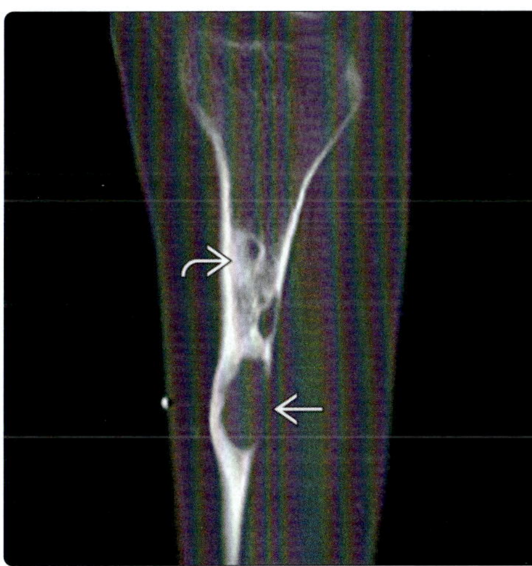

(Left) *Axial bone CT in the same patient shows the cortical location to best advantage ➡. The anterior rim is not distinctly seen as being osseous, but contains the lesion.* **(Right)** *Coronal reformatted bone CT shows the major portion of the lesion with its excessively thin containment ➡. There are other lesions ↗ that are either separate or a proximal conglomerate extension of the original lesion. Any one of the lesions in the differential (OFD, intracortical fibrous dysplasia, adamantinoma) may have this appearance.*

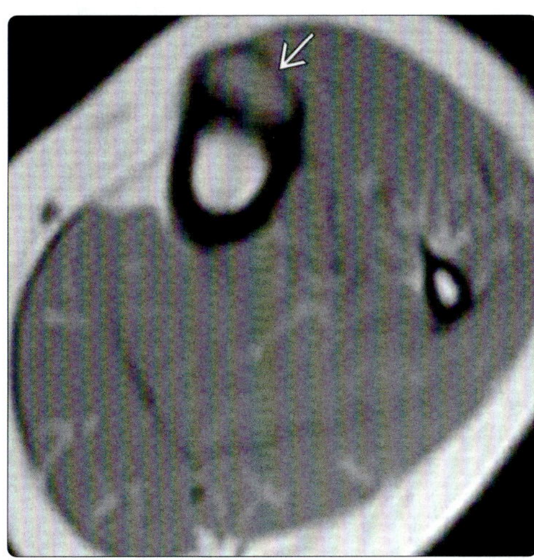

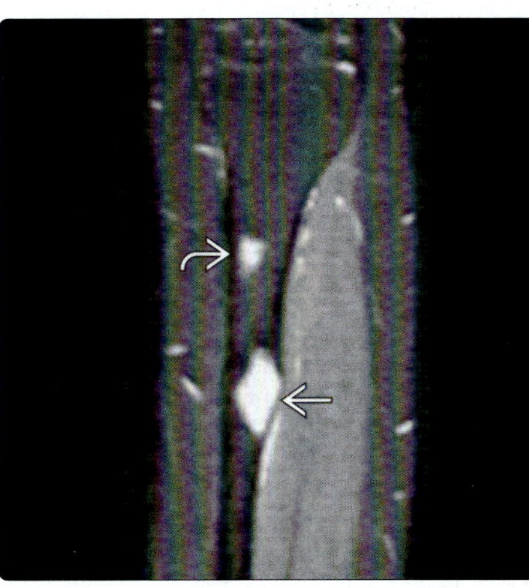

(Left) *Axial T1WI MR shows that the lesion has a thin rim of bone rather than true cortical breakthrough ➡. The lesion is homogeneous and isointense with muscle.* **(Right)** *Coronal STIR MR shows the primary lesion to be high signal ➡, as is the proximal extension or 2nd lesion ↗. The overall appearance is of a moderately aggressive tibial process. The imaging does not differentiate the possible diagnoses of adamantinoma, OFD, or cortical fibrous dysplasia. Careful biopsy of the center of the primary lesion proved it to be OFD.*

Simple Bone Cyst

KEY FACTS

TERMINOLOGY

- Benign fluid-filled (serous or serosanguinous fluid) cystic osseous lesions

IMAGING

- In children, 90% occur in long bones
  - Humerus (proximal) most common site
  - Arise in metaphysis, adjacent to physeal plate
  - With skeletal growth, physis grows away from lesion
- In adults, simple bone cyst (SBC) occurs in other sites
  - Calcaneus > iliac wing > distal radius, patella
- Radiograph: Lytic lesion arising centrally in medullary cavity
  - May contain pseudotrabeculations
  - No periosteal reaction in absence of fracture
  - May contain "fallen fragment"
- MR: Cystic nature of lesion confirmed
  - Fluid-fluid levels often seen on various sequences; need not be present
  - Fibrous septations may be present
  - Pathologic fracture may complicate MR appearance
  - Postcontrast imaging: Central low signal, surrounded by rim which often enhances (80%)
  - Central enhancement may occur in part of lesion (27%)

CLINICAL ISSUES

- 85% occur in first 2 decades
- Many spontaneously resolve as patients approach skeletal maturity
- No consensus of best treatment

DIAGNOSTIC CHECKLIST

- < 50% of proven SBC meet all criteria of "simple" cysts
  - Lesion may contain septa, be loculated, and show inhomogeneous contents not fully meeting criteria of fluid
  - Complex MR features should not deter consideration of SBC diagnosis

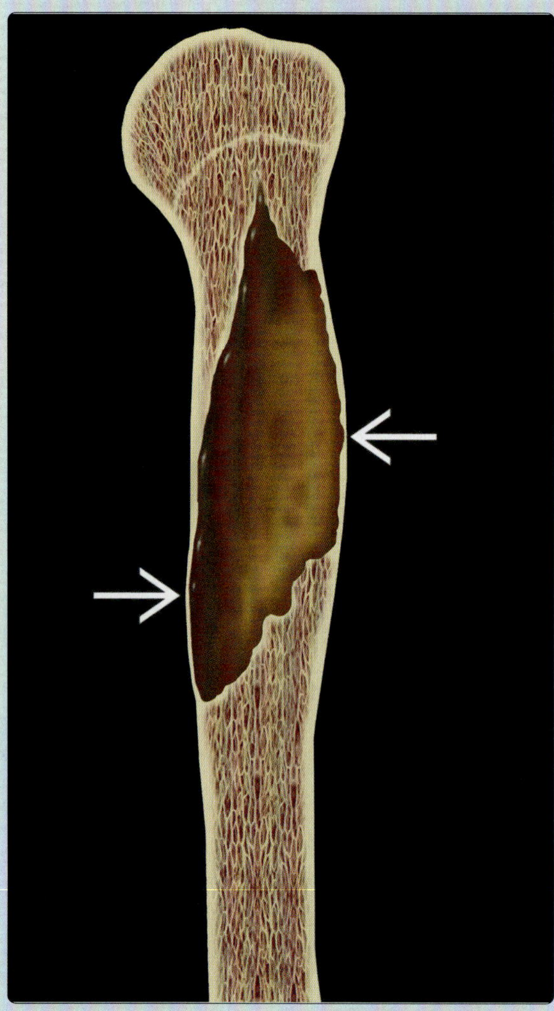

Graphic depicting simple bone cyst (SBC) in the typical proximal humeral location. The cystic cavitation is well demarcated, with cortical thinning and mild expansion ➡. The lesions usually contain a clear, serous-like fluid; the glistening cystic lining is seen here.

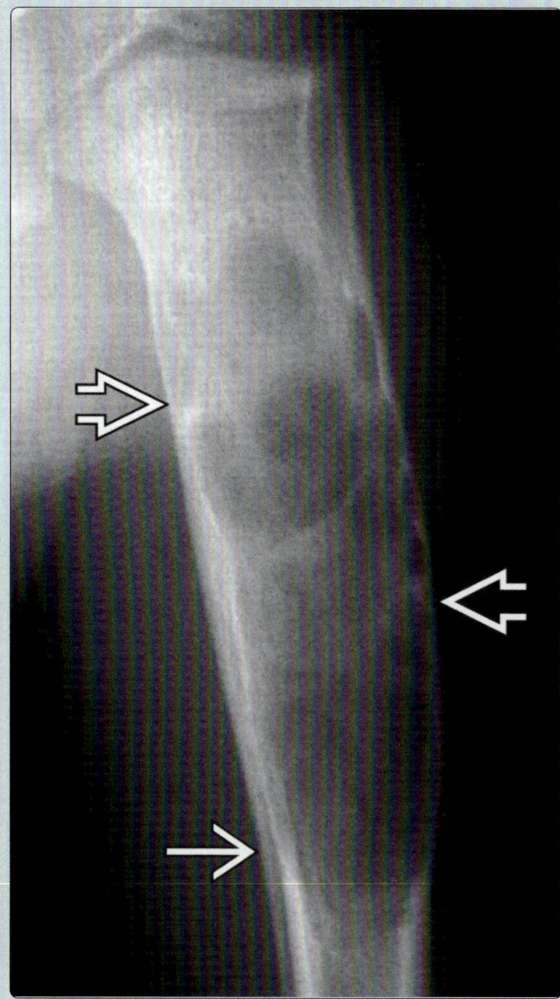

AP radiograph of a typical SBC, showing a central lytic lesion that has expanded the bone mildly and thinned the cortex ➡. Periosteal reaction ➡ relates to prior pathologic fracture. The proximal metaphyseal location in the humerus is classic.

TERMINOLOGY

Abbreviations

- Simple bone cyst (SBC)

Synonyms

- Solitary bone cyst, unicameral bone cyst, juvenile bone cyst, essential bone cyst

Definitions

- Benign fluid-filled (serous or serosanguinous fluid) cystic osseous lesions

IMAGING

General Features

- Location
  - 90% occur in long bones
    - Humerus (proximal) most common site
      - Followed by proximal femur, then proximal tibia in children
    - Arise in metaphysis, adjacent to physeal plate
      - With skeletal growth, physis grows away from lesion
      - Lesion appears to "migrate" into metadiaphysis or even diaphysis as child grows
      - Does not cross growth plate
  - In adults, SBC occurs in other sites
    - Calcaneus > iliac wing > distal radius, patella

Radiographic Findings

- Lytic lesion arising centrally in medullary cavity
- Long axis parallel to length of host bone
- Geographic, with thin sclerotic margin
- May contain pseudotrabeculations or septa
- Cortical thinning
- Mild circumferential expansion of bone
- No periosteal reaction in absence of fracture
  - Reaction to fracture is smooth, linear
- No cortical breakthrough in absence of fracture
- May contain "fallen fragment"
  - Fractured fragment of bone, which moves in dependent position as patient position is changed
- May see SBC in healing phase
  - Sclerosis healing of part of lesion
  - Some lucent regions often remain
  - Often signs of mild malalignment from pathologic fracture

CT Findings

- Centrally located; cortex thinned but intact
- 15-20 HU
- No enhancement
- May show fluid-fluid level
- "Fallen fragment" of bone floats within cystic fluid following fracture, in dependent position
- Bubble of gas in nondependent portion of lytic lesion suggests SBC with pathologic fracture
  - "Rising bubble" sign

MR Findings

- Cystic nature of lesion confirmed
  - T1WI: Majority of lesions homogeneous, low to intermediate signal intensity
    - 40% show heterogeneity and may contain small regions of high signal
      - High signal presumed related to blood products from fracture
  - Fluid-sensitive sequences: High fluid signal intensity
    - May be inhomogeneous, with some loculated areas less hyperintense than others (up to 60%)
  - Postcontrast imaging: Central low signal, surrounded by rim which often enhances (80%)
    - Central enhancement may occur in part of lesion (27%)
- Fluid-fluid levels often seen on various sequences but need not be present
- Fibrous septations may be present
  - Thin, low signal with surrounding high signal on fluid-sensitive sequences
  - Septations may enhance following contrast (36%)
  - Septa may be only partial and fluid may track through entire lesion
    - 75-83% may have loculated regions
- "Rising bubble" sign may be seen; unlikely that "floating fragment" will be noted on MR
- Pathologic fracture may complicate MR appearance

Nuclear Medicine Findings

- Bone scan
  - May be normal
  - May have peripheral ↑ uptake; central photopenia
- FDG-active; may mimic metastasis on PET/CT

DIFFERENTIAL DIAGNOSIS

Fibrous Dysplasia

- Central lesion in metadiaphysis or diaphysis
- Same age group
- Usually contains "ground-glass" density
  - Partially healed SBC may mimic "ground-glass"

Aneurysmal Bone Cyst

- Lytic, metadiaphyseal lesion
  - Aneurysmal bone cyst (ABC) usually eccentric rather than central like SBC
- ABC usually shows aneurysmal expansion of cortex rather than mild concentric expansion
- ABC may appear identical to SBC in phalanx or metacarpal/metatarsal

Enchondroma

- Central proximal metaphysis of humerus is most common location, as in SBC
- Usually (not invariably) contains chondroid matrix
- Generally less sclerotic margination than seen in SBC
- Lytic enchondroma in hand or foot may be indistinguishable from SBC

Langerhans Cell Histiocytosis

- Similar age group
- Lytic lesion occupying central metaphysis or diaphysis of long bones; other sites (skull, pelvis) more common

- May appear either highly aggressive or nonaggressive; latter appearance may mimic SBC

Osteomyelitis

- Metaphyseal location most frequent in child
- Lytic, but generally elicits sclerotic bone reaction
- Periosteal reaction often present
- MR may show osseous or soft tissue abscess

Brown Tumor of Hyperparathyroidism

- Lytic, central in long bones
- Other findings of hyperparathyroidism will be present
  - Abnormal bone density
  - Various resorptive patterns

PATHOLOGY

General Features

- Etiology
  - Unknown; multiple theories
    - Possibly these are intraosseous synovial cysts
      - Based on electron microscopy
    - Possibly related to trauma
    - Elevation of prostaglandin levels in cyst fluid suggests possible role in pathogenesis
    - Venous congestion of intramedullary space

Gross Pathologic & Surgical Features

- Cystic cavity: Serous or serosanguineous fluid
- Inner surface of cyst shows ridges separating depressed zones, covered by thin membrane
- Partial septa

Microscopic Features

- Inner lining and septa: Connective tissue
  - May contain reactive new bone formation, hemosiderin, and giant cells
- 63% show cementum-like material in lining: Specific
  - Can be seen maturing into reparative bone
- Fracture callus may be present
- Blood products in cyst if prior fracture

CLINICAL ISSUES

Presentation

- Most common signs/symptoms
  - Usually asymptomatic unless fractured
    - Humeral lesions may be seen on chest radiograph
  - 66% with pathologic fracture

Demographics

- Age
  - 10-20 years of age most common
  - 85% occur in first 2 decades
- Gender
  - Male > female (3:1)
- Epidemiology
  - 3% of primary bone lesions
  - 1/3 of 752 lesions of hip in children < 14 years of age were found to be SBC in 1 study

Natural History & Prognosis

- Many spontaneously resolve as patients approach skeletal maturity
  - 7-15% of symptomatic cases; likely more in asymptomatic cases
- Conservative treatment leads to resolution in 30%
  - Fracture appears to increase or advance spontaneous resolution in some cases
  - Case study of 20 treated conservatively; of those that resolved, 5 had fractured, 2 had not
- Fracture, risk of fracture, or continued pain → treatment
- Growth arrest (up to 10% of patients) may occur following pathologic fracture or curettage
- Rare osteonecrosis of femoral head following pathologic fracture

Treatment

- No consensus on best treatment
  - Wide reported range of failure (recurrence or fracture) with various treatments
    - Failure after curettage (22-47%)
    - Failure after steroid injection (41-78%)
      - Success rate may be higher in calcaneus than long bones
- Various treatments compared in 1 large study
  - Injection of corticosteroids
    - 84% failed after 1 treatment
  - Curettage and bone grafting
    - 64% failed after 1 treatment
    - Lowest rate of pathologic fracture following treatment
    - Highest rate of pain following treatment
  - Injection of combination of steroid, demineralized bone matrix, and bone marrow aspirate
    - 50% failed after 1 treatment
- Percutaneous injection of osteoconductive apatetic calcium phosphate (α-BSM) seems promising
- Fractures with allogenic bone graft and platelet-rich plasma appears promising in 1 study

DIAGNOSTIC CHECKLIST

Image Interpretation Pearls

- < 50% of proven SBC meet all criteria of "simple" cysts
  - Lesion may contain septa, be loculated, and show inhomogeneous contents not fully meeting criteria of fluid
  - Complex MR features should not deter consideration of SBC diagnosis

SELECTED REFERENCES

1. Pretell-Mazzini J et al: Unicameral bone cysts: general characteristics and management controversies. J Am Acad Orthop Surg. 22(5):295-303, 2014
2. Tariq MU et al: Cementum-like matrix in solitary bone cysts: a unique and characteristic but yet underrecognized feature of promising diagnostic utility. Ann Diagn Pathol. 18(1):1-4, 2014
3. Pedzisz P et al: Treatment of solitary bone cysts with allogenic bone graft and platelet-rich plasma. A preliminary report. Acta Orthop Belg. 76(3):374-9, 2010
4. Jordanov MI: The "rising bubble" sign: a new aid in the diagnosis of unicameral bone cysts. Skeletal Radiol. 38(6):597-600, 2009
5. Wootton-Gorges SL: MR imaging of primary bone tumors and tumor-like conditions in children. Magn Reson Imaging Clin N Am. 17(3):469-87, vi, 2009

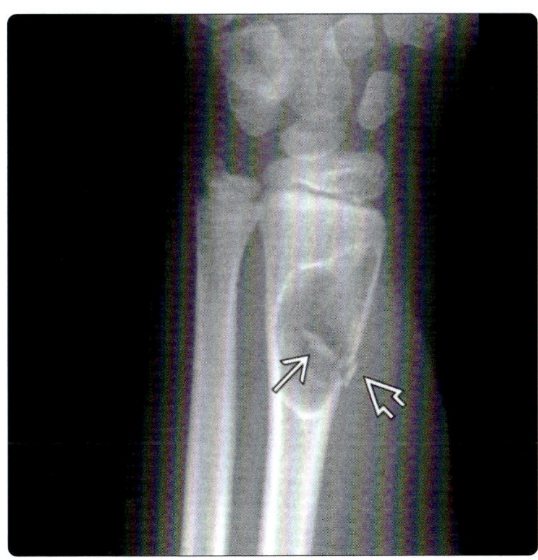

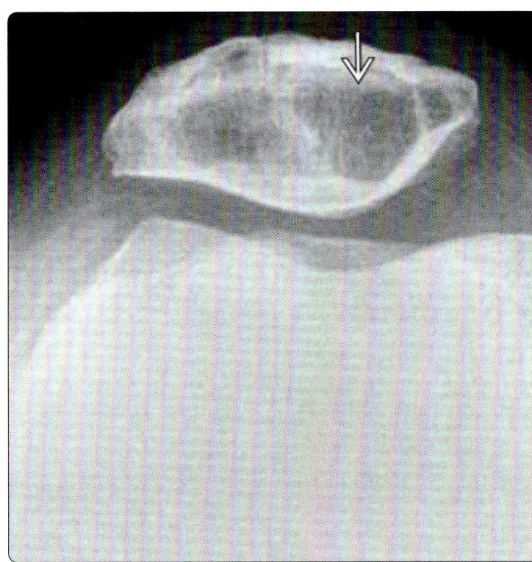

(Left) *Oblique radiograph shows a central lytic metaphyseal lesion with a thin sclerotic margin. There is a pathologic fracture ➡ as well as a "fallen bone" fragment ➡. This is pathognomonic for a SBC.* **(Right)** *Axial radiograph of the patella in a 35 year old shows a lytic lesion ➡, likely containing septa. The appearance is nonspecific, but in patients under 40 years of age, the differential includes SBC, aneurysmal bone cyst (ABC), giant cell tumor (GCT), and chondroblastoma.*

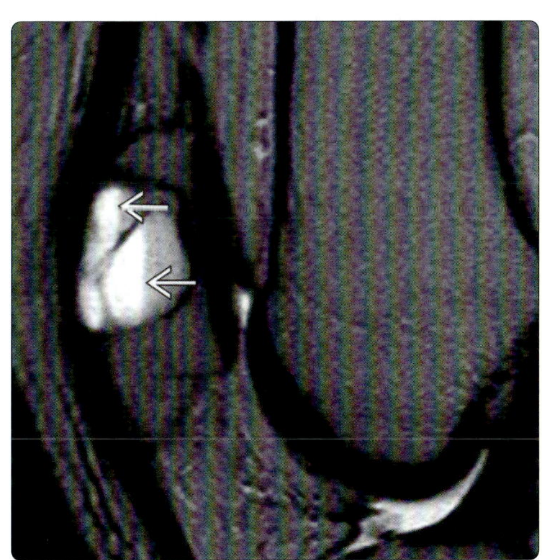

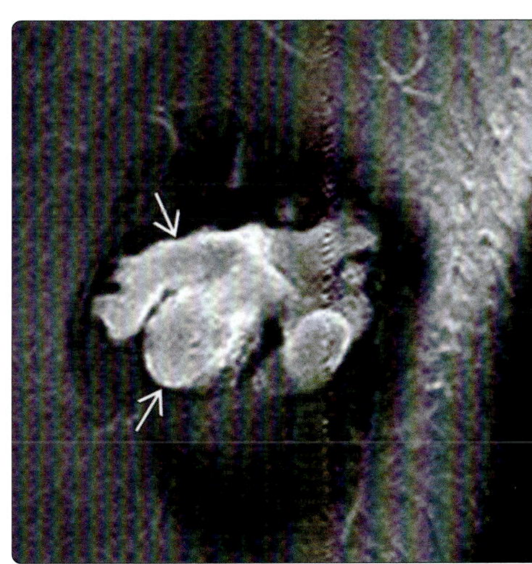

(Left) *Sagittal T2 FS MR in the same patient shows fluid levels ➡. Of the diagnostic considerations, this makes SBC or ABC more likely. Fluid levels in either lesion are neither specific nor required.* **(Right)** *Coronal T1 C+ FS MR in the same patient shows a strongly enhancing rim ➡, with mild enhancement centrally. The lesion proved to be a SBC.*

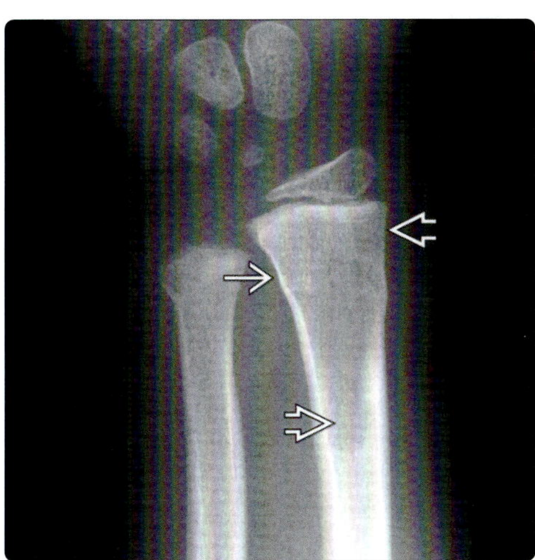

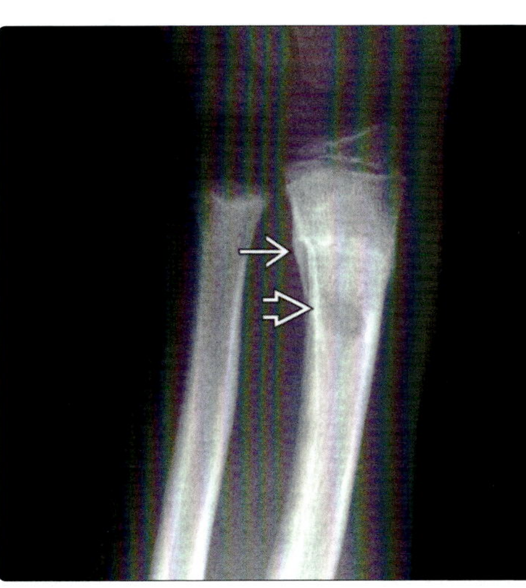

(Left) *AP radiograph shows a torus fracture ➡ of the radial metaphysis. There is a subtle lytic lesion, which is not well marginated, extending over the whole metaphyseal region ➡. The fracture must be considered pathologic, and the lesion proved to be a SBC.* **(Right)** *AP radiograph obtained 2 months later shows fracture healing ➡. A portion of the SBC remains and is better delineated ➡. The remainder of the cyst has healed; it is speculated that a fracture accelerates a healing response in a SBC.*

(Left) *Lateral radiograph shows a well-marginated lesion arising in the anterior body of calcaneus ➡. The differential by radiograph is a SBC vs. intraosseous lipoma.* **(Right)** *Axial PD FS FS MR in the same case shows high signal, indicating an SBC rather than lipoma. Note that the cyst has thin septa separating regions of slightly different signal intensity ➡. Such septa may enhance following contrast administration. It is not unusual to see regions of different signal intensity within a SBC.*

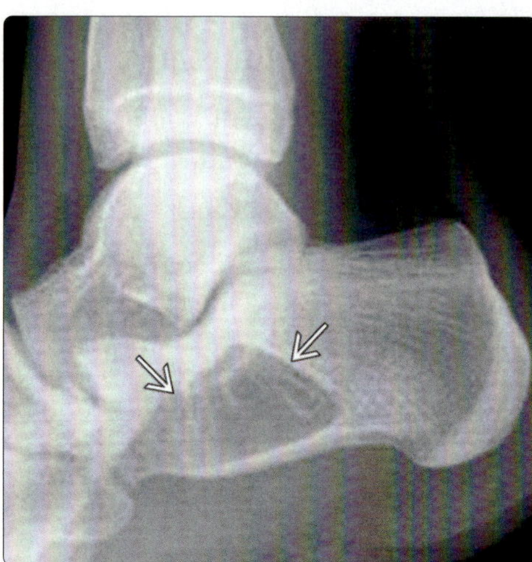

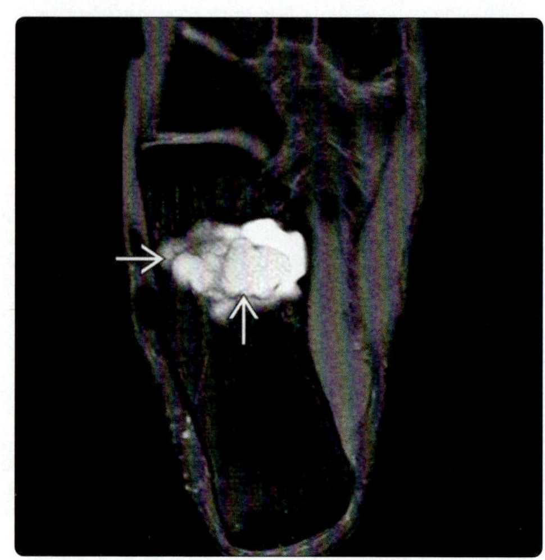

(Left) *Lateral bone scan shows peripheral uptake around a photopenic lesion in the calcaneus ➡. Bone scan of a SBC may be normal or may have this peripheral uptake pattern.* **(Right)** *Sagittal T1WI MR in the same patient shows a low signal lesion ➡ in a typical location for SBC. There is subtle inhomogeneity but the majority of the lesion shows signal nearly isointense to muscle. Perhaps surprisingly, T1 imaging may be quite inhomogeneous in a SBC, even containing high signal regions.*

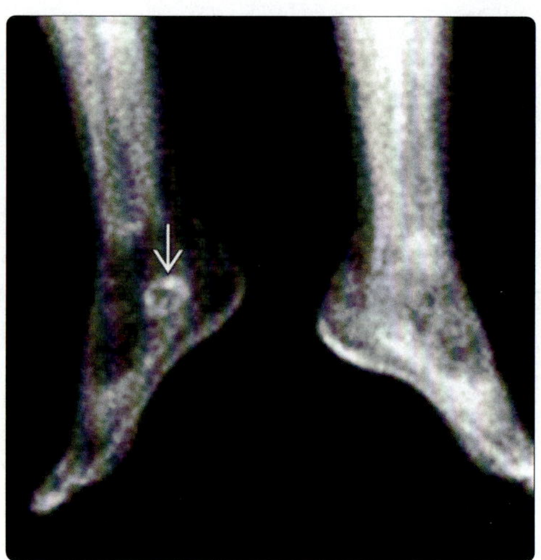

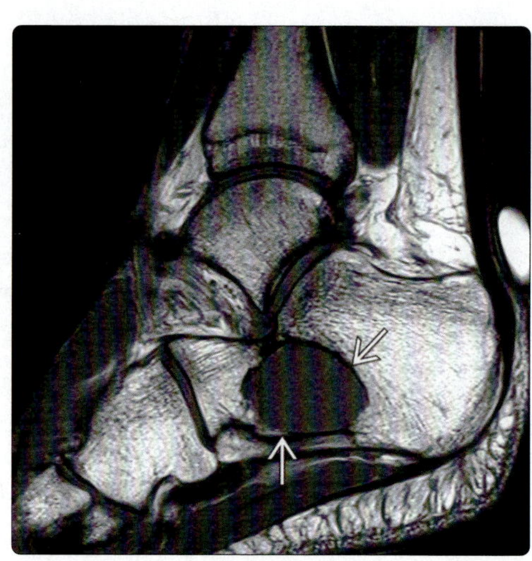

(Left) *Axial T2WI FS MR shows the lesion to be nearly homogeneous high signal. There is a fluid-fluid level, as is fairly frequently seen in SBC lesions ⇨. Note also that there is a thin incomplete septum ➡; septa are often present within these lesions.* **(Right)** *Sagittal T1 C+ FS MR demonstrates a moderately enhancing central fluid collection; the fluid need not enhance but occasionally may do so. There is an enhancing rim ➡, which correlates with the peripheral uptake on bone scan.*

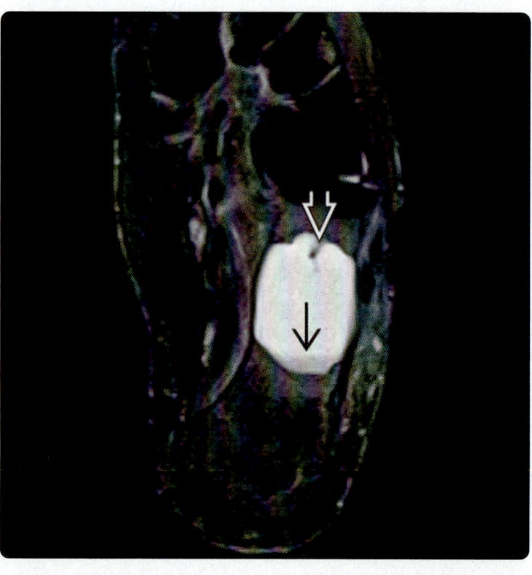

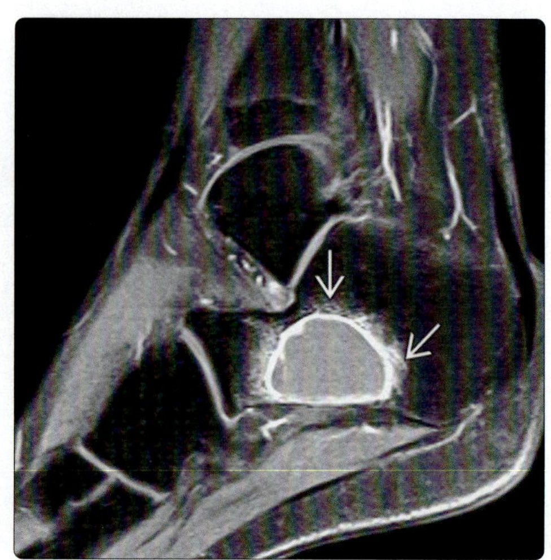

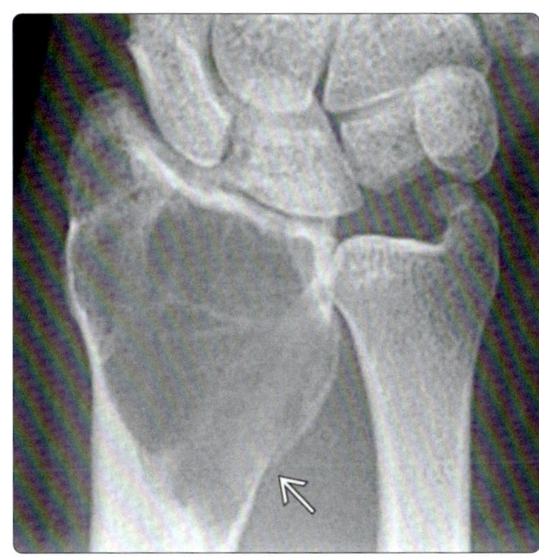

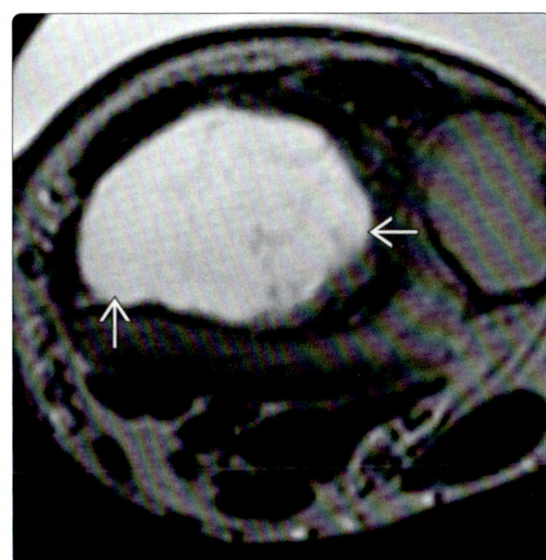

(Left) *AP radiograph shows a lytic lesion at the end of the bone in a 35 year old, typical of GCT. There is a pathologic fracture ➡. Remember, however, that SBC might also be considered with a nonaggressive central lesion in adult.* **(Right)** *Axial T2WI FS MR in the same patient demonstrates the lesion to be somewhat inhomogeneous, with regions of slightly different high signal intensity ➡. There are several thin lower signal partial septa within the lesion, partially separating the cystic regions.*

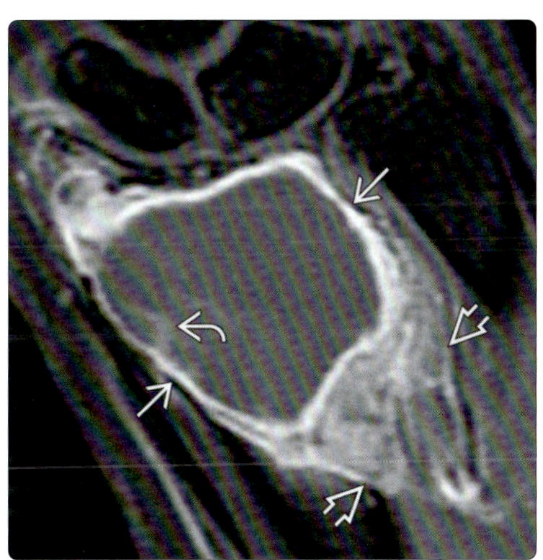

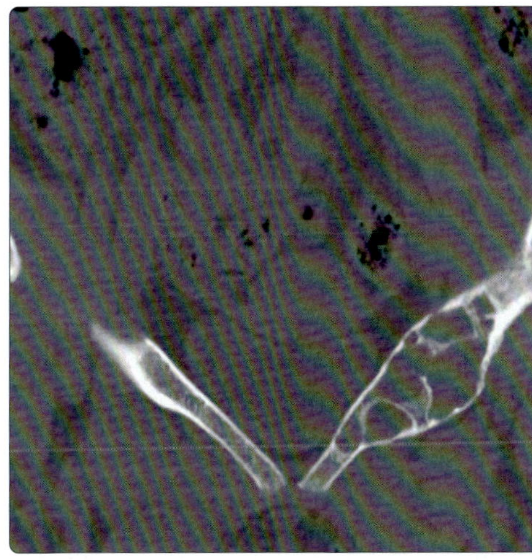

(Left) *Coronal T1WI C+ FS MR in the same patient shows the lesion to be low signal fluid, with an enhancing rim ➡. Small internal enhancing septa are seen ➡. Finally, there is inhomogeneous enhancement at the site of fracture ➡; if one were unaware of the fracture, this might be a confusing picture.* **(Right)** *Coronal bone CT in an adult woman shows an expansile lytic lesion containing septa. The lesion has the typical appearance of a SBC.*

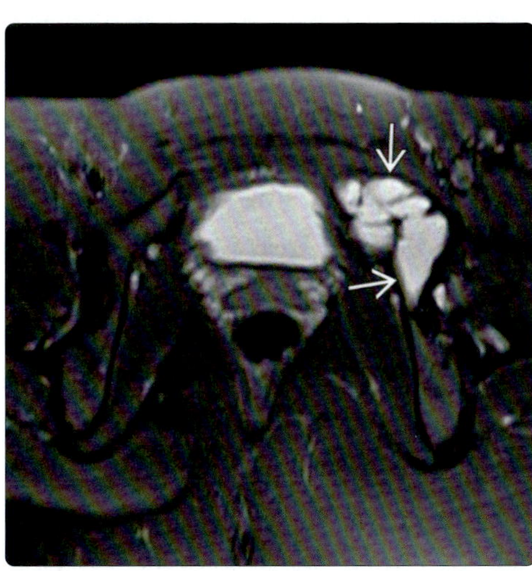

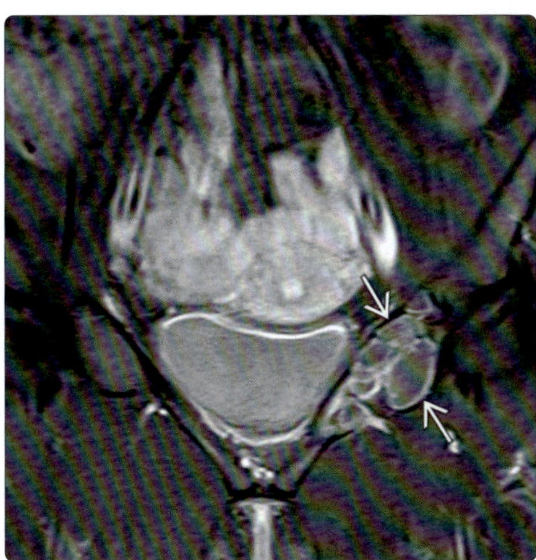

(Left) *Axial T2 FS MR, same patient, shows high signal within the lesion ➡, along with septa. There are no fluid levels on this image; however, this appearance need not be present for the diagnosis of a SBC.* **(Right)** *Coronal T1 C+ FS MR, same patient, shows the lesion ➡ to have variable mild central enhancement, with more pronounced rim enhancement. The entire imaging pattern is typical of a SBC. Although uncommon in adults, when a SBC occurs in this age group, the pelvis, calcaneus, and patella are the most common locations.*

KEY FACTS

TERMINOLOGY

- Benign cystic lesion of bone composed of blood-filled spaces separated by connective tissue septa
- May arise as primary or secondary lesion
  - 70% of aneurysmal bone cysts (ABCs) are primary
  - Secondary ABCs arise in various tumors

IMAGING

- Vertebrae: 15% of cases
  - Generally arise in posterior elements; often extend into body
- Usually metaphyseal in long bone (70-90%)
- Eccentric location
  - If large or in gracile bone, may appear central
- Lytic expanded lesion
  - Since usually eccentric, expands into soft tissues
- Geographic; narrow zone of transition
  - Sclerotic margin generally thin
  - Margin appears complete in only 63%
- MR: Cysts of different signal intensity seen on all sequences (different stages of blood products)
- MR: Fluid-fluid levels seen on all sequences, but most obvious on fluid-sensitive sequences
- Uncommonly appear solid (5%)

CLINICAL ISSUES

- Most common in first 2 decades (range: 5-30 years)
- Recurrence rate following curettage is variable in different series (20-50%)

DIAGNOSTIC CHECKLIST

- ABC may have phase of rapid growth
  - May be mistaken for more aggressive lesion
- Watch for any red flags in diagnosis of ABC
  - Any regions of wide zone of transition
  - Small area of cortical breakthrough/soft tissue mass may be sign of telangiectatic osteosarcoma

(Left) *PA radiograph of the wrist in a young adult shows an eccentrically placed lytic lesion, mildly expanded ➡, arising in the metaphysis and extending towards the subchondral bone. There is only a mildly sclerotic margin. Based on this image, a giant cell tumor might be the favored diagnosis.* **(Right)** *Lateral radiograph of the same lesion shows a greater degree of expansion ➡ on the volar aspect of the wrist. Both a giant cell tumor and an aneurysmal bone cyst (ABC) should be considered.*

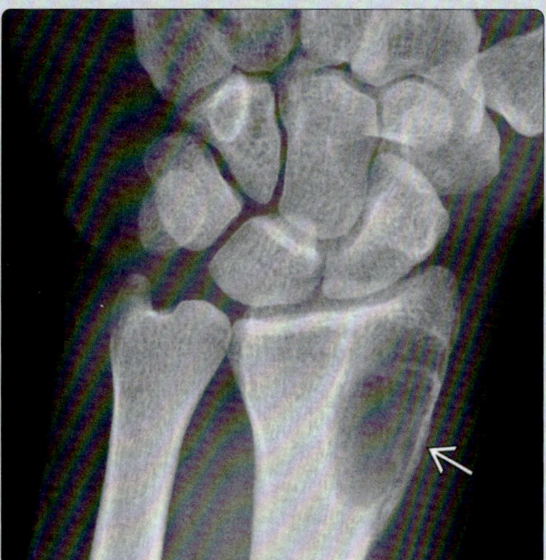

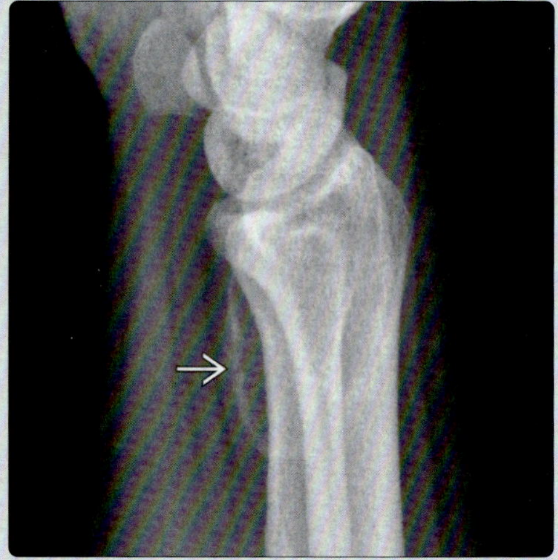

(Left) *Sagittal T2 FS MR of the same lesion confirms the diagnosis of ABC. The lesion consists entirely of fluid, with pronounced fluid-fluid levels ➡. Note the different signal intensities of the layering fluid.* **(Right)** *Sagittal T1 C+ FS MR confirms the findings of fluid-fluid levels ➡ and of nonenhancing cysts. Again, as with the T2 FS sequence, different signal intensity within the cysts relates to different stages of blood products. There is no suggestion of a solid component of the lesion.*

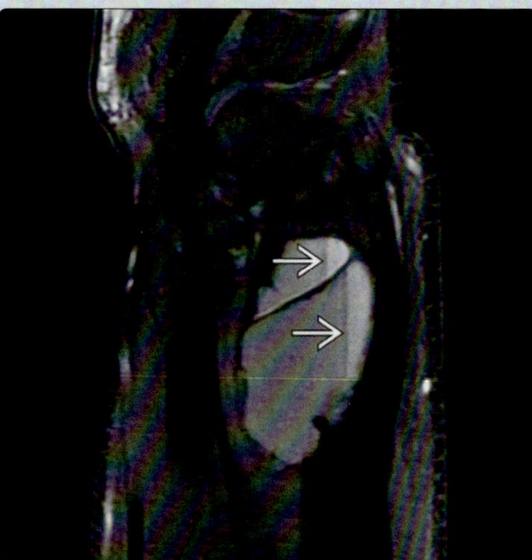

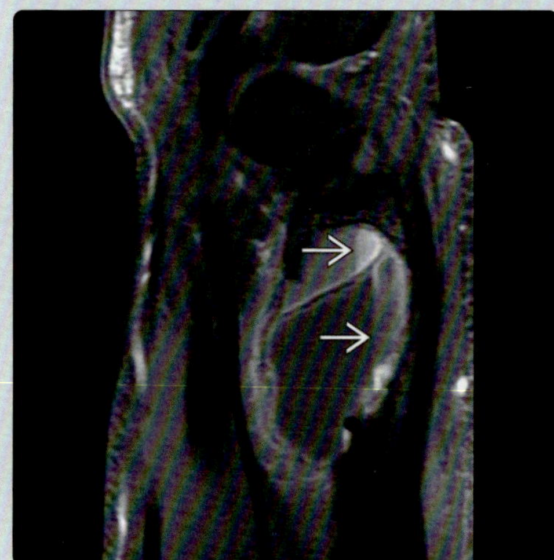

TERMINOLOGY

Abbreviations

- Aneurysmal bone cyst (ABC)

Definitions

- Benign cystic lesion of bone composed of blood-filled spaces separated by connective tissue septa
- May arise as primary or secondary lesion
  - 70% of ABCs are primary
  - Secondary ABCs arise in various tumors

IMAGING

General Features

- Best diagnostic clue
  - Eccentric metaphyseal lytic lesion composed nearly entirely of fluid-fluid levels
- Location
  - Usually metaphyseal in long bone
    - Physis grows away from lesion, leaving it in metadiaphyseal position
    - Few (10%) are truly diaphyseal
  - Eccentric location
    - If large or in gracile bone, may appear central
  - Long bones: 70-80%
    - Femur, tibia, humerus most common
  - Vertebrae: 15%
    - Generally arise in posterior elements; often extend into body
    - May cross disc to involve adjacent vertebra
  - Hands: 10-15%
  - Rare in flat bones; 50% of these are in pelvis
  - Uncommon intracortical (12-18%) or surface (7-8%) origin; rare soft tissue lesions

Radiographic Findings

- Radiography
  - Lytic expanded lesion
    - May have trabeculation, but internal matrix exceedingly rare (seen more commonly histologically than by imaging)
  - Usually eccentric so expands into soft tissues
  - Geographic; narrow zone of transition
    - Sclerotic margin generally thin
    - Margin appears complete in only 63%
  - Periosteal reaction variable

MR Findings

- Septa visible
- Cysts of different signal intensity seen on all sequences (different stages of blood products)
- Fluid-fluid levels seen on all sequences but most obvious on fluid-sensitive sequences
  - Different densities of blood products
- No enhancement of cystic components
  - Septa may enhance; honeycomb appearance
- Geographic, with thin low signal sclerotic margin
- Surrounding edema, both in bone and soft tissue
  - Evaluate carefully to be certain this is not permeative tumor, such as telangiectatic osteosarcoma
- Majority of lesions show loculated regions of fluid levels throughout, but there are exceptions
  - Uncommonly, majority of lesion may be solid (5%)
    - Isointense to skeletal muscle on T1
    - Fairly uniform ↑ SI on fluid-sensitive sequences
    - Intense enhancement with adjacent edema
    - Cystic portions may be present
  - Some ABCs contain small regions of solid tumor
  - Secondary ABC shows 2 distinctly different regions
    - Solid focus of underlying lesion, with signal characteristics of that lesion
    - Loculated fluid-fluid levels in ABC portion

Nuclear Medicine Findings

- Bone scan may show doughnut sign (64%)
  - Photopenic center, peripheral increased uptake

DIFFERENTIAL DIAGNOSIS

Telangiectatic Osteosarcoma

- Most important differential, since treatment and prognosis are different
- Radiographically similar: Eccentric, metaphyseal, mostly geographic
- Similar fluid-fluid levels on MR
- May have suggestions of greater degree of aggressiveness
  - Incomplete margination
  - Small area of cortical breakthrough/soft tissue mass
  - Significant solid regions

Giant Cell Tumor

- Eccentric, metaphyseal lytic lesion
- Often extends to subchondral bone; ABC rarely does
- May be as expanded and bubbly as ABC
- MR: Solid lesion with significant ↓ SI on T2WI
- MR may show fluid-fluid levels, as does ABC
- ABC may arise in giant cell tumor (GCT), showing fluid levels
  - MR should show solid tumor (GCT) as well as ABC

Simple Bone Cyst

- Lytic, expanded, metaphyseal or metadiaphyseal
- Generally more central in location than ABC
- Pseudotrabeculations on radiograph
- MR shows less complex cystic structure
  - Fluid-fluid levels may be present but less complex loculations and layering of blood products

Osteoblastoma

- Differential difficulty primarily in vertebral lesions
- Arises in posterior elements, as does ABC
- Moderately aggressive: Expanded with thin cortex
- If matrix is present, serves as differentiating factor
- MR: Generally solid mass; may contain fluid levels
- ABC may arise in osteoblastoma (OB), showing fluid levels
  - MR should show solid tumor (OB) as well as ABC component

Metastases

- Some may be hemorrhagic, such as renal cell

DDx of Aneurysmal Bone Cyst Arising in Phalanx

- All of these may appear identical on radiograph

- MR with fluid-fluid levels may be only differentiating feature for ABC
- Enchondroma protuberans
  - Often lytic and bubbly in phalanx
- Simple bone cyst
- Giant cell tumor

PATHOLOGY

General Features

- Etiology
  - May be related to trauma-induced vascular process
    - Possible osseous arteriovenous malformation, venous obstruction
  - 2° ABC (up to 1/3 of cases) related to prior lesions, including
    - Giant cell tumor (19-39% of 2° ABC)
    - OB
    - Chondroblastoma
    - Less common: Fibrous dysplasia, chondromyxoid fibroma, fibroxanthoma, solitary bone cyst
    - Some malignant lesions have ABC components
      - Osteosarcoma, chondrosarcoma, malignant fibrous histiocytoma
- Genetics
  - Rearrangement of chromosome 17 short arm; many variations
    - Assumed to result from acquired aberrations, arising in cytogenetically normal precursor cells

Gross Pathologic & Surgical Features

- Multiloculated mass of blood-filled cystic spaces
- Septa: Tan-white gritty material
- Solid regions may be seen
  - Solid portion of ABC
  - Underlying lesion with characteristics of 1° tumor

Microscopic Features

- Blood-filled cystic spaces
- Lined by single layer of flat undifferentiated cells
  - Endothelial lining rarely seen
- Connective tissue septa: Moderately dense cellular proliferation
  - Fibroblasts
  - Osteoclast-type giant cells
  - Reactive woven bone rimmed by osteoblasts
- Solid portions
  - Same components as septa
  - Similar to giant cell reparative granuloma

CLINICAL ISSUES

Presentation

- Most common signs/symptoms
  - Pain, swelling
  - Pathologic fracture uncommon (20%)
    - Most common in spine
  - Neurologic symptoms if in vertebra
  - May have history of trauma

Demographics

- Age
  - Most common in first 2 decades (range: 5-30 years old)
    - 76% occur in patients < 20 years old
    - Median age at diagnosis: 13 years
- Gender
  - M = F, or minimal female predominance
- Epidemiology
  - 6% of primary bone tumors

Natural History & Prognosis

- Recurrence rate following curettage is variable in different series (20-50%)
  - Recurrence generally within 2 years
  - Risk of recurrence greatest in children with juxtaphyseal lesions
- Rare reports of malignant transformation
  - Controversial; primary lesion may not have been recognized in those cases

Treatment

- Identify underlying lesion if present; appropriate treatment for that underlying tumor
- Treatment for 1° ABC
  - Curettage, cryosurgery, bone graft
  - Sclerotherapy is used with reported success
  - Consider preoperative embolization
    - Osteonecrosis may complicate embolotherapy
  - Denosumab and doxycycline show promise

DIAGNOSTIC CHECKLIST

Consider

- ABC may be mistaken for more aggressive lesion
  - May have phase of rapid growth
    - Marked bone destruction with periosteal reaction
    - Not clearly contained by thin peripheral cortex
- Watch for any red flags in diagnosis of ABC
  - Any regions of wide zone of transition
  - Small area of cortical breakthrough/soft tissue mass
  - Substantial regions of solid mass among areas of fluid-fluid levels
  - All of above may be signs of telangiectatic osteosarcoma
    - Biopsy must be directed to solid regions
    - All tissue must be carefully evaluated by pathologist for osteosarcoma

SELECTED REFERENCES

1. Boriani S et al: Aneurysmal bone cysts of the spine: treatment options and considerations. J Neurooncol. 120(1):171-8, 2014
2. Pauli C et al: Response of an aggressive periosteal aneurysmal bone cyst (ABC) of the radius to denosumab therapy. World J Surg Oncol. 12:17, 2014
3. Reddy KI et al: Aneurysmal bone cysts: do simple treatments work? Clin Orthop Relat Res. 472(6):1901-10, 2014
4. Burch S et al: Aneurysmal bone cysts of the spine. Neurosurg Clin N Am. 19(1):41-7, 2008
5. Cottalorda J et al: Modern concepts of primary aneurysmal bone cyst. Arch Orthop Trauma Surg. 127(2):105-14, 2007
6. Kransdorf MJ et al: Aneurysmal bone cyst: concept, controversy, clinical presentation, and imaging. AJR Am J Roentgenol. 164(3):573-80, 1995

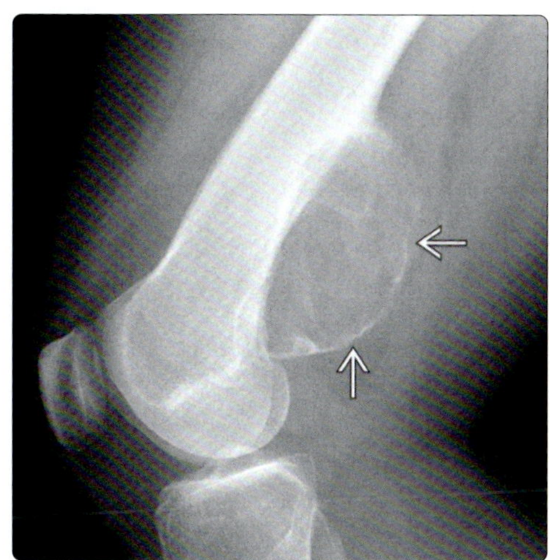

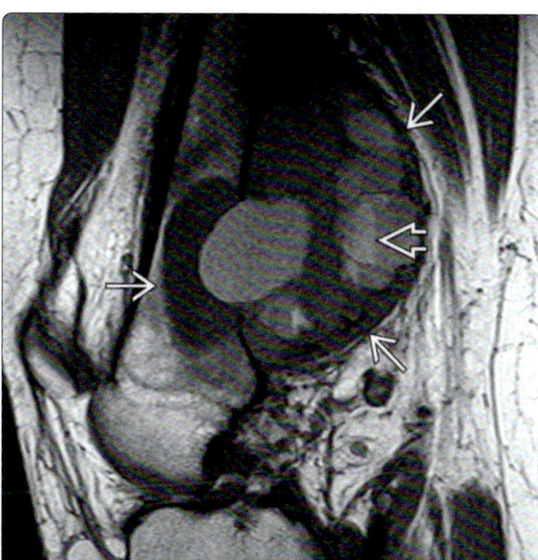

(Left) *Lateral radiograph shows a highly expanded lesion of the posterior femur* ➡. *The cortex is extremely thin but intact. There is no evidence of permeative change or cortical breakthrough. In a patient of this age, the appearance is most typical of ABC. However, telangiectatic osteosarcoma must be considered as a possibility.* **(Right)** *Sagittal T1WI MR in the same patient shows regions of high signal representing blood, with surrounding low signal* ➡. *Fluid levels are present* ➡.

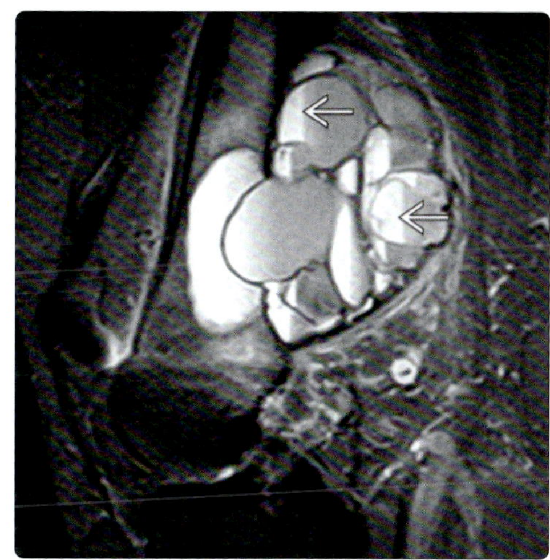

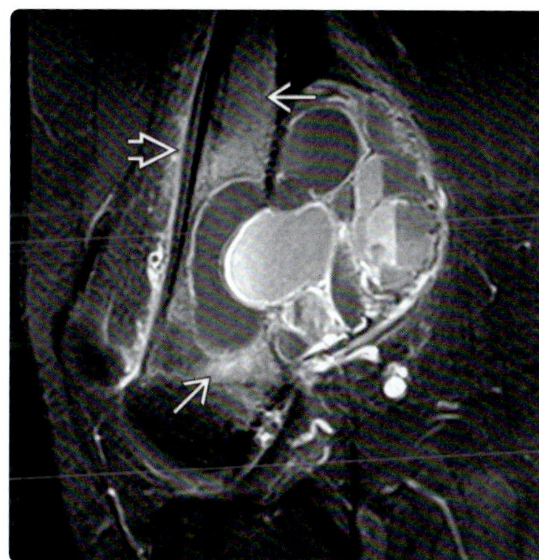

(Left) *Sagittal T2WI FS MR shows fluid levels much more prominently* ➡. *The lesion appears well circumscribed, but direct involvement of the femur is greater than suggested on radiograph. Note marrow edema.* **(Right)** *Sagittal T1WI C+ FS MR shows enhancement of bone adjacent to the lesion* ➡ *and periosteal reaction* ➡. *This may be reactive, but one must be concerned about permeative extension of a subtle telangiectatic osteosarcoma. At surgery, the lesion was found to be ABC.*

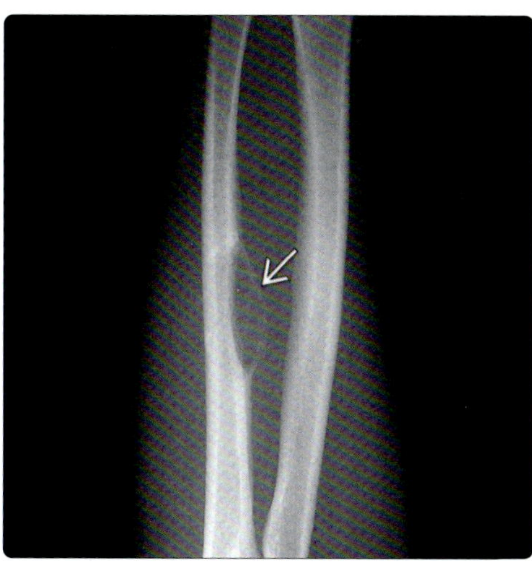

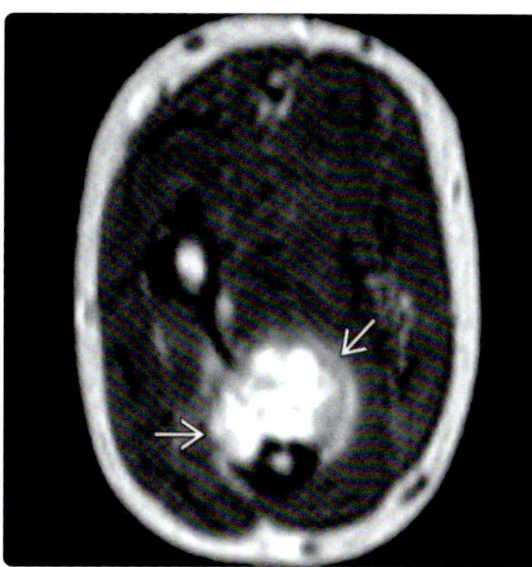

(Left) *AP radiograph demonstrates an eccentric middiaphyseal lesion of the ulna. The lesion is extremely expanded but appears to have a thin intact cortex* ➡. *This radiographic finding is fairly typical for ABC, though diaphyseal location is less frequent than metaphyseal.* **(Right)** *Axial T2WI MR in the same patient shows the lesion to be quite large, appearing to have broken through the cortical rim* ➡ *seen on the radiograph. There are no fluid levels. This proved to be a solid variant of ABC.*

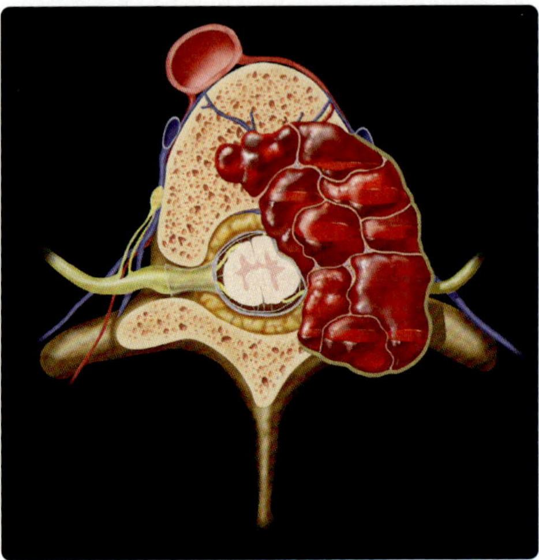

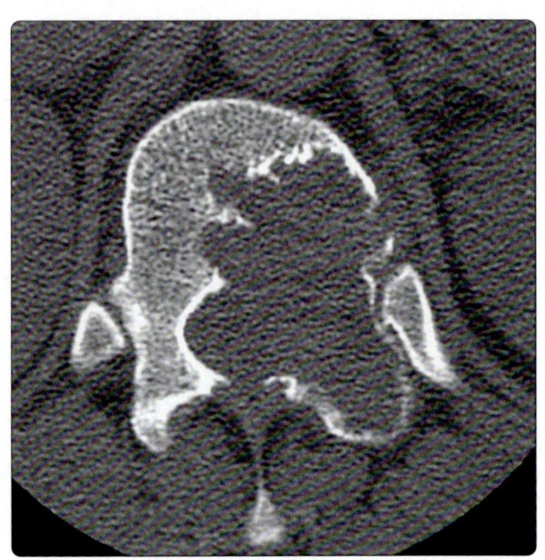

(Left) *Axial graphic through the spine demonstrates a ABC, with the blood-filled lesion originating in the posterior elements and extending into the vertebral body. There is a small epidural component.* **(Right)** *Axial bone CT shows a lytic expanded mass with a thin "eggshell" rim of cortex peripherally but extensive destruction of cortex around 1/2 of the spinal canal. It is not clear in this case whether the lesion originated in the vertebral body or posterior elements.*

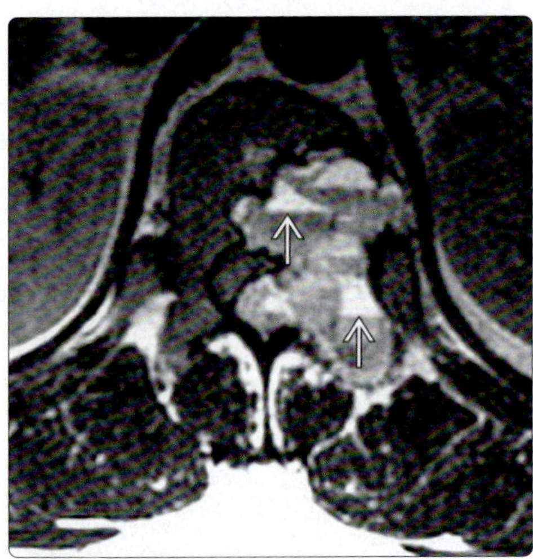

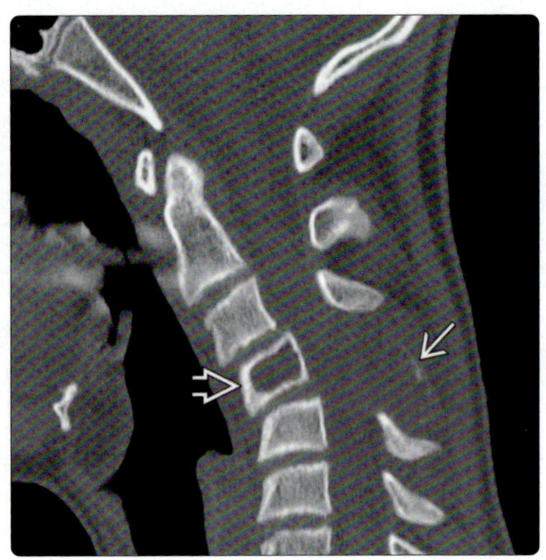

(Left) *Axial T2WI MR in the same patient shows a multiloculated mass containing multiple fluid-fluid levels ➡. Mixed signal intensity reflects the presence of blood products. The appearance is typical of ABC, though other lesions may also contain fluid levels.* **(Right)** *Sagittal bone CT in the midline shows a lytic lesion significantly expanding the spinous process ➡ of C4. There is less severe involvement of the vertebral body ➡. This is the typical location and appearance of ABC of the spine.*

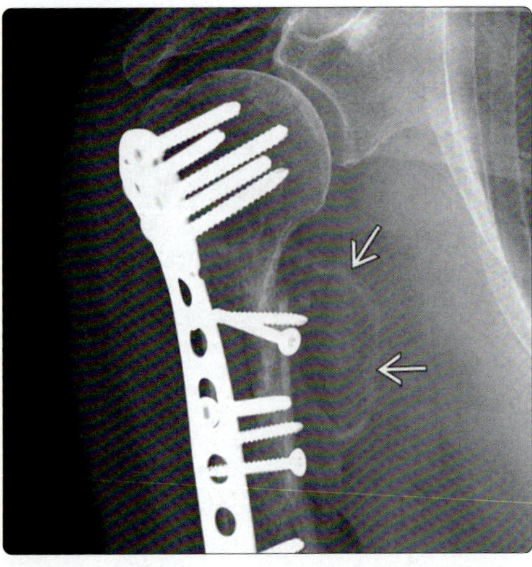

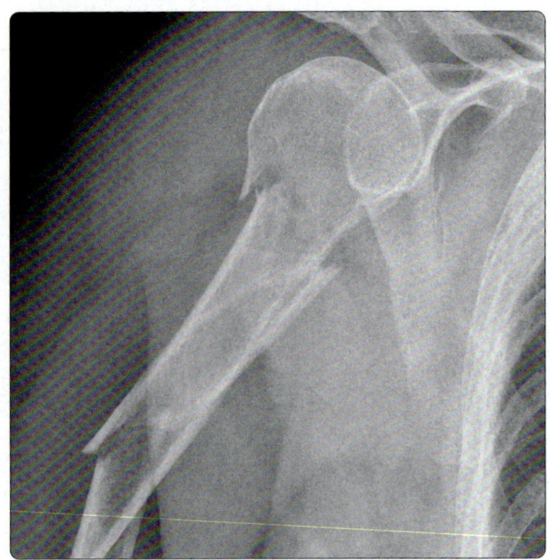

(Left) *AP radiograph obtained as follow-up for fracture fixation is shown. Besides the healing fracture, there is an expanded lytic lesion ➡. Given the timing relative to the fracture, this represents an example of ABC arising secondary to trauma.* **(Right)** *AP radiograph of the same patient obtained at the time of injury is shown. Note that although the fracture is significantly comminuted, there is no evidence of underlying bone lesion. This confirms the traumatic origin of the ABC seen on the previous image.*

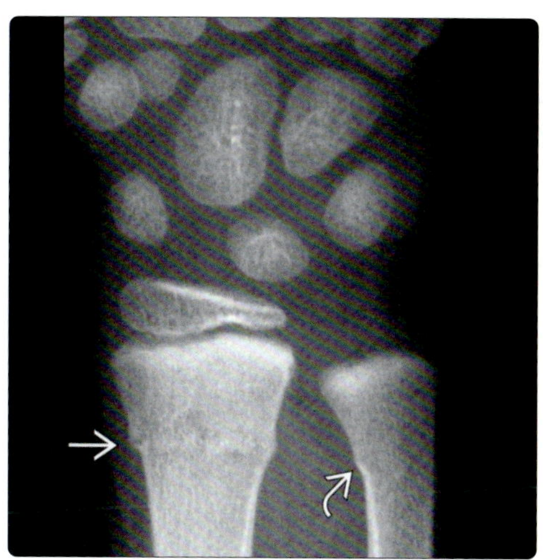

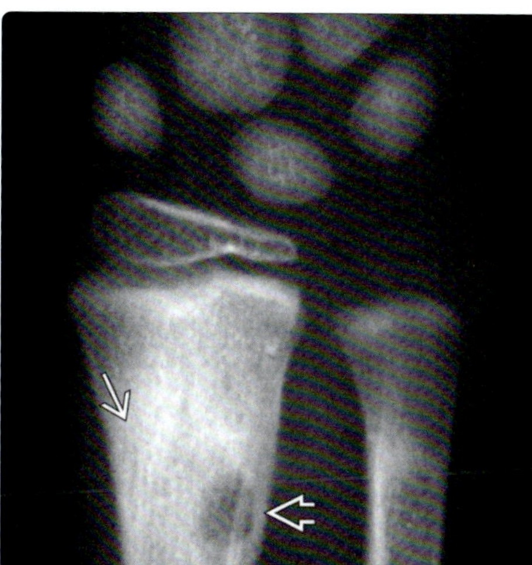

(Left) *AP radiograph shows a buckle (torus) fracture of the forearm (distal radius ➡ and ulna ➡). These normally heal without complication, remodeling to normal-appearing bone.* **(Right)** *AP radiograph in the same patient 3 months later shows fracture healing ➡ but also a new lytic lesion ➡ developing adjacent to the trauma. This was proven to be ABC. It is interesting that occasionally ABC develops following trauma or else within another otherwise unrelated neoplasm.*

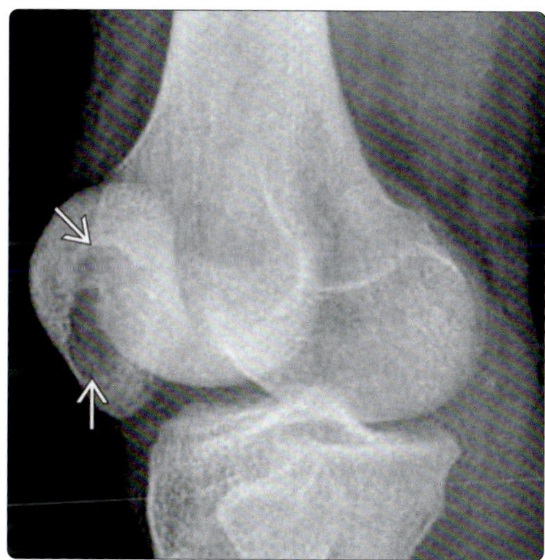

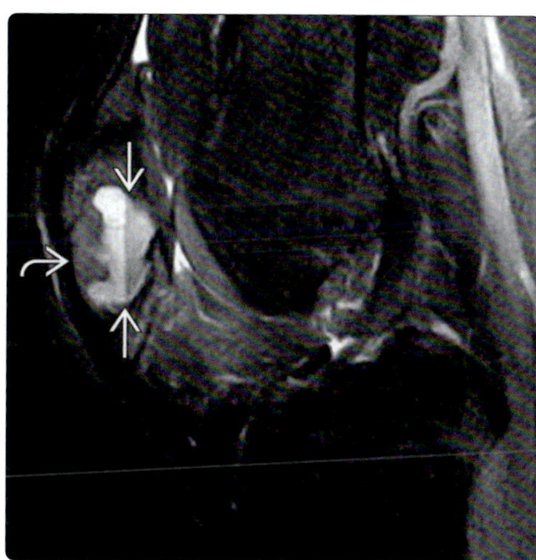

(Left) *Oblique radiograph shows a lytic lesion with a thin sclerotic margin ➡, sans aggressive features. Giant cell tumor, ABC, or chondroblastoma (CB) should be considered.* **(Right)** *Sagittal T2WI FS MR in the same patient shows the anterior portion as solid and only mildly hyperintense ➡, while the posterior portion contains a fluid level ➡. The location and patient age are typical for CB, which may serve as an underlying focus for development of ABC, proven at biopsy. (Courtesy K. Suh, MD.)*

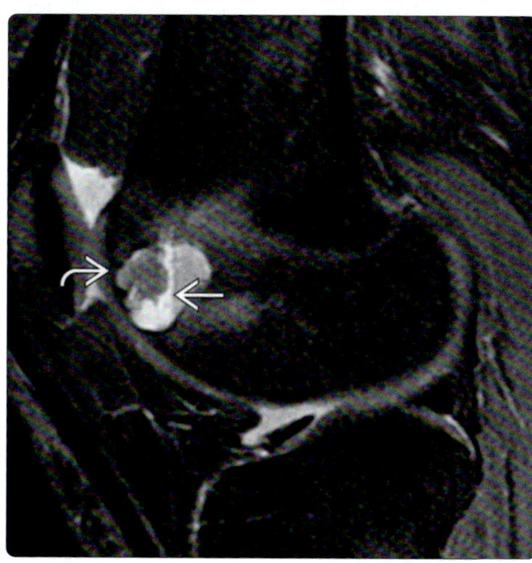

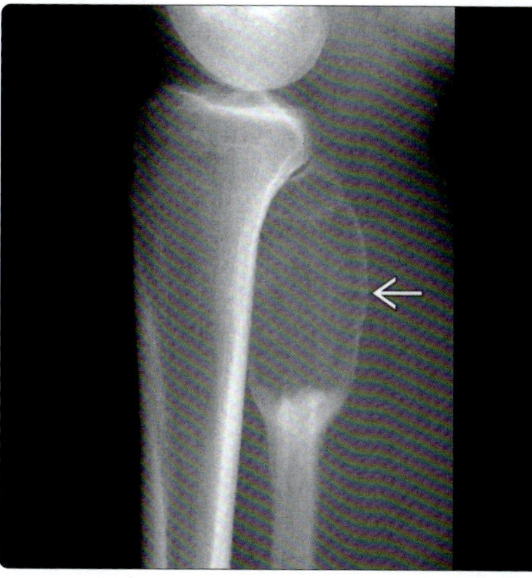

(Left) *Sagittal FS MR (different patient with CB and superimposed ABC) demonstrates the epiphyseal lesion to be heterogeneous; the mildly hyperintense lobulated anterior CB portion ➡ is different in appearance than fluid levels in posterior ABC portion ➡.* **(Right)** *Lateral radiograph shows a highly expanded lesion occupying the entire proximal fibula ➡. Though ABC usually arises in an eccentric position, it usually appears central in gracile bones, such as the fibula or ulna; pathology proved ABC.*

Fibroxanthoma

KEY FACTS

TERMINOLOGY

- Synonymous with nonossifying fibroma (NOF)
- Definition: Benign fibrous lesion composed of spindle cells in collagenous matrix
  - Considered by some to be developmental defect rather than true neoplasm
  - Benign fibrous cortical defect is histologically identical to NOF, so considered same lesion here

IMAGING

- Location: Most common around knee and in distal tibia
- Cortically based, except
  - Appears central in gracile bones (fibula, ulna)
  - Appears central when NOF is large
- Early radiographic appearance: Lytic, geographic, with thin sclerotic margin
- Beginning healing phase radiographic appearance: Thicker sclerotic margin, forming peripheral bone
- Late radiographic appearance: Entirely sclerotic; usually remodels to normal
- Fluid-sensitive MR sequences: Inhomogeneous, with areas of low signal and others that are hyperintense
  - ~ 80% show hypointensity in at least part of lesion
  - Septa seen on T2WI in majority of cases
  - Avid peripheral and septal enhancement; some central enhancement, depending on degree of sclerosis
- FDG PET: Mild to intense uptake in NOF

CLINICAL ISSUES

- Childhood and adolescence (first 2 decades)
- Most lesions naturally heal and involute

DIAGNOSTIC CHECKLIST

- NOF is one of the few "leave me alone" lesions
- Seldom presents as diagnostic dilemma unless very large
- Frequently seen incidentally on MR of knee

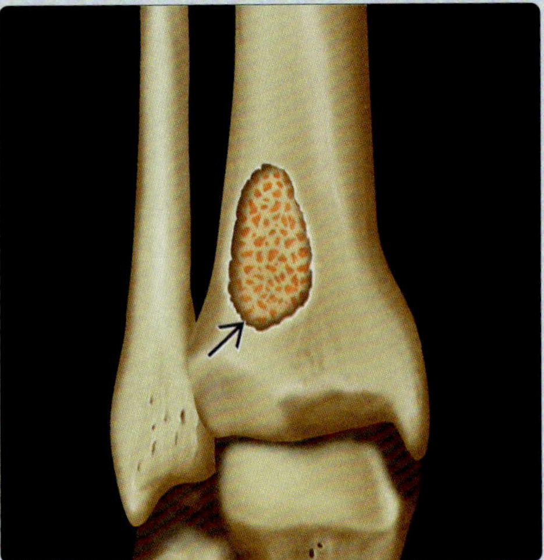

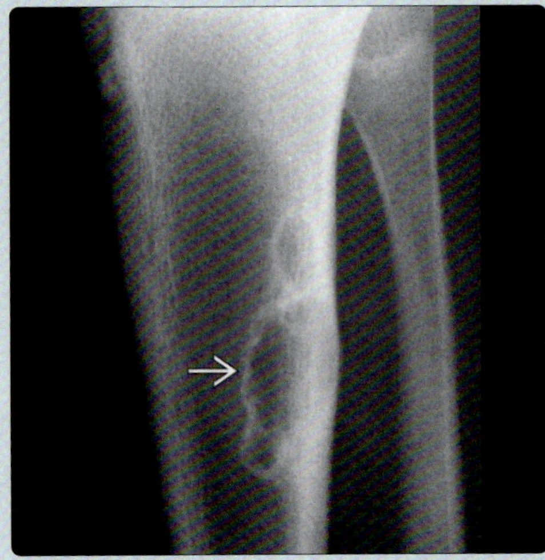

(Left) *Coronal graphic depicts fibroxanthoma as a cortically based lesion with geographic sclerotic margin ➡. The most frequent location is metaphysis. Note that this lesion is also popularly termed nonossifying fibroma (NOF).* **(Right)** *Lateral radiograph shows a typical fibroxanthoma (NOF), cortically based and located in the metaphysis or metadiaphysis of a child. There is no question that the lesion is completely geographic. There is a thick sclerotic margin ➡ surrounding the lesion entirely.*

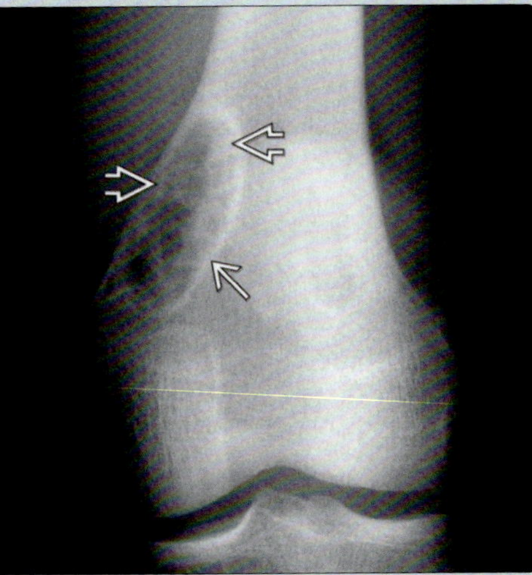

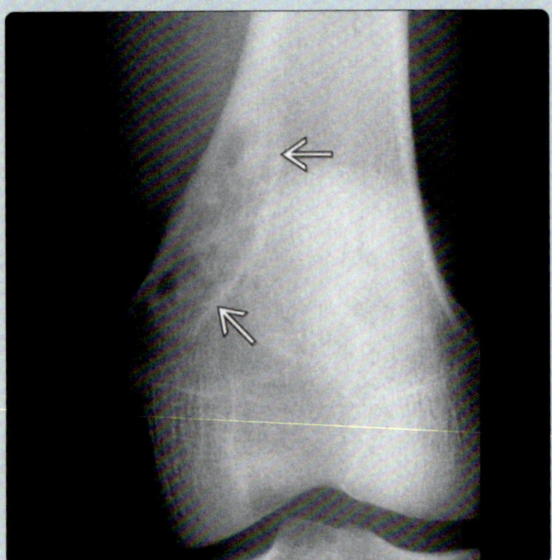

(Left) *AP radiograph shows a typical NOF in a young adult. Note the metaphyseal and cortical location of the lesion, as well as the densely sclerotic margin ➡. Though much of the lesion is lytic, there are peripheral regions that show a smooth sclerosis ➡, indicating healing of the lesion about the periphery.* **(Right)** *AP radiograph in the same patient 3 years later shows the lesion to be nearly completely healed ➡. With time, it will remodel until it is not visible. This is a common occurrence for NOF.*

TERMINOLOGY

Synonyms

- Nonossifying fibroma (NOF), benign fibrous cortical defect (BFCD), nonosteogenic fibroma, metaphyseal defect, histiocytic xanthogranuloma

Definitions

- Benign fibrous lesion composed of spindle cells in collagenous matrix
  - Considered by some to be developmental defect rather than true neoplasm
  - BFCD is histologically identical to NOF, so considered same lesion here

IMAGING

General Features

- Location
  - Most common around knee and in distal tibia
  - Cortically based, except
    - Appears central in gracile bones (fibula, ulna)
    - Appears central when NOF is large
  - Originates in metaphysis
    - With increasing age, physis grows away from lesion, leaving it in metadiaphyseal position
  - Multifocal in 8%
- Size
  - BFCD: Generally < 3 cm in greatest dimension
  - NOF: Generally > 3 cm in greatest dimension; may become very large

Radiographic Findings

- Appearance depends on morphologic age of lesion
  - Early: Lytic, geographic, with thin sclerotic margin
  - Beginning healing phase: Thicker sclerotic margin, forming peripheral bone
  - Late: Entirely sclerotic; usually remodels to normal

MR Findings

- Hypointense to skeletal muscle on T1WI; may have heterogeneous ↓ SI, depending on areas of sclerosis
- Fluid-sensitive sequences: Inhomogeneous, with low signal areas and hyperintense areas
  - Regions of low signal are fibrous elements and hemosiderin; appearance relates to relative amounts
  - ~ 80% show hypointensity in at least part of lesion
  - Septa seen on T2WI in majority of cases
- Avid peripheral and septal enhancement; some central enhancement, depending on degree of sclerosis
- Low signal sclerotic margin, complete around lesion
  - No cortical breakthrough or soft tissue mass

Nuclear Medicine Findings

- Bone scan: Minimal to mild increased activity
- FDG PET: Mild to intense uptake in NOF

DIFFERENTIAL DIAGNOSIS

Desmoplastic Fibroma

- Generally central
- Variable degrees of fibrous material affects MR SI

Large Central Nonossifying Fibroma

- Simple bone cyst (SBC)
  - Central and may appear multiloculated
  - MR differentiates SBC: Cystic lesion defined on fluid-sensitive and post-contrast sequences
- Aneurysmal bone cyst (ABC)
  - Eccentric lytic metaphyseal lesion
  - MR differentiates ABC by fluid-fluid levels

PATHOLOGY

General Features

- Genetics
  - Generally thought to represent developmental defect rather than neoplasm
  - 2 reports of clonally aberrant NOF cases
- Associated abnormalities
  - Multifocal NOF may be associated with neurofibromatosis (Jaffe-Campanacci syndrome)

CLINICAL ISSUES

Presentation

- Most common signs/symptoms
  - Usually asymptomatic
  - Rare pathologic fracture

Demographics

- Age
  - Childhood and adolescence (first 2 decades)
- Gender
  - Male > female (2:1)
- Epidemiology
  - Common: BFCD occurs in 30% of normal children

Natural History & Prognosis

- Most lesions naturally heal and involute
  - Progression of sclerosis from periphery of lesion to obliteration of entire lesion with mild sclerosis
  - Remodels to normal bone
- Some continue to grow, becoming large and occupying entire diameter of bone

Treatment

- None required in vast majority of cases
- If at risk of pathologic fracture, curettage and bone graft

DIAGNOSTIC CHECKLIST

Reporting Tips

- NOF is one of the few "leave me alone" lesions
  - Diagnosis secure on basis of radiographs in majority
  - In most cases, should be able to recommend that neither further imaging nor biopsy required

SELECTED REFERENCES

1. Wadhwa V et al: Enlarging nonossifying fibroma mimicking aggressive bone tumour. Indian J Cancer. 50(4):301, 2013
2. Sakamoto A et al: Nonossifying fibroma accompanied by pathological fracture in a 12-year-old runner. J Orthop Sports Phys Ther. 38(7):434-8, 2008

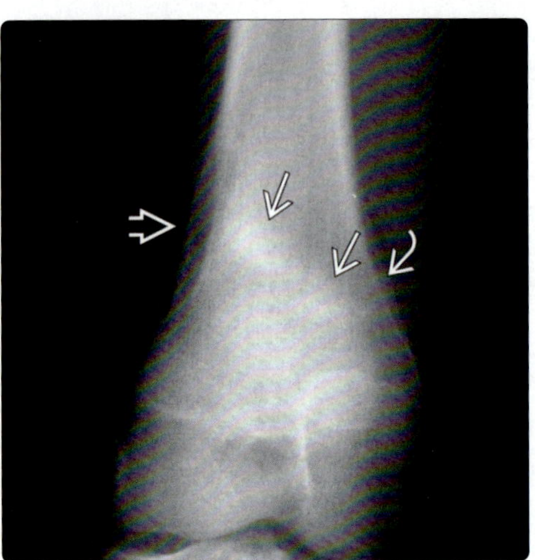

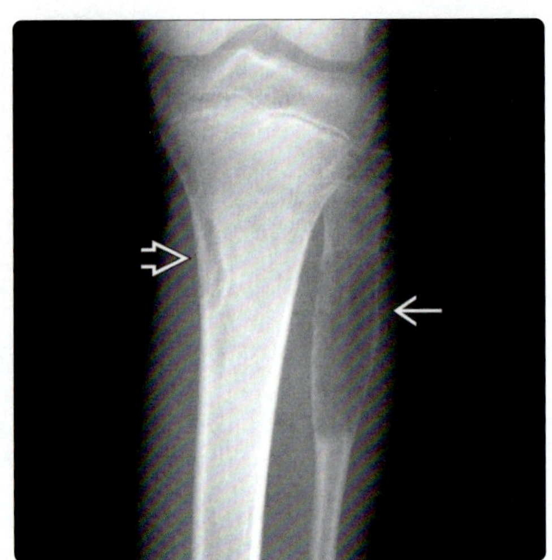

(Left) *AP radiograph shows linear sclerosis across the metaphysis ➡, representing a healing fracture line, extending from a cortically based lytic lesion, which is nonaggressive and typical in appearance for NOF ➡. Note that the periosteal reaction is very regular and dense ➡, relating to the healing of the fracture.* **(Right)** *AP radiograph shows a typical benign fibrous cortical defect in the tibia ➡. The metaphyseal lesion of the proximal fibula is centrally located ➡, typical of NOF arising in thin bones.*

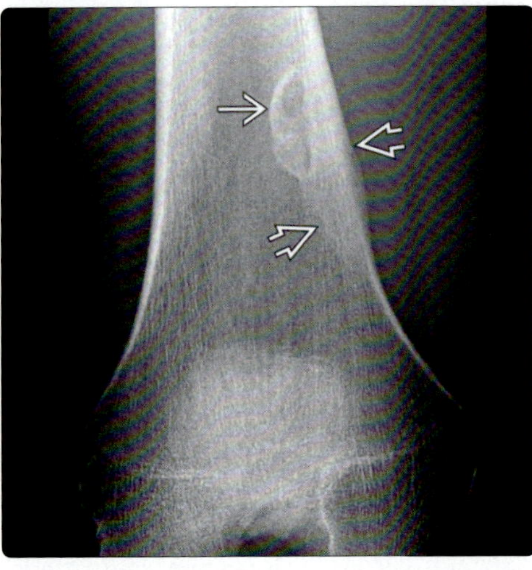

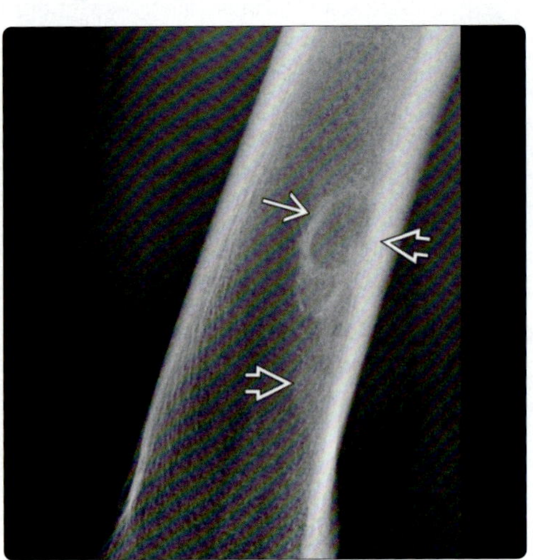

(Left) *AP radiograph of the knee in a patient who has recently become skeletally mature shows a cortically based lytic lesion with a sclerotic margin ➡ that also has filled in with normal bone in its peripheral portions ➡.* **(Right)** *Lateral radiograph of the same lesion confirms the lytic, well-marginated portion ➡ as well as the normal bone formation in the healing portion ➡. This is a typical fibroxanthoma (NOF) undergoing its natural healing evolution upon skeletal maturation.*

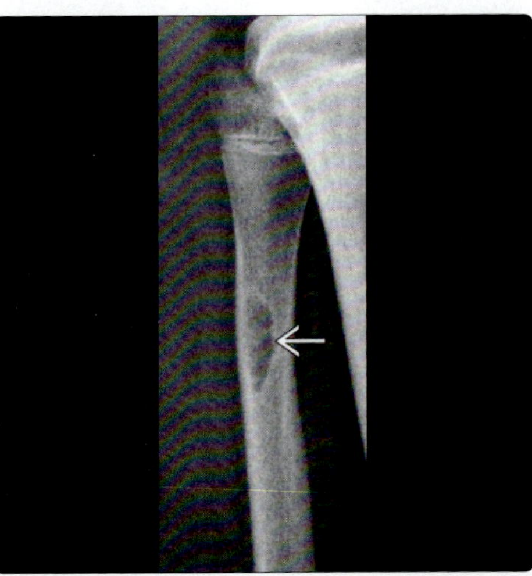

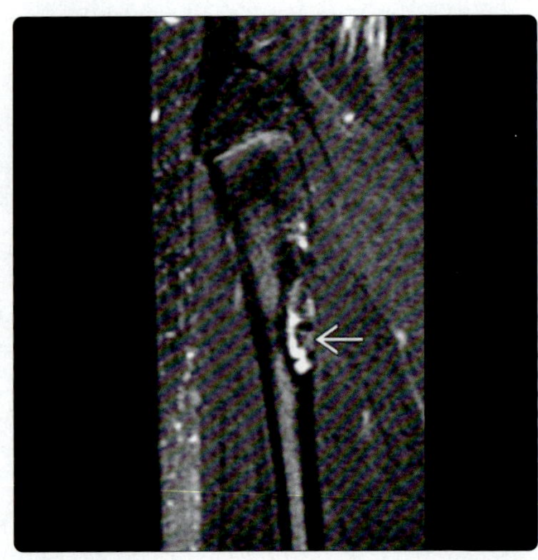

(Left) *AP oblique radiograph shows a fibular lesion with a sclerotic margin ➡ arising eccentrically. This is an early appearance of NOF; as the lesion grows, it will appear to be more centrally located in this gracile bone.* **(Right)** *Coronal STIR MR in the same patient shows heterogeneous signal with septation, containing hypointense signal ➡ representing either fibrous or hemosiderin deposition, as well as hyperintense portions. It is unusual to MR this lesion, as it is usually diagnosed based on radiograph.*

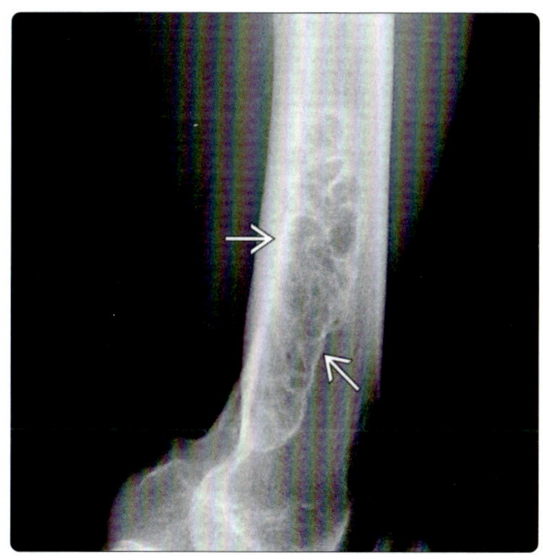

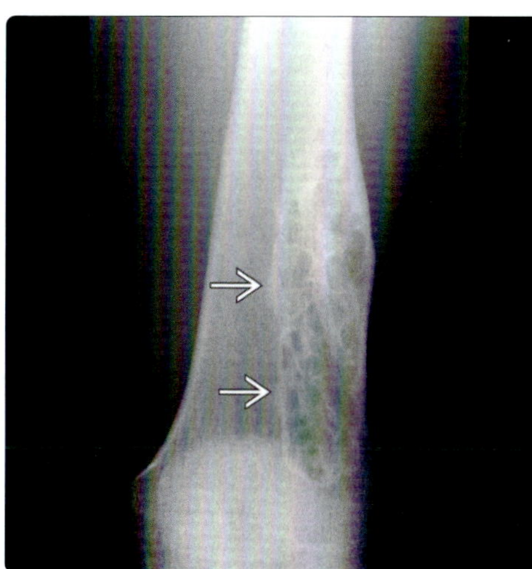

(Left) *Lateral radiograph shows a large (otherwise classic) NOF. This geographic lesion is located in the metaphysis and is cortically based. It has a narrow zone of transition, sclerotic margination ➡, and no periosteal reaction.* **(Right)** *AP radiograph in the same patient shows the classic appearance of NOF. Even though it is a large lesion, it is asymptomatic and should be left alone. The sclerosis around the outer margins ➡ suggests that it is starting to fill in with normal bone.*

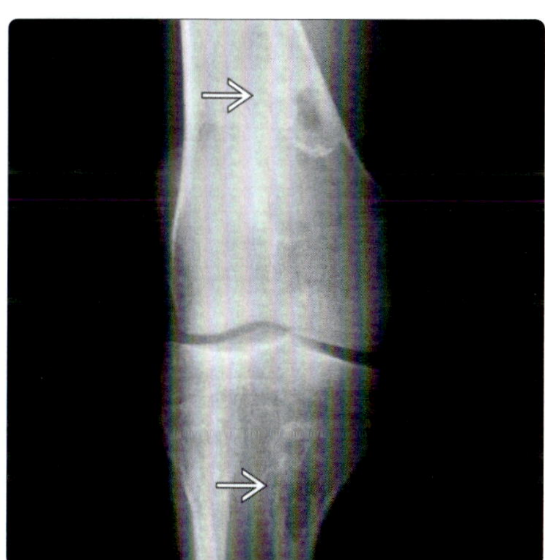

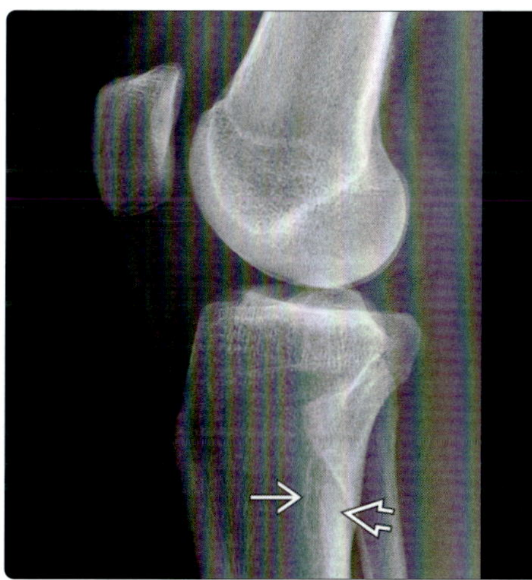

(Left) *Oblique radiograph shows multiple NOF with peripheral sclerosis, indicating partial healing ➡. Multiple NOF is most frequently seen with neurofibromatosis.* **(Right)** *Lateral radiograph shows an asymptomatic lesion that is cortically based in the metaphysis of the tibia ➡. There is normal bone healing in a portion of the lesion ➡ and the patient is becoming skeletally mature. The lesion is a typical NOF and needs no further imaging or follow-up.*

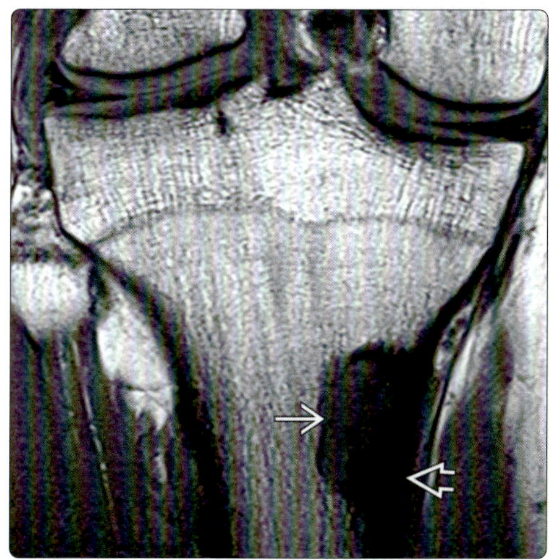

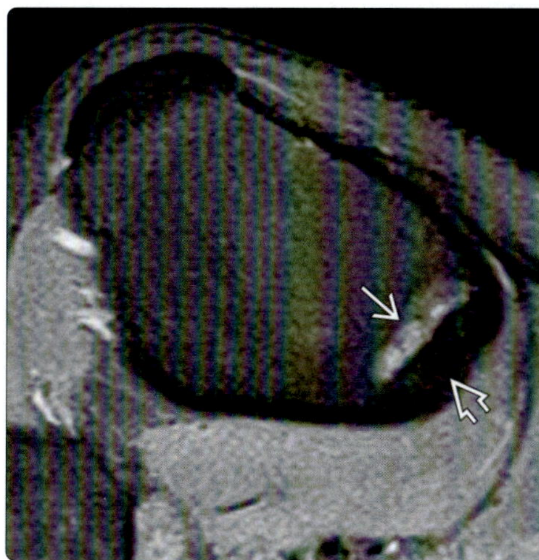

(Left) *Coronal T1WI MR in the same patient (obtained to evaluate the menisci) confirms the expected appearance of NOF, with a hypointense center ➡ and low signal in the healing region that matches the cortex ➡.* **(Right)** *Axial T2FS MR in the same patient shows the hyperintense portion of the NOF ➡ that is still active and the dense low signal of the peripheral healing portion ➡. The lesion is following the most common natural history, with normal bone replacement as the patient becomes skeletally mature.*

Trevor Fairbank

KEY FACTS

TERMINOLOGY

- Synonyms: Dysplasia epiphysealis hemimelica, Trevor disease
- Definition: Intraarticular osteochondroma-like lesion arising from epiphysis

IMAGING

- Location: Usually unilateral and single side of that extremity
  - Lower > upper extremity
  - Ankle most common site (talus, distal tibia, or fibula)
- 3 forms
  - Localized (monoarticular): Usually ankle
  - Classic (2/3 of cases): > 1 joint, unilateral, usually knee and ankle
  - Generalized form: Entire (usually lower) extremity
- Radiographic appearance
  - Premature epiphyseal ossification
  - Abnormal morphology, with lobulations, overgrowth, asymmetry
  - Stippled calcification may be seen
- MR: Confirms lesion is cartilaginous
  - Signal matches that of adjacent epiphysis at various stages of growth

CLINICAL ISSUES

- Presentation
  - Limb length discrepancy (premature physeal closure)
  - Malalignment (usually varus/valgus)
  - Joint mass
  - Early osteoarthritis
- Demographics
  - Developmental; arises in childhood
  - Males > females (3:1)
  - Rare: 1/1,000,000 population
- Treatment is surgical
  - Surgical resection → reestablishing congruity of joint
  - Osteotomy may address malalignment of limb

(Left) *AP radiograph shows a lobulated intraarticular ossification arising from the medial femoral condyle ➡. Since it is clearly ossification and is not loose within the joint, this must represent Trevor Fairbank, an osteochondroma-like intraarticular lesion.* **(Right)** *AP radiograph in the same patient at a younger age shows a lobulated osseous mass arising from the talus ➡, with associated deformity of the distal tibial epiphysis. It is not unusual for this process to be polyarticular, but it is usually unilateral.*

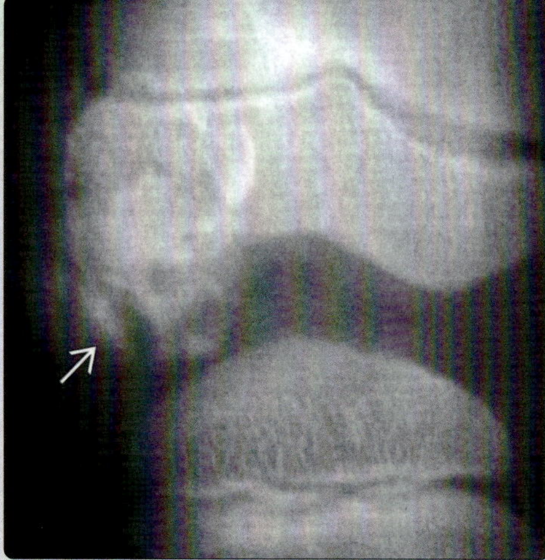

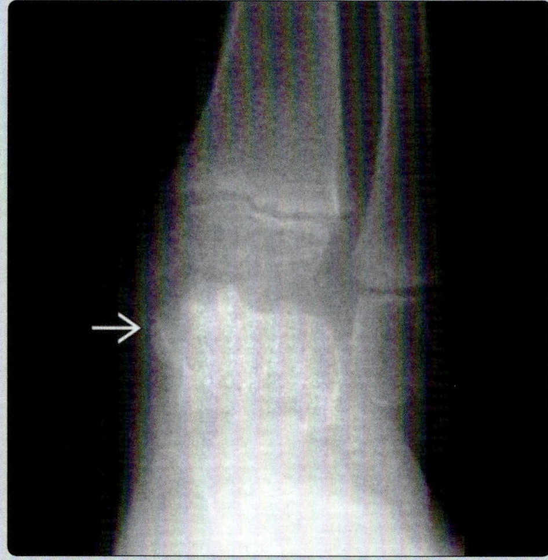

(Left) *AP radiograph demonstrates lateral subluxation of the femoral head and a metallic implant from prior varus-producing osteotomy ➡ aimed at improving joint contiguity in a patient thought to have hip dysplasia. There is a hint of abnormal calcification within the joint ➡.* **(Right)** *Coronal T2WI MR in the same case shows multiple bodies displaying MR characteristics of cartilage ➡ attached to the acetabulum. This is Trevor disease, presenting radiographically and initially treated as hip dysplasia.*

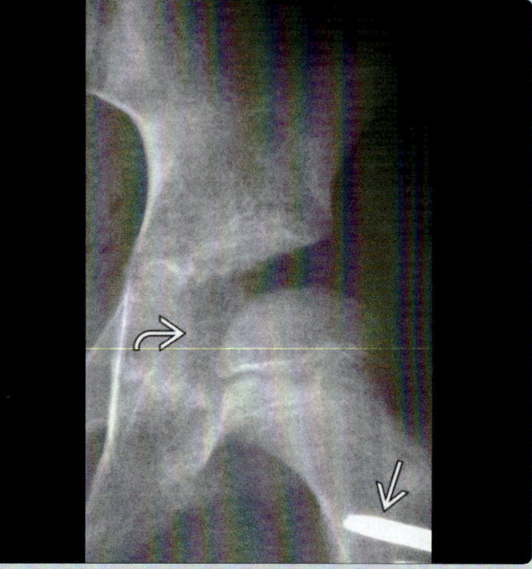

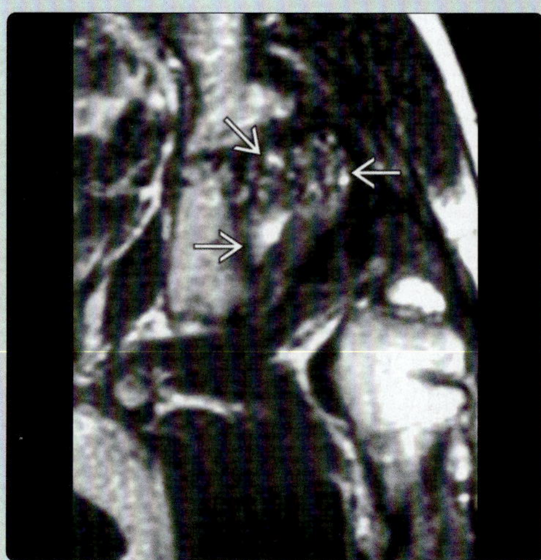

TERMINOLOGY

Synonyms

- Dysplasia epiphysealis hemimelica, Trevor disease

Definitions

- Intraarticular osteochondroma-like lesion arising from epiphysis

IMAGING

General Features

- Best diagnostic clue
  - Rounded intraarticular bodies attached to epiphysis
- Location
  - Usually unilateral and single side of that extremity
    - Medial > lateral side of limb
  - Lower > upper extremity
    - Ankle most common site (talus, distal tibia, or fibula)
  - 3 forms
    - Localized (monoarticular): Usually ankle
    - Classic (2/3 of cases): > 1 joint, unilateral, usually knee and ankle
    - Generalized form: Entire (usually lower) extremity

Radiographic Findings

- Premature epiphyseal ossification
- Advanced bone age due to hyperemia
- Abnormal morphology, with lobulations, overgrowth, asymmetry
- Stippled calcification may be seen
- Eventual merger with adjacent epiphysis
- Continuity with adjacent normal bone not as apparent as with metaphyseal exostosis
- Rare involvement of metaphysis → undertubulation

MR Findings

- Demonstrates deformity in 3 planes for surgical planning
- Confirms lesion is cartilaginous
  - Signal matches that of adjacent epiphysis at various stages of growth
    - Cartilage portion intermediate on T1, high on T2
    - Areas of low signal → calcification

DIFFERENTIAL DIAGNOSIS

Loose Bodies

- Osseous matrix
- Older individuals

Synovial Chondromatosis

- Multiple intraarticular rounded bodies of similar size
- Not attached to epiphysis, as in Trevor disease
- May be seen in children, though more frequently found in adults

Hip Dysplasia (DDH)

- Epiphyseal asymmetric exostoses in Trevor disease result in incongruity of femoral head and acetabulum
  - Incongruity of components of joint mimic DDH

PATHOLOGY

General Features

- Etiology
  - Thought to be developmental disorder
  - Hypothesis: Abnormal cellular activity at cartilaginous ossification center, disturbing normal sequence of development
- Genetics
  - Normal expression levels of *EXT1* and *EXT2* genes
    - Helps to differentiate from osteochondroma, which has low levels of these (gene mutation)
- Associated abnormalities
  - Reported to be rarely associated with Ollier disease and mixed sclerosing dysplasia

Gross Pathologic & Surgical Features

- Lobulated mass protruding from epiphysis
- Cartilage cap

Microscopic Features

- Subtle differences from osteochondroma
  - In infancy: Osteochondral nodules that resemble secondary ossification centers
  - By 4-5 years of age: Osteochondroma-like
    - Contain bands of cartilage separating areas of cancellous bone; not seen in osteochondromas

CLINICAL ISSUES

Presentation

- Most common signs/symptoms
  - Painful gait
  - Limb length discrepancy (premature physeal closure)
  - Malalignment (usually varus/valgus)
  - Joint mass; may develop loose bodies & progressive symptoms
- Other signs/symptoms
  - Early osteoarthritis

Demographics

- Age
  - Developmental; arises in childhood
- Gender
  - Males > females (3:1)
- Epidemiology
  - Rare: 1/1,000,000 population

Treatment

- Surgical resection → reestablishing congruity of joint
- Osteotomy may address malalignment of limb

SELECTED REFERENCES

1. Wheeldon G et al: Dysplasia epiphysealis hemimelica of the knee: an unusual presentation with intra-articular loose bodies and literature review. J Pediatr Orthop B. ePub, 2015
2. Arealis G et al: Trevor's disease: a literature review regarding classification, treatment, and prognosis apropos of a case. Case Rep Orthop. 2014:940360, 2014
3. Bahk WJ et al: Dysplasia epiphysealis hemimelica: radiographic and magnetic resonance imaging features and clinical outcome of complete and incomplete resection. Skeletal Radiol. 39(1):85-90, 2010

KEY FACTS

TERMINOLOGY

- Spectrum of osseous abnormalities related to radiation
  - Acute nonneoplastic marrow abnormalities
  - Chronic red marrow replacement
  - Radiation-induced fragility fractures
  - Radiation osteonecrosis
  - Radiation-induced growth deformities
  - Radiation-induced osteochondroma
  - Radiation-induced sarcoma

IMAGING

- Location: Any radiation port; most common include
  - Lumbar spine (radiation for Wilms tumor)
  - Pelvis (radiation for genitourinary or GI cancers)
  - Shoulder girdles (axillary node radiation for breast cancer or mantle radiation for Hodgkin disease)
  - Long bone at focal site of radiation
  - Long bones (whole-bone radiation for Ewing sarcoma or lymphoma)
- MR of acute marrow changes after local radiation
  - Multiple focal rounded regions in 37%, diffuse in bones included in radiation port in 10% of cases
  - Low T1, high T2, mild enhancement
  - Increases or fluctuates in size over time; may become large; nonmass-like configuration
- MR of chronic marrow changes following radiation
  - Marrow replacement by fat; high SI on T1

TOP DIFFERENTIAL DIAGNOSES

- DDx of trabecular disturbance in radiated bone
  - Radiation osteonecrosis
  - Recurrent tumor
  - Radiation-induced sarcoma

DIAGNOSTIC CHECKLIST

- Key to picking up on diagnosis of radiation change is often distribution of abnormality
  - Square "port" with normal surrounding tissues

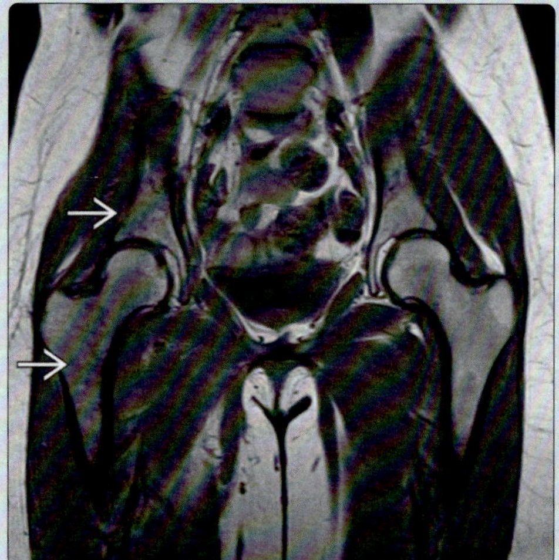

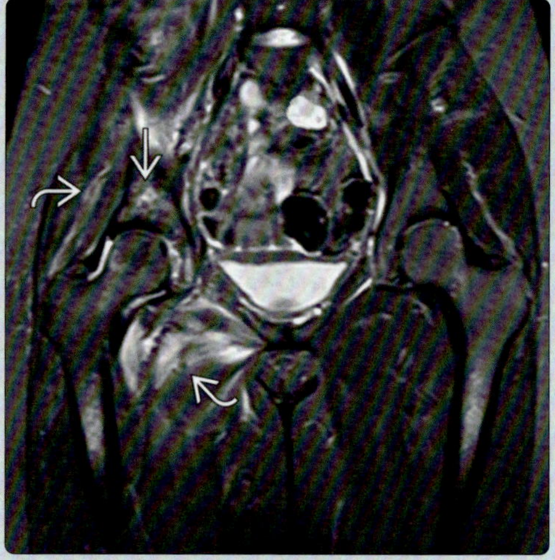

(Left) *Coronal T1WI MR shows an inhomogeneous low signal in the right acetabulum and femoral neck/metadiaphysis ➡. Compare this to the normal left hip with patchy replacement of red marrow by yellow marrow expected in a middle-aged woman.* **(Right)** *Coronal STIR MR in the same patient shows high signal in the acetabular region ➡, as well as in the glutei and adductor muscles ⮫. Note that the abnormalities are in a square, port-like configuration; they are all due to radiation damage to these tissues.*

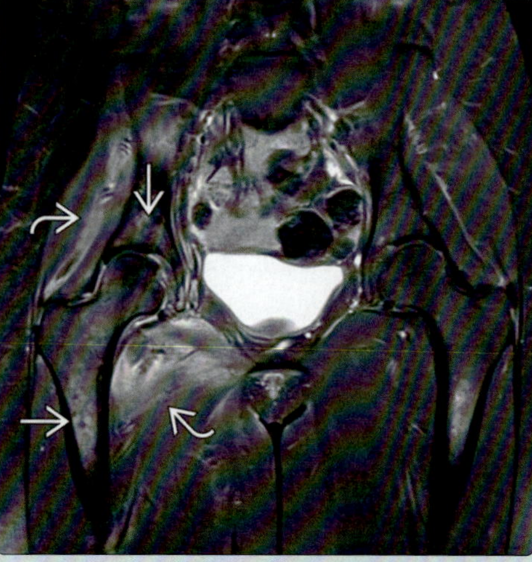

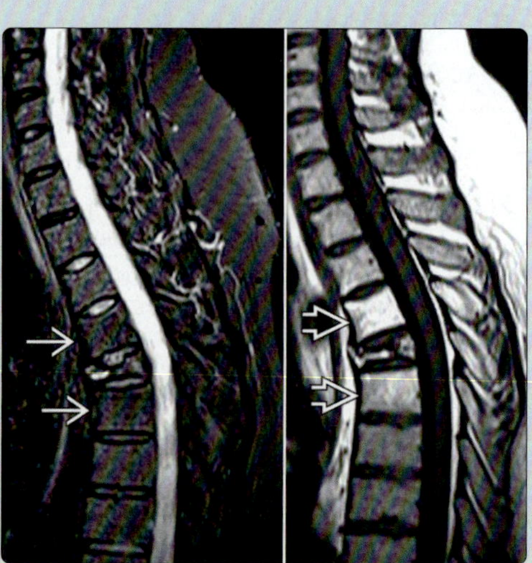

(Left) *Coronal T1WI C+ FS MR shows enhancement in the right acetabulum and femoral marrow ➡, as well as in the previously mentioned muscles ⮫. Typically radiation injury shows modest enhancement, as in this case.* **(Right)** *Sagittal STIR and T1MR in T5 compression fracture due to myeloma treated with radiation is shown. Adjacent T4 and T6 bodies show hypointensity on STIR ➡ and high signal intensity on T1 ➡ relative to other vertebral bodies. This signal is due to fat replacement of the marrow within the radiation port.*

TERMINOLOGY

Definitions

- Spectrum of osseous abnormalities related to radiation
  - Acute nonneoplastic marrow abnormalities
    - Focal or diffuse, fluctuating over time
  - Chronic red marrow replacement with fatty marrow
  - Radiation osteonecrosis
  - Radiation-induced growth deformities
  - Radiation-induced osteochondroma
  - Radiation-induced sarcoma
  - Fragility fractures

IMAGING

General Features

- Best diagnostic clue
  - Any change listed (osteonecrosis, growth deformity, osteochondroma, sarcoma) **located in square, port-like configuration**
- Location
  - Any radiation port; most common include
    - Lumbar spine (radiation for Wilms tumor)
    - Pelvis (radiation for genitourinary or GI cancers)
    - Shoulder girdles (axillary node radiation for breast cancer or mantle radiation for Hodgkin disease)
    - Long bones (whole-bone radiation for Ewing sarcoma or lymphoma)

Radiographic Findings

- Acute marrow changes: No radiographic findings
- Radiation osteonecrosis
  - Disturbance of normal trabecular pattern
  - Mixed lytic and sclerotic pattern of bone destruction
  - Generally no cortical breakthrough, but may appear rather aggressive
  - Femoral and humeral heads: Collapse in weight-bearing regions
- Radiation-induced growth deformities
  - Found only if radiation occurred prior to skeletal maturation and full achievement of growth
  - Spine: Appearance depends on whether radiation field involved entire vertebral body
    - Bone-within-bone seen at 9-12 months
    - If only 1/2 of vertebral bodies (in coronal plane) are radiated, scoliosis develops with concavity on side of hypoplastic (short) radiated vertebral bodies
      - Progression of scoliosis with growth spurts
    - If entire width of vertebral bodies is radiated, symmetric hypoplasia of those involved bodies
    - Adjacent levels of spine show normal height and alignment of bodies
  - Pelvis or shoulder girdle: Hypoplasia of radiated portion; normal adjacent bones
  - Long bone: If whole bone radiation, entire bone is short compared to adjacent normal bones
    - Radiation of physis → widening of growth plate, fragmentation at metaphysis
      - May develop dense metaphyseal bands
    - Periosteal new bone formation → undertubulation
- Radiation-induced osteochondroma
  - Identical to other exostoses
    - Stalk of normal cortex and bone arising from normal underlying bone with cartilage cap
  - May be multiple; rare transformation to chondrosarcoma
- Cortical thickening and associated fragility fracture
- Radiation-induced sarcoma
  - Underlying changes of radiation osteonecrosis (50%)
  - New destructive osseous change in radiated field
    - May be difficult to recognize
    - Permeative bone destruction, periosteal reaction
    - Cortical breakthrough, soft tissue mass
    - Osteoid formation common since osteosarcoma is most frequent cell type of radiation sarcoma

MR Findings

- Acute marrow changes after local radiation
  - Multiple focal rounded regions in 37%, diffuse in bones included in radiation port in 10% of cases
  - Focal: Linear, curvilinear, patchy, mixed
  - T1WI: Low signal intensity, between muscle and fat
  - Fluid-sensitive sequences: High signal intensity
  - Heterogeneous mild enhancement
  - Increases or fluctuates in size over time; may become large; nonmass-like configuration
- Chronic marrow changes following radiation
  - Marrow replacement by fat; high SI on T1
- Radiation osteonecrosis
  - Femoral or humeral head: Normal pattern of osteonecrosis (double line sign)
    - Flattening in weight-bearing region
  - Other sites: Loss of normal trabecular pattern
    - Mixed low and high signal, matching sclerotic and lytic regions on radiograph
- Radiation-induced growth deformities
  - Early physeal fusion
- Radiation-induced osteochondroma
  - Normal MR appearance of osteochondroma
    - Normal cortex and marrow in stalk, arising from normal underlying bone
      - Underlying bone may have chronic marrow changes of fat replacement
    - Cartilage cap: High signal containing septa seen on fluid-sensitive sequences
  - Generally occur at periphery of radiated field
- Radiation-induced sarcoma
  - Underlying radiation osteonecrosis (50%)
  - Change in marrow to infiltrative pattern
  - Cortical breakthrough, soft tissue mass: Heterogeneously high on T2
  - Periosteal reaction, soft tissue and marrow edema
  - Diffuse enhancement of bone and soft tissue mass and reactive edema

DIFFERENTIAL DIAGNOSIS

DDx of Trabecular Disturbance in Radiated Bone

- Radiation osteonecrosis
  - May be nidus for superimposed osteomyelitis
- Recurrent tumor
  - Usually occurs within first 2 years posttherapy
- Radiation-induced sarcoma

- Usually has latent period of 7-20 years

PATHOLOGY

General Features

- Etiology
  - Radiation-induced marrow changes
    - Likely radiation osteonecrosis
  - Fragility fractures related to ↓ osteoclasts and unopposed cortical mineral apposition
  - Radiation-induced osteonecrosis
    - Impaired osteoblast function
  - Radiation-induced growth deformities
    - Radiation destroys microvascular supply to epiphyses → early fusion of physes → short or hypoplastic bone
    - May also have direct cellular damage to osteocytes
  - Radiation-induced osteochondroma
    - Thought to be radiation-caused migration of undifferentiated cartilage into metaphysis from epiphyseal plate

Gross Pathologic & Surgical Features

- Radiation-induced osteochondroma
  - Histologically identical to other exostoses
- Radiation-induced sarcoma
  - Underlying changes of osteonecrosis in most
  - High-grade osteosarcoma and malignant fibrous histiocytoma predominate

CLINICAL ISSUES

Presentation

- Most common signs/symptoms
  - Radiation osteonecrosis
    - Pain, → osteoarthritis if in femoral or humeral head
    - Pathologic fracture
  - Radiation-induced growth deformity
    - Scoliosis or limb length discrepancy
  - Radiation-induced osteochondroma
    - Mass, impingement
  - Radiation-induced sarcoma
    - New onset pain, swelling, pathologic fracture

Demographics

- Epidemiology
  - Nonneoplastic marrow abnormalities
    - 45% of radiated bone
    - Mean latency 9 and 24 months in 2 studies
    - Mean radiation dose 5,900 cGy
  - Radiation-induced osteochondroma
    - 6-24% prevalence in 2 reported series
    - Osteochondroma occurs 10x more frequently in irradiated than nonirradiated bone
    - Most frequently found in patients treated for Wilms tumor or neuroblastoma
      - Generally radiated between ages of 8 months and 11 years (usually < 2 years old)
      - Radiation dose usually 1,500-5,500 cGy
      - Latency of 3-17 years (mean: 5-12 years in different studies)
  - Radiation-induced sarcoma
    - Risk in irradiated bone is 0.03-0.8%
      - Children treated with high-dose radiation and chemotherapy are at greatest risk
      - Prevalence of postradiation sarcomas is increasing as children survive initial malignancy and treatment
    - 50-60% are osteosarcoma; radiation is etiology of 3.4-5.5% of osteosarcomas
    - Radiation doses usually > 2,000 cGy; most commonly 5,500 cGy
    - Latency generally many years (median: 11 years) but may be as short as 2 years
      - Inversely related to radiation dose

Natural History & Prognosis

- Acute and chronic marrow changes after local radiation for soft tissue mass
  - Eventual recovery of marrow elements, or else complete replacement by fatty marrow
- Radiation osteonecrosis
  - Abnormal bone; at increased risk for fracture and as nidus for infection
- Radiation-induced growth deformity
  - Early onset osteoarthritis related to abnormal alignment
- Radiation-induced osteochondroma
  - No different from natural history of routine exostosis
  - Rare reports of transformation to chondrosarcoma
- Radiation-induced sarcoma
  - 5-year survival 62% for extremity lesions
  - 5-year survival 27.3% for axial lesions

Treatment

- Acute and chronic marrow changes after local radiation for soft tissue mass: No treatment
- Radiation osteonecrosis
  - Arthroplasty where appropriate
- Radiation-induced osteochondroma
  - Marginal resection if painful
- Radiation-induced sarcoma
  - Aggressive chemotherapy and wide resection

DIAGNOSTIC CHECKLIST

Image Interpretation Pearls

- Key to picking up on diagnosis of radiation change is often distribution of abnormality
  - Watch for square "port" of abnormality, with normal surrounding tissues

SELECTED REFERENCES

1. Oest ME et al: Long-term loss of osteoclasts and unopposed cortical mineral apposition following limited field irradiation. J Orthop Res. ePub, 2014
2. Zbojniewicz AM et al: Posttreatment imaging of pediatric musculoskeletal tumors. Radiographics. 34(3):724-40, 2014
3. Pacheco R et al: Effects of radiation on bone. Curr Osteoporos Rep. 11(4):299-304, 2013
4. Hwang S et al: Local changes in bone marrow at MRI after treatment of extremity soft tissue sarcoma. Skeletal Radiol. 38(1):11-9, 2009
5. Mitchell MJ et al: Radiation-induced changes in bone. Radiographics. 18(5):1125-36; quiz 1242-3, 1998

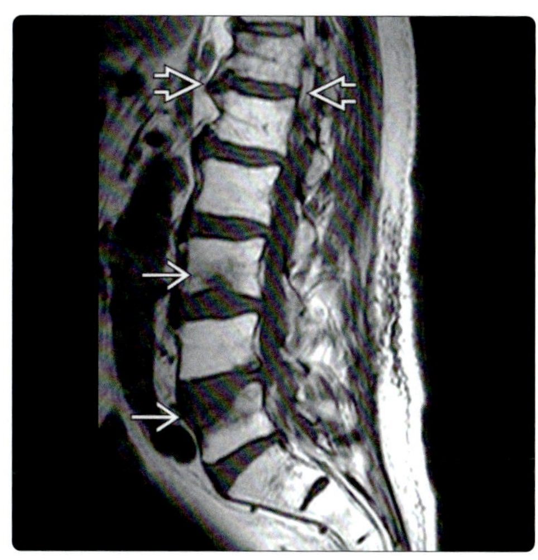

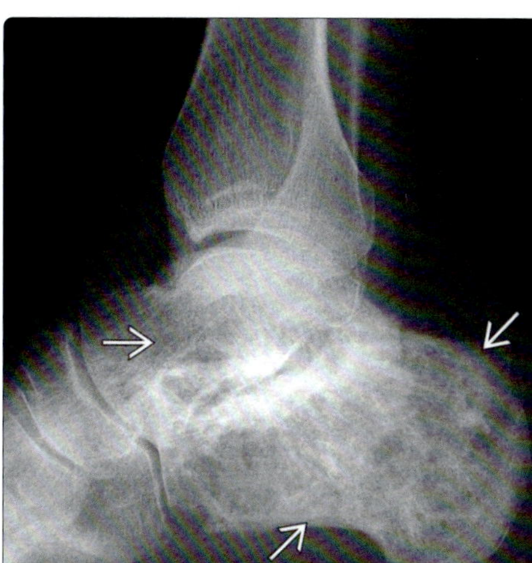

(Left) *Sagittal T1WI MR shows marked increased marrow fat in the lumbar vertebra segments and sacrum, resulting from radiation therapy with a distinct portal margin at T12-L1* ➡. *Insufficiency fractures in the inferior endplate of L3 and superior endplate of L5* ➡ *are secondary to the fragile necrotic bone.* **(Right)** *Lateral radiograph shows a port-like distribution of mixed lytic and sclerotic bone, involving the calcaneus and the plantar portion of the talus* ➡. *This is typical radiation osteonecrosis.*

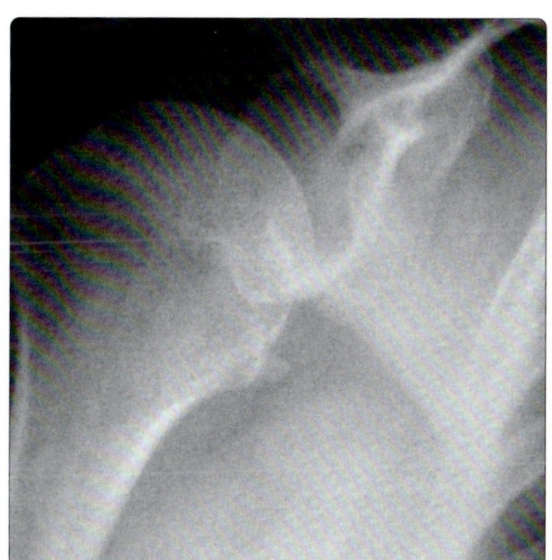

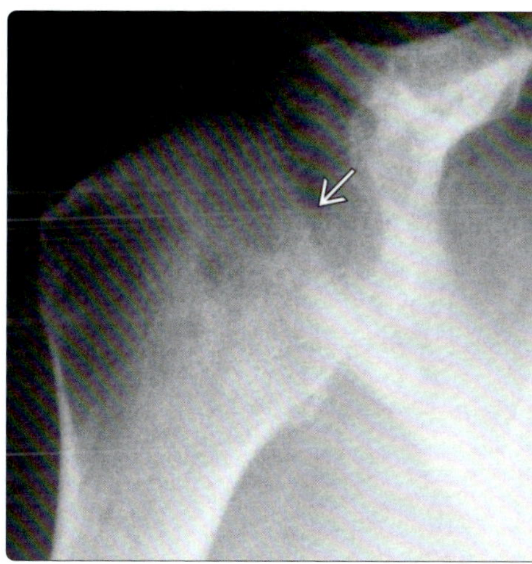

(Left) *AP radiograph obtained several months following radiation of axillary nodes in a patient with breast cancer shows mild osteopenia in the humeral head and glenoid.* **(Right)** *AP radiograph in the same patient, obtained 3 years later, shows frank bone destruction at the articular surface* ➡ *and more pronounced mixed lytic and sclerotic density within the humeral head, glenoid, and coracoid process. The involvement of these bones forms a square "port," typical of radiation osteonecrosis.*

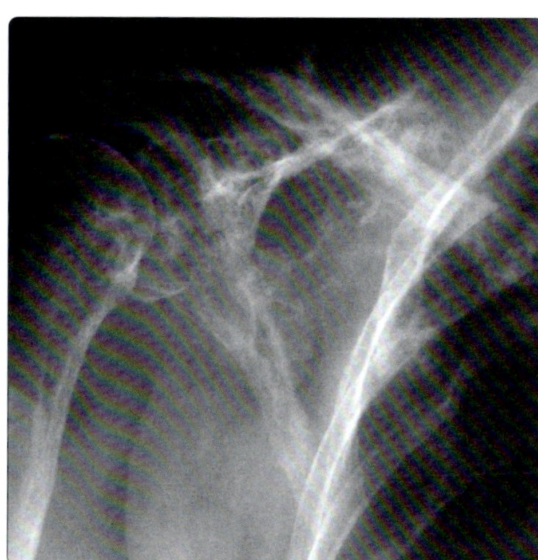

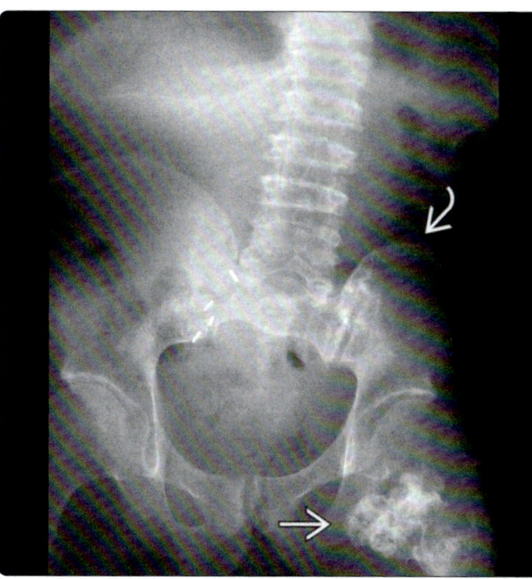

(Left) *AP radiograph shows mixed lytic and sclerotic lesions occupying the scapula, clavicle, and a portion of the humeral head and adjacent ribs. The scapular lesions appear moderately aggressive. This is osteonecrosis from axillary node radiation.* **(Right)** *AP radiograph shows an osteochondroma arising from the left proximal femoral neck* ➡. *Additionally, there is hypoplasia of the left iliac wing* ⮐, *sacral ala, and lumbar vertebral bodies. The affected areas form a radiation "port."*

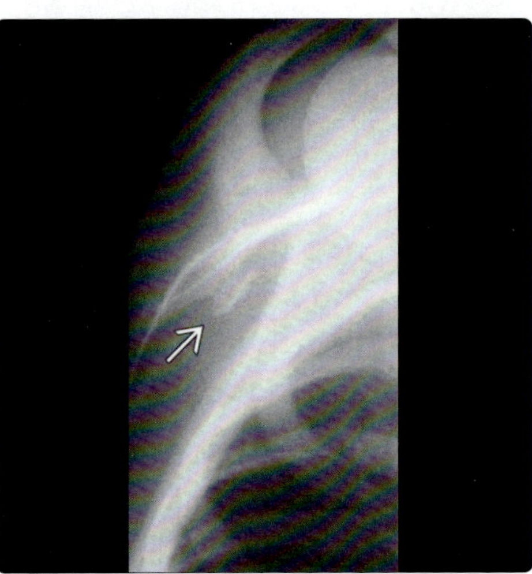

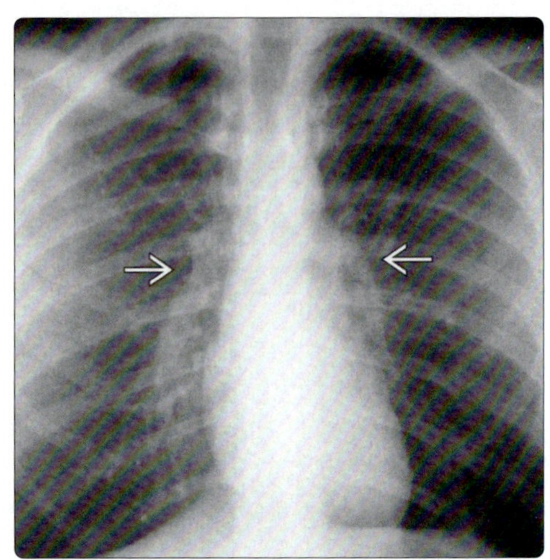

(Left) *Oblique radiograph of the scapula demonstrates an exostosis arising from the undersurface of the body ➡. This patient had mantle radiation for Hodgkin disease several years earlier.* **(Right)** *PA radiograph of the chest in the same patient shows retracted hila ➡, another change 2° to mantle radiation. Osteochondromas can arise in a radiation field, generally peripherally. This patient is older than usual for osteochondroma formation; generally, the patients are younger than 2 years of age at the time of their radiation.*

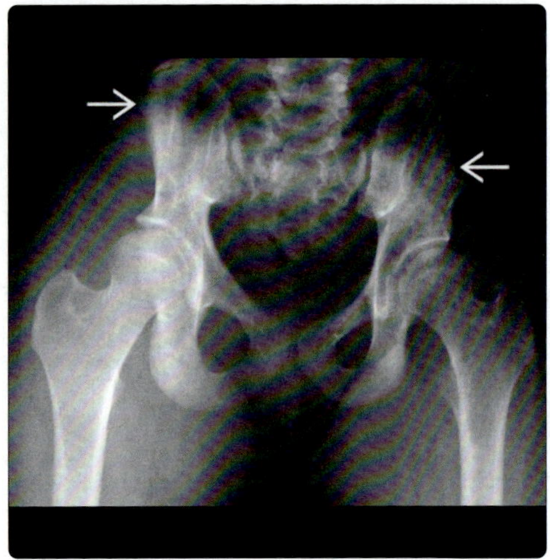

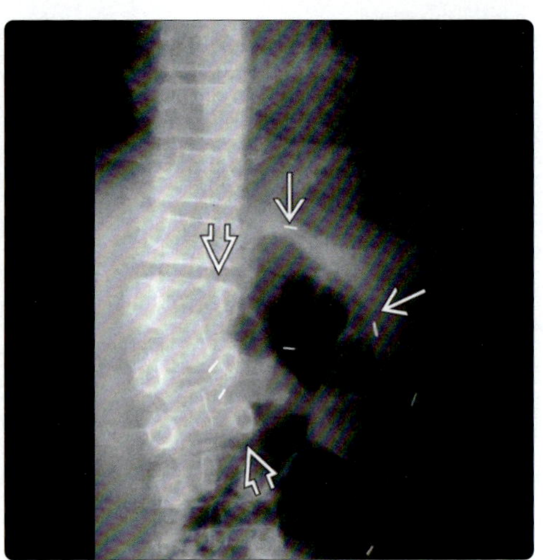

(Left) *AP radiograph shows a differential growth deformity with significant hypoplasia of the sacrum, lower lumbar spine, and iliac wings ➡, including acetabulae. However, the ischii and femora are normal. This patient had radiation for a pelvic tumor at a young age.* **(Right)** *AP radiograph shows relative hypoplasia of the left side of the T12, L1, L2, and L3 vertebral bodies creating an asymmetric platyspondyly and scoliosis ➡. This results from radiation of the left Wilms tumor; note the clips in the renal fossa ➡.*

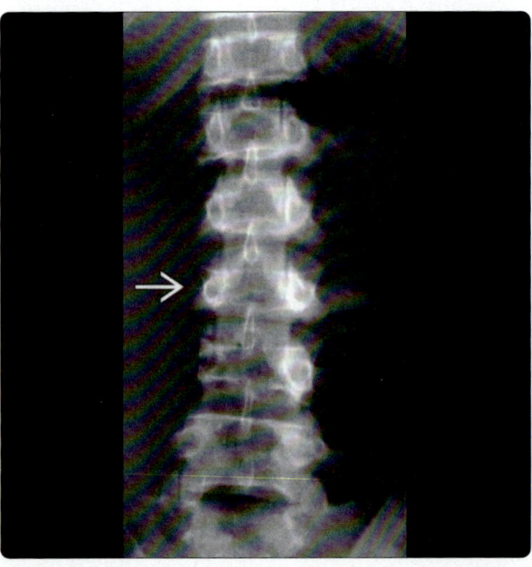

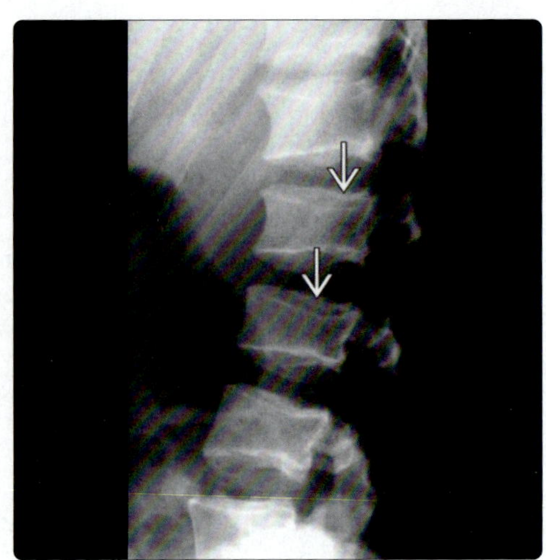

(Left) *AP radiograph of the lumbar spine shows a mild scoliosis concave to the right ➡. This is due to a mild asymmetric platyspondyly with the right side of the lumbar vertebral bodies shorter than the left.* **(Right)** *Lateral radiograph in the same patient confirms the asymmetric platyspondyly with "double" endplates seen at each level ➡. The growth deformity is secondary to earlier radiation of the right renal fossa. Note on both radiographs that T12 and L5 are normal in height.*

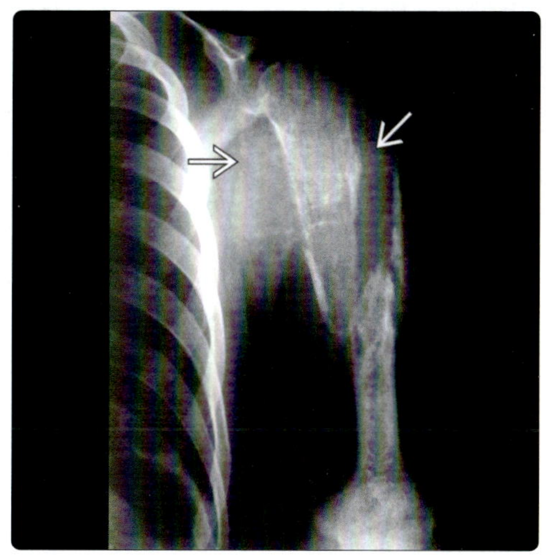

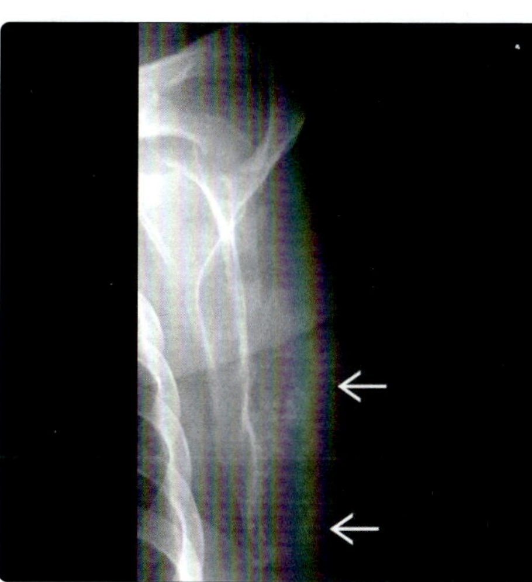

(Left) *AP radiograph shows an aggressive lesion with a large soft tissue mass containing osteoid ➡. The overall density is mixed lytic and sclerotic, and the humerus is extremely short relative to the thorax. These findings are typical of radiation osteonecrosis with 2° osteosarcoma.* **(Right)** *Scapular Y-view radiograph shows a large soft tissue mass containing tumor matrix ➡. This patient was radiated 10 years earlier for breast cancer; the scapula is within the radiation field. She has developed radiation osteosarcoma.*

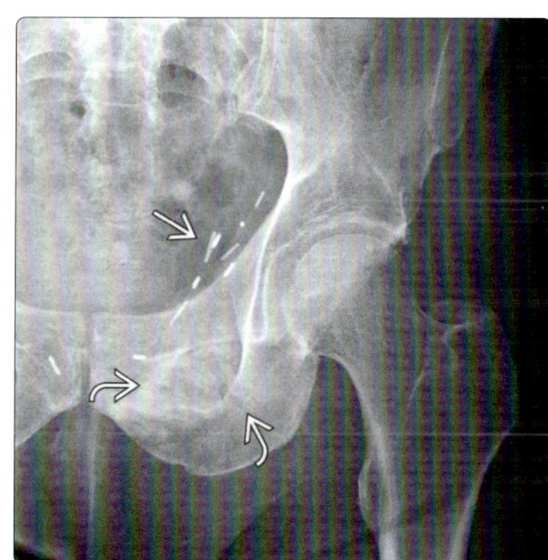

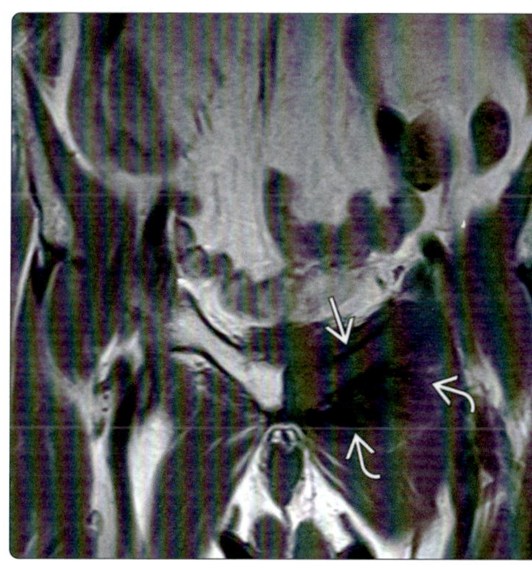

(Left) *AP radiograph shows clips ➡ in a distribution typical of lymph node resection for prostate cancer. Additionally, there is amorphous sclerosis superimposed over the region of the obturator foramen ⮫.* **(Right)** *Coronal T1 MR in the same patient shows marrow replacement in the left pubic ramus ➡. In addition, there is ill-defined hypointensity in the region of the obturator foramen ⮫ (area noted to be sclerotic on radiograph), confirming the presence of tumor osteoid in a soft tissue mass.*

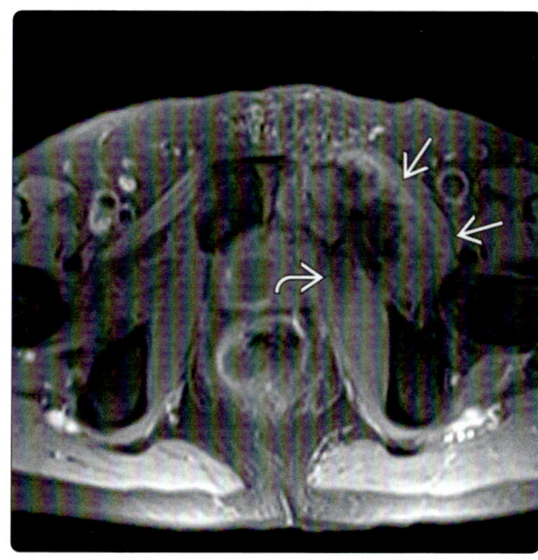

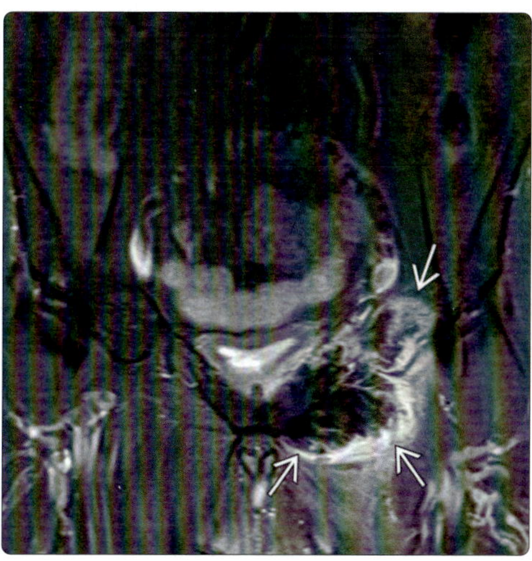

(Left) *Axial PDFS MR in the same patient through the obturator foramen shows a large soft tissue mass containing tumor osteoid ➡ extending posteriorly into the obturator internus muscle ⮫.* **(Right)** *Coronal postcontrast T1 FS MR in the same patient confirms the large osteoid-containing mass ➡. In this 75-year-old man who has been treated for prostate cancer, it is reasonable to diagnose a radiation-induced osteosarcoma. Prognosis for this type of secondary osteosarcoma is poor.*

SECTION 3

Soft Tissue Tumors

Introduction and Overview

Adipocytic Tumors

Fibroblastic/Myoblastic Tumors

So-Called Fibrohistiocytic Tumors

Smooth Muscle Tumors

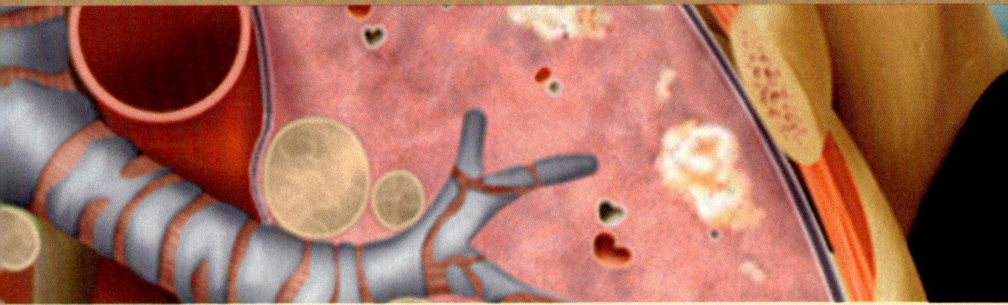

Introduction

Soft tissue masses are very common and have an exceptionally large number of potential etiologies. The World Health Organization recognizes nine different categories of soft tissue tumors. Within each category, these tumors are further separated into benign, intermediate (locally aggressive), and malignant types. The categories are as follows.

- Adipocytic tumors
- Fibroblastic/myofibroblastic tumors
- So-called fibrohistiocytic tumors
- Smooth muscle tumors
- Pericytic (perivascular) tumors
- Skeletal muscle tumors
- Vascular tumors
- Chondroosseous tumors
- Tumors of uncertain differentiation

Malignant soft tissue tumors (sarcomas) are relatively uncommon, representing less than 1% of all malignancies. Soft tissue sarcomas are associated with a high mortality rate. There are over 50 different soft tissue sarcoma subtypes as defined by the World Health Organization. The most common soft tissue sarcomas in adults are liposarcoma, leiomyosarcoma, and undifferentiated pleomorphic sarcoma.

The World Health Organization classifies neurogenic tumors and skin and appendage tumors separately from soft tissue tumors. In addition to the very large number of neoplastic causes of soft tissue masses, many soft tissue masses are nonneoplastic. These tumor-like entities are reviewed in the soft tissue tumor mimics chapters. The tumor mimics chapters are separated into infection/inflammation, vascular, crystal disease, and other causes.

Differentiating Benign From Malignant Soft Tissue Tumors

Differentiating many soft tissue masses as benign vs. malignant with imaging alone can be exceptionally difficult. Some soft tissue sarcomas have a deceptively bland appearance with well-defined, smooth borders and homogeneous signal intensity. If a lesion is not pathognomonic for a specific benign entity, then it should be regarded as a potentially malignant mass. Superficial soft tissue masses larger than 5 cm in greatest dimension have a 10% chance of being a sarcoma.

Predicting Grade or Prognosis by Imaging

Predicting the grade of a soft tissue sarcoma using imaging is not reliable. The presence of a large, necrotic, and infiltrative mass suggests a high-grade lesion. However, high-grade lesions may be small and have a homogeneous, encapsulated appearance.

Patient prognosis is most directly related to the presence of nodal and distant metastatic disease. The sites of soft tissue sarcoma metastatic disease are highly dependent on the tumor type. There is a relatively low incidence of lymph node metastasis, although some sarcoma subtypes are more prone to lymph node metastases. These include rhabdomyosarcoma, angiosarcoma, clear cell sarcoma, synovial sarcoma, and epithelioid sarcoma. The presence of nodal metastases indicates stage III disease. This has an overall 56% 5-year survival rate. Lymph nodes are considered suspicious for tumor involvement by imaging if they are greater than 1 cm in short-axis dimension with obliteration of the fatty hilum, as identified on CT or MR. PET/CT demonstrates increased F18 FDG tracer uptake in malignant lymph nodes. Since nodal involvement is uncommon in soft tissue sarcomas, its presence should initiate further work-up for distant metastases.

The majority of distant metastases involve the lung. Myxoid liposarcoma has an unusual tendency to metastasize to other soft tissue sites. Retroperitoneal sarcomas have an increased incidence of metastasis to liver. The presence of distant metastases confers stage IV disease. This has an overall 10-20% 5-year survival rate.

Predicting Histologic Type of Soft Tissue Tumors

Most soft tissue tumors have a nonspecific, heterogeneous signal intensity on both T1-weighted and fluid-sensitive MR sequences. Some tissue signal types can help suggest a specific type of tumor. Adipocytic tumors contain fat and thus may have visible foci of high signal on T1-weighted MR with corresponding low signal on fat-suppressed sequences. Fibroblastic tumors often contain intermediate to low signal regions on both T1-weighted and fluid-sensitive MR sequences. Fibrohistiocytic tumors often have marked heterogeneity of signal.

The presence of a mass in a typical location may also help suggest a diagnosis. These typical locations include the plantar fascia (plantar fibromatosis), second or third intermetatarsal space (Morton neuroma), nailbed (glomus tumor), between the tip of the scapula and chest wall (elastofibroma), and between the medial head of the gastrocnemius and semimembranosus tendon (popliteal synovial cyst).

Several outstanding books and review papers listed in the selected references contain tables, figures, and flow charts that can assist in limiting the exceptionally large potential differential diagnosis of soft tissue lesions.

Staging of Soft Tissue Sarcoma

There are two main staging systems for soft tissue sarcomas. The most commonly utilized staging system is the American Joint Committee on Cancer (AJCC) staging system. The seventh edition was published in 2010. Staging is based on histologic grade (three-grade system), primary tumor size and depth, and presence of nodal disease and distant metastases. This staging system does not take into account anatomic site or whether tumor extends outside the compartment of origin.

Several soft tissue tumors are not included in the AJCC staging system: Extraskeletal osteosarcoma, extraskeletal Ewing sarcoma, angiosarcoma, dermatofibrosarcoma protuberans, extraskeletal chondrosarcoma, Kaposi sarcoma, rhabdomyosarcoma, desmoid tumor, mesothelioma, infantile fibrosarcoma, inflammatory myofibroblastic tumor, and gastrointestinal stromal tumor. This staging system is also not applicable to sarcomas arising from the dura matter, brain, parenchymal organs, or hollow viscera. Skin carcinoma and melanoma have entirely separate staging systems.

An alternate staging system is the Surgical Staging System of the Musculoskeletal Tumor Society (a.k.a. Enneking staging system). This staging system emphasizes whether tumor is confined to the compartment of origin and is commonly used by orthopedic oncologic surgeons. Although this information is useful for surgical planning, it has not been proven as a predictor of survival. Only two histologic grades (low or high) are utilized. This staging system does not take into account tumor size, tumor location, or nodal status. Stage Ia is low grade and intracompartmental. Stage Ib is low grade and extracompartmental. Stage IIa is high grade and intracompartmental. Stage IIb is high grade and extracompartmental. Stage IIIa is low or high grade and intracompartmental with metastases. Stage IIIb is low or high grade and extracompartmental with metastases.

Rhabdomyosarcoma has a separate staging system. The most commonly utilized staging system is the Soft Tissue Sarcoma Committee of the Children's Oncology Group, which was formerly known as the Intergroup Rhabdomyosarcoma Study Group. In this staging system, patients are separated into four clinical groups based on complete resection vs. varying degrees of partial resection, extent of tumor beyond the muscle or organ of origin, nodal involvement, and distant metastases.

Biopsy Considerations

Computed tomography and ultrasound are the best imaging modalities to guide percutaneous biopsy. CT provides excellent demonstration of compartmental anatomy. This helps avoid iatrogenic spread of tumor into adjacent tissue compartments. The borders of tissue compartments can be difficult to assess with ultrasound if the user does not have a definitive sense of the mass location and approach. Both CT and ultrasound can assist in directing biopsy to the most viable portion of the lesion, as it is important to avoid areas of necrosis. These viable tumor regions enhance on CT and show increased blood flow on color Doppler ultrasound.

Ideally, prebiopsy consultation with an oncologic surgeon will allow the biopsy trajectory to correspond to any potential definitive surgical approach needed in the future. Remember that the primary goal when performing a biopsy is first to do no harm and second to provide diagnostic material. Poorly planned biopsies can be devastating to the patient.

Treatment Options for Soft Tissue Sarcoma

The ultimate therapy chosen for a soft tissue sarcoma has significant variation based on individual tumor characteristics and the treatment facility. Surgical excision is the mainstay of treatment in patients with localized disease. The type of surgery chosen is based on a balance of both maximizing survival and preserving limb function. Limb-sparing surgery is usually preferred. Amputations are undertaken for very large tumors, extensive neurovascular involvement, and nonfunctional extremities. Chemotherapy &/or radiotherapy is administered based on tumor size, type, location, and spread. Radiotherapy is particularly helpful in decreasing local recurrence rate. Chemotherapy is considered for tumor types that have a known high response rate, such as rhabdomyosarcoma. Chemotherapy may also be considered in patients who have a high risk of metastasis.

In stage IV disease with limited organ involvement, surgical removal of metastases can be considered. Better outcomes are seen with slow-growing sarcomas and long disease-free intervals since diagnosis. In stage IV disease with disseminated involvement, palliative surgery, chemotherapy, &/or radiotherapy can be considered. Local control or pain relief may be provided by the use of radiofrequency ablation, cryoablation, or embolization. The treatment is otherwise supportive.

Major Treatment Roadblocks

Adjacent soft tissues or tissue compartments may be contaminated due to percutaneous biopsy or initial subtotal resection. Known contamination or microscopically positive margins that are discovered postoperatively all require reexcision of the operative bed. Sarcomas involving the retroperitoneal region remain some of the most technically challenging tumors for complete resection. Treatment may also result in complications. Head and neck tumor treatment may cause cataracts, dental abnormalities, and growth or intellectual delay in children. Treatment of abdominal and retroperitoneal tumors may result in bowel obstruction. Adjuvant radiation therapy involving the extremities can result in osteonecrosis, osteochondromas, and osteitis. All primary tumor locations have an increased risk of secondary malignancy.

Follow-Up of Soft Tissue Sarcoma

Posttreatment follow-up of soft tissue sarcomas is complicated and based on several variables. Foremost is the initial success of the tumor excision (whether clear wide margins were achieved or not). The risk of metastasis based on tumor type is also a variable for consideration. For example, leiomyosarcoma and malignant peripheral nerve sheath tumors have an increased risk of metastasis over other soft tissue sarcomas. The risk of metastatic disease is also based on the tumor size, with progressive risk associated with tumor size greater than 5 cm. Higher tumor histologic grade also puts the patient at higher risk for metastasis. Finally, individual practice patterns will also alter management.

Common follow-up for a low-risk patient includes an MR of the soft tissue sarcoma resection area with a chest CT every 6 months for the first two years after treatment. Annually thereafter, the patient will undergo an MR of the sarcoma resection area and a CT of the chest. Recurrence is unlikely after 10 years and routine surveillance discontinuation can be considered.

High-risk patients have lifetime follow-up. Every three months for the first two years after resection, the patient will undergo an MR of the area and a chest CT. For the next three years, the patient will have an MR of the area and a chest CT every six months. Annually thereafter, the patient will continue to have an MR of the area and a chest CT.

Soft Tissue Tumor Reporting Checklist

When reporting the imaging appearance of a potentially malignant soft tissue tumor, the following characteristics are helpful to describe: Maximum tumor dimension (three-plane measurements ideal), involved body part with laterality, anatomic compartment involved, craniocaudad location in reference to an anatomic landmark, relationship to/involvement of superficial fascia, neurovascular invasion, bone invasion or periosteal reaction, any signal characteristics suggesting tumor type, and estimation of the percent of the mass that is nonviable.

Selected References

1. Del Grande F et al: Detection of soft-tissue sarcoma recurrence: added value of functional MR imaging techniques at 3.0 T. Radiology. 271(2):499-511, 2014
2. Subhawong TK et al: Diffusion-weighted MR imaging for characterizing musculoskeletal lesions. Radiographics. 34(5):1163-77, 2014
3. Surov A et al: Malignant and benign lesions of the skeletal musculature. Semin Ultrasound CT MR. 35(3):290-307, 2014

AJCC Classification

TNM	Definitions
Primary Tumor (T)	
TX	Primary tumor cannot be assessed
T0	No evidence of primary tumor
T1	Tumor ≤ 5 cm in greatest dimension
T1a	Superficial tumor ≤ 5 cm in greatest dimension
T1b	Deep tumor ≤ 5 cm in greatest dimension
T2	Tumor > 5 cm in greatest dimension
T2a	Superficial tumor > 5 cm in greatest dimension
T2b	Deep tumor > 5 cm in greatest dimension
Regional Lymph Nodes (N)	
NX	Regional lymph nodes cannot be assessed
N0	No regional lymph node metastasis
N1	Regional lymph node metastasis
Distant Metastasis (M)	
M0	No distant metastasis
M1	Distant metastasis
Histologic Grade (G)	
GX	Grade cannot be assessed
G1	Grade 1 (FNCLCC score 2-3)
G2	Grade 2 (FNCLCC score 4-5)
G3	Grade 3 (FNCLCC score 6-8)

The American Joint Committee on Cancer (AJCC) prefers the use of the Fédération Nationale des Centres de Lutte Contre le Cancer (FNCLCC) histologic grading method. Additional descriptors that can be utilized include residual tumor (R) and combined lymph-vascular invasion (LVI). Residual tumor is coded as cannot be assessed = RX, is not present = R0, is microscopically present = R1, or is macroscopically present = R2. Lymph-vascular invasion is described as not present/not identified, present/identified, not applicable, or unknown/indeterminate. Adapted from 7th edition AJCC Staging Forms.

AJCC Stages/Prognostic Groups

Stage	T	N	M	G
IA	T1a, T1b	N0	M0	G1, GX
IB	T2a, T2b	N0	M0	G1, GX
IIA	T1a, T1b	N0	M0	G2, G3
IIB	T2a, T2b	N0	M0	G2
III	T2a, T2b	N0	M0	G3
	Any T	N1	M0	Any G
IV	Any T	Any N	M1	Any G

The AJCC staging system shown above is commonly utilized, as well as the Surgical Staging System of the Musculoskeletal Tumor Society. Adapted from 7th edition AJCC Staging Forms.

4. Zhao F et al: Can MR imaging be used to predict tumor grade in soft-tissue sarcoma? Radiology. 272(1):192-201, 2014
5. Manaster BJ: Soft-tissue masses: optimal imaging protocol and reporting. AJR Am J Roentgenol. 201(3):505-14, 2013
6. Rakheja R et al: Necrosis on FDG PET/CT correlates with prognosis and mortality in sarcomas. AJR Am J Roentgenol. 201(1):170-7, 2013
7. Subhawong TK et al: Proton MR spectroscopy in metabolic assessment of musculoskeletal lesions. AJR Am J Roentgenol. 198(1):162-72, 2012
8. American Joint Committee on Cancer: AJCC Cancer Staging Manual. 7th ed. New York: Springer. 291-6, 2010
9. Charest M et al: FDG PET/CT imaging in primary osseous and soft tissue sarcomas: a retrospective review of 212 cases. Eur J Nucl Med Mol Imaging. 36(12):1944-51, 2009
10. Garner HW et al: Benign and malignant soft-tissue tumors: posttreatment MR imaging. Radiographics. 29(1):119-34, 2009
11. Stacchiotti S et al: High-grade soft-tissue sarcomas: tumor response assessment--pilot study to assess the correlation between radiologic and pathologic response by using RECIST and Choi criteria. Radiology. 251(2):447-56, 2009
12. Kransdorf MJ et al: Imaging of Soft Tissue Tumors. 2nd ed. Philadelphia: Lippincott Williams & Wilkins, 2006

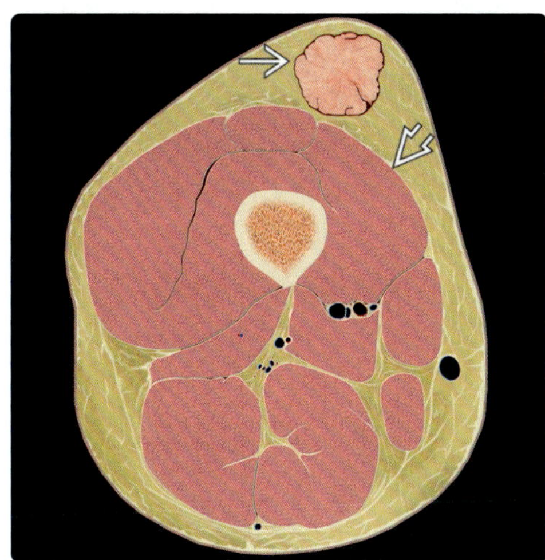

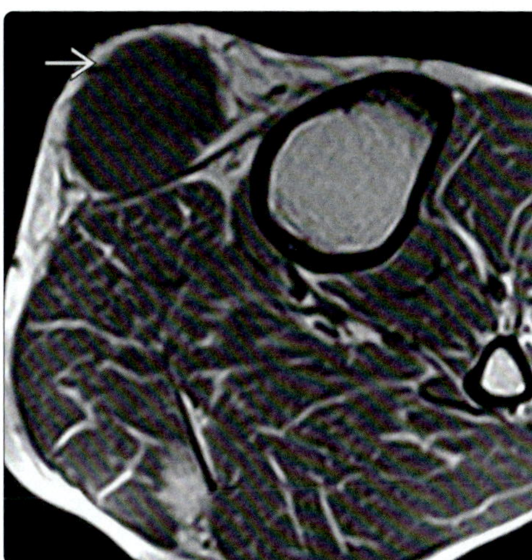

(Left) *Axial graphic shows a T1a ➔ soft tissue sarcoma. These tumors must be ≤ 5 cm in greatest dimension. The "a" designation refers to the tumor being located superficial to, and not involving, the superficial fascia ⇨.* **(Right)** *Axial T1WI MR shows a low-grade myxoid liposarcoma ➔. The mass is well defined and located in the subcutaneous fat of the proximal medial calf. It did not invade or involve the superficial fascia. This is stage IA (T1a N0 M0 G1) disease.*

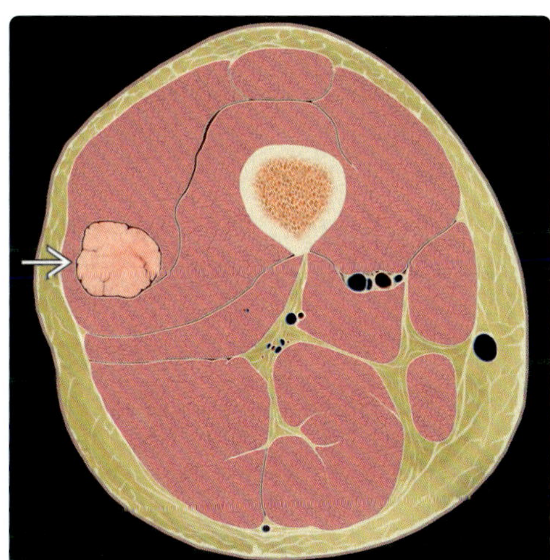

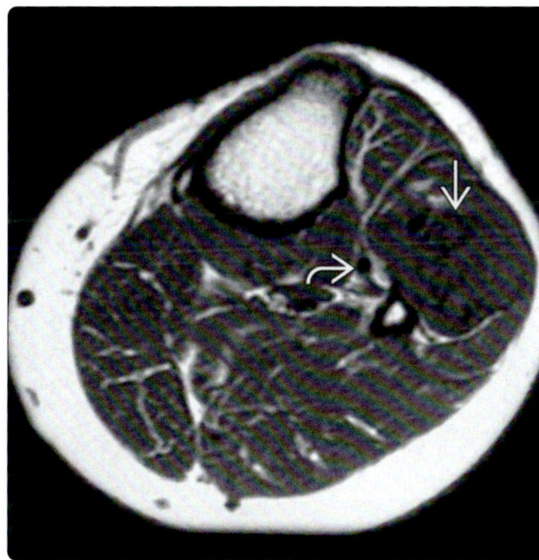

(Left) *Axial graphic shows a T1b ➔ soft tissue sarcoma. These lesions must be ≤ 5 cm in diameter. The "b" designation refers to a deep lesion. Any involvement of the superficial fascia or a location exclusively deep to the fascia is defined as a deep tumor.* **(Right)** *Axial T1WI MR shows a heterogeneous, low signal malignant peripheral nerve sheath tumor ➔ in the calf located deep to the fascia and adjacent to a neurovascular bundle ↪. The deep location makes it a T1b lesion.*

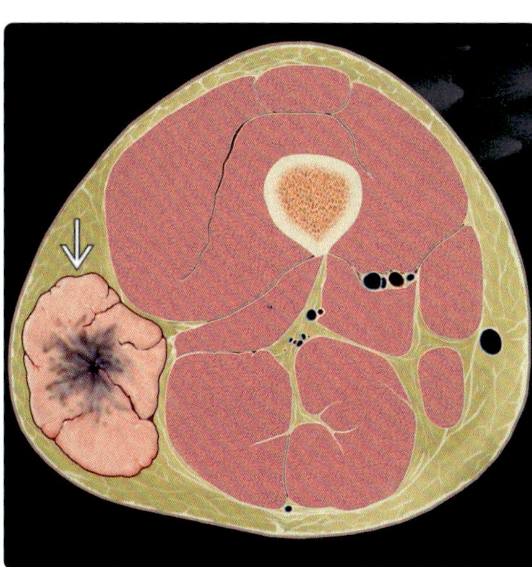

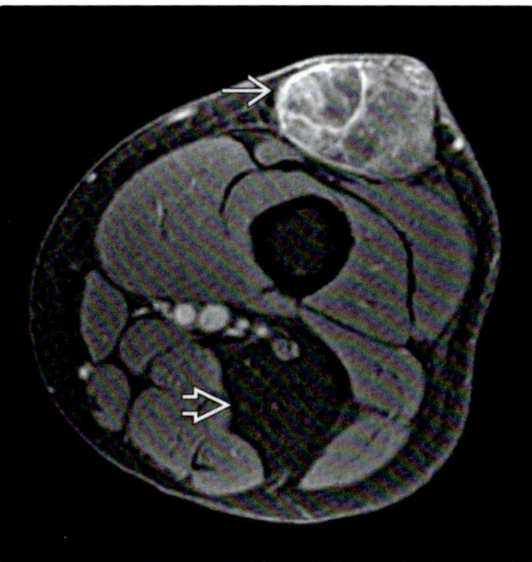

(Left) *Axial graphic shows a T2a ➔ soft tissue sarcoma. These tumors are > 5 cm in greatest dimension. The "a" designation indicates that the mass is located superficial to the superficial fascia, without any fascial involvement.* **(Right)** *Axial T1WI C+ FS MR shows a high-grade myxoid sarcoma ➔ in the subcutaneous fat of the anterior thigh. The lesion has heterogeneous enhancement. An unrelated benign lipoma ⇨ was shown to be stable and without aggressive features over several years.*

(Left) *Axial graphic shows a T2b soft tissue sarcoma ➡. This tumor measures > 5 cm. Although it is predominantly located superficial to the fascia, fascial invasion ➡ causes this to be designated a deep lesion.* **(Right)** *Axial T1WI MR shows a dedifferentiated liposarcoma ➡ appearing as a complex, heterogeneous mass that invaded the superficial fascia of the gluteal region. The very large size of this mass necessitated imaging the patient in a prone position. This is stage III (T2b N0 M0 G3) disease.*

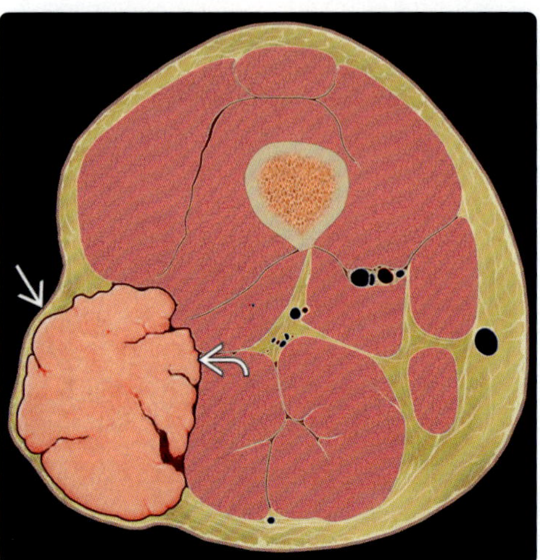

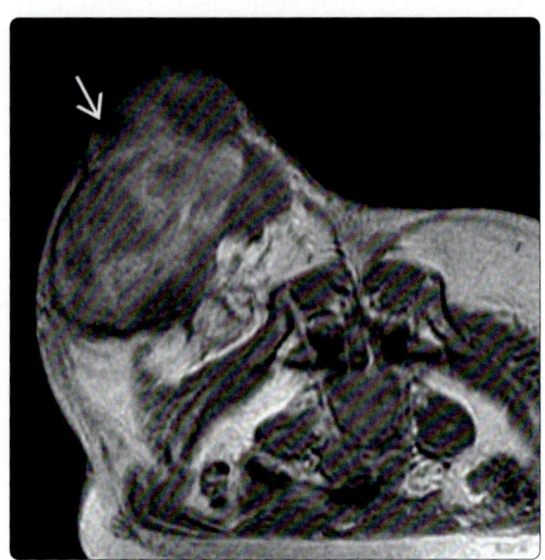

(Left) *Axial graphic shows another type of T2b ➡ soft tissue sarcoma. This tumor is > 5 cm and is deep to the superficial fascia. Note that this tumor abuts adjacent neurovascular structures ➡. Neurovascular involvement was included in earlier staging systems but is not currently included.* **(Right)** *Axial T2WI FS MR shows a pleomorphic liposarcoma ➡ in the posterior thigh. Lesion size > 5 cm plus location deep to the fascia makes this a T2b lesion. With histologic grade 3, it is stage III disease.*

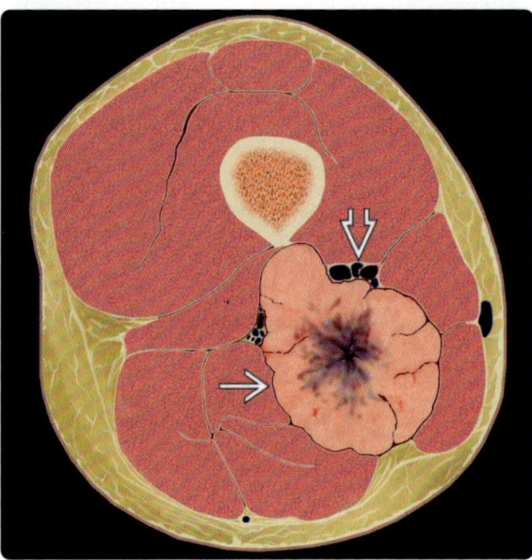

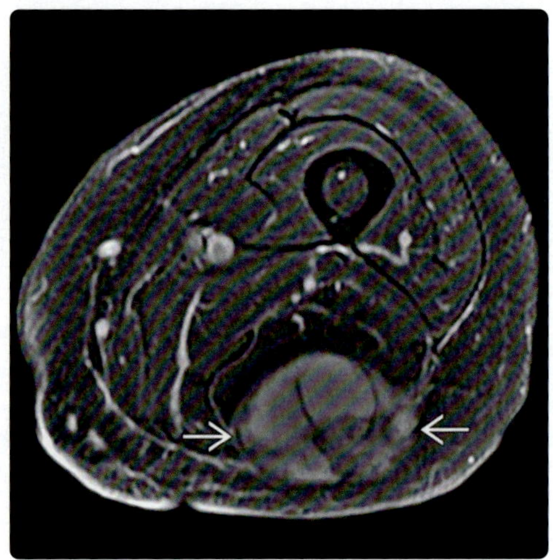

(Left) *Axial graphic of a stage I soft tissue sarcoma. The key characteristic of a stage I soft tissue sarcoma is that the lesion is low grade. An example of low-grade pathology is inset. Stage I tumors can be any size and may be located either superficial or deep to the fascia. A T1a mass ➡ is shown in this example.* **(Right)** *Axial T1WI MR shows a fibromyxoid sarcoma ➡ in the subcutaneous fat of the medial knee. The mass has a bland homogeneous appearance. This is stage IA (T1a N0 M0 G1) disease.*

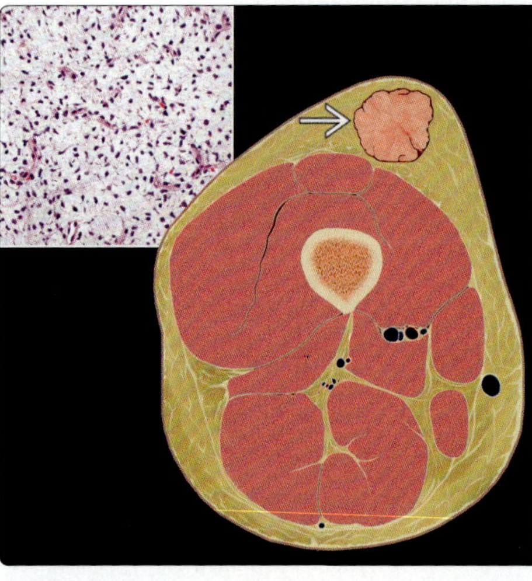

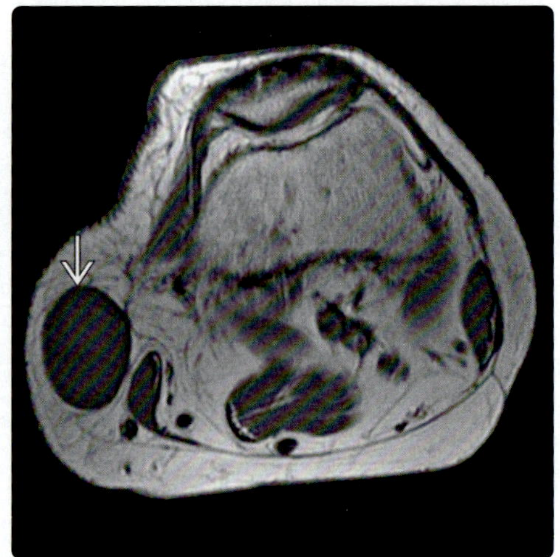

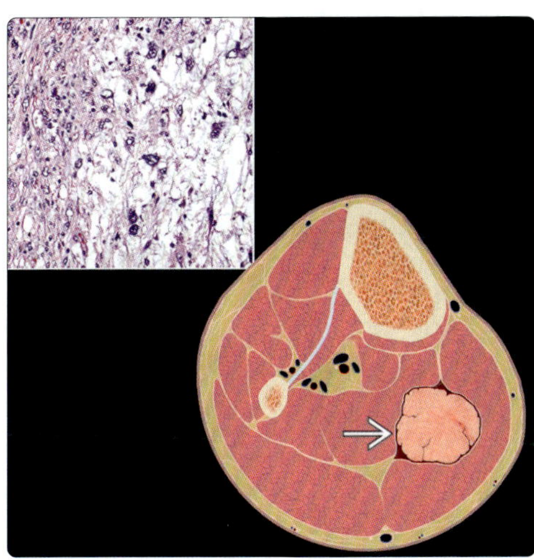

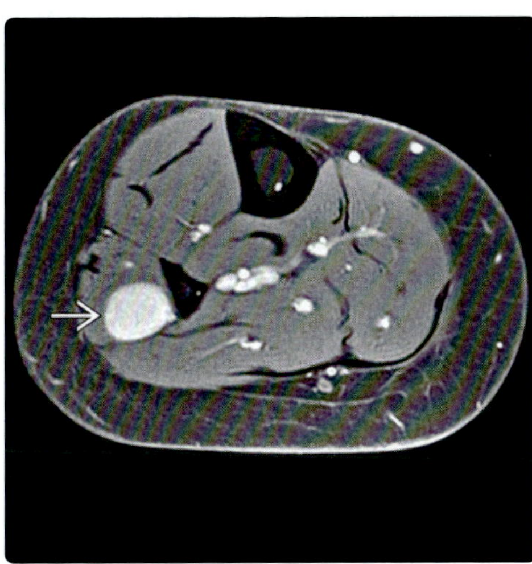

(Left) *Axial graphic shows a stage II soft tissue sarcoma. These lesions are all G2 or G3 tumors. An example of high-grade pathology is inset. If the mass is ≤ 5 cm, it may be either G2 or G3 and may be located superficial (T1a) or deep (T1b, ➔) to the fascia. However, if the mass is larger than 5 cm, then it must be G2 to qualify for stage II.* **(Right)** *Axial T1WI C+ FS MR shows a synovial sarcoma ➔ abutting the cortex of the fibula. This mass homogeneously enhances. This is stage IIA (T1b N0 M0 G2) disease.*

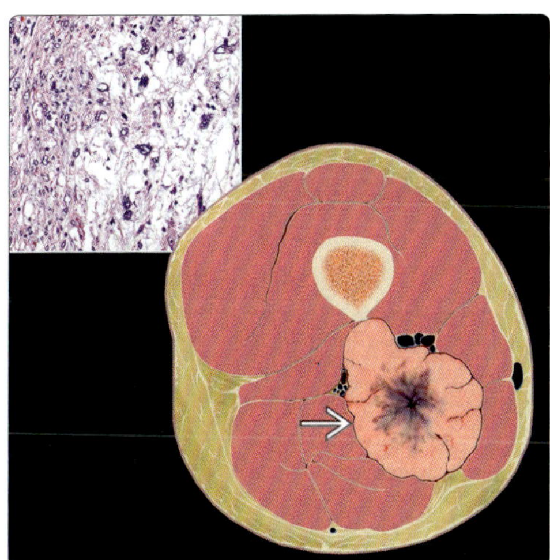

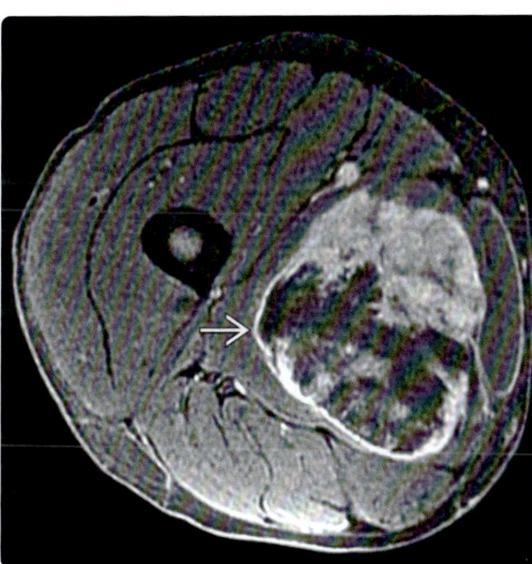

(Left) *Axial graphic shows a stage III soft tissue sarcoma. These tumors measure > 5 cm and may be superficial (T2a) or deep (T2b, ➔) to the superficial fascia and are high-grade (G3) tumors. An example of high-grade pathology is inset. Nodal metastases, with any lesion size, location, or grade, also confer stage III disease.* **(Right)** *Axial T1WI C+ FS MR shows a heterogeneously enhancing high-grade myxofibrosarcoma ➔ in the posterior compartment of the thigh. This is stage III (T2b N0 M0 G3) disease.*

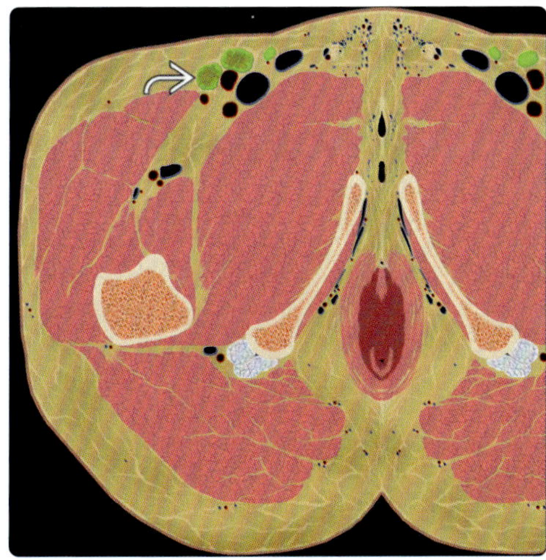

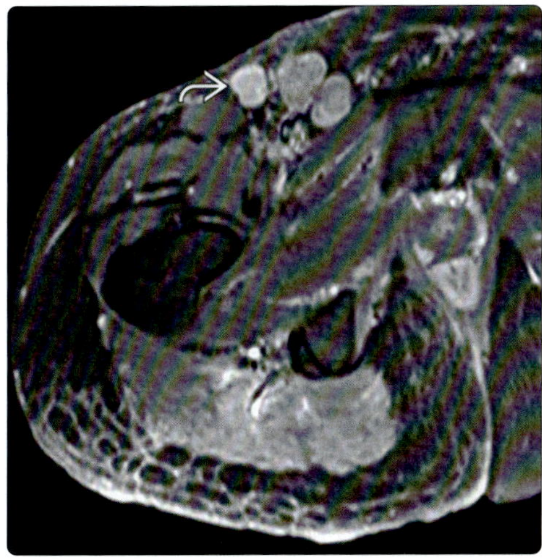

(Left) *Axial graphic in a patient with soft tissue sarcoma shows inguinal adenopathy ↪. The presence of lymph nodes involved with tumor makes this stage III disease. The primary tumor can be any size, located at any depth, and have any histologic grade. The previous staging system designated nodal metastases as stage IV disease.* **(Right)** *Axial T1WI C+ FS MR shows enlarged inguinal lymph nodes ↪ in a patient with a gluteal epithelioid sarcoma. This is stage III (T2b N1 M0 G3) disease.*

(Left) *Coronal graphic through the lungs shows bilateral metastases ➡. The presence of distant metastases confers stage IV disease. Stage IV primary sarcomas can be any size, have any depth, and have any histologic grade. Over 75% of soft tissue sarcoma metastases involve the lung.* **(Right)** *Coronal MIP CECT shows bilateral pulmonary metastases ➡ in a patient with a high-grade liposarcoma in the thigh. The presence of distant metastases makes this stage IV (T2b N0 M1 G3) disease.*

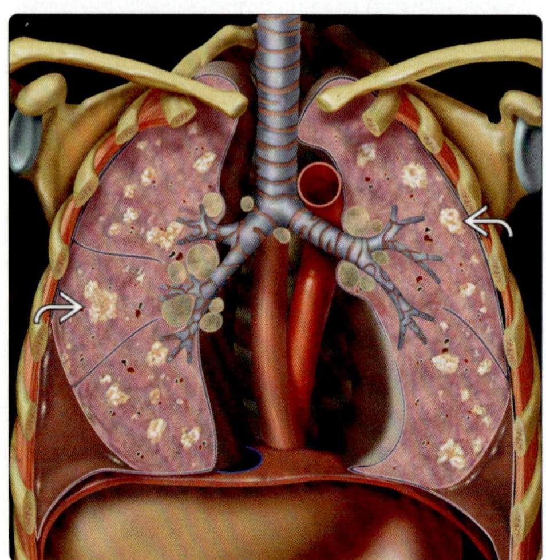

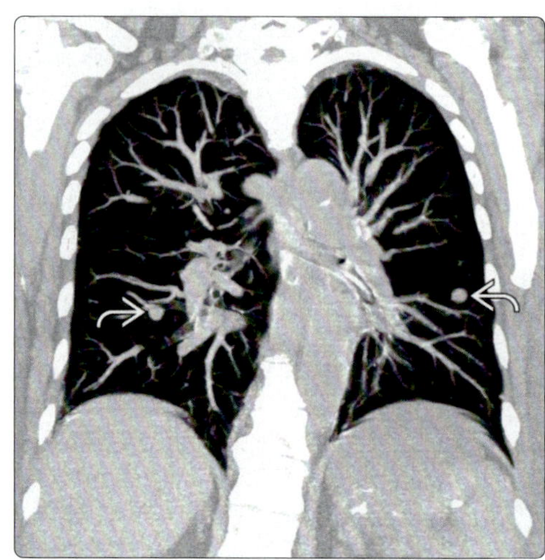

(Left) *Axial graphic shows the muscle compartments in the upper thigh, as outlined in different colors. It is important to not contaminate an additional muscular compartment when performing a percutaneous soft tissue mass biopsy, as this may necessitate a more extensive surgical resection.* **(Right)** *Axial noncontrast CT shows a needle biopsy ➡ of a mass ➡ in the pectineus muscle. This mass had unusually low signal intensity on fluid-sensitive sequences. Biopsy revealed a desmoplastic fibroma.*

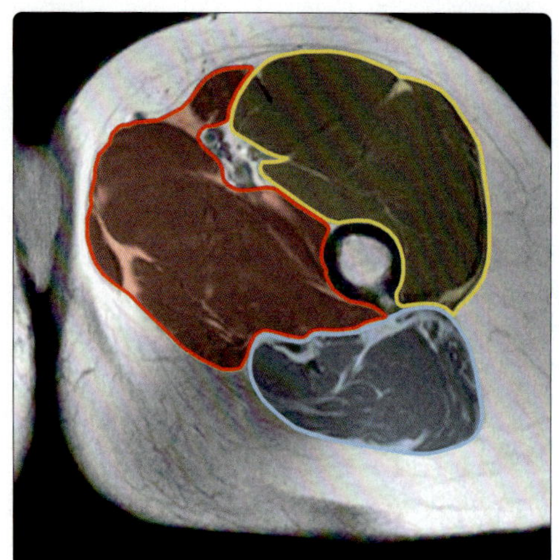

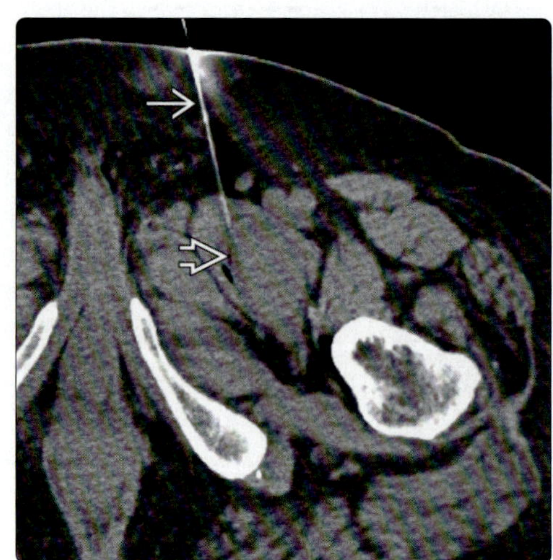

(Left) *Axial T1WI MR of the forearm shows a benign lipoma ➡. The mass has the same signal as the subcutaneous fat without nodules or thick septa. An even, thin capsule surrounds the mass. This mass was painful and tethered on physical examination.* **(Right)** *Axial T1WI MR shows a chest wall mass ➡ that is nearly isointense to muscle. This is in a classic location for an elastofibroma, being between the lower tip of the scapula ➡ and the rib cage. The mass contains small foci of high signal fat ➡.*

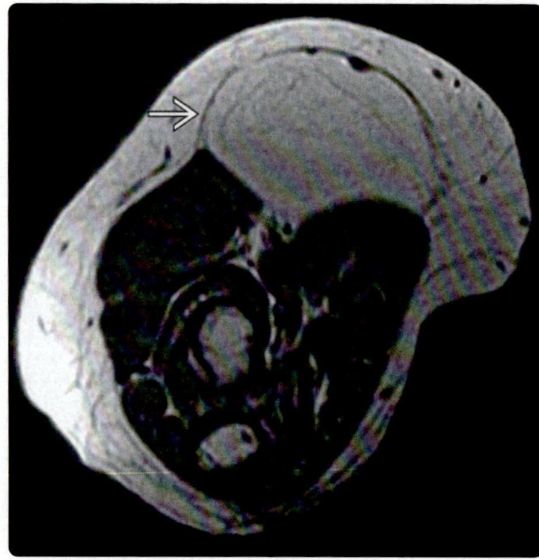

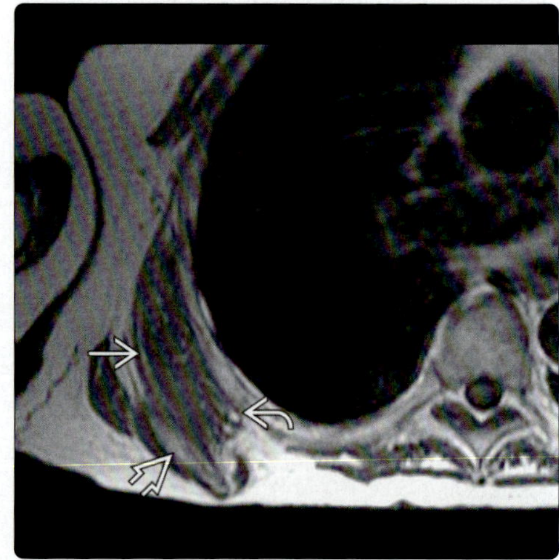

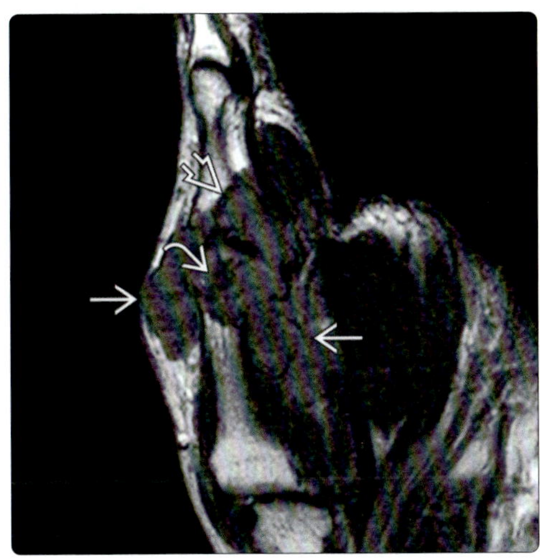

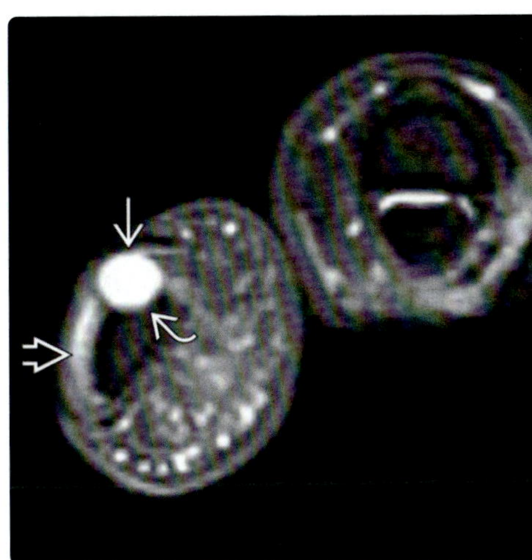

(Left) *Oblique T2WI MR of the thumb shows a giant cell tumor of tendon sheath ➡. The mass is slightly hyperintense relative to the adjacent muscle and contains scattered septa and low signal foci ➡. Bone erosion ➡ is demonstrated and is not unusual for large lesions.* **(Right)** *Axial T2WI FS MR shows a well-circumscribed glomus tumor ➡ in the nailbed with homogeneously hyperintense signal. This lesion is higher in signal than the adjacent nailbed tissue ➡ and erodes the underlying bone ➡.*

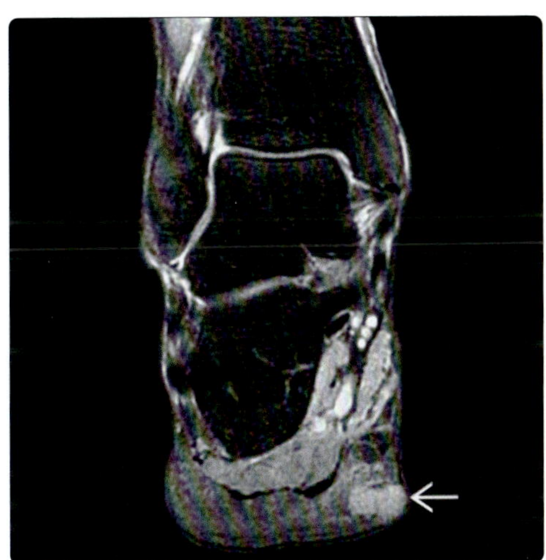

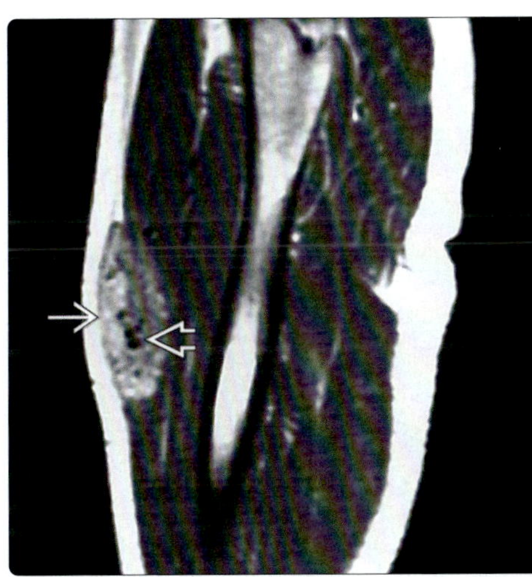

(Left) *Coronal PDWI FS MR shows an angioleiomyoma ➡ in the medial aspect of the heel. The mass has intermediate signal intensity and showed mild enhancement. The overall appearance is nonspecific, and other entities, such as foreign body granuloma and sarcoma, are in the differential diagnosis.* **(Right)** *Sagittal T1WI C+ FS MR shows an intramuscular hemangioma ➡ with intense enhancement. High signal fat tissue is obscured by the enhancement. Note that there is a large draining vessel ➡.*

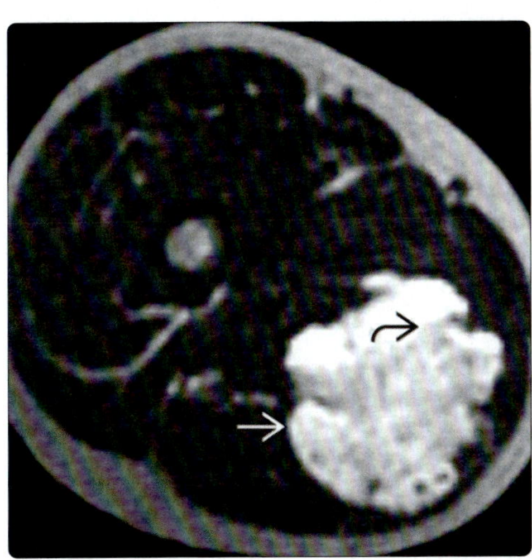

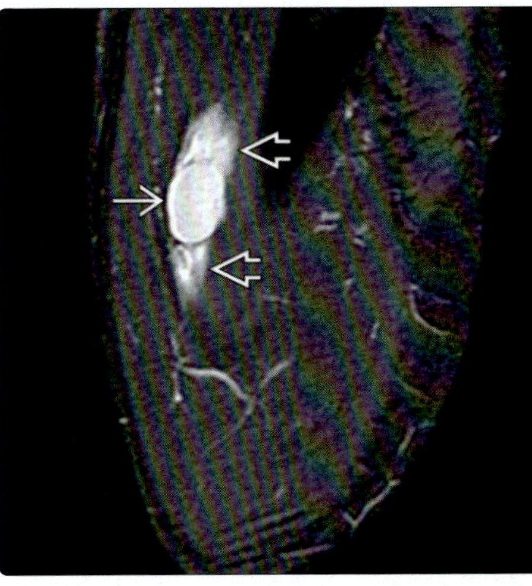

(Left) *Axial T2WI MR shows a lymphangioma ➡ in the thigh of a child. The mass has heterogeneous high signal with internal septa ➡. This mass has a nonspecific appearance for a pediatric patient. Hemangioma and lymphangioma would both be reasonable to include in the differential diagnosis.* **(Right)** *Sagittal STIR MR shows an intramuscular myxoma ➡ in the thigh. Flame-shaped high signal ➡ in the surrounding soft tissues adjacent to the proximal and distal poles of the lesion is a typical finding.*

KEY FACTS

TERMINOLOGY

- Benign lipomatous tumor, representing almost 50% of soft tissue masses

IMAGING

- Mass has same imaging appearance as subcutaneous fat
  - Septa measuring < 2 mm in diameter
  - Capsule may be incomplete or absent (nonvisible)
- Fat attenuation of mass on CT -65 to -120 HU
- MR is best imaging modality for lipoma
- Lipomas will follow intensity of SQ fat on every MR imaging sequence
  - High signal on T1WI
  - Compare to normal fat located a similar distance from coil
  - Signal of mass should become hypointense with fat suppression
  - Mild increased T2 signal can occasionally be present, possibly due to increased vascularity
  - Thin, low signal peripheral capsule is typical
  - May have fine peripheral enhancement of capsule
- Classic appearance can be complicated by infarction, calcification, and hemorrhage
- US: Most are hyperechoic relative to muscle
  - Compressible and without posterior acoustic enhancement
  - No flow on color Doppler sonography

DIAGNOSTIC CHECKLIST

- Should be similar to SQ fat on any imaging modality
- Most important to differentiate from atypical lipomatous tumor/well-differentiated liposarcoma
- Comment on presence or absence of aggressive features, such as soft tissue nodules or thick septa
- Mineralization possible but should raise question of malignant neoplasm
- Even simple fatty mass in retroperitoneum should be regarded with suspicion

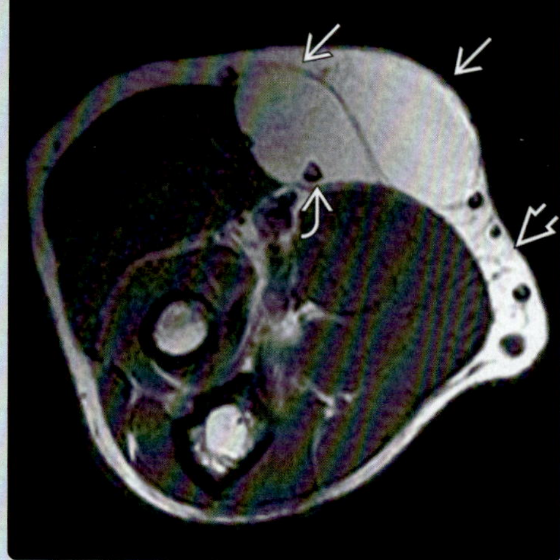

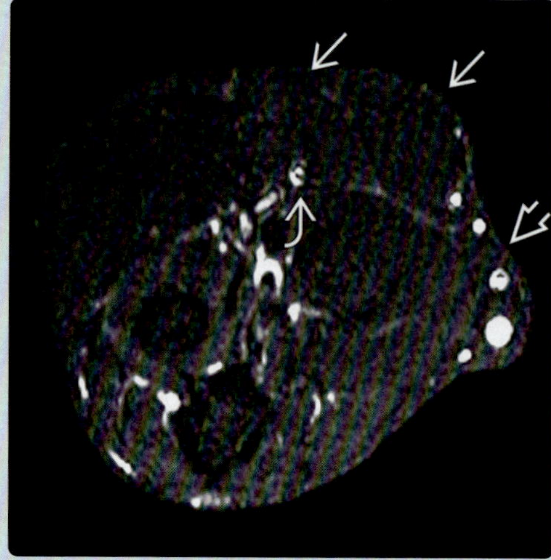

(Left) *Axial T1WI MR shows a homogeneous, high signal, bilobed fatty mass ➡ along the volar surface of the proximal forearm. The mass has the same signal intensity as the adjacent subcutaneous fat ➡. There are no nodules or thick septa. A blood vessel ➡ is present along the deep border of the mass.* **(Right)** *Axial T2WI FS MR shows the signal intensity of the lipoma ➡ to entirely suppress, just as the subcutaneous fat ➡ does, to become homogeneously low. The single high signal focus ➡ is vascular.*

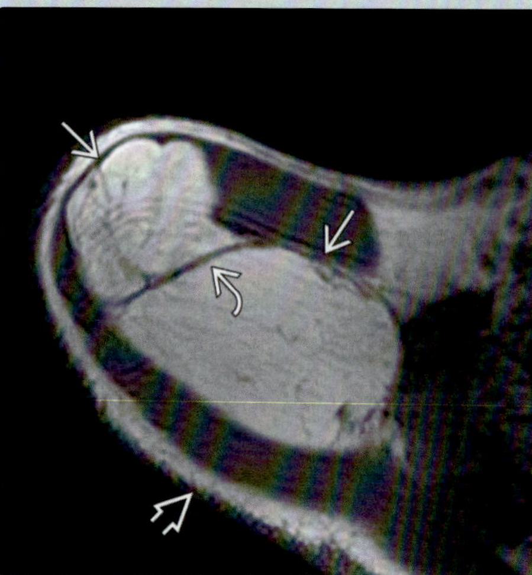

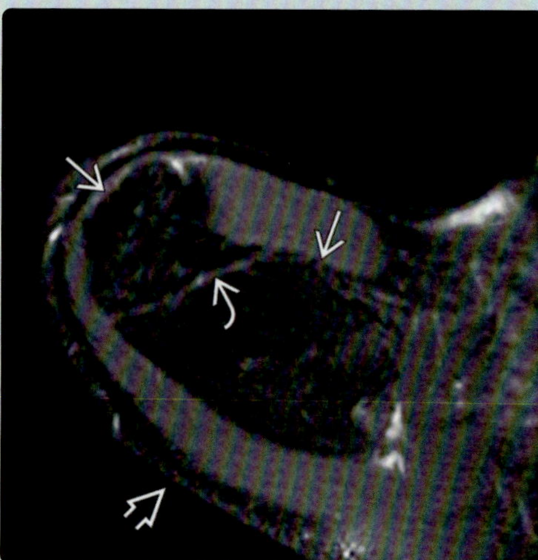

(Left) *Axial T1WI MR of the superior shoulder shows a lobulated fatty mass ➡ composed of high signal that is the same as SQ fat ➡. Fine septa are scattered throughout the mass. Despite a mildly prominent fibrous ➡ septation, this proved to be a lipoma rather than an atypical lipomatous tumor.* **(Right)** *Axial T2WI FS MR in the same patient shows the mass ➡ to have diffusely low signal, following the intensity of the SQ fat ➡. The dominant septation ➡ and scattered fine septa have mildly increased T2 signal.*

TERMINOLOGY

Definitions

- Benign lipomatous tumor, representing almost 50% of soft tissue masses

IMAGING

General Features

- Best diagnostic clue
  - Mass has same appearance as subcutaneous (SQ) fat regardless of imaging modality
    - Fine internal septa measuring < 2 mm in diameter may be present
  - Classic appearance can be complicated by infarction, calcification, and hemorrhage
    - Histologic diagnosis needed in cases where typical imaging findings are not present
  - Underlying bone cortex thickening or erosion is rare
- Location
  - Characterized as being superficial or deep
  - Majority are superficially located in SQ fat
    - Trunk > shoulder > upper arm > neck
  - Intramuscular/intermuscular location is 2nd most common location
    - Intramuscular lipomas predominate in lower extremity
  - Spindle cell lipoma most frequently located in posterior neck
    - Usually elderly male
    - Internal fat content may be scant, making diagnosis difficult
  - Deep lipomas
    - < 1% have deep location
      - Chest wall, deep tissues of hands and feet, and retroperitoneal locations
      - Some literature conflicts and may include intra-/intermuscular lipomas
    - Since benign retroperitoneal lipomas are rare, well-differentiated liposarcoma should always be in differential diagnosis
    - Fatty masses in deep location tend to have more aggressive behavior
- Size
  - 80% are < 5 cm
  - Uncommon to be > 10 cm
  - Deep lipomas are usually larger at presentation than superficial lipomas
- Morphology
  - Palpable, mobile, doughy soft tissue mass

Radiographic Findings

- Radiography
  - Small lesions may not be visible
  - Larger masses correspond to area of radiolucency, similar to SQ fat
    - Density may be higher than SQ fat due to overlapping structures
    - Fine peripheral or coarse central calcification is uncommon

CT Findings

- Fat attenuation of mass, -65 to -120 HU
- Capsule attenuation similar to muscle
- No enhancement
- May have chondroid or osteoid mineralization but presence should raise question of intermediate or malignant fatty neoplasm
- May have adjacent cortical thickening
- Erosion of underlying bone is rare

MR Findings

- T1WI
  - Homogeneous, high signal fatty mass with similar intensity to SQ fat
    - Compare mass to normal fat located similar distance from coil
  - Thin, low signal internal septa and peripheral capsule is typical
    - Capsule may be incomplete or absent (nonvisible)
- T2WI FS
  - Signal of mass should become hypointense with fat suppression
  - Capsule has low signal on all unenhanced imaging sequences
  - Mild increased T2 signal can occasionally be present, possibly due to increased vascularity
- T1WI C+ FS
  - May have fine peripheral capsular enhancement
  - Should never have central, nodular, or mass-like enhancement
    - If present, consider atypical lipoma or liposarcoma

Imaging Recommendations

- Best imaging tool
  - MR is best imaging modality for lipoma
  - Lipomas will follow intensity of SQ fat on every unenhanced MR imaging sequence
  - Utilize MR-compatible markers to indicate proximal and distal borders of palpable mass in case lesion is nonencapsulated
- Protocol advice
  - T1WI sequence in 2 planes
    - Best defines anatomic location
    - Intramuscular lipomas often contain strands of normal muscle tissue, which need to be differentiated from nodules and thickened septa
  - T2WI with fat suppression
    - Either in 2 planes or in 1 plane with alternate plane STIR sequence
  - Gadolinium-enhanced images are not necessary for diagnosis of simple lipoma
    - Enhancement is useful when lesions have components other than pure fat and thin septa or if they are in a deep location
    - Subtraction postprocessing (T1WI FS postgadolinium minus T1WI FS pregadolinium) highlights enhancing regions
    - Must be performed with fat suppression due to intrinsic high T1WI signal

Ultrasonographic Findings

- Most are hyperechoic relative to muscle
  - Isoechoic and hypoechoic appearances are also normal but less common
- Septa are seen as thin, echogenic lines parallel to skin surface
- Compressible and without posterior acoustic enhancement
- No flow on color Doppler sonography

DIFFERENTIAL DIAGNOSIS

Atypical Lipomatous Tumor

- a.k.a. well-differentiated liposarcoma
- Can be very difficult to differentiate from lipoma
  - Histologic examination may be necessary
  - Molecular pathology useful in differentiating
- Look for soft tissue nodules with enhancement and septa > 2 mm thick

Fat Necrosis

- Thicker, more irregular, low signal rim on MR imaging
- Have more variable calcification, enhancement, and cystic appearance
- Found in characteristic locations over pressure points or bony protuberances

Lipomatosis

- Not as well defined as lipoma
- Diffuse overgrowth and infiltration of fat

Hibernoma

- Has similar but not identical appearance to SQ fat
- Hyperintense on STIR MR images due to vascularity
- CT attenuation is between SQ fat and muscle

PATHOLOGY

General Features

- Etiology
  - Mesenchymal neoplasm vs. local fat hyperplasia
- Genetics
  - Familial multiple lipomas is multifactorial
    - More common in males
    - Few to several hundred lipomas
    - Predilection for extensor surfaces
  - Cytogenetic abnormalities in 50-80% of lipomas
    - *MDM2* and *CDK4* gene overexpression related to amplification of 12q13-15 chromosomal region observed in atypical lipomatous tumor/well-differentiated lipoma
      - May be useful in differentiating large lipoma from more aggressive lesions

Gross Pathologic & Surgical Features

- Soft, well-circumscribed mass
- Pale yellow to orange or tan
- Usually has capsule or pseudocapsule
- Greasy, lobular surface

Microscopic Features

- Mature, uniform lipocytes
  - No nuclear hyperchromasia
- Identical to normal adult fat
- Can contain mesenchymal elements
  - Fibrous tissue is most common
- Well vascularized but vessels compressed by fat cells

CLINICAL ISSUES

Presentation

- Most common signs/symptoms
  - Palpable superficial mass
  - Usually painless
    - Can be mildly tender to palpation
  - May cause neuropathy from nerve compression
- Other signs/symptoms
  - May limit range of motion when located near joint
  - Usually freely mobile
    - Tethering to underlying tissue is less common
  - Slowly enlarges over time then stabilizes
    - May increase in size during weight gain
  - May seem to increase in size with severe weight loss
    - Fat in lipoma is protected from metabolism

Demographics

- Age
  - 5th-7th decades of life most frequent
- Gender
  - Studies conflict, with some reporting male predominance and others reporting female predominance
  - Deep lipomas more common in men
- Epidemiology
  - No racial predilection

Natural History & Prognosis

- < 5% recur after surgery
  - Deep lipomas more likely to recur
- Rare reported cases of malignant transformation, likely due to malignant features being initially overlooked

Treatment

- Marginal excision for cosmesis or definitive diagnosis

DIAGNOSTIC CHECKLIST

Consider

- Most important to differentiate from atypical lipomatous tumor/well-differentiated liposarcoma

Image Interpretation Pearls

- Lipomas should not contain soft tissue nodules or thick septa
- Should have same appearance as SQ fat on any imaging modality
- Retroperitoneal location or internal calcification should raise suspicion of intermediate-grade or malignant tumor

Reporting Tips

- Comment on presence or absence of aggressive features, such as soft tissue nodules or thick septa

SELECTED REFERENCES

1. Brisson M et al: MRI characteristics of lipoma and atypical lipomatous tumor/well-differentiated liposarcoma: retrospective comparison with histology and MDM2 gene amplification. Skeletal Radiol. 42(5):635-47, 2013

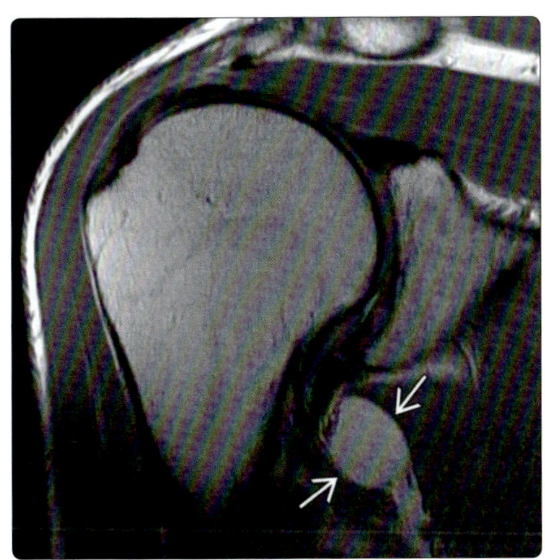

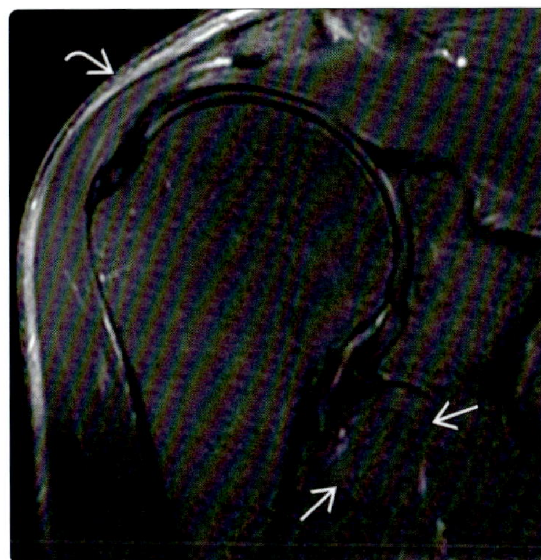

(Left) *Coronal T1 shows a small fat-density lesion ➡ located in the quadrilateral space. Findings are typical of lipoma; further imaging with fat saturation should be confirmatory.* **(Right)** *Coronal T2 FS MR in the same patient shows the lesion ➡ within the quadrilateral space to be completely saturated out. In this case, comparison with subcutaneous fat ➡ is not useful since peripheral fat saturation in the shoulder often fails. The lesion, however, behaves as a typical lipoma in its imaging characteristics.*

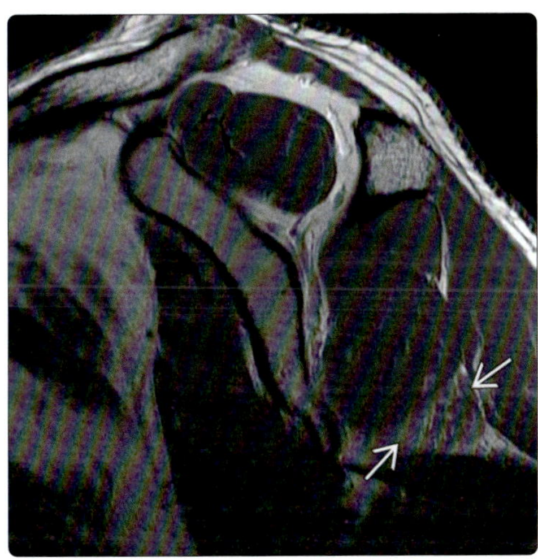

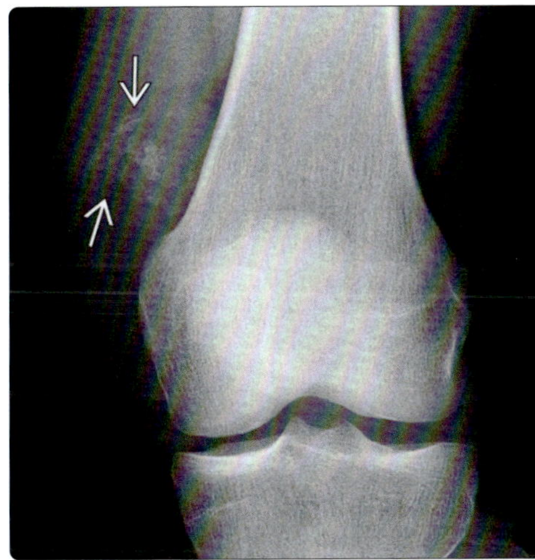

(Left) *Sagittal T1 MR in the same patient is located medial to the lesion, but shows denervation atrophy of the teres minor ➡, which may occur with lesions in the quadrilateral space.* **(Right)** *AP radiograph in a young adult female shows dystrophic calcification ➡ within a lesion adjacent to the knee. No other abnormal density is seen. The most likely diagnosis, given this appearance, is synovial sarcoma. MR imaging is required.*

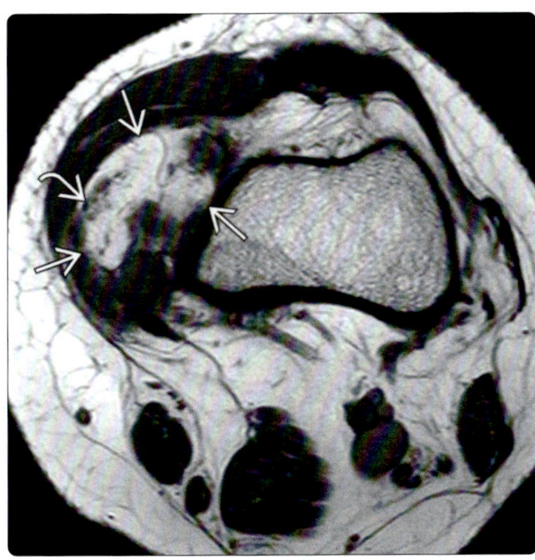

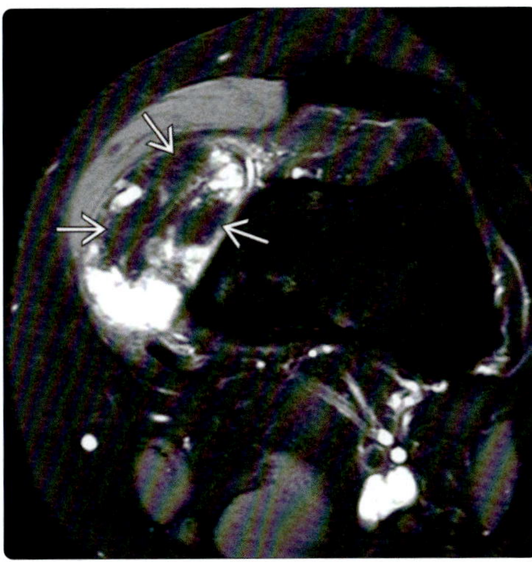

(Left) *Axial T1 MR in the same patient shows the lesion to be intraarticular and to contain a significant amount of fat ➡; neither of these findings is characteristic of synovial sarcoma. The dystrophic calcification is punctate ➡ and seen throughout the lesion.* **(Right)** *Axial T2 FS MR in the same patient shows the fatty portion of the lesion ➡ to saturate out, becoming hypointense. The remainder of the lesion is hyperintense. This is a case of intraarticular chondroid lipoma, containing metaplastic chondroid tissue.*

(Left) *Longitudinal US of the posterior chest wall shows a well-defined, predominantly hypoechoic mass ➡. It contains linear, hyperechoic septa ➡ at right angles to the US beam. There is no increased through transmission.* **(Right)** *Axial T1WI MR shows a well-defined fat signal mass ➡ in the radial aspect of the carpal tunnel. The median nerve ➡ is slightly flattened. There is mild volar bowing of the flexor retinaculum ➡. This lipoma produced carpal tunnel syndrome.*

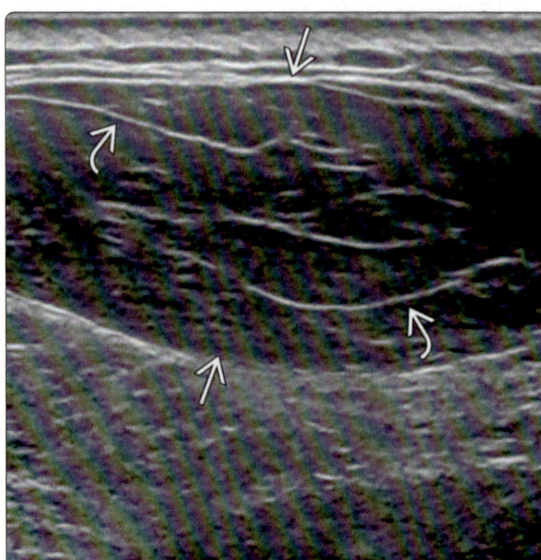

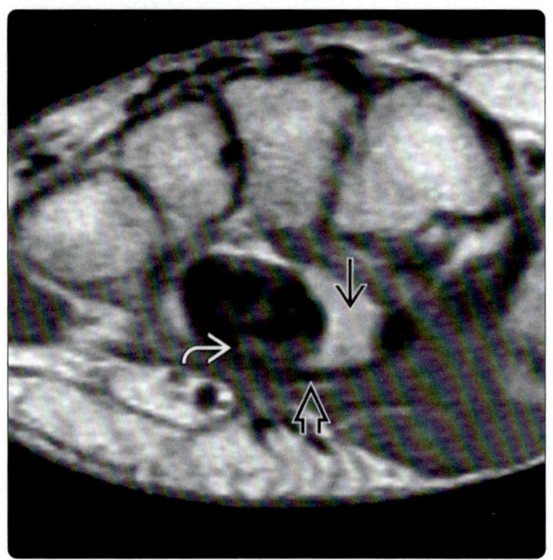

(Left) *Coronal T1WI MR shows normal-appearing subcutaneous fat ➡ in the region of a skin marker ➡ that denotes the location of a palpable mass. The pattern of septa in the subcutaneous fat is relatively even.* **(Right)** *Axial T2WI FS MR in the same patient again shows normal-appearing fat ➡ adjacent to the skin marker. When the location of a palpable mass is confidently known and other etiologies for a mass have been excluded, the diagnosis of a nonencapsulated lipoma can be suggested.*

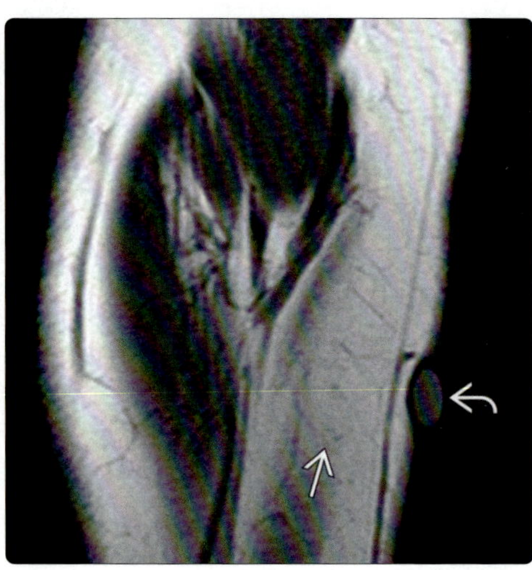

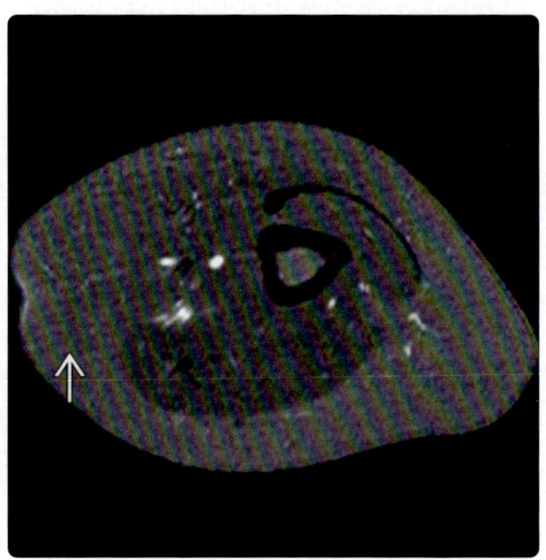

(Left) *Axial T1WI MR through the upper arm shows a fatty mass ➡ within the deltoid muscle. This mass contains numerous entrapped muscle fibers ➡.* **(Right)** *Axial PDWI FS MR in the same patient shows the fat signal intensity of the mass ➡ to suppress similar to the subcutaneous fat. The entrapped muscle fibers ➡ are isointense to the remainder of the deltoid muscle. Intramuscular lipomas often contain muscle fibers, which can simulate thick septa or nodularity.*

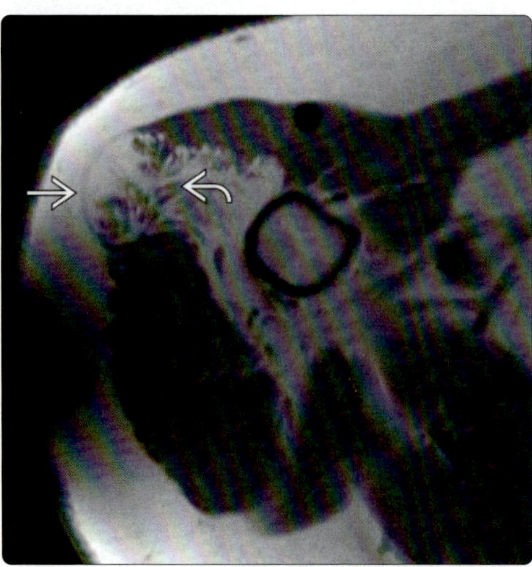

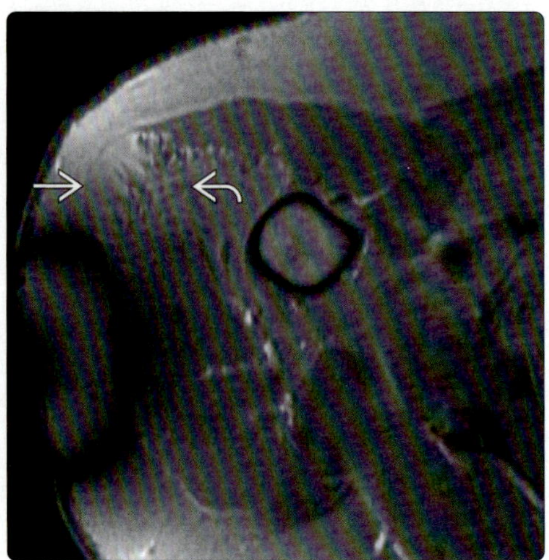

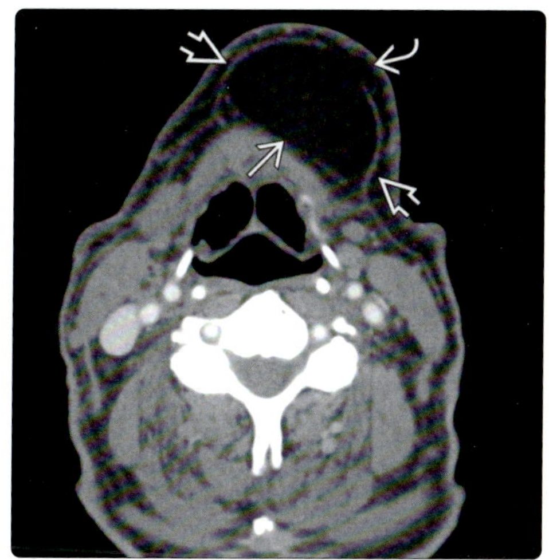

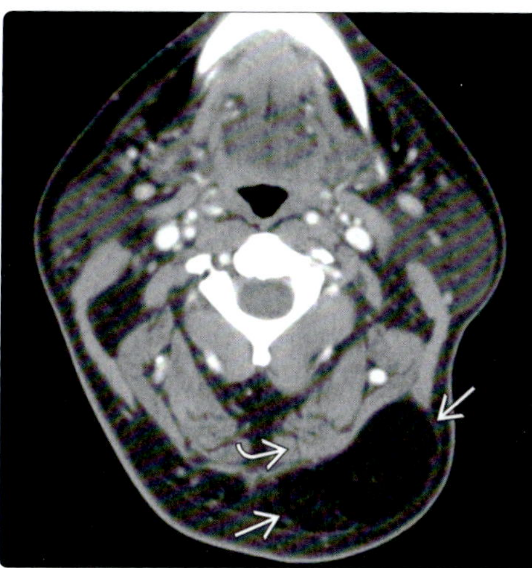

(Left) *Axial CECT shows a large, homogeneous, fat-attenuation mass ➡ in the anterior neck, beneath the platysma muscle ➡. This submandibular space lipoma partially herniates through a rent in the platysma muscle ➡.* **(Right)** *Axial CECT demonstrates a fat-attenuation mass ➡ in the posterior left neck, located superficial to the paraspinous musculature ➡. The mass is homogeneous fat density with fine septations and lacks nodularity. The features are pathognomonic of a benign lipoma.*

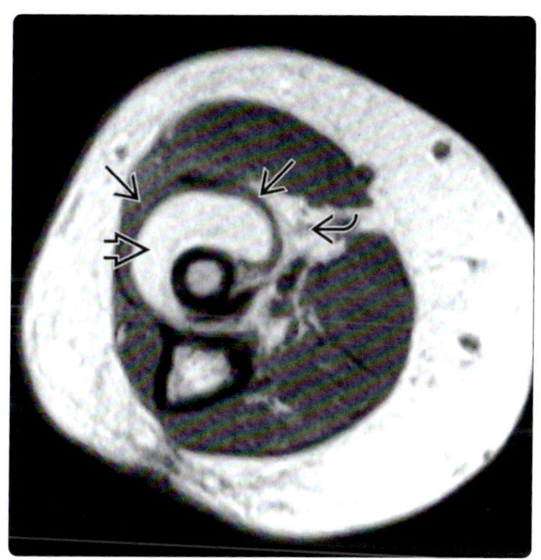

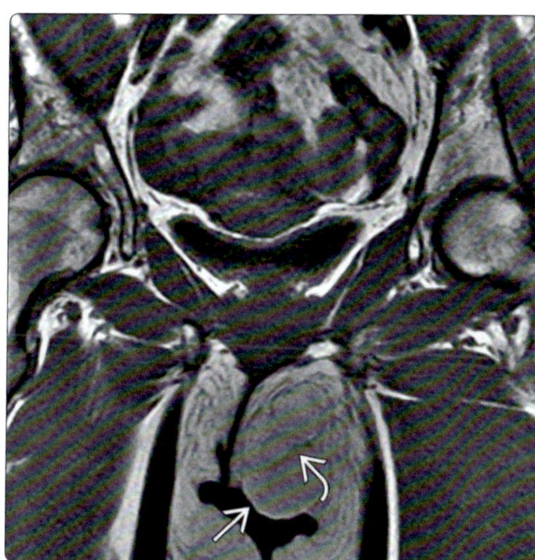

(Left) *Axial T1 MR shows a lipoma causing impingement of the posterior interosseous branch of the radial nerve. The mass ➡ within the belly of the supinator muscle ➡ has uniform fat signal, consistent with a lipoma. The radial nerve ➡ is compressed by the mass during supination.* **(Right)** *Coronal T1 MR shows a lobulated, high signal fatty mass ➡ in the left perineal region. It contains a few thin septa ➡, as does the adjacent SQ fat. The mass has no aggressive features. It was removed for cosmetic reasons and confirmed to be a lipoma.*

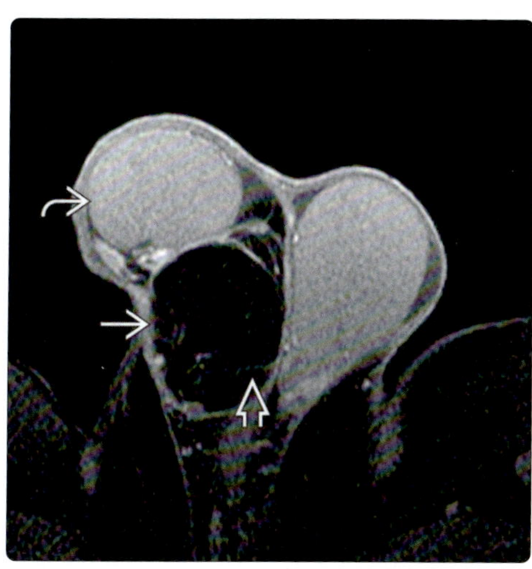

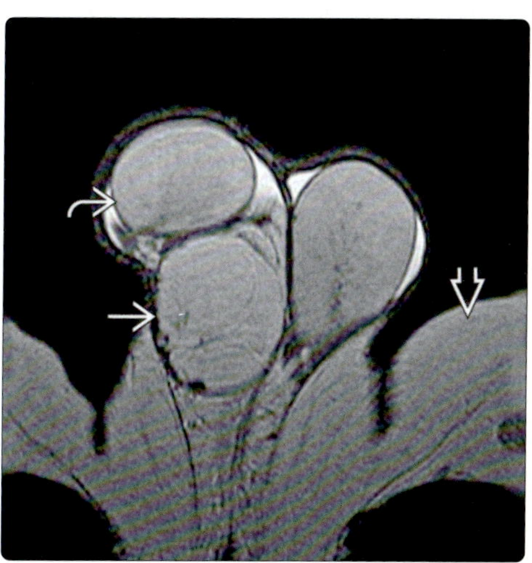

(Left) *Axial T1WI C+ FS MR through the scrotum shows a right spermatic cord lipoma ➡ located posterosuperior to the right testicle ➡. It followed fat signal intensity on all series and contained a few enhancing septa ➡.* **(Right)** *Axial T2WI MR in the same patient shows the lipoma ➡ to have similar signal as the right testicle ➡ and SQ fat ➡. Fat-suppressed images are important to confirm fat content. It is also important to exclude a hernia when fat is seen in the scrotum, as was done in this case.*

Lipomatosis

KEY FACTS

TERMINOLOGY

- Diffuse overgrowth or regional deposition of mature adipose tissue
- Found in multiple clinical situations and syndromes
- Variety of body parts affected

IMAGING

- Distribution defines clinical type of lipomatosis
- CT and MR are diagnostic
  - Confirms fatty composition of mass
  - Axial imaging defines distribution of fat
- Protocol MR sequences ± fat suppression
- Contrast not usually necessary for CT or MR
- Radiographs show nonspecific soft tissue prominence
  - ± mottled lucent regions

PATHOLOGY

- Poorly circumscribed aggregates of soft yellow fat
- Described entities based on location are histologically identical

CLINICAL ISSUES

- Accumulation of fat may mimic neoplasm
- Usually painless, except adiposis dolorosa
  - May rarely cause spinal cord or nerve root compression
  - Neck: Laryngeal obstruction, rarely resulting in death
  - Abdomen/chest: Cough, vena cava compression
  - Pelvis: Urinary frequency, constipation, pain
- Treatment with surgical excision or liposuction
  - High local recurrence rate

DIAGNOSTIC CHECKLIST

- Numerous entities can produce focal, regional, and diffuse fat accumulation
- Location and extent of involvement is key to identifying etiology

(Left) *Axial T1WI MR through the wrist demonstrates massive overgrowth of the fat ➡ in this young child with diffuse lipomatosis. The contours of the wrist are grossly distorted. The carpal tunnel contents ➡ are displaced away from the bone.* **(Right)** *Axial T1WI MR shows that the diffuse lipomatosis extends into the forearm. Proliferation of fat involves all regions of soft tissue, including the musculature ➡. Tendons are significantly displaced away from their normal positions.*

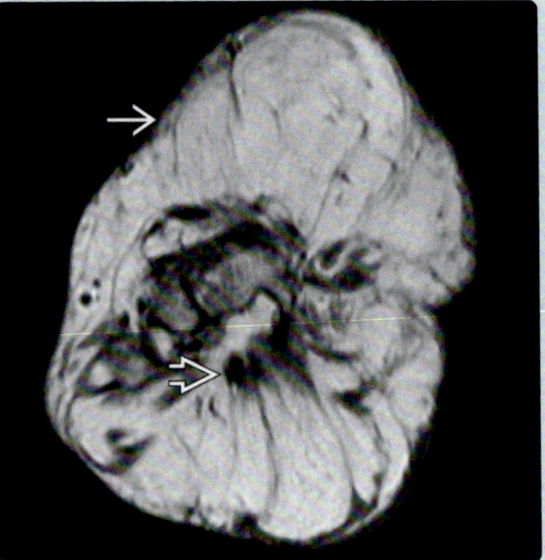

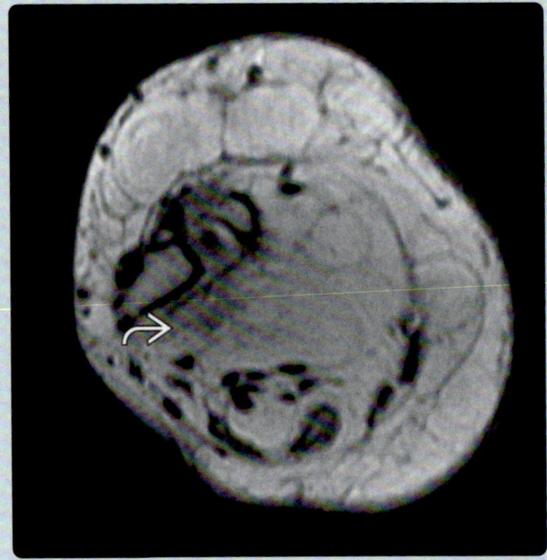

(Left) *Axial T2WI FS MR in the same patient demonstrates that the markedly overgrown fat ➡ has normal decreased signal on this fat-suppressed sequence.* **(Right)** *Coronal T1WI MR in the same patient with diffuse lipomatosis demonstrates markedly overgrown and proliferated subcutaneous fat ➡. The musculature ➡ is also diffusely invaded with fat. The bones of the thumb were relatively overgrown compared with the young age of the patient.*

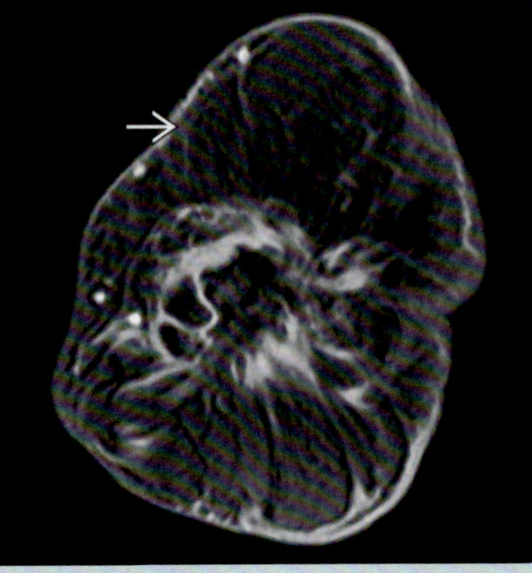

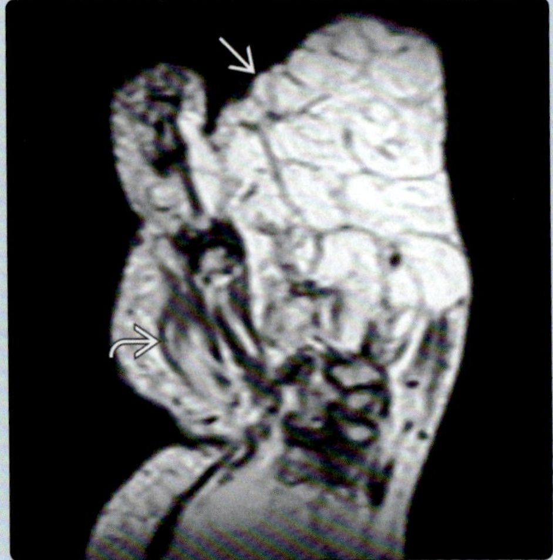

TERMINOLOGY

Synonyms

- Infiltrating lipoma, diffuse congenital lipomatosis, Madelung disease, Launois-Bensaude syndrome, Dercum syndrome

Definitions

- Diffuse overgrowth or regional deposition of mature adipose tissue
- Found in multiple clinical situations and syndromes
  - Variety of body parts potentially involved

IMAGING

General Features

- Location
  - Distribution defines clinical type of lipomatosis

Imaging Recommendations

- Best imaging tool
  - CT and MR are diagnostic
    - Confirm fatty composition of mass
    - Define distribution of fat
- Protocol advice
  - MR sequences ± fat suppression
  - Contrast not usually necessary for CT or MR

Radiographic Findings

- Radiography
  - Nonspecific soft tissue prominence
    - ± mottled lucent regions

DIFFERENTIAL DIAGNOSIS

Diffuse Lipomatosis (Clinical Type)

- Adipose tissue that infiltrates extremity or trunk
  - Less commonly involves head/neck, intestine, abdominal cavity
- Involves subcutaneous fat and muscles
- Usually occurs in children under 2 years old
  - Reported in adolescents and adults
- Rare association with tuberous sclerosis
- Radiography shows soft tissue overgrowth
  - ± osseous hypertrophy
- Large fatty deposits may severely limit function

Mediastinal Lipomatosis (Clinical Type)

- Diffuse deposition of adipose tissue in mediastinum
- Patients are usually obese with cushingoid features
  - Associated endogenous or exogenous steroid excess
- Usually produces only mild symptoms
  - May cause dyspnea, dysphonia, or cough
  - Electrocardiogram = low voltage complexes
  - May complicate placement of internal jugular or subclavian catheters
- Chest radiography shows mediastinal widening
  - Double contour effect from shadows of fat and normal mediastinal structures
  - Can simulate hemorrhage, aortic dissection, mass, pericardial effusion

Renal Sinus Lipomatosis (Clinical Type)

- Fat proliferation in peripelvic region of kidney
  - Associated with chronic inflammation or any entity causing atrophy of renal tissue
  - Worsened by ↑ exogenous or endogenous steroids
- Excretory urography demonstrates effacement and stretching of pelvicalyceal system
- CT and MR demonstrate fat proliferation in peripelvic region and renal parenchymal atrophy
- Rarely symptomatic

Pelvic Lipomatosis (Clinical Type)

- Perirectal and perivesical fat accumulation
- Most common in 3rd-4th decade of life
  - Any age can be affected (9-80 years)
- Predominance in males of African descent
- Compresses bladder and rectosigmoid colon
  - 75% with cystitis cystica or cystitis glandularis
- Findings on excretory urography and barium enema
  - Pear- or gourd-shaped bladder
  - Medially displaced ureters
  - Elevated prostate gland and bladder base
  - Straightened, narrowed rectosigmoid colon

Multiple Symmetric Lipomatosis (Clinical Type)

- a.k.a. Madelung disease
- Multiple well-circumscribed, nonencapsulated lipomas, which may infiltrate adjacent tissue
- Symmetric fat deposition most commonly involving cervical region and upper trunk
  - Spares distal arms and legs
- Typically seen in middle-aged men
  - ↑ frequency in those of Mediterranean descent
- High association with alcoholism
  - 50% have history of excessive alcohol intake
- Associated with diabetes, hypertriglyceridemia, hyperuricemia, and ↑ HDL cholesterol
- Peripheral motor and sensory neuropathy is common
  - 86% have axonal sensorimotor neuropathy
  - 50% have central nervous system involvement
    - Hearing loss, optic nerve atrophy, cerebellar ataxia

Shoulder Girdle Lipomatosis (Clinical Type)

- Unilateral accumulation of fat involving chest wall, shoulder, and upper arm
- Leads to slowly progressive enlargement of soft tissues
  - May cause airway compression
  - Neuromyopathy common
- Female predominance

HIV-Associated Lipodystrophy (Clinical Type)

- Features of lipoatrophy and lipohypertrophy
  - Abdominal obesity
  - Buffalo hump
  - Decreased facial and subcutaneous fat
- Attributed to use of protease inhibitor and other antiretroviral drugs
- Predominantly problem of cosmesis
- May be symptomatic involving Hoffa fat pad
  - ↑ signal intensity on fluid-sensitive MR sequences

Epidural Lipomatosis (Clinical Type)

- Overgrowth of normal epidural fat
- Associated with obesity and exogenous steroid use > endogenous steroid overproduction
- May result in pain, radicular symptoms, and spinal cord compression
- Surgical intervention when neurologic signs present

Intramuscular Lipomas

- Lipoma confined to muscle or intermuscular tissue
  - Can have infiltrative appearance
  - Often contain entrapped muscle fibers
- Does not involve subcutaneous fat

Multiple Lipomas

- 5-8% of patients with lipomas have multiple tumors
- Each mass is identical to solitary lipoma

Adiposis Dolorosa

- a.k.a. Dercum syndrome
- Tender, diffuse, or nodular accumulations of subcutaneous fat
  - Extremities > trunk
- Affects postmenopausal women
  - Obese, easily fatigued
  - Psychiatric disturbances
  - Endocrine and lipid metabolic dysfunction
- Treatment with lidocaine infusion and steroids or surgery

Infiltrating Congenital Lipomatosis of Face

- Subcutaneous fatty masses involving face and cheek
  - Infiltrates muscles, fibrous tissue, parotid gland
  - ± osseous hypertrophy
- Rare, congenital disorder
- Associated with macroglossia, mucosal neuromas, cutaneous capillary blush
- Fatty infiltration of face occurs in other entities
  - Proteus syndrome
  - Encephalocraniocutaneous lipomatosis
  - Facial hemangioma
- Local recurrence common

Diffuse Angiomatosis

- Regional or disseminated distribution of capillary or cavernous hemangiomas
  - Pronounced vascular proliferation is key finding
- Associated with fat and osseous overgrowth

Atypical Lipomatous Tumor

- Solitary fatty mass in adult patient
  - Variable presence of thickened septa and nodularity
- Histologically shows cellular atypia

Encephalocraniocutaneous Lipomatosis

- a.k.a. Fishman syndrome, Haberland syndrome
- Unilateral cutaneous, ocular, and neurologic malformations
  - Subcutaneous, cranial, and spinal lipomas
- Patients present with seizures and mental retardation

PATHOLOGY

Gross Pathologic & Surgical Features

- Poorly circumscribed aggregates of soft yellow fat

Microscopic Features

- Clinical types are histologically identical
- Mature adipose tissue
  - No atypia, lipoblasts, or cellular pleomorphism
- Lobules and sheets of adipocytes may infiltrate muscle, depending on type of lipomatosis
- Positive stains for vimentin and S100, like normal fat

CLINICAL ISSUES

Presentation

- Most common signs/symptoms
  - Accumulation of fat in affected area
    - May mimic neoplasm
  - Usually painless, except adiposis dolorosa
- Other signs/symptoms
  - Extremity: Limited range of motion
  - Neck: Laryngeal obstruction
  - Abdomen/chest: Cough, vena cava compression
  - Pelvis: Urinary frequency, constipation, pain

Natural History & Prognosis

- All idiopathic forms have tendency to recur locally
- Massive accumulation of fat in neck may rarely cause death from laryngeal obstruction

Treatment

- Surgical excision or liposuction for excess fat removal

DIAGNOSTIC CHECKLIST

Consider

- Numerous entities can produce focal, regional, and diffuse fat accumulation

Image Interpretation Pearls

- Location and extent of involvement is key to identifying etiology

SELECTED REFERENCES

1. Concepcion E et al: Mediastinal lipomatosis presenting as persistent pneumonia. J Pediatr. 167(2):493-493.e1, 2015
2. Garcia-Ortega DY et al: Parapharyngeal space lipomatosis with secondary dyspnea, disphagia and disphonia. Int J Surg Case Rep. 15:54-56, 2015
3. Michael GA et al: Neuroimaging findings in encephalocraniocutaneous lipomatosis. Pediatr Neurol. ePub, 2015
4. Park KH et al: Multiple symmetric lipomatosis presenting with bilateral brachial plexopathy. J Clin Neurol. ePub, 2015
5. Al-Khawaja D et al: Spinal epidural lipomatosis–a brief review. J Clin Neurosci. 15(12):1323-6, 2008
6. Puttarajappa C et al: Mediastinal lipomatosis as a cause of low voltage complexes on electrocardiogram and widened mediastinum: A case report. Cases J. 1(1):171, 2008
7. Weiss SW et al: Benign lipomatous tumors. In Weiss SW et al: Enzinger and Weiss' Soft Tissue Tumors. 5th ed. Philadelphia: Elsevier. 461-5, 2008
8. Dhawan SS et al: Atypical mediastinal lipomatosis. Heart Lung. 36(3):223-5, 2007
9. Kransdorf MJ et al: Lipomatous tumors. In Kransdorf MJ et al: Imaging of Soft Tissue Tumors. 2nd ed. Philadelphia: Lippincott Williams & Wilkins. 109-17, 2006

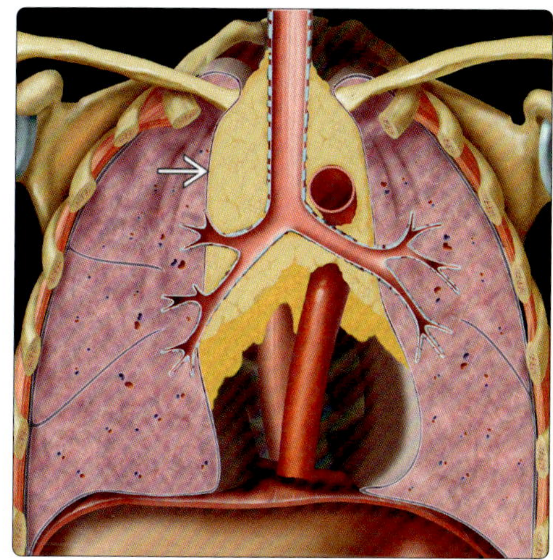

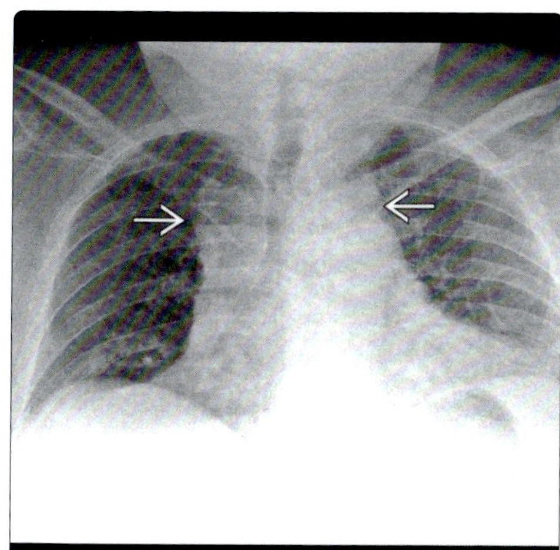

(Left) *Coronal graphic shows diffuse deposition of adipose tissue ➡ within the chest mediastinum. The fat smoothly surrounds the mediastinal structures and laterally displaces the medial border of each lung.* **(Right)** *Frontal radiograph shows typical radiographic features of mediastinal widening ➡ due to lipomatosis. The patient has a large body habitus.*

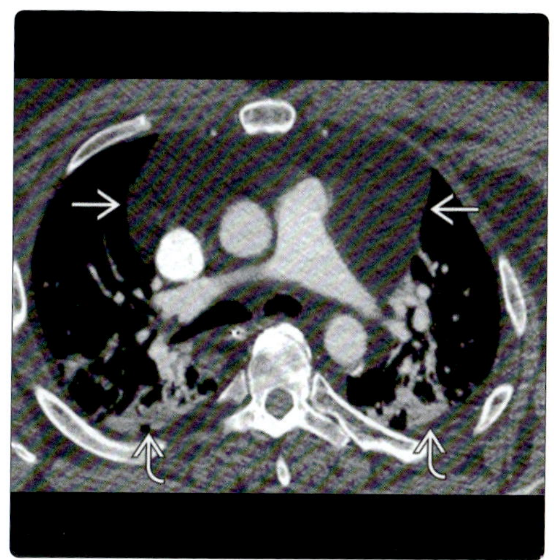

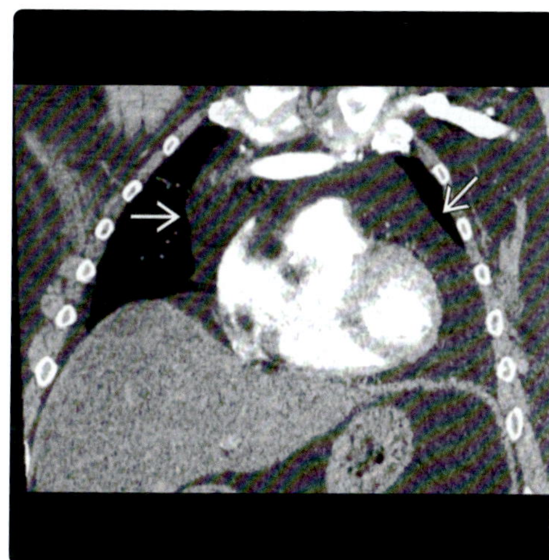

(Left) *Axial CECT in the same patient shows that the widened mediastinum was due to diffuse deposition of fat ➡. Dependent pulmonary atelectasis ➡ was also present.* **(Right)** *Coronal reformatted enhanced CT best demonstrates the correlative appearance of diffuse mediastinal widening from fat ➡, as compared with the previous chest radiograph.*

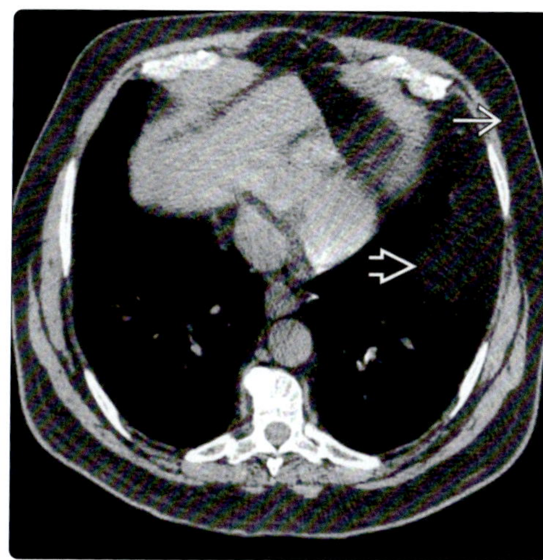

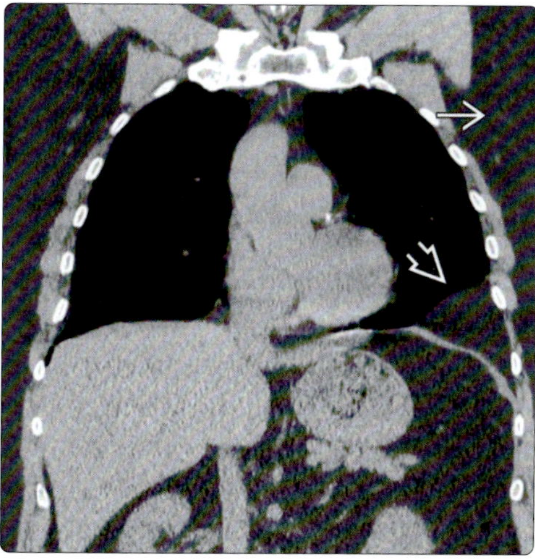

(Left) *Axial HRCT shows a fatty mass ➡ located at the left costophrenic angle in a patient with lipomatosis. The attenuation of the mass is similar to the subcutaneous fat ➡.* **(Right)** *Coronal reconstructed HRCT in this same lipomatosis patient better delineates the fatty mass ➡ in the left costophrenic angle. Again, this mass has an attenuation that is the same as subcutaneous fat ➡.*

(Left) *Anteroposterior excretory urogram shows medial deviation of both the left and right ureters ➡ and a pear-shaped bladder ➡. In this case, the medial displacement and contour deformity proved to be due to pelvic lipomatosis.* **(Right)** *Axial NECT in a patient with pelvic lipomatosis shows a compressed bladder ➡ and a straightened sigmoid colon ➡. This patient had a large amount of retroperitoneal, mesenteric, and pelvic fat, but not excessive subcutaneous fat.*

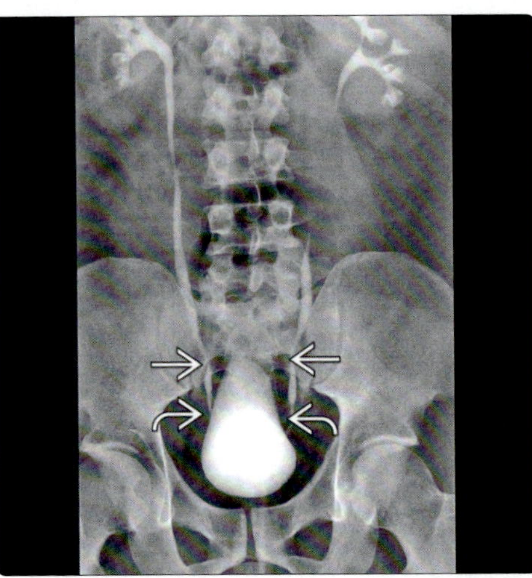

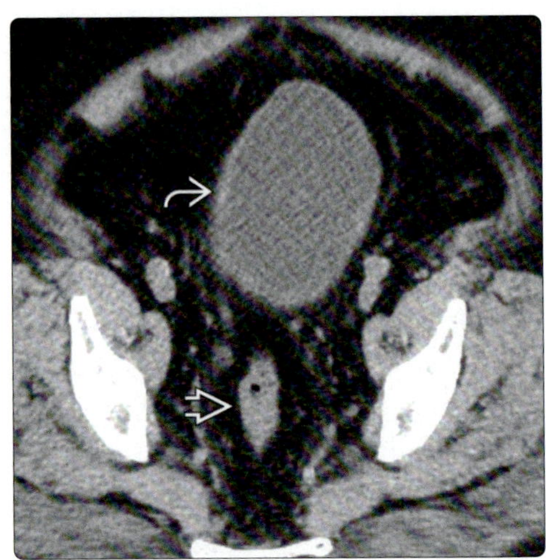

(Left) *Axial CECT shows left side renal cortical loss, dilated calices ➡, and markedly proliferated renal sinus fat ➡. The caliectasis and renal scarring were the result of multiple and chronic episodes of renal and ureteral calculi and infection.* **(Right)** *Axial CECT shows a large stone ➡ in the right renal pelvis and a small, deformed kidney ➡. Proliferation of fat and an inflammatory process ➡ represent findings of both renal lipomatosis and xanthogranulomatous pyelonephritis.*

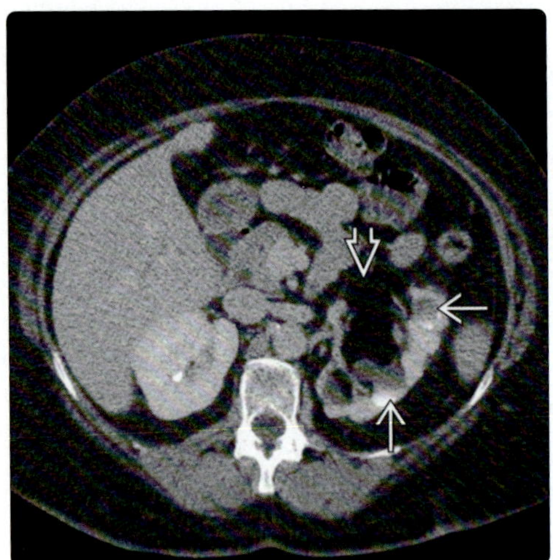

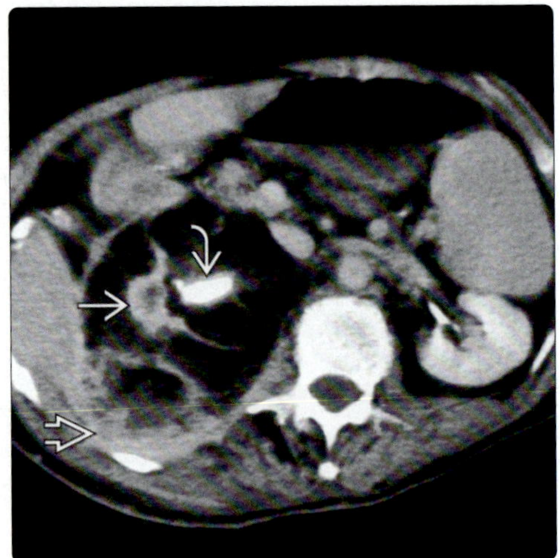

(Left) *Axial NECT shows a dramatic case of gastric lipomatosis. There are many fat-containing masses in the wall of the stomach ➡. The hepatic lesion was a simple cyst ➡. Lipomas uncommonly arise in the submucosa of the intestine. They have no malignant potential.* **(Right)** *Coronal T1WI MR through the hand shows multiple lipomas ➡ within the volar soft tissues. These lipomas had no aggressive features. A small percentage of patients with lipomas have multiple tumors.*

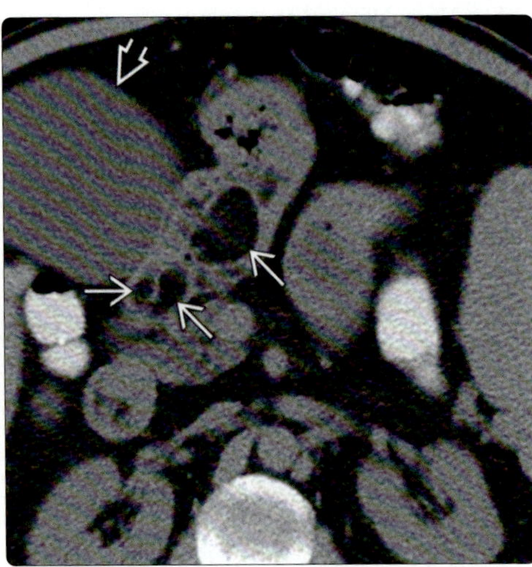

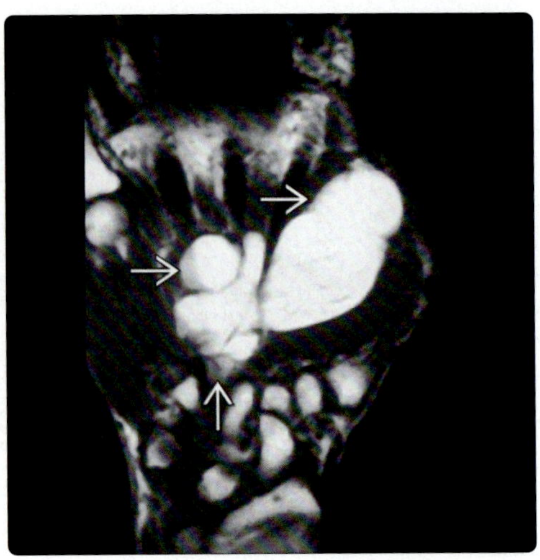

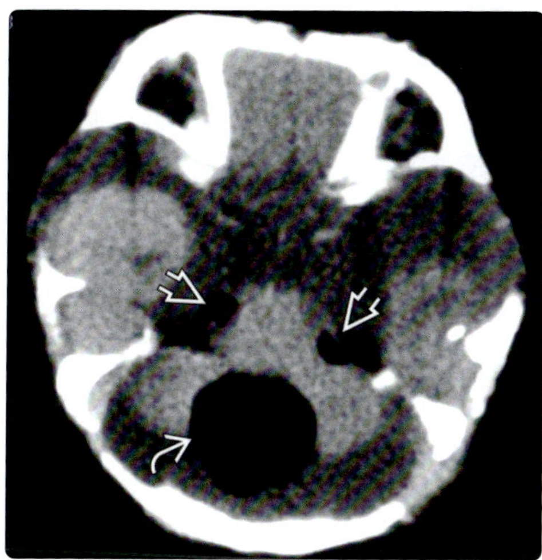

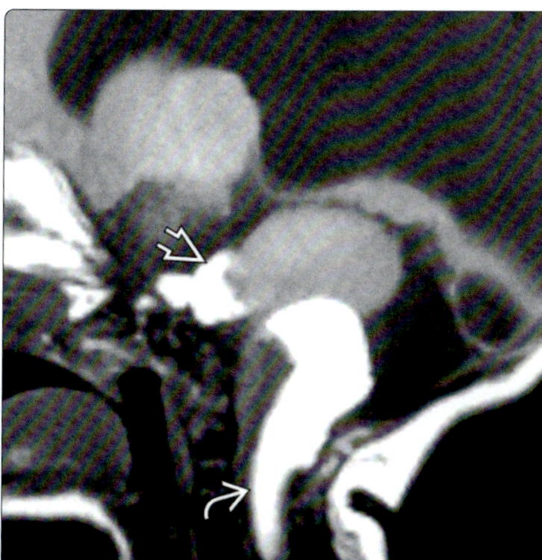

(Left) *Axial CECT in a patient with encephalocraniocutaneous lipomatosis shows a very low-density mass in the midline posterior fossa* ➡ *with smaller masses in both cerebellopontine angles* ➡. **(Right)** *Sagittal T1WI MR in the same patient shows a moderate-sized lipoma that extends into the upper cervical canal* ➡ *and another lipoma in the cerebellopontine angle cistern* ➡.

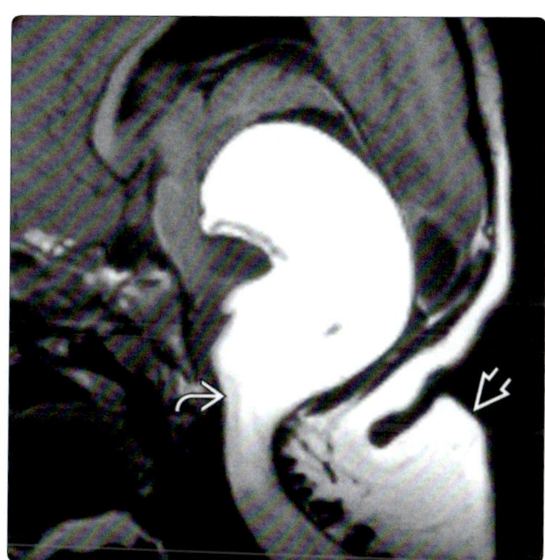

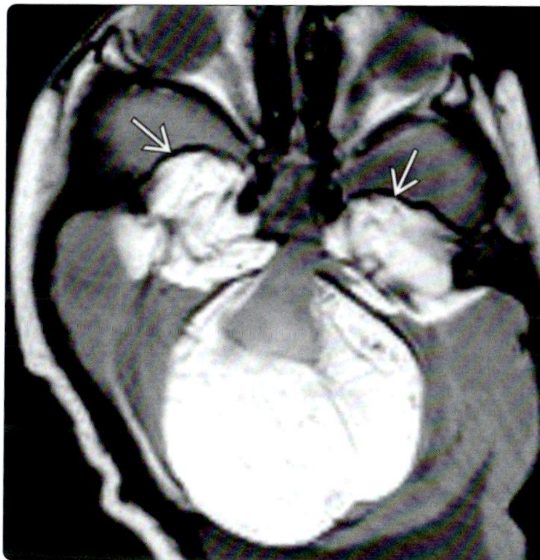

(Left) *Sagittal T1WI MR in the same patient 2 years later shows that the cervical lipoma* ➡ *is much more extensive. Note the large subcutaneous lipoma* ➡. **(Right)** *Axial PD/intermediate MR in the same patient 2 years later confirms an increase in the size of the lipomas. The cerebellopontine angle lipomas now extend anteriorly into the middle cranial fossae. There is a striking chemical shift artifact* ➡ *on the anterior margins of the lipomas.*

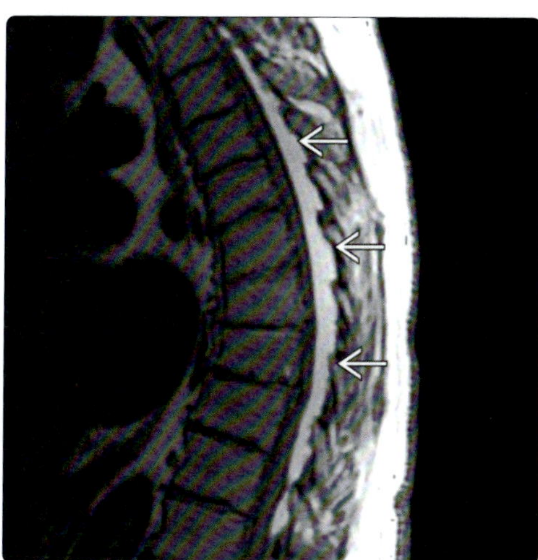

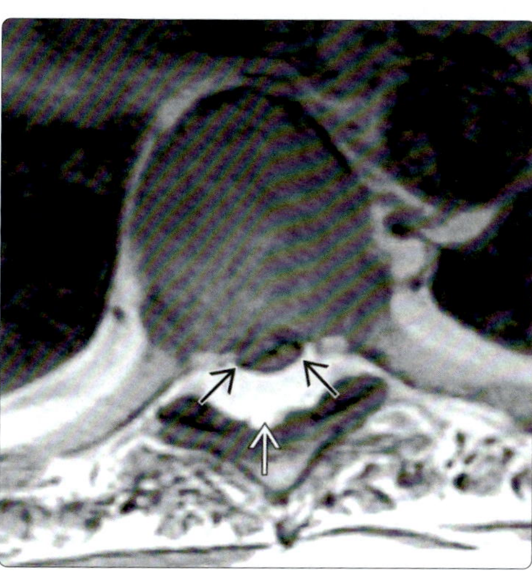

(Left) *Sagittal T1WI MR in a typical case of epidural lipomatosis demonstrates abundant dorsal epidural fat* ➡. *This fat followed the signal intensity of subcutaneous fat on all sequences, including having decreased signal intensity on fat-suppressed sequences.* **(Right)** *Axial T1WI MR in the same patient demonstrates that the epidural lipomatosis* ➡ *is producing significant mass effect on the thoracic spinal cord* ➡.

Lipomatosis: Nerve

KEY FACTS

TERMINOLOGY

- Neural fibrolipoma, fibrolipomatous hamartoma of nerve, lipofibromatous hamartoma of nerve, neurolipomatosis, perineural lipoma, fatty infiltration of nerve, intraneural lipoma
- Fibrofatty nerve infiltration resulting in fusiform enlargement

IMAGING

- 78-96% in upper extremity
  - 80% of these in median nerve distribution
- Left hand > right hand
- CT shows increased fat along course of nerve
- MR shows collection of enlarged cylindrical fascicles along course of nerve
  - Each fascicle has central intermediate signal focus (nerve + fibrosis) surrounded by high signal fat
  - Has coaxial cable or spaghetti-like appearance
- Nerve bundles are punctate on cross section and wavy longitudinally
- Additional fibrofatty masses may arise in soft tissues near enlarged nerve
- Can be confused with liposarcoma, especially if involving lumbosacral plexus or other unusual location

PATHOLOGY

- Associated macrodystrophia lipomatosa in 27-67%
- Appearance is same regardless of whether macrodactyly is present

CLINICAL ISSUES

- Soft, slowly enlarging mass
  - Pain and tenderness
  - Decreased sensation or paresthesia
  - Late compression neuropathy
- Surgical decompression to relieve symptoms

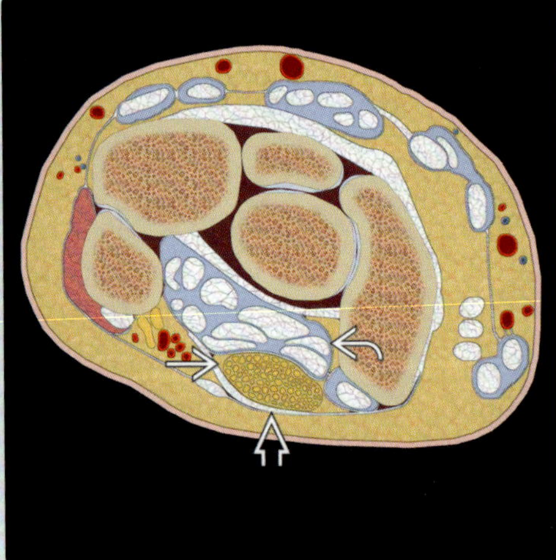

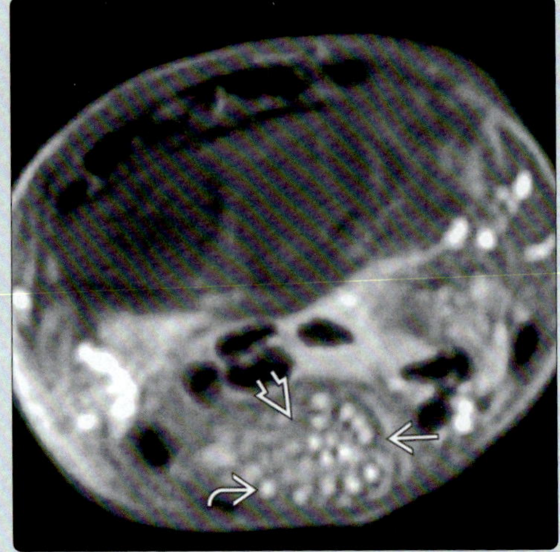

(Left) *Axial graphic through the level of carpal tunnel demonstrates lipomatosis of the median nerve ➡ causing flattening of the flexor tendons ↪ and volar bulging of the flexor retinaculum ⇨.* **(Right)** *Axial T1WI FS MR shows marked enlargement of the median nerve ➡ with fat signal ⇨ filling the spaces between individual nerve fascicles ↪, creating the classic telephone or coaxial cable appearance. The fascicles appear relatively bright due to decreased fat signal on this fat-saturated sequence.*

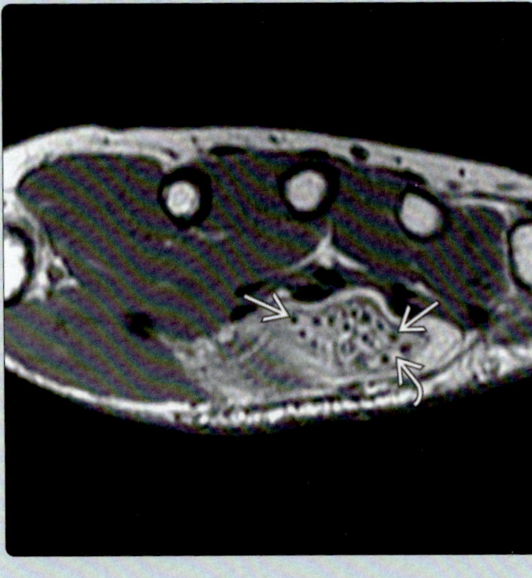

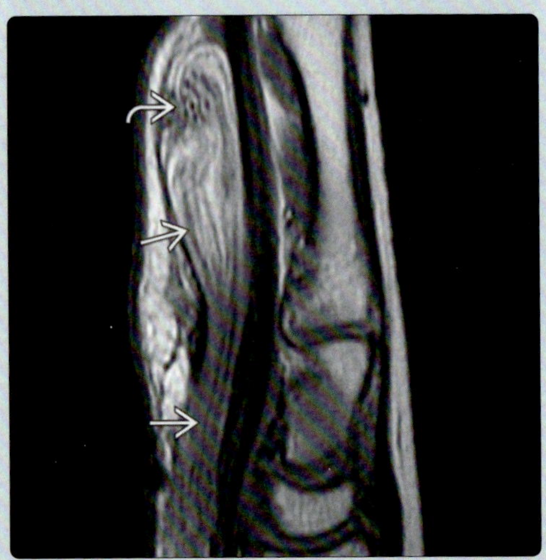

(Left) *Axial T1 MR shows lipomatosis of the median nerve, with mild enlargement of intermediate-signal nerve fascicles ➡ and surrounding fatty deposits ↪ showing high signal. Note that both the degree of enlargement of the nerve/fibrous tissue and the amount/distribution of surrounding fat can be variable.* **(Right)** *Sagittal T1 MR in the same case shows the mildly enlarged nerve fascicles both in longitudinal ➡ and cross section ↪, giving the classic appearance of spaghetti strands and coaxial cable, respectively.*

Lipomatosis: Nerve

TERMINOLOGY

Synonyms

- Neural fibrolipoma, fibrolipomatous hamartoma of nerve, lipofibromatous hamartoma of nerve, neurolipomatosis, perineural lipoma, fatty infiltration of nerve, intraneural lipoma

Definitions

- Fibrofatty nerve infiltration resulting in fusiform enlargement

IMAGING

General Features

- Best diagnostic clue
  - Fusiform fibrofatty infiltration of nerve
- Location
  - 78-96% in upper extremity
    - 80% in median nerve distribution
    - Median nerve > median nerve digital branches > ulnar > radial > brachial plexus > peroneal > cranial nerves
  - Left hand > right hand
  - Preferentially involves volar nerves

CT Findings

- Increased fat along course of nerve
- Mass effect on local structures
- Metaplastic bone is rare
- Can be confused with liposarcoma, especially when involving unusual location or if nerve fascicles are misinterpreted as soft tissue masses or nodules

MR Findings

- T1WI
  - Collection of enlarged cylindrical fascicles along course of nerve
    - Each fascicle has central intermediate signal focus (nerve + fibrosis) surrounded by high signal fat
    - Fatty distribution and extent may be variable
  - Has coaxial cable or spaghetti-like appearance
  - Nerve bundles are punctate on cross section and wavy longitudinally
  - Additional fibrofatty masses may arise in soft tissues near enlarged nerve
    - Can have similar appearance to simple lipomas or discrete soft tissue nodules
- T2WI FS
  - High signal punctate (axial) or wavy (longitudinal) nerve bundles surrounded by low signal fat
- T1WI C+ FS
  - Increased signal of nerve bundles
  - Suppressed (low) signal of surrounding fat

Ultrasonographic Findings

- Alternating hyperechoic and hypoechoic bands
- Cable-like appearance

DIFFERENTIAL DIAGNOSIS

Nerve Sheath Lipoma

- Focal fatty mass within nerve sheath eccentrically displaces nerve
- Individual nerve bundles not involved
- Lacks infiltrative appearance of nerve lipomatosis

Liposarcoma, Soft Tissue

- Will not have branching or longitudinally cylindrical appearance
- Older patients, usually 6th-7th decade

PATHOLOGY

General Features

- Etiology
  - Etiology unclear
  - May be hypertrophy of mature fat and fibroblasts
- Associated abnormalities
  - Macrodystrophia lipomatosa in 27-67%
  - Neurofibromatosis

Gross Pathologic & Surgical Features

- Soft, gray-yellow mass within nerve sheath
  - Large nerve and branches are involved
- Fusiform, sausage-shaped enlargement of nerve

Microscopic Features

- Fibroadipose tissue infiltration of epi- and perineurium
- Nerve fascicles normal or atrophied (late)
- Appearance is same regardless of whether macrodactyly is present or not

CLINICAL ISSUES

Presentation

- Most common signs/symptoms
  - Soft, slowly enlarging mass in volar hand, wrist, or forearm
- Other signs/symptoms
  - Pain and tenderness
  - Late compression neuropathy

Demographics

- Age
  - Most lesions present at birth or infancy
  - Also seen in 2nd-4th decades
- Gender
  - No overall gender predilection
  - Female predominance when macrodactyly present

Natural History & Prognosis

- Progressive, slow growth over many years

Treatment

- Surgical resection risks sensory and motor nerve damage
- Surgical decompression, e.g., carpal tunnel release, to relieve symptoms

SELECTED REFERENCES

1. Mahan MA et al: Occult radiological effects of lipomatosis of the lumbosacral plexus. Skeletal Radiol. 43(7):963-8, 2014
2. Weiss SW et al: Benign lipomatous tumors. In Weiss SW et al: Enzinger and Weiss' Soft Tissue Tumors. 5th ed. Philadelphia: Elsevier. 460-1, 2008
3. Wong BZ et al: Lipomatosis of the sciatic nerve: typical and atypical MRI features. Skeletal Radiol. 35(3):180-4, 2006
4. Kransdorf MJ et al: Lipomatous tumors. In Kransdorf MJ et al: Imaging of Soft Tissue Tumors. 2nd ed. Philadelphia: Lippincott Williams & Wilkins. 103-5, 2006

(Left) *Axial T1WI MR shows a fibrofatty mass ➡ involving the median nerve, which extended from the level of the wrist into the palm of the hand. The flexor tendons ⇨ are flattened dorsally. High signal fat ➡ surrounds the thickened nerve fascicles.* **(Right)** *Axial T1WI C+ FS MR in the same patient shows mild increased signal in the nerve bundles ↪ of the volar wrist mass ➡ with surrounding areas of low signal fat. Mass effect at the level of the wrist produced carpal tunnel syndrome.*

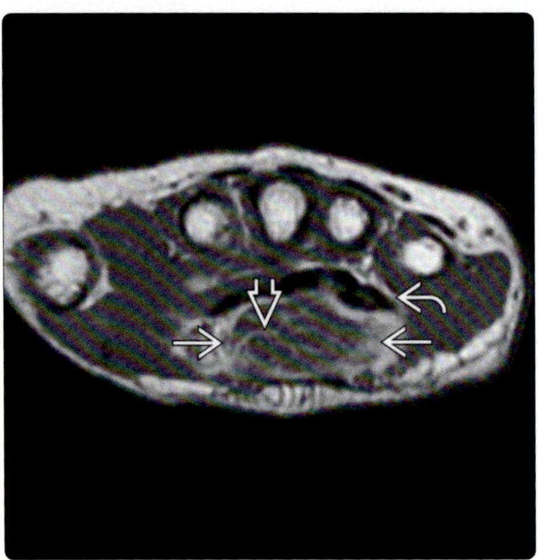

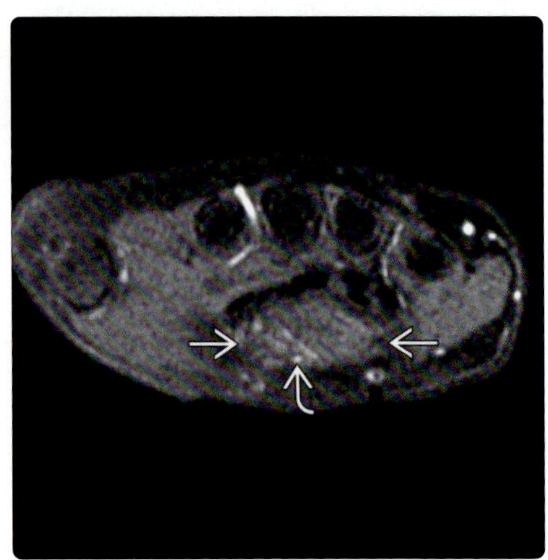

(Left) *Axial T1 MR shows lipomatosis of the median nerve in the midforearm. The fascicles of the nerve ➡ are markedly enlarged with surrounding fat signal ↪. Note that the intermediate signal of the nerve fascicles is inhomogeneous, indicating the combined nerve and fibrous tissue.* **(Right)** *Coronal T1 MR in the same patient shows the longitudinal extent of the thickened nerve fascicles ➡ with their fibrous content.*

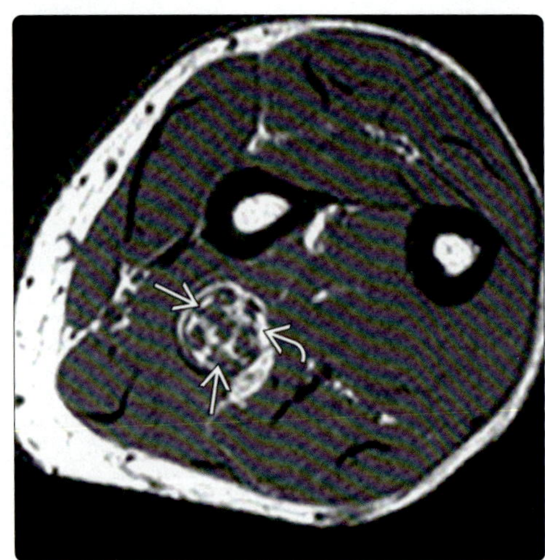

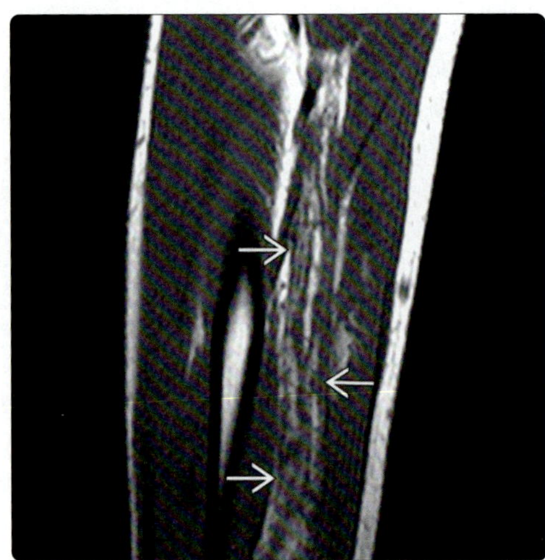

(Left) *Axial T1WI MR through the level of the wrist shows a markedly enlarged median nerve ➡. The nerve fascicles ↪ are disproportionately enlarged with a relative paucity of surrounding fat.* **(Right)** *Axial T2WI FS MR in the same patient shows the enlarged nerve ➡ with a relatively small amount of fat surrounding the nerve fascicles ↪. Compare this to the prior case. Variability in nerve fascicle size and fat content is normal and should not dissuade one from this diagnosis.*

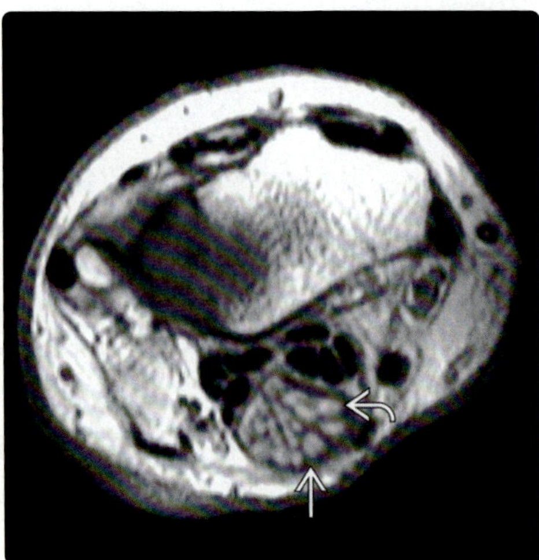

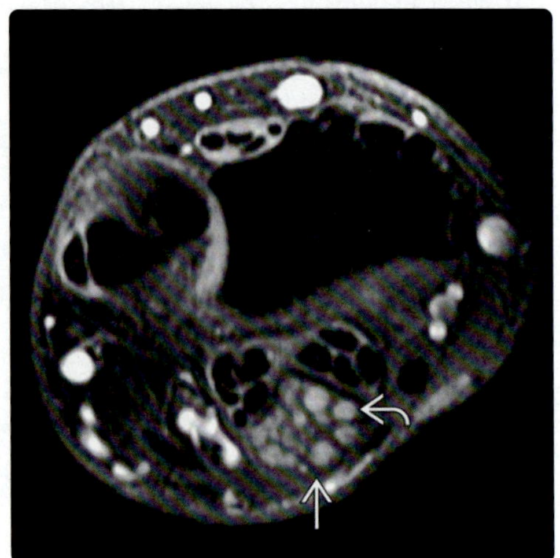

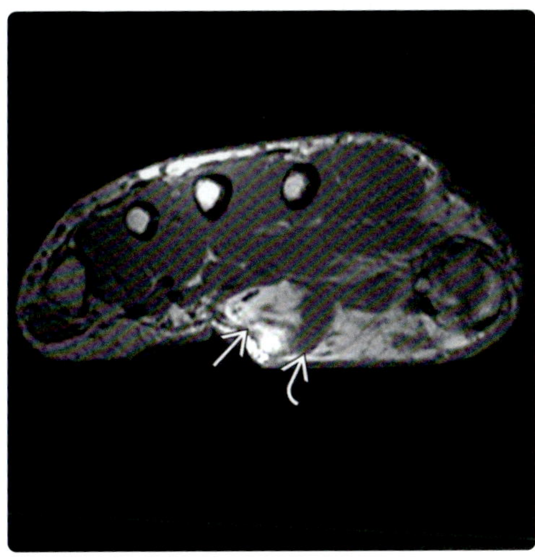

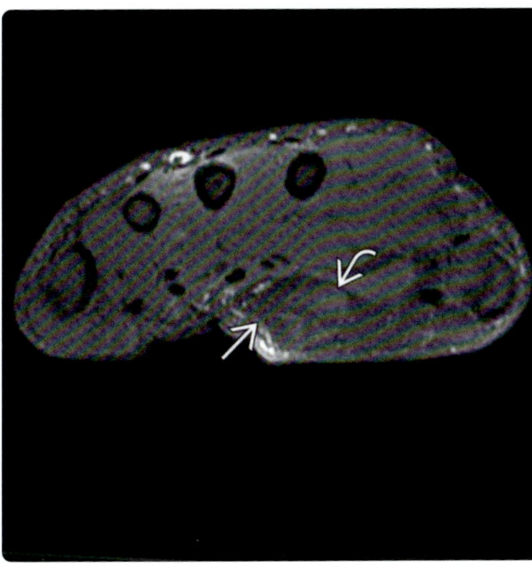

(Left) *Axial T1WI MR shows a median nerve digital branch mass ➡ due to fatty overgrowth and mild nerve fascicle enlargement. An unusual, but normal finding is an adjacent fibrofatty mass ➦. Additional areas of fibrofatty proliferation can sometimes raise concern for a liposarcoma, although this location is classic for lipomatosis.* **(Right)** *Axial T1WI C+ FS MR shows mild enhancement of the fibrofatty mass ➦ adjacent to the median nerve branch lipomatosis ➡.*

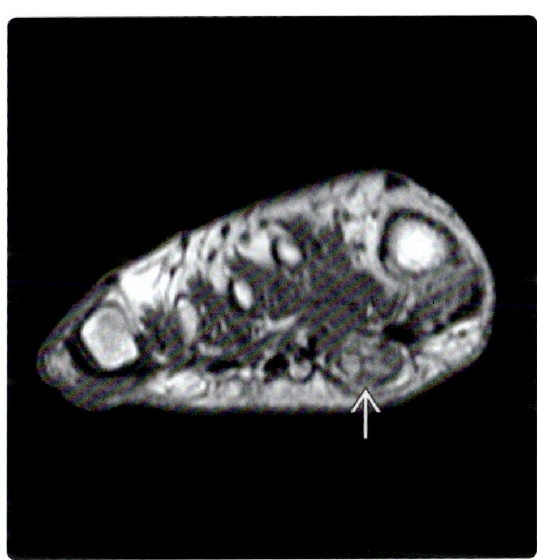

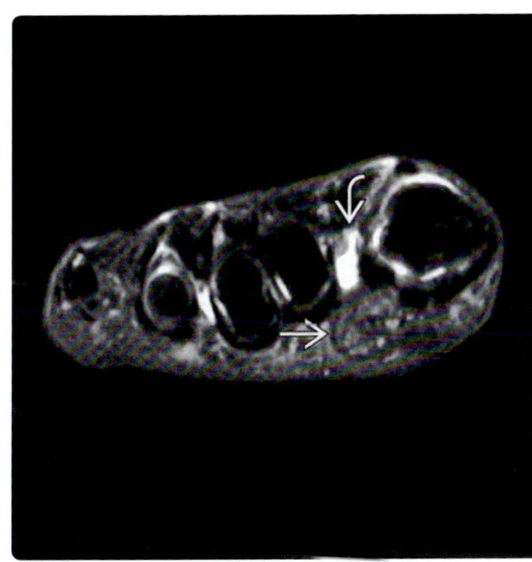

(Left) *Axial T1WI MR through the forefoot demonstrates markedly enlarged plantar digital nerve fascicles ➡ with mild interspersed fat. Involvement of the foot is rare with up to 96% of cases involving the upper extremity.* **(Right)** *Axial T2WI FS MR in the same patient shows nerve enlargement ➡ and adjacent intermetatarsal bursitis ➦. The differential diagnosis of a plantar foot mass could include a Morton neuroma, but the 1st intermetatarsal space would be a rare location for that entity.*

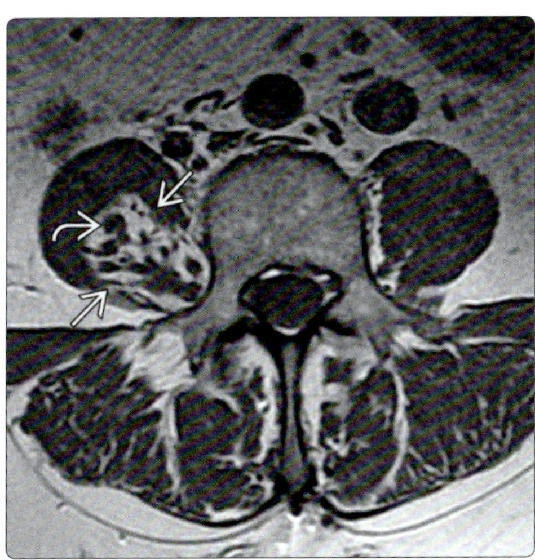

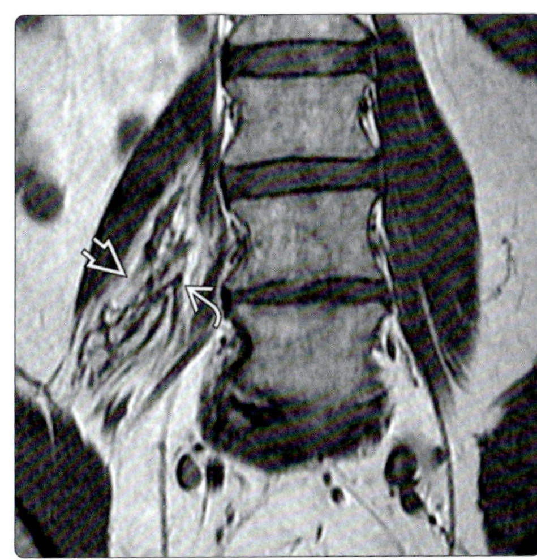

(Left) *Axial T1WI MR shows a fat-containing mass in the right psoas muscle ➡. Central areas of nodularity ➦ and retroperitoneal location would typically raise suspicion for a liposarcoma.* **(Right)** *Coronal T1WI MR in the same patient best illustrates the wavy branching appearance of the lumbar plexus nerve fascicles ➦ that produced the appearance of nodularity on axial images. High signal fat ➡ surrounding the nerve fascicles is a classic appearance for nerve lipomatosis.*

Macrodystrophia Lipomatosa

KEY FACTS

TERMINOLOGY

- Progressive overgrowth of bone and adipose tissue (local gigantism) of single or multiple digits

IMAGING

- 2nd and 3rd digits of hand or foot most commonly involved
  - Median nerve distribution in hand
  - Plantar nerve distribution in foot
- Overgrowth of bone and fatty soft tissue
  - Preferentially distal and either volar or plantar
  - Bone overgrowth can produce bowing
- Long, broad phalanges with splayed distal tufts
- Early osteoarthritis
- High signal fat overgrowth on T1WI becomes low signal on T2WI FS and STIR
- Lipomatosis of nerve may be associated
  - Coaxial cable appearance in cross section, wavy linear nerve fascicles in longitudinal plane

PATHOLOGY

- Upper extremity macrodactyly most commonly associated with lipomatosis of nerve
  - Less commonly idiopathic or associated with vascular malformation or neurofibromatosis
- Lower extremity macrodactyly is most commonly idiopathic or vascular
  - Nerve lipomatosis is least common cause of lower extremity macrodactyly

CLINICAL ISSUES

- Present at birth or infancy
- Female > male
- 27-67% of patients with lipomatosis of nerve
- Bony overgrowth ceases after puberty in majority
  - Rare reported cases of bone growth in adulthood
- Soft tissue proliferation continues into adulthood

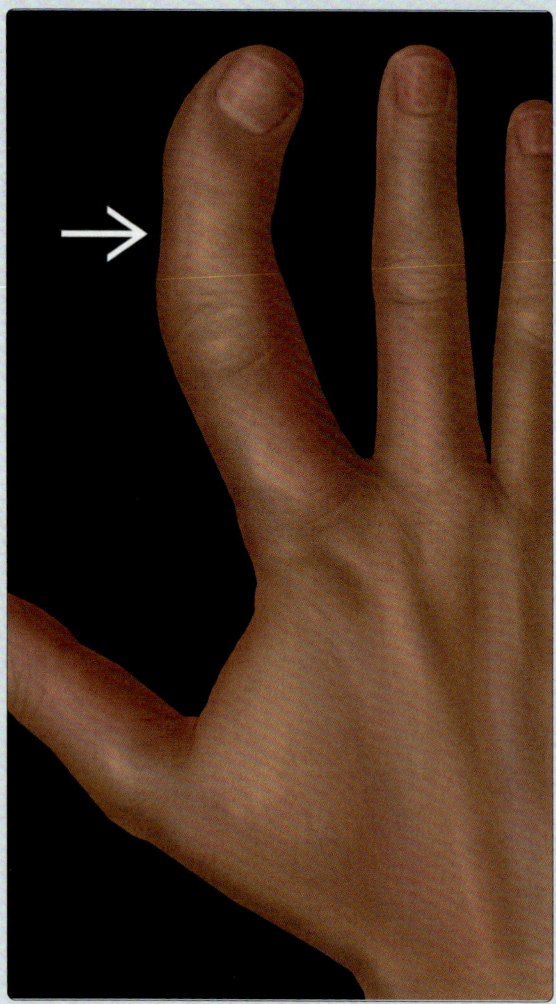

Graphic drawing of the dorsum of the hand shows that the index finger ➡ is overgrown and bowed, typical for macrodystrophia lipomatosa. This entity causes enlargement of both the bones and soft tissues.

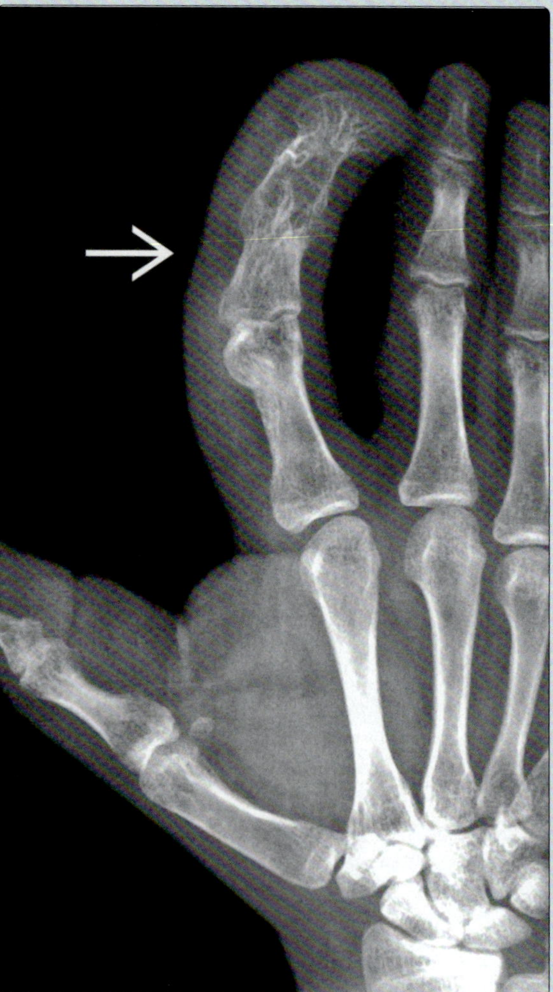

Posteroanterior radiograph shows focal giantism, involving a single ray of the hand ➡. The remainder of the hand is normal. Focal overgrowth, such as this, may result from a variety of entities, including macrodystrophia lipomatosa.

TERMINOLOGY

Synonyms

- Nerve territory-oriented macrodactyly, neural fibrolipoma with macrodactyly

Definitions

- Progressive overgrowth of bone and adipose tissue (local gigantism) of single or multiple digits

IMAGING

General Features

- Best diagnostic clue
  - Enlargement of single or multiple digits
    - Localized overgrowth occurs in both axial and longitudinal planes
- Location
  - 2nd and 3rd digits of hand or foot usually involved
  - Distribution of median nerve in hand or plantar nerve in foot commonly involved
- Morphology
  - Overgrowth is preferentially distal and either volar or plantar

Radiographic Findings

- Osseous overgrowth of digits
  - Long, broad phalanges
  - Splayed distal tufts
  - Early osteoarthritis
  - Bowing often present
- Enlarged soft tissues
  - Density similar to subcutaneous fat

MR Findings

- Overgrown osseous structures
- Prominent high signal fat on T1WI MR
  - Fatty tissue has low signal on fat-suppressed and STIR
- Lipomatosis of nerve has coaxial cable appearance in axial plane, wavy enlarged nerve fascicles in longitudinal plane

DIFFERENTIAL DIAGNOSIS

Localized Gigantism

- Vascular malformation
- Maffucci syndrome
- Neurofibromatosis type 1
- Klippel-Trenaunay-Weber syndrome
- Proteus syndrome
- Osteoid osteoma
- Melorheostosis
- Amyloidosis

Triphalangeal Thumb

- Clinically appears as elongated thumb
- Diagnostic radiographic appearance showing 3 phalanges

Diffuse Lipomatosis With Overgrowth of Bone

- Can be difficult to differentiate from macrodystrophia
- Primarily affects subcutis and muscles
- Secondary nerve involvement

Hemiplegia From Cerebral Palsy

- Can cause localized tissue overgrowth
- Correlate with clinical history

PATHOLOGY

General Features

- Etiology
  - Unknown
- Genetics
  - No hereditary cause
- Associated abnormalities
  - Upper extremity macrodactyly most commonly associated with lipomatosis of nerve
    - Less commonly idiopathic or associated with vascular malformation or neurofibromatosis
  - Lower extremity macrodactyly is most commonly idiopathic or vascular
    - Nerve lipomatosis is least common cause of lower extremity macrodactyly

CLINICAL ISSUES

Presentation

- Most common signs/symptoms
  - Progressively enlarging digits
- Other signs/symptoms
  - Limited range of motion
  - Osteoarthritis disproportionately severe for age

Demographics

- Age
  - Present at birth or infancy
- Gender
  - Female > male
- Epidemiology
  - Occurs in 27-67% of patients with lipomatosis of nerve

Natural History & Prognosis

- Bone overgrowth ceases after puberty
  - Rare reported cases of bone growth in adulthood
- Predisposes to premature osteoarthritis

Treatment

- Redundant, hypertrophied fatty tissue can be surgically debulked
- Enlarged digits may be completely or partially amputated

SELECTED REFERENCES

1. Prasetyono TO et al: A Review of Macrodystrophia Lipomatosa: Revisitation. Arch Plast Surg. 42(4):391-406, 2015
2. Siddiqui MA et al: Macrodystrophia lipomatosa with ulnar distribution in hand: MR evaluation of a rare disorder. JBR-BTR. 98(1):43-4, 2015
3. Weiss SW et al: Benign lipomatous tumors. In Weiss SW et al: Enzinger and Weiss' Soft Tissue Tumors. 5th ed. Philadelphia: Elsevier. 460-1, 2008
4. Fritz TR et al: Macrodystrophia lipomatosa extending into the upper abdomen. Pediatr Radiol. 37(12):1275-7, 2007
5. Ho CA et al: Long-term follow-up of progressive macrodystrophia lipomatosa. A report of two cases. J Bone Joint Surg Am. 89(5):1097-102, 2007
6. Turkington JR et al: MR imaging of macrodystrophia lipomatosa. Ulster Med J. 74(1):47-50, 2005
7. Murphey MD et al: From the archives of the AFIP: benign musculoskeletal lipomatous lesions. Radiographics. 24(5):1433-66, 2004

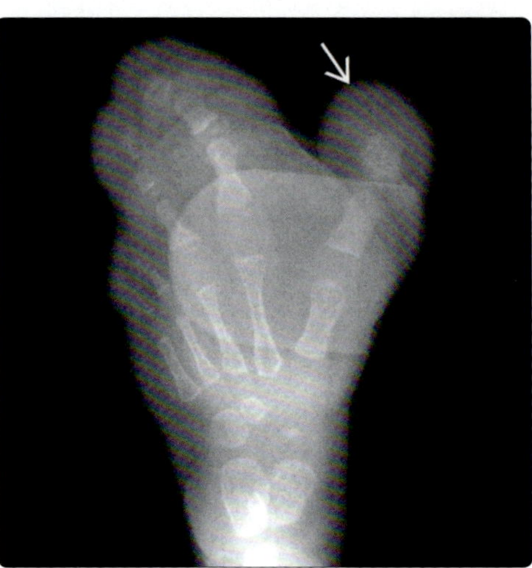

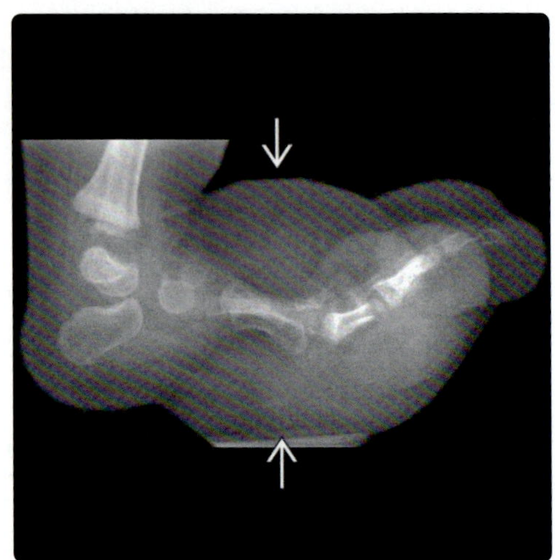

(Left) *Anteroposterior radiograph of the foot shows a normal hindfoot, midfoot, and lateral 2 toes. However, the 1st, 2nd, and 3rd toes ➡ show giantism of both the soft tissues and osseous structures. Involvement of the medial rays is typical.* **(Right)** *Lateral radiograph in the same patient shows massive soft tissue overgrowth ➡. This overgrowth can be seen in multiple disorders, including vascular malformations, neurofibromatosis, and macrodystrophia lipomatosa.*

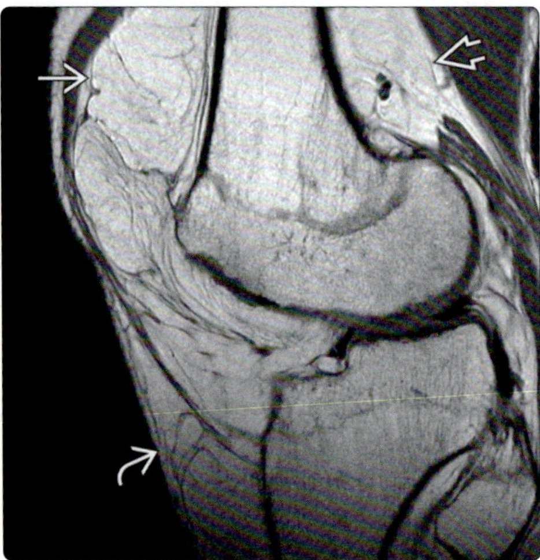

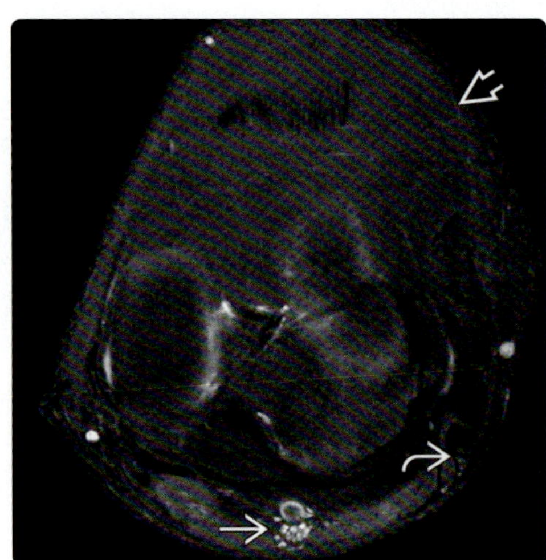

(Left) *Sagittal PD MR of the knee in the same patient with below-knee amputation several years earlier is shown. MR shows ongoing process, with large regions of fat in the subcutaneous ➡, intraarticular ➡, and extraarticular ➡ sites.* **(Right)** *Axial T2FS MR in the same patient shows the large regions of fat ➡ to have diffusely low signal. Note the hyperintensity and enlargement of multiple nerve fascicles in both the tibial nerve ➡ and peroneal nerve ➡. Nerves may become enlarged in this disease.*

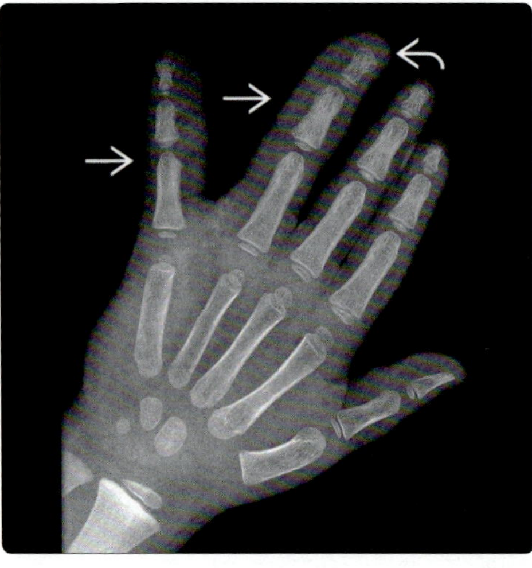

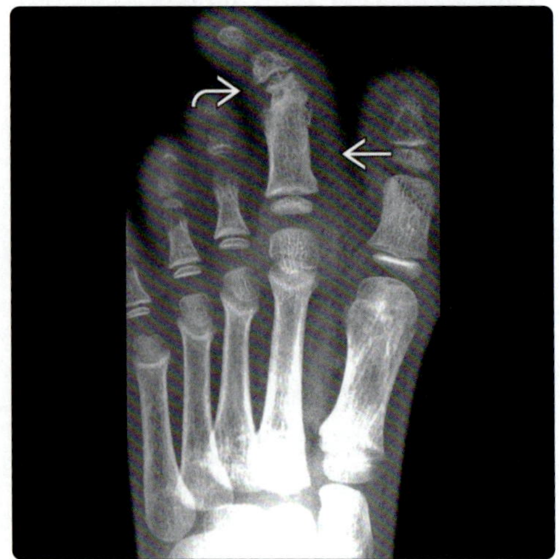

(Left) *Posteroanterior radiograph shows diffuse enlargement ➡ of the 4th and 5th fingers. The bones and soft tissues are enlarged. The 4th digit has a mild curvature ➡. Involvement of the ulnar digits is relatively uncommon.* **(Right)** *AP radiograph shows a single enlarged toe ➡. Overgrowth of bone and lipomatous soft tissue has resulted in a bowing deformity. The proximal interphalangeal joint ➡ is severely narrowed. Involvement of the 2nd digit is typical.*

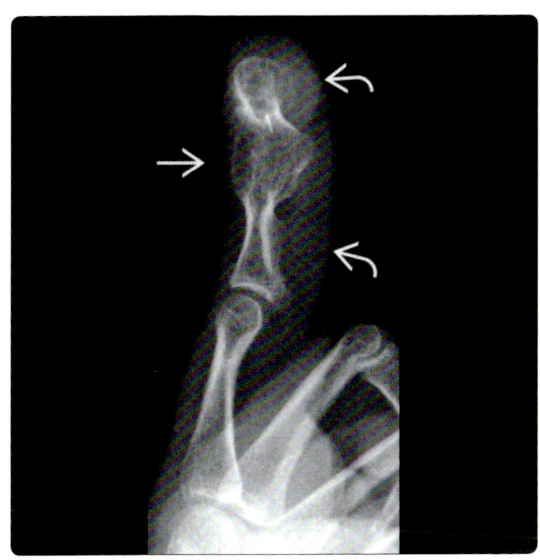

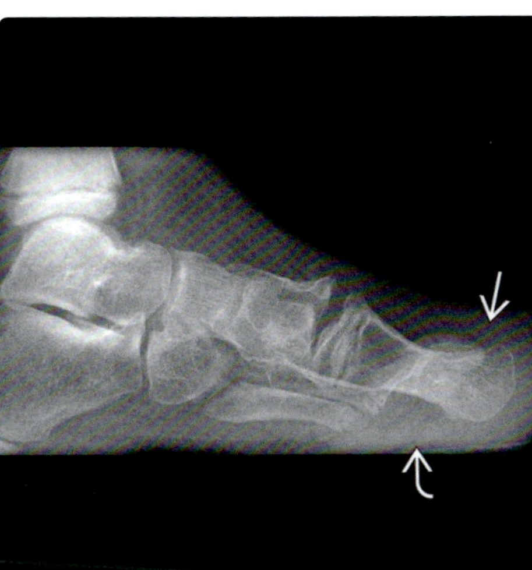

(Left) *Lateral radiograph of the hand shows an enlarged index finger. The distal interphalangeal joint* ➔ *is fused. Note that the soft tissue prominence* ➔ *preferentially involves the volar soft tissues in the hand.* **(Right)** *Lateral radiograph shows gigantism of the 1st ray* ➔*. The great toe has been resected, as have the 2nd and 3rd rays, to allow the foot to approach normal size. Soft tissue proliferation* ➔ *is predominantly along the plantar aspect of the foot.*

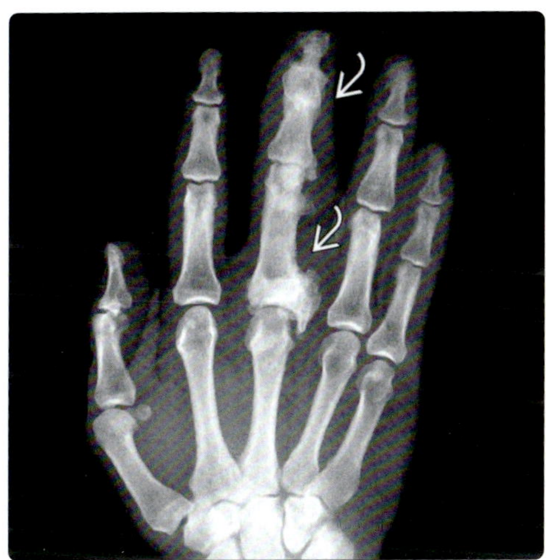

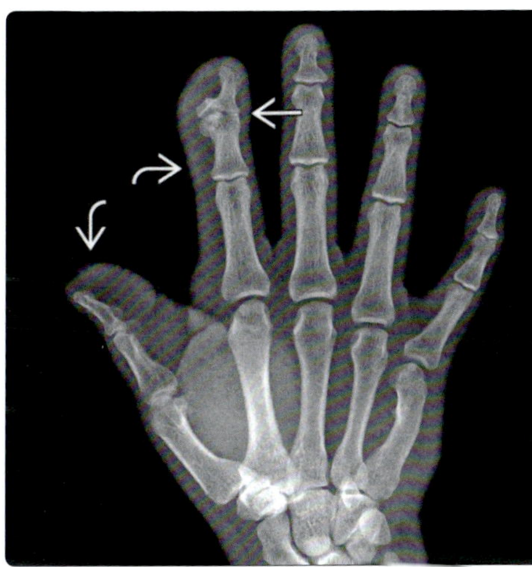

(Left) *Posteroanterior radiograph shows soft tissue prominence and associated bone overgrowth* ➔ *involving the right long finger. Dystrophic bone formation in macrodystrophia lipomatosa as seen in this case is an uncommon finding.* **(Right)** *Posteroanterior radiograph shows soft tissue and bone enlargement* ➔ *involving the right thumb and index finger. Advanced osteoarthritis* ➔ *of the distal interphalangeal joint is a commonly associated complication. Deformity of the right 5th metacarpal may be due to old trauma.*

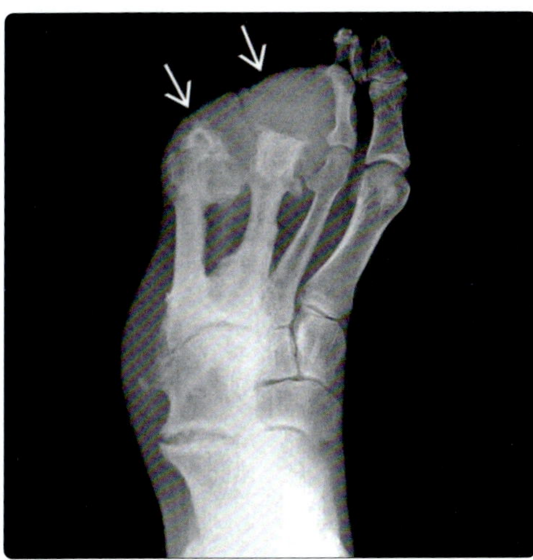

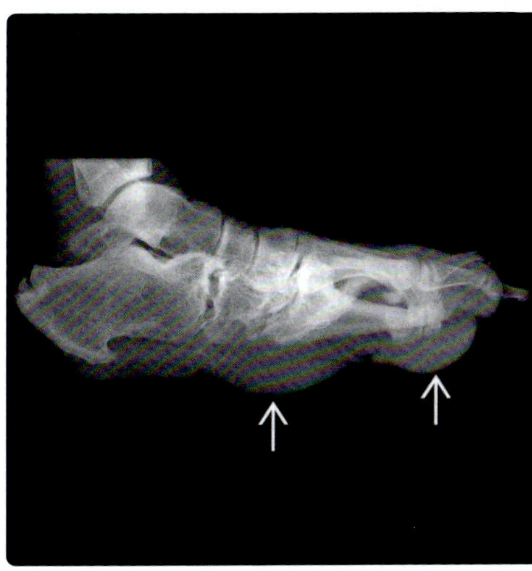

(Left) *Anteroposterior radiograph of the foot shows overgrowth of the lateral 2 digits* ➔*. The toes and 1 ray have been previously amputated. Involvement of the lateral rays is unusual.* **(Right)** *Lateral radiograph of the foot in the same patient again shows the focal gigantism. Note that the soft tissue overgrowth* ➔ *more prominently involves the plantar aspect of the foot. These patients require custom shoes to accommodate the significant deformities associated with this entity.*

Lipoma Arborescens: Knee

KEY FACTS

TERMINOLOGY

- Infiltration of fat tissue in synovium and subsynovial tissue forming frond-like masses
- a.k.a. diffuse synovial lipoma or villous lipomatous proliferation of synovial membrane

IMAGING

- Frond-like intraarticular (rarely bursal or within tendon sheath) masses that follow fat signal intensity on all MR sequences
  - High T1WI signal intensity
  - Low signal on any fat-suppressed sequence
  - Compare to subcutaneous fat
- Inflamed overlying synovium may enhance
- Most common in suprapatellar recess of knee joint
- Can be multifocal and bilateral
- Fronds progressively enlarge to form globular, rounded masses

PATHOLOGY

- Probably reactive process secondary to chronic synovial irritation
  - Chronic joint pathology: Osteoarthritis, rheumatoid arthritis, or prior trauma
- Mature adipocytes within subsynovium and enlarged synovial fronds
- Osseous or chondroid metaplasia in some cases
- Chronic inflammatory reaction

CLINICAL ISSUES

- Seen in children to adults
  - Male predilection
- Intermittent clinical exacerbations
- Painless synovial thickening/swelling
  - Joint effusion
- Treated with synovectomy, but may recur

(Left) *Sagittal graphic shows diffuse villous fatty infiltration of the synovium throughout the joint. This results in distention of the joint capsule both anteriorly ➡ and posteriorly ➘.* **(Right)** *Sagittal T1WI MR shows a grossly distended knee joint. This distension is due to high signal fatty proliferation of the synovium ➡ and a low signal joint effusion ➘. Note the frond-like, multilobulated, papillary appearance of the intraarticular fatty masses.*

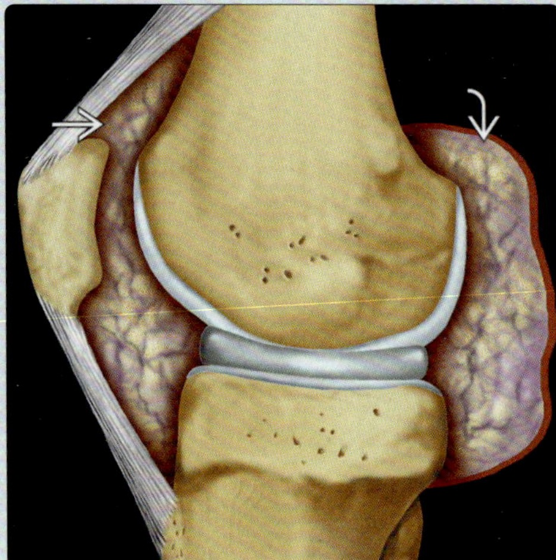

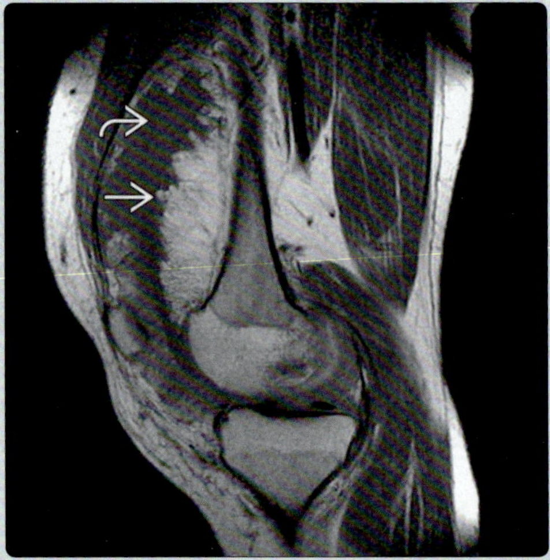

(Left) *Sagittal PDWI FS MR in the same patient shows the frond-like fatty masses ➡ to have suppressed signal similar to the subcutaneous fat. The large joint effusion ➘ has high signal on this fluid-sensitive sequence.* **(Right)** *Sagittal T1WI C+ FS MR shows peripheral enhancement of the fatty masses ➡. This represents the superficial synovium, which normally enhances, but is likely inflamed. The deeper, subsynovial fatty infiltration maintains a similar intensity to subcutaneous fat.*

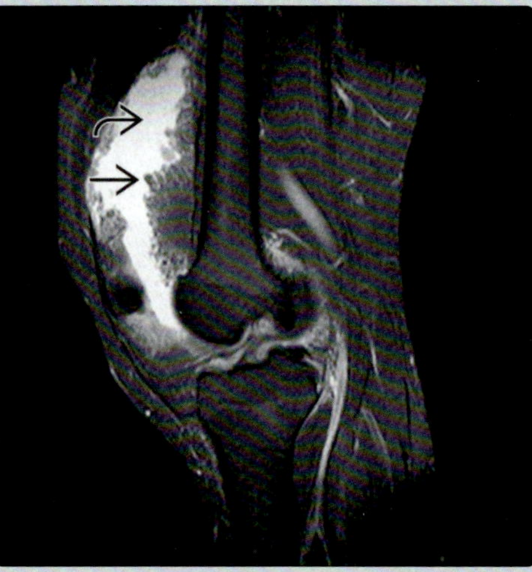

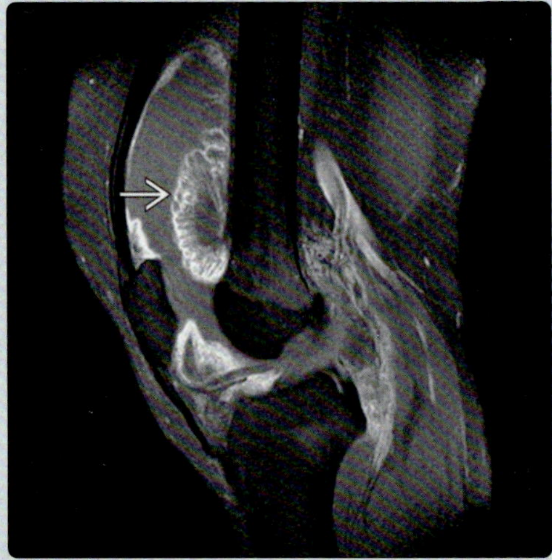

TERMINOLOGY

Synonyms

- Diffuse synovial lipoma
- Villous lipomatous proliferation of synovial membrane

Definitions

- Infiltration of fat tissue in synovium and subsynovial tissue forming frond-like masses

IMAGING

General Features

- Best diagnostic clue
  - Frond-like intraarticular masses that follow fat signal intensity on all MR sequences
- Location
  - Intraarticular
    - Rarely bursal or within tendon sheath
  - Usually knee joint, most common in suprapatellar recess
  - May be bilateral (unilateral in 94%)
- Size
  - Variable: Small to large fronds
- Morphology
  - Progressive enlargement of delicate fronds to form globular, rounded masses

Radiographic Findings

- Joint distension ± visible fat density

CT Findings

- Fat density synovial masses
- Frond-like morphology more difficult to appreciate

MR Findings

- T1WI
  - High signal intensity synovial masses that match intensity of subcutaneous fat
- T2WI FS
  - Low signal intensity on any fat-suppressed sequence
  - Signal intensity decreases as with subcutaneous fat
- STIR
  - Low signal synovial masses
- T1WI C+ FS
  - Overlying synovium enhances; mass SI hypointense

DIFFERENTIAL DIAGNOSIS

Synovial Lipoma

- Single fatty mass, usually in suprapatellar bursa

Synovial Chondromatosis

- Intraarticular cartilaginous masses
- May calcify or ossify

Synovitis

- Visualized as thickened synovium but without saturation on fat-saturation techniques
- ± synovial fronds

Loose Bodies

- Low MR signal structures, most often calcified
- ± cortical rim
- ± marrow fat vs. sclerotic hypointense signal

Normal Fat Around Joint

- Volume averaging of normal prefemoral or suprapatellar fat

PATHOLOGY

General Features

- Etiology
  - Probably reactive process secondary to chronic synovial irritation
- Associated abnormalities
  - Joint effusion
  - Chronic joint pathology: Osteoarthritis, rheumatoid arthritis, or prior trauma
  - Some cases do not have associated chronic joint disease

Gross Pathologic & Surgical Features

- Frond-like fibrofatty synovial enlargement

Microscopic Features

- Mature adipocytes within subsynovium and enlarged synovial fronds
- Chronic inflammatory reaction
- Osseous or chondroid metaplasia in some cases

CLINICAL ISSUES

Presentation

- Most common signs/symptoms
  - Painless synovial thickening
  - Intermittent effusion

Demographics

- Age
  - Children to adults
- Gender
  - Male predilection
- Epidemiology
  - Rare

Natural History & Prognosis

- Painless swelling with intermittent exacerbations

Treatment

- Synovectomy, but may recur

DIAGNOSTIC CHECKLIST

Consider

- Other causes of synovial proliferation when intraarticular masses are nonfatty

Image Interpretation Pearls

- Saturation of synovial masses (especially frond-like) on fat-suppressed images is diagnostic

SELECTED REFERENCES

1. White EA et al: Lipoma arborescens of the biceps tendon sheath. Skeletal Radiol. 42(10):1461-4, 2013
2. Coll JP et al: Best cases from the AFIP: lipoma arborescens of the knees in a patient with rheumatoid arthritis. Radiographics. 31(2):333-7, 2011

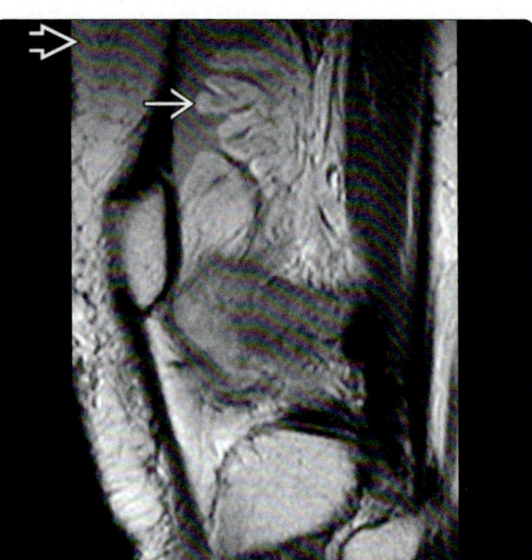

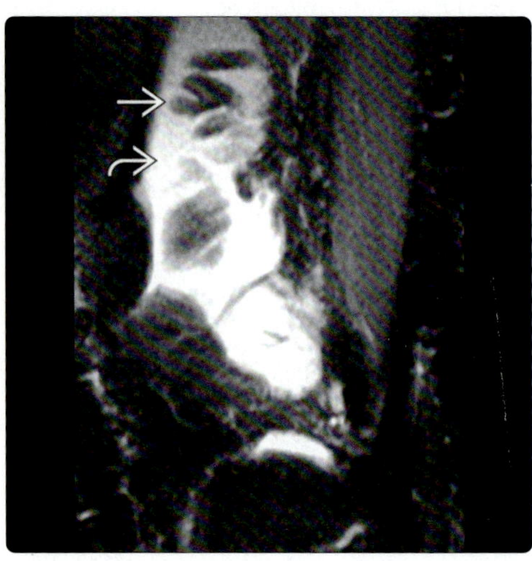

(Left) *Sagittal PD FSE MR shows large, frond-like excrescences ➡ arising from the prefemoral fat pad. These excrescences extend into the suprapatellar bursa and follow the signal intensity of subcutaneous fat ➡.* **(Right)** *Sagittal T2WI FS MR in the same patient shows the frond-like excrescences ➡ to have low signal intensity due to fat suppression. The fatty fronds are highlighted by the high signal large joint effusion ➡.*

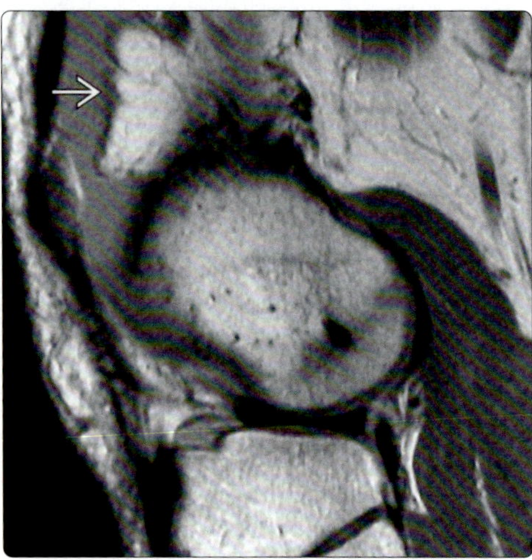

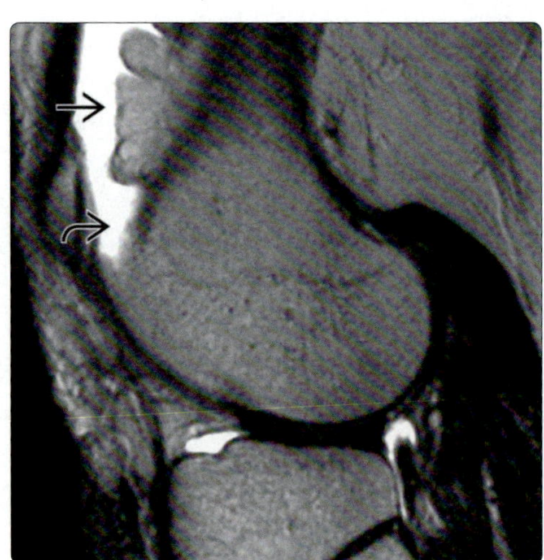

(Left) *Sagittal T1WI MR shows lipoma arborescens localized in the suprapatellar bursa. A lobulated fatty mass ➡ within the suprapatellar bursa is outlined by low signal effusion.* **(Right)** *Sagittal T2WI FS MR in the same patient shows the mass ➡ in the suprapatellar bursa to have signal intensity that saturates out. The effusion ➡ has typical high signal intensity. Note that the lobulations can be rounded, as opposed to being exclusively frond-like.*

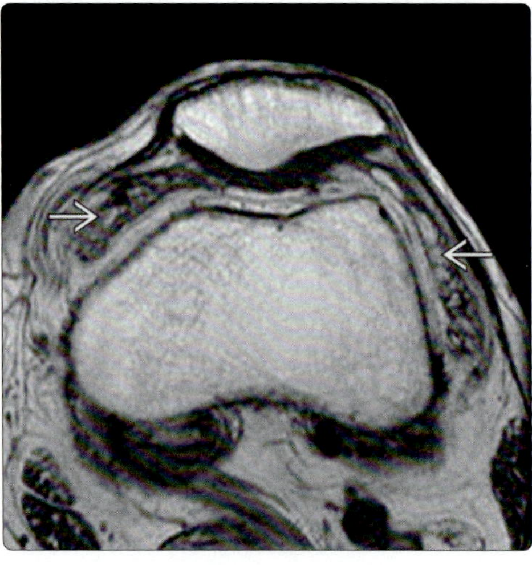

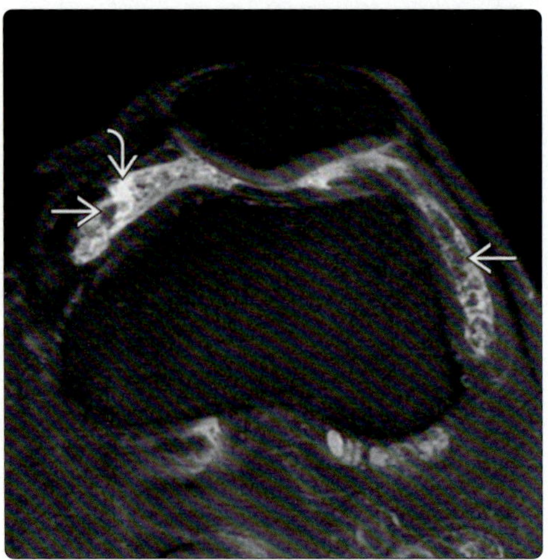

(Left) *Axial T1WI MR shows the typical appearance of lipoma arborescens. Numerous high signal intensity fatty fronds ➡ are present in the knee joint. There is no distention of the joint and the underlying bony structures are normal.* **(Right)** *Axial T2WI FS MR in the same patient shows that the fatty fronds of synovium ➡ become low signal intensity on fat-suppressed sequences. There is a normal amount of high signal joint fluid ➡. Note the tiny size of the fronds.*

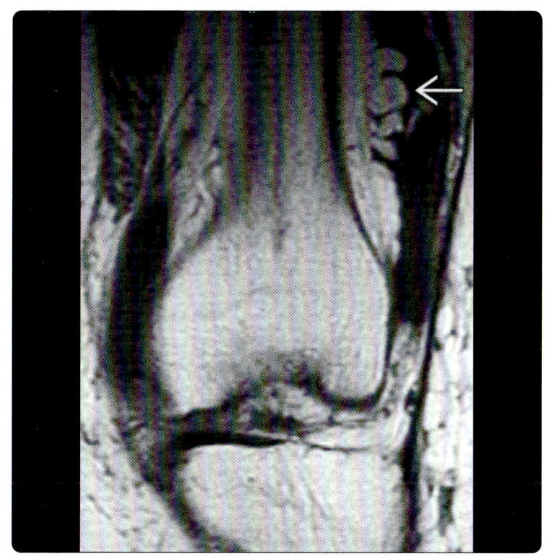

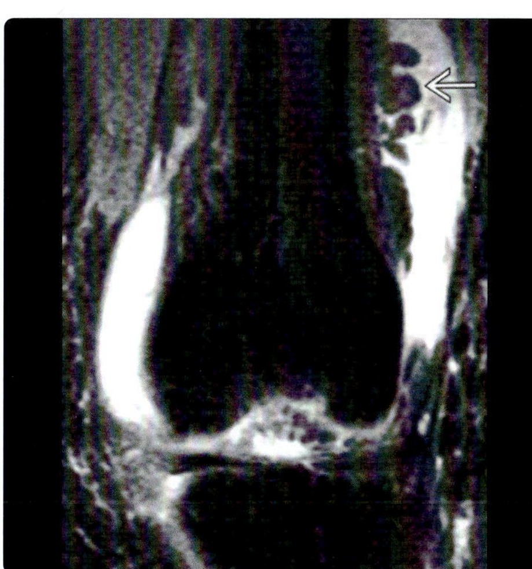

(Left) *Coronal T1WI MR shows papillary masses ➔ in the knee joint. Although marked synovial proliferation can produce intraarticular masses, the fat signal intensity is typical for lipoma arborescens.* **(Right)** *Coronal T2WI FS MR in the same patient confirms that the previously high signal T1WI intraarticular masses ➔ saturate to low signal, confirming fat composition. The large surrounding joint effusion is typical, as many of these cases are a response to chronic joint inflammation.*

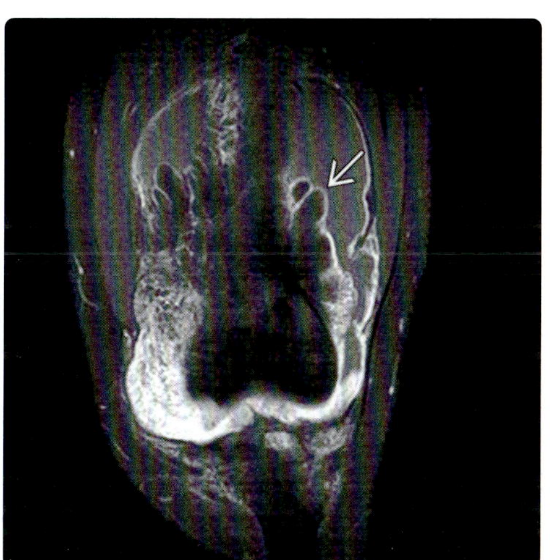

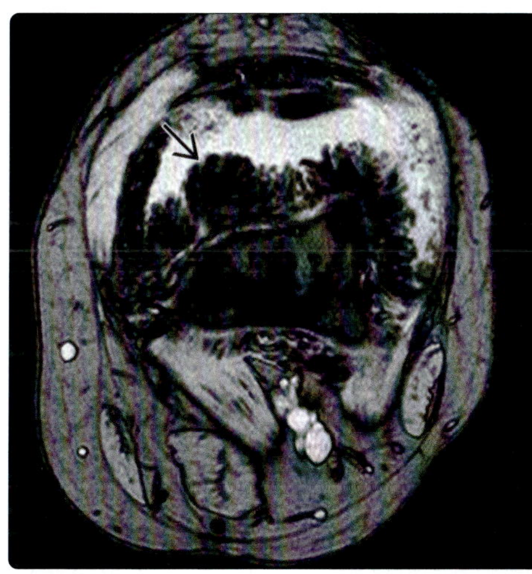

(Left) *Coronal T1WI C+ FS MR shows lobulated fronds of fatty tissue ➔ extending into the suprapatellar bursa. The fronds and joint have peripheral synovial enhancement. Note the large surrounding joint effusion.* **(Right)** *Axial gradient-echo MR in the same patient shows low signal villous masses ➔ in the prefemoral region. These masses had the same intensity as subcutaneous fat on other sequences, but have a similar intensity to marrow fat on gradient-echo.*

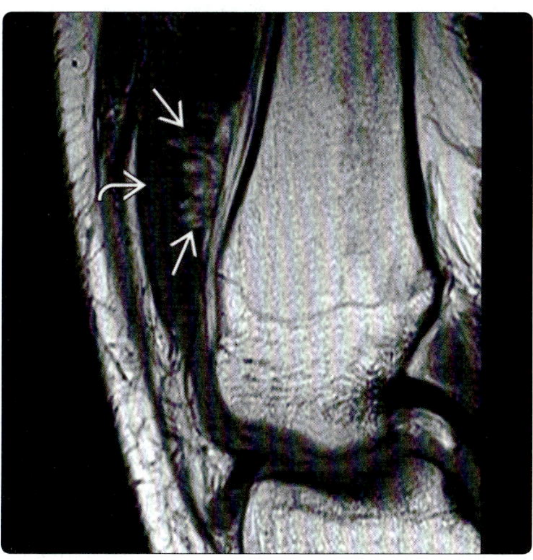

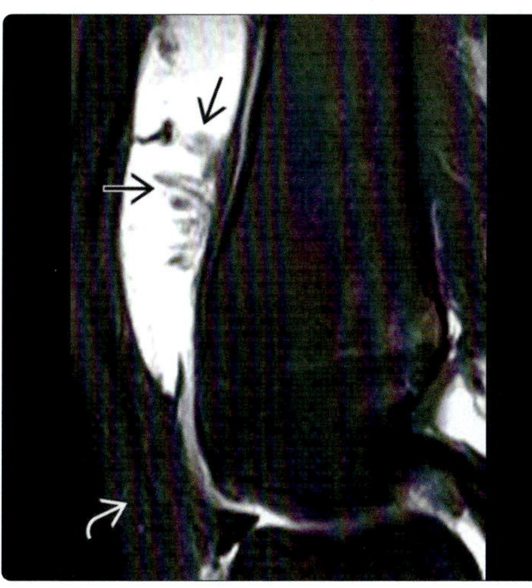

(Left) *Sagittal T1 MR in a 20-year-old woman with recurrent effusions shows small, frond-like fatty excrescences ➔ extending from the synovium. There is a low signal effusion ➔.* **(Right)** *Sagittal T2 FS MR in the same patient shows that the frond-like extensions ➔ follow the signal of the fat-suppressed subcutaneous fat ➔, while the effusion is hyperintense. This lesion is relatively small and easily overlooked. This patient had no other intraarticular abnormality to explain her symptoms.*

Lipoblastoma/Lipoblastomatosis

KEY FACTS

TERMINOLOGY

- Circumscribed (lipoblastoma) and diffuse (lipoblastomatosis) forms of benign pediatric tumor composed of immature fat cells

IMAGING

- Fatty mass with varying complexity in very young patient
  - Fat component follows subcutaneous fat signal intensity on all sequences
  - Septa and nodules isointense to muscle
- Masses in very young patients more likely to have predominantly myxoid composition with little fat
- ~ 2/3 in upper and lower extremities
  - Most are 2-5 cm in size

PATHOLOGY

- Resembles fetal adipose tissue
- Lipoblasts may have range of developmental stages
- Mucinous material inversely related to differentiation

CLINICAL ISSUES

- Painless slowly growing mass or nodule
  - Similar clinical presentation to lipoma, but more complex imaging features
  - Uncommonly, rapid growth
- May compress neurovascular or other structures
- Typically presents within first 3 years of age
  - May be present at birth
- Local recurrence in 9-25%
- No reported malignant transformation or metastasis
- Incomplete excision is more common in lipoblastomatosis

DIAGNOSTIC CHECKLIST

- Young age of patient should suggest this entity
- Imaging cannot definitively diagnose these lesions, necessitating histologic examination
- Report full extent of tumor to help avoid recurrence
- Be vigilant for invasion or potential invasion of critical structures, such as spinal canal or airway

(Left) *Lateral radiograph demonstrates a moderately large lucency ➔ within the mid calf. Minimal contour deformity of the proximal fibula is likely due to chronic changes from mass effect. No periosteal reaction or soft tissue calcification is present.* **(Right)** *Axial T1WI MR shows a large fatty mass ➔ in the proximal calf. The mass has predominantly fat signal intensity, which is high signal on T1WI and matches the subcutaneous fat. There are prominent septa ➔. Note the immature growth plates in this young child ➔.*

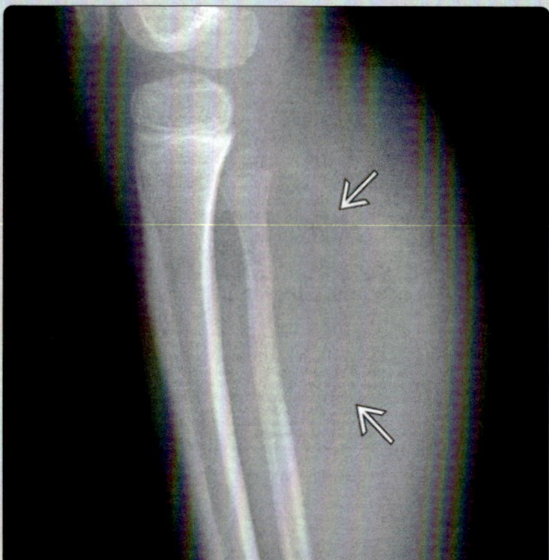

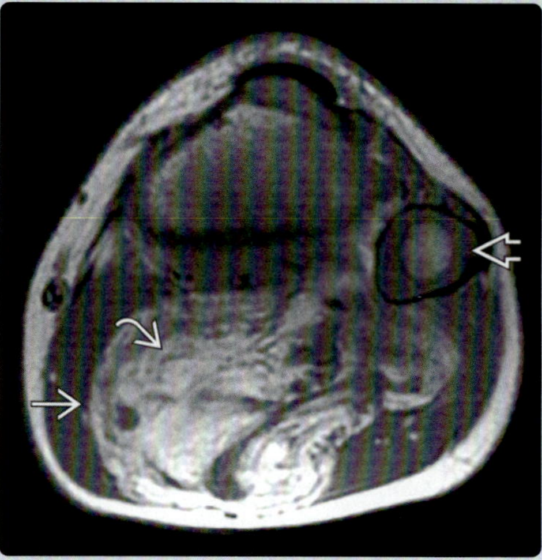

(Left) *Axial T2WI FS MR in the same patient shows the fatty components of the mass ➔ to partially suppress, as the subcutaneous fat does. The septa ➔ and nodularity remain isointense to muscle.* **(Right)** *Axial T1WI C+ FS MR shows the mass ➔ to have peripheral and hazy central regions of enhancement. The soft tissue nodularity and enhancement would suggest a malignant fatty tumor in an adult, but in a child raises the question of a lipoblastoma, which was confirmed histologically.*

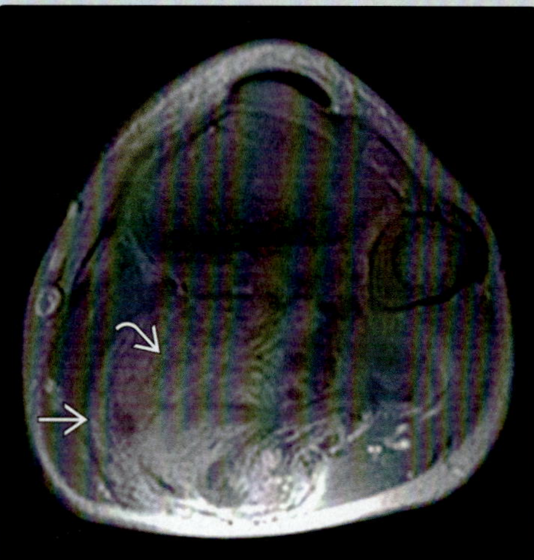

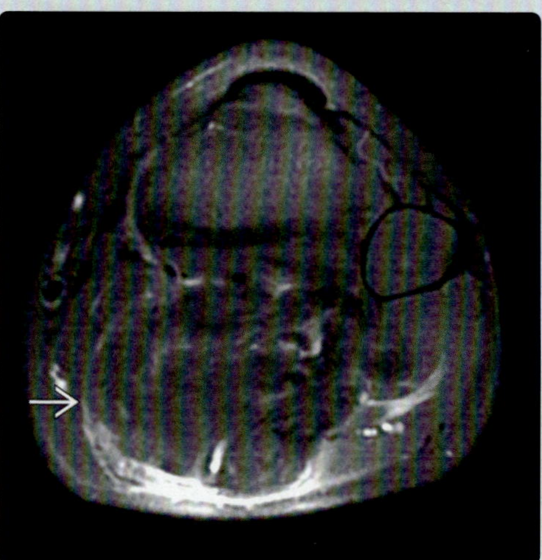

TERMINOLOGY

Synonyms

- Benign lipoblastoma, diffuse lipoblastomatosis, fetal lipoma, embryonic lipoma, infantile lipoma

Definitions

- Circumscribed (lipoblastoma) and diffuse (lipoblastomatosis) forms of benign pediatric tumor composed of immature fat cells

IMAGING

General Features

- Best diagnostic clue
  - Fatty mass with varying complexity, septa, and nodularity in very young patient
- Location
  - ~ 2/3 in extremities
    - Also reported in head/neck, axilla, supraclavicular region, trunk, mediastinum, mesentery, omentum, scrotum, spinal canal, and retroperitoneum
    - May involve organs: Lung, heart, parotid gland
  - Subcutaneous fat (lipoblastoma) or subcutaneous fat and muscle (lipoblastomatosis)

Radiographic Findings

- Focal soft tissue mass ± fat density

MR Findings

- Complex fatty mass
  - Fat component follows subcutaneous fat signal intensity
  - Septa and nodules isointense to muscle
- Masses in very young patients more likely to have predominantly myxoid composition with little fat

DIFFERENTIAL DIAGNOSIS

Lipoma

- Older patient population
- Lacks complex imaging appearance
- Histologically more mature than lipoblastoma

Hibernoma

- Histologically composed of brown fat cells

Atypical Lipomatous Tumor

- Older patient population
- Can have similar imaging appearance

Liposarcoma

- Would be extremely rare in childhood
- Myxoid liposarcoma can have almost identical histologic appearance to lipoblastoma

PATHOLOGY

General Features

- Etiology
  - Variant of lipoma and lipomatosis
    - Almost all found during infancy and early childhood
  - Resembles fetal adipose tissue

Gross Pathologic & Surgical Features

- Pale color compared with lipoma
- Myxoid or gelatinous cut surface

Microscopic Features

- Irregular lobules of immature fat cells
  - Lipoblasts may have range of developmental stages
    - Each tumor may have single or multiple degrees of differentiation
  - Differs from mature fat of lipomas
- Connective tissue septa with variable thickness
- Myxoid mesenchymal areas
  - Mucinous material amount inversely related to differentiation
- Plexiform vascularity in some may mimic myxoid liposarcoma

CLINICAL ISSUES

Presentation

- Most common signs/symptoms
  - Painless mass or nodule
  - Slow growing
    - Uncommonly, period of rapid growth
  - Similar clinical presentation to lipoma
- Other signs/symptoms
  - May compress neurovascular or other structures
    - Spinal cord compression when in spinal canal
    - Respiratory distress when in neck

Demographics

- Age
  - Infancy and early childhood
    - Typically presents within first 3 years of life
- Epidemiology
  - 2% of pediatric soft tissue tumors

Natural History & Prognosis

- Excellent overall prognosis
  - Local recurrence in 9-25%
    - Incomplete excision is more common in lipoblastomatosis

DIAGNOSTIC CHECKLIST

Consider

- Painless fatty mass in pediatric patient

Image Interpretation Pearls

- Young age of patient should suggest this entity
- Imaging cannot definitively diagnose these lesions, necessitating histologic examination

Reporting Tips

- Report full extent of tumor
- Be vigilant for invasion or potential invasion of critical structures, such as spinal canal or airway

SELECTED REFERENCES

1. Dadone B et al: Molecular cytogenetics of pediatric adipocytic tumors. Cancer Genet. ePub, 2015
2. Salem R et al: Lipoblastoma: a rare lesion in the differential diagnosis of childhood mediastinal tumors. J Pediatr Surg. 46(5):e21-3, 2011

Hibernoma

KEY FACTS

TERMINOLOGY

- Rare, benign tumor of brown adipose tissue

IMAGING

- Most common in thigh (30%)
- On CT, mass has density between fat and muscle
- Range of MR signal intensity depending on subtype
  - T1WI intensity ranges from fat to fluid
  - Hyperintense on fluid-sensitive sequences
  - Internal low signal septa
  - Enhancement due to prominent vascularity

PATHOLOGY

- 4 variants of hibernoma
  - Typical > myxoid > lipoma-like > spindle cell

CLINICAL ISSUES

- Slow-growing, mobile, painless subcutaneous mass
  - 10% are intramuscular
- Peak incidence in 3rd decade of life
- Benign tumor without potential for malignant transformation

DIAGNOSTIC CHECKLIST

- Well-defined mass in middle-aged patient
- Must exclude atypical lipomatous tumor/well-differentiated liposarcoma and liposarcoma when considering any complex fatty mass
  - Often not possible based on imaging alone
  - Needle biopsy usually sufficient to diagnose hibernoma preoperatively
- Increased vascularity produces characteristics that help differentiate from intermediate-grade or malignant lipomatous tumors
  - Increased signal on fluid-sensitive MR sequences
  - Variable diffuse enhancement
  - Vascular blush on angiography
  - Avid tracer uptake on PET/CT

(Left) *Axial T1WI MR shows a large, lobulated mass ➡ in the right retroperitoneum. This mass medially displaces the right psoas muscle ⇨. Note that the signal intensity of the mass is slightly lower than subcutaneous fat.* **(Right)** *Axial T2WI FS MR in the same patient again shows the large retroperitoneal mass ➡. The majority of the mass decreases in signal on this fat-suppressed sequence, although the signal intensity remains slightly higher than the subcutaneous fat.*

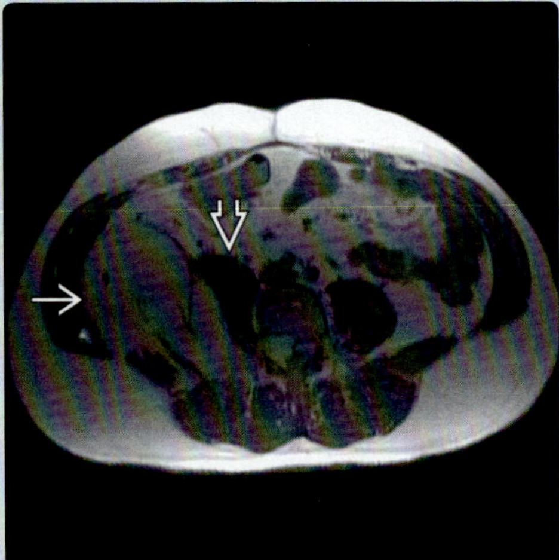

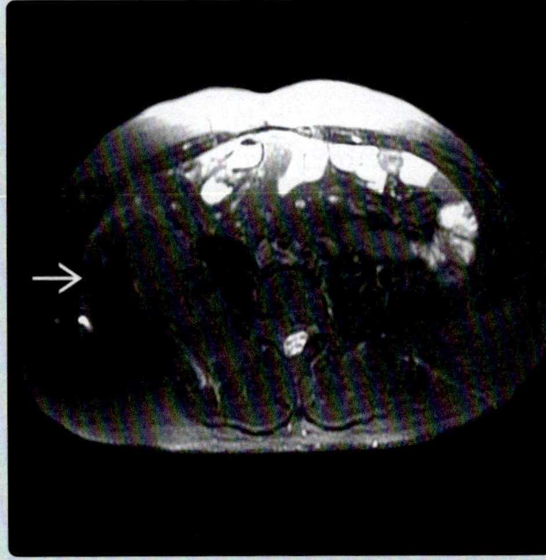

(Left) *Axial T1WI C+ FS MR in the same patient shows mild heterogeneous enhancement of the retroperitoneal mass ➡. Note the large vessels ↪ along the periphery and within the mass. This increased vascularity is typical for hibernoma, but liposarcoma cannot be excluded.* **(Right)** *Axial CECT shows the mass ➡ to have a density between subcutaneous fat and muscle. The vessels ↪ are well demonstrated and were seen to stream through the mass on additional images in the series.*

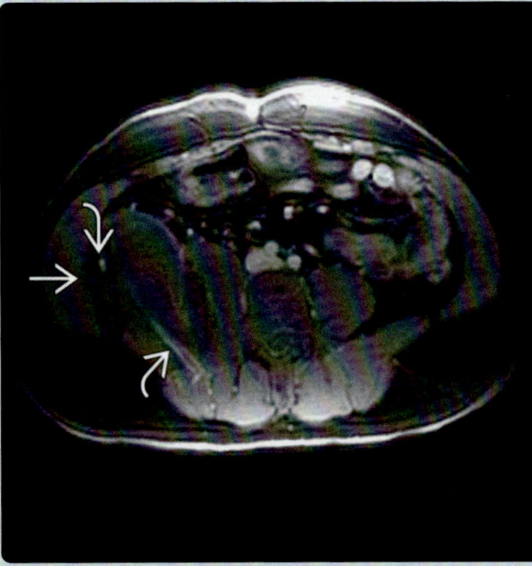

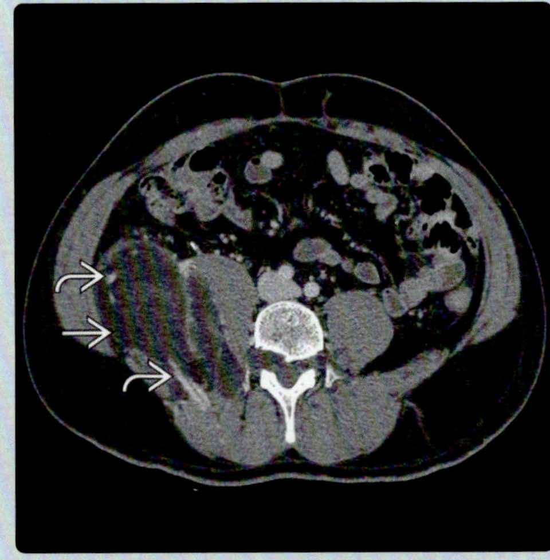

TERMINOLOGY

Synonyms

- Lipoma of immature adipose tissue, lipoma of embryonic fat, fetal lipoma

Definitions

- Rare, benign tumor of brown adipose tissue
- Composed at least in part of brown fat cells with granular, multivacuolated cytoplasm

IMAGING

General Features

- Best diagnostic clue
  - Hypervascular mass with signal intensity similar to fat on MR
- Location
  - Most common in thigh (30%)
    - Shoulder > back > neck > chest > arm > abdominal cavity/retroperitoneum
    - Rare reported locations in mediastinum, breast, adrenal gland
  - May arise in body locations that do not typically have brown fat
- Size
  - 5-15 cm in diameter
  - Reported as large as 24 cm
- Morphology
  - Macrolobulated

Imaging Recommendations

- Best imaging tool
  - MR best evaluates these soft tissue masses
- Protocol advice
  - T1WI + fluid-sensitive sequence with fat suppression + enhanced T1WI FS series
  - 2 planes ± single sequence in 3rd plane

CT Findings

- Mass is composed of density between fat and muscle
- Variable appearance related to amount of fat
- Variable enhancement

MR Findings

- T1WI
  - Range of signal intensity depending on subtype
    - Typical = signal intensity similar to, but not exactly matching, subcutaneous fat
    - Myxoid = fluid signal intensity
    - Lipoma-like = subcutaneous fat signal intensity
  - Prominent low signal septa
- T2WI FS
  - Signal intensity varies by subtype, as it does on T1WI
  - Prominent low signal septa
- STIR
  - Hyperintense to muscle
- T1WI C+ FS
  - Variable enhancement
- Key MR imaging features
  - Prominent septa
  - Branching vessels
- Variant: Intraosseous hibernoma
  - Sclerotic bone lesion on radiograph
  - T1 hypointense to subcutaneous fat, hyperintense to muscle
  - T2 variable hyperintensity

Ultrasonographic Findings

- Grayscale ultrasound
  - Hyperechoic, well-defined mass
  - May have similar appearance to lipoma
- Color Doppler
  - Prominent vascularity

Angiographic Findings

- Hypervascular
- Intense blush
- Arteriovenous shunting

Nuclear Medicine Findings

- Bone scan
  - Moderate uptake on blood-pool
  - Mild uptake on static imaging
- PET/CT
  - Intense uptake of FDG due to hypervascularity and glucose metabolism

DIFFERENTIAL DIAGNOSIS

Imaging Differential Diagnosis

- Liposarcoma, soft tissue
  - Has fat signal intensity and septa similar to hibernoma
  - Less vascular than hibernoma
  - Older patient age than hibernoma
- Atypical lipomatous tumor
  - Will not have intense uptake on F-18 FDG PET, as hibernoma does
  - Less vascular than hibernoma
  - Older patient age than hibernoma
- Lipoma, soft tissue
  - Has less complex appearance than hibernoma
  - Signal intensity matches subcutaneous fat on all MR imaging sequences
  - Older patient age than hibernoma
  - No septations > 2 mm in diameter
  - No enhancement

Pathology Differential Diagnosis

- Rhabdomyoma
  - Larger cells than hibernoma
  - Contain glycogen, crystals, and cross striations
- Granular cell tumor
  - Similar superficial appearance
  - Intracellular lipid vacuoles absent
- Lipoma, spindle cell/pleomorphic
  - Easily confused with spindle cell variant of hibernoma due to very similar histologic appearance
- Liposarcoma, round cell
  - Questionable reports of malignant hibernomas likely represent misdiagnosed round cell liposarcomas containing eosinophilic lipoblasts
  - Differentiate using cytogenetics or molecular analysis

PATHOLOGY

General Features

- Etiology
  - Tumor of brown fat
  - Brown fat is separate entity from white adipose tissue
    - Formerly thought to be early stage of white fat development due to similar histologic appearance
    - Assists in nonshivering thermogenesis
    - Axillary and subpleural locations in fetus and newborn
  - 4 variants of hibernoma
    - Typical > myxoid > lipoma-like > spindle cell
      - Intramuscular lesions are predominantly "typical" variant
      - Myxoid variants preferentially involve men
      - Lipoma-like variant is usually in thigh
      - Spindle cell variant is usually in posterior neck or scalp
- Genetics
  - Cytogenetic abnormalities involve 11q13-21 and 10q22

Staging, Grading, & Classification

- None for this benign tumor

Gross Pathologic & Surgical Features

- Encapsulated, soft, lobulated mass
- Greasy, soft, and spongy cut surface
- Color ranges from yellow to tan to red-brown
  - Varies by lipid content and vascularity

Microscopic Features

- Appearance differs by variant
  - Typical = distinct lobular pattern
    - Cells have varying degrees of differentiation
      - Round to ovoid, granular eosinophilic cells
      - Multivacuolated cells with lipid droplets and centrally placed nuclei
      - CD34(-)
  - Myxoid = prominent myxoid change
    - Thick bundles of collagen fibers, scattered mast cells, and mature adipose tissue
  - Lipoma-like = univacuolated lipocytes with rare hibernomatous features
  - Spindle cell = variety contains spindle cells, similar to those in spindle cell lipoma
    - CD34-positive spindle cell component
- Stain strongly for S100
- Usually mixed with lipocytes
  - Pure hibernomas without lipomatous components are rare
  - Lipomas may have hibernoma components
  - Unclear at which proportion mass is designated, hibernoma or lipoma, when mixed tissue components are present
- Increased vascularity compared with lipoma
- Lobular, well-demarcated, and vary in color from yellow to brown

CLINICAL ISSUES

Presentation

- Most common signs/symptoms
  - Slow-growing, mobile, painless subcutaneous mass
    - 10% are intramuscular
  - Overlying skin may be warm due to hypervascularity
- Other signs/symptoms
  - Often noted for years before removal
  - May cause symptoms from nerve compression or limit range of motion depending on location

Demographics

- Age
  - Peak incidence in 3rd decade of life
    - 60% occur in 3rd and 4th decades
    - 5% occur in children 2-18 years old
    - 7% occur in adults over 60 years old
- Gender
  - Mild female predominance

Natural History & Prognosis

- Benign tumor without potential for malignant transformation
- No recurrence, even if incompletely excised

Treatment

- Surgical excision

DIAGNOSTIC CHECKLIST

Consider

- Must exclude atypical lipomatous tumor and liposarcoma when considering any complex fatty mass
  - Often not possible based on imaging alone
  - Needle biopsy is usually sufficient to diagnose hibernoma preoperatively

Image Interpretation Pearls

- Well-defined mass in middle-aged patient
- Imaging characteristics similar to fat but also containing septa and branching vessels
- Increased vascularity produces characteristics that help differentiate from intermediate grade or malignant lipomatous tumors
  - Increased signal on fluid-sensitive sequences
  - Variable enhancement
  - Vascular blush + arteriovenous shunting on angiography
  - Avid tracer uptake on PET/CT

Reporting Tips

- Report location of dominant feeding vessels for surgical planning
- Emphasize need for tissue diagnosis

SELECTED REFERENCES

1. Bonar SF et al: Intraosseous hibernoma: characterization of five cases and literature review. Skeletal Radiol. 43(7):939-46, 2014
2. Botchu R et al: Intraosseous hibernoma: a case report and review of the literature. Skeletal Radiol. 42(7):1003-5, 2013
3. Liu W et al: Hibernoma: comparing imaging appearance with more commonly encountered benign or low-grade lipomatous neoplasms. Skeletal Radiol. 42(8):1073-8, 2013
4. Kransdorf MJ et al: Lipomatous tumors. In Kransdorf MJ et al: Imaging of soft tissue tumors. 2nd ed. Philadelphia: Lippincott Williams & Wilkins. 117-20, 2006
5. Lewandowski PJ et al: Hibernoma of the medial thigh. Case report and literature review. Clin Orthop Relat Res. (330):198-201, 1996

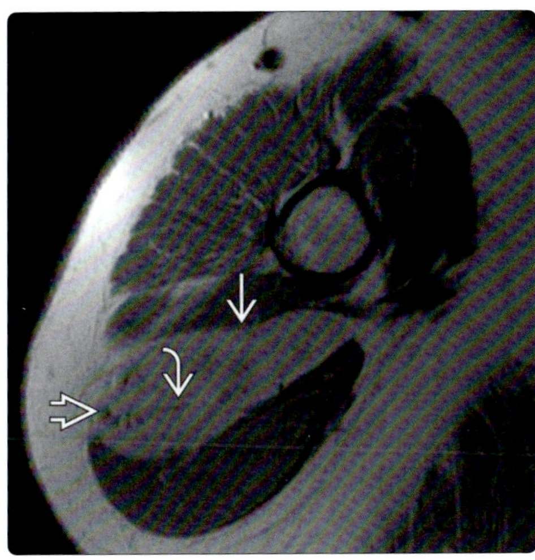

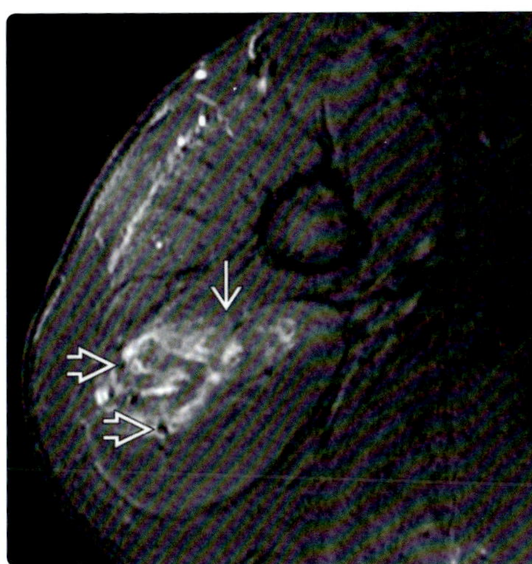

(Left) *Axial T1WI MR shows a mass ➡ in the posterior compartment of the upper arm. The mass contains regions of signal intensity similar to subcutaneous fat but has a predominantly complex appearance containing septa ↪ and enlarged vessels ⇨.* **(Right)** *Axial STIR MR in the same patient reveals the mass ➡ to have signal intensities ranging from isointense to fat to hyperintense relative to muscle. Multiple low signal vessels ⇨ are now apparent.*

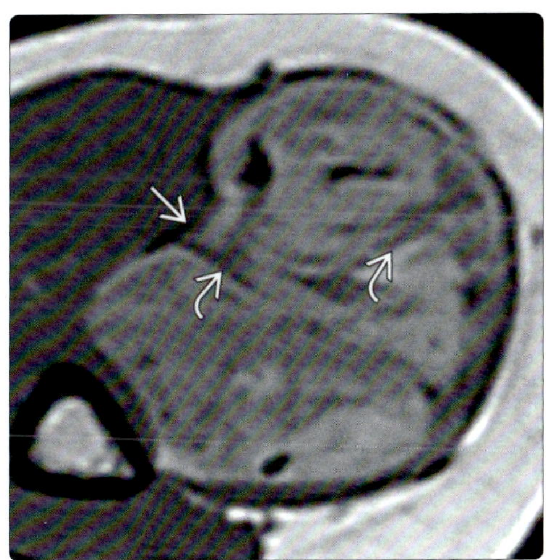

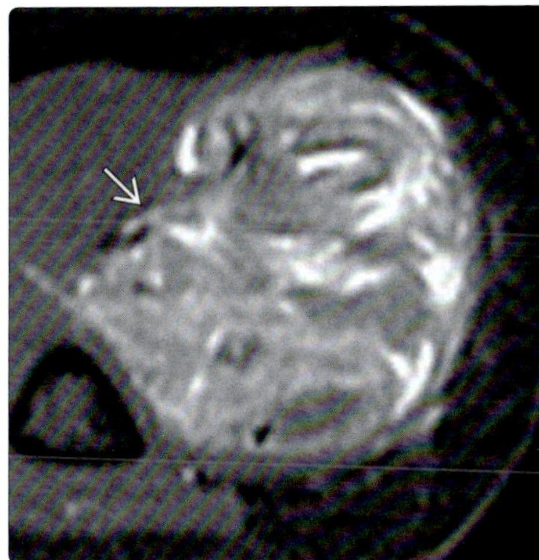

(Left) *Axial T1WI MR shows a large heterogeneous mass ➡ within the lateral aspect of the arm musculature. The signal intensity of the mass is higher than muscle but not as high as the adjacent subcutaneous fat. Note the numerous internal septa ↪.* **(Right)** *Axial T2WI FSE MR shows the mass ➡ to have markedly heterogeneous signal intensity, with areas ranging from low to high intensity. The appearance of the mass on this sequence alone would raise the question of a sarcoma.*

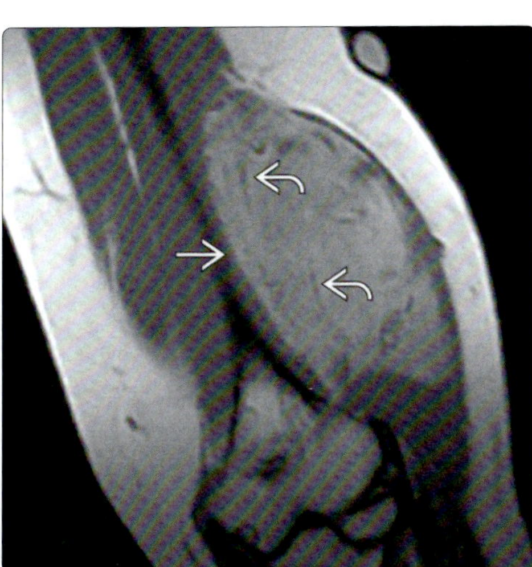

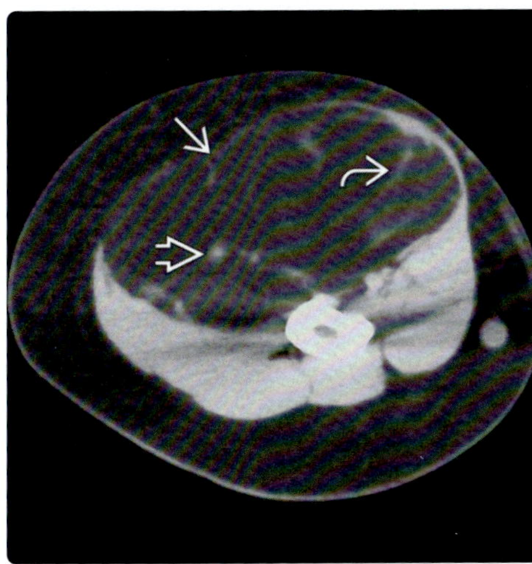

(Left) *Coronal T1WI MR in the same patient again shows the mass ➡ to be hyperintense to muscle. Internal septa ↪ are well demonstrated. Increased signal intensity on T1WI sequences should cause one to consider a hibernoma.* **(Right)** *Axial NECT shows a mass ➡ with a density that is similar to, but slightly higher than, the subcutaneous fat. The mass contains both septa ↪ and vessels ⇨. An atypical lipoma or liposarcoma could have an identical appearance.*

KEY FACTS

TERMINOLOGY

- Fatty lesion arising from bone surface

IMAGING

- ~ 33% adjacent to femur
- Radiolucent/fat density soft tissue mass
  - ± septa
  - ± calcification
  - ± ossification
- Changes in adjacent bone
  - Osseous excrescence in 67-100%
  - ± thickened cortex
  - ± solid or spiculated periosteal new bone
  - ± cortical saucerization
- MR findings
  - Majority of soft tissue mass follows fat signal intensity on all MR sequences
  - May have increased signal on fluid-sensitive sequences in regions of septation or cartilage
    - Thin, internal septa, peripheral fibrous tissue
    - Foci of hyaline cartilage
  - Septa and fibrous tissue may enhance
- Increased radiotracer uptake seen on bone scan in regions of new bone formation

PATHOLOGY

- Benign neoplasm of adipocytes
- Strongly adherent to underlying periosteum
- Gritty bone spicules or firm cartilage nodules
- Can be identical to soft tissue lipoma
  - Diagnosis made on relationship of lesion to bone

CLINICAL ISSUES

- Asymptomatic soft tissue mass
  - Can produce nerve compression
- Adults in 5th-6th decades of life
- Represents 0.3% of all lipomas
- No potential for malignant degeneration

(Left) *Axial T1WI MR shows a mass ➡ with the same signal intensity as subcutaneous fat. The mass abuts ~ 1/3 of the femoral shaft circumference where the cortex is seen to be thickened and has an ossific protuberance ⮫.* **(Right)** *Axial T1WI C+ FS MR shows the signal of the mass ➡ to completely suppress, as does the subcutaneous fat. Minimal enhancement is present between the fatty mass and osseous excrescence ⮫. There are no thick enhancing septa or nodules.*

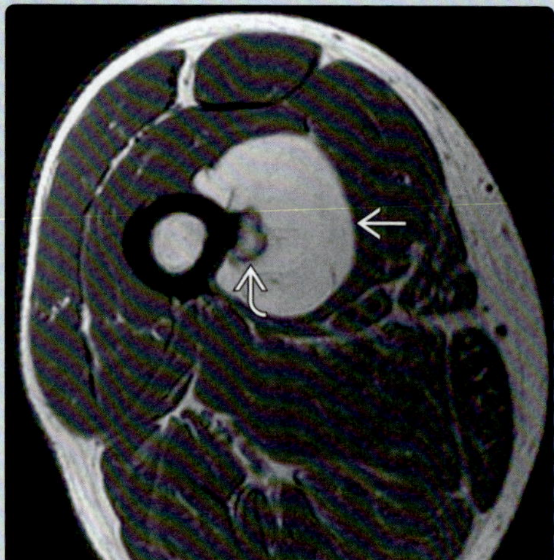

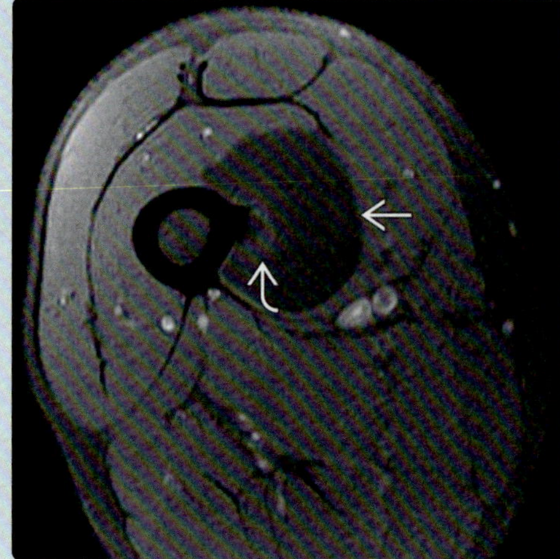

(Left) *Coronal T1WI MR demonstrates the intimate location of the lipoma ➡ with respect to the underlying femur. Grossly, these masses are firmly adherent to the bone. Note the "tail" ⇨ of lipomatous tissue that is present at the proximal and distal aspects of the lesion.* **(Right)** *Coronal STIR MR shows that the signal intensity of the mass ➡ matches subcutaneous fat. Linear high signal is present at the interface of the mass and overlying musculature. Faint internal increased signal is associated with fine septa.*

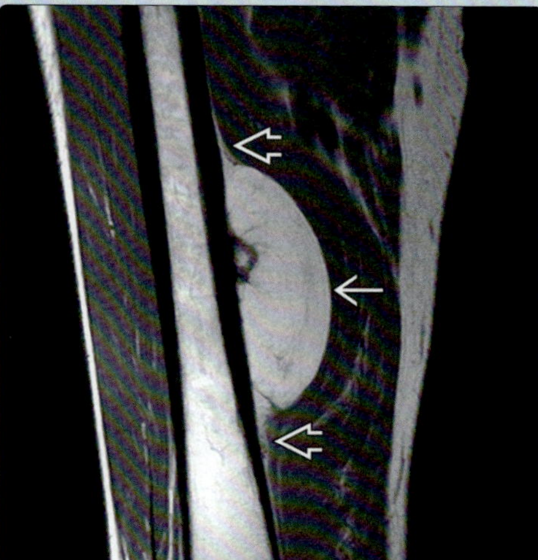

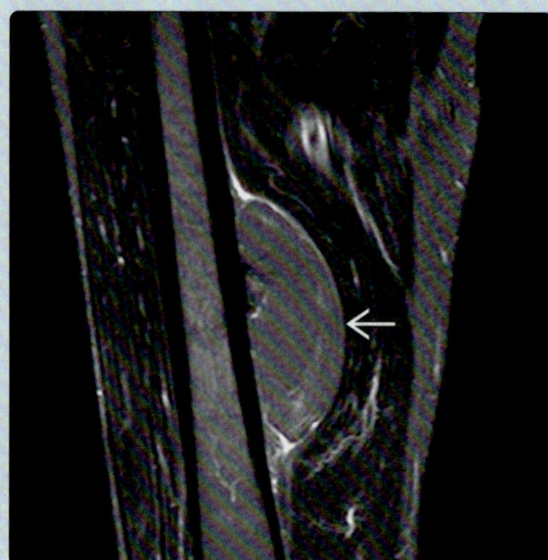

TERMINOLOGY

Synonyms

- Periosteal lipoma, ossifying lipoma

Definitions

- Fatty lesion arising from bone surface

IMAGING

General Features

- Location
  - Femur > forearm > tibia and humerus
    - ~ 33% adjacent to femur
  - Diaphyseal or metadiaphyseal
- Size
  - Typically 4-10 cm

Radiographic Findings

- Radiolucent soft tissue mass
  - Well defined
  - Variable internal septa
- Changes in adjacent bone
  - Osseous excrescence in 67-100%
  - ± thickened cortex
  - ± solid or spiculated periosteal new bone
  - ± cortical saucerization

CT Findings

- Fat density mass abutting bone
  - ± septa
  - ± calcification
  - ± ossification
- Bone cortex changes, as listed above

MR Findings

- Majority of soft tissue mass follows fat signal intensity on all sequences
- May have areas of increased signal on fluid-sensitive sequences
  - Thin, internal septa, peripheral fibrous tissue
  - Foci of hyaline cartilage
- Septa and fibrous tissue may enhance

Nuclear Medicine Findings

- Increased tracer uptake on bone scan in regions of new bone formation

DIFFERENTIAL DIAGNOSIS

Osteochondroma

- Smooth bony excrescence
- Oriented away from joint
- Cortex and medullary space contiguous between native bone and excrescence
- Lacks associated fatty soft tissue mass

Lipoma, Soft Tissue

- Microscopically identical to soft tissue portion of parosteal lipoma
- Not firmly adherent to adjacent bone

PATHOLOGY

General Features

- Etiology
  - Benign neoplasm of adipocytes
  - Site of origin unknown; no fat cells in periosteum

Gross Pathologic & Surgical Features

- Soft, yellow mass
- Strongly adherent to underlying periosteum
- Gritty bone spicules or firm cartilage nodules possible

Microscopic Features

- Mature white adipocytes
  - No cellular atypia
- Islands of hyaline cartilage, fibrocartilage, or bone
- Fibrovascular tissue septa may be present
- Can be identical to soft tissue lipoma
  - Diagnosis made on relationship of lesion to bone

CLINICAL ISSUES

Presentation

- Most common signs/symptoms
  - Asymptomatic soft tissue mass
  - May be mildly tender to palpation
- Other signs/symptoms
  - Can produce nerve compression
    - More common in upper extremity
    - May result in muscle atrophy
    - Proximal radius involvement → posterior interosseous nerve palsy
    - Radial, ulnar, median, and sciatic nerve compression reported

Demographics

- Age
  - 5th-6th decades of life
    - Reported in children and adolescents
- Gender
  - Slight male predilection
- Epidemiology
  - Represents 0.3% of all lipomas
  - < 0.1% of primary bone neoplasms

Natural History & Prognosis

- Benign process without potential for malignant degeneration
- No local recurrence

Treatment

- No treatment necessary
- Surgical resection if symptomatic

SELECTED REFERENCES

1. Aoki S et al: Large Parosteal Lipoma without Periosteal Changes. Plast Reconstr Surg Glob Open. 3(1):e287, 2015
2. Greco M et al: Parosteal lipoma. Report of 15 new cases and a review of the literature. Ann Ital Chir. 84(2):229-35, 2013
3. Kransdorf MJ et al: Parosteal lipoma. In Kransdorf MJ et al: Imaging of Soft Tissue Tumors. 2nd ed. Philadelphia: Lippincott Williams & Wilkins. 120-3, 2006
4. Murphey MD et al: Parosteal lipoma: MR imaging characteristics. AJR Am J Roentgenol. 162(1):105-10, 1994

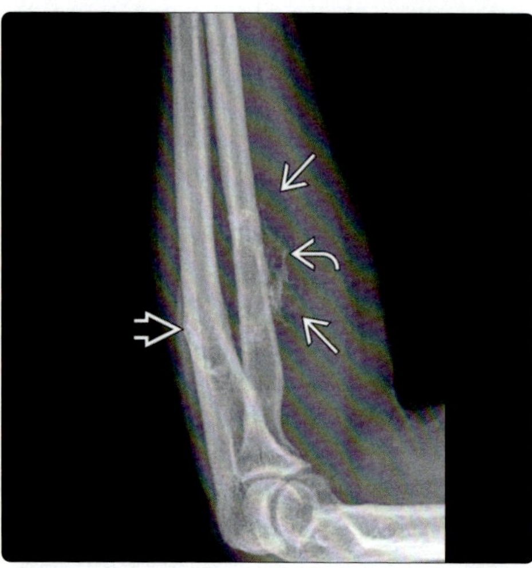

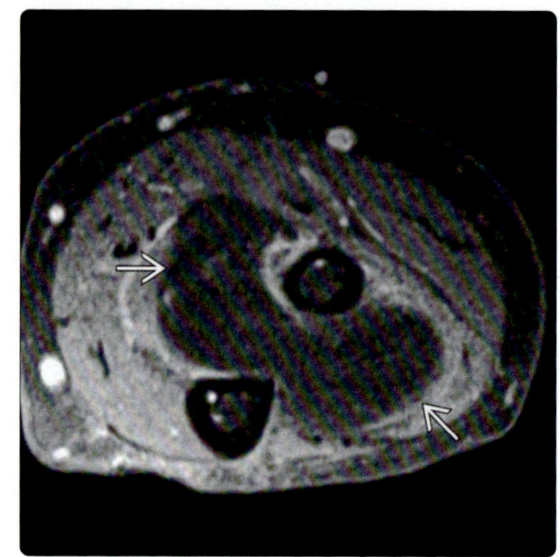

(Left) *Lateral radiograph shows a large fat density mass ➡. New bone formation is localized as being associated with the underlying bone periosteum ↷. Cortical thickening ➡ is also present.* **(Right)** *Axial PD FSE FS MR in the same patient shows the fat signal mass ➡. The branching new bone formation is difficult to appreciate. The lipoma completely saturates out, similar to the subcutaneous fat.*

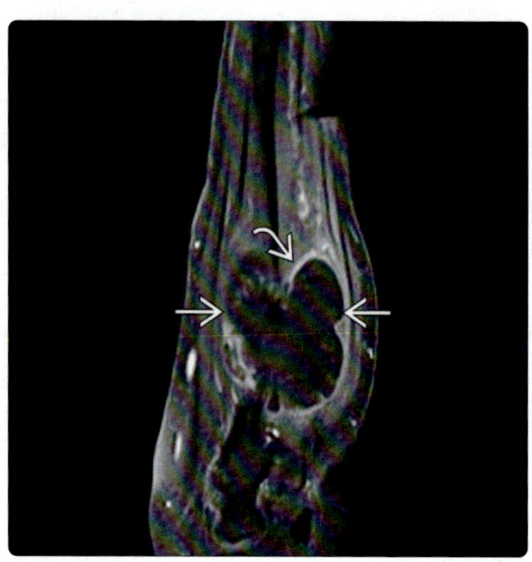

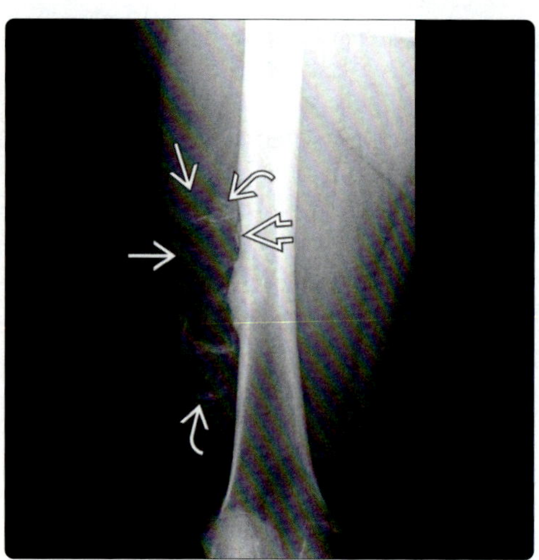

(Left) *Coronal T1WI C+ FS MR, same patient, shows a relative paucity of enhancement of the parosteal lipoma ➡. Septa in the periphery of the mass have thin linear enhancement. There is also enhancement ↷ along the border of the mass likely due to fibrous tissue.* **(Right)** *AP radiograph shows fat density soft tissue mass in the thigh ➡ that elicits bizarre periosteal bone formation ↷ perpendicular to the shaft. There is both cortical thickening and mild scalloping ➡. Both the location and appearance are classic for parosteal lipoma.*

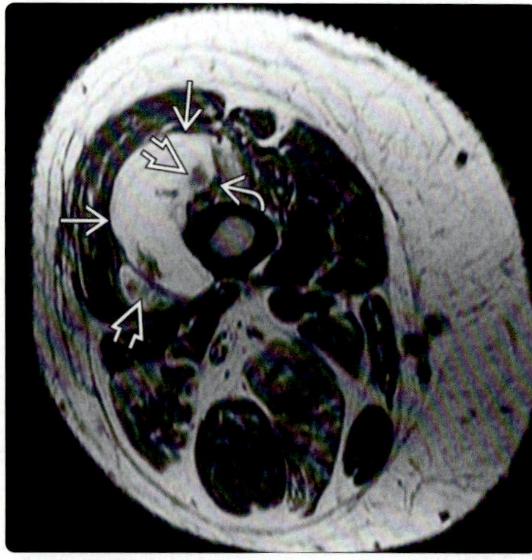

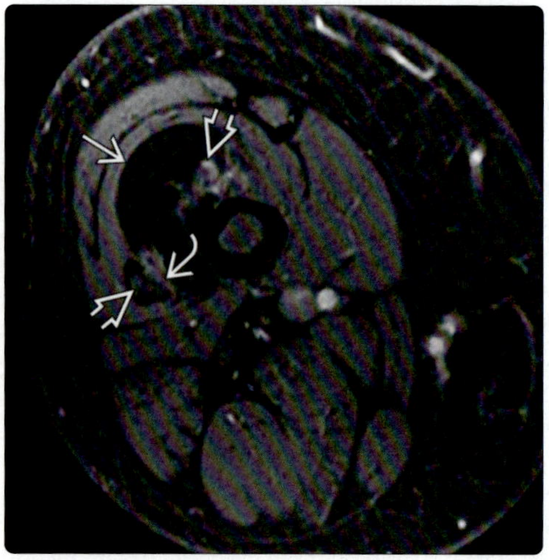

(Left) *Axial T1WI MR in the same patient shows SI similar to subcutaneous fat comprising the majority of the lesion ➡. Note also the lower SI parosteal bone formation ↷. Small nodular regions ➡ and a single septum are noted to have intermediate SI.* **(Right)** *Axial T1WI C+ FS MR in the same patient shows the fatty portion of the lesion ➡ saturates out. The septum ↷ and nodular portions ➡ noted on the T1 scan now show mild to moderate enhancement. This tissue can make a parosteal lipoma appear complicated and raise concern.*

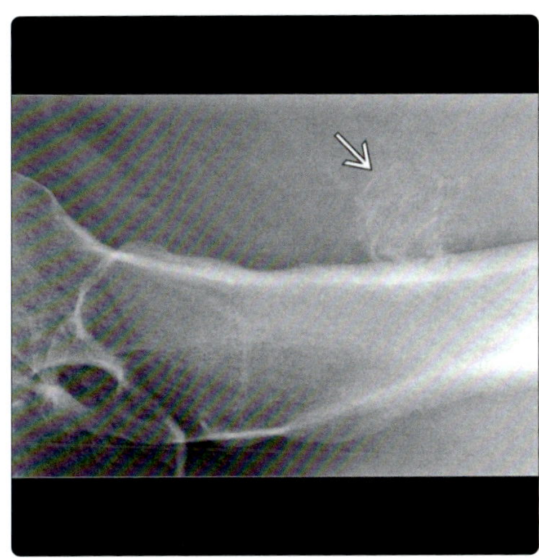

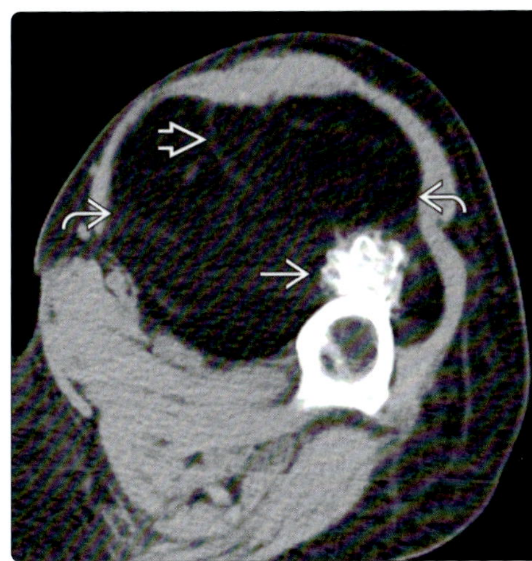

(Left) *Lateral radiograph of the femur shows a bony excrescence ➡ arising from the anterior cortex of the proximal femoral diaphysis. An associated soft tissue mass was not clearly evident on the radiograph.* **(Right)** *Axial bone CT in the same patient again shows a bony excrescence ➡ arising from the femoral cortex. A large fat attenuation mass ➡ surrounds the bony excrescence and abuts the femoral cortex. A few thin septa ➡ are present within the parosteal lipoma.*

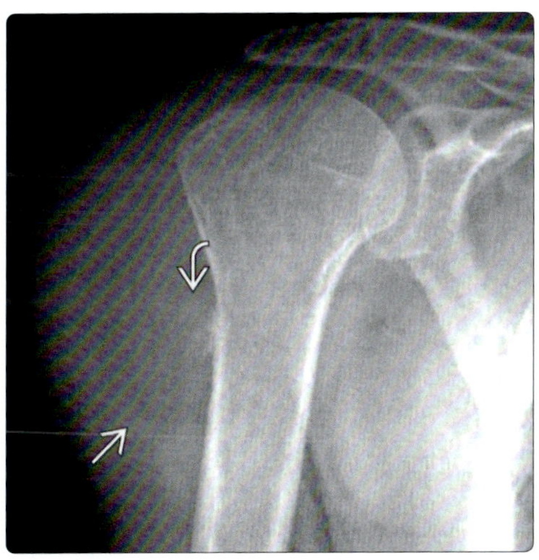

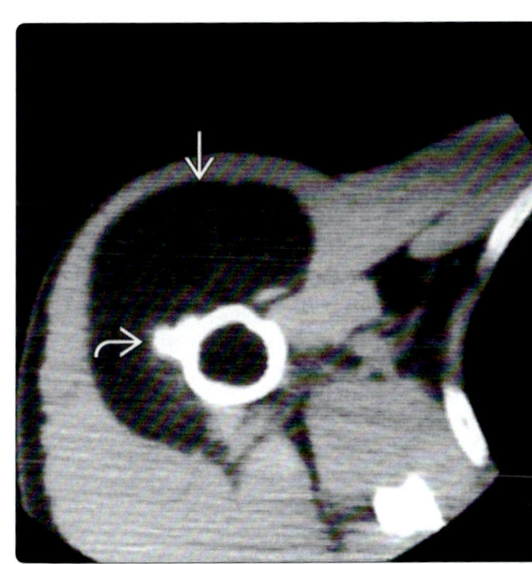

(Left) *AP radiograph of the humerus shows a soft tissue mass ➡ in the upper arm. The mass has low density that is typical for fat. An osseous excrescence ➡ is present, extending from the underlying humeral diaphysis into the fatty mass.* **(Right)** *Axial NECT in the same patient confirms that the mass ➡ consists of low-attenuation, simple-appearing fat. The osseous excrescence ➡ seen arising from the humeral shaft is a typical finding.*

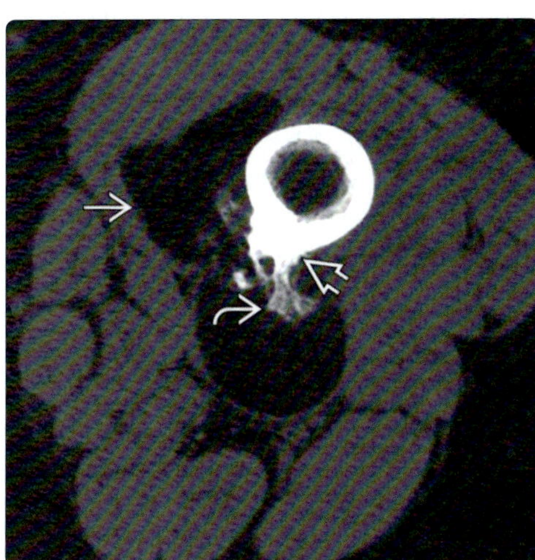

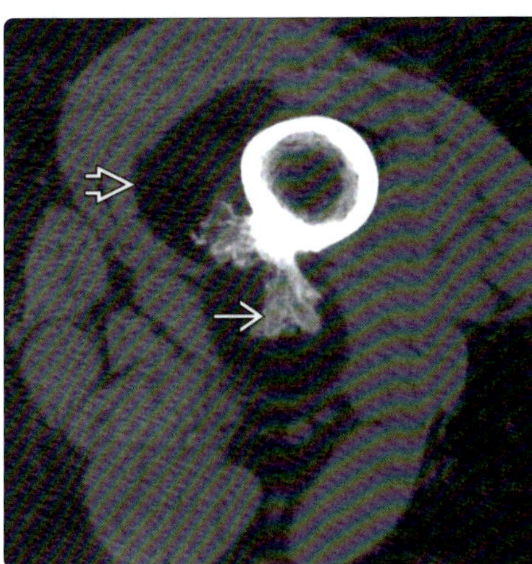

(Left) *Axial NECT shows a lobulated fat collection ➡ abutting ~ 50% of the circumference of the femoral shaft. Frond-like areas of reactive bone ➡ extend into the fatty mass. The femoral cortex ➡ is thickened.* **(Right)** *Axial NECT in the same patient shows continuation of the fatty mass ➡ and reactive bone formation ➡. This is a classic appearance of a parosteal lipoma. There are no therapeutic implications beyond a potential for nerve compression.*

KEY FACTS

TERMINOLOGY

- Intermediate, locally aggressive neoplasm predominantly composed of fat
- WHO designation: Atypical lipomatous tumor/well-differentiated liposarcoma
  - Use of either or both terms acceptable

IMAGING

- Soft tissue mass, typically composed of > 75% fat with septa and variable nodularity
- 75% in deep extremities (thigh is most common)
- Radiographs may show mass to have visibly lower density than adjacent muscle
- CT: Low-attenuation mass with negative HU measurements
  - Often contains septa and nodules
- MR best for lesion characterization
  - T1WI MR to define lesion extent and content
  - Utilize sequences ± fat suppression
  - Nodules and septa often have ↑ T2WI MR signal intensity and mild to marked enhancement

PATHOLOGY

- Multilobular, deep-yellow to ivory mass
- Mature adipocytes of different sizes

CLINICAL ISSUES

- Painless extremity mass that has been enlarging over months to years
- Retroperitoneal lesions may be found incidentally
  - Location suggests lesion should be looked at with high degree of suspicion
- 5th-7th decades of life
- Most common form of liposarcoma (40-50%)
- Locally aggressive tumor that does not metastasize
- Risk of local recurrence based on anatomic location
- Prognosis significantly worsens if lesion dedifferentiates (a.k.a. dedifferentiated liposarcoma)

(Left) *Axial T1WI MR demonstrates a fatty mass ➡ located deep in posterior compartment of the thigh. It is located between and significantly displaces the posterior compartment musculature. This mass contains multiple low signal septa ➡.* **(Right)** *Axial T1WI C+ FS MR (same patient) shows mild enhancement of the septa ➡. Mass ➡ abuts neurovascular bundle ➡. Greater than 75% of mass is composed of fat, typical for atypical lipomatous tumor (ALT)/well-differentiated liposarcoma (WDL).*

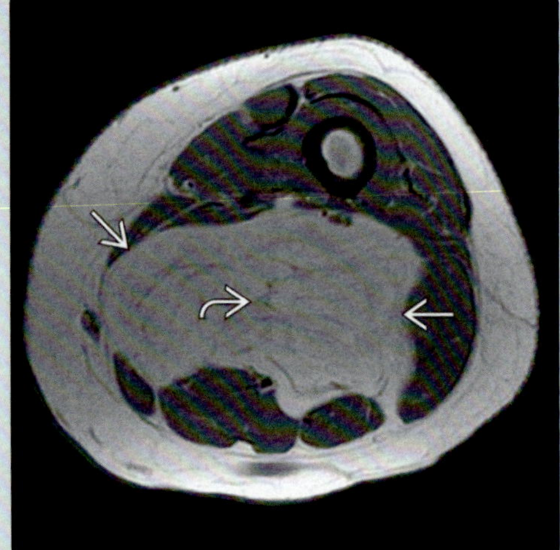

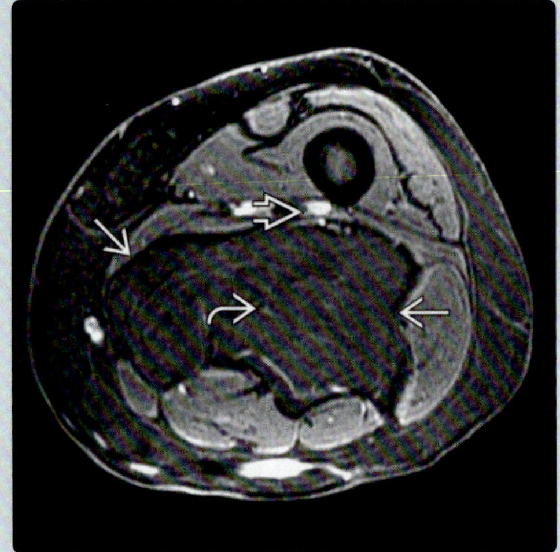

(Left) *Coronal T1WI MR in the same patient shows the very large extent of the fatty mass ➡, which involves almost the entire length of the thigh. This lobulated mass contains numerous septa ➡ that have a flowing, whorled pattern.* **(Right)** *Coronal STIR MR in the same patient shows the predominantly fatty mass ➡ to have surprisingly high signal intensity. The increased signal involves both the septa ➡ and fatty-appearing regions.*

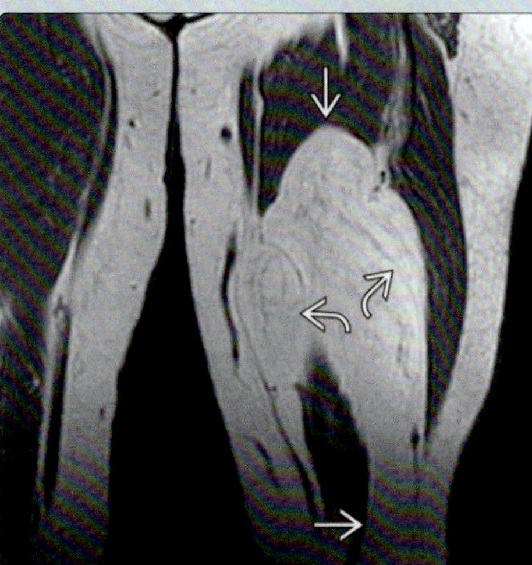

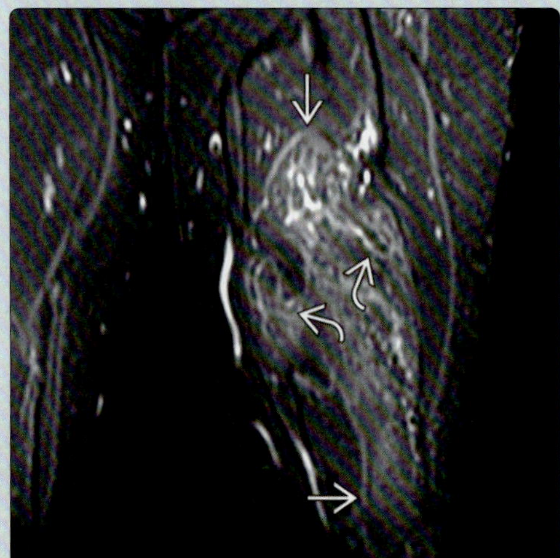

TERMINOLOGY

Abbreviations

- Atypical lipomatous tumor (ALT)
- Well-differentiated liposarcoma (WDL)

Synonyms

- Atypical lipoma, atypical lipomatous neoplasm, adipocytic liposarcoma, lipoma-like liposarcoma, sclerosing liposarcoma, spindle cell liposarcoma, inflammatory liposarcoma

Definitions

- Intermediate, locally aggressive neoplasm composed predominantly of fat
- WHO designation: ALT/WDL
  - Use of either or both terms is acceptable
  - Some reserve WDL to indicate deep tumors that cannot be completely resected

IMAGING

General Features

- Best diagnostic clue
  - Soft tissue mass, typically composed of > 75% fat
- Location
  - 75% in deep soft tissues of extremities (thigh is most common)
  - 20% in retroperitoneum, peritesticular, mediastinum (decreasing order of frequency)
- Size
  - Lesions located in retroperitoneum or deep in extremities can reach very large size

Imaging Recommendations

- Best imaging tool
  - MR best evaluates fatty soft tissue tumors
- Protocol advice
  - T1WI best assesses lesion contents
  - Utilize sequences with and without fat suppression
  - IV gadolinium enhancement useful to evaluate nonfatty elements

Radiographic Findings

- Nonspecific soft tissue mass
- May have visibly lower density than adjacent muscle

MR Findings

- T1WI
  - Majority of lesion will have signal intensity similar to subcutaneous fat
    - Septa and nodularity variably present
- T2WI FS
  - Fatty components will suppress or have low signal
  - Nodules and septa often have ↑ signal intensity
- T1WI C+ FS
  - Nodules and septa show mild to marked enhancement

DIFFERENTIAL DIAGNOSIS

Lipoma

- Simple fatty mass ± capsule
- Lacks thickened septa and nodularity

Fat Necrosis

- Focal fat collection with thick irregular capsule
- Variable presence of septa or calcification
- May be indistinguishable from ALT/WDL on imaging

PATHOLOGY

General Features

- Genetics
  - *MDM2* and *CDK4* gene overexpression related to amplification of 12q13-15 chromosomal region observed in ALT/WDL
    - May be useful in differentiating large lipoma from more ALT/WDL

Gross Pathologic & Surgical Features

- Multilobular, deep-yellow to ivory mass
  - Retroperitoneal masses may be discontiguous

Microscopic Features

- Mature adipocytes of different sizes
  - Focal nuclear atypia
  - ± foci of hemorrhagic, myxoid, or fibrous tissue
- Subtypes: Lipoma-like, sclerosing, and inflammatory
- Fat necrosis common in large lesions

CLINICAL ISSUES

Presentation

- Most common signs/symptoms
  - Painless extremity mass that has been enlarging over months to years
  - Retroperitoneal lesions may be found incidentally
- Other signs/symptoms
  - Pain, tenderness, or nerve compression in 1/4

Demographics

- Age
  - 5th-7th decades of life
- Epidemiology
  - Most common form of liposarcoma (40-50%)

Natural History & Prognosis

- Locally aggressive tumor that does not metastasize
  - 0% mortality for lesions in extremities
  - 80% mortality for retroperitoneal lesions
- Sclerosing variant
  - Less likely to be composed predominantly of fat
  - ↑ propensity to dedifferentiation
- Prognosis significantly worsens if lesion dedifferentiates (a.k.a. dedifferentiated liposarcoma)
- Risk of local recurrence based on anatomic location
  - 25-43% recurrence in extremities
  - 90-100% recurrence in retroperitoneum

Treatment

- Surgical excision with clear margins
- Radiotherapy utilized if excision is not possible

SELECTED REFERENCES

1. Bestic JM et al: Sclerosing variant of well-differentiated liposarcoma: relative prevalence and spectrum of CT and MRI features. AJR Am J Roentgenol. 201(1):154-61, 2013

(Left) *Axial T1WI MR shows a large fatty mass ➙ within the adductor compartment of the thigh. The mass contains irregular, thickened septa ➙. The size, deep location, and complexity of this lesion make it worrisome for a liposarcoma.* **(Right)** *Axial T1WI C+ FS MR in the same patient shows the majority of the complex fatty mass ➙ to suppress in signal intensity. There is linear and nodular enhancement in the periphery and in the regions where the septa were suspicious ➙.*

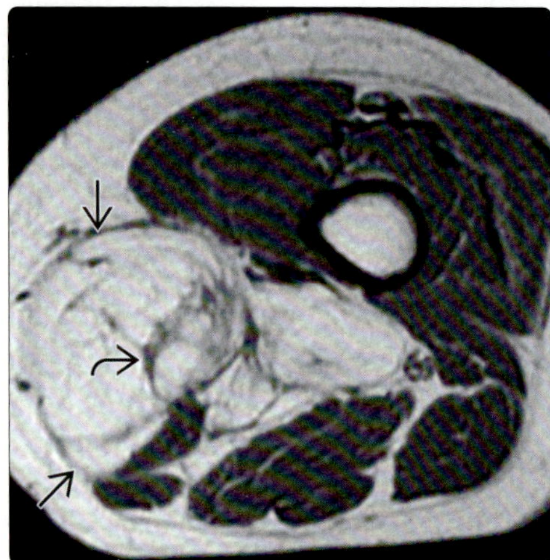

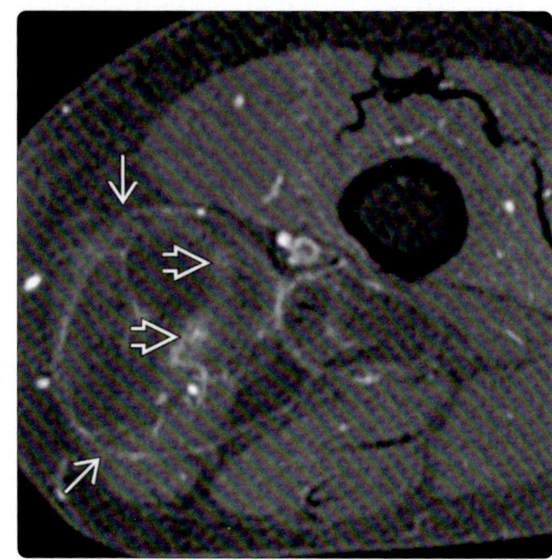

(Left) *Coronal T1WI MR shows a large mass ➙ in the right gluteal region, which is almost entirely composed of fat signal intensity. However, the mass contains regions of nodularity ➙ and fine septations ➙. This lesion recurred after prior resection, as seen by adjacent foci of metal artifact ➙.* **(Right)** *Coronal T1WI C+ FS MR in the same patient shows the large fatty gluteal mass ➙. There is faint enhancement within the septate ➙ and nodular ➙ portions of the mass, making it suspicious for ALT.*

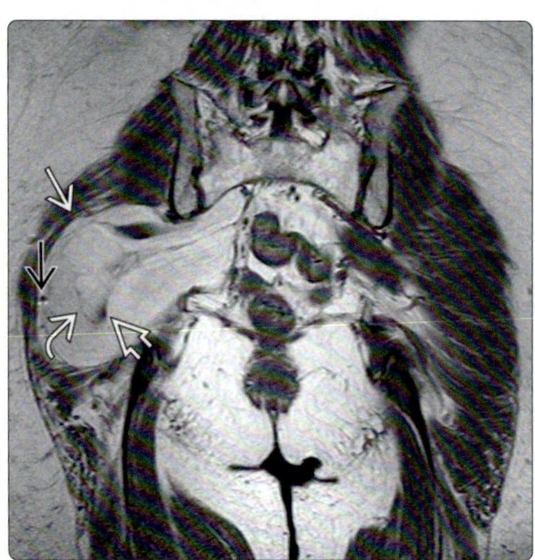

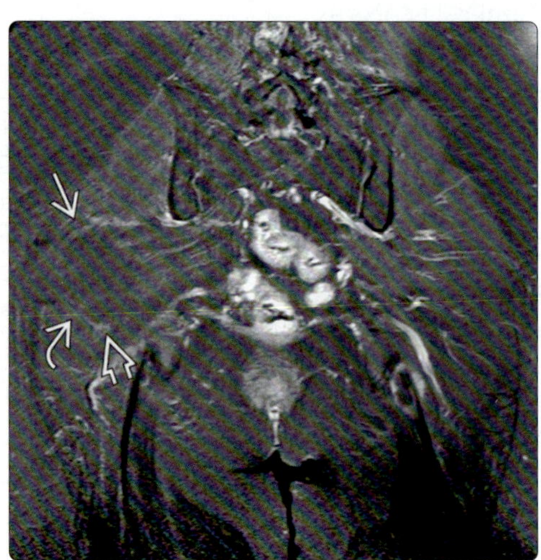

(Left) *Axial T1WI FSE MR shows an incompletely encapsulated fatty mass ➙ that mildly deforms the underlying muscle ➙. The lesion does not contain nodules or particularly thick septa. ALT/WDL can range from simple to very complex in appearance.* **(Right)** *Axial T1WI C+ FS MR in the same patient shows the fatty mass ➙ to contain a few enhancing septa ➙. This should raise suspicion that the lesion may not be a simple lipoma. The pathologist should be alerted to look for atypical tissue.*

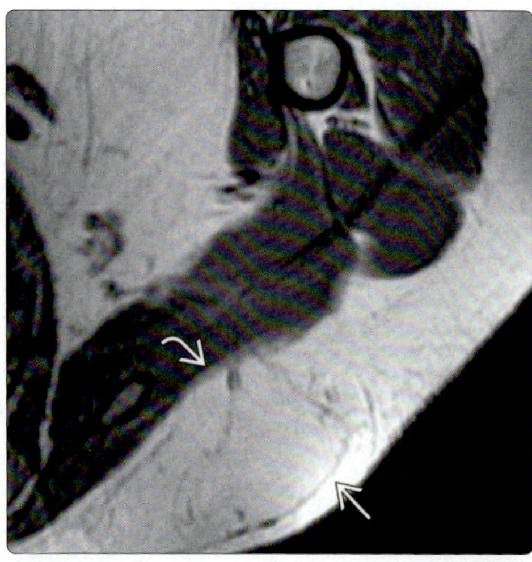

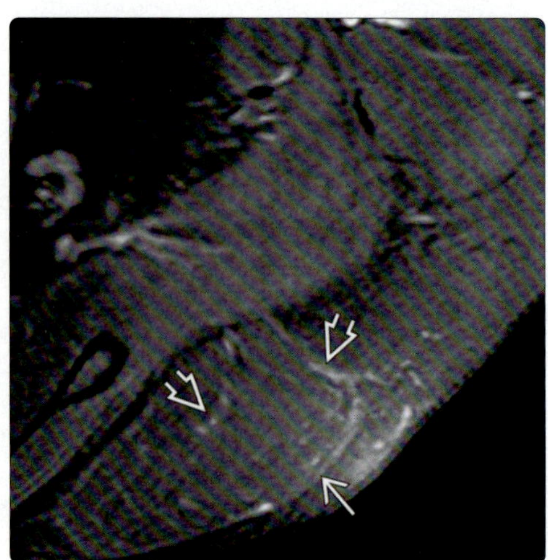

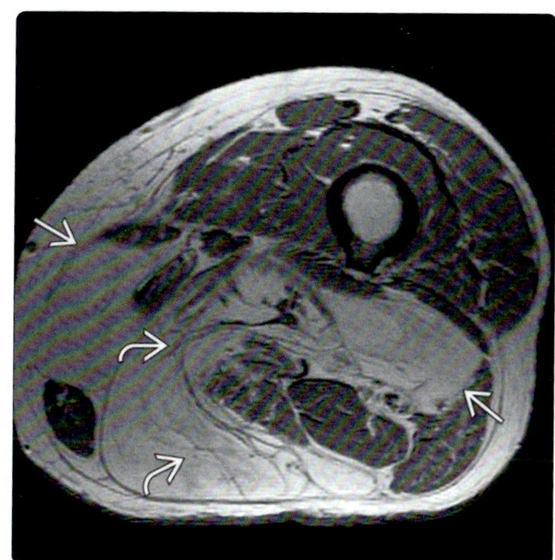

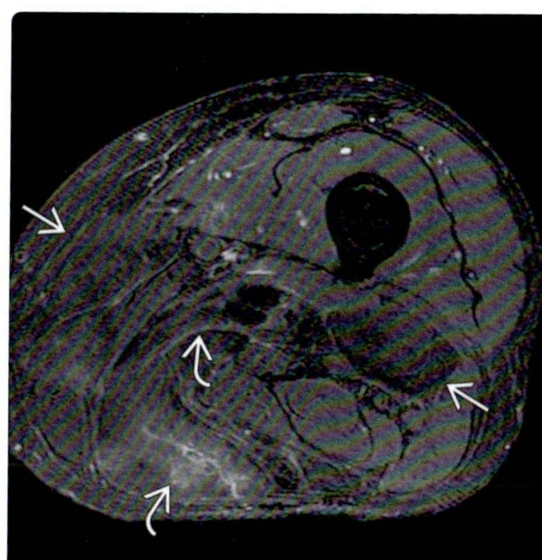

(Left) *Axial T1WI MR shows a large mass ➡ insinuating itself between and within the musculature of the thigh posterior compartment. The mass has signal intensity that is the same as subcutaneous fat with swirling, flowing septa ↪.* **(Right)** *Axial T1WI C+ FS MR in the same patient shows the majority of the mass ➡ to have low signal intensity due to fat suppression. Areas of enhancement correspond to regions of septa ↪. The complexity of this lesion suggests ALT/WDL.*

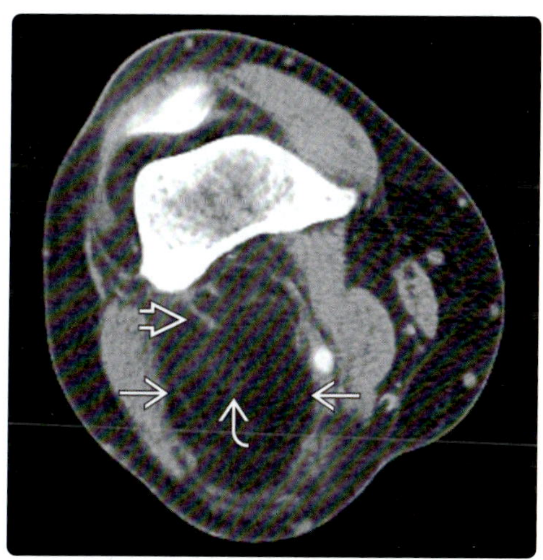

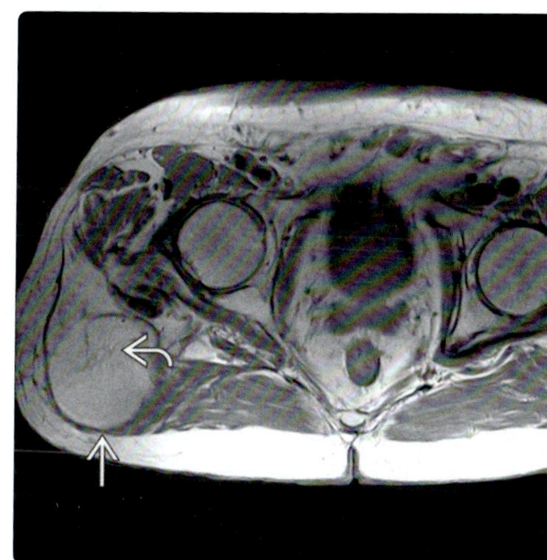

(Left) *Axial CECT shows a mass ➡ with the same attenuation as subcutaneous fat located deep in the popliteal fossa. There are fine septa within the mass ↪. Along the anterior border of the mass, there are foci of what could be thick septa but are actually entrapped muscle fibers ⇨.* **(Right)** *Axial T1WI MR shows a complex fatty mass ➡ in the right gluteal region. The mass lies within and anterior to the gluteus medius muscle. Internal septa ↪ measure < 2 mm in thickness, but the lesion proved to be ALT/WDL.*

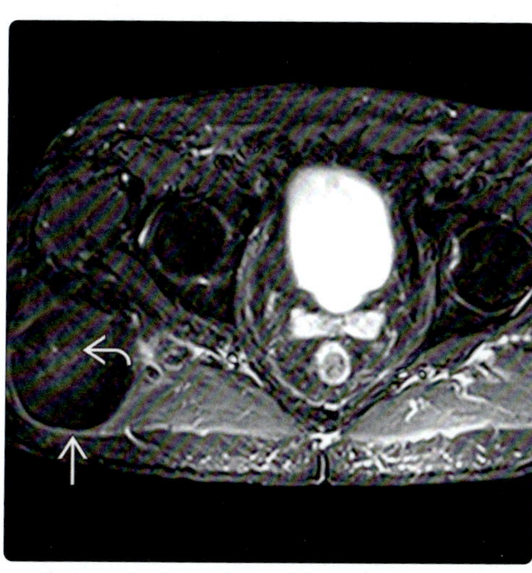

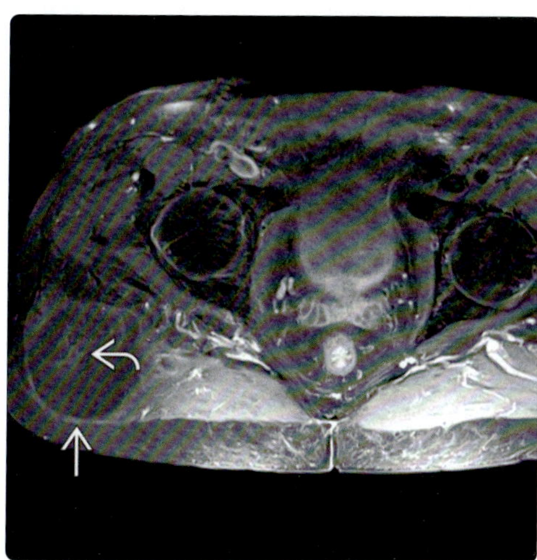

(Left) *Axial T2WI FS MR in the same patient shows the majority of the mass ➡ to suppress in signal, as does the subcutaneous fat. A small area in the central portion of the mass, corresponding to fine septa ↪, has increased T2 signal.* **(Right)** *Axial T1WI FS C+ MR in the same patient shows the mass ➡ to lack enhancement, except for the small, central region of fine septa ↪. The septa are not unusually thick but are increased in number compared with a lipoma.*

KEY FACTS

TERMINOLOGY

- Malignant tumor encompassing continuum from highly differentiated myxoid tissue with lipoblasts to poorly differentiated round cells

IMAGING

- Myxoid and fat tissue mass in deep extremity tissues
  - Typically < 25% fat
  - May have no lipomatous tissue visible on imaging
- 75% in lower extremity; deep thigh > popliteal
- Well-defined mass with CT attenuation higher than fat but lower than muscle
  - Calcification uncommon
- Round cell components have variable appearance
- Contrast essential to differentiate from cyst on MR
  - Low signal on T1WI
  - High signal on T2WI
  - Heterogeneous to homogeneous enhancement

PATHOLOGY

- Similar to developing fetal fat: Primitive nonlipogenic mesenchymal cells + signet ring lipoblasts
  - Characteristic chicken wire vascular pattern
  - Low cellularity with prominent myxoid stroma
- ± solid sheets of primitive round cells
- Areas of osseous or cartilaginous differentiation

CLINICAL ISSUES

- 4th and 5th decades of life
- Most common liposarcoma in patients < 20 yr old
- 2nd most common liposarcoma subtype
- Relatively poor prognosis even when low grade
  - Survival rates are better in children
  - Prognosis worsens with round cell component
- Unusual predilection for metastasizing to other soft tissues or bone

(Left) *Coronal T1 MR in a 65-year-old woman shows a lesion in which the majority of the tissue ➡ is hypointense to muscle but which shows fat signal both superiorly and inferiorly ➦. With peripheral fat, this could represent intramuscular myxoma; however, the distal fat should make myxoid liposarcoma a consideration.* **(Right)** *Coronal PDFS MR in the same patient shows the fat to saturate out ➦ while the myxoid portion of the lesion and tail ➡ are hyperintense.*

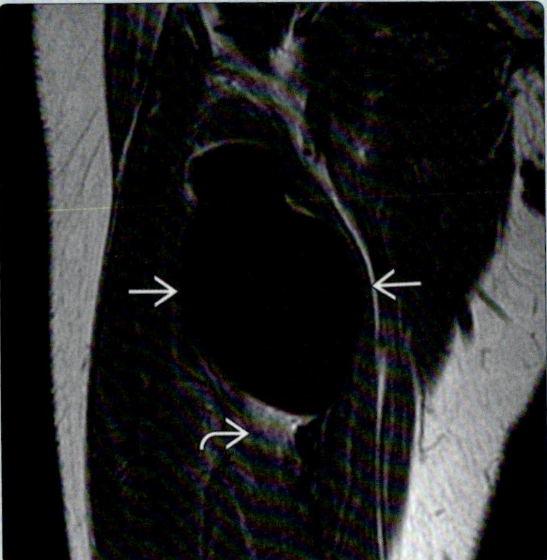

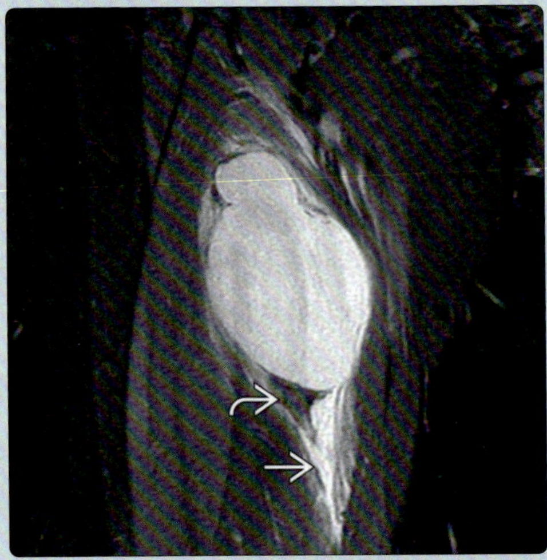

(Left) *Coronal postcontrast T1FS in the same patient shows significant enhancement of the majority of the lesion ➡, with some hypointense areas suggesting necrosis ➦. This pattern strongly pushes the diagnosis towards myxoid liposarcoma rather than myxoma.* **(Right)** *Axial CT shows the slightly hypodense lesion ➡ with the appropriate approach of the biopsy needle, which avoids the rectus femoris while staying within a single compartment. Biopsy proved myxoid liposarcoma.*

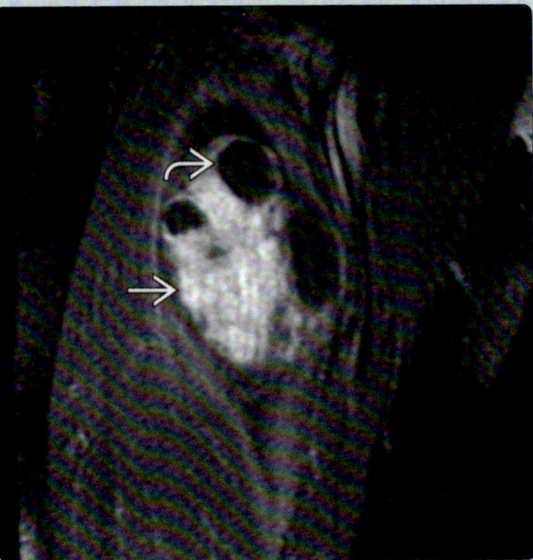

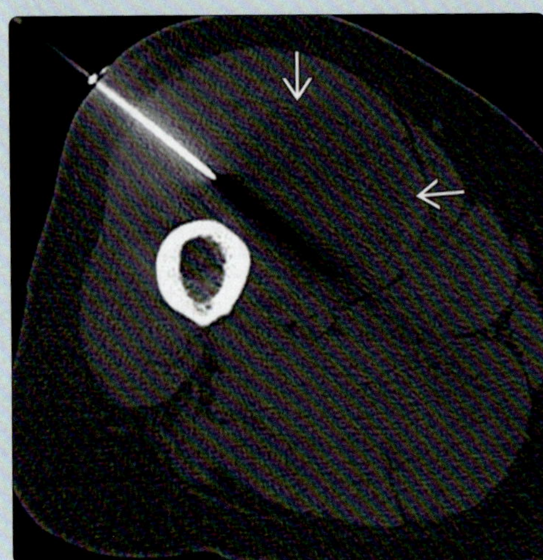

TERMINOLOGY

Synonyms

- Round cell liposarcoma

Definitions

- Malignant tumor encompassing continuum from highly differentiated myxoid tissue with lipoblasts to poorly differentiated round cells

IMAGING

General Features

- Best diagnostic clue
  - Soft tissue mass in deep tissues of extremity with myxoid and fat tissue
    - Typically < 25% fat
    - May have no lipomatous signal visible on imaging
- Location
  - 75% in lower extremity; deep thigh > popliteal
    - Retroperitoneum less common

Imaging Recommendations

- Protocol advice
  - IV contrast is essential to differentiate from cyst

Radiographic Findings

- Nonspecific soft tissue mass with density greater than fat

CT Findings

- Well-defined mass with attenuation higher than fat but lower than muscle
  - May lack or have only small amount of purely fat-attenuation tissue
  - Calcification uncommon
- Round cell region attenuation similar to muscle

MR Findings

- Can simulate cyst if contrast is not utilized
  - Low signal on T1WI
  - High signal on T2WI
- Heterogeneous to homogeneous enhancement
  - More intense enhancement associated with worse prognosis
- Lesions with round cell components have more variable appearance

Ultrasonographic Findings

- Complex hypoechoic mass
- Internal vascularity on Doppler sonography

DIFFERENTIAL DIAGNOSIS

Myxoid Malignant Fibrous Histiocytoma

- Significant atypia and coarse vasculature

Intramuscular Myxoma

- Peripheral rim of fat and surrounding edema
- Globular enhancement pattern

Ganglion Cyst

- Lacks enhancement and fat signal intensity on MR

PATHOLOGY

General Features

- Genetics
  - 90% have t(12;16)(q13; p11) translocation

Gross Pathologic & Surgical Features

- Well-circumscribed, gelatinous, multinodular mass
- Round cell component: Fleshy, white to yellow

Microscopic Features

- Similar to developing fetal fat: Primitive nonlipogenic mesenchymal cells and signet ring lipoblasts
  - Low cellularity with prominent myxoid stroma
  - Characteristic chicken wire vascular pattern
  - Rare to absent mitotic activity
- ± round cell component (solid sheets of primitive round cells)
- Areas of osseous or cartilaginous differentiation
- High grade: > 5% round cell component, necrosis, p53 overexpression

CLINICAL ISSUES

Presentation

- Most common signs/symptoms
  - Nontender soft tissue mass in deep extremity soft tissues

Demographics

- Age
  - 4th and 5th decades of life
    - Younger presentation than other liposarcomas
  - Most common liposarcoma in patients < 20 years old
- Gender
  - No gender predilection
- Epidemiology
  - 2nd most common liposarcoma subtype
    - 1/3 of all liposarcomas
    - Exceeded in number by atypical lipomatous tumor/well-differentiated liposarcoma
  - 10% of adult soft tissue sarcomas

Natural History & Prognosis

- Relatively poor prognosis even when low grade
  - 10-year survival: 70%
  - Survival rates are better in children
- Prognosis worsens with round cell component
  - 10-year survival: 40%
- Unusual predilection for metastatic disease to other soft tissues or bone
  - Soft tissue sarcomas usually metastasize to lung

SELECTED REFERENCES

1. Wortman JR et al: Neoadjuvant radiation in primary extremity liposarcoma: correlation of MRI features with histopathology. Eur Radiol. ePub, 2015
2. Mankin HJ et al: Liposarcoma: a soft tissue tumor with many presentations. Musculoskelet Surg. 98(3):171-7, 2014
3. Petscavage-Thomas JM et al: Soft-tissue myxomatous lesions: review of salient imaging features with pathologic comparison. Radiographics. 34(4):964-80, 2014
4. Craig WD et al: Fat-containing lesions of the retroperitoneum: radiologic-pathologic correlation. Radiographics. 29(1):261-90, 2009

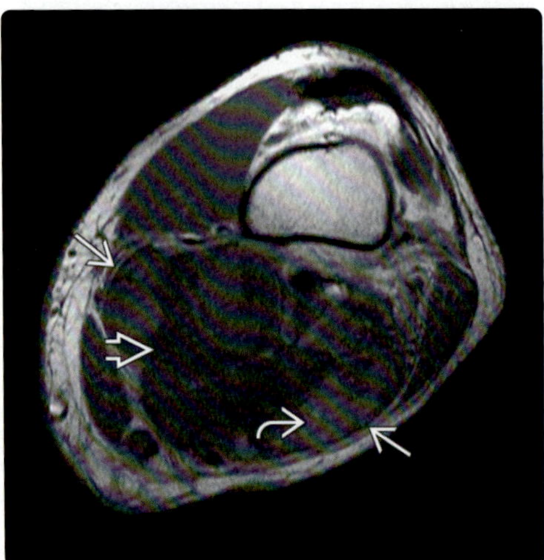

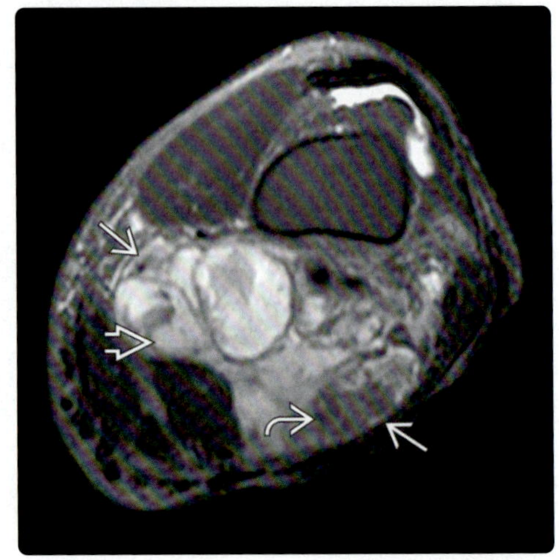

(Left) *Axial T1WI MR shows a heterogeneous soft tissue mass ➡ in the distal thigh with multiple regions of differing signal intensity. A small area of fat ➡ has high signal intensity and a myxoid region ➡ shows relatively homogeneous low signal intensity.* **(Right)** *Axial T2WI FS MR in the same patient shows the mass ➡ in the distal thigh to have high signal in myxoid regions ➡ and low signal in regions of fat ➡. This deeply located, infiltrating, complex mass is clearly malignant.*

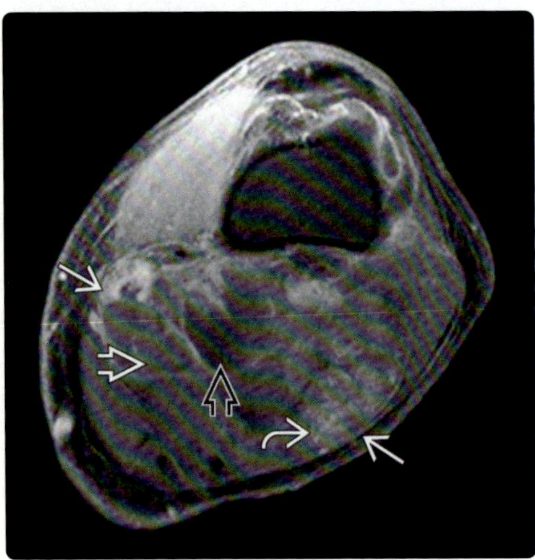

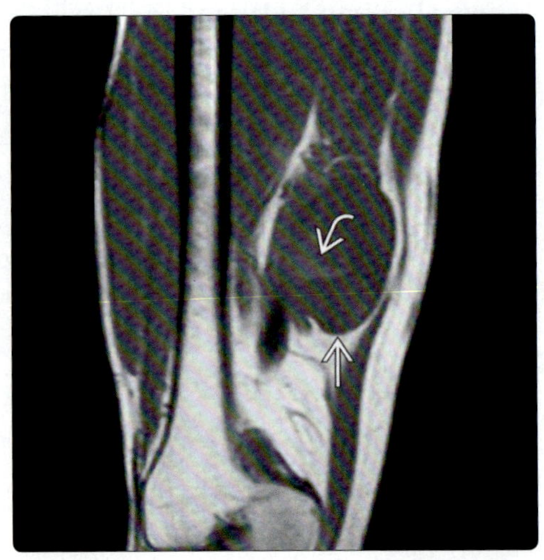

(Left) *Axial T1WI C+ FS MR in the same patient shows prominent enhancement of the mass ➡. The myxoid ➡ and fatty ➡ tissue show enhancement. An area of hypoenhancement ➡ may represent complex fluid, hemorrhage, or necrosis.* **(Right)** *Coronal T1WI MR shows an oval, low signal mass ➡ in the distal thigh, with a small region of high signal suggesting lipomatous tissue ➡. Myxoid liposarcomas usually contain < 25% fat, as in this case.*

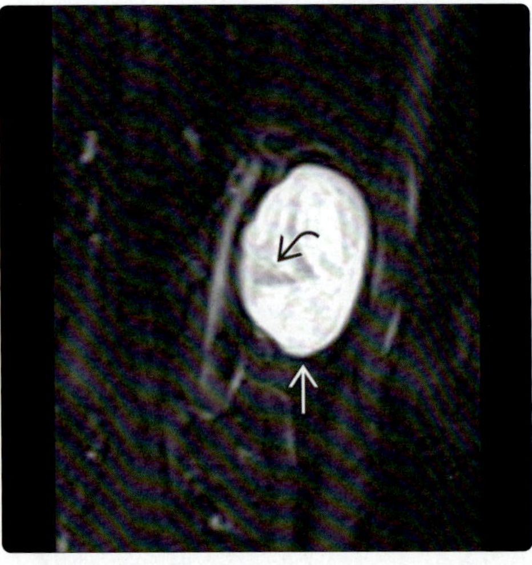

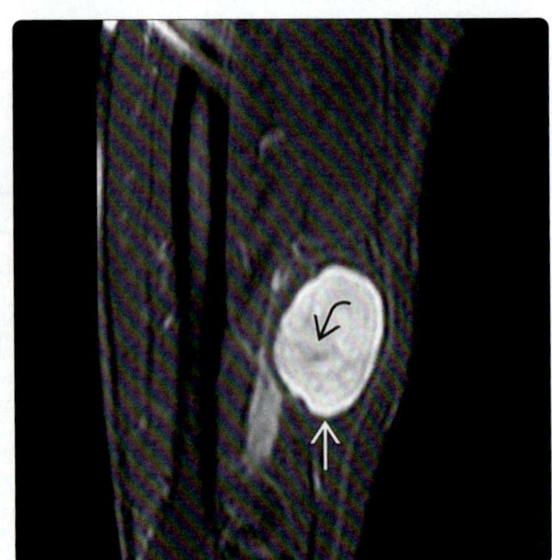

(Left) *Coronal STIR MR in the same patient shows the majority of the lesion ➡ to be high signal, but the regions of fat are now low signal ➡.* **(Right)** *Coronal T1WI C+ FS MR in the same patient shows diffuse enhancement of the posterior thigh mass ➡. The enhancement is intense, involving most of the lesion. The small area of fat ➡ shows less intense enhancement. Prominent enhancement has been shown to reflect a worse clinical prognosis.*

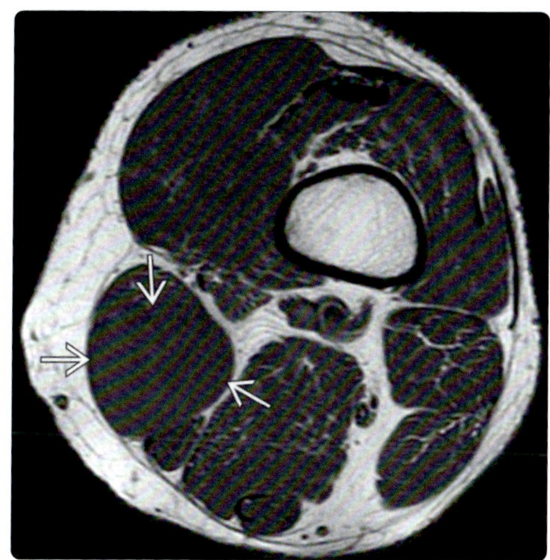

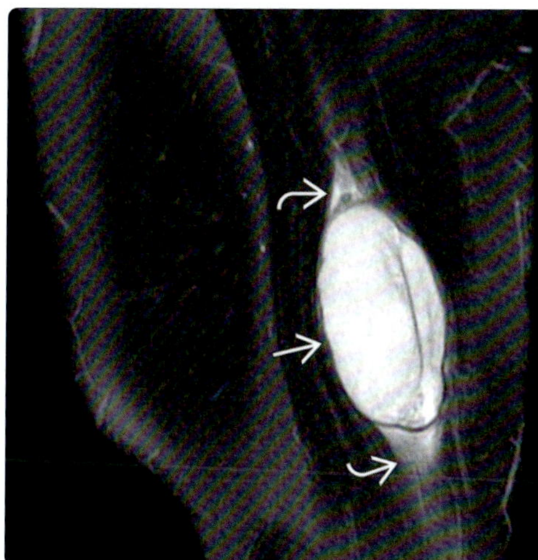

(Left) *Axial T1MR shows an intramuscular mass ➡ in a 44-year-old man that is isointense with skeletal muscle. There is no high signal within the mass to suggest adipose tissue.* **(Right)** *Sagittal T2FS MR in the same patient shows the lesion ➡ to be hyperintense, appearing myxoid, and containing thin septa. There are tails of material extending from the lesion ↪. The lack of fat and presence of these tails are typical of intramuscular myxoma, making this the leading diagnostic consideration.*

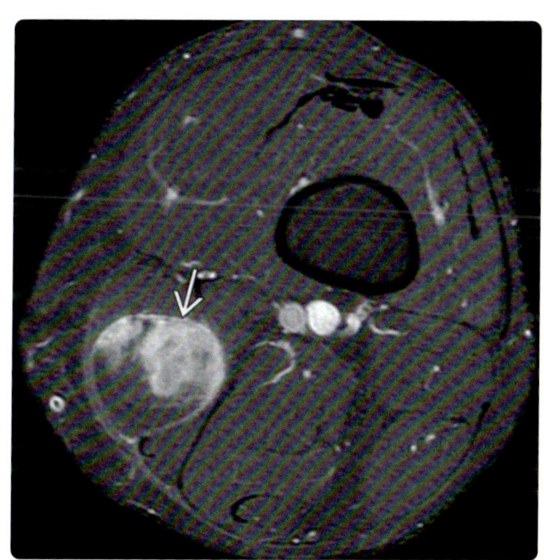

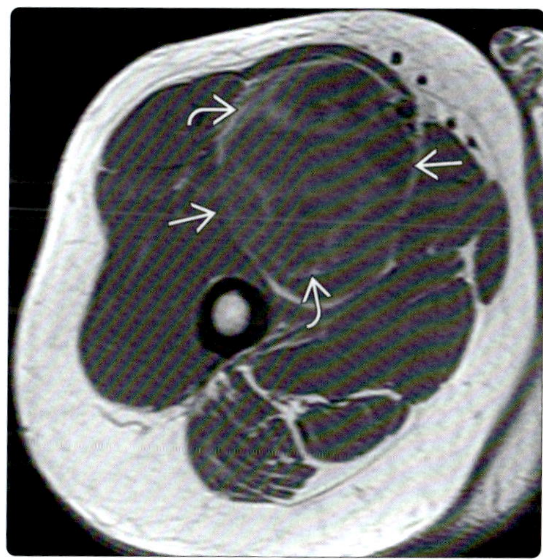

(Left) *Axial postcontrast T1FS MR in the same patient shows significant enhancement ➡, greater than expected in myxoma. Biopsy proved the lesion to be myxoid liposarcoma; it is worth remembering that this lesion need not show significant fat on imaging.* **(Right)** *Axial T1MR of the thigh in a 32-year-old man shows small amounts of hyperintensity suggesting fat ↪ within a lesion ➡ that is predominantly isointense with muscle.*

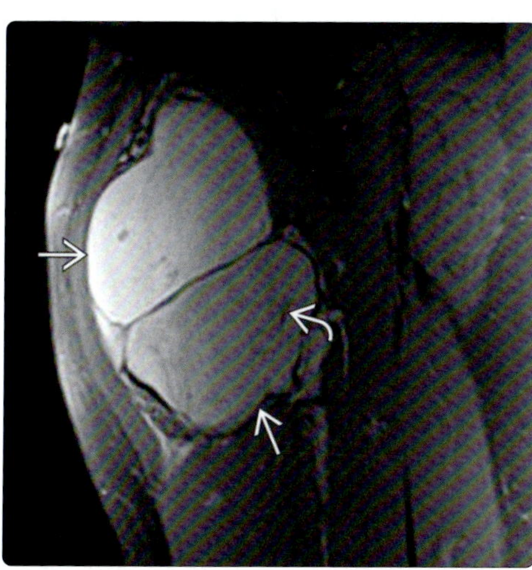

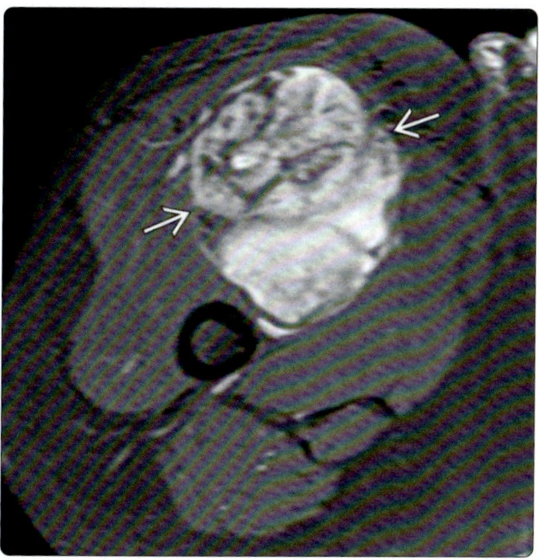

(Left) *Sagittal PDFS MR in the same patient shows heterogeneous hyperintensity of the lesion ➡ with small regions of hypointensity suggesting fat ↪. The more proximal portion of the lesion has a myxoid appearance.* **(Right)** *Axial postcontrast T1FS MR in the same patient shows heterogeneous enhancement of the lesion ➡. At biopsy the lesion proved to be a myxoid liposarcoma. There were prominent round cell components, which leads to a worse prognosis.*

Pleomorphic Liposarcoma

KEY FACTS

TERMINOLOGY

- High-grade sarcoma having variable number of pleomorphic lipoblasts
  - Rarest subtype (~ 5-10% of liposarcomas)

IMAGING

- Most arise in deep soft tissues of extremities or retroperitoneum
- Median diameter > 10 cm
- Contains < 25% fat tissue
- Markedly heterogeneous signal intensity
  - Isointense to muscle with small regions of hyperintense fat or hemorrhage on T1WI
  - Heterogeneous high signal intensity on fluid-sensitive sequences
- Contrast enhancement present but variable due to proportion of myxoid tissue and necrosis

CLINICAL ISSUES

- Painless, firm, enlarging mass
  - Pain in ~ 15% of patients
- 5th decade of life and above
- No sex predilection
- Metastatic rate: 30-50%
  - Metastatic disease most commonly to lung
- 5-year survival rate: 40-65%
  - Aggressive clinical course
  - Worse outcome predicted by older patient age, large tumor size, and deep location
  - Superficial lesions have better prognosis
- Chemotherapy, radiotherapy, and surgical excision
  - Local recurrence extremely high with retroperitoneal tumors
  - Local recurrence in 25-43% of extremity liposarcomas overall

(Left) *Axial CECT shows a large, heterogeneously enhancing mass ➔ in the adductor compartment of the proximal left thigh. An unrelated simple, benign intramuscular lipoma ➔ is located within the left vastus lateralis muscle.* **(Right)** *Axial T2WI FS MR in the same patient shows the pleomorphic liposarcoma ➔ and the benign intramuscular lipoma ➔. The liposarcoma has markedly heterogeneous signal intensity. Only a few small areas had signal intensity similar to subcutaneous fat.*

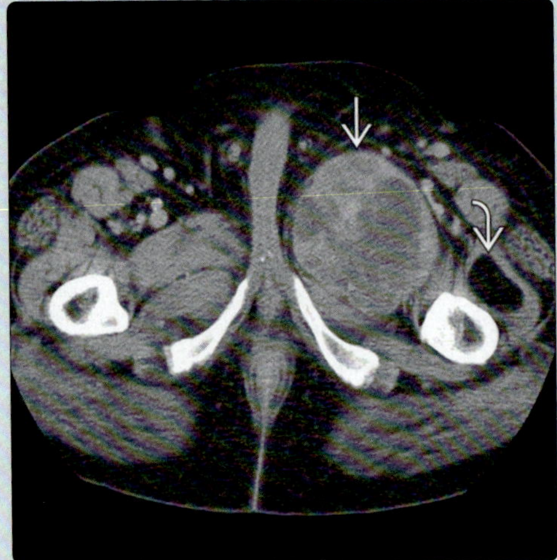

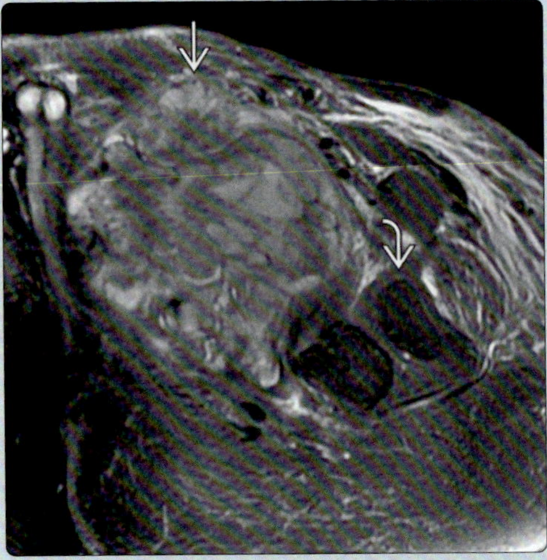

(Left) *Coronal T1WI MR demonstrates a well-defined oval mass ➔ in the posterior thigh. The mass is predominantly isointense to muscle with a small area of increased signal suggesting hemorrhage ➔, which is common in pleomorphic liposarcoma.* **(Right)** *Coronal STIR MR shows the mass ➔ to have heterogeneous high signal that approaches fluid signal intensity in some regions. There were no convincing regions of mature fat, as is typically seen with other liposarcoma subtypes.*

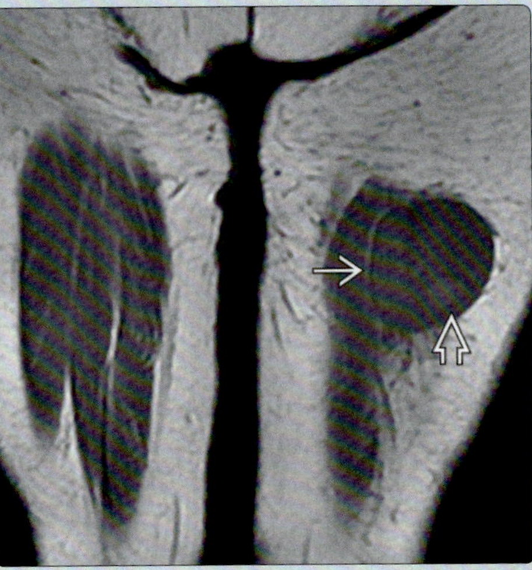

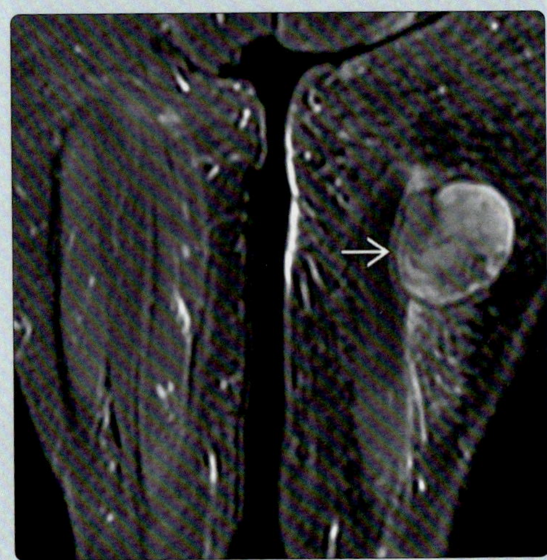

KEY FACTS

TERMINOLOGY

- Malignant fatty tumor with dedifferentiation from well-differentiated liposarcoma to nonlipogenic sarcoma

IMAGING

- Retroperitoneum > deep extremities (3:1)
  - < 20% in spermatic cord, head, neck, and trunk
- Nonspecific soft tissue mass on radiographs
- CT shows bimorphic mass containing areas of complex fatty tissue and nonfatty solid tissue
- Complex, predominantly fat-attenuation mass on MR containing variable septa and nodularity
  - Additional area of mass without lipomatous foci

PATHOLOGY

- Histologic areas of atypical lipomatous tumor/well-differentiated liposarcoma + areas of histologically different sarcoma
  - Undifferentiated pleomorphic sarcoma or fibrosarcoma in 90%
  - Low- or high-grade dedifferentiated region
- Dedifferentiated areas often contain necrosis

CLINICAL ISSUES

- Large painless mass
  - Recent change in longstanding mass
- Peak incidence in 7th decade
- Dedifferentiation occurs 7-8 years after presentation
  - 5% risk of dedifferentiation for extremity tumors
  - 15% risk of dedifferentiation for retroperitoneum
- Less aggressive clinical course compared to high-grade pleomorphic sarcoma
  - 40% have local recurrence
  - 15-20% have metastases
  - 28-30% mortality at 5-year follow-up
- Retroperitoneal tumors have worst prognosis

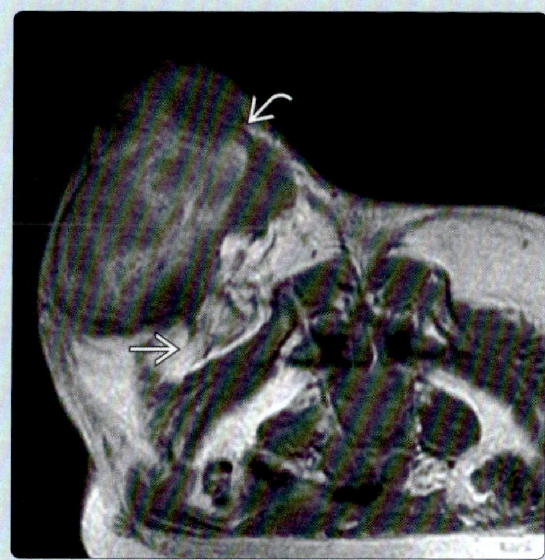

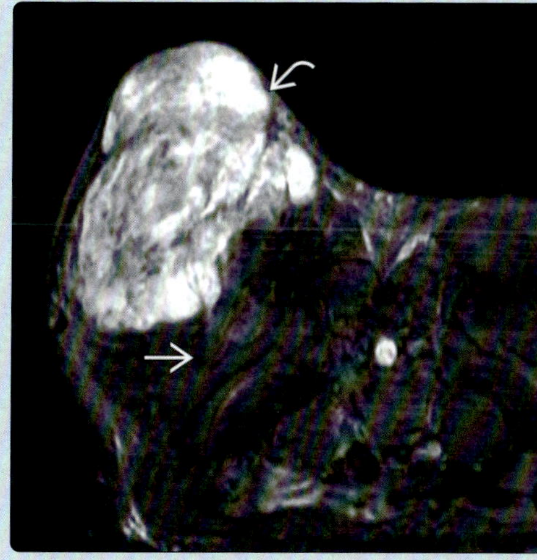

(Left) *Axial T1WI MR shows a heterogeneous mass lying both deep ➡ and superficial ↗ in the gluteal region, which appeared to arise deep to the gluteus maximus muscle. Increased complexity of the superficial component suggests that it is a higher grade sarcoma.* **(Right)** *Axial T2WI FS MR in the same patient shows the bimorphic character of the lesion with differing appearances to the deep ➡ and superficial ↗ portions. The deep component has a more typical appearance for liposarcoma.*

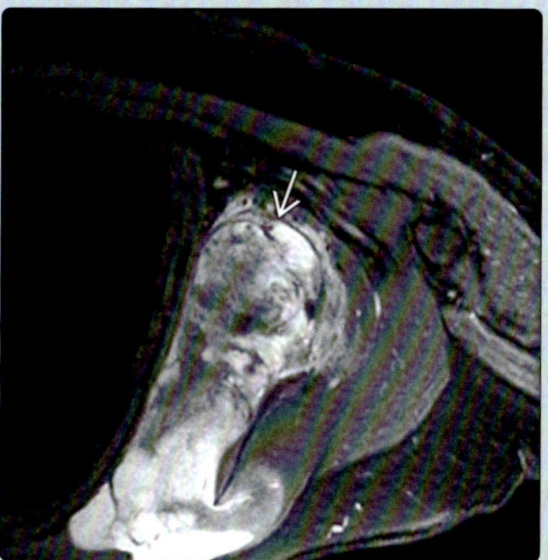

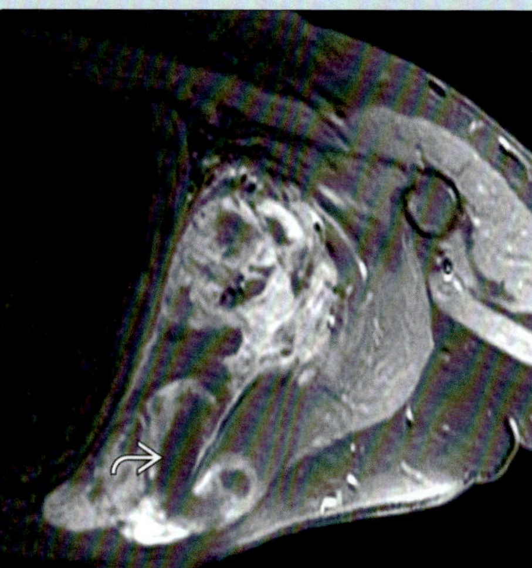

(Left) *Axial T2WI FS MR shows a large, aggressive-appearing mass ➡ lying between the scapula and lateral ribs and replacing most of the the subscapularis muscle. The mass has markedly heterogeneous signal intensity ranging from high to low.* **(Right)** *Axial T1WI C+ FS MR in the same patient shows irregular regions of solid enhancement with interspersed areas of hypo- and absent enhancement ↪. The regions of absent enhancement likely represent areas of necrosis in this dedifferentiated liposarcoma.*

Nodular and Proliferative Fasciitis

KEY FACTS

TERMINOLOGY

- Mass-forming fibrous proliferation
- Most common benign tumor mistaken for sarcoma

IMAGING

- Nodular fasciitis location
  - Upper extremity > thigh > head/neck > chest wall, back
  - Most common in volar aspect of forearm
- Proliferative fasciitis location
  - Upper extremity > lower extremity > trunk
- Predominantly subcutaneous location
- Borders of mass may be well defined or infiltrative
  - Subcutaneous type
    - Well-circumscribed round nodule attached to fascia extending into superficial fat
  - Fascial type
    - Poorly circumscribed fascial mass with stellate growth pattern
  - Intramuscular type
    - Round to ovoid intramuscular mass attached to fascia ± infiltrative borders
- CT shows nonspecific mass ~ density to muscle
  - Myxoid lesions: ↓ attenuation than muscle
- MR appearance
  - T1WI: Similar intensity to skeletal muscle
  - T2WI: Intermediate to high signal intensity
  - Mild surrounding edema
  - Enhancement varies with content of lesion
- Ossification and calcification rare (ossifying fasciitis)
- Extension of mass along fascia suggests diagnosis

CLINICAL ISSUES

- Tender mass, rapidly growing over 1-2 weeks
- Most commonly seen during adulthood
- May spontaneously resolve
- Surgical excision usually curative
  - Local recurrence < 2% after incomplete excision

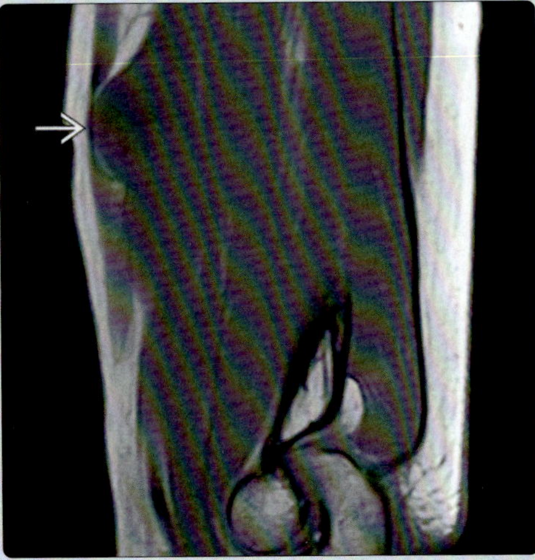
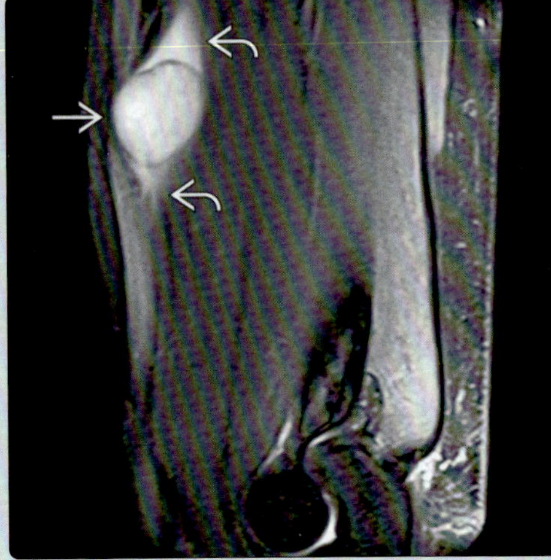

(Left) *Sagittal T1WI MR of nodular fasciitis shows a mass ➡ in the distal aspect of the upper arm lying between the biceps and brachialis muscles. The mass is slightly hypointense to muscle.* **(Right)** *Sagittal T2WI FS MR in the same patient shows the mass ➡ to be hyperintense to skeletal muscle. Flame-shaped regions of high signal ↩ lie along the proximal and distal borders of the mass. Differential diagnosis includes a benign peripheral nerve sheath tumor, myxoma, or less likely, a sarcoma.*

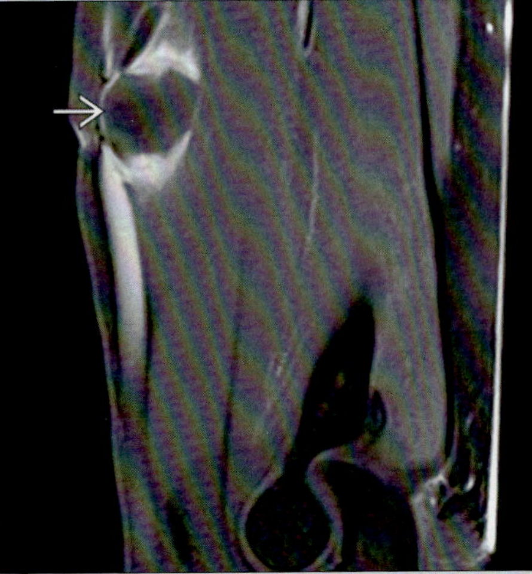
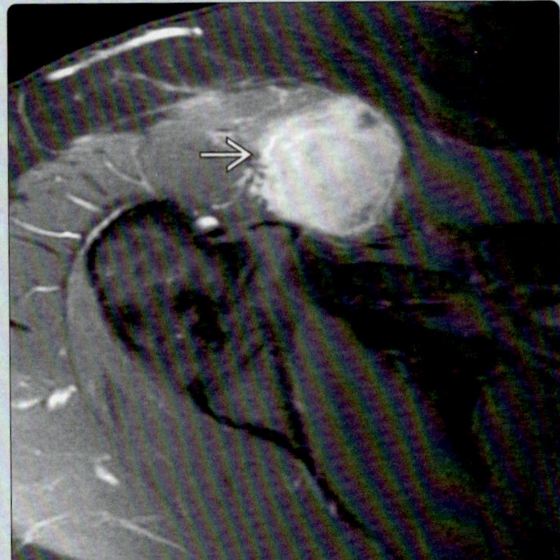

(Left) *Sagittal T1WI C+ FS MR in the same patient shows the enhancement of the mass ➡ to be predominantly peripheral, with mild heterogeneous central enhancement. Enhancement characteristics of these lesions are quite variable based on the cellular content.* **(Right)** *Axial PD FS MR shows a large, heterogeneous mass with infiltrative margins ➡ that could easily be mistaken for a malignant process. The mass location, at the intersection of muscle and fascia, suggests the diagnosis of nodular fasciitis.*

KEY FACTS

TERMINOLOGY

- Bizarre parosteal osteochondromatous proliferation
- Synonym: Nora lesion
- Disordered mass of bone, cartilage, and fibrous tissue
  - May be part of continuum from fibroosseous pseudotumor of digits to acquired osteochondroma

IMAGING

- Mineralized mass on bone surface without marrow continuity
  - Hands (55%), long bones (27%), feet (15%)
- Radiographs and CT are helpful to delineate mass morphology and mineralization
  - MR has somewhat nonspecific appearance
- Radiographs show pedunculated or sessile mass
  - ± cleavage plane between mass and bone cortex
  - Lacks periosteal reaction
- CT best defines ossified mass
  - Cortex and medullary space from mass and from underlying bone are discontinuous
- Nonspecific MR appearance
  - Variable signal on T1WI
  - High signal on fluid-sensitive sequences
  - Mild, heterogeneous enhancement
  - ± edema in marrow and surrounding soft tissues

TOP DIFFERENTIAL DIAGNOSES

- Fibroosseous pseudotumor of digits
  - Similar pathologic process
  - Can lack ossification
- Myositis ossificans
  - Circumscribed, ossified soft tissue mass
  - Matures from peripheral to central
  - Usually involves large muscles
- Periosteal chondroma
  - Surface lesion with chondroid matrix
  - May cause cortical scalloping
- Osteochondroma
  - Medullary space and bone cortex flow from underlying bone into ossified mass
  - Apex of lesion is oriented away from physis
  - Has cartilage cap
- Parosteal osteosarcoma
  - Would be very rare in hand

PATHOLOGY

- May be related to trauma
- Similar gross appearance to osteochondroma
- Histologic findings
  - Bizarre and binucleate chondrocytes
  - Irregular bone-cartilage interface
  - Marked proliferative activity
  - May have cartilaginous cap
- Benign but may be misinterpreted as malignant

CLINICAL ISSUES

- Mildly painful mass
  - Grows over weeks to months
  - ± history of trauma
- Mean patient age in 4th decade
  - Also seen in children and older adults
- No gender predominance
- Local recurrence in up to 58%
- Treatment = surgical excision

DIAGNOSTIC CHECKLIST

- Radiographs and CT are more helpful than MR
  - Cortical or marrow continuity between bone and lesion should suggest osteochondroma
- Consider other entities in differential diagnosis
- Histologic examination is often needed
  - If malignancy is suggested on histology, confirm that imaging findings were shared with pathologist, and consider subspecialty 2nd opinion before definitive therapy

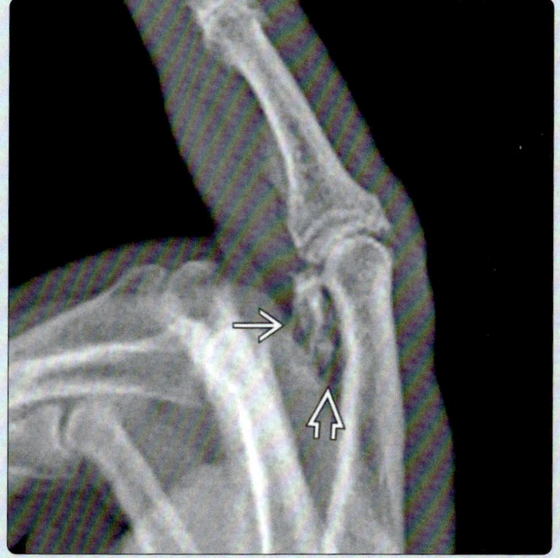

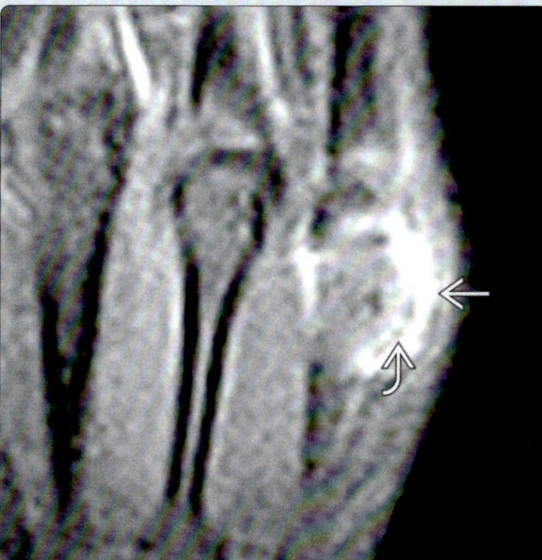

(Left) *Lateral radiograph shows an ossified mass ➡ lying along the volar aspect of the index finger proximal phalanx. There is a partial cleavage plane ⇨ between the mass and the underlying bone cortex.* **(Right)** *Coronal STIR MR demonstrates a mass ➡ with high signal intensity partially surrounding the distal 5th metacarpal. A surface-based lesion ⮫ is subtly visible on this sequence. The overall appearance is entirely nonspecific and could be related to neoplasm, infection, or trauma.*

Elastofibroma

KEY FACTS

TERMINOLOGY

- Benign fibroelastic tumor-like lesion primarily arising between scapula and chest wall

IMAGING

- Morphology: Crescentic or lenticular fibrous mass with entrapped regions of linear fat
- Location: Between lower scapula and chest wall in 95%
  - Deep to latissimus dorsi and rhomboid major
- CT and MR are equally diagnostic
- Bone erosion is exceedingly rare
- Well-defined to ill-defined borders
- CT attenuation of mass is similar to muscle with interspersed streaks of low-attenuation fat
- MR appearance
  - T1WI: Intermediate signal intensity of collagen and elastic fibers + high signal fat
  - T2WI: Intermediate to high signal intensity of collagen and elastic fibers + high signal fat
    - Fat suppression: Low signal lipomatous regions
  - Heterogeneous enhancement
- Ultrasound: Echogenic background with curvilinear hypoechoic strands
  - No significant blood flow on Doppler

PATHOLOGY

- Reactive lesion that is not neoplastic
- Likely due to mechanical friction between scapula and chest wall

CLINICAL ISSUES

- Usually painless, slowly growing mass
  - Bilateral in 10-60%
- Peak: 7th-8th decades
  - Female predominance
- No malignant transformation
- Treatment: Surgical excision if symptomatic
  - < 10% with local recurrence

(Left) *Axial graphic just distal to the tip of the scapula shows an elastofibroma ➡. The crescentic mass is composed of linear and curvilinear fibrous tissue with interspersed fat. The mass is located deep to the chest wall musculature ➡.* **(Right)** *Axial T1WI MR demonstrates a chest wall mass ➡ that is nearly isointense to muscle. This is in a classic location for an elastofibroma, between the lower tip of the scapula ➡ and the rib cage. The mass contains small foci of high signal fat ➡.*

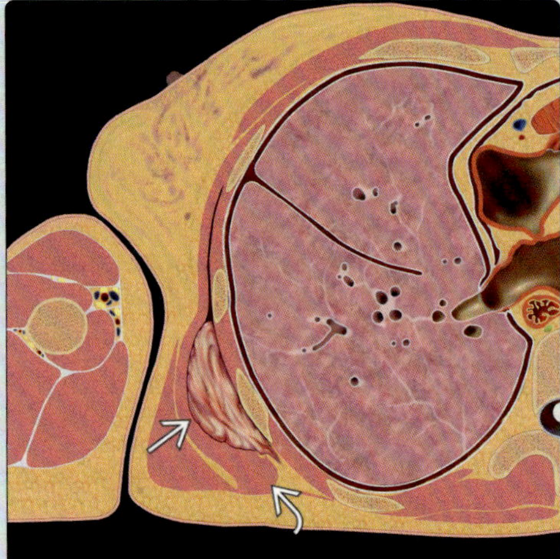

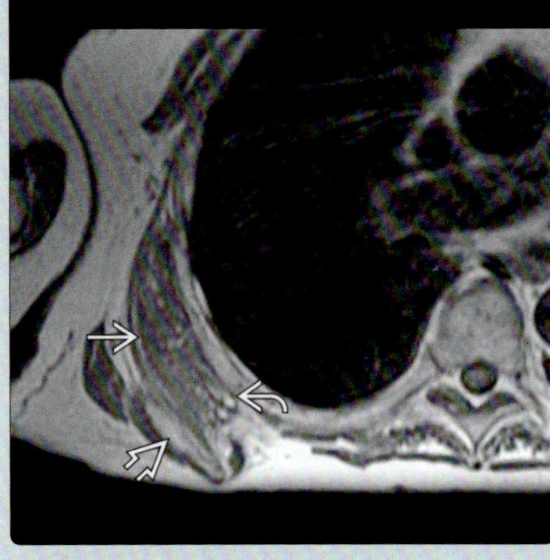

(Left) *Axial T2WI MR in the same patient demonstrates the chest wall mass ➡ to again be isointense to muscle. The small regions of fat ➡ and fat within the lower tip of the scapula ➡ have similar intensity to the subcutaneous fat.* **(Right)** *Coronal T1WI MR in the same patient demonstrates the elastofibroma ➡ to have a crescentic shape. The adjacent bone and soft tissues are normal, with the exception of mass effect ➡. There is no surrounding edema.*

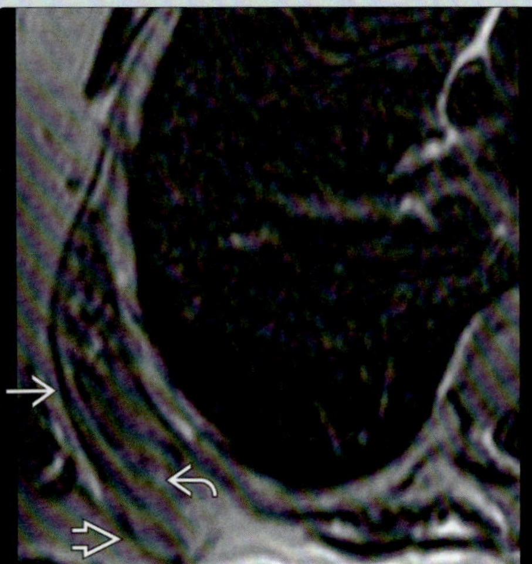

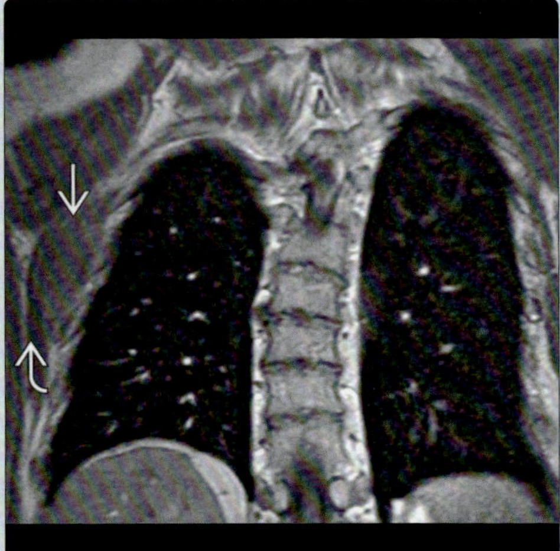

TERMINOLOGY

Synonyms

- Elastofibroma dorsi

Definitions

- Benign fibroelastic tumor-like lesion primarily arising between scapula and chest wall

IMAGING

General Features

- Best diagnostic clue
  - Crescentic soft tissue mass containing fat
- Location
  - Between lower scapula and chest wall in 95%
    - Deep to latissimus dorsi and rhomboid major muscles
    - Attached to periosteum and ligaments of ribs 6-8
  - Elbow 2nd most common location
  - Bilateral in 10-60%
- Size
  - 2-15 cm in diameter
    - Reported up to 20 cm
- Morphology
  - Crescentic, lenticular, or spherical mass

Nuclear Medicine Findings

- Mild to moderate uptake of 18F-FDG on PET/CT

Imaging Recommendations

- Best imaging tool
  - CT and MR are equally diagnostic

Radiographic Findings

- Bone erosion is exceedingly rare

CT Findings

- Attenuation of mass is similar to muscle with interspersed streaks of low-attenuation fat
- May be incidentally found on chest CT

MR Findings

- T1WI: Intermediate signal intensity of collagen and elastic fibers + high signal fat
- T2WI: Low to mildly increased signal intensity of collagen and elastic fibers + high signal fat
- Fat suppression causes lipomatous regions to have low signal
- Mild heterogeneous enhancement

Ultrasonographic Findings

- Echogenic background with curvilinear hypoechoic strands
- No significant blood flow on Doppler
- Well-defined to ill-defined borders

DIFFERENTIAL DIAGNOSIS

Liposarcoma, Soft Tissue

- Fat containing soft tissue mass
- Location around scapular tip is uncommon
- Variable myxoid or necrotic regions
- May have areas of intense enhancement

PATHOLOGY

General Features

- Etiology
  - Reactive lesion that is not neoplastic
  - Likely due to mechanical friction between scapula and chest wall
  - Abnormal development of elastic fibers rather than degeneration of existing tissue
- Genetics
  - Possible genetic predisposition

Gross Pathologic & Surgical Features

- Ill-defined, rubbery, gray-white mass of fibrous tissue with entrapped yellow fat

Microscopic Features

- Paucicellular collagenous tissue and elastic fibers
  - Entrapped mature fat + mucoid stroma
  - Occasional fibroblasts
- Positive elastic stains show central dense core with branched and unbranched fibers

CLINICAL ISSUES

Presentation

- Most common signs/symptoms
  - Painless, slowly growing mass
- Other signs/symptoms
  - 25% have decreased range of motion
  - 10% have pain
  - Rare scapular snapping

Demographics

- Age
  - Peak: 7th-8th decades
  - Rarely reported in children
- Gender
  - Female predominance
- Epidemiology
  - 11-24% of elderly patients (autopsy series)

Natural History & Prognosis

- < 10% with local recurrence
  - May have been incompletely excised
- No malignant transformation

Treatment

- Surgical excision if symptomatic

SELECTED REFERENCES

1. Fang N et al: Characteristics of elastofibroma dorsi on PET/CT imaging with ^{18}F-FDG. Clin Imaging. ePub, 2015
2. Kakudo N et al: Elastofibroma dorsi: a case report with an immunohistochemical and ultrastructural studies. Med Mol Morphol. ePub, 2015
3. Clinckemaillie G et al: Bilateral elastofibroma dorsi: typical CT and MRI features. JBR-BTR. 97(1):45, 2014
4. Tambasco D et al: Elastofibroma: management and surgical outcome. Ann Ital Chir. 85(ePub), 2014
5. Kransdorf MJ et al: Benign fibrous and fibrohistiocytic tumors. In Kransdorf MJ et al: Imaging of Soft Tissue Tumors. 2nd ed. Philadelphia: Lippincott Williams & Wilkins.196-203, 2006

(Left) *Axial T1WI MR of the posterosuperior right chest wall demonstrates a mass ➡ lying between the deep margin of the rhomboid muscle and the chest wall that has a classic striated appearance with mixed fat intensity ➡ and fibrous elements.* **(Right)** *Axial T1WI C+ FS MR shows the mass ➡ to have heterogeneous enhancement of the fibrous portions of the mass. Enhancement is usually mild. Areas of fat have low signal intensity, as does the subcutaneous fat.*

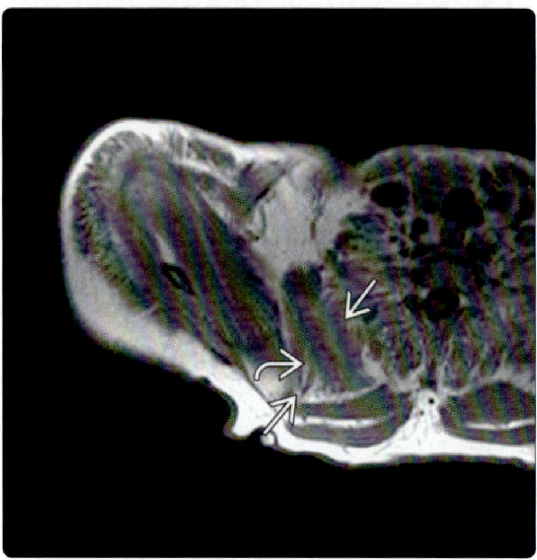

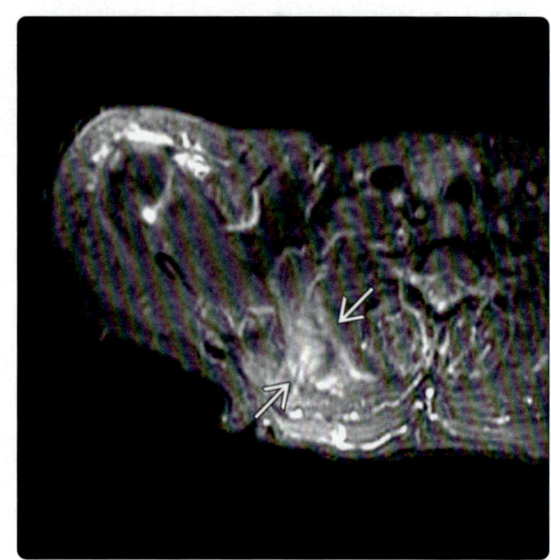

(Left) *Coronal T1WI MR in the same patient demonstrates the striated pattern of the elastofibroma ➡. These masses usually have a predominance of fibrous tissue with a small amount of fat ➡.* **(Right)** *Coronal STIR MR shows the mass ➡ to have mixed low to intermediate signal and high signal intensity. Some elastofibromas have low signal overall on fluid-sensitive, fat-suppressed sequences. This location is slightly higher than is normally seen.*

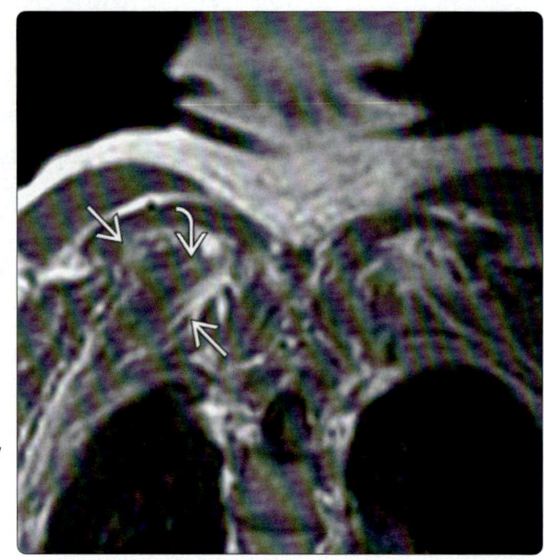

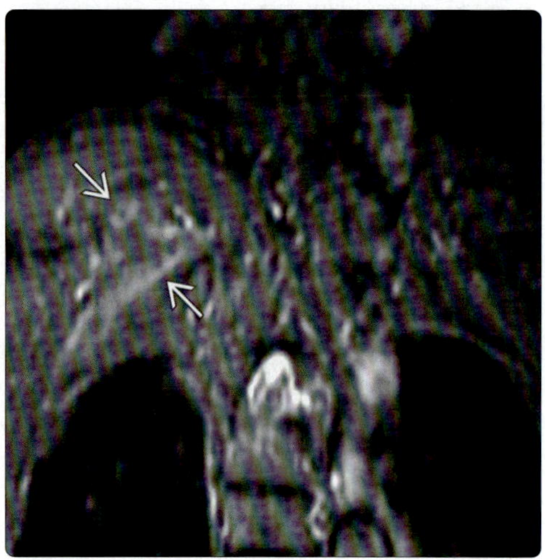

(Left) *Coronal T1WI MR shows a striated mass ➡ in the posterolateral chest wall. The mass is isointense to muscle with areas of interspersed fat. The mass is partially ill-defined and appears contiguous with the intercostal muscles.* **(Right)** *Coronal T2WI MR in the same patient shows the nonadipose portions of the mass ➡ to be isointense to muscle. The fatty regions ➡ remain high signal, similar to the subcutaneous fat since this sequence is not fat suppressed.*

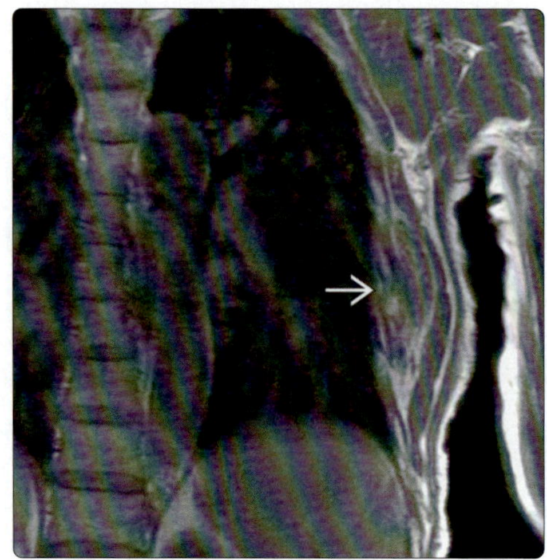

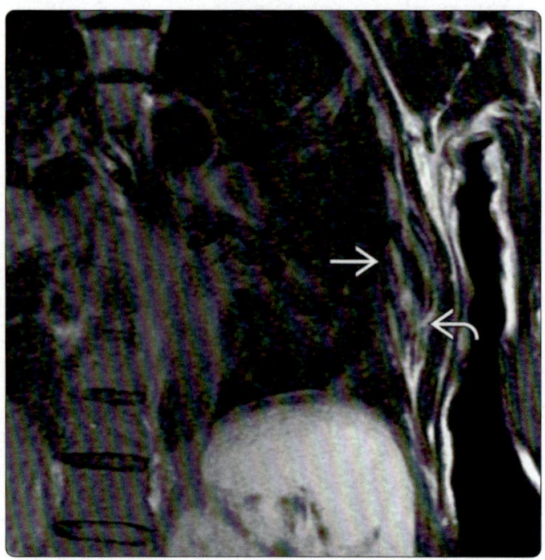

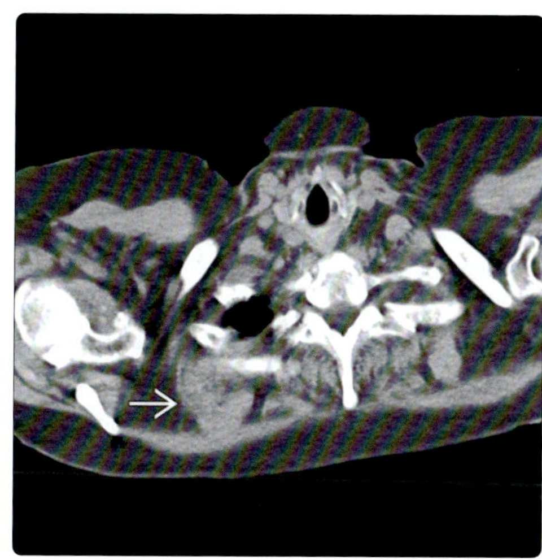

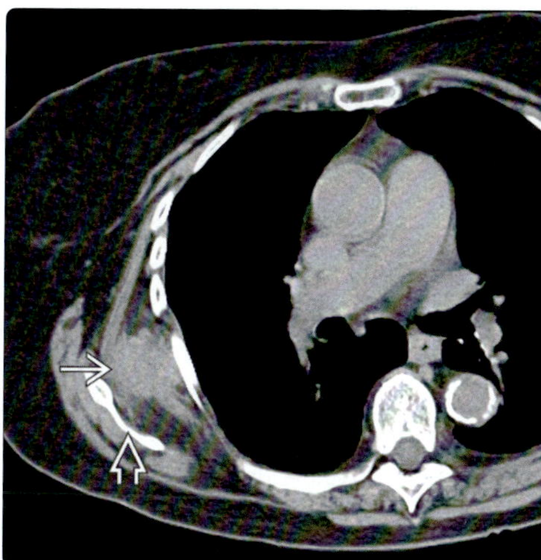

(Left) *Axial bone CT through the upper chest shows a mass ➡ against the posterior chest wall. Note the asymmetry with the opposite chest wall. The attenuation of the mass is similar to muscle with small foci of fat.* **(Right)** *Axial bone CT shows a mass ➡ between the scapula ➡ and ribs. The mass has relatively homogeneous central attenuation similar to muscle. Ill-defined borders and a spherical shape could raise the question of a sarcoma, but this typical location still favors an elastofibroma.*

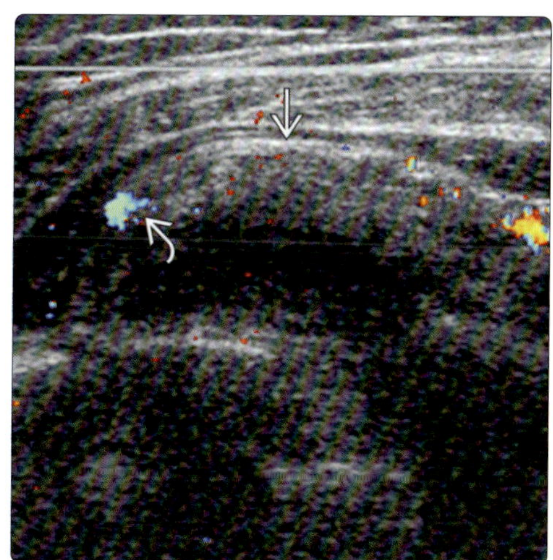

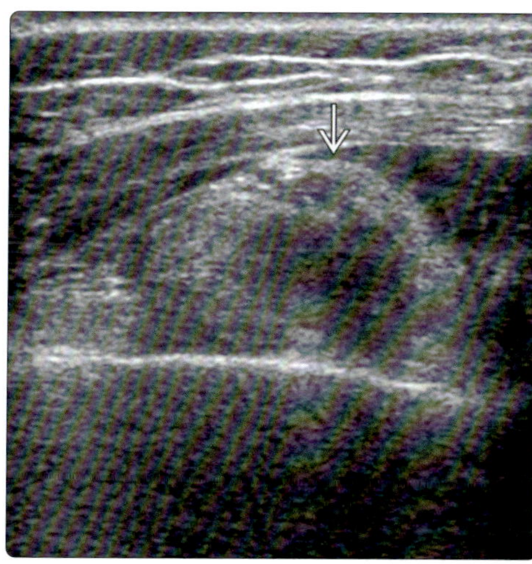

(Left) *Longitudinal Doppler ultrasound of the posterior chest wall shows a mass ➡ with a heterogeneous echotexture. This biopsy-proven elastofibroma shows internal blood flow ➡, which is uncommon.* **(Right)** *Transverse ultrasound in the same patient shows the elastofibroma ➡ to have hypoechoic regions superimposed on the hyperechoic mass. If this lesion had a more typical appearance, the hypoechoic regions would have a more curvilinear contour.*

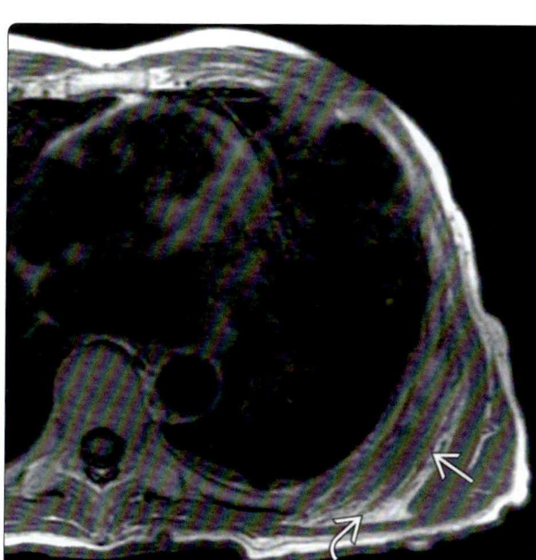

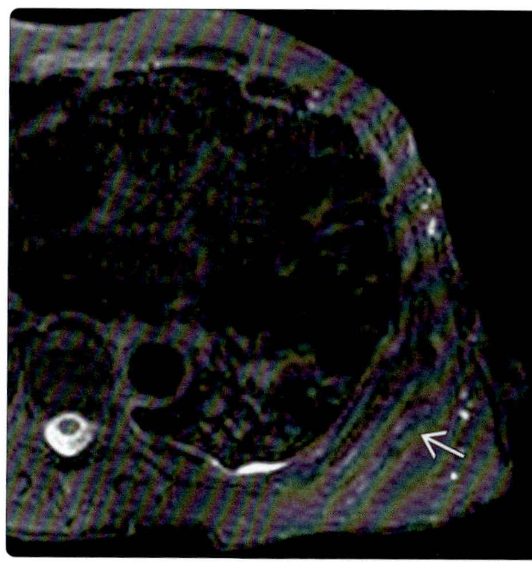

(Left) *Axial T1WI MR of a classic elastofibroma ➡ shows a crescentic mass of mixed linear isointense ➡ and hyperintense signal, corresponding to fibrous and fat tissue respectively, located in the posterolateral chest wall of an elderly patient.* **(Right)** *Axial T2WI FS MR in the same patient shows the mass ➡ to be almost indistinguishable, due to low signal of the fibrous tissue and low fat signal from fat suppression. Variable signal on fluid-sensitive sequences is normal.*

Fibrous Hamartoma of Infancy

KEY FACTS

TERMINOLOGY

- Subdermal fibromatous tumor of infancy
- Benign soft tissue mass in infant composed of fibrocollagenous tissue, primitive mesenchymal cells, and mature fat

IMAGING

- Rapidly growing, subcutaneous mass in soft tissues adjacent to shoulder in infant
- Axilla > upper arm, shoulder > neck, thigh, back, forearm
  - Reported in perineal and inguinal regions
  - Rare in hands and feet
- Usually < 5 cm
  - Rarely > 10 cm
- Radiographs are normal or show soft tissue fullness
  - No calcification or other matrix
- Nonspecific soft tissue mass on CT
  - Usually infiltrative
- MR reveals soft tissue mass containing variable amount of fat
  - Remainder of mass is isointense to hypointense relative to skeletal muscle on both T1WI and T2WI MR sequences
  - May show organized arrangement of fat interspersed among heterogeneous soft tissue bands composed of mesenchymal and fibrous tissue
    - Mirrors histology; if present, fairly diagnostic
- US: Heterogeneously hyperechoic mass with serpentine pattern and ill-defined or lobulated margin

TOP DIFFERENTIAL DIAGNOSES

- Infantile fibromatosis
  - Arises in muscle rather than subcutis
  - Lacks organoid histologic pattern
- Diffuse myofibromatosis
  - Nodular or multinodular
  - Contains hemangiopericytoma-like vascular areas
- Calcifying aponeurotic fibroma
  - Occurs in older children
  - Typical location in palm of hand or sole of foot
  - Similar histologic pattern early, before calcifications develop
- Infantile fibrosarcoma
  - Cytologic atypia
- Embryonal rhabdomyosarcoma, spindle cell variant
  - Both may occur in scrotal region
  - Occurs in older children
  - Cytologic atypia

PATHOLOGY

- Hamartomatous lesion likely, but reparative process has been suggested
  - No increased familial incidence
  - No malignant transformation
- 3 classic histologic components in typical organoid pattern
  - Dense fibrocollagenous tissue composed of spindle-shaped cells
  - Primitive mesenchymal cells in myxoid matrix with delicate vessels
  - Mature fat, variable small to large amount

CLINICAL ISSUES

- Solitary, freely mobile subcutaneous mass
  - Rapid growth is common; may simulate malignancy
  - May be adherent to fascia
  - Rarely invades underlying muscle
- Most commonly occurs during first 2 years of life
  - Present at birth: 15-25% of cases
- Male predominance (2-3:1)
- Rare overall: 0.02% of all soft tissue tumors
  - Relatively common fibrous tumor of childhood
- Benign
  - Lacks potential for malignant degeneration
- Treatment consists of surgical excision
  - No reports of spontaneous resolution
  - Local recurrence: 10-16% of cases

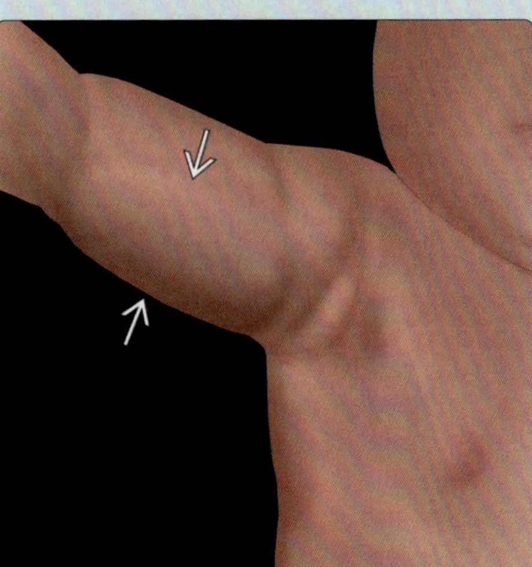

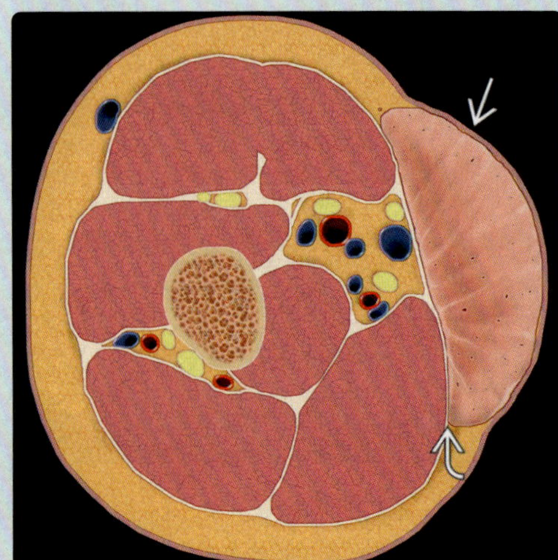

(Left) *Frontal graphic of an infant demonstrates a large, bulging mass ➡ involving the medial aspect of the upper arm. The location involving the subcutaneous tissues near the shoulder joint, most commonly the axilla or upper arm, is typical.* **(Right)** *Axial graphic of the upper arm shows a subcutaneous mass ➡ that abuts the fascia ➡. Invasion of the underlying musculature is rare. The rapid growth of these lesions can be clinically alarming.*

KEY FACTS

TERMINOLOGY

- Most common fibrous tumor of infancy, comprised of contractile myoid cells surrounding thin-walled blood vessels
  - Solitary lesion = myofibroma
  - Multicentric lesions = myofibromatosis

IMAGING

- ~ 50% of solitary lesions are in cutaneous or subcutaneous tissues
  - Head and neck > lower extremity, upper extremity
- Lesions also involve muscle, aponeurosis, viscera, and bone
  - Osseous lesions may be primary or related to soft tissue lesions
    - Soft tissue lesions can erode into bone
    - Long bones and skull most common primary osseous locations
- Involved viscera = lungs, heart, gastrointestinal tract, liver, kidney, pancreas, central nervous system
- Wide variety of sizes with average being 2.5 cm
- Radiographs may be normal or show soft tissue mass with calcifications
  - Bone involvement typically consists of eccentric, elongated, metaphyseal lucent lesions
  - Region of bone immediately adjacent to physis often not involved
  - Mature lesions have central calcification and well-defined sclerotic border
  - Early lesions may show periosteal reaction or cortical erosion
  - Presence of multiple scattered lytic lesions in child can falsely suggest metastatic neuroblastoma
- CT shows soft tissue mass, commonly containing calcifications
  - Usually has higher attenuation than adjacent musculature
  - Borders of mass may be well defined to infiltrative
- Sonographic findings are nonspecific
- MR is imaging procedure of choice for follow-up of visceral lesions
- Normal or increased radiotracer uptake on bone scan

PATHOLOGY

- Familial predilection suggests possible autosomal dominant and recessive inheritance patterns
- Superficial lesions tend to be more well defined than deep lesions
- Commonly contain regions of necrosis, cystic change, or hemorrhage
- Plump myofibroblasts in fascicles or whorls
- Nodules or whorls of myxoid material may simulate chondroid matrix
- Blood vessels have similar appearance to hemangiopericytoma
  - Thin walls + irregular branching
- No malignant transformation

CLINICAL ISSUES

- Can occur at any age
  - Usually identified before 2 years of age
- Male predominance (2:1)
- Painless, freely mobile subcutaneous mass
  - Deep lesions may be tethered
- Skin lesions appear as red to purple nodule
- Visceral involvement causes organ-associated symptoms
- Visceral lesions, especially pulmonary lesions, have worse prognosis
  - Cardiopulmonary or gastrointestinal complications can lead to death
- May regress spontaneously
- Surgical excision is most common treatment
  - Chemotherapy or radiation may be utilized to reduce size of aggressive tumors preoperatively
  - 10% recurrence rate for solitary lesions
- Observation can be considered for nonaggressive tumors that do not involve vital organs

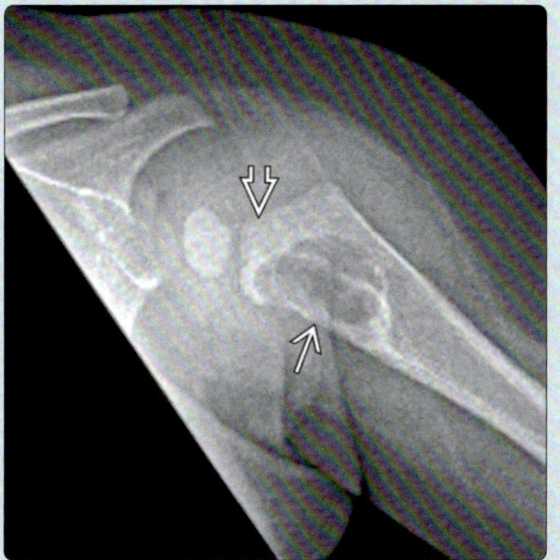

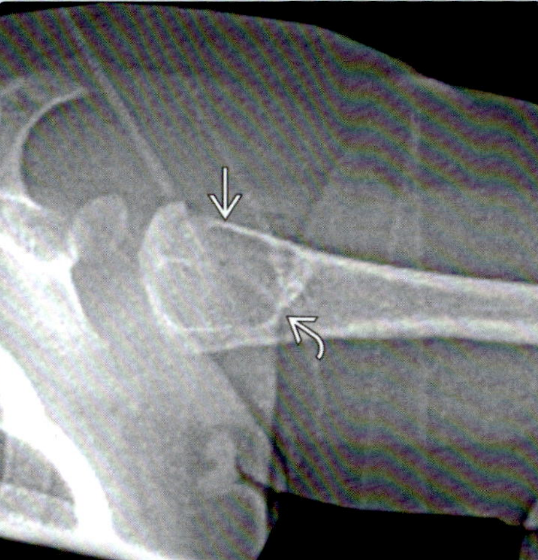

(Left) *Radiograph of the left shoulder with the arm in external rotation demonstrates a lobulated lucent lesion ➡ in the metaphysis. Sparing ➡ of the metaphyseal region immediately adjacent to the physis and an eccentric location is typical.* **(Right)** *Radiograph of the same patient with the arm internally rotated demonstrates the lobulated metaphyseal lesion ➡. The sclerotic, well-defined border ➡ is typical. Faint central calcification is difficult to appreciate without magnification.*

Fibromatosis Colli

KEY FACTS

TERMINOLOGY

- Synonyms: Congenital muscle torticollis, pseudotumor of infancy, sternocleidomastoid tumor of infancy
- Definition: Fibrous proliferation (fibromatosis) in sternocleidomastoid muscle of infant

IMAGING

- Ultrasound is imaging modality of choice
  - Shows diffusely enlarged muscle or focal mass within muscle, which can be isoechoic, hyperechoic, or hypoechoic
  - Mass moves with action of muscle
- CT shows fusiform muscle enlargement with similar attenuation to normal muscle
- MR typically shows increased signal intensity on fluid-sensitive sequences
  - Lesions with low signal intensity have been reported
  - Enhancement of lesions can inappropriately raise question of malignancy

CLINICAL ISSUES

- Firm mass in lower neck of infant
  - Lower 1/3 of sternocleidomastoid
- Scar-like reaction to trauma
  - Usually abnormal intrauterine positioning or traumatic birth
- Majority are diagnosed before 6 months of age
  - Usually presents within first 2-4 weeks of life
- Clinical presentation
  - Torticollis
  - Elevated clavicle and shoulder
  - Facial deformities
- 0.4% of all births
- 90% have normal appearance and function if treated before 1 year of age
  - Spontaneous regression in 70%
  - Conservative treatment with stretching and exercise
  - Surgical tenotomy utilized in 10-15%

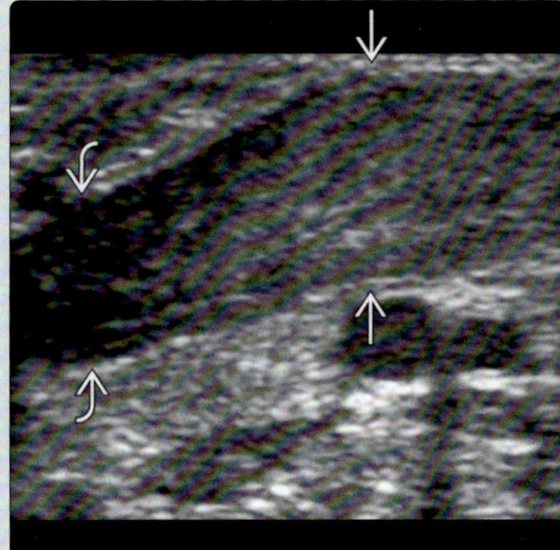

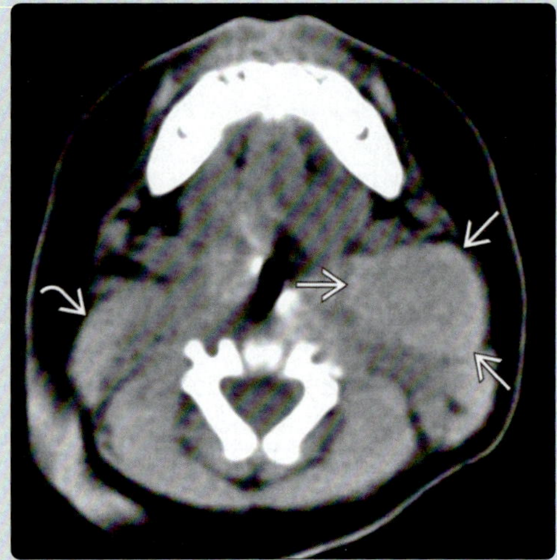

(Left) *Longitudinal oblique ultrasound of the lateral neck shows fusiform thickening ➡ of the distal sternocleidomastoid muscle with a normal appearance ➡ of the proximal aspect of the muscle.* **(Right)** *Axial NECT demonstrates fusiform enlargement of the left sternocleidomastoid muscle ➡, which has similar to slightly increased attenuation relative to the normal sternocleidomastoid muscle ➡. The mass follows the course of the muscle, without heterogeneity or calcification.*

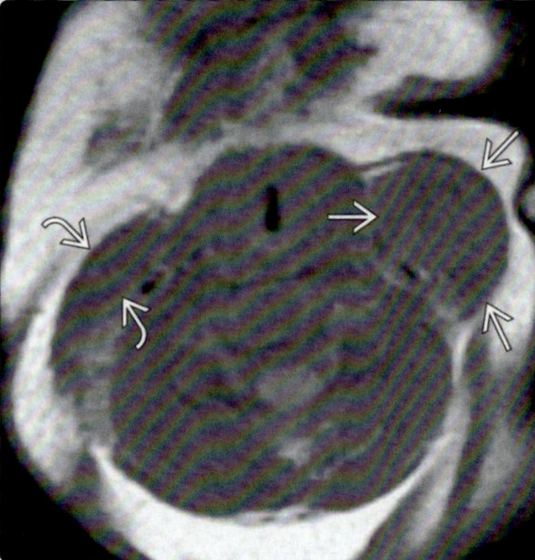

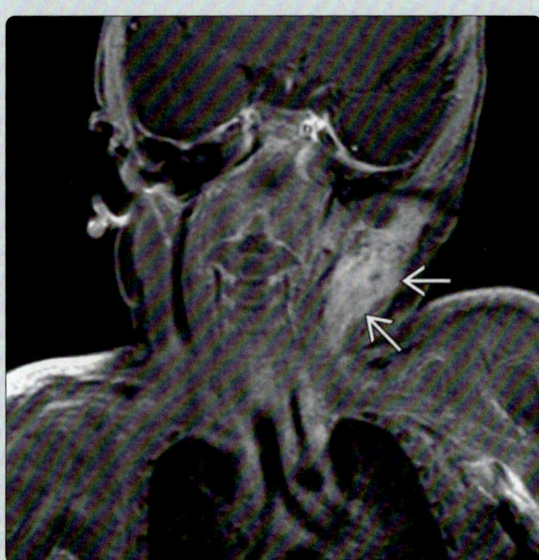

(Left) *Axial T1WI MR demonstrates fusiform enlargement of the left sternocleidomastoid muscle, corresponding to fibromatosis colli ➡, which has isointense signal relative to the normal contralateral muscle ➡.* **(Right)** *Coronal T1 C+ MR shows enlargement and heterogeneous diffuse enhancement of the left sternocleidomastoid muscle from fibromatosis colli ➡ without a discreet mass. Notice the typical finding of the head tilting to the side of the sternocleidomastoid enlargement.*

Juvenile Hyaline Fibromatosis

KEY FACTS

TERMINOLOGY

- Synonyms: Molluscum fibrosum, mesenchymal dysplasia, fibromatosis hyalinica multiplex juvenilis, puretic syndrome, systemic hyalinosis
- Definition: Rare congenital disease producing subcutaneous tumors, gingival hypertrophy, osteolytic bone lesions, and flexion joint contractures

IMAGING

- Location
  - Skin or subcutaneous papules, nodules, or masses
    - Especially face and neck
    - Soft tissue lesions may arise intraarticularly
  - 60% have multiple discrete lytic bone lesions
    - Skull
    - Long bones
    - Phalanges
      - Distal phalanges may be severely involved
  - Gingival hyperplasia
- Imaging: Radiography
  - Generalized osteoporosis
  - Flexion joint contractures
- Imaging: MR
  - Nonspecific heterogeneous soft tissue mass
  - Predominantly isointense to muscle on T1WI
  - Hyperintense on fluid-sensitive sequences
  - Nonspecific enhancement

TOP DIFFERENTIAL DIAGNOSES

- Multicentric infantile myofibromatosis
  - Nodules present at birth
  - No involvement of gums or bone
- Neurofibromatosis
  - Café au lait spots
- Gingival fibromatosis
  - Limited to gum involvement
- Cylindromas
  - Involvement limited to head
- Winchester syndrome
  - Short stature
  - Small joint contractures
  - Corneal opacities
  - Carpal bone resorption

PATHOLOGY

- Unknown, possibly related to decreased type III collagen
- Gross pathology: Solid, white or waxy nodules
- Microscopic features: Plump fibroblastic cells + extracellular homogeneous eosinophilic material
  - Vague fascicular pattern of fibroblasts
  - Old lesions are less cellular
  - No atypia or necrosis

CLINICAL ISSUES

- Genetics: Autosomal recessive disease
- Etiology: Unknown
- Gender: Slight male predilection
- Age: Usually presents in infancy
  - Lesions continue to appear and grow into adulthood
- Epidemiology
  - Extremely rare
  - Patients often have consanguineous parents
- Clinical presentation
  - Slowly growing, painless skin papules
  - Limited range of motion
  - Gingival hyperplasia results in poor feeding and malnutrition
    - May produce airway obstruction
- Lifespan is to 2nd or 3rd decade of life
  - Severely limited mobility due to joint contractures
- Treatment
  - Surgical excision is mainstay of therapy
    - Local recurrence is common despite wide margins
  - Radiotherapy, chemotherapy, and endocrine therapy sometimes used, but not proven

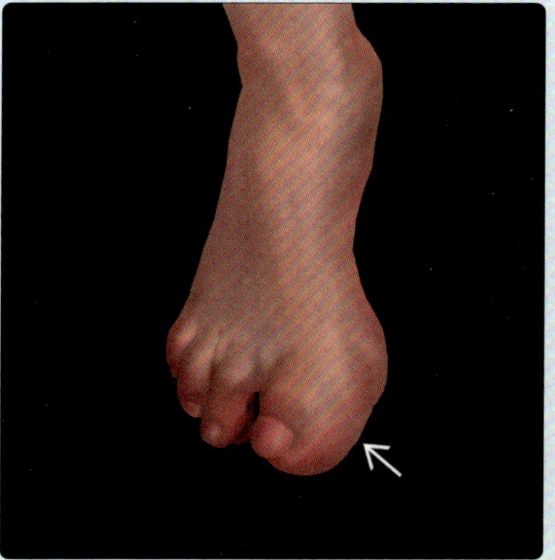

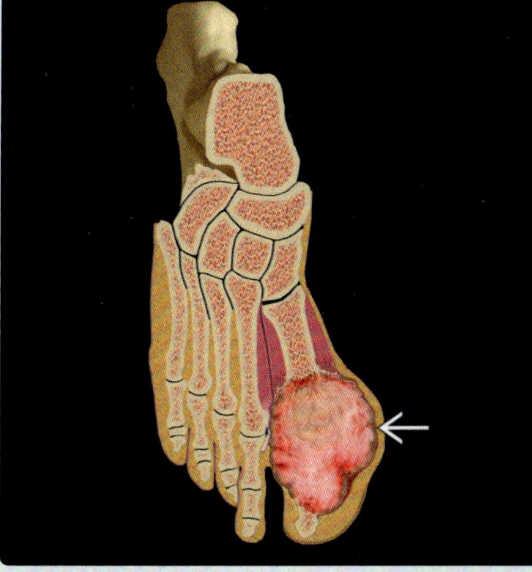

(Left) *Graphic of the dorsum of the foot shows an enlarged, deformed great toe ➡ on an otherwise normal foot.* **(Right)** *Axial graphic shows a lobulated soft tissue mass ➡ causing enlargement of the soft tissues and erosion of the surrounding bones. The appearance of this lesion is nonspecific by any imaging means. Location, multiplicity of lesions, presentation, and similar lesions in parents may help suggest the correct diagnosis.*

Fibroma of Tendon Sheath

KEY FACTS

TERMINOLOGY

- Dense, slowly growing benign soft tissue nodule located adjacent to tendon sheath

IMAGING

- Location: Upper extremity > lower extremity
  - Most common: 1st-3rd digits of hand with volar hand and wrist
- Size: Typically < 3 cm
- Radiographs show soft tissue mass or are normal
  - Bone erosion is uncommon
- MR signal not specific
  - Heterogeneous low to intermediate signal on T1WI
  - Heterogeneous low to high signal on T2WI
  - Variable mild to intense enhancement

PATHOLOGY

- Unknown; possibly reactive lesion
  - History of trauma in only 10%
- Well-defined, firm, rubbery mass
  - Multilobulated and may be multinodular
  - May contain cystic or myxoid regions
- Paucicellular nodules containing spindle-shaped cells resembling fibroblasts
  - Slit-like vascular channels

CLINICAL ISSUES

- Painless, slowly growing, firm mass
  - May have mild pain or tenderness
- Decreased range of motion or trigger finger
- Nerve impingement, carpal tunnel syndrome
- Age: Any age; most common in 4th decade of life
- Gender: Male predominance
- Treatment: Surgical excision with preservation of tendon
  - Local recurrence in 1/4 of cases; can occur months to years after resection
  - No malignant potential

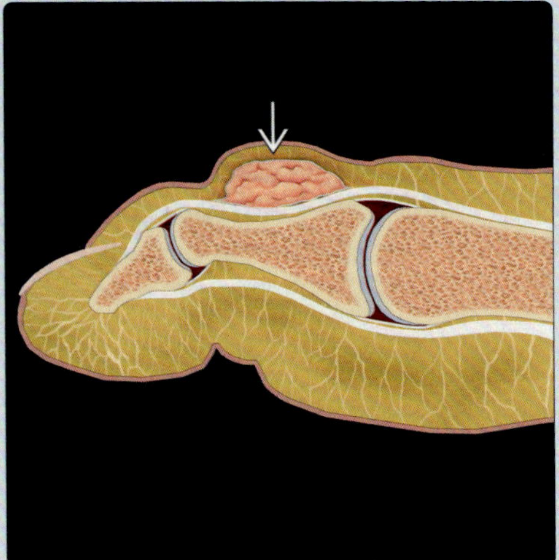

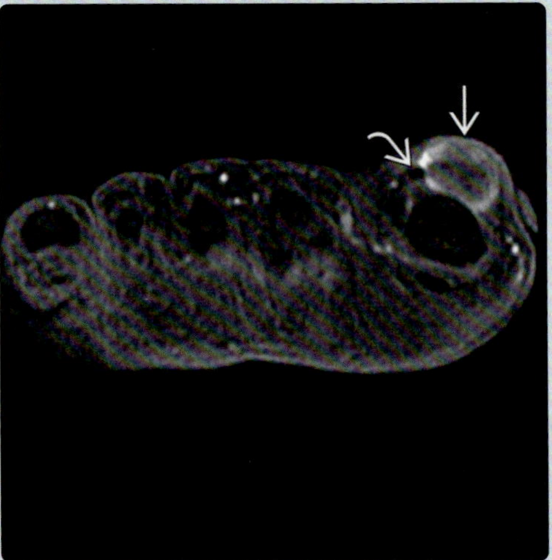

(Left) *Sagittal graphic of the great toe demonstrates a well-defined, mildly lobulated, oval soft tissue mass ➡. This mass has a subcutaneous location and, along its deep surface, abuts the great toe extensor tendon.* **(Right)** *Coronal T1WI C+ FS MR demonstrates a dorsally located mass ➡ involving the great toe. The mass has mild, predominantly peripheral enhancement and an irregular central region that lacks enhancement. It is intimately associated with the extensor hallucis longus tendon ↪.*

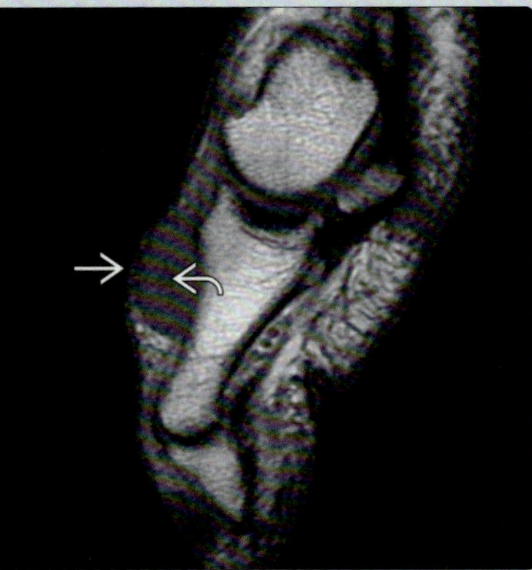

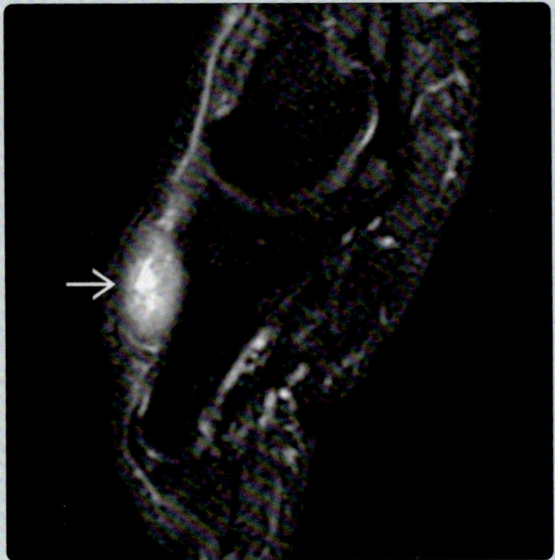

(Left) *Sagittal T1WI MR in the same patient shows the well-defined, ovoid morphology of the mass ➡, which abuts the cortex of the great toe proximal phalanx without underlying bone erosion. The mass is isointense to skeletal muscle and has a small, central focus of low signal ↪.* **(Right)** *Sagittal T2WI FSE MR shows the mass ➡ to have very high signal intensity centrally, surrounded by intermediate to high heterogeneous signal. The central high signal region was due to cystic degeneration.*

TERMINOLOGY

Synonyms

- Tenosynovial fibroma

Definitions

- Benign fibrous nodule that arises near tendinous structures

IMAGING

General Features

- Best diagnostic clue
  - Dense, slowly growing soft tissue nodule located adjacent to tendon sheath
- Location
  - Upper extremity > lower extremity
    - Most common: 1st-3rd digits of hand with volar hand and wrist
  - Adjacent tendon sheath most common
    - Intraarticular origin reported
  - Right > left side of body
- Size
  - Typically < 3 cm

Radiographic Findings

- Radiographs show soft tissue mass or are normal
- Bone erosion is uncommon

MR Findings

- Well-defined, oval mass abutting tendon sheath
- Heterogeneous low to intermediate signal intensity on T1WI
  - Central band-like hypointense regions reported
- Heterogeneous low to high signal intensity on fluid-sensitive sequences
- Variable mild to intense enhancement
- No decrease in signal intensity on GRE imaging

DIFFERENTIAL DIAGNOSIS

Fibrous Histiocytoma

- Similar location and clinical presentation

Fasciitis, Nodular

- May have very similar histologic appearance
- Not associated with tendon sheath

Giant Cell Tumor Tendon Sheath

- More common than fibroma of tendon sheath
- Occurs in similar location
- More cellular, contains multinucleated giant cells

Inflammatory Myxohyaline Tumor

- Contains bizarre cells similar to Reed-Sternberg cells

PATHOLOGY

General Features

- Etiology
  - Unknown; possibly reactive lesion
    - History of trauma in only 10%
- Genetics
  - Single case with clonal chromosomal abnormality, t(2;11)(q31-32;q12)

Gross Pathologic & Surgical Features

- Well-defined, firm, rubbery mass
- Multilobulated and may be multinodular
- Homogeneous pale gray or pearl white color
- May contain cystic or myxoid regions

Microscopic Features

- Common features
  - Paucicellular nodules containing spindle-shaped cells resembling fibroblasts
  - Slit-like vascular channels
  - Collagenous stroma
  - Mitotic activity depends on cellularity
  - Positive smooth muscle actin and vimentin
- Less common features
  - Bizarre pleomorphic or stellate cells
  - Cystic or myxoid change
  - Dense hyalinization
  - Chondroid or osseous metaplasia

CLINICAL ISSUES

Presentation

- Most common signs/symptoms
  - Painless, slowly growing, firm mass
- Other signs/symptoms
  - Mild pain or tenderness in ~ 1/3 of patients
  - Decreased range of motion or trigger finger
  - Nerve impingement, including carpal tunnel syndrome

Demographics

- Age
  - Any age; most common in 4th decade of life
- Gender
  - Male predominance
- Epidemiology
  - No familial or racial predilection

Natural History & Prognosis

- Local recurrence in 1/4 of cases; can occur months to years after resection
- No malignant potential

Treatment

- Surgical excision with preservation of adjacent tendon

SELECTED REFERENCES

1. De Maeseneer M et al: Fibroma of the tendon sheath of the long head of the biceps tendon. Skeletal Radiol. 43(3):399-402, 2014
2. Glover M et al: Intra-articular fibroma of tendon sheath arising in the acromioclavicular joint. Skeletal Radiol. 43(5):681-6, 2014
3. Nishio J et al: Fibroma of tendon sheath with 11q rearrangements. Anticancer Res. 34(9):5159-62, 2014
4. Weiss SW et al: Benign fibroblastic/myofibroblastic proliferations. In Weiss SW et al: Enzinger and Weiss' Soft Tissue Tumors. 5th ed. Philadelphia: Elsevier. 203-06, 2008
5. Kransdorf MJ et al: Benign fibrous and fibrohistiocytic tumors. In Kransdorf MJ et al: Imaging of Soft Tissue Tumors. 2nd ed. Philadelphia: Lippincott Williams & Wilkins. 195-6, 2006
6. Farshid G et al: Elastofibroma. In Fletcher CDM et al: World Health Organization Classification of Tumours. Pathology and Genetics of Tumours of Soft Tissue and Bone. Lyon: IARC Press. 66, 2002

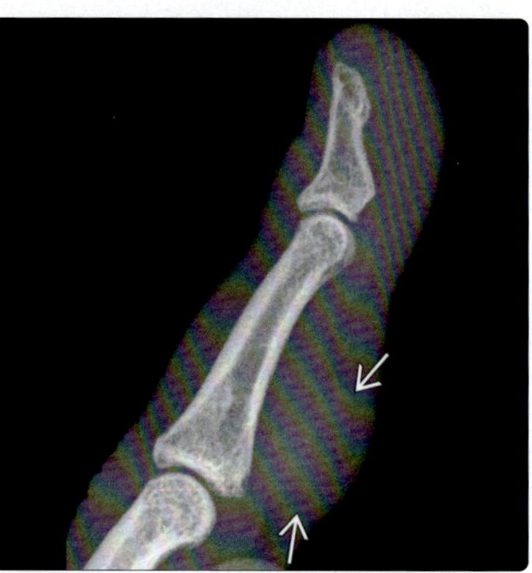

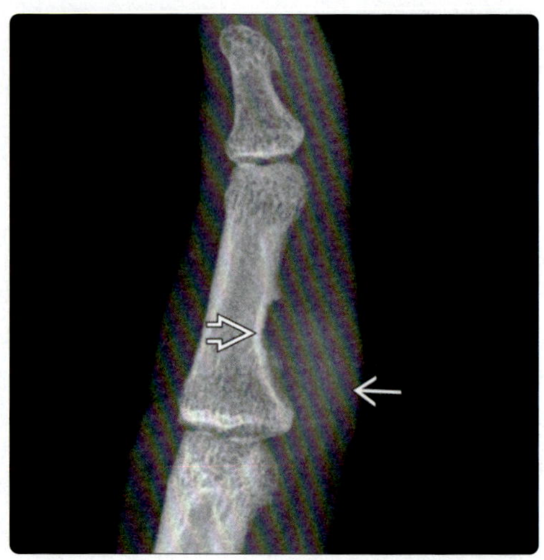

(Left) *Lateral radiograph shows an oval soft tissue mass ➡ on the volar aspect of a middle phalanx. There are no other characterizing features.* **(Right)** *Oblique radiograph in the same patient shows the mass ➡ as well as prominent erosion of the adjacent bone ⇨. The latter is an unusual feature of fibroma of the tendon sheath. The process appears to be slow, since there is cortical thickening at the site of erosion.*

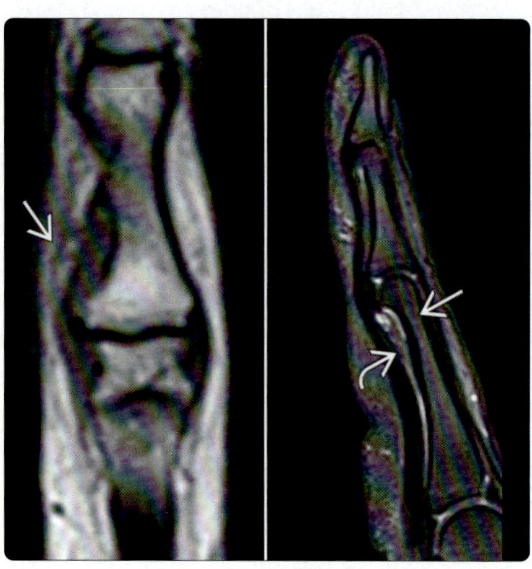

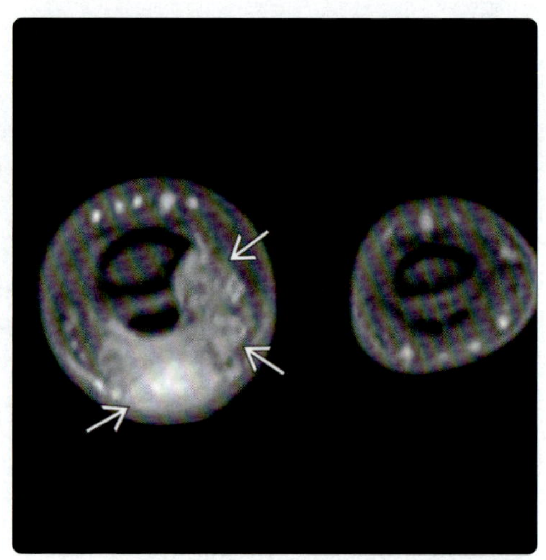

(Left) *Coronal T1 MR (left) and sagittal T2FS MR (right) show the mass ➡ to be hypointense on T1 and inhomogeneously hyperintense on T2. On the sagittal image, note the adjacency to the flexor tendon ↪. The bone erosion is well seen on both images.* **(Right)** *Axial postcontrast T1FS MR in the same patient shows the lesion ➡ to enhance moderately and to be mildly inhomogeneous, typical of fibroma of tendon sheath. The lesion is indistinguishable from giant cell tumor of the tendon sheath by imaging characteristics.*

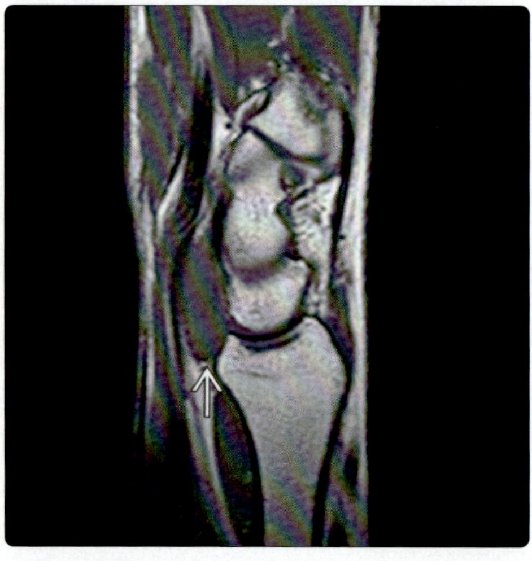

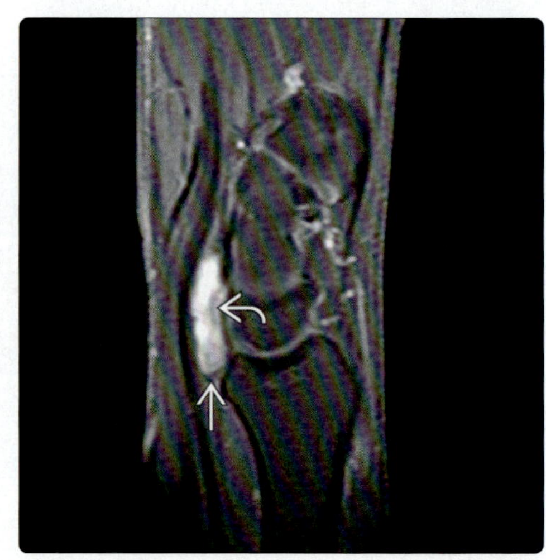

(Left) *Sagittal T1WI MR shows a nonspecific, oval mass ➡ lying in the volar aspect of the wrist. This mass has homogeneous signal that is isointense to skeletal muscle.* **(Right)** *Sagittal T2WI FS MR shows the lobulated oval mass ➡ to have relatively homogeneous high signal intensity. There is a faint suggestion of undulating collagenous tissue ↪. Without contrast, this lesion would be difficult to differentiate from a ganglion cyst; however, solid enhancement of the lesion was confirmed (not shown).*

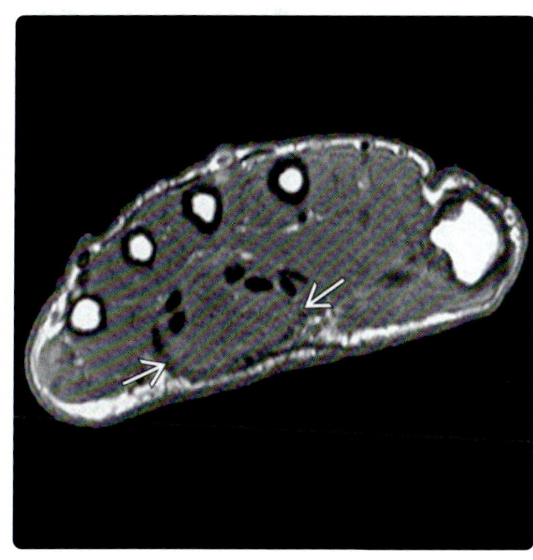

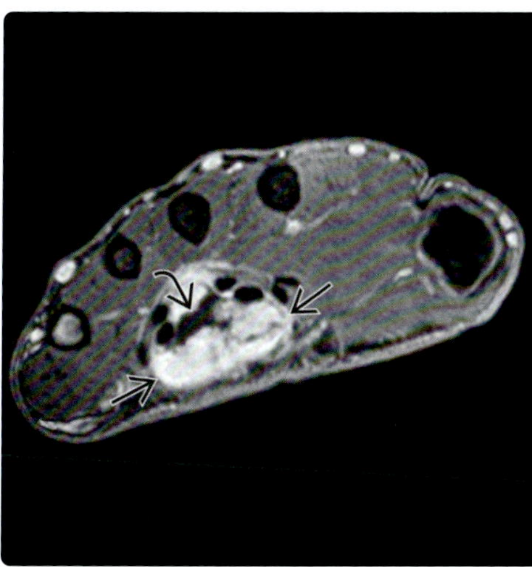

(Left) *Axial T1WI MR demonstrates a mildly inhomogeneous mass ➡ that is similar in intensity to the adjacent skeletal muscle. The mass lies deep in the palm of the hand and displaces both the flexor tendons and median nerve.* **(Right)** *Axial T1WI C+ FS MR shows the mass ⇨ to have an intense, nodular enhancement with a central region of hypoenhancement ↷. At surgical excision, this area of hypoenhancement corresponded to a region of myxoid change, which is relatively uncommon.*

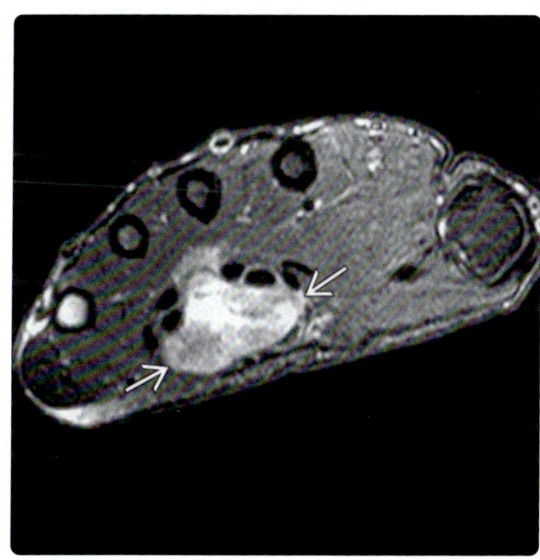

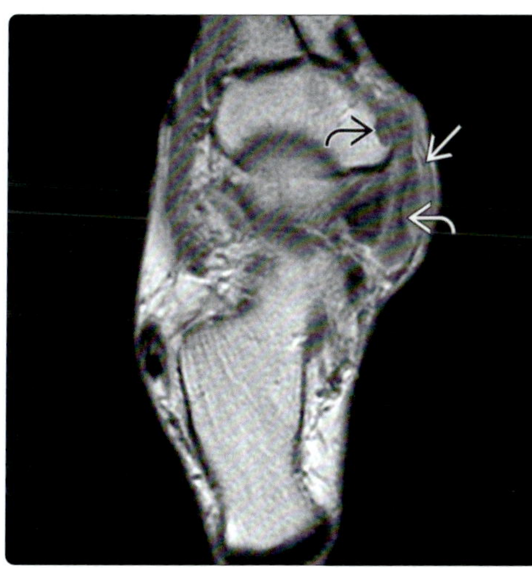

(Left) *Axial T2WI FS MR in the same patient shows the fibroma of tendon sheath ➡ to have heterogeneous, predominantly high signal intensity, along with a few areas that are isointense to skeletal muscle.* **(Right)** *Axial PDWI MR of the hindfoot shows a nonspecific medially located mass ➡ with a signal intensity that is similar to skeletal muscle with a central region of undulating hypointensity ↷. A small erosion ↷ involves the medial navicular bone.*

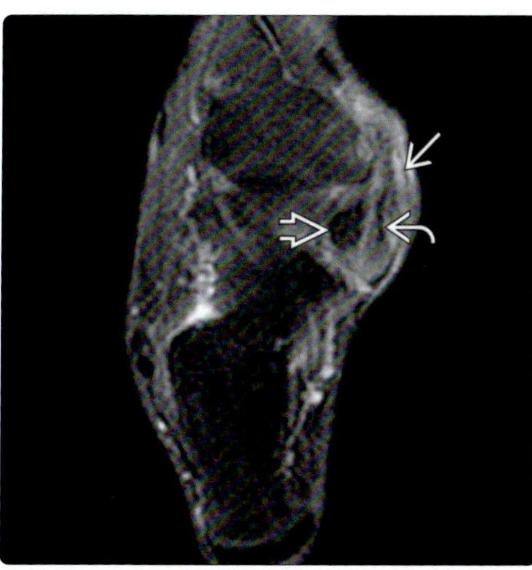

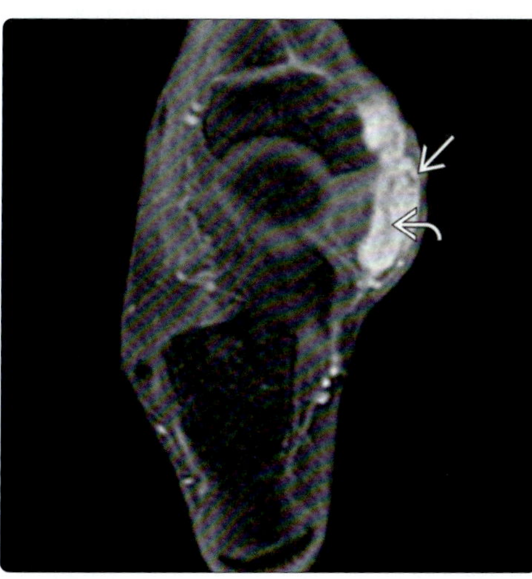

(Left) *Axial T2WI FS in the same patient shows the mass ➡ to be hyperintense to skeletal muscle, with a persistently low signal central region ↷. The mass abuts the posterior tibialis tendon ⇨, which is diffusely enlarged due to tendinosis.* **(Right)** *Axial T1WI C+ FS MR shows the fibroma of tendon sheath ➡ to have intense enhancement, with the exception of the region of persistently low signal ↷, likely representing dense collagenous tissue.*

KEY FACTS

TERMINOLOGY

- a.k.a. collagenous fibroma
- Benign paucicellular soft tissue tumor

IMAGING

- Usually located peripherally in body
  - Arm, shoulder, calf, back, forearm, hands, and feet
  - Rare reports in abdominal wall, parotid, lacrimal gland, and palate
- Subcutaneous location most common
  - Often involves fascia
  - Skeletal muscle involvement not uncommon (25%)
- Most commonly 1-4 cm in diameter
  - Reported up to 20 cm
- Best imaging tool: MR
  - Regions of low signal intensity on T1WI and T2WI due to collagen and low cellularity
  - Mild enhancement
- Associated bone erosion rarely reported

PATHOLOGY

- Well circumscribed and sometimes lobulated
  - Smooth, round to elongated contour
  - Homogeneous, firm pearl-gray tissue
- Prominent collagenous stroma with low cellularity
  - Scattered fibroblasts and myofibroblasts
  - Few, thin-walled vessels
- Positive vimentin

CLINICAL ISSUES

- Asymptomatic mass (unless it compresses nearby neurovascular structures)
- Slowly growing
- Male predominance (3-5:1)
- Usually seen in 5th-7th decades of life
  - Reported in adolescents
- Treatment is surgical excision
- No propensity for local recurrence or metastasis

(Left) *Axial T1WI MR of the distal forearm demonstrates a mass ➡ in the region of the interosseous membrane located between the metadiaphyseal regions of the distal ulna and radius. The mass has mixed intermediate and low ➡ signal relative to skeletal muscle.* **(Right)** *Axial T2WI FS MR shows the mass ➡ to have predominantly low signal intensity ➡ with intermixed regions of intermediate signal intensity. The mass abuts the adjacent bones, without evidence of osseous erosion or invasion.*

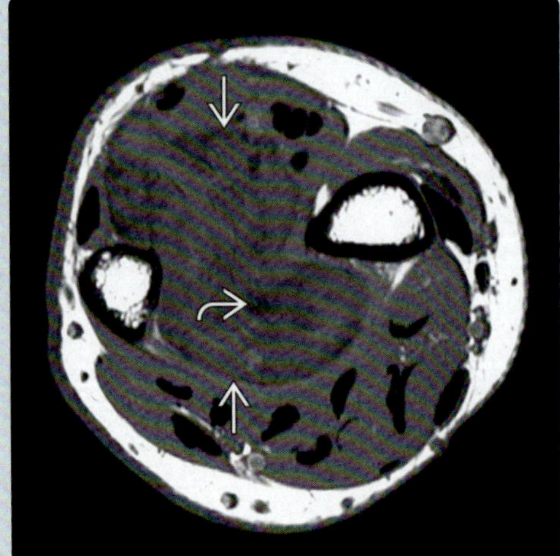

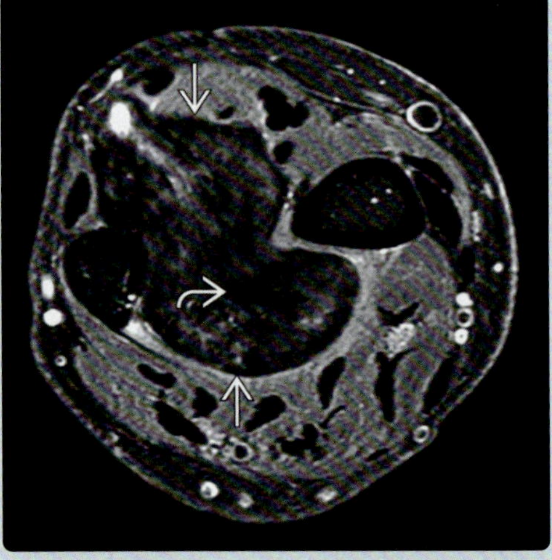

(Left) *Axial T1WI C+ FS MR demonstrates mild enhancement of the mass ➡ with interspersed regions of persistently low signal intensity ➡.* **(Right)** *Coronal T1WI C+ FS MR shows the well-defined, lobulated borders of the mass ➡. Mild enhancement is predominantly peripheral. Central regions of low signal intensity on all sequences are suggestive of dense fibrous tissue, which can be seen in several entities, including desmoplastic fibroblastoma, desmoid tumor, and fibroma of the tendon sheath.*

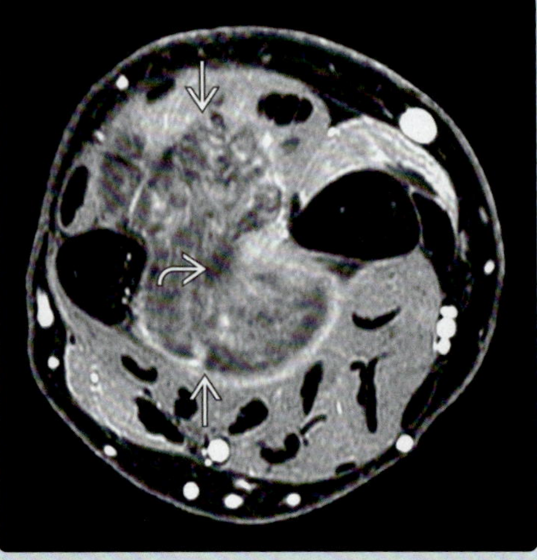

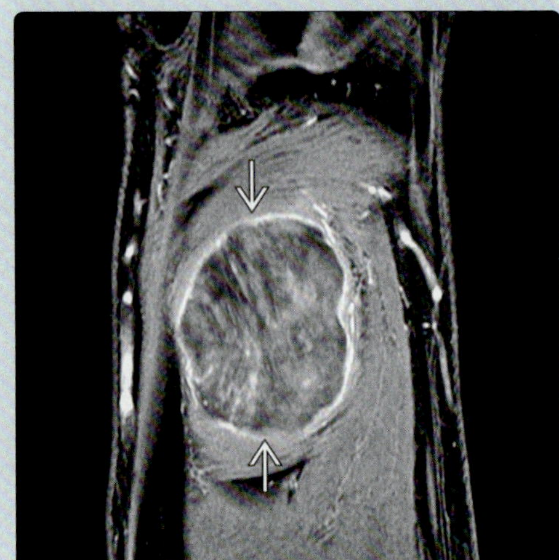

TERMINOLOGY

Synonyms

- Collagenous fibroma

Definitions

- Benign paucicellular soft tissue tumor

IMAGING

General Features

- Location
  - Usually located peripherally in body
    - Arm (24%), shoulder (19%), calf, back, forearm, hands, and feet
    - Rare reports in abdominal wall, parotid, lacrimal gland, and palate
  - Subcutaneous location most common
    - Often involves fascia
    - Skeletal muscle involvement (25%)
- Size
  - Most commonly 1-4 cm in diameter
    - Reported up to 20 cm

CT Findings

- Inhomogeneous mass with inhomogeneous enhancement

Ultrasonographic Findings

- Solid mass, isoechoic to muscle, with smooth and lobulated margins
- Power Doppler: Rich diffuse vascularization

Imaging Recommendations

- Best imaging tool
  - MR for tumor extent and characterization

Radiographic Findings

- Associated bone erosion rarely reported

MR Findings

- Regions of low signal intensity on T1WI and T2WI due to collagen and low cellularity
- Mild enhancement
  - Rim enhancement appeared characteristic in one small study

DIFFERENTIAL DIAGNOSIS

Neurofibroma

- Similar fusiform morphology
- Wavy pattern of cells in myxoid and collagenous stroma
- Shredded carrot bundles of collagen

Desmoid-Type Fibromatosis

- More infiltrative appearance
- More cellular, vascular tumor

Calcifying Fibrous Tumor

- Children and young adults
- Contains psammomatous calcifications and lymphoplasmacytic infiltrate

Low-Grade Fibromyxoid Sarcoma

- Whorled collection of cells in fibromyxoid stroma

Elastofibroma

- Located between scapula and chest wall
- Contains elastic fibers

Fasciitis, Nodular

- Usually in subcutaneous location
- More cellular tumor

Fibroma of Tendon Sheath

- Contains low T1 and T2 signal foci
- Location abuts tendon sheath

PATHOLOGY

General Features

- Genetics
  - t(2;11) and breakpoint at 11q12

Gross Pathologic & Surgical Features

- Smooth, round to elongated contour
- Well circumscribed and sometimes lobulated
- Homogeneous, firm pearl-gray tissue
- Lacks hemorrhage and necrosis

Microscopic Features

- Prominent collagenous or myxocollagenous stroma with low cellularity
  - Scattered fibroblasts and myofibroblasts
  - Few, thin-walled vessels
- Rare or absent mitotic figures
- Positive vimentin
- Variably positive for smooth muscle actin and keratins AE1/AE3
- Negative desmin, epithelial membrane antigen, S100 protein, CD34

CLINICAL ISSUES

Presentation

- Most common signs/symptoms
  - Asymptomatic mass unless it compresses nearby neurovascular structures
  - Slowly growing

Demographics

- Age
  - Usually seen in 5th-7th decades of life
    - Reported in adolescents
- Gender
  - Male predominance (3-5:1)

Natural History & Prognosis

- No propensity for local recurrence or metastasis

Treatment

- Surgical excision

SELECTED REFERENCES

1. Bonardi M et al: US and MRI appearance of a collagenous fibroma (desmoplastic fibroblastoma) of the shoulder. J Ultrasound. 17(1):53-6, 2014
2. Yamamoto A et al: Three cases of collagenous fibroma with rim enhancement on postcontrast T1-weighted images with fat suppression. Skeletal Radiol. 42(1):141-6, 2013

Calcifying Aponeurotic Fibroma

KEY FACTS

TERMINOLOGY

- a.k.a. juvenile aponeurotic fibroma
- Benign, locally aggressive fibroblastic lesion of childhood

IMAGING

- Small, slowly growing mass in child
  - Typically < 3 cm in diameter
- Most common sites: Palms, soles, wrists, and ankles
  - Associated with tendons, fascia, and aponeuroses
  - Rare in back, arms, legs, neck, and abdominal wall
- Ill-defined, solitary mass on all imaging
- Radiographic findings
  - Nonspecific, infiltrative soft tissue mass that may erode adjacent bone
  - May contain stippled calcifications
- MR best delineates location and extent of lesion
  - Nonspecific, infiltrative soft tissue mass
  - May contain stippled calcifications
  - Regions of low signal on T1WI and T2WI MR
  - Intense, heterogeneous enhancement

PATHOLOGY

- Firm or rubbery infiltrative mass
  - Gray-white, gritty calcified cut surface
- Nodular calcific deposits
- Spindle cells in collagenous stroma

CLINICAL ISSUES

- Asymptomatic, freely mobile mass
- Median age: 12 years
  - Majority within first 2 decades of life
  - Reported from birth to 6th decade of life
- Slight male predominance
- Local recurrence in ~ 50%
  - Usually occurs within 3 years of excision
  - More common in patients < 5 years old
- Treatment is surgical resection and reexcision with attention to preservation of function

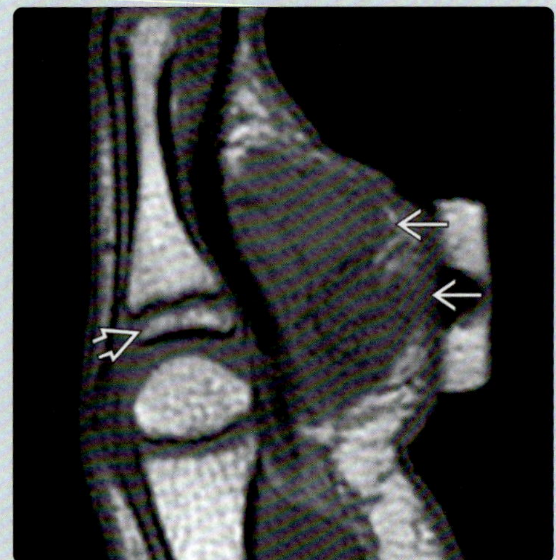

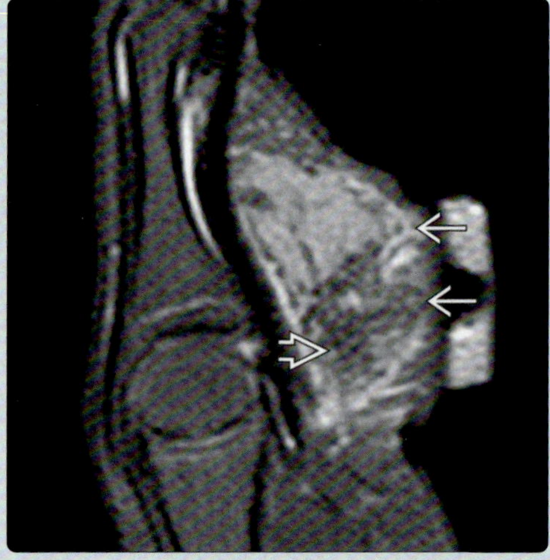

(Left) *Sagittal T1WI MR shows a mass ➡ along the palmar aspect of the metacarpophalangeal joint. This mass has an irregular, infiltrative border. The signal intensity is similar to skeletal muscle with foci of low signal intensity. Note the open growth plate ➡ in this child.* **(Right)** *Sagittal T2WI FS MR shows the infiltrative mass ➡ to have heterogeneous hyperintense signal, again with superimposed, speckled foci of low signal ➡ intensity, which corresponds to calcification.*

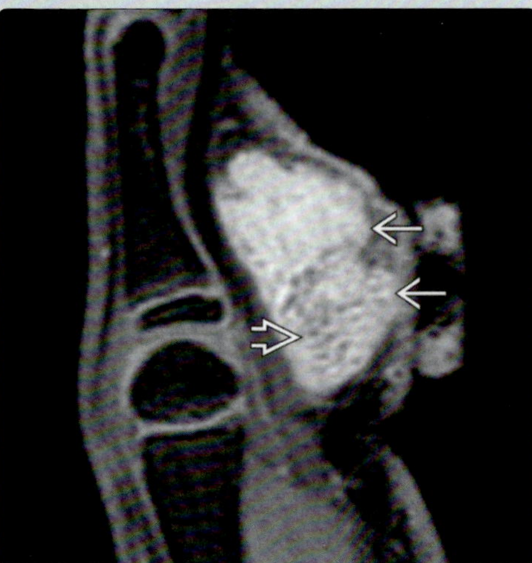

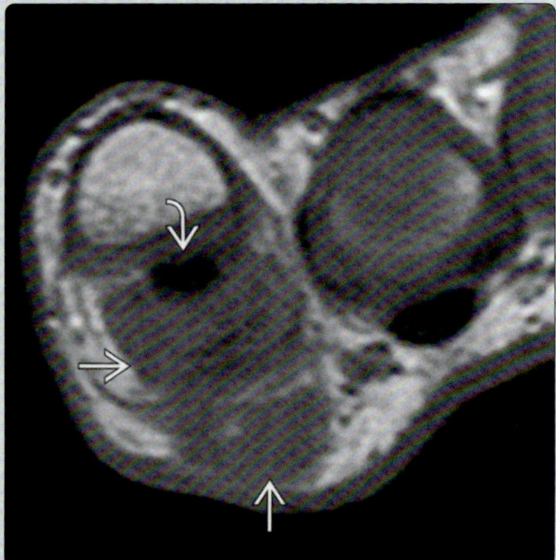

(Left) *Sagittal T1WI C+ FS MR demonstrates heterogeneous, relatively intense contrast enhancement of the mass ➡. The small foci of calcification ➡ do not enhance.* **(Right)** *Axial T1WI MR of the calcifying aponeurotic fibroma ➡ demonstrates the infiltrative, ill-defined nature of the lesion. This lesion abuts the flexor tendon ➡, which would also suggest giant cell tumor or fibroma of the tendon sheath, both of which would normally be well-defined masses.*

TERMINOLOGY

Synonyms

- Juvenile aponeurotic fibroma

Definitions

- Benign, locally aggressive fibroblastic lesion of childhood

IMAGING

General Features

- Best diagnostic clue
  - Small tumor in palm or sole of child
- Location
  - Palms, soles, wrists, and ankles
    - Rare in back, arms, legs, neck, and abdominal wall
  - Associated with tendons, fascia, and aponeurotic tissue
- Size
  - Typically < 3 cm in diameter
- Morphology
  - Ill-defined, solitary mass

Imaging Recommendations

- Best imaging tool
  - MR best delineates location and extent of lesion

Radiographic Findings

- Radiography
  - Nonspecific, infiltrative soft tissue mass that may erode adjacent bone
  - May contain stippled calcifications

MR Findings

- Regions of low signal on T1WI and T2WI MR
- Intense, heterogeneous enhancement

DIFFERENTIAL DIAGNOSIS

Fibrous Hamartoma of Infancy

- Located in axillary fold, upper arm, shoulder predominantly
- Has 3 distinct histologic components
- Involvement of hands or feet is rare
- Calcification or ossification is rare

Giant Cell Tumor Tendon Sheath

- Occurs most commonly between 30-50 years of age
- Well-circumscribed mass, most commonly in hand
- May erode into adjacent bone

Fibroma of Tendon Sheath

- Most common in 4th decade of life
- Well-defined mass, most commonly in volar hand and wrist

Superficial Fibromatoses

- Occurs more commonly in older patients
- More nodular or ellipsoid contour
- No calcification or chondroid tissue

Soft Tissue Chondroma

- Occurs in older adults
- Prominent chondroid differentiation
- Less likely to recur

PATHOLOGY

General Features

- Genetics
  - No genetic association

Gross Pathologic & Surgical Features

- Firm or rubbery infiltrative mass
- Gray-white, gritty calcified cut surface

Microscopic Features

- Nodular calcific deposits
  - Surrounded by parallel chondrocyte-like cells or osteoclastic giant cells
- Spindle cells between calcified nodules
- Hyalinized or chondroid stroma
- Neurovascular structures may lie within lesion
- No necrosis or significant atypia
- Rare, more infiltrative variant seen in very young children
  - Less calcification and more cellularity
- Variably positive vimentin, smooth muscle actin, muscle-specific actin, CD99, and S100 protein

CLINICAL ISSUES

Presentation

- Most common signs/symptoms
  - Asymptomatic, slowly growing mass

Demographics

- Age
  - Median: 12 years
    - Majority within first 2 decades of life
    - Reported from birth to 6th decade of life
- Gender
  - Slight male predominance
- Epidemiology
  - Very rare
  - No racial predisposition

Natural History & Prognosis

- Local recurrence in ~ 50%
  - Usually occurs within 3 years of excision
  - More common in patients < 5 years old
- Single report of malignant transformation

Treatment

- Treatment is surgical resection, and often reexcision, with attention to preservation of function

SELECTED REFERENCES

1. Cho YH et al: Calcifying aponeurotic fibroma of the dorsum of the foot: radiographic and magnetic resonance imaging findings in a four-year-old boy. Iran J Radiol. 12(2):e23911, 2015
2. Kim OH et al: Calcifying aponeurotic fibroma: case report with radiographic and MR features. Korean J Radiol. 15(1):134-9, 2014
3. Murphey MD et al: From the archives of the AFIP: musculoskeletal fibromatoses: radiologic-pathologic correlation. Radiographics. 29(7):2143-73, 2009
4. Weiss SW et al: Fibrous tumors of infancy and childhood. In Weiss SW et al: Enzinger and Weiss' Soft Tissue Tumors. 5th ed. Philadelphia: Elsevier. 289-93, 2008

KEY FACTS

TERMINOLOGY

- Infiltrative, fibroblastic lesions most commonly found arising from palmar or plantar fascia or aponeuroses

IMAGING

- Location
  - Palmar (volar surface of hands): 50% bilateral
  - Plantar (nonweight bearing plantar aponeurosis, usually medial): 20-50% bilateral
- Radiographs may demonstrate flexion deformities of fingers due to flexor tendon contraction
- MR appearance
  - Isointense to hypointense nodules relative to skeletal muscle on T1WI
  - Isointense to hyperintense nodules relative to skeletal muscle on fluid-sensitive sequences
  - Postcontrast MR imaging: Variable enhancement
    - Mature lesions are more likely to have low signal intensity on all sequences and are less likely to recur
  - Can invade muscles or neurovascular bundles
  - MR shows lentiform lesion that often blends with plantar aponeurosis at proximal and distal ends
- Ultrasound shows small, superficial, hypoechoic to mixed echogenicity masses

CLINICAL ISSUES

- Age: Affects adults, incidence increases with age
  - Unusual in patients < 30 yr old
- Gender: Palmar fibromatosis 4x more common in males
- Clinical symptoms
  - Painless, firm nodule on palmar aspect of hand
    - Cord-like induration between nodules with flexion contractures of fingers
    - 4th and 5th fingers are most commonly affected
  - Firm, tender nodule on plantar aspect of foot
- Treatment
  - Plantar lesion treatment = modified footwear
  - Tendon release or resection for palmar lesions

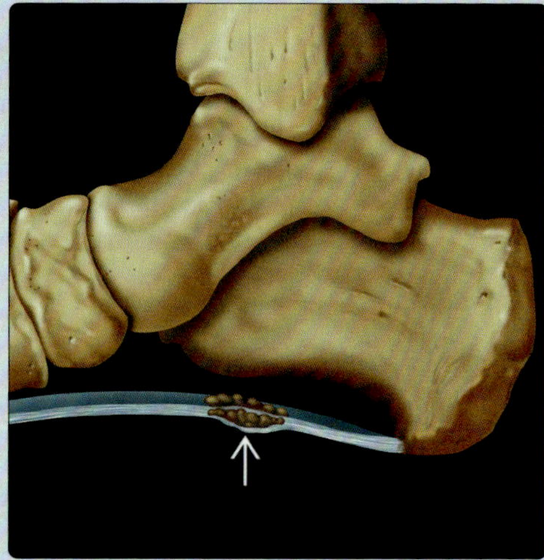

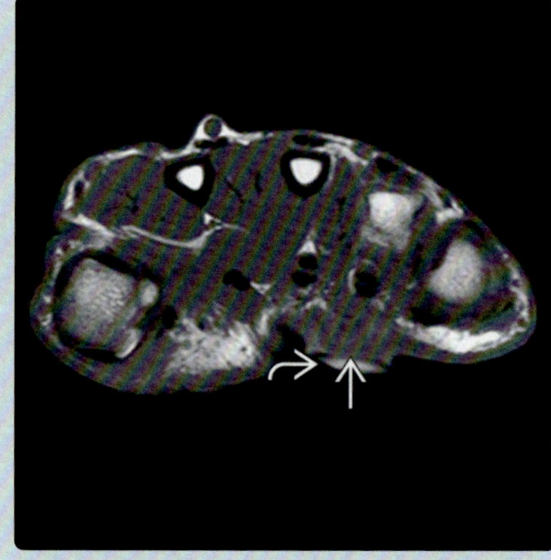

(Left) *Lateral graphic of the hindfoot shows a mass ➡ involving the plantar fascia. The proximal and distal ends of the mass smoothly blend with the fascia, which is a typical finding.* **(Right)** *Axial T1WI MR shows a poorly defined soft tissue mass ➡ in the hypothenar region of the palm of the hand. The mass is isointense to slightly hyperintense relative to skeletal muscle. A marker ➡ placed on the skin mildly deforms the superficial border of the mass.*

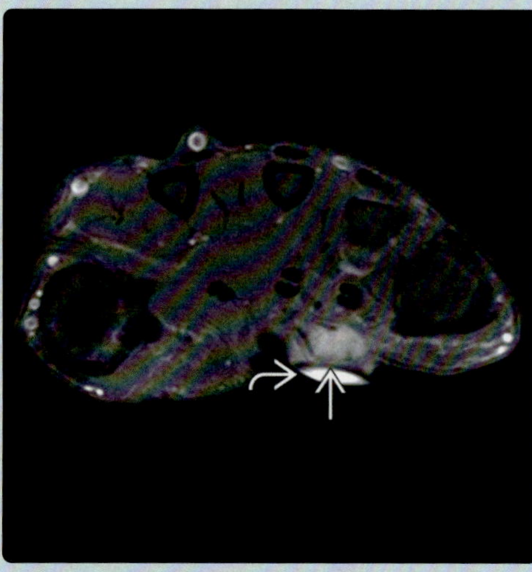

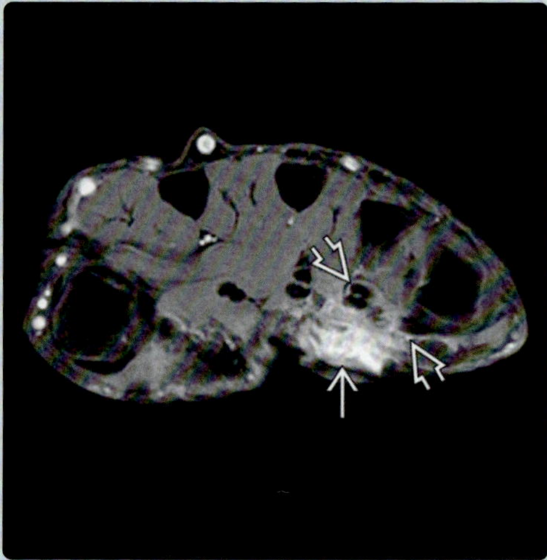

(Left) *Axial T2WI FS MR in the same patient shows a hypothenar soft tissue mass ➡ to be heterogeneously hyperintense to skeletal muscle. The mass is located in the region of the palmar aponeurosis. A skin marker ➡ is not part of the mass.* **(Right)** *Axial T1WI C+ FS MR in the same patient shows significant enhancement of the palmar soft tissue mass ➡. Enhancement also involves the 4th and 5th digit superficial flexor tendons ➡. Enhancement varies with the maturity of the mass.*

TERMINOLOGY

Synonyms

- Palmar fibromatosis: Dupuytren disease/contracture
- Plantar fibromatosis: Ledderhose disease
- Penile fibromatosis: Peyronie disease

Definitions

- Infiltrative, fibroblastic lesions most commonly found arising from palmar or plantar fascia or aponeuroses

IMAGING

General Features

- Location
  - Palmar fibromatosis
    - Volar surface of hands, 50% bilateral
    - 4th > 5th > 3rd > 2nd finger
    - Right hand slightly ↑ involvement than left
  - Plantar fibromatosis
    - Nonweight bearing plantar aponeurosis
      - Medial location is most common
      - 20-50% bilateral
- Size
  - Palmar lesions < 1 cm typically
  - Plantar lesions = 2-3 cm

Radiographic Findings

- Radiographs may demonstrate flexion deformities of fingers due to flexor tendon contraction
- Soft tissue masses are rarely visible

MR Findings

- Palmar
  - Nodular lesions intimately associated with palmar fascia
  - Isointense to hypointense relative to skeletal muscle on T1WI and T2WI
  - Mature lesions are more likely to have low signal intensity on all sequences and are less likely to recur
- Plantar
  - Nodular lesion that blends with plantar aponeurosis at proximal and distal ends
  - Isointense to hypointense relative to skeletal muscle on T1WI and T2WI
  - Can invade muscles or neurovascular bundles
- Variable, heterogeneous enhancement relates to degree of maturity of lesion
  - ↑ enhancement = ↓ maturity = ↑ recurrence rate

Ultrasonographic Findings

- Mixed echogenicity to hypoechoic small masses

PATHOLOGY

General Features

- Etiology
  - Multifactorial etiology including genetic predisposition and trauma
- Genetics
  - Near diploid karyotypes, often chromosome 7 or 8
- Associated abnormalities
  - Epilepsy, diabetes, alcohol-induced liver disease

Gross Pathologic & Surgical Features

- Nodular mass or conglomerate of masses with white or yellow-gray cut surface

Microscopic Features

- Proliferative phase (immature) lesions have homogeneous fibroblasts with moderate collagen
- Mature lesions are hypocellular and contain predominantly dense collagen
- Presence of mitotic figures is normal and does not indicate malignancy

CLINICAL ISSUES

Presentation

- Most common signs/symptoms
  - Palmar fibromatosis
    - Painless, firm nodule on palmar aspect of hand
      - Overlying skin puckered
    - Cord-like induration between nodules with flexion contractures of fingers
      - 4th & 5th fingers are most commonly affected
  - Plantar fibromatosis
    - Firm, tender nodule on plantar aspect of foot
      - Contracture deformities of toes are uncommon
- Other signs/symptoms
  - Associated with other forms of fibromatosis
    - Up to 4% of patients have penile fibromatosis
    - 5-20% of palmar fibromatosis patients also have plantar fibromatosis
    - Up to 50% of plantar fibromatosis patients have palmar fibromatosis

Demographics

- Age
  - Adults; incidence increases with age
  - Unusual in patients < 30 yr old
    - Plantar lesions more common in young patients
- Gender
  - Palmar fibromatosis: 4x more common in males
  - Plantar fibromatosis: Mild male predominance
- Epidemiology
  - Palmar fibromatosis = 1-2% of population
  - Plantar fibromatosis = 0.23% of population
  - Northern European descent most common
    - Rare in non-Caucasian populations

Natural History & Prognosis

- Local recurrence is more common after resection of immature lesions or incomplete surgical excision

Treatment

- Palmar lesion treatment = surgical tendon release &/or mass resection
- Plantar lesion treatment = modified footwear

SELECTED REFERENCES

1. Lennox L et al: Superficial plantar fibromatosis. Cutis. 92(5):220, 225, 226, 2013
2. Kransdorf MJ et al: Benign fibrous and fibrohistiocytic tumors. In Kransdorf MJ et al: Imaging of Soft Tissue Tumors. 2nd ed. Philadelphia: Lippincott Williams & Wilkins. 217-23, 2006

(Left) *Sagittal T1WI MR shows a large plantar fibroma ➡. The mass is isointense to muscle with a region of low signal ⮫ along the plantar aspect of the mass. The mass arose from the deep surface of the plantar fascia.* **(Right)** *Sagittal T2WI FS MR in the same patient shows the plantar fibroma ➡ to have slightly hyperintense signal relative to muscle and a persistently low-signal region ⮫. This is a typical appearance and location along the medial, nonweight bearing plantar fascia.*

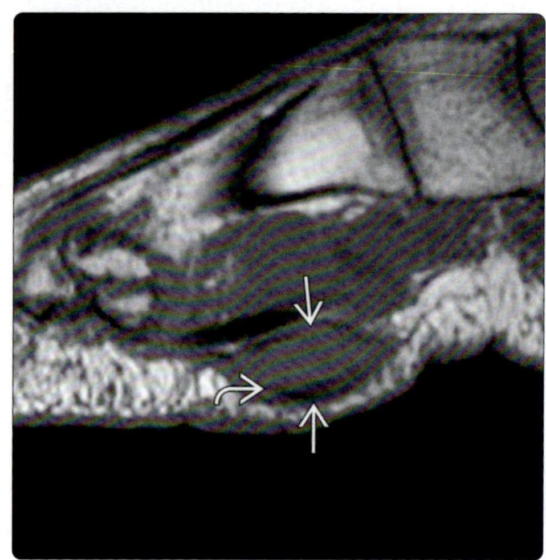

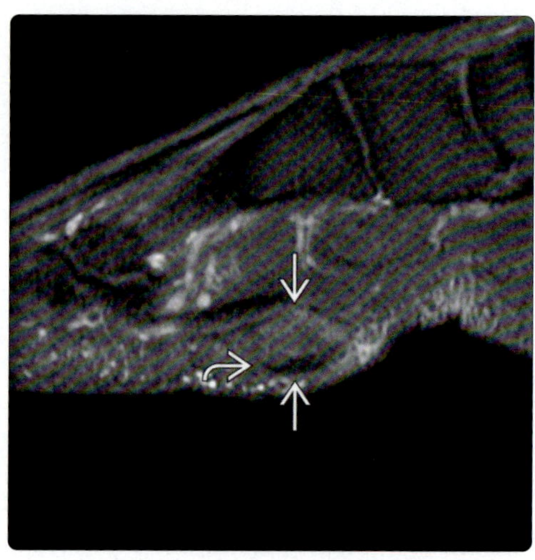

(Left) *Coronal T1WI MR shows a palpable mass along the plantar aspect of the midfoot with a classic appearance for plantar fibromatosis ➡. The mass has diffusely low signal and arises from the plantar aponeurosis ⮫.* **(Right)** *Coronal T1WI C+ FS MR in the same patient shows the mass ➡ to have heterogeneous enhancement. Although the mass had low signal on T1WI and fluid-sensitive sequences, the enhancement suggests that this lesion is still relatively immature.*

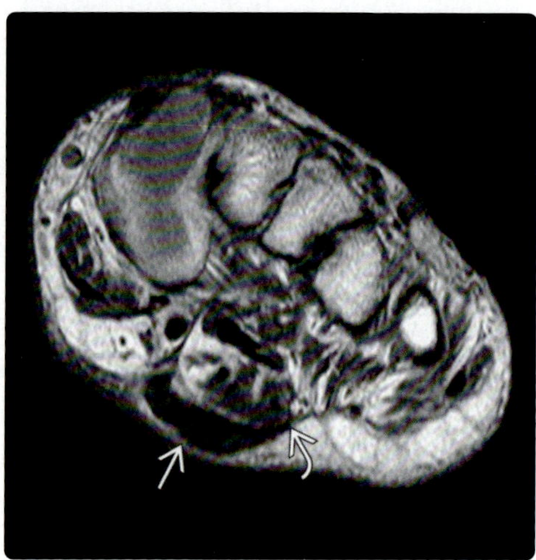

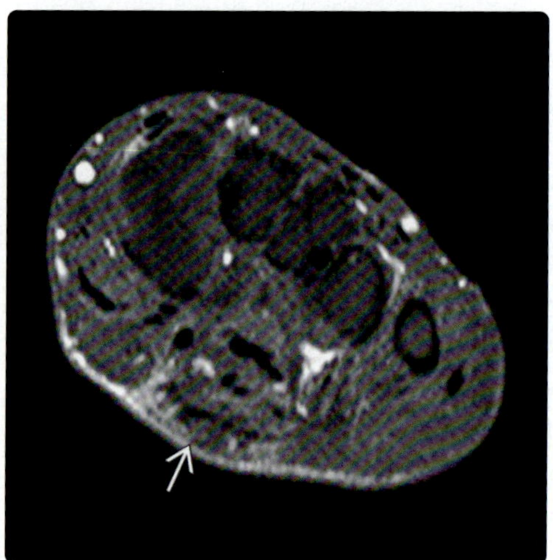

(Left) *Sagittal T1WI MR in the same patient shows midfoot plantar fibromatosis ➡. The mass has low signal relative to muscle. Note how the mass smoothly blends ⮫ to the normal-caliber plantar fascia.* **(Right)** *Sagittal FSE STIR MR in the same patient shows midfoot plantar fibromatosis ➡ to have diffusely low signal intensity. Signal intensity of these lesions vary based on the cellular contents of the lesion, with low-signal lesions containing more dense collagen.*

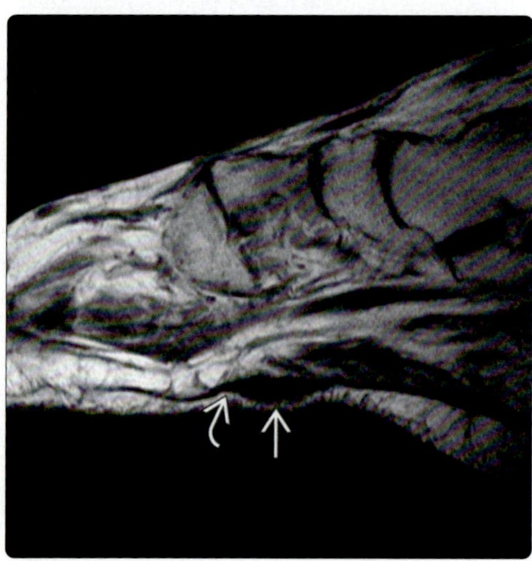

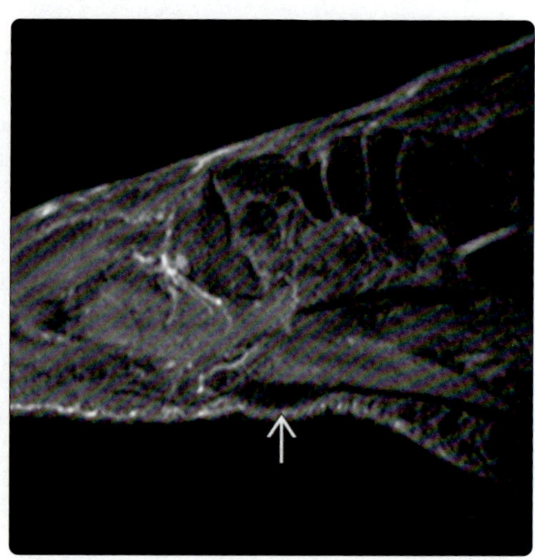

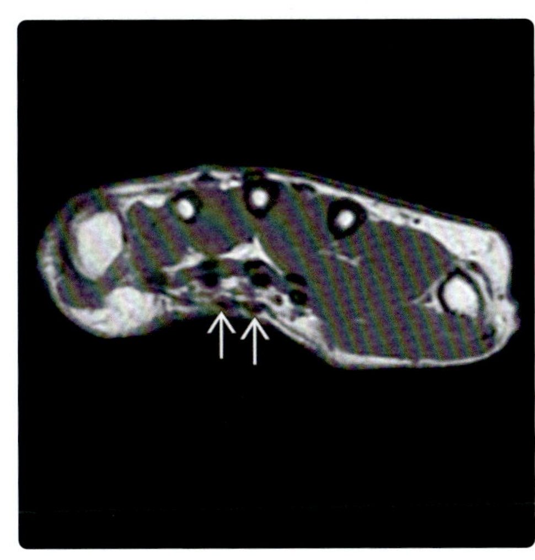

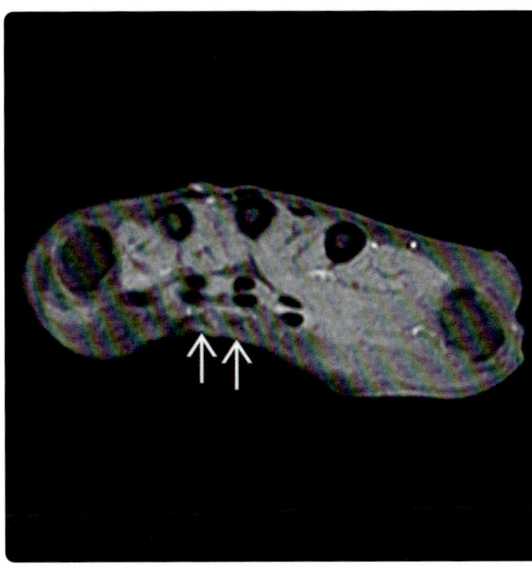

(Left) *Axial T1WI MR shows small nodules ➡ involving the palmar fascia of the hand that have a signal intensity that is slightly lower than the muscle. On T2-weighted, fat-suppressed MR, the nodules had persistently low signal intensity (not shown).* **(Right)** *Axial T1WI C+ FS MR in the same patient demonstrates that the small nodules ➡ have mild peripheral enhancement. Additional similar small nodules were seen along the palmar fascia and extending into the fingers, causing finger flexion deformities.*

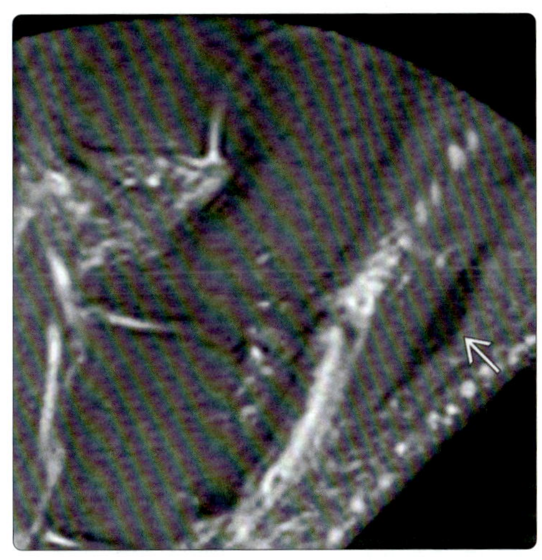

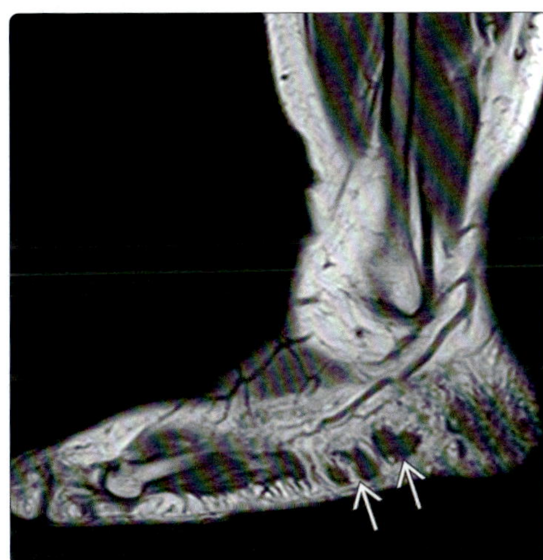

(Left) *Sagittal STIR MR shows the dominant focus of plantar fibromatosis ➡ to have homogeneous ↓ SI. The lentiform shape that blends with the plantar fascia is typical. Involvement of the plantar fascia lateral band is less common than the medial band.* **(Right)** *Sagittal T1 MR, different patient, shows multiple nodules ➡ in the superficial soft tissues, lateral and plantar aspect of the foot. The signal intensity is isointense to skeletal muscle.*

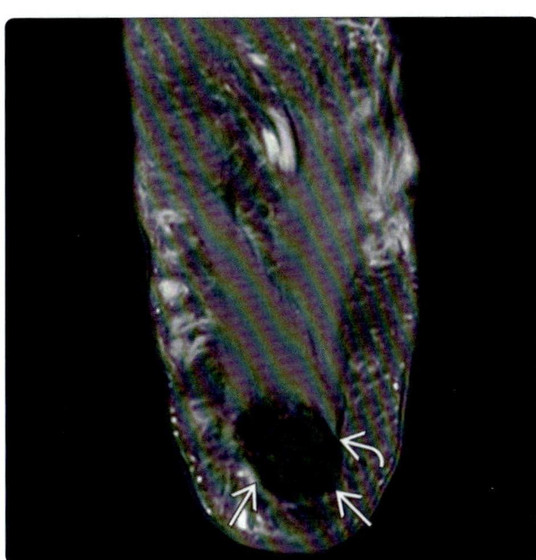

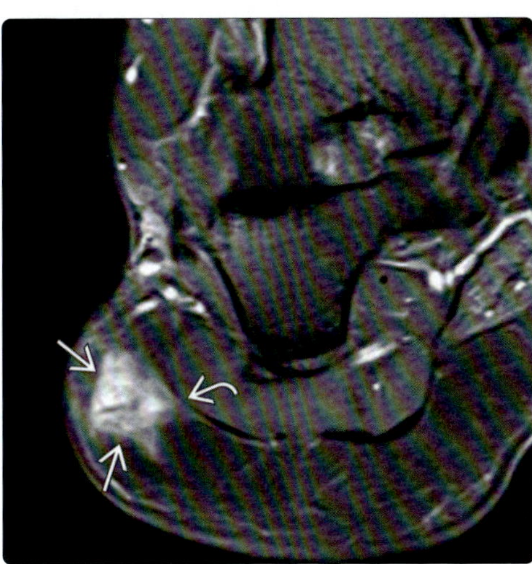

(Left) *Axial PD FS MR, same case, shows the lesion ➡ to be fairly homogeneously hypointense, suggesting fibromatosis. Note the adjacent fascial tissue ↪.* **(Right)** *Coronal T1WI C+ FS MR, same case, shows one of the nodules ➡ to enhance significantly. Note again the adjacent fascial tissue ↪. Note also the infiltrative nature of the lesion, indicating one reason for the high recurrence rate following surgical resection.*

Desmoid-Type Fibromatosis

KEY FACTS

TERMINOLOGY

- Benign, but locally aggressive, clonal fibroblastic proliferation

IMAGING

- Extraabdominal location → 70% in extremities, intermuscular
- Abdominal wall muscles and fascia → common location in female patients 20-30 years old
- Intraabdominal location → small bowel mesentery is most common site of origin
- Nonspecific, ill-defined soft tissue mass
  - Bone involvement is uncommon, but can cause erosion or periosteal reaction
  - Variable CT attenuation: Higher, lower, or similar to muscle
  - MR appearance
    - Low to intermediate signal on T1WI MR
    - Low, intermediate, or hyperintense signal on T2WI MR
    - Usually moderate to marked enhancement, but may lack enhancement
- Generally more locally infiltrative than sarcomas

PATHOLOGY

- Multifactorial pathogenesis
  - Genetic, as with familial adenomatous polyposis
  - Endocrine, as associated with pregnancy
  - Trauma also implicated

CLINICAL ISSUES

- Most common in adults 25-35 years old
  - Local recurrence in 19-88%
- Can be fatal due to invasion of local structures and poor ability to stop progression
- Treated by wide local surgical excision
  - Radiotherapy as adjunct or primary therapy
  - Chemotherapy, antiinflammatory, and antiestrogen therapy have also been utilized

(Left) *Coronal T1WI FSE MR shows a large, highly infiltrative lesion ➡ located in the posterior thigh. The mass has uniformly low signal intensity. There is no identifiable pseudocapsule.* **(Right)** *Coronal STIR MR in the same patient better demonstrates the extent of the infiltrative lesion ➡ in the posterior thigh. The mass has relatively homogeneous high signal on fluid-sensitive sequences with a few central regions of low signal intensity, likely representing collagen.*

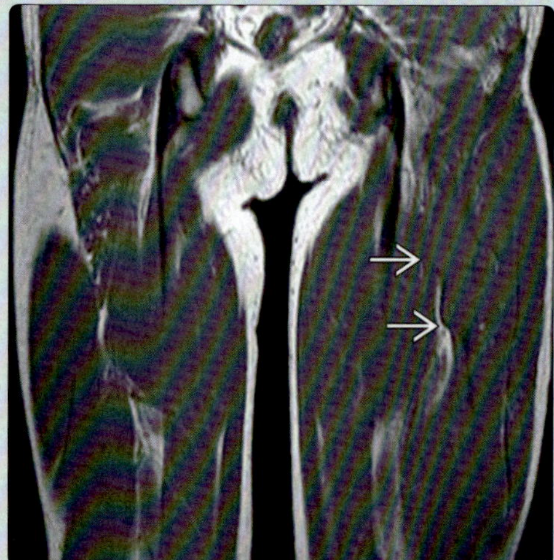

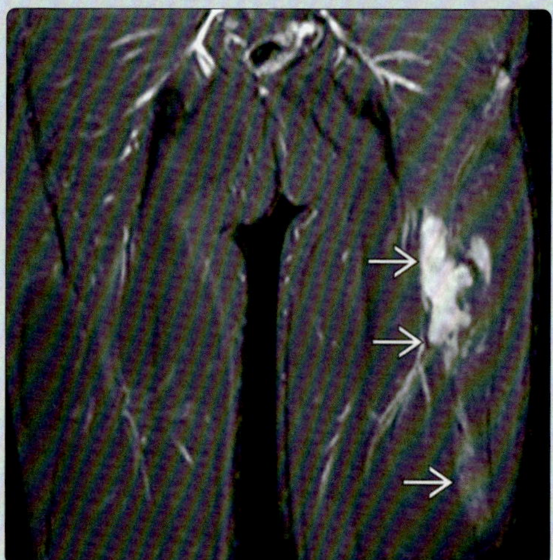

(Left) *Axial T2WI FS MR in the same patient shows the uniformly high signal mass ➡ in the posterior thigh, which contains central foci of low signal ⇨. The mass abuts the posterior cortex of the femur and is causing mild periosteal thickening ➡.* **(Right)** *Sagittal T1WI C+ FS MR shows significant enhancement of the posterior thigh mass ➡, typical of fibromatosis, which has variable low signal on T2WI but prominently enhances and, in general, is more locally infiltrative than is usually seen in sarcomas.*

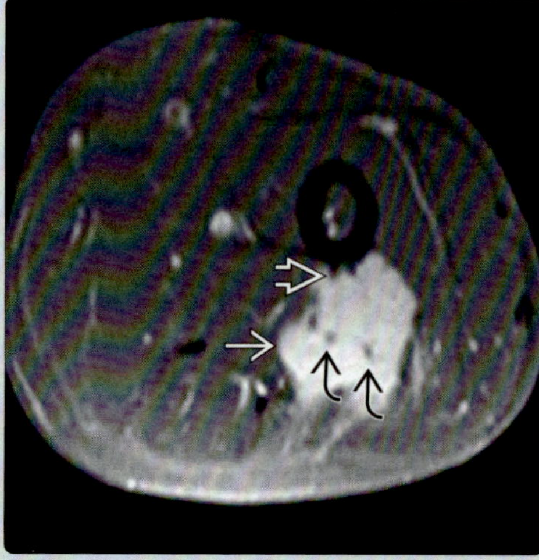

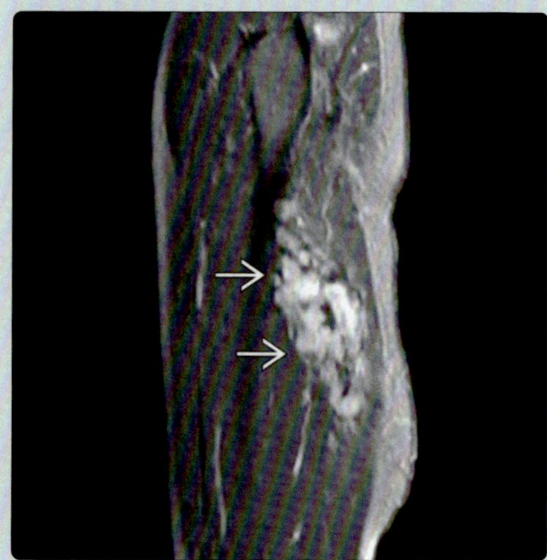

TERMINOLOGY

Synonyms

- Extraabdominal desmoid, desmoid tumor, aggressive fibromatosis, musculoaponeurotic fibromatosis, well-differentiated nonmetastasizing fibrosarcoma

Definitions

- Benign, but locally aggressive, clonal fibroblastic proliferation
  - Formerly histologically divided by location (extraabdominal, abdominal, intraabdominal)

IMAGING

General Features

- Location
  - Extraabdominal location
    - 70% in extremities
      - Shoulder region, upper arm: 28%
      - Chest wall and back: 17%; thigh: 12%; head and neck: 8%
    - Usually intermuscular
  - Abdominal location
    - Abdominal wall muscles and fascia
      - Rectus abdominis and internal oblique muscles
    - Common location in female patients 20-30 years old
  - Intraabdominal location
    - Small bowel mesentery is most common site of origin
    - Encompasses pelvic, retroperitoneal, and mesenteric regions
    - 13% of patients with mesenteric fibromatosis have familial adenomatous polyposis (Gardner syndrome)
      - Remainder are sporadic
- Size
  - Extraabdominal lesions usually measure 5-10 cm
  - Abdominal wall lesions are smaller, being 3-7 cm
  - Intraabdominal lesions are largest, being 10-25 cm
- Morphology
  - Ill-defined, infiltrative mass
  - Usually single, but may be multiple synchronous lesions
    - Multiple intraabdominal lesions are more common in patients with familial adenomatous polyposis

Imaging Recommendations

- Best imaging tool
  - MR best demonstrates location and extent of lesions
    - Most useful modality for follow-up after treatment

Radiographic Findings

- Radiography
  - Radiographs are usually normal
    - Calcification or ossification is rare
    - Bulging or puckering of overlying skin
  - Bone involvement is uncommon (6-37%) but can include erosion or periosteal reaction
    - Increased with recurrent tumors
  - Intraabdominal involvement may cause displacement of small bowel loops or mass effect on other structures, such as bladder

CT Findings

- Nonspecific, ill-defined soft tissue mass
- Variable attenuation: Higher, lower, or similar to muscle
- Mild, heterogeneous enhancement with IV contrast is typical
  - Enhancement may be absent

MR Findings

- Heterogeneous soft tissue mass that may extend along fascial plane
  - Locally invasive (46-51%), with linear extension along fascial planes (83%) or crossing compartmental lines
- Variable signal intensity based on amount of collagen
  - Low to intermediate signal on T1WI
  - Low, intermediate, or hyperintense signal on T2WI
  - Regions with low T1WI and T2WI signal suggest mature collagen
    - Early lesions more cellular, with ↑ T2 SI; more mature lesions more heterogeneous, with foci of ↓ T2 SI; highly mature lesions have ↑ in fibrous tissue and ↓ T2 SI
    - More mature lesions have lower recurrence rates
- Lesions show variable enhancement
  - Usually moderate to marked, but enhancement may be absent
  - Lesions without CT enhancement may still show enhancement on MR
  - Myxoid lesions have least enhancement
- Intermuscular location results in rim of fat (split fat sign)
  - Not seen with local invasion of muscle

Ultrasonographic Findings

- Color Doppler
  - Blood flow visible within these hypervascular lesions
- Ill-defined hypoechoic soft tissue lesion
- Posterior acoustic shadowing

Angiographic Findings

- Normal or hypervascular depending on lesion

Nuclear Medicine Findings

- Increased radiotracer uptake on blood pool and delayed imaging
  - May suggest bone involvement

DIFFERENTIAL DIAGNOSIS

Fibrosarcoma, Soft Tissue

- More uniformly cellular than fibromatosis
- Fascicular or herringbone growth pattern of cells
- Hyperchromatic, atypical nuclei with more prominent nucleoli

Sarcoma, Soft Tissue

- Similar appearance on imaging
- Biopsy necessary for diagnosis
- Histologically malignant

Elastofibroma

- Typical location between tip of scapula and chest wall
- Lacks locally aggressive characteristics
- Usually contains areas of fat, unlike desmoid-type fibromatosis

- Has areas of low signal on T1WI and T2WI MR

Lymphoma

- Involvement of bowel walls and solid intraabdominal masses can have same appearance on imaging
- Histologically distinct entity

Intramuscular Myxoma

- Prominent myxoid matrix with few cells
- Intramuscular location rather than intermuscular location

Solitary Fibrous Tumor and Hemangiopericytoma

- Imaging appearance very similar to intraabdominal fibromatosis
- Multiple lesions less common than intraabdominal desmoid
- Not associated with familial adenomatous polyposis

PATHOLOGY

General Features

- Etiology
  - Multifactorial pathogenesis
    - Similar pathogenesis in all forms: Activation of β-catenin signaling pathway
    - Genetic causes, as seen with familial adenomatous polyposis
    - Endocrine factors implicated by association with pregnancy
    - Trauma also implicated as cause
- Genetics
  - Trisomy 8, 20 in up to 30% of cases
- Associated abnormalities
  - Skeletal dysplasia
  - 83% of familial adenomatous polyposis patients have history of abdominal surgery

Staging, Grading, & Classification

- Divided by extraabdominal, abdominal wall, and intraabdominal locations

Gross Pathologic & Surgical Features

- Firm, glistening, white trabeculated lesion
  - Resembles scar tissue
- Margins are poorly circumscribed and infiltrating in extraabdominal and abdominal wall locations
  - Intraabdominal lesions are well circumscribed

Microscopic Features

- Uniform, spindle-shaped fibroblasts
  - No atypia or hyperchromasia
  - Bland nuclei with small nucleoli
  - Flowing bundles of cells
  - Variable mitotic rate
- Variable collagen stroma
  - May be extensively hyalinized, have myxoid change, or contain keloid-like collagen
  - ± perivascular edema, hemorrhage, inflammation
- Intraabdominal form insinuates in or through bowel wall muscularis propria
- Strongly positive stain for vimentin
- Variably positive for muscle-specific and smooth muscle actin, desmin, and S100 protein

CLINICAL ISSUES

Presentation

- Most common signs/symptoms
  - Extraabdominal location
    - Painless, slowly growing mass
    - Firm and ill defined
    - Rarely cause pain or decreased range of motion
  - Abdominal wall location
    - Painless mass arising during or after pregnancy
  - Intraabdominal location
    - Asymptomatic mass
    - Rare cause of bowel perforation, bowel obstruction, fistula formation, and gastrointestinal bleeding
- Other signs/symptoms
  - Intraabdominal lesions can be mistaken for malignancy
  - Patients with familial adenomatous polyposis have numerous colon polyps or evidence of colectomy

Demographics

- Age
  - Seen from puberty through adulthood
    - Most common in adults 25-35 years old
    - Intraabdominal location: Mean: 41 years
- Gender
  - Female predisposition in patients < 40 years old
- Epidemiology
  - 700-900 new cases per year
  - Less common than superficial fibromatoses

Natural History & Prognosis

- Local recurrence in 19-77% (average 30-40%)
  - Recurrence increases with ↑ size, patient age < 30 years, female gender, incomplete resection
    - Local invasiveness may make complete resection difficult
  - Intraabdominal lesions associated with familial adenomatous polyposis are most likely to recur
  - Abdominal wall lesions are least likely to recur
- Can be fatal due to invasion of local structures and poor ability to stop progression
  - Invasion of neurovascular structures, ureters, bowel
- Spontaneous regression has been reported
- No potential for metastatic disease

Treatment

- Treated by wide local surgical excision
  - Amputation may be necessary for local control
- Radiotherapy as adjunct or primary therapy
- Chemotherapy, antiinflammatory, and antiestrogen therapy have also been utilized

SELECTED REFERENCES

1. Lee CH et al: Lipomatosis of the sciatic nerve secondary to compression by a desmoid tumor. Skeletal Radiol. 42(12):1751-4, 2013
2. Oweis Y et al: Extra-abdominal desmoid tumor with osseous involvement. Skeletal Radiol. 41(4):483-7, 2012
3. Ilaslan H et al: Radiofrequency ablation: another treatment option for local control of desmoid tumors. Skeletal Radiol. 39(2):169-73, 2010
4. Murphey MD et al: From the archives of the AFIP: musculoskeletal fibromatoses: radiologic-pathologic correlation. Radiographics. 29(7):2143-73, 2009

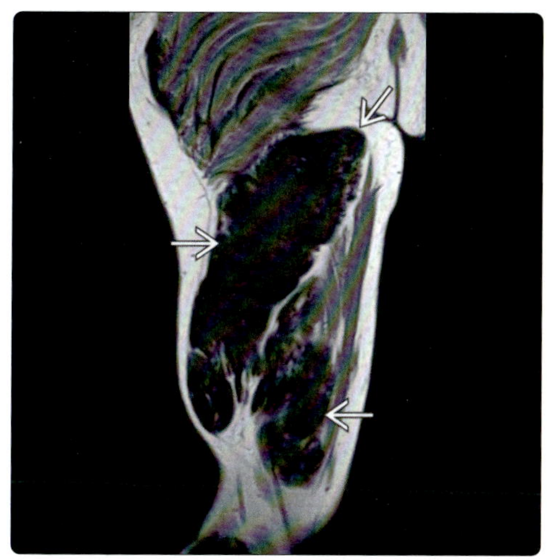

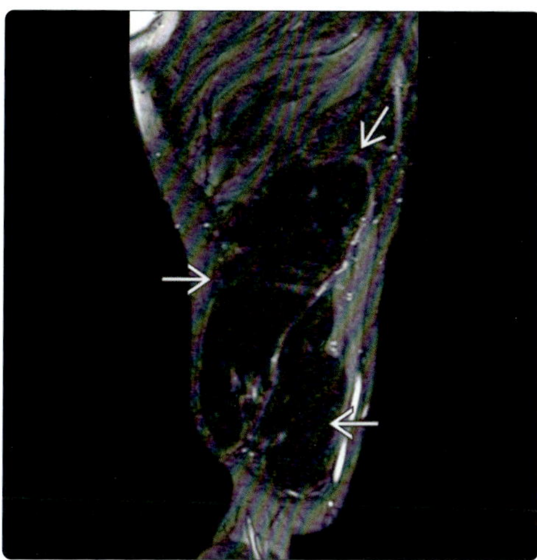

(Left) *Coronal T1WI MR shows a very large posterior thigh mass →, which is highly infiltrative. The mass has a homogeneous low signal. Cortically based osteomas were present in the adjacent femur.* **(Right)** *Coronal STIR MR in the same patient shows the large posterior thigh mass to have persistently low signal →. Desmoid-type fibromatosis need not be quite this densely low signal and homogeneous, but this was the diagnosis in this patient with familial adenomatous polyposis.*

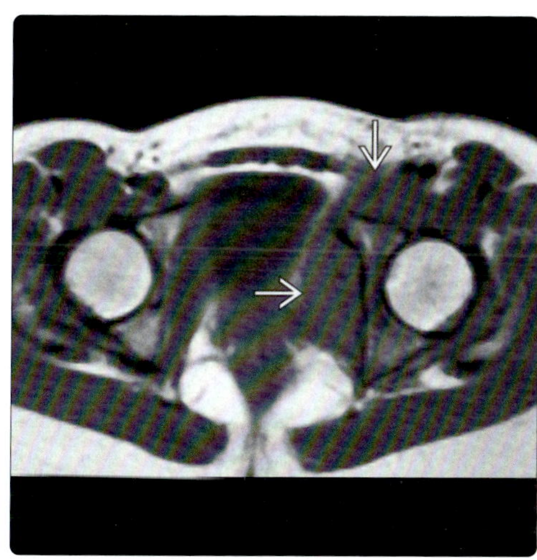

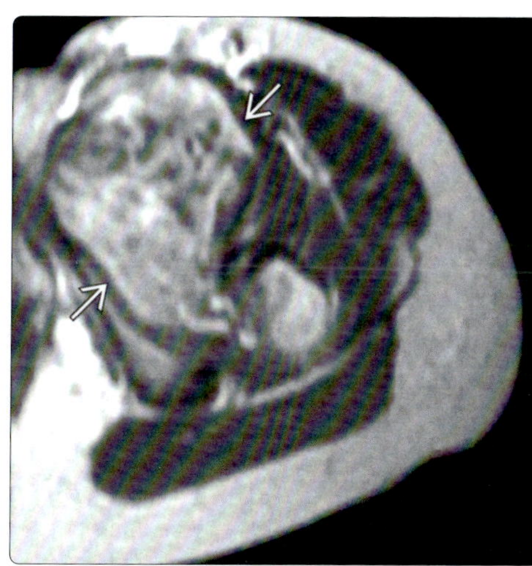

(Left) *Axial T1WI MR demonstrates a very large mass → arising in the adductor muscles that has slightly higher signal intensity than muscle. This mass extends through the obturator foramen to surround the ischial tuberosity both anteriorly and posteriorly.* **(Right)** *Axial T2WI MR in the same patient shows the large inhomogeneous mass → to have considerably higher signal than muscle with central areas of low signal. The mass displaces but does not invade the neurovascular bundle.*

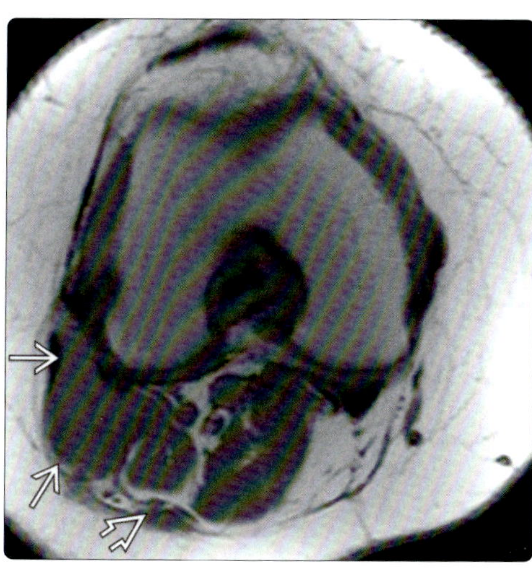

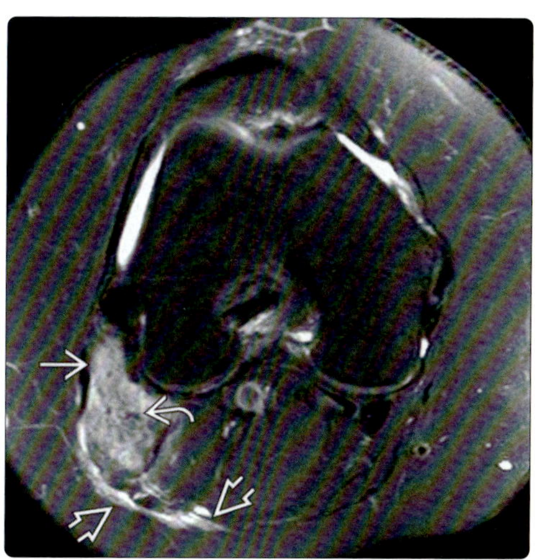

(Left) *Axial T1WI MR shows an infiltrative mass involving the biceps femoris →. The lesion is similar in SI to muscle, though inhomogeneous. Note that the lesion extends beyond the predominant mass, along fascial planes ⇨.* **(Right)** *Axial T2WI FS MR in the same patient shows the mass → to be hyperintense, but containing low-signal foci ↪. The extension along fascial planes ⇨ is more obvious on this sequence. This finding is important since such extension and infiltration makes complete resection difficult.*

(Left) *Sagittal T2WI MR shows a paraspinal mass ➡ that is markedly heterogeneous with signal intensity ranging from low to high. The mass appears well circumscribed. Desmoid-type fibromatosis may mimic malignant head and neck tumors, such as sarcoma and lymphoma.* **(Right)** *Sagittal T1WI C+ MR in the same patient shows heterogeneous enhancement of the paraspinal mass ➡. The heterogeneity on the T2 and postcontrast T1 sequences would raise the question of a malignant process.*

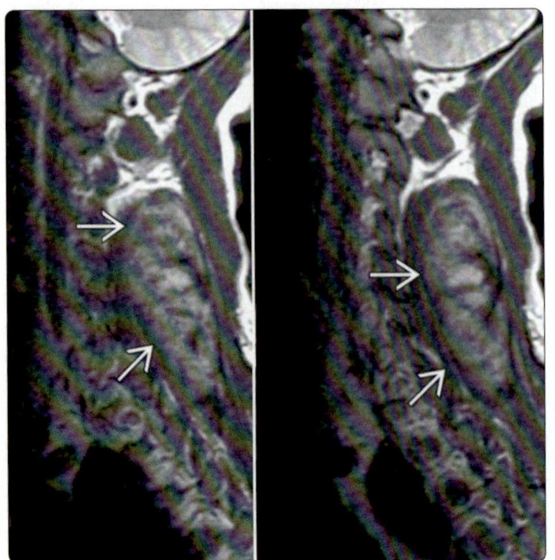

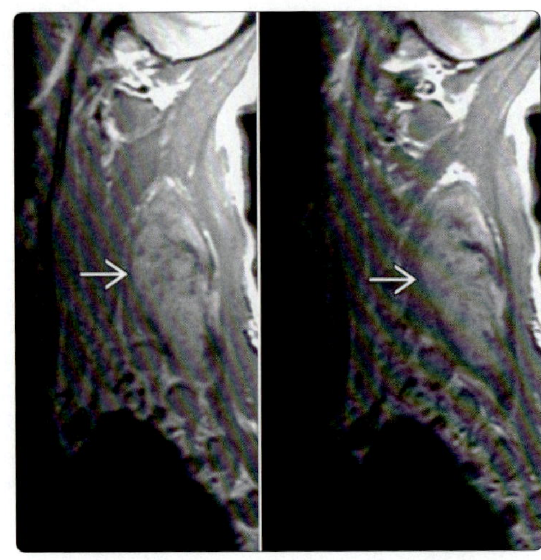

(Left) *Axial CECT shows mesenteric masses ➡ in a patient with Gardner syndrome. The masses are isointense to muscle and were shown to rapidly grow over several months. Recurrence after resection is common and patients frequently develop short gut syndrome as a result.* **(Right)** *Coronal CECT in a young adult female shows a slightly enhancing mass arising in the rectus abdominis ➡. This location, appearance, and the gender and age of the patient are typical of desmoid-type fibromatosis.*

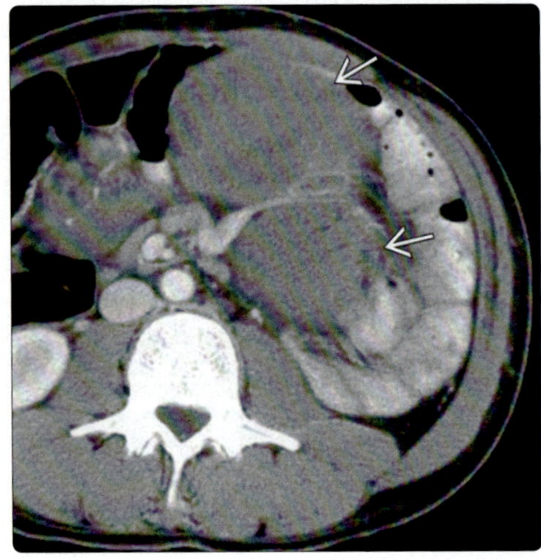

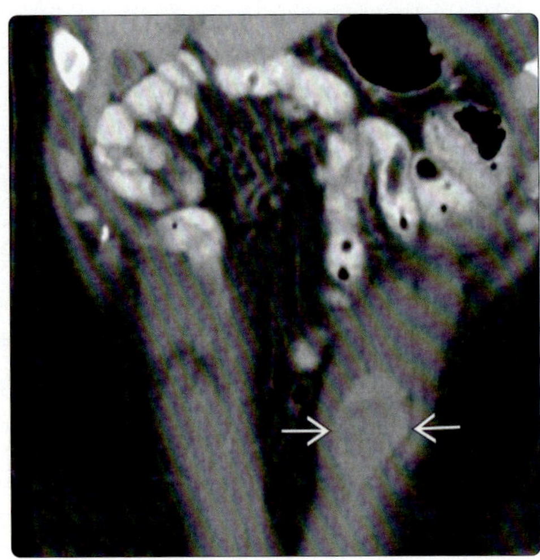

(Left) *Coronal T1WI MR, same patient but obtained 9 months later, shows the mass ➡ to have enlarged significantly. Given the rapid enlargement of the mass, the clinicians were concerned that this may represent sarcoma rather than the original diagnosis of desmoid.* **(Right)** *Sagittal T1WI C+ FS MR shows enhancement of the mass ➡. In this case, the clinical history of a failed pregnancy 5 months earlier is important. Desmoid tumors can enlarge significantly during pregnancy. The lesion is typical of desmoid; sarcoma need not be considered.*

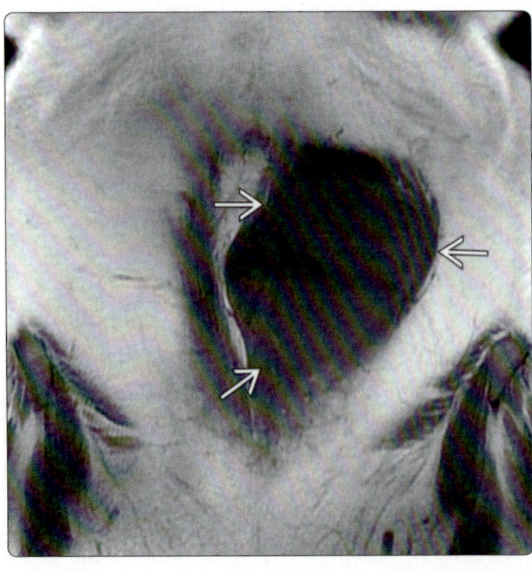

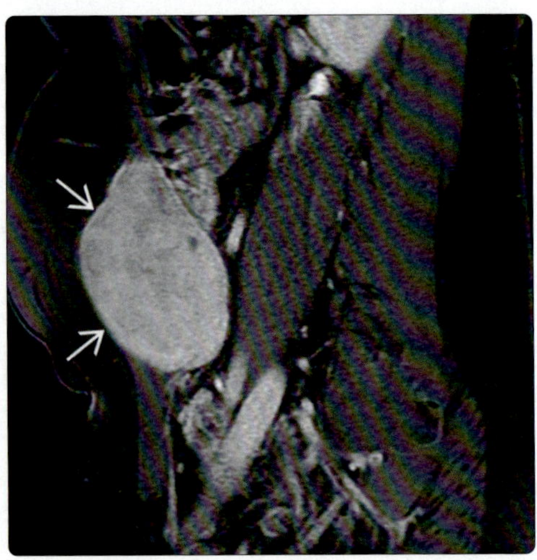

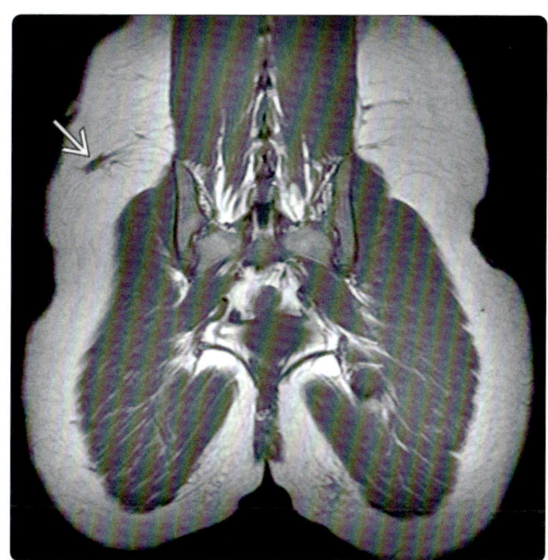

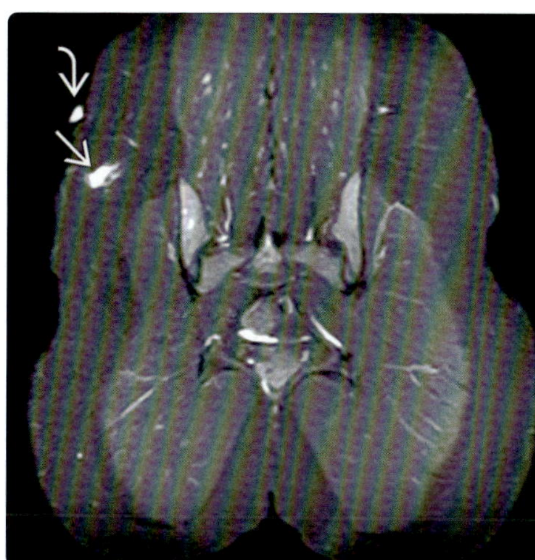

(Left) *Coronal T1WI MR demonstrates a somewhat unimpressive, ill-defined, small focus* ➡ *of abnormal signal intensity, similar to skeletal muscle, that lies just deep to a region of the skin puckering in the subcutaneous fat.* **(Right)** *Coronal STIR MR in the same patient shows the ill-defined, small mass* ➡ *to have diffusely high signal. The borders of the mass are infiltrative. A skin marker* ➦ *denotes the location of the slowly growing mass reported by this young adult female.*

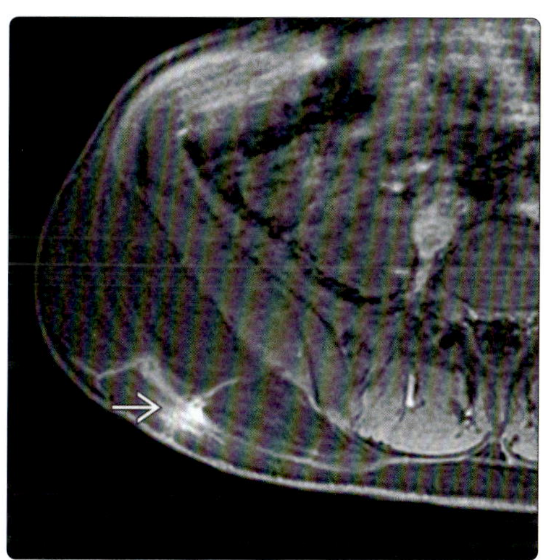

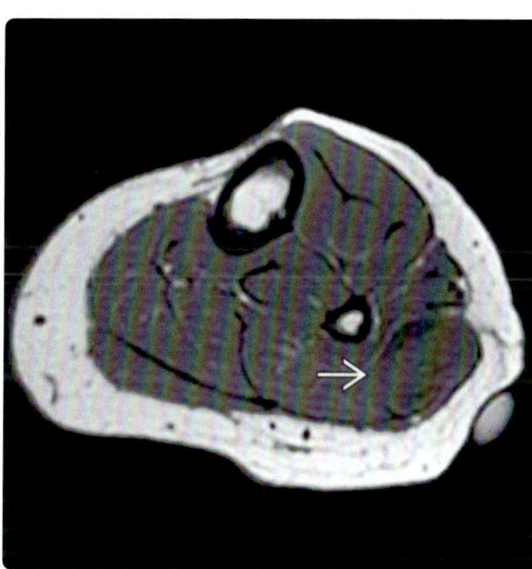

(Left) *Axial T1WI C+ FS MR in the same patient shows intense enhancement of the palpable mass* ➡*. The intense, solid enhancement favors fibromatosis. An area of prior subcutaneous medication injection or traumatic scarring would not be expected to show this degree of solid enhancement.* **(Right)** *Axial T1WI MR shows a homogeneous low-signal mass* ➡ *along the far lateral aspect of the soleus muscle. The mass is well defined, which is unusual for the typically infiltrative desmoid-type fibromatosis.*

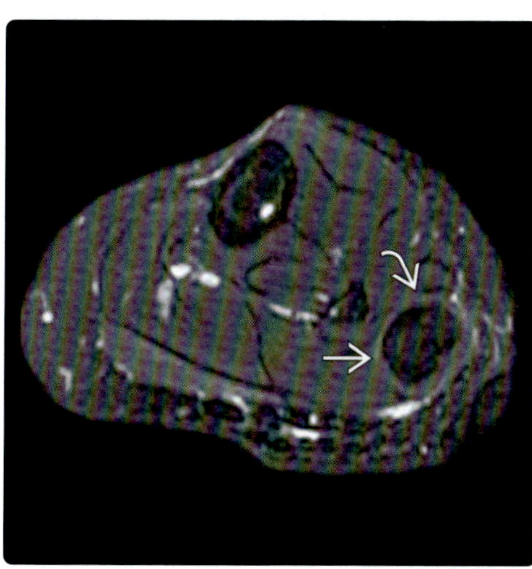

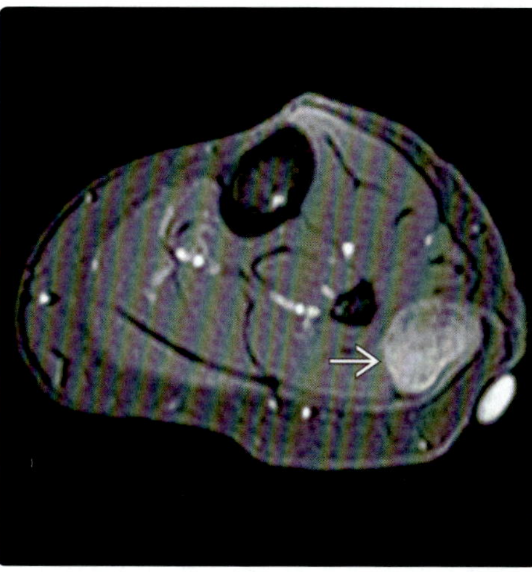

(Left) *Axial T2WI FS MR shows the mass* ➡ *to have homogeneous low signal with mild surrounding edema* ➦*. An intermuscular location for desmoid-type fibromatosis is more common than lesions that are entirely intramuscular.* **(Right)** *Axial T1WI C+ FS MR shows the mass* ➡ *to have mildly heterogeneous enhancement after gadolinium administration. The variable cellular content of desmoid-type fibromatosis produces the variable signal and enhancement characteristics on MR.*

KEY FACTS

TERMINOLOGY

- Solitary fibrous tumor and hemangiopericytoma are terms that are used almost interchangeably

IMAGING

- May be found in any location
  - Chest, extremities, retroperitoneum, abdomen/pelvis, orbit, head and neck
  - 40% subcutaneous
- Wide range of sizes (1-25 cm)
- Pleural lesions may be visible on chest radiographs
  - Well-circumscribed mass associated with pleura
  - Lesion may change location based on patient position, if mass is on pedicle
  - Erosion or saucerization of bone is uncommon
- Unenhanced CT shows heterogeneous attenuation similar to muscle
  - May contain areas of hypoattenuation secondary to myxoid change, necrosis, or hemorrhage
- Prominent vascularity may be evident as intense enhancement &/or visible blood vessels
- Abdominal lesions may demonstrate secondary bowel or bladder obstruction
- MR findings
  - T1WI: Heterogeneous hypo- to hyperintense (blood) SI
  - T2WI: Heterogeneous hypo-to hyperintense SI
  - Homogeneous to heterogeneous enhancement
  - Feeding vessels may be prominent

CLINICAL ISSUES

- Painless, slowly growing mass
- Symptoms from compression of adjacent structures
  - Intestinal, urinary, neurovascular, orbital
- May cause paraneoplastic syndromes
  - Insulin-like growth factor = hypoglycemia
- Aggressive behavior in 15-20% of SFT-HPC
- Long-term follow-up necessary to evaluate for delayed recurrence and metastases

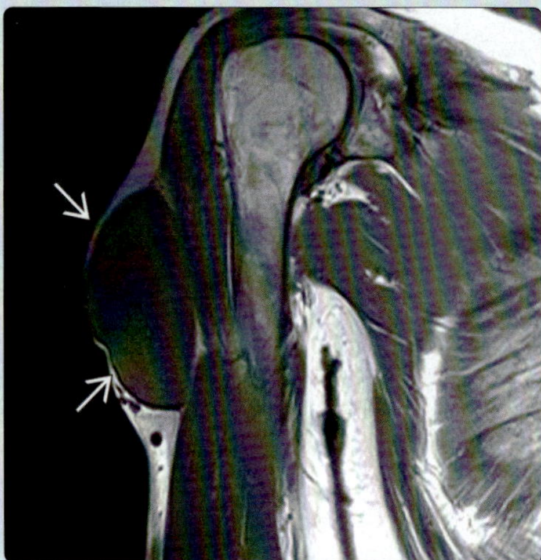
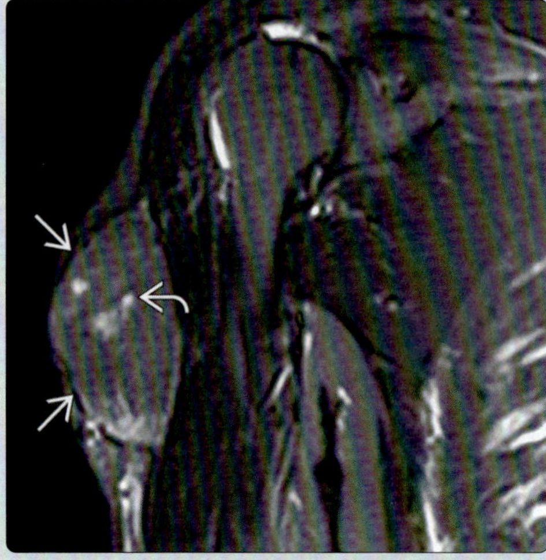

(Left) *Coronal T1WI MR of a solitary fibrous tumor (SFT) demonstrates a lobulated, ovoid mass ➡, which is confined to the subcutaneous space. The mass is homogeneously isointense to muscle. There is no invasion of the underlying deltoid muscle.* **(Right)** *Coronal STIR MR in the same patient shows inhomogeneous signal intensity of the subcutaneous mass ➡, which is relatively low but contains branching high-signal vessels ↪.*

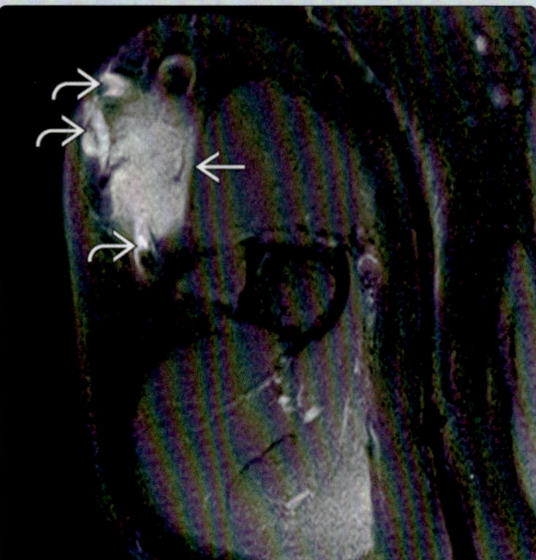
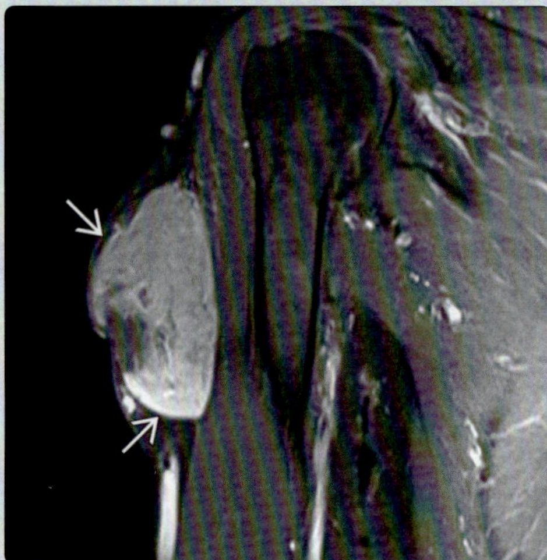

(Left) *Axial PDWI FS MR in the same patient shows the lesion ➡ to be relatively high signal but to have very large feeding vessels ↪, which continued into the lesion with a typical branching pattern. At histologic examination, multiple thin-walled branching vessels were confirmed, as are typically seen in this entity.* **(Right)** *Coronal T1WI C+ FS MR in the same patient shows the majority of the lesion ➡ to enhance intensely. At surgery the lesion was confirmed to be well encapsulated.*

TERMINOLOGY

Abbreviations

- Solitary fibrous tumor (SFT)
- Hemangiopericytoma (HPC)

Definitions

- Solitary fibrous tumor
  - Mesenchymal tumor, likely fibroblastic type, with hemangiopericytoma-like branching vessels
- Hemangiopericytoma
  - Formerly used to describe wide variety of neoplasms with thin-walled branching vessels
    - Most were histologically similar to solitary fibrous tumor and may represent same lesion
  - Also refers to distinct entity arising from pericytes
- Solitary fibrous tumor and hemangiopericytoma are currently used almost interchangeably

IMAGING

General Features

- Location
  - Solitary fibrous tumor
    - May be found in any location
    - Most typically found in body cavity, especially pleura
      - ☐ Chest wall, mediastinum, and pericardium
      - ☐ Deep soft tissues of extremities, retroperitoneum, and abdomen/pelvis
      - ☐ Orbit, head and neck
      - ☐ Rare in spinal cord, meninges, solid and hollow visceral organs
    - 40% subcutaneous
  - Hemangiopericytoma
    - Lower extremity > retroperitoneum > head/neck > trunk > upper extremity
      - ☐ More likely to be in extremity than SFT
- Size
  - SFT
    - Large range of sizes (1-25 cm)
    - Usually 5-8 cm
  - Hemangiopericytoma
    - Usually 5-15 cm
- Morphology
  - Rounded, well-circumscribed, solitary mass
  - Pleural lesions may have pedicle
  - Plaque-like lesions are uncommon

Imaging Recommendations

- Best imaging tool
  - MR is typically best imaging modality
  - CT preferred for masses in chest

Radiographic Findings

- Pleural-based lesions may be visible on chest x-ray
  - Well-circumscribed mass associated with pleura
  - Lesion may change location based on patient position if mass has pedicle
- Erosion or saucerization of bone is uncommon

CT Findings

- Rounded, homogeneous to heterogeneously enhancing mass
  - Prominent vascularity may be evident as intense enhancement
- Unenhanced imaging demonstrates heterogeneous attenuation similar to muscle
  - May contain areas of hypoattenuation secondary to myxoid change, necrosis, or hemorrhage
- Abdominal lesions may demonstrate secondary findings of bowel or bladder obstruction
- Calcification is not uncommon

MR Findings

- Heterogeneous isointense to hypointense signal relative to muscle on T1WI
  - Areas of hemorrhage may demonstrate hyperintense signal on T1WI
- Heterogeneous hypo- to hyperintense signal on fluid-sensitive sequences depending on cellular content
- Homogeneous to heterogeneous enhancement
  - Tubular flow voids seen with large vessels
- May contain small amount of fat

Ultrasonographic Findings

- Well-defined mass with mixed echogenicity
- Internal blood flow demonstrable on Doppler exam

DIFFERENTIAL DIAGNOSIS

Liposarcoma, Myxoid

- May contain only small amount of fat, as can SFT
- Prominent myxoid tissue is similar to SFT
- SFT lacks lipoblasts

Liposarcoma, Soft Tissue

- Well-differentiated liposarcoma may have similar histologic appearance to lipomatous HPC-SFT
- Imaging usually shows component of fatty tissue

Deep Benign Fibrous Histiocytoma

- May have similar histologic appearance, especially in orbit

Synovial Sarcoma

- More likely to occur near joint
- More likely to contain calcification than SFT
- May contain hemangiopericytoma-like vessels

PATHOLOGY

General Features

- Etiology
  - Neoplasm with variable aggressiveness
- Genetics
  - SFT
    - Lesions larger than 10 cm often have cytogenetic aberrations
      - ☐ Frequent genomic gains and losses
      - ☐ Trisomy 21
  - Hemangiopericytoma
    - Variable chromosome aberrations
      - ☐ Breakpoints in 12q13-15 and 19q13
      - ☐ Balanced t(12;19)(q13;q13)

- Near diploid karyotype

Gross Pathologic & Surgical Features

- SFT
  - Well-circumscribed, lobulated, or multinodular mass
  - Firm, whitish cut surface
  - Partially encapsulated
  - May contain hemorrhage or myxoid change
  - Aggressive tumors may show necrosis or infiltrative margins
- Hemangiopericytoma
  - Well-circumscribed mass
  - Cut surface is spongy to fleshy with yellowish-tan to red-brown surface ± apparent large vessels
  - Hemorrhagic change is common
  - Necrosis is rare

Microscopic Features

- SFT
  - Round to spindle-shaped tumor cells with fibroblastic, myofibroblastic, or potentially pericytic differentiation
    - Cellular areas are separated from hypocellular areas by collagen and hemangiopericytoma-like vessels
      - Vascular pattern is more focal compared with diffuse finding in hemangiopericytoma
    - Prominent hyalinization
    - Mitoses are usually < 3 per 10 HPF
    - Fibrosis, mast cells, & myxoid change are common
  - Malignant SFT = cytologic atypia, necrosis, > 4 mitoses per 10 HPF, hypercellular, infiltrative margins
  - Immunophenotype
    - 90-95% immunoreactive for CD34 and CD99
  - Other findings
    - Presence of giant multinucleated stromal cells has overlapping appearance with giant cell angiofibroma
- Hemangiopericytoma
  - Characteristic thin-walled branching, staghorn configuration of vessels
  - Fusiform-to-round cells with indistinct margins
    - Lacks varying cellularity of SFT
    - Lacks convincing pericytic differentiation
    - Stromal hyalinization uncommon, unlike SFT
    - Variable mitotic rate
  - Most are positive for CD34 and CD99
  - Usually negative endothelial markers, actin, and desmin
  - Presence of mature adipocytes suggests lipomatous hemangiopericytoma
    - Controversial whether this represents separate entity or lesion that has engulfed fat

CLINICAL ISSUES

Presentation

- Most common signs/symptoms
  - Painless, slowly growing mass
  - May cause symptoms from compression of adjacent structures
    - Intestinal or urinary
    - Neurovascular
    - Orbital
- Other signs/symptoms
  - May cause paraneoplastic syndromes
    - Insulin-like growth factor = hypoglycemia
      - Hypoglycemia common in HPC
      - Hypoglycemia in 25% of SFT

Demographics

- Age
  - SFT
    - Middle-aged adults: Range 20-70 years
    - Children and adolescent involvement rare
  - Hemangiopericytoma
    - Most common in 5th decade of life
    - Rare infantile type is probably better classified as infantile myofibromatosis
- Gender
  - No sex predilection
- Epidemiology
  - SFT is uncommon
  - Hemangiopericytoma
    - Rare lesions without dependable incidence rates due to changing terminology
      - Myopericytoma: Most common of HPC subsets

Natural History & Prognosis

- Overall prognosis is good
  - 54-89% 10-yr survival
- SFT
  - Unpredictable behavior that is not always correlated with histologic appearance
    - Most do not recur or metastasize
    - 10-15% recur or metastasize
      - Metastases to lungs, liver, and bone
      - Recurrences seen > 10 yr from excision
  - Aggressive behavior is more common in mediastinal, abdomen/pelvis, and retroperitoneal locations
- Hemangiopericytoma
  - 70% benign
- Hypoglycemia resolves after tumor removal

Treatment

- Complete surgical excision
- Insensitive to cytotoxic chemotherapy & radiotherapy
  - Antiangiogenic therapy may be useful
- Long-term follow-up necessary to evaluate for delayed recurrence and metastases

SELECTED REFERENCES

1. Frazier AA: The Yin and Yang of solitary fibrous tumor. Radiographics. 34(2):294, 2014
2. Garcia-Bennett J et al: Soft tissue solitary fibrous tumor. Imaging findings in a series of nine cases. Skeletal Radiol. 41(11):1427-33, 2012
3. Musyoki FN et al: Solitary fibrous tumor: an update on the spectrum of extrapleural manifestations. Skeletal Radiol. 41(1):5-13, 2012
4. Shanbhogue AK et al: Somatic and visceral solitary fibrous tumors in the abdomen and pelvis: cross-sectional imaging spectrum. Radiographics. 31(2):393-408, 2011
5. Aftab S et al: Fat-forming solitary fibrous tumour (lipomatous haemangiopericytoma) of the spine: case report and literature review. Skeletal Radiol. 39(10):1039-42, 2010
6. Wignall OJ et al: Solitary fibrous tumors of the soft tissues: review of the imaging and clinical features with histopathologic correlation. AJR Am J Roentgenol. 195(1):W55-62, 2010

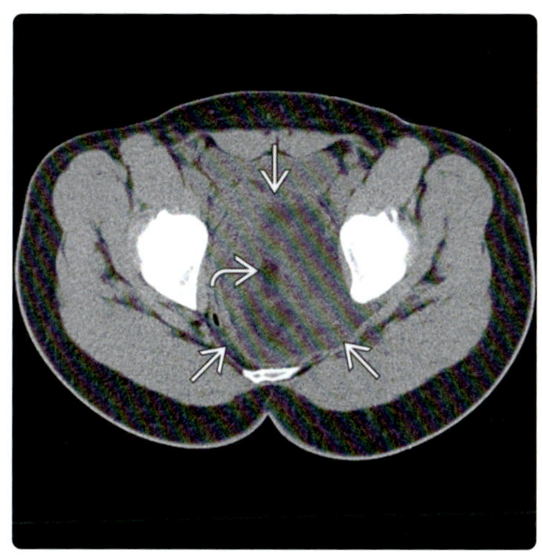

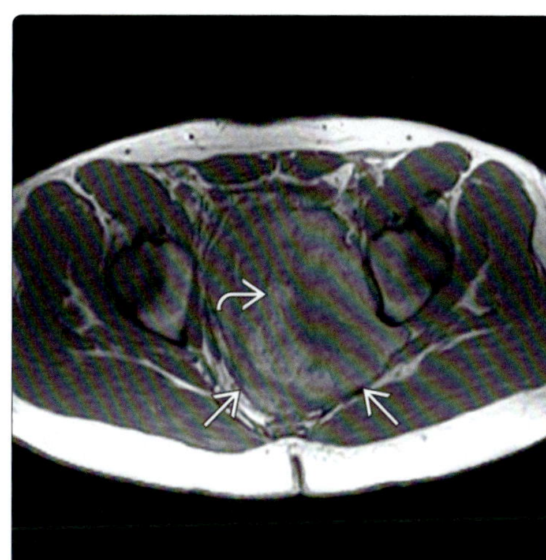

(Left) *Axial noncontrast CT of a lipomatous hemangiopericytoma shows a very large mass ➡ in the low pelvis. The mass is composed of soft tissue attenuation similar to muscle mixed with fat attenuation ↪.* **(Right)** *Axial T1WI MR in the same patient shows the large pelvic mass ➡ to have both fat signal intensity ↪ and signal intensity similar to muscle. The presence of fat within the mass and complex appearance would favor a liposarcoma over an uncommon lipomatous hemangiopericytoma.*

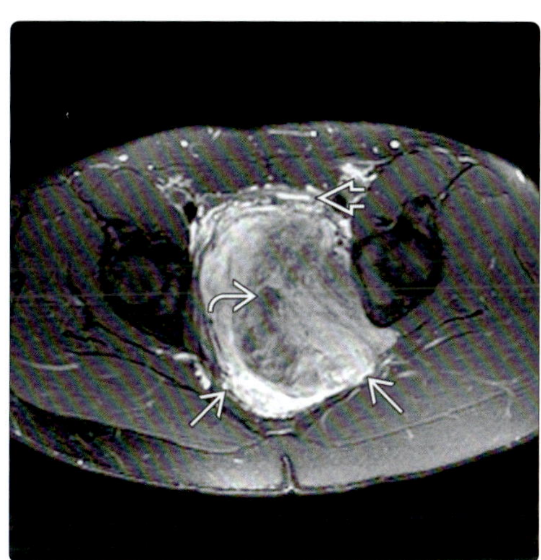

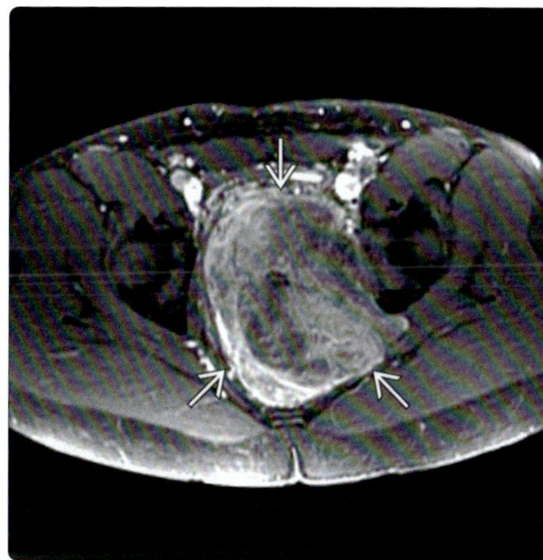

(Left) *Axial T2WI FS MR in the same patient shows the large pelvic mass ➡ to have heterogeneously high signal with admixed low-signal fat ↪. The bladder ➡ is compressed along the anterior wall of the pelvis.* **(Right)** *Axial T1WI C+ FS MR in the same patient shows heterogeneous enhancement on the pelvic floor mass ➡. The imaging appearance of this lesion strongly suggests a malignant lipomatous tumor. Tissue diagnosis of hemangiopericytoma was essential for appropriate surgical planning.*

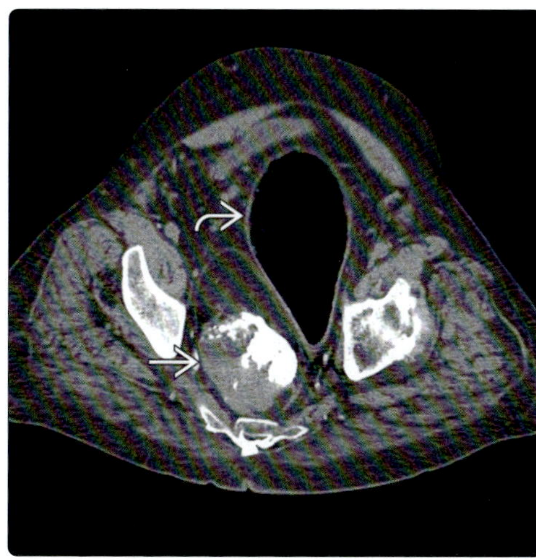

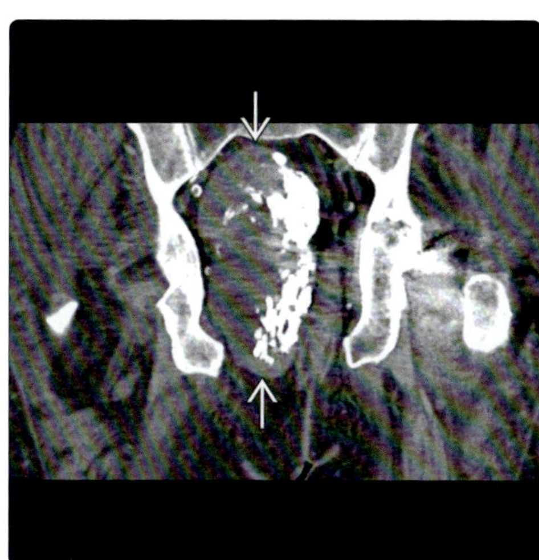

(Left) *Axial NECT demonstrates a mass ➡ in the low right pelvis being composed of both soft tissue and relatively dense peripheral calcification. It is located in the presacral region. Sigmoid colon distention ↪ due to compression from the mass is also evident.* **(Right)** *Coronal NECT in the same patient shows the large size of the pelvic mass ➡, which extends from the midsacrum through the inferior sciatic notch and into the proximal thigh. This mass had been asymptomatic for decades.*

(Left) *Coronal T1WI MR shows a rounded soft tissue mass ➡ in the low left pelvis. The mass is predominantly isointense to muscle, although there are a few tiny scattered foci of low signal intensity.* **(Right)** *Axial T2WI FS MR in the same patient shows the SFT ➡ to be predominantly hyperintense to muscle. The appearance of the mass on the fluid-sensitive sequences also includes scattered small foci of both low signal and very high signal intensity.*

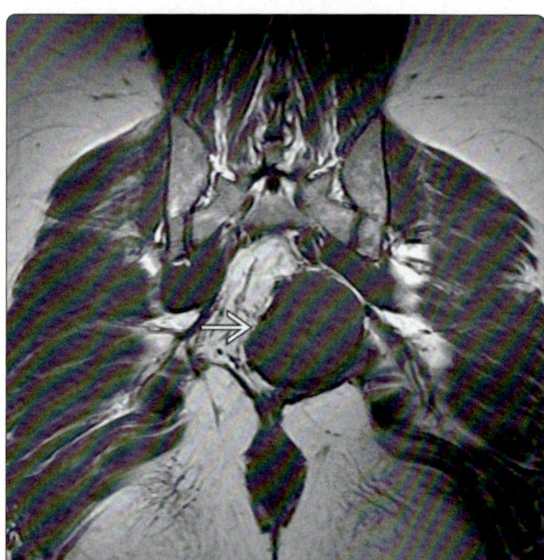

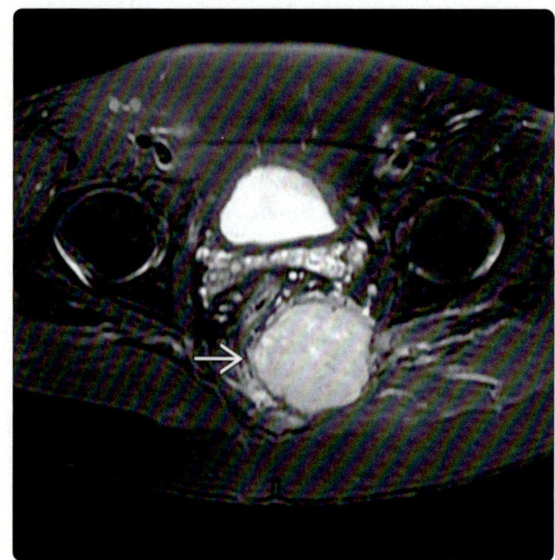

(Left) *Axial T1WI C+ FS MR in the same patient shows heterogeneous enhancement of the mass ➡. The sciatic nerve, coccygeus muscle, puborectalis muscle, and the rectum were displaced but not invaded by tumor. This lesion was histologically malignant.* **(Right)** *Axial T1WI MR in a 35-year-old woman shows a subcutaneous lesion ➡ that is isointense with skeletal muscle. The lesion has abundant peripheral feeding vessels ➡.*

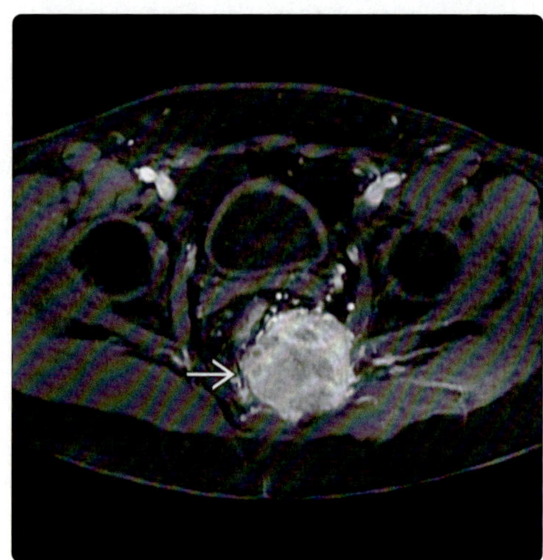

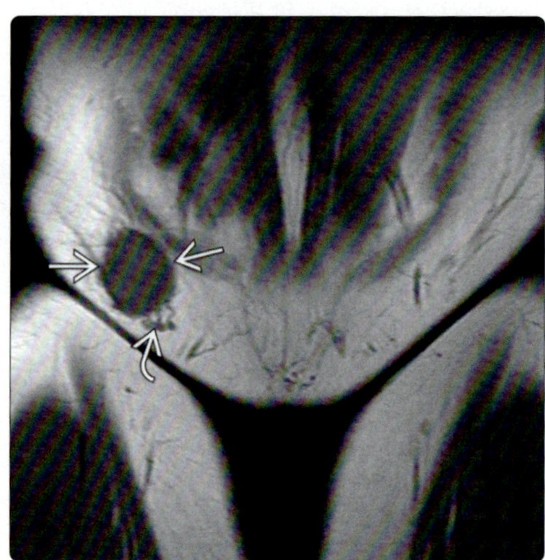

(Left) *Coronal PD FS MR, same case, shows the lesion ➡ to be hyperintense. Note all the feeding vessels ➡. The subcutaneous location, along with the abundant vessels, is typical of SFT.* **(Right)** *Axial T1 C+ FS MR shows the lesion ➡ to enhance intensely. The feeding vessels ➡ are well seen around the lesion; note also that the lesion is intimately associated with the common femoral vein ➡.*

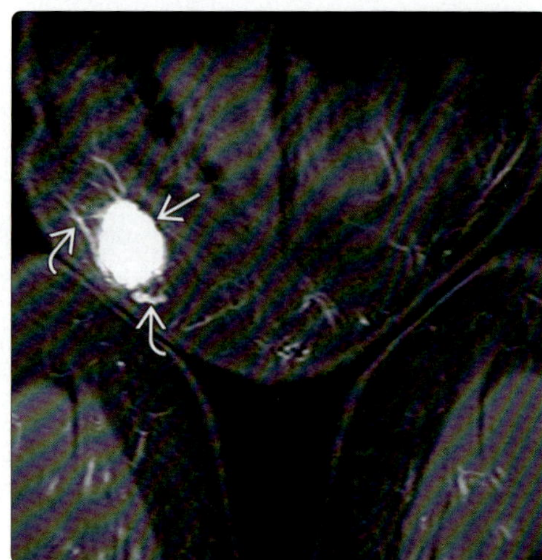

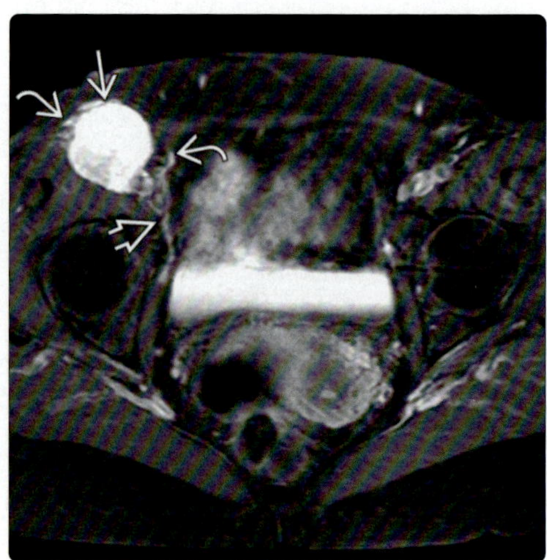

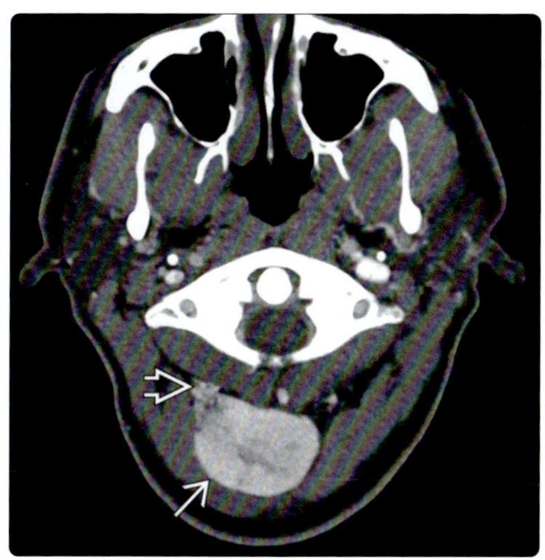

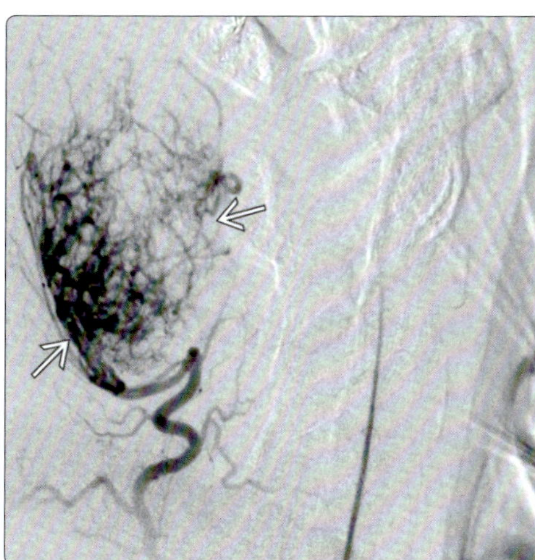

(Left) *Axial CECT of paraspinal hemangiopericytoma shows an intensely enhancing mass → in the suboccipital musculature with prominent vasculature → adjacent to the lesion.* **(Right)** *Lateral angiography in the same patient shows a paraspinal hemangiopericytoma → during injection of the ascending cervical artery, which reveals typical hypervascularity of these lesions.*

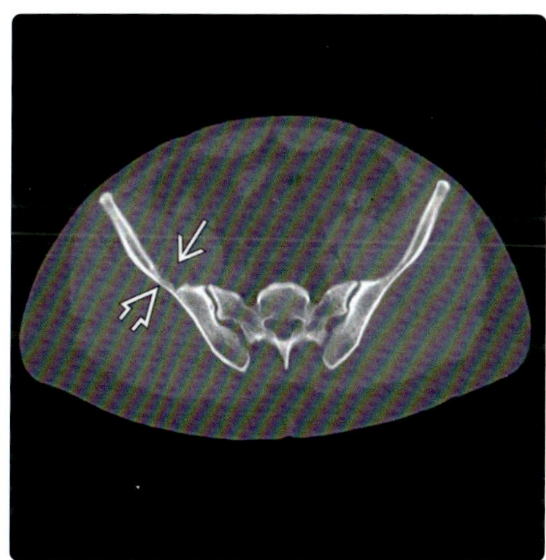

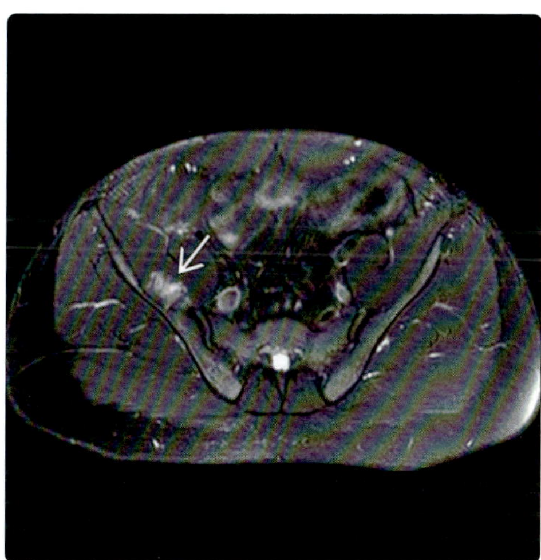

(Left) *Axial noncontrast CT shows a focal region of anterior cortical destruction → involving the right ilium. A soft tissue mass → in the region of the iliopsoas muscle is faintly visible.* **(Right)** *Axial T2WI FS MR in the same patient shows the SFT → to have heterogeneously hyperintense signal. Cortical scalloping of the underlying bone is an uncommon finding.*

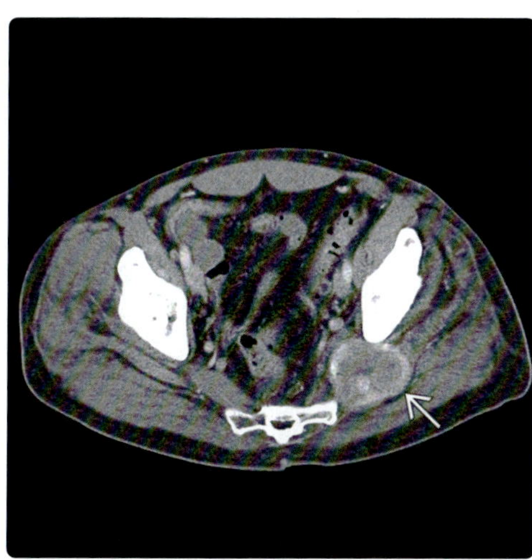

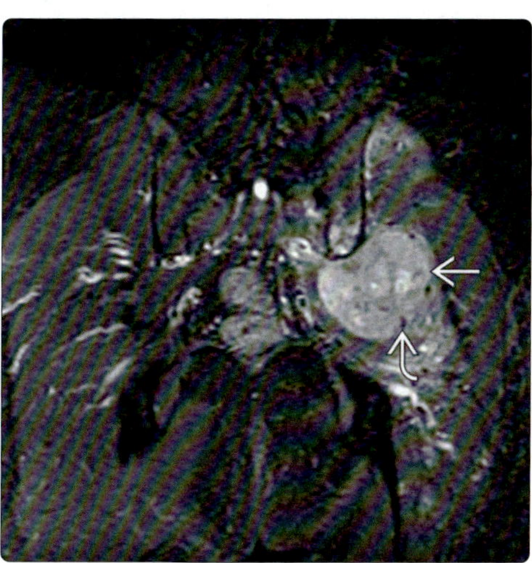

(Left) *Axial CECT through the pelvis shows a rounded mass → within the left sciatic notch. The mass has heterogeneous attenuation. Enhancement is predominantly peripheral.* **(Right)** *Coronal STIR MR in the same patient best shows the heterogeneous high signal of the SFT →, with low-signal vessels → located peripherally. On histologic examination, the mass contained neither significant mitoses nor necrosis but was considered malignant due to hypercellularity.*

Inflammatory Myofibroblastic Tumor

KEY FACTS

TERMINOLOGY

- Synonyms: Numerous, with most common being inflammatory pseudotumor
- Definition: Myofibroblastic spindle cell neoplasm with associated inflammatory infiltration of plasma cells, eosinophils, lymphocytes, and histiocytes

IMAGING

- Found throughout body
  - Most common in lung and orbit
  - 43% of extrapulmonary lesions are in mesentery and omentum
  - Other sites: Soft tissues, mediastinum, gastrointestinal tract, bladder, skin, nerve, bone, pancreas, adrenal, breast, mouth, brain, ventricle, meninges, spine, prostate, urethra, scrotum, lymph nodes
- Nonspecific soft tissue mass
  - ± calcification
  - May have infiltrative borders
- Homogeneous to heterogeneous mass on CT and MR
  - Usually isointense to muscle or brain on T1WI MR
  - May show low signal on T2WI MR depending on degree of fibrosis
  - Prominent enhancement with persistent enhancement visible on delayed imaging

CLINICAL ISSUES

- Symptoms
  - Fever, night sweats, weight loss
  - Symptoms from compression of local structures
- Age: Affects children and young adults typically
  - Can be found at any age
- Natural history
  - 15-25% of extrapulmonary lesions recur
  - Metastatic disease in < 5%
  - If systemic clinical symptoms reappear after treatment, work-up for recurrent or metastatic disease
- Treatment is complete surgical excision

(Left) *Axial excretory phase CECT shows a large mass ➡ arising from the anterolateral wall of the bladder in a 25-year-old woman having irritative voiding symptoms. The mass has persistent heterogeneous enhancement on delayed imaging.* **(Right)** *Axial T1WI MR in the same patient shows the anterior bladder mass ➡ to be isointense to muscle. The mass extends into the lumen of the bladder but does not invade through the bladder wall.*

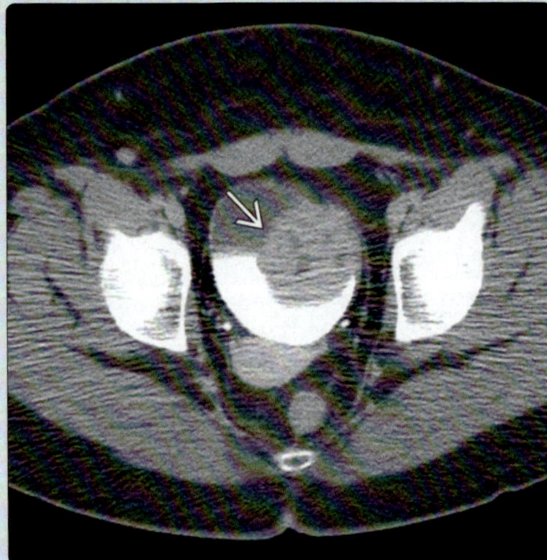

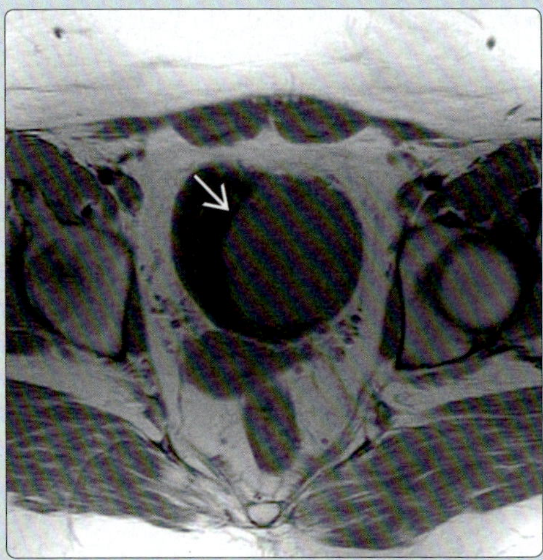

(Left) *Axial T2WI FS MR in the same patient shows the mass ➡ to have very high signal intensity that is mildly heterogeneous. A thick, irregular, low-signal rim surrounds the lesion.* **(Right)** *Axial T1WI C+ FS MR in the same patient shows the inflammatory myofibroblastic tumor ➡ to have heterogeneous central enhancement similar to the pattern seen on CT. Areas of intense enhancement alternate with regions of hypoenhancement. The thick rim has mild enhancement.*

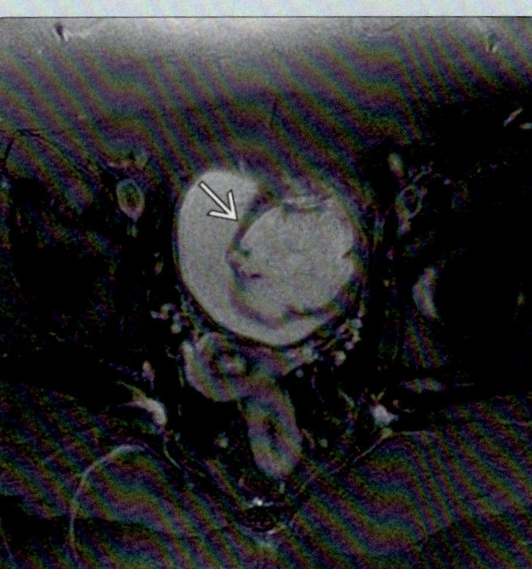

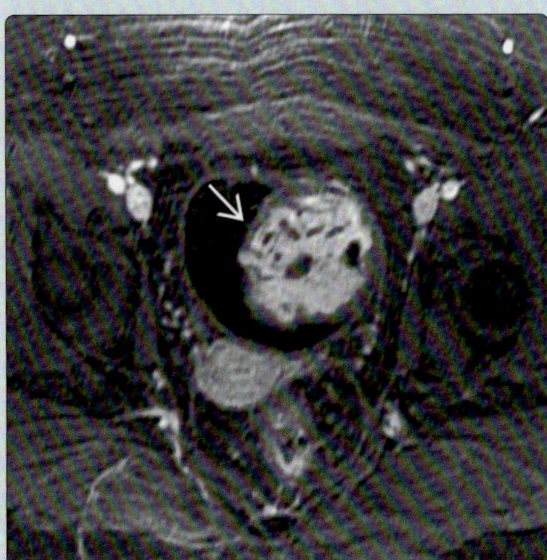

TERMINOLOGY

Abbreviations

- Inflammatory myofibroblastic tumor (IMT)

Synonyms

- Inflammatory pseudotumor, plasma cell granuloma, plasma cell pseudotumor, inflammatory myofibrohistiocytic proliferation, omental mesenteric myxoid hamartoma, xanthomatous pseudotumor, pseudosarcomatous myofibroblastic proliferation, myofibroblastoma

Definitions

- Myofibroblastic spindle cell neoplasm with associated inflammatory infiltration of plasma cells, eosinophils, lymphocytes, and histiocytes

IMAGING

General Features

- Location
  - Found throughout body, most commonly in lung and orbit
  - 43% of extrapulmonary lesions in mesentery and omentum
  - Soft tissues, mediastinum, gastrointestinal tract, bladder, skin, nerve, bone, pancreas, adrenal, breast, mouth, brain, ventricle, meninges, spine, prostate, urethra, scrotum, lymph nodes
- Size
  - 2-20 cm (average: 6 cm)

Radiographic Findings

- Nonspecific soft tissue mass ± calcification

CT Findings

- Homogeneous to heterogeneous mass
- May have infiltrative borders
- Prominent enhancement with persistent enhancement visible on delayed imaging

MR Findings

- Homogeneous to heterogeneous soft tissue mass
- Usually isointense to muscle or brain on T1WI
- May show low signal on T2WI depending on fibrotic lesion contents
- Intense gadolinium enhancement

Ultrasonographic Findings

- Hypoechogenic to hyperechogenic mass
- Doppler exam reveals prominent vascularity

DIFFERENTIAL DIAGNOSIS

Inflammatory Leiomyosarcoma

- Can be histologically similar when having a fascicular growth pattern
- Associated with paraneoplastic symptoms
- Can be found in any location

Gastrointestinal Stromal Tumor

- Can be histologically similar to IMT when it occurs in gastrointestinal tract
- CD117 and CD34 positive
- ALK negative

PATHOLOGY

General Features

- Etiology
  - Unknown origin

Gross Pathologic & Surgical Features

- Whitish-gray to tan-yellow or red multinodular mass
  - May contain central scar
- Variable texture of cut surface being hard, gritty, rubbery, fleshy, or myxoid

CLINICAL ISSUES

Presentation

- Most common signs/symptoms
  - Fever, night sweats, weight loss
  - Symptoms from compression of local structures
    - Chest pain, shortness of breath, bowel obstruction, increased abdominal girth, bladder obstruction, urinary frequency, hematuria
- Other signs/symptoms
  - Elevated ESR, anemia, thrombocytosis, polyclonal hyperglobulinemia
  - Amenorrhea from adrenal tumors
  - Dural venous sinus thrombosis
  - Rarely, dermatomyositis or obliterative phlebitis

Demographics

- Age
  - Typically affects children and young adults
    - Usually diagnosed before age 20
    - Can be found at any age
- Gender
  - Mild female predominance

Natural History & Prognosis

- Extrapulmonary lesions have 15-25% recurrence rate
  - Central nervous system lesions have up to 40% recurrence rate
- Metastatic disease in < 5%
- Systemic symptoms resolve after tumor removal

Treatment

- Complete surgical excision
- Rare reported response to nonsteroidal antiinflammatory agents and corticosteroids
- If systemic clinical symptoms reappear after treatment, additional work-up should be performed to evaluate for recurrent or metastatic disease

SELECTED REFERENCES

1. Cheng KJ et al: A case report of an inflammatory myofibroblastic tumor of the neck: A focus on the computed tomography and magnetic resonance imaging findings. Oncol Lett. 10(1):518-522, 2015
2. Chung EM et al: Solid tumors of the peritoneum, omentum, and mesentery in children: radiologic-pathologic correlation: from the radiologic pathology archives. Radiographics. 35(2):521-46, 2015
3. Höhne S et al: Inflammatory pseudotumor (IPT) and inflammatory myofibroblastic tumor (IMT): a representative literature review occasioned by a rare IMT of the transverse colon in a 9-year-old child. Tumori. 101(3):249-56, 2015

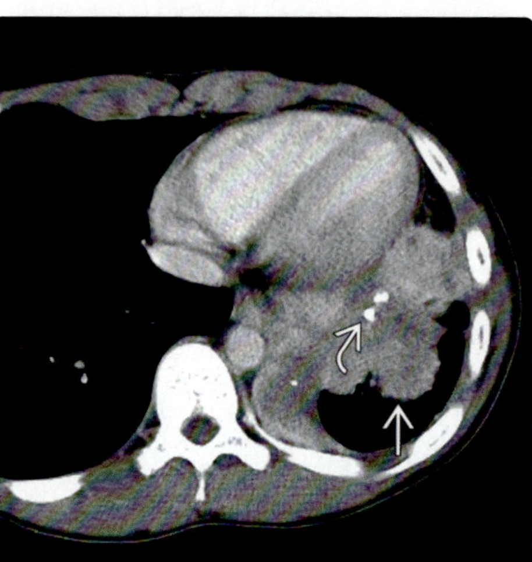
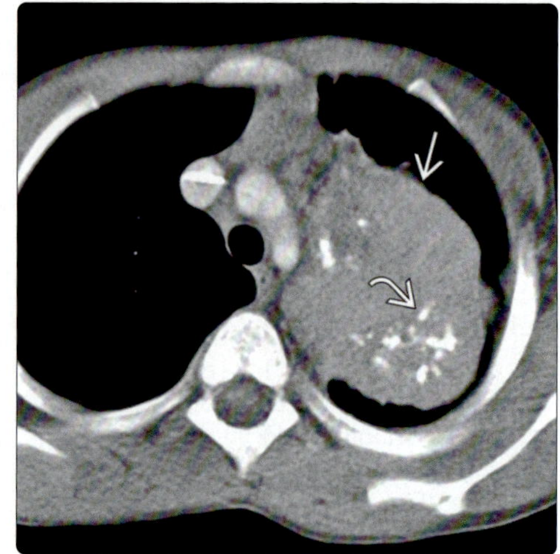

(Left) *Axial CECT of the lower chest shows a pleural-based mass containing calcifications. The mass is inseparable from the pericardium and partially encases the aorta and esophagus.* **(Right)** *Axial CECT in a different patient shows a large inflammatory myofibroblastic tumor in the left upper lobe of the lung. The mass abuts the superior mediastinum and contains multiple coarse calcifications.*

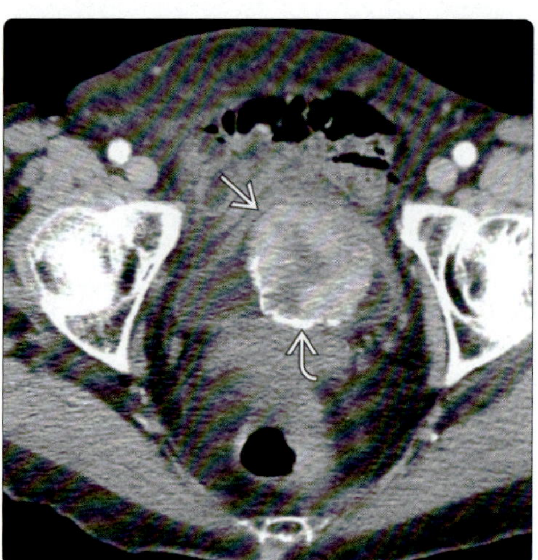
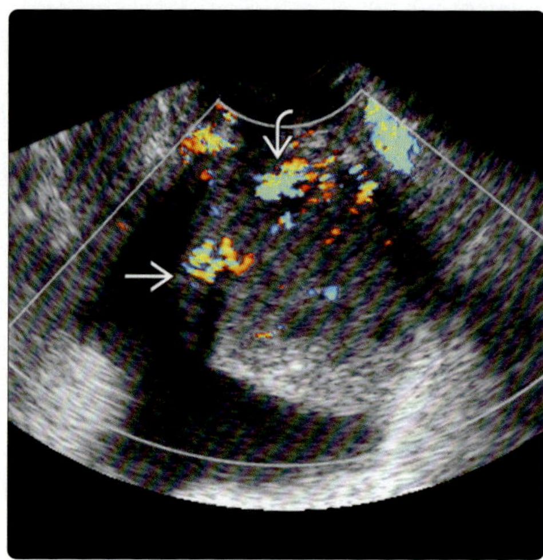

(Left) *Axial CECT shows a large, heterogeneously enhancing mass located within the bladder that has a partially calcified surface.* **(Right)** *Longitudinal Doppler ultrasound of the pelvis demonstrates a large mass within the bladder. The intravesicular mass has moderate vascularity. Additional imaging confirmed lack of invasion through the bladder wall and lack of adenopathy.*

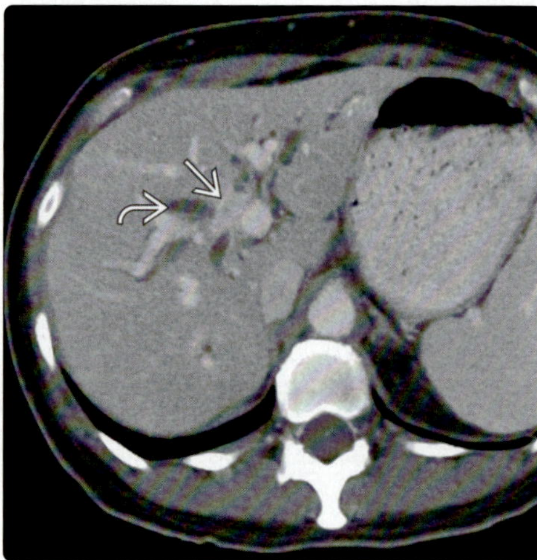
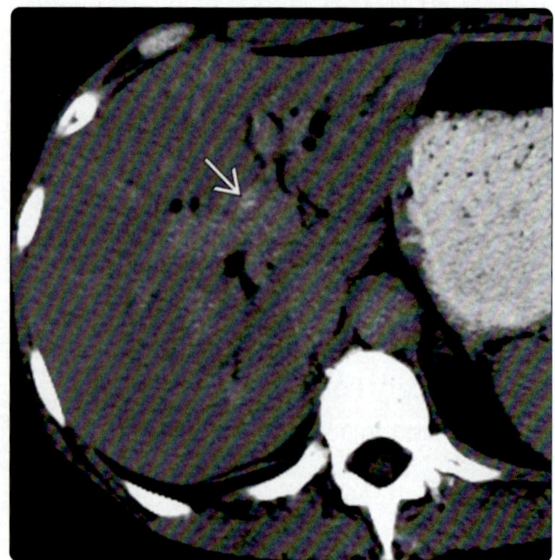

(Left) *Axial CECT through the upper abdomen shows dilation of the intrahepatic bile ducts and a poorly defined mass at the duct bifurcation.* **(Right)** *Axial delayed phase CECT in the same patient shows persistent increased retention of contrast material within the hepatic hilar mass that is producing biliary obstruction at the bifurcation. Findings were considered to indicate a Klatskin tumor, but surgery proved it to be an inflammatory myofibroblastic tumor.*

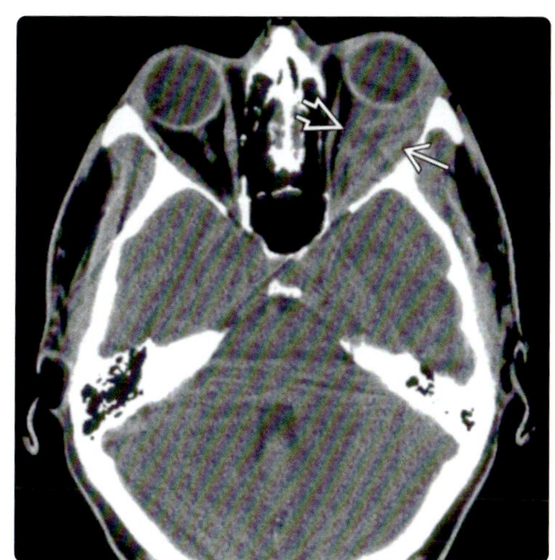

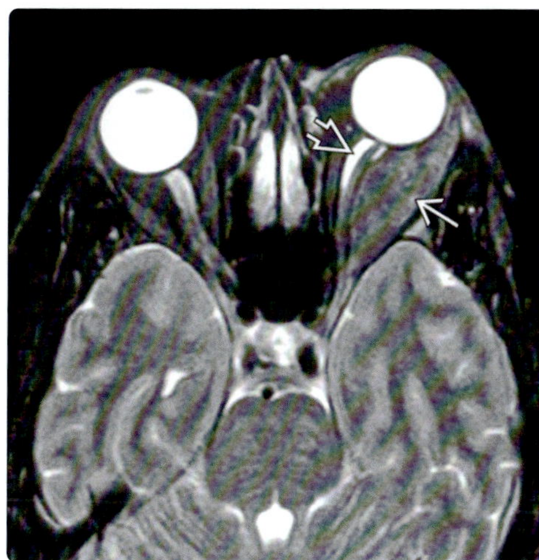

(Left) *Axial NECT shows an isodense mass located laterally in the left orbit, which displaces the optic nerve sheath complex medially.* **(Right)** *Axial STIR MR in the same patient shows that the mass involves the lateral rectus muscle. The mass is relatively hypointense, suggesting a highly cellular infiltrate or fibrosis. The displaced optic nerve sheath shows increased trapped cerebrospinal fluid due to mass effect.*

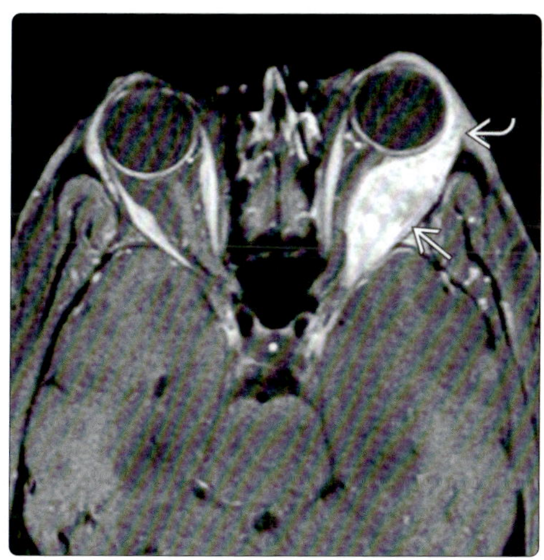

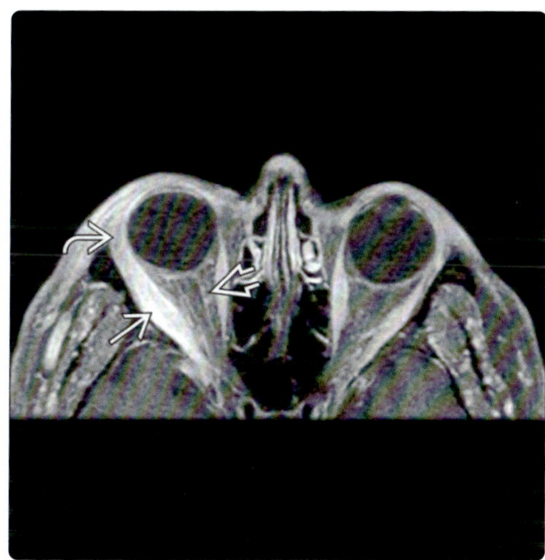

(Left) *Axial T1WI C+ MR in the same patient shows marked enhancement of the orbital mass. Note that the anterior tendinous insertion is involved, which is a typical finding for inflammatory myofibroblastic tumor (pseudotumor) of the orbit.* **(Right)** *Axial T1WI C+ MR shows isolated enlargement of the right lateral rectus muscle with anterior tendinous insertion involvement. Mild irregular enhancement along the optic nerve sheath indicates intraconal inflammation.*

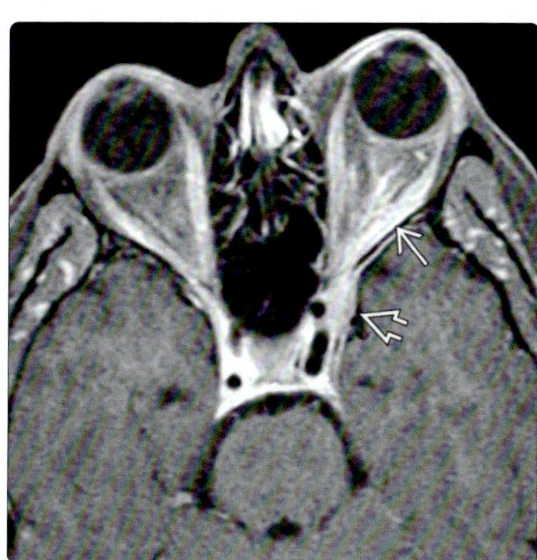

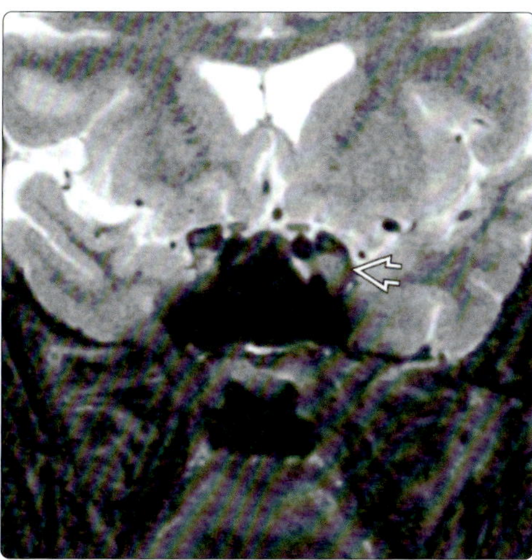

(Left) *Axial T1WI C+ FS MR of inflammatory myofibroblastic tumor (pseudotumor) shows enhancing tissue involving the left orbital apex and lateral rectus muscle with contiguous involvement of the ipsilateral anterior cavernous sinus.* **(Right)** *Coronal T2WI MR in the same patient shows that the tumor in the cavernous sinus is hypointense. Low signal on T2 with enhancement on T1WI C+ MR suggests meningioma with calcification or intracranial inflammatory myofibroblastic tumor.*

KEY FACTS

TERMINOLOGY

- Rare, malignant neoplasm of infancy histologically similar to adult fibrosarcoma but with different molecular alterations and more favorable clinical course

IMAGING

- Painless, rapidly enlarging mass in extremity of infant
  - May become disproportionately large relative to size of child
- MR best evaluates tumor extent and vital structure involvement
  - Nonspecific, heterogeneously enhancing soft tissue mass with encapsulated or infiltrative appearance
    - < 5% with cortical thickening, bowing, erosion, or destruction of underlying bone
    - Focal regions of hemorrhage or necrosis
- Enlarged blood vessels with rapid blood flow may be visible with MR or Doppler US
  - Hypervascularity may mimic neoplasm of vascular origin on angiography

PATHOLOGY

- No predisposing factors or hereditary susceptibility

CLINICAL ISSUES

- Age: Vast majority of cases occur in 1st yr of life
- Gender: Slight male predominance
- Clinical symptoms
  - Enlarging, painless mass lesion in infant
  - Overlying skin may become red and ulcerated
- Natural history
  - Less aggressive behavior than adult fibrosarcoma
  - Similar behavior to fibromatosis
  - 4-25% mortality rate from hemorrhage or vital structure invasion
- Treated by complete surgical excision
  - May require limb amputation

(Left) *Anteroposterior angiography shows a large, noncalcified soft tissue mass ➔ that distorts the left femoral vessels and has a highly vascular tumor bed.* **(Right)** *Axial CECT shows a heterogeneously enhancing soft tissue mass ➔ extending from the iliac crest into the posteromedial thigh. Low-density regions ➔ suggest necrosis. The differential diagnosis is broad and includes many soft tissue tumors, such as those of muscle, fibrous tissue, synovium, vascular, or lymphatic origin.*

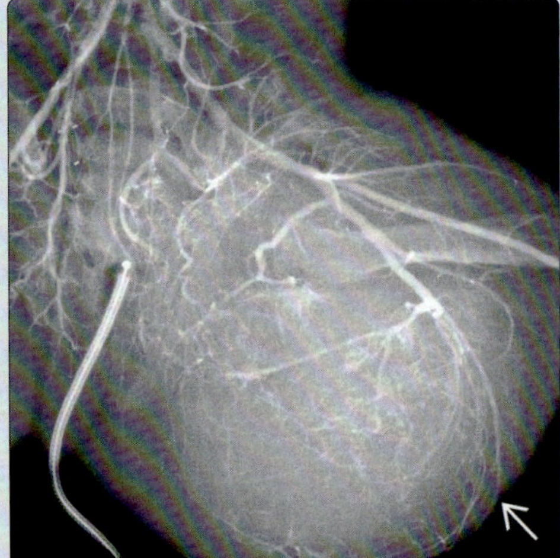

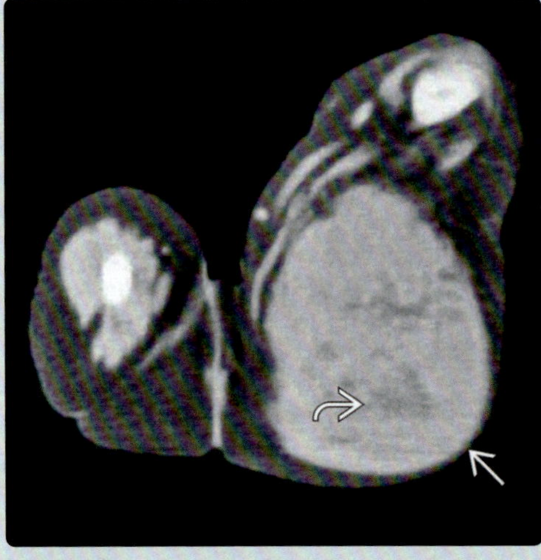

(Left) *Axial T1WI MR shows a large soft tissue mass ➔ in the forearm of an infant that infiltrates the flexor tendons as well as the muscles. The signal intensity of the mass is isointense to slightly hyperintense relative to skeletal muscle.* **(Right)** *Axial T2WI MR in the same patient shows inhomogeneous mixed low and high signal of the forearm mass ➔. This mass is more infiltrative than juvenile aponeurotic fibromatosis. Other types of sarcoma could have a similar appearance.*

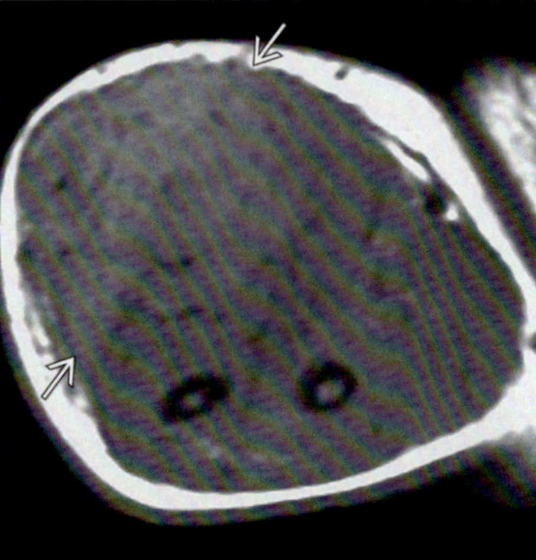

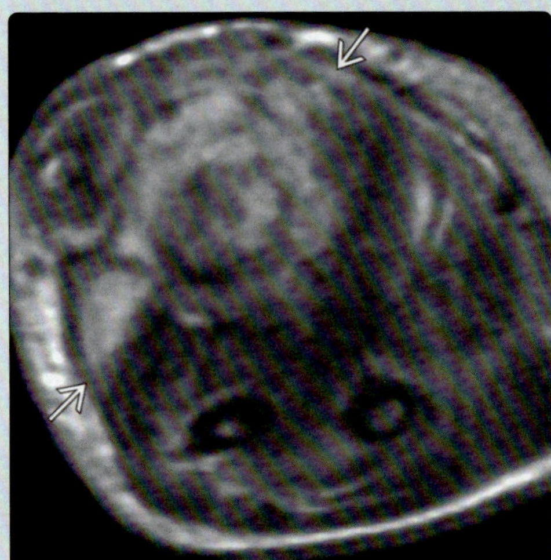

TERMINOLOGY

Synonyms

- Congenital fibrosarcoma, desmoplastic fibrosarcoma of infancy, congenital infantile fibrosarcoma, juvenile fibrosarcoma, medullary fibromatosis of infancy, aggressive infantile fibromatosis, congenital fibrosarcoma-like fibromatosis, medullary fibromatosis of infancy

Definitions

- Rare, malignant neoplasm of infancy histologically similar to adult fibrosarcoma but with different molecular alterations and more favorable clinical course

IMAGING

General Features

- Best diagnostic clue
  - Painless, rapidly enlarging mass in extremity of infant
- Location
  - 61% in distal extremities
    - Superficial or deep
  - 19% in trunk
  - 16% in head and neck
  - Rare in mesentery and retroperitoneum
- Size
  - May become disproportionately large relative to size of child
    - Reported up to 30 cm
- Morphology
  - Lobulated soft tissue mass that may invade adjacent structures

Imaging Recommendations

- Best imaging tool
  - MR best evaluates tumor extent and vital structure involvement

Radiographic Findings

- Nonspecific soft tissue mass
- < 5% with cortical thickening, bowing, erosion, or destruction of underlying bone

CT Findings

- Nonspecific, heterogeneously enhancing soft tissue mass

MR Findings

- Nonspecific, heterogeneous soft tissue mass
- Heterogeneous enhancement
  - Focal regions of hypoenhancement due to hemorrhage or necrosis
- Enlarged blood vessels with rapid blood flow may be visible

Ultrasonographic Findings

- Useful for in utero tumor evaluation
- Heterogeneous, hypervascular mass
- Enlarged blood vessels may be visible on Doppler

Angiographic Findings

- Hypervascularity may mimic neoplasm of vascular origin

PATHOLOGY

General Features

- Etiology
  - Unknown
  - No predisposing factors or hereditary susceptibility
- Genetics
  - Typical translocation t(12;15)(p13;q26)

Gross Pathologic & Surgical Features

- Soft to firm, gray-tan, lobulated mass
  - ± hemorrhage, necrosis, cystic/myxoid changes
- Pseudocapsule from adjacent tissue compression

Microscopic Features

- Infiltrative margins despite pseudocapsule
- Herringbone pattern or cords/sheets of primitive ovoid and spindle cells are typical
- May engulf regions of muscle or fat
- 100% positive vimentin

CLINICAL ISSUES

Presentation

- Most common signs/symptoms
  - Enlarging, painless mass in infant
  - Overlying skin may become red and ulcerated

Demographics

- Age
  - Vast majority of cases occur in 1st yr of life
  - Lesions occurring after 2 yr of age should have cytogenetic confirmation
- Gender
  - Slight male predominance
- Epidemiology
  - 12% of infantile soft tissue malignancies
  - 13% of childhood/adolescent fibroblastic-myofibroblastic tumors

Natural History & Prognosis

- Similar behavior to fibromatosis
- Less aggressive behavior than adult fibrosarcoma
  - Local recurrence in 5-50%
  - Rarely metastasizes
- 4-25% mortality rate
  - Invasion of vital structures or hemorrhage

Treatment

- Complete surgical excision
  - May require limb amputation

SELECTED REFERENCES

1. Suzuki T et al: Sonographic features of congenital infantile fibrosarcoma that appeared as a sacrococcygeal teratoma during pregnancy. J Obstet Gynaecol Res. 41(8):1282-6, 2015
2. Ainsworth KE et al: Congenital infantile fibrosarcoma: review of imaging features. Pediatr Radiol. 44(9):1124-9, 2014
3. Hu Z et al: Infantile fibrosarcoma-a clinical and histologic mimicker of vascular malformations: case report and review of the literature. Pediatr Dev Pathol. 16(5):357-63, 2013

Fibrosarcoma: Soft Tissue

KEY FACTS

TERMINOLOGY

- Malignant fibroblastic/myofibroblastic neoplasm with predilection for deep soft tissues of extremities

IMAGING

- Mass with similar density as muscle on CT
  - Low-density myxoid, cystic, or necrotic regions
  - High-density hemorrhage
  - Calcification or bone erosion is uncommon
- Solid tumor elements are typically isointense on T1WI and hyperintense on fluid-sensitive MR sequences
  - Enhancement ↓ with myxoid, cystic, or necrotic change
  - Thin, low-signal pseudocapsule may be visible
- Gadolinium enhancement characteristics useful to differentiate surrounding, nonenhancing edema from enhancing tumor
  - Can direct biopsy to region of viable tumor
- US: Variably low echogenicity

PATHOLOGY

- Uniform spindle cells in classic herringbone pattern with variable amount of collagen
- Higher incidence in patients with prior therapeutic radiation exposure
- Trauma, thermal injury, and foreign material implants suggested as contributing factors
- May arise within another soft tissue neoplasm

CLINICAL ISSUES

- Painless, slowly enlarging soft tissue mass
  - Most common in 3rd to 5th decades of life
- Prognosis estimates vary due to changing tumor classification
  - Estimated 39-54% 5-year survival
  - Preferentially metastasizes to lung and axial skeleton
- Treatment with wide surgical excision
  - ± adjuvant radiotherapy and chemotherapy

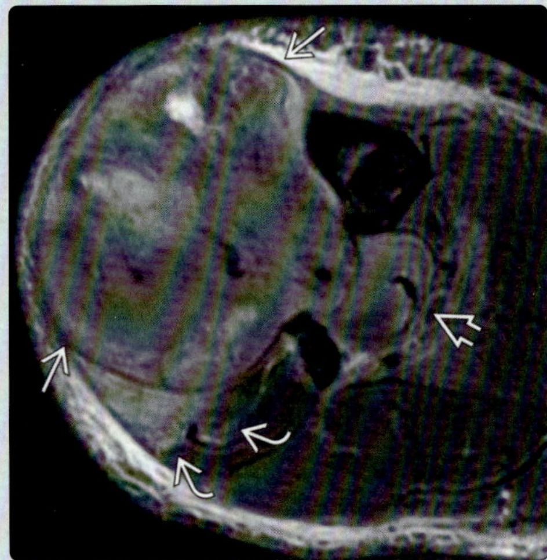

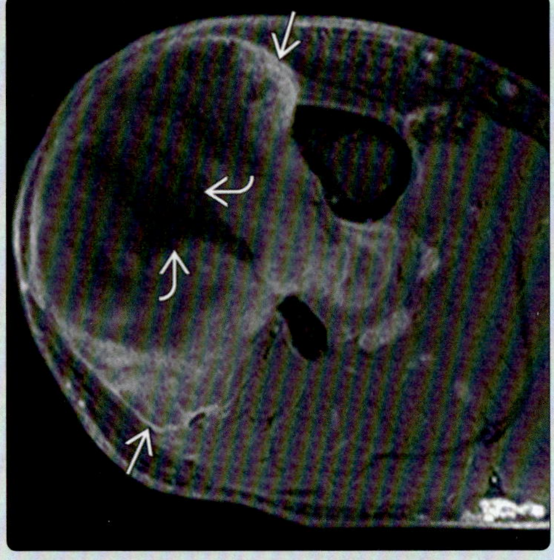

(Left) *Axial T2WI FS MR in a 39-year-old man demonstrates a large, heterogeneous fibrosarcoma centered in and involving all of the muscles in the anterior compartment* ➡ *of the lower leg. The peroneus longus and brevis muscles* ➡ *and the tibialis posterior muscle* ➡ *are also involved.* **(Right)** *Axial T1WI C+ FS MR in the same patient shows heterogeneous enhancement of the large lower leg mass* ➡*. Irregular regions within the mass that lack enhancement* ➡ *are consistent with necrosis.*

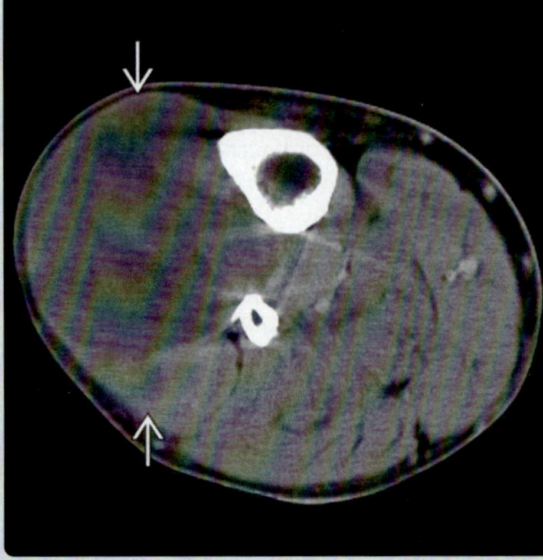

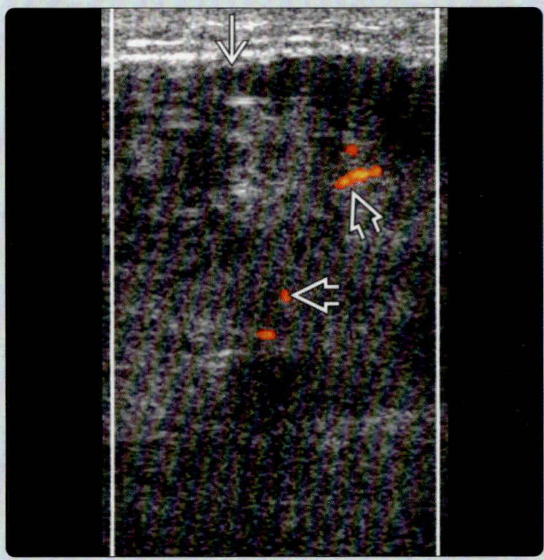

(Left) *Axial NECT in the same patient shows the mass* ➡ *to have heterogeneous attenuation that is both similar to and lower than skeletal muscle. This mass was painless and had been growing for over 8 months.* **(Right)** *Doppler US of the anterolateral calf demonstrates a mildly vascular* ➡*, heterogeneous mass* ➡ *that is highly suspicious for a soft tissue neoplasm. An US-guided biopsy performed at that time revealed spindle-shaped cells in a streaming or herringbone pattern.*

TERMINOLOGY

Definitions

- Malignant fibroblastic/myofibroblastic neoplasm with typical herringbone histologic pattern

IMAGING

General Features

- Location
  - Deep soft tissues of extremities; lower > upper
  - Trunk, head and neck
  - Retroperitoneal location is rare

Radiographic Findings

- Normal or nonspecific soft tissue prominence
- Calcification or bone erosion is uncommon

CT Findings

- Mass with similar density to muscle
  - Low-density myxoid, cystic, or necrotic regions
  - High-density hemorrhage
- Enhancement depends on cellular contents
  - ↓ with myxoid, cystic, or necrotic change

MR Findings

- Heterogeneous low to high signal intensity relative to muscle on T1WI and fluid-sensitive sequences
  - Solid tumor elements are typically isointense on T1WI and hyperintense on fluid-sensitive sequences
  - Thin, low-signal pseudocapsule may be visible
  - Heterogeneous enhancement

Ultrasonographic Findings

- Variably low echogenicity

Imaging Recommendations

- Protocol advice
  - Gadolinium enhancement characteristics useful to differentiate surrounding, nonenhancing edema from enhancing tumor
    - Can direct biopsy to region of viable tumor

PATHOLOGY

General Features

- Etiology
  - Higher incidence in patients with prior therapeutic radiation exposure, latency up to 15 years
    - *RET* oncogene rearrangement implicated
  - Trauma and burns suggested as contributing factors
    - Cicatricial fibrosarcoma → arising within scar
  - Suggested association with foreign material implants
  - May arise within another soft tissue tumor
    - Dermatofibrosarcoma (10% of cases), solitary fibrous tumor, and well-differentiated liposarcoma
- Genetics
  - Complex, inconsistent chromosome rearrangements
  - Lacks characteristic chromosomal translocation found in infantile fibrosarcoma

Staging, Grading, & Classification

- American Joint Committee on Cancer staging system or Surgical Staging System of Musculoskeletal Tumor Society
- Low-grade lesions have orderly collections of cells, prominent collagen, and low mitotic activity
- High-grade lesions have > 2 mitoses per HPF, necrosis, high cellularity, and little collagen

Gross Pathologic & Surgical Features

- White to tan-yellow lobulated mass
  - Degree of firmness related to collagen content

Microscopic Features

- Uniform spindle cells in fascicular, herringbone pattern with variable amount of collagen
  - Mitotic activity present but variable
  - ± osseous or chondroid metaplasia
- Positive vimentin staining

CLINICAL ISSUES

Presentation

- Most common signs/symptoms
  - Painless, slowly enlarging soft tissue mass
- Other signs/symptoms
  - Compression of local structures
  - Hypoglycemia reported

Demographics

- Age
  - May be found at any age
  - Most common in 3rd-5th decades of life
- Gender
  - Male predilection
- Epidemiology
  - Estimated at 1-3% of sarcomas in adults

Natural History & Prognosis

- Difficult to definitively estimate due to changing tumor classification
  - Estimated 39-54% 5-year survival
  - Local recurrence in 12-79%
  - Metastases in 9-63%
    - Usually < 2 years, but can occur late
    - Lung and axial skeleton preferentially involved
    - Spread to lymph nodes in < 8%
- Prognosis worse with large tumors, high-grade tumors, tumors that are incompletely excised initially, and those arising in prior radiation field

Treatment

- Wide surgical excision
  - ± adjuvant radiotherapy
- Chemotherapy utilized in patients with poor prognostic factors

SELECTED REFERENCES

1. Verschoor AJ et al: Radiation-induced Sarcomas Occurring in Desmoid-type Fibromatosis Are Not Always Derived From the Primary Tumor. Am J Surg Pathol. ePub, 2015

(Left) *Coronal NECT of the thigh demonstrates a large soft tissue mass ➡ centered in the vastus medialis with areas of low-attenuation necrosis centrally ➡. This mass is nonspecific. In an older adult, an undifferentiated pleomorphic sarcoma or liposarcoma would be more common.* **(Right)** *Axial NECT shows a heterogeneous mass ➡ in the medial thigh. Biopsy was directed to the periphery to avoid the central areas of necrosis. Note how portions of the tumor blend with the surrounding musculature.*

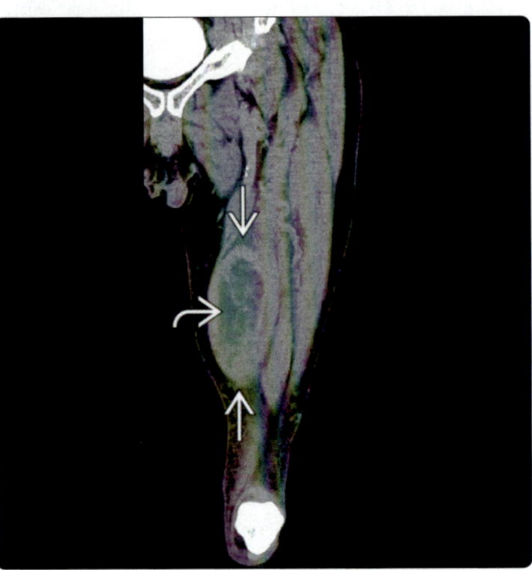

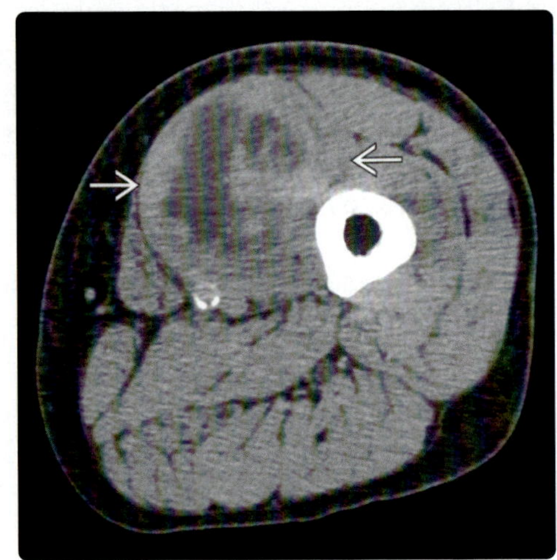

(Left) *Axial T1WI MR shows a rounded mass ➡ in the adductor brevis muscle of the thigh. This mass is isointense to slightly decreased in signal compared with muscle. The mass was painless and had been slowly enlarging.* **(Right)** *Axial T1WI C+ FS in the same patient shows inhomogeneous, predominantly peripheral enhancement of the mass ➡. This lesion was not resected, due to metastatic disease to the same thigh and bilateral buttocks. The patient was treated with chemotherapy for this high-grade tumor.*

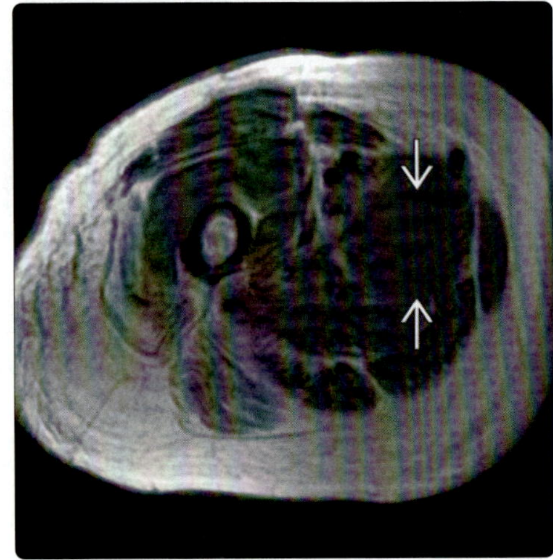

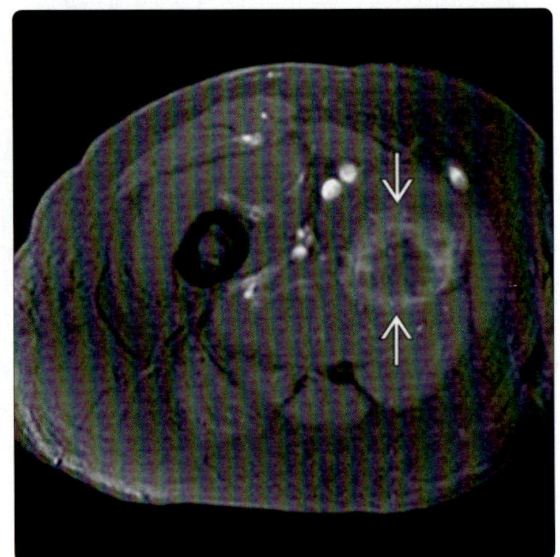

(Left) *Axial T1WI MR in the same patient 1 year after chemotherapy shows mild increase in the size of the lobulated medial thigh mass ➡.* **(Right)** *Axial T2WI FS MR in the same patient 1 year after chemotherapy shows mixed high to low signal intensity of the still viable and enlarging fibrosarcoma ➡. Metastatic disease to the soft tissues, as was present in this patient, is unusual. Metastatic tumor usually involves the lungs and axial skeleton.*

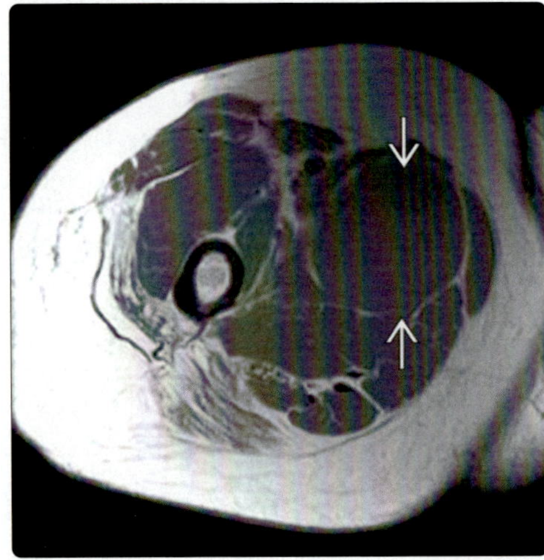

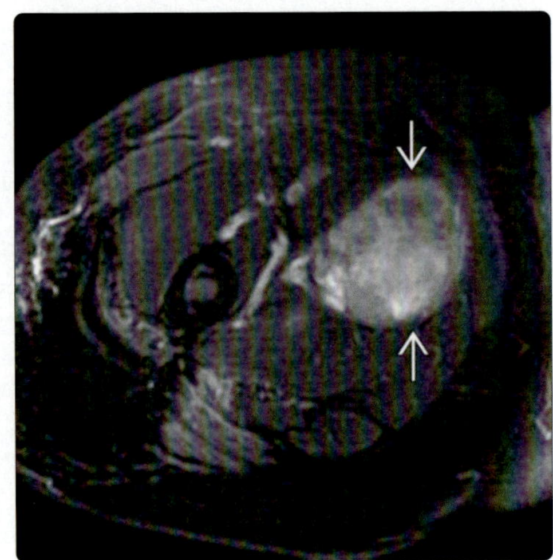

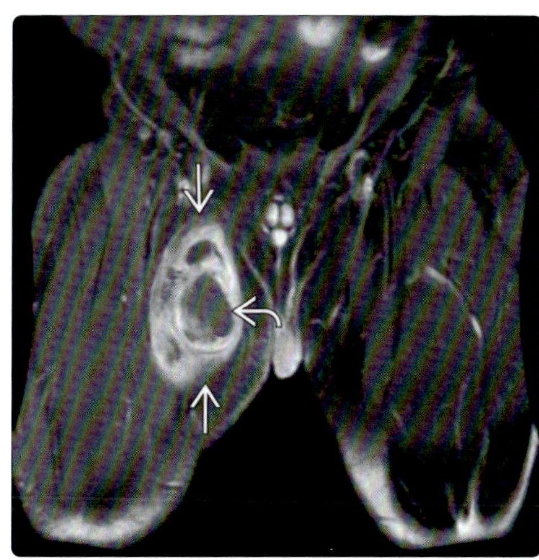

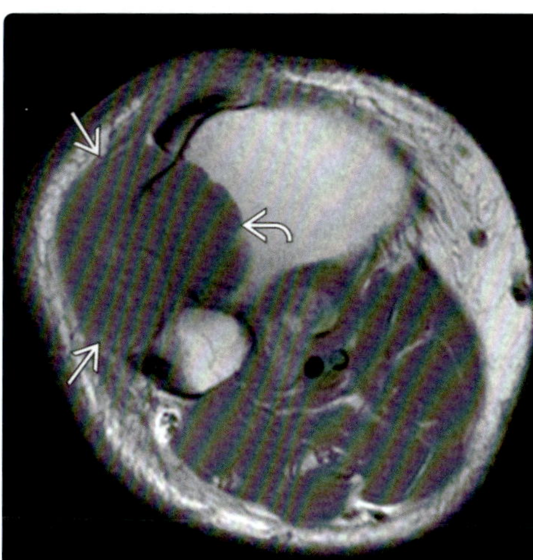

(Left) *Coronal T1WI C+ FS MR shows a large heterogeneously enhancing mass ➔ with large areas of necrosis ➔ centered in the right adductor compartment of the thigh.* **(Right)** *Axial T1WI MR shows a soft tissue mass ➔ in the the upper leg with signal intensity similar to muscle, with invasion of the tibia ➔. This is likely secondary invasion, as opposed to primary bone involvement, because the bulk of the tumor lies outside of the bone and clinical symptoms appeared late in the course of the disease.*

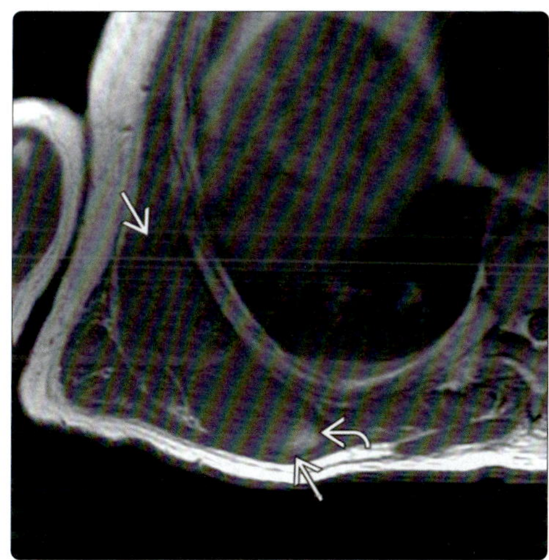

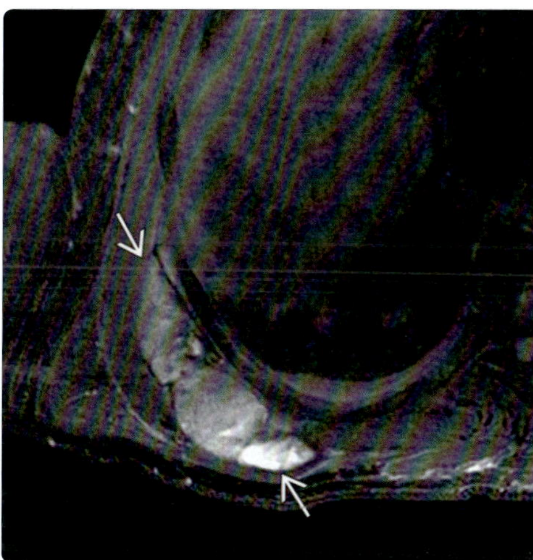

(Left) *Axial T1WI MR shows a large heterogeneous soft tissue mass ➔ in the posterolateral chest wall. The mass is predominantly isointense to muscle, although there is a peripherally located region of high-signal hemorrhage ➔.* **(Right)** *Axial T2WI FS MR shows heterogeneity of the lentiform ➔ chest wall mass located distal to the scapular tip. The signal intensity of the mass ranges from low-signal rim to hyperintense signal similar to fluid. The trunk is the 2nd most common location of fibrosarcoma.*

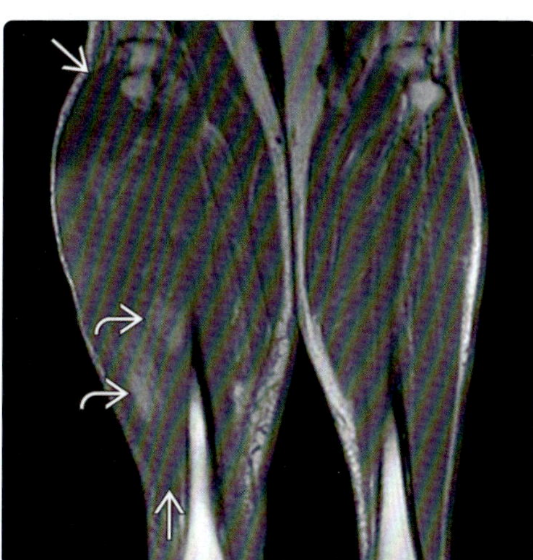

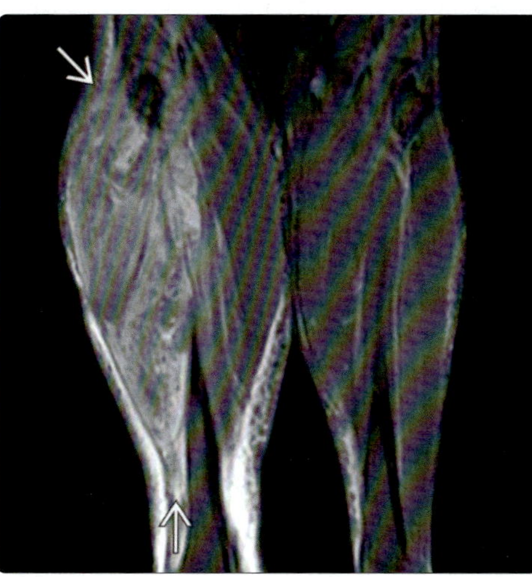

(Left) *Coronal T1WI MR shows tumor ➔ in the calf extending from the knee joint line to the level of the distal 1/3 of the tibial diaphysis. Regions of high T1 signal within the mass are due to hemorrhage ➔.* **(Right)** *Coronal STIR MR in the same patient shows the very large size and extent of the tumor ➔. The signal intensity is heterogeneous but lacks gross cystic or necrotic change, even with such a large area of involvement. Many soft tissue sarcomas could have a similar appearance.*

Myxofibrosarcoma

KEY FACTS

TERMINOLOGY

- Common fibroblastic soft tissue sarcoma involving elderly patients, with wide range of appearances depending on cellularity and myxoid content

IMAGING

- Subcutaneous > intramuscular location
  - Lower extremity > upper extremity > > trunk
- CT attenuation lower than muscle in low-grade lesions with high myxoid content
  - Attenuation similar to muscle with ↑ grade
- MR findings
  - Low-grade, high myxoid lesions → homogeneous low T1, high T2, low-level enhancement
    - May mimic cyst or old hematoma if faint enhancement is not appreciated
  - High-grade, high cellularity lesions → heterogeneous intermediate T1, high T2, intense enhancement
    - ± hemorrhage, necrosis

PATHOLOGY

- Morphologic spectrum of lesions from hypocellular to hypercellular with varying proportion of myxoid material and fibrous septa

CLINICAL ISSUES

- Most common in 6th-8th decades of life
  - Slight male predilection
- High local recurrence rate (38-79%)
  - Significant even with superficial, low-grade tumors
- Poor prognostic factors: Necrosis > 10%, size > 5 cm, < 75% myxoid tissue, > 20 mitoses per 10 HPF, incomplete initial resection

DIAGNOSTIC CHECKLIST

- Lesions may have cyst-like appearance with very subtle central enhancement
  - Watch for any red flags to avoid misinterpreting as benign lesion

(Left) *Axial T1WI MR demonstrates a very large soft tissue mass ➡ in the posterior compartment of the thigh. The mass has mildly heterogeneous signal intensity that is lower than skeletal muscle. There was no adenopathy or evidence of distant metastases.* **(Right)** *Axial T2WI FS MR in the same patient shows heterogeneity of the soft tissue mass ➡ in the posterior compartment of the thigh. The mass has predominantly high signal intensity with regions of linear low-signal fibrous septa. This high-grade tumor was painful.*

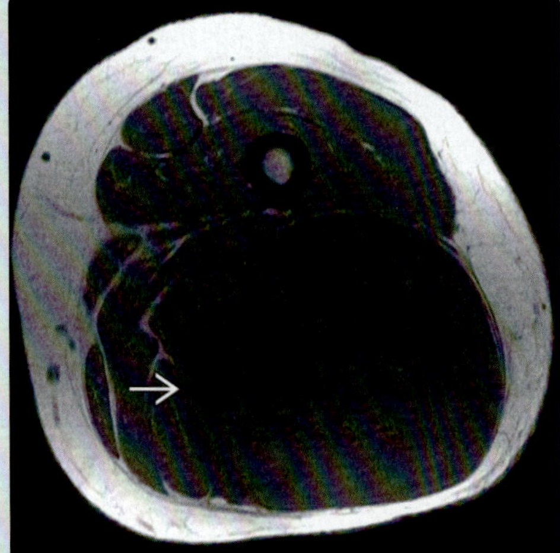

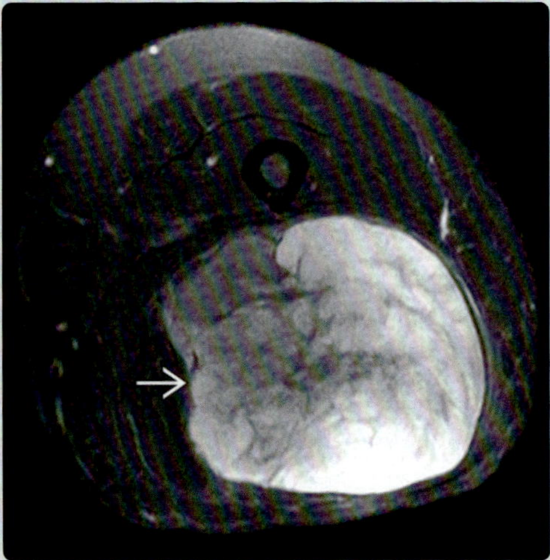

(Left) *Axial T1WI C+ FS MR in the same patient shows the mass ➡ to have slightly nodular peripheral enhancement with very low-level internal enhancement. The relative paucity of central enhancement is typical and is secondary to the large myxoid component of this tumor.* **(Right)** *Axial NECT in the same patient shows the mass ➡ to have mildly heterogeneous low attenuation. The more rounded contour of the lesion on CT imaging was due to the patient being positioned prone for biopsy.*

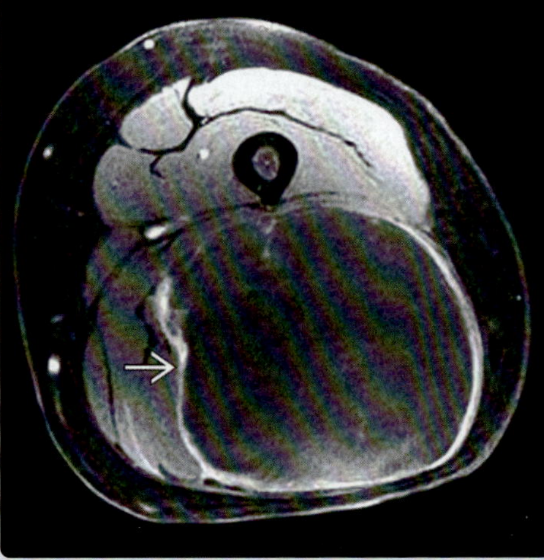

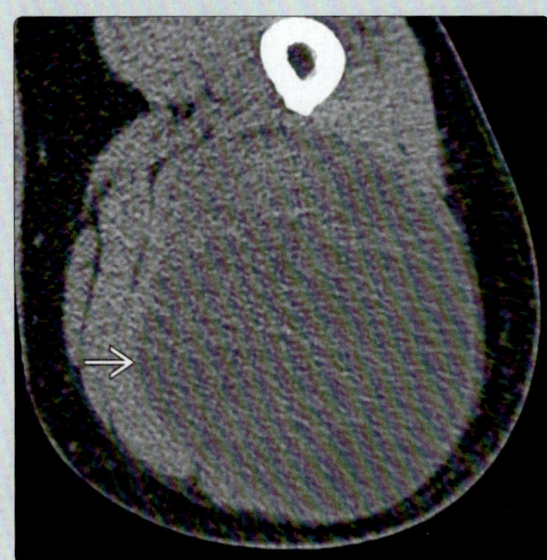

TERMINOLOGY

Synonyms

- Myxoid malignant fibrous histiocytoma; fibrosarcoma, myxoid type

Definitions

- Common fibroblastic soft tissue sarcoma involving elderly patients, with wide range of appearances depending on cellularity and myxoid content
  - Reclassified as distinct entity by World Health Organization in 2002
  - Formerly malignant fibrous histiocytoma variant
  - Not same entity as fibromyxoid sarcoma

IMAGING

General Features

- Location
  - Subcutaneous > intramuscular
  - Lower extremity > upper extremity > > trunk > head and neck
    - Should exclude dedifferentiated liposarcoma if found in retroperitoneum

Radiographic Findings

- Nonspecific soft tissue mass
- No calcified matrix or bone involvement

CT Findings

- Attenuation lower than muscle in low-grade lesions with high myxoid content
- Attenuation similar to muscle with higher grade lesions

MR Findings

- Low-grade, high myxoid content lesions → homogeneous low T1, high T2, mild enhancement
  - May mimic cyst or old hematoma if faint enhancement is not appreciated
- High-grade, high cellularity lesions → heterogeneous intermediate T1, high T2, intense enhancement
  - ± hemorrhage, necrosis
- Infiltrative appearance = ↑ risk of local recurrence
- Tail-like pattern on T2 & postcontrast imaging has sensitivity of 64-77% and specificity of 74-90%
  - Curvilinear fascial tumor extension
  - More frequently seen in superficial lesions

DIFFERENTIAL DIAGNOSIS

Low-Grade Fibromyxoid Sarcoma

- Younger patient age
- More likely to be found in muscle

Liposarcoma, Myxoid

- Middle-aged adults
- Deep thigh location is most common
- Contains lipoblasts

Nodular Fasciitis

- Rapidly growing, painful mass in middle-aged patient
- Found adherent to fascia
- Mitoses may be mistaken for malignancy

Intramuscular Myxoma

- Located within muscle
- Curvilinear central vessels absent
- Fewer mitoses

PATHOLOGY

Gross Pathologic & Surgical Features

- Subcutaneous → gelatinous multinodular mass
- Deep → firm, infiltrative solitary mass

Microscopic Features

- Morphologic spectrum of lesions from hypocellular to hypercellular with varying proportion of myxoid material and fibrous septa
  - Low grade → hypocellular, spindle cells in prominent myxoid stroma, rare mitoses
  - High grade → hypercellular, pleomorphic cells, necrosis, hemorrhage, numerous mitoses
- Elongated capillaries with cells aligned along vessels
- Strong positive vimentin stain
- Lacks true lipoblasts seen in myxoid liposarcoma

CLINICAL ISSUES

Presentation

- Most common signs/symptoms
  - Painless, slowly enlarging mass

Demographics

- Age
  - Most common in 6th-8th decades of life
  - Rare < 20 yr
- Gender
  - Slight male predilection
- Epidemiology
  - Common type of sarcoma in elderly

Natural History & Prognosis

- High local recurrence rate (38-79%)
  - Significant even with superficial, low-grade tumors
- High-grade lesions are associated with higher mortality
  - Poor prognostic factors: Necrosis > 10%, size > 5 cm, < 75% myxoid tissue, > 20 mitoses per 10 HPF, incomplete initial resection

Treatment

- Complete surgical excision with wide margins

DIAGNOSTIC CHECKLIST

Image Interpretation Pearls

- Lesions may have cyst-like appearance with very subtle central enhancement
  - Do not misinterpret as benign lesion

SELECTED REFERENCES

1. Kikuta K et al: An analysis of factors related to the tail-like pattern of myxofibrosarcoma seen on MRI. Skeletal Radiol. 44(1):55-62, 2015
2. Lefkowitz RA et al: Myxofibrosarcoma: prevalence and diagnostic value of the "tail sign" on magnetic resonance imaging. Skeletal Radiol. 42(6):809-18, 2013

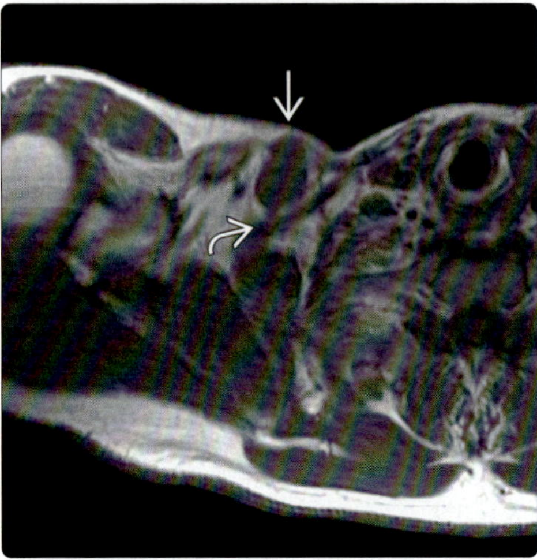

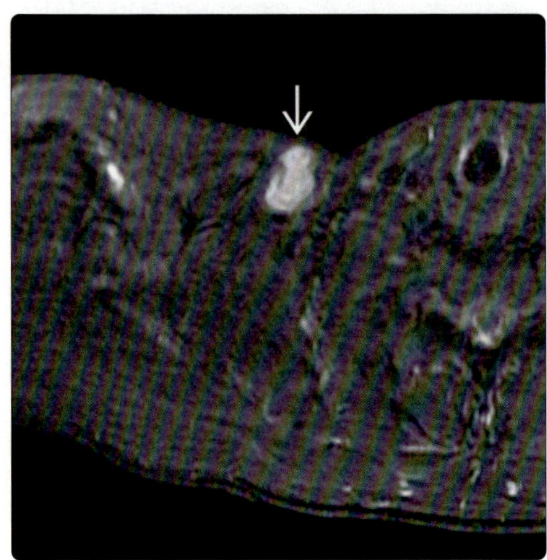

(Left) *Axial T1WI MR shows a typical myxofibrosarcoma ➡ in a 71-year-old man. This slowly growing, painless supraclavicular mass shows mildly inhomogeneous low T1 signal. This mass is anterior to and abuts the omohyoid muscle ➡.* **(Right)** *Axial T2WI FS MR in the same patient shows the mass ➡ to have mildly inhomogeneous high signal. There was no lymphadenopathy or distant metastasis. The subcutaneous location is a typical finding.*

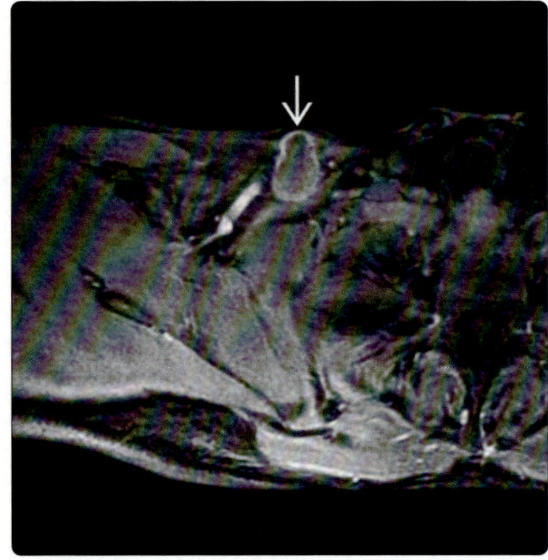

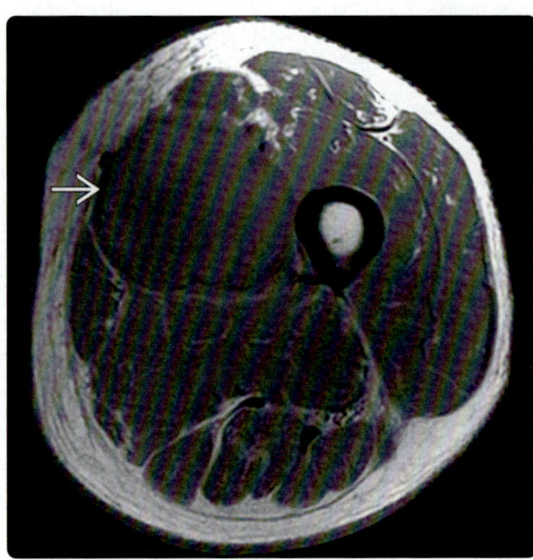

(Left) *Axial T1WI C+ FS MR in same patient shows the enhancement to be predominantly a thin peripheral rim with only mild central enhancement of the mass ➡. Even with hypoenhancement of the central portion of the lesion, this was still a high-grade lesion.* **(Right)** *Axial T1WI MR demonstrates a large, rounded mass ➡ in the adductor longus muscle of the thigh. The mass is mildly heterogeneous, with areas that are isointense to minimally hyperintense relative to skeletal muscle.*

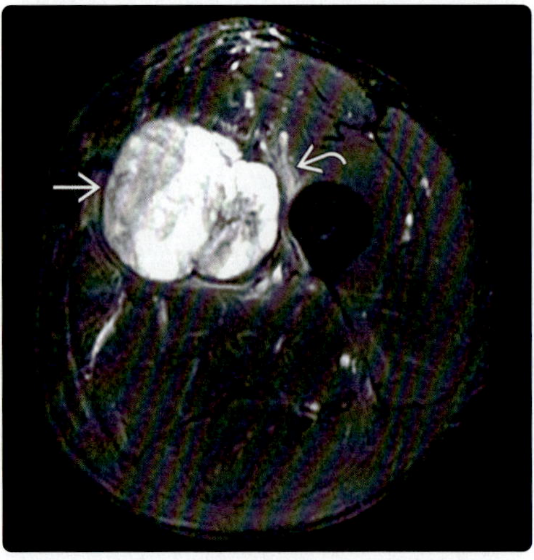

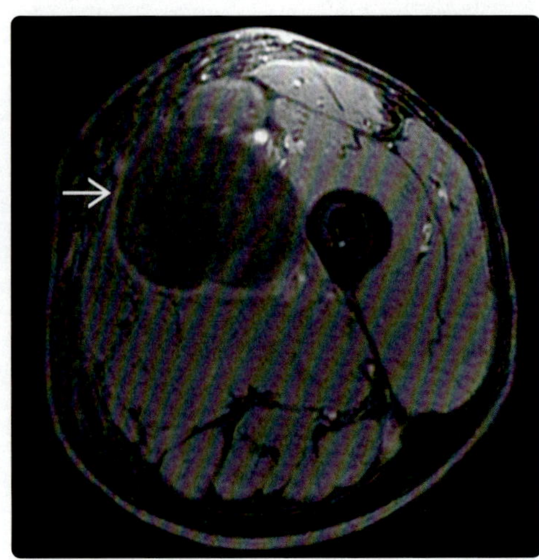

(Left) *Axial T2WI FS MR in the same patient shows the lobulated mass ➡ to have heterogeneously high signal with irregular regions of low signal. Mild edema ➡ surrounds the lesion.* **(Right)** *Axial T1WI C+ FS MR in the same patient is somewhat unimpressive, with low-level enhancement that is most prominent at the periphery of the mass ➡. This lesion could be mistaken for a hematoma or an intramuscular myxoma if the central enhancement were misinterpreted or disregarded.*

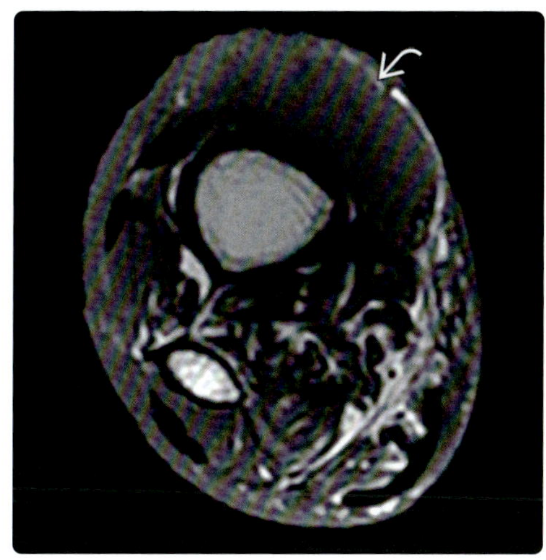

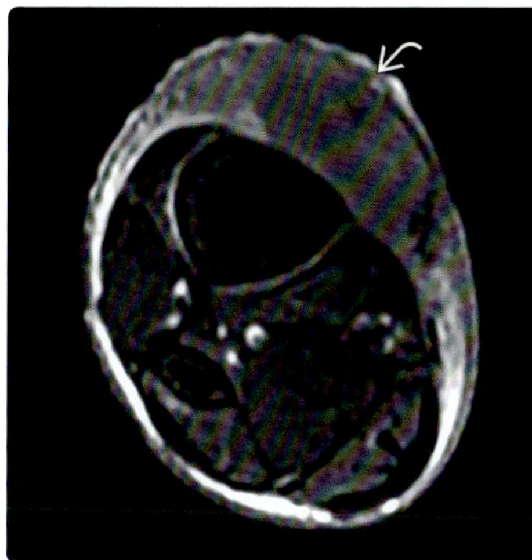

(Left) *Axial T1WI MR shows a lobulated subcutaneous mass that had been slowly growing in the lower leg of an 82-year-old woman. The mass has homogeneous signal intensity similar to muscle. The mass abuts but does not invade the anteromedial cortex of the tibia.* **(Right)** *Axial T2WI FS MR in the same patient shows that the mass is mildly hyperintense to muscle and predominantly homogeneous, with a few scattered foci of T2 hypointensity.*

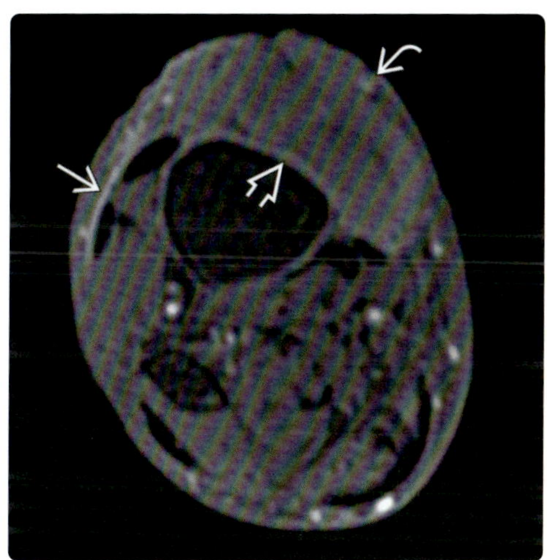

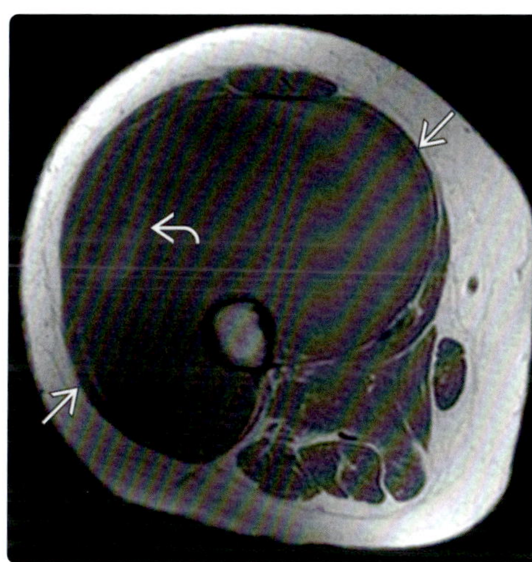

(Left) *Axial T1WI C+ FS MR in the same patient shows moderate, diffuse enhancement of the mass. The anterior compartment fascia and tibial periosteum also show mild enhancement.* **(Right)** *Axial T1WI MR shows a large mass in the vastus intermedius muscle of the thigh. The majority of the mass has lower signal intensity than muscle, suggesting fluid or myxoid tissue. An area with higher signal, likely representing hemorrhage, is present near the periphery.*

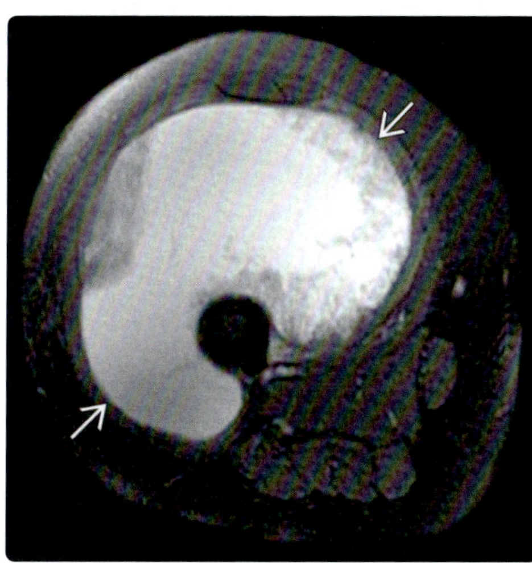

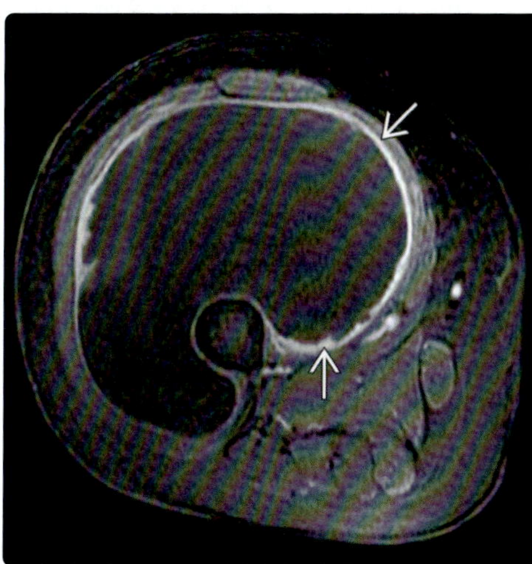

(Left) *Axial T2WI FS MR in the same patient shows the majority of the mass to have high signal with mild peripheral heterogeneity.* **(Right)** *Axial T1WI C+ FS MR in the same patient shows nodular peripheral enhancement of the mass, suggesting malignancy. The mild central enhancement, combined with T1 and T2 signal characteristics similar to fluid, suggests myxoid tissue. If an enhanced sequence had not been obtained, this could be mistaken for a chronic hematoma.*

Low-Grade Fibromyxoid Sarcoma

KEY FACTS

TERMINOLOGY

- Rare malignant fibrosarcoma variant found in young to middle-aged adults with deceivingly bland histologic appearance

IMAGING

- Subfascial > > subcutaneous > dermal location
- Lower extremity > chest wall/axilla > shoulder > inguinal region > buttock
  - Most common location is thigh
  - Typically 8-12 cm
- Intramuscular soft tissue mass with attenuation similar to or lower than muscle on CT
- Mildly heterogeneous low T1 and high T2 MR signal
  - Heterogeneous enhancement
- May contain nonenhancing regions of cystic degeneration or hypoenhancing myxoid tissue
  - No necrosis or hemorrhage

PATHOLOGY

- Well-circumscribed yellow-white mass with microscopic infiltration
- Bland spindle cells in whorls with fibrous and myxoid regions, few mitoses

CLINICAL ISSUES

- Very slowly enlarging, painless soft tissue mass
  - 15% with > 5 years of growth before presentation
- Young adults, median age of 34 yr
  - 19% are < 18 yr
  - Equal gender distribution to slight male predominance reported
- Local recurrence in 9%
- Metastases in 6%, may be delayed for decades
  - Preferentially spreads to lung and pleura
- Mortality rate: 2%
- Wide surgical excision and lifetime follow-up

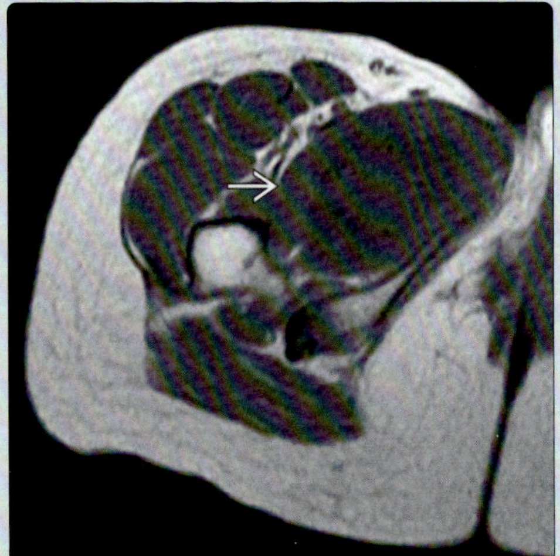

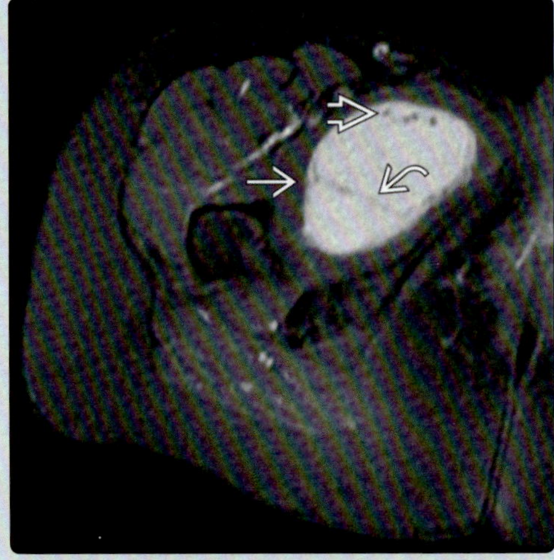

(Left) *Axial T1WI MR shows a heterogeneous, isointense to hypointense mass ➡ in the right adductor brevis muscle. Regions of myxoid tissue and cystic degeneration have lower signal intensity than skeletal muscle. This low signal can also be seen with areas of necrosis, uncommon in this diagnosis.* **(Right)** *Axial T2WI FS MR in the same patient shows the mass ➡ to have predominantly high signal with a low-signal septation ⬏ and punctate foci ⇨. The deep soft tissue of the thigh is the most common location.*

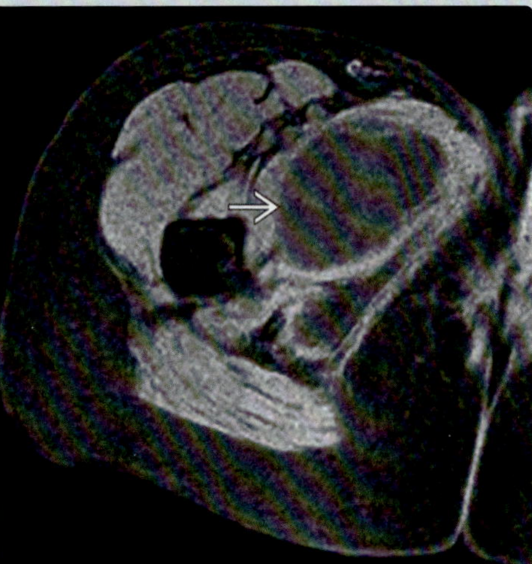

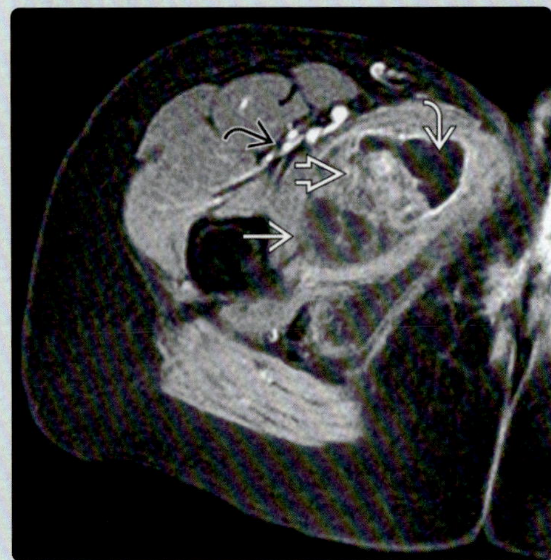

(Left) *Axial T1WI FS MR in the same patient, obtained before IV gadolinium, shows the mass ➡ to be heterogeneously hypointense relative to muscle.* **(Right)** *Axial T1WI C+ FS MR shows the mass ➡ to have both solidly enhancing ⇨ and non- or hypoenhancing myxoid regions ⬏. There was no involvement of the adjacent neurovascular structures ⬏. Other myxoid tumors, such as myxoid liposarcoma and myxofibrosarcoma, can have similar MR imaging characteristics.*

TERMINOLOGY

Synonyms

- Fibrosarcoma, fibromyxoid type; hyalinizing spindle cell tumor with giant rosettes

Definitions

- Rare malignant fibrosarcoma variant found in young to middle-aged adults with deceivingly bland histologic appearance

IMAGING

General Features

- Location
  - Subfascial > > subcutaneous > dermal location
  - Lower extremity > chest wall/axilla > shoulder > inguinal region > buttock
    - Most common location is thigh
    - Head and retroperitoneum are uncommon
- Size
  - Typically 8-12 cm
- Morphology
  - Lobulated soft tissue mass

Imaging Recommendations

- Protocol advice
  - Gadolinium-enhanced MR to direct biopsy of most solid region of tumor

CT Findings

- Intramuscular soft tissue mass with attenuation similar to or lower than muscle

MR Findings

- Mildly heterogeneous low T1 and high T2 signal
- Heterogeneous enhancement
  - May contain nonenhancing regions of cystic degeneration or hypoenhancing myxoid tissue
  - Gyriform pattern of enhancing and hyperintense regions has been described
- No necrosis or hemorrhage

DIFFERENTIAL DIAGNOSIS

Myxofibrosarcoma

- Elderly patients
- Subcutaneous > intramuscular location
- More homogeneous imaging appearance
- Less likely to metastasize

Liposarcoma, Myxoid

- May have similar imaging appearance when fat content is not visible
- Similar age range and anatomic location
- Contains lipoblasts

Intramuscular Myxoma, Cellular

- More homogeneous imaging appearance
- Peripheral rim of fat and surrounding edema

Fasciitis, Nodular

- Similar patient age
- Painful, rapidly growing mass adherent to fascia
- May contain some histologically similar areas

Liposarcoma, Spindle Cell

- Subcutaneous location
- Uniform spindle cells in parallel orientation
- Contains lipoblasts
- Very rare

PATHOLOGY

Gross Pathologic & Surgical Features

- Glistening yellow-white mass
- Well-circumscribed, though microscopically infiltrative

Microscopic Features

- Bland spindle cells in whorls with fibrous and myxoid regions, few mitoses
  - Prominent vessels in myxoid regions
  - 10-20% have foci of intermediate-grade fibrosarcoma
  - 40% have rosettes of collagen bordered by epithelioid fibroblasts
- Positive vimentin stain
- Negative desmin, S100 protein, cytokeratin, CD34, and epithelial membrane antigen stains
- MUC4 expression is highly sensitive and specific immunohistochemical marker

CLINICAL ISSUES

Presentation

- Most common signs/symptoms
  - Very slowly enlarging, painless soft tissue mass
    - 15% with > 5 yr of growth before presentation

Demographics

- Age
  - Young adults, median age of 34 yr
    - 19% are < 18 yr
- Gender
  - Equal distribution to slight male predominance reported

Natural History & Prognosis

- Local recurrence in 9%
- Metastases in 6%, may be delayed for decades
  - Preferentially spreads to lung and pleura
- Mortality rate: 2%
- Early studies overestimated aggressiveness due to primary misdiagnosis as benign lesion

Treatment

- Wide surgical excision with lifetime follow-up

SELECTED REFERENCES

1. Yamashita H et al: Intramuscular myxoma of the buttock mimicking low-grade fibromyxoid sarcoma: diagnostic usefulness of MUC4 expression. Skeletal Radiol. 42(10):1475-9, 2013
2. Hwang S et al: Imaging features of low-grade fibromyxoid sarcoma (Evans tumor). Skeletal Radiol. 41(10):1263-72, 2012
3. Weiss SW et al: Fibrosarcoma. In Weiss SW et al: Enzinger and Weiss' Soft Tissue Tumors. 5th ed. Philadelphia: Elsevier. 316-25, 2008
4. Kransdorf MJ et al: Malignant fibrous and fibrohistiocytic tumors. In Kransdorf MJ et al: Imaging of Soft Tissue Tumors. 2nd ed. Philadelphia: Lippincott Williams & Wilkins. 276, 2006
5. Folpe A et al: Low grade fibromyxoid sarcoma. In Fletcher CDM et al: World Health Organization Classification of Tumours. Pathology and Genetics of Tumours of Soft Tissue and Bone. Lyon: IARC Press. 104-5, 2002

Sclerosing Epithelioid Fibrosarcoma

KEY FACTS

TERMINOLOGY

- Rare fibrosarcoma variant that is histologically similar to poorly differentiated carcinoma and sclerosing lymphoma

IMAGING

- Intramuscular, lower extremity > trunk > upper extremity > head and neck
  - Rarely invades underlying bone
  - 2-22 cm in size (mean: 7-10 cm)
- Similar attenuation to muscle on CT
  - Low-attenuation myxoid or cystic degeneration foci; necrosis uncommon
  - May contain calcification
- Majority of lesion is heterogeneously isointense to muscle on T1 & hyperintense to muscle on T2WI MR
  - Geographic foci of low signal on T1WI & T2WI MR is most distinctive finding

PATHOLOGY

- Often appears well circumscribed but is histologically infiltrative
- Prominent dense, hyalinized stroma with variably patterned cords or nests of epithelioid-like cells
  - Microscopic regions of necrosis in up to 33%
- Low cellularity may mimic benign lesion

CLINICAL ISSUES

- Slowly enlarging, deep soft tissue mass
  - Painful in 33%
- > 50% with local recurrence
- 43% with metastatic disease, usually within 5-8 yr
  - Lung, bone, and pleura/chest wall
- 50% mortality rate
- Treatment with wide surgical excision
  - Adjuvant radiotherapy frequently utilized

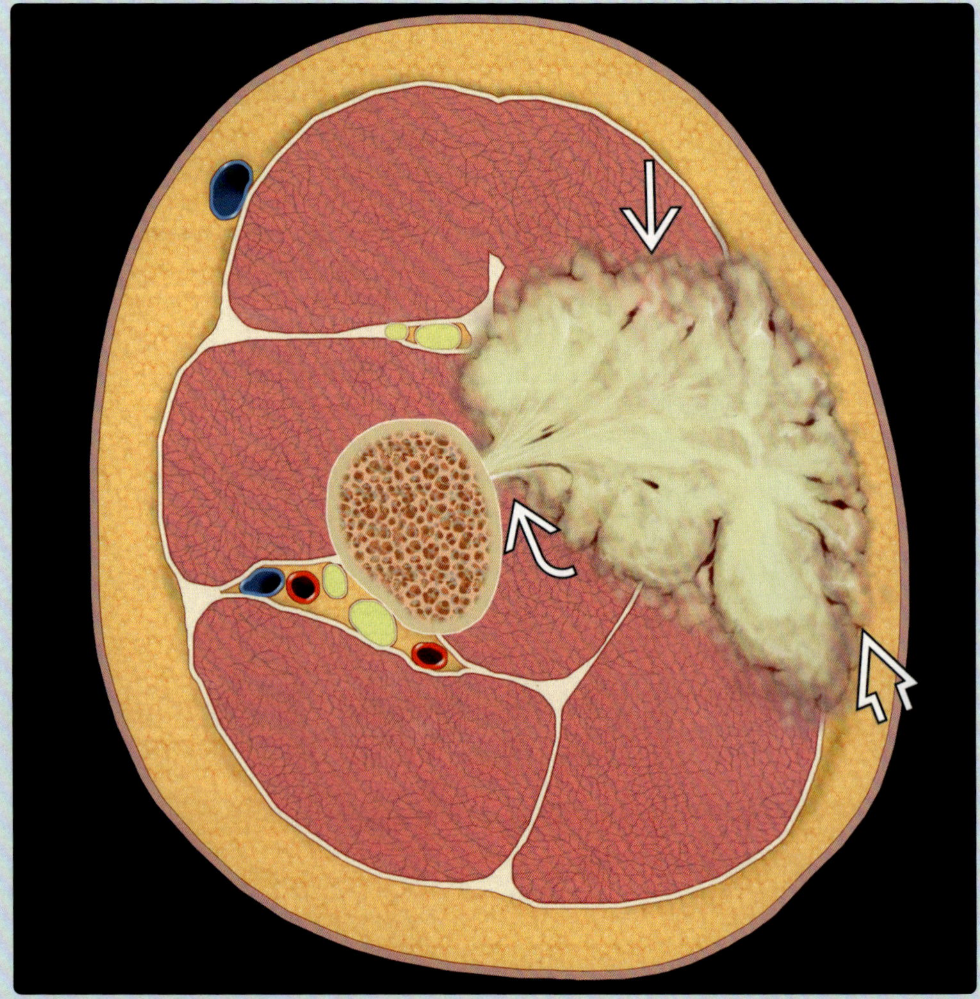

Axial graphic of the upper arm demonstrates a lobulated, infiltrative mass ➡ that is centered intramuscularly, but extends to involve the subcutaneous fat ➡ and abuts the underlying bone ↪. The dense collagenous stroma of these lesions gives them a firm, whitish cut surface.

TERMINOLOGY

Definitions

- Rare fibrosarcoma variant that is histologically similar to poorly differentiated carcinoma and sclerosing lymphoma

IMAGING

General Features

- Best diagnostic clue
  - Circumscribed to infiltrative deep soft tissue mass with geographic regions of low signal on T1WI and T2WI MR
- Location
  - Intramuscular, lower extremity > trunk > upper extremity > head and neck
  - Rare in pelvis, retroperitoneum, bone, and ovary
- Size
  - 2-22 cm in size (mean: 7-10 cm)
- Morphology
  - Lobulated to multinodular mass

Radiographic Findings

- Rarely invades underlying bone

CT Findings

- Deep mass with similar attenuation to muscle
  - Low-attenuation regions of myxoid tissue or cystic degeneration
- May contain calcification

MR Findings

- Majority of lesion is heterogeneously isointense to muscle on T1WI and hyperintense to muscle on T2WI MR
  - Geographic foci of low signal on T1WI and T2WI MR is most distinctive, but not specific, finding

Nuclear Medicine Findings

- PET/CT shows variably abnormal FDG accumulation in small series
  - Closely related to histopathologic characteristics of aggressiveness

DIFFERENTIAL DIAGNOSIS

Undifferentiated Adenocarcinoma

- Positive immunoreactivity to epithelial membrane antigen can also be present with sclerosing epithelioid fibrosarcoma
- May not be possible to differentiate histologically

Synovial Sarcoma

- Predilection for periarticular regions
- Similar patient demographics
- Cytogenetic studies can assist identification

Sclerosing Lymphoma

- Positive immunoreactivity for leukocyte common antigen, which is not present with sclerosing epithelioid fibrosarcoma

Malignant Peripheral Nerve Sheath Tumor

- Contiguous with nerve or nerve sheath
- Central low signal on MR can have similar appearance

PATHOLOGY

Gross Pathologic & Surgical Features

- Firm mass with whitish cut surface
- Appears well circumscribed but is histologically infiltrative

Microscopic Features

- Prominent dense, hyalinized stroma with variably patterned cords or nests of epithelioid-appearing cells
  - Invasive tumor margins
  - Vessels may be similar to hemangiopericytoma
  - Variable mitotic rate: Ranging from very low to > 5 per 10 HPF
  - May contain myxoid regions, cystic degeneration, metaplastic bone, and calcification
  - Microscopic regions of necrosis in up to 33%
- Appearance can be similar to sclerosing lymphoma, myxofibrosarcoma, & poorly differentiated carcinoma
  - Low cellularity may mimic benign lesion
- Strong positive vimentin stain
- 50% weakly positive epithelial membrane antigen

CLINICAL ISSUES

Presentation

- Most common signs/symptoms
  - Slowly enlarging, deep soft tissue mass
    - Painful in 33%

Demographics

- Age
  - Adolescents to elderly, median age: 45 yr
- Gender
  - Mild male predominance
- Epidemiology
  - Very rare fibrosarcoma variant

Natural History & Prognosis

- Highly aggressive tumor
  - > 50% with local recurrence
  - 43% with metastatic disease, usually 5-8 yr
    - Lung, bone, and pleura/chest wall
  - 50% mortality rate
- Prognosis worse if head and neck involved

Treatment

- Wide surgical excision
  - Adjuvant radiotherapy frequently utilized

SELECTED REFERENCES

1. Righi A et al: Sclerosing epithelioid fibrosarcoma of the thigh: report of two cases with synchronous bone metastases. Virchows Arch. 467(3):339-44, 2015
2. Luo Y et al: ^{18}F-fluorodeoxyglucose PET/CT features and correlations with histopathologic characteristics in sclerosing epithelioid fibrosarcoma. Int J Clin Exp Pathol. 7(10):7278-85, 2014
3. Ossendorf C et al: Sclerosing epithelioid fibrosarcoma: case presentation and a systematic review. Clin Orthop Relat Res. 466(6):1485-91, 2008
4. Weiss SW et al: Fibrosarcoma. In Weiss SW et al: Enzinger and Weiss' Soft Tissue Tumors. 5th ed. Philadelphia: Elsevier. 310-2, 2008
5. Kransdorf MJ et al: Malignant fibrous and fibrohistiocytic tumors. In Kransdorf MJ et al: Imaging of Soft Tissue Tumors. 2nd ed. Philadelphia: Lippincott Williams & Wilkins. 276, 2006

(Left) *Axial T1WI MR shows a rounded axillary mass ➡ with a signal intensity similar to skeletal muscle.* **(Right)** *Axial T1WI MR obtained slightly distal to the previous image shows the rounded axillary mass ➡ to lie between the proximal humeral shaft and rib cage, without evidence of underlying bone invasion. This mass was engulfing portions of the brachial plexus, explaining the patient's reported progressive pain and arm weakness. The majority of these lesions are painless.*

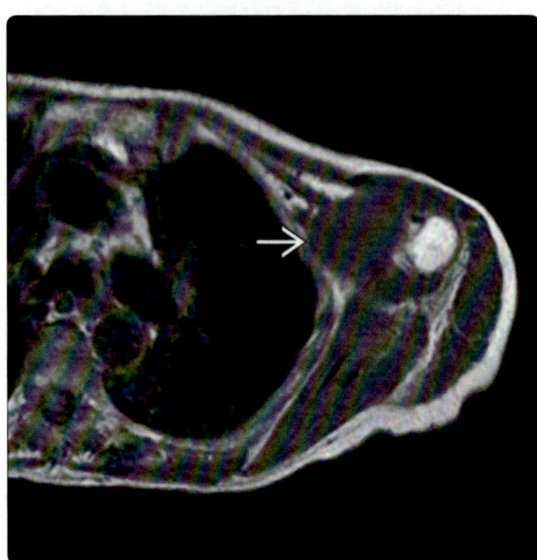

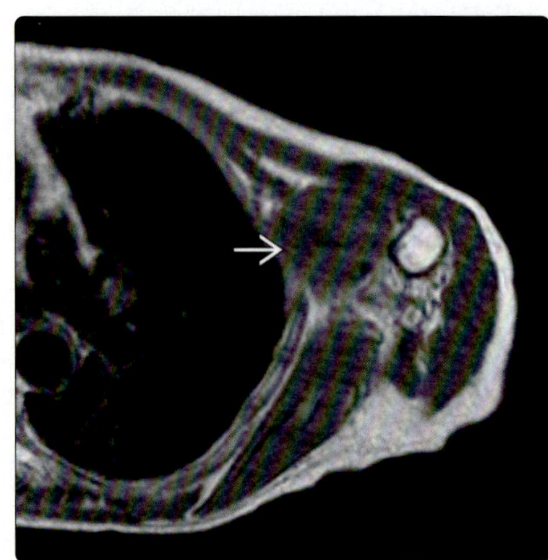

(Left) *Axial STIR MR shows the mass ➡ to be predominantly hyperintense but contain geographic regions of hypointensity ⮕. These low-intensity regions are not specific for this diagnosis but are the most distinctive finding of this otherwise nonspecific soft tissue mass.* **(Right)** *Axial STIR MR obtained slightly distal to the previous image shows the mass ➡ to have peripheral hyperintense signal with a low signal intensity center ⮕. Infiltrative margins and surrounding edema ➡ are also evident.*

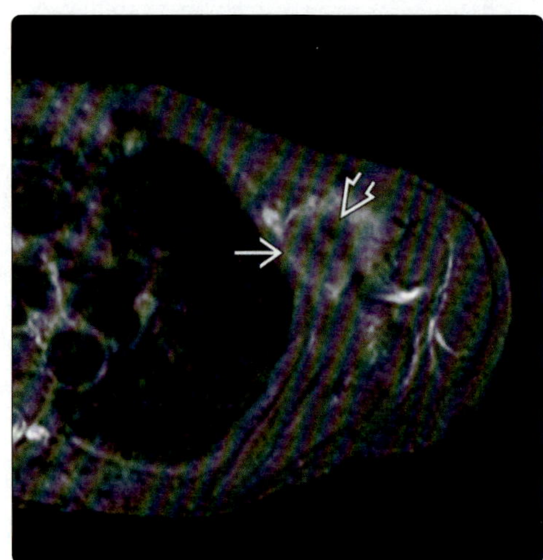

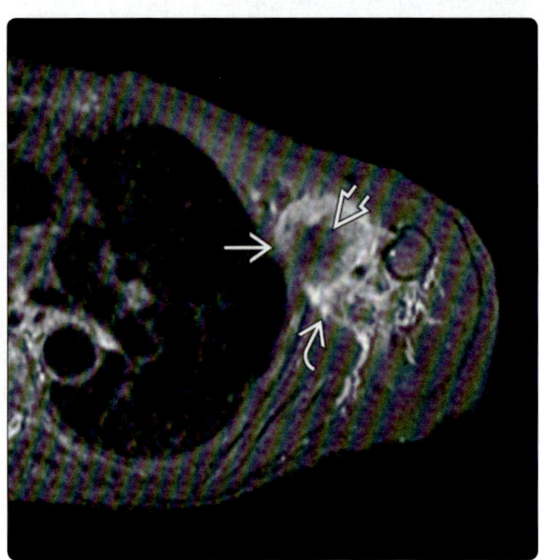

(Left) *Axial CECT shows the axillary mass ➡ to have similar density to muscle and to lie deep to the pectoralis major muscle ➡. The mass posteriorly displaces the left subclavian artery ⮕.* **(Right)** *Axial CECT obtained slightly distal to the previous image shows the mass ➡ to engulf small blood vessels ➡. Although this lesion may appear relatively well circumscribed on CT, the margins of these lesions are usually quite infiltrative. Prognosis is poor due to local recurrences and metastases.*

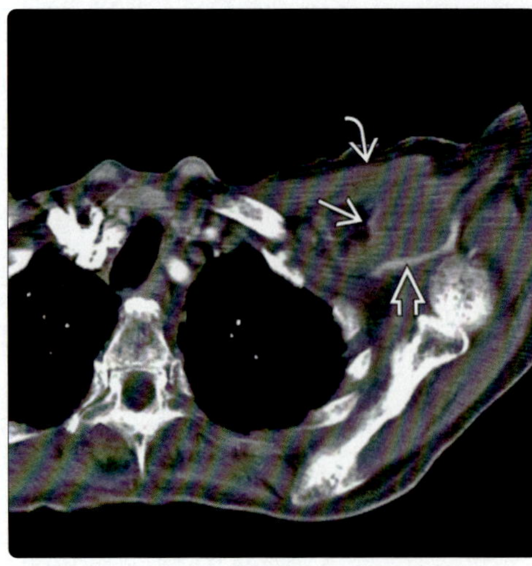

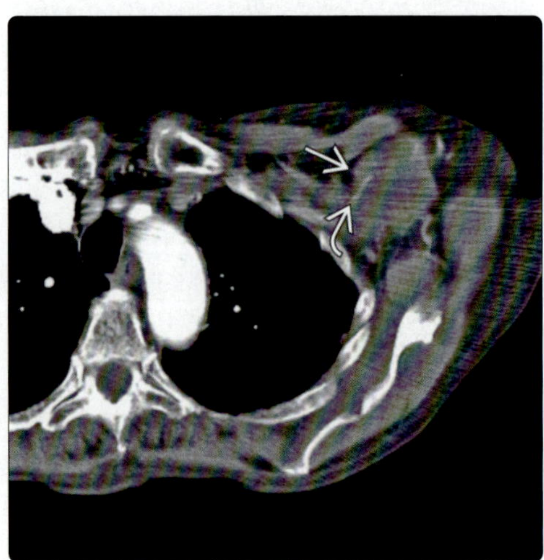

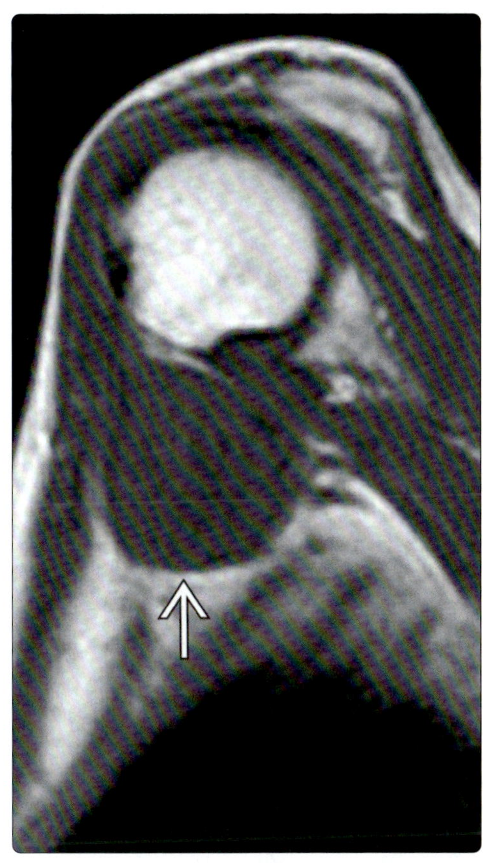

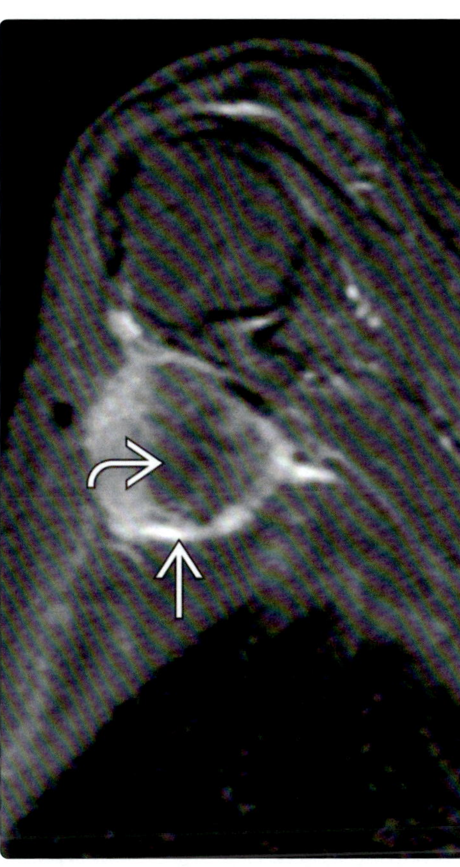

(Left) *Sagittal oblique T1WI MR shows a rounded axillary mass ➡ to have a signal intensity similar to skeletal muscle. No local invasion is evident.* **(Right)** *Sagittal oblique STIR MR shows the rounded axillary mass ➡ to be predominantly hyperintense relative to skeletal muscle, with geographic central regions of hypointensity ➡. This hypointensity is frequently seen in sclerosing epithelioid fibrosarcoma but is not specific. It can be reminiscent of the target sign in peripheral nerve sheath tumors.*

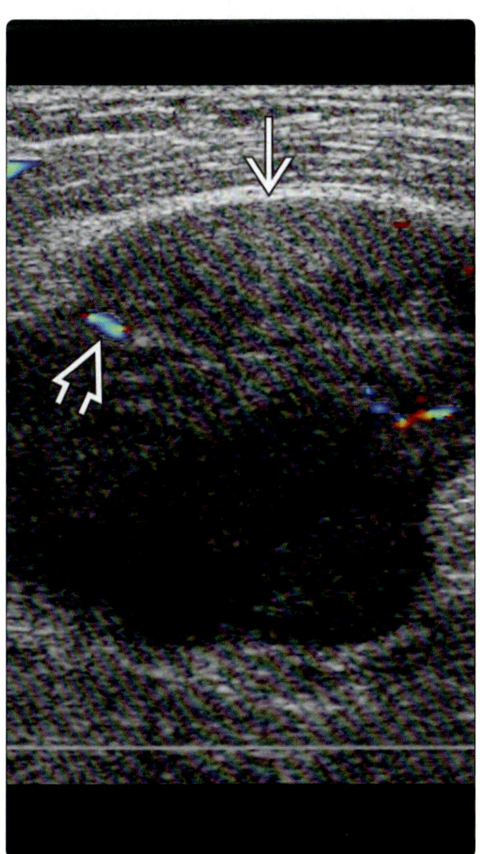

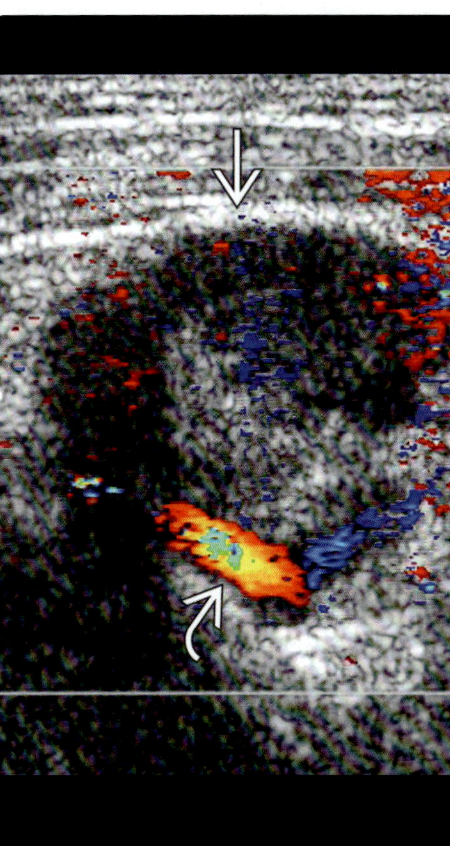

(Left) *Longitudinal Doppler ultrasound demonstrates a mixed echogenicity, lobulated mass ➡ with mild internal blood flow ➡.* **(Right)** *Longitudinal Doppler ultrasound obtained slightly more proximal to the prior image demonstrates more prominent mixed echogenicity of the mass ➡ than was seen on the prior image. A portion of the left axillary artery ➡ is visible lying deep to the mass.*

Giant Cell Tumor Tendon Sheath

KEY FACTS

TERMINOLOGY

- a.k.a. tenosynovial giant cell tumor, localized type; nodular tenosynovitis
- Benign synovial proliferation within tendon sheath, most commonly involving fingers
  - Represents same pathologic entity as pigmented villonodular synovitis (PVNS)

IMAGING

- 85% in fingers
- Nonspecific soft tissue fullness on radiographs
  - Adjacent cortical erosion in 10-28%
  - Periosteal reaction, intraosseous invasion, and cystic/degenerative change are uncommon
  - Calcification & chondroid metaplasia uncommon
- Lobulated mass with low to intermediate signal intensity on T1WI and T2WI MR
  - ± hypointense fibrous septations
  - Lacks surrounding edema
  - Low signal hemosiderin foci "bloom" on gradient-echo imaging
- Intense enhancement which may be heterogeneous

PATHOLOGY

- Etiology controversial: Neoplastic process is supported by chromosomal abnormalities and autonomous lesion growth

CLINICAL ISSUES

- Age: 30-50 years (peak: 40-50)
  - Slight female predominance (2:1)
- Painless mass growing for weeks to years
  - ± distal numbness, functional limitation
  - Prior trauma reported in 1-5%
- Treatment with surgical excision
  - Local recurrence in 4-44%
  - Following local recurrence, likely to have multiple relapses; poor surgical curative potential

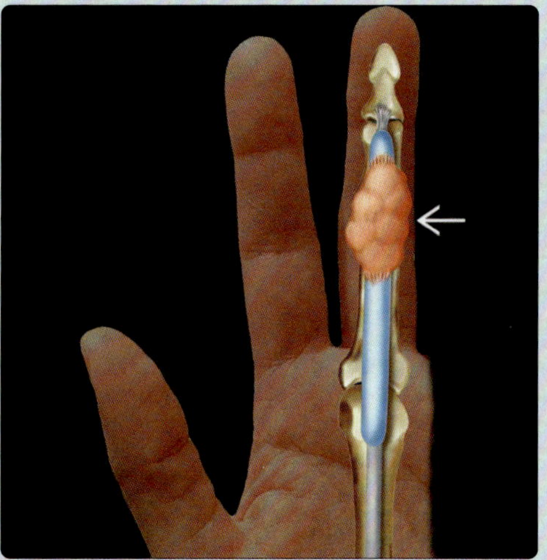

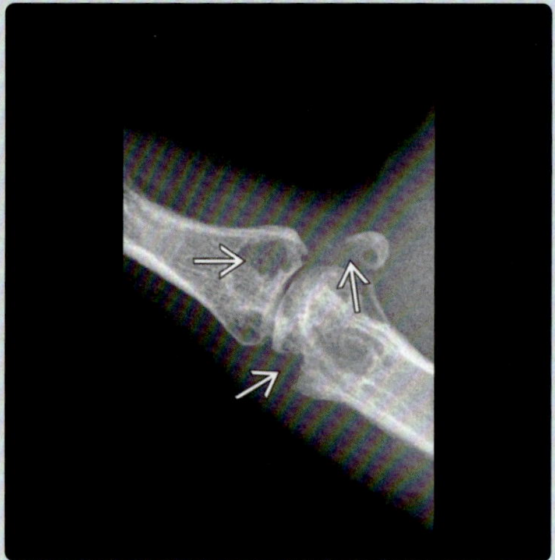

(Left) *Coronal graphic shows a giant cell tumor involving the 3rd digit flexor tendon sheath ➡. Characteristic lobulations are also present.* **(Right)** *Oblique radiograph of the thumb demonstrates prominent erosions ➡ of the 1st metacarpal, adjacent phalanx, and even the adjacent sesamoid bone. The appearance is of a joint-based process. However, there is also a nonspecific soft tissue mass, and given the location, giant cell tumor of the tendon sheath (GCTTS) should be considered.*

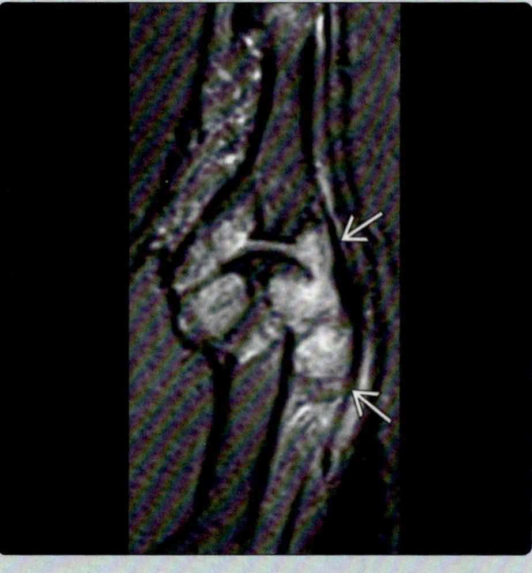

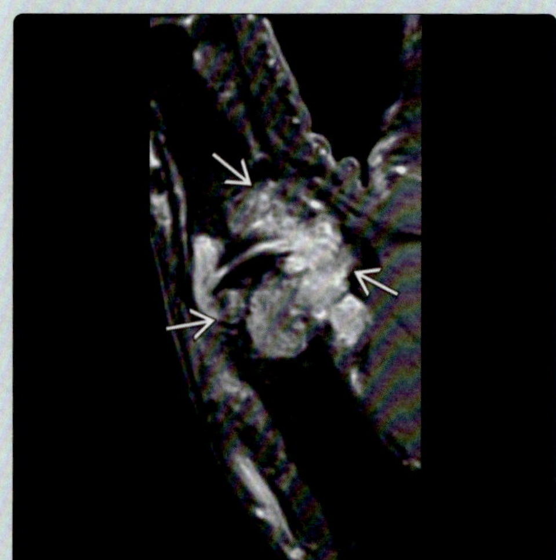

(Left) *Sagittal PD FS MR, same patient, shows bowing of the extensor tendon ➡, with a intermediate/hyperintense mass surrounding this structure and extending to surround and erode adjacent bones. The morphology is diagnostic of giant cell tumor of tendon sheath (GCTTS).* **(Right)** *Coronal T1 C+ FS MR, same case, shows intensely enhancing nodular masses ➡ causing pressure erosion on the adjacent bones, reflecting the erosions seen on radiograph. Findings are typical of GCTTS.*

TERMINOLOGY

Abbreviations

- Giant cell tumor of tendon sheath (GCTTS)

Synonyms

- Tenosynovial giant cell tumor, localized type; nodular tenosynovitis

Definitions

- Benign synovial proliferation within tendon sheath, most commonly involving fingers
  - Same pathologic entity as pigmented villonodular synovitis (PVNS) but in a different location

IMAGING

General Features

- Best diagnostic clue
  - Lobulated soft tissue mass immediately adjacent to tendon
- Location
  - Hand > wrist > ankle/foot > knee > elbow > hip
  - 85% in fingers
    - Initially reported to have predilection for volar/flexor surfaces
      - Additional studies report equal volar and dorsal distribution with additional locations being lateral and circumferential
    - Commonly located superficially and near interphalangeal joints
      - Less common origin deep to tendon (between tendon and bone)
    - Index and long fingers are most common
  - Slight predominance for right hand
  - Occasionally multifocal along tendon sheath
- Size
  - Usually small (0.5-5 cm)
- Morphology
  - Well-circumscribed lobulated mass
  - Lesions in feet are larger and more irregular than in hands

Radiographic Findings

- Radiography
  - Nonspecific soft tissue fullness
  - Adjacent cortical erosion in 10-28%
    - Uncommon bone changes include periosteal reaction, intraosseous invasion, and cystic/degenerative change
  - Calcification and chondroid metaplasia are uncommon

MR Findings

- T1WI
  - Lobulated mass with hypointense to intermediate signal intensity
    - ± hypointense fibrous septations
    - ± inhomogeneous signal
    - ± bone erosion or invasion
  - Convex bowing/bulge toward skin from tendon sheath
  - Extension in longitudinal plane most prominent
- T2WI
  - Inhomogeneous low to intermediate signal intensity
    - ± hypointense fibrous septations
  - Hypointense hemosiderin foci
    - Peripheral hypointense foci (± clumped)
    - Small hypointense foci throughout lesion
  - Lacks surrounding edema
- T2* GRE
  - Low signal hemosiderin foci "bloom" on gradient-echo imaging
- T1WI C+
  - Intense enhancement ± inhomogeneity

Imaging Recommendations

- Best imaging tool
  - MR to document size, morphology, and extent
- Protocol advice
  - T1WI C+ can be useful to define extent of tumor, especially when lesion has intermediate to low signal on both T1-weighted and fluid-sensitive sequences

Ultrasonographic Findings

- Solid, homogeneously hypoechoic
- Internal blood flow visible on Doppler

Nuclear Medicine Findings

- PET
  - May demonstrate high accumulation of 18-F FDG, similar to malignant neoplasm

DIFFERENTIAL DIAGNOSIS

Fibroma of Tendon Sheath

- Similar location and appearance on MR
  - May contain wavy low-signal regions of collagen
- Typically enhances less intensely than GCTTS

Ganglion Cyst

- Thin-walled; fluid intensity lesion near joint
- Hypointense on T1WI
- Hyperintense on fluid-sensitive sequences
- Nonenhancing except peripherally

Hemangioma & Vascular Malformations, Soft Tissue

- Poorly circumscribed compared with GCTTS
- Low to intermediate signal on T1WI
- Hyperintense serpiginous vessels on FS PD FSE
- Hypointense foci secondary to hemosiderin

Foreign Body

- Intermediate signal intensity of granulomatous reaction (T1WI and T2WI)
- Adjacent subcutaneous tissue edema
- ± peripheral rim-like enhancement
- Gradient-echo to emphasize susceptibility artifacts from metallic foreign bodies

Lipoma, Soft Tissue

- Follows fat signal intensity on all imaging sequences
- ± thin septa
- Presence of nodules or enhancement should suggest atypical lipomatous tumor or liposarcoma

Synovial Sarcoma

- 15-35 years of age

- Close proximity to joints, however most are extraarticular in location
- Calcification in approximately 1/3 of cases
- Aggressive tracking along tendons is possible
- Thick septations are unusual
- ± central necrosis

PATHOLOGY

General Features

- Etiology
  - Controversial: Neoplastic process supported by chromosomal abnormalities and autonomous lesion growth
  - Initially suggested to be reactive or regenerative hyperplasia associated with inflammatory process due to frequent trauma history and predilection for 1st 3 fingers of right hand
  - Other theories
    - Disturbed lipid metabolism
    - Osteoclastic proliferation
    - Infection
    - Vascular disturbances
    - Immune mechanisms
    - Inflammation
    - Neoplasia
    - Metabolic disturbances
- Genetics
  - Short arm of chromosome 1
    - Recurrent t(1;2)(p11;q35-36) abnormalities
  - Several other translocation partners reported

Staging, Grading, & Classification

- Localized, nodular synovitis, and diffuse types of PVNS
  - Localized type is most common
  - Nodular synovitis reflects solitary intraarticular nodule
  - Diffuse type is extraarticular, soft tissue mass

Gross Pathologic & Surgical Features

- Firm, well-circumscribed lobulated mass
  - Nodular and villous morphology
- Mottled pink-gray with yellow or brown regions
- Grooves along surface may be secondary to pressure from adjacent tendons

Microscopic Features

- Synovial-like mononuclear rounded or polygonal cells: Lipid-laden histiocytes and multinucleated giant cells
  - Variable number of giant cells, inflammatory cells, foamy macrophages, and siderophages
  - Hemosiderin-containing xanthoma cells in periphery of lesion
  - Necrosis is rare
- Variable mitotic activity from 3-20 mitoses per 10 HPF

CLINICAL ISSUES

Presentation

- Most common signs/symptoms
  - Usually painless slow-growing mass, presents weeks to years
  - Prior trauma reported in 1-5%
- Clinical profile
  - May cause occasional distal numbness
  - May cause limited function of digit due to size of lesion
  - Mass is nontransilluminating

Demographics

- Age
  - 30-50 years (peak: 40-50)
    - Rare < 10 or > 60 years
- Gender
  - Mild female predominance (M:F = 1:2)
- Epidemiology
  - 2nd most common mass of hand after ganglion cyst

Natural History & Prognosis

- Slowly growing lesions
- Late stage = exuberant, heavily pigmented villous synovial overgrowth
- Osseous erosions related to lesion hypervascularity
- Complications
  - Satellite lesions are common after incomplete resection
  - Puncturing lesions may seed operative bed
  - Tendon reconstruction may be necessary
  - No malignant degeneration reported
- Local recurrence in 4-44%

Treatment

- Treatment is surgical excision
  - Morphology of lesion usually results in marginal excision
  - Complete excision can be difficult depending on extent
  - Bony debridement may be necessary
- Following 1st recurrence, surgical curative rate decreases significantly
- Researching use of tyrosine kinase inhibitors for target potential

DIAGNOSTIC CHECKLIST

Consider

- True bone invasion rather than focal erosion is not typical and is suggestive of aggressive neoplasm
- Reactive soft tissue edema is atypical
- T2* gradient-echo to document hemosiderin

SELECTED REFERENCES

1. Palmerini E et al: Tenosynovial giant cell tumour/pigmented villonodular synovitis: Outcome of 294 patients before the era of kinase inhibitors. Eur J Cancer. ePub, 2014
2. Bancroft LW et al: Imaging of benign soft tissue tumors. Semin Musculoskelet Radiol. 17(2):156-67, 2013
3. Zeinstra JS et al: Multifocal giant cell tumor of the tendon sheath: case report and literature review. Skeletal Radiol. 42(3):447-50, 2013
4. Fotiadis E et al: Giant cell tumour of tendon sheath of the digits. A systematic review. Hand (N Y). 6(3):244-9, 2011

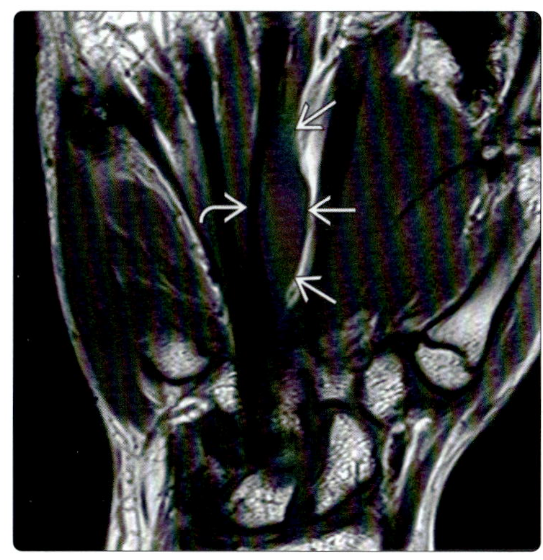

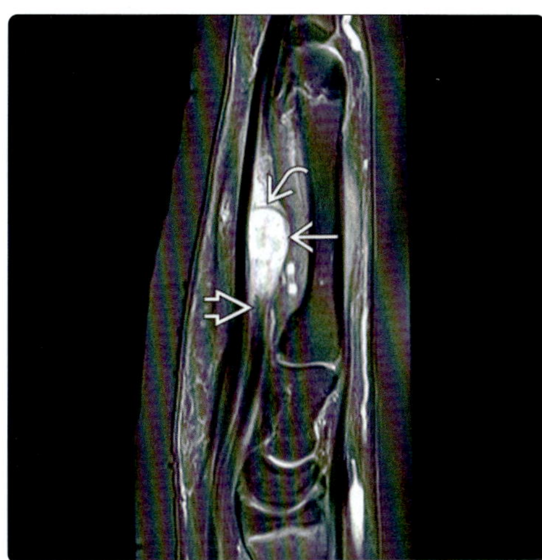

(Left) *Coronal T1 MR in a patient with a palmar mass shows the flexor tendon ➔ to be bowed in an ulnar direction. The displacement of the tendon is caused by an elongated mass ➔ that is isointense to muscle.* **(Right)** *Sagittal PD FS MR, same patient, shows the mass ➔ to be inhomogeneously hyperintense. It contains low-signal fibrous septa ➔ and arises from the adjacent tendon sheath ➔. All these findings are typical of giant cell tumor of tendon sheath.*

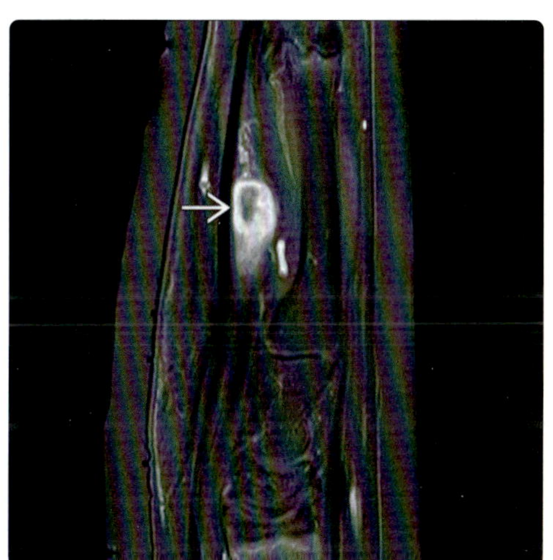

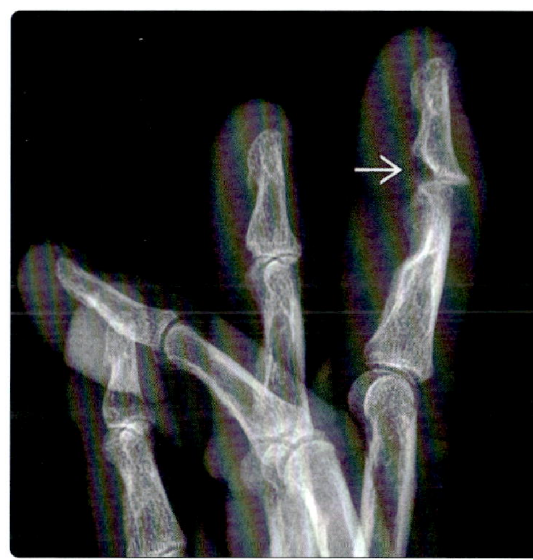

(Left) *Sagittal T1 C+ FS MR in the same patient shows the lesion to enhance peripherally ➔ around low-signal material. Inhomogeneity in the enhanced areas may be seen in GCTTS.* **(Right)** *Lateral radiograph shows a solitary abnormality in the digit of a 58 year old. There is soft tissue swelling around the DIP, and a single well-marginated erosion of the distal phalanx ➔. There is mild dorsal subluxation at the joint. This might make one consider trauma, with resorption of a volar fracture fragment.*

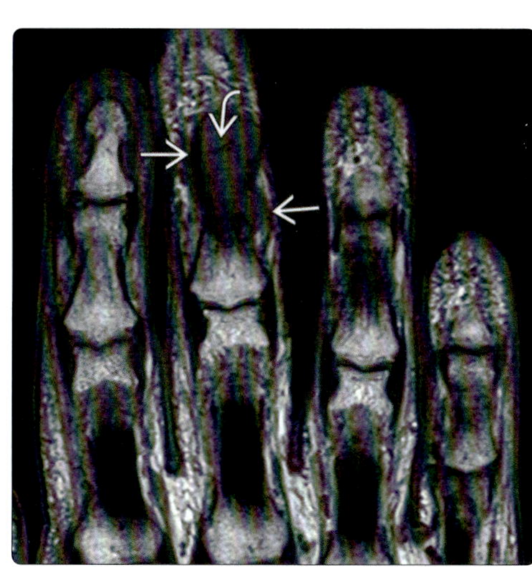

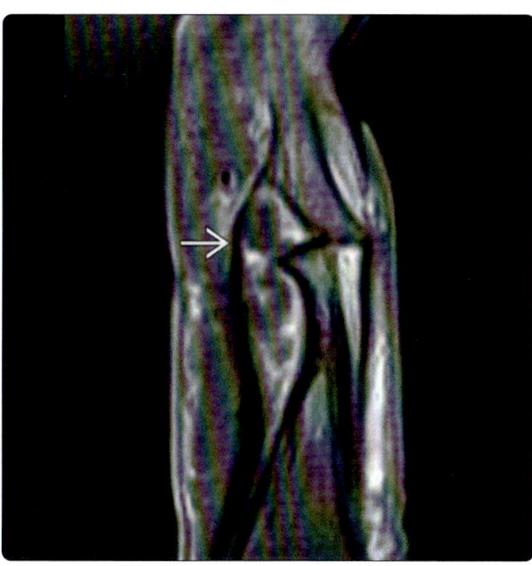

(Left) *Coronal T1 MR, same patient, shows a homogeneous hypointense mass ➔ that contains a single septum ➔. It is on the volar aspect of the DIP joint.* **(Right)** *Sagittal T1 C+ FS MR, same patient, shows the longstanding erosion, bowed flexor tendon ➔, and enhancement around a wavy hypointense mass. The latter suggests fibroma of tendon sheath. This lesion is in the differential, but is less common than GCTTS. However, at surgery this lesion proved to be GCTTS.*

(Left) *Axial T1 MR demonstrates an intermediate to hypointense soft tissue mass ➡ arising from the flexor hallucis longus tendon sheath at the level of the great toe interphalangeal joint.* **(Right)** *Axial T2 FS MR in the same patient best demonstrates the lobulated nature of the mass ➡. Note the increased signal centrally and peripheral areas of low signal intensity corresponding to hemosiderin deposition.*

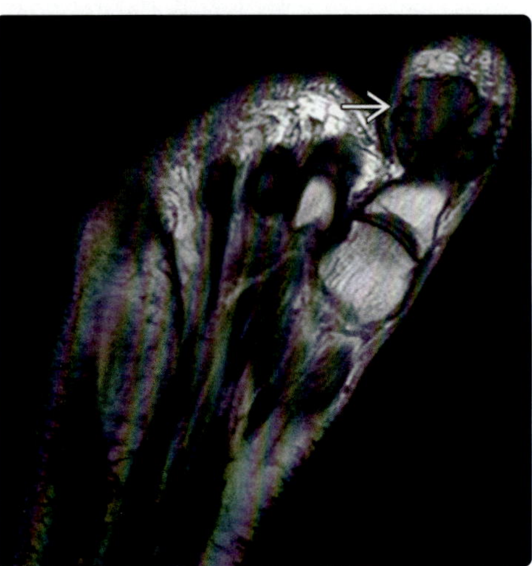

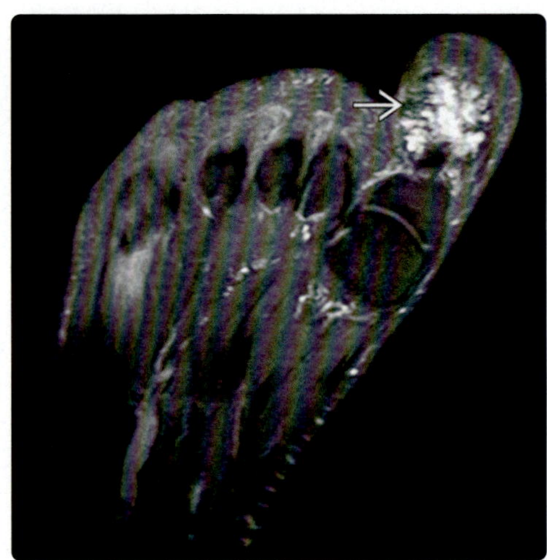

(Left) *Axial T1 C+ FS MR in the same patient shows intense, inhomogeneous enhancement of the mass ➡. The peripheral rim of the lesion remains low in signal.* **(Right)** *Axial T1 C+ FS MR demonstrates a large soft tissue mass ➡ involving the palm of the hand, which extended proximally from the volar aspect of one finger. The mass heterogeneously enhances and surrounds all of the flexor tendons at the proximal metacarpal level.*

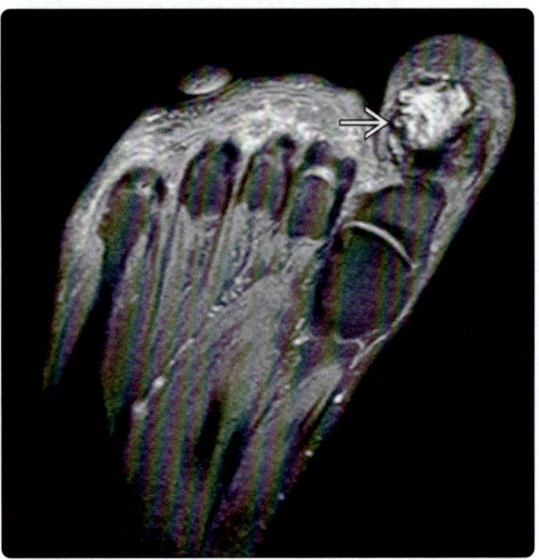

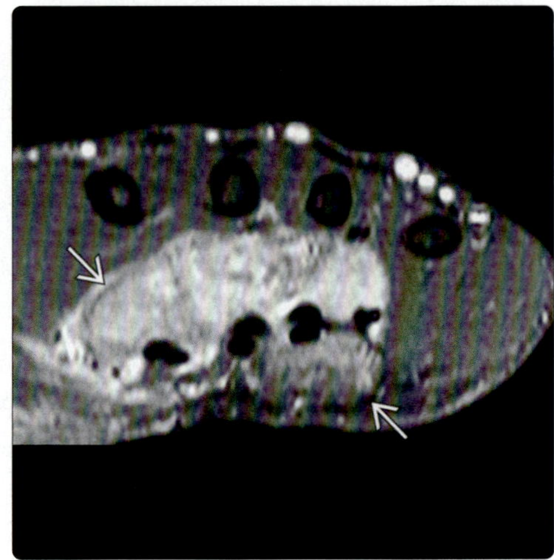

(Left) *Axial T1 C+ MR shows mildly inhomogeneous enhancement of a giant cell tumor of tendon sheath ➡. The location of this mass along the superficial surface of the tendon sheath is typical.* **(Right)** *Axial T1WI C+ MR shows intense enhancement of a giant cell tumor of tendon sheath ➡ arising between the tendon and bone. This is a less common origin (deep to tendon).*

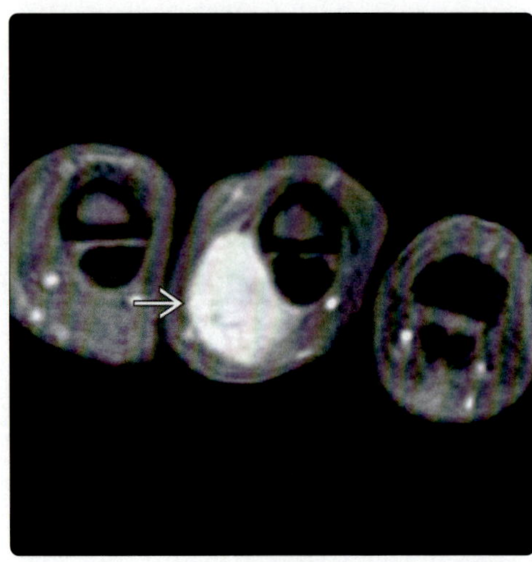

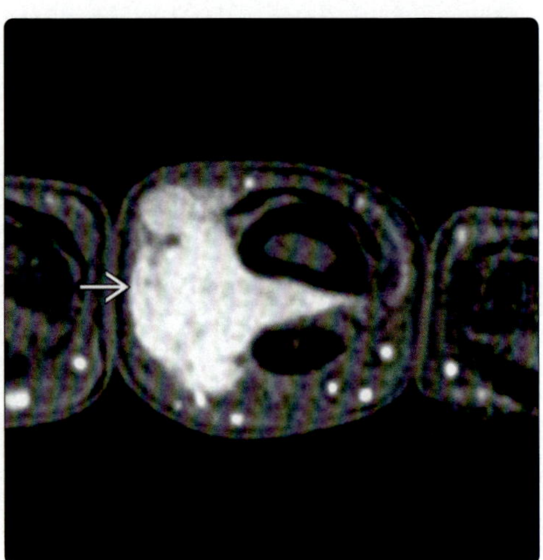

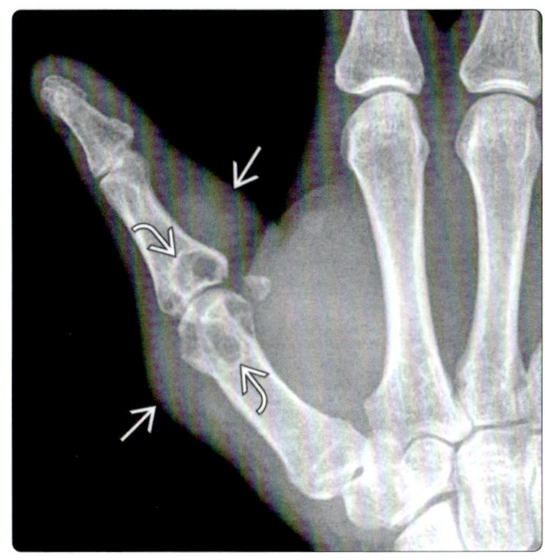

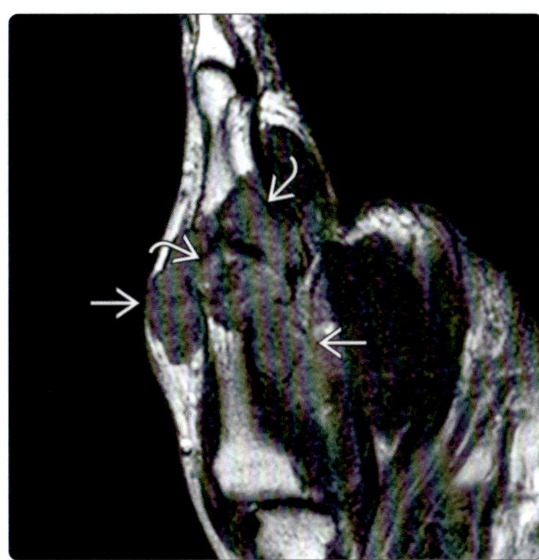

(Left) *Posteroanterior radiograph of the hand shows erosions ➔ on both sides of the MCP joint and asymmetric soft tissue swelling ➔. This asymmetric soft tissue prominence strongly suggests that the process is a soft tissue mass causing local erosion.* **(Right)** *Oblique T2 MR shows the soft tissue mass ➔ to be slightly hyperintense relative to the adjacent muscle, with scattered septa and low-signal foci. Bone erosion ➔ is again demonstrated. It is not unusual for large lesions to erode the underlying bone.*

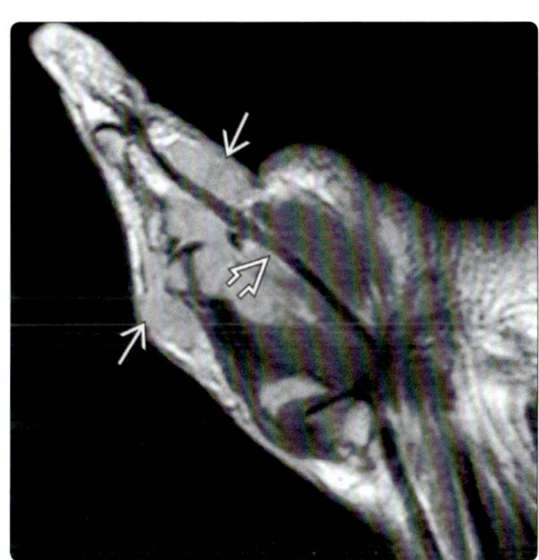

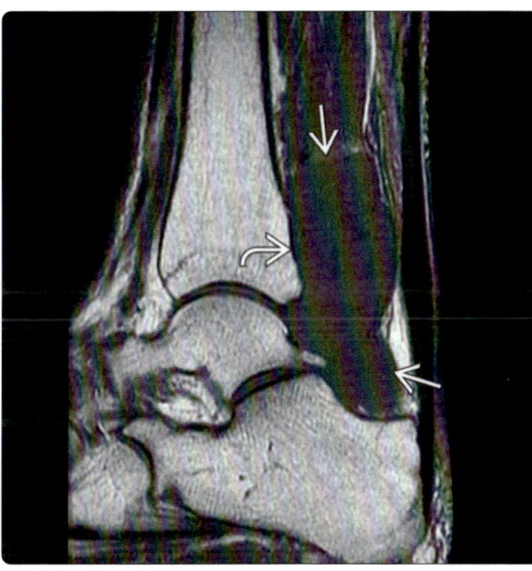

(Left) *Sagittal T1 C+ MR in the same patient shows the mass ➔ to diffusely enhance. Note that the mass surrounds the flexor tendon of the thumb ➔. In this particular case, the erosions on either side of the joint are potentially confusing, suggesting an arthritic process, but the distribution of the mass should dissuade one from misdiagnosis.* **(Right)** *Sagittal T1 MR shows a large soft tissue mass ➔ virtually replacing the Kager fat pad and causing mild erosion of the posterior tibia ➔. The mass is isointense to muscle.*

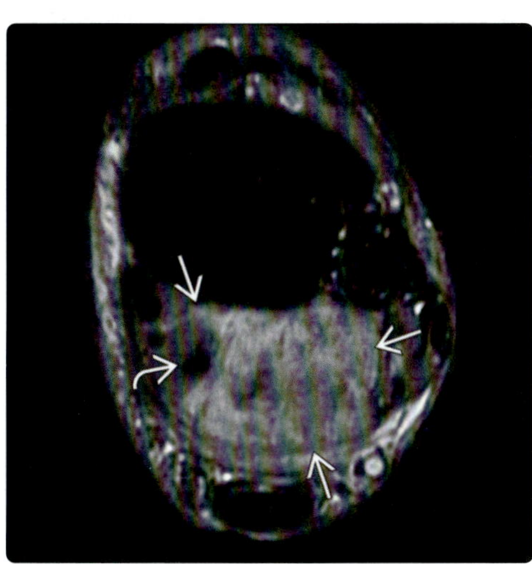

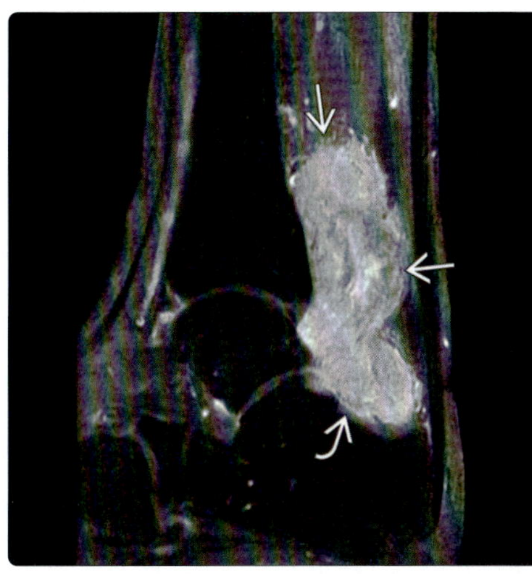

(Left) *Axial T2 FS MR, same case, shows the mildly hyperintense soft tissue mass ➔ surrounding the flexor hallucis tendon ➔ and occupying the space normally filled with the Kager fat pad.* **(Right)** *Sagittal T1 C+ FS MR, same patient, shows the mass ➔ to enhance. There is mild erosion on the adjacent calcaneus ➔. Although GCTTS involves the hand far more frequently than the ankle, in this case the location and morphology of the mass arising from a tendon, as well as the signal and adjacent erosions, make the diagnosis.*

Diffuse-Type Giant Cell Tumor (Extraarticular PVNS)

KEY FACTS

TERMINOLOGY

- Uncommon, rarely metastasizing fibrohistiocytic tumor representing extraarticular soft tissue form of pigmented villonodular synovitis (PVNS)

IMAGING

- Periarticular soft tissues of knee > thigh > foot
  - Intramuscular or subcutaneous locations are less common
- Nonspecific soft tissue mass near joint on radiographs or CT
  - ± calcification
- MR findings
  - Majority of mass is isointense to muscle on T1WI MR
  - Majority of mass isointense to hyperintense to muscle on fluid-sensitive tissues
  - Foci of low signal on T1WI and T2WI MR are typical, but not diagnostic
  - With enhancement
  - Hemorrhage is less evident than with intraarticular PVNS
- Reported high accumulation of F-18 FDG on PET imaging, similar to malignant neoplasm

CLINICAL ISSUES

- Clinical symptoms
  - Pain, tenderness, or swelling
  - May limit joint range of motion when large or multiple lesions are present
  - May be asymptomatic, incidental discovery on imaging
- Age: Wide range; most patients < 40 years
- Gender: Mild female predominance
- Natural history
  - More aggressive clinical behavior than localized giant cell tumor of tendon sheath
    - Local recurrence in up to 50%
    - Atypical histologic features do not predict recurrence
    - Malignant variant, malignant transformation, and metastases have been rarely reported
- Treatment: Wide surgical excision

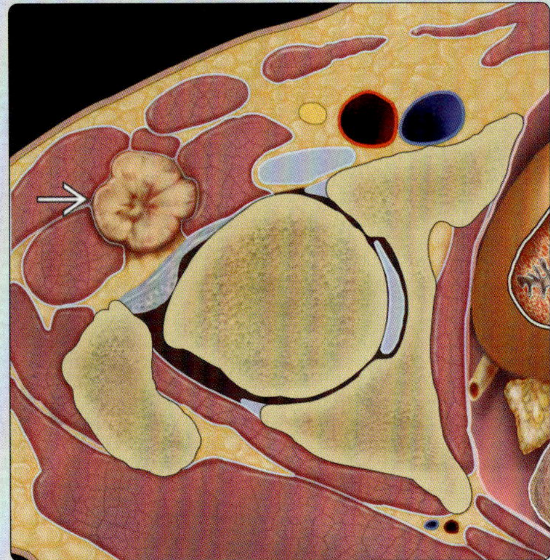

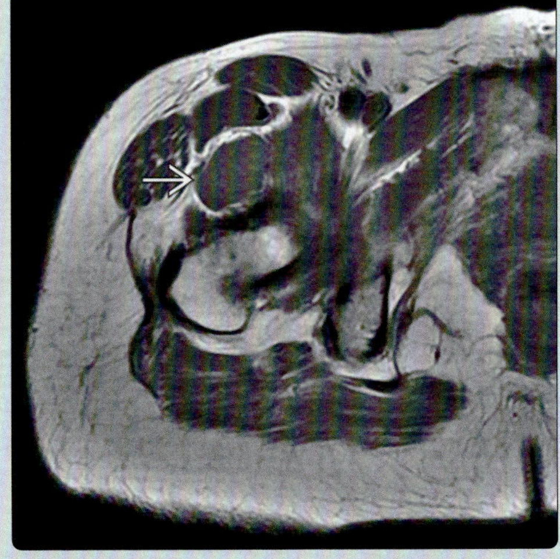

(Left) *Axial graphic shows a lobulated mass ➡ in the periarticular soft tissues of the hip. These periarticular lesions lack the villous pattern seen with intraarticular pigmented villonodular synovitis (PVNS).* **(Right)** *Axial T1WI MR shows a lobulated, oval mass ➡ located in the extraarticular soft tissues anterior to the right femoral neck. The mass is homogeneously isointense relative to muscle. This mass is not intimately associated with any tendon sheath.*

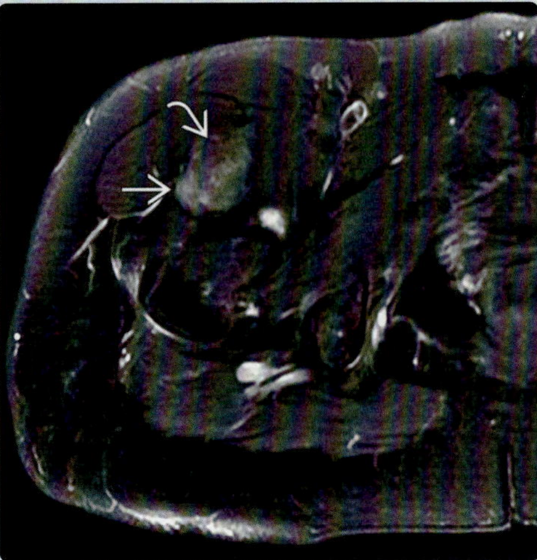

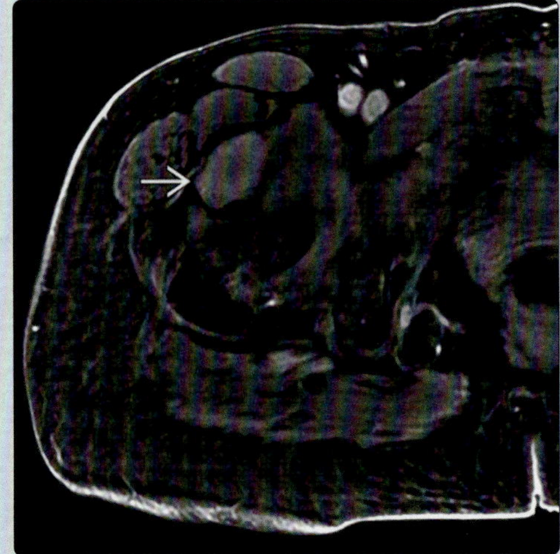

(Left) *Axial T2WI FS MR shows the mass ➡ to be heterogeneously hyperintense to muscle, with an eccentric area of low signal ➡. The mass is located in an intermuscular space, bordered by the tensor fascia lata, rectus femoris, and iliopsoas muscles.* **(Right)** *Axial T1WI C+ FS MR shows relatively homogeneous enhancement of the mass ➡. The appearance of the mass is nonspecific, and entities such as sarcoma, lymphoma, and desmoid would be considered more likely than diffuse-type giant cell tumor.*

TERMINOLOGY

Synonyms

- Extraarticular pigmented villonodular synovitis (PVNS), tenosynovial giant cell tumor (diffuse type), proliferative synovitis, florid synovitis

Definitions

- Uncommon, rarely metastasizing fibrohistiocytic tumor representing extraarticular soft tissue form of PVNS

IMAGING

General Features

- Location
  - Periarticular soft tissues of knee > thigh > foot
    - Found rarely in finger, groin, wrist, elbow, toe, and paravertebral region
    - May involve adjacent joint
  - Intramuscular or subcutaneous locations are less common
- Size
  - Usually > 5 cm

CT Findings

- Nonspecific soft tissue mass near joint
  - ± calcification

MR Findings

- Majority of mass is isointense to muscle on T1WI and isointense to hyperintense relative to muscle on fluid-sensitive MR sequences
  - Foci of low signal on T1WI and T2WI MR are typical, but not diagnostic
    - Hemorrhage is less evident than with intraarticular PVNS
  - + enhancement

Nuclear Medicine Findings

- PET
  - Reported high accumulation of F-18 FDG, similar to malignant neoplasm

DIFFERENTIAL DIAGNOSIS

Synovial Sarcoma

- Predilection for periarticular regions, especially lower limbs
- May contain cystic, hemorrhagic, and solid elements
- Up to 33% with calcification or ossification
- Most common: 15-35 years

Pigmented Villonodular Synovitis: Intraarticular

- Joint capsule distention
- Hemorrhagic effusion
- Underlying bone erosion

Low-Grade Fibromyxoid Sarcoma

- Most common location is thigh
- Young adults; median age: 34 years
- Mildly heterogeneous low T1 and high T2 MR signal
- May contain nonenhancing regions of cystic degeneration or hypoenhancing myxoid tissue

PATHOLOGY

General Features

- Etiology
  - Neoplastic nature suggested by identified clonal anomalies and autonomous growth

Staging, Grading, & Classification

- Localized type, nodular synovitis, and diffuse PVNS
  - Localized type (giant cell tumor of tendon sheath) is most common type
  - Nodular synovitis reflects solitary intraarticular nodule
  - Diffuse type is extraarticular soft tissue mass

Gross Pathologic & Surgical Features

- Spongy or firm, multinodular soft tissue mass
  - Lacks villous pattern of intraarticular PVNS

Microscopic Features

- Synovial-like mononuclear cells with foam cells, multinucleated giant cells, inflammatory cells, and siderophages
  - Fewer giant cells than in giant cell tumor of tendon sheath
  - Mitoses may be > 5 per 10 HPF

CLINICAL ISSUES

Presentation

- Most common signs/symptoms
  - Pain, tenderness, or swelling
  - May be asymptomatic, incidental discovery on imaging
- Other signs/symptoms
  - May limit joint range of motion when large or multiple lesions are present

Demographics

- Age
  - Wide range; most patients < 40 years
- Gender
  - Slight female predominance
- Epidemiology
  - Rare

Natural History & Prognosis

- More aggressive than localized giant cell tumor of tendon sheath
  - Local recurrence in up to 50%
  - Atypical histologic features do not predict recurrence
  - Malignant variant, malignant transformation, and metastases have been rarely reported

Treatment

- Treated with wide surgical excision

SELECTED REFERENCES

1. van der Heijden L et al: Functional outcome and quality of life after the surgical treatment for diffuse-type giant-cell tumour around the knee: a retrospective analysis of 30 patients. Bone Joint J. 96-B(8):1111-8, 2014
2. Yun SJ et al: Intramuscular diffuse-type tenosynovial giant cell tumor of the deltoid muscle in a child. Skeletal Radiol. 43(8):1179-83, 2014
3. Sanghvi DA et al: Diffuse-type giant cell tumor of the subcutaneous thigh. Skeletal Radiol. 36(4):327-30, 2007

Deep Benign Fibrous Histiocytoma

KEY FACTS

TERMINOLOGY

- Rare, benign, fibrohistiocytic neoplasm located in subcutaneous tissue, deep soft tissue, or organs
- Benign fibrous histiocytoma is separated into cutaneous and deep subtypes
  - Cutaneous subtype referred to as benign fibrous histiocytoma or dermatofibroma
  - Lesions within or deep to subcutaneous region are considered deep

IMAGING

- Mass in subcutaneous tissue of extremities > head and neck > trunk > visceral soft tissue
  - Deeper lesions most often found in extremity or paraspinal muscles
  - Visceral organs may be affected
- Range: 0.5-25 cm (median: 3 cm)
- Similar attenuation to muscle on CT
- MR findings
  - Low to intermediate signal intensity on T1WI MR
  - Variable low to high signal intensity on fluid-sensitive MR sequences
  - ± heterogeneity
  - ± hemorrhage

PATHOLOGY

- Bland ovoid to spindle-shaped cells in prominent storiform pattern with hemangiopericytoma-like regions containing lymphocytes with mitoses < 5 per 10 HPF

CLINICAL ISSUES

- Painless, slowly growing mass
- Most common in young to middle-aged adult men
- High risk of local recurrence (22-60%)
- Occasional metastatic potential that is not predicted by histologic features
- Treatment is complete surgical excision

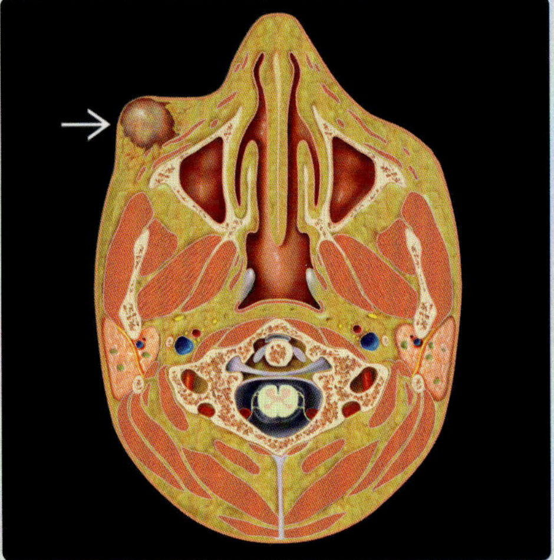

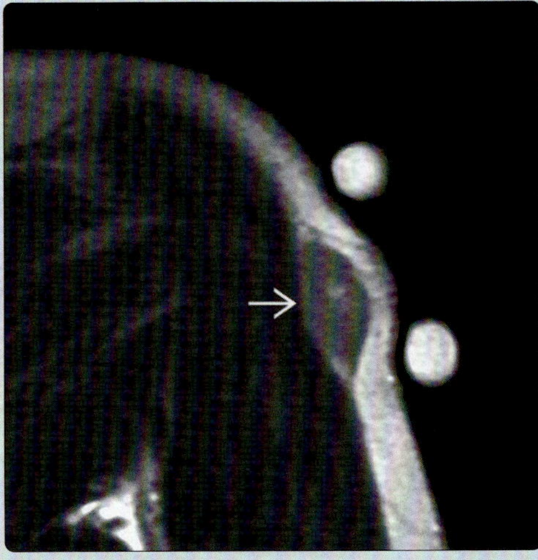

(Left) *Axial graphic shows a mass ➡ in the subcutaneous tissues of the face. The head and neck is the 2nd most common location of these lesions after the extremities.* **(Right)** *Coronal T2WI MR of the shoulder shows a deep benign fibrous histiocytoma ➡ in the subcutaneous tissues. The mass is heterogeneously hyperintense relative to skeletal muscle and has a nonspecific appearance. It is not possible to completely exclude malignant soft tissue tumors; biopsy is required.*

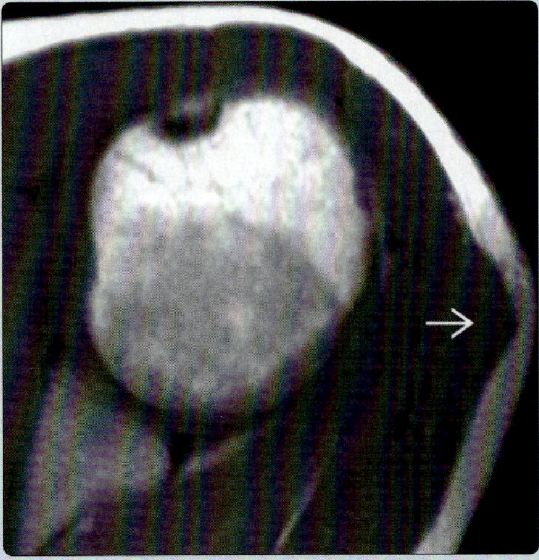

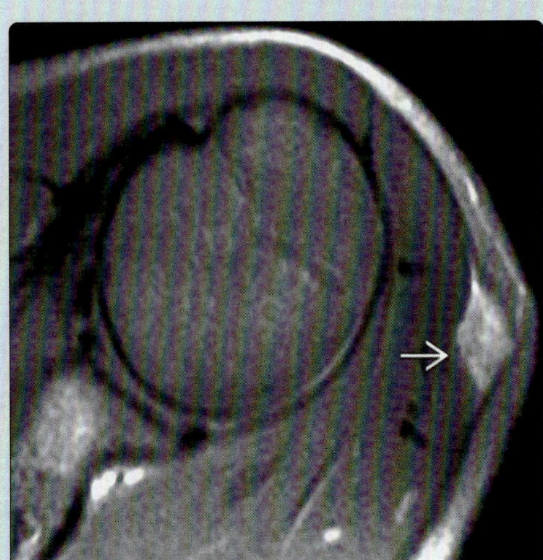

(Left) *Axial T1WI MR shows a mass ➡, isointense to muscle, which displaces the subcutaneous fat and cannot be completely delineated from the deltoid muscle.* **(Right)** *Axial T1WI C+ FS MR in the same patient shows the mass ➡ to have inhomogeneous enhancement. Benign fibrous lesions tend to have low signal on both T1WI and T2WI MR, which is not seen in this case. At least mild enhancement is typical. Note that although the lesion is subcutaneous, the location is considered deep for this diagnosis.*

TERMINOLOGY

Synonyms

- Fibroxanthoma, dermatofibroma, sclerosing hemangioma, dermal histiocytoma, histiocytoma cutis, and nodular subepidermal fibrosis

Definitions

- Rare, benign fibrohistiocytic neoplasm located in subcutaneous tissue, deep soft tissue, or organs
  - Cutaneous form referred to as benign fibrous histiocytoma or dermatofibroma

IMAGING

General Features

- Location
  - Subcutaneous tissue of extremities > head and neck > trunk > visceral soft tissue
    - Deeper lesions most often found in extremity or paraspinal muscles
      - Visceral organs may be affected
  - Cutaneous lesions most often found in limbs
- Size
  - Range: 0.5-25 cm (median: 3 cm)
    - More deeply located lesions tend to be larger than superficial lesions (> 5 cm)
  - Cutaneous lesions are usually < 1 cm
- Morphology
  - Subcutaneous and more deeply located lesions are well-circumscribed masses
  - Cutaneous lesions are less well-defined masses that may be multiple

CT Findings

- Similar attenuation to muscle

MR Findings

- Low to intermediate signal intensity on T1WI MR
- Variable low to high signal intensity on fluid-sensitive MR sequences
- ± heterogeneity
- ± hemorrhage

DIFFERENTIAL DIAGNOSIS

Solitary Fibrous Tumor and Hemangiopericytoma

- Histologically very similar due to hemangiopericytoma-like vascular pattern with hyalinized stroma
- Many lesions previously diagnosed as deep benign fibrous histiocytoma would now be classified as solitary fibrous tumors

Dermatofibrosarcoma Protuberans

- Young to middle-aged adults
- Trunk > proximal extremities
- Dermal-based, infiltrating subcutaneous tissues

Nodular Fasciitis

- Painful, rapidly growing mass in young to middle-aged adult
- Mass intimately associated with fascia
- Fibroblasts in loose bundles with myxoid regions and extravasated red blood cells

PATHOLOGY

Staging, Grading, & Classification

- Benign fibrous histiocytoma is separated into cutaneous and deep subtypes
  - Subcutaneous lesions are considered deep, along with those in deep soft tissues and visceral organs

Gross Pathologic & Surgical Features

- Well-circumscribed, yellow to white mass
  - ± hemorrhage
- Cutaneous lesions are red-brown papules or nodules

Microscopic Features

- Bland ovoid to spindle-shaped cells in prominent storiform pattern with hemangiopericytoma-like regions with lymphocytes
  - Similar to cutaneous fibrous histiocytoma cellular variant
  - Multinucleated giant cells, osteoclastic giant cells, foam cells in 59%
  - Myxoid or hyalinized stroma
  - Rare metaplastic ossification, necrosis, lymphovascular invasion

CLINICAL ISSUES

Presentation

- Most common signs/symptoms
  - Painless, slowly growing mass

Demographics

- Age
  - Found in children to elderly
    - Most common in young to middle-aged adults
- Gender
  - Male predominance
- Epidemiology
  - Subcutaneous and more deeply located lesions are rare (< 1% of fibrohistiocytic tumors)
  - Cutaneous benign fibrous histiocytoma is common skin mesenchymal neoplasm

Natural History & Prognosis

- Subcutaneous and more deeply located lesions have high risk of local recurrence (22-60%)
- Cutaneous lesions rarely recur
  - Some subtypes are more prone to recurrence
    - Atypical, aneurysmal, and cellular fibrous histiocytoma
- Occasional metastatic potential that is not predicted by histologic features

Treatment

- Complete surgical excision

SELECTED REFERENCES

1. Yamasaki F et al: Benign fibrous histiocytoma arising at the temporal bone of an infant-case report and review of the literature. Childs Nerv Syst. ePub, 2015
2. Doyle LA et al: Metastasizing "benign" cutaneous fibrous histiocytoma: a clinicopathologic analysis of 16 cases. Am J Surg Pathol. 37(4):484-95, 2013
3. Gleason BC et al: Deep "benign" fibrous histiocytoma: clinicopathologic analysis of 69 cases of a rare tumor indicating occasional metastatic potential. Am J Surg Pathol. 32(3):354-62, 2008

Undifferentiated Pleomorphic Sarcoma

KEY FACTS

TERMINOLOGY

- Term undifferentiated high-grade pleomorphic sarcoma is used synonymously with pleomorphic malignant fibrous histiocytoma

IMAGING

- Thigh > leg > > upper extremity > retroperitoneum > trunk
- 5% are extensively hemorrhagic, presenting as fluctuant mass often misdiagnosed as hematoma
- May erode or invade bone
- Calcification present peripherally in 5-20%
- Peripheral ossification can mimic myositis ossificans
- Similar signal intensity to muscle on T1WI MR
    - High SI on T1WI MR if hemorrhage
- Heterogeneously hyperintense to muscle on fluid-sensitive sequences
    - Fluid-fluid levels from hemorrhage
- Heterogeneously intense enhancement on CT & MR

PATHOLOGY

- Prior radiation exposure ↑ risk
- Possible association with metal devices and shrapnel

CLINICAL ISSUES

- Large, painless, growing mass
- > 40 yr old with peak in 6th-7th decades
- 50-70% 5-yr survival
- 19-31% local recurrence rate
- 5% with metastases at presentation
    - Metastatic disease involves lung in 90%
- Prognosis worse with ↑ tumor size, ↑ depth, high grade, and presence of necrosis

DIAGNOSTIC CHECKLIST

- Underlying malignancy must be excluded in every patient thought to have spontaneous musculoskeletal hemorrhage
    - Postcontrast MR differentiates tumor from hemorrhage in most cases

(Left) *Axial T1WI MR of the arm shows a mass ➡ with signal intensity similar to muscle and scattered foci of slightly higher signal intensity. The mass abutted but did not definitively invade the superficial fascia on any imaging sequence.* **(Right)** *Axial T2WI FS MR best shows the heterogeneity of the mass ➡ with predominately high signal and lobulated areas of varying intensity. Irregularity of the skin surface ➡ was secondary to prior attempted drainage of the lesion.*

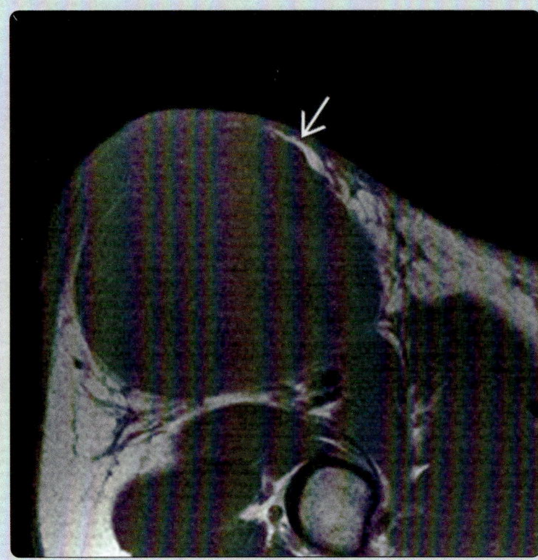

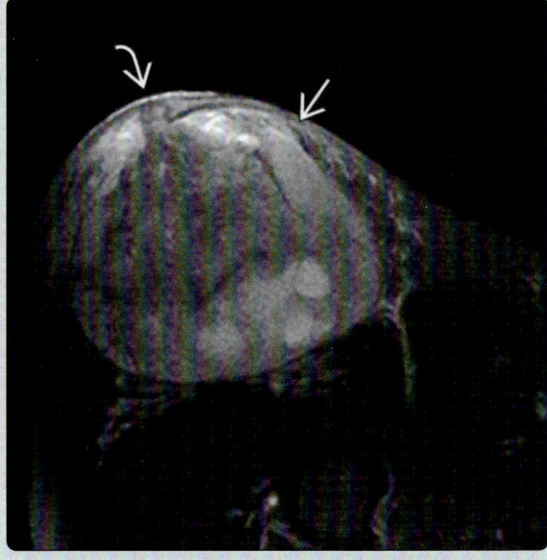

(Left) *Coronal STIR MR with the arm positioned over the head shows the very large mass ➡ to be centered in the axilla and measure over 10 cm in greatest dimension. The mass is markedly heterogeneous in signal intensity and has extensive septa.* **(Right)** *Axial T1WI C+ FS MR of the mass ➡ shows intense irregular peripheral enhancement and mild central enhancement. This rapidly growing axillary lesion was initially misdiagnosed as an abscess in this middle-aged man but proved to be pleomorphic sarcoma.*

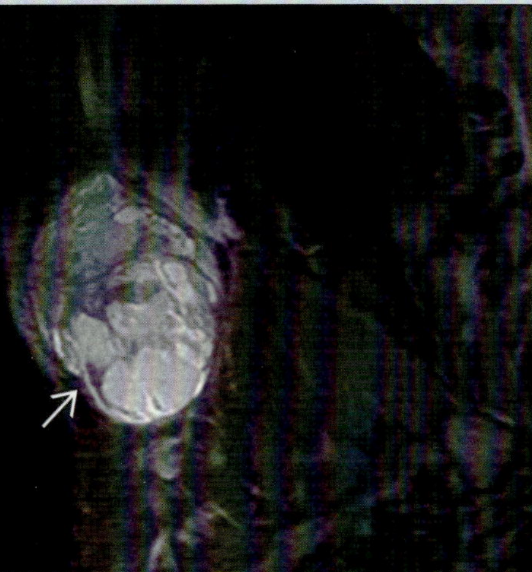

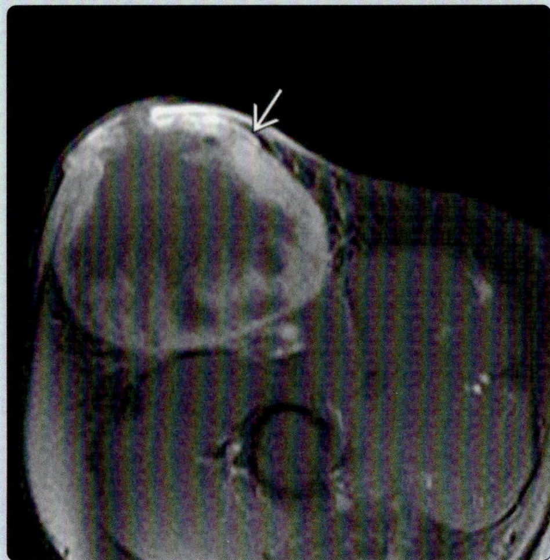

TERMINOLOGY

Synonyms

- Malignant fibrous histiocytoma (MFH), storiform or fibroblastic type; malignant fibrous xanthoma; atypical fibroxanthoma (when involving skin); fibroxanthosarcoma

Definitions

- Term undifferentiated high-grade pleomorphic sarcoma is used synonymously with pleomorphic malignant fibrous histiocytoma
  - Terminology updated by World Health Organization in 2002 due to lack of histiocytic differentiation
  - Formerly considered common, distinct sarcoma subtype but now is diagnosis of exclusion
  - Terminology usage varies by institution

IMAGING

General Features

- Location
  - Thigh > leg > > upper extremity > retroperitoneum > trunk
    - 90% in deep soft tissues
- Size
  - 5-15 cm; retroperitoneal lesions > 20 cm
- Morphology
  - Most appear as solid, lobulated mass
  - 5% are extensively hemorrhagic, presenting as fluctuant mass often misdiagnosed as hematoma

Radiographic Findings

- Nonspecific soft tissue mass
- May erode or invade bone
- Calcification present peripherally in 5-20%
  - Peripheral ossification can mimic myositis ossificans

CT Findings

- Heterogeneously enhancing mass with attenuation similar to muscle
  - Hemorrhage or necrosis common

MR Findings

- Similar signal intensity to muscle on T1WI
- Heterogeneously hyperintense to muscle on fluid-sensitive sequences
  - Fluid-fluid levels from hemorrhage
- Heterogeneously intense enhancement

Ultrasonographic Findings

- Heterogeneous intermediate- to low-echogenicity mass due to varied tumor contents
  - Hypervascular to hypovascular on Doppler

Nuclear Medicine Findings

- PET/CT
  - Lesions are glucose avid

DIFFERENTIAL DIAGNOSIS

Sarcoma, Unspecified Soft Tissue

- Imaging appearance has considerable overlap between different types of sarcomas
- Tissue diagnosis necessary

PATHOLOGY

General Features

- Etiology
  - Prior radiation exposure ↑ risk
    - May worsen prognosis
  - Possible association with metal devices and shrapnel
- Genetics
  - Genomic imbalances, complex karyotypes
    - Amplified protooncogenes at 12q13-15

Gross Pathologic & Surgical Features

- Pseudoencapsulated pale fleshy mass
  - ± hemorrhage, necrosis, myxoid change

Microscopic Features

- Broad range of appearances of these poorly differentiated tumors with few cells demonstrating specific lineage
  - Pleomorphic cells and nuclei
  - Storiform pattern around vessels
  - Chronic inflammatory cells, giant cells, hemorrhage, fibrous stroma, necrosis

CLINICAL ISSUES

Presentation

- Most common signs/symptoms
  - Large, painless, growing mass
  - More likely to be painful if rapidly enlarging
- Other signs/symptoms
  - Fever and leukocytosis are rare
  - Hypoglycemia is rare
  - Retroperitoneal lesions → weight loss, malaise

Demographics

- Age
  - > 40 yr old with peak in 6th-7th decades
    - Rare in children and young adults
- Gender
  - Male predominance
- Epidemiology
  - 1-2 cases per 100,000 population annually

Natural History & Prognosis

- 50-70% 5-yr survival
- 19-31% local recurrence rate
- 5% with metastases at presentation
  - Metastatic disease involves lung in 90%
- Prognosis worse with ↑ tumor size, ↑ depth, high grade, and presence of necrosis

Treatment

- Wide surgical excision
  - Adjuvant chemotherapy and radiotherapy based on clinical presentation

SELECTED REFERENCES

1. Delisca GO et al: MFH and high-grade undifferentiated pleomorphic sarcoma-what's in a name? J Surg Oncol. 111(2):173-7, 2015

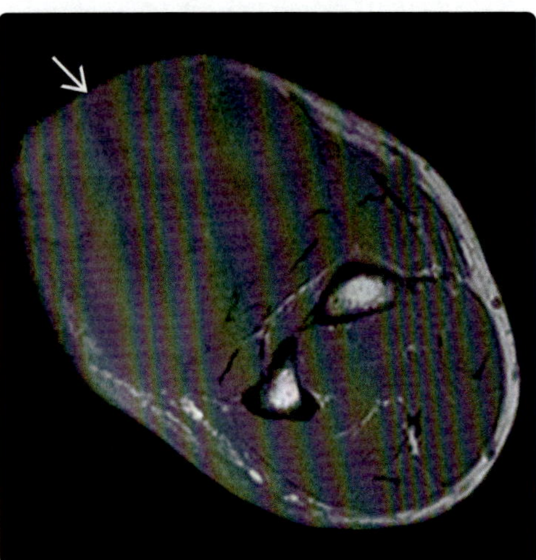

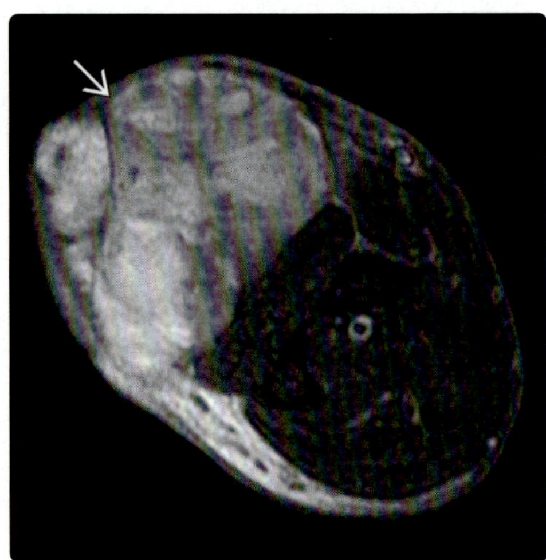

(Left) *Axial T1WI MR shows a large soft tissue mass ➡ in the proximal, dorsal aspect of the forearm. The mass has heterogeneous signal intensity, with regions isointense to muscle and regions hyperintense to muscle, possibly representing hemorrhage.* **(Right)** *Axial STIR MR shows the mass ➡ to be heterogeneously hyperintense with lobulated borders. Note that the signal intensity is not as high as would be expected for fluid. The mass abuts and displaces the forearm musculature, without convincing invasion.*

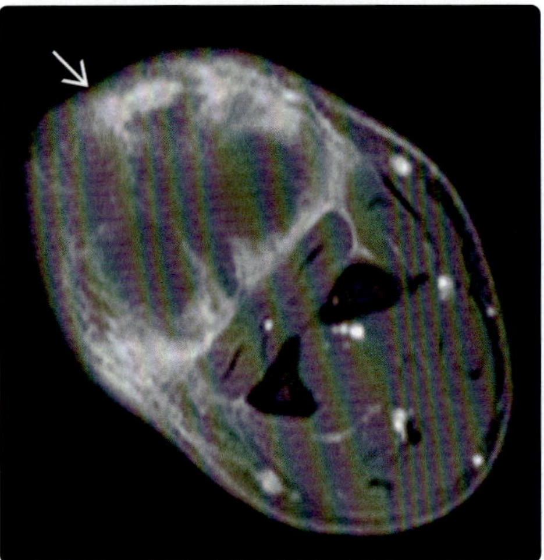

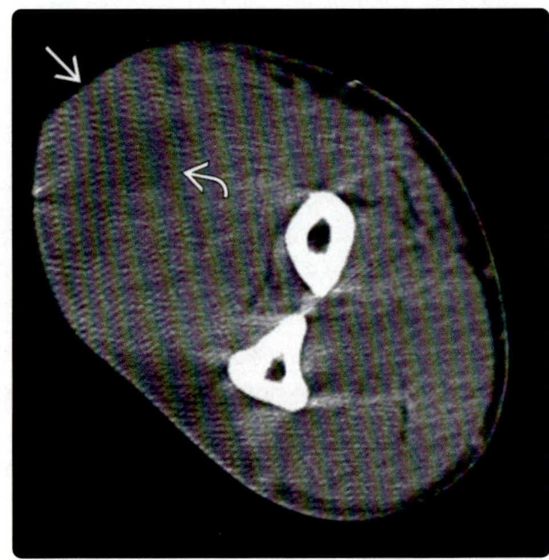

(Left) *Axial T1WI C+ FS MR shows a large soft tissue mass ➡ to have irregular, peripheral nodular enhancement. The central portion of the mass is relatively hypoenhancing although it is not clearly cystic or hemorrhagic on the T1- and T2-weighted sequences.* **(Right)** *Axial CECT shows the majority of the mass ➡ to be isointense to muscle with a central region of irregular hypoenhancement ↩. The lesion is centered in the subcutaneous space, which is less common than arising in the deep soft tissues.*

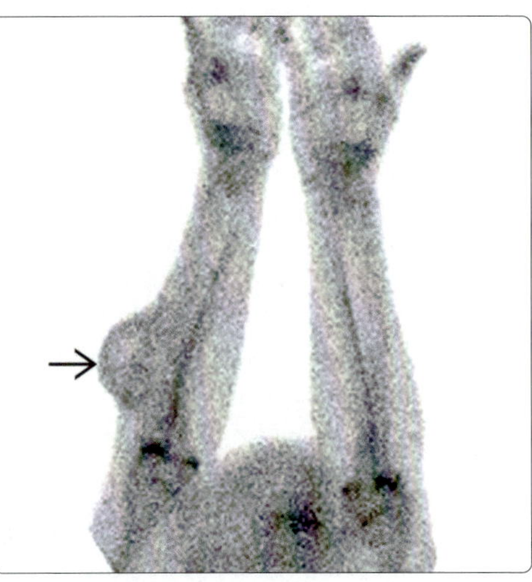

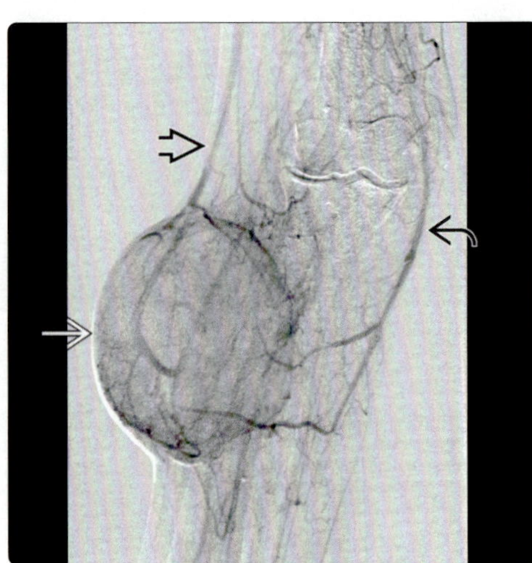

(Left) *AP bone scan in the same patient shows increased radiotracer uptake in the forearm mass ➡ consistent with a soft tissue neoplasm. There was no evidence of abnormal uptake in the underlying bones or in the remainder of the skeleton.* **(Right)** *AP angiography in the venous phase demonstrates the forearm mass ➡ to be hypervascular. The tumor is supplied by branches from the radial and common interosseous arteries. Blood flow from the tumor drains into both the cephalic ⇨ and basilic ↩ veins.*

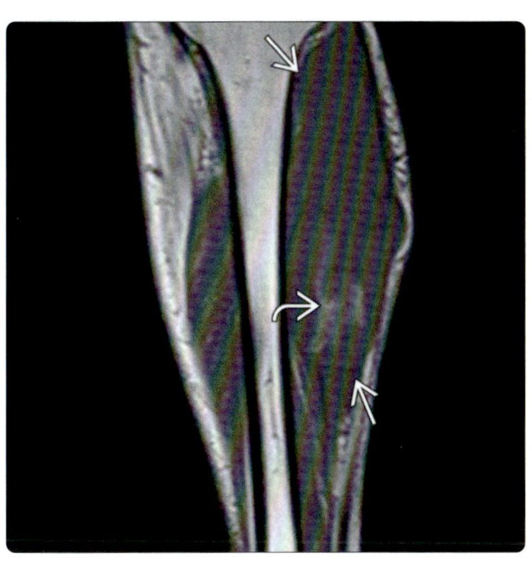

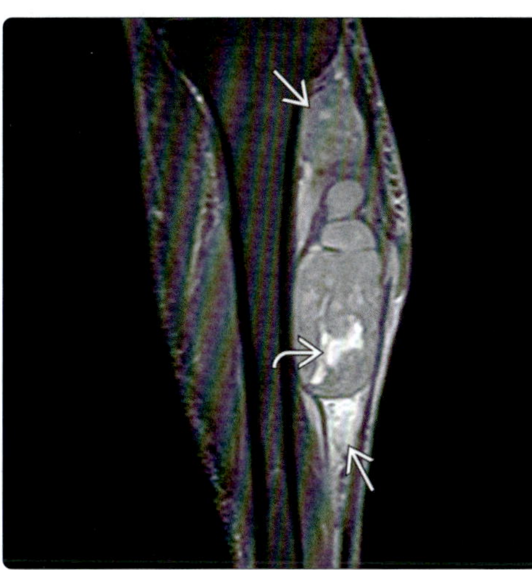

(Left) *Coronal T1WI MR, obtained in an elderly woman who noted a mass 4 days following a fall where she fractured the ipsilateral, shows the mass ➔ to be isointense to skeletal muscle, but to contain a substantial amount of high-signal material ➔. It is important to work-up this mass for tumor, despite clinical history pointing toward hemorrhage from trauma.* **(Right)** *On coronal STIR MR, the mass ➔ is heterogeneously hyperintense with differentially high SI in region that was high signal on T1 ➔.*

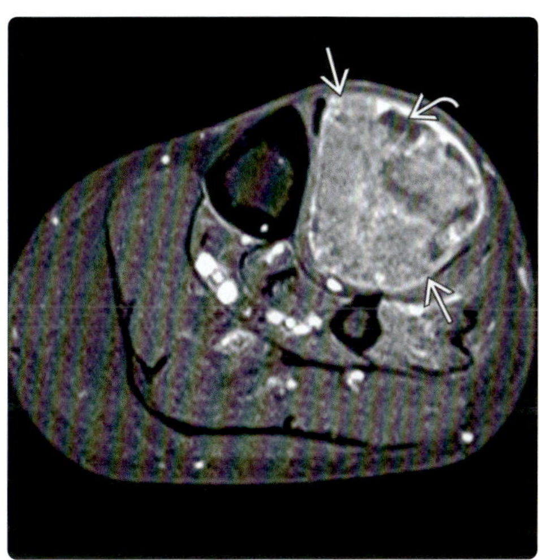

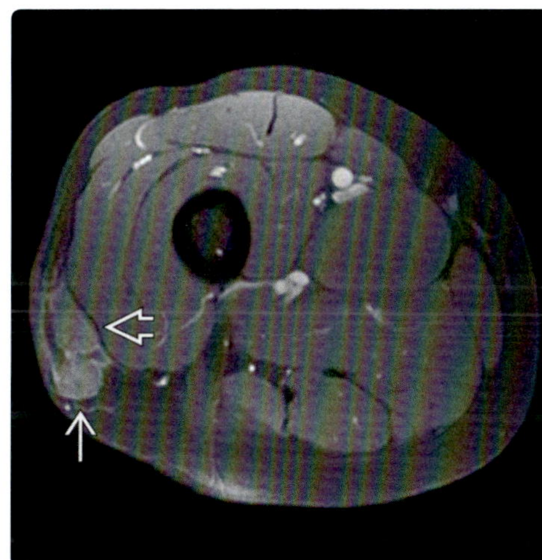

(Left) *Axial T1 C+ FS MR in the same case shows the lesion ➔ to enhance, with foci of low signal ➔ representing necrosis. Despite the history of trauma, the lesion proved to be undifferentiated pleomorphic sarcoma.* **(Right)** *Axial T1WI C+ FS MR shows a mass ➔ that heterogeneously enhances. The mass abuts the superficial fascia ➔. Undifferentiated pleomorphic sarcomas have a nonspecific MR imaging appearance due to variable amounts of fibrous tissue, myxoid tissue, calcification, hemorrhage, and necrosis.*

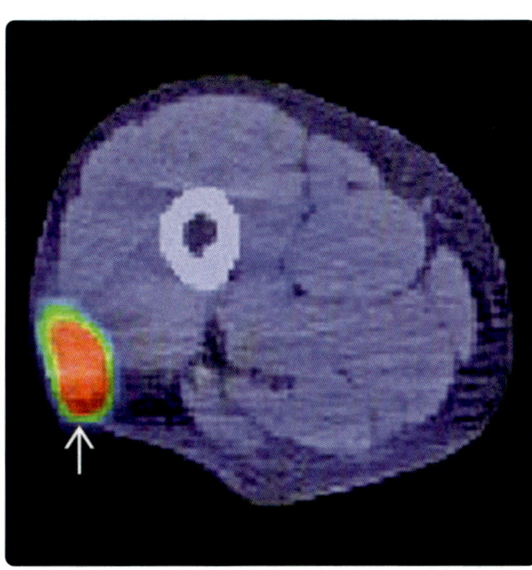

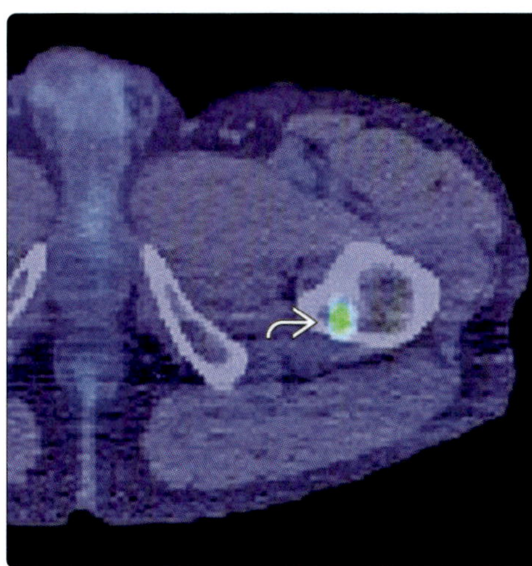

(Left) *Axial PET/CT in the same patient shows intense uptake of F-18 FDG by the mass ➔.* **(Right)** *Axial PET/CT in the same patient also shows metastases to the lung, rib, and contralateral lesser trochanter ➔ from the primary lesion in the opposite thigh, which measured ~ 5 cm in greatest dimension. There were no lymph node metastases. The tumors have heterogeneous signal and enhancement on MR imaging and are glucose avid on PET.*

Undifferentiated Pleomorphic Sarcoma With Prominent Inflammation

KEY FACTS

TERMINOLOGY

- Malignant sarcoma composed of malignant and benign xanthomatous cells, atypical spindle cells, and both acute and chronic inflammatory cells
  - Most rare type of undifferentiated pleomorphic sarcoma

IMAGING

- Retroperitoneum > > intraabdominal > extremity deep soft tissues
  - Large at time of diagnosis
- Very rare tumor without specific imaging findings beyond solid, soft tissue mass
- Heterogeneously isointense to muscle on T1WI MR
- Heterogeneously hyperintense to muscle on fluid-sensitive MR sequences
- Heterogeneous enhancement
- Internal vascularity visible on Doppler examination
- High-uptake value of lesion on PET

PATHOLOGY

- Originally thought to be variant of malignant fibrous histiocytoma
  - May actually be dedifferentiated liposarcoma
- Yellow mass due to xanthoma cells on gross exam
- Few atypical large cells with hyperchromatic, irregular nucleoli in background of benign xanthoma cells
  - Rare hemorrhage or necrosis

CLINICAL ISSUES

- > 40 yr old without sex predilection
- Signs and symptoms suggesting infection caused by cytokine production
  - Fever, leukocytosis, eosinophilia, leukemoid reaction, weight loss
- Poor prognosis
  - ~ 1/2 with recurrent or persistent disease causing death
  - ~ 33% with metastatic disease

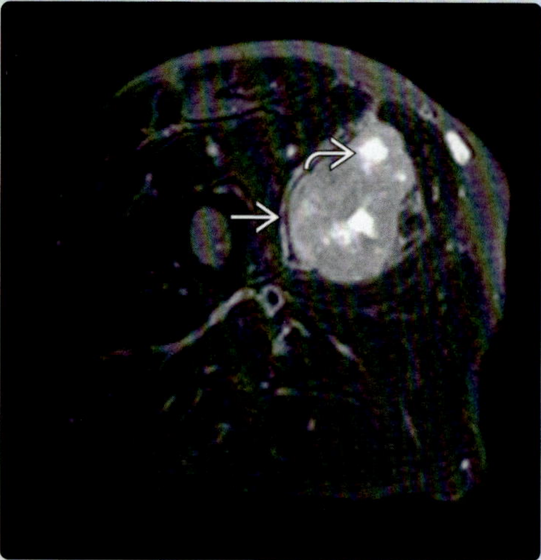

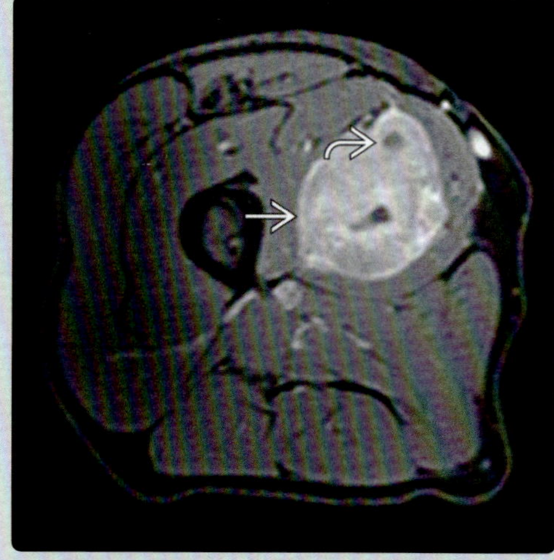

(Left) *Axial T2WI FS MR reveals an oval mass ➔ in the proximal thigh that is hyperintense to muscle with central foci of fluid-intensity signal ➔. The extent of the mass is well defined since it does not blend in with the muscles it abuts.* **(Right)** *Axial T1WI C+ FS MR shows the mass ➔ in the proximal thigh to have heterogeneous enhancement, with lack of enhancement in the previously described foci that are suggestive of cystic change or necrosis ➔.*

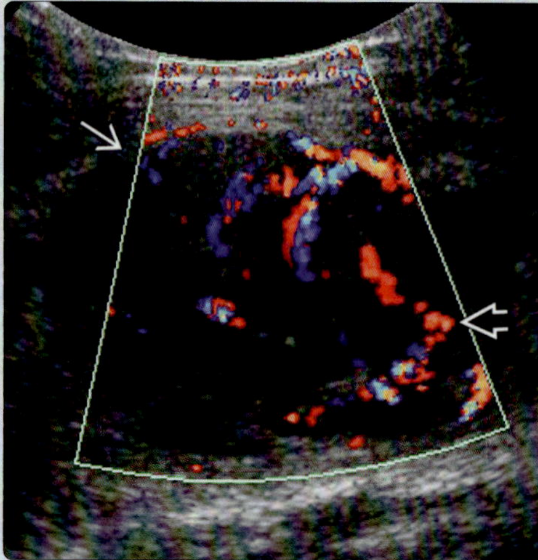

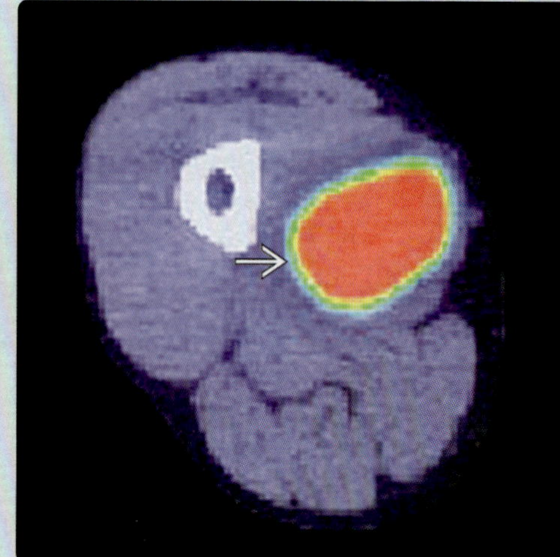

(Left) *Longitudinal Doppler ultrasound shows the predominantly hypoechoic mass ➔ to have prominent vascularity ➔.* **(Right)** *Axial fused PET/CT shows the mass ➔ to have intense radiotracer uptake. The mass abuts and may invade the vastus medialis, sartorius, and adductor musculature. The size of the lesion plus the location deep to the superficial fascia makes this a T2b lesion on TNM staging. No nodal or distant metastases were present, giving the tumor an overall stage III (T2b N0 M0).*

TERMINOLOGY

Synonyms

- Xanthomatous malignant fibrous histiocytoma, malignant xanthogranuloma, malignant fibrous xanthoma, xanthosarcoma, retroperitoneal xanthogranuloma

Definitions

- Very rare malignant sarcoma composed of malignant and benign xanthomatous cells, atypical spindle cells, and both acute and chronic inflammatory cells

IMAGING

General Features

- Location
  - Retroperitoneum > > intraabdominal > extremity deep soft tissues
- Size
  - Large at time of diagnosis

Imaging Recommendations

- Best imaging tool
  - MR best evaluates extent of soft tissue mass involvement
  - Very rare tumor without specific imaging findings beyond solid, soft tissue mass

Radiographic Findings

- Normal or soft tissue swelling

MR Findings

- Heterogeneously isointense to muscle on T1WI
- Heterogeneously hyperintense to muscle on fluid-sensitive sequences
- Heterogeneous enhancement

Ultrasonographic Findings

- Internal vascularity visible on Doppler examination

Nuclear Medicine Findings

- PET/CT
  - High uptake value in lesion

DIFFERENTIAL DIAGNOSIS

Pleomorphic MFH/Undifferentiated Pleomorphic Sarcoma

- Same imaging appearance and patient demographics
- Differentiated by pathologic criteria

Liposarcoma, Dedifferentiated

- Contains region of atypical lipomatous tumor/well-differentiated liposarcoma
- Does not produce systemic symptoms
- Theorized to represent variant of same entity

PATHOLOGY

General Features

- Etiology
  - Unknown: Single case reported post radiation
- Genetics
  - Helpful to exclude other etiologies

Staging, Grading, & Classification

- Originally thought to be variant of malignant fibrous histiocytoma/pleomorphic sarcoma
  - May actually be dedifferentiated liposarcoma

Gross Pathologic & Surgical Features

- Yellow mass due to xanthoma cells
  - Rare hemorrhage or necrosis

Microscopic Features

- Few atypical large cells with hyperchromatic, irregular nucleoli in background of benign xanthoma cells
  - Atypical cells phagocytize neutrophils
  - Prominent component of inflammatory cells
    - Neutrophils, eosinophils comprise majority
    - Few plasma cells and lymphocytes
- Mixed areas of typical pleomorphic sarcoma
- Positive MDM2, CDK4, and vimentin
  - Negative CD15, CD20, CD30, CD43, and CD45

CLINICAL ISSUES

Presentation

- Most common signs/symptoms
  - Signs and symptoms suggesting infection caused by cytokine production
    - Fever, leukocytosis, eosinophilia, leukemoid reaction, weight loss

Demographics

- Age
  - > 40 yr old
- Gender
  - No gender predilection
- Epidemiology
  - Most rare type of undifferentiated pleomorphic sarcoma

Natural History & Prognosis

- Poor prognosis
  - ~ 1/2 with recurrent or persistent disease causing death
  - ~ 33% with metastatic disease

Treatment

- Surgical resection, if possible

SELECTED REFERENCES

1. Weiss SW et al: Malignant fibrous histiocytoma (Pleomorphic undifferentiated sarcoma). In Weiss SW et al: Enzinger and Weiss' Soft Tissue Tumors. 5th ed. Philadelphia: Elsevier. 422-5, 2008
2. Kransdorf MJ et al: Malignant fibrous and fibrohistiocytic tumors. In Kransdorf MJ et al: Imaging of Soft Tissue Tumors. 2nd ed. Philadelphia: Lippincott Williams & Wilkins. 279, 2006
3. Hallor KH et al: Two genetic pathways, t(1;10) and amplification of 3p11-12, in myxoinflammatory fibroblastic sarcoma, haemosiderotic fibrolipomatous tumour, and morphologically similar lesions. J Pathol. 217(5):716-27, 2009
4. Coindre JM et al: Inflammatory malignant fibrous histiocytomas and dedifferentiated liposarcomas: histological review, genomic profile, and MDM2 and CDK4 status favour a single entity. J Pathol. 203(3):822-30, 2004
5. Coindre JM: Inflammatory malignant fibrous histiocytoma/Undifferentiated pleomorphic sarcoma with prominent inflammation. In Fletcher CDM et al: World Health Organization Classification of Tumours. Pathology and Genetics of Tumours of Soft Tissue and Bone. Lyon: IARC Press. 125-6, 2002

Dermatofibrosarcoma Protuberans

KEY FACTS

TERMINOLOGY

- Low-grade sarcoma of dermis and subcutis

IMAGING

- 50% involve chest, back, and abdominal wall
  - Proximal extremities in 35-40%
  - Head and neck, especially scalp, also common
- Nonspecific, superficial soft tissue mass on radiographs, without mineralization
- Exophytic, nodular mass involving skin and subcutis with similar attenuation to muscle on CT
- Isointense to hyperintense to muscle on T1WI MR
- Hyperintense to muscle on fluid-sensitive MR
  - ± satellite nodules
  - ± skin surface involved beyond nodular mass
  - Heterogeneity more common in larger lesions
- Moderate enhancement
- Mildly to moderately hypervascular

PATHOLOGY

- Indurated plaque or nodule involving subcutis and dermis with firm, gray-white cut surface
  - Some cases do not involve overlying skin
  - Lacks muscle involvement, unless recurrent/large
- Necrosis and hemorrhage rare

CLINICAL ISSUES

- 6% of soft tissue sarcomas
  - Young to middle-aged adults
  - Male predominance
- Slowly growing and evolving cutaneous mass
  - Ulceration and satellite nodules in advanced lesions
- Wide surgical excision with at least 3-cm margins
  - Local recurrence in 18-55% depending on completeness of initial excision
- May develop fibrosarcomatous transformation
- Metastatic disease in 3-6%, usually pulmonary

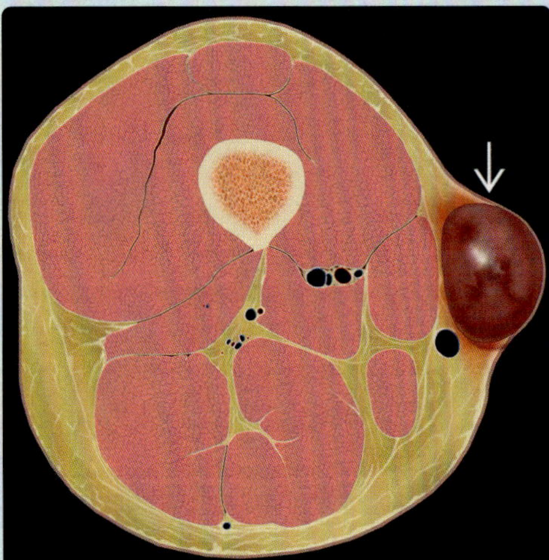

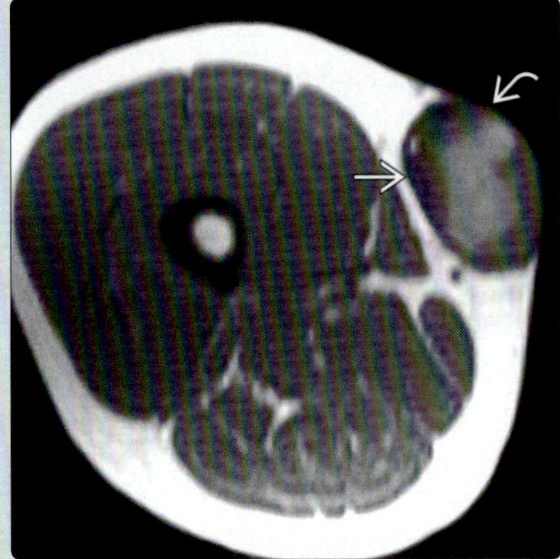

(Left) *Axial graphic demonstrates a protuberant mass ➡ centered in the subcutaneous tissues and involving the skin. Involvement of the proximal extremities is the 2nd most common location behind the trunk.* **(Right)** *Axial T1WI MR shows a superficial mass ➡ located entirely within the soft tissues and abutting the skin. Low-signal peripheral tissue ➡ surrounds a central portion, which is slightly higher signal intensity than muscle.*

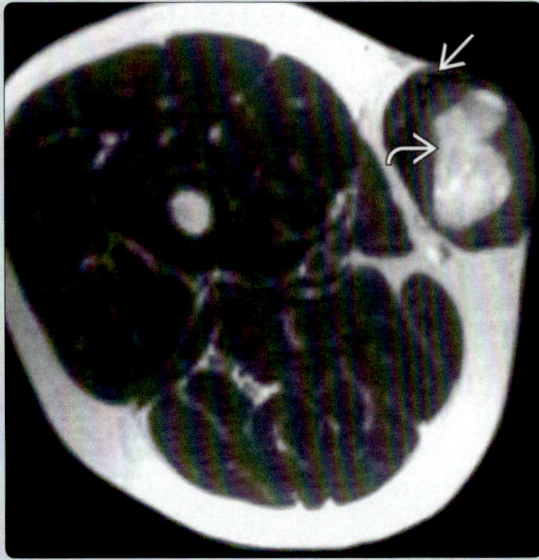

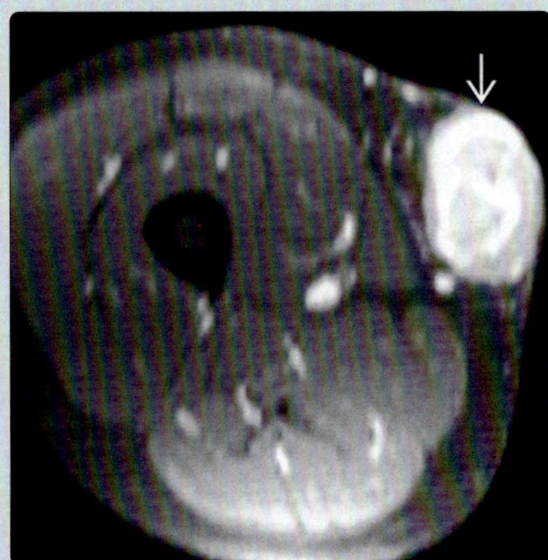

(Left) *Axial T2WI MR in the same patient shows the peripheral portion of the mass to have low signal ➡ and the heterogeneous central portion to have high signal ➡.* **(Right)** *Axial T1WI C+ FS MR shows the superficial mass ➡ in the thigh to have prominent, inhomogeneous enhancement of much of the peripheral portion, as well as the entire central portion. The location and appearance is typical for dermatofibrosarcoma protuberans.*

TERMINOLOGY

Abbreviations

- Dermatofibrosarcoma protuberans (DFSP)

Synonyms

- Progressive and recurring dermatofibroma

Definitions

- Low-grade mesenchymal sarcoma of dermis and subcutis

IMAGING

General Features

- Location
  - 50% involve chest, back, and abdominal wall
    - Proximal extremities in 35-40%
    - Head and neck, especially scalp, also common
- Size
  - Averages 5 cm at time of excision

CT Findings

- Exophytic, nodular mass involving skin and subcutaneous fat with similar attenuation to muscle

MR Findings

- Isointense to hyperintense relative to muscle on T1WI
- Hyperintense relative to muscle on fluid-sensitive sequences
- Moderate enhancement
- Heterogeneity more common in larger lesions
- ± satellite nodules
- ± skin surface involvement beyond nodular mass

Angiographic Findings

- Mildly to moderately hypervascular

DIFFERENTIAL DIAGNOSIS

Fibrohistiocytic Neoplasm, Unspecified

- Can be histologically challenging to differentiate from other fibrohistiocytic neoplasms

Deep Benign Fibrous Histiocytoma

- More likely to involve extremities
- Has similar histologic appearance to superficial portions of DFSP
- Less CD34 immunoreactivity than DFSP

Giant Cell Fibroblastoma

- Usually found before 4 years of age
- Histologically similar to DFSP
- Same chromosomal anomalies as DFSP

PATHOLOGY

General Features

- Etiology
  - Suggested association with prior trauma, surgical scars, vaccination sites, acanthosis nigricans, acrodermatitis, arsenism, and burns
- Genetics
  - Typical t(17;22) (q22;q13) translocation
  - May have ring chromosomes (↑ in adult cases)

Gross Pathologic & Surgical Features

- Indurated plaque or nodule involving subcutis and dermis with firm, gray-white cut surface
  - Some cases do not involve overlying skin
  - Lacks muscle involvement, unless recurrent or large
  - ± ulceration of skin, central gelatinous change

Microscopic Features

- Histopathology varies by location within lesion
  - Central regions contain spindle-shaped cells in storiform pattern with myxoid change
  - Peripheral regions are hypocellular with dermal collagen separating spindle cells
  - Deep regions contain spindle cells expanding fibrous septa and interdigitating with fat
- Myxoid change not uncommon
- Necrosis and hemorrhage rare
- Diffuse, strongly positive CD34 reactivity
- Negative S100 protein

CLINICAL ISSUES

Presentation

- Most common signs/symptoms
  - Slowly growing and evolving cutaneous mass
    - Plaque-like indurated region progressing to single or multiple protuberant nodules
      - May originate as small nodule
    - Surrounding red to blue skin discoloration
    - Ulceration and satellite nodules in advanced lesions
- Other signs/symptoms
  - Pain and bleeding with large lesions

Demographics

- Age
  - Young to middle-aged adults
    - Peak in 3rd to 5th decades of life
    - Some lesions may arise during childhood
- Gender
  - Male predominance
- Epidemiology
  - 6% of soft tissue sarcomas

Natural History & Prognosis

- Local recurrence in 18-55% depending on completeness of initial excision
  - Usually seen < 3 years after resection
    - Head and neck lesions more likely to recur
- May develop fibrosarcomatous transformation
- Metastatic disease in 3-6%
  - Metastases involve lungs in 75%

Treatment

- Wide surgical excision, with at least 3-cm margins

SELECTED REFERENCES

1. Basu S et al: Aggressive clinical course of dermatofibrosarcoma protuberans: 18F-FDG PET-CT predictive of tumor biology. J Nucl Med Technol. ePub, 2015
2. Kuzel P et al: A clinicopathologic review of a case series of dermatofibrosarcoma protuberans with fibrosarcomatous differentiation. J Cutan Med Surg. 19(1):28-34, 2015

(Left) *Coronal T1WI MR shows a large, superficial soft tissue mass ➡ involving the superior soft tissues of the shoulder. The mass has uniformly low signal, similar to muscle. Note the exceptionally large size of this mass, which had been growing for many years.* **(Right)** *Coronal STIR MR in the same patient shows the mass ➡ to have a medial region of higher signal ⇨, while much of the lesion remains inhomogeneously low signal.*

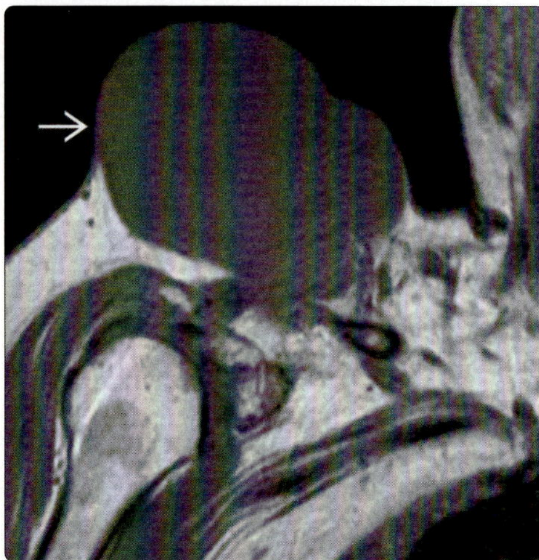

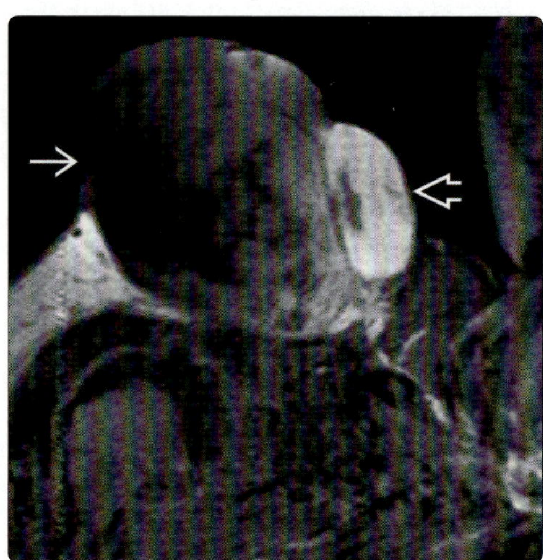

(Left) *Sagittal T2WI MR in the same patient shows the mass ➡ to be inhomogeneous, with areas of slightly higher signal intensity than muscle, but no regions of distinctly high signal. The mass extends near, but does not appear to invade, the underlying musculature.* **(Right)** *Sagittal T1WI C+ FS MR in the same patient shows the majority of the lesion ➡ to have mild diffuse enhancement, while there is a central ↩ nonenhancing portion as well.*

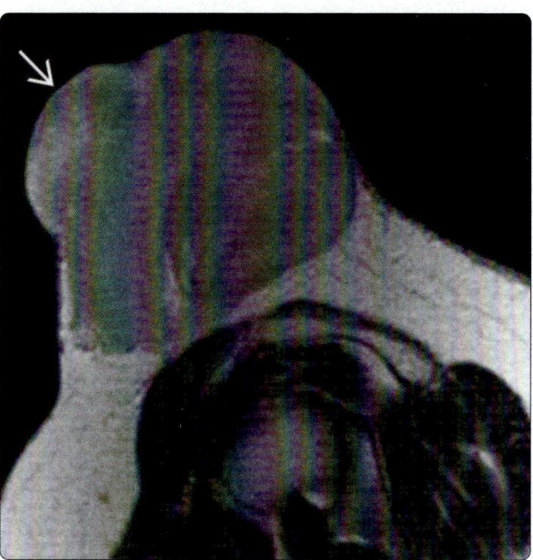

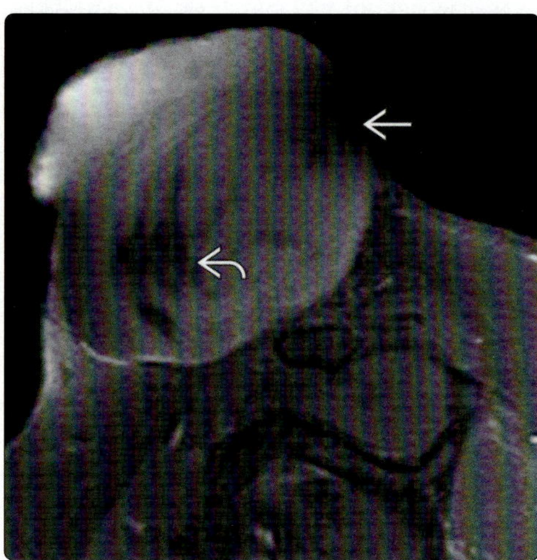

(Left) *Axial T1WI MR shows an unusual case of dermatofibrosarcoma protuberans. This lesion ↘ is in a deeper location than is usually seen. These lesions typically involve the skin, but may be confined to the subcutaneous tissues. This lobulated lesion has a signal intensity similar to that of skeletal muscle.* **(Right)** *Axial T1WI C+ FS MR in the same patient shows inhomogeneous enhancement of the lobulated lesion ↘. There is no invasion of the underlying muscle.*

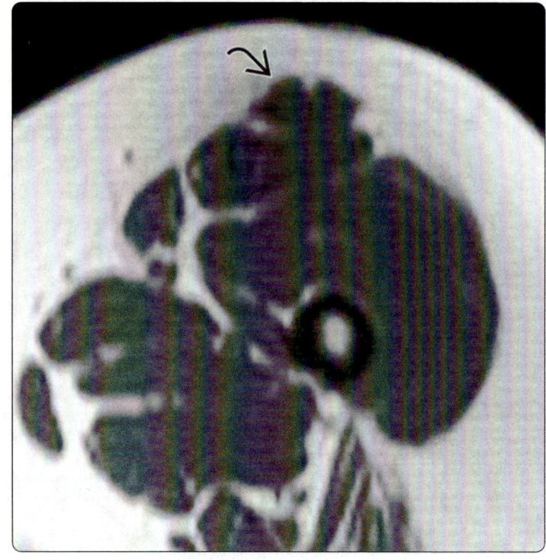

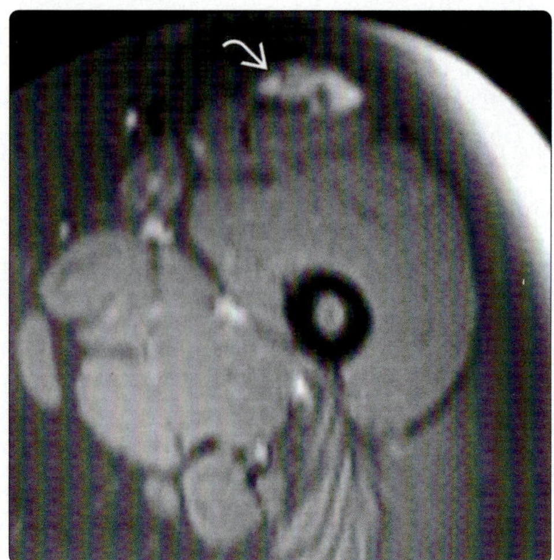

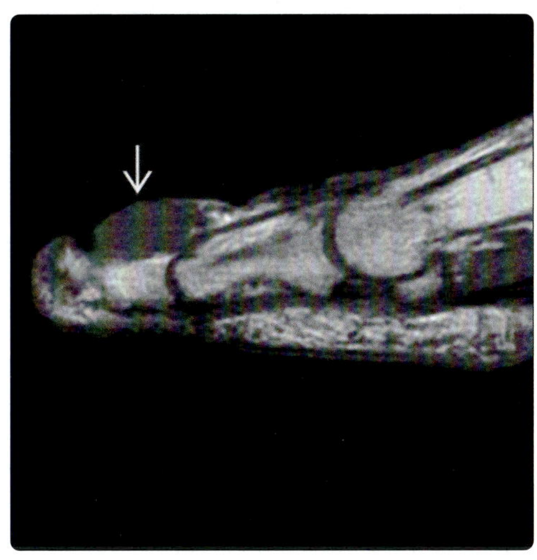

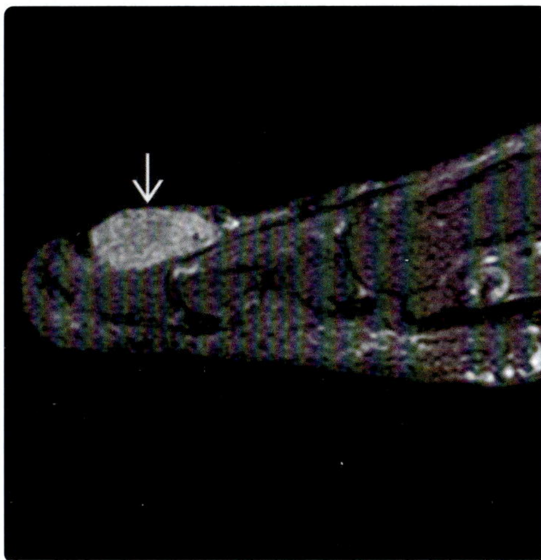

(Left) *Sagittal T1WI MR of the great toe shows a well-defined ovoid mass ➡ in the subcutaneous tissues that extend from the distal aspect of the proximal phalanx to the region of the nailbed. This mass is homogeneously isointense to muscle.* **(Right)** *Sagittal STIR MR shows the dorsal toe mass ➡ to have mildly inhomogeneous, hyperintense signal relative to muscle. There is no erosion of the underlying bone. The location in a distal extremity is unusual.*

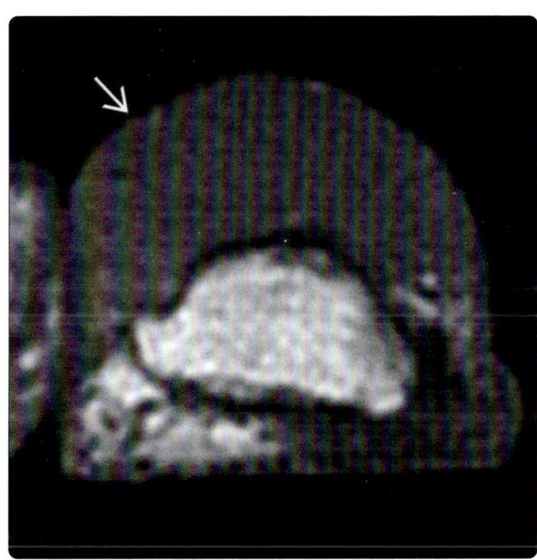

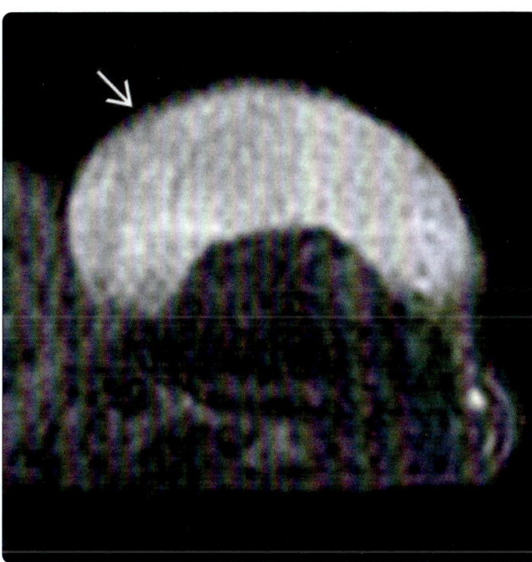

(Left) *Coronal T1WI MR in the same patient shows the great toe mass ➡ to have homogeneous signal that is isointense to muscle.* **(Right)** *Coronal T2WI FS MR shows mildly inhomogeneous hyperintense signal of the mass ➡. Coronal images at this level have an appearance somewhat similar to a very large glomus tumor. However, there is no erosion of the underlying bone, as would often be seen with a glomus tumor.*

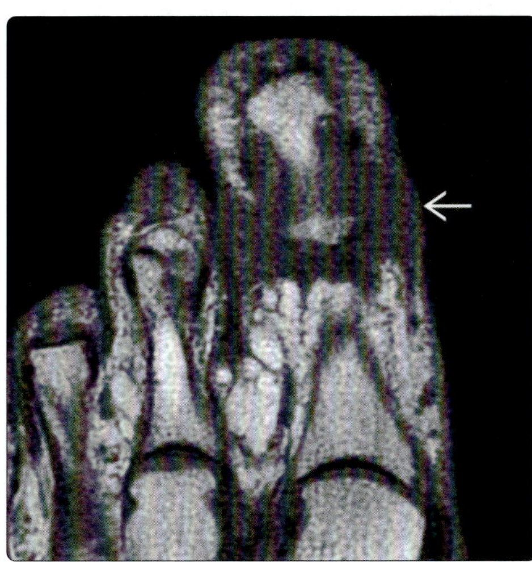

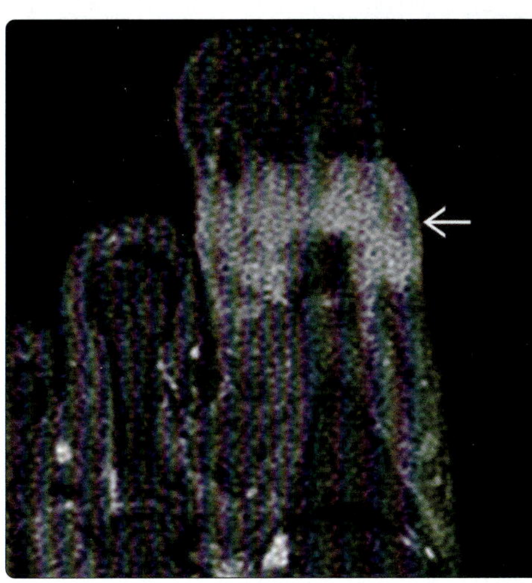

(Left) *Axial T1WI MR in the same patient shows the intermediate signal intensity mass ➡ to have lobulated borders and extend across the entire width of the toe.* **(Right)** *Axial T2WI FS MR shows the DFSP ➡ to have mildly heterogeneous hyperintense signal. This case is unusual not only in location, but also in patient demographics. These patients are usually 30- to 50-year-old men, but this case occurred in an elderly woman.*

Angioleiomyoma

KEY FACTS

TERMINOLOGY

- Benign, often painful, smooth muscle neoplasm preferentially occurring in superficial soft tissues

IMAGING

- Lower leg > thigh > upper extremity
  - Head and trunk in < 10%
- SQ fat > deep dermis > superficial fascia > > muscle
- Size: Usually < 2 cm in diameter
- Often excised without imaging
- Radiographs normal or show mild soft tissue swelling or bone scalloping
- MR findings
  - Homogeneous or heterogeneously isointense to mildly hyperintense to muscle on T1WI
  - Heterogeneously hyperintense to muscle on fluid-sensitive sequences
  - Variable enhancement, homogeneously intense to mild peripheral, likely dependent on subtype
  - Well-defined mass with similar attenuation to muscle
    - Low-signal fibrous pseudocapsule surrounds lesion on T1WI and T2WI sequences
    - ± adjacent vessels or internal branching structures
    - Small internal foci of fat and hemorrhage reported

PATHOLOGY

- Solitary, pseudoencapsulated, gray-white mass
- Proliferation of mature smooth muscle cells and thin- to thick-walled vascular channels

CLINICAL ISSUES

- Clinical symptoms
  - Superficial mass that slowly grows over several years
  - Lesions are painful or tender in most cases
- Age: Arises in 4th-6th decades of life
- Gender: Female predominance
- Natural history: Benign lesion that rarely recurs
- Treatment: Marginal excision; recurrence rare

(Left) *Axial graphic through the knee depicts an angioleiomyoma as an ovoid gray-white mass ➡ in the superficial soft tissues of the knee.* **(Right)** *Sagittal T1WI MR shows a mass ➡, which was clinically palpable, located at the medial aspect of the right heel, corresponding to a bilobed lesion with mildly infiltrative borders that is homogeneously isointense to muscle. This lesion abuts the skin but otherwise lies within the subcutaneous fat.*

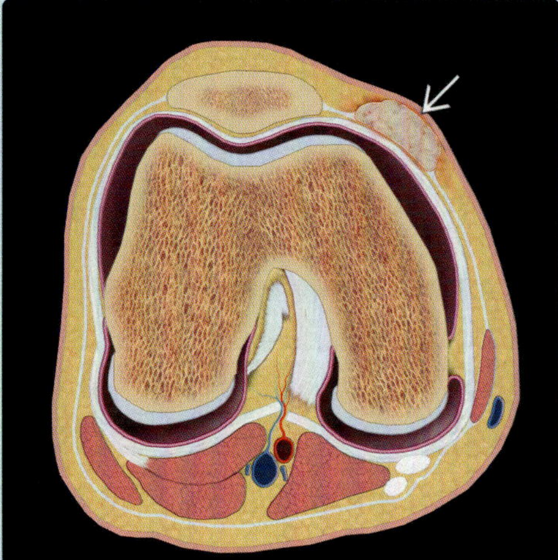

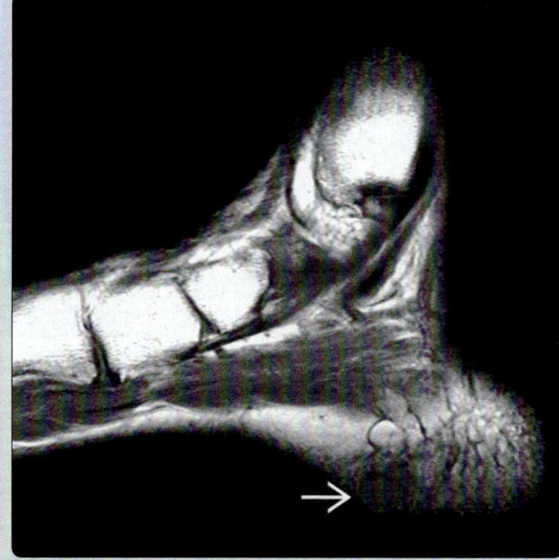

(Left) *Sagittal STIR MR in the same patient shows the mass ➡ to have heterogeneously isointense to hyperintense signal on this fluid-sensitive sequence.* **(Right)** *Coronal T1WI C+ FS MR shows the mass ➡ to have mild, heterogeneous internal enhancement. The overall appearance is nonspecific, and other entities, such as foreign body granuloma and sarcoma, are included in the differential diagnosis for this superficial lesion.*

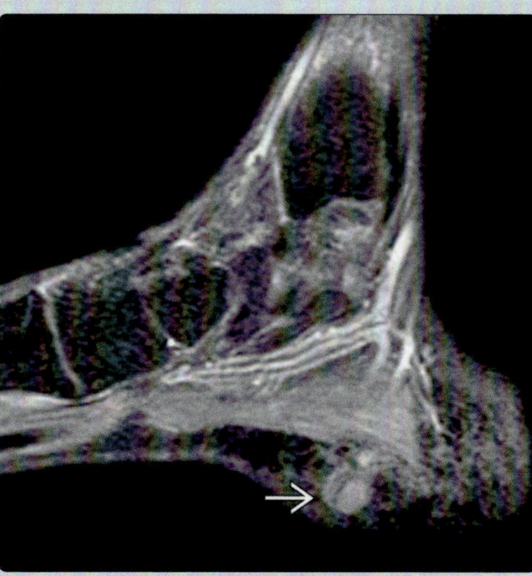

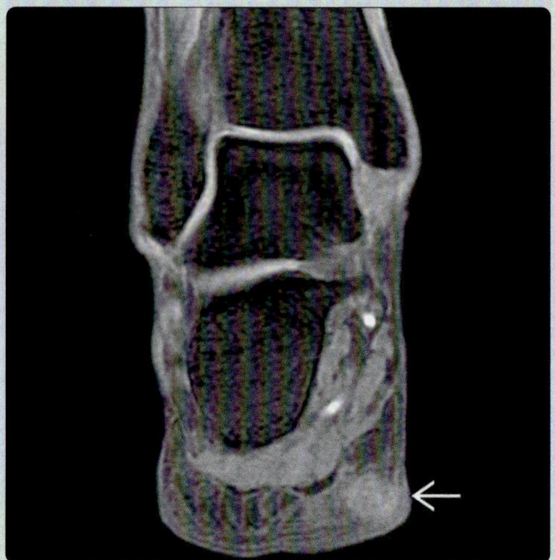

TERMINOLOGY

Synonyms

- Angiomyoma, vascular leiomyoma

Definitions

- Benign, often painful, smooth muscle neoplasm preferentially occurring in superficial soft tissues of lower extremity

IMAGING

General Features

- Location
  - Lower leg > thigh > upper extremity
    - Head and trunk in < 10%
  - Subcutaneous fat > deep dermis > superficial fascia > > muscle
- Size
  - Usually < 2 cm in diameter
- Morphology
  - Spherical to ovoid nodule

Ultrasonographic Findings

- Homogeneously hypoechoic echotexture with circumscribed margin
- Color Doppler: Straight and linear vessels with convergence to one point

Imaging Recommendations

- Best imaging tool
  - None; often excised without imaging

Radiographic Findings

- Normal or mild soft tissue prominence
- May cause scalloping of underlying bone cortex

CT Findings

- Well-defined mass with similar attenuation to muscle
  - May calcify

MR Findings

- Similar appearance to peripheral nerve sheath tumor
- Isointense to mildly hyperintense to muscle on T1WI
  - Homogeneous or heterogeneous
- Heterogeneously hyperintense to muscle on fluid-sensitive sequences
- Low signal surrounding fibrous pseudocapsule on T1WI and T2WI sequences
- Variable enhancement (homogeneously intense to mild peripheral) dependent on subtype
- ± adjacent vessels or internal branching structures
- Small internal foci of fat and hemorrhage reported

DIFFERENTIAL DIAGNOSIS

Benign Peripheral Nerve Sheath Tumor

- Similar imaging appearance
- Lacks intimately associated vascular channels

Giant Cell Tumor Tendon Sheath

- Painless mass abutting tendon sheath
- More likely to have low signal on T1 and T2WI MR

Leiomyosarcoma

- Similar appearance on MR when small

Synovial Sarcoma

- Similar appearance on MR when small
- More likely to arise near joint

PATHOLOGY

General Features

- Etiology
  - Benign smooth muscle neoplasm proposed as arising from vein tunica media or arteriovenous anastomoses
- Genetics
  - No consistent chromosomal abnormality
    - Near diploid karyotypes

Gross Pathologic & Surgical Features

- Solitary, pseudoencapsulated, gray-white myxoid mass
  - May be blue or red

Microscopic Features

- Proliferation of mature smooth muscle cells and thin- to thick-walled vascular channels
  - ± calcification, hemorrhage, fat, myxoid change, hyalinization
  - Absent or rare mitoses
- 3 histologic subtypes with differing amounts of smooth muscle and types of vessels (solid, venous, cavernous)

CLINICAL ISSUES

Presentation

- Most common signs/symptoms
  - Small, superficial mass; slowly grows over years
  - Lesions are painful or tender in most cases
    - Paroxysmal with worsening by light touch, temperature, or hormonal changes
    - Upper extremity lesions are less likely to be painful than lower extremity lesions

Demographics

- Age
  - Arise in 4th-6th decades of life
- Gender
  - Female predominance
    - Lesions in upper extremity and head are more commonly seen in men
- Epidemiology
  - ~ 5% of benign soft tissue tumors

Natural History & Prognosis

- Benign lesion that rarely recurs

Treatment

- Marginal surgical excision

SELECTED REFERENCES

1. Park HJ et al: Sonographic appearances of soft tissue angioleiomyomas: differences from other circumscribed soft tissue hypervascular tumors. J Ultrasound Med. 31(10):1589-95, 2012
2. Yoo HJ et al: Angioleiomyoma in soft tissue of extremities: MRI findings. AJR Am J Roentgenol. 192(6):W291-4, 2009

Leiomyoma: Superficial and Deep

KEY FACTS

TERMINOLOGY

- Benign neoplasm originating from smooth muscle

IMAGING

- May arise in skin, subcutaneous tissues, or deep soft tissues, including abdomen and retroperitoneum
  - Does not include uterine or GI leiomyomas
- Radiographs and CT show soft tissue mass or masses that are commonly calcified
  - Punctate, plaque-like, or "popcorn" calcifications
  - May mimic cartilaginous matrix
- Well-defined, soft tissue mass or masses on MR
  - Calcified foci have low signal on all imaging sequences
- MR findings in subcutaneous lesions
  - Isointense to slightly hyperintense relative to muscle on T1WI
  - Homogeneous to heterogeneous hyperintense signal on fluid-sensitive sequences
  - Prominent contrast enhancement
- MR findings in deep soft tissue lesions
  - Isointense to muscle on T1WI
  - Heterogeneous, hypointense to hyperintense signal on fluid-sensitive sequences
  - Heterogeneous or mostly peripheral enhancement

PATHOLOGY

- Orderly fascicles of cells similar to smooth muscle
- Calcification, hyalinization, and myxoid changes common

CLINICAL ISSUES

- Epidemiology
  - Subcutaneous lesions are relatively common but not commonly imaged before excision
  - Deep lesions are very rare
- Age: Occurs in young to middle-aged adults
- Treatment: Surgical excision
- Natural history: Recurrence of subcutaneous lesions uncommon; deep lesions recur more commonly

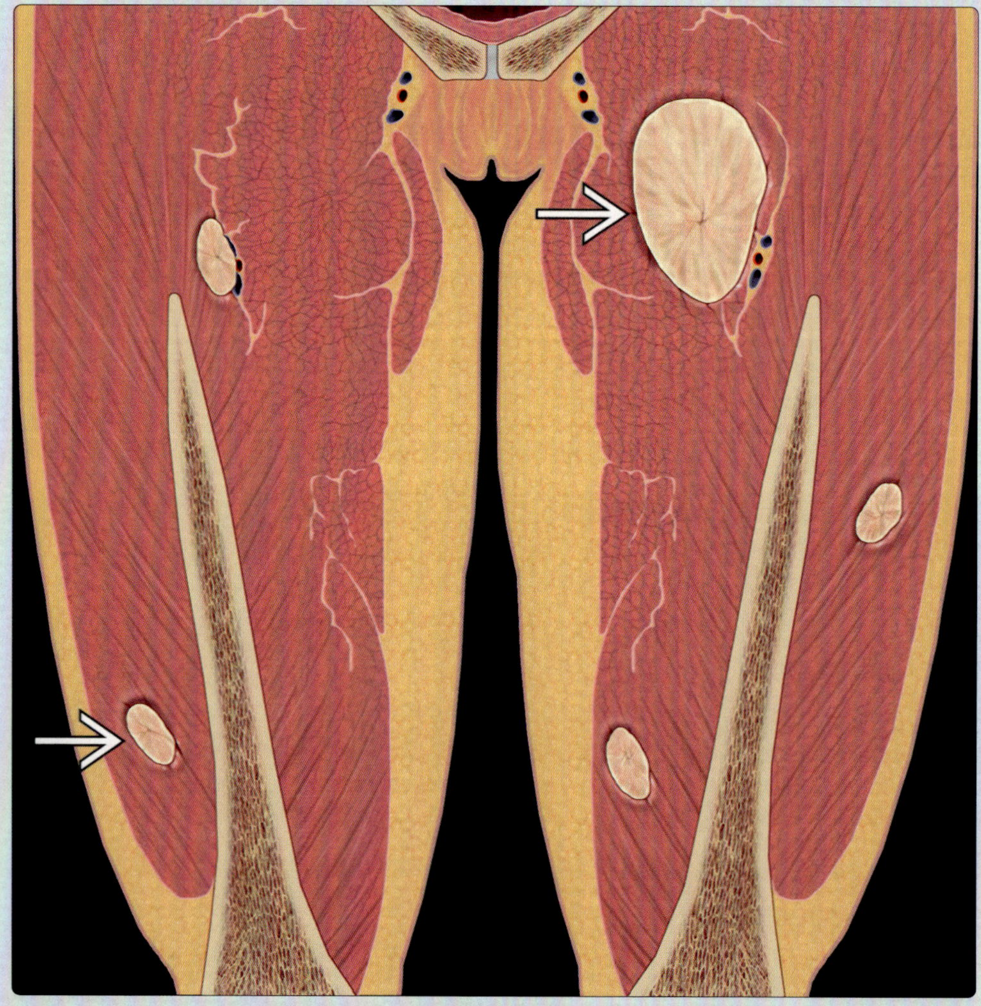

Coronal graphic of the bilateral thighs demonstrates multiple well-defined, round to oval masses ➡ in the deep soft tissues. Extrauterine leiomyomas may occur in the skin, subcutis, muscles, abdomen, and retroperitoneum. These lesions typically lack surrounding edema unless they are in a location that undergoes mechanical irritation.

TERMINOLOGY

Definitions

- Benign neoplasm originating from smooth muscle

IMAGING

General Features

- Location
  - May arise in skin, subcutaneous tissues, or deep soft tissues, including abdomen and retroperitoneum
    - Does not include leiomyomas of uterine or gastrointestinal origin
- Size
  - Cutaneous lesions measure a few mm to 2 cm
  - Subcutaneous lesions usually < 2 cm
  - Deep lesions reported up to 37 cm, weighing 5.4 kg
- Morphology
  - Skin lesions may be clustered papules or solitary nodules

Imaging Recommendations

- Best imaging tool
  - Superficial lesions are often not imaged
  - MR is best modality to evaluate deep lesions

Radiographic Findings

- Soft tissue mass or masses that are commonly calcified
  - Punctate, plaque-like, or "popcorn" calcifications

CT Findings

- Calcified, solitary or multiple soft tissue masses
  - May mimic cartilaginous matrix

MR Findings

- T1WI
  - Subcutaneous → isointense to slightly hyperintense relative to muscle
  - Deep soft tissue → isointense to muscle
- T2WI
  - Subcutaneous → homogeneous to heterogeneous signal hyperintense to muscle
  - Deep soft tissue → heterogeneous hypointense to hyperintense signal
- T1WI C+ FS
  - Subcutaneous → prominent contrast enhancement
  - Deep soft tissue → heterogeneous or predominantly peripheral enhancement
- Well-defined soft tissue mass or masses
- Internal calcified foci have low signal on all imaging sequences

DIFFERENTIAL DIAGNOSIS

Schwannoma, Calcifying

- May have same appearance as leiomyoma on imaging
- Found near neurovascular bundle
- Nerve may be visibly contiguous with mass

Extraskeletal Osteosarcoma

- Soft tissue mass with central ossification
- Middle-aged adults to elderly
- Predilection for buttocks, shoulder girdle, trunk, retroperitoneum

Synovial Sarcoma

- Hypervascular, calcified mass near joint
- May have same appearance on imaging as leiomyoma when small

Soft Tissue Chondroma

- Most commonly found in fingers
- Arises near joints and tendons
- Positive S100 protein

Extraskeletal Myxoid Chondrosarcoma

- Soft tissue mass with chondroid matrix
- Less intense enhancement

Myositis Ossificans/Heterotopic Ossification

- Progressive peripheral ossification
- Lacks origin in abdomen/retroperitoneum

PATHOLOGY

Gross Pathologic & Surgical Features

- Well-circumscribed, gray-white mass

Microscopic Features

- Orderly fascicles of cells similar to smooth muscle
  - Calcification, hyalinization, and myxoid changes common
  - Uncommon clear cell change, ossification, psammoma bodies, and fatty differentiation
  - No atypia or necrosis
  - Low or no mitotic activity
- Focally positive for actin, desmin, and HCAD
- Negative S100 protein

CLINICAL ISSUES

Demographics

- Age
  - Young to middle-aged adults
- Gender
  - No predominance
- Epidemiology
  - Subcutaneous lesions are relatively common but not commonly imaged before excision
  - Deep lesions are very rare

Natural History & Prognosis

- Local recurrence reported with deep lesions

Treatment

- Surgical excision

SELECTED REFERENCES

1. Arleo EK et al: Review of Leiomyoma Variants. AJR Am J Roentgenol. 205(4):912-21, 2015
2. Fasih N et al: Leiomyomas beyond the uterus: unusual locations, rare manifestations. Radiographics. 28(7):1931-48, 2008
3. Weiss SW et al: Benign tumors of smooth muscle. In Weiss SW et al: Enzinger and Weiss' Soft Tissue Tumors. 5th ed. Philadelphia: Elsevier. 522-8, 2008
4. Kransdorf MJ et al: Muscle tumors. In Kransdorf MJ et al: Imaging of Soft Tissue Tumors. 2nd ed. Philadelphia: Lippincott Williams & Wilkins. 298-303, 2006
5. Hashimoto H et al: Leiomyoma of deep soft tissue. In Fletcher CDM et al: World Health Organization Classification of Tumours. Pathology and Genetics of Tumours of Soft Tissue and Bone. Lyon: IARC Press. 130, 2002

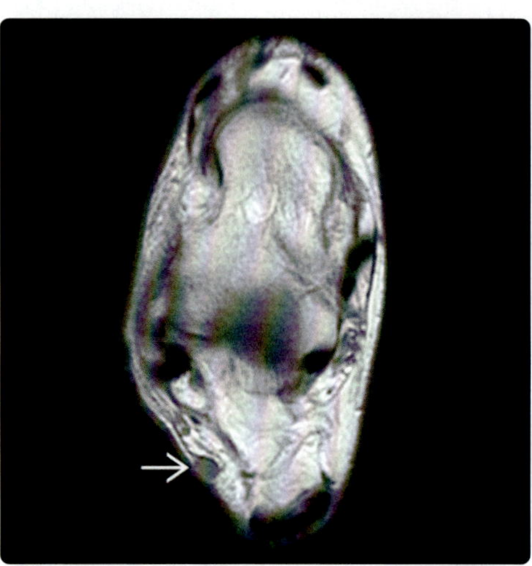

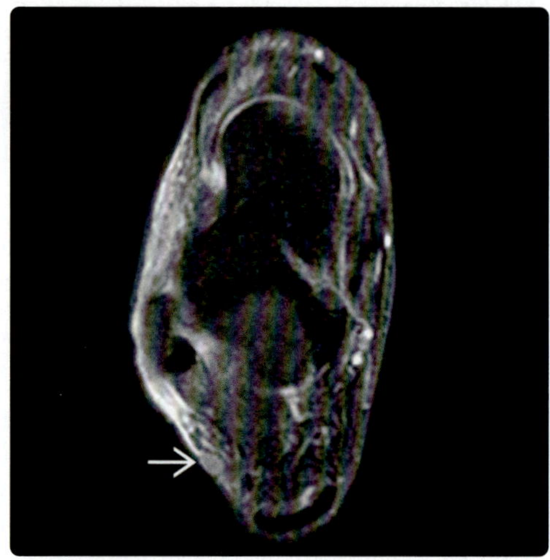

(Left) *Axial PDWI MR shows a mass ➡ in the subcutaneous tissues of the posterolateral ankle. The mass is well defined and has mildly hyperintense signal relative to skeletal muscle.* **(Right)** *Axial T2WI FS MR shows the soft tissue leiomyoma ➡ to have homogeneously hyperintense signal relative to muscle. An additional, similar lesion was present more distally.*

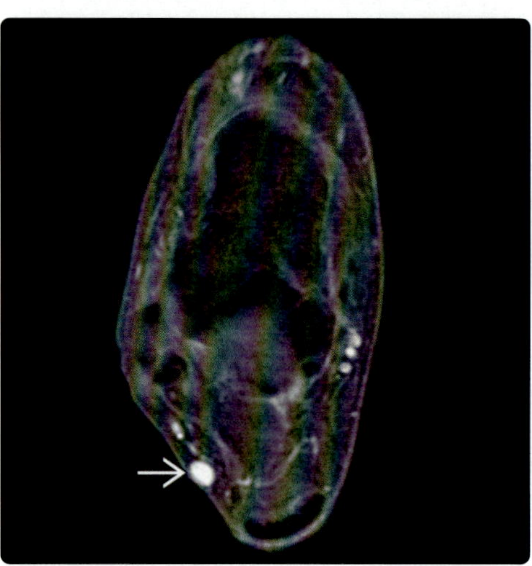

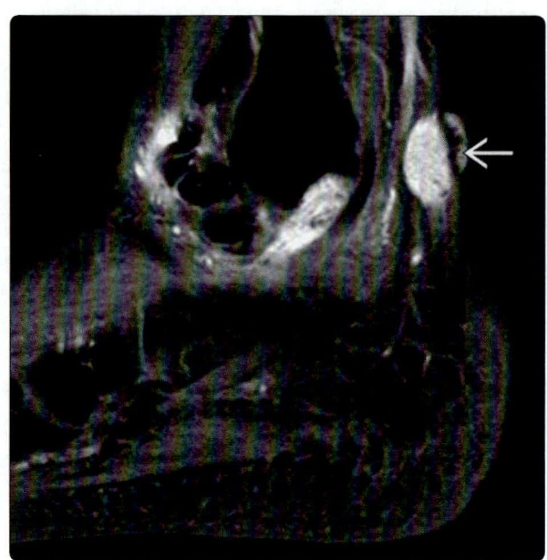

(Left) *Axial T1WI C+ FS MR in the same patient shows the well-defined, oval soft tissue leiomyoma ➡ to intensely enhance. The differential diagnosis for this small lesion includes benign nerve sheath tumors and malignant sarcomas.* **(Right)** *Sagittal T1WI C+ FS MR shows a well-defined oval mass ➡ in the subcutaneous fat of the posterolateral ankle, which was bordered by the Achilles tendon medially and the neurovascular bundle laterally. The mass shows intense enhancement.*

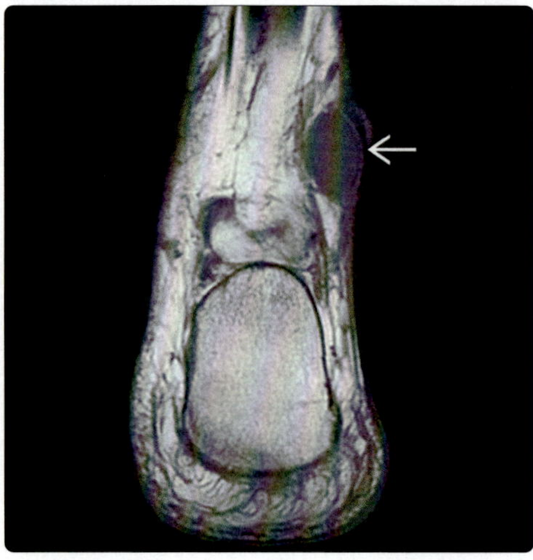

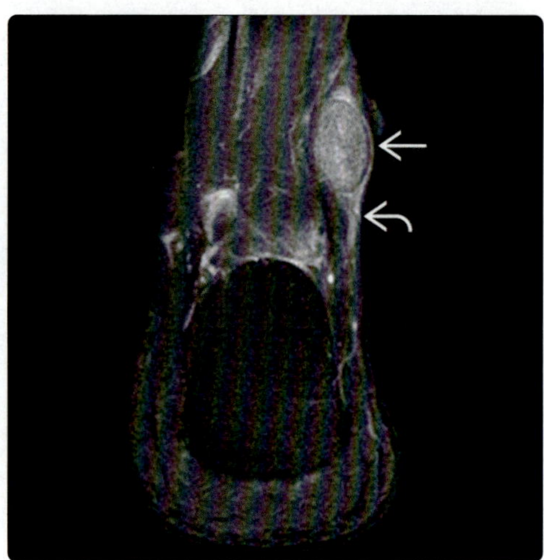

(Left) *Coronal T1WI MR in the same patient shows the mass ➡ to have homogeneous signal intensity that is slightly higher than muscle.* **(Right)** *Coronal T2WI FS MR shows the mass ➡ to have mildly heterogeneous high signal intensity. Mild surrounding edema ↪ was presumed to be due to mechanical irritation.*

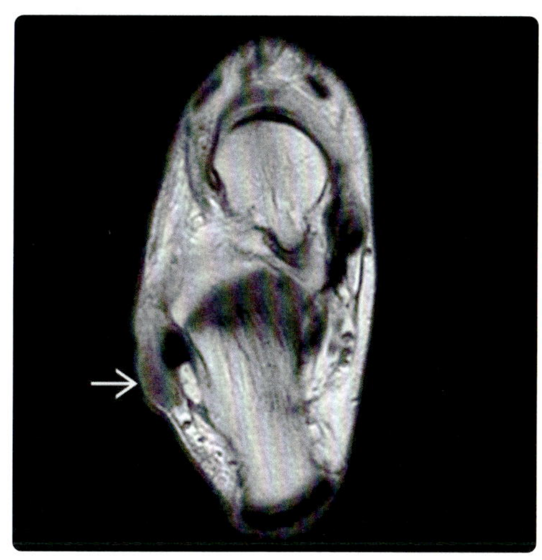

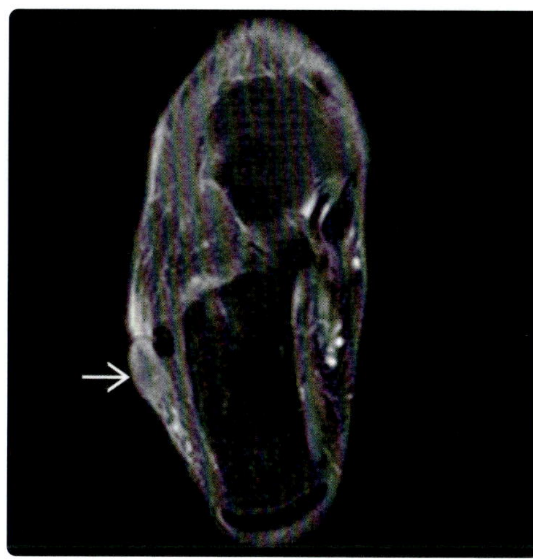

(Left) *Axial PDWI MR shows an oval mass ➡ in the subcutaneous fat of the ankle. The mass has heterogeneous, mildly hyperintense signal relative to skeletal muscle.* **(Right)** *Axial T2WI FS MR shows the mass ➡ to have heterogeneous, hyperintense signal. Note that the lesion has a target appearance, similar to that often seen with benign nerve sheath tumors.*

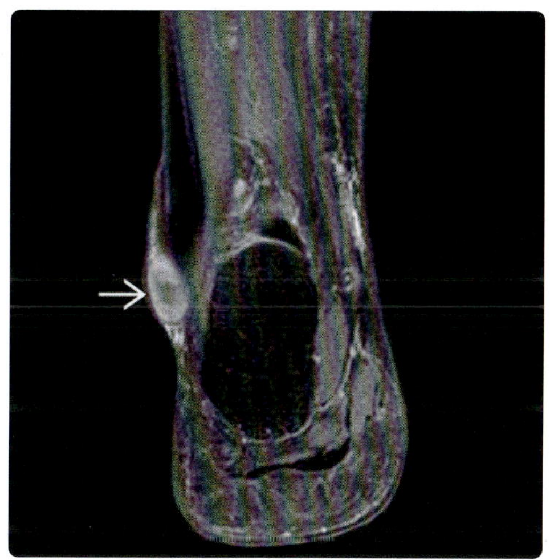

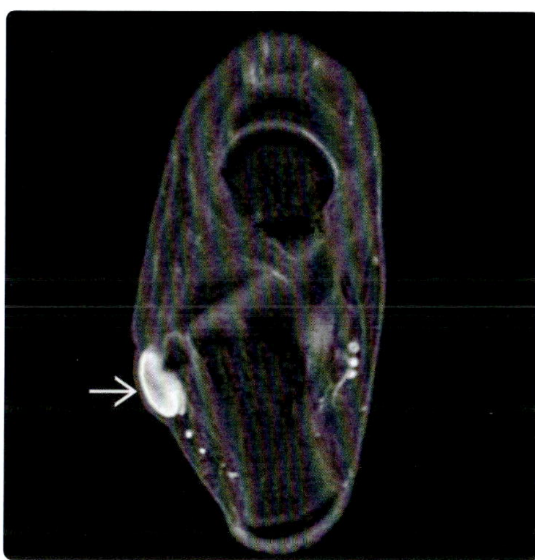

(Left) *Coronal PDWI FS MR in the same patient again shows the well-defined, oval soft tissue leiomyoma ➡ with the target appearance and a hyperintense rim surrounding a relatively hypointense center.* **(Right)** *Axial T1WI C+ FS MR in the same patient shows the soft tissue leiomyoma ➡ to have intense peripheral enhancement with a hypoenhancing central region.*

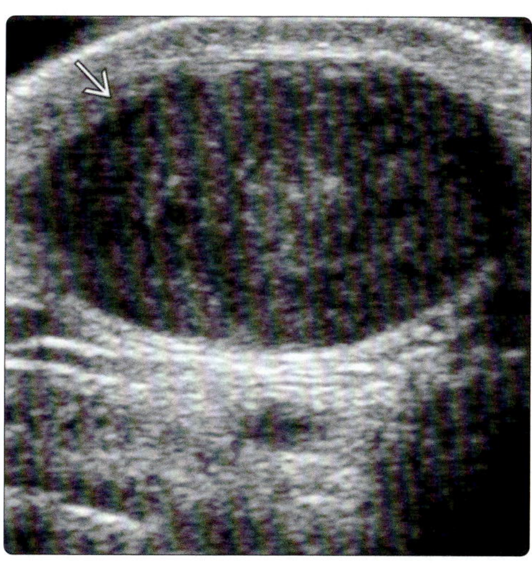

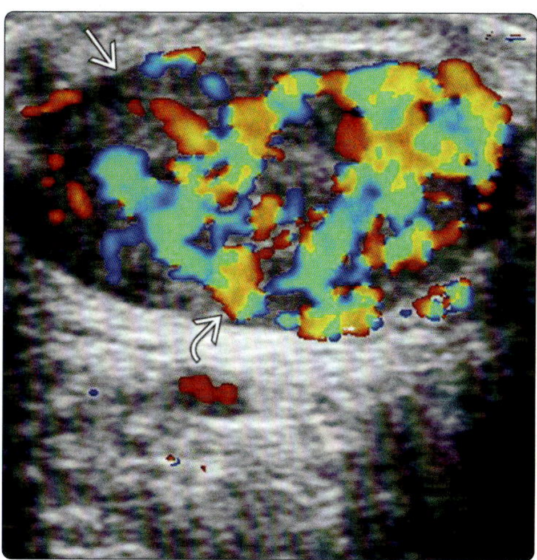

(Left) *Longitudinal ultrasound in a patient with leiomyoma shows a well-circumscribed, subcutaneous mass ➡ with heterogeneous echogenicity.* **(Right)** *Longitudinal Doppler ultrasound in the same patient demonstrates the leiomyoma ➡ to have high vascularity ➦.*

KEY FACTS

TERMINOLOGY

- Malignant neoplasm arising from smooth muscle

IMAGING

- Arises in skin, soft tissue, blood vessel
  - 12-41% occur in peripheral extremity soft tissue, most commonly thigh
- Radiographs may be normal or show soft tissue mass
  - Calcification or ossification in up to 17%
  - May invade underlying bone
- CT: Nonspecific soft tissue mass ± calcification
  - Low-attenuation regions may reflect necrosis, hemorrhage, or cystic change
- MR: Nonspecific soft tissue mass with deceptively encapsulated appearance
  - T1WI: Homogeneous to heterogeneous, hypointense to slightly hyperintense signal
  - T2WI: Heterogeneously hyperintense to muscle
  - May contain fluid-fluid levels from hemorrhage
  - Intense, heterogeneous enhancement
- Moderately vascular or hypervascular tumor on Doppler US or angiography

PATHOLOGY

- Approximately 1/3 of soft tissue leiomyosarcomas arise from small vein
- Degree of mitotic activity ranges from high to low (< 1 per 10 HPF)

CLINICAL ISSUES

- Nontender, enlarging soft tissue mass
- Age: Most common in middle-aged adults or elderly
- 3rd most common soft tissue sarcoma
- Natural history
  - Highest overall mortality for sarcomas
  - Prognosis worse with retroperitoneal location, high mitotic rate, and size > 5 cm
  - Metastases often present at presentation

(Left) *Axial T1WI MR shows a high-grade soft tissue leiomyosarcoma ➡. This large, heterogeneous thigh mass has mixed intensity, being both isointense and hypointense relative to muscle. On T2WI FS MR, the hypointense regions had signal intensity similar to fluid (not shown).* **(Right)** *Axial T1WI C+ FS MR shows the nodular and septate regions of the mass ➡ to demonstrate intense enhancement. Lack of enhancement in the areas of presumed fluid on T2WI fat-suppressed MR is consistent with necrosis ⮌.*

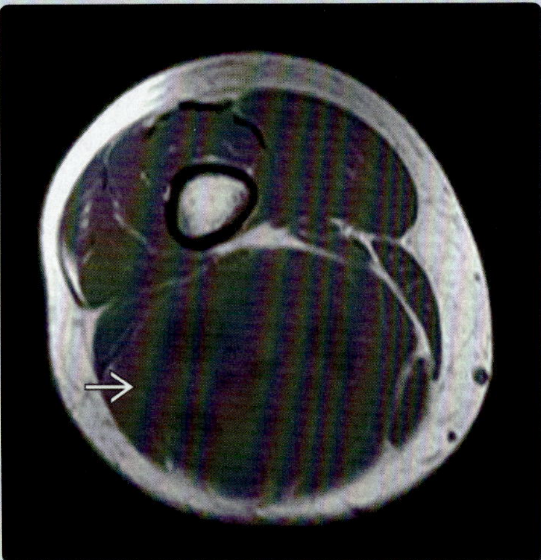

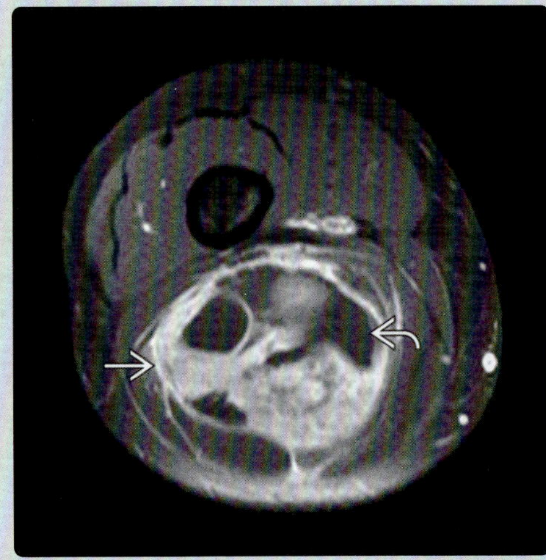

(Left) *Axial NECT in the same patient, obtained for radiation treatment planning purposes, shows the mixed attenuation of the mass ➡ and low-attenuation regions consistent with necrosis ⮌.* **(Right)** *Transverse color Doppler US in the same patient shows the mass ➡ to be heterogeneously hypoechoic with predominantly peripheral blood flow. Areas of hemorrhage and necrosis lack demonstrable vascularity. Both hemorrhage and necrosis are common in large lesions.*

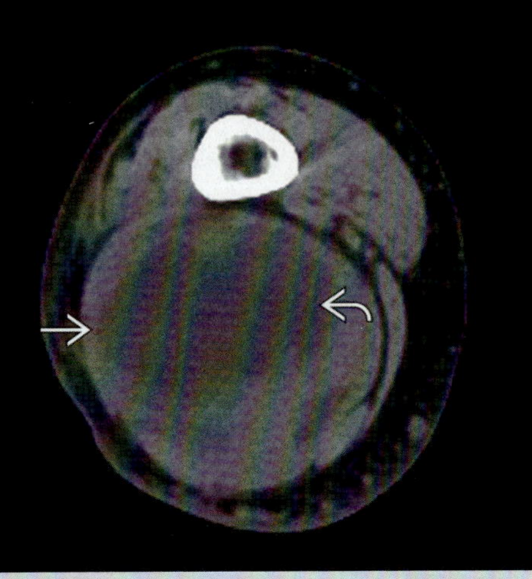

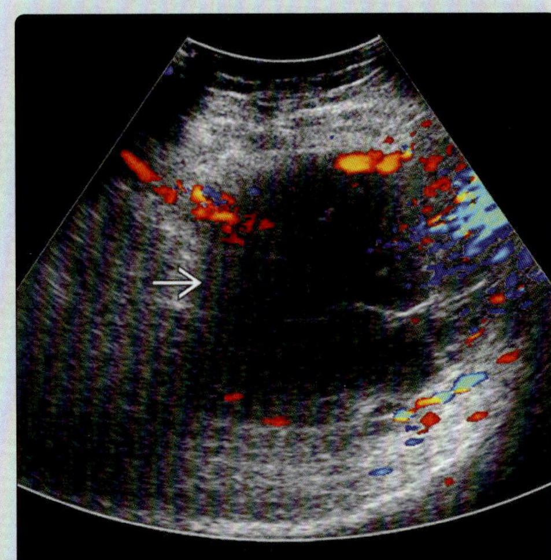

TERMINOLOGY

Definitions

- Malignant neoplasm arising from smooth muscle cells

IMAGING

General Features

- Location
  - Skin, soft tissue, blood vessels
    - Soft tissue lesions divided into somatic soft tissue and retroperitoneal/abdominal locations
    - 12-41% occur in peripheral extremity soft tissue, most commonly thigh
      - 50:50 distribution of superficial vs. deep location in extremity
- Size
  - Cutaneous lesions usually < 2 cm
  - Somatic soft tissue lesions ~ 6 cm
  - Retroperitoneal lesions usually > 10 cm
- Morphology
  - Nodular cutaneous lesions often cause ulceration and discoloration of overlying skin
  - Somatic soft tissue lesions are multinodular and better circumscribed than retroperitoneal lesions
  - Vascular lesions are polypoid and extend along lumen or surface of blood vessel

Imaging Recommendations

- Best imaging tool
  - MR is most helpful in evaluating relationship to anatomic compartments and vital structures

Radiographic Findings

- Radiographs may be normal or demonstrate soft tissue mass
  - Calcification or ossification in up to 17%
  - May invade underlying bone

CT Findings

- Nonspecific soft tissue mass ± calcification
  - Low-attenuation regions may reflect necrosis, hemorrhage, or cystic change

MR Findings

- T1WI
  - Homogeneous to heterogeneous signal ranging from hypointense to slightly hyperintense relative to skeletal muscle
- T2WI
  - Heterogeneously hyperintense to muscle
  - May contain fluid-fluid levels from hemorrhage
- T1WI C+ FS
  - Intense, heterogeneous enhancement
- Nonspecific soft tissue mass with deceptively encapsulated appearance
- Calcifications have low signal on all imaging sequences

Ultrasonographic Findings

- Heterogeneous echogenicity
- Hypervascular on Doppler imaging
  - Hypovascular necrotic and hemorrhagic regions
- ± shadowing calcification, hypoechoic cystic, or necrotic regions

Angiographic Findings

- Moderately vascular or hypervascular tumor
  - Arteriovenous shunting

DIFFERENTIAL DIAGNOSIS

Fibrosarcoma

- Similar imaging appearance as leiomyosarcoma
- Histologically similar, moderately differentiated spindle cells in fascicles
  - Cells have more tapered appearance than leiomyosarcoma
  - Less likely to have intersecting fascicles

Malignant Peripheral Nerve Sheath Tumor

- Histologically similar moderately differentiated spindle cells in fascicles
  - Wavy, buckled cells

Inflammatory Myofibroblastic Tumor

- Located in parenchymal organs, especially lung, orbit, and bladder
- Fibrotic contents may produce low signal on T1WI and T2WI MR
- Prominent enhancement visible even on delayed imaging

Calcifying Aponeurotic Fibroma

- Small, slowly growing mass in child
- Palms, soles, wrists, and ankles
- Stippled calcifications

Fasciitis, Nodular and Proliferative

- Painful, rapidly growing mass in young to middle-aged adult
- Mass intimately associated with fascia

Solitary Fibrous Tumor and Hemangiopericytoma

- Prominent vascularity may be evident as intense enhancement &/or visible blood vessels
- Hemangiopericytoma-like vascular pattern + hyalinized stroma
- Painless, slowly growing mass ± calcification

Low-Grade Fibromyxoid Sarcoma

- Similar mass location and overall appearance, but lacking necrosis and hemorrhage
- Young adults; median age: 34 yr

Pleomorphic MFH/Undifferentiated Pleomorphic Sarcoma

- Markedly heterogeneous appearance
  - Fluid-fluid levels from hemorrhage
  - May erode or invade bone
- > 40 yr old with peak in 6th-7th decades
- Calcification present peripherally in 5-20%

Myxofibrosarcoma

- Elderly patients
- Subcutaneous > intramuscular location
- More homogeneous imaging appearance
- High local recurrence rate

Deep Benign Fibrous Histiocytoma

- More likely to have low signal on T1WI MR
- Well-circumscribed subcutaneous or deep mass

Synovial Sarcoma

- Propensity to occur near joints
- Well-defined mass often containing calcification

PATHOLOGY

General Features

- Etiology
  - Malignant neoplasm of unknown etiology
  - Suggested association with radiation exposure
- Genetics
  - Complex karyotypes without consistent abnormality
    - Loss involving 3p21-23, 8p21-pter, 13q12-13, 13q32-qter
    - Gain involving 1q21-31 region
- Associated abnormalities
  - Possible association with *RB1* retinoblastoma gene

Staging, Grading, & Classification

- American Joint Committee on Cancer (AJCC) staging system and Surgical Staging System of Musculoskeletal Tumor Society are commonly utilized

Gross Pathologic & Surgical Features

- Gray-white to tan, fleshy mass
  - Grossly encapsulated although microscopically invasive
  - May have whorled appearance
- ± areas of hemorrhage, cystic change, or necrotic tissue
- May invade adjacent organs or bone

Microscopic Features

- ~ 1/3 of somatic soft tissue leiomyosarcomas arise from small vein
- Elongated spindle cells with cigar-shaped nuclei
  - Fascicular growth pattern
  - Variable pleomorphism
  - Multinucleated giant cells common
  - May demonstrate nuclear palisading
- Degree of mitotic activity ranges from high to low (< 1 per 10 HPF)
- Positive for smooth muscle actin, desmin, and h-caldesmon
  - Focally positive for keratin, epithelial membrane antigen, CD34, and S100 protein

CLINICAL ISSUES

Presentation

- Most common signs/symptoms
  - Nontender, enlarging soft tissue mass
    - Pain in 10% of retroperitoneal tumors
  - Tumors involving blood vessels may result in vascular insufficiency
- Other signs/symptoms
  - Retroperitoneal → increase in abdominal girth, weight loss, nausea
  - Hepatic vein obstruction → Budd-Chiari syndrome (hepatomegaly, jaundice, ascites)
  - Renal vein obstruction → renal insufficiency
  - Lower inferior vena cava obstruction → lower extremity edema

Demographics

- Age
  - Most common in middle-aged adults or elderly
    - May arise in children and young adults
- Gender
  - Female predominance for retroperitoneal and inferior vena cava lesions
  - Male predominance for peripheral soft tissue and cutaneous lesions
- Epidemiology
  - 3rd most common soft tissue sarcoma
    - 9% of all classified sarcomas
  - Large blood vessel origin is rare

Natural History & Prognosis

- Highest overall mortality for sarcomas
  - Medial survival: 4.2 yr
  - Prognosis worse with retroperitoneal location, high mitotic rate, and size > 5 cm
- Metastases often present at presentation
  - Lung most common
  - Liver, bone, soft tissue, lymph nodes
  - Most common sarcoma to metastasize to brain (rare overall)
- Retroperitoneal leiomyosarcoma
  - Local recurrence common
- Cutaneous leiomyosarcoma
  - Better prognosis
  - Less likely to metastasize
  - Metastases often involve lymph nodes

Treatment

- Surgical excision with wide margins
  - Complete excision difficult with retroperitoneal tumors
- Adjuvant chemotherapy or radiation therapy

SELECTED REFERENCES

1. Gordon RW et al: MRI, MDCT features, and clinical outcome of extremity leiomyosarcomas: experience in 47 patients. Skeletal Radiol. 43(5):615-22, 2014
2. Weiss SW et al: Leiomyosarcoma. In Weiss SW et al: Enzinger and Weiss' Soft Tissue Tumors. 5th ed. Philadelphia: Elsevier. 545-64, 2008
3. Efstathopoulos N et al: Inflammatory leiomyosarcoma of the ankle: a case report and review of the literature. J Foot Ankle Surg. 45(2):127-30, 2006
4. Kransdorf MJ et al: Muscle tumors. In Kransdorf MJ et al: Imaging of Soft Tissue Tumors. 2nd ed. Philadelphia: Lippincott Williams & Wilkins. 306-12, 2006
5. Massi D et al: Prognostic factors in soft tissue leiomyosarcoma of the extremities: a retrospective analysis of 42 cases. Eur J Surg Oncol. 30(5):565-72, 2004
6. Evans HL et al: Leiomyosarcoma. In Fletcher CDM et al: World Health Organization Classification of Tumours. Pathology and Genetics of Tumours of Soft Tissue and Bone. Lyon: IARC Press. 131-4, 2002
7. Abdelwahab IF et al: Radiation-induced leiomyosarcoma. Skeletal Radiol. 24(1):81-3, 1995
8. Kransdorf MJ: Malignant soft-tissue tumors in a large referral population: distribution of diagnoses by age, sex, and location. AJR Am J Roentgenol. 164(1):129-34, 1995
9. Hartman DS et al: From the archives of the AFIP. Leiomyosarcoma of the retroperitoneum and inferior vena cava: radiologic-pathologic correlation. Radiographics. 12(6):1203-20, 1992

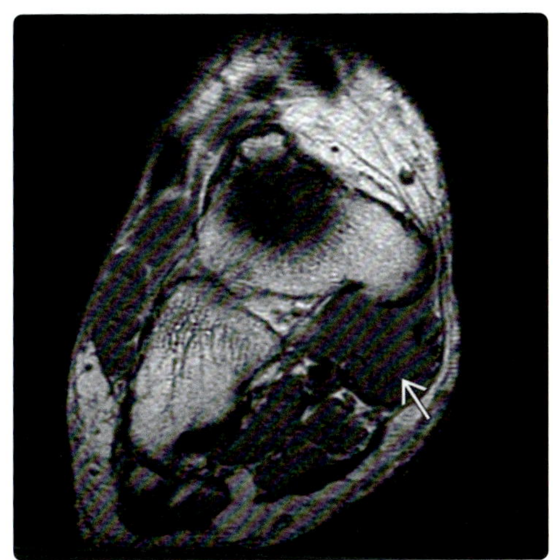

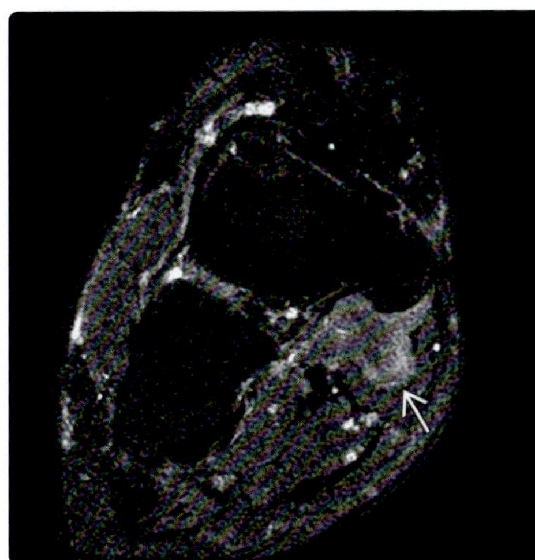

(Left) *Coronal T1WI MR of the midfoot at the level of the sustentaculum tali has an unremarkable appearance. A mass ➡ is best demonstrated on additional imaging sequences, since on this sequence the mass is isointense to muscle, without a visible border.* **(Right)** *Coronal T2WI FS MR shows the mass ➡ to be mildly hyperintense to muscle with a lobulated contour. Small lesions are more difficult to detect due to having signal intensity similar to the surrounding muscle.*

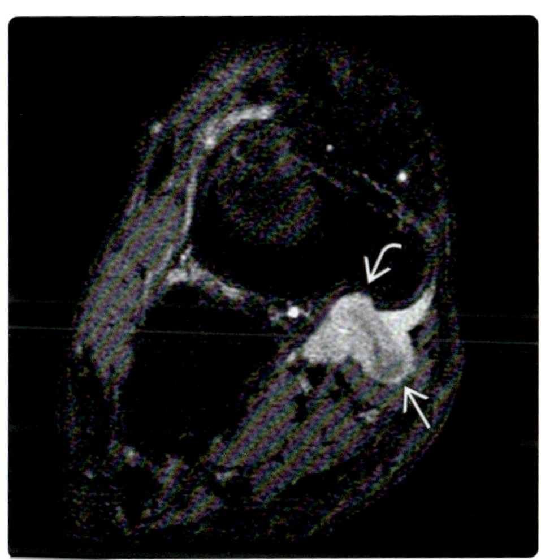

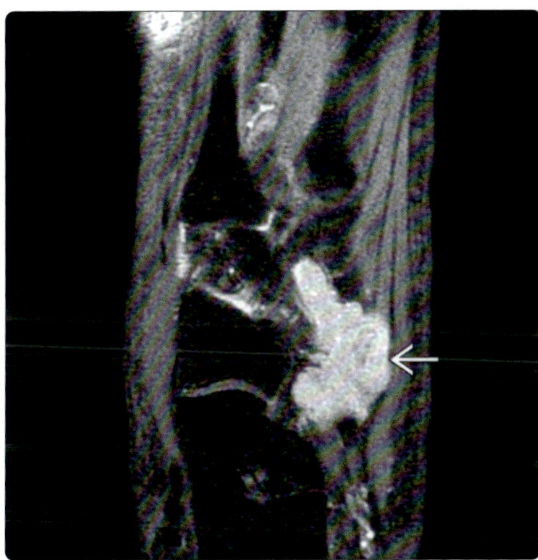

(Left) *Coronal T1WI C+ FS MR in the same patient best demonstrates the lobulated leiomyosarcoma ➡ due to the prominent, relatively homogeneous enhancement. The mass is eroding ➡ the adjacent bone. The foot is a relatively uncommon location for this tumor.* **(Right)** *Axial T1WI C+ FS MR shows the enhancing mass ➡ to have lobulated borders and extend along the long axis of the foot. This low-grade tumor was producing tarsal tunnel syndrome, which was confirmed on EMG.*

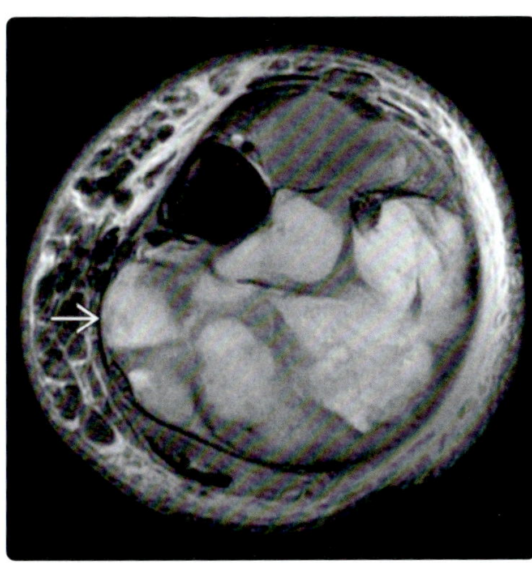

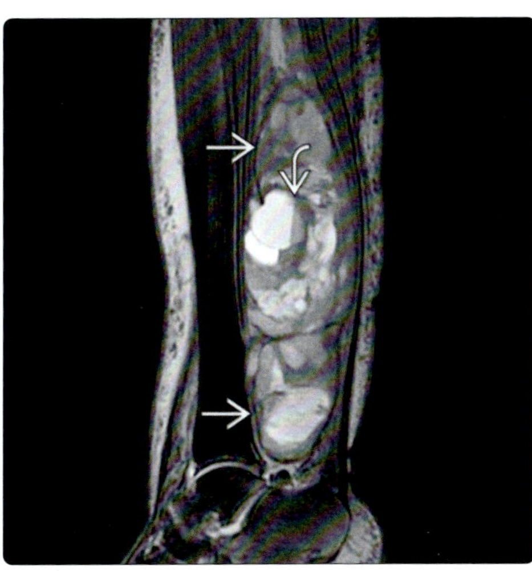

(Left) *Axial T2WI FS MR shows tumor ➡ involving all muscle compartments of the lower leg in a 48-yr-old woman. The mass shows heterogeneous signal intensity that is predominantly hyperintense relative to skeletal muscle.* **(Right)** *Sagittal T2WI FS MR shows the mass ➡ extending from the proximal calf to the ankle. Hemorrhagic regions of the mass are evident by fluid-fluid levels ➡. The overall imaging appearance suggests an aggressive sarcoma, but is otherwise nonspecific.*

(Left) *Coronal T1WI MR was obtained in a 64-yr-old woman who fell off an exercise ball. She has had multiple evacuations of hematoma, but the mass recurs. Note that the majority of the mass ➡ is hyperintense, representing blood. However, there are also multiple nodules along the wall of the mass ➡ that are hypointense. A simple hematoma should not have such nodularity.* **(Right)** *Coronal STIR MR in the same case shows the hemorrhage ➡ to retain its hyperintense signal. The nodules ➡ show a nonspecific heterogeneity.*

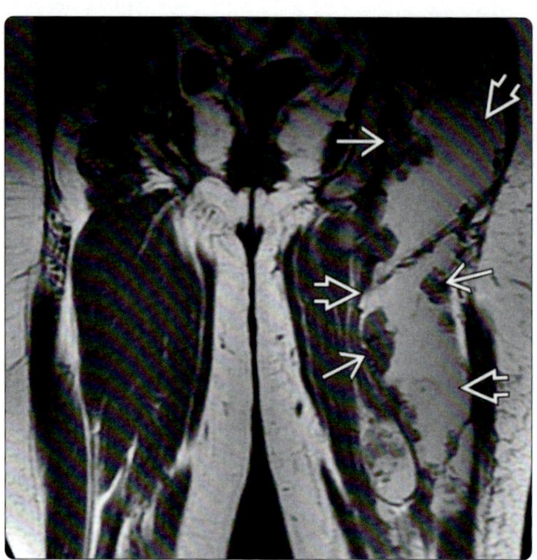

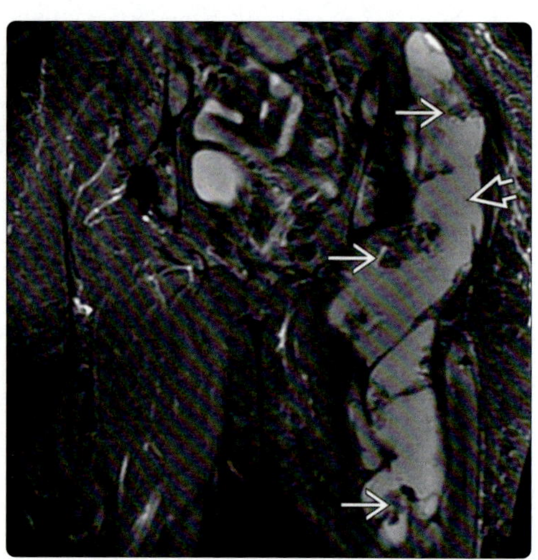

(Left) *Sagittal PD FS MR, same case, shows multiple fluid levels ➡ throughout the mass, with differing signal in the blood products. The nodules ➡ show heterogeneity and must lead to biopsy to determine the type of underlying tumor results in this impressive hemorrhage.* **(Right)** *Axial T1WI C+ FS MR shows enhancing tissue ➡ surrounding nonenhancing hemorrhage ➡. Note that some of the nodules show enhancement ➡, while others do not. Biopsy directed at enhancing nodules is required.*

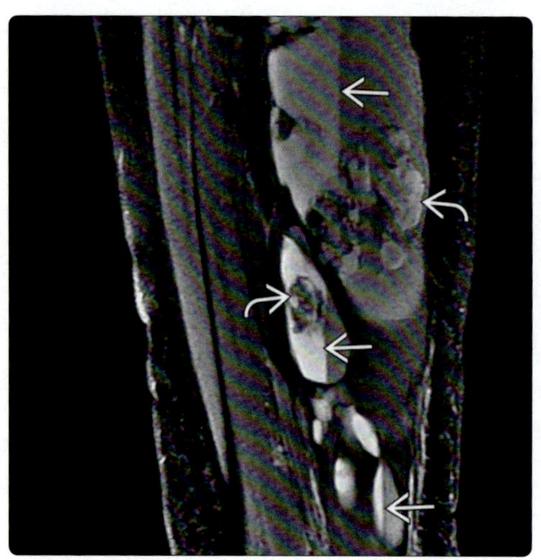

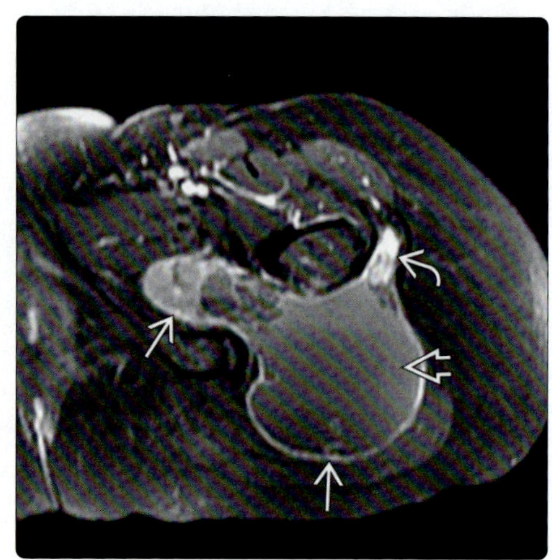

(Left) *Axial CT obtained at time of biopsy shows punctate calcifications ➡ within the mass lesion ➡.* **(Right)** *Axial CT obtained more distally shows calcifications ➡ as well as erosion of the femoral neck ➡ by the mass lesion ➡. This case shows many common features of leiomyosarcoma, including location in the thigh, large size of lesion, heterogeneity, necrosis, calcifications, erosion of bone, hemorrhage, and fluid levels. The diagnosis was proven at biopsy.*

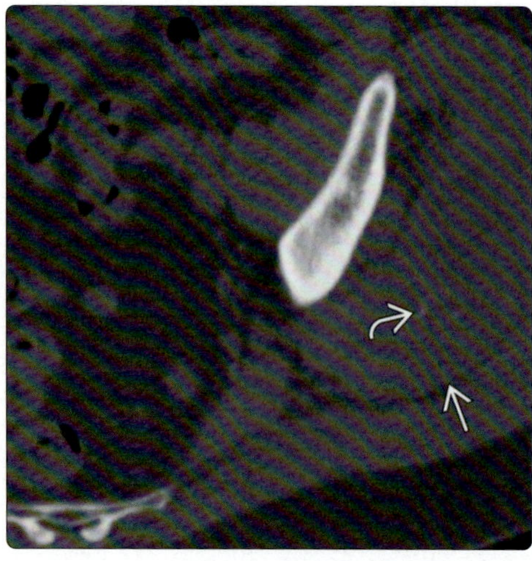

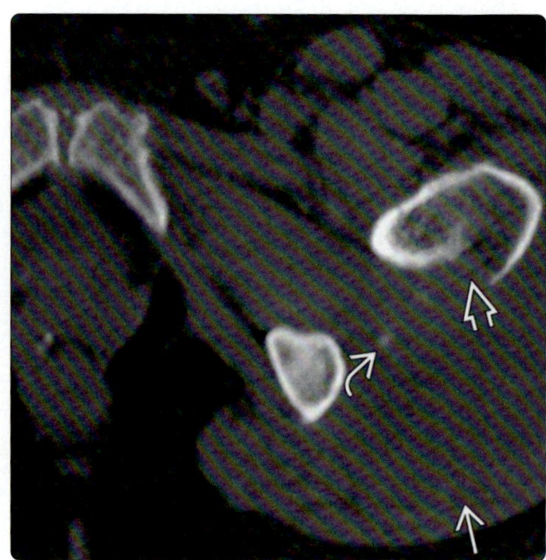

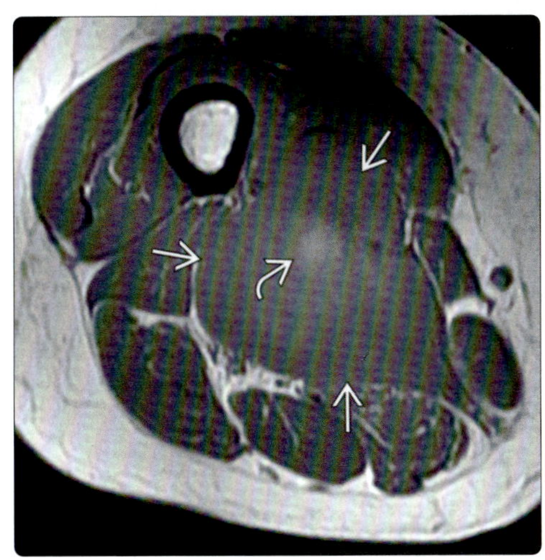

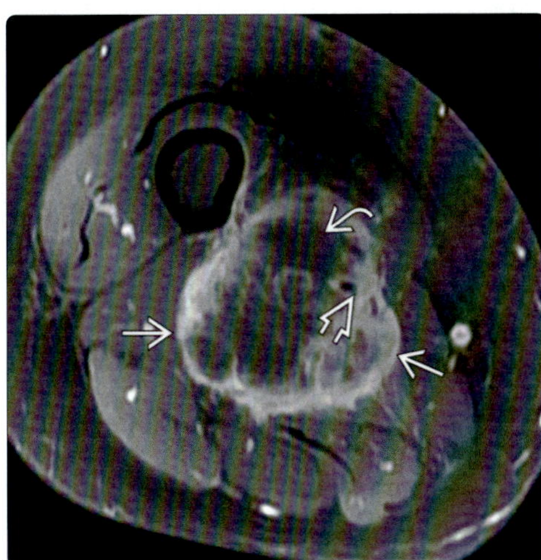

(Left) *Axial T1WI MR shows a large mass ➡ within the posterior compartment of the thigh. The majority of the signal is slightly hyperintense relative to skeletal muscle. Centrally, there is hyperintensity ➡ that is suggestive of hemorrhage.* **(Right)** *Axial T1WI C+FS MR in the same case shows enhancement of much of the lesion ➡ with extensive central necrosis ➡. Note vascular involvement ➡ by the lesion. The thigh is the most common site for leiomyosarcoma; hemorrhage is relatively common.*

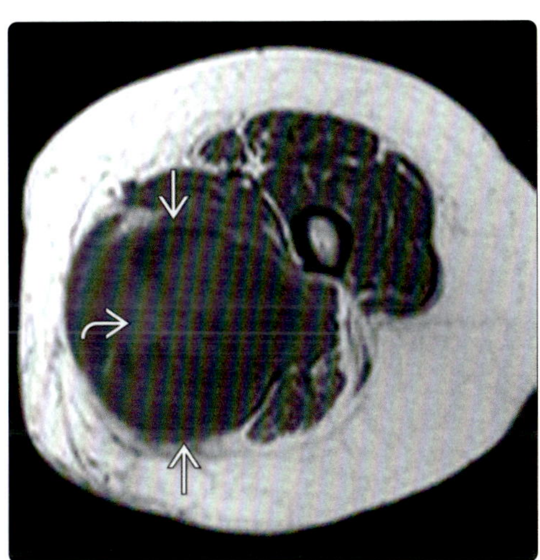

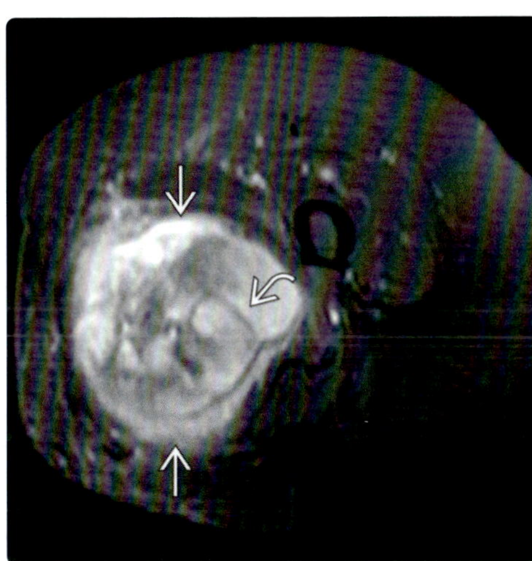

(Left) *Axial T1WI MR shows a well-circumscribed mass ➡ in the thigh with heterogeneous signal ranging from isointense to hyperintense ➡ relative to muscle. The hyperintense signal is due to hemorrhage.* **(Right)** *Axial T2WI FS MR shows the mass ➡ to have heterogeneously hyperintense signal with internal septa ➡. The thigh is the most common extremity location. These lesions are prone to local recurrence and metastatic disease. Metastatic sites most commonly involved are the lungs and liver.*

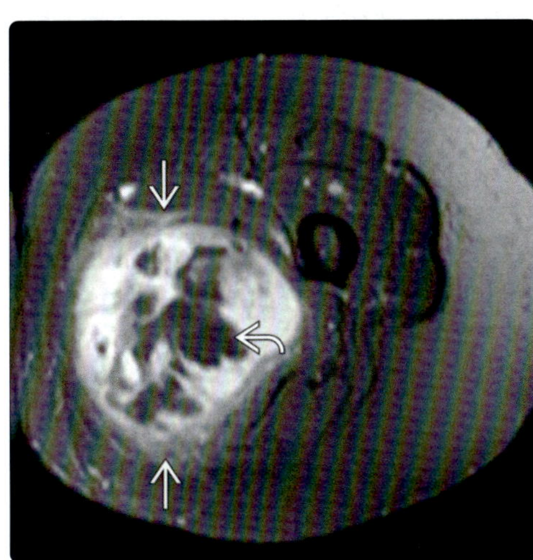

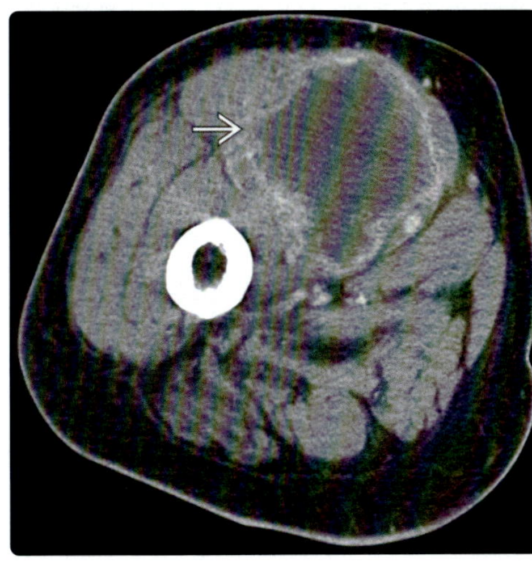

(Left) *Axial T1WI C+ FS MR in the same patient demonstrates thick, irregular enhancement of the mass ➡ with central areas of hypoenhancement ➡ likely representing regions of necrosis.* **(Right)** *Axial soft tissue algorithm CT with contrast in a different patient shows an irregular, deep mass ➡ in the thigh. The infiltrative appearance of the mass borders is a less common appearance than a well-circumscribed mass. The mass has mild peripheral enhancement.*

Glomus Tumor

KEY FACTS

TERMINOLOGY

- Usually benign, mesenchymal neoplasm of smooth muscle cells similar to glomus body cells

IMAGING

- Propensity to involve subungual region
  - Distal extremities (fingers and toes) most common
  - Reported throughout body
- Radiographs
  - Soft tissue mass may or may not be evident on radiographs
  - Subungual lesions commonly produce scalloped defect with sclerotic border involving dorsal aspect of terminal phalanx
- MR appearance
  - Homogeneously isointense to muscle or adjacent nail bed on T1WI MR
  - Homogeneous to mildly heterogeneous, hyperintense signal on fluid-sensitive MR sequences
  - Intense enhancement with gadolinium is typical

PATHOLOGY

- Solid glomus tumor is most common subtype
- Glomuvenous malformation (glomangioma)
  - Less circumscribed; more likely to be extradigital
- Glomangiopericytoma = associated branching, hemangiopericytoma-like vasculature
- Glomangiomatosis = diffuse, infiltrating glomus tumor that can be deep and difficult to excise
- Malignant glomus tumor (glomangiosarcoma)
  - 25-40% mortality rate due to metastases

CLINICAL ISSUES

- Superficial lesions are usually painful and sensitive to cold temperature and touch
- < 2% of soft tissue tumors overall
- > 99% of glomus tumors are benign
- Benign lesions are treated with surgical excision

(Left) *Sagittal graphic shows a well-circumscribed mass ➡ in the subungual region. This mass is producing smooth, extrinsic erosion ↪ of the underlying distal phalanx dorsal cortex. This type of bone erosion typically has a sclerotic border when seen on radiographs.* **(Right)** *Sagittal T2WI FS MR shows a well-circumscribed oval mass ➡ located eccentrically beneath the nail of the thumb. The mass has homogeneously hyperintense signal.*

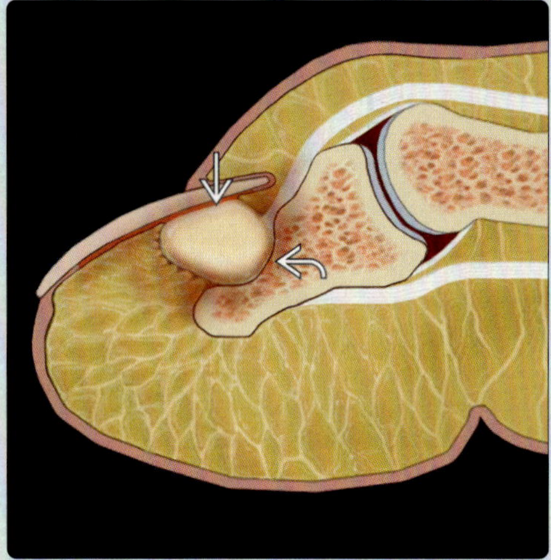

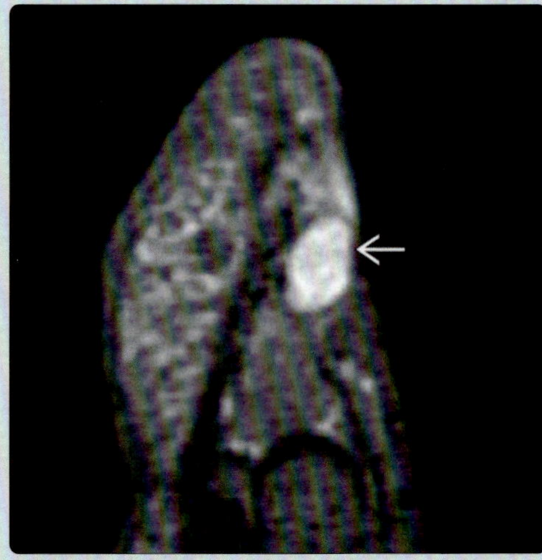

(Left) *Axial T1WI MR in the same patient shows the mass ➡ to be located within the nail bed, homogeneously isointense to the nail bed tissue, causing mild extrinsic scalloping of the underlying cortex of the distal phalanx ↪.* **(Right)** *Axial T2WI FS MR in the same patient shows the well-circumscribed mass ➡ to have homogeneously hyperintense signal. This lesion is higher in signal than the adjacent nail bed tissue. Erosion ↪ of the underlying bone is again demonstrated.*

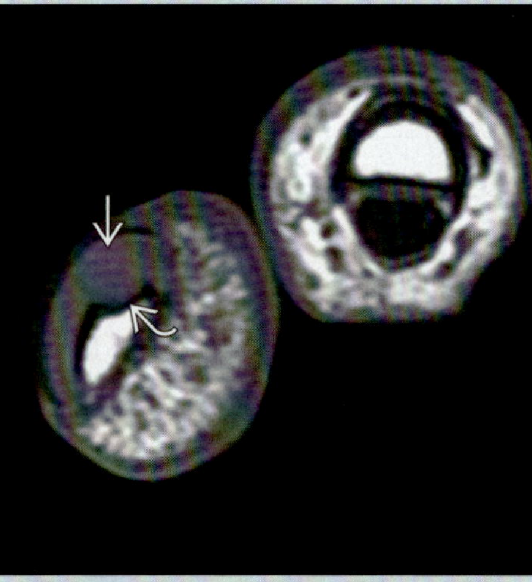

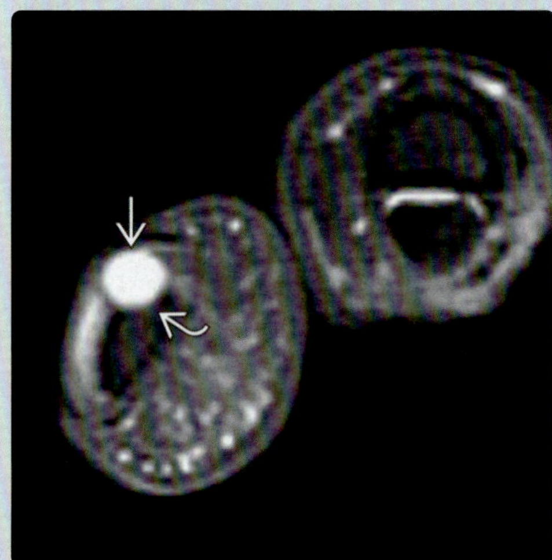

TERMINOLOGY

Definitions

- Usually benign, mesenchymal neoplasm of smooth muscle cells similar to glomus body cells

IMAGING

General Features

- Best diagnostic clue
  - Soft tissue mass in subungual region that erodes underlying bone
- Location
  - Propensity to involve subungual region
    - Almost always in superficial soft tissues
    - Rare in deep soft tissues or organs
      - Malignant glomus tumors more likely to have deep location
  - Distal extremities (fingers and toes) most common
    - Also common in palm, wrist, foot, forearm
    - Upper extremity 48%, lower extremity 48%
    - Reported throughout body (much less common)
- Size
  - Typically < 2 cm; mean 13 mm

Imaging Recommendations

- Best imaging tool
  - MR best for detecting and assessing for recurrence

Radiographic Findings

- Soft tissue mass may or may not be evident
- Subungual lesions produce scalloped defect with sclerotic border involving dorsal aspect of terminal phalanx in 22-80%

CT Findings

- May blend with nail bed or muscle on unenhanced CT

MR Findings

- Homogeneously isointense to adjacent nail bed or muscle on T1WI MR
- Homogeneous to mildly heterogeneous, hyperintense signal on fluid-sensitive sequences
  - Low signal on fluid-sensitive sequences reported
- Intense enhancement with gadolinium is typical

Ultrasonographic Findings

- Hypoechoic mass; marked vascularity on color Doppler

DIFFERENTIAL DIAGNOSIS

Epidermal Inclusion Cyst

- Posttraumatic intradermal or intraosseous cyst from penetrating trauma
- Deforms bone of distal phalanx
- Less well defined than glomus tumor
- Male predominance

PATHOLOGY

General Features

- Etiology
  - Neoplasm arising from neuromyoarterial plexus
- Genetics
  - ↑ subungual tumors with neurofibromatosis type 1
  - Multiple inherited glomus tumors: Autosomal dominant localized to chromosome 1p21-22

Gross Pathologic & Surgical Features

- Soft, well-defined red to purple nodule

Microscopic Features

- Typical glomus tumor has 3 subcategories
  - Solid glomus tumor
    - Most common (~ 75% of cases)
    - Nests of round to cuboidal glomus cells around capillaries, which may extend outside main mass
  - Glomuvenous malformation (glomangioma)
    - ~ 20% of cases
    - Glomus cell clusters around dilated veins
    - Less likely to occur in subungual location
    - Less circumscribed than solid glomus tumors
    - Multiple lesions are often of this type
  - Glomangiomyoma
    - Rarest subtype of typical glomus tumor
    - Contains elongated cells similar to smooth muscle
    - When branching, hemangiopericytoma-like vasculature is present = **glomangiopericytoma**
- Malignant glomus tumor (glomangiosarcoma)
  - < 1% of glomus tumors
  - Poor prognosis
    - 25-40% mortality rate due to metastases
  - Located deep to fascia or in viscera; > 2 cm in size; moderate to high nuclear grade; atypical mitotic figures and high mitotic activity

CLINICAL ISSUES

Presentation

- Most common signs/symptoms
  - Superficial lesions are usually painful and sensitive to cold temperature and touch (mean duration 7.2 years)

Demographics

- Age
  - Most common in adults but found at any age
  - Multiple glomus tumors are more likely to occur in childhood or adolescence
- Gender
  - Subungual lesions more common in women
  - Extradigital location more common in men
- Epidemiology
  - < 2% of soft tissue tumors overall
    - Approximately 10% are multiple

Natural History & Prognosis

- Vast majority of glomus tumors are benign

Treatment

- Benign lesions are treated with surgical excision
  - 10% local recurrence rate

SELECTED REFERENCES

1. Glazebrook KN et al: Imaging features of glomus tumors. Skeletal Radiol. 40(7):855-62, 2011

(Left) *Sagittal T1WI MR of a glomangiopericytoma* ➔ *shows multiple masses in the soft tissues that extend from the distal calf into the foot. These masses are heterogeneously isointense to hyperintense relative to muscle on T1WI and were present in the subcutaneous fat and in the deep musculature.* **(Right)** *Sagittal T1WI C+ FS MR in the same patient shows intense, heterogeneous enhancement of the dominant mass* ➔ *and best demonstrates the large associated blood vessels* ⇨.

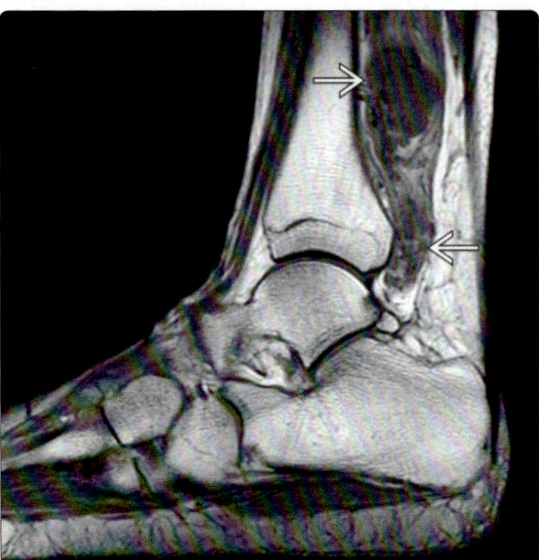

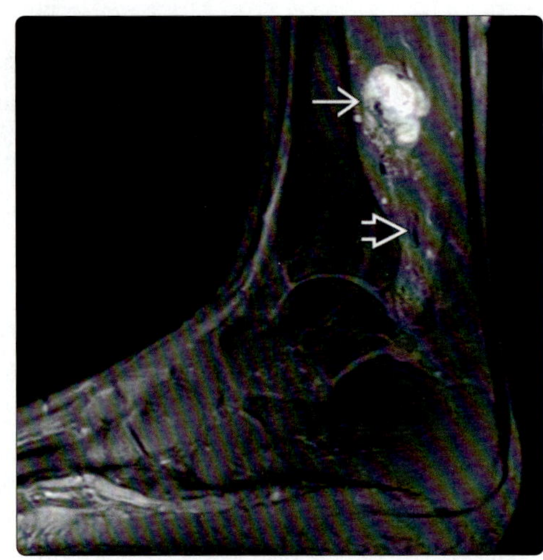

(Left) *Longitudinal color Doppler ultrasound of the glomangiopericytoma in the same patient shows an ill-defined, hypoechoic lesion* ➔ *with prominent blood flow.* **(Right)** *Axial noncontrast CT shows a round, mildly hyperdense mass* ➔ *within the posterolateral aspect of the deltoid muscle of a 39-year-old man. This lesion was painful. Percutaneous biopsy confirmed a glomus tumor. Although these lesions are typically subungual, glomus tumors have been reported throughout the body.*

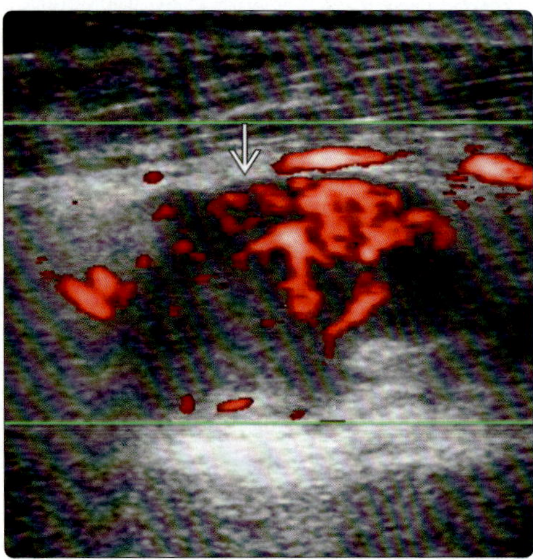

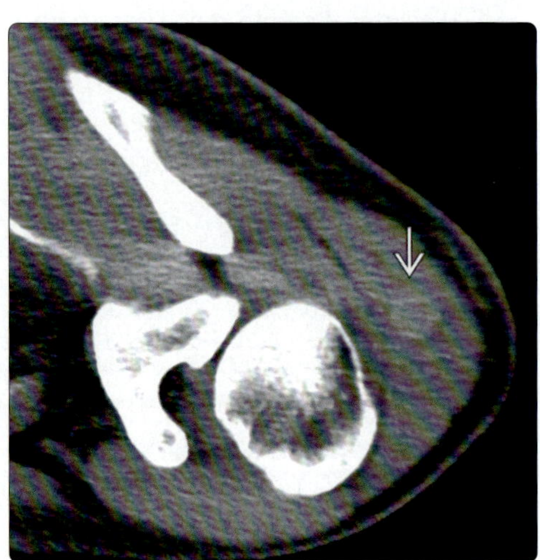

(Left) *Axial T1WI MR of a glomuvenous malformation (glomangioma) demonstrates a lobulated mass* ➔ *in the anterolateral subcutaneous fat of the knee. The mass is isointense to skeletal muscle and abuts the dermis.* **(Right)** *Axial T2WI FS MR demonstrates homogeneously hyperintense signal of the lobulated mass* ➔. *There is no edema surrounding the mass, which intensely enhanced (not shown). The differential diagnosis for this lesion includes a foreign body granuloma and posttraumatic neuroma.*

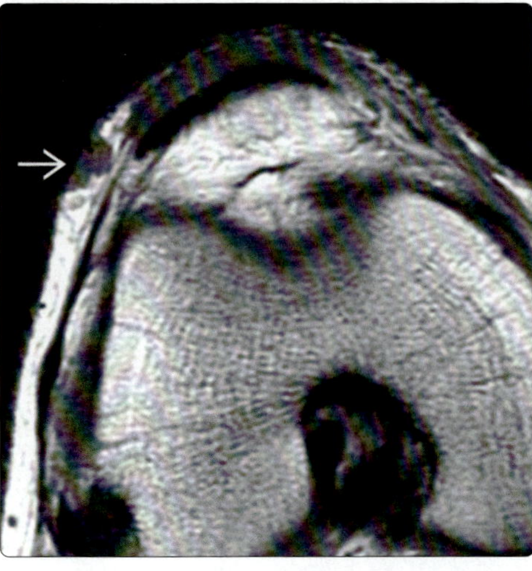

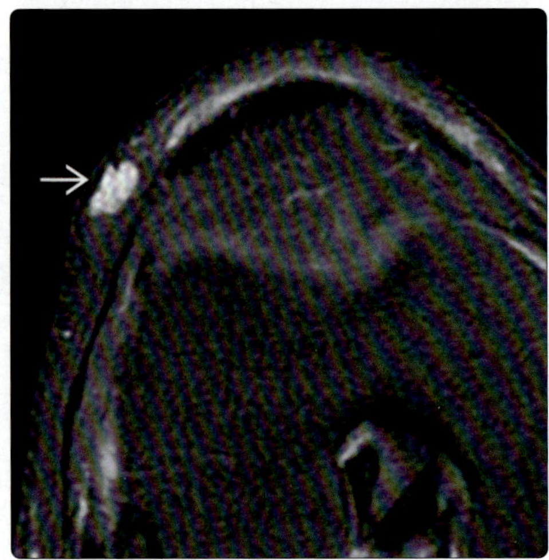

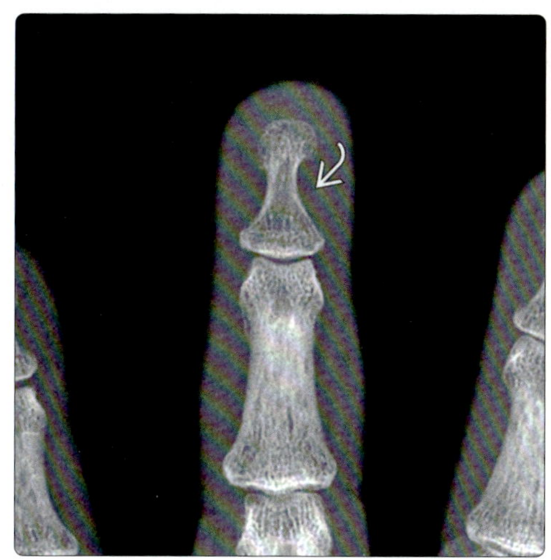

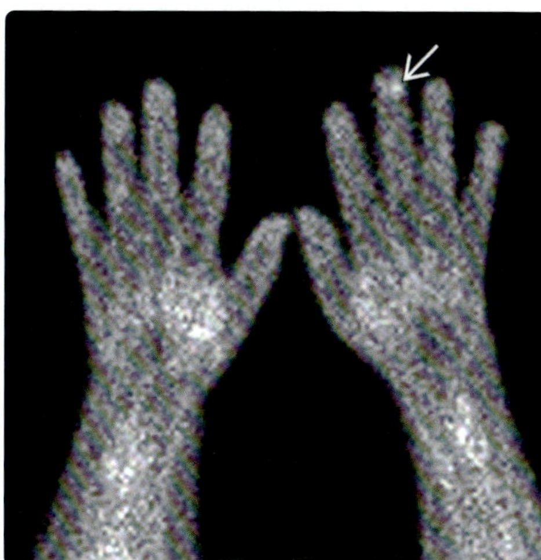

(Left) *PA radiograph of a classic glomus tumor shows smooth erosion ➡ of the ulnar side of the middle finger distal phalanx. The borders of the erosion are sclerotic and well defined, suggesting a longstanding lesion. No soft tissue mass was evident. This 60-year-old woman reported fingertip pain for several years.* **(Right)** *PA blood pool image from a bone scan shows increased tracer activity in the soft tissues ➡ immediately adjacent to the region of bone erosion seen on the previous radiograph.*

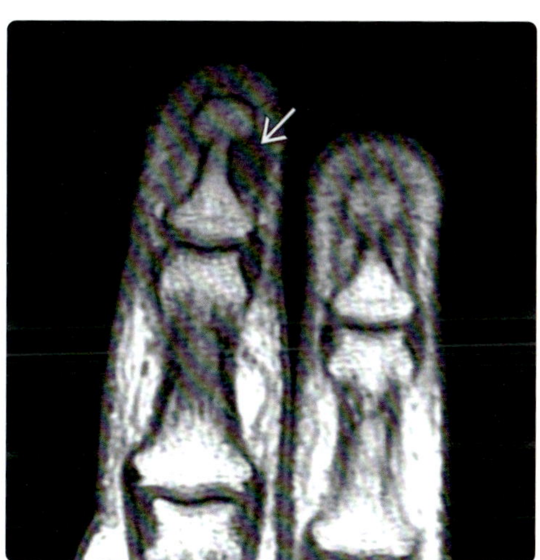

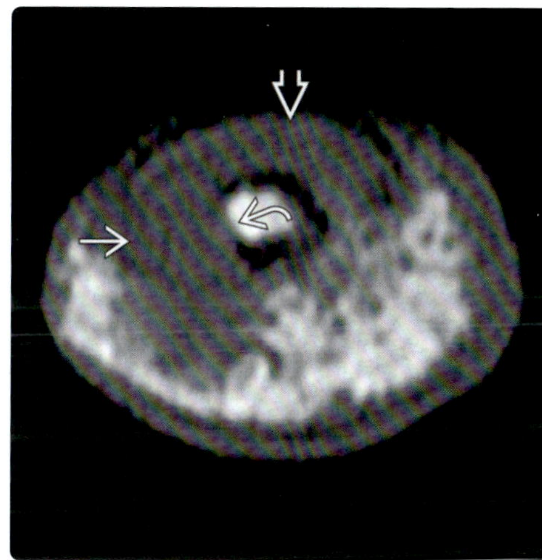

(Left) *Coronal T1WI MR in the same patient shows a soft tissue mass ➡ extending around the ulnar side of the distal phalanx shaft and producing underlying bone erosion.* **(Right)** *Axial T1WI MR shows the soft tissue mass ➡ to be located within the ulnar border of the long finger nail bed. The mass is isointense to the normal nail bed soft tissue ➡ located anteriorly. The mass smoothly erodes ➡ the underlying bone cortex.*

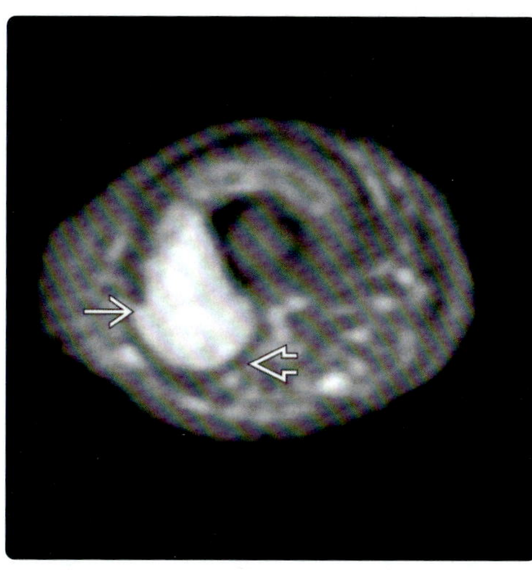

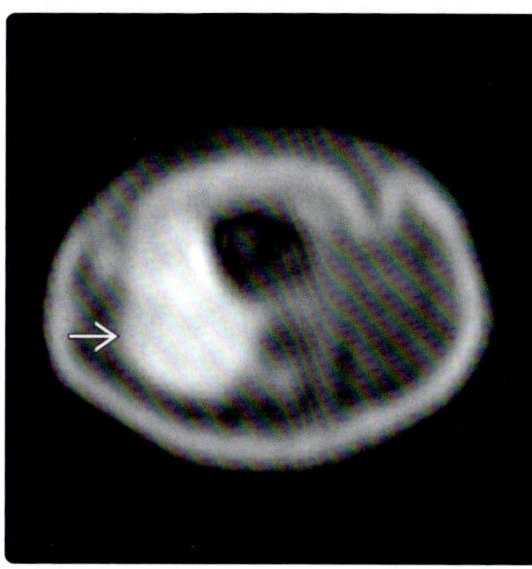

(Left) *Axial T2WI FS MR in the same patient shows the nail bed mass ➡ to be mildly hyperintense to the remainder of the nail bed tissue. The mass extends into the soft tissues ➡ of the distal phalanx.* **(Right)** *Axial T1WI C+ FS MR shows intense, homogeneous enhancement of the mass ➡, typical for a glomus tumor. An epidermal inclusion cyst could also erode the distal phalanx but would not be expected to have well-circumscribed, intense enhancement.*

KEY FACTS

IMAGING

- Adult and fetal RM → 90% in soft tissues/mucosa of head and neck
- Genital RM: Vagina, vulva, and cervix
  - Rare in paratesticular region and epididymis
- Cardiac RM: Left ventricle and septum
  - 30% in right ventricle or in atria
- RM involving mucosal surface may be visible as filling defect on contrast fluoroscopy studies
- Similar CT attenuation as muscle, + enhancement
- Echocardiography shows well-circumscribed echogenic myocardial masses
- MR: Homogeneous to mildly heterogeneous signal
  - Isointense or hyperintense to skeletal muscle on T1WI and fluid-sensitive sequences
  - Hemorrhage or necrosis is uncommon
  - Extracardiac lesions mildly enhance
    - Cardiac lesions are hypointense to myocardium postgadolinium

CLINICAL ISSUES

- Slowly growing solitary mass may be asymptomatic
  - Upper airway obstruction not uncommon
- Cardiac RM are most symptomatic
  - Dysrhythmias, hydrops, low cardiac output, respiratory distress, congestive heart failure, cyanosis, death
  - Associated with tuberous sclerosis
- 2% of muscle tumors
- Adult and genital RM: Middle-aged adults
- Fetal and cardiac RM: Children
- No aggressive behavior or metastases
  - May locally recur
- Adult, fetal, and genital RM: Surgical excision
- Cardiac RM: Spontaneously regress; surgical resection only if causing serious clinical symptoms

(Left) *Axial CECT in a patient with adult rhabdomyoma shows a homogeneously enhancing, well-circumscribed mass ➡ in the right parapharyngeal space. The neck was otherwise normal.* **(Right)** *Axial T1WI MR shows the parapharyngeal mass ➡ to be slightly hyperintense relative to muscle. The adult rhabdomyoma in this case produced a typical clinical presentation, typified by a middle-aged man with a slowly growing mass in the head and neck.*

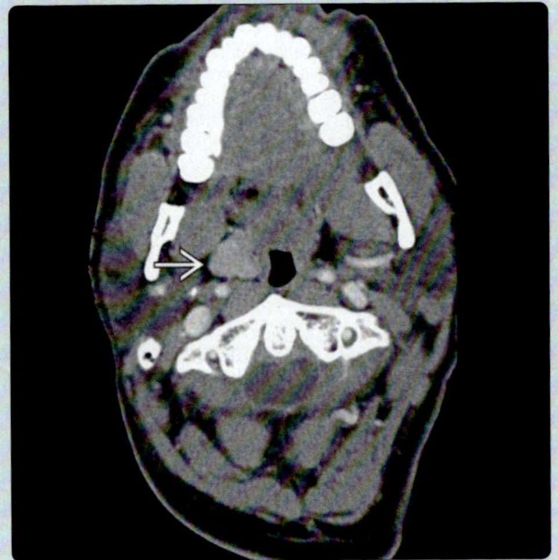

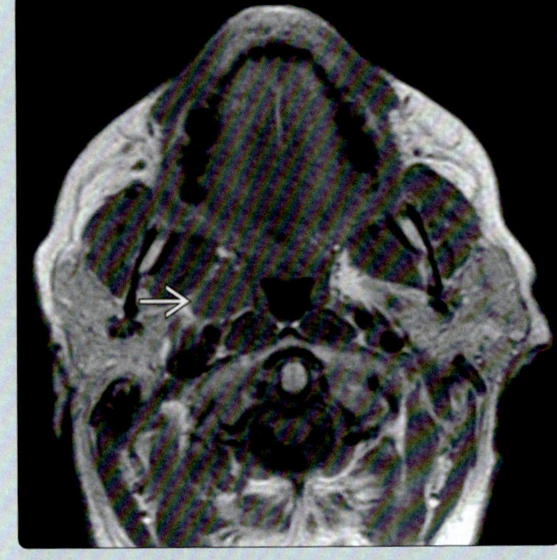

(Left) *Axial T2WI FS MR in the same patient demonstrates the mass ➡ to be heterogeneously hyperintense to muscle.* **(Right)** *Axial T1WI C+ FS MR shows the parapharyngeal mass ➡ to have mild enhancement with peripheral foci of more intense enhancement. MR imaging of adult rhabdomyomas usually reveals a well-defined mass that is isointense to hyperintense to muscle on T1 and T2WI. Enhancement is typical and may be homogeneous or heterogeneous.*

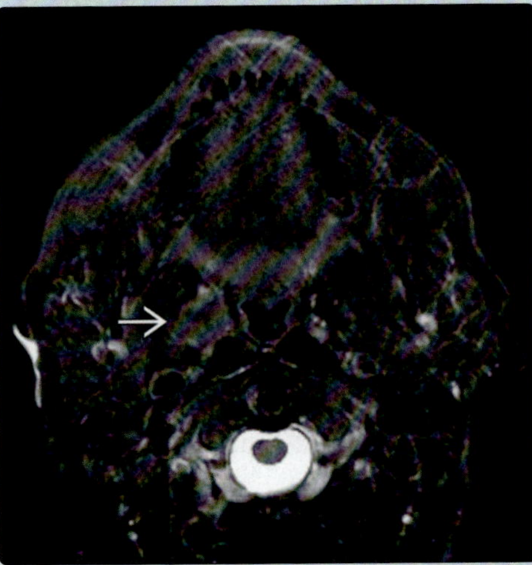

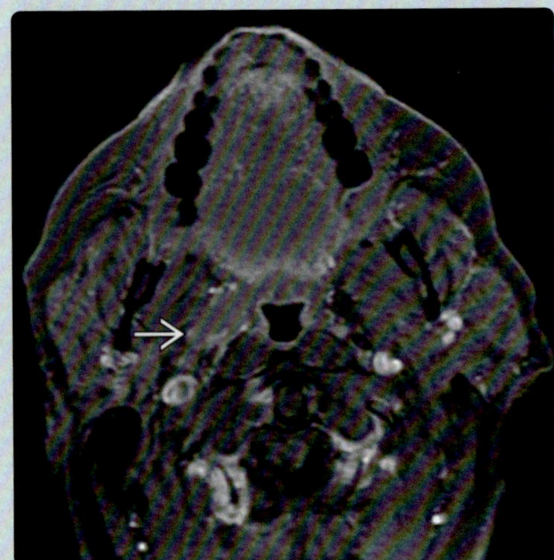

TERMINOLOGY

Abbreviations

- Rhabdomyoma (RM)
- Fetal rhabdomyoma (F-RM)
- Adult rhabdomyoma (A-RM)
- Genital rhabdomyoma (G-RM)
- Cardiac rhabdomyoma (C-RM)

IMAGING

General Features

- Location
  - Adult and fetal RM: 90% in soft tissues/mucosa of head and neck
    - Postauricular soft tissues in fetal RM
  - Genital RM: Vagina, vulva, and cervix
    - Rare in paratesticular region and epididymis
  - Cardiac RM: Left ventricle and septum
    - 30% in right ventricle or in atria
- Size
  - A-RM, F-RM, G-RM: median size 2-3 cm
  - Sporadic solitary cardiac lesions: Median size 3.4 cm
    - Multiple miliary cardiac nodules < 1 mm each

Radiographic Findings

- RM involving mucosal surface may be visible as filling defect on contrast fluoroscopy studies

CT Findings

- Similar attenuation as muscle, + enhancement

MR Findings

- Homogeneous to mildly heterogeneous signal that is isointense or hyperintense to skeletal muscle on T1WI and fluid-sensitive sequences
  - Extracardiac lesions mildly enhance
  - Cardiac lesions are hypointense to myocardium postgadolinium
- Hemorrhage or necrosis is uncommon

Ultrasonographic Findings

- Echocardiography shows well-circumscribed echogenic myocardial masses

DIFFERENTIAL DIAGNOSIS

Rhabdomyosarcoma

- Poorly differentiated, pleomorphic round to spindle-shaped cells
- Nuclear atypia and ↑ mitotic activity differentiate from rhabdomyoma

Granular Cell Tumor

- Commonly arises in skin, tongue, larynx
- Historically confused with rhabdomyoma due to histologic similarity
  - Cells are not vacuolated

Salivary Gland Oncocytoma

- Benign epithelial neoplasm most common in parotid gland of elderly females
- Polyhedral epithelial oncocytes with granular eosinophilic cytoplasm
- Negative staining for actin or desmin

PATHOLOGY

General Features

- Genetics
  - Cardiac RM associated with tuberous sclerosis
    - 30% of patients with tuberous sclerosis develop cardiac RM
      - 90% have miliary morphology
  - Fetal RM associated with nevoid basal cell carcinoma syndrome

Microscopic Features

- Adult RM: Large polygonal cells with little stroma
  - "Spider cells" in A-RM and C-RM, when strands of cytoplasm stretch from peripheral cell membrane to central nucleus
- Fetal RM: Bland fetal myotubules and primitive spindle cells in myxoid stroma
- Genital RM: Strap-like rhabdomyoblasts with dilated vessels in fibrous stroma
- Cardiac RM: Enlarged cardiac myocytes with vacuolization and prominent intracellular glycogen

CLINICAL ISSUES

Presentation

- Most common signs/symptoms
  - Slowly growing solitary mass may be asymptomatic
    - Upper airway obstruction not uncommon
  - Cardiac RM are most symptomatic
    - Dysrhythmias, hydrops, low cardiac output, respiratory distress, congestive heart failure, cyanosis, death

Demographics

- Age
  - Adult and genital RM: Middle-aged adults
  - Fetal and cardiac RM: Children
- Gender
  - Male predominance in A-RM and F-RM
  - Female predominance in G-RM
- Epidemiology
  - 2% of muscle tumors

Natural History & Prognosis

- No aggressive behavior or metastases
- May locally recur

Treatment

- Adult, fetal, and genital RM: Surgical excision
- Cardiac RM: Spontaneously regress; surgical resection only if causing serious clinical symptoms
  - Non-life-threatening arrhythmias treated medically

SELECTED REFERENCES

1. Sciacca P et al: Rhabdomyomas and tuberous sclerosis complex: our experience in 33 cases. BMC Cardiovasc Disord. 14:66, 2014

Rhabdomyosarcoma

KEY FACTS

TERMINOLOGY

- Malignant tumor showing skeletal muscle differentiation
- Most common soft tissue malignancy in childhood
  - 19% of all childhood sarcomas
  - 5-8% of all cancers in childhood

IMAGING

- Head & neck > > genitourinary system > extremities
  - Rhabdomyosarcoma (RMS) reported throughout body
- Average size: 3-4 cm
- Permeative bone invasion in approximately 1/4
  - ± periosteal reaction
- Bone metastases lytic, or mixed sclerotic and lytic
- CT: Circumscribed to infiltrative soft tissue mass
  - ± necrosis &/or hemorrhage
- MR findings
  - Isointense to hyperintense relative to skeletal muscle on T1WI
  - Hyperintense on fluid-sensitive sequences
  - Heterogeneous enhancement dependent on vascularity and hemorrhage/necrosis
    - High-flow vessels, especially in alveolar type

CLINICAL ISSUES

- Painless, rapidly growing mass
  - Symptoms are related to mass effect
- Age: Predominantly infants to adolescents, most < 5 years of age → embryonal RMS
  - Children to young adults → alveolar RMS
  - Least common in adults → almost exclusively pleomorphic RMS
- Non-Hispanic Caucasian (70%) > > African American > Asian
- Gender: Mild male predominance overall
- Treatment: Combination of surgery, chemotherapy, and radiotherapy based on patient's risk of disease recurrence
- Natural history: Prognosis related to age, size at presentation, location, histologic variant of lesion, completeness of resection

(Left) *Axial graphic shows a mass ➡ in the lateral aspect of the distal thigh that erodes ↪ into the distal femur.* **(Right)** *Coronal T1WI MR shows a large soft tissue mass ➡ with heterogeneous signal ranging from hyperintense to isointense relative to skeletal muscle. The femoral cortex is eroded and the marrow space is extensively involved with tumor ⇨. Coronal imaging serves to identify an external landmark (knee joint line) from which to measure proximal and distal extent of tumor.*

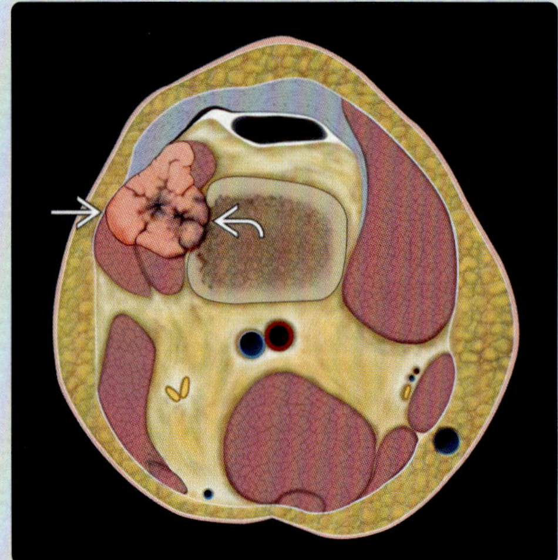

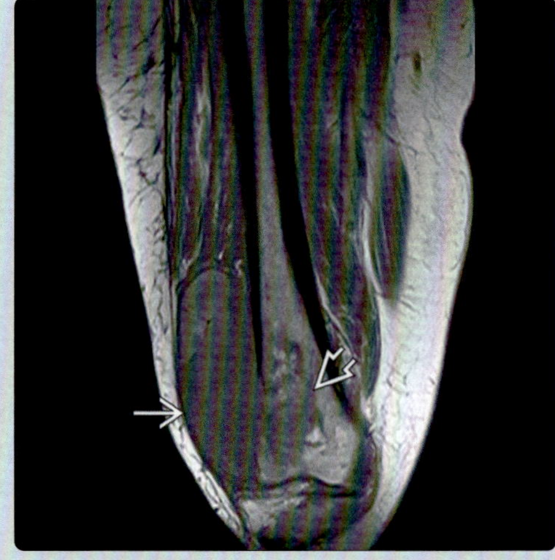

(Left) *Axial PDWI FS MR shows the mass ➡ to have heterogeneously high signal. Tumor involves the anterior compartment and the bone ↪, but does not invade the posterior compartment or neurovascular bundle. It does extend to involve the joint, which is unusual.* **(Right)** *Coronal T1WI C+ FS MR shows inhomogeneous enhancement of the mass ➡. Enhancing tumor, as opposed to edema, which would not enhance, is confirmed to involve the marrow space ⇨ where the femoral cortex has been breached.*

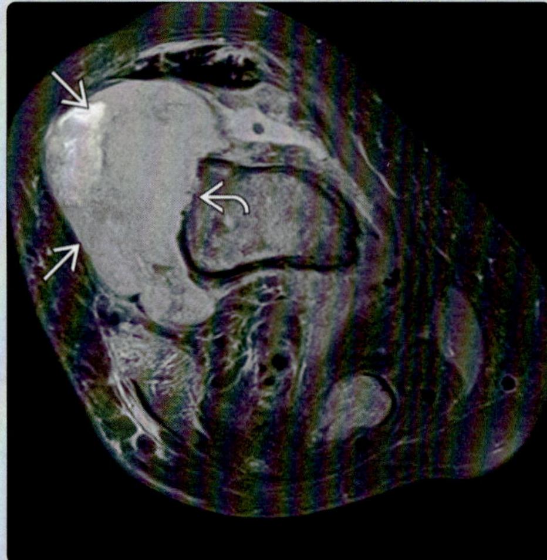

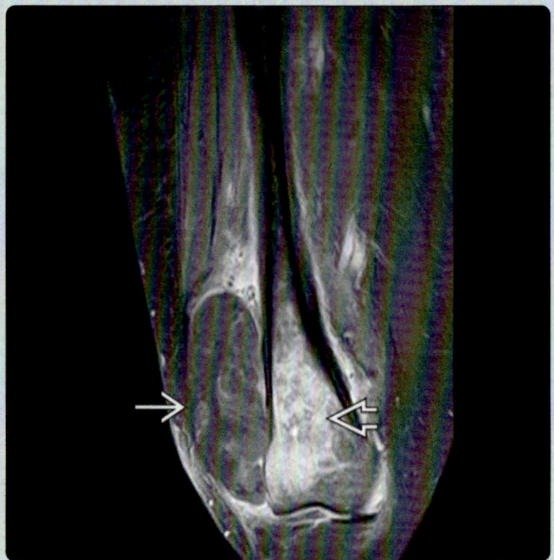

TERMINOLOGY

Abbreviations

- Rhabdomyosarcoma (RMS)

Synonyms

- Embryonal RMS → malignant rhabdomyoma, rhabdomyosarcoma, myosarcoma, rhabdopoietic sarcoma, rhabdosarcoma, embryonal sarcoma
- Alveolar RMS → monomorphous round cell rhabdomyosarcoma, rhabdomyoblastoma, rhabdomyopoietic sarcoma

Definitions

- Malignant tumor showing skeletal muscle differentiation, with 3 main subtypes being embryonal, alveolar, and pleomorphic

IMAGING

General Features

- Best diagnostic clue
  - Aggressive-appearing soft tissue mass in child
- Location
  - Head and neck > > genitourinary system > extremities
    - RMS reported throughout body
    - Head and neck and genitourinary lesions are usually embryonal, which is most common type
    - Extremity soft tissue lesions are usually alveolar
- Size
  - Average: 3-4 cm
    - Pleomorphic lesions usually 5-15 cm
- Morphology
  - Well-circumscribed, multinodular masses

Radiographic Findings

- Permeative bone invasion in approximately 1/4
  - ± periosteal reaction
- Bone metastases lytic or mixed sclerotic and lytic

CT Findings

- Circumscribed to infiltrative soft tissue mass
  - Heterogeneously enhances
  - ± necrosis &/or hemorrhage

MR Findings

- Isointense to hyperintense relative to skeletal muscle on T1WI
- Hyperintense to skeletal muscle on fluid-sensitive sequences
- Hypointensity on T1WI and fluid-sensitive sequences
- Heterogeneous enhancement dependent on vascularity and hemorrhage/necrosis
  - High-flow vessels, especially alveolar type

Ultrasonographic Findings

- Heterogeneous echogenicity
- ± prominent vascularity on Doppler

Nuclear Medicine Findings

- Bone scan
  - Useful for detection of bone invasion and bone marrow metastases
- PET
  - F-18 FDG-avid tumors

DIFFERENTIAL DIAGNOSIS

Infantile Fibrosarcoma

- Painless, rapidly enlarging mass in extremity of infant
- Most common in 1st year of life
- Bone destruction, erosion, cortical thickening in < 5%
- ± hemorrhage &/or necrosis
- Can be prominently hypervascular

Infantile Rhabdomyofibrosarcoma

- Resembles infantile fibrosarcoma with rhabdomyoblastic differentiation
- Distinct monosomy 19 and 22 cytogenetic alterations
- Similar age range and imaging appearance

Malignant Extrarenal Rhabdoid Tumor

- Perirenal location in child < 1 year old
- Hemorrhage and necrosis common
- < 50% 5-year survival rate

Fasciitis, Nodular and Proliferative

- Most common in adults
- Rapidly growing, tender mass associated with fascia
- Heterogeneous imaging appearance depending on cellular composition

Fibrous Hamartoma of Infancy

- Rapidly growing soft tissue mass predominately involving shoulder girdle of infants
- Contains variable amount of fat on MR imaging
- Benign clinical course, but may locally recur

PATHOLOGY

General Features

- Etiology
  - Primary malignant mesenchymal tumor with rhabdomyoblastic differentiation
    - Embryonal RMS may arise from chromosomal mutations (sporadic or inherited)
- Genetics
  - Embryonal → allelic loss on chromosome 11p15
- Associated abnormalities
  - Associated with neurofibromatosis type 1, Beckwith-Wiedemann syndrome, Costello syndrome, Li-Fraumeni syndrome, and maternal illicit drug use

Staging, Grading, & Classification

- Soft Tissue Sarcoma Committee of the Children's Oncology Group (formerly known as Intergroup Rhabdomyosarcoma Study Group)
  - Complete resection vs. varying degrees of partial resection
  - Extent of tumor beyond muscle or organ of origin
  - Nodal involvement
  - Distant metastases

Gross Pathologic & Surgical Features

- Embryonal and alveolar RMS → poorly circumscribed, pale tan, fleshy lesions

- Spindle cell type → tan-yellow firm, fibrous lesion with whorled cut surface
- Botryoid type → grape-like nodular growth involving mucosal-lined hollow organ
- Pleomorphic RMS → pseudoencapsulated, firm white mass

Microscopic Features

- Embryonal RMS → variable pattern from poorly differentiated to well-differentiated embryonic muscle tissue in mucoid stroma
  - Botryoid type has "cambium layer" of tumor cells abutting epithelial surface
  - Spindle cell type has storiform architecture
  - Anaplastic type has large, atypical cells with hyperchromatic nuclei
- Alveolar RMS → nests of rhabdomyoblasts and undifferentiated tumor cells with collagenous fibrovascular septa
  - Round cell cytological features similar to lymphoma
  - Histologic subtypes based on typical features, solid pattern, or mixed embryonal & alveolar features
    - Giant cells common in typical subtype
    - Fibrovascular stroma absent in solid pattern
    - Embryonal histology present in mixed subtype
- Pleomorphic RMS → least common type containing bizarre spindle, round, and polygonal cells with skeletal muscle differentiation
  - Predominately lacks cross striations that are common in embryonal RMS
  - Ultrastructurally contains rudimentary sarcomeres
- MYOD1 and myogenin antibodies highly sensitive and specific for RMS

CLINICAL ISSUES

Presentation

- Most common signs/symptoms
  - Painless, rapidly growing mass
  - Symptoms are related to mass effect
    - Abdominal → bowel obstruction
    - Head and neck → cranial nerve deficits, proptosis, sinusitis, diplopia, unilateral deafness
    - Genitourinary → hydronephrosis, urinary retention
    - Paraspinal → hyperesthesia, paresthesia, paresis
    - Biliary → jaundice

Demographics

- Age
  - Predominantly infants to adolescents; most < 5 years of age → embryonal RMS
  - Children to young adults; median 16 years of age → alveolar RMS
  - Least common in adults; median 5th to 6th decade of life → almost exclusively pleomorphic RMS
- Gender
  - Mild male predominance overall
- Ethnicity
  - Non-Hispanic Caucasian (70%) > > African American > Asian
- Epidemiology
  - Most common soft tissue malignancy in childhood
    - 19% of all childhood sarcomas
    - 5-8% of all cancers in childhood
    - 4.6 per 1 million children < 15 years old in USA

Natural History & Prognosis

- Favorable prognostic factors
  - Presentation in infancy or childhood
  - Location in orbit or genitourinary system
  - Size < 5 cm
  - Botryoid or spindle cell variant of embryonal RMS
  - Complete initial resection of localized tumor
  - No lymph node or distant metastases
- Unfavorable prognostic factors
  - Presentation in adulthood
  - Location outside of orbit or genitourinary system
  - Size > 5 cm
  - Alveolar RMS or pleomorphic RMS
    - Alveolar RMS are often high-stage lesions at presentation
  - Incomplete initial resection
  - Local tumor recurrence
  - Lymph node involvement or distant metastases (lung most common)

Treatment

- Combination of surgery, chemotherapy, and radiotherapy based on patient's risk of recurrence

DIAGNOSTIC CHECKLIST

Consider

- Percutaneous biopsies should mimic definitive surgical approach to allow resection of track

Reporting Tips

- Maximum diameter of tumor, with 3-plane measurements useful for follow-up
- Anatomic compartment(s) or organs involved
- Craniocaudad location referenced to anatomic landmark
- Neurovascular or bone invasion
- Appearance of regional lymph nodes
- Evidence of distant metastasis

SELECTED REFERENCES

1. Chung EM et al: Solid tumors of the peritoneum, omentum, and mesentery in children: radiologic-pathologic correlation: from the radiologic pathology archives. Radiographics. 35(2):521-46, 2015
2. Karunanithi S et al: Spectrum of physiologic and pathologic skeletal muscle (18)F-FDG uptake on PET/CT. AJR Am J Roentgenol. 205(2):W141-9, 2015
3. Saboo SS et al: Imaging features of primary and secondary adult rhabdomyosarcoma. AJR Am J Roentgenol. 199(6):W694-703, 2012
4. National Cancer Institute: Childhood Rhabdomyosarcoma Treatment. http://www.cancer.gov/cancertopics/pdq/treatment/childrhabdomyosarcoma/HealthProfessional/page6. Updated August 5, 2015. Accessed October 22, 2009
5. Weiss SW et al: Rhabdomyosarcoma. In Weiss SW et al: Enzinger and Weiss' Soft Tissue Tumors. 5th ed. Philadelphia: Elsevier. 595-631, 2008
6. Kransdorf MJ et al: Muscle Tumors. In Kransdorf MJ et al: Imaging of Soft Tissue Tumors. 2nd ed. Philadelphia: Lippincott Williams & Wilkins. 312-24, 2006
7. Breneman JC et al: Prognostic factors and clinical outcomes in children and adolescents with metastatic rhabdomyosarcoma—a report from the Intergroup Rhabdomyosarcoma Study IV. J Clin Oncol. 21(1):78-84, 2003
8. Montgomery E et al: Pleomorphic rhabdomyosarcoma. In Fletcher CDM et al: World Health Organization Classification of Tumours. Pathology and Genetics of Tumours of Soft Tissue and Bone. Lyon: IARC Press. 153-4, 2002

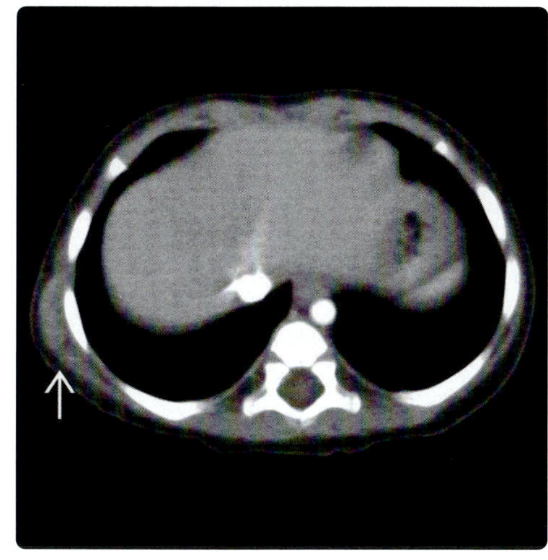

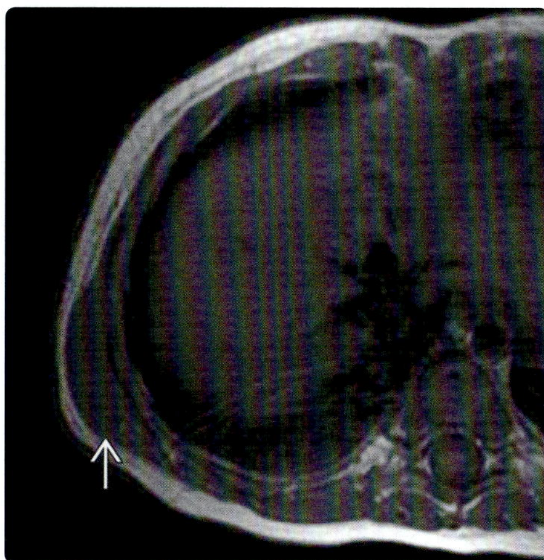

(Left) *Axial CECT demonstrates a nonspecific soft tissue mass ➡ involving the lateral aspect of the right lower chest. This nontender mass in a 1-year-old boy was noted by the patient's mother. The mass has mixed attenuation ranging from hypodense to slightly hyperdense relative to skeletal muscle.* **(Right)** *Axial T1WI MR in the same patient shows the mass ➡ to be slightly hypointense relative to skeletal muscle. The borders of this mass are ill-defined.*

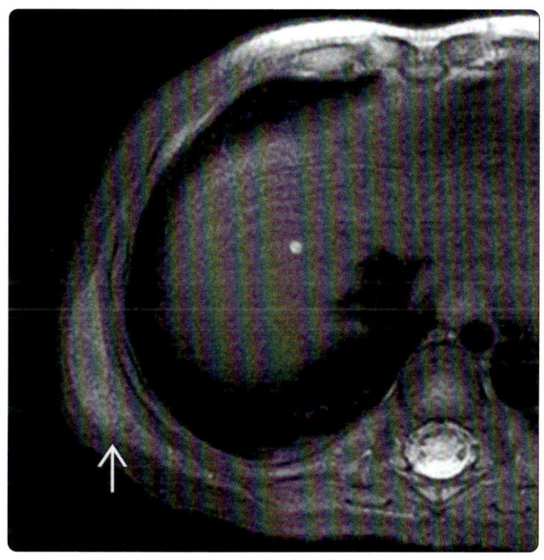

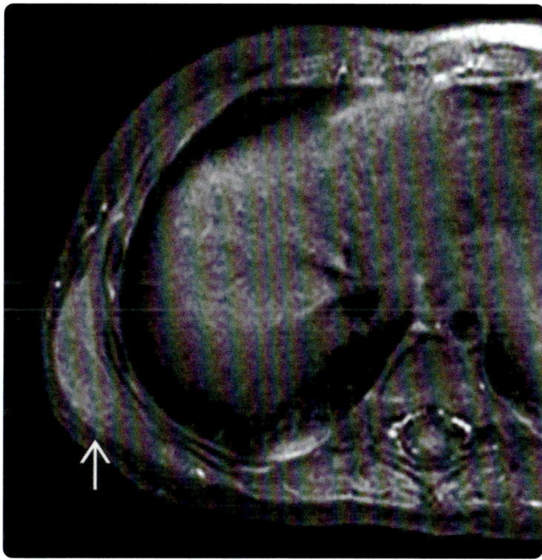

(Left) *Axial T2WI FS MR in the same patient shows the mass ➡ to have mildly heterogeneous signal that is hyperintense relative to skeletal muscle. There is no involvement of the underlying ribs.* **(Right)** *Axial T1WI C+ FS MR in the same patient shows heterogeneous mild enhancement of the mass ➡. There were no areas of hemorrhage, necrosis, or enlarged vessels, which can sometimes be present. There was no evidence of lymph node involvement or distant metastasis.*

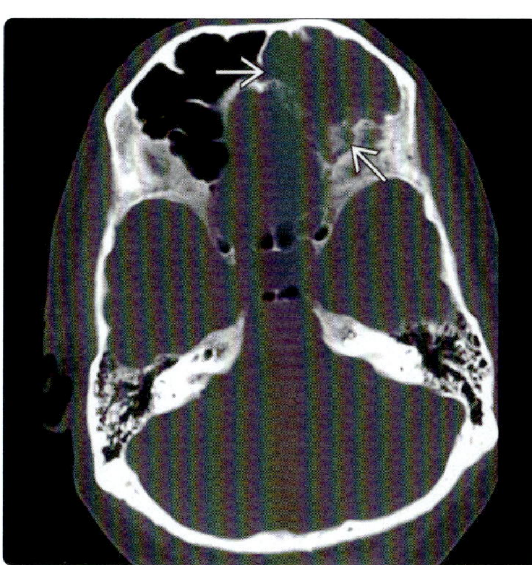

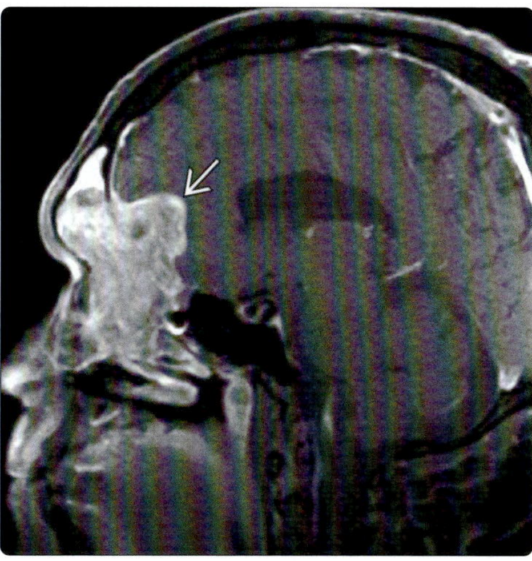

(Left) *Axial NECT through paranasal sinuses demonstrates a mass ➡ centered in left frontal-ethmoid junction, with invasion of left frontal sinus, and significant bone destruction.* **(Right)** *Sagittal T1WI C+ MR shows that the large, heterogeneously enhancing mass ➡ destroys frontal bone, transgresses the dura, and invades the anterior cranial fossa. A squamous cell carcinoma, lymphoma, or esthesioneuroblastoma was initially favored in this adult patient with proven rhabdomyosarcoma (RMS).*

(Left) *Axial soft tissue algorithm CT through the pelvis of an infant shows an extremely large, heterogeneously enhancing mass ➔ occupying the majority of the pelvis. The mass has a large central region of low attenuation that is consistent with necrosis ⇨. The bladder ↶ is laterally displaced.* **(Right)** *Transverse Doppler US in the same patient shows the heterogeneous, aggressive-appearing mass ➔ to be moderately vascular and contain hypoechoic necrotic regions ⇨.*

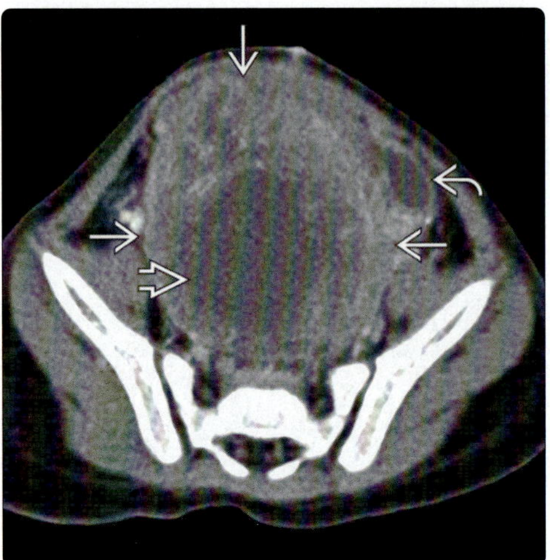

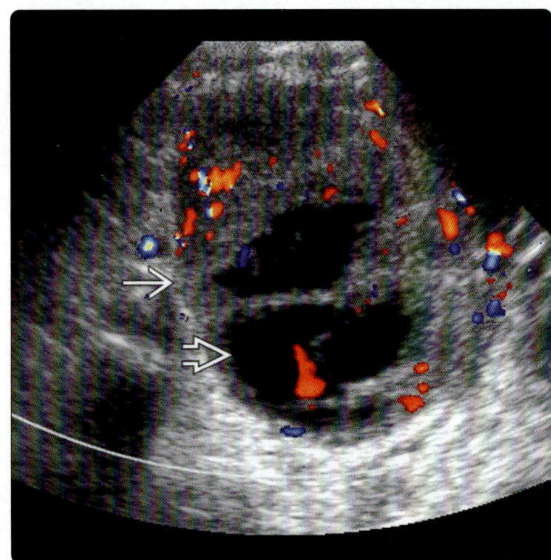

(Left) *Coronal T1WI MR demonstrates a large soft tissue mass ➔ centered in the right upper thigh. The mass has a variable signal intensity ranging from fluid-like low signal to signal that is mildly hyperintense relative to skeletal muscle. On T2WI MR (not shown), the lesion was heterogeneously hyperintense with surrounding edema.* **(Right)** *Coronal T1WI C+ FS MR shows the mass ➔ to heterogeneously enhance. Regions lacking enhancement ↶ likely represent necrosis. This was a sclerosing type of RMS.*

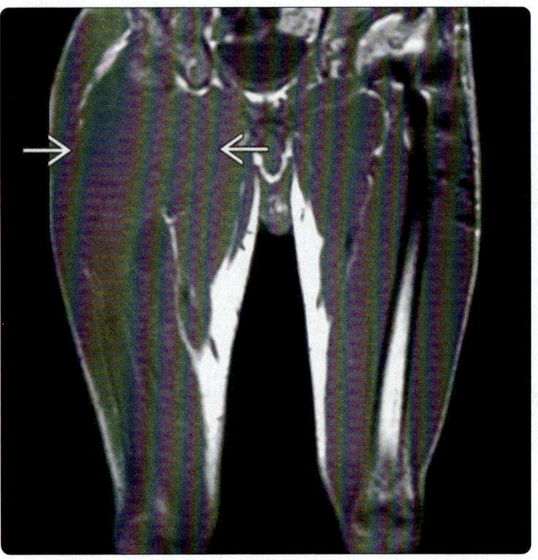

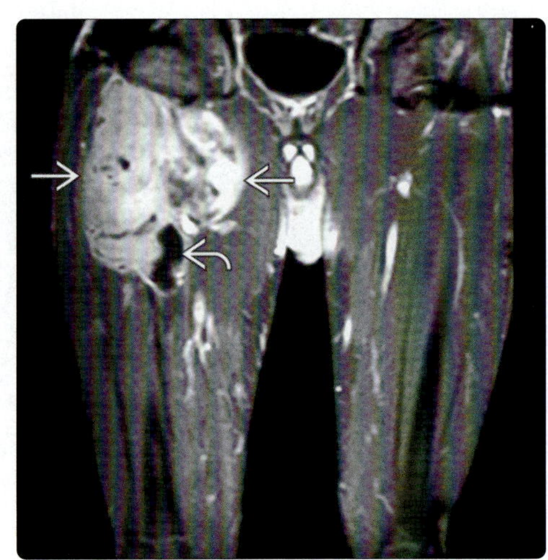

(Left) *Axial NECT with a bone algorithm shows a homogeneously low-attenuation, nonspecific soft tissue mass ⇨ involving the hypothenar region of the hand.* **(Right)** *Axial T1WI C+ MR shows the mass ⇨ to have prominent, mildly heterogeneous enhancement. The mass is relatively well defined and involves the palmaris brevis and flexor digitorum minimi muscles. There is no involvement of the neurovascular bundle or carpal tunnel. The imaging findings are nonspecific, but RMS was proven at biopsy.*

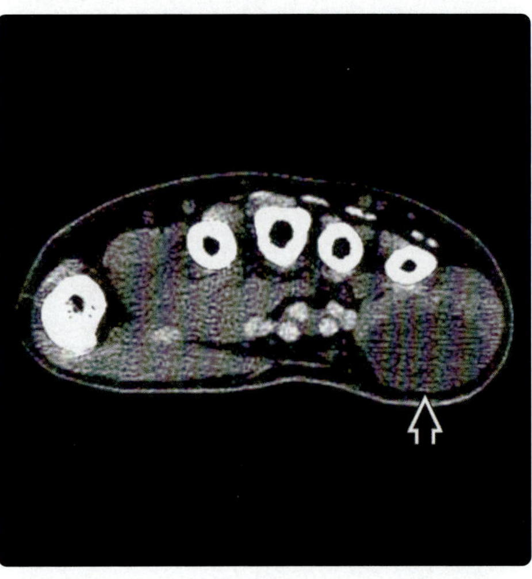

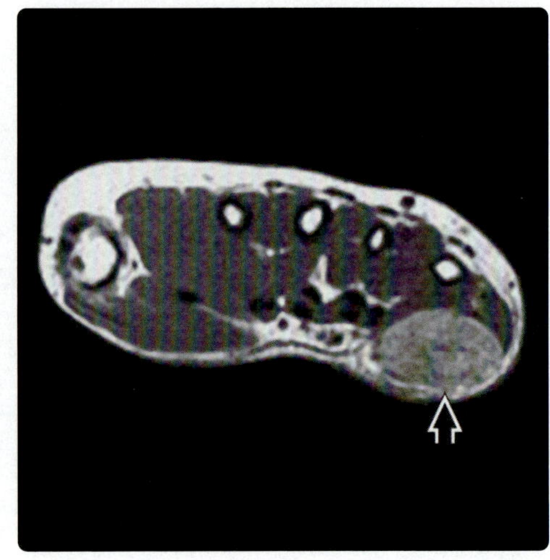

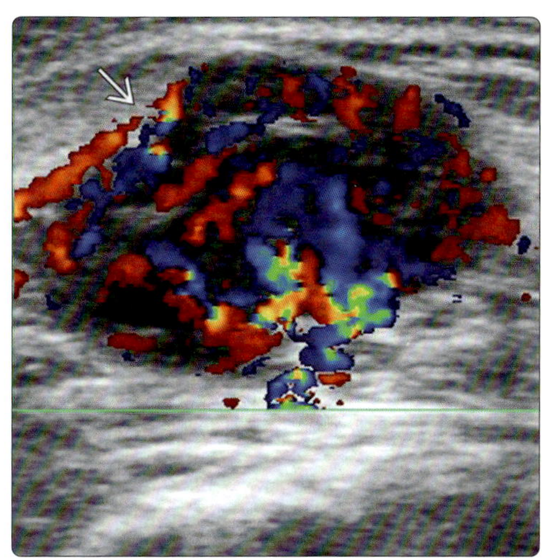

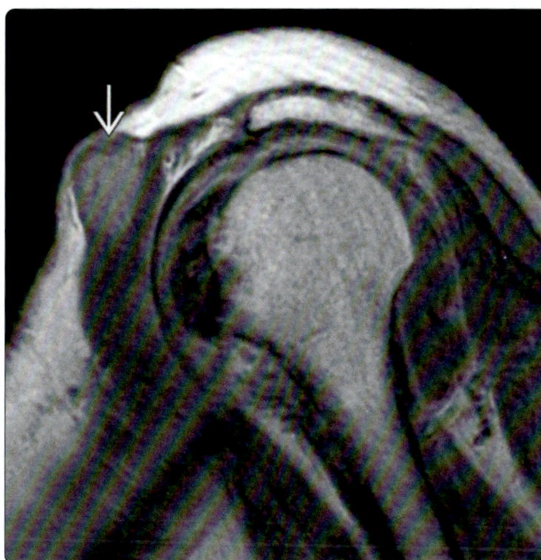

(Left) *Longitudinal Doppler US shows an ovoid hypervascular mass ➡. The mass was superficially located in this adult patient.* **(Right)** *Sagittal PDWI MR in the same patient shows a circumscribed mass ➡ in the anterior aspect of the deltoid muscle. The mass is hyperintense to skeletal muscle on this fluid-sensitive sequence and was isointense to muscle on T1WI, and had prominent enhancement with IV gadolinium. The mass has a nonspecific appearance, but proved to be RMS.*

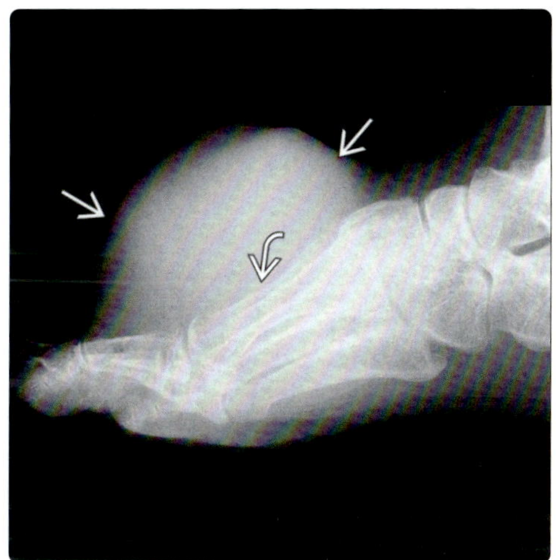

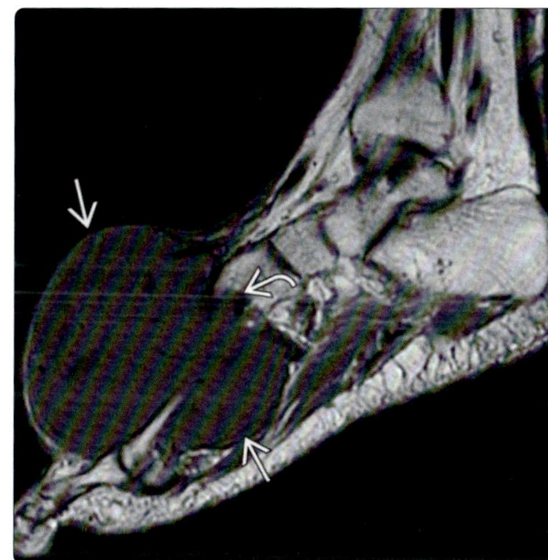

(Left) *Lateral radiograph of the foot in a 43-year-old woman with a rapidly growing mass shows a nonspecific mass lesion ➡. Erosion of the dorsum of a metatarsal ↪ is seen.* **(Right)** *Sagittal T1WI MR shows the large lesion ➡ to be mildly heterogeneous, though mostly isointense, to skeletal muscle. There is osseous erosion ↪ that is likely underestimated on this slice.*

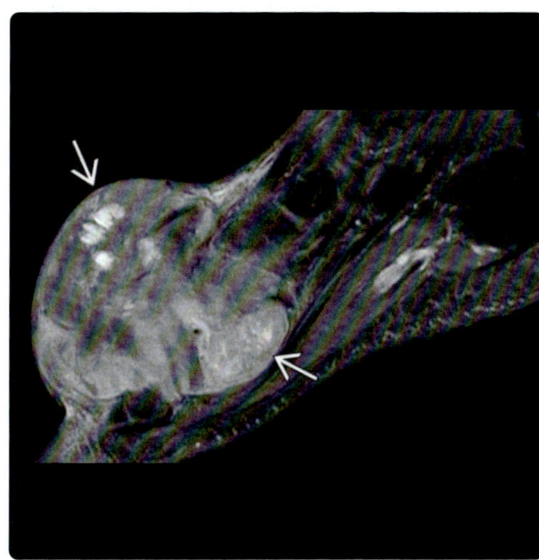

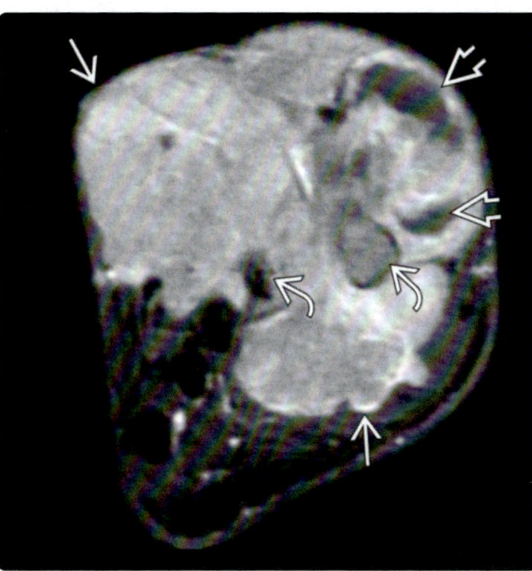

(Left) *Sagittal T2WI FS MR, same case, shows heterogeneous hyperintensity of the mass ➡.* **(Right)** *Axial T1WI C+ FS MR shows avid enhancement of the large, invasive mass ➡. There are areas of necrosis ➡ and invasion of both the 1st and 2nd metatarsals ↪. The features of the lesion are of a nonspecific highly aggressive lesion that proved to be RMS. Osseous invasion is seen in 25% of RMS cases in the extremities, but the adult age is unusual.*

Hemangioma and Vascular Malformations: Soft Tissue

KEY FACTS

TERMINOLOGY

- Benign lesions closely resembling normal blood vessels, classified by predominant vessel type
- One of most common soft tissue tumors overall
  - Most common tumor in infancy and childhood

IMAGING

- Can be difficult/impossible to definitively identify type of vascular malformation on imaging alone
- Radiographs show low-density soft tissue mass
  - Calcifications are common
  - Changes involving underlying bone often evident
- Well-defined to ill-defined mass on CT
  - Similar or ↓ attenuation relative to skeletal muscle
  - Prominent enhancement of vessels
  - Hemorrhage may produce fluid-fluid levels
- Isointense to hypointense relative to skeletal muscle on T1WI MR
- Foci of high T1 signal corresponding to adipose tissue or slow-flow blood
  - Adipose tissue follows subcutaneous fat signal on all imaging sequences
- Hyperintense vascular regions on T2WI MR for slow-flow lesions; signal voids in high-flow lesions
- Calcifications have low signal on all sequences
- Ultrasound shows heterogeneous echogenic mass
  - Thrombosis may limit detection of blood flow
- Angiography confirms vascular origin of most lesions

CLINICAL ISSUES

- May enlarge and progressively discolor during day (or while in dependent position), then decrease in size and coloration overnight
- Capillary hemangioma is most common type, followed by cavernous hemangioma
- Multiple different treatment options available

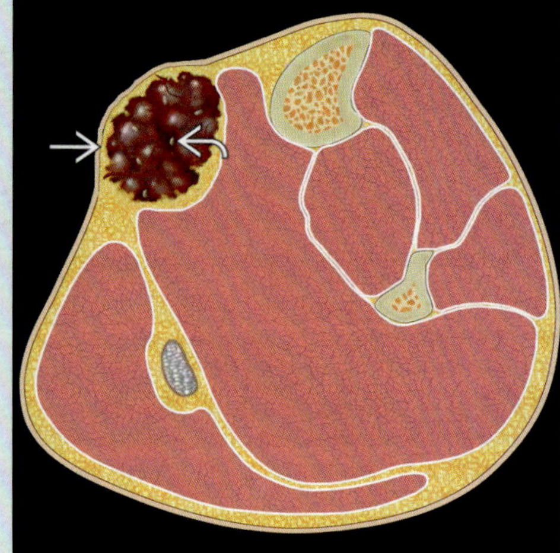

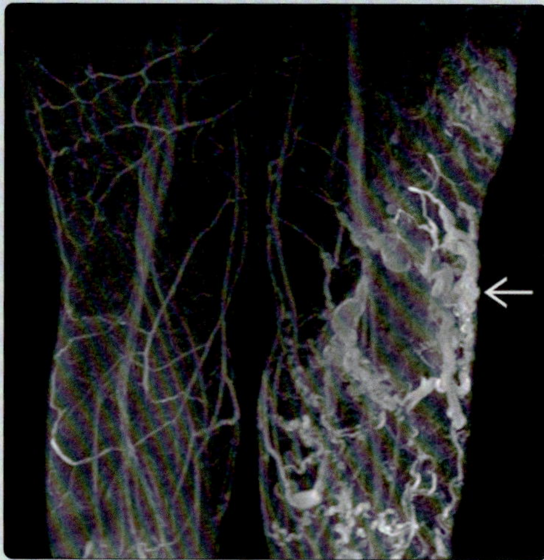

(Left) *Axial graphic shows a lobulated mass ➡ superficially located in the soft tissues of the calf. The mass has a reddish coloration and corresponds to a clinically elevated lesion. Foci of fat ➡ are present within the mass and there is hypertrophy of fat around the lesion.* **(Right)** *Coronal MRA of the thighs shows the left thigh to have an extensive arteriovenous hemangioma ➡. This large vascular malformation was predominantly confined to the subcutaneous fat. There was no bone hypertrophy.*

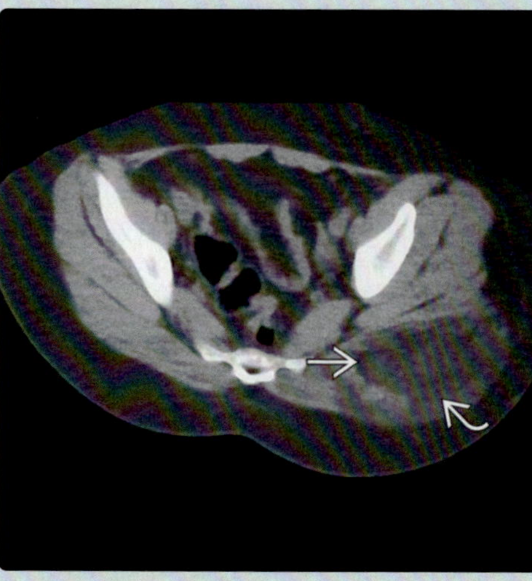

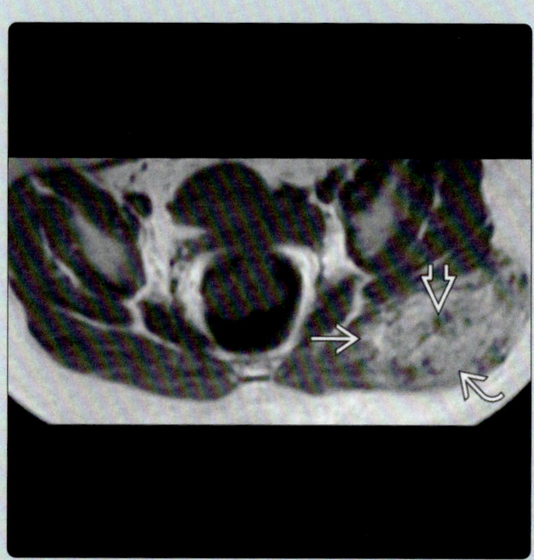

(Left) *Axial soft tissue algorithm CT shows an intramuscular hemangioma ➡ in the left gluteal region, containing a great amount of fat density tissue ➡ with soft tissue density intermingled. There may be some phleboliths identifiable by CT, but it is not definitive in this case.* **(Right)** *Axial T2WI FS MR best shows the infiltrative nature of the hemangioma ➡. Fat signal intensity ➡ is confirmed on this sequence. Tubular structures ➡ with flow voids corresponding to high-flow vessels are clearly identified.*

TERMINOLOGY

Abbreviations

- Capillary hemangioma (CapH)
- Cavernous hemangioma (CavH)
- Venous hemangioma or malformation (VH)
- Arteriovenous hemangioma or malformation (AVH)
- Synovial vascular malformation (SVM) (a.k.a. synovial hemangioma)
- Intramuscular hemangioma (IMH)

Definitions

- Benign lesions closely resembling normal blood vessels, classified by predominant vessel type and location

IMAGING

General Features

- Best diagnostic clue
  - Can be difficult or impossible to definitively identify type of vascular malformation on imaging alone
  - Most commonly appears as superficial lesion involving head and neck region
    - Superficial lesions often not imaged
- Location
  - CapH → most in skin or SQ fat of upper body
    - Deep lesions usually found in head and neck
  - CavH → more likely to involve deep tissues
  - VH → subcutaneous or deep soft tissues, limbs predominantly affected (40%) or head & neck (40%)
    - Also affects mesentery and retroperitoneum
  - AVH → head and neck > limbs
  - SVM → knee > elbow > hand; joint or bursa
  - IMH → lower extremity musculature, especially thigh
    - Followed by head and neck > upper limb > trunk
    - Mediastinum and retroperitoneum rarely involved

Radiographic Findings

- Inhomogeneous low-density soft tissue mass
- Curvilinear or amorphous calcifications, phleboliths
  - Phleboliths in 20-67% of cavernous hemangiomas, 30% of venous hemangiomas
- Bone overgrowth, cortical thickening, cortical tunneling, osteopenia, periosteal reaction, or erosion
- Medullary space sclerosis, invasion, or osteopenia

CT Findings

- NECT
  - Well-defined to ill-defined mass
  - Similar to ↓ attenuation relative to skeletal muscle
  - May contain areas of fat signal intensity
  - Calcifications are common
- CECT
  - Prominent enhancement of vessels

MR Findings

- T1WI
  - Isointense to hypointense relative to skeletal muscle
  - Foci of high signal corresponding to adipose tissue or slow-flow blood
    - Adipose tissue follows subcutaneous fat signal on all imaging sequences
- T2WI
  - Hyperintense vascular regions in slow-flow lesions (VH); may show signal void in high-flow lesions (AVH)
- T1WI C+
  - Vascular regions intensely enhance
  - Little or no early enhancement due to slow flow in larger cavitary lesions; consider delayed imaging
- CapH and small lesions have more homogeneous imaging appearance
- Calcifications have low signal on all sequences
- Hemorrhage may produce fluid-fluid levels
- AVH: Tangle of vessels with no prominent soft tissue component
  - Vascular shunting: Draining vein enhances before venous phase of contrast enhancement
- SVM may show hemosiderin arthropathy due to repeated bleeds into joint

Ultrasonographic Findings

- Mass with heterogeneous echogenicity
- Thrombosis may limit detection of blood flow
- Acoustic shadowing from calcification
- AVH: Vascular shunting; low-resistance waveforms in feeding artery
- VH: Variable US appearance
  - Focal dilatation of vein ("phlebectasia")
  - Dysplastic ectatic type: Multiple tortuous veins clumped together
  - Cavitary spongiform type: Multiple fluid-filled, cystic-appearing structures
  - Blood flow may be sluggish → absent Color Doppler flow

Angiographic Findings

- Confirms vascular origin of most lesions
  - Can identify large feeding vessels
  - Contrast pooling
- VH may only be visible on venous phase imaging
- Variable arteriovenous shunting and early draining veins seen with AVH
- Early venous run off and striated pattern with IMH

Imaging Recommendations

- Best imaging tool
  - MR best detects blood vessels and fat overgrowth
  - CT best detects calcifications

DIFFERENTIAL DIAGNOSIS

Hemangioendothelioma, Soft Tissue

- Tumor of intermediate aggressiveness that can metastasize
- Occurs throughout adulthood
- May invade bone
- Epithelioid variant histologically distinctive from other vascular tumors
  - Superficial and deep lesions are painful

Angiosarcoma, Soft Tissue

- Imaging shows vascular component and nonspecific solid regions of mass
- Peak incidence in 7th decade of life
- Male predilection
- 50% 1-year survival rate

PATHOLOGY

General Features

- Etiology
  - Vascular malformations, as opposed to neoplasms
    - Trauma often reported but not likely causative
  - Craniospinal cavernous hemangiomas can be radiation-induced
- Associated abnormalities
  - Klippel-Trenaunay-Weber syndrome = bone and soft tissue hypertrophy, varicose veins, cutaneous hemangioma
  - Maffucci syndrome = multiple cavernous hemangiomas + enchondromas
  - Kasabach-Merritt syndrome = thrombocytopenia purpura complicating giant cavernous hemangioma
  - Blue rubber nevus syndrome (sporadic and autosomal dominant) = superficial and gastrointestinal cavernous hemangiomas, often producing anemia
  - Turner syndrome associated with VH
  - Osler-Weber-Rendu syndrome = fibrovascular dysplasia of vessels producing arteriovenous hemangiomas, telangiectasias, and aneurysms with propensity for bleeding

Microscopic Features

- CapH → proliferation of capillary-sized vessels served by feeder vessel
  - Several different subtypes, with juvenile and senile hemangiomas being most common
- CavH → dilated, blood-filled spaces lined by flattened endothelium with scattered inflammatory cells
  - Calcification common
  - May contain mature bone
- VH → variably sized, slow-flow veins with thick muscular walls
- AVH → variably sized arteries and veins with arteriovenous shunting
- SVM → vessel proliferation deep to synovial surface
  - Similar appearance to cavernous hemangioma
- IMH → blood vessel proliferation within skeletal muscle with associated adipose tissue

CLINICAL ISSUES

Presentation

- Most common signs/symptoms
  - Vascular lesions in general may enlarge and progressively discolor during the day (or while in dependent position), then decrease in size and coloration overnight
  - CapH → superficial mass with variable presentation based on subtype
    - Juvenile hemangioma: Rapid ↑ in size; color intensifies with crying or straining
  - CavH → deep intramuscular mass
  - VH → slowly growing mass
  - AVH → pain, limb hypertrophy, cardiac failure, coagulopathy
  - SVM → painful joint with limited range of motion and associated joint effusion, ± limb overgrowth
  - IMH → may become painful after exercise, especially when in long narrow muscle
    - Rarely impedes muscle function
- Other signs/symptoms
  - Capillary and cavernous hemangiomas may change size during pregnancy and menarche
  - Seizures from intracranial cavernous hemangiomas
  - Superficial arteriovenous hemangiomas can mimic Kaposi sarcoma
  - Repetitive hemarthrosis from synovial vascular malformation may mimic hemophiliac arthropathy

Demographics

- Age
  - CapH and CavH → young children or adults
    - Cherry angioma arises during adult life
  - VH → adults
  - AVH and SVM → children to young adults
  - IMH → adolescents and young adults most common; wide age range
- Gender
  - Female predilection with CapH and CavH
  - Male predilection with synovial vascular malformation
  - No sex predilection with IMH
- Epidemiology
  - One of most common soft tissue tumors overall
    - Most common tumor in infancy and childhood
  - Capillary hemangioma most common, followed by cavernous hemangioma
    - Juvenile hemangioma occurs in 1/200 live births
  - VH and SVM → rare
  - AVH → deep-seated form uncommon
  - IMH → most common form of hemangioma in muscle but still relatively uncommon
    - 0.8% of all benign vascular tumors

Natural History & Prognosis

- Untreated lesions have limited growth potential
  - Juvenile hemangioma form of CapH usually spontaneously involutes by age 7
- No malignant transformation

Treatment

- Multiple different treatment options based on lesion type and location
  - Observation, systemic steroids, intralesional steroids, topical steroids, vincristine, interferon alpha, propranolol, pulsed dye laser, embolization, surgical removal
- Treatment decision based on psychosocial issues and avoidance of life-/function-threatening complications
  - Balanced against resultant disfigurement and other potential adverse effects from treatment

SELECTED REFERENCES

1. Behr GG et al: Vascular anomalies: hemangiomas and beyond–part 1, Fast-flow lesions. AJR Am J Roentgenol. 200(2):414-22, 2013
2. Behr GG et al: Vascular anomalies: hemangiomas and beyond–part 2, Slow-flow lesions. AJR Am J Roentgenol. 200(2):423-36, 2013
3. Flors L et al: MR imaging of soft-tissue vascular malformations: diagnosis, classification, and therapy follow-up. Radiographics. 31(5):1321-40; discussion 1340-1, 2011
4. Navarro OM et al: Pediatric soft-tissue tumors and pseudotumors: MR imaging features with pathologic correlation: part 1. Imaging approach, pseudotumors, vascular lesions, and adipocytic tumors. Radiographics. 29(3):887-906, 2009

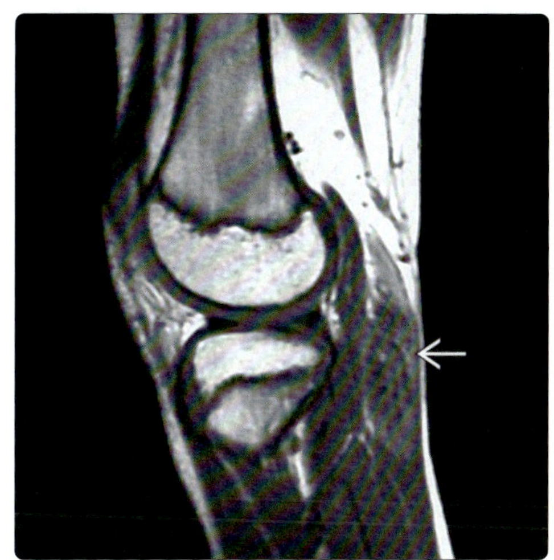

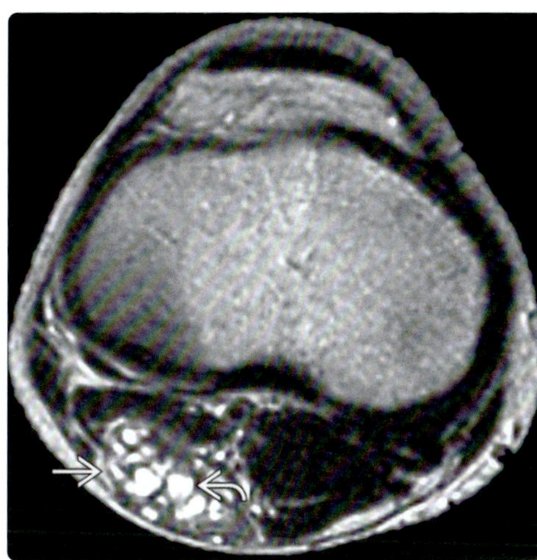

(Left) *Sagittal T1WI MR shows a hemangioma ➡ infiltrating the lateral gastrocnemius muscle. The mass is composed of tortuous vessels in a stroma that is slightly higher SI than muscle. Note however that this is not the most typical appearance of hemangioma, in that little interdigitating lacy fat signal areas providing the stroma are seen.* **(Right)** *Axial T2WI MR in the same patient shows multiple tubular structures ➡ with mixed low and high signal, quite typical for a hemangioma ➡.*

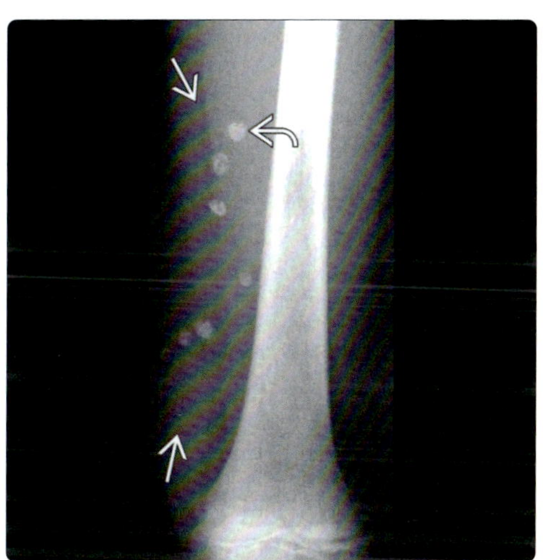

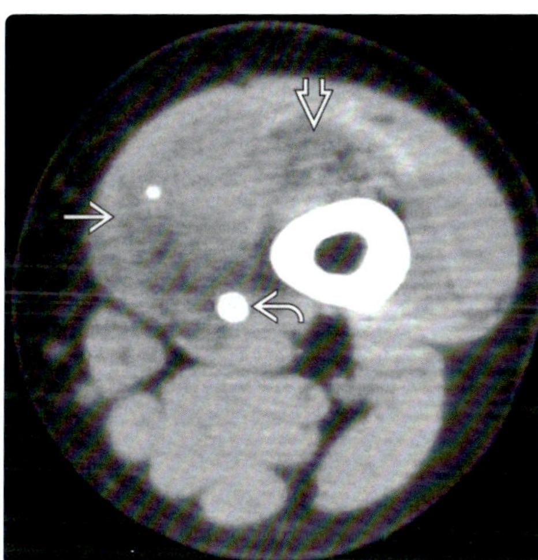

(Left) *Anteroposterior radiograph shows a poorly defined mass ➡ in the thigh containing multiple calcific densities with central lucency (phleboliths) ➡. This is highly suggestive of soft tissue hemangioma.* **(Right)** *Axial bone CT shows the mass ➡ to contain phleboliths ➡ and fatty stroma ➡. This mass is ill-defined and diffusely infiltrates the muscle, as opposed to displacing it. Although there can be a variety of changes in the adjacent bone, the underlying bone in this case was normal.*

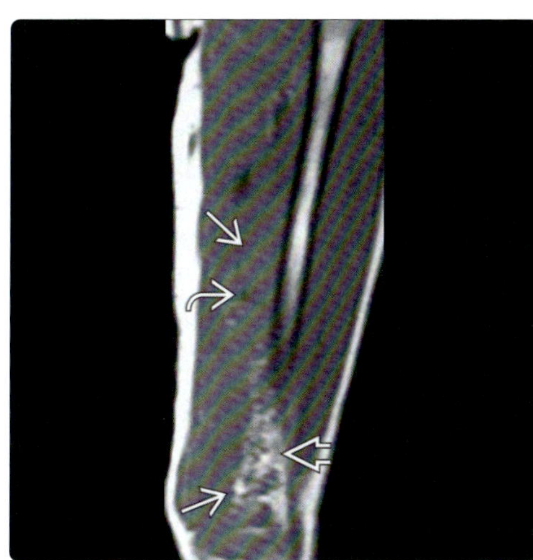

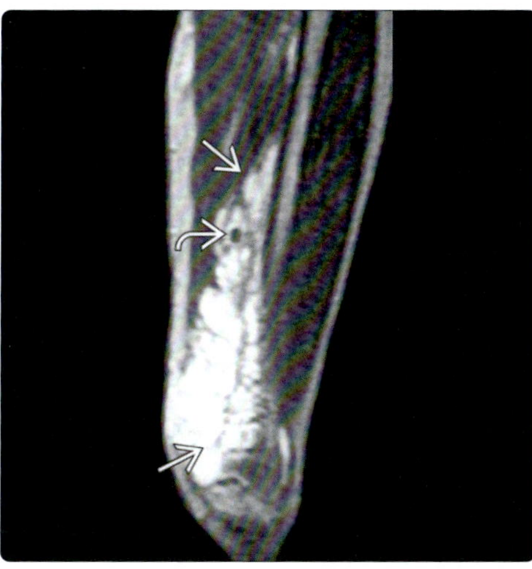

(Left) *Coronal T1WI MR in the same patient confirms the previous findings. The phleboliths ➡ are low signal on all sequences. The mass ➡ has heterogeneous isointense to hyperintense signal, with high-signal fatty stroma ➡ anterior to the femur, corresponding to that seen on the CT.* **(Right)** *Coronal T2WI MR shows the majority of the soft tissue mass ➡ to have lobulated high signal on this fluid-sensitive sequence. The intense high signal indicates a slow-flowing malformation. A low-signal phlebolith ➡ is again identified.*

(Left) *Coronal MR angiography shows multiple hemangiomas ➡ involving the fingers and wrist. The finger hemangiomas had early filling on the arterial phase. The index finger and 5th digit hemangiomas were associated with flexion deformities of the digits.* **(Right)** *Axial T2WI FS MR at the level of the wrist shows a lobulated hyperintense mass ➡ surrounding the extensor tendons. This extensive hemangioma had somewhat slow filling, best seen on venous and delayed phase imaging.*

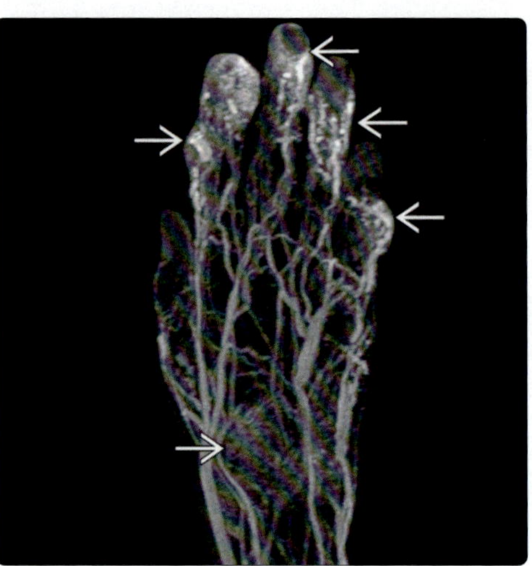

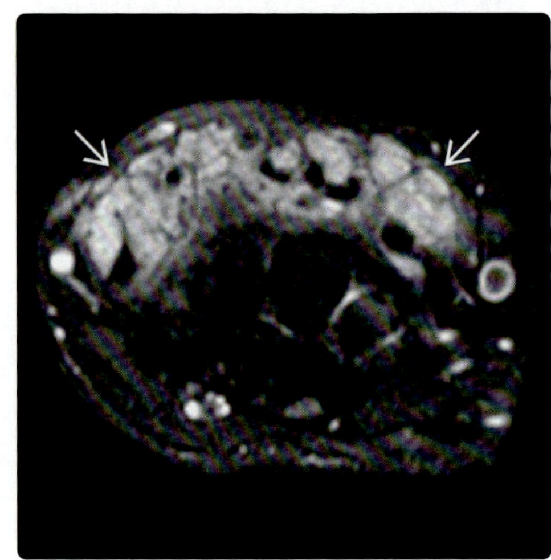

(Left) *AP radiograph in a 36-year-old woman shows small phleboliths ➡ within a soft tissue mass ➡. Note erosion of tibial cortex ➡ as well as intramedullary reactive bone change ➡. The appearance is typical of hemangioma. Bone involvement can take many forms, including erosion and reaction as seen here.* **(Right)** *Coronal T1WI MR in the same case shows tubular structures ➡ isointense to muscle with some surrounding fatty stroma ➡. The phleboliths are round and low signal ➡. Findings are typical of hemangioma.*

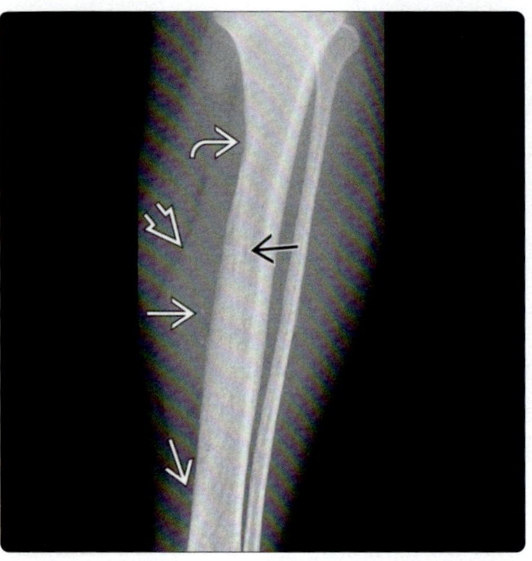

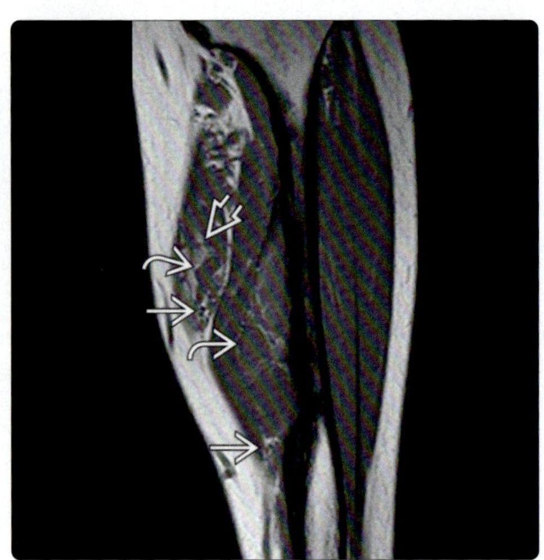

(Left) *Axial T2WI FS MR in the same case shows the dilated, almost cystic vessels to contain fluid-fluid levels ➡. These levels are often seen when the vessels in a vascular malformation are particularly dilated, as in this case.* **(Right)** *Coronal T1WI C+ FS MR in the same patient shows many of the vessels to enhance ➡. Degree of enhancement in vascular malformations varies with blood flow; slow-flow lesions may not appear to enhance without having delayed imaging.*

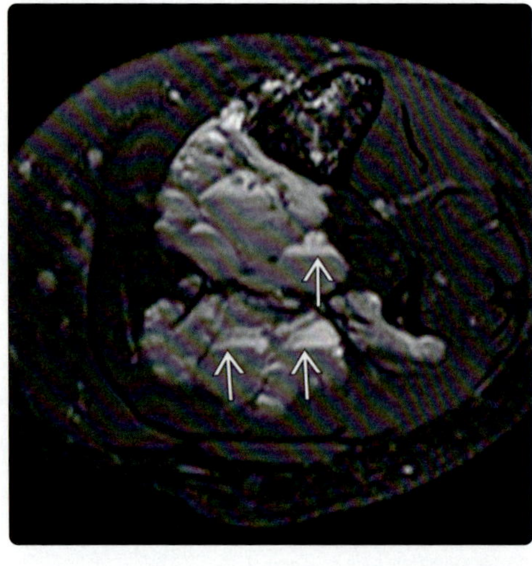

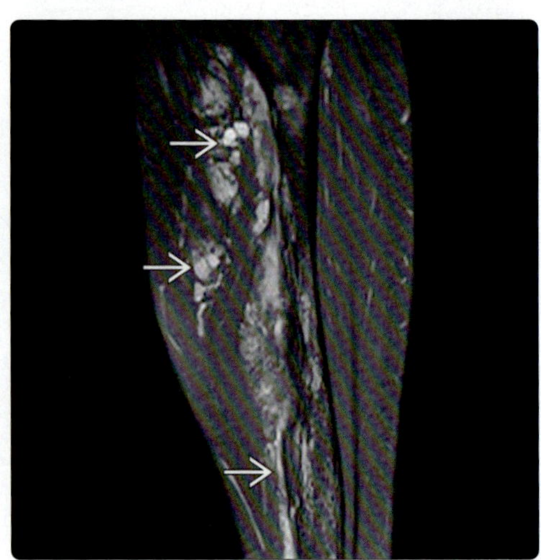

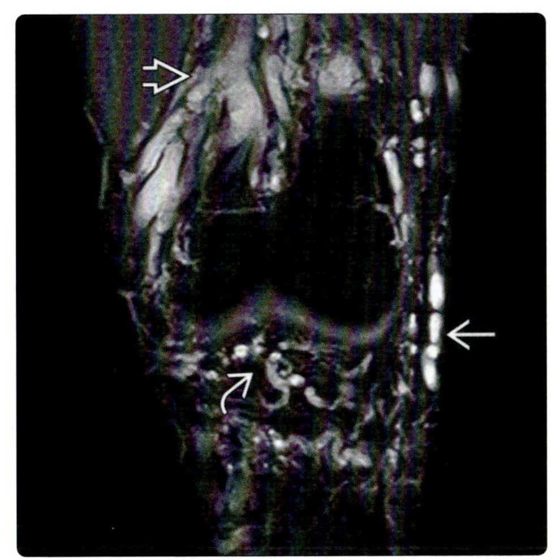

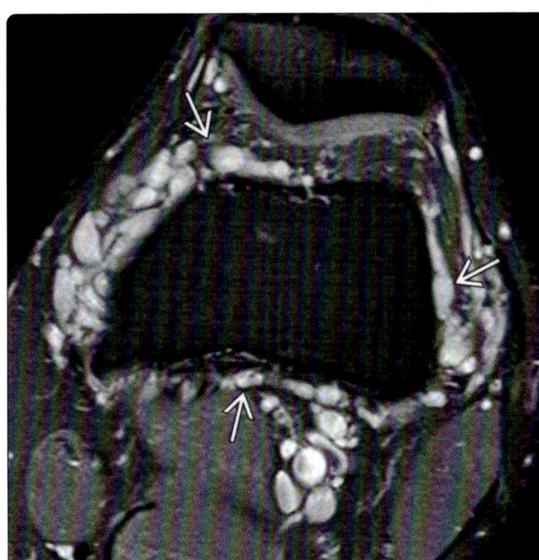

(Left) *Coronal T2WI FS MR of knee in a young woman shows massively dilated tubular structures, some within Hoffa fat pad ➡ and others that appear to be extraarticular ➡ or within subcutaneous fat ➡. Although vascular malformation is presumed, axial imaging allows better localization of process.* **(Right)** *Axial T2WI FS MR in the same patient shows the majority of the dilated vessels ➡ to be intraarticular, while extraarticular feeding vessels are also enlarged. This is a synovial vascular malformation.*

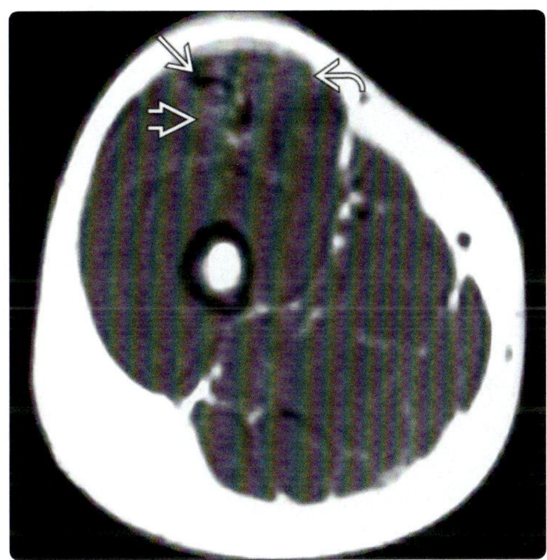

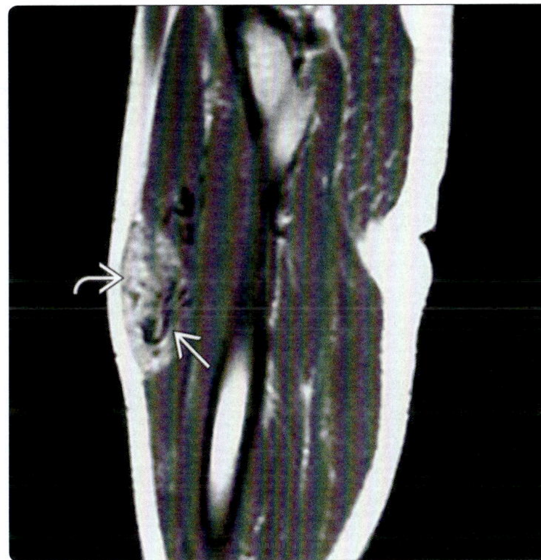

(Left) *Axial T1WI MR demonstrates an intramuscular lesion ➡, which has multiple tortuous vessels within it ➡ and has infiltrating fat signal throughout ➡.* **(Right)** *Sagittal T1WI C+ MR in the same patient shows the mass ➡ to have an overall increase in signal due to enhancement. Note that there is a large draining vessel ➡. The combination of infiltrating fat around multiple tangled vessels is a classic appearance for a hemangioma.*

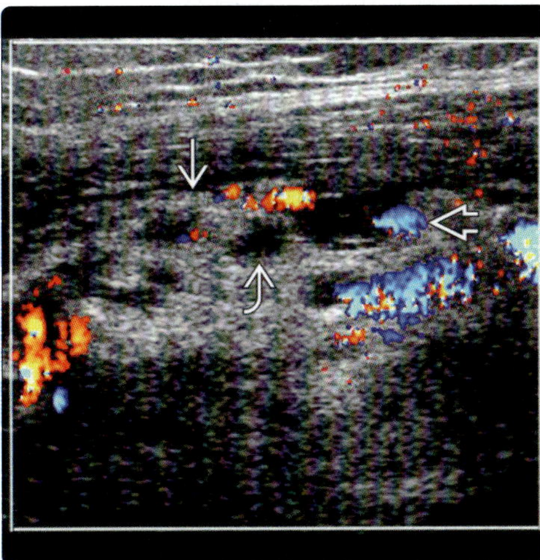

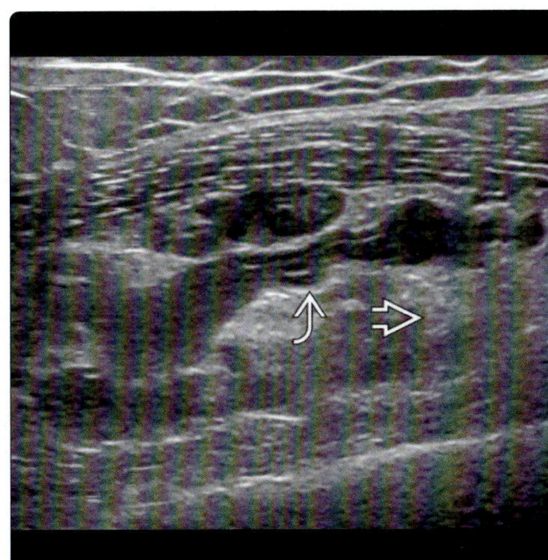

(Left) *Longitudinal Doppler ultrasound of a mass ➡ involving the vastus lateralis muscle shows that it consists of multiple vascular channels ➡ that have thrombosed. Only a mild amount of blood flow ➡ is present with augmentation performed on the more distal veins.* **(Right)** *Longitudinal ultrasound shows elongated, vascular-appearing structures ➡ with mixed solid components ➡. The appearance suggests a hemangioma, but hemangioendothelioma and angiosarcoma cannot be excluded.*

Angiomatosis

KEY FACTS

TERMINOLOGY

- Rare, benign, diffuse hemangioma contiguously affecting large segment of body

IMAGING

- Same imaging characteristics as hemangioma but involving larger area
- Lower extremity > > chest wall > abdomen > upper extremity
  - May involve either single tissue type (e.g., muscle) or multiple soft tissue types
- Average 10-20 cm in diameter
- Soft tissue prominence or ill-defined mass on radiographs
  - Bones involved may be lytic or sclerotic
- CT shows ill-defined mass often containing fat
  - May contain identifiable vessels
  - Prominent enhancement
- Isointense to hypointense relative to skeletal muscle on T1WI MR
  - High-signal adipose tissue or slowly flowing blood
- Hyperintense vascular regions on T2WI MR
  - Can simulate appearance of sarcoma

CLINICAL ISSUES

- Soft tissue swelling that may vary in size relative to physical activity
  - Lesions can be painful
  - May produce reddish discoloration of skin
  - Hypertrophy or gigantism due to arteriovenous shunting is rare
- Most develop within first 2 decades of life
  - Majority diagnosed by 4th decade of life
- Attempted surgical resection often results in incomplete excision or local recurrence
- Natural history
  - No malignant transformation or metastasis
  - Angiomatous syndromes may carry increased risk of malignancy

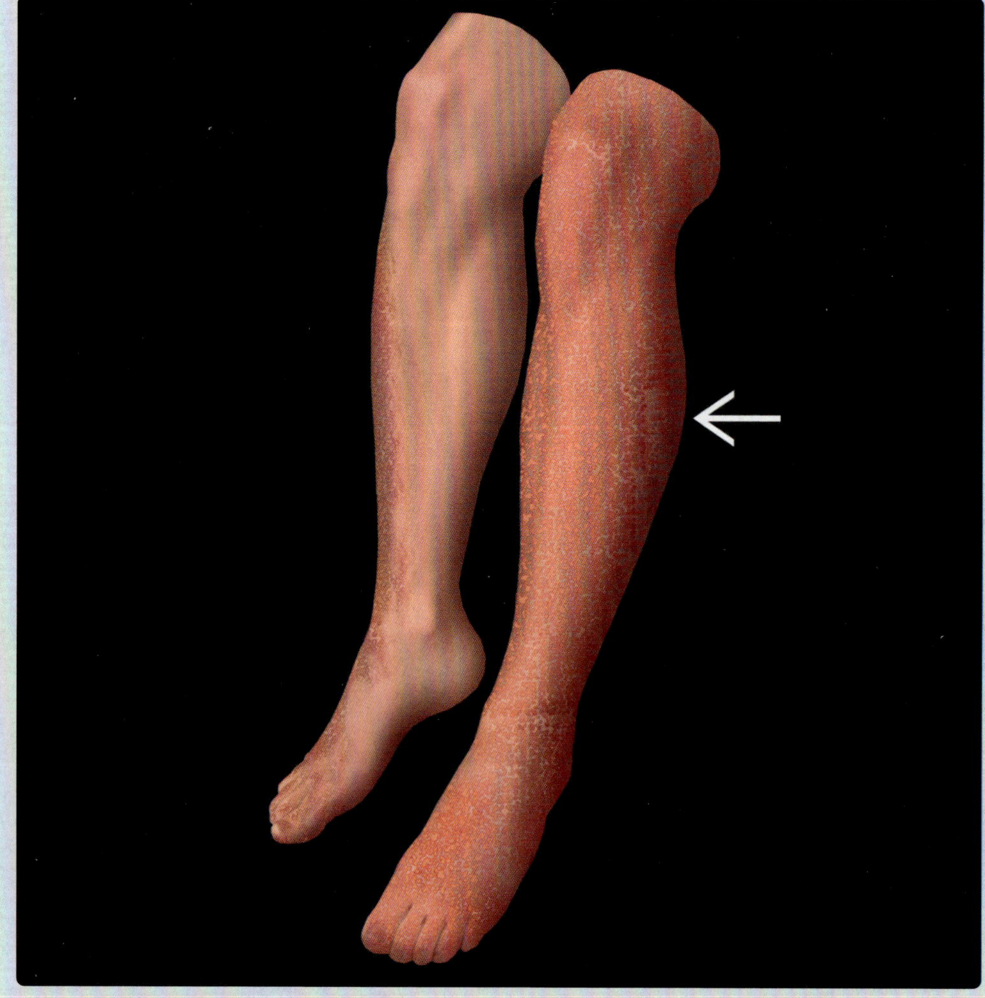

Graphic shows the left leg ➡ to be diffusely enlarged compared to the right. Skin discoloration is secondary to involvement of the subcutaneous tissues. The lower extremity is most commonly involved. Imaging findings in angiomatosis are similar to hemangioma but require a large contiguous region of the body to be affected for this clinicopathologic diagnosis to be made.

TERMINOLOGY

Synonyms

- Vascular malformation, arteriovenous malformation, venous malformation, infiltrating angiolipoma

Definitions

- Rare, benign, diffuse hemangioma contiguously affecting large segment of body

IMAGING

General Features

- Best diagnostic clue
  - Same imaging characteristics as hemangioma but involving large body region
- Location
  - Lower extremity is involved in over 50%
    - Chest wall > abdomen > upper extremity
  - May involve either single tissue type (e.g., muscle) or multiple soft tissue types
    - Limited to bone involvement in ~ 1/3 of cases
- Size
  - Average 10-20 cm in diameter

Radiographic Findings

- Soft tissue prominence or ill-defined mass
- Bones involved may be lytic or sclerotic

CT Findings

- Ill-defined mass often containing fat
- May contain identifiable vessels
- Can simulate appearance of sarcoma

MR Findings

- T1WI
  - Isointense to hypointense relative to skeletal muscle
  - High signal regions of adipose tissue or slowly flowing blood
- T2WI FS
  - Hyperintense vascular regions
- T1WI C+ FS
  - Prominent enhancement

Angiographic Findings

- Rare arteriovenous shunting

DIFFERENTIAL DIAGNOSIS

Soft Tissue Liposarcoma

- Fat-containing neoplasm with variable nodularity and septa
- Calcification or ossification uncommon
- Lacks large, enhancing vessels
- Middle-aged to elderly adults

Soft Tissue Hemangioma and Vascular Malformations

- Same pathologic entity as angiomatosis but with less extensive involvement
- Differentiation from angiomatosis is often based on clinical criteria

PATHOLOGY

General Features

- Etiology
  - Developmental malformation, as opposed to neoplastic entity

Gross Pathologic & Surgical Features

- Lesion often has pale coloration due to prominent fat content

Microscopic Features

- Mix of variably sized vessels irregularly located throughout affected tissue
  - Thick-walled veins may have clustered small vessels located in or adjacent to vein wall
- Less common appearance is similar to infiltrating capillary hemangioma
- If prominent glomus cells are present, then lesions are classified as glomangiomatosis
- If lesion has predominant lymphatic differentiation, then it is classified as lymphangiomatosis

CLINICAL ISSUES

Presentation

- Most common signs/symptoms
  - Soft tissue swelling that may vary in size relative to physical activity
- Other signs/symptoms
  - Lesions can be painful
  - May produce reddish discoloration of skin
  - Hypertrophy or gigantism due to arteriovenous shunting is rare

Demographics

- Age
  - Most develop within first 2 decades of life
    - Majority diagnosed by 4th decade of life
- Gender
  - Mild female predilection

Natural History & Prognosis

- No malignant transformation or metastasis
  - Angiomatous syndromes may carry increased risk of malignancy

Treatment

- Attempted surgical resection often results in incomplete excision or local recurrence

SELECTED REFERENCES

1. Crickx E et al: Diffuse dermal angiomatosis associated with severe atherosclerosis: two cases and review of the literature. Clin Exp Dermatol. 40(5):521-4, 2015
2. Khan S et al: Angiomatosis: a rare vascular proliferation of head and neck region. J Cutan Aesthet Surg. 8(2):108-10, 2015
3. Luks VL et al: Lymphatic and other vascular malformative/overgrowth disorders are caused by somatic mutations in PIK3CA. J Pediatr. 166(4):1048-54.e1-5, 2015
4. Weiss SW et al: Benign tumors and tumor-like lesions of blood vessels. In Weiss SW et al: Enzinger and Weiss' Soft Tissue Tumors. 5th ed. Philadelphia: Elsevier. 665-6, 2008
5. Kransdorf MJ et al: Vascular and lymphatic tumors. In Kransdorf MJ et al: Imaging of Soft Tissue Tumors. 2nd ed. Philadelphia: Lippincott Williams & Wilkins. 168-9, 2006

Klippel-Trenaunay-Weber Syndrome

KEY FACTS

IMAGING

- Classic triad
  - Bone and soft tissue hypertrophy
  - Cutaneous hemangioma
  - Congenital varicose veins
- Usually involves single limb
  - Lower limb in 3/4 of patients
  - Can be limited to digits
- 70% have incompetent vein extending from ankle to infrainguinal region
- MR is very useful to evaluate vascular malformations in soft tissues, without disadvantage of using ionizing radiation
- Common findings identifiable using radiography, CT, and MR
  - Limb hypertrophy &/or macrodactyly
  - Thickening of cortical bone
  - Abnormal superficial to deep vein connections
  - Lack of venous valves
  - Phleboliths
  - Subcutaneous fat hypertrophy
- Prenatal ultrasound can demonstrate peripheral and visceral vascular anomalies, cardiomegaly, nonimmune hydrops, macrocephaly, hemihypertrophy, and umbilical cord hemangioma
- Lymphoscintigraphy may demonstrate lymphatic hyperplasia, abnormal dermal flow, aplasia, and hypoplasia
- Radionuclide venography and arteriography may demonstrate radionuclide uptake in affected extremity, collateral venous channels, venous occlusion, and pulmonary emboli

CLINICAL ISSUES

- Abnormalities can be identified prenatally
- Elastic support garments for venous insufficiency and lymphatic stasis
- Surgery for serious deformity or bleeding
  - Venous ligation may worsen deep venous malformations

(Left) *Axial CECT through the thighs shows the soft tissues of the right leg to be diffusely enlarged ➡. Soft tissue enlargement is secondary to multiple vascular malformations ➡ and fat hypertrophy. A phlebolith ➡ is present within one of the vascular malformations.* **(Right)** *Axial T1WI MR shows numerous, tortuous dilated vessels ➡ in the subcutaneous and deep muscle regions of the calf. Fat hypertrophy ➡ is also evident, contributing to the overall enlargement of the extremity.*

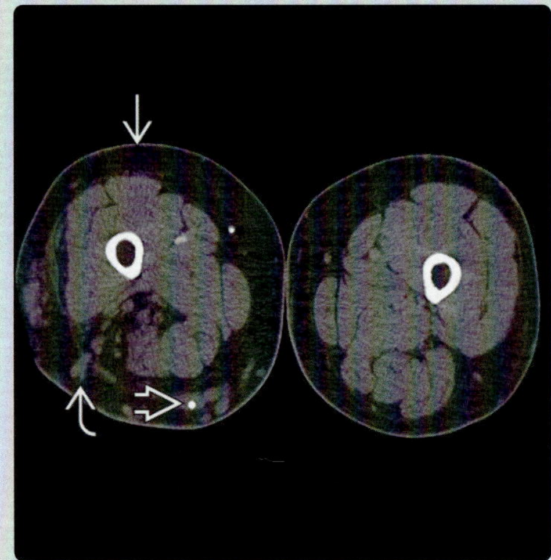

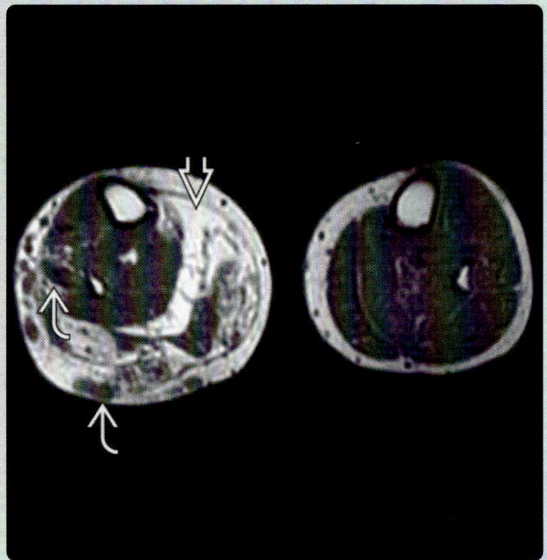

(Left) *Axial T2WI FS MR in the same patient shows the majority of the vascular malformations ➡ to have high signal intensity. The underlying bones were not involved in this patient. The left leg is normal.* **(Right)** *Transverse Doppler ultrasound of the thigh demonstrates numerous tubular structures ➡ in the soft tissues with variable high to absent blood flow. Klippel-Trenaunay-Weber syndrome is relatively uncommon and tends to involve a single lower extremity.*

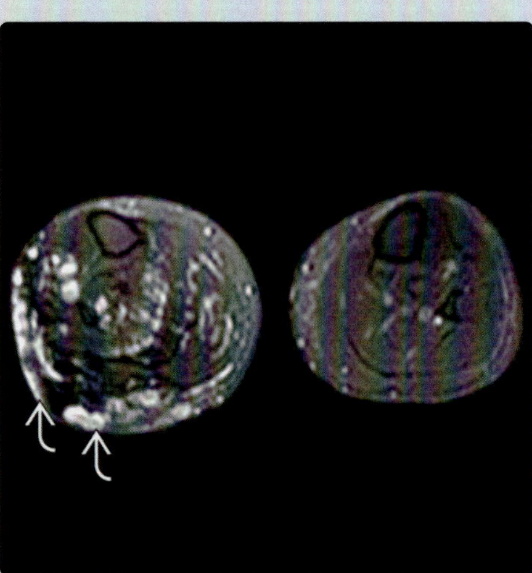

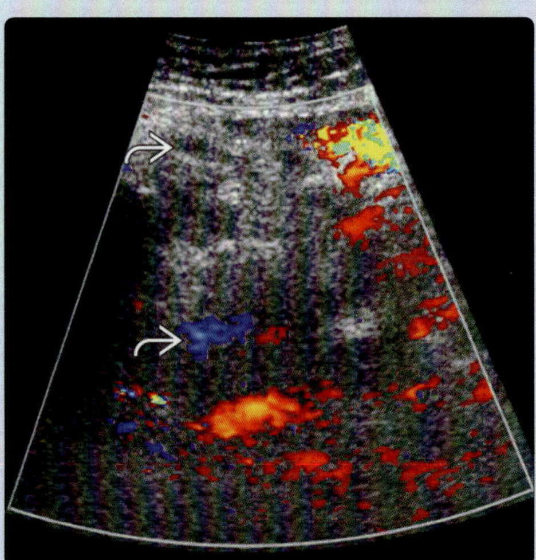

TERMINOLOGY

Abbreviations

- Klippel-Trenaunay-Weber (KTW)

Synonyms

- Angio-osteohypertrophy syndrome, Klippel-Trenaunay syndrome, nevus vasculosus osteohypertrophicus

IMAGING

General Features

- Best diagnostic clue
  - Classic triad of bone and soft tissue hypertrophy, cutaneous hemangioma, and congenital varicose veins
- Location
  - Usually involves single limb
    - Lower limb in 3/4 of patients
  - Can be limited to digits

Common Multimodality Findings

- Limb hypertrophy &/or macrodactyly
- Thickening of cortical bone
- Subcutaneous fat hypertrophy
- Abnormal superficial to deep vein connections
  - Lack of venous valves
- Phleboliths
- 70% of patients have incompetent vein extending from ankle to infrainguinal region

Less Common Multimodality Findings

- Bone anomalies: Syndactyly, polydactyly, hip dislocation, kyphosis, scoliosis
- Internal organ anomalies: Hemangiomas, vesicoureteral reflux, polycystic kidney disease, hydronephrosis, pericardial effusion, pleural effusion
- Various vascular anomalies: Aplasia, malformation, dilatation or duplication of major vessels; arteriovenous fistula
- Central nervous system anomalies: Myelopathy, cerebral atrophy, cerebral hemihypertrophy, cerebellar hemihypertrophy, cerebral calcification, leptomeningeal enhancement

Ultrasonographic Findings

- Prenatal ultrasound can demonstrate peripheral and visceral vascular anomalies, cardiomegaly, nonimmune hydrops, macrocephaly, hemihypertrophy, and umbilical cord hemangioma

Nuclear Medicine Findings

- Lymphoscintigraphy may demonstrate lymphatic hyperplasia, abnormal dermal flow, aplasia, and hypoplasia
- Radionuclide venography and arteriography may demonstrate radionuclide uptake in affected extremity, collateral venous channels, venous occlusion, and pulmonary emboli

DIFFERENTIAL DIAGNOSIS

Parkes-Weber Syndrome

- Classic findings of KTW plus arteriovenous fistula
- Sometimes considered same entity as KTW

Neurofibromatosis

- Plexiform growth pattern may result in enlarged extremity with hypertrophy of underlying bone
- Additional signs of neurofibromatosis will be present
- Lacks vascular malformations

Macrodystrophia Lipomatosa

- Bone and adipose tissue overgrowth
- Usually involves digits
- No vascular malformations

PATHOLOGY

General Features

- Genetics
  - Occasionally autosomal dominant
- Associated abnormalities
  - Fabry disease
  - Sturge-Weber syndrome

CLINICAL ISSUES

Presentation

- Most common signs/symptoms
  - Soft tissue and bone hypertrophy
  - Cutaneous hemangioma
  - Varicose veins
  - Port-wine telangiectatic nevi
  - Pain
- Other signs/symptoms
  - Internal organs: Visceral vascular malformations, protein-losing enteropathy, rectal bleeding, hematuria, chronic renal failure, pulmonary emboli
  - Peripheral: Deep venous thrombosis, limb atrophy, lymphatic insufficiency
  - Craniofacial: Early eruption of permanent teeth, malocclusion, congenital nystagmus, anisomyopia, hemimegalencephaly, hemifacial hypertrophy
  - Miscellaneous: Hypertension, thrombocytopenia, renal artery aneurysm, hypospadias, basal cell carcinoma, squamous cell carcinoma, pseudo-Kaposi sarcoma

Demographics

- Age
  - Abnormalities can be identified prenatally
- Gender
  - No sex predilection
- Epidemiology
  - < 1,000 reported cases, likely underreported

Treatment

- Elastic support garments for venous insufficiency and lymphatic stasis
- Surgery for serious deformity or bleeding
  - Venous ligation may worsen deep venous malformations

SELECTED REFERENCES

1. Luks VL et al: Lymphatic and other vascular malformative/overgrowth disorders are caused by somatic mutations in PIK3CA. J Pediatr. 166(4):1048-54.e1-5, 2015
2. Lacerda Lda S et al: Differential diagnoses of overgrowth syndromes: the most important clinical and radiological disease manifestations. Radiol Res Pract. 2014:947451, 2014

(Left) *Sagittal T1WI MR shows multiple rounded and serpiginous masses ➡ that have a similar intensity to muscle. These foci represent vascular malformations.* **(Right)** *Sagittal T2WI FS MR best demonstrates the extensively infiltrating nature of the vascular malformations. These involve all of the soft tissues, both extraarticular and intraarticular ↪. Additionally, osseous involvement ⇨ of the femur, tibia, and fibula is demonstrated.*

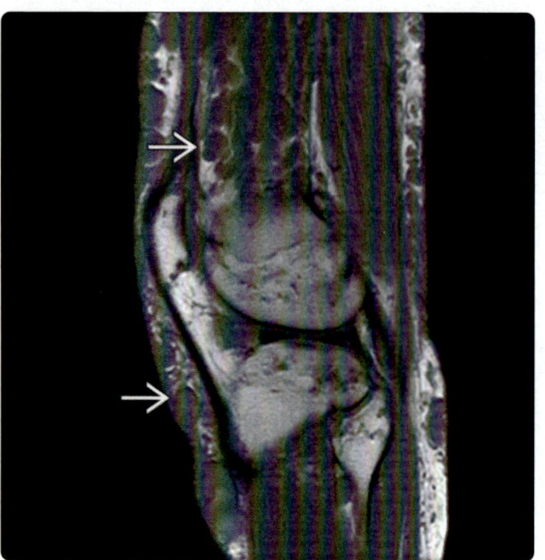

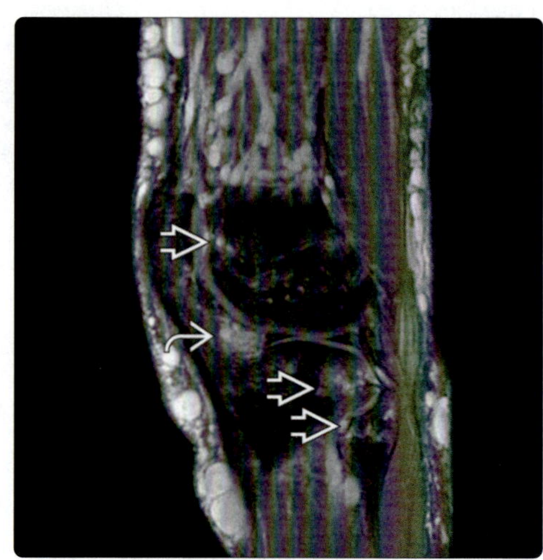

(Left) *Transverse Doppler ultrasound of the thigh musculature in the same patient shows multiple foci of blood flow ↪. The presence of thrombus in these vascular malformations sometimes limits visualization of flowing blood on Doppler examination.* **(Right)** *AP radiograph shows the left leg to be diffusely enlarged. Soft tissue varicosities ➡ are visible as areas of serpiginous increased attenuation. Note the leg length discrepancy and disproportionally advanced osteoarthritis ⇨.*

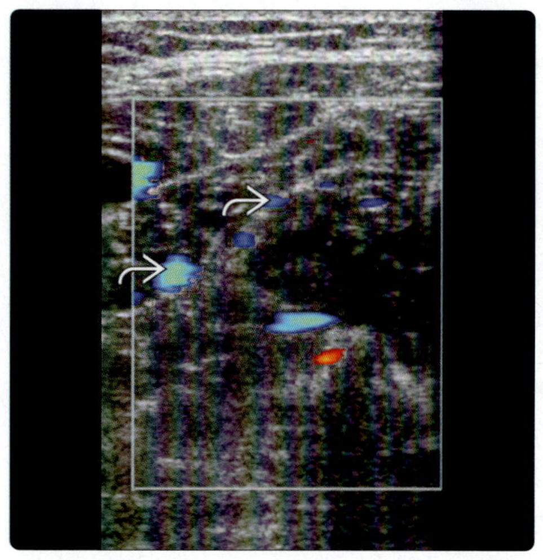

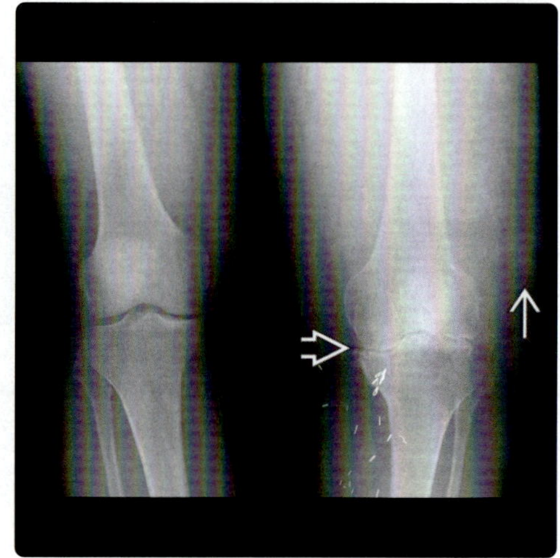

(Left) *Axial T1WI MR shows hemangiomas ↪ extending from near the skin surface, through the musculature, and down to the bone. Note that the subcutaneous fat is also hypertrophied ⇨, contributing to the overall enlarged left lower extremity.* **(Right)** *Axial STIR MR shows hyperintense hemangiomas ↪ involving the subcutaneous fat, muscle, and likely extending into the bone. A below-knee amputation performed for pain also revealed venous thrombosis, which is common.*

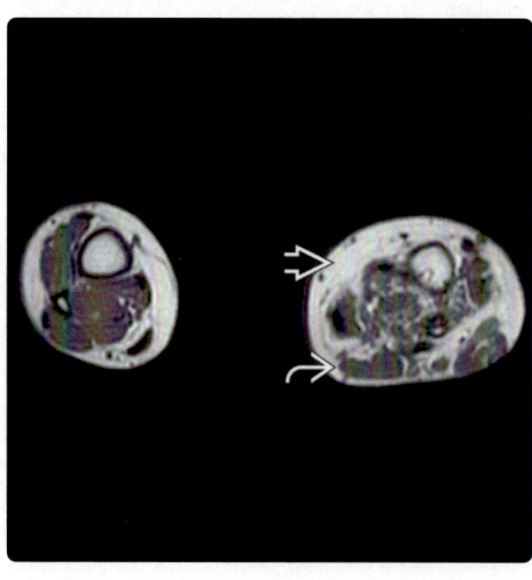

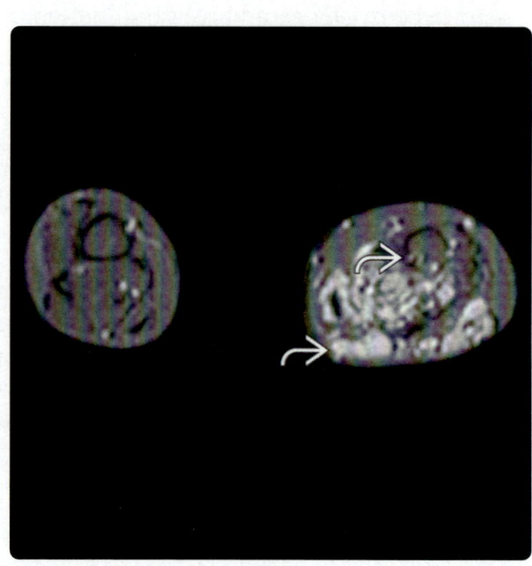

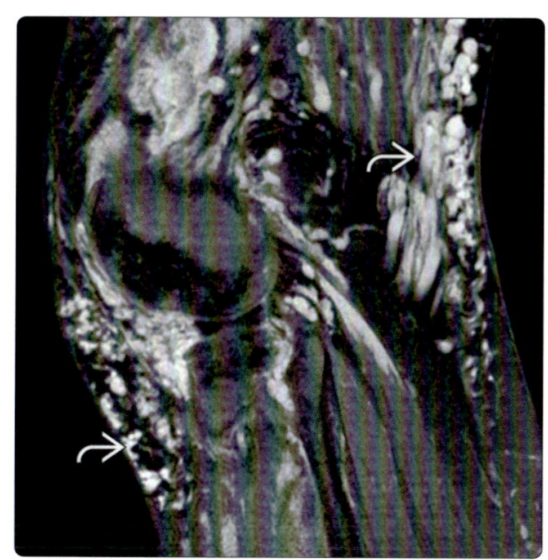

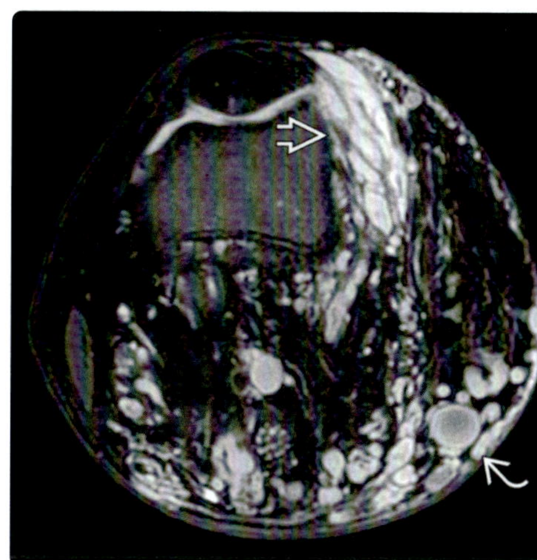

(Left) *Sagittal PD FS MR through the knee shows extensive vascular malformations throughout all of the soft tissues ➔, producing a diffusely enlarged leg.* **(Right)** *Axial T2WI FS MR shows extensive vascular malformations ➔ extending from the level of the skin, through the musculature, and down into the joint ➔. Involvement of the intraarticular regions with hemangiomas places this patient at increased risk for hemarthrosis.*

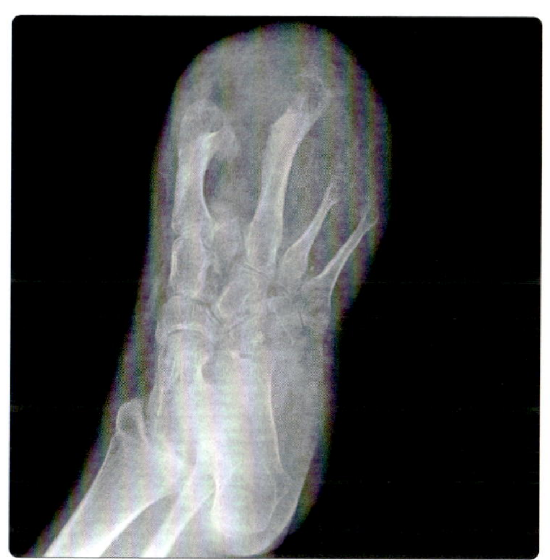

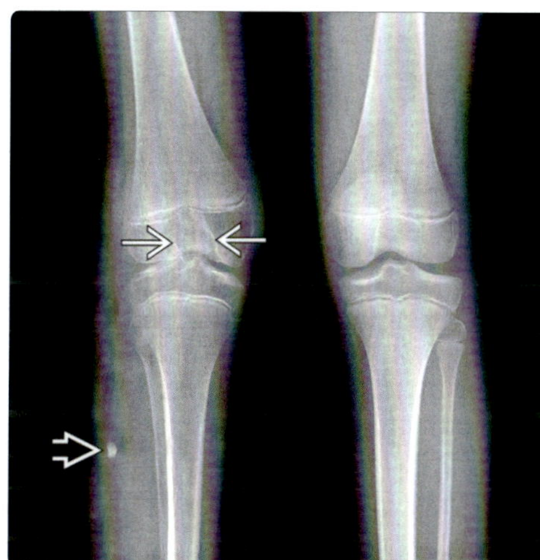

(Left) *Oblique radiograph of the foot shows the soft tissues and bones to be diffusely overgrown. The patient has undergone prior amputation of her toes and partial amputation of the metatarsals for debulking purposes.* **(Right)** *AP radiograph of the knees shows overgrowth of the bones and soft tissues of the right lower extremity. Note the widened intercondylar notch ➔, which has a similar imaging appearance to hemophilia. A phlebolith ➔ is present in the calf.*

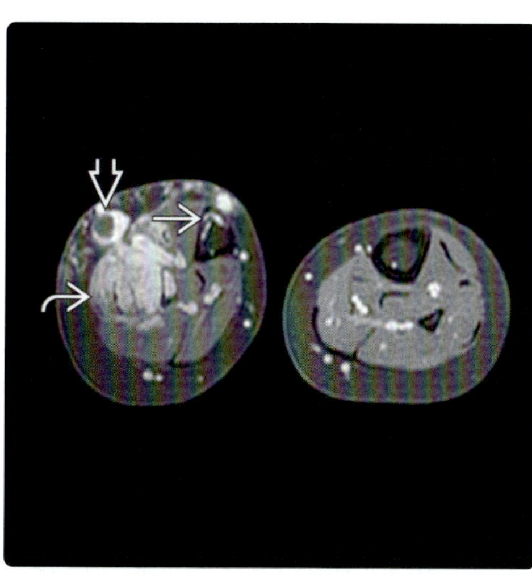

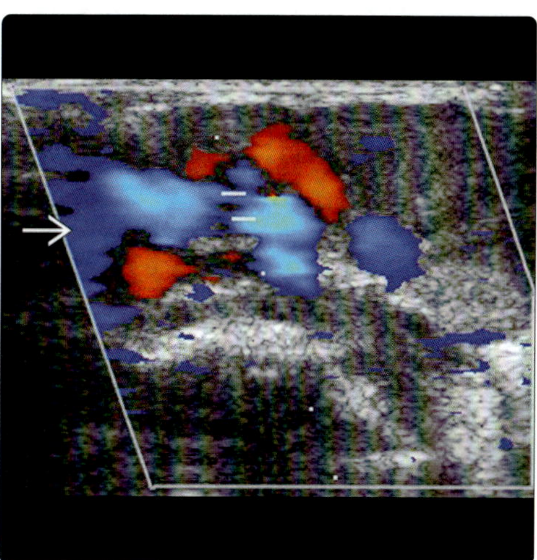

(Left) *Axial T1WI C+ FS MR through the calf shows numerous nodular and serpiginous enhancing regions consistent with vascular malformations ➔. Enlarged blood vessels also involve the tibia ➔. The phlebolith ➔ from the previous image is seen to have developed in one of the slow-flow, superficial vascular malformations.* **(Right)** *Transverse Doppler ultrasound of the calf in the same patient demonstrates extensive active blood flow ➔ in one of the previously documented hemangiomas.*

Lymphangioma

KEY FACTS

TERMINOLOGY

- Benign developmental lesion composed of dilated lymphatic channels

IMAGING

- Up to 75% in head, neck, and axilla
- Cystic lymphangiomas in neck are most common overall
- May invade or displace adjacent organs
- CT: Low-attenuation, lobulated mass
  - Well-circumscribed to ill-defined mass
  - Cystic areas lack enhancement
  - Rare calcification
- MR findings
  - Multiloculated mass with septations having heterogeneous signal intensity
    - Majority of mass follows fluid signal intensity
  - Hyperintense signal on T1WI can be caused by hemorrhage or proteinaceous fluid
  - Fluid-fluid levels from layering debris in cystic spaces
  - Mass wall and internal septa have intermediate to low signal intensity and show mild enhancement
- US: Anechoic to hypoechoic cystic spaces depending on debris in fluid
- Lymphangiography: May demonstrate mass continuity with normal lymphatic channels

PATHOLOGY

- Lesions contain serous, chylous, or proteinaceous fluid

CLINICAL ISSUES

- Usually identified within 1st 2 years of life
- Painless mass that may wax and wane in size
- Natural history
  - Morbidity and mortality from compression of vital structures, especially trachea and esophagus
  - High death rate when identified in utero
- Surgical excision has 15% recurrence rate
- Sclerotherapy has 76% long-term response rate

(Left) *AP graphic shows a large, multiloculated mass ➯ involving the head, neck, upper arm, and trunk of an infant. These lesions tend to be palpably soft and fluctuant. Propensity for these lesions to vary in size over time is not uncommon.* **(Right)** *Anteroposterior radiograph of an infant shows a massive soft tissue lesion ➯ involving the left chest wall and left upper extremity. The underlying bone is normal. There is no identifiable mineralization within the lesion.*

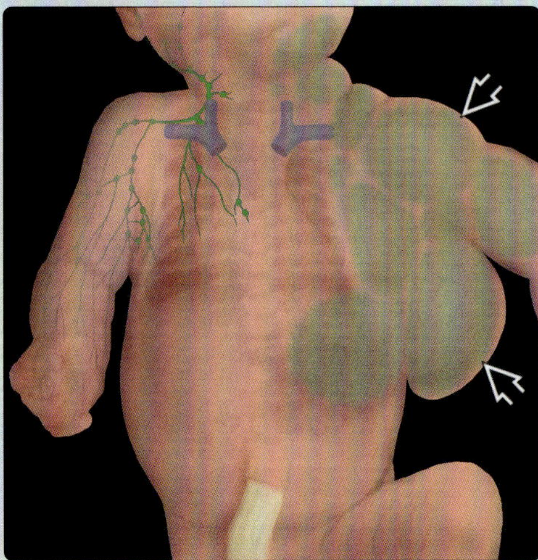

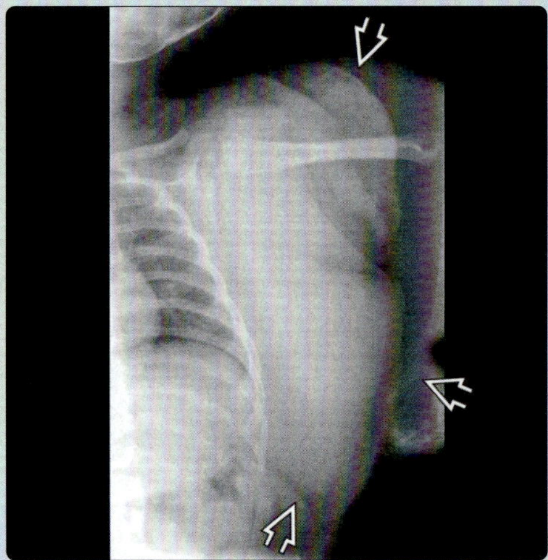

(Left) *Coronal T2WI FS MR in the same patient shows the large mass ➯ involving the left hemithorax and left upper extremity to be centered in the subcutaneous tissues and to infiltrate the chest wall musculature. The lesion can also be seen to extend into the neck ➯.* **(Right)** *Axial T2WI FS MR shows the highly infiltrative mass ➯ to have high signal intensity similar to fluid. Note the extensive septa ➙ within the lesion. This lesion produced significant mass effect on the brachial plexus.*

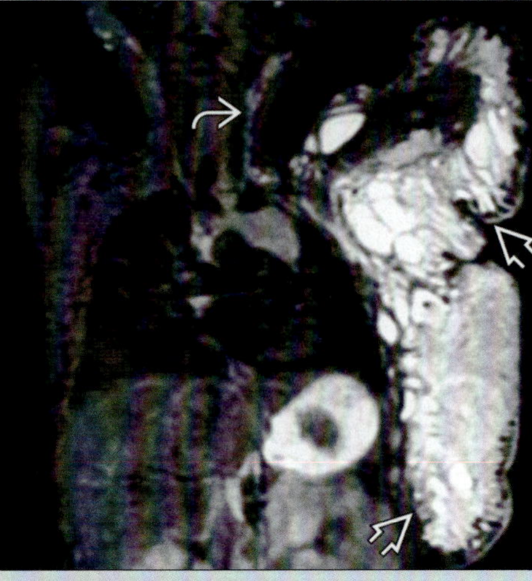

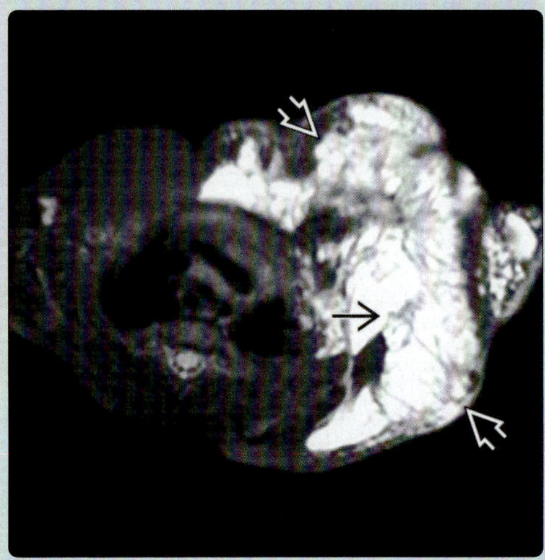

TERMINOLOGY

Synonyms

- Cystic hygroma

Definitions

- Benign developmental lesion composed of dilated lymphatic channels

IMAGING

General Features

- Location
  - Up to 75% in head, neck, and axilla (20%)
  - May be found throughout body: Subcutaneous tissues, soft tissues, organs, and bones
    - Cystic lymphangiomas in neck are most common overall
    - Cutaneous location is overall uncommon
    - Intraabdominal location is overall rare
  - Cystic lymphangioma: Neck, axilla, and groin
  - Cavernous lymphangioma: Oral cavity, upper trunk, limbs, bones, organs, mesentery, and retroperitoneum
  - Capillary lymphangioma: Subcutaneous tissue

Radiographic Findings

- Nonspecific soft tissue mass
- Rare adjacent bone hypertrophy

CT Findings

- Well-circumscribed to ill-defined mass
- Lobulated with low-attenuation cystic regions
  - Cystic areas lack enhancement
- May invade or displace adjacent organs
- Rare calcification

MR Findings

- Multiloculated mass with heterogeneous signal intensity
- Majority of mass follows fluid signal intensity
  - Hyperintense signal on T1WI can be caused by hemorrhage or proteinaceous fluid
  - Fluid-fluid levels from layering debris in cystic spaces
- Mass wall and internal septa have intermediate to low signal intensity and show mild enhancement

Ultrasonographic Findings

- Unilocular or multilocular cystic mass with posterior acoustic enhancement
- Anechoic to hypoechoic depending on debris in fluid

Angiographic Findings

- Low vascularity differentiates from hemangioma

DIFFERENTIAL DIAGNOSIS

Hemangioma & Vascular Malformations

- Contrast confirms vascular nature of lesions

Hematoma

- May have history of trauma
- Complex internal debris from hemorrhage
- Enhancement of hematoma wall; no central enhancement

Abscess

- Thick, shaggy-enhancing abscess wall
- Surrounding inflammatory change
- Systemic symptoms of infection

PATHOLOGY

General Features

- Etiology
  - Developmental malformation
  - Genetic aberrations contribute to development
- Genetics
  - Turner syndrome and chromosomal aneuploidies are associated with cystic lymphangioma (cystic hygroma) of neck
- Associated abnormalities
  - Cystic lymphangioma: Noonan syndrome, fetal alcohol syndrome, hydrops fetalis, familial pterygium coli
  - Commonly associated with other vascular malformations
    - Occur with hemangiomas in Maffucci syndrome

Gross Pathologic & Surgical Features

- Multicystic or spongy lesions containing white-tan or translucent vesicles

Microscopic Features

- Dilated lymphatic vessels of varying size with flattened endothelial lining
- Cavities contain serous, chylous, or proteinaceous fluid

CLINICAL ISSUES

Presentation

- Most common signs/symptoms
  - Painless mass that may wax and wane in size
    - Palpably soft and fluctuant (but unlike vascular malformations, non-compressible
  - Respiratory distress and feeding problems
- Other signs/symptoms
  - Lesion rupture, secondary infection or hemorrhage

Demographics

- Age
  - Usually identified within 1st 2 years of life
    - Can be identified in utero
  - Cutaneous lymphangioma may arise in adults after trauma, surgery, or irradiation
- Epidemiology
  - Less common than hemangiomas

Natural History & Prognosis

- Morbidity from vital structure compression
  - High death rate when identified in utero
- Rare reports of spontaneous resolution

Treatment

- Surgical excision has 15% recurrence rate
- Sclerotherapy has 76% long-term response rate

SELECTED REFERENCES

1. Behr GG et al: Vascular anomalies: hemangiomas and beyond–part 2, Slow-flow lesions. AJR Am J Roentgenol. 200(2):423-36, 2013

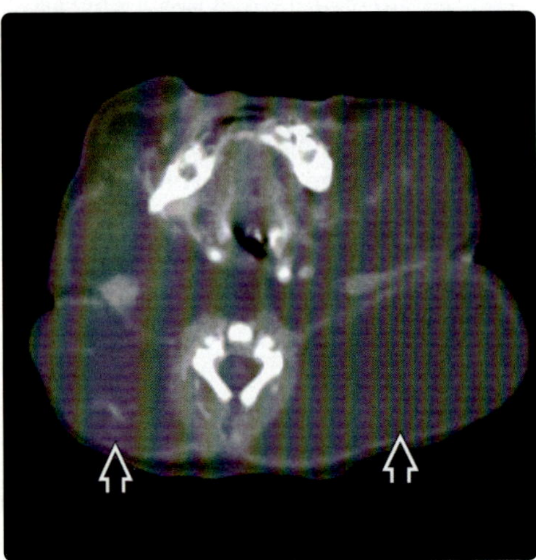

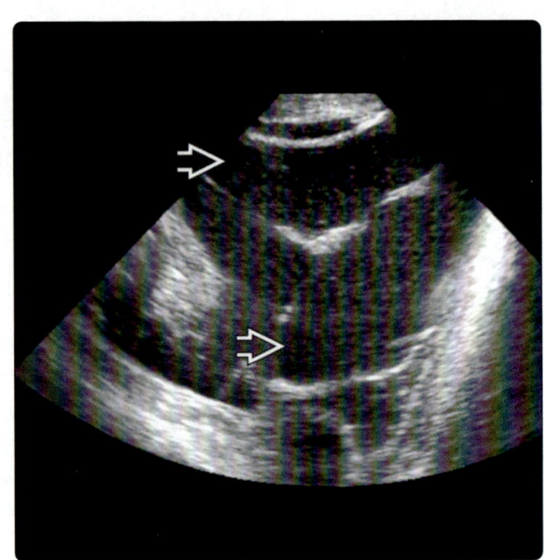

(Left) *Axial CECT shows a large, multicystic, bilateral neck mass ➔ replacing almost all normal tissues circumferentially. This 2-day-old male infant was imaged to evaluate the extent of the lesion for percutaneous sclerotherapy.* **(Right)** *Ultrasound in the same patient, obtained for imaging guidance during percutaneous sclerotherapy, shows multiple fluid-filled cysts ➔ containing various amounts of echogenic material.*

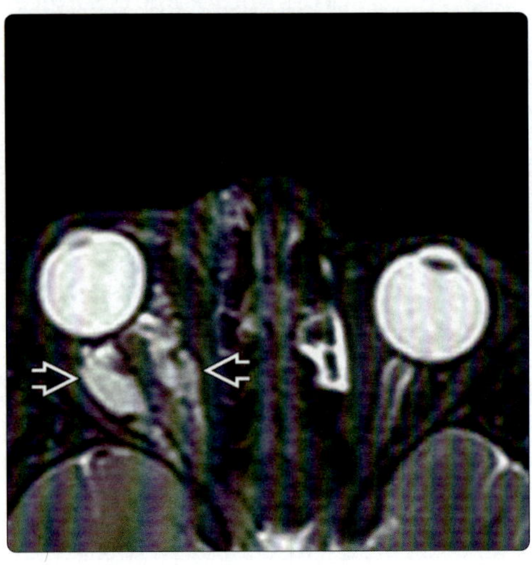

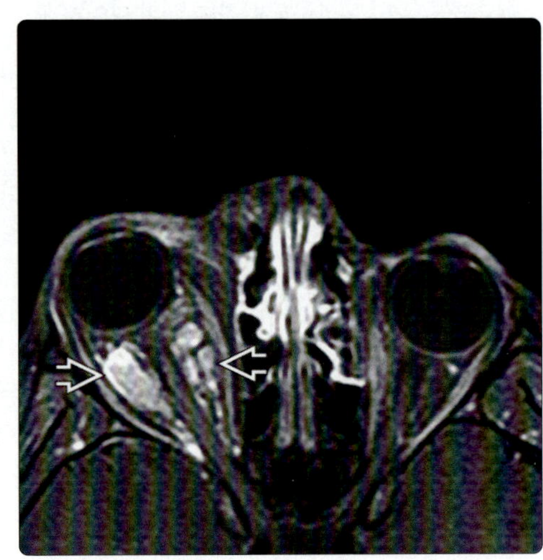

(Left) *Axial T2WI FS MR shows a lobulated intraconal mass ➔ to be hyperintense to muscle. The mass surrounds the optic nerve and is producing proptosis of the right globe, along with bowing of the medial and lateral rectus muscles.* **(Right)** *Axial T1WI C+ MR demonstrates mild enhancement involving the borders and septa of the mass ➔. High signal within the cystic portions of the mass were present pregadolinium and presumably secondary to elevated protein content.*

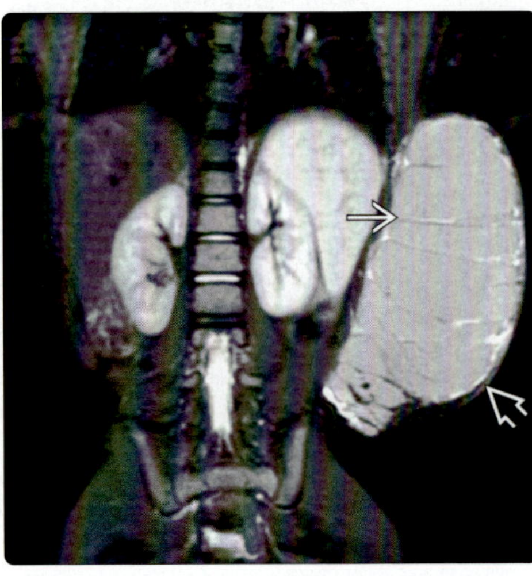

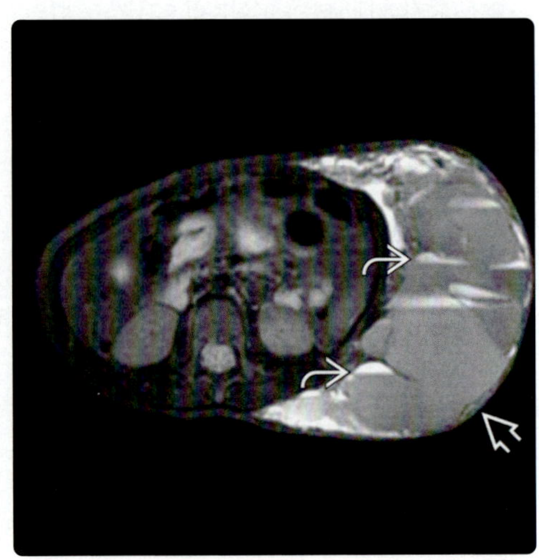

(Left) *Coronal T2WI FS MR shows a very large, exophytic mass ➔ protruding from the left lateral aspect of the chest and abdomen. The mass contains multiple septa ➔. The overall signal intensity is high but not as high as would be expected with simple fluid.* **(Right)** *Axial T2WI FS MR in the same patient shows the large mass ➔ to have heterogeneously hyperintense signal. Multiple fluid-fluid levels ➔ are present. This mass rapidly increased in size during a viral illness.*

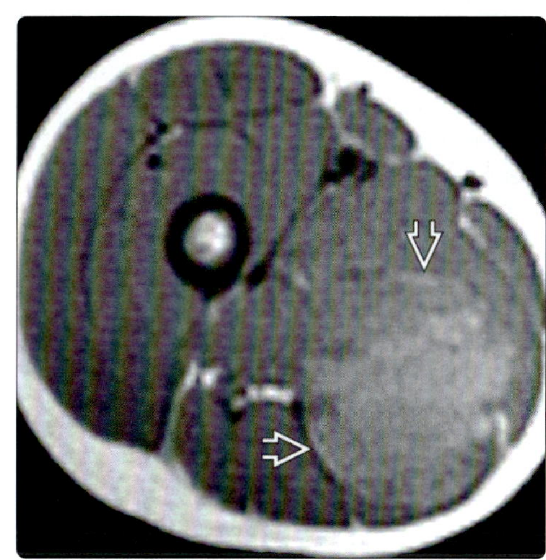

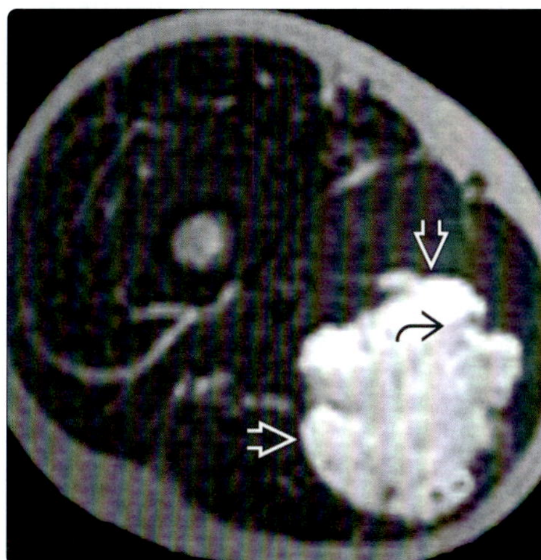

(Left) *Axial T1WI MR shows a large soft tissue mass ➡ in the thigh of a child. The mass is isointense to mildly hyperintense relative to muscle. There were no reactive changes in the surrounding tissues.* **(Right)** *Axial T2WI MR shows the mass ➡ to have heterogeneous high signal intensity. Thin internal septa ↗ are visible. This lesion has a somewhat nonspecific appearance for a pediatric patient. Hemangioma and lymphangioma would both be reasonable to include in the differential diagnosis.*

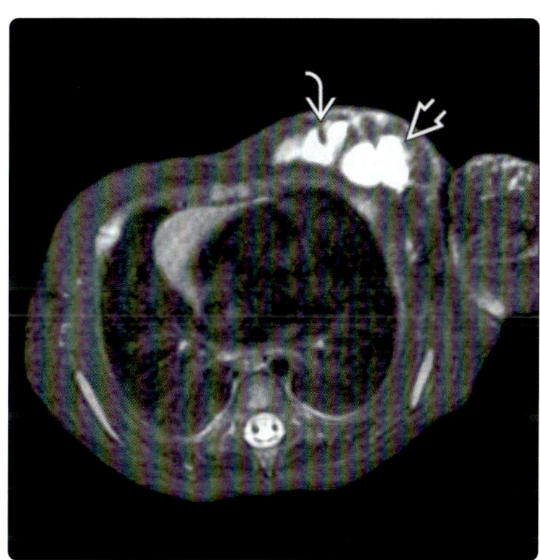

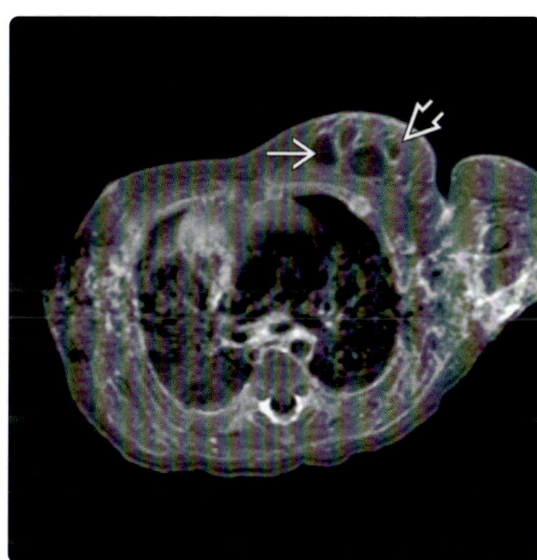

(Left) *Axial T2WI FS MR shows a large mass ➡ in the region of the left breast in an infant. The majority of the lesion has high signal intensity similar to fluid. The lesion has a multiloculated appearance, with a few incomplete septa ➡ visible on this image.* **(Right)** *Axial T1WI C+ FS MR in the same patient demonstrates that only the walls and septa of the mass ➡ enhance. The regions having fluid signal intensity ➡ on T2WI MR lack any identifiable enhancement.*

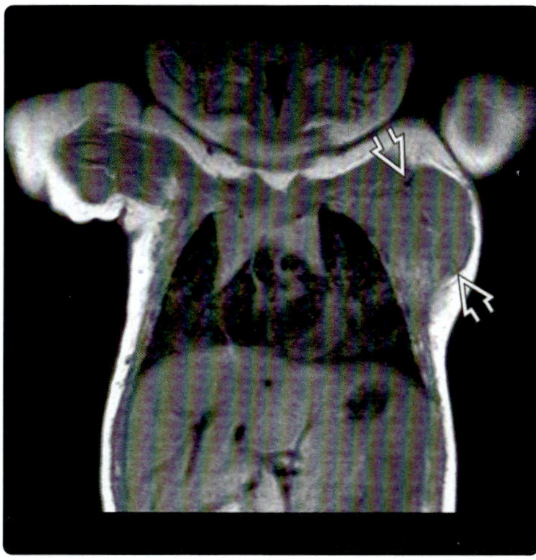

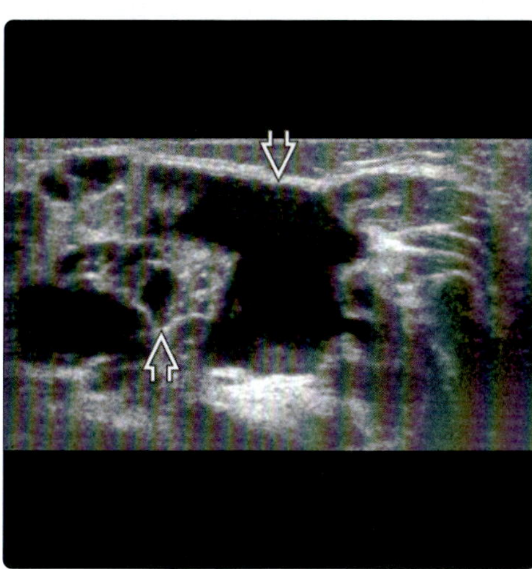

(Left) *Coronal T1WI MR shows a large, lobulated mass ➡ involving the left axillary region of an infant. This mass has similar signal intensity to muscle. The lobulated regions had high signal intensity on T2WI FS MR and lacked central enhancement, consistent with fluid-filled regions. The increased T1 signal is likely due to proteinaceous or hemorrhagic fluid contents.* **(Right)** *Ultrasound obtained during localization for percutaneous sclerosis shows multiple irregularly sized, cystic lesions ➡.*

Kaposi Sarcoma

KEY FACTS

TERMINOLOGY

- Rarely metastasizing endothelial neoplasm associated with human herpesvirus 8 (HHV-8)

IMAGING

- Typically involves skin of lower legs
  - Also mucosal membranes, lymph nodes, and organs
  - Rarely centered in bone, muscle, brain, and kidney
- Radiographs: Nonspecific soft tissue enlargement
  - Osseous encroachment uncommon
    - Periosteal reaction, erosion, cortical destruction
- CT: Nodular enhancing mass
  - ± skin thickening and subcutaneous edema
  - Hyperattenuating adenopathy
- T1WI MR: Isointense to muscle
- T2WI MR: Hyperintense to muscle
- Positive thallium-201 and red blood cell pooling
- Negative gallium-67 scintigraphy

TOP DIFFERENTIAL DIAGNOSES

- Hemangioma & vascular malformations
  - Cutaneous arteriovenous malformations sometimes called "pseudo-Kaposi sarcoma"
- Soft tissue angiosarcoma
  - May have similar imaging appearance
- Lymphoma, non-Hodgkin
  - Positive gallium-67 scintigraphy

CLINICAL ISSUES

- Classic KS: Usually indolent with 10-20% mortality
- Endemic KS: Indolent in adults, aggressive in children (lymphadenopathic form)
- Iatrogenic KS: Unpredictably indolent or aggressive
- AIDS-related KS: Most aggressive type
- Treatment options include surgery, cryotherapy, intralesional injection, radiotherapy, and chemotherapy
- Widespread visceral involvement has worse prognosis

(Left) *Sagittal T1WI MR of the forefoot shows an extensive, nodular mass ➔ involving the soft tissues. The mass has heterogeneous signal that is isointense to mildly hyperintense relative to skeletal muscle.* **(Right)** *Sagittal STIR MR shows the mass ➔ to have heterogeneously hyperintense signal. Numerous, fine septa ↪ are present within the mass. This patient has typical demographics for the classic form of Kaposi sarcoma, that being an older adult man of Mediterranean descent.*

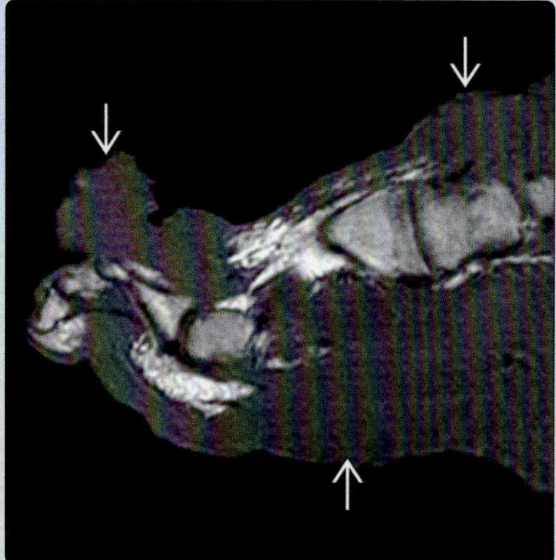

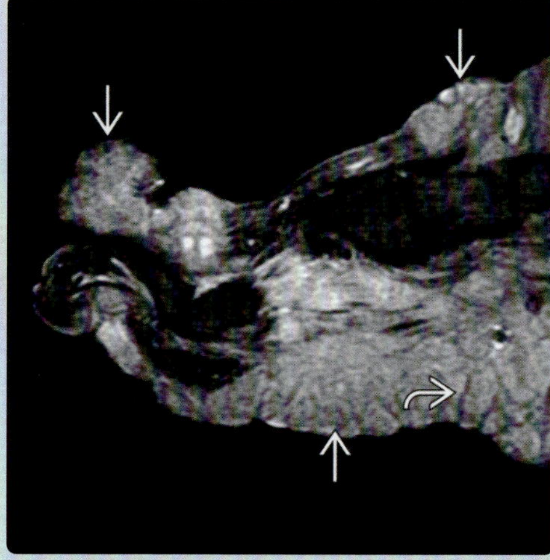

(Left) *Coronal T1WI MR best demonstrates the massive, circumferential involvement of the foot soft tissues by the nodular mass ➔. The mass infiltrates subcutaneous fat, fascia, and muscle. The bones were abutted, but not definitively invaded, by tumor.* **(Right)** *Coronal STIR MR shows heterogeneous hyperintensity of the mass ➔, which is composed of nodules of varying sizes. This patient had been treated for over 10 years, utilizing different treatment modalities, without disease control.*

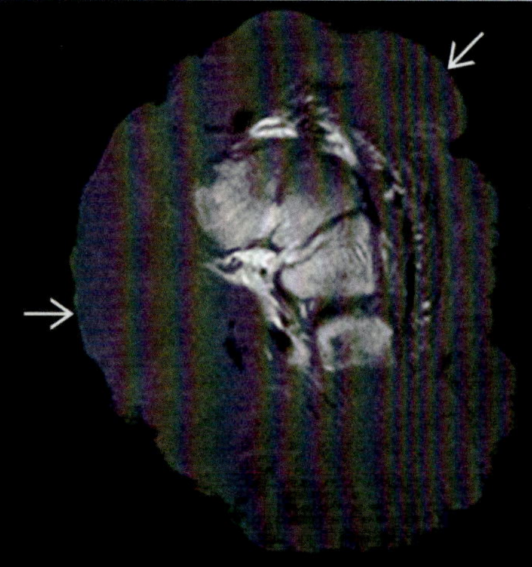

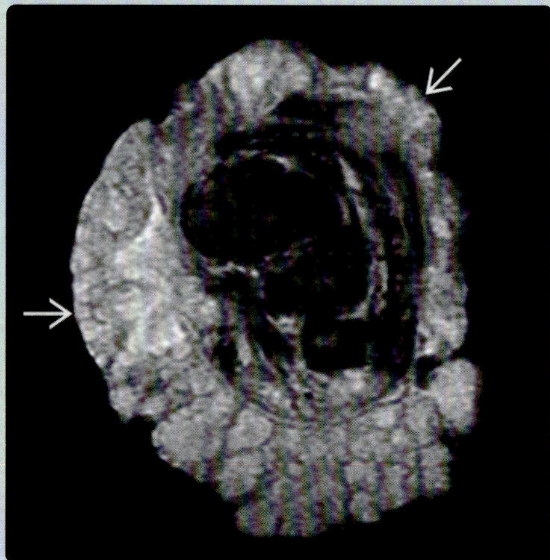

TERMINOLOGY

Abbreviations

- Kaposi sarcoma (KS)

Definitions

- Rarely metastasizing endothelial neoplasm associated with human herpesvirus 8 (HHV-8)

IMAGING

General Features

- Location
  - Typically involves skin of lower legs
    - Also mucosal membranes, lymph nodes, & organs
    - Rarely centered in bone, muscle, brain, kidney
  - AIDS-related KS also involves face and genitalia

Imaging Recommendations

- Imaging appearance discussion is limited to skin and musculoskeletal findings

Radiographic Findings

- Nonspecific soft tissue enlargement
- Osseous encroachment uncommon
  - Periosteal reaction, erosion, cortical destruction

CT Findings

- Nodular enhancing mass
  - ± skin thickening and subcutaneous edema
  - Hyperattenuating adenopathy

MR Findings

- Isointense to muscle on T1WI
- Hyperintense to muscle on T2WI
- Heterogeneous enhancement

Ultrasonographic Findings

- Nonspecific intermediate echogenicity mass

Angiographic Findings

- Lesions demonstrate ↑ vascularity

Nuclear Medicine Findings

- Positive thallium-201 and red blood cell pooling
- Negative gallium-67 scintigraphy

DIFFERENTIAL DIAGNOSIS

Hemangioma & Vascular Malformations

- Cutaneous arteriovenous malformations sometimes called pseudo-Kaposi sarcoma
- Angiography confirms vascular malformation

Soft Tissue Angiosarcoma

- May have similar imaging appearance
- Biopsy may be necessary for diagnosis

Lymphoma, Non-Hodgkin

- Extranodal, disseminated disease can involve musculoskeletal system
- Osseous involvement is better defined than KS
- Positive gallium-67 scintigraphy

Lymphedema

- Lacks focal enhancing nodules found in KS

PATHOLOGY

General Features

- Etiology
  - HHV-8 produces all epidemiological-clinical types of Kaposi sarcoma

Microscopic Features

- Lesions from 4 epidemiological-clinical types of KS have same histologic appearance
- HHV-8, CD34, and FLI1 positive

CLINICAL ISSUES

Presentation

- Most common signs/symptoms
  - Classic KS: Lower leg lesions ± lymphedema
    - ↑ risk of lymphoma, myeloma, and leukemia
  - Endemic KS: Extremity skin lesions with common visceral involvement
  - Iatrogenic KS: Lower leg lesions with fairly common visceral involvement
    - Organ transplant or immunosuppressive therapy initiated months to years prior to presentation
  - AIDS-related KS: Face, genitalia, and leg lesions
    - Visceral involvement may be silent or symptomatic

Demographics

- Age
  - Classic KS: Elderly men
  - Endemic KS: Middle-aged adults and children
  - Iatrogenic KS: Any age
  - AIDS-related KS: Younger adult men
- Epidemiology
  - Classic KS: Mediterranean/East European descent
  - Endemic KS: Equatorial Africa (not HIV infected)
  - Iatrogenic KS: Transplant and other medically immunosuppressed patients
  - AIDS-related KS: Homosexual or bisexual HIV-1 infected men predominately

Natural History & Prognosis

- Depends on epidemiological-clinical type
  - Classic KS: Usually indolent with 10-20% mortality
  - Endemic KS: Indolent in adults, aggressive in children (lymphadenopathic form)
  - Iatrogenic KS: Unpredictably indolent or aggressive
    - May spontaneously resolve if immunosuppressive therapy discontinued
  - AIDS-related KS: Most aggressive type

Treatment

- Treatment options include surgery, cryotherapy, intralesional injection, radiotherapy, and chemotherapy

SELECTED REFERENCES

1. Kransdorf MJ et al: Vascular and lymphatic tumors. In Kransdorf MJ et al: Imaging of Soft Tissue Tumors. 2nd ed. Philadelphia: Lippincott Williams & Wilkins. 177-83, 2006

(Left) *Axial CECT through the vertex reveals an intensely enhancing soft tissue mass ➡ within the scalp.* **(Right)** *Axial CECT more inferior to the previous image shows the mass ➡ to extend from the subcutis into the muscle and have a mildly nodular contour. Differential considerations would include lymphoma, scalp vascular malformation, neurofibroma, and metastasis. Knowing the patient's history of AIDS makes Kaposi sarcoma the likely diagnosis in this case.*

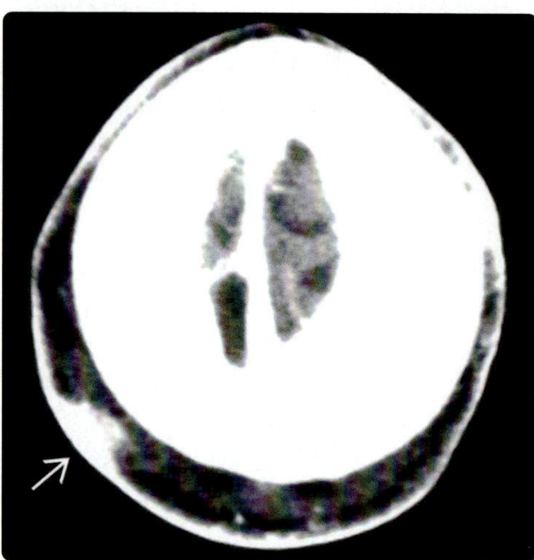

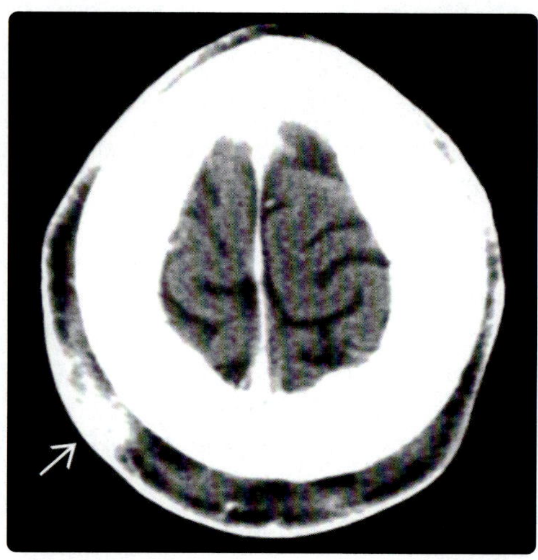

(Left) *Axial soft tissue algorithm CT shows multiple infiltrating soft tissue nodules ➡ in the skin and subcutaneous areas. These nodules moderately enhance. Their appearance is suspicious for malignancy but is otherwise fairly nonspecific.* **(Right)** *Axial soft tissue algorithm CT shows an infiltrating mass ➡ located just deep to the subcutaneous fat. There are also enlarged high deep cervical lymph nodes ➢. This immunocompromised patient had biopsy-proven Kaposi sarcoma.*

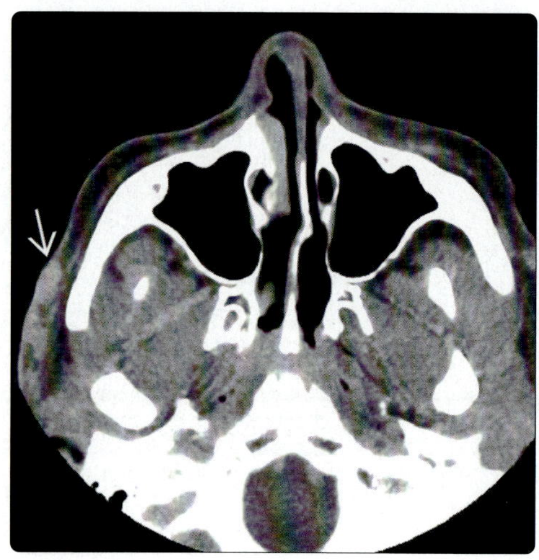

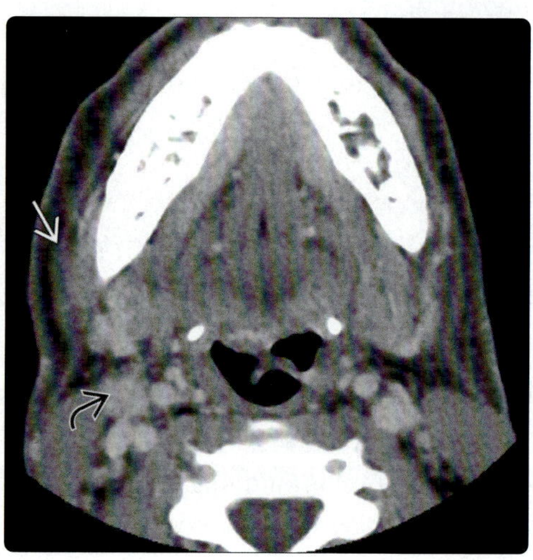

(Left) *Axial CECT demonstrates enlarged enhancing bilateral axillary adenopathy ➡ and a single enhancing mediastinal lymph node ➡. These findings were secondary to Kaposi sarcoma.* **(Right)** *Axial soft tissue algorithm CT in a different patient shows widespread lymphadenopathy. Some of the lymph nodes ➡ in the groin show intense enhancement, a common feature seen with Kaposi sarcoma involvement.*

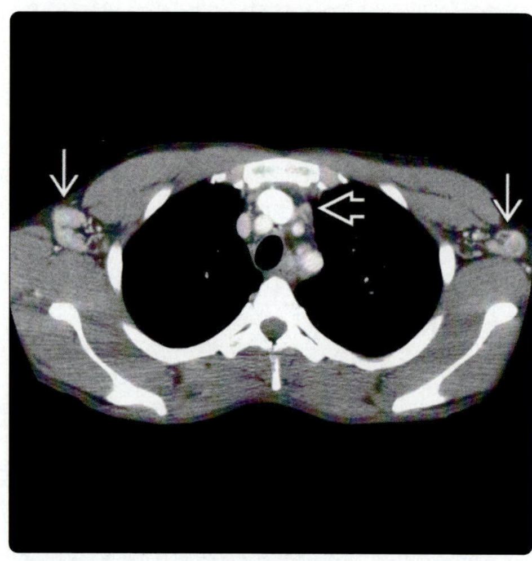

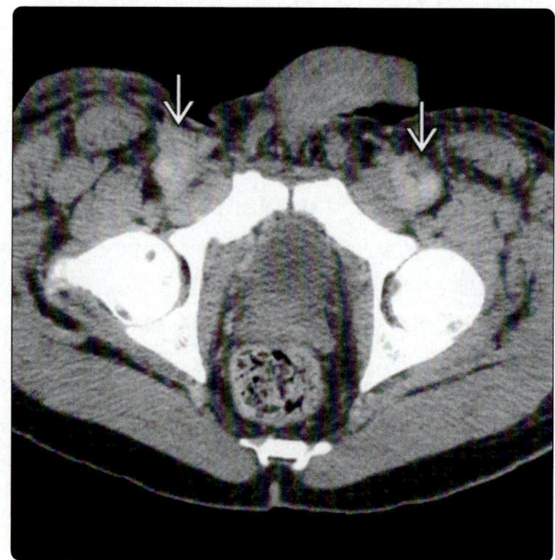

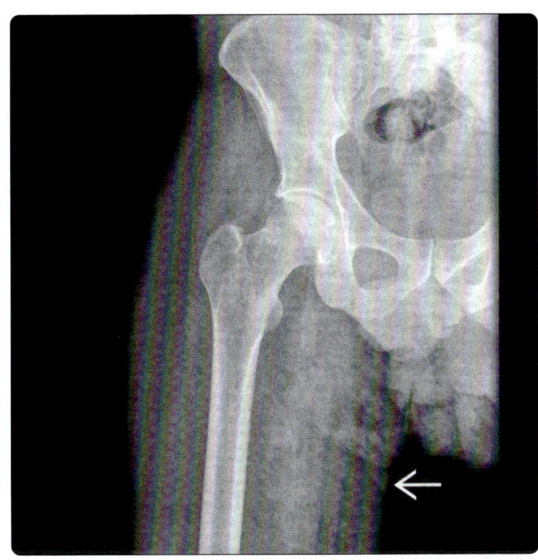

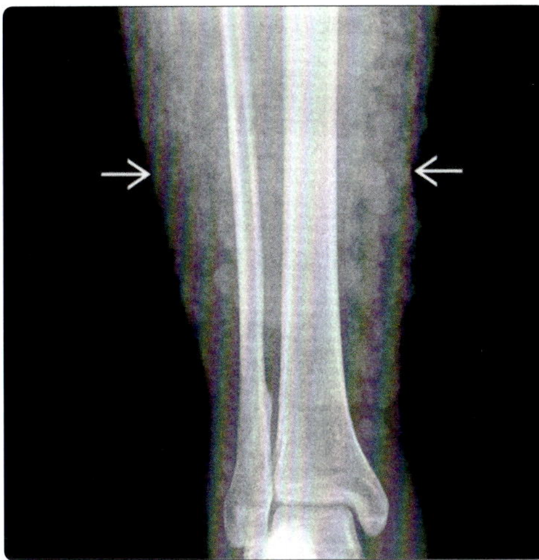

(Left) *AP radiograph of the hip in an HIV-positive patient demonstrates numerous variably sized, rounded foci of increased attenuation ➡ projected over the medial thigh. The underlying bones are normal.* **(Right)** *AP radiograph of the lower leg demonstrates diffuse, plaque-like soft tissue thickening ➡. The soft tissues are circumferentially involved. Kaposi sarcoma in HIV-infected patients often involves the skin. Radiographic imaging shows nonspecific nodular soft tissue thickening.*

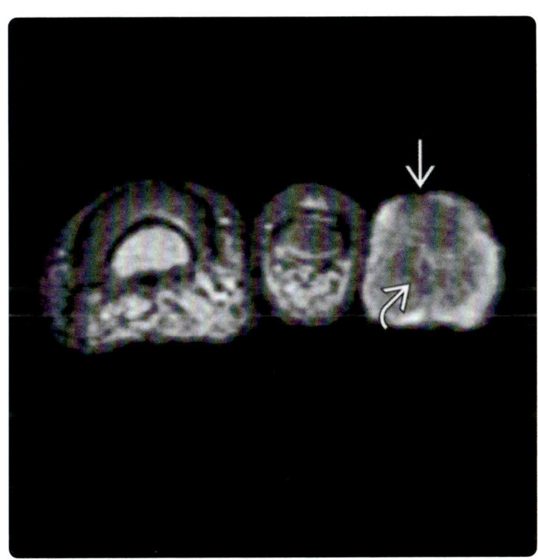

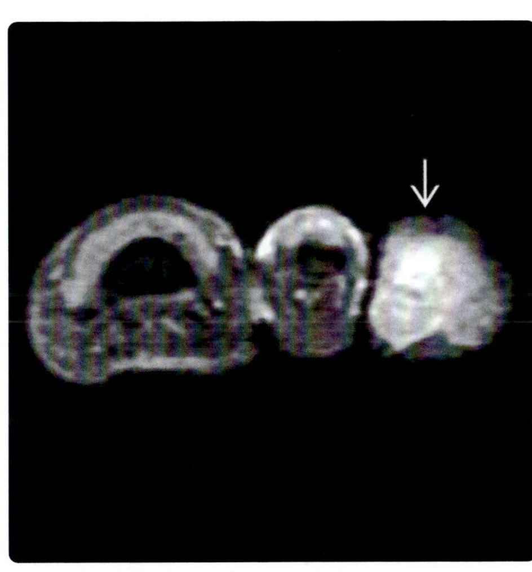

(Left) *Coronal T1WI MR through the forefoot of an HIV-positive patient shows the soft tissues of the 3rd toe ➡ to be diffusely enlarged. The enlarged soft tissues have heterogeneously isointense to slightly hyperintense signal relative to skeletal muscle. There is a suggestion of a low-signal septation ➡.* **(Right)** *Coronal T1WI C+ FS MR shows the thickened soft tissues ➡ of the 3rd toe to have diffuse, heterogeneous enhancement.*

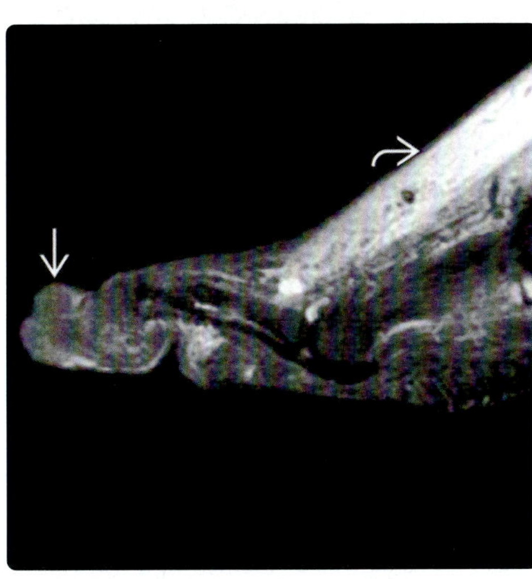

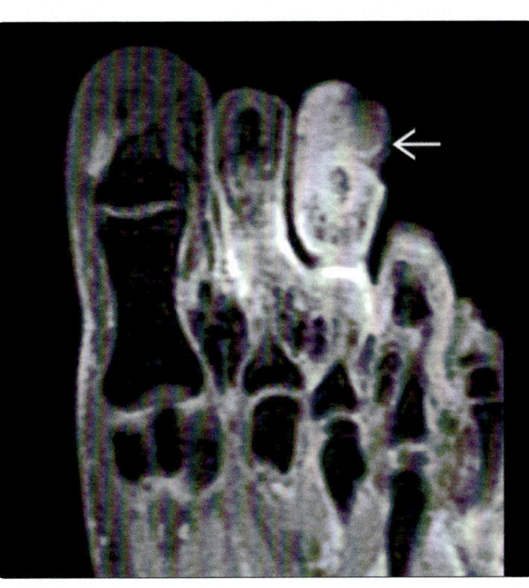

(Left) *Sagittal T2WI FS MR shows the 3rd toe tissues ➡ to have heterogeneous signal that is isointense to mildly hyperintense to muscle. Subcutaneous edema ➡ involves the dorsum of the foot.* **(Right)** *Axial T1WI C+ FS MR shows the thickened, enhancing soft tissues involving the 3rd toe ➡. MR imaging of Kaposi sarcoma usually demonstrates nonspecific nodular masses with isointense signal on T1WI MR, hyperintense signal on fluid-sensitive sequences, and heterogeneous enhancement.*

KEY FACTS

TERMINOLOGY

- Group of intermediate to malignant vascular neoplasms with less aggressive behavior than angiosarcoma

IMAGING

- Epithelioid hemangioendothelioma (EH): Superficial or deep extremity soft tissues
  - Also occur in bone, lung, and liver
- Kaposiform hemangioendothelioma (KH): Most common in retroperitoneum and skin
  - Also occur in head and neck, mediastinum, trunk, and extremities
- Retiform hemangioendothelioma (RH) and papillary intralymphatic angioendothelioma (PILA): Skin and subcutaneous tissue of distal extremities
- Composite hemangioendothelioma (CH): Distal extremities
- Radiographs show soft tissue mass that may contain calcification and erode underlying bone
- CT: Ill-defined mass ± calcification or hemorrhage
- MR shows nonspecific, infiltrative soft tissue mass
  - Signal is intermediate on T1WI and heterogeneously hyperintense on T2WI MR
    - Low-signal foci may be caused by calcification or high-flow vessels
  - \+ enhancement

CLINICAL ISSUES

- Thrombophlebitis or edema from vascular obstruction
- May have history of radiotherapy or lymphedema
- Kasabach-Merritt syndrome with large KH lesions
- Abdominal KH may present with bowel obstruction, jaundice, or ascites
- Lesion types have different biologic behavior
  - Locally aggressive → KH
  - Rarely metastasizing → RH, CH, PILA
  - Malignant → EH
- Surgical excision with wide margins

(Left) *Axial T1WI MR of distal forearm shows a composite hemangioendothelioma ➡ involving the subcutaneous fat. The mass is isointense to slightly hyperintense relative to skeletal muscle.* **(Right)** *Axial T2WI FS MR demonstrates the ill-defined soft tissue mass ➡ to have mildly heterogeneous, hyperintense signal. The extent of the lesion appears larger compared with the T1WI MR due to surrounding edema. This adult male reported the mass had been present for several decades but recently enlarged.*

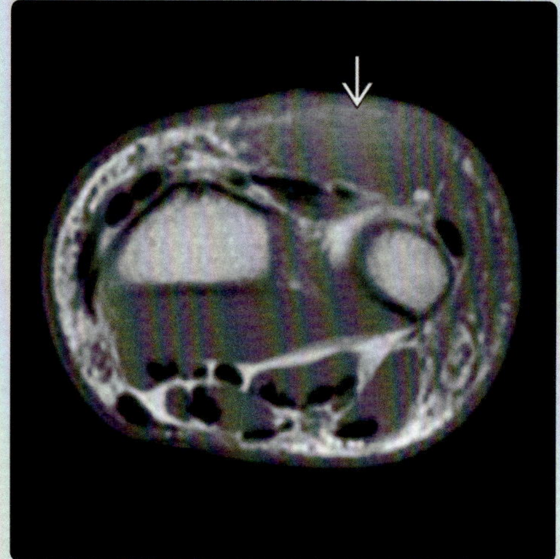

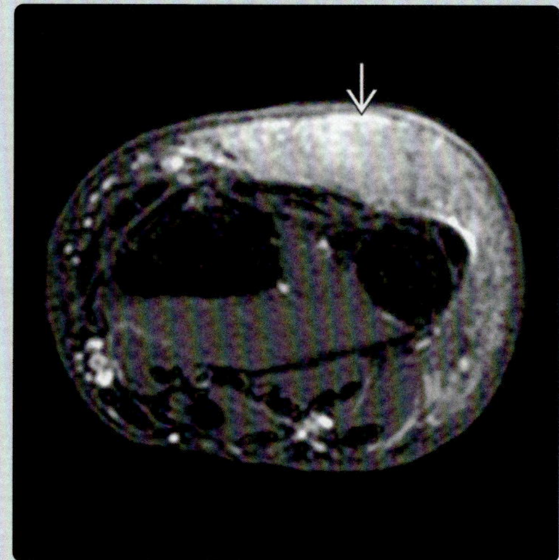

(Left) *Axial T1WI FS MR after IV contrast shows mildly heterogeneous enhancement of the mass ➡. The skin is also seen to enhance, consistent with tumor involvement.* **(Right)** *Axial NECT shows an ill-defined mass ➡ in the left suprascapular region. The majority of this mass is isointense to skeletal muscle with low-attenuation regions suggestive of fat or myxoid material ➡ and high-attenuation, dystrophic-appearing calcifications ➡. Biopsy revealed an epithelioid hemangioendothelioma.*

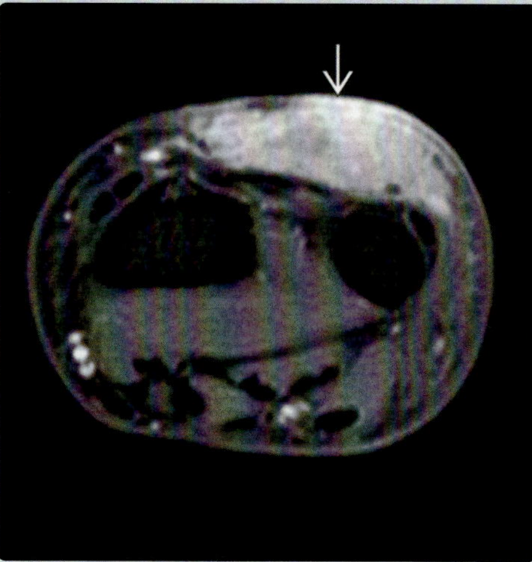

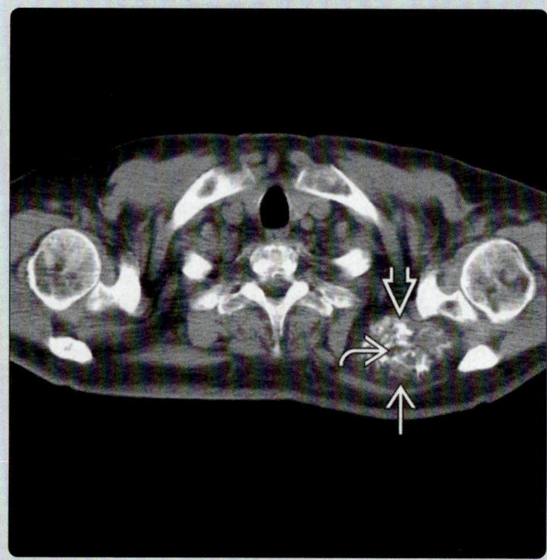

TERMINOLOGY

Abbreviations

- Epithelioid hemangioendothelioma (EH)
- Kaposiform hemangioendothelioma (KH)
- Retiform hemangioendothelioma (RH)
- Composite hemangioendothelioma (CH)
- Papillary intralymphatic angioendothelioma (PILA)

Definitions

- Group of intermediate to malignant vascular neoplasms with less aggressive behavior than angiosarcoma
  - Epithelioid hemangioendothelioma is malignant
  - Other forms have intermediate biologic behavior with local aggressiveness ± rare metastases

IMAGING

General Features

- Location
  - EH: Superficial or deep extremity soft tissues
    - 50-70% arise near vessel and may be occlusive
    - Also occur in bone, lung, and liver
  - KH: Most common in retroperitoneum and skin
    - Superficial or deep soft tissues
    - Also occur in head and neck, mediastinum, trunk, and extremities
  - RH and PILA: Skin and subcutaneous tissue of distal extremities
  - CH: Distal extremities
- Size
  - RH: < 3 cm in maximum dimension

Radiographic Findings

- Soft tissue mass that may contain calcification and erode underlying bone

CT Findings

- Ill-defined soft tissue mass ± calcification or hemorrhage

MR Findings

- Nonspecific, infiltrative soft tissue mass
- Signal is intermediate on T1WI and heterogeneously hyperintense on T2WI
- Low-signal foci may be caused by calcification or high-flow vessels
- + enhancement

DIFFERENTIAL DIAGNOSIS

Angiosarcoma, Epithelioid

- Histologically highly malignant-appearing lesion
- Necrosis common

Kaposi Sarcoma

- + human herpes virus 8 (HHV-8)
- Regions of KH may be histologically identical
- Older patient population than KH

Sarcoma, Epithelioid

- Histologically similar appearance
- Immunohistochemistry helpful for differentiation from EH

PATHOLOGY

General Features

- Etiology
  - Vascular neoplasm of unknown etiology
    - No association with HHV-8

Gross Pathologic & Surgical Features

- Infiltrative, variably nodular gray to reddish blue lesions

Microscopic Features

- Overall appearance and vascular components vary with different types
  - Myxoid, hyaline, or sclerotic stroma
- Positive CD31 and CD34

CLINICAL ISSUES

Presentation

- Most common signs/symptoms
  - EH: Painful, superficial or deep nodular mass
  - KH: Well-defined cutaneous plaque
  - RH: Reddish blue plaque or nodule
  - CH: Variably nodular superficial lesion
    - May be present > 10 years before diagnosis
  - PILA: Painless, slowly growing plaque or nodule involving skin
- Other signs/symptoms
  - Thrombophlebitis or edema from vascular obstruction
  - May have history of radiotherapy or lymphedema
  - Kasabach-Merritt syndrome with large KH lesions
  - Abdominal KH may present with bowel obstruction, jaundice, or ascites

Demographics

- Age
  - Adults → EH, CH, 25% of PILA
  - Young adults → RH
  - Infants and children → KH, PILA

Natural History & Prognosis

- Lesion types have different biologic behavior
  - Locally aggressive → KH
    - Recurrence of superficial lesions is rare
    - Deep, invasive lesions may lead to death
  - Rarely metastasizing → RH, CH, PILA
    - High local recurrence rate of up to 60%
    - PILA metastasizes to regional lymph nodes
  - Malignant → EH
    - Prognosis worse with mitoses > 1 per 10 HPF, spindling of cells, necrosis, and marked nuclear atypia

Treatment

- Surgical excision with wide margins
  - Invasive lesions in deep soft tissues may be unresectable

SELECTED REFERENCES

1. Kransdorf MJ et al: Vascular and lymphatic tumors. In Kransdorf MJ et al: Imaging of Soft Tissue Tumors. 2nd ed. Philadelphia: Lippincott Williams & Wilkins. 177-88, 2006

KEY FACTS

TERMINOLOGY

- Malignant endothelial neoplasm with exceptionally poor prognosis

IMAGING

- Majority involve skin and subcutis
  - < 25% are located deep to subcutis
  - Deep muscles of lower extremities > > arm > trunk > head
  - Rare in bone, head and neck, breast, liver, spleen, heart
- Nodular, infiltrative soft tissue mass on CT
  - Attenuation is similar to muscle
- Nonspecific infiltrative mass on MR
  - Isointense to hyperintense relative to skeletal muscle on T1WI
  - Hemorrhage produces high signal on T1WI
  - Hemorrhage may also produce fluid-fluid levels
  - Hyperintense to muscle on fluid-sensitive sequences
  - Prominent enhancement

CLINICAL ISSUES

- Cutaneous lesions initially appear similar to bruise that does not resolve
  - Lesions later become nodular ± ulceration
- Associated with chronic lymphedema, radiotherapy, foreign bodies, environmental exposures, and both benign and malignant tumors
- Found throughout life (considering all types of angiosarcoma)
  - Peak incidence in 7th decade
- M > F (2:1)
- Poor prognosis for these highly aggressive tumors
  - > 50% death rate within 1 year
  - Prognosis worsens with older age, size > 5 cm, retroperitoneal location, and high Ki-67 proliferation antigen expression
- Surgical excision often combined with radiotherapy
  - Adjuvant chemotherapy has evolving role

(Left) *Axial graphic shows an aggressive-appearing nodular, hemorrhagic mass ➡ involving the thigh. Note that this infiltrative tumor is superficially located, involving the skin and subcutis. This lesion lacks fat overgrowth, which helps differentiate it from a benign vascular tumor.* **(Right)** *Axial soft tissue algorithm CT shows an infiltrative mass ➡ located predominately anterior to the heart. Enhancing vessels ➡ are present peripherally. The lesion has metastasized ➡ to the lung and pleura.*

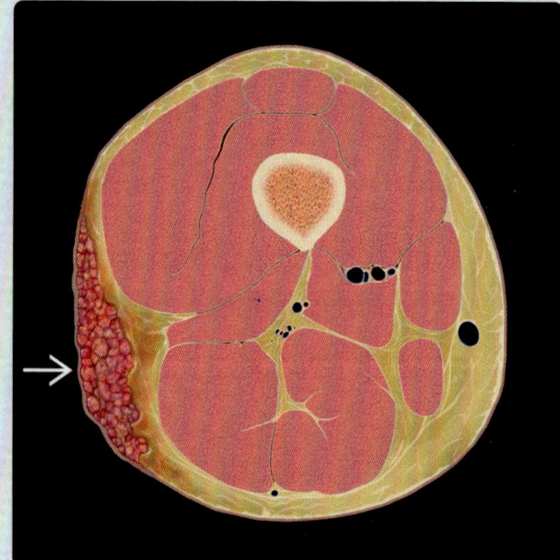

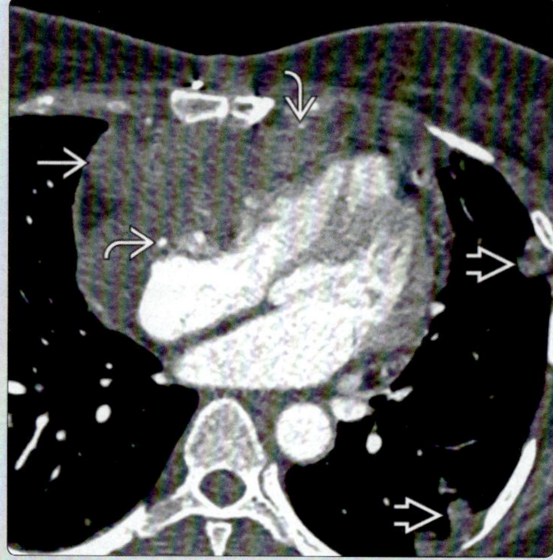

(Left) *Coronal T1WI MR shows a large mass ➡ involving the thigh. This mass has heterogeneous signal intensity that is isointense to hyperintense relative to skeletal muscle, with serpiginous low-signal foci ➡ around the periphery of the lesion. There was an intact fat plane between the mass and the underlying fascia.* **(Right)** *Coronal STIR MR shows the mass ➡ to have markedly heterogeneous signal intensity. The previously identified low-signal serpiginous foci ➡ correspond to enlarged blood vessels.*

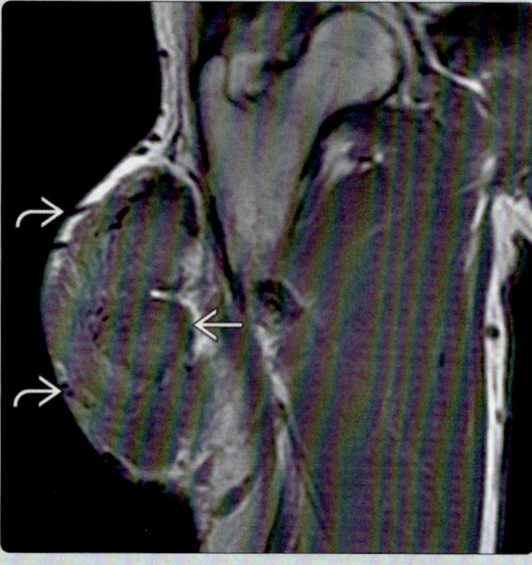

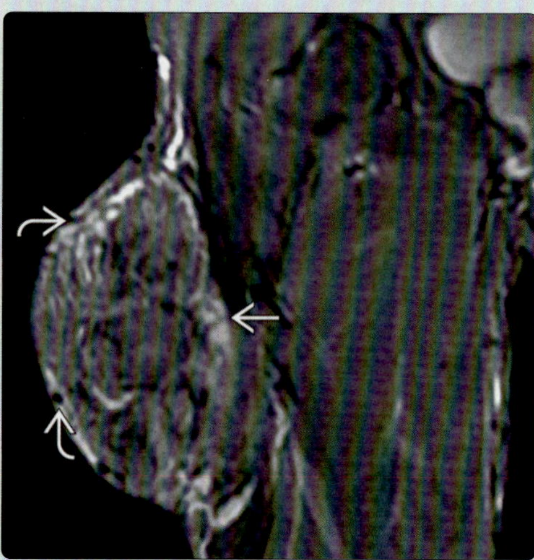

TERMINOLOGY

Synonyms

- Hemangiosarcoma, malignant hemangioendothelioma, lymphangiosarcoma, hemangioblastoma, malignant angioendothelioma

Definitions

- Malignant endothelial neoplasm with exceptionally poor prognosis

IMAGING

General Features

- Location
  - Majority involve skin and subcutis
  - < 25% are located deep to subcutis
    - Deep muscles of lower extremities > > arm > trunk > head
    - Significant proportion arise in abdominal cavity
  - Rare in bone, head and neck, breast, liver, spleen, and heart
- Size
  - Several centimeters in diameter
- Morphology
  - Multinodular but rarely multifocal

CT Findings

- Nodular, infiltrative soft tissue mass
- Attenuation is similar to muscle

MR Findings

- Nonspecific infiltrative mass
  - Isointense to hyperintense relative to skeletal muscle on T1WI
    - Hemorrhage produces high signal on T1WI
  - Hyperintense to muscle on fluid-sensitive sequences
    - Hemorrhage may also produce fluid-fluid levels
- Skin thickening with superficial lesions
- Prominent enhancement
  - Serpiginous enhancing vessels relatively common in periphery of deep lesions

Nuclear Medicine Findings

- PET/CT
  - F-18 FDG PET CT useful to demonstrate local recurrence &/or distant metastasis

DIFFERENTIAL DIAGNOSIS

Hematoma

- Extensive hemorrhage of angiosarcoma may mimic chronic hematoma

Hemangioma and Vascular Malformations

- Contains fat overgrowth, which is not present in angiosarcoma

Hemangioendothelioma, Soft Tissue

- Similar imaging appearance as angiosarcoma
- Lacks necrosis

Fibrosarcoma, High Grade

- Angiosarcoma having predominantly spindled cells may be similar histologically

Kaposi Sarcoma

- Spindled cells cluster around vessels, unlike angiosarcoma
- Positive human herpesvirus 8 (HHV-8)

Squamous Cell Carcinoma, Pseudovascular

- May have similar histologic appearance to angiosarcoma due to variable morphology

Carcinoma, Undifferentiated

- Angiosarcoma with epithelioid appearance may be similar histologically

PATHOLOGY

General Features

- Genetics
  - Complex cytogenetic aberrations within tumors
    - Diploid, tetraploid, and aneuploid patterns do not correlate with prognosis
  - Multiple angiogenic growth factors expressed; possible combination treatment targeting
    - Fibroblastic growth receptor 1 correlated with angiopoietin 2F
    - Tie2
    - Hepatocyte growth factor and *NOTCH1* expression ($P = 0.001$, $P = 0.001$, $P < 0.001$, and $P < 0.001$ respectively)
  - *MYC* amplification may distinguish postradiation cutaneous angiosarcomas from atypical vascular lesions following radiotherapy
    - Immunohistochemical stainings for myc useful for mapping of lesions for tumor margin control
- Associated abnormalities
  - Chronic lymphedema
    - Stewart-Treves syndrome: Chronic lymphedema resulting in development of angiosarcoma
    - Presumed mechanism: Immunocompromised district of affected area
    - Formation of collateral lymphatic and vascular vessels in response to lymphedema produces environment rich in growth factors; may also play role
  - Prior radiotherapy for both benign and malignant processes
  - Implanted foreign material, including vascular grafts, shrapnel, and surgical sponges
  - Nerve sheath tumors, benign or malignant, in patients with neurofibromatosis
  - Benign hemangiomas in Maffucci syndrome and Klippel-Trenaunay-Weber syndrome
  - Vinyl chloride and thorium dioxide (Thorotrast) exposure → liver angiosarcoma

Gross Pathologic & Surgical Features

- Infiltrative, hemorrhagic mass
- Sponge-like with blood-filled spaces

Microscopic Features

- Initial nonspecific histologic appearance in many cases

- Suggestive of metastatic carcinomas, malignant mesothelioma, melanoma, anaplastic lymphoma, epithelioid peripheral nerve sheath malignancies, epithelioid sarcoma
- Must also distinguish from malignancies with apparent vascular differentiation such as less aggressive vascular neoplasms, including epithelioid hemangioendothelioma

- Variable morphology containing spindled to epithelioid cells
  - Epithelioid areas usually more prominent
    - Large rounded cells with high nuclear grade
  - Difficult to differentiate vascular from lymphatic elements
- Rudimentary vascular channels, nests, sheets, or cords of cells
  - Vascular channels are irregular and communicate in sinusoidal fashion
  - Intravascular papillation of cells
- Prominent areas of hemorrhage
- Endothelial markers may be important in immunohistochemical analysis to avoid misdiagnosis
  - Positive von Willebrand factor, CD31, and CD34
    - von Willebrand factor is most specific and least sensitive
    - CD31(+) in 90%
- HHV-8(-)

CLINICAL ISSUES

Presentation

- Most common signs/symptoms
  - Cutaneous lesions initially appear similar to bruise that does not resolve
    - Lesions later become nodular ± ulceration
  - Enlarging deep mass
- Other signs/symptoms
  - Lymphedema
  - Coagulopathy, anemia, or bruisability
  - Hemorrhage or hematoma
  - Stewart-Treves syndrome after mastectomy
  - High-output cardiac failure from arteriovenous shunting

Demographics

- Age
  - All ages; peak incidence in 7th decade
    - Rare in childhood
- Gender
  - M > F (2:1)
- Epidemiology
  - Very rare soft tissue neoplasm
    - < 1% of sarcomas

Natural History & Prognosis

- Poor prognosis for these highly aggressive tumors
  - > 50% death rate within 1 year
  - Local recurrence in approximately 20%
  - Approximately 50% with hematogenous metastasis
    - Lung > > lymph node, bone, and soft tissue
- Prognosis worsens with older age, size > 5 cm, retroperitoneal location, and high Ki-67 proliferation antigen expression
  - High mitotic rate and extensive necrosis also related to poor prognosis

Treatment

- Surgical excision often combined with radiotherapy
  - Adjuvant chemotherapy has evolving role

SELECTED REFERENCES

1. Chen YR et al: Distant metastases in a young woman with Stewart-Treves syndrome demonstrated by an FDG-PET/CT scan. Clin Nucl Med. 39(11):975-6, 2014
2. Lee R et al: Lymphedema-related angiogenic tumors and other malignancies. Clin Dermatol. 32(5):616-20, 2014
3. Young RJ et al: Angiogenic growth factor expression in benign and malignant vascular tumours. Exp Mol Pathol. 97(1):148-53, 2014
4. Cox CA et al: Angiosarcoma presenting with minor erythema and swelling. Case Rep Ophthalmol. 4(1):59-63, 2013
5. Fisher C: Unusual myoid, perivascular, and postradiation lesions, with emphasis on atypical vascular lesion, postradiation cutaneous angiosarcoma, myoepithelial tumors, myopericytoma, and perivascular epithelioid cell tumor. Semin Diagn Pathol. 30(1):73-84, 2013
6. Sharma P et al: Detection of recurrent cutaneous angiosarcoma of lower extremity with (18)F-fluorodeoxyglucose positron emission tomography-computed tomography: report of three cases. Indian J Dermatol. 58(3):242, 2013
7. Mentzel T et al: Postradiation cutaneous angiosarcoma after treatment of breast carcinoma is characterized by MYC amplification in contrast to atypical vascular lesions after radiotherapy and control cases: clinicopathological, immunohistochemical and molecular analysis of 66 cases. Mod Pathol. 25(1):75-85, 2012
8. Chen Y et al: Epithelioid angiosarcoma of bone and soft tissue: a report of seven cases with emphasis on morphologic diversity, immunohistochemical features and clinical outcome. Tumori. 97(5):585-9, 2011
9. Hart J et al: Epithelioid angiosarcoma: a brief diagnostic review and differential diagnosis. Arch Pathol Lab Med. 135(2):268-72, 2011
10. Mentzel T: Sarcomas of the skin in the elderly. Clin Dermatol. 29(1):80-90, 2011
11. Sakemi M et al: A case of postirradiation angiosarcoma of the greater omentum with hemorrhage. Clin J Gastroenterol. 4(5):302-6, 2011
12. Suchak R et al: Primary cutaneous epithelioid angiosarcoma: a clinicopathologic study of 13 cases of a rare neoplasm occurring outside the setting of conventional angiosarcomas and with predilection for the limbs. Am J Surg Pathol. 35(1):60-9, 2011
13. Tokmak E et al: F18-FDG PET/CT scanning in angiosarcoma: report of two cases. Mol Imaging Radionucl Ther. 20(2):63-6, 2011
14. Moukaddam H et al: MRI characteristics and classification of peripheral vascular malformations and tumors. Skeletal Radiol. 38(6):535-47, 2009
15. Weiss SW et al: Malignant vascular tumors. In Weiss SW et al: Enzinger and Weiss' Soft Tissue Tumors. 5th ed. Philadelphia: Elsevier. 703-19, 2008
16. Kransdorf MJ et al: Vascular and lymphatic tumors. In Kransdorf MJ et al: Imaging of Soft Tissue Tumors. 2nd ed. Philadelphia: Lippincott Williams & Wilkins. 177-188, 2006
17. Weiss SW et al: Angiosarcoma of soft tissue. In Fletcher CDM et al: World Health Organization Classification of Tumours. Pathology and Genetics of Tumours of Soft Tissue and Bone. Lyon: IARC Press. 175-7, 2002
18. Murphey MD et al: From the archives of the AFIP. Musculoskeletal angiomatous lesions: radiologic-pathologic correlation. Radiographics. 15(4):893-917, 1995

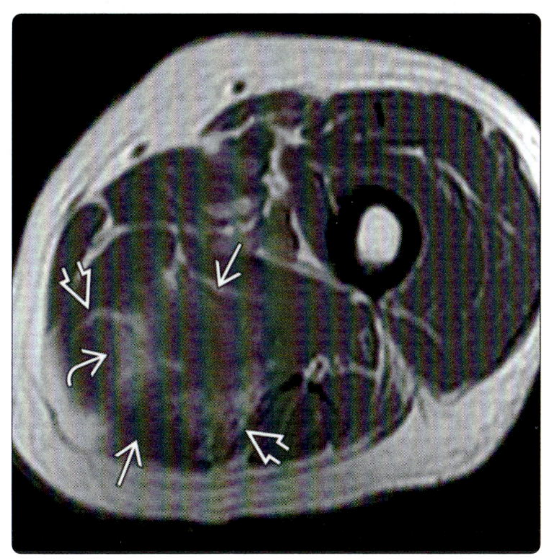

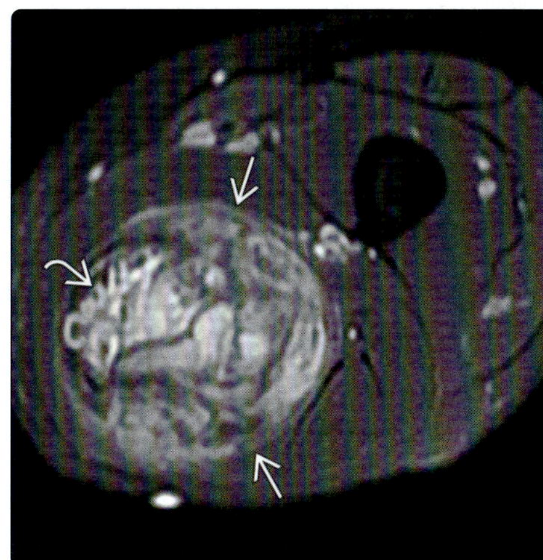

(Left) *Axial T1 MR of the thigh of an 83-year-old man shows a mass ➡ that is mostly isointense to skeletal muscle. There is high signal within parts of the mass ➡ that could represent either fat or blood (other imaging proved blood rather than fat). Tortuous higher signal vessels are also seen ➡.* **(Right)** *Axial T2 FS MR, same case, shows hyperintense tortuous vessels ➡, but otherwise highly heterogeneous hyperintense mass ➡. Blood and abnormal vessels in a large heterogeneous lesion suggests angiosarcoma.*

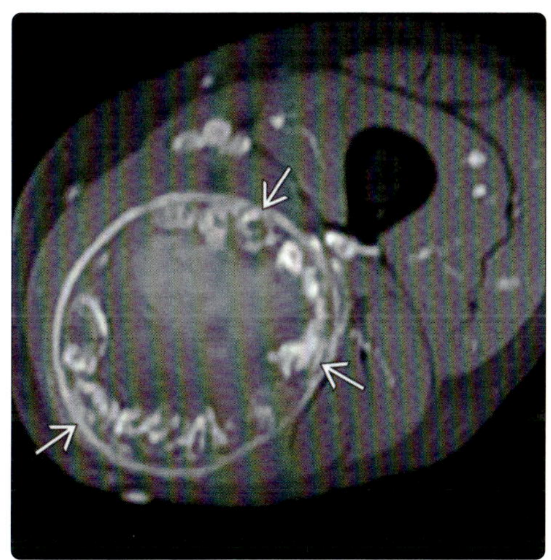

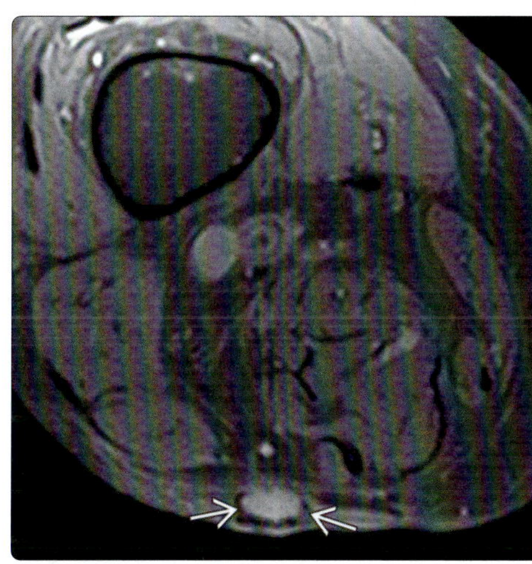

(Left) *Axial post-contrast T1 FS MR, same case, shows enhancing rim and peripheral vessels ➡ with nonenhancing center representing necrosis. This high-grade angiosarcoma has an extremely poor prognosis.* **(Right)** *Axial T2 FS MR in an 89-year-old woman shows hyperintensity in a subcutaneous lesion ➡. This lesion had bothered the patient as an unresolving "bruise." This clinical scenario is typical of subcutaneous angiosarcoma, which the lesion proved to be.*

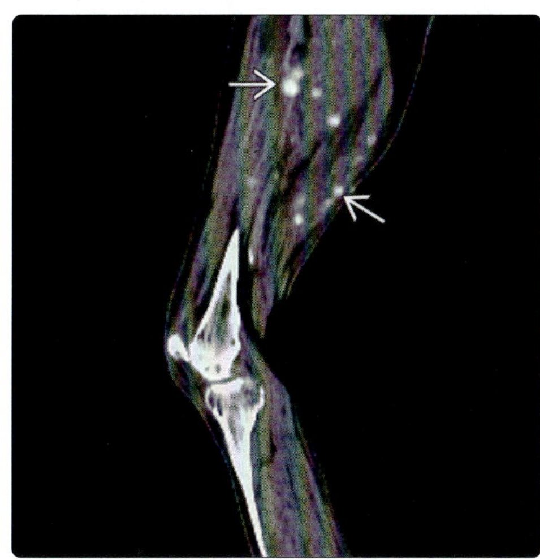

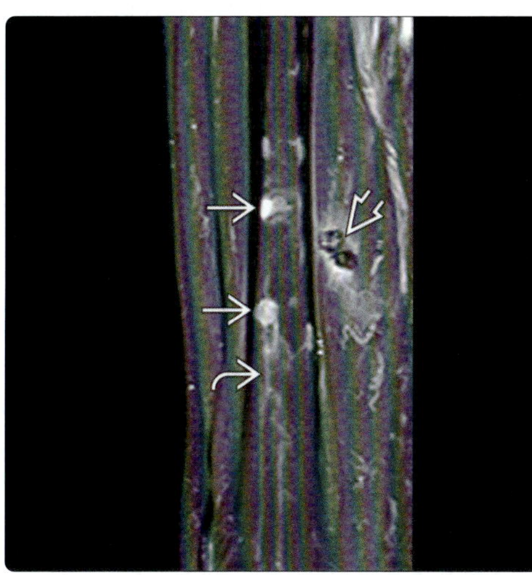

(Left) *Sagittal FDG PET/CT, same case, shows multiple foci ➡ of abnormal uptake, indicating metastatic disease.* **(Right)** *Coronal STIR MR of the thigh, same case, shows metastatic foci within the bone ➡ that have prominent associated intraosseous vessels ➡. Soft tissue metastases ➡ with edema and associated vessels are seen as well. Angiosarcoma may often arise from a small subcutaneous lesion; nonetheless the metastatic potential is significant and prognosis is extremely poor.*

KEY FACTS

TERMINOLOGY

- Benign soft tissue lesion composed of mature hyaline cartilage, excluding periosteal and synovial locations
  - a.k.a. extraskeletal chondroma (fibrochondroma, myxochondroma, osteochondroma), chondroma of soft parts

IMAGING

- Majority arise in hands and feet (84%)
  - Typically near tendon or joint
- Calcifications usually present (33-70%)
  - Central or peripheral calcification
  - Chondroid rings and arcs, coarse or curvilinear
  - Finger lesions less likely to be calcified
- ± ossification
- ± bone erosion and remodeling
- Well-defined, round to oval soft tissue mass
  - Isodense to hypodense relative to muscle on CT
- T1WI MR: Intermediate intensity
  - Calcified regions have low signal intensity on all imaging sequences
- Fluid-sensitive MR sequences: Hyperintense to muscle
- Enhances with contrast
- US: Well-defined, heterogeneously hypoechoic mass

PATHOLOGY

- May be misdiagnosed as chondrosarcoma
- Extensive calcification may obscure cartilage (33%)
- ± hemorrhage, myxoid areas, or cystic change

CLINICAL ISSUES

- Painless, slowly growing, solitary soft tissue mass
  - Uncommonly tender or painful
- Found throughout life, from infants to elderly
  - Mean: 44 years old
- Benign lesion
  - Local recurrence in 15-25%
- Local surgical excision

(Left) *Lateral radiograph shows a densely calcified mass ➡ dorsal to metacarpophalangeal joint. Calcification is most dense around periphery, raising the possibility of myositis ossificans. However, dots of dystrophic calcification are pathognomonic for cartilage calcification.* **(Right)** *Axial CECT shows a rounded mass ➡ lying between the carotid ➡ and vertebral ➡ arteries. The mass has low attenuation when compared to skeletal muscle. There is no matrix and no reactive change in the adjacent bone.*

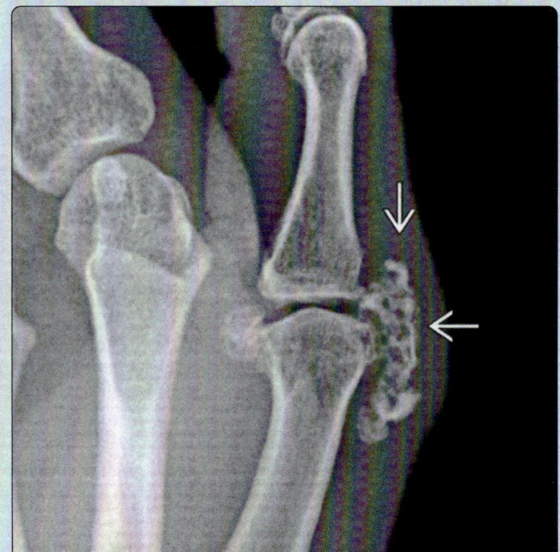

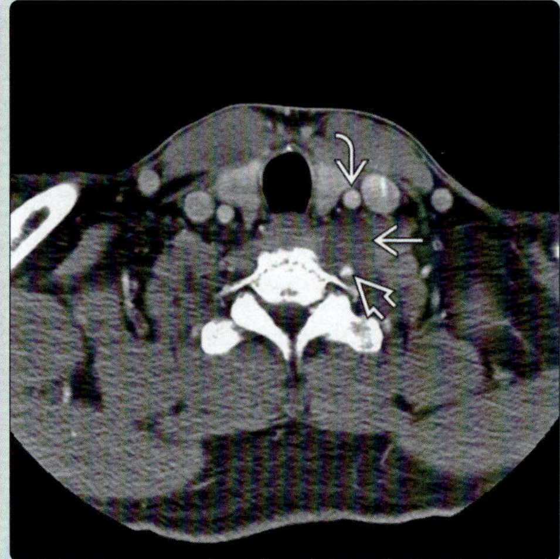

(Left) *Sagittal T1WI MR shows lobulated soft tissue masses ➡ causing erosion of the bones of the midfoot. The masses have signal intensity similar to muscle.* **(Right)** *Sagittal T2WI MR shows the midfoot masses ➡ to be lobulated and have high signal. This MR appearance is typical of benign or low-grade cartilage lesions. The lesions were resected and confirmed to be soft tissue chondroma, locally invading bone. This lesion later degenerated into a low-grade chondrosarcoma, which is exceptionally unusual for these lesions.*

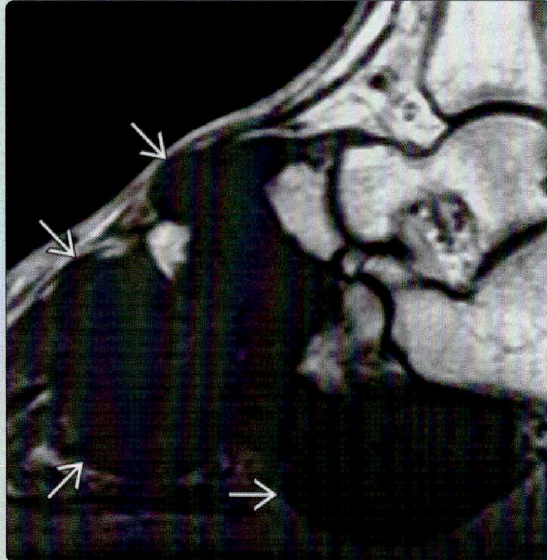

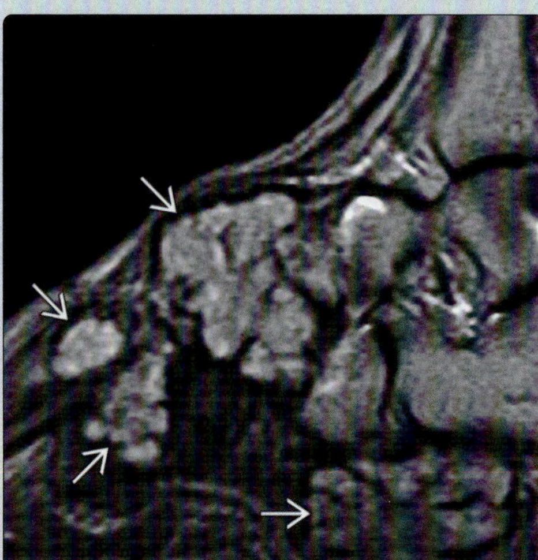

TERMINOLOGY

Synonyms

- Extraskeletal chondroma (fibrochondroma, myxochondroma, osteochondroma), chondroma of soft parts

Definitions

- Benign soft tissue lesion composed of mature hyaline cartilage, excluding periosteal and synovial locations

IMAGING

General Features

- Location
  - Majority arise in hands and feet (84%)
    - Most common in fingers (up to 80%); may be subungual
    - Uncommon in head and neck
  - Typically near tendon or joint
    - May be attached to tendon or tendon sheath
  - Lesions involving periosteum or synovial-lined surface are classified separately
- Size
  - Usually < 3 cm in diameter
- Morphology
  - Lobulated, round to oval mass

Ultrasonographic Findings

- Well-defined, heterogeneously hypoechoic mass

Radiographic Findings

- Soft tissue mass
- Calcifications usually present (33-70%)
  - Central or peripheral calcification
  - Chondroid rings and arcs, coarse or curvilinear
  - Finger lesions less likely to be calcified
- ± ossification
- ± bone erosion and remodeling

CT Findings

- Well-defined, round to oval soft tissue mass
  - Isodense to hypodense relative to skeletal muscle

MR Findings

- Nonspecific soft tissue mass
- Intermediate intensity on T1WI MR
- Hyperintense to muscle on fluid-sensitive sequences
- Calcified regions have low signal intensity on all imaging sequences

DIFFERENTIAL DIAGNOSIS

Giant Cell Tumor Tendon Sheath

- Typically found in adults 30-50 years old
- Intimately associated with tendon sheath
- May erode underlying bone
- Calcification or ossification uncommon

Bizarre Parosteal Osteochondromatous Proliferation

- Mean patient age: 4th decade
- Mineralized mass on bone surface
- Predilection for hands (55%)

Gout

- Periarticular tophi with amorphous calcification
- Bone erosions with overhanging edges

Calcifying Aponeurotic Fibroma

- Patients are usually < 25 years old (median: 12 years)
- Predilection for volar hand and plantar foot
- May contain stippled calcifications

Synovial Sarcoma

- Soft tissue mass, usually near joint
- Predilection for deep soft tissues of extremity
- Calcification in 33%

PATHOLOGY

General Features

- Etiology
  - Controversial, may be neoplastic or metaplastic

Gross Pathologic & Surgical Features

- Firm, well-circumscribed mass
- Cartilaginous cut surface
- ± hemorrhage, myxoid areas, or cystic change

Microscopic Features

- May be misdiagnosed as chondrosarcoma due to variable histology
- Lobules of mature hyaline cartilage
- 33% have cartilage obscured by extensive calcification
- 15% have multinucleated giant cells and epithelioid cells peripherally
- No atypical mitotic figures

CLINICAL ISSUES

Presentation

- Most common signs/symptoms
  - Painless, slowly growing, solitary soft tissue mass
    - Infrequently tender or painful
    - Firm, rubbery, often mobile on palpation

Demographics

- Age
  - Found throughout life, from infants to elderly
    - Mean: 44 years; range: 30-60 years
- Gender
  - Slight male predominance
- Epidemiology
  - 1.5% of benign soft tissue tumors

Natural History & Prognosis

- Benign lesion
  - Degeneration to chondrosarcoma more common with osseous and synovial cartilaginous tumors
- Local recurrence in 15-25%

Treatment

- Local surgical excision

SELECTED REFERENCES

1. Baek HJ et al: Subungual tumors: clinicopathologic correlation with US and MR imaging findings. Radiographics. 30(6):1621-36, 2010

Extraskeletal Mesenchymal Chondrosarcoma

KEY FACTS

TERMINOLOGY

- Rare malignant cartilaginous tumor

IMAGING

- Head and neck, especially periorbital
  - Cranial and spinal dura/meninges > posterior neck > lower extremity (thigh)
  - Reported throughout body
- Soft tissue mass with chondroid matrix
  - ± reactive change in underlying bone (erosion, periosteal reaction, or invasion)
- CT and MR show nonspecific soft tissue mass
  - Calcifications common: Oval to chondroid to fine granular configuration
  - Isointense to muscle on T1WI
  - Hyperintense to muscle on fluid-sensitive MR sequences
  - Intense, heterogeneous enhancement
  - ± necrosis
- Neovascularity, especially peripheral

TOP DIFFERENTIAL DIAGNOSES

- Synovial sarcoma
- Extraskeletal myxoid chondrosarcoma
- Myositis ossificans

PATHOLOGY

- Bimorphic appearance with well-differentiated cartilage surrounded by sheets of closely packed undifferentiated cells
  - ± hemorrhagic and necrotic regions
  - ± hemangiopericytoma-like vessels

CLINICAL ISSUES

- Extremity lesions usually painless and slow growing
  - May produce symptoms from mass effect
- Young adults: 15-35 years of age most common
- Approximately 25% 10-year survival rate
- Common metastases to lymph nodes, lung, and bone
- Wide surgical excision ± radiotherapy or chemotherapy

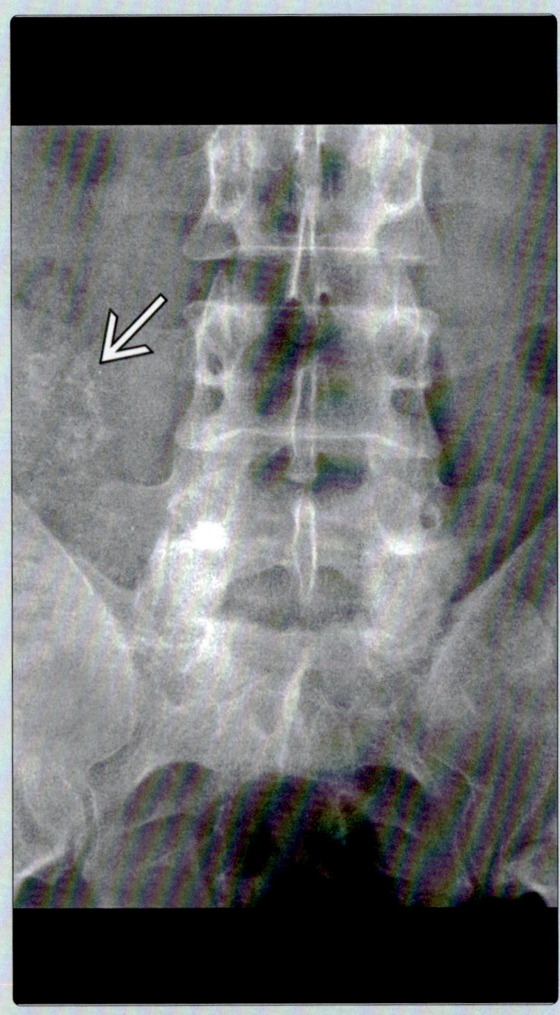

Anteroposterior radiograph shows punctate chondroid calcifications ➡ in the right lower quadrant of the abdomen. The adjacent bones are normal. This lesion proved to be extraskeletal mesenchymal chondrosarcoma. It requires cross-sectional imaging for further evaluation.

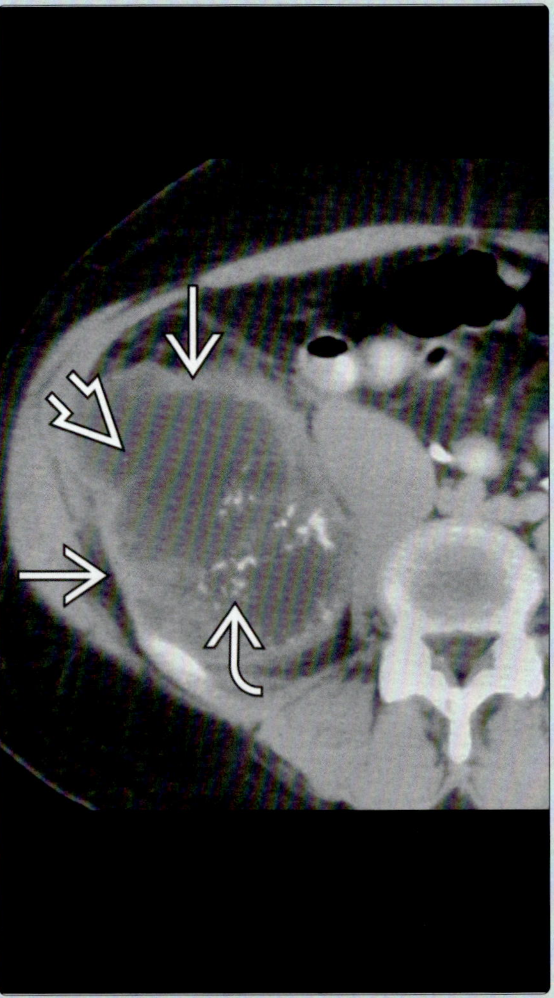

Axial CECT shows a large mass arising in the retroperitoneum ➡, which displaces the psoas muscle toward the midline. The lesion peripherally enhances, contains chondroid matrix ➡, and shows extensive regions of low attenuation ➡.

TERMINOLOGY

Definitions

- Rare malignant cartilaginous tumor

IMAGING

General Features

- Location
  - Head and neck, especially periorbital
    - Cranial and spinal dura/meninges > posterior neck > lower extremity (thigh)
    - Reported throughout body
- Size
  - Variable (2.5-37 cm)

Radiographic Findings

- Soft tissue mass with chondroid matrix
- ± reactive change in underlying bone (erosion, periosteal reaction or invasion)

CT Findings

- Soft tissue mass with similar attenuation to muscle
  - Mineralization best demonstrated with CT
    - Central or eccentric location
    - Large oval to chondroid to fine granular configuration
  - ± necrosis
- Heterogeneous enhancement

MR Findings

- Nonspecific soft tissue mass containing variable low signal mineralization
  - Isointense to muscle on T1WI MR
  - Hyperintense to muscle on fluid-sensitive sequences
- Intense, heterogeneous enhancement

Angiographic Findings

- Neovascularity, especially peripheral

DIFFERENTIAL DIAGNOSIS

Synovial Sarcoma

- Predilection for periarticular regions
- Commonly contains stippled calcifications
- May contain hemangiopericytoma-like vessels

Myositis Ossificans/Heterotopic Ossification

- Early findings may have similar calcifications to mesenchymal chondrosarcoma
- Mature lesions demonstrate typical peripheral calcification

Extraskeletal Myxoid Chondrosarcoma

- Less likely to demonstrate cartilaginous matrix than extraskeletal mesenchymal chondrosarcoma

Solitary Fibrous Tumor & Hemangiopericytoma

- Malignant form may have similar histologic appearance
- Most common in middle-aged adults
- Does not contain cartilage
- May be calcified

PATHOLOGY

General Features

- Etiology
  - Malignant cartilaginous neoplasm typically considered chondrosarcoma variant
  - May be related to extraskeletal Ewing sarcoma/primitive neuroectodermal tumor
- Genetics
  - t(11;22)(q24;q12) in 1 case
  - Robertsonian t(13;21) in 2 cases

Gross Pathologic & Surgical Features

- Well-defined, fleshy gray-white, multilobulated mass
- Foci of cartilage and bone
- ± hemorrhagic and necrotic regions

Microscopic Features

- Bimorphic appearance with well-differentiated cartilage surrounded by sheets of closely packed undifferentiated cells
- ± hemangiopericytoma-like vessels
- Positive S100, neuron-specific enolase, and Leu-7
- Negative actin, epithelial membrane antigen, and cytokeratin

CLINICAL ISSUES

Presentation

- Most common signs/symptoms
  - Extremity lesions usually painless and slow growing
  - May produce symptoms from mass effect
    - Orbit: Visual disturbance, exophthalmos, and pain
    - Intracranial/intraspinal: Headache, vomiting, and motor or sensory deficits

Demographics

- Age
  - Young adults: 15-35 years
    - May arise in young children
      - Rarely present at birth
- Gender
  - Slight female predominance
- Epidemiology
  - Very rare cartilaginous neoplasm
    - Occurs 2-3x more commonly in bone

Natural History & Prognosis

- Poor clinical prognosis
  - Approximately 25% 10-year survival rate
- High rate of metastasis to lymph nodes, lung, and bone
- Local recurrence and metastases may occur early or late

Treatment

- Wide surgical excision ± radiotherapy, chemotherapy

SELECTED REFERENCES

1. Gupta SR et al: A rare case of extraskeletal mesenchymal chondrosarcoma with dedifferentiation arising from the buccal space in a young male. J Maxillofac Oral Surg. 14(Suppl 1):293-9, 2015
2. Herrera A et al: Primary orbital mesenchymal chondrosarcoma: case report and review of the literature. Case Rep Med. 2012:292147, 2012

Extraskeletal Osteosarcoma

KEY FACTS

TERMINOLOGY

- Malignant mesenchymal soft tissue tumor that synthesizes osteoid, bone, or chondroid material

IMAGING

- Deep soft tissues, not arising from bone
  - Uncommon in dermis or subcutis (< 10%)
- Thigh most common location (42-50%)
  - Shoulder girdle (12-23%)
  - Retroperitoneum (8-17%)
- Well-circumscribed soft tissue mass on CT with overall attenuation similar to or lower than muscle
- Variable mineralization: Cloud-like to dense
  - Mineralization apparent in 50% of cases
  - Most prominent in center of lesion
- Necrosis and hemorrhage are common
- ± secondary involvement of periosteum, cortex, or medullary canal (rare)
- Nonspecific, heterogeneous soft tissue mass on MR
  - Mineralization has low signal on all sequences
  - Fluid-fluid levels from hemorrhage
- Increased radiotracer uptake on bone scintigraphy

PATHOLOGY

- Up to 31% with prior radiotherapy or trauma
- Well circumscribed or infiltrating

CLINICAL ISSUES

- Older patient age than bone osteosarcoma
  - 5th-7th decades of life
- Usually painless, enlarging deep soft tissue mass
  - ~ 33% are painful
- ↑ serum alkaline phosphatase with metastatic disease
- 1-2% of soft tissue sarcomas
- Extremely poor clinical prognosis
  - ~ 25% 5-year survival rate
  - Local recurrence and metastases very common
- Treatment: Wide excision, radiotherapy, and chemotherapy

(Left) *Axial NECT shows a large mass ➡ between the right gluteus maximus and medius muscles with an attenuation similar to skeletal muscle. The mass contains hyperattenuating foci of dense calcification or ossification ➡ and central low-attenuation regions ➡.* **(Right)** *Axial T1WI MR shows the mass ➡ to have heterogeneous signal that is isointense and hypointense relative to muscle. The irregular central region of low signal intensity ➡ is consistent with fluid from necrosis or remote hemorrhage.*

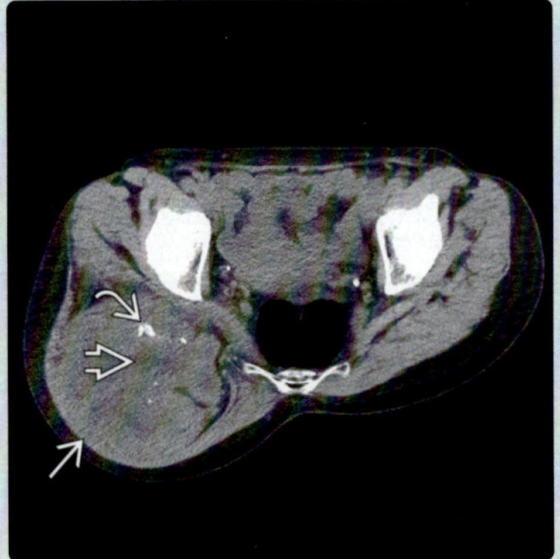

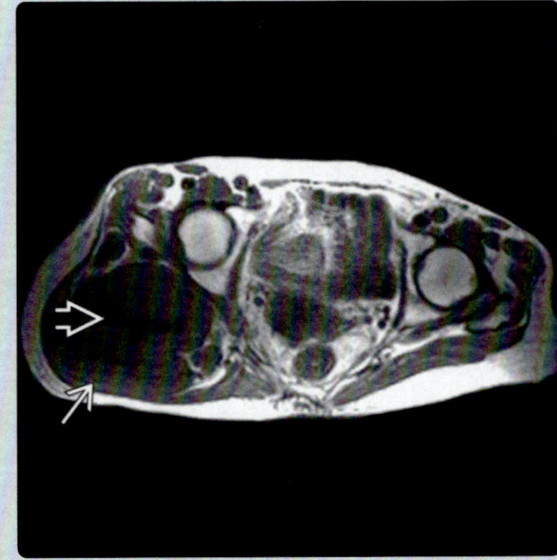

(Left) *Axial T2WI FS MR in the same patient shows the gluteal mass ➡ to have heterogeneous signal ranging from low to high, with the majority of the lesion being hyperintense. Persistently low-signal areas are calcified ➡.* **(Right)** *Axial T1WI C+ FS MR shows the mass ➡ to have intense, heterogeneous enhancement, except for the foci of calcification or ossification ➡, which remain low in signal. This mass was separate from the underlying bone along its entire length. Metastases were present at the time of diagnosis.*

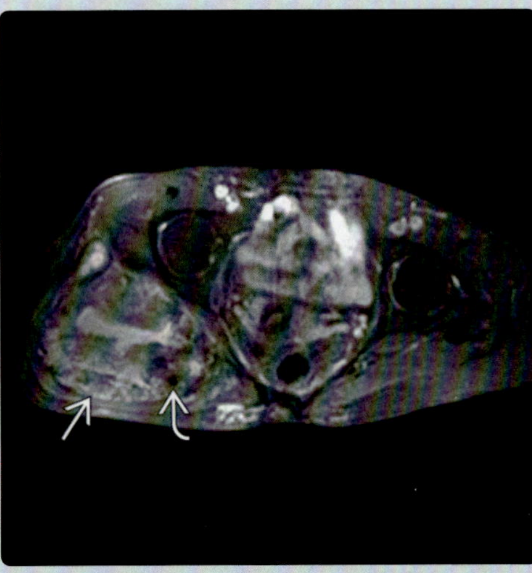

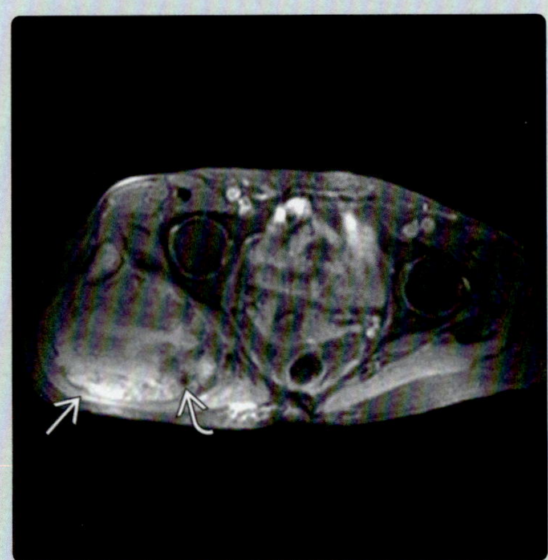

TERMINOLOGY

Synonyms

- Soft tissue osteosarcoma

Definitions

- Malignant mesenchymal soft tissue tumor that synthesizes osteoid, bone, or chondroid material, excluding similar lesions that arise from bone

IMAGING

General Features

- Location
  - Deep soft tissues, not arising from bone
    - Uncommon in dermis or subcutis (< 10%)
  - Thigh most common location (42-50%)
    - Shoulder girdle (12-23%)
    - Retroperitoneum (8-17%)
    - Gluteal region
    - Rare reports in pleura, colon, central nervous system, tongue, mediastinum, genitourinary tract
- Size
  - Wide range (1-50 cm)
    - Mean: 8-10 cm

Radiographic Findings

- Soft tissue mass with variable calcification or ossification
  - Mineralization apparent in 50% of cases

CT Findings

- Well-circumscribed soft tissue mass with overall attenuation similar to or lower than muscle
- Variable mineralization: Cloud-like to dense
  - Most prominent in center of lesion
    - Pattern opposite of myositis ossificans
- Necrosis and hemorrhage are common
- ± secondary involvement of periosteum, cortex, or medullary canal (rare)

MR Findings

- Heterogeneous, deep soft tissue mass
- T1WI: Isointense to hypointense relative to skeletal muscle
- T2WI: Predominantly hyperintense relative skeletal muscle
- Prominent, heterogeneous enhancement
- Mineralization has low signal on all sequences
- Fluid-fluid levels from hemorrhage

Nuclear Medicine Findings

- Increased radiotracer uptake on bone scintigraphy

Angiographic Findings

- Hypervascular focal mass

DIFFERENTIAL DIAGNOSIS

Synovial Sarcoma

- Extremity deep soft tissues near joint or tendon sheath
- Calcification in ~ 33%
- Most common around knee
- Younger patient age (15-35 years)

Undifferentiated Pleomorphic Sarcoma

- Histologically similar when contains metaplastic bone
- Peak age: 6th and 7th decades of life
- May have similar imaging appearance

Myositis Ossificans/Heterotopic Ossification

- Mineralization matures peripheral to central
- Muscles of lower or upper extremity
- Peak age: 2nd-3rd decades life
- Development of extraskeletal osteosarcoma reported

PATHOLOGY

General Features

- Etiology
  - Up to 31% with prior radiotherapy or trauma
    - At least 4 year latency from radiotherapy or use of radioactive thorium dioxide (Thorotrast)
    - Reported to arise in myositis ossificans or region of intramuscular injection

Gross Pathologic & Surgical Features

- Well circumscribed with pseudocapsule or infiltrating

Microscopic Features

- Same histologic subtypes seen in bone osteosarcoma
  - All contain neoplastic osteoid, bone, or cartilage
  - Typically high-grade lesions

CLINICAL ISSUES

Presentation

- Most common signs/symptoms
  - Usually painless enlarging deep soft tissue mass
    - ~ 33% are painful
- Other signs/symptoms
  - ↑ serum alkaline phosphatase with metastases

Demographics

- Age
  - 5th to 7th decades of life
    - Rare before 4th decade of life
- Gender
  - Male predominance (M:F = 1.9:1)
- Epidemiology
  - 1-2% of soft tissue sarcomas
  - 2-4% of all osteosarcomas
  - Annual incidence: 2-3 cases per million population

Natural History & Prognosis

- Extremely poor clinical prognosis
  - ~ 25% 5-year survival rate
  - Local recurrence and metastases very common
    - Lung > > liver, bones, lymph nodes, soft tissue
    - Lung metastases ± calcification, even if tumor mineralized

Treatment

- Wide excision, radiotherapy, and chemotherapy

SELECTED REFERENCES

1. Mc Auley G et al: Extraskeletal osteosarcoma: spectrum of imaging findings. AJR Am J Roentgenol. 198(1):W31-7, 2012

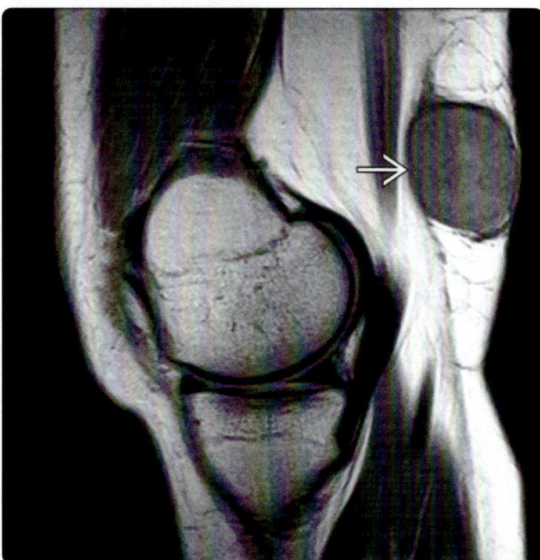

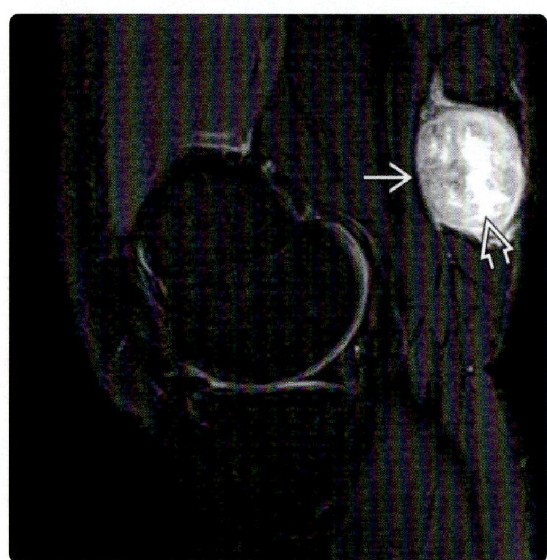

(Left) *Sagittal PDWI MR demonstrates a nonspecific, well-defined mass ➡ in the subcutaneous fat of the popliteal fossa. The mass has heterogeneous, intermediate to high signal. There is no visible mineralization.* **(Right)** *Sagittal T2WI FS MR shows the mass ➡ to have heterogeneous high signal with a central region likely representing necrosis ➡. The appearance and location of the lesion in this young adult initially favored synovial sarcoma, but extraskeletal osteosarcoma was proven on excision.*

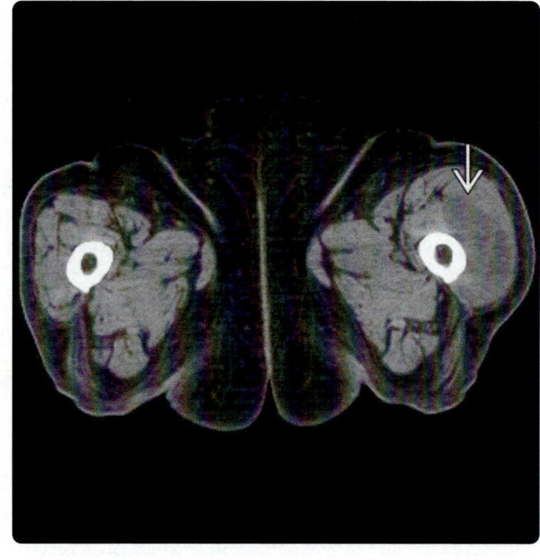

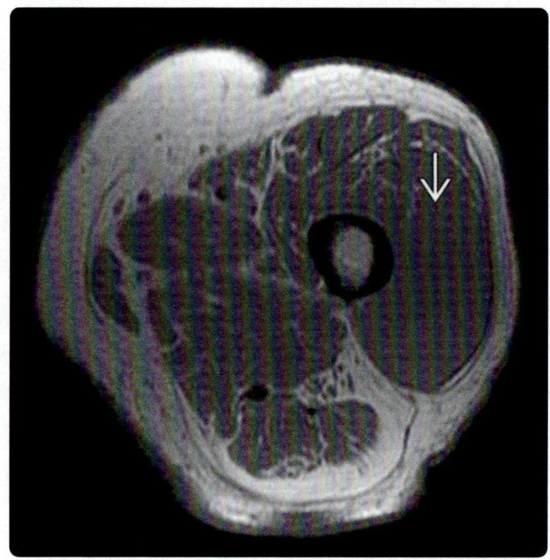

(Left) *Axial NECT shows a heterogeneous mass ➡ involving the proximal thigh. The mass has mixed attenuation being similar to and lower than skeletal muscle. No mineralization is evident. The underlying bone was not involved.* **(Right)** *Axial T1WI MR shows the mass ➡ to have mildly heterogeneous signal, being predominantly isointense to skeletal muscle. The mass involves the vastus lateralis and intermedius muscles. The lesion abuts bone, but there is no periosteal reaction or cortical involvement.*

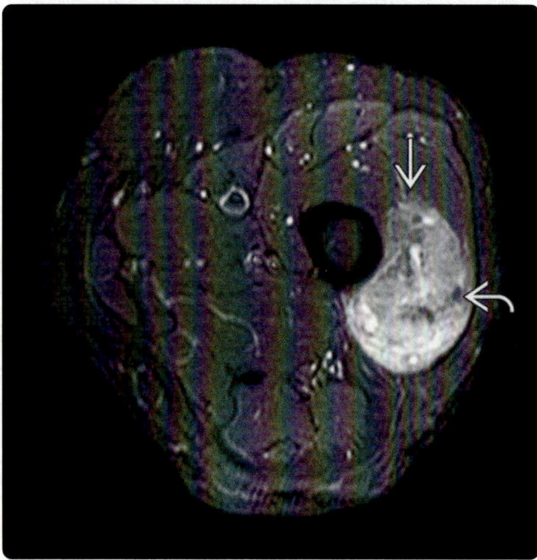

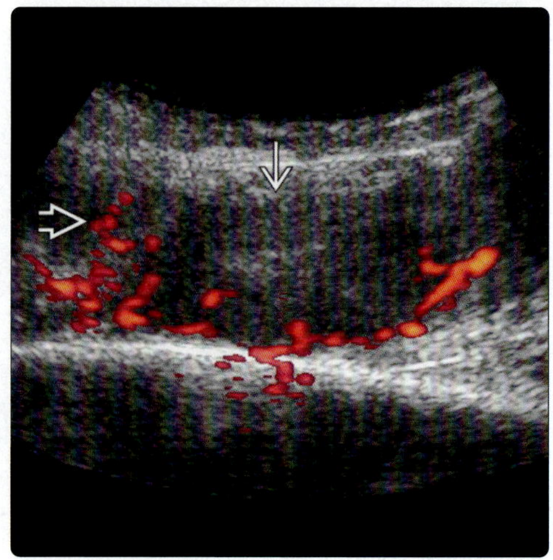

(Left) *Axial STIR MR shows the mass ➡ to be heterogeneously hyperintense. There are scattered small foci of hypointensity ➡ that may represent faint mineralization, since no overt mineralization was visible on additional imaging.* **(Right)** *Longitudinal power Doppler ultrasound shows the mass ➡ to have heterogeneous echogenicity. Neovascularity ➡ is predominately peripheral in location. This patient had no evidence of metastases but died within 1 year.*

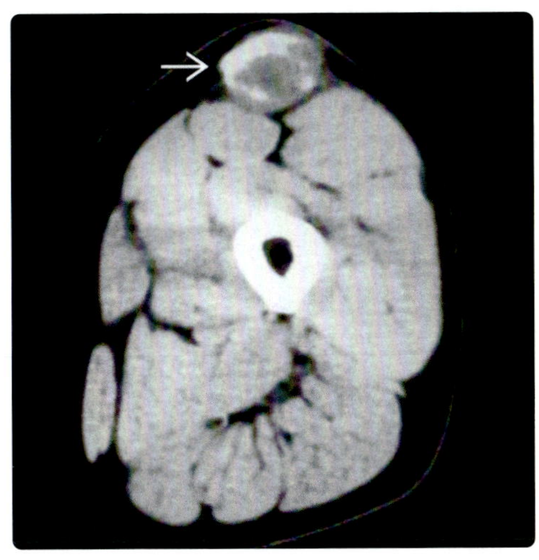

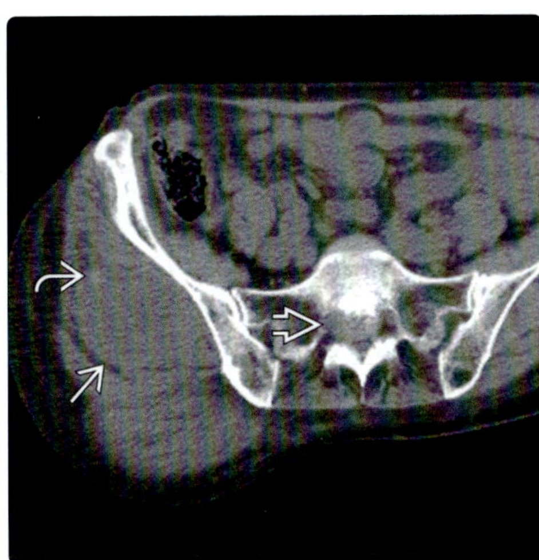

(Left) *Axial bone CT shows a rounded mass ➡ in the subcutaneous fat of the thigh. It contains soft tissue, mostly centrally, with ossification seen mostly peripherally. Myositis ossificans could have this appearance, but extraskeletal osteosarcoma proved to be the diagnosis. Superficial location is rare.* **(Right)** *Axial NECT shows a nonspecific soft tissue mass ➡ in the gluteal region. There is a suggestion of faint calcification ➡. An additional mass ➡ at S1 proved to be a metastasis.*

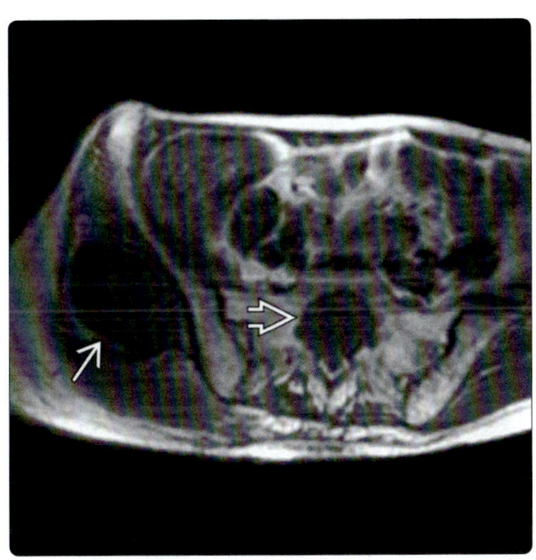

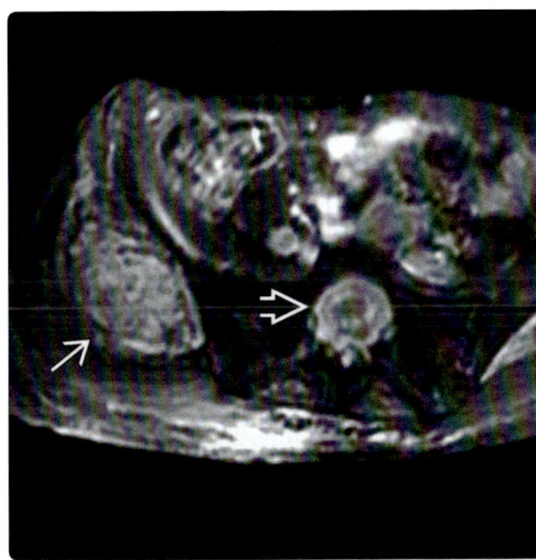

(Left) *Axial T1WI MR shows a nonspecific soft tissue mass ➡ in the gluteal region. The mass is homogeneously hypointense relative to skeletal muscle. A metastasis to the bone ➡ has similar imaging characteristics.* **(Right)** *Axial T2WI MR shows the gluteal mass ➡ to have heterogeneously hyperintense signal. Again, the focus of metastatic disease in S1 ➡ has similar nonspecific imaging characteristics to the primary lesion. Undifferentiated pleomorphic sarcoma would be more common in an elderly patient.*

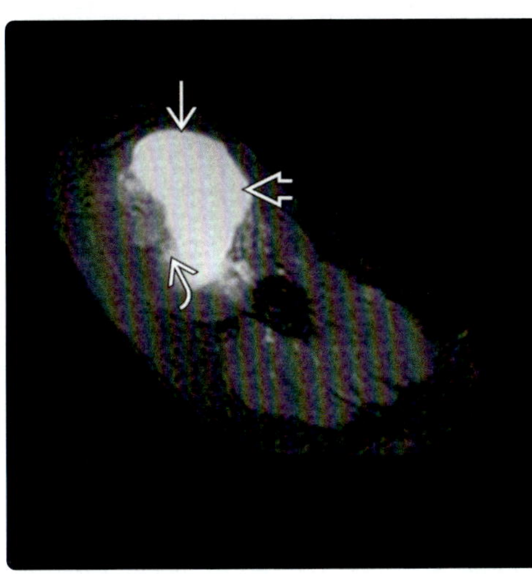

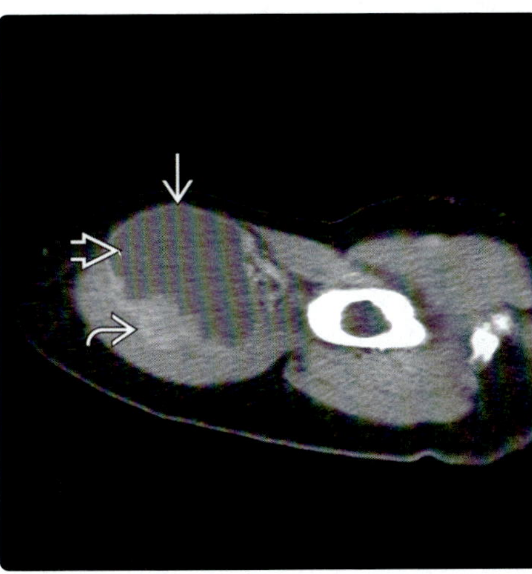

(Left) *Oblique T2WI FS MR shows a biphasic mass ➡ in the upper arm. The nodular, solid component ➡ is eccentrically located and has a similar attenuation to skeletal muscle. The cystic component ➡ is homogeneously hyperintense, typical for fluid.* **(Right)** *Oblique CECT confirms the mass ➡ to have 2 distinct components: An unenhancing cystic portion ➡ and a heterogeneously enhancing solid, nodular component ➡. This appearance of extraskeletal osteosarcoma is very unusual.*

Intramuscular Myxoma

KEY FACTS

IMAGING

- Predilection for large muscles
  - Thigh, buttocks, and shoulder girdle/upper arm
- CT attenuation of mass is between fluid and muscle
- MR appearance
  - Low to intermediate signal intensity on T1WI MR
    - Homogeneous to mildly heterogeneous
    - Characteristic rim of fat, especially around superior and inferior poles of lesion
  - High signal intensity on fluid-sensitive MR sequences
    - High signal surrounding lesion from leakage of myxomatous tissue is common
    - ± septa and purely cystic foci
  - Mild to moderate enhancement
- US: Heterogeneously hypoechoic to near anechoic
  - Increased through transmission
  - Mild to absent internal vascularity
- Changes in underlying bone rarely present

PATHOLOGY

- Mazabraud syndrome = intramuscular myxomas with skeletal fibrous dysplasia
- Lobulated, well-circumscribed mass
  - May have subtly infiltrative borders
  - ± fluid-filled cysts

CLINICAL ISSUES

- Painless soft tissue mass
  - < 25% report tenderness
- Age: 40-70 years
- Gender: ~ 57- 66% in female patients
- Benign, without risk of malignant degeneration

DIAGNOSTIC CHECKLIST

- Review all MR imaging planes to assess for characteristic thin rim of fat and surrounding edema
- Biopsy usually necessary to exclude malignancy

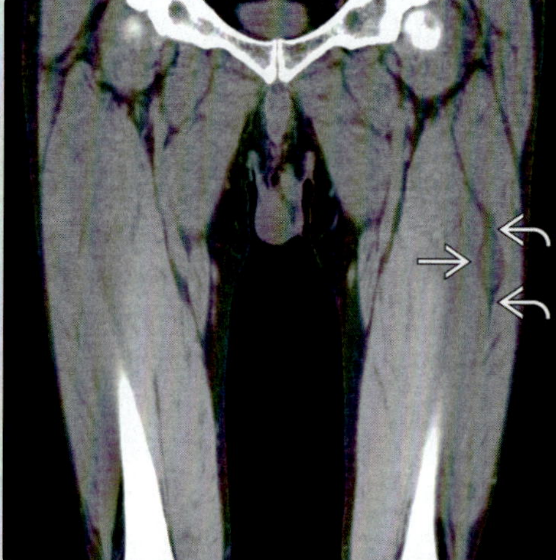

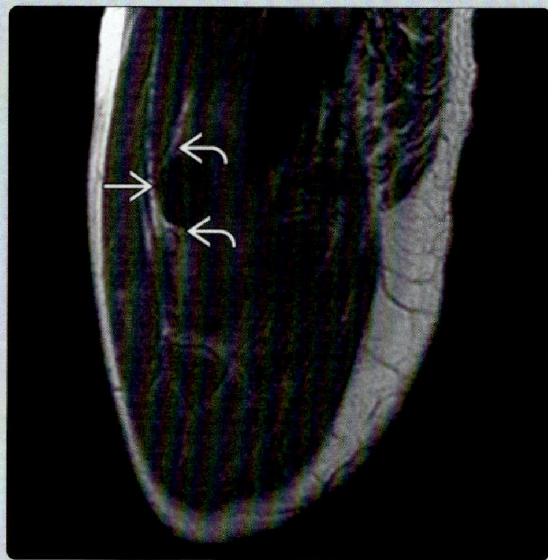

(Left) *Coronal NECT of the thighs shows a well-defined, low-attenuation mass ➡ located within the vastus intermedius muscle. Triangular regions of fat ⮌ are located along the proximal and distal poles of the lesion.* **(Right)** *Sagittal T1WI MR demonstrates the well-defined, ovoid, intramuscular mass ➡ to be homogeneously hypointense relative to skeletal muscle. A small amount of high-signal fat ⮌ is present involving the periphery of the mass, predominantly involving the proximal and distal poles.*

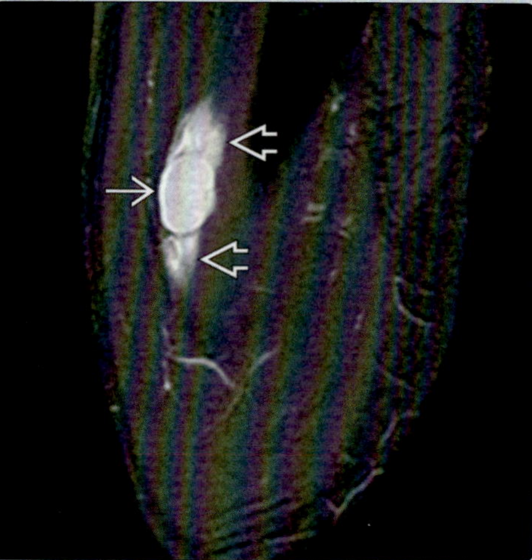

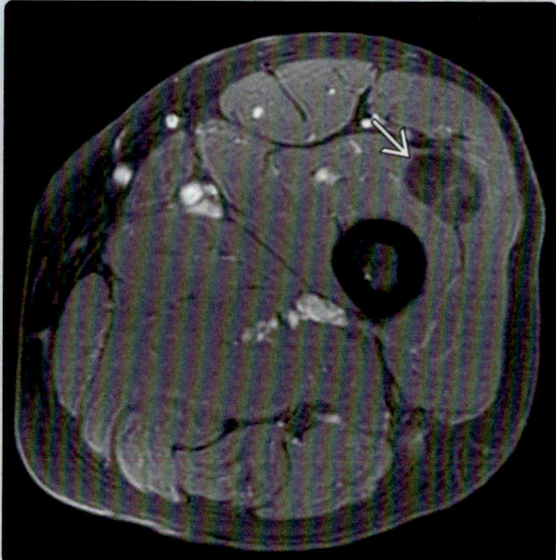

(Left) *Sagittal STIR MR shows the mass ➡ to have high signal intensity, simulating fluid, and flame-shaped high signal in the surrounding soft tissues ⇨ arising from the proximal and distal poles of the lesion.* **(Right)** *Axial T1WI C+ FS MR demonstrates heterogeneous mild to moderate enhancement of the mass ➡. Although the imaging appearance of this lesion was typical for an intramuscular myxoma, percutaneous biopsy was performed to exclude malignancy.*

TERMINOLOGY

Definitions

- Benign, soft tissue neoplasm with prominent myoid stroma

IMAGING

General Features

- Location
  - Usually intramuscular (82%)
    - Predilection for large muscles
      - Thigh (51%), buttocks (7%)
      - Shoulder girdle/upper arm (9%)
- Size
  - 5-10 cm average diameter
    - Up to 20 cm
- Morphology
  - Well-circumscribed, ovoid mass
    - Fluid-sensitive MR sequences often show flame-shaped extension of signal, especially along long muscle axis
  - Multiple tumors more likely to be seen in Mazabraud syndrome

Imaging Recommendations

- Best imaging tool
  - MR best evaluates these intramuscular lesions
- Protocol advice
  - Use of gadolinium controversial due to enhancement of benign and malignant myxoid lesions

Radiographic Findings

- Usually normal (55%)
- Focal area of decreased density in soft tissues (45%)
- Calcification uncommon
- Changes in underlying bone rare

CT Findings

- Attenuation of mass is between fluid and muscle
- Mild diffuse enhancement or peripheral and septal enhancement in 50%

MR Findings

- Homogeneous to mildly heterogeneous
  - ± septa
  - ± cystic foci
- Low (81-100%) to intermediate (0-19%) signal intensity on T1WI MR
  - Characteristic rim of fat, especially around superior and inferior poles of lesion
    - May represent atrophy of adjacent muscle
- High signal intensity on fluid-sensitive sequences
  - High signal surrounding lesion from leakage of myxomatous tissue is common (79-100%)
    - Often flame-shaped or brush-like, along longitudinal muscle fascicles
    - Best seen on coronal or sagittal images
    - Thought to represent leakage of myxomatous tissue
  - Cystic areas in 50%
- Mild (76%) to moderate (24%) enhancement
  - Usually less enhancement than malignant lesions
  - Enhancement pattern diffuse (57%) or shows thick peripheral and septal pattern (43%)
  - Regions of globular enhancement have been described

Ultrasonographic Findings

- Well-circumscribed mass
- Heterogeneously hypoechoic to near anechoic
  - Increased through transmission
  - Small anechoic cystic areas in 85%
- Bright rim sign of increased echogenicity around lesion (83%), corresponding to fat surrounding rim seen on MR
- Mild to absent internal vascularity, with surrounding vessels

Angiographic Findings

- Hypovascular to avascular mass

Nuclear Medicine Findings

- Minimal or absent uptake on bone scintigraphy

DIFFERENTIAL DIAGNOSIS

Liposarcoma, Myxoid

- Malignant soft tissue tumor with predilection for deep soft tissues of thigh
- May have no visible lipomatous tissue on imaging
- Heterogeneous to homogeneous enhancement
- Most common in 4th and 5th decades of life

Myxofibrosarcoma

- Subcutaneous > intramuscular location
- Lower extremity > upper extremity
- Mild enhancement may be difficult to appreciate
- 6th-8th decades of life

Ganglion Cyst

- Simple to complex fluid contents on imaging
- Lacks central enhancement

Hematoma, Chronic

- Lacks internal enhancement
- Heterogeneous signal intensity on MR
- May have peripheral and internal calcification

Soft Tissue Abscess

- Unilocular to multiloculated mass
- Irregular, thick peripheral enhancement
- Inflammatory changes in surrounding soft tissues

Lymphangioma

- Well-defined to infiltrative multiloculated masses
- May erode or resorb adjacent bone
- Rarely contain calcifications

Metastases, Soft Tissue

- Cystic or mucinous adenocarcinoma metastases
  - Low CT attenuation, MR signal similar to fluid, variable enhancement

Nerve Sheath Myxoma

- a.k.a neurothekeoma
- Dermis and subcutis of head, neck, and shoulder
- Found in children and young adults
- Rare in deep soft tissue

Benign Peripheral Nerve Sheath Tumor

- Fusiform mass along course of nerve
- ± peripheral rim of fat
- Hypodense to muscle on CT
- ± target sign on T2WI MR
- Variable enhancement pattern

PATHOLOGY

General Features

- Etiology
  - Characterized as tumor of uncertain differentiation
- Genetics
  - Point mutations of *GNAS1* gene
- Associated abnormalities
  - Mazabraud syndrome
    - Monostotic or polyostotic fibrous dysplasia with intramuscular myxomas (often multiple)

Gross Pathologic & Surgical Features

- Lobulated, well-circumscribed mass
  - May have subtly infiltrative borders
  - ± fluid-filled cysts
- Gelatinous cut surface

Microscopic Features

- Bland spindle and stellate cells, prominent myxoid stroma ± fibrous capsule
  - Sparse capillaries
- Surrounding muscle may be infiltrated or atrophic
- No necrosis, mitoses, or atypia
- Cellular myxoma if hypercellular with ↑ collagen fibers and ↑ vascularity
- Positive vimentin
  - Variable CD34, desmin, and actin positivity
- Negative S100

CLINICAL ISSUES

Presentation

- Most common signs/symptoms
  - Painless soft tissue mass
    - 25-51% report tenderness
  - Slowly enlarging

Demographics

- Age
  - 40-70 years
- Gender
  - ~ 57-66% in female patients
- Epidemiology
  - Reported incidence 1 per 1 million people

Natural History & Prognosis

- Benign, without risk of malignant degeneration
  - Cellular myxoma has mild risk of local recurrence
- Variable growth rate if left in situ

Treatment

- Simple excision is curative
  - Typically no recurrence
- May elect to observe once malignancy is ruled out

DIAGNOSTIC CHECKLIST

Image Interpretation Pearls

- Review all MR imaging planes to assess for characteristic thin rim of fat and myxoid tissue leakage
- Biopsy usually necessary to exclude malignancy
  - Many malignant soft tissue tumors develop prominent myxoid regions and may mimic myxoma

SELECTED REFERENCES

1. Petscavage-Thomas JM et al: Soft-tissue myxomatous lesions: review of salient imaging features with pathologic comparison. Radiographics. 34(4):964-80, 2014
2. Yamashita H et al: Intramuscular myxoma of the buttock mimicking low-grade fibromyxoid sarcoma: diagnostic usefulness of MUC4 expression. Skeletal Radiol. 42(10):1475-9, 2013
3. Weiss SW et al: Benign soft tissue tumors and pseudotumors of uncertain type. In Weiss SW et al: Enzinger and Weiss' Soft Tissue Tumors. 5th ed. Philadelphia: Elsevier. 1066-75, 2008
4. Kransdorf MJ et al: Tumors of uncertain histogenesis. In Kransdorf MJ et al: Imaging of Soft Tissue Tumors. 2nd ed. Philadelphia: Lippincott Williams & Wilkins. 485-8, 2006
5. Bancroft LW et al: Intramuscular myxoma: characteristic MR imaging features. AJR Am J Roentgenol. 178(5):1255-9, 2002
6. Murphey MD et al: Imaging of soft-tissue myxoma with emphasis on CT and MR and comparison of radiologic and pathologic findings. Radiology. 225(1):215-24, 2002
7. Nielsen G et al: Intramuscular myxoma. In Fletcher CDM et al: World Health Organization Classification of Tumours. Pathology and Genetics of Tumours of Soft Tissue and Bone. Lyon: IARC Press. 186-7, 2002

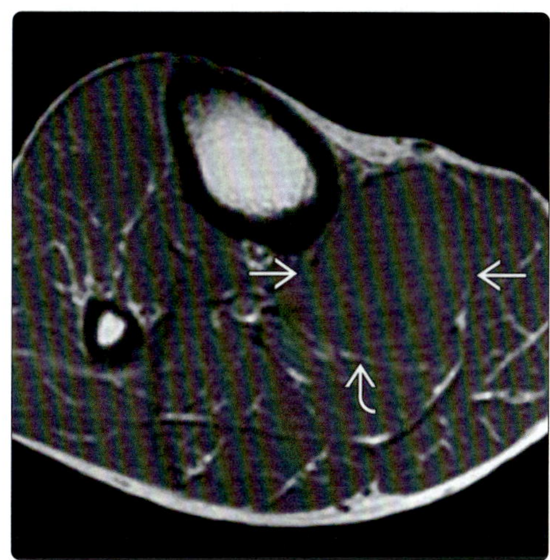

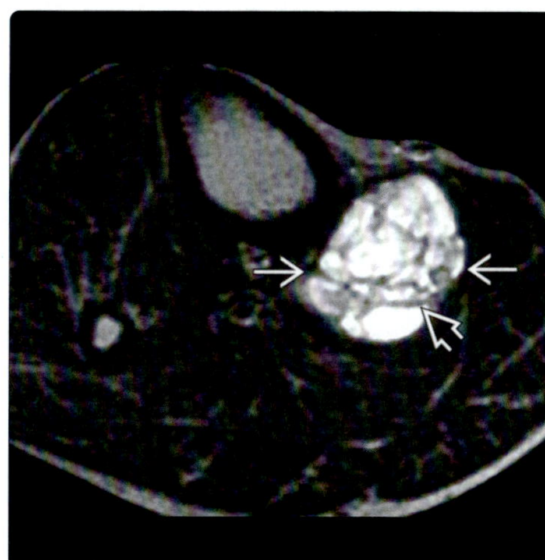

(Left) *Axial T1WI MR of the calf shows an intramuscular mass ➡ in this 38-year-old man. The mass has isointense to low signal relative to skeletal muscle. There is a discontinuous thin rim of high signal fat ➡.* **(Right)** *Axial T2WI MR demonstrates the mass ➡ to have predominantly high signal intensity and to contain numerous septa ➡ of variable thickness. This mass is unusually heterogeneous for an intramuscular myxoma.*

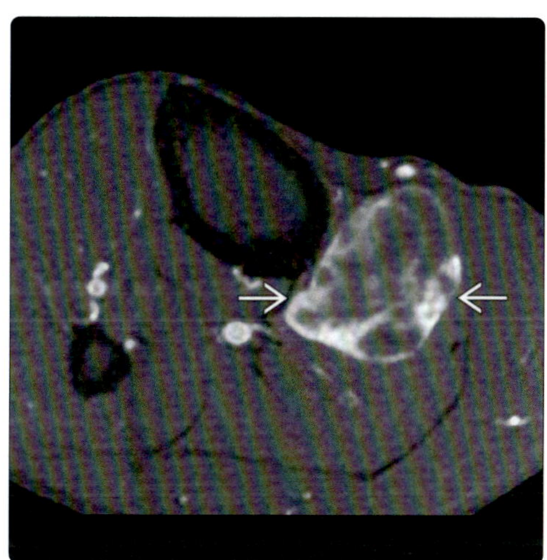

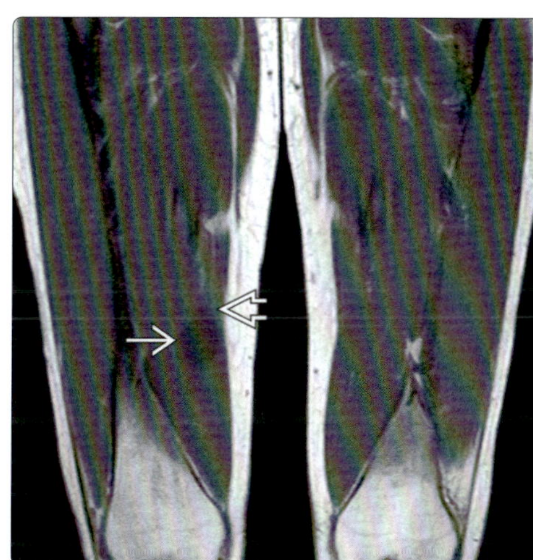

(Left) *Axial T1WI C+ FS MR in the same patient shows moderate heterogeneous enhancement of the mass ➡. Some of the areas of enhancement appear globular, which has been reported in the literature.* **(Right)** *Coronal T1WI MR in a different patient shows an intramuscular mass ➡ with homogeneously hypointense signal. There is a faint suggestion of fat signal intensity ➡ adjacent to the proximal pole of the lesion. This palpable mass was nontender.*

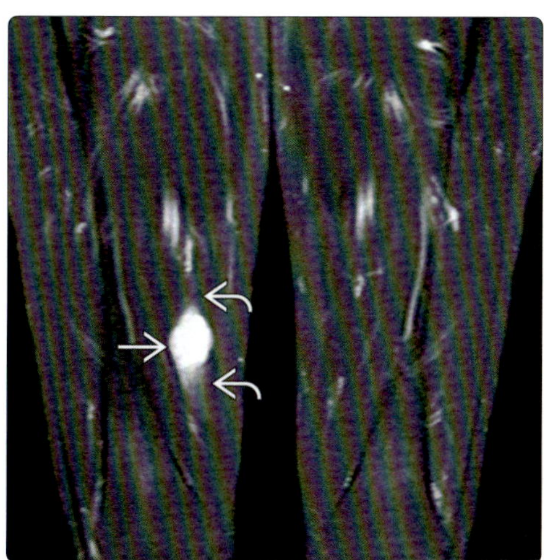

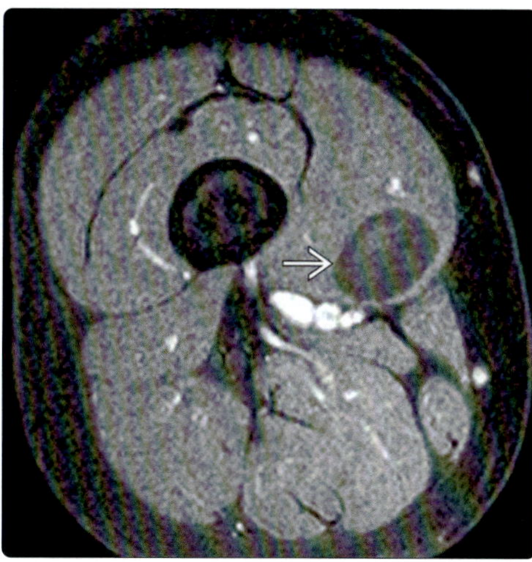

(Left) *Coronal STIR MR shows the intramuscular mass ➡ to have very high signal intensity simulating fluid. This sequence and plane best demonstrate high signal adjacent to the proximal and distal poles of the lesion ➡, which is a typical finding in these lesions and likely reflects leakage of myxomatous tissue.* **(Right)** *Axial T1WI C+ FS MR shows the well-circumscribed, rounded mass ➡ to be in the vastus medialis muscle and have mild heterogeneous enhancement.*

(Left) *Coronal T1WI MR shows a well-circumscribed, oval mass ➡ in the medial thigh. The mass is homogeneous hypointense to muscle. A thin peripheral rim of high-signal fat ➡ is seen at the distal pole of the mass.* **(Right)** *Axial T2WI FS MR shows the well-defined, intramuscular mass ➡ to have homogeneous hyperintensity. High signal in the soft tissues adjacent to the proximal and distal poles of the lesion (best seen on longitudinal images), without edema involving the midportion of the lesion, is typical.*

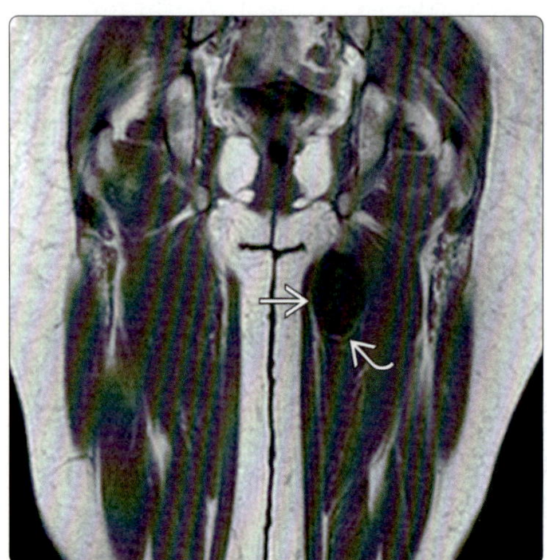

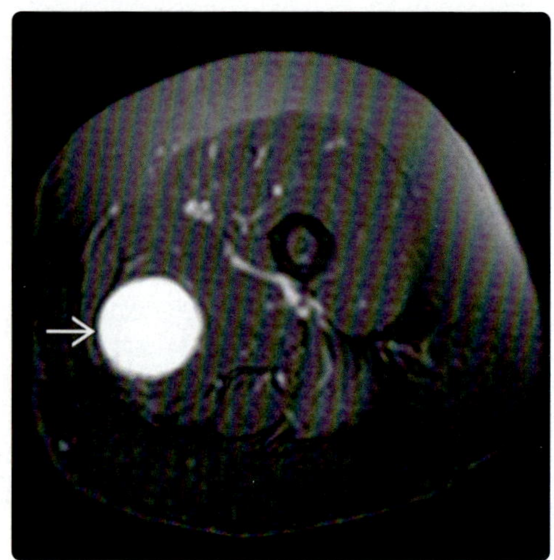

(Left) *Coronal T1WI MR in a 65-year-old man shows a low-signal ovoid mass ➡ within the sartorius muscle. There is some fatty atrophy in the muscle ➡ adjacent to the lesion.* **(Right)** *Coronal T2WI FS MR in the same patient shows the mass itself ➡ to be homogeneously high signal. There is high signal, flame-shaped extravasation from the mass extending proximally and distally along the muscle fascicles ➡. This appearance is typical of intramuscular myxoma.*

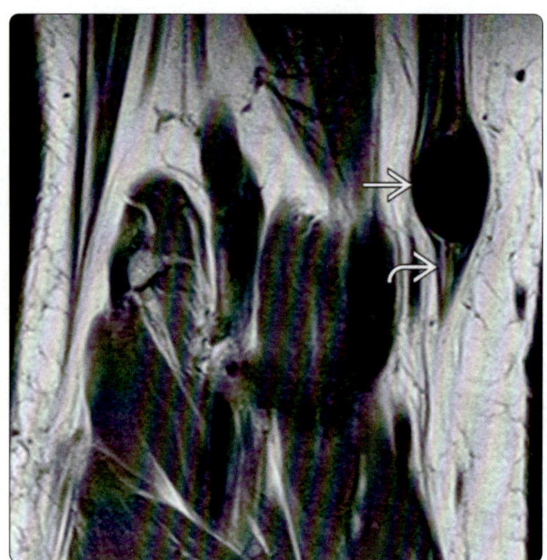

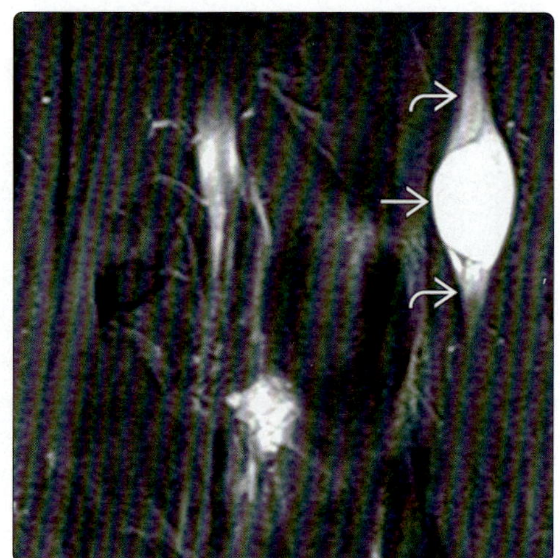

(Left) *Longitudinal ultrasound of an intramuscular myxoma ➡ shows a well-circumscribed, heterogeneously hypoechoic mass with increased through transmission ➡.* **(Right)** *Longitudinal power Doppler ultrasound of the mass ➡ demonstrates mild internal vascularity ➡. Ultrasound examination of these lesions is typically nonspecific, with common findings being heterogeneous hypoechogenicity, increased through transmission, focal cystic regions, and absent to mild internal vascularity.*

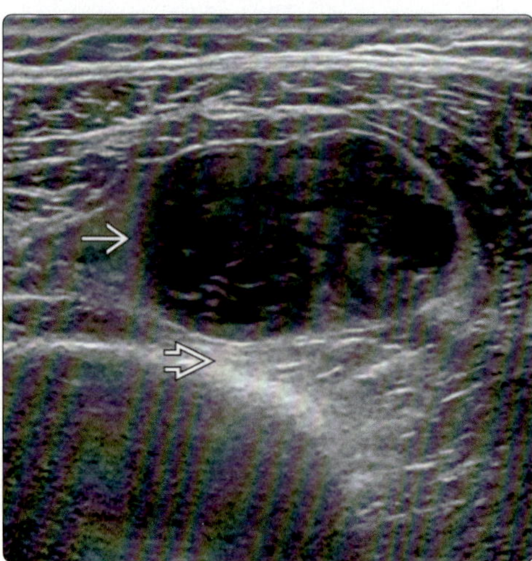

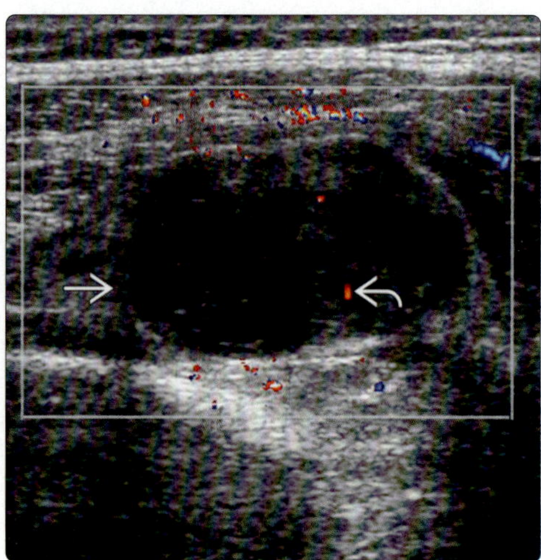

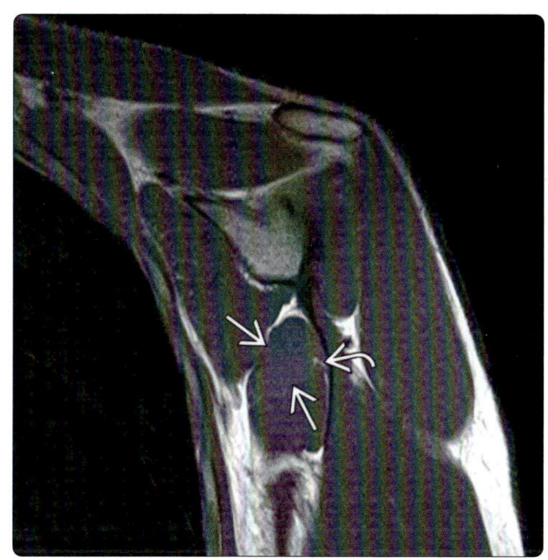

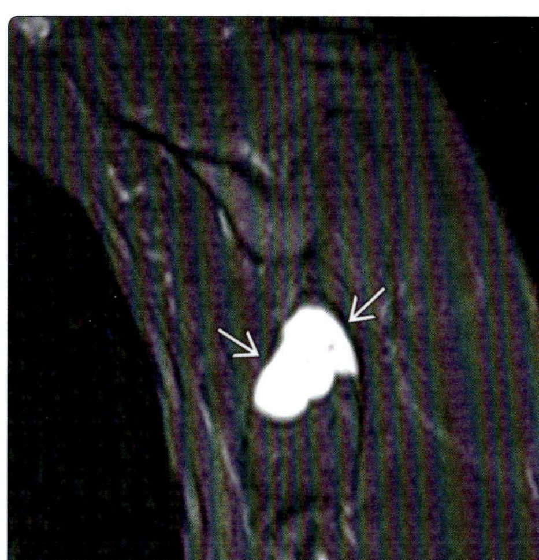

(Left) *Coronal T1WI MR shows a lesion* → *within the triceps muscle that is minimally hyperintense relative to the adjacent muscle. Note the small rim of fat* ↷ *at one edge of the lesion.* **(Right)** *Coronal T2WI FS MR in the same patient shows the lesion* → *to be homogeneously hyperintense. This is so homogeneous that it may suggest fluid. Contrast MR is required before the assumption of fluid can be made.*

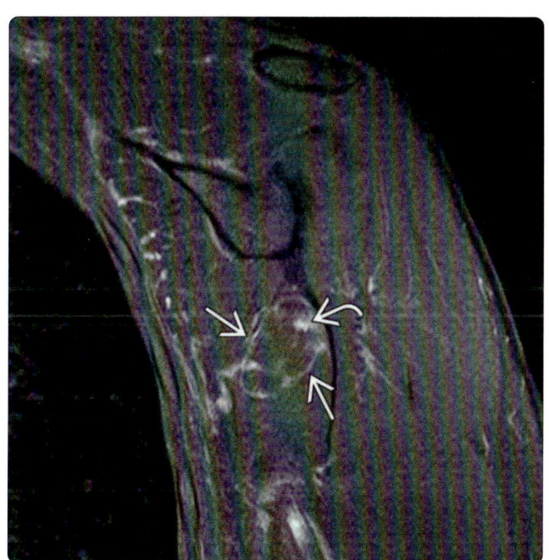

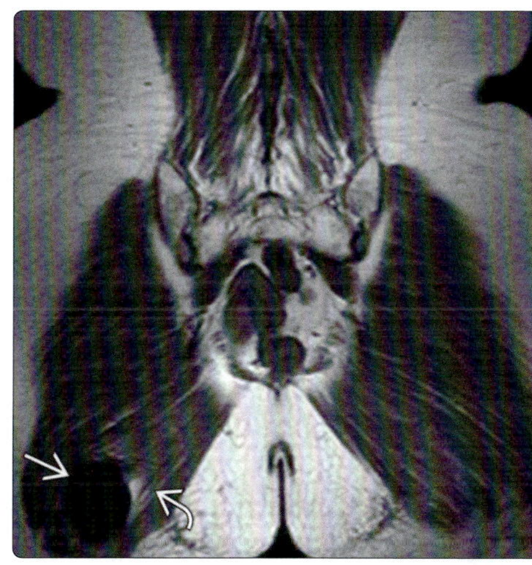

(Left) *Coronal postcontrast T1WI FS MR shows peripheral* →*, as well as mild globular* ↷*, enhancement. This pattern precludes fluid and is typical for intramuscular myxoma.* **(Right)** *Coronal T1WI MR shows a lesion* → *that is hypointense to adjacent muscle. There is adjacent fat signal and fatty muscle atrophy* ↷*. This pattern is suspicious for, but not diagnostic of, intramuscular myxoma.*

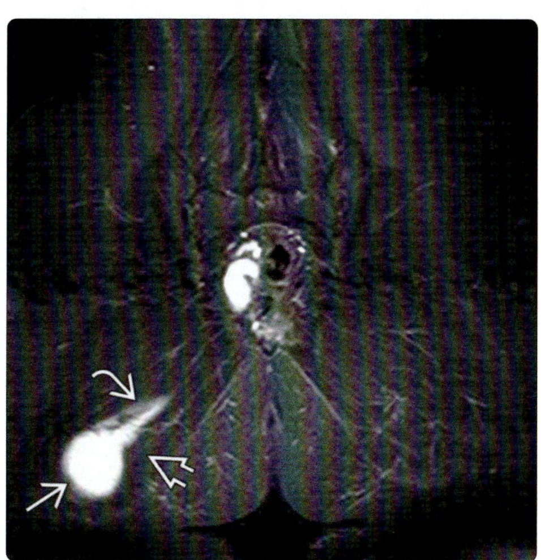

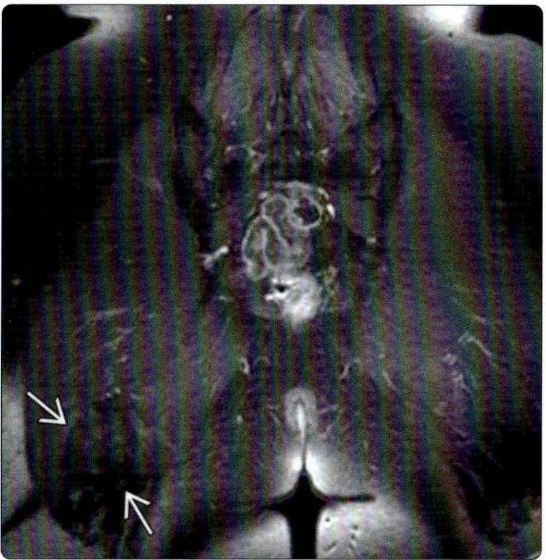

(Left) *Coronal STIR MR in the same patient shows the mass* → *to be homogeneously high signal, with flame-shaped extension* ↷ *along muscle fascicles. The area of fat* ⇨ *seen on the T1 image is now saturated out. These findings further suggest the diagnosis should be intramuscular myxoma.* **(Right)** *Coronal postcontrast T1WI FS MR in the same patient shows minimal inhomogeneous enhancement of the lesion* →*. This is the final diagnostic element for intramuscular myxoma.*

Ossifying Fibromyxoid Tumor

KEY FACTS

TERMINOLOGY

- Rare tumor of uncertain differentiation with intermediate (rarely metastasizing) aggressiveness

IMAGING

- Extremities (70%) > head/neck > trunk
  - Most common in lower extremities
  - Subcutis > muscle > > dermis (10%)
  - Typically 3-5 cm; median: 4 cm
- Soft tissue mass with central and peripheral calcification/ossification
  - 80% calcified; degree of calcification varies widely
  - Nonossifying variant (20%) lacks calcification
- ± periosteal reaction or erosion of underlying bone
- Heterogeneous signal intensity on T1WI, fluid-sensitive, and enhanced sequences
  - Regions of calcification & ossification have low signal on all sequences
  - ± foci of high T1 signal fatty marrow in regions of ossification
- Hypoechoic avascular mass on ultrasound

PATHOLOGY

- Well-circumscribed, nodular mass with thick fibrous pseudocapsule
  - May be tethered to fascia, muscle, or tendon
  - Incomplete peripheral shell of bone

CLINICAL ISSUES

- Majority have benign clinical course
- Painless, slowly growing mass in extremity
  - Median: 50 yr of age (range: 14-79 yr)
  - Male predominance
- Treated with wide surgical excision
- Malignant or atypical tumors may receive adjuvant radiotherapy and chemotherapy

(Left) *Coronal graphic shows a well-circumscribed mass ➡ in the subcutaneous fat of the shoulder. This lesion is tethered to the underlying fascia ↗. (Right) Axial NECT at the level of the hip shows a large, well-circumscribed soft tissue mass ➡. This mass contains discontinuous foci of mineralization ↗. There are no changes in the adjacent bone. The surrounding musculature is displaced but not invaded. Regional lymph nodes were increased in number but not pathologically enlarged in size.*

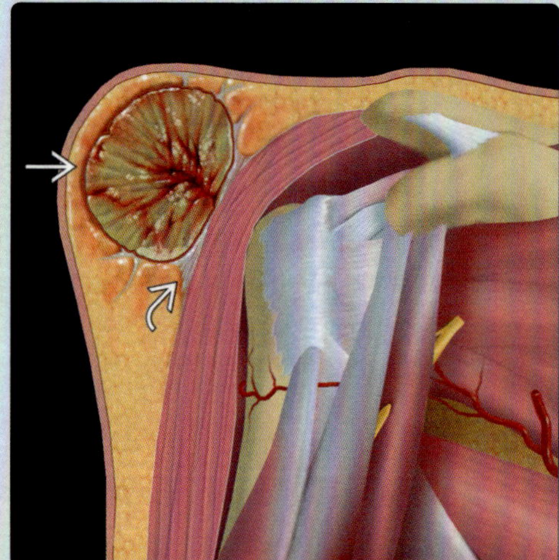

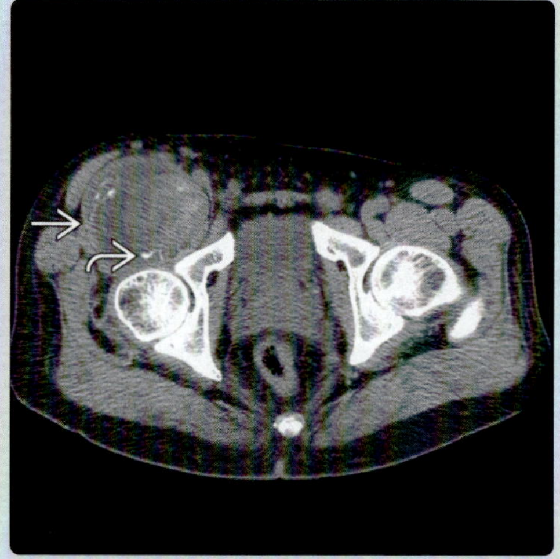

(Left) *Coronal STIR MR in the same patient shows marked heterogeneity of the large anterior thigh mass ➡, which has signal intensity ranging from hypointense to hyperintense. This includes low-signal regions of mineralization and fibrous tissue ↗. On T1WI MR (not shown), the mass was predominately isointense to muscle. (Right) Coronal T1WI C+ FS MR shows the mass ➡ to have heterogeneous enhancement ⇨. Regions of persistently low-signal mineralization ↗ do not enhance.*

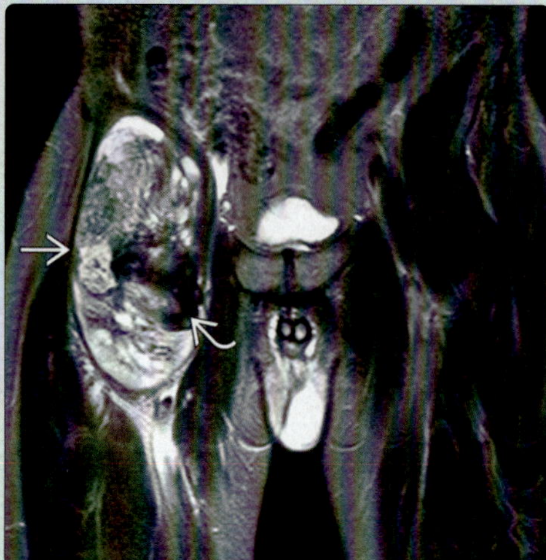

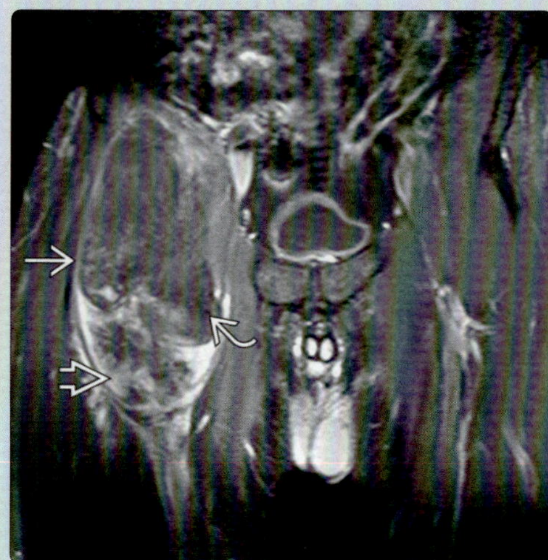

TERMINOLOGY

Definitions

- Rare tumor of uncertain differentiation with intermediate (rarely metastasizing) aggressiveness

IMAGING

General Features

- Location
  - Extremities (70%) > head/neck > trunk
    - Most common in lower extremities
    - Rare in mediastinum and retroperitoneum
  - Subcutis > muscle > > dermis (10%)
- Size
  - Typically 3-5 cm; median: 4 cm
    - Reported > 17 cm
- Morphology
  - Well-circumscribed, lobulated soft tissue mass

Radiographic Findings

- Soft tissue mass with central and peripheral calcification/ossification
  - 80% calcified; degree of calcification varies widely
    - Nonossifying variant (20%) lacks calcification
- ± periosteal reaction or erosion of underlying bone

CT Findings

- Mass with variable peripheral & central mineralization

MR Findings

- Heterogeneous signal intensity on T1WI, fluid-sensitive, and enhanced sequences
- Calcification & ossification low signal on all sequences
  - ± foci of high T1 signal fatty marrow in regions of ossification

Ultrasonographic Findings

- Well-demarcated, hypoechoic avascular mass
  - Shadowing marginal calcification

Nuclear Medicine Findings

- Marked Tc-99m MDP radiotracer uptake
- Avid uptake of F-18 FDG on PET

DIFFERENTIAL DIAGNOSIS

Myositis Ossificans/Heterotopic Ossification

- Zonal ossification progresses peripherally to centrally
- May contain high-signal fat on T1WI MR

Hematoma

- Heterogeneous mass without central enhancement
- Peripheral calcification when chronic

Extraskeletal Osteosarcoma

- Variably mineralized soft tissue mass
- Necrosis and hemorrhage are common

Synovial Sarcoma

- Soft tissue mass near a joint
- Calcification in 25-30%

Osteosarcoma, Parosteal

- Variably mineralized with broad attachment to bone
- Zonal ossification is most mature centrally

Sclerosing Epithelioid Fibrosarcoma

- Very rare deep soft tissue mass that may calcify
- Can be histologically similar

Schwannoma

- Elongated mass in region of neurovascular bundle
- May have target sign on T2WI MR

Malignant Peripheral Nerve Sheath Tumor

- Ill-defined, heterogeneous mass > 5 cm
  - Central necrosis is common

PATHOLOGY

Gross Pathologic & Surgical Features

- White to tan, well-circumscribed, nodular mass
  - May be tethered to fascia, muscle, or tendon
  - Incomplete peripheral shell of bone
- Firm, gritty to hard with thick fibrous pseudocapsule

Microscopic Features

- Uniform, round to spindle-shaped cells distributed in nests, sheets, or cords
  - Variably myxoid to collagenous stroma
  - Common incomplete rim of lamellar bone
  - ± central calcification, osteoid, and metaplastic cartilage
  - Low mitotic activity: < 2 per 50 HPF
- Malignant features: Hypercellularity, high nuclear grade, > 2 mitoses per 50 HPF

CLINICAL ISSUES

Presentation

- Most common signs/symptoms
  - Painless, slowly growing mass in extremity
    - Can be present for > 20 yr (median: 4 yr)

Demographics

- Age
  - Median: 50 yr (range: 14-79 yr)
    - Can be found at any age
- Gender
  - Male predominance

Natural History & Prognosis

- Majority have benign clinical course
- Single or multiple local recurrences in 17-27%
- Metastases, usually to lung or soft tissue, in 5%

Treatment

- Wide surgical excision
- Malignant or atypical tumors may receive adjuvant radiotherapy and chemotherapy

SELECTED REFERENCES

1. Atanaskova Mesinkovska N et al: Ossifying fibromyxoid tumor: a clinicopathologic analysis of 26 subcutaneous tumors with emphasis on differential diagnosis and prognostic factors. J Cutan Pathol. 42(9):622-31, 2015

KEY FACTS

TERMINOLOGY

- Malignant soft tissue tumor of uncertain differentiation

IMAGING

- Location
  - Up to 95% in extremities (lower > > upper)
  - Often near joint (especially popliteal fossa of knee) or tendon sheath but almost never intraarticular
- Calcification in 1/3 but variable in extent
- Changes involving adjacent bone in 11-25%
- CT attenuation is similar or ↓ relative to muscle
- Heterogeneous signal intensity on MR
  - Hemosiderin, cystic change, fluid-fluid levels relatively common
  - Prominent heterogeneous enhancement
- Split fat sign, triple sign, bowl of grapes sign on MR
- May have deceptively bland, well-defined, homogeneous appearance on imaging

PATHOLOGY

- Does **not** arise from synovium
- Specific chromosomal translocation t(X;18) in 90%

CLINICAL ISSUES

- Most commonly found at 15-40 years of age
- Most common lower extremity malignancy in 6- to 35-year-old patients
- Slowly growing soft tissue mass that may be either painful or asymptomatic
- Guarded prognosis
  - 5-year survival rate: 27-76%
  - Local recurrence in up to 50%
  - Metastases in up to 41%

DIAGNOSTIC CHECKLIST

- Enhancing soft tissue mass near joint, especially containing calcification, should not be dismissed as being benign without definitive work-up

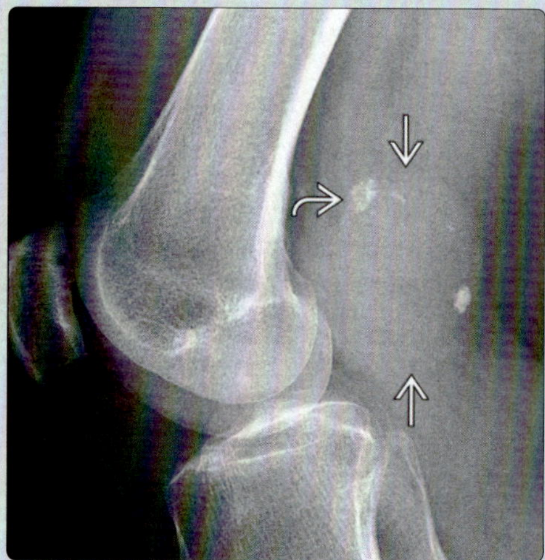

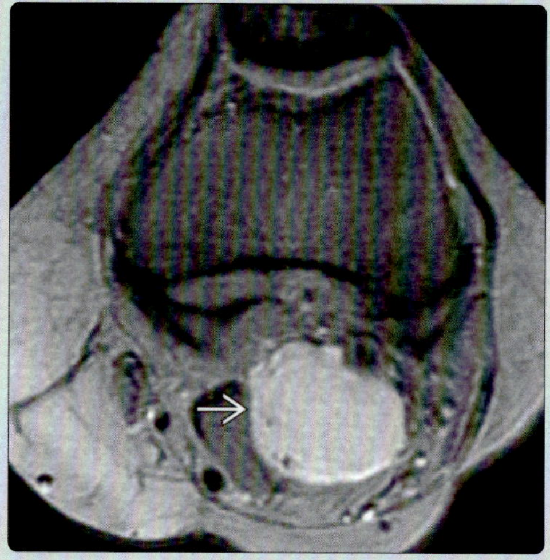

(Left) *Lateral radiograph shows a soft tissue mass ➡ posterior to the knee. Eccentrically located calcifications ➡ have a dystrophic appearance. These calcifications were initially thought to represent synovial chondromatosis in a popliteal cyst. However, these calcifications do not have the rounded appearance expected for synovial chondromatosis.* **(Right)** *Axial T2* GRE MR shows the soft tissue mass ➡ to be extraarticular and located lateral to the expected position of a popliteal cyst.*

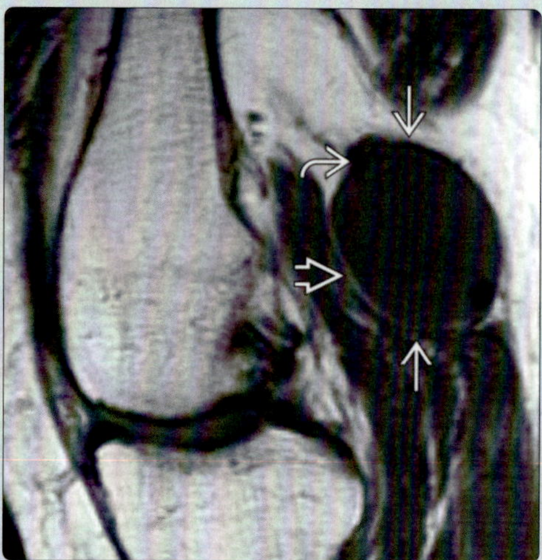

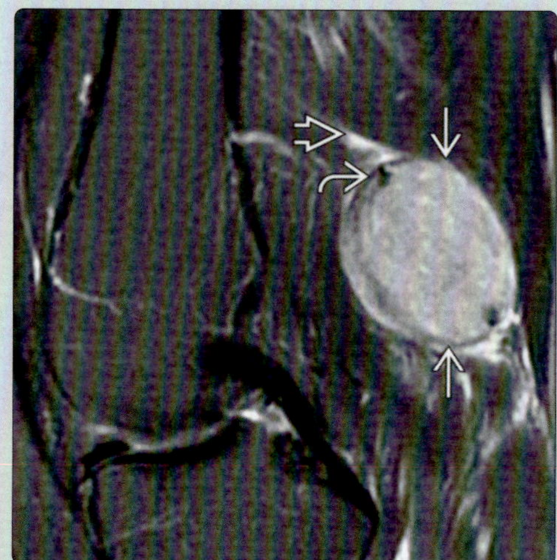

(Left) *Sagittal T1WI MR in the same patient shows the popliteal fossa mass ➡ to have a relatively homogeneous signal similar to muscle, with calcified foci ➡ showing expected low signal. Note the thin peripheral rim of fat ➡, the so-called split fat sign.* **(Right)** *Sagittal T2WI FS MR shows the mass ➡ to have heterogeneous high signal with low-signal calcification ➡. The lesion showed prominent enhancement with a small region of central necrosis. Peripheral edema ➡ is more common post treatment.*

TERMINOLOGY

Abbreviations

- Synovial sarcoma (SS)

Synonyms

- Carcinosarcoma, spindle cell carcinoma of soft tissue
- Archaic: Synovial cell sarcoma, tendosynovial sarcoma, synovioma, malignant synovioma, synovioblastic sarcoma, synovial endothelioma

Definitions

- Malignant soft tissue tumor of uncertain differentiation with predilection for juxtaarticular regions of young patients

IMAGING

General Features

- Location
  - Up to 95% in extremities (lower > > upper)
    - Most common near joint (especially popliteal fossa of knee) or tendon sheath
      - < 10% arise within joint or bursa
      - Joint involvement, if present, usually due to local invasion
  - 5% in head and neck, 2.6% in abdominal wall, 0.5% in retroperitoneum
  - Found throughout body: Skin, genitourinary system, breast, intrathoracic, intravascular, intraneural, intracranial, intraosseous
  - Deep > > subcutis > > dermis
- Size
  - Usually < 5 cm (range: 3-15 cm)
- Morphology
  - Rounded to oval, nodular mass with either circumscribed or infiltrative borders

Radiographic Findings

- Radiography
  - Normal (50%) or soft tissue mass
  - Calcification in 1/3 but variable in extent
    - Peripheral or eccentric location more common than central
    - Ossification is uncommon
  - Changes involving adjacent bone in 11-25%
    - Pressure erosion or periosteal reaction
    - Bone invasion in 5%

CT Findings

- Well-defined to partially infiltrative soft tissue mass ± calcification
  - Density is similar to or slightly lower than muscle
    - May contain cystic or hemorrhagic regions
  - Heterogeneous enhancement
- Pulmonary metastases may calcify

MR Findings

- T1WI
  - Homogeneous or heterogeneous soft tissue mass with signal intensity similar to or lower than skeletal muscle
    - Small tumors have more homogeneous appearance
  - Split fat sign = thin rim of fat around mass due to intermuscular origin near neurovascular bundle
- T2WI
  - Heterogeneously hyperintense to skeletal muscle
    - Homogeneous, isointense lesions reported
  - Hemosiderin, cystic change, fluid-fluid levels relatively common
    - Triple sign = multiple signal intensities due to hemorrhage, necrosis, solid tissue, and calcification
    - Bowl of grapes sign = multiloculated appearance of mass with internal septa
    - Cystic component may be dominant feature of lesion
  - Edema surrounding mass is most commonly seen post radiotherapy
- Prominent heterogeneous enhancement
- Mineralization has low signal intensity on all MR sequences
- MR of synovial sarcoma may appear deceptively nonaggressive in children

Angiographic Findings

- Hypervascular mass that displaces native vessels
- Arteriovenous shunting in 24%

Nuclear Medicine Findings

- Bone scan
  - Mineralization shows normal or ↑ uptake of Tc-99m MDP on scintigraphy
  - Hypervascularity causes ↑ tracer uptake in solid portions of lesion on flow and blood-pool images
- PET
  - 80% sensitivity for F-18 FDG PET
  - Pretherapy tumor SUV may predict survival

DIFFERENTIAL DIAGNOSIS

Malignant Peripheral Nerve Sheath Tumor

- Infiltrative mass ± hemorrhage
- Calcification common
- Arises from large or medium deep nerves
- Can be histologically similar to synovial sarcoma

Extraskeletal Osteosarcoma

- Peak age: 5th to 7th decades of life
  - Older patient population than SS
- Most common in deep soft tissues of thigh
- Variably mineralized soft tissue mass
- May have fluid-fluid levels

Hematoma

- Lacks solid regions of enhancing tissue
- May calcify when chronic
- Fluid-fluid levels common

Extraskeletal Mesenchymal Chondrosarcoma

- Similar peak age (15-35 years) as synovial sarcoma
- Soft tissue mass with chondroid matrix
- Most common in head and neck

Myositis Ossificans/Heterotopic Ossification

- Mineralization matures peripheral to central
- Muscles of upper or lower extremity
- Peak age: 2nd to 3rd decades of life

Solitary Fibrous Tumor and Hemangiopericytoma

- Wide age range: 2nd to 7th decade of life
  - Most common in middle-aged adults
- May have mineralization, necrosis, or hemorrhage

PATHOLOGY

General Features

- Etiology
  - Does **not** arise from synovium
  - No specific proven predisposing factors
    - Reported association with metal joint prosthesis and radiotherapy
- Genetics
  - Specific chromosomal translocation t(X;18) (p11;q11) in 90%

Gross Pathologic & Surgical Features

- Soft to firm, tan or gray nodular mass
  - Circumscribed or infiltrative
  - ± multinodular, multicystic, or hemorrhagic
  - May be adherent to tendon, tendon sheath, joint capsule, bursa, fascia, ligament, or interosseous membrane

Microscopic Features

- Biphasic SS: Contains both epithelial and spindle cell components (classic form)
- Monophasic SS: Contains only spindle cells in dense sheets or fascicles
  - Focal hemangiopericytoma-like vessels
- Purely glandular monophasic SS: Histologically identical to adenocarcinoma
- Monophasic epithelial SS: Consists of plump epithelioid cells
- Calcifying SS: Shows calcification ± ossification
- Ossifying SS: Contains lamellar and trabecular bone
- Poorly differentiated SS: Highly cellular with high mitotic activity and necrosis
- Immunohistochemistry
  - Cytokeratin (CK) &/or epithelial membrane antigen should be positive in SS
    - CK positive in 90% of SS with epithelial component
      - Differentiate from malignant peripheral nerve sheath tumor and Ewing sarcoma/PNET (CK negative)
  - Epithelial membrane antigen more widely positive than CK in monophasic and poorly differentiated SS

CLINICAL ISSUES

Presentation

- Most common signs/symptoms
  - Slowly growing soft tissue mass that may be painful or asymptomatic
    - Duration present: 2-4 years on average, up to 20 years; insidious onset may cause delay in diagnosis
    - May cause symptoms due to mass effect
  - Mass is usually < 5 cm at presentation
- Other signs/symptoms
  - Systemic symptoms, such as weight loss, are unusual
    - More common with poorly differentiated SS
  - More likely to report prior trauma to region with calcifying SS

Demographics

- Age
  - Most common: 15-40 years (mean: 32 years)
    - Up to 90% occur before age 50
    - Reported from birth to 89 years of age
- Gender
  - Conflicting studies report equal incidence, mild male predominance, and mild female predominance
- Epidemiology
  - Most common lower extremity malignancy in 6- to 35-year-old patients
  - 2.5-10% of all soft tissue sarcomas
  - Incidence 2.75 per 100,000 population
  - No ethnic predilection

Natural History & Prognosis

- Guarded prognosis
  - 5-year survival rate: 27-76%
  - 10-year survival rate: 20-63%
  - Calcifying SS has better survival rate: 5 year: 83%, 10 year: 66%
- Local recurrence in up to 50%
  - Mean of 3.6 years after diagnosis (range: 0.5-14.9 years)
  - Reported up to 30-year delay
- Metastases in up to 41%
  - Metastases at presentation in 16-25%
  - Mean of 5.7 years after diagnosis (range: 0.5-16 years in 1 study)
    - Indicates follow-up required for > 10 years
  - 59-94% of metastases are to lung, > > lymph nodes > bone > soft tissue
- Improved outcome: Patient age < 25 years, extensive calcification, tumor < 5 cm, < 10 mitoses per 10 HPF, complete local resection, *SYT/SSX2* variant gene (in monophasic fibrous subtype)
- Poor prognostic factors: Tumor ≥ 5 cm, > 50% necrosis, poorly differentiated subtype, rhabdoid cells, hemorrhage, location other than extremity, patient age > 40 years

Treatment

- Wide surgical excision
  - Limb amputation when wide excision not possible or limb function cannot be preserved
- Adjuvant radiotherapy for local control ± chemotherapy depending on clinical situation

SELECTED REFERENCES

1. Bakri A et al: Synovial sarcoma: imaging features of common and uncommon primary sites, metastatic patterns, and treatment response. AJR Am J Roentgenol. 199(2):W208-15, 2012
2. Krieg AH et al: Synovial sarcomas usually metastasize after >5 years: a multicenter retrospective analysis with minimum follow-up of 10 years for survivors. Ann Oncol. 22(2):458-67, 2011
3. Bixby SD et al: Synovial sarcoma in children: imaging features and common benign mimics. AJR Am J Roentgenol. 195(4):1026-32, 2010

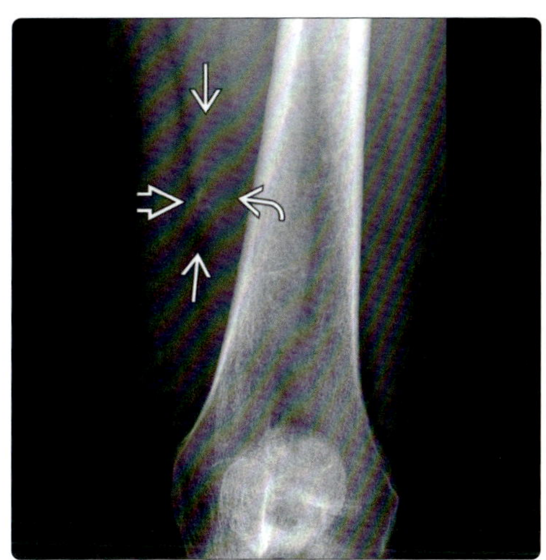

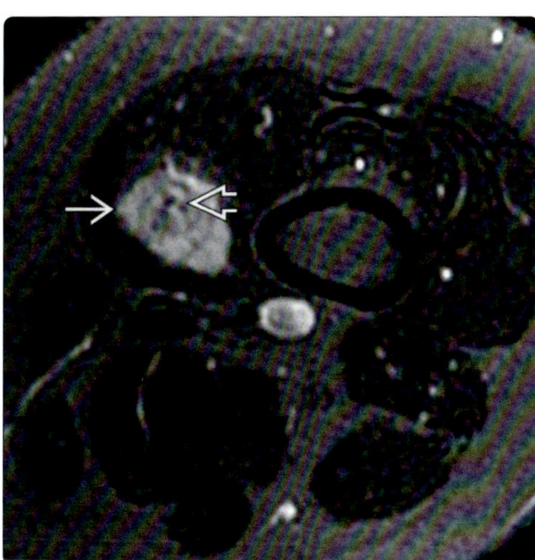

(Left) *AP radiograph in a 28-year-old woman shows a soft tissue mass ➡ that displaces fat ➡ & contains calcification ➡. Given the calcification, the patient's age and location of the lesion, synovial sarcoma must be strongly considered.* **(Right)** *Axial STIR MR in the same patient shows a relatively homogeneous hyperintense mass ➡ that contains low-signal calcifications ➡. Postcontrast imaging is not shown, but the lesion showed intense enhancement with a small region of central necrosis, typical of synovial sarcoma.*

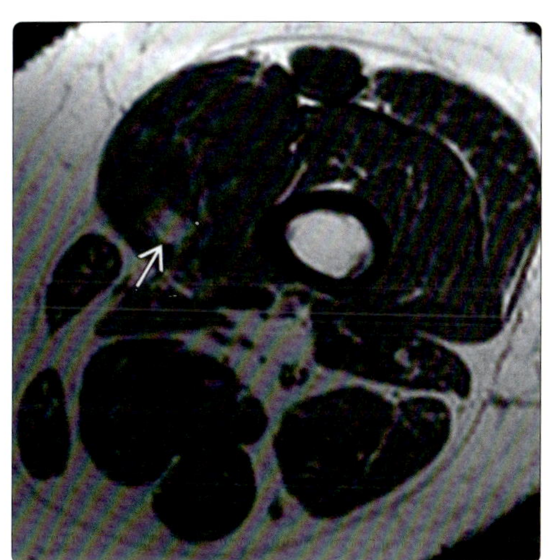

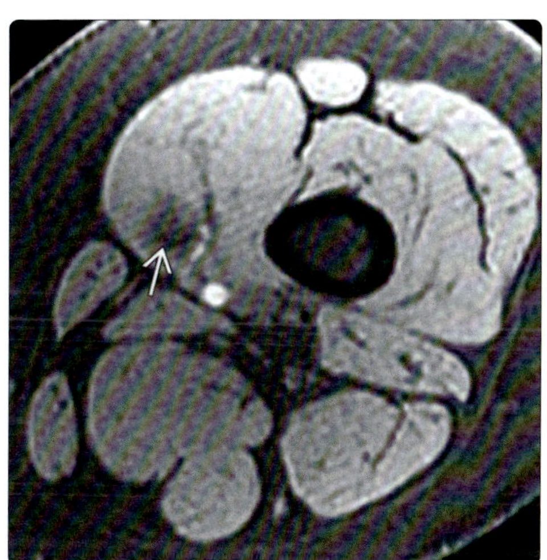

(Left) *Axial T1WI MR in the same case, obtained at a different level of the lesion, shows a region of fat ➡ at the periphery of the lesion.* **(Right)** *Axial T1WI FS MR, matched in level to the prior image, shows that the peripheral focus of fat saturates out ➡, proving its adipose nature. This represents the split fat sign, or displaced fat, that may be seen in synovial sarcomas.*

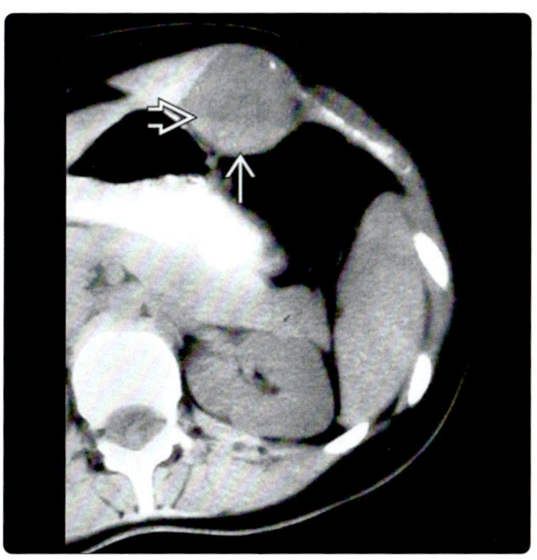

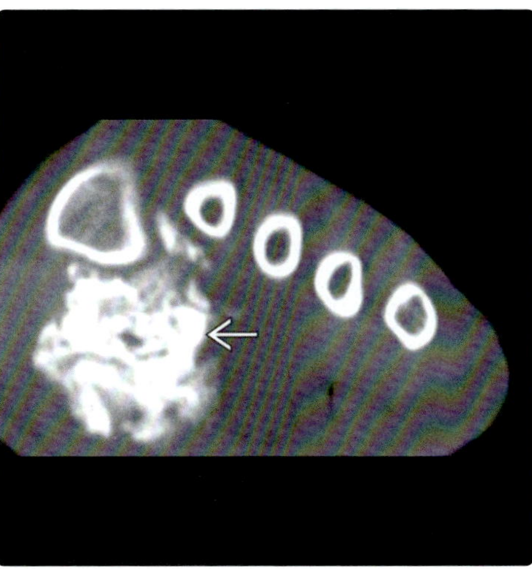

(Left) *Axial CT shows an anterior abdominal wall soft tissue mass ➡ that contains a prominent fluid level ➡. Synovial sarcomas often contain cystic areas, which may show fluid levels. This lesion should not be mistaken for a hematoma.* **(Right)** *Short-axis CT shows irregular, dense mineralization of a plantar foot mass ➡. Synovial sarcomas can both calcify and ossify. Extensively calcified synovial sarcomas have a better prognosis than those that are noncalcified or contain a small amount of calcification.*

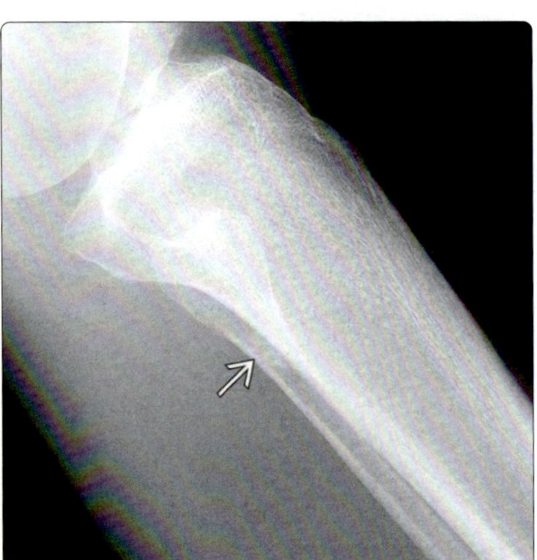

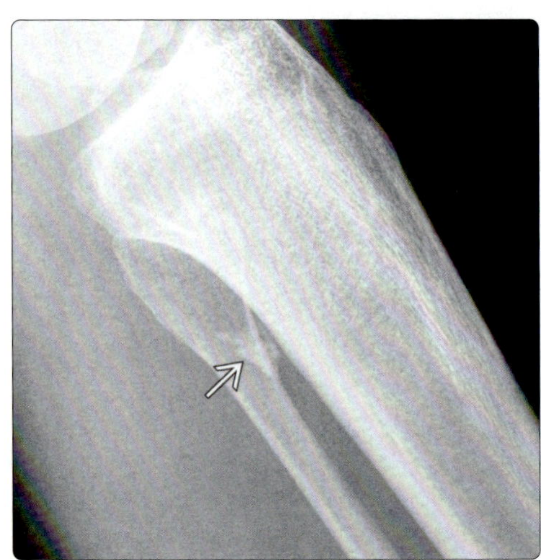

(Left) *Lateral radiograph shows a small focus of dystrophic calcification ➡ in the region of the interosseous membrane. There is no other characterizing feature.* **(Right)** *Lateral radiograph obtained several months later shows enlargement of the dystrophic calcification ➡. This is worrisome, especially because of the periarticular location in a 20 year old. It is too deep for myositis ossificans and lacks the characteristic zoning seen in that process. One must be concerned that this represents tumor that contains mineralization.*

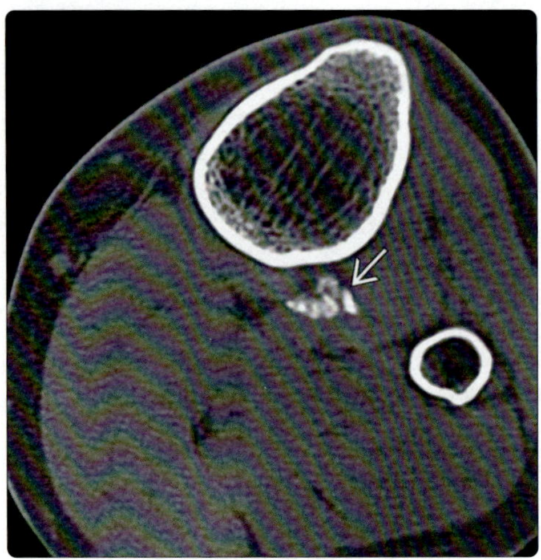

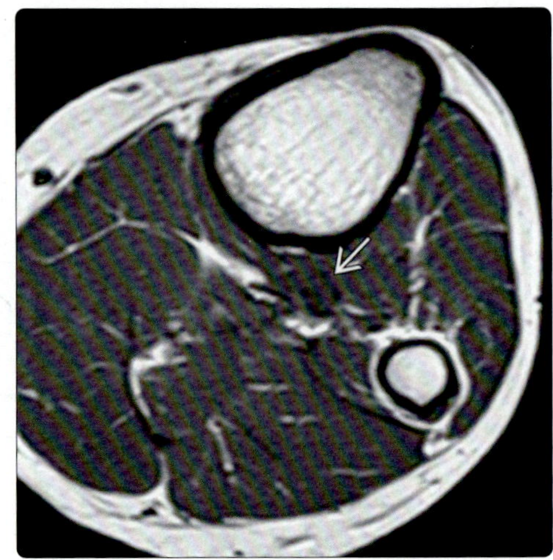

(Left) *Axial bone CT shows the calcification to have a dystrophic character ➡ and to either involve or lie adjacent to the tibialis posterior muscle. It is also adjacent to the neurovascular bundle. This location near a neurovascular bundle is typical. As these lesions enlarge, they can produce the split fat sign by peripherally displacing the normal fat that is present in this region.* **(Right)** *Axial T1WI MR shows a tiny mass ➡ that is isointense to muscle and contains low-signal calcification.*

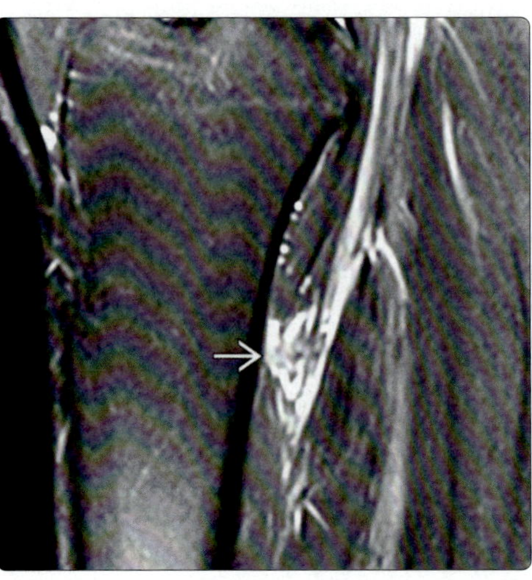

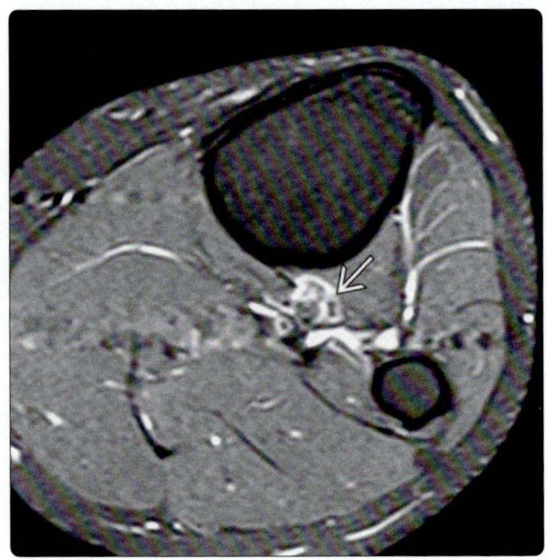

(Left) *Sagittal T2WI FS MR in the same patient shows the mass ➡ to have heterogeneous high signal.* **(Right)** *Axial T1WI C+ FS MR shows intense enhancement of the soft tissue portions of the mass ➡. Because the lesion was not easily surgically accessible, the oncologic surgeons were not eager to biopsy or resect it. However, the typical clinical and imaging appearance favoring synovial sarcoma pushed the issue. At surgery, the lesion was confirmed to be a synovial sarcoma.*

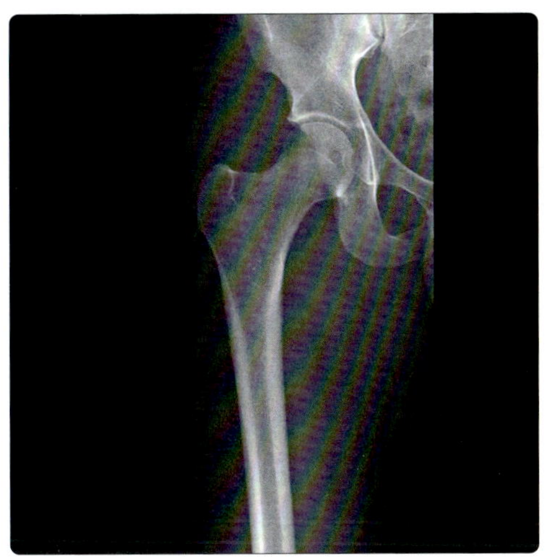

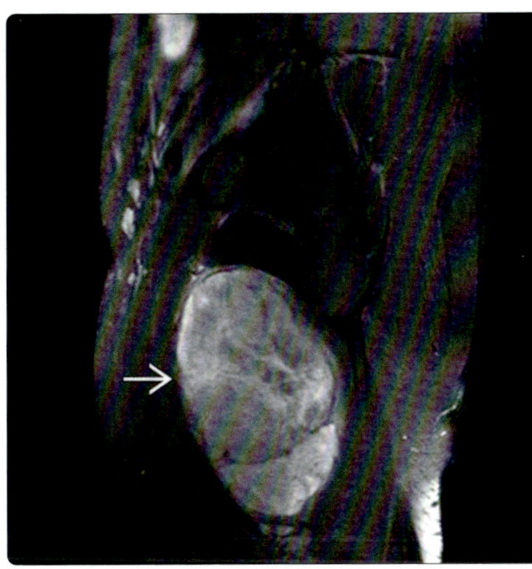

(Left) *AP radiograph obtained in a young adult male with a palpable thigh mass shows no calcification or other feature.* **(Right)** *Sagittal T2WI FS MR in the same case shows a large, inhomogeneous mass ➡. Given the patient's age and the location of the lesion in the lower extremity, synovial sarcoma must be strongly considered, even in the absence of calcifications. Although synovial sarcoma is the most frequent sarcoma to contain calcification, it is worth remembering that 2/3 of cases do not have this feature.*

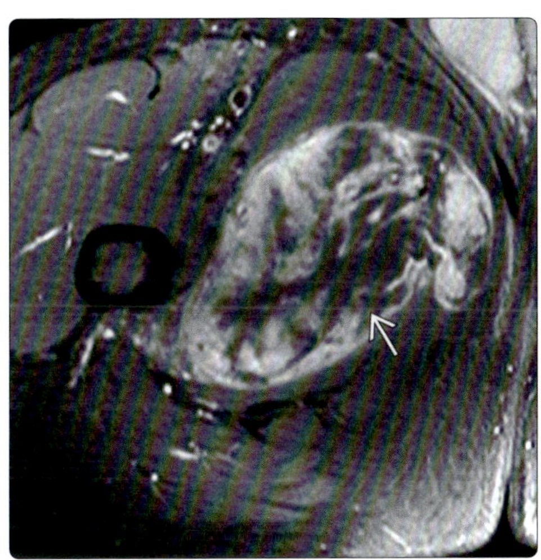

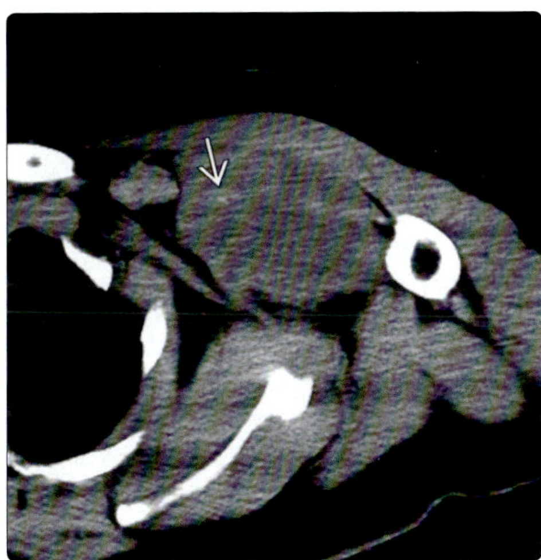

(Left) *Axial T1WI C+ FS MR in the same case shows extensive central necrosis ➡. At biopsy, this aggressive lesion proved to be synovial sarcoma.* **(Right)** *Axial bone CT shows a large mass with density slightly lower than muscle that contains a small focus of calcification ➡. The patient is a young adult; with the presence of calcification, synovial sarcoma must be strongly suspected.*

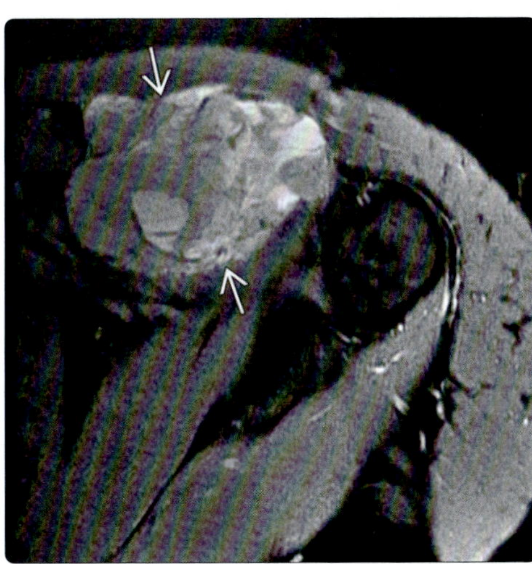

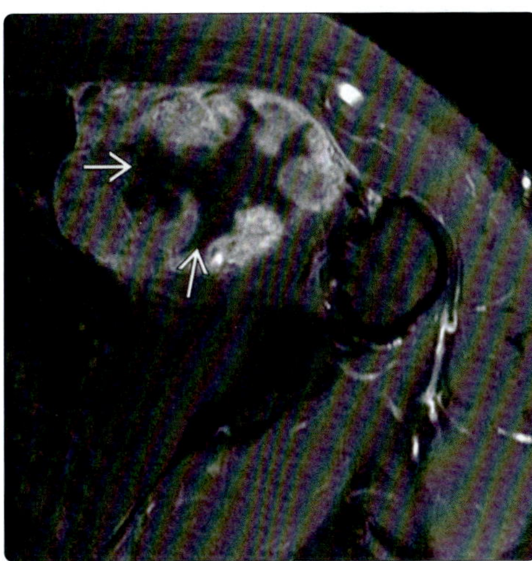

(Left) *Axial T2WI FS MR in the same patient shows the mass ➡ to arise near a neurovascular bundle, as synovial sarcoma frequently does. The mass appears highly complex, with 3 different signal intensities. This triple sign is often seen in synovial sarcoma and is due to the combination of areas of solid tumor, hemorrhage, and necrosis.* **(Right)** *Axial T1WI C+ FS MR in the same patient shows the mass to contain a large region of central necrosis ➡. At surgery, this lesion proved to be synovial sarcoma.*

Epithelioid Sarcoma

KEY FACTS

TERMINOLOGY

- Aggressive soft tissue sarcoma of uncertain differentiation, which propagates along fascia, tendon sheaths, nerve sheaths, and lymphatics

IMAGING

- Conventional (distal)-type epithelioid sarcoma (ES): 60% involve flexor surface of distal upper extremity
- Proximal-type ES: Pelvis > > perineum > genital tract (pubis, vulva, penis)
- Nodular to ill-defined soft tissue mass
  - Calcification or ossification in 8-28%
- Homogeneously isointense to muscle on T1WI MR
  - May contain high signal hemorrhage
- Heterogeneously hyperintense on fluid-sensitive MR sequences with necrosis common
- Peripheral edema
- Heterogeneous enhancement

CLINICAL ISSUES

- Most common hand/wrist malignancy in patients ages 6-25 years
- Solitary or multiple firm, painless nodules
  - Tenderness in 25%
  - Skin ulceration in 10%
- Slowly growing with mean duration: 2.5 years
- Conventional (distal) type ES: 10-35 years of age
  - Proximal-type ES: Older adults
- Local recurrence up to 77%, metastases 45%
- Radical surgical excision or amputation
  - Regional lymph node dissection
  - Adjuvant radiotherapy and chemotherapy commonly utilized

DIAGNOSTIC CHECKLIST

- Do not misinterpret as infection/inflammation or sequelae of trauma

(Left) *Axial T1WI MR shows an ill-defined, infiltrative mass ➡ in the subcutaneous fat of the anterior lower leg. This 18-year-old man reported painful swelling in this region for 1 year and an injury to this area 4 years prior. The mass is predominantly isointense to muscle with a focus of high signal ↪, likely representing hemorrhage.* **(Right)** *Axial T2WI FS MR shows the mass ➡ to have heterogeneous high signal intensity. Note the surrounding edema ⇨ and extent along the fascia.*

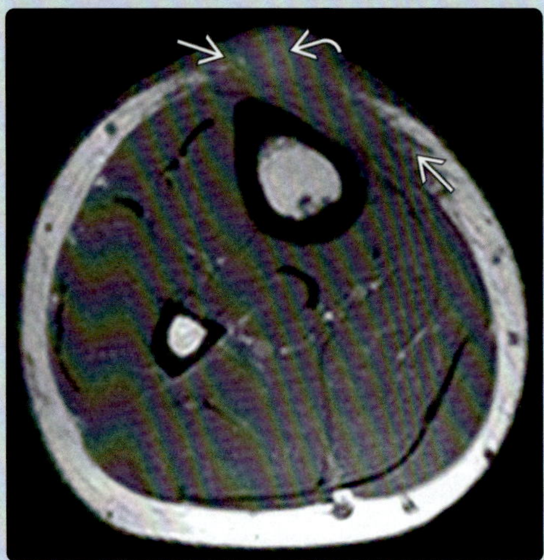

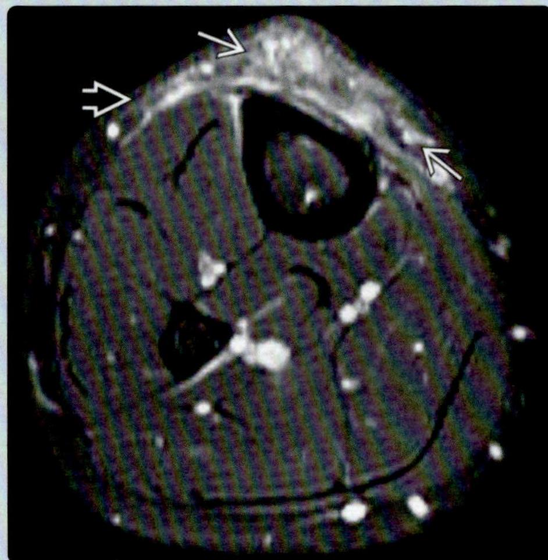

(Left) *Sagittal T1WI C+ FS MR shows heterogeneous enhancement of the mass ➡ with foci lacking enhancement ↪, likely representing necrosis or hemorrhage.* **(Right)** *Axial PET/CT performed for tumor staging shows ↑ tracer uptake involving a right inguinal lymph node ➡. There was no evidence of tumor at surgical excision, thus this finding was presumed to be reactive. Despite surgical resection, node-positive status, and adjuvant radiotherapy and chemotherapy, this patient died 1 year later.*

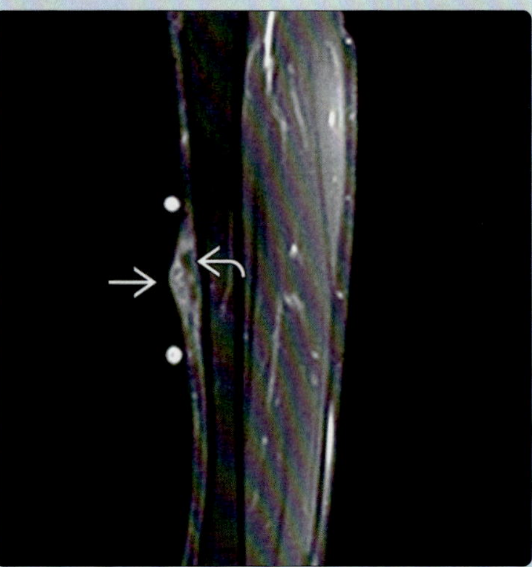

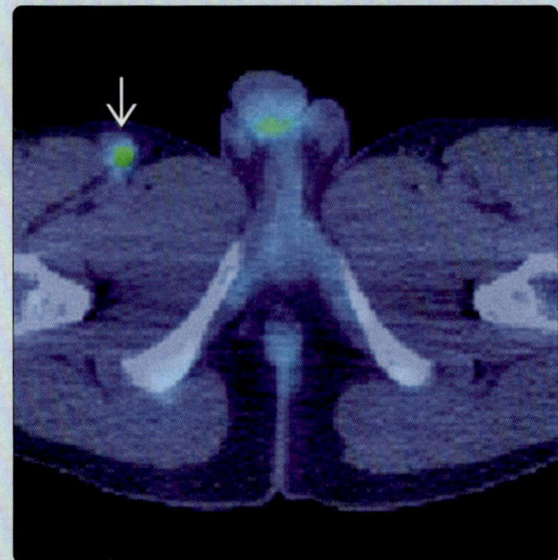

TERMINOLOGY

Abbreviations

- Epithelioid sarcoma (ES)

Definitions

- Aggressive soft tissue sarcoma of uncertain differentiation with tendency to propagate along fascia, tendon sheaths, nerve sheaths, and lymphatics

IMAGING

General Features

- Location
  - Conventional (distal)-type ES
    - 60% involve flexor surface of distal upper extremity: Finger, hand > wrist, forearm
    - Less common in knee/lower leg > buttock/thigh > shoulder/arm > ankle, foot, and toe
    - Rare in trunk and head and neck
  - Proximal-type ES: Pelvis > > perineum > genital tract (pubis, vulva, penis)
- Size
  - Superficial lesions: Few mm to 6 cm
  - Deep lesions: 15 ≥ cm

CT Findings

- Nodular to ill-defined soft tissue mass
- Calcification or ossification in 8-28%
- Osseous involvement or periosteal reaction uncommon

MR Findings

- Homogeneously isointense to muscle on T1WI
  - May contain high-signal hemorrhage
- Heterogeneously hyperintense on fluid-sensitive sequences with necrosis common
  - Fluid-fluid levels reported
  - Peripheral high-signal edema
- Heterogeneous enhancement
- Extension along fascial planes common

DIFFERENTIAL DIAGNOSIS

Squamous Cell Carcinoma

- Clinical mimic of ulcerating, superficially located ES
- Histologic mimic of ES due to epithelioid cells
- CD5/6(+) and cyclin-D1 (nuclear) negative

Soft Tissue Ulcer

- Clinical mimic of ulcerated superficial ES
- Chronic inflammatory cells in ES can mimic infections

Foreign Body Granuloma

- ES mimic on imaging and focally on histology
- Look for embedded foreign body

Angiosarcoma of Soft Tissue

- Histologic and imaging overlap with ES
- CD31 and von Willebrand factor positive

Schwannoma

- ES may mimic nerve sheath tumor when extending along course of nerve

PATHOLOGY

General Features

- Etiology
  - Trauma may contribute to development
    - Reported in up to 25%
  - Reported after exposure to chemicals and plutonium

Microscopic Features

- Conventional (distal)-type ES
  - Nodular growth pattern of eosinophilic epithelioid and spindle cells with prominent intercellular collagen and surrounding chronic inflammation
  - Necrosis may mimic granulomatous change
  - Cytokeratins, EMA, and vimentin positive
  - CD34(+) in up to 60%

CLINICAL ISSUES

Presentation

- Most common signs/symptoms
  - Superficial lesions
    - Solitary or multiple firm, painless nodules
      - Tenderness in 25%
    - Slowly growing with mean duration: 2.5 years
    - Skin ulceration in 10%
  - Deep-seated lesions
    - Mass ± discomfort or limited range of motion
    - Mass effect on neurovascular structures

Demographics

- Age
  - Conventional (distal)-type ES
    - 10-35 years of age (median: 26 years)
  - Proximal-type ES: Older adults
- Gender
  - Male predominance (2:1)
- Epidemiology
  - 1.4% of all soft tissue sarcomas
  - Most common hand/wrist malignancy in patients age 6-25 years

Natural History & Prognosis

- Conventional (distal)-type ES
  - Local recurrence: Up to 77%
  - Metastases: 45% (lung ~ lymph nodes > > scalp > bone and brain > liver)
  - 10-year survival rate: 41-73%
- Proximal-type ES
  - More aggressive than conventional type
  - Resistant to multimodal therapy

Treatment

- Radical surgical excision or amputation
  - Regional lymph node dissection
- Adjuvant radiotherapy and chemotherapy commonly utilized

SELECTED REFERENCES

1. Wadhwa V et al: Epithelioid sarcoma presenting as radial mononeuropathy: anatomical, magnetic resonance neurography and diffusion tensor imaging appearances. Skeletal Radiol. 42(6):853-8, 2013

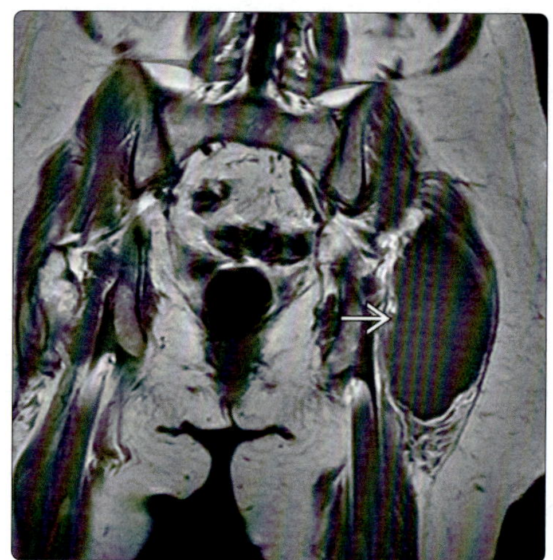

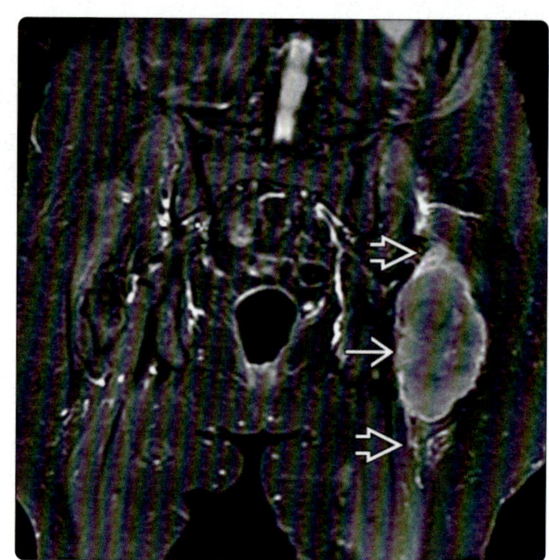

(Left) *Coronal T1WI MR of the pelvis shows a lobulated, ovoid mass ➡ posterior to the left hip with homogeneous signal intensity similar to muscle. This mass extended along the fascial plane between the gluteus medius and gluteus minimus muscles.* **(Right)** *Coronal STIR MR shows the lobulated heterogeneous mass ➡ to have mild surrounding edema ⇨. This proximal-type epithelioid sarcoma has a predilection to arise in the pelvis, genital tract, and perineum.*

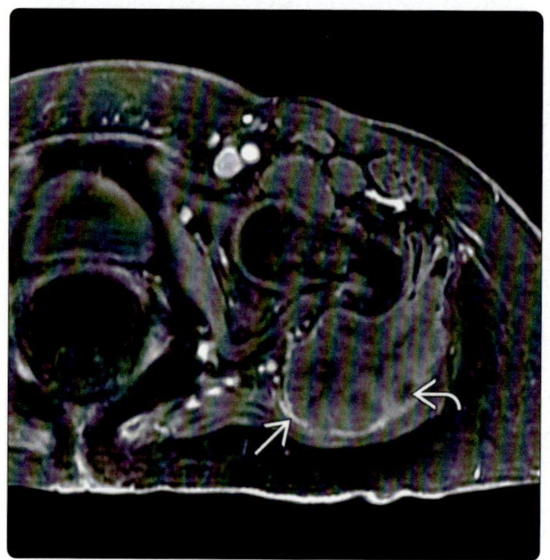

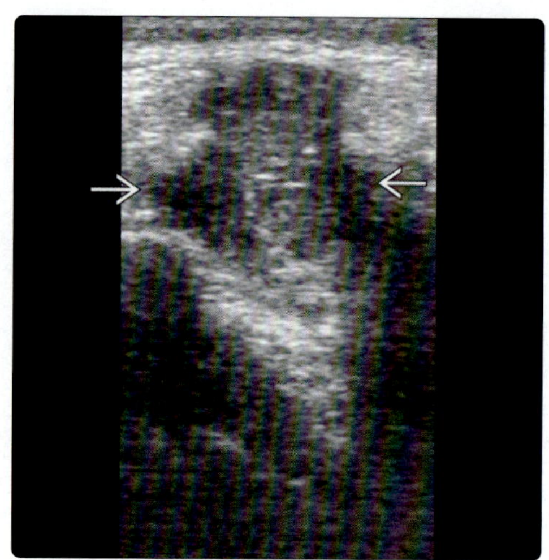

(Left) *Axial T1WI C+ FS MR shows mild to moderate heterogeneous enhancement of the mass ➡ with presumed necrotic foci that lack enhancement ↪. The mass abutted the greater trochanter and iliotibial band.* **(Right)** *Longitudinal ultrasound of the scrotum in a 24-year-old man shows an irregular mass ➡ with heterogeneous echogenicity. Mild internal blood flow was demonstrated on Doppler. This mass extended from the region of the spermatic cord into the subcutis and measured less than 2 cm.*

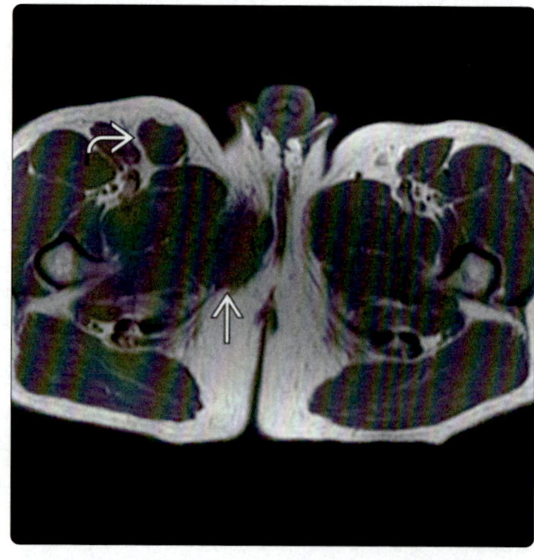

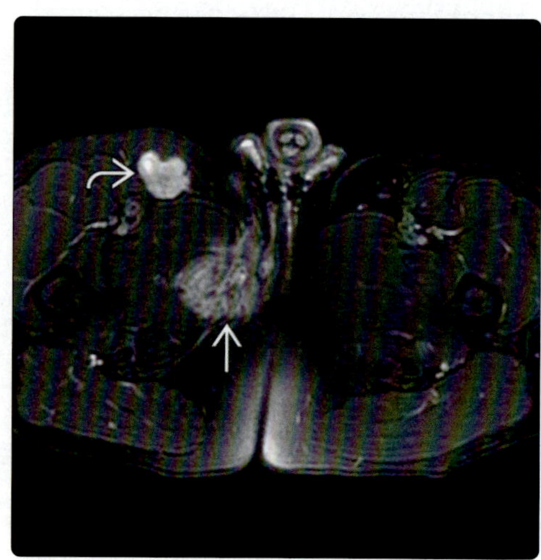

(Left) *Axial T1WI MR of a 37-year-old man who presented for evaluation of swelling in his right groin, which corresponded to adenopathy ↪, is shown. Also identified is an ill-defined right perineal mass ➡ that is isointense to muscle.* **(Right)** *Axial T2WI FS MR shows the ill-defined right perineal mass ➡ to have signal ranging from hypointense to hyperintense. Adenopathy ↪ is again noted. Treatment included resection, radiotherapy, and chemotherapy. No evidence of recurrent disease has been seen in 3 years of follow-up.*

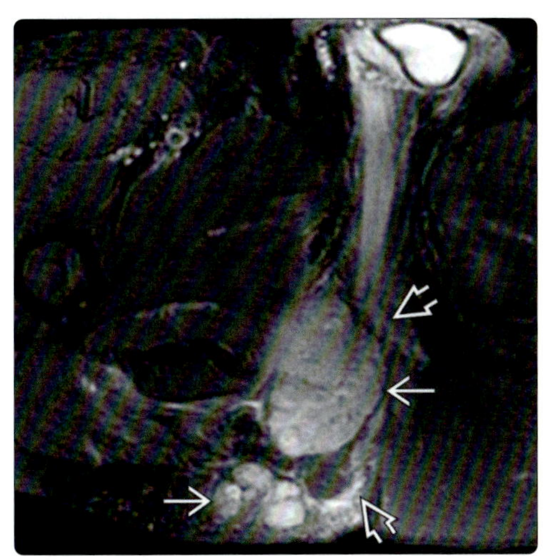

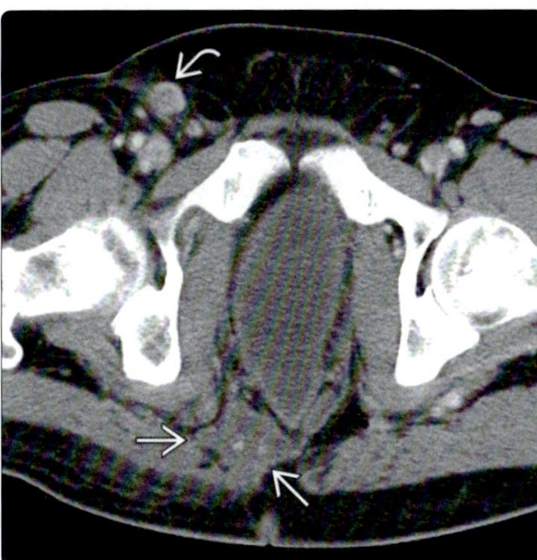

(Left) *Axial T2WI FS MR shows a heterogeneously hyperintense, multilobulated mass ➡ in the gluteal/perineal region of a 51-year-old man. Note the surrounding edema ➡. The patient had a painless mass excised from this region 8 years prior with unclear pathology.* **(Right)** *Axial CECT in the same patient shows the more proximal extent of the mass ➡ extending into the pelvis. An inguinal lymph node ➡ was positive for tumor. This was a high-grade, proximal-type epithelioid sarcoma.*

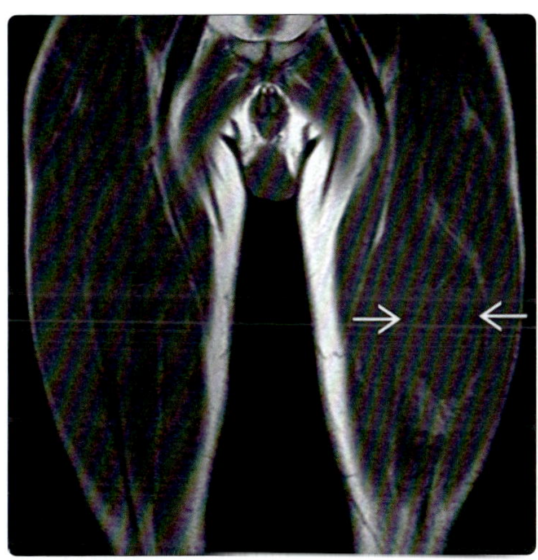

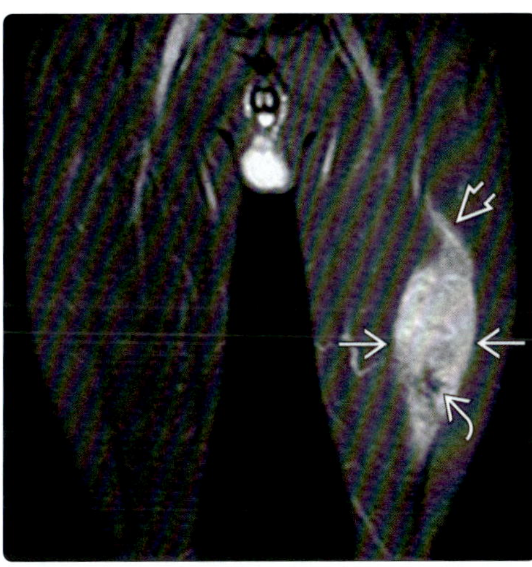

(Left) *Coronal T1WI MR shows an oval mass ➡ in the anterior left thigh that is homogeneously isointense to muscle. This 43-year-old man reported a slightly tender mass present for 4 months.* **(Right)** *Coronal STIR MR in the same patient shows the mass ➡ to be heterogeneously hyperintense with a small pathologically proven focus of fibrosis ➡. A mild amount of edema ➡ surrounds the lesion. A left inguinal lymph node was positive for tumor. This patient died within 3 years of diagnosis.*

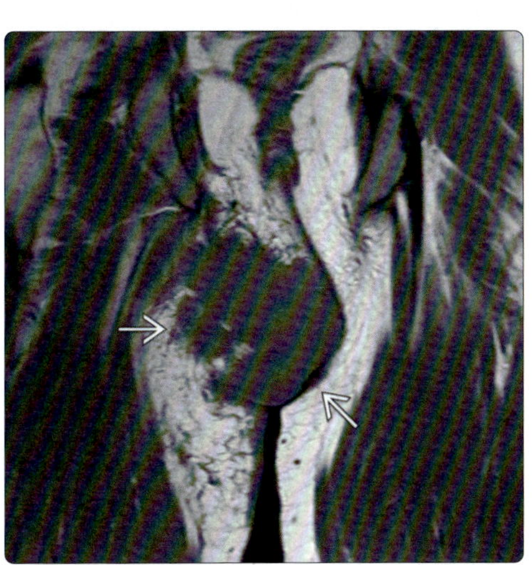

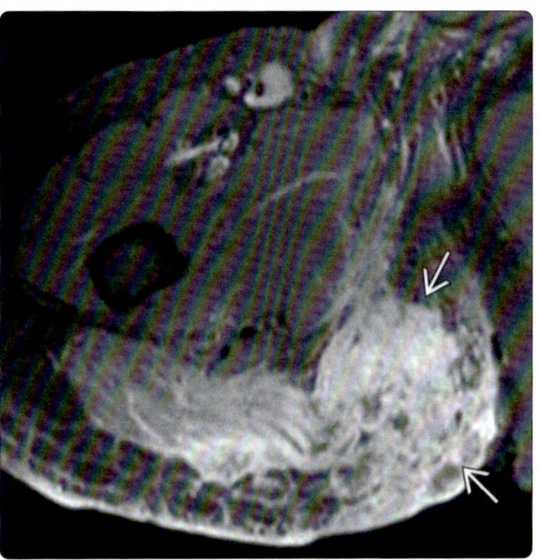

(Left) *Coronal T1WI MR shows a large, highly invasive mass ➡ within the buttock. The lesion is isointense to muscle.* **(Right)** *Axial T2WI FS MR in the same patient shows the mass ➡ to have heterogeneous high signal and extend to the skin. Despite the fact that the lesion arises in a subcutaneous position, it does not have other characteristics of the more circumscribed dermatofibrosarcoma protuberans. This lesion proved on biopsy to be epithelioid sarcoma.*

KEY FACTS

TERMINOLOGY

- Rare malignant soft tissue tumor of uncertain differentiation with hemorrhagic, multinodular appearance

IMAGING

- Proximal extremity/limb girdle (thigh most common) > trunk > paraspinal
- Well-circumscribed, multinodular mass with overall lower attenuation than muscle on CT
  - ± periosteal reaction, bone erosion or invasion
  - Calcification is uncommon
- MR appearance
  - Heterogeneously isointense to muscle on T1WI MR
    - Foci of high-signal hemorrhage common
  - Heterogeneously hyperintense on T2WI MR
    - Regions of homogeneous high-signal myxoid tissue or necrosis
    - Fluid-fluid levels reported
  - ± incomplete low-signal rim around nodules
  - Homogeneous or heterogeneous enhancement more intense at periphery, corresponding to ↑ cellularity

PATHOLOGY

- No convincing evidence for cartilaginous differentiation, despite name
- Pseudoencapsulated mass of gelatinous nodules separated by fibrous septa
- Hemorrhage, both recent and remote, is common and may be extensive

CLINICAL ISSUES

- Slowly enlarging soft tissue mass
- Peak age: 5th to 6th decade
- Male predominance (2:1)
- Natural history: High risk (≤ 50%) of local recurrence and metastases
  - May have prolonged survival with metastatic disease
- Treatment: Radical local excision ± adjuvant radiotherapy

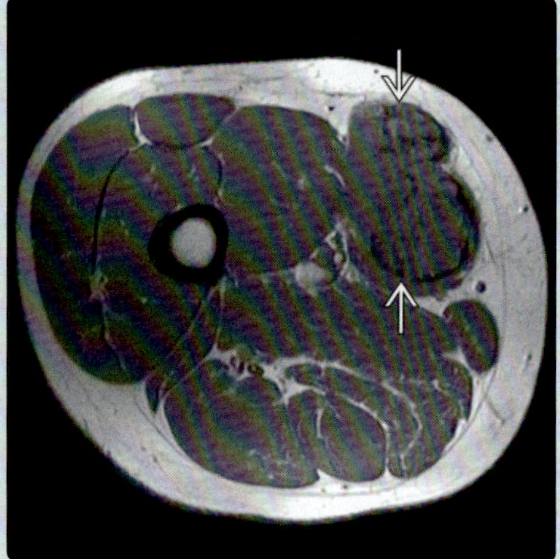

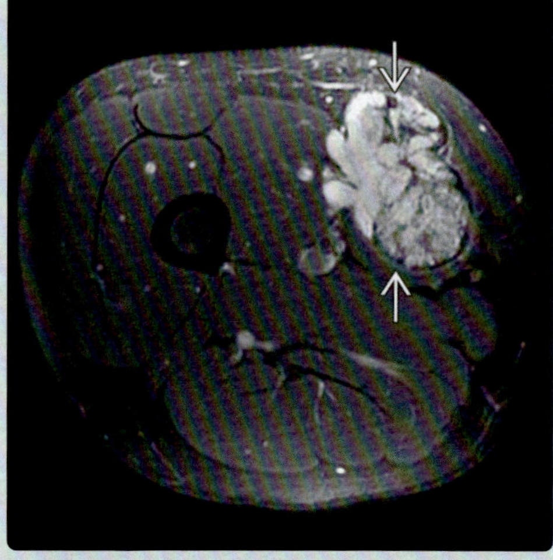

(Left) *Axial T1WI MR demonstrates a lobulated mass ➡ in the medial thigh of a 51-year-old man. This mass had been growing for approximately 7 years. He did not seek treatment because he was told it was clinically benign. This mass is predominantly isointense to muscle. It contains low-signal septa and an incomplete low-signal peripheral rim.* **(Right)** *Axial T2WI FS MR shows the mass to be heterogeneously hyperintense ➡. Again, the peripheral rim and multiple internal septa have low signal intensity.*

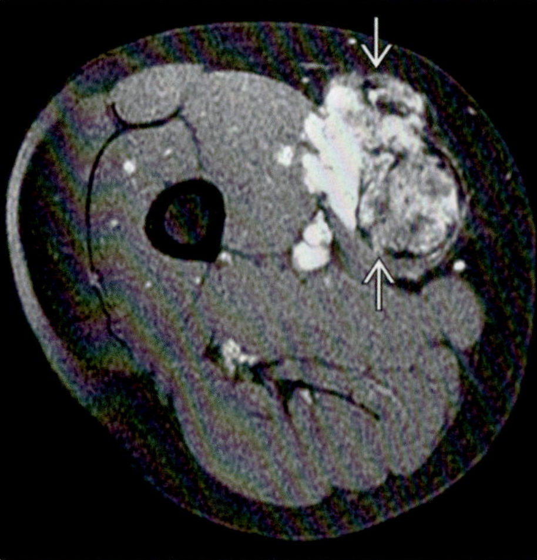

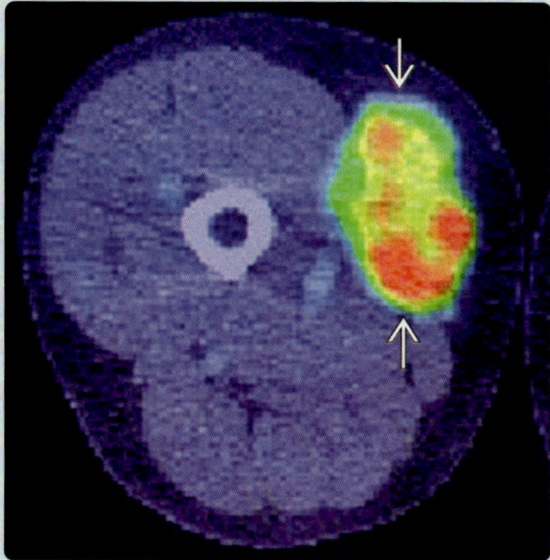

(Left) *Axial T1WI C+ FS MR shows moderate to intense, heterogeneous enhancement of the mass ➡. These lesions often contain hemorrhage of varying ages and necrosis, giving them a variable appearance on imaging. The adjacent neurovascular bundle was not involved by tumor.* **(Right)** *Axial fused PET/CT shows the thigh mass ➡ to be an F-18 FDG-avid tumor. This tumor had metastasized to the intraabdominal soft tissues and lymph nodes at the time of presentation. The metastases were also F-18 FDG avid.*

TERMINOLOGY

Synonyms

- Chordoid sarcoma, tendosynovial sarcoma

Definitions

- Rare malignant soft tissue tumor of uncertain differentiation with hemorrhagic, multinodular appearance

IMAGING

General Features

- Location
  - Proximal extremity/limb girdle (thigh most common) > trunk > paraspinal > foot > head and neck
    - Rare in finger, retroperitoneum, pleura, bone, central nervous system, vulva, intraarticular, vein
  - 75% in deep soft tissues
- Size
  - Median size: 7 cm (up to 25 cm)
- Morphology
  - Well-defined soft tissue mass composed of nodules of varying size

CT Findings

- Well-circumscribed, multinodular mass, with overall lower attenuation than muscle
- ± periosteal reaction, bone erosion or invasion
- Calcification is uncommon

MR Findings

- T1WI
  - Heterogeneously isointense to muscle
  - Foci of high-signal hemorrhage common
- T2WI FS
  - Heterogeneously hyperintense to muscle
  - Regions of homogeneous high-signal myxoid tissue or necrosis
  - Fluid-fluid levels reported
- T1WI C+ FS
  - Homogeneous or heterogeneous enhancement more intense at periphery, corresponding to ↑ cellularity
- ± incomplete low-signal rim around nodules

Nuclear Medicine Findings

- PET/CT
  - F-18 FDG-avid tumors

DIFFERENTIAL DIAGNOSIS

Pleomorphic Malignant Fibrous Histiocytoma/Undifferentiated Pleomorphic Sarcoma

- Heterogeneous appearance on imaging
- Hemorrhage and necrosis common

Liposarcoma, Soft Tissue

- Intratumoral fat may be misinterpreted as hemorrhage
- Confirm ↑ T1 signal fat has corresponding decrease in signal on fat-suppressed sequences

Hematoma

- Lacks solid regions of enhancement

PATHOLOGY

General Features

- Etiology
  - No convincing evidence for cartilaginous differentiation, despite name
- Genetics
  - Reciprocal translocation t(9;22)(q22;q12) in 50%
    - t(9;17)(q22;q11) less commonly identified

Gross Pathologic & Surgical Features

- Pseudoencapsulated mass of gelatinous nodules separated by fibrous septa
  - Hemorrhage, both recent and remote, is common and may be extensive
  - Necrosis or cystic change common

Microscopic Features

- Chondroblast-like cells in cords, clusters, or delicate network within abundant myxoid matrix
  - ± epithelioid cells or rhabdoid cells
  - Rare hyaline cartilage
- Fibrous septa divide nodules of myxoid or chondromyxoid stroma
  - ↑ cellularity at periphery of nodules
- < 2 mitotic figures per 10 HPF
- Vimentin is only consistently positive marker

CLINICAL ISSUES

Presentation

- Most common signs/symptoms
  - Slowly enlarging soft tissue mass
    - 1/3 with pain or tenderness
    - ↓ range of motion if near joint
  - Superficial tumors may ulcerate

Demographics

- Age
  - Peak: 5th-6th decade
    - Range: 4-92 years
    - Rare in childhood or adolescence
- Gender
  - Male predominance (2:1)
- Epidemiology
  - < 3% of soft tissue sarcomas

Natural History & Prognosis

- High risk (≤ 50%) of local recurrence and metastases
  - Metastases: Lung > soft tissue > lymph node
    - Reports of initial metastases to bone
- May have prolonged survival with metastatic disease
  - 10-year survival rate: 70-88%
- Poor prognostic factors are controversial

Treatment

- Radical local excision ± adjuvant radiotherapy

SELECTED REFERENCES

1. Oike N et al: Extraskeletal myxoid chondrosarcoma arising in the femoral vein: a case report. Skeletal Radiol. 43(10):1465-9, 2014
2. Bhamra JS et al: Intra-articular extraskeletal myxoid chondrosarcoma of the ankle. Skeletal Radiol. 41(8):1017-20, 2012

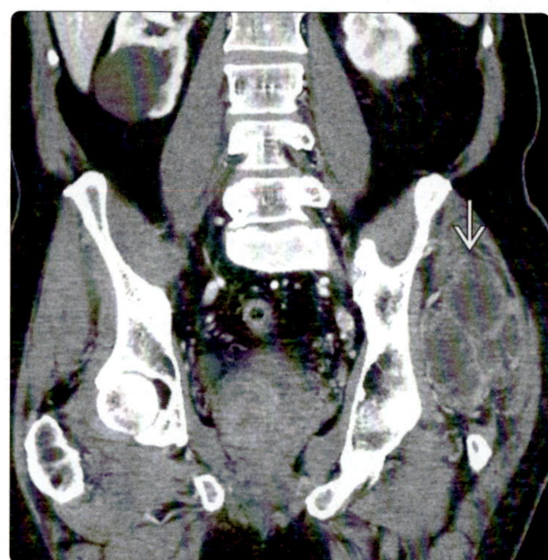

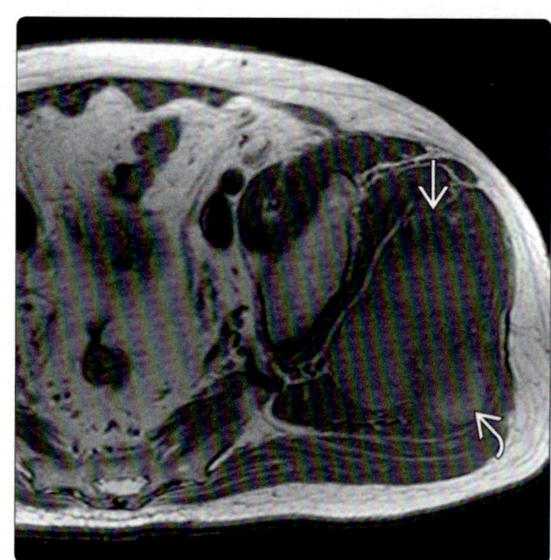

(Left) *Coronal reformatted CECT shows a lobulated mass ➡ in the left gluteal musculature. The mass has heterogeneous attenuation that is predominantly lower than skeletal muscle with peripheral enhancement of the lobulations. This was an incidental finding on a study performed for other reasons.* **(Right)** *Axial T1WI MR in the same patient shows the mass ➡ to have heterogeneous signal. Areas of high signal ➡ likely represent hemorrhage. The remainder of the mass is isointense to muscle.*

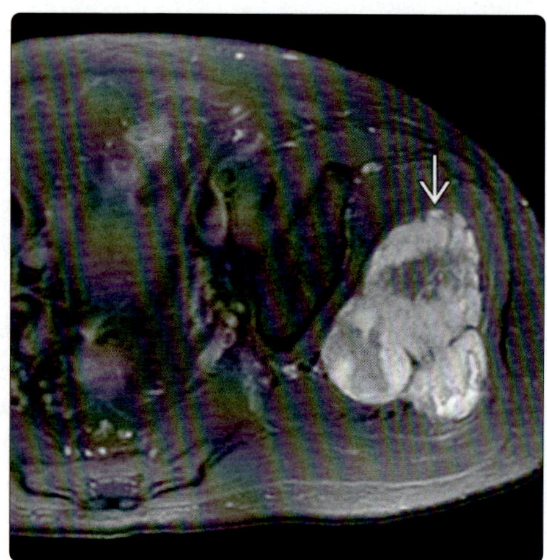

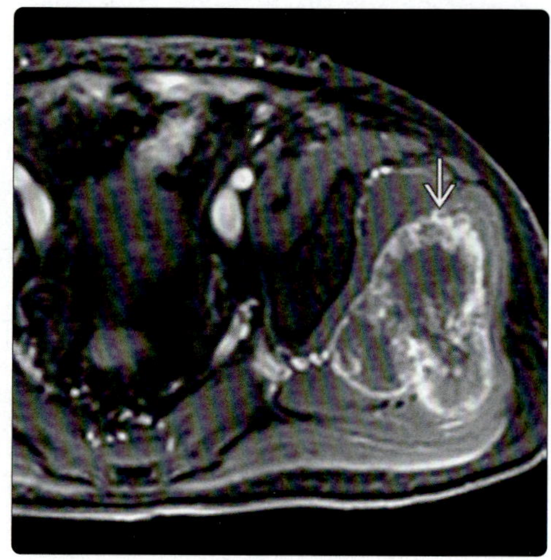

(Left) *Axial T2WI FS MR in the same patient shows the lobulated gluteal mass ➡ to have nonspecific, heterogeneous signal intensity, which ranges from low to high.* **(Right)** *Axial T1WI C+ FS MR in the same patient shows nodular intense enhancement involving the periphery of the mass ➡. The central regions lacking enhancement histologically corresponded to prominent areas of infarct-like necrosis. Despite the large size of this lesion, no metastases were evident at presentation.*

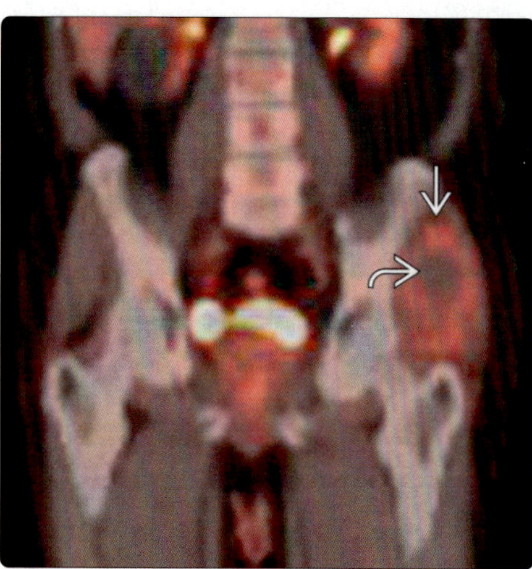

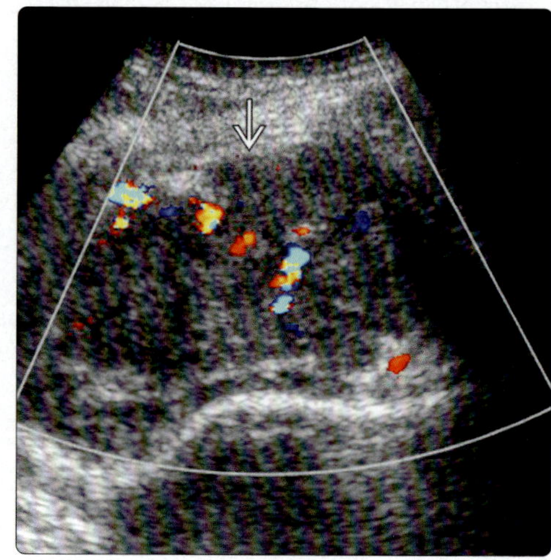

(Left) *Coronal fused PET/CT in the same patient shows the mass ➡ to be F-18 FDG avid with a maximum SUV of 3.8. The central portion of the mass that corresponded to necrosis ➡ is photopenic.* **(Right)** *Longitudinal color Doppler US in the same patient shows the mass ➡ to be heterogeneously hypoechoic with moderate vascularity. This 77-year-old man had been aware of a painless, slowly growing mass for many years, but did not seek medical attention.*

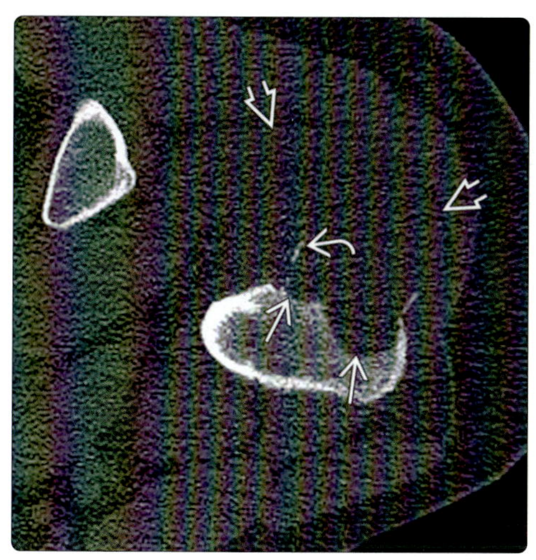

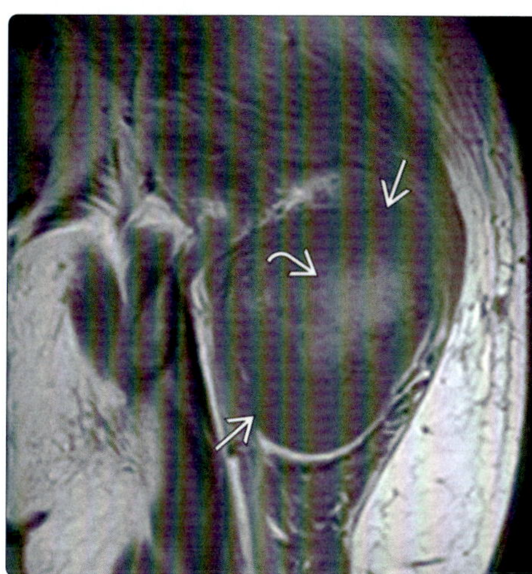

(Left) *Axial CT in a middle-aged man shows erosion of the femoral neck/trochanter ➡ by a large mass ➡ that has slightly lower attenuation than skeletal muscle. The mass contains matrix ➡, which is uncommon for extraskeletal myxoid chondrosarcoma.* **(Right)** *Coronal T1 MR shows the large mass ➡ to be isointense to skeletal muscle. It contains hyperintense material ➡ centrally, likely representing hemorrhage (frequently seen in this lesion).*

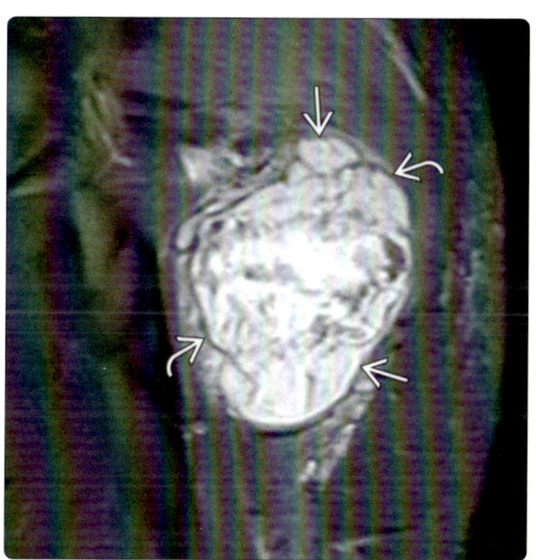

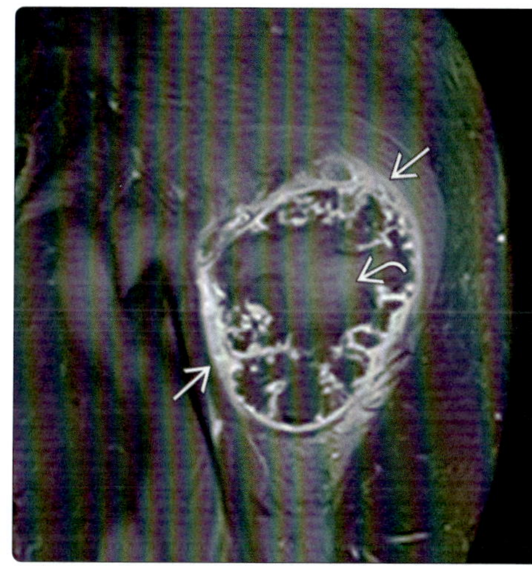

(Left) *Coronal STIR MR, same case, shows the lobulated nature of the lesion ➡ with inhomogeneous hyperintensity. Low-signal septa ➡ and rims are noted and are typical of this tumor.* **(Right)** *Coronal T1 C+ FS MR shows intense enhancement of the rim and peripheral portions of the lesion ➡, with central hypointensity ➡ representing a combination of hemorrhage and necrosis. All findings are typical of extraskeletal myxoid chondrosarcoma.*

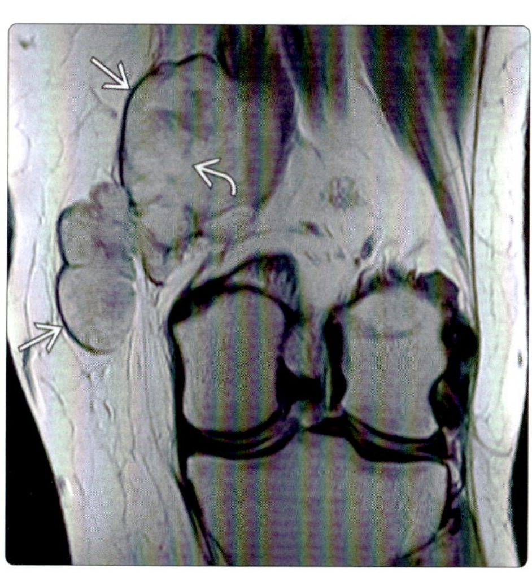

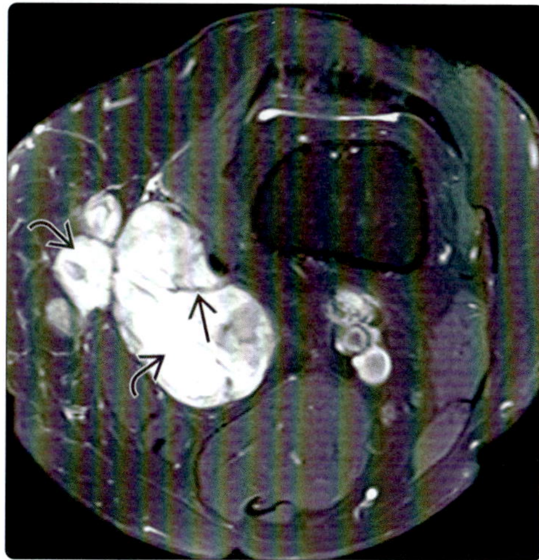

(Left) *Coronal T1 MR of extraskeletal myxoid chondrosarcoma shows low-signal rim ➡ around much of the periphery of the lobulated lesion. There is central high signal in a portion of the lesion ➡ that likely represents hemorrhage.* **(Right)** *Axial T2 FS MR, same case, shows heterogeneous hyperintensity with focally hyperintense areas ➡ that likely are myxoid in nature. Low-signal rim and septa ➡ are noted. The thigh is the most common location of this lesion, and the lobulated appearance is typical.*

KEY FACTS

IMAGING

- Well-circumscribed to infiltrative, multilobulated mass in deep soft tissue of extremity most common
  - Upper thigh, buttock > upper arm, shoulder
  - Less common in paravertebral soft tissues, chest wall (Askin tumor), and retroperitoneum
- Nonspecific soft tissue mass with similar to ↓ attenuation relative to skeletal muscle on CT
  - Adjacent bone involvement uncommon, except with chest wall lesions (50% show bone abnormalities)
  - Calcification uncommon
- Isointense to ↓ signal on T1WI MR ± hemorrhage
- Heterogeneous intermediate to ↑ signal on fluid-sensitive MR sequences
  - High-signal foci of fluid common
  - ± fluid-fluid levels
- ± high-flow vascular channels peripherally or centrally
- Prominent homogeneous to heterogeneous enhancement

PATHOLOGY

- Initially thought to represent different entities, but genetics suggests same family of tumor
- Monotonous proliferation of solidly packed small blue round cells
  - Necrosis, cystic change, and hemorrhage common
  - Chondroid or osseous differentiation rare
- Rich vascularity visible in cystic or necrotic regions, a.k.a. filigree pattern
- Hemorrhage may mimic vascular neoplasm

CLINICAL ISSUES

- Most common: 10-30 years of age
- Rapidly growing deep soft tissue mass usually present for < 1 year before diagnosis (1/3 painful)
- 25% with metastatic disease at presentation
  - Metastases to lung and bone
- Treatment: Preoperative chemotherapy and surgical resection ± stem cell reinfusion, radiotherapy

(Left) *Axial T1WI MR shows a soft tissue mass ➡ within the right iliopsoas muscle of a 9-year-old girl. The mass is heterogeneously isointense to hyperintense relative to skeletal muscle. There is no involvement of the adjacent bone.* **(Right)** *Axial STIR MR shows the mass ➡ to have heterogeneous signal intensity that is isointense to hyperintense relative to skeletal muscle. A fluid-fluid level is present ➡. Hemorrhage, necrosis, and cystic change are common in these tumors.*

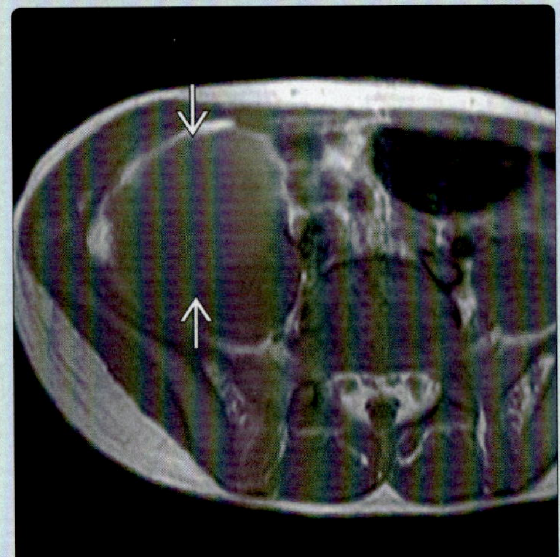

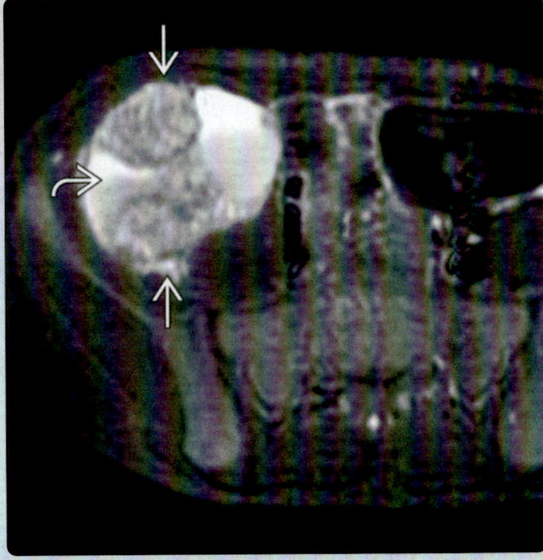

(Left) *Axial T1WI C+ FS MR in the same patient shows prominent, heterogeneous enhancement of the mass ➡. The cystic regions ➡ do not enhance.* **(Right)** *Axial T2WI MR of the mass ➡ obtained more distally shows an additional fluid-fluid level ➡. These imaging findings are relatively nonspecific. High vascularity of these tumors can produce intense enhancement, hemorrhage, and flow voids (not present in this case) on MR imaging.*

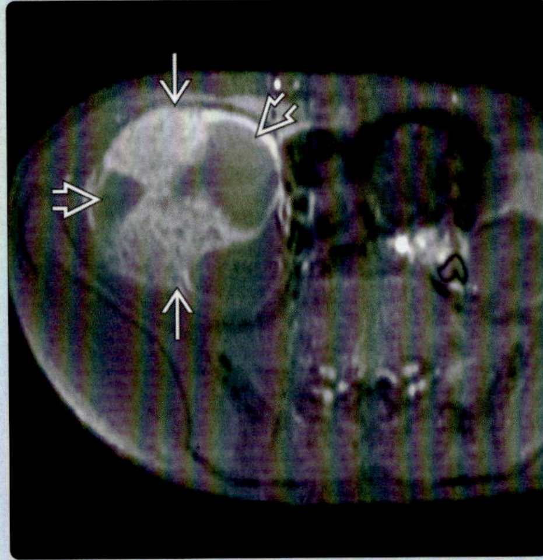

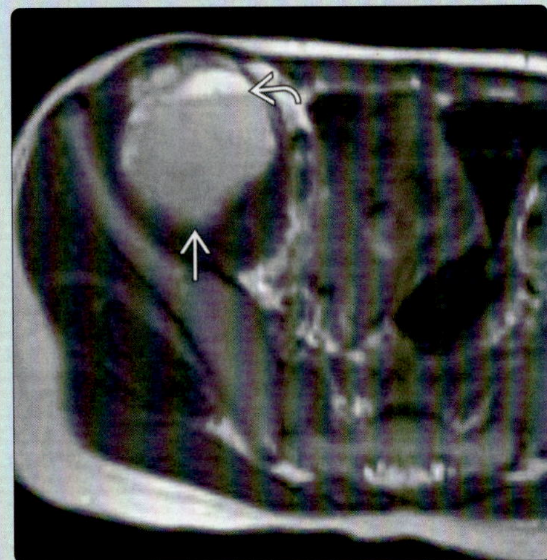

TERMINOLOGY

Abbreviations

- Primitive neuroectodermal tumor/extraskeletal Ewing sarcoma (PNET/EES)

Synonyms

- Peripheral neuroepithelioma, peripheral neuroblastoma, extraosseous Ewing sarcoma

IMAGING

General Features

- Location
  - Deep soft tissues of extremities most common
    - Upper thigh, buttock > upper arm, shoulder
      - Less common in paravertebral soft tissues, chest wall (Askin tumor), and retroperitoneum
      - Can be found throughout body
  - Superficially located lesions uncommon
- Morphology
  - Well circumscribed to infiltrative, multilobulated

CT Findings

- Nonspecific soft tissue mass with similar to ↓ attenuation relative to skeletal muscle
  - Adjacent bone involvement uncommon, except with chest wall lesions (50%)
  - Calcification uncommon

MR Findings

- T1WI
  - Isointense to ↓ signal relative to skeletal muscle
  - ± hyperintense hemorrhage
- T2WI FS
  - Heterogeneous intermediate to ↑ signal
  - High-signal foci of fluid common
  - ± fluid-fluid levels
- T1WI C+ FS
  - Prominent homogeneous to heterogeneous enhancement
- ± high-flow vascular channels peripherally or centrally

Ultrasonographic Findings

- Heterogeneous, hypoechoic mass

Angiographic Findings

- Hypervascular mass

DIFFERENTIAL DIAGNOSIS

Rhabdomyosarcoma

- Most common soft tissue malignancy in childhood
- Painless, rapidly growing mass
- Alveolar subtype has similar age distribution and can be histologically similar to PNET/EES

Synovial Sarcoma

- Most common lower extremity malignancy in patients 6-35 years old
- Slowly growing mass with predilection for juxtaarticular regions

PATHOLOGY

General Features

- Etiology
  - Family of tumors with neuroectodermal origin
- Genetics
  - Reciprocal translocation t(11;22)(q24;q12) in ≤ 95%

Gross Pathologic & Surgical Features

- Gray-yellow or gray-tan, soft multilobulated mass
  - Necrosis, cystic change, and hemorrhage common

Microscopic Features

- Monotonous proliferation of solidly packed small blue round cells
  - Intracellular glycogen vacuoles may indent nuclei
  - Rich vascularity visible in cystic or necrotic regions, a.k.a. filigree pattern
- Hemorrhage may mimic vascular neoplasm
- PNET pattern (15%): Small round cells in Homer Wright or Flexner-Wintersteiner rosettes
- CD99 positive in 95%

CLINICAL ISSUES

Presentation

- Most common signs/symptoms
  - Rapidly growing, deep soft tissue mass usually present for < 1 year before diagnosis
    - 1/3 painful
  - Sensory or motor abnormalities with nerve or spinal cord involvement
- Other signs/symptoms
  - Askin tumor: ± fever, weight loss

Demographics

- Age
  - PNET/EES most common: 10-30 years of age
    - PNET has wider range: Birth to 81 years of age
- Gender
  - Mild male predominance
- Epidemiology
  - Predilection for Caucasians

Natural History & Prognosis

- 75% have localized disease at presentation
  - 10-year survival rate: 90%
  - 75% long-term cure rate
- 25% with metastatic disease at presentation
  - Metastases to lung and bone
  - < 30% long-term cure rate

Treatment

- Preoperative chemotherapy and surgical resection ± stem cell reinfusion, radiotherapy

SELECTED REFERENCES

1. Murphey MD et al: From the radiologic pathology archives: ewing sarcoma family of tumors: radiologic-pathologic correlation. Radiographics. 33(3):803-31, 2013
2. Carvajal R et al: Ewing's sarcoma and primitive neuroectodermal family of tumors. Hematol Oncol Clin North Am. 19(3):501-25, vi-vii, 2005

KEY FACTS

TERMINOLOGY

- Nonneoplastic, painful, fibrosing process of plantar digital nerve

IMAGING

- Well-demarcated, fusiform soft tissue mass
  - Vast majority are unifocal and unilateral
  - > normal interdigital nerve diameter (2 mm)
- Plantar digital nerve
  - 3rd intermetatarsal space (between 3rd and 4th metatarsal heads) most common
  - 2nd intermetatarsal space 2nd most common
  - Plantar side of transverse metatarsal ligament
- MR: Hypointense to isointense to muscle on T1WI
- MR: Isointense to hyperintense to muscle on T2WI FS
  - Signal varies due to maturity of fibrosis
  - ± associated intermetatarsal fluid collection > 3 mm transverse diameter (bursitis)
- MR: Variable enhancement, absent to prominent
- Ultrasound: Ovoid mass with variable echogenicity ranging from homogeneously anechoic to heterogeneously hypoechoic
  - ± vascularity on power Doppler
  - ± sonographic Mulder sign

PATHOLOGY

- Ill-fitting shoes, hindfoot valgus, or intermetatarsal bursitis may cause nerve compression or traction
  - Ischemia also suggested as etiology

CLINICAL ISSUES

- Marked female predominance (18:1)
- Focal tenderness without palpable mass
  - Worse with exercise, improves with rest
- Positive Mulder sign
- Asymptomatic prevalence up to 33%
- Conservative treatment: Modify footwear
- Most successful treatment: Surgical resection

(Left) *Axial graphic through the forefoot shows a Morton neuroma ➡ with localized enlargement of the interdigital nerve branch between the 3rd and 4th metatarsal heads. This 3rd intermetatarsal space is the most common location for Morton neuromas.* **(Right)** *Coronal T1WI MR shows a large mass ➡ arising from the plantar aspect of the 3rd intermetatarsal space. This mass has a typical teardrop configuration. The signal intensity of the mass is homogeneously isointense to skeletal muscle.*

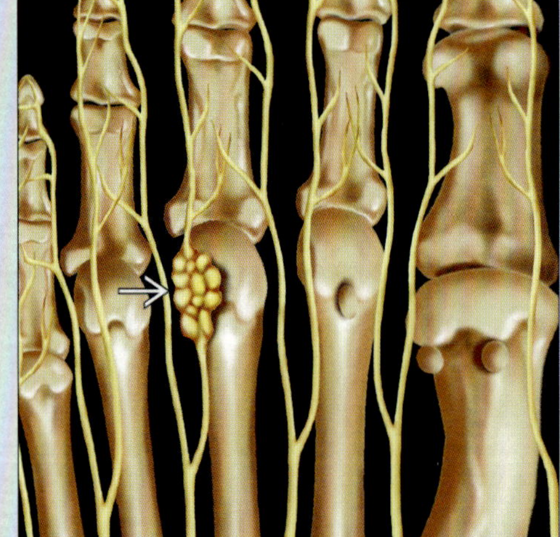

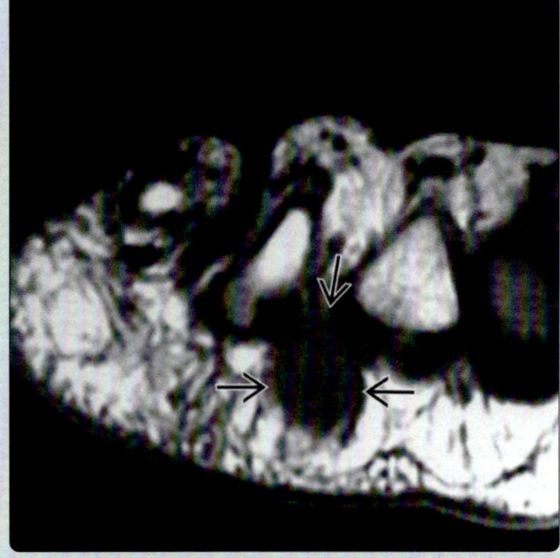

(Left) *Coronal T2WI FS MR in the same patient shows the mass ➡ to have heterogeneous signal that is difficult to differentiate from the adjacent suppressed fat signal.* **(Right)** *Coronal T1WI C+ FS MR shows heterogeneous enhancement of the intermetatarsal mass ➡ after the intravenous administration of gadolinium contrast. Note that the neuroma in this location is much more conspicuous on T1WI or post-contrast imaging than on T2WI FS MR sequences.*

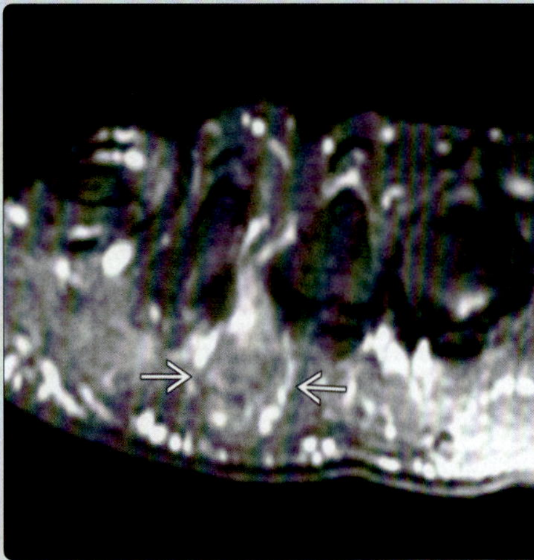

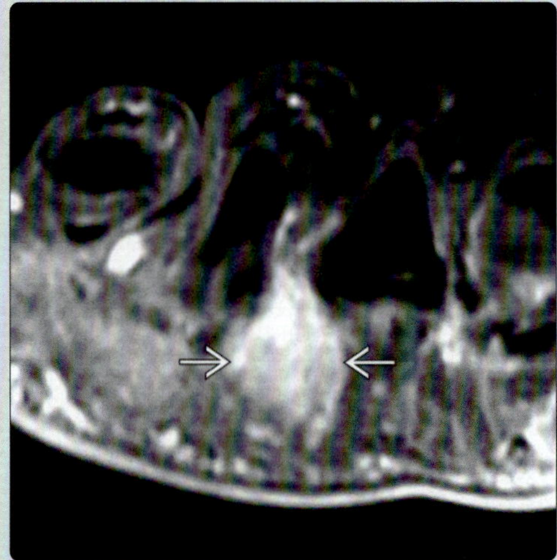

TERMINOLOGY

Synonyms

- Plantar neuroma, localized interdigital neuritis, Morton toe, Morton node, interdigital neuralgia, Morton metatarsalgia

Definitions

- Nonneoplastic, painful, fibrosing process of plantar digital nerve

IMAGING

General Features

- Location
  - Plantar digital nerve in 3rd intermetatarsal space (between 3rd and 4th metatarsal heads)
    - 2nd intermetatarsal space 2nd most common
    - 1st intermetatarsal space uncommon
    - 4th intermetatarsal space rare
  - Plantar side of transverse metatarsal ligament
  - Vast majority are unifocal and unilateral
    - 2 intermetatarsal spaces of 1 foot < 4%
    - Bilateral in 0-12%
- Size
  - > normal interdigital nerve diameter (2 mm)
- Morphology
  - Well-demarcated, fusiform soft tissue mass

Radiographic Findings

- ± increased intermetatarsal angle
- May identify other cause for forefoot pain

MR Findings

- Mass plantar to intermetatarsal space
- Hypointense to isointense to muscle on T1WI
- Isointense to hyperintense to muscle on T2WI FS
  - Signal varies due to maturity of fibrosis
- Variable enhancement, absent to prominent
- ± intermetatarsal fluid collection > 3 mm transverse diameter (bursitis)

Imaging Recommendations

- Best imaging tool
  - MR and ultrasound have high sensitivity and specificity
- Protocol advice
  - Coronal MR sequences most helpful
  - Consider MR imaging in prone position
  - Longitudinal ultrasound with and without manual interdigital compression

CT Findings

- Limited utility for Morton neuroma imaging

Ultrasonographic Findings

- Ovoid mass with variable echogenicity ranging from homogeneously anechoic to heterogeneously hypoechoic
- Continuity with interdigital nerve in up to 56%
- ± vascularity on power Doppler
- ± associated intermetatarsal bursal distension
- ± sonographic Mulder sign (palpable click from enlarged digital nerve moving beneath transverse intermetatarsal ligament with transverse compression of forefoot and vertical compression of symptomatic interspace)

DIFFERENTIAL DIAGNOSIS

Intermetatarsal Bursitis

- No soft tissue mass
- Focal fluid collection between metatarsal heads

Rheumatoid Arthritis of Ankle and Foot

- Soft tissue rheumatoid nodule
- Associated findings of erosions and synovitis

PATHOLOGY

General Features

- Etiology
  - Reactive, fibrosing process of plantar digital nerve
  - Ill-fitting shoes, hindfoot valgus, or intermetatarsal bursitis may cause nerve compression or traction
  - Ischemia also suggested as etiology

Microscopic Features

- Concentric fibrosis of epineurium and perineurium
- Fibrosis involves vessels ± surrounding soft tissue
- Edema of nerve fascicles

CLINICAL ISSUES

Presentation

- Most common signs/symptoms
  - Focal tenderness of plantar forefoot, no palpable mass
    - Worse with exercise
    - Improves with rest
  - Positive Mulder sign
  - Symptoms may be present years before diagnosis
  - Neurogenic pain may radiate proximally or distally
  - Asymptomatic prevalence up to 33%

Demographics

- Age
  - Teenagers to elderly adults
- Gender
  - Marked female predominance (18:1)

Treatment

- Conservative: Modify footwear
- Most successful: Surgical resection of interdigital nerve
  - Subsequent risk of developing traumatic neuroma
- Alternate: Transverse metatarsal ligament release, steroid injection, neurolysis, ultrasound therapy

SELECTED REFERENCES

1. Yablon CM: Ultrasound-guided interventions of the foot and ankle. Semin Musculoskelet Radiol. 17(1):60-8, 2013
2. Weiss SW et al: Benign tumors of peripheral nerves In Weiss SW et al: Enzinger and Weiss' Soft Tissue Tumors. 5th ed. Philadelphia: Elsevier. 832-3, 2008

(Left) *Coronal T1WI MR demonstrates a mass ➡ extending into the plantar subcutaneous fat from the level of the 2nd intermetatarsal space. This is the 2nd most common location for a Morton neuroma. The signal intensity is homogeneously isointense to muscle.* **(Right)** *Coronal T1WI C+ FS MR in the same patient shows heterogeneous enhancement of the 2nd intermetatarsal space mass ➡.*

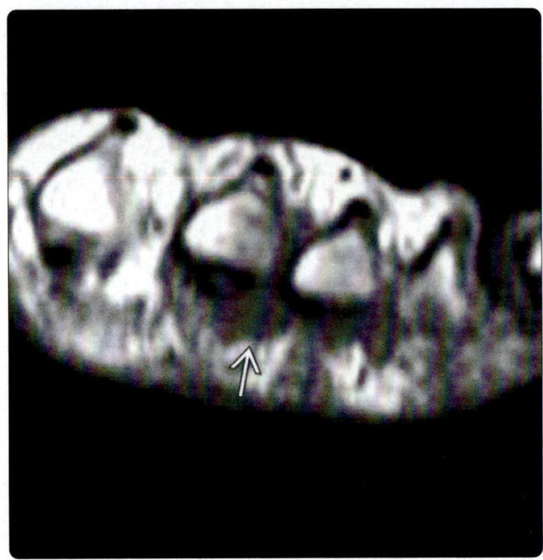

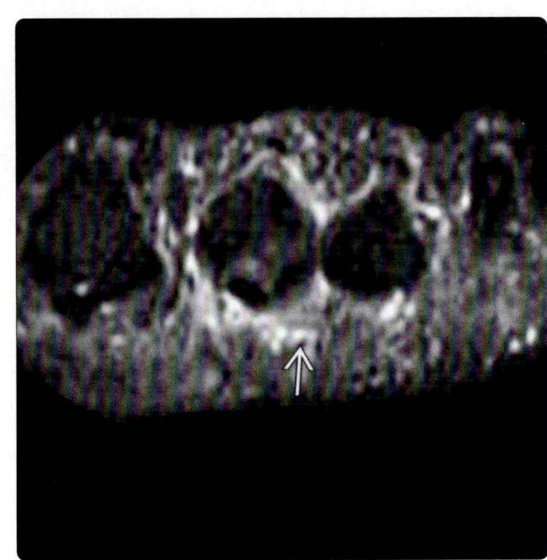

(Left) *Axial T1WI MR in the same patient shows the 2nd intermetatarsal mass ➡ that is partially outlined by subcutaneous fat along the plantar aspect of the foot. The degenerative, fibrosing changes that involve the plantar digital nerve can also involve the surrounding soft tissue, thus obscuring the borders of the mass.* **(Right)** *Axial T1WI C+ FS MR in the same patient best demonstrates the mildly heterogeneous, moderately intense gadolinium enhancement of the mass ➡.*

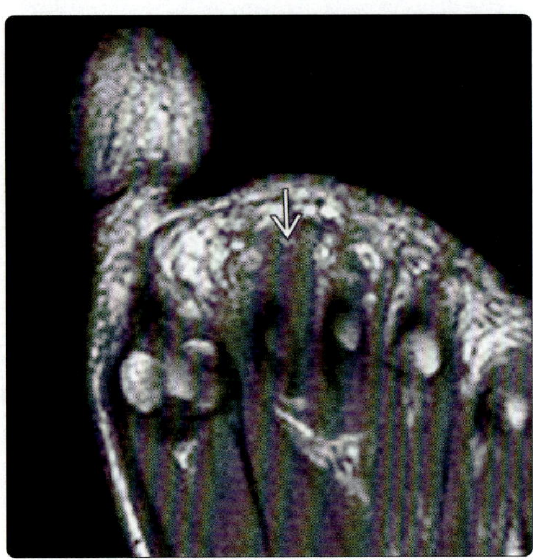

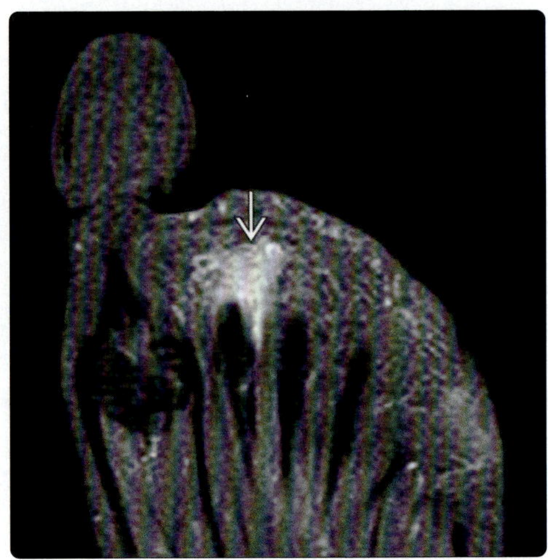

(Left) *Axial T1WI MR reveals a bulbous soft tissue mass ➡ between the 3rd and 4th metatarsal heads. This is centered in the location of the 3rd common digital branch of the medial plantar nerve. The mass is isointense to skeletal muscle. Note that the space between the metatarsal heads ➡ is slightly widened by the mass.* **(Right)** *Axial T1WI C+ FS MR in the same patient shows mild heterogeneous enhancement of the Morton neuroma ➡.*

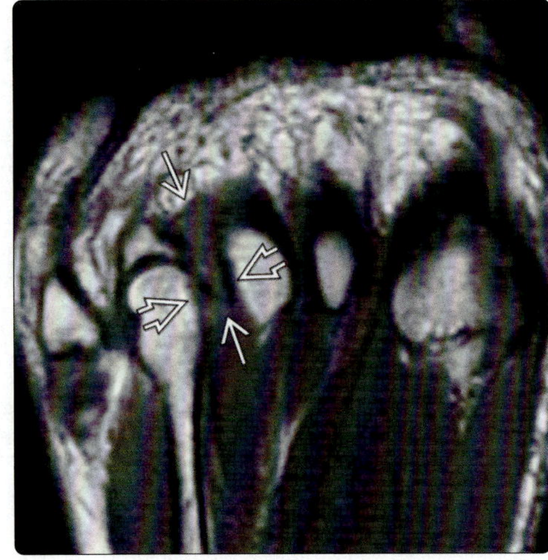

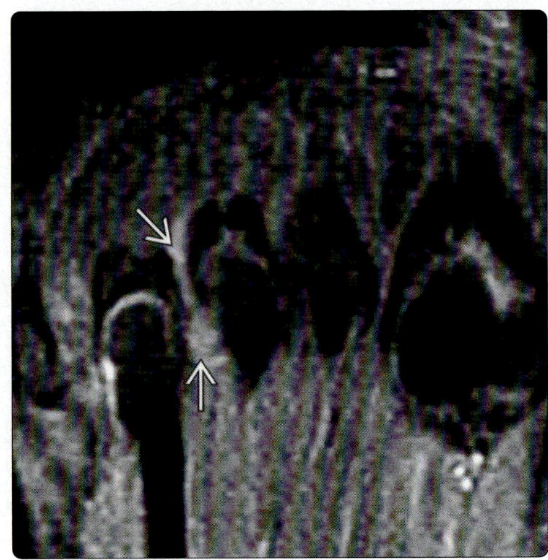

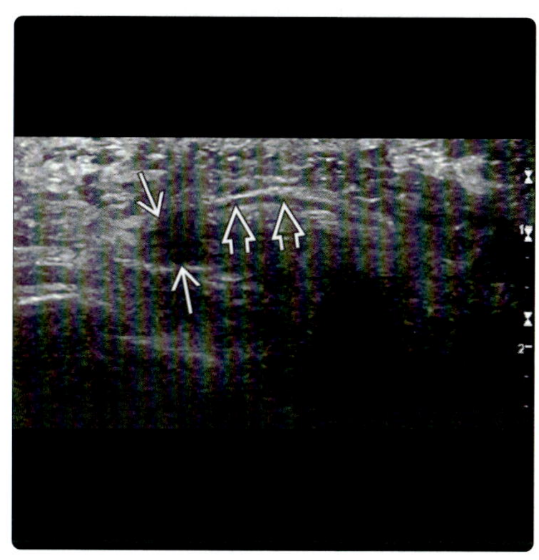

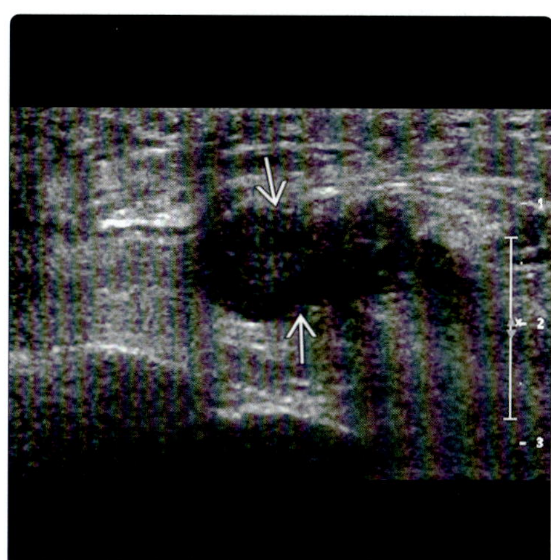

(Left) *Longitudinal ultrasound of the forefoot shows a hypoechoic mass ➡ between the 2nd and 3rd metatarsal heads representing a Morton neuroma. The plantar interdigital nerve ➡ can be seen in continuity with the neuroma.* **(Right)** *Longitudinal oblique ultrasound shows a hypoechoic, noncompressible mass ➡ within the 2nd interspace representing a Morton neuroma.*

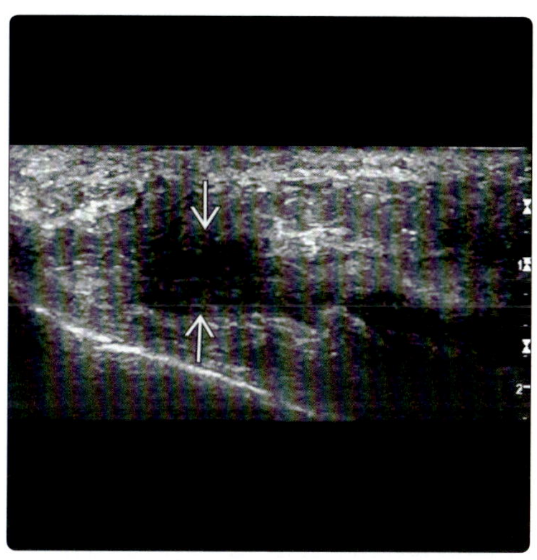

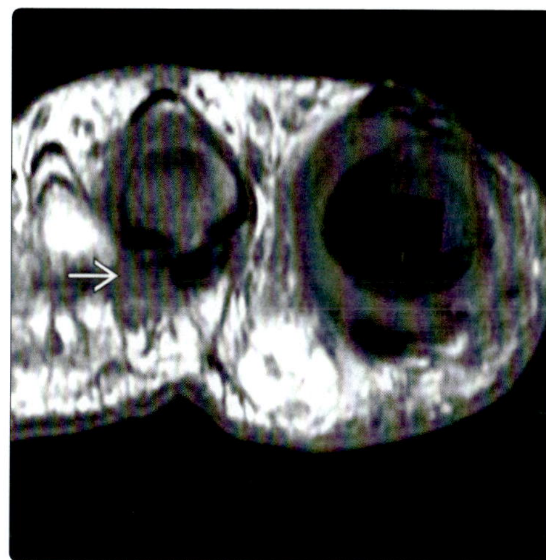

(Left) *Longitudinal ultrasound shows a hypoechoic, noncompressible mass ➡ within the 3rd interspace representing a Morton neuroma. Compression is useful for distinguishing between a neuroma and bursitis, as bursal fluid will dissipate with compression.* **(Right)** *Coronal T1WI MR reveals a teardrop-shaped plantar mass ➡ arising between the 2nd and 3rd metatarsal heads. This mass has mildly heterogeneous signal that is isointense to skeletal muscle.*

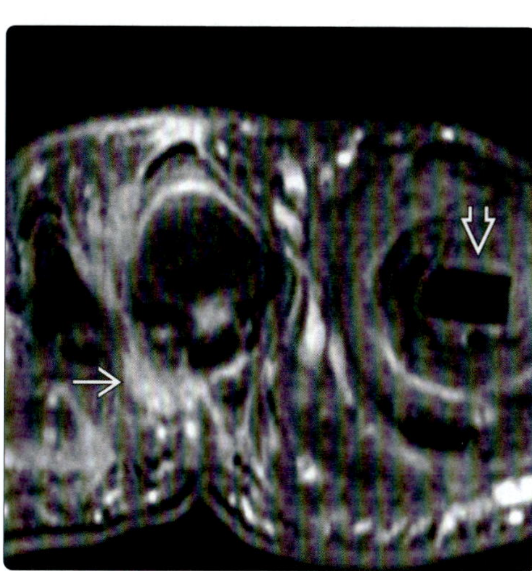

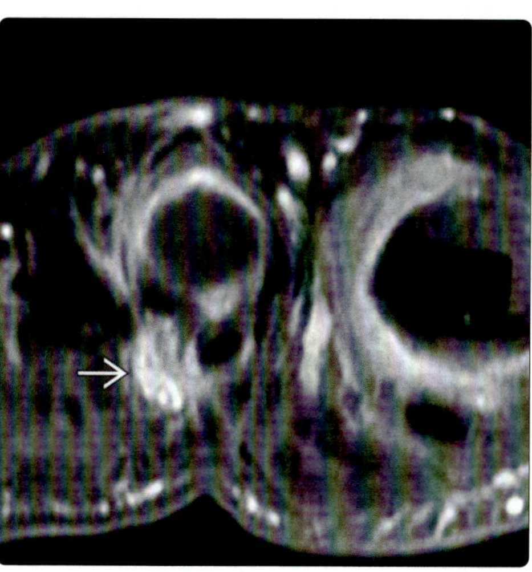

(Left) *Coronal T2WI FS MR in the same patient reveals mild hyperintense signal of the 2nd intermetatarsal mass ➡. Note the 1st metatarsophalangeal Silastic implant ➡. Altered weight-bearing, related to the implant placement, may have contributed to the development of the neuroma.* **(Right)** *Coronal T1WI C+ FS MR in the same patient reveals intense enhancement of the Morton neuroma between the 2nd and 3rd metatarsal heads ➡, markedly increasing the conspicuity of the lesion.*

Traumatic Neuroma

KEY FACTS

TERMINOLOGY

- Nonneoplastic proliferative nerve response to injury
  - Nerve transection, disruption, or avulsion → bulbous mass at nerve end (terminal/lateral type)
  - Chronic irritation, friction, or compression of intact nerve → fusiform enlargement away from nerve end (spindle type)

IMAGING

- Mass, may be visibly contiguous with normal nerve
- CT: Central low-density mass with hyperdense rim
- MR
  - Isointense to muscle on T1WI
  - Hyperintense to muscle on fluid-sensitive sequences
    - ± ring-like or telephone cable appearance from enlarged nerve fascicles (fascicular sign)
  - Hypointense peripheral rim reported on T1WI and T2WI
  - Variable enhancement, mild to marked
- US: Hypoechoic to isoechoic mass
  - Internal parallel heterogeneous hyperechogenicity
  - ± central hyperechoic focus
  - Mass borders may be irregular
- Lesions are exquisitely painful when biopsied

PATHOLOGY

- Disordered nerve fascicle proliferation in collagen
- May be adherent to skin, bone, or soft tissue

CLINICAL ISSUES

- Usually forms 1-12 months after injury
- Firm, palpable mass ± pain
  - Tinel sign = pain with percussion
- ↓ pain with local lidocaine injection
- No risk of malignant transformation
- Multiple treatment options
  - Surgical: Simple resection with translocation of proximal nerve stump away from scar

(Left) *Coronal oblique T1WI MR of the upper arm shows a bulbous soft tissue mass ➡ near the level of a mid humerus amputation site. The mass is homogeneously isointense to skeletal muscle. This mass is contiguous with a nerve ➡. It had mild enhancement.* **(Right)** *Coronal oblique STIR MR demonstrates the soft tissue mass ➡ to be heterogeneously hyperintense relative to skeletal muscle. The bulbous mass contour and location at the end of a transected nerve make this typical for a terminal type traumatic neuroma.*

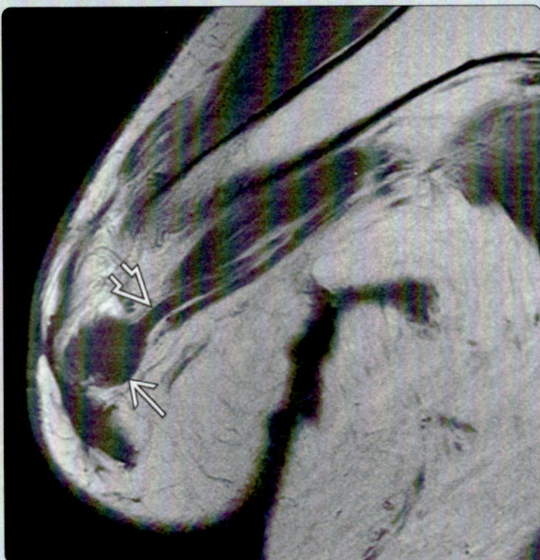

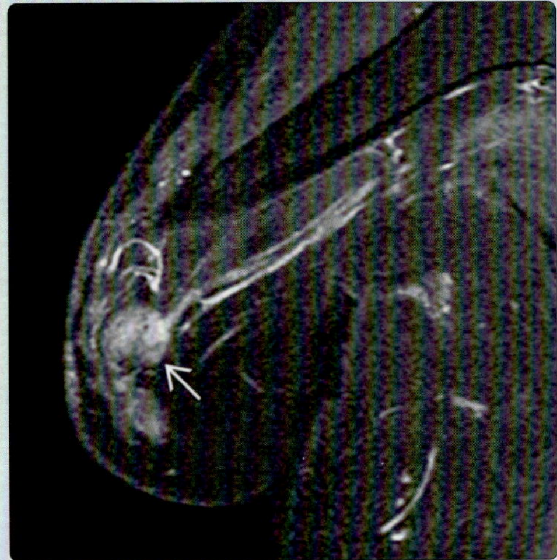

(Left) *Axial T1WI MR through the tibial plateau shows diffuse enlargement of the tibial nerve ➡ proximal to a below knee amputation. The enlarged nerve is isointense to skeletal muscle.* **(Right)** *Axial T2WI FS MR shows the enlarged nerve ➡ to have heterogeneous high signal intensity and a low-signal rim. The enlarged nerve fascicles are faintly visible, giving it a telephone cable or fascicular appearance. Fusiform nerve enlargement over a several centimeter segment of intact nerve is typical for a spindle type traumatic neuroma.*

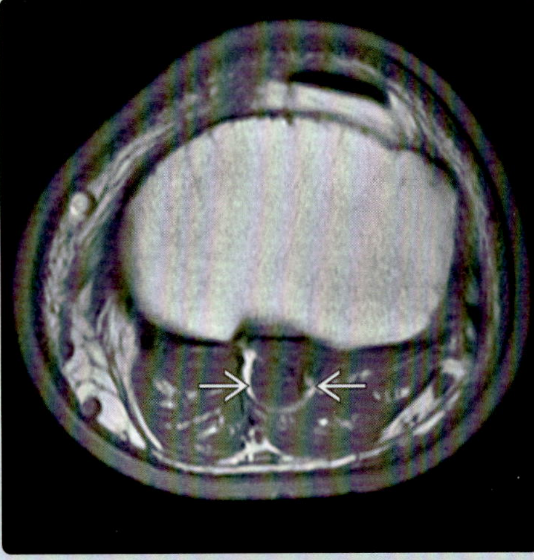

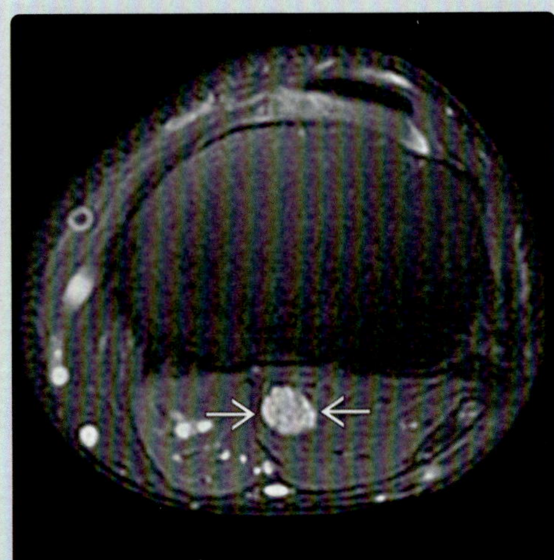

TERMINOLOGY

Synonyms

- Postamputation neuroma, stump neuroma

Definitions

- Nonneoplastic proliferative nerve response to injury

IMAGING

General Features

- Location
  - Contiguous with nerve
  - Lower extremity > head and neck > other
- Size
  - Usually < 5 cm
- Morphology
  - Fusiform nerve thickening = spindle type
  - Bulbous mass = terminal (or lateral) type

Radiographic Findings

- Soft tissue mass or normal

CT Findings

- Mass with central low density and hyperdense rim

MR Findings

- T1WI
  - Isointense to muscle
- T2WI FS
  - Hyperintense to muscle
  - ± ring-like or telephone cable appearance from enlarged nerve fascicles
    - a.k.a. fascicular sign
- Hypointense peripheral rim reported
- Mass may or may not be visibly contiguous with normal nerve
- Variable enhancement, mild to marked

Ultrasonographic Findings

- Hypoechoic to isoechoic mass with internal parallel heterogeneous hyperechogenicity
  - ± mass visibly contiguous with transected nerve
- ± central hyperechoic focus
- Mass borders may be irregular

Image-Guided Biopsy

- Lesions are exquisitely painful when biopsied

DIFFERENTIAL DIAGNOSIS

Benign Peripheral Nerve Sheath Tumor

- Nerve enters and exits mass
- Histologically ordered nerve fascicles

Metastases, Soft Tissue

- Recurrence or spread of original tumor
- Obliterates fatty hilum in lymph node
- Lacks continuity with nerve

Morton Neuroma

- Location between metatarsal heads
- Histologic degenerative change of nerve
  - Traumatic neuroma → proliferative change

PATHOLOGY

General Features

- Etiology
  - Reactive change secondary to nerve injury commonly associated with amputation or trauma
    - Nerve transection, disruption, or avulsion → bulbous mass at nerve end (terminal/lateral type)
    - Chronic irritation, friction, or compression of intact nerve → fusiform enlargement away from nerve end (spindle type)

Gross Pathologic & Surgical Features

- Well-defined, white-gray mass
- May be adherent to skin, bone, or soft tissue

Microscopic Features

- Disordered nerve fascicle proliferation in collagen
  - Myelinated axons, endoneurial cells, perineurial cells, and Schwann cells; peripheral fibroblasts
- Prominent myxoid areas may mimic neurofibroma

CLINICAL ISSUES

Presentation

- Most common signs/symptoms
  - Firm, palpable mass ± pain
    - Tinel sign = pain with percussion
- Other signs/symptoms
  - ↓ pain with local lidocaine injection
- Clinical profile
  - Clinical differential diagnosis for stump pain: Improper alignment or fit of prosthesis, traumatic neuroma, abscess, bursitis, hematoma, adenopathy, fat necrosis, scar formation, osteomyelitis, aneurysm, heterotopic ossification, protruding bone edge, tumor recurrence, soft tissue inflammation, muscle atrophy, stress or insufficiency fracture, sinus tract squamous cell carcinoma, chronic lymphedema-associated angiosarcoma

Demographics

- Epidemiology
  - Usually forms 1-12 months after injury

Natural History & Prognosis

- No risk of malignant transformation

Treatment

- Surgical: Simple resection with translocation of proximal nerve stump away from scar
- Conservative: Physical therapy, steroid injection, nerve stimulation, acupuncture, prosthesis reshaping
- Avoidance: Approximation of severed nerve ends to promote healing or nerve graft placement

SELECTED REFERENCES

1. Ahlawat S et al: MRI features of peripheral traumatic neuromas. Eur Radiol. ePub, 2015
2. Zeidenberg J et al: The utility of ultrasound in the assessment of traumatic peripheral nerve lesions: report of 4 cases. Neurosurg Focus. 39(3):E3, 2015
3. Kransdorf MJ et al: Neurogenic tumors. In Kransdorf MJ et al: Imaging of Soft Tissue Tumors. 2nd ed. Philadelphia: Lippincott Williams & Wilkins. 328-3, 2006

Neurofibroma

KEY FACTS

TERMINOLOGY

- Benign peripheral nerve sheath tumor with neoplastic tissue inseparable from normal nerve

IMAGING

- Localized neurofibroma (NF): Well-defined, fusiform mass
  - Hypodense relative to muscle on CT
  - Isointense to mildly hyperintense relative to muscle on T1WI MR
  - Hyperintense to muscle on fluid-sensitive MR
  - Target sign = central low signal focus
  - Fascicular sign = multiple, small ring-like structures
  - Split-fat sign = thin peripheral rim of fat
  - Homogeneous hypoechoic mass with mild posterior acoustic enhancement on ultrasound
- Diffuse NF: Ill-defined plaque-like or infiltrative expansion of subcutaneous tissue
  - Nonspecific MR signal characteristics
- Plexiform NF: Long segments of diffusely and irregularly enlarged nerves and nerve branches
  - Multilobulated masses with low attenuation on CT
  - Bag of worms appearance on MR

PATHOLOGY

- Localized & diffuse NF arise sporadically (90%) much more commonly than in association with NF1
- Plexiform NF highly associated with NF1

CLINICAL ISSUES

- ~ 5% of benign soft tissue neoplasms
- Localized NF: Painless, slowly growing nodule
- Diffuse NF: Plaque-like skin elevation
- Plexiform NF: Limb disfigurement, enlarging mass, weakness, dysesthesia, pain
  - High risk of malignant transformation of plexiform NF (8-12%)

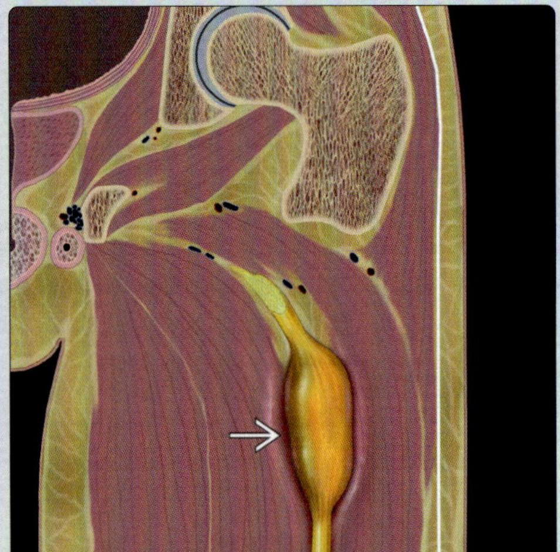

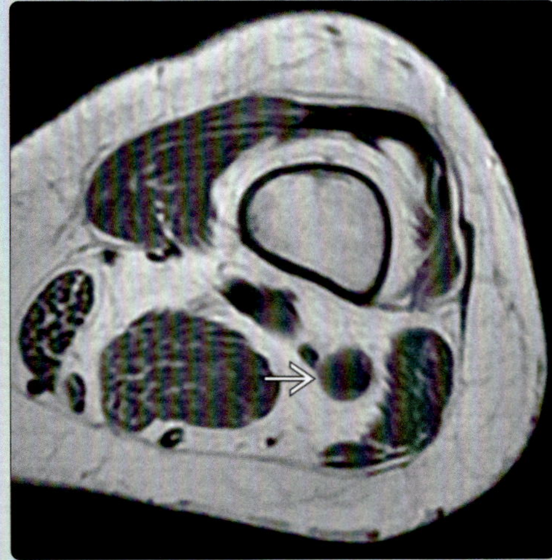

(Left) *Coronal graphic shows a well-defined, fusiform mass ➡ involving the sciatic nerve, typical of neurofibroma. The mass is in an intermuscular location, without invasion of the surrounding structures. The mass is inseparable from intermixed nerve fibers.* **(Right)** *Axial T1WI MR shows a well-defined, round mass ➡ in the distal thigh. The mass has mixed signal intensity, being isointense to muscle centrally with a peripheral rim that is faintly hyperintense to muscle. This asymptomatic lesion was incidentally found during staging for lymphoma.*

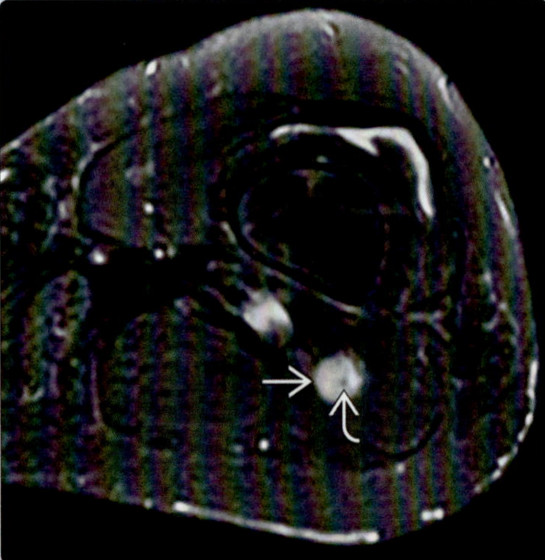

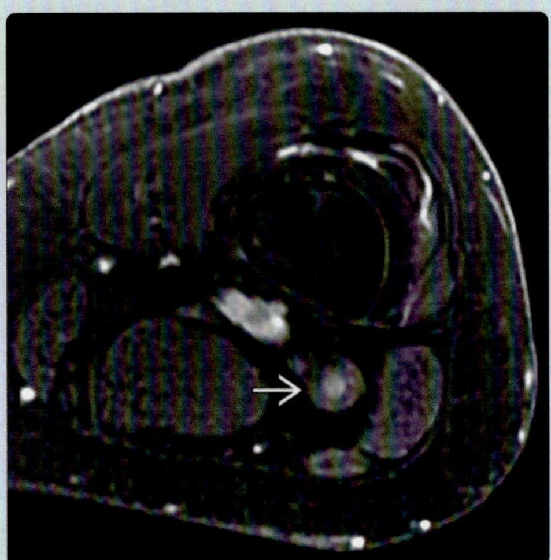

(Left) *Axial T2WI FS MR in the same patient shows the distal thigh mass ➡ to be heterogeneously hyperintense. There is a small focus of decreased signal intensity ➡ located eccentrically, but this is not large enough to reflect the target sign that can be seen with these lesions.* **(Right)** *Axial T1WI C+ FS MR in the same patient demonstrates heterogeneous enhancement of the mass ➡. The central portion of the mass more intensely enhances compared with the peripheral portion of the mass. Biopsy showed neurofibroma.*

TERMINOLOGY

Abbreviations

- Neurofibroma (NF)
- Neurofibromatosis type 1 (NF1)

Definitions

- Benign peripheral nerve sheath tumor with neoplastic tissue interspersed with normal nerve bundles

IMAGING

General Features

- Location
  - Localized NF: Dermis or subcutis anywhere in body, 90% of cases
    - Deep location uncommon
    - Intraosseous location rare
  - Diffuse NF: Trunk > limbs > head and neck
  - Plexiform NF: Trunk > limbs > head and neck
    - Organ involvement includes colon and bladder
- Size
  - Localized NF: < 5 cm
- Morphology
  - Localized NF: Solitary, well-defined nodule
  - Diffuse NF: Ill-defined plaque-like or infiltrative expansion of subcutaneous tissue
  - Plexiform NF: Bag of worms enlargement of multiple nerve branches

Radiographic Findings

- Mineralization uncommon
- Bone erosion or invasion rare

CT Findings

- Localized NF: Well-defined mass hypodense to muscle
  - Central focus of ↑ attenuation produces target sign
  - + enhancement
- Diffuse NF: Nonspecific infiltration of subcutis
- Plexiform NF: Multilobulated masses having low attenuation

MR Findings

- Localized NF: Well-defined, fusiform mass
  - Isointense to mildly hyperintense relative to muscle on T1WI MR
    - Hypointensity relative to muscle also possible
    - Split-fat sign = peripheral rim of fat
  - Hyperintense to muscle on fluid-sensitive MR
    - Variable heterogeneity
    - Target sign = central low signal focus
    - Fascicular sign = multiple, small ring-like structures
  - + enhancement, most prominent centrally
  - ± subtle surrounding or distal muscle atrophy
  - Characteristic dumbbell shape with spinal nerve involvement in foramina
- Diffuse NF: Nonspecific MR signal characteristics of plaque-like or infiltrative neoplasm involving subcutis
  - Areas of low signal on fluid-sensitive MR sequences likely related to collagen content
  - Prominent internal vascularity corresponds to prominent enhancement
- Plexiform NF: Long segments of diffusely and irregularly enlarged nerves and nerve branches
  - Similar MR signal characteristics as localized NF
  - Superficial lesions more likely to involve skin, lack nodular morphology, and lack target-like signal intensity

Ultrasonographic Findings

- Localized NF: Well-defined, homogeneous hypoechoic mass with mild posterior acoustic enhancement
  - ± hyperechoic center with hypoechoic periphery (target appearance), coarse echotexture, pseudocystic appearance, or foci of increased echogenicity
  - Complete or incomplete internal echogenic ring is highly suggestive but rare
  - Normal nerve entering and exiting center of mass may be visible
- Diffuse NF: Hyperechoic masses with multiple hypoechoic nodular or tubular structures
  - Hypoechogenicity reported in deep masses
  - Increased blood flow
- Plexiform NF: Multinodular mass

Nuclear Medicine Findings

- F-18 FDG PET suggested to be helpful for differentiating from malignant peripheral nerve sheath tumor (MPNST) using cut-off point of ≤ 6.1 standard uptake valve (max)

DIFFERENTIAL DIAGNOSIS

Schwannoma

- a.k.a. neurilemoma
- May be impossible to differentiate from NF on imaging
- More likely than NF to contain cysts, hemorrhage, fibrosis, or calcification
- Eccentrically located tumor can be separated from nerve
- Contains histologic Antoni A and B areas

Lymph Node

- Contains fatty hilum when not involved with tumor

Nerve Sheath Myxoma

- a.k.a. neurothekeoma
- Dermal or subcutaneous mass in head > face > neck > shoulders
  - Deep lesions are rare
- Childhood to early adult age with female predominance
- Isointense on T1WI MR, hyperintense on T2WI FS MR
- Benign lesion treated with excision

Perineurioma

- Subcutaneous mass most commonly involving upper extremity
- Intraneural
  - Bundles of perineural cells surrounding fibers of single nerve
    - 2-10 cm in length
  - Adolescents to young adults, no sex predilection
  - Will lose nerve function if resected
- Extraneural
  - Well-circumscribed mass of perineural cells
    - 30% are deep or visceral
  - Does not involve a nerve
  - Treatment with surgical excision

- Sclerosing subtype → hands of young men
- Usually benign, but there is malignant form

Malignant Peripheral Nerve Sheath Tumor

- Enlarging mass involving major nerve trunk
- More likely to contain hemorrhage and necrosis than NF or schwannoma
- ± invasion of surrounding soft tissues
- May not be able to differentiate from NF; however, more likely MPNST if 2 of following features are present
  - Large size of mass
  - Peripheral enhancement of mass
  - Perilesional edema zone
  - Intratumoral cysts

PATHOLOGY

General Features

- Etiology
  - Localized & diffuse NF arise sporadically (90%) much more frequently than in association with NF1
  - Plexiform NF highly associated with NF1
- Genetics
  - NF1 from mutation on chromosome 17 long arm

Gross Pathologic & Surgical Features

- Localized NF: Fusiform enlargement of nerve with glistening tan-white cut surface
  - Normal nerve at each end of mass
  - ± capsule
- Diffuse NF: Firm, grayish tissue expanding subcutaneous space
  - Extends along connective tissue septa, envelops fat
- Plexiform NF: Convoluted mass of irregularly enlarged nerve branches

Microscopic Features

- Localized NF: Bundles of wavy, elongated cells in fascicles, whorls or cartwheel patterns interspersed with normal nerve tissue
  - Collagen strands appearing like "shredded carrots"
  - Variable amount of mucoid material
    - Highly myxoid lesions mimic myxomas
    - Absent myxoid tissue in cellular variant containing Schwann cells in dense collagen background
- Diffuse NF: Schwann cells suspended in uniform fine collagen matrix
  - Meissner body-like structures helps differentiate from dermatofibrosarcoma protuberans
- Plexiform NF: Increased endoneurial matrix separating normal nerve fascicles
  - Propensity to extend into surrounding soft tissues
  - ± nuclear atypia
- Pigmented NF: Melanin-bearing dendritic or epithelioid-shaped cells in superficial regions
  - < 1% of NF, usually diffuse type
  - Positive S100 protein and melanin markers
  - Dispersed throughout tumors but have tendency to cluster & localize toward superficial portions of lesion

CLINICAL ISSUES

Presentation

- Most common signs/symptoms
  - Localized NF: Painless, slowly growing nodule
  - Diffuse NF: Plaque-like skin elevation
  - Plexiform NF: Limb disfigurement, enlarging mass, weakness, dysesthesia, pain
  - Symptoms vary based on compression of other structures
- Other signs/symptoms
  - Other manifestations of NF1 involving central nervous system, skin, and bones
  - Elephantiasis neuromatosa
    - Plexiform NF enlarging entire extremity
    - Loose, hyperpigmented skin ± bone hypertrophy

Demographics

- Age
  - Localized NF: Arises in 2nd to 3rd decades of life
  - Diffuse NF: Arises in children to adults
  - Plexiform NF: Arises in early childhood
- Gender
  - Equal gender distribution
- Epidemiology
  - Slightly > 5% of benign soft tissue neoplasms

Natural History & Prognosis

- High risk of malignant transformation of plexiform NF (8-12%)
- Low risk of malignant transformation of localized NF (though more common with deep lesions)

Treatment

- Simple excision but may sacrifice function of nerve
- Routine surveillance for malignant transformation of plexiform NF

DIAGNOSTIC CHECKLIST

Image Interpretation Pearls

- Significant overlap in appearance between localized NF and schwannoma precludes definitive diagnosis with imaging alone

SELECTED REFERENCES

1. Schaefer IM et al: Malignant peripheral nerve sheath tumor (MPNST) arising in diffuse-type neurofibroma: clinicopathologic characterization in a series of 9 cases. Am J Surg Pathol. ePub, 2015
2. Ravi AK et al: Diffuse infiltrative neurofibroma: a clinical, radiological, and histological conundrum. Skeletal Radiol. 43(12):1773-8, 2014
3. Patel NB et al: Musculoskeletal manifestations of neurofibromatosis type 1. AJR Am J Roentgenol. 199(1):W99-106, 2012
4. Wasa J, Nishida Y, Tsukushi S, et al. MRI features in the differentiation of malignant peripheral nerve sheath tumors and neurofibromas. AJR Am J Roentgenol. 194(6):1568-74., 2010
5. Hassell DS et al: Imaging appearance of diffuse neurofibroma. AJR Am J Roentgenol. 190(3):582-8, 2008
6. Bredella MA et al: Value of PET in the assessment of patients with neurofibromatosis type 1. AJR Am J Roentgenol. 189(4):928-35, 2007
7. Kransdorf MJ et al: Neurogenic tumors. In Kransdorf MJ et al: Imaging of Soft Tissue Tumors. 2nd ed. Philadelphia: Lippincott Williams & Wilkins. 335, 349-51, 2006
8. Reynolds DL Jr et al: Sonographic characteristics of peripheral nerve sheath tumors. AJR Am J Roentgenol. 182(3):741-4, 2004

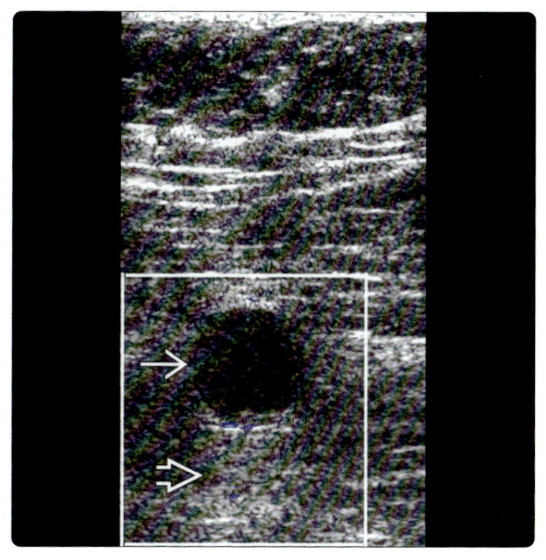

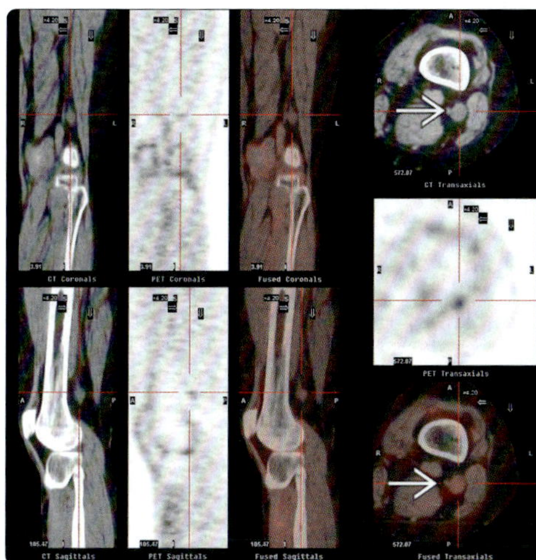

(Left) *Transverse color Doppler ultrasound shows a homogeneously hypoechoic mass ➡ that is well defined. Note the posterior acoustic enhancement ⇨. No internal blood flow was visible, nor was the mass clearly contiguous with a nerve.* **(Right)** *Composite PET/CT in the same patient shows the soft tissue mass ➡ to have F-18 FDG uptake with a maximum SUV of 2.2. It has been suggested that an SUV (max) of ≤ 6.1 can help differentiate neurofibroma from malignant peripheral nerve sheath tumors.*

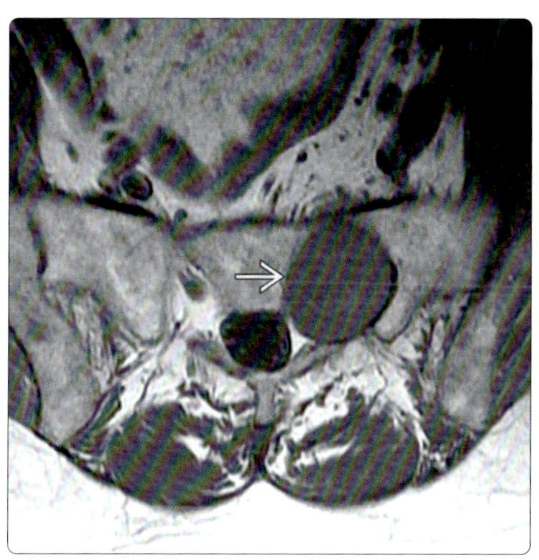

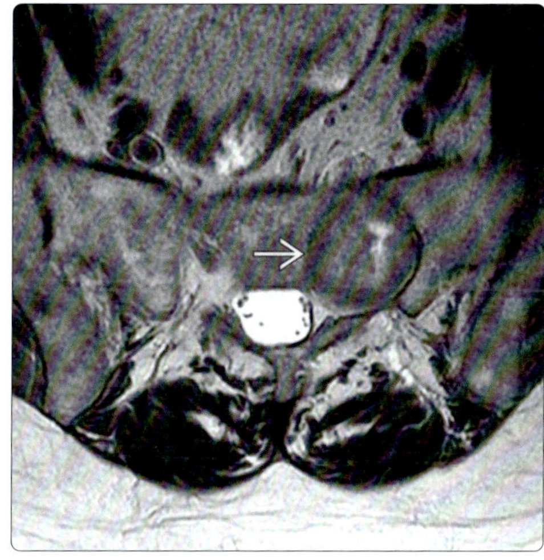

(Left) *Axial T1WI MR through the sacrum demonstrates a round, homogeneous mass ➡. The signal intensity of this mass is similar to skeletal muscle. This mass is smoothly expanding the left S1 neural foramen. The sclerotic border of the expansion suggests a longstanding process.* **(Right)** *Axial T2WI MR in the same patient demonstrates heterogeneous hyperintense signal of the mass ➡. The mass was contiguous with the exiting S1 nerve root. This lesion was found during work-up for anterior pelvis pain.*

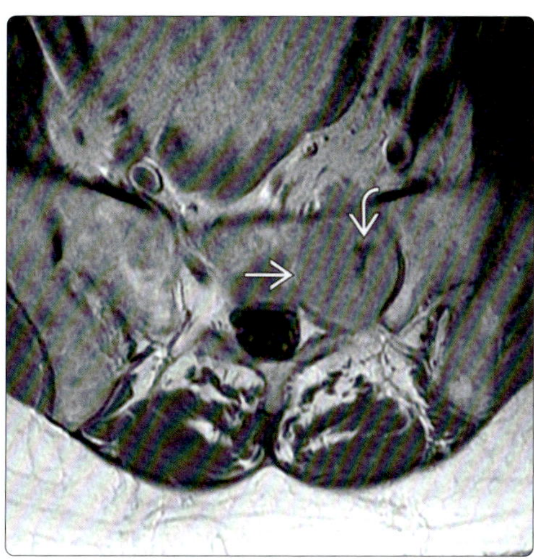

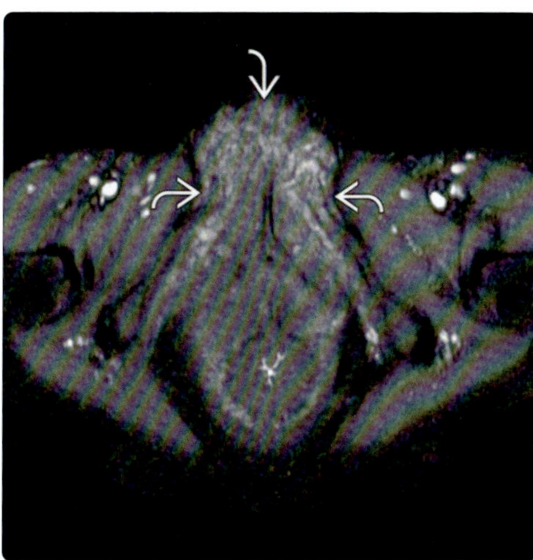

(Left) *Axial T1WI C+ FS MR after IV contrast in the same patient shows homogeneous enhancement of the mass ➡ with the exception of a small focus ↪ that lacks enhancement and had corresponding fluid intensity signal on the T2-weighted image, suggestive of mucoid or cystic degeneration.* **(Right)** *Axial STIR MR shows a large, plexiform neurofibroma ↪ involving the perineum. This lesion has the typical bag of worms appearance. The mass originated in the lumbosacral plexus.*

(Left) *Axial T1WI MR shows a nonspecific, infiltrating mass ➡ in the subcutaneous fat of the right superior gluteal region, extending from the level of the skin to the fascia. A small cutaneous nodule ➡ is isointense to skeletal muscle.* **(Right)** *Axial T2WI FS MR shows the subcutaneous mass ➡ to be heterogeneously hyperintense. Additionally, the cutaneous lesion ➡ also has hyperintense signal. These lesions represent diffuse and localized neurofibromas in a patient with known neurofibromatosis type 1.*

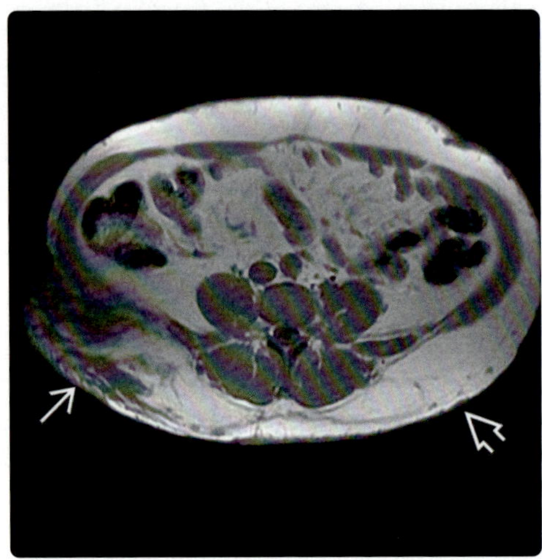

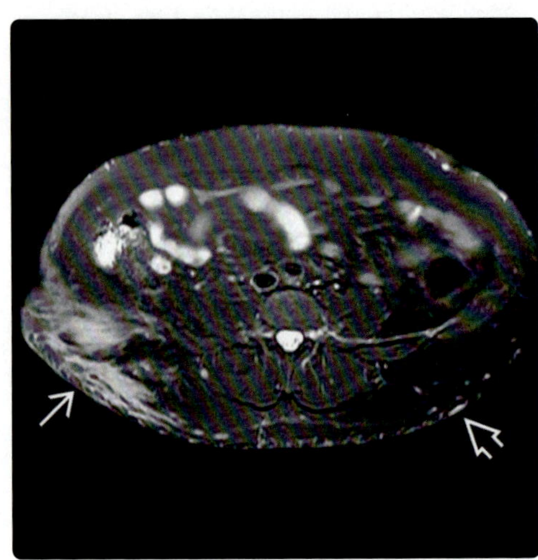

(Left) *Axial T1WI C+ FS MR in the same patient shows intense enhancement of the diffuse ➡ and localized ➡ neurofibromas, which is a typical finding. Diffuse neurofibromas have a tendency to spread along connective tissue septa ➡.* **(Right)** *Axial T1WI MR of the upper arm demonstrates plexiform neurofibromas ➡ appearing as multiple lobulated masses conforming to distribution of the radial, median, and ulnar nerves. These masses are mildly hyperintense relative to muscle.*

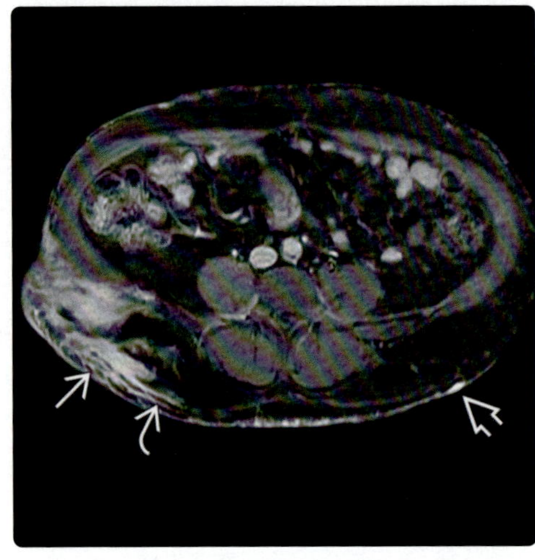

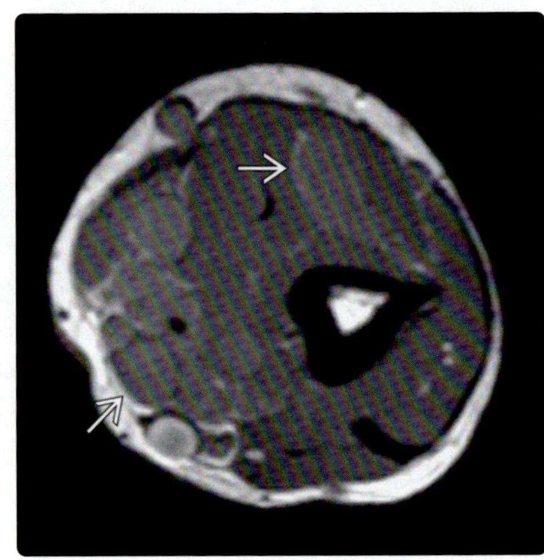

(Left) *Axial T2WI FS MR in the same patient confirms abnormal, heterogeneously hyperintense signal characteristics of the plexiform neurofibromas ➡. One of the masses has a central focus of decreased signal ➡, consistent with a target sign. The surrounding structures are displaced, rather than invaded.* **(Right)** *Axial T1WI C+ FS MR in the same patient depicts mild heterogeneous enhancement of the plexiform neurofibromas ➡. Note the lack of surrounding edema.*

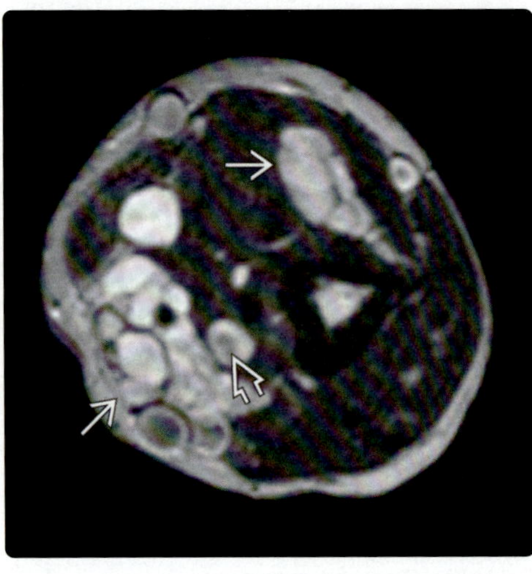

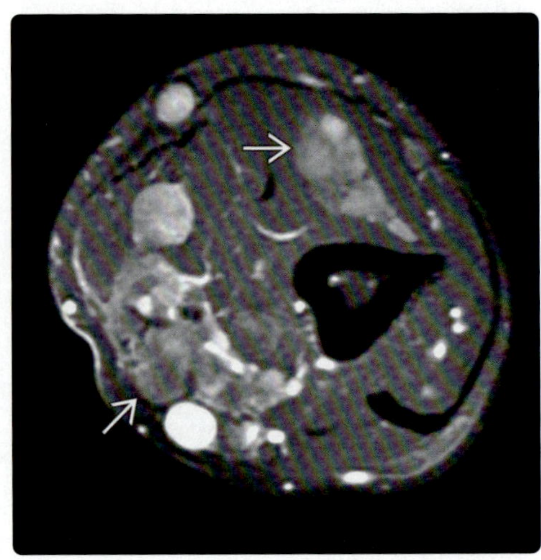

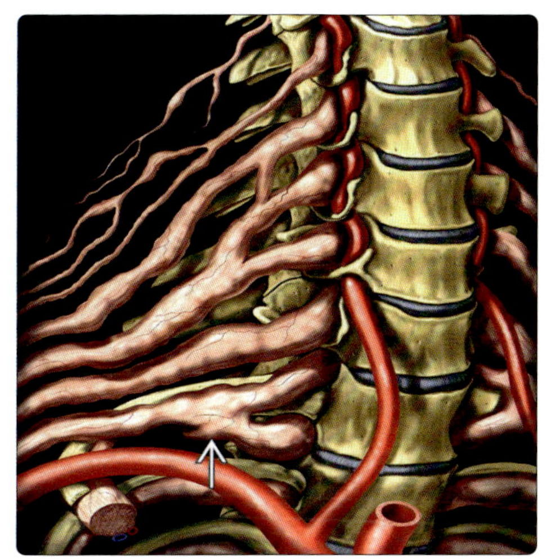

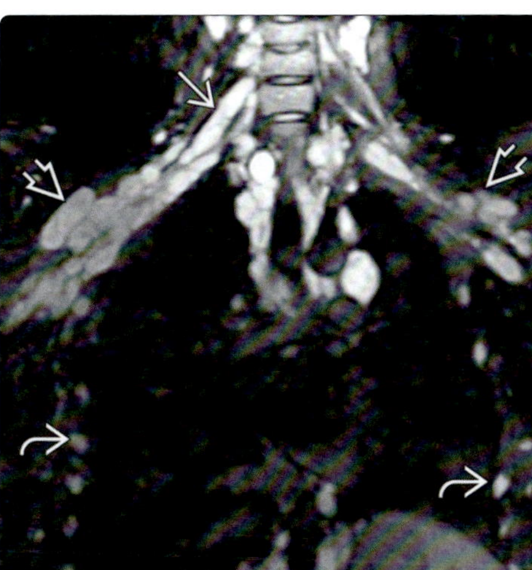

(Left) *Oblique graphic of the brachial plexus shows irregular, nodular enlargement of multiple nerves and nerve branches, consistent with a plexiform neurofibroma* ➔*. This type of neurofibroma is highly associated with NF1.* **(Right)** *Coronal STIR MR shows innumerable plexiform neurofibromas involving bilateral spinal nerves* ➔*, sympathetic chains, and brachial plexus* ➔*, as well as involvement of multiple intercostal nerves* ➔*. These masses have mildly heterogeneous high SI.*

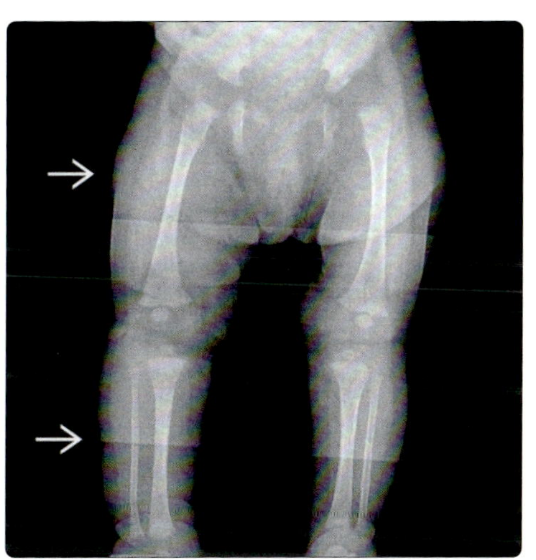

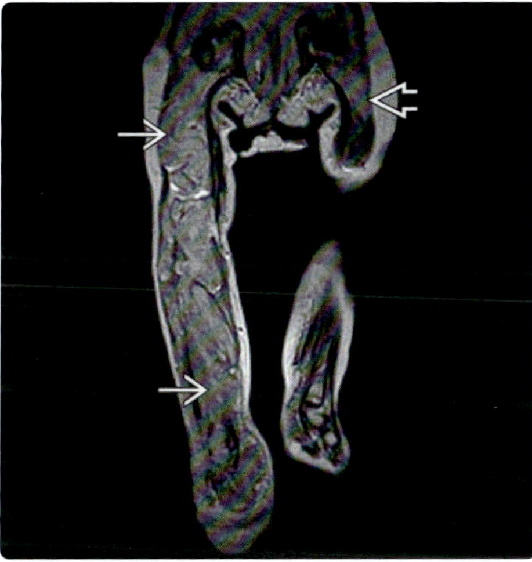

(Left) *Frontal radiograph of both lower extremities shows asymmetric increased soft tissue about the right lower extremity* ➔ *along with mild limb length discrepancy, with the right leg slightly longer than the left. This patient has neurofibromatosis type 1.* **(Right)** *Coronal T2WI FSE MR in the same patient shows a giant plexiform neurofibroma* ➔ *involving the right leg from the level of the sacral foramen to the medial foot. Also seen is a smaller plexiform neurofibroma along the posterior left thigh* ➔*.*

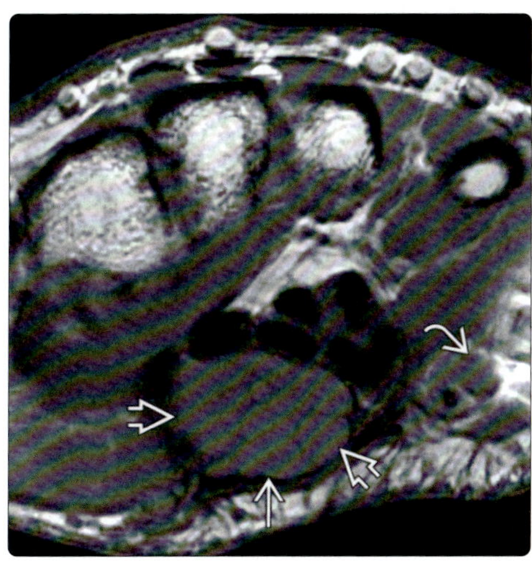

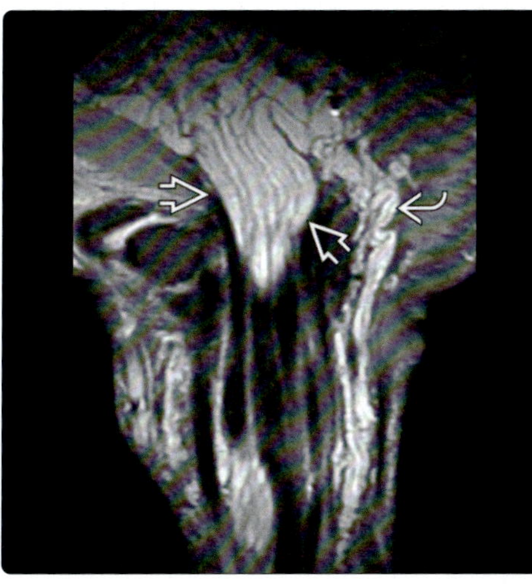

(Left) *Axial T1WI MR shows fairly uniform but significantly enlarged nerve fascicles of the median* ➔ *and ulnar* ➔ *nerves. These plexiform neurofibromas are mildly hyperintense to muscle. There is prominent bowing of the flexor retinaculum* ➔ *and displacement of the flexor tendons.* **(Right)** *Coronal PD FSE FS MR in the same patient shows the plexiform neurofibromas of the median* ➔ *and ulnar* ➔ *nerves to have high signal intensity, with the typical bag of worms appearance.*

KEY FACTS

TERMINOLOGY

- Encapsulated benign peripheral nerve sheath tumor typically located eccentrically on normal nerve

IMAGING

- Upper and lower extremity flexor surface nerves
- Well-defined, solitary fusiform mass
- Bone involvement uncommon
- CT: Fusiform, low-attenuation (5-30 HU) mass
  - ± central focus of higher attenuation
- MR appearance
  - Similar to slightly increased signal relative to muscle on T1WI MR
    - Split-fat sign = thin peripheral rim of fat
    - May have subtle muscle atrophy distal to lesion
  - Hyperintense to muscle on fluid-sensitive MR
    - Target sign = central low-signal region
    - Fascicular sign = multiple small, ring-like structures
  - Thin, hyperintense rim more suggestive of schwannoma than neurofibroma
  - More likely to have cystic change than neurofibroma
  - Diffuse enhancement is typical
- US: Well-defined, hypoechoic mass with mild posterior acoustic enhancement
  - Echogenic capsule usually present
- F-18 FDG PET **not** helpful for differentiation from malignant peripheral nerve sheath tumor

PATHOLOGY

- Classic histologic appearance of schwannoma consists of alternating Antoni A and B areas
- Ancient schwannoma: ↑ calcification, hemorrhage, cystic change, and hyalinization
- Cellular schwannoma: ↑ cellularity and mitoses can cause misdiagnosis of malignancy in > 25% of cases
- Slightly less common than neurofibroma

(Left) *Coronal T1WI MR demonstrates a fusiform mass ➡ located along the path of the peroneal nerve. The nerve can be seen extending from the mass distally ➡, and the mass deviates the lateral head of the gastrocnemius muscle ➡. The mass has heterogeneous signal intensity ranging from isointense to slightly hyperintense to skeletal muscle.* **(Right)** *Axial T2WI FSE MR shows the mass ➡ to have heterogeneous signal intensity that is slightly higher along the periphery of the mass.*

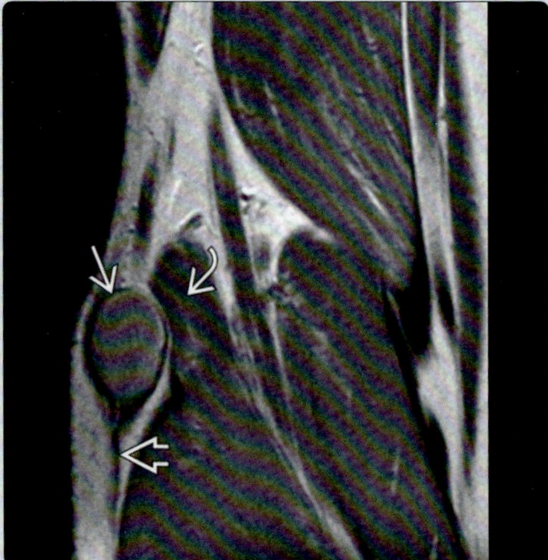

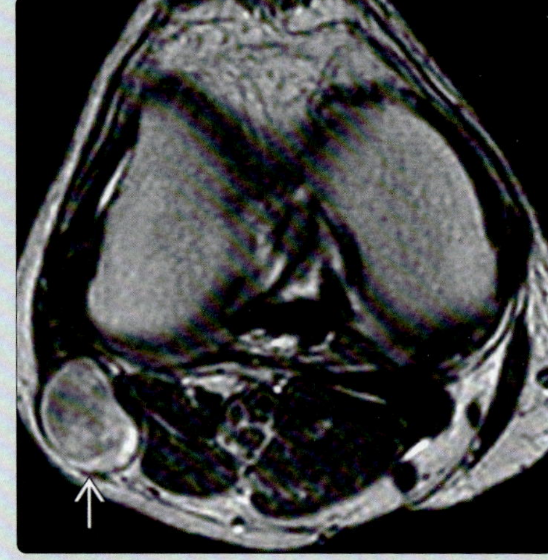

(Left) *Sagittal T2WI FS MR shows the mass ➡ to be heterogeneously hyperintense. The central low signal is again noted. This is a variant of a target sign, often seen in peripheral nerve sheath tumors.* **(Right)** *Axial T1WI C+ FS MR shows heterogeneous enhancement of the well-defined mass ➡. The location of the mass along the course of the peroneal nerve gives a hint to the tumor's origin. Only a single core biopsy was obtained since the mass was exquisitely painful. Biopsy confirmed a schwannoma.*

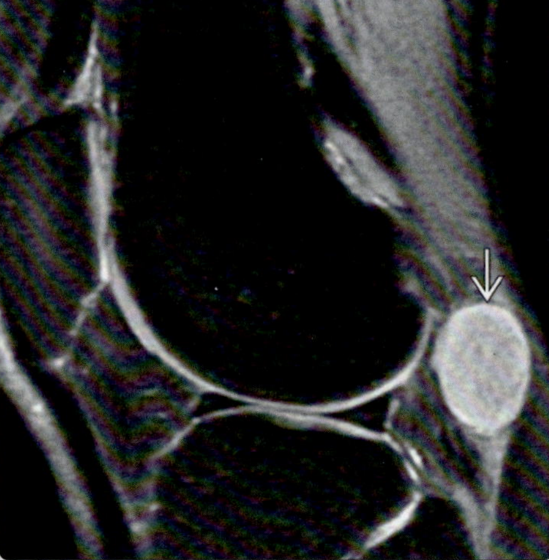

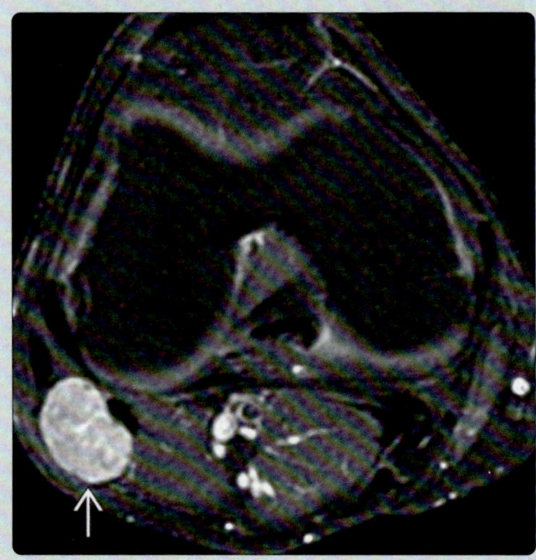

TERMINOLOGY

Synonyms

- Neurilemoma

Definitions

- Encapsulated benign peripheral nerve sheath tumor typically located eccentrically on nerve

IMAGING

General Features

- Location
  - Upper and lower extremity flexor surface nerves
    - Peroneal and ulnar nerves most common
  - Spinal, sympathetic, and cutaneous nerves of head and neck region
    - Predilection to involve sensory nerves
  - Subperiosteal and intraosseous locations rare
  - Ancient and cellular schwannomas most common in retroperitoneum and posterior mediastinum
    - 25% of cellular schwannomas in deep extremities
  - Multiple schwannomas or schwannomatosis may have segmental distribution
- Size
  - Usually < 5 cm
    - Larger tumors found in retroperitoneum and mediastinum
      - Reported up to 15 cm
- Morphology
  - Well-defined, solitary fusiform mass
    - Multiple masses in 5% of cases

Radiographic Findings

- Mineralization uncommon
- Bone involvement uncommon

CT Findings

- Fusiform, low-attenuation (5-30 HU) mass
  - ± central focus of higher attenuation
- + enhancement

MR Findings

- Fusiform mass eccentrically positioned in relation to parent nerve
  - Similar to slightly increased signal relative to muscle on T1WI
    - Split-fat sign = thin peripheral rim of fat
    - May have subtle muscle atrophy distal to lesion
  - Hyperintense to muscle on fluid-sensitive sequences
    - Target sign = central low-signal region
    - Fascicular sign = multiple small, ring-like structures
  - Diffuse enhancement (often greater than neurofibroma) is typical, but absent enhancement reported
- Imaging appearance may be similar to neurofibroma
  - More likely to have cystic change than neurofibroma
  - Thin, hyperintense rim on T2WI more suggestive of schwannoma

Ultrasonographic Findings

- Well-defined, hypoechoic mass with mild posterior acoustic enhancement
  - May contain foci of ↑ echogenicity or cystic spaces
  - Complete or incomplete internal echogenic ring is highly suggestive of diagnosis but rare
  - Parent nerve may be visible associated with periphery of mass
- Echogenic capsule usually present
- Increased blood flow on color Doppler

Nuclear Medicine Findings

- F-18 FDG PET not helpful for differentiation from malignant peripheral nerve sheath tumor due to high tumor-to-background ratio
  - Widely variable SUV based on tumor cellularity
  - Average SUV may be > 6
- Increased radiotracer uptake on bone scan with ancient schwannoma
- Lack of tracer uptake on Ga-67 citrate imaging may differentiate from malignant peripheral nerve sheath tumor

Angiographic Findings

- Variably present but characteristic corkscrew-type vessels at upper and lower pole of lesion

DIFFERENTIAL DIAGNOSIS

Neurofibroma

- More likely to have target sign and central enhancement on MR imaging
  - May not be possible to differentiate from schwannoma
- Mass is intermingled with normal nerve fibers
- Lacks histologic Antoni A and B areas
- S100 protein focally positive, as opposed to intensely positive with schwannoma

Synovial Sarcoma

- Well-defined to partially infiltrative mass with predilection for periarticular regions
- On MR, may have split-fat sign, triple sign, and bowl of grapes sign
- Prominent heterogeneous enhancement on CT and MR imaging
- More likely to contain mineralization than schwannoma

Malignant Peripheral Nerve Sheath Tumor

- Enlarging mass involving major nerve trunk
- ± invasion of surrounding structures
- Hemorrhage and necrosis more common than in neurofibroma or schwannoma

Hematoma

- Lacks solid regions of enhancing tissue
- May chronically calcify

Melanotic Schwannoma

- Distinct neoplasm from classic schwannoma
- Predilection to involve spinal or midline autonomic nerves
- 55% associated with Carney complex
- Black-brown to gray-blue encapsulated mass
  - Psammoma bodies common
- Mild female predominance
- Increased risk of metastatic disease (13-26%)

PATHOLOGY

General Features

- Genetics
  - Arises sporadically in most cases
  - Commonly aberration of chromosome 22
- Associated abnormalities
  - May arise in association with neurofibromatosis type 1 (NF1) or type 2 (NF2)
    - Association with NF1 is rare

Gross Pathologic & Surgical Features

- Encapsulated pink, white, or yellow mass
- Mass located eccentrically to nerve
  - Small nerves may be engulfed

Microscopic Features

- Classic schwannoma appearance consists of alternating Antoni A and B areas
  - Antoni A = highly ordered cellular component
    - Compact spindle cells with twisted nuclei in fascicles or short bundles
      - ± Verocay bodies, nuclear palisading, whorling of cells, clear intranuclear vacuoles
    - Occasional mitotic figures
  - Antoni B = hypocellular loose myxoid component
    - Haphazard spindle or oval cells, inflammatory cells, microcystic change, and collagen
      - ± glands and benign epithelial structures
    - Large vessels have thickened walls and may be filled with thrombus
  - S100 protein intensely positive
- Ancient schwannoma
  - Large, longstanding tumors with calcification, hemorrhage, cystic change, and hyalinization
    - Siderophages and histiocytes common
  - Marked nuclear atypia but absent mitotic figures
- Cellular schwannoma
  - Predominantly Antoni A areas
    - Hemorrhage common, but cystic degeneration uncommon
    - Lacks Verocay bodies
    - Up to 10% with necrosis
  - ↑ cellularity and mitoses can cause misdiagnosis of malignancy in > 25% of cases
    - Usually < 4 mitoses per 10 HPF
  - 25% in deep soft tissues of extremities
  - ± associated bone destruction
  - Circumscribed tan mass, sometimes multinodular
  - S100 protein strongly positive
- Plexiform schwannoma
  - Plexiform or multinodular mass most commonly arising from skin or subcutaneous tissue
    - Deep lesions rare but reported
  - Variant of cellular schwannoma
  - 5% of all schwannomas
- Epithelioid schwannoma
  - Superficial, encapsulated mass
  - Small, round epithelioid Schwann cells in clusters or cords ± atypical cells
    - Collagenous or myxoid stroma
    - Lacks mitotic figures
  - S100 protein strongly positive
  - Type IV collagen immunostain positive

CLINICAL ISSUES

Presentation

- Most common signs/symptoms
  - Painless, slowly growing mass
    - Percussion produces painful Tinel sign
    - Pain more common with large, multiple, or deep lesions
  - Mass tethered along longitudinal axis but mobile transverse to nerve
- Other signs/symptoms
  - 2% have schwannomatosis
    - Distinct from NF2
    - Multiple schwannomas without involvement of vestibular apparatus
  - 3% associated with NF2
  - 5% have multiple meningiomas ± NF2

Demographics

- Age
  - Most common in 2nd-5th decades of life
    - Found at all ages
- Gender
  - No gender predominance
- Epidemiology
  - ~ 5% of benign soft tissue tumors
  - Slightly less common than neurofibroma

Natural History & Prognosis

- Benign without local recurrence
- Malignant degeneration rare

Treatment

- Nerve function can usually be preserved with surgical excision, unlike neurofibroma

SELECTED REFERENCES

1. Khoo M et al: Melanotic schwannoma: an 11-year case series. Skeletal Radiol. ePub, 2015
2. Ahlawat S et al: Schwannoma in neurofibromatosis type 1: a pitfall for detecting malignancy by metabolic imaging. Skeletal Radiol. 42(9):1317-22, 2013
3. Kashima TG et al: Intraosseous schwannoma in schwannomatosis. Skeletal Radiol. 42(12):1665-71, 2013
4. Koontz NA et al: Schwannomatosis: the overlooked neurofibromatosis? AJR Am J Roentgenol. 200(6):W646-53, 2013
5. Hamada K et al: (18)F-FDG PET analysis of schwannoma: increase of SUVmax in the delayed scan is correlated with elevated VEGF/VPF expression in the tumors. Skeletal Radiol. 38(3):261-6, 2009
6. Kransdorf MJ et al: Neurogenic tumors. In Kransdorf MJ et al: Imaging of Soft Tissue Tumors. 2nd ed. Philadelphia: Lippincott Williams & Wilkins. 334, 338-4, 2006
7. Beaulieu S et al: Positron emission tomography of schwannomas: emphasizing its potential in preoperative planning. AJR Am J Roentgenol. 182(4):971-4, 2004
8. Isobe K et al: Imaging of ancient schwannoma. AJR Am J Roentgenol. 183(2):331-6, 2004
9. Reynolds DL Jr et al: Sonographic characteristics of peripheral nerve sheath tumors. AJR Am J Roentgenol. 182(3):741-4, 2004
10. Lin J et al: Cross-sectional imaging of peripheral nerve sheath tumors: characteristic signs on CT, MR imaging, and sonography. AJR Am J Roentgenol. 176(1):75-82, 2001

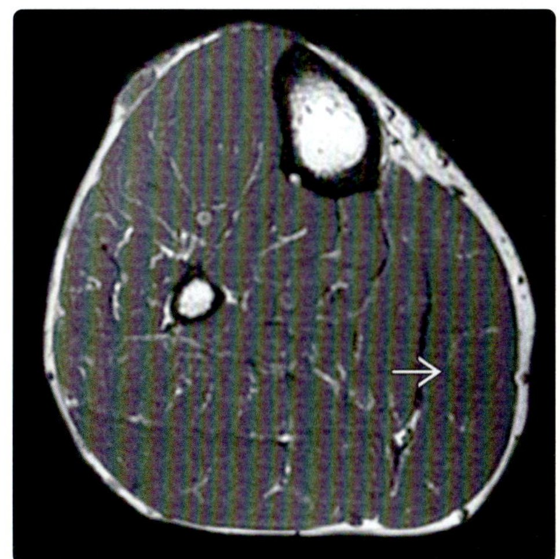

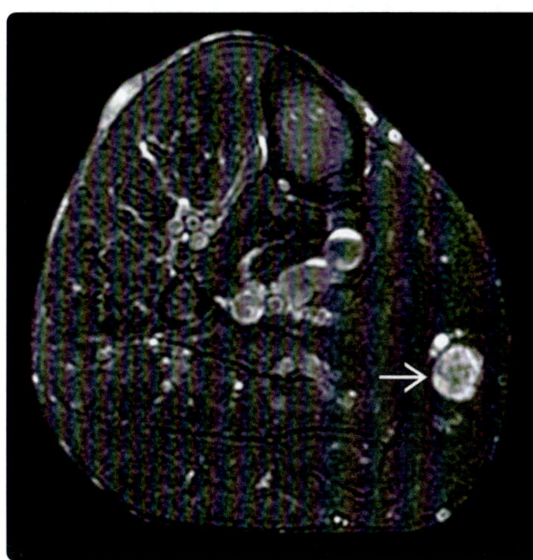

(Left) *Axial T1WI MR shows a small oval mass ➡ located in the medial head of the gastrocnemius muscle of the calf. The mass is isointense to slightly hypointense to the adjacent muscle, making it difficult to delineate.* **(Right)** *Axial T2WI FS MR in the same patient shows the mass ➡ to be heterogeneously hyperintense to muscle. The mass lacks the classic target appearance (high peripheral signal with low central signal) of nerve sheath tumors that is often seen on fluid-sensitive MR sequences.*

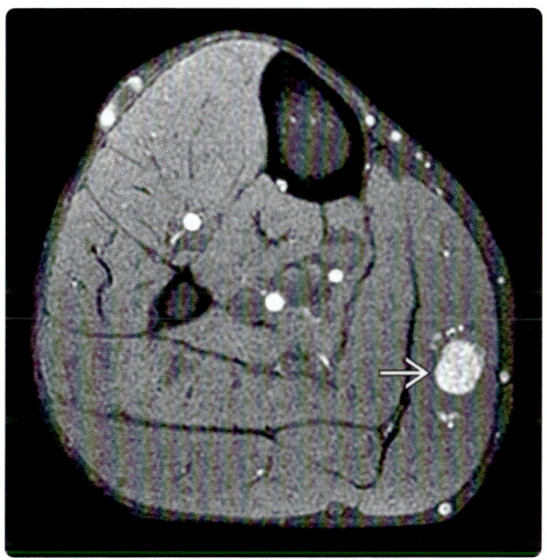

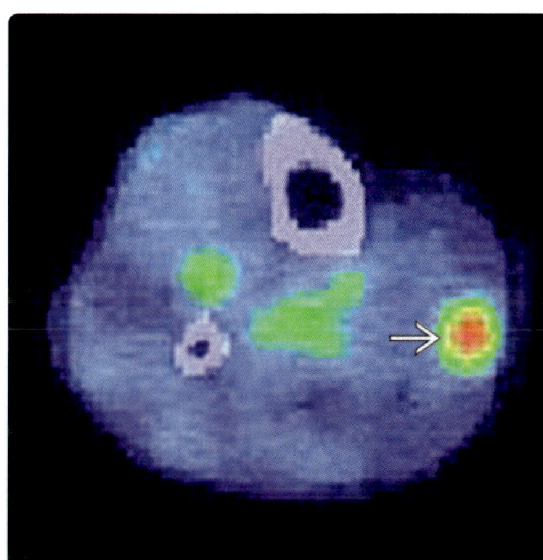

(Left) *Axial T1WI C+ FS MR shows homogeneous enhancement of the mass ➡. Schwannoma enhancement varies from absent to intense and may be homogeneous or inhomogeneous. Diffuse enhancement seen here is more typical of schwannoma than neurofibroma.* **(Right)** *Axial PET/CT shows increased F-18 FDG uptake of the mass ➡. This study initially prompted work-up of this lesion. Biopsy was required to exclude a metastasis from an undifferentiated pleomorphic sarcoma located in the patient's ipsilateral thigh.*

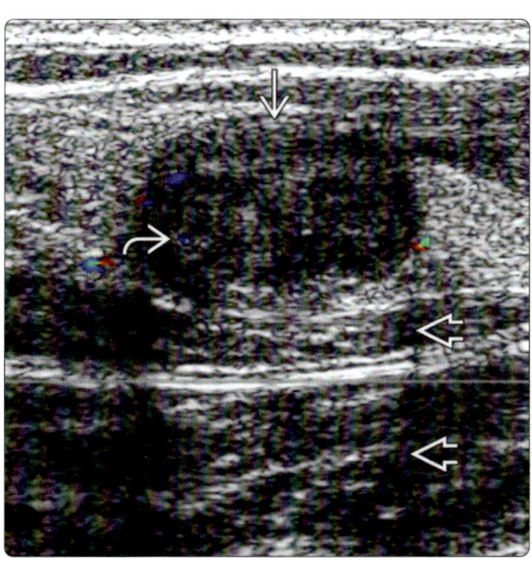

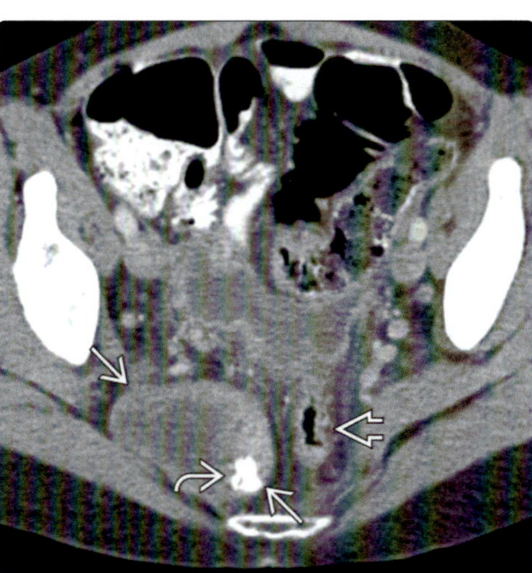

(Left) *Longitudinal color Doppler ultrasound in the same patient performed for biopsy guidance shows a well-defined, heterogeneous oval mass ➡ with posterior acoustic enhancement ➡ and mild internal blood flow ➡.* **(Right)** *Axial NECT demonstrates a mass ➡ within the right sciatic notch, displacing the rectum ➡. A coarse calcification ➡ is eccentrically located within the mass. The right sciatic nerve is not identified as a separate structure, and proved to be intimately related to this schwannoma.*

(Left) *Axial CT shows a large mass that erodes the sacrum and adjacent L5 vertebrae ➡. Note that the iliac artery ➡ has been significantly displaced.* **(Right)** *Left parasagittal T1WI MR, same case, shows the mass to have an axial origin, extending to involve L5 ➡, S1 ➡, and the pelvis ➡. It is homogeneously low signal intensity. Given the location, giant cell tumor or neurofibroma are likely diagnoses, though schwannoma and chordoma should be considered as well.*

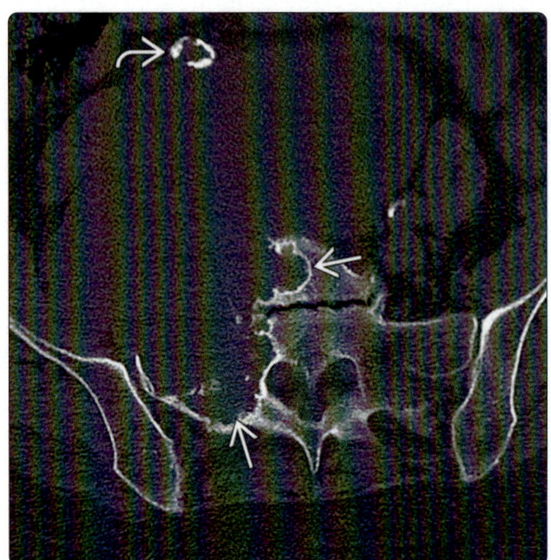

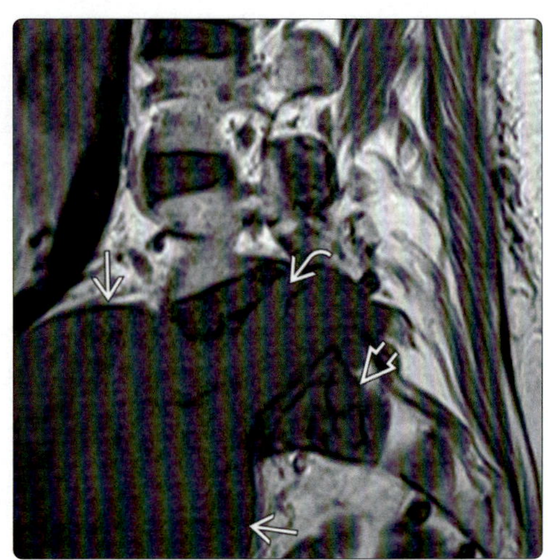

(Left) *Axial T2WI MR shows the mass ➡ to be markedly heterogeneous with hypointensity suggesting giant cell tumor as a leading diagnosis. The lesion also involves the neural foramen ➡, increasing the likelihood of nerve sheath tumor; schwannoma was proven.* **(Right)** *AP radiograph shows a mass ➡ within the thigh that contains dystrophic calcification. Although this may be seen in any soft tissue tumor, it occurs most often in synovial sarcoma, the most likely working diagnosis.*

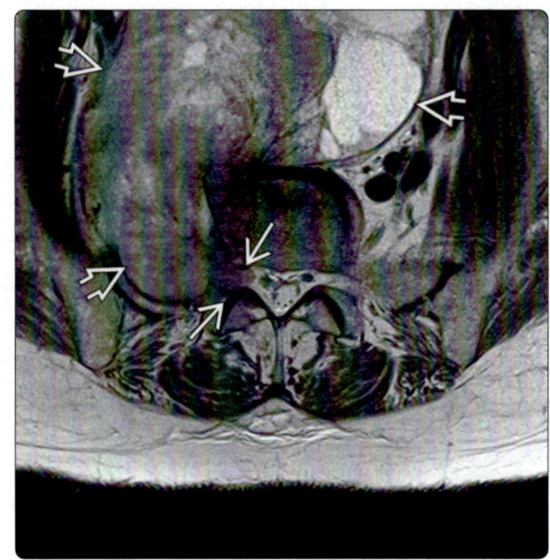

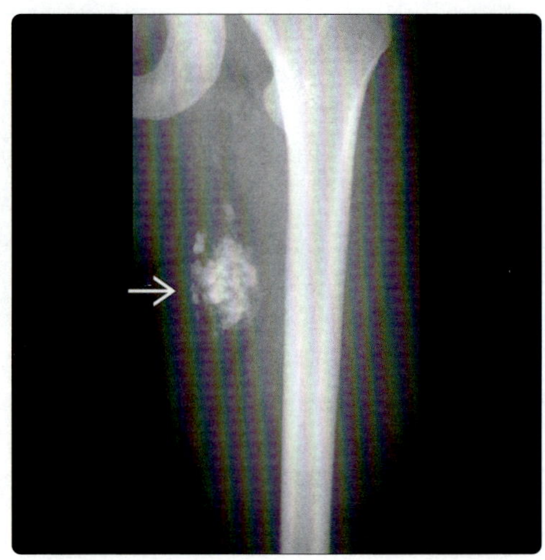

(Left) *Axial T1WI MR in the same patient shows the large mass ➡ to contain low-signal calcification ➡.* **(Right)** *Axial T2WI MR in the same patient shows the mass ➡ to have heterogeneously high signal with persistently low-signal central calcifications ➡. It is significant that the lesion is in the path of a branch of the femoral nerve. Longstanding schwannomas are more likely to have heterogeneous signal from calcification and other degenerative change.*

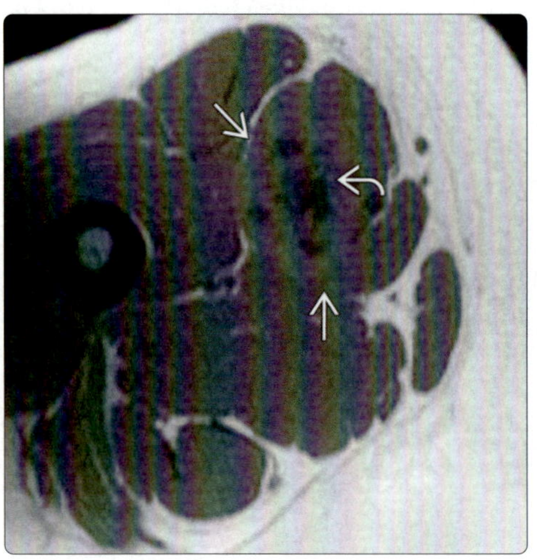

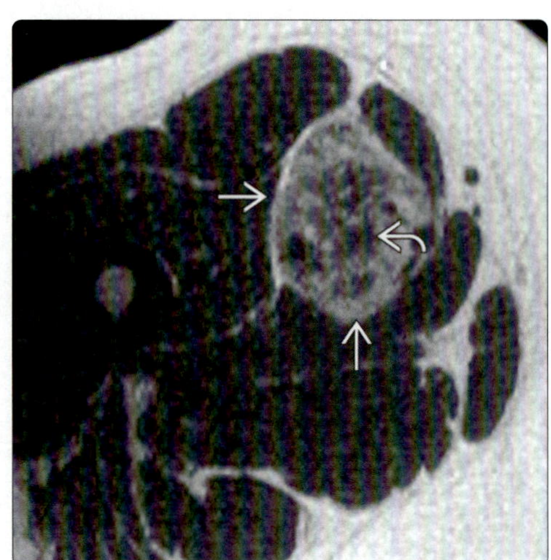

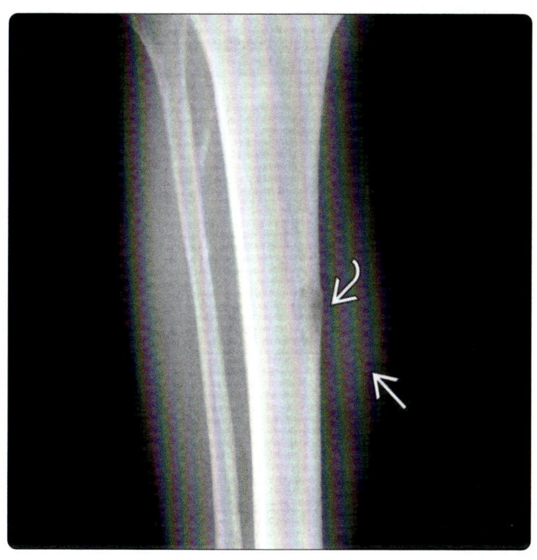

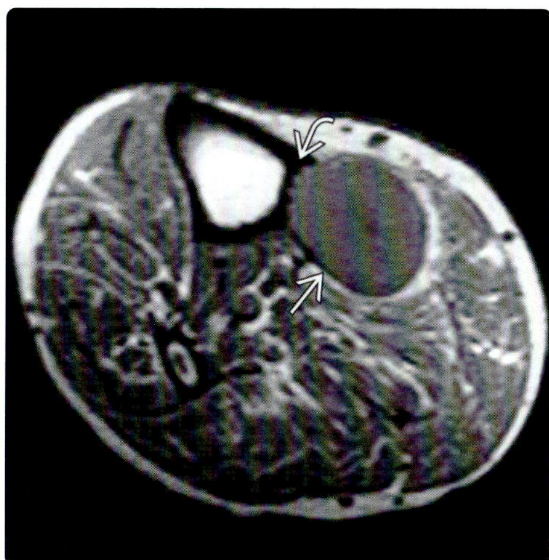

(Left) *Anteroposterior radiograph demonstrates a soft tissue mass ➡ in the midcalf, which appears to be excavating the underlying tibia ↪. The center of the lesion is soft tissue rather than parosteal or osseous.* **(Right)** *Axial T1WI MR in the same patient confirms that the center of the lesion is in soft tissue ➡, with local saucerization and invasion of the cortex of the tibia ↪. The mass is heterogeneously isointense to skeletal muscle with a small central focus of decreased signal.*

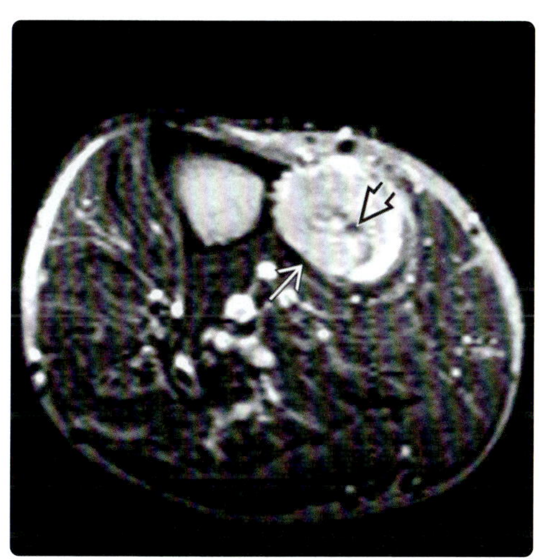

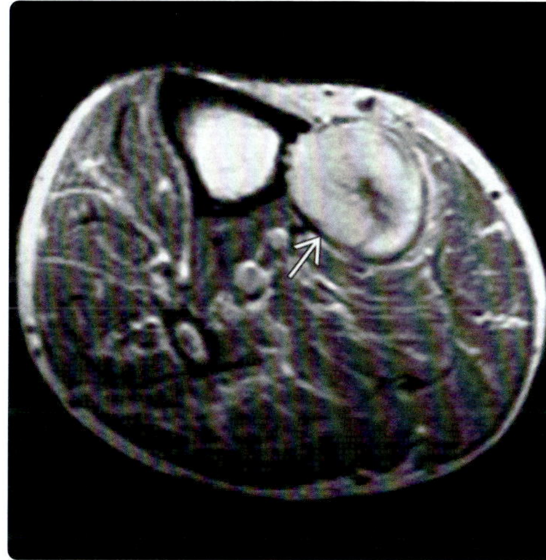

(Left) *Axial T2WI MR in the same patient shows the mass ➡ to be predominantly high in signal intensity with a central region of decreased signal intensity ⇨. The marrow space of the partially invaded tibia is normal.* **(Right)** *Axial T1WI C+ MR shows the mass ➡ to heterogeneously enhance. This lesion is quite elongated, measuring 7 cm from proximal to distal, while it is only 3 cm in diameter. The slow erosion of the tibia is a tip-off that this is a benign lesion.*

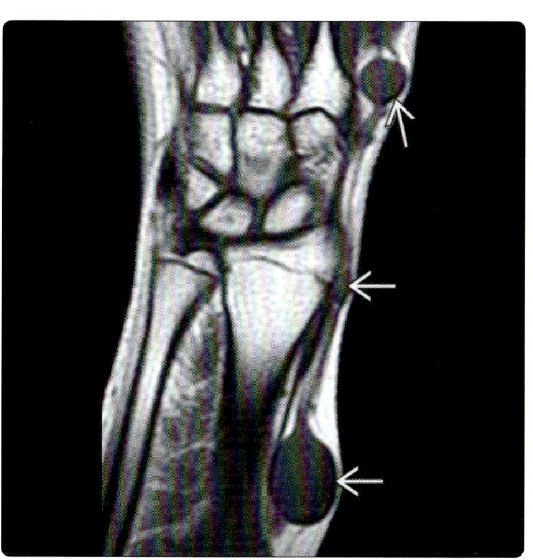

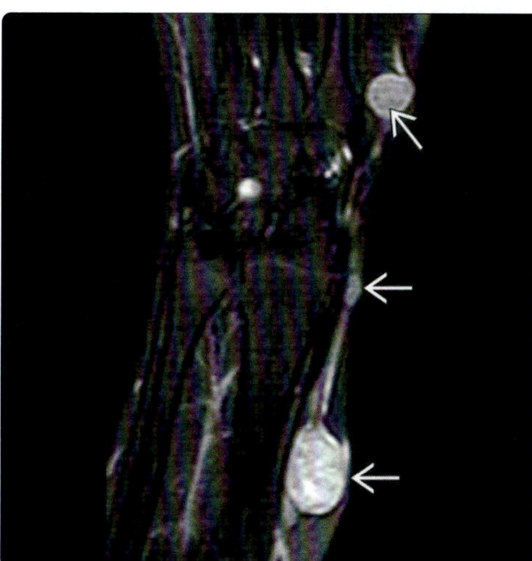

(Left) *Coronal T1WI MR shows 3 fusiform or rounded masses ➡ intimately associated with and extending along the course of the radial nerve. This is a case of schwannomatosis.* **(Right)** *Coronal T2WI FS in the same case shows inhomogeneous hyperintensity in the 3 schwannomas ➡. It should be remembered that schwannomatosis is a distinct entity from NF2.*

Malignant Peripheral Nerve Sheath Tumor

KEY FACTS

IMAGING

- Ill-defined, fusiform mass > 5 cm
  - Large to medium deep nerves
  - Proximal extremities, retroperitoneum, posterior mediastinum
- CT: Infiltrative mass with heterogeneous attenuation secondary to hemorrhagic or necrotic contents
  - ± calcification or bone involvement
- MR appearance
  - Heterogeneously hypo- to hyperintense on T1WI MR
  - Heterogeneously hyperintense on fluid-sensitive MR
  - Intense heterogeneous enhancement, especially peripherally
  - May contain interlesional cysts
  - May have peripheral edema
- US: Heterogeneous echogenicity mass with infiltrative borders + posterior acoustic enhancement
  - Hyperemic on color and power Doppler
- Bone scan: ↑ Tc-99m uptake
- ↑ F-18 FDG PET uptake, SUV ≥ 6.1
- Corkscrew vessels at proximal and distal poles of mass on angiography

PATHOLOGY

- Malignant spindle cell sarcoma of neural origin
  - 25-50% associated with NF1
  - 10-20% radiation-induced
- 3-10% of all soft tissue sarcomas

CLINICAL ISSUES

- Pain, weakness, sensory deficit
- Sudden enlargement of preexisting neurofibroma
- Radiation-induced lesions have 10-20 yr latency
- Poor long-term prognosis
  - Local recurrence: 40-65%
  - Distant metastases: 40-68% (lung > bone > pleura)
  - 5-year survival rate: 23-44%

(Left) *Coronal graphic of the pelvis shows a malignant peripheral nerve sheath tumor ➡ arising from the sciatic nerve. The mass has a typical fusiform shape and is contiguous with the nerve. Origin in a large, deep-seated nerve is typical.* **(Right)** *Axial T1WI MR of the lower leg shows a mass ➡ anterior to the fibula with heterogeneous signal intensity that is isointense to hypointense relative to skeletal muscle. There is adjacent scalloping of the fibular cortex ➡. The marrow space of the fibula remains normal.*

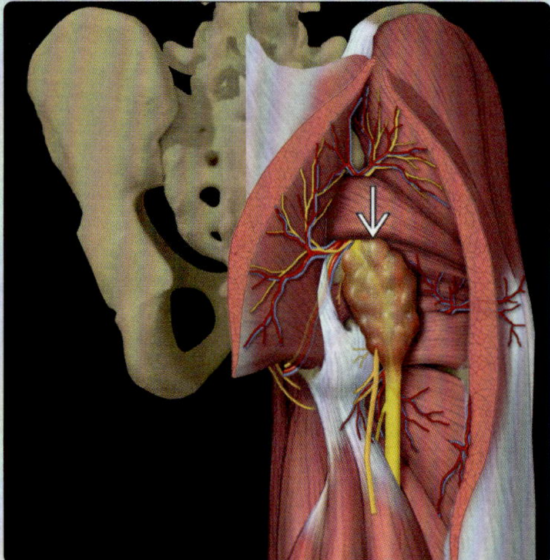

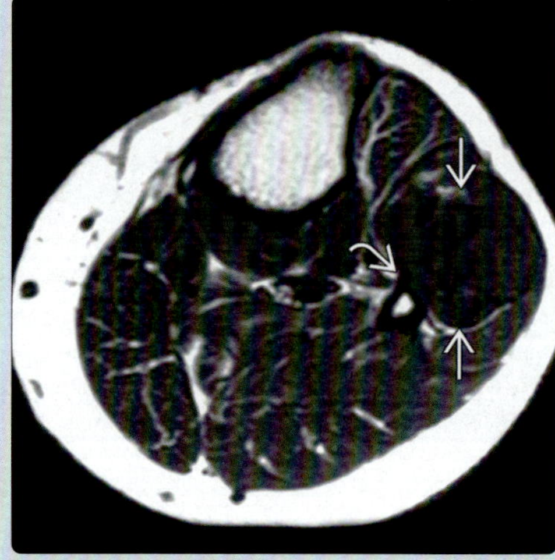

(Left) *Axial STIR MR in same patient shows the mass ➡ to have markedly heterogeneous signal with a broad range of signal intensities. Persistently low-signal regions likely represent calcification, which is more common in MPNST than in benign peripheral nerve sheath tumors. Regions of very high signal can be due to hemorrhage, cyst, or necrosis, both of which are common.* **(Right)** *Axial T1WI C+ MR shows the mass ➡ to have prominent but inhomogeneous enhancement. An incomplete rim of fat is present posteriorly ➡.*

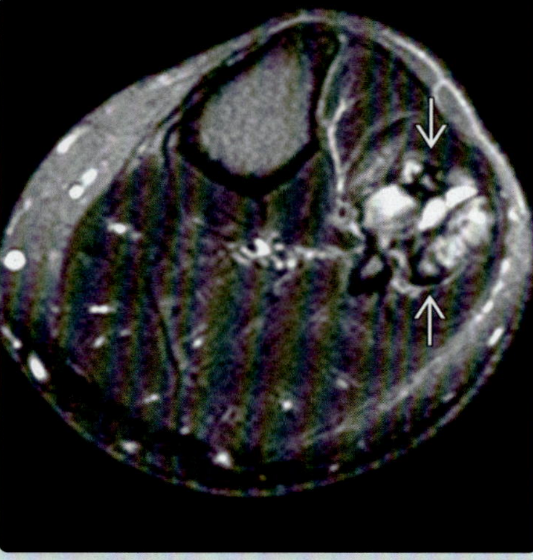

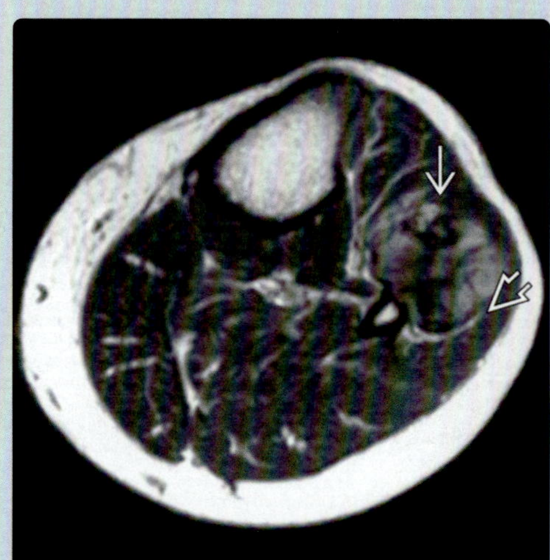

TERMINOLOGY

Abbreviations

- Malignant peripheral nerve sheath tumor (MPNST)

Synonyms

- Malignant schwannoma, neurogenic sarcoma, malignant neurilemmoma, neurofibrosarcoma

IMAGING

General Features

- Location
  - Large to medium deep nerves
    - Sciatic nerve > brachial plexus, sacral plexus
  - Proximal extremities, retroperitoneum, posterior mediastinum
    - Skin or bone (mandible) origin rare
- Size
  - > 5 cm
- Morphology
  - Ill-defined, fusiform mass

Radiographic Findings

- Radiography
  - Normal or soft tissue mass
    - ± calcification (more frequently seen than in neurofibroma) or bone involvement

CT Findings

- Infiltrative mass with heterogeneous attenuation secondary to hemorrhage or necrosis

MR Findings

- Heterogeneously hypo- to hyperintense on T1WI MR
  - Heterogeneity more frequent in MPNST than neurofibroma
- Heterogeneously hyperintense on fluid-sensitive MR
  - ± hemorrhagic fluid-fluid levels, cysts
- Intense heterogeneous enhancement
  - Diffuse, peripheral, or nodular patterns
- Differentiating features from neurofibroma (2 of 4 features should be considered highly suspicious for MPNST)
  - Large size
  - Peripheral enhancement pattern
  - Perilesional edema zone
  - Presence of intratumoral cystic lesion

Nuclear Medicine Findings

- Bone scan
  - ↑ blood pool and delayed Tc-99m uptake
  - ↑ Ga-67 citrate uptake
- PET
  - ↑ F-18 FDG uptake, SUV ≥ 6.1
  - 11C-methionine PET increases specificity

Ultrasonographic Findings

- Heterogeneous echogenicity mass with infiltrative borders and posterior acoustic enhancement
- Lacks target appearance seen in benign peripheral nerve sheath tumor
- Hyperemic on color and power Doppler

DIFFERENTIAL DIAGNOSIS

Benign Peripheral Nerve Sheath Tumor

- Well-circumscribed mass along course of nerve
- Less likely to produce pain at rest
- Smaller, better defined lesions than MPNST
- More likely to have target sign and fascicular sign
- Less likely to calcify, except ancient schwannoma

Pleomorphic MFH/Undifferentiated Pleomorphic Sarcoma

- Heterogeneous mass on MR ± fluid-fluid levels
- Less likely to be along course of nerve

PATHOLOGY

General Features

- Etiology
  - Malignant spindle cell sarcoma of neural origin
- Associated abnormalities
  - 25-50% associated with NF1
    - Yet only ~ 10% of NF1 patients develop MPNST
  - 10-20% radiation-induced (10-20 yr latency)

Microscopic Features

- Diagnostic criteria disagreement complicates diagnosis
- MPNST if meets 1 of following 3 criteria
  - Sarcoma arising from peripheral nerve
  - Sarcoma arising from preexisting benign peripheral nerve sheath tumor
  - Sarcoma reflecting Schwann cell differentiation

CLINICAL ISSUES

Presentation

- Most common signs/symptoms
  - Pain, weakness, sensory deficit
  - Sudden enlargement of preexisting neurofibroma

Demographics

- Age
  - 2nd-5th decades of life
  - In NF1: Earlier presentation and wider age range
- Gender
  - Slight female predilection
    - MPNST with NF1: Marked male predominance
- Epidemiology
  - 3-10% of all soft tissue sarcomas

Natural History & Prognosis

- Poor long-term prognosis
  - Local recurrence: 40-65%
  - Distant metastases: 40-68% (lung > bone > pleura)
  - 5-yr survival rate: 23-44%

Treatment

- Surgical excision ± chemotherapy &/or radiotherapy

SELECTED REFERENCES

1. Schaefer IM et al: Malignant peripheral nerve sheath tumor (MPNST) arising in diffuse-type neurofibroma: Clinicopathologic Characterization in a Series of 9 Cases. Am J Surg Pathol. ePub, 2015

(Left) *Coronal T1WI MR shows a large mass ➡ exiting the pelvis through the sciatic notch. The mass has similar signal intensity to normal muscle. Note expansion of the right sacral foramen ⇨. There is chronic denervation of the right gluteus muscles with fatty infiltration ↷.* **(Right)** *Coronal T2WI FS MR shows the sacral plexus/sciatic nerve MPNST ➡ to be heterogeneously hyperintense to muscle. Again seen is right sacral foramen expansion ⇨ and gluteal muscle atrophy ↷.*

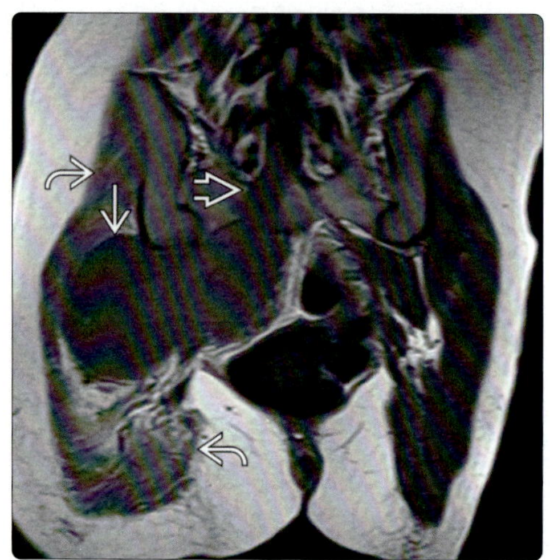

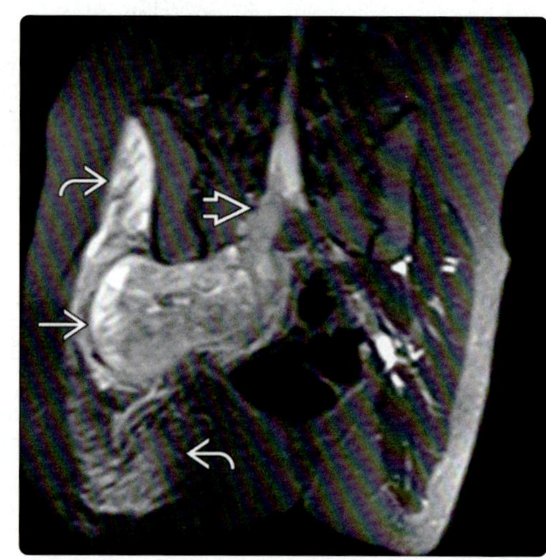

(Left) *Coronal T1WI C+ FS MR in the same patient shows heterogeneous enhancement of the mass ➡ as well as enhancement of the denervated muscles ↷. Tumor extends into the spinal canal ⇨. This patient also had hepatic metastases.* **(Right)** *Coronal T1WI MR of the knee shows a large, relatively well-circumscribed subcutaneous mass ➡, which contains low-signal calcification ↷. The majority of the lesion is isointense to skeletal muscle. This lesion extends very near the skin surface.*

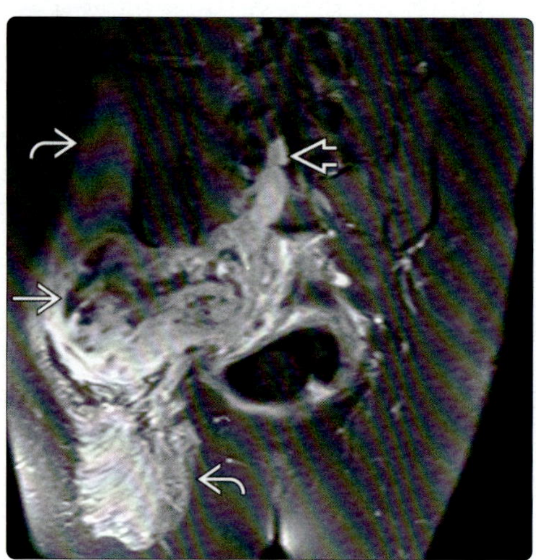

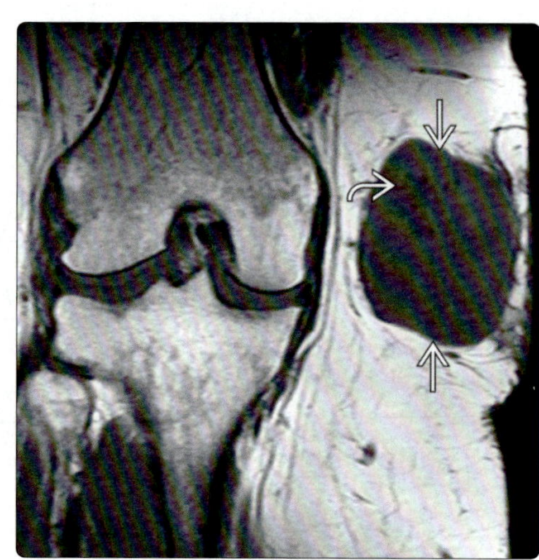

(Left) *Axial PDWI FS MR in the same patient shows the mass ➡ to have heterogeneous high signal, with nodular regions of dystrophic calcification ↷.* **(Right)** *Axial T1WI C+ FS MR, same patient, shows the mass ➡ to have heterogeneous intense enhancement, predominantly peripherally, a feature more often seen in MPNST than neurofibroma. Nonenhancing regions likely represent a combination of necrosis, old hemorrhage, or calcification. Tumor origin from a small, superficial nerve is uncommon for MPNST.*

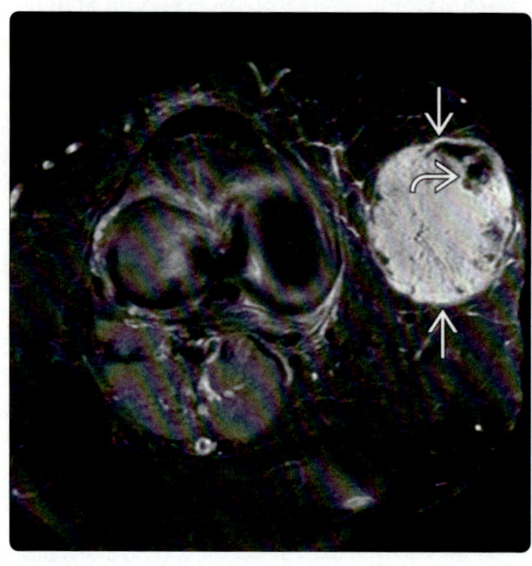

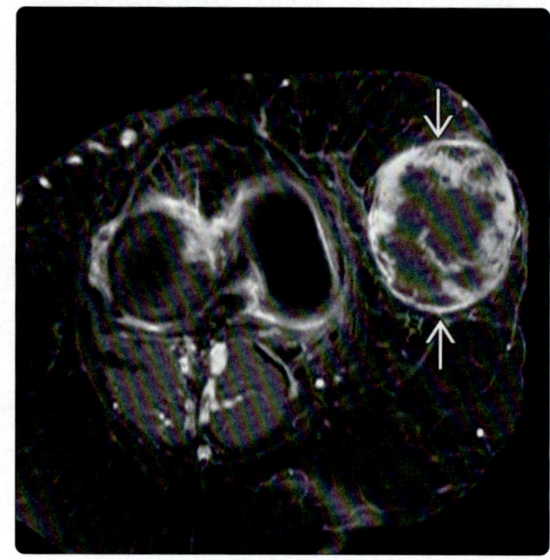

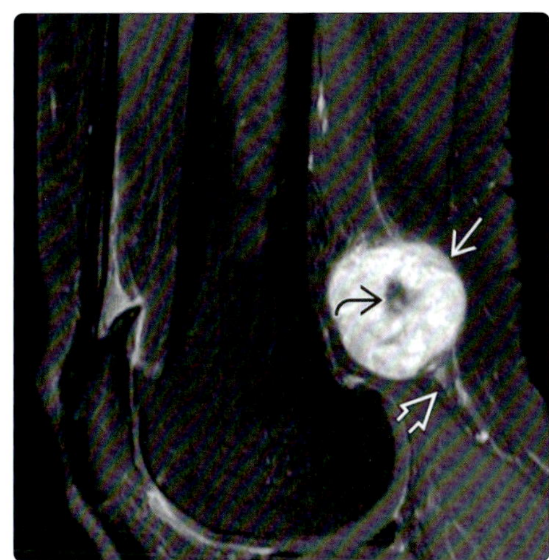

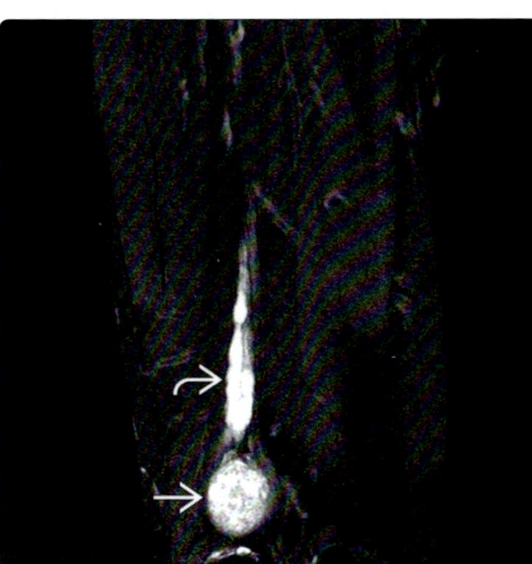

(Left) *Sagittal T2WI FS MR shows a heterogeneously hyperintense lesion ➡ associated with a deep nerve ➡. The lesion contains a central hypointense focus ➡; targets have been described in all peripheral NSTs, but are more frequently seen in benign than malignant lesions.* **(Right)** *Coronal STIR MR, same case, shows the large lesion ➡ relative to smaller neurofibromas ➡ beading the peroneal nerve. There is no peripheral edema or other feature to differentiate benign from malignant, but it proved to be MPNST.*

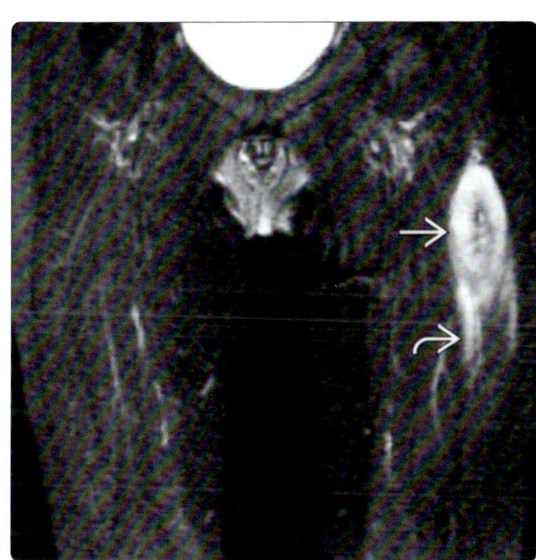

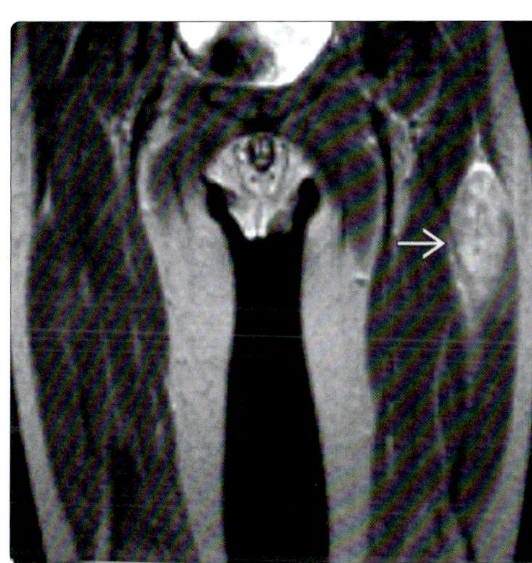

(Left) *Coronal T2WI FS MR reveals a spindle-shaped, heterogeneous, hyperintense mass ➡ in the anterior left thigh. Hyperintense signal in adjacent soft tissues ➡ likely represents surrounding edema, which is more frequently seen in MPNST than neurofibroma.* **(Right)** *Coronal T1WI C+ MR in the same patient shows prominent, mildly heterogeneous enhancement of the anterior thigh mass ➡. This mass was along the course of a neurovascular bundle and was confirmed to represent a MPNST.*

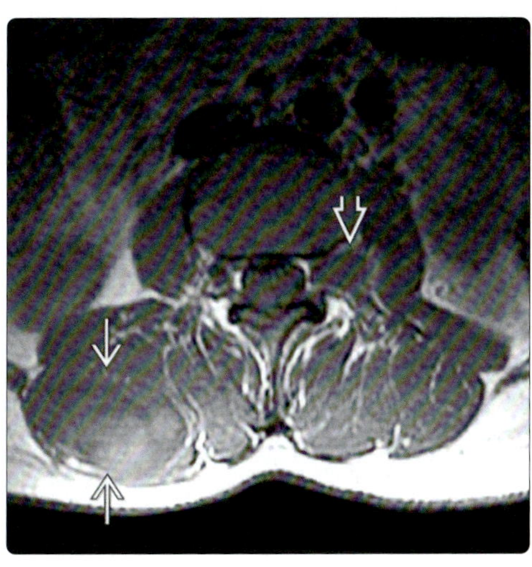

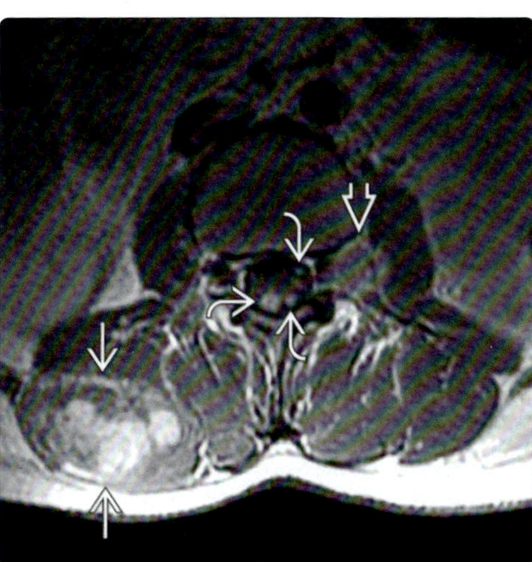

(Left) *Axial T1WI MR in a patient with NF1 shows a large mass ➡ within the right paraspinous muscles. This mass is slightly inhomogeneous, with signal intensity similar to and slightly higher than skeletal muscle. A 2nd smaller mass resides in left neural foramen ➡.* **(Right)** *Axial T1WI C+ MR shows heterogeneous enhancement of the right paraspinous mass ➡, which represented a MPNST upon biopsy. The left neurofibroma ➡ also enhances, as well as other additional intrathecal neurofibromas ➡.*

Epidermal Inclusion Cyst

KEY FACTS

TERMINOLOGY

- Common benign lesion of cutis and subcutis that arises from obstruction of hair follicle or deep implantation of epidermis

IMAGING

- Scalp > face > neck > trunk
  - < 10% involve extremities
- Osseous lesions appear lytic with sclerotic margin ± soft tissue swelling
- CT: Soft tissue density mass in subcutaneous fat
- MR findings
  - Isointense to muscle with mild heterogeneous signal ranging from low to high on T1WI
  - Hyperintense signal plus ↑ or ↓ signal debris (cholesterol crystals or keratin) on T2WI FS
    - Debris may be positionally dependent
- US: Well-circumscribed, heterogeneously hypoechoic to hyperechoic mass

PATHOLOGY

- Traumatic or developmental nonneoplastic lesion
- Additional findings associated with cyst rupture
  - Granulomatous reaction, granulation tissue, foreign body reaction, abscess, meningitis (intracranial)

CLINICAL ISSUES

- Majority are incidental findings
- Firm, slowly growing, painless mass
- Simple excision is curative

DIAGNOSTIC CHECKLIST

- May be difficult to differentiate intrinsic high T1 signal from enhancement on T1WI C+ FS MR if pregadolinium T1WI FS MR not obtained
- Imaging appearance varies based on lesion contents and hydration

(Left) *Axial T1WI MR of the distal thigh shows a well-circumscribed mass ➡ in the posterior superficial soft tissues. The mass is relatively homogeneous with a signal intensity that is slightly hyperintense relative to skeletal muscle.* **(Right)** *Axial T2WI FS MR shows the mass ➡ to be heterogeneously hyperintense relative to muscle. The mass contains scattered foci of debris that have slightly decreased signal intensity. MR imaging of these lesions is variable based on cyst contents and degree of hydration of the lesion.*

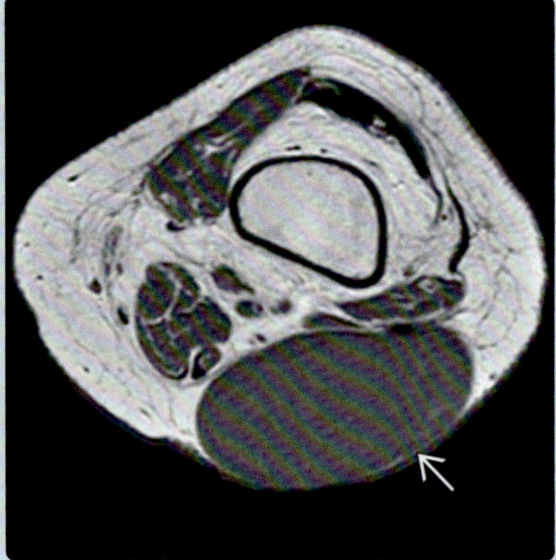

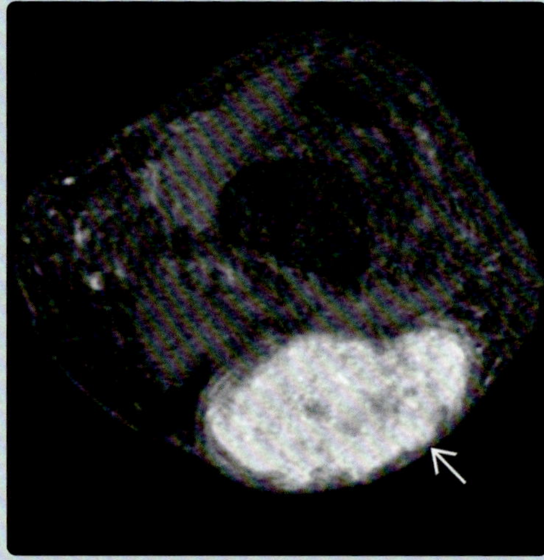

(Left) *Axial T1WI C+ FS MR shows the mass ➡ to have peripheral enhancement. Internal enhancement is difficult to assess due to the intrinsic T1 hyperintensity of the lesion. A subtraction postprocessed MR confirmed only peripheral enhancement.* **(Right)** *Transverse ultrasound shows the mass ➡ to be well-circumscribed with heterogeneous hypoechogenicity. Internal foci of debris ➡ are visible and were composed of keratin on excision. Color Doppler ultrasound showed no blood flow within the mass.*

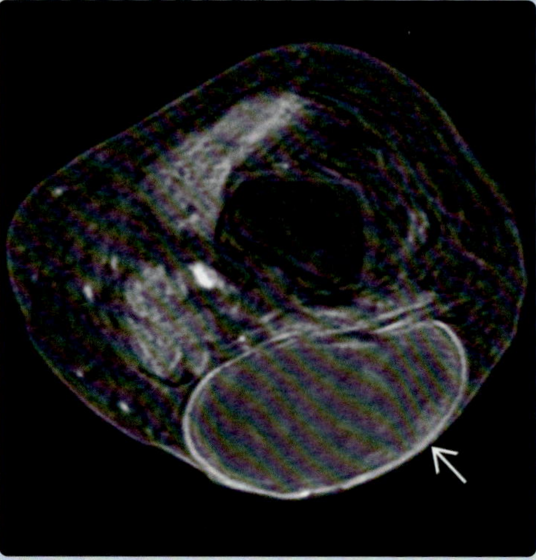

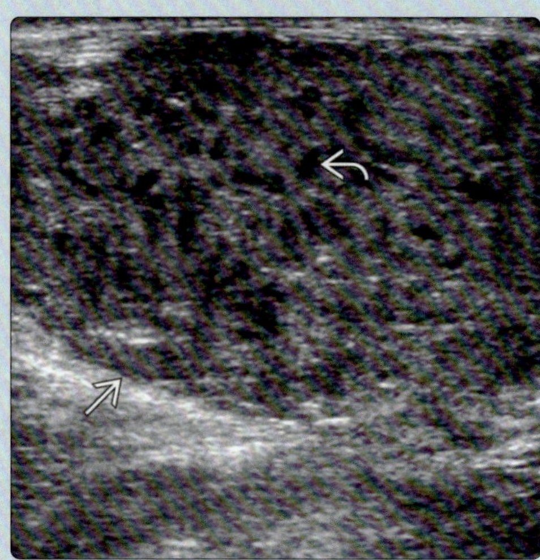

TERMINOLOGY

Synonyms

- Epidermal cyst, epidermoid cyst, infundibular cyst

Definitions

- Common benign lesion of cutis and subcutis that arises from obstruction of hair follicle or deep implantation of epidermis

IMAGING

General Features

- Location
  - Scalp > face > neck > trunk
    - < 10% involve extremities
  - Soft tissue > > bones (fingers and toes)
- Size
  - Small lesions, usually 0.2-5.0 cm
  - May uncommonly grow > 14 cm
- Morphology
  - Well-circumscribed subcutaneous mass

Radiographic Findings

- Radiographically occult soft tissue mass
- Osseous lesions appear lytic with sclerotic margin ± soft tissue swelling

CT Findings

- Soft tissue attenuation mass in subcutaneous fat
  - High lipid content can produce low attenuation

MR Findings

- T1WI
  - Predominantly isointense to muscle with mild heterogeneous signal ranging from low to high
- T2WI FS
  - Hyperintense signal plus ↑ or ↓ signal debris
    - Low signal debris = keratin (may calcify)
    - High signal debris = cholesterol crystals
    - Debris may be positionally dependent
    - Debris may be linear to rounded
  - Fluid-fluid levels reported
- T1WI C+ FS
  - Absent to low-level central enhancement with enhancing capsule
- Imaging appearance dependent on cyst contents

Ultrasonographic Findings

- Well-circumscribed, heterogeneously hypoechoic to hyperechoic mass
- Claw sign of dermis surrounding superficial portion of lesion suggests intradermal location
- Posterior acoustic enhancement common
- Inflamed lesions may demonstrate blood flow

DIFFERENTIAL DIAGNOSIS

Sebaceous Cyst

- Arises from obstructed sebaceous gland
- Similar imaging appearance

Hematoma

- Lacks central enhancement
- Fluid-fluid levels

Glomus Tumor

- Nailbed location may erode distal phalanx producing similar radiographic appearance

Soft Tissue Abscess

- Thick, irregularly enhancing walls
- Can be associated with epidermal inclusion cyst rupture

PATHOLOGY

General Features

- Etiology
  - Ectopic implantation of epidermal tissue
    - Traumatic or developmental
  - Cystic ectasia of hair follicle infundibulum
    - Causes: Obstruction, inflammation, scarring
- Associated abnormalities
  - Gardner syndrome has ↑ risk of multiple lesions

Microscopic Features

- Simple cyst with walls resembling follicular infundibular or stratified squamous epithelium
- Laminated keratin or cholesterol cyst contents
- Additional findings associated with cyst rupture
  - Granulomatous reaction, granulation tissue, foreign body reaction, abscess, meningitis (intracranial)

CLINICAL ISSUES

Presentation

- Most common signs/symptoms
  - Majority are incidental findings
  - Firm, slowly growing, painless mass
    - Mobile or tethered to skin
- Other signs/symptoms
  - May report history of trauma, puncture, or injection

Demographics

- Age
  - 3rd-5th decades of life
- Gender
  - Mild male predominance

Natural History & Prognosis

- No local recurrence if completely resected

Treatment

- Simple excision is curative

DIAGNOSTIC CHECKLIST

Image Interpretation Pearls

- May be difficult to differentiate intrinsic high T1 signal from enhancement on T1WI C+ FS MR if pregadolinium T1WI FS MR not obtained

SELECTED REFERENCES

1. Melamud K et al: Diagnostic imaging of benign and malignant osseous tumors of the fingers. Radiographics. 34(7):1954-67, 2014

Rheumatoid Nodule

KEY FACTS

TERMINOLOGY

- Nonneoplastic soft tissue nodule that is most common extraarticular manifestation of rheumatoid arthritis

IMAGING

- Solitary or multiple nodules
- Well-defined rounded to infiltrative borders
- Subcutaneous, between skin & bony prominence
  - Most commonly found over olecranon and remainder of upper extremity extensor surface
- Soft tissue mass ± adjacent bone erosion
  - Calcification uncommon
- Continuity with adjacent bursa supports diagnosis
- Homogeneous to heterogeneous signal intensity ranging from isointense to ↓ signal compared with muscle on T1WI MR
- Heterogeneous ↓ to ↑ signal intensity on T2WI MR
- Diffuse homogeneous to predominantly peripheral heterogeneous enhancement
- Moderate FDG uptake (SUV max: 4.2) reported on PET/CT, mimicking tumor

PATHOLOGY

- Histologically similar nodules in systemic lupus erythematosus, Jaccoud arthropathy, ankylosing spondylitis, and agammaglobulinemia

CLINICAL ISSUES

- Nontender, palpable mass
  - Adherent to deep tissues or freely mobile
- Risk of infection and skin ulceration
- Rheumatoid factor seropositivity very common
  - Patients need not have rheumatoid arthritis to have rheumatoid nodules
- Epidemiology: 20-35% of patients with rheumatoid arthritis
  - Increased incidence in patients taking methotrexate
- Treatment with surgical excision, rheumatoid arthritis drugs, or intralesional corticosteroids

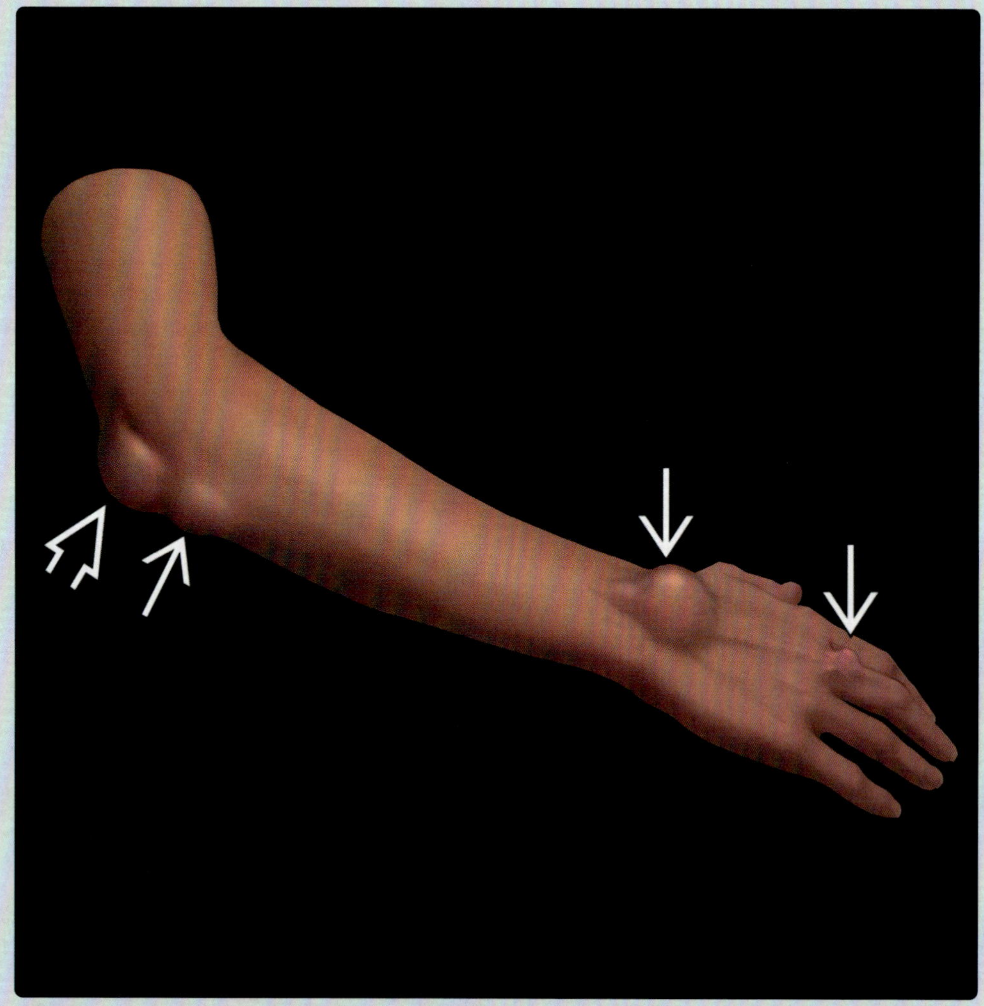

Graphic of the upper extremity shows multiple soft tissue nodules. The most common location for a rheumatoid nodule is over the olecranon process ➲. Location along the extensor surface of the remainder of the upper extremity is the 2nd most common site; additional nodules ➡ are shown involving the dorsal wrist, and dorsal finger. The firm, fleshy superficial nodules may be adherent to underlying structures or freely mobile. Imaging of these lesions can mimic a soft tissue neoplasm, abscess, crystal disease, and foreign body granuloma. Positive serum rheumatoid factor and additional imaging findings of arthropathy can help suggest the diagnosis.

TERMINOLOGY

Definitions

- Nonneoplastic soft tissue nodule that is most common extraarticular manifestation of rheumatoid arthritis

IMAGING

General Features

- Location
  - Subcutaneous, between skin & bony prominence
    - Most commonly found over olecranon and remainder of upper extremity extensor surface
    - Also found in gluteal region, Achilles tendon region, femoral trochanter, ischial tuberosity, occiput, and heel pad
  - Noncutaneous locations less common
    - Lungs, synovium, dura matter, mesentery, sclera, retropharyngeal tissue, and heart
    - Arthroplasty cement-bone interface
- Size
  - Few millimeters to > 6 cm
- Morphology
  - Rounded, well-defined to infiltrative borders
  - Solitary or multiple nodules

Radiographic Findings

- Soft tissue mass ± adjacent bone erosion
- Calcification uncommon

MR Findings

- T1WI FS
  - Homogeneous to heterogeneous signal intensity ranging from isointense to ↓ signal compared with muscle
- T2WI FS
  - Heterogeneous low to high signal intensity
    - ± very high-signal cystic regions
- T1WI C+ FS
  - Diffuse homogeneous to predominantly peripheral heterogeneous enhancement
- Continuity with adjacent bursa supports diagnosis

Nuclear Medicine Findings

- PET/CT
  - Moderate FDG uptake (SUV max: 4.2) reported

DIFFERENTIAL DIAGNOSIS

Soft Tissue Abscess

- Irregular peripheral enhancement
- Systemic symptoms of infection

Soft Tissue Neoplasm

- Benign and malignant soft tissue neoplasms may have similar imaging appearance
- Giant cell tumor of tendon sheath is most common mimic
- Other mimics include ganglion/synovial cyst, lymphoma, and sarcoma

Foreign Body

- Intermediate signal of granulomatous reaction
- Low signal foreign body may be visible on MR

Gout

- Calcification of tophi helps differentiate from rheumatoid nodule

Rheumatoid Nodulosis

- Atypical variant of rheumatoid disease (controversial)
- Multiple subcutaneous nodules without systemic manifestations of rheumatoid arthritis
  - a.k.a. pseudorheumatoid nodules
- Imaging reveals osseous defects with preservation of joint spaces and mineralization

PATHOLOGY

General Features

- Etiology
  - Pathogenesis controversial
    - Trauma/pressure and vasculitis suggested

Microscopic Features

- Soft tissue mass with 3 histologic zones
  - Central necrosis ± cyst formation
  - Intermediate zone of elongated histiocytic-like cells
  - Peripheral granulation tissue

CLINICAL ISSUES

Presentation

- Most common signs/symptoms
  - Nontender, palpable mass
    - Often adherent to deep fascia or periosteum
    - May be freely mobile
  - Rheumatoid factor seropositivity very common
  - Histologically identical nodules found in systemic lupus erythematosus, Jaccoud arthropathy, ankylosing spondylitis, and agammaglobulinemia
- Other signs/symptoms
  - ± severe articular symptoms & vasculitis

Demographics

- Gender
  - Male predominance for rheumatoid nodules
    - Rheumatoid arthritis has overall female predominance (3:1)
- Epidemiology
  - 20-35% of patients with rheumatoid arthritis
  - Increased incidence in patients taking methotrexate

Natural History & Prognosis

- Risk of infection and skin ulceration

Treatment

- May spontaneously regress
- Antirheumatic drugs, intralesional corticosteroids
- Surgical excision for infection, neurovascular compression or ↓ range of motion

SELECTED REFERENCES

1. Plymale M et al: Isolated intra-articular pseudorheumatoid nodule of the knee. Skeletal Radiol. 40(4):463-6, 2011
2. Sanders TG et al: Rheumatoid nodule of the foot: MRI appearances mimicking an indeterminate soft tissue mass. Skeletal Radiol. 27(8):457-60, 1998

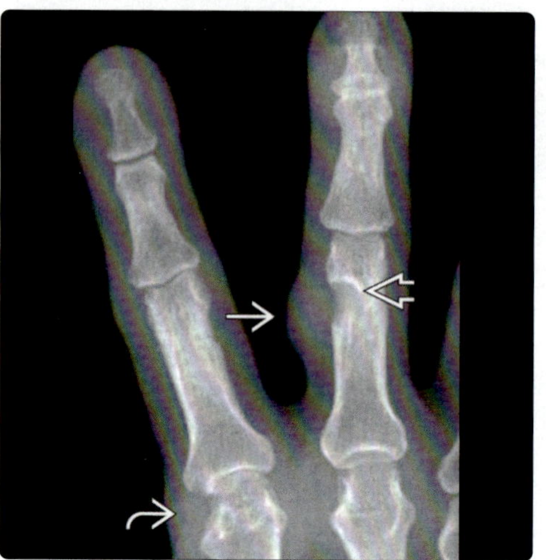

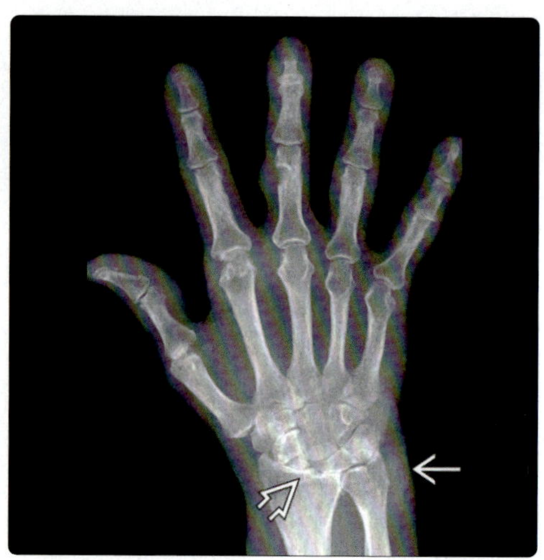

(Left) *Posteroanterior radiograph of the fingers shows a focal soft tissue nodule ➡, which causes scalloping of the underlying bone ➡. Note the decreased cartilage width at the 2nd MCP joint, along with the marginal erosion ➡.* **(Right)** *Posteroanterior radiograph in the same patient shows soft tissue swelling over the ulnar styloid ➡, complete loss of cartilage at the radiocarpal joint, with erosive changes and ulnar translocation of the carpus ➡. This is typical for rheumatoid arthritis.*

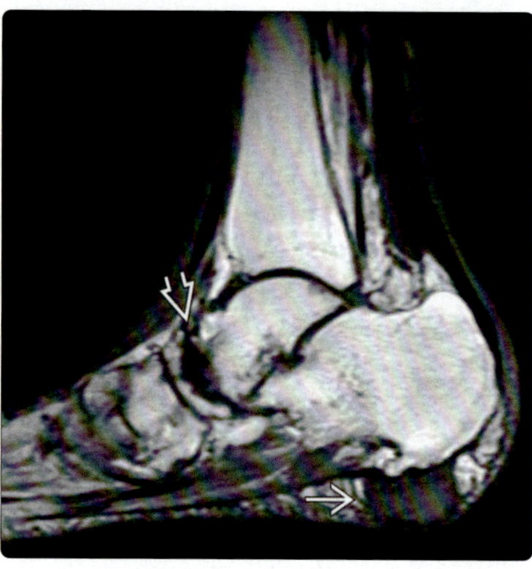

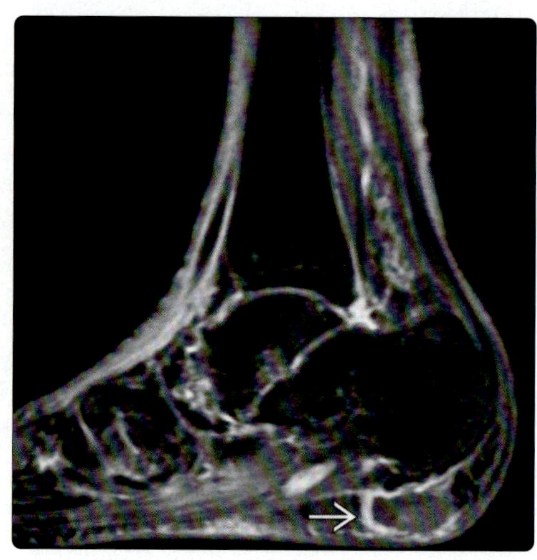

(Left) *Sagittal T1WI MR shows an ovoid mass ➡ in the subcutaneous fat plantar to the calcaneus. This mass has signal intensity that is similar to skeletal muscle. The mass borders are well defined. Extensive erosions and joint space narrowing ➡ involve the hindfoot and midfoot that are typical for rheumatoid arthritis.* **(Right)** *Sagittal T1WI C+ FS MR shows heterogeneous enhancement of the mass ➡, which is predominantly peripheral in location. Less than 1% of rheumatoid nodules occur in the foot.*

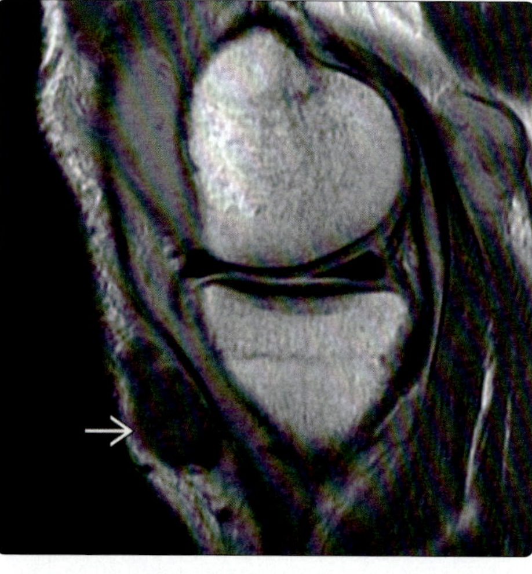

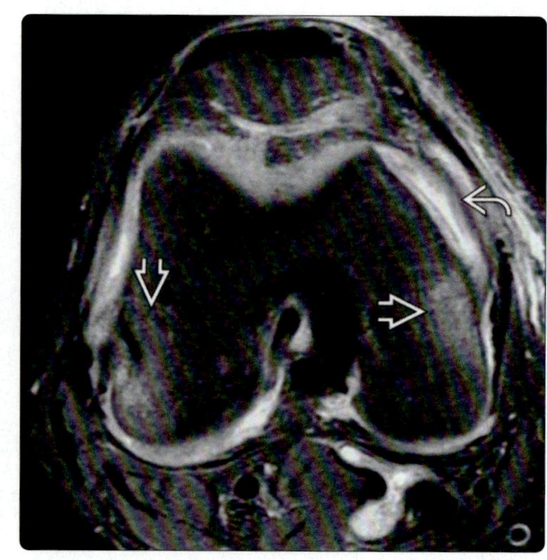

(Left) *Sagittal PDWI MR of the knee shows a rheumatoid nodule ➡ at the level of the tibial tubercle in a patient with known rheumatoid arthritis. The lobulated nodule is isointense to slightly hypointense relative to skeletal muscle. Lower extremity location is uncommon, but origin near a bony prominence is typical.* **(Right)** *Axial PDWI FS MR in the same patient shows additional findings of rheumatoid arthritis, including an effusion, synovitis ➡, and reactive bone edema ➡.*

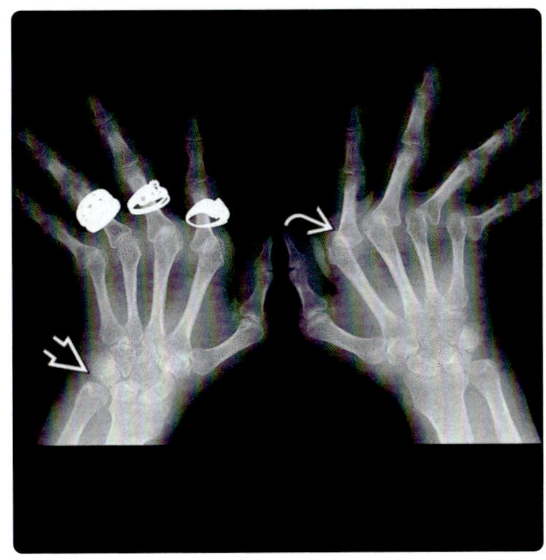

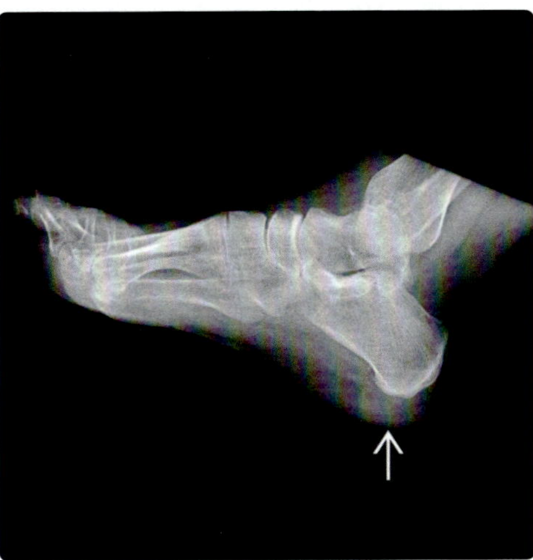

(Left) *PA radiograph of the hands shows metacarpophalangeal joint space narrowing and ulnar deviation ➡ of the fingers. Pan-carpal joint space narrowing involving the wrists and erosion of each ulnar styloid tip ➡ is seen bilaterally. The appearance is typical for rheumatoid arthritis.* **(Right)** *Lateral radiograph of the foot in the same patient demonstrates a nonspecific, rounded soft tissue mass ➡ in the subcutaneous fat between the skin of the heel and the calcaneal tuberosity.*

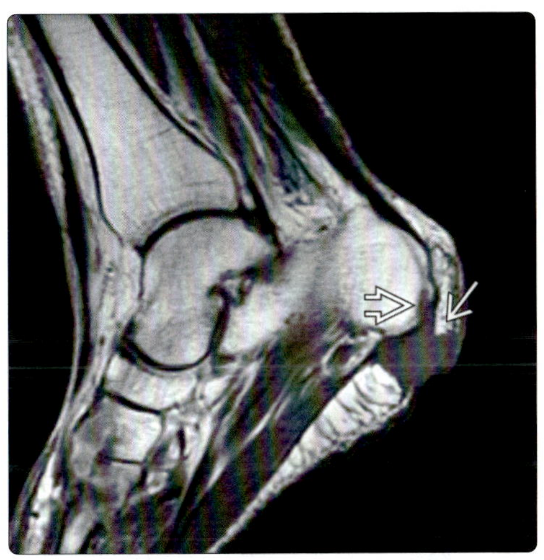

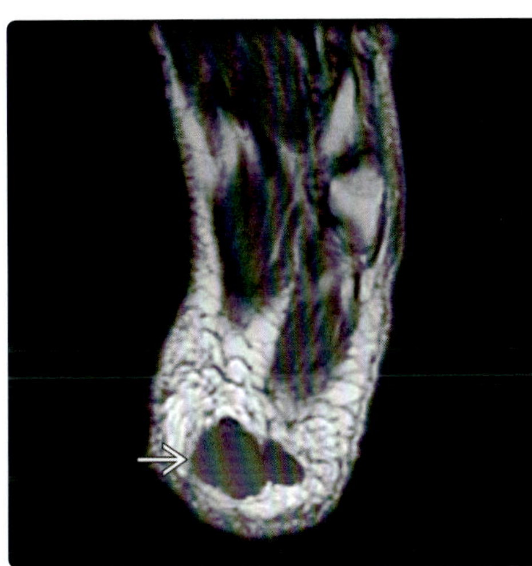

(Left) *Sagittal T1WI MR in the same patient demonstrates a well-defined mass ➡ with signal intensity similar to skeletal muscle. A small erosion ➡ is present in the adjacent calcaneal bone. No additional erosions were present involving the hindfoot or midfoot.* **(Right)** *Axial T1WI MR in the same patient shows the relatively homogeneous subcutaneous mass ➡ to have a bilobed contour. The findings typical for rheumatoid arthritis seen in the hands are most helpful for suggesting rheumatoid nodule.*

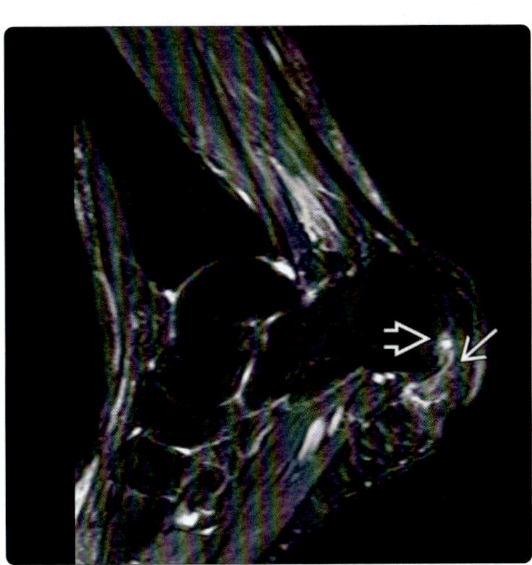

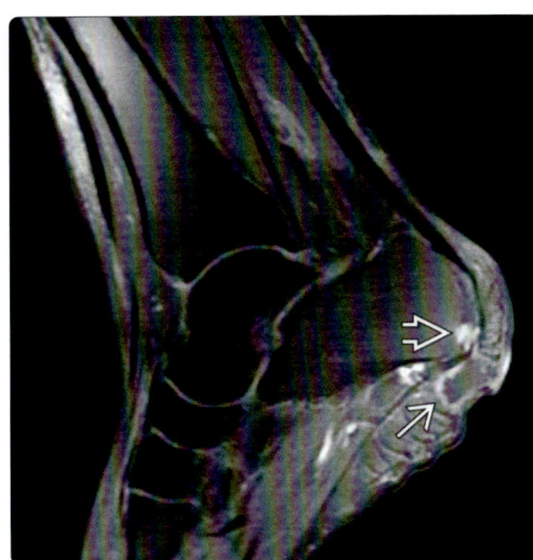

(Left) *Sagittal STIR MR in the same patient shows the nodule ➡ to have heterogeneous signal ranging from hypointense to hyperintense relative to skeletal muscle. The small erosion ➡ involving the calcaneal tuberosity is high in signal.* **(Right)** *Sagittal T1WI C+ FS MR in the same case shows the mass ➡ to have predominantly peripheral enhancement. The small calcaneal erosion ➡ also enhances. An abscess with associated osteomyelitis would be in the differential diagnosis for this lesion.*

KEY FACTS

TERMINOLOGY

- Relatively uncommon cause of soft tissue mass

IMAGING

- Abdominal wall > back and periscapular region > thigh > chest wall
- Primary tumor of origin: Skin ≥ lung, breast > kidney, colon, rectum
    - Primary site of origin unknown in 13.5%
- Metastasis location does not correlate with primary tumor location
- Imaging appearance is nonspecific
    - Well-defined to infiltrative mass
    - Biopsy necessary for diagnosis
- Isodense to hypodense to muscle on CT
- Isointense to hypointense to muscle on T1WI
    - Metastatic melanoma may have ↑ signal on T1WI MR due to paramagnetic effect of melanin
- Heterogeneously hyperintense on fluid-sensitive MR
- Homogeneous to heterogeneous enhancement on CT and MR

PATHOLOGY

- Tumor type: Carcinoma > > malignant melanoma > sarcoma and carcinosarcoma
- Metastasis may be misidentified as primary soft tissue malignancy
- Primary epithelioid sarcoma may be misidentified as metastatic carcinoma at pathology

CLINICAL ISSUES

- Median age: 53 yr
- Patients may or may not have history of primary malignancy
- < 2% of all soft tissue tumors
    - Solitary late metastasis in 70%
    - Initial manifestation of malignancy in 27%
    - Disseminated metastases in 2.5%
- More likely to be painful than sarcoma

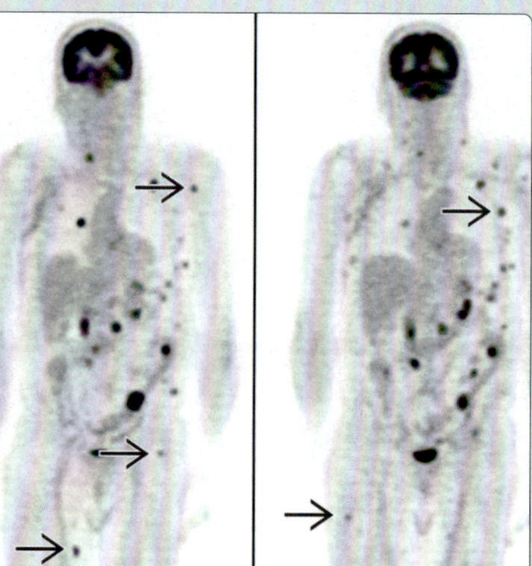

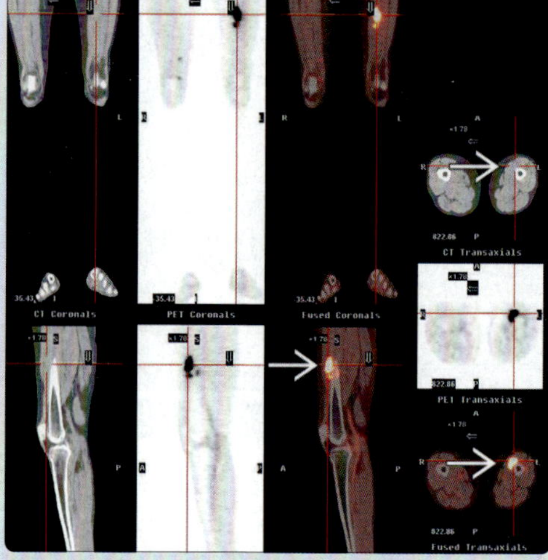

(Left) *Coronal PET shows innumerable foci of abnormal tracer uptake predominantly involving the soft tissues ➡ and organs. This elderly man underwent this exam for staging of a newly discovered forearm malignant melanoma. He was asymptomatic.* **(Right)** *Multiplanar fused PET/CT shows a dominant focus of metastatic melanoma ➡ involving the musculature of the left thigh. This lesion had a maximum SUV of 18.7. The lesion is slightly hypodense to skeletal muscle on the unenhanced CT images.*

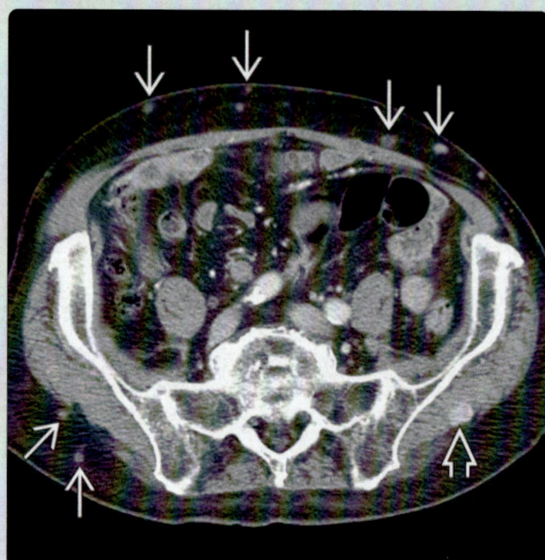

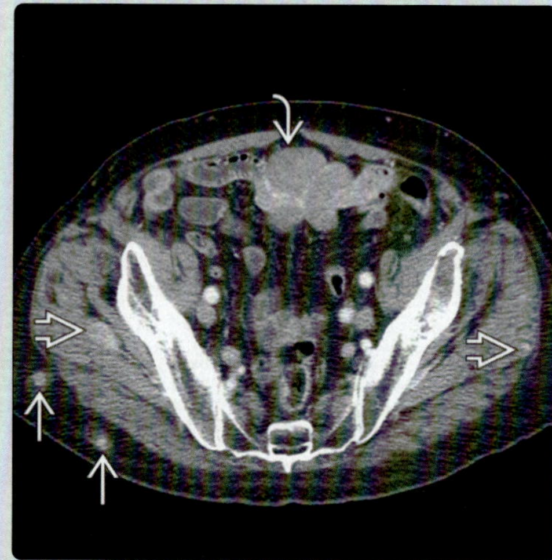

(Left) *Axial CECT in the same patient shows numerous metastatic lesions, which involve the subcutaneous fat ➡ and skeletal muscle ➡. The subcutaneous metastases are isodense to skeletal muscle.* **(Right)** *Noncontiguous axial CECT shows subcutaneous ➡, mesenteric ➡, and skeletal muscle ➡ metastases. The skeletal muscle metastases enhance more intensely than the muscle metastases. In this case, melanoma had also spread to the lymph nodes, lungs, mediastinum, bones, and pancreas.*

IMAGING

General Features

- Location
  - Abdominal wall > back and periscapular region > thigh > chest wall
    - Discussion excludes organ metastases, direct extension from primary lesion, adenopathy, lymphoma, leukemia, and myeloma
  - Deep > superficial to fascia
  - Primary tumor of origin: Skin ≥ lung, breast > kidney, colon, rectum
    - May spread from any primary tumor location
      - Metastasis location does not correlate with primary tumor location
    - Primary site of origin unknown in 13.5%
      - Most commonly poorly differentiated adenocarcinoma
- Size
  - Variable; mean: 8.3 mm
- Morphology
  - Well-defined to infiltrative mass

Imaging Recommendations

- Imaging appearance is nonspecific
- Biopsy necessary for diagnosis

CT Findings

- Isodense to hypodense to muscle
- Variable enhancement

MR Findings

- Isointense to hypointense to muscle on T1WI
  - Metastatic melanoma may have ↑ signal on T1WI MR due to paramagnetic effect of melanin
- Heterogeneously hyperintense on fluid-sensitive MR
- Homogeneous to heterogeneous enhancement
- Diffusion-weighted imaging shows different apparent diffusion coefficient (ADC) values in intramuscular masses
  - Metastases show broad range ADC values
  - Metastases & sarcoma significantly higher than lymphoma

DIFFERENTIAL DIAGNOSIS

Soft Tissue Sarcoma

- Can have similar imaging appearance
- Epithelioid sarcoma
  - Histologic mimic of metastatic carcinoma

Benign Soft Tissue Neoplasm

- Can have similar imaging appearance
- ↑ F18 FDG PET uptake by schwannoma may mimic metastatic disease on tumor staging studies

Lymph Node

- Has fatty hilum when not involved with tumor

Hematoma

- Heterogeneous mass due to degrading blood products
- Lacks internal enhancement

Soft Tissue Abscess

- Irregular peripheral enhancement
- Systemic signs of infection

PATHOLOGY

General Features

- Etiology
  - Tumor type: Carcinoma > > malignant melanoma > sarcoma and carcinosarcoma
    - Soft tissue sarcomas uncommonly metastasize to soft tissues
      - Leiomyosarcoma is primary sarcoma most likely to metastasize to other soft tissues
  - Relative paucity of metastases to skeletal muscle postulated due to variable blood flow, changing tissue pressure, low tissue oxygen tension, and changes in pH
    - Trauma may ↑ risk of skeletal muscle metastasis due to altering normal muscle physiology

Microscopic Features

- Histologic diagnosis can be challenging
  - Metastasis may be misidentified as primary soft tissue malignancy
  - Primary epithelioid sarcoma may be misidentified as metastatic carcinoma
- Use of immunohistochemical markers important

CLINICAL ISSUES

Presentation

- Most common signs/symptoms
  - Patients may or may not have history of primary malignancy
  - More painful than primary soft tissue sarcoma
    - Peripheral nerve sheath tumors also painful

Demographics

- Age
  - Median: 53 yr
    - Range: 20-87 yr
- Epidemiology
  - < 2% of all soft tissue tumors
    - Solitary late metastasis in 70%
    - Initial manifestation of malignancy in 27%
    - Disseminated metastases in 2.5%

Natural History & Prognosis

- Denotes stage IV disease regardless of primary tumor type or location

Treatment

- Treatment of metastatic disease highly variable based on tumor type and clinical presentation

SELECTED REFERENCES

1. Surov A et al: Comparison of ADC values in different malignancies of the skeletal musculature: a multicentric analysis. Skeletal Radiol. 44(7):995-1000, 2015
2. Abed R et al: Soft-tissue metastases: their presentation and origin. J Bone Joint Surg Br. 91(8):1083-5, 2009

(Left) *Coronal T1WI MR shows a focus of metastatic renal cell carcinoma ➡ to be located entirely within the subcutaneous fat. This mass has similar signal intensity to skeletal muscle.* **(Right)** *Coronal STIR MR in the same patient shows the metastasis ➡ to have mildly heterogeneous high signal. Note the absence of surrounding edema. The appearance of this mass is nonspecific. This patient also had metastatic renal carcinoma involving the lungs, lymph nodes, bones, and brain.*

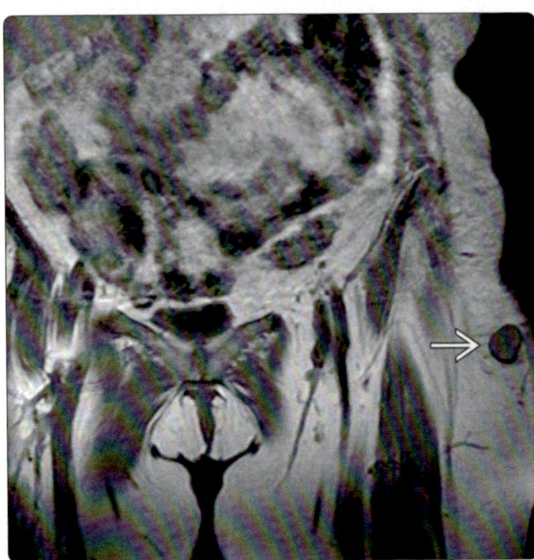

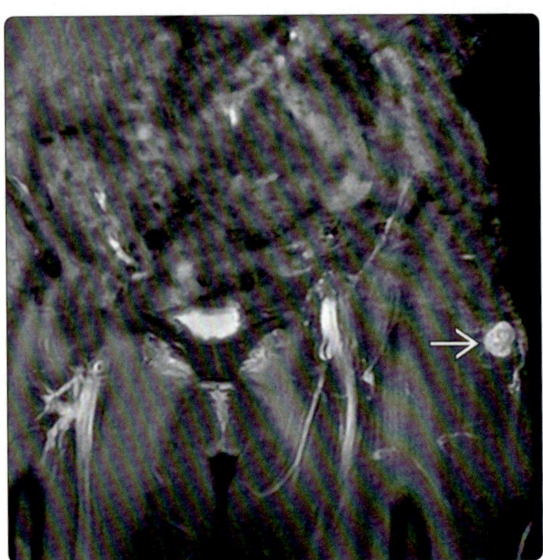

(Left) *Axial CECT in the same patient shows a rounded mass ➡ in the subcutaneous fat anterolateral to the left hip. This mass shows intense peripheral enhancement.* **(Right)** *Axial T2WI MR shows a heterogeneously hyperintense superficial mass ➡ in the left paraspinal region. Percutaneous biopsy confirmed metastatic poorly differentiated adenocarcinoma consistent with the patient's previous primary esophageal carcinoma. This patient died in less than 6 months.*

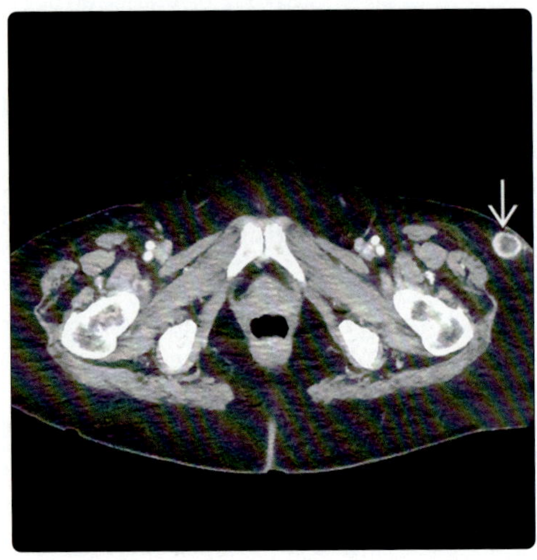

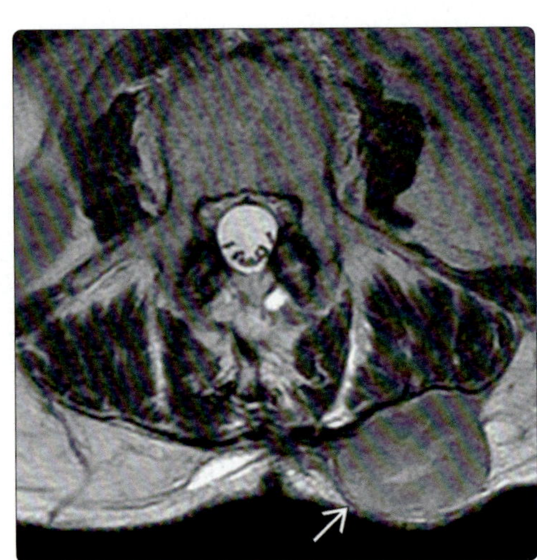

(Left) *Axial T1WI MR of the calf shows a mass ➡ within the medial head of the gastrocnemius muscle. The mass is homogeneous and slightly hypointense relative to skeletal muscle.* **(Right)** *Axial T2WI MR in the same patient shows the mass ➡ to have heterogeneous high signal intensity. On this sequence, the lesion appears more infiltrative than mass-like, which was a hint that it is not a sarcoma. Biopsy proved metastatic adenocarcinoma.*

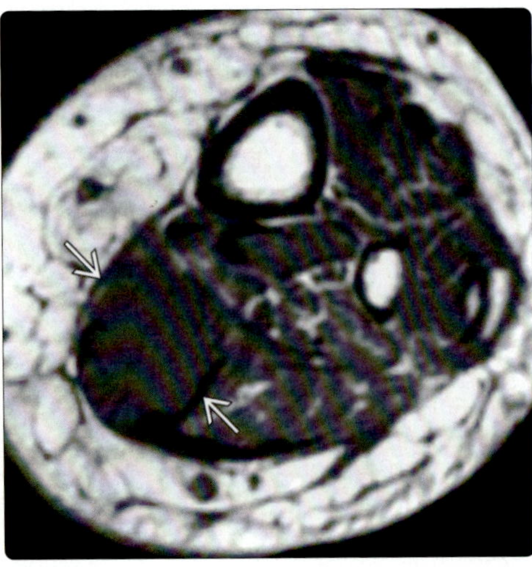

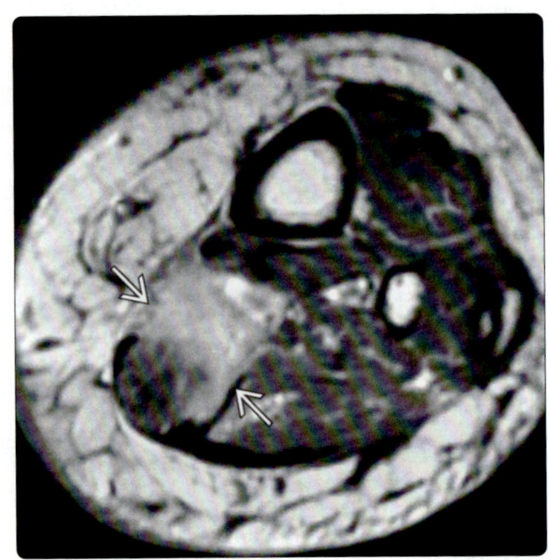

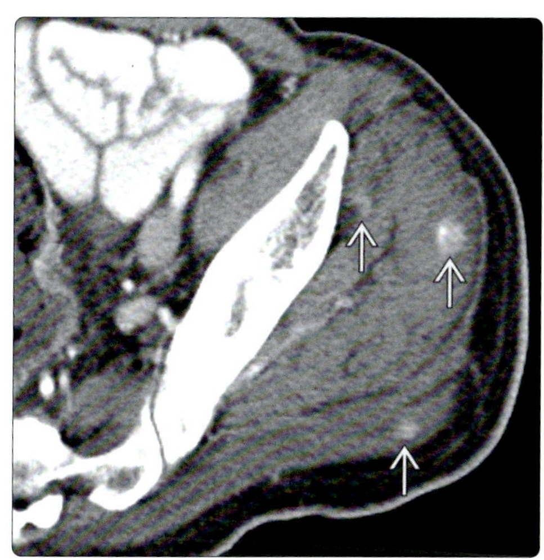

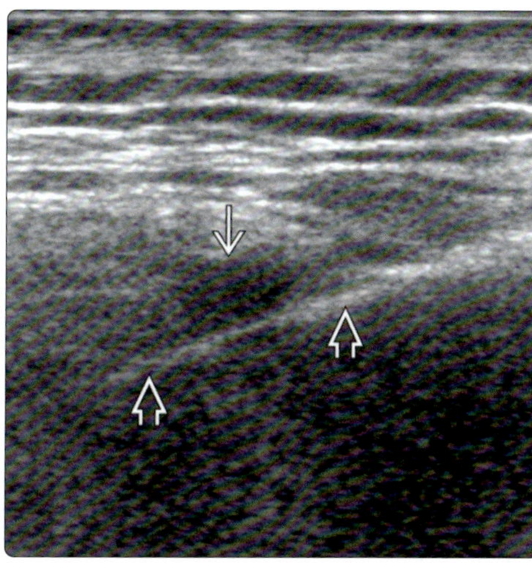

(Left) *Axial CECT of the left hemipelvis shows 3 enhancing intramuscular masses ➡. This patient had numerous similar skeletal muscle lesions throughout his body and later developed brain and adrenal metastases.* **(Right)** *Longitudinal oblique ultrasound in the same patient shows one of the left gluteal lesions ➡ to be homogeneously hypoechoic. The needle biopsy ➡ confirmed metastatic esophageal carcinoma in this patient who was status post esophagectomy.*

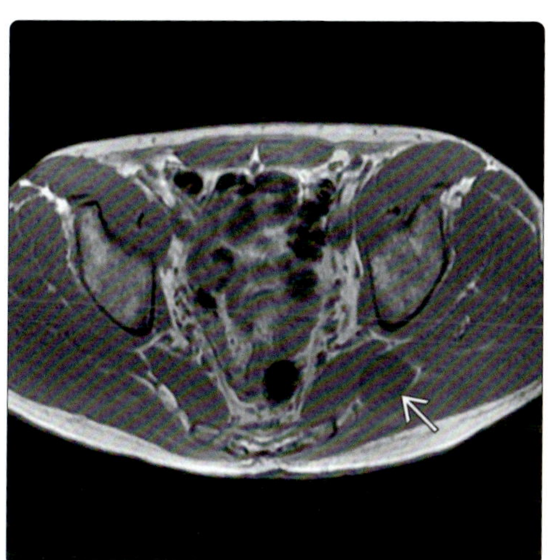

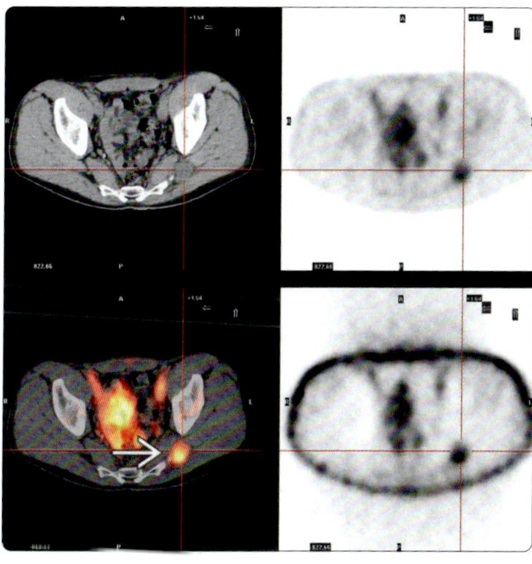

(Left) *Axial T1WI MR shows a homogeneously hypointense mass ➡ lying between the left piriformis and left gluteus maximus muscles. This patient had myxoid liposarcoma resected from a different site > 3 years prior. This is either a soft tissue or lymph node metastasis.* **(Right)** *Axial-fused PET/CT in the same patient shows F-18 FDG uptake of the lesion ➡ with a maximum SUV of 2.8. Myxoid liposarcomas are one of the few soft tissue sarcomas that have a propensity to metastasize to other soft tissues.*

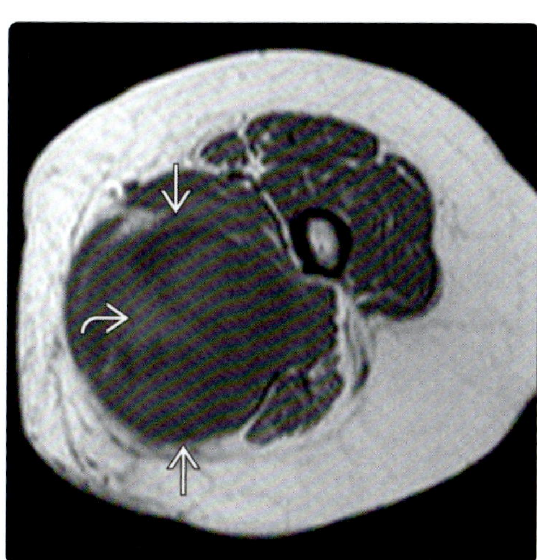

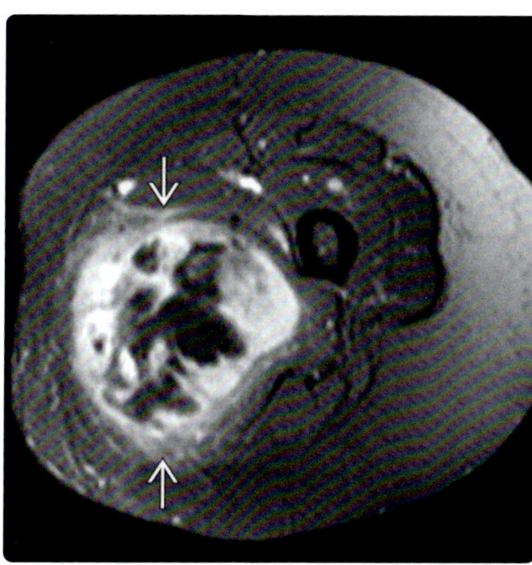

(Left) *Axial T1WI MR shows a leiomyosarcoma ➡ that has metastasized from the uterus to the soft tissues of the proximal thigh. This heterogeneous mass has regions of increased signal intensity relative to muscle ➡ due to hemorrhage.* **(Right)** *Axial T1WI C+ FS MR shows heterogeneous enhancement of the mass ➡. The appearance of this mass is nonspecific, with sarcomas having a similar appearance. The history of prior uterine leiomyosarcoma removal is key in suggesting the correct diagnosis for this case.*

Melanoma

KEY FACTS

TERMINOLOGY

- Malignant tumor of melanocytes usually appearing as skin lesion that is asymmetric, with irregular border, uneven color, and diameter > 6 mm

IMAGING

- Primary lesions are uncommonly imaged
- MR or ultrasound to evaluate for satellite (< 2-3 cm from primary) or in-transit metastases
- F-18 FDG PET/CT for whole body staging
  - Use nonattenuation corrected PET images to evaluate skin
- CT superior to PET for lung metastases < 6 mm
- Primary lesions and soft tissue metastases appear as masses isodense to skeletal muscle on CT
- MR findings
  - Isointense to skeletal muscle on T1WI MR ± hyperintense signal secondary to paramagnetic effect of melanin
    - Metastases often hemorrhagic, thus also having ↑ T1WI MR signal
  - Homogeneous to heterogeneously hyperintense to hypointense relative to skeletal muscle on T2WI MR
- Bone metastases usually lytic but may be sclerotic or mixed lytic and sclerotic
- US: Well-defined hypoechoic lesion beneath echogenic epidermis ± ↑ through-transmission

CLINICAL ISSUES

- 1 in 55 lifetime risk for melanoma in USA
- Majority of melanomas arise de novo
- Metastases can involve any tissue in any part of body

DIAGNOSTIC CHECKLIST

- Number and location of suspicious lymph nodes important for staging
- Document size and specific location of all satellite and in-transit disease for surgical resection

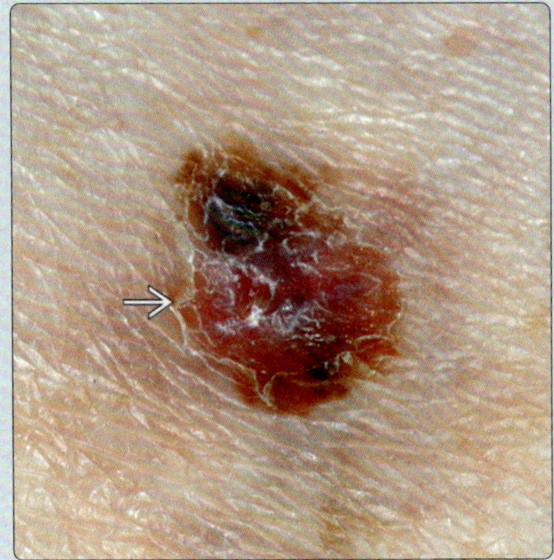
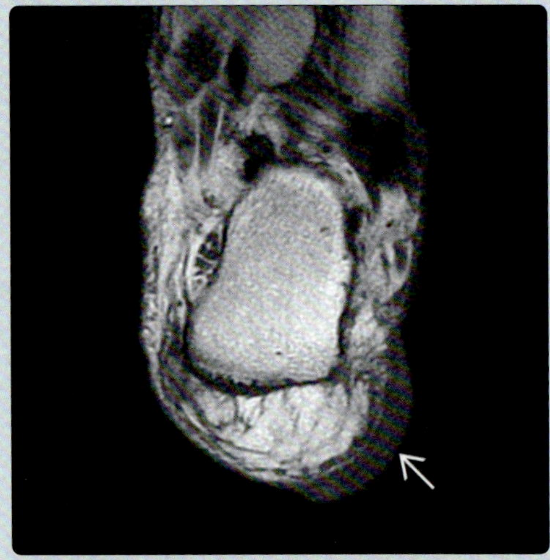

(Left) *Clinical photograph of a melanoma ➡. This skin lesion is asymmetric, having an irregular border, uneven color, and a size > 6 mm. Initial biopsy would involve only a portion of the lesion or narrow margins so as not to disrupt the lymphatic drainage for future sentinel lymph node identification.* **(Right)** *Coronal T1WI MR of the hindfoot shows a raised lesion ➡ involving the lateral aspect of the heel. This lesion is contiguous with the skin surface and has a signal intensity similar to skeletal muscle.*

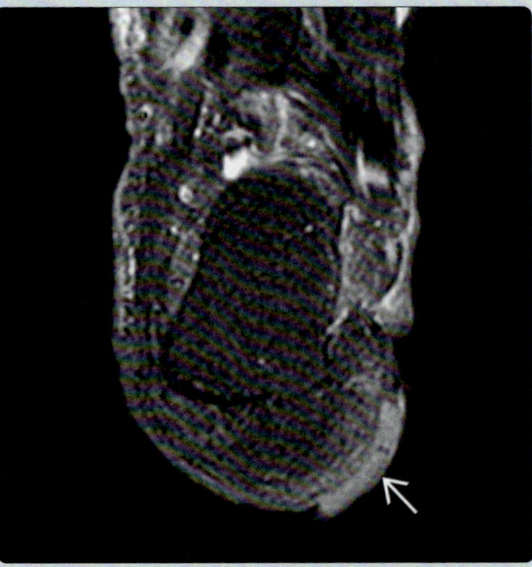
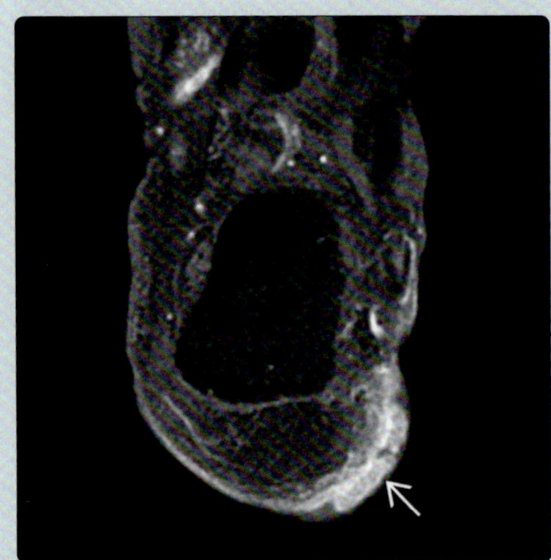

(Left) *Coronal T2WI FS MR in the same patient shows the skin lesion ➡ to be hyperintense relative to muscle. The MR appearance is nonspecific.* **(Right)** *Coronal T1WI C+ FS MR in the same patient shows heterogeneous enhancement of the lesion ➡, which was biopsy-proven to represent a melanoma. This 85-year-old woman had been initially treated in a wound clinic due to ulceration of this mass. Despite the large size of this lesion, sentinel lymph node biopsy was negative.*

TERMINOLOGY

Synonyms

- Malignant melanoma

Definitions

- Malignant tumor of melanocytes usually appearing as skin lesion that is asymmetric, with irregular border, uneven color, and diameter > 6 mm

IMAGING

General Features

- Location
  - Face area is overall most common location for males and females
    - Females also have high incidence on lower extremities
    - Males also have high incidence on ear, head, neck, back, and shoulders
    - Non-Caucasian patients more likely to develop melanomas in nonpigmented skin areas
- Size
  - Typically > 6 mm
- Morphology
  - Asymmetric superficial skin lesion with uneven pigmentation and irregular border

Imaging Recommendations

- Best imaging tool
  - Primary lesions are uncommonly imaged
  - MR or ultrasound to evaluate for locoregional lymphatic metastases
    - Satellite (< 2 cm from primary)
    - In-transit (> 2 cm from primary but not beyond regional node basin)
  - F-18 FDG PET/CT for whole body staging
  - CT superior to PET for lung metastases < 6 mm
- Protocol advice
  - Use nonattenuation corrected PET images to evaluate skin
  - Extend PET imaging to cover entire body

CT Findings

- Primary lesions and soft tissue metastases appear as masses isodense to skeletal muscle
- Bone metastases usually lytic but may be sclerotic or mixed lytic and sclerotic

MR Findings

- Primary lesions appear as mass contiguous with skin
  - Isointense to skeletal muscle on T1WI MR; may have areas of hyperintense signal secondary to paramagnetic effect of melanin
  - Variable: Homogeneous to heterogeneously hyperintense to hypointense relative to skeletal muscle on T2WI MR
  - Intense enhancement with variable pattern
    - Homogeneous, heterogeneous, nodular, or ring enhancement
- Soft tissue metastases have similar imaging characteristics as primary lesion, except lesions often not contiguous with skin surface
  - Metastases commonly hemorrhagic, resulting in ↑ T1WI MR signal

Ultrasonographic Findings

- Useful for evaluation of primary melanoma, in-transit metastasis, satellite metastasis, and lymphadenopathy
- Primary melanoma: Well-defined hypoechoic lesion beneath echogenic epidermis ± mild ↑ through-transmission
- Soft tissue metastases: Hypoechoic nodule with irregular to lobulated margin ± low-level internal echoes and ↑ through-transmission

Image-Guided Biopsy

- Biopsy of primary lesions usually performed by dermatologist
  - Important that initial biopsy does not interfere with subsequent lymphatic mapping and sentinel lymph node biopsy (avoid wide tumor margins)

Nuclear Medicine Findings

- PET/CT
  - Primary and metastatic melanoma F-18 FDG avid

DIFFERENTIAL DIAGNOSIS

Congenital Nevus

- Round to oval skin lesion with homogeneous pigmentation and even, well-circumscribed border

Granuloma Pyogenicum

- Clinical mimic of ulcerated melanoma

Seborrheic Keratosis and Common Wart

- Clinical mimics of verrucous melanoma

PATHOLOGY

General Features

- Etiology
  - Environmental factors: Sun exposure (UV radiation), agricultural chemical exposure
    - Childhood sun exposure is main risk factor for melanoma development
      - Multiple sunburns and high sun exposure in adulthood also contributes to risk
    - Head and neck melanomas usually related to sun exposure
    - Acral melanoma related to agricultural chemical and UV radiation exposure
  - Genetic/familial factors: Family history of skin cancer, clinically atypical nevi, ↑ number of nevi, skin type, immune deficiency
    - Trunk melanomas usually associated with multiple melanotic nevi
  - Majority of melanomas arise de novo
    - 20-30% arise within preexisting melanocytic nevus
- Genetics
  - Familial melanoma (< 1% of cases): *CDKN2A/p16* on chromosome 9p21, *CDK4* on chromosome 12

Staging, Grading, & Classification

- American Joint Committee on Cancer staging
  - Clinical and pathologic staging tables

- Includes primary tumor thickness, regional lymph node, and distant metastatic disease status
  - Primary tumor thickness established histologically
  - Regional lymph node involvement grading depends on number of nodes and macrometastasis vs. micrometastasis
  - Distant metastasis grading varies by location
    - Metastases to skin, subcutaneous tissue, and distant lymph nodes is denoted differently than metastases to lung or other viscera
- Histologic grade not utilized
- Staging studies utilized varies by institution
  - Sentinel lymph node biopsy, PET/CT, MR, CT
  - Brain imaging recommended for even minimal central nervous system findings

Gross Pathologic & Surgical Features

- Irregular dermal lesion with indistinct borders and color ranging from whitish to gray &/or black

Microscopic Features

- 4 main histologic subtypes
  - Superficial spreading melanoma, nodular melanoma, lentigo maligna melanoma, and acral lentiginous melanoma
- Atypical intraepithelial melanocytes
  - Epithelioid, fusiform, or mixture of both cell types
  - Dispersed and sporadic arrangement
- Abnormal mitotic activity
- Surrounding inflammatory reaction common

CLINICAL ISSUES

Presentation

- Most common signs/symptoms
  - Begins as flat brown macule progressing to unevenly pigmented plaque with irregular nodules
  - "ABCD" mnemonic
    - **A**symmetry, irregular **b**order, uneven **c**olor, **d**iameter > 6 mm
  - Some melanomas are small, homogeneous lesions with sharp margins
- Other signs/symptoms
  - Pain, bleeding, itching, or ulceration
- Clinical profile
  - Nodular melanoma is most aggressive type
  - Superficial spreading melanoma more common in younger patients
  - Acral lentiginous melanoma most common melanoma in patients with heavily pigmented skin
    - Palms of hands, soles of feet, under nails
  - Lentigo maligna melanoma most common in head and neck of elderly patients
  - Amelanotic melanoma most common on face
  - Mucosal melanoma often multifocal
  - Subungual melanoma often associated with pigmented longitudinal streak

Demographics

- Age
  - Children to elderly patients
    - Median age: 59 years
- Gender
  - 16th most common cancer in men
  - 15th most common cancer in women
- Epidemiology
  - Most common in Caucasians
    - ↑ incidence with personal or family history of melanoma, skin type 1 or 2, multiple melanocytic nevi, giant congenital nevi, and xeroderma pigmentosa
      - 4-8% lifetime risk of developing 2nd primary
  - Highest incidence in Australia
  - Overall lifetime risk for melanoma in USA is 1 in 55
    - > 8,000 USA patients die of melanoma per year

Natural History & Prognosis

- 5-year survival rates improving
  - 90% for localized disease, primary tumor < 1 mm deep
    - 50-90% if primary tumor > 1 mm deep
  - 20-70% for regional disease (stage III)
  - < 10% for distant metastatic disease (stage IV)
- Positive sentinel lymph node biopsy has ↓ prognosis
  - 55% recurrence rate within 42 months
  - 0.5-3.7% have concurrent clinically occult distant metastatic disease
- Metastases can involve any tissue in any part of body
  - Metastases to lymph nodes and skin common (55%)
  - Visceral metastases and high number of lymph node metastases have worse clinical prognosis
  - Can metastasize with unpredictable pattern
  - Metastases may present up to 25 years after diagnosis
- Spontaneous regression of primary melanoma is poor prognostic sign associated with metastatic disease

Treatment

- Treatment varies by surgical stage
- Wide surgical excision ± sentinel lymph node biopsy
  - Additional options for in-transit disease include surgical resection, complete lymph node dissection, hyperthermic perfusion/infusion with melphalan, intralesional injection, and radiotherapy
- Higher stages of disease offered clinical trial participation or interferon alfa

DIAGNOSTIC CHECKLIST

Reporting Tips

- Number and location of suspicious lymph nodes important for staging
- Accurate, comprehensive documentation of size and location of satellite and in-transit disease important because surgical resection may be undertaken, unlike metastases in most other diseases

SELECTED REFERENCES

1. Rahim S et al: Correlation of PUV and SUV in the extremities while using PEM as a high-resolution positron emission scanner. Skeletal Radiol. 43(4):453-8, 2014
2. Catalano O et al: Locoregional spread of cutaneous melanoma: sonography findings. AJR Am J Roentgenol. 194(3):735-45, 2010
3. Melanoma of the skin staging form. In AJCC Cancer Staging Manual. 7th ed. New York: Springer. 341-4, 2010

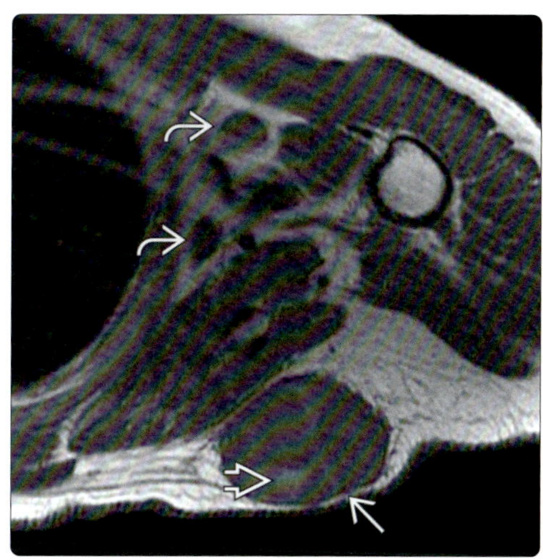

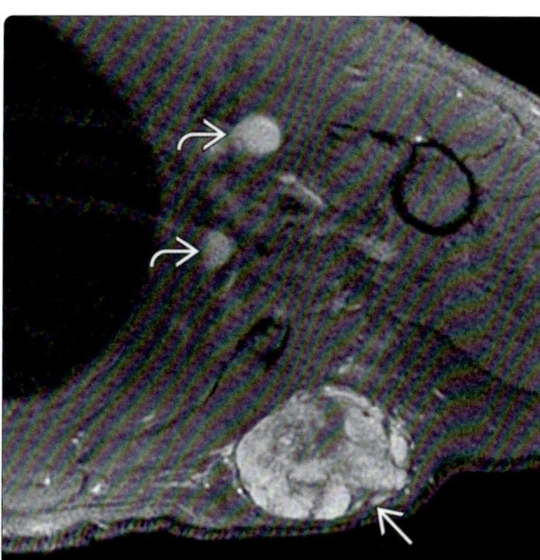

(Left) *Axial T1WI MR shows a large, rounded mass in the subcutaneous fat of the upper back. The mass is isointense to muscle with regions of hyperintense signal. Axillary lymph nodes are enlarged.* **(Right)** *Axial T2WI FS MR shows the dominant mass to have heterogeneously hyperintense signal. Enlarged axillary lymph nodes are homogeneously hyperintense. The patient had noted fullness in these regions for 18 months. Four years prior, he had several skin lesions removed from his arm.*

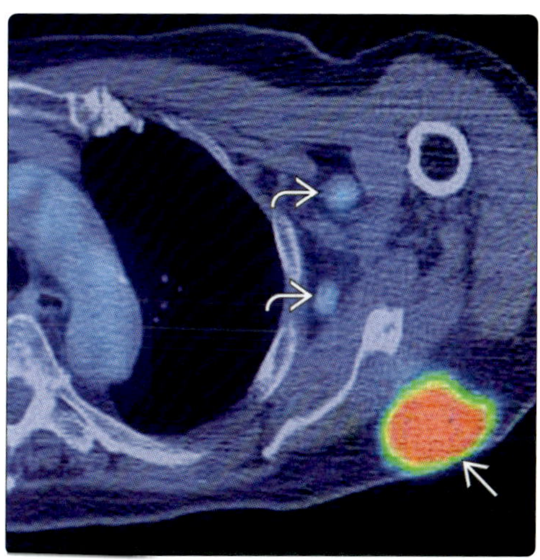

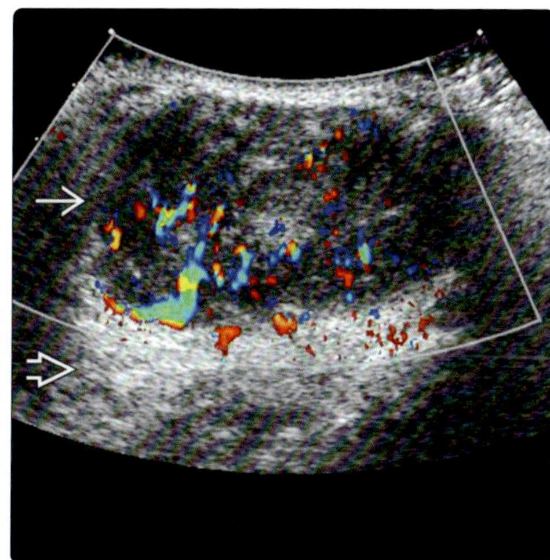

(Left) *Axial fused PET/CT in the same patient shows avid F-18 FDG uptake within the mass. Less intense radiotracer uptake involves axillary lymph nodes, which were proven to reflect additional metastatic disease.* **(Right)** *Longitudinal color Doppler ultrasound in the same patient shows the left posterior chest wall mass to have heterogeneous echogenicity. Prominent color Doppler reflects hypervascularity of the lesion. There is mild increased through-transmission.*

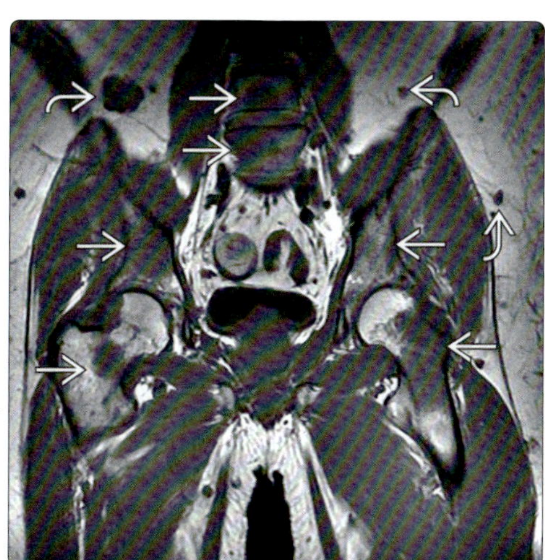

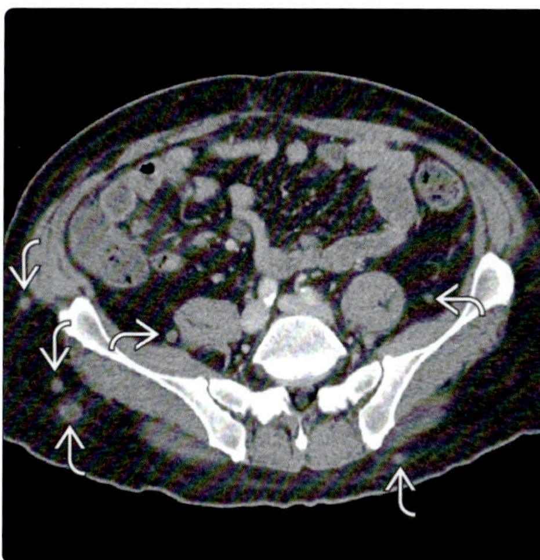

(Left) *Coronal T1WI MR shows extensive metastatic melanoma. Metastases involved the bones and soft tissues, having a similar signal intensity as skeletal muscle. This patient presented with painless jaundice due to a pancreatic metastasis. The remainder of his metastatic disease was asymptomatic.* **(Right)** *Axial CECT shows numerous soft tissue metastases that are isodense to slightly hypodense relative to skeletal muscle. The primary site of melanoma was never discovered.*

(Left) *Axial T1WI MR shows an ill-defined mass ➡ predominantly located in the subcutaneous fat of the medial calf. The mass has mildly heterogeneous signal intensity, which is isointense to slightly hyperintense relative to skeletal muscle.* **(Right)** *Axial T1WI C+ FS MR shows the mass ➡ to have heterogeneous intense enhancement. The mass invades the superficial fascia to involve the underlying calf musculature ↪. The appearance of this mass suggests a malignant process but is otherwise nonspecific.*

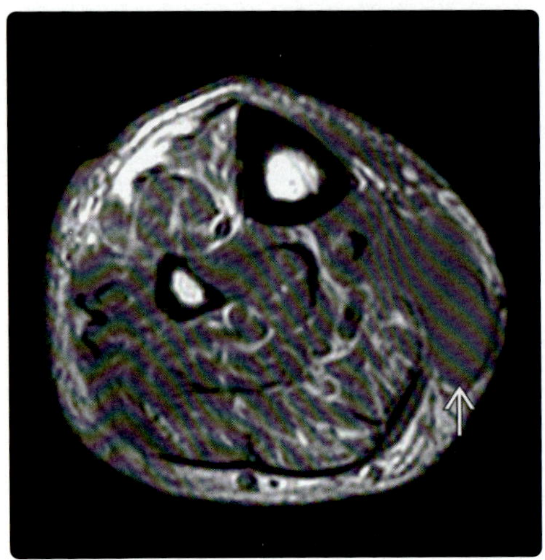

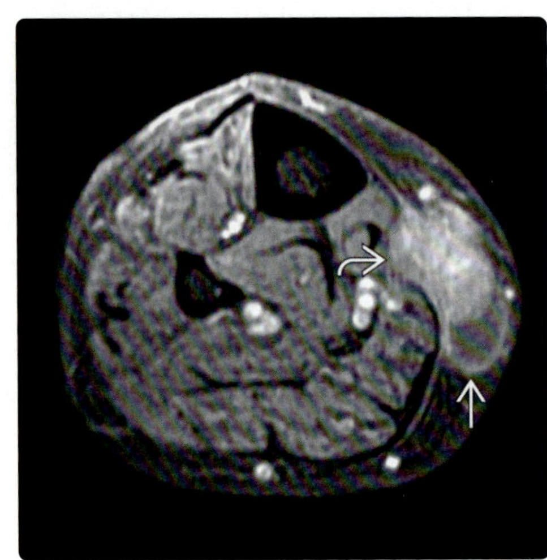

(Left) *Axial NECT obtained as part of a PET/CT study shows the mass ➡ to be isodense to muscle. This painless calf mass had been growing for the prior 2 years.* **(Right)** *Axial fused PET/CT shows the calf mass ➡ to have intense F-18 FDG uptake with a maximum SUV of 25.9. The PET scan also identified metastasis to a popliteal lymph node. Biopsy proved metastatic melanoma. This patient had a melanoma removed from his forearm 10 years prior. He died < 1 year after diagnosis of metastatic disease.*

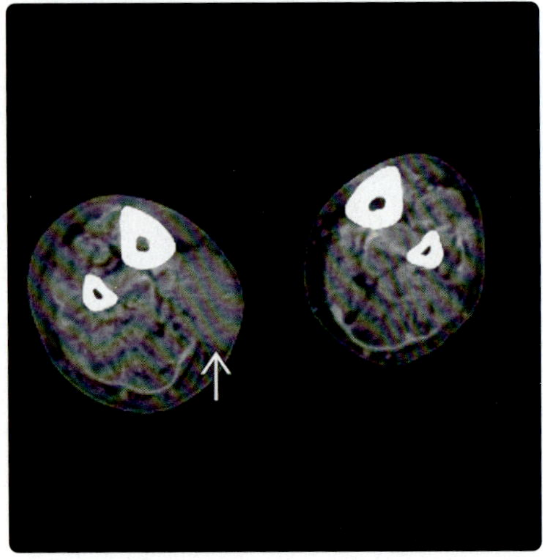

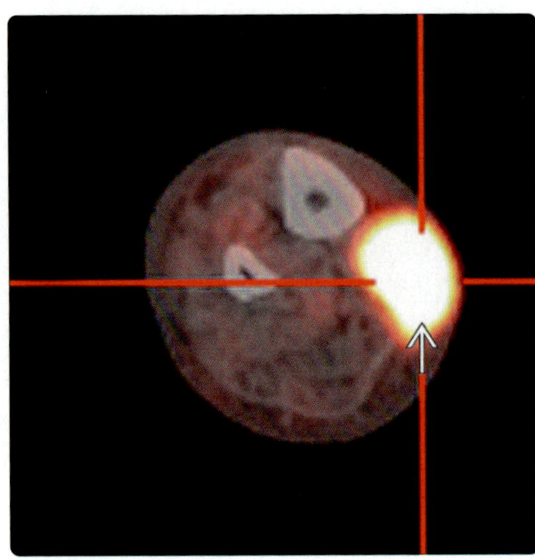

(Left) *Axial CECT of the sacrum shows a melanoma metastasis ➡ that is peripherally sclerotic with central lucency.* **(Right)** *Axial CECT in the same patient shows 2 thoracic spine melanoma metastases ➡. The more anterior lesion is sclerotic. The laterally located lesion has a target pattern with central low attenuation. This is a somewhat unusual appearance since metastatic melanoma to bone is usually lytic. Additional metastases involved the liver, peritoneum, and spleen.*

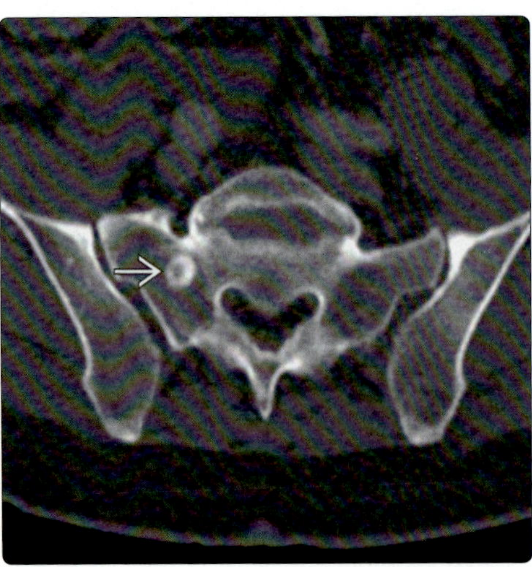

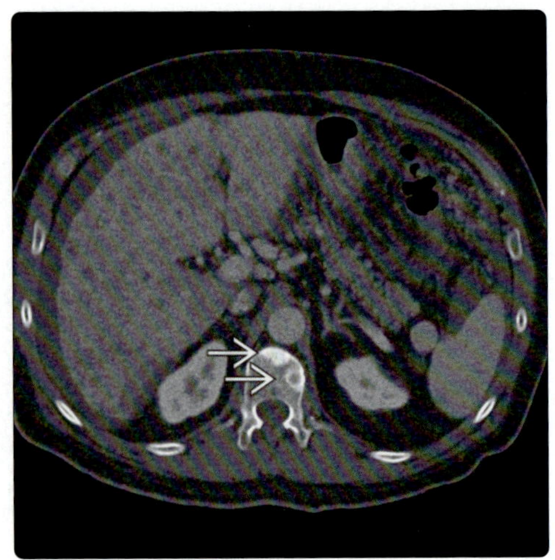

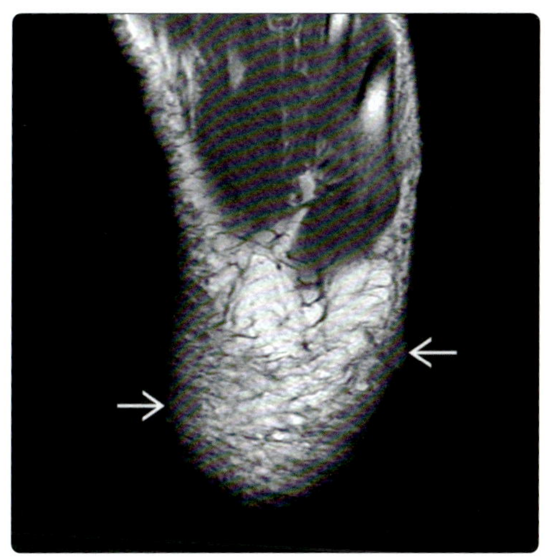

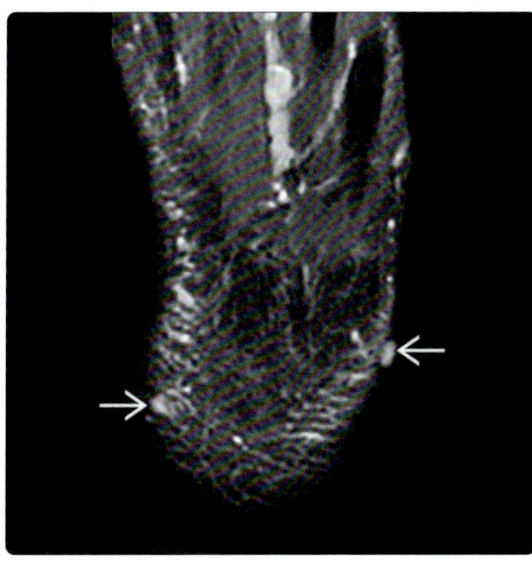

(Left) *Axial T1WI MR through the plantar aspect of the heel demonstrates tiny, ovoid, superficial nodules ➡ that are slightly hyperintense to skeletal muscle.* **(Right)** *Axial T2WI FS MR in the same patient shows these small nodules ➡ to have hyperintense signal. These nodules are satellite lesions from a primary melanoma that was "burnt off" by a podiatrist several years prior. Although these lesions were clinically evident, MR was performed to identify all regional lesions for surgical excision.*

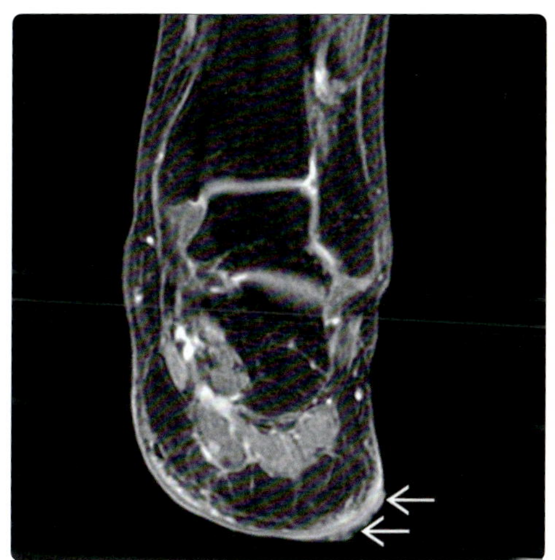

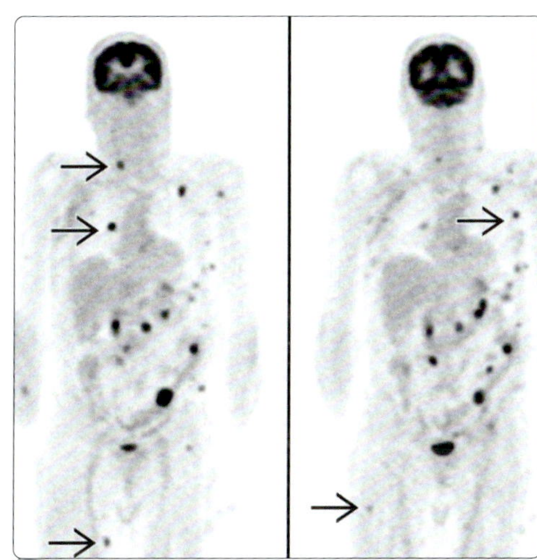

(Left) *Coronal T1WI C+ FS MR in the same patient shows the small satellite melanoma nodules ➡ to enhance. Although this patient had an otherwise normal staging PET/CT, she developed an in-transit metastasis involving her ipsilateral thigh 1 year later.* **(Right)** *Coronal PET shows innumerable foci of abnormal tracer uptake ⇨ representing metastatic melanoma. This finding was unexpected since this was an initial staging study for an 8-mm forearm melanoma in an asymptomatic patient.*

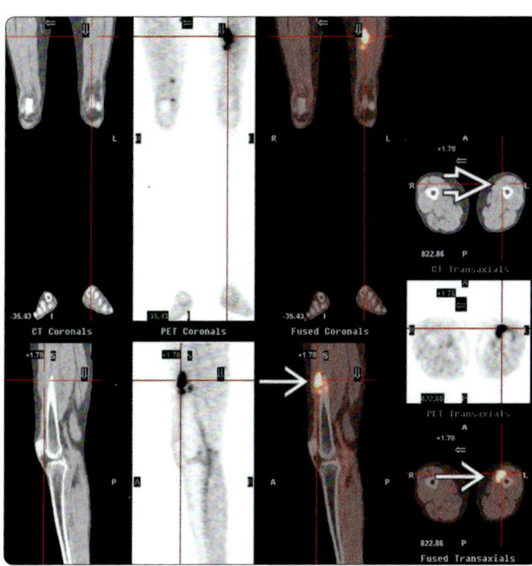

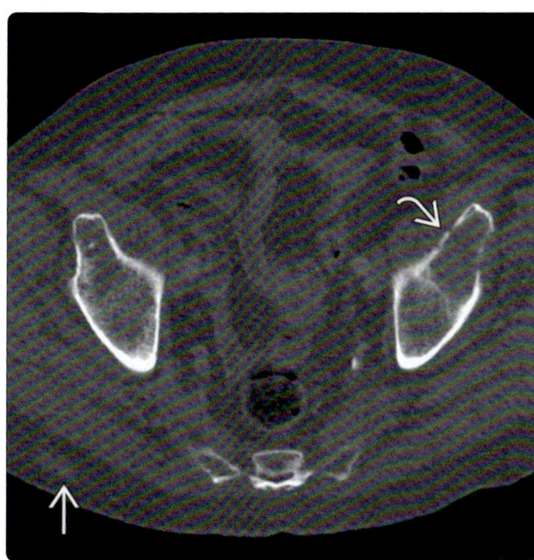

(Left) *Multiplanar fused PET/CT in the same patient shows a focus of metastatic melanoma involving the musculature of the left thigh. This lesion had a maximum SUV of 18.7 ➡. The lesion is slightly hypointense to skeletal muscle on the unenhanced CT image ➡.* **(Right)** *Axial CECT in the same patient shows the dominant skeletal metastasis ↷ involving the left supraacetabular region. This metastasis is lytic and has traversed the bone cortex. A subcutaneous metastasis ➡ is also evident.*

Soft Tissue Tumor Mimics: Infection/Inflammation

KEY FACTS

TERMINOLOGY

- Group of infectious or inflammatory processes that can mimic soft tissue neoplasm

TOP DIFFERENTIAL DIAGNOSES

- Soft tissue abscess
  - Collection of bacteria, white cells, and necrosis
  - MR: Homogeneous to heterogeneous ↓ T1 and ↑ T2 signal, with variable wall signal
  - Thick, irregular abscess wall enhancement
- Bursitis
  - Bursa contains ↑ fluid ± debris
  - Misdiagnosis avoided by knowledge of anatomy
- Synovitis
  - May have associated bone erosion from inflammatory arthropathy
- Arthroplasty component wear/particle disease
  - Erosion/resorption of bone surrounding prosthesis
- Foreign body granuloma
  - MR: Isointense on T1WI, heterogeneously hyperintense on T2WI ± signal void
- Myositis
  - Most likely to involve fusiform region of muscle, except with nodular or focal myositis
  - MR: Enlarged muscle having ↓ T1 and ↑ T2 signal ± focal fluid collection or abscess
- Cat scratch disease
  - Enlarged lymph node(s) with surrounding edema
  - Epitrochlear, cervical, and inguinal most common
- Denervation hypertrophy
  - Muscle denervation with prominent fat infiltration resulting in enlargement

DIAGNOSTIC CHECKLIST

- Radiographs helpful for initial mass evaluation
  - Lesion mineralization and changes in adjacent bone may help limit differential diagnosis

(Left) *Sagittal T2WI MR of the knee shows a large posterior soft tissue mass ➾, which has eroded into the posterior cortex of the femur ➾. The mass has nonspecific mildly heterogeneous hyperintense signal.* **(Right)** *Sagittal T1WI C+ MR in the same patient shows the mass ➾ to have thick, irregular peripheral enhancement surrounding a nonenhancing central fluid collection. The appearance is typical for an abscess with adjacent osteomyelitis. This infection was due to an uncommon organism, Yersinia pestis.*

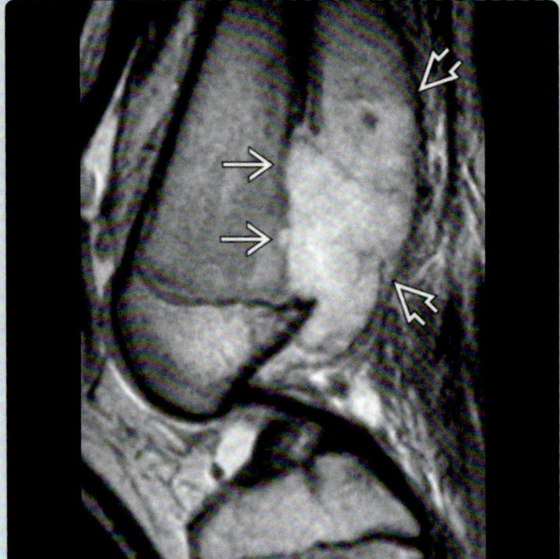

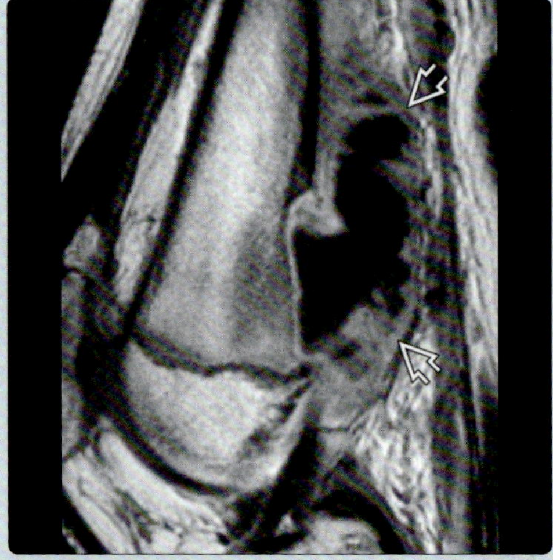

(Left) *Axial CECT demonstrates a low-density lesion with a thin enhancing rim ➾ within the deltoid muscle. This is the typical appearance of an intramuscular abscess.* **(Right)** *Axial T1WI C+ FS MR of a septic shoulder joint shows a thick enhancing rind surrounding nonenhancing fluid collections within the glenohumeral joint ➾ and subdeltoid bursa. Additional abscesses are present within the anterior deltoid muscle ➾, as well as surrounding the ruptured pectoralis major tendon ➾.*

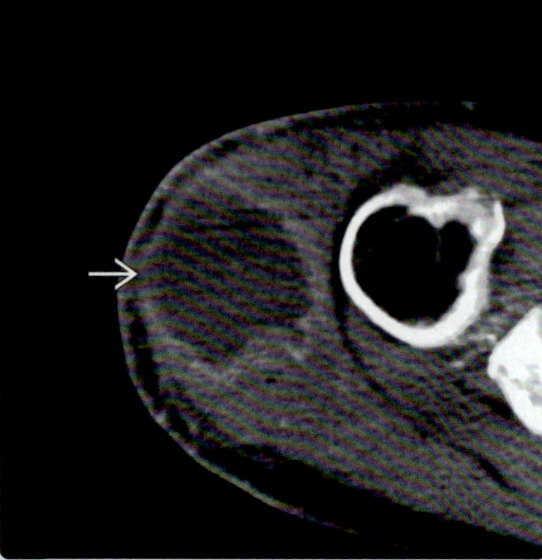

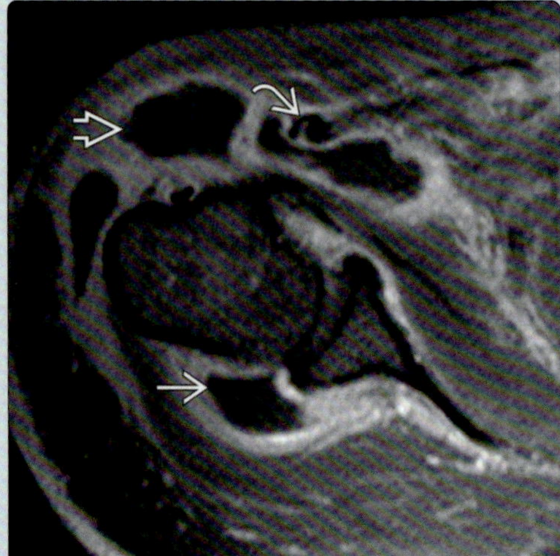

TERMINOLOGY

Definitions

- Group of infectious or inflammatory processes that can mimic soft tissue neoplasm

DIFFERENTIAL DIAGNOSIS

Soft Tissue Abscess

- Focal collection of bacteria, white cells, and necrosis
  - Clinically swollen and painful
- CT: Fluid density soft tissue mass ± gas
  - Peripheral calcification may develop chronically
- MR: Homogeneous to heterogeneous low T1 signal and high T2 signal, with variable wall signal
  - Thick, irregular abscess wall enhancement
  - Marked surrounding edema
- US: Variable echogenicity depending on abscess contents

Bursitis

- Inflammation or infection of synovial-lined bursae; distended bursa may mimic a mass
- Bone erosion or marrow edema suggests infection
- Bursa contains ↑ fluid ± debris
- Misdiagnosis avoided by knowledge of anatomy
  - Iliopsoas, prepatellar, trochanteric, subacromial/subdeltoid, olecranon, and ischiogluteal common

Synovitis

- Thickened, inflamed synovial tissue
- May have associated bone erosion
- MR: Hyperintense joint synovium on T2WI with prominent enhancement

Arthroplasty Component Wear/Particle Disease

- Erosion/resorption of bone surrounding prosthesis
  - ± lobulated fluid collections of varying density
- Fluid collections do not centrally enhance

Foreign Body Granuloma

- Inflammatory reaction to embedded foreign material
- Mass with well-defined or ill-defined margins
- MR: Isointense on T1WI, heterogeneously hyperintense on T2WI ± signal void of foreign body

Myositis

- Infectious and noninfectious etiologies
  - Pyomyositis usually due to *Staphylococcus aureus*
- Most likely to involve fusiform region of muscle
  - Exception is nodular or focal myositis (mass-like)
- CT: Heterogeneous attenuation of enlarged muscle
- MR: Enlarged muscle having ↓ T1 and ↑ T2 signal ± focal fluid collection or abscess
  - Skin thickening, subcutaneous edema, and thickening of fascia
  - Irregular wall enhancement of fluid collections

Compartment Syndrome

- Increased pressure within a muscle compartment resulting in muscle necrosis
  - Late peripheral calcification (calcific myonecrosis)
- Radiographs and CT: Peripherally calcified mass in expected region of muscle

Fasciitis

- Inflammatory fascial process; abscess may mimic mass
- MR: Thick deep fascia with ↓ T1 and ↑ T2 signal
  - Absent enhancement suggests necrotizing fasciitis

Elastofibroma

- Lentiform mass between scapula and chest wall
  - Older patients, commonly bilateral
- Not neoplasm, likely reaction to friction/repetitive trauma
- MR: Isointense to muscle with strand-like regions of fat signal, mild enhancement

Cat Scratch Disease

- *Bartonella henselae* lymphatic infection
- Due to cat exposure; not necessarily scratch
- Most patients ≤ 21 years old
- Enlarged lymph node(s) with surrounding edema may mimic tumor
  - Epitrochlear, cervical, and inguinal most common
  - More extensive in immunocompromised patients
- Rare associated lytic bone lesions

Denervation Hypertrophy

- Muscle denervation with prominent fat infiltration resulting in enlargement

Dermatomyositis

- Idiopathic inflammatory myopathy
- Muscle edema, calcification, and fatty atrophy
- Involves multiple muscles, usually bilaterally symmetric

Mycotic Aneurysm

- Necrosis of vessel wall due to intraluminal or extraluminal spread of infection

Cellulitis

- Infection of skin and subcutaneous tissue
  - More likely to be diffuse than focal (mass-like)
- Red, warm, and painful superficial soft tissues
- MR: Strand-like fluid signal in subcutaneous fat and adjacent fascia; contrast helps exclude fluid collections

Hydatid (Echinococcal) Disease

- *Echinococcus granulosus* infection
- Hydatid cysts uncommon in skeletal muscle; when present, mimic mass lesion
- MR: Variable appearance from multivesicular cysts to solid-appearing masses; thin peripheral rim enhancement

DIAGNOSTIC CHECKLIST

Image Interpretation Pearls

- Radiographs helpful for initial mass evaluation
- Lesion mineralization and involvement or changes in adjacent bone may help limit differential diagnosis

SELECTED REFERENCES

1. Chaudhry AA et al: Necrotizing fasciitis and its mimics: what radiologists need to know. AJR Am J Roentgenol. 204(1):128-39, 2015
2. McKenzie G et al: Pictorial review: Non-neoplastic soft-tissue masses. Br J Radiol. 82(981):775-85, 2009

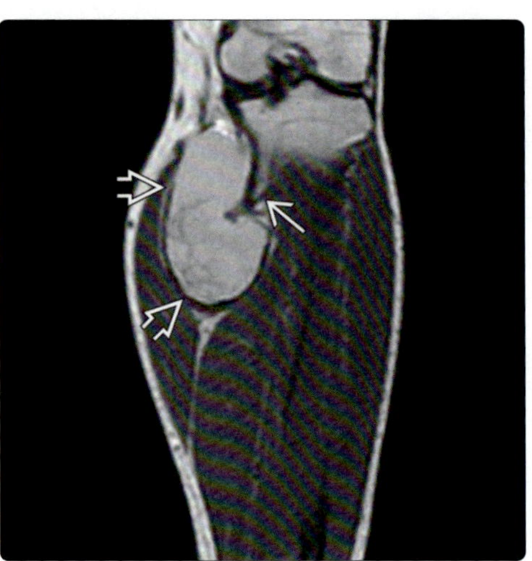

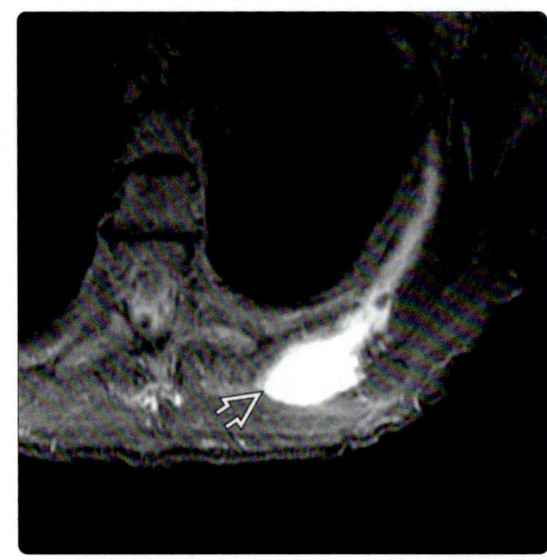

(Left) *Coronal T1WI MR shows a large bursa ➡ complicating an osteochondroma ➡. This bursa has complex high signal. The osteochondroma marrow space is contiguous with the underlying tibia. This bursa was aspirated due to pain.* **(Right)** *Axial T2WI FS MR shows a complex fluid collection ➡ located deep to the left scapula. This was scapulothoracic bursitis but seroma, lymphocele, and cystic neoplasm are in the differential diagnosis. This lesion was aspirated/biopsied under ultrasound guidance.*

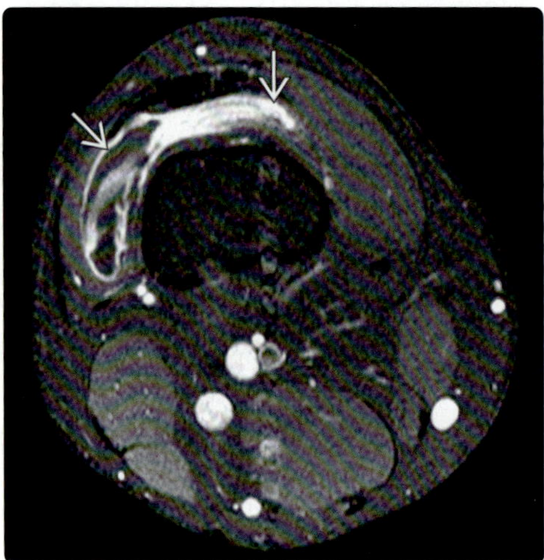

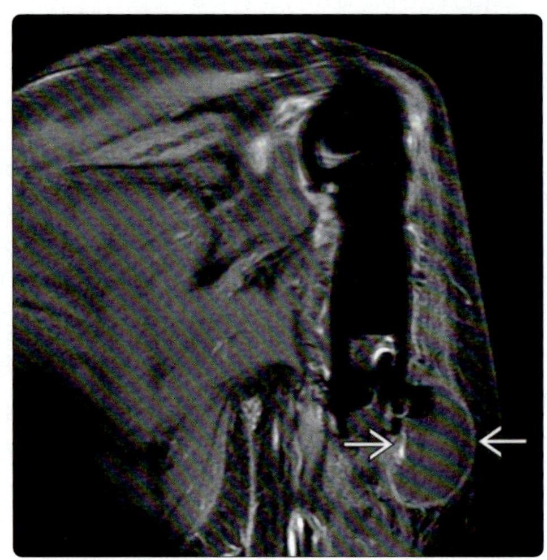

(Left) *Axial T1WI C+ FS MR shows irregular, mildly thickened and enhancing synovium ➡ of the knee joint. This appearance is classic for synovitis, although it is nonspecific. This patient's knee aspirate showed no organisms or culture growth.* **(Right)** *Coronal T1WI C+ FS MR shows a soft tissue mass ➡ adjacent to the distal aspect of a custom left shoulder endoprosthesis. This patient had previous resection of the proximal humerus due to giant cell tumor. Surgical resection of the mass revealed particle disease.*

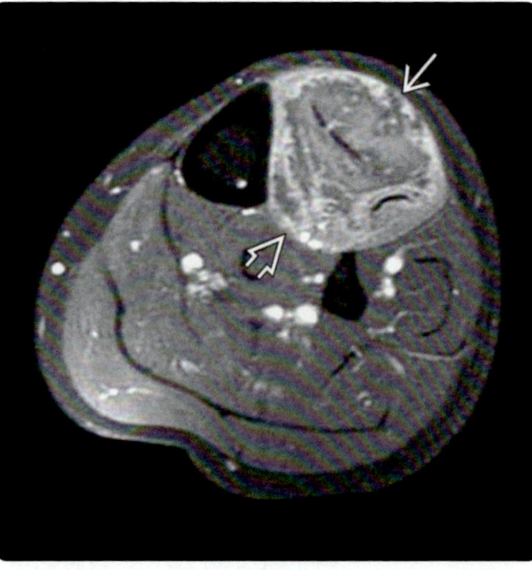

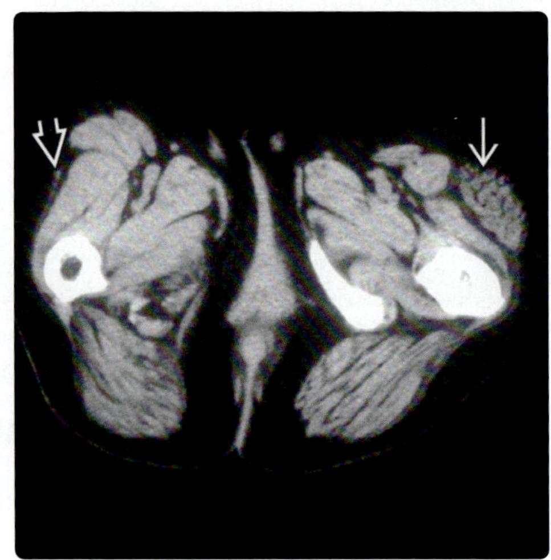

(Left) *Axial T1WI C+ FS MR demonstrates patchy diffuse enhancement of the swollen anterior compartment of the lower leg ➡. Note the posterior bowing of the interosseous membrane ➡ in this typical case of compartment syndrome.* **(Right)** *Axial NECT shows enlargement of the left tensor fascia lata muscle ➡ compared to the right ➡. An increase in intramuscular fat is present within the enlarged muscle. No soft tissue mass is present. This constellation of findings is consistent with denervation hypertrophy.*

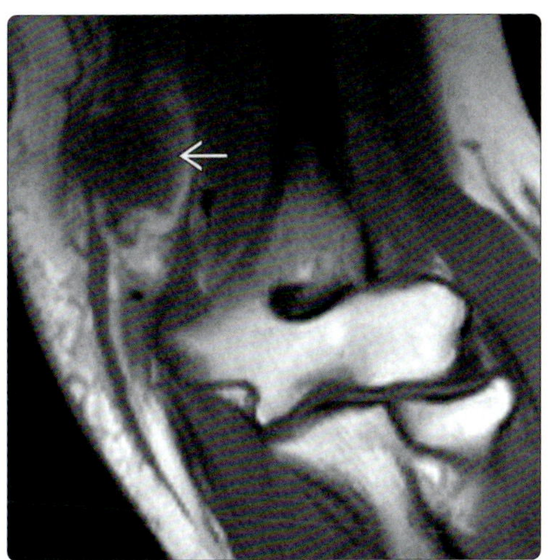

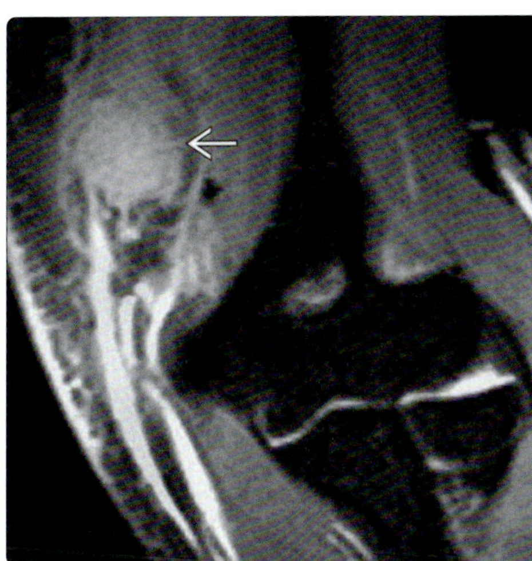

(Left) *Coronal T1WI MR of the elbow shows an ill-defined mass ➡ in the epitrochlear region. The mass has similar signal intensity to skeletal muscle with surrounding inflammatory change.* **(Right)** *Coronal T2WI FS MR in the same patient shows the epitrochlear mass ➡ to have very high signal intensity with prominent surrounding inflammatory edema. Surrounding edema would be unusual for a primary soft tissue neoplasm. This is benign regional lymphadenitis due to cat scratch disease.*

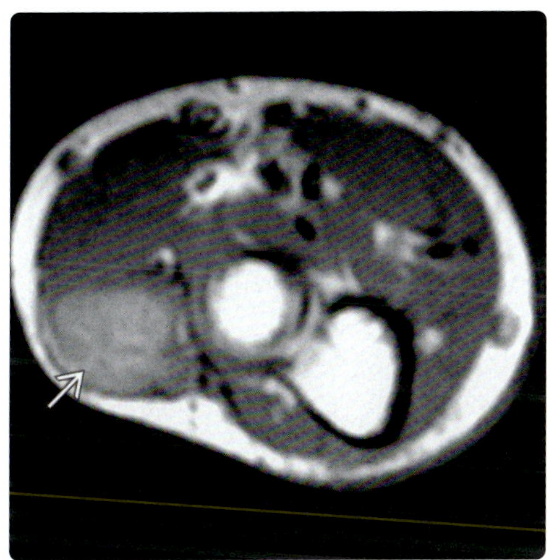

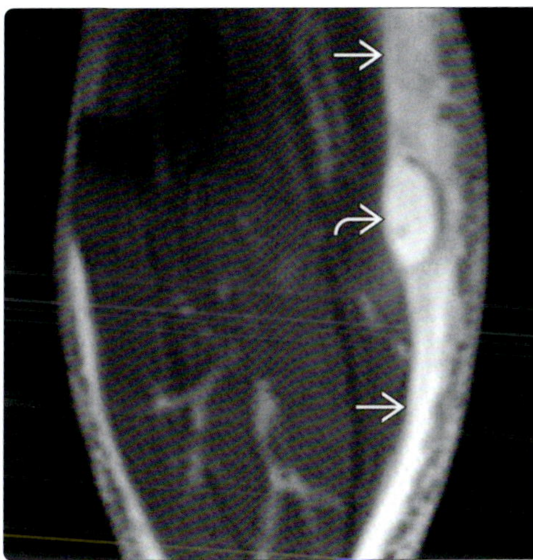

(Left) *Axial T1WI C+ MR shows an enhancing mass ➡ within the extensor digitorum muscle. The appearance is nonspecific, and sarcoma must be considered. This is a case of focal myositis, which may be a precursor to polymyositis. It may be mistaken for a soft tissue sarcoma by imaging and at surgery.* **(Right)** *Coronal T2WI FS MR of the calf shows extensive edema involving the fascia ➡ with a focal fluid collection ➡. No air was evident. At surgery, this was diagnosed as necrotizing fasciitis, with a small abscess.*

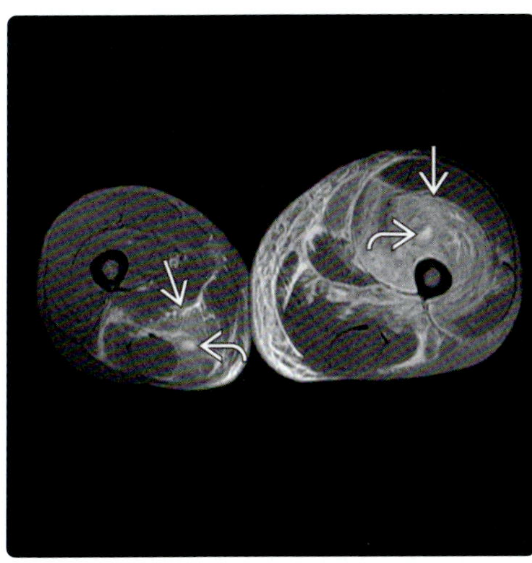

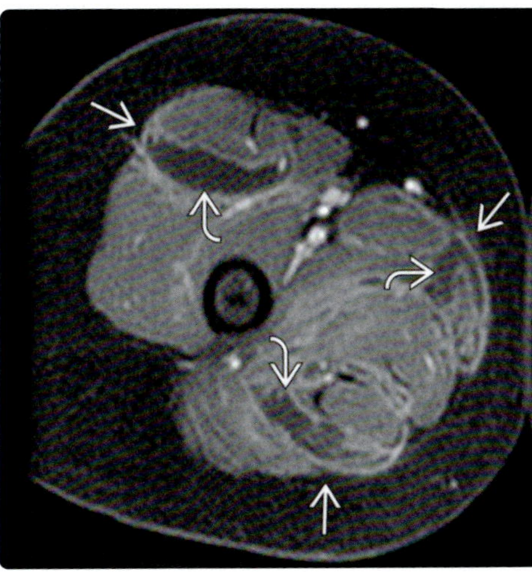

(Left) *Axial T2WI FS MR shows bilateral thigh muscle edema and enlargement ➡ with preserved muscular architecture, compatible with inflammation rather than mass. Also note small areas of high signal compatible with bilateral small abscesses ➡. This was Staphylococcus aureus infectious myositis in an HIV-positive patient.* **(Right)** *Axial T1WI C+ FS MR shows irregular enhancement of the thigh musculature ➡. Several small fluid collections ➡ are present within the muscle. These findings were due to dermatomyositis.*

KEY FACTS

TERMINOLOGY

- Group of vascular-related abnormalities that may mimic soft tissue neoplasm

TOP DIFFERENTIAL DIAGNOSES

- Hematoma
  - High signal on T1WI MR can mimic fat signal of lipomatous neoplasm
  - High signal on T1WI MR also complicates assessment of postgadolinium imaging
  - Remain vigilant for hemorrhagic sarcoma
- Aneurysm
  - Popliteal artery aneurysm most common in extremities
  - MR: Flow void when nonthrombosed; heterogeneous signal intensity due to turbulence and variably aged thrombosis
  - ± pulsation artifact or lamellated appearance
- Pseudoaneurysm
  - Eccentrically located to parent vessel
  - Ultrasound: Characteristic yin-yang swirling blood flow pattern; to-and-fro flow of blood entering in systole and exiting on diastole
- Cystic adventitial disease
  - Typical patient is young to middle-aged man with sudden onset of calf pain or claudication
  - MR: Fluid signal intensity lobulated collections involving artery wall (usually popliteal) with thin peripheral enhancement
- Morel-Lavallée lesion
  - Closed degloving injury resulting in collection of blood and lymph

DIAGNOSTIC CHECKLIST

- Soft tissue sarcomas are not uncommonly misdiagnosed as hematomas at presentation
  - Either short-term interval follow-up documenting near resolution or convincing lack of central enhancement is needed for imaging diagnosis of hematoma

(Left) *Axial T1WI MR of the lateral thigh shows a round lesion ➡ in the subcutaneous fat. This lesion has a faintly visible fluid-fluid level ➢. The dependent portion of the lesion has a similar signal intensity to muscle. The antidependent portion of the lesion is hyperintense to muscle due to the presence of blood products.* **(Right)** *Axial T2WI FS MR in the same patient more clearly demonstrates the fluid-fluid level ➢ in the rounded mass ➡. This diabetic patient recalled no trauma to this area.*

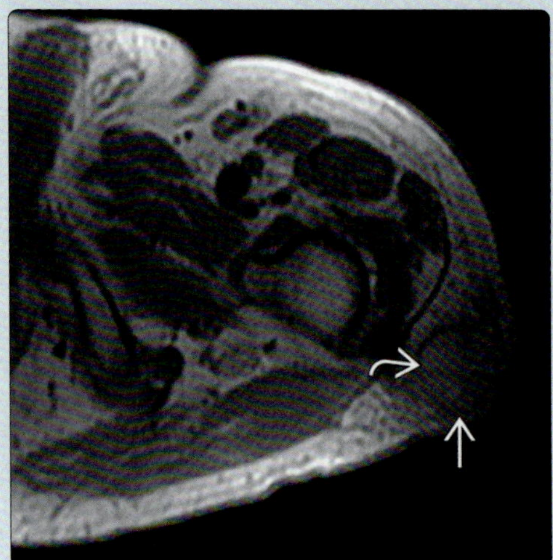

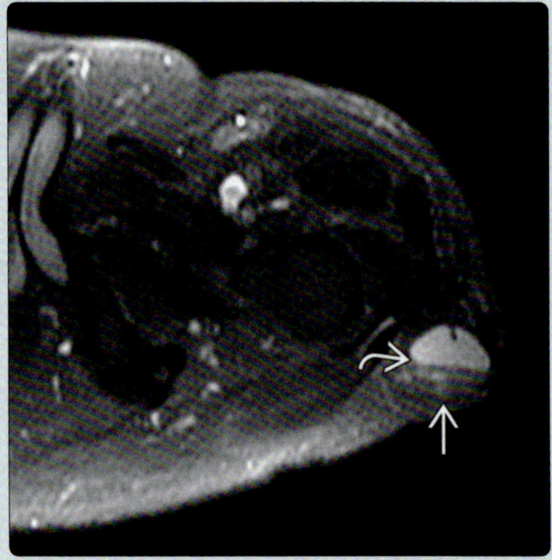

(Left) *Axial T1WI C+ FS MR shows that the mass ➡ has only smooth peripheral enhancement. Lack of central enhancement was further confirmed with the use of subtraction postprocessing images, yielding diagnosis of hematoma.* **(Right)** *Axial T1WI C+ MR shows a mass ➡ in the medial thigh that appears to have diffuse enhancement but was hyperintense on the unenhanced T1WI (not shown). Thus, it is not possible to differentiate enhancing tumor from blood products. Follow-up confirmed hematoma.*

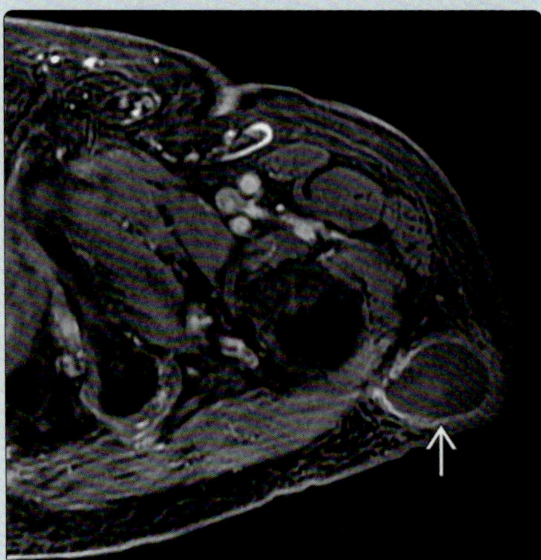

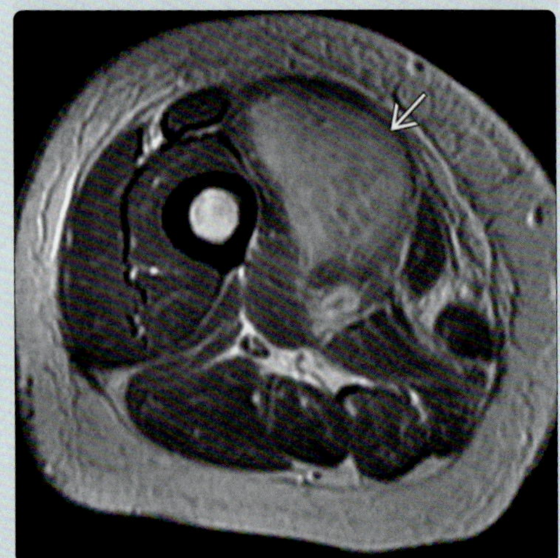

TERMINOLOGY

Definitions

- Group of vascular-related abnormalities that may mimic soft tissue neoplasm

DIFFERENTIAL DIAGNOSIS

Hematoma

- Focal soft tissue mass with heterogeneous appearance on CT and MR depending on lesion contents and acuity
- High signal on T1WI MR can mimic fat signal of lipomatous neoplasm
- High signal on T1WI MR also complicates assessment of postgadolinium imaging
  - Consider utilizing postprocessing subtraction (T1WI FS postgadolinium image minus T1WI FS pregadolinium image)
- Remain vigilant for underlying sarcoma that has hemorrhaged
  - Short-term interval follow-up usually necessary unless postgadolinium imaging definitively demonstrates lack of central enhancement
  - Patients with soft tissue sarcomas often notice them after or attribute them to minor trauma
- Ultrasound: Acutely anechoic; irregular echoic regions develop chronically

Aneurysm

- Involves all 3 layers of vessel
- Mass is fusiform & contiguous with long axis of vessel
- Popliteal artery aneurysm most common extremity aneurysm
  - Often bilateral and associated with abdominal aortic aneurysm
- Variable imaging appearance due to varying degrees of thrombosis
- CT: Prominent enhancement when nonthrombosed; thrombosis has similar attenuation to muscle
  - Leaking will produce surrounding ill-defined soft tissue attenuation
- MR: Flow void when nonthrombosed; heterogeneous signal intensity due to turbulence and variably aged thrombosis
  - ± pulsation artifact or lamellated appearance
- Angiography: Fusiform widening of artery, mural thrombus, and wall calcification

Pseudoaneurysm

- Involves only adventitial layer of vessel
  - Supported by surrounding soft tissues
- Multiple causes including iatrogenic, posttraumatic, and intravenous drug abuse
- Lesion is eccentrically located with respect to parent vessel
- Ultrasound: Characteristic yin-yang swirling blood flow pattern; to-and-fro flow of blood entering in systole and exiting on diastole

Cystic Adventitial Disease

- Typical patient is young to middle-aged man with sudden onset of calf pain or claudication
- Collection of mucin in adventitial layer of artery of unknown cause
  - Narrows, occludes, or causes rupture of artery
  - Predominantly affects popliteal artery
- MR: Fluid signal intensity lobulated collections involving artery wall with thin peripheral enhancement
- Angiography: Eccentrically located, smooth extrinsic narrowing of vessel lumen

AV Fistula

- Acquired abnormal communication between artery and vein
  - Penetrating trauma, surgical placement for dialysis

Muscle Infarction

- Diabetic myonecrosis
  - Acute onset of severe muscle pain in patient with poorly controlled diabetes
  - Typically involves bilateral thighs
  - Advanced arteriosclerosis present histologically
- Thromboembolic disease
  - Distal embolization of thrombus, usually from atherosclerotic disease, resulting in tissue death
- Calcific myonecrosis
  - Follows ischemic necrosis, usually due to compartment syndrome
  - Anterior compartment of lower leg most common
  - Radiographs and CT: Peripherally calcified mass in expected region of muscle
    - Lacks mass effect due to atrophy of muscle

Morel-Lavallée Lesion

- Closed degloving injury
- Detachment of subcutaneous fat from fascia due to violent sheer stress
  - Tears perforating vessels and lymphatics
  - Results in mobile skin and subcutaneous fat
- Most common involving thigh, lumbar region, and periscapular region
- MR: Fluid collection superficial to fascia of variable complexity

DIAGNOSTIC CHECKLIST

Image Interpretation Pearls

- Soft tissue sarcomas are not uncommonly misdiagnosed as hematomas at presentation
  - Either short-term interval follow-up documenting near resolution or convincing lack of central enhancement is needed for imaging diagnosis of hematoma

SELECTED REFERENCES

1. Manaster BJ: Soft-tissue masses: optimal imaging protocol and reporting. AJR Am J Roentgenol. 201(3):505-14, 2013
2. McKenzie G et al: Pictorial review: Non-neoplastic soft-tissue masses. Br J Radiol. 82(981):775-85, 2009
3. Stacy GS et al: Pitfalls in MR image interpretation prompting referrals to an orthopedic oncology clinic. Radiographics. 27(3):805-26; discussion 827-8, 2007
4. Kransdorf MJ et al: Masses that may mimic soft tissue tumors. In Kransdorf MJ et al: Imaging of Soft Tissue Tumors. 2nd ed. Philadelphia: Lippincott Williams & Wilkins. 532-9, 2006
5. Jelinek J et al: MR imaging of soft-tissue masses. Mass-like lesions that simulate neoplasms. Magn Reson Imaging Clin N Am. 3(4):727-41, 1995

(Left) *Axial PD FSE FS MR shows a focus of high signal ➡ in the deltoid muscle that was elongated along the superior-to-inferior extent of the muscle and had a feathery pattern extending into the adjacent muscle fibers. This palpable lesion was a hematoma.* **(Right)** *Axial T1WI MR shows a heterogeneously hyperintense mass ➡ located in the medial head of the gastrocnemius muscle. This mass was heterogeneously hyperintense on T2WI MR and represented a capsular hematoma.*

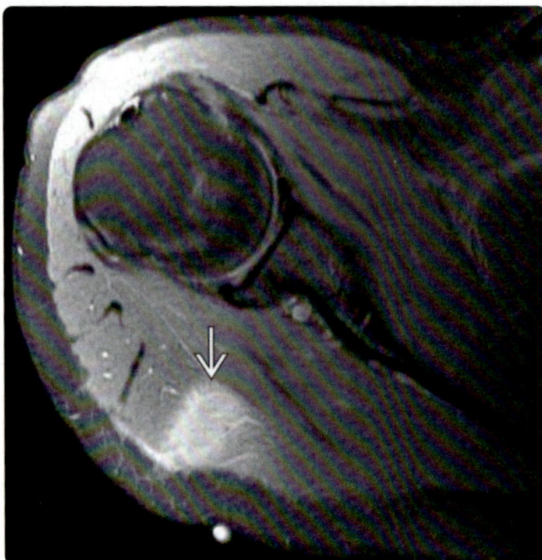

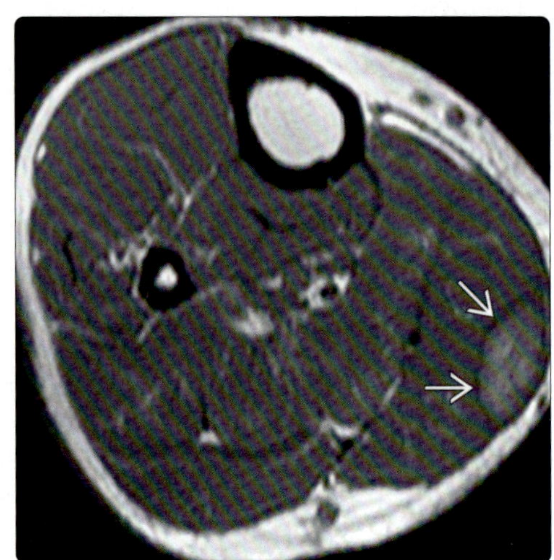

(Left) *Axial T1WI MR shows a well-defined mass ➡ in the gastrocnemius muscle. Central decreased signal intensity ➡ is surrounded by a rim of increased T1 signal suggesting hemorrhage. This was a hematoma.* **(Right)** *Sagittal PDWI FS MR shows a mass ➡ in the popliteal fossa of the knee. The key to the diagnosis of an aneurysm is noting the fusiform shape and that it is contiguous with the popliteal artery. Thrombosis and turbulent blood flow may give these lesions a highly complex appearance.*

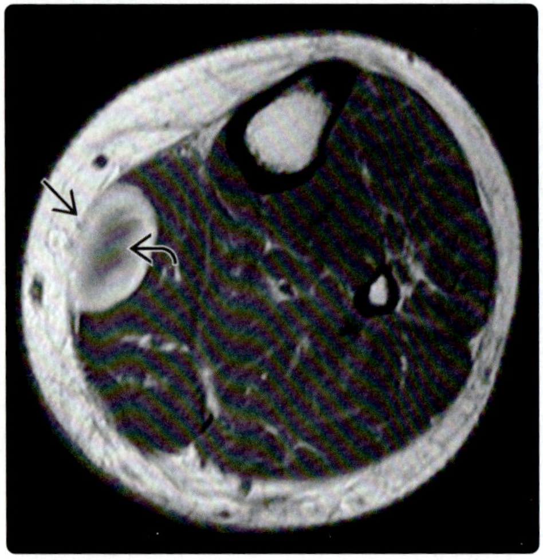

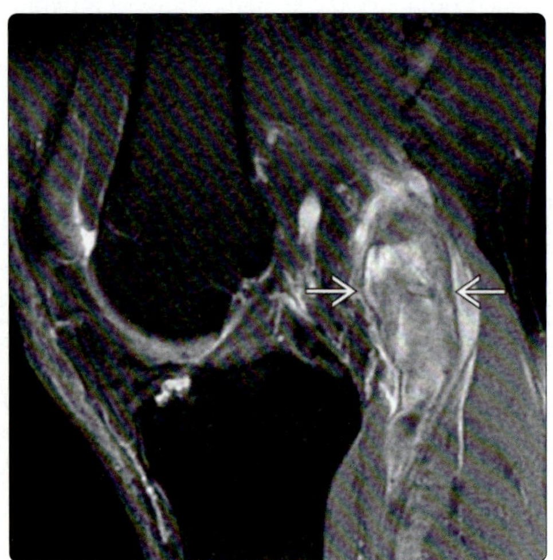

(Left) *Axial contrast-enhanced soft tissue algorithm CT shows a 4.3 cm left popliteal artery aneurysm ➡. The aneurysm has mural thrombus with a 2.5 cm diameter residual opacified lumen. Atherosclerotic calcification ➡ involves the aneurysm wall.* **(Right)** *Coronal MR angiogram MIP shows a posttraumatic pseudoaneurysm ➡ of the ulnar artery. On axial imaging, this appeared as a well-defined, multiloculated mass in the Guyon canal, which could have been mistaken for a ganglion cyst.*

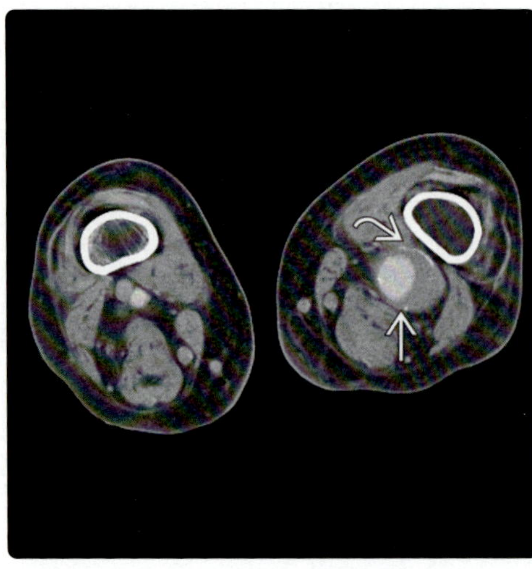

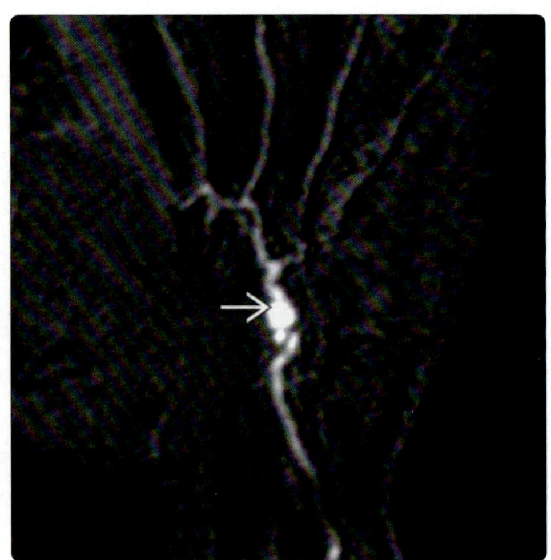

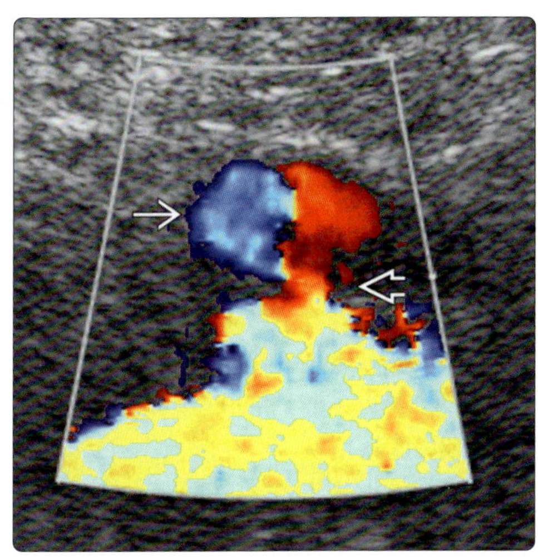

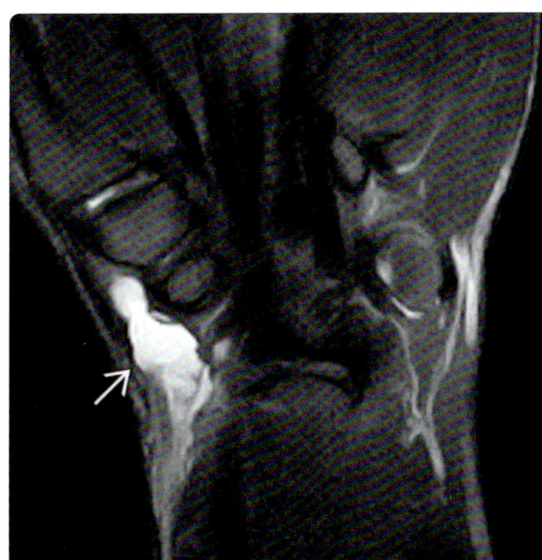

(Left) *Transverse color Doppler ultrasound to evaluate a mass that developed after femoral artery puncture demonstrates a pseudoaneurysm ➡. This pseudoaneurysm shows a typical yin-yang appearance of swirling blood flow and has a small neck ➡.* **(Right)** *Coronal STIR MR shows a lobulated, high-signal mass ➡ along the radial side of the wrist. While a ganglion cyst would be the most common etiology in this location, this lesion was cystic adventitial disease associated with the radial artery.*

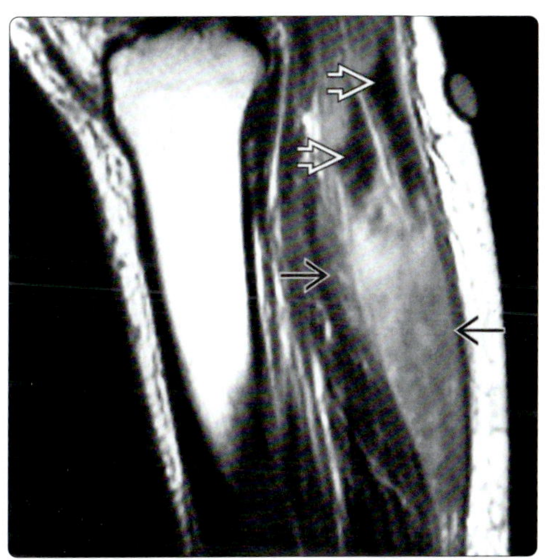

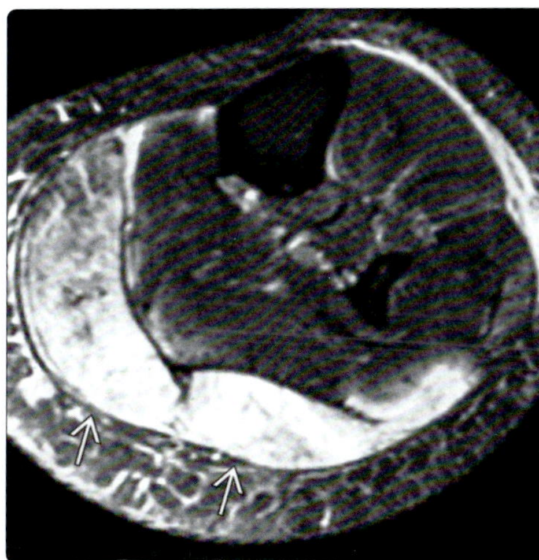

(Left) *Sagittal T1WI C+ FS MR shows mild diffuse enhancement involving the gastrocnemius and soleus muscles of the calf ➡. There are additional regions of diffuse low signal ➡ that lack rim enhancement, suggesting necrosis rather than abscess.* **(Right)** *Axial T2WI FS MR in the same patient shows high signal intensity predominantly involving posterior calf muscles ➡. Given the history of poorly controlled diabetes and severe pain, the diagnosis is spontaneous diabetic muscle necrosis.*

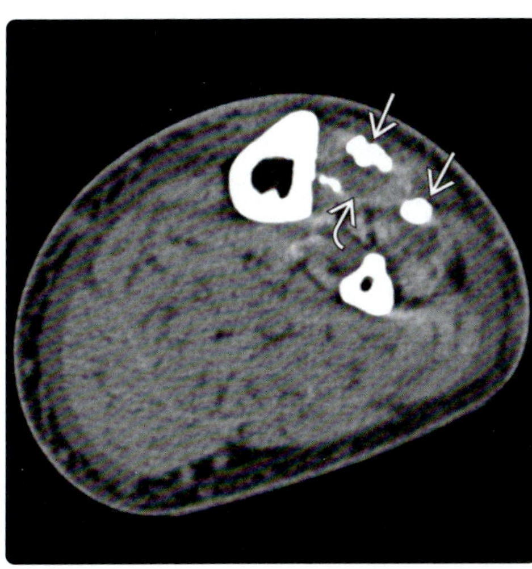

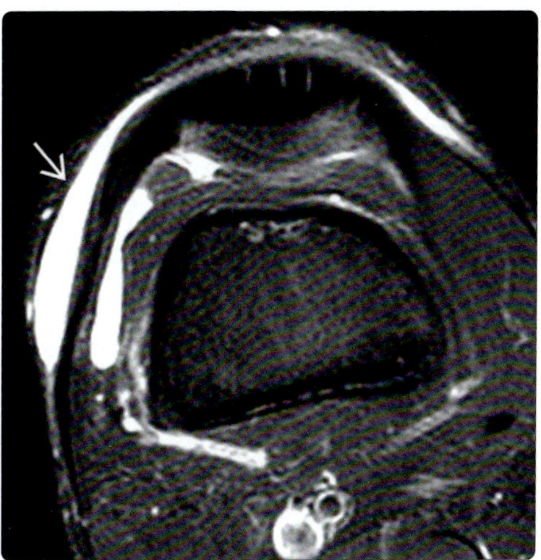

(Left) *Axial NECT with soft tissue windows shows calcifications ➡ and atrophy of the anterior compartment musculature ➡. The finding of muscle atrophy is especially useful in discounting this appearance as malignancy. This is calcific myonecrosis.* **(Right)** *Axial T2WI FS MR shows a crescentic fluid collection ➡ tracking along the fascia of the anterolateral knee. This fluid collection was not contiguous with the bursa and was secondary to a traction injury. This is a Morel-Lavallée lesion.*

Soft Tissue Tumor Mimics: Crystal Disease

KEY FACTS

TERMINOLOGY

- Group of entities due to crystal deposition that may appear mass-like, mimicking soft tissue tumor

TOP DIFFERENTIAL DIAGNOSES

- Gout
  - Juxtaarticular soft tissue mass ± calcification
  - Usually have concurrent findings of gout arthropathy
  - Intense homogeneous or heterogeneous enhancement can mimic neoplasm
- Calcium pyrophosphate dihydrate deposition disease
  - Mimics neoplasm when presenting as monoarticular calcified mass
  - Well-defined, calcified mass ± bone erosion
- Hydroxyapatite deposition disease
  - Radiographs: Well-defined, globular calcification progressing to well-defined calcified focus
  - ± comet tail configuration
  - CT: Bone erosion may appear aggressive, especially involving proximal humerus (pectoralis major insertion) and femoral diaphysis
- Tumoral (idiopathic) calcinosis
  - Early presentation in 1st and 2nd decades of life
  - Radiographs and CT: Large, multilobulated, amorphous, and cystic periarticular masses
  - Fluid-fluid levels (sedimentation sign) common
- Calcinosis of chronic renal failure
  - a.k.a. metastatic calcification, secondary tumoral calcinosis
  - Abnormal serum calcium and phosphate levels
  - Identical imaging appearance as tumoral calcinosis

DIAGNOSTIC CHECKLIST

- Attention to changes in adjacent bones/joints, available lab values, and clinical history helps narrow differential diagnosis

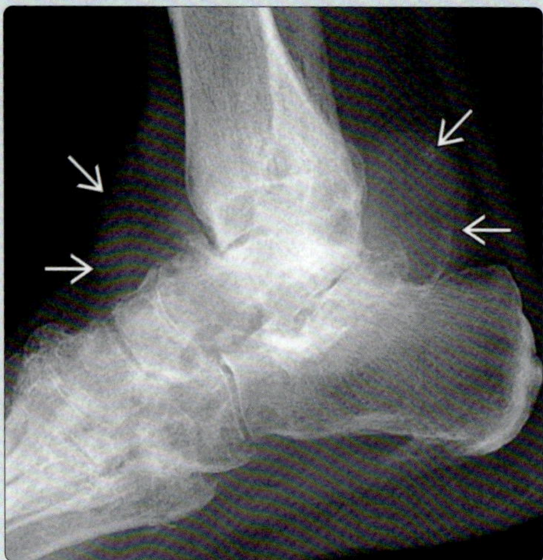

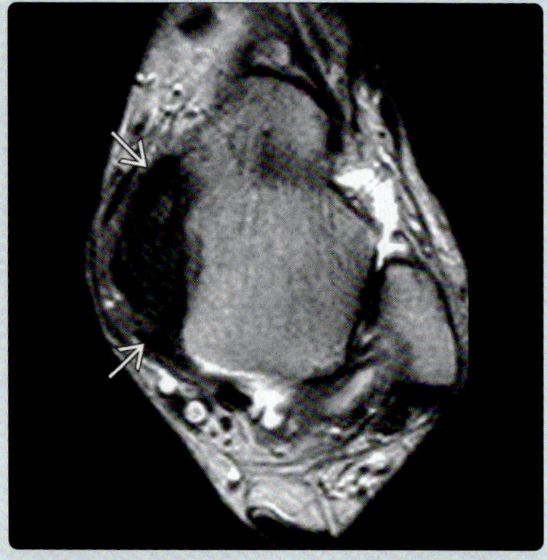

(Left) *Lateral radiograph of the ankle shows an extremely large soft tissue mass ➡ in the distribution of a distended tibiotalar joint. This mass is dense, suggesting mineral deposition in tophus. Additional images showed large juxtaarticular erosions typical for gout.* **(Right)** *Axial T2WI MR of the ankle shows a low-signal mass ➡ distal to the medial malleolus. This mass also had low signal on T1W images. The persistently low signal on all sequences is typical of the sodium urate deposition in gout.*

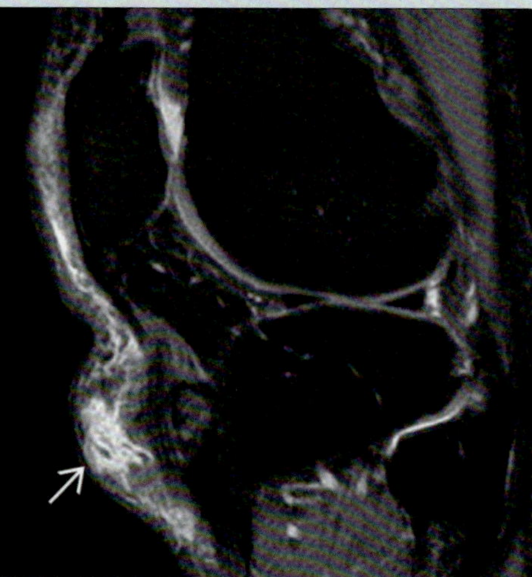

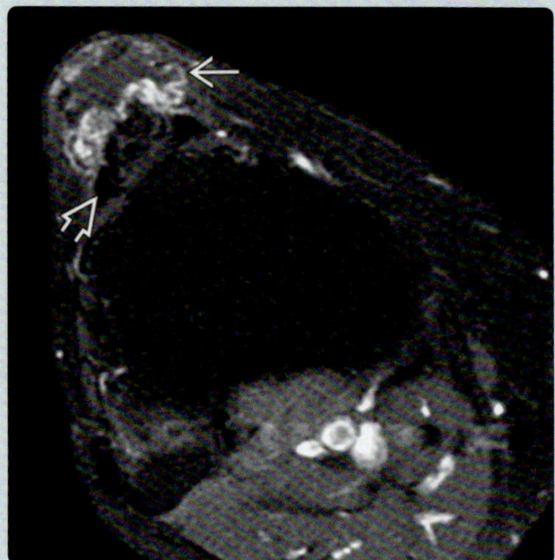

(Left) *Sagittal T2WI FS MR of the knee shows a poorly defined, irregularly shaped heterogeneous signal intensity lesion ➡ in the region of the superficial infrapatellar bursa. The mass has high signal centrally with low to intermediate signal peripherally.* **(Right)** *Axial T1WI C+ FS MR in the same patient shows heterogeneous, predominantly peripheral enhancement of the mass ➡. The majority of the enhancement is seen along the deep margin, adjacent to the low-signal patellar tendon ➡. This is surgically proven gout.*

TERMINOLOGY

Definitions

- Group of entities due to crystal deposition that may appear mass-like, mimicking soft tissue tumor

IMAGING

General Features

- Best diagnostic clue
  - Changes in adjacent joints or bones can be useful for differentiation
  - Laboratory values may also be helpful for differentiation of entities

Imaging Recommendations

- Best imaging tool
  - Radiographs and CT most useful for assessing characteristics of calcified mass and associated findings in adjacent bone
  - Enhanced MR occasionally useful to differentiate from tumor when findings are equivocal

DIFFERENTIAL DIAGNOSIS

Gout

- Metabolic disease resulting in hyperuricemia
- Soft tissue deposits of monosodium urate = tophi
- Feet, hands, ankles, elbows, knees, and spine
- Radiographs: Juxtaarticular soft tissue mass ± calcification
  - Concurrent findings of gout arthropathy
- CT: Improved detection of calcification within tophi
  - Pressure erosion of adjacent bone
- MR: Intermediate to low T1WI and T2WI signal mass
  - May have high signal on fluid-sensitive sequences
  - Intense homogeneous to heterogeneous enhancement can mimic neoplasm

Calcium Pyrophosphate Dihydrate Deposition Disease

- a.k.a. tophaceous pseudogout
- Calcium pyrophosphate dihydrate crystal deposition in juxtaarticular and articular soft tissues
- Mimics neoplasm when presenting as monoarticular calcified mass
- Radiographs and CT: Well-defined calcified mass ± bone erosion
- MR: Low to intermediate T1 and T2 signal mass

Hydroxyapatite Deposition Disease

- a.k.a. calcium hydroxyapatite disease, calcific tendonitis, calcific bursitis
- Focal calcified deposit in tendon, bursa, and periarticular soft tissues
  - Shoulder and hip most common
- Radiographs: Well-defined, globular calcification progressing to well-defined calcified focus
  - ± comet tail configuration
- CT: Bone erosion may appear aggressive
  - Proximal humerus (especially involving pectoralis major insertion) and proximal femoral diaphysis
  - Upper cervical spine location can have particularly aggressive appearance
  - Lacks fluid-fluid levels
- MR: Calcium deposit has low signal on all sequences
  - Surrounding edema in acute phase
- Bone scan: Increased radiotracer uptake

Tumoral (Idiopathic) Calcinosis

- Inherited disorder producing painless, densely calcified periarticular masses
  - Calcium hydroxyapatite crystals, amorphous calcium carbonate, and calcium phosphate
  - Normocalcemia and hyperphosphatemia (normal phosphate less common)
- Autosomal dominant with variable expressivity
  - Early presentation in 1st and 2nd decades of life
  - Most common in patients of African descent
- Predilection for extensor surface of joint
  - Hip > elbow > shoulder > foot > wrist
- Radiographs and CT: Large, multilobulated, amorphous, and cystic periarticular masses
  - Fluid-fluid levels (sedimentation sign) common
    - Homogeneous calcifications suggest ↓ metabolic activity
  - Commonly contiguous with bursa
  - Adjacent bone reaction uncommon
- MR: Low T1 signal, low to high T2 signal

Calcinosis of Chronic Renal Failure

- a.k.a. metastatic calcification, secondary tumoral calcinosis
- Dystrophic and metabolic calcification associated with chronic renal failure
  - Abnormal serum calcium and phosphate levels
  - Abnormal glomerular filtration rate
  - Patient undergoing hemodialysis
- Identical imaging appearance as tumoral calcinosis

Calcinosis Universalis

- Sheet-like calcium deposition involving muscle, fascia, and subcutaneous tissues
- Associated with polymyositis, dermatomyositis, and less commonly systemic lupus erythematosus

Calcinosis Circumscripta

- Nodular calcium deposits in dermis or subcutis
- Produced by connective tissue diseases and any cause of metabolic calcification

DIAGNOSTIC CHECKLIST

Image Interpretation Pearls

- Attention to available lab values and clinical history helps narrow differential diagnosis

SELECTED REFERENCES

1. McKenzie G et al: Pictorial review: Non-neoplastic soft-tissue masses. Br J Radiol. 82(981):775-85, 2009
2. Kransdorf MJ et al: Masses that may mimic soft tissue tumors. In Kransdorf MJ et al: Imaging of Soft Tissue Tumors. 2nd ed. Philadelphia: Lippincott Williams & Wilkins. 524-9, 2006
3. Olsen KM et al: Tumoral calcinosis: pearls, polemics, and alternative possibilities. Radiographics. 26(3):871-85, 2006
4. Flemming DJ et al: Osseous involvement in calcific tendinitis: a retrospective review of 50 cases. AJR Am J Roentgenol. 181(4):965-72, 2003

(Left) *Lateral radiograph of the elbow shows a large soft tissue mass ➡ in the expected region of the olecranon bursa. The mass contains scattered, coarse calcifications. The appearance and location are typical for a gouty tophus.* **(Right)** *Axial PDWI FS MR of the wrist shows prominent fluid surrounding the volar tendon sheaths ➡. A focus of amorphous material ➡ could be mistaken for a soft tissue neoplasm. This represents a nodular collection of calcium pyrophosphate dihydrate crystals.*

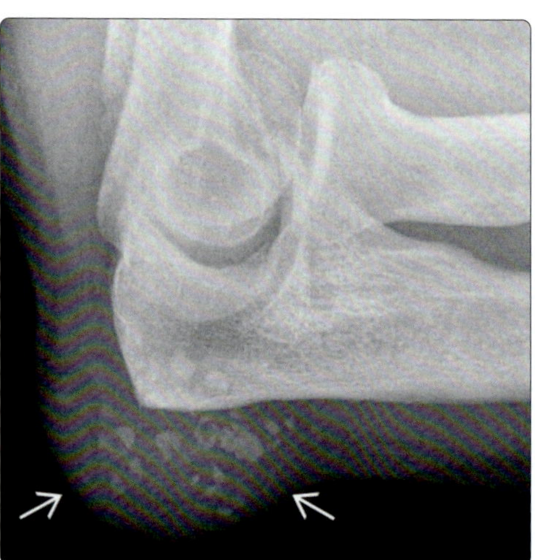

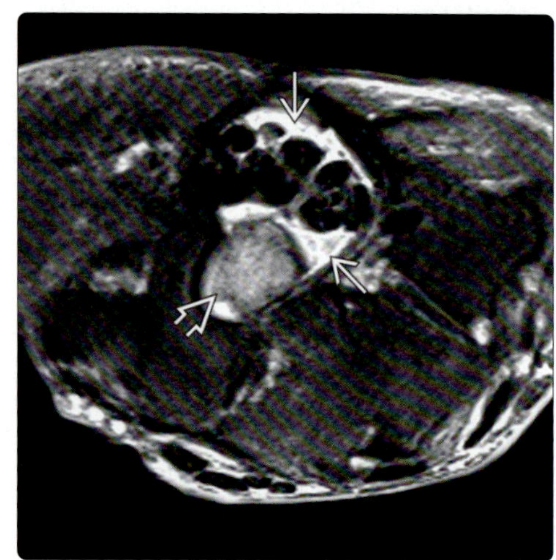

(Left) *Coronal bone CT through the hindfoot shows hyperdense punctate foci of calcium ➡ within muscle, deep to the subcutaneus tissue. No mass is evident.* **(Right)** *Coronal PDWI FS MR in the same patient shows low-signal calcifications ➡ in the flexor digitorum brevis muscle, with surrounding inhomogeneous high signal in the muscle, fascia, and subcutaneous fat. MR confirms the absence of a mass. At biopsy, the lesion was calcium pyrophosphate dihydrate deposition without other abnormality.*

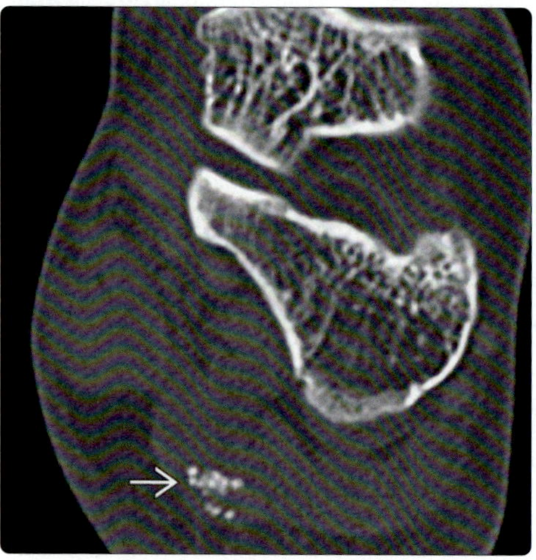

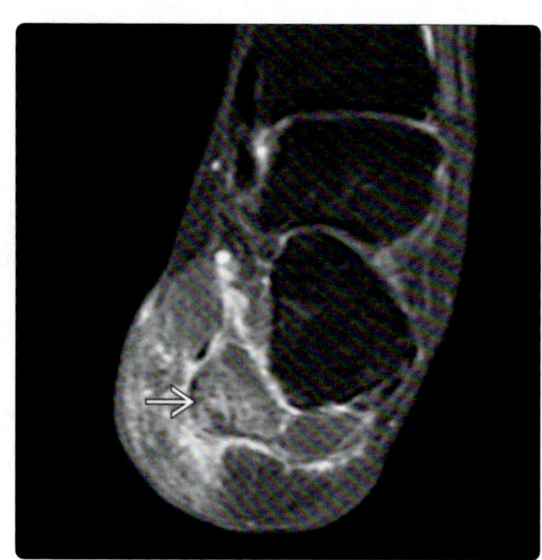

(Left) *Sagittal STIR MR shows a markedly enlarged hypointense peroneus longus tendon ➡. While one might consider a diagnosis such as xanthofibroma, it is important to consider the possibility that the low signal represents calcification.* **(Right)** *Lateral radiograph in the same patient confirms the source of low MR signal, showing dense, fairly homogeneous calcification following the expected path of the peroneus tendon ➡. This was due to hydroxyapatite deposition within the tendon.*

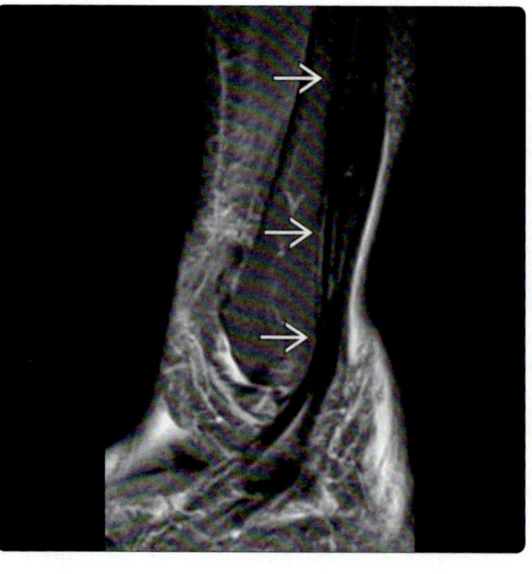

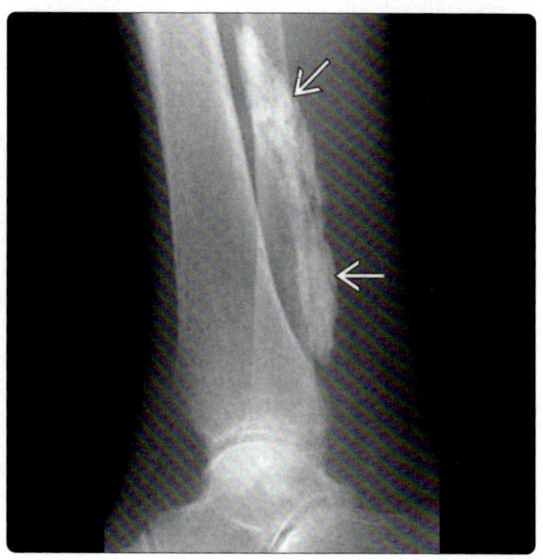

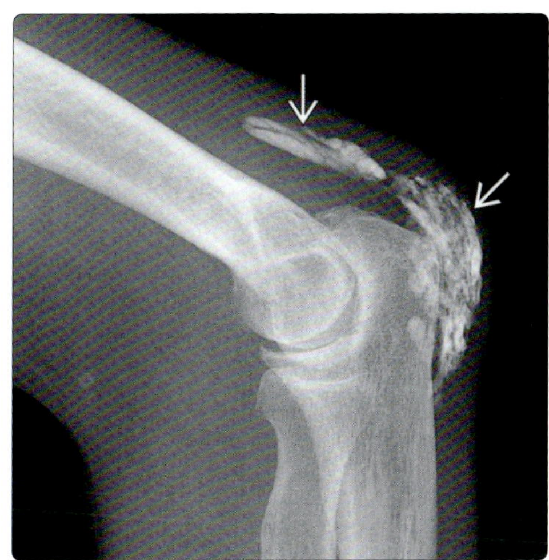

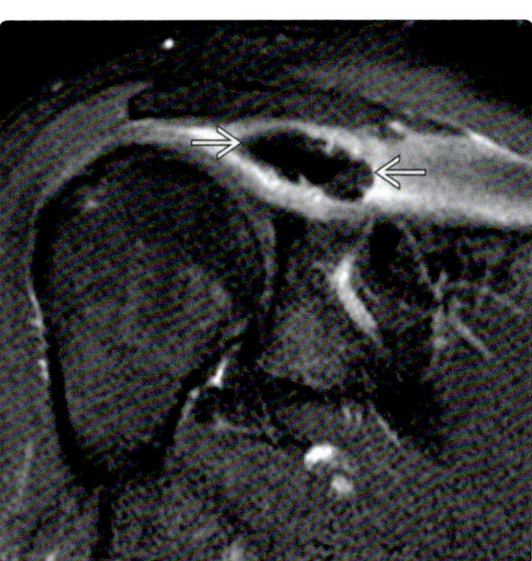

(Left) *Lateral radiograph shows extensive dense mineralization in the region of the olecranon bursa ➡ due to hydroxyapatite deposition disease. The dense and well-defined nature of the mineralization indicates longstanding involvement of the bursa.* **(Right)** *Coronal oblique T1WI C+ FS MR shows globular low-signal material ➡ within the supraspinatus muscle and tendon. Intense surrounding enhancement indicates prominent inflammation. The low signal is hydroxyapatite deposition disease.*

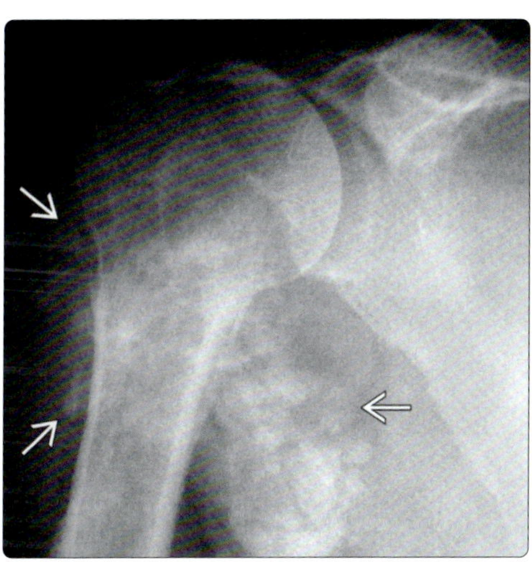

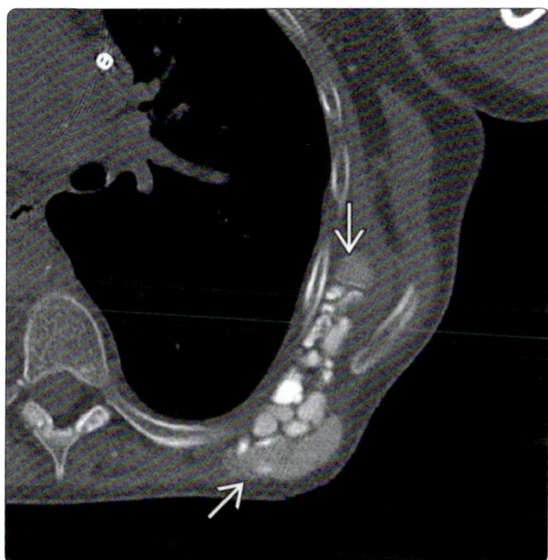

(Left) *Anteroposterior radiograph shows dense, cloud-like calcification ➡ surrounding an otherwise normal-appearing shoulder. While the more common etiology of this appearance is calcinosis of chronic renal failure, this was tumoral (idiopathic) calcinosis.* **(Right)** *Axial CT through the posterior chest in a patient on chronic hemodialysis shows a multicystic mass ➡ between the scapula and ribs. These cysts contain varying density of calcification. This is calcinosis of chronic renal failure.*

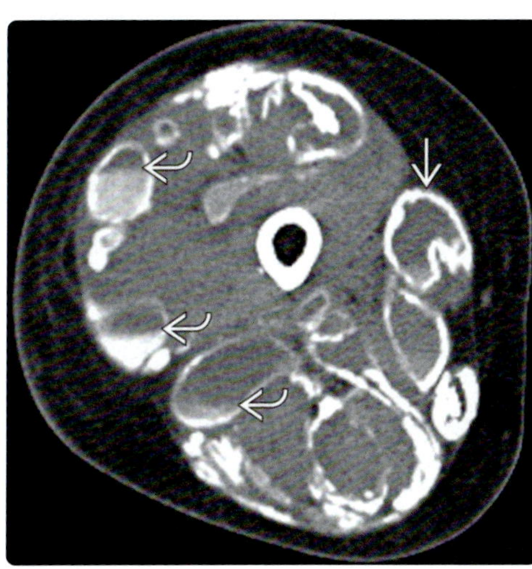

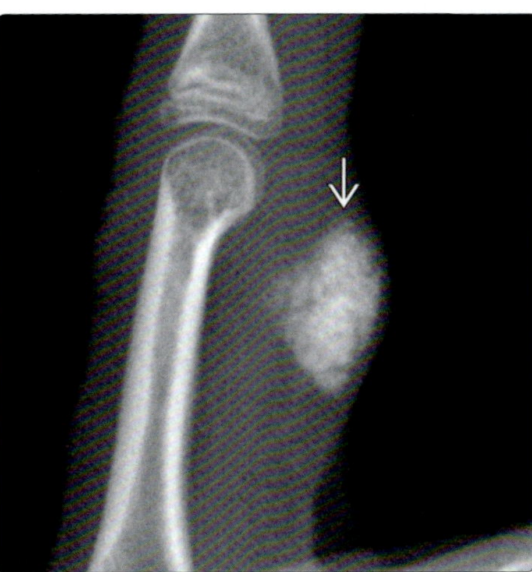

(Left) *Axial NECT shows extensive, sheet-like calcification ➡ of the muscles and fascial planes of the thigh with scattered fluid-fluid levels ➡. This type of calcium deposition is termed calcinosis universalis and was due to dermatomyositis.* **(Right)** *Lateral radiograph of the index finger shows a superficial globular calcification ➡. This type of calcium deposition is termed calcinosis circumscripta and was due to scleroderma. Metabolic causes of calcium deposition can have a similar appearance.*

Soft Tissue Tumor Mimics: Other

KEY FACTS

TERMINOLOGY

- Various entities that may mimic soft tissue neoplasm

TOP DIFFERENTIAL DIAGNOSES

- Myositis ossificans/heterotopic ossification
  - Heterotopic bone and cartilage formation
  - No identifiable cause in 40%
  - Typical zonal maturation: Peripheral to central
- Ganglion cyst
  - May not be connected to joint
  - MR: Fluid signal intensity with thin peripheral enhancement
- Synovial cyst
  - Lined by synovium, usually contiguous with joint
  - MR: Fluid signal intensity with thin peripheral enhancement
  - Complex signal with hemorrhage &/or debris
- Fat necrosis
  - Range of appearances from nonspecific soft tissue stranding to mimicking lipoma or liposarcoma
  - Well-defined nodule usually between skin and bony prominence
- Rheumatoid nodule
  - Assess for associated bone erosions and synovitis of rheumatoid arthritis
- Amyloid deposition
  - Abnormal protein deposition, often around joints
  - CT: Mass isodense to muscle ± bone erosion
  - Common clinical association: Dialysis
- Muscle injury
  - Palpable contour abnormality ± hematoma

DIAGNOSTIC CHECKLIST

- If imaging findings are not pathognomonic for specific entity, then biopsy or short-term follow-up may be necessary to exclude neoplasm

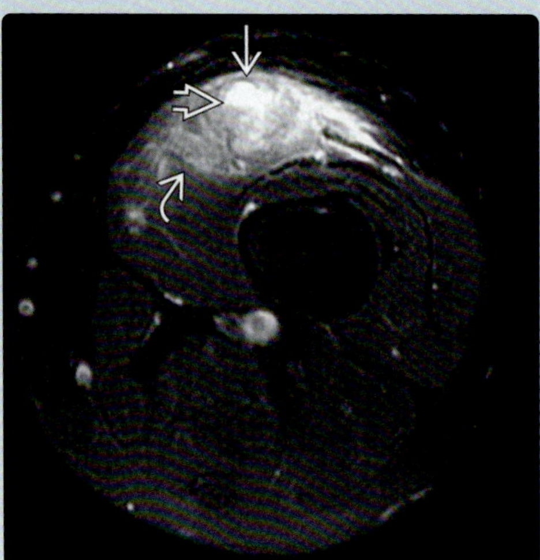

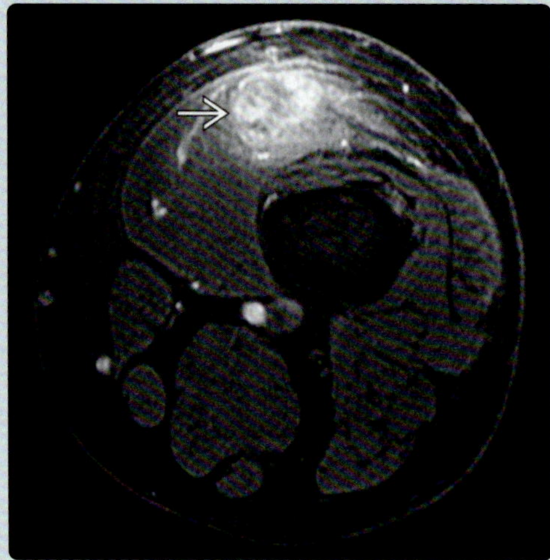

(Left) *Axial T2WI FS MR shows heterotopic ossification (myositis ossificans) ➡ in the thigh. This oval lesion has intermediate to high signal with surrounding edema ➡ and a suggestion of a fluid-fluid level ➡.* **(Right)** *Axial T1WI C+ FS MR in the same patient shows the thigh lesion ➡ to have inhomogeneous enhancement. Heterotopic ossification, also referred to as myositis ossificans when occurring in muscle, can enhance and have an aggressive appearance on MR.*

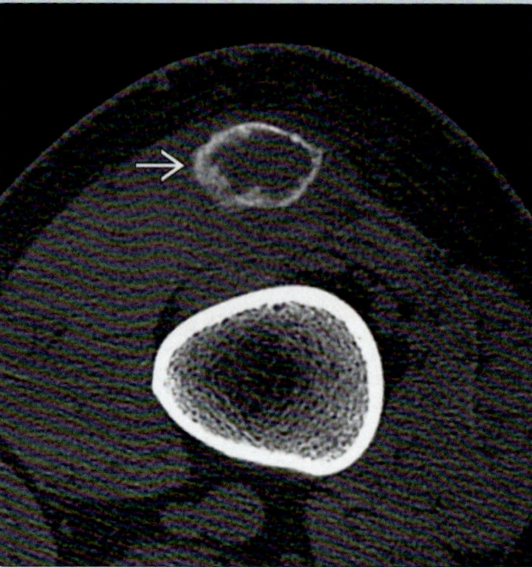

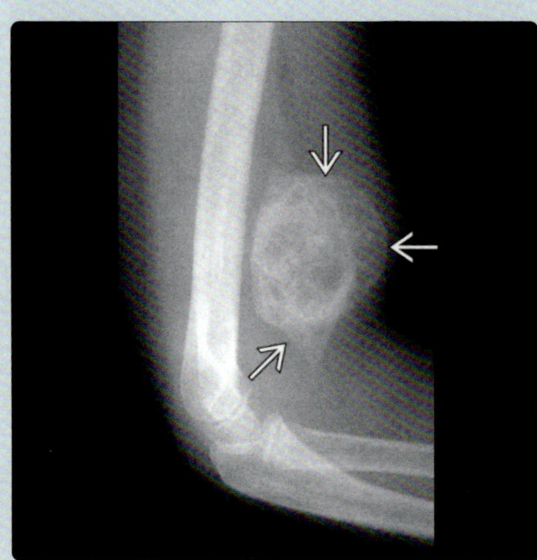

(Left) *Axial NECT in the same patient best demonstrates the peripheral zonal ossification pattern that is typical of heterotopic ossification ➡. If peripheral ossification is suggested on radiographs, CT may be useful in confirming the characteristic appearance of heterotopic ossification.* **(Right)** *Lateral radiograph of the elbow in a different patient shows a mature case of myositis ossificans ➡ in the distal aspect of the upper arm. The mass has a distinct, smooth outer cortex with a less-defined center.*

TERMINOLOGY

Definitions

- Various entities that may mimic soft tissue neoplasm

IMAGING

Imaging Recommendations

- Best imaging tool
  - MR most helpful for mass characterization, although radiographs useful for mineralization and associated bone findings
- Protocol advice
  - Skin markers useful to denote site of palpable abnormality and thus confirm complete assessment of area

DIFFERENTIAL DIAGNOSIS

Myositis Ossificans/Heterotopic Ossification

- Heterotopic bone and cartilage formation
  - Trauma, cerebrospinal disorder, and burns are most common causes
  - No identifiable cause in 40%
- Usually involves muscle
  - Less commonly occurs around ligament, fascia, tendon, joint capsule, and aponeurosis
- Typical zonal maturation → peripheral to central
  - Faint calcification (early) progressing to well-circumscribed osseous mass (late)
- MR: Heterogeneously hyperintense on T2WI with intense surrounding edema (early) and low signal rim of bone with internal fatty marrow (late)
  - Surrounding edema is uncommon in untreated soft tissue sarcomas

Ganglion Cyst

- Focal mucin collection with flat pseudosynovial cell lining
- May not be contiguous with joint
- Postulated to be response to repetitive microtrauma
- MR: Fluid signal intensity
  - Thin peripheral enhancement

Synovial Cyst

- Lined by synovium, usually contiguous with joint
- Popliteal cyst has typical location between medial head of gastrocnemius and semimembranosus tendon
- MR: Fluid signal intensity
  - Complex signal with hemorrhage &/or debris
  - Thin peripheral enhancement

Fat Necrosis

- Classic location over pressure point or bony protuberance
- Range of appearances from nonspecific soft tissue stranding to mimicking lipoma or liposarcoma
  - Early lesions show inflammatory stranding of fat
  - Mature lesions have central fat with thick peripheral capsule ± calcification
  - May contain nodular elements mimicking liposarcoma

Lymph Node

- Normal lymph nodes usually measure < 1 cm on short axis diameter
  - Inguinal lymph nodes have wider range of normal size
- Nonneoplastic nodes contain fatty hilum

Rheumatoid Nodule

- Well-defined nodule usually between skin and bony prominence
- Most common extraarticular manifestation of rheumatoid arthritis
  - Patients do not need to have rheumatoid arthritis to have rheumatoid nodules
- Radiographs: Nonspecific soft tissue mass that is uncommonly calcified
  - Assess for associated bone erosions and synovitis of rheumatoid arthritis
- MR: Nonspecific mass with variable signal intensity and variable enhancement
- F-18 FDG PET: Moderate uptake (SUV max 4.2) may mimic tumor

Amyloid Deposition

- Abnormal protein deposition, often around joints
  - Soft tissue masses distant from joints are rare
- Primary or secondary causes
  - Secondary causes: Hemodialysis, multiple myeloma, rheumatoid arthritis
- CT: Soft tissue masses isodense to muscle ± bone erosion
- MR: Intermediate signal on T1WI, low to intermediate signal mass on T2WI, + enhancement

Morton Neuroma

- Nonneoplastic fibrosing process of plantar digital nerve
- Plantar mass in intermetatarsal space
  - 3rd and 2nd intermetatarsal spaces most common
  - Marked female predominance (18:1)
- MR: Hypointense to isointense on T1WI, isointense to hyperintense on T2WI FS MR, with variable enhancement
  - ± associated intermetatarsal fluid collection > 3 mm transverse diameter (bursitis)
- Ultrasound: Ovoid mass with variable echogenicity ranging from homogeneously anechoic to heterogeneously hypoechoic
  - ↑ vascularity on color Doppler

Epidermal Inclusion Cyst

- Nonneoplastic subcutaneous mass containing keratin or cholesterol
  - Cystic ectasia of hair follicle infundibulum or deep traumatic implantation of epidermis
- Majority of lesions are found in scalp, face, neck, and trunk
- MR: Well-defined subcutaneous mass with variable signal dependent on internal debris
  - ↑ T1 signal pregadolinium complicates interpretation of postgadolinium images
- Cyst rupture associated with granulomatous reaction, granulation tissue, foreign body reaction, abscess, and meningitis (intracranial)

Sebaceous Cyst

- Arises from obstructed sebaceous gland
- Similar imaging appearance as epidermal inclusion cyst

Muscle Injury

- Full-thickness and partial-thickness tears of muscle and tendon
  - Palpable contour abnormalities
  - Associated hematomas

Muscle Atrophy

- Focal atrophy from any cause (denervation, trauma, diabetes) may cause adjacent or contralateral muscle to appear enlarged
- Hypertrophic muscle atrophy is associated with fat infiltration that enlarges muscle

Accessory Muscles

- Lower extremity: Accessory soleus, flexor digitorum longus, peroneus quartus
- Upper extremity: Accessory flexor carpi ulnaris, accessory abductor digiti minimi, duplicated hypothenar muscle, anomalous extensor tendon
- Appearance is same as other muscles/tendons on all imaging modalities

Postinjection Fibrosis of Skeletal Muscle

- Irregular area of muscle fibrosis after repeated intramuscular injections
  - Patient may or may not report injections
- Commonly involves thigh, shoulder, and gluteal regions
- MR: Ill-defined intramuscular mass with low T1WI and T2WI signal

Postoperative/Posttreatment Changes

- Normal disruption of soft tissue neoplasm operative bed from treatment
  - Seroma, hematoma, myocutaneous flap, and granulation tissue
- Radiation-induced pseudotumor: Ill-defined focus of heterogeneous enhancement lacking significant mass effect

Hemophilia

- Pseudotumor: Nonneoplastic mass lesion that occurs with repeated focal intraosseous, subperiosteal, or soft tissue bleeding
- Radiographs and CT: Soft tissue mass ± calcifications and extrinsic bone scalloping
  - May have unusual periosteal reaction (perpendicular to bone)
- MR: Heterogeneous signal on T1WI and T2WI ± fluid-fluid levels

Traumatic Neuroma

- Proliferative response of nerve to injury, usually associated with amputation
- ± mass visibly contiguous with normal nerve
- MR: Isointense to muscle on T1WI, hyperintense on fluid-sensitive MR
  - ± ring-like or telephone cable appearance from enlarged nerve fascicles
  - Mild to marked enhancement
- May be mistaken for tumor recurrence when amputation performed for malignancy

Fascial Hernia

- Herniation of muscle through fascia
- Mass more prominent during muscle contraction
- Most common involving anterior compartment of lower leg and tensor fascia lata
- Appearance is same as other muscles on all imaging modalities

Sarcoidosis, Soft Tissue Masses

- Nodular sarcoid myopathy uncommon
- Found with systemic disease
- MR: Irregular nodules isointense on T1WI, hyperintense on T2WI

Primary Bone Tumor

- Primary bone tumors may have disproportionately large soft tissue extension mimicking primary soft tissue tumor

Brown Tumor

- Associated with hyperparathyroidism and renal osteodystrophy
- Typically presents as lytic, geographic bone lesion
  - Look for additional findings of bone resorption
- Lesions involving soft tissues extend from underlying bone

Granuloma Annulare

- Uncommon subcutaneous mass
  - Usually found in children
- MR: Ill-defined mass with low T1 signal, low to intermediate T2 signal, and with enhancement

Melorheostosis

- Uncommon bone dysplasia
- Typical bone changes of "flowing candle wax" in sclerotome distribution
  - 27-53% with soft tissue mass ± mineralization
- MR: Nonspecific enhancing mass, may contain fat

Hoffa Disease

- Infrapatellar fat pad impingement resulting in scar tissue
- Scar may mimic tumor when containing foci of metaplastic bone and cartilage

DIAGNOSTIC CHECKLIST

Image Interpretation Pearls

- If imaging findings are not pathognomonic for specific entity, then biopsy or short-term follow-up may be necessary to exclude neoplasm

SELECTED REFERENCES

1. Czeyda-Pommersheim F et al: Amyloidosis: modern cross-sectional imaging. Radiographics. 35(5):1381-92, 2015
2. Garner HW et al: Benign and malignant soft-tissue tumors: posttreatment MR imaging. Radiographics. 29(1):119-34, 2009
3. McKenzie G et al: Pictorial review: Non-neoplastic soft-tissue masses. Br J Radiol. 82(981):775-85, 2009
4. Moore LF et al: Radiation-induced pseudotumor following therapy for soft tissue sarcoma. Skeletal Radiol. 38(6):579-84, 2009
5. Stacy GS et al: Pitfalls in MR image interpretation prompting referrals to an orthopedic oncology clinic. Radiographics. 27(3):805-26; discussion 827-8, 2007
6. Kransdorf MJ et al: Masses that may mimic soft tissue tumors. In Kransdorf MJ et al: Imaging of Soft Tissue Tumors. 2nd ed. Philadelphia: Lippincott Williams & Wilkins. 529-69, 2006

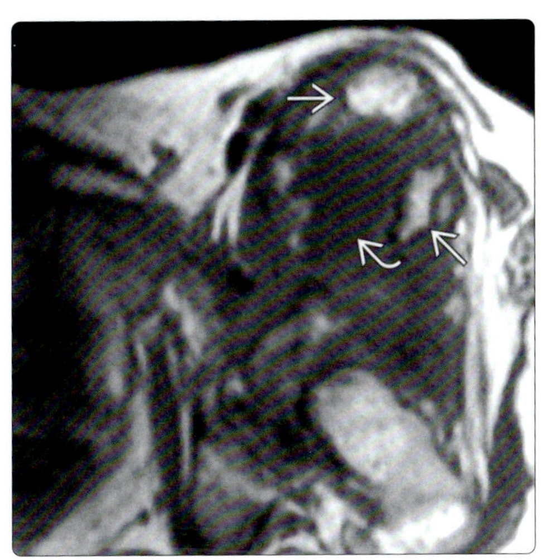

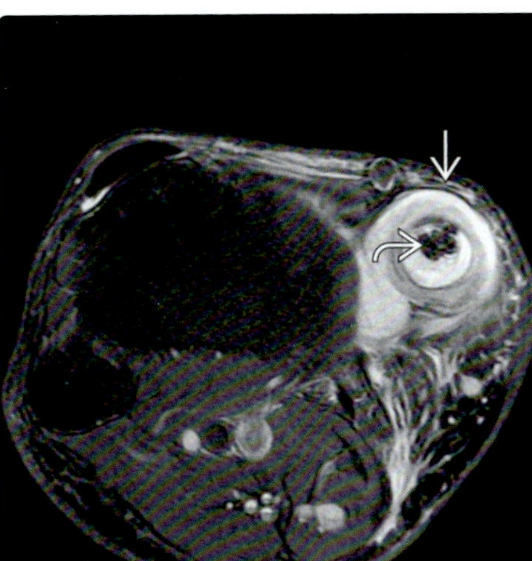

(Left) *Axial T1WI MR shows myositis ossificans anterior to the left hip in a paraplegic patient. Foci of mature bone ➡ are characterized by marrow signal matching that of the femur. The myositis lies anterior to a fluid collection ↪, which can be seen in mature myositis as well.* **(Right)** *Axial T1WI C+ FS MR shows a complex mass ➡ in the medial soft tissues of the knee. The cyst contains small foci of air ↪ and has a laminated wall. There was minimal peripheral enhancement. Excision revealed a ganglion cyst.*

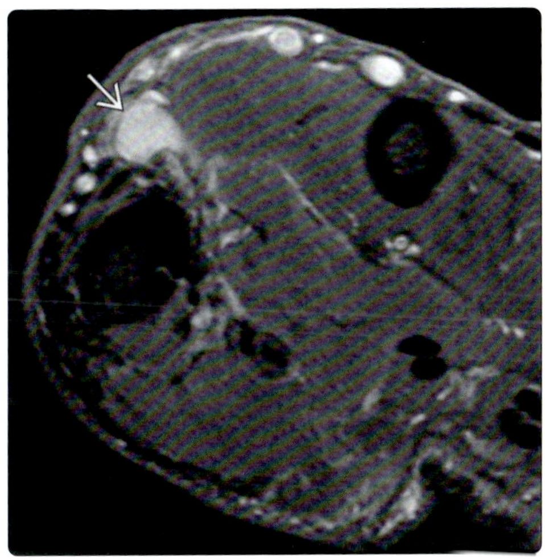

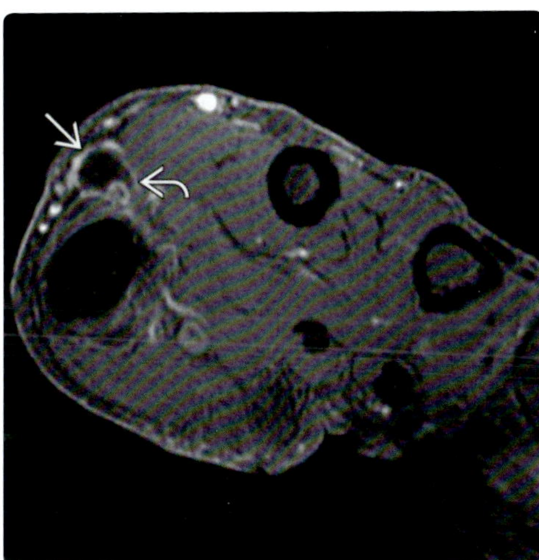

(Left) *Axial T2WI FS MR of the wrist shows a small ganglion cyst ➡ within the radial soft tissues adjacent to the right thumb metacarpal bone. The mass is homogeneously hyperintense.* **(Right)** *Axial T1WI C+ FS MR in the same patient shows only thin peripheral enhancement of the lesion ➡. This differentiates a benign cyst from a solid soft tissue tumor. Note that a small tail ↪ arises from the mass. This finding is often present when a ganglion cyst extends from a joint.*

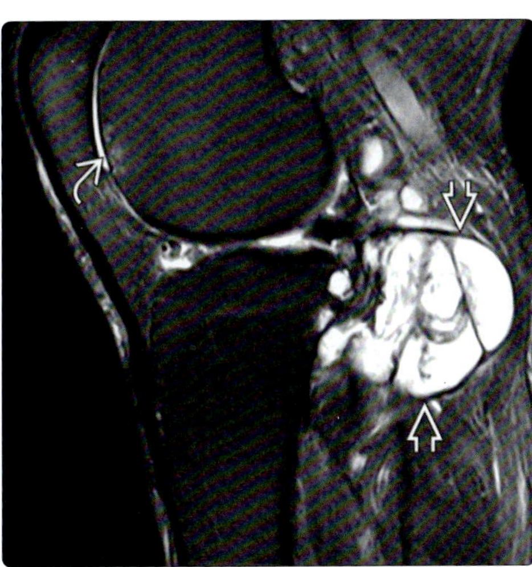

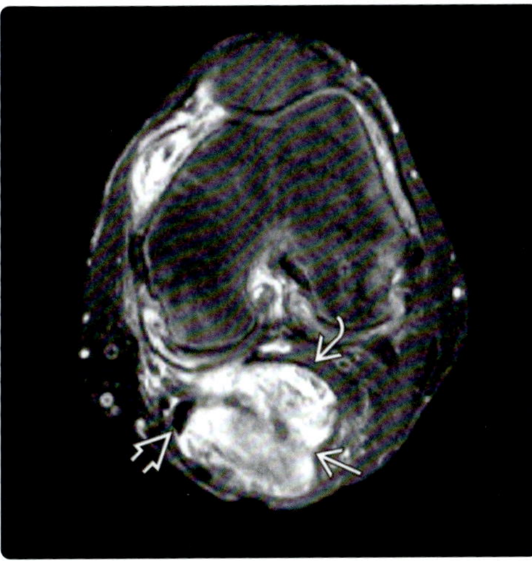

(Left) *Sagittal T2WI FS MR shows a complex synovial cyst ⇨. This was not in the typical location for a popliteal cyst. Severe degenerative change of the patellofemoral joint ↪ is typical for pyrophosphate arthropathy.* **(Right)** *Axial T2WI FS MR shows a complex popliteal synovial cyst ➡ in a patient with rheumatoid arthritis. The mass has heterogeneous high signal. The mass is situated in the typical location, between the semimembranosus tendon ⇨ and the medial head of gastrocnemius muscle ↪.*

(Left) *Axial NECT of the chest shows early changes of fat necrosis ➡. This focal area of nonspecific increased density with surrounding inflammatory change has a nonspecific appearance. The lesion developed acutely and was painful. Biopsy was performed to exclude neoplasm or infection.* **(Right)** *Axial NECT of the low pelvis shows chronic fat necrosis ➡ appearing as an ill-defined mass with similar attenuation to skeletal muscle and coarse calcification. Prone positioning was in preparation for biopsy.*

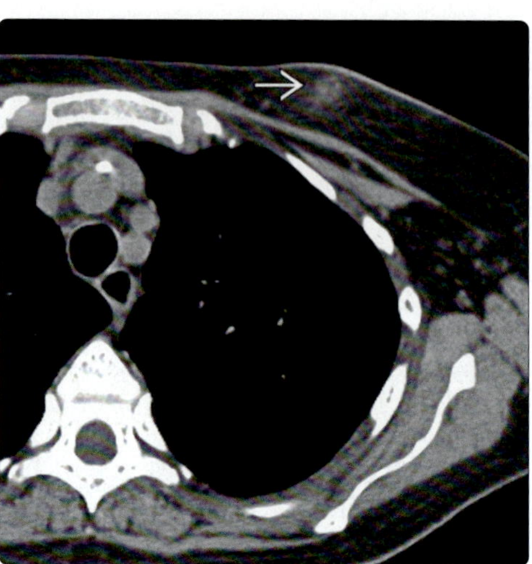

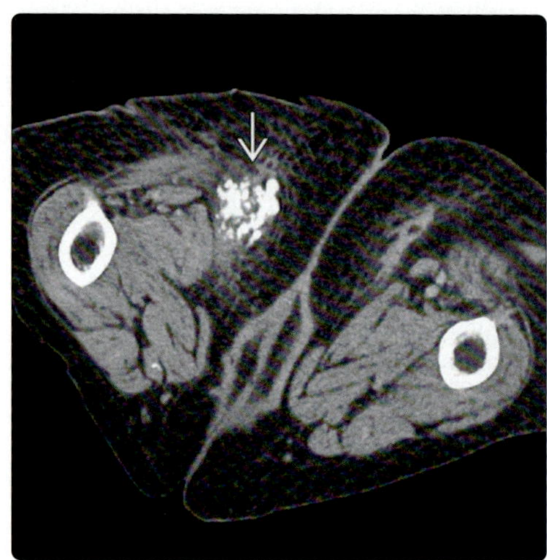

(Left) *Lateral radiograph of the ankle shows a large anterior soft tissue mass ➡ without underlying osseous abnormalities. The soft tissue mass has no further defining characteristics, such as matrix or abnormal density. This was due to amyloid deposition.* **(Right)** *Axial T1WI MR shows a low signal intensity mass ➡ arising from the plantar aspect of the 3rd intermetatarsal space. The mass stayed low in signal intensity on the T2WI FS MR and had heterogeneous enhancement. This is a Morton neuroma.*

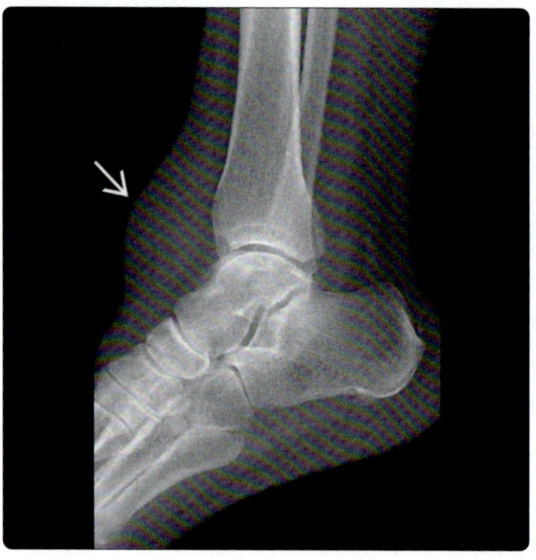

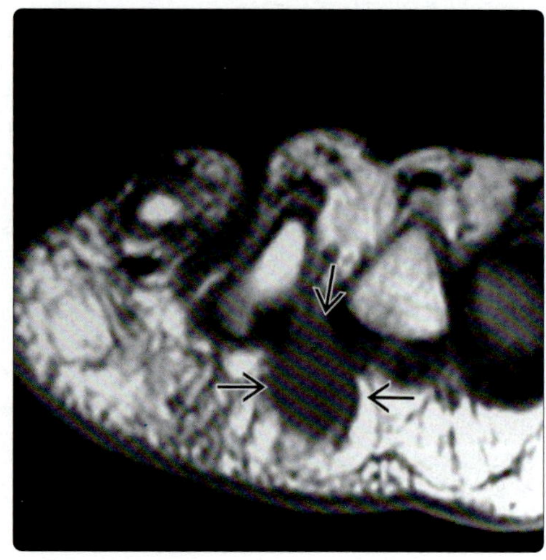

(Left) *Axial T1WI MR of the distal thigh shows an epidermal inclusion cyst ➡. This superficial mass is relatively homogeneous with a signal intensity slightly hyperintense relative to skeletal muscle, which can mimic enhancement on T1WI C+ FS MR.* **(Right)** *Axial T1WI MR shows a focal area of atrophy ➡ involving the lateral aspect of the lateral gastrocnemius muscle. There is no mass effect, thus excluding an intramuscular lipoma. The patient reported a palpable abnormality at the distal edge of this atrophy.*

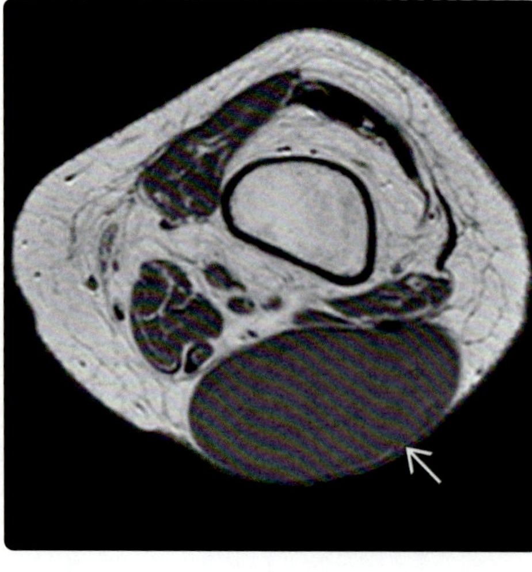

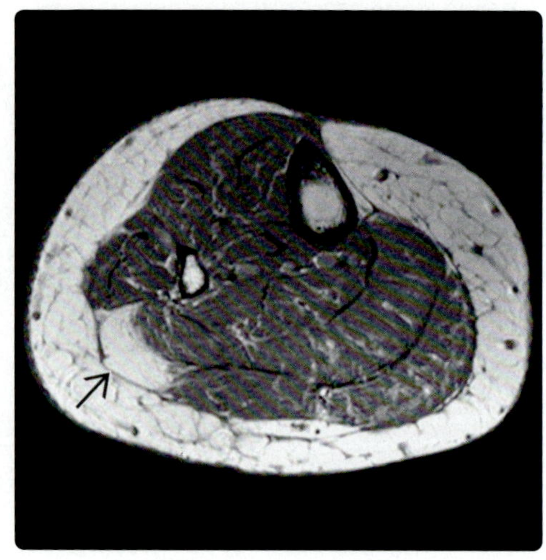

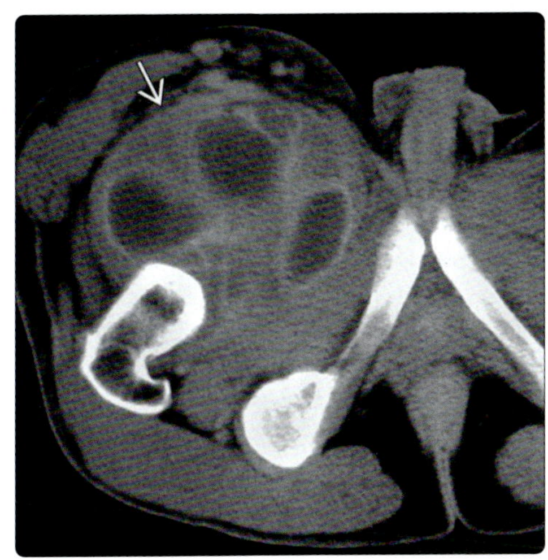

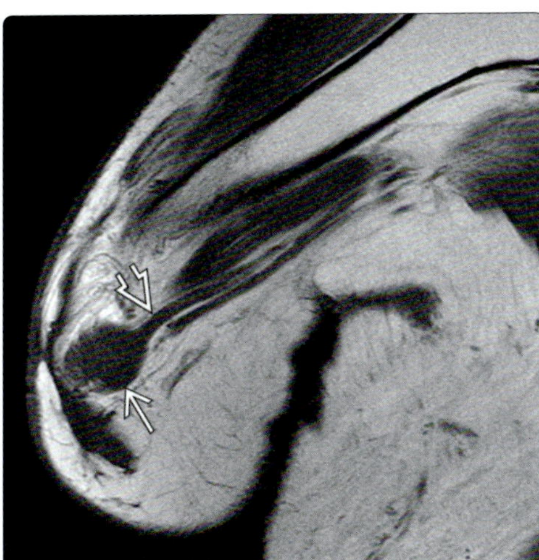

(Left) *Axial CECT shows a pseudotumor* ➡ *in a patient with hemophilia. This mass contains loculated fluid collections with enhancing rims. The mass resulted from repeated hemorrhage that produced pressure erosion of the bone and extended into the surrounding soft tissues.* **(Right)** *Coronal oblique T1WI MR shows a traumatic neuroma* ➡ *near the level of an upper arm amputation site. The mass is homogeneously isointense to skeletal muscle. The mass is also seen to be contiguous with an enlarged nerve* ➡*.*

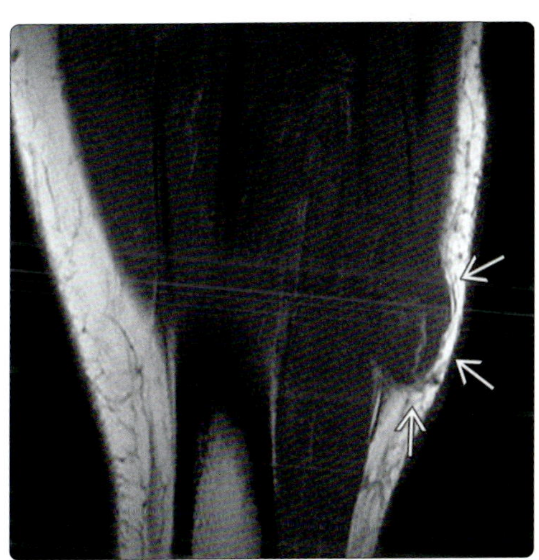

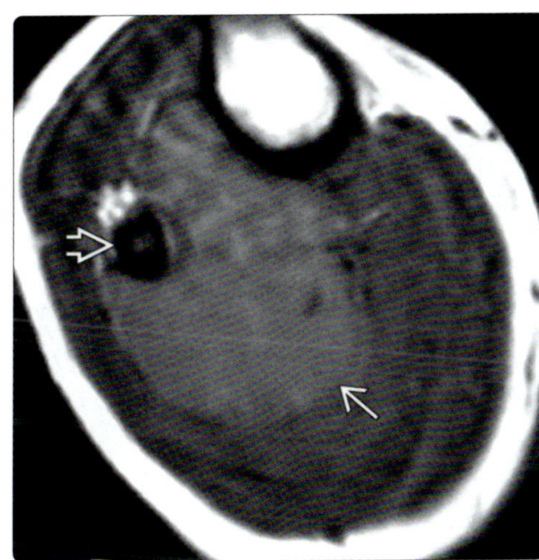

(Left) *Coronal T1WI MR shows a fascial herniation* ➡*. The mass-like appearance of the muscle is caused by bulging through a fascial defect. Many myofascial herniations become more apparent with exercise due to increased blood volume.* **(Right)** *Axial T1WI MR shows an Ewing sarcoma of the fibula* ➡ *with a prominent soft tissue mass* ➡*. The mass could be mistaken for a primary soft tissue tumor if the changes in the fibular marrow space were not appreciated or misinterpreted as invasion.*

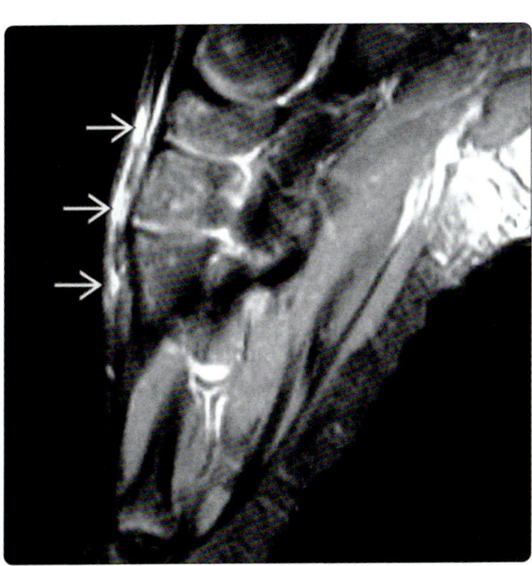

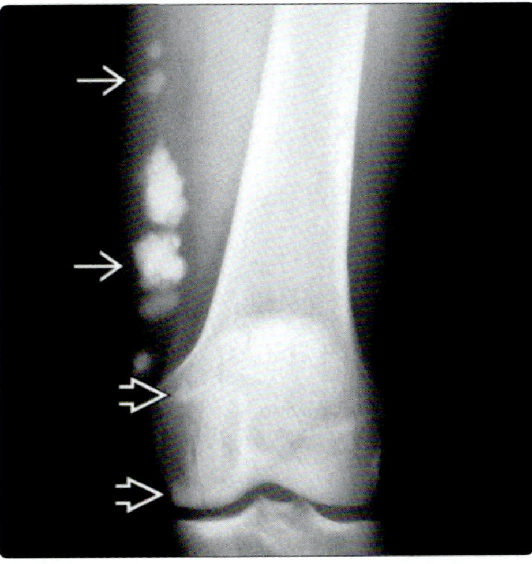

(Left) *Sagittal T1WI C+ FS MR in a child shows granuloma annulare* ➡*. Small subcutaneous nodules involving the dorsum of the foot show intense enhancement. The nodules are not contiguous and do not invade the underlying tissue.* **(Right)** *AP radiograph of the knee shows soft tissue melorheostosis* ➡ *as several small, densely mineralized masses in a linear orientation. Small sclerotic foci within the adjacent femoral condyle* ➡ *have a more rounded appearance than is typical for melorheostosis.*

KEY FACTS

TERMINOLOGY

- Heterotopic formation of bone and cartilage in soft tissue
  - Benign, solitary, self-limiting

IMAGING

- Classic appearance: Mature bone formation within soft tissues, seen in later stages of disease
  - Earlier stages are confusing: Bone is amorphous and appears similar to tumor bone formation
- Radiographic appearance distinctive and related to time following trauma
  - 0-2 weeks: Soft tissue mass with indistinct surrounding soft tissue planes
  - 3-4 weeks: Amorphous osteoid forms within mass; adjacent periosteal reaction may be seen
  - 6-8 weeks: Sharper cortex begins to form about lacy central osseous mass
  - 5-6 months: Mature bone formation
  - During 2-6 month period, osseous maturation assumes distinctive zoning pattern diagnostic of MO: Mature cortical bone peripherally, less mature bone centrally
  - Toward end of this period, size may begin to ↓
  - ≥ 7 months: Mass may continue to decrease in size; trabeculae may be seen enclosed by mature cortex
- CT: Peripheral rim of more organized mineralization seen by 4-6 weeks, earlier than radiograph
- MR: Appearance relates to age of lesion, paralleling other imaging
  - May show marrow edema, periosteal reaction, and peripheral edema at any stage

DIAGNOSTIC CHECKLIST

- History of trauma and timing relative to imaging are crucial to diagnosis, though trauma may be denied
- Must avoid biopsy during early stages to avoid misdiagnosis of tumor

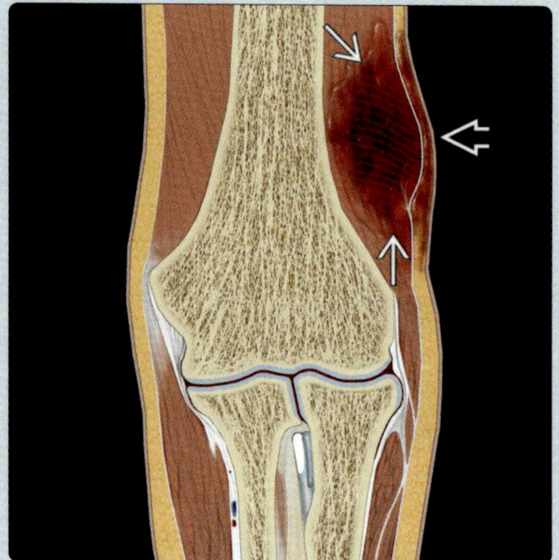

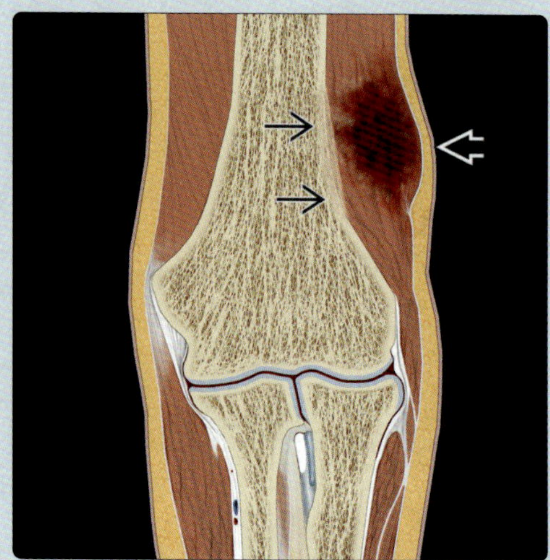

(Left) *Coronal graphic shows the earliest appearance of myositis ossificans (MO). There is a doughy mass ➡, which distorts the subcutaneous fat plane. Edema is seen in the subcutaneous tissues ➡, but the adjacent bone is normal.* **(Right)** *Coronal graphic shows MO at 3-4 weeks. Note that the mass itself is slightly smaller and that the subcutaneous edema ➡ has resolved. However, there is new development of periosteal reaction and cortical edema ➡. This is the stage at which MO may be most confusing on imaging.*

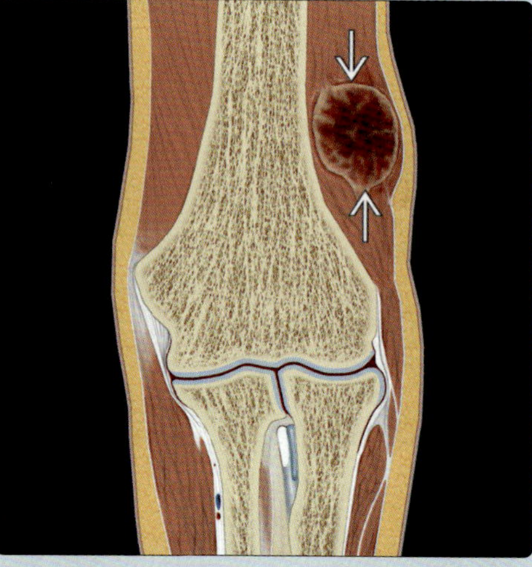

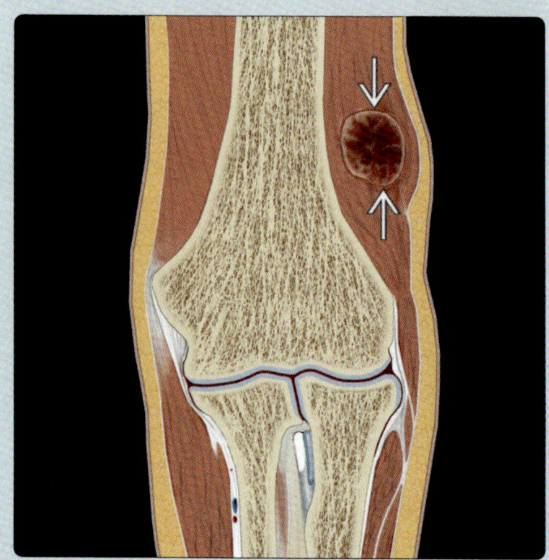

(Left) *Coronal graphic shows MO at 6-8 weeks. There is now newly organized mature bone seen peripherally about the lesion ➡ with less mature bone centrally.* **(Right)** *Coronal graphic depicts MO at 5-6 months. By this time, the peripheral bone is clearly mature ➡. There may be trabeculae within the lesion, but the lesion generally retains a less mature appearance centrally, particularly on axial imaging. There is no surrounding soft tissue mass. The entire lesion often begins to decrease in size.*

TERMINOLOGY

Abbreviations

- Myositis ossificans (MO)
- Heterotopic ossification (HO)

Definitions

- Heterotopic formation of bone and cartilage in soft tissue: Benign, solitary, self-limiting
- Term myositis is misleading
  - Most frequently occurs in muscle
  - May also be found in fascia, tendons, and fat
  - Heterotopic ossification is more correct term and is same entity; however, myositis ossificans continues to be in popular usage at this time

IMAGING

General Features

- Best diagnostic clue
  - Mature bone formation within soft tissues, seen in later stages of disease
  - Earlier stages are confusing: Bone is amorphous and appears similar to tumor bone formation
- Location
  - Common in areas prone to trauma
    - Antecubital fossa following elbow dislocation
    - Anterolateral thigh in football players
    - Fat adjacent to adductors in horseback riders
  - Shoulder and elbows in burn patients
  - Formed about pelvis and hips in spinal cord or brain injured patients
- Size
  - May be several cm in length or diameter
- Morphology
  - Distinctive and related to time following trauma
  - All imaging modalities reflect progressive changes

Radiographic Findings

- Distinctive and related to time following trauma
- 0-2 weeks: Soft tissue mass with indistinct surrounding soft tissue planes
- 3-4 weeks: Amorphous osteoid forms within mass; adjacent periosteal reaction may be seen
- 6-8 weeks: Sharper cortex begins to form about lacy central osseous mass
- 5-6 months: Mature bone formation
  - During 2-6 month period, osseous maturation assumes distinctive zoning pattern diagnostic of MO: Mature cortical bone peripherally, less mature bone centrally
  - Toward end of this period, size may begin to ↓
- ≥ 7 months: Mass may continue to decrease in size; trabeculae may be seen enclosed by mature cortex

CT Findings

- Appearance relates to age of lesion, paralleling histology and other imaging
- Earliest findings: Low-attenuation soft tissue mass
- Amorphous bone density seen by 3-4 weeks, more prominently than on radiograph
- Peripheral rim of more organized mineralization seen by 4-6 weeks, earlier than radiograph
- Mature lesions show peripheral cortical rim and central decreased attenuation (may contain trabeculae)

MR Findings

- Appearance relates to age of lesion, paralleling histology and other imaging
- May show marrow edema, periosteal reaction, and peripheral edema at any stage
- Early stages
  - T1: Signal intensity isointense to muscle
  - Fluid-sensitive sequences: Hyperintense, markedly inhomogeneous
- Intermediate stages
  - T1: Normal, isointense to muscle, perhaps with local distortion of fat planes
  - Fluid-sensitive sequences: Hyperintense mass, with curvilinear and irregular areas of decreased signal intensity surrounding lesion
    - This low-signal halo may be incomplete and difficult to visualize but serves to differentiate MO from tumor bone formation
    - Earliest equivalent to well-organized cortical rim visualized on radiograph or CT
    - Curvilinear density occasionally seen in early lesions but fairly reliably seen by 3-4 weeks
  - Marked enhancement with contrast
- Late stages
  - Well-defined inhomogeneous masses with signal approximating bone, without associated edema

Imaging Recommendations

- Best imaging tool
  - Depending on age of lesion, may need combination of radiograph + CT or MR

DIFFERENTIAL DIAGNOSIS

Tumoral Calcinosis

- Periarticular calcified (not ossified) soft tissue mass
- Separate from underlying bone

Parosteal Osteosarcoma

- Well-organized bone formation mostly in soft tissues, though osseous attachment is present
- Opposite zoning pattern
  - Parosteal osteosarcoma has organized bone centrally, less mature bone peripherally

High-Grade Surface or Soft Tissue Osteosarcoma

- Less well-organized tumor bone formation within soft tissues
- May have very similar appearance to MO in its early amorphous stages
- Opposite zoning pattern
  - More mature osteoid centrally, less mature bone peripherally, less organized overall

Osteochondroma (Exostosis)

- Normally organized bone arising from metaphyseal region of underlying bone
- "Stalk" of marrow, outlined by cortex, cartilage cap
- Careful evaluation shows no true similarity to MO

Fibrodysplasia Ossificans Progressiva

- Autosomal dominant mesodermal disorder with wide range of expressivity
- Target is interstitial tissues, with muscle involvement secondary to pressure atrophy
- Progressive ossification of striated muscle, tendons, ligaments, and fascial planes

Proliferative Myositis

- Benign inflammatory myopathy
- Present with rapidly enlarging firm, painful soft tissue mass, similar to MO
- T1 SI hypo-/isointense to muscle
- T2 hyperintense; enhancement is intense
- No differentiation by MR from early stage MO; does not develop ossification

PATHOLOGY

General Features

- Etiology
  - Progenitor stem cells for osteoid production exist within affected soft tissues
  - With proper stimulus, stem cells differentiate into osteoblasts and form osteoid
  - Experiments suggest that bone morphogenic proteins can stimulate HO and may play role
  - Overt stimulus is usually traumatic, though it may be inapparent or forgotten by patient
  - Avulsion fracture, especially around pelvis, may result in heterotopic bone formation
    - Bone forms between donor site and avulsed bone
    - Follows same timing and zoning pattern as MO
    - Ages 14-25 particularly at risk: Ranges from period of apophyseal ossification to fusion
    - Most frequent sites: Anterior superior iliac spine, anterior inferior iliac spine, ischial apophysis, adductor apophysis
  - Burn patients at additional risk
  - Brain injury patients at additional risk
    - Extent and functional severity directly related to severity of intracranial injury
  - Spinal cord injury patients at risk
    - Strong propensity to recur following resection
  - Other causes of neurologic compromise may be associated: Tetanus, poliomyelitis, Guillain-Barré
  - Total hip arthroplasty patients at risk for local HO

Microscopic Features

- Histologic evolution of MO parallels that of imaging, with progression and similar zoning phenomenon
  - Weeks 1-4: Pseudosarcomatous appearance in central zone, giving appearance of tumor bone
  - Weeks 4-8: Centrifugal pattern, with periphery of amorphous osteoid, surrounding cellular center
  - Following week 8: Gradual organization into mature peripheral bone surrounding cellular center

CLINICAL ISSUES

Presentation

- Most common signs/symptoms
  - First 2 weeks: Painful soft tissue mass
    - Warm, doughy
    - Patient may not recall episode of trauma (particularly if child or teenager)

Demographics

- Age
  - Any age
- Gender
  - M > F, particularly in spinal cord injury patients
- Epidemiology
  - 20-30% of patients with neurologic deficits → HO
  - 33-49% of paraplegics show HO
  - 5% of total hip patients develop HO; 1% severe

Natural History & Prognosis

- Single traumatic lesion may stabilize and regress
  - Residual: Symptomatic based on size/location
- Brain/spinal cord HO tends not to regress
  - May cause decreased range of motion
  - May develop ulceration if in weight-bearing area

Treatment

- Following maturation of lesion, surgical resection may be considered if lesion is symptomatic
- May prophylax total hip patients at high risk for HO with low-dose radiation
- Long-term oral etidronate may be useful for early HO

DIAGNOSTIC CHECKLIST

Consider

- History of trauma and timing relative to imaging is crucial to diagnosis, though trauma may be denied
- Must avoid biopsy during early stages to avoid misdiagnosis of tumor
- Radiologist, oncologic surgeon, and pathologist must work as team to avoid misdiagnosis

Image Interpretation Pearls

- Do not overinterpret early amorphous osteoid formation as tumor bone
- Periosteal reaction &/or cortical, marrow, and soft tissue edema commonly associated with MO
- Watch for peripheral organization, either as organized bone on radiograph or CT, or as "halo" on MR

SELECTED REFERENCES

1. Demir MK et al: Case 118: proliferative myositis. Radiology. 244(2):613-6, 2007
2. Balboni TA et al: Heterotopic ossification: pathophysiology, clinical features, and the role of radiotherapy for prophylaxis. Int J Radiat Oncol Biol Phys. 65(5):1289-99, 2006
3. Eid K et al: Systemic effects of severe trauma on the function and apoptosis of human skeletal cells. J Bone Joint Surg Br. 88(10):1394-400, 2006
4. Hudson SJ et al: Heterotopic ossification–a long-term consequence of prolonged immobility. Crit Care. 10(6):174, 2006
5. McCarthy EF et al: Heterotopic ossification: a review. Skeletal Radiol. 34(10):609-19, 2005
6. Kransdorf MJ et al: Myositis ossificans: MR appearance with radiologic-pathologic correlation. AJR Am J Roentgenol. 157(6):1243-8, 1991

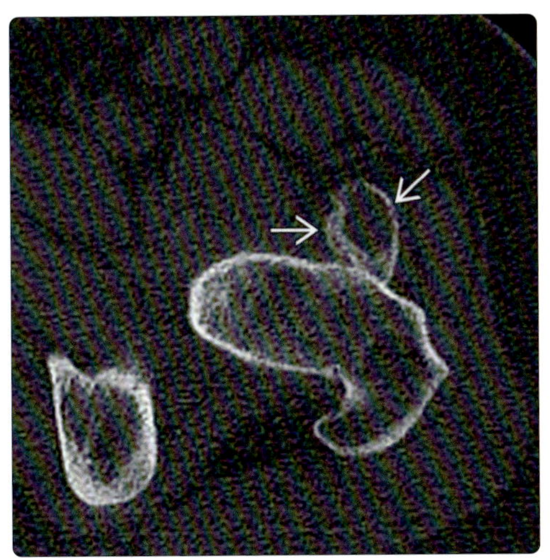

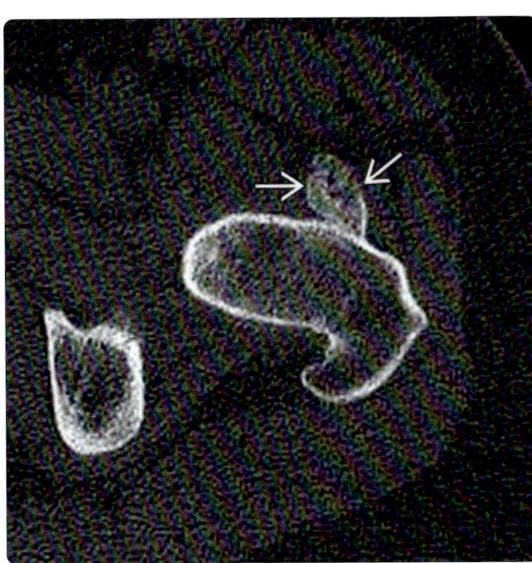

(Left) *Axial CT through the proximal femur of a 30 year old shows well-defined bone matrix ➡ peripherally, surrounding a hypodense center. This zoning pattern is typical of myositis ossificans and is the opposite of parosteal osteosarcoma (central ossific density, peripheral soft tissue). In this case, the CT was obtained 22 weeks post trauma.* **(Right)** *Axial CT in the same case, but obtained 20 weeks following the previous image, shows the lesion ➡ to be decreasing in size while retaining the benign myositis ossific zoning.*

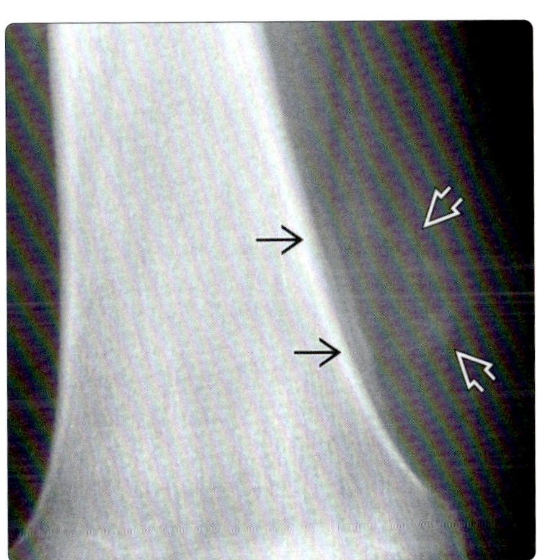

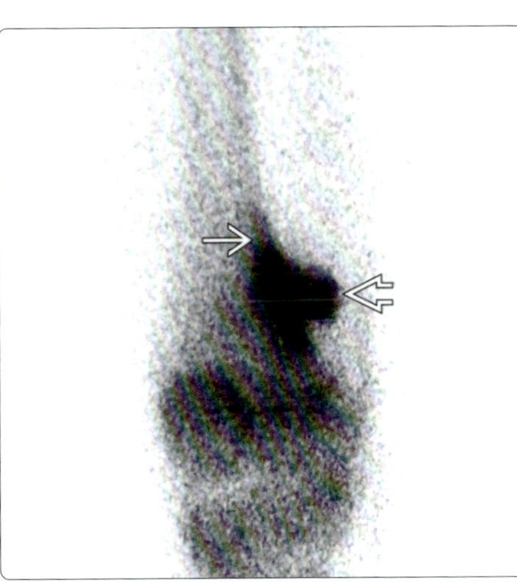

(Left) *AP radiograph appearance in this case may be alarming; it shows periosteal reaction ➡ and faint osseous matrix in the adjacent soft tissues ➡. This appearance could represent either early myositis ossificans or early surface osteosarcoma.* **(Right)** *AP Tc-99m bone scan shows intense uptake at the lesion ➡ as well as periosteum ➡, but it is entirely nonspecific. This demonstrates that bone scan is often not a cost-effective diagnostic exam, as it often does not provide additional information.*

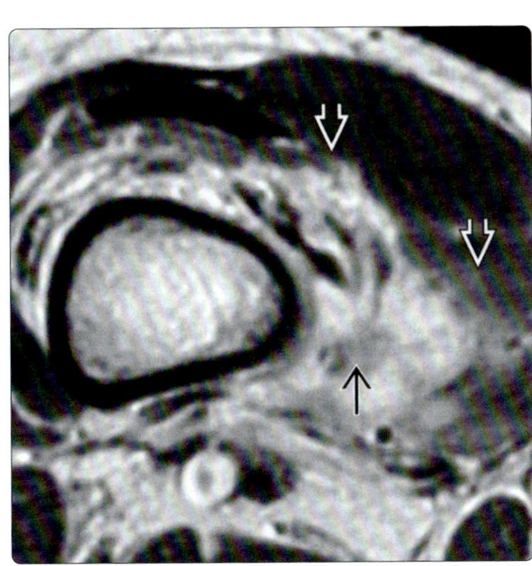

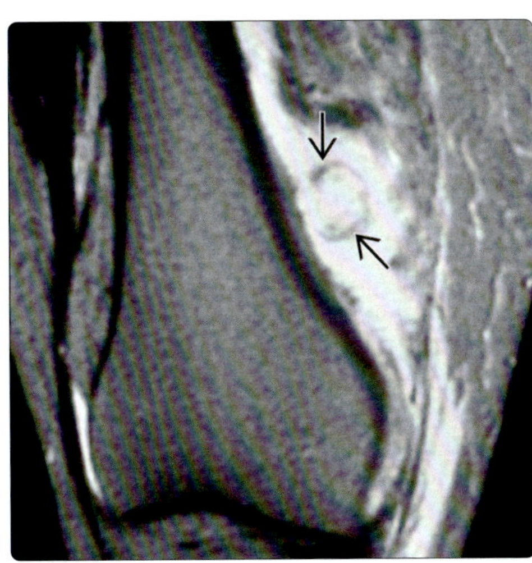

(Left) *Axial T1WI FS C+ MR in the same case shows low signal centrally in the area of the soft tissue mass ➡, surrounded by edema ➡, but this is an expected appearance and does not differentiate between myositis and surface osteosarcoma.* **(Right)** *Coronal T2WI FS MR shows a halo of low signal ➡ with central and surrounding high signal at the site of the mass. This is an early representation of the zoning phenomenon, showing early peripheral maturity in MO. It may be considered diagnostic and should preclude biopsy.*

(Left) *Axial T2WI FS MR shows an oval lesion with intermediate to high signal intensity and a suggestion of a fluid-fluid level ➡. There is surrounding edema ↪. This is a nonspecific appearance.* **(Right)** *Axial T1WI C+ FS MR of the same lesion shows inhomogeneous enhancement ➡. The lesion appears rather aggressive, but findings are nonspecific. Myositis ossificans should be one of the lesions under consideration. The patient had denied trauma, but trauma around the thigh is often forgotten.*

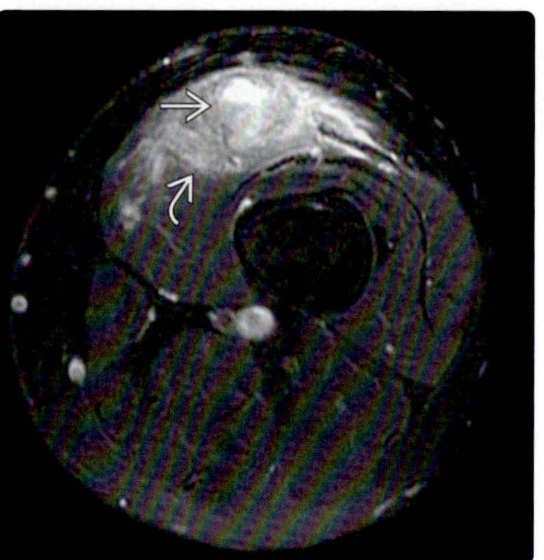

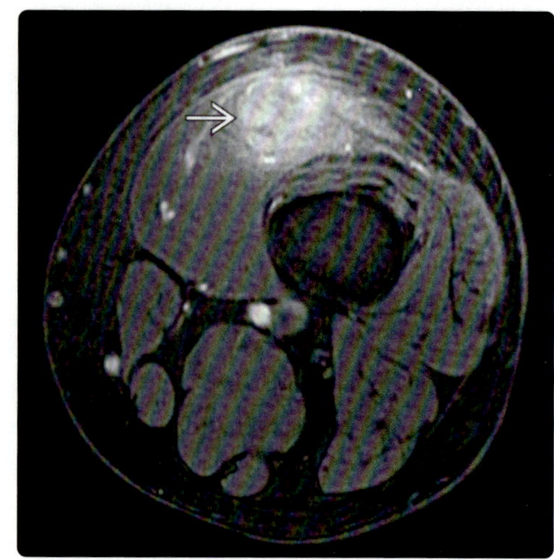

(Left) *Coronal T1WI MR in the same case demonstrates the central SI of the lesion to be similar to muscle, with a low-signal periphery ➡. This suggests peripheral zoning.* **(Right)** *Sagittal reformatted CT best demonstrates the peripherally ossified focus of MO ➡, confirming the diagnosis. Remember that MO can enhance and have an aggressive appearance on MR. If radiographs are negative, CT may be useful in demonstrating the typical appearance of early amorphous or peripheral ossification.*

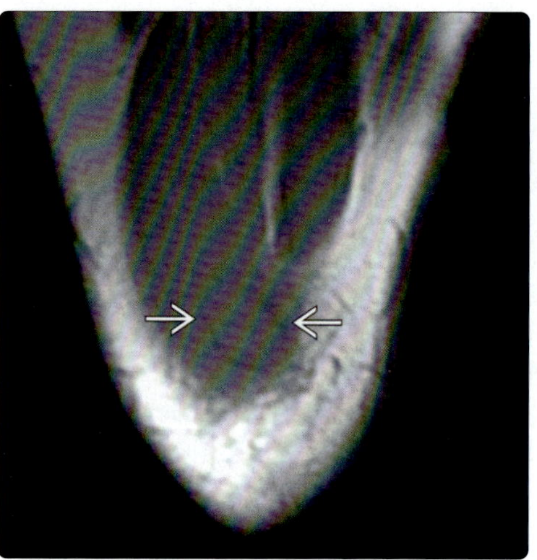

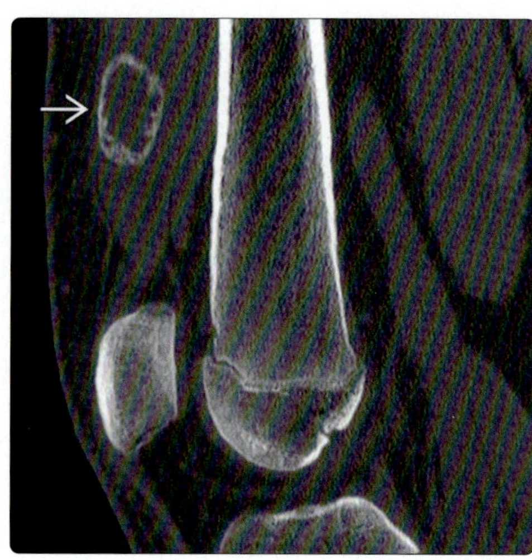

(Left) *Axial T2WI FS MR obtained in a patient with a palpable mass and normal x-ray (not shown) demonstrates an inhomogeneously hyperintense mass ➡ with periosteal edema ➡ but no cortical edema. Note the suggestion of a curvilinear ossific pattern ↪ that raises possibility of myositis ossificans.* **(Right)** *Frog-leg lateral x-ray obtained 9 weeks later shows peripheral ossification ➡, diagnostic of myositis ossificans. Given the appearance and timing of progression, the diagnosis is secure.*

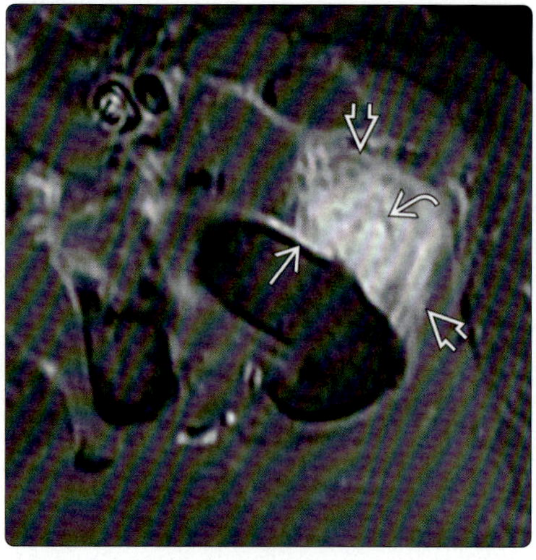

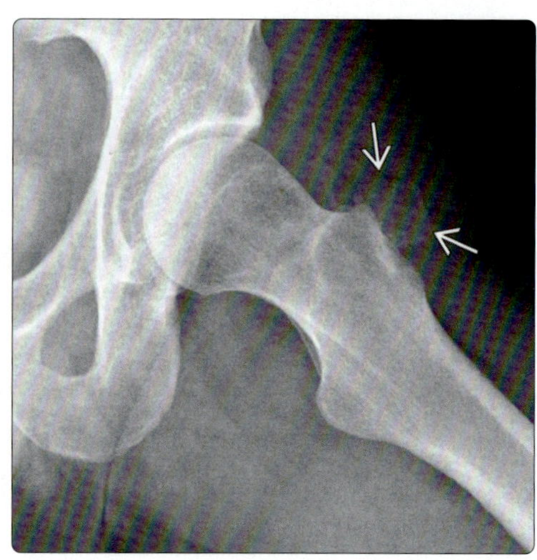

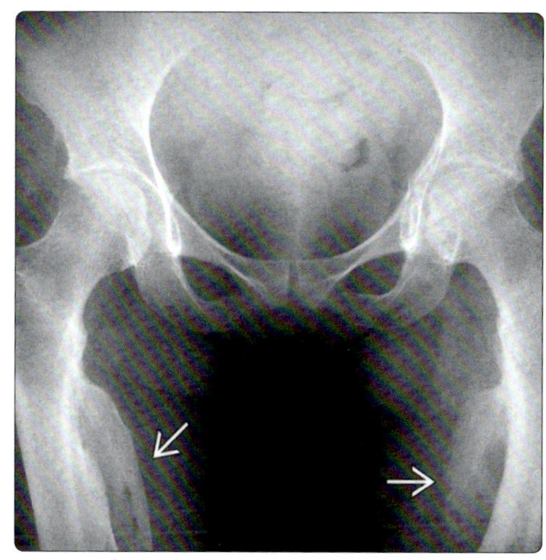

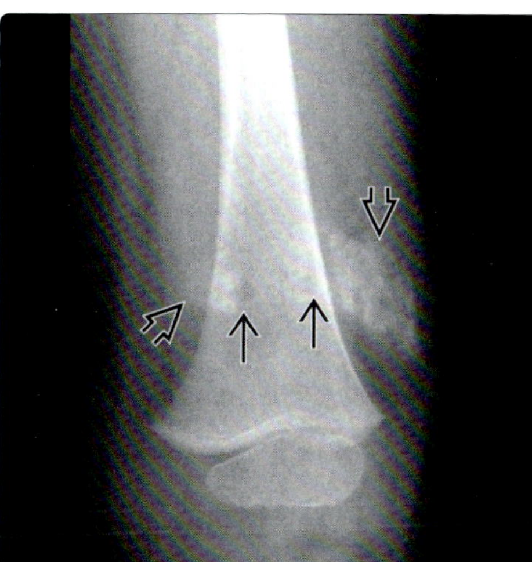

(Left) *Anteroposterior radiograph shows mature MO within the adductors bilaterally ➡. Maturity is judged by the development of peripheral cortex and central trabeculae. This patient is an avid horseback rider.* **(Right)** *AP radiograph demonstrates a pin tract through the distal femoral diaphysis ⇨; the pin was placed for suspension of a burned extremity. There is classic myositis ossificans ⇨ surrounding the pin tract. Burn patients are particularly prone to developing myositis ossificans.*

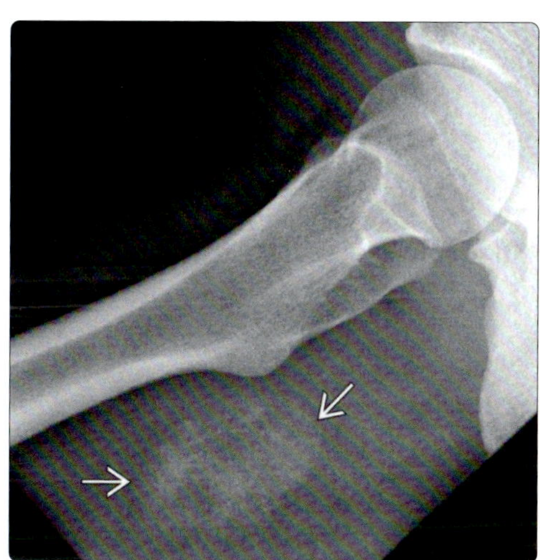

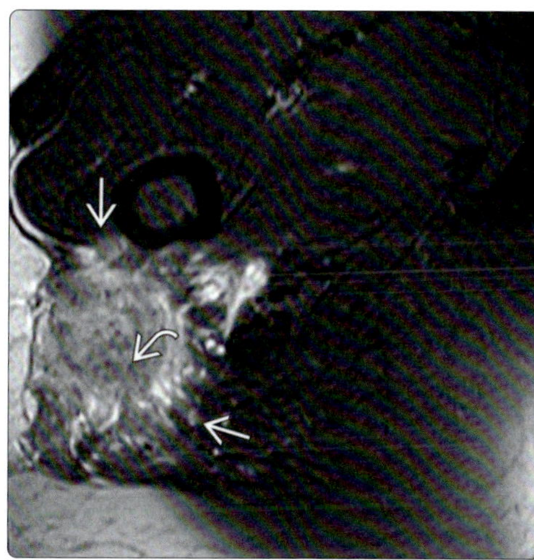

(Left) *Frog-leg lateral radiograph obtained in a 26-year-old cowgirl shows immature osteoid within a soft tissue mass ➡. The clinical scenario suggests myositis ossificans, but surface osteosarcoma cannot be ruled out based on this appearance at this stage of the lesion's evolution.* **(Right)** *Axial T2WI FS MR, same patient, shows an aggressive-appearing lesion ➡ with peripheral infiltration and edema. Note the small low-signal ossific foci ➡.*

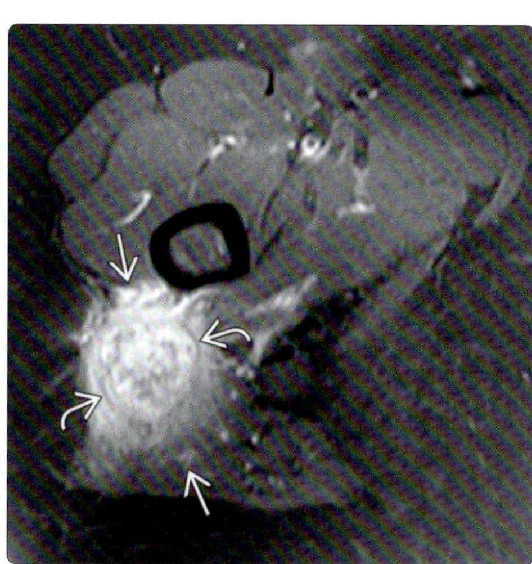

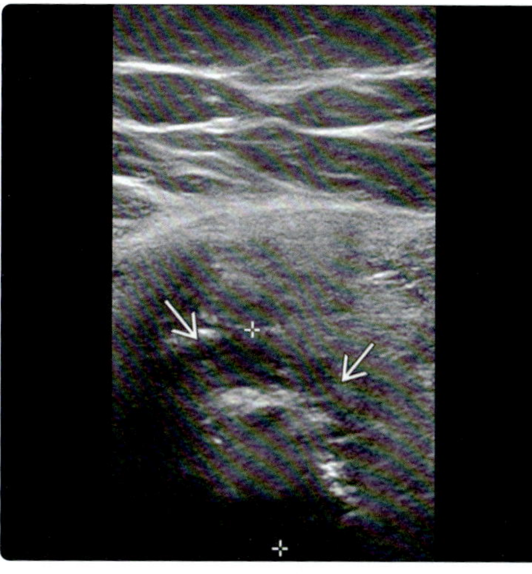

(Left) *Axial T1WI C+ FS MR, same case, shows intense enhancement of the lesion ➡ but a more distinct rounded appearance of the ossification ➡. This ossific "halo" increases the likelihood that the lesion represents myositis ossificans rather than tumor.* **(Right)** *Longitudinal ultrasound of the lesion confirms the peripheral circumferential calcification ➡; the diagnosis of myositis ossificans was presumed and patient followed with radiographs to prove the expected evolution of the lesion.*

Xanthoma

KEY FACTS

TERMINOLOGY

- Nonneoplastic collection of lipid-laden histocytes due to hyperlipoproteinemia

IMAGING

- Skin, subcutis, tendons, fascia, synovium, bone, brain, spinal cord, and lungs
    - Achilles is most common tendon involved
- Skin and subcutaneous lesions not usually imaged
- Soft tissue mass ± bone erosion on radiographs
    - Bone erosion most commonly seen in digits
- Intracranial abnormalities in cerebrotendinous xanthomatosis on CT include hypodense white matter changes, hyperdense focal cerebellar lesions, and diffuse atrophy
- Tendon xanthomas on MR show intermediate T1 and T2 signal material between low-signal tendon bundles → speckled appearance on axial images
- Although lesions contain lipid, they do not typically demonstrate fat signal intensity on MR
    - Small foci of fat reported with intracranial lesions
- Ultrasound shows diffuse hypoechoic tendon enlargement with heterogeneous echotexture or focal hypoechoic nodules

PATHOLOGY

- Sheets of foamy histiocytes with giant cells
- Birefringent extracellular cholesterol collections

CLINICAL ISSUES

- Painless, slowly growing nodules
- Medical therapy to ↓ hyperlipidemia
    - Chenodeoxycholic acid + statins
- Large lesions may be surgically excised
    - Tendon reconstruction to preserve function
- May recur after treatment

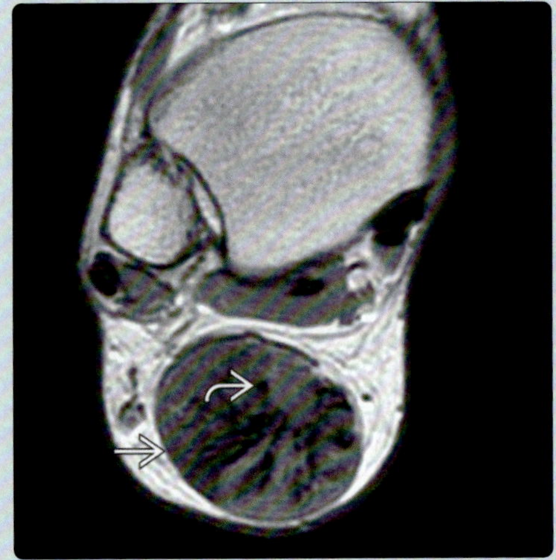

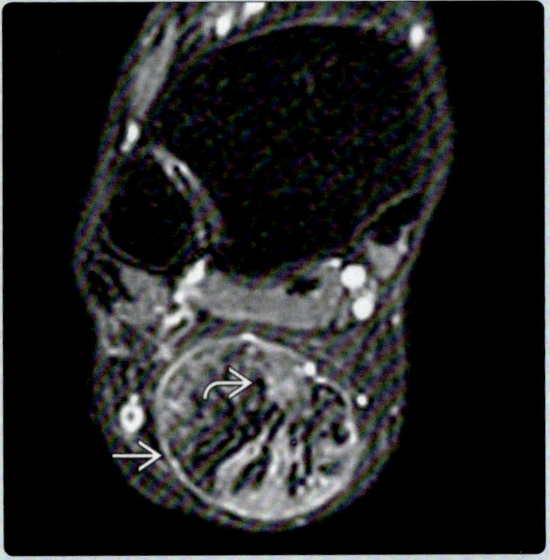

(Left) *Axial PDWI MR shows a tendon xanthoma in a patient with cerebrotendinous xanthomatosis. The diffusely enlarged Achilles tendon ➡ has overall similar signal intensity to muscle with interspersed, longitudinally oriented low-signal tendon fibers ➡.* **(Right)** *Axial T2WI FS MR shows that the Achilles tendon ➡ is predominately hyperintense relative to skeletal muscle and again contains longitudinally oriented low-signal tendon fibers ➡, which remained low signal on all imaging sequences.*

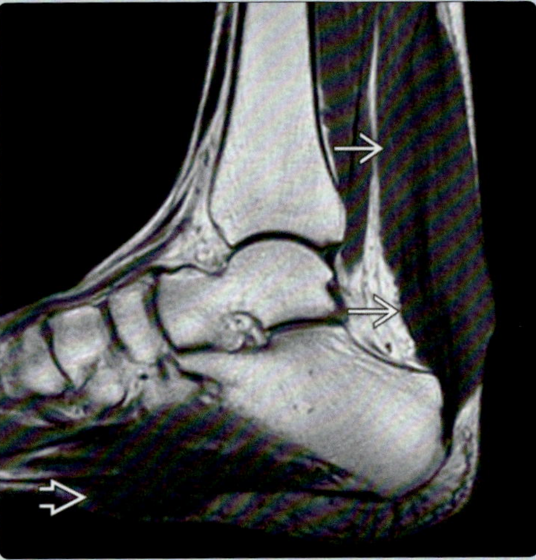

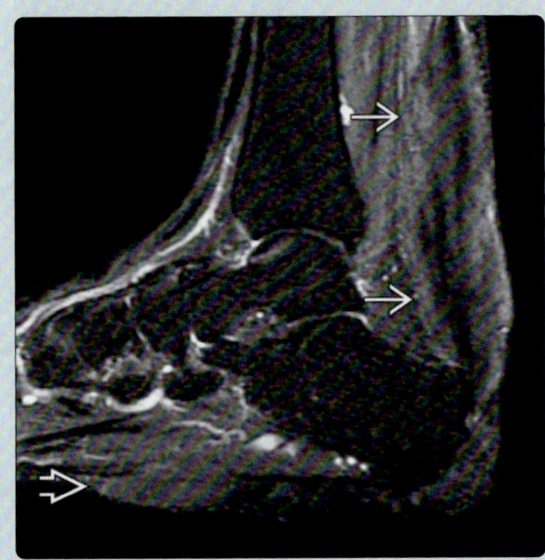

(Left) *Sagittal T1WI MR in the same patient shows the Achilles tendon ➡ to be markedly enlarged over a long segment. An additional xanthomatous mass ➡ is located within the plantar fascia.* **(Right)** *Sagittal STIR MR shows the xanthomatous tissue in the Achilles tendon ➡ to be similar in intensity to muscle. An additional xanthoma ➡ in the plantar fascia has similar imaging characteristics as the Achilles tendon xanthoma, with the exception of the internal tendon fibers.*

TERMINOLOGY

Abbreviations

- Cerebrotendinous xanthomatosis (CTX)

Definitions

- Nonneoplastic collection of lipid-laden histocytes due to hyperlipoproteinemia

IMAGING

General Features

- Location
  - Skin, subcutis, tendons, fascia, synovium, bone, brain, spinal cord, and lungs
    - Achilles is most common tendon involved
- Size
  - Several centimeters or less
- Morphology
  - Tendinous = infiltrating tissue causes diffuse tendon enlargement
  - Tuberous = plaque-like subcutaneous lesions, often in fingers, elbows, buttocks, and knees
  - Eruptive = cutaneous lesions, often in buttocks
  - Plane = palmar skin creases

Radiographic Findings

- Soft tissue mass ± bone erosion
  - Bone erosion most commonly seen in digits
- Bone lesions → well-defined to ill-defined borders

CT Findings

- Intracranial abnormalities in CTX include hypodense white matter changes, hyperdense focal cerebellar lesions, and diffuse atrophy
  - Focal lesions may erode skull

MR Findings

- Although lesions contain lipid, they do not typically demonstrate fat signal intensity on MR
  - Small foci of fat reported with intracranial lesions
- Tendon xanthomas show intermediate T1 & T2 signal material between low-signal tendon bundles
  - Speckled appearance on axial images
- Brain lesions demonstrate hyperintense signal in globus pallidus, substantia nigra, and inferior olive on fluid-sensitive sequences
  - Dentate nucleus may have hyperintense or hypointense signal due to calcification or hemorrhage
  - Lesion enhancement reported
- Spinal cord involvement shows abnormal signal involving lateral and dorsal columns

Ultrasonographic Findings

- Diffuse hypoechoic tendon enlargement with heterogeneous echotexture
- Focal hypoechoic nodules

DIFFERENTIAL DIAGNOSIS

Deep Lesions

- Tendon injury
  - Chronic partial-thickness tearing and tendinosis results in ↑ tendon size and signal intensity
- Giant cell tumor tendon sheath
  - Focal mass associated with tendon sheath
  - ± associated bone erosion
  - Intense enhancement typical
  - Doppler ultrasound shows internal blood flow
- Synovial sarcoma
  - Late adolescence through young adulthood
  - Mass in close proximity to joint
  - Intense enhancement
  - May aggressively track along tendons

PATHOLOGY

General Features

- Etiology
  - Reactive lesions due to hyperlipoproteinemia
    - Familial hypercholesterolemia, essential hyperlipidemia, diabetes mellitus, primary biliary cirrhosis, cerebrotendinous xanthomatosis
- Genetics
  - CTX = autosomal recessive lipid storage disease due to bile acid synthesis disruption

Gross Pathologic & Surgical Features

- Cutaneous → small, yellow papules
- Deep → whitish yellow to brown

Microscopic Features

- Tuberous and tendinous
  - Sheets of foamy histiocytes with giant cells
  - Birefringent extracellular cholesterol collections
  - ± hemorrhage, inflammation, and fibrosis

CLINICAL ISSUES

Presentation

- Most common signs/symptoms
  - Painless, slowly growing nodules
  - CTX = diarrhea in infancy, childhood cataracts, teenage tendon xanthomas, neurologic dysfunction

Demographics

- Age
  - CTX xanthomas develop in 2nd to 4th decade of life

Natural History & Prognosis

- May recur after treatment

Treatment

- Medical therapy to ↓ hyperlipidemia
  - Chenodeoxycholic acid + statins
- Large lesions may be surgically excised
  - Tendon reconstruction to preserve function

SELECTED REFERENCES

1. Weiss SW et al: Benign fibrohistiocytic tumors. In Weiss SW et al: Enzinger and Weiss' Soft Tissue Tumors. 5th ed. Philadelphia: Elsevier. 355-8, 2008
2. Kransdorf MJ et al: Benign fibrous and fibrohistiocytic tumors. In Kransdorf MJ et al: Imaging of Soft Tissue Tumors. 2nd ed. Philadelphia: Lippincott Williams & Wilkins. 236-40, 2006

(Left) *Axial T2WI MR demonstrates globular areas of increased signal within the dentate nuclei* ➡. **(Right)** *Axial FLAIR MR in the same patient again demonstrates globular areas of increased signal within the dentate nuclei* ➡. *In this patient with cerebrotendinous xanthomatosis, the inherited disorder of cholesterol metabolism leads to accumulation of cholestanol within body tissues. Serum cholestanol levels were elevated, thus confirming the diagnosis.*

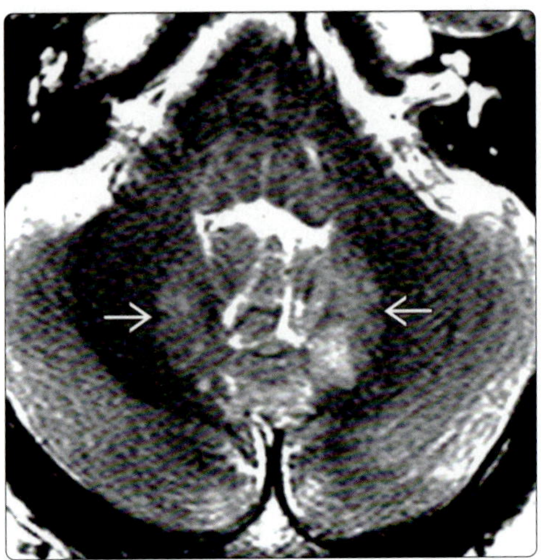

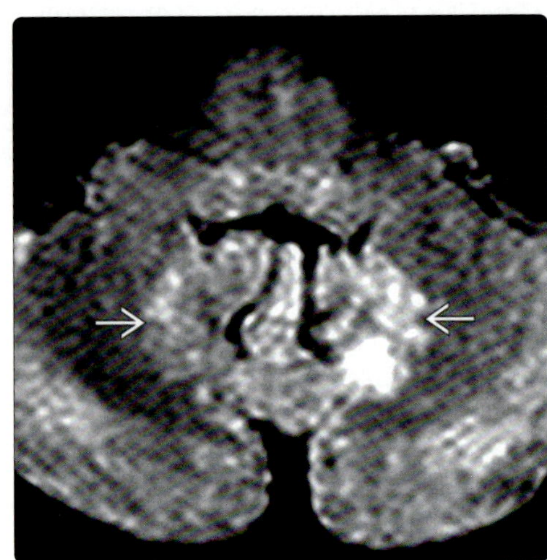

(Left) *Sagittal T1WI MR in the same patient demonstrates fusiform enlargement of the Achilles tendon* ➡ *with striated increased signal between the normal low-signal tendon fibers.* **(Right)** *Axial T1WI MR shows the abnormally round configuration of the Achilles tendon* ➡ *resulting from deposition of xanthomatous tissue. The Achilles tendon normally has a crescent shape with a concave anterior surface. Development of a more round configuration is more commonly due to chronic tendinosis.*

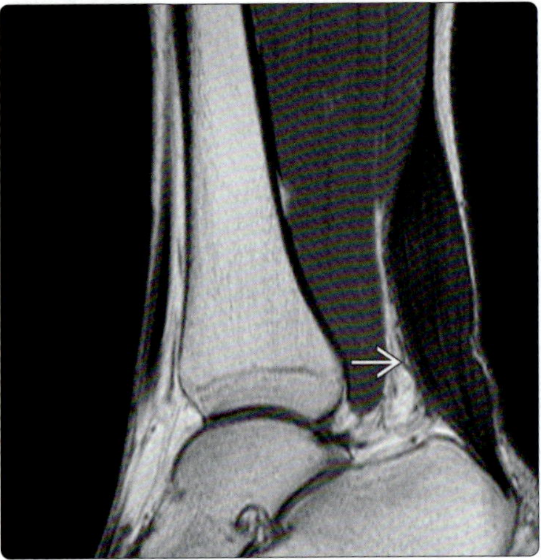

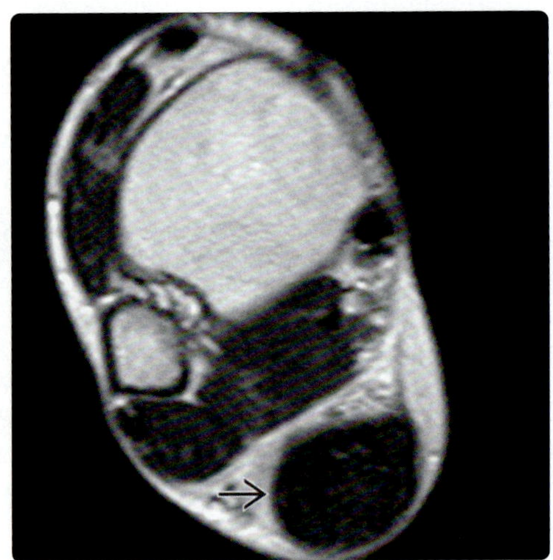

(Left) *Axial T1WI MR shows a very large mass involving the Achilles tendon* ➡, *which was heterogeneously isointense to muscle to low in signal on all sequences. Note also there is a similar appearing mass in the posterior tibial tendon* ➡. **(Right)** *Axial T1WI MR obtained more distally in the same patient again shows the diffusely enlarged Achilles tendon* ➡ *and posterior tibial tendon* ➡. *These findings are quite typical of xanthomas. This patient had hypercholesterolemia.*

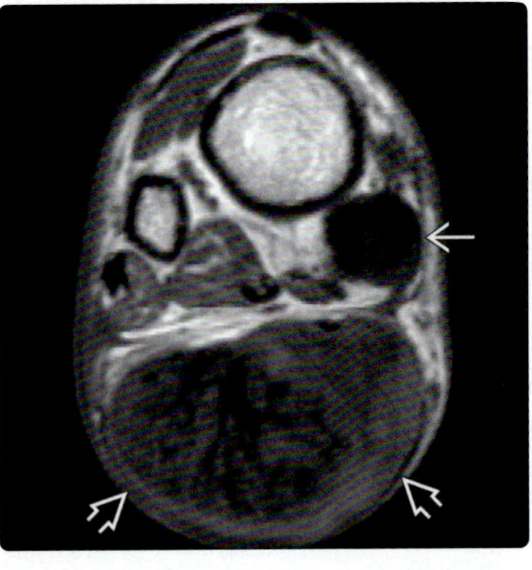

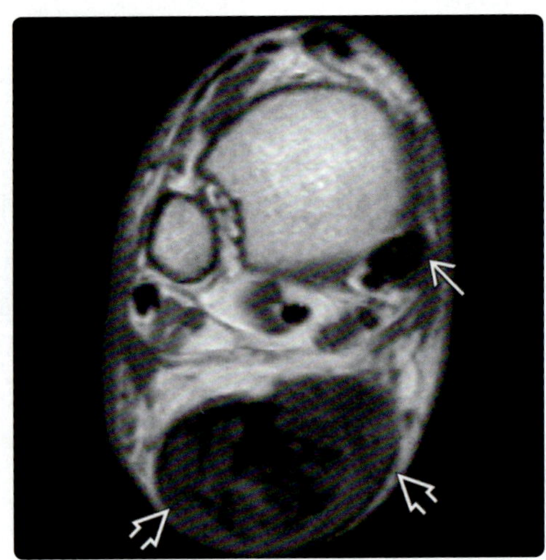

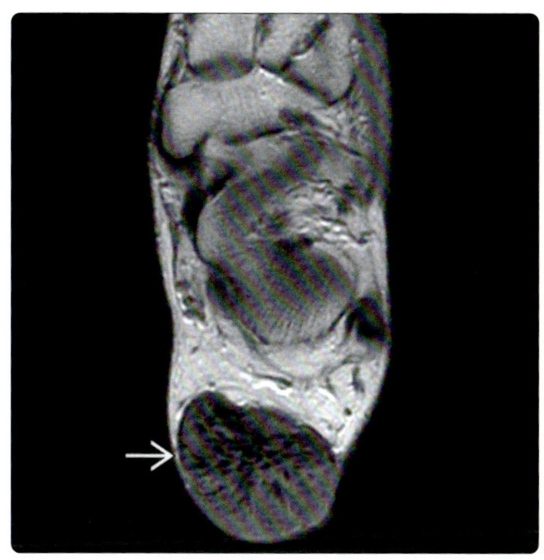

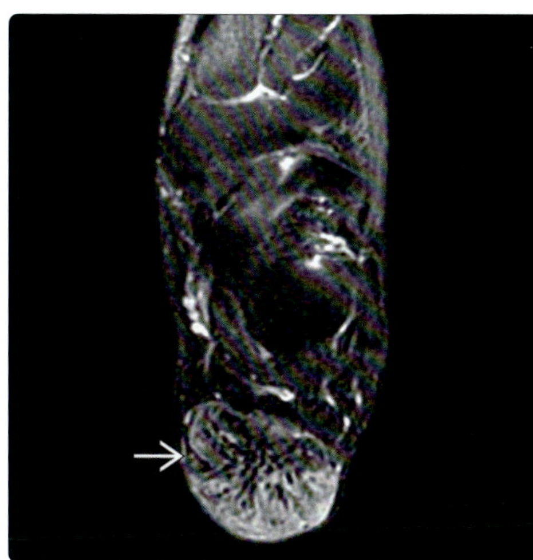

(Left) *Axial PDWI MR shows a markedly enlarged Achilles tendon ➡. A normal Achilles tendon measures approximately 6-7 mm in thickness. This tendon measured several centimeters.* **(Right)** *Axial T2WI FS MR shows the enlarged Achilles tendon ➡ to have low-signal foci in a background of tissue that is hyperintense to muscle. MR imaging typically shows a diffusely enlarged tendon with a speckled pattern on axial images due to interspersed, normal, low-signal tendon fibers.*

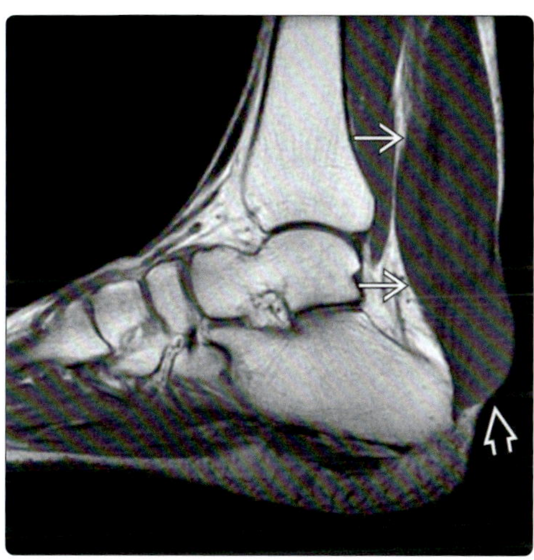

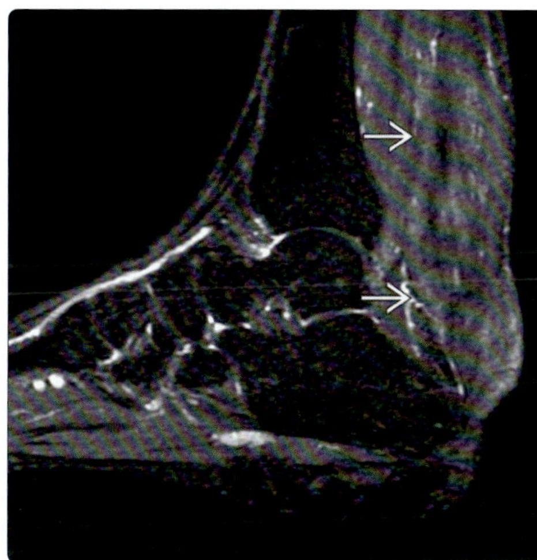

(Left) *Sagittal T1WI MR in the same patient shows the enlarged Achilles tendon ➡. The tendon has a somewhat wavy contour when viewed on sagittal images. The protuberant nature ➡ of these lesions causes difficulty with footwear.* **(Right)** *Sagittal STIR MR shows the Achilles tendon xanthoma ➡ to have heterogeneous low and intermediate signal intensity. This young female patient with known cerebrotendinous xanthomatosis presented requesting surgical excision of multiple similar xanthomas.*

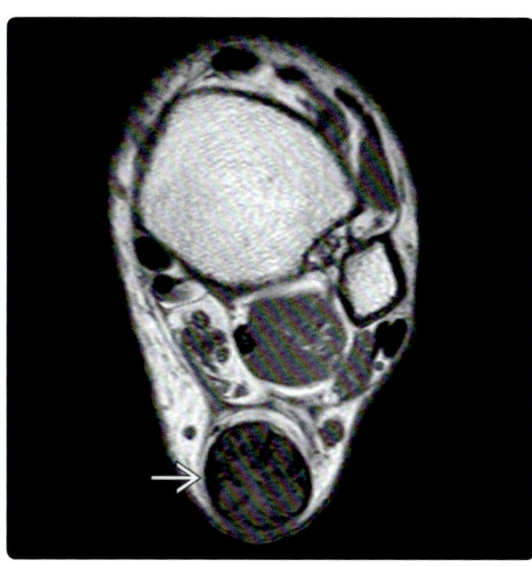

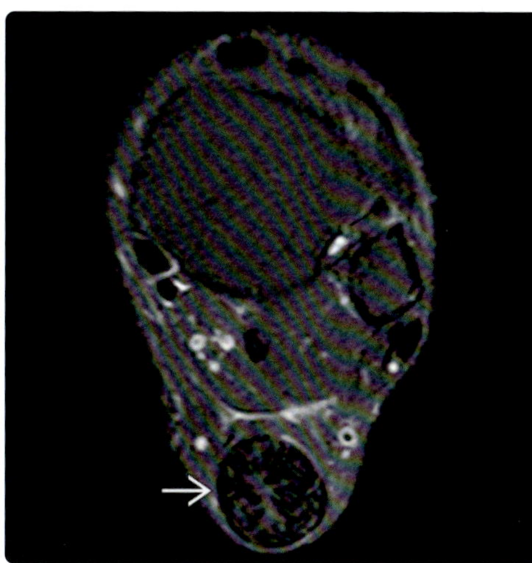

(Left) *Axial T1WI MR shows the Achilles tendon ➡ to have an abnormally round contour. Regions of signal intensity similar to muscle correspond to abnormal xanthomatous tissue accumulation. Punctate low-signal regions are the normal, low-signal Achilles tendon fibers.* **(Right)** *Axial T2WI FS MR shows the large Achilles tendon ➡ to have central signal that is hyperintense to muscle with persistently low-signal tendon fibers located peripherally. This patient had cerebrotendinous xanthomatosis.*

SECTION 4

Congenital and Developmental Abnormalities

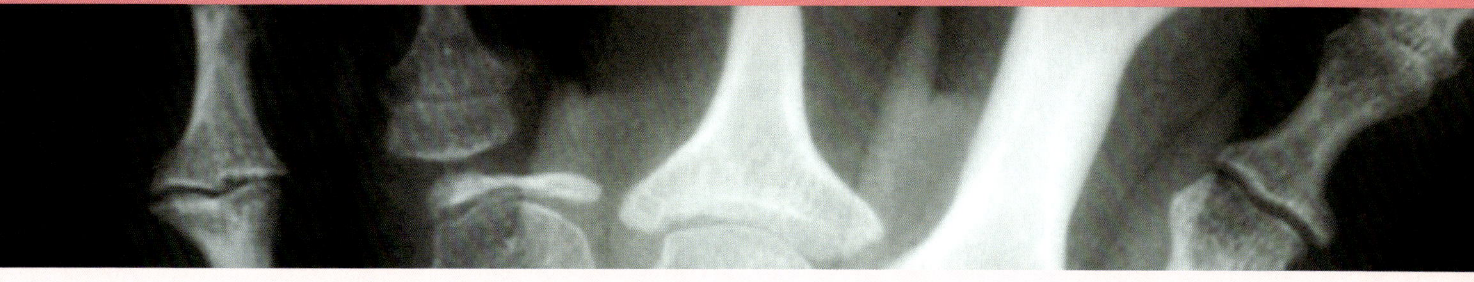

General

Upper Extremity

Lower Extremity

Arthrogryposis

KEY FACTS

TERMINOLOGY

- Definition: Heterogeneous group of disorders that have in common fixed joint contractures

IMAGING

- Location: Spine, lower > upper extremities
- Spine: Long C-shaped neurogenic scoliosis
- Limbs
  - Gracile tubular bones
  - Muscles not developed
- Joints
  - Appear relatively dense
  - Due to density of cartilage and arthrofibrosis
  - Density highlighted due to ↓ normal muscle
- Pelvis
  - Hypoplastic due to nonweight bearing
  - Fixed hip joint deformity
  - Hip dislocation
- Knee
  - Extension contracture
  - Patella subluxated superiorly and laterally
- Foot: Clubfoot
  - Equinus, varus hindfoot, varus forefoot
- Associated abnormalities
  - Polyhydramnios, pulmonary hypoplasia, micrognathia

PATHOLOGY

- Multiple causes (usually neuropathic)
- No motion in utero (fetal akinesis)
  - → joint contractures, which become fixed
  - → muscles do not develop normally
- Most cases not genetically caused (30% genetic)

CLINICAL ISSUES

- 1/3,000 live births
- Abnormality present at birth; nonprogressive
- Aggressive management may result in ambulatory status for majority

(Left) *AP radiograph shows a long, C-shaped neurogenic scoliosis. It is evident that the patient does not walk, as the pelvis is hypoplastic compared with the size of the thorax.* **(Right)** *AP radiograph in the same patient shows a fixed abducted right hip ➡ and chronically dislocated left hip ⇨. Note that the hip capsules are relatively dense. Fixed neurogenic scoliosis is commonly seen, as in this case, but nonspecific. Hip contractures and dislocations are common, as is clubfoot deformity.*

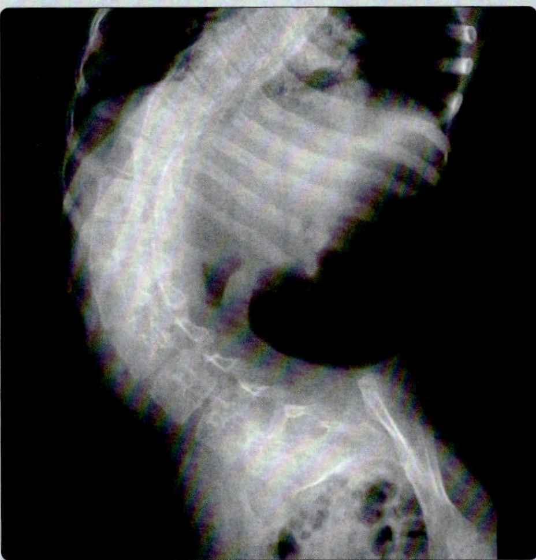

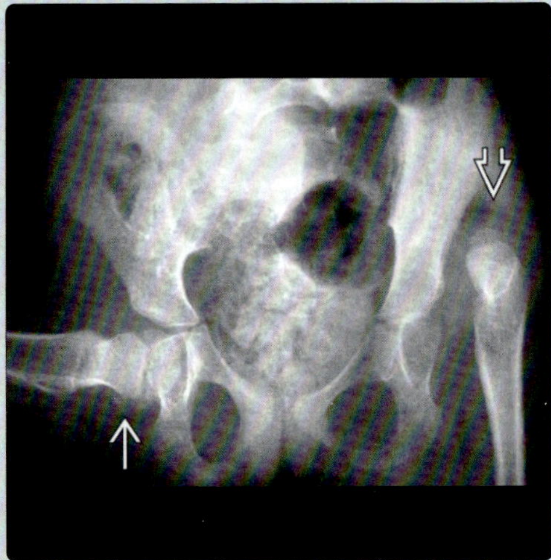

(Left) *AP radiograph in the same patient shows a clubfoot deformity. There is varus hindfoot ➡ as well as varus forefoot ⇨. Equinus was confirmed on the lateral (not shown). The abnormality was bilateral.* **(Right)** *Lateral radiograph of the knee in a different patient shows a fixed contracture. Note the relatively dense joint capsule ➡. This is not an effusion but represents the relatively dense cartilage and fibrous tissue of the capsule compared with the absence of muscle. The finding is considered fairly specific for arthrogryposis.*

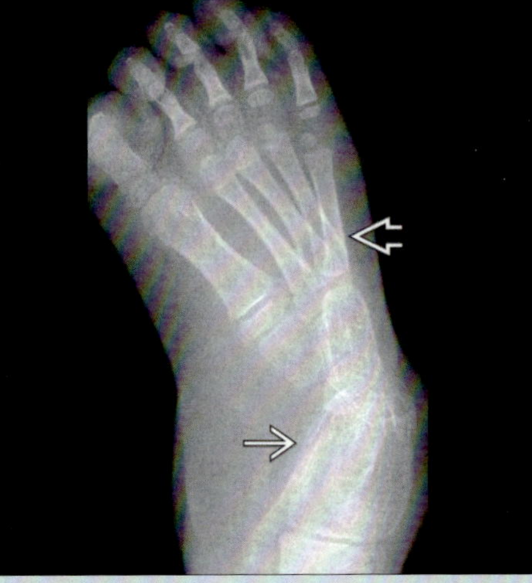

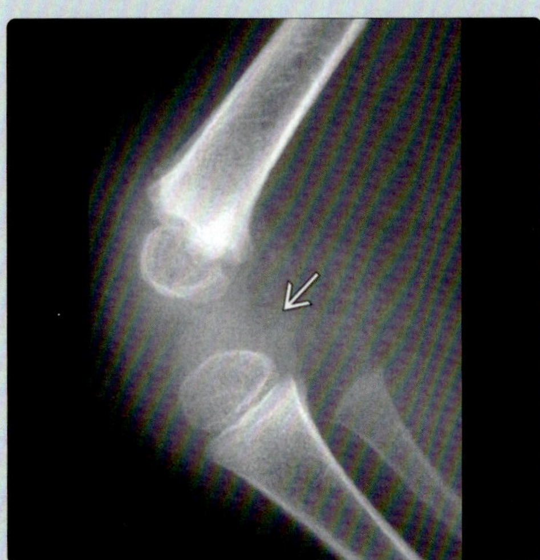

KEY FACTS

TERMINOLOGY

- Definition: Constriction of fetal body parts by amniotic strands resulting in array of body part deletions and deformities

IMAGING

- Primarily affects distal extremities
- Range of transverse abnormalities
  - Digital ring constrictions
  - Distal atrophy of soft tissues and bone
  - Lymphedema
  - Acrosyndactyly, clubfoot
  - Intrauterine amputation
- Ultrasound: Cleft or absence of extremity parts
  - Bands often tightly adherent to fetus and not explicitly seen by ultrasound
  - Abnormal but present blood flow detected by power Doppler may suggest those bands that are amenable to prenatal surgery
  - Other abnormalities may overshadow extremity defects (acrania, cleft palate, bowel extrusion)

TOP DIFFERENTIAL DIAGNOSES

- Neonatal compartment syndrome
- Congenital pseudarthrosis, tibia

PATHOLOGY

- Early amnion rupture
  - Not always present; may relate to prior percutaneous intervention
  - Entanglement of fetal parts in amniotic strands
    - Subsequent constriction and loss of blood supply

CLINICAL ISSUES

- Prenatal fetoscopic surgery may release bands and restore blood supply to extremity
  - Umbilical cord involvement must be sought; may not be diagnosed preoperatively
- Postnatal treatment directed at restoring function

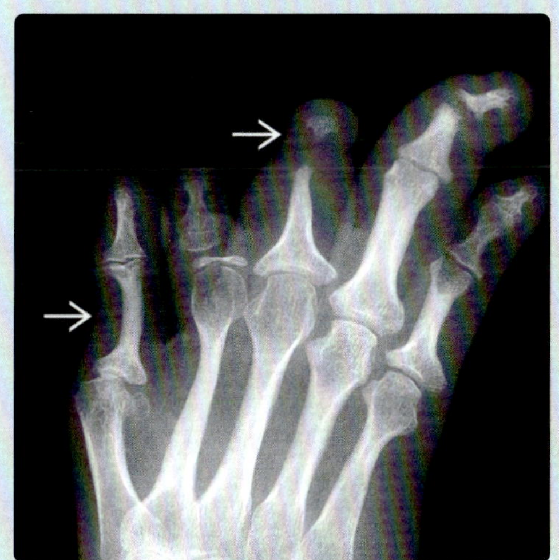

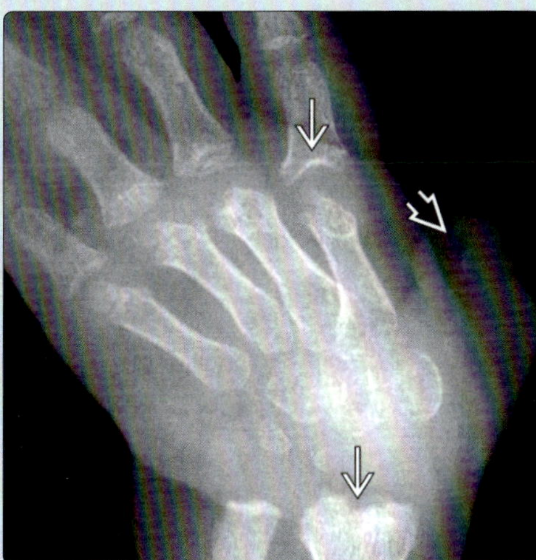

(Left) *PA radiograph shows severe acroosteolysis, with constriction of the soft tissues ➡ and incomplete development of some of the phalanges. This was the only extremity that was involved. Findings are typical of amniotic band syndrome; the soft tissue constrictions are particularly diagnostic.* **(Right)** *PA radiograph shows multiple coned epiphyses ➡, with premature fusion at many of these sites, typical of loss of blood supply in this patient with amniotic band syndrome. The thumb suffered intrauterine amputation ➡.*

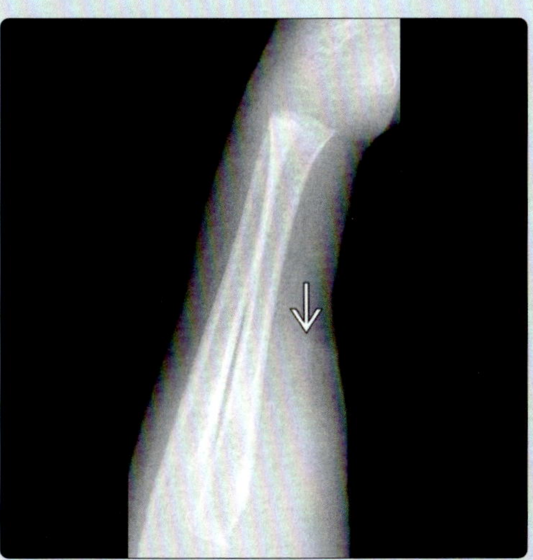

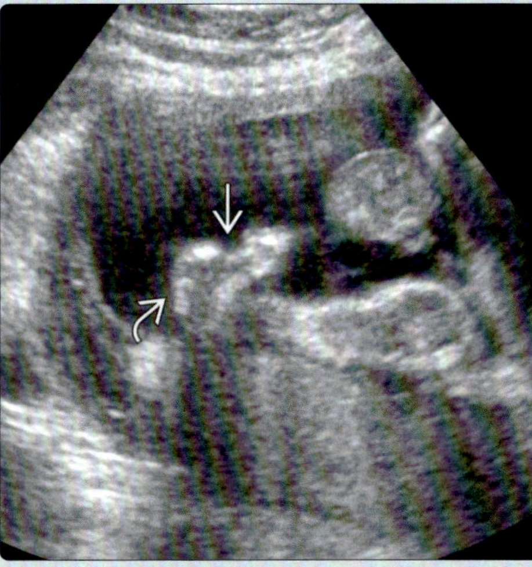

(Left) *Lateral radiograph of the forearm shows a sudden change in caliber of the soft tissues ➡, which formed a ring. Such rings may be seen in digits or more proximally in amniotic band syndrome.* **(Right)** *Coronal prenatal ultrasound of the right lower extremity shows a clubbed foot ➡ with a cleft being created by missing amputated toes ➡. Multiple other extremity deformities were also seen. The patient unfortunately also had several other abnormalities, including abdominal wall defect, acrania, and cleft lip.*

Cerebral Palsy

KEY FACTS

TERMINOLOGY

- Cerebral palsy (CP)

IMAGING

- Scoliosis: 15-61% of spastic CP
  - Often long, C-shaped neuromuscular type of curve
  - Results in pelvic obliquity
  - Scoliosis may also be S-shaped double-curve or appear similar to idiopathic scoliosis curve
  - Associated thoracic hyperkyphosis and lumbar hyperlordosis
    - Increased incidence of spondylolysis with exaggerated lumbar lordosis
  - Deformity initially positional; becomes fixed
  - Progresses rapidly; may continue to progress post skeletal maturation
- Hip involvement
  - 28% of spastic CP (17% bilateral)
  - Flexion contracture of hip
  - Pelvis may have "windswept" appearance (28%): Hip adduction deformity on 1 side, abduction on contralateral
  - External rotation of hip, with prominent lesser trochanter
  - Coxa valga and anteverted femoral neck (average: 55° in CP; normal adult: 8-15°)
  - Eventual superolateral subluxation/dislocation
  - Secondary acetabular dysplasia
  - Secondary flattening or notching of femoral head
  - Longstanding disease → osteoarthritis and pseudoacetabulum formation
- Knee involvement: 58-72% of spastic CP
  - Flexion deformity secondary to hamstring contracture
  - → patella alta
  - Elongated patella
  - May have fragmentation of inferior pole
  - C-shaped patella on lateral view
  - → chondromalacia patella
  - Genu recurvatum (knee hyperextension in gait): Secondary to rectus femoris contraction in conjunction with gastrocnemius weakness
- Foot findings
  - Equinus
  - Combination of hindfoot and forefoot deformities, which suggests spasticity
  - Often hindfoot valgus combined with forefoot varus
  - Equinovalgus most common; equinovarus seen as well
  - Talonavicular subluxation

TOP DIFFERENTIAL DIAGNOSES

- Meningomyelocele
  - Spinal dysraphism and associated abnormalities on MR
- Polio
  - Usually unilateral limb involvement
  - Generally lower extremity, progressive muscle weakness
- Muscular dystrophy
  - Fatty atrophy in enlarged muscles
  - Different muscle groups preferentially

PATHOLOGY

- Etiology of CP: Intrapartum asphyxia
- Alternative etiology of CP: Prenatal injury
  - Intrauterine asphyxia
  - Congenital or placental infection
  - Cerebral venous or arterial occlusion
- Etiology of osseous deformities in CP
  - Spasticity → muscle power imbalance on growing bones
  - Spasticity develops between 6-18 months
  - Muscles most likely to display spasticity: Paraspinal, hip flexors, hip adductors, hamstrings, gastrocnemius, soleus
  - Progressive alteration of skeletal anatomy

CLINICAL ISSUES

- Epidemiology: 1-5 per 1,000 live births
  - Most → spastic diplegia, predominantly lower limbs
- Spasticity develops between 6-18 months

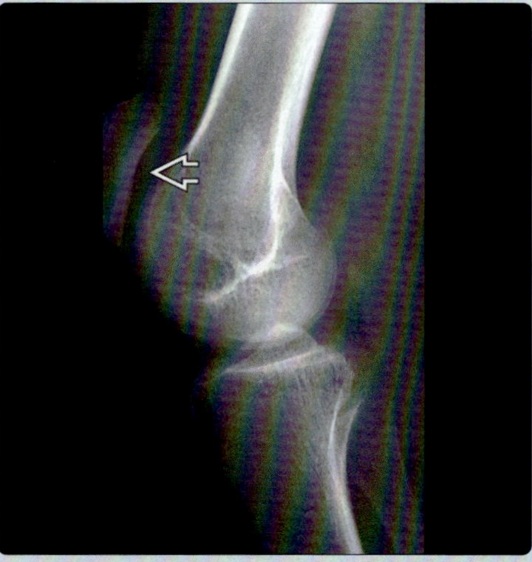

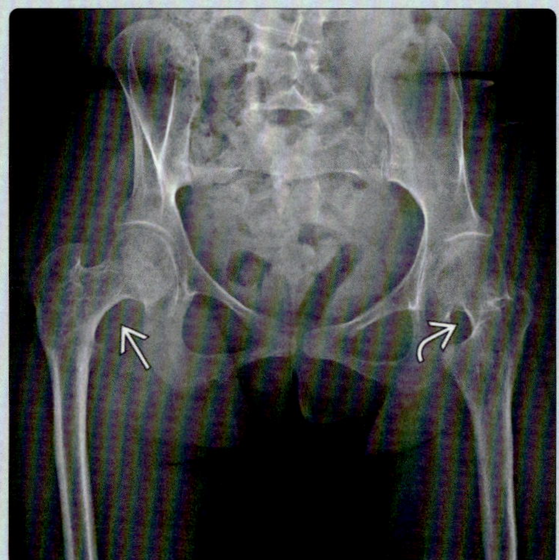

(Left) *Lateral radiograph shows a gracile femur and patella alta in a patient with cerebral palsy. Note the concave "C" shape of the elongated patella ⇒; this abnormal morphology is virtually only seen in CP knees.* **(Right)** *AP radiograph in a patient with severe CP shows gracile femora, hypoplastic iliac wings, and osteopenia suggesting limited ambulation. There is a typical valgus left hip ⇒. The right hip has been treated with varus-producing osteotomy ⇒.*

Down Syndrome (Trisomy 21)

KEY FACTS

IMAGING

- Skull
  - Brachycephaly, flat occiput
- Spine
  - Hypoplastic C1 arch
  - Atlantoaxial subluxation with instability
  - Neurologic complications uncommon
- Chest
  - 11 pairs of ribs
  - Double ossification center for manubrium
- Pelvis
  - Flared iliac wings compared to elephant ears
  - Decreased sacrosciatic notch
  - Decreased acetabular index (horizontal roof)
- Hands
  - Clinodactyly, brachydactyly
- Axial CT: Iliac wings divergent (↑ iliac angle)
  - Increased iliac length
- US: Antenatal diagnosis
  - Increased nuchal translucency
  - Decreased length of nasal bone
  - Cystic hygroma

PATHOLOGY

- Trisomy 21 chromosomal disorder
  - Secondary to nondisjunction in 90%
  - Secondary to translocation or mosaicism in remaining 10%
- Associated congenital heart disease (classically atrioventricular septal defect)
- Associated gastrointestinal tract disease
  - Duodenal atresia
  - Annular pancreas
  - Hirschsprung disease

CLINICAL ISSUES

- 1/1,000 live births

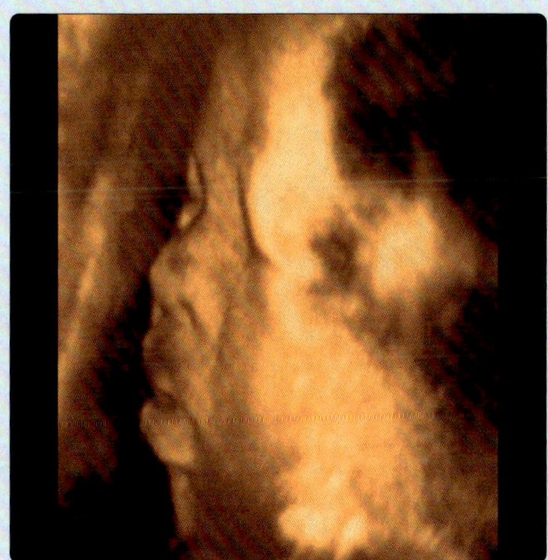

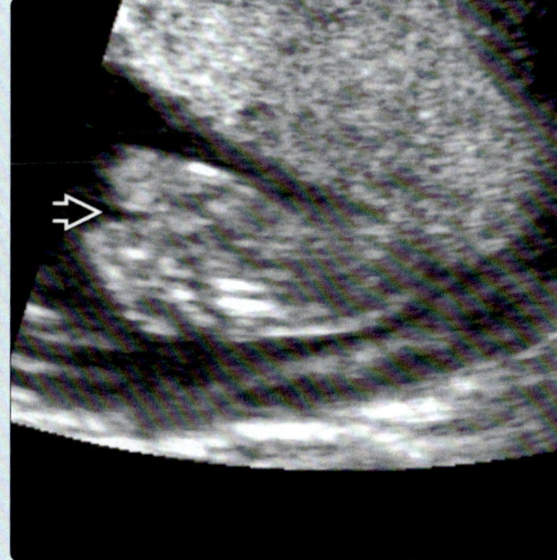

(Left) *3D ultrasound shows an abnormal fetal face with a flattened nose and midface. No other anomalies were seen. Bone rendered 3D views confirmed the presence of 2 nasal bones, which were diminished in length. The baby was born with the typical facies of Down syndrome.* **(Right)** *Axial ultrasound shows a sandal gap deformity of the foot ➡, which is a minor sign of Down syndrome.*

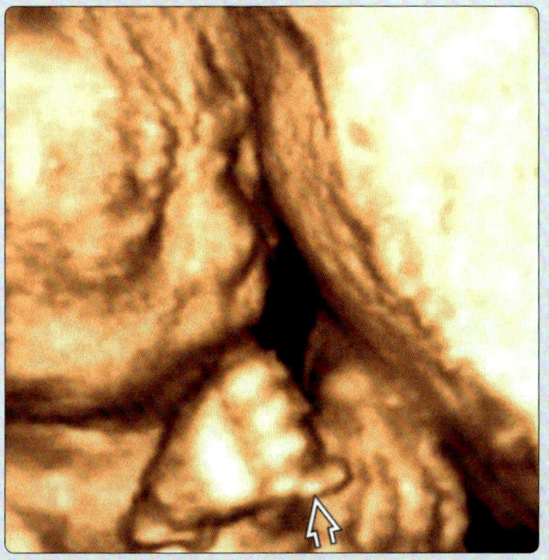

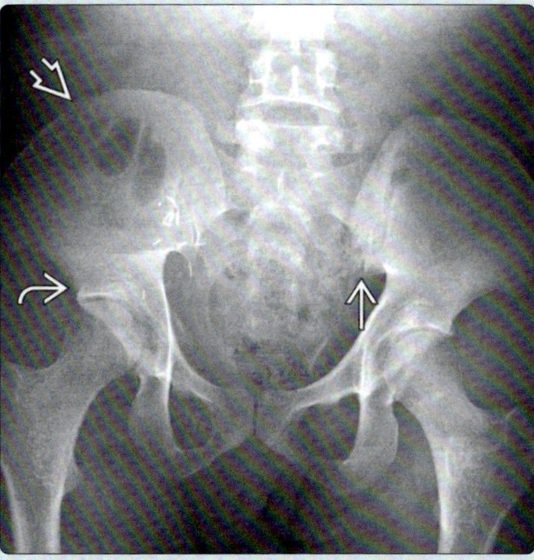

(Left) *3D ultrasound shows a somewhat flattened midface as well as 5th finger clinodactyly ➡. Trisomy 21 was confirmed after delivery.* **(Right)** *AP radiograph demonstrates broad iliac wings ➡ and narrow sacrosciatic notches ➡. Note that the acetabular roofs are nearly horizontal ➡, typical of the pelvis in Down syndrome. While this description may also fit achondroplasia, this case shows no evidence of narrowed interpediculate distance, as one would expect in that form of dwarfism.*

Fibrodysplasia Ossificans Progressiva

KEY FACTS

TERMINOLOGY

- Hereditary mesodermal disorder resulting in mature ossification within soft tissues, bridging between osseous structures

IMAGING

- Sternocleidomastoid often initial site
  - Progresses to shoulder girdle, upper arms, spine, and pelvis
  - End result is bridging between extremities and torso, between ribs, and between thorax and pelvis
- Radiograph: Follows same pattern of development as myositis ossificans (progressive zonal ossification)
  - Early: Mass and edema distorting fat planes
  - 3-4 weeks: Amorphous bone formation in mass
  - 6-8 weeks: Distinct cortex forms around outer margin of mass
  - 5-6 months: Mature bone formation
  - Malformation of great toes, short thumb
- CT: Ossification visible earlier than on radiograph
  - Demonstrates lesion develops adjacent to and extending around muscles
- MR early in process: Mass, low T1 signal intensity (SI), high SI on fluid-sensitive sequences, intense enhancement
  - May be misinterpreted as tumor; correlation with radiograph or CT essential
- MR late in process: Mature bone, may contain marrow signal as well as cystic regions

PATHOLOGY

- Autosomal dominant with wide range of expressivity
- Target is interstitial tissues, with muscle involvement secondary to pressure atrophy
  - Progressive ossification of muscle, tendons, and ligaments

CLINICAL ISSUES

- Average age at onset: 5 years
- Progresses to significant bridging between bone

(Left) *Posterior graphic depicts fibrodysplasia ossificans progressiva (FOP). Note the mature bone that bridges between the ribs, along the spine, from the thorax to the proximal humerus, and from the thorax to the pelvis ➡.* **(Right)** *AP radiograph shows FOP (a.k.a. myositis ossificans progressiva) with mature bone bridging between osseous structures. This is a case that is far advanced, showing bone bridging between ribs, as well as between the humerus and rib cage ➡. The end result is complete loss of motion.*

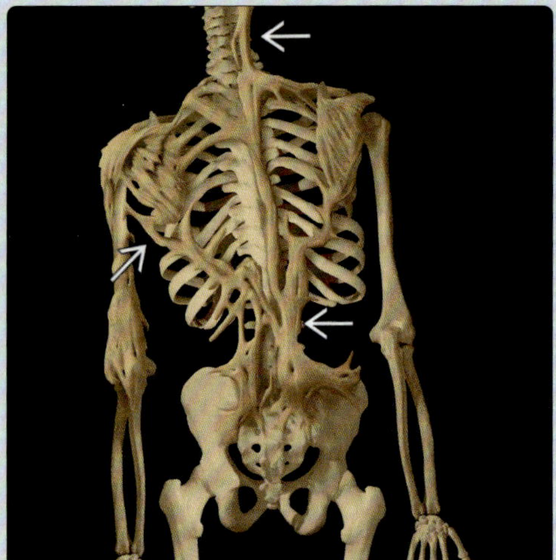

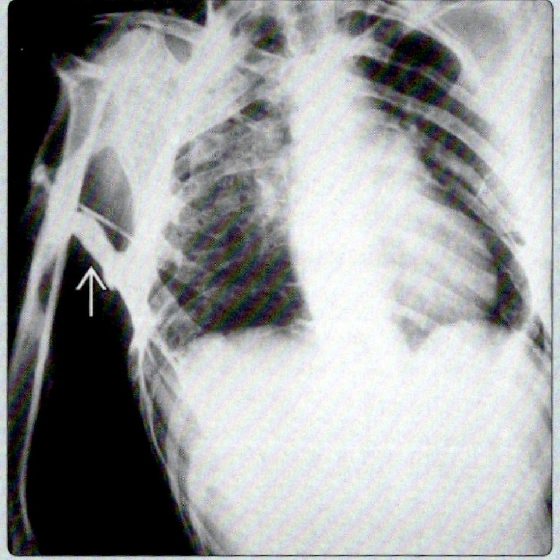

(Left) *AP radiograph demonstrates mature ossification within the soft tissues of the back ➡. A similar ossification was present at the anterior thigh. This child shows early signs of FOP.* **(Right)** *Lateral radiograph in the same case shows ossification in the anterior thigh ➡. The patient had been treated with a chelator to help resorb the dystrophic bone. Unfortunately, the heterotopic bone did not resorb, but there is resorption of bone in the form of a rickets-like pattern at the growth plate ➡.*

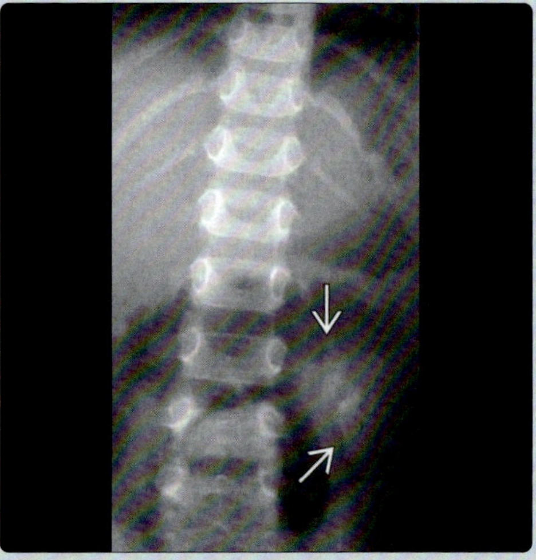

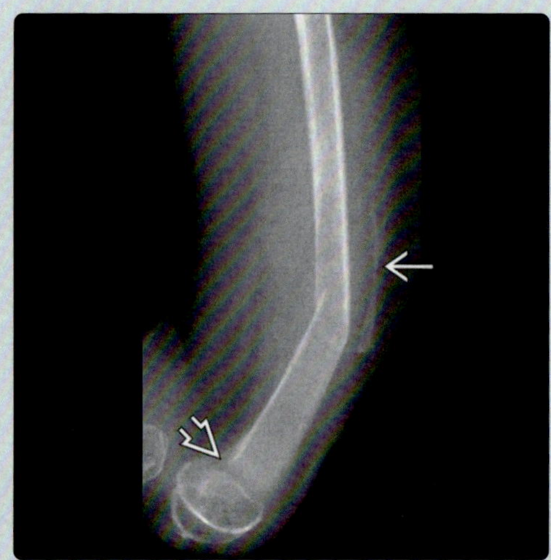

KEY FACTS

TERMINOLOGY

- Group of inherited myopathies; Duchenne variety most commonly affects musculoskeletal system

CLINICAL ISSUES

- Duchenne muscular dystrophy
  - X-linked recessive inheritance pattern (only males)
  - Clinically apparent by 5 years of age
  - Rapid progression; incapacitated by adolescence
  - Highly elevated serum creatine kinase
  - Clinical exam: Muscles large, firm, rubbery
  - Early weakness is proximal (hips, shoulders)
  - Foot deformities (pes planus, equinovarus) due to early tightening of Achilles tendon
  - Progressive knee and hip contractures
  - Scoliosis, kyphosis; late cardiac myopathy
  - Imaging: Muscles enlarged but replaced by fatty (majority) and fibrous tissue
  - Relative sparing of sartorius, gracilis, semimembranosus, semitendinosus
- Becker muscular dystrophy: Similar to Duchenne but later onset and less severe symptoms
- Facioscapulohumeral dystrophy
  - Autosomal dominant (affects males and females)
  - Proximal weakness, especially shoulders
  - Slow progression
- Limb-girdle dystrophy
  - Autosomal recessive (affects males and females)
  - Waddling gait from pelvic girdle weakness
  - Variable progression
- Myotonic dystrophy
  - Autosomal dominant (males and females affected)
  - Variable age of onset and degree of severity
  - Weakness predominantly distal (hands, face, sternocleidomastoid)

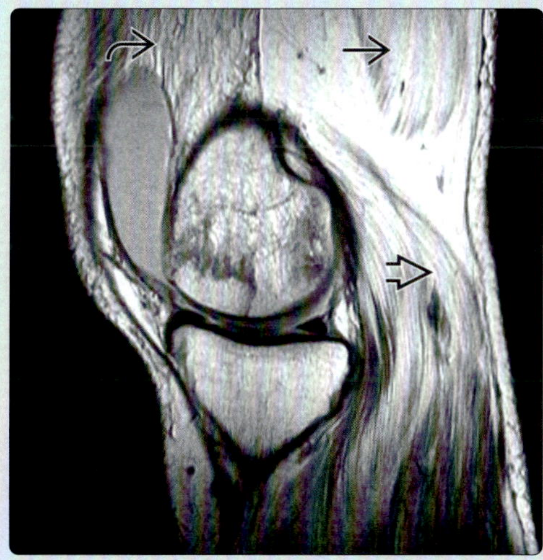

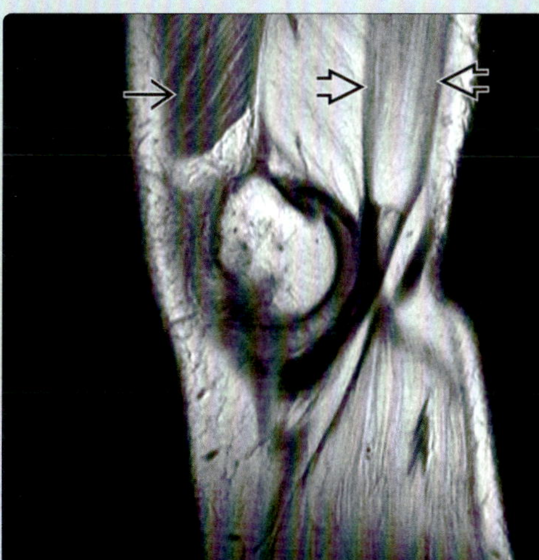

(Left) *Sagittal PD MR in a patient with Duchenne muscular dystrophy, located in the mid medial compartment, demonstrates severe fatty replacement of the majority of the muscles about the knee, including semimembranosus ➙, gastrocnemius ➯, and vastus medialis ➯. Incidental note is made of incomplete fracture in the medial femoral condyle resulting from patient's recent fall.* **(Right)** *Sagittal PD MR, same patient, located far medially, shows a few remaining fibers in semimembranosus ➯ & more within vastus medialis ➙.*

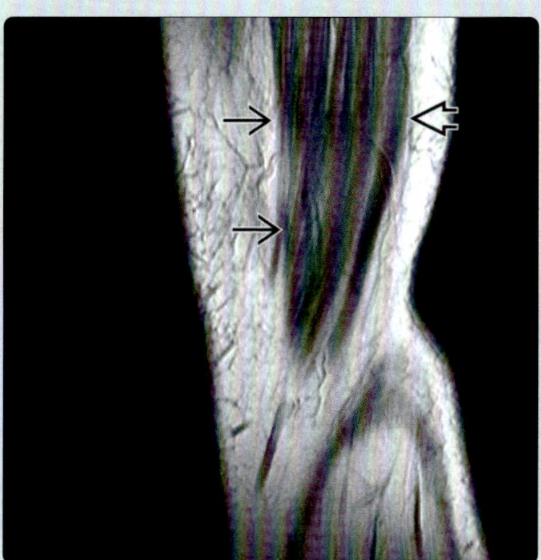

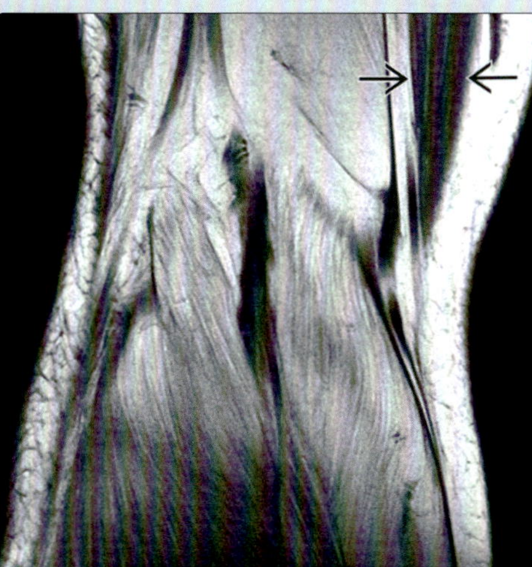

(Left) *Sagittal PD MR in the same patient, located in the farthest medial aspect of the knee, shows that the atrophy is not uniform; the sartorius ➙ and gracilis ➯ show some residual muscle fibers.* **(Right)** *Coronal T1WI MR confirms the nonuniform fatty atrophy; note the relatively normal sartorius ➙. It has been established that the least affected muscles include gracilis, semimembranosus, semitendinosus, and sartorius in patients with muscular dystrophy, and this patient generally follows that pattern.*

Neurofibromatosis

KEY FACTS

TERMINOLOGY

- Congenital and familial disorder that involves neuroectoderm, mesoderm, and endoderm
- Neurofibromatosis type 1 (NF1): 85-90% of patients
- Neurofibromatosis type 2 (NF2): 10-15% of patients

IMAGING

- Skull: Macrocrania and skull markings if severe
  - Lambdoid suture calvarial defect
  - Absence of greater or lesser wing of sphenoid or orbital floor
- Spine: Kyphoscoliosis
  - Other curve patterns, including that of idiopathic scoliosis often present
  - Posterior vertebral body scalloping: Dural ectasia or neurofibroma
- Ribs: Ribbon deformity
- Pelvis: Protrusio acetabuli in 32%
- Tibial dysplasia
  - Pseudarthrosis
  - Thinning, with transverse fractures
  - Severe bowing deformity
- Nonossifying fibroma (NOF): May be multiple
- Nerve sheath tumors
  - Elongated along length of nerve
  - Chain of beads appearance
  - Generally low T1 signal, high T2 signal, showing enhancement
  - Target sign: Low signal in center of lesion
- Whole-body MR imaging suggested to determine tumor burden

CLINICAL ISSUES

- 1/3,000-4,000 individuals
- Usually diagnosed by age 4
- 50-70% of NF patients have skeletal abnormalities
- 3-15% of NF patients develop malignant peripheral nerve sheath tumor (MPNST)

(Left) *Coronal T2WI FS MR shows multiple tubular neurofibromas arising from the right cervicothoracic nerve roots ➡. Other smaller neurofibromas are seen on the left side, further distally along the thoracic spine, and in the axilla. This is a patient with neurofibromatosis type 1 (NF1).* **(Right)** *Sagittal T2WI MR of the lumbar spine in a different patient with NF shows extensive dural ectasia that results in pressure erosion of the posterior bodies ➡ of L4, L5, and the sacrum. No spinal neurofibromas are seen.*

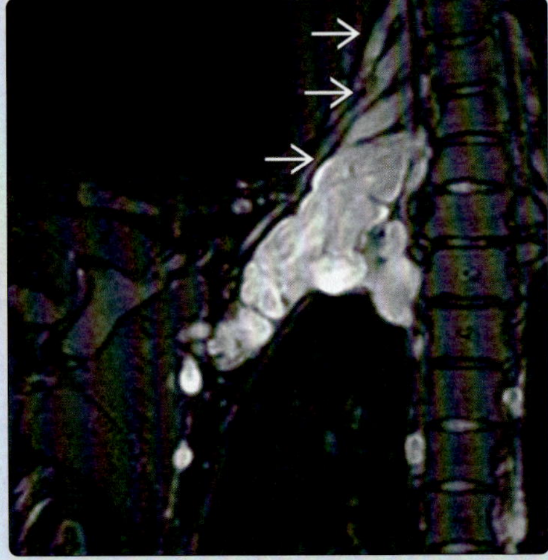

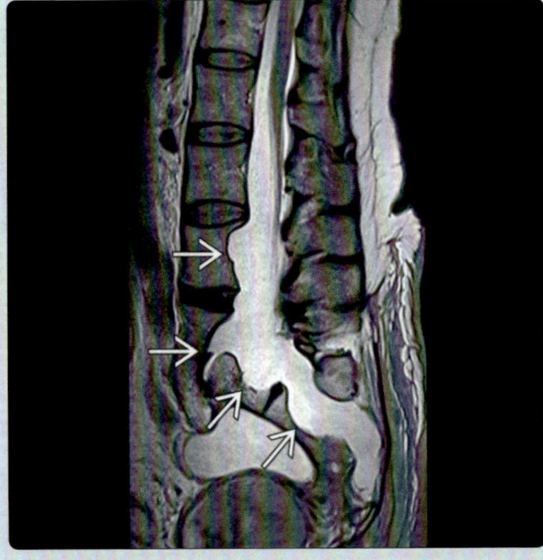

(Left) *Lateral radiograph shows well-defined pressure erosion of the posterior elements of L1-L2 ➡. This may be secondary to either dural ectasia or nerve sheath tumor in this patient with NF.* **(Right)** *Axial T2WI FS MR in the same patient shows both posterior element and posterior body scalloping ➡. There is a large adjacent soft tissue tumor ➡ causing erosion and displacing the kidney ➡. This proved to be a malignant peripheral nerve sheath tumor. In addition, there are innumerable small neurofibromas ➡.*

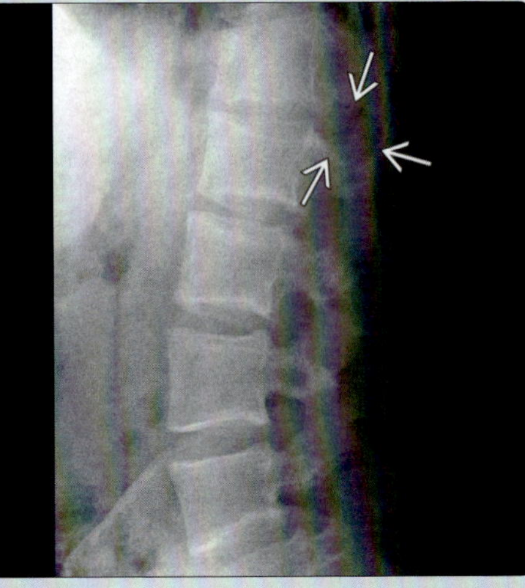

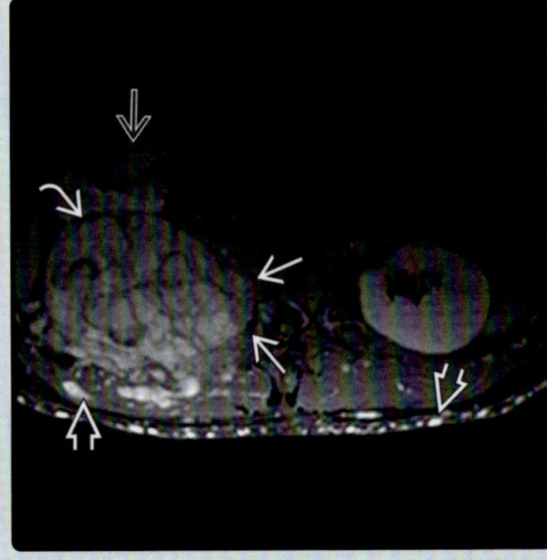

TERMINOLOGY

Abbreviations

- Neurofibromatosis (NF)

Synonyms

- Recklinghausen disease [neurofibromatosis type 1 (NF1)]

Definitions

- Congenital and familial disorder that involves neuroectoderm, mesoderm, and endoderm
  - 8 subtypes proposed but only 2 commonly used
    - NF1: 85-90% of patients
    - Neurofibromatosis type 2 (NF2): 10-15% of patients (bilateral acoustic neuromas/vestibular schwannomas)

IMAGING

General Features

- Location
  - Skull, spine, ribs, tubular bones (particularly tibia)

Radiographic Findings

- Skull
  - Hydrocephalus
    - Macrocrania and skull markings if severe
    - May see shunt and associated tubing
  - Lambdoid suture calvarial defect
    - Lytic region within lambdoid suture, usually left
  - Absence of greater or lesser wing of sphenoid
  - Absence of orbital floor or enlargement of orbit
  - Widening of foramina with cranial nerve involvement: Optic, auditory
  - J-shaped sella
- Spine
  - Kyphoscoliosis
    - High thoracic short angular scoliosis fairly specific to NF1
    - Other curve patterns, including that of idiopathic scoliosis, often present
  - Posterior vertebral body scalloping
    - Often associated with deformity of pedicle and lamina → wide neural foramina
    - Associated with either dural ectasia or neurofibroma
  - Neurofibroma or malignant peripheral nerve sheath tumor (MPNST)
    - Widening of neural foramen &/or excavation of vertebral body
    - Bubbly expanded lesion in sacrum
    - Generally nonaggressive in appearance for neurofibroma
    - Destructive process may appear more aggressive for MPNST
    - Rarely contain dystrophic calcification
- Ribs: Ribbon deformity (thin, attenuated, twisting, inferior notching)
  - Generally, dysplasia rather than secondary to intercostal neurofibroma
- Pelvis: Protrusio acetabuli in 32%
  - Often mild but may progress to severe
- Tubular bones
  - Dysplasia
    - Tibial dysplasia
      - Pseudarthrosis
      - Thinning, with transverse fractures (complete or incomplete)
      - Severe bowing deformity
  - Nonossifying fibroma (NOF or fibroxanthoma)
    - May be multiple when associated with NF
    - Cortically based geographic lesion
    - Metaphyseal or metadiaphyseal
    - Sclerotic margin; over time may resolve spontaneously
      - Fills in with mildly sclerotic bone, generally from periphery
  - True intraosseous neurogenic tumors extremely rare
  - Extrinsic erosion may occur from adjacent soft tissue neurofibroma
  - Cortical or surface "lesion" rarely seen
    - Periosteal dysplasia, hemorrhage → elevated periosteum
    - Rare severe subperiosteal hemorrhage resulting in ossification and widening of bone
- Soft tissue masses
  - Noted by distortion of fat planes if lesion is large enough
  - May contain dystrophic calcification
- Limb length discrepancy, local gigantism
- Overall osteoporosis

CT Findings

- Osseous abnormalities well seen, particularly in spine
- Fusiform solid soft tissue masses, often with "tail" of nerve
  - Occasional dystrophic calcification within mass
- Dural ectasia, dumbbell-shaped spine neurofibromas

MR Findings

- Tubular bones
  - NOF
    - Expanded, cortically based
    - No cortical breakthrough or soft tissue mass
    - Low signal rim on all sequences
    - T1WI: Low signal throughout, fairly homogeneous
    - Fluid-sensitive sequences show variety of signal, depending on stage of lesion filling in with bone
      - Ranges from uniform high signal to heterogeneous low signal
      - Avid peripheral and septal enhancement; central enhancement variable, depending on ossification
  - Rare "cyst" at surface of bone
    - Elevated periosteum; may have osseous periosteal reaction
    - Hemorrhage, fluid collects beneath; not true neoplasm
- Nerve sheath tumors
  - Elongated along length of nerve
    - Chain of beads appearance
  - Nerve may be seen extending from ends of lesion
  - Generally low T1 signal, high T2 signal, showing enhancement
  - Target sign: Low signal in center of lesion
    - Best seen on T2 and postcontrast imaging
    - May be seen in neurofibroma, schwannoma, MPNST; does not differentiate among these

- In NF, may have large focal lesion, with many other smaller lesions in vicinity
- Spine
  - Extent of posterior body and posterior element scalloping better seen than on radiograph
    - Most often 2° to dural ectasia but may also be due to nerve sheath tumors
      - MR differentiates between these etiologies
- Whole-body MR imaging suggested to determine tumor burden

Nuclear Medicine Findings

- FDG PET useful in detecting MPNST
  - 95% sensitive, 72% specific, 71% positive predictive value, 95% negative predictive value, 82% accuracy
- In equivocal cases, addition of 11C methionine PET may add specificity

DIFFERENTIAL DIAGNOSIS

Polyostotic Fibrous Dysplasia

- Could mimic NOF in NF, but fibrous dysplasia lesions are central
- Café au lait spots (coast of Maine rather than coast of California spots of NF)

PATHOLOGY

General Features

- Etiology
  - Most bone deformities thought to be mesodermal dysplasia
    - Dysplastic bone is fragile, resulting in fractures and bowing
- Genetics
  - Both NF1 and NF2 autosomal dominant with variable expression
  - 50% of cases result from new mutation
  - NF1: 17q11 locus on *NF1* gene
    - Mutation rate in *NF1* among highest known
  - NF2: 22q12 locus on *NF2* gene
- Associated abnormalities
  - NF1-associated tumors
    - Neurofibroma
    - MPNST
  - NF2-associated tumor: Schwannoma
  - Association with subungual glomus tumors reported
  - Association with soft tissue angiosarcoma reported

Microscopic Features

- Reduced trabecular bone volume, increased osteoid volume within dysplastic bone
- Decreased calcium content in NF1 bone

CLINICAL ISSUES

Presentation

- Most common signs/symptoms
  - Neuroectodermal (skin and nervous system)
    - Café au lait spots, skin hyperpigmentation
    - Skin and subcutaneous neurofibromas, generally developing after puberty
    - Intracranial manifestations
      - Optic pathway glioma (most common intracranial tumor associated with NF1)
      - Cerebral glioma, hydrocephalus, schwannoma of cranial nerve, vascular dysplasia
  - Scoliosis
  - Tibial deformity
- Other signs/symptoms
  - Endodermal (endocrine gland)

Demographics

- Age
  - Generally diagnosed by age 4, earlier if parent is affected
    - Plexiform neurofibromas of face rarely occur after age 1
    - Plexiform neurofibromas of other sites rarely occur after adolescence
  - MPNST: Adolescent and adult
- Gender
  - M = F
- Epidemiology
  - 1/3,000-4,000 individuals
  - 50-70% of NF patients have skeletal abnormalities
  - 5% of patients with multiple NOF have coexistent NF
  - 3-15% of NF patients develop MPNST

Natural History & Prognosis

- Scoliosis may progress rapidly, resulting in loss of function
- Wide resection of MPNST is difficult, with high recurrence rate
- Mean age of death: 54 years (20 years younger than normal population); generally related to MPNST

Treatment

- Treatment of complications
  - Restoration of function of dysplastic bone
  - Stabilization of spine as needed
  - Treatment of benign tumors affecting function
  - Aggressive treatment of malignant tumors
- Treatment of underlying osteoporosis is now being explored (cholecalciferol, vitamin D)

DIAGNOSTIC CHECKLIST

Image Interpretation Pearls

- When multiple NOF are noted, consider NF
- Dysplastic tibia, even without bowing, should raise possibility of NF

SELECTED REFERENCES

1. Al Kaissi A et al: Bilateral and symmetrical anteromedial bowing of the lower limbs in a patient with neurofibromatosis type-I. Case Rep Orthop. 2015:425970, 2015
2. Meneses-Quintero D et al: Dystrophic thoracic spine dislocation associated with type-1 neurofibromatosis: Case report and rationale for treatment. J Craniovertebr Junction Spine. 6(2):79-82, 2015
3. Ueda K et al: Computed tomography (CT) findings in 88 neurofibromatosis 1 (NF1) patients: Prevalence rates and correlations of thoracic findings. Eur J Radiol. 84(6):1191-5, 2015
4. Ahlawat S et al: Schwannoma in neurofibromatosis type 1: a pitfall for detecting malignancy by metabolic imaging. Skeletal Radiol. 42(9):1317-22, 2013
5. Cai W et al: Tumor burden in patients with neurofibromatosis types 1 and 2 and schwannomatosis: determination on whole-body MR images. Radiology. 250(3):665-73, 2009

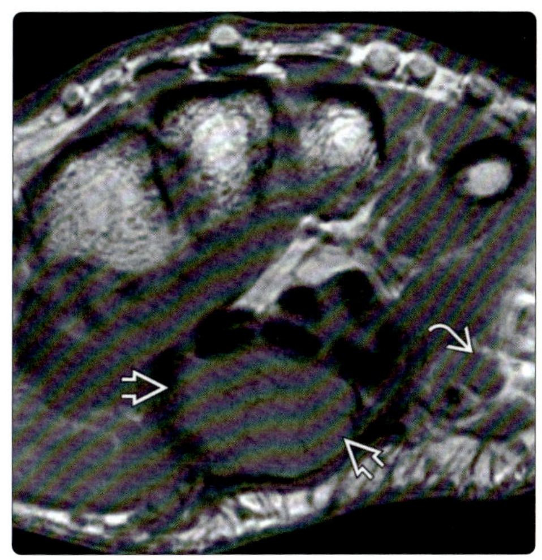

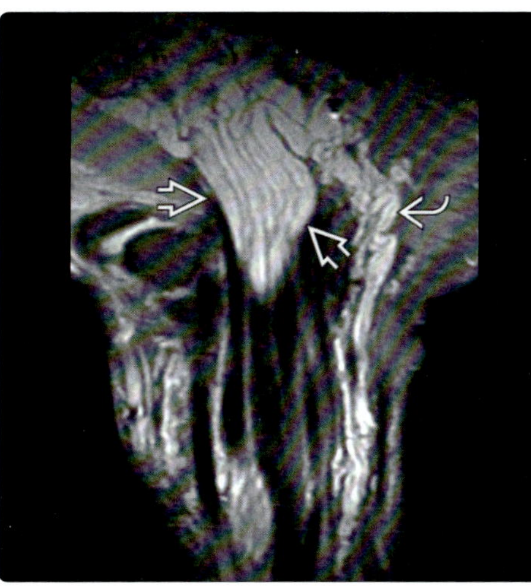

(Left) *Axial T1WI MR shows uniform but significantly enlarged nerve fascicles of the median ➡ and ulnar ➡ nerves. There is prominent bowing of the flexor retinaculum at the carpal tunnel and displacement of the flexor tendons.* **(Right)** *Coronal PD FS MR of the same hand shows high signal within the enlarged median ➡ and ulnar ➡ nerves. This neural enlargement is due to NF.*

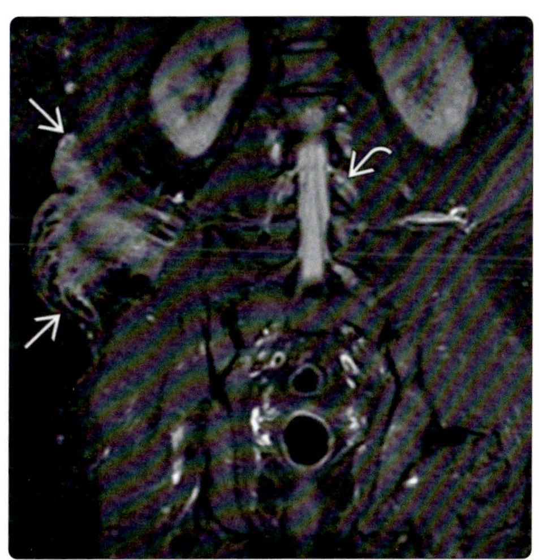

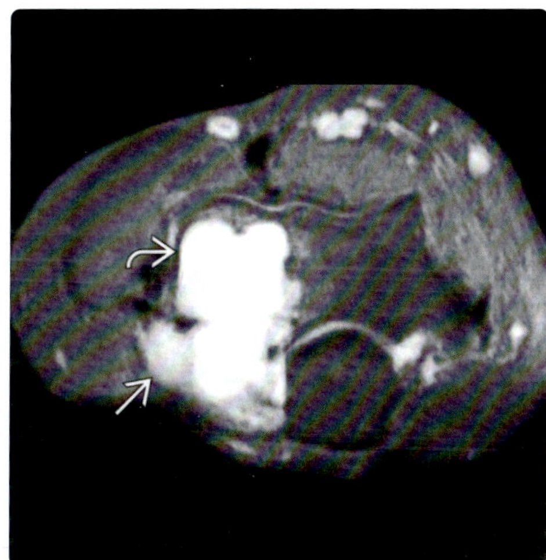

(Left) *Coronal T2WI FS MR shows a soft tissue lesion extending from the skin to the right iliac crest ➡; this is a plexiform neurofibroma. Bilateral, focal soft tissue fusiform thickening, along multiple nerve roots of the mid and lower lumbar spine, suggest multiple small neurofibromas ➡.* **(Right)** *Axial T2WI FS MR shows a large, high-signal mass ➡, which appears to have originated at or near the ulnar nerve. The lesion invades the distal humerus ➡; on radiograph, this appeared as a lytic lesion.*

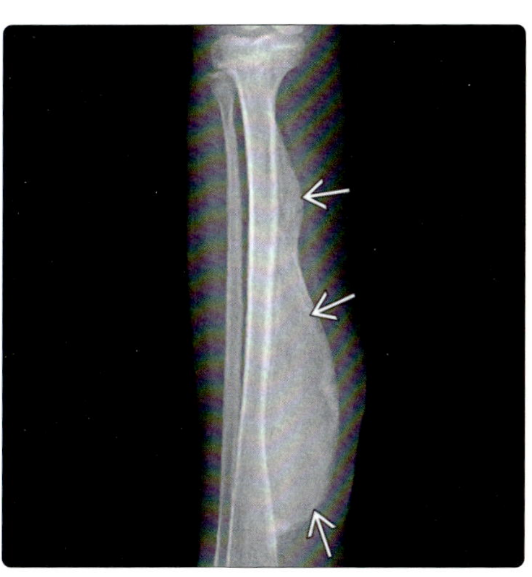

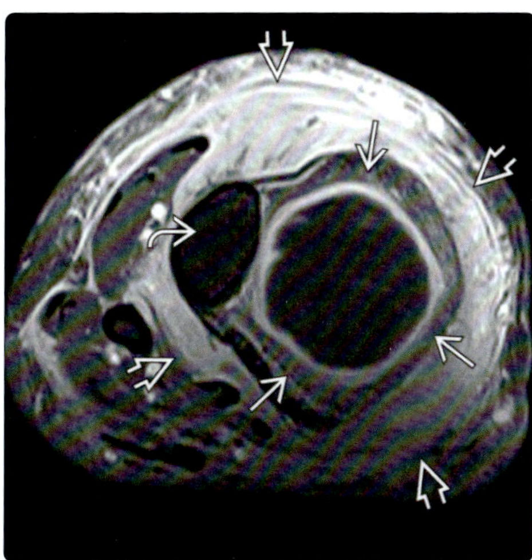

(Left) *AP radiograph in a 13 year old with NF shows an osseous surface lesion of the tibia ➡. This is not the typical dysplastic tibia seen in NF but suggests chronic subperiosteal hemorrhage with surrounding ossification.* **(Right)** *Axial T1WI C+ FS MR in the same patient shows the tibia ➡ with a fluid-filled surface lesion ➡ surrounded by bone, proving chronic subperiosteal hemorrhage. More importantly, there is a huge circumferential malignant nerve sheath tumor ➡.*

(Left) *Axial T2WI MR in a patient with ulnar neuropathy due to NF shows fusiform enlargement of the ulnar nerve with elevated T2 signal ⇒. A neurofibroma of the median nerve is also present ↪.* **(Right)** *Sagittal T2WI MR in the same patient shows fusiform enlargement of portions of the ulnar nerve ⇒, with normal caliber of the intervening portion of the nerve in the cubital tunnel →. This string of beads configuration is typical of neurofibromatosis.*

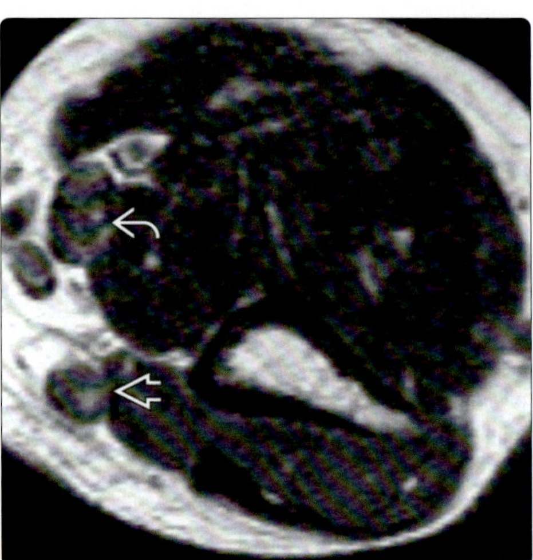

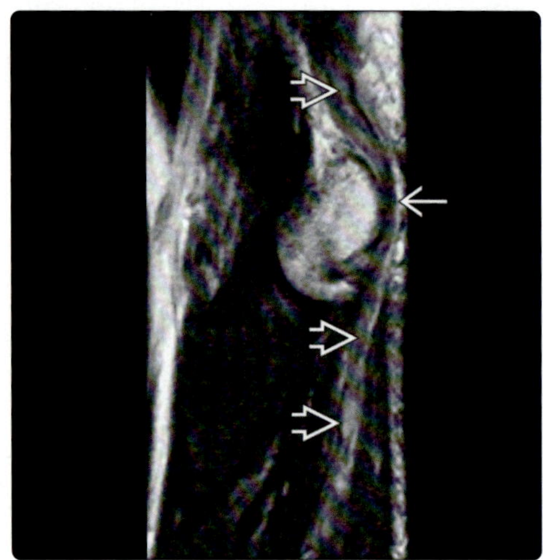

(Left) *Lateral radiograph shows a large, cortically based lytic lesion typical of nonossifying fibroma (NOF) →. Additionally, there is a mass within the popliteal fossa ↪.* **(Right)** *Axial PD FS MR in the same patient shows the large popliteal mass ⇒. It is high signal and contains a central region of lower signal intensity ↪; this is a target sign, which may be seen in neural lesions. This proved to be MPNST. Note also the multiple neurofibromas lining the common peroneal and tibial nerves ↪, as well as in other locations →.*

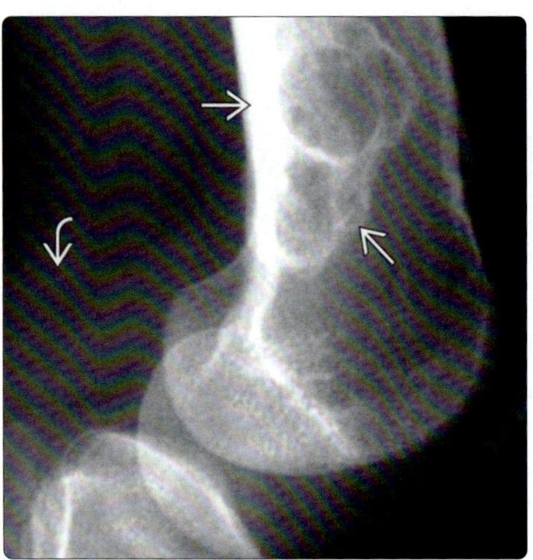

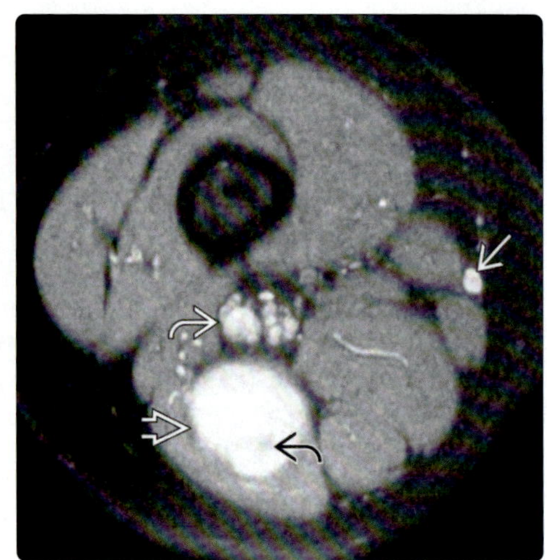

(Left) *This case demonstrates a recurrence of a MPNST, extending proximally as well as distally from a resected sciatic nerve. Sagittal T2WI FS MR shows a large, hyperintense, lobulated mass involving the entire length of the tibial nerve →.* **(Right)** *Coronal oblique T1WI C+ FS MR of the sacrum in the same patient shows each of the nerve roots of the sacrum to be enlarged on the affected left side → compared with the normal right. This is a devastating recurrence, both proximally and distally.*

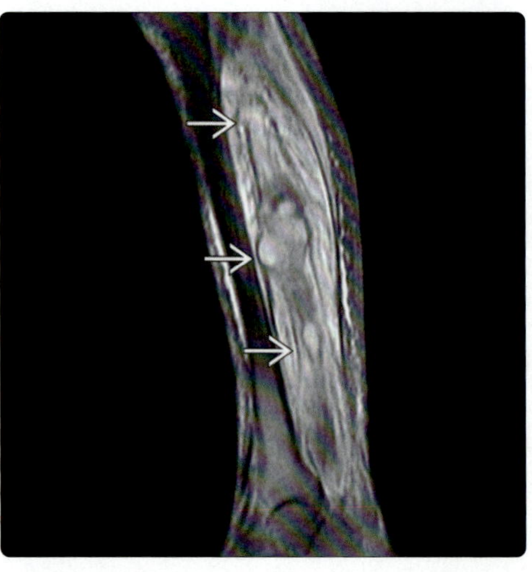

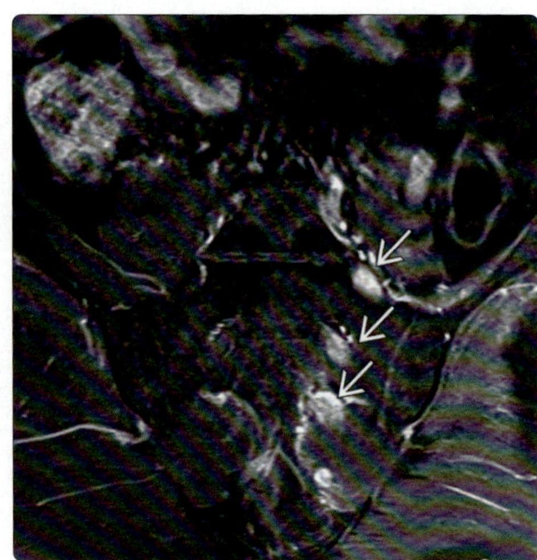

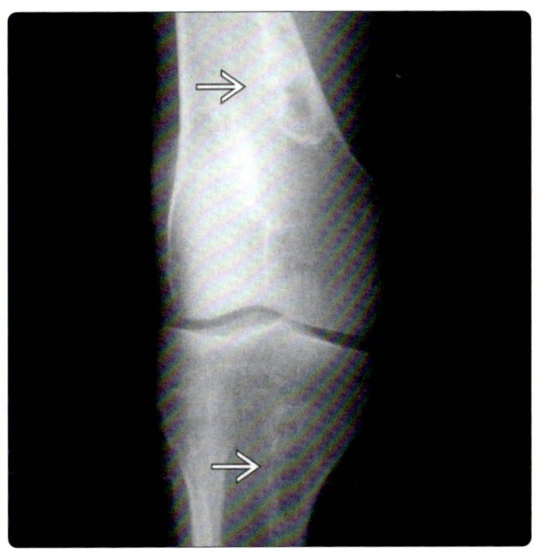

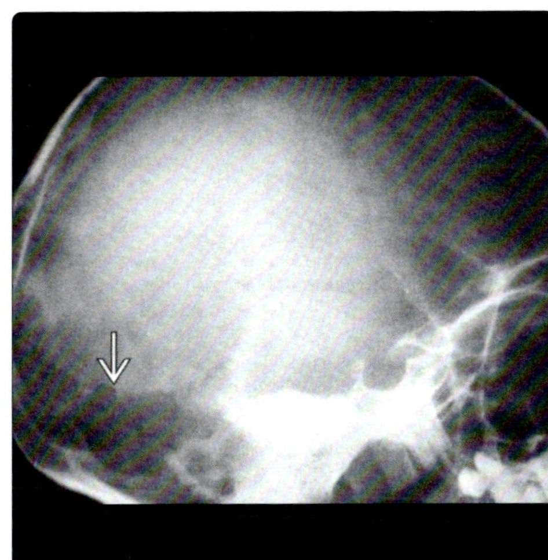

(Left) *Oblique radiograph shows multiple NOFs in a patient with NF. The natural history of these lesions is to heal, often with mild sclerosis prior to developing normal trabeculation. In this case, the healing is at a midpoint, with peripheral sclerosis but central residual lucency ➡.* **(Right)** *Lateral radiograph shows a defect in the lambdoid suture ➡, one of the skull dysplasias described for NF. Others include absence of the greater &/or lesser wings of the sphenoid or the orbital floor.*

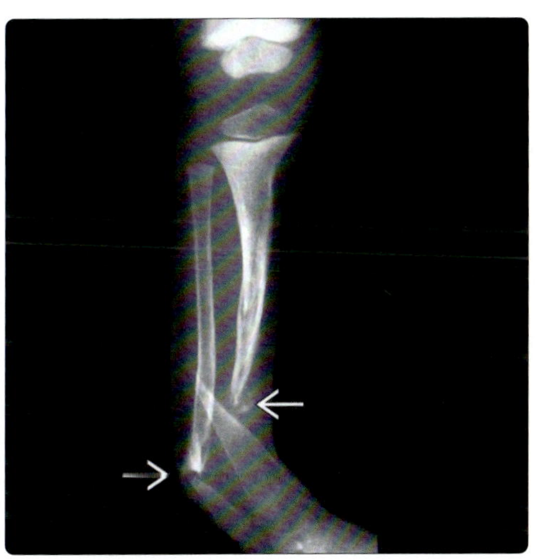

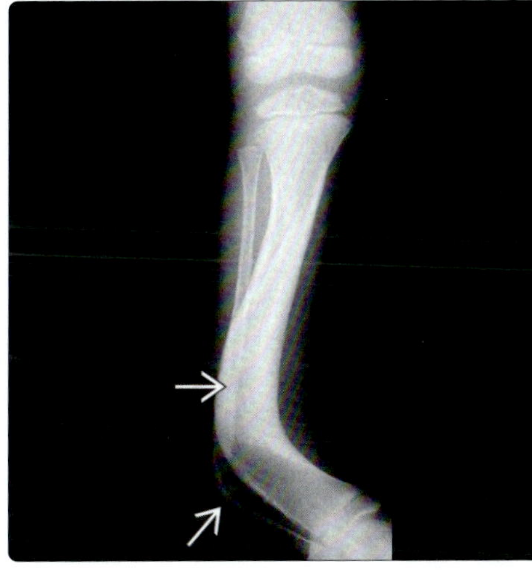

(Left) *AP radiograph demonstrates complete fracture through the tibia and fibula at the junction of the mid and distal 1/3 of the diaphyses ➡. The fracture margins are smoothly tapered; no callus is seen. This appearance is classic for pseudoarthrosis, often associated with NF.* **(Right)** *AP radiograph demonstrates a prominently bowed tibia and fibula ➡. The fibula is quite gracile, though the tibia shows normal thickness. This is another form of tibial dysplasia found in NF.*

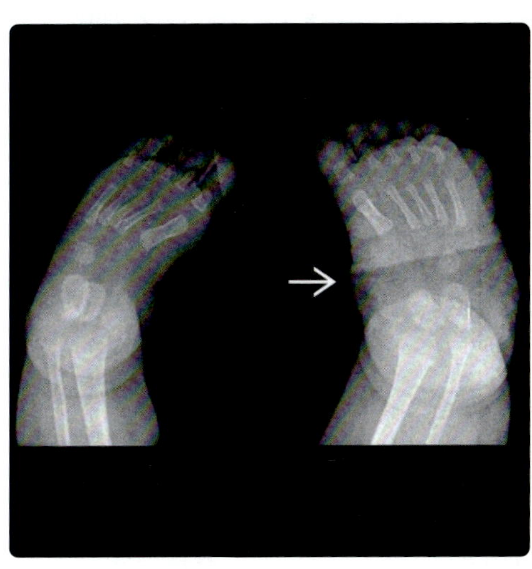

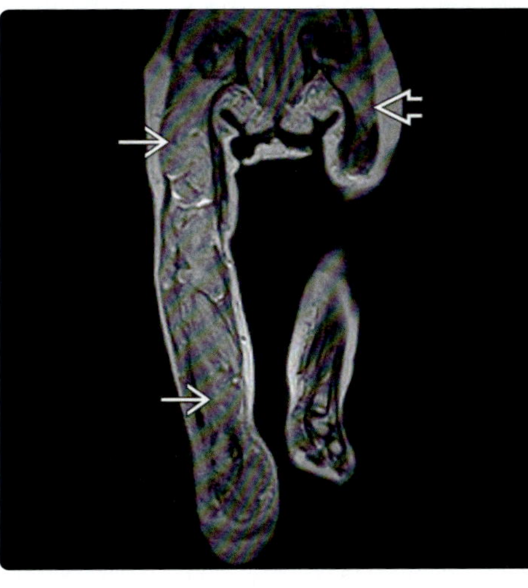

(Left) *AP radiograph shows localized gigantism. Note the asymmetric increased soft tissue about the right lower extremity/foot ➡ along with mild osseous overgrowth.* **(Right)** *Coronal T2WI MR in the same patient better shows the asymmetric soft tissue prominence and limb length discrepancy. MR also reveals a giant plexiform neurofibroma ➡ along the posterior right leg. A smaller plexiform neurofibroma along the posterior left thigh ➡ is seen as well. NF is in the differential for focal gigantism.*

Osteogenesis Imperfecta

KEY FACTS

TERMINOLOGY

- Genetic defect in type I collagen resulting in multiple fractures with little trauma
- Several subtypes: All have varying degrees of bone fragility, fractures, and deformities

IMAGING

- US prenatal diagnosis if severe; radiograph thereafter
- Types I and IV most likely imaged for routine fracture evaluation
- Type II may be imaged at birth; quickly lethal
- Type III is most likely to be imaged by radiographs
  - Most severe type that survives into childhood
- Tubular bone and rib morphology varies
  - Least severe: Thin, gracile, nearly normal length
  - Severe: Short, thick, bowed; callus formation gives crumpled appearance
- Skull involvement varies
  - Less severe: Normal or wormian bones
  - Severe: Delayed/absent calvarial ossification
  - Basilar impression of skull possible in any type, more common in type IV
- Kyphoscoliosis 40% overall; varies among types
- Multiple fractures in severe form result in small chest with broad, deformed ribs
  - "Beading" from healed fractures variable in extent

CLINICAL ISSUES

- Associated findings depend on type of OI
  - Blue sclera, hearing loss
  - Tooth abnormalities (dentinogenesis imperfecta)
- Prognosis
  - Types I and IV may have normal lifespan
  - Type II lethal in perinatal period
  - Type III has high childhood mortality
- Treatment
  - Bisphosphonates (less useful post skeletal maturation)
  - Surgical correction of bone deformity

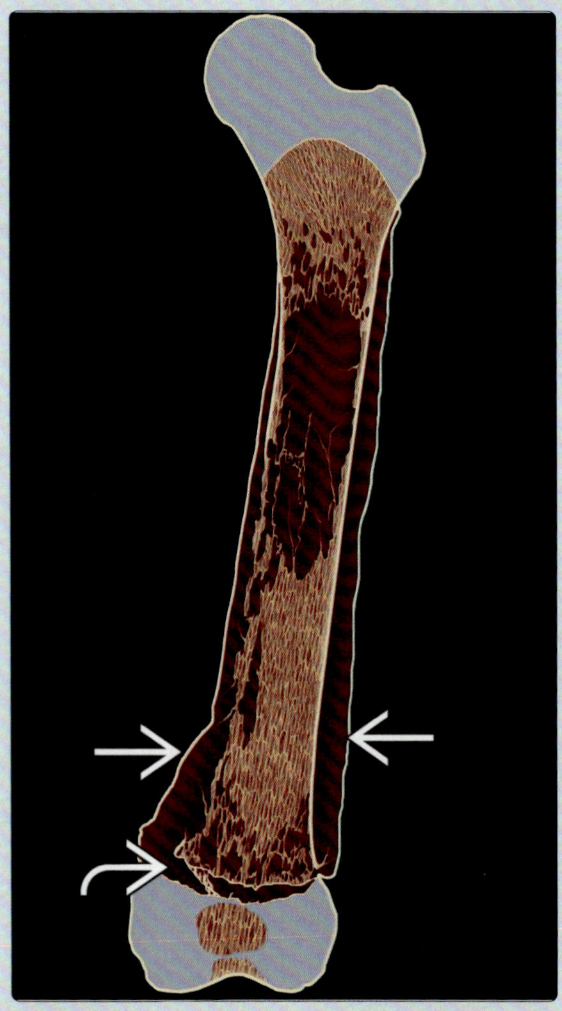

Graphic depicts a sectioned femur showing abnormal trabeculae in a patient with osteogenesis imperfecta. There is a physeal fracture distally ➲, with associated subperiosteal hemorrhage ➡, typical of injury in these fragile bones.

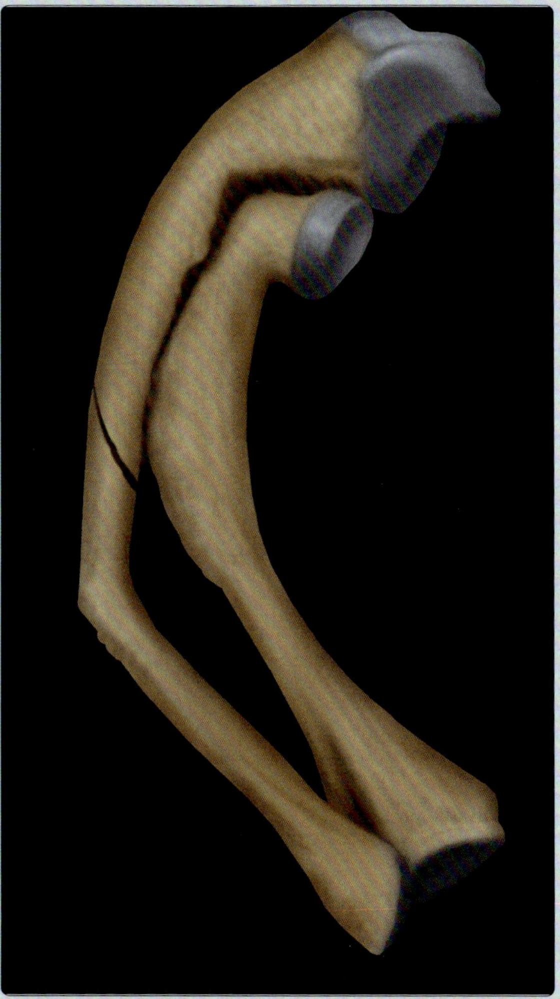

Graphic depicts bowing and callus from multiple fractures of different ages in a patient with OI. The appearance is of gracile bones with moderate deformity typically seen in OI type IV rather than the short, crumpled bones expected in types II/III.

TERMINOLOGY

Abbreviations

- Osteogenesis imperfecta (OI)

Definitions

- Genetic defect in type I collagen resulting in multiple fractures with little trauma
- Several subtypes: All have varying degrees of bone fragility, fractures, and deformities
  - Sillence classification is most commonly used
    - Based on clinical and radiological findings

IMAGING

General Features

- Best diagnostic clue
  - Osteopenia & multiple fractures; fracture number varies
    - Tubular bone and rib morphology varies
      - Thin, gracile, nearly normal length
      - Severely short, thick, bowed
      - Callus formation gives crumpled appearance

Imaging Recommendations

- Best imaging tool
  - US for prenatal diagnosis; radiograph thereafter

Radiographic Findings

- Types I & IV likely imaged for routine fracture evaluation
  - Fractures more common than normal population but much less common than in OI types II and III
  - Systemic disease may not be recognized on x-ray
    - Osteopenia, mildly gracile shape and deformities from prior fractures may be overlooked
- Type II may be imaged at birth
  - Usually diagnosed prenatally by ultrasound
  - Lethal at or soon after birth
- Type III most likely to be imaged by radiographs
  - Most severe type that survives into childhood
  - Evaluated for surgical correction of fx, dwarfism
- Long bones
  - Mild types of OI (I and IV)
    - Thin, gracile bones
    - Relatively few fractures
    - Only mild shortening: Normal height or within 2 or 3 standard deviations (SD) of mean
  - Severe types of OI (II and III)
    - Short, thick bones
    - Multiple fractures
    - Often hypertrophic fracture callus
    - Prone to nonunion or malunion
    - Deformities: Bowing, protrusio, coxa vara
    - Severe dwarfism (10 SD below mean)
- Skull
  - Mild types may be normal
  - Wormian bones (less severe types), delayed/absent calvarial ossification (severe types)
  - Basilar impression of skull possible in any type, more common in type IV
- Spine
  - Platyspondyly
  - Kyphoscoliosis 40% overall; varies among types
- Ribs
  - Multiple fractures in severe form result in small chest with broad, deformed ribs
  - "Beading" from healed fractures variable in extent

CT Findings

- Thin osseous cortices
- Basilar invagination; associated neuroradiological abnormalities
- Otosclerosis

MR Findings

- Fetal MR may add information to prenatal ultrasound
  - Lung capacity
  - Other soft tissue abnormalities

Ultrasonographic Findings

- Most cases identified at prenatal US are type II
  - Presence of fractures differentiates from other short-limbed dwarfs
    - Shortening with angulation, pseudarthroses
    - Crumpled appearance 2° to callus
    - Osteopenia: No shadowing from anterior cortex so may see posterior cortex
  - Small circumference chest, rib beading
  - Poorly mineralized skull; no reverberation artifact
    - Skull deformation from transducer pressure
- Type III or IV may be recognized by bent femur

DIFFERENTIAL DIAGNOSIS

Nonaccidental Trauma

- Most important differential consideration; differentiated by normal bone density
- Skeletal injury common, especially classic metaphyseal (corner) fracture
- Head and visceral injuries

Temporary Brittle Bone Disease

- Controversial transient form of OI
- Radiologically identical to nonaccidental trauma

Hypophosphatasia

- Rickets-like, with wide and frayed metaphyses
- Osteopenia, with short fragile bone, fx, bowing
- Severe and tarda forms

Idiopathic Juvenile Osteoporosis

- Transient osteoporosis
- Develop more fractures than expected for age
- Self-limited

PATHOLOGY

General Features

- Etiology
  - Disturbance in synthesis of type I collagen
    - Major constituent of bone, dentin, sclerae, ligaments, blood vessels, skin
- Genetics
  - 90% of OI have mutations in either of genes encoding pro-alpha1 or pro-alpha2 chains of type I collagen

Sillence Classification of Osteogenesis Imperfecta

Type	Inheritance Pattern	Relative Frequency	Severity of Bone Fragility	Bone Morphology	Sclerae	Dentinogenesis Imperfecta	Hearing Loss
Type I	Autosomal dominant	Most common	Least severe (+)	Thin, gracile tubular bones	Blue	Depends on subtype	Yes
Type IA		Common				No	
Type IB		Rare				Yes	
Type II	Autosomal dominant (mutation or mosaic parent)	2nd most common	Most severe (++++)	Depends on subtype	Blue	No	No
Type IIA			(++++)	Short, thick tubular bones; ribs short, broad, with continuous beading			
Type IIB			(++++)	Short, thick tubular bones; ribs short, broad, with little beading			
Type IIC			(+++ to ++++)	Tubular bones longer & thinner than types IIA or IIB; ribs thin with beading			
Type III	Autosomal dominant; rarely recessive	3rd most common	2nd most severe (most severe to survive childhood) (+++)	Short, thick tubular bones	May be pale blue at birth but → normal	No	No
Type IV	Autosomal dominant	Least common	2nd least severe (+ to ++)	Thin, gracile bones with mild to moderate deformity; basilar skull impression more common than in other types	Normal	Depends on subtype	Yes (less common than type I)
Type IVA		Rare				No	
Type IVB		More common than IVA				Yes	

CLINICAL ISSUES

Presentation

- Most common signs/symptoms
  - Depends on type of OI
    - Multiple fractures of different ages
    - Bone pain, joint laxity
    - Kyphoscoliosis, short stature
- Other signs/symptoms
  - Depend on type of OI
    - Blue sclera, hearing loss
    - Tooth abnormalities (dentinogenesis imperfecta)

Demographics

- Age
  - Types II and III present prenatally or at birth
  - Types I and IV present in childhood

Natural History & Prognosis

- Types I and IV may have normal lifespan
- Type II lethal in perinatal period
- Type III high childhood mortality

Treatment

- Bisphosphonates
  - ↑ bone mineral density
  - May improve stature when given during infancy
  - Some studies suggest pain modification
  - ↓ incidence fracture in some, but not all, studies
  - Less effective after skeletal maturation
  - Experimental in maternal OI (preconception)
- Surgical correction of bone deformity
- Bone marrow transplant being investigated
- Human mesenchymal stem cell therapy promising

DIAGNOSTIC CHECKLIST

Consider

- Consider OI type I or IV in patient with mild osteopenia, deformity, and slightly ↑ number of fx than expected

SELECTED REFERENCES

1. Lindahl K et al: Genetic epidemiology, prevalence, and genotype-phenotype correlations in the Swedish population with osteogenesis imperfecta. Eur J Hum Genet. ePub, 2015

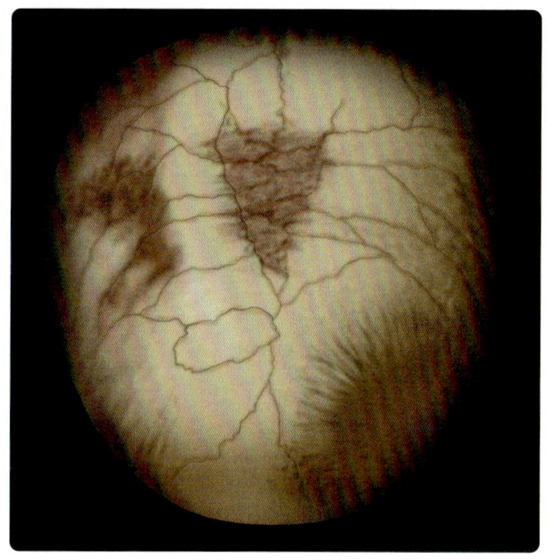

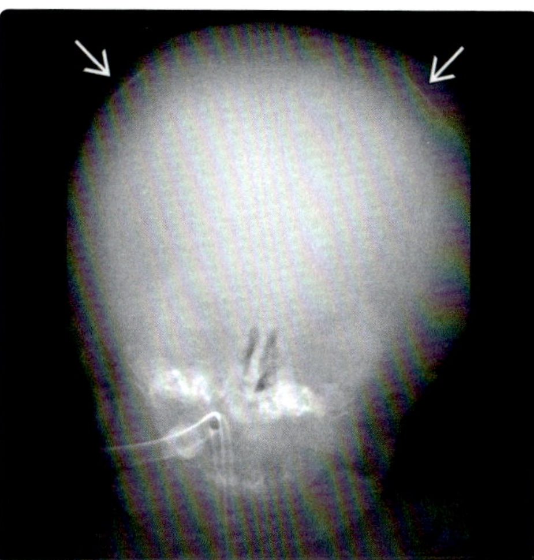

(Left) *Graphic depicts wormian bones and thin calvaria in a patient with osteogenesis imperfecta. This appearance is seen with the severe forms of OI types II and III.* **(Right)** *AP radiograph of a skull shows ossification of the facial bones and two small regions of the cranium ➡. The severe lack of calcification is reminiscent of hypophosphatasia, but the presence of even a small amount of calcification in the skull makes the diagnosis of osteogenesis imperfecta type II. This is the most severe form.*

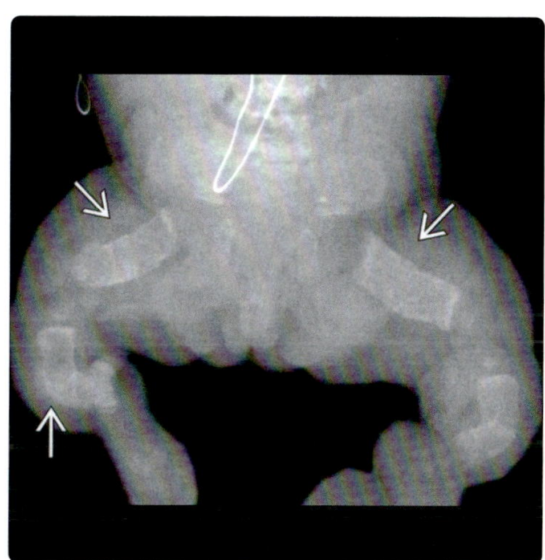

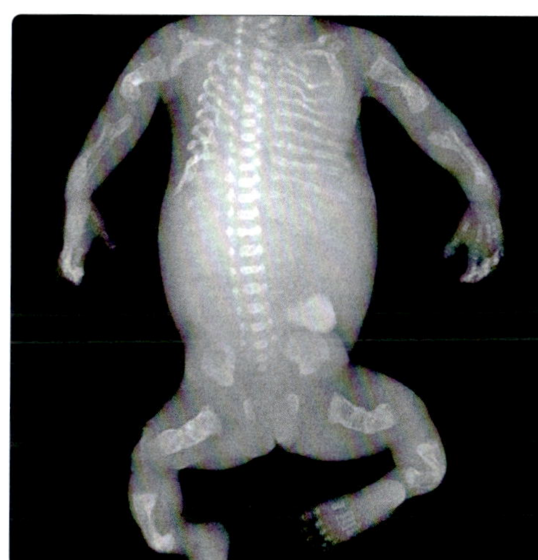

(Left) *AP radiograph of the pelvis in the same patient shows the long bones of lower extremities to be short and broad, with multiple fractures ➡. The severity of the osteoporosis should not allow confusion with a dwarf syndrome. This type II OI is lethal in the perinatal period.* **(Right)** *AP radiograph shows a typical case of osteogenesis imperfecta type II in a newborn with innumerable fractures. The arms and legs are short due to angulation and deformity resulting from the fractures. Note the small chest 2° to rib fractures.*

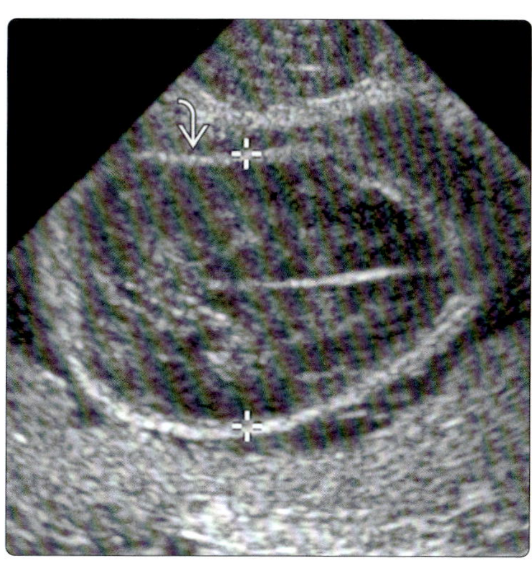

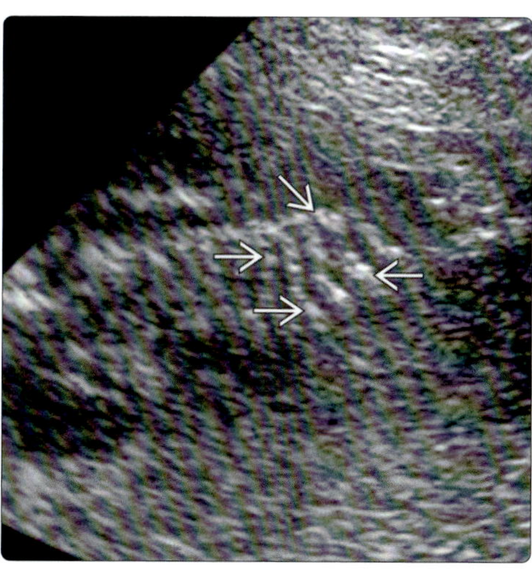

(Left) *Axial prenatal US shows a typical example of osteogenesis imperfecta. The skull is poorly mineralized and is deformed by transducer pressure ➡. The near field structures of the brain are also well seen due to the lack of reverberation.* **(Right)** *Longitudinal oblique US in the same case shows the chest is small in circumference. The ribs are short and angulated ➡. They appear beaded, relating to healed fractures. This is type II OI; the perinatal lethal episode is usually due to pulmonary compromise.*

(Left) *AP radiograph shows extremely thin, gracile, osteoporotic bones which are deformed, relating to multiple fractures.* **(Right)** *AP radiograph in the same case also shows multiple fractures with residual bowing. The gracile appearance may be seen in OI type IIC or type IV. Type IV generally shows less severe bone fragility than seen here, but type IIC rarely survives into childhood. Type III generally shows severe disease but survives into childhood; however, the bones are usually short & thick.*

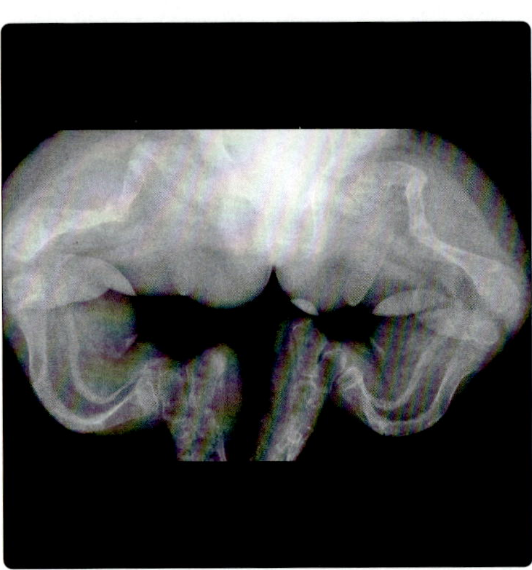

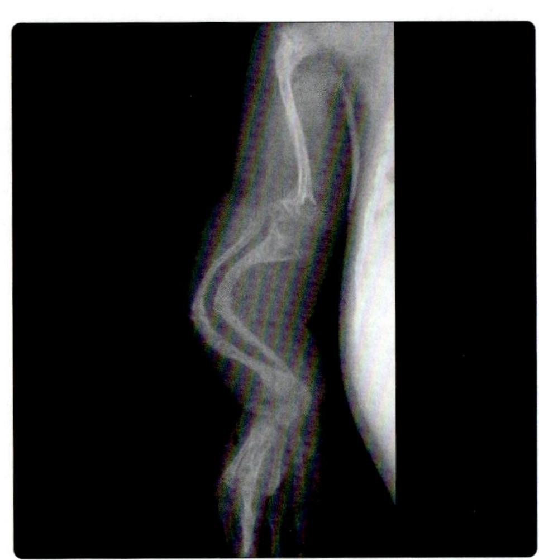

(Left) *AP radiograph shows typical coxa vara ➡ along with osteoporosis, seen in osteogenesis imperfecta. There is shortening and thickening of the right femur ⇨. This is a case of OI type III, with the patient demonstrating severe disease but surviving into childhood.* **(Right)** *Lateral radiograph of the skull shows osteopenia along with wormian bones, too numerous to count ↗. Wormian bones may be seen in any form of OI.*

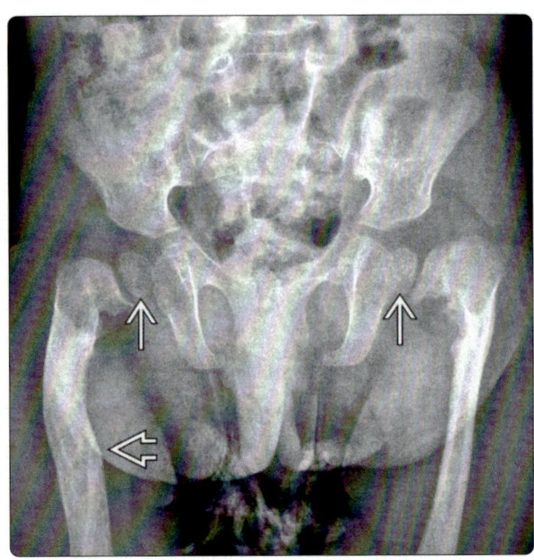

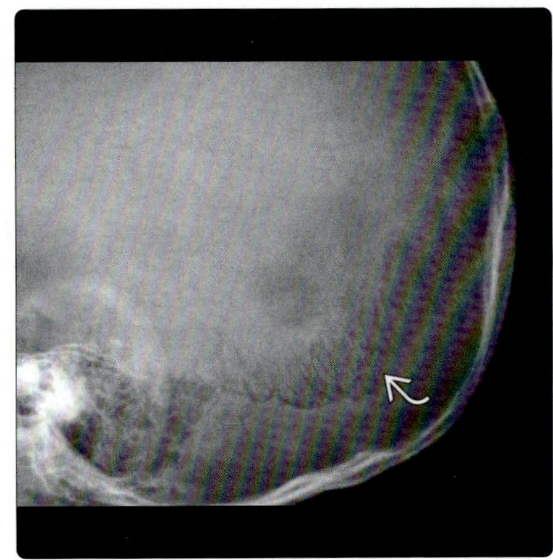

(Left) *AP radiograph shows the femur in a child with gracile limbs of normal length but severe osteopenia. There have been prior fractures, and a new mid diaphyseal fracture is seen ➡. This morphology is typical of OI type I or IV.* **(Right)** *AP radiograph in a child shows severe osteopenia & an old, healed, slightly angulated fracture ➡. The bone is gracile but of normal length. This represents radiographic findings typical of either OI type I or IV; clinical findings are required for further differentiation.*

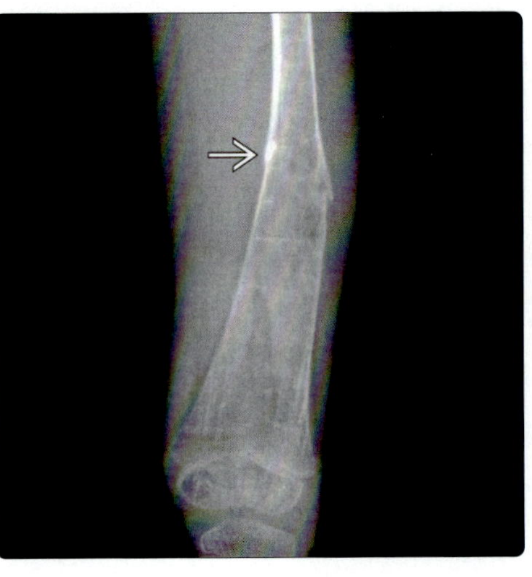

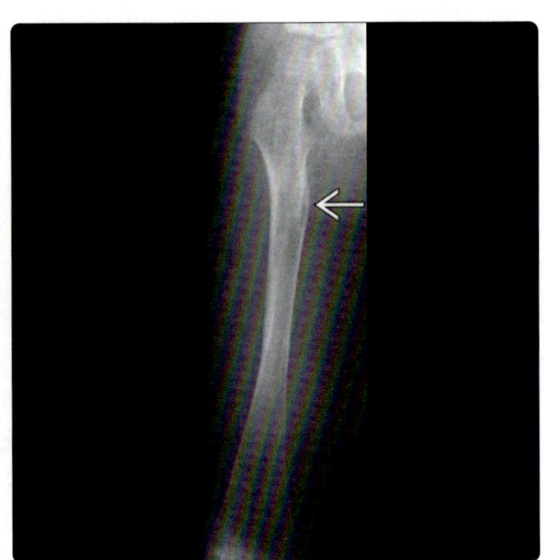

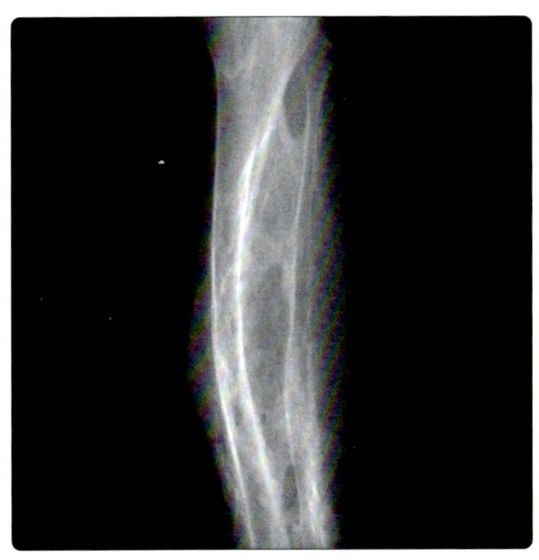

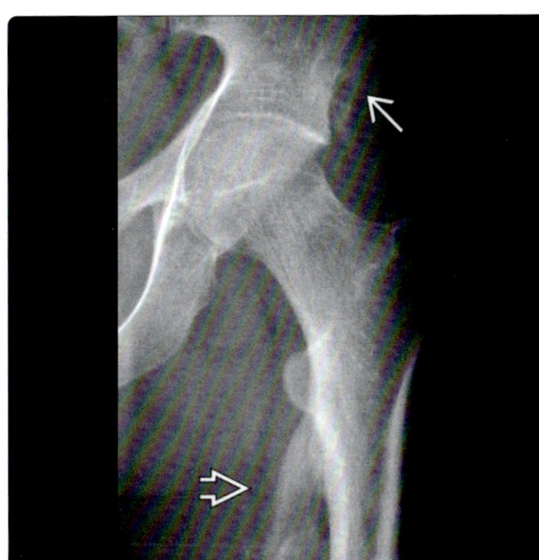

(Left) *AP radiograph shows osteopenia, bowing, and evidence of prior fractures in this leg. Additionally, there is prominent hypertrophic callus formation across malunited fractures. The bones are of normal length, though thin.* **(Right)** *AP radiograph in the same patient shows enthesopathy at the inferior iliac spine ➡, as well as extensive callus crossing a site of previous femoral fracture ➡. Given the normal length but osteopenic, gracile, fragile bones, the diagnosis is OI type I or IV.*

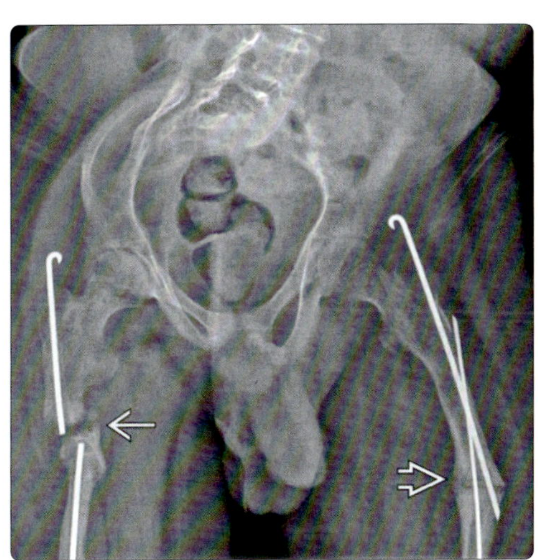

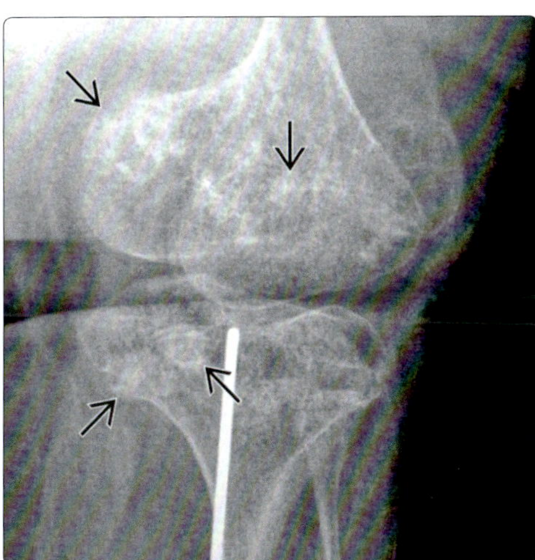

(Left) *AP radiograph in an adolescent, who is unable to walk, shows pelvic deformity, severe osteopenia, and multiple fractures. Intramedullary rods have been used to correct deformities and stabilize fractures; there is a malunion on the left ➡ and nonunion on the right ➡. This is OI type III in a patient who survived childhood.* **(Right)** *AP radiograph shows severe osteogenesis imperfecta with popcorn calcifications within the long bone epiphyses ➡; these must not be confused with tumor matrix.*

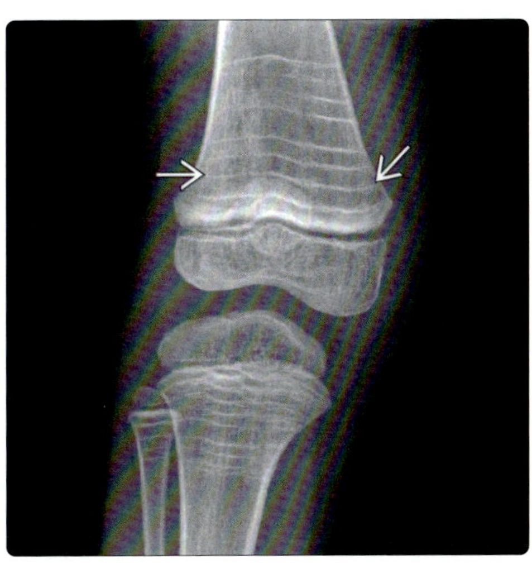

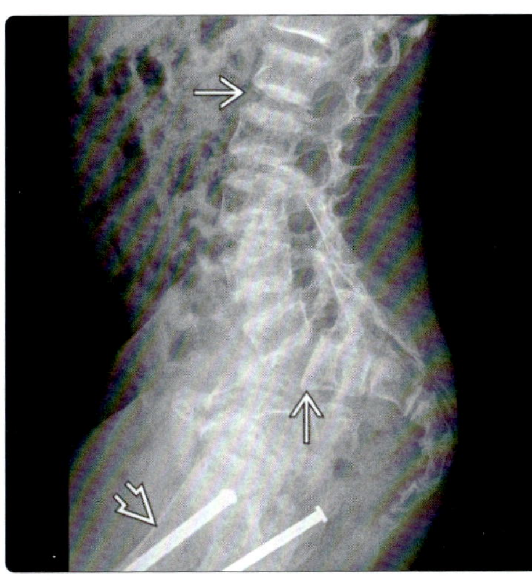

(Left) *AP radiograph shows a case of OI with osteoporosis but normal length, indicating OI type I or IV. There are at least 8 sclerotic metaphyseal lines ➡, a result of cyclic bisphosphonate therapy.* **(Right)** *Lateral radiograph in type III OI shows intramedullary rods from treatment of tubular bones ➡. There is mild platyspondyly & exaggerated lumbar lordosis & sacral curvature. Sclerotic bands ➡ are due to bisphosphonate therapy. Combined therapies improve patient morbidity/mortality.*

Turner Syndrome

KEY FACTS

TERMINOLOGY

- Syndrome of female phenotype with 45,XO chromosome complement

IMAGING

- Osteoporosis
- Delayed epiphyseal fusion (often 3rd decade)
- Morphologic abnormalities of hand and wrist
  - Shortening of metacarpals (particularly 4th)
  - Drumstick morphology of phalanges
  - Decreased carpal angle; Madelung deformity
- Deformity at knee
  - Flattening/downsloping of medial tibial plateau
  - Overgrowth medial femoral condyle
  - May have mild varus deformity
  - Excrescence or beaking at medial proximal tibial metaphysis
- Cubitus valgus
- Thin clavicles and ribs
- Vertebral body irregularities
- Skull
  - Brachycephaly
  - Small facial bones
  - Prominent mandible
  - Enlarged sinuses

PATHOLOGY

- Associated extraosseous abnormalities
  - Pituitary gland hyperplasia or neoplasm
  - Coarctation of aorta
  - Hemangiomas
  - Intestinal telangiectasia
  - Renal anomalies
  - Short stature
  - Laterally displaced nipples on shield-like chest
  - Lymphedema in 60%
- Premature mortality, usually cardiovascular-related

(Left) *PA radiograph of the wrist in a patient with Turner syndrome is shown. The distal radius shows abnormal ulnar tilt ➔ and widened distal radioulnar joint, resulting in proximal migration of the lunate, decreased carpal angle, and a triangular-shaped carpus.* **(Right)** *Lateral radiograph in the same patient shows exaggerated volar tilt of the radius ➔. The carpus maintains alignment with the radius, while the ulna is overgrown and dorsally dislocated ➔. This typical Madelung deformity may be seen with Turner syndrome.*

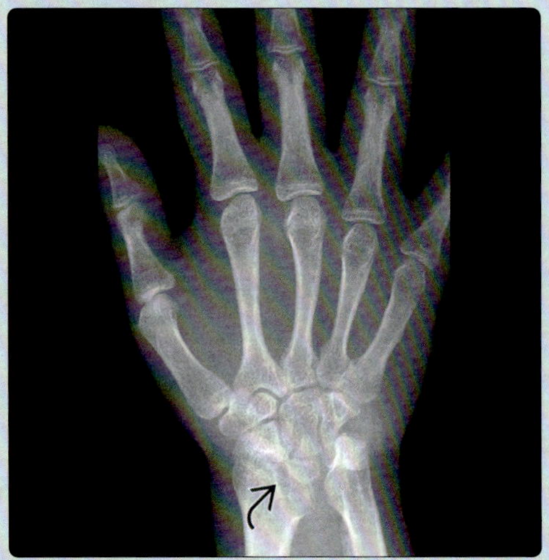

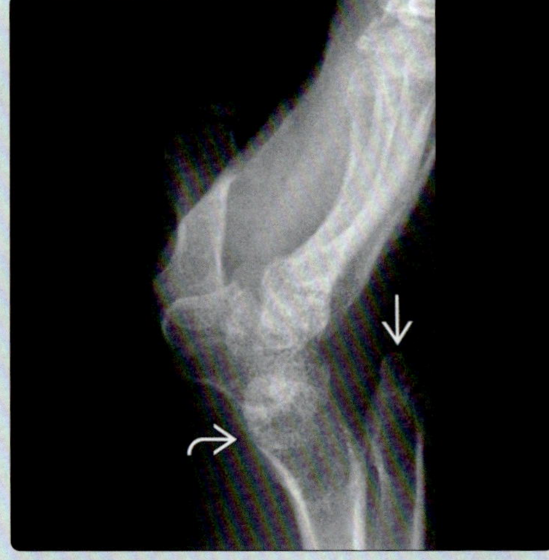

(Left) *AP radiograph shows underdevelopment (flattening) of the medial tibial plateau ➔, with relative overgrowth of the medial femoral condyle. This can result in a varus deformity. There is beaking at the proximal medial tibial metaphysis ➔. The findings were bilateral and are typical of Turner syndrome.* **(Right)** *PA radiograph shows short metacarpals 3-5. There is no other morphologic abnormality. Short metacarpals are nonspecific, seen in many syndromes (including Turner).*

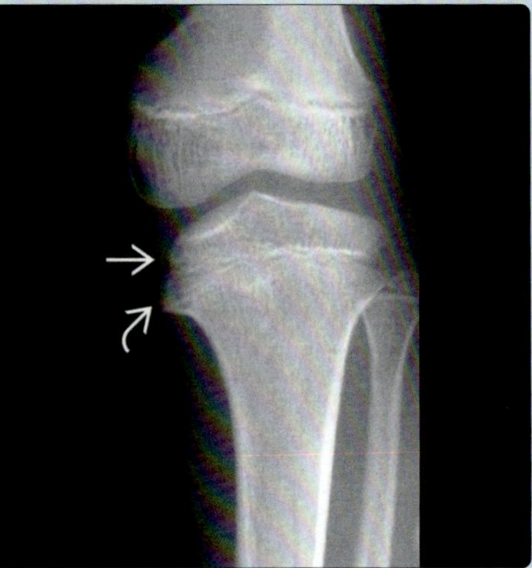

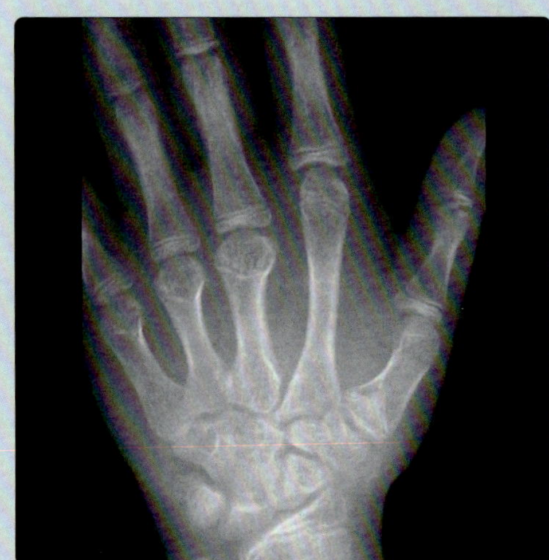

KEY FACTS

TERMINOLOGY

- Congenital anomaly resulting in dysplasia of posteroinferior glenoid &/or scapular neck

IMAGING

- Location: Inferior & posterior glenoid of scapula
  - Often bilateral & symmetric
- Notched appearance of inferior articular surface of glenoid
  - Surface may be irregular, or shallow & smooth
  - Rare associated hypoplasia (flattening) of humeral neck &/or head
  - Rare associated hyperplasia & bowing of acromion &/or clavicle
- Axial imaging (CT or MR)
  - Posterior inferior insufficiency of glenoid
  - Posterior subluxation of humeral head may be seen, but not invariable
- Additional MR findings
  - Glenoid defect filled by tissue with either fibrocartilage or fat MR signal characteristics
  - Posterior labral abnormalities common: Enlarged, detached, torn, degenerated, perilabral cyst
  - Findings of shoulder instability: Patulous capsule, rotator cuff, or glenohumeral ligament injury

TOP DIFFERENTIAL DIAGNOSES

- Luxatio erecta with fracture
- Reverse Bankart fracture

PATHOLOGY

- Congenital failure of ossification of lower 2/3 of glenoid & adjacent scapular apophysis

CLINICAL ISSUES

- May be incidental finding
- Multidirectional instability in ≥ 1/3

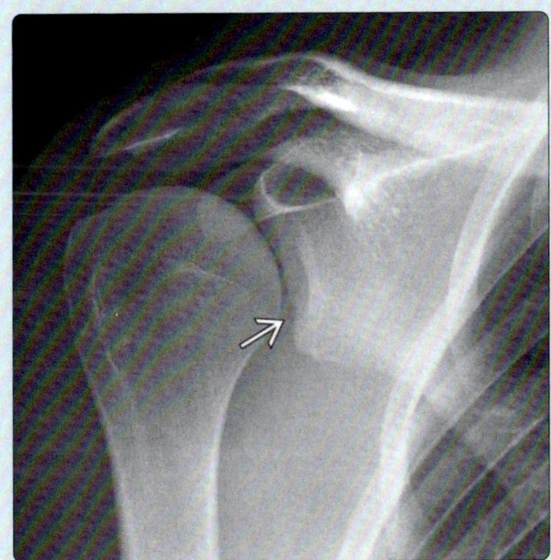

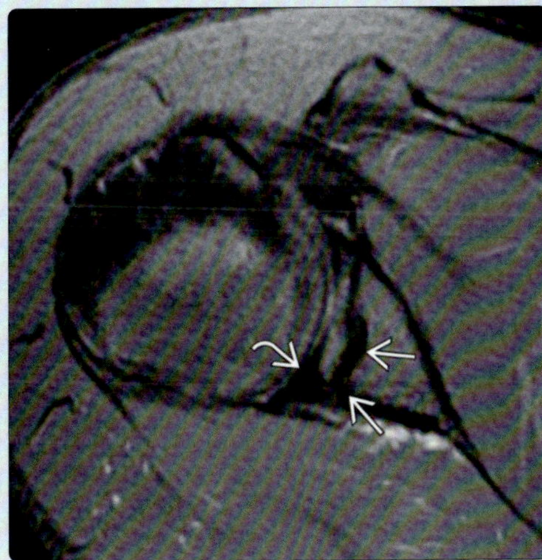

(Left) *AP radiograph shows hypoplasia of the inferior glenoid ➡. The humeral head and neck appear unaffected. This relatively mild dysplasia is easily overlooked, but the patient had multidirectional instability.* **(Right)** *Axial PD FS MR, same case, shows the defect at the mid- and posterior glenoid ➡. There is associated mild hyperplasia of the posterior glenoid labrum ➡, with incomplete detachment.*

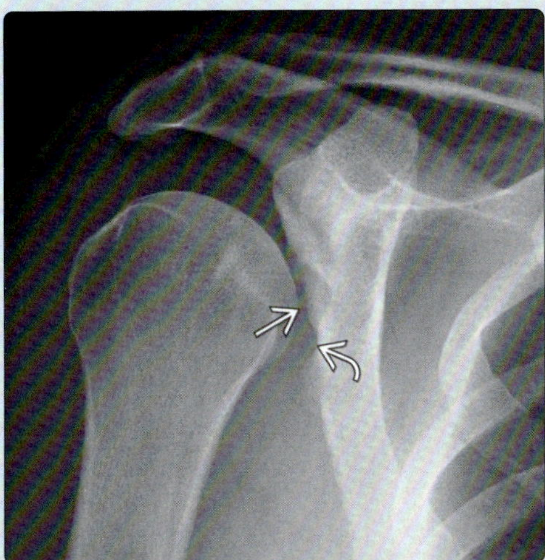

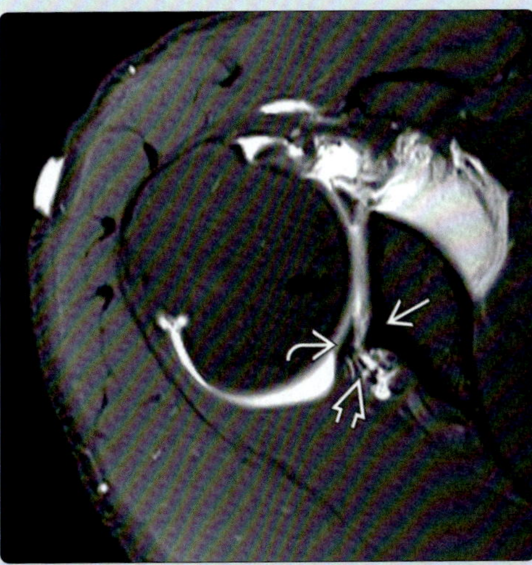

(Left) *AP radiograph, different case, shows significant inferior glenoid hypoplasia ➡. In addition to the glenoid defect, there is a mild defect in the adjacent axillary border of the scapula ➡.* **(Right)** *Axial T2WI FS MR, same case, shows the posterior angular deformity of the glenoid ➡. The inferior glenoid labrum ➡ is not significantly hypertrophied, but is detached from the underlying abnormal bone. There is fibrous tissue ➡ that partially fills the defect.*

KEY FACTS

TERMINOLOGY

- Developmental wrist bowing deformity resulting from growth disturbance of distal radial physis

IMAGING

- Morphology on all imaging
  - Ulnar and volar tilt of distal radius
  - Decreased carpal angle
  - Elongated, dorsally subluxated ulna
  - Triangularization of lunate
  - Absent lunate facet on triquetrum
  - Absent sigmoid notch at distal radius
- Bilateral more frequent than unilateral
- Severity may be asymmetric
- MR
  - Radial physeal bar on volar/ulnar aspect
  - Abnormality of metadiaphysis of radius at ulnar side osseous excrescence or cyst
  - Anomalous extrinsic ligament (radiotriquetral) tethers carpus to radius (thick, low signal)
  - Hypertrophy of short radiolunate (Vickers) ligament: Originates from ulnar border of radius, inserts on volar border of lunate
  - Triangular fibrocartilaginous complex (TFCC) thinned, with oblique radial attachment

TOP DIFFERENTIAL DIAGNOSES

- Dyschondrosteosis (Leri-Weill)
- Turner syndrome
- Distal radial fracture in child
- Multiple hereditary exostoses

CLINICAL ISSUES

- Develops in childhood, deformity worsens throughout adolescence
- Male < female (ratio: 1:3-5)
- Treatment usually conservative

(Left) *PA radiograph shows a typical Madelung deformity, with relatively long straight ulna & radius with ulnar tilt. There is a decreased carpal angle. Note the excrescence at the medial aspect of the radial metaphysis ➡, due to the large anomalous attaching ligament.* **(Right)** *In the same patient, coronal T1WI MR in dorsal region of wrist shows the anomalous radiotriquetral ligament ➡ attaching to the medial radial metaphysis. Note the medial portion of the radial physis ➡ shows early fusion, contributing to the osseous deformity.*

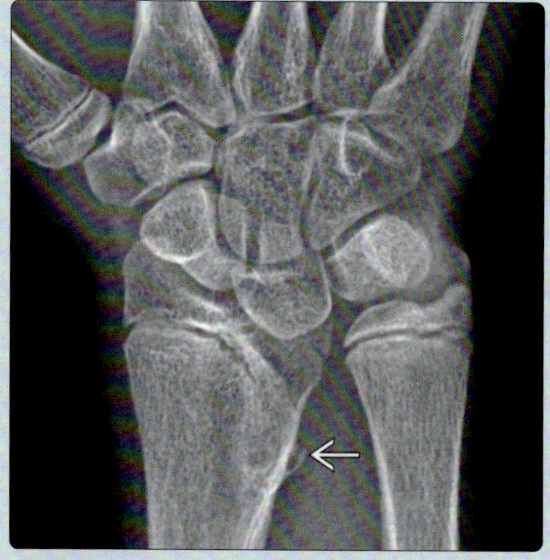

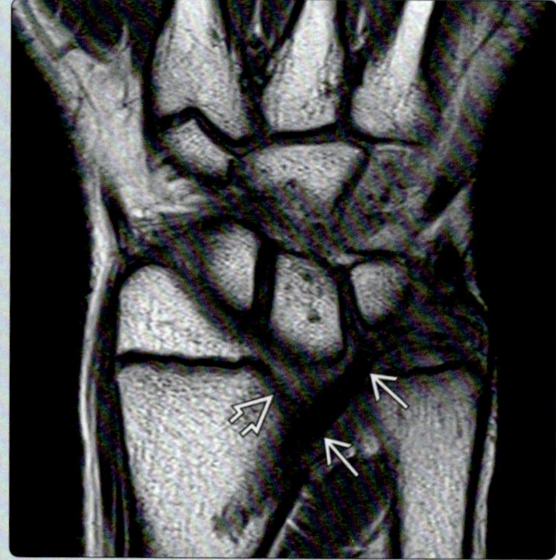

(Left) *Sagittal T2WI FS MR at midjoint shows the radiotriquetral ligament ➡ approaching the medial radial metaphysis.* **(Right)** *Axial T2WI FS MR, same case, shows the thick radiotriquetral ligament ➡ and Vickers ligament attaching to the medial radius at an abnormal sigmoid notch ➡. Note that the ulnar-sided extensor ligaments ➡ are thinned and stretched over the dorsally subluxed ulna. The findings were bilateral, as is commonly the case with Madelung deformity.*

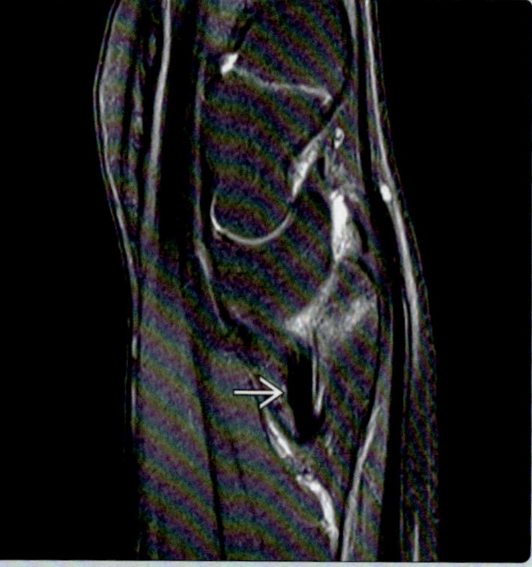

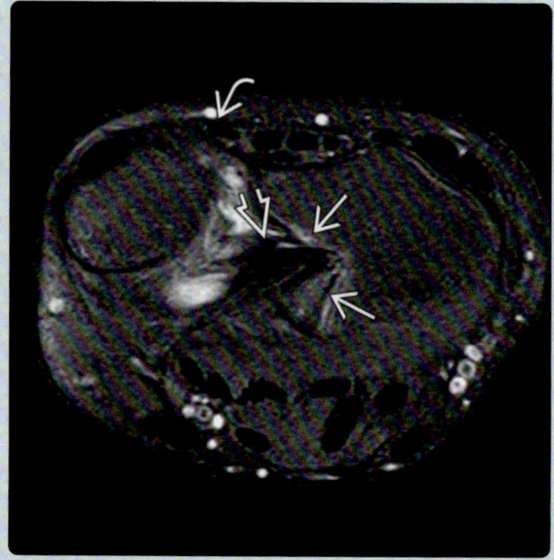

TERMINOLOGY

Definitions

- Developmental wrist bowing deformity resulting from growth disturbance of distal radial physis

IMAGING

General Features

- Best diagnostic clue
  - Ulnar and volar tilt of distal radius
    - Decreased carpal angle
    - Elongated, dorsally subluxated ulna
- Location
  - Bilateral more frequent than unilateral
    - Severity may be asymmetric
- Morphology
  - Range of severity and associated deformity

Radiographic Findings

- Madelung deformity
  - Radius
    - Epiphysis relatively short on medial (ulnar) aspect, giving triangular appearance
      - Medial (ulnar) portion of radial epiphysis may fuse prematurely
    - Exaggerated ulnar tilt of distal radial articular surface (lateral curvature of distal radius)
    - Exaggerated volar tilt of distal radial articular surface (dorsal curvature of distal radius)
    - Osseous excrescence or cyst may develop on ulnar aspect of radial metaphysis, ~ 3 cm proximal to radiocarpal joint line
    - Widening at distal radioulnar joint (DRUJ)
    - Absent sigmoid notch of distal radius precludes normal articulation with ulna
  - Ulna
    - Normal or increased length; appears elongated relative to radius
    - Subluxated dorsally; lacks normal articulation at distal radioulnar joint
    - Overgrowth of ulnar head may occur
  - Carpus
    - Decreased carpal angle for articulation with radius and ulna (normal is 130-137°)
    - Carpus maintains articulation with radius, not ulna (follows radius on lateral radiograph)
    - Entire carpus assumes triangular configuration, with apex at lunate
    - Lunate migrates proximally, articulating with short deformed medial portion of distal radial epiphysis
      - If radioulnar diastasis is wide, proximally migrated lunate appears wedged between them
    - Lunate facet on triquetrum is absent, deformed
    - Various degrees of osteoarthritis: Joint space narrowing, sclerosis
- Reverse Madelung variant
  - Radial articular surface tilted dorsally
  - Carpus shifts dorsally, maintaining articulation with radius
  - Ulna subluxates volarly
- Chevron carpus variant
  - Triangulation of carpus, lunate wedged between radius and ulna
  - No dorsal or volar subluxation of distal ulna
  - No clinical deformity

CT Findings

- Infrequently used but allows 3D evaluation of osseous relationships

MR Findings

- Osseous structures
  - Normal signal on all sequences
    - Physis hyperintense on fluid-sensitive sequences
  - Malalignment as noted on radiograph
    - Axial plane especially useful to evaluate radioulnar alignment and proximal migration of lunate
  - Distorted morphology
    - Triangularization of lunate
    - Absent lunate facet on triquetrum
    - Absent sigmoid notch at distal radius
  - Radial physeal abnormalities
    - Physeal bar or premature fusion on volar and ulnar aspect
  - Abnormality of metadiaphysis of radius at ulnar side
    - At site of attachment of extrinsic radiotriquetral ligament
      - May be osseous excrescence
      - May result in cyst formation
  - Osteonecrosis of lunate (rare)
  - Varying degrees of osteoarthritis
    - Cartilage thinning
    - Marrow edema
    - Subchondral cyst formation
    - Osteophytes
- Ligaments
  - Anomalous extrinsic ligament (radiotriquetral) tethers carpus to radius
    - Thick, low-signal ligament, seen best on coronals
    - Extends from deformed lunate facet of triquetrum, across proximal ulnar aspect of lunate, to insert on ulnar aspect of radial metadiaphysis
  - Hypertrophy of short radiolunate (Vickers) ligament: Originates from ulnar border of radius, inserts on volar border of lunate
    - Likely contributes to pyramidalization of carpus
  - Triangular fibrocartilaginous complex (TFCC)
    - Thinned, with oblique radial attachment
- Tendons
  - Tendinopathy or rupture of extensor tendons (rare)

Imaging Recommendations

- Best imaging tool
  - Diagnosis established on radiograph
  - MR used to evaluate for physeal bar and abnormal tethering ligaments

DIFFERENTIAL DIAGNOSIS

Dyschondrosteosis (Leri-Weill)

- Mesomelic variety of dwarfism with Madelung deformity

- Characterized by wrist deformity, which appears identical to Madelung on radiograph
  - On CT, early cases show no ulnar subluxation and relative pronation of carpus (opposite of case in early Madelung)
  - Advanced disease: Lack of proximal lunate support by radius
- Male > > female
- Some believe isolated Madelung deformity to be at minor end of spectrum of dyschondrosteosis

Turner Syndrome

- Madelung deformity common
- Other osseous abnormalities
  - Flattening, undergrowth of medial tibial plateau with mild overgrowth of medial femoral condyle
  - Short metacarpals
- Mental deficits

Mucopolysaccharidoses

- Morquio and Hurler syndrome may have Madelung deformity
- Other osseous abnormalities
  - Fan-shaped metacarpals
  - Constricted acetabulum, wide sacrosciatic notch
  - Hypoplastic L1 body with anterior beaking
  - Oar-shaped posterior ribs

Distal Radial Fracture in Child

- Salter fracture through distal radial physis with early fusion leads to deformity
- Differential medial fusion of radial physis may lead to deformity similar to Madelung

Multiple Hereditary Exostoses

- Sessile exostoses in forearm may result in disruption of distal radioulnar joint, triangular-shaped distal radial epiphysis
- May result in decreased carpal angle
- Radial head may be dislocated at elbow
- Widespread exostoses elsewhere are diagnostic

PATHOLOGY

General Features

- Genetics
  - Reports of it being dominant, familial deformity
    - Incomplete penetrance

Microscopic Features

- Normal chondrocytes in physis
- Abnormal arrangement of columns of cells

CLINICAL ISSUES

Presentation

- Most common signs/symptoms
  - Visible deformity
  - Pain, fatigue of wrist
  - Limited range of motion (especially dorsal extension, ulnar deviation, supination)
- Other signs/symptoms
  - Carpal tunnel symptoms (uncommon)
    - Due to obliquity of carpal tunnel and consequent susceptibility of median nerve to trauma
  - Extensor tendon rupture (uncommon)
    - Thinned over enlarged and dorsally subluxated ulnar head

Demographics

- Age
  - Develops in childhood, deformity worsens throughout adolescence
  - Clinical presentation generally during adolescence or early adulthood, as wrist becomes painful
- Gender
  - Male < female (1:3-5)
- Epidemiology
  - Rare
  - Increased incidence reported in West Indies

Natural History & Prognosis

- Symptoms may correlate poorly with degree of abnormality seen on imaging
- Pain and limitations may stabilize in adulthood
- Eventual progression to early and often severe osteoarthritis

Treatment

- Conservative is most frequent
  - Bracing
- Surgical infrequently used
  - Indications: Persistent pain, weakness of grip, and severe deformity
  - Ulnar shortening
    - Report ulnar variance, lunate subsidence, & carpal palmar displacement
  - DRUJ fusion and ulnar osteotomy (Sauve-Kapandji procedure)
  - Radial osteotomy (open or closed)
  - Excision of physeal bar
  - Epiphysiodesis (either radius or ulna)
  - Arthrodesis

DIAGNOSTIC CHECKLIST

Reporting Tips

- Report status of radial physis
  - Physeal bar or early closure may alter surgical plan
- Report status of ligaments
  - TFCC, scapholunate, lunate triquetral usually intact, though TFCC may be stretched and thinned
  - Thick tethering volar radiolunate ligament
  - Thick tethering anomalous radiotriquetral ligament

SELECTED REFERENCES

1. Farr S et al: Radiographic criteria for undergoing an ulnar shortening osteotomy in Madelung deformity: a long-term experience from a single institution. J Pediatr Orthop. ePub, 2015
2. Ghatan AC et al: Madelung deformity. J Am Acad Orthop Surg. 21(6):372-82, 2013
3. Stehling C et al: High resolution 3.0 Tesla MR imaging findings in patients with bilateral Madelung's deformity. Surg Radiol Anat. 31(7):551-7, 2009
4. Zebala LP et al: Madelung's deformity: a spectrum of presentation. J Hand Surg Am. 32(9):1393-401, 2007

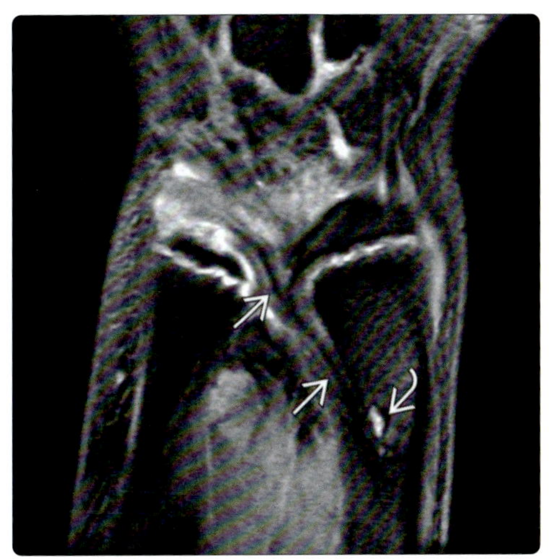

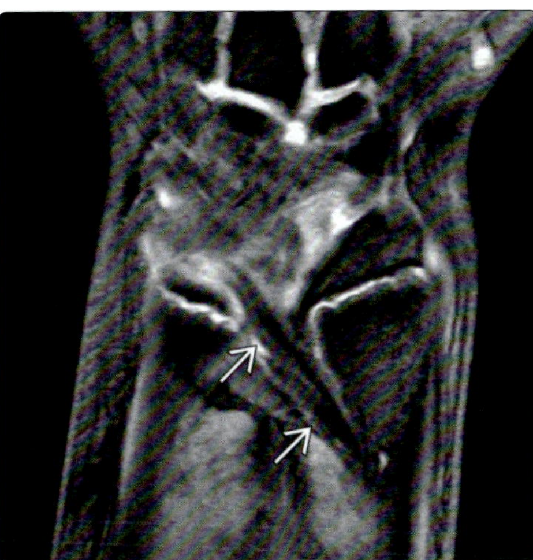

(Left) *Coronal T2* GRE MR, 1st in a series of 4, shows a dorsal cut through a Madelung deformity. The ulna is prominent dorsally; the dorsal-most portion of the radius is seen, and the carpals are not visualized since they are located more volarly. A portion of the anomalous radiotriquetral ligament is seen →, along with cyst formation at its insertion at the radial metadiaphysis →.* **(Right)** *Coronal T2* GRE MR, adjacent cut, shows the thick anomalous radiotriquetral ligament tethering the triquetrum to the radius →.*

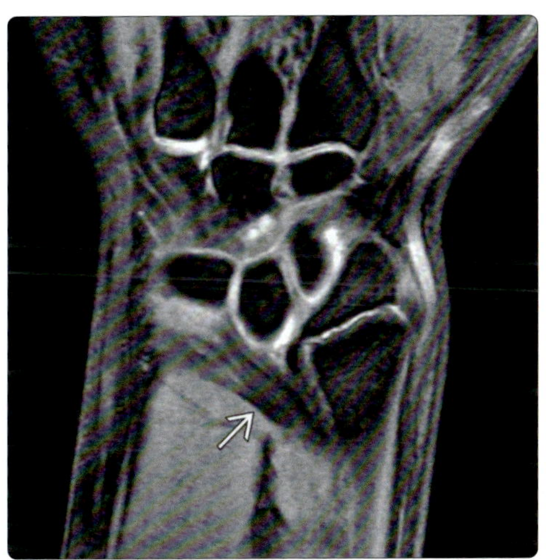

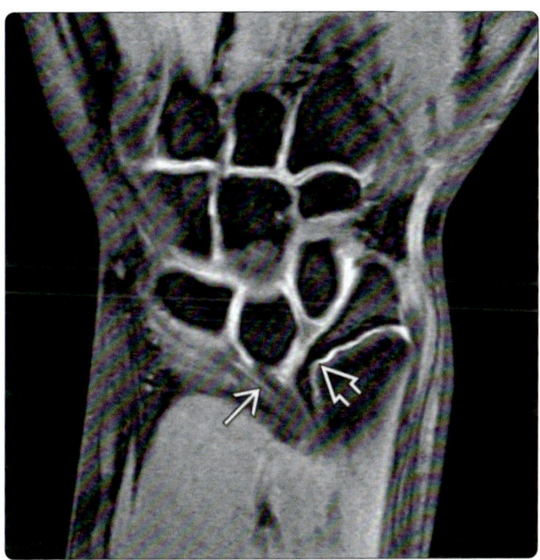

(Left) *Coronal T2* GRE MR, cut through the carpals, shows their triangular configuration, with ↓ carpal angle. A portion of the thick radiotriquetral ligament → is still seen.* **(Right)** *Coronal T2* GRE MR, more volar in position, shows the thick volar radiolunate ligament →. Note the triangular shape of the lunate and the intact scapholunate ligament. The distal radial physis → remains entirely open in this case; note the triangular shape of the epiphysis and how it wraps around the medial radial metaphysis.*

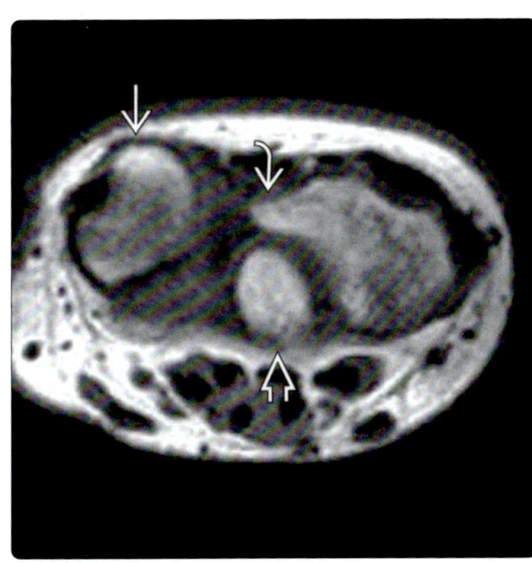

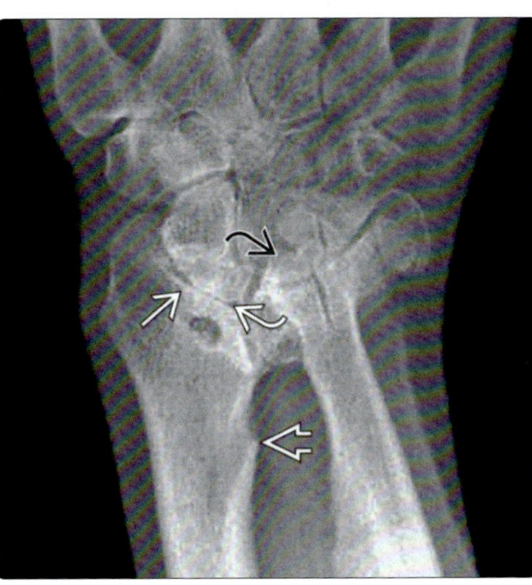

(Left) *Axial T1WI MR shows dorsal displacement of the ulna → and absent sigmoid notch on the radius →. The lunate → is proximally migrated. Extensor tendons are thinned and stretched over the ulna.* **(Right)** *PA radiograph demonstrates medially angulated distal radial articular surface → and long distal ulna →. The radiocarpal joint space is severely narrowed with associated subchondral sclerosis →, indicating advanced osteoarthritis. Note the typical excrescence at the radial metadiaphysis →.*

KEY FACTS

TERMINOLOGY

- Abnormal length of ulna relative to distal radius → adjacent soft tissue and osseous abnormalities
  - Associated abnormalities related to abnormal load-bearing through ulna
- Measurement of ulnar length
  - Ulnar neutral: Ulna 0-2 mm shorter than radius
  - Ulnar negative: Ulna > 2 mm shorter than radius
  - Ulnar positive: Ulna longer than radius

IMAGING

- Associated abnormalities found in triangular fibrocartilage (TFC), lunate-triquetral ligament, lunate, triquetrum, hyaline cartilage, adjacent ulnar aspect of radius
- Findings associated with ulnocarpal abutment
  - Ulnar positive variance
  - Marrow edema lunate, triquetrum, ulnar head
  - Sclerosis of proximal pole lunate (± triquetrum)
  - Subchondral cysts proximal lunate (± triquetrum)
  - Cartilage thinning, lunate (occasionally ulna, triquetrum, radius)
  - Thinned, elongated TFC draped over elongated ulna (may be perforated)
  - Lunate-triquetral ligament perforation
  - Osteophytes at proximal lunate/triquetrum
  - Late changes of ulnar column osteoarthritis
- Findings associated with lunate malacia (Kienböck)
  - May have ulnar minus variance
  - Sclerosis of lunate on radiograph
  - Marrow edema on MR
  - ± fracture line and collapse
- Findings associated with ulnar impingement
  - Ulnar negative variance
  - Ulnar head curved toward distal radial metaphysis
  - Scalloped concavity of radius at site of impingement; subchondral cysts & osteophytes

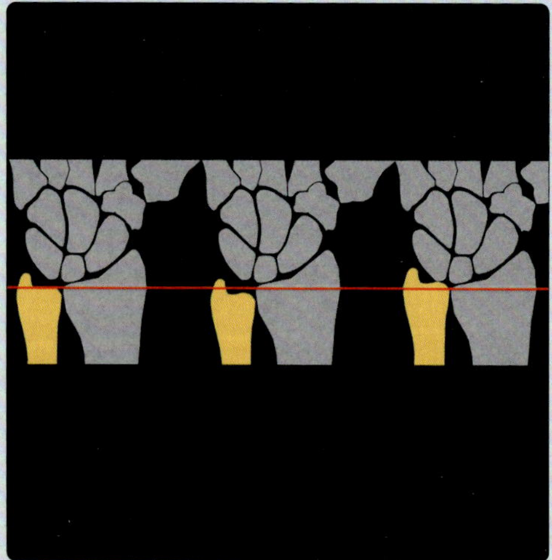

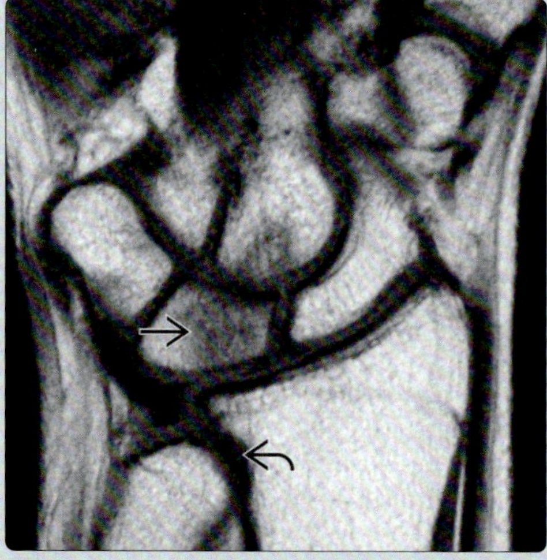

(Left) *Ulnar variance is measured as the length of the distal ulna (radial aspect) compared to the distal radius (ulnar aspect). Drawing on left represents ulnar neutral (ulna 0-2 mm shorter than radius). The middle drawing depicts ulnar negative variance (ulna > 2 mm shorter than radius). The drawing on the right shows ulnar positive variance, with the ulna longer than the radius.* **(Right)** *Coronal T1WI MR shows ulnar negative variance, with the ulna > 2 mm shorter than the radius ⮫. There is associated ↓ SI in the lunate ➙.*

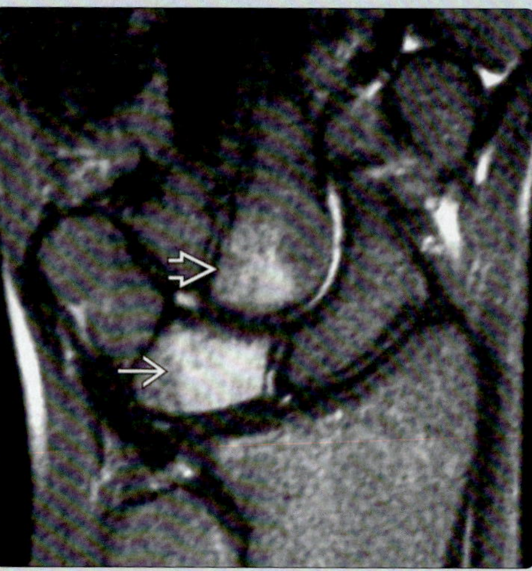

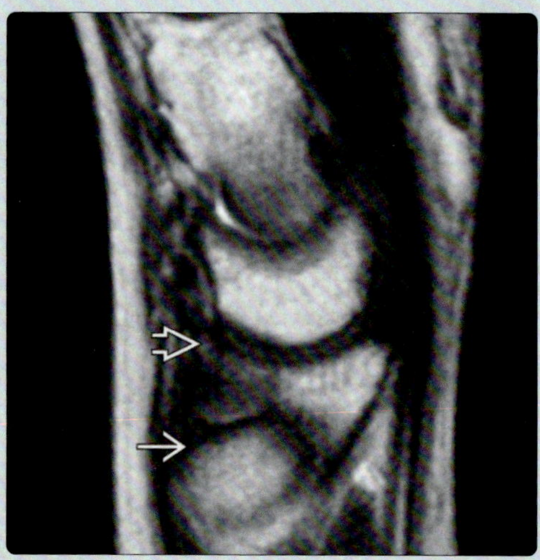

(Left) *Coronal T2WI FS MR in same patient shows edema within the lunate ➙, indicating stage I Kienböck disease, which has significant statistical association with negative ulnar variance. There is also edema in the proximal capitate ➙, a finding that may be related to the altered axial loading mechanics due to the severe ulnar minus.* **(Right)** *Sagittal T2WI MR (same patient) shows partial volume of the radius ➙ and ulna ➙ and confirms ulnar minus variance. The TFCC was thickened but intact (not shown).*

TERMINOLOGY

Definitions

- Abnormal length of ulna relative to distal radius → adjacent soft tissue and osseous abnormalities
  - Related to abnormal load-bearing through ulna
  - Measurement of ulnar length
    - Ulnar neutral: Ulna 0-2 mm shorter than radius
    - Ulnar negative: Ulna > 2 mm shorter than radius
    - Ulnar positive: Ulna longer than radius

IMAGING

General Features

- Best diagnostic clue
  - Abnormal length of ulna relative to radius should initiate search for associated abnormalities
- Location
  - Besides ulnar length, other abnormalities may be found
    - Triangular fibrocartilage (TFC), lunatotriquetral ligament, lunate, triquetrum, hyaline cartilage, adjacent ulnar aspect of radius

Imaging Recommendations

- Best imaging tool
  - Ulnar variance and some of its complications diagnosed on radiograph
  - Soft tissue/cartilage complications diagnosed on MR
- Protocol advice
  - MR arthrography (either direct or indirect) useful to evaluate hyaline cartilage

Radiographic Findings

- Ulnar positive variance
  - Ulna longer than radius
  - Findings associated with ulnocarpal abutment
    - Sclerosis of proximal pole lunate (± triquetrum)
    - Subchondral cysts in proximal lunate (± triquetrum)
    - Osteophytes at proximal lunate/triquetrum
    - Late changes of ulnar column osteoarthritis
- Ulnar negative variance
  - Ulna > 2 mm shorter than adjacent radius
  - Findings associated with lunate malacia (Kienböck)
    - Sclerosis of lunate
    - Fracture, flattening of lunate
    - Late changes of ulnar column osteoarthritis
  - Findings associated with ulnar impingement
    - Ulnar head curved toward distal radial metaphysis
    - Scalloped concavity of ulnar aspect distal radius at site of impingement
    - Subchondral cyst at site of impingement
    - Osteophyte formation late in process

MR Findings

- Ulnar positive variance
  - Marrow edema in lunate, triquetrum, ulnar head
  - Cyst formation in lunate, triquetrum
  - Cartilage thinning along lunate (occasionally ulna, triquetrum, radius)
  - Thinned, elongated TFC draped over elongated ulna
    - May be perforated
  - Lunatotriquetral ligament perforation
  - Subchondral low SI sclerosis, lunate > triquetrum
- Ulnar negative variance
  - Lunate malacia
    - Marrow edema
    - ± fracture line and collapse
  - Correlation with extensor carpi ulnaris pathology
  - Ulnar impingement
    - Curved morphology short distal ulna, scalloped adjacent radial cortex
    - Marrow edema, cyst formation

DIFFERENTIAL DIAGNOSIS

Madelung Deformity

- Elongated ulna, subluxated dorsally
- Associated ulnar and volar tilt distal radius and decreased carpal angle

Multiple Hereditary Exostoses

- Sessile osteochondromas often → short ulna

PATHOLOGY

Microscopic Features

- Significantly higher number of apoptotic cells in degenerative lesions of TFC in ulnar positive patients

CLINICAL ISSUES

Presentation

- Most common signs/symptoms
  - Relate to complications of abnormal ulnar variance
    - Lunate malacia
      - ▫ Dorsal tenderness about lunate
      - ▫ Pain, weakness, decreased range of motion
    - Ulnocarpal abutment
      - ▫ Chronic or subacute dorso-ulnar pain
      - ▫ Pain worsens with extremes of rotation and ulnar deviation
      - ▫ Clicking, weakness, decreased range of motion
    - Ulnar impingement
      - ▫ Distal forearm pain with pronation/supination

Natural History & Prognosis

- Either lunate malacia or ulnar abutment progress to osteoarthritis if untreated

Treatment

- Conservative: ↓ activity, antiinflammatory Rx
- Ulnar shortening or lengthening to alter load transmission through ulna
  - Resection of distal ulna (Darrach) may result in weakness, instability
  - Hemiresection of distal ulna may result in impingement
- ± TFC debridement, repair
- If late-stage lunate malacia or abutment, salvage procedures

SELECTED REFERENCES

1. Chang CY et al: Association between distal ulnar morphology and extensor carpi ulnaris tendon pathology. Skeletal Radiol. 43(6):793-800, 2014

(Left) *AP radiograph shows ulnar positive variance ➡, with a long ulna relative to the radius. This puts the TFCC and lunatotriquetral ligaments at risk for disruption. It also leads to impaction on the lunate. Early osteophytes are seen at the lunate and triquetrum ➡.* **(Right)** *Oblique radiograph in the same patient shows a cyst within the lunate ➡ as well as sclerosis and osteophyte formation in both the lunate and triquetrum ➡. This results from the abnormal weight-bearing on these bones due to the long ulna.*

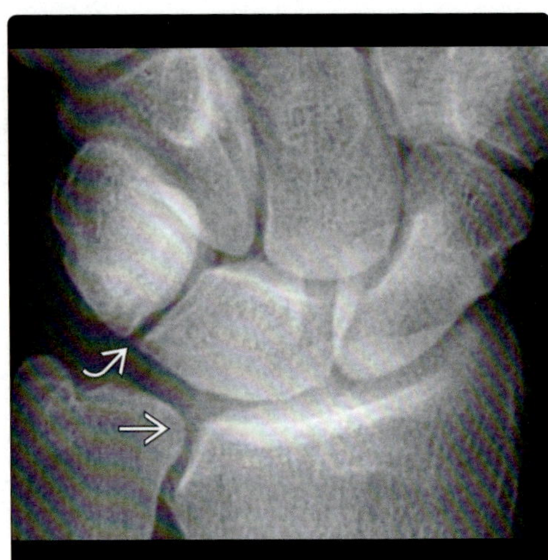

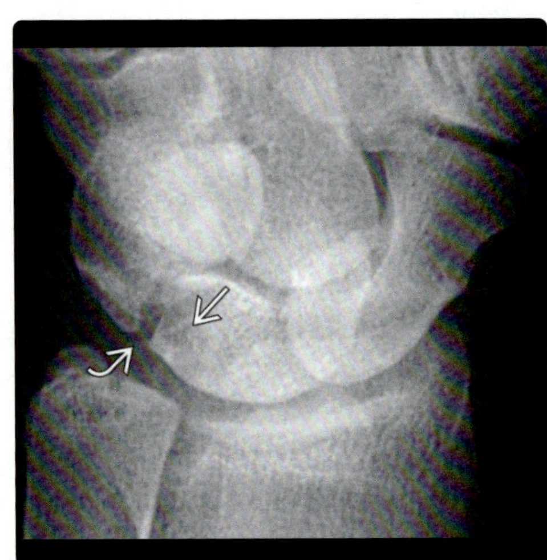

(Left) *PA radiograph during radiocarpal joint arthrogram shows mild positive ulnar variance. There is a defect in the central aspect of the TFC ➡, with contrast flow into the distal radioulnar joint.* **(Right)** *Coronal T1WI MR arthrogram show full-thickness cartilage loss in the distal ulna ➡ and proximal lunate ➡. Central triangular fibrocartilage perforation is confirmed adjacent to the ulnar cartilage loss. Contrast is noted in both radiocarpal and distal radioulnar joints. Lunatotriquetral ligament is intact.*

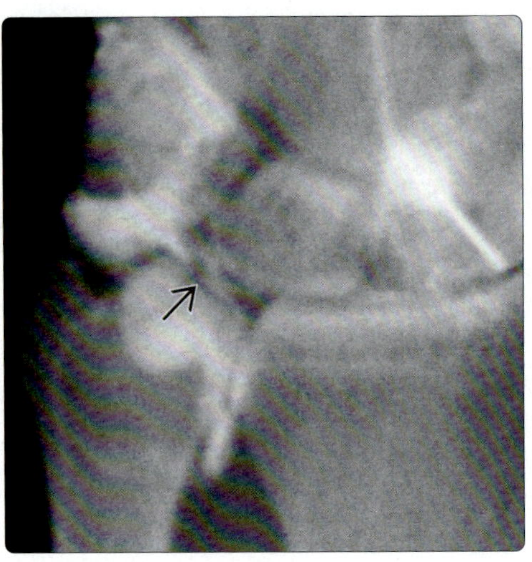

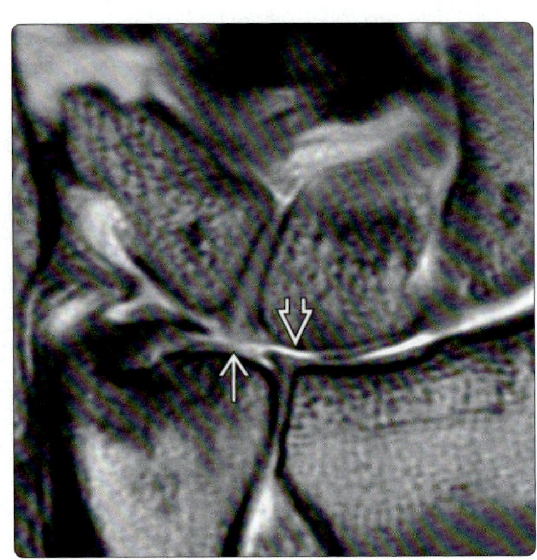

(Left) *Coronal T2* GRE MR, post arthrogram, shows cyst formation within the triquetrum ➡ and lunate ➡. There is marrow edema in the distal ulna ➡, which is slightly long relative to the radius. The TFC perforation is easily seen; lunatotriquetral and scapholunate ligaments are intact.* **(Right)** *Coronal T2WI FS MR, located more dorsally, shows significant marrow edema in the distal ulna ➡ and contrast in the distal radioulnar joint ➡. Radiocarpal cartilage is thinned ➡ as part of the degenerative change.*

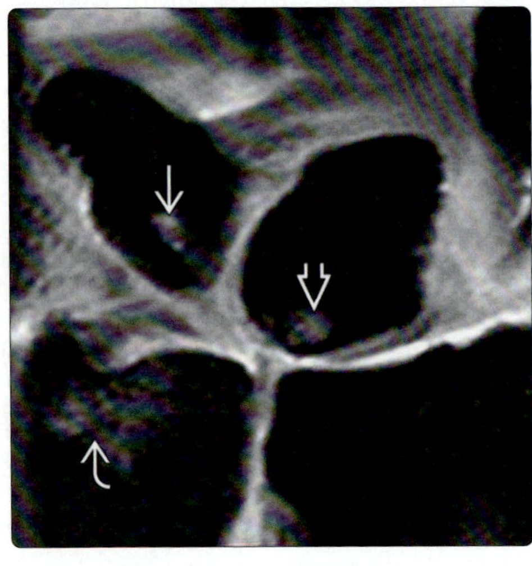

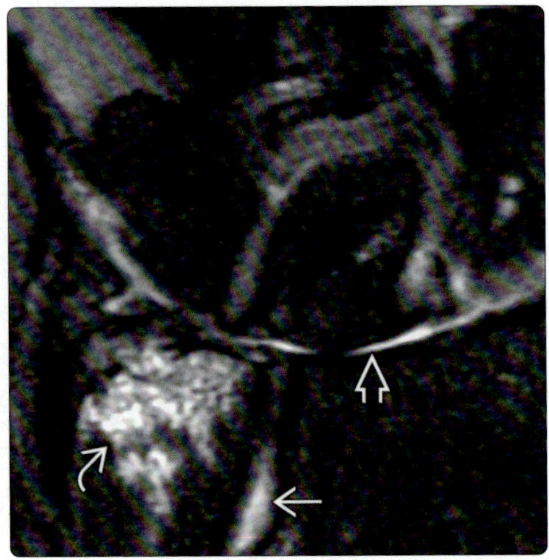

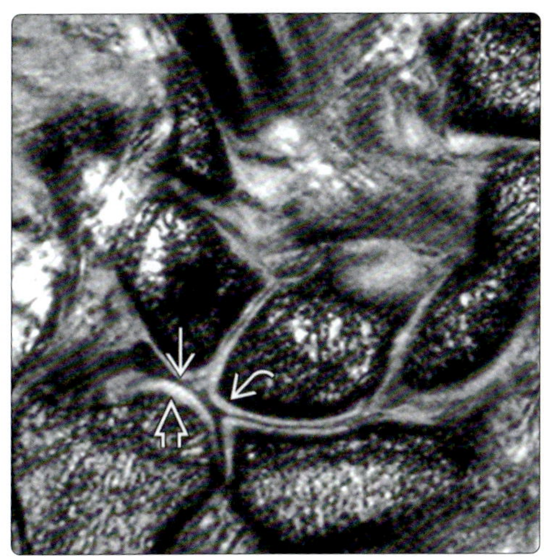

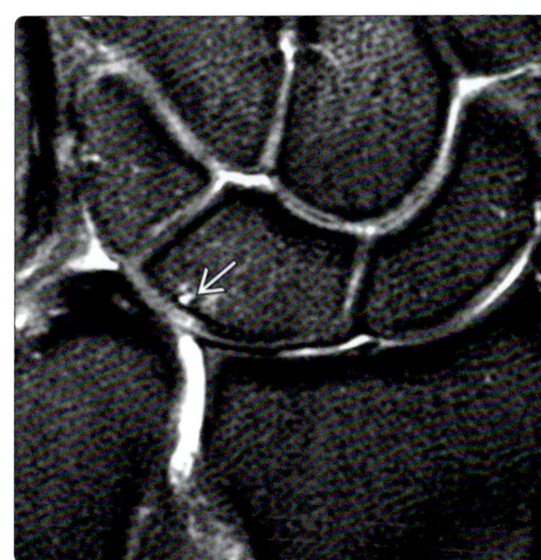

(Left) *Coronal T2* GRE MR shows positive ulnar variance and diffuse thinning of the triangular fibrocartilage ➡. There is no tear of the ligament. Chondral surfaces of the ulna ➡ & lunate ➡ are normal. Thinning of the TFC is a common finding in association with positive ulnar variance and probably is a precursor to TFC tears and chondromalacia of the lunate & ulna.* **(Right)** *Coronal T2WI FS MR shows early ulnolunate abutment with lunate cyst formation ➡. There is a radial-sided TFC tear and ulnar plus variance.*

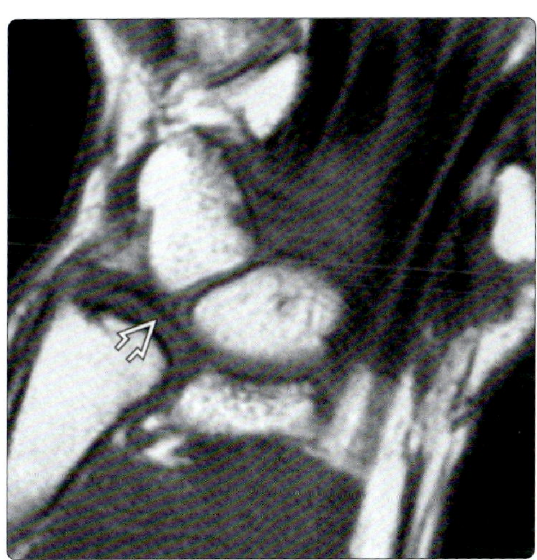

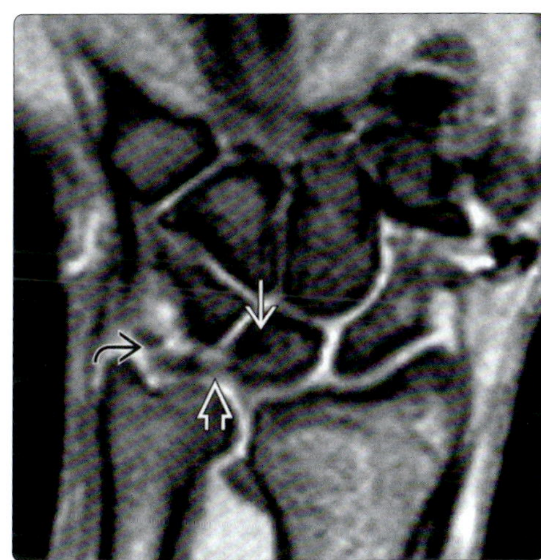

(Left) *Coronal T1WI MR shows ulnocarpal abutment with mild positive ulnar variance and thinned but intact TFC ➡.* **(Right)** *Coronal T2* GRE MR demonstrates positive ulnar variance. There are sclerotic low-signal foci in the proximal aspect of the lunate ➡, and there is irregular morphology and signal in the triangular fibrocartilage ➡. There is a small ossicle in the ulnar aspect of the TFC ➡, likely the result of previous avulsion of the tip of the ulnar styloid.*

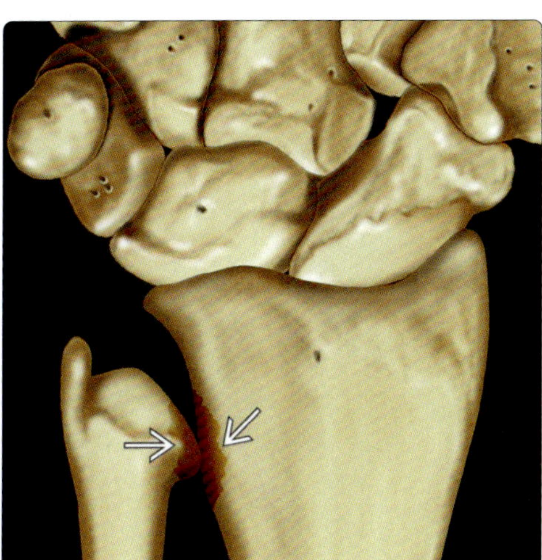

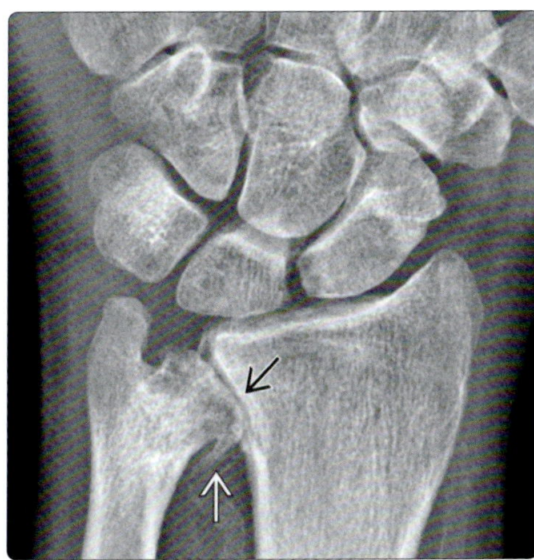

(Left) *AP graphic depicts ulnar impingement resulting from negative ulnar variance. Short, dysmorphic ulna impinges on the ulnar surface of the distal radius, resulting in marrow edema & degenerative changes ➡.* **(Right)** *PA radiograph shows ulnar impingement. The ulna is short and curved toward the radial metaphysis. There is scalloping and sclerosis of the radius ➡, along with subchondral cyst and osteophyte formation on the ulna ➡. (Courtesy R. Hastings, MD.)*

KEY FACTS

TERMINOLOGY

- Wide spectrum of disease, based on modeling failure of acetabulum and subsequently femoral head

IMAGING

- Bilateral in 20%
- US method of Graf for evaluation of infants
  - Acetabular morphology, angle of acetabular roof (alpha angle), femoral head coverage, dynamic subluxation during stress maneuvers
- Radiograph in child
  - Femoral epiphysis not located within lower inner quadrant formed by Hilgenreiner and Perkins lines
  - Disruption of Shenton line
  - Acetabular roof angle > 30° indicates DDH
- Radiograph in adult
  - Acetabulum retroverted in 37%
  - Least severe: Upturning of lateral acetabular roof
  - More severe: Center-edge angle of Wiberg < 25° [(borderline 20-25°; normal 20 [or 25]-40°)]
  - Vertical center-edge angle < 25°
- MR arthrogram in adult
  - Labral hypertrophy, ↑ mucoid degeneration or tear
  - Hypertrophied ligamentum teres and pulvinar
  - Acetabular/femoral head dysplasia, retroversion
  - Associated cartilage defect or delamination
  - Significant ↑ incidence of perilabral cysts

CLINICAL ISSUES

- Clinical presentation
  - Child: Hip click, limb length discrepancy
  - Adult: Symptoms of acetabular rim overload
- Male < female (1:5-8)
- 1/1,000 live births in North America
- 25-50% will develop early osteoarthritis
- Early treatment to improve acetabular coverage

(Left) *Coronal ultrasound of the left hip in an infant shows a shallow acetabulum ➡, fatty pulvinar between the femoral head and deepest acetabulum ➡, and lateral subluxation of the femoral head ➡.* **(Right)** *Transverse ultrasound confirms the shallow acetabulum ➡, fatty pulvinar ➡, and lateral subluxation of the femoral head ➡. Dynamic investigation is used to demonstrate whether or not the femoral head is reducible or unstable. Ultrasound is the imaging modality of choice for DDH in an infant.*

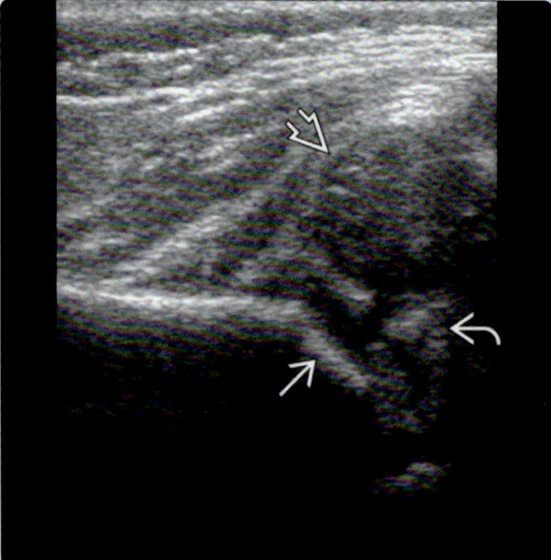

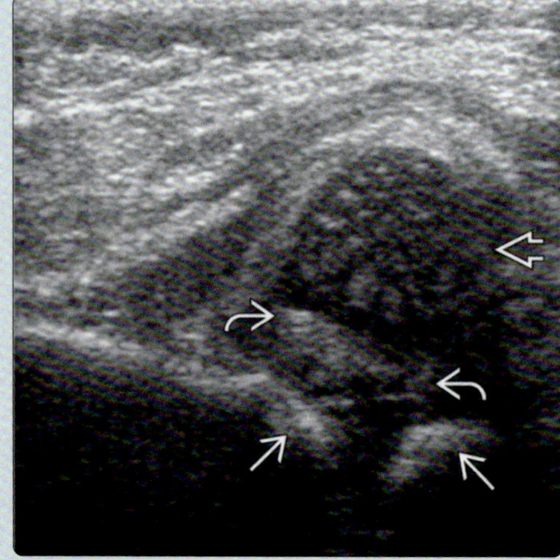

(Left) *AP radiograph shows a right total hip arthroplasty in a 30 year old. The left hip shows a shallow acetabulum ➡, with upturned sourcil and decreased center-edge angle of Wiberg, diagnostic of subtle DDH. In young adults with hip pain and early OA, look carefully for subtle DDH.* **(Right)** *Frog leg lateral in a patient with DDH, as shown by shallow acetabulum, shows calcified labrum ➡ as well as faint calcification within a perilabral cyst ➡. These are secondary degenerative changes.*

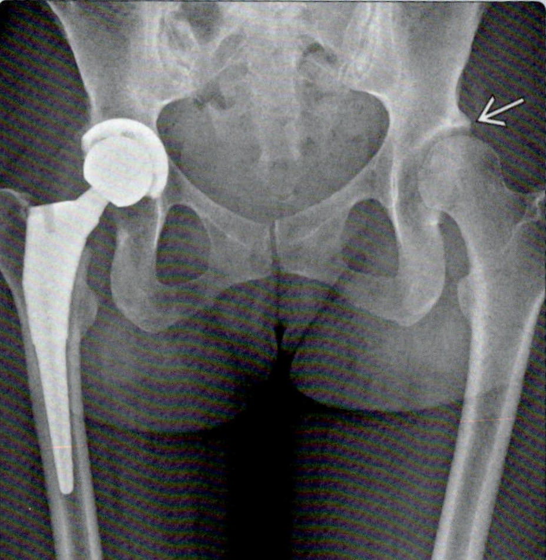

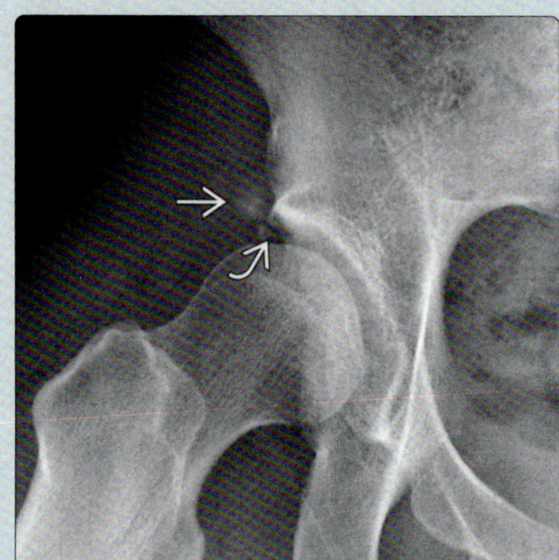

TERMINOLOGY

Abbreviations

- Developmental dysplasia of hip (DDH)

Definitions

- Wide spectrum of disease, based on modeling failure of acetabulum and subsequently femoral head

IMAGING

General Features

- Best diagnostic clue
  - Noncongruent femoral head and acetabulum or subtle lack of coverage of head by acetabulum
- Location
  - Bilateral in 20%

Radiographic Findings

- Infant or child (ultrasound should preferentially be used in infant to avoid radiation)
  - Femoral epiphysis not located within lower inner quadrant formed by Hilgenreiner and Perkins lines
  - Disruption of Shenton line (continuous curve around obturator foramen to medial femoral metaphysis)
  - Acetabular roof angle > 30° indicates DDH
  - Delayed ossification of femoral head
  - May develop osteonecrosis in childhood
- Adult acetabulum
  - Least severe: Upturning of lateral acetabular roof (sourcil), or harlequin sign
  - Intermediate: Shallow acetabulum, increased acetabular angle
  - More severe: Inadequate coverage of lateral &/or anterior femoral head
    - Vertical center-edge angle < 25° on false profile
  - Most severe: No formed acetabulum, with femoral head articulating in iliac pseudoacetabulum
  - Acetabulum also retroverted in 37%
- Adult femoral head
  - Ranges from spherical to nonspherical
  - Congruent or noncongruent with acetabulum
  - May be broadened, with short wide femoral neck (coxa magna)
  - Up to 40% also show cam-type of femoral deformity

MR Findings

- Osseous abnormalities
  - Acetabular/femoral head dysplasia, retroversion
  - Associated cartilage defect or delamination
- Labral hypertrophy
  - High frequency mucoid degeneration or tear
- Hypertrophied ligamentum teres and pulvinar (fibrofatty tissue filling space in medial acetabulum)
- Significant ↑ incidence of perilabral cysts

Ultrasonographic Findings

- Cartilaginous portions of hip directly visualized, including position and depth of acetabulum
- Method of Graf: Acetabular morphology, angle of acetabular roof (alpha angle), femoral head coverage, dynamic subluxation during stress maneuvers

DIFFERENTIAL DIAGNOSIS

Osteoarthritis

- Should be suspicious of underlying DDH in young adult with signs of early osteoarthritis (OA)

PATHOLOGY

General Features

- Etiology
  - Femoral head and acetabulum must be congruent for normal development
    - Dislocated or subluxated femoral head results in incomplete development of acetabulum
    - Conversely, incomplete coverage of femoral head results in dysplasia of that structure
  - ↑ incidence in DDH with oligohydramnios, breech position, 1st gestation
  - DDH ↑ in arthrogryposis, cerebral palsy, trisomy 21, neuromuscular disease, ligamentous laxity

CLINICAL ISSUES

Presentation

- Most common signs/symptoms
  - Child: Hip click, limb length discrepancy
  - Adult: Symptoms of acetabular rim overload

Demographics

- Gender
  - Male < female (1:5-8)
- Epidemiology
  - 1/1,000 live births in North America

Natural History & Prognosis

- 25-50% will develop early osteoarthritis

Treatment

- Early treatment to improve acetabular coverage
  - Reduce sheer stress on labrum and decrease likelihood of early cartilage damage
- Initial treatment in infant: Pavlik harness, hip spica
- Childhood reconstruction: Salter acetabular ± varus rotational hip osteotomy
- Adult reconstruction: Periacetabular osteotomy
- Salvage procedure: Chiari osteotomy

DIAGNOSTIC CHECKLIST

Image Interpretation Pearls

- Radiographic signs of OA in young adult should prompt search for subtle acetabular dysplasia

SELECTED REFERENCES

1. Ida T et al: Prevalence and characteristics of cam-type femoroacetabular deformity in 100 hips with symptomatic acetabular dysplasia: a case control study. J Orthop Surg Res. 9(1):93, 2014
2. Mabee M et al: Reproducibility of Acetabular Landmarks and a Standardized Coordinate System Obtained from 3D Hip Ultrasound. Ultrason Imaging. 37(4):267-76, 2014
3. Sakellariou VI et al: Reconstruction of the Acetabulum in Developmental Dysplasia of the Hip in total hip replacement. Arch Bone Jt Surg. 2(3):130-6, 2014
4. Starr V et al: Imaging update on developmental dysplasia of the hip with the role of MRI. AJR Am J Roentgenol. 203(6):1324-35, 2014

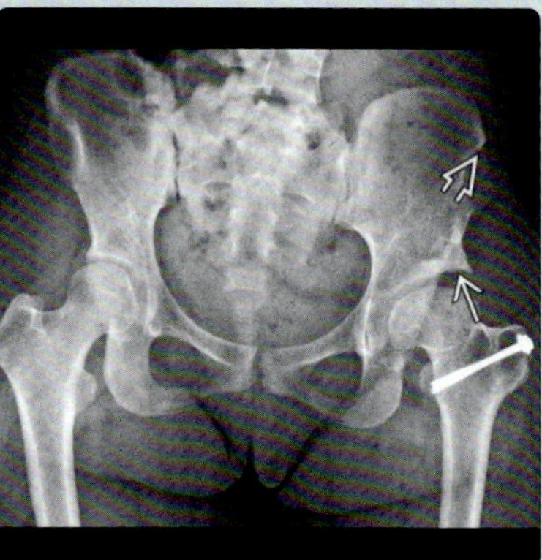

Adult patient who had a Salter opening wedge osteotomy for DDH as a child is shown. The graft was harvested from the iliac wing ➡ and placed at the superior acetabulum, providing adequate lateral coverage of the femoral head ➡.

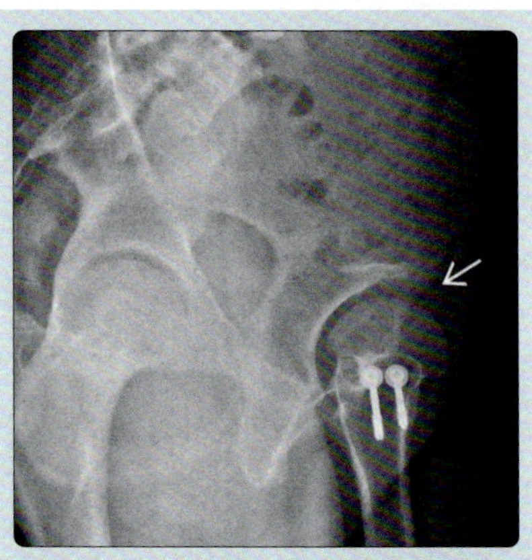

False profile view in the same patient shows that the osteotomy does not provide adequate anterior coverage of the femoral head ➡. The coxa magna deformity of the head puts the patient at risk for femoral acetabular impingement and early OA.

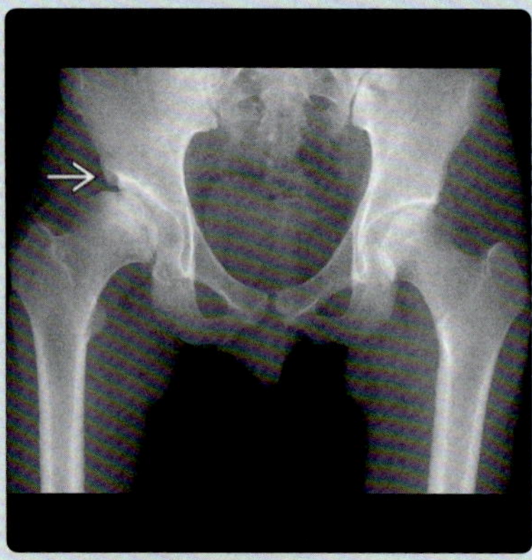

Young adult has mild dysplasia of the right hip, indicated by an upturned sourcil ➡ (harlequin sign) and mildly abnormal center-edge angle of Wiberg. The patient was developing early symptoms of OA.

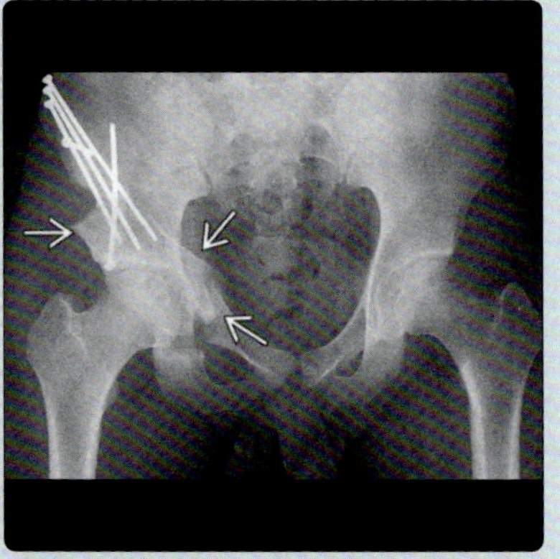

Periacetabular osteotomy in the same patient is dome-shaped ➡ and provides significant improvement of lateral femoral head coverage. This procedure is generally performed in a young adult.

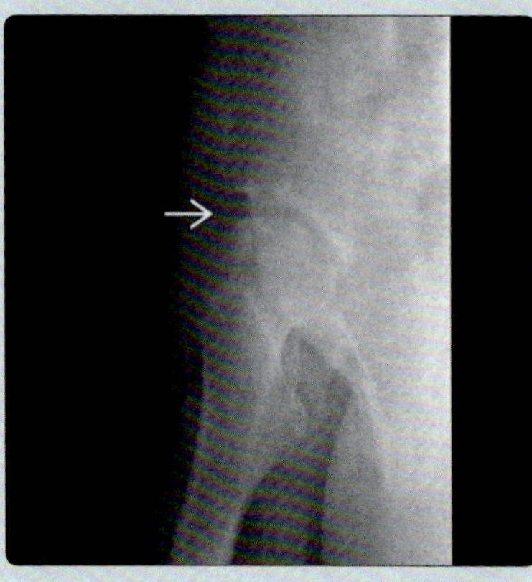

False profile view in the same patient seen preoperatively shows inadequate coverage of the anterior femoral head ➡.

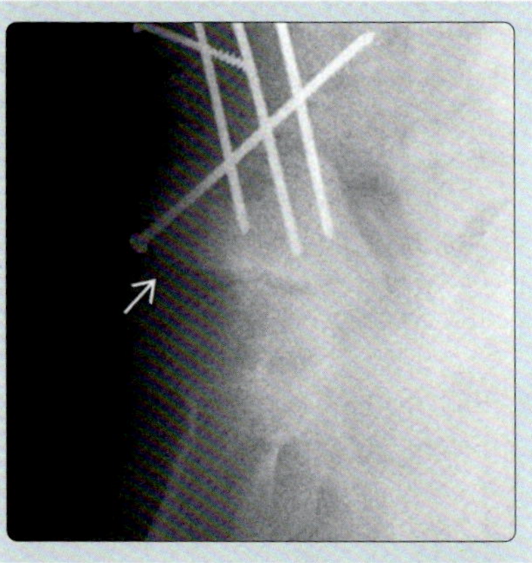

Periacetabular osteotomy, false profile view, now provides improved coverage of the anterior femoral head ➡. Periacetabular osteotomy may allow several years of pain-free activity before development of OA.

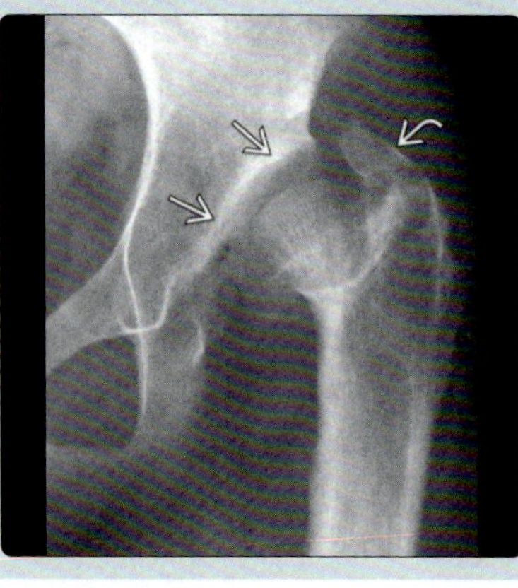

Long-term DDH has resulted in shallow vertical acetabulum ➡, which does not cover the femoral head adequately. There is proximal displacement of the trochanter ➡, making the gluteal muscles inefficient. The patient has symptoms of OA.

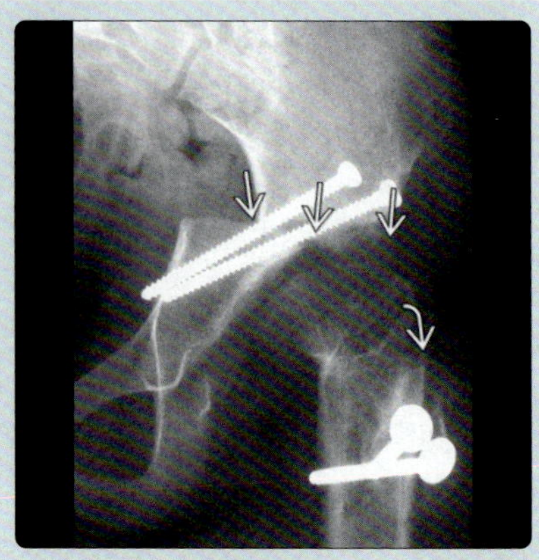

Chiari osteotomy is a salvage procedure, with an intraarticular displacement osteotomy ➡. Femoral head coverage is improved. Greater trochanteric transfer ➡ completes the procedure.

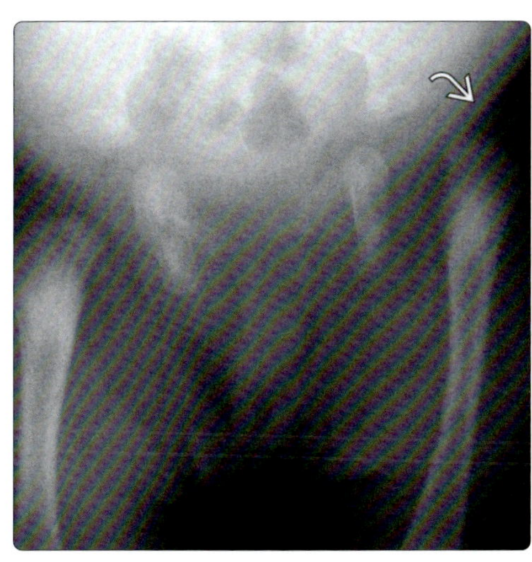

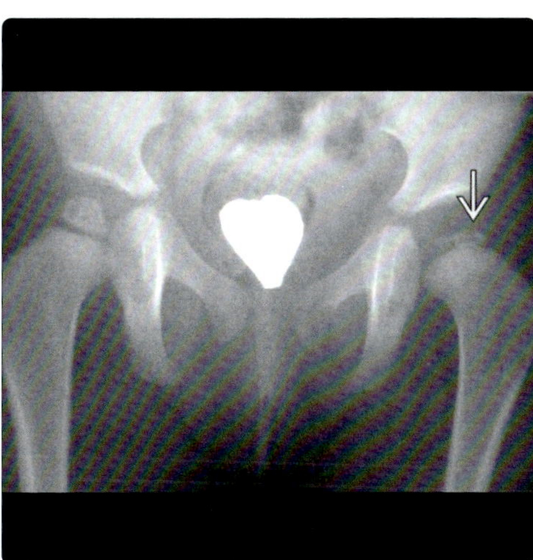

(Left) *AP radiograph shows superior and lateral dislocation of the left femoral head ➡, compared to the normal right. The left head would fall in the upper outer, rather than the lower inner, quadrant formed by Hilgenreiner and Perkin lines, and the Shenton line is interrupted. Hip was reduced and child was treated with casting.* **(Right)** *AP radiograph obtained 2 years later shows a complication of DDH, development of osteonecrosis of the femoral head ➡. Note that the acetabular coverage is now normal.*

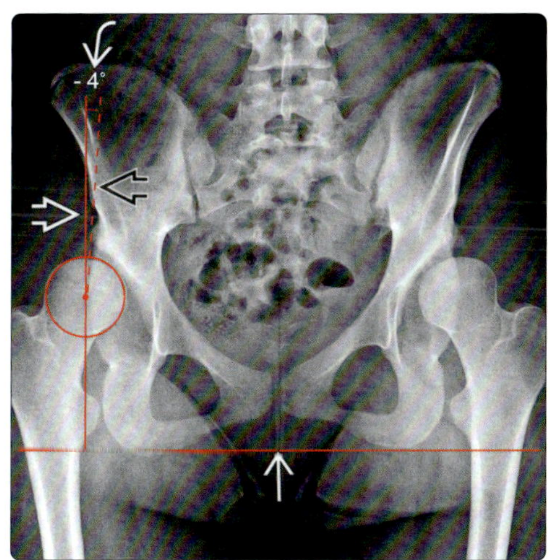

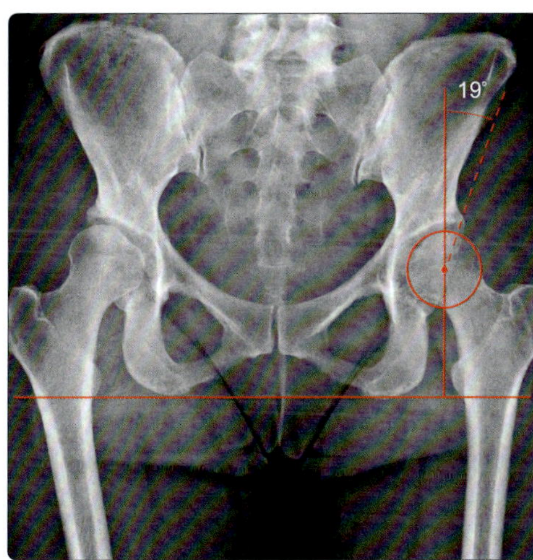

(Left) *AP radiograph shows obvious bilateral DDH. The method of measurement for center-edge angle of Wiberg is shown. Line of reference is transischial ➡; a perpendicular line is drawn through the center of the femoral head ➡. Finally, a line is drawn from the center of femoral head to lateral edge of acetabulum ➡; angle between these 2 lines is the center-edge angle of Wiberg. It is negative in this case ➡; normal is 20-40°.* **(Right)** *AP radiograph in a subtle case of DDH shows the center-edge angle of Wiberg to be 19°.*

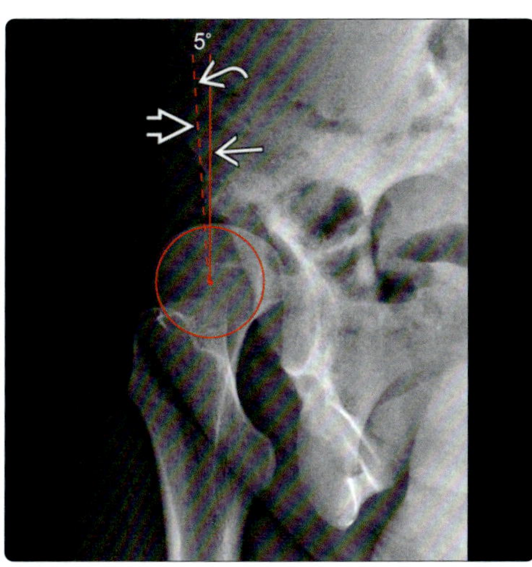

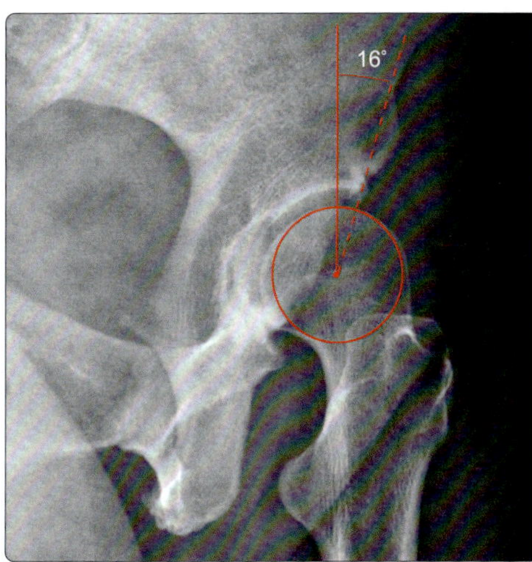

(Left) *False profile radiograph in a case of severe DDH shows the vertical center-edge angle. A vertical line ➡ is drawn from the center of the femoral head. A 2nd line is drawn from the center head to the anterior edge of acetabulum ➡. The angle between the 2 ➡ is the vertical center-edge angle, which estimates the amount of anterior coverage of the femoral head by the acetabulum. A normal vertical center-edge angle is ≥ 25°.* **(Right)** *Vertical center-edge angle is shown in case of subtle DDH with incomplete anterior coverage.*

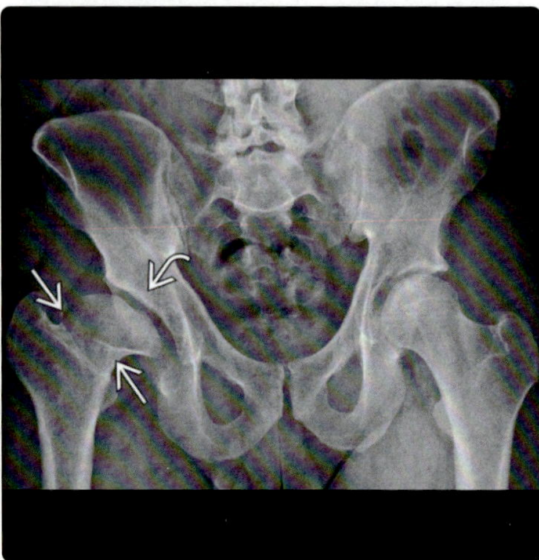

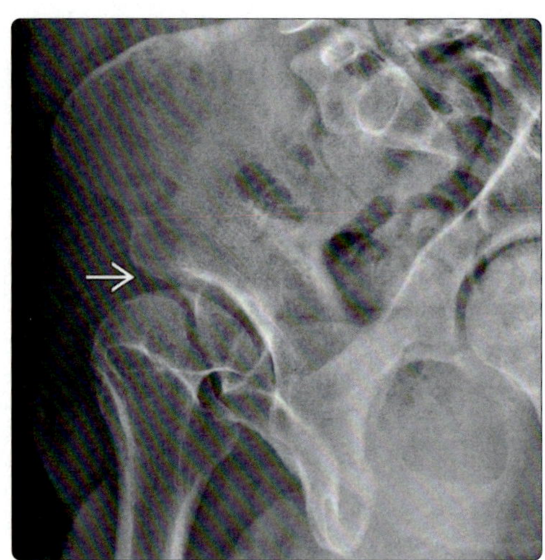

(Left) *AP radiograph shows a coxa magna deformity of the right hip, with a short wide femoral neck ➔ and mushroom-shaped head. The coxa magna deformity is secondary to DDH; the shallow acetabulum with insufficient femoral head coverage is seen ↪. Note that the right leg is relatively short (compare lesser trochanter placement relative to opposite side).* **(Right)** *False profile radiograph in the same patient shows insufficient anterior head coverage ➔. The hip and acetabulum are concentric but not spherical.*

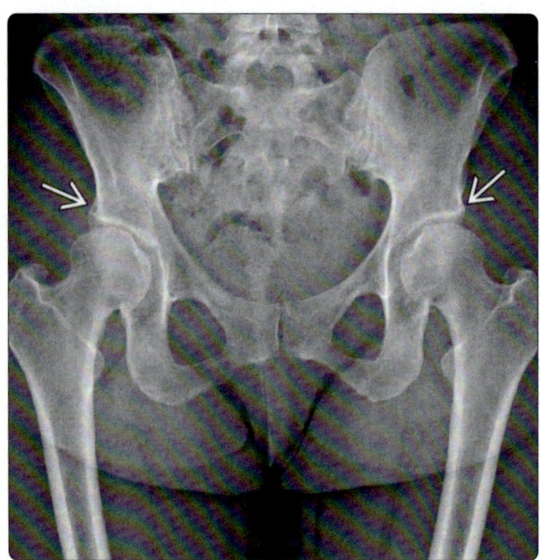

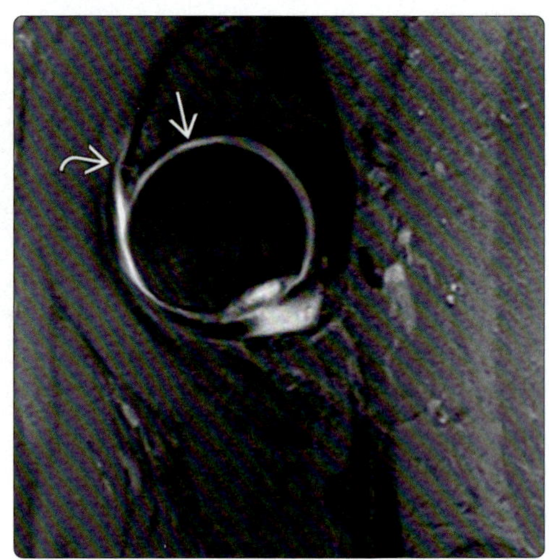

(Left) *AP radiograph shows subtle bilateral DDH, with upturned sourcil ➔. The left hip center-edge angle of Wiberg measures < 25°.* **(Right)** *Sagittal MR arthrogram, same case, shows adequate anterior coverage but a tear through the degenerated labrum ↪. In addition, there is severe thinning of cartilage ➔ in the weight-bearing segment of the hip. Although there is no radiographic OA in this young adult, the cartilage damage suggests early-onset OA is inevitable.*

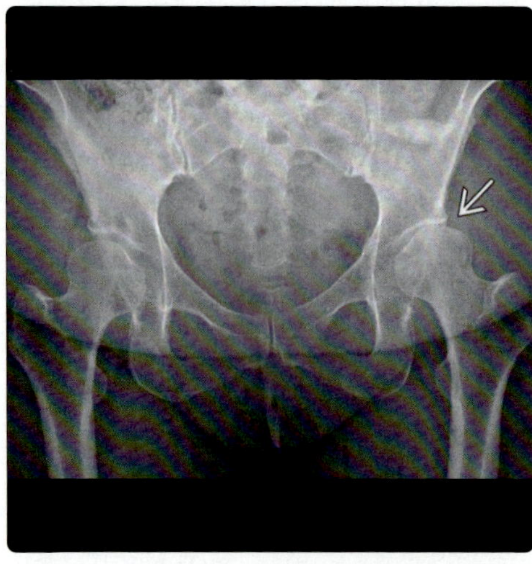

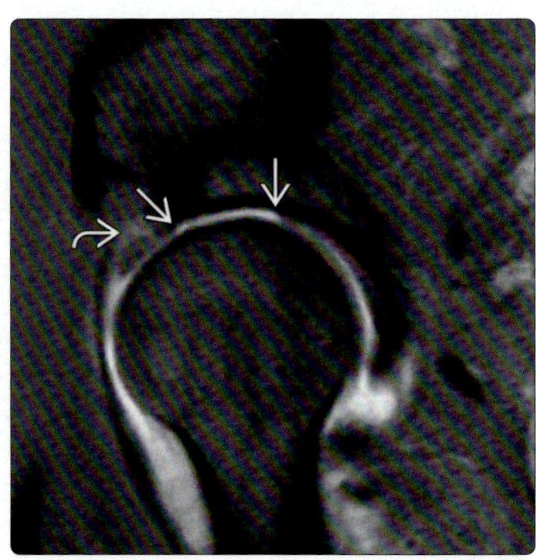

(Left) *AP radiograph shows bilateral DDH, left ➔ worse than right. Center-edge angle of Wiberg is abnormal for both hips; the left shows joint space narrowing. The patient is only 30 years old and had complained of mild hip pain for several years, with recent worsening.* **(Right)** *Sagittal MR arthrogram T1WI FS in the same patient shows a hypertrophied anterior labrum with tear ↪ as well as inadequate anterior coverage of the femoral head. A large cartilaginous defect extending across the weight-bearing surface ➔ indicates OA.*

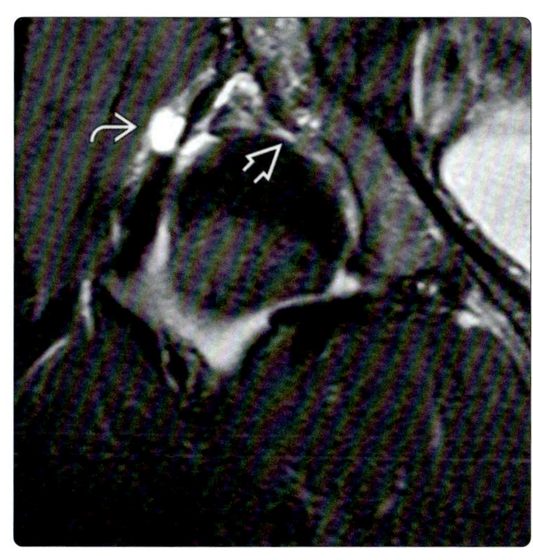

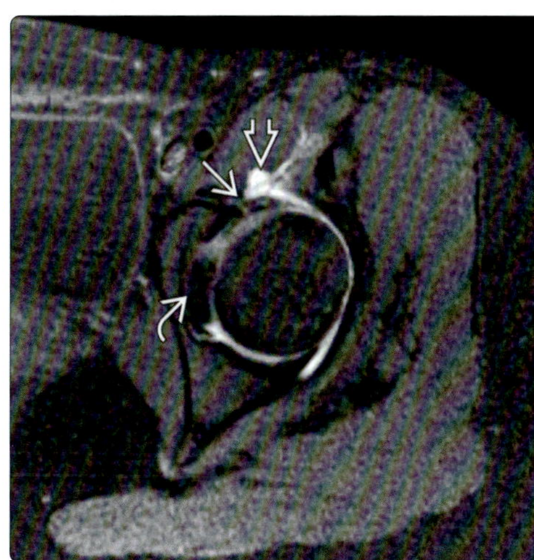

(Left) *Coronal T2WI FS MR arthrogram in a patient with DDH shows a paralabral cyst, a common finding in DDH. Note focal hyaline cartilage defect and increased signal in labrum due to degenerative changes. The severity of dysplasia is noted; the center-edge angle of Wiberg is negative.* **(Right)** *Axial T1WI FS MR arthrogram in DDH shows hypertrophied torn labrum with adjacent paralabral cyst. Note the hypertrophied ligamentum teres, a common secondary finding in DDH.*

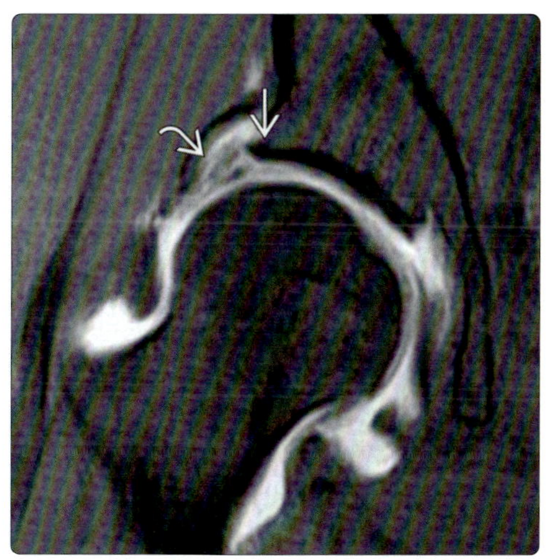

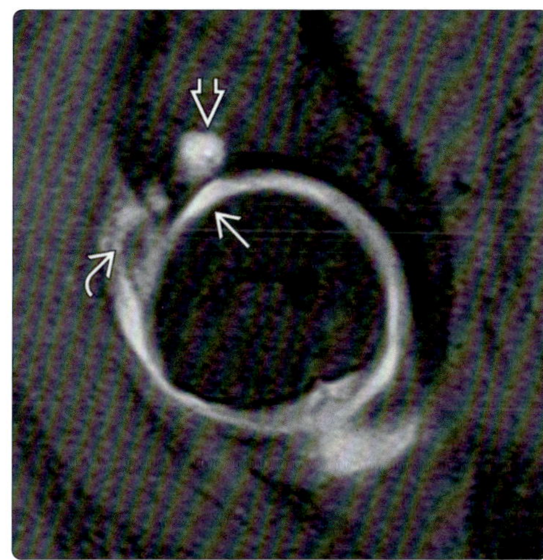

(Left) *Coronal MR arthrogram T1WI FS shows mild acetabular dysplasia. However, the labrum is significantly hypertrophied, detached, and torn.* **(Right)** *Sagittal MR arthrogram in the same case shows findings that unfortunately are common even in mild DDH. The hypertrophied labrum has a complex tear. There is a significant cartilage defect as well as subchondral cyst formation, indicating OA.*

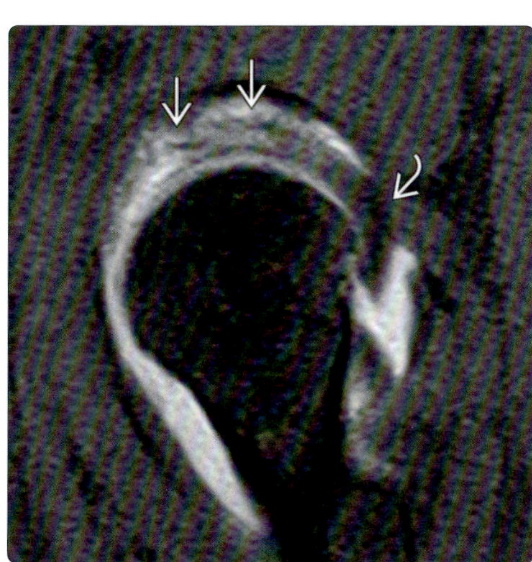

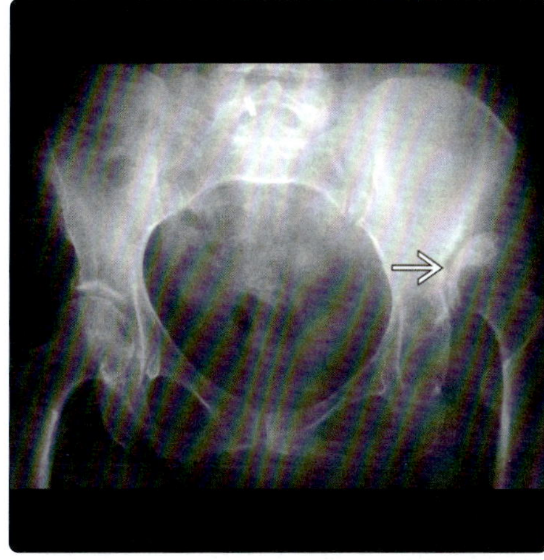

(Left) *Sagittal image from the same MR arthrogram, located slightly more laterally, shows the full extent of the hypertrophied labrum and its nearly circumferential tear. Only the posterior labrum appears intact, though it also is enlarged.* **(Right)** *AP radiograph demonstrates longstanding DDH. The hip has been dislocated for this patient's entire life, and she has developed a pseudoarticulation at the iliac wing. The left acetabulum is unformed, as it has never contained a head.*

KEY FACTS

TERMINOLOGY

- Displaced Salter I fracture of femoral capital epiphysis, related to sheer stress

IMAGING

- Bilateral in 20-40%
- AP radiograph
  - Earliest change: Mild widening and irregularity
  - Later: Epiphysis slips posteriorly and medially
  - Klein line: Line drawn parallel to lateral femoral neck should intersect femoral epiphysis
- Frog-lateral radiograph: More sensitive than AP
  - Southwick head/shaft angular displacement
  - Wilson percent linear epiphyseal displacement
- MR is more sensitive in early disease
  - Physeal widening, even without slip
  - ↑ SI at physis, adjacent marrow edema if active
  - ± periosteal sleeve avulsion if traumatic

PATHOLOGY

- Majority of cases thought to have mechanical etiology, due to sheer stress
  - Angled physis at risk for Salter I fracture, resulting in SCFE, particularly in period of active growth
  - Growth spurt coincides with age at which femoral neck-shaft angle ↑ to achieve adult angle
  - Obesity contributes added sheer stress

CLINICAL ISSUES

- Girls: Average 11-12 yr; range 8-15 yr
- Boys: Average 13-14 yr; range 10-17 yr
- Male > female (2.5:1)
- SCFE most common adolescent hip condition
  - Incidence may be increasing with worsening frequency of obesity in children
- Complications: FAI (32%), chondrolysis (7-10%), osteonecrosis (1%)

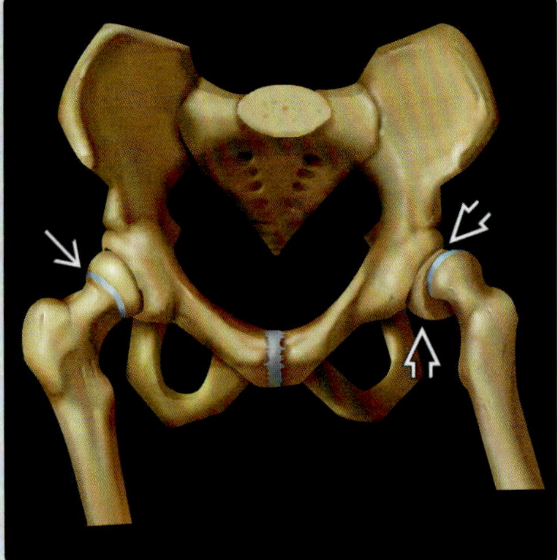

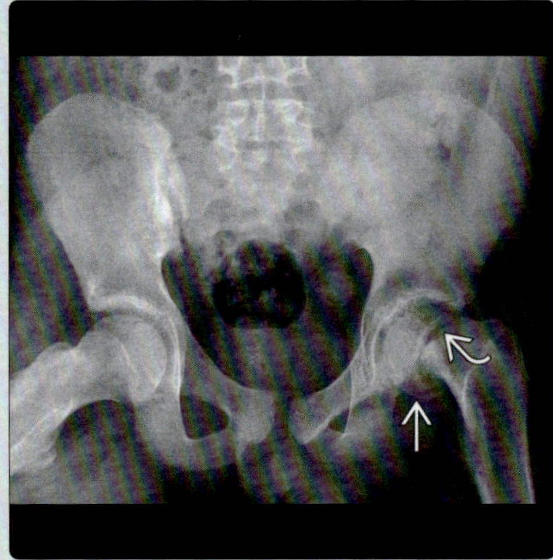

(Left) *AP graphic depicts a slipped capital femoral epiphysis (SCFE) on the left. Note the normal femoral head/neck cutback on the right hip ➡; this is reduced on the left, where the epiphysis has slipped both medially and posteriorly ➡.* **(Right)** *AP radiograph shows posterior, medial, and inferior slipping of the left femoral capital epiphysis ➡, compared to the normal right side. There is apparent widening of the left physis ➡. The left limb is shorter than the right (compare levels of the trochanters).*

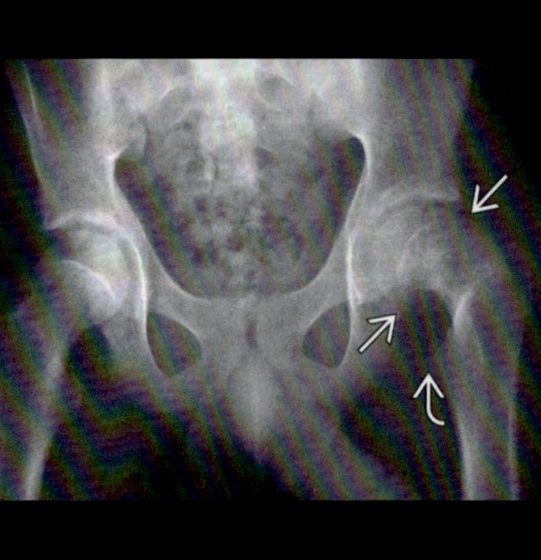

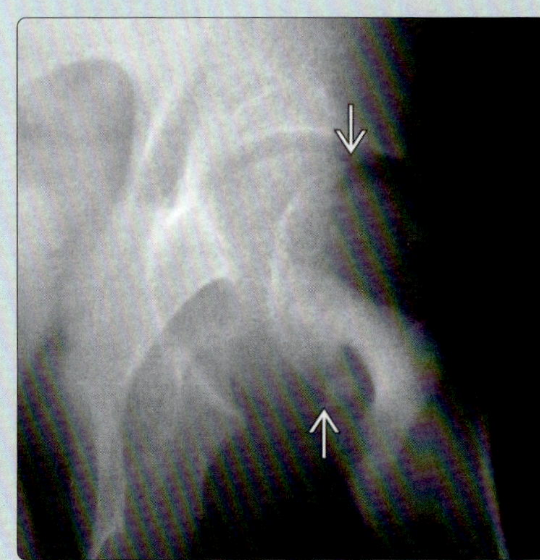

(Left) *AP radiograph of a 15 year old who falls within the expected age group for SCFE shows that the left capital epiphysis has slipped medially and posteriorly ➡. Because of the slip, the limb shortens; note the level of the left lesser trochanter ➡ compared to the normal right side. This is a severe SCFE; the image obtained at initial presentation was normal.* **(Right)** *False profile x-ray in the same patient emphasizes the posterior slip of the capital epiphysis ➡. Degree of slip visualized on AP radiograph may be deceptively small.*

TERMINOLOGY

Synonyms

- Slipped femoral capital epiphysis (SCFE)

Definitions

- Displaced Salter I fracture of femoral capital epiphysis, related to sheer stress

IMAGING

General Features

- Best diagnostic clue
  - Posteromedial displacement of femoral capital epiphysis
- Location
  - Bilateral in 20-40% (contralateral preslip demonstrated on MR may increase this percentage)
    - Contralateral slip usually occurs within 2 years of initial diagnosis

Imaging Recommendations

- Best imaging tool
  - Usually diagnosed on radiograph (frog-lateral more sensitive than AP)
  - MR is more sensitive in early disease (subtle or preslip)

Radiographic Findings

- Radiography
  - AP radiograph
    - Earliest change: Mild widening and irregularity of physis
    - Later abnormality: Femoral capital epiphysis slips posteriorly and medially
    - Klein line: Line drawn parallel to lateral femoral neck should intersect femoral epiphysis
      - Lack of intersection with epiphysis indicates medial displacement of structure
      - May be subtle, difficult to detect: 60% missed
    - Modified Klein line suggested
      - Measure width of epiphysis lateral to Klein line; difference of 2 mm between hips indicates slip
      - Improves sensitivity to 79%
    - Epiphysis appears short 2° to posterior slip
  - Frog-lateral radiograph
    - Southwick head/shaft angular displacement
      - Method: Bisect femoral shaft on frog-lateral; bisect epiphysis; measure angle formed
      - Diaphyseal-epiphyseal angle > 0° in SCFE
      - ↑ angle even prior to slip in higher risk groups, such as obese or patients taking growth hormone replacement; may be predictive
    - Wilson percent linear epiphyseal displacement
      - Measure metaphyseal width at level of physis
      - Measure amount of epiphyseal displacement
      - Grade by percent displacement
  - Metaphyseal scalloping and posterior beaking

MR Findings

- Physeal widening, even without slip, allows earlier diagnosis than on radiograph
  - Preslip: Subtle physeal irregularity
- Slip seen in 3 planes
  - SCFE extent often underestimated on radiograph
- Active slip shows high SI at physis with adjacent marrow edema on fluid-sensitive sequences
- Effusion generally present with active slip
- If patient had trauma, periosteal sleeve avulsion may be present
- Evaluate for complications
  - Chondrolysis
    - Cartilage thinning
    - Marrow edema
    - Effusion and synovitis
  - Osteonecrosis
    - Double line sign on fluid-sensitive sequences
    - Subchondral fracture, flattening in weight-bearing portion of head
    - Effusion

Nuclear Medicine Findings

- Osteonecrosis: Central ↓ uptake on blood pool
- Chondrolysis: ↑ uptake both sides joint

DIFFERENTIAL DIAGNOSIS

Traumatic Salter I Fracture

- Unequivocal history of trauma

PATHOLOGY

General Features

- Etiology
  - Majority of cases thought to have mechanical etiology, with elevated sheer stress
    - Physis at risk for Salter I fracture, resulting in SCFE, particularly in period of active growth
    - Growth spurt often coincides with age at which femoral neck-shaft angle increases to achieve adult morphology
    - Obesity contributes added sheer stress
  - Abnormal collagen in growth plate cartilage is postulated
    - Abnormalities found that could affect quality, distribution, and organization of growth plate
      - Type II collagen mRNA in slip specimen only 13% of normal expected amount
      - Aggrecan in slip specimen only 26% of normal
      - Both could be either cause or result of SCFE
  - Growth hormone replacement represents ↑ risk
  - Rickets puts patient at risk for SCFE
    - Widened zone of provisional calcification: Weak physis, at risk for Salter I fracture
  - Osteomyelitis/septic hip puts patient at risk for SCFE
    - Infection often at metaphysis, extending to physis
    - Weakens physis, at increased risk for Salter I fracture
- Associated abnormalities
  - Rare association with panhypopituitarism, hypothyroidism, Down syndrome
  - May have ↑ risk with prior radiation or chemotherapy

Staging, Grading, & Classification

- Loder classification of physeal stability
  - Stable: Able to bear weight on affected extremity, ± crutches (85% at presentation)

- Unstable: Pain too severe to bear weight on affected extremity
- Southwick head/shaft angular displacement on frog-lateral view
  - Normal, or preslip: 0°
  - Mild slip: ≤ 29°
  - Moderate slip: 30-50°
  - Severe slip: ≥ 51°
- Wilson linear displacement of head on neck, measured on frog-lateral
  - Mild (grade 1): < 1/3 epiphyseal displacement relative to metaphyseal width
  - Moderate (grade 2): 1/3-2/3 epiphyseal displacement
  - Severe (grade 3): > 2/3 epiphyseal displacement

Microscopic Features

- Fracture occurs in zone of hypertrophic chondrocytes

CLINICAL ISSUES

Presentation

- Most common signs/symptoms
  - Gradual onset of hip pain
  - Uncommonly (15%) presents as knee pain
  - Severe pain and inability to bear weight if slip becomes unstable
  - Clinical exam
    - Limited internal rotation
    - Obligatory external rotation in flexion

Demographics

- Age
  - Girls: Average 11-12 yr; range 8-15 yr
  - Boys: Average 13-14 yr; range 10-17 yr
  - SCFE 2° to rickets or infection often occurs at younger age (variable)
- Gender
  - Male > female (2.5:1)
- Ethnicity
  - Slightly more common in African Americans than Caucasians or Hispanics
- Epidemiology
  - SCFE most common adolescent hip condition
  - 3.4-10.8 cases per 100,000 individuals
  - Incidence may be increasing with worsening frequency of obesity in children

Natural History & Prognosis

- 80% of grade 3 (severe) slips, treated with adequate (uncomplicated) in situ pinning, had good to excellent **midterm** results (5.5 yr post surgery)
- Femoral acetabular impingement (FAI) may develop in young adult 2° to SCFE
  - 32% of patients with SCFE develop clinical signs of FAI once they are skeletally mature
    - Southwick angle of > 35° appears associated with development of impingement
      - May be basis of surgical decision regarding in situ fixation vs. partial reduction
  - Medial slip of epiphysis usually pinned in situ
    - Results in loss of normal cutback at femoral head-neck junction
    - Morphology analogous to bump of cam FAI
  - Patients at risk for labral tear, cartilage loss, and OA
  - Grade of slip in adolescence not predictive of development of FAI
- Chondrolysis (7-10%)
  - Most often results from pinning of SCFE
  - Chondrolysis also seen posttrauma and with hip spica casting
- May be complicated by osteonecrosis (ON) (1%)
  - Slip pinned in situ rather than reduced in order to avoid putting head at further risk for ON
  - Increased incidence with open reduction, use of multiple pins, or pin extension into superolateral quadrant of epiphysis

Treatment

- In situ surgical pinning for moderate SCFE
- Partial capital realignment to moderate slip is attempted for severe SCFE
- Prophylactic pinning of contralateral hip: Controversial
  - Previously strongly advocated
  - Current treatment generally careful observation, follow-up with MR may be reasonable
  - One study suggests posterior sloping angle of 15° as threshold for prophylactic pinning

DIAGNOSTIC CHECKLIST

Consider

- If SCFE seen in patient younger than expected 8-14 yr, look for evidence of rickets or infection as etiology for slip

SELECTED REFERENCES

1. Albers CE et al: Twelve percent of hips with a primary cam deformity exhibit a slip-like morphology resembling sequelae of slipped capital femoral epiphysis. Clin Orthop Relat Res. 473(4):1212-23, 2015
2. Bellemore JM et al: Biomechanics of slipped capital femoral epiphysis: evaluation of the posterior sloping angle. J Pediatr Orthop. ePub, 2015
3. Kitano T et al: Closed reduction of slipped capital femoral epiphysis: high-risk factor for avascular necrosis. J Pediatr Orthop B. 24(4):281-5, 2015
4. Nectoux E et al: Evolution of slipped capital femoral epiphysis after in situ screw fixation at a mean 11 years' follow-up: a 222 case series. Orthop Traumatol Surg Res. 101(1):51-4, 2015
5. Thawrani DP et al: Current practice in the management of slipped capital femoral epiphysis. J Pediatr Orthop. ePub, 2015
6. Georgiadis AG et al: Slipped capital femoral epiphysis: how to evaluate with a review and update of treatment. Pediatr Clin North Am. 61(6):1119-35, 2014
7. Miese FR et al: MRI morphometry, cartilage damage and impaired function in the follow-up after slipped capital femoral epiphysis. Skeletal Radiol. 39(6):533-41, 2010
8. Castañeda P et al: Functional outcome of stable grade III slipped capital femoral epiphysis treated with in situ pinning. J Pediatr Orthop. 29(5):454-8, 2009
9. Clarke NM et al: Slipped capital femoral epiphysis. BMJ. 339:b4457, 2009
10. de Andrade AC et al: Southwick's angle determination during growth hormone treatment and its usefulness to evaluate risk of epiphysiolysis. J Pediatr Orthop B. 18(1):11-5, 2009
11. Dodds MK et al: Femoroacetabular impingement after slipped capital femoral epiphysis: does slip severity predict clinical symptoms? J Pediatr Orthop. 29(6):535-9, 2009
12. Dwek JR: The hip: MR imaging of uniquely pediatric disorders. Magn Reson Imaging Clin N Am. 17(3):509-20, vi, 2009
13. Gholve PA et al: Slipped capital femoral epiphysis update. Curr Opin Pediatr. 21(1):39-45, 2009
14. Green DW et al: A modification of Klein's Line to improve sensitivity of the anterior-posterior radiograph in slipped capital femoral epiphysis. J Pediatr Orthop. 29(5):449-53, 2009
15. Tins B et al: The role of pre-treatment MRI in established cases of slipped capital femoral epiphysis. Eur J Radiol. 70(3):570-8, 2009

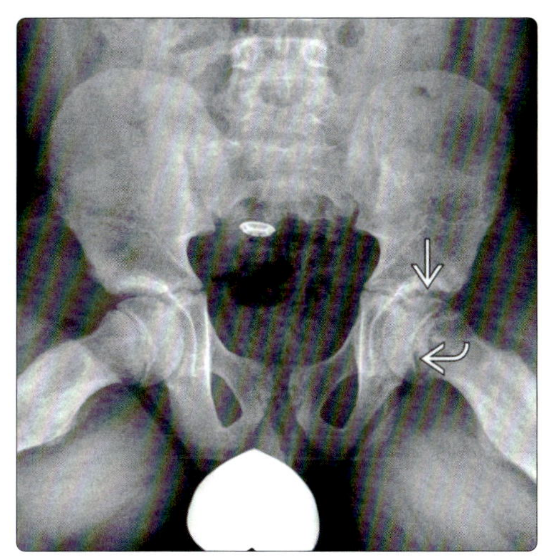

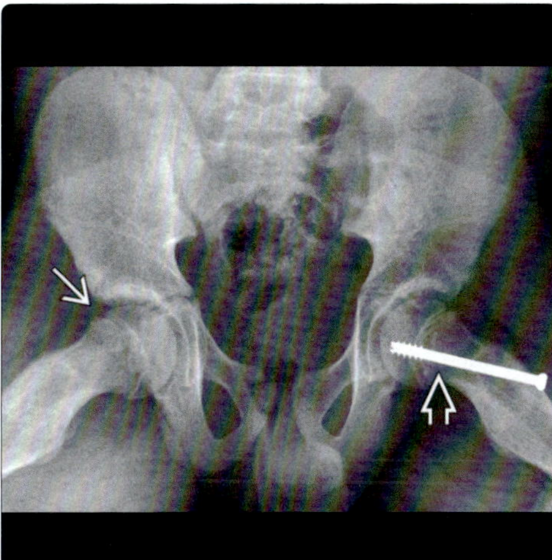

(Left) *Frog-lateral radiograph shows a subtle SCFE, with posterior slipping of the femoral head ➡ and slight widening of the physis ➡. There is osteopenia and decreased thigh musculature on the left, compared with the right side.* **(Right)** *Frog-lateral radiograph in the same patient 3 weeks later is shown. The left SCFE was treated in situ with internal fixation (cannulated screw) ➡. Note that the patient has now developed SCFE of the right hip ➡, which is subtle but appears distinctly different from the prior image.*

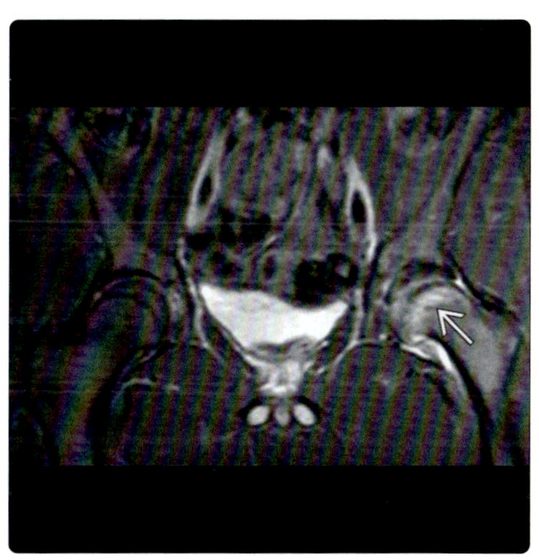

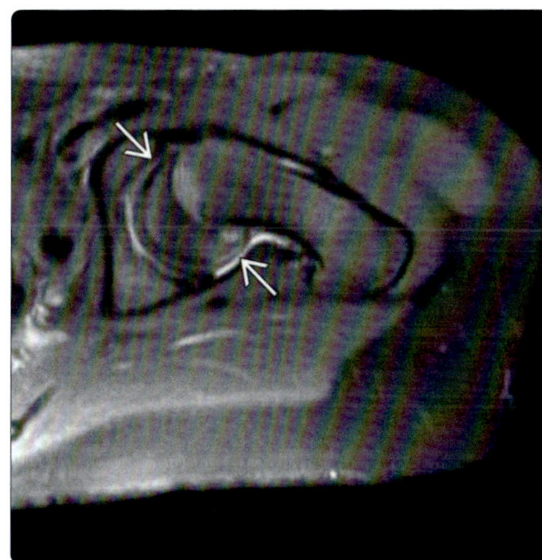

(Left) *Coronal STIR MR shows bilateral slipped capital femoral epiphyses. Both epiphyses appear "short," indicating posterior displacement. Additionally, there is medial slip, left hip worse than right. There is high signal at the left physis ➡ and effusion, indicating continued activity. Neither hip shows osteonecrosis as a complication.* **(Right)** *Axial oblique PD FS MR shows the degree of posterior slip of the left hip ➡. This posterior and medial direction of the slipped epiphysis is expected.*

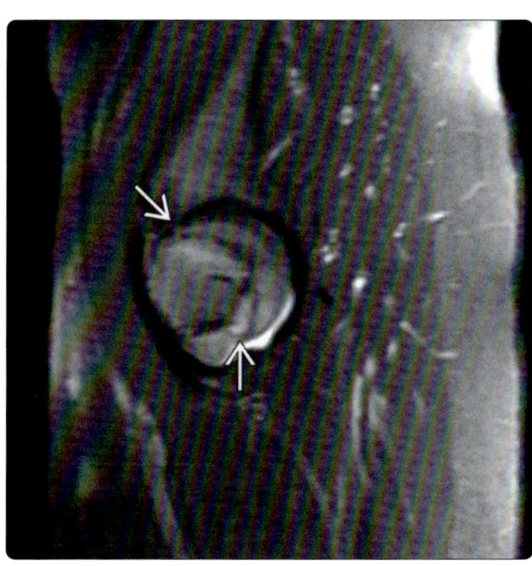

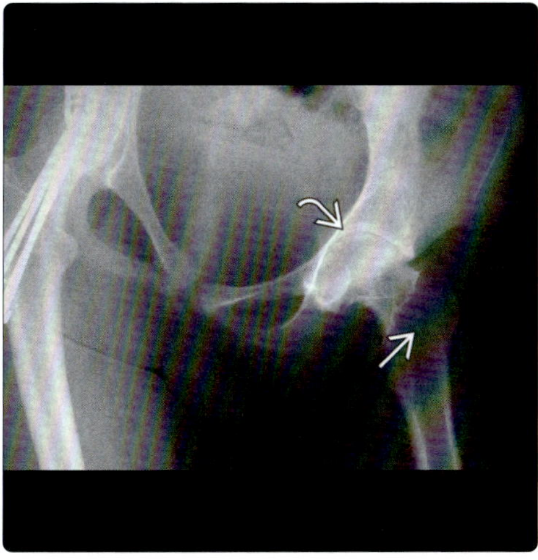

(Left) *Sagittal PD FS MR shows posterior slip of the femoral capital epiphysis ➡. This posterior displacement explains the short appearance of a slipped epiphysis on AP radiograph.* **(Right)** *AP radiograph shows pin tracks ➡ for left SCFE, evidenced by medial displacement of the head. Unfortunately, the patient developed chondrolysis, a known complication of this process. Note the complete loss of cartilage ➡, resulting in a fixed flexion and abduction. Prophylactic right hip pinning is seen.*

(Left) *AP radiograph shows diffusely abnormal bone density as well as widened zone of provisional calcification and frayed metaphyses ➡. This represents the rickets contribution to renal osteodystrophy. The capital femoral epiphyses are distinctly small, and the right one has slipped ➡.* **(Right)** *AP radiograph, 2.5 years later shows both femoral capital epiphyses have slipped further ➡. This is due to the weakened physeal plate secondary to the patient's rickets.*

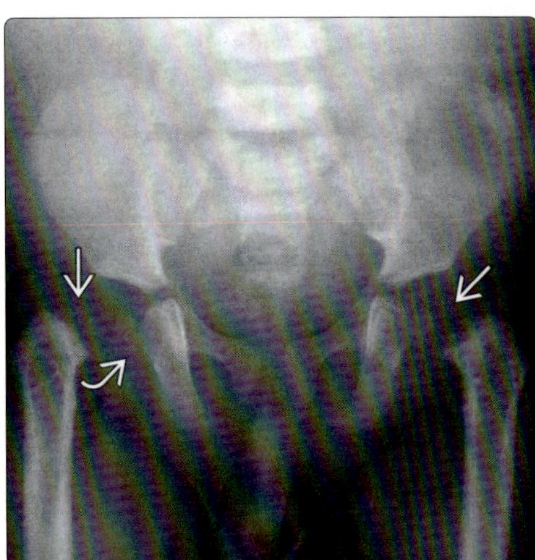

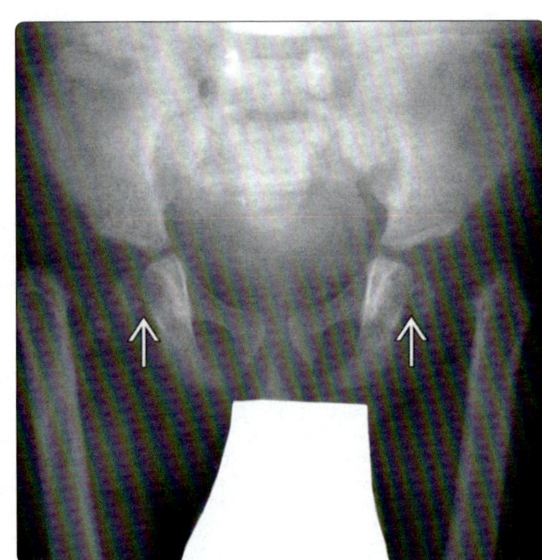

(Left) *AP radiograph shows an unusually severely displaced capital femoral epiphysis ➡. Surgeons do not reduce the Salter I fracture because of the risk of further disturbing the fragile blood supply to the epiphysis, thereby causing femoral head osteonecrosis (ON). Thus, the severely slipped SCFE was fixed in position.* **(Right)** *AP radiograph in the same case obtained 6 months postop shows sclerosis of the superior 1/2 of the head compatible with ON ➡, contrasting with a more radiolucent inferior head ➡.*

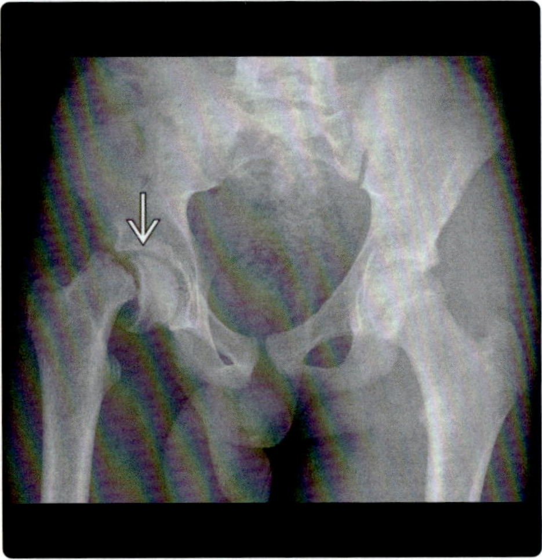

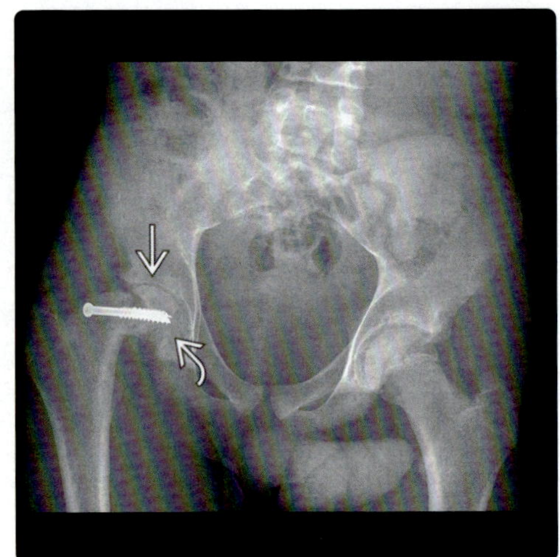

(Left) *AP radiograph shows femoroacetabular impingement (FAI) related to prior SCFE. The screw was placed when the patient was young, as judged by the screw being buried in the femoral neck. The femoral head is somewhat medial and posterior relative to the neck, resulting in an abnormal head/neck relationship, with a ridge of bone ➡ located at the site of the bump that is seen in FAI.* **(Right)** *Frog-lateral emphasizes the bump ➡ resulting in FAI, acquired from fixation of the SCFE in situ.*

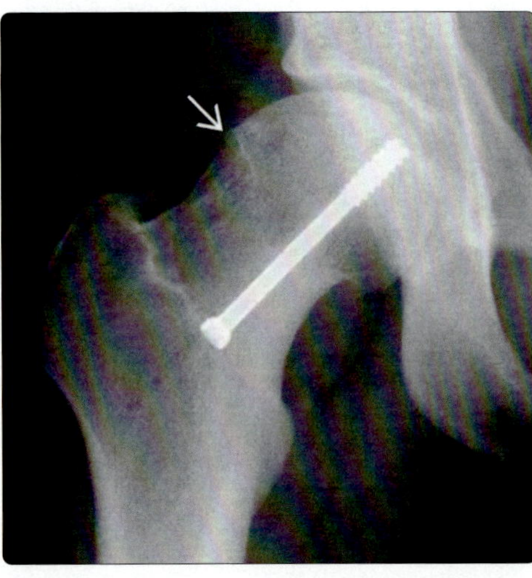

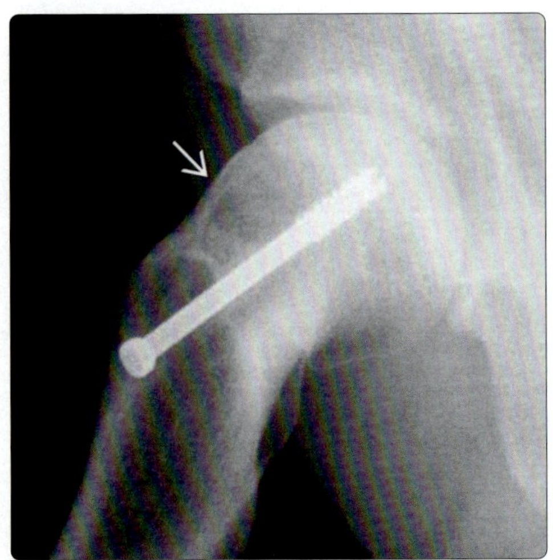

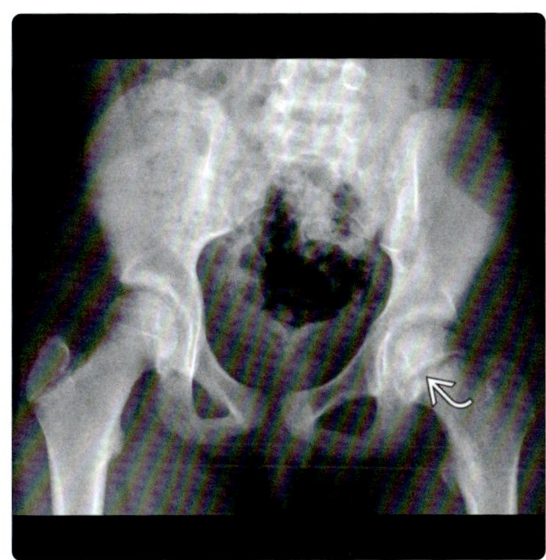

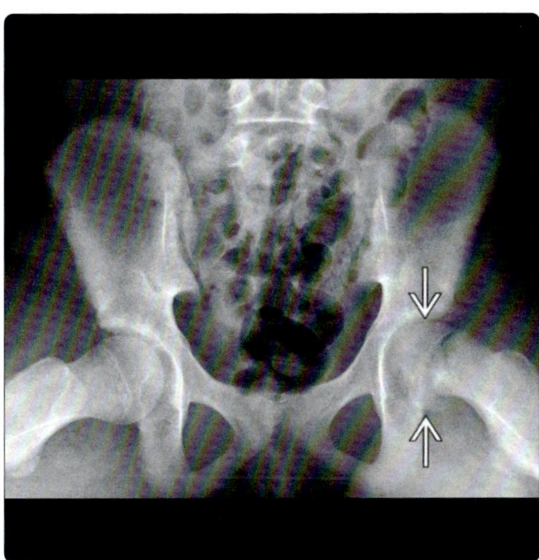

(Left) *AP radiograph shows a typical mild case of slipped capital femoral epiphysis. There is femoral and acetabular osteopenia on the left. The physis is widened but slip is not clearly evident on this AP. It might erroneously be classified as a preslip if only the AP is evaluated.* **(Right)** *Frog-lateral radiograph in the same case better shows the posterior slip of the femoral head. SCFE may be underdiagnosed or its severity undergraded if evaluation is based only on an AP radiograph.*

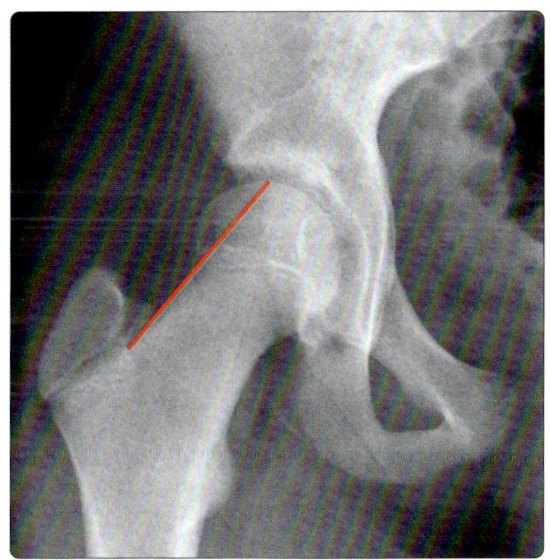

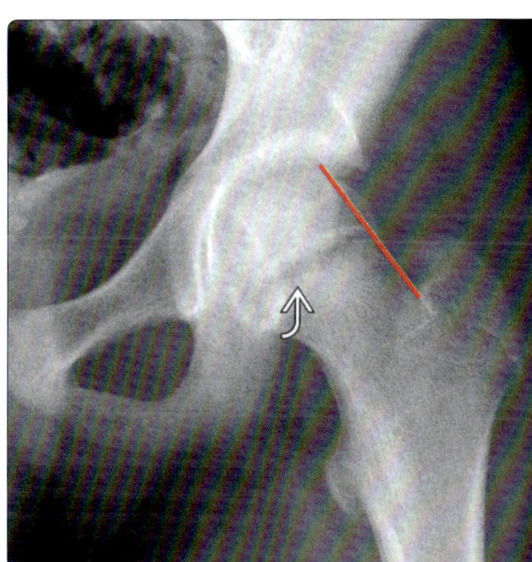

(Left) *AP radiograph of a normal right hip shows the femoral epiphysis transected by Klein line extended along the lateral cortex of the femoral neck.* **(Right)** *AP radiograph of abnormal left hip shows the widened and irregular physis. Note that Klein line does intersect the epiphysis, but much less of the epiphysis is transected when compared with the normal side. If the amount of epiphysis transected is measured, taking a side-to-side difference of 2 mm as indicating SCFE, this sign becomes more sensitive.*

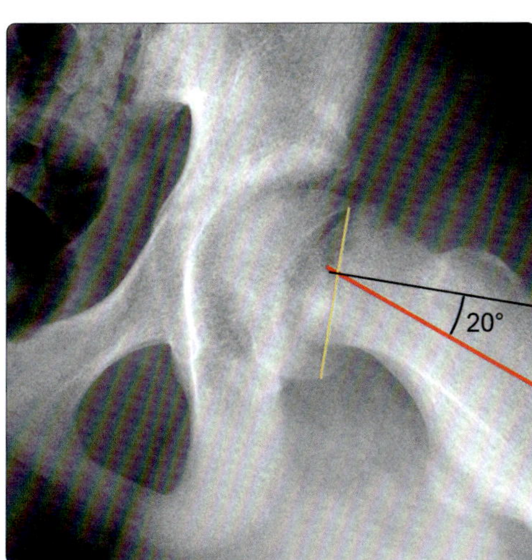

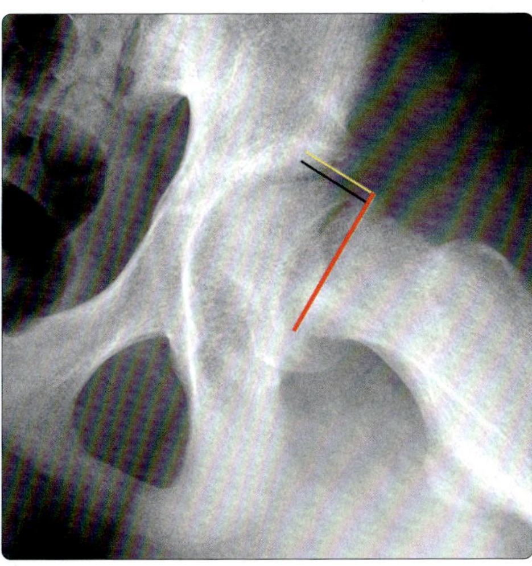

(Left) *Frog-lateral in the same case shows Southwick head-shaft angular displacement. Red line bisects shaft; black line perpendicular to yellow line bisects the head. The head-shaft angle is less than 29°, indicating a mild SCFE.* **(Right)** *Frog-lateral shows the method of determining linear epiphyseal displacement. Red line = metaphyseal width; space between black and yellow lines = epiphyseal displacement. By the Wilson grading system, displacement is < 1/3 the metaphyseal width, making it a mild or grade 1 SCFE.*

Proximal Femoral Focal Deficiency

KEY FACTS

TERMINOLOGY

- Rare skeletal disorder characterized by failure of development of proximal femur
- Spectrum ranges from mild proximal femoral shortening and varus to complete absence of acetabulum and majority of femoral shaft

IMAGING

- Initial diagnosis with fetal US
  - Fetal US: Short femur with normal echogenicity
  - Bone may be absent or short and bowed
  - Other abnormalities of limb and elsewhere
- Radiograph confirmation of diagnosis
  - Acetabular dysplasia ranges from normal through dysplastic to absent
  - Femoral capital epiphysis dysplasia ranges from delayed ossification of normal head through absent femoral head
  - Femoral shaft deficiency ranges from mild delay in ossification through absence of nearly entire shaft
- MR essential for full evaluation; radiographs during infancy overestimate osseous deficiency
  - Unossified acetabular cartilage may be identified
  - Femoral capital epiphysis, if present but unossified, seen on MR
  - Cartilaginous, but unossified, portions of proximal femoral shaft may be seen
  - All muscles about hip present; many hypoplastic
  - Instability of knee: Absent cruciate ligaments and menisci

CLINICAL ISSUES

- M:F = 2:1
- Treatment highly individualized
  - Aimed at providing functional ambulation; depends on type of deficiency

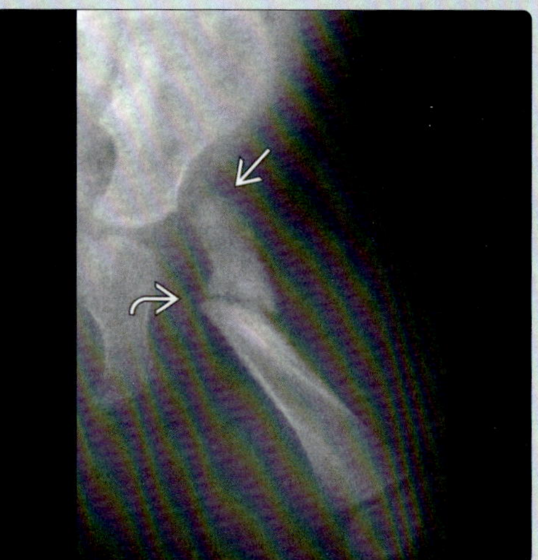

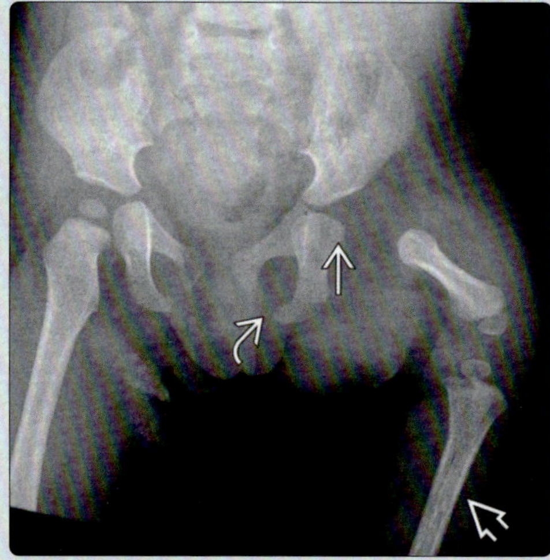

(Left) *AP radiograph demonstrates a short, dislocated femur. The femoral capital epiphysis as well as much of the neck are absent ➡. There is also a pseudarthrosis in the mid femoral diaphysis ➡. Full evaluation by MR is necessary to determine whether there is any cartilaginous structure at the site of defect.* **(Right)** *AP radiograph shows a short left femur and dysplastic left acetabulum. A hypoplastic capital femoral ossification center ➡ is present. The obturator foramen is enlarged ➡, & left fibula is absent ➡.*

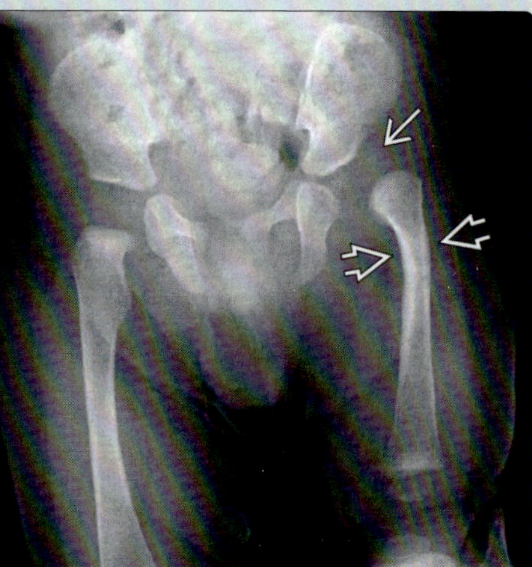

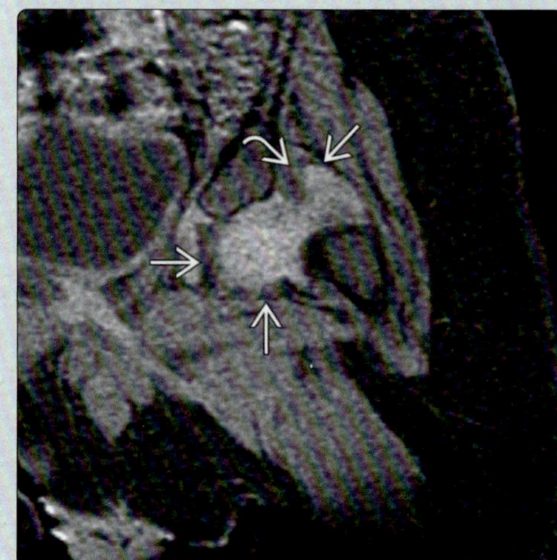

(Left) *AP radiograph shows a left femur to be markedly shorter than the right. There is proximal varus angulation ➡. The acetabulum is shallow, and the femoral head is dislocated superolaterally ➡.* **(Right)** *Coronal GRE MR in the same patient shows a dysmorphic subluxated femoral head. The deformed cartilage ➡ is high signal in this sequence; tiny ossified capital epiphysis is low signal ➡. Note the shallow acetabular roof conforms to the shape of the epiphyseal cartilage of the femoral head. This is Aitken class A PFFD.*

TERMINOLOGY

Abbreviations

- Proximal femoral focal deficiency (PFFD)

Definitions

- Rare skeletal disorder characterized by failure of development of proximal femur, with varying degrees of shortening
  - Spectrum ranges from mild proximal femoral shortening and varus to complete absence of acetabulum and majority of femoral shaft

IMAGING

General Features

- Best diagnostic clue
  - Short proximal femur ± dysplastic/absent femoral head and acetabulum
- Location
  - 15% bilateral

Imaging Recommendations

- Best imaging tool
  - Initial diagnosis with fetal US, confirmed by radiograph
  - MR essential for full evaluation; radiographs during infancy overestimate osseous deficiency
- Protocol advice
  - Optimize visualization of cartilage

Radiographic Findings

- Acetabular dysplasia ranges from normal through dysplastic to absent
  - Dysplastic acetabular characteristics
    - ↓ center-edge angle of Wiberg
    - Acetabular retroversion
    - Adjacent obturator foramen may be enlarged
- Femoral capital epiphysis dysplasia ranges from delayed ossification of normal head through absent femoral head
  - If present, but delayed ossification, femoral capital epiphysis usually ossifies by 25 months in PFFD
  - Femoral capital epiphysis, separated from short femoral shaft, may be either fixed to acetabulum or freely mobile
- Femoral shaft deficiency ranges from mild delay in ossification through absence of nearly entire shaft
  - Mild proximal femoral neck or subtrochanteric deficiency may have intact unossified cartilage, which ossifies normally with skeletal maturation
  - Coxa vara
  - Patients with more severe proximal femoral shaft deficiency develop pseudarthrosis
  - Proximally deficient shaft may be bulbous, pencil-pointed, or have only small tuft present if severe
- Distal (rather than proximal) femoral focal deficiency associated with hip dislocation also described

Arthrography

- May be utilized to judge size, shape, and mobility of femoral capital epiphysis
  - Note: Capital epiphysis may appear fixed in acetabulum when pseudarthrosis of shaft is present

CT Findings

- CTA may identify abnormal vascular morphology preoperatively

MR Findings

- Additive to radiographic findings; degree of deficiency often downgraded from that seen on radiograph; affects treatment plan and prognosis
  - Unossified acetabular cartilage may be identified
  - Femoral capital epiphysis, if present but unossified, seen on MR
  - Cartilaginous, but unossified, portions of proximal femoral shaft may be seen
- All muscles about hip present; many hypoplastic
  - Sartorius may be hypertrophied (explains flexion, abduction, external rotation of hip)
  - Aitken class A: Hip external rotators larger, abductors smaller, obturator externus muscle is straight
  - Aitken class B-C: Obturator externus is L-shaped
- Instability of knee: Absent cruciate ligaments and menisci

Ultrasonographic Findings

- Fetal US: Short femur with normal echogenicity
  - Bone may be absent or short and bowed
  - Other abnormalities of limb and elsewhere may be identified
- In infants, identifies femoral capital epiphysis and assesses its mobility within acetabulum

DIFFERENTIAL DIAGNOSIS

Developmental Dysplasia of Hip

- Severe acetabular dysplasia plus dislocation of femoral head may mimic PFFD
  - Femoral capital epiphysis may show delayed ossification
- Limb shortening
- Normal length of femoral shaft is differentiating feature

Traumatic Capital Femoral Epiphysiolysis

- Seen in newborn
- Edema of inguinal crease and proximal thigh soft tissues

Congenital Short Femur

- Congenital coxa vara should be considered
- Neither has specific abnormalities of acetabulum, head, neck, or shaft

Meningococcemia

- Embolic episodes result in ischemia, often involving proximal femur
- Fragmented, deformed femoral head and neck
- Limb shortening
- Usually other sites involved, serving as differentiating factor

PATHOLOGY

General Features

- Etiology
  - Unknown
    - Sclerotome subtraction theory: Injury to neural crest cells that form precursors to peripheral sensory nerves of L4 and L5

- Possible defect in proliferation and maturation of chondrocytes in proximal femoral growth plate
  - Anoxia, ischemia, radiation, infection, toxins (thalidomide), thermal injury may be agents
- Genetics
  - Several familial cases reported; no known genetic cause
- Associated abnormalities
  - Fibular deficiency: 70-80%
    - Suspect PFFD if lateral malleolus is absent
  - Other limb anomalies (including valgus foot deformity): 50%
  - Other anomalies (congenital heart anomalies, spinal anomalies, cleft palate, Hirschsprung, femuro-fibula-ulna complex): Rare

Staging, Grading, & Classification

- Aitken classification most widely used: Based on radiographic findings of presence and location of femoral head and neck
  - Class A (38%): Acetabulum and femoral head present; deficient proximal femoral shaft
    - Femoral shaft unconnected with head in infant; osseous connection develops by skeletal maturity
  - Class B (32%): Acetabulum and femoral head present, but capital femoral epiphysis shows delayed ossification; deficient proximal femoral shaft
    - No cartilaginous connection between head and shaft; elements move independently and do not show osseous connection at skeletal maturity
  - Class C (17%): Acetabulum severely dysplastic, femoral head does not develop; deficient proximal femoral shaft
  - Class D (13%): Acetabulum and femoral head absent; femoral shaft extremely short, with knee abnormality
- Anton classification
  - Milder dysplasia: Aitken classes A and B (femoral head is present in acetabulum)
    - 70% of cases fall into this category
  - Severe dysplasia: Aitken classes C and D (no femoral head, and acetabulum either severely dysplastic or absent)
    - 30% of cases fall into this category
- Multiple other classifications, but none frequently used

Gross Pathologic & Surgical Features

- Varying degrees of connection between shaft and head
  - Osteocartilaginous connection
  - Discontinuity: Subtrochanteric (27%), femoral neck (15%), both subtrochanteric and femoral neck (4%)

Microscopic Features

- Failure of organization of proliferative hypertrophic chondrocytes into longitudinal columns
- Disorganized vascular invasion with honeycomb rather than columnar pattern of trabeculae

CLINICAL ISSUES

Presentation

- Most common signs/symptoms
  - Femur short, flexed, abducted, externally rotated
  - Flexion contractures of hip and knee
  - Hip and knee often unstable
  - Limb shortening

Demographics

- Age
  - Identified in fetus or at birth
- Gender
  - M:F = 2:1
- Epidemiology
  - 0.5-2.0 cases per 100,000 individuals

Natural History & Prognosis

- Prognosis relates to severity and location of deficiency
  - Pseudarthrosis of cervical portion of femoral neck often fails to fuse
  - Pseudarthrosis of subtrochanteric portion of femoral shaft may fuse spontaneously and responds well to surgery

Treatment

- Treatment highly individualized, based on extent of process
- Aimed at providing functional ambulation; depends on type of deficiency
  - Stability of hip and knee joints with reconstructive surgery
  - Limb lengthening if adjacent joints are stable
  - Severe cases require rotationplasty, amputation, and use of prosthesis
- Early treatment generally beneficial
  - MR visualization of anatomy provides early and accurate assessment

DIAGNOSTIC CHECKLIST

Consider

- If radiographs show normally formed acetabulum, it is likely that (cartilaginous) femoral capital epiphysis exists

SELECTED REFERENCES

1. Bergère A et al: Imaging features of lower limb malformations above the foot. Diagn Interv Imaging. ePub, 2015
2. Canavese F et al: Rotationplasty as a salvage of failed primary limb reconstruction: up to date review and case report. J Pediatr Orthop B. 23(3):247-53, 2014
3. Ackman J et al: Long-term follow-up of Van Nes rotationplasty in patients with congenital proximal focal femoral deficiency. Bone Joint J. 95-B(2):192-8, 2013
4. Lin TH et al: Prenatal diagnosis of proximal femoral focal deficiency: a case report and literature review. Taiwan J Obstet Gynecol. 52(2):267-9, 2013
5. Biko DM et al: Proximal focal femoral deficiency: evaluation by MR imaging. Pediatr Radiol. 42(1):50-6, 2012
6. Chomiak J et al: Cruciate ligaments in proximal femoral focal deficiency: arthroscopic assessment. J Pediatr Orthop. 32(1):21-8, 2012
7. Chomiak J et al: Computed tomographic angiography in proximal femoral focal deficiency. J Bone Joint Surg Am. 91(8):1954-64, 2009
8. Taylor BC et al: Distal focal femoral deficiency. J Pediatr Orthop. 29(6):576-80, 2009
9. Westberry DE et al: Proximal focal femoral deficiency (PFFD): management options and controversies. Hip Int. 19 Suppl 6:S18-25, 2009
10. Oh KY et al: Unilateral short femur–what does this mean? Report of 3 cases. Ultrasound Q. 24(2):89-92, 2008
11. Maldjian C et al: Efficacy of MRI in classifying proximal focal femoral deficiency. Skeletal Radiol. 36(3):215-20, 2007
12. Bernaerts A et al: Value of magnetic resonance imaging in early assessment of proximal femoral focal deficiency (PFFD). JBR-BTR. 89(6):325-7, 2006
13. Dora C et al: Morphologic characteristics of acetabular dysplasia in proximal femoral focal deficiency. J Pediatr Orthop B. 13(2):81-7, 2004
14. Court C et al: Radiological study of severe proximal femoral focal deficiency. J Pediatr Orthop. 17(4):520-4, 1997

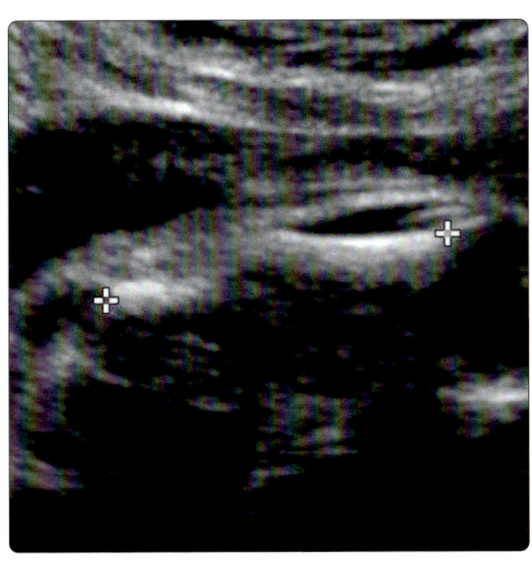

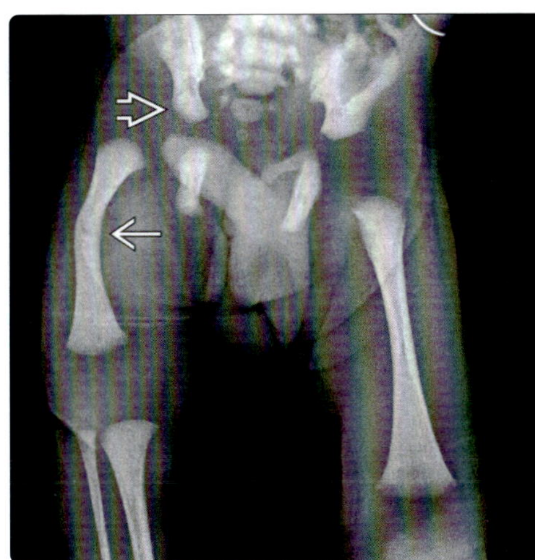

(Left) *Long-axis fetal ultrasound shows this right femur is shorter than the left and appears bowed. Ultrasound suggests the diagnosis of PFFD. It is also utilized to evaluate for the presence of the femoral capital epiphysis.* **(Right)** *AP postnatal radiograph confirms the short and bowed right femur. The right femoral capital epiphysis is not ossified, and the shallow acetabulum suggests the epiphysis is either absent or deformed. If MR confirms cartilaginous epiphysis, this is Aitken class B PFFD.*

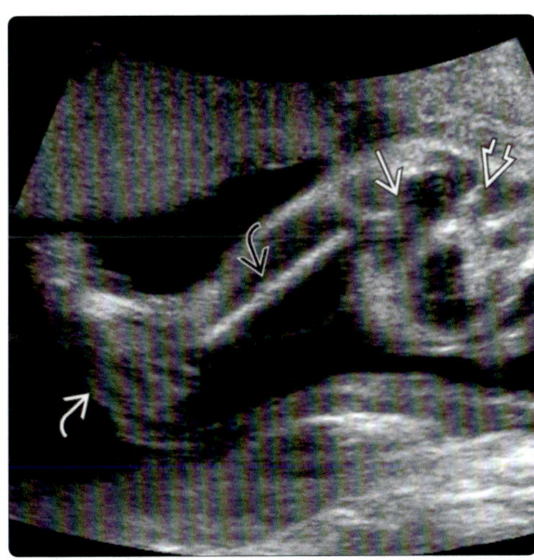

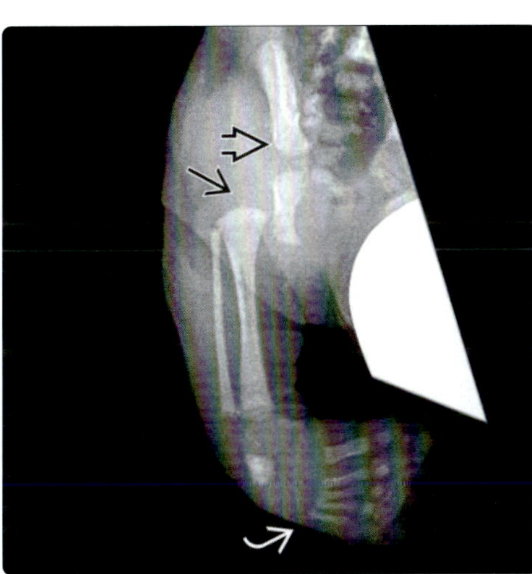

(Left) *Long-axis fetal ultrasound shows the absence of the femur in its expected location between the iliac bone and the tibia. In addition, the foot is inverted. This appears to be severe PFFD.* **(Right)** *AP postnatal radiograph confirms an absent right femur, absent acetabulum, and club foot. This completely matches the prenatal ultrasound. This is an extremely severe case of PFFD, Aitken class D.*

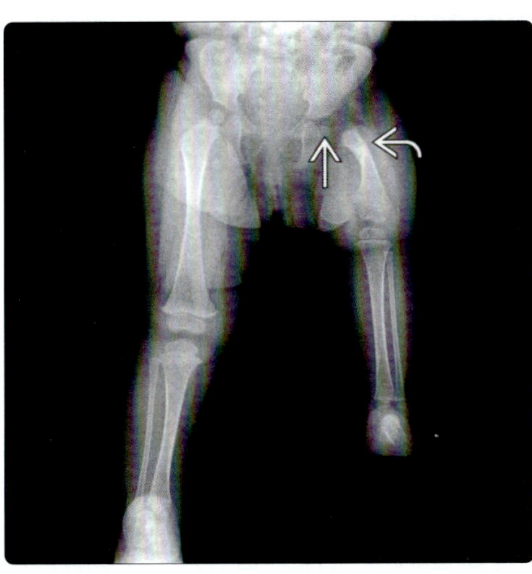

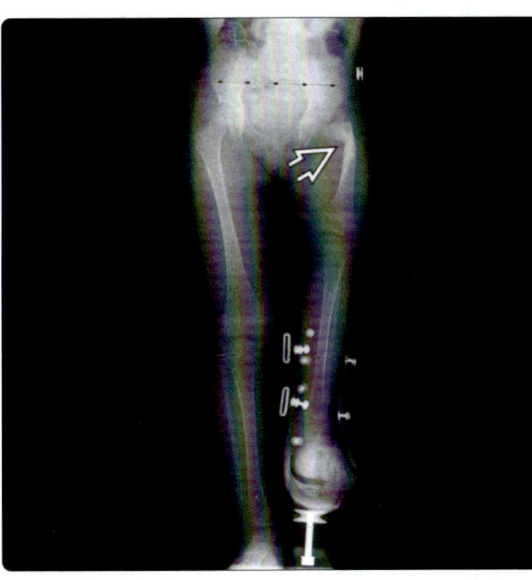

(Left) *AP radiograph shows a short left femoral diaphysis with a bulbous proximal end of the shaft. A capital femoral ossification center is seen. Despite the severe shortening of the shaft, the presence of the epiphysis makes this an Aitken class A case.* **(Right)** *AP radiograph of same patient was obtained 3 years later (age 4). The severe femoral varus deformity was subsequently corrected surgically. The child was radiographed wearing her leg-extension prosthesis. The goal of functional ambulation was achieved.*

KEY FACTS

TERMINOLOGY

- Traction apophysitis of patellar ligament insertion on tibial tubercle

IMAGING

- Bilateral in 25-50%
- Radiograph/CT
  - Ossification & thickening inferior patellar tendon adjacent to tibial tubercle
  - Irregular, fragmented ossification of tibial tubercle
  - Adjacent soft tissue swelling
  - Fragmentation remains following resolution of clinical symptoms; no associated swelling
- MR findings
  - Bone marrow edema in fragments and adjacent tibial tubercle
  - Edema of thickened infrapatellar tendon and surrounding soft tissues
  - Distended deep infrapatellar bursa

PATHOLOGY

- Repetitive microtrauma during phase of skeletal maturation of tibial tubercle
  - Stress on tibial tubercle → traction osteochondritis & eventual partial avulsion fracture

CLINICAL ISSUES

- Presentation: Visible & painful bump anterior tibial metaphysis
- Age: Adolescents in period of rapid growth (male 10-15, female 8-13 years old)
- Gender: Male > female
- Common in jumping sports: Basketball, volleyball
- Natural history: Usually self-limited
  - Symptoms relieved when either osseous or fibrous union develops
- Treatment: Rest, immobilization

(Left) *Lateral radiograph shows fragmentation of the tibial tubercle ➔ and adjacent soft tissue swelling ➔, typical for Osgood-Schlatter disease. There is no effusion.* **(Right)** *Sagittal reformatted NECT show soft tissue swelling ➔ overlying fragmentation of the tibial apophysis. The patient is an active adolescent, as is expected with Osgood-Schlatter disease. Note that Hoffa fat pad is not disturbed, and there is no effusion.*

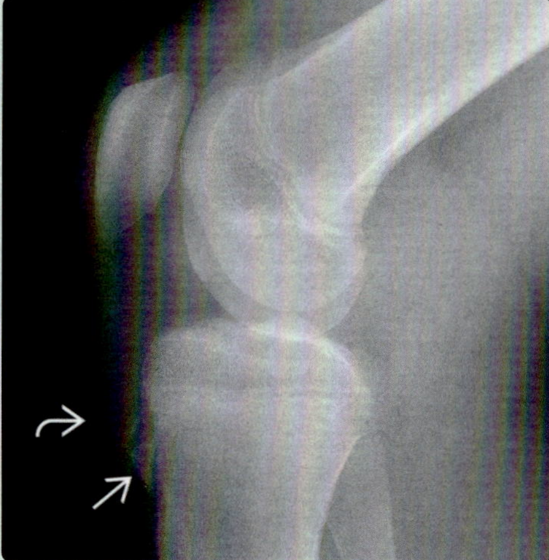

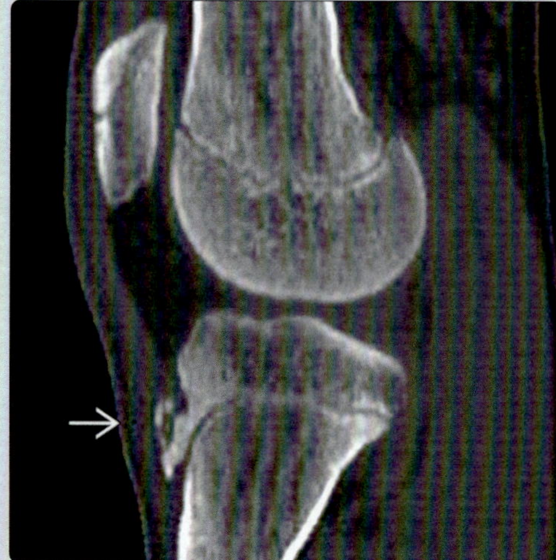

(Left) *Sagittal T1 FS MR shows marrow edema in the anterior proximal tibial epiphysis and tibial tubercle ➔. There is fluid interposed between the proximal tibia and the distal patellar tendon in the deep infrapatellar bursa ➔. Mild soft tissue swelling ➔ is seen anterior to the distal patellar tendon.* **(Right)** *Sagittal ultrasound of symptomatic (left) and asymptomatic (right) patellar tendons show a thickened left patellar tendon as well as intratendinous ossicles ➔ in this 18-year-old basketball player. The right side is normal.*

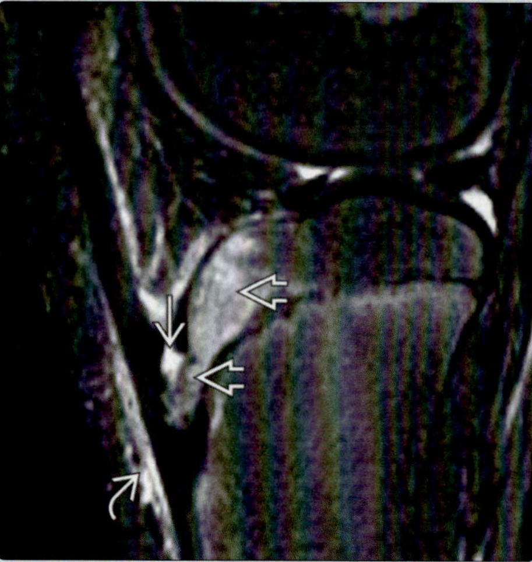

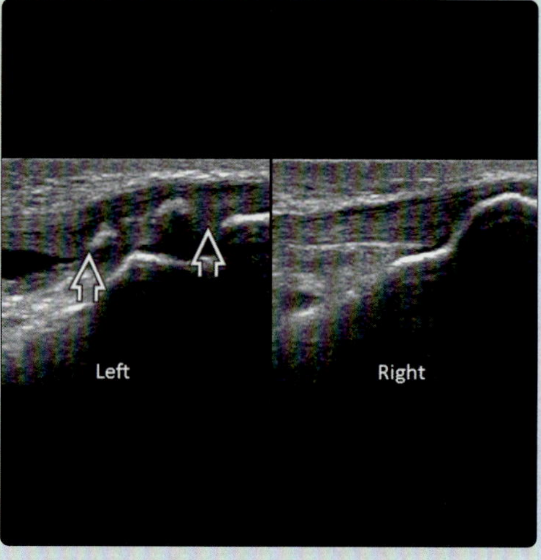

KEY FACTS

TERMINOLOGY

- Traction tendinitis at inferior pole of patella
  - Results in ossification within proximal portion of inferior patellar tendon

IMAGING

- Radiograph/CT
  - Calcification or ossification of proximal inferior patellar tendon
  - Adjacent to inferior pole of patella
  - May be fragmented
  - Variable in size
  - No donor site seen at inferior pole of patella
  - Soft tissue swelling in inferior patellar tendon
  - No associated effusion
- Fragments may eventually coalesce
  - May become incorporated into inferior pole of patella
  - Inferior pole appears prominent but otherwise normal
- MR: Ossific fragments at inferior pole patella or within proximal inferior patellar tendon
  - Edema in involved tissues (low SI on T1WI, high SI on fluid-sensitive sequences)
    - Inferior pole of patella
    - Within ossific fragments large enough to be visualized
    - Surrounding soft tissues
    - Proximal portion of inferior patellar tendon
    - Adjacent Hoffa fat pad

TOP DIFFERENTIAL DIAGNOSES

- Patellar sleeve avulsion
  - Occurs in child or adolescent with unossified cartilage at inferior pole of patella
  - Cartilage of inferior pole of patella avulsed, often with small bone fragment
  - Extent of cartilage damage underestimated by radiograph
  - MR for both diagnosis and evaluation of extent of cartilaginous injury
  - Patella alta
  - May have effusion
  - Clinical scenario is of single traumatic event rather than chronic microtrauma
  - Occurs with vigorous contraction of quadriceps on flexed knee
- Normal variation of ossification
  - Accessory ossification centers

PATHOLOGY

- Repetitive microtrauma at attachment of patellar tendon on inferior pole of patella
- Likely traction phenomena; 2 possible scenarios
  - Tendinosis in proximal attachment of inferior patellar tendon leads to calcification/ossification
  - Patellar avulsion results in ossification
- Associations
  - May coexist with Osgood-Schlatter disease
  - May be seen in patients with spastic paralysis

CLINICAL ISSUES

- Presentation
  - Point tenderness inferior pole of patella
  - Soft tissue swelling over lower pole of patella
  - Aggravated by activity
- Age
  - 10-14 years old most common age at presentation
- Natural history
  - Generally 3-12 months of duration of symptoms
- Treatment
  - Rest, immobilization

DIAGNOSTIC CHECKLIST

- MR may serve to differentiate Sinding-Larsen-Johansson from patellar sleeve avulsion
  - Extent of cartilage injury in patellar sleeve avulsion underestimated by radiograph but well seen on MR

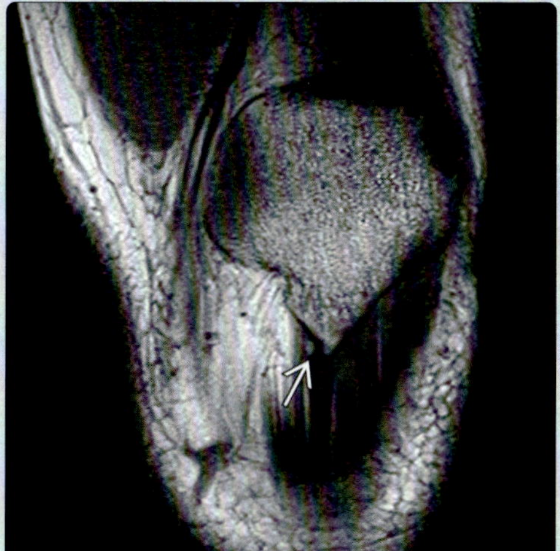

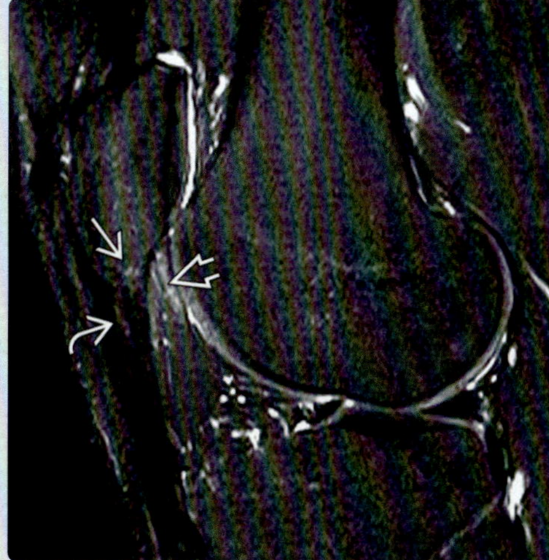

(Left) *Coronal T1 MR shows mild fragmentation as well as deformity at the distal pole of the patella ➡ typical of Sinding-Larsen-Johannson disease. The deformity arises from coalescence of other fragments.* **(Right)** *Sagittal T2WI FS MR in the same patient shows mild edema at the distal pole of the patella ➡. The small fragment is not seen on this cut, but a thickened and edematous inferior patellar tendon is seen ➡. Finally, edema within Hoffa fat pad ➡ adjacent to the tendinopathy is noted.*

Blount Disease

KEY FACTS

TERMINOLOGY

- Developmental condition characterized by disordered endochondral ossification of posteromedial portion of proximal tibial physis
  - Results in multiplanar deformities of lower limb
- Clinically distinct forms
  - Early onset (infantile): Onset ≤ 4 years of age
  - Juvenile type: Onset 4-10 years of age
  - Adolescent type (late onset): Onset > 10 years of age

IMAGING

- Tibial varus, centered at proximal metaphysis
- Tibial procurvatum (apex anterior)
- Internal rotation of tibia
- Widening and irregularity of medial growth plate
- Beaking of medial proximal metaphysis
- Medial sloping and irregular ossification of medial epiphysis
- CT: Abnormal torsion of tibia and femur, best seen on gunsight evaluation
- MR: Unossified portion of medial tibial metaphysis, physis, and epiphysis is low signal on T1WI
  - Hypertrophied medial tibial epiphyseal cartilage
  - Medial meniscus hypertrophy
  - Growth plate irregularities and physeal bars
  - Occasional distal femoral epiphysis/physis abnormalities
- Bilateral involvement is common, especially with early-onset type (50-75%)
  - Bilaterality may be as little as 10-30% in late onset

TOP DIFFERENTIAL DIAGNOSES

- Developmental (physiologic) bowing
  - Associated metaphyseal fragmentation
- Focal fibrocartilaginous dysplasia

PATHOLOGY

- Unknown, probably multifactorial
- Presumed mechanical in many cases, given association with obesity and early walking

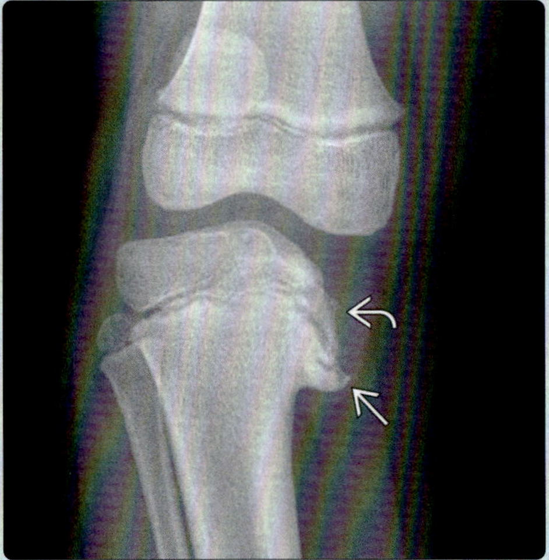

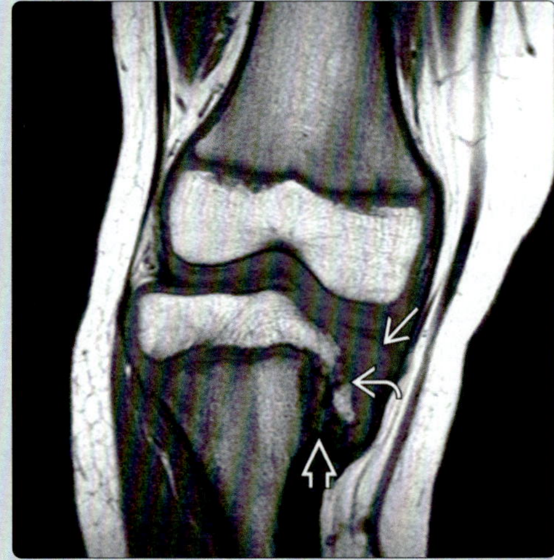

(Left) *AP radiograph shows an advanced case of early-onset Blount disease. The medial growth plate is more vertically oriented and irregular than normal, resulting in a beak-like appearance of the proximal tibial metaphysis ➔. Note the poorly formed and down-sloping medial epiphysis ➔.* **(Right)** *Coronal T1WI MR in the same patient shows low SI and beaking of the proximal tibial metaphysis ➔, narrowing and irregularity of the ossified medial tibial epiphysis ➔, and hypertrophy of the medial tibial plateau cartilage ➔.*

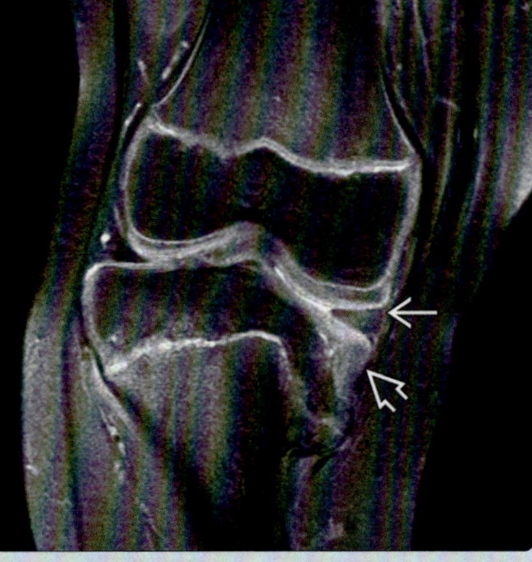

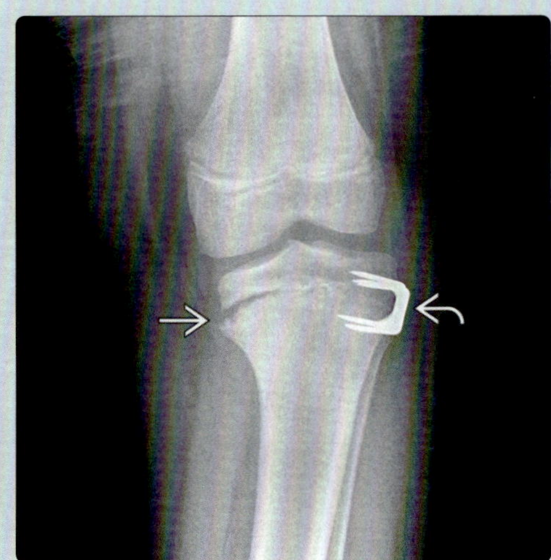

(Left) *Coronal PD FS MR emphasizes the hypertrophy of the medial tibial plateau cartilage ➔. Note also the mild hypertrophy of the medial femoral condyle and more pronounced medial meniscal hypertrophy ➔.* **(Right)** *AP x-ray shows early changes in a late-onset Blount disease, with beaking of the proximal tibial metaphysis and widening and irregularity of the physis ➔. There is mild medial femoral overgrowth and varus deformity. The patient has undergone lateral epiphysiodesis ➔ to slow lateral tibial growth.*

TERMINOLOGY

Definitions

- Developmental condition characterized by disordered endochondral ossification of posteromedial portion of proximal tibial physis
  - Results in multiplanar deformities of lower limb
- Clinically distinct forms
  - Early onset (infantile): Onset ≤ 4 years of age
  - Juvenile type: Onset 4-10 years of age
  - Adolescent type (late onset): Onset > 10 years of age

IMAGING

General Features

- Location
  - Bilateral involvement is common, especially with early-onset type (50-75%)
    - Bilaterality may be as little as 10-30% in late onset

Radiographic Findings

- Angular deformities: Multiplanar
  - Tibial varus, centered at proximal metaphysis
    - Mean metaphyseal-diaphyseal angle 16° ± 4.3
    - Range: 8-22°
  - Tibial procurvatum (apex anterior)
  - Internal rotation of tibia
- Widening and irregularity of medial growth plate
- Beaking of medial proximal metaphysis
- Medial sloping, irregular ossification medial epiphysis

CT Findings

- Abnormal torsion of tibia and femur, best seen on gunsight CT evaluation
  - Internal tibial version
  - Internal femoral version: Anteversion averages 26°

MR Findings

- Unossified portion of medial tibial metaphysis, physis, and epiphysis is low signal on T1WI
- Medial meniscus hypertrophy
- Medial tibial epiphyseal cartilage hypertrophy
- Growth plate irregularities and physeal bars if traumatic etiology

DIFFERENTIAL DIAGNOSIS

Developmental (Physiologic) Bowing

- Normal development
  - Neonates and infants normally genu varus
  - Gradual correction: Fully corrected within 6 months of walking or by 18-24 months of age
- Developmental bowing
  - Varus angulation seen during 2nd year of life
    - Mean metaphyseal-diaphyseal angle 5 ± 2.8°
  - Mild posteromedial proximal tibial metaphyseal beaking; no fragmentation
  - Patients tend to be obese, African American, and to walk early (similar to Blount profile)
- Metaphyseal fragmentation associated with physiologic bowing
  - Distal femoral &/or proximal tibial metaphyseal irregularities found in 11% of patients with physiologic bowing
  - Mean age of patients: 18 months
  - Tibial site identical to early Blount disease
  - Lacks gross fragmentation, sclerosis, downward sloping of medial physis of Blount disease

PATHOLOGY

General Features

- Associated abnormalities
  - Early-onset Blount disease
    - Obesity, but lower BMI than late-onset disease
    - More severe varus and procurvatum deformities than late-onset disease
  - Late-onset Blount disease associated with complicated additional abnormalities, which may make realignment difficult
    - Morbid obesity
    - Distal femoral varus
    - Proximal tibial procurvatum
    - Distal tibial valgus

CLINICAL ISSUES

Demographics

- Gender
  - Male = female
- Ethnicity
  - Predisposition for all types of Blount disease in obese African American children and children of Scandinavian descent
- Epidemiology
  - Early onset 5-8x more frequent than late onset

Natural History & Prognosis

- Infantile tibial vara progressing to Blount disease may be predicted based on
  - Tibial metaphyseal-diaphyseal angle ≥ 10°
  - BMI ≥ 22
- Residual malalignment results in
  - Abnormal gait
  - Increased risk of early osteoarthritis

Treatment

- Leg orthoses to unload medial weight bearing
- Double osteotomy: Medial tibial plateau elevation and concurrent gradual tibial osteotomy
- External fixation with gradual correction
- When angulation persists into adolescence, hemiepiphysiodesis (physeal stapling) may prevent progression of angular deformity

SELECTED REFERENCES

1. Sabharwal S: Blount disease: an update. Orthop Clin North Am. 46(1):37-47, 2015
2. Gill KG et al: Magnetic resonance imaging of the pediatric knee. Magn Reson Imaging Clin N Am. 22(4):743-63, 2014
3. Ho-Fung V et al: MRI evaluation of the knee in children with infantile Blount disease: tibial and extra-tibial findings. Pediatr Radiol. 43(10):1316-26, 2013

Pes Planus (Flatfoot)

KEY FACTS

TERMINOLOGY

- Group of foot disorders having in common a flattened longitudinal arch
  - May have several contributing factors

IMAGING

- Hindfoot malalignment may contribute to flatfoot
  - Decreased calcaneal pitch (normal: 20-30°)
  - Hindfoot valgus: Increased talocalcaneal angle
- Midfoot malalignment may contribute to flatfoot
  - Midfoot sag
  - Midfoot Lisfranc ligament disruption
- Forefoot malalignment may contribute to flatfoot
  - Pronation, valgus, abduction
- Osseous malalignment may be masked on MR since not performed in weight-bearing position
- Evaluate MR for
  - Tendon abnormalities, particularly posterior tibial tendon
  - Ligament disruption or stretching resulting in malalignment

PATHOLOGY

- Support of arch depends on several factors, both dynamic and static; 1 or more may fail, resulting in flatfoot
  - Osseous architecture
  - Intrinsic and extrinsic musculature/tendons
  - Fascia and ligaments
- Etiologies of pes planus
  - Idiopathic (flexible flatfoot)
    - Seen only on weight-bearing radiographs
    - Reduces to normal appearance if not weight-bearing
  - Tibialis posterior tendon (PTT) tear
  - Charcot (neuropathic) joint
  - Traumatic Lisfranc ligament disruption
  - Tarsal coalition
  - Rheumatoid arthritis
  - Defective collagen synthesis

(Left) *AP radiograph, weight-bearing, shows increased talocalcaneal angle (talus ➡, calcaneus ⇨), indicating hindfoot valgus. Note that the talus points medial to the base of the 1st metatarsal (MT). Additionally, there is pronation and mild abduction of the forefoot, resulting in decreased convergence (overlap) at the bases of the MTs.* **(Right)** *AP radiograph, same patient/day, non-weight-bearing, shows normal talocalcaneal angle. The talus ➡ now points to the base of the 1st MT, & there is normal overlap of MT bases.*

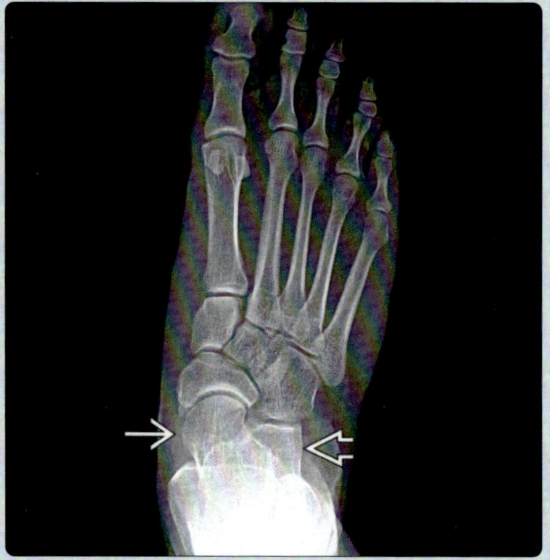

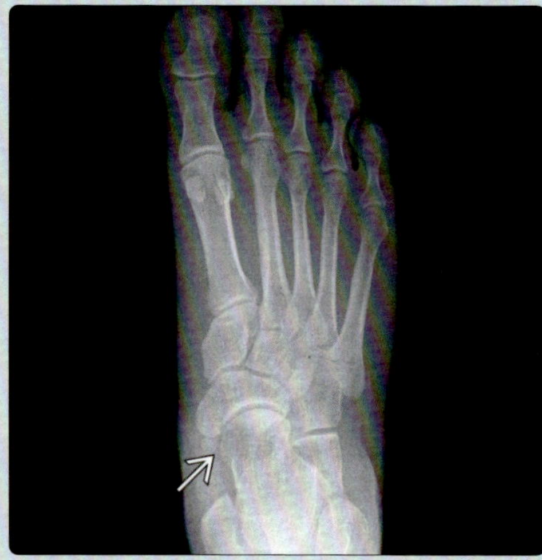

(Left) *Lateral radiograph, same patient, weight-bearing, shows mild increased talocalcaneal angle (hindfoot valgus) and pronation of the forefoot (overlap of the MTs ➡). The longitudinal arch is decreased.* **(Right)** *Lateral x-ray, same patient/day, non-weight-bearing, shows normal talocalcaneal angle and MT alignment ➡. This patient has a typical flexible flatfoot, with hindfoot and forefoot valgus/pronation seen only on weight-bearing images. The differences between normal and abnormal may be subtle, as in this case.*

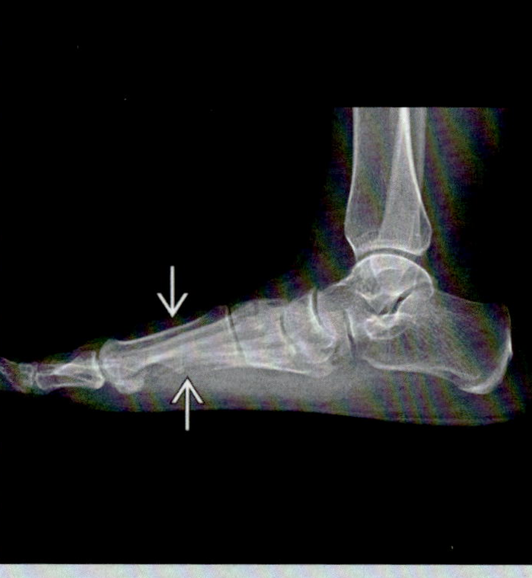

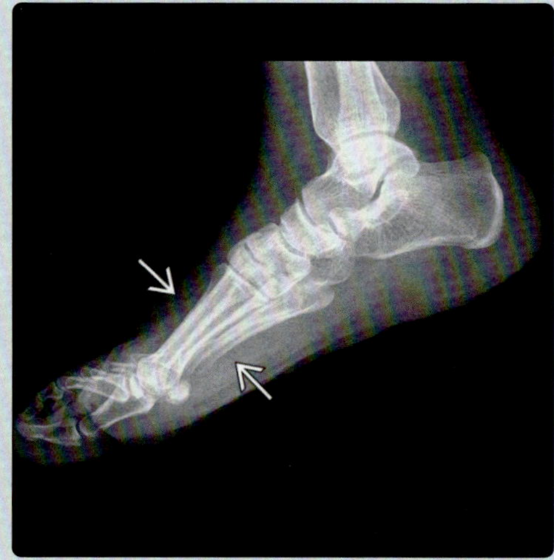

TERMINOLOGY

Synonyms

- Pes planus, pes valgus, congenital hypermobile flatfoot, talipes calcaneovalgus, compensated talipes equinus collapsing pes valgo planus

Definitions

- Group of foot disorders having in common a flattened longitudinal arch; may have several contributing factors
- Clinically, foot is recognized as having some or all of the following
  - Everted heel
  - Abduction of forefoot on hindfoot
  - Collapse of medial column
  - Flexibility of foot with reducibility of deformity

IMAGING

Imaging Recommendations

- Protocol advice
  - **Radiographs must be weight-bearing**

Radiographic Findings

- Abnormalities in hindfoot, midfoot, &/or forefoot may contribute to flatfoot deformity
- Hindfoot malalignment
  - Decreased calcaneal pitch (normal 20-30°)
  - Hindfoot valgus: Increased talocalcaneal angle
    - Lateral talocalcaneal angle > 50°
      - Normal adult mean: 35° (range: 25-50°)
    - AP talocalcaneal angle > 45°
      - Normal adult mean: 35° (range: 15-45°)
    - Standing PA hindfoot alignment view
      - If distance from lowest point of calcaneus (if it were normally aligned) > 8 mm lateral to line bisecting tibia, indicates hindfoot valgus
- Midfoot malalignment/dorsolateral talonavicular subluxation
  - Midfoot sag
    - Lateral midfoot sag
      - Articular surface angle of talonavicular, naviculocuneiform, and 1st tarsometatarsal joints are normally approximately parallel
      - Midfoot sag results in loss of parallelism of these articular surfaces with one another
    - AP talonavicular subluxation
      - If distance between midpoints of talus and navicular ≥ 7 mm, indicates subluxation
  - Midfoot Lisfranc ligament disruption
    - Disruption of tarsometatarsal joints
      - Displacement of 1st MT relative to medial cuneiform
      - Displacement of 2nd MT relative to middle cuneiform
      - Displacement of 3rd MT relative to lateral cuneiform
      - Displacement of 4th and 5th MT relative to cuboid
    - Over long term, results in midfoot sag on lateral
- Forefoot malalignment
  - Pronation, valgus, abduction
    - Lateral radiograph
      - Superimposition of metatarsals on one another
      - Angle of inclination decreases for MT 1-4
    - AP radiograph
      - Divergence of bases of metatarsals from one another
      - Abduction of forefoot relative to hindfoot

MR Findings

- Osseous abnormalities
  - Osseous malalignment may be masked since MR not performed in weight-bearing position
  - Tarsal coalition may be noted
    - Usually talocalcaneal (medial facet) or calcaneonavicular
    - Broadening and irregularity of involved articulation
    - Edema, sclerosis on fluid-sensitive sequences
- Tendon abnormalities
  - Posterior tibial tendinopathy
    - Disruption ± retraction
    - Partial tear/tendinopathy
      - Altered morphology (hypertrophic or thinned)
      - High central signal on fluid-sensitive sequences indicating split
- Ligament abnormalities
  - Disruption or stretching of any supporting ligaments resulting in osseous displacement
  - Fluid signal within osseous diastasis
- Other soft tissue abnormalities
  - Diabetic Charcot foot usually shows large joint effusions ± osseous fragments

Ultrasonographic Findings

- High-resolution US useful and accurate for diagnosis of posterior tibial tendon injury
  - 87% concordance with MR in one study

DIFFERENTIAL DIAGNOSIS

Congenital Vertical Talus (Rocker-Bottom Foot)

- Rigid, nonreducible convex plantar surface
- Hindfoot valgus and forefoot valgus, as in other etiologies of pes planus
- Additionally has dislocation of talonavicular joint, with head of talus at apex of rocker bottom
- Equinus is part of the deformity; not seen with pes planus

PATHOLOGY

General Features

- Etiology
  - Support of arch depends on several factors, both dynamic and static; 1 or more may fail, resulting in flatfoot
    - Osseous architecture
    - Intrinsic and extrinsic musculature/tendons
    - Fascia and ligaments
  - Flexible flatfoot
    - Most common etiology of flatfoot in children and young adults
    - Valgus hindfoot + valgus pronated forefoot on weight-bearing radiographs

- Reduces completely when not bearing weight
- Tibialis posterior tendon (PTT) tear
  - Most common etiology of new onset flatfoot deformity in middle-aged to elderly women
  - PTT is most important supinator of foot
    - Stabilizes arch by its many deep plantar insertions
    - Damaged tendon prevents normal re-supination of foot when walking
    - Leads to pronated foot and flexible pes planovalgus
  - Gliding ability of PTT is reduced with flatfoot deformity
    - Preexisting flatfoot aggravates tendency of PTT to develop tendinopathy
- Charcot (neuropathic) joint
  - Lisfranc joint
    - Tarsometatarsal joint disruption
    - If not stabilized, result is midfoot collapse
  - Chopart joint
    - Subluxation and collapse at talonavicular and calcaneocuboid joints produces flattened midfoot
  - Osseous fragmentation and large fluid collections help make diagnosis
- Traumatic Lisfranc ligament disruption
  - Progressive disruption of tarso-metatarsal joints
  - Patients develop pronation of forefoot, with collapse of longitudinal arch
- Tarsal coalition
  - Spastic peroneal flatfoot
    - ↓ mobility in hindfoot/midfoot from coalition results in spastic peroneal muscle contraction
    - Pulls forefoot/midfoot into pronation
  - Most common etiology of painful flatfoot in 2nd and 3rd decades
- Rheumatoid arthritis
  - Long-term disease results in ligamentous disruption and laxity
  - Ligamentous laxity → abnormal osseous motion and eventual collapse
- Diseases with defective collagen synthesis
  - Marfan, Ehlers-Danlos
  - Ligamentous laxity allows foot structure to stretch and relax
  - Hypermobility results in flatfoot when weight-bearing

CLINICAL ISSUES

Presentation

- Most common signs/symptoms
  - May be asymptomatic
  - Deformity
  - Eventual pain, limitation in activity
  - Tarsal coalition may result in lateral leg pain along course of peroneal tendons

Demographics

- Age
  - Flexible flatfoot: Childhood
  - Tarsal coalition: Present at birth but presents in adolescence or young adulthood
  - Marfan or Ehlers-Danlos: Adolescence
  - PTT-related flatfoot: Middle-aged to elderly
- Epidemiology
  - 20% of otherwise normal adults have flatfoot deformity
  - Flexible flatfoot affects 4% of population
  - Tarsal coalition affects 1% of population

Natural History & Prognosis

- Some forms are nonprogressive
- Others progress to significant osseous collapse, with associated deformity and disability

Treatment

- Orthotics
- Physical therapy
- Arthroereisis may be used in childhood flexible flatfoot
  - Implant of various shapes inserted in sinus tarsus
    - Designed to limit eversion at subtalar joint
  - May be difficult to control placement
  - May develop reactive synovitis, osteolysis
- Lateral column (calcaneal) lengthening in adults
  - Some develop abnormal lateral pressure and pain following procedure
- Posterior tibial tendon dysfunction
  - Medial calcaneal displacement osteotomy
  - Flexor digitorum longus transfer
- Resection of coalition
- Other reconstructive surgical procedures

SELECTED REFERENCES

1. Arnoldner MA et al: Imaging of posterior tibial tendon dysfunction-Comparison of high-resolution ultrasound and 3T MRI. Eur J Radiol. ePub, 2015
2. Erol K et al: An important cause of pes planus: the posterior tibial tendon dysfunction. Clin Pract. 5(1):699, 2015
3. Meyr AJ et al: Descriptive Quantitative Analysis of Rearfoot Alignment Radiographic Parameters. J Foot Ankle Surg. ePub, 2015
4. Shah NS et al: 2013 Subtalar Arthroereisis Survey: The Current Practice Patterns of Members of the AOFAS. Foot Ankle Spec. 8(3):180-5, 2015
5. Toullec E: Adult flatfoot. Orthop Traumatol Surg Res. 101(1 Suppl):S11-7, 2015
6. Blitz NM et al: Flexible pediatric and adolescent pes planovalgus: conservative and surgical treatment options. Clin Podiatr Med Surg. 27(1):59-77, 2010
7. Blitz NM: Pediatric & adolescent flatfoot reconstruction in combination with middle facet talocalcaneal coalition resection. Clin Podiatr Med Surg. 27(1):119-33, 2010
8. Chen YC et al: Effects of foot orthoses on gait patterns of flat feet patients. Clin Biomech (Bristol, Avon). 25(3):265-70, 2010
9. Ellis SJ et al: Plantar pressures in patients with and without lateral foot pain after lateral column lengthening. J Bone Joint Surg Am. 92(1):81-91, 2010
10. Arangio GA et al: A biomechanical analysis of posterior tibial tendon dysfunction, medial displacement calcaneal osteotomy and flexor digitorum longus transfer in adult acquired flat foot. Clin Biomech (Bristol, Avon). 2009 May;24(4):385-90. Epub 2009 Mar 9. Erratum in: Clin Biomech (Bristol, Avon). 24(6):530, 2009
11. Fujii T et al: The influence of flatfoot deformity on the gliding resistance of tendons about the ankle. Foot Ankle Int. 30(11):1107-10, 2009
12. Hirano T et al: Effects of foot orthoses on the work of friction of the posterior tibial tendon. Clin Biomech (Bristol, Avon). 24(9):776-80, 2009
13. Jerosch J et al: The stop screw technique--a simple and reliable method in treating flexible flatfoot in children. Foot Ankle Surg. 15(4):174-8, 2009
14. Koning PM et al: Subtalar arthroereisis for pediatric flexible pes planovalgus: fifteen years experience with the cone-shaped implant. J Am Podiatr Med Assoc. 99(5):447-53, 2009
15. Kulig K et al: Effect of eccentric exercise program for early tibialis posterior tendinopathy. Foot Ankle Int. 30(9):877-85, 2009
16. Jacobs AM: Soft tissue procedures for the stabilization of medial arch pathology in the management of flexible flatfoot deformity. Clin Podiatr Med Surg. 24(4):657-65, vii-viii, 2007

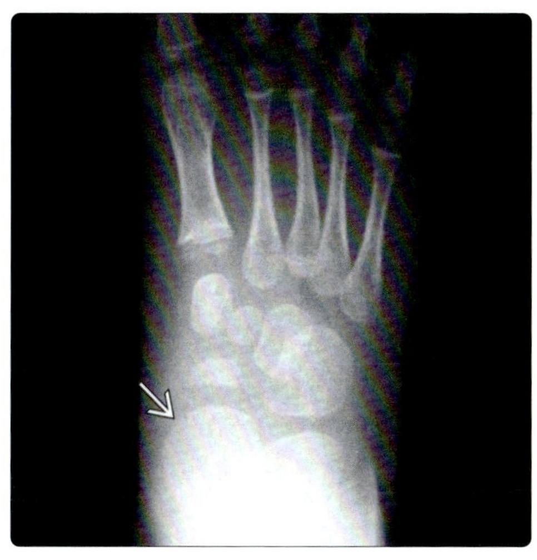

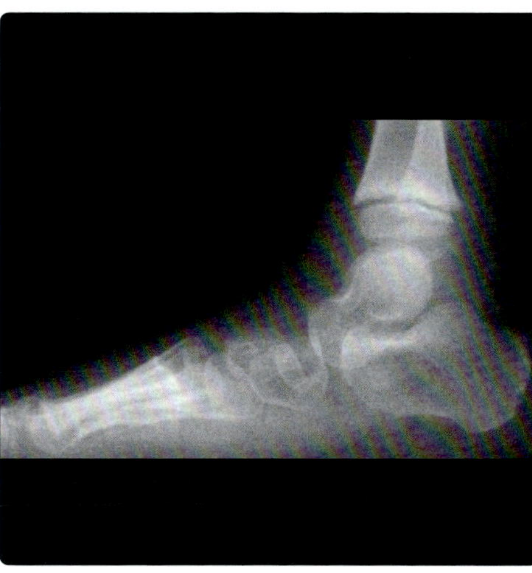

(Left) *AP radiograph, weight-bearing, in a child shows hindfoot valgus, with the talus ➡ pointing medial of the 1st MT. The bases of the MTs show ↓ convergence, indicating forefoot valgus/pronation.* **(Right)** *Lateral radiograph, weight-bearing, in same patient shows abnormal talar plantarflexion and resultant talocalcaneal angle ↑ with longitudinal arch ↓. Pronation/valgus of forefoot (superimposition of the MTs) contributes to the flatfoot. Alignment returned to normal when not weight-bearing.*

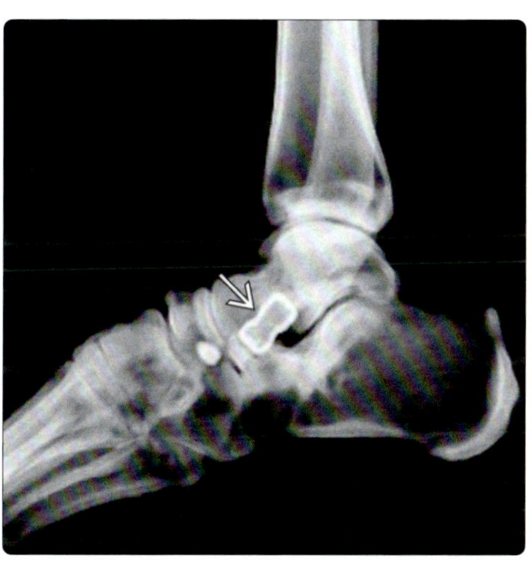

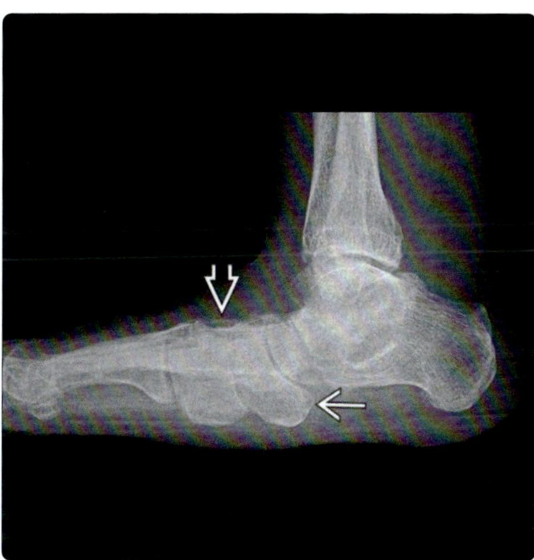

(Left) *3D CT shows arthroereisis implant in the sinus tarsi ➡ of a child with flexible flatfoot. There was progressive painful collapse; CT demonstrated the plug subluxated laterally, resulting in mechanical erosion of anterior calcaneus.* **(Right)** *Lateral radiograph shows severe pes planus with midfoot sag ➡ & forefoot pronation in a middle-aged woman. The hindfoot valgus is so severe it is difficult to see how plantarflexed the talus is; the navicular ➡ is subluxated & forms the medial plantar weight-bearing surface.*

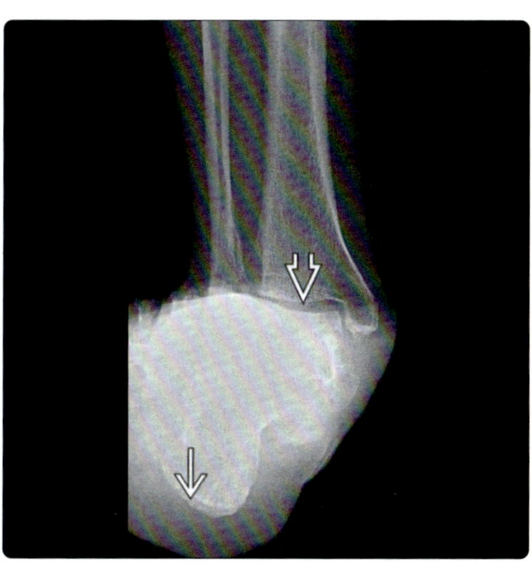

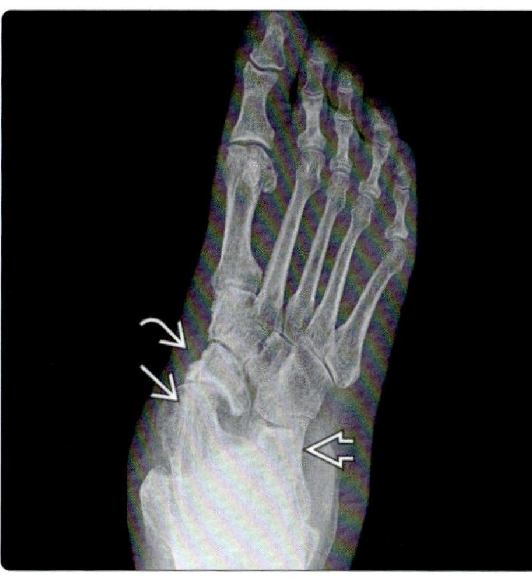

(Left) *PA hindfoot alignment radiograph, same patient, shows the plantar-most aspect of the calcaneus ➡ to fall > 8 mm lateral to a line that would bisect the tibia (line would extend through ➡). This confirms severe hindfoot valgus.* **(Right)** *AP radiograph also shows hindfoot valgus, with talo ➡, calcaneal ➡ angle significantly increased. Note the subluxation of the navicular ➡ and the pronation/abduction of the forefoot. This is a typical, though severe, acquired pes planus in an adult.*

(Left) *Lateral radiograph shows midfoot sag; note that the talonavicular joint line ➡ is not parallel with the naviculocuneiform joint line ➡. This appearance in a middle-aged woman should suggest posterior tibial tendon dysfunction.* **(Right)** *Axial PDWI FS MR, same patient, shows central hyperintensity within the posterior tibial tendon ➡, as well as mild hypertrophy. PTT dysfunction is a common etiology of new-onset flatfoot deformity in adults, especially older women.*

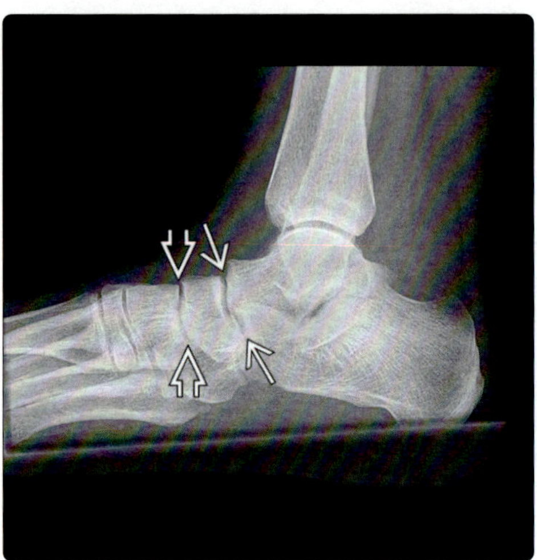

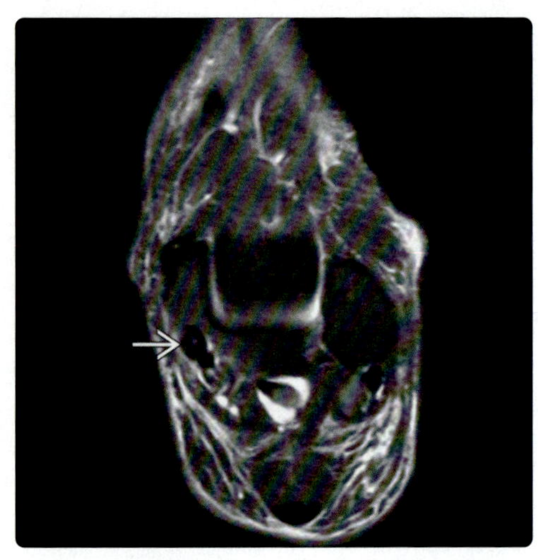

(Left) *AP radiograph shows a flatfoot deformity. Note the increased talocalcaneal angle, with the talus pointing medially ➡. A middle-aged woman with new-onset flatfoot deformity will frequently have a disrupted PTT.* **(Right)** *Sagittal T2WI MR shows the PTT tendon to have a complete disruption at the level of the posterior talus, with retraction of the fibers ➡. Additionally noted is tear with retraction of tibialis anterior tendon ➡; this is an unassociated injury.*

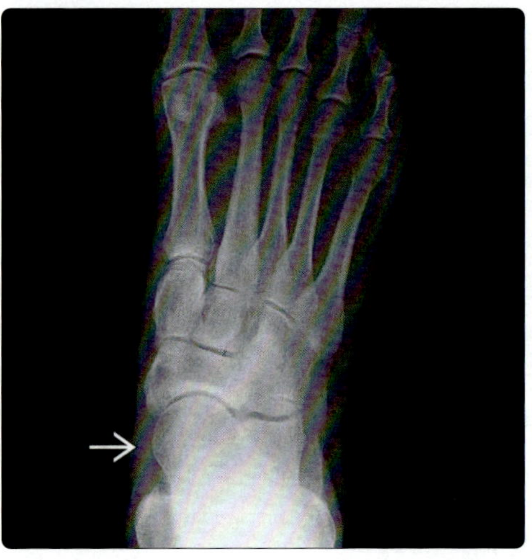

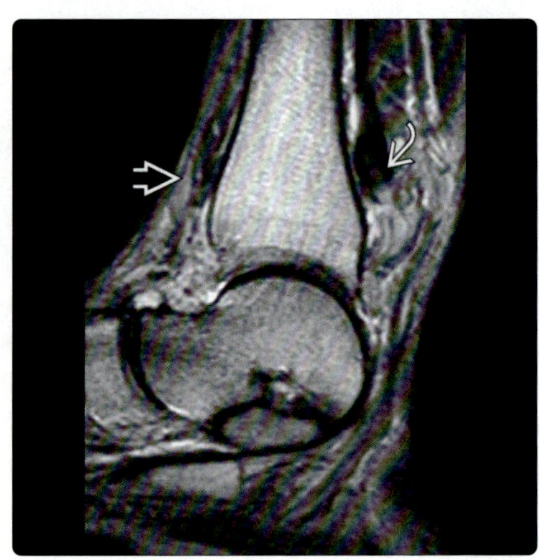

(Left) *Sagittal radiograph shows a typical Charcot midfoot (Chopart) joint in a diabetic patient. The dislocated talonavicular joint shows with erosive change and debris in a dorsal effusion ➡. The result is collapse of the midfoot ➡ and clinical flatfoot.* **(Right)** *Lateral radiograph shows a flatfoot deformity ➡ in a teenager. There is elongation of the anterior process of the calcaneus ➡, indicating calcaneonavicular coalition. Tarsal coalition is the most common cause of painful flatfoot in a teenager.*

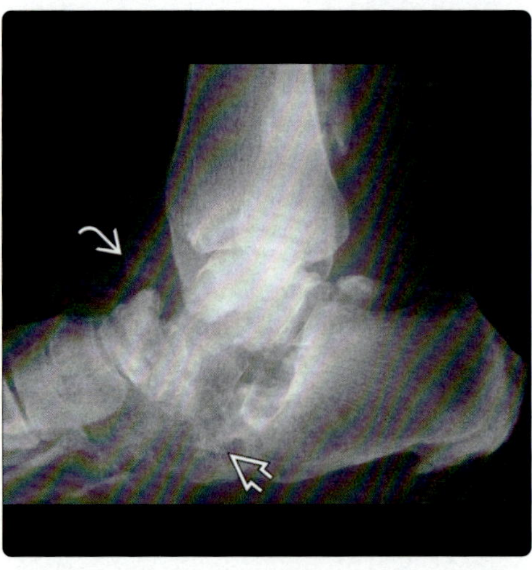

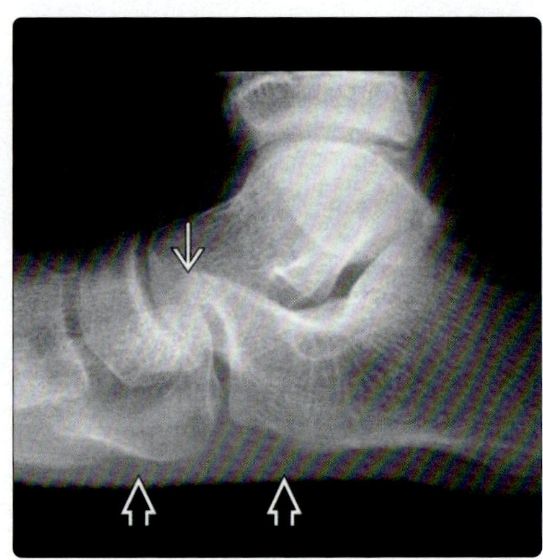

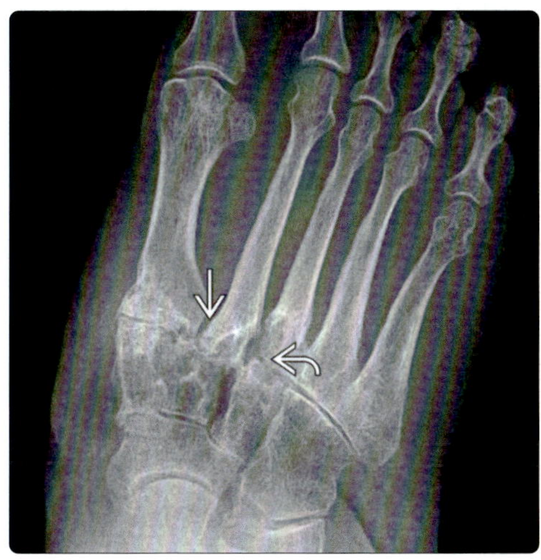

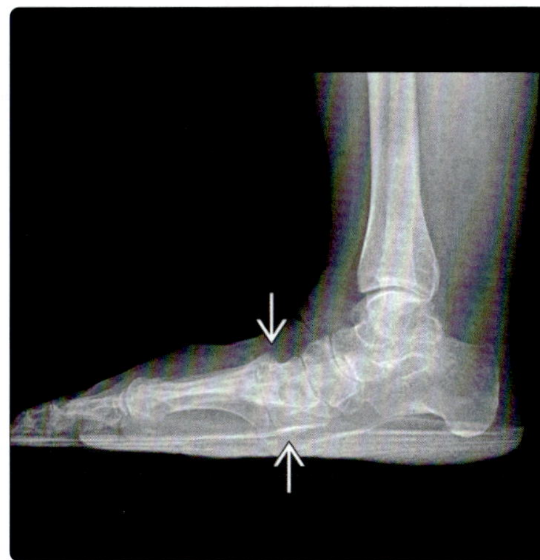

(Left) *AP radiograph shows a posttraumatic Lisfranc fracture subluxation, with lateral subluxation of the 2nd MT relative to middle cuneiform ➔, as well as 3rd MT relative to the lateral cuneiform ↪. The injury went unnoticed and was not treated.* **(Right)** *Lateral radiograph, same patient, shows a midfoot sag ➔ and forefoot pronation, resulting in pes planus. Note that the hindfoot is normal. Untreated Lisfranc injury may result in midfoot collapse and pes planus.*

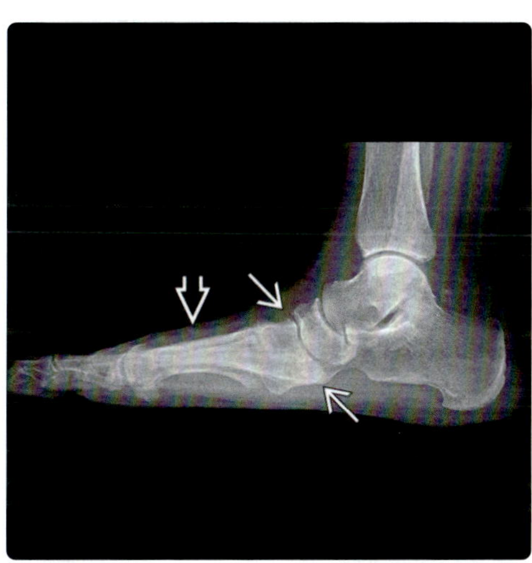

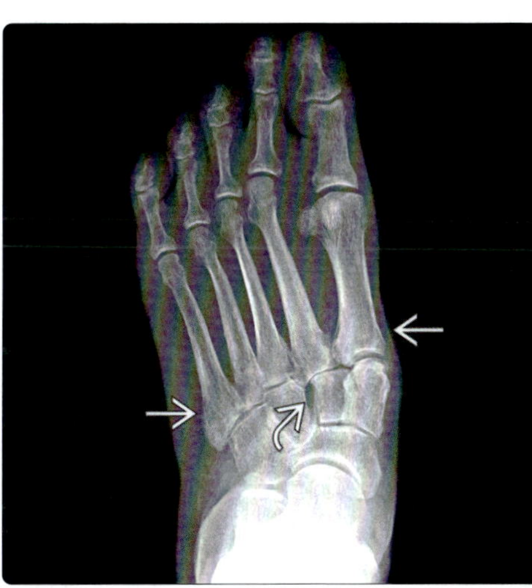

(Left) *Lateral radiograph shows a flatfoot deformity due to Marfan disease; note the arachnodactyly. There is forefoot pronation, with complete overlap of the metatarsals ⇨. There is a sag of the midfoot, with the apex at the naviculocuneiform joint ➔. The hindfoot is normal.* **(Right)** *AP radiograph, same case, shows pronation of the forefoot, indicated by the ↓ convergence of the bases of metatarsals ➔. There is also a gap between cuneiforms ↪. Again, the hindfoot appears normal.*

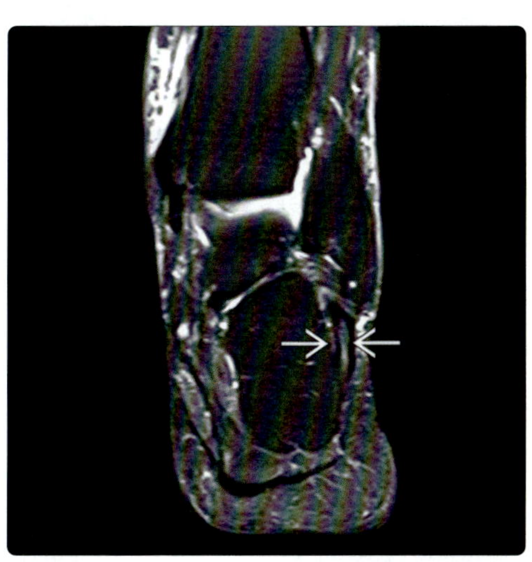

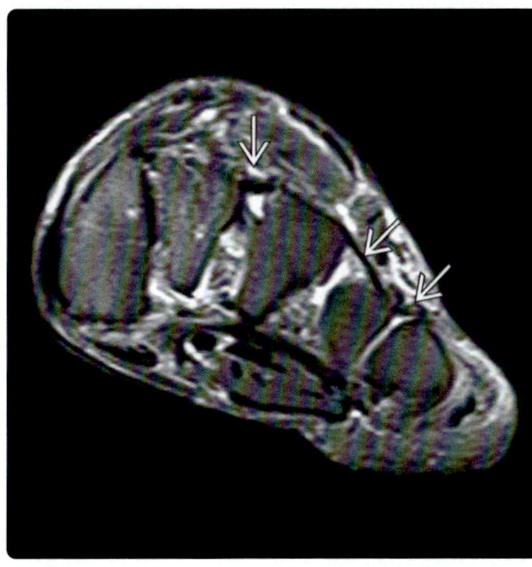

(Left) *Coronal T2WI FS MR of this case of Marfan disease shows a wide split in the peroneus longus tendon ➔. In other cuts, the PTT tendon was abnormal as well (not shown).* **(Right)** *Coronal T2WI FS MR, more anteriorly, shows the intercuneiform and intermetatarsal ligaments are stretched ➔, allowing an abnormal gap to form between cuneiforms and metatarsals. This matches the gap seen on radiograph. The collagen abnormality in Marfan disease allows ligament and tendon laxity and resultant pes planus.*

Club Foot (Talipes Equinovarus)

KEY FACTS

TERMINOLOGY

- Congenital fixed-foot deformity consisting of hindfoot equinus and varus plus forefoot varus

IMAGING

- Idiopathic congenital: 50% bilateral
- **Radiographs must be weight-bearing**
- Hindfoot equinus
  - Calcaneotibial angle > 90°
  - Calcaneal pitch is negative
- Hindfoot varus: Decrease in talocalcaneal angle
  - Lateral talocalcaneal (Kite) angle < 23° in newborn, < 30° in adult
  - AP talocalcaneal angle < 27° in newborn, < 25° in adult
- Forefoot varus, adducted and supinated
  - Lateral: Metatarsals appear stacked
  - AP: Increased convergence at metatarsal bases with adducted metatarsals
- MR useful to assess nonossified bone position
- MRA: Evaluate anterior tibial artery
  - Hypoplastic or absent in 85% if severe clubfeet
- Prenatal US: Abnormal orientation of foot and ankle
  - Coronal metatarsals in same plane as leg bones
  - Plantarflexed foot appears short
  - Bilateral clubfoot: 60% have other abnormalities
  - Up to 15% false-positive on prenatal US

PATHOLOGY

- Family history of club foot in 24%
- Siblings: 30x increased risk

CLINICAL ISSUES

- Associated anomalies in 50-60%
  - Chronic oligohydramnios
  - Spina bifida (24% have clubfoot)
  - Arthrogryposis akinesia deformation sequence
  - Myotonic dystrophy
- M > F (2-3:1); 1-2 per 1,000 live births

(Left) *Lateral radiograph shows hindfoot varus deformity in a patient with clubfoot. The longitudinal axes of the talus ➡ and calcaneus ➡ are nearly parallel, measuring 0°; normal talocalcaneal angle in this plane is 23-55° in a newborn.* **(Right)** *AP radiograph in the same patient shows near parallelism of the talus ➡ and calcaneus ➡ (angle of 5°), indicating hindfoot varus. The normal AP talocalcaneal angle measures 27-56° in the newborn.*

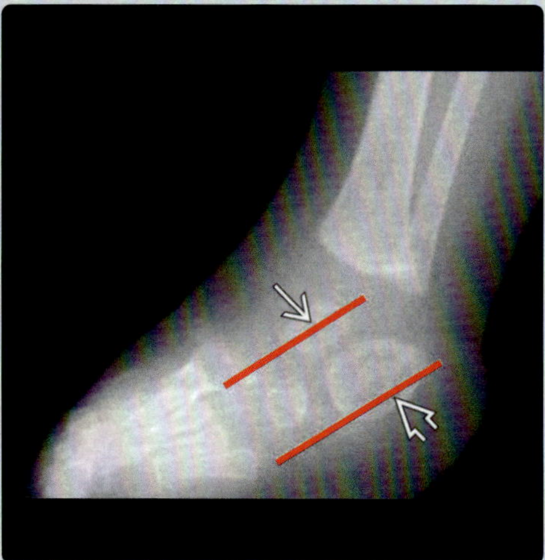

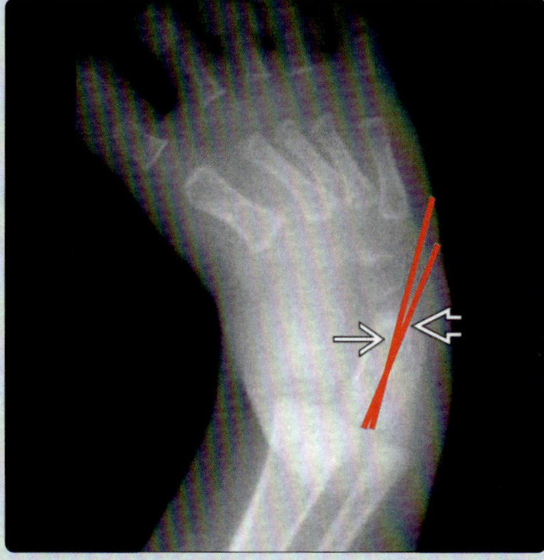

(Left) *Lateral radiograph shows the typical forefoot deformity of clubfoot. The foot is in simulated weight-bearing. The metatarsals appear stacked, without any significant overlap. The 1st metatarsal ➡ is in the dorsal-most position, and the 5th metatarsal (circled) is in the plantar-most position.* **(Right)** *AP radiograph in the same case shows the forefoot deformity typical of clubfoot. The metatarsals are adducted and show increased convergence (overlap) at their bases, as shown by the bisecting lines.*

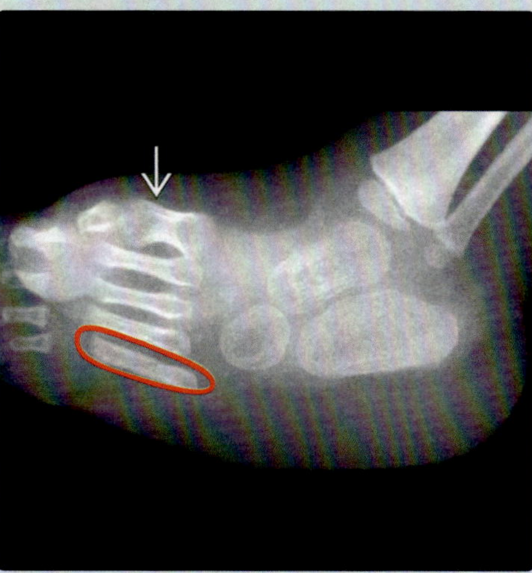

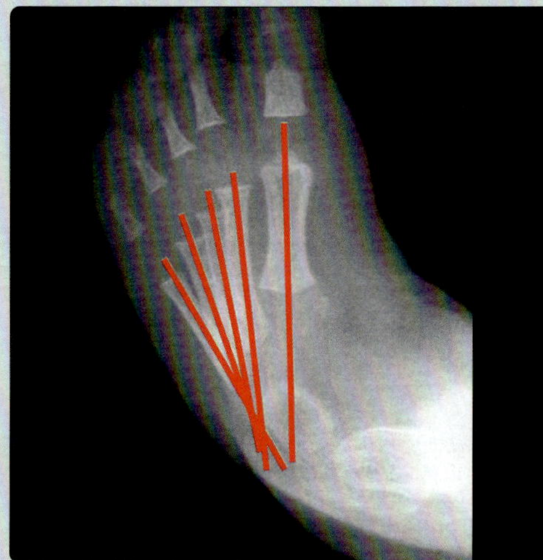

Club Foot (Talipes Equinovarus)

TERMINOLOGY

Definitions

- Congenital fixed foot deformity consisting of
  - Hindfoot equinus (plantarflexion of calcaneus relative to tibia)
  - Inversion of calcaneus relative to talus (hindfoot varus)
  - Adduction and supination of metatarsals (forefoot varus)

IMAGING

General Features

- Location
  - May be bilateral or unilateral
    - Idiopathic congenital: 50% bilateral

Imaging Recommendations

- Best imaging tool
  - Diagnosed by prenatal US or on weight-bearing radiographs

Radiographic Findings

- **Radiographs must be weight-bearing** (simulated in infant)
- Hindfoot equinus
  - Fixed plantarflexion of calcaneus
    - Calcaneotibial angle > 90°
    - Calcaneal pitch is negative
- Hindfoot varus: Decrease in talocalcaneal angle
  - Talus and calcaneus appear nearly parallel to one another on both AP and lateral radiographs
    - Lateral talocalcaneal (Kite) angle < 23° in newborn, < 30° in adult
      - Generally -10° to 20° in clubfoot
    - AP talocalcaneal angle < 27° in newborn, < 25° in adult
      - Generally 0-10° in clubfoot
- Forefoot varus, metatarsals adducted and supinated
  - Lateral: Metatarsals appear stacked
    - 5th metatarsal in plantar-most position
  - AP: Increased convergence at metatarsal bases
    - Metatarsals adducted
- Hindfoot-midfoot malalignment
  - Talonavicular joint: Medial subluxation of navicular on talus
  - Calcaneocuboid joint: Medial subluxation of cuboid on calcaneus
- Corrected clubfoot has altered appearance
  - Achilles lengthening reduces equinus deformity
  - May develop rocker-bottom deformity if equinus not corrected
  - Navicular may appear wedged, mildly subluxated
  - Usually some residual hindfoot and forefoot varus
  - Associated distal tibial abnormalities following surgery
    - Anteflexion in 48%
    - Valgus deformity in 56%
    - Abnormal lateral talocalcaneal angle in 42%
    - Flattened talar dome

CT Findings

- Reformatted and 3D useful in older children for surgical planning

MR Findings

- Useful to assess nonossified bone position
- Assessment of arteries
  - Anterior tibial artery hypoplastic or absent in 85% of patients with severe clubfoot
  - Sporadic reports of absent posterior tibial artery

Ultrasonographic Findings

- Clubfoot develops in 1st trimester
- Most recognized on prenatal US
- Abnormal orientation of foot and ankle
  - Coronally aligned metatarsals seen in same plane as coronal tibia/fibula
- Plantarflexed foot appears short
  - Normal foot length = femur length
- Bilateral clubfoot: 60% have other abnormalities
  - Up to 15% false-positive on prenatal US
- Unilateral clubfoot: 40% have other anomalies
  - Up to 29% false-positive on prenatal US
- Associated anomalies in 50-60%
  - Chronic oligohydramnios
  - Spina bifida (24% have clubfoot)
  - Arthrogryposis akinesia deformation sequence
    - Multiple limb contractures
    - Intrauterine growth restriction
    - Polyhydramnios
  - Myotonic dystrophy

DIFFERENTIAL DIAGNOSIS

Congenital Vertical Talus

- Superficial similarity because of hindfoot equinus
- Differentiated by hindfoot and forefoot valgus, dislocated talonavicular joint

Metatarsus Adductus

- Adducted forefoot, no equinus or varus deformity
- Common abnormality, self-correcting

Rocker-Bottom Foot

- Foreshortened, plantar convex foot (Persian slipper)
- May be associated with prior clubfoot repair
- 70% bilateral
- Association with trisomy 18

Vertical Calcaneus in Myelodysplasia

- Calcaneus is vertical; forefoot does not contact plantar surface
- Heel ulceration
- Decreased knee extension

Congenital Diastasis Distal Tibiofibular Joint

- Talus wedged between tibia and fibula

PATHOLOGY

General Features

- Etiology
  - Likely multifactorial; possible contributing factors
    - Ligamentous imbalance 2° to defective connective tissue
    - Muscle imbalance

- Intrauterine positional deformity
- Persistence of early normal fetal relationship
- Fetal akinesia deformation sequence seen with
  - Arthrogryposis
  - Amyoplasia
  - Pena-Shokeir syndrome, type 1
- Intrauterine growth retardation
- Polyhydramnios
- Oligohydramnios (renal hypoplasia)
- Following amniocentesis performed during 77-90 days' gestation
- Spinal dysraphism, sacral agenesis
- Fetal muscle disease: Myotonic dystrophy

- Genetics
  - Family history of clubfoot in 24%
  - Siblings: 30x increased risk
    - Monozygotic twins: 33% risk of both being affected
    - Dizygotic twins: 3% risk of both being affected
- Associated abnormalities
  - Trisomy 18: Clubfoot in 23% (rocker bottom in 10%)
  - Trisomy 21: Clubfoot usually bilateral

Staging, Grading, & Classification

- Classified as
  - Idiopathic congenital
  - Teratologic
    - Myelodysplasia
    - Arthrogryposis
    - Amyoplasia
  - Syndromic
    - Diastrophic dysplasia
    - Larson syndrome
    - Craniocarpotarsal dysplasia (Freeman-Sheldon syndrome)
    - Wolf-Hirschhorn syndrome
    - Antley-Bixler syndrome
  - Acquired
    - Cerebral palsy: Onset after birth, often after 5 years of age
    - Present in 22% hemiplegic, 8% diplegic, 8% quadriplegic cerebral palsy patients

CLINICAL ISSUES

Presentation

- Most common signs/symptoms
  - Foot deformity
  - Underdeveloped calf muscles
  - Stiffness of ankle and foot

Demographics

- Gender
  - M > F (2-3:1)
- Ethnicity
  - Polynesians > > Caucasians > Chinese
- Epidemiology
  - 1-2 per 1,000 births

Natural History & Prognosis

- If mild or adequately treated, residual asymmetry
  - Foot foreshortened (average 1.6 cm)
  - Limb shortened (average 0.6 cm)
  - Decreased calf circumference (average 2.5 cm)

Treatment

- Idiopathic clubfoot
  - Birth to 3-12 months
    - Ponseti method: Serial manipulation and corrective casting
      - Corrects forefoot and hindfoot varus initially, followed by equinus
      - 78% excellent or good results
    - Other methods of stretching and manipulation: French, Kite, and Lovell
    - Botulinum toxin injection to relax muscles
  - May require more significant surgical correction
    - Generally after 3-12 months
    - Combination of soft tissue releases, osteotomies, tendon transfers
      - Medial plantar release: Abductor hallucis, flexor hallucis longus and brevis, peroneus longus attachments, relaxing incisions of calcaneocuboid and medial talocalcaneal joint capsules, division of posterior tibial tendon slips to cuneiforms and metatarsal bases 2-4
      - Posterior release: Z-plasty of Achilles, relaxing incision of posterior talocalcaneal and tibiotalar joints, division of calcaneofibular and posterior talofibular ligaments
      - Lateral release to rotate calcaneus laterally: Talonavicular and calcaneocuboid capsulotomy, division of lateral talocalcaneal interosseous ligament
      - Reduction of osseous structures, pinning
  - Persistent severe hindfoot deformities may require triple arthrodesis
    - 68% excellent or good results
- Nonidiopathic clubfoot treatment
  - Generally requires more procedures, with generally less satisfactory results
- Myelodysplastic clubfoot
  - Treatment goal: Plantigrade foot that can be braced and is free of pain and ulceration
  - Charcot arthropathy may be complication

DIAGNOSTIC CHECKLIST

Consider

- Do not attempt to evaluate congenital foot deformities on nonweight-bearing radiographs
- Foot deformities seen in adult patients may not follow rules of angular measurement since they may be postoperative and partially corrected
- Beware of tendency to overcall clubfoot in prenatal US

SELECTED REFERENCES

1. Atanda AA et al: Prognostic Value of the Radiologic Appearance of the Navicular Ossification Center in Congenital Talipes Equinovarus. J Foot Ankle Surg. 54(5):844-7, 2015
2. Burghardt RD et al: Growth Disturbance of the Distal Tibia in Patients With Idiopathic Clubfeet: Ankle Valgus and Anteflexion of the Distal Tibia. J Pediatr Orthop. ePub, 2015

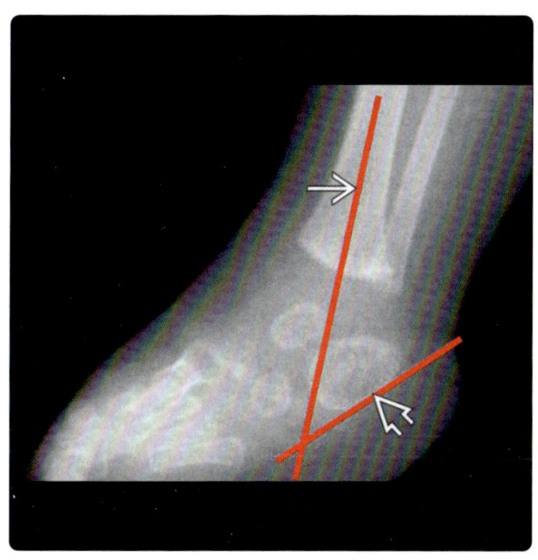

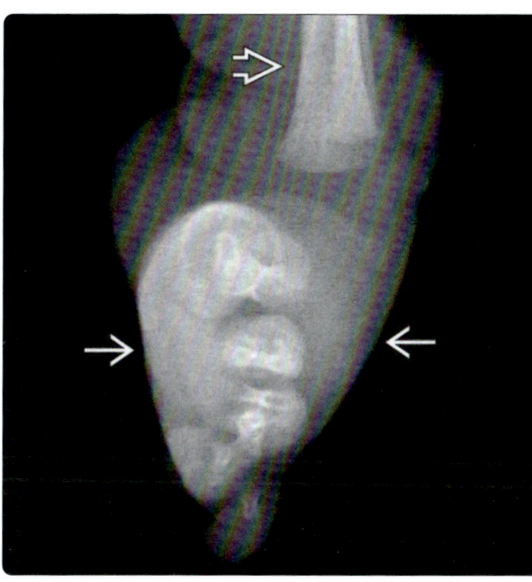

(Left) *Lateral radiograph shows a typical equinus deformity of clubfoot. The foot is in simulated weight-bearing position; no further dorsiflexion was possible. The angle formed by line bisecting the tibia ➡ and line extending along the base of calcaneus ➡ is > 90°, indicating equinus.* **(Right)** *AP oblique radiograph of the ankle shows almost 90° inversion of plantar aspect of foot ➡ relative to long axis of tibia ➡ in a 5-day-old infant.*

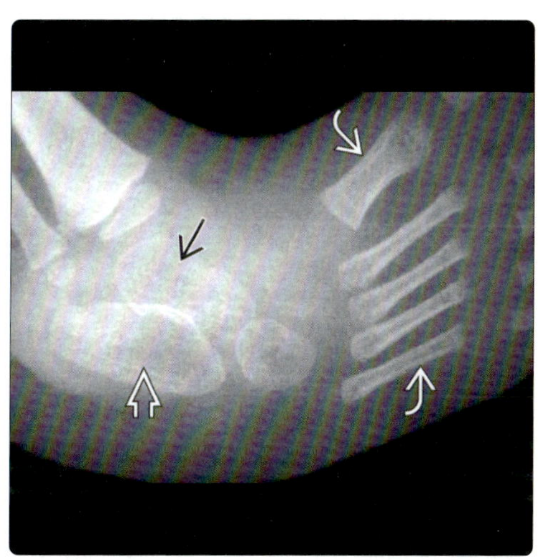

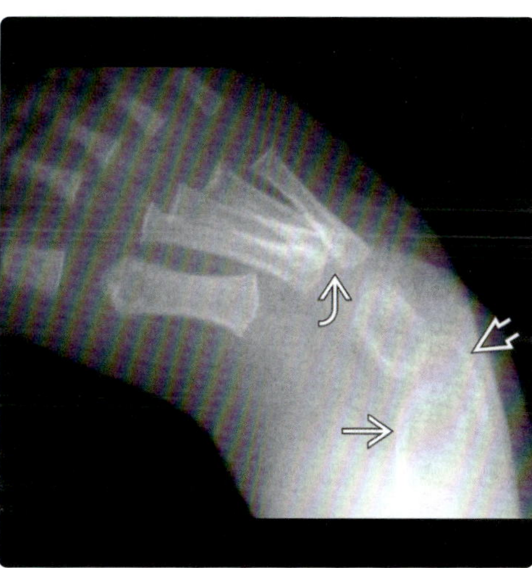

(Left) *Lateral radiograph of a young child's foot in simulated weight-bearing position shows equinus of the calcaneus ➡ (excessive plantar flexion). Note the parallelism of the talus ➡ and calcaneus, indicating hindfoot varus. The forefoot shows stacked metatarsals ➡.* **(Right)** *AP radiograph confirms near parallelism of the talus ➡ and calcaneus ➡ (hindfoot varus). Metatarsals show overconvergence at the bases ➡ (forefoot varus with supination) and adduction.*

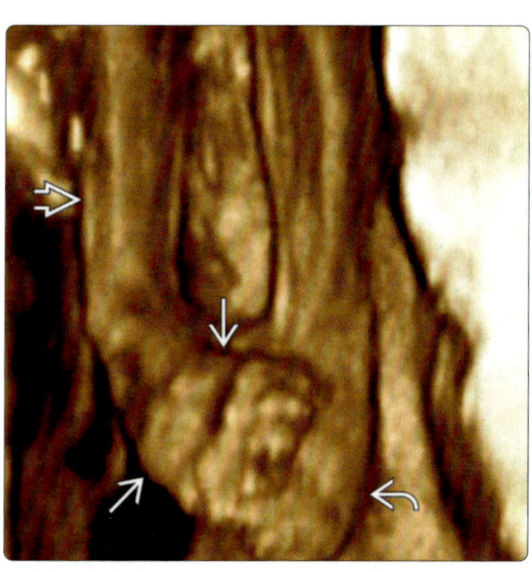

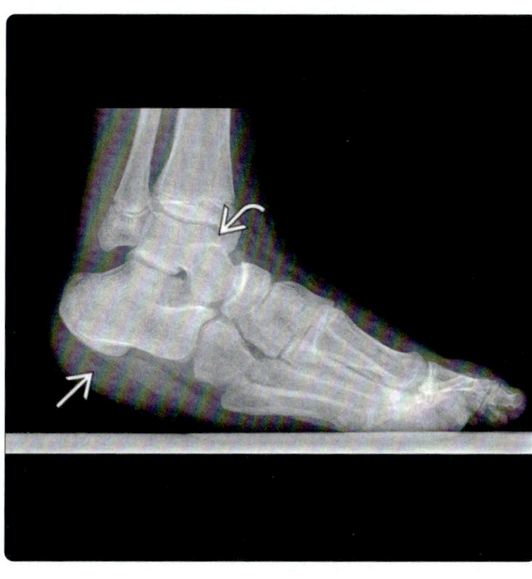

(Left) *3D reformation prenatal US shows bilateral clubfoot, with a coronal plane of the adducted forefoot ➡ seen on the same image as the coronal plane of the leg bones ➡. The contralateral foot is plantarflexed ➡ and adducted.* **(Right)** *Lateral radiograph of an incompletely corrected clubfoot shows that the calcaneal equinus has not been corrected ➡. The result is a rocker bottom deformity. Note that the dome of the talus ➡ appears rather flattened. There is residual hindfoot and forefoot varus.*

Congenital Vertical Talus (Rocker-Bottom Foot)

KEY FACTS

TERMINOLOGY

- Rigid foot deformity with convex plantar surface (rocker-bottom foot)

IMAGING

- **Radiographs must be weight-bearing**
- Hindfoot equinus
  - Plantarflexion of calcaneus such that anterior calcaneotibial angle > 90° or calcaneal pitch is negative
- Severe plantarflexion of talus
  - Dislocated from navicular
  - Apex of rocker bottom is head of navicular
- Hindfoot valgus
  - Lateral talocalcaneal angle (Kite) > 55° in newborn, > 50° in adult
  - AP talocalcaneal angle > 56° in newborn, > 45° in adult
- Forefoot pronated and valgus
  - Lateral: Metatarsals superimposed, 1st in plantar-most position
  - AP: Divergence of bases of metatarsals
- MRA: May show absence of posterior tibial artery
- US: May visualize alignment of nonossified navicular relative to talus in newborn

TOP DIFFERENTIAL DIAGNOSES

- Corrected clubfoot
  - May appear to be rocker bottom but has residual hindfoot and forefoot varus
- Malunited calcaneal fracture
  - Will have decreased Boehler angle

PATHOLOGY

- May be isolated; 50% associated with various syndromes or genetic abnormalities
  - Meningomyelocele
  - Arthrogryposis
  - Sacral agenesis
- Trisomy 18 is most common genetic association

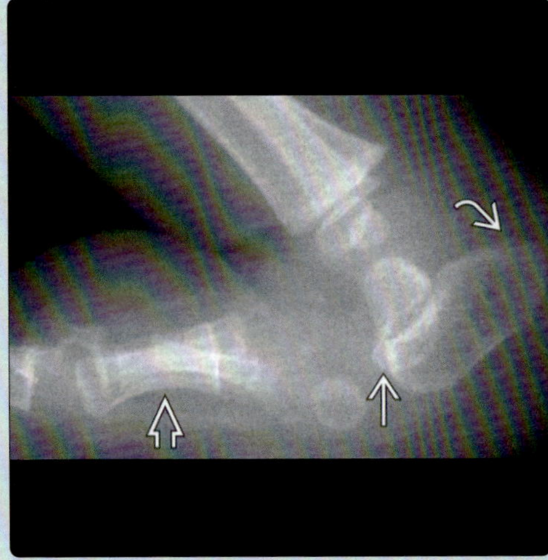

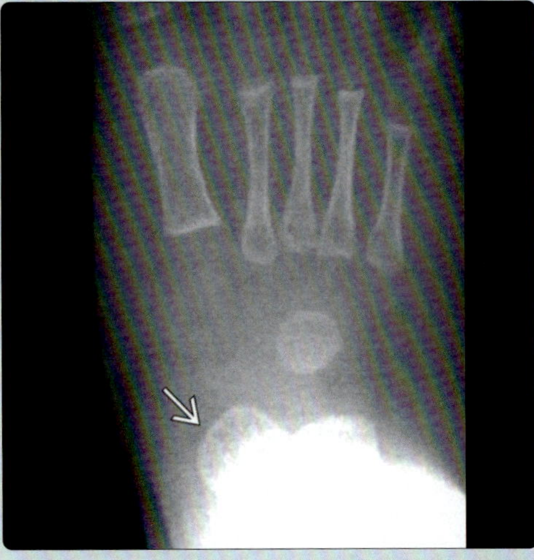

(Left) *Lateral radiograph is classic for the diagnosis of congenital vertical talus. The elements include calcaneus equinus ➡, plantarflexion of the talus ➡ (dislocated from the navicular, which is not yet ossified) resulting in hindfoot valgus, and forefoot valgus/pronation ➡.* **(Right)** *AP radiograph shows hindfoot valgus, with the talus angled medially ➡ relative to the 1st metatarsal, and increased talocalcaneal angle. It shows lack of convergence of the bases of the metatarsals, indicating forefoot pronation/valgus.*

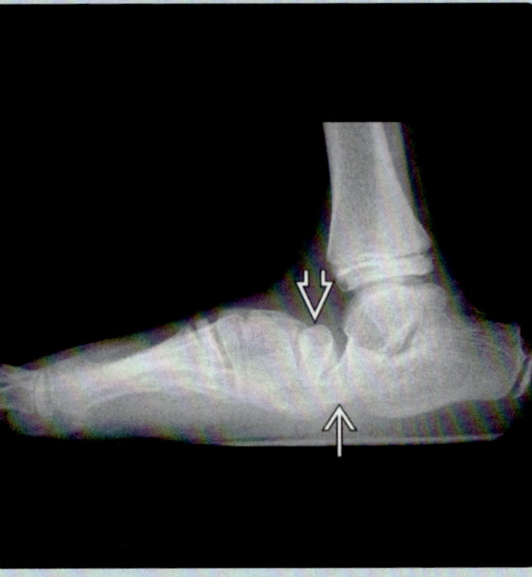

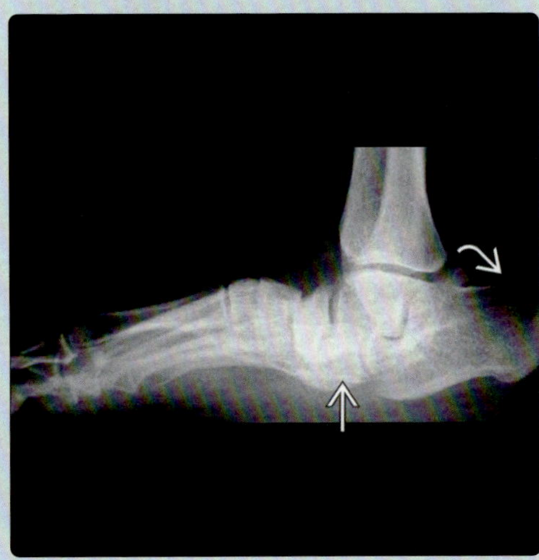

(Left) *Lateral radiograph shows a mild equinus (plantarflexion of the calcaneus). There is also significant plantarflexion of the talus ➡, with dislocation from the navicular ➡. There is pronation and valgus of the forefoot. These features make the diagnosis of congenital vertical talus. It is a rigid deformity.* **(Right)** *Lateral radiograph in an adult shows congenital vertical talus, with calcaneus equinus ➡, severe plantarflexion of the talus ➡ (with talonavicular dislocation), and forefoot pronation.*

KEY FACTS

TERMINOLOGY

- Deformities that have in common a high longitudinal arch of foot
  - Deformity may occur at hindfoot, midfoot, forefoot, or combination
  - May be fixed or relatively flexible

IMAGING

- Hindfoot abnormality that contributes to pes cavus: Dorsiflexion of calcaneus
  - Calcaneotibial angle < 60°
  - Calcaneal pitch > 30°
  - Generally results in rotated talus and abnormal profile on lateral radiograph
  - May have associated varus or valgus (less common) deformity
- Forefoot abnormalities that contribute to pes cavus
  - Plantarflexion of metatarsals ± varus deformity
  - Claw toe deformities

PATHOLOGY

- Idiopathic (20%): Nonprogressive
- Trauma
  - Malunion of calcaneal or talar fracture
  - Burn
  - Sequela of compartment syndrome
  - Chinese bound foot
- Residual clubfoot deformity following surgical treatment
- Neuromuscular (imbalance of intrinsic and extrinsic muscles ± contraction of plantar fascia)
  - Muscular dystrophy (MD)
  - Charcot-Marie-Tooth (CMT): Cavovarus deformity
  - Spinal dysraphism, spinal cord injury: High arch, claw toes
  - Poliomyelitis: Weak gastrocnemius
  - Cerebral palsy: Equinovalgus hindfoot most common, often with forefoot varus
- Genetics: CMT is most common inherited neurological disorder

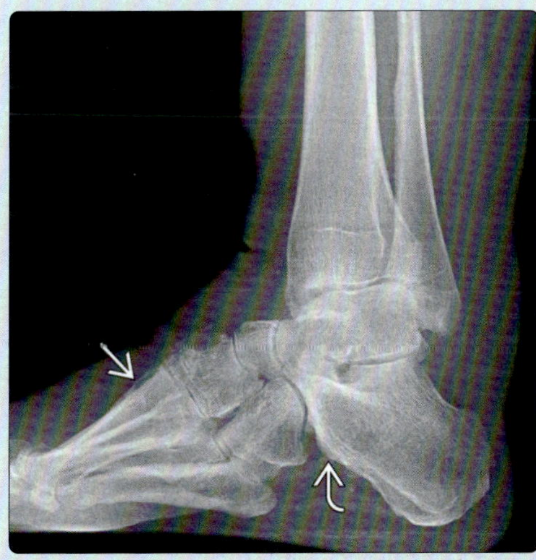

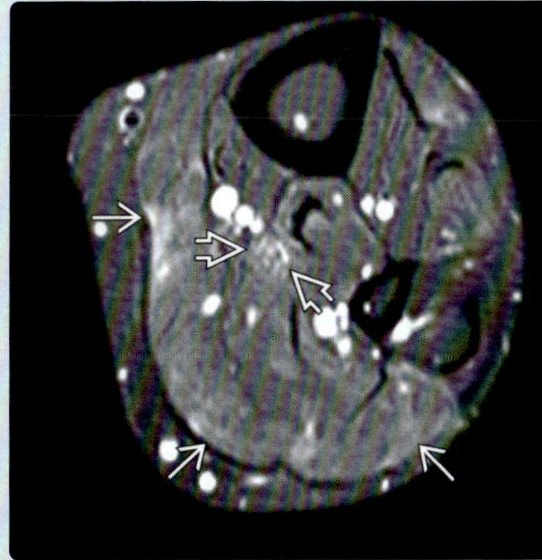

(Left) *Lateral radiograph shows the typical CMT cavovarus foot. There is excessive dorsiflexion of the calcaneus ➡. The forefoot is in varus, seen as supination, with ↓ overlap of the metatarsal bases and ↑ inclination angle of the 1st metatarsal ➡.* **(Right)** *Axial PD FS MR shows denervation edema of all the muscles, particularly in the posterior compartment ➡. There is also hyperintensity and enlargement of the tibial nerve fascicles ➡. This is typical of CMT, though there may be variations.*

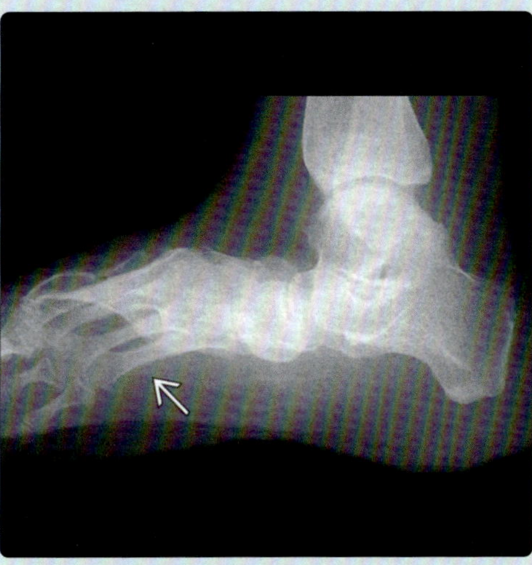

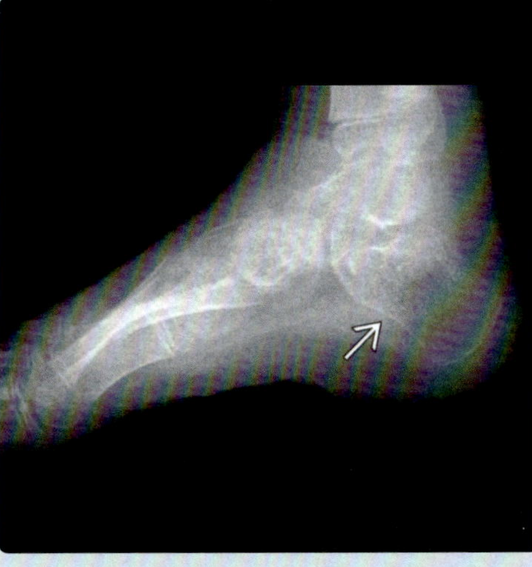

(Left) *Lateral radiograph in a patient with polio shows pes cavus formed by both hindfoot and forefoot abnormalities. The dorsiflexed calcaneus with hindfoot valgus partly contributes to the deformity, as does the varus forefoot ➡ with plantarflexed metatarsals. This combination of varus and valgus deformity is often seen in neuromuscular diseases.* **(Right)** *Lateral radiograph shows a cavus foot deformity and diffuse osteopenia. Note the high calcaneal pitch ➡ and atrophied soft tissues in this child with muscular dystrophy.*

KEY FACTS

TERMINOLOGY

- Abnormal bridging between tarsal bones, usually 2° to failure of embryological segmentation
  - Bridging may be osseous, cartilaginous, or fibrous

IMAGING

- Calcaneonavicular (CN) ~ 45%
- Talocalcaneal (TC) ~ 45%
  - Intraarticular: Usually entire middle facet
  - Extraarticular: Usually involves interval at posterior margin of sustentaculum and talus
- Widespread coalition: Rare
- Morphology of involved articulation is altered
  - Joint morphology is broadened
  - Articular surfaces irregular if coalition not bony
  - Orientation of joint may be altered
- Direct visualization of coalition on radiograph
  - Calcaneonavicular seen best on internal oblique
  - Talocalcaneal coalition limited to middle facet seen best on axial view of calcaneus (Harris Beath)
- Indirect signs of coalition on radiograph
  - Talar beak on dorsum of talus
  - Anteater sign: Elongated anterior process of calcaneus, suggesting calcaneonavicular coalition
  - C sign: Sclerosis in an inverted C shape on lateral
- Ball and socket joint
- Directly visualized and best characterized on MR or CT

CLINICAL ISSUES

- Discovered during adolescence or young adulthood
- 1% of population (likely an underestimate)

DIAGNOSTIC CHECKLIST

- 25% bilateral, even if clinical suspicion is unilateral
- Since direct visualization of single site coalitions is not possible on 2-view radiographs (AP and lateral), watch for subtle 2° signs

(Left) *Lateral radiograph shows elongation of the anterior process of the calcaneus ➔. There is a subchondral cyst formation ➔ as well. Although the calcaneonavicular coalition is not directly seen, it can be inferred from these findings.* **(Right)** *Axial NECT (bone window) in the same case shows the CN joint on the left to be broadened and irregular as well as sclerotic ➔, while the normal right side is shown for comparison ➔. The altered morphology is typical; the coalition is fibrous.*

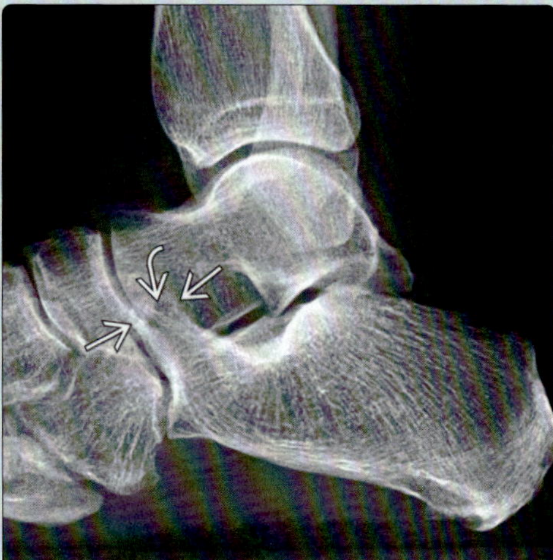

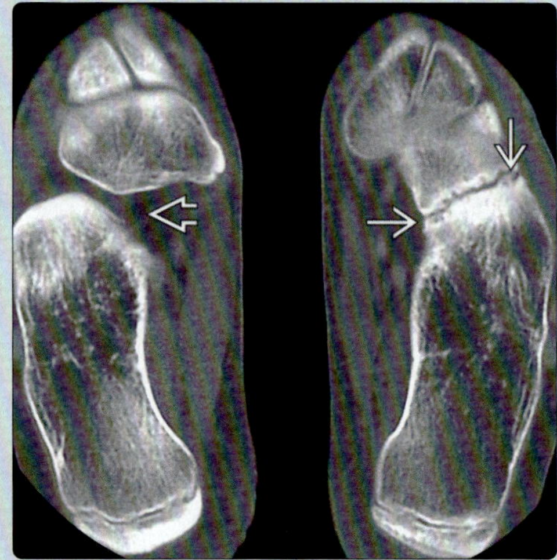

(Left) *Sagittal T1WI MR shows a CN coalition. There is a small talar beak ➔, indicating abnormal motion at the talonavicular joint. The cause of that abnormal motion is seen on the same image, as a CN coalition ➔.* **(Right)** *Axial T1WI MR in the same case shows the CN joint to be irregular and broad ➔, a typical coalition morphology. There is no bony bridging; this is a fibrous or cartilaginous coalition. Though MR does not show the bone in as exquisite detail as CT, it shows associated abnormalities better.*

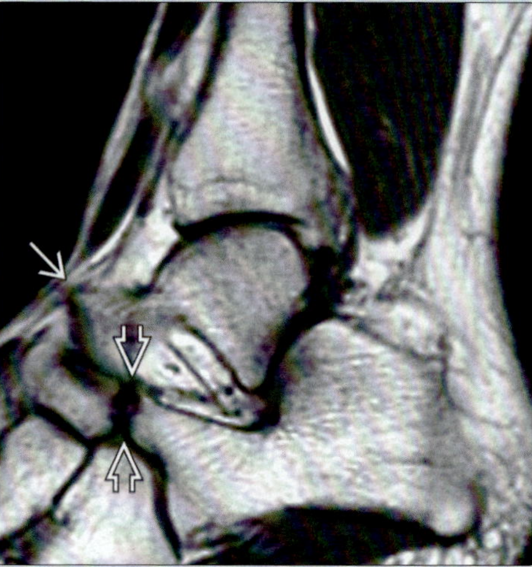

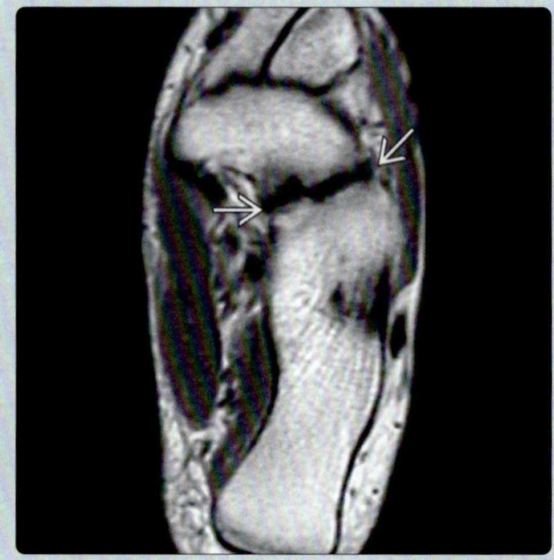

TERMINOLOGY

Synonyms

- Spastic peroneal flatfoot

Definitions

- Abnormal bridging between tarsal bones, usually 2° to failure of embryological segmentation
  - Bridging may be osseous, cartilaginous, or fibrous

IMAGING

General Features

- Best diagnostic clue
  - Secondary signs on radiograph of pes planus in teenager or young adult
    - Should stimulate search for other secondary signs: Talar beak, anteater, C signs
  - Direct visualization of broad, abnormal articulation on CT or MR
- Location
  - Most common articular coalitions (90%, ~ equal distribution between them)
    - Calcaneonavicular
    - Talocalcaneal, classified as intra- or extraarticular
      - Intraarticular: Usually entire middle facet
      - Extraarticular: Usually involves interval between posterior margin of sustentaculum and posteromedial process of talus
  - Widespread coalition: Rare
    - May involve majority of subtalar joint ± calcaneonavicular, talonavicular, calcaneocuboid joints
  - Bilateral in 25%
- Morphology
  - Morphology of involved articulation is altered
    - Joint is broadened
    - Articular surfaces irregular if coalition is not osseous
    - Joint orientation is altered (particularly medial talocalcaneal coalition, with tilt of middle facet toward posterior facet)

Radiographic Findings

- Direct visualization of coalition
  - Calcaneonavicular seen best on internal oblique
  - Talocalcaneal coalition limited to middle facet seen best on axial view of calcaneus (Harris Beath)
- Indirect signs of coalition
  - Talar beak on dorsum of talus, adjacent to articulation with navicular
  - Anteater sign: Elongated anterior process of calcaneus, suggesting calcaneonavicular coalition
  - C sign: Sclerosis in an inverted C shape on lateral view of calcaneus near angle of Gissane
- Pes planus in teenager or young adult
  - Fairly rigid; does not return to normal alignment on non-weight-bearing radiographs
- Ball-and-socket tibiotalar joint
  - With widespread coalition, talar dome assumes rounded shape
  - Ankle mortise accommodates ball of talus, forming a rounded socket; converts from expected hinge tibiotalar joint

CT Findings

- Mimic radiographic findings, with superior definition of location and extent of coalition
- Osseous bridging: Marrow and trabecular continuation across articulation
- Fibrous or cartilaginous bridging: Sclerosis, irregularity at articulation
  - Subchondral cysts may develop
- Secondary signs: Talar beak

MR Findings

- Morphologic abnormality at site of coalition
  - Articulation is broadened transversely, often significantly, at any site of coalition
  - Middle facet talocalcaneal coalition (most frequent)
    - Broadened, downsloping medial facet
  - Anterior facet talocalcaneal coalition: Rare
    - Usually associated with middle facet coalition
  - Posterior facet talocalcaneal coalition
    - Rare, usually cartilaginous
    - When isolated, may be incomplete, involving posteromedial aspect of posterior facet
    - Bony overgrowth may protrude into tarsal tunnel
  - Extraarticular talocalcaneal coalition
    - Located immediately posterior to sustentaculum
    - Normal or hypoplastic middle talocalcaneal facet
    - Broadening of posterior margins of sustentaculum and posteromedial talar process in both sagittal and coronal planes
    - May have osseous or fibrous protrusion into tarsal tunnel
- Osseous coalition
  - Osseous bridging, with trabeculae crossing coalition
    - High SI marrow on T1WI, gray SI on T2WI
    - Marrow suppression on STIR or FS sequences
  - Solid fusion precludes abnormal motion at coalition
    - No marrow edema seen at coalition if solid
- Fibrous/cartilaginous coalition
  - Irregular broadened articulation
  - Articular ends often sclerotic: Low SI all sequences
  - May see variable amounts of cartilaginous tissue
  - With motion, marrow edema occurs
    - ↓ SI on T1WI, ↑ SI on fluid-sensitive sequences
  - With enough abnormal motion across fibrous coalition, degenerative changes develop
    - Subchondral cyst formation, sclerosis
- Alignment abnormality of hindfoot
  - Coronal may show valgus tilt of calcaneus
- Secondary abnormalities
  - Beaking of dorsal talus
    - May see as edema within a small excrescence
    - If mature, beak contains normal marrow signal
  - Osseous edema at sites of abnormal motion
    - Most common: Talus and navicular, along talonavicular joint
  - Occasional ganglion formation (cystic appearance)
    - May decompress into tarsal tunnel or tarsal sinus
  - Ligamentous thickening from abnormal motion at joints adjacent to fused joints
  - Inflammatory change adjacent to fibrous unions

- Sinus tarsus with adjacent fibrous coalition

Imaging Recommendations

- Best imaging tool
  - Radiographic diagnosis; best characterized on MR or CT
- Protocol advice
  - Reformatted CT: Reformat perpendicular to coalition site
  - Acquire images of both feet simultaneously to check for bilateral abnormalities

DIFFERENTIAL DIAGNOSIS

Pes Planus (Flatfoot)

- Flexible flatfoot: Valgus hindfoot and forefoot, reduced on non-weight-bearing images

Normal Variant: Medial Talocalcaneal Ligament

- Variably present (~ 2% ankles)
- Mimics fibrous extraarticular talocalcaneal coalition
- Originates from posteromedial process of talus and inserts onto posterior aspect of sustentaculum tali
- May be a narrow bundle or multifascicular
- Smooth cortical attachments, location, and absence of osseous deformity help distinguish from coalition

Normal Variant: Thickened Ligaments

- Anterior capsular ligament of posterior subtalar joint (thickening of anterior capsule, located just posterior to interosseous talocalcaneal ligament)
- Interosseous talocalcaneal ligament may mimic extraarticular fibrous talocalcaneal coalition on sagittal images

Normal Variant: Accessory Articular Facet

- Medial extension of articular margins: Facet located between posterior margin of sustentaculum and anteroinferior margin of posteromedial process of talus
- Anterior extension of articular margins: Base of anterior process of calcaneus and anterior margin of lateral process of talus and talar body

Arthrodesis

- Surgical subtalar fusion: Entire subtalar joint
  - Triple arthrodesis also fuses talonavicular and calcaneocuboid joints
- Screws/plates or their tracks will be visible

PATHOLOGY

General Features

- Etiology
  - Usually congenital, due to lack of segmentation during fetal development
    - Foot normally develops from block, which then segments into individual osseous elements
    - Coalition → decreased hindfoot/midfoot mobility
    - Decreased mobility of 1 segment promotes increased mobility at others (initially talonavicular)
    - Develops shortening with persistent or intermittent spasm of peroneal muscles
  - Rarely may be a part of syndromes
    - Hereditary symphalangism
    - Apert syndrome
    - Hand-foot-uterus syndrome

CLINICAL ISSUES

Presentation

- Most common signs/symptoms
  - May be asymptomatic or minimally painful
  - Painful, stiff flatfoot
  - Lateral leg pain from peroneal muscle spasm
  - ↓ hindfoot motion on clinical exam
  - Uncommonly may present with tarsal sinus or tarsal tunnel symptoms
  - Patients with bilateral involvement may present with unilateral symptoms
    - Always consider contralateral foot, whether or not symptomatic
    - Even if asymptomatic, contralateral foot may have minor morphologic abnormalities

Demographics

- Age
  - Discovered during adolescence or young adulthood
    - Present at birth, but symptoms develop later, coinciding with progressive coalition ossification
- Gender
  - Male > female (slight)
- Epidemiology
  - 1-13% of population by various reports

Natural History & Prognosis

- Progressive pain, stiffness

Treatment

- Conservative (orthotics, casting, NSAIDs)
- Surgical resection of coalition with fat or muscle interposition
- With failure of other treatment, triple arthrodesis

DIAGNOSTIC CHECKLIST

Consider

- 25% bilateral, even if clinical suspicion is unilateral
- Since direct visualization of single site coalitions may not be possible on 2-view radiographs (AP and lateral), watch for subtle 2° signs

SELECTED REFERENCES

1. Lawrence DA et al: Tarsal Coalitions: Radiographic, CT, and MR Imaging Findings. HSS J. 10(2):153-66, 2014
2. Bixby SD et al: Unilateral subtalar coalition: contralateral sustentaculum tali morphology. Radiology. 257(3):830-5, 2010
3. Sperl M et al: Preliminary report: resection and interposition of a deepithelialized skin flap graft in tarsal coalition in children. J Pediatr Orthop B. 19(2):171-6, 2010
4. Linklater J et al: Anatomy of the subtalar joint and imaging of talo-calcaneal coalition. Skeletal Radiol. 38(5):437-49, 2009
5. Mubarak SJ et al: Calcaneonavicular coalition: treatment by excision and fat graft. J Pediatr Orthop. 29(5):418-26, 2009
6. Yoo JH et al: Tarsal coalition as a cause of failed tarsal tunnel release for tarsal tunnel syndrome. Orthopedics. 32(4), 2009
7. Crim J: Imaging of tarsal coalition. Radiol Clin North Am. 46(6):1017-26, vi, 2008
8. Philbin TM et al: Results of resection for middle facet tarsal coalitions in adults. Foot Ankle Spec. 1(6):344-9, 2008

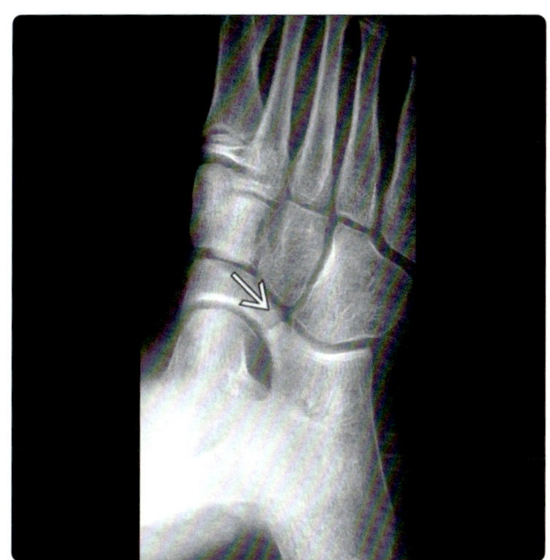

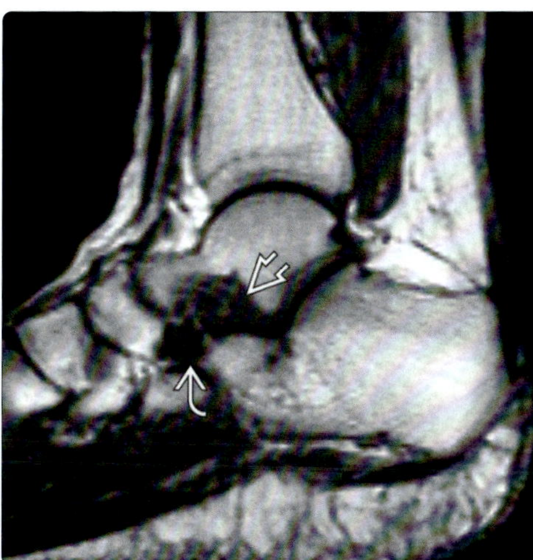

(Left) *AP oblique radiograph gives direct visualization of a calcaneonavicular coalition ➡. This is an osseous coalition; no sclerosis, fragmentation, or irregularity is seen.* **(Right)** *Sagittal T1WI MR shows extensive low signal and broadened morphology of a CN coalition ➡. There is an additional abnormality; low signal is seen replacing the expected fat within the tarsal sinus ➡. This suggests reactive change in the sinus tarsi, related to the adjacent coalition.*

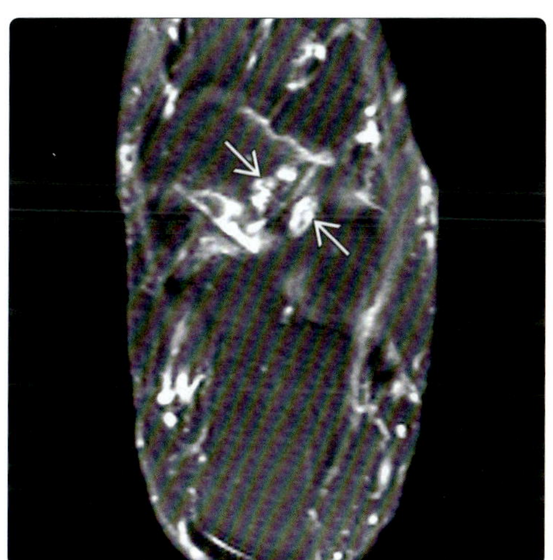

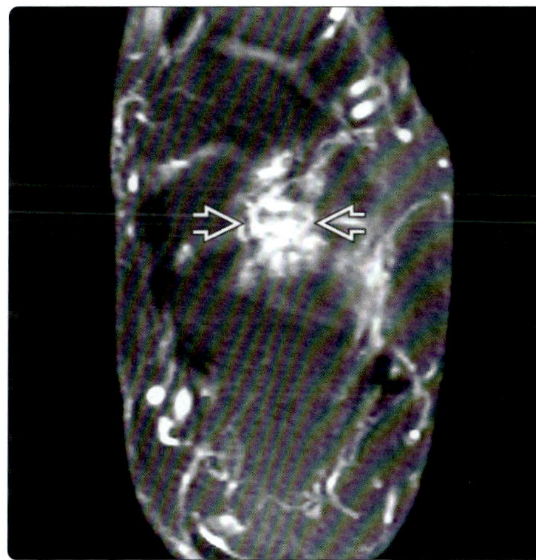

(Left) *Axial T2WI FS MR in the same case shows an abnormal, broad, and irregular calcaneonavicular joint. There is prominent subchondral cyst formation ➡; this is a fibrous coalition, which allows some abnormal motion and resultant degenerative changes.* **(Right)** *Axial T2WI FS MR in the same case shows the adjacent sinus tarsi with severe inflammatory change ➡ surrounding its ligaments. This patient's sinus tarsi syndrome developed secondary to the CN fibrous coalition.*

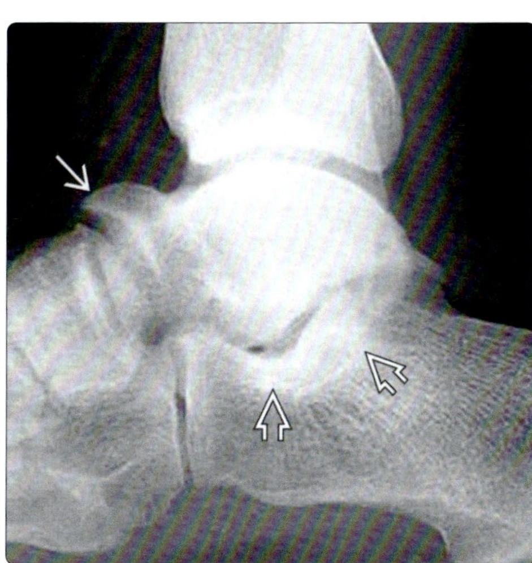

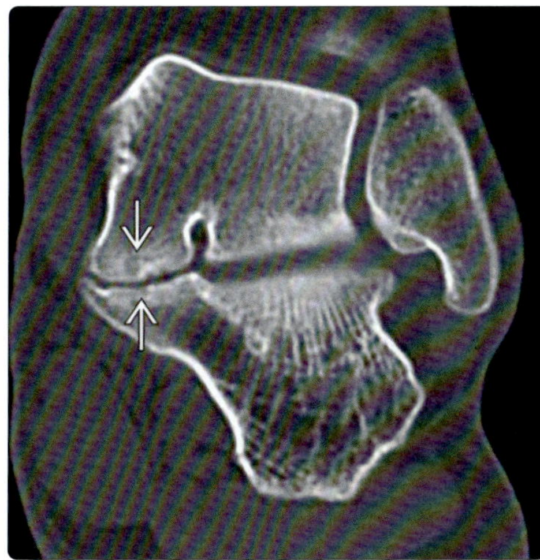

(Left) *Lateral radiograph is distinctly abnormal, showing a large talar beak ➡. There is C-shaped sclerosis at the subtalar joint ➡. Both findings are secondary signs of a talocalcaneal (TC) coalition.* **(Right)** *Axial oblique bone CT through the subtalar joint confirms the broad and irregular talocalcaneal joint ➡; there is no osseous bridging, and this is a fibrous or cartilaginous TC coalition. The medial facet of the subtalar joint is the most frequently involved in this type of coalition.*

(Left) *Sagittal bone CT shows an osseous fusion across the medial facet of the subtalar joint ➡, indicating talocalcaneal coalition. Note the normal posterior facet ➡ of the subtalar joint. There is a talar beak ➡, as is often seen as a secondary sign of TC coalition.* **(Right)** *Coronal bone CT in the same case confirms the fused medial facet of the subtalar joint ➡, while the posterior facet ➡ remains normal. This is a typical intraarticular TC coalition, which usually only involves the medial facet.*

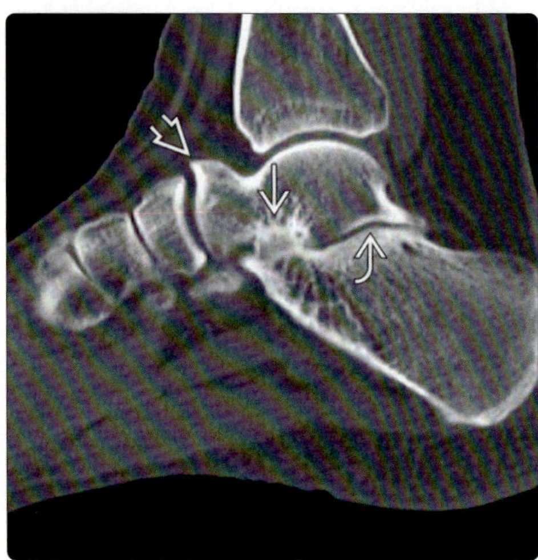

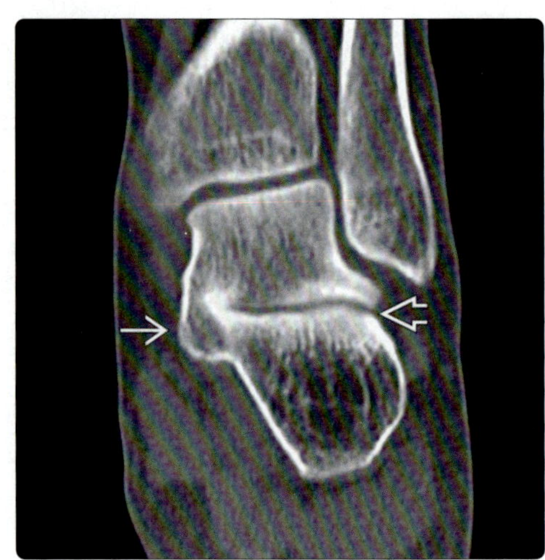

(Left) *Lateral radiograph shows a widely sclerotic C sign ➡ superimposed on the subtalar joint, indicating subtalar coalition. The absence of any hint of a talar beak is a bit unusual, but should not dissuade one from the proper diagnosis.* **(Right)** *Sagittal T2WI FS MR in the same case shows the extremely broad morphology of the medial facet ➡. There is no osseous fusion, and edema ➡ indicates some degree of motion. This is a fibrous subtalar coalition.*

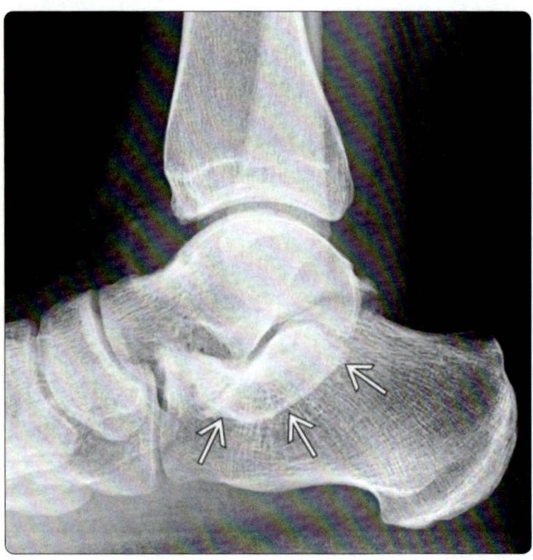

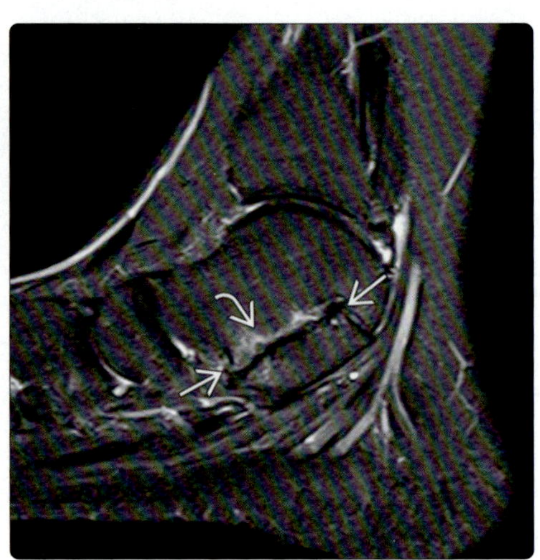

(Left) *Coronal T1WI MR in a different patient shows broadening and irregularity of the posterior sustentaculum talus and adjacent medial process of talus ➡. The plane cuts through the normal posterior facet ➡ of the subtalar joint.* **(Right)** *Sagittal T1WI MR, same case, shows the morphologic abnormality of the broadened bone ➡ located posterior to the medial facet of the subtalar joint. Since the medial facet ➡ is normal (though slightly hypoplastic), this represents extraarticular TC coalition. (Courtesy J. Linklater, MD.)*

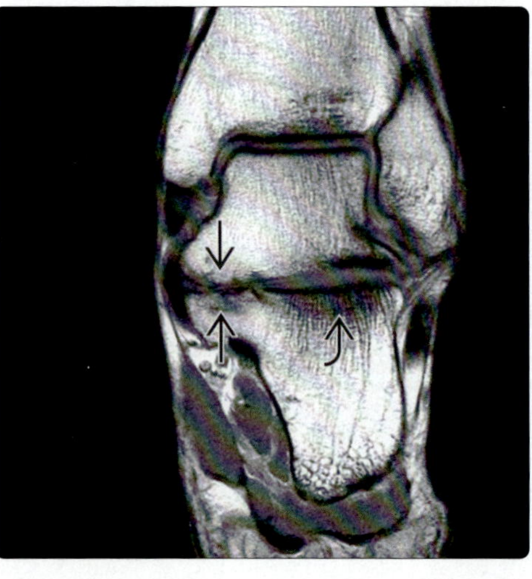

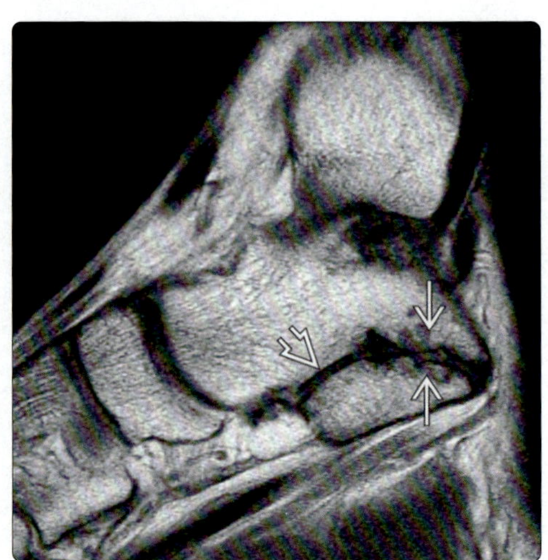

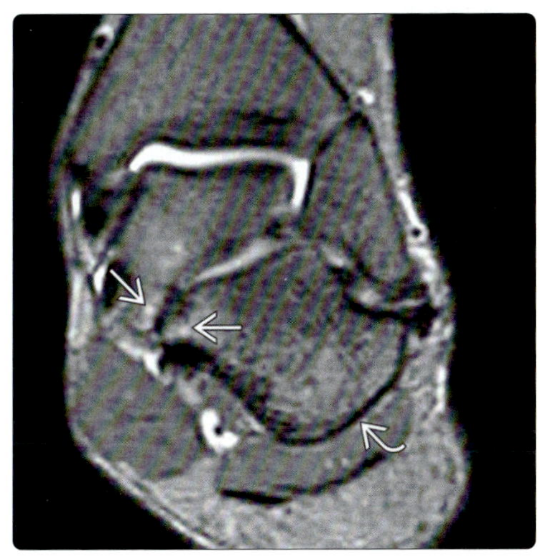

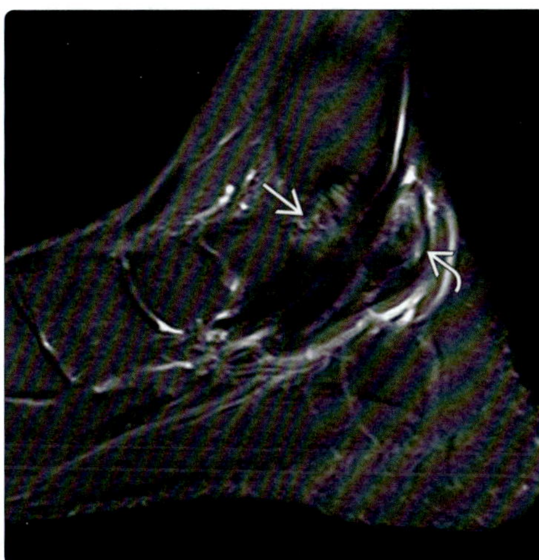

(Left) *Coronal PD FS MR shows a typical obliquely oriented talocalcaneal coalition ➡. Note the valgus pronated position of the calcaneus ➡. It is not surprising this patient presents with painful flatfoot.* **(Right)** *In a different patient, sagittal T2WI FS MR located far medially shows edema in the medial ST joint ➡. There is also a mixed signal "mass" ➡ located posterior to the flexor hallucis tendon. The patient presented with burning and tingling on the bottom of her foot.*

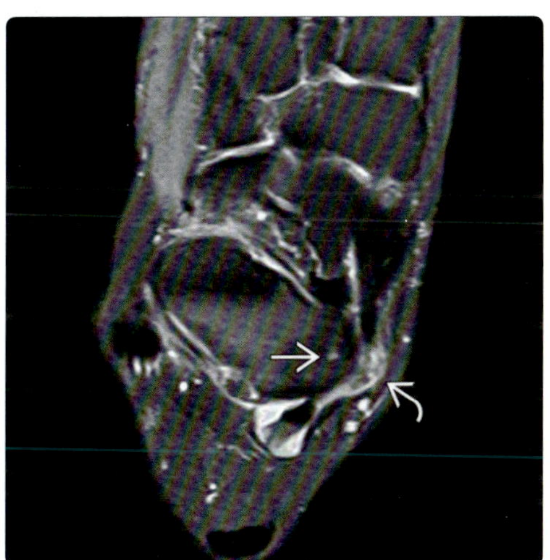

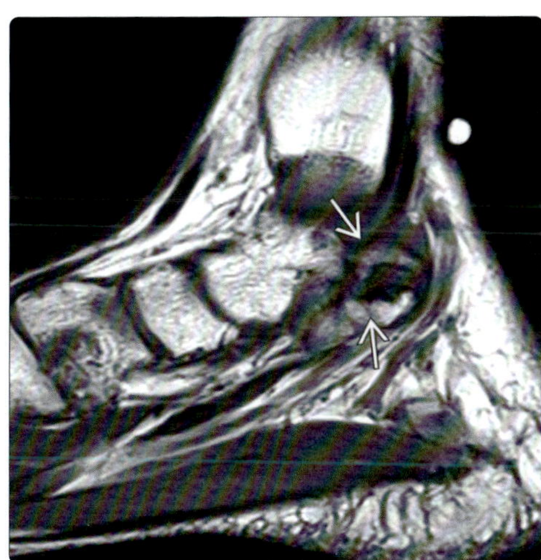

(Left) *Long-axis T2WI FS MR in the same patient shows mixed signal "mass" ➡ that deviates the inferior flexor retinaculum. The medial talus is elongated, protruding toward the mass, and showing cystic changes ➡.* **(Right)** *Sagittal T1WI MR in the same patient shows the enlarged posterior aspect of the medial facet, subtalar joint ➡. This represents a fibrous coalition that has resulted in osseous protrusion and fibrous tissue "mass" extending posteromedially, resulting in tarsal tunnel symptoms.*

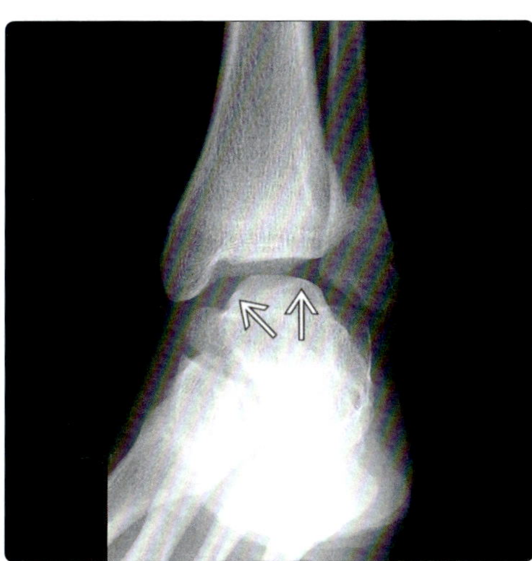

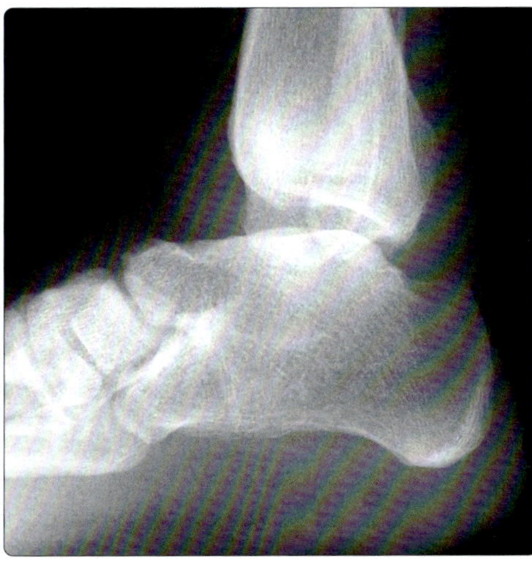

(Left) *AP radiograph shows a ball-and-socket tibiotalar joint. Note that the dome of the talus is rounded ➡, with rounding of the plafond as well, accommodating the abnormal shape of the talus.* **(Right)** *Lateral radiograph shows the rounded tibiotalar joint, as well as the very extensive tarsal coalition, with fusion at the talocalcaneal as well as talonavicular and calcaneocuboid joints. With this extensive coalition, the patient develops a ball-and-socket tibiotalar joint to provide more universal motion at that site.*

SECTION 5

Dysplasias

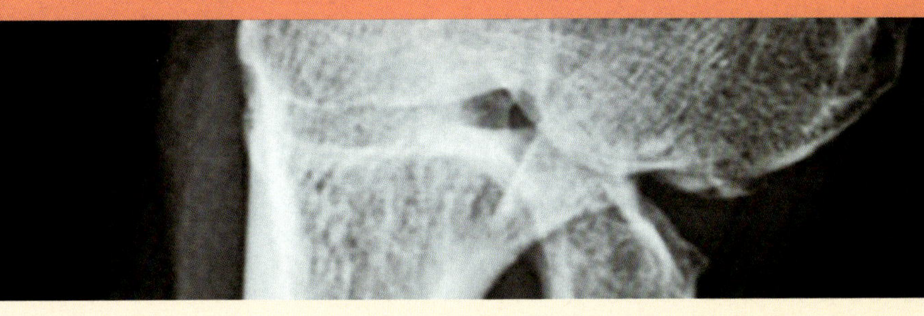

Skeletal Dysplasia

Dwarfism Dysplasia

Nondwarfing Dysplasias

Sclerosing Dysplasias

General Comments

Dwarfing dysplasias are abnormalities of cartilage and bone that result in short stature, defined as 3 standard deviations below the mean for age, race, and sex. Short limb dysplasia is a term that is gaining favor. Socially, the term little people is commonly used. These dysplasias include a broad spectrum of disorders, most of which are quite rare. Achondroplasia is the most common and well known. The reported frequency is less than 2/10,000 live births. Short limb dysplasias are divided along several different lines, the most important division being into **lethal** and **nonlethal** forms. This division has implications for continuation of a pregnancy or institution of life-saving measures after birth.

Terminology

Several terms are used to describe the pattern of limb shortening. Distinguishing among the different forms of limb shortening is a key step in characterizing a dwarfing dysplasia. **Rhizomelic** dwarfs have shortening at the "root," femur, and humerus. Achondroplasia is the classic rhizomelic dwarfing dysplasia. Shortening in the "middle," tibia/fibula, and radius/ulna is known as **mesomelic** shortening. A typical example is chondroectodermal dysplasia. **Acromelic** shortening refers to shortening at the "end," hands, and feet. Lastly, **micromelic** refers to shortening of the entire limb, such as seen with achondrogenesis.

Imaging Anatomy

The common underlying pathogenesis of abnormal bone &/or cartilage development leads to many similarities among these dysplasias. However, each dysplasia has a relatively characteristic spectrum of skeletal abnormalities. Careful consideration of each anatomic site is necessary to narrow the diagnostic possibilities and establish a diagnosis.

Skull and face may be abnormal. When abnormal, these features are usually nonspecific.

Spine involvement is a key feature that helps narrow the differential diagnosis. An abnormal spine differentiates spondyloepiphyseal dysplasia from multiple epiphyseal dysplasia. Chondroectodermal dysplasia is another short limb dysplasia that does not involve the spine. Abnormal vertebral morphology includes platyspondyly as well as bullet-shaped vertebra and vertebra with anterior beaking or tongue-like projections. Congenital diffuse platyspondyly is a key finding in several short limb dysplasias. Poor or absent mineralization distinguishes achondrogenesis. Involvement of the spine, especially the craniovertebral junction, can be a significant cause of morbidity.

Thoracic cavity abnormalities, especially shortening of the ribs, with subsequent respiratory insufficiency is a key feature of the lethal dwarfing dysplasias. Nonlethal dysplasia may also have thoracic abnormalities, although they are obviously less severe.

Pelvis abnormalities are frequently found in dwarfing dysplasia, although the findings are relatively nonspecific. A common nonspecific constellation of findings is small iliac wings, narrow sacrosciatic notches, and flattened acetabular roofs. Spikes of bone from the acetabulum have been noted in several of these dysplasias.

Extremity shortening is another defining feature of these dysplasias. Differentiation between rhizomelic, mesomelic, and micromelic shortening is crucial. Malformation of the long bones may also be a distinguishing feature. The "telephone receiver" femurs of thanatophoric dysplasia are instantly recognizable. Widespread epiphyseal abnormalities are present in spondyloepiphyseal dysplasia as well as multiple epiphyseal dysplasia. Polydactyly is a defining feature of the short rib polydactyly syndromes, including asphyxiating thoracic dystrophy and chondroectodermal dysplasia.

Pathologic Issues

The underlying genetic mutation has been discovered for many of these dysplasias. Understanding the underlying defect will hopefully, in the future, produce a cure, although that possibility currently remains elusive. The mode of transmission is known for most of these dysplasias. The role of genetics is invaluable in family planning. However, the vast majority of cases are the result of spontaneous mutations.

Imaging Protocols

Radiographs are the preferred imaging modality for characterization of these dysplasias. For the neonate, AP and lateral babygram will provide sufficient information to establish a diagnosis. Additional imaging evaluation is usually directed by clinical symptoms. Radiographs are also useful to monitor the progression of bone growth and to assess for secondary changes, such as degenerative joint disease. Head CT may be used to characterize craniofacial abnormalities and brain malformations. MR of the spine is frequently used to evaluate craniovertebral anomalies and the degree of spinal stenosis.

Prenatal Evaluation: Prenatal US may be used to evaluate a fetus at risk for dwarfing dysplasia. A thorough knowledge of the timetable for detection of abnormalities is required. If such abnormalities are being sought, referral to a high-risk obstetrical sonographer is a wise decision. Critical features to identify include small thoracic cavity, platyspondyly, short limbs, and abnormal bone mineralization.

Clinical Implications

The most clinically relevant component of characterizing a dwarfing dysplasia is determining whether or not the dysplasia is one of the lethal forms. This distinction is obviously crucial in the prenatal evaluation and in the first few hours and days of life. The diagnosis of a nonlethal dwarfing dysplasia has both medical and social implications. As a generalization, intelligence is normal and life expectancy is not limited. However, the skeletal abnormalities can lead to a host of problems, including premature arthritis, spinal stenosis, and craniovertebral junction instability.

Family planning when one or both parents are affected by a short limb dysplasia requires consideration of several factors. First and foremost is an understanding of the genetics of the dysplasia and the likelihood of having an affected child. Consideration of this possibility is a highly personal decision. If the mother is affected, the risks of a pregnancy must be considered,as well as the potential risk to the fetus.

Selected References

1. Orphanet: the portal for rare diseases and orphan drugs. www.orpha.net. Updated December 2015
2. Panda A et al: Skeletal dysplasias: A radiographic approach and review of common non-lethal skeletal dysplasias. World J Radiol. 6(10):808-25, 2014

Skeletal Features of Dwarfing Dysplasias

Dysplasias	Lethal	Skull and Face	Spine	Chest	Pelvis	Long Bones	Hands and Feet
Achondrogenesis	Yes	Large head; flat forehead & nasal bridge; cleft palate; micrognathia	Absent or poor ossification	Short & narrow (bell- or barrel-shaped); thin ribs	Small iliac wings; ischia poorly mineralized	Severe micromelia; flipper-like limbs (type I)	Phalanges poorly mineralized
Achondroplasia (heterozygous)	No	Frontal bossing; midface hypoplasia; small skull base	Posterior scalloping; bullet-shaped vertebra; ↓ interpediculate distance distally; congenital canal stenosis; narrowed foramen magnum; craniocervical instability	↓ AP diameter; flared rib ends	Champagne pelvis; flat acetabular roof	Rhizomelic shortening; metaphyseal cupping & fraying	Trident hands; metacarpals all equal in length
Asphyxiating thoracic dystrophy	Yes	Normal	Normal	Short, horizontal ribs; narrow & elongated chest; handle bar clavicles	Small iliac wings; flat acetabular roof; acetabular spikes of bone	Mild micromelia; cone-shaped epiphyses	Shortening phalanges, metacarpals, metatarsals; polydactyly
Chondroectodermal dysplasia	No	Normal	Normal	Normal	Small iliac wings, narrow sacrosciatic notch; acetabular spikes of bone	Rhizomelic & mesomelic shortening	Short phalanges; polydactyly (hands); carpal anomalies; dysplastic nails
Multiple epiphyseal dysplasia	No	Normal	Normal or minimally involved	Normal	Normal	Epiphyseal irregularity	Carpal & tarsal irregularity (recessive form); mild brachydactyly
Pseudoachondroplasia	No	Normal	Tongue-like projections; oval or biconcave shape	Normal	Delayed development pubic bones & triradiate cartilage; flat acetabular roofs; acetabular spikes of bone	Rhizomelic shortening; small flat epiphyses & wide metaphyses	Short & broad
Spondyloepiphyseal dysplasia	No	Normal	Variable platyspondyly; odontoid hypoplasia; craniocervical instability	Bell-shaped chest; flared ribs	Small iliac wings; flattened acetabular roofs; delayed ossification pubic bones	Rhizomelic & mesomelic shortening; abnormal epiphyses; metaphyseal flaring	Normal
Thanatophoric dwarf	Yes	Enlarged head; frontal bossing; flattened nasal bridge; small skull base; cloverleaf skull (type II)	Severe platyspondyly	Short, horizontal ribs; narrow long chest	Small iliac wings, narrow sacrosciatic notch, flat acetabular roof	Severe rhizomelic shortening; "telephone receiver" femurs	Short, broad hands & feet

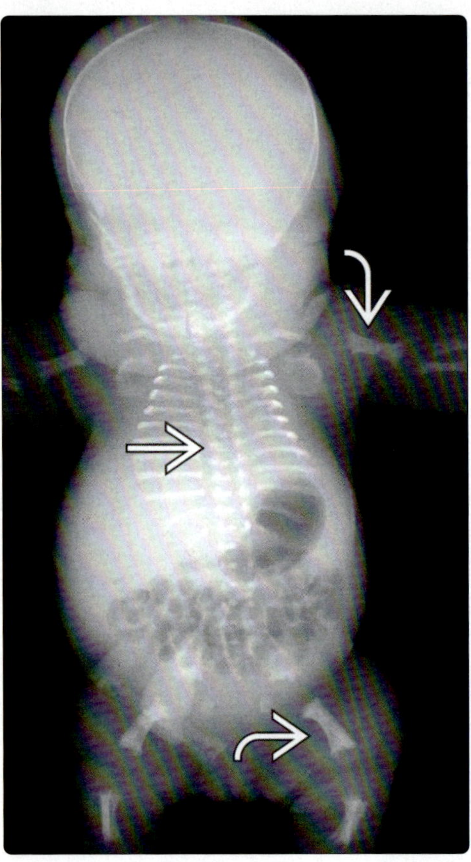

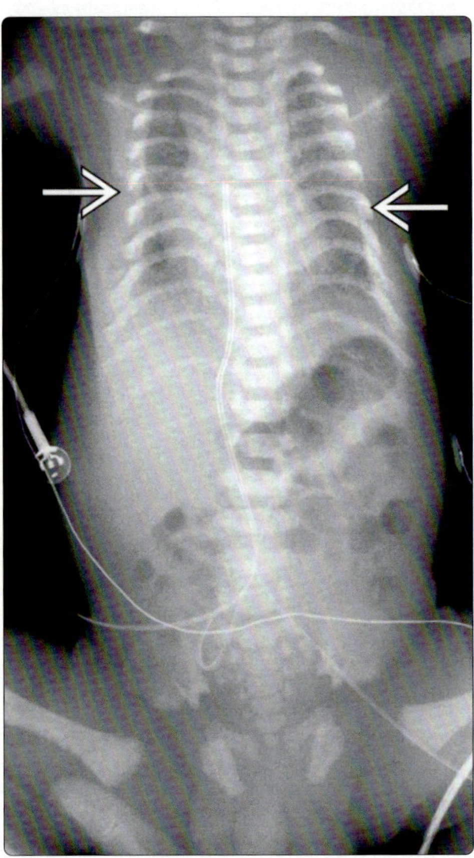

(Left) *AP radiograph of an infant with achondrogenesis reveals classic findings. Note the micromelia with severe shortening of femur and humerus ➡ as well as the tibia/fibula and radius/ulna. The vertebra are poorly mineralized and barely visible ➡. The thoracic cavity is small, characteristic of the lethal short limb dysplasias. The large head and protuberant abdomen are nonspecific findings. Note the small square iliac wings.* **(Right)** *AP radiograph demonstrates characteristic findings of asphyxiating thoracic dystrophy of Jeune. The most characteristic and diagnostic finding is the markedly shortened ribs and extremely small thoracic cavity ➡. The spine is normal. Mild micromelic extremity shortening is present and involves both the femurs and tibia/fibula. Note the nonspecific constellation of abnormalities in the pelvis.*

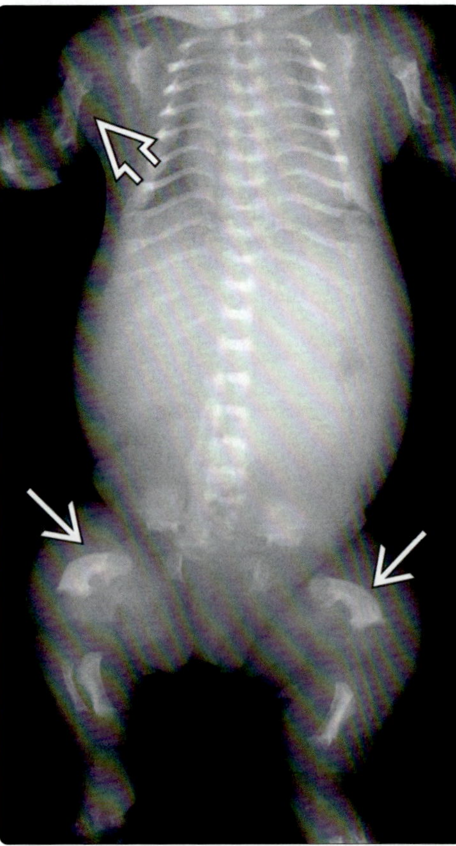

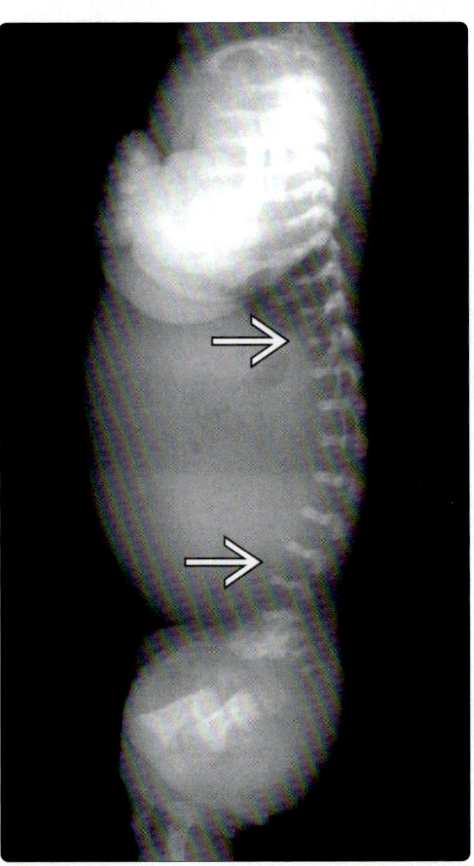

(Left) *AP radiograph shows classic manifestations of thanatophoric dwarfism. The upper and lower extremities are markedly shortened with fairly symmetric shortening of both the femurs and tibia/fibula. Note the incredibly short humeri ➡. The curved femurs, resembling telephone receivers ➡, are pathognomonic. The thoracic cavity is small, and in this patient, has a bell shape.* **(Right)** *Lateral radiograph reveals severe diffuse congenital platyspondyly ➡. This severity of spinal involvement is a key feature of thanatophoric dwarfism and may also be seen with homozygous achondroplasia and spondyloepiphyseal dysplasia (SED). Differential features include abnormal epiphyses of SED, other spinal manifestations of achondroplasia, and the different patterns of long bone shortening.*

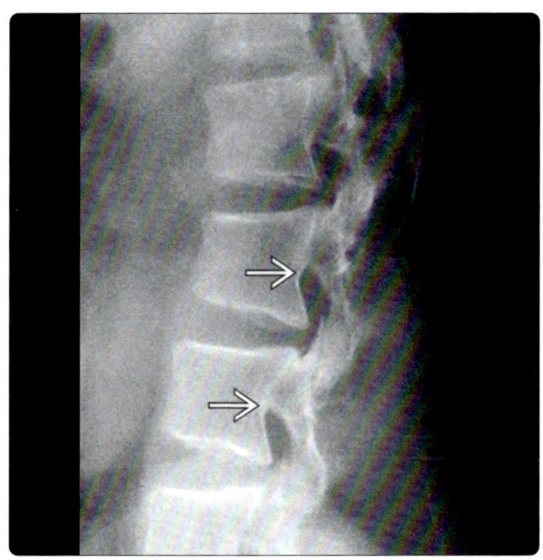

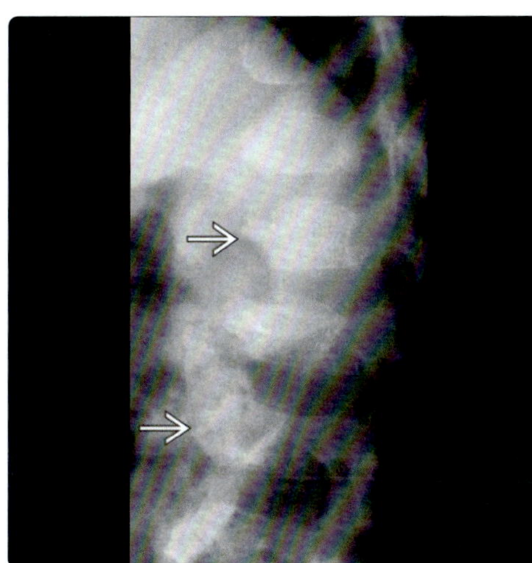

(Left) *Lateral radiograph shows vertebra with posterior scalloping ➡. This finding is seen in achondroplastic dwarfs, but has a large differential diagnosis and may be a normal variant.* **(Right)** *Lateral radiograph shows vertebra with tongue-like projections ➡ in a patient with pseudoachondroplasia. Various anomalies of the vertebral bodies, including bullet shapes and anterior beaking, have been associated with achondroplasia, pseudoachondroplasia, and other nondwarfing conditions.*

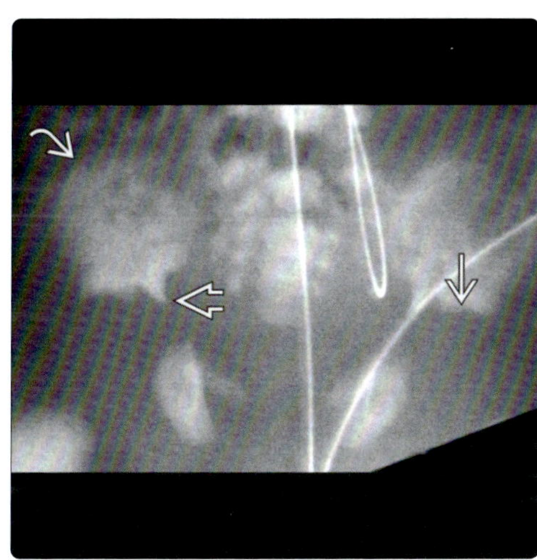

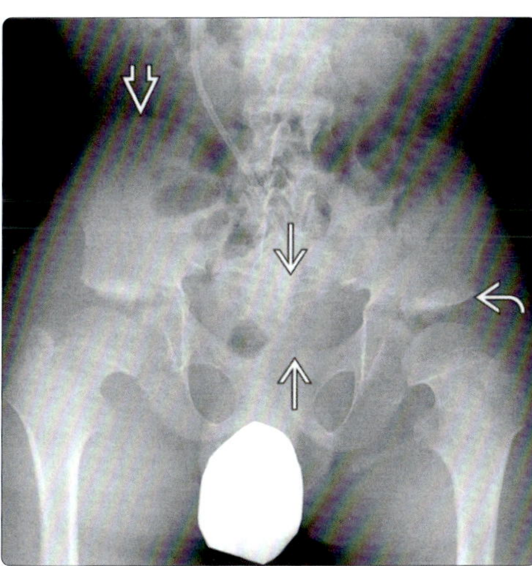

(Left) *AP radiograph shows the pelvis with the constellation of nonspecific findings seen in many dysplasias. The findings include small square iliac wings ➡, flattened acetabular roofs ➡, and spikes of bone arising from the acetabulum ➡.* **(Right)** *AP radiograph shows a pelvis with the characteristic champagne glass pelvis appearance ➡. Other features include squared iliac wings ➡ and flattened acetabular roofs ➡. The proximal femoral epiphyses are normal.*

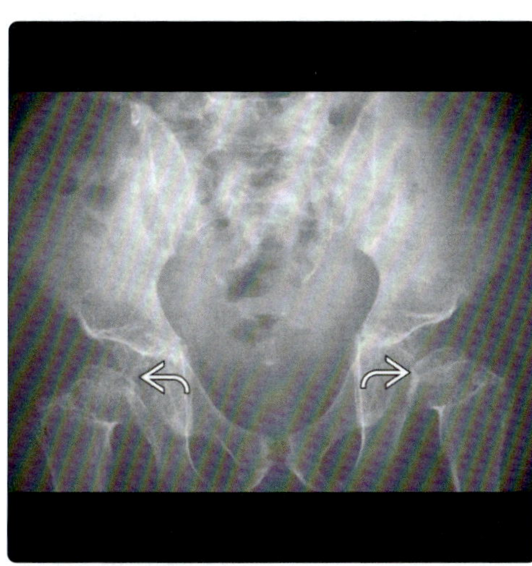

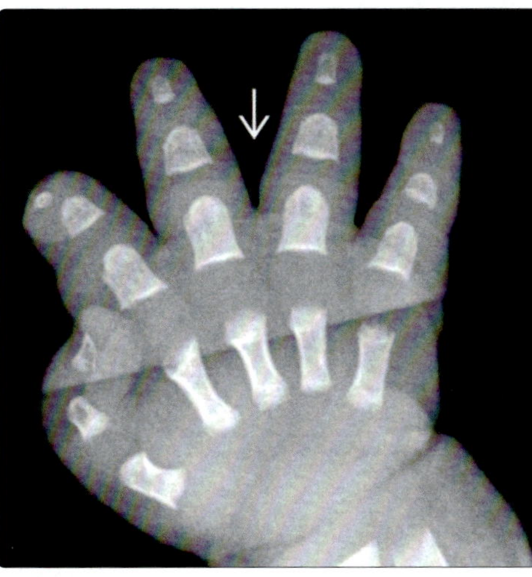

(Left) *AP radiograph shows a patient with a mild SED. The epiphyses are slightly irregular ➡. Other dwarfing dysplasias to consider include multiple epiphyseal dysplasia and pseudoachondroplasia. In this case, identification of spinal abnormalities helped confirmed the diagnosis.* **(Right)** *AP radiograph shows an infant hand with short metacarpals that are of equal length. The division between the 3rd and 4th fingers ➡ leads to the trident hand appearance.*

KEY FACTS

TERMINOLOGY

- Rhizomelic dwarfism with normal trunk, large head, and midface hypoplasia
- Most common nonlethal skeletal dysplasia

IMAGING

- Craniofacial
  - Enlarged head with frontal bossing
  - Hydrocephalus
  - Midface hypoplasia
- Spine and pelvis
  - Bullet-shaped vertebra at thoracolumbar junction
  - Posterior vertebral body scalloping
  - Congenital canal stenosis 2° to short pedicles
  - Narrowed interpediculate distance distal L spine
  - Thoracolumbar gibbus in infancy
  - Increased lumbar lordosis once walking
- Pelvis and extremities
  - Narrow sacroiliac notches
  - Shallow acetabular angle
  - Trident hand
  - Genu varum

PATHOLOGY

- Abnormal fibroblastic growth factor receptor gene 3
- Autosomal dominant transmission
- Most cases are spontaneous mutations

CLINICAL ISSUES

- Heterozygous: Normal intelligence and life expectancy
- Homozygous: Fatal in infancy/early childhood
- Narrow foramen magnum and cervical instability may lead to brainstem compression
- Obstructive apnea secondary to midface hypoplasia
- Obesity and premature osteoarthritis
- No gender predilection
- No race predilection
- 1/15,000-40,000 births worldwide

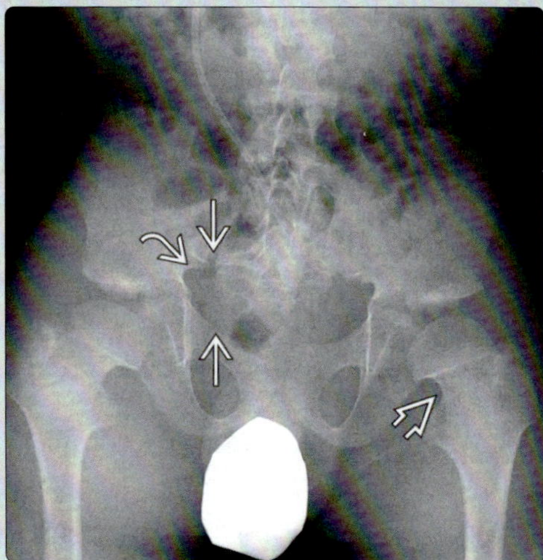

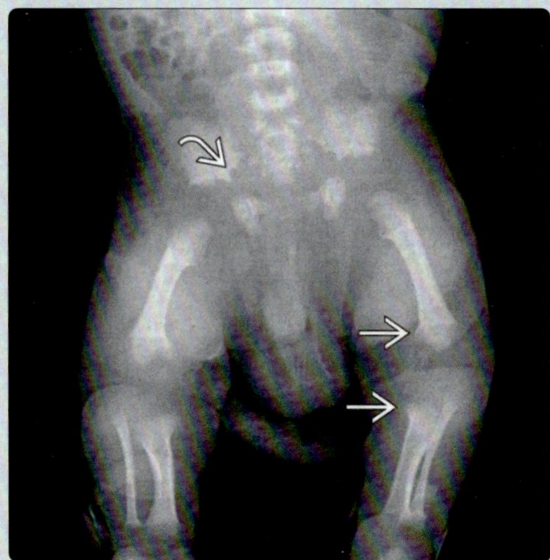

(Left) *Anteroposterior radiograph of the pelvis in a patient with achondroplasia shows a broad, flat pelvic inlet ➡, narrow sacrosciatic notches ➡, short femoral necks ➡, and wide iliac wings. Ventriculoperitoneal shunt is also present.* **(Right)** *Anteroposterior radiograph of the pelvis and lower extremities reveals characteristic narrow sacrosciatic notch ➡, short femurs and tibias/fibulas. Metaphyseal flaring is evident in the distal femurs and proximal tibias ➡.*

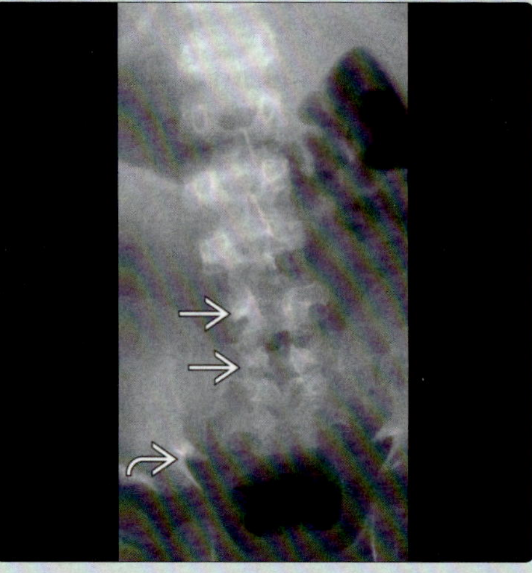

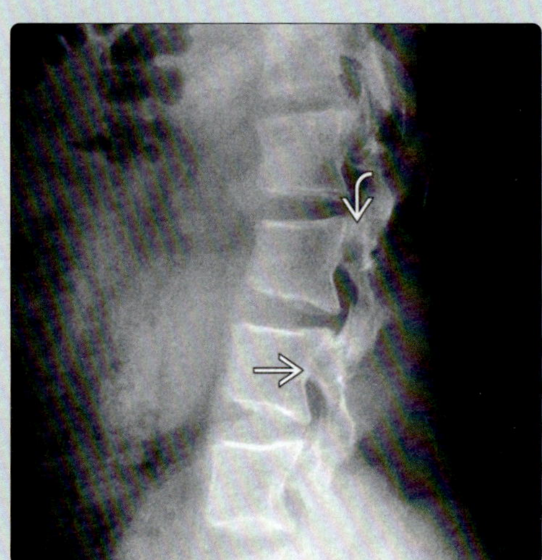

(Left) *AP radiograph of the lower lumbar spine is pathognomonic for achondroplasia. There is progressive narrowing of the interpediculate distance ➡ from L1 to L5 as well as narrowing of the sacrosciatic notch ➡.* **(Right)** *Lateral radiograph shows short pedicles ➡, which are responsible for congenital spinal stenosis in achondroplasia. Characteristic but nonspecific posterior vertebral body scalloping is present ➡. A very mild thoracolumbar kyphosis is seen as well.*

TERMINOLOGY

Synonyms

- Dwarf; term being replaced by "dysplasia"
- Little person

Definitions

- Rhizomelic ("root") dwarfism
  - In this dwarfism, shortening is greatest proximally, or at root (meaning humerus, femur)
- Most common nonlethal short-limbed skeletal dysplasia

IMAGING

General Features

- Best diagnostic clue
  - Narrow lumbar interpediculate distance is key radiographic finding in rhizomelic dwarf with otherwise normal trunk and large head

Imaging Recommendations

- Best imaging tool
  - Radiographs provide best demonstration of full spectrum of anatomic abnormalities
  - MR most useful for detailed assessment of specific anatomic abnormalities, such as narrowing of foramen magnum or spinal stenosis

Radiographic Findings

- Radiography
  - Skull & face
    - Enlarged head
    - Frontal bossing
    - Midface hypoplasia
    - Small skull base, shortened clivus
    - Malalignment and crowding of teeth
  - Chest
    - Flaring of rib ends
    - Decreased anterior to posterior diameter
  - Pelvis
    - Flared iliac wings
    - Narrow sacroiliac (sacrosciatic) notches
    - Champagne pelvis
      - Flattened pelvic inlet
    - Shallow acetabular angle
  - Thoracic and lumbar spine
    - Narrowing of interpediculate distance from upper to lower lumbar spine
    - Congenital canal stenosis 2° to short pedicles
    - Posterior vertebral body scalloping
    - Bullet-shaped vertebra at thoracolumbar junction
    - Thoracolumbar kyphosis in infancy
    - Increased lumbar lordosis once walking
      - Leads to horizontal sacrum
  - Upper extremity
    - Humeral shortening > shortening of radius and ulna
    - Metaphyseal cupping and fraying
    - Decreased elbow extension
      - Due to posteriorly bowed humerus ± radial head dislocation
    - Metacarpals all have equal length
    - Trident hand
      - Divergence of middle and ring fingers
    - Brachydactyly
      - Shortening greatest in proximal and middle phalanges
  - Lower extremity
    - Femoral shortening > shortening tibia and fibula
    - Metaphyseal cupping & fraying
    - Short femoral neck
    - Long fibula
    - Genu varum, patella baja
    - Discoid meniscus
- Prenatal ultrasound
  - Normal scan in 1st trimester
  - Long bone shortening evident after 22 weeks
  - Thoracolumbar kyphosis
  - Megalencephaly
  - Depressed nasal bridge
  - Normal ossification
  - No fractures, angular deformities of long bones
  - Polyhydramnios is not common
    - Mild when present
  - Homozygous disease
    - More severe changes
    - Evident earlier in pregnancy

CT Findings

- Head CT
  - Narrow foramen magnum
  - Hydrocephalus
  - Malformation of middle ear
- Spine CT
  - Vertebral body anomalies
  - Congenital spinal stenosis
    - Short pedicles limit anteroposterior dimension
    - Narrow interpediculate distance narrows medial to lateral dimension
  - Compression of cervicomedullary junction

MR Findings

- Brain
  - Narrow foramen magnum
  - Hydrocephalus
  - Prominent subarachnoid space over frontal lobes
- Spine
  - Vertebral body anomalies
  - Congenital spinal stenosis
    - Short pedicles
    - Narrow interpediculate distance
  - Compression of cervicomedullary junction

DIFFERENTIAL DIAGNOSIS

Hypochondroplasia

- Findings similar to and less severe than achondroplasia
  - Significant overlap with mild achondroplasia
- May require gene typing to differentiate

Osteogenesis Imperfecta

- Osteopenia
- Multiple fractures that may mimic rhizomelic dwarfism

- Blue sclera
- Abnormal teeth
- Thin beaded ribs

Thanatophoric Dwarfism

- Lacks interpediculate narrowing
- Diffuse platyspondyly present
- Bowed "telephone receiver" femurs
- Significant overlap with homozygous achondroplasia
- Lethal in infancy

PATHOLOGY

General Features

- Etiology
  - Most common nonlethal skeletal dysplasia
  - Form of chondrodysplasia
    - Failure of conversion of cartilage to bone
  - Mutation of *FGFR3*
    - Fibroblastic growth factor receptor gene 3
- Genetics
  - Autosomal dominant transmission
  - Most cases are spontaneous mutations
    - Associated with increasing age of father

Gross Pathologic & Surgical Features

- Failure of enchondral ossification

CLINICAL ISSUES

Presentation

- Most common signs/symptoms
  - Rhizomelic dwarf with normal trunk, large head, and midface hypoplasia
  - Findings are evident at birth
  - May be detected prenatally
    - Large head may require cesarean section
- Other signs/symptoms
  - Hypotonia in infancy common
  - Delayed motor milestones
    - Separate developmental charts have been created
  - Redundant skin folds on extremities
  - Limited elbow extension
  - Genu varum
  - Joint laxity (except elbow and hip)
  - Waddling gait

Demographics

- Gender
  - No predilection
- Ethnicity
  - No predilection
- Epidemiology
  - 1/15,000-40,000 births worldwide

Natural History & Prognosis

- Heterozygous disease
  - Normal intelligence and life expectancy
- Homozygous disease
  - Fatal in infancy/early childhood
    - Respiratory insufficiency
- Complications
  - Narrow foramen magnum and cervical instability may lead to brainstem compression
    - Increases risk of death in infancy
    - May require decompression later in life
      - Symptoms include hyperreflexia, clonus, central apnea
  - Obstructive apnea secondary to midface hypoplasia
  - Otitis media secondary to middle ear malformation
  - Obesity
  - Premature osteoarthritis
  - Spinal stenosis
  - Hydrocephalus
    - Secondary to venous obstruction at sigmoid sinus
    - Not related to macrocephaly
  - Women with achondroplasia will require cesarean section for delivery

Treatment

- Directed at relieving symptoms related to structural abnormalities
  - Cervicomedullary decompression
  - Lumbar spinal decompression
  - Ventricular shunting
  - Limb lengthening procedures
    - Controversial
  - Weight management to prevent obesity
  - Adenoidectomy and tonsillectomy, continuous positive airway pressure by mask to relieve sleep apnea
    - May require tracheostomy
  - Early studies of growth hormone &/or statins promising

DIAGNOSTIC CHECKLIST

Image Interpretation Pearls

- Nonspecific constellation of findings among dysplasias
  - Underdeveloped pelvis
    - Small, squared iliac wings
    - Narrow sacroiliac (sacrosciatic) notch
    - Flat acetabular roof
  - Craniofacial abnormalities
    - Frontal bossing
    - Dental anomalies
  - Small chest
    - Rib cage abnormalities have different descriptions yet appearance is usually not distinctive enough to establish diagnosis
- Spine is key differentiating feature among dysplasias with rhizomelic limb shortening

SELECTED REFERENCES

1. Chitty LS et al: Non-invasive prenatal diagnosis of achondroplasia and thanatophoric dysplasia: next generation sequencing allows for a safer, more accurate and comprehensive approach. Prenat Diagn. ePub, 2015
2. Panda A et al: Skeletal dysplasias: A radiographic approach and review of common non-lethal skeletal dysplasias. World J Radiol. 6(10):808-25, 2014

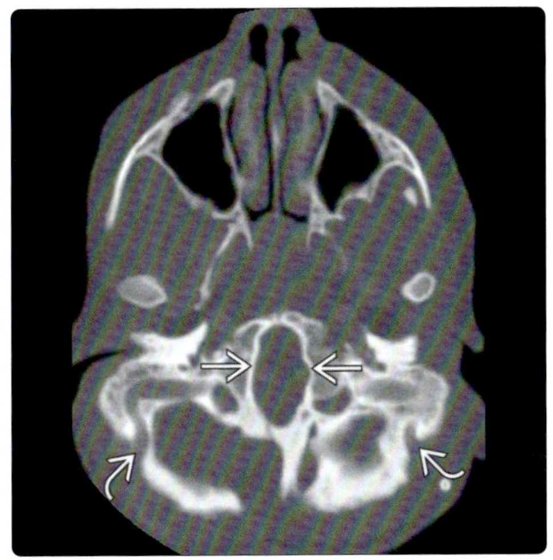

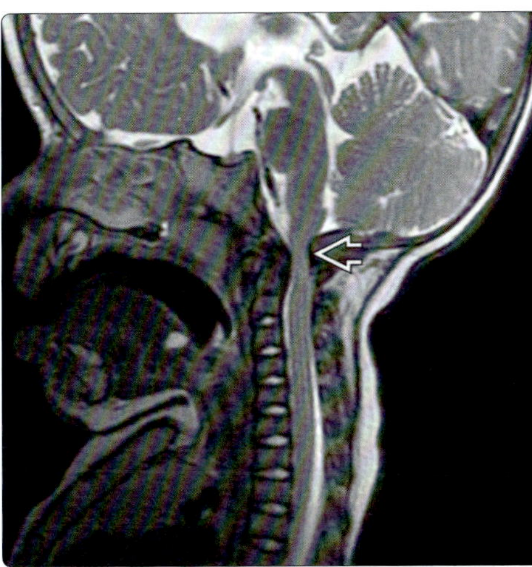

(Left) *Axial CECT shows the dysplasia of the skull base and cranio-cervical junction associated with achondroplasia. The foramen magnum is narrowed* ➡*, and enlarged emissary veins* ➡ *are present.* **(Right)** *Sagittal T2WI MR shows marked osseous narrowing of the spinal canal at the craniovertebral junction, with compression and caliber change of the upper cervical spinal cord* ➡*.*

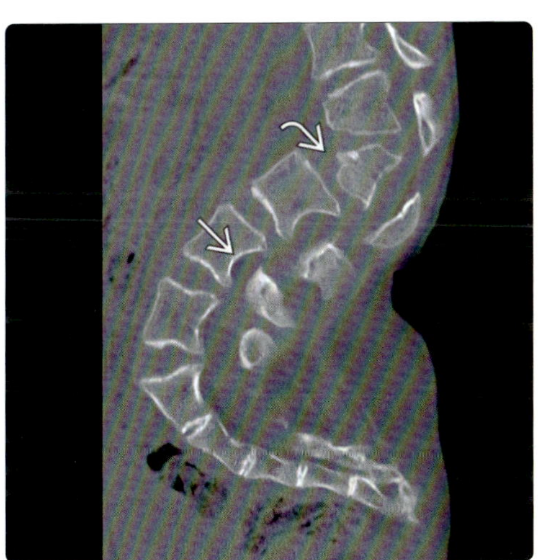

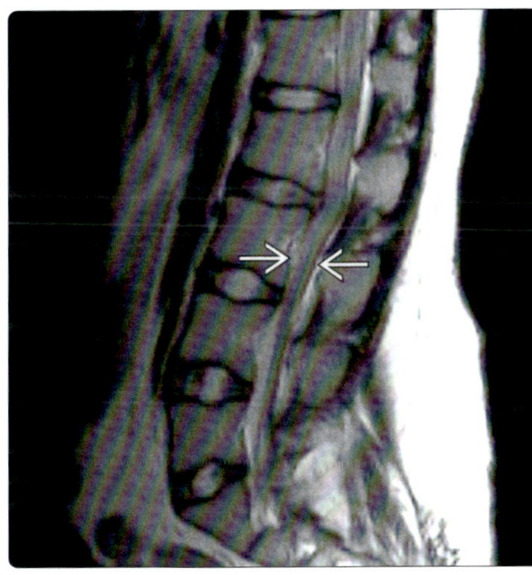

(Left) *Sagittal bone CT of the lumbar spine depicts congenital hypoplasia of the anterior L2 vertebral body with central beaking* ➡ *producing focal kyphosis. The kyphosis accentuates congenital spinal stenosis from short pedicles. The remaining lumbar vertebral bodies show characteristic posterior vertebral scalloping* ➡*.* **(Right)** *Sagittal T2WI MR demonstrates congenital lumbar spinal stenosis* ➡ *secondary to shortening of the pedicles, typical of achondroplasia.*

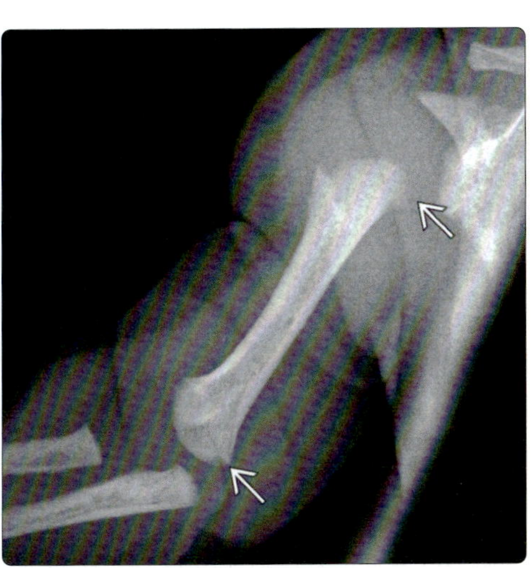

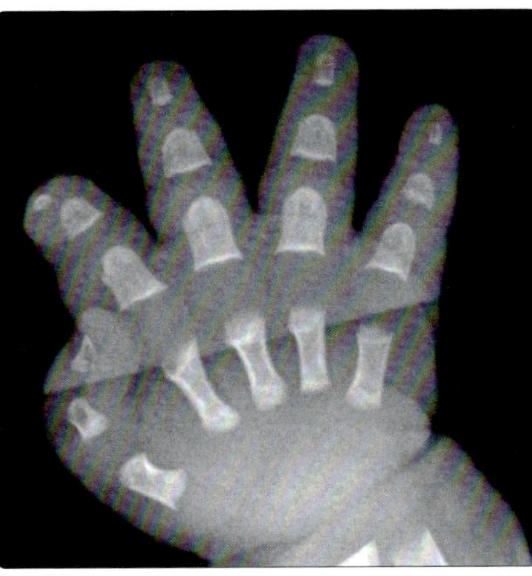

(Left) *Anteroposterior radiograph reveals the typical shortening of the humerus seen with achondroplasia. Mild proximal and distal metaphyseal flaring are also present* ➡*.* **(Right)** *Anteroposterior radiograph of the hand shows diffuse brachydactyly. Separation between the 3rd and 4th fingers creates the typical trident (3-pronged) hand.*

KEY FACTS

TERMINOLOGY

- Synonyms
  - Pseudoachondroplastic dysplasia
  - Pseudoachondroplastic spondyloepiphyseal dysplasia

IMAGING

- Radiographs essential to identify underlying epiphyseal and metaphyseal abnormalities
- Abnormal epiphyses and metaphyses in spine, pelvis, and lower extremity > upper extremity
- Changes are age-related
  - Normal in infancy, most pronounced in childhood, less severe in adulthood
- Pelvis
  - Underdeveloped, especially pubic bones
  - Characteristic delayed development of triradiate cartilage, flattened acetabular angles
  - Spikes of bone from medial and lateral borders of acetabulum
- Spine
  - Childhood vertebra: Anterior tongue-like projections, oval or biconcave shape
  - Adult vertebra: Wedged, flattened, or normal
  - Odontoid hypoplasia, atlantoaxial instability
  - Increased lumbar lordosis ± scoliosis
- Extremities
  - Rhizomelic shortening
  - Shortening, widening tubular bones, especially hands and feet
  - Epiphyses small, flattened in child; remain irregular in adult leading to premature osteoarthritis
  - Metaphyseal flaring persists into adulthood as widening of distal end of bones
  - Coxa vara; genu varum and valgum

TOP DIFFERENTIAL DIAGNOSES

- Achondroplasia
  - Large head, abnormal face, narrow interpediculate distance
  - Present at birth
  - Metaphyseal flaring with normal epiphysis
- Vitamin D resistant rickets
  - Similar bowing deformities
  - Epiphyses normal, growth plates irregular
  - Low serum phosphorus
- Spondyloepiphyseal dysplasia
  - Present in infancy, delayed milestones
  - Craniofacial abnormalities, respiratory abnormalities
- Morquio
  - Craniofacial abnormalities
  - Normal pubic ossification

PATHOLOGY

- Abnormal collagen oligomeric matrix protein 3 gene (*COMP*) on short arm chromosome 19
- Develop "soft cartilage," which deforms in regions of high stress, explains prevalence findings spine, pelvis, and lower extremities
- Autosomal dominant (types I, III) or autosomal recessive (types II, IV); most are spontaneous mutations

CLINICAL ISSUES

- M = F; ~ 1 in 30,000 births
- Normal growth in infancy with subsequent slowed growth or fall off growth chart in toddler years
- Development of gait abnormalities, such as waddling, or lower extremity deformities, such as bowing
- Hypermobile joints of hand and wrist, knee, ankle
- Scoliosis, kyphosis, and increased lumbar lordosis
- Limited ROM elbow and hips
- Hands and feet → short and broad
- Premature osteoarthritis is most significant sequelae
- Elective limb lengthening
- Treatment directed at joint abnormalities and symptoms arising from scoliosis and lumbar hyperlordosis

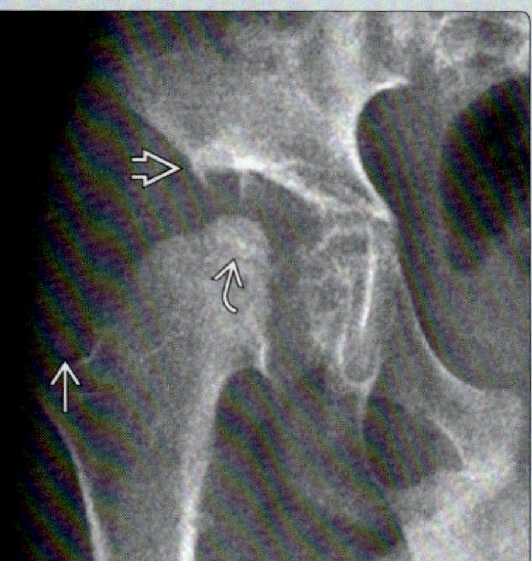

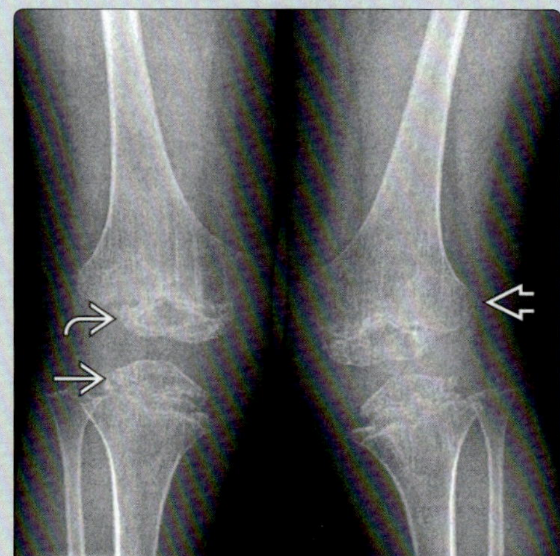

(Left) *AP radiograph of the pelvis reveals small proximal femoral epiphyses ➡ and greater trochanteric apophyses ➡, commonly seen in patients with pseudoachondroplasia. Small spikes of bone are present along the lateral acetabular borders ➡, and the acetabular angles are flattened.* **(Right)** *AP radiograph of the knees demonstrates genu valgum deformities. The distal femoral ➡ and proximal tibial ➡ epiphyses are flattened and irregular. The metaphyses are widened ➡.*

Achondrogenesis

KEY FACTS

TERMINOLOGY

- Heterogeneous group that includes most severe chondrodysplasias
  - Type 1A: Houston-Harris
  - Type 1B: Parenti-Fraccaro
  - Type 2: Langer-Saldino

IMAGING

- Skull and face
  - Large head
- Chest
  - Short and narrow
  - Thin ribs with multiple fractures (type 1)
  - Barrel shaped (type 1)
  - Bell shaped (type 2)
- Axial skeleton
  - Absent or poor ossification of spine (type 1A and type 2)
  - Small iliac bones, may only be mineralized superiorly
  - Ischia poorly mineralized
- Extremities
  - Severe micromelia
  - Long bones misshapen
  - Extremely short femur, humeri
  - Poorly mineralized fibula
  - Phalanges poorly mineralized, appear to be absent
  - Metaphyseal spurring

TOP DIFFERENTIAL DIAGNOSES

- Lethal (type II) osteogenesis imperfecta
  - Short long bones secondary to multiple fractures
  - Blue sclera
  - Intracranial hemorrhage
- Thanatophoric dwarfism
  - Long narrow thorax
  - "Telephone receiver" femur
  - "Cloverleaf" skull
  - Severe platyspondyly
- Short rib polydactyly syndrome

PATHOLOGY

- Abnormal collagen formation
  - Type 1A: Unknown genetics
  - Type 1B: *SLC26A2* mutation (DDST diastrophic dysplasia sulfate transporter gene)
  - Type 2: *COL2A1*; type II collagenopathy
- Genetics
  - Type 1A and 1B: Autosomal recessive
  - Type 2: Autosomal dominant
- No race or sex predilection

CLINICAL ISSUES

- ~ 1 in 40,000-60,0000
- Type 1 more common and more severe than type 2
- Prenatal
  - Hydrops
  - Polyhydramnios
  - Short femora may be evident by 13-14 weeks
  - Breech
- Premature, stillborn, or die shortly after birth from respiratory failure
- Craniofacial
  - Large head, flat forehead
  - Flat nasal bridge, prominent philtrum
  - Micrognathia
  - Cleft palate (type 2)
- Chest and abdomen
  - Lung hypoplasia
  - Cardiac anomalies (type 1)
  - Protuberant abdomen
  - Anasarca-like appearance due to abundant soft tissues and short neck
  - Umbilical and inguinal hernias (type 1B)
- Extremities
  - Short limbs evident at birth
  - Extremely short, flipper-like in type 1

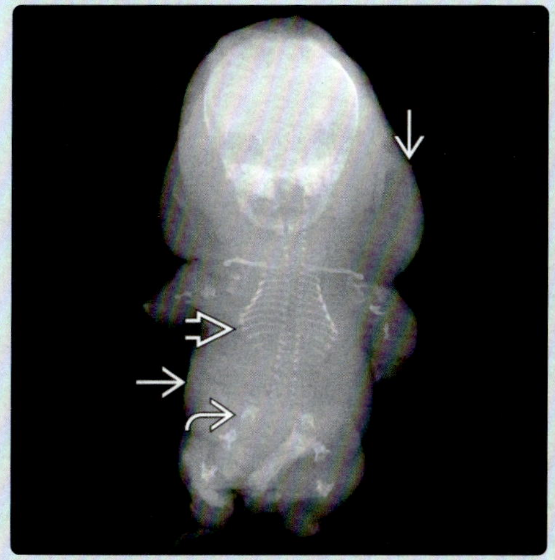

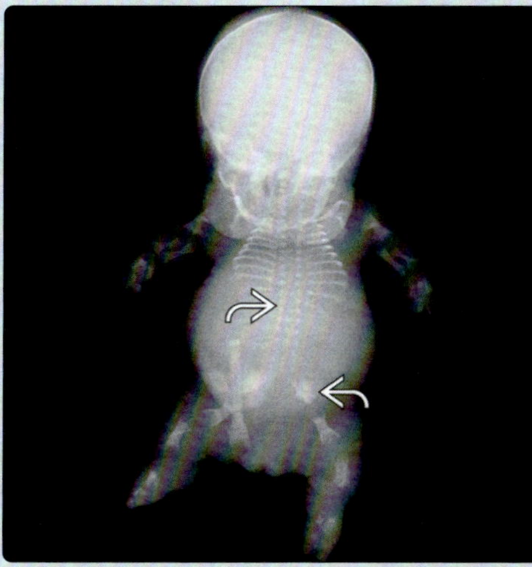

(Left) *AP radiograph of a stillborn infant shows the most severe manifestations of achondrogenesis, including anasarca-like appearance 2° to excessive skin folds ➡, flipper-like limbs, poorly mineralized vertebra and pelvic bones ➦, and extremely short ribs ➡.* **(Right)** *AP radiograph shows moderately severe skeletal abnormalities of achondrogenesis. Severe micromelia with misshapen long bones is present. The vertebra, pelvic bones, and small bones of the hands and feet are poorly mineralized ➦.*

Thanatophoric Dwarfism

KEY FACTS

TERMINOLOGY

- Synonym: Death-bearing dwarf
- Most common lethal skeletal dysplasia
  - Type I: "Telephone receiver" femurs
  - Type II: "Cloverleaf" skull (Kleeblattschädel)

IMAGING

- Radiographs are sufficient to confirm diagnosis
  - Severe rhizomelic limb shortening & bowing
  - Severe platyspondyly, increased disc space height
  - Short horizontal ribs
  - Narrow, relatively long chest
  - "Cloverleaf" skull
  - Enlarged head with frontal bossing
  - Narrow sacroiliac notch
  - Flat acetabular roof
  - Small squared iliac wings
  - Outwardly bowed ("telephone receiver") femurs
  - Megalencephaly, especially temporal lobes
  - Ventriculomegaly
- Prenatal ultrasound: Diagnose as early as 14 weeks
  - Severe micromelia & platyspondyly
  - Severe polyhydramnios 2nd trimester

TOP DIFFERENTIAL DIAGNOSES

- Homozygous achondroplasia
- Osteogenesis imperfecta
- Short rib polydactyly
- Diastrophic dysplasia

PATHOLOGY

- Abnormal fibroblastic growth factor receptor gene 3

CLINICAL ISSUES

- Uniformly fatal within hours to days from respiratory insufficiency
- M:F = 2:1
- 1/20,000-50,000 live births

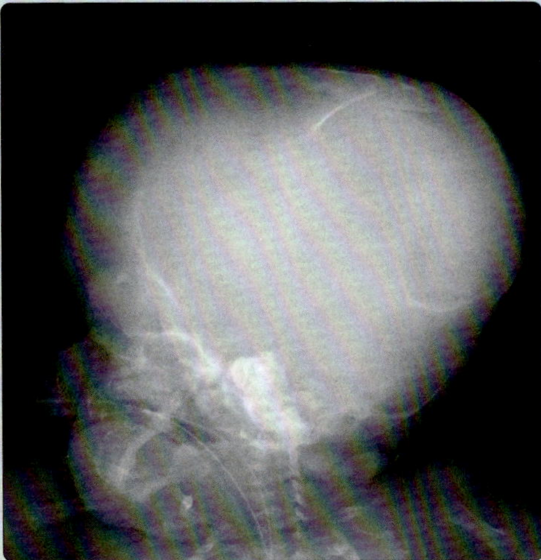

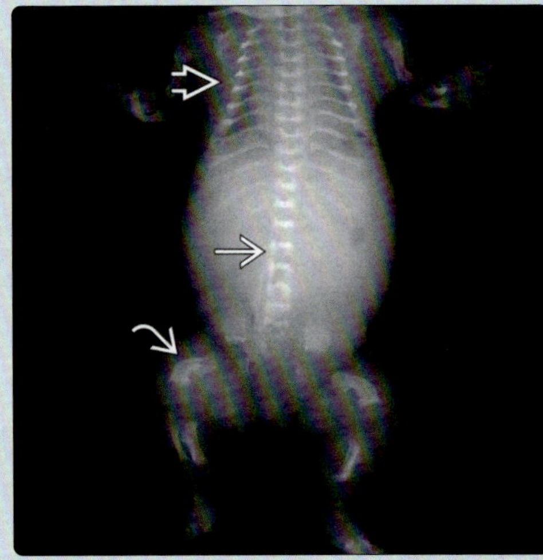

(Left) *Lateral radiograph of the skull shows the self-explanatory "cloverleaf" appearance, which is a variable feature of thanatophoric dwarfism (type II).* **(Right)** *AP radiograph shows severe micromelia involving all the long bones. There is characteristic marked bowing of the femur ➔, an appearance often called "telephone receiver," indicating type I thanatophoric dwarfism. The chest cavity is narrow, and the ribs are short and horizontal ➔. Diffuse flattening of the vertebral bodies ➔ is present.*

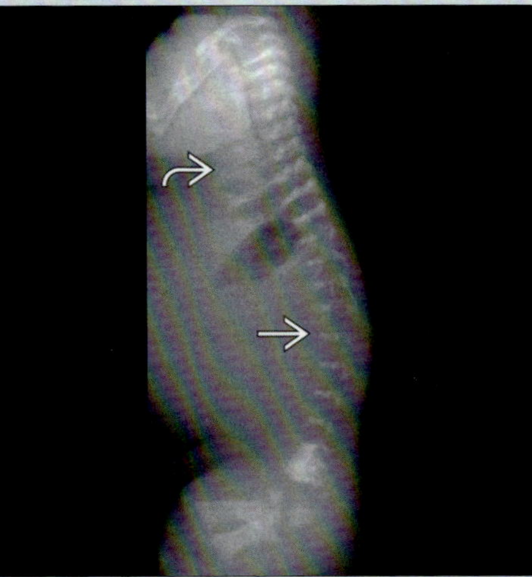

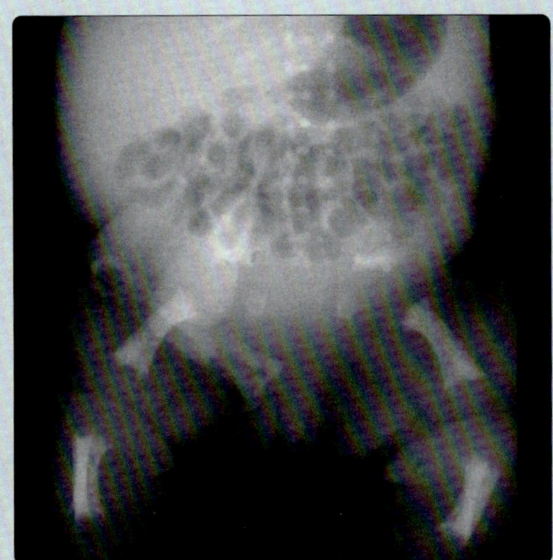

(Left) *Lateral radiograph shows severe platyspondyly of the entire thoracolumbar spine ➔ and a relatively increased disc space height. The ribs are markedly shortened ➔, and the abdomen is protuberant.* **(Right)** *Anteroposterior radiograph demonstrates the severely shortened bones of the lower extremity. The femur is markedly shortened relative to the tibia and fibula. Note also the abnormal morphology of the pelvis, including small squared iliac wings, narrowed sacrosciatic notch, & flat acetabular roof.*

TERMINOLOGY

Synonyms

- Death-bearing dwarf

Definitions

- Most common lethal skeletal dysplasia

IMAGING

General Features

- Best diagnostic clue
  - Severe micromelia and platyspondyly
    - Type I: "Telephone receiver" femurs
    - Type II: "Cloverleaf" skull (Kleeblattschädel)

Imaging Recommendations

- Best imaging tool
  - Radiographs are sufficient to confirm diagnosis

Radiographic Findings

- Skull & face
  - "Cloverleaf" skull (type II)
  - Enlarged head with frontal bossing
  - Depressed nasal bridge
  - Small skull base
- Chest
  - Short horizontal ribs
  - Narrow, relatively long chest
- Spine
  - Severe platyspondyly, increased disc space height
- Pelvis
  - Small squared iliac wings
  - Narrow sacroiliac notch
  - Flat acetabular roof
- Extremities
  - Severe rhizomelic shortening
  - Outwardly bowed femurs (type I)
    - Telephone receiver appearance
  - Metaphyseal flaring
  - Short, broad phalanges

Head CT & Brain MR

- Megalencephaly
  - Especially temporal lobes
- Ventriculomegaly
- Narrowed foramen magnum
- Polymicrogyria

Prenatal Ultrasound

- Can be diagnosed as early as 14 weeks
- Increased nuchal translucency
- Severe micromelia
- Platyspondyly
- Severe polyhydramnios 2nd trimester

DIFFERENTIAL DIAGNOSIS

Homozygous Achondroplasia

- Narrow interpediculate distance from upper to lower lumbar spine
- At least 1 parent has achondroplasia

Short Rib Polydactyly

- Includes asphyxiating thoracic dystrophy & Ellis-van Creveld
- Polydactyly

Osteogenesis Imperfecta

- Congenital platyspondyly seen with type IIA

Diastrophic Dysplasia

- Cleft palate
- Club foot, hitchhiker thumb
- Swelling of the ears

PATHOLOGY

General Features

- Genetics
  - Abnormal fibroblastic growth factor receptor gene 3
    - 1 mutated gene required for transmission
    - All cases are spontaneous mutations

Staging, Grading, & Classification

- Type I
  - More severe limb shortening, bowing, & platyspondyly
    - Outwardly bowed femurs known by telephone receiver appearance
- Type II
  - Less severe limb shortening, bowing, & platyspondyly
  - Pronounced "cloverleaf" skull

CLINICAL ISSUES

Presentation

- Most common signs/symptoms
  - Severe rhizomelic limb shortening with bowing
- Other signs/symptoms
  - Enlarged head with wide set eyes
  - Narrow chest
  - Protuberant abdomen
  - Abducted, externally rotated legs
  - Extra skin on arms and legs

Demographics

- Gender
  - M:F = 2:1
- Epidemiology
  - 1/20,000-50,000 live births

Natural History & Prognosis

- Nearly uniformly fatal within hours to days from respiratory insufficiency
- For those few that survive, complications of progressive seizures, craniocervical stenosis, ventilator dependence, & limitations in motor & cognitive abilities

SELECTED REFERENCES

1. Chitty LS et al: Non-invasive prenatal diagnosis of achondroplasia and thanatophoric dysplasia: next generation sequencing allows for a safer, more accurate and comprehensive approach. Prenat Diagn. ePub, 2015
2. Zhen L et al: Increased first-trimester nuchal translucency associated with thanatophoric dysplasia type 1. J Obstet Gynaecol. 1-3, 2015

Asphyxiating Thoracic Dystrophy of Jeune

KEY FACTS

TERMINOLOGY

- Short-limbed dwarfism with respiratory and renal abnormalities
- 1 congenital form of thoracic insufficiency syndrome
- Synonyms
  - Jeune syndrome
  - Thoracic-pelvic-phalangeal dystrophy
  - Asphyxiating thoracic chondrodystrophy

IMAGING

- Chest
  - Elongated, narrow, rectangular or bell-shaped chest
  - Short, horizontal ribs
  - Bulbous enlargement of costochondral junctions
  - Horizontal "handlebar" clavicles
- Pelvis
  - Triradiate acetabulum: Flat acetabular roof, medial spikes of bone (also described as spurs of inferolateral sacrosciatic notch)
  - Small, square iliac wings
- Extremities: Micromelia
  - Shortening acromelic or mesomelic
  - Shortening mild to severe, usually mild
  - Cone-shaped epiphyses
  - Short phalanges, metacarpals, metatarsals
  - Polydactyly
  - Premature ossification of proximal femoral epiphysis
- Spine
  - Normal vertebral bodies
- No significant craniofacial abnormalities
- Prenatal imaging
  - May not be evident in 1st trimester
  - Small chest, short ribs
  - Decreased respiratory motion
  - Limb shortening not always apparent
  - Cystic renal disease
  - Oligohydramnios may be seen

TOP DIFFERENTIAL DIAGNOSES

- Chondroectodermal dysplasia
  - a.k.a. Ellis-van Creveld syndrome
  - More pronounced nail abnormalities
  - Less renal and hepatic disease
  - Ribs not as short
  - Cardiac anomalies common
- Short rib polydactyly syndrome
  - Type III (Verma-Naumoff)
  - More severe than Jeune
  - Jeune & this syndrome may be spectrum of same disease

PATHOLOGY

- Autosomal recessive
- Genetically heterogeneous
- Mutation of *IFT80* gene
  - Regulates cilia function

CLINICAL ISSUES

- 1/100,000-130,000 births
- No racial or sex predilection
- Normal intelligence
- Main clinical issue is pulmonary status
  - Spectrum of pulmonary hypoplasia
  - Small inflexible chest impacts pulmonary function
  - Recurrent pulmonary infections
- Microcystic renal disease
- Hepatic fibrosis may lead to cirrhosis
- Variable cardiac and gastrointestinal abnormalities
- Most do not survive to adulthood
  - Lung hypoplasia associated with early death
  - End-stage renal disease seen in those who survive infancy
- Respiratory status may improve in those who survive infancy 2° to growth of rib cage
- Rib expansion techniques
  - Normalize shape of chest cavity & increase volume
  - Improve pulmonary development and function

(Left) *Anteroposterior radiograph of the chest demonstrates a narrow, elongated, bell-shaped chest, short horizontally oriented ribs, and "handlebar" clavicles characteristic of asphyxiating thoracic dystrophy.* **(Right)** *Anteroposterior radiograph of the pelvis reveals small, squared iliac wings and the triradiate acetabulum with flat acetabular roof and inferiorly projecting spikes of bone along the medial aspect* ➡.

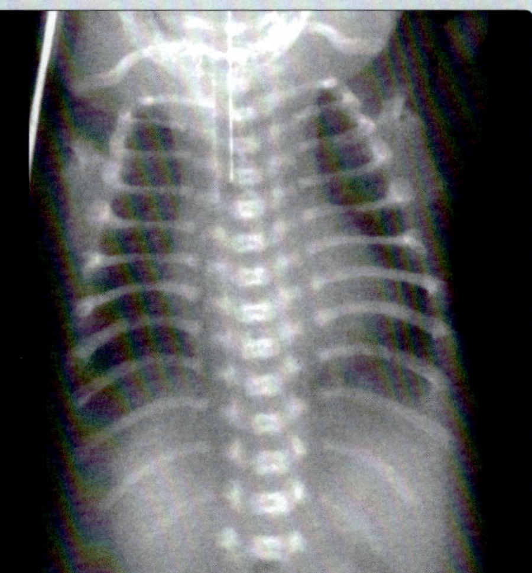

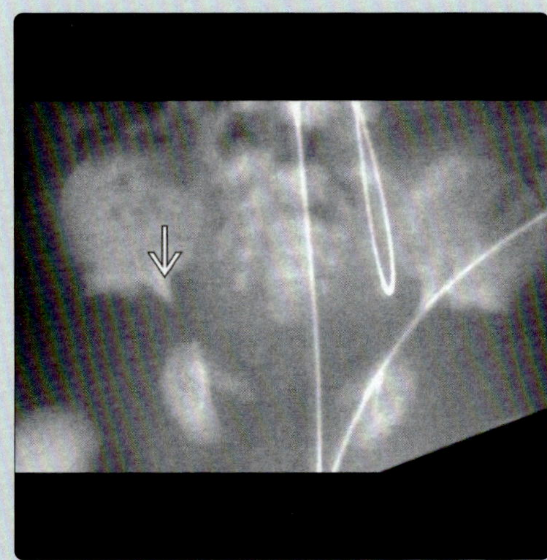

Chondroectodermal Dysplasia (Ellis-van Creveld)

KEY FACTS

TERMINOLOGY

- Chondro (cartilage) plus ectodermal (nails and teeth) dysplasia
- Belongs to spectrum of short rib polydactyly syndromes

IMAGING

- Pelvis
  - Small iliac crests
  - Narrow sacrosciatic notches
  - Spike of bone from triradiate cartilage
- Extremities
  - Disproportionate dwarfism: Limb shortening more severe distally than proximally
  - Greater shortening of tibia/fibula and radius/ulna relative to femur and humerus, respectively
  - Greater shortening of middle and distal phalanges relative to proximal phalanges
  - Cubitus valgus
  - Carpal anomalies, including accessory carpal bones and fusions, especially capitohamate
  - Bilateral post-axial polydactyly of hand (ulnar polydactyly); extra finger on ulnar side of little finger
  - Polydactyly in feet uncommon
  - Valgus deformity of knee secondary to deformity of proximal tibial epiphysis
- Craniofacial and spine
  - Normal development and mineralization
- Thorax: Short ribs
- Delayed skeletal maturation
- Prenatal diagnosis may be made after 18 weeks gestation
  - Short limbs
  - Polydactyly
  - Cardiac anomalies
  - Short ribs
  - Increased nuchal translucency after 13 weeks

TOP DIFFERENTIAL DIAGNOSES

- Other short rib polydactyly syndromes
- Asphyxiating thoracic dystrophy (Jeune)
  - Lacks ectodermal dysplasia: Hair, teeth, nails
  - Lacks cardiac defects
- McKusick-Kaufman dysplasia
  - Lacks ectodermal dysplastic changes

PATHOLOGY

- Autosomal recessive
- *EVC* and *EVC2* mutations identified

CLINICAL ISSUES

- 1/60,000-200,000 live births
- 5/1,000 births in Old Order Amish of Lancaster, PA
- 50% die in infancy secondary to congenital heart disease or respiratory insufficiency
- Chondrodystrophy, ectodermal dysplasia, congenital heart disease, polydactyly
  - Dwarfism at birth; may have normal height if survive to adulthood
  - Dysplastic finger and toe nails
  - Sparse hair
  - Dental anomalies
  - Oral deformities include partial harelip and other lip deformities
  - Congenital heart disease in 50-60%; especially atrial septal defects
  - Other anomalies include CNS, GU (epispadias, undescended testicle)
  - Small chest with respiratory difficulties
  - Normal intelligence
- Treatment in neonatal period directed at support for respiratory and cardiac anomalies
- Treatment post infancy directed at repairing anatomic anomalies
  - Repair cardiac defects
  - Resection of extra digit
  - Osteotomy to repair genu valgum
  - Appropriate dental care

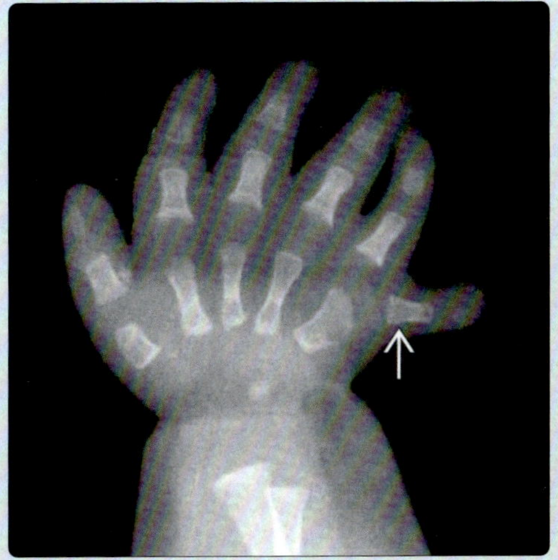

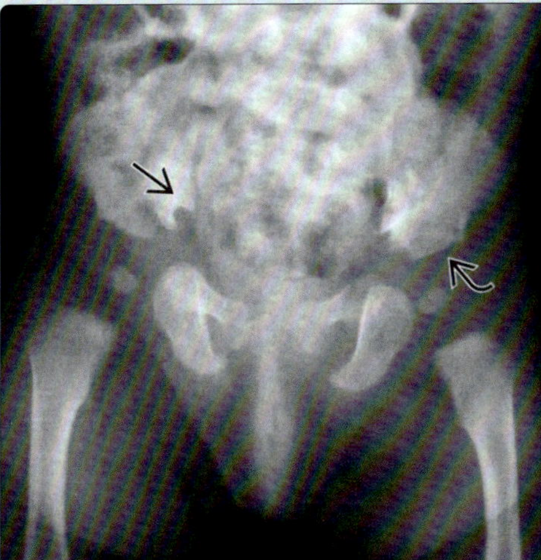

(Left) *AP radiograph of the hand demonstrates ulnar polydactyly with a 6th digit ➡ arising from the little finger. The hands are broad. Progressive shortening is noted from the proximal phalanges to the distal phalanges.* **(Right)** *AP radiograph of the pelvis demonstrates hypoplastic iliac wings, small sciatic notches ➡, and horizontal acetabulae ➡. There is mild thickening and bowing of the femoral diaphyses. These findings are nonspecific and may be present in many different skeletal dysplasias.*

KEY FACTS

TERMINOLOGY

- Dwarfism with disproportionately short trunk
  - Trunk shortening > extremity shortening

IMAGING

- Radiographs most useful for establishing diagnosis
  - Abnormal epiphyses (absent, poorly mineralized, flat, irregular, &/or fragmented)
  - Platyspondyly
- Congenita form
  - Delayed development of ossification centers with subsequent deformity
  - Hips, knees most severely involved
  - Coxa vara, hip dislocation
  - Genu valgum, overgrowth medial femoral condyle
  - Varying degrees of platyspondyly
  - Odontoid hypoplasia
  - Abnormal spine curvature
- Tarda form
  - Short stature (not always dwarf)
  - Odontoid hypoplasia, abnormal spine curvature
  - Shoulder, hip, knee most severely affected
  - Mimics Legg-Calvé-Perthes disease in hip

PATHOLOGY

- Congenita: Autosomal dominant
- Tarda: X-linked autosomal recessive

CLINICAL ISSUES

- Tarda manifests at puberty with slowed growth, development of spine deformities, joint pain
- Normal life expectancy
- Morbidities: Spine deformities, premature osteoarthritis
- Treatment
  - Spine deformity: Instrumentation/stabilization
  - Joint replacement

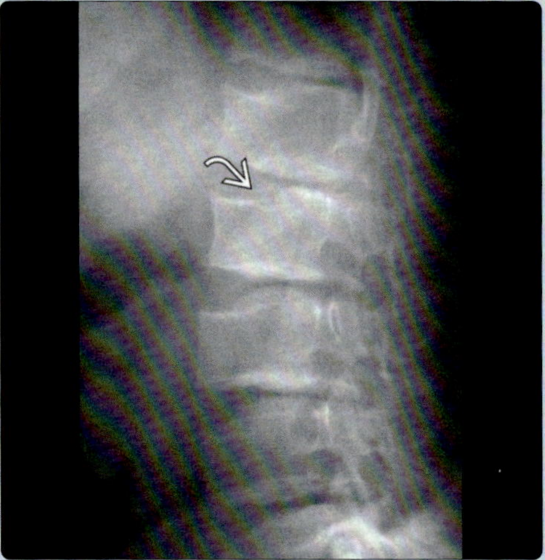

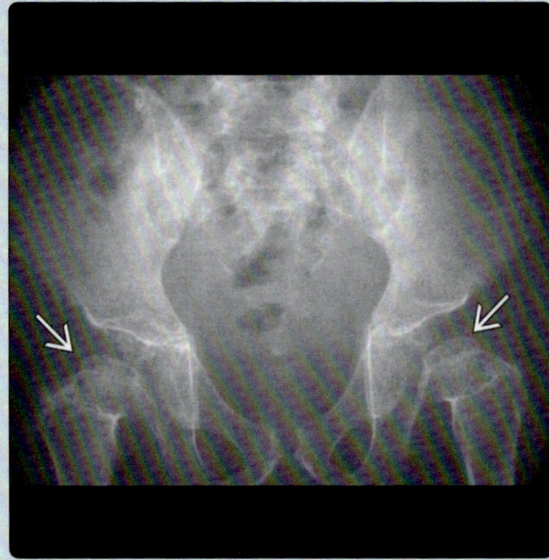

(Left) *Lateral radiograph reveals mild diffuse platyspondyly of all vertebral bodies in a patient with SED tarda. Prominent humps are present along the superior endplates ➲. These humps are the result of abnormal development of the vertebral apophyseal ring.* **(Right)** *AP radiograph demonstrates mild changes of SED. The femoral heads are symmetrically involved with flattening and broadening ➔. In this case, the iliac wings and pubic bones appear normal, though they may not in more severe disease.*

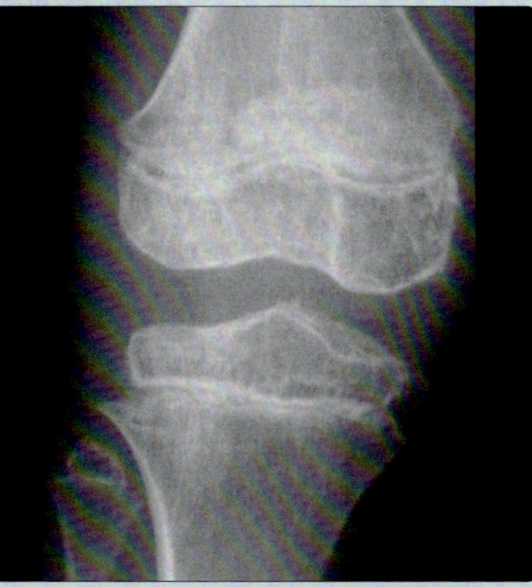

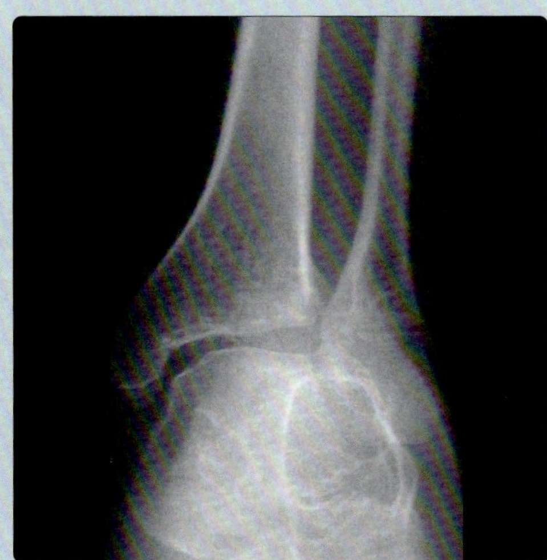

(Left) *Anteroposterior radiograph reveals irregularity of the epiphyses in a patient with mild SED. These changes are subtle and nonspecific. In this patient, the diagnosis was established only after examining the spine.* **(Right)** *AP radiograph demonstrates significant irregularity and flattening of articular surfaces of the distal tibia and the talar dome in a patient with more severe SED. The joint surfaces are incongruent; narrowing along the medial tibiotalar space heralds the onset of osteoarthritis.*

TERMINOLOGY

Abbreviations

- Spondyloepiphyseal dysplasia (SED)
- Spondyloepiphyseal dysplasia congenita (SDC)

Definitions

- Dwarfism with disproportionately short trunk
  - Trunk shortening > extremity shortening
- Heterogeneous group of disorders involving spine & epiphyses; divided into congenital & tarda forms

IMAGING

General Features

- Best diagnostic clue
  - Platyspondyly & abnormal epiphyses (absent, poorly mineralized, flat, irregular, fragmented)

Imaging Recommendations

- Best imaging tool
  - Radiographs most useful for establishing diagnosis

Radiographic Findings

- Radiography
  - Congenita
    - Short trunk & limbs; normal hands/feet & head
    - Delayed development of ossification centers with subsequent flattening, irregularity
      - Involves apophyses of spine
      - Hips, knees most severely involved, with 2° progressive deformity created by weight bearing on abnormal epiphyses
    - Chest: Bell-shaped with flared ribs
    - Spine: Varying degrees of platyspondyly
      - Odontoid hypoplasia ± atlantoaxial instability ± spinal cord compression
      - ↑ thoracic kyphosis, scoliosis, lumbar lordosis
    - Pelvis: Small iliac wings, horizontal acetabular roofs, delayed ossification of pubic bones
    - Extremity: Rhizomelic & mesomelic shortening
      - Short broad tubular bones, metaphyseal flaring
      - Coxa vara, hip dislocation
      - Genu valgum secondary to overgrowth medial femoral condyle; equinovarus foot
  - Tarda
    - Short stature (not always dwarf)
    - Spine: Odontoid hypoplasia ± atlantoaxial instability ± spinal cord compression
      - Superior & inferior hump on vertebral endplates
      - ↑ thoracic kyphosis, scoliosis, lumbar lordosis
    - Extremities: Flattened, irregular epiphyses
      - Shoulder, hip, knee most severely affected
      - Mimics Legg-Calvé-Perthes disease in hip

CT Findings

- Reconstructions useful for preoperative planning

MR Findings

- Evaluate cord compression & unossified epiphyses

DIFFERENTIAL DIAGNOSIS

Morquio

- Anterior vertebral beaking, thoracolumbar gibbus
- Pointed proximal metacarpals

Achondroplasia (Homozygous)

- Normally shaped & mineralized epiphyses
- Posterior vertebral body scalloping
- Narrowed interpediculate distance lower lumbar spine
- Short pedicles

PATHOLOGY

General Features

- Etiology
  - Type II collagenopathy
- Genetics
  - Congenita: Autosomal dominant
    - *COL2A1* gene: Produces abnormal type II collagen
    - Most cases are spontaneous mutations
    - Associated with advanced paternal age
  - Tarda: X-linked autosomal recessive (males only)
    - Mutation in SED late (*SEDL*) gene

CLINICAL ISSUES

Presentation

- Most common signs/symptoms
  - Congenita: At birth, disproportionately short trunk, rhizomelic & mesomelic limb shortening
  - Tarda: Manifests around puberty
    - Slowed growth, development of spine deformities
    - Joint pain, mainly hip, knee
- Other signs/symptoms
  - Congenita
    - Flat face, wide set eyes, cleft palate, retinal detachment, cataracts
    - Short neck, barrel chest, protuberant abdomen
    - Abnormal gait 2° to hip/knee malalignment &/or spinal cord compression
    - Normal intelligence, delayed motor milestones

Demographics

- Epidemiology
  - 1 in 100,000 live births

Natural History & Prognosis

- Normal life expectancy
- Morbidity 2° to spine deformities & premature osteoarthritis

Treatment

- Instrumentation for correction of spine deformities
- Joint replacement

SELECTED REFERENCES

1. Panda A et al: Skeletal dysplasias: A radiographic approach and review of common non-lethal skeletal dysplasias. World J Radiol. 6(10):808-25, 2014

(Left) *Lateral radiograph demonstrates mild platyspondyly of the cervical vertebra ➡ with delayed ossification, most recognizable within the odontoid process ↪.* **(Right)** *Sagittal T2WI MR demonstrates severe canal stenosis at the foramen magnum. There is associated spinal cord compression and intramedullary T2 signal abnormality in the brainstem and cervicomedullary junction ↩. Note also the prominent pectus carinatum deformity ➡.*

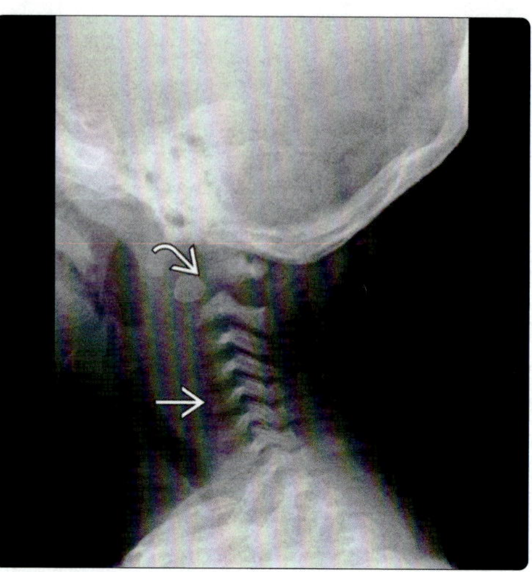

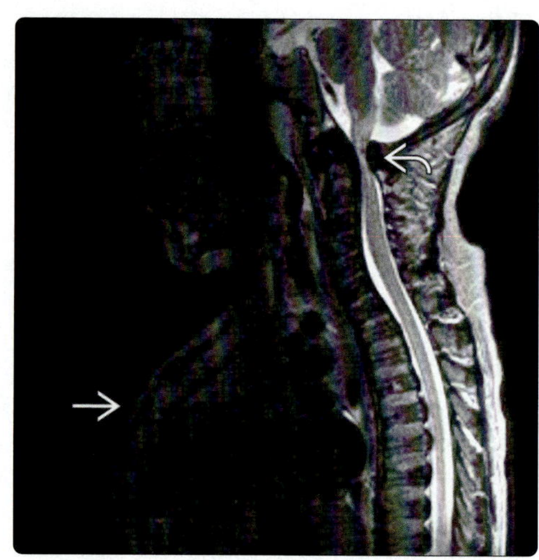

(Left) *Anteroposterior radiograph shows a patient with a mild form of spondyloepiphyseal dysplasia. Mild generalized flattening of vertebral bodies is present.* **(Right)** *Lateral radiograph shows a patient with a mild form of spondyloepiphyseal dysplasia. Generalized mild flattening of the vertebral bodies is present. Subtle humps are present on the endplates.*

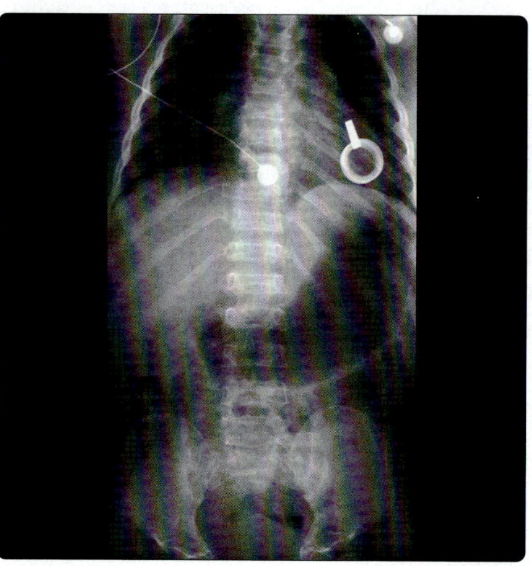

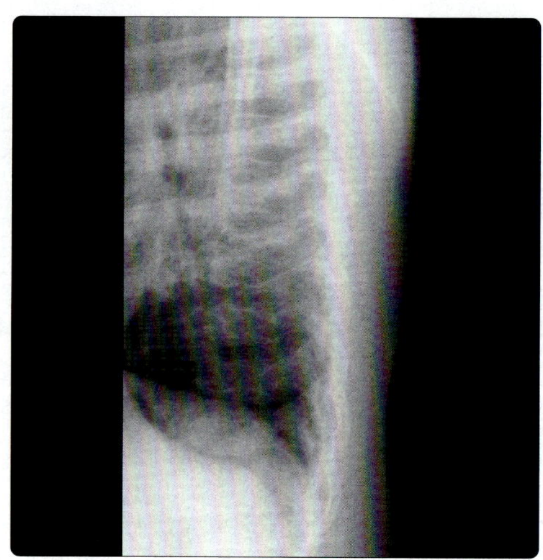

(Left) *AP radiograph of the hips shows subtly abnormal femoral heads. They have an aspherical shape and are slightly flattened. Loss of cartilage space is an early finding of osteoarthritis.* **(Right)** *AP radiograph shows a patient with severely deformed epiphyses, including marked fragmentation of the femoral heads ➡. The abnormalities are so severe that they have lead to metaphyseal deformity as well as joint malalignment. The plates relate to a femoral lengthening procedure.*

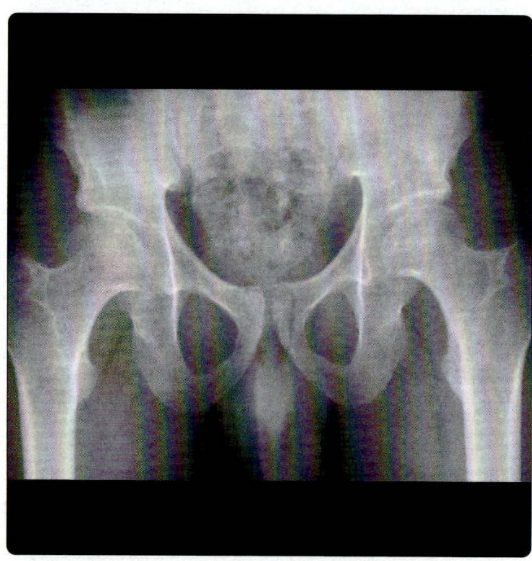

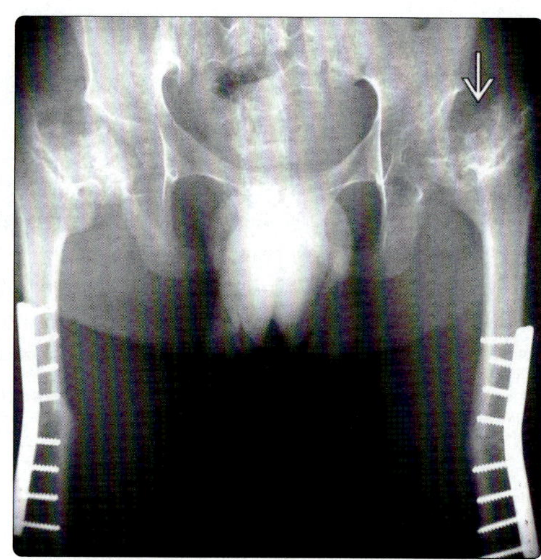

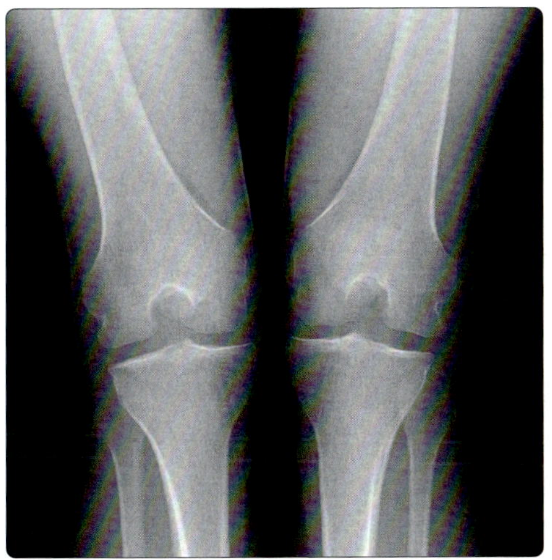

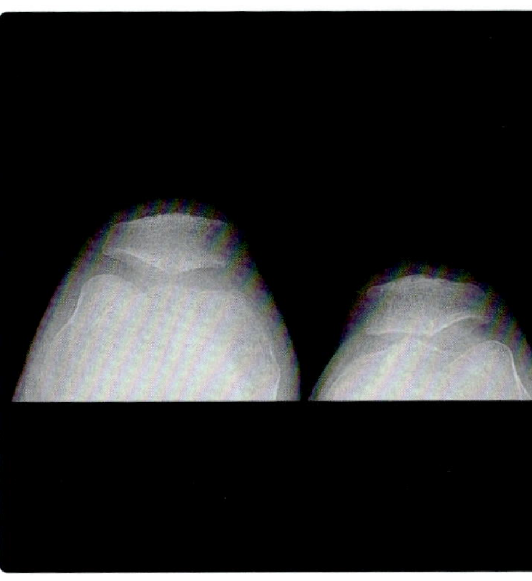

(Left) *Anteroposterior radiograph demonstrates morphologically abnormal knees. The changes are symmetric and include enlargement of the femoral condyles and flattening of the tibial articular surfaces. These findings are nonspecific.* **(Right)** *Sunrise radiograph demonstrates abnormal patella. The patella are slightly enlarged, and the articular facets have a slightly flattened appearance. The diagnosis can be established only through correlation with other skeletal findings in this patient with SED.*

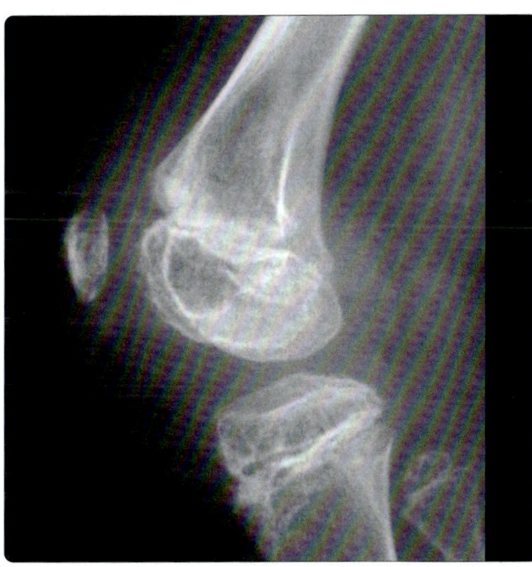

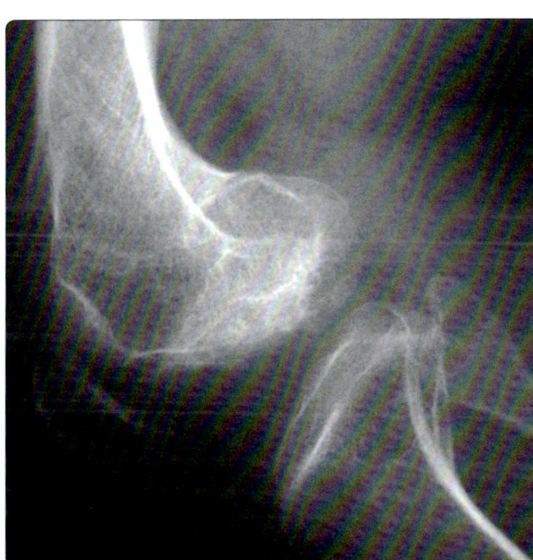

(Left) *Lateral radiograph shows the irregularity and flattening of the epiphyses in a patient with mild spondyloepiphyseal dysplasia.* **(Right)** *Lateral radiograph of the knee demonstrates extensive fragmentation of the femoral condyles and flattening of the tibial articular surface in a more severe case of SED congenita. Development of early osteoarthritis in such cases is not surprising.*

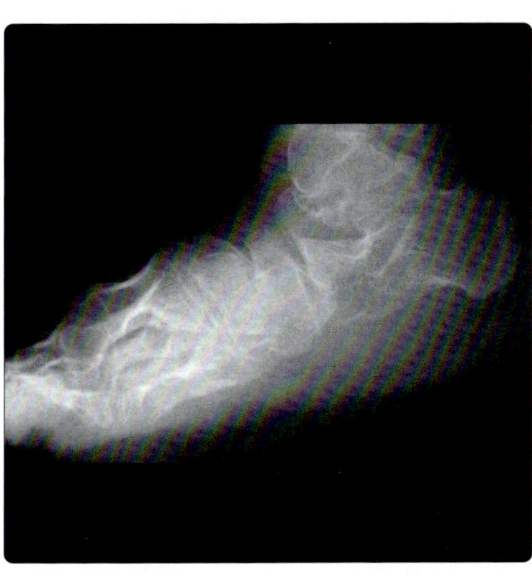

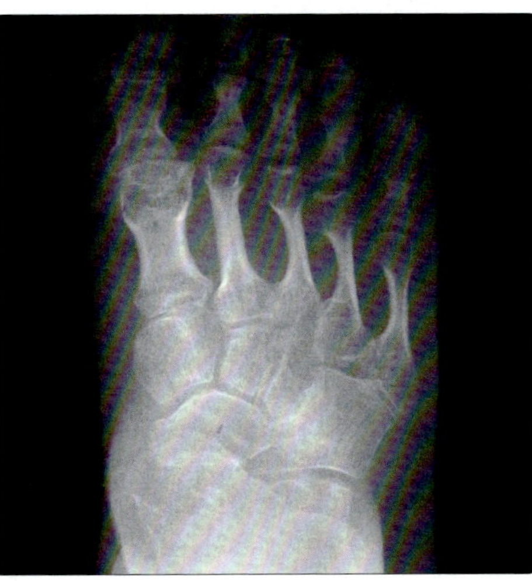

(Left) *Lateral radiograph shows markedly abnormal foot. The bones are misshapen with irregular articular surfaces, and the metatarsals are short.* **(Right)** *Anteroposterior radiograph of the foot shows brachydactyly resulting from the epiphyseal growth deformities. Malformation of the articular surfaces of the metatarsal heads is also present. Involvement of the foot is uncommonly seen in spondyloepiphyseal dysplasia.*

Multiple Epiphyseal Dysplasia

KEY FACTS

IMAGING

- Radiographs sufficient to establish diagnosis
  - Requires evaluation of all joints plus spine
- Autosomal dominant form
  - Epiphyseal irregularity that is bilateral, symmetric
    - Epiphyseal appearance initially delayed → small and fragmented → flattened
    - Most severely involved: Hip, knees, ankles, wrists
  - Minimal involvement of spine
- Recessive form
  - Hands, feet, spine also involved
  - Primarily carpal and tarsal bones
  - Mild brachydactyly
- Delayed bone age
- Alignment abnormalities

TOP DIFFERENTIAL DIAGNOSES

- Pseudoachondroplasia
  - More severe spine involvement
  - Rhizomelic limb shortening with short wide tubular bones
- Spondyloepiphyseal dysplasia
  - More severe spine involvement, including platyspondyly
  - Rhizomelic and mesomelic limb shortening
- Hypothyroidism
  - Severely delayed bone age

PATHOLOGY

- Abnormal enchondral ossification in physes/epiphyses
- Autosomal dominant form more common
- Autosomal recessive form less common

CLINICAL ISSUES

- Waddling gait, joint pain common
- Usually present in childhood; mild cases may not be diagnosed until young adulthood
- Develop premature osteoarthritis
- Treatment is symptomatic

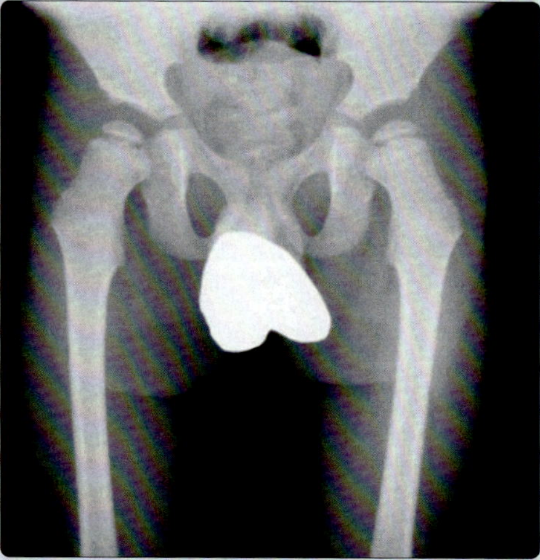

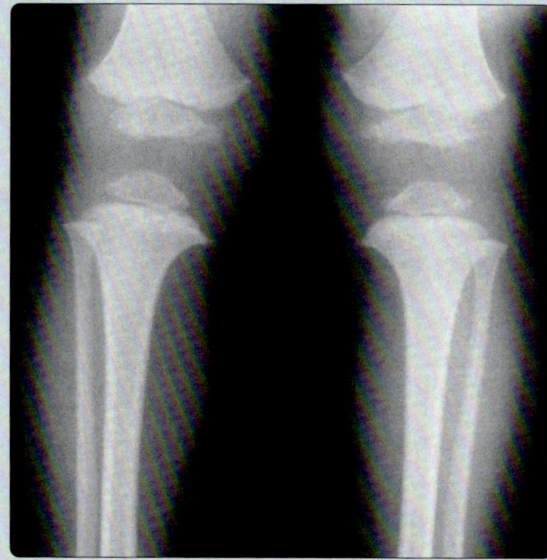

(Left) *AP radiograph reveals mild changes of the proximal femoral capital epiphyses. Both are slightly small and mildly flattened; neither shows fragmentation or stippling. When combined with a normal spine and similar abnormalities in other epiphyses, the diagnosis of multiple epiphyseal dysplasia is established.* **(Right)** *AP radiograph of the knees shows mild abnormality of the epiphyses of the distal femurs and proximal tibias. The epiphyses are small, and the margins are irregular. The growth plates appear normal.*

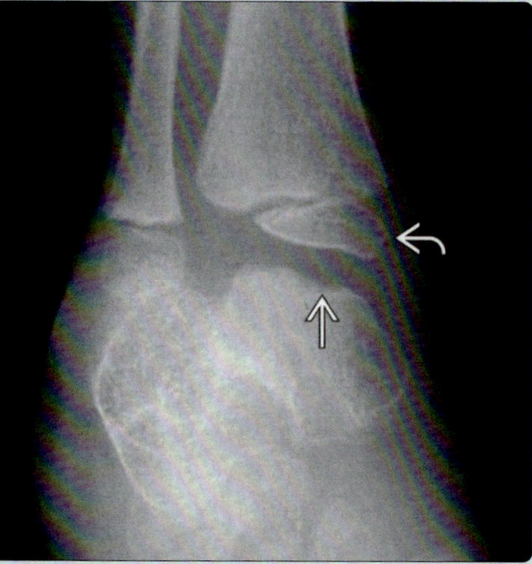

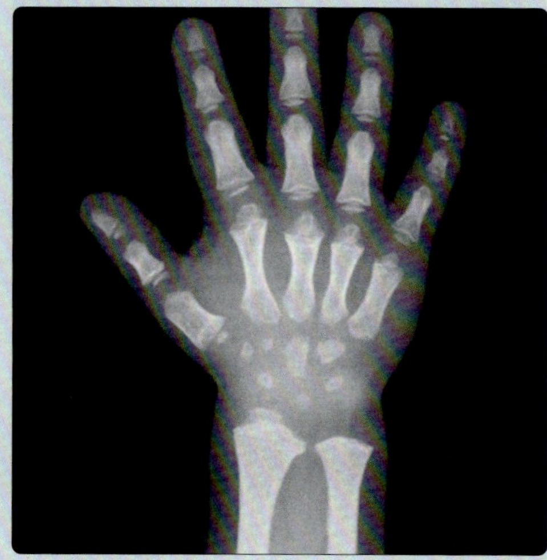

(Left) *Oblique radiograph is most remarkable for flattening of the talar dome ➔. Recognition of the small, mildly irregular distal tibial epiphysis ➔ helps direct the differential diagnosis to a systemic process.* **(Right)** *PA radiograph shows a hand with multiple manifestations of MED. The carpal bones and epiphyses are small with irregular margins, and the metacarpals are short and broad. These manifestations are more common with the autosomal recessive form of MED.*

TERMINOLOGY

Abbreviations

- Multiple epiphyseal dysplasia (MED)
- Epiphyseal dysplasia multiple (EDM)

IMAGING

General Features

- Best diagnostic clue
  - Epiphyseal irregularity, which is bilateral, symmetric
- Location
  - Most severe: Hip, knees, ankles, wrists
  - Minimal involvement of spine

Imaging Recommendations

- Best imaging tool
  - Radiographs sufficient to establish diagnosis
- Protocol advice
  - Requires evaluation of all joints plus spine

Radiographic Findings

- Radiography
  - Bilateral, symmetric abnormal epiphyses
    - Delayed ossification
    - Small and fragmented epiphyses
    - Flattening of epiphyses as skeletal matures
    - Normal metaphyses
  - Delayed bone age
  - Alignment abnormalities
    - Coxa vara
    - Genu valgum
    - Tibiotalar slant
      - Upward, outward tilt of tibiotalar joint
    - Abnormal elbow carrying angle
    - Madelung deformity
  - Hips
    - May mimic Legg-Calvé-Perthes disease
    - May mimic Meyer dysplasia (focal hypoplasia of capital femoral epiphysis)
  - Dominant forms
    - Spine typically normal, although mild endplate irregularity may be seen
  - Recessive form
    - Hands, feet, spine also involved
      - Primarily carpal and tarsal bones
      - Mild brachydactyly
      - Double patella
      - Deformed apophyses, especially T12 and L1

DIFFERENTIAL DIAGNOSIS

Pseudoachondroplasia

- Rhizomelic limb shortening with short, wide tubular bones
- More severe spine involvement
- Small iliac wings, acetabular spikes of bone

Spondyloepiphyseal Dysplasia

- More severe spine involvement, including platyspondyly
- Rhizomelic and mesomelic limb shortening
- Small iliac wings, horizontal acetabular roofs

Hypothyroidism

- Severely delayed bone age
- Mental retardation

PATHOLOGY

General Features

- Etiology
  - Abnormal enchondral ossification in epiphyses and growth plates
- Genetics
  - Multiple different genes involved, most commonly *COMP*
    - Other genes: *COL9A1*, *COL9A2*, *COL9A3*, *MATN3*
    - Involved with formation of type IX collagen
  - Autosomal dominant
    - Fairbanks type: More severe
    - Ribbing type: Less severe
  - Autosomal recessive form less common

CLINICAL ISSUES

Presentation

- Most common signs/symptoms
  - Difficulty walking: Waddling gait common
  - Joint pain
  - Fatigue after exercise
  - Short stature, but not dwarfism
  - Autosomal recessive form
    - 50% have abnormality evident at birth
    - Clubfoot, cleft palate, ear swelling, clinodactyly, scoliosis

Demographics

- Age
  - Usually present in childhood; mild cases may not be diagnosed until young adulthood
- Epidemiology
  - 1 in 10,000 for autosomal dominant type
  - Incidence of autosomal recessive form unknown

Natural History & Prognosis

- Premature osteoarthritis, limited range of motion

Treatment

- Symptomatic: Analgesics, joint replacement

SELECTED REFERENCES

1. Anthony S et al: Multiple Epiphyseal Dysplasia. J Am Acad Orthop Surg. 23(3):164-172, 2015
2. Jeong C et al: Novel COL9A3 mutation in a family diagnosed with multiple epiphyseal dysplasia: a case report. BMC Musculoskelet Disord. 15:371, 2014
3. Panda A et al: Skeletal dysplasias: A radiographic approach and review of common non-lethal skeletal dysplasias. World J Radiol. 6(10):808-25, 2014
4. Park KW et al: Assessment of skeletal age in multiple epiphyseal dysplasia. J Pediatr Orthop. 34(7):738-42, 2014
5. Unger SL et al: Multiple epiphyseal dysplasia: radiographic abnormalities correlated with genotype. Pediatr Radiol. 31(1):10-8, 2001
6. Haga N et al: Stature and severity in multiple epiphyseal dysplasia. J Pediatr Orthop. 18(3):394-7, 1998
7. Silverman FN: C. John Hodson Lecture. Reflections on epiphyseal dysplasias. AJR Am J Roentgenol. 167(4):835-42, 1996

(Left) *Lateral radiograph of the spine shows relatively normal findings, except for mild irregularity of the endplates. The vertebral bodies are otherwise unremarkable; there is no beaking, tongue-like projection, or height loss. Findings such as the latter are more commonly seen with entities such as spondyloepiphyseal dysplasia than MED, which usually has a nearly normal spine, as in this case.* **(Right)** *AP radiograph shows an elbow in a young adult. The radial head and capitellum are both malformed and lack congruity. The medial condyle is also irregular, although more difficult to see. Note the more AP angulation of the forearm relative to the humerus, which clinically manifests as an increased carrying angle.*

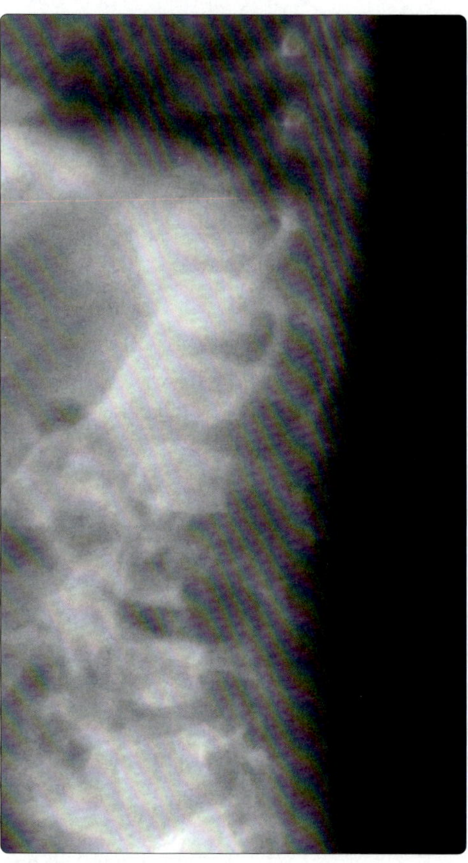

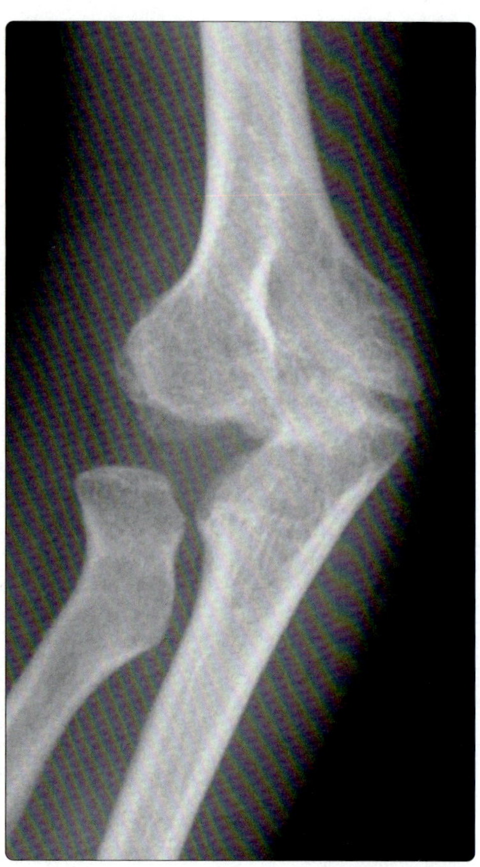

(Left) *AP radiograph shows a right hip with marked abnormality of the femoral epiphysis. The epiphysis is small, with collapse of the articular surface. The acetabulum is normally formed and oriented. The femoral and acetabular articular surfaces are incongruent, which will contribute to premature osteoarthritis.* **(Right)** *AP radiograph of the contralateral (left) hip in the same patient shows femoral epiphysis that is markedly flattened. Interestingly, in this hip the acetabular roof is slightly upturned, likely unrelated to the epiphyseal dysplasia. In both hips, the growth plates and the femoral necks appear normal.*

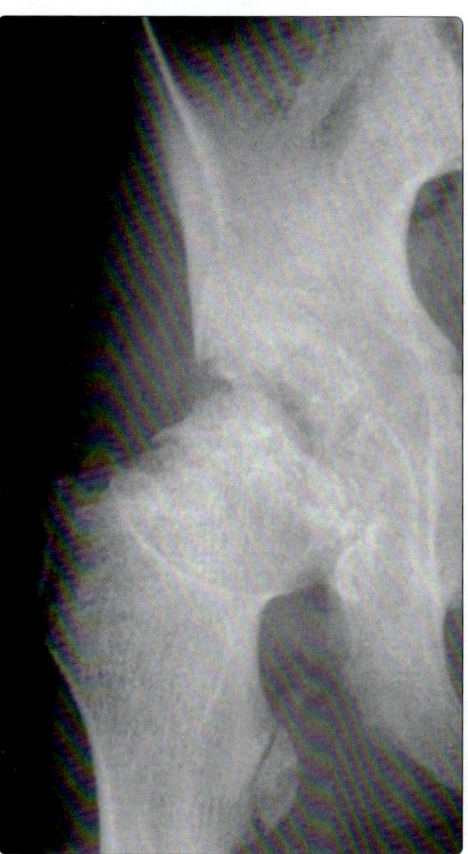

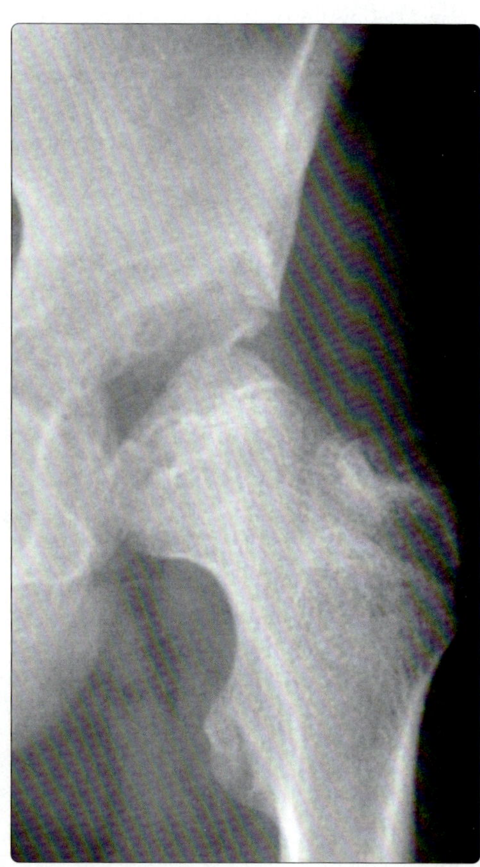

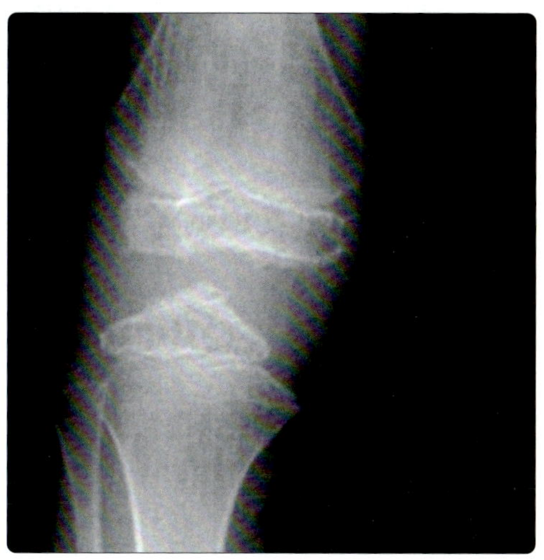

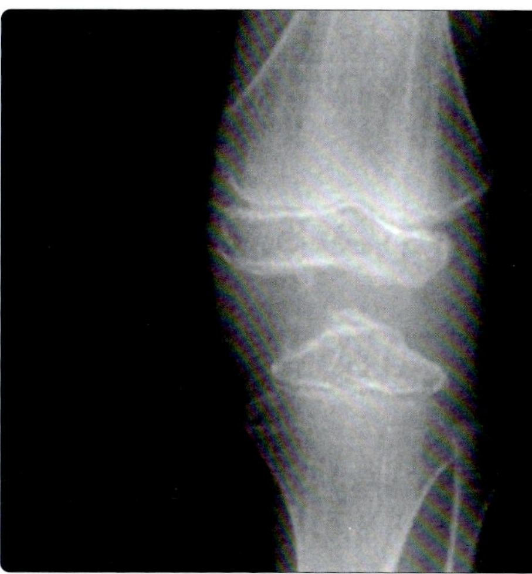

(Left) *AP radiograph of the right knee shows mild changes of multiple epiphyseal dysplasia. The distal femoral epiphysis & proximal tibial epiphysis are small with margin irregularity. The epiphyses should be more mature in this 13 year old; remember to interpret pediatric images within the context of patient age.* **(Right)** *AP radiograph of the opposite (left) knee reveals the bilateral symmetric nature of the epiphyseal abnormalities in MED. Note the absence of the proximal fibular epiphysis.*

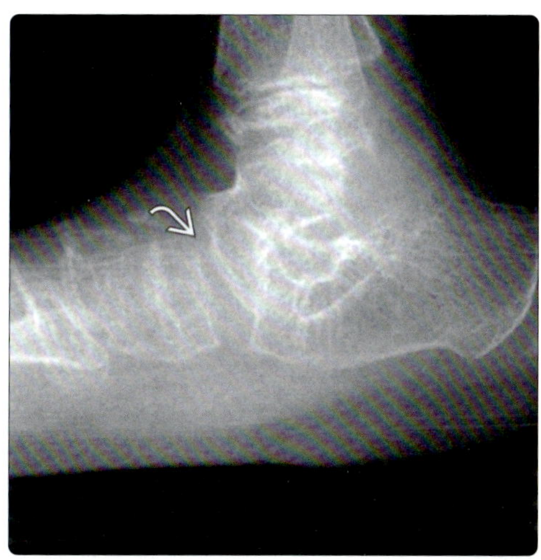

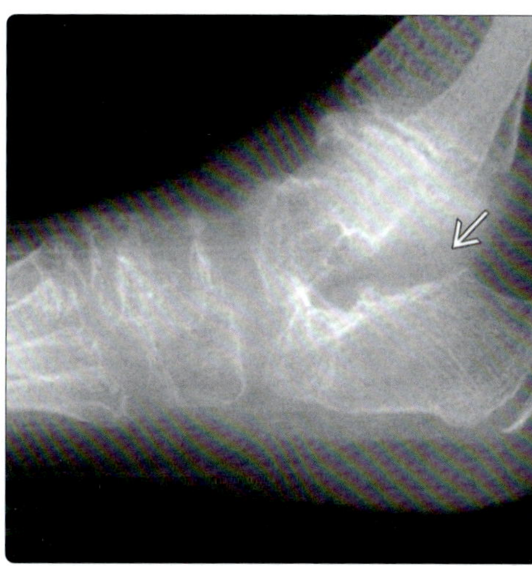

(Left) *Lateral radiograph of the midfoot shows moderate changes of MED. All of the visualized articular surfaces are abnormal. Most dramatic is the articular surface of the talar head ➔, which is flattened and broadened, lacking congruity with the navicular bone.* **(Right)** *Lateral radiograph of the opposite midfoot shows marked distortion of the subtalar articular surfaces ➔. The epiphyses of the metatarsals are significantly delayed for a 13 year old.*

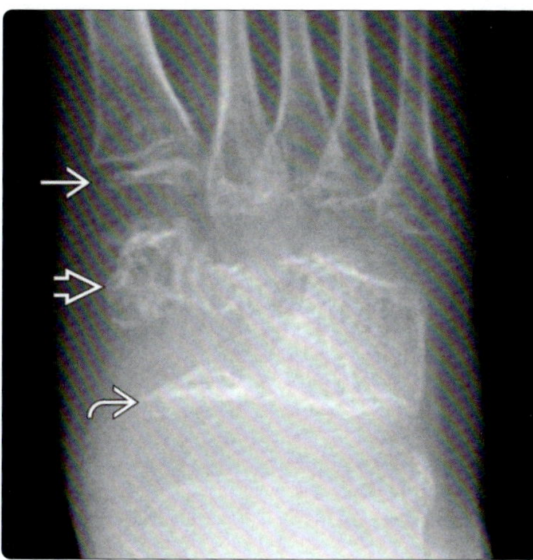

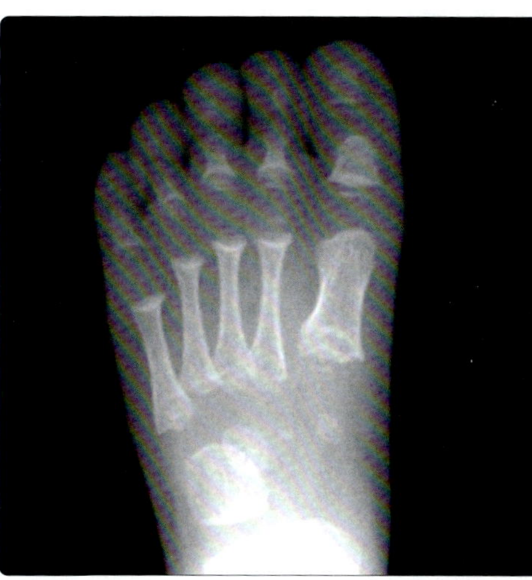

(Left) *AP view of the midfoot demonstrates a small, irregular 1st metatarsal epiphysis ➔ appearing to belong to a younger child, not a patient already 13 years of age. The medial cuneiform ➔ and navicular bone ➔ are particularly small and malformed.* **(Right)** *PA view of the forefoot in a 4 year old shows that the epiphyses of the 3rd through 5th metatarsals are absent, and the head of the 2nd metatarsal is quite small. At this age, the tarsal bones are quite immature; irregularity is not yet apparent.*

Ollier Disease

KEY FACTS

TERMINOLOGY

- Ollier disease: Dysplasia involving predominantly metaphyses, containing chondroid matrix
  - Typically unilateral or asymmetric distribution
  - Spares skull and spine
- Disease is dysplasia, not simply multiple enchondromas

IMAGING

- Lesion characteristics
  - Multiple expansile metaphyseal lytic lesions
  - Osseous expansion; greatest in hands and feet
  - Geographic sclerotic margins
  - Chondroid mineralization: Arcs and whorls, popcorn, ground-glass
  - Spiral or streaky growth pattern from physis into metaphysis
- Pathologic fracture common in hands and feet
- Bone scan may have mild uptake
  - Difficult to confirm malignant transformation to low-grade malignancy

TOP DIFFERENTIAL DIAGNOSES

- Generalized enchondromatosis
  - Diffuse distribution, including skull
- Polyostotic fibrous dysplasia

CLINICAL ISSUES

- Earlier disease onset = more severe deformities
- Palpable mass(es) that enlarge through childhood
- Deformities: Madelung, extremity shortening, limb length discrepancy, angular deformities
- Lesions stabilize or regress with skeletal maturation
- Intervention to treat deformities
- ↑ risk of malignant degeneration to chondrosarcoma
  - Requires surveillance
  - Watch for destructive change, especially after skeletal maturation

(Left) *PA radiograph of the digits in a patient with Ollier disease shows the variety of appearance the dysplasia may display. At one end of the spectrum, the lesions can be extremely expanded ➔ while at the other they may be central and only discernible by the presence of punctate matrix ➔. Although most lesions are central or eccentric, some may be cortically based ➔.* **(Right)** *Lateral radiograph of the same digits shows the bizarre expansion that can occur in this dysplasia ➔. Punctate and whorled matrix is seen.*

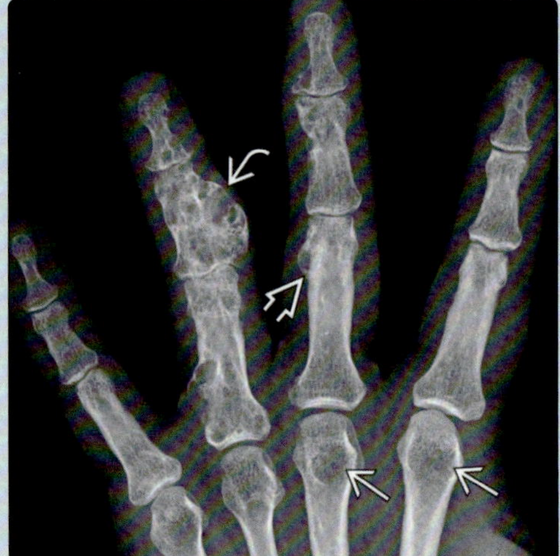

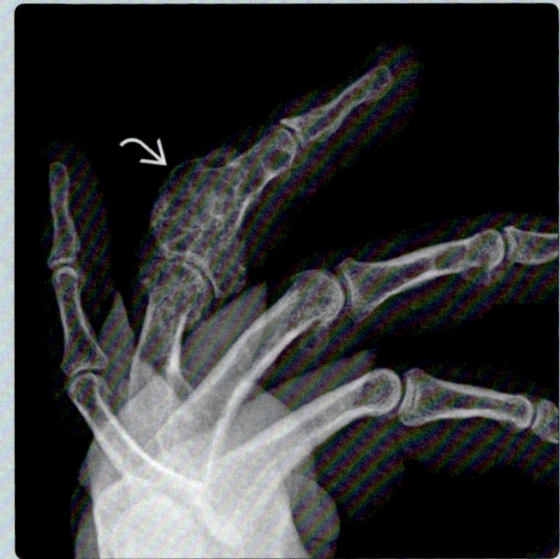

(Left) *AP x-ray shows bizarre expansion and extensive chondroid mineralization of the phalanges of the 4th toe ➔ and prominent expansion and mineralization of the 3rd toe phalanges ➔. The chondroid mineralization provides a diagnostic clue. The 4th metacarpal is shortened secondary to prior pathologic fracture.* **(Right)** *AP x-ray demonstrates a lytic lesion within the proximal femoral metaphysis. The lesion has the streaky or striated appearance ➔ that is commonly seen in the lesions of enchondromatosis.*

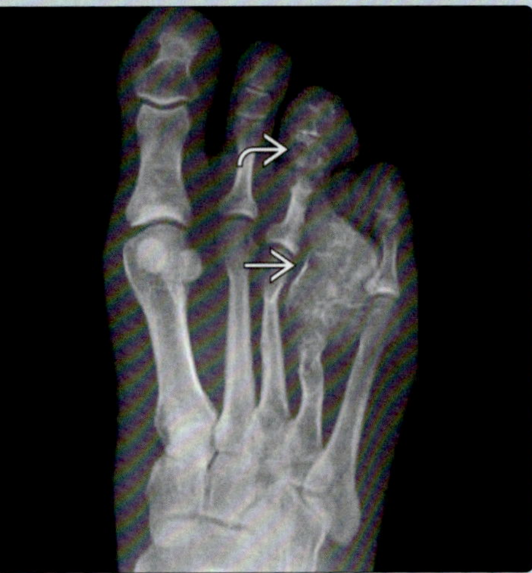

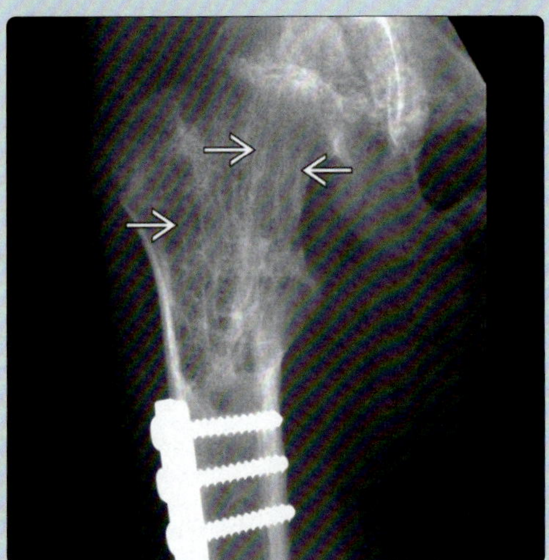

TERMINOLOGY

Synonyms

- Enchondromatosis
- Dyschondroplasia

Definitions

- Ollier disease: Dysplasia involving predominantly metaphyses, containing chondroid matrix
  - Dysplasia, not simply multiple enchondromas

IMAGING

General Features

- Location
  - Predominantly metaphyseal; spares skull and spine
  - Number of lesions and location highly variable
  - Tends to be unilateral or asymmetric
  - Typically central medullary lesions arising near growth plate oriented along long axis of bone
  - Long tubular bones especially femur and tibia > short tubular bones hands and feet > flat bones
  - Other sites: Cortex, periosteum, soft tissues

Imaging Recommendations

- Best imaging tool
  - Radiographs display characteristic appearance

Radiographic Findings

- Radiography
  - Lytic lesion with geographic sclerotic margins
  - Chondroid mineralization
    - Arcs and whorls, popcorn, ground-glass
  - Osseous expansion; greatest in hands and feet
  - Lesion often contains distinct longitudinal streaks
  - Spiral, striated, or streaky growth pattern crosses physis
  - No cortical destruction, periosteal new bone, or soft tissue mass
  - Pathologic fracture common in hands and feet
    - In long bones consider malignant transformation
  - Malignant transformation
    - Pain, cortical destruction, soft tissue mass
    - Loss of previously seen calcifications
    - Enlargement or change after skeletal maturation

CT Findings

- Sensitive for identifying mineralization

MR Findings

- Lesions follow cartilage signal on all sequences
  - Lobulated high signal on fluid-sensitive sequences
- ± low-signal matrix on all sequences
- Lobulated margins characteristic of cartilage lesions
- Aids identification of soft tissue mass associated with malignant transformation

Nuclear Medicine Findings

- Bone scan
  - Lack of uptake excludes malignant transformation
  - May have mild uptake; difficult to confirm malignant transformation to low-grade malignancy

DIFFERENTIAL DIAGNOSIS

Polyostotic Fibrous Dysplasia

- Lesions diaphyseal, lack chondroid mineralization
- Involves facial bones, skull, spine, pelvis

Multiple Enchondromas

- Confined to hands, rarely feet; lacks growth deformities

Generalized Enchondromatosis

- Diffuse distribution, including vertebrae (often platyspondyly), skull, metaphyses
- Inherited process (M > F), variable expressivity

Maffucci Syndrome

- Enchondromatosis with soft tissue hemangiomas

PATHOLOGY

General Features

- Genetics
  - Sporadic, nonfamilial

Microscopic Features

- Intraosseous foci of hyaline cartilage
- Increased cellularity mimics grade I chondrosarcoma, limits role of histopathology especially for determining malignant transformation
  - Imaging plays more significant role

CLINICAL ISSUES

Presentation

- Most common signs/symptoms
  - Palpable mass(es), which enlarge through childhood
  - Limb length discrepancy, angular deformities

Demographics

- Age
  - Typically diagnosed during childhood
- Gender
  - M < F
- Epidemiology
  - Estimated prevalence 1/100,000

Natural History & Prognosis

- Earlier disease onset = more severe deformities
- Lesions stabilize or regress with skeletal maturation
- ↑ risk of malignancy, most common chondrosarcoma
  - 25% at age 40 years

Treatment

- Intervention to treat angular or limb length deformities
- Surveillance for malignant transformation of lesions

SELECTED REFERENCES

1. Herget GW et al: Insights into Enchondroma, Enchondromatosis and the risk of secondary Chondrosarcoma. Review of the literature with an emphasis on the clinical behaviour, radiology, malignant transformation and the follow up. Neoplasma. 61(4):365-78, 2014
2. Le BB et al: Ollier disease with digital enchondromatosis: anatomic and functional imaging. Clin Nucl Med. 39(8):e375-8, 2014
3. Silve C et al: Ollier disease. Orphanet J Rare Dis. 1:37, 2006

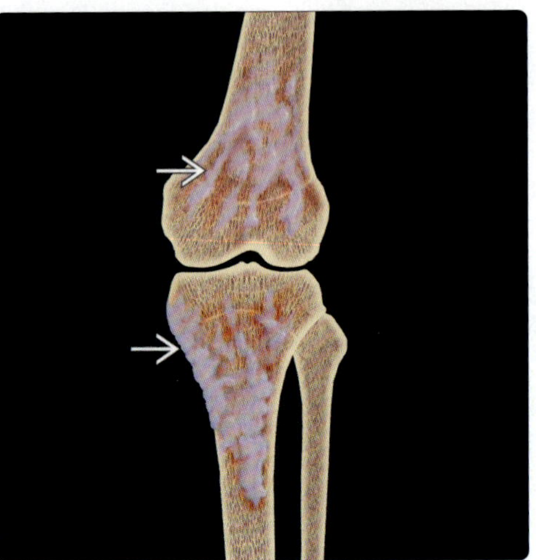

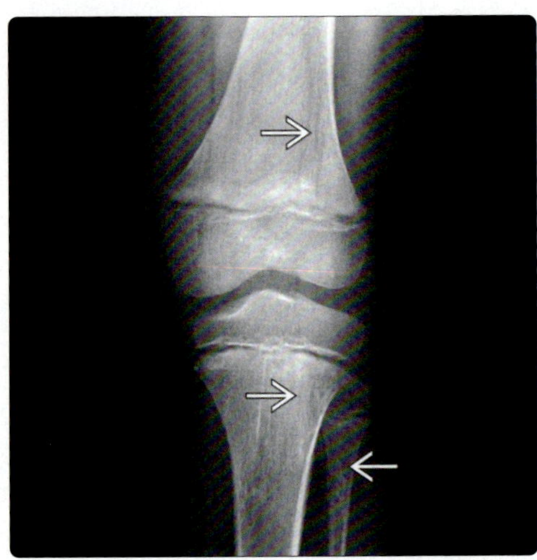

(Left) *Graphic depicts the gross pathologic appearance of Ollier disease. Note the vertical columns of cartilage that cross from the metaphysis into the epiphysis. These columns result in the striated appearance of the lesions in long bones. Cartilage matrix may or may not be present. Crossing the physis often results in growth abnormalities and a unilateral short limb. The diaphysis remains normal.* **(Right)** *AP x-ray shows subtle radiolucent streaks in the metaphyses due to cartilage columns in a patient with Ollier disease.*

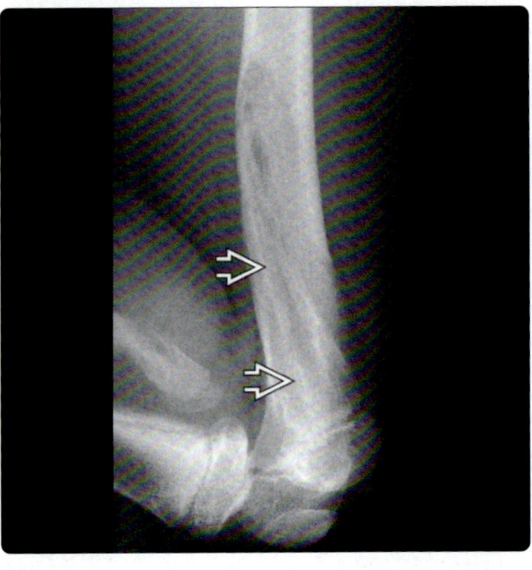

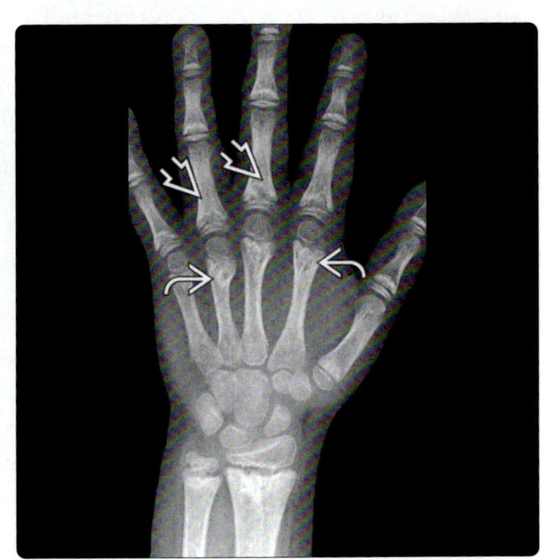

(Left) *Lateral x-ray shows a well-defined femoral lytic lesion. Typical linear lucencies are evident within the lesion. These linear abnormalities have a spiral orientation, which is a variant growth pattern of the cartilage columns that cross the physis in Ollier disease. Note that similar lesions are present in the ipsilateral fibula, and a small lesion is seen within the tibia. The contralateral limb was normal.* **(Right)** *PA x-ray shows a hand with multiple minimally expanded metacarpal and phalangeal enchondromas.*

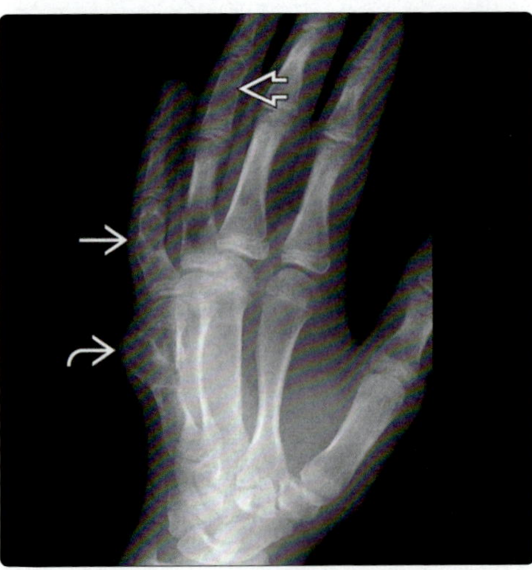

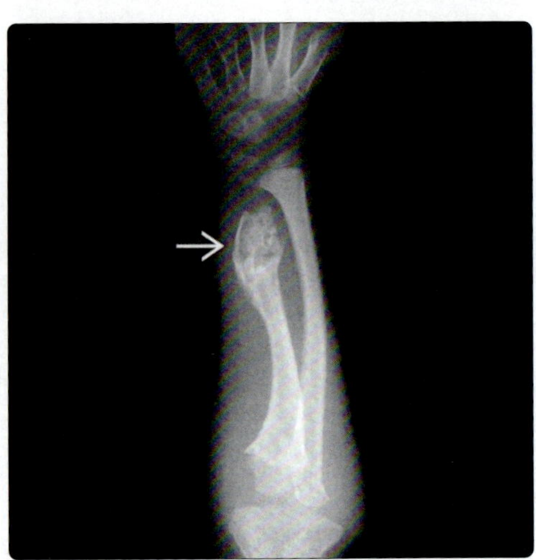

(Left) *Oblique radiograph shows multiple enchondromas. 5th metacarpal lesion is quite expanded, & 5th proximal phalanx lesion is less expansile. A minimally expanded lesion is present in 4th middle phalanx. Each lesion has ground-glass matrix with faint stippled mineralization.* **(Right)** *AP radiograph shows deformity of the ulna. Expanded lytic lesion with arcs & whorls mineralization typical of chondroid matrix is seen in the distal metaphysis. Abnormal carpal angle simulates Madelung deformity.*

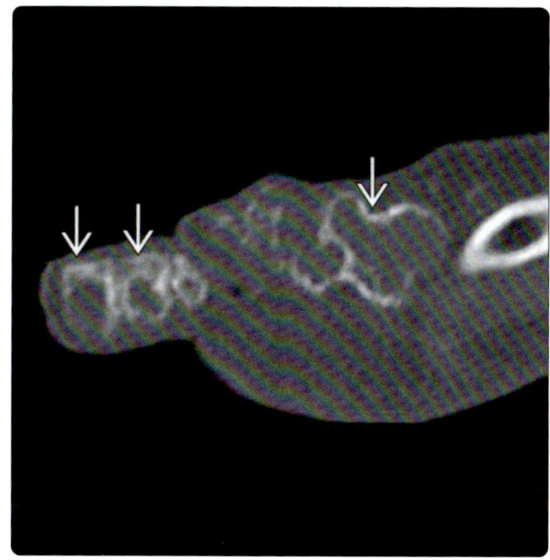

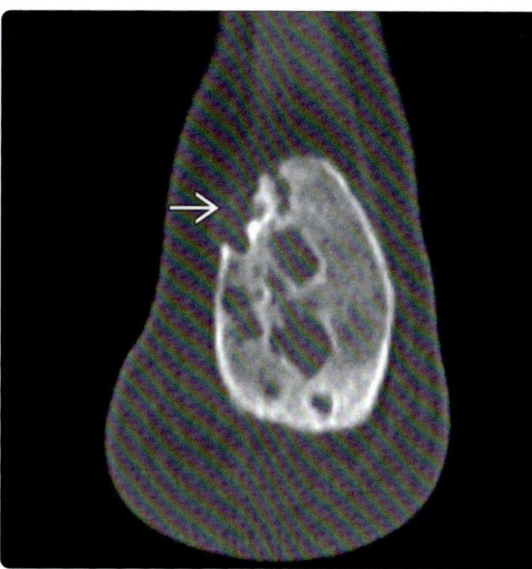

(Left) *Sagittal bone CT of the toes displays multiple expansile lytic lesions involving all of the visualized phalanges* ➡*. No cortical destruction is visible. Chondroid matrix is not evident.* **(Right)** *Coronal bone CT reveals several lytic lesions within the calcaneus. A subperiosteal lesion is present causing pressure erosion on the adjacent cortex* ➡*. Speckled foci of mineralization are faintly seen within the lesion. A subperiosteal location is not unusual for lesions of enchondromatosis.*

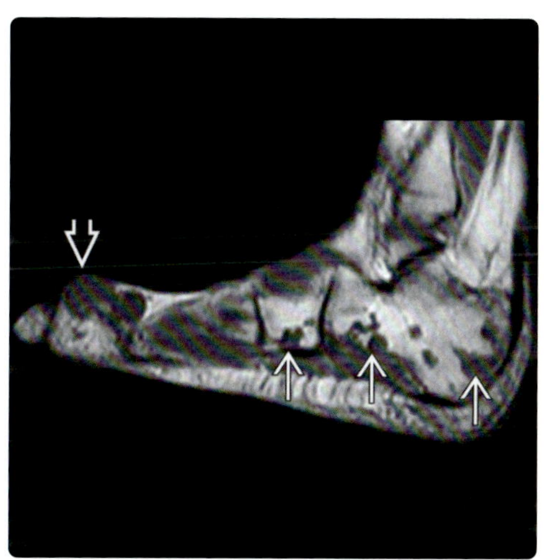

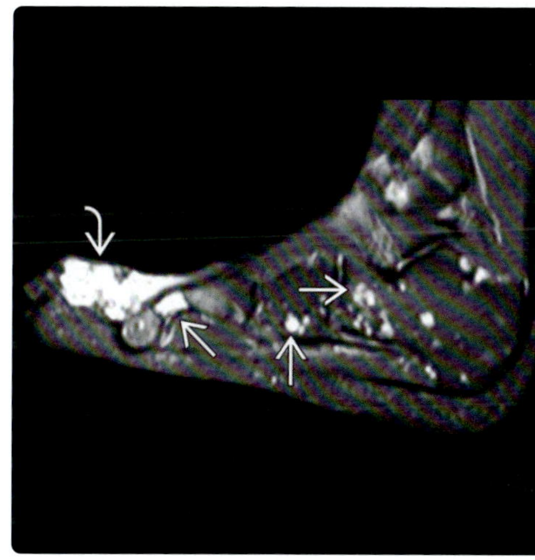

(Left) *Sagittal T1WI MR shows multiple low-intensity lesions with the calcaneus and cuboid* ➡ *as well as a soft tissue mass* ➡ *of similar intensity. Correlation with the radiographic appearance helps establish the diagnosis of multiple enchondromatosis.* **(Right)** *Sagittal T2WI FS MR reveals multiple hyperintense intraosseous lesions* ➡ *as well as a large soft tissue mass* ➡*. Several of the lesions, especially the soft tissue mass, have the lobulated appearance typical of chondroid lesions.*

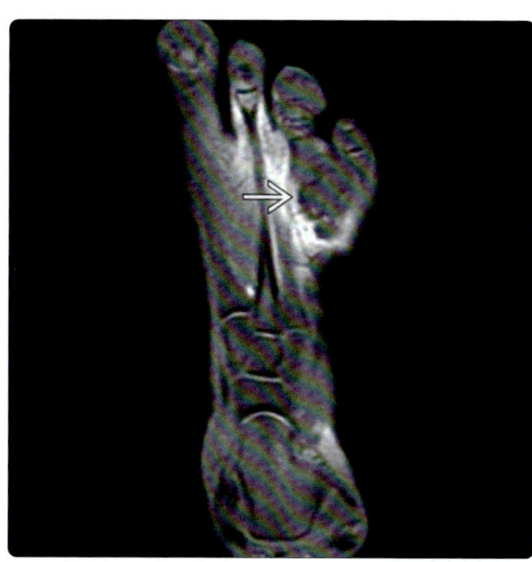

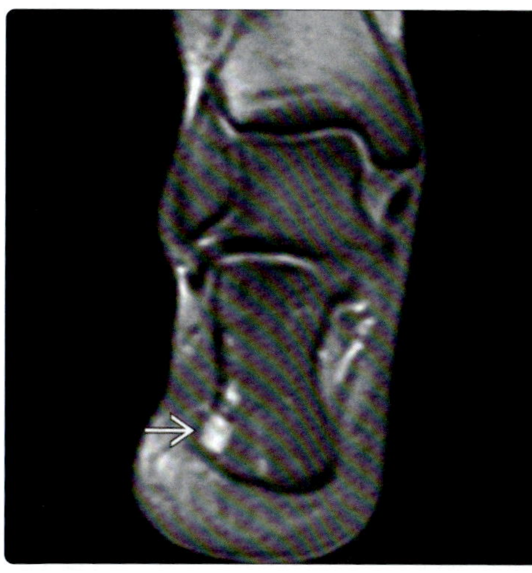

(Left) *Axial T1WI C+ FS MR is shown through a soft tissue mass adjacent to the 4th metatarsal* ➡*. The mass has lobulated margins, which is a common finding among lesions of cartilage origin. This mass did not enhance; enhancement within the lesions of enchondromatosis is variable.* **(Right)** *Coronal T1WI C+ FS MR demonstrates diffuse enhancement of the intraosseous lesions of the calcaneus* ➡ *in this patient with multiple enchondromatosis. These lesions have no defining characteristics.*

Maffucci Syndrome

KEY FACTS

TERMINOLOGY

- Multiple enchondromas with associated soft tissue masses, most commonly hemangiomas
- Hemangiomas distinguish this condition from Ollier disease

IMAGING

- Asymmetric distribution of lesions: Up to 50% unilateral
- Lesions favor upper extremity
- All imaging reflects underlying disease processes
- Enchondromas
  - Multiple expanded metaphyseal lytic lesions with geographic sclerotic margins and chondroid mineralization
  - Lesions typically medullary, central, or eccentric in location; may be intracortical; subperiosteal location uncommon
  - Favor tubular bones, especially phalanges, metacarpals, metatarsals
  - May also appear as tubular lesions extending from growth plate to diaphysis; these lesions may demonstrate striated columnar growth pattern
  - Chondroid mineralization: Arcs and whorls, stippled, popcorn, ground-glass
- Soft tissue masses
  - CT and MR hemangiomas: Intralesional fat, serpentine tubular flow voids that enhance, located subcutaneously or intramuscularly
  - Phleboliths help identify lesions: Appear as calcific foci on radiographs and CT scans; low signal intensity on all MR sequences

PATHOLOGY

- Condition is a form of mesodermal dysplasia
- Enchondromas
  - Abnormal cartilage growth
  - Cartilage tissue extends from growth plate into metaphysis
  - In metaphysis cartilage tissue continues to grow
  - Histology: Lobules of hyaline and myxoid chondroid tissue with enchondral ossification, varying degrees of cellularity, no cellular atypia
- Soft tissue masses
  - Spindle cell hemangioma most common
  - Lymphangiomas less common but may be seen

CLINICAL ISSUES

- Sporadic, nonfamilial
- < 160 reported cases in English literature
- Present with multiple soft tissue and bony masses
  - Over time progress in size and number
- Age at presentation
  - 25% congenital
  - Most manifest in early childhood
  - Almost always present before puberty
- Bone abnormalities secondary to enchondromatosis
  - Angular deformities
  - Limb length discrepancy
  - Pathologic fracture
- Soft tissue masses
  - Bluish hue
  - Decompress with pressure
  - Not limited to extremities; may occur anywhere in body
- Associated malignancy
  - 25% of enchondromas undergo malignant transformation to chondrosarcoma by 40 years old, transformation to fibrosarcoma rare
  - Malignant transformation of hemangiomas
  - Other malignancies may be seen, including pancreas, GI, ovary, glioma
  - Present with pain
  - Imaging: Aggressive bone destruction, change in previously seen mineralization
- Treatment aimed at correction of bone deformities and fractures
- Require ongoing screening for malignant transformation of lesions & associated treatment planning

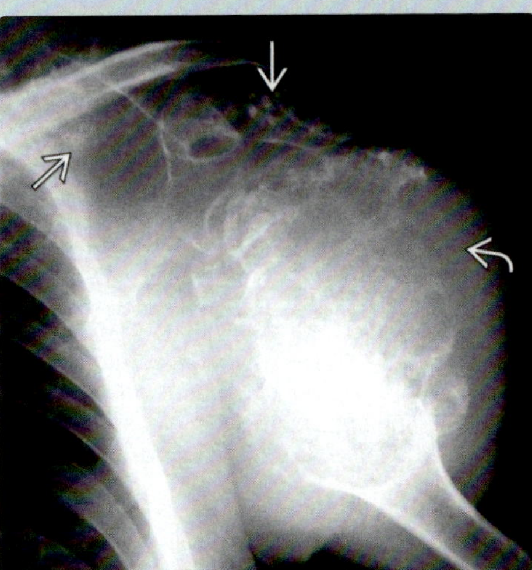

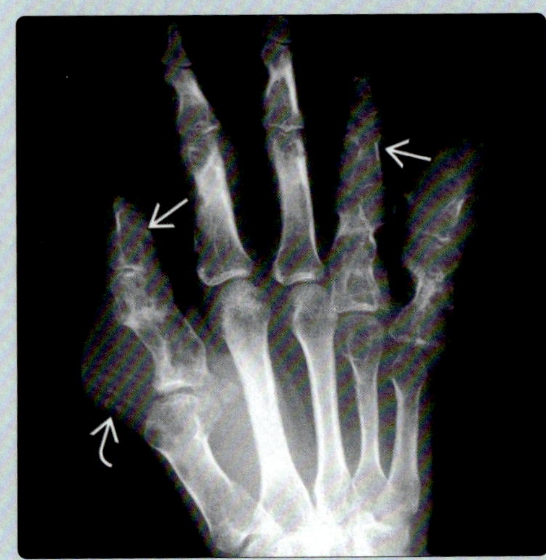

(Left) *AP x-ray shows an aggressive humeral lesion ➢. It represents transformation of enchondroma to chondrosarcoma, as seen in Maffucci syndrome. Multiple phleboliths are in the associated soft tissue hemangioma ➡. (Previously published in Musculoskeletal Imaging: The Requisites. 2nd ed. Philadelphia, PA: Mosby, Elsevier; 2002.)* **(Right)** *PA x-ray, same patient with Maffucci syndrome, shows multiple enchondromas ➡ & phleboliths in a soft tissue hemangioma ➢.*

KEY FACTS

TERMINOLOGY

- Definition: Bone dysplasias with common feature of stippled epiphyses
  - Congenital stippled epiphyses
  - Dysplasia epiphysealis punctata
  - Chondrodystrophia calcificans congenita
  - Conradi-Hünermann disease
  - Curry disease

IMAGING

- Extremities: Stippled epiphyses characteristic
  - Limb shortening, which may be asymmetric
  - Congenital hip dysplasia, clubfoot, clinodactyly
- Spine: Scoliosis, vertebral cleft, or wedging
- Larynx, trachea may calcify; may cause stenosis

TOP DIFFERENTIAL DIAGNOSES

- Warfarin embryopathy: Appropriate history should differentiate
- Hypothyroidism: Thyroid hormone levels obtained at birth and appropriate treatment should prevent
- Spondyloepiphyseal dysplasia: Short trunk differentiates

PATHOLOGY

- Autosomal recessive: Most common; rhizomelic limb shortening, enzyme defect in peroxisomes
- X-linked dominant: Conradi-Hünermann
  - Lethal in males
- X-linked recessive: Curry disease

CLINICAL ISSUES

- 1 in 100,000 births
- Craniofacial: Downward sloping palpebral fissures, flat nasal bridge, high arched palate, frontal bossing, hypertelorism
- Dermatologic: Dry, coarse hair; abnormal nails, hyperkeratosis, ichthyosiform erythroderma
- Congenital cataracts, microphthalmia, microcornea
- Spinal stenosis

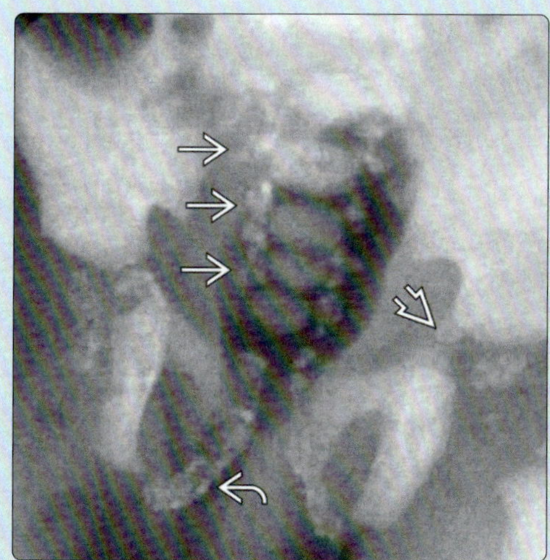

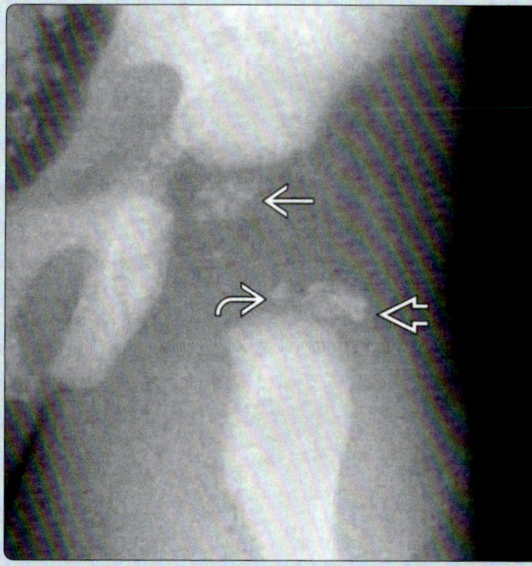

(Left) *AP radiograph reveals extensive stippling in the cartilaginous ossification centers, including the sacral and coccygeal segments ➔, inferior pubic rami ➔, femoral heads, and acetabulum ➔.* **(Right)** *AP radiograph of the left hip reveals stippling of chondrodysplasia punctata. Stippling within the acetabulum ➔ should not be confused with the femoral head. In this patient, the femur is dislocated. The femoral epiphysis ➔ and greater trochanteric apophysis ➔ are stippled.*

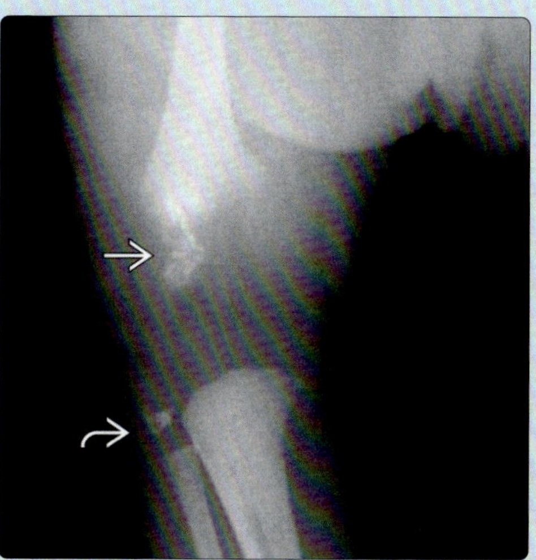

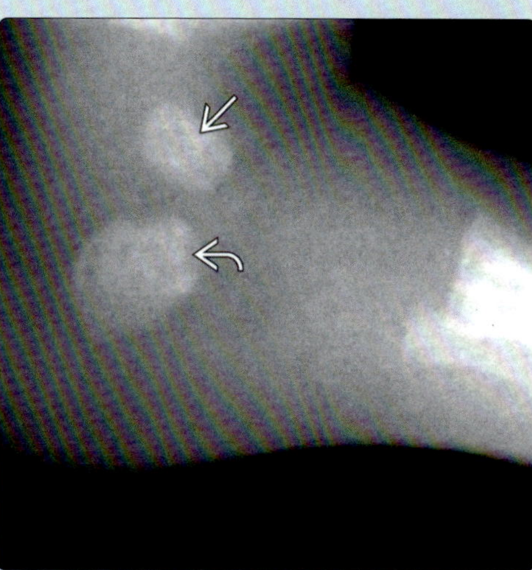

(Left) *AP radiograph of the right knee shows involvement of the epiphyses of the distal femur ➔ and proximal fibula ➔, indicative of chondrodysplasia punctata. Involvement of the entire epiphysis and the patient's young age help differentiate this entity from others associated with stippled epiphyses.* **(Right)** *Lateral radiograph of the foot shows that the stippling in chondrodysplasia punctata involves not only the epiphyses but many sites of enchondral ossification, including the talus ➔ and calcaneus ➔.*

Cleidocranial Dysplasia

KEY FACTS

TERMINOLOGY

- Delayed ossification of midline structures formed through intramembranous ossification
- Synonym: Cleidocranial dysostosis, Marie-Sainton disease

IMAGING

- Radiographs of chest, pelvis diagnostic
- Clavicles
  - Absent or hypoplastic
  - Another appearance: Loss of central 1/3
- Hypoplastic central superior and inferior pubic rami
  - Mimics widened symphysis pubis
- Skull: Wormian bones, wide sutures, premature closure coronal suture, persistent metopic suture, thin calvaria in infancy, persistent fontanelle
- Face: Hypertelorism, frontal bossing, protruding jaw with malocclusion, high arched or cleft palate, dental anomalies
- Hypoplastic glenoid
- Narrow chest
- Coxa vara
- Hand: Short middle and distal phalanges, pointed distal phalanges; accessory metacarpal ossification centers, elongated 2nd metacarpal
  - Short middle phalanx, especially 2 and 5 digits
  - Accessory ossification centers metacarpals 2 and 5
  - Elongated 2nd metacarpal
  - Coned epiphyses

TOP DIFFERENTIAL DIAGNOSES

- Pycnodysostosis: Bones diffusely sclerotic

PATHOLOGY

- Autosomal dominant
- Abnormality in transcription factor gene *RUNX2* (*CBFA1*)

CLINICAL ISSUES

- Short stature
- Able to touch shoulders together in front of chest
- Recurrent otitis media, hearing loss

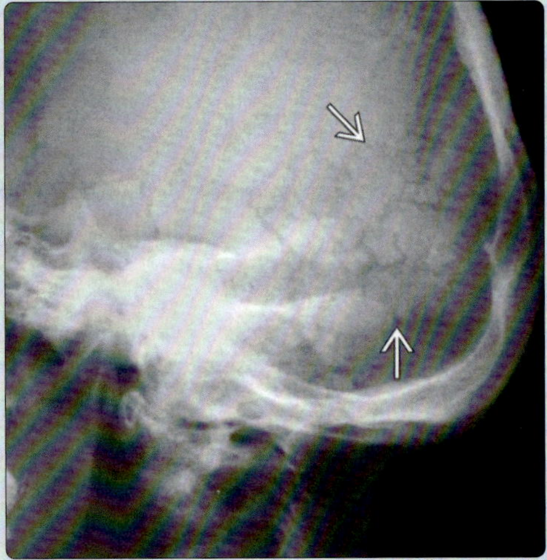

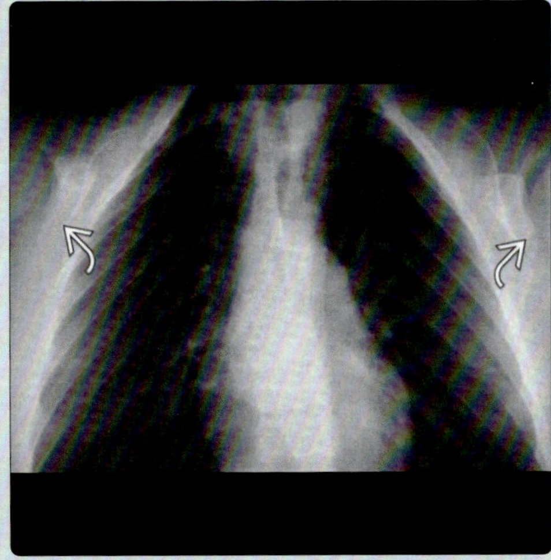

(Left) *Lateral radiograph demonstrates multiple wormian bones ➡. A nonspecific finding, wormian bones are common in patients with cleidocranial dysplasia.* **(Right)** *Anteroposterior radiograph of the chest is diagnostic, demonstrating absence of both clavicles, as well as hypoplastic glenoid fossae ➡. Clavicular anomalies, such as these, lead to the clinical appearance of drooping shoulders and the ability to touch the shoulders together in front of the chest.*

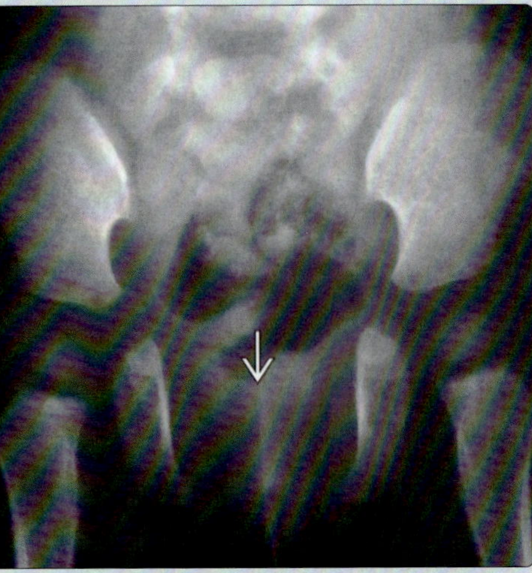

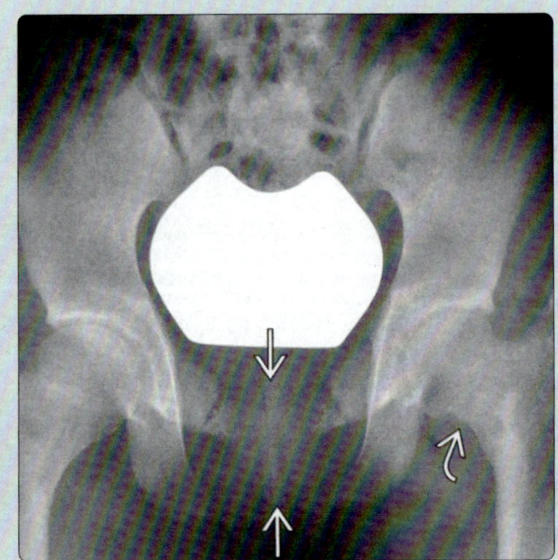

(Left) *AP radiograph of the pelvis demonstrates near-complete absence of midline structures ➡ due to poor ossification within the pubic bodies and rami.* **(Right)** *Anteroposterior radiograph of the pelvis in a skeletally mature individual shows the characteristic midline defect associated with cleidocranial dysplasia ➡. Evaluation of the left hip suggests a coxa vara deformity ➡ with a decreased femoral neck-shaft angle. This femoral anomaly may be seen in patients with cleidocranial dysplasia.*

KEY FACTS

TERMINOLOGY

- Infantile cortical hyperostosis

IMAGING

- Asymmetric, polyostotic cortical hyperostosis
  - Mandible involved > 80% cases
  - Favors ribs, clavicles, scapula, skull, ilium
  - Diaphyses, ± metaphyses, spares epiphyses
  - As periostitis is incorporated into cortical bone → medullary cavity widening, bowing
  - Bowing can persist for years, resolves with remodeling during growth

TOP DIFFERENTIAL DIAGNOSES

- Prostaglandin therapy for congenital heart disease
- Metastatic disease: Neuroblastoma, Ewing sarcoma
- Osteomyelitis: Variable distribution of process
- Trauma: Accidental and nonaccidental
  - Variable distribution ± metaphyseal corner fx
- Physiologic: Asymptomatic, bilateral, resolves by 6 months of age

PATHOLOGY

- Autosomal dominant transmission reported
  - Genetically heterogeneous
  - Mutations in type 1 collagen
- Acute: Inflammation in periosteum ± soft tissues
  - Periosteal new bone ± cortical resorption
- Subacute stage: Periostitis ossifies, incorporated into cortical bone

CLINICAL ISSUES

- Triad: Fever, soft tissue swelling, hyperirritability
- < 5 months of age; may occur in utero
- M = F; no racial/ethnic predilection
- Natural history: Usually self-limited condition
  - Resolves without sequelae after 6-9 months
  - Rarely protracted course with multiple relapses

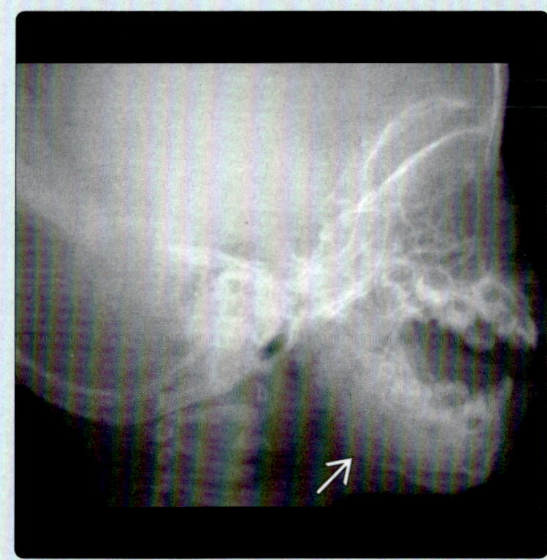

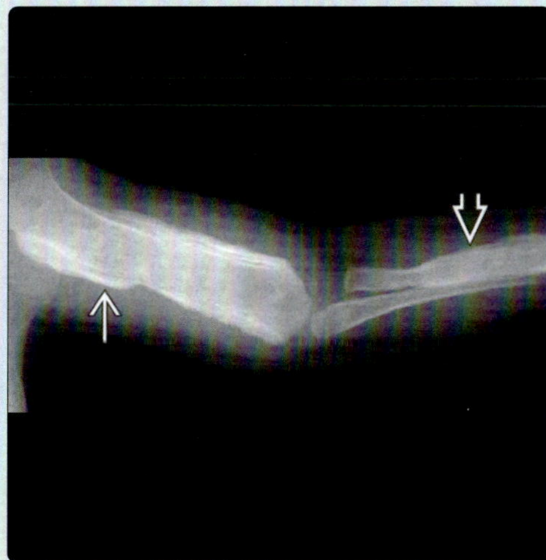

(Left) *Lateral x-ray shows the mandible of a 1 month old. The mandible appears enlarged; note the distance from the tooth roots to the cortex. The cortical margin is wavy ➡. Periosteal changes have a variable appearance throughout the disease course.* **(Right)** *Lateral x-ray shows the upper extremity with exuberant periostitis. Osseous involvement is variable. In this case, the humerus ➡ and radius ➡ are involved, and the ulna is spared. Widening of the medullary canal of the involved bones is already evident.*

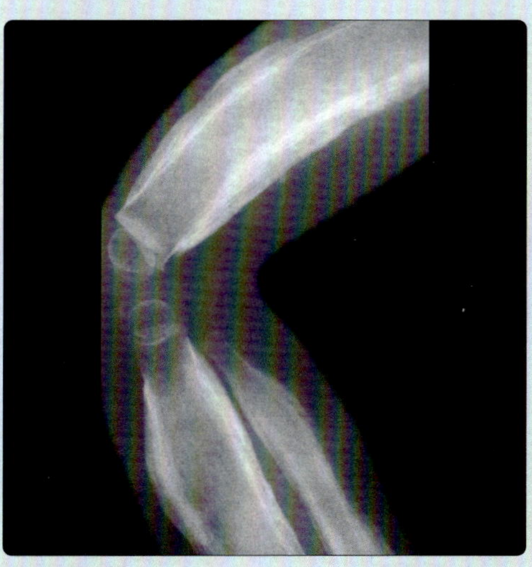

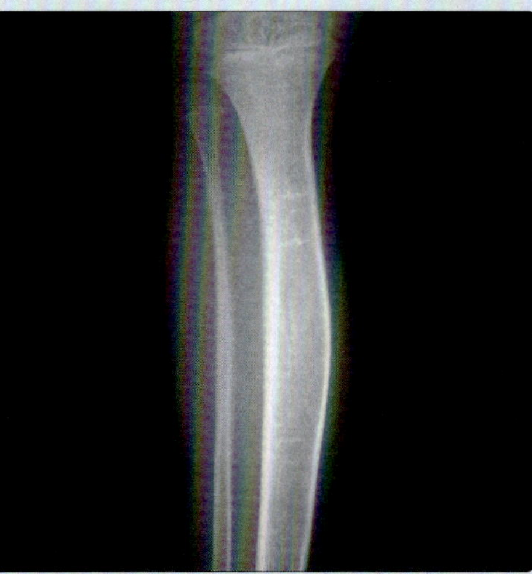

(Left) *Lateral radiograph of the lower extremity reveals marked involvement of the diaphyses of all bones, sparing of the metaphyses of the tibia and fibula and all epiphyses. The medullary cavities are widened and anterior bowing of the femur is evident.* **(Right)** *Anteroposterior radiograph shows the lower extremity at 5 years of age. The periostitis has resolved. Slight medial bowing remains, and the diaphysis is mildly widened. As the child continues to grow, the bones will remodel to a more normal appearance.*

Fong Disease (Nail Patella Syndrome)

KEY FACTS

TERMINOLOGY

- Hereditary osteo-onychodysplasia (HOOD) disease
- Iliac horn syndrome

IMAGING

- Radiographs in conjunction with clinical findings sufficient to establish diagnosis
- Iliac horns (symmetric)
  - Pathognomonic
  - Present in 80%
  - Palpable, asymptomatic
- Absent/hypoplastic patella (asymmetric)
  - Superolateral dislocation
  - Overgrowth medial femoral condyle
  - Hypoplastic lateral femoral condyle
- Absent/hypoplastic radial head (asymmetric)
  - Radial head may sublux or dislocate
- Hypoplastic changes shoulder, hip
- Talipes equinovarus and other foot deformities

TOP DIFFERENTIAL DIAGNOSES

- Nail dysplasia and patellar abnormalities are characteristic; no significant differential considerations

PATHOLOGY

- Autosomal dominant
- *LMX1B* mutation

CLINICAL ISSUES

- 1 in 50,000 live births
- Spectrum of findings is highly variable
- Nail deformities characteristic
  - Bilateral and symmetric
  - Absent, hypoplastic, or malformed
  - Most severe at thumb and along ulnar side of nail
- Renal disease
  - Spectrum from proteinuria to nephrotic syndrome
- Glaucoma
- Joint deformities lead to osteoarthritis

(Left) *Anteroposterior radiograph of the pelvis shows distinct iliac "horns" ➡. These horns are relatively small. Note also the broad horizontal acetabulae ➡ seen in a multitude of skeletal dysplasias.* **(Right)** *Sunrise radiograph shows typical dysplastic changes of the patella. The abnormalities are asymmetric, more severe on the left knee. On the left, the lateral femoral condyle is flattened, and the medial femoral condyle is enlarged. Early osteoarthritic changes are present.*

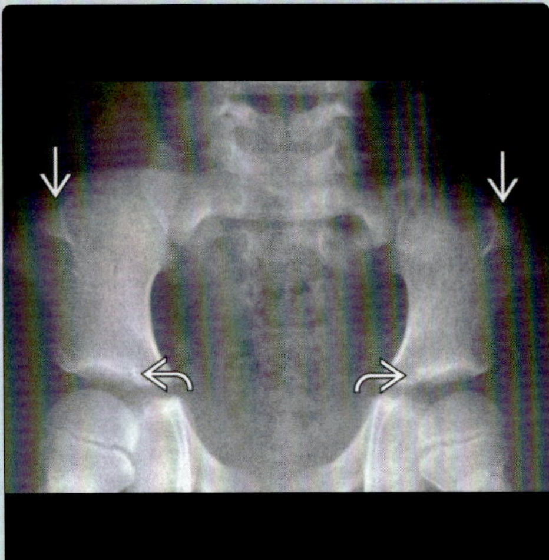

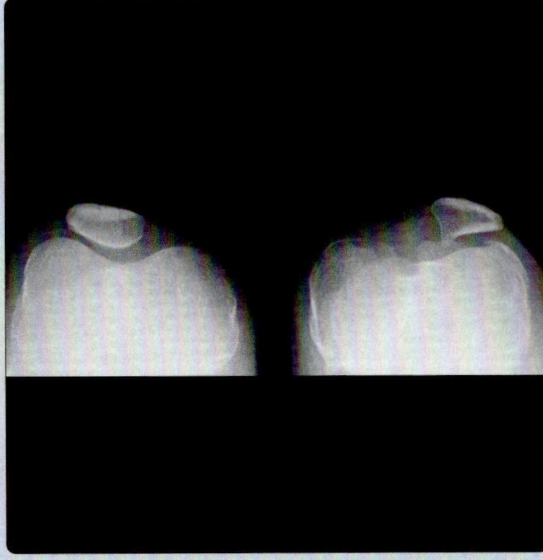

(Left) *Anteroposterior radiograph shows characteristic congenital radial head dislocation. The lateral aspect of the joint is abnormal with morphologic distortion of both the radial head ➡ and capitellum ➡.* **(Right)** *Anteroposterior radiograph reveals hypoplasia of the glenoid and humeral head. While the knee and elbow are most commonly involved in nail patella syndrome, hypoplastic changes may be identified in any joint.*

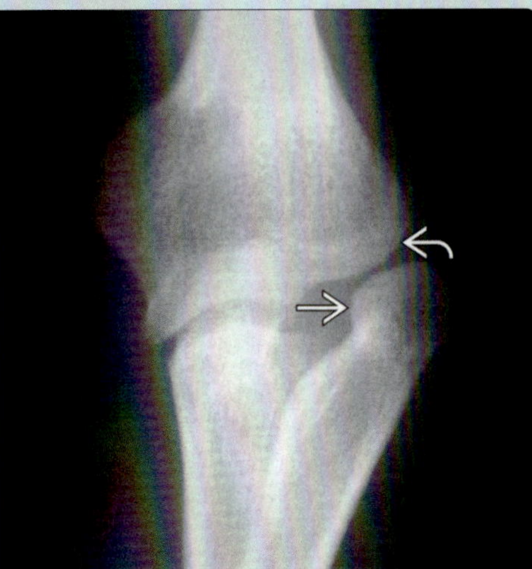

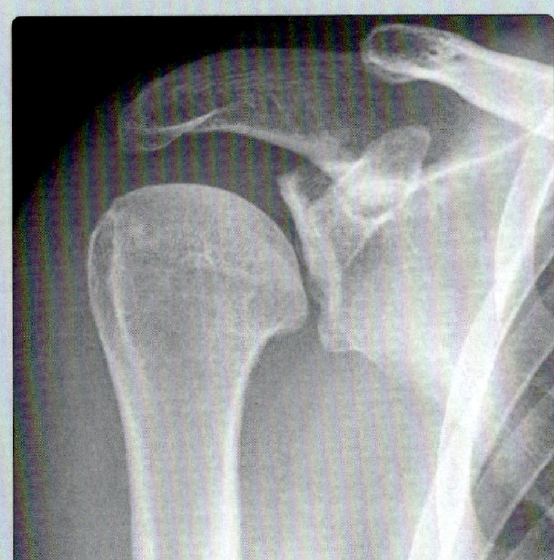

TERMINOLOGY

Synonyms

- Hereditary osteo-onychodysplasia (HOOD) disease
- Iliac horn syndrome
- Turner-Kieser syndrome

IMAGING

General Features

- Best diagnostic clue
  - Iliac horns are pathognomonic

Imaging Recommendations

- Best imaging tool
  - Radiographs in conjunction with clinical findings sufficient to establish diagnosis

Radiographic Findings

- Iliac horns
  - Symmetric
  - Present in 80% of cases
  - Project posterior and lateral from central ilium
  - Palpable
  - Asymptomatic
- Absent/hypoplastic patella
  - Asymmetric
  - Superolateral dislocation
  - Knees appear flattened
  - Overgrowth medial femoral condyle
  - Hypoplastic lateral femoral condyle
  - Enlarged tibial tubercle
- Absent/hypoplastic radial head
  - Asymmetric
  - Radial head may sublux or dislocate
  - Hypoplastic capitellum and lateral condyle
  - Prominent medial condyle
  - Creates ulna positive deformity at wrist
  - Cubitus valgus
  - Limited motion
- Hypoplastic changes shoulder, hip
- Talipes equinovarus and other foot deformities

DIFFERENTIAL DIAGNOSIS

Nail Dysplasia and Patellar Abnormalities

- Characteristic; no significant differential considerations

PATHOLOGY

General Features

- Genetics
  - Autosomal dominant
    - Most individuals have affected parent
  - *LMX1B* mutation

CLINICAL ISSUES

Presentation

- Most common signs/symptoms
  - Spectrum of findings is highly variable
  - Typically complaint of knee pain or instability
    - Limited extension
    - Locking, clicking
  - Nail deformities characteristic
    - Bilateral
    - Symmetric
    - Abnormal lunula
      - Malformed or triangular
      - Triangular lunula may be only manifestation of syndrome
    - Absent, hypoplastic, or malformed
      - Discolored, ridges, pitted, split, thickened
    - Most severe at thumb
      - Lessening severity toward little finger
    - Changes more severe along ulnar side of nail
    - Fingers more affected than toes
  - Renal disease
    - Spectrum from proteinuria to nephrotic syndrome
    - Develops in 40%
    - Cause of most significant syndrome-related morbidity
  - Glaucoma
- Other signs/symptoms
  - Lester iris (hyperpigmentation of pupillary margin of iris)
  - Pterygium (skin webs) at elbow
  - Lean body habitus
    - Poor muscle development in upper arms and thighs
  - Absent skin creases over DIP joints
  - Limited motion DIP and PIP joints
  - Poor hair growth
    - Hair tends to be fine
    - Male pattern baldness
  - Irritable bowel syndrome

Demographics

- Epidemiology
  - 1 in 50,000 live births

Natural History & Prognosis

- Joint deformities lead to osteoarthritis

Treatment

- Symptomatic treatment of joint disease
  - Realignment of patella; resection of synovial band
- Ongoing screening
  - Hypertension
  - Renal disease
  - Glaucoma

SELECTED REFERENCES

1. Lo Sicco K et al: Nail-patella syndrome. J Drugs Dermatol. 14(1):85-6, 2015
2. Albishri J: Arthropathy and proteinuria: nail-patella syndrome revisited. Ger Med Sci. 12:Doc16, 2014
3. Lippacher S et al: Correction of malformative patellar instability in patients with nail-patella syndrome: a case report and review of the literature. Orthop Traumatol Surg Res. 99(6):749-54, 2013
4. Sweeney E et al: Nail patella syndrome: a review of the phenotype aided by developmental biology. J Med Genet. 40(3):153-62, 2003
5. Karabulut N et al: Imaging of "iliac horns" in nail-patella syndrome. J Comput Assist Tomogr. 20(4):530-1, 1996
6. Falvo KA et al: Osteo-onychodysplasia. Clin Orthop Relat Res. 81:130-5, 1971

KEY FACTS

IMAGING

- 1 bone or multiple bones of single extremity
- Favors lower extremity, spares skull and face, rarely involves spine
- Hyperostosis
  - Predominately periosteal; undulating appearance along cortex likened to dripping candle wax
  - May be endosteal with intramedullary extension
- Linear intraosseous sclerosis
- Rounded osteoma-like foci of sclerosis
- Soft tissue masses (uncommon)
  - Periarticular; varying degrees of mineralization

TOP DIFFERENTIAL DIAGNOSES

- Progressive diaphyseal dysplasia
- Osteopathia striata
- Intramedullary osteosclerosis
- Myositis ossificans

PATHOLOGY

- Nonhereditary, sporadic distribution
- Hyperostosis: Lamellar and woven bone
- Soft tissue masses: Varying combinations of fibrovascular, osteocartilaginous, and adipose tissue

CLINICAL ISSUES

- Usually incidental finding
- Symptomatic disease: Pain and stiffness
  - Presents in teenage years or early adulthood
  - Slowly progressive, eventually stabilizes in adulthood
  - Severe symptoms may be treated with bisphosphonates
- Associated soft tissue changes
  - Involved dermatome in same distribution as osseous changes
  - Vascular tumors and malformations: Hemangioma, arteriovenous malformations, glomus tumors

(Left) *AP x-ray shows a mixed pattern of sclerosis common in melorheostosis. Multiple foci of thick linear sclerosis are seen, accompanied by multiple rounded osteoma-like foci.* **(Right)** *AP x-ray shows a sclerotomal pattern of sclerosis seen in melorheostosis. There is intramedullary sclerosis throughout the great toe and the bones along the medial aspect of the midfoot and hindfoot. Involvement of the 2nd toe and the middle cuneiform is confined to the medial aspect of those bones.*

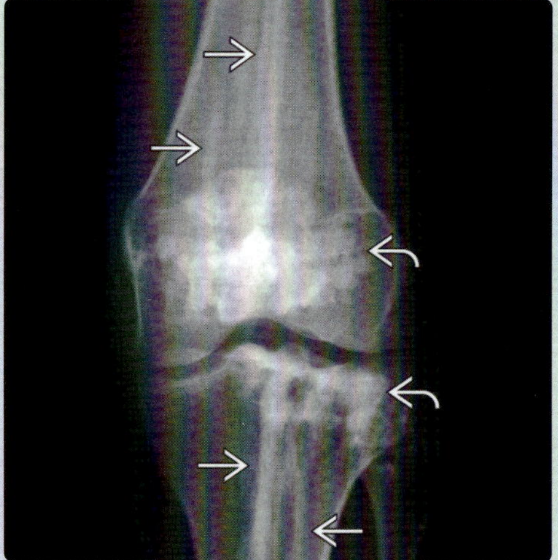

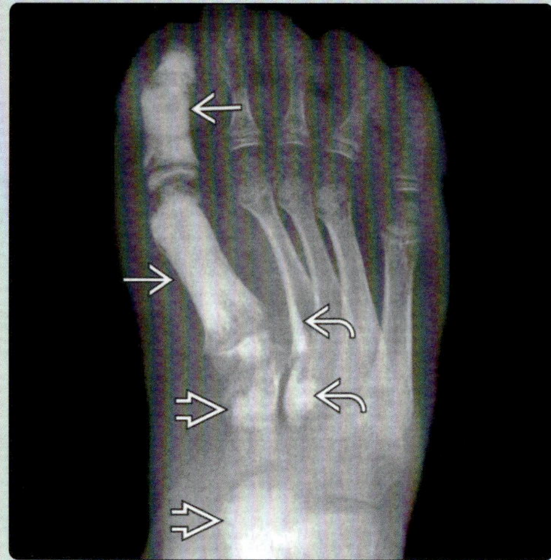

(Left) *Sagittal T1WI MR of an uncommon upper extremity case of melorheostosis shows the undulating pattern of periosteal hyperostosis, which has been likened to dripping candle wax. Note the mild involvement of the endosteum.* **(Right)** *Anterior view of the forearm from a bone scan reveals an intense focus of uptake in the proximal ulna. The uptake is along the surface of the bone, consistent with periosteal hyperostosis. Even on this study, with its low resolution, the dripping candle wax appearance is easily appreciated.*

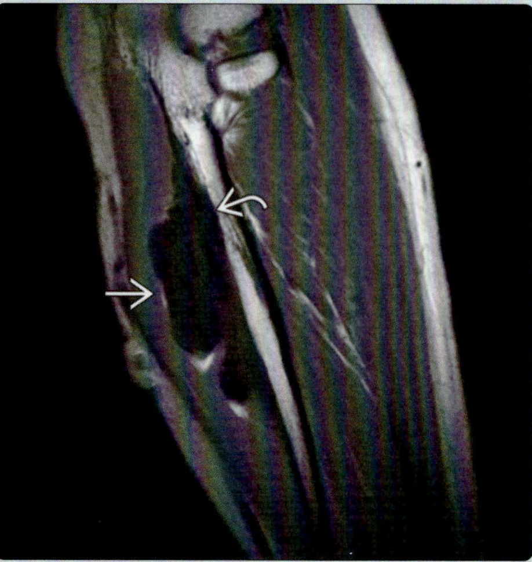

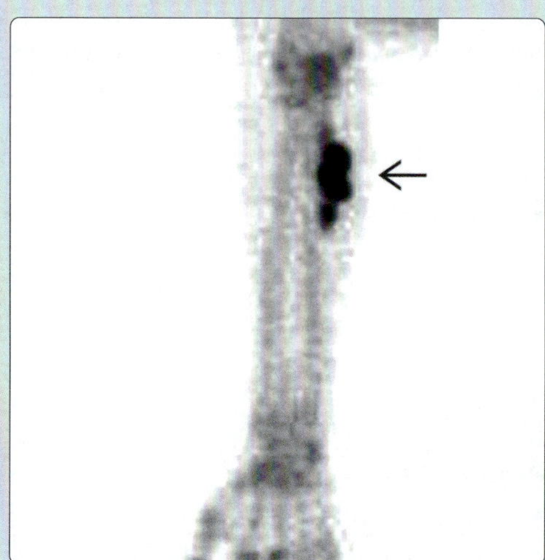

TERMINOLOGY

Synonyms

- Leri disease
- Flowing periosteal hyperostosis

IMAGING

General Features

- Best diagnostic clue
  - Dripping candle wax appearance of cortical hyperostosis or linear intraosseous sclerosis
- Location
  - 1 bone or multiple bones of single extremity
    - Occurs in sclerotomal distribution
  - Favors lower extremity, spares skull and face, rarely involves spine

Imaging Recommendations

- Best imaging tool
  - Radiographs are sufficient to establish diagnosis

Radiographic Findings

- Radiography
  - Hyperostosis
    - Cortical thickening, predominately periosteal
      - □ May be endosteal with intramedullary extension
    - Undulating appearance along cortex likened to dripping candle wax
    - Rarely extends beyond margins of bone into joint
    - Linear intraosseous sclerosis &/or rounded osteoma-like sclerosis
  - Soft tissue masses uncommon
    - Periarticular distribution
    - May be mineralized
      - □ No zoning pattern; should not be mistaken for myositis ossificans

MR Findings

- Hyperostosis
  - Low signal on all imaging sequences
  - No enhancement
- Bursa over hyperostosis
- Muscle atrophy secondary to nerve compression
- Soft tissue mass: Appearance depends on composition
  - T1WI: Low to intermediate signal
  - T2WI: Variable, depending on maturity
  - Contrast enhanced: Variable enhancement

Nuclear Medicine Findings

- Bone scan
  - Intense uptake in skeletal lesions
  - Uptake may be seen in mineralized soft tissue masses

DIFFERENTIAL DIAGNOSIS

Progressive Diaphyseal Dysplasia

- Symmetric bilateral distribution, diaphysis
- No soft tissue involvement

Osteopathia Striata

- Centered around joints, lacks sclerotome distribution
- May coexist with melorheostosis

Intramedullary Osteosclerosis

- Confined to intramedullary location
- Tibia almost always involved

Myositis Ossificans

- Soft tissue masses of melorheostosis may mimic myositis ossificans (MO)
  - MO has distinctive zoning pattern not seen on melorheostosis

PATHOLOGY

General Features

- Etiology
  - Error in intramembranous bone formation
  - Abnormal angiogenesis may also play role
- Genetics
  - Alteration in *LEMD3* gene
  - Nonhereditary, sporadic distribution

Microscopic Features

- Hyperostosis
  - Lamellar and woven bone
- Soft tissue masses
  - Fibrovascular, osteocartilaginous, and adipose tissue

CLINICAL ISSUES

Presentation

- Most common signs/symptoms
  - Usually incidental finding
  - When symptomatic presents with pain or stiffness
- Other signs/symptoms
  - Soft tissue abnormalities
    - Same dermatomal distribution as osseous changes
    - Vascular tumors and malformations: Hemangioma, arteriovenous malformations, glomus tumors
  - Physical deformity uncommon
    - Limb length discrepancy; joint contractures

Demographics

- Age
  - Presents in teenage years or early adulthood

Natural History & Prognosis

- Slowly progressive, stabilizes in adulthood

Treatment

- Aimed at reducing pain and stiffness if present
- Bisphosphonates reported to relieve symptoms

SELECTED REFERENCES

1. Kadhim M et al: Melorheostosis: segmental osteopoikilosis or a separate entity? J Pediatr Orthop. 35(2):e13-7, 2015
2. Slimani S et al: Successful treatment of pain in melorheostosis with zoledronate, with improvement on bone scintigraphy. BMJ Case Rep. 2013, 2013
3. Judkiewicz AM et al: Advanced imaging of melorheostosis with emphasis on MRI. Skeletal Radiol. 30(8):447-53, 2001

(Left) *AP x-ray shows diffuse cortical thickening, a typical finding of melorheostosis. Extensive periosteal new bone formation is seen along the medial cortex ➡. Diffuse endosteal sclerosis is present, encroaching on the medullary canal ➡. Linear sclerosis can be seen proximally ➡.* **(Right)** *AP x-ray shows endosteal sclerosis confined to the medial aspect of the tibia ➡ and ankle ➡. The sclerosis appears to flow along the bone. The lateral tibia and fibula are spared, typical of the sclerotomal distribution seen with this dysplasia.*

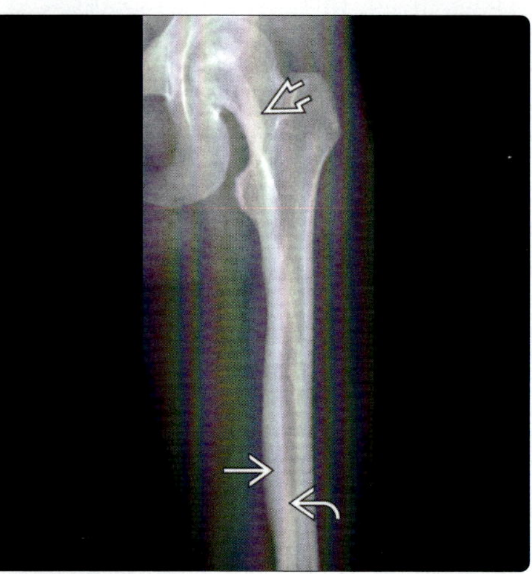

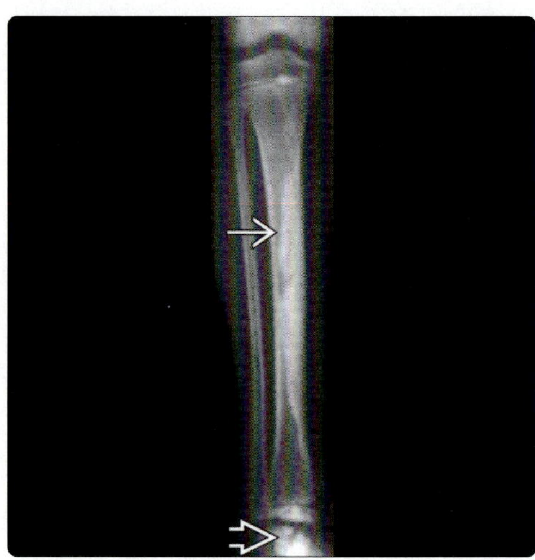

(Left) *Lateral radiograph in a young woman shows a fluffy sclerotic mass ➡ in posterior thigh, with normal underlying bone. Importantly, there is no zoning phenomenon to suggest myositis ossificans. The various etiologies of heterotopic ossification vs. an extremely rare extraosseous osteosarcoma could be considered.* **(Right)** *Lateral radiograph in same patient was taken following biopsy and partial excision. Pathology showed myositis ossificans; this diagnosis should have been disputed, given the lack of zoning pattern on the x-ray.*

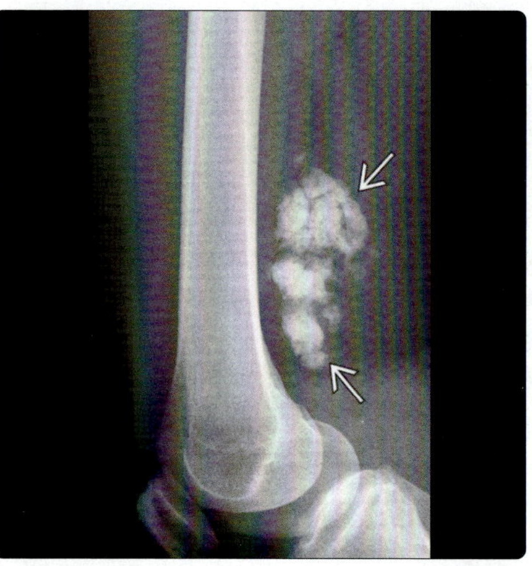

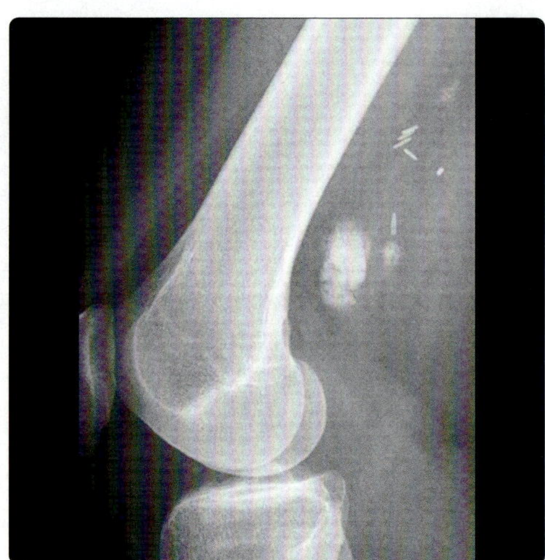

(Left) *Lateral radiograph obtained 6 years later shows mild recurrence of the ossification. It does not appear to be aggressive.* **(Right)** *AP radiograph of the tibia in the ipsilateral extremity obtained at the same time as the follow-up distal thigh shows findings typical of melorheostosis. There is periosteal osseous thickening ➡, with little endosteal involvement. This proves the overall diagnosis of melorheostosis involving both bone and soft tissues, initially misdiagnosed as myositis ossificans.*

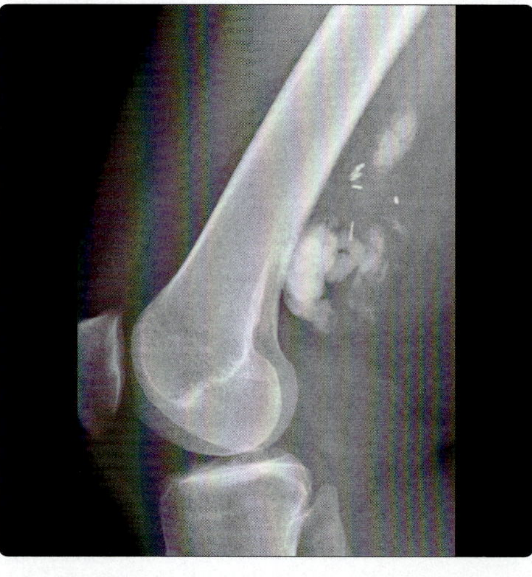

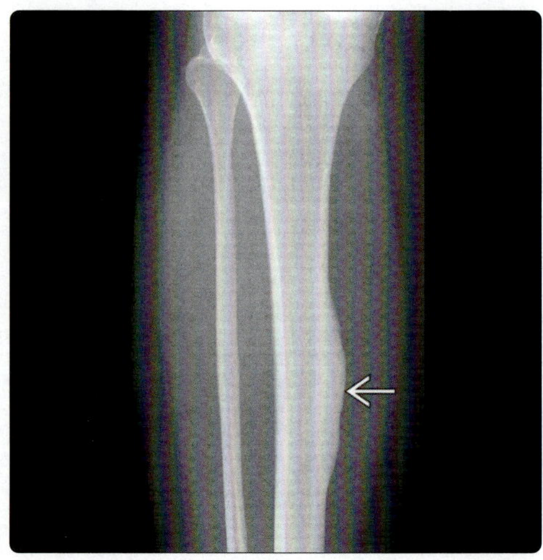

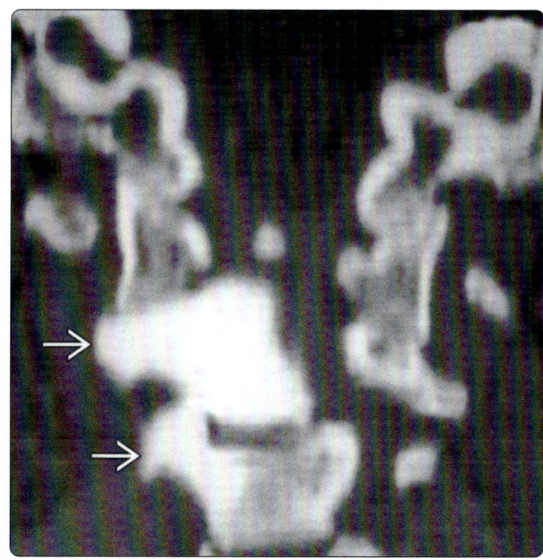

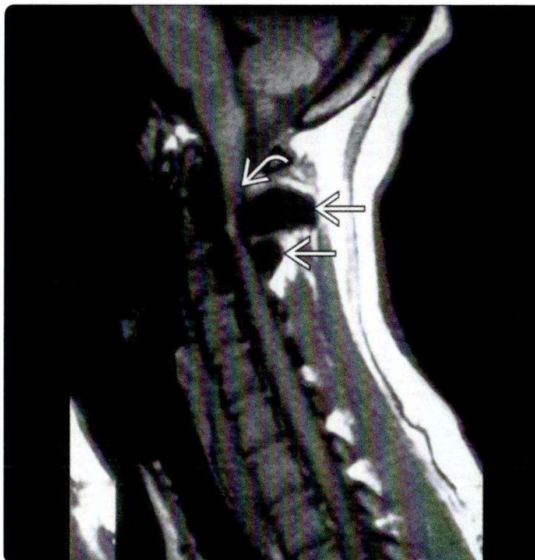

(Left) *Coronal reformatted CT reveals extensive C2 & C3 endosteal and periosteal hyperostosis with loss of the intervening marrow. The changes are confined to the right side of contiguous vertebral bodies.* **(Right)** *Sagittal T1WI MR reveals the low signal that is typical for the lesions of melorheostosis. In addition, the marked canal stenosis with spinal cord compression is easily appreciated.*

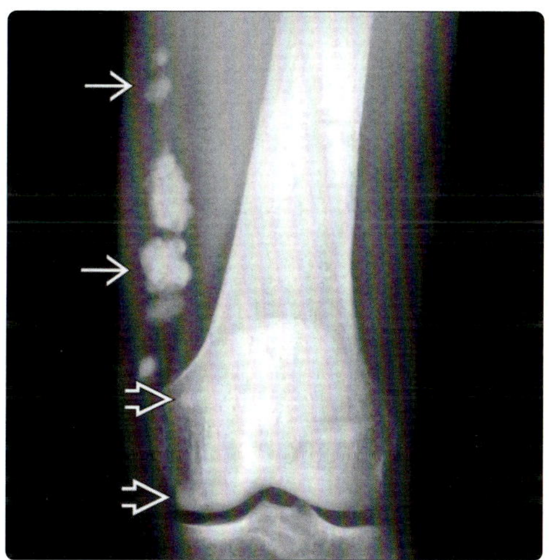

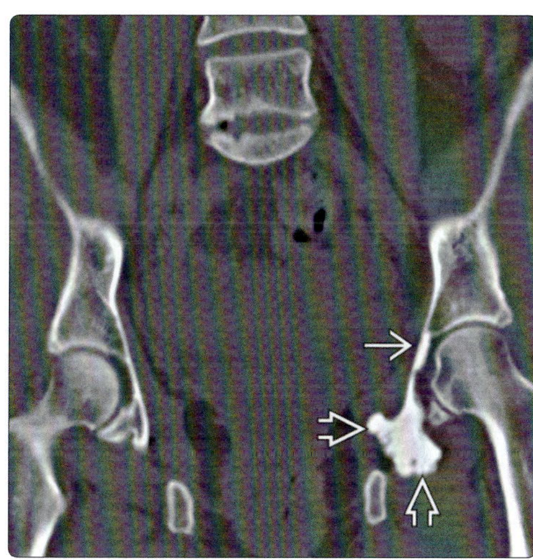

(Left) *AP radiograph reveals an uncommon pattern of melorheostosis. In this case the soft tissue changes dominate. Multiple rounded, completely mineralized soft tissue masses are present in a linear distribution. The osseous changes are less conspicuous.* **(Right)** *Coronal CT demonstrates dense endosteal bone formation extending along the medial plate of the acetabulum. Associated periosteal hyperostosis extends into the adjacent musculature. There are no aggressive features.*

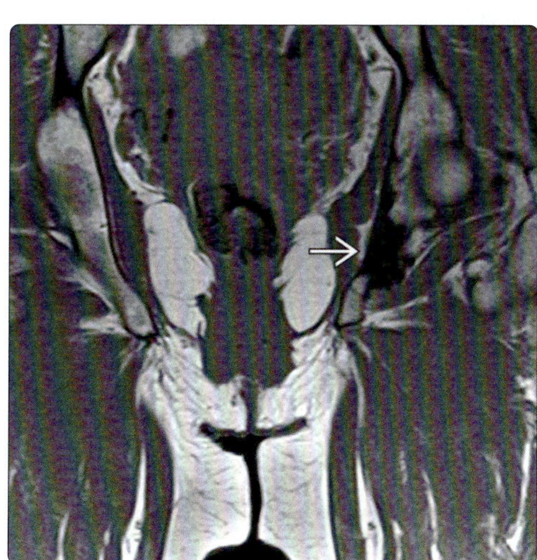

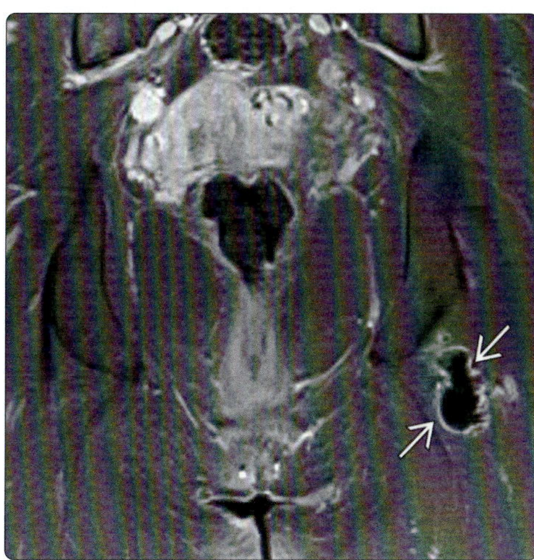

(Left) *Coronal T1WI MR in the same patient reveals the homogeneous low signal intensity of the endosteal and periosteal hyperostosis of melorheostosis. The sclerotic regions remained low signal on all sequences.* **(Right)** *Coronal T1WI C+ FS MR demonstrates an adjacent, extraosseous focus of ossification. The ossified body is low signal on all sequences, with thin surrounding enhancement. This large separate body was asymptomatic. Extraosseous involvement by melorheostosis is uncommon.*

Progressive Diaphyseal Dysplasia

KEY FACTS

TERMINOLOGY

- Progressive diaphyseal dysplasia (PDD)
- Engelmann-Camurati disease (ECD) is synonymous
- Belongs to group of craniotubular hyperostoses

IMAGING

- Symmetric, irregular endosteal and periosteal diaphyseal hyperostosis
  - Long bones, skull, vertebra
  - Starts in femur and tibia
- Hyperostosis symmetrically distributed within body, irregular thickness along bone
  - Begins within diaphysis
  - Encroaches upon & may obliterate medullary canal
  - Severe cases extend to metaphysis
- Skull changes range from no involvement → skull base sclerosis → sclerosis entire skull with hyperostosis
  - Severe disease encroaches on cranial vault, paranasal sinuses, & neural foramina

TOP DIFFERENTIAL DIAGNOSES

- Ribbing disease (many think same disease)
- van Buchem disease
- Craniodiaphysial dysplasia

PATHOLOGY

- Autosomal dominant: Variable expressivity, low penetrance, more severe and earlier onset observed in subsequent generations

CLINICAL ISSUES

- Often asymptomatic
- Pain, proximal muscle weakness, waddling gait, fatigue
- Usually presents in childhood, always before age 30
- Treatment: Corticosteroids, analgesics
- Natural history: Progressive disease
  - Degree of progression quite variable, greatest during adolescence

(Left) *AP radiograph of the right tibia in a typical case of progressive diaphyseal dysplasia shows endosteal and periosteal thickening restricted to the diaphysis ➡. Note that the metaphyses are spared ➡.* **(Right)** *AP radiograph in the same patient shows the left tibia to have symmetric distribution involving the diaphysis of the tibia ➡, though the involvement is less severe. Symmetric distribution is typical of progressive diaphyseal dysplasia.*

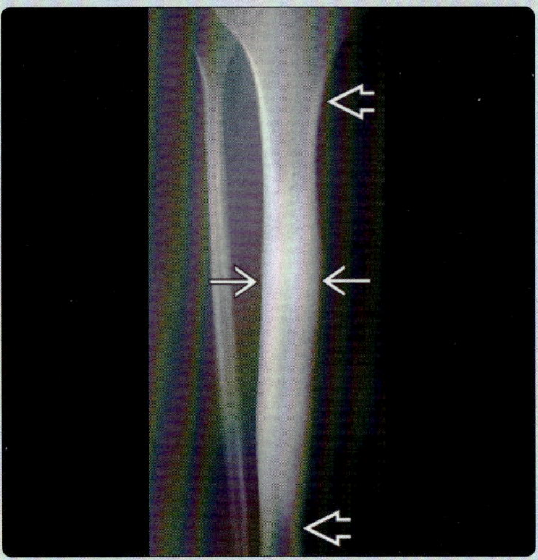

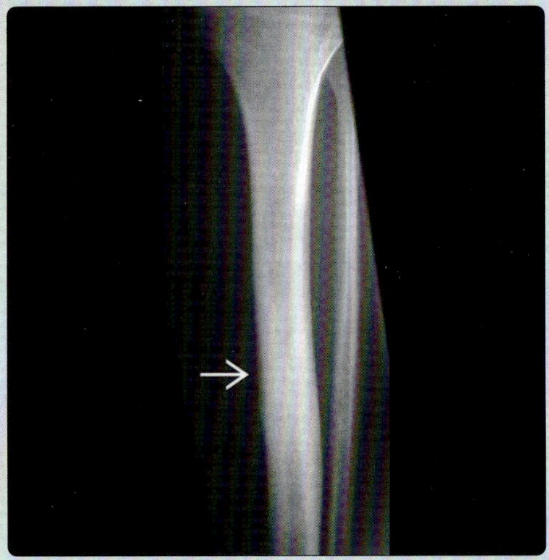

(Left) *Axial T1WI MR in the same patient demonstrates both endosteal and periosteal thickening of the tibia ➡. The residual marrow cavity is tiny.* **(Right)** *Posterior view from a bone scan shows intense uptake along the endosteal and periosteal regions of the diaphyses of both tibias. Note the difference in severity of the right ➡ vs. left ➡, which may occur during maturation. Other entities, such as Ribbing disease, appear similar. Distribution throughout the skeleton will aid differentiation.*

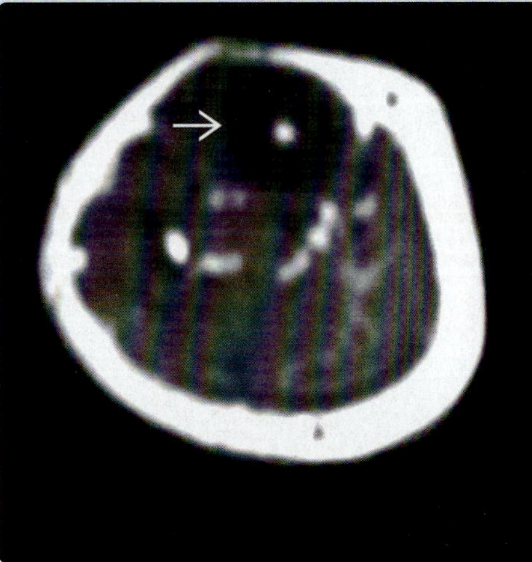

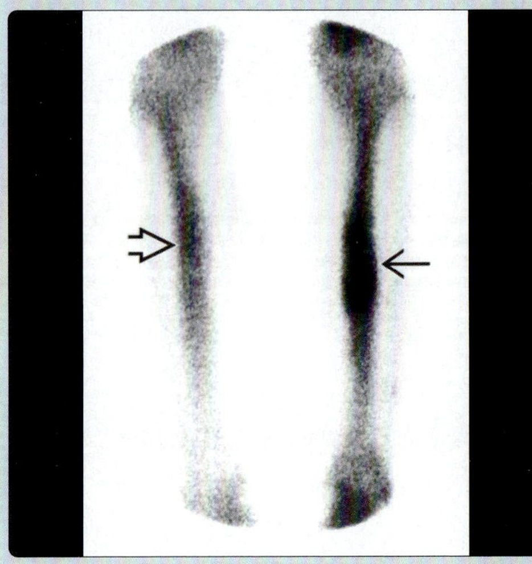

Progressive Diaphyseal Dysplasia

TERMINOLOGY

Abbreviations

- Progressive diaphyseal dysplasia (PDD)

Synonyms

- Engelmann-Camurati disease (ECD)
- Camurati-Engelmann disease or syndrome (CED)

Definitions

- Belongs to group of craniotubular hyperostoses

IMAGING

General Features

- Best diagnostic clue
  - Symmetric, irregular endosteal and periosteal diaphyseal hyperostosis in long bones
- Location
  - Starts in femur and tibia; progresses to other long bones, skull, vertebra
    - Lower extremity > upper extremity
    - Skull and pelvis involved in > 50%
- Morphology
  - Hyperostosis symmetrically distributed within body, irregular thickness along bone

Imaging Recommendations

- Best imaging tool: Radiographs are diagnostic

Radiographic Findings

- Severity of radiographic changes highly variable
- Long bones
  - Extensive periosteal and endosteal hyperostosis
    - Encroaches upon & may obliterate medullary canal
    - Mild disease limited to endosteal surface
  - Hyperostosis begins in diaphysis
    - Spares epiphysis; severe cases involve metaphysis
    - Results in undertubulation
  - Severe disease has associated joint deformities
- Skull
  - Spectrum: No involvement → skull base sclerosis → sclerosis entire skull with hyperostosis
    - Severe disease encroaches on cranial vault, paranasal sinuses, and neural foramina
- Spine
  - Sclerosis of posterior vertebral body & neural arch
  - Spares transverse and spinous processes

CT Findings

- Better demonstrates hyperostosis extent, irregularity

MR Findings

- Hyperostosis: Low signal all imaging sequences

Nuclear Medicine Findings

- Bone scan: Intense uptake within hyperostosis

DIFFERENTIAL DIAGNOSIS

Ribbing Disease

- Many think same disease
- Asymmetric or unilateral hyperostosis and sclerosis
- Confined to diaphyses: Presents after puberty

van Buchem Disease

- Autosomal recessive, hyperostosis endosteal only

Craniodiaphysial Dysplasia

- Facial changes more severe
- Hyperostosis of diaphysis only

Osteopetrosis/Pycnodysostosis

- Bone-in-bone appearance
- Skull and axial skeleton show earlier and more common involvement

PATHOLOGY

General Features

- Genetics
  - Autosomal dominant: Variable expressivity, low penetrance, more severe and earlier onset observed in subsequent generations

Microscopic Features

- Decreased trabecular bone; ↑ thickness lamellar bone

CLINICAL ISSUES

Presentation

- Most common signs/symptoms
  - Often asymptomatic
  - Proximal muscle weakness, waddling gait, fatigue
  - Pain: ± worsening by physical stress (activity, cold)
- Other signs/symptoms
  - Mandibular enlargement
  - Joints: Arthritis, dislocations, contractures
  - Tenderness over affected bones
  - Decreased muscle bulk

Demographics

- Age
  - Usually presents in childhood, always before age 30
- Gender
  - No racial or sex predilection
- Epidemiology
  - *TGFβ1* gene (transforming growth factor β) abnormal in 90%; CED type II lacks gene mutation

Natural History & Prognosis

- Progressive disease: Degree of progression quite variable, greatest during adolescence

Treatment

- Corticosteroids to decrease bone formation
- NSAID, aspirin for pain control
- Improvement with angiotensin II type 1 receptor antagonist reported
- Bone decompression can alleviate pain

SELECTED REFERENCES

1. Ayyavoo A et al: Elimination of pain and improvement of exercise capacity in Camurati-Engelmann disease with losartan. J Clin Endocrinol Metab. 99(11):3978-82, 2014

(Left) *AP radiograph shows a typical case of mature progressive diaphyseal dysplasia. There is both endosteal thickening ➡ and periosteal thickening ➡. The bone appears quite mature. Note that it involves the diaphysis and the thickening extends into the metaphysis, but there is no epiphyseal involvement. It is interesting that the cross-sectional involvement of the diaphysis does not appear symmetric; this may occasionally be seen.* **(Right)** *AP radiograph in a different patient shows mature progressive diaphyseal dysplasia. Note that, as with the previous patient, there is mature endosteal and periosteal thickening of bone ➡. However, the distribution is more symmetric in this case, involving the medial and lateral sides of the bone equally. As is typical with this process, the metaphyses and epiphyses are spared.*

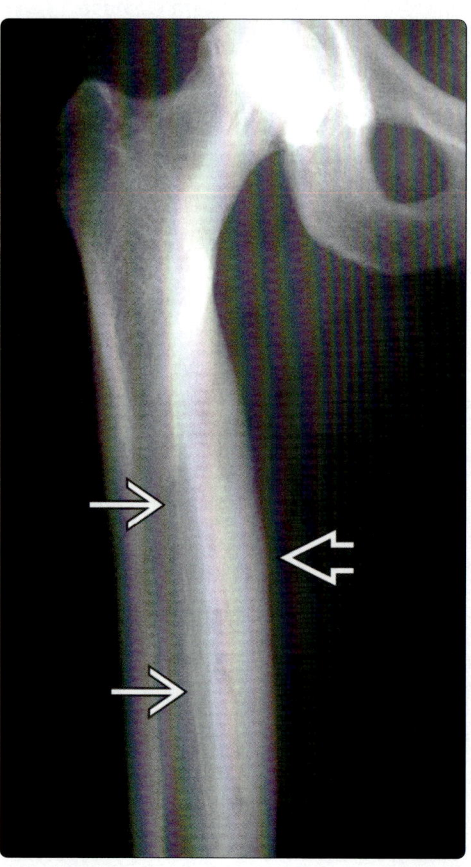

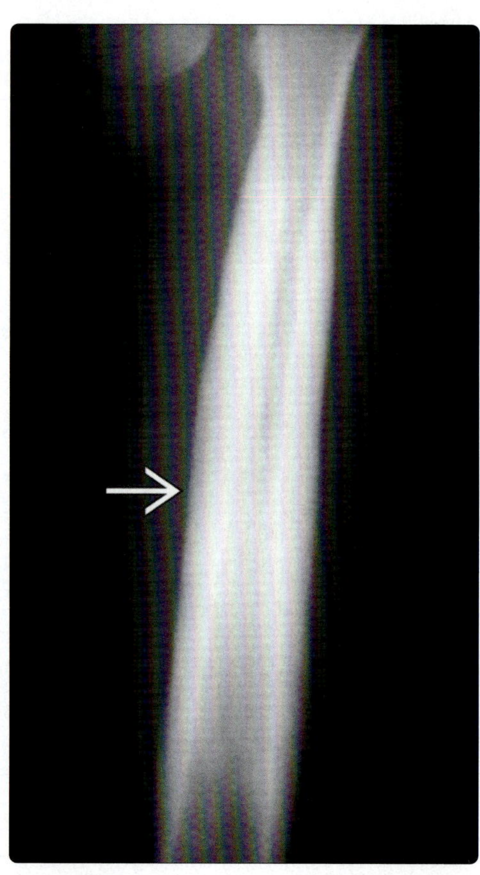

(Left) *AP radiograph of the forearm in the same patient shows mature hyperostosis involving the diaphysis of the radius ➡, with normal metaphysis and epiphysis. Interestingly, only the proximal diaphysis of the ulna was involved (not shown). Thin bones, such as the ulna and fibula, may show later and less complete involvement.* **(Right)** *AP radiograph shows the tibia in the same patient. As in the femur, the hypertrophy of the endosteal and periosteal bone is circumferential ➡, leaving little marrow centrally. The metaphyses are absolutely normal (proximal included in this image ➡). Although only the left femur, forearm, and tibia are shown in this case, the contralateral bones were symmetrically involved. This is a classic case of progressive diaphyseal dysplasia.*

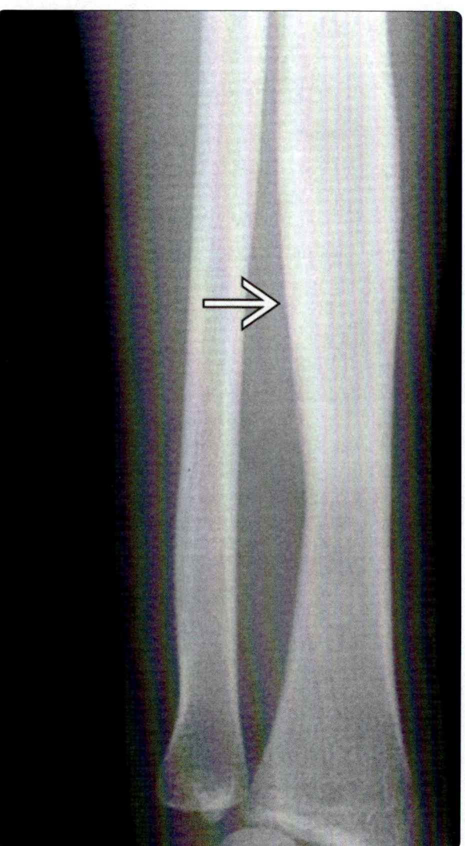

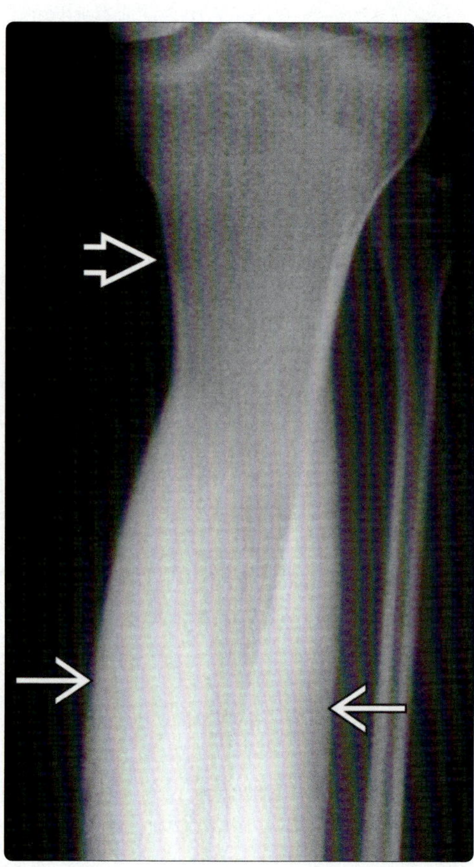

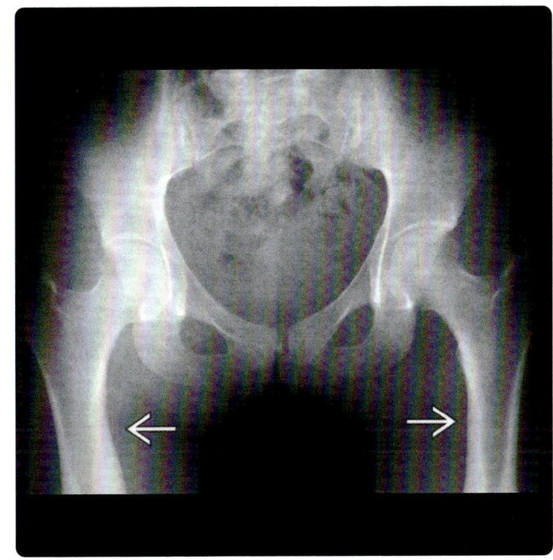

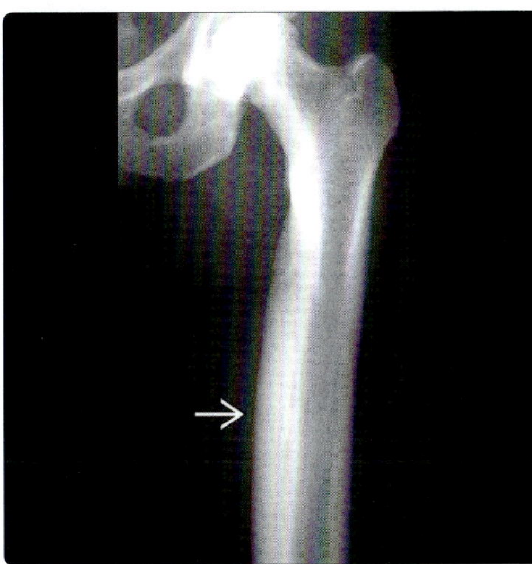

(Left) *AP radiograph shows a nice example of Camurati-Engelmann disease. The bilaterally symmetric sclerosis & thickening of both the endosteum & periosteum, resulting in severe cortical thickening, is limited to the diaphyses of the femora ➡, leaving the epiphyses & metaphyses with a normal appearance.* **(Right)** *AP radiograph shows cortical thickening ➡, which involves the entire length of the diaphyses, leaving the metaphyses & epiphyses unaffected, typical of Camurati-Engelmann disease.*

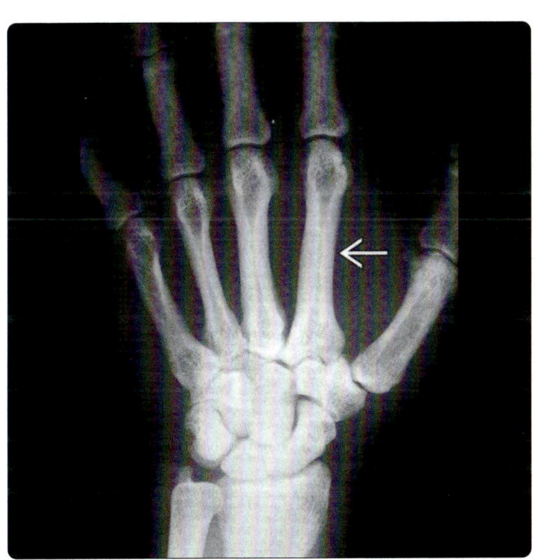

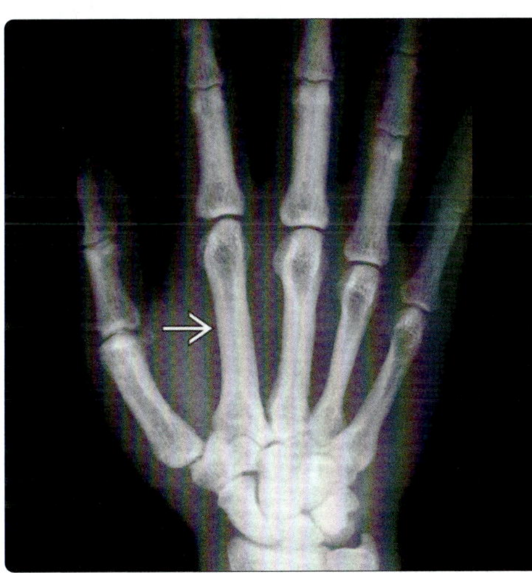

(Left) *PA radiograph shows the hand in a patient with mature progressive diaphyseal dysplasia. Involvement of the hands is a late finding. However, the appearance is unmistakable, with all the long bones of the hand showing both periosteal and endosteal cortical thickening ➡.* **(Right)** *PA radiograph of the contralateral side in the same patient shows that the expected symmetry is maintained ➡. Since this is a mature process, the femora and tibias showed mature diaphyseal involvement as well.*

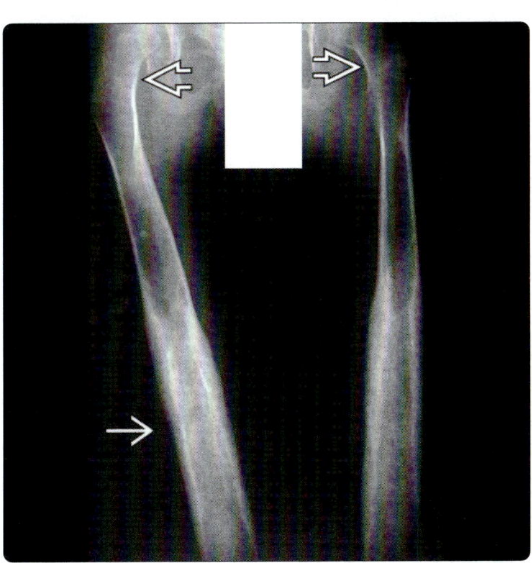

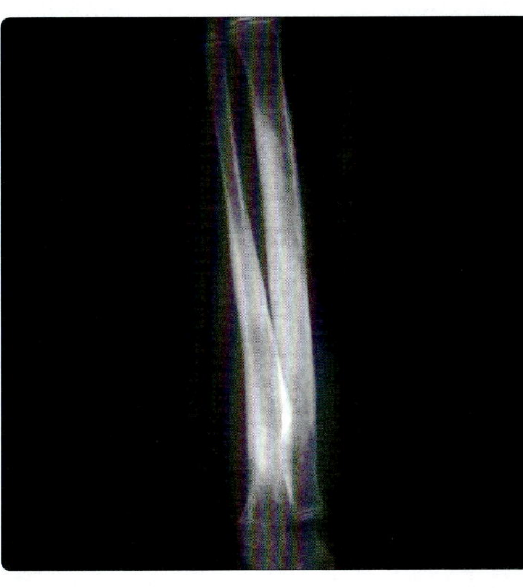

(Left) *AP radiograph shows early PDD in a child, manifested as disordered cortical and endosteal bone, which results in a cortical thickening. The process is restricted to the diaphyses ➡. Note the normal metaphyses and epiphyses ➡. The proximal femora are not yet involved, but the process will become more smooth, thick, and will involve the entire diaphysis as the child matures.* **(Right)** *AP radiograph in the same patient shows the disordered hyperostosis of early Camurati-Engelmann.*

KEY FACTS

TERMINOLOGY

- Albers-Schönberg disease
- Marble bone disease

IMAGING

- Radiographs reveal characteristic hyperostosis and sclerosis: Distribution in skull and spine helps differentiate types
- Undertubulation of metaphyses
- Bone within bone appearance
- Rugger jersey or sandwich vertebrae
- MR: "Black bone"
- Bone scan: SuperScan

TOP DIFFERENTIAL DIAGNOSES

- Pycnodysostosis
  - Short stature, acroosteolysis, obtuse mandibular angle, delayed closure of sutures
- Progressive diaphyseal dysplasia
  - Irregular cortical and endosteal thickening; primarily diaphysis, spares epiphyses
  - Variable manifestations in skull

PATHOLOGY

- Abnormal osteoclast function creates imbalance between bone formation and resorption
- Genetics
  - Infantile type: Autosomal recessive
  - Adult types: Autosomal dominant
  - Intermediate type: Autosomal recessive
  - Sly disease: Autosomal recessive

CLINICAL ISSUES

- Infantile type: Failure to thrive, marrow failure
- Adult types: Often incidentally discovered
- Intermediate type: Variable
- Carbonic anhydrase type II deficiency (Sly disease)
  - Cerebral calcifications, renal tubular acidosis

(Left) *Lateral radiograph reveals classic changes of osteopetrosis in the skull. The cranial vault is diffusely thickened ➡, and the vault and skull base ➡ are extremely dense.* **(Right)** *Lateral radiograph depicts rugger jersey spine. Within the vertebral bodies, sclerosis extends from the endplate almost to the center of the vertebral body ➡. This appearance is typically associated with the adult type II form of osteopetrosis.*

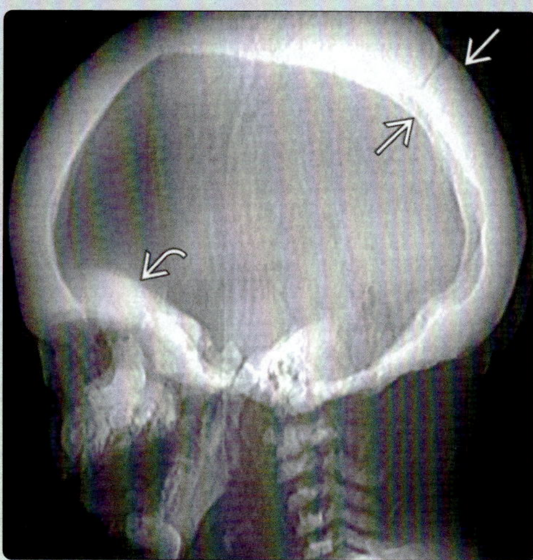

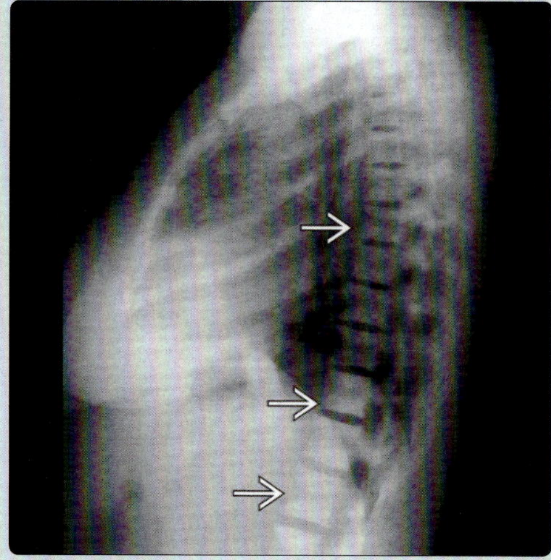

(Left) *AP radiograph shows typical bone-in-bone appearance seen in osteopetrosis ➡. The endobone appearance occurs because the osteoclasts do not remodel properly during skeletal maturation.* **(Right)** *AP radiograph reveals the most extreme changes of autosomal recessive osteopetrosis. Bones are diffusely and densely sclerotic. Femurs are undertubulated with relative widening of the distal metadiaphyses ➡. This appearance explains the frequently used marble bone terminology.*

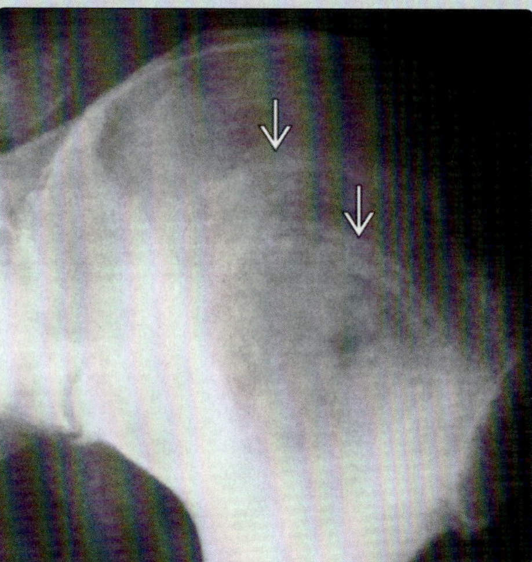

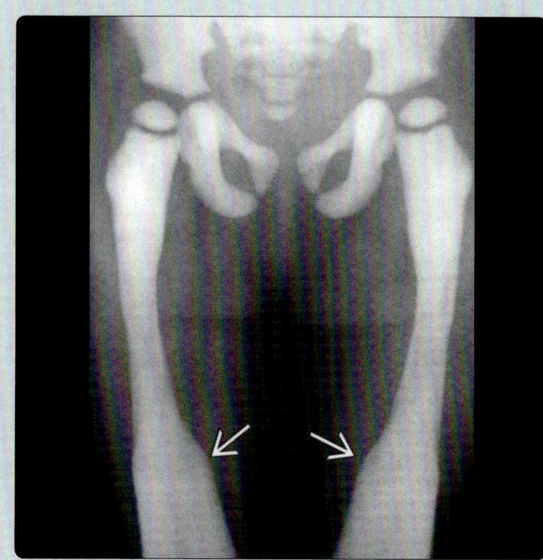

TERMINOLOGY

Abbreviations

- Autosomal recessive osteopetrosis (AROP)
- Autosomal dominant osteopetrosis (ADOP)

Synonyms

- Albers-Schönberg disease
- Marble bone disease

Definitions

- Malignant (infantile) type
- Benign (adult) type
- Intermediate type
- Carbonic anhydrase isoenzyme type II deficiency (Sly disease)

IMAGING

General Features

- Best diagnostic clue
  - Diffusely dense bones
- Location
  - Pattern of involvement of skull: Cranial vault, skull base, or both differs among different types
  - Involvement of vertebrae varies between 2 types of adult variety

Imaging Recommendations

- Best imaging tool
  - Radiographs reveal characteristic findings
    - Sufficient to establish diagnosis
- Protocol advice
  - Radiographic assessment should include skull, spine, and extremities

Radiographic Findings

- Radiography
  - Infantile type
    - Skull
      - Cranial vault and skull base affected
    - Diffuse involvement of entire skeleton
    - Transverse metaphyseal lucencies
  - Adult type I
    - Skull
      - Cranial vault sclerosis and hyperostosis
      - Skull base not involved
    - Appendicular skeleton
      - No (or limited) involvement
    - Spine
      - No (or limited) involvement
  - Adult type II
    - Skull
      - Skull base sclerosis and hyperostosis
      - Cranial vault spared
    - Spine
      - Rugger jersey or sandwich vertebrae secondary to endplate hyperostosis
  - Intermediate type
    - Variable manifestations in spectrum between infantile and adult forms
  - General
    - Sclerotic bones
      - Bones are uniformly dense
      - Smooth margins: No irregular periosteal new bone
      - Loss of normal corticomedullary differentiation
      - Involves epiphysis, metaphysis, diaphysis
    - Undertubulation of metaphyses
      - Most prominent in distal femur
      - Manifestation of inability of defective osteoclasts to normally remodel bone during growth
    - Cranial vault involvement
      - Diffuse thickening and sclerosis
      - Loss of diploic space
      - Seen in infantile and adult type I forms
    - Skull base involvement
      - Hyperostosis and sclerosis
      - Seen in infantile and adult type II forms
    - Bone within bone appearance
      - Most evident in spine
      - Endobone seen in ilium
      - Like undertubulation, endobone is manifestation of inability to remodel bone
      - As growth occurs, cortical bone is not resorbed and remains visible within larger (more adult) bone

CT Findings

- Not necessary for disease diagnosis
- Demonstrates extent of involvement and complications of cranial vault and skull base disease
  - Infantile form has clinical sequelae of hyperostosis
    - Stenosis of neural and vascular foramina
    - Hydrocephalus secondary to aqueduct stenosis
    - Encroachment on paranasal sinuses and mastoid air cells
- Sly disease
  - Cerebral calcifications

MR Findings

- Primarily used to assess degree of marrow involvement
  - May be useful to assess response to therapy
    - Especially useful following bone marrow transplant
  - Infantile type: "Black bones"
    - Complete absence of marrow due to replacement by dense bone
- Demonstrates extent and complications of cranial vault and skull base involvement
  - Hydrocephalus secondary to aqueduct stenosis
  - Optic nerve atrophy
    - Seen in infantile, adult type II
  - Tonsillar ectopia, optic nerve sheath dilatation
    - Seen in infantile, adult type I
  - Ventriculomegaly, subarachnoid space dilatation
    - Seen in infantile, adult type I

Nuclear Medicine Findings

- Bone scan
  - SuperScan
    - Uptake of radioisotope throughout skeleton
    - Fingers and toes are visible
    - Reduced or absent renal and soft tissue uptake

DIFFERENTIAL DIAGNOSIS

Pycnodysostosis

- Short stature
- Acroosteolysis
- Wormian bones
- Delayed closure of skull sutures
- Obtuse mandibular angle

Progressive Diaphyseal Dysplasia

- Irregular cortical and endosteal thickening
- Spares epiphyses
- Vertebral involvement confined to posterior body and neural arch
- Variable manifestations in skull

PATHOLOGY

General Features

- Etiology
  - Abnormal osteoclast function
    - Results in imbalance between bone formation and resorption
    - Bone production is not impaired
      - Continue to produce bone, which cannot be remodeled, leading to hyperostosis
    - Unable to remodel bone at endosteum to create medullary space
      - Leads to diffusely sclerotic bones
      - Results in failure to create normal marrow spaces
    - Predisposes to fractures
      - At sites of stress, bone develops and does not remodel appropriately
      - e.g., osseous protrusion lateral cortex femur in subtrochanteric region (similar mechanism seen with bisphosphonate therapy)
    - Leads to poor fracture healing
- Genetics
  - Infantile type: Autosomal recessive
  - Adult types: Autosomal dominant
  - Intermediate types: Autosomal recessive
  - Sly disease: Autosomal recessive

Microscopic Features

- Thick trabeculae with central foundation of cartilage
- Osteoclasts increased, decreased, or normal in number

CLINICAL ISSUES

Presentation

- Most common signs/symptoms
  - Infantile type
    - Failure to thrive
    - Growth retardation
    - Cranial nerve deficits, especially poor vision
  - Adult types
    - Usually incidentally found
    - May have pain, fractures
  - Intermediate types
    - Variable manifestations and severity
- Other signs/symptoms
  - Short stature
  - Hearing and visual loss
    - Most common in infantile type
    - Seen in 5% adult disease
  - Mandible osteomyelitis (especially adult types)
  - Fractures (especially adult types)
  - Abnormal dentition, dental caries
  - Frontal bossing
  - Infantile type
    - Increased intracranial pressure
    - Hematologic deficiencies due to lack of marrow
      - Anemia, thrombocytopenia, leukopenia
      - Hepatosplenomegaly, extramedullary hematopoiesis
    - Nasal obstruction
    - Hypocalcemia
      - Secondary to hyperparathyroidism
      - May lead to seizures
    - Blindness, deafness, facial nerve palsy
    - Stroke
  - Sly disease
    - Renal tubular acidosis

Demographics

- Age
  - Malignant type: Congenital or presents in infancy
  - Benign types: Present in adults
  - Intermediate type: Presents in childhood
  - Sly disease: Onset in infancy
- Epidemiology
  - AROP: 1/250,000 births
  - ADOP: 1/20,000 births

Natural History & Prognosis

- Infantile type
  - Death usually occurs during childhood secondary to complications of bone marrow failure
- Adult types
  - Normal life span
- Intermediate types
  - Variable clinical sequelae

Treatment

- Bone marrow transplant to cure infantile type
- Otherwise directed at complications, such as fractures

SELECTED REFERENCES

1. Florido Angulo A et al: The sandwich vertebral body sign. Osteopetrosis: Report of a case. Arthritis Rheumatol. ePub, 2015
2. Machado Cde V et al: Infantile osteopetrosis associated with osteomyelitis. BMJ Case Rep. 2015, 2015
3. van Hove RP et al: Autosomal dominant type I osteopetrosis is related with iatrogenic fractures in arthroplasty. Clin Orthop Surg. 6(4):484-8, 2014
4. Jenkins PF et al: Osteopetrosis. Am Orthopt J. 63:107-11, 2013
5. Nour M et al: Infantile malignant osteopetrosis. J Pediatr. 163(4):1230-1230.e1, 2013
6. Fotiadou A et al: Type II autosomal dominant osteopetrosis: radiological features in two families containing five members with asymptomatic and uncomplicated disease. Skeletal Radiol. 38(10):1015-21, 2009
7. Stark Z et al: Osteopetrosis. Orphanet J Rare Dis. 4:5, 2009

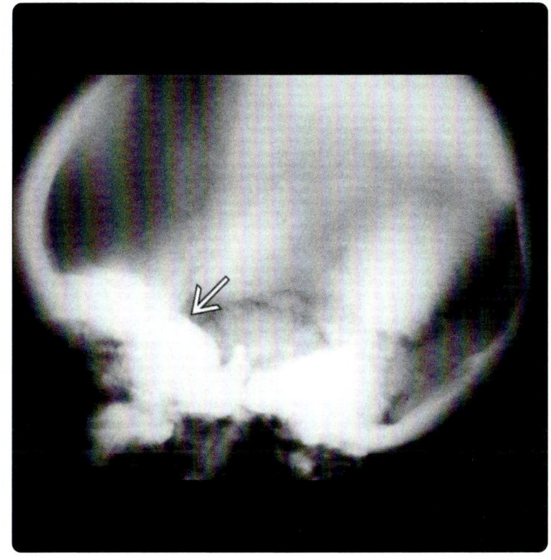

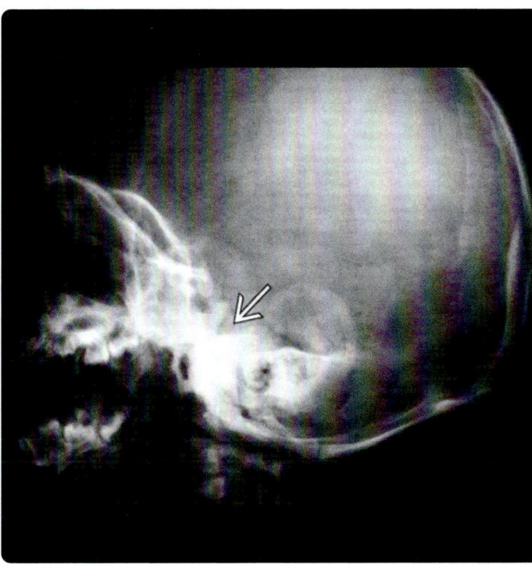

(Left) *Lateral radiograph reveals the marked involvement of the skull seen with infantile (autosomal recessive) osteopetrosis. The cranial vault and the skull base are diffusely sclerotic. Note the severe hyperostosis of the skull base ➡.* **(Right)** *Lateral radiograph shows the less severe end of the spectrum of osteopetrosis. In this case, the cranial vault is spared. The skull base, however, is dense and hyperostotic ➡. This pattern of skull involvement is most commonly seen with adult type II disease.*

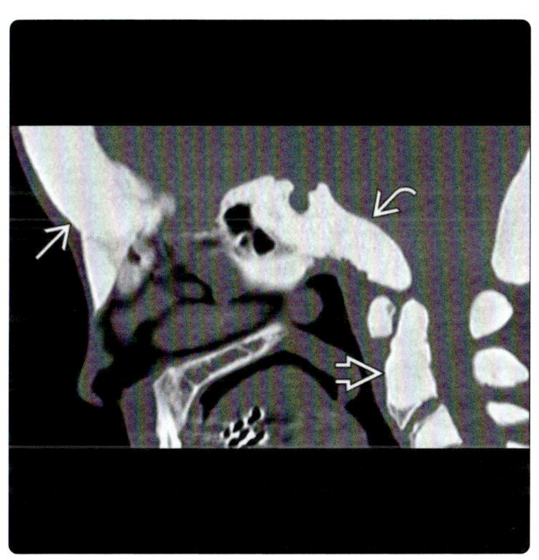

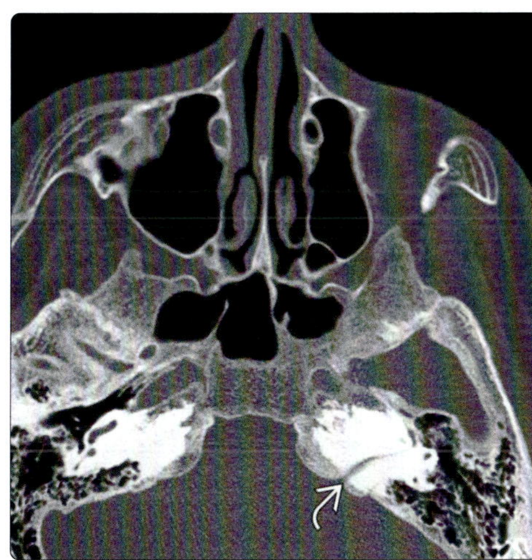

(Left) *Sagittal bone CT demonstrates severe bone thickening involving the skull base and cranial vault. Observe how thick the clivus has become ➡. The skull ➡ and vertebral bodies ➡ are extremely dense. Note the sparing of the maxilla.* **(Right)** *Axial bone CT of a patient with autosomal recessive osteopetrosis shows dense sclerosis and thickening of the temporal bone and skull base. The hyperostosis has lead to encroachment upon and narrowing of the internal auditory canal ➡.*

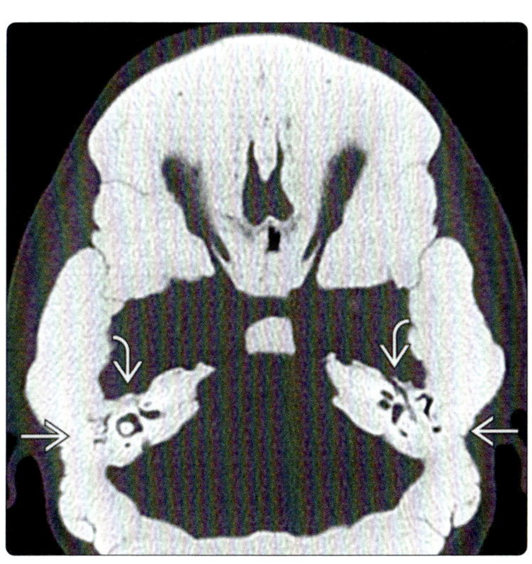

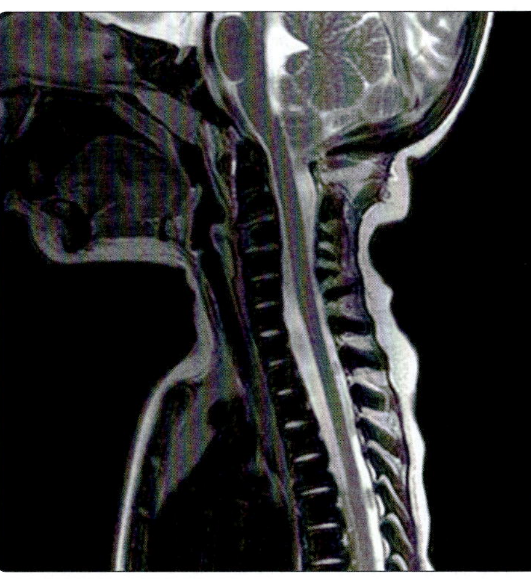

(Left) *Axial bone CT shows massive hyperostosis and sclerosis of osteopetrosis. The marrow spaces are completely obliterated. The external auditory canals are completely occluded ➡, and the middle ears are narrowed ➡. These changes result in deafness.* **(Right)** *Sagittal T2WI MR shows the black bone appearance seen with osteopetrosis. This appearance is the result of complete replacement of the marrow space by dense bone. Marrow failure is a cause of death in the infantile form of this disease.*

(Left) *Sagittal T2WI MR shows dense, sharply demarcated bands of low signal intensity due to bony sclerosis involving all the vertebral bodies* ➡. *This appearance is the MR equivalent of the rugger jersey spine. Note that sclerosis and trabecular thickening are also present centrally in the vertebral bodies* ➡. **(Right)** *Lateral radiograph in a case of infantile osteopetrosis shows diffuse marked sclerotic bone density in all imaged bones, including the vertebral bodies, neural arches, and ribs.*

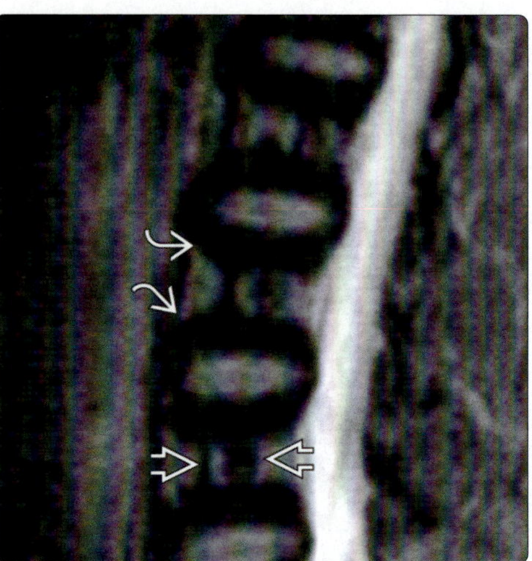

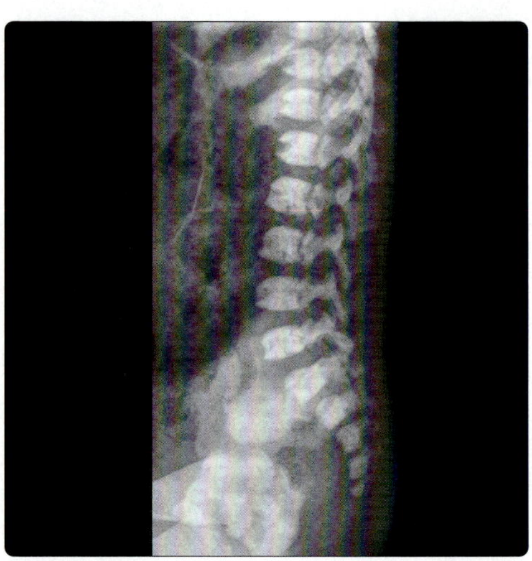

(Left) *Lateral radiograph close-up view of L4 shows a classic bone-in-bone appearance* ➡. **(Right)** *Axial bone CT shows a vertebra with the bone-in-bone appearance. Without the benefit of radiographs, this finding may not be recognized for what it is. Note how the shape of the apparent sclerotic lesion* ➡ *exactly mirrors the cortical margin.*

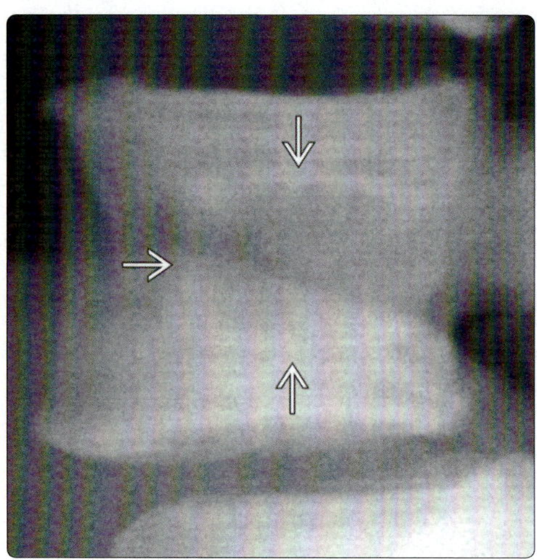

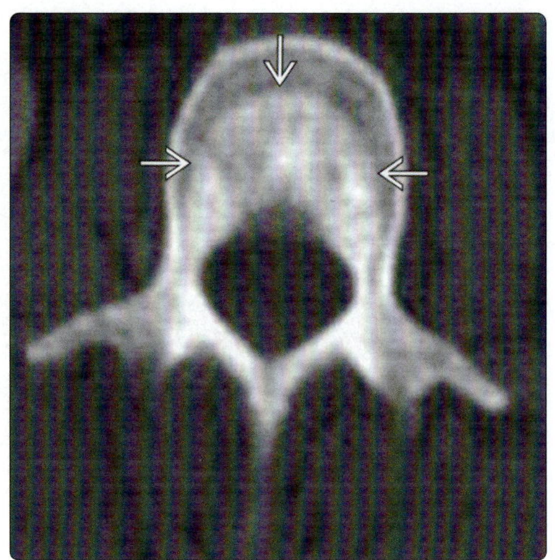

(Left) *AP radiograph shows a patient with osteopetrosis complicated by subtrochanteric fracture* ➡. *Note iliac wing endobone* ➡ *and typical thickened endosteal femoral cortex.* **(Right)** *AP radiograph of the contralateral femur after prophylactic rodding shows a bump along the lateral femoral cortex* ➡. *This bump, also seen with bisphosphonate therapy, results from weight-bearing stresses. However, there is insufficient osteoclast activity to effectively remodel it. Thus, the site is weak and at risk for fracture.*

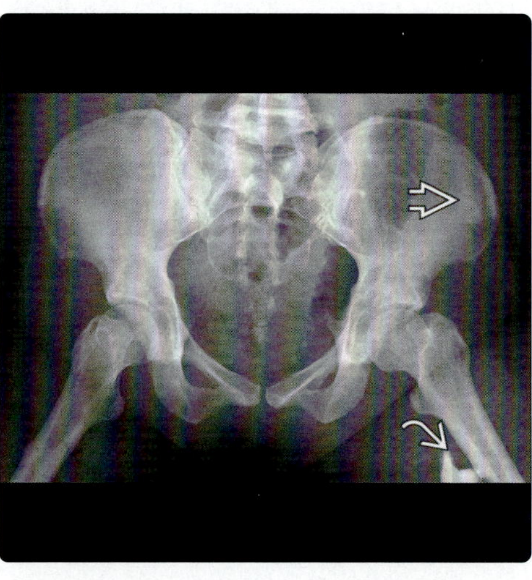

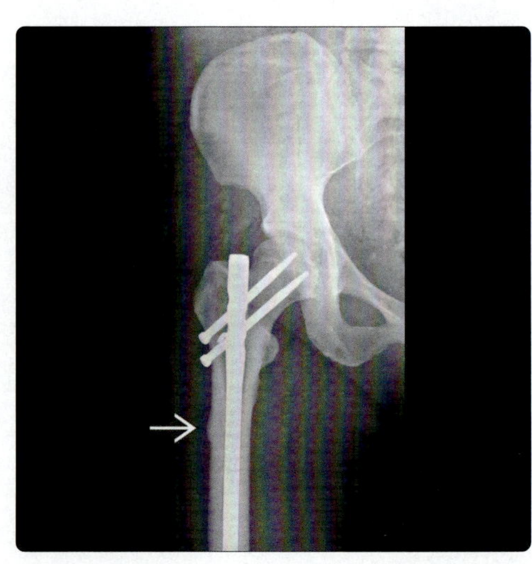

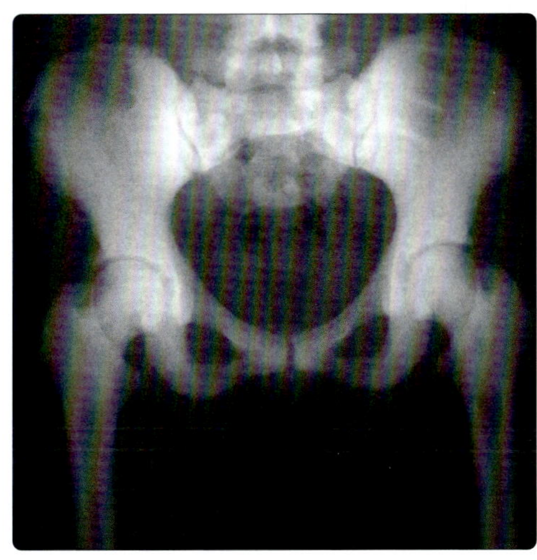

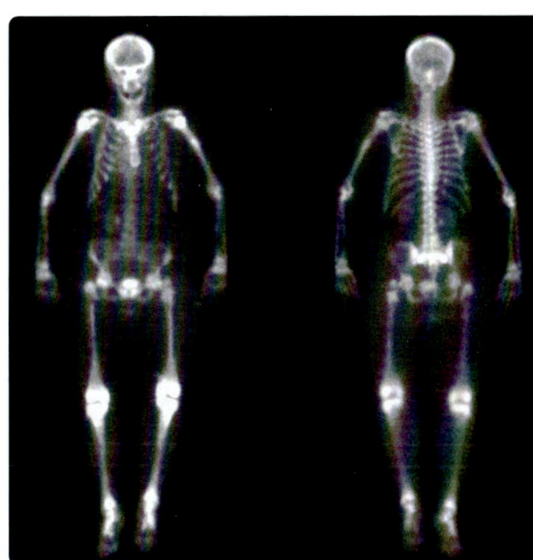

(Left) *AP radiograph shows an adult with severe sclerosis from osteopetrosis. Note the severely restricted medullary space; it is not surprising that these patients develop complications of anemia.* **(Right)** *Anterior and posterior bone scans show diffusely increased radiotracer accumulation throughout the entire skeleton due to osteopetrosis. There is diminished visualization of the kidneys and bladder due to the diffuse increased uptake in the skeleton (SuperScan).*

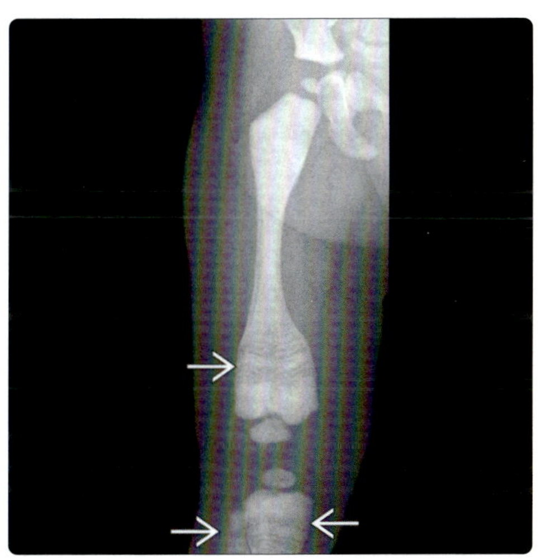

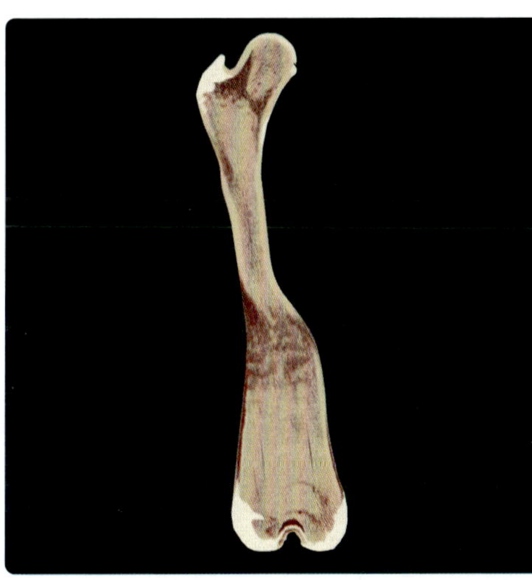

(Left) *AP radiograph reveals diffusely sclerotic bones. The distal metadiaphysis is widened secondary to impaired remodeling by defective osteoclasts. Transverse metaphyseal bands are present around the knee* ➔ *and are associated with the infantile form of this disease.* **(Right)** *Coronal graphic shows a bisected femur depicting the changes of osteopetrosis. Corticomedullary differentiation is absent. Dense bone extends into medullary space. There is undertubulation distally.*

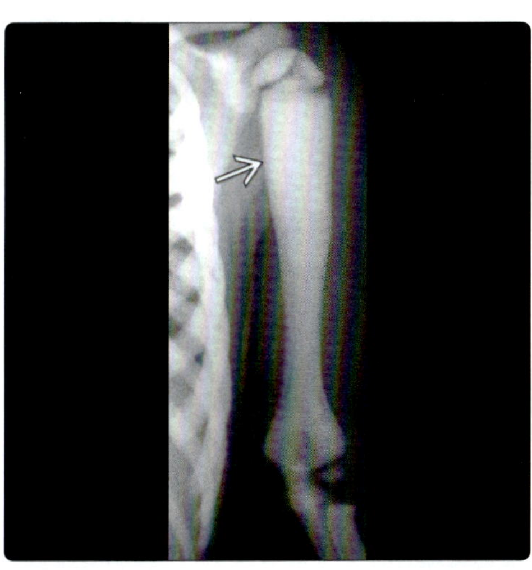

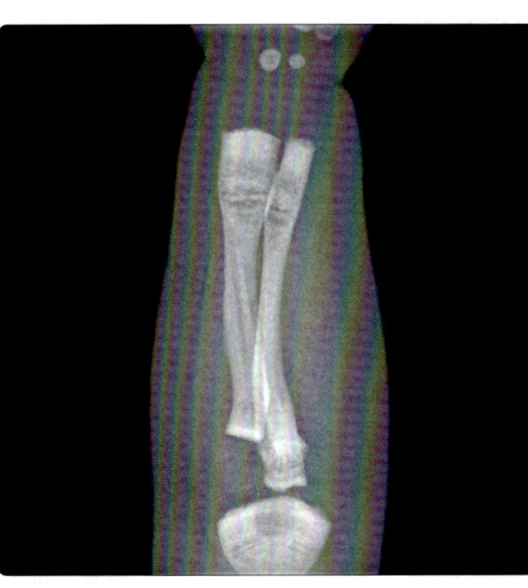

(Left) *AP radiograph reveals typical findings of severe autosomal recessive osteopetrosis. The bones are all diffusely and densely sclerotic. The sclerosis involves the epiphysis, metaphysis, and diaphysis. The proximal humerus is undertubulated* ➔. **(Right)** *AP radiograph shows a typical case of osteopetrosis with abnormal increased bone density and undertubulation of the distal radius and ulna. A bone-in-bone appearance is noted in each of the bones. Minimal trauma was needed to fracture these bones.*

Pycnodysostosis

KEY FACTS

TERMINOLOGY

- Lysosomal storage disease resulting in dense bones

IMAGING

- Dense bones with short stature, acroosteolysis, decreased angle of mandible
  - Osteosclerosis is dominant radiographic finding
- Skull
  - Wormian bones
  - Thick skull base
  - Thin cranial vault
  - Delayed closure of calvarial sutures
  - Persistent anterior fontanelle
- Poorly developed midface
  - Obtuse mandibular angle
- Hypoplastic/malformed clavicles
- Fragility fractures
  - Spondylolysis
- Acroosteolysis terminal phalanges

TOP DIFFERENTIAL DIAGNOSES

- Osteopetrosis
  - Primary differential diagnostic consideration
  - Bone-in-bone appearance
  - Obliterates marrow space
  - No acroosteolysis or mandibular deformity
- Progressive diaphyseal dysplasia
  - Cortical thickening
  - Bilateral symmetric distribution
  - Typically confined to diaphyses

PATHOLOGY

- Mutation in cathepsin K enzyme
- Autosomal recessive

CLINICAL ISSUES

- Osteomyelitis of mandible; abnormal tooth development
- Midface hypoplasia with associated sleep apnea
- Transverse fragility fractures of long bones

(Left) *Lateral radiograph shows an abnormal mandibular angle ➡. The normal angle is 110° to 120°. In pyknodysostosis, the angle becomes more obtuse, approaching 180°. This mandibular anomaly leads to complications, such as sleep apnea.* **(Right)** *AP radiograph shows severe thickening of the endosteum of the femora ➡. In isolation, this finding is nonspecific. When associated with resorption of the terminal tufts of the phalanges (not shown), the radiographs are diagnostic of pycnodysostosis.*

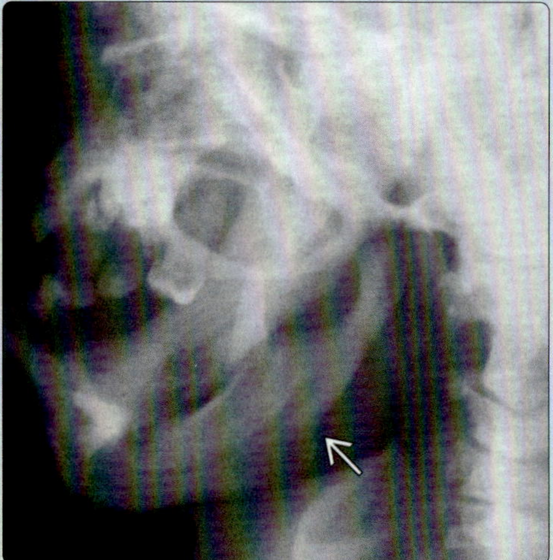

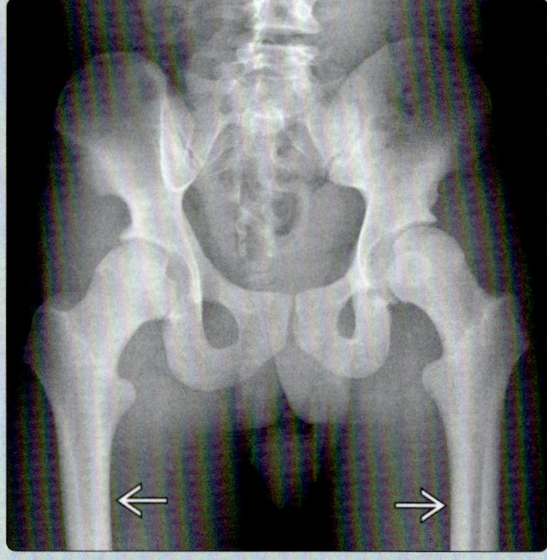

(Left) *AP radiograph reveals diffuse sclerosis of the radius and ulna accompanied by diffuse endosteal thickening ➡. Mild undertubulation of the distal radius is present ➡. Undertubulation is more pronounced and prevalent in osteopetrosis and is an inconsistent finding in pycnodysostosis.* **(Right)** *PA x-ray shows diffuse sclerosis and significant resorption of the terminal tufts of all of the distal phalanges ➡. In this case, the osteolysis is severe and uniformly distributed. Acroosteolysis is typical in pycnodysostosis.*

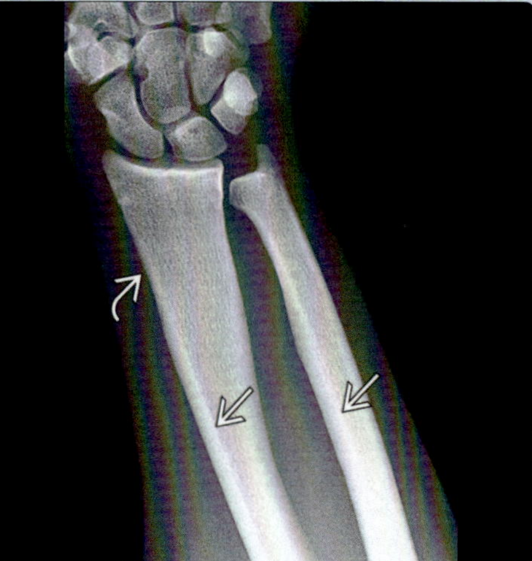

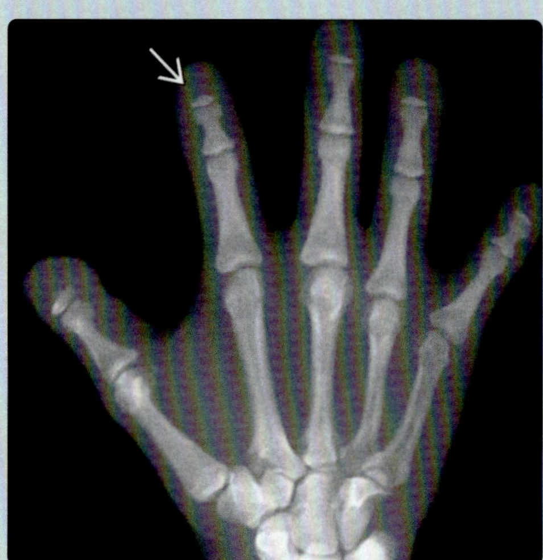

TERMINOLOGY

Synonyms

- Maroteaux-Lamy

Definitions

- Lysosomal storage disease resulting in dense bones

IMAGING

General Features

- Best diagnostic clue
  - Dense bones with short stature, acroosteolysis, decreased angle of mandible
- Location
  - Involves entire skeleton

Imaging Recommendations

- Best imaging tool
  - Radiographs are diagnostic

Radiographic Findings

- Osteosclerosis is dominant radiographic finding
  - Does not obliterate marrow space
- Acroosteolysis
  - Resorption or band-like lucency in terminal tuft
  - Asymmetric distribution
  - May not involve all digits
  - May be progressive
- Skull
  - Wormian bones
  - Thick skull base
  - Thin cranial vault
  - Delayed closure of calvarial sutures
    - Persistent anterior fontanelle
- Face
  - Poorly developed midface
  - Hypoplastic mandible
    - Obtuse mandibular angle
  - Hypoplastic paranasal sinuses
- Minimal undertubulation of long bones
- Hypoplastic/malformed clavicles, especially laterally
- Fragility fractures
  - Transverse in long bones
  - Poor healing
  - Spondylolysis

CT Findings

- Depict same changes identified on radiographs
- May be used to assess fracture healing
- Useful to detail anomalies, especially dental and facial

MR Findings

- May be useful to evaluate fracture healing/pseudoarthrosis

DIFFERENTIAL DIAGNOSIS

Osteopetrosis

- Primary differential diagnostic consideration
- Undertubulation may be marked, especially distal femur
- Bone-in-bone appearance
- Obliterates marrow space
  - Clinical symptoms of marrow failure

Progressive Diaphyseal Dysplasia

- Cortical thickening
  - Bilateral symmetric distribution
  - Typically confined to diaphyses
- Spares spine
- Thick calvaria

Ribbing Disease

- Endosteal sclerosis confined to lower extremities

PATHOLOGY

General Features

- Etiology
  - Mutation in cathepsin K enzyme
    - Enzyme required for bone turnover
    - Abnormal enzyme results in abnormal osteoclast activity, decreased bone resorption/turnover
    - Results in brittle bones, similar to osteopetrosis
- Genetics
  - Autosomal recessive

CLINICAL ISSUES

Presentation

- Most common signs/symptoms
  - Short stature
  - Hands are characteristic
    - Short and broad, irregular shortening secondary to acroosteolysis, wrinkled skin
- Other signs/symptoms
  - Large head
    - Frontal and occipital bossing
  - Hypoplastic nails
  - Fractures, often with minor trauma
    - Poor healing
  - Osteomyelitis of mandible
  - Abnormal tooth development
  - Midface hypoplasia with associated sleep apnea
  - Grooved palate
  - Prominent/beaked nose
  - No sequelae of marrow failure, in contrast to osteopetrosis
  - Probably condition of artist Toulouse-Lautrec

Demographics

- Epidemiology
  - Rare

SELECTED REFERENCES

1. S R et al: Osteomyelitis in pycnodysostosis - report of 2 clinical cases. J Clin Diagn Res. 9(1):ZD15-7, 2015
2. Yates CJ et al: An atypical subtrochanteric femoral fracture from pycnodysostosis: a lesson from nature. J Bone Miner Res. 26(6):1377-9, 2011
3. Bathi RJ et al: Pyknodysostosis—a report of two cases with a brief review of the literature. Int J Oral Maxillofac Surg. 29(6):439-42, 2000
4. Vanhoenacker FM et al: Sclerosing bone dysplasias: genetic and radioclinical features. Eur Radiol. 10(9):1423-33, 2000

(Left) *Lateral radiograph demonstrates a shallow mandibular angle ➡, a characteristic finding in pyknodysostosis. Generalized thinning of the cranial vault ➡ can also be observed. Wormian bones are present although they are difficult to visualize on this image ➡.* **(Right)** *AP radiograph shows uniformly dense bone, which is a nonspecific finding. This may be seen in several sclerosing dysplasias, including osteopetrosis and pyknodysostosis. The latter was the diagnosis in this case.*

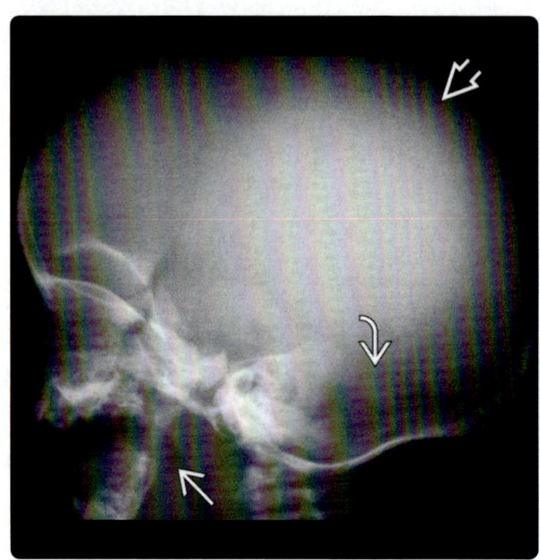

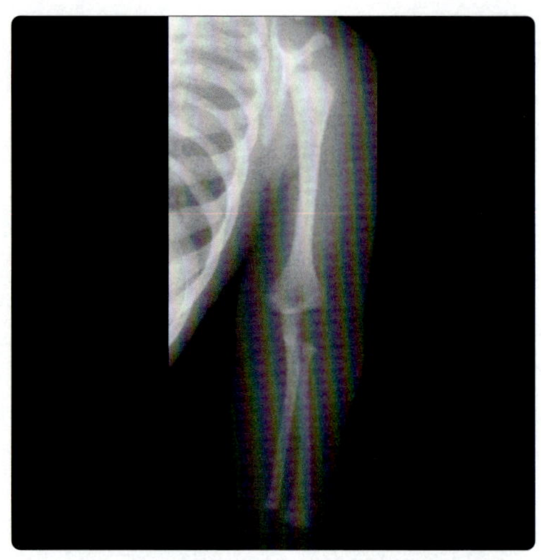

(Left) *PA radiograph shows diffusely dense bones associated with acroosteolysis ➡. In this young child, the resorption is minimal. Acroosteolysis may be a progressive process and can be more severe in adults.* **(Right)** *Lateral radiograph demonstrates acroosteolysis. Note that the resorption is not uniform, sparing the 3rd and 4th distal phalanges. Two patterns of resorption can be seen: Band-like resorption in the index finger ➡ and tuftal resorption of the 1st and 5th distal phalanges ➡.*

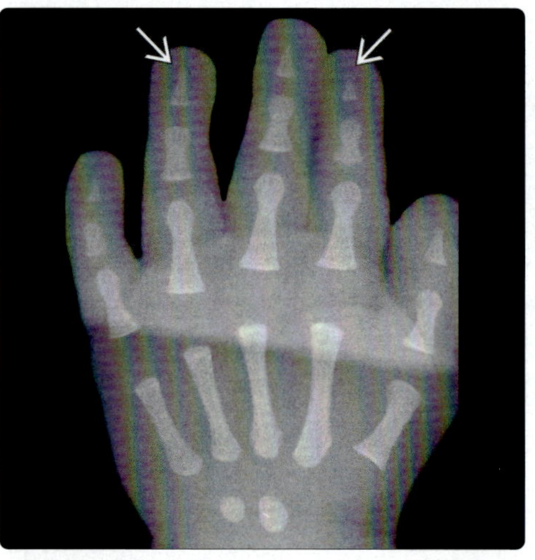

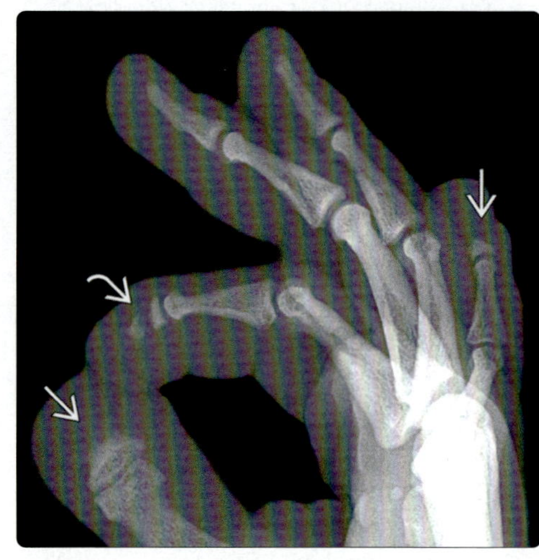

(Left) *AP radiograph is remarkable for diffusely dense bones, resorption of the terminal tufts of the distal phalanges ➡, and a fragility fracture at the base of the 5th metatarsal ➡. This combination of findings is diagnostic for pyknodysostosis.* **(Right)** *Sagittal bone CT reveals increased density throughout all of the vertebra. Multiple pars interarticularis defects are visible ➡. These fractures are one of the manifestations of bone fragility.*

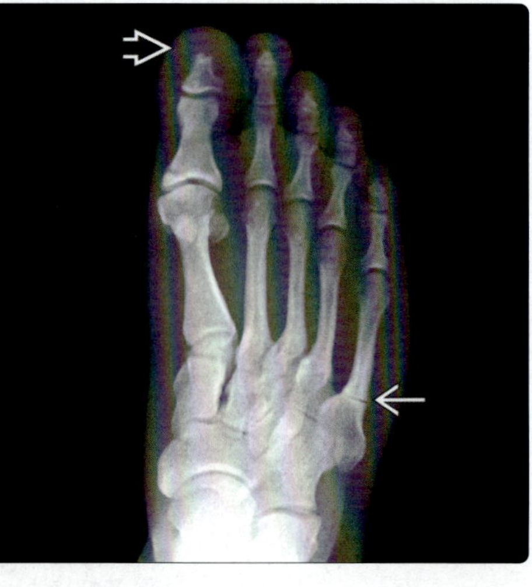

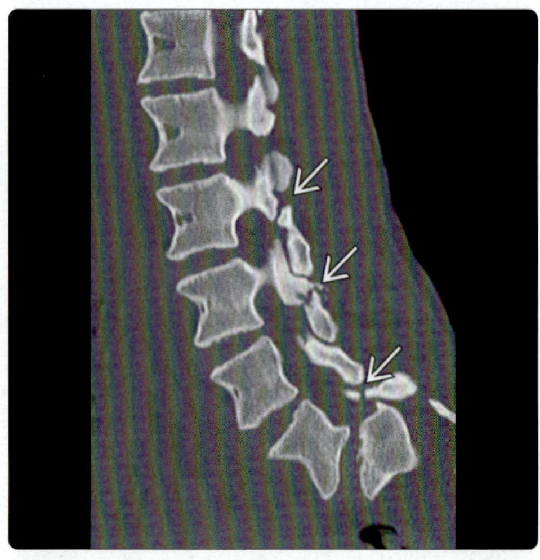

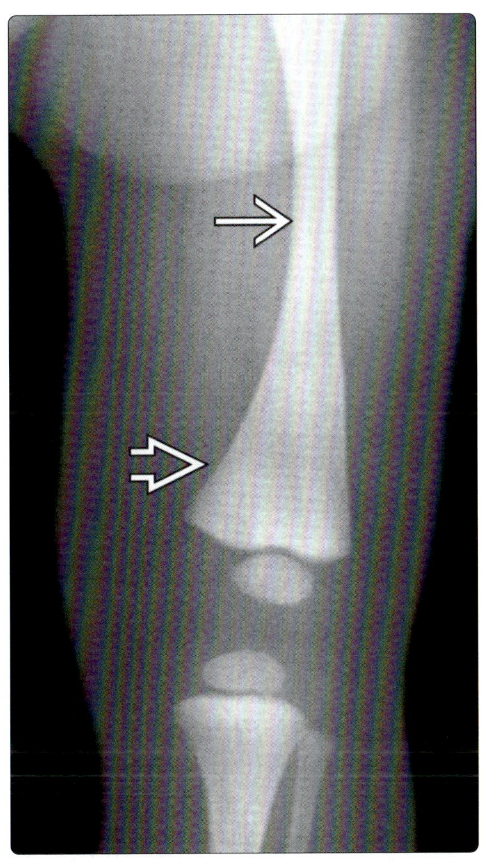

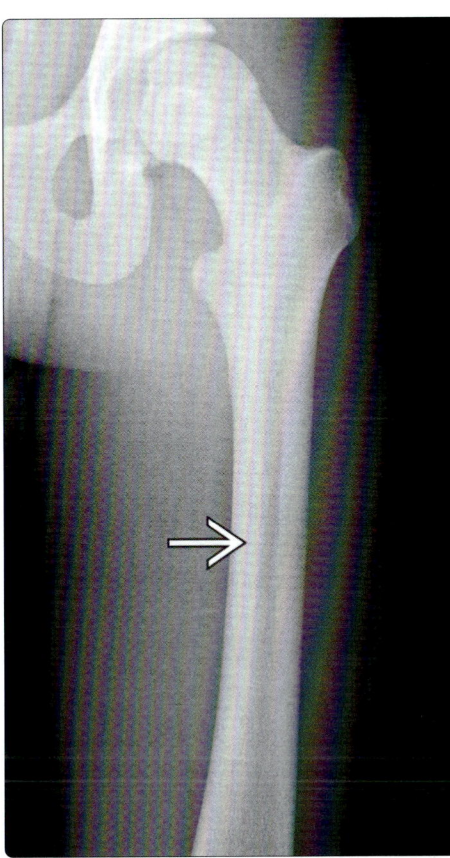

(Left) *AP radiograph demonstrates diffusely dense bones of the lower extremity with poor cortical-medullary differentiation ➡. Mild undertubulation of the distal femur is present ➡. The appearance is nonspecific and leads to a diagnosis of sclerosing dysplasia. Pycnodysostosis and osteopetrosis are the leading diagnoses.* **(Right)** *AP radiograph nicely reveals diffuse endosteal thickening ➡, which is one of the manifestations of pyknodysostosis. The spectrum of dense bones in this disease ranges from endosteal thickening, as in this case, to diffusely dense bones, which mimic osteopetrosis. Evaluation of the hands and feet as well as the skull will help to differentiate these entities.*

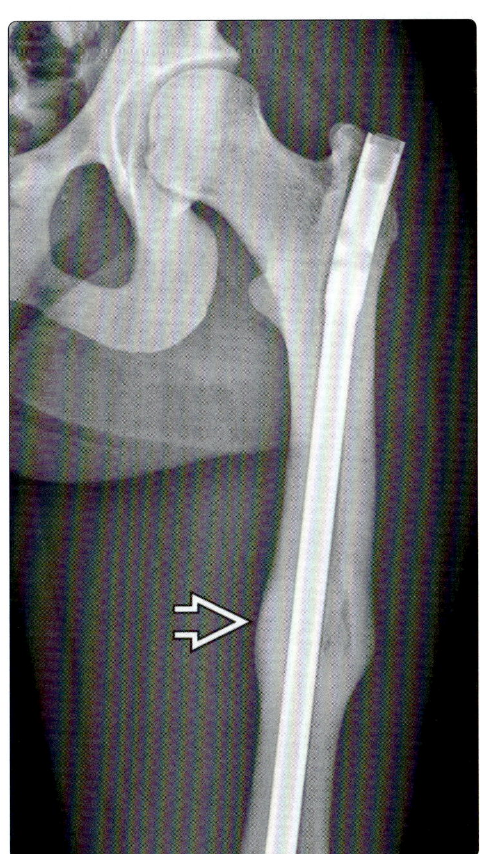

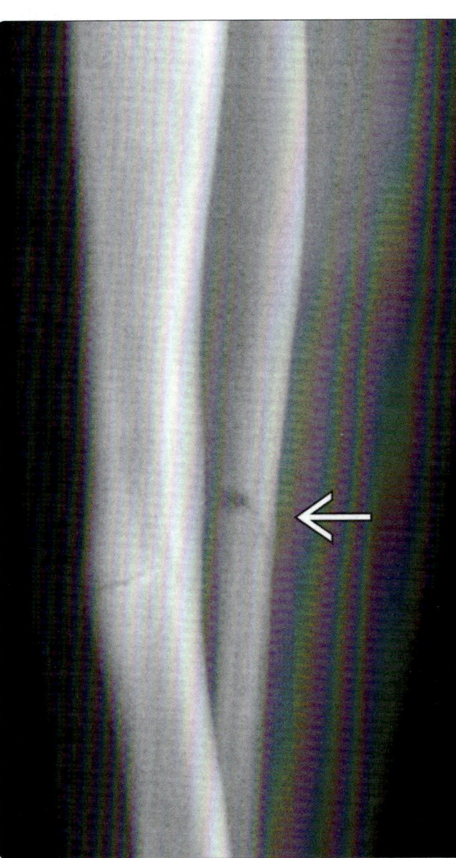

(Left) *AP radiograph shows a femur with diffuse sclerosis and prominent endosteal thickening. Despite the thickened cortex, fracture has occurred (now healed) ➡. Even though the bone is dense, the disorganized architecture and the inability to properly remodel in response to normal stresses places these bones at ↑ risk for fracture.* **(Right)** *Lateral radiograph of the leg shows dense bone, as well as transverse fractures ➡. Transverse fractures either occur from significant trauma (not the case here), or in abnormal bone. Note how the fracture has occurred along the anterior tibial cortex at the junction of mid and distal 1/3, a site of tension stresses. This location is a common site for adult tibial stress fractures. Normal stress on dense but abnormally remodeled bone in this case of pycnodysostosis has resulted in pathologic fracture.*

Osteitis Condensans

KEY FACTS

IMAGING

- Osteitis condensans ilii
  - Bilateral, symmetric sclerosis of ilium along sacroiliac joint
  - Sclerosis; triangular shape with apex cephalad; follows iliac articular surface, extends variable distance into adjacent marrow
  - No changes along sacral articular surface
  - Absence of other findings, such as subchondral cysts, erosions, joint space narrowing
- Osteitis condensans of clavicle
  - Typically unilateral
  - Sclerosis along inferomedial aspect of clavicle head
  - May have small inferomedial osteophyte
  - May have adjacent soft tissue edema on CT, MR

TOP DIFFERENTIAL DIAGNOSES

- Metastatic disease
  - Lesions identified elsewhere in skeleton
- Osteoarthritis
  - Joint space narrowing, subchondral cysts, osteophytes
- Sternoclavicular hyperostosis (SAPHO)
  - Favors teenagers and young adults
  - More common in men
  - May involve sternum, 1st costochondral junction
- Friedrich disease (osteonecrosis, clavicle head)
  - Diffuse involvement clavicle head
- Sacroiliitis
  - Joint space narrowing, erosions
  - Sclerosis on both sides of joint
  - More likely to be asymmetric

PATHOLOGY

- Response to mechanical stress

CLINICAL ISSUES

- Usually incidental finding, occasionally symptomatic
- M < F; 20-60 yr of age

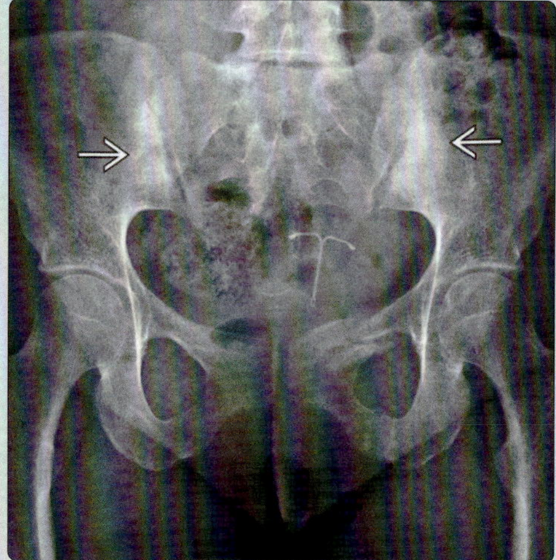

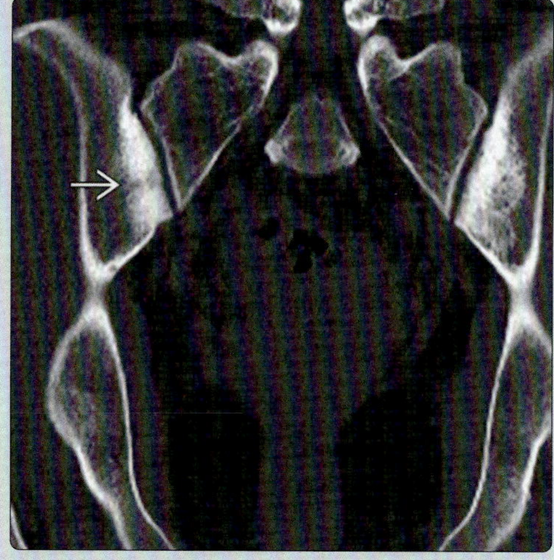

***(Left)** AP radiograph in a young woman being evaluated for trauma shows an incidental finding of osteitis condensans ilii. There is bilateral sclerosis limited to the iliac wings ➡ adjacent to normal sacroiliac joints. The sclerosis is roughly triangular shaped, with the apex of the triangle pointed cephalad. **(Right)** Coronal CT shows the triangular shape of the iliac wing sclerosis ➡, clearly delineating the morphology of the abnormality. This young woman had undergone several pregnancies and was asymptomatic.*

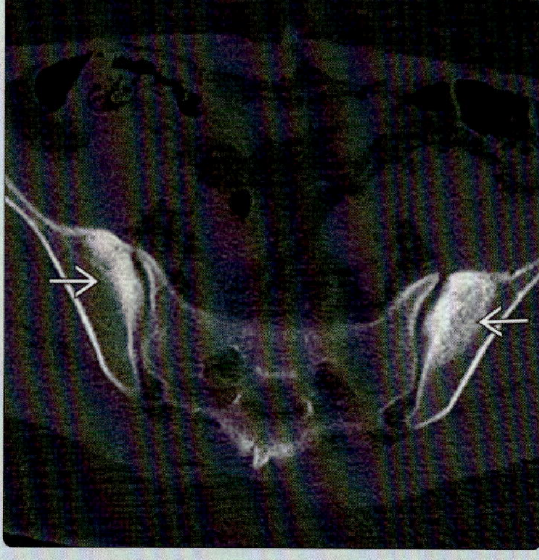

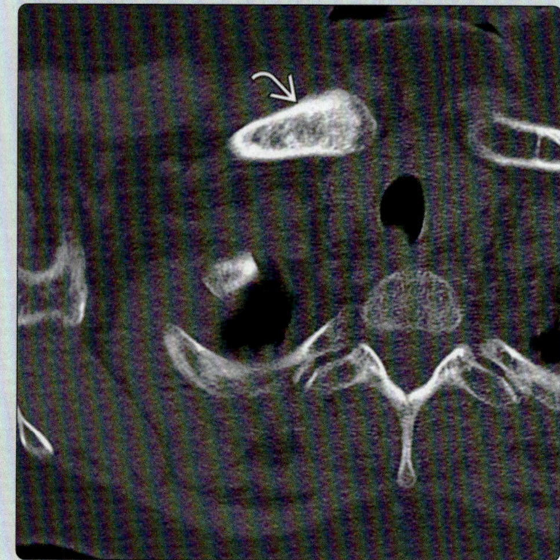

***(Left)** Axial CT in the same case confirms the sclerosis to be isolated to the iliac wings ➡ and that both the sacrum and sacroiliac joints are normal. No further imaging or follow-up of osteitis condensans ilii is required. **(Right)** Axial bone CT of a patient with pain over the right sternoclavicular joint reveals diffuse sclerosis in the right clavicular head ➡. The sternum (not shown) is normal. No other lesions were present in the skeleton. Osteitis condensans of the clavicle is a top diagnostic consideration.*

TERMINOLOGY

Abbreviations

- Osteitis condensans ilii (OCI)
- Osteitis condensans of clavicle (OCC)

IMAGING

General Features

- Best diagnostic clue
  - OCI: Bilateral, symmetric, triangular-shaped sclerosis of ilium at sacroiliac joint
  - OCC: Sclerosis of inferomedial clavicle head

Imaging Recommendations

- Best imaging tool
  - In most cases, radiographs are sufficient

Radiographic Findings

- Radiography
  - Osteitis condensans ilii
    - Sclerosis: Arises along iliac articular surface, extending variable distance into adjacent marrow
    - Triangular appearance; apex points cephalad
    - No changes along sacral articular surface
    - Absence of other findings, such as subchondral cysts, erosions, joint space narrowing
    - Typically bilateral and symmetric
    - Asymmetric disease is less common
    - Unilateral disease is rare
  - Osteitis condensans clavicle
    - Typically unilateral
    - Involves inferomedial aspect of clavicular head
    - May have small inferomedial osteophyte
    - Extends to subchondral bone
    - Absence of other findings, such as subchondral cysts, erosions, joint space narrowing

CT Findings

- CT better shows findings seen on radiography

MR Findings

- Areas of sclerosis will appear as areas of low signal intensity on all imaging sequences
- Distribution of findings as outlined under radiography
- Osteitis condensans clavicle may have adjacent soft tissue edema

Nuclear Medicine Findings

- Bone scan: Demonstrates intense uptake; may mimic arthritis
  - Helps exclude multifocal diseases, such as metastases
- FDG PET shows uptake; coregistered CT avoids misdiagnosis

DIFFERENTIAL DIAGNOSIS

Metastases, Bone Marrow

- Lesions identified elsewhere in skeleton
- Lacks bilateral, symmetric appearance and triangular shape of OCI
- Single focus of uptake in clavicular head unlikely to be solitary metastasis

Osteoarthritis

- Lacks triangular morphology and extension into marrow
- Joint space narrowing, subchondral cysts, osteophytes

Sternoclavicular Hyperostosis (SAPHO)

- Favors teenagers and young adults
- More common in men
- Unilateral or bilateral
- Enthesitis is more extensive
- May involve sternum, 1st costochondral junction

Sacroiliitis

- Joint space narrowing, erosions
- Sclerosis more irregular, lacks triangular shape, involves both sides of joint
- More likely to be symptomatic
- More likely to be asymmetric

Friedrich Disease (Osteonecrosis, Clavicle Head)

- Some believe it is same process
- Rare, patients younger (teenage to early adult)

PATHOLOGY

General Features

- Etiology
  - Response to mechanical stress

Microscopic Features

- Increase in number and size of trabeculae
- Obliteration of normal marrow space

CLINICAL ISSUES

Presentation

- Most common signs/symptoms
  - Incidental finding
  - Occasionally may be symptomatic
    - Stiffness, arthralgia
    - Compression testing of sacroiliac joint may be painful

Demographics

- Age
  - 20-60 yr
- Gender
  - M < F
    - ↑ incidence of OCI following pregnancy

Natural History & Prognosis

- Nonprogressive disease; no significant sequelae

Treatment

- If symptomatic, treat with over-the-counter analgesics
- Excision/stabilization required in rare cases
- Core decompression suggested in one small study

SELECTED REFERENCES

1. Jans L et al: MRI of the SI joints commonly shows non-inflammatory disease in patients clinically suspected of sacroiliitis. Eur J Radiol. 83(1):179-84, 2014

KEY FACTS

TERMINOLOGY

- Abnormal appearance of symphysis pubis in nonathletic individual
- In this context, findings are typically seen in middle-aged to elderly population

IMAGING

- Narrowing of symphysis pubis
  - Occasional appearance of widening due to resorption
- Subchondral sclerosis and cysts
- Osteophytes
- Vacuum phenomenon
- Chondrocalcinosis, periarticular mineralization
- Osseous fragmentation
- Capsular hypertrophy
- Fluid within symphysis
- MR: Subchondral marrow changes
  - Ranges from edema (↓ T1 signal, ↑ signal fluid-sensitive sequences) to sclerosis (↓ signal all sequences)

TOP DIFFERENTIAL DIAGNOSES

- Infection
  - Always consider if symphysis pubis is painful, especially if there are clinical signs of infection
  - May require aspiration to exclude
  - MR: Extensive edema in adjacent soft tissues
- Osteoblastic metastatic disease
  - Demonstrates multiple lesions
- Hyperparathyroidism
  - Subchondral bone resorption

PATHOLOGY

- Secondary osteoarthritis, crystal deposition disease

CLINICAL ISSUES

- Usually incidental finding
- Occasionally symptomatic
- Incidence increases with age
- Treatment usually conservative

(Left) *AP radiograph shows abnormal symphysis pubis with subchondral sclerosis and subchondral cysts ➡. There is no bone destruction.* **(Right)** *Axial NECT nicely demonstrates changes of crystal deposition disease. Changes include periarticular mineralization ➡, subchondral cyst formation ↪, and capsular hypertrophy ⇨. Similar changes are also present within the right ischiogluteal bursa ⇨.*

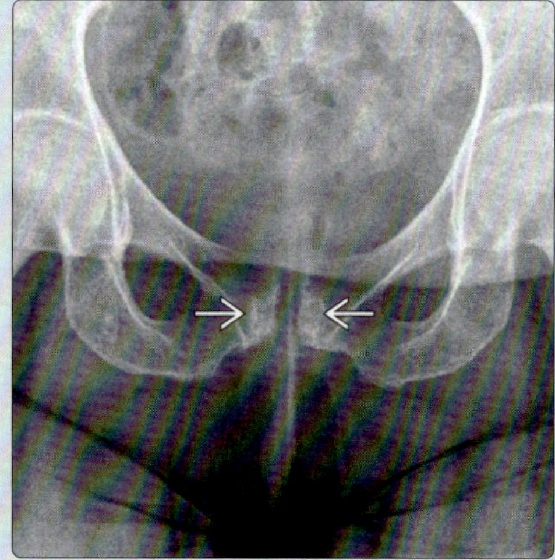

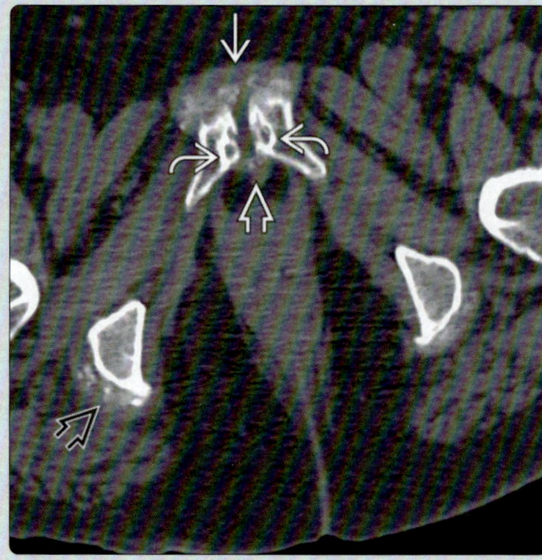

(Left) *Frontal bone scan shows a common finding of increased uptake along both sides of the symphysis pubis ➡. Unless symptoms arise from this region, this finding is typically attributed to degenerative disease.* **(Right)** *Coronal STIR MR reveals fluid within the symphysis ↪ with inflammatory changes in the joint capsule and adjacent soft tissues ➡. Mild bone marrow edema is present on both sides of the articulation. These findings are not uncommon in the elderly population.*

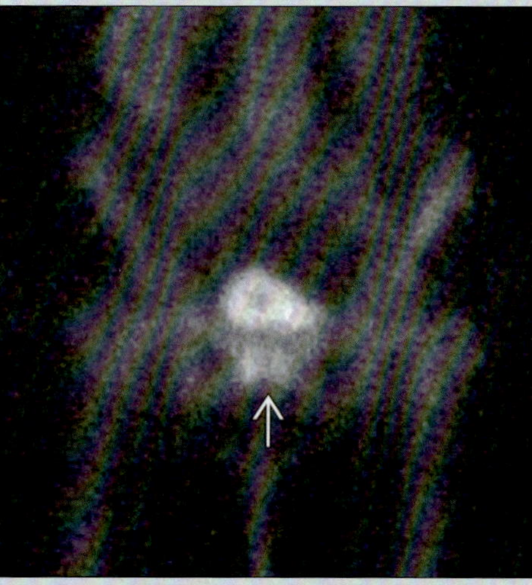

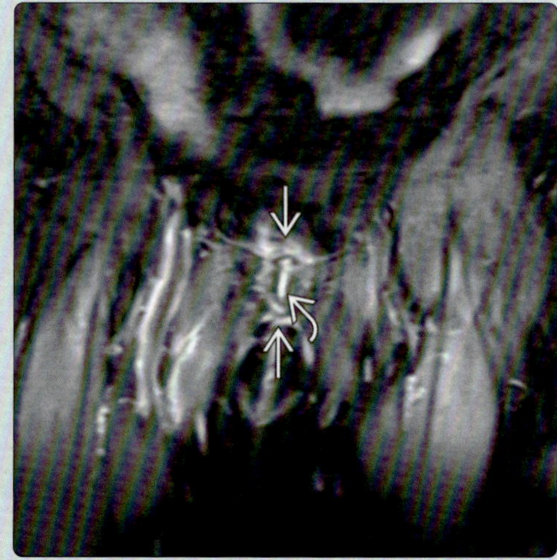

TERMINOLOGY

Definitions

- Abnormal imaging appearance of symphysis pubis in nonathletic individual
- In this context, findings are typically seen in middle-aged to elderly population
- Differentiate this diagnosis from traumatic osteitis pubis, which presents in younger, athletic (usually high-performance) individuals (athletic pubalgia)

IMAGING

General Features

- Best diagnostic clue
  - Subchondral sclerosis, cysts, articular surface irregularity or resorption at symphysis pubis

Imaging Recommendations

- Best imaging tool
  - Incidental finding on radiographs, CT, MR, bone scan

Radiographic Findings

- Radiography
  - Narrowing of symphysis pubis
    - May also appear widened, with resorption
  - Subchondral sclerosis and cysts
  - Osteophytes and osseous fragmentation
  - Vacuum phenomenon
  - Chondrocalcinosis and periarticular mineralization

CT Findings

- Mimics radiography
- Capsular hypertrophy may be seen
- Joint distention from fluid
- ↑ sensitivity for chondrocalcinosis, capsular calcification

MR Findings

- Cartilage thinning, irregularity
- Subchondral marrow signal changes
  - Unilateral or bilateral
  - Symmetric or asymmetric
  - Ranges from edema (↓ T1 signal, ↑ signal fluid-sensitive sequences) to sclerosis (↓ signal all sequences)
- Subchondral cysts, osteophytes
- Capsular hypertrophy
- Fluid within symphysis
- Mild edema in adjacent soft tissues (fat and muscle)
  - If extensive edema, need to consider infection

Nuclear Medicine Findings

- Bone scan
  - Increased radiopharmaceutical uptake
    - Typically on both sides of symphysis
    - Symmetric or asymmetric
    - If unilateral uptake consider other diagnoses
      - Stress fracture, metastases

DIFFERENTIAL DIAGNOSIS

Infection

- Always consider if
  - Recent genitourinary instrumentation
  - Constitutional symptoms of infection
- Bone destruction, gas bubbles
- Immature, irregular new bone formation
- MR may show extensive edema in adjacent soft tissues
- In appropriate clinical setting, may require aspiration to confirm/exclude infection

Osteoblastic Metastatic Disease

- Typically multifocal disease
- Unilateral uptake may be with pubic rami metastases
  - Radiographs help; metastases not subchondral

Rheumatologic Disease

- Rheumatoid, ankylosing spondylitis, psoriatic arthritis
- Erosions, excessive periostitis suggest this etiology
- Manifestations of arthritis seen elsewhere in skeleton

Hyperparathyroidism

- Subchondral bone resorption

PATHOLOGY

General Features

- Etiology
  - Multiple etiologies
    - Secondary osteoarthritis
      - Mechanical disease as sequelae of microinstability: Injury in younger years (traumatic osteitis pubis), multiparous women
      - Late stage of arthritides that involve symphysis pubis: Rheumatoid, ankylosing spondylitis, psoriatic arthritis
    - Crystal deposition disease
    - Previous instrumentation in pelvis, especially GU, gynecologic

CLINICAL ISSUES

Presentation

- Most common signs/symptoms
  - Incidental finding
- Other signs/symptoms
  - Occasionally may be symptomatic
  - No specific imaging findings help to confirm or exclude abnormal symphysis as cause of pain
  - If symptomatic must consider infection

Demographics

- Age
  - Middle-aged to elderly population
    - Incidence increases with age

SELECTED REFERENCES

1. Budak MJ et al: There's a hole in my symphysis – a review of disorders causing widening, erosion, and destruction of the symphysis pubis. Clin Radiol. 68(2):173-80, 2013

KEY FACTS

IMAGING

- Process only described in lower extremities
  - Tibia most common; also seen in femur, fibula
  - Usually bilateral asymmetric, may be unilateral
  - Located within diaphysis, usually midshaft
- Bone scan: Intense radiopharmaceutical uptake
  - Not all lesions will be radiographically evident
  - Distribution helps differentiate sclerosing dysplasias
- CT and MR: Homogeneous and continuous sclerosis
  - Sclerosis extends from endosteal bone into medullary canal, may obliterate canal
  - Limited periosteal cortical thickening
  - ± soft tissue edema/enhancement; no mass

TOP DIFFERENTIAL DIAGNOSES

- Ribbing disease may be indistinguishable
- Progressive diaphyseal dysplasia
  - Boys more common; presents in childhood
  - Skull and vertebral involvement
  - Periosteal and endosteal hyperostosis
- Sclerotic metastasis: Usually older population
  - More patchy, discontinuous in appearance
- Melorheostosis: Dripping candle wax appearance
  - Unilateral distribution; upper or lower extremity
  - May have mineralized soft tissue mass
- Stress fracture: Sclerosis more focal
  - Periosteal new bone formation

PATHOLOGY

- Mixture of irregular woven bone and interspersed lamellar bone within medullary space
- Does not differentiate from other sclerosing dysplasias

CLINICAL ISSUES

- Nonhereditary
- Pain exacerbated by activity; more common in women
- Wide age range, from childhood to late middle age
- Decompression of medullary canal may relieve symptoms

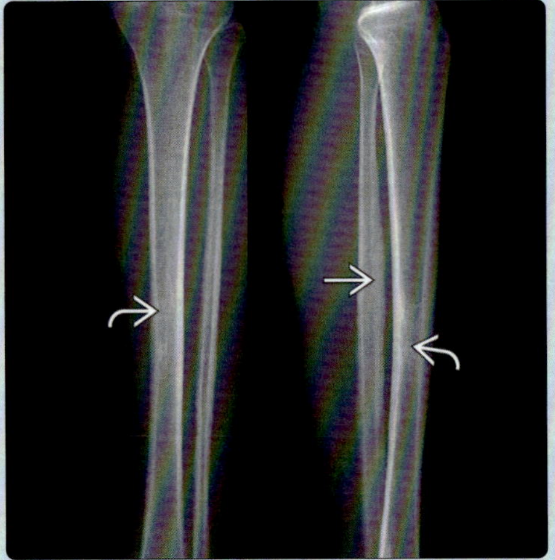

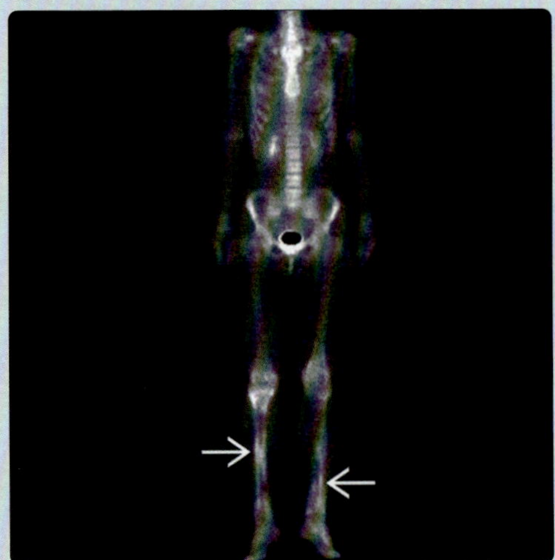

(Left) *AP and lateral radiographs show the left leg of a 34-year-old woman who has had leg pain for 7 months. Sclerosis is shown within the medullary canal* ➡ *of both the tibia and fibula. Endosteal thickening is more prominent in the fibula* ➡ *than the tibia.* **(Right)** *AP bone scan shows that the abnormality is bilateral within the legs* ➡*. There is also mild abnormality seen in the distal femora bilaterally. No other bones are involved. This bilateral and predominantly leg abnormality is typical of intramedullary osteosclerosis.*

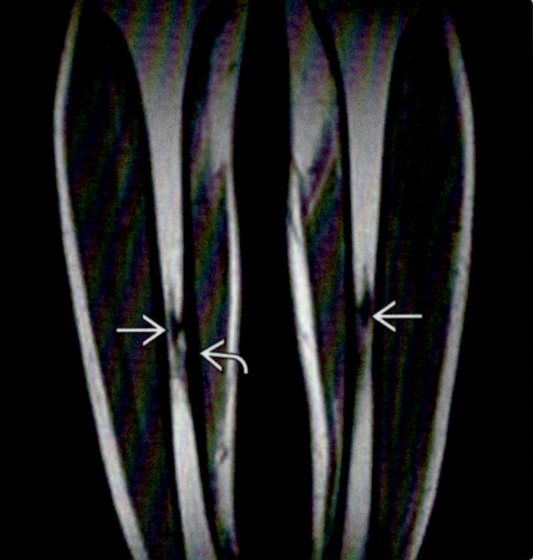

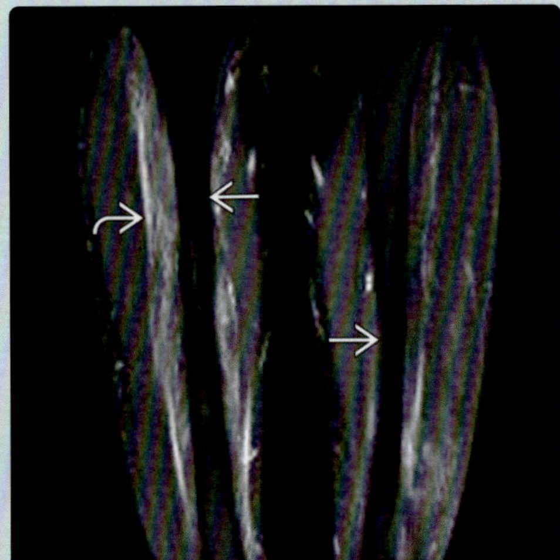

(Left) *Coronal T1WI MR in the same patient shows the low signal of the intramedullary sclerosis* ➡*, as well as the endosteal thickening* ➡*. This signal is expected in all MR sequences in bones affected by intramedullary osteosclerosis.* **(Right)** *Coronal STIR MR shows the dense osteosclerosis of both tibiae* ➡*. In addition, there is extensive edema within the soft tissues* ➡*. This latter finding need not be present in all cases of intramedullary osteosclerosis.*

KEY FACTS

IMAGING

- Radiographs sufficient to establish diagnosis
- **Osteopoikilosis (OPK)**: Bone polka dots
  - Multiple uniform ovoid/round sclerotic foci
  - Range in number from 1 or 2 to numerous
  - Metaphyseal and subarticular; multiple locations
  - Favors appendicular skeleton, generally spares spine, skull, ribs
  - Associated cutaneous lesions in 25%
  - May ↑ or ↓ size & number in children; static in adults
- **Osteopathia striata (Voorhoeve disease)**: Striped bones
  - Vertical striations in metaphyses extending to diaphysis of long bones; usually bilateral
  - Flat bones have sunburst appearance
  - Temporal bone sclerosis with hearing loss
- **Mixed sclerosing bone dysplasia**: Combination of osteopoikilosis, osteopathia striata, melorheostosis
- Bone scan: Typically not detected, ± mild uptake
- MR: Low signal on all imaging sequences; no soft tissue changes, marrow edema, or enhancement

TOP DIFFERENTIAL DIAGNOSES

- Osteopoikilosis
  - Sclerotic metastases: Random distribution, irregular (non-feathery) margins, spares epiphyses
  - Mastocytosis: Rare, random distribution, skin rash
- Osteopathia striata
  - Enchondromatosis: Unilateral, striated pattern
  - Rubella: Celery stalk metaphysis

PATHOLOGY

- OPK: Compact lamellar bone in medullary canal
- Autosomal dominant transmission reported
- Osteopoikilosis associated with *LEMD3*

CLINICAL ISSUES

- 80-85% asymptomatic, incidental, no treatment required
- 15-20% mild articular symptoms, ± effusion

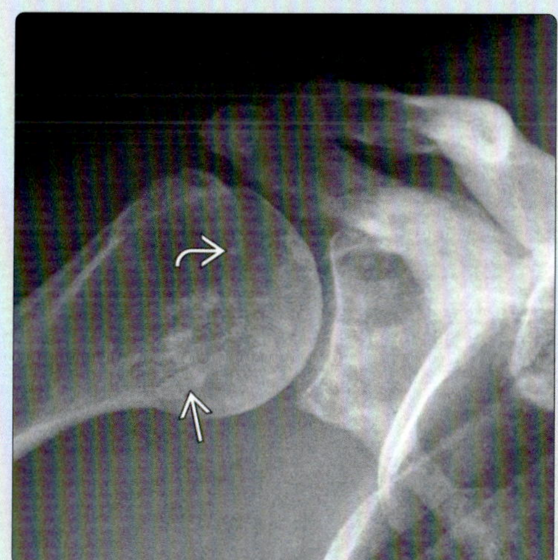

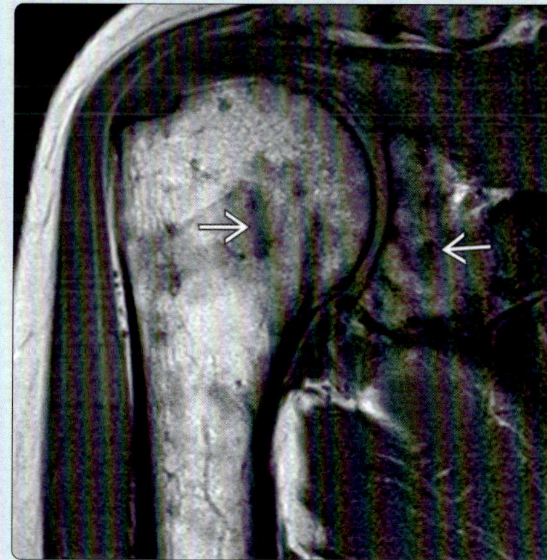

(Left) *AP radiograph shows multiple small, sclerotic lesions that range in shape from round ➙ to oval ➙. Given the concentration in the metaphyses and subchondral regions, this is pathognomonic for osteopoikilosis. Other sclerosing diseases, such as osteoblastic metastases or mastocytosis, are not this uniform and typically spare the epiphyses.* **(Right)** *Coronal T1WI MR in the same patient shows all the lesions ➙ to have low signal, with surrounding normal marrow.*

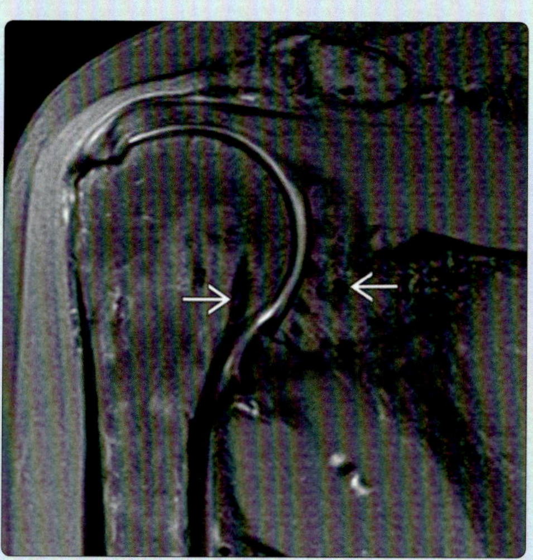

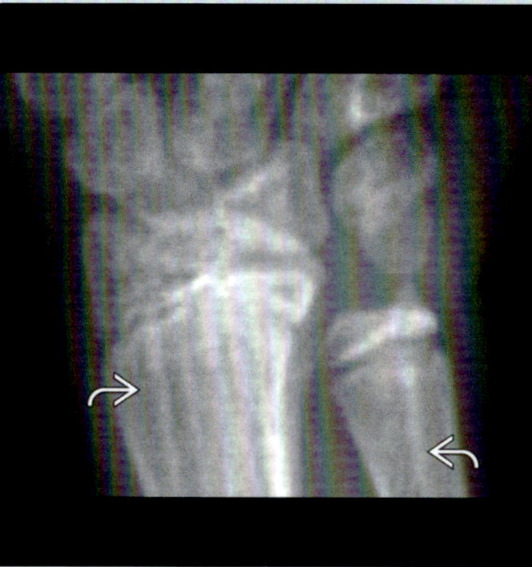

(Left) *Coronal T2WI FS MR confirms that all the lesions ➙ show hypointense signal, with surrounding normal marrow. There is no diagnosis to consider other than osteopoikilosis.* **(Right)** *AP radiograph reveals classic changes of osteopathia striata. Multiple sclerotic lines are oriented along the long axis of the radius and ulna ➙. The lines begin in the metaphysis and extend into the diaphysis. Similar findings were present in the opposite wrist. This process is typically bilateral.*

SECTION 6

Systemic Diseases With MSK Involvement

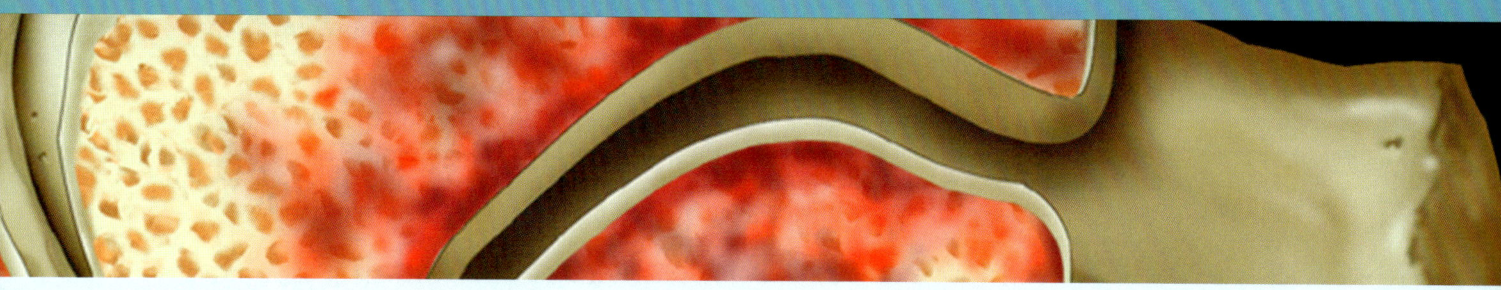

General

Storage Disorders

Connective Tissue Disorders

Connective Tissue Disorder With Arachnodactyly

Soft Tissue Disorders

Vascular

KEY FACTS

TERMINOLOGY

- Musculoskeletal complications related to paraplegia

IMAGING

- Decubitus ulcers
  - At risk: Sacrum, ischial tuberosity, greater trochanter
  - Air seen in sinus track; ± extension to bone
- Osteoporosis
  - Increased risk for fracture, particularly around joints of lower extremity from vigorous physical therapy
  - May initially appear aggressive in young, recent paraplegic patient
    - Subchondral linear lucency or metaphyseal bands
    - Moth-eaten pattern may mimic infection/tumor
- Osteomyelitis
  - Associated with decubitus ulcers
  - Vertebral osteomyelitis/discitis: High risk 2° to neurogenic bladder, chronic low-grade infection, and venous plexus leading up posterior vertebral bodies
- Heterotopic ossification
  - Develops in 16-53% of paraplegic patients
  - Periarticular, especially at joints surrounded by spastic muscles
  - Adult: Generally appears 2-6 months post paralysis
  - Child: Appears on average 1 year following trauma
- Neuropathic joint
  - Spine particularly at risk in paraplegic patients
  - Location: Below level of stabilizing instrumentation
  - Generally no associated paraspinous soft tissue mass; should help differentiate from discitis
- Squamous cell carcinoma
  - Rare osseous tumor, related to long-term sinus track at decubitus ulcer extending into bone
  - Differential diagnosis is osteomyelitis; size of soft tissue mass with carcinoma helps to differentiate
- Cartilage atrophy
  - Synovial fluid production ↓ with immobilization
  - Sacroiliac joints abnormal in 61% of paraplegics

(Left) *Axial bone CT shows a soft tissue mass within the iliacus muscle ➡. There is central amorphous calcific density ➡. No other abnormality is seen on this image.* **(Right)** *Axial bone CT in same patient 6 weeks earlier was obtained 2 weeks after the patient suffered trauma resulting in paraplegia. The image is normal. Given the time sequence from normal to development of mass with calcification (6 weeks), this is diagnostic of immature heterotopic bone formation in a patient at risk secondary to paraplegia.*

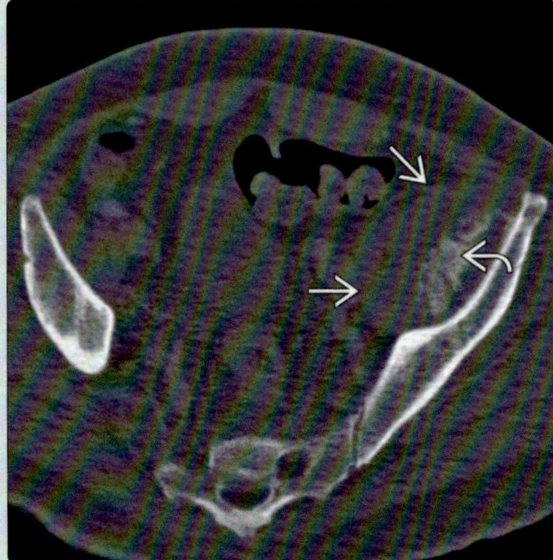

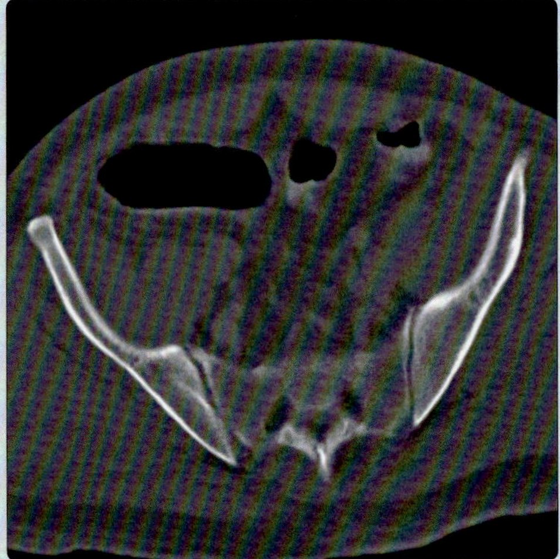

(Left) *Axial CT in the same patient was obtained at the same level, 2 weeks post trauma. There is amorphous calcification seen within masses of the left psoas ➡ as well as bilateral obturator internus ➡.* **(Right)** *Axial CT shows no abnormality of the muscles. There is a rectal tube and bladder catheter placed in this patient with new paraplegia. The multiplicity of abnormalities 6 weeks later and the patient's risk factor of paraplegia makes the diagnosis of heterotropic ossification, despite the immature zoning.*

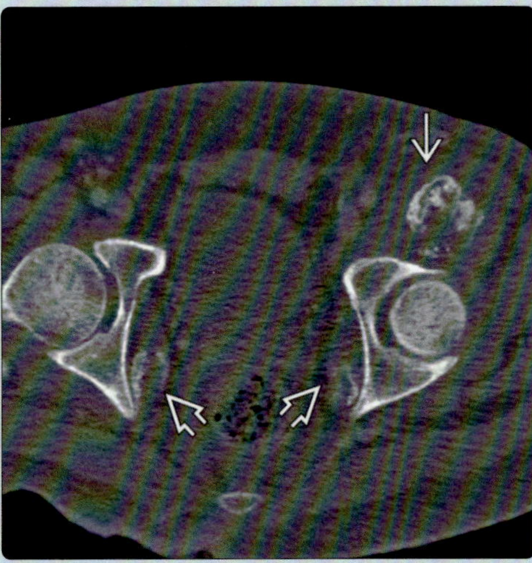

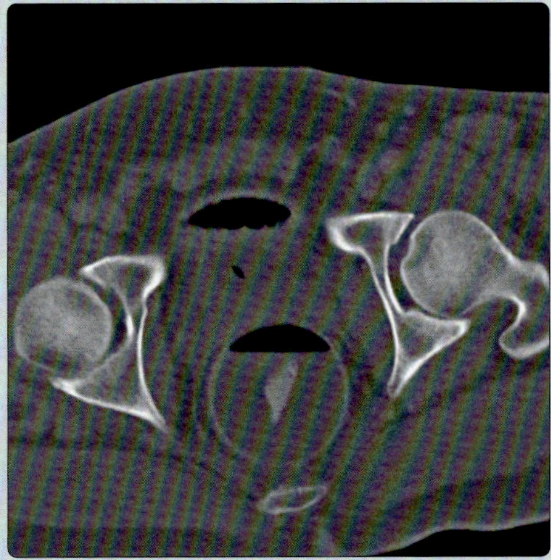

TERMINOLOGY

Definitions

- Musculoskeletal complications related to paraplegia

IMAGING

Radiographic Findings

- Decubitus ulcers
  - At risk: Sacrum, ischial tuberosity, greater trochanter
  - Air seen in sinus track; ± extension to bone
- Osteoporosis
  - May initially appear aggressive in young, recent paraplegic patient
    - Subchondral linear lucency or metaphyseal bands
    - Moth-eaten pattern may suggest infection/tumor
  - With chronicity, develops diffuse ↓ bone density
  - Increased risk for fracture, particularly around joints of lower extremity from vigorous physical therapy
- Heterotopic ossification (HO)
  - Common complication of spinal cord disorders
    - Develops in 16-53% of paraplegic patients
    - More frequent in spastic than flaccid paralysis
  - Periarticular, especially at joints surrounded by spastic muscles
  - Generally appears 2-6 months post paralysis in adult
    - Later in child, on average 1 year following trauma
    - Progression of ossification follows timing of HO elsewhere
      - 0-2 weeks after onset: Soft tissue mass with indistinct surrounding soft tissue planes
      - 3-4 weeks: Amorphous osteoid forms within mass; adjacent periosteal reaction may be seen
      - 6-8 weeks: Sharper cortex begins to form about lacy central osseous mass
      - 5-6 months: Mature bone formation
  - HO maturation: Distinctive zoning pattern over 2-6 months
    - Mature cortical bone peripherally
    - Centrally, less mature bone, ± soft tissue, cystic regions
  - MR of heterotopic ossification
    - As with CT/x-ray, appearance relates to lesion age
    - May show marrow edema, periosteal reaction, and peripheral edema at any stage
    - Early stage
      - T1: Signal intensity isointense to muscle
      - Fluid-sensitive sequences: Hyperintense, markedly inhomogeneous
    - Intermediate stage
      - T1: Isointense to muscle, perhaps with local distortion of fat planes
      - Fluid-sensitive sequences: Hyperintense mass, with curvilinear and irregular areas of decreased SI surrounding lesion
      - Low signal "halo" on T2WI may be incomplete but serves to differentiate HO from tumor bone formation
      - Earliest equivalent to well-organized cortical rim visualized on radiograph or CT
    - Late stage
      - Well-defined inhomogeneous osseous mass
      - Central cystic regions may be seen
      - No associated edema
- Osteomyelitis
  - Associated with decubitus ulcers
    - May see sinus track ± air leading to region of osseous destruction
    - Permeative bone change, cortical destruction
    - Periosteal reaction
    - Appearance may be complicated by prior debridement/resection of bone
  - Spine osteomyelitis/disc space infection
    - High risk 2° to neurogenic bladder, chronic low-grade infection, and venous plexus leading up posterior vertebral bodies
    - Disc space narrowing, adjacent vertebral body endplate destruction
    - Paravertebral soft tissue mass
  - MR of osteomyelitis
    - Early: May see only confluent low SI on T1, high SI on T2, enhancement
    - Later: Destructive osseous change with periosteal reaction (low SI T1, high SI T2)
    - Adjacent abscesses, demonstrated by enhancing rim around low signal fluid on contrast imaging
    - ± low signal air, likely enhancing sinus track
- Neuropathic joint
  - Spine particularly at risk in paraplegic patients
    - Occurs below level of stabilizing instrumentation
  - Unprotected motion of spine below paraplegic level leads to fragmentation of osteoporotic bone, breakdown of restraining ligaments
    - Disc space loss
    - Osseous fragmentation
    - Subluxation, often at multiple levels
    - Generally no associated paraspinous soft tissue mass; should help differentiate from discitis
- Squamous cell carcinoma
  - Rare osseous tumor, related to long-term sinus track at decubitus ulcer; carcinoma develops along sinus track, extends to adjacent bone
  - Extremely rapid bony destruction, poor prognosis
  - Differential diagnosis is osteomyelitis; size of soft tissue mass with carcinoma helps to differentiate
- Cartilage atrophy
  - Synovial fluid production ↓ with immobilization
  - Fibrillation, erosion, and resorption of cartilage
  - Sacroiliac, hip, knee joint space narrowing
    - Sacroiliac (SI) joints abnormal in 61% of paraplegics
      - Periarticular osteoporosis, joint space narrowing, occasional ankylosis
      - Suggested etiology of SI joint process: Chronic low-grade pelvic sepsis from neurogenic bladder via paravertebral venous plexus
      - Others suggest it is 2° to chronic osteoporosis, cartilage atrophy, and mechanical stress

SELECTED REFERENCES

1. Aebli N et al: Characteristics and surgical management of neuropathic (Charcot) spinal arthropathy after spinal cord injury. Spine J. 14(6):884-91, 2014

(Left) *Axial T1WI MR shows mature bone ➡ located within the soft tissues around the hip, characterized by marrow signal that matches that of the femur. There is a more central low signal focus ➡.* **(Right)** *Axial T2WI MR in the same patient shows mature bone ➡ anterior to a fluid collection ➡. It should be remembered that neurologically injured patients, particularly paraplegics, are at high risk for developing HO, especially around the hips. Mature heterotopic bone formations may contain fluid centrally.*

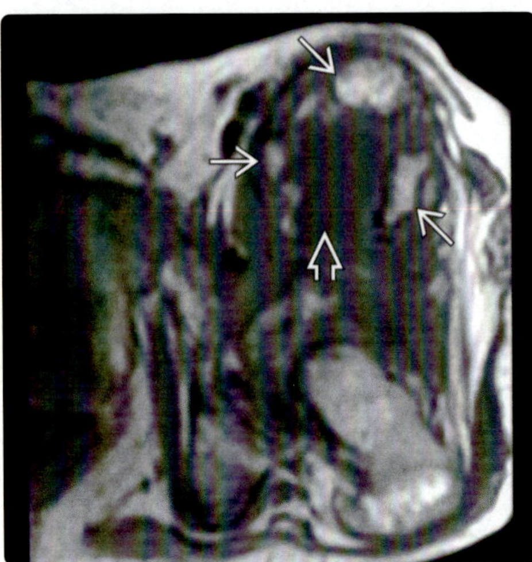

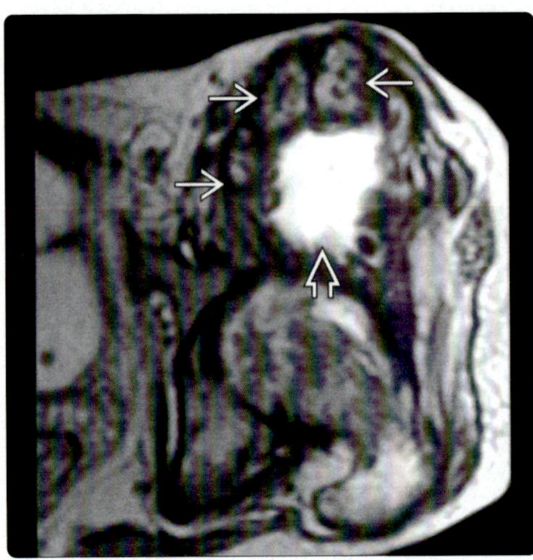

(Left) *Coronal T1WI MR obtained in a paraplegic patient with sacral decubitus shows low signal within the soft tissues ➡ leading to confluent low signal in the ischium ➡. Confluent rather than hazy reticulated low signal on T1 strongly suggests osteomyelitis rather than reactive marrow change. Note the muscle atrophy.* **(Right)** *Coronal T1WI C+ FS MR in the same patient shows enhancement of both the soft tissue and ischial tuberosity ➡. No abscess is seen, but this is biopsy-proven osteomyelitis.*

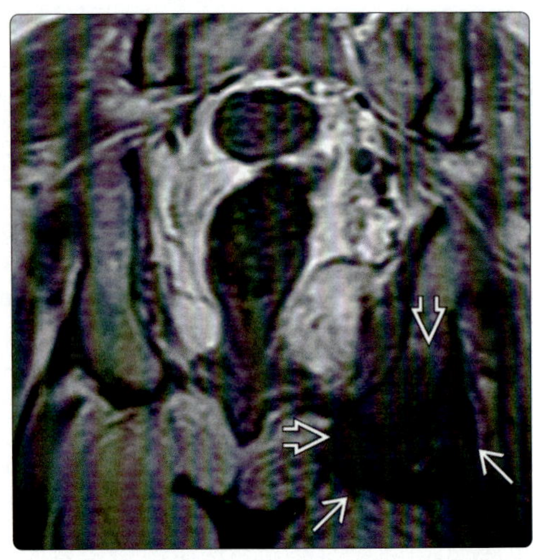

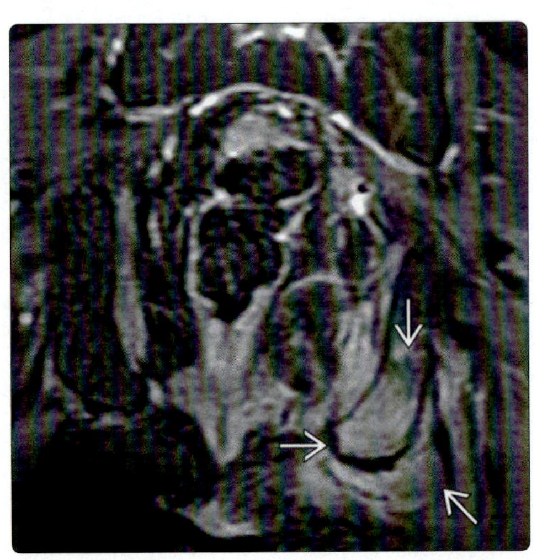

(Left) *AP radiograph in this paraplegic patient shows air in the soft tissues ➡ from a chronic ischial decubitus ulcer. There is a clean edge along the ischium from surgical resection of previously infected bone ➡.* **(Right)** *AP radiograph obtained 6 weeks later shows aggressive dissolution of bone ➡ with permeative change. Although this may represent rapid osteolysis from infection, the rapidity of bone destruction should make one also consider squamous cell carcinoma, which was proven at biopsy.*

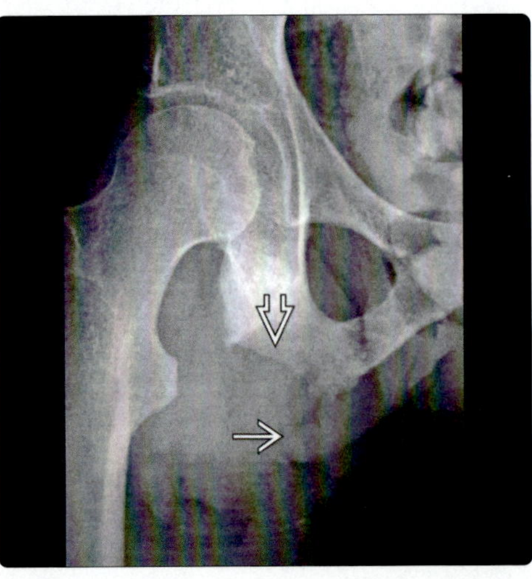

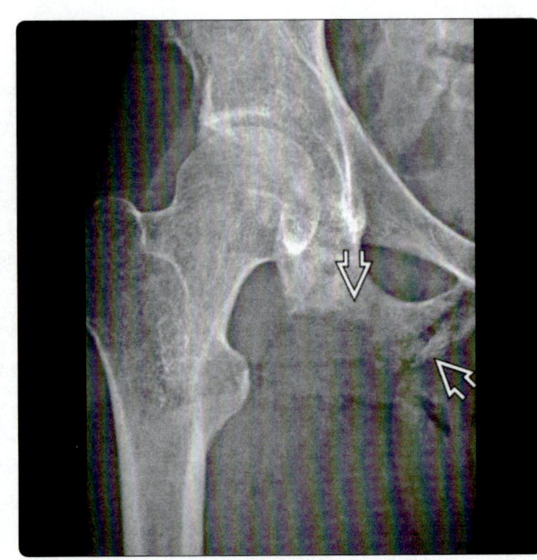

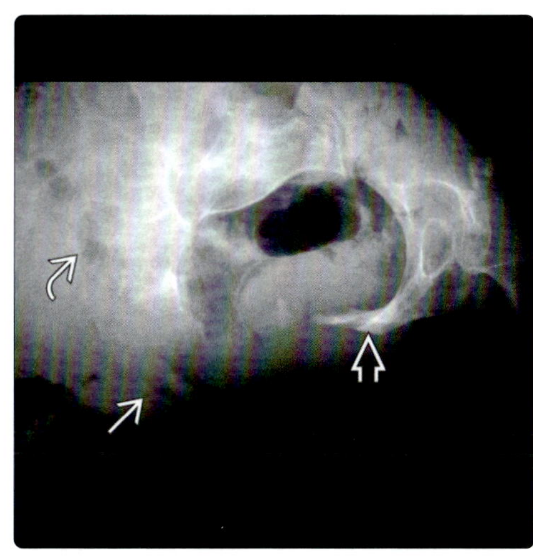

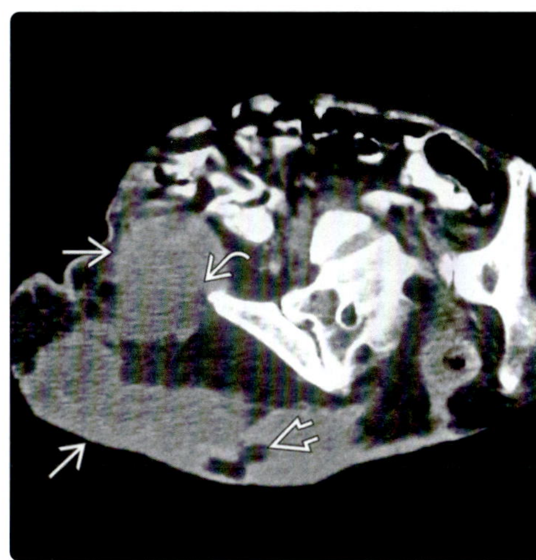

(Left) *AP radiograph of the pelvis shows a rare case of squamous cell carcinoma complicating chronic infection in a long-term paraplegic patient. There are chronic changes typical of paraplegia, including resection of the ischii related to chronic osteomyelitis ➡, air in the soft tissues from ongoing infection ➡, and destruction of the iliac wing ⇨.* **(Right)** *Axial CT in the same patient shows a mass ➡, iliac wing destruction ⇨, and air within a chronic sinus track ➡. This squamous cell tumor carries a grave prognosis.*

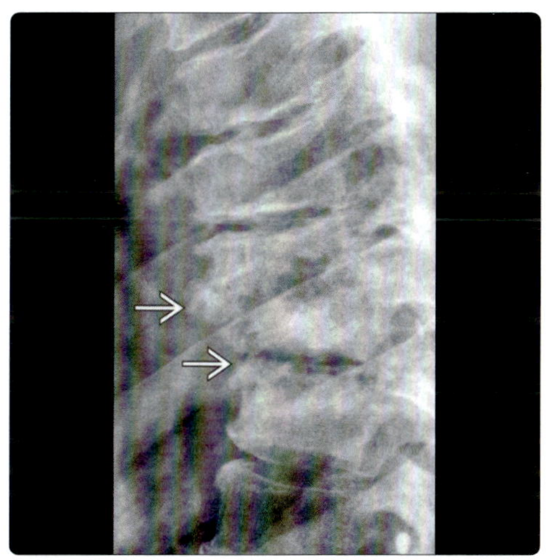

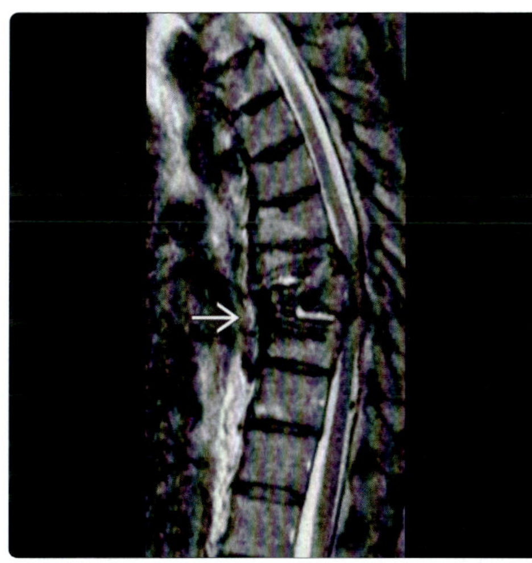

(Left) *Lateral radiograph shows significant subluxation and destruction of vertebral endplates with osseous debris at 2 adjacent levels ➡. This paraplegic patient is unstable at this level of the thoracic spine.* **(Right)** *Sagittal T2WI MR in the same patient shows the instability of the spine across this interval ➡, which causes cord compression. However, there is no paraspinous or epidural soft tissue mass to suggest infection. This is a neuropathic spine 2° to a more proximal paraplegic level.*

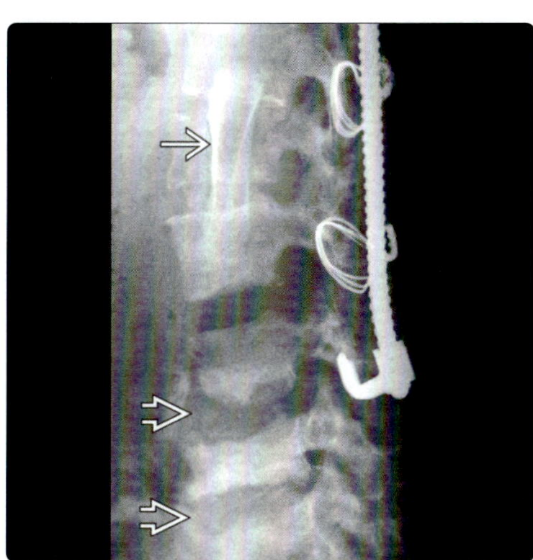

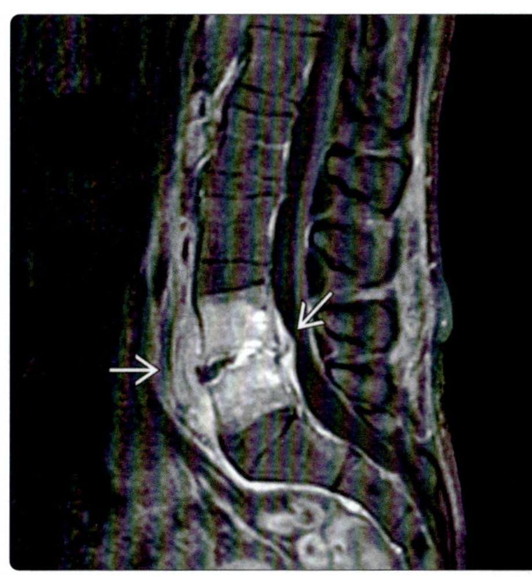

(Left) *Lateral radiograph in a paraplegic patient with burst fracture of L1 stabilized by rods and strut graft ➡ is shown. There is osseous destruction and instability of 2 lower levels ➡; these are adjacent sites of neuropathic joints.* **(Right)** *Sagittal T1 C+ FS MR shows extensive enhancement of L5 and S1 bodies, intervertebral disc, and prevertebral and epidural extension ➡, typical of disc space infection. The spine in paraplegic patients are at risk for both infection and neuropathic changes; differentiation must be made.*

Acroosteolysis

KEY FACTS

TERMINOLOGY

- Group of processes with shortening of distal phalanges as common feature

IMAGING

- Short phalanges due to variety of forms of osteolysis

TOP DIFFERENTIAL DIAGNOSES

- Resorptive etiologies
  - Hyperparathyroidism
  - Progressive systemic sclerosis
- Vascular etiologies
  - Frostbite
  - Vasculitis
  - Diabetes
  - Meningococcemia
  - Amniotic band syndrome
- Traumatic etiologies
  - Burn
  - Congenital insensitivity/indifference to pain
  - Occupational acroosteolysis
- Inflammatory etiologies
  - Psoriatic arthritis
  - Multicentric reticulohistiocytosis
- Infectious etiology: Leprosy
- Congenital (genetic) etiologies
  - Pycnodysostosis
  - Hajdu-Cheney
  - Lesch-Nyhan

DIAGNOSTIC CHECKLIST

- Watch for associated findings to help determine etiology of acroosteolysis
  - Presence and distribution of soft tissue changes, calcification, arthritic changes
- Osseous injury to distal phalanges may take different forms
  - Tuft or midshaft lucency, premature fusion of physis

(Left) *PA radiograph shows multiple findings of HPTH related to renal osteodystrophy. Subperiosteal resorption is seen at many sites ➔, along with a brown tumor ➔. There is tuft resorption ➔. It is important to remember that HPTH is a common cause of acroosteolysis.* **(Right)** *PA radiograph of a patient with HPTH shows how severe acroosteolysis may become in this disease. There is near complete resorption of distal phalanges 2 and 5 ➔ and a band-like pattern of osteolysis in phalanges 3 and 4 ➔.*

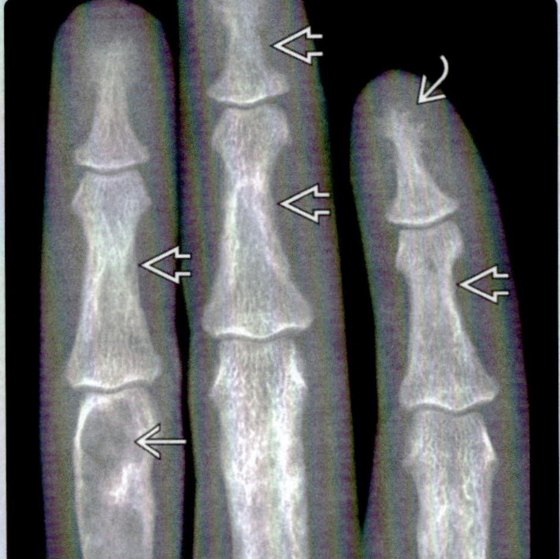

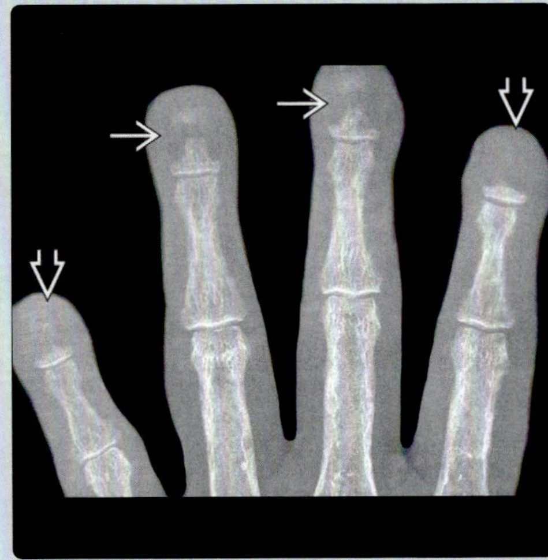

(Left) *PA radiograph shows findings typical of progressive systemic sclerosis, or scleroderma. There is osseous acroosteolysis ➔ as well as soft tissue tapering ➔. Note the prominent soft tissue calcification; this feature helps to secure the diagnosis.* **(Right)** *PA radiograph shows acroosteolysis ➔ with normal adjacent soft tissues. However, there are numerous lytic lesions of the phalanges that have the lacy pattern of sarcoidosis. Though these lacy lesions are most typical, acroosteolysis may be seen in sarcoid.*

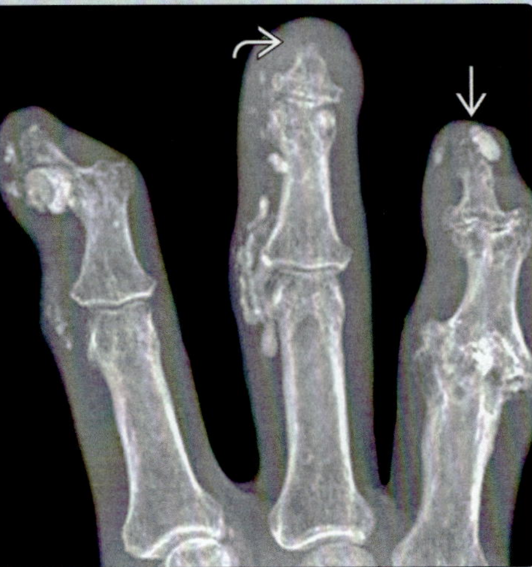

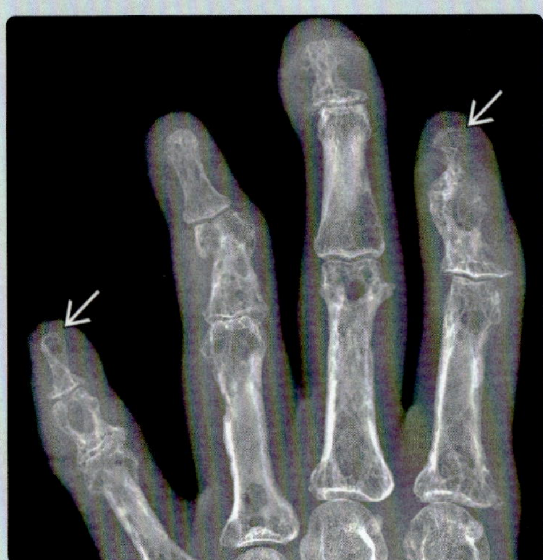

TERMINOLOGY

Definitions

- Group of processes with shortening of distal phalanges as common feature

IMAGING

General Features

- Best diagnostic clue
  - Short phalanges, with variety of forms of osteolysis
    - Associated features provide best clue as to etiology; watch for character and distribution

Radiographic Findings

- Osteolysis may take different forms
  - Subtle tuft resorption
  - Tuft destruction
  - Lucent line crossing mid distal phalanx, overall shortening of phalanx
  - Sharp cut-off of osseous shaft
  - Short, stubby distal phalanx, otherwise morphologically normal
- Bone abnormalities associated with various etiologies
  - Arthritis: Erosions, osteophytes, periostitis, cartilage narrowing
  - Resorption elsewhere: Subperiosteal, subligamentous, subchondral
- Soft tissue may provide clue as to etiology
  - Tapering of soft tissues of distal phalanx
  - Ulcerations of soft tissues
  - Soft tissue nodules
  - Contractures or other deformities
  - Soft tissue calcification: Dystrophic, digital nerve, or vascular

DIFFERENTIAL DIAGNOSIS

Hyperparathyroidism (HPTH)

- Acroosteolysis at tufts is frequent in both HPTH and renal osteodystrophy
- Generalized resorption, including subperiosteal, subchondral, trabecular sites
- Soft tissue calcification (vascular, juxtaarticular, other)

Progressive Systemic Sclerosis (PSS)

- Resorption tufts with tapering of distal soft tissues
- Globular soft tissue calcification is prominent feature

Thermal Injury

- Burn
  - Osteolysis, with associated soft tissue defects
  - Often have contractures, soft tissue scarring
  - Dystrophic soft tissue calcification may be present
- Frostbite
  - Frostbite in child: Epiphyses are at greatest risk for vascular compromise from vasoconstriction
    - With physeal damage, epiphyses fuse prematurely (no longer present in affected digits)
    - Results in short, stubby distal phalanges with normal shape of soft tissues
  - Frostbite in adult
    - If injury occurred during childhood, distal phalanges are disproportionately short
    - If injury during adulthood, resorption of tufts
  - Primary differentiating feature: Thumbs are normal

Psoriatic Arthritis (PSA)

- Acroosteolysis ranges from subtle to prominent
- IP mixed erosive/productive arthritis, often with periostitis and ankylosis

Vasculitis

- Any type of vasculitis (especially Raynaud, lupus)
- Osseous and soft tissue tapering
- Soft tissue ulceration

Pycnodysostosis

- Osteosclerosis, narrowing of medullary canal
  - Multiple fragility fractures: Tubular bones, spine

Congenital Insensitivity/Indifference to Pain

- Neuropathic process
- Nonsymmetric joint destruction
- Corneal abrasions, scarring, and burns on skin

Leprosy

- Severe acroosteolysis, which may involve entire digits
- Associated digital nerve calcification (linear)

Multicentric Reticulohistiocytosis (MR)

- Soft tissue nodules, predominantly IP arthritis

Occupational Acroosteolysis

- Polyvinylchloride (PVC) workers: Usual pattern is lucent band across phalanx with shortening
- Guitar players: Lucent phalangeal band, mimics PVC

PATHOLOGY

General Features

- Etiology
  - Resorptive: HPTH, PSS (scleroderma)
  - Vascular: Vasculitis (Raynaud, lupus), frostbite, amniotic band, meningococcemia
  - Traumatic: Amputation, burn, diabetes (neuropathic), congenital insensitivity to pain, occupational
  - Inflammatory: PSA, MR
  - Infectious: Leprosy, diabetes
  - Genetic: Hajdu-Cheney (autosomal dominant), pycnodysostosis (autosomal recessive), Lesch-Nyhan (X-linked)

DIAGNOSTIC CHECKLIST

Image Interpretation Pearls

- Watch for associated findings to help determine etiology of acroosteolysis
  - Presence and distribution of soft tissue changes, calcification, arthritic changes

SELECTED REFERENCES

1. Canalis E et al: Hajdu-Cheney syndrome: a review. Orphanet J Rare Dis. 9(1):200, 2014
2. Freire V et al: Hand and wrist involvement in systemic sclerosis: US features. Radiology. 269(3):824-30, 2013

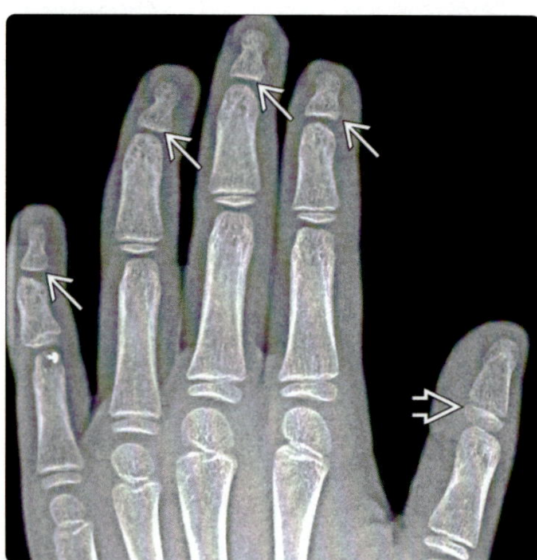

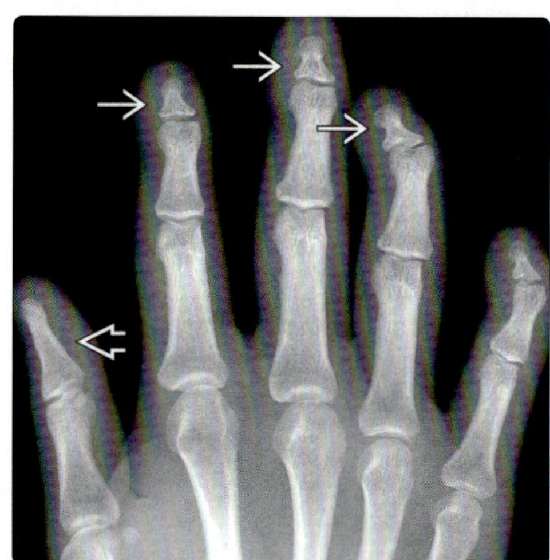

(Left) *PA radiograph shows acroosteolysis resulting from frostbite. Each of the distal phalanges of digits 2-5 is short ➡ and has fused the epiphysis far earlier than expected, while the physis of the thumb remains open ➡ and its distal phalanx is normal in length. The physis is at risk for thermal injury, and resulting shortening is a form of acroosteolysis.* **(Right)** *PA radiograph shows terminal phalanges of digits 2-5 to be short ➡, while the thumb is normal ➡. This is the adult sequelae of frostbite during childhood.*

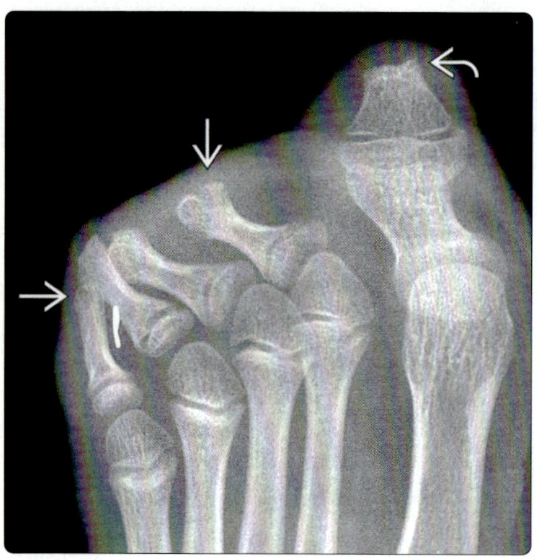

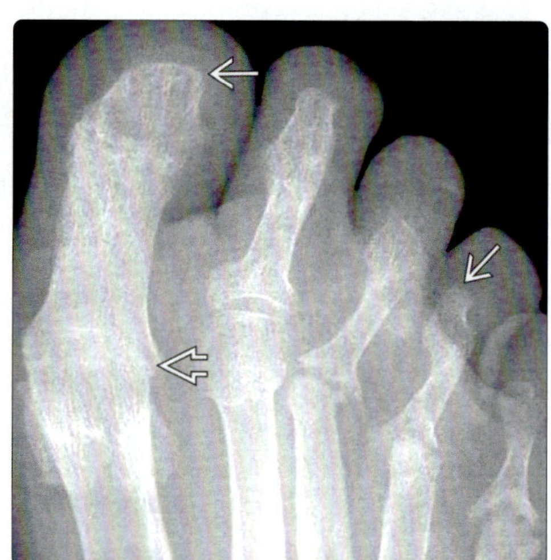

(Left) *AP radiograph shows acroosteolysis with complete resorption of middle and distal phalanges of digits 2-5 ➡ and partial resorption of the tuft of digit 1 ➡. There are contractions of the lateral digits and likely scarring of the web space. This combination of acroosteolysis and contraction/scarring is typical of burn injury.* **(Right)** *AP radiograph shows severe acroosteolysis of all digits ➡ in a patient with psoriatic arthritis. In addition, there are typical psoriatic findings of IP joint erosions and 1st MTP joint ➡ fusion.*

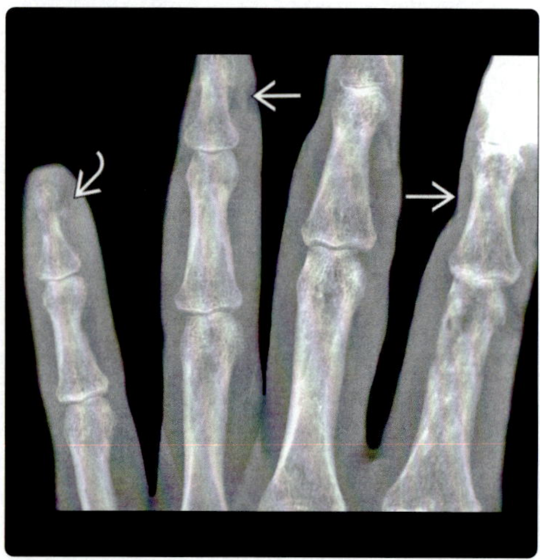

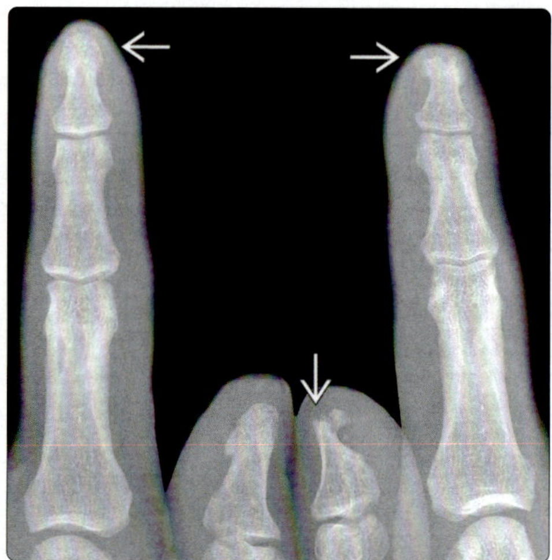

(Left) *PA radiograph shows mild acroosteolysis ➡ and soft tissue tapering with ulceration ➡. This patient has lupus vasculitis and dry gangrene, which may result in acroosteolysis.* **(Right)** *PA radiograph shows both thumbs and index fingers of a patient with Raynaud disease. There is tapering of the soft tissues of the distal phalanges, along with acroosteolysis of the right terminal phalanx of the thumb and index finger ➡. Vascular insufficiency is one etiology of acroosteolysis.*

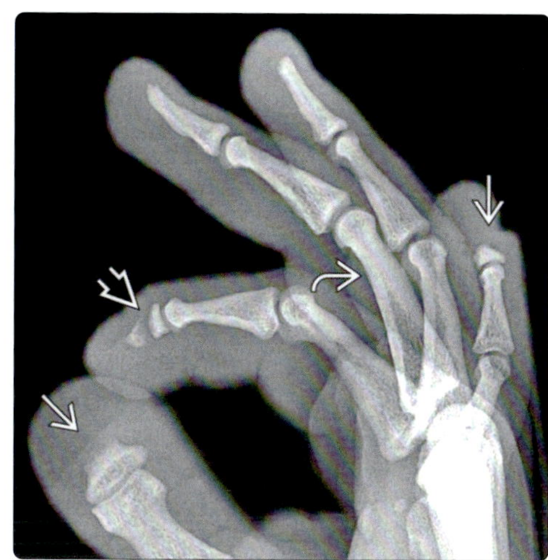

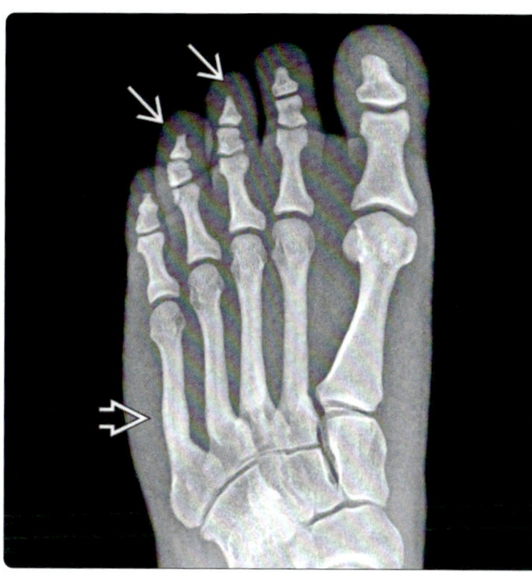

(Left) *Lateral radiograph is remarkable for severe but nonuniform acroosteolysis of the terminal phalanges ➡, as well as a lucent band at one site ➡. Moreover, the bones are dense ➡ with thick endosteal bone. The combination of dense bones and acroosteolysis is seen in pycnodysostosis.* **(Right)** *AP radiograph shows acroosteolysis at several terminal phalanges ➡. There is evidence of osseous fragility, with an old transverse fracture through dense bone of the 5th metatarsal ➡, all typical of pycnodysostosis.*

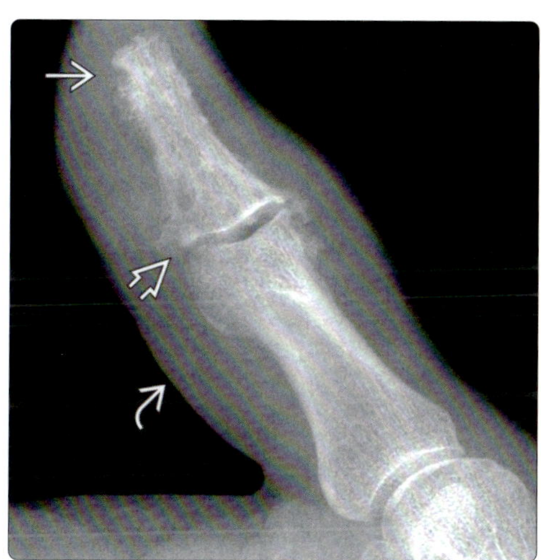

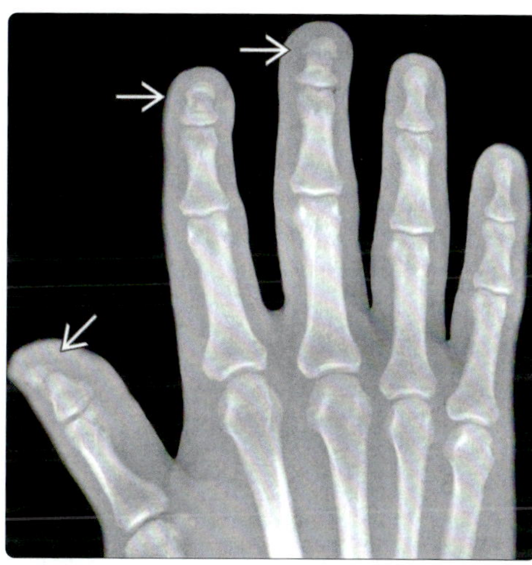

(Left) *Oblique radiograph shows acroosteolysis ➡ associated with soft tissue nodularity ➡ and erosive change at the IP joint ➡. The latter 2 findings might suggest gout, but with acroosteolysis, the diagnosis is multicentric reticulohistiocytosis.* **(Right)** *PA radiograph shows acroosteolysis with shortening of 3 distal phalanges and transverse lucencies ➡. The pattern is typical of acroosteolysis seen in polyvinylchloride workers; it can also be seen in work-related lysis (guitar players).*

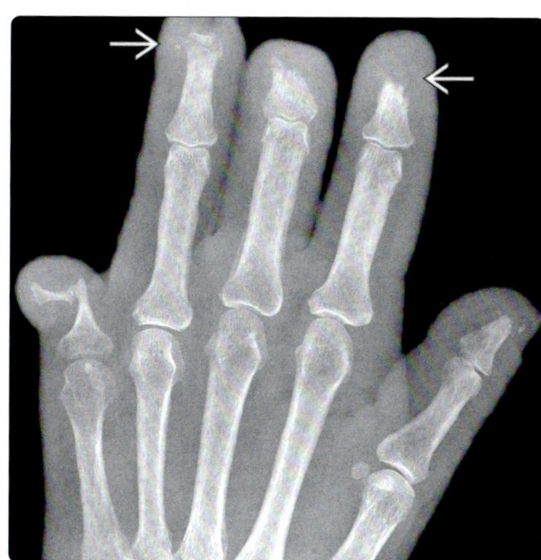

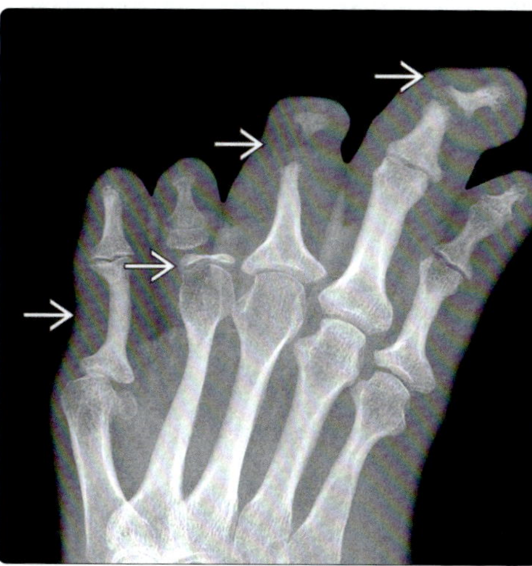

(Left) *PA radiograph shows acroosteolysis due to leprosy. There is destruction of all the distal phalanges, as well as the middle phalanges of digits 2-5 ➡. The remaining bones are completely normal. This incredible amount of acroosteolysis should make one consider the diagnosis of leprosy vs. Lesch-Nyhan disease.* **(Right)** *PA radiograph shows severe acroosteolysis and pressure erosion in a pattern extending obliquely across the hand ➡. The patient is otherwise normal; the deformity is due to amniotic band.*

Sickle Cell Anemia

KEY FACTS

TERMINOLOGY

- Homozygous HbSS (autosomal recessive) inherited hemoglobinopathy
- Musculoskeletal imaging findings reflect one or both of the following processes
  - Chronic hemolytic anemia
  - Microvascular occlusion created by sickled red blood cells when exposed to low oxygen tension

IMAGING

- Infarct may occur in any bone
  - Long bones: Femur 96%, humerus 48%
  - Small tubular bones of hands and feet: 20-50%
  - Spine: 43-70%; skull: 25%
- Osteonecrosis (ON): Femoral head > humeral head > vertebral bodies > other sites
  - 50% of patients develop ON by age 35
- Bone infarct on radiograph
  - Acute: Normal; rare lysis or periosteal reaction
  - Focal (subacute/chronic): Serpiginous calcification
  - Diffuse (chronic): Patchy diffuse sclerosis
- MR may have complicated signal due to combination of factors
  - Marrow repopulation
  - Marrow infarct
  - Marrow fibrosis
  - Superimposed infection
- Infection (18% develop osteomyelitis, 7% septic arthritis)

DIAGNOSTIC CHECKLIST

- Pay attention to marrow signal
  - Bone marrow edema may be 1st sign of impending osteonecrosis
    - Nonspecific, but patients at such high risk that it must be considered
- Acute infarction & osteomyelitis can be indistinguishable on imaging
  - Fat-saturated T1 sequence may differentiate

(Left) *Coronal graphic depicts the tibia in sickle cell (SC) disease. There is extensive necrosis, seen as an opaque yellow coloration ➡. Living bone is seen more proximally ➡; between these 2 regions, a focus of osteomyelitis is seen ➡.* **(Right)** *AP radiograph demonstrates patchy areas of increased ➡ and decreased ➡ density. Chronic osseous infarction, often with superimposed fibrosis, presents with this patchy sclerotic pattern. The radiographic appearance is nonspecific, but SC disease should be considered.*

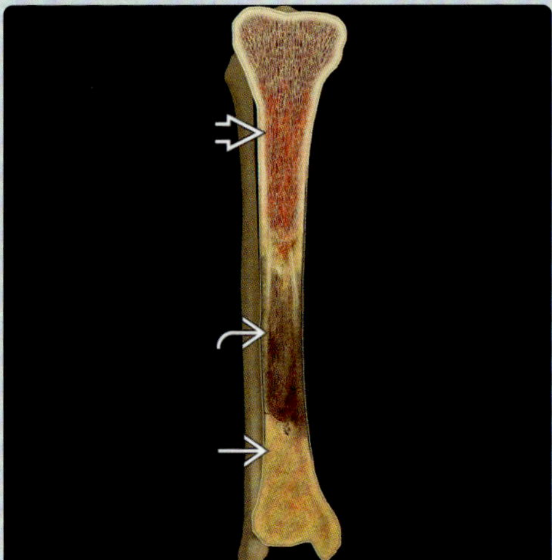

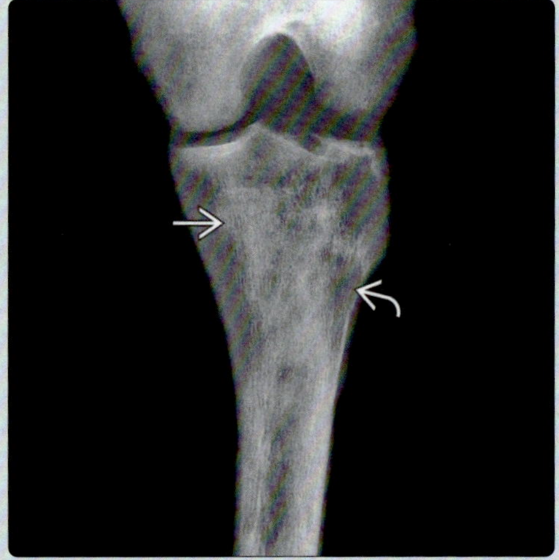

(Left) *Coronal STIR MR shows typical high signal subacute serpiginous bone infarcts ➡. This pattern indicates chronicity. In addition, there is a more diffuse hyperintense region occupying the posterior acetabulum and ischium ➡. This region is acutely painful and could represent either acute infarct or osteomyelitis in this SC patient.* **(Right)** *Coronal T1WI C+ MR (same patient) shows enhancement about the rim of the subacute infarct ➡ and more diffuse enhancement at the other site ➡ (biopsy-proven acute infarct, not infection).*

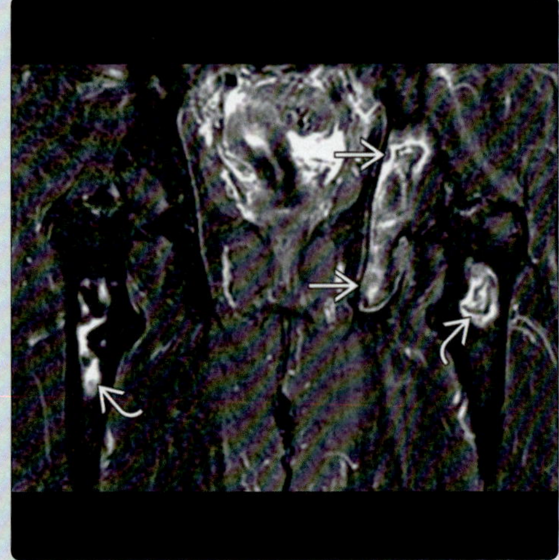

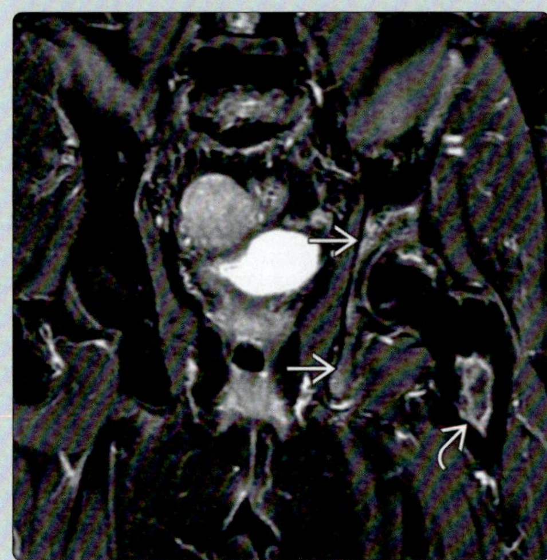

TERMINOLOGY

Abbreviations

- Sickle cell (SC) disease

Definitions

- Homozygous HbSS (autosomal recessive) inherited hemoglobinopathy
  - Musculoskeletal imaging findings reflect one or both of the following processes
    - Chronic hemolytic anemia
    - Microvascular occlusion created by sickled red blood cells when exposed to low oxygen tension
- Heterozygous: HbSA (sickle cell trait), HbSC (↓ severity)

IMAGING

General Features

- Best diagnostic clue
  - Generalized patchy bone density on radiograph, reflecting chronic diffuse bone infarcts
  - Osteonecrosis (ON), especially of femoral head, humeral head, or vertebral bodies
  - May have other associated findings on imaging
    - Chest: Cardiomegaly, pulmonary infarct
    - Abdomen: Gallstones, absence or calcified spleen (splenic infarct with eventual autosplenectomy)
- Location
  - Any bone may be involved with infarct
    - Long bones: Femur 96%, humerus 48%
    - Small tubular bones of hands & feet: 20-50%
    - Spine: 43-70%, skull: 25%
  - ON: Femoral head > humeral head > vertebral bodies > other sites

Radiographic Findings

- Bone infarct
  - Long bones
    - Acute: Normal; rare lysis or periosteal reaction
    - Subacute/chronic, focal: Serpiginous calcification
    - Chronic, diffuse: Patchy diffuse sclerosis
    - Occasional associated periosteal reaction
  - Tubular bones of hands & feet (dactylitis)
    - Periosteal reaction initially
    - Patchy sclerosis later
- ON (50% of patients by age 35)
  - Femoral and humeral heads: Initially, central ↑ density
    - Weight-bearing portion: Anterosuperior head
    - Subchondral lucent fracture line, paralleling cortex in weight-bearing region
    - Flattening, with mixed lytic & sclerotic density
  - Vertebral body: Initial sub-endplate sclerosis
    - Collapse is of central endplates, either in biconcave pattern or more sharp "H" shape
- Marrow repopulation
  - Uncommon radiographic findings or often so subtle as to not be noted, unless anemia is severe
  - Skull may show mild widening of diploic space, with thinning of calvaria
    - Hair on end appearance uncommon or subtle in SC anemia, as opposed to thalassemia
    - Mandible may show coarse trabeculae
- Infection: 18% develop osteomyelitis, 7% septic arthritis
  - Periosteal reaction
  - Blurring/obliteration of fat planes
  - Eventual permeative osseous change
- Growth abnormalities: Premature epiphyseal closure (→ growth discrepancy), coned epiphyses
- Splenic autoinfarction
  - Splenic shadow in left posterior upper quadrant replaced by bowel gas; small spleen may be calcified

MR Findings

- Bone infarct
  - Acute: Focal areas of low signal on T1WI and high signal intensity on T2WI MR (edema); may be subtle
    - T1FS often shows focal high SI at site of acute infarct
      - Due to sequestered erythrocytes; may differentiate acute infarct from infection
    - T1 C+: Thin linear rim enhancement
  - Chronic: Patchy or focal, classic serpiginous pattern
    - T1WI MR: Serpiginous very low signal pattern outlining red marrow
    - T2WI MR: High signal serpiginous outline; often double line appearance of low and high signal
- Osteonecrosis
  - May present initially as bone marrow edema
  - Later presentation
    - T1WI MR: Low signal in weight-bearing region
    - T2WI MR: Double density (low and high signal) serpiginous rim around region of necrosis in weight-bearing portion of bone
    - Eventual subchondral fracture and flattening
- Marrow repopulation
  - T1WI MR: Low signal red marrow (↓ or isointense to muscle or disc) replaces fatty marrow; may have focal or patchy retained yellow marrow
  - T2WI MR: Marrow retains low signal of red marrow, slightly hyperintense to muscle
  - Gradient-echo: Sites of repopulation may bloom 2° to hemosiderin deposits from chronic transfusions
  - Opposed-phase imaging: Sites of repopulation ↓ SI > 20% since regions of fat retained in marrow
  - Repopulated marrow enhances only ~ 10%
  - Pattern of repopulation is same as all causes of marrow repopulation, reconversion, or stimulation
    - Axial, followed by distal appendicular skeleton
    - Large tubular bones: Metaphyses, followed by diaphysis, followed by epiphyses
- Osteomyelitis
  - T1WI: Confluent low signal; may not differentiate from low signal of red marrow hyperplasia
  - Fluid-sensitive sequences: High signal intensity; adjacent soft tissue edema, cellulitis, or abscess
  - T1 C+: Geographic, thick, irregular rim enhancement of marrow, adjacent soft tissue reaction or abscess
- Extramedullary hematopoiesis (less common in SC than other sickle variants)
  - Hepatomegaly, deposits in thorax and skin
- Myonecrosis: Rare; hyperintensity on fluid-sensitive sequences and enhancement of muscle & fascia

Imaging Recommendations

- Best imaging tool
  - Diagnosis generally made on radiograph
  - MR may be required to diagnose early infarct/ON
  - MR may differentiate acute infarct/osteomyelitis

DIFFERENTIAL DIAGNOSIS

Thalassemia

- Marrow hyperplasia in long bones
- Skull: Severe hyperplasia of marrow, sparing occiput
- Extramedullary hematopoiesis (usually paravertebral)
- Osteonecrosis & diaphyseal infarcts much less frequent than in sickle cell anemia

Sickle Cell Trait (Heterozygous, HbSA)

- Few musculoskeletal findings
- Bone infarcts relatively rare

Sickle Cell Hemoglobin C (HbSC)

- Marrow hyperplasia of skull
- Osteonecrosis, few bone infarcts
- Splenomegaly rather than splenic infarction

PATHOLOGY

General Features

- Etiology
  - Structural defect in hemoglobin HbS: Glutamic acid in position 6 substituted with valine
  - Order of events leading to infarct
    - Lowered oxygen tension →
    - Altered shape & plasticity of red blood cells →
    - Increased blood viscosity, stasis →
    - Occlusion of microvasculature by sickled cells
      - Small terminal vessels in femoral head and humeral head are particularly at risk
      - In vertebral bodies, terminal vessels loop under endplates; with focal osteonecrosis at endplates, there is collapse of central 75% of endplates, resulting in "H" shape
  - Dactylitis
    - Ambient cold temperatures → vasoconstriction in hematopoietic marrow of digits → bone infarct
    - Often 1st manifestation of SC (6 months to 2 years)
    - Periosteal reaction can make infarct impossible to differentiate from osteomyelitis
  - Risk for osteomyelitis is high
    - Majority of cases caused by *Staphylococcus*
    - *Salmonella* osteomyelitis more common than in normal population
  - Children are protected for first 6 months by elevated levels of fetal Hb (HbF)
- Genetics
  - Hemoglobin S (HbS) in all forms
    - Defective form of hemoglobin (HbS) results from a single amino acid substitution in β globin gene on chromosome 11
  - Sickle cell anemia (HBSS): Homozygous; both β globin genes are HbS
  - Sickle C (HbSC): Heterozygous; 1 HbS, 1 hemoglobin C
  - Sickle cell trait (HbSA): Heterozygous; 1 HbS, 1 normal gene
- Associated abnormalities
  - Thrombosis/infarction
    - Renal papillary necrosis, cholelithiasis, splenic autoinfarction, cardiomegaly, pulmonary infarction, stroke
  - May coexist with thalassemia

CLINICAL ISSUES

Presentation

- Most common signs/symptoms
  - Sickle cell crisis
    - Sudden onset severe bone, abdominal, chest pain
    - Often as result of infection, cold temperature, or hypoxia related to altitude/plane flight
    - ± fever, leukocytosis
    - Time course: Hours to days
  - Hand/foot syndrome
    - Often initial manifestation, in child 0.5-2 years
    - Swelling, decreased range of motion of digits
    - Occurs with new onset of cold temperatures & resultant vasoconstriction
    - Self-limiting, days to weeks

Demographics

- Age
  - Initial manifestation in first 2 years of life; symptoms persist lifelong
- Epidemiology
  - 0.2-1% of African Americans, 0.1% of Hispanic American population; rarely seen in Mediterranean
  - 8-13% of African Americans carry sickle factor (HbS)

Natural History & Prognosis

- Repeated episodes lead to progressive bone infarction
- ON leads to arthritis and requirement for surgery
- Repeated hospitalizations due to crisis or infection
- Poor prognostic factors: Dactylitis before 1 year of age, Hb levels < 7 g/dL, leukocytosis without infection
- Early death (average prior to 48 years of age)
  - Pneumonia, meningitis, stroke are leading causes

DIAGNOSTIC CHECKLIST

Image Interpretation Pearls

- Pay attention to marrow signal
  - Bone marrow edema may be 1st sign of impending osteonecrosis
  - Marrow signal in SC may be complicated
    - Combination of repopulation, infarct, and fibrosis
- Acute infarction & osteomyelitis can be indistinguishable on imaging
  - Fat-saturated T1 sequence may differentiate (acute infarcts show ↑ SI)

SELECTED REFERENCES

1. Walters MC: Update of hematopoietic cell transplantation for sickle cell disease. Curr Opin Hematol. 22(3):227-33, 2015
2. Wood JC: Estimating tissue iron burden: current status and future prospects. Br J Haematol. ePub, 2015

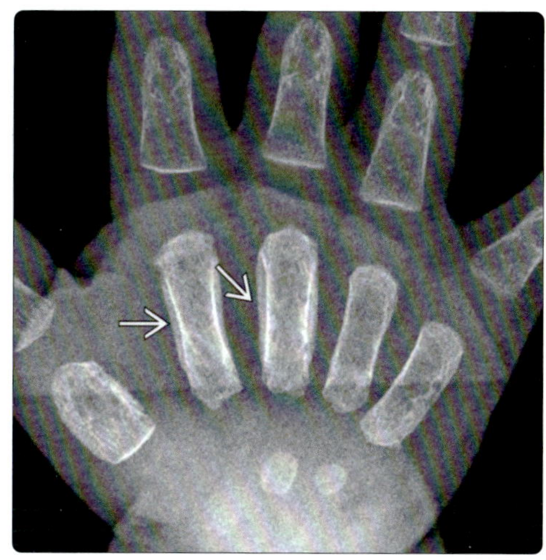

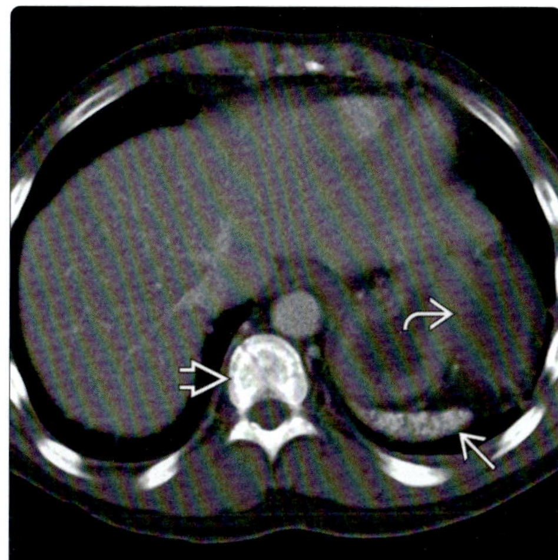

(Left) *AP radiograph shows a periosteal reaction* ➡ *involving several metacarpals in a baby. These represent infarcts in hand-foot syndrome, often the initial indication of sickle cell anemia.* **(Right)** *Axial bone CT shows patchy bone infarcts in a vertebral body* ➡*. Additionally, there is a calcified hypoplastic spleen resulting from infarction* ➡*; a loop of colon occupies the normal location of the spleen* ➡*. Autoinfarction of the spleen is a common finding in sickle cell anemia.*

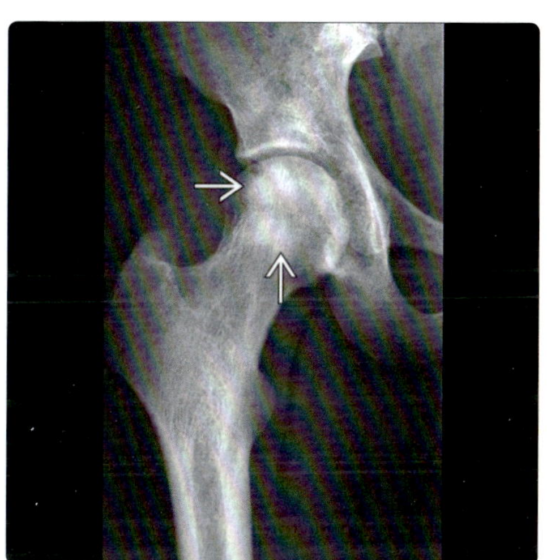

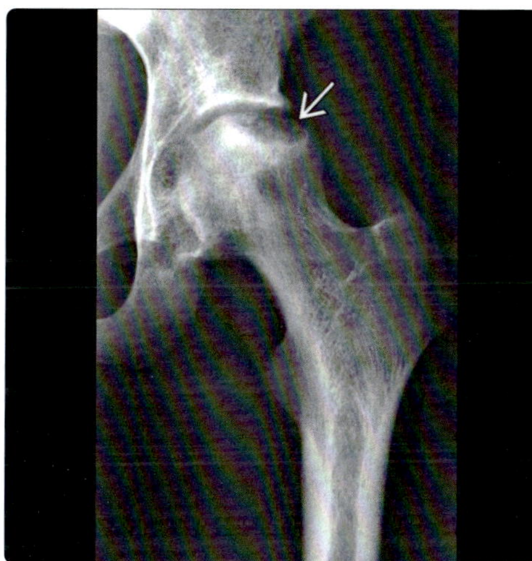

(Left) *AP radiograph shows diffuse infarcts in the femur and acetabulum. In addition, the femoral head shows signs of early osteonecrosis, with increased density centrally in the weight-bearing portion* ➡*. There is not yet collapse in the right femoral head.* **(Right)** *AP radiograph in same patient, who is young and has sickle cell anemia, shows much more advanced osteonecrosis in the contralateral hip, with subchondral fracture and collapse of the weight-bearing portion of the femoral head* ➡*.*

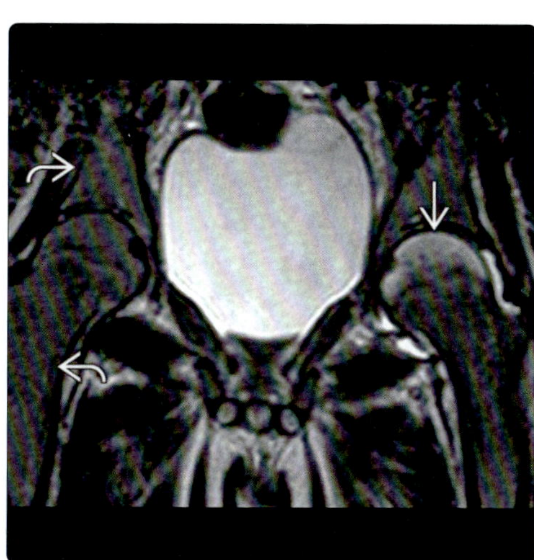

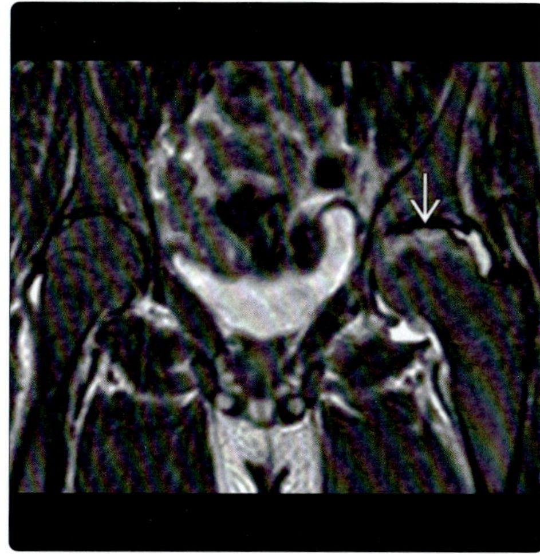

(Left) *Coronal T2WI MR shows diffuse low signal red marrow repopulation* ➡ *in a sickle cell patient. Painful left hip shows marrow edema* ➡ *as well as effusion. This could represent a septic hip; aspirate showed a sterile effusion.* **(Right)** *Coronal T2WI MR 7 months later shows flattening of the femoral head* ➡*. This is osteonecrosis, with subchondral fracture. This is a common complication of sickle cell anemia. The edema seen earlier was an early but nonspecific indicator of osteonecrosis.*

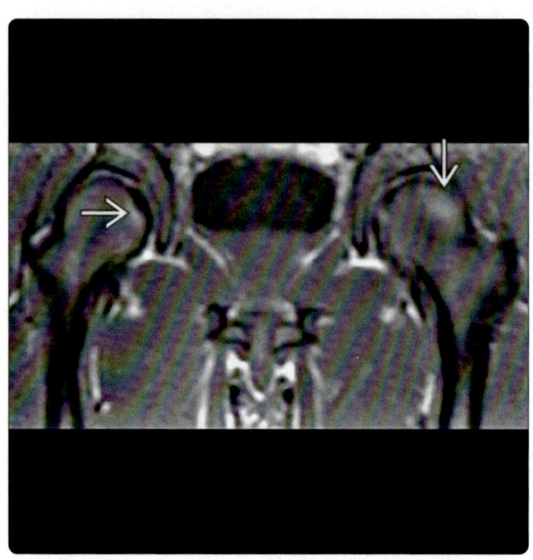

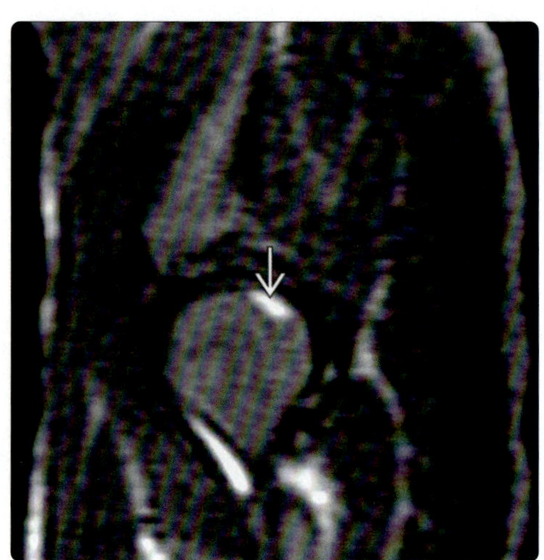

(Left) *Coronal T1WI MR in a sickle cell patient being evaluated for osteonecrosis shows low signal throughout the visualized bones, indicating diffuse marrow repopulation. A small region of high signal is seen in each femoral head ➡. This high T1 signal is not expected to represent infarct.* **(Right)** *Sagittal T2WI MR (same case) shows the same high signal ➡ to be located posteriorly, not an expected site for necrosis. It represents a small area of normal residual fatty marrow. There was no progression to osteonecrosis.*

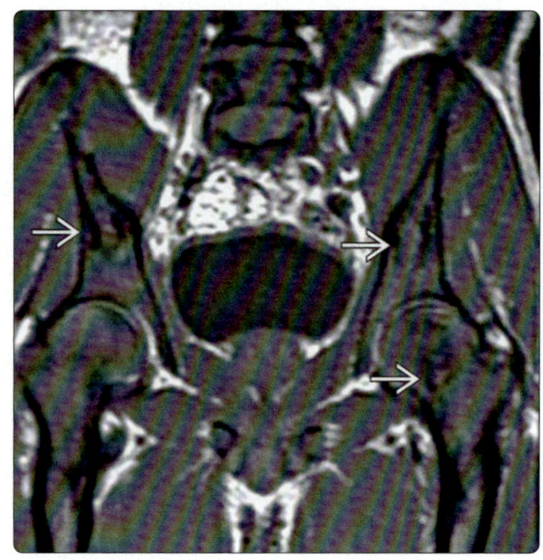

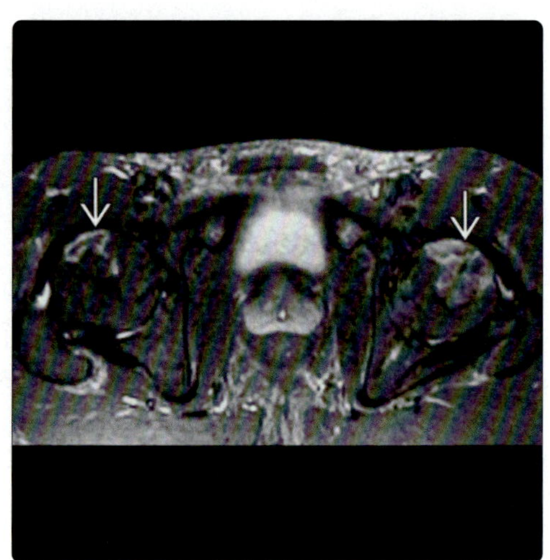

(Left) *Coronal T1WI MR shows red marrow repopulation of the pelvis & proximal femora. Fibrosis and hemosiderin deposition also contribute to the low SI. Serpiginous low signal bone infarcts are superimposed on this abnormal marrow ➡.* **(Right)** *Axial STIR MR confirms the serpiginous bone infarcts in the heads & metaphyses of the femora ➡. Infarcts are a common complication of SC anemia and may be seen either as discrete serpiginous foci, as in this case, or as diffuse patchy bone density changes.*

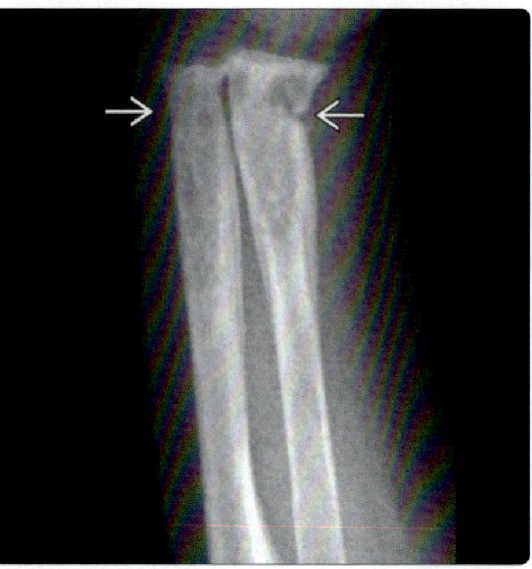

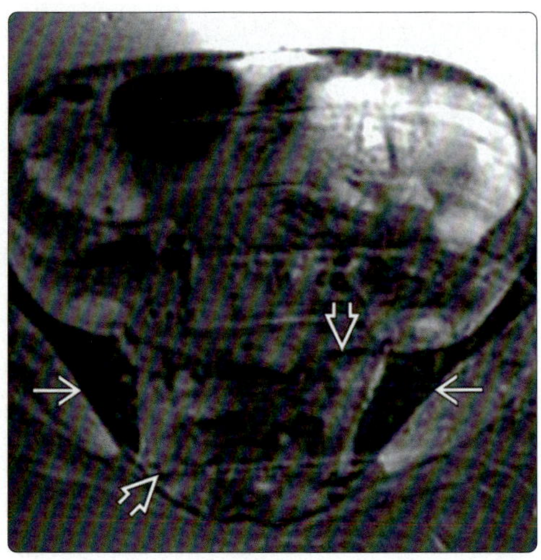

(Left) *AP radiograph in a child with sickle cell anemia, fever, and leukocytosis shows lytic lesions ➡ with periosteal reaction and cortical destruction of the distal radius and ulna. This was found to represent osteomyelitis due to salmonella.* **(Right)** *Coronal T2WI FS MR in a sickle cell anemia patient shows increased signal of the entire sacrum ➡ proven to be osteomyelitis. Acute bone infarct might look the same. The signal of the iliac bones ➡ is low due to a combination of marrow repopulation and iron deposition.*

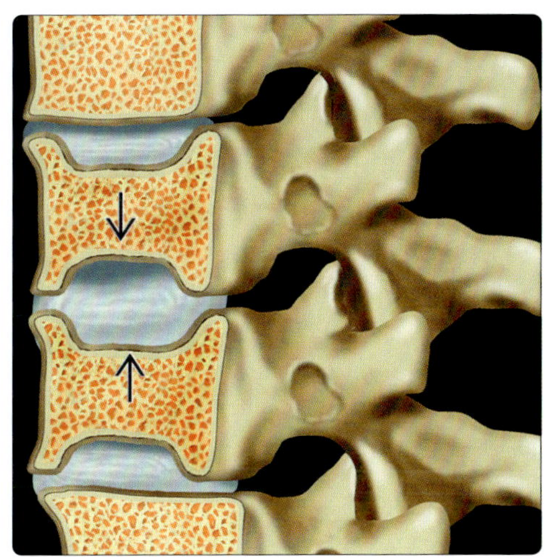

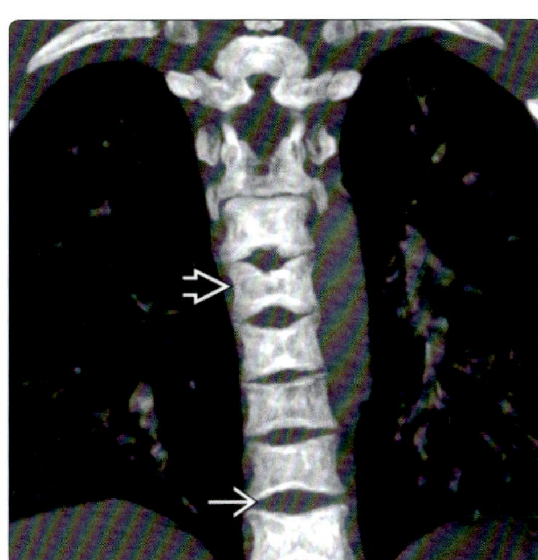

(Left) *Sagittal graphic shows step-like endplate depression ⇨ of the vertebral bodies resulting in an "H" shape of the body. The infarct occurs at the central endplate and bone collapses at that site. Vertebral body osteonecrosis may also result in a biconcave appearance.* **(Right)** *Coronal bone CT shows vertebral body sclerosis from multiple bone infarcts. There is concave ➡ as well as H-shaped ➡ endplate collapse. Both patterns are seen with vertebral endplate osteonecrosis.*

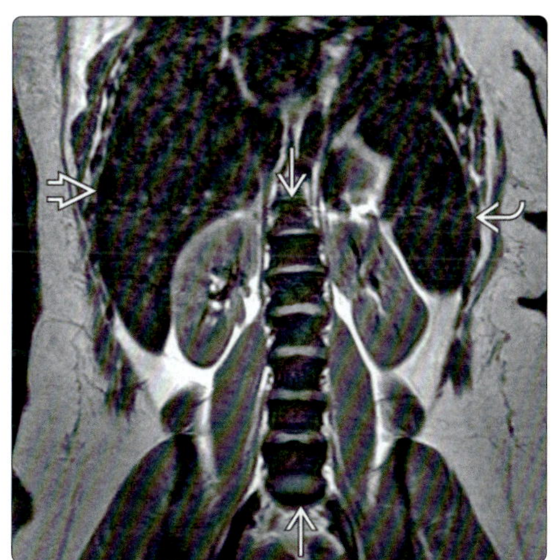

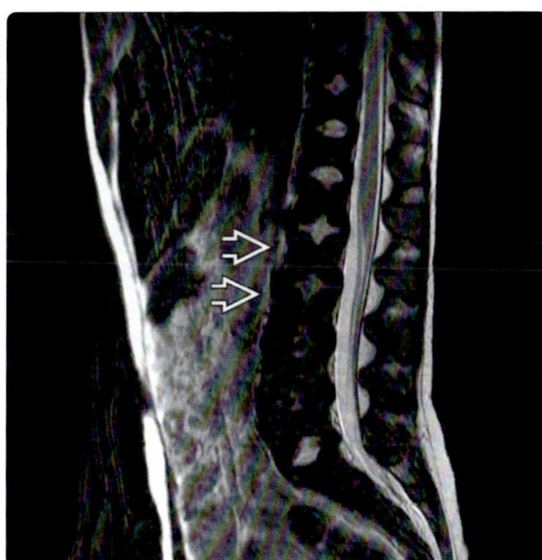

(Left) *Coronal T1WI MR shows typical findings of transfusion hemosiderosis in the bone marrow ➡, liver ➡, and spleen ➡, with ↓ SI in all these. Hemosiderin deposition occurs due to chronic transfusions. Gradient echo imaging would show blooming.* **(Right)** *Sagittal T2WI MR shows multiple H-shaped vertebrae in the spine ➡. Note diffuse low signal in the vertebral bodies; it is lower than is usually seen with marrow repopulation and is characteristic of hemosiderin deposition due to transfusions in this patient with sickle cell.*

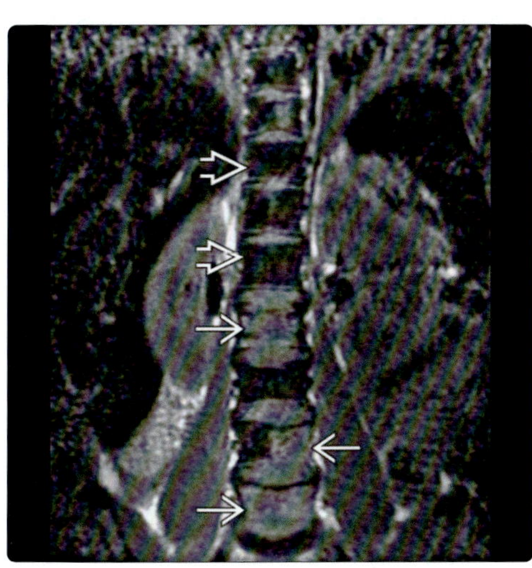

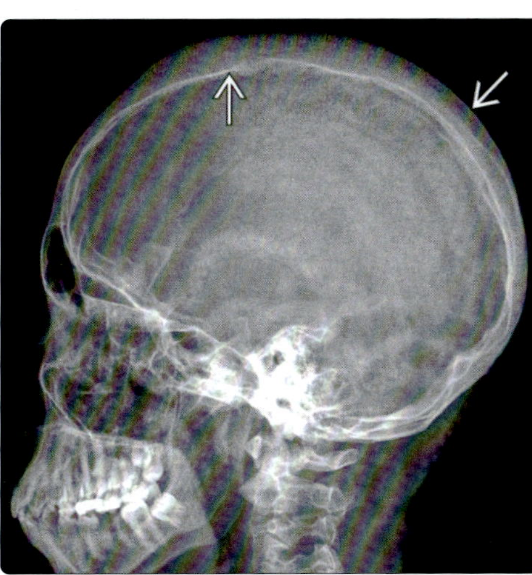

(Left) *Coronal T1WI MR shows ↓ SI portions of the vertebrae due to iron deposition and repopulation ➡. There are also extensive regions of old marrow infarction ➡, now replaced by gray SI fibrous tissue. Marrow signal in SC anemia can be complex 2° to combinations of marrow infarct, repopulation, and fibrosis.* **(Right)** *Lateral radiograph shows mildly widened diploic space ➡ in a 16 year old with sickle cell anemia. The widening is not as prominent as is seen in thalassemia.*

Thalassemia

KEY FACTS

TERMINOLOGY

- Hemoglobinopathy resulting in ↑ red blood cell (RBC) destruction and ↑ marrow production of RBCs

IMAGING

- Location: Affects virtually all marrow since anemia demand is severe, even in infancy
  - Spine, pelvis, long and short tubular bones, skull
- Best imaging clue: Expansion of medullary cavity, osteopenia, extramedullary hematopoiesis
  - Expanded medullary cavity results in loss of normal tubulation of long bones
- Osseous complications of iron chelation therapy
  - Treatment-related spondylometaphyseal dysplasia
  - Treatment-related arthropathy
- Extramedullary hematopoiesis, particularly paraspinous
- Marrow abnormalities: Combination of findings due to anemia, hemosiderin deposition, fibrosis
  - Marrow repopulation secondary to anemia
    - ↓ SI foci (early) or diffuse (later) on T1WI/T2WI
  - Marrow hemosiderin deposition
    - ↓ SI marrow on all sequences; GRE → blooming

PATHOLOGY

- Thalassemia of various types caused by mutations at globin gene foci on chromosomes 16 and 11
  - Affects production of α or β globin, respectively
- > 200 disease-causing mutations identified; majority are single nucleotide substitutions, deletions, or insertions

CLINICAL ISSUES

- Thalassemia major diagnosed during infancy
- Male = female
- Epidemiology
  - Thalassemia major: 10% in high-risk regions (Southeast Asia, Northeast India, Mediterranean)
  - Thalassemia minor: 2.5% of Italian Americans, 7-10% of Greek Americans

(Left) *Graphic demonstrates thalassemia in the cranium. There is marked thinning of the cortices ➡, widening of the diploic space, and open porotic cancellous bone ➡. The mahogany brown color ➡ results from extensive iron deposition in the marrow.* **(Right)** *Axial NECT shows marked thickening of the diploic marrow space ➡. Sparing of the occipital bone ➡, relative to the frontal region, is typical.*

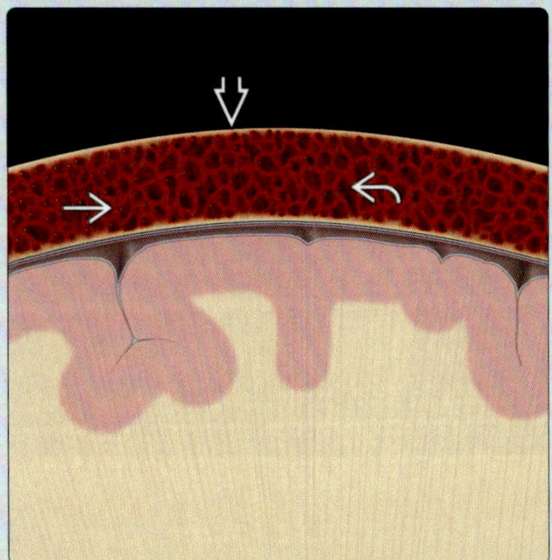

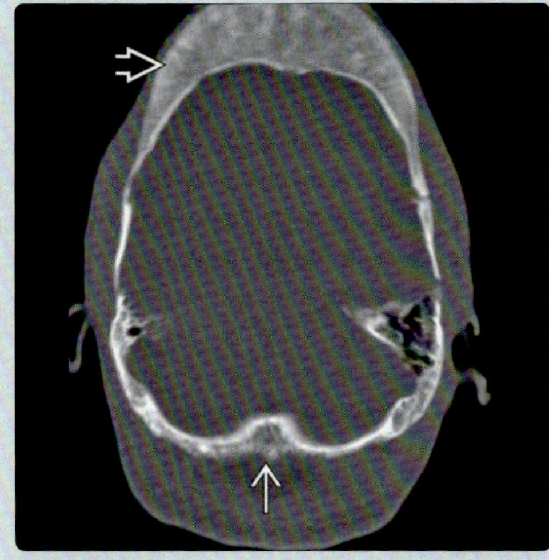

(Left) *Axial NECT in the same case shows the severely widened diploic space ➡ involving both the frontal and parietal regions of the skull. The cortices of both tables of the skull are thinned to the point of being indistinct.* **(Right)** *Coned lateral radiograph of the skull in a thalassemia major patient shows severe widening of the diploic space, with the typical hair on end ➡ appearance of the cancellous bone located between the severely thinned cortices of the inner and outer tables of the skull.*

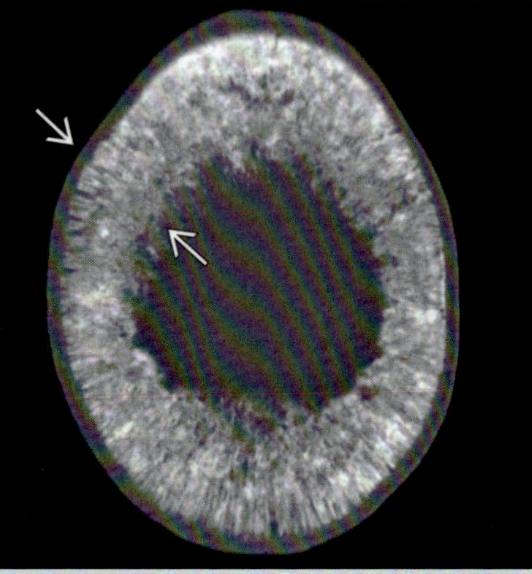

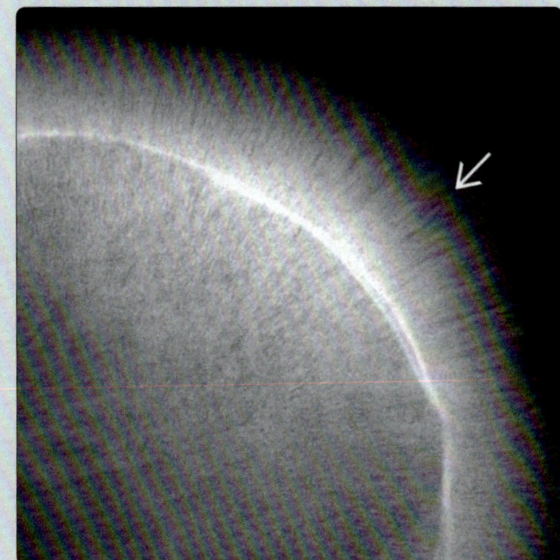

TERMINOLOGY

Abbreviations

- Thalassemia major (TM)

Synonyms

- β-thalassemia major, Cooley anemia, Mediterranean anemia, hereditary leptocytosis, erythroblastic anemia

Definitions

- Hemoglobinopathy resulting in ↑ red blood cell (RBC) destruction and ↑ marrow production of RBCs
- 3 clinical and hematological conditions of increasing severity recognized
  - β-thalassemia carrier state
    - Heterozygosity for β-thalassemia
    - Clinically asymptomatic; defined by hematological features
  - Thalassemia intermedia
    - Clinically and genotypically heterogeneous group of thalassemia-like disorders
    - Ranges from asymptomatic carrier to severe transfusion-dependent type
  - TM
    - Severe transfusion-dependent anemia
    - Anemia-related and treatment-related musculoskeletal abnormalities

IMAGING

General Features

- Best diagnostic clue
  - Expansion of medullary cavity, osteopenia, extramedullary hematopoiesis
- Location
  - All sites of hematopoietic marrow
    - TM affects virtually all marrow since anemia demand is severe, even in infancy
      - Spine, pelvis, long and short tubular bones, skull
- Morphology
  - Expanded medullary cavity results in loss of normal tubulation of long bones

Radiographic Findings

- Osteopenia
- Medullary space of all tubular bones is widened
  - Thin cortices with coarse trabeculation
  - Squaring of tubular bones, absence of tubulation
- Skull
  - Widened diploic space
    - Ranges from moderate to severe
    - Thickened trabeculae cause hair on end appearance
    - Occiput relatively spared
  - Marrow packing obliterates paranasal sinuses
    - Enlarged, contain marrow, no aeration
  - Rodent facies: Facial bones relatively small compared with expansion of skull and sinuses
- Spine
  - Thickened vertebral trabeculae, paucity of horizontal trabeculae (striated appearance)
  - Compression fractures
  - Paraspinal masses from extramedullary hematopoiesis
- Ribs
  - Posterior rib expansion; rib within rib appearance
- Treatment-related spondylometaphyseal dysplasia
  - Associated with deferoxamine (iron chelator)
  - Appears to preferentially affect growth centers
    - Metaphyseal widening
    - Sclerotic longitudinal trabeculation
    - Irregularity of metaphyseal zone with sclerotic and lucent cystic areas
    - Growth plate widening
  - Results in angular deformity (especially genu valgum) and limb shortening
- Treatment-related arthropathy
  - Associated with deferiprone (L1, iron chelator)
  - Effusion
  - Subchondral bone irregularity, flattening
  - Broad "beak" at superior patellar articular surface
- Extramedullary hematopoiesis
  - Widening of paraspinous line when paravertebral

CT Findings

- Parallels and better defines radiographic abnormalities
  - Character of osseous abnormalities better defined
  - Extramedullary hematopoiesis sites better visualized

MR Findings

- Marrow abnormalities: Combination of findings due to anemia, hemosiderin deposition, fibrosis
  - Marrow repopulation secondary to anemia
    - ↓ SI foci (early) or diffuse (later) on T1WI/T2WI
  - Marrow hemosiderin deposition
    - ↓ SI marrow on all sequences; GRE → blooming
    - May have interspersed regions of retained marrow fat (high signal T1, gray T2WI)
- Extramedullary hematopoiesis
  - Active regions: Intermediate T1 SI, marked enhancement
  - Inactive regions: Low signal 2° to hemosiderin, high SI if fatty replacement
  - Evaluate for cord compression
- Treatment-related spondylometaphyseal dysplasia
  - Present in 100% of cases in small study
  - Irregular ↓ SI T1 and ↑ SI T2 foci at epiphysis, metaphysis, or metadiaphysis
  - Physeal indistinctness or widening
  - Tongue-like extensions from hyperintense physis into metaphysis on fluid-sensitive sequences
    - May appear pseudocystic in more severe cases
- Treatment-related arthropathy
  - Present in 86% of cases treated by L1 in 1 study
  - Synovial thickening and intense enhancement
  - Cartilage irregular thickening, extending into subchondral bone defects
    - May contain irregular high T2 signal
  - Hypointense bands (hemosiderin) in Hoffa fat pad
  - Subchondral erosions
- May be used to detect and quantify iron deposition in soft tissues
  - Low signal on all sequences

DIFFERENTIAL DIAGNOSIS

Gaucher Disease

- Undertubulation of long bones related to storage disease may mimic early TM

Leukemia

- Diffuse osteopenia, leukemic lines
- Osseous destruction but generally no expansion

Myelofibrosis

- Low signal on all MR sequences is typical
- Should not bloom on GRE since no hemosiderin deposition

Rickets

- Osteopenia and widened, irregular zone of provisional ossification mimics treatment-related spondylometaphyseal dysplasia of TM

PATHOLOGY

General Features

- Etiology
  - Rapid erythrocyte destruction due to free radical mediated injury
  - Arthropathy related to chelation treatment
- Genetics
  - Various types caused by mutations at globin gene foci on chromosomes 16 and 11
    - Affects production of α or β globin, respectively
  - Severity of β-thalassemia related to extent of imbalance between α and nonα globin chains
  - > 200 disease-causing mutations identified; majority are single nucleotide substitutions, deletions, or insertions

Gross Pathologic & Surgical Features

- Hyperplastic hematopoietic bone marrow
- Marrow spaces filled with clotted blood

CLINICAL ISSUES

Presentation

- Most common signs/symptoms
  - Presents with hypochromic microcytic anemia
  - Hepatosplenomegaly
  - Skin hyperpigmentation
  - Joint pain ranges from mild to severe
    - Knees most frequent, but other joints may be involved
    - Appears dose-related to L1 chelator
  - Thalassemia intermedia may be asymptomatic except for periods of stress (infection, pregnancy)
- Other signs/symptoms
  - Myocardial dysfunction related to iron load, cardiomyopathy
  - Spinal cord compression from extramedullary hematopoiesis
  - Endocrine toxicity related to iron (thyroid, pituitary, pancreas)
  - Cholelithiasis, biliary sludge

Demographics

- Age
  - TM diagnosed during infancy
- Gender
  - Male = female
- Epidemiology
  - Thalassemia major: 10% in high-risk regions (Southeast Asia, Northeast India, Mediterranean)
  - Thalassemia minor: 2.5% of Italian Americans, 7-10% of Greek Americans
  - α-thalassemia: 30% in Southeast Asia and Africa

Natural History & Prognosis

- TM: Death in infancy or early childhood if not treated
- Leading cause of death in treated patients is cardiac and complications of hemosiderin deposition
- Thalassemia intermedia: Longer life expectancy than TM, clinically less severe
- Thalassemia minor: Normal life expectancy

Treatment

- No treatment for heterozygote patients
- Lifelong blood transfusions for TM
  - Intermittent transfusions for thalassemia intermedia
- Survival improves with iron chelation therapy
  - Toxic side effects: Agranulocytosis, gastrointestinal symptoms, arthropathy
  - MR & CT useful in assessing organ iron burden
- Bone marrow transplant may be curative
- Stem cell gene therapy being investigated
- Partial splenectomy (may be by radiofrequency ablation) for thalassemia intermedia

DIAGNOSTIC CHECKLIST

Consider

- Imaging important to detect serious complications from extramedullary hematopoiesis (cord compression) or chronic transfusions (hemosiderosis)

SELECTED REFERENCES

1. Inati A et al: Endocrine and bone complications in β-thalassemia intermedia: current understanding and treatment. Biomed Res Int. 2015:813098, 2015
2. Wood JC: Estimating tissue iron burden: current status and future prospects. Br J Haematol. ePub, 2015
3. Orphanidou-Vlachou E et al: Extramedullary hemopoiesis. Semin Ultrasound CT MR. 35(3):255-62, 2014
4. Aypar E et al: The efficacy of tissue Doppler imaging in predicting myocardial iron load in patients with beta-thalassemia major: correlation with T2* cardiovascular magnetic resonance. Int J Cardiovasc Imaging. 26(4):413-21, 2010
5. Cao A et al: Beta-thalassemia. Genet Med. 12(2):61-76, 2010
6. Chakraborty I et al: Non-haem iron-mediated oxidative stress in haemoglobin E beta-thalassaemia. Ann Acad Med Singapore. 39(1):13-6, 2010
7. Cunningham MJ: Update on thalassemia: clinical care and complications. Hematol Oncol Clin North Am. 24(1):215-27, 2010
8. Chand G et al: Deferiprone-induced arthropathy in thalassemia: MRI findings in a case. Indian J Radiol Imaging. 19(2):155-7, 2009
9. Rasekhi AR et al: Radiofrequency ablation of the spleen in patients with thalassemia intermedia: a pilot study. AJR Am J Roentgenol. 192(5):1425-9, 2009
10. Wood JC et al: Magnetic resonance imaging assessment of excess iron in thalassemia, sickle cell disease and other iron overload diseases. Hemoglobin. 32(1-2):85-96, 2008
11. Kellenberger CJ et al: Radiographic and MRI features of deferiprone-related arthropathy of the knees in patients with beta-thalassemia. AJR Am J Roentgenol. 183(4):989-94, 2004
12. Chan Y et al: Deferoxamine-induced bone dysplasia in the distal femur and patella of pediatric patients and young adults: MR imaging appearance. AJR Am J Roentgenol. 175(6):1561-6, 2000

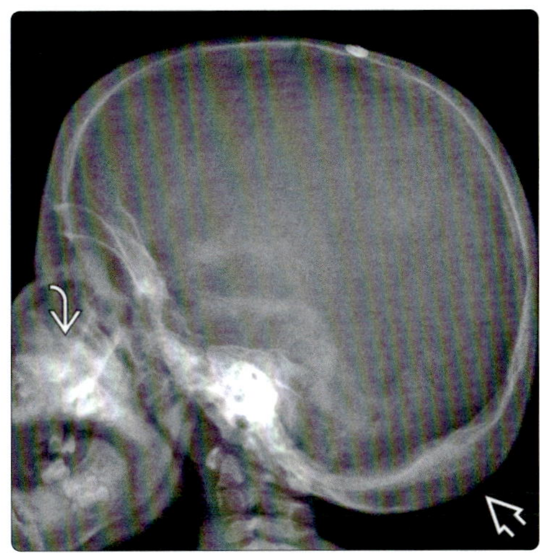

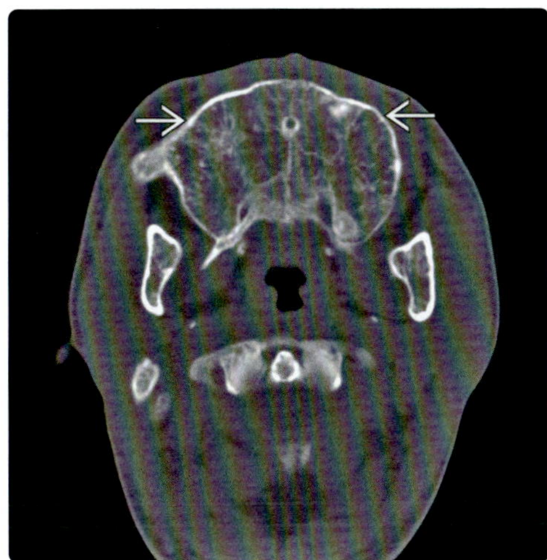

(Left) *Lateral radiograph of the skull shows the diploic space is quite widened, most prominently posteriorly ➡. It is unusual for the occiput to show the predominant involvement in thalassemia, but that is the case here. The paranasal sinuses, which should be aerated by this age, are quite solidly replaced by marrow ➡.* **(Right)** *Axial NECT shows widening and obliteration of the paranasal sinuses ➡ secondary to marrow hyperplasia in a patient with thalassemia major.*

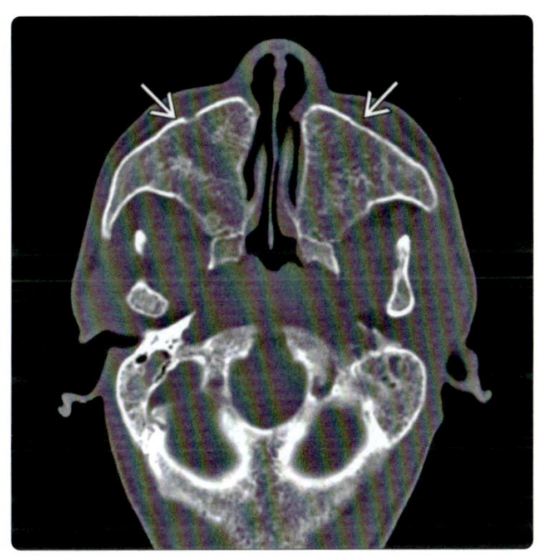

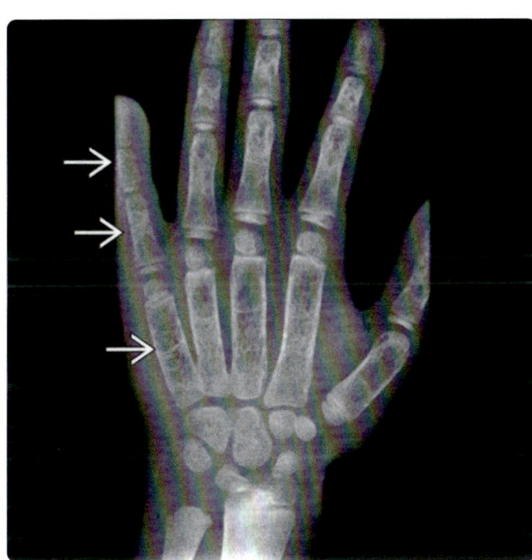

(Left) *Axial NECT in the same case shows hyperplasia of the maxillary sinuses ➡. There is no aeration. The expansion of paranasal sinuses in this disease leads to a distortion of the facial features, which is typical of thalassemia and is known as rodent facies.* **(Right)** *PA radiograph shows the typical appearance of the tubular bones of the hand in thalassemia, in which a preponderance of marrow hyperplasia is seen. All the bones show squaring, or loss of their normal morphology ➡, due to marrow packing.*

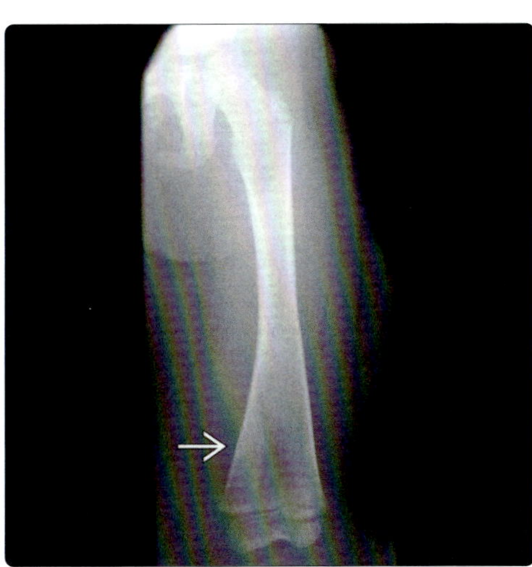

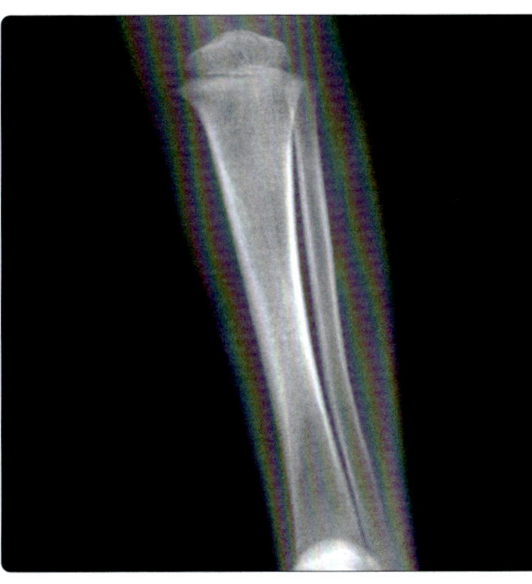

(Left) *AP x-ray of a child's femur shows lack of normal tubulation of the distal metaphysis ➡. This is reminiscent of the Erlenmeyer flask appearance of Gaucher, a storage disease. In this case the marrow is packed with hematopoietic cells.* **(Right)** *AP x-ray of the leg shows some cortical thinning and a rather squared morphology and undertubulation, consistent with a marrow replacement in thalassemia. Interestingly, bone infarcts are much less frequent in this disease than sickle cell anemia.*

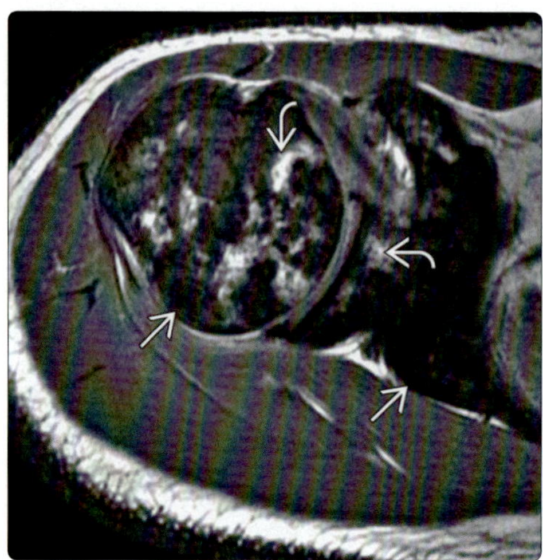

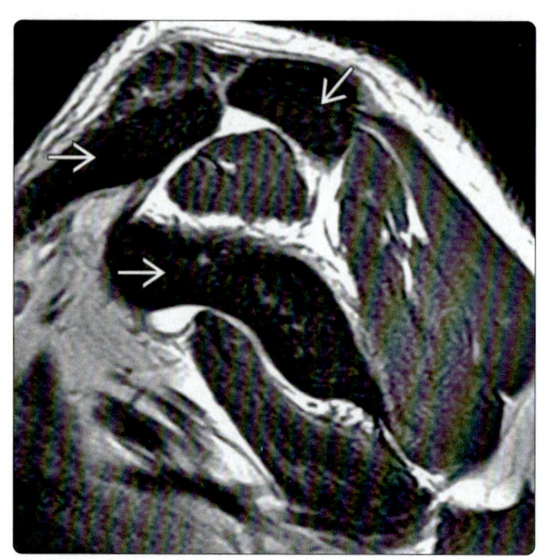

(Left) *Axial PDWI MR shows significantly lower than expected SI within the humeral head and scapula ➡. There are some foci of interspersed fat cells ➡, but the overall low SI is very abnormal for a middle-aged man.* **(Right)** *Sagittal T2WI MR in the same case shows extraordinarily low SI within the bones of the shoulder girdle ➡. The contralateral shoulder had a similar signal. It is not surprising that this patient has thalassemia; the low SI relates to both marrow hyperplasia and hemosiderin deposition.*

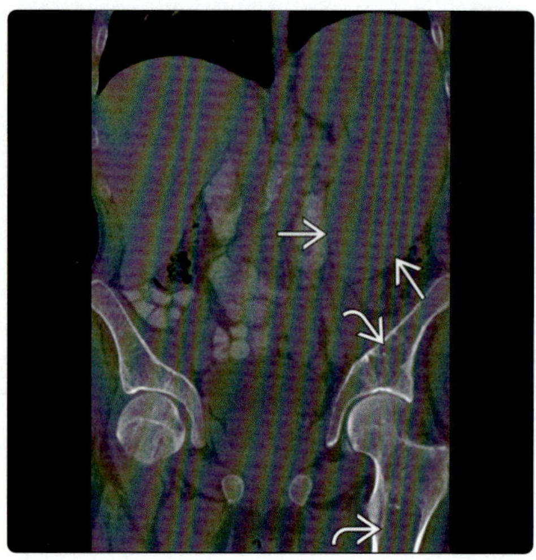

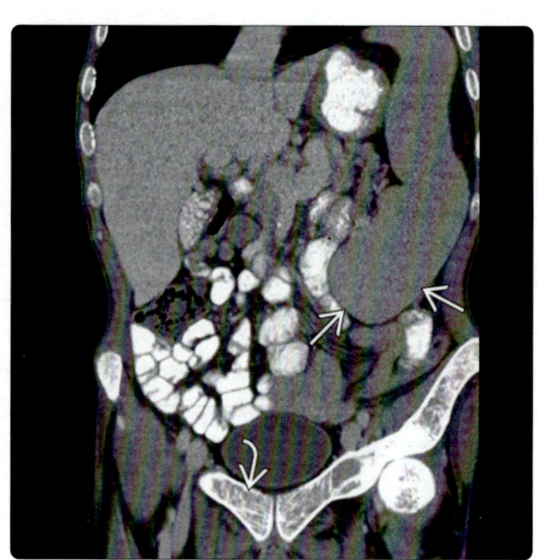

(Left) *Coronal bone CT in a 37-year-old man with thalassemia shows diffuse osteopenia, to the point of having lytic foci ➡. The remaining trabeculae are coarsened and the endosteal cortex is thinned. The other finding suggestive of thalassemia is splenomegaly ➡.* **(Right)** *Coronal CT in the same case emphasizes both the splenomegaly ➡ and the coarsened trabeculae ➡.*

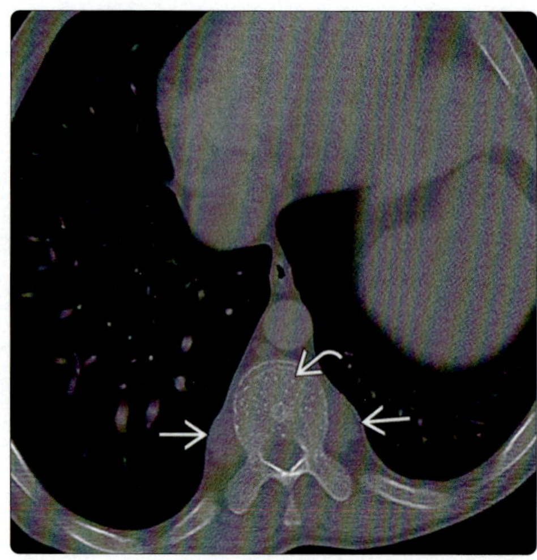

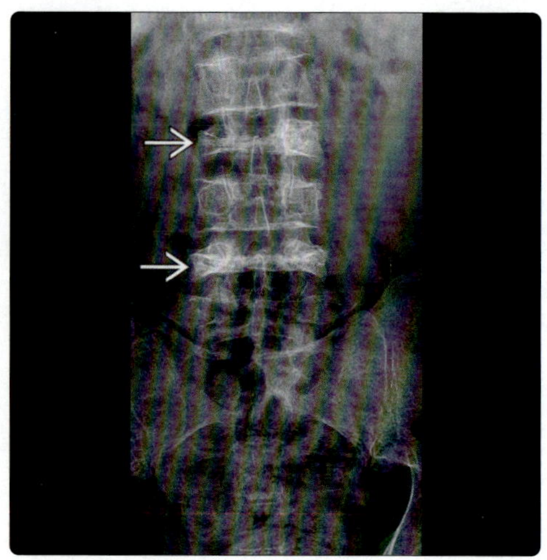

(Left) *Axial CT in the same case shows the remaining vertical trabeculae of the vertebral body as thin polka dots ➡. The paraspinal soft tissue masses ➡ represent extramedullary hematopoiesis, also typical of thalassemia.* **(Right)** *AP radiograph in the same case shows this patient's terrible axial osteopenia and resultant multiple compression fractures of the spine ➡.*

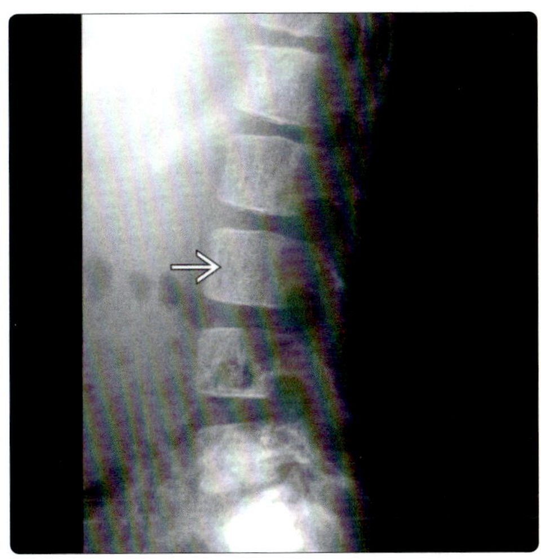

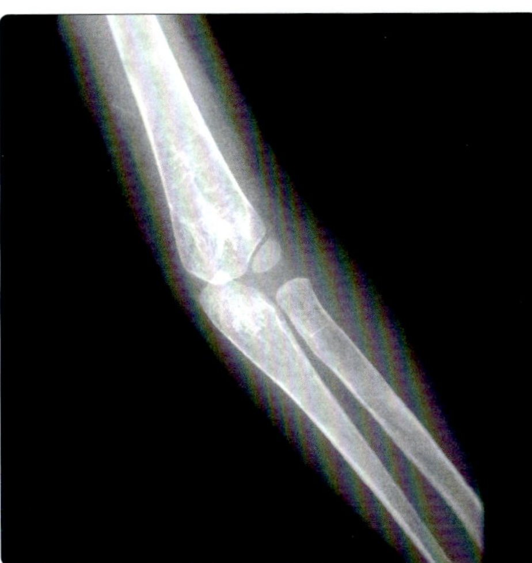

(Left) *Lateral radiograph shows thickened vertical trabeculae* ➡ *with paucity of horizontal trabeculae resulting in a striated appearance, typical of thalassemia. Note expansion of the medullary cavity.* **(Right)** *Anteroposterior radiograph shows expansion of the medullary cavity with coarsened trabeculae and cortical thinning in a child with thalassemia.*

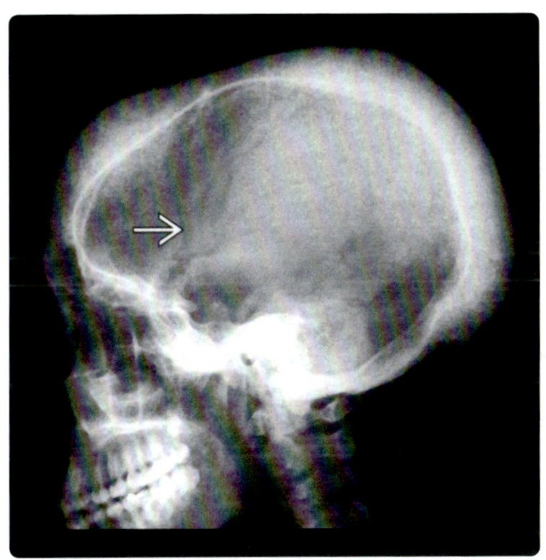

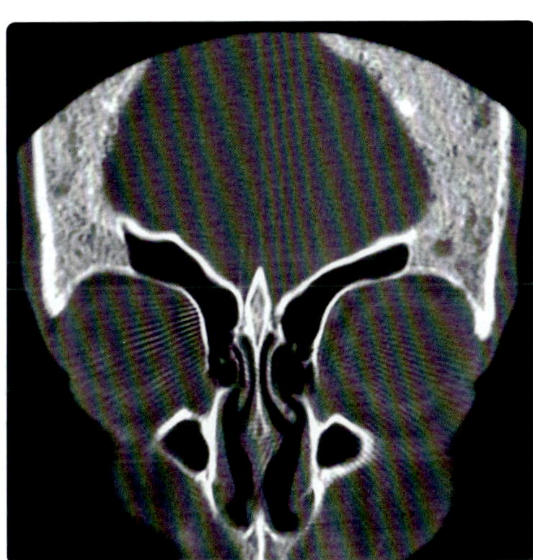

(Left) *Lateral radiograph shows marked expansion of the calvaria and hair on end appearance. Note the enlarged impressions of the calvarial vessels* ➡. **(Right)** *Coronal bone CT shows a typical example of generalized skull thickening in a patient with thalassemia.*

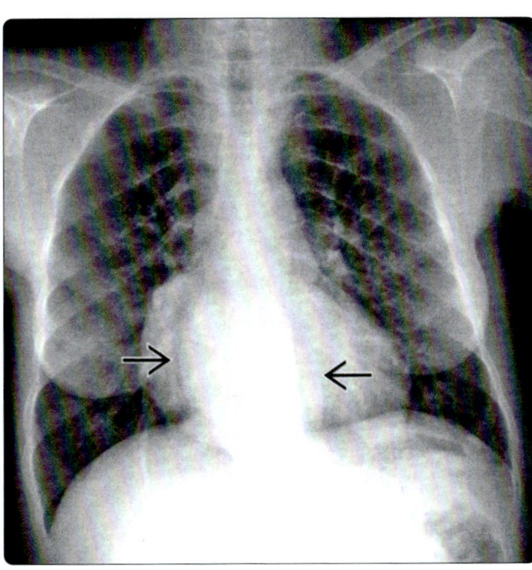

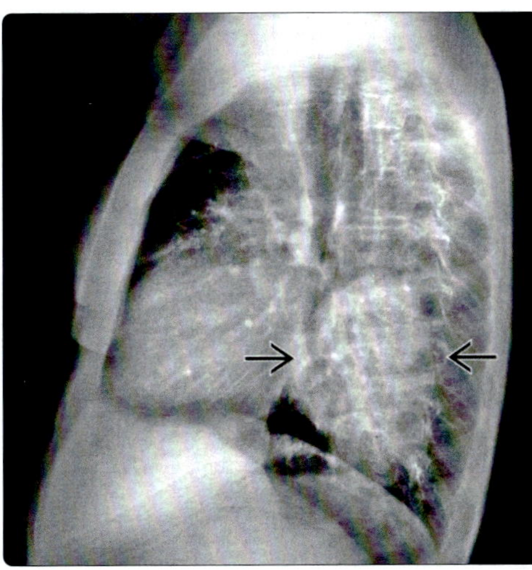

(Left) *PA radiograph shows cardiomegaly as well as a large mediastinal mass* ➡. **(Right)** *Lateral chest radiograph in the same case demonstrates that the mass is paravertebral in location* ➡. *This mass is a focus of site of extramedullary hematopoiesis in a patient with thalassemia and is found in the most common location for this process. The mass was subtle when the patient was 1st seen at age 9, but is much larger and more obvious 12 years later.*

Myelofibrosis

KEY FACTS

TERMINOLOGY

- Chronic myeloproliferative disorder resulting in marrow fibrosis
- Most cases are secondary to other processes
  - Malignant: Leukemia or lymphoma
  - Essential thrombocytopenia
  - Multiple nonmalignant etiologies
- Primary myelofibrosis: 2 classes
  - Agnogenic myeloid metaplasia with myelofibrosis: Indolent myeloproliferative syndrome (usually has splenomegaly)
  - Acute myelofibrosis (usually no splenomegaly)

IMAGING

- Location
  - Axial skeleton, including pelvis and shoulder girdles
  - Long tubular bones, proximal > distal
- Radiograph/CT
  - Marrow sclerosis (or normal)
  - Hepatosplenomegaly
  - May have extramedullary hemopoiesis
- MR
  - T1WI: Very low signal (lower than disc or muscle)
  - SI remains low on T2WI or STIR
  - No enhancement of marrow
  - Fat in marrow is replaced; opposed-phase imaging does not show ↓ in SI

TOP DIFFERENTIAL DIAGNOSES

- Osteoblastic metastases
- Sclerotic multiple myeloma
- Chronic sickle cell anemia
- Marrow regeneration or stimulation
- Leukemia/lymphoma

DIAGNOSTIC CHECKLIST

- If myelofibrosis has no obvious cause, search for lymphoproliferative disease

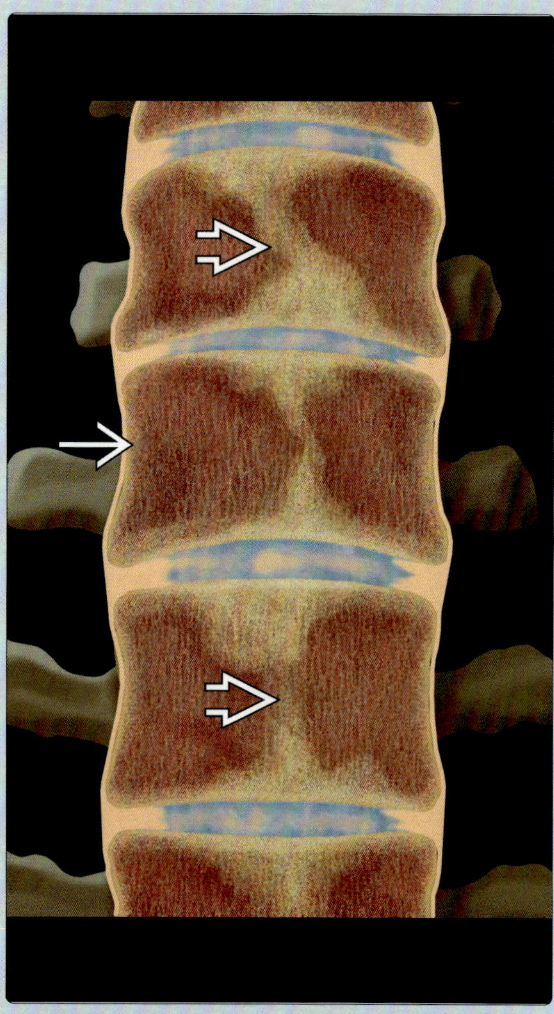

Graphic depicts myelofibrosis, with new bone formation giving a dense appearance of the trabeculae, seen radiographically as sclerosis. The marrow also contains fibrosis ➡; fatty marrow is compressed and displaced ➡.

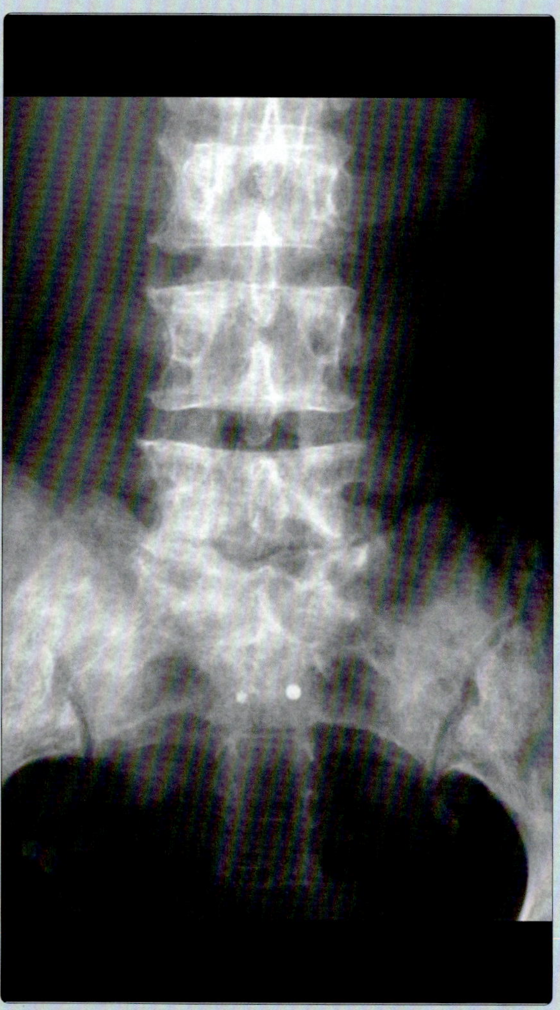

AP radiograph of myelofibrosis shows diffuse sclerosis, predominantly involving the medullary space, without thickening of the cortex. The process is prominent in this case; the bones in cases of early myelofibrosis may appear normal.

TERMINOLOGY

Definitions

- Chronic myeloproliferative disorder → marrow fibrosis
- Most cases are secondary to other processes
  - Leukemia (myelofibrosis may be diagnosed either prior to or at time of diagnosis of leukemia)
  - Non-Hodgkin lymphoma and Hodgkin disease
  - Essential thrombocythemia
  - Nonmalignant causes (including infections, renal osteodystrophy, systemic lupus erythematosus, juvenile idiopathic arthritis, pernicious anemia, Gaucher disease, exposure to radiation, toxins)
- Primary myelofibrosis: 2 classes
  - Agnogenic myeloid metaplasia with myelofibrosis: Indolent myeloproliferative syndrome (usually has splenomegaly)
  - Acute myelofibrosis (usually no splenomegaly)

IMAGING

General Features

- Best diagnostic clue
  - Sclerotic bone marrow, ↓ SI on all MR sequences
- Location
  - Axial skeleton, including pelvis and shoulder girdles
  - Long tubular bones, proximal > distal

Radiographic Findings

- Marrow sclerosis (or normal)
- Generally no endosteal cortical thickening
- Hepatosplenomegaly
- Pleural, paraspinous sites of extramedullary hematopoiesis

MR Findings

- Very low SI on T1WI (lower than disc or muscle)
- SI remains low on T2WI or STIR
- No enhancement of marrow
- Marrow replacement of fat; opposed-phase imaging does not show ↓ in SI

DIFFERENTIAL DIAGNOSIS

Osteoblastic Metastases/Sclerotic Myeloma

- Low signal on all sequences; usually show at least minimal enhancement (> 35% ↑ in SI)
- Generally not as diffusely homogeneous involvement

Sickle Cell Anemia

- Combination of low marrow signal from regeneration secondary to anemia and more serpiginous bone infarction

Marrow Regeneration/Stimulation

- Low SI on all MR sequences; may be diffuse or focal
- Does not replace fat; opposed-phase imaging serves to differentiate; shows ↓ in SI because fat suppresses

Leukemia/Lymphoma

- Fluid-sensitive sequences may be only moderately high SI but greater than myelofibrosis
- Enhancement of involved marrow > 35% ↑ in SI

PATHOLOGY

General Features

- Etiology
  - Either primary or secondary
    - Secondary may be due to malignant or nonmalignant causes
    - Primary form may be precursor to polycythemia vera and chronic myeloid leukemia
- Genetics
  - V617F-*JAK2*, *JAK2* exon 12, and W515-*MPL* mutations found in majority of myeloproliferative disorders (polycythemia vera, essential thrombocythemia, primary myelofibrosis); felt to be oncogenic events driving disorders

Microscopic Features

- Marrow fibrosis, variable degree of hyperplasia
- Increased reticulin staining

CLINICAL ISSUES

Presentation

- Most common signs/symptoms
  - Fatigue, weight loss, fever, night sweats
  - Easy bruising, anemia
  - Hepatosplenomegaly
  - Asymptomatic in 25%
- Other signs/symptoms
  - Gout, renal failure secondary to high cell turnover

Demographics

- Age
  - Mean: 60 years at time of diagnosis; rare in children
- Epidemiology
  - 1 per 100,000

Natural History & Prognosis

- Primary indolent form: Median life expectancy 10 years from time of diagnosis
- Primary acute onset form: Rapidly fatal
- Leukemic conversion (5-20%)
- Complications of overwhelming infection, hemorrhage, or renal or liver failure

Treatment

- Allogenic marrow transplantation
- Reduce anemia with androgens ± steroids, thalidomide
- *JAK2* inhibitors under development

DIAGNOSTIC CHECKLIST

Consider

- Cannot exclude concomitant tumor by MR; requires biopsy
- If myelofibrosis has no obvious cause, search for lymphoproliferative disease

SELECTED REFERENCES

1. Kröger N et al: Impact of allogeneic stem cell transplantation on survival of patients less than 65 years with primary myelofibrosis. Blood. 125(21):3347-50, 2015
2. Ihde LL et al: Sclerosing bone dysplasias: review and differentiation from other causes of osteosclerosis. Radiographics. 31(7):1865-82, 2011

(Left) *Sagittal T1WI MR shows diffuse, homogeneous marrow replacement. The vertebrae ➡ are lower signal than the intervertebral discs, except for residual fat around the vertebral veins ↪. (Right) Sagittal T1WI C+ MR, same case, shows enhancement of the veins and adjacent fat ➡ but no enhancement of the remainder of the vertebral bodies. The homogeneity of the marrow changes and lack of enhancement after gadolinium administration distinguish this case from diffuse marrow replacement by tumor.*

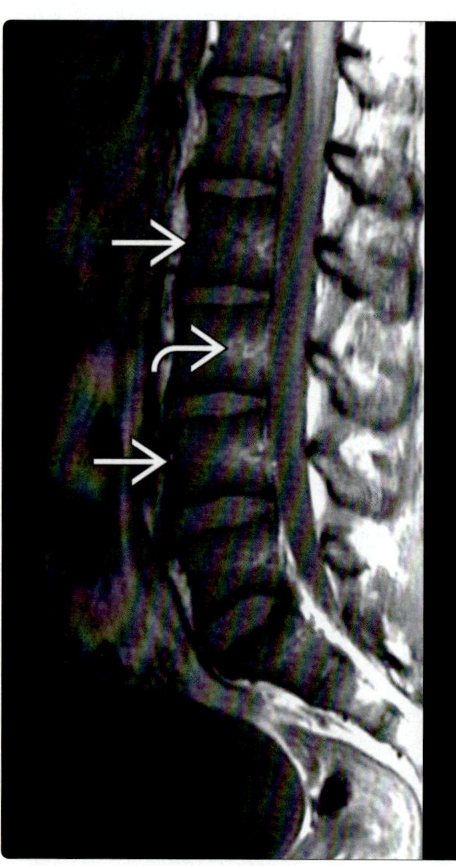

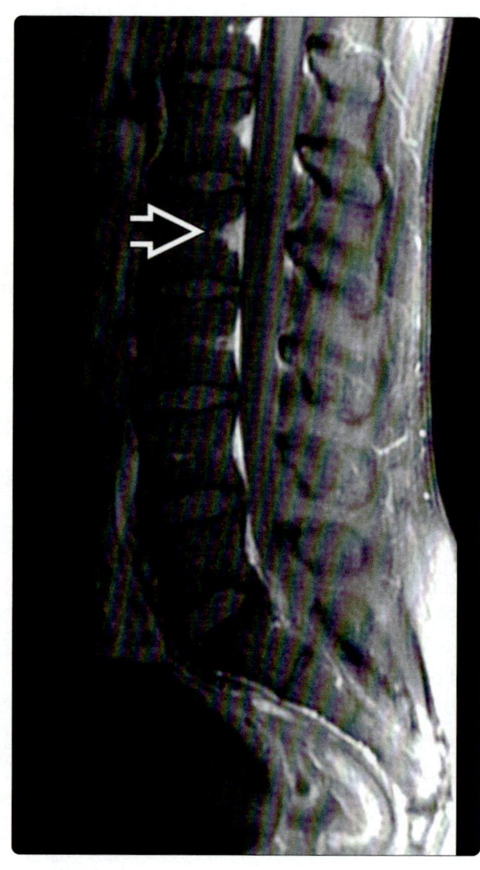

(Left) *AP chest radiograph of a patient with myelofibrosis shows bilateral pleural disease, which proved to be involvement by extramedullary hematopoiesis.* **(Right)** *AP radiograph demonstrates diffuse osteosclerosis of the tubular bones. The abnormality predominantly involves the medullary space, without thickening of the endosteal cortex. This is typical of myelofibrosis, which results from replacement of the fatty marrow with fibrous tissue.*

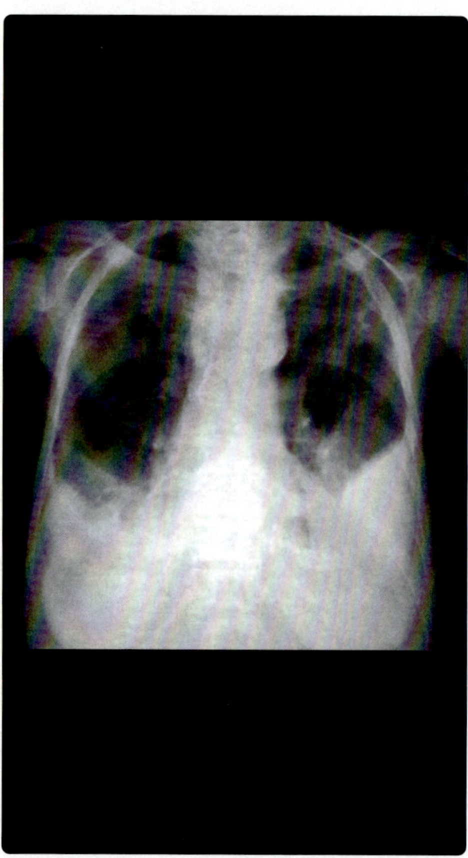

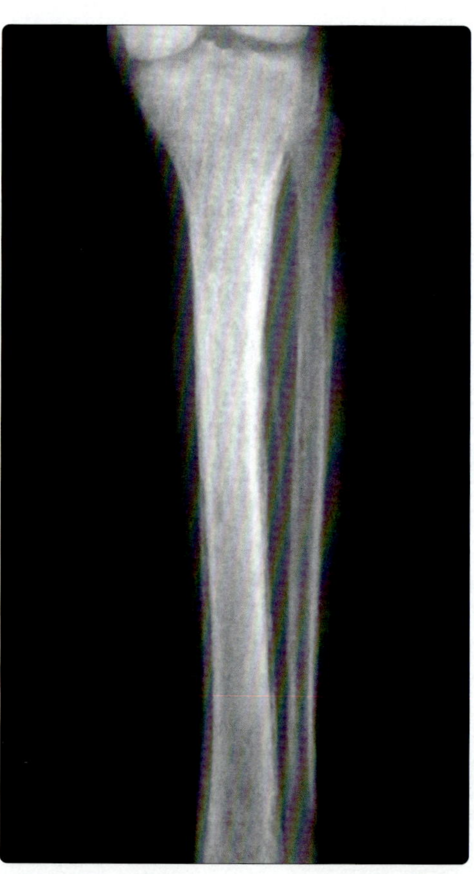

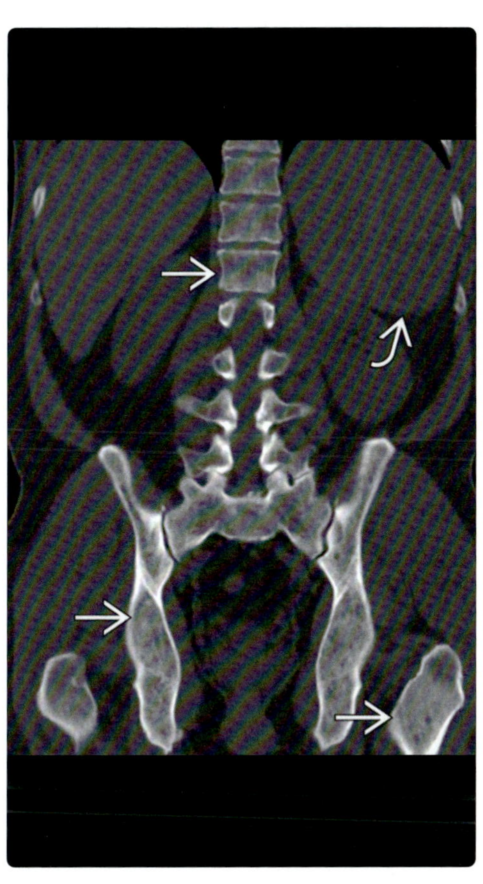

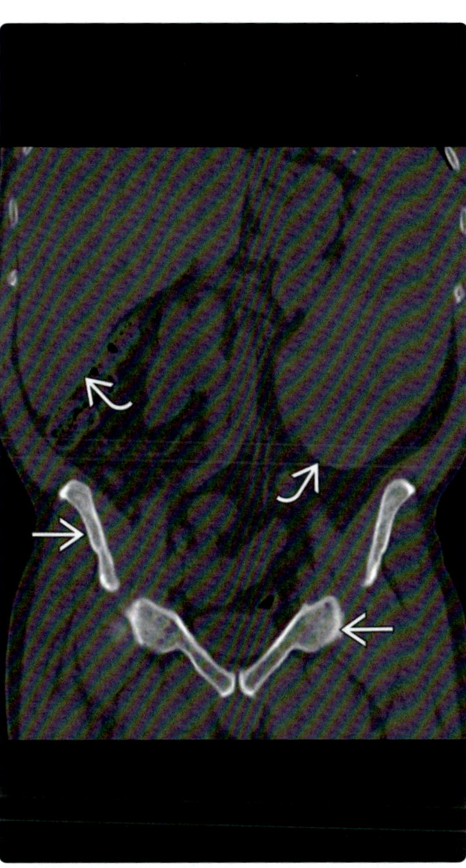

(Left) *Coronal CT in a 57-year-old man with an elevated hematocrit shows splenomegaly ➡ and diffuse sclerosis of the bones ➡ of the pelvis, spine, and proximal femora.* **(Right)** *Coronal CT, same patient, more anteriorly located, shows the extent of the hepatosplenomegaly ➡. Diffuse sclerosis of the pelvis, without cortical thickening, is seen ➡. The findings are typical of myelofibrosis that, in this case, developed secondary to the patient's underlying disease polycythemia vera.*

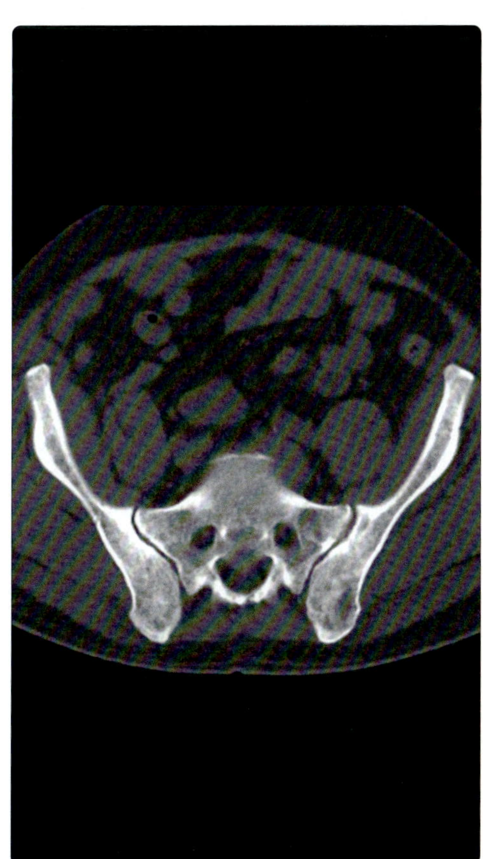

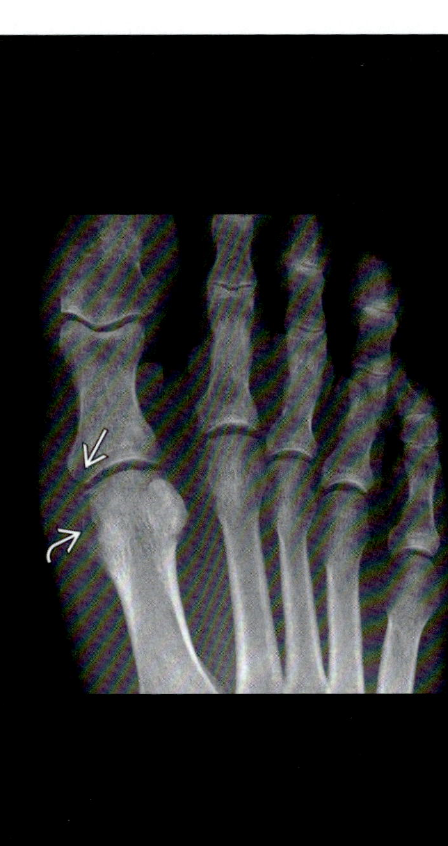

(Left) *Axial CT, same patient, shows the diffuse and somewhat patchy sclerosis, without alteration of the size of the bones or cortex, that is typical of myelofibrosis.* **(Right)** *AP radiograph, same patient, shows the cause of the patient's painful foot. There is soft tissue swelling at the 1st metatarsophalangeal joint as well as both marginal ➡ and juxtaarticular ➡ erosions. This patient has developed gout secondary to the increased cellular turnover of his underlying disease process.*

KEY FACTS

TERMINOLOGY

- X-linked recessive bleeding disorder resulting from clotting factor deficiencies
- Pseudotumor of hemophilia: Nonneoplastic mass lesion that occurs with repeated focal intraosseous, subperiosteal, or soft tissue bleeding

IMAGING

- Location of arthropathy: Knee > elbow > ankle > hip
- Location of pseudotumor: Soft tissue > bone
  - Intraosseous pseudotumor: Femur > pelvis > tibia > small bones of hand > calcaneus
- Radiograph: Hemophilic arthropathy
  - Inflammatory synovitis causes cartilage destruction, erosions, and subchondral cysts
  - Generally, epiphyses and metaphyses show overgrowth (ballooning) due to hyperemia; diaphyses are gracile
  - Large effusion, ↑ density if chronic bleeding results in hemosiderin deposits in synovium
- Radiograph: Pseudotumor
  - If intraosseous, extremely expanded lytic lesion; endosteal scalloping, cortical thinning
  - If subperiosteal or soft tissue in origin, extrinsic bony scalloping with sharp margin, bizarre periosteal reaction
- MR: Hemophilic arthropathy
  - Effusion heterogeneous on both T1 and T2: Due to blood products in various stages
  - Hemosiderin deposits along synovial lining
  - May contain fluid-fluid levels (blood products)

TOP DIFFERENTIAL DIAGNOSES

- Juvenile idiopathic arthritis
- Tuberculosis arthritis
- Pigmented villonodular synovitis

CLINICAL ISSUES

- Treatment: Aggressive use of synthetic clotting factors
  - Chronic: Synovectomy; if end stage, arthroplasty

(Left) *Graphic demonstrates the most frequent distribution of hemophilic arthropathy. The knee is the most frequently involved joint, followed by the elbow and ankle. Pseudotumor of hemophilia has a different distribution, seen most frequently in the femur/thigh and pelvis.* **(Right)** *Lateral x-ray of a child's knee shows a large, dense effusion ➡, along with erosions ➡ and cartilage narrowing. The epiphyses are significantly overgrown and the diaphysis is gracile. This is a typical hemophilic knee with advanced disease.*

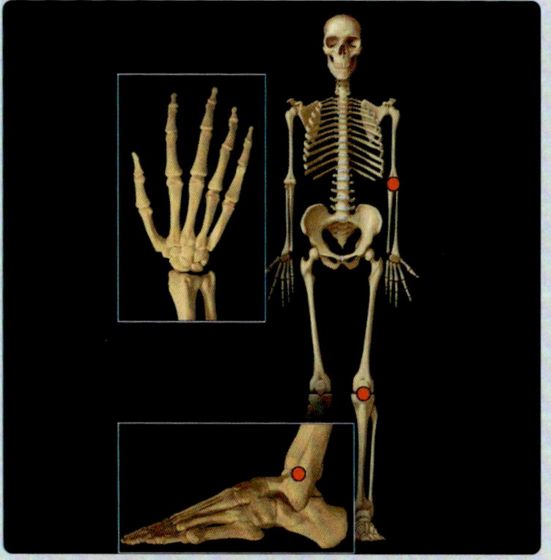

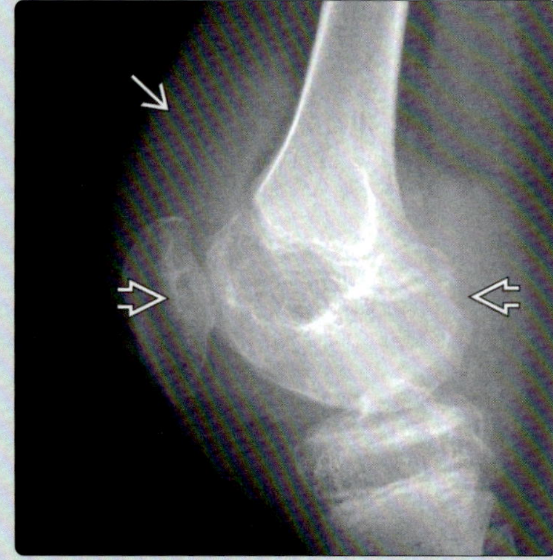

(Left) *Lateral radiograph of a teenager's knee shows a huge effusion ➡. Note also the enlargement of the femoral condyles (ballooning) relative to the femoral diaphysis.* **(Right)** *AP radiograph in the same patient shows the hypertrophied femoral condyles and widening of the intercondylar notch ➡. The process is relatively early, since cartilage narrowing and erosions have not yet developed. The findings are typical of either hemophilic arthropathy or juvenile idiopathic arthritis; the patient is known to be hemophilic.*

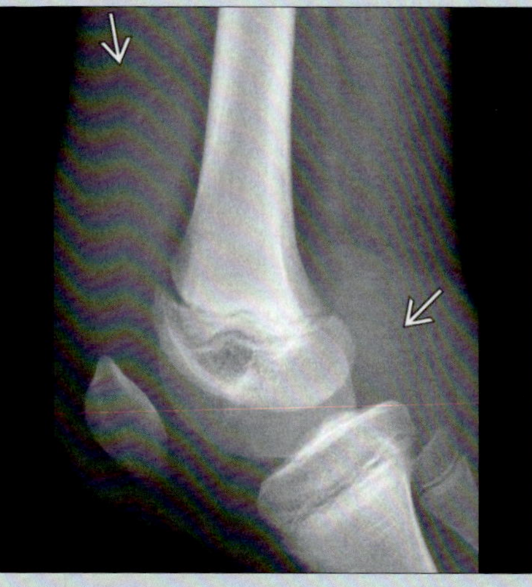

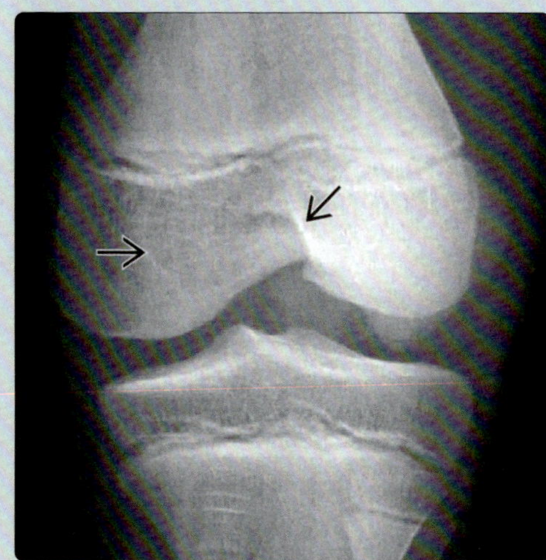

TERMINOLOGY

Synonyms

- Hemophilia A (factor VIII deficiency), hemophilia B (factor IX deficiency, Christmas disease)

Definitions

- X-linked recessive bleeding disorder resulting from clotting factor deficiencies
- Pseudotumor of hemophilia: Nonneoplastic mass lesion that occurs with repeated focal intraosseous, subperiosteal, or soft tissue bleeding

IMAGING

General Features

- Best diagnostic clue
  - Dense hemarthrosis, arthropathy, growth deformity
  - MR: Blooming nodules of hemosiderin deposits
- Location
  - Arthropathy: Knee > elbow > ankle > hip > shoulder
    - May be polyarticular but usually not symmetric
  - Pseudotumor: Soft tissue > bone > subperiosteal
    - Intraosseous pseudotumor: Femur > pelvis > tibia > small bones of hand > calcaneus
    - Soft tissue pseudotumor: Thigh > gluteal region > iliopsoas muscle
- Size
  - Pseudotumors may become extremely large
- Morphology
  - Chronic hemarthroses and hyperemia → growth deformities
    - Overgrowth epiphyses/metaphyses (ballooning)
    - Early fusion results in limb length discrepancy

Radiographic Findings

- Hemophilic arthropathy
  - Large effusion
    - Increased density if chronic bleeding results in hemosiderin deposits in synovium
  - Overgrowth pattern
    - Generally, epiphyses and metaphyses show overgrowth (ballooning) due to hyperemia; diaphyses are gracile
    - In elbow, radial head is particularly enlarged
  - Premature physeal fusion results in limb shortening
  - Osteoporosis
  - Pannus causes erosion and widening of intercondylar notch in knee, trochlear notch in elbow
  - Inflammatory synovitis causes cartilage destruction, erosions, and subchondral cysts
  - Eventual secondary osteoarthritis
- Hemophilic pseudotumor
  - If intraosseous, extremely expanded lytic lesion
    - Appears bizarre due to its size but is geographic
    - May be single lytic lesion or multiloculated
    - Daughter cysts often seen
    - May contain septa
    - Rarely, dystrophic calcification present
    - Endosteal scalloping, cortical thinning
    - Well-marginated sclerotic rim
    - Adjacent reactive bone formation
  - If subperiosteal or soft tissue in origin
    - Soft tissue density ± internal calcifications
    - Extrinsic scalloping on bone, with sharp margin
    - Periosteal reaction may be unusual in appearance, with sharp bony excrescences extending perpendicularly from bone

CT Findings

- Valuable in evaluation of septa and thin cortical rim in pseudotumor
- Enhanced CT can define outlines and wall thickness of peripheral capsule
- Central variable attenuation, representing different stages of hemorrhage

MR Findings

- Hemophilic arthropathy
  - Hemosiderin deposits along synovial lining of joint
    - May be nodular
    - Low signal on all sequences, bloom on gradient-echo
  - Effusion heterogeneous on both T1 and T2: Blood products in various stages
    - Acute: Isointense on T1, hypointense on T2
    - > 1 week: SI progressively ↑ on both T1 and T2
    - May contain fluid-fluid levels
  - Cartilage destruction, subchondral erosions, and cysts
- Hemophilic pseudotumor
  - Intramedullary cystic lesion
    - Thin low signal rim
    - May have low signal periosteal reaction and adjacent reactive bone formation
    - Low signal hemosiderin deposits within wall
    - Contains fluid components, best seen on T2 and postcontrast T1; may have fluid-fluid levels
    - Complex internal signal (remote and recurrent hemorrhage, clot organization): Mixed high and low signal regions on all sequences
  - Soft tissue/subperiosteal pseudotumor
    - Hemosiderin nodular deposits along capsule of lesion (low signal on all sequences, blooms)
    - Pressure erosions (scalloping) on adjacent bone
    - Low signal bony excrescences extending several centimeters perpendicularly to long bone
    - Pressure may lead to pain, skin necrosis, and eventually infection
    - Soft tissue mass heterogeneous on both T1 and T2, representing blood products of various ages
    - May have fluid-fluid levels

Ultrasonographic Findings

- US to follow progression/resolution of pseudotumor

Imaging Recommendations

- Best imaging tool
  - Radiographs make initial diagnosis
  - MR used to confirm presence of hemosiderin and evaluate any mass lesion and adjacency to peripheral nerves
- Protocol advice
  - Gradient-echo sequences show blooming of hemosiderin deposits in synovium

DIFFERENTIAL DIAGNOSIS

DDx of Hemophilic Arthropathy

- Juvenile idiopathic arthritis (JIA)
  - JIA occurs in skeletally immature patient, so hyperemia results in overgrowth and early fusion
  - Pannus and synovitis causes similar pattern of erosion and cartilage/bone destruction
  - Hemophilia may be distinguished from JIA if hemosiderin deposits can be demonstrated either by radiographic density or blooming on MR
- Tuberculosis arthritis (TB)
  - Same growth disturbance may occur in TB arthritis of skeletally immature patient
  - Cartilage destruction and erosions tend to develop and progress slower in TB than in pyogenic septic joint
  - Erosions may have more sclerotic and well-defined rim
- Pigmented villonodular synovitis (PVNS)
  - Both show low signal intraarticular synovium on all sequences, which blooms on gradient-echo
  - PVNS often has more focal nodular pattern
  - If PVNS occurs in skeletally immature patient, it could result in overgrowth, though typically not to same extent as hemophilia
  - Erosive pattern in PVNS is more focal, related specifically to nodular lesions

DDx of Pseudotumor of Bone

- May simulate multiple 1° or 2° tumors
  - Giant cell tumor
  - Desmoplastic fibroma
  - Plasmacytoma
  - Metastasis
  - Simple or aneurysmal bone cyst

PATHOLOGY

General Features

- Etiology
  - Hemophilic arthropathy
    - Joints whose stability depends on adjacent soft tissues seem to be most at risk
    - Initial bleed predisposes to recurrent bleed
    - Recurrent bleeding results in hyperemia → osseous overgrowth and early physeal fusion
    - Hypertrophy and inflammation in synovial membrane → cartilage and osseous damage
  - Pseudotumor of hemophilia
    - Recurrent hemorrhage in extraarticular location of musculoskeletal system →
    - Chronic, slowly expanding encapsulated mass →
    - Depending on site, osseous reaction to mass

Gross Pathologic & Surgical Features

- Altered synovial membrane: Inflammatory tissue, pannus, with brownish color
- Discoloration of cartilage, focal areas of fibrillation, erosion, and necrosis

CLINICAL ISSUES

Presentation

- Most common signs/symptoms
  - Acute hemarthrosis: Tense, swollen, red, painful
    - May have leukocytosis and fever
  - Subacute or chronic hemarthrosis: Contractures, severely restricted range of motion
  - Pseudotumor presents with mass and occasionally
    - Neuropathy
    - Pathologic fracture
    - Compartment syndrome

Demographics

- Age
  - 1st episode of joint hemorrhage by 2-3 years of age
  - Repeated hemarthrosis through adolescence and childhood
  - Hemarthrosis occurrence decreases in older patients
- Gender
  - Male only (x-linked recessive abnormality)
  - Extremely rare female manifestations seen with various chromosomal abnormalities
- Epidemiology
  - Hemophilia A: 1:10,000 males in USA (> 80% of cases)
  - Hemophilia B: 1:100,000 males in USA
  - Hemarthrosis occurs in 70-90% of hemophiliacs
    - 50% of hemophilic patients develop permanent arthropathy
  - Pseudotumor occurs in 1-2% of patients with severe hemophilia (clotting factor level < 1% of normal)

Natural History & Prognosis

- Severity varies
  - Least severe: Bleed excessively with surgery/trauma
  - Most severe: Spontaneous or minor trauma → bleeding
- Repeated intraarticular bleeding results in joint contracture and destruction
- Pseudotumor may spontaneously resolve but usually continues to enlarge; rare malignant degeneration

Treatment

- Hemophilic arthropathy
  - Acute: Administer appropriate clotting factor
  - Chronic: Synovectomy; if end stage, arthroplasty
  - Note: Patients should routinely receive aggressive treatment with synthetic clotting factors
- Hemophilic pseudotumor: Goal of preserving function
  - Conservative: Immobilization
  - Radical: Resection or radiation

DIAGNOSTIC CHECKLIST

Consider

- Early MR of arthropathy should be obtained; allows early assessment, which leads to aggressive prophylaxis and delays joint complications

SELECTED REFERENCES

1. de Almeida AM et al: Arthroscopic partial anterior synovectomy of the knee on patients with haemophilia. Knee Surg Sports Traumatol Arthrosc. 23(3):785-91, 2015

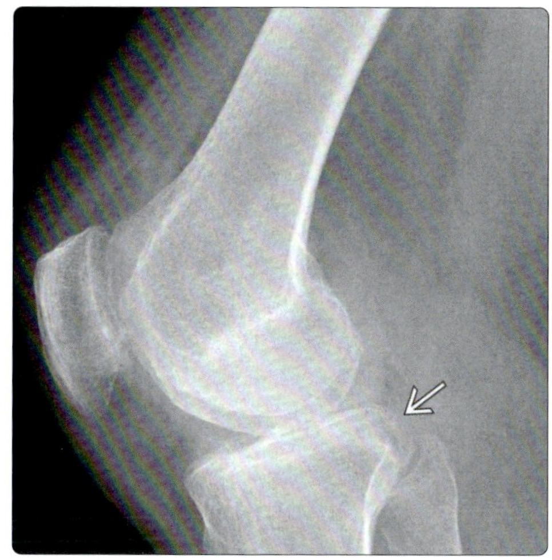

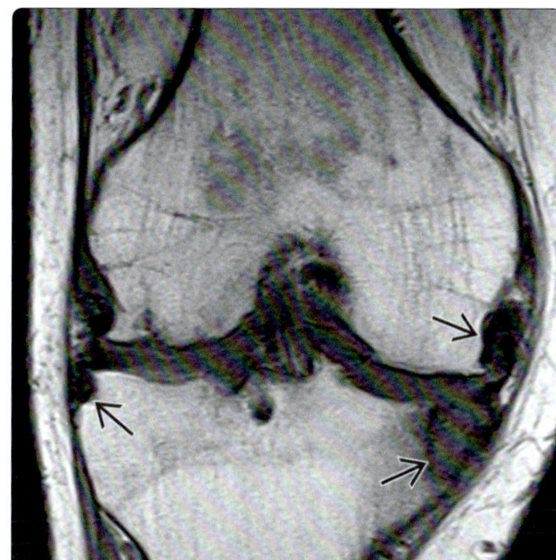

(Left) *Lateral radiograph in a 31-year-old man shows cartilage thinning at the patellofemoral joint with articular irregularity and a posterior tibial erosion ➡. There is overgrowth (ballooning) of the epiphyses relative to gracile diaphyses.* **(Right)** *Coronal T1 MR in the same patient shows extensive erosive disease ➡. Given the morphology and patient gender, diagnosis of hemophilic arthropathy is probable.*

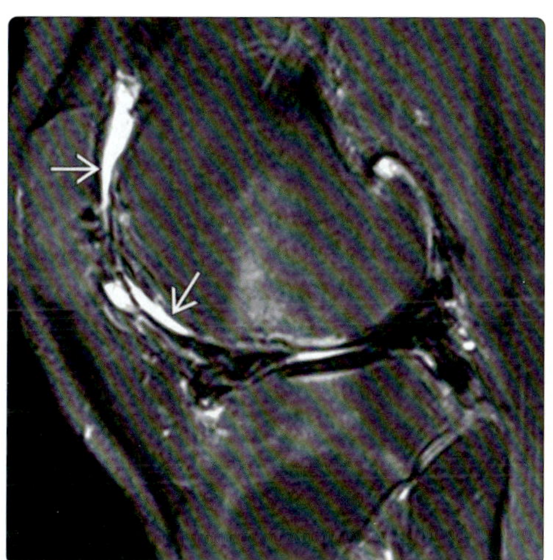

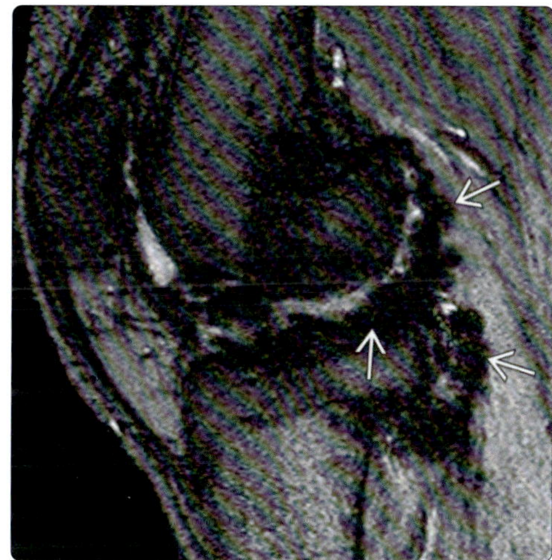

(Left) *Sagittal T2 FS MR in the same patient shows the extent of cartilage destruction, full thickness on all surfaces ➡, along with bone marrow edema. The severe arthropathy is typical of hemophilic arthropathy.* **(Right)** *Sagittal GRE MR in the same patient shows blooming within the synovium ➡. This is indicative of hemosiderin deposits and proves the diagnosis of hemophilic arthropathy.*

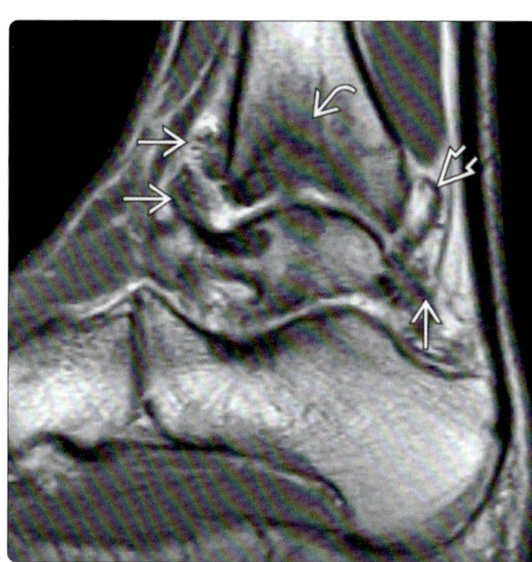

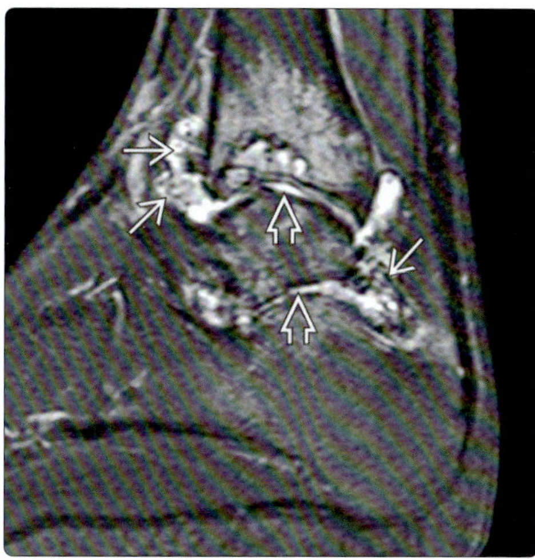

(Left) *Sagittal T1WI MR arthrogram shows low signal intensity hemosiderin deposits ➡, synovial thickening ➡, cartilage irregularity, and bone marrow edema surrounding a large subchondral cyst ➡.* **(Right)** *Sagittal T2WI MR arthrogram also shows low signal intensity hemosiderin deposits ➡ with synovial thickening. The bone marrow edema is even more apparent. Cartilage is absent in both the tibiotalar and subtalar joints ➡. All findings are typical of hemophilic arthropathy.*

(Left) *AP radiograph shows enormous subchondral cysts on both sides of the joint but particularly within the talus ➡. On these coned images, the degree of overgrowth is not apparent, but the cartilage narrowing and erosive disease is impressive. This young man has significant arthropathy and is a known hemophilic patient.* **(Right)** *Oblique radiograph shows an overgrown radial head ➡ and mild subchondral cyst formation in the ulna and humerus ➡, findings of early hemophilic arthropathy.*

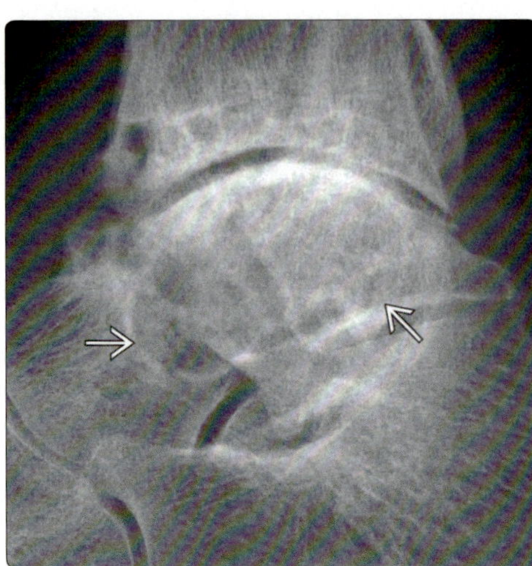

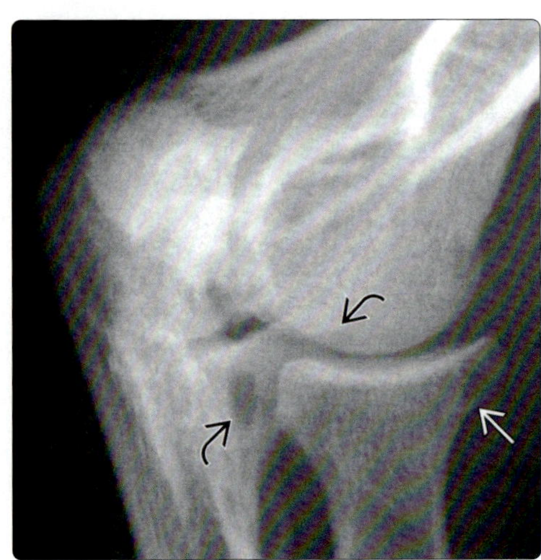

(Left) *AP radiograph shows typical advanced hemophilic arthropathy of the elbow. There is large subchondral cyst formation ➡, widened trochlear notch ➡, and significant overgrowth of the radial head ➡.* **(Right)** *Coronal T1WI MR shows erosive change in the humeral head ➡. Glenohumeral cartilage is completely absent ➡. Even though this is a T1 image, one can see that there is a rotator cuff tear. Additionally, there is a low signal mass lining the subdeltoid bursa ➡.*

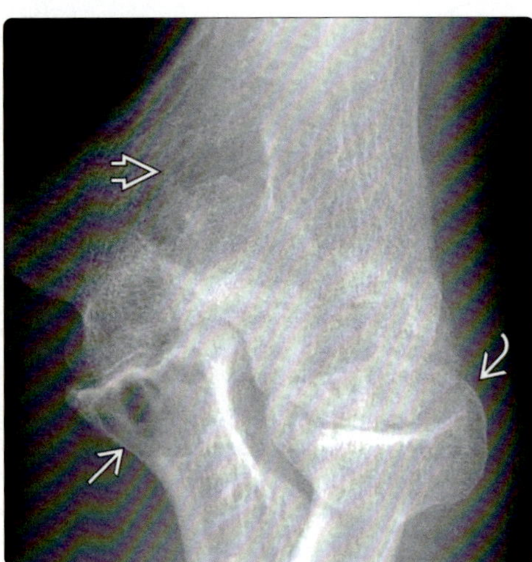

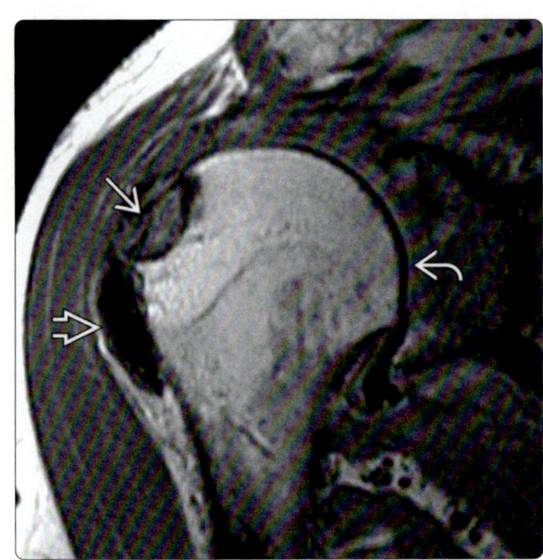

(Left) *Axial PD MR obtained at the lower portion of the glenohumeral joint shows the densely low signal mass lining the subdeltoid bursa ➡, matching that seen on the prior image. Low signal material is also seen intraarticularly ➡.* **(Right)** *Axial gradient-echo image at the same level shows blooming of the mass within the subdeltoid bursa ➡ as well as the intraarticular masses ➡. This strongly supports the diagnosis of hemophilic arthropathy with hemosiderin deposition.*

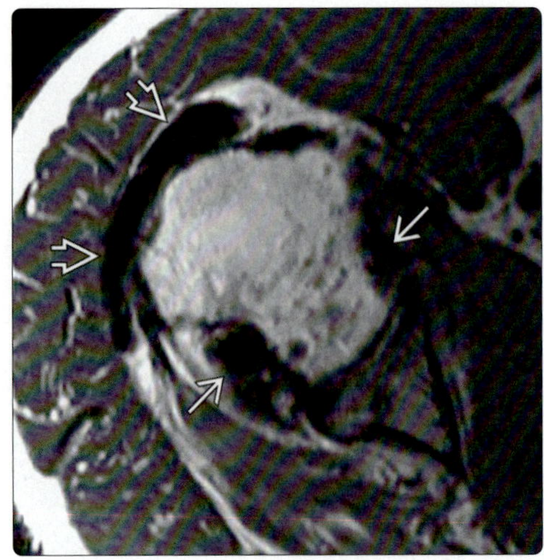

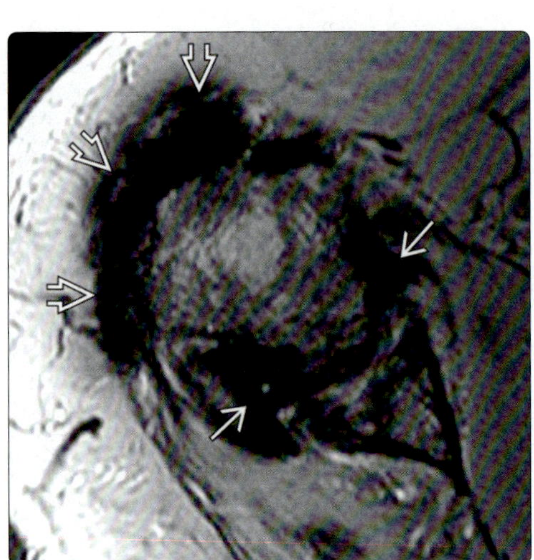

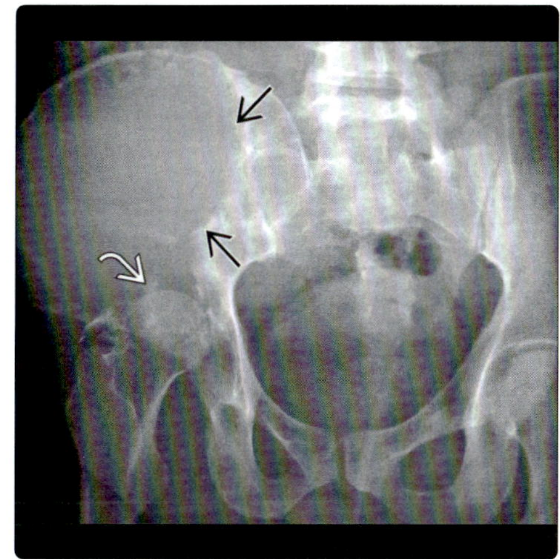

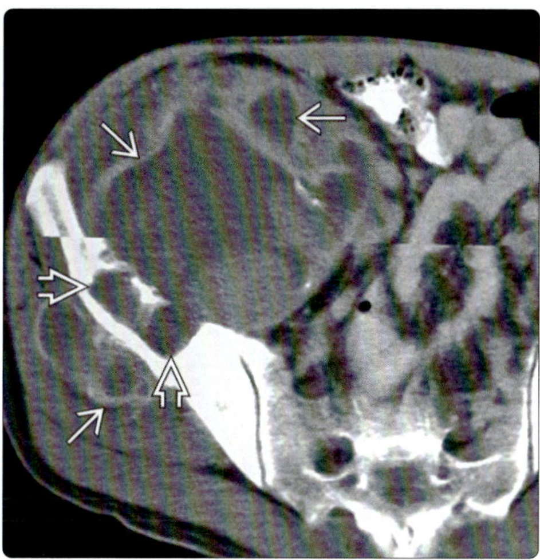

(Left) *AP radiograph shows a highly expanded lytic lesion of the right iliac wing. However, the margins of the lesion → are fairly geographic. This is typical of hemophilic pseudotumor, despite the extensive destructive change. The lesion had been stable prior to the recent pathologic fracture →.* **(Right)** *Axial CT shows smooth margins of bone destruction → within an intraosseous pseudotumor. The mass extends into soft tissues as multiple lobulated fluid collections with enhancing rims →.*

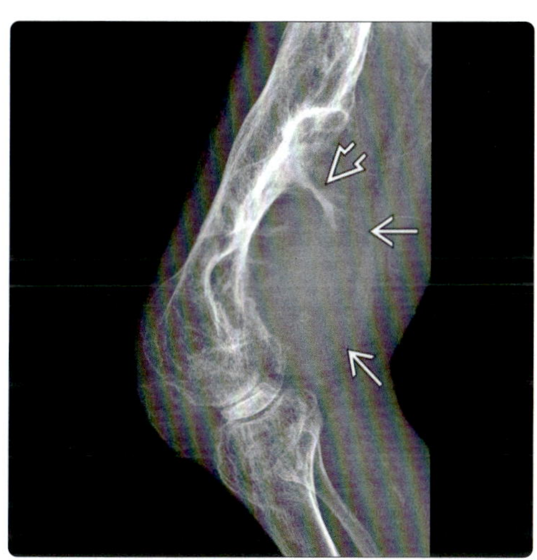

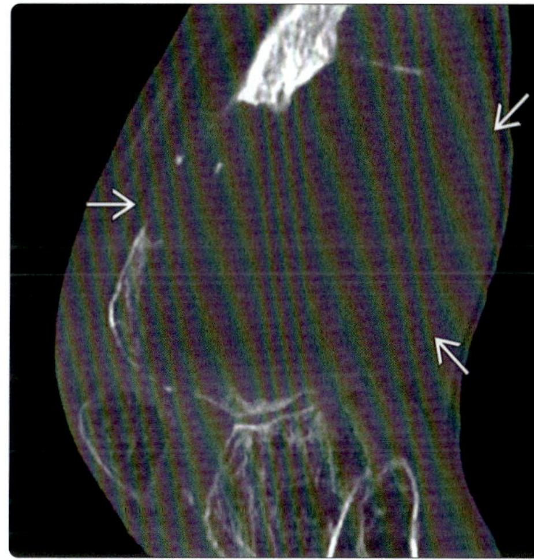

(Left) *Lateral radiograph shows a subperiosteal pseudotumor. The soft tissue mass → scallops the adjacent bone; the osseous destruction is geographic with transverse osseous excrescences →. This is a typical appearance, 2° to repeated bleeding, pressure erosion, and periosteal lifting.* **(Right)** *Sagittal CT in the same patient several years later shows new osseous destruction and a soft tissue mass →. This could be due to recurrent bleeding but biopsy showed transformation to malignant hemangioendothelioma.*

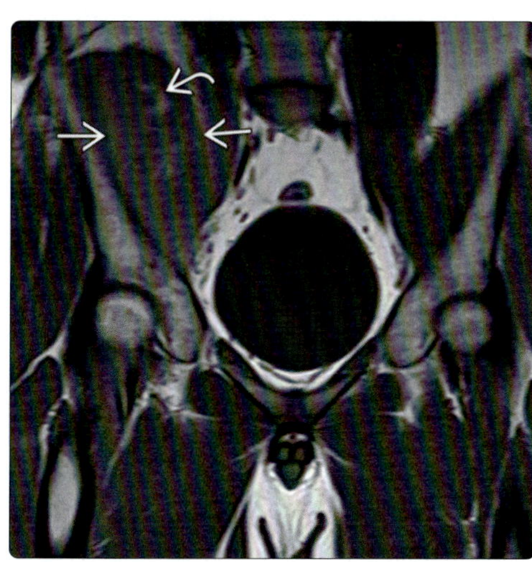

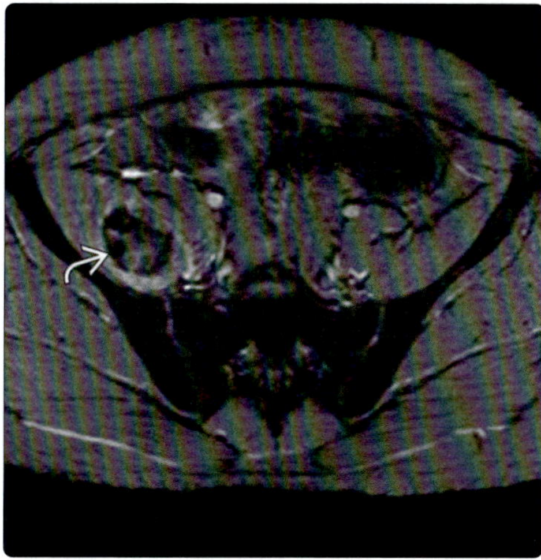

(Left) *Coronal T1 MR in a 21-year-old hemophilic with a pelvic mass → shows inhomogeneity with foci of hyperintensity → suggesting blood. T2 and postcontrast imaging demonstrated nonspecific hyperintensity and enhancement, respectively (not shown).* **(Right)** *Axial GRE in the same patient shows blooming → within the mass. This evidence of hemosiderin secures the diagnosis of pseudotumor of hemophilia.*

Diabetes

KEY FACTS

TERMINOLOGY

- Symptomatic abnormalities of skin, bones, joints, and tendons associated with type 1 or 2 diabetes

IMAGING

- Osteopenia/insufficiency fracture
  - Posterior calcaneal tuberosity insufficiency fracture thought to be specific for diabetes
- Osteomyelitis
  - Air in soft tissues with adjacent osseous destruction
  - MR: Confluent ↓ T1 SI, enhancement, abscess
  - Location: Particularly foot, at sites of pressure, such as 1st or 5th MTP, 1st distal phalanx, or heel
- Septic joint
  - Effusion and intraarticular deossification in appropriate setting
  - Any joint at risk, particularly sacroiliac joint, hip, and foot
  - 1/3 of patients with pedal osteomyelitis have adjacent septic joints
- Neuropathic (Charcot) joint
  - **5D**s: Normal bone **d**ensity, joint **d**istension, bony **d**ebris, joint **d**isorganization, **d**islocation
  - Lisfranc (tarsometatarsal) > talonavicular > Chopart (hindfoot-midfoot) > intertarsal joints
- Muscle infarction
  - Hyperintense muscle swelling on MR with adjacent soft tissue reaction
  - Thigh in ≥ 80%; calf is 2nd most common site
- Renal osteodystrophy (end-stage renal disease) secondary to diabetes
  - Altered bone density and various resorptive patterns
  - All bones, but particularly notable in hands, cranium, distal clavicles
- Crystal and amyloid deposition
  - Nodular soft tissue density, generally periarticular
  - Sodium urate, hydroxyapatite, amyloid
    - Amyloid deposition extremely common in patients on dialysis

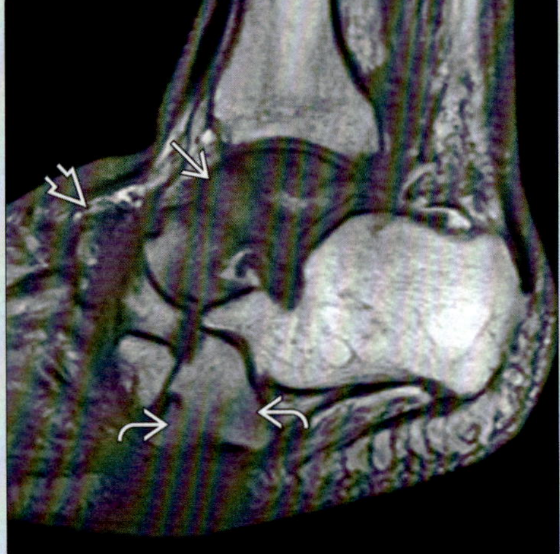

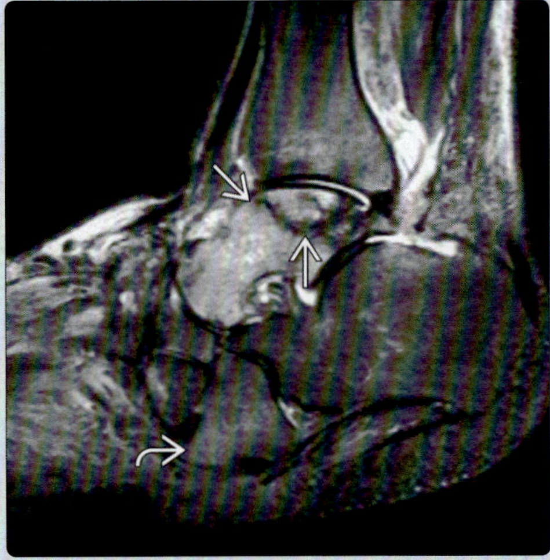

***(Left)** Sagittal T1WI MR in a diabetic foot shows dorsal subluxation of the navicular ➡ relative to both the talus and cuneiforms, part of a neuropathic midfoot. There is confluent gray signal in the cuboid ➡ adjacent to low SI in plantar soft tissues, suggesting osteomyelitis. The low SI in the talus ➡ was unexpected. **(Right)** Sagittal STIR MR further defines the talar abnormality as an insufficiency fracture of the dome of the talus ➡, with some degree of flattening and surrounding edema. The cuboid shows diffuse ↑ SI ➡.*

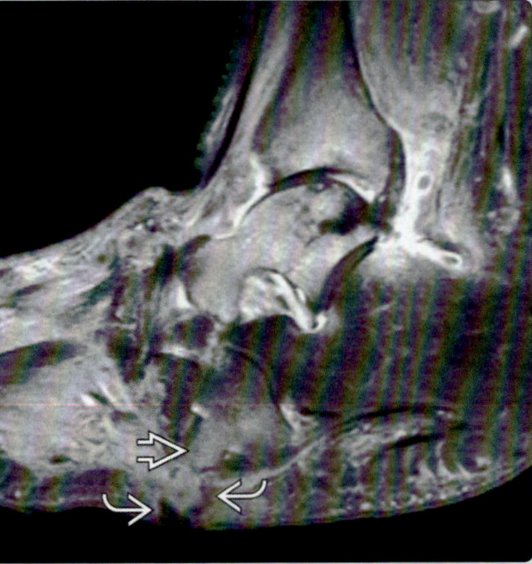

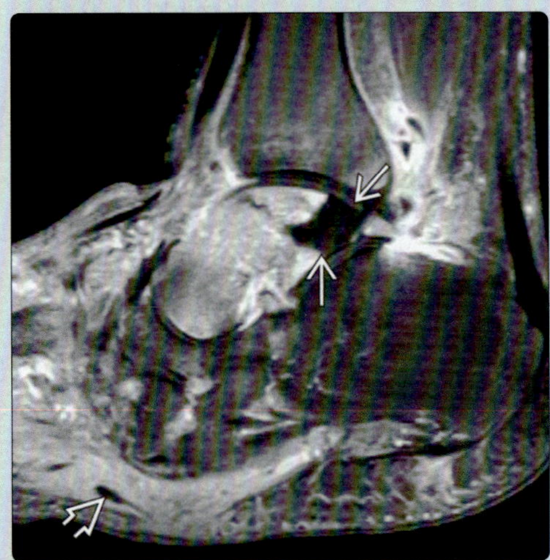

***(Left)** Sagittal T1WI C+ FS MR, same case, shows small abscesses ➡ extending from a sinus track to the high signal in the cuboid ➡ confirming osteomyelitis. **(Right)** Sagittal T1WI C+ FS MR, same case, shows the talar fracture but also a wedge-shaped region of hypointensity ➡, representing a segment of osteonecrosis (ON) in the body of talus. It should be remembered that the talus is prone to ON and that the tarsal bones are prone to insufficiency fracture in diabetic feet. Small extension of plantar abscess ➡ is seen.*

TERMINOLOGY

Definitions

- Symptomatic abnormalities of skin, bones, joints, and tendons associated with type 1 or 2 diabetes

IMAGING

General Features

- Best diagnostic clue
  - Osteopenia/insufficiency fracture
  - Infection
    - Osteomyelitis: Air in soft tissues with adjacent osseous destruction
    - Septic joint: Effusion and intraarticular deossification in appropriate setting
  - Neuropathic (Charcot) joint
    - **5D**s: Normal bone **d**ensity, joint **d**istension, bony **d**ebris, joint **d**isorganization, **d**islocation
  - Muscle infarction: Hyperintense muscle swelling with adjacent soft tissue reaction on MR, particularly thigh
  - Renal osteodystrophy (end-stage renal disease) secondary to diabetes: Nonspecific but altered bone density plus various resorptive patterns
  - Crystal and amyloid deposition: Nodular soft tissue density, generally periarticular, often low SI on fluid-sensitive MR sequences
- Location
  - Insufficiency fracture: Posterior tuberosity of calcaneus most frequent; other sites also common
  - Osteomyelitis: Particularly foot, at sites of pressure, such as 1st or 5th MTP, 1st distal phalanx, or heel
  - Septic joint
    - Particularly in foot (1/3 of patients with pedal osteomyelitis have adjacent septic joints)
    - Any joint at risk, sacroiliac & hip common
  - Neuropathic (Charcot) joint
    - Charcot foot: Lisfranc (tarsometatarsal) > talonavicular > Chopart (hindfoot-midfoot) > intertarsal joints
  - Renal osteodystrophy: All bones but particularly notable in hands, cranium, distal clavicles
  - Diabetic muscle infarction: Thigh in ≥ 80%; calf is 2nd most common site
    - Within thigh, usually vasti complex
    - Often more than 1 compartment
    - Bilateral in 40%

Radiographic Findings

- Calcaneal insufficiency avulsion (CIA fracture)
  - Posterior tuberosity of calcaneus at Achilles insertion
  - Extraarticular, with proximal displacement of large tongue of posterior tuberosity by Achilles
- Osteomyelitis
  - Air in sinus tract
  - Osseous destruction or periosteal reaction
- Septic joint
  - Some joints demonstrate effusion by displacement of fat pads (particularly hip & elbow)
  - Deossification of subarticular cortex may be seen earlier than frank osseous destruction
- Neuropathic (Charcot) joint
  - Large effusion
  - Debris (hypertrophic type); debris may resorb (atrophic)
  - Subluxation/dislocation
- Renal osteodystrophy
  - Generalized osteopenia, often with regions of sclerosis (vertebral body endplates)
  - Various resorptive patterns
    - Subperiosteal: Particularly radial aspect of middle phalanges & medial cortex of proximal metaphyses of long bones
    - Subligamentous: Particularly distal inferior clavicle & ischial tuberosity
    - Subchondral: Particularly distal clavicle, sacroiliac joint, subchondral regions of phalanges
    - Endosteal: Particularly small bones of hand
    - Trabecular: Salt and pepper pattern on skull
- Crystal deposition
  - Soft tissue mass; gouty tophus may have ↑ density
    - May erode adjacent bone
  - Periarticular dialysis-related calcification
- Radiography unlikely to show abnormality with diabetic muscle infarction
- DISH: Anterior bridging ossification of vertebral bodies

MR Findings

- Calcaneal insufficiency avulsion
  - Low signal fracture line on T1 with displacement of posterior tuberosity fragment
  - High signal fracture line with surrounding edema on fluid-sensitive sequences
- Osteomyelitis
  - Air in soft tissue sinus tracts, leading to osseous destruction
  - T1: Areas of confluent low signal in bone
  - Fluid-sensitive sequences: Hyperintense regions of bone with adjacent & subcutaneous edema
  - Diffuse enhancement following contrast administration; may have adjacent abscess
- Septic joint: Nonspecific findings
  - Effusion
  - Thickening of synovium with contrast enhancement
  - Aspiration required to confirm diagnosis
- Neuropathic (Charcot) joint
  - Large effusion, often containing debris
  - Disruption of joint, with osseous reaction
    - T1: Subcortical bone shows finely reticulated low signal regions
    - Fluid-sensitive sequences: Hyperintense regions of bone, particularly adjacent to disrupted regions
    - Enhancement in areas of osseous reaction
- Diabetic neuropathy
  - Acute & subacute: T2 hyperintensity & fascicular enlargement
  - Chronic: Atrophic-appearing fascicles with intraepineurial fat deposition
- Renal osteodystrophy: Patchy nonspecific osseous signal
- Crystal and amyloid deposition
  - Mass generally is low signal on both T1 and fluid-sensitive sequences (inhomogeneous in latter)
  - Mass generally shows inhomogeneous enhancement
- Diabetic muscle infarction

- Acute: Marked muscle swelling
    - T1: Isointense compared with skeletal muscle
        - If hemorrhage present, high signal foci
    - Fluid-sensitive sequences: Hyperintense
    - Diffuse enhancement following contrast administration; may have foci with only rim enhancement indicating necrosis
    - Diffuse subcutaneous edema
    - Fascial fluid frequently seen
- Chronic: Atrophic, fibrotic, or necrotic muscle

- Adhesive capsulitis, especially glenohumeral joint

Imaging Recommendations

- Protocol advice
    - If attempting to differentiate osteomyelitis from osseous reaction in Charcot joint, obtain T1 in at least 2 planes and use contrast if possible

DIFFERENTIAL DIAGNOSIS

DDx of Pedal Osteomyelitis

- Charcot joint: Osseous reaction can be virtually indistinguishable from osteomyelitis on MR

DDx of Septic Arthritis

- Noninfectious inflammation: Reactive or arthritic

DDx of Diabetic Muscle Infarction

- Soft tissue abscess
- Pyomyositis
- Necrotizing fasciitis
- Other causes of myositis (dermatomyositis, nodular myositis, proliferative myositis)
- Diagnosis relies on combined clinical & imaging findings; may require histologic confirmation

PATHOLOGY

General Features

- Etiology
    - Pedal osteomyelitis results almost exclusively from contiguous soft tissue ulcer or skin defect
        - Foot ulceration results from combination of peripheral neuropathy, peripheral arterial disease, and susceptibility to infection
    - Neuropathic (Charcot) joint
        - ↓ proprioception → recurrent trauma → progressive destruction → disorganization of joint
    - Renal osteodystrophy: Combination of osteomalacia & secondary hyperparathyroidism
    - Deposition disease: Generally sodium urate (gout) or dialysis-related amyloid; may also be hydroxyapatite or pyrophosphate crystals
    - Diabetic muscle infarction: Extensive thrombosis of medium and small arterioles
    - Diabetic neuropathy: Nerve ischemia; thickening and hyalinization of walls of small blood vessels

CLINICAL ISSUES

Presentation

- Most common signs/symptoms
    - CIA
        - May be painful, but proprioception likely reduced
        - Deformity of posterior heel, with bulbous osseous prominence at usual site of distal Achilles
    - Osteomyelitis: Deep ulceration
    - Septic joint: Swelling, decreased range of motion
    - Neuropathic joint: Swollen, warm, deformed joint
    - Diabetic muscle infarction
        - Sudden onset of severe pain & tenderness, with or without palpable mass (34-44%)
        - Pain more severe than in other etiologies of myositis
        - Bilateral in ~ 40%
        - Generally in patients with longstanding, poorly controlled diabetes, either type 1 or 2
    - Adhesive capsulitis
        - Shoulder pain, limited range of motion
    - DISH: Far higher prevalence in patients with type 2 diabetes than in general population

Demographics

- Epidemiology
    - 15% of diabetics in USA have neuropathic joints
    - MSK manifestations most common in patients with longstanding type 1 diabetes

Natural History & Prognosis

- Calcaneal insufficiency avulsion
    - Shows progressive displacement
    - Healing slow and poor, whether treated with cast or surgically
- Osteomyelitis: Progressive destruction
- Septic joint: Progressive destruction
- Neuropathic: Progressive destruction and deformity
- Diabetic muscle infarction
    - Symptoms resolve over several weeks
    - Patients often have other complications of diabetes and have high rate of mortality in short term

DIAGNOSTIC CHECKLIST

Consider

- Diabetic muscle infarct when severity of pain seems disproportionate in poorly controlled diabetic

Image Interpretation Pearls

- **Osteomyelitis & osseous reaction to Charcot joints may be indistinguishable by MR**
    - Both show hyperintense enhancing osseous signal
    - Both may have associated fluid collections
    - Presence of sinus tract leading to osseous destruction can define abnormality as osteomyelitis
    - Character of T1 regions of hypointensity (confluent vs. reticulated) may help differentiate
    - Presence of osseous debris more suggestive of neuropathic joint than osteomyelitis

SELECTED REFERENCES

1. Baker JC et al: Diabetic musculoskeletal complications and their imaging mimics. Radiographics. 32(7):1959-74, 2012
2. Thakkar RS et al: Spectrum of high-resolution MRI findings in diabetic neuropathy. AJR Am J Roentgenol. 199(2):407-12, 2012
3. Donovan A et al: Use of MR imaging in diagnosing diabetes-related pedal osteomyelitis. Radiographics. 30(3):723-36, 2010

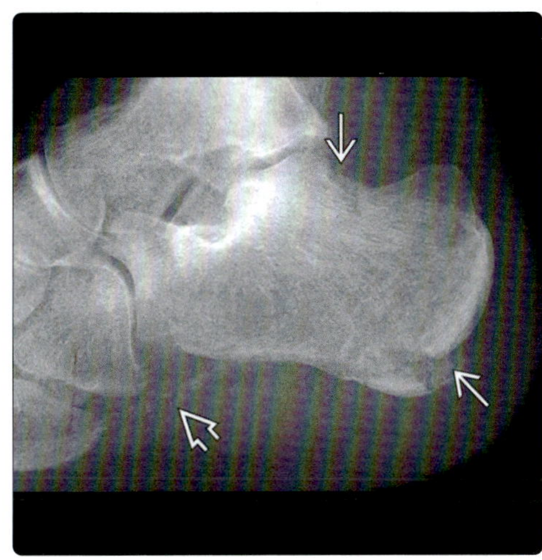

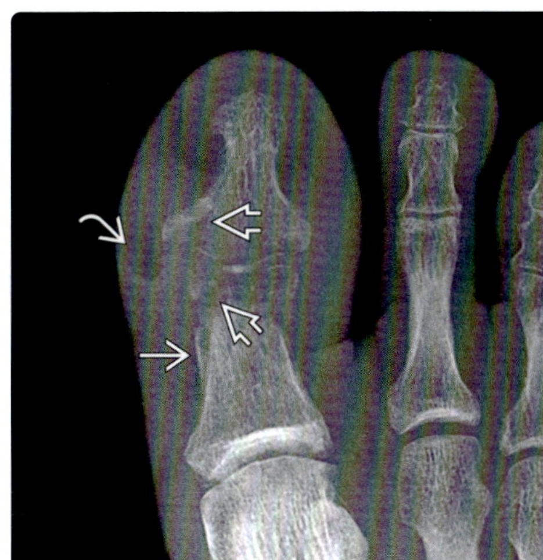

(Left) *Lateral radiograph shows a calcaneal insufficiency avulsion (CIA) fracture ➡ with the Achilles elevating the posterior tubercle. It occurs in diabetic patients (note the vascular calcification ➡) and is very difficult to treat.* **(Right)** *AP radiograph shows air in the soft tissues ➡ leading to osseous destruction within both the proximal and distal phalanges ➡ with associated periosteal reaction ➡. This constellation of findings is classic for septic arthritis/osteomyelitis.*

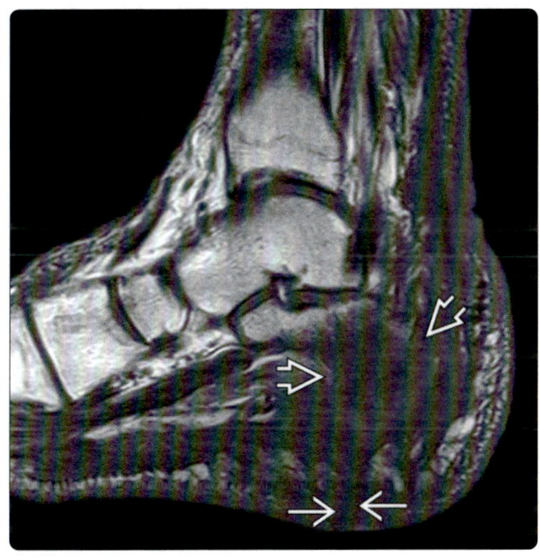

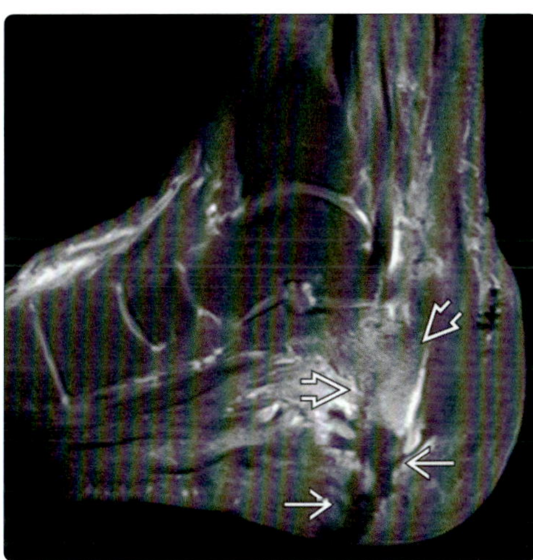

(Left) *Sagittal T1WI MR shows a plantar ulcer containing ↓ SI air ➡. The calcaneus ➡ shows highly confluent ↓ SI, much more suggestive of osteomyelitis than simple osseous reactive edema.* **(Right)** *Sagittal T1WI C+ FS MR shows the sinus track ➡ very clearly leading to the enhancing calcaneus ➡. Although bone may show reactive edema to nearby soft tissue infection and may be difficult to differentiate from osteomyelitis, the sinus track leading to confluent marrow abnormality is diagnostic.*

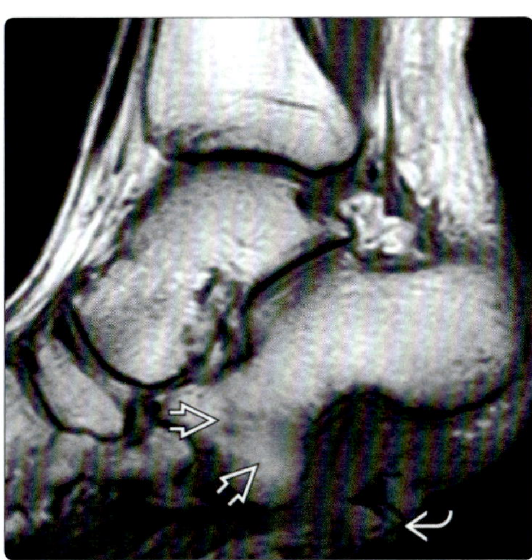

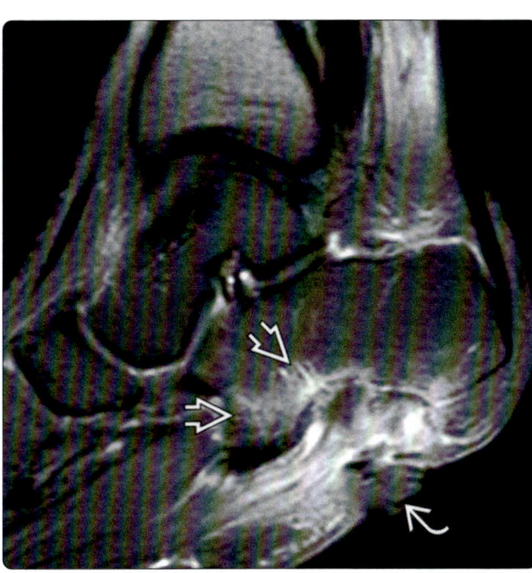

(Left) *Sagittal T1WI MR shows plantar ulceration ➡ with air approaching a morphologically abnormal calcaneus. There is a fine reticulated pattern of ↓ T1 SI ➡, which usually does not represent osteomyelitis, but rather osseous reaction.* **(Right)** *Sagittal T1 C+ FS MR shows the same ulceration ➡ and surrounding soft tissue infection. The calcaneus shows ↑ SI ➡, but this proved to be reactive bone rather than osteomyelitis. The T1 signal pattern is more specific for osteomyelitis than is the enhancement.*

(Left) *AP radiograph of a painful hip in a diabetic man shows distended fat pads indicating effusion. There is deossification both on the femoral head (note that the cortex has lost its crisp distinctness) and acetabulum. These are all signs of septic joint, proven at aspiration.* **(Right)** *Axial T1WI C+ FS MR shows high SI in the osseous structures on both sides of the pubic symphysis as well as a collection of fluid, representing septic joint in a diabetic patient with end-stage renal disease.*

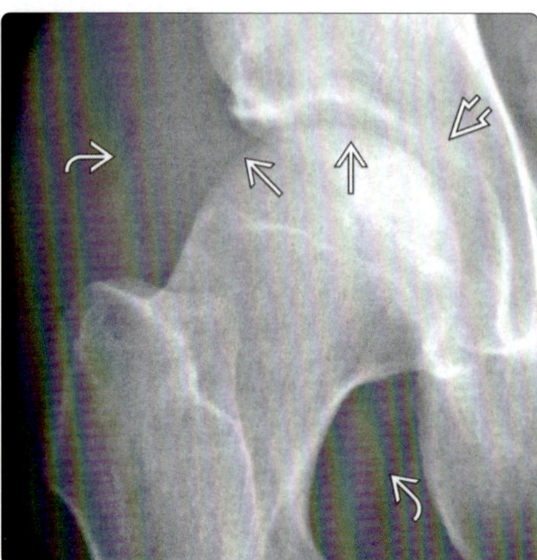

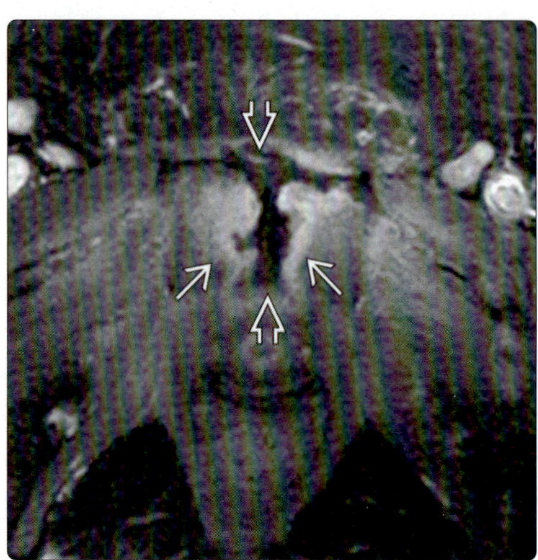

(Left) *Lateral radiograph shows an old, healed calcaneal insufficiency fracture in this diabetic patient. There is also destruction of the talonavicular joint and debris contained within a large joint effusion. These findings are typical of Charcot joint; talonavicular is a common site in diabetic patients.* **(Right)** *Axial CT through the tarsometatarsal (Lisfranc) joints in a different patient shows tiny fragments of osseous debris floating in distended joint spaces, indicating an early Charcot joint.*

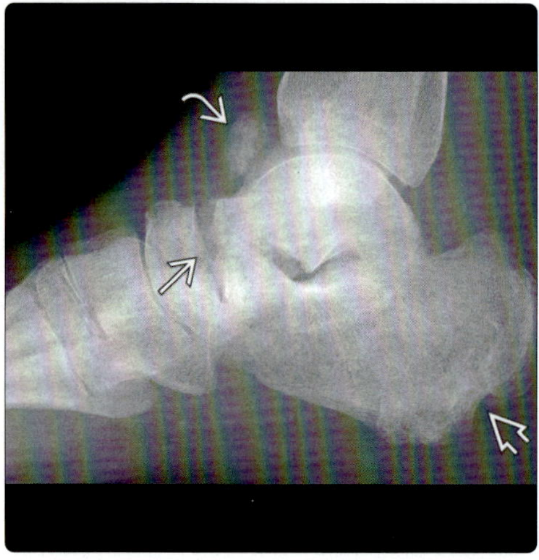

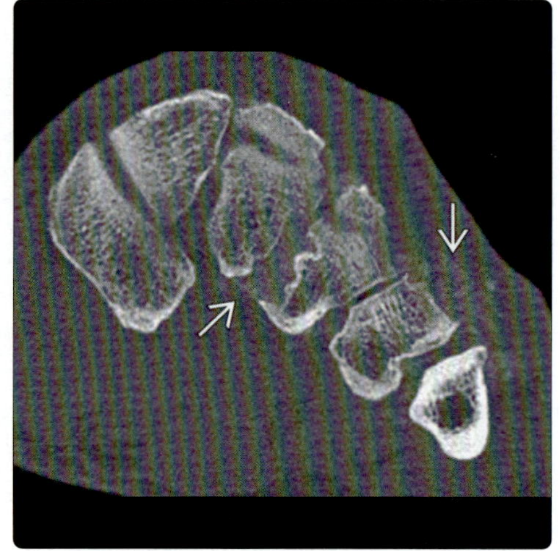

(Left) *Lateral radiograph shows a failed triple arthrodesis in a diabetic. There is tremendous soft tissue swelling and destruction of the tibiotalar and talonavicular joints, with debris seen anteriorly, indicating Charcot joint.* **(Right)** *Sagittal T1 C+ FS MR, same patient, shows (despite metal artifact) soft tissue fluid collections, some containing debris, along with high signal in the tibia. These abnormalities are typical of Charcot joint, & in its presence should not be misinterpreted as infection.*

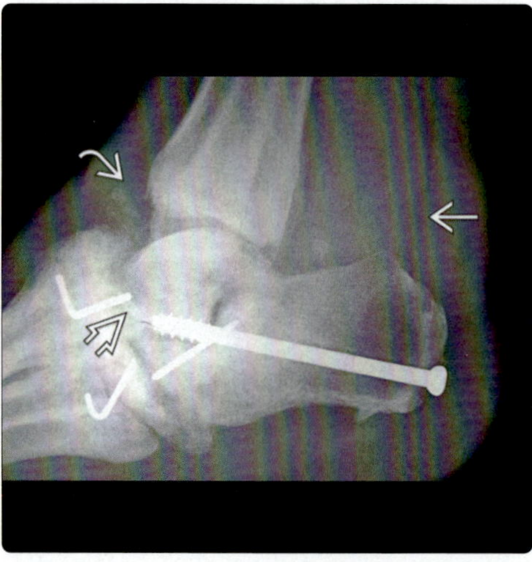

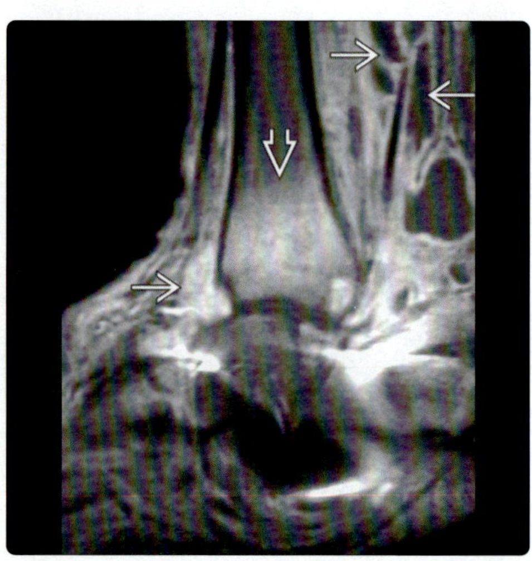

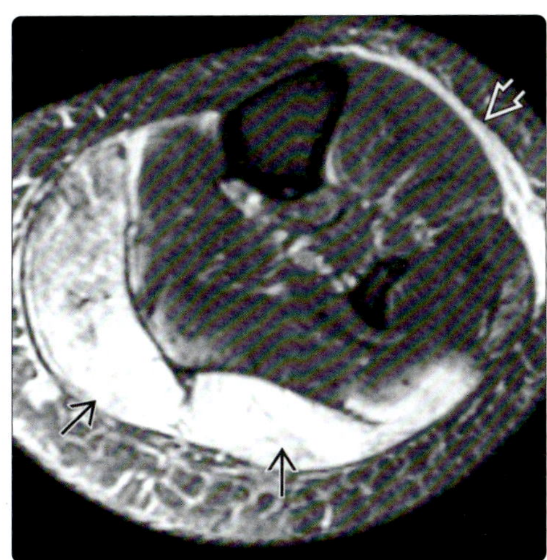

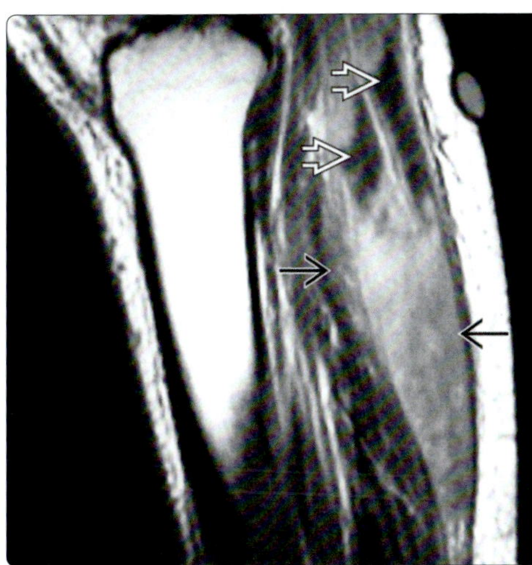

(Left) *Axial T2WI FS MR shows high signal involving the gastrocnemius and soleus muscles* ⇨*. There is fascial fluid present in subcutaneous planes as well* ➡*. This patient has poorly controlled diabetes.* **(Right)** *Sagittal T1WI C+ MR, same patient, shows mild diffuse enhancement throughout the same muscles* ⇨*, along with central diffuse low signal regions* ➡*. There is no enhancing rim around the low signal areas; therefore they represent spontaneous diabetic muscle necrosis rather than abscess.*

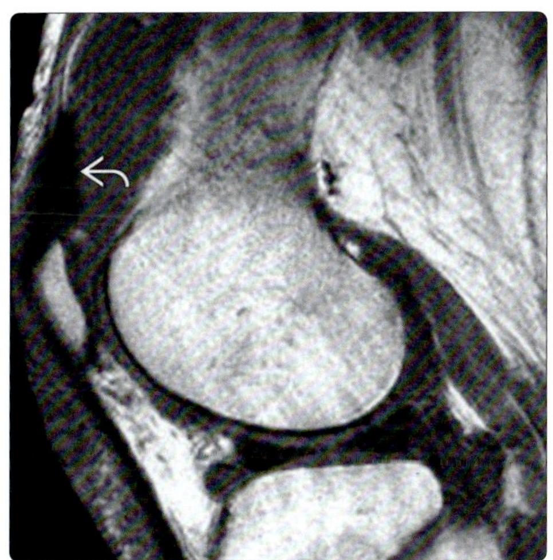

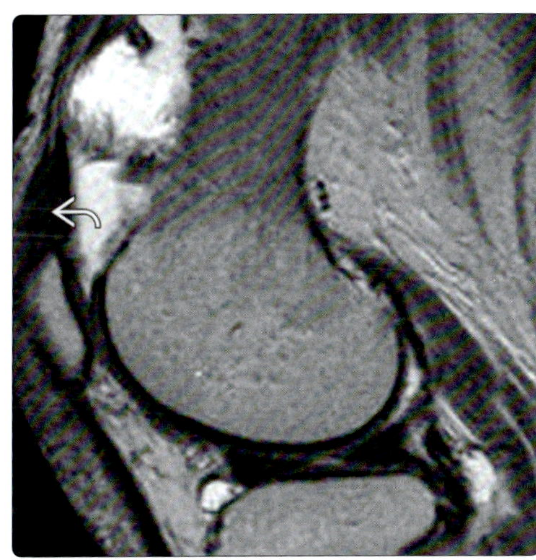

(Left) *Sagittal T1WI MR in a diabetic on long-term dialysis shows low signal thickening of the quadriceps tendon* ➡ *outlined by effusion.* **(Right)** *Sagittal T2WI MR, same patient, shows the quadriceps thickening maintains its low signal* ➡*. Other cuts showed similar signal material filling the intercondylar notch and surrounding the cruciates. This is typical of amyloid deposition, proven by biopsy. Amyloid is very commonly found in patients on long-term dialysis, as is the case with so many diabetics.*

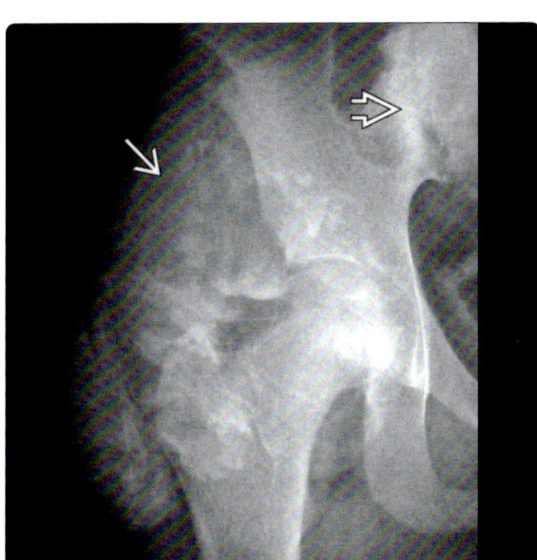

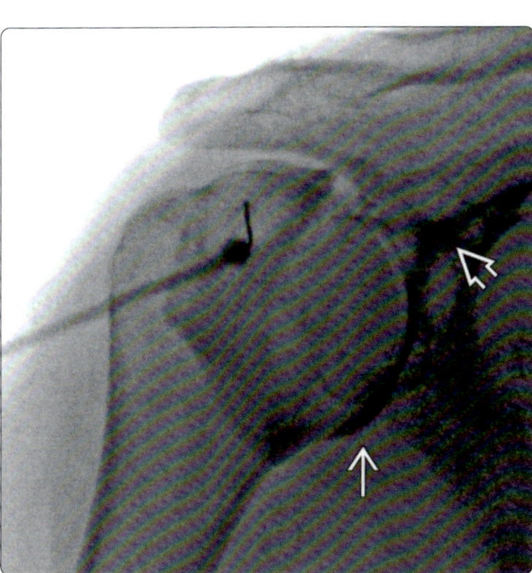

(Left) *AP x-ray shows renal osteodystrophy, (secondary to diabetes in this case), including abnormal bone density with smudgy trabeculae and subchondral resorption of the iliac side of the sacroiliac joint* ➡*. There is prominent cloudy periarticular calcific density* ➡*, typical of the dystrophic calcification that may form following long-term dialysis.* **(Right)** *AP shoulder arthrogram reveals a remarkably tight joint capsule. There is loss of normal axillary* ➡ *and subscapularis* ➡ *recesses in this diabetic with adhesive capsulitis.*

HIV-AIDS

KEY FACTS

TERMINOLOGY

- Set of symptoms and infections resulting from damage to human immune system caused by HIV

IMAGING

- Osteopenia (46-67%)
  - Associated insufficiency fracture
- Infection
  - Osteomyelitis
  - Septic joint
  - Cellulitis: Limited to subcutaneous tissues
  - Necrotizing fasciitis
  - Pyomyositis
- Osteonecrosis
- Tumor: May be osseous or soft tissue
  - Most frequently Kaposi sarcoma or non-Hodgkin lymphoma
- HIV-related arthritis
  - Including CRA, psoriatic, RA or SLE post HAART
- HIV-related marrow abnormalities
  - Repopulated marrow, 2° to anemia of chronic disease
  - Serous atrophy (depletion of red & yellow marrow)
- Inflammatory & noninflammatory myopathy
- HIV-related lipodystrophy

CLINICAL ISSUES

- Musculoskeletal manifestations throughout course of HIV infection; more common with development of AIDS
  - 72% with HIV experience noninfectious MSK symptoms
- Arthralgias & arthritis: Most common complaint; several distinct syndromes

DIAGNOSTIC CHECKLIST

- MSK complaints in HIV patients may stem from
  - Underlying immunodeficiency, directly or indirectly (complications of treatment)
  - Secondary infection
  - Complication of medications used to treat HIV

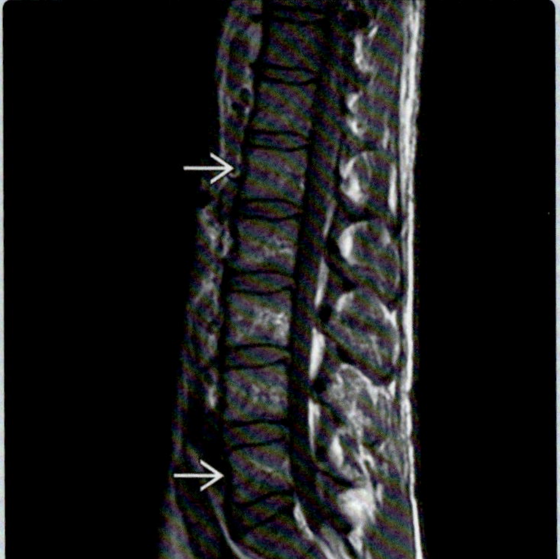

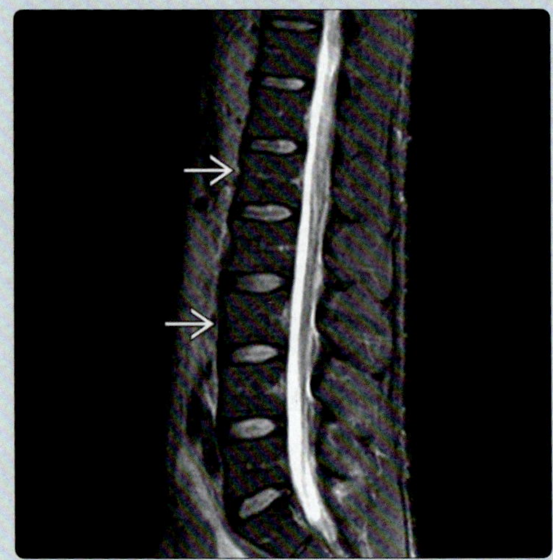

(Left) *Sagittal T1WI MR shows marrow that is lower in SI than is expected ➡. Remember this general rule: With T1 imaging, the marrow should be higher in SI than the disc. This low signal suggests marrow repopulation or infiltration.* **(Right)** *Sagittal STIR MR, same case, shows no significant ↑ SI ➡, making tumor or infection unlikely. Another consideration is a dysplasia affecting 1 of the blood cell lines (erythroid dysplasia resulting from chronic anemia is the most frequent, affecting over 50% of HIV-infected patients).*

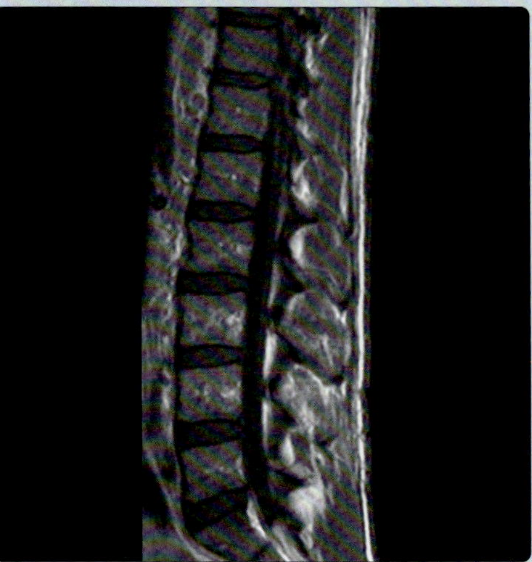

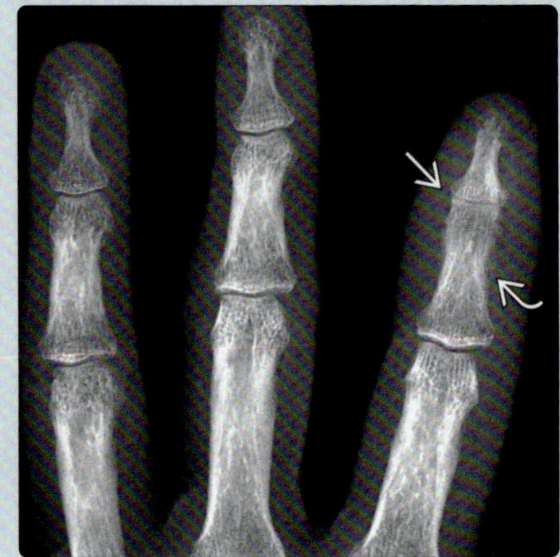

(Left) *Sagittal T1WI C+ FS MR, same patient, shows no significant enhancement of the vertebral bodies, further confirming that infection and tumor need not be considered. It is not uncommon to see this marrow pattern in HIV patients.* **(Right)** *PA radiograph shows soft tissue swelling of the index finger, as well as cartilage narrowing in the DIP ➡. Additionally, there is periostitis that is prominent at the middle phalanx ➡. This is a typical pattern of HIV-related arthritis, similar to that seen in CRA or psoriatic arthritis.*

TERMINOLOGY

Definitions

- Set of symptoms and infections resulting from damage to human immune system caused by HIV
  - Most common musculoskeletal complications include infection, arthritis syndromes, marrow abnormalities, myositis, and tumor formation

IMAGING

Radiographic Findings

- Osteopenia (46-67%); insufficiency fracture
- Osteomyelitis
  - Periosteal reaction
  - Permeative osseous destruction
  - Reactive bone formation
  - Bacillary angiomatosis: Well-defined lytic lesion
- Septic joint
  - Effusion
  - Subchondral bone loss (osteopenic, less sharp)
- Osteonecrosis
  - Early relative sclerosis in central femoral head
  - Later subchondral lucent fracture line & collapse
- Tumor: May be osseous or soft tissue
  - Permeative lytic osseous destruction
  - Periosteal reaction, cortical breakthrough
  - Deep soft tissue mass: Distorts fat planes
  - Kaposi sarcoma: Plaque-like mucocutaneous lesions
    - Rarely contiguous osseous involvement
- HIV-related arthritis
  - Soft tissue swelling, periostitis
  - Juxtaarticular osteopenia
  - Cartilage narrowing, erosions

MR Findings

- HIV-related marrow abnormalities
  - Repopulated marrow, 2° to anemia of chronic disease
    - Focal or diffuse, moderately hypointense SI on T1
    - Remains hypointense on fluid-sensitive sequences
    - Minimal enhancement following contrast
    - Signal dropout > 20% on opposed-phase imaging due to residual marrow fat
  - Marrow replacement by tumor
    - Focal marked hypointense SI on T1
    - Inhomogeneously ↑ SI on T2WI
    - Enhancement > 35% following contrast
    - No signal dropout on opposed-phase imaging
    - Lymphoma is most frequent
      - Circumferential permeation through cortex
  - Serous atrophy (depletion of red & yellow marrow)
    - Generally cachectic patient (minimal subcutaneous fat), related to starvation
    - Focal gray signal T1, ↑ SI on fluid-sensitive sequences
    - Usually coalescent (initially several small foci)
- Soft tissue infection
  - Cellulitis: Limited to subcutaneous tissues
  - Necrotizing fasciitis
    - Extensive high SI T2 fascial fluid
    - ± air in soft tissues, ± muscle necrosis
  - Pyomyositis
    - Low T1 signal (± hyperintense rim, relating to blood products), high T2 signal, rim enhancement
- Osteomyelitis
  - Low SI T1 (confluent)
  - High SI on fluid-sensitive sequences
  - Involved marrow enhances, plus enhancing rim
- Septic arthritis
  - Marrow edema in juxtaarticular bone
  - Effusion, with enhancing synovitis
- Osteonecrosis
  - Typical double line sign; not specific for HIV
- HIV-related arthritis
  - Effusion, juxtaarticular marrow edema
  - Uncommon erosions and periostitis
- Inflammatory myopathy
  - Hyperintense on fluid-sensitive sequences
  - Involved muscles show enhancement
- HIV-related lipodystrophy
  - Normal fat signal, abnormal distribution (↓ or ↑)
  - When symptomatic in Hoffa fat pad, may show ↑ SI on T2 FS imaging

PATHOLOGY

General Features

- Etiology
  - Osteomyelitis, septic arthritis, & pyomyositis result from immunodeficiency 2° to CD4 T-cell depletion
    - Musculoskeletal infectious agents in HIV patients
      - > 70% are *Staphylococcus aureus*
      - Pyogenic sacroiliitis & myositis usually *S. aureus*
      - With advanced CD8 T-cell depletion, fungal & mycobacterial septic arthritis may be seen
  - Lymphocytic infiltrative syndromes result from host response to chronic antigenic stimulation by HIV-1
  - Diffuse infiltrative lymphocytosis syndrome: CD8 T-cell infiltration
  - Immune dysregulation with abnormal cytokine production may be responsible for inflammatory arthritis
    - CD8-dependent diseases, such as reactive arthritis & psoriasis, have more aggressive course in HIV
  - ↑ risk of developing malignancies associated with Epstein-Barr and human herpesvirus 8
    - Kaposi sarcoma (KS): HIV-encoded proteins can directly induce tumor angiogenesis and enhance Kaposi sarcoma-associated herpesvirus transmission to target cells
      - Osseous KS usually 2° to direct extension from mucocutaneous site
      - Skull > vertebrae > pelvis > ribs, sternum
    - Non-Hodgkin lymphoma (NHL): 60x normal incidence
      - Extranodal NHL common in advanced AIDS: Marrow, muscle

CLINICAL ISSUES

Presentation

- Most common signs/symptoms
  - MSK manifestations throughout course of HIV infection but more common with development of AIDS

- 72% of HIV patients → noninfectious MSK symptoms
- Arthralgias & arthritis: Most common complaint; several distinct syndromes
  - HIV painful articular syndrome
    - Severe arthritic pain; often brings patient to emergency department
    - Oligoarticular, asymmetric
    - Knee, elbow, shoulder most common
    - No sign of inflammation on exam; however, must consider septic arthritis
    - Resolves spontaneously, usually within 24 hours
  - HIV-associated arthritis
    - Asymmetric oligoarthritis involving large joints
    - 3-25% prevalence in HIV(+) cohorts
    - Thought to be secondary to HIV itself; viral particles found in synovium
    - Self-limited course; mean duration 6-12 weeks
  - Immune reconstitution inflammatory syndrome
    - Develops in patients receiving highly active antiretroviral therapy (HAART)
    - Paradoxical worsening in clinical status caused by improved inflammatory response to organisms present before initiation of therapy
    - Often in response to mycobacterial infections
  - Spondyloarthropathies [chronic rheumatoid arthritis (CRA) & psoriatic arthritis]
    - Prevalence greater in HIV(+) patients (5-10% have CRA, 6% have psoriatic)
    - Arthritis behaves aggressively in HIV(+) patients
- Osteonecrosis
  - Prevalence of 4.4% in HIV patients
  - Femoral head > knees, shoulders, elbows
  - Protease inhibitors (cause hyperlipidemia) + traditional risk factors considered causative
- Osteoporosis in 46% → risk for fracture
- Hypertrophic osteoarthropathy 2° to pulmonary infections
- Osteomyelitis
  - 1% incidence in HIV patients
  - Patients are often also IV drug users
  - Most common organism *S. aureus*; others *Salmonella*, *Pseudomonas*, *Streptococcus*
  - Pre-HAART, *Bartonella* species often present with lytic bone lesions
  - If CD4 count < 100 μL, consider atypical *Mycobacterium* & fungal diseases
- Septic arthritis
  - Prevalence < 1% of HIV patients
    - Increased risk as CD4 count decreases
  - Patients are often also IV drug users
  - *S. aureus* most common
- Diffuse infiltrative lymphocytosis syndrome: Similar to Sjögren syndrome
  - Bilateral ↑ parotid gland (often massive)
  - Sicca symptoms
  - Extraglandular sites of lymphocytic infiltration
- Muscle complaints
  - Myalgias in 30% HIV(+) patients
  - Polymyositis occurs early in disease
    - Proximal muscle weakness, ↑ creatine kinase
    - May indicate acute HIV seroconversion in patients who have terminated HAART
  - Pyomyositis clinically indistinguishable from polymyositis; MR with contrast makes diagnosis
  - Noninflammatory myopathy associated with zidovudine therapy
  - Rhabdomyolysis 2° to protease inhibitors, alcohol, substance abuse
- HIV-associated lipodystrophy
  - Features of lipoatrophy and lipohypertrophy
    - Abdominal obesity
    - "Buffalo hump"
    - Decreased facial and subcutaneous fat
  - 2° to protease inhibitor & other antiretroviral drugs
  - Predominantly problem of cosmesis
  - May be symptomatic involving Hoffa fat pad

Demographics

- Epidemiology
  - 75% of AIDS patients develop MSK complications
    - Occur later in disease or in those with AIDS
  - Arthralgia/myalgia: 1/3 of patients with HIV
  - Tumors: Kaposi sarcoma (KS) > NHL
    - KS seen in up to 20% of patients with AIDS
    - Lymphoma 60x more frequent in HIV patients than normal population
    - Increase in prevalence of NHL in AIDS population since introduction of HAART therapy
  - Osteonecrosis in 4.4% HIV patients, osteoporosis in 46%

Natural History & Prognosis

- HIV infection can be latent for many years
- Progression from HIV to AIDS ~ 11 years after infection
- Sarcoid & autoimmune diseases (rheumatoid arthritis, SLE) reappear or worsen with HAART

Treatment

- Optimize HAART
- Septic joint: Antimicrobial therapy tailored to organism
- Arthritis: Same as for CRA/psoriatic arthritis (DMARDS, perhaps TNF inhibitors)
- Polymyositis: Prednisone
- Diffuse infiltrative lymphocytosis syndrome: Prednisone; may respond to antiretroviral Rx alone

DIAGNOSTIC CHECKLIST

Consider

- MSK complaints in HIV patients may stem from
  - Underlying immunodeficiency, directly or indirectly
    - Secondary infection
    - Complication of medications used to treat HIV

SELECTED REFERENCES

1. Booth TC et al: Update on imaging of non-infectious musculoskeletal complications of HIV infection. Skeletal Radiol. 41(11):1349-63, 2012
2. Nguyen BY et al: Rheumatic manifestations associated with HIV in the highly active antiretroviral therapy era. Curr Opin Rheumatol. 21(4):404-10, 2009
3. Marquez J et al: HIV-associated musculoskeletal involvement. AIDS Read. 14(4):175-9, 183-4, 2004

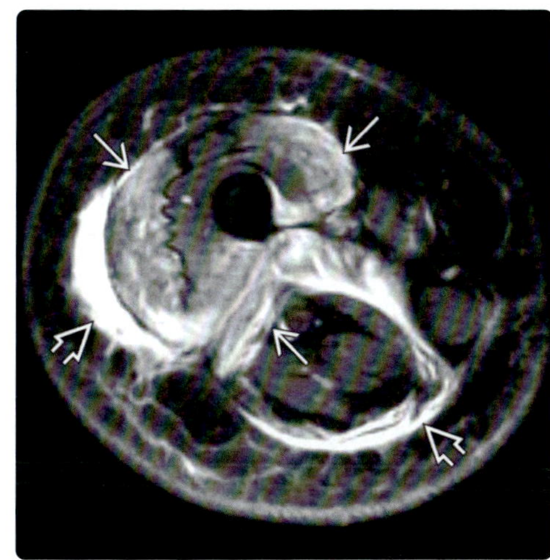

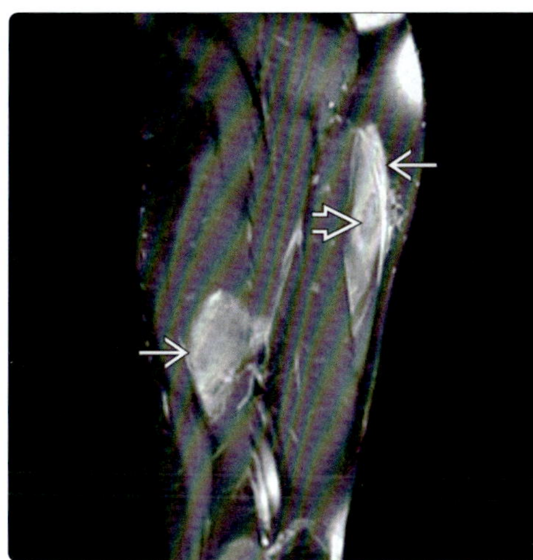

(Left) *Axial PDWI FS MR in an AIDS patient with myositis and fasciitis shows enlargement and increased T2 signal in the vastus musculature ➡ extending posteriorly. Fluid is tracking along the fascial planes ➡.* **(Right)** *Coronal T1WI C+ FS MR shows abnormal enhancement of the vastus lateralis and semimembranosus ➡. This AIDS patient has myositis. Note the focal nonenhancing area ➡, indicating myonecrosis.*

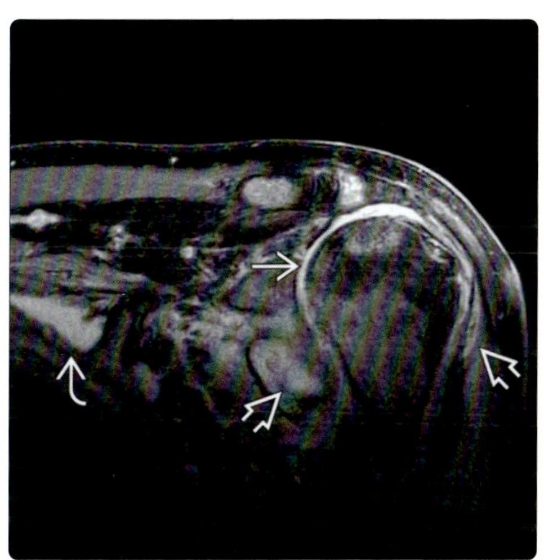

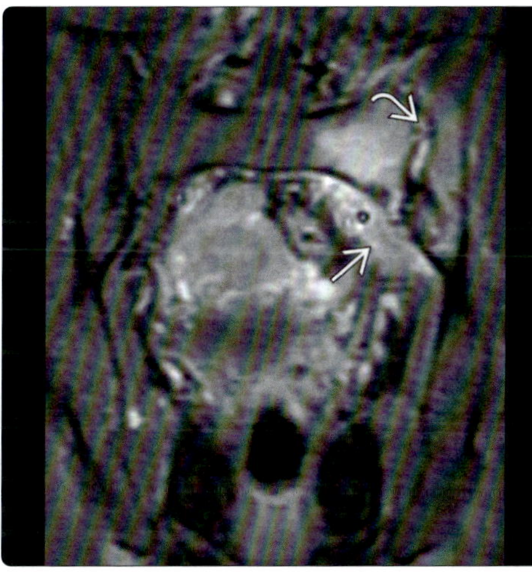

(Left) *Coronal PDWI FS MR shows septic arthritis with destruction of the glenohumeral joint ➡ and inflammatory changes in the surrounding soft tissues ➡ in an HIV-infected IV drug abuser. Note the soft tissue abscess in the chest wall ➡.* **(Right)** *Coronal T2WI FS MR shows fluid within the left sacroiliac joint ➡ and high signal within the adjacent bones. Note the swollen iliacus ➡. This is septic arthritis in a patient with HIV. S. Aureus is the most common infecting agent.*

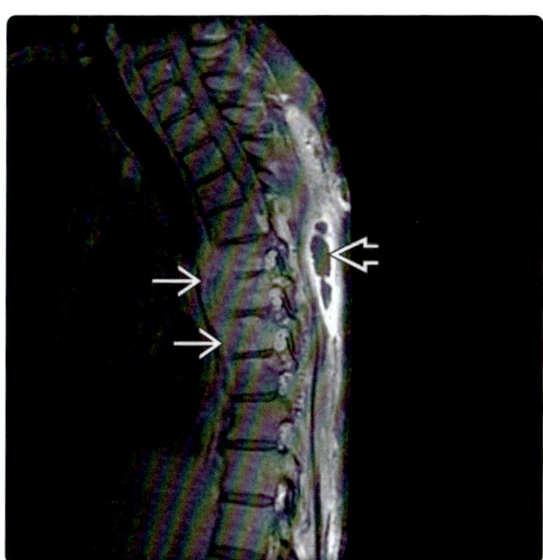

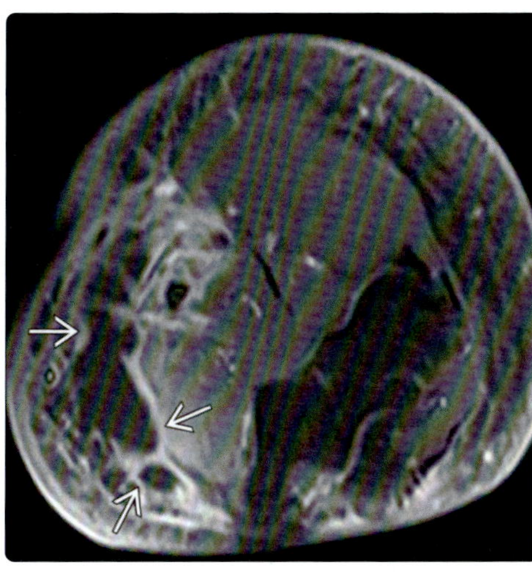

(Left) *Sagittal T1WI C+ FS MR shows subligamentous spread of tuberculous discitis/osteomyelitis of the thoracic spine ➡, extending across multiple vertebrae. Note the large posterior soft tissues abscess ➡.* **(Right)** *Axial postcontrast T1FS MR in a patient with HIV shows diffuse soft tissue swelling and subcutaneous edema. There is also a multiloculated fluid collection ➡ surrounded by a thick enhancing rim. This pyomyositis is at an injection site.*

(Left) *AP radiograph of the right lower extremity shows diffuse, plaque-like soft tissue thickening ➡ with circumferential involvement. The appearance is nonspecific, but this proved to be a typical case of AIDS-related Kaposi sarcoma.* **(Right)** *Coronal T1WI MR shows the soft tissues of the 3rd toe ➡ to be diffusely enlarged. The mass appears nodular, with nonspecific signal nearly isointense to skeletal muscle; this is Kaposi sarcoma. Rarely, this mucocutaneous sarcoma may result in extrinsic invasion of the adjacent bone.*

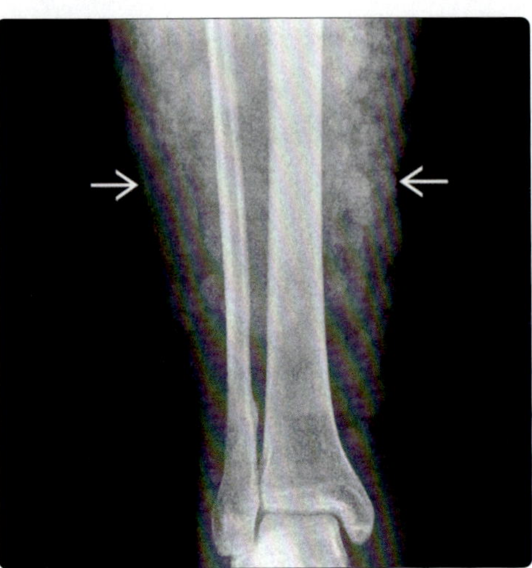

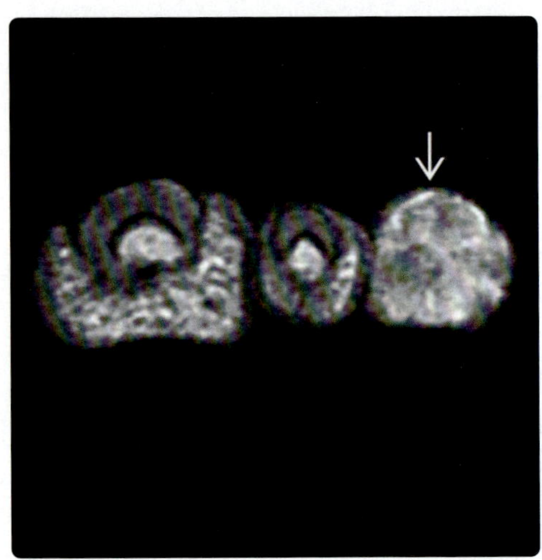

(Left) *Sagittal T1WI C+ FS MR shows a typical case of AIDS-related Kaposi sarcoma. Nodular thickened soft tissues about the great toe ➡ show diffuse enhancement. Kaposi sarcoma allows a definitive diagnosis of AIDS.* **(Right)** *Axial T2WI FS MR shows lymphoma in a patient with HIV-AIDS. ↑ SI marrow replaces the acetabulum, with a small associated soft tissue mass ➡. Lymphoma typically shows tumor cells percolating through small defects in the cortex to form a circumferential mass, as in this case.*

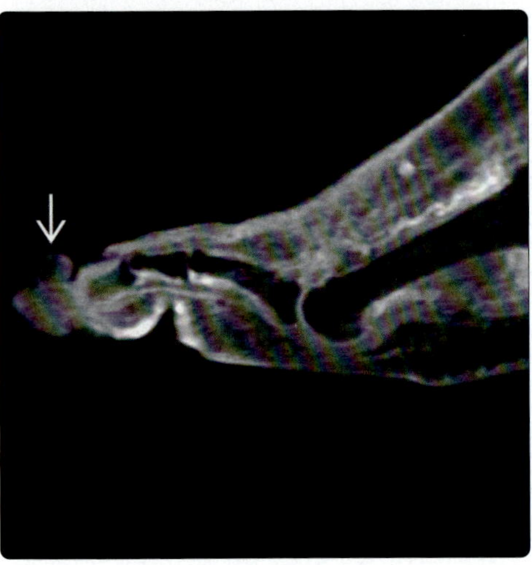

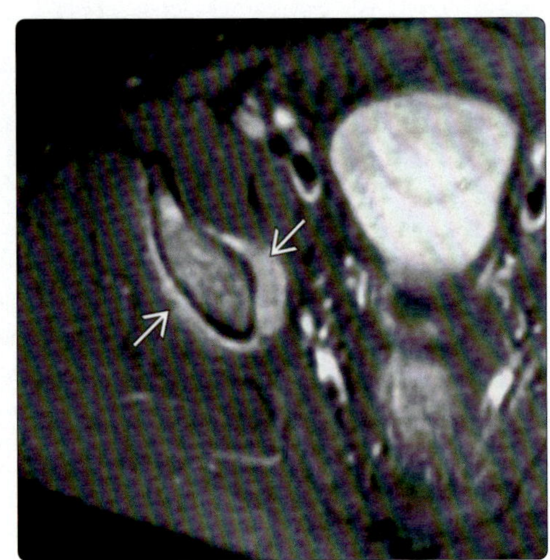

(Left) *Coronal T1WI MR shows hypointense marrow replacement of the left acetabulum ➡ in this AIDS patient with lymphoma. Note the osteonecrosis on the right ➡, a common complication from AIDS.* **(Right)** *Frogleg lateral radiograph, different patient, shows an extensive subchondral lucency ➡ with minimal flattening, indicating osteonecrosis. This process develops in 4% of patients with HIV, likely related to treatment along with concomitant factors such as alcohol abuse.*

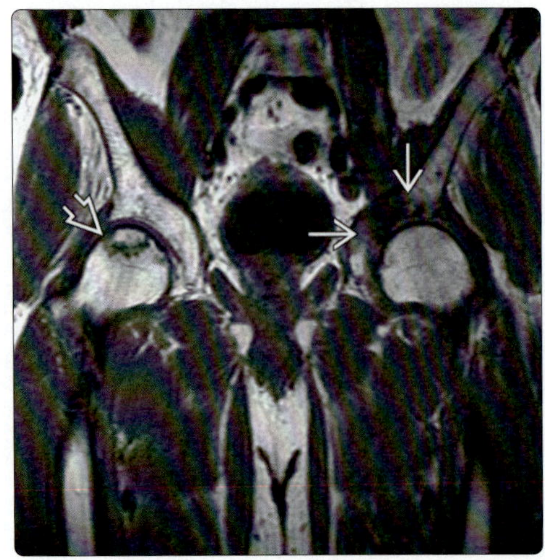

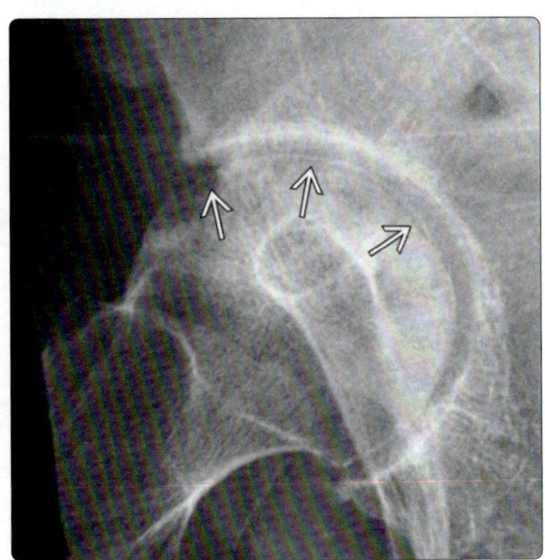

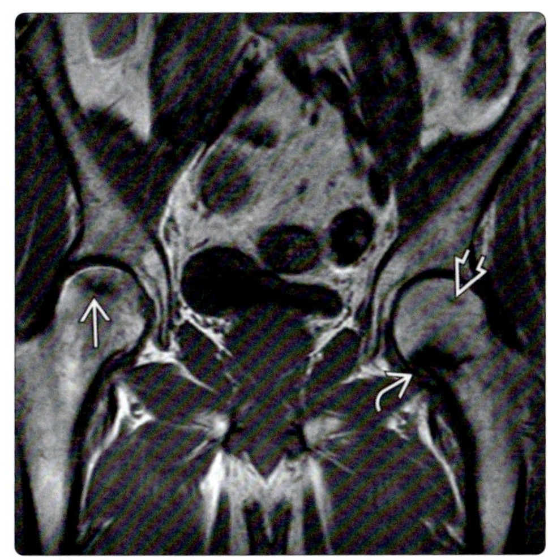

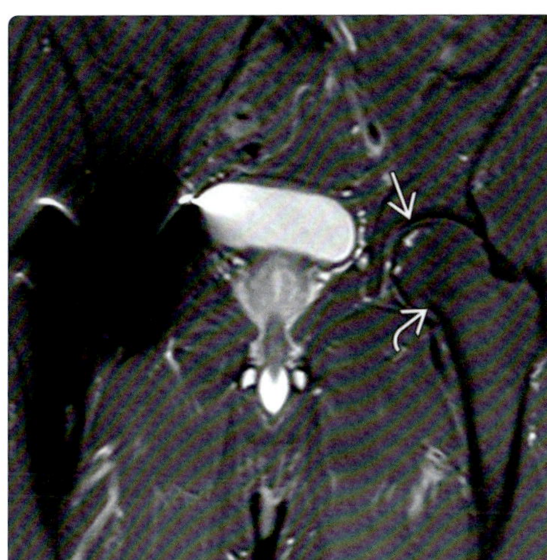

(Left) *Coronal T1 MR in a patient with HIV-AIDS shows a subchondral fracture indicating osteonecrosis of the right hip. There is also an incomplete insufficiency fracture of the left hip and a small focus of abnormality in the left femoral head. Nearly half of HIV patients develop osteoporosis and are at risk for fracture.* **(Right)** *Coronal T2 FS MR, same patient 1 year later, shows right hip arthroplasty. The left hip subcapital fracture has healed, but there is new evidence of left hip osteonecrosis.*

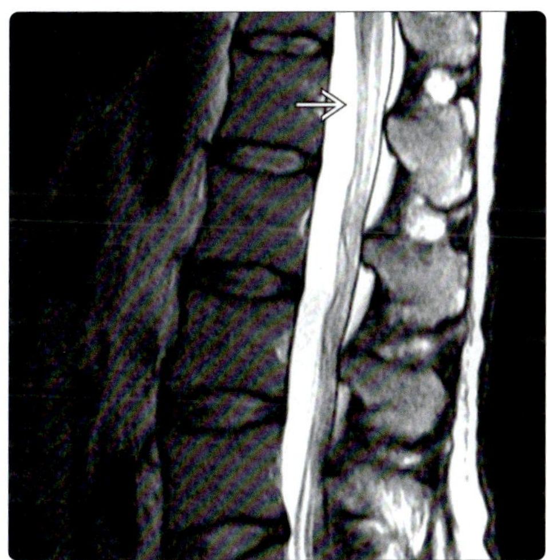

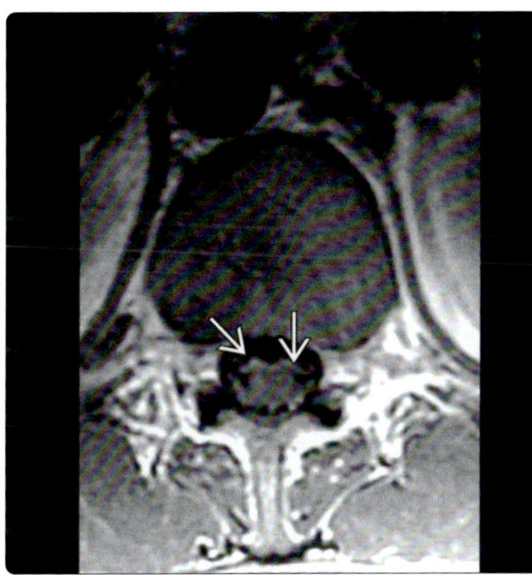

(Left) *Sagittal T2WI MR demonstrates very mild thickening of the proximal cauda equina. This patient has HIV-AIDS and contrast administration is essential to evaluate for subtle opportunistic infection or neoplasm.* **(Right)** *Axial T1WI C+ MR, same case, shows diffuse enhancement of the cauda equina; this is proven CMV radiculitis.*

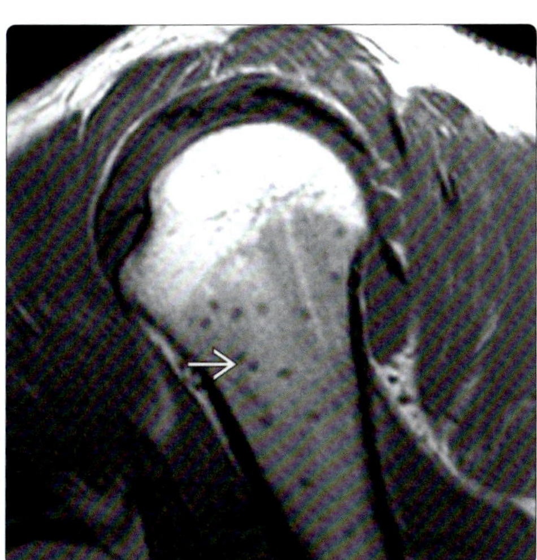

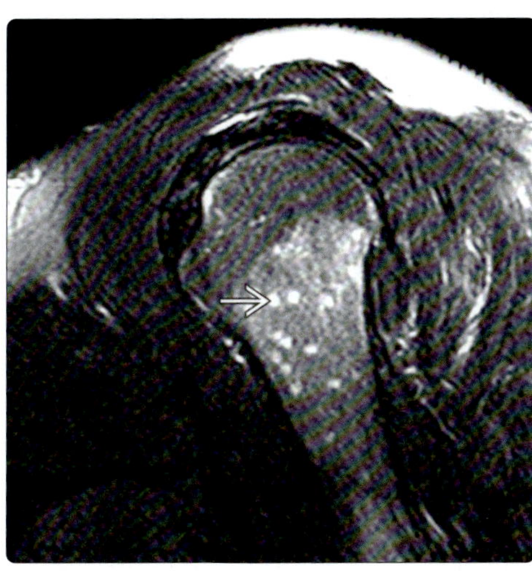

(Left) *Sagittal T1WI MR shows multiple low signal foci on a background of low signal marrow repopulation in a young HIV(+) man. This is a nonspecific appearance; biopsy proved early serous atrophy.* **(Right)** *Sagittal T2WI FS MR, same case, shows the small foci to be hyperintense. This early case of serous atrophy is atypical; generally the lesions are coalescent and the patient is more cachectic than is apparent in this case. (Courtesy S. Moore, MD.)*

KEY FACTS

TERMINOLOGY

- Inflammatory disorder of unknown cause resulting in noncaseating granulomatous deposits in tissues, including bone

IMAGING

- Radiographic findings: Lacy lytic bone lesions in hands and feet
  - Virtually pathognomonic in setting of clinical sarcoidosis
- Large lesions may occur, without lacy pattern
  - Surprisingly often occult on radiograph
  - When visible, geographic
  - May be lytic, sclerotic, or mixed density
- Small lesions in long bones or axial skeleton usually occult on radiograph
- MR imaging nonspecific
  - T1WI: Low signal, homogeneous
  - Fluid-sensitive sequences: Homogeneous, ↑ SI
  - Enhances with contrast

CLINICAL ISSUES

- Associated with pulmonary lesions in ~ 90% of cases
  - Small bone sarcoidosis lesions associated with sarcoidosis skin lesions
- Peak incidence: 20-39 years
- In USA, preponderance in African Americans relative to Caucasians (3-4x risk)

DIAGNOSTIC CHECKLIST

- Consider sarcoidosis in differential diagnosis of patients with history of malignancy who develop lymphadenopathy or bone lesions
- Discriminators allowing confident differentiation of sarcoidosis bone lesions from osseous metastases on MR not established
  - Presence of fat in lesion suggests sarcoidosis
  - Biopsy required for definitive diagnosis

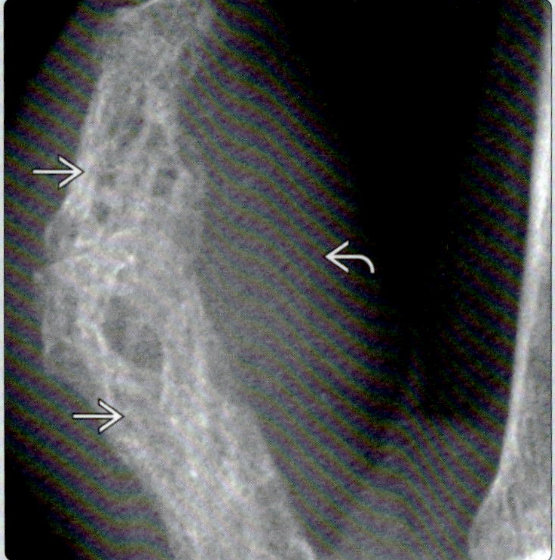

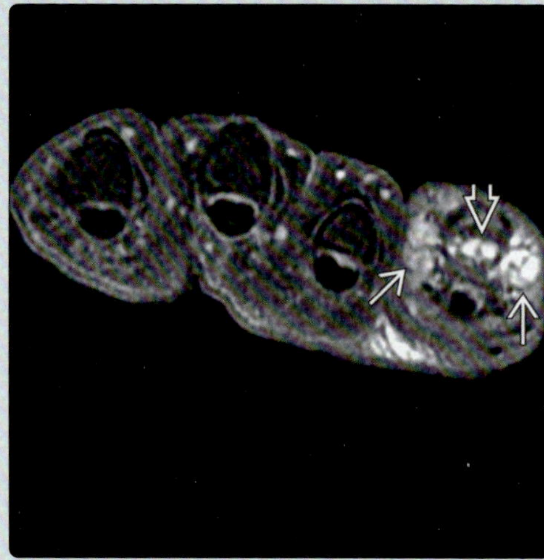

(Left) *Oblique radiograph of the thumb in a patient with sarcoidosis demonstrates the characteristic lacy osteolysis and trabecular thickening of small bone sarcoidosis ➡. Granulomas extend into the soft tissues, causing diffuse swelling ➡.* **(Right)** *Axial PDWI FS MR demonstrates fluid signal granulomata within the medullary space of the 5th proximal phalanx ➡, and lobulated granulomatous deposits in the surrounding soft tissues ➡. Conglomerate lesions of the phalanges may break through cortex, as seen in this case.*

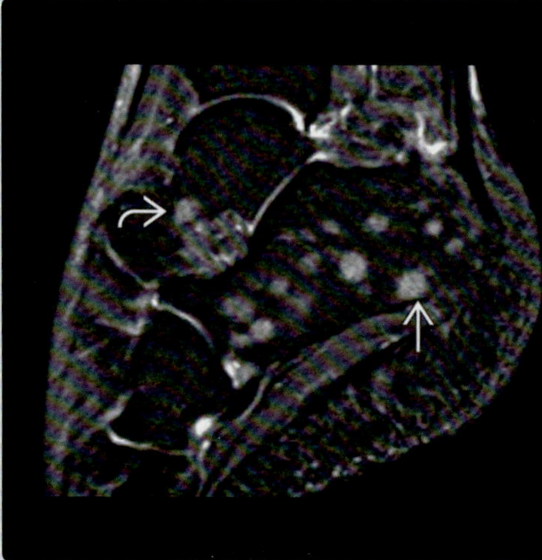

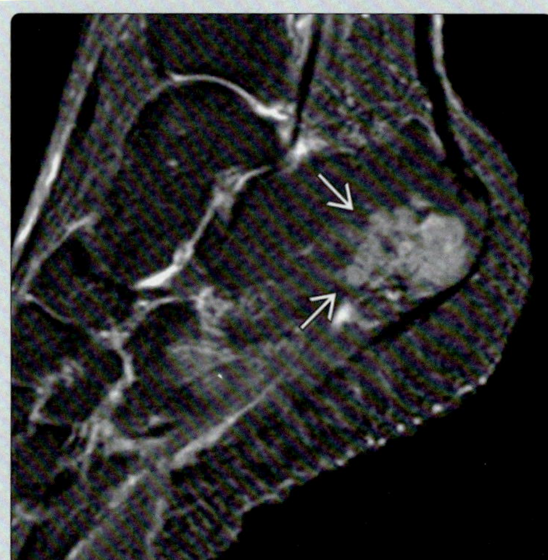

(Left) *Sagittal PDWI FS MR demonstrates multiple cannonball-like bright foci in the calcaneus ➡ and talar neck ➡. Some of the calcaneal lesions demonstrate a brush-like border. Radiographs were negative.* **(Right)** *Sagittal PDWI FS MR in the same patient shows the contralateral calcaneus with a coalescent lesion ➡, also intermediate to bright on fluid-sensitive images. Coalescent lesions may have a much more irregular border than individual small lesions.*

TERMINOLOGY

Definitions

- Inflammatory disorder of unknown cause resulting in noncaseating granulomatous deposits in tissues
  - Lungs/lymph nodes most frequently affected
  - Wide variety of musculoskeletal manifestations
    - Bone, muscle, joint, soft tissue; bone discussed in this section

IMAGING

General Features

- Best diagnostic clue
  - Lacy lytic bone lesions in hands and feet
    - Virtually pathognomonic in setting of clinical sarcoidosis
    - Large lesions may occur, without lacy pattern
  - Lesions in long bones and axial skeleton may be radiographically and scintigraphically occult; best detected on MR
    - Often multiple, with imaging features that mimic osseous metastases or multiple myeloma
- Location
  - Can occur in any bone
    - Lesions often favor more distal extremities
      - Acral location may help differentiate from metastases
- Size
  - Most range from 2 mm to 1 cm in diameter
  - Coalescent lesions may be larger
- Morphology
  - Lesions often discrete and may be irregularly shaped or round (cannonball-like)
    - Indistinctly marginated sarcoidosis bone lesions likely reflect regressing lesions
      - Often contain central fat if regressing
  - Coalescent lesions may have highly irregular contour

Imaging Recommendations

- Best imaging tool
  - Radiographs usually suffice for hand and foot sarcoidosis lesions
    - MR may reveal more extensive involvement
  - Large lesions occasionally radiographically occult
    - Axial lesions occult as well
    - Revealed by MR
- Protocol advice
  - Routine marrow sequences (T1 and fluid sensitive, fat saturated)
    - Contrast imaging not required
      - Lesions enhance, but conspicuity or specificity not improved

Radiographic Findings

- Lesions in digits generally lytic, geographic
  - Lacy trabecular configuration considered pathognomonic
  - Characteristically no periosteal reaction
  - Generally no cortical breakthrough
    - Cortical breech may occur when coalescent granulomata in digit becomes large
- Large bone lesions
  - Surprisingly often occult on radiograph
  - When visible, geographic
  - May be lytic, sclerotic, or mixed density

CT Findings

- Bone CT
  - Phalangeal lesions mimic radiographic appearance
  - Large bone lesions
    - As with radiograph, may not be visible on CT
      - May demonstrate faint, cloud-like sclerosis
      - Makes CT-guided biopsy (of lesion detected on MR) challenging
    - May be discrete sclerotic or lytic lesions

MR Findings

- MR imaging nonspecific
  - T1WI: Low signal, homogeneous, though may contain fatty foci (presumed involuting)
  - Fluid-sensitive sequences: Homogeneous, high signal
  - Enhance with contrast
  - When multifocal, scattered throughout skeleton, but most common at metaphyses
    - Presumed hematogenous dissemination
- Opposed-phase sequences
  - Variable findings: May or may not drop significantly in signal intensity

Nuclear Medicine Findings

- TcMDP bone scan
  - Variable uptake but may appear normal
- PET/CT
  - Sarcoid shows FDG uptake (frequency unknown)
    - May be false-positive for metastatic disease

DIFFERENTIAL DIAGNOSIS

Enchondroma

- Extremely common lesion in tubular bones
  - Especially hand and foot
- Often lytic and expanded
- Does not have lacy pattern of sarcoid
  - If lacy pattern present, differential not difficult

Tuberous Sclerosis

- Lytic geographic lesion, often in phalanges
- Should not contain lacy trabeculae or internal matrix
- Clinical differentiation from sarcoid

Metastases, Bone Marrow

- Lytic or sclerotic, usually rather geographic
- Generally not acral in position
- MR signal intensity or enhancement characteristics identical to sarcoid
- Biopsy may be required for definitive differentiation in lesions of large bones

Multiple Myeloma

- Generally multiple lytic lesions, usually not acral
- May not be visible on radiograph

- Same MR imaging characteristics as sarcoid; biopsy, laboratory findings required for differentiation

PATHOLOGY

General Features

- Etiology
  - Multiple disease/risk factor associations proposed
    - Interactions between environment and genetic factors are implicated
- Genetics
  - Familial clusters suggest genetic susceptibility
  - ACCESS study suggests genetic heterogeneity of sarcoidosis risk among different populations
  - Candidate genes for sarcoidosis susceptibility are emerging from genomics research
    - Linkages to chromosome 5 (in African Americans) and chromosome 6 (in Germans)
- Associated abnormalities
  - Small bone sarcoidosis lesions associated with sarcoidosis skin lesions

Staging, Grading, & Classification

- No system for grading musculoskeletal lesions
  - Whole body marrow MR imaging: Useful estimate of granulomatous load

Gross Pathologic & Surgical Features

- Granulomas: Well-circumscribed soft tissue lesions
  - May resemble metastatic tumor

Microscopic Features

- Sarcoid granulomas
  - Well-circumscribed collections of epithelioid histiocytes and multinucleated histiocytic giant cells
  - Surrounded by fibrous tissue, sometimes containing lymphocytes
  - Central necrosis common
- Note: Nonnecrotizing granulomas may also be found in
  - Fungal infections
  - Leprosy
  - Atypical mycobacteriosis
  - Foreign body reactions
  - Occasionally tuberculosis

CLINICAL ISSUES

Presentation

- Most common signs/symptoms
  - May be asymptomatic
  - May cause musculoskeletal symptoms
    - Pain, arthralgias
  - Large bone sarcoidosis often incidental finding in studies performed for other indications
- Other signs/symptoms
  - Associated with pulmonary lesions in ~ 90% of cases

Demographics

- Age
  - Usually develops < 50 years
  - Peak incidence: 20-39 years
    - Disease presents later in African Americans
- Gender
  - Female preponderance (< 2x)
- Ethnicity
  - In USA, preponderance in African Americans relative to Caucasians (3-4x risk)
    - Generally more severe manifestations of sarcoid, including marrow involvement
    - Siblings of patients with sarcoidosis have 5x risk of developing sarcoid
- Epidemiology
  - Incidence of sarcoidosis varies worldwide
  - Bone lesions occur in 5-13% of sarcoidosis patients
    - Estimate based on radiographic data
    - Likely underestimates large bone and axial lesions

Natural History & Prognosis

- Clinical course highly variable
  - Up to 2/3 have spontaneous remission within 3-10 years of onset
- Sarcoidosis of large bone and axial skeletal lesions detected on MR may involute → fibrofatty "ghost"

Treatment

- To ameliorate symptoms &/or if organ function is threatened
- Corticosteroids: Standard and efficacious
  - Suppress TNF-α and other cytokines
  - Uncertain if steroids provide long-term modification
  - Side affects may confound assessment of lesions
- TNF antagonists (used in treatment of rheumatoid arthritis) used in some cases of sarcoidosis

DIAGNOSTIC CHECKLIST

Consider

- Large bone lesions have differential diagnosis of metastases or multiple myeloma
  - Consider sarcoidosis in differential diagnosis of patients with history of malignancy who develop lymphadenopathy or bone lesions
  - If clinical diagnosis of sarcoidosis, imperative to obtain tissue diagnosis prior to instituting therapy for presumed metastases
- Discriminators allowing confident differentiation of sarcoidosis bone lesions from osseous metastases on MR not established
  - Presence of fat within (or replacing) lesions suggests involuting granulomata, and in patients with known sarcoidosis, strongly suggests diagnosis of sarcoidosis rather than metastasis (excellent specificity but poor sensitivity)
  - Biopsy may be required for definitive diagnosis
- When large bone lesions are encountered on MR, diagnosis of osseous sarcoidosis should be advanced with caution if sarcoidosis diagnosis has not been otherwise established

SELECTED REFERENCES

1. Lew PP et al: Imaging of disorders affecting the bone and skin. Radiographics. 34(1):197-216, 2014
2. Vardhanabhuti V et al: Sarcoidosis–the greatest mimic. Semin Ultrasound CT MR. 35(3):215-24, 2014
3. Moore SL et al: Can sarcoidosis and metastatic bone lesions be reliably differentiated on routine MRI? AJR Am J Roentgenol. 198(6):1387-93, 2012

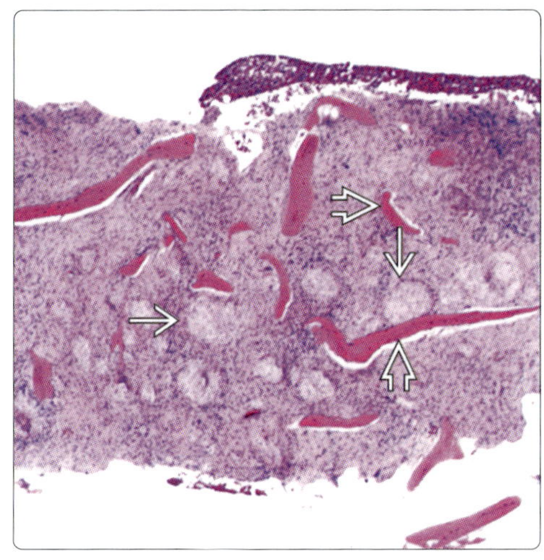

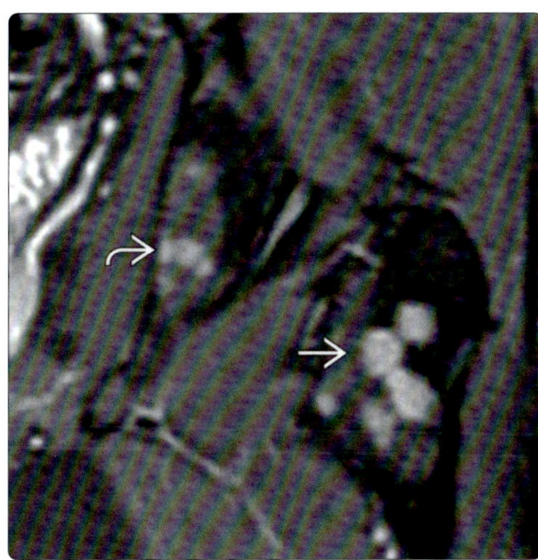

(Left) *Low-power micrograph of a core biopsy specimen of sarcoidosis shows a noncaseating granulomata ➡ insinuating between the trabeculae ➡. (Courtesy M. Klein, MD.)* **(Right)** *Coronal PDWI FS MR of the left proximal femur in a 45-year-old man with sarcoidosis demonstrates cannonball-like lesions in the left intertrochanteric region ➡. Also note ischial lesions ➡. Each of 2 biopsies were nondiagnostic. These lesions were occult on radiographs, and had nearly vanished on 6-month follow-up MR.*

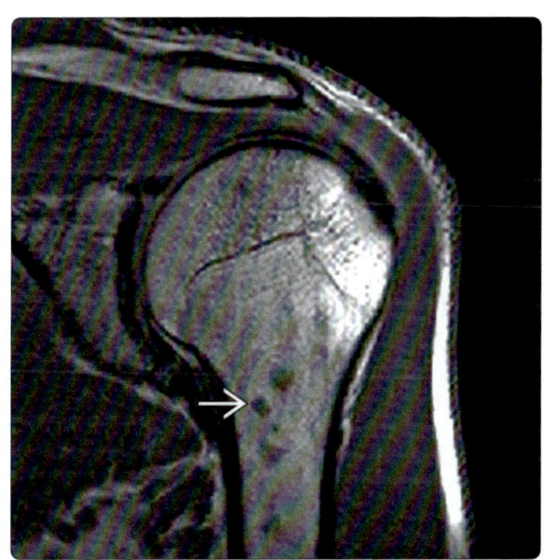

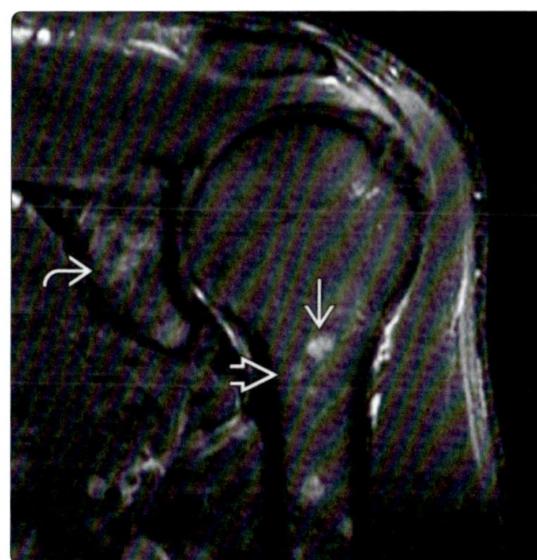

(Left) *Coronal T1WI MR demonstrates rounded and irregular intramedullary lesions ➡ in a 48-year-old man with biopsy-proven noncaseating granulomata of the left humerus. These are low signal but slightly hyperintense to muscle.* **(Right)** *Coronal T2WI FS MR in the same patient shows lesions with faintly increased ➡ to bright ➡ T2 signal intensity. Involvement of the glenoid is also noted ➡. Without clinical information or biopsy, differentiation from metastases or multiple myeloma is not possible.*

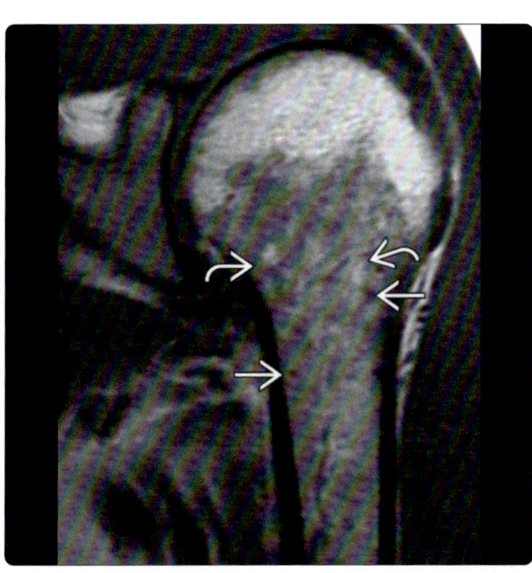

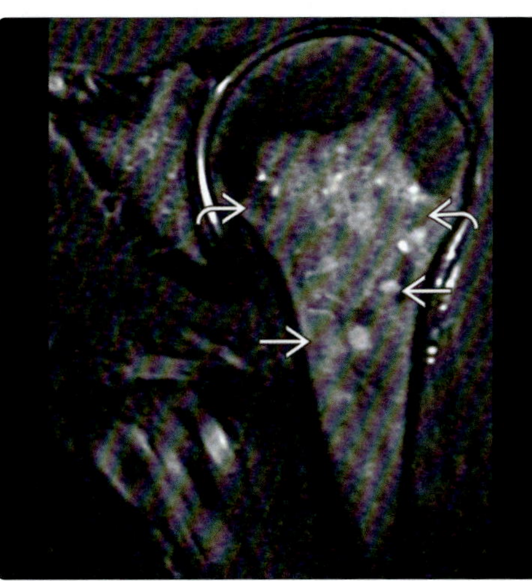

(Left) *Coronal T1 MR in a different patient with known sarcoidosis shows hypointense small foci ➡. Note also that there are some foci that contain fat signal ➡.* **(Right)** *Coronal T2 FS MR, same patient, shows that most of the lesions that were hypointense on T1 now are hyperintense ➡. However, those lesions that appeared fatty on T1 are now saturated out, confirming adipose tissue ➡. The presence of fat within some of the lesions suggests sarcoid granulomata (in the appropriate clinical setting) as opposed to metastatic disease.*

KEY FACTS

TERMINOLOGY

- Sarcoidosis muscle involvement may present as
  - Granulomatous nodules
  - Myositis
  - Myopathy
- Muscle lesions reported in 1.4% of sarcoidosis cases
- 50-80% of sarcoidosis patients if biopsied demonstrate skeletal muscle granulomata
  - Usually asymptomatic

IMAGING

- Muscle granulomata
  - MR findings
    - Present as fusiform, longitudinally oriented (cord-like) intramuscular nodules on sagittal and coronal views
    - May have central low-signal umbilication (dark star appearance) most conspicuous on T2WI and postcontrast imaging due to peripheral bright signal
    - Subtle or occult on T1WI, isointense with muscle
  - CT findings
    - Muscle granulomata may be occult; use of contrast may enhance conspicuity of lesions
    - Comparison of bilateral lower extremities helps identify lesions
- Sarcoidosis myositis
  - Diffuse intramuscular high T1 feathering or complete fatty replacement of muscle
  - Muscle edema on fluid-sensitive sequences
  - Enhancement of regions of muscle sarcoidosis
  - Proximal > distal muscle involvement
  - MR appearance nonspecific relative to other inflammatory myopathy etiologies

TOP DIFFERENTIAL DIAGNOSES

- Corticosteroid therapy may result in muscle atrophy
  - Differentiation of sarcoid from corticosteroid myopathy based on clinical grounds

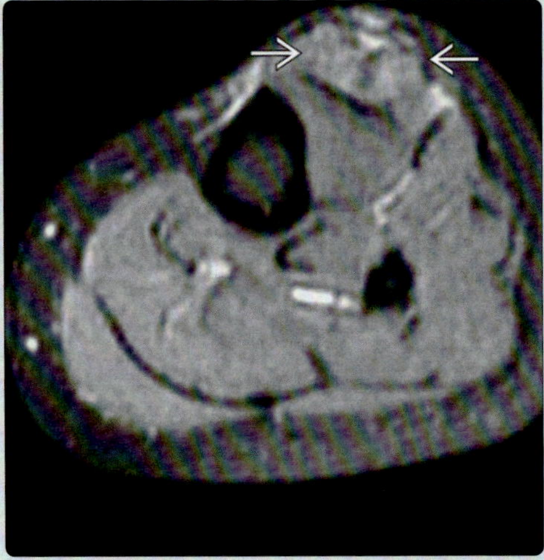

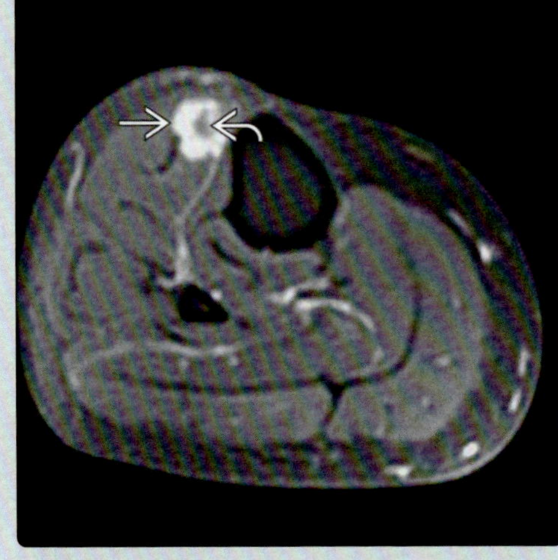

(Left) *Axial T2WI FS MR shows a muscle nodule in the anterior compartment* ➡ *of the left calf. There is mild muscle fullness, and the lesion is faintly bright on T2WI. This middle-aged woman with sarcoidosis complained of tender calf masses.* **(Right)** *Axial T1WI C+ FS MR is from the same patient. Sarcoidosis muscle nodules were also seen in the contralateral calf. Contrast administration reveals peripheral enhancement* ➡ *& low-signal umbilication; the dark star* ➡ *appearance is characteristic of sarcoidosis muscle nodules.*

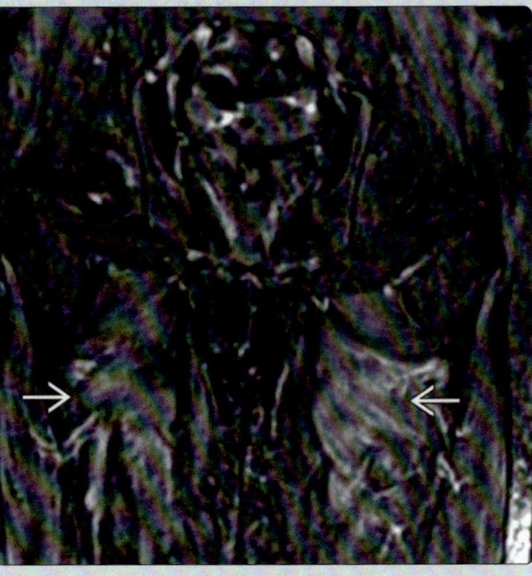

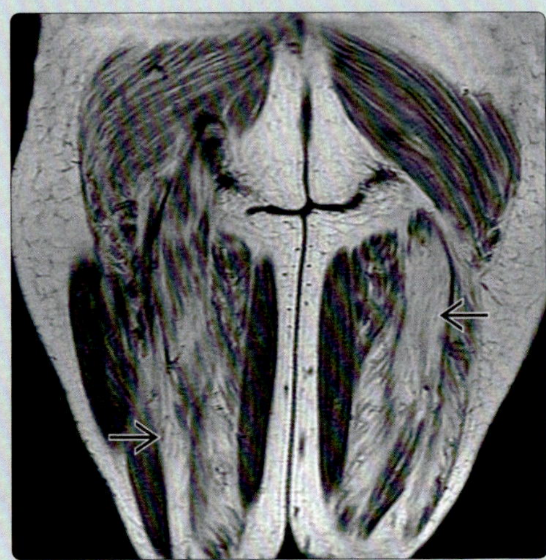

(Left) *Coronal STIR MR demonstrates muscle edema in the bilateral adductor compartments* ➡ *in a middle-aged woman with sarcoidosis. The muscle edema enhanced on postcontrast image (not shown). The MR appearance is nonspecific.* **(Right)** *Coronal T1WI MR in a woman with sarcoidosis and proximal thigh weakness shows fatty replacement greatest in the posterior compartments* ➡*. Histologic examination of the tissue revealed noncaseating granulomata. Corticosteroid treatment may cause an identical appearance.*

TERMINOLOGY

Definitions

- Sarcoidosis muscle involvement that may manifest as
  - Intramuscular granulomatous nodules
  - Myositis
  - Myopathy

IMAGING

General Features

- Best diagnostic clue
  - Sarcoidosis muscle nodules
    - Longitudinally oriented nodules at musculotendinous junction in patient with sarcoidosis
  - Sarcoidal myositis
    - Muscle edema that enhances with contrast administration in patient with sarcoidosis
    - Noncaseating granulomata found at biopsy
  - Sarcoidosis myopathy: Proximal muscle atrophy with fatty replacement
- Location
  - Sarcoid nodules
    - Generally in region of musculotendinous junction
    - Usually lower extremities
  - Sarcoid myositis/myopathy
    - Usually lower extremities, proximal > distal
- Size
  - Sarcoid muscle nodules: Variable, 1- to 2-cm range
    - Larger if nodules are coalescent
- Morphology
  - Sarcoid muscle nodules: Intramuscular, longitudinally oriented fusiform masses
  - Sarcoid myositis/myopathy: Feathery pattern along length of involved muscle

CT Findings

- CT is limited for assessment of sarcoidosis myositis
  - Muscle nodules isodense with muscle and occult on CT
    - Bilateral asymmetry may be useful in diagnosis
    - Contrast increases conspicuity
  - Myositis: May enhance; myopathy: Fatty atrophy

MR Findings

- Sarcoid muscle nodules
  - Fusiform, longitudinally oriented nodules
  - May be isointense with muscle on T1WI
  - Inhomogeneous increased SI on T2WI
  - Conspicuity increases with contrast enhancement
  - May contain central low signal umbilication (dark star appearance) on T2WI or T1WI C+ FS
  - Coronal and sagittal planes may show elongated, cord-like appearance of nodules
- Sarcoidosis myositis
  - MR appearance nonspecific
    - T1WI appears normal
    - Fluid-sensitive sequences show ↑ SI muscle edema
    - Enhancement of involved muscles
- Sarcoidosis myopathy
  - Diffuse intramuscular high T1 SI with "feathering"
  - Complete fatty atrophy of muscle

DIFFERENTIAL DIAGNOSIS

Steroid Therapy

- Muscle atrophy may appear identical to sarcoid myopathy
- Differentiation may be made on clinical grounds

Polymyositis

- May have identical MR appearance to sarcoid myositis
- Clinical presentation may be identical

Soft Tissue Tumor

- Sarcoid granuloma with low SI center may resemble target sign of nerve sheath tumors; umbilicated appearance may help differentiation
- Tumor is generally better defined relative to surrounding muscle than sarcoidal nodules

PATHOLOGY

Microscopic Features

- Typical sarcoid granulomata if muscle nodular form
- Discrete mass not evident with sarcoid myopathy
  - Meticulous histologic examination of tissue reveals noncaseating granulomata

CLINICAL ISSUES

Presentation

- Most common signs/symptoms
  - Sarcoid muscle nodules
    - Palpable mass, often multiple and bilateral
    - May be tender
  - Generalized sarcoid myopathy
    - Resembles polymyositis clinically
      - □ Symmetric proximal weakness
      - □ Elevated serum creatine kinase and aldolase
      - □ Myopathy by EMG evaluation

Demographics

- Epidemiology
  - Discrete muscle sarcoidosis lesions reported in 1.4% of known sarcoidosis cases
  - 50-80% of sarcoidosis patients, if biopsied, demonstrate skeletal muscle granulomata but usually asymptomatic

Natural History & Prognosis

- Sarcoidosis muscle granulomata may resolve over time ± treatment

Treatment

- Sarcoid muscle nodules may be treated with steroids

DIAGNOSTIC CHECKLIST

Consider

- Differential diagnosis for each form of muscle sarcoid may not have distinctive features for differentiation
  - Clinical history important to lead to correct Dx

SELECTED REFERENCES

1. Vardhanabhuti V et al: Sarcoidosis–the greatest mimic. Semin Ultrasound CT MR. 35(3):215-24, 2014
2. Schulze M et al: MRI findings in inflammatory muscle diseases and their noninflammatory mimics. AJR Am J Roentgenol. 192(6):1708-16, 2009

Sarcoidosis: Joint

KEY FACTS

TERMINOLOGY

- Sarcoidosis arthropathy due to granulomas forming in synovium, inciting synovitis and bone erosion
- 2 principal manifestations: **Acute** (resolving) and **chronic** (transient/relapsing)
  - **Acute** sarcoidosis arthropathy
    - Presents as painful, stiff joints and may be associated with fever
    - Polyarticular, involving ankles, knees, PIP joints, wrists, elbows
    - Usually self-limiting, remitting in 4-6 weeks
    - Termed Löfgren syndrome if present with arthralgias (often of bilateral ankles), erythema nodosum, and bilateral hilar lymphadenopathy
    - Generally younger patients than chronic variety
  - **Chronic/relapsing** sarcoidosis arthropathy
    - ≥ 6 months after sarcoidosis is diagnosed
    - Usually involves 2-3 joints (knee, ankle, PIP, occasionally wrist and shoulder)

IMAGING

- Radiograph: Soft tissue swelling (sausage dactylitis)
  - Subchondral cyst and erosions occasionally seen
- MR: Synovitis, subchondral cysts or erosions

TOP DIFFERENTIAL DIAGNOSES

- Rheumatoid arthritis (erosion, subchondral cysts may mimic)
- Gout (patients may be hyperuricemic and can be clinically misdiagnosed with gout)

CLINICAL ISSUES

- Joint symptoms manifested in 10-35% of patients with sarcoidosis
- Males < females
- Prognosis for acute joint sarcoidosis (including Löfgren syndrome): Excellent
- Prognosis for chronic joint sarcoidosis: Good, though disease may wax and wane

(Left) *AP radiograph in a 35-year-old man with sarcoidosis and chronic knee pain shows a subchondral cyst ➡ or erosion.* **(Right)** *Coronal PDWI FS MR in the same patient confirms a subchondral erosion ➡. Patients with sarcoidosis may be hyperuricemic, and these changes can be clinically misdiagnosed as gout. Radiographic considerations include rheumatoid arthritis. Occasionally the erosions or cysts may become very large.*

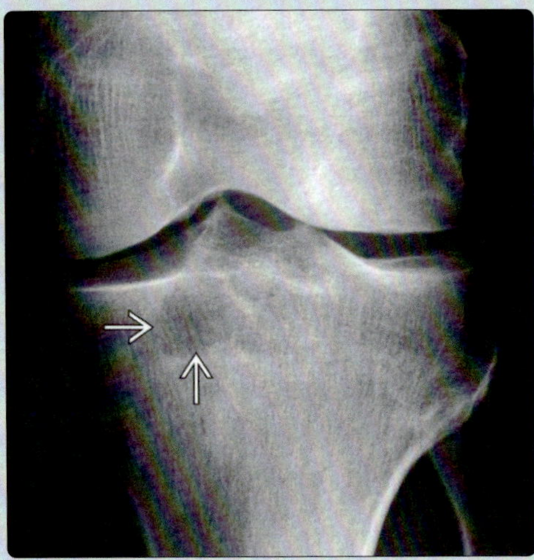

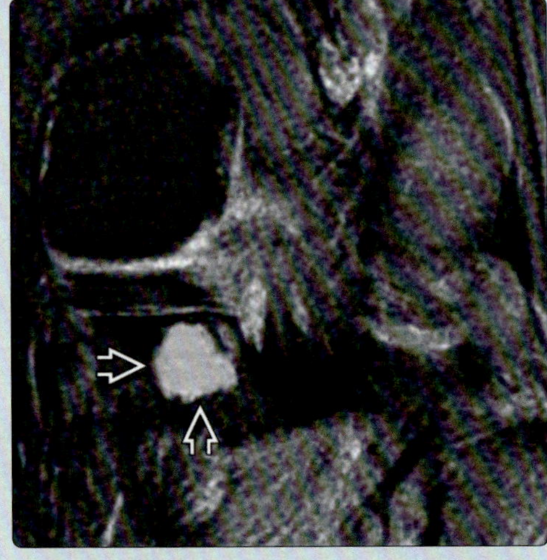

(Left) *Coronal T1WI MR in a woman in her 30s with sarcoidosis and severe hip pain shows marked superolateral joint space narrowing and subchondral erosions ➡. This appearance raises consideration of coexistent RA with secondary OA, but chronic sarcoidosis arthritis should also be considered.* **(Right)** *Coronal T1WI C+ FS MR in a middle-aged woman with sarcoidosis and wrist "mass" shows tenosynovitis ➡. This is nonspecific, and synovial biopsy may be required to establish the granulomatous etiology.*

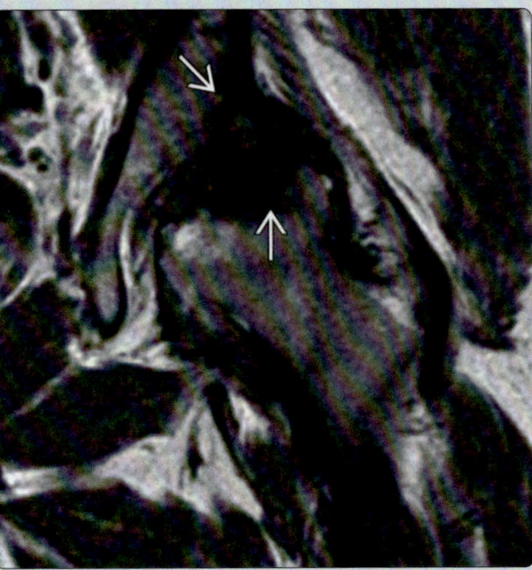

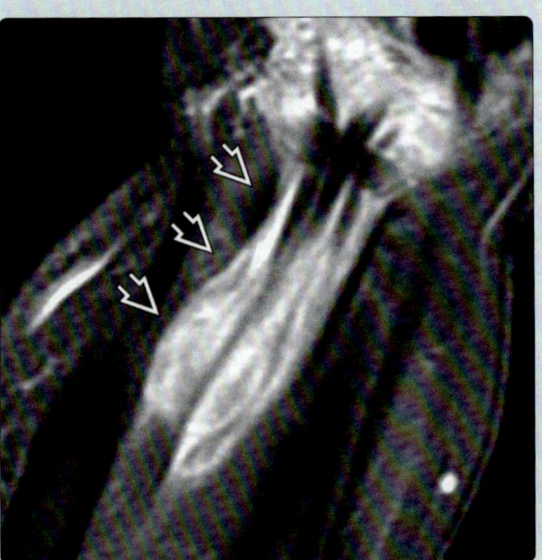

KEY FACTS

TERMINOLOGY

- Sarcoidal noncaseating granulomata located within soft tissues
  - Soft tissue mass
  - Skin nodules
  - Subcutaneous infiltration
- Associated with lymphadenopathy

IMAGING

- Best diagnostic clue
  - Mass or soft tissue reticulation in patient known to have sarcoidosis
- Location
  - Anywhere in soft tissues
  - Most common in ankles, feet, and hands
- Morphology: Variable
  - May be discrete nodule
  - May be reticulated, indistinctly marginated
- Size: Highly variable
- Radiographic appearance: Unlikely to be detected
- CT imaging
  - Nonspecific soft tissue or subcutaneous mass
  - Usually isodense with muscle
  - Surrounding fat in subcutaneous tissue increases conspicuity in that site
- MR imaging
  - Nonspecific signal characteristics
  - Generally similar to other solid mesenchymal masses
  - T1WI: Low signal intensity, isointense to skeletal muscle
  - Fluid-sensitive sequences: Variable high signal
  - Postcontrast imaging: Variable enhancement
  - MR useful in identifying biopsy site
- Nuclear medicine findings
  - FDG PET relatively sensitive but nonspecific
  - FDG PET range of standardized uptake volume (SUV) for sarcoidosis soft tissue lesions overlaps with that of benign and malignant masses

TOP DIFFERENTIAL DIAGNOSES

- DDx of soft tissue sarcoidosis in hands or feet
  - Ganglion cyst
  - Giant cell tumor of tendon sheath
  - Fibrous histiocytoma
  - Gouty tophys
- DDx of subcutaneous infiltrative sarcoidosis
  - Malignant melanoma
  - Hemangioma
  - Fibroma of tendon sheath
  - Epithelioid sarcoma
  - Fibromatosis

CLINICAL ISSUES

- Soft tissue swelling or lump
  - May coexist with lacy lytic changes in hands or feet
- Cutaneous sarcoidosis occurs in 25-33% of patients with systemic sarcoidosis
- Mimics other diseases in dermatology because of varied presentation
  - Erythema nodosum: Nonspecific finding
    - Associated with benign self-limiting acute sarcoidosis, such as Löfgren syndrome
  - Papules and plaques: Fairly sarcoid-specific
    - Asymptomatic pink-yellow or red-brown
    - Favor face, posterior neck, areas of prior trauma
  - Lupus pernio
    - Red-brown or violaceous papules/plaques on nasal alae, cheeks, ear lobes, digits
    - Associated with more severe systemic involvement

DIAGNOSTIC CHECKLIST

- As MR findings are nonspecific, differential diagnosis includes usual gamut of benign and malignant mesenchymal masses
- In setting of established sarcoidosis diagnosis, sarcoidal mass is in differential for soft tissue masses

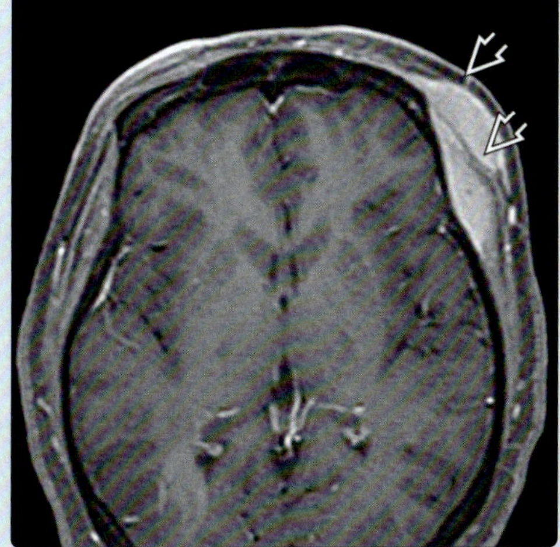

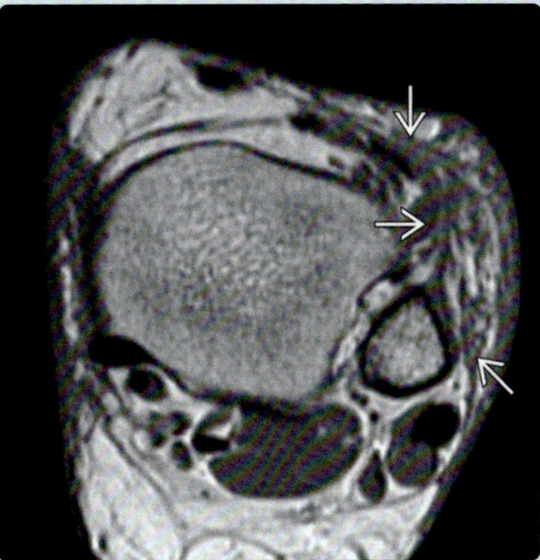

(Left) *Axial T1WI C+ FS MR of a patient with sarcoidosis and left temporal swelling demonstrates an enhancing soft tissue mass insinuating into the left temporal muscle ➾. Biopsy of an adjacent mass (not depicted) revealed noncaseating granulomata. No erosion of the underlying calvaria was demonstrated.* **(Right)** *Axial PDWI MR of a woman with sarcoidosis and ankle "mass" demonstrates soft tissue reticulation about the anterior lateral ankle ➾. Biopsy revealed noncaseating granulomata.*

Mastocytosis

KEY FACTS

TERMINOLOGY

- Heterogeneous neoplastic disorder that results from clonal mast cell proliferation in various organs

IMAGING

- Osseous abnormalities in 70%
- Bone lesions may be focal or diffuse
  - Focal lesions can progress to diffuse
- 2 distinct appearances of osseous structures
  - Osteosclerosis
  - Osteoporosis
- Pathologic fracture, particularly in spine
- MR: Low SI on T1WI
  - Hyperintense SI on fluid-sensitive sequences unless lesion is densely sclerotic

CLINICAL ISSUES

- Constellation of symptoms
  - Flushing
  - Abdominal pain
  - Diarrhea
  - Unexplained syncope
  - Classic urticaria pigmentosa
  - Bone pain in as many as 28%
- Age of onset
  - Generally begins in adulthood
  - Uncommon childhood mastocytosis usually restricted to skin manifestations
- Gender: Male = female
- Natural history, prognosis, and treatment
  - Diagnosis established by bone biopsy
  - Indolent mastocytosis: Normal life expectancy
  - Patients assessed for tumor burden and end-organ damage
    - Cytoreductive therapy only if significantly symptomatic
  - Kyphoplasty may cause hypotension 2° to pressure-induced release of allergy mediator histamine

(Left) *Lateral radiograph of the thoracic spine shows a classic ivory vertebra ➡ with dense bone replacing the entire body but no change in size. Focal sclerosis, such as this, is one appearance found in mastocytosis.* **(Right)** *Lateral x-ray, same patient, shows mixed lysis and sclerosis but also enlargement of the vertebra ➡. This may suggest Paget disease, but this is a case of polyostotic mastocytosis. This diagnosis can present a radiographically confusing picture, presenting as osteopenia, sclerosis, or mixed disease.*

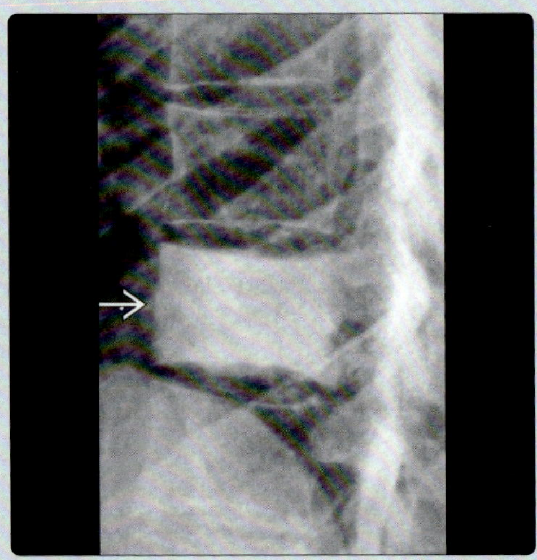

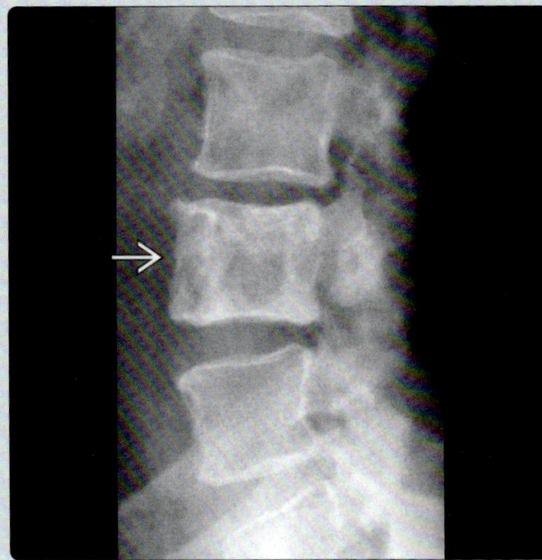

(Left) *AP radiograph shows diffuse and severe osteoporosis with multiple fractures. The appearance is nonspecific, but biopsy proved mastocytosis. It is unusual for childhood mastocytosis to have osseous abnormalities.* **(Right)** *AP radiograph shows a densely sclerotic isolated lesion, with enlargement of the diaphysis of the clavicle ➡. There is a wide differential for this appearance. This patient had GI difficulties that appeared episodically, as well as a rash, which helps narrow the diagnosis to mastocytosis.*

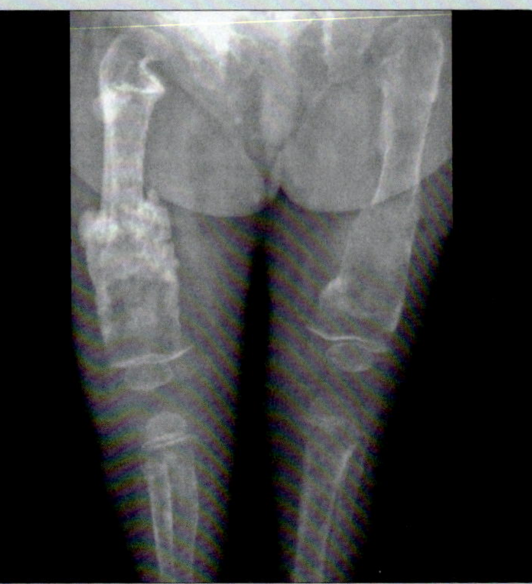

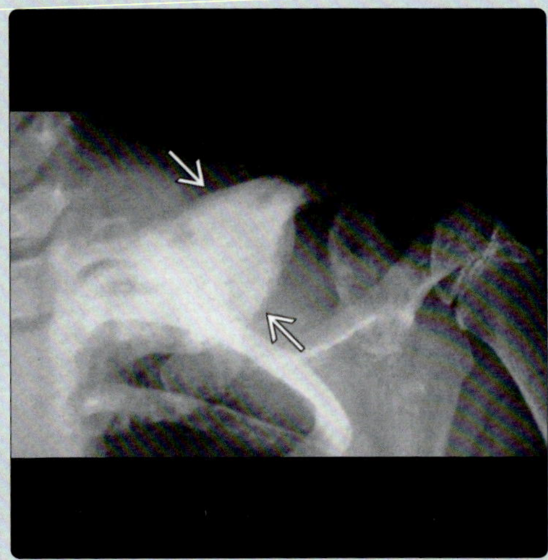

TERMINOLOGY

Definitions

- Heterogeneous neoplastic disorder that results from clonal mast cell proliferation in various organs

IMAGING

General Features

- Location
  - Osseous lesions may be focal or diffuse
    - Focal lesions can progress to diffuse

Radiographic Findings

- Primary radiographic findings
  - 2 distinct appearances of osseous structures
    - Osteosclerosis
    - Osteoporosis
- Secondary radiographic findings
  - Pathologic fracture, particularly in spine

CT Findings

- Low dose whole body CT may be useful in assessing osseous lesion burden
- Nonskeletal CT findings seen in 19% of patients in one study
  - Hepatosplenomegaly
  - Retroperitoneal adenopathy
  - Periportal adenopathy
  - Mesenteric adenopathy
  - Thickening of omentum and mesentery
  - Ascites
  - Less common findings
    - Hepatofugal portal venous flow
    - Budd-Chiari syndrome
    - Cavernous transformation of portal vein
    - Ovarian mass

MR Findings

- T1WI MR
  - Low SI if sclerotic type
- Fluid-sensitive sequences
  - Hyperintense SI
    - Unless lesion is densely sclerotic
- Whole-body MR may be useful in assessing lesion burden

Nuclear Medicine Findings

- Lesions show abnormal uptake on bone scan

CLINICAL ISSUES

Presentation

- Most common signs/symptoms
  - Constellation of symptoms
    - Flushing
    - Abdominal pain
    - Diarrhea
    - Unexplained syncope
    - Classic urticaria pigmentosa
  - Bone pain in as many as 28%

Demographics

- Age
  - Generally begins in adulthood
    - Uncommon childhood mastocytosis usually restricted to skin manifestations
- Gender
  - Male = female
- Epidemiology
  - Osseous abnormalities in 70%

Natural History & Prognosis

- Indolent mastocytosis
  - Normal life expectancy

Treatment

- Diagnosis is established by bone biopsy
- Patients are assessed for tumor burden and end-organ damage
- Cytoreductive therapy is performed only if significantly symptomatic
- Kyphoplasty may cause hypotension secondary to pressure-induced release of allergy mediator histamine

SELECTED REFERENCES

1. Alpay Kanıtez N et al: Osteoporosis and osteopathy markers in patients with mastocytosis. Turk J Haematol. 32(1):43-50, 2015
2. Arock M et al: Current treatment options in patients with mastocytosis: status in 2015 and future perspectives. Eur J Haematol. ePub, 2015
3. Gasljevic G et al: Hodgkin's lymphoma is a rare form of clonal haematological non-mast cell disease in systemic mastocytosis. Diagn Pathol. 10(1):5, 2015
4. Pardanani A: Systemic mastocytosis in adults: 2015 update on diagnosis, risk stratification, and management. Am J Hematol. 90(3):250-62, 2015
5. Fritz J et al: Advanced imaging of skeletal manifestations of systemic mastocytosis. Skeletal Radiol. 41(8):887-97, 2012
6. Bains SN et al: Current approaches to the diagnosis and treatment of systemic mastocytosis. Ann Allergy Asthma Immunol. 104(1):1-10; quiz 10-2, 41, 2010
7. Pardanani A et al: Systemic mastocytosis in adults: a review on prognosis and treatment based on 342 Mayo Clinic patients and current literature. Curr Opin Hematol. 17(2):125-32, 2010
8. Krüger A et al: Multimodal therapy for vertebral involvement of systemic mastocytosis. Spine (Phila Pa 1976). 34(17):E626-8, 2009
9. Lim KH et al: Systemic mastocytosis in 342 consecutive adults: survival studies and prognostic factors. Blood. 113(23):5727-36, 2009
10. Mathew R et al: Systemic mastocytosis presenting as osteoporosis–a case report. Clin Rheumatol. 28(7):865-6, 2009
11. Nguyen BD: CT and scintigraphy of aggressive lymphadenopathic mastocytosis. AJR Am J Roentgenol. 178(3):769-70, 2002
12. Zettinig G et al: FDG positron emission tomography in patients with systemic mastocytosis. AJR Am J Roentgenol. 179(5):1235-7, 2002
13. Avila NA et al: Systemic mastocytosis: CT and US features of abdominal manifestations. Radiology. 202(2):367-72, 1997

KEY FACTS

TERMINOLOGY

- Tuberosis sclerosis complex (TSC): Multiorgan genetic neurocutaneous syndrome characterized by development of hamartomas

IMAGING

- Osseous abnormalities (3rd most common abnormality)
  - Focal sclerotic lesions (occasionally lytic)
    - Generally multiple (> 4 lesions)
    - Round, oval, or occasionally flame-shaped
  - Hyperostosis of inner table of calvaria + sclerotic foci (40%)
  - Hypertrophic osteoarthropathy, especially hands/feet (66%)
- Intracranial abnormalities (most common abnormality)
  - Cortical or subependymal tubers (95-100%)
  - White matter abnormalities (40-90%)
  - Subependymal giant cell astrocytoma
- Cardiac rhabdomyoma (50-65%)
  - Majority (70%) show spontaneous regression, leaving fatty foci along ventricular septum
  - Single or multiple, located on ventricular septum
- Pulmonary abnormalities
  - Lymphangioleiomyomatosis: Round, thin-walled cysts
  - Multifocal micronodular pneumocyte hyperplasia
- Renal abnormalities (2nd most common abnormality)
  - Renal angiomyolipoma (70-90%): Intratumoral fat may be obscured by bleeding from rupture
  - Renal cysts
  - Renal cell carcinoma: When associated with TSC, tends to occur in younger patients and to grow more slowly

PATHOLOGY

- Autosomal dominant; 2/3 cases have sporadic mutations

CLINICAL ISSUES

- 1 case per 6,000-12,000
- 40% mortality by age 35

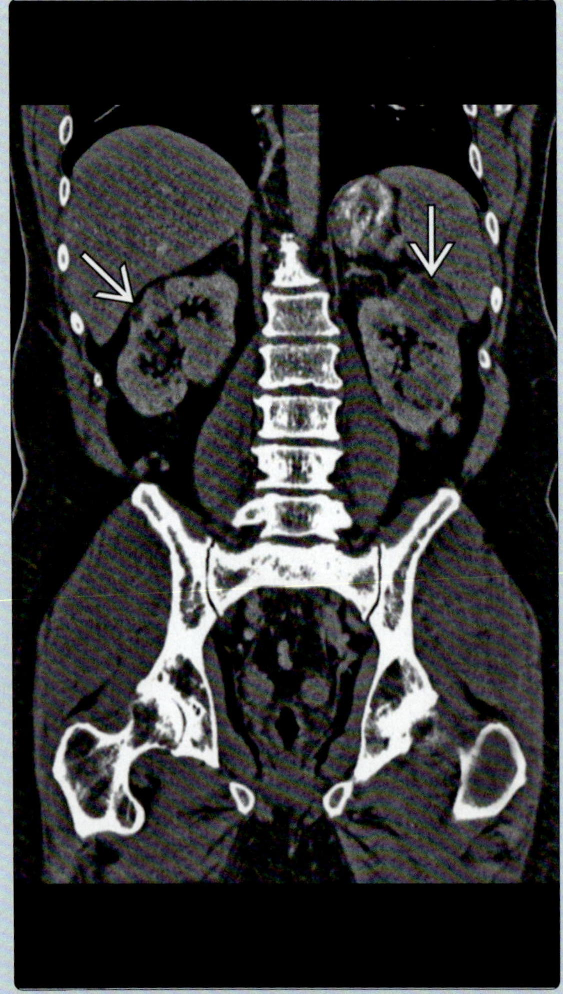

Coronal CT shows polyostotic sclerotic lesions throughout the axial skeleton. Additionally, there are multiple solid as well as fat-attenuation ➡ lesions within the kidneys. The kidney lesions are typical of angiomyolipomas and had not changed in character over several years.

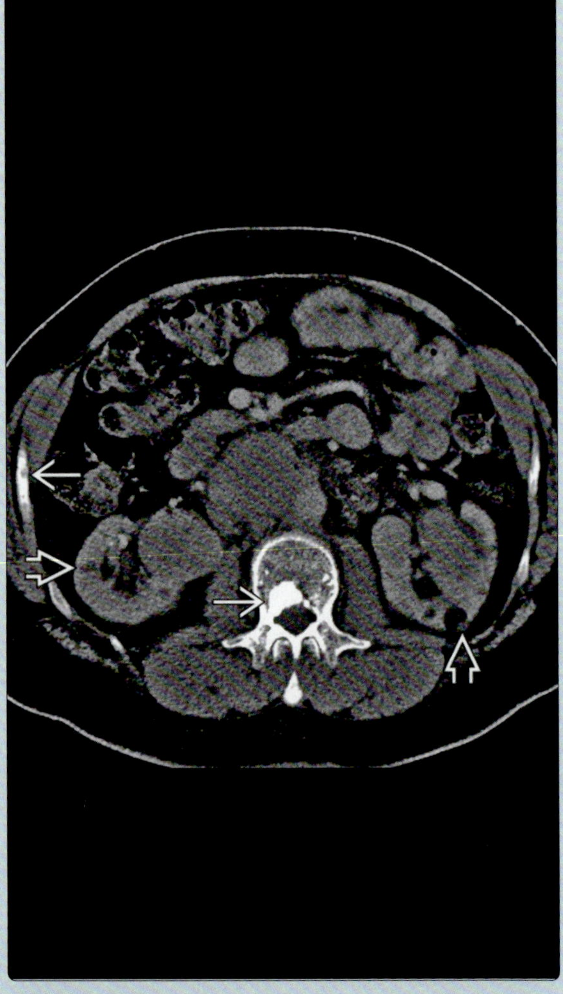

Axial CT, same patient, shows typical angiomyolipomas within the kidneys ➡. The sclerotic osseous lesions are found throughout the axial skeleton and ribs ➡. There is incidental retroperitoneal follicular cell lymphoma.

TERMINOLOGY

Definitions

- Tuberosis sclerosis complex (TSC): Multiorgan genetic neurocutaneous syndrome characterized by development of hamartomas

IMAGING

Radiographic Findings

- Osseous abnormalities
  - Focal sclerotic lesions
  - Lytic lesions may occur
  - Hyperostosis of inner table of calvaria + sclerotic foci (40%)
  - Hypertrophic osteoarthropathy, especially hands/feet (66%)

MR Findings

- Intracranial abnormalities
  - Cortical or subependymal tubers (95-100%)
  - White matter abnormalities (40-90%)
  - Subependymal giant cell astrocytoma
- Cardiac rhabdomyoma (50-65%)
  - Conversely, 40-80% of patients with cardiac rhabdomyoma have TSC
  - Single or multiple, located on ventricular septum
  - Majority (70%) show spontaneous regression, leaving fatty foci along ventricular septum
- Pulmonary abnormalities
  - Lymphangioleiomyomatosis: Rare diffuse interstitial proliferation of smooth muscle cells seen as round, thin-walled cysts
  - Multifocal micronodular pneumocyte hyperplasia
- Renal abnormalities
  - Renal angiomyolipoma (55-75%): Intratumoral fat may be obscured by bleeding from rupture
  - Renal cysts
  - Renal cell carcinoma: When associated with TSC, tends to occur in younger patients and to grow more slowly

DIFFERENTIAL DIAGNOSIS

Bone Island (Enostosis)

- Hamartomatous lesions of no clinical importance
- Clinical setting differentiates from TSC

Osteoblastic Metastasis

- Clinical setting may help differentiate

Osteopoikilosis

- Distribution (metaphyseal prominence) different than TSC
- Dysplasia has no associated findings, differentiating it from TSC

Sclerotic Multiple Myeloma

- Generally POEMS syndrome; associated findings should help differentiate
  - Polyneuropathy, organomegaly, endocrinopathy, myeloma, skin findings

PATHOLOGY

General Features

- Genetics
  - Mutations in *TSC1* or *TSC2* genes
    - Hamartin and tuberin encoded on separate chromosomes
    - Single mutation in either gene, coupled with inevitable loss of heterozygosity, sufficient to cause tuberous sclerosis
      - Defective tuberin causes more severe phenotype
  - Autosomal dominant; 2/3 cases have sporadic mutations

Staging, Grading, & Classification

- Classical clinical criteria triad
  - Epilepsy, mental retardation, adenoma sebaceum
    - 1/2 have normal intelligence
    - 1/4 do not have epilepsy

CLINICAL ISSUES

Presentation

- Most common signs/symptoms
  - Severe neurological disease (90%)
    - Epilepsy
    - Developmental delay
    - Autism
    - Psychiatric abnormalities
  - Renal disease
    - Multiple angiomyolipomas
    - Occasional malignant tumor within field of benign tumors
  - Cardiac disease
    - Intracardiac fatty foci
    - Rhabdomyoma
  - Cutaneous lesions (90%)
    - "Ash-leaf" macules
    - "Shagreen" patches
    - Facial angiofibromas (up to 80% of patients)
    - Periungual fibromas

Demographics

- Epidemiology
  - 1 case per 6,000-12,000

Natural History & Prognosis

- 40% mortality by age 35

SELECTED REFERENCES

1. Lew PP et al: Imaging of disorders affecting the bone and skin. Radiographics. 34(1):197-216, 2014
2. Avila NA et al: CT of sclerotic bone lesions: imaging features differentiating tuberous sclerosis complex with lymphangioleiomyomatosis from sporadic lymphangioleiomymatosis. Radiology. 254(3):851-7, 2010
3. Ess KC: Tuberous sclerosis complex: a brave new world? Curr Opin Neurol. 23(2):189-93, 2010
4. Adriaensen ME et al: Fatty foci in the myocardium in patients with tuberous sclerosis complex: common finding at CT. Radiology. 253(2):359-63, 2009
5. Bonsib SM: Renal cystic diseases and renal neoplasms: a mini-review. Clin J Am Soc Nephrol. 4(12):1998-2007, 2009
6. Napolioni V et al: Genetics and molecular biology of tuberous sclerosis complex. Curr Genomics. 9(7):475-87, 2008
7. Umeoka S et al: Pictorial review of tuberous sclerosis in various organs. Radiographics. 28(7):e32, 2008

(Left) *Coronal CT shows multiple round sclerotic lesions scattered throughout the axial skeleton ➡. In addition, there is abnormal fat-density distribution within the retroperitoneum that requires further review.* **(Right)** *Coronal CT, same patient, shows the enlarged kidneys containing innumerable angiomyolipomas. The combination of kidney and bone findings makes the diagnosis of tuberous sclerosis.*

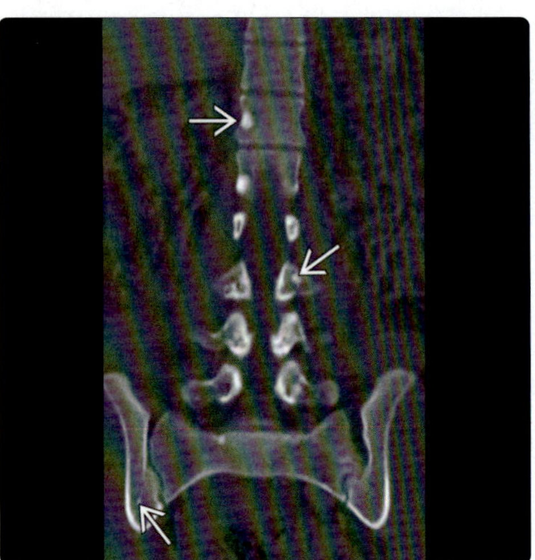

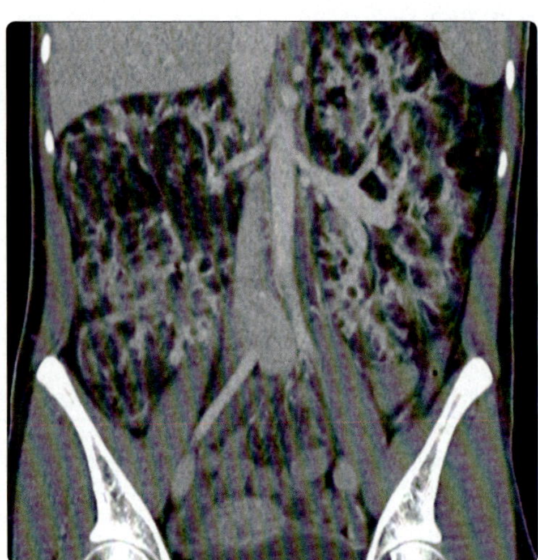

(Left) *Axial CT, same patient, shows multiple round sclerotic lesions within the body and posterior elements of the spine ➡. These lesions do not appear aggressive, are entirely homogeneous, and have no other characterizing features.* **(Right)** *Axial CT through the sacrum shows sclerotic lesions ➡. However, there are also a few lytic lesions ➡. Either appearance is typical of the osseous lesions of tuberous sclerosis. Either could be seen in metastatic disease or myeloma as well, but the kidney disease secures the diagnosis of tuberous sclerosis.*

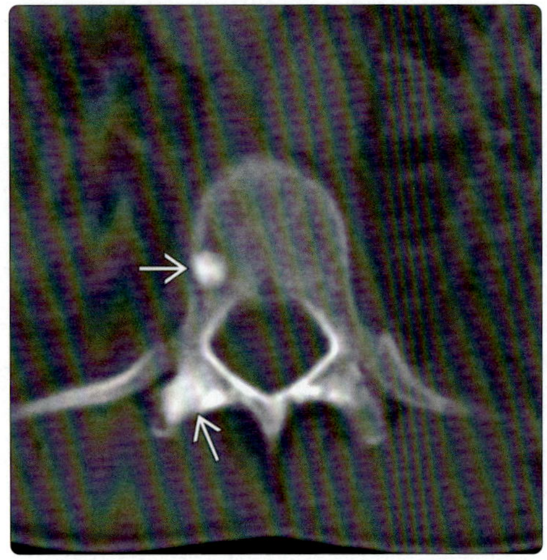

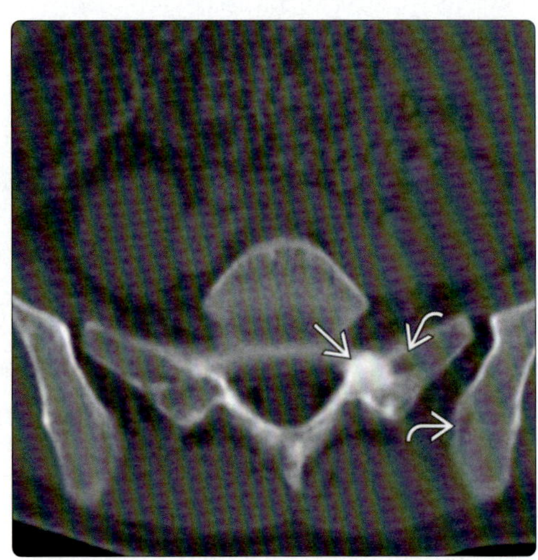

(Left) *Axial FLAIR MR, same patient, shows typical subcortical tubers ➡. Neurologic findings are the most frequent in tuberous sclerosis, followed by the kidney, and then osseous lesions.* **(Right)** *Oblique radiograph shows thick, wavy periosteal reaction involving all the metatarsals ➡. This is a typical appearance of hypertrophic osteoarthropathy, most frequently seen in association with lung disease but rarely associated with tuberous sclerosis, as in this case.*

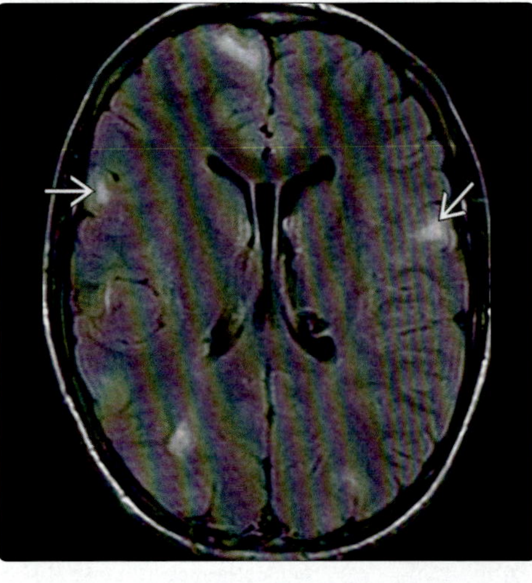

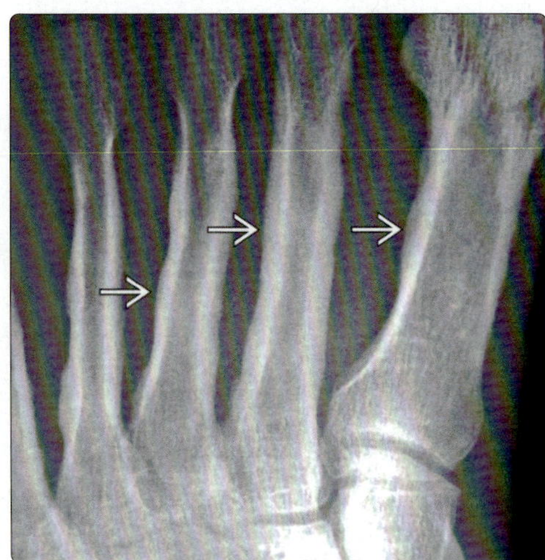

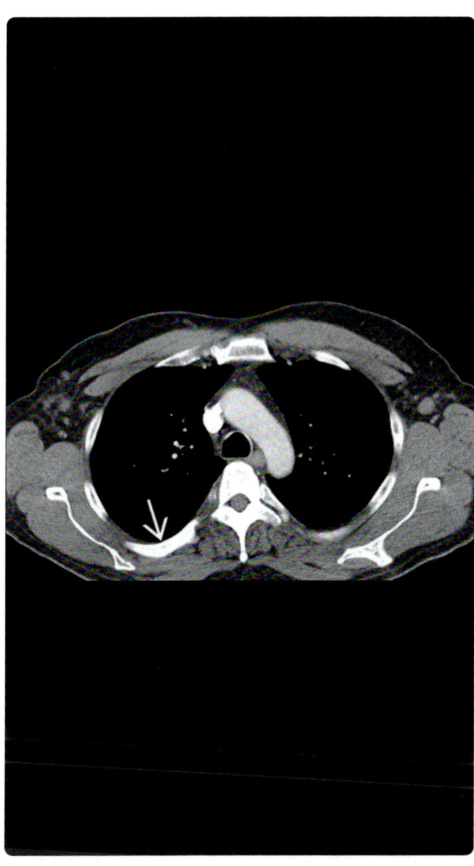

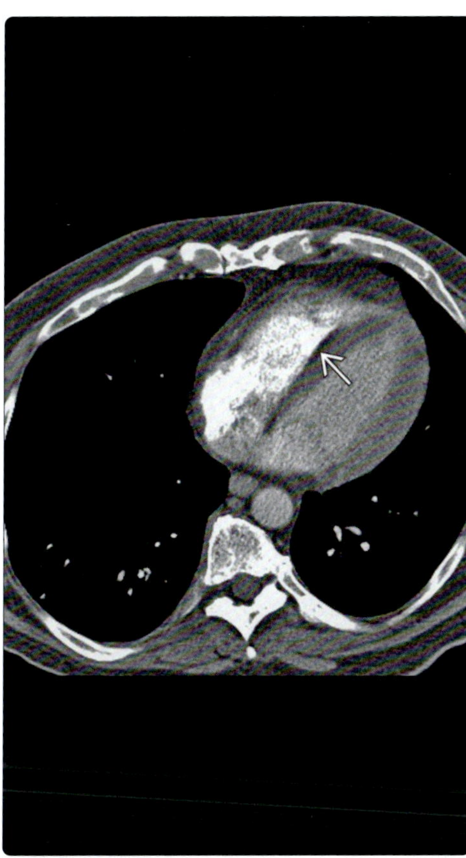

(Left) *Axial CT, same case, shows a dense, slightly expanded rib lesion ➡, one of many sclerotic osseous lesions in this patient with tuberous sclerosis.* **(Right)** *Axial CECT, same case, shows a focal fatty streak along the interventricular septum ➡. This is thought to be residual fat from a fetal or infantile rhabdomyoma, which spontaneously regresses; this is a typical behavior pattern. (Courtesy R. Hastings, MD.)*

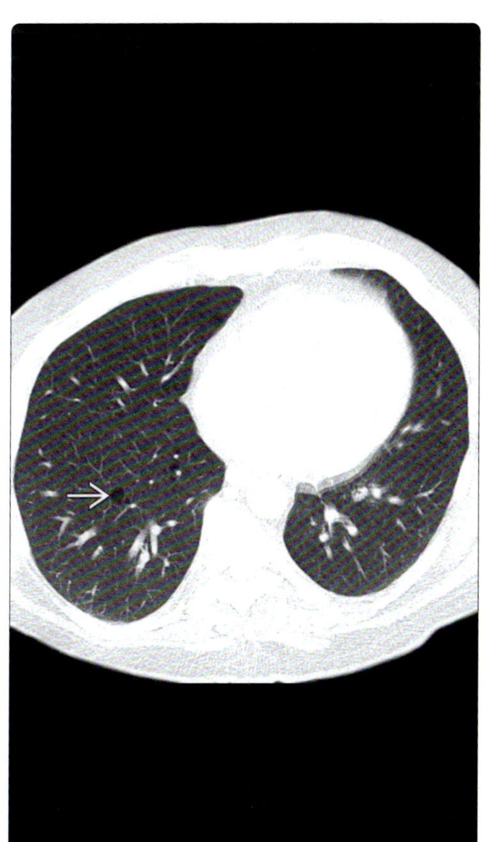

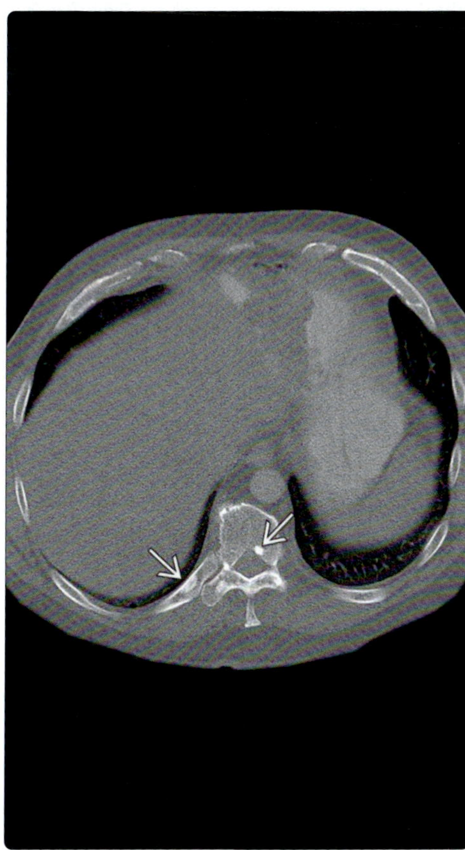

(Left) *Axial CT shows a thin-walled cyst ➡ within the lower lung field, typical of angiomyolipoma in a patient with tuberous sclerosis.* **(Right)** *Axial CT in the same patient shows 2 sclerotic osseous lesions ➡. These are nonspecific in appearance but, in the company of visceral findings of tuberous sclerosis, are considered typical of that disease.*

KEY FACTS

TERMINOLOGY

- Lysosomal storage disorder resulting in deposition of glucocerebroside in cells of reticuloendothelial system, including bone marrow

IMAGING

- Initial involvement is in axial skeleton
  - Later (often irreversible) involvement in long bones
- Generalized osteopenia, trabecular coarsening
  - Later, superimposed sclerosis 2° to bone infarction
- Erlenmeyer flask deformity: Cortical thinning, widening of distal femoral metadiaphysis
- Osteonecrosis, femoral (20%) and humeral (10%)
- Marrow replacement seen by MR
  - Early focal, later diffuse
  - Low SI on T1WI
  - Acute disease: Intermediate to high SI on T2
  - Chronic replacement disease: Low SI on fluid-sensitive sequences
  - < 35% ↑ SI with contrast if chronic, > 35% ↑ if acute

TOP DIFFERENTIAL DIAGNOSES

- Sickle cell anemia
- Niemann-Pick
- Osteopetrosis

CLINICAL ISSUES

- Most common lysosomal storage disease
- M = F
- Bone symptoms in 75%
  - Bone crises (infarction), osteonecrosis, atypical bone pain, pathologic fracture
- Hepatosplenomegaly
- Adult type 1 patients with mild manifestations may show slow progression or even spontaneous regression
  - Up to 20% with type 1 develop impaired mobility
- Bone crises with severe pain and swelling may mimic osteomyelitis

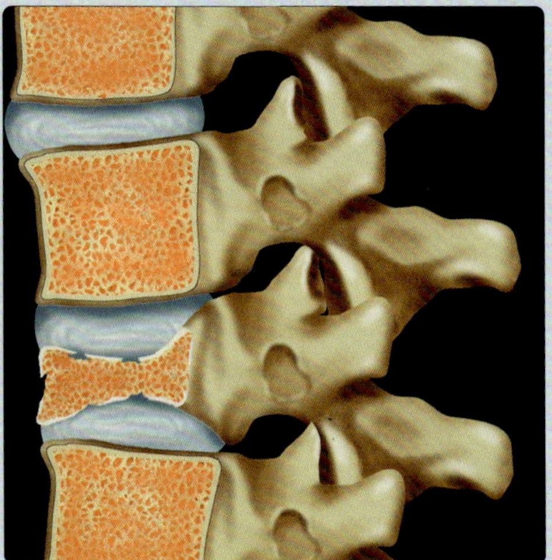

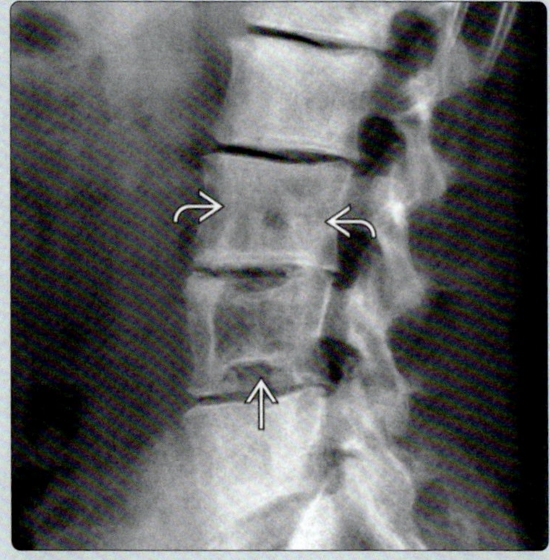

(Left) *Sagittal graphic portrays vertebral bodies as having diffuse marrow replacement. Fractures are related to bone infarct and may take the form of biconcavity, single endplate compression, or H-shaped vertebral bodies.* **(Right)** *Lateral lumbar spine x-ray shows sclerotic vertebral bodies. Centrally, each body shows a sclerotic, serpentine line ➔ surrounding regions of mottled density, an appearance pathognomonic for bone infarct. The infarct has progressed to central vertebral body collapse at L4 ➔.*

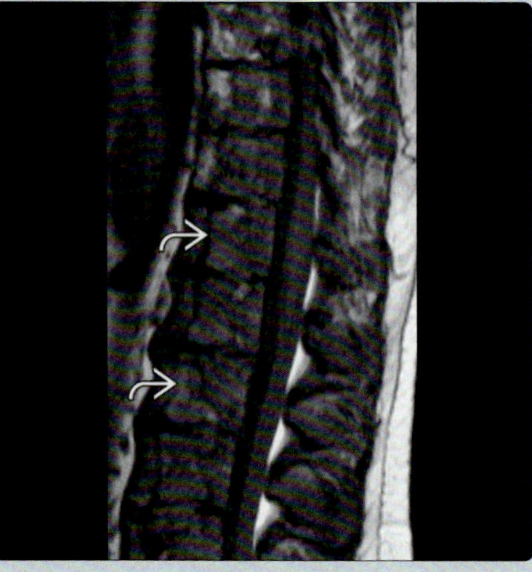

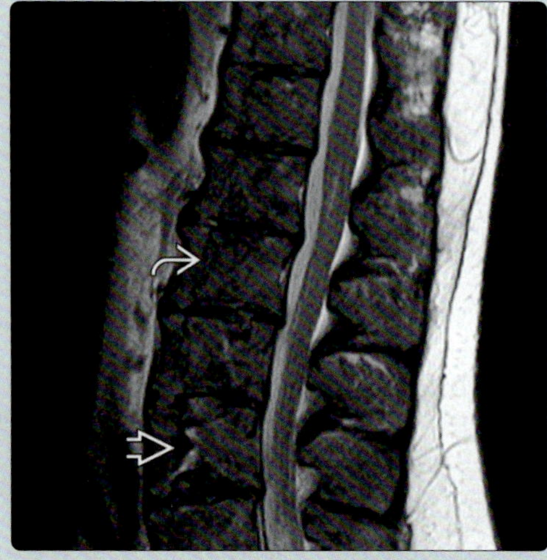

(Left) *Sagittal T1WI MR shows low-signal intensity bone marrow replacement diffusely and superimposed infarcts ➔. This is severe involvement; no fat is preserved, even around basivertebral vessels.* **(Right)** *Sagittal T2WI MR in the same patient shows persistent low signal of the replaced bone marrow. Many of the bone infarcts remain low signal ➔, but others show the double line sign of both high and low signal intensity ➔. Mild endplate compression is seen at one level, but no significant compression fractures are seen, despite diffuse disease.*

TERMINOLOGY

Definitions

- Gaucher disease: Lysosomal storage disorder resulting in deposition of glucocerebroside in cells of reticuloendothelial system, including bone marrow

IMAGING

General Features

- Location
  - Initial involvement is in axial skeleton
  - Later (often irreversible) involvement in long bones

Radiographic Findings

- Bone density
  - Generalized osteopenia, trabecular coarsening
    - May have multiple lytic regions, which appear somewhat circumscribed
  - Later, superimposed sclerosis 2° to bone infarction
    - Serpiginous pattern most common
    - May have double endosteal cortical density
- Modeling deformity
  - Erlenmeyer flask deformity: Cortical thinning, widening of distal femoral metadiaphysis
  - Undertubulation not limited to distal femur; metadiaphyses of all long bones may be involved
- Osteonecrosis, femoral (20%) and humeral (10%) heads
  - Initial relative increased density, followed by subchondral lucent fracture
  - With collapse, eventual 2° osteoarthritis
- Pathologic fracture
  - Long bones
  - Spine (10%); pattern may be biconcave, collapse of single endplate, or H-shaped collapse of central endplates

MR Findings

- Marrow replacement
  - Early focal, later diffuse
  - Low SI on T1WI
  - Fluid-sensitive sequences
    - Acute disease: Intermediate to high SI
    - Chronic disease: Low SI
  - Post contrast: < 35% ↑ SI if chronic, > 35% ↑ if acute
  - Opposed-phase imaging: Signal dropout depends on stage of diffuse marrow replacement
    - If some fat remains (often around basivertebral vessels in vertebra), will show ↓ in SI
- Bone infarcts
  - Low SI; hyperintense rim on fluid-sensitive sequences
  - Serpiginous pattern most frequent; may be focal or elongated along cortex
- Osteonecrosis
  - Low SI on T1WI, double line sign with high SI rim on fluid-sensitive sequences
- Extraosseous cellular deposits rare but may mimic tumor
- MR may be used to quantify disease progression (along with blood values)
  - Bone marrow fat content (quantitative chemical shift imaging used)
  - Liver ratio (mL/kg body weight), splenic volume

DIFFERENTIAL DIAGNOSIS

Sickle Cell Anemia

- Marrow repopulation may mimic marrow replacement
- Osteonecrosis (infarct shaft, femoral/humeral heads)
- Generally no Erlenmeyer flask deformity
- Splenic infarcts are differentiating factor

Niemann-Pick

- Erlenmeyer flask deformity
- Severe mental retardation

PATHOLOGY

General Features

- Etiology
  - Deficient activity of enzyme glucocerebrosidase
  - Leads to accumulation of glucosylceramide within cells of reticuloendothelial system
    - Storage in bone, liver, spleen, lungs
- Genetics
  - Autosomal recessive
  - Gene for glucocerebrosidase: Chromosome 1q21

Staging, Grading, & Classification

- 3 major phenotypes
  - Type 1: Most common
    - Variable hepatosplenomegaly
    - Cytopenia
    - Bone disease
    - No neurologic manifestations
  - Types 2 and 3: Varying degrees of neurologic involvement

CLINICAL ISSUES

Presentation

- Most common signs/symptoms
  - Bone symptoms in 75%
    - Bone crises (infarction), atypical bone pain, osteonecrosis, pathologic fracture
  - Hepatosplenomegaly

Demographics

- Age
  - Type 1: Presents in either childhood or adulthood
- Ethnicity
  - Type 1 has strong predilection for Ashkenazi Jewish population (60% are homozygotes)

Natural History & Prognosis

- Adult type 1 patients with mild manifestations may show slow progression or even spontaneous regression
- Up to 20% with type 1 develop impaired mobility

Treatment

- Mild disease: May watch for progression prior to Rx
- Enzyme-replacement therapy
- Pharmacological chaperone therapy

SELECTED REFERENCES

1. Meyer BJ et al: Extraosseous Gaucher cell deposition without adjacent bone involvement. Skeletal Radiol. 43(10):1495-8, 2014

(Left) *AP radiograph of the distal femur shows abnormal modeling (undertubulation) of the distal diaphysis ➡, secondary to marrow packing with Gaucher cells in this sphingolipid disorder. This has been termed the Erlenmeyer flask deformity and is seen in 40-50% of Gaucher patients.* **(Right)** *Coronal T2WI FS MR shows diffuse hypointense signal in Gaucher disease. The low signal is due to chronic sphingolipid storage in reticuloendothelial cells. If there were acute disease, it would appear as high signal.*

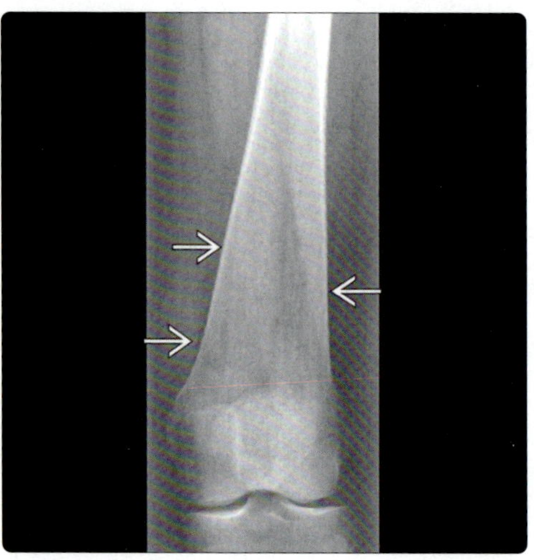

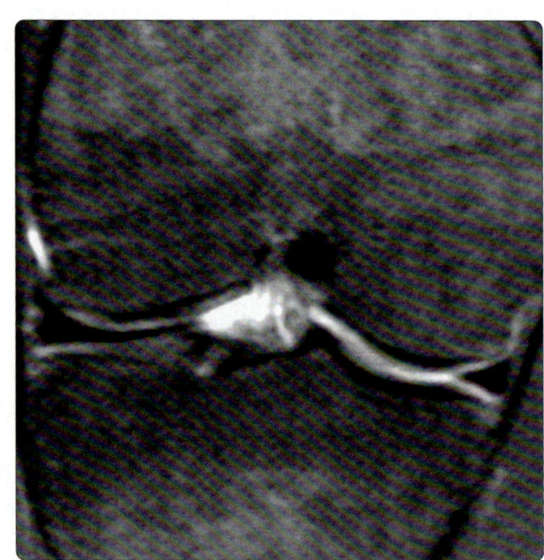

(Left) *Lateral radiograph shows a widened metaphyses from marrow packing. Serpentine lines of bone sclerosis ➡ are indicative of bone infarcts. Endosteal splitting ➡ is a less commonly recognized sign of bone infarct. Bone infarcts in Gaucher disease are secondary to increased marrow pressure from the Gaucher cells.* **(Right)** *Coronal T1WI MR in the same patient shows a serpentine contour ➡ of reparative bone outlining the bone infarct. Some residual high-signal marrow fat remains.*

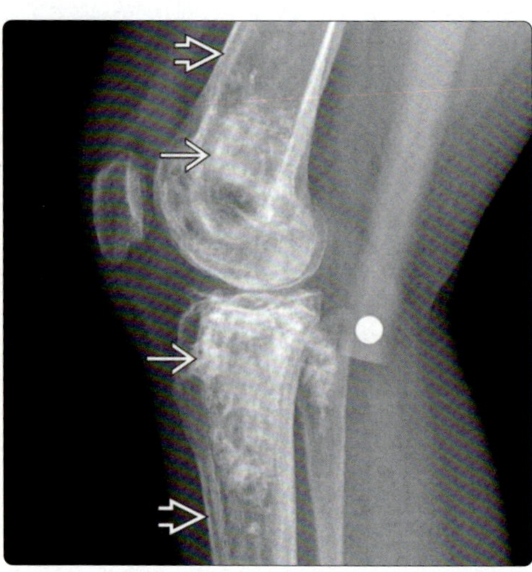

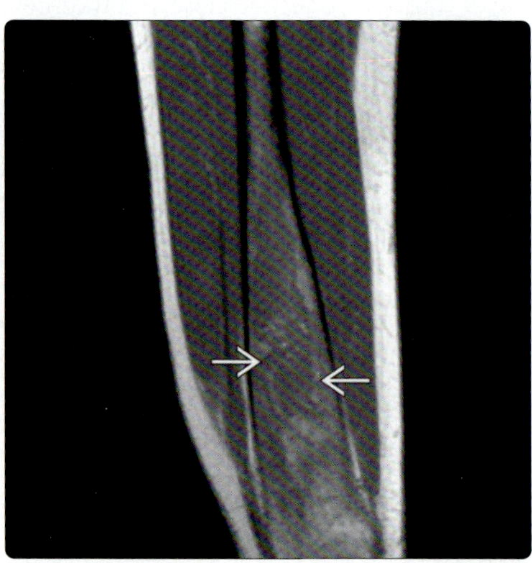

(Left) *Coronal STIR MR shows the margin of the infarct with a double rim of low and high signal intensity ➡ reparative bone. Around the infarct, intermediate signal intensity marrow replacement is seen throughout the entire shaft distal to the right total hip replacement.* **(Right)** *Coronal T1WI C+ FS MR in the same patient shows a rim of enhancement ➡ around the bone infarcts. The marrow abnormalities in both the spine and the long bones result from a combination of marrow replacement (partial or complete) and infarct.*

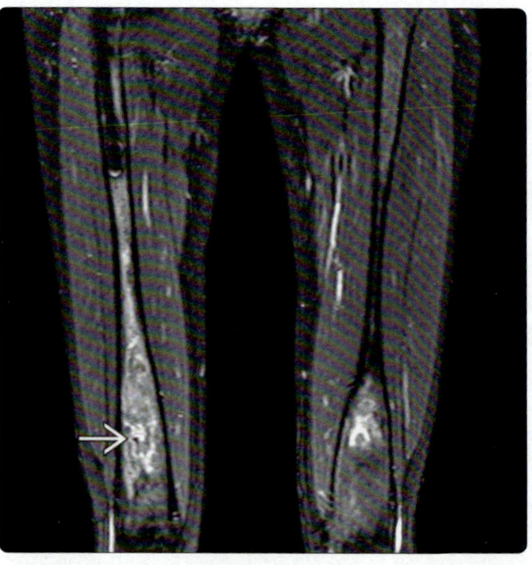

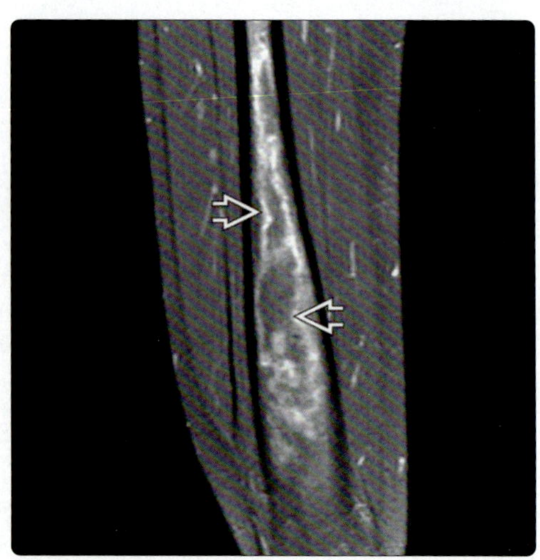

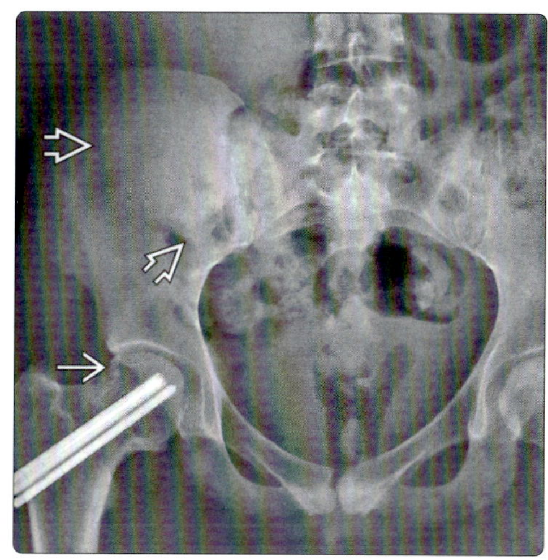

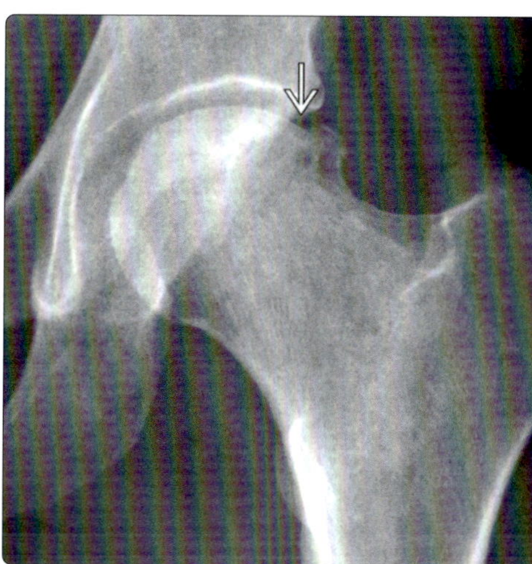

(Left) *AP radiograph shows pinning of a flattened femoral head ➡ along with hepatomegaly ➡; the enlarged liver displaces the bowel gas toward the center of the abdomen. Osteonecrosis (ON) in conjunction with hepatosplenomegaly is diagnostic of Gaucher disease.* **(Right)** *AP x-ray of left hip in the same patient shows old collapse of the weight-bearing portion of the femoral head ➡, healed with abnormal morphology. Femoral head ON is found in 20% of Gaucher patients.*

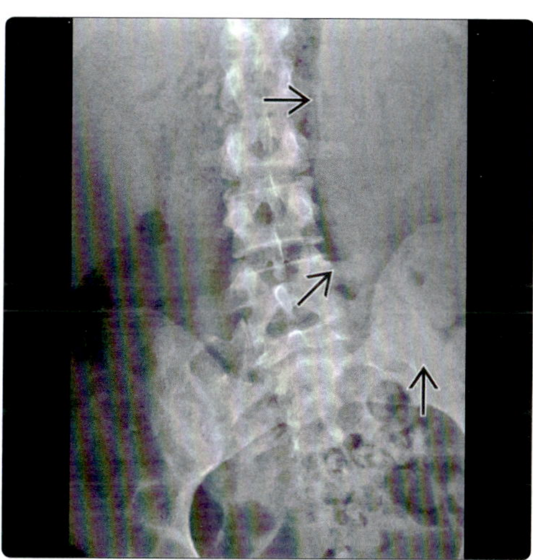

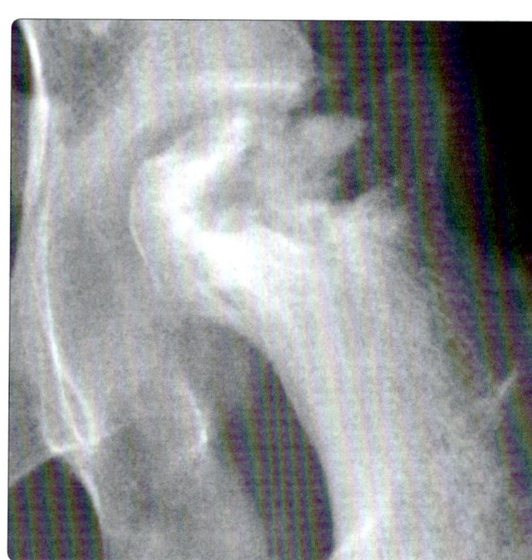

(Left) *AP radiograph shows tremendous splenomegaly ➡; the liver outline appears large as well. Additionally, the bones appear abnormally dense, suggesting diffuse infarction. This combination of findings is seen in Gaucher disease.* **(Right)** *AP radiograph in the same patient shows severe ON of the femoral head, with collapse of the femoral head and secondary osteoarthritis. Note the generalized increase in bone density, typical of Gaucher disease.*

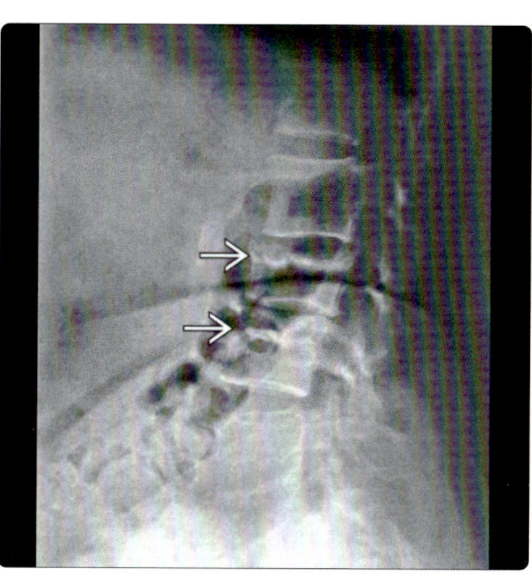

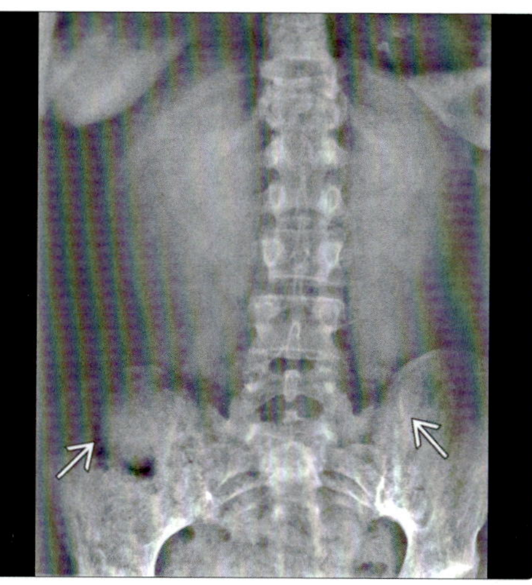

(Left) *Lateral radiograph shows ON and collapse of the superior endplates of 2 vertebral bodies ➡, which has resulted in half of an H shape. Organomegaly is seen, with bowel compressed posteriorly by an enlarged liver.* **(Right)** *AP radiograph shows a typical case of Gaucher disease, with an enlarged liver and spleen ➡ causing centralization and depression of bowel gas into the lower abdomen. Diffuse increased bone density is seen, typical of osseous infarction in this process.*

KEY FACTS

TERMINOLOGY

- Inherited metabolic disorders caused by single gene defects leading to progressive cellular accumulation of glycosaminoglycans and damage to multiple organs
- Radiographic abnormalities are mostly shared by different disorders; termed dysostosis multiplex

IMAGING

- Posterior vertebral body scalloping
- Hypoplastic vertebral bodies: Oval, slightly flattened; L1 most commonly affected
  - Thoracolumbar kyphosis, centered at this level
  - Anterior beaking, involved vertebral bodies
- Ribs: Posterior constriction, oar-shaped
- Pelvis: Constricted, narrow superior acetabulum
- Hand: Constricted base of metacarpals 2-5
  - Fan-shaped on PA view
- MR: Noninflammatory joint contractures
- Spine MR: Dural thickening → cervical myelopathy

PATHOLOGY

- Most autosomal recessive; Hunter is X-linked recessive
- Short, with lumbar kyphosis, sternal protrusion, joint contractures, hepatosplenomegaly, corneal opacification, normal intelligence

CLINICAL ISSUES

- Most detected at birth
  - Mild forms, such as Schele (MPS I-S), may have diagnosis delayed until contractures noted in early adulthood
- Natural history/prognosis: Varies with MPS form
- Treatment depends on type and severity

DIAGNOSTIC CHECKLIST

- Severity of dysostosis multiplex is variable, even intrafamilially
  - Related to phenotypic expression in individual
  - Not possible to differentiate between MPS types based on imaging characteristics

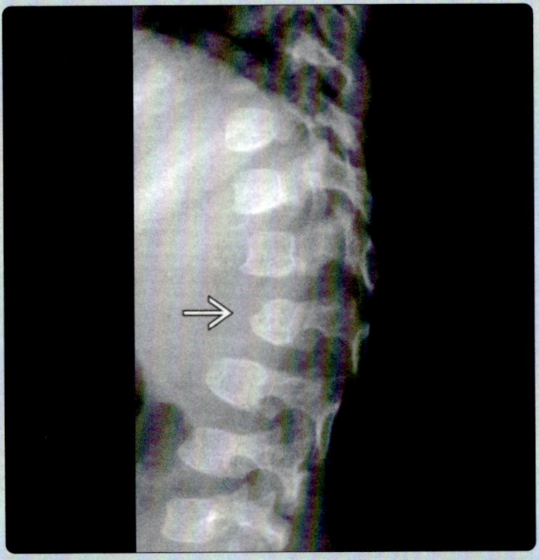

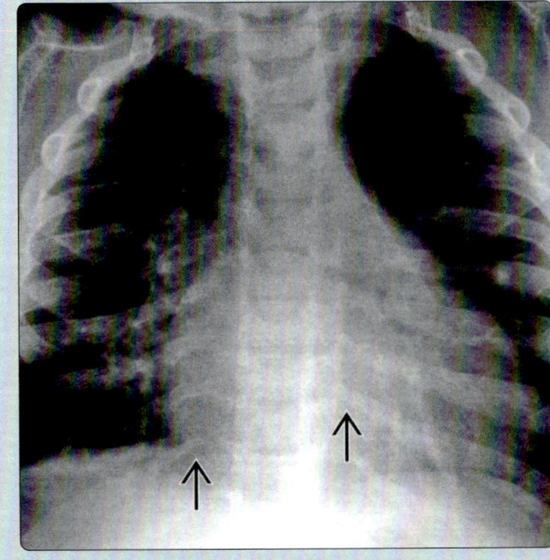

(Left) *Lateral radiograph findings are typical of the thoracolumbar spine in mucopolysaccharidosis. There is hypoplasia of L1, with an anterior beak ➡, resulting in thoracolumbar kyphosis. This is itself not a specific abnormality, as it may be seen in some dwarfs.* **(Right)** *AP chest radiograph in a patient with mucopolysaccharidosis shows ribs that are constricted at the costovertebral junction, giving the appearance of handles on a boat oar (oar-shaped ribs ➡). This is a specific appearance.*

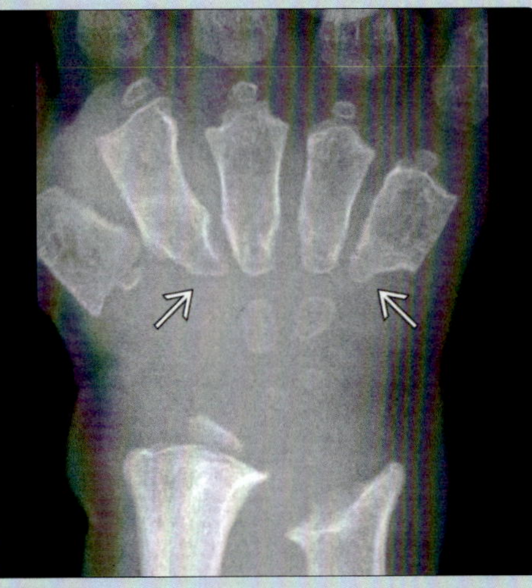

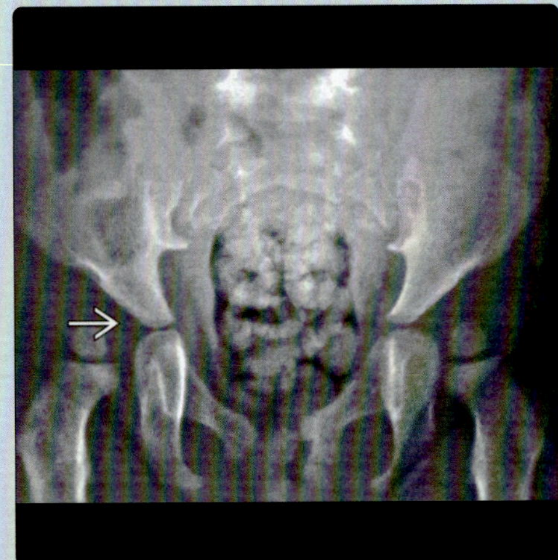

(Left) *PA radiograph shows metacarpals that are short, broad, and constricted proximally. This morphology yields a fan-shaped appearance ➡, which is typical in mucopolysaccharidosis.* **(Right)** *AP radiograph of the pelvis shows a widened sacrosciatic notch due to the narrow and constricted superior acetabulum ➡, which is seen in all types of mucopolysaccharidoses.*

TERMINOLOGY

Abbreviations

- Mucopolysaccharidosis (MPS)

Definitions

- Inherited metabolic disorders caused by single gene defects leading to progressive cellular accumulation of glycosaminoglycans and damage to multiple organs
  - Radiographic abnormalities are mostly shared by different disorders; termed dysostosis multiplex

IMAGING

Radiographic Findings

- Spine
  - Posterior vertebral body scalloping
  - Hypoplastic vertebral bodies: Oval, slightly flattened
    - L1 most commonly affected; adjacent levels may show similar abnormality
    - Thoracolumbar kyphosis, centered at this level
  - Anterior beaking, involved vertebral bodies
  - In addition, Morquio shows hypoplasia of odontoid process and atlantoaxial instability; also more severe flattening and irregularity of vertebral bodies; anterior sternal bowing may result
- Ribs
  - Widened over most of rib but constriction of posterior ribs at costovertebral junction
    - Termed oar-shaped
- Pelvis
  - Constricted, narrow superior acetabulum
    - Results in wide sacrosciatic notch
  - Coxa valga, delayed development femoral heads
- Tubular bones
  - Mild metadiaphyseal expansion, cortical thinning
  - Delay in epiphyseal ossification
  - Upper > lower extremities
- Hand
  - Narrowed, constricted base of metacarpals 2-5
    - Results in fan-shaped metacarpal morphology
  - Short, wide phalanges
  - Delay in carpal ossification
  - Carpal angle may be altered
- Skull
  - Dolichocephalic, macrocephaly
  - Elongated, J-shaped sella

MR Findings

- Joint MR
  - Joint and soft tissue manifestations may be earliest in mild forms of MPS
    - Noninflammatory joint contractures
    - Carpal tunnel syndrome
- Brain MR
  - White matter lesions
  - Dilated perivascular spaces, with prominent involvement of corpus callosum
  - Hydrocephalus
  - Spinal canal stenosis
- Spine MR: Dural thickening → cervical myelopathy

DIFFERENTIAL DIAGNOSIS

Achondroplasia

- Posterior vertebral scalloping
- May have hypoplastic bullet-shaped vertebra at thoracolumbar junction
- Narrow sacrosciatic notch
- Narrowing of interpediculate distance from L1-L5 on AP

PATHOLOGY

General Features

- Etiology
  - Hurler (MPS I-H)
    - Most severe form of MPS I
    - Mental retardation, deafness, dwarfism, hepatosplenomegaly, cardiomegaly, corneal clouding
  - Schele (MPS I-S)
    - Mildest form of MPS I; may have delayed diagnosis
      - □ Stiff joints, flexion deformities may point toward diagnosis
    - Normal mentation, normal or slightly short height, aortic regurgitation, corneal clouding
  - Hunter disease (MPS II)
    - Differentiated from Hurler by less severe hearing impairment, absence of corneal cloudiness, and generally more benign course
    - Cerebral manifestations range widely from mild to severe disability
  - Sanfilippo syndrome (MPS III)
    - Hepatosplenomegaly, ↓ joint mobility, mental retardation
  - Morquio syndrome (MPS IV)
    - Variable severity of clinical manifestations & life span
    - Severe dwarfism, short spine with kyphoscoliosis, joint laxity, corneal clouding, deafness, normal intelligence
      - □ Hypoplastic odontoid and atlantoaxial instability is additional feature

CLINICAL ISSUES

Treatment

- Enzyme replacement therapy beneficial in some
- Allogenic hematopoietic stem cell transplant may help those with cognitive disorders

DIAGNOSTIC CHECKLIST

Reporting Tips

- Severity of dysostosis multiplex is variable, even intrafamilially
  - Related to phenotypic expression in individual
  - Not possible to differentiate between MPS types based on imaging characteristics

SELECTED REFERENCES

1. Lachman RS et al: Mucopolysaccharidosis IVA (Morquio A syndrome) and VI (Maroteaux-Lamy syndrome): under-recognized and challenging to diagnose. Skeletal Radiol. 43(3):359-69, 2014
2. Lachman R et al: Radiologic and neuroradiologic findings in the mucopolysaccharidoses. J Pediatr Rehabil Med. 3(2):109-18, 2010
3. Prasad VK et al: Transplant outcomes in mucopolysaccharidoses. Semin Hematol. 47(1):59-69, 2010

KEY FACTS

TERMINOLOGY

- Histiocytosis characterized by infiltration of skeleton and viscera by lipid-laden histiocytes
  - Leads to fibrosis and osteosclerosis

IMAGING

- Tubular bones (98%)
  - Upper extremities less commonly and less severely involved than lower extremities
- Bilaterally symmetric (98%)
- Patchy or diffuse sclerosis of medullary cavity
  - Heterogeneous (65%) or homogeneous (35%) sclerosis in majority
  - 1/3 mixed lytic/sclerotic
- Cortical thickening
  - Periostitis (66%): Wavy contour of cortex
  - Endosteal thickening (94%)
  - Blurring of corticomedullary differentiation
- Relative epiphyseal sparing, at least subchondrally
- MR appearance
  - Heterogeneous low signal on T1WI
  - Mixed inhomogeneous signal on T2WI/STIR
  - Intense enhancement, heterogeneous
  - Periostitis visualized as high signal along cortices
  - Bone infarcts may be present

TOP DIFFERENTIAL DIAGNOSES

- Langerhans cell histiocytosis
- Myelofibrosis
- Progressive diaphyseal dysplasia
- Intramedullary osteosclerosis

CLINICAL ISSUES

- Classic triad: Bone pain, exophthalmos, diabetes
- Age range: 7-84 years; mean age: 53 years
- Majority of patients die within 3 years
  - Renal, cardiovascular, pulmonary, or central neurologic complications

(Left) *AP radiograph shows sclerotic coarsened trabeculae with regions of lysis occupying the metaphyses & much of the diaphyses of the long tubular bones ➡. Sclerosis fills the medullary canal, with no distinct margin between the cortex and canal. The pattern is symmetric, & the epiphyses are spared ➡. Waviness of the cortex ➡ indicates periosteal involvement.* **(Right)** *Frontal bone scan in the same patient shows involvement of distal radius ⇨ & facial bones →; axial skeleton is normal. Pattern is classic Erdheim-Chester (EC).*

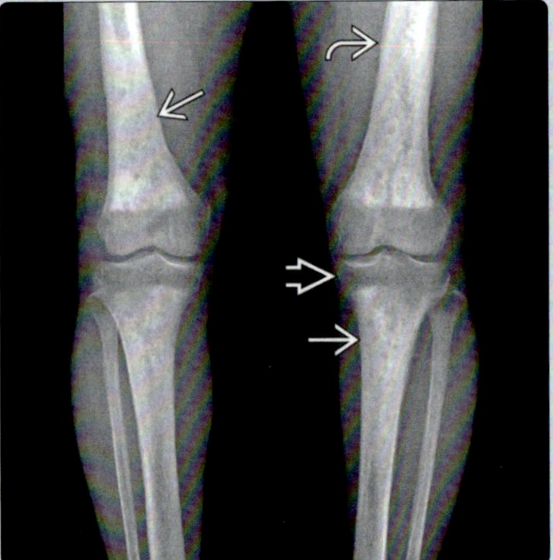

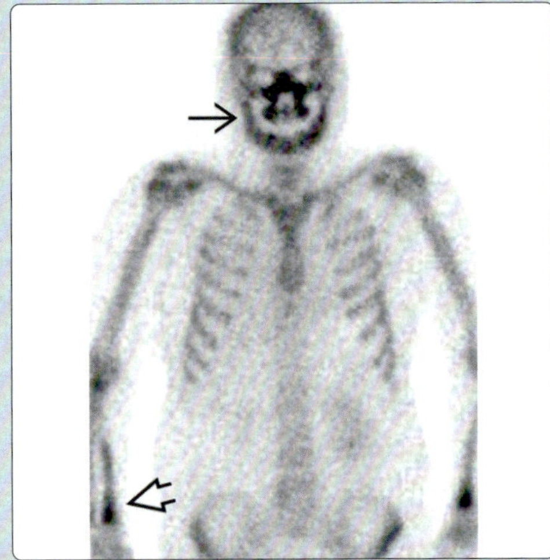

(Left) *Coronal T1WI MR in a 79 year old shows patchy ↓ SI replacing normal fatty marrow in the diaphyses ➡ and homogeneous ↓ SI in the distal metadiaphysis ➡. The distal femoral epiphyses contain normal fatty marrow.* **(Right)** *Coronal T2WI FS MR, same patient, shows mostly homogeneous low signal in the distal metadiaphysis ➡, corresponding to the dense sclerosis seen on T1. The mid diaphyses show inhomogeneous high signal ➡, indicating active marrow replacement process, which proved at biopsy to be EC.*

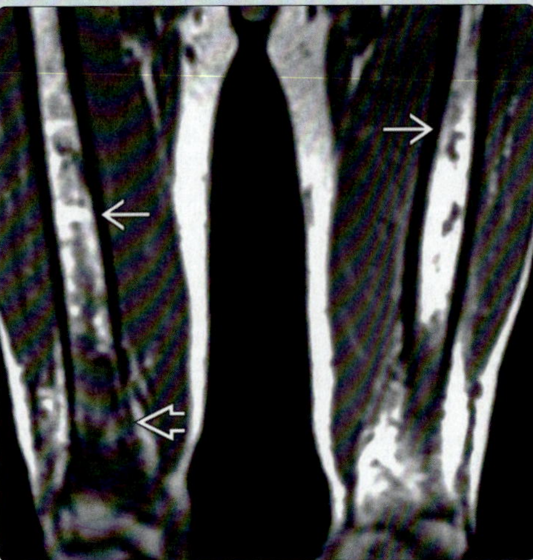

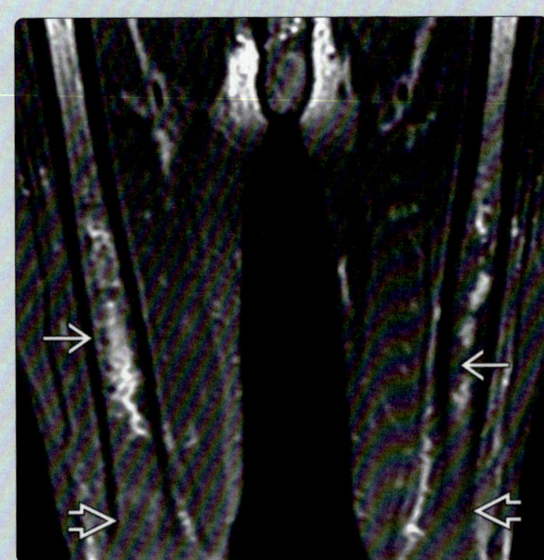

TERMINOLOGY

Abbreviations

- Erdheim-Chester (EC)

Definitions

- Histiocytosis characterized by infiltration of skeleton and viscera by lipid-laden histiocytes
  - Leads to fibrosis and osteosclerosis

IMAGING

General Features

- Best diagnostic clue
  - Diffuse intramedullary sclerosis of tubular bones, bilaterally symmetric and generally lower extremities
- Location
  - Predominantly large long bones
    - Upper extremities less commonly and less severely involved than lower extremities
    - Diaphysis (100%), metaphysis (83%)
    - Epiphyses classically said to be spared
      - Actually, subchondral bone spared; partial epiphyseal involvement in 45%
  - Flat bones can be involved
  - Rare vertebral involvement

Radiographic Findings

- Tubular bones (98%)
  - Bilaterally symmetric (98%)
  - Patchy or diffuse sclerosis of medullary cavity
    - Heterogeneous (65%) or homogeneous (35%) sclerosis in majority
    - 1/3 mixed lytic/sclerotic
    - Purely lytic lesions in only 5-8% of cases
  - Coarse trabeculae
  - Cortical thickening
    - Periostitis (66%): Wavy contour of cortex
    - Endosteal thickening (94%)
      - Blurring of corticomedullary differentiation
      - Marrow cavity may be obliterated
  - Relative epiphyseal sparing, at least subchondrally
    - May have metaepiphyseal lucent line
- Vertebra (rare)
  - Lytic lesions with sclerotic margin
  - Virtually always have coexisting long bone disease
- Focal pseudotumoral lesion (rare)
  - Variably lytic, cortical destruction, soft tissue mass

MR Findings

- Heterogeneous low signal on T1WI
- Mixed inhomogeneous signal on T2WI/STIR
- Intense enhancement, heterogeneous
- Periostitis visualized as high signal along cortices
- Bone infarcts may be present

Nuclear Medicine Findings

- Abnormal increased uptake on bone scan
  - Bilateral, symmetric in tubular bones
- PET/CT shows variable sensitivity
  - Orbital (60%), bones (55%), pulmonary (37%), retroperitoneal (7%)

DIFFERENTIAL DIAGNOSIS

Langerhans Cell Histiocytosis (LCH)

- Reports of biopsy-proven LCH and radiographic findings classic for EC, rarely vice versa
- Other reports of biopsy-proven LCH + EC and radiographic findings of EC or both diseases

Myelofibrosis

- Sclerosis of tubular bones has similar appearance to EC
- Axial skeleton involvement differentiates from EC

Progressive Diaphyseal Dysplasia

- Younger patient population
- Distinct endosteal and periosteal thickening; residual marrow cavity is clearly distinguished from cortex

Intramedullary Osteosclerosis

- Confined to diaphysis; may obliterate canal
- May be unilateral or bilaterally asymmetric

PATHOLOGY

Microscopic Features

- Diffuse infiltration of marrow by foamy histiocytes
  - Associated with dense fibrosis, lymphocytes, plasma cells, Touton giant cells

CLINICAL ISSUES

Presentation

- Most common signs/symptoms
  - Bone pain, rarely with soft tissue swelling
- Other signs/symptoms
  - Extraskeletal manifestations in > 50%
    - Hypothalamus-pituitary axis: Diabetes insipidus
    - Orbit: Exophthalmos, periorbital xanthomas
    - Retroperitoneum: Particularly perirenal
  - Classic triad: Bone pain, exophthalmos, diabetes
  - Serum lipid profile usually relatively normal

Demographics

- Age
  - Peak incidence 5th-7th decades
- Gender
  - Slight male predominance

Natural History & Prognosis

- Prognosis worse with visceral involvement
- Majority of patients die within 3 years
  - Renal, cardiovascular, pulmonary, or central neurologic complications

Treatment

- Interferon-α
- Steroids
- Bisphosphonates

SELECTED REFERENCES

1. Campochiaro C et al: Erdheim-Chester disease. Eur J Intern Med. ePub, 2015
2. Bindra J et al: Erdheim-Chester disease: an unusual presentation of an uncommon disease. Skeletal Radiol. 43(6):835-40, 2014
3. Zaveri J et al: More than just Langerhans cell histiocytosis: a radiologic review of histiocytic disorders. Radiographics. 34(7):2008-24, 2014

KEY FACTS

TERMINOLOGY

- Autoimmune disease characterized by inflammation in multiple organ systems

IMAGING

- Symmetric, polyarticular joint disease
- Most frequent finding: Nonerosive joint deformities
  - Deformities are reducible
- Tenosynovitis
  - Common presenting sign
  - Most common in flexor tendons of hand
- Tendon ruptures: Often large tendons
- Arthritis
  - Symptoms of polyarthralgia common
  - Radiographic abnormalities uncommon
    - Soft tissue swelling, periarticular
    - Juxtaarticular osteopenia
    - Occasional true erosions & cartilage narrowing
- At ↑ risk for septic joint
- Osteoporosis; at risk for insufficiency fractures
- Osteonecrosis (6-40%)
- Inflammatory myositis (4%)

TOP DIFFERENTIAL DIAGNOSES

- Rheumatoid arthritis (RA)
  - Subluxation, deformities of hand may be identical though not reducible
  - Generally RA shows much more impressive marginal erosions & cartilage destruction
  - Rarely SLE results in such significant erosive disease as to completely mimic RA by imaging

CLINICAL ISSUES

- Peak incidence: 15-40 years of age
- F > M (10:1 ratio); 25-50 per 100,000
- Patients of African descent have greater incidence & more severe disease
- MSK system involved in 90% of SLE

(Left) *Sagittal T2WI MR obtained in a patient with systemic lupus erythematosus (SLE) shows abundant ↑ SI fluid, containing ↓ SI debris, surrounding a flexor tendon ➡, which itself is intact. The other soft tissue structures appear normal.* **(Right)** *Axial T1WI C+ FS MR, same case, shows the synovitis as low signal, with high signal lining tendon sheath ➡ and tendons themselves. It is uncommon for patients with SLE to exhibit true arthritis. However, tenosynovitis, particularly of the hand flexors, is a relatively common clinical complaint.*

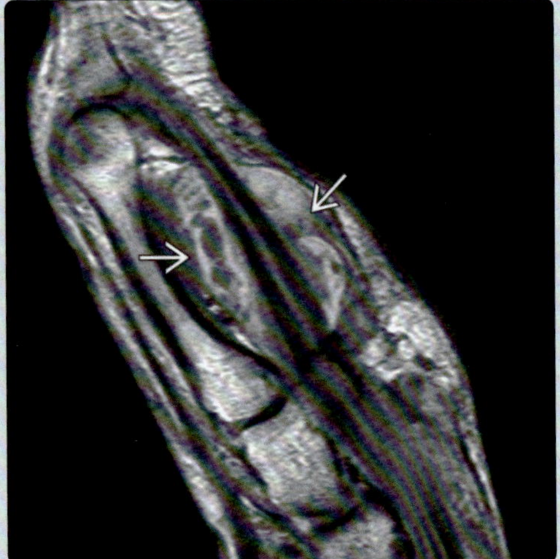

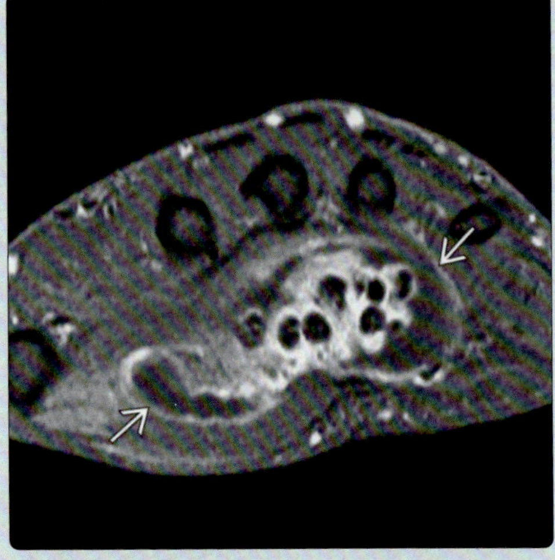

(Left) *PA x-ray demonstrates long-term SLE with severe deformities overshadowing erosive disease. There is volar subluxation and ulnar deviation of the MCP joints ➡. For the degree of deformity, there is little erosive disease seen.* **(Right)** *Oblique x-ray, same case, shows exaggerated deformities now that the hand is no longer supported on the cassette. This is typical of the reducible deformities of SLE. Note also that there is cartilage narrowing and mild erosive disease at 2 of the MCPs ➡.*

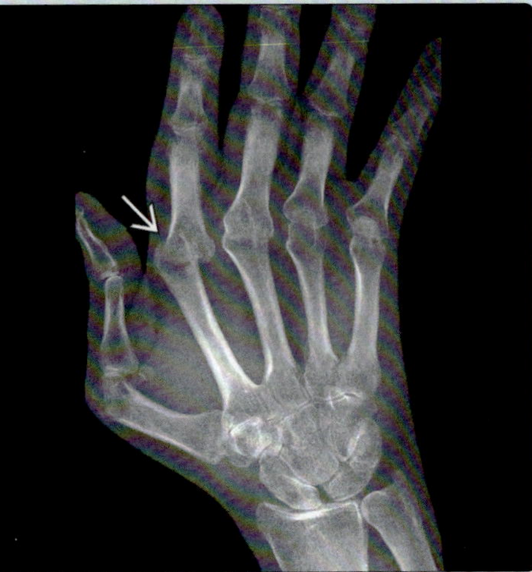

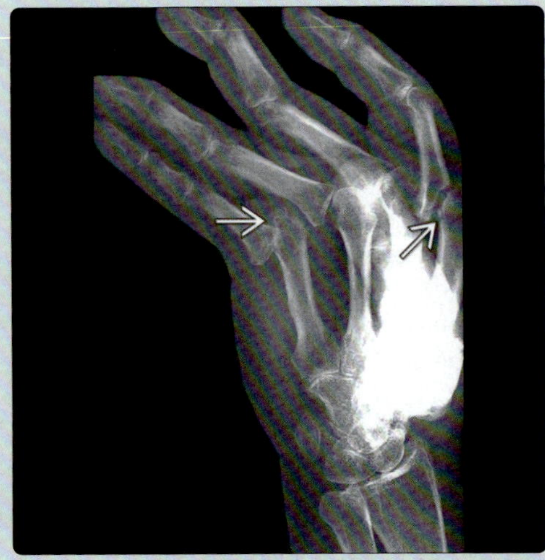

TERMINOLOGY

Abbreviations

- Systemic lupus erythematosus (SLE)

Synonyms

- Lupus; lupus erythematosus

Definitions

- Autoimmune disease characterized by inflammation in multiple organ systems
- Drug-induced lupus: Uncommon complication of several commonly used medications
  - Characterized by development of lupus-like symptoms, ANA positivity

IMAGING

General Features

- Best diagnostic clue
  - Nonerosive reducible deformity of digits
  - Osteoporosis, high rate of osteonecrosis (ON)
- Location
  - Symmetric
  - Polyarticular
  - Small joints of hand, knee, wrist, shoulder

Imaging Recommendations

- Best imaging tool
  - MR for complications (ON, septic joint)

Radiographic Findings

- Subcutaneous tissues
  - Lupus vasculitis involving skin: Ulceration
    - May have associated tuft osteolysis
  - Calcification (uncommon)
    - More often involves lower than upper extremities
- Joints
  - Most frequent: Nonerosive joint deformities (5-40%)
    - Hands, feet
    - Subluxations at MCP, MTPs
    - Swan neck or Boutonnière deformities of digits
    - Deformities most apparent when hand/foot not supported on radiographic cassette
      - Oblique, open book views rather than PA of hands
    - Deformities are reducible
      - Rarely develop into true contractures
    - Atlantoaxial subluxation reported in 10%
      - More common in those patients with nonerosive joint deformities
  - Arthritis (symptoms of polyarthralgia common; radiographic abnormalities less so)
    - Soft tissue swelling, periarticular
    - Juxtaarticular osteopenia
    - Occasional true erosions & cartilage narrowing
  - At ↑ risk for septic joint
    - Effusion
    - Deossification along subchondral bone
- Osteoporosis
  - Insufficiency fractures, especially spine
- ON (6-40%)
  - ON very common in SLE, both in frequency & involving less common locations
    - Not only femoral & humeral heads, but also femoral condyles, tibial plateaus, scaphoid, lunate, talus, MTs
    - Widespread ON in unusual locations should suggest SLE as etiology
  - Abnormal density, subchondral fracture
  - Eventual collapse & development of osteoarthritis

MR Findings

- Subcutaneous tissues
  - Tissue edema: Low T1, high T2, enhancing
  - Rare calcification, low or heterogeneous signal on all sequences; surrounding edema if active
- Tenosynovitis (common presenting MSK sign)
  - Most common in flexor tendons of hand
  - Fluid within tendon sheath: High T2 SI, enhancing tissue around fluid in sheath
- Tendon ruptures
  - May be associated with steroid therapy &/or lupus renal disease
  - Often large tendons (quadriceps, inferior patellar, Achilles)
  - MR signs of partial tendon rupture
    - Abnormal cross-sectional morphology (thickened or thinned)
    - Abnormal high T2 signal within tendon
- Myositis (4%)
  - Nonspecific high signal intensity on fluid-sensitive sequences, especially STIR, with enhancement
  - SLE patients with myositis: Earlier diagnosis, worse prognosis
  - May develop drug-induced myopathy
- Joints
  - Arthritis
    - Effusion
    - Marrow edema
    - Subtle erosions, cartilage loss
      - One study shows small erosions more common in SLE than expected
  - Septic arthritis
    - Marrow edema
    - Effusion; thick enhancing synovium surrounding fluid
    - May see debris within joint
    - Aspiration required for diagnosis
- ON
  - Both central marrow & subchondral infarction
  - Early: Marrow edema, effusion
  - Later: Typical double line sign at site of infarcted bone
- Brain: Small white matter lesions, atrophy

Ultrasonographic Findings

- Tenosynovitis well shown
- May show synovitis, early erosions

DIFFERENTIAL DIAGNOSIS

Rheumatoid Arthritis (RA)

- Subluxation, deformities of hand may be identical to SLE
- Generally RA shows much more impressive marginal erosions & cartilage destruction than SLE

- Rarely, SLE results in such significant erosive disease as to completely mimic RA by imaging

PATHOLOGY

General Features

- Etiology
  - Autoantibodies react with components of cell nucleus (ANA)
    - End organs: Deposition of immune complexes
  - Drug-induced lupus
    - Most commonly involved: Procainamide, hydralazine, isoniazid, quinidine, sulfasalazine, chlorpromazine
- Genetics
  - Likely susceptible genetic background
    - Monozygotic twins concordant for SLE in 30%; dizygotic twins in 5%
    - Likely environmental factors superimposed (most commonly UV light)
  - Certain histocompatibility complex alleles (HLA-B8, DR2, DR3) associated with ↑ risk of SLE

Criteria for Classification of SLE (ARCheum)

- Must have ≥ 4 of following criteria at any time
  - Malar rash
  - Discoid rash
  - Photosensitivity
  - Oral ulcers
  - Arthritis
  - Serositis
  - Renal disorder [persistent proteinuria (> 0.5 g/day) or cellular casts]
  - Neurologic disorder (seizures or psychosis)
  - Hematologic disorder (hemolytic anemia, leukopenia, lymphopenia, thrombocytopenia)
  - Immunologic disorder (anti-DNA antibodies, anti-Sm antibodies, positive LE cell preparation)
  - ANA

CLINICAL ISSUES

Presentation

- Most common signs/symptoms
  - Musculoskeletal system involved in 90% of SLE
    - Arthralgias in most (75-90%)
    - Synovitis less frequent than arthralgias; erosions uncommon
      - Anti-CCP antibodies may be marker for more severe joint disease in SLE
    - Myalgias (30-50%)
    - Reducible deformities of joints
    - ON if treated with steroids, high prolonged dose; ON likely, also related to SLE itself
  - Drug-induced lupus: Milder symptoms
- Other signs/symptoms
  - Autoantibodies
    - Drug-induced lupus has fewer & different autoantibodies
    - ANA(+) equally in SLE & drug-induced lupus
  - Constitutional symptoms: Fever, malaise, weakness, anorexia, weight loss
  - Pleuritis & pericarditis: Both SLE & drug-induced lupus
  - CNS, renal abnormalities in SLE, less frequent in drug-induced lupus
    - Lupus nephritis common; may have severe morbidity
    - Neuropsychiatric findings common & varied
      - Brain MR abnormalities in 25% of newly diagnosed SLE (focal lesions or cerebral atrophy)
  - Lupus skin findings
    - Malar rash, oral ulcers, photosensitivity, vasculitic skin lesions
    - Uncommon in drug-induced lupus
  - Vascular: Common
    - Hypertension: Predictor of ↓ patient survival
    - Atherosclerotic cardiovascular disease

Demographics

- Age
  - Peak incidence: 15-40 years
  - Drug-induced lupus: Older patient age group
- Gender
  - F > M (10:1 ratio)
  - Female preponderance ↓ in older patient age group
- Epidemiology
  - 25-50 per 100,000
  - Patients of African descent have greater incidence & more severe disease
    - Among African American females, prevalence of 4 per 1,000
  - ON in SLE may have some relation to age at which steroids started
    - One study shows, in 1-year follow-up for ON by MR, only 6% of pediatric patients developed ON, while 49% of adolescents & 41% of adults did

Natural History & Prognosis

- Frequency of end-organ involvement varies widely, as does associated prognosis
- Most common is flare pattern: Relapsing-remitting
  - Others have continuous symptoms
  - Minority have long quiescent periods
- 50% develop permanent damage in at least 1 organ system
- 80% survival 10 years after diagnosis
  - Major cause of death is accelerated atherosclerosis
- Opportunistic infections relatively common
- ↑ risk of malignancy suggested from cohort studies

Treatment

- Guided by specific end-organ involvement
  - Lupus nephritis: Steroids & cytotoxic agents
  - Arthralgias: NSAIDs & hydroxychloroquine
    - If severe, may treat as RA
  - Corticosteroids widely used for multiple manifestations of SLE
- Drug-induced lupus: Resolves with withdrawal of offending drug

SELECTED REFERENCES

1. Chiara T et al: MRI pattern of arthritis in systemic lupus erythematosus: a comparative study with rheumatoid arthritis and healthy subjects. Skeletal Radiol. 44(2):261-6, 2015
2. Nakamura J et al: Age at time of corticosteroid administration is a risk factor for osteonecrosis in pediatric patients with systemic lupus erythematosus: A prospective magnetic resonance imaging study. Arthritis Rheum. 62(2):609-615, 2010

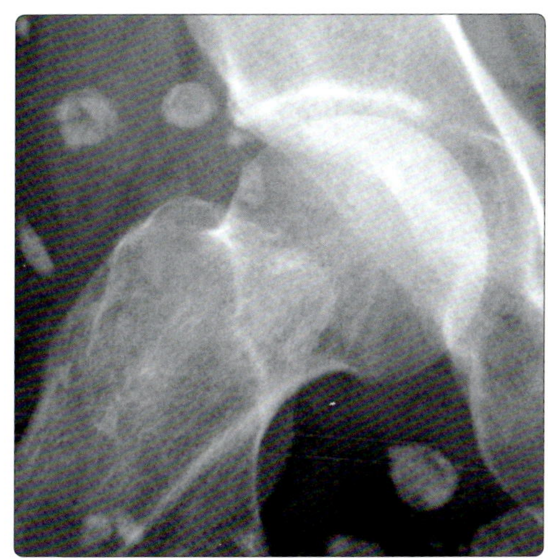
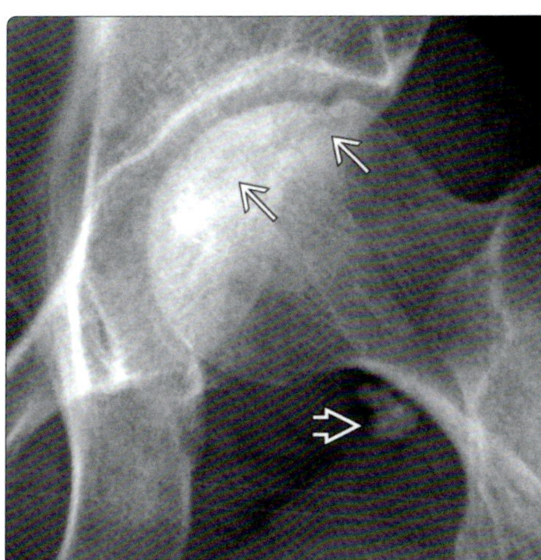

(Left) *Frog leg lateral radiograph shows multiple sites of dense globular soft tissue calcification. Occasionally patients with SLE, as in this case, develop soft tissue calcification; lower extremities are more often involved than upper.* **(Right)** *Frog leg lateral radiograph, in the contralateral hip of the same patient, shows osteonecrosis (ON) of the femoral head, seen as a subchondral fracture ➡. A focus of soft tissue calcification is also seen ➡. ON is not a surprising finding in patients with SLE.*

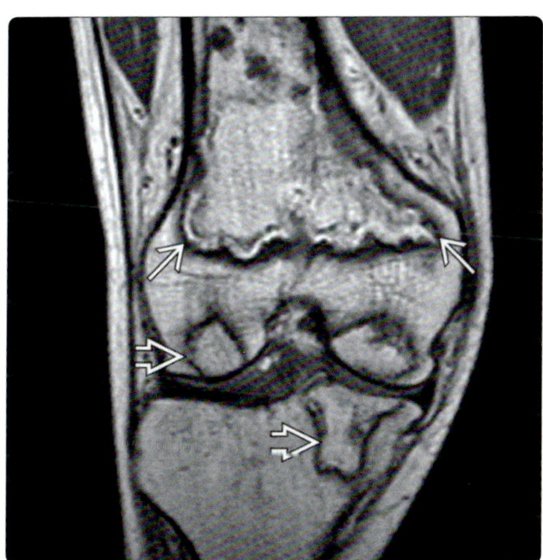
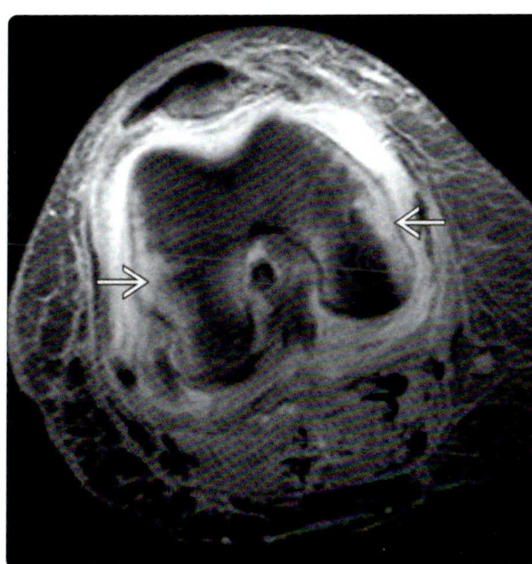

(Left) *Coronal T1WI MR demonstrates serpiginous low signal geographic abnormalities in the femoral metaphysis ➡ and subchondral bone of both the femur and tibia ➡. Bone infarct is a common complication of SLE.* **(Right)** *Axial T1WI C+ FS MR in a patient with known SLE shows bone enhancement ➡, more than expected for reactive marrow edema from a noninfective synovitis. Joint aspirate proved infection. Patients with SLE are at greater than normal risk for septic joint.*

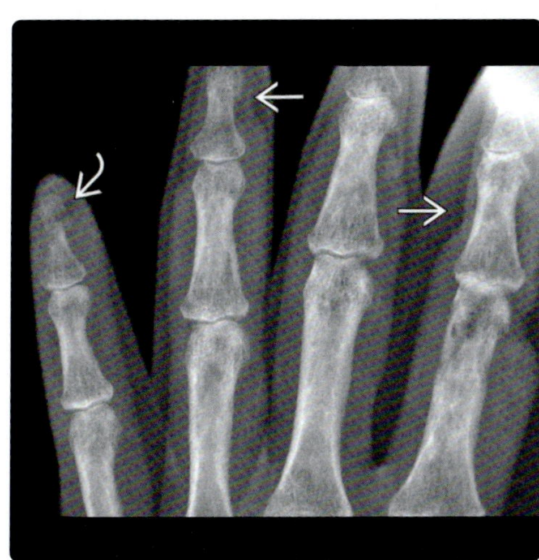
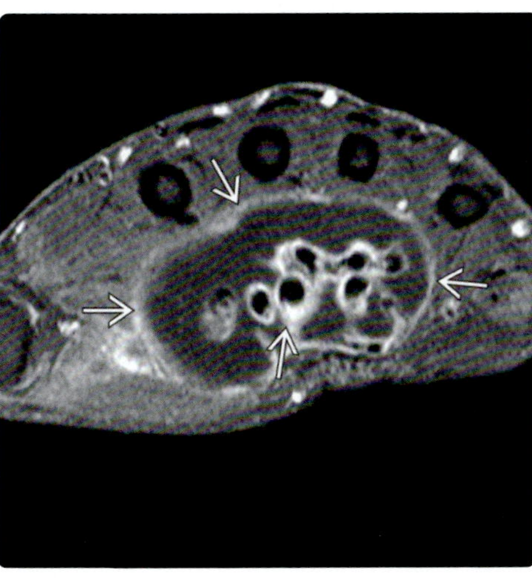

(Left) *PA radiograph shows soft tissue tapering and ulceration along the terminal portions of the digits ➡. There is early osteolysis of the tufts, best seen at the 5th digit ➡. The findings are typical of a vasculitis but otherwise nonspecific. This patient had lupus vasculitis and dry gangrene.* **(Right)** *Axial postcontrast T1FS MR shows hypointense fluid within the tendon sheaths surrounded by a hyperintense rim ➡. This is typical tenosynovitis and is often the 1st imaging finding of SLE.*

Progressive Systemic Sclerosis

KEY FACTS

TERMINOLOGY

- Progressive systemic sclerosis (PSS): Multisystem disorder characterized by skin thickening and fibrosis

IMAGING

- Skin changes
  - Early: Swelling
  - Mid-disease: Tapering of skin at ends of digits
  - Late: Contractures
- Calcinosis
  - May be punctate, globular, even sheet-like
  - 73-86% of patients with calcinosis have it in hand
- Acroosteolysis (40-80%)
  - Resorption of tufts, pencilling, eventual resorption of entire distal phalanx
- Arthritis (uncommon early in disease)
  - Late in disease may develop erosions and cartilage narrowing
  - Subluxation and erosion at 1st carpometacarpal thought to be hallmark of PSS
- HRCT used to evaluate lung fibrosis
  - Dilated esophagus with air-fluid levels
- MR of MSK abnormalities
  - Tenosynovitis often early finding (fibrotic nodules on tendon may be seen, outlined by synovial fluid)
  - Muscle: Late atrophy and fibrosis
  - Early myopathy, not distinguishable from other etiologies

CLINICAL ISSUES

- 50% present before age 40
- PSS: 80% are female
  - CREST syndrome: Male < female (M:F =1:3)
- Rare: Prevalence of 250 patients per million in USA
- Prognosis closely related to internal organ involvement
  - 5-year survival rate of 50% with renal involvement
  - 5-year survival 70% with pulmonary involvement

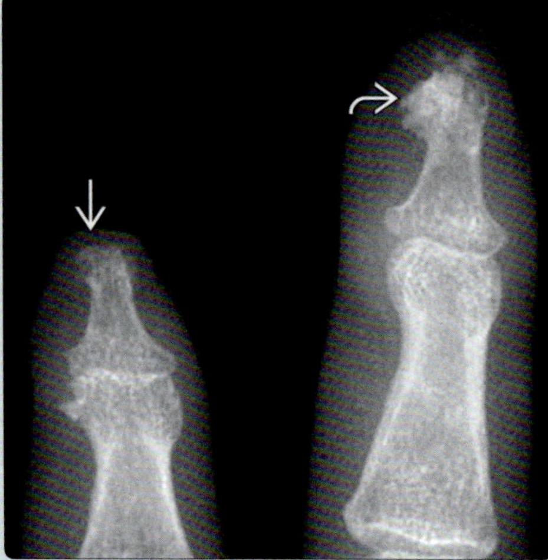

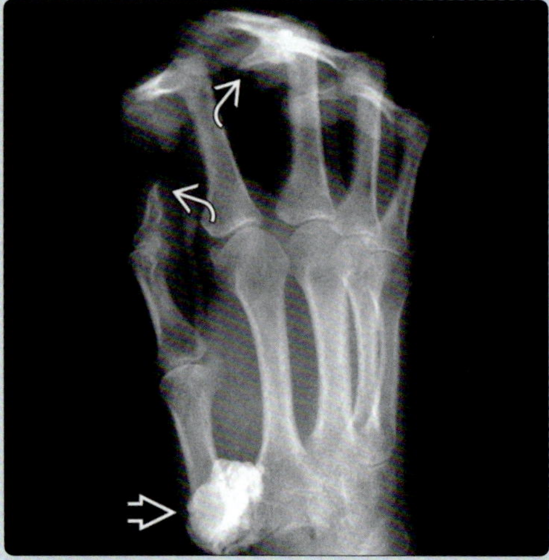

(Left) *PA radiograph of the digits shows early acroosteolysis with associated soft tissue tapering → as well as globular soft tissue calcification →. Although both findings may be seen in HPTH, there is no evidence of subperiosteal resorption, making PSS the most likely diagnosis.* **(Right)** *Oblique radiograph in late PSS shows acroosteolysis → and globular calcification within soft tissues →. There are contractures of digits 2-4. This constellation of findings might be seen with burn injury, but the proven diagnosis is PSS.*

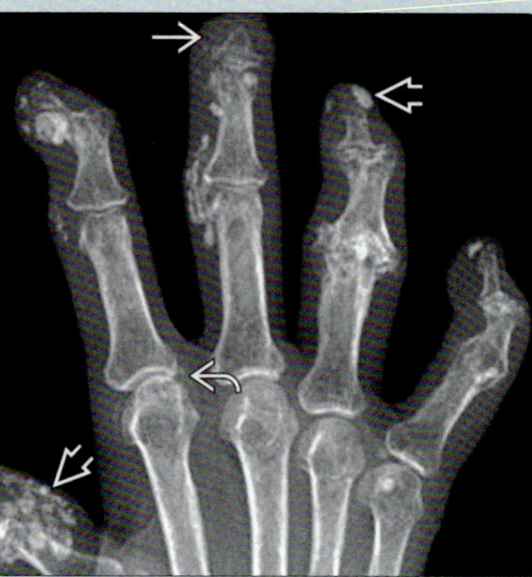

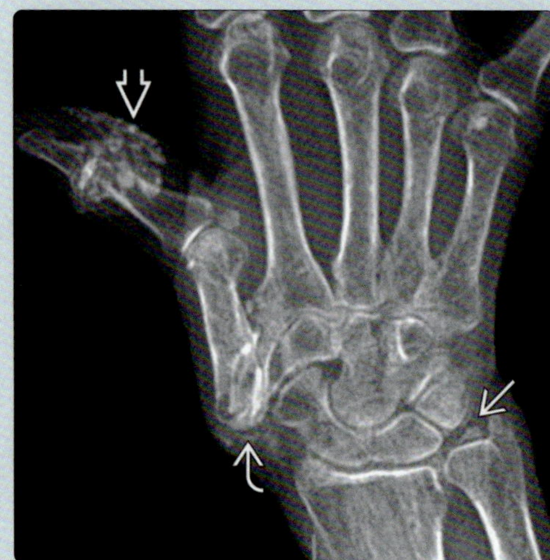

(Left) *PA radiograph shows classic advanced progressive systemic sclerosis (PSS), or scleroderma. There is prominent soft tissue calcinosis, both in the subcutaneous tissues → and periarticular regions →. Note the acroosteolysis, most prominently seen in the 3rd digit →. There are DIP erosions, often a late feature in PSS.* **(Right)** *PA x-ray of wrist shows subcutaneous → and TFC → calcification. The 1st CMC → shows resorption at the joint and significant subluxation. This is thought to be a hallmark of PSS.*

TERMINOLOGY

Synonyms

- Scleroderma, diffuse scleroderma
  - CREST syndrome (calcifications, Raynaud phenomenon, esophageal hypomobility, sclerodactyly, telangiectasia) = limited scleroderma

Definitions

- Progressive systemic sclerosis (PSS): Multisystem disorder characterized by skin thickening and vasculitis
  - Triad of widespread microangiopathy, fibrosis, and autoimmunity

IMAGING

General Features

- Best diagnostic clue
  - Acroosteolysis with soft tissue calcification

Imaging Recommendations

- Best imaging tool
  - For MSK abnormalities, radiograph often diagnostic
  - MR for subtle MSK abnormalities: erosions, tenosynovitis, myositis, and problem solving
  - MR, CT for screening for internal organ involvement (lung, cardiac, GI)

Radiographic Findings

- Skin changes
  - Early: Swelling
  - Mid-disease: Tapering of skin at ends of digits
  - Late: Contractures
  - May develop ulcerations
- Calcinosis
  - May be seen at any stage
  - May be punctate, globular, even sheet-like
  - 73-86% of patients with calcinosis have it in hand
    - Conversely, frequency of digital calcification in patients with PSS 10-30%
- Acroosteolysis (40-80%)
  - Resorption of tufts, pencilling, eventual resorption of entire distal phalanx
- Arthritis
  - Uncommon early in disease
  - Late in disease: Erosions and cartilage narrowing
    - May become severe, → ankylosis, especially of DIPs
  - Subluxation at 1st carpometacarpal joint thought to be hallmark of disease
    - Resorption of trapezium and base of 1st metacarpal, radial and proximal subluxation of thumb

Ultrasonographic Findings

- Synovitis, tenosynovitis, calcinosis, distal vascularization assessment

CT Findings

- HRCT used to evaluate lung fibrosis
  - Honeycomb pattern of fibrosis (basilar)
  - Ground-glass pattern with alveolitis
- Dilated esophagus with air-fluid levels
- Abdomen
  - Wide-mouthed colonic diverticula
  - Antimesenteric small bowel pseudosacculation
  - Rare pneumatosis

MR Findings

- Calcinosis
  - Low signal on all sequences
- Skin changes
  - Early: Edema, with high SI on fluid-sensitive sequences
  - Subcutaneous septal thickening (65%)
  - Later: Fibrosis, with low SI and disturbance of normal subcutaneous architecture
- Tenosynovitis
  - Often early finding (21%)
  - Fluid-filled synovial sheaths
    - Fluid: Low SI on T1WI
    - Fluid: High SI on fluid-sensitive sequences
      - □ May contain low signal synovial thickening or fibrinous nodules on tendons
    - With contrast, synovium enhances around ↓ SI fluid
  - Tendons themselves usually normal
- Arthritis
  - Marrow edema
  - Synovitis (43%)
  - Small erosions, cartilage thinning
- Fascial changes
  - Thickening (60%) and enhancement (53%)
  - Perifascial enhancement (16%)
- Myopathy (14%)
  - Early bland myopathy due to muscle fibrosis
    - Generally not true for inflammatory myopathy
    - High signal on STIR, with enhancement
  - Atrophy: Decreased muscle mass, ↑ fat signal
- Myocardial fibrosis demonstrated by contrast-enhanced MR

DIFFERENTIAL DIAGNOSIS

Hyperparathyroidism

- Acroosteolysis and soft tissue calcification similar
- Hyperparathyroidism (HPTH) should show other findings of bone resorption
  - Subperiosteal, subchondral, subligamentous

Thermal Injury, Burns

- Acroosteolysis and soft tissue calcification similar
- Often have contractures (may be seen late in PSS)

Psoriatic Arthritis

- May have acroosteolysis
- Increased density in tuft (ivory tuft) may mimic calcinosis
- DIP erosions are similar though occur earlier in psoriatic than PSS disease process

PATHOLOGY

General Features

- Etiology
  - Unknown; immunologic abnormality suggested by characteristic antibodies
    - ANA, anti-centromere, anti-Scl-70
  - Possible environmental trigger in susceptible individuals

- Scleroderma-like syndromes with epidemic exposure to toxins
- Vascular damage may be primary event
  - Endothelial cell activation/damage and apoptosis, intimal thickening, delamination, vessel narrowing, and obliteration
  - Impaired angiogenic response
- Genetics
  - Multiple genes involved in immune regulation are susceptibility genes for PSS

Microscopic Features

- Early dermal changes: Lymphocytic infiltrates consisting primarily of T cells
- Major abnormality: Collagen accumulation/fibrosis
  - Increased fibrotic tissue in dermis accompanied by loss of normal skin appendages, such as hair follicles
  - Skeletal muscle and myocardium show atrophy of muscle fibers and replacement by fibrotic tissue

CLINICAL ISSUES

Presentation

- Most common signs/symptoms
  - Skin changes are hallmark of disease (63%)
    - Early stages: Thickening, swelling; normal skin folds over knuckles may be obliterated
    - No hair in affected areas
    - In PSS, involves acral regions, plus proximal extremity and truncal and facial skin
    - Raynaud phenomenon, loss of digital pulp; hyperkeratosis under nails; open ulcerations
    - Subcutaneous calcinosis
    - Late disease: Contractures
  - MSK symptoms
    - Arthralgias and joint stiffness common
    - Occasionally, initially appear rheumatoid-like, with synovitis
    - Palpable tendon friction rubs
    - Muscle weakness from atrophy, fibrosis
  - Gastrointestinal symptoms
    - Esophageal dysmotility; substernal dysphagia
    - Symptomatic reflux
    - Involvement of small bowel (smooth muscle atrophy) less common
    - Recurrent bouts of alternating diarrhea and constipation; pseudo-obstruction uncommon
  - Cardiopulmonary symptoms
    - Interstitial lung disease → restrictive abnormality on pulmonary function tests
    - Increased pulmonary pressures may contribute to right-sided heart failure
    - 80% have interstitial lung disease (ILD); 10-20% develop progressive ILD
    - Myocardial fibrosis may develop
  - Kidney symptoms
    - Renal hypertensive crisis may result in rapidly progressive renal failure
  - Hypothyroidism (fibrosis of thyroid gland) in 25%
  - CREST syndrome (limited scleroderma)
    - Calcinosis is least common of findings
    - Nearly all develop sclerodactyly and Raynaud phenomenon
      - Should prompt search for esophageal dysmotility or cutaneous telangiectasia
      - Sclerodactyly: Skin thickening distal to elbows/knees
      - Rarely affects face or neck
    - Arthralgia/arthritis rare
    - Pulmonary fibrosis in 1/3
- Other signs/symptoms
  - Majority are ANA(+)
  - Anticentromere antibodies: Positive in > 50% patients with CREST, fewer with PSS

Demographics

- Age
  - 50% present before 40 years
- Gender
  - PSS: 80% are female
  - CREST syndrome: Male < female (M:F = 1:3)
- Ethnicity
  - Possible higher incidence and severity in African American women than Caucasians
  - 100x ↑ prevalence in Choctaw Native Americans
- Epidemiology
  - Rare: Prevalence of 250 patients per million in USA
  - Possibly higher prevalence in USA than in northern Europe or Asia
  - CREST (limited scleroderma) more common than diffuse scleroderma (PSS)

Natural History & Prognosis

- Prognosis closely related to internal organ involvement
  - 5-year survival without organ involvement > 90%
  - 5-year survival 70% with pulmonary involvement
    - Even mild pulmonary arterial hypertension may result in severe morbidity
  - 5-year survival rate of 50% with renal involvement
    - 20% mortality if renal hypertensive crisis occurs

Treatment

- No proven disease-modifying medication exists
- Vasodilating agents may be used for Raynaud
- Prednisone may be useful in early stages of disease
- Penicillamine: Possible reduction in skin thickening and pulmonary, gastrointestinal abnormalities
- CREST treatment directed toward symptomatic relief
  - Hand warmers
  - Smoking cessation
  - Hand/foot skin care
- Yearly screening to detect internal organ involvement

SELECTED REFERENCES

1. Freire V et al: Hand and wrist involvement in systemic sclerosis: US features. Radiology. 269(3):824-30, 2013
2. Hachulla E et al: Diagnosis and classification of systemic sclerosis. Clin Rev Allergy Immunol. 40(2):78-83, 2011
3. Schanz S et al: Localized scleroderma: MR findings and clinical features. Radiology. 260(3):817-24, 2011
4. Agarwal SK et al: The genetics of scleroderma (systemic sclerosis). Curr Opin Rheumatol. 22(2):133-8, 2010

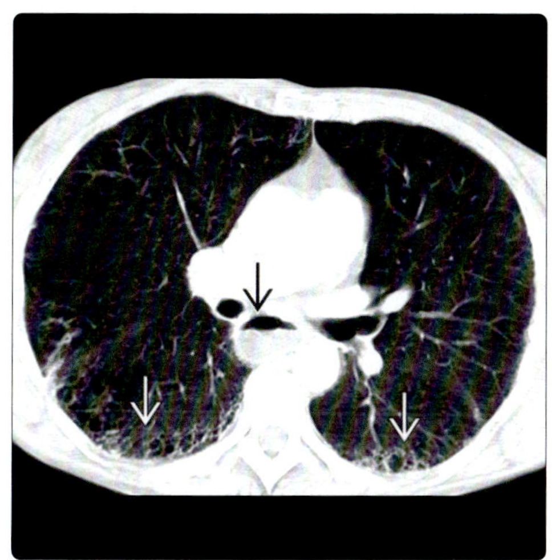

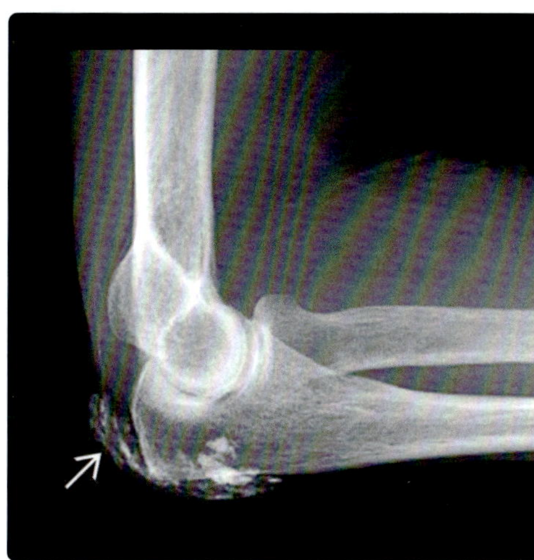

(Left) *Axial high-resolution CT shows a dilated esophagus with the air-fluid level ➔ indicating dysmotility, as well as interstitial disease involving the lung bases ➔. Lung involvement may result in severe morbidity in PSS, and patients should be routinely screened for this.* **(Right)** *Lateral radiograph, same patient, shows dense sheet-like calcification in the subcutaneous tissues ➔. While this pattern may be seen in inflammatory myositis, it is also seen in PSS, the diagnosis this patient carries.*

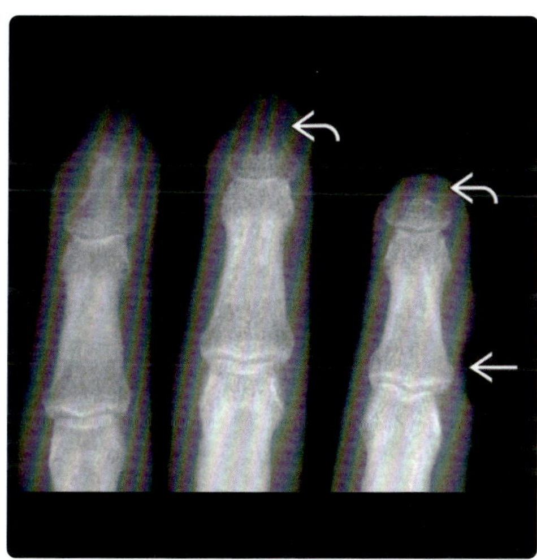

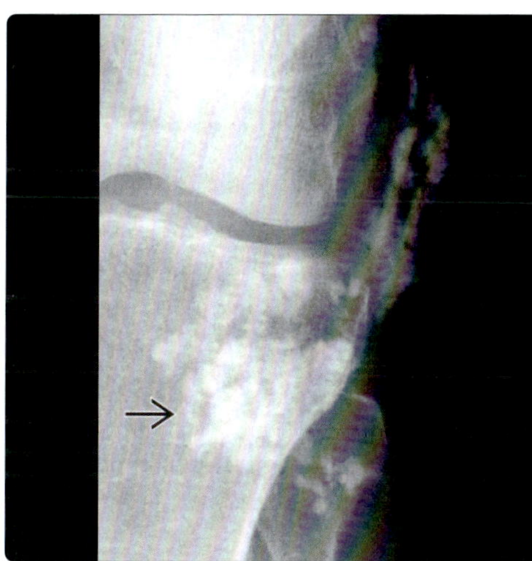

(Left) *PA radiograph shows ulceration of the soft tissue ➔ but also shows tapering of the soft tissues of the digits along with acroosteolysis ➔. The soft tissues are tapered as well. This severe degree of acroosteolysis may develop at mid or late disease in PSS.* **(Right)** *AP radiograph shows soft tissue calcinosis ➔ in a patient with PSS, which appears almost sheet-like, as one might expect in dermatomyositis. This appearance is nonspecific.*

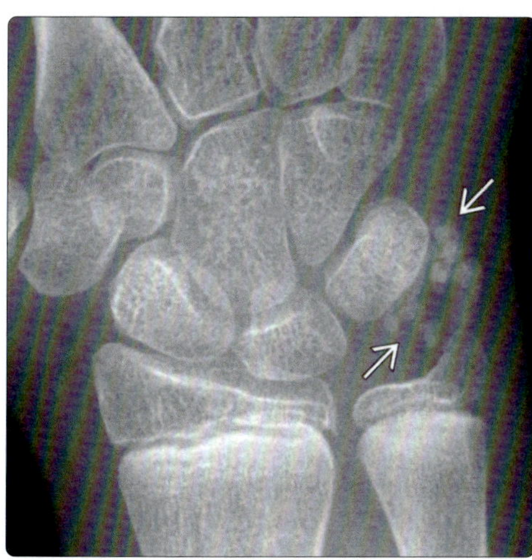

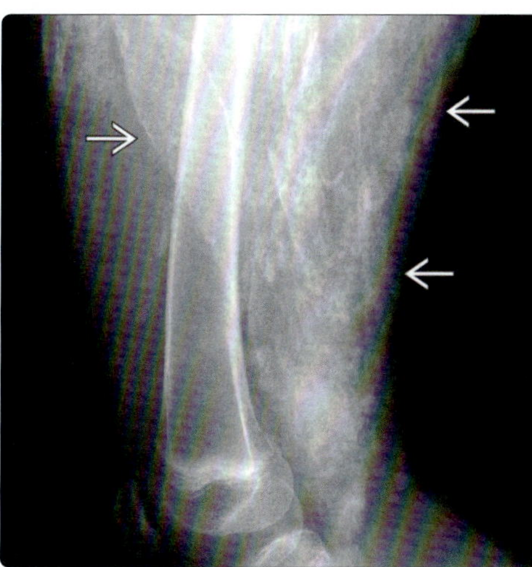

(Left) *AP radiograph shows globular calcifications ➔ in the soft tissues of the wrist. There was also globular calcification along the volar aspect of 1 finger (not shown), both suggesting the diagnosis of PSS.* **(Right)** *Lateral radiograph, same case, shows sheet-like calcifications ➔ that are more suggestive of dermatomyositis. While both patterns may be seen in either PSS or dermatomyositis, the combination makes one consider mixed connective tissue disorder (overlap syndrome).*

Inflammatory Myopathy

KEY FACTS

TERMINOLOGY

- Inflammation and damage to skeletal muscle, with ↑ in muscle-derived proteins (creatine kinase)
  - Includes polymyositis (PM), dermatomyositis (DM), focal myositis, inclusion body myositis

IMAGING

- DM, PM bilaterally symmetric
  - Early location: Proximal lower extremities; usually vasti
  - Progresses to upper extremity, neck, and pharyngeal muscles
- Diagnosis and complications suggested on radiograph
  - Soft tissue calcification (20-50%)
    - Classic description is sheet-like
    - Many cases are globular or amorphous
  - Osteopenia, related to steroid therapy
  - Osteonecrosis, related to steroid therapy
- MR preferred imaging (early diagnosis, choice of biopsy site, cost-effective follow-up)
  - Whole body MR may show areas of involvement not clinically suspected
  - Muscle inflammation shows ↑ SI fluid-sensitive sequences; STIR highly sensitive
  - Abnormalities seen in muscle body; may also have myofascial distribution
- Subcutaneous edema
  - May detect DM prior to clinical evidence of skin rash
- CT: Shows distribution of soft tissue calcification
  - Shows rare fluid-calcium levels

TOP DIFFERENTIAL DIAGNOSES

- Infectious myositis and pyomyositis
- Diabetic spontaneous myonecrosis

PATHOLOGY

- Underlying connective tissue disease in 33%
- Underlying malignancy in 10% of DM and PM

(Left) *Coronal STIR MR shows bilateral, symmetric abnormally high signal intensity involving all the muscles ➡ of the anterior and adductor compartments of the thighs. In this case, the muscles are diffusely involved.* **(Right)** *Coronal T1WI C+ FS MR in the same patient shows diffuse and apparently symmetric enhancement ➡ in a typical case of polymyositis. Even though there appears to be diffuse involvement, clinical signs may be less impressive. MR often shows earlier and more widespread involvement than is expected clinically.*

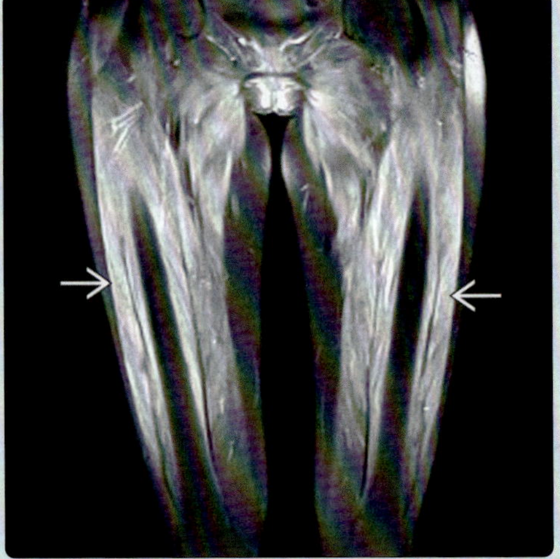

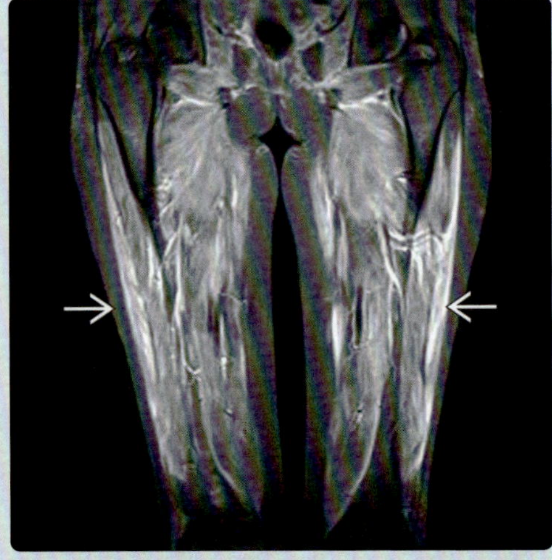

(Left) *Axial T1WI C+ FS MR shows mostly symmetric enhancement. However, the vastus lateralis shows differential enhancement ➡; this was chosen for biopsy, confirming polymyositis. It is not uncommon for the vasti to show the earliest and most prominent disease. (Courtesy J. Linklater, MD.)* **(Right)** *Axial T2WI FS MR reveals asymmetric disease. Note the patchy edema in several muscles ➡ and in the subcutaneous and fascial planes ➡. Findings suggest early myositis and require biopsy for definitive diagnosis.*

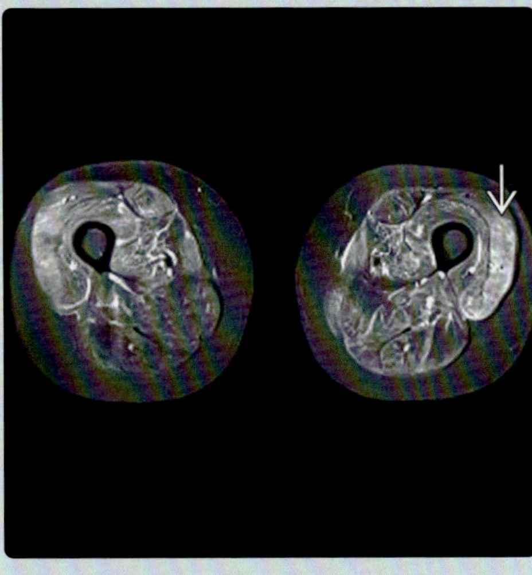

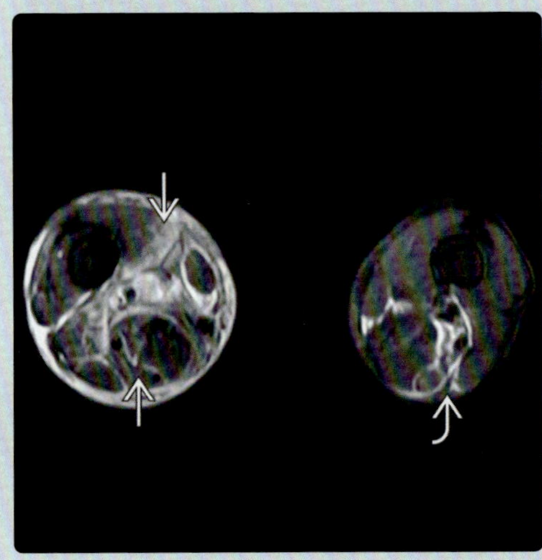

TERMINOLOGY

Synonyms

- Idiopathic inflammatory myopathy

Definitions

- Inflammation and damage to skeletal muscle with ↑ in muscle-derived proteins (creatine kinase)
  - Diffuse: Polymyositis (PM), dermatomyositis (DM)
  - Focal patterns: Inclusion body myositis (IBM), focal myositis (FM; may progress to PM)

IMAGING

General Features

- Location
  - DM, PM bilaterally symmetric
    - Early: Proximal lower extremities; usually vasti
      - Progresses to upper extremity, neck, and pharyngeal muscles
  - IBM, FM: Focal involvement

Imaging Recommendations

- Best imaging tool
  - Diagnosis and complications suggested on radiograph
  - MR is preferred imaging modality: Early diagnosis, choice of biopsy site, cost-effective follow-up
    - Whole body MR may show areas of involvement not clinically suspected

Radiographic Findings

- Soft tissue calcification (20-50% of DM)
  - Classic description is sheet-like
  - Many cases are globular or amorphous
- Osteopenia, related to steroid therapy
  - Associated insufficiency fracture, especially in spine
- Osteonecrosis, related to steroid therapy
  - Intramedullary infarct: Patchy or serpiginous
  - Subchondral infarct: Relative sclerosis, surrounding osteopenia, followed by subchondral fracture line

CT Findings

- Shows distribution of soft tissue calcification
- Shows rare fluid-calcium levels

MR Findings

- Subcutaneous edema
  - Prominent on fluid-sensitive sequences
  - May detect DM prior to clinical evidence of skin rash
- Fasciitis
  - Common finding; hyperintense fascia surrounding muscle on fluid-sensitive or postcontrast imaging
  - Often predates findings of myositis, both on MR and histology
    - Suggests fasciitis contributes to muscle symptoms in patients who have not yet progressed to true myositis
      - May explain why blind biopsy of symptomatic muscle may not show inflammation of muscle tissue
- Inflammatory myositis
  - Calcification low signal on all sequences
  - Abnormalities seen in muscle body; may also have myofascial distribution
  - ↑ SI fluid-sensitive sequences; STIR highly sensitive
    - Individual muscle edema ranges from patchy to diffuse
    - May have ring-like hyperintensity at muscle periphery
  - No mass or architectural distortion
  - MR preferred to identify muscles for directed biopsy
  - Sequelae: ↓ muscle bulk (atrophy) and ↑ T1W signal (fat infiltration)
- Focal myositis
  - T1 ↓ SI, T2 ↑ SI, enhances inhomogeneously
  - Generally does not show encapsulation
- Osteonecrosis
  - Typical double line sign on T2WI

DIFFERENTIAL DIAGNOSIS

Infectious Myositis and Pyomyositis

- Focal abscess within abnormal muscle signal; thick enhancing rim
- Elevated white blood cell count

Diabetic Spontaneous Myonecrosis

- History of poorly controlled diabetes; develops muscle infarction
- May show vascular disease inappropriate for patient age

Crohn Disease Granuloma

- May rarely develop focal granulomas within muscle
- Responds to therapy directed at underlying disease

Sarcoidosis of Muscle

- Nodular (central region hypointensity) or myopathic (diffuse nonspecific signal abnormality)

Behçet Syndrome

- Rare vasculitic disease (venous)
- Rarely develops focal necrotizing myositis

Familial Mediterranean Fever

- Fever plus serositis, synovitis, or skin rash
- May develop short-lasting myalgia with nonspecific myositis on MR

Drug-Induced Rhabdomyalgia

- Generally due to cholesterol-lowering agents or glucocorticoids
- HIV treatment (zidovudine)
- D-penicillamine
- Illicit drugs

Chronic Graft-vs.-Host Disease

- Following allogenic stem cell transplantation
- Focal muscle necrosis with massive lymphocytic infiltration

Radiation-Recall Myositis

- Uncommon reaction in which administration of chemotherapeutic agent induces inflammatory reaction in previously irradiated tissues
- Often weeks to years after radiation therapy

PATHOLOGY

General Features

- Etiology
  - Crohn disease patients rarely may develop focal granulomas within muscle
  - Possible viral etiology in genetically susceptible patient
- Genetics
  - Some DM associated with major histocompatibility complex alleles HLA-DR3 and DRw52
- Associated abnormalities
  - Underlying connective tissue disease in 33%
    - Systemic lupus erythematosus (SLE), Sjögren syndrome, systemic sclerosis, overlap syndromes, mixed connective tissue disease may be accompanied by inflammatory myositis
    - SLE may have associated true myositis
      - Generally diagnosed at earlier age and have poorer prognosis
    - SLE patients may develop drug-induced myopathy
    - Sjögren syndrome patients rarely may have lesions similar to IBM
    - Progressive sclerosis patients may have myalgias and bland myopathy due to muscle fibrosis (generally not true inflammation)
    - Overlap syndromes: 83% have associated myositis
  - Underlying malignancy in 10% of DM and PM; risk is greater in older patients

Microscopic Features

- Mononuclear cell infiltrate, predominately lymphocytes, surrounding or invading muscle fibers
  - PM: Predominant cells are cytotoxic CD8 T cells, endomysial in location
  - DM: Predominant cells are CD4 T cells and B cells, perimysial in location
- Intramuscular vasculature may be primary target
  - Microvascular deposition of immunoglobulin, complement, and membrane attack complex hypothesized
    - Deposits induce endothelial cell edema, vacuolization, capillary necrosis, and perivascular inflammation
  - Inflammatory infiltrates predominantly perivascular or clustered in interfascicular septa surrounding rather than within muscle fascicles
- Muscle fiber necrosis, degeneration, phagocytosis, regeneration
- Fasciitis: Inflammatory infiltrates around fascial small blood vessels
- Late findings: Atrophy, fibrosis, fat replacement
- If biopsy < 2 months following onset of muscle symptoms, vascular inflammation of fascia >> that of muscle
  - Biopsy ≥ 2 months following onset of muscle symptoms shows no difference in vascular inflammation of fascia and muscle
  - Suggests process of inflammation progression, involving fascia prior to muscle

CLINICAL ISSUES

Presentation

- Most common signs/symptoms
  - Symmetric, proximal muscle weakness in DM/PM
    - Difficult to climb stairs, rise from tub or toilet, exit from car, raise arms over head
  - Skin findings in DM
    - Scaly nontender lesions over MCPs, PIPs, knees
      - Calcinosis, more common in children
    - Heliotrope rash over eyelids
    - Violaceous shawl pattern rash on sun-exposed areas (upper chest, back, neck)
- Other signs/symptoms
  - Rare pharyngeal muscle involvement → dysphagia, risk of aspiration
  - Rare respiratory muscle involvement → dyspnea, respiratory failure
  - Cardiac involvement in 50%, rarely symptomatic
  - Pulmonary involvement (interstitial lung disease, bronchiolitis obliterans, respiratory failure)

Demographics

- Age
  - PM: Peak incidence: 40-60 years
  - DM: Onset in early adulthood
    - Juvenile DM: 5-15 years
- Gender
  - Female > male (2:1 for PM, DM)
  - Male > female for IBM
- Epidemiology
  - 5-10 cases per million
  - PM more common than DM in adults (1.5:1); opposite in children [DM > PM (20:1)]

Natural History & Prognosis

- Focal myositis
  - Confused with soft tissue tumors; usually biopsied
  - May spontaneously regress; 1/3 progress to PM
- Fasciitis may predate myositis, yet patients present with muscle symptoms
  - May explain negative results in blind muscle biopsy
  - In these cases, MR assists in choosing biopsy site
- With early recognition and adequate treatment, may return to full function
  - 25% complete response, 60% partial response, 15% no response to initial steroid therapy
- Without early treatment, irreversible muscle damage
- Osteonecrosis/osteoporosis: Steroid complications
- Associated malignancies
  - 9% PM; > 15% DM
  - Same cancers as those in general population
  - No evidence to suggest screening is efficacious (beyond normal physical and screening exams)

Treatment

- Glucocorticosteroids over period of several months
  - If no response, methotrexate/azathioprine 2° agents
- Physical therapy to improve function

SELECTED REFERENCES

1. Delavan JA et al: Gemcitabine-induced radiation recall myositis. Skeletal Radiol. 44(3):451-5, 2015
2. Yoshida K et al: Fasciitis as a common lesion of dermatomyositis, demonstrated early after disease onset by en bloc biopsy combined with magnetic resonance imaging. Arthritis Rheum. 62(12):3751-9, 2010

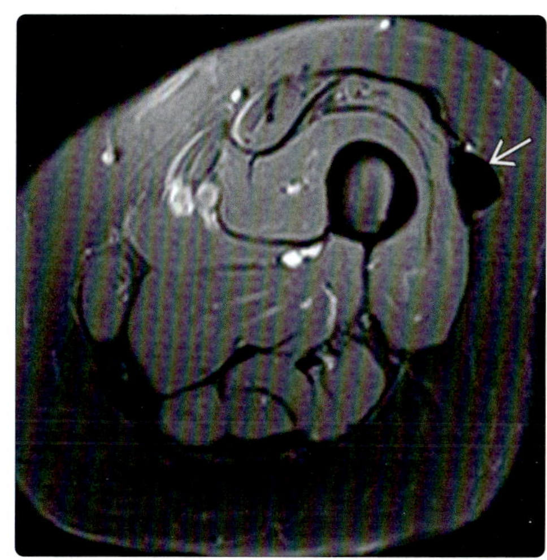

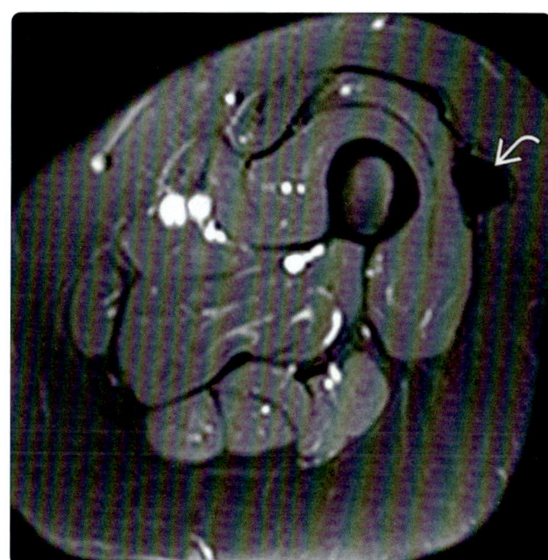

(Left) *Axial T2 FS MR was obtained in a middle-aged woman who complained of a lump in her thigh. The exam demonstrates a hypointense nodular lesion ➡ applied to the fascia of vastus lateralis. This signal suggests several possible diagnoses, including amyloid, metastatic melanoma, and fibromatosis (desmoid).* **(Right)** *Axial postcontrast T1 FS MR in the same patient shows no lesion enhancement ➡. This makes the suggested diagnoses unlikely. Radiograph should be obtained to evaluate for calcification.*

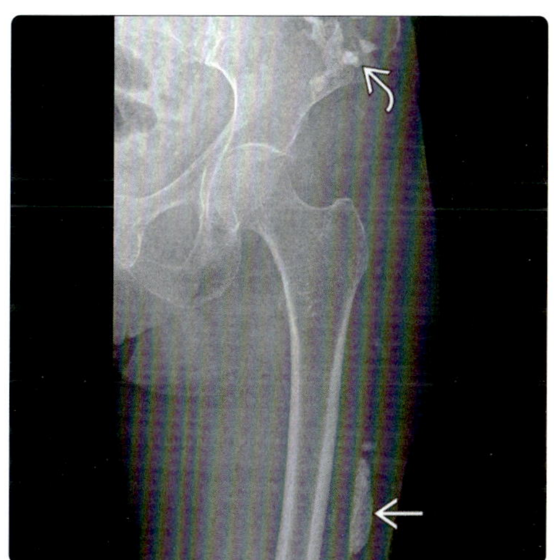

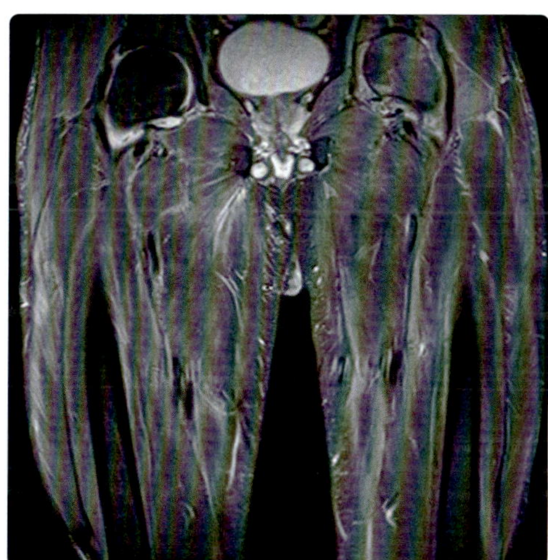

(Left) *AP radiograph in the same patient shows somewhat globular calcification corresponding to the lesion ➡. There are other sites of soft tissue calcification as well ➡. The patient proved to have dermatomyositis without active inflammation at the time of imaging.* **(Right)** *This 57-year-old man had thigh muscle pain and weakness, with elevated ESR and creatine kinase (CK). Coronal T2FS MR through the anterior portion of the thigh shows diffuse hyperintensity of the muscles.*

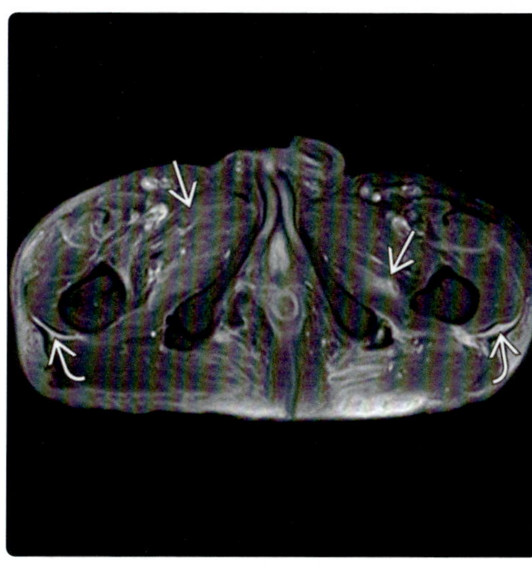

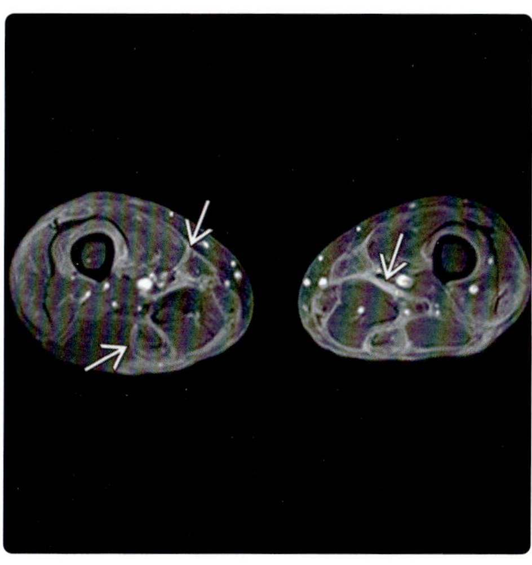

(Left) *Axial T2 FS MR in the same patient shows diffuse muscle hyperintensity, particularly within the adductors ➡ but in other muscles as well. There is also prominent fascial hyperintensity ➡.* **(Right)** *More distally in the thigh, axial T2 FS MR shows thick fascial hyperintensity ➡ surrounding most of the muscles. Fascial inflammation is a prominent feature of inflammatory myositis, often predating the myositis itself.*

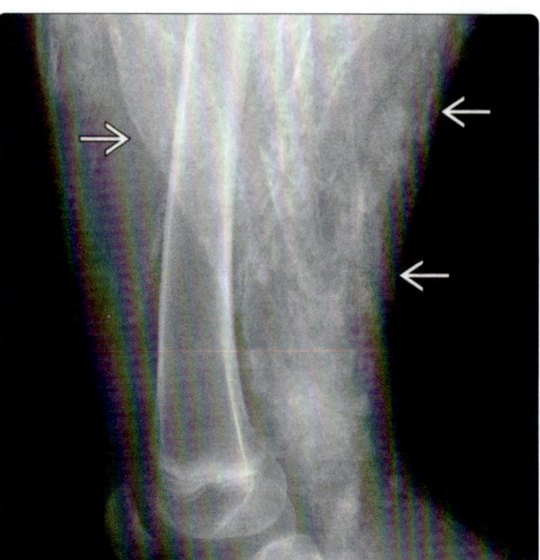
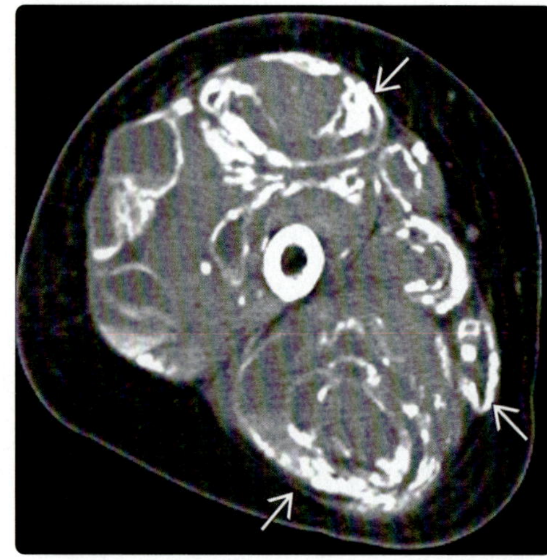

(Left) *Lateral radiograph shows extensive, sheet-like calcification of the muscles and fascial planes ➡.* **(Right)** *Axial NECT in the same patient confirms myofascial calcification ➡. The calcification, which appeared sheet-like on the radiograph, in fact is formed in a circumferential pattern both surrounding and within individual muscles. The calcification in this case of dermatomyositis is extremely prominent.*

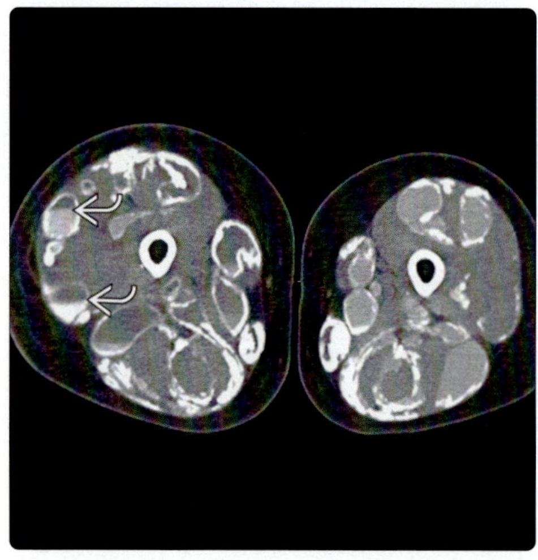
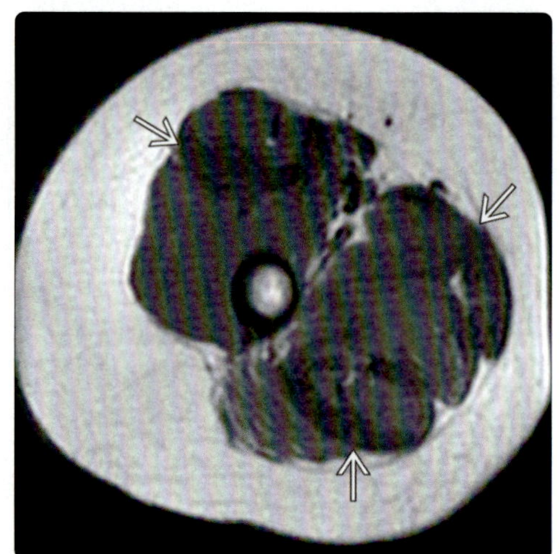

(Left) *Axial NECT in the same patient shows a rare finding of fluid-calcium levels ➡ within the myofascial calcific collections.* **(Right)** *Axial T1WI MR, performed 1 year prior to the CT, shows the involved areas ➡ to have low signal. The interval progression is impressive.*

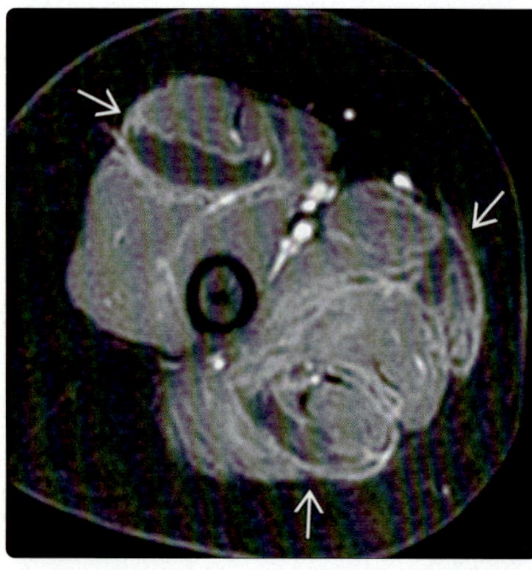
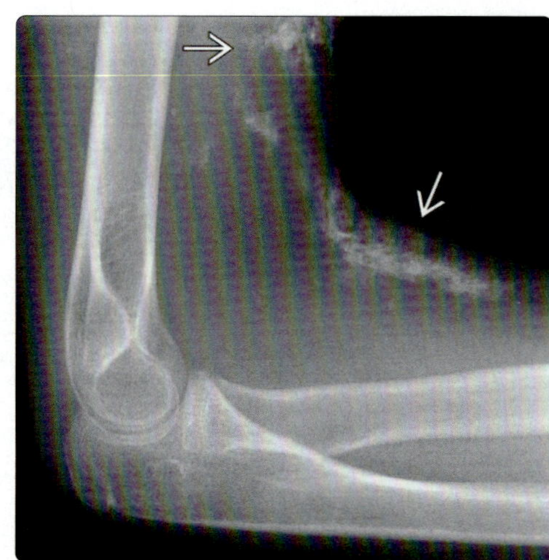

(Left) *Axial T1WI C+ FS MR in the same patient shows enhancement surrounding the low signal areas of calcification ➡. There are other sites of myofascial enhancement, indicating activity of disease.* **(Right)** *Lateral elbow radiograph in the same patient shows additional areas of sheet-like calcification ➡. Globular calcifications (not shown) were seen along the ulnar side of the wrist. It is worthwhile to remember that the pattern of calcification in DM may not always fit the classic description.*

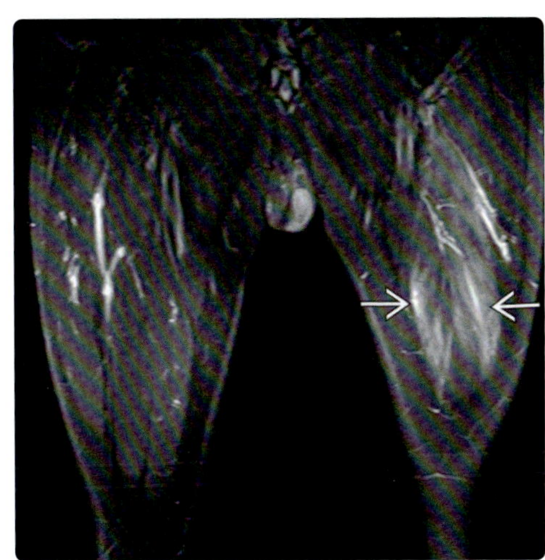

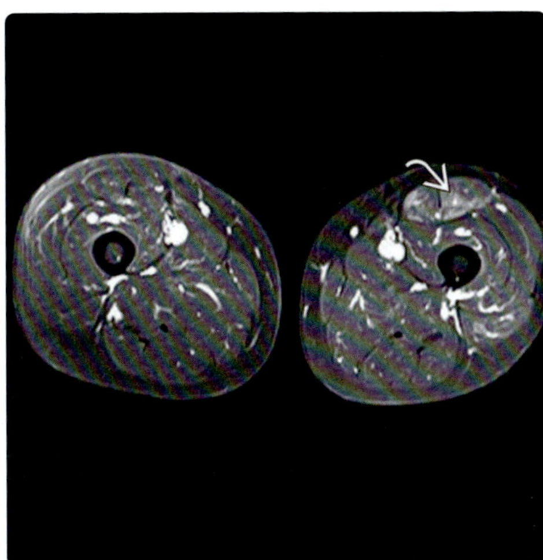

(Left) *This patient undergoing chemotherapy had right thigh pain, presumed to be rhabdomyolysis. Coronal STIR MR shows no abnormality on the right but left quadriceps hyperintensity* ➡*.* **(Right)** *Axial postcontrast T1 FS MR in the same patient shows patchy hyperintensity in the rectus femoris* ➡ *of the left thigh. Note, despite symptoms on the right side, there is no MR abnormality. In this case, MR was instrumental in guiding the clinicians to a productive muscle biopsy, confirming their clinical diagnosis of rhabdomyolysis.*

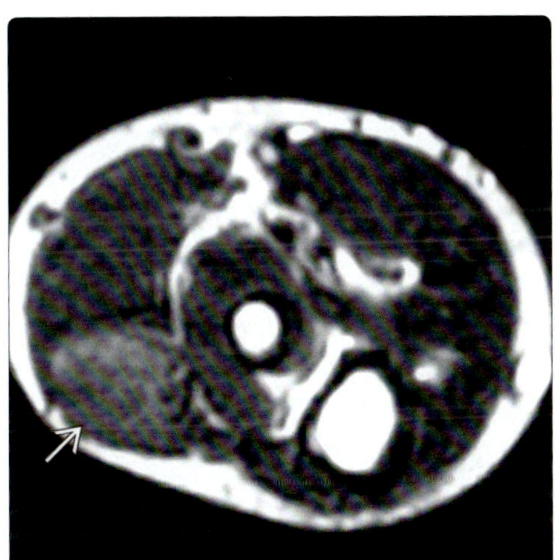

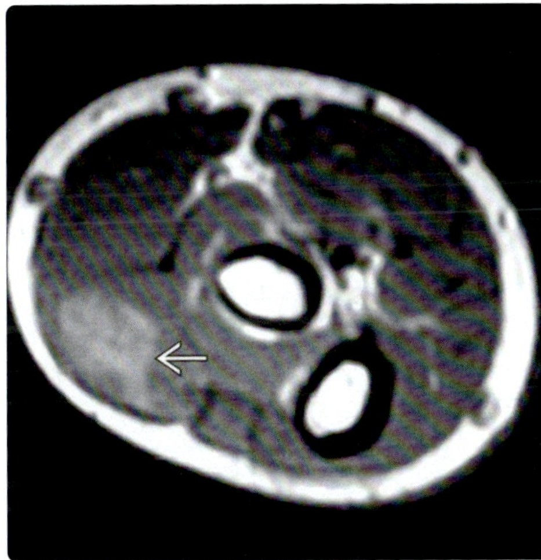

(Left) *Axial T2WI MR shows a lesion that is mildly hyperintense to muscle* ➡*. It was isointense to muscle on T1WI (not shown).* **(Right)** *Axial T1WI C+ MR in the same patient shows inhomogeneous mild enhancement of the mass* ➡*. Note that the mass does not appear to be encapsulated. This is a case of focal myositis; these lesions are often mistaken for a soft tissue sarcoma by imaging criteria and at surgery. The lesion may resolve spontaneously; 33% progress to polymyositis.*

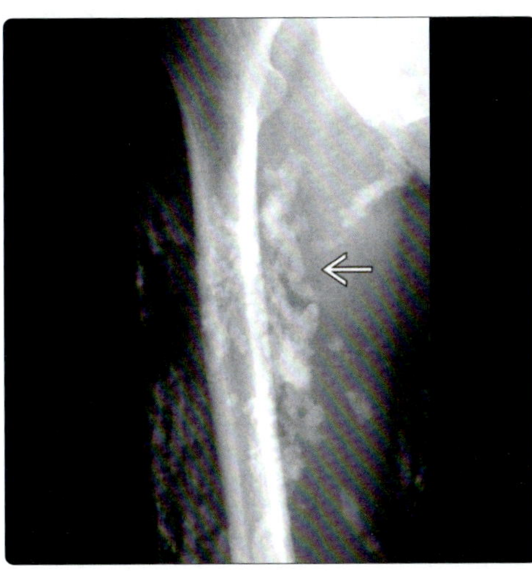

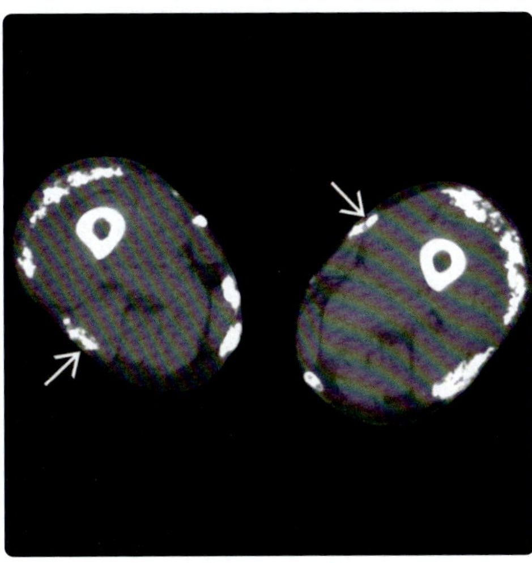

(Left) *AP radiograph shows dense, sheet-like calcification in the thigh* ➡*. This sheet-like character of the calcification is typical of dermatomyositis, though not specific. It may be seen in progressive systemic sclerosis and overlap syndrome as well. Conversely, the calcification pattern of dermatomyositis is not always sheet-like but may rather be globular.* **(Right)** *Axial CT in the same patient shows that the calcification occupies the periphery of several muscles of the thigh, as well as the adjacent fascial planes* ➡*.*

KEY FACTS

TERMINOLOGY

- Combination or overlap of clinical symptoms plus high titers of serum antibodies that react with nuclear ribonuclear protein (U1-RNP)
  - Overlap syndrome: Systemic sclerosis (PSS) & inflammatory myositis
  - Mixed connective tissue disease (MCTD): Systemic lupus erythematosus (SLE) and PSS and polymyositis

IMAGING

- Soft tissue calcification
  - Globular or sheet-like
- Acroosteolysis: Osseous, plus soft tissue tapering
- Joint effusions
- Nonspecific marrow edema; rarely erosions
- Nonspecific myositis in 83%: ↑ SI fluid sequences, enhancement along length of involved muscles
- Chest: Interstitial lung disease, air-fluid levels in distended esophagus

CLINICAL ISSUES

- Overlap of signs & symptoms resembling several rheumatic diseases
  - Arthritis, myalgias
  - Dactylitis (sausage digits)
  - Raynaud phenomenon, sclerodactyly
  - Dysphagia
  - Pleuritis/pericarditis
  - Interstitial lung disease
- Originally thought to be unique disease state
  - May have similar symptoms early in disease
- When followed over time, patients with MCTD evolve into single identifiable condition
  - Usually systemic sclerosis but may evolve into SLE or inflammatory myopathy (dermatomyositis/polymyositis)
  - 2° to this evolution, no unique prognosis; prognosis relates to disease they evolve into
- Treated according to symptoms or features present

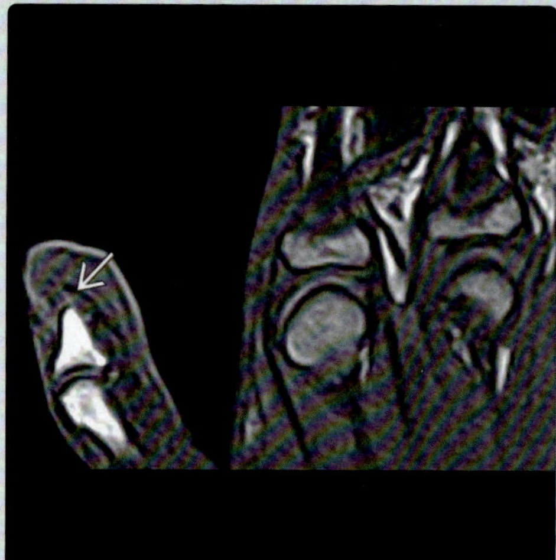

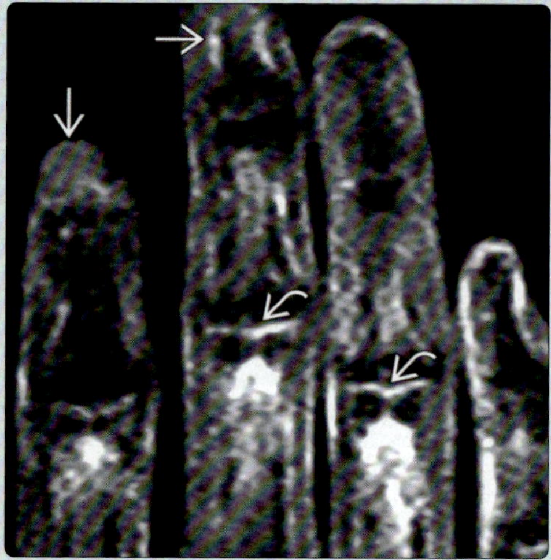

(Left) *Coronal 3D GRE MR demonstrates the expected high signal fat within the terminal phalanx of the thumb as well as acroosteolysis ➡.* **(Right)** *Coronal STIR MR, same patient, shows edema in the soft tissues and tufts of 2 involved digits ➡ and lack of edema in the adjacent ring finger tuft. Additionally, there is joint fluid, indicating mild synovitis at 2 proximal interphalangeal joints ➡. This patient shows a combination or overlap of symptoms of systemic sclerosis (scleroderma) and synovitis, both clinically and by imaging.*

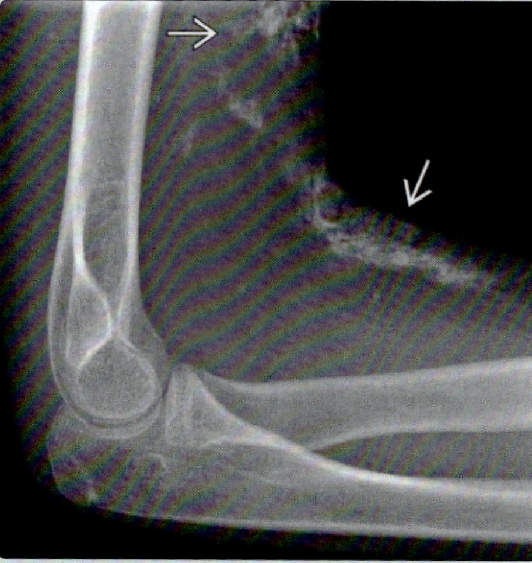

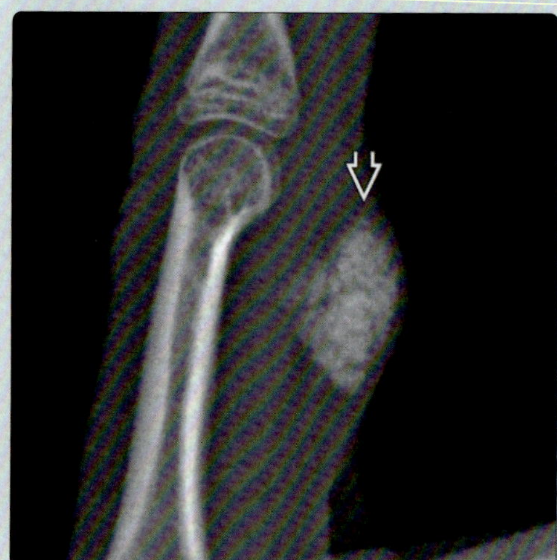

(Left) *Lateral radiograph shows subcutaneous sheet-like calcifications ➡ typical of dermatomyositis; such findings were present at other sites in this patient as well.* **(Right)** *Lateral x-ray, same patient, shows a globular calcification ➡ along the volar aspect of the index finger, which is more typical for scleroderma. Findings of dermatomyositis and scleroderma (or progressive systemic sclerosis) often coexist in mixed connective tissue disorder or overlap syndrome. The majority also have an inflammatory myopathy.*

Homocystinuria

KEY FACTS

TERMINOLOGY

- Group of disorders that have inborn errors in methionine metabolism and excessive homocysteine in body fluids

IMAGING

- Musculoskeletal abnormalities in 25-65% of patients
- Generalized osteoporosis
- Appendicular skeleton
    - Disproportionately long extremities; particularly arachnodactyly
    - Multiple growth recovery lines
    - Mild flattening of epiphyses, broadening of metaphyses
    - Joint laxity, often with multiple contractures
- Spine
    - Scoliosis
    - Biconcave endplates, compression fractures
- Pectus excavatum
- Skull: Variety of inconstant findings
    - Enlargement paranasal sinuses, widened diploic space

TOP DIFFERENTIAL DIAGNOSES

- Marfan syndrome, Ehlers-Danlos
    - All have arachnodactyly and joint laxity
    - Neither has degree of osteopenia seen in homocystinuria
    - Neither has extent of joint contractures seen in homocystinuria
    - Differ in pattern of vascular abnormality
    - Marfan has bilateral dislocated lens but develops later and with different pattern (upward)

CLINICAL ISSUES

- Associated abnormalities
    - Neurologic: Seizures, mental retardation
    - Ocular: Bilateral lens dislocation (downward)
    - Vascular thromboses often cause of early death
- 23% mortality by age 30 if untreated (usually thrombotic event)
    - 4% mortality by age 30 if responsive to treatment

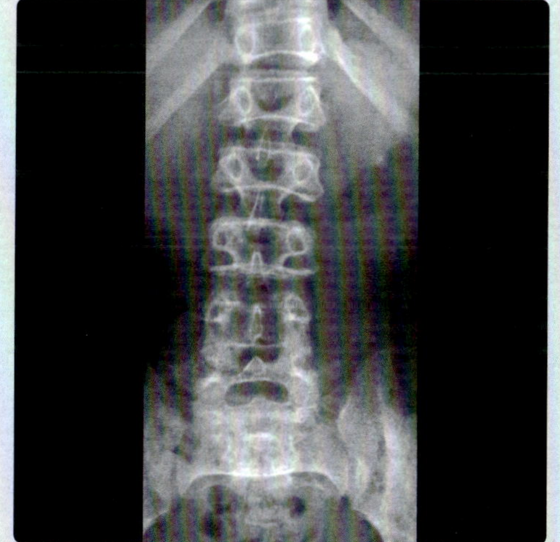

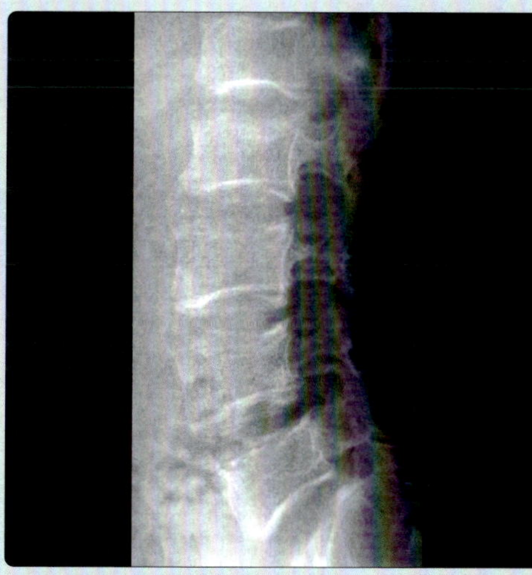

(Left) *AP radiograph shows diffuse osteopenia and mild platyspondyly in a 12-year-old patient. These are nonspecific findings.* **(Right)** *Lateral radiograph in the same patient confirms severe osteopenia and multiple mild compression fractures, with biconcavity seen at some vertebral endplates. Though posterior scalloping has been described in homocystinuria, it is not seen in this case.*

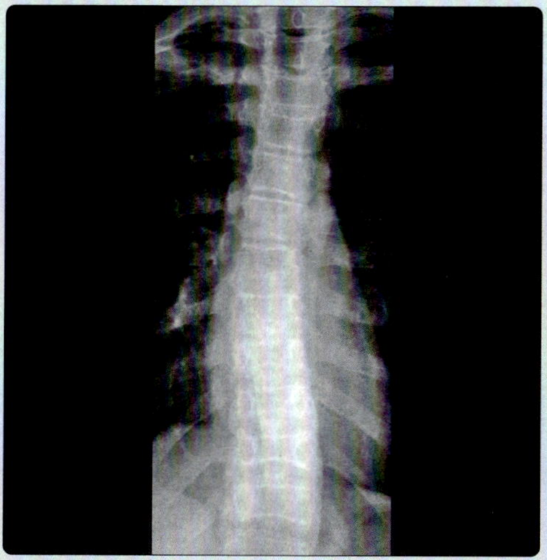

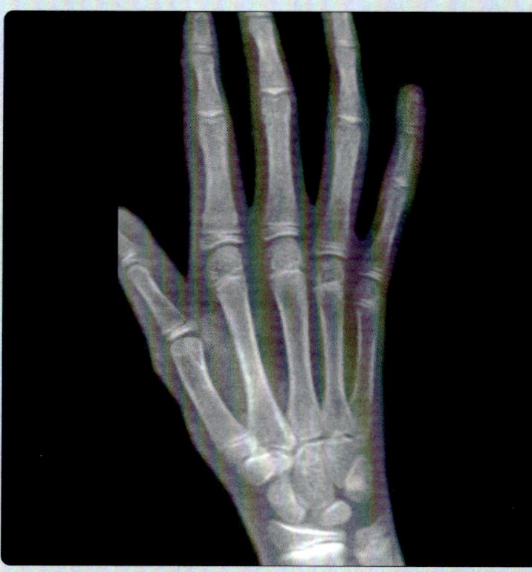

(Left) *AP radiograph in the same patient shows mild thoracic scoliosis, but the overwhelming impression is of osteopenia. The spine findings are nonspecific; radiographic diagnosis depends on the disproportionate length of the extremities.* **(Right)** *PA hand x-ray adds specificity by showing significant arachnodactyly. The combination of osteopenia and arachnodactyly is seen with homocystinuria. These patients may have laxity of the joints, as in Marfan, but more frequently develop contractures.*

Marfan and Ehlers-Danlos Syndrome

KEY FACTS

TERMINOLOGY

- Marfan syndrome (MF): Familial disorder of connective tissue with MSK, ocular, and vascular manifestations but variable phenotypic expression
- Ehlers-Danlos syndrome (ED): Hereditary disorder of connective tissue with various phenotypes (multiple syndromes)

IMAGING

- Disproportionate limb lengthening
  - Especially hands and feet (arachnodactyly) in 89% of cases (MF, ED)
- Ligamentous laxity (MF, ED)
  - Abnormal angulation possible at multiple sites
  - Pes planus, hallux valgus, hammertoes
- Joint dislocations (patella, hip, mandible, clavicle, digit) ED > MF
- Normal bone density
- Scoliosis (40-60%)
- Posterior vertebral body scalloping with dural ectasia
- Spondylolysis with spondylolisthesis
- Chest: Pectus excavatum or carinatum
- Soft tissues: Different manifestation in ED, MF
  - MF: Thin, muscular atrophy, sparse subcutaneous fat
  - ED: Subcutaneous calcifications (fat necrosis) plus increased incidence of heterotopic ossification

CLINICAL ISSUES

- Marfan syndrome
  - Disproportionate limb length relative to trunk
  - Vascular: Aortic dissection
  - Ocular: Bilateral lens dislocation
- Ehlers-Danlos diagnosis rests on clinical triad
  - Skin & vascular fragility, hyperelasticity of joints
- Age: Findings often do not manifest until childhood
- Gender: Male = female
- Epidemiology: Marfan: 4-6 per 100,000 live births

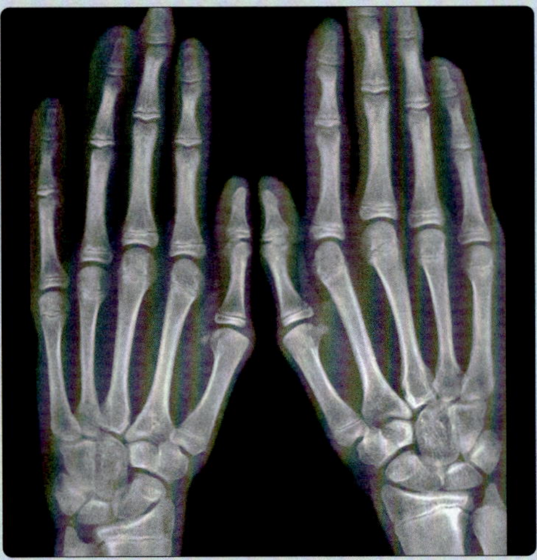

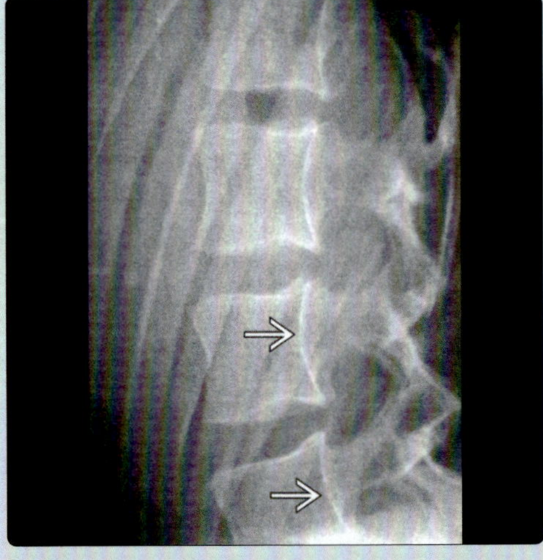

(Left) *PA radiograph of the hands shows arachnodactyly but no other abnormality. The metacarpal index is abnormal.* **(Right)** *Lateral radiograph in the same patient shows posterior vertebral body scalloping ➡. The bone density is normal. At the level of L5-S1, there was bilateral spondylolysis with grade IV spondylolisthesis (not shown). The spine abnormalities combined with arachnodactyly may be seen in either Marfan or Ehlers-Danlos; diagnosis in this case was Marfan syndrome.*

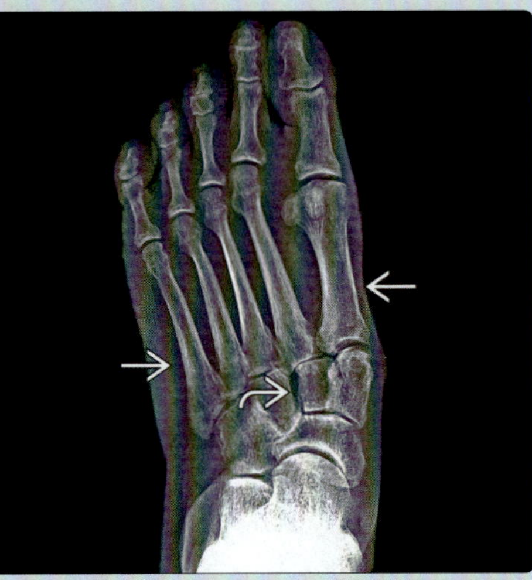

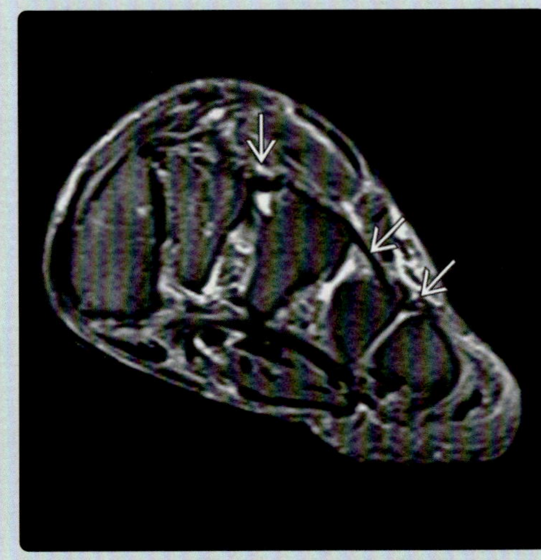

(Left) *AP radiograph shows pes planus due to Marfan disease. There is pronation of the forefoot, indicated by the divergence of the bases of metatarsals ➡. There is also a gap between cuneiforms ➡ suggesting ligamentous laxity.* **(Right)** *Coronal T2FS MR, same case, shows stretched intercuneiform and intermetatarsal ligaments ➡, resulting in an abnormal gap between cuneiforms and MTs. Other images (not shown) demonstrated tendon ruptures, all contributing to clinical flatfoot deformity typical of Marfan disease.*

TERMINOLOGY

Definitions

- Marfan syndrome (MF): Familial disorder of connective tissue with MSK, ocular, and vascular manifestations but variable phenotypic expression
- Ehlers-Danlos syndrome (ED): Hereditary disorder of connective tissue with various phenotypes (multiple syndromes)

IMAGING

Disproportionate Limb Lengthening (MF, ED)

- Especially hands, feet (arachnodactyly) in 89% of cases

Ligamentous Laxity (MF, ED)

- Abnormal angulation possible at multiple sites
  - 90° flexion deformity of 5th digit is most common
  - Genu recurvatum, patella alta
- Less commonly, carpal instability
- Pes planus, hallux valgus, hammertoes
- Joint instability likely responsible for chronic abnormalities
  - Repeated subclinical trauma
  - Effusions, hemarthrosis (ED > MF)
  - Early osteoarthritis (ED > MF)
- Joint dislocations (patella, hip, mandible, clavicle, digit) ED > MF
- Protrusio acetabulae

Soft Tissues: Different Manifestation in MF, ED

- MF: Thin, muscular atrophy, sparse subcutaneous fat
- ED: Subcutaneous calcifications (fat necrosis) plus increased incidence of heterotopic ossification
- MR demonstrates ligament laxity, redundancy
- MR demonstrates tendon ruptures, tendinopathy

Spine (MF, ED)

- Scoliosis (40-60%)
  - Similar pattern to idiopathic scoliosis
- Posterior body scalloping with dural ectasia (63%)
  - May also have widened foramina, sacral morphologic abnormalities
- Spondylolysis with spondylolisthesis
- Atlantoaxial subluxation (rare)

Chest (MF, ED)

- Pectus excavatum or carinatum

Other Findings

- Bone density (MF, ED): Normal
- Slipped capital femoral epiphysis (MF, ED): ↑ incidence

DIFFERENTIAL DIAGNOSIS

Homocystinuria

- Similar disproportionately long limbs, arachnodactyly, and joint laxity
- Mental retardation is clinical differentiator
- Diffuse osteopenia in homocystinuria, not in others
- Greater number of joint contractures
- Different pattern of ocular disease: Downward dislocation of bilateral lenses, occurring early in life
- Different pattern of vascular disease: Thromboembolic

PATHOLOGY

General Features

- Genetics
  - Marfan: Usually autosomal dominant; 20-30% spontaneous mutations
    - 1 or more mutations in locus (15q15-15q21) of long arm of chromosome 15 (*MFS1*)
  - ED: Complex classification systems
    - Multiple genetic defects apply to collagen synthesis (at least 19 foci on at least 12 genes)

CLINICAL ISSUES

Presentation

- Most common signs/symptoms
  - Marfan syndrome
    - Tall, thin appearance (> 95th percentile)
    - Disproportionate limb length relative to trunk
      - Hands, feet > lower extremities > upper
    - Vascular abnormalities
      - Cystic medial necrosis with aortic dissection and rupture
      - Dilation of proximal ascending aorta → incompetence of aortic valve and dilation of coronary sinuses
      - Medial necrosis of main pulmonary artery (less common)
      - Aortic and mitral valve insufficiency
    - Ocular abnormalities
      - Abnormality in suspensory ligaments → bilateral lens dislocation (upward direction) in 57% of cases
      - Strabismus and retinal detachments also seen
  - Ehlers-Danlos diagnosis rests on clinical triad
    - Skin fragility
      - Skin can be raised in high folds; with time, folds become permanent; skin scars easily
    - Hyperelasticity of joints
    - Vascular fragility
      - Bleeding in GI tract, skin, bronchopulmonary
      - Spontaneous dissections of aorta or major vessels may lead to bleeding death
    - Ocular abnormalities occur, but bilateral lens dislocation less frequent than in MF

Demographics

- Age
  - Findings often do not manifest until childhood
- Epidemiology
  - Marfan: 4-6 per 100,000 live births

Natural History & Prognosis

- Mean Marfan syndrome age of death: 28 yr; related to cardiovascular event

Treatment

- Address cardiovascular & ocular issues
- Reconstruction of unstable lax ligaments

SELECTED REFERENCES

1. Hammarstedt JE et al: Arthroscopic ligamentum teres reconstruction of the hip in Ehlers-Danlos syndrome: a case study. Hip Int. 0, 2015

Denervation Hypertrophy

KEY FACTS

TERMINOLOGY

- **Pseudohypertrophy**: Generalized enlargement of muscle with increase in intramuscular fat
- **True hypertrophy**: Generalized enlargement of muscle due to increase in muscle tissue

IMAGING

- Best diagnostic clue: Generalized enlargement of muscle without architectural distortion ± edema
- Most commonly involves lower extremity
  - Usually isolated pseudohypertrophy in lower extremity; tensor fascia lata and semimembranosus muscles commonly involved
- MR or CT demonstrates changes in muscle bulk and depicts preservation of architecture
  - Enlargement easiest to recognize in axial plane
  - T1WI best to identify ↑ intramuscular fat in pseudohypertrophy
  - Fluid-sensitive sequences to identify edema

TOP DIFFERENTIAL DIAGNOSES

- Overuse hypertrophy
- Compensatory hypertrophy
- Delayed-onset muscle soreness
- Lymphoma

PATHOLOGY

- Etiology: Partial loss of innervation leads to overstimulation of remaining innervated muscle fibers, which enlarge
- Underlying insults
  - Spine disease, i.e., disc herniation, most common; usually involves S1
  - Peripheral nerve injury
  - Muscular dystrophy, especially Duchenne

CLINICAL ISSUES

- Painless enlargement
- Clinical relevance is derived from identifying underlying cause of denervation

(Left) *Coronal T1WI MR of both lower legs demonstrates diffuse enlargement of the right gastrocnemius muscle* ➡*. On this image, the intramuscular signal is increased secondary to an increase in intramuscular fat. This appearance is characteristic of pseudohypertrophy.* **(Right)** *Coronal STIR MR in the same patient shows increased intramuscular signal within the right gastrocnemius muscle* ➡*. This edematous change is seen with both true hypertrophy and pseudohypertrophy.*

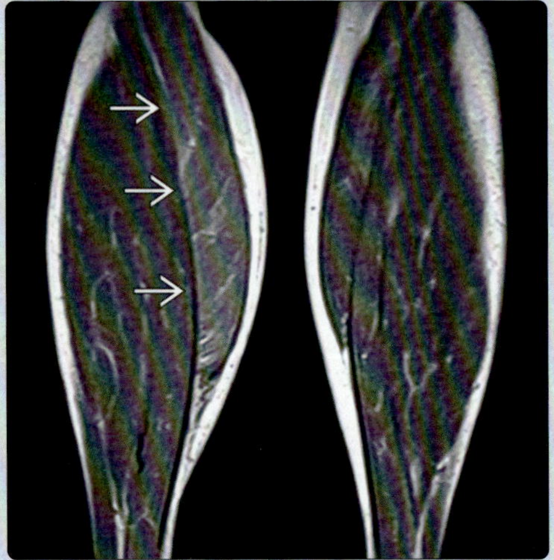

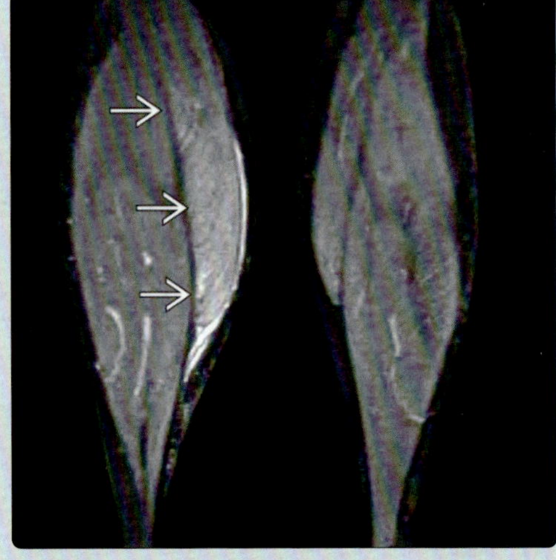

(Left) *Sagittal MR shows a patient with muscular dystrophy. Note the diffuse fat replacement of the gastrocnemius* ➡ *& semimembranosus* ➡ *muscles. Interestingly, these muscles are not diminished in size & appear enlarged. These changes contribute to the prominent calves typical of affected children.* **(Right)** *Axial CT shows denervation hypertrophy of the tensor fascia lata. The muscle is enlarged with an increase in intramuscular fat* ➡*. No architectural distortion is seen.*

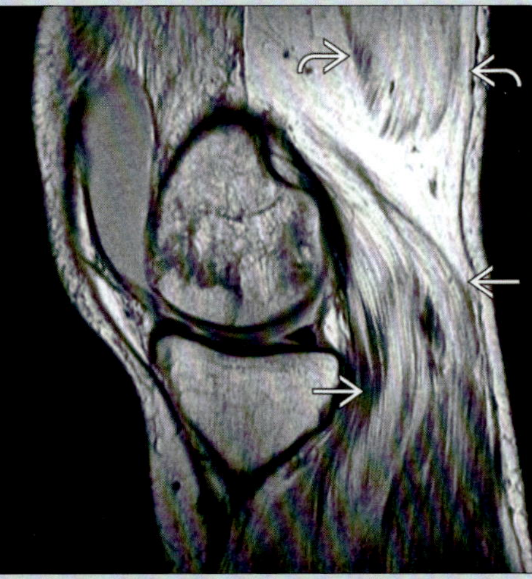

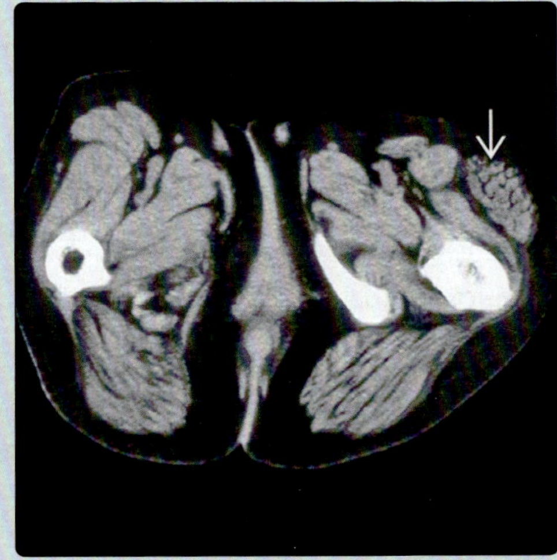

TERMINOLOGY

Synonyms

- Neurogenic muscular hypertrophy

Definitions

- **Pseudohypertrophy**: Generalized enlargement of muscle with increase in intramuscular fat
- **True hypertrophy**: Generalized enlargement of muscle due to increase in muscle tissue

IMAGING

General Features

- Best diagnostic clue
  - Generalized enlargement of muscle without architectural distortion
- Location
  - Most commonly involves lower extremity
    - Isolated denervation involvement most common
      - Usually pseudohypertrophy in lower extremity
      - Tensor fascia lata and semimembranosus muscles commonly involved
    - Duchenne muscular dystrophy is classic example
      - Bilateral symmetric pseudohypertrophy of calf muscles
- Morphology
  - Enlarged with smooth margins, normal shape

Imaging Recommendations

- Best imaging tool
  - MR or CT demonstrates changes in muscle bulk and depicts preservation of architecture
- Protocol advice
  - Enlargement easiest to recognize in axial plane
  - Inclusion of opposite extremity may be helpful
  - T1WI best to identify ↑ intramuscular fat
  - Fluid-sensitive sequences to identify edema

CT Findings

- Increased size of entire muscle
- No contour abnormalities or discrete mass
- Normal internal architecture preserved
  - Feathery pattern of intramuscular fat not distorted
- Pseudohypertrophy has increased intramuscular fat
  - Normal feathery pattern more prominent

MR Findings

- Same findings as described under CT
- Increased signal seen on T1WI in pseudohypertrophy
- ± intramuscular edema: Patchy or diffuse
  - Seen with both pseudo- and true hypertrophy

DIFFERENTIAL DIAGNOSIS

Overuse Hypertrophy

- Weightlifters are typical example
- Edema seen if associated delayed-onset muscle soreness
- Usually involves > 1 muscle
  - Often bilateral and symmetric

Compensatory Hypertrophy

- Form of true hypertrophy, different etiology
- Look for causative muscle deficiency or damage
- e.g., levator scapula hypertrophy following radical neck dissection

Delayed-Onset Muscle Soreness

- Lacks muscle enlargement, increased intramuscular fat
- Usually involves > 1 muscle
- Painful: Onset following activity

Lymphoma

- Muscle infiltration with architectural distortion
- Enlargement generally focal

Idiopathic, Benign Enlargement of Masseter

- Confined to muscles of mastication

PATHOLOGY

General Features

- Etiology
  - Partial loss of innervation leads to overstimulation of remaining innervated muscle fibers, which enlarge
  - Increased intramuscular fat in pseudohypertrophy is from unknown mechanism
  - Underlying insults
    - Spine disease, i.e., disc herniation, most common; usually involves S1
    - Peripheral nerve injury
    - Muscular dystrophy, especially Duchenne

Microscopic Features

- True hypertrophy: Spectrum of small angulated muscle fibers, normal fibers, hypertrophied fibers
  - Type 1 and 2 fibers affected
- Pseudohypertrophy: Same spectrum as above and ↑ in adipose and other connective tissue between fibers

CLINICAL ISSUES

Presentation

- Most common signs/symptoms
  - Painless enlargement
- Other signs/symptoms
  - EMG confirms denervation

Natural History & Prognosis

- Hypertrophy itself is of no clinical significance
- Clinical relevance is derived from identifying underlying cause of denervation

Treatment

- Directed at underlying cause of denervation

DIAGNOSTIC CHECKLIST

Reporting Tips

- Recommend search for underlying cause if none clinically apparent

SELECTED REFERENCES

1. Evertsson K et al: p38 mitogen-activated protein kinase and mitogen-activated protein kinase-activated protein kinase 2 (MK2) signaling in atrophic and hypertrophic denervated mouse skeletal muscle. J Mol Signal. 9(1):2, 2014

Embolic Disease

KEY FACTS

TERMINOLOGY

- Material traveling by way of vessels to other body parts, in this case affecting MSK system
  - Blood clots
  - Septic emboli
  - Air emboli
  - Tumor emboli

IMAGING

- Involvement of multiple sites in single extremity suggests etiology is embolus from catheter
  - Umbilical artery catheter thrombi may result in limb length discrepancy
- Blood clot emboli
  - Osteonecrosis
  - Acroosteolysis
  - In growing skeleton, coned epiphyses
- Septic emboli
  - Locations at risk relate to site of infection and its related vascular anatomy
  - Vertebral bodies/discs particularly at risk
  - Metaphyses, especially in children
- Air emboli
  - Caisson disease (dysbaric osteonecrosis)
  - Results from rapid decompression following hyperbaric environment
  - Tissues supersaturated with nitrogen; may release into bloodstream
  - Air emboli thought to occlude small vessels, leading to osteonecrosis
- Tumor emboli
  - Tumor cells separate from primary tumor, gain vascular access, attach to endothelium of distant capillary bed, exit vessel, and develop supporting blood supply at new site

(Left) *AP radiograph shows a coned epiphysis at the distal femur ➡ and mild coning of the proximal tibia resulting in limb shortening. There is a long differential for coned epiphyses; most are eliminated since the contralateral knee was normal.* **(Right)** *AP radiograph, same patient, shows osteonecrosis of the left femoral capital epiphysis ➡, with a normal right side. Given the unilaterality of the process, the diagnosis is most likely embolic disease due to umbilical artery catheter in this child who had spent several weeks in the NBICU.*

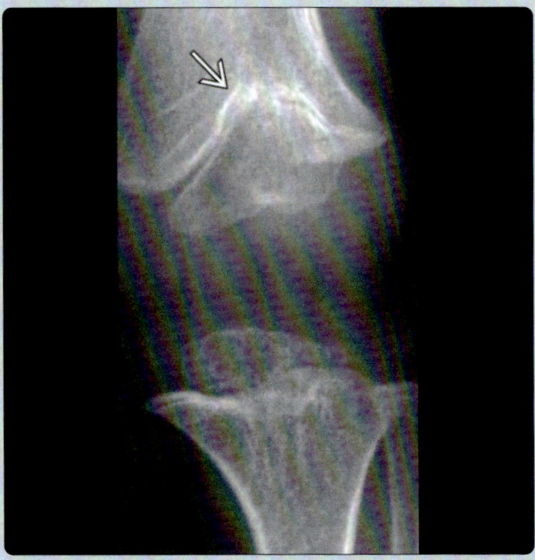

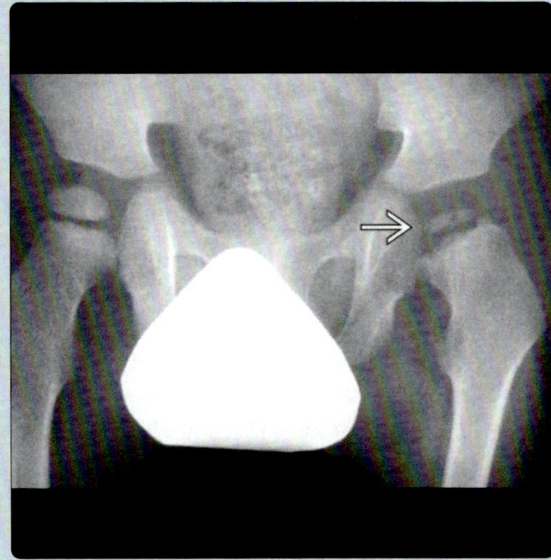

(Left) *AP radiograph shows advanced osteonecrosis ➡ in the typical location within the humeral head and secondary osteoarthritis ➡. This patient had Caisson disease, and the osteonecrosis is thought to develop from air emboli, which block small blood vessels.* **(Right)** *Lateral radiograph shows impressive prevertebral soft tissue swelling ➡ with disc and vertebral body destruction ➡. This young woman with an IV drug habit had bacterial endocarditis, with discitis 2° to embolization from the cardiac vegetation.*

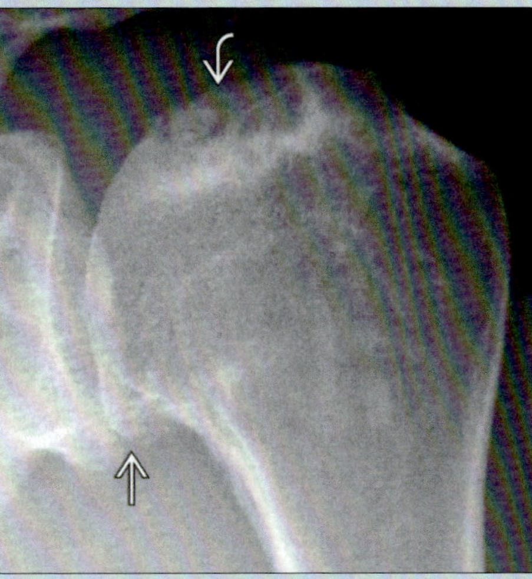

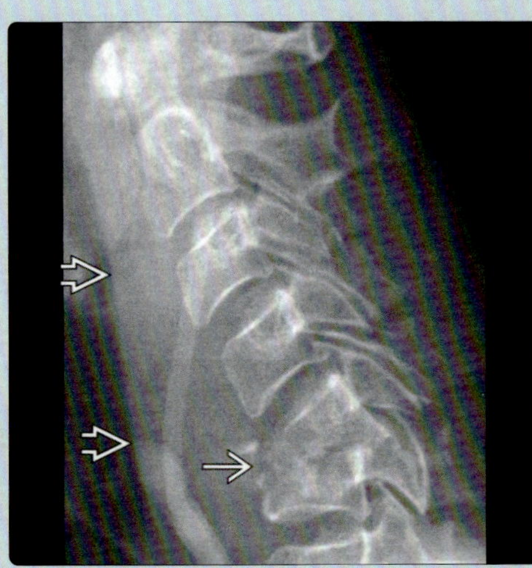

KEY FACTS

TERMINOLOGY

- Infection caused by *Neisseria meningitidis*

IMAGING

- Musculoskeletal signs and symptoms at time of infection
  - Tenosynovitis
  - Arthritis
    - Acute transient polyarthritis: Pain and tenderness occurring simultaneously with petechial rash
    - Purulent arthritis (often knee), occurring after 5th day of illness (5-10%)
- Skeletal abnormalities developing in children following survival of significant disease
  - Premature fusion of physes, often in central part, leading to appearance of coned epiphyses/metaphyses
  - Epiphyseal fragmentation, abnormal morphology → bowing and angular deformities
  - Shortening and limb length discrepancy
  - Polyostotic but not symmetric; lower > upper extremity

TOP DIFFERENTIAL DIAGNOSES

- DDx of coned epiphyses
  - Embolic disease
  - Disseminated infection

PATHOLOGY

- Etiology of osseous abnormalities: Timing and appearance makes infection unlikely; thought to be vascular insult

CLINICAL ISSUES

- Varies in severity, from benign and asymptomatic to fulminant and fatal
  - Fever, shaking chills, skin eruption, petechiae, myalgias
- Fulminant cases (Waterhouse-Friderichsen syndrome)
  - Hypotension, confusion, tachypnea, peripheral cyanosis, disseminated intravascular coagulation (DIC)
    - DIC → diffuse bleeding from mucosal surfaces, small vessel occlusion with necrosis in skin, brain, kidney, adrenal glands

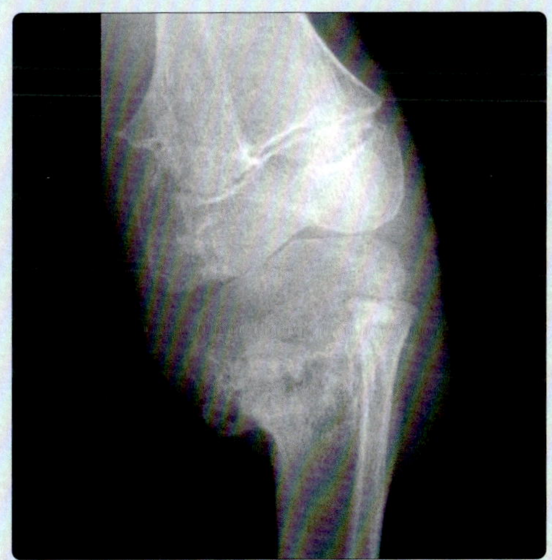

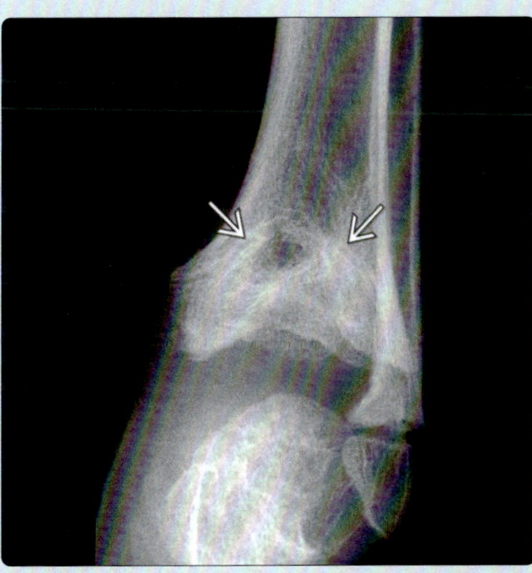

(Left) *AP radiograph shows abnormal early fusion of the central and medial portions of the distal femoral and proximal tibial physes. This results in abnormal epiphyseal morphology and a varus deformity of the knee. The contralateral knee was normal.* **(Right)** *AP radiograph in the same patient shows a similar abnormality involving the distal tibial physis, which has resulted in a more distinct coned epiphysis morphology ➡. The talus is also abnormal, with a rounded dome.*

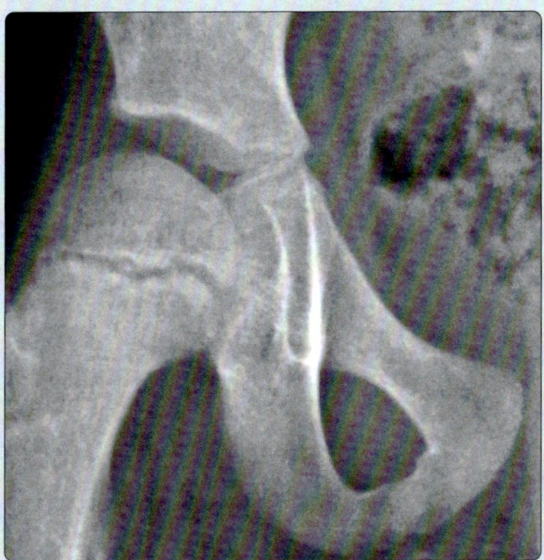

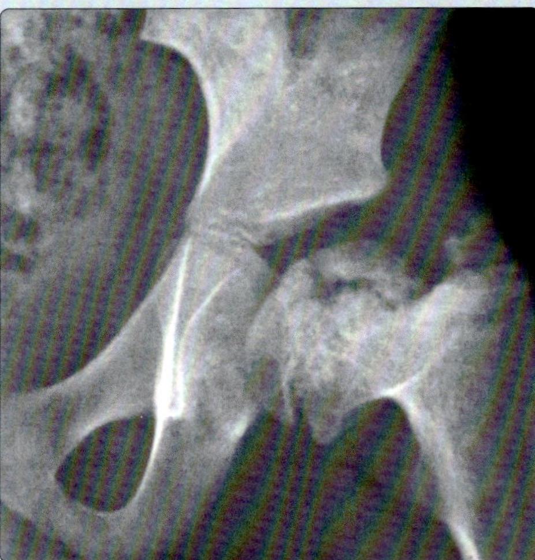

(Left) *AP radiograph in the same patient shows a normal right hip. This indicates that the abnormality is not a diffuse metaphyseal or epiphyseal dysplasia.* **(Right)** *AP x-ray, left hip, shows an abnormally widened physis and fragmentation of the epiphysis, with resultant varus deformity. Overall, the appearance is typical of either an embolic process or sequelae of meningococcemia coagulopathy and subsequent vascular insult, affecting the entire extremity. History indicated the latter process in this case.*

SECTION 7

Orthopedic Implants or Arthrodesis

Arthroplasties and Arthrodesis

Internal Fixation

Introduction: Arthroplasty Terminology

Arthroplasties have much in common with one another, despite being performed at different joints and with different constructs. Although each joint has unique attributes that must be assessed, each is also at risk for a common set of complications that have a similar imaging appearance, no matter which joint is being assessed. Developing a standard search pattern for complications should result in good patient care.

It is extremely difficult to keep up with the different manufacturers' names for the implants. Often it is most convenient to refer to them by name of joint [i.e., total hip arthroplasty (THA) or total knee arthroplasty (TKA)] or else by a commonly used descriptive name (i.e., reverse shoulder arthroplasty or Silastic arthroplasty for small joint implants).

Since some components may be secured by cement, they may be referred to as cemented arthroplasty. Others are secured by bone ingrowth into an irregular surface. The type of surface is not always obvious on radiographs. A beaded interface (tiny microspheres secured to the surface) is visible, while an etched surface is not. Hence, acceptable terminology for these includes cementless arthroplasty or, if one component is cemented and the other is not, hybrid arthroplasty.

Components for the major joints are usually metal, but portions may be polyethylene (acetabular cup, patellar button, glenoid, occasionally tibial tray). Metal-on-metal THAs are relatively commonly seen, but many THAs and most other joints have a polyethylene gliding interface between the metal components.

Initial Placement of Components

Initial placement of the arthroplasty components is crucial to their long-term success. Generally speaking, the components are placed such that they mimic the placement of the original nonpathologic joint, allowing stabilizing structures and muscles to exert their normal stresses across the components. However, some constructs, even when appropriately placed, may not appear to be "anatomically" located. It is crucial to properly understand and evaluate the expected postoperative location and angulation of components as well as associated osteoplasties, which may be required to decrease the probability of impingement. This will be discussed in later sections on a joint-specific basis.

Implant Fracture

Fracture of a component may occur because of instability or abnormal stress. Incorrect placement of a component may be a contributing factor. While a fractured implant might be obvious, it is usually subtle. A discontinuity of a metallic stem may be visualized only by a slight buckle; it is usually not displaced.

Fractures of a cemented polyethylene component are usually visualized by a fracture in the cement or distortion of the component shape (a spherical acetabular cup may become more oval). If the implant is polyethylene with thin metal backing (patellar buttons are one example), the metal backing may fragment or fracture and may carry the polyethylene attachment with it when it separates. When there is fragmentation of metal backing, the tiny pieces may coalesce along a synovial or polyethylene surface; this is termed metallosis. Prominent synovitis and eventual osteolysis may be associated with metallosis.

Silastic components are particularly prone to fracture when they have thin mobile portions or are abnormally stressed by ligamentous instability, as at the "hinges" of an interphalangeal or MCP arthroplasty. Watch for these fractures by noting an abrupt change in alignment of phalanges, since the implant itself is difficult to see.

Dislocation

Joint dislocation, or lack of continuity between expected sites of articulation, may occur when the joint is placed out of its expected range of motion. Some joints, such as the hip, are prone to dislocate when placed in certain positions, such as significant adduction (as in crossing the legs) or extreme abduction. Joints are also at risk of dislocation if the components are not placed in appropriate position and alignment.

Implants may dislocate from the underlying bone. This may occur by means of cement dissociating from the bone or by stress on an implant that has not developed bony or fibrous ingrowth to a cementless component. Glenoid and patellar components appear to be at particular risk. Other implants, such as Silastic carpal replacements, have no osseous fixation. Abnormal motion or stress may result in their dislocation.

A polyethylene component that is attached to a metal tray may dissociate from the metal and dislocate within the joint. The etiology of these dislocations is likely abnormal stress &/or joint instability; polyethylene wear may add to joint instability. Since the polyethylene is radiolucent, it may be surprisingly difficult to see. If there are small bits of cement or metal attached to it, the displaced component will be more easily seen. Otherwise, the displacement may be seen as a radiolucency (slightly lower density than soft tissue or effusion) in the shape of the component, displacing other structures, or wedged between a part of the joint, resulting in locking or widening.

Stress Shielding

Arthroplasties alter weight-bearing through the bones in which they are placed. Areas through which there is more stress produce bone, and those with less stress lose bone density through resorption. The process and appearance is termed stress shielding. It occurs in predictable locations and should not be misdiagnosed as a pathologic osteolytic process. Stress shielding has not been shown to correlate with arthroplasty failure or with pain and is considered normal.

Infection

Risk of infection in orthopedic procedures requiring surgical instrumentation or placement of hardware ranges from 3-6%. The risk increases with prolonged operative time as well as with multiple incisions and operative sites.

Arthroplasties are at increased risk for infection. The symptoms usually bring the patient to medical attention prior to developing radiographic changes. If there are radiographic abnormalities, they include effusion, serpiginous osseous destruction, periosteal reaction, and endosteal bone reaction. Rarely, air is seen in the soft tissues. Fluffy, immature, periarticular heterotopic bone formation can be suggestive of the diagnosis. However, the majority of cases appear normal on radiograph; if there is clinical suspicion of an infected arthroplasty, aspiration should be performed.

MR imaging may be useful in diagnosing fistula or abscess formation, with T1 weighted imaging as well as contrast administration aiding the differentiation of abscess from hematoma or seroma. Metal artifact reduction techniques are required; one might also consider utilizing multislice CT with reconstruction to better identify bony sequestra or periosteal reaction.

An infected arthroplasty usually must be removed. All cement from the arthroplasty should be removed as well since it could remain as a nidus for chronic infection. The defect is then filled with antibiotic-impregnated cement. The cement may be shaped in beads connected by a string or may be shaped as a spacer to maintain normal spacing between residual bone surfaces. An infected hip may be left with the residual femoral shaft in a muscle sling, termed a Girdlestone. Once the full treatment for infection is completed, the patient may be re-imaged or reaspirated to rule out residual infection prior to placement of a revision arthroplasty.

Loosening

One of the more common complications of arthroplasties is loosening. The most specific sign of loosening is change in position of the implant. This change in position may be surprisingly difficult to notice. A component may "subside" into the underlying bone, moving superiorly (acetabular cup, patellar button), inferiorly (femoral or tibial components), or in a medial-lateral direction. With this subsidence, there may be no obvious lucency surrounding the component. New tilt of a component is another indication of loosening. Subtle tilt or subsidence may be noted only when the image is compared with an older index image obtained soon after the placement of the components.

Loosening of a component may also be seen as a lucency at the interface between bone and cement or the interface between bone and component. Not every lucency indicates loosening, however. A cemented component may normally show a slight lucency at the bone-cement interface, but it is not considered to be loose unless the lucency measures ≥ 2 mm and surrounds the majority of the component. A less significant lucency should be watched for stability. Fractured cement also indicates significant component motion and associated loosening.

Loosening of a cementless component may be more complicated to diagnose. These components are expected to have osseous ingrowth, though this ingrowth cannot be discerned radiographically. If there is bead shedding from the ingrowth surface, loosening is presumed. Interestingly, it has been demonstrated in autopsy series that, in patients whose THA had been asymptomatic prior to death, 1/3 showed no bony ingrowth and 2/3 showed ingrowth in only 2-10% of the available surface. These hips, however, were not loose; they showed fibrous ingrowth. The fibrous ingrowth may result in some lucency at the bone-component interface. The lucency is not considered diagnostic of loosening unless it measures ≥ 2 mm and surrounds the majority of the component. There is often a sclerotic line surrounding the lucency. Another finding that is unique to a cementless femoral component may be endosteal &/or cortical hypertrophy, which form near the tip of the stem. This is considered normal unless the bone hypertrophy is so extensive that it bridges the medullary canal; in that case, loosening should be suggested. Overall, it is recommended that if bone-component lucency and hypertrophic change are judged to not represent true loosening, the findings should be followed to see if stability is maintained. Progressive change without stabilization is considered evidence of loosening.

Component Wear

Theoretically, arthroplasty components should not show enough wear to cause significant problems (0.06 mm/year). However, wear can be seen in both polyethylene acetabular cups and tibial polyethylene in TKAs. It may be accentuated in components that are not placed in anatomic position. It is also believed that there is in vivo degradation of polyethylene due to oxidation where there is contact with joint fluid. Mechanical friction against metal abrades microscopic particles.

Polyethylene wear is diagnosed by observation of differential thinning in the weight-bearing region compared with other regions of the component. Specifically, acetabular polyethylene wear usually occurs differentially at the superolateral and anterior portions of the component compared to the inferomedial portion. Differential wear of a tibial component may be either medial or lateral. Although the wear characteristics of metal-on-metal THA are improved compared to metal-on-polyethylene, the former have also been shown to release metal particles and ions into the joint.

Silastic implants used in small joints of the hand and foot are often not anchored to bone. Abnormal motion as well as the thinness of parts of these components frequently results in breakdown of the implants.

Particle Disease

Particle disease results from debris of a critical size triggering an inflammatory reaction and synovitis, which in turn may trigger soft tissue necrosis &/or massive osteolysis. The origin of the particles seems immaterial; osseous debris, cement fragments, metal particles (including beads), and polyethylene or Silastic particles may all be of the appropriate size to initiate the reaction. The particles incite an inflammatory response in periprosthetic tissues, resulting in secretion of cytokines, growth factors, and enzymes; these promote formation of osteolytic granulomas. Activated macrophages express osteoprotegerin ligands (RANKL), which activate osteoclasts, resulting in lysis. The repetitive hydraulic effect of joint fluid brings reactive tissue in contact with susceptible bone.

Synovitis may be demonstrated by MR or ultrasound. Osteolysis is usually a radiographic diagnosis, but its extent is usually greater than suspected; CT may demonstrate the true extent. Osteolysis may be elongated, due to debris and its reactive tissue tracking along a screw or along cement-bone or metal-bone interfaces. Alternatively, osteolysis may be massive, lytic, and rounded, giving the appearance of a tumor.

Osteolysis has a differential diagnosis that includes metastases or multiple myeloma. Most patients with arthroplasties are older adults, and therefore the tumor differentials must be strongly considered. Osteolysis becomes a much stronger consideration if the source of the particles can be demonstrated. Polyethylene particles are the most frequent source of osteolysis, and it is worthwhile to look carefully for evidence of component wear.

Particle disease may also result in development of large necrotic soft tissue masses. These are often mistaken for soft tissue tumors. As with osteolysis, imaging of soft tissue masses accompanying arthroplasties should be evaluated for sources of particles which may explain the mass as reactive rather than tumor.

Periprosthetic Fracture

Periprosthetic fracture may occur at the time of surgery, either because of abnormal morphology, osteoporosis, slight oversizing of components, or bad luck. The surgeon is usually aware of these fractures as they occur. The fracture is often incomplete and nondisplaced; the surgeon will usually protect the bone and construct by placement of a cerclage wire. The fracture may not be visible postoperatively, but the wire indicates that one is likely present. Postoperative radiographs must include the entire construct so that fractures beyond the tip of the prosthesis can be visualized. Orthogonal views should be obtained as soon as possible in the postoperative period. Specific sites are particularly prone to intraoperative fracture, such as at the tip of a longstem femoral component of a THA or at the patella of a TKA; these regions should be evaluated particularly carefully.

Periprosthetic fractures also occur following rehabilitation, when the patient becomes physically active. Some patients, particularly those who are osteoporotic (for example the elderly, those with RA or ankylosing spondylosis, or those on steroid therapy) are particularly prone to fracture. The most common fracture locations may be similar to those that occur in the immediately perioperative period (such as the patella in a TKA) or may be located in different (but characteristic) sites (for example, distal femoral or proximal tibial metaphyseal fractures adjacent to a TKA). An acute fracture may be seen as only a slight buckle; subacute fractures are seen as linear sclerosis. It is important to have good quality follow-up radiographs and a knowledgeable search pattern so that these fractures, which may be subtle and incomplete, are not missed.

Imaging Recommendations

With correct positioning, proper exposure, and orthogonal views, most complications of arthroplasties can be detected on radiograph. The entire prosthesis must be included in the images.

CT may be selectively used to confirm complications, particularly osseous destruction related to component loosening or massive osteolysis resulting from particle disease. It is important for the surgeon to understand the extent of bony defects as part of the surgical planning process prior to arthroplasty revision, including amount and quality of residual bone stock. CT is also useful for image-guided biopsy or aspiration of iliopsoas fluid collections from THA complications.

Even large, metallic prostheses can be successfully imaged on CT. Selective consideration should be made for increasing kVp and mAs, which improves image resolution. Improvements can also be seen by using soft tissue image acquisition, narrowed collimation, and decreased pitch. Coronal and sagittal reformations are essential to minimize metallic artifact. There is ongoing and encouraging research with cone beam CT and dual energy CT technology that promises improved diagnostic capability.

MR is generally not required for evaluation of orthopedic implant failure. However, it may be selectively useful to diagnose fluid collections or soft tissue mass related to infection or particle disease. Fluid-sensitive sequences may show Silastic-related synovitis extremely well. If the prosthesis is placed following tumor resection, MR may be used to demonstrate tumor complications of seroma or recurrence.

Metallic artifact can be substantial, but there are some adjustments that may modify it: Thin section imaging, increased frequency-encoding gradient strength, increased receiver bandwidth, decreased interecho spacing, decreased effective echo times, use of intermediate-weighted fast spin-echo sequences, and STIR rather than fat-saturated imaging are all useful.

Ultrasound may be useful for detection and aspiration of fluid collections, provided they are not too deep. It is also selectively used to follow tumor patients for recurrence or other complications if MR of the region is too distorted by metallic artifact.

Bone scan seems insufficiently sensitive for evaluation of arthroplasty complications. The components themselves are photopenic, with expected surrounding uptake. There is significant variability in the length of time following surgery that the uptake is significant; therefore, there is overlap between normal expected uptake and pathologic uptake. One report suggests a specificity of 90% using triple phase bone scan to differentiate THA loosening from infection. Another shows specificity of FDG PET to be similar to that of triple-phase bone scan, but both to be significantly less sensitive than radiography. Most clinicians agree that if there is a question of arthroplasty infection, aspiration of the joint is required.

Conclusion

Imaging can be instrumental in evaluating arthroplasties. A careful search pattern for abnormalities, including malposition, subtle fractures, infection, loosening, and particle disease, should be a part of every examination. Comparison with an older index radiograph for any change is instrumental in diagnosing early change in component position and associated loosening. Recognition of common patterns of failure for each type of arthroplasty should assist in visualizing subtle abnormalities. CT, MR, and ultrasound can be valuable adjuncts to the radiograph in problem-solving situations.

Selected References

1. Müller GM et al: Evaluation of metal artifacts in clinical MR images of patients with total hip arthroplasty using different metal artifact-reducing sequences. Skeletal Radiol. 44(3):353-9, 2015
2. Fritz J et al: MR imaging of hip arthroplasty implants. Radiographics. 34(4):E106-32, 2014
3. Pessis E et al: Virtual monochromatic spectral imaging with fast kilovoltage switching: reduction of metal artifacts at CT. Radiographics. 33(2):573-83, 2013
4. Tuominen EK et al: Weight-bearing CT imaging of the lower extremity. AJR Am J Roentgenol. 200(1):146-8, 2013
5. Roth TD et al: CT of the hip prosthesis: appearance of components, fixation, and complications. RadioGraphics. 32:1089-1107, 2012
6. Sutter R et al: Reduction of metal artifacts in patients with total hip arthroplasty with slice-encoding metal artifact correction and view-angle tilting MR imaging. Radiology. 265(1):204-14, 2012
7. Hargreaves BA et al: Metal-induced artifacts in MRI. AJR Am J Roentgenol. 197(3):547-55, 2011
8. Squire MW: Imaging of metal-on-metal hip prostheses. AJR Am J Roentgenol. 197(3):556-7, 2011
9. Heffernan EJ et al: The imaging appearances of metallosis. Skeletal Radiol. 37(1):59-62, 2008
10. Nagoya S et al: Diagnosis of peri-prosthetic infection at the hip using triple-phase bone scintigraphy. J Bone Joint Surg Br. 90(2):140-4, 2008

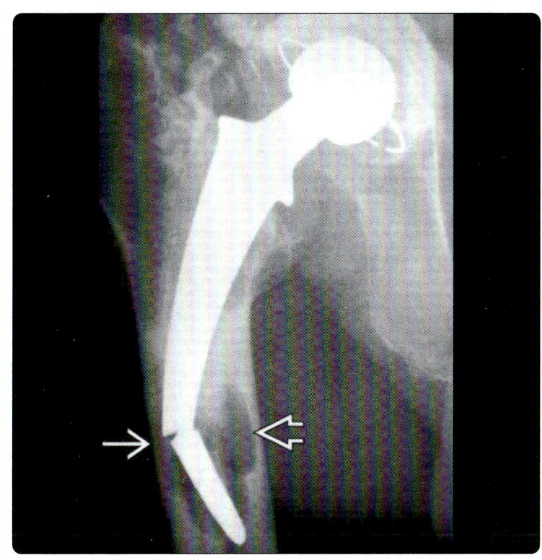

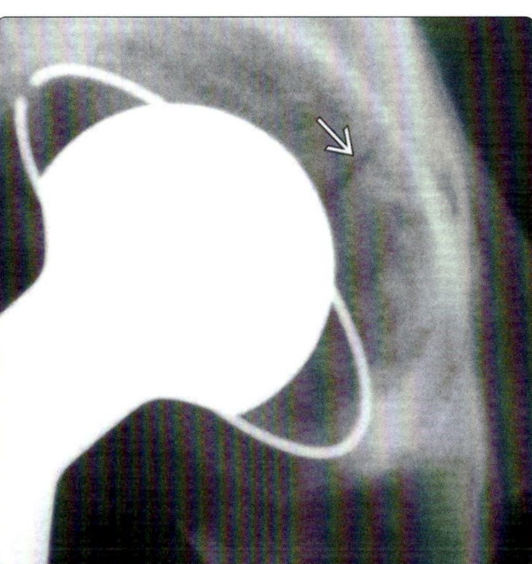

(Left) *AP radiograph shows a cemented total hip arthroplasty (THA) with an obvious fracture of the shaft ➡. Fractures are not usually as obvious as this one but are seen as a subtle buckle of the metal. It is likely that this component has been fractured for some time, as there is evidence of motion and lysis ⇨ about the fragment.* **(Right)** *AP radiograph shows a cemented polyethylene acetabular component. There is a fracture in the lucent component, seen because the cement has fractured as well ➡.*

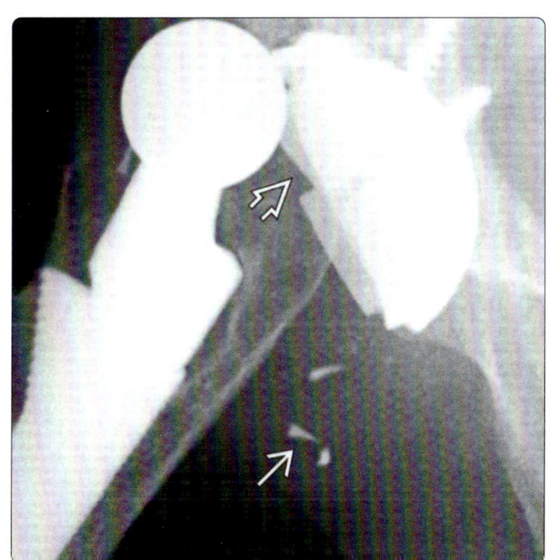

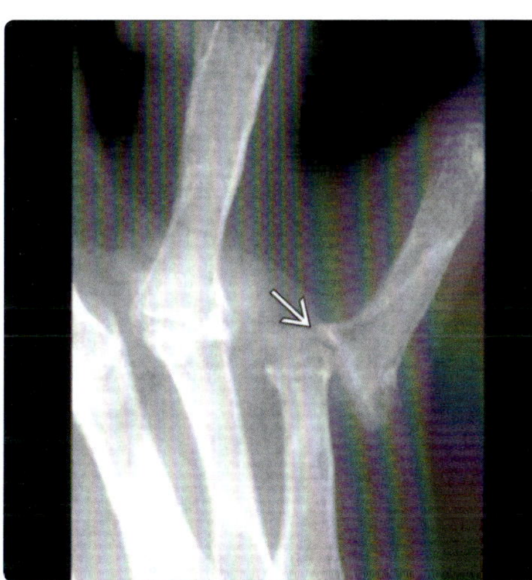

(Left) *Oblique radiograph shows a dislocated THA. There are several wedge-shaped metallic densities (tines) in the soft tissues ➡. These are used to secure the polyethylene liner in the cup, and their presence in the soft tissues indicates failure. The metallic cup itself is fractured as well ⇨.* **(Right)** *PA radiograph shows Silastic arthroplasties placed at MCPs 4 and 5. The 5th MCP arthroplasty has fractured ➡ at the junction of the body and flange. This is a typical site of prosthesis fracture in patients with RA.*

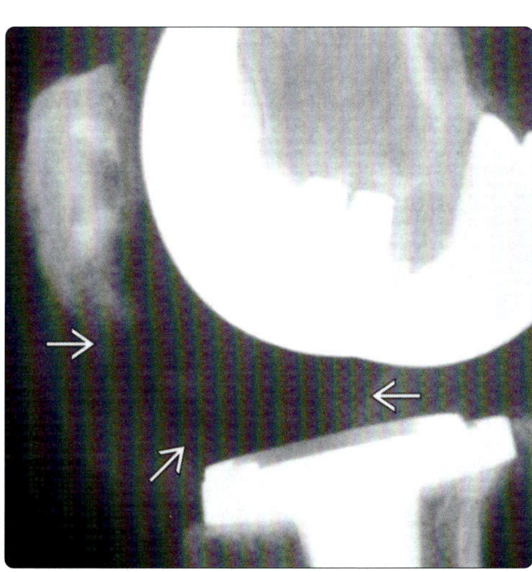

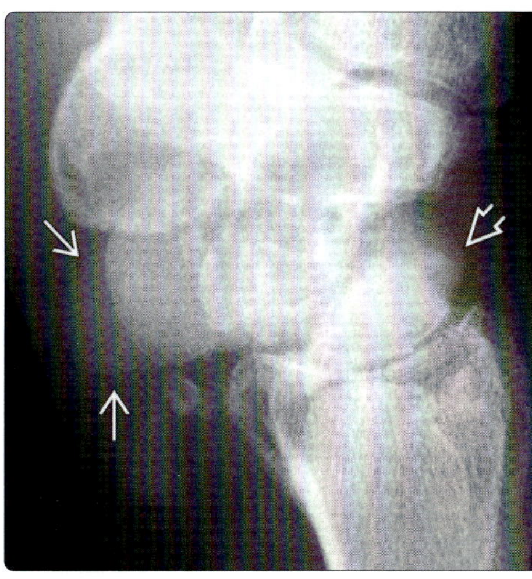

(Left) *Lateral radiograph shows a lucent structure shaped like the tibial liner, dislocated anteriorly within the joint ➡. It has come loose from the tibial tray and has caused the joint to lock.* **(Right)** *Lateral radiograph shows a Silastic scaphoid that is dislocated volarly ➡. There is also a Silastic lunate ⇨ that articulates with the radius but is dislocated from the capitate. Carpal replacements frequently fail, with consequent synovitis and osteolysis due to particle disease.*

(Left) *AP radiograph shows a dislocated acetabular cup. The implant has disrupted the medial acetabular wall and protrudes into the pelvis ➡. It is no longer able to contain the head of the femoral implant; that implant is dislocated and has migrated superiorly, creating a pseudoacetabulum ➡. Prominent metallosis ➡ is present, which likely results in reactive change.* **(Right)** *AP radiograph shows fracture of the outer rim of the patellar button, with the metal backing of the button separating ➡.*

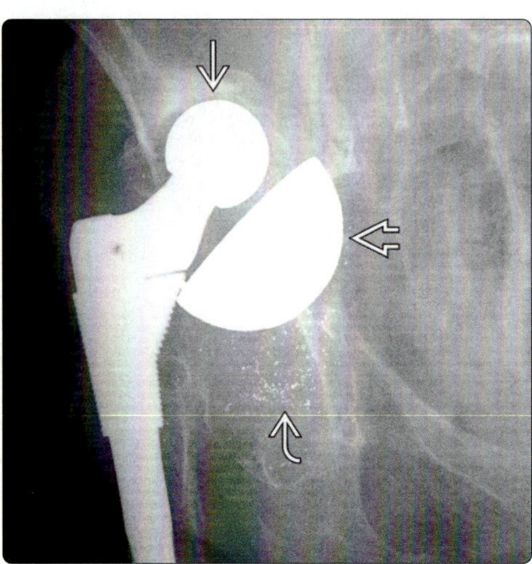

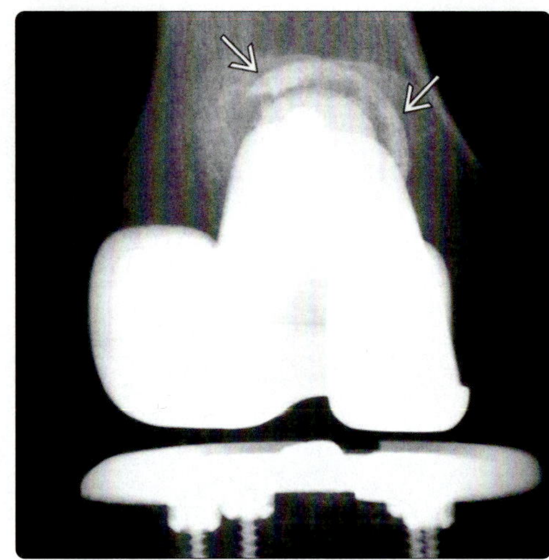

(Left) *Lateral radiograph obtained 7 years after total knee arthroplasty (TKA). There is a lucency in the anterior distal femoral metaphysis ➡, as well as a linear sclerosis "streaming" from the posterior cortex to the posterior part of the condylar component ➡.* **(Right)** *Lateral radiograph 2 years later shows both the lucency ➡ and sclerosis ➡ to be even more prominent. This represents stress shielding where the major stress of weight-bearing is transferred posteriorly in a TKA with an anterior flange (most common design).*

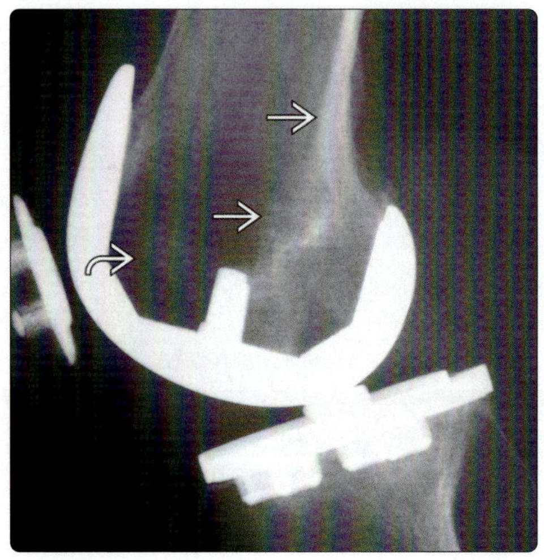

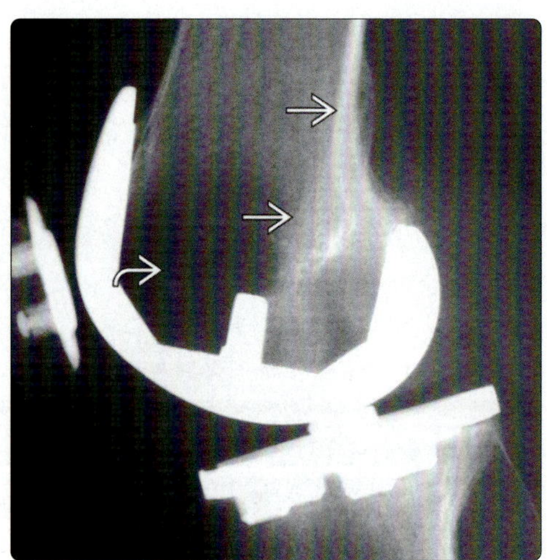

(Left) *AP radiograph of an acetabular component shows serpiginous tracking and lytic destruction ➡ within the bone. There is sclerotic reactive change ➡; the findings are of infection.* **(Right)** *AP radiograph shows a nonsymmetric lucency ➡ surrounding the tip of a femoral prosthesis. The nearby shaft shows tremendous endosteal and cortical reactive change ➡. This is osteomyelitis and an infected THA. Though one always seeks them, it is uncommon for the signs of infection to be so obvious.*

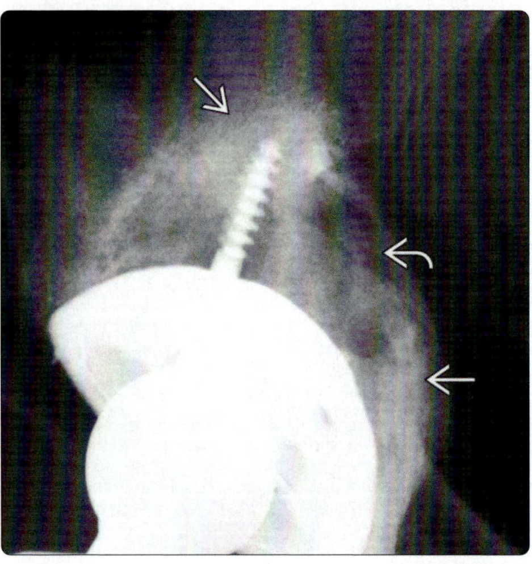

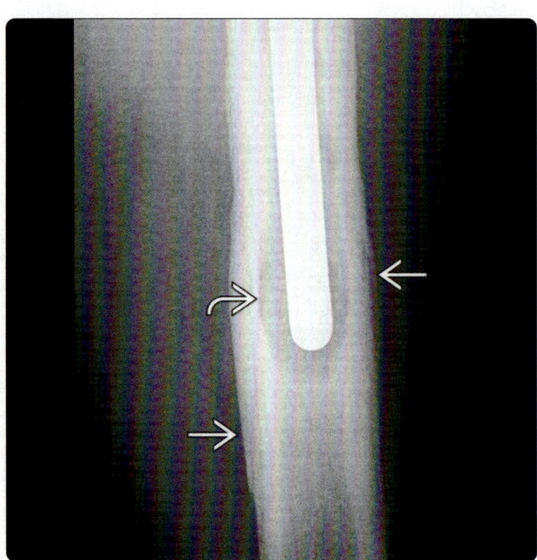

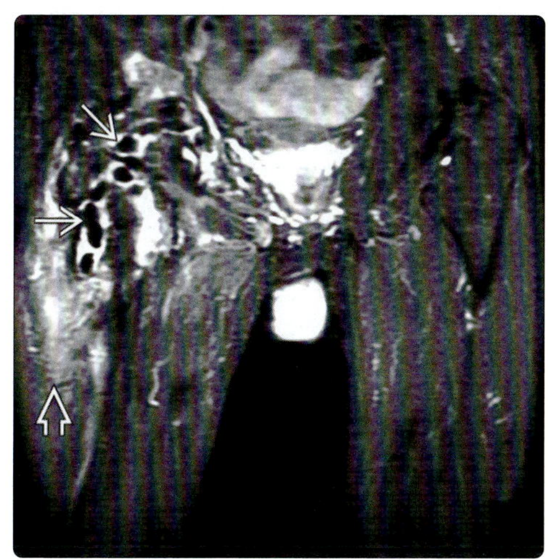

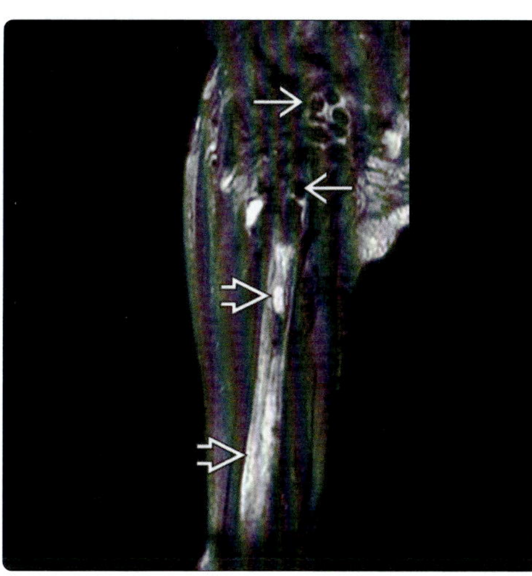

(Left) *Coronal T2WI MR shows typical antibiotic-impregnated beads ➡ placed in the defect left by removal of right THA. The soft tissue surrounding the beads is thickened and hyperintense ➡, suggesting ongoing infection.* **(Right)** *Sagittal PD FS MR, same case, shows the extent of the ongoing chronic osteomyelitis in the right femoral shaft with edema and small focal fluid pockets ➡. Note the antibiotic-impregnated beads ➡ located more proximally, at the original site of THA.*

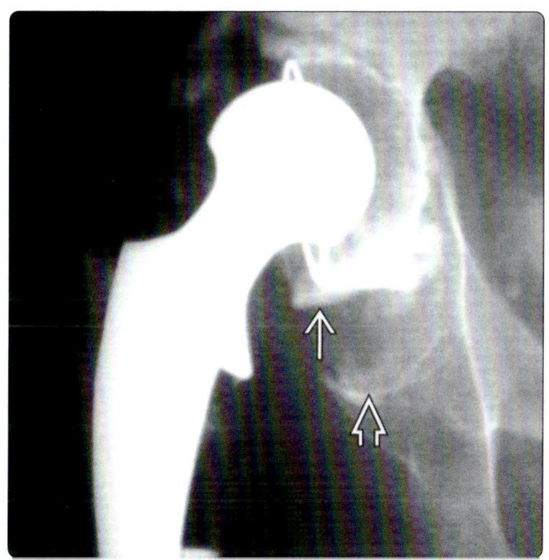

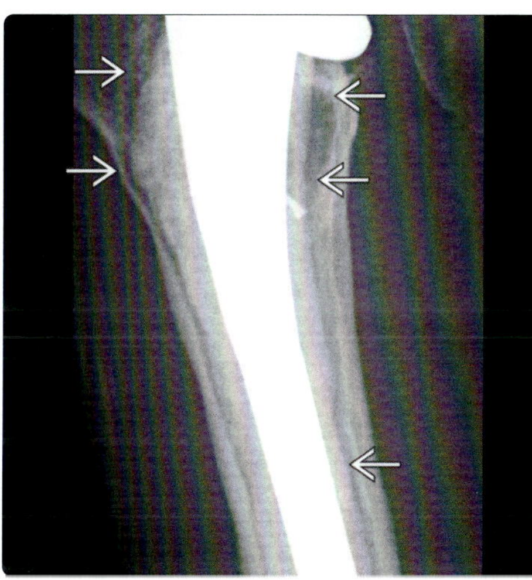

(Left) *AP radiograph shows gross loosening of a cemented acetabular component. There is superior subsidence of the cup by 2 cm ➡ relative to its original position ➡, as well as abnormal lateral opening (tilt).* **(Right)** *AP radiograph shows loosening of a cemented femoral stem. There is a lucency surrounding the majority of the stem ➡, which measures more than 2 mm. The entire stem is not included on the image, but the lucency extended distally. Note the cortical endosteal thinning.*

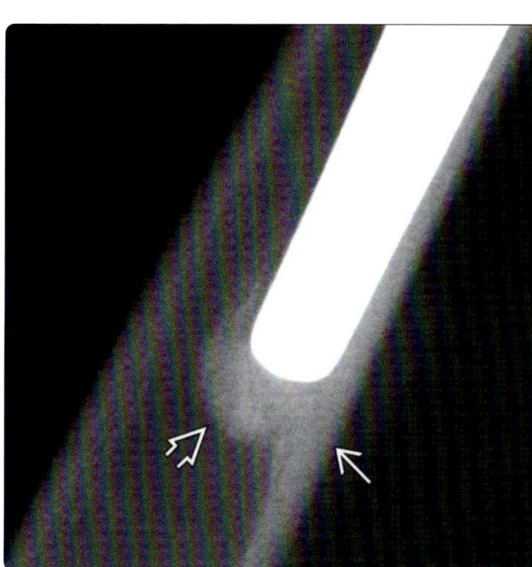

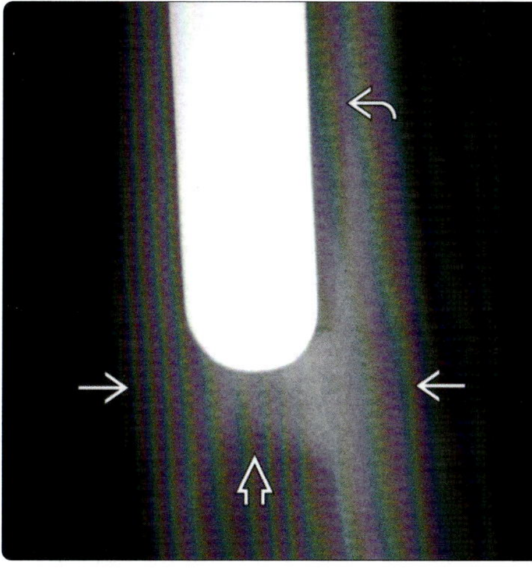

(Left) *Lateral radiograph shows mild cortical hypertrophy ➡ and prominent endosteal hypertrophy ➡ at the tip of a femoral stem. These findings are considered normal, as long as the hypertrophy does not become excessive but should be watched for stability.* **(Right)** *AP radiograph shows excessive cortical ➡ and endosteal ➡ hypertrophy, bridging across the tip of the femoral stem. There is also a wide lucency at the bone-component interface ➡. This is a loose femoral component.*

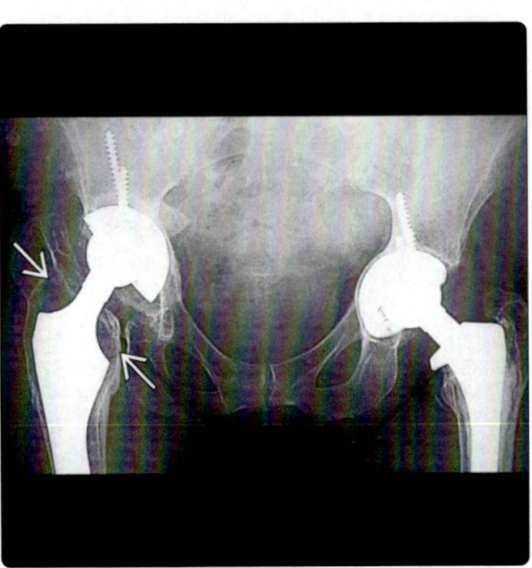

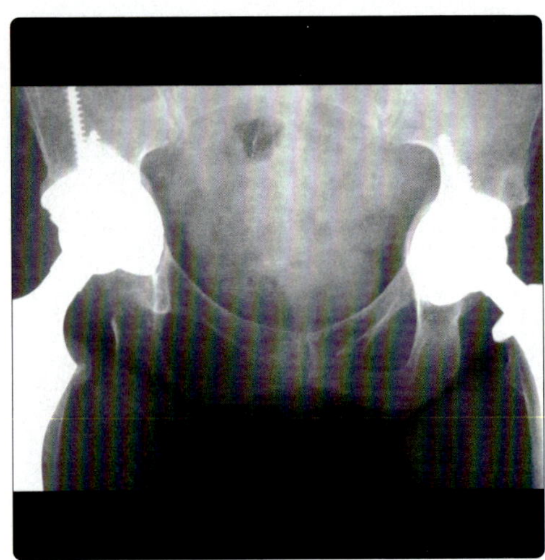

(Left) *AP radiograph obtained 4 years following THA shows gross loosening of the femoral component, with inferior subsidence by 1.5 cm ➡. At 1st glance, the acetabular cup does not appear loose since there is no surrounding lucency. However, compared to the index image, the cup has subsided superiorly (note its relation to teardrop) and shows an increased lateral tilt. This change in position is diagnostic of loosening.* **(Right)** *AP radiograph shows normal placement of the THA, shown to compare the acetabular position.*

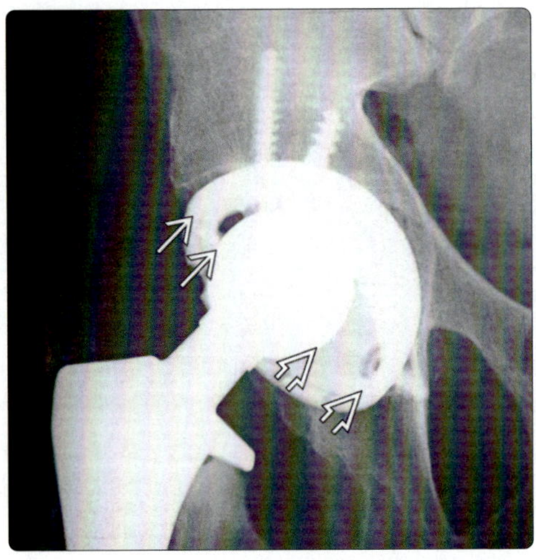

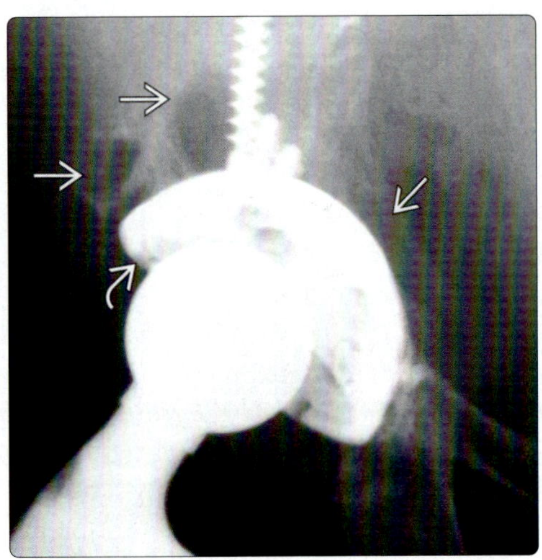

(Left) *AP radiograph shows evidence of polyethylene cup wear. The width of the superolateral polyethylene (between ➡) is significantly smaller than the width inferomedially (between ➡). Polyethylene wear can result in a painful prosthesis as well as particle disease.* **(Right)** *AP radiograph shows massive osteolysis ➡ of the acetabulum secondary to particle disease. The source of particles is wear of the polyethylene acetabular liner, indicated by offset of the head relative to cup ➡.*

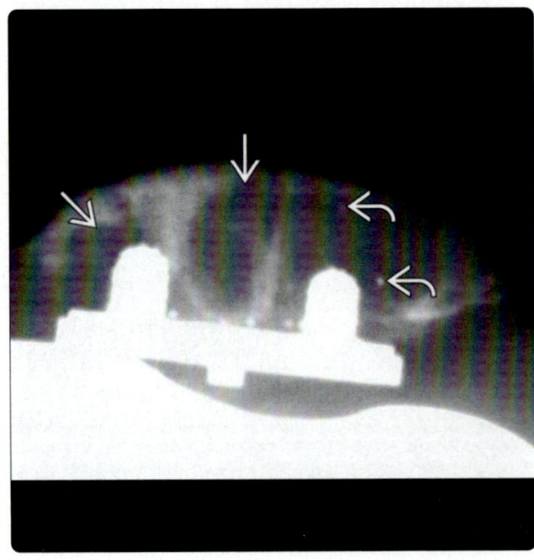

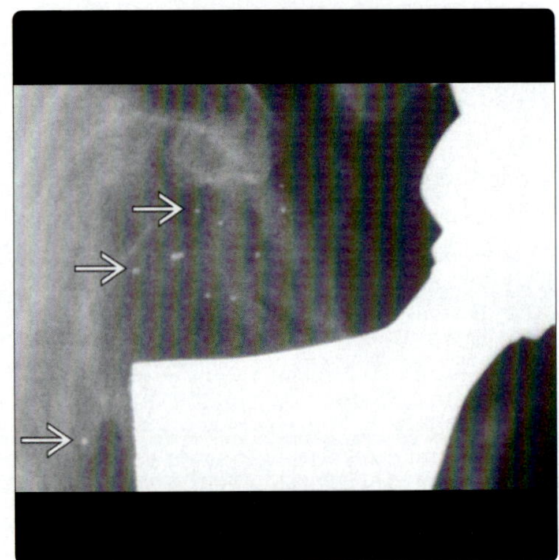

(Left) *Sunrise radiograph of a patella with TKA shows massive osteolysis ➡. The particles that triggered the inflammatory reaction in this case are metallic beads ➡, which were shed as the component loosened.* **(Right)** *AP radiograph shows prominent bead shedding ➡, which may be taken as a secondary sign of loosening of this femoral component. Though these metal beads are the right size to incite particle disease, this had not occurred at the time of the examination.*

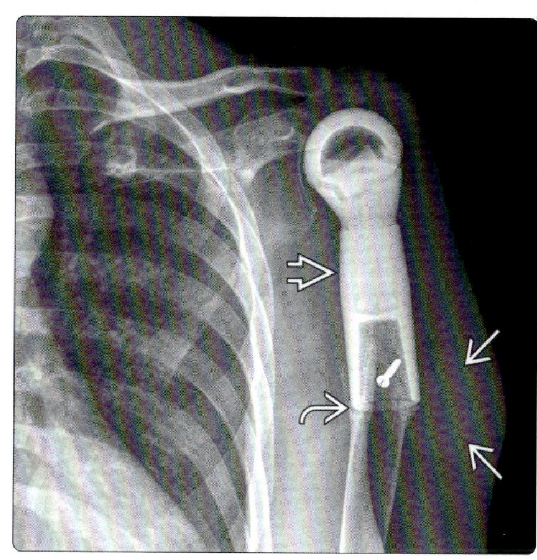

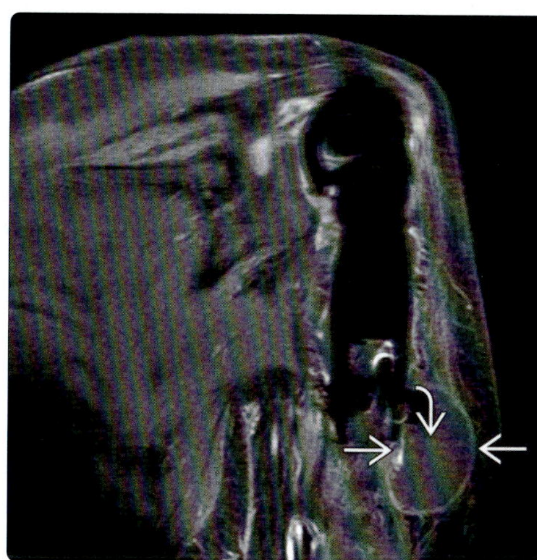

(Left) *AP radiograph shows a customized left shoulder endoprosthesis ➡, placed following resection of the proximal humerus for tumor. There is a fracture at the interface with the host bone ➡ and an adjacent soft tissue mass ➡.* **(Right)** *Coronal T1WI C+ FS MR shows the mass ➡ to have mild heterogeneous enhancement ➡. This is less enhancement than would be expected for tumor recurrence. Particle disease with granuloma and necrosis was proven, developed 2° to the fracture.*

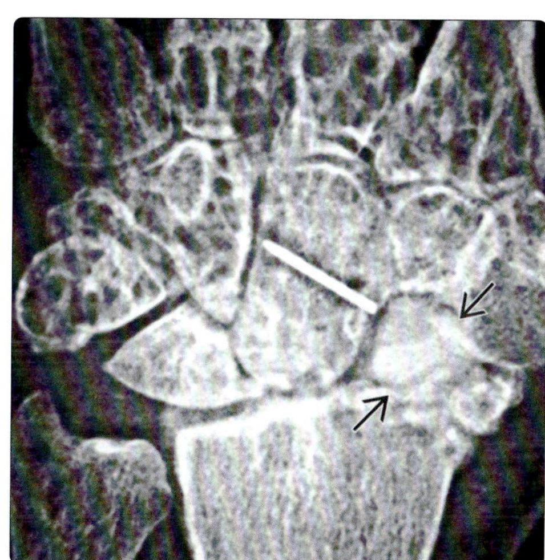

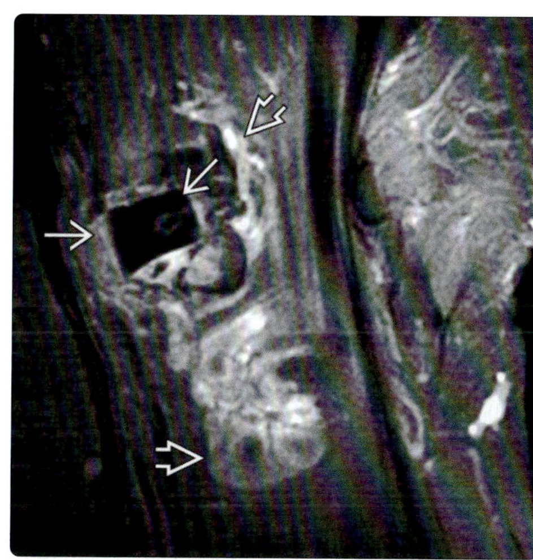

(Left) *PA radiograph shows osteolysis of all carpal bones as well as the base of metacarpals 2-5. The source of the particles inciting this massive osteolysis is a Silastic scaphoid prosthesis ➡ that has fractured, rotated, and worn down. The fractured K-wire was originally placed to stabilize the prosthesis.* **(Right)** *Coronal STIR MR demonstrates a trapezium prosthesis ➡ and extensive synovitis seen extending throughout carpal recesses ➡. This synovitis is seen in reaction to breakdown of the Silastic prosthesis.*

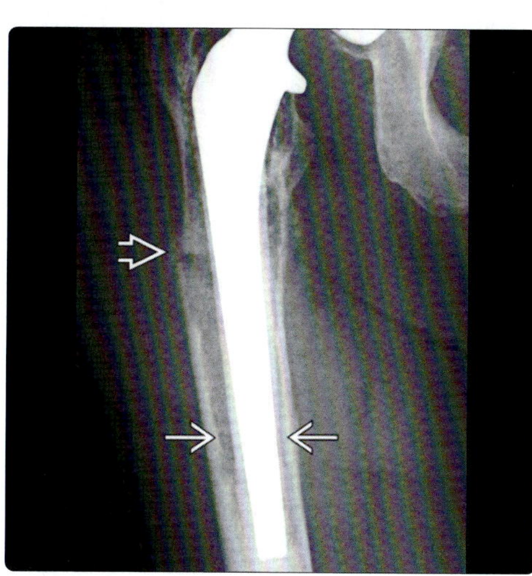

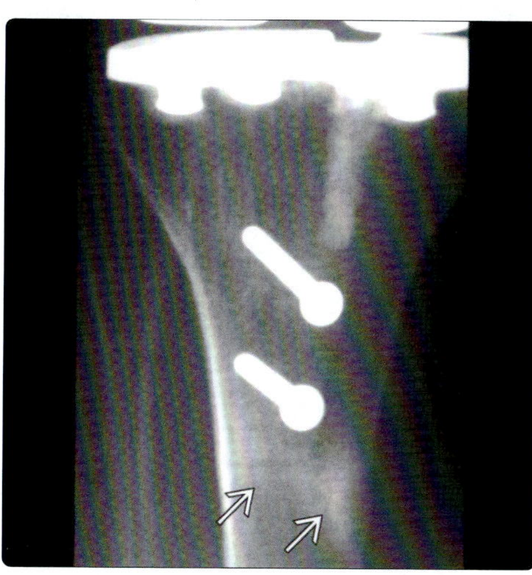

(Left) *AP radiograph shows gross loosening of a cemented THA femoral component, with wide lucency surrounding the cement-bone interface ➡. It is not surprising that a periprosthetic fracture ➡ has occurred at the excessively thin cortex.* **(Right)** *AP radiograph shows linear sclerosis, indicating a periprosthetic fracture of the tibia ➡. Patients are at risk for periprosthetic fracture following TKA, particularly if they have also had a tibial tubercle transfer, as in this case.*

Hip Implant

KEY FACTS

TERMINOLOGY

- Total hip arthroplasty: Replacement of both acetabulum and femoral head
- Hemiarthroplasty or endoprosthesis: Replacement of femoral head only
- Hip resurfacing: Replacement of surface of femoral head, retaining stump of head, with short stem

IMAGING

- Evaluate initial placement of components
  - Length equal to contralateral side
  - Lateral opening cup angle: 40° ± 10°
  - Cup anteversion: 15° ± 10° on groin lateral
  - Horizontal center of rotation should be similar to that of normal hip
- Infection
  - Radiographs usually normal; requires aspiration if clinically suspected
- Loosening
  - Change in component position: Tilt or subsidence
    - Acetabular component subsides superiorly or medially
    - Femoral component subsides inferiorly
  - Cemented: ≥ 2-mm lucency at bone-cement interface surrounding majority of component indicates loosening; often has sclerotic margin
  - Cementless: ≥ 2-mm lucency at bone-component interface, often with sclerotic margin, surrounding majority of component indicates loosening
- Component wear: Offset of femoral head in cup
- Particle disease: Polyethylene, bone, metal, cement particles incite massive osteolysis
  - Search for source of particles to establish diagnosis
- Periprosthetic fracture
- CT used to evaluate
  - Version of cup in recurrent dislocators
  - Periprosthetic loosening or osteolysis
- MR used for problem solving; suggested for evaluation of painful metal-on-metal implants

(Left) *Normal positioning of a THA with transischial line (TL) of reference ➡ is shown. Angle (B) (nl 40° ± 10°) is the lateral opening of the cup. Limb length (A) is evaluated by a landmark (usually lesser trochanter) relative to TL.* **(Right)** *AP radiograph shows a patient with repeated left hip dislocations. Note the left hip is relatively long compared with the right (distance from transischial line to lesser trochanter: L > R). Increased length puts a THA at risk for dislocation. One should search for component malposition in chronic dislocators.*

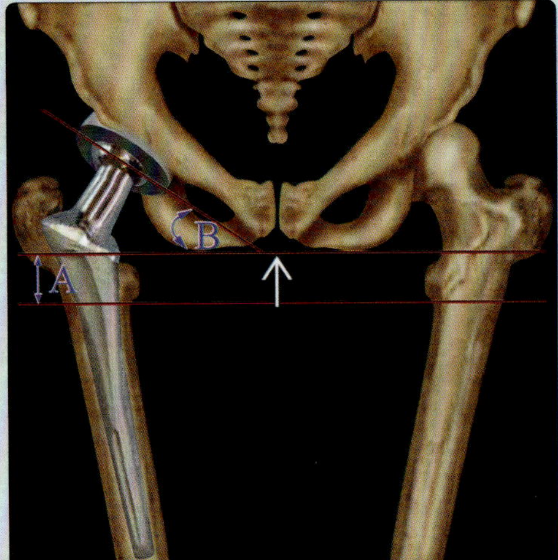

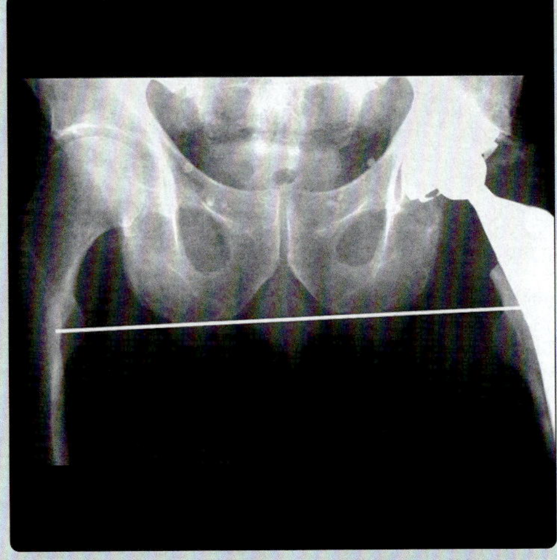

(Left) *AP radiograph shows a lateral opening angle of the acetabular component ➡ < 30°, the lower limit. This puts the hip at risk for dislocation when it is placed in forced abduction.* **(Right)** *AP radiograph shows a dislocated THA in a repeating dislocator. The reason is clear on the radiograph; the lateral opening angle ➡ of the acetabular component is significantly > 50°, which is considered the upper limit of normal. Poor positioning of the cup is the most common reason for nonpositional THA dislocations.*

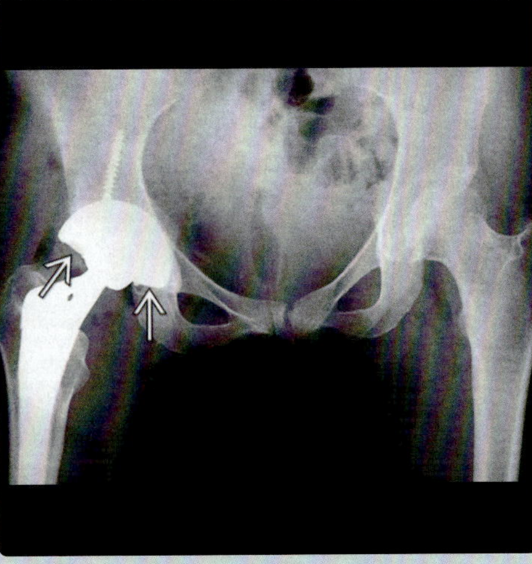

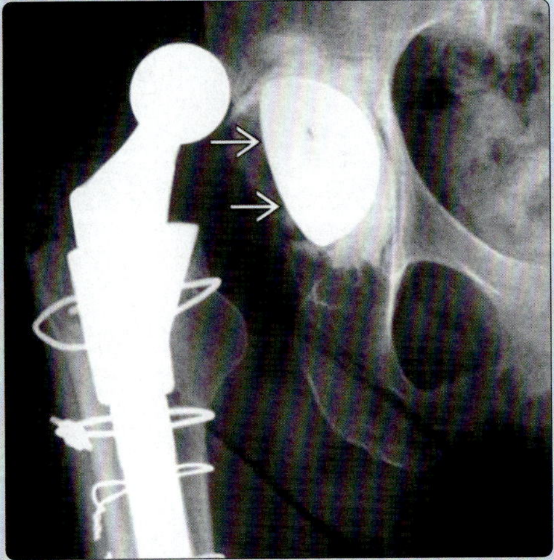

TERMINOLOGY

Definitions

- Total hip arthroplasty (THA): Replacement of both acetabulum and femoral head
- Hemiarthroplasty or endoprosthesis: Replacement of femoral head only
  - Used in cases of osteonecrosis or displaced subcapital fracture without associated arthritis of hip
- Hip resurfacing: Replacement of surface of femoral head, retaining stump of head, with short stem or peg
  - Used in younger patient population
  - Theoretically maximizes THA life available to patient by maintaining bone stock, allowing revision to standard THA

IMAGING

Radiographic Findings

- Evaluate initial placement of components
  - Length equal to contralateral side
    - Length can be affected by position of cup, femoral stem, or size of neck, head, or polyethylene
    - Evaluation: Draw transischial line, measure distance to landmark (such as greater or lesser trochanter), then compare sides
    - Overlengthening: Muscle spasm → dislocation
    - Shortening: Hip muscles ineffective, leaving hip at risk for dislocation
  - Acetabular cup position
    - Lateral opening angle: 40° ± 10°
      - Measured on AP radiograph, open (flat) surface angled relative to transischial line
      - ↑ lateral opening → ↑ risk of dislocation
      - Excessive lateral opening correlated with ↑ serum levels of metal in metal-on-metal THA, likely due to ↑ edge loading
      - ↓ lateral opening → torquing head out when hip is fully abducted
    - Anteversion of cup
      - AP: Can tell if there is version but cannot determine if it is anteverted or retroverted
      - Aligns with bony acetabulum on Lauenstein
      - Normally measures 15° ± 10° on groin lateral
      - Groin lateral measurement depends on patient position; affected by rotation of pelvis (may be minimized by imaging with knee flexed over end of table)
      - Retroversion or excessive anteversion predisposes hip to dislocation
    - Medial-lateral position of cup
      - Horizontal center of rotation should be similar to that of normal hip
      - Lack of medialization puts hip at risk for dislocation if center of rotation falls lateral to iliopsoas muscle pull
      - Too much medialization puts medial acetabulum at risk for fracture
  - Femoral component position
    - Neutral to slightly valgus (implant resting against lateral endosteum proximally and against medial endosteum distally)
    - Varus position predisposes implant to loosening
- Implant fracture
  - Cup may fracture anywhere around its convexity
    - Polyethylene cup fracture seen by fracture of surrounding cement
  - Stem fracture usually near distal tip
    - May be displaced but usually subtle buckle
- Dislocation
  - Femoral head dislocated from acetabular cup
    - Look for predisposing component malposition
      - Abnormal lateral opening angle (> 50° or < 30°)
      - Abnormal version of cup (retroverted or anteverted > 25°)
      - Lack of medialization of cup
      - Abnormal limb length (either long or short)
  - Polyethylene dislocation
    - May become dissociated from metal backing
      - Tines or metal wedges, which hold it in place, may be seen in soft tissues
      - Polyethylene seen as lucency separate from cup's backing
- Stress shielding
  - Most frequently in lateral metaphysis of proximal femur, including greater trochanter
  - Resorbed bone: Relative lucency, thinned cortex
- Infection
  - Radiographs usually normal; requires aspiration if clinically suspected
    - If chronic infection, serpiginous bony destruction with reactive bone ± periosteal reaction may be seen
- Loosening
  - Change in component position
    - Altered alignment (tilt)
    - Change in superior-inferior position (subsidence)
      - Cup subsides superiorly, possibly medially; femoral component subsides inferiorly down shaft
    - Subsidence and tilt often occur without lucency surrounding component
      - Comparison with index postoperative radiograph essential to avoid missing loosening
  - Cemented component
    - ≥ 2-mm lucency at bone-cement interface surrounding majority of component indicates loosening; often has sclerotic margin
    - ≥ 2-mm lucency at cement-component interface may result from motion at time of placement
    - Fractured cement
  - Cementless component
    - ≥ 2-mm lucency at bone-component interface, often with sclerotic margin, surrounding majority of component indicates loosening
    - Extensive sclerosis at femoral tip, both cortical and endosteal hypertrophy
      - Bridging bone across medullary canal considered secondary sign of loosening
      - Less extensive bone formation considered normal in cementless stem but should be watched for progression

- Component wear
  - With loosening, beaded surface of cementless arthroplasty may separate (bead shedding)
  - Polyethylene wear shown by differential width between femoral head and acetabulum
    - Wear generally in weight-bearing superolateral portion compared with inferomedial portion
- Particle disease
  - Morphology
    - Focal lytic bone destruction; may mimic tumor
    - May extend along component, with bone destruction appearing more elongated
    - May extend into soft tissues as mass or bursal collection
  - Search for source of particles to establish diagnosis
    - Polyethylene wear
    - Cement fracture or osseous debris
    - Metallosis (bead shedding or other metal debris)
    - Metal-on-metal THA may develop reactive, necrotic soft tissue or bursal masses (pseudotumors)
- Periprosthetic fracture
  - Acetabulum: Medial wall
  - Femoral shaft: Usually anterior cortex, extending from tip of prosthesis
    - Metaphyseal cracks may occur during surgery; noted during surgery and treated with cerclage wiring

CT Findings

- Evaluation of version of cup in recurrent dislocators
  - Accurate, independent of patient position
  - Method: Reformat image to standardize pelvis for rotation and pelvic tilt
    - Directly measure angle of anteversion, referencing off vertical line
- Evaluation of periprosthetic loosening or osteolysis
  - Presence and extent of osteolysis better evaluated by CT than radiograph
  - Used to evaluate location of lysis and adequacy of bone stock prior to revision

MR Findings

- Generally used for problem solving; suggested for evaluation of painful metal-on-metal implants
- Umbrella terms: Adverse reaction to metal debris or adverse local tissue reaction
  - Include metallosis, aseptic lymphocytic vasculitis-associated lesions (ALVAL), and pseudotumors
- MR predictive model for adverse local tissue reaction (reactions to arthroplasty-related metal products)
  - Best predictors for diagnosis of moderate to severe adverse local tissue reaction (ALVAL > 5): Maximal synovial thickness (> 7 mm) and mixed solid-cystic synovial pattern
  - Best predictors for intraoperative tissue damage: Pseudocapsular dehiscence, mixed pattern of synovitis, and decompression of synovitis into adjacent soft tissues

Imaging Recommendations

- Protocol advice
  - Metal artifact reduction techniques for CT
    - Soft tissue image acquisition
    - ↑ kVp (140) and mAs (350-450 if 1 THA, 450-600 if 2)
    - Narrowed collimation
    - ↓ pitch (0.3)
    - Image reconstruction at 1-mm section width with 0.5-mm reconstruction increment
    - Dual-energy CT reduces beam-hardening artifacts
  - Metal artifact reduction techniques for MR
    - ↑ receiver bandwidth
    - ↓ interecho spacing
    - ↓ effective echo times
    - Use intermediate-weighted fast spin echo sequences with high spatial resolution
    - STIR rather than fat-saturation techniques

PATHOLOGY

General Features

- Etiology
  - Femoral shaft fractures: Related to cross-sectional diameter and length of stem
  - Dislocation
    - Positional: Joint placed beyond expected range
    - Incorrect surgical positioning of components
  - Stress shielding: Altered weight-bearing through implant reduces stress on regions of bone
  - Massive osteolysis: Particles of critical size → inflammatory reaction
  - ALVAL: Associated with metal-on-metal THA
    - Possibly toxic reaction to metal-wear debris
    - Possibly hypersensitivity reaction to normally expected amount of metal debris

CLINICAL ISSUES

Natural History & Prognosis

- 80% of THAs last 20 years without revision
- Uncemented acetabular components with polyethylene liners undergo silent lysis and merit regular long-term radiological review
- Rate of development of abnormal soft tissue reaction and mass in metal-on-metal THA is unknown

DIAGNOSTIC CHECKLIST

Consider

- Watch for subsidence of components to indicate loosening, even without obvious lucency
- Compare follow-up image with index radiograph for change in component position
- With dislocation, search for malposition of components
- With osteolysis, search for evidence of particle disease

SELECTED REFERENCES

1. Fritz J et al: MR imaging of hip arthroplasty implants. Radiographics. 34(4):E106-32, 2014
2. Awan O et al: Imaging evaluation of complications of hip arthroplasty: review of current concepts and imaging findings. Can Assoc Radiol J. 64(4):306-13, 2013
3. Pessis E et al: Virtual monochromatic spectral imaging with fast kilovoltage switching: reduction of metal artifacts at CT. Radiographics. 33(2):573-83, 2013
4. Chang EY et al: Metal-on-metal total hip arthroplasty: do symptoms correlate with MR imaging findings? Radiology. 265(3):848-57, 2012

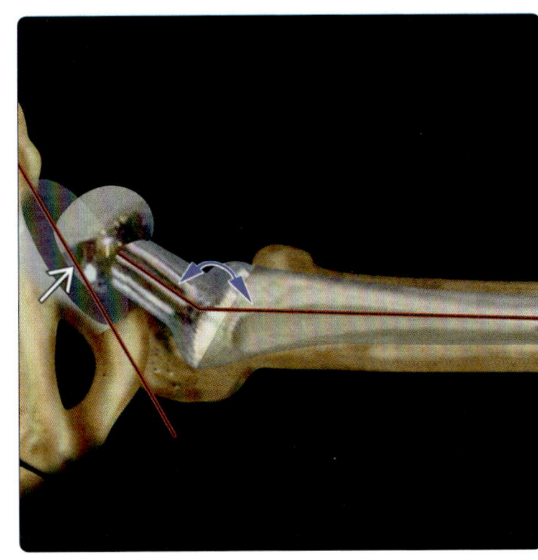

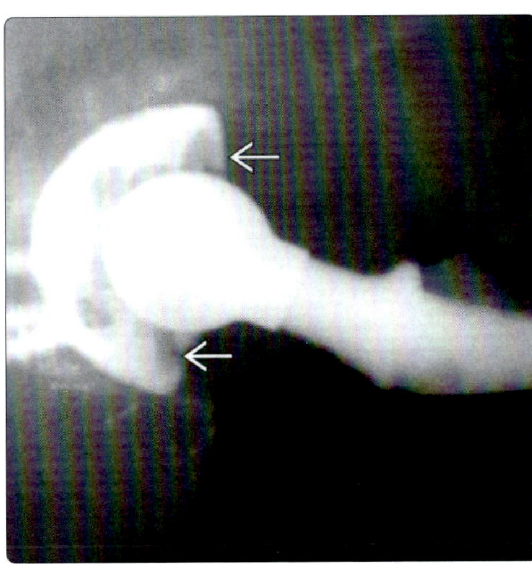

(Left) *Groin lateral graphic shows the expected anterior tilt (anteversion) of the acetabular component ➡. The angle on the femoral component describes the neck-shaft angle.* **(Right)** *Groin lateral view of a THA in a patient with recurrent dislocations shows retroversion of the acetabular component ➡ (compare with graphic). One cannot determine retroversion vs. anteversion on AP radiograph; groin lateral or CT is required. Retroversion puts a THA at risk for dislocation.*

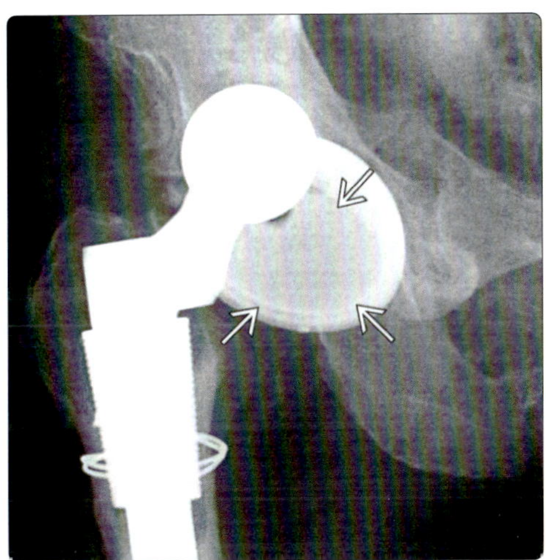

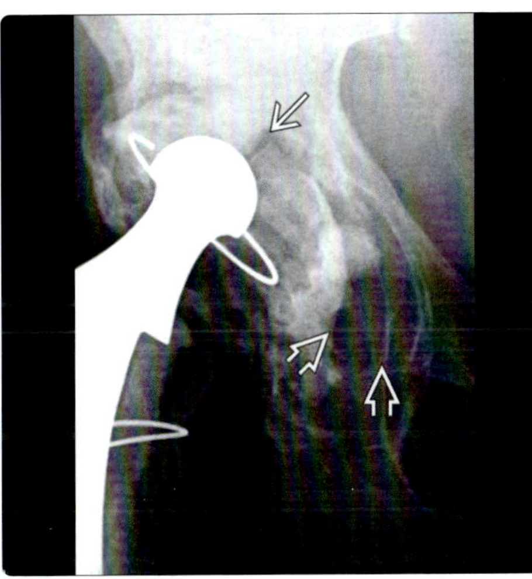

(Left) *AP radiograph shows a hip dislocation. The acetabular component shows normal lateral tilt. However, there is excessive version ➡ (opening either anterior or posterior). The groin lateral (not shown) confirmed excessive anteversion. While anteversion of the cup is expected, this degree puts the hip at risk for dislocation.* **(Right)** *AP radiograph shows gross loosening of the cup with superior subsidence (note distance from original site ➡). The cup is fractured ➡ and shows a wide lucency relative to cement.*

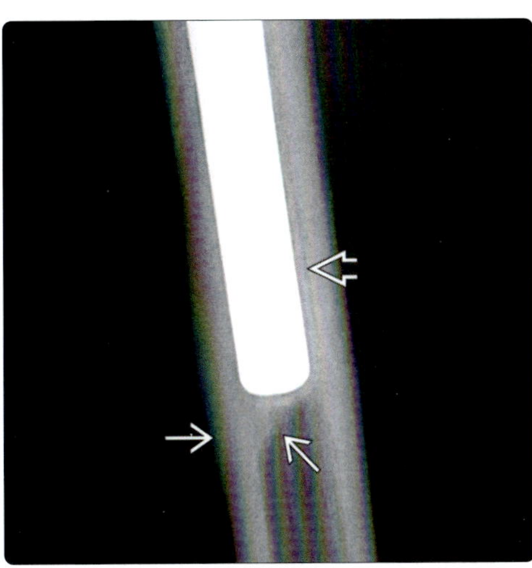

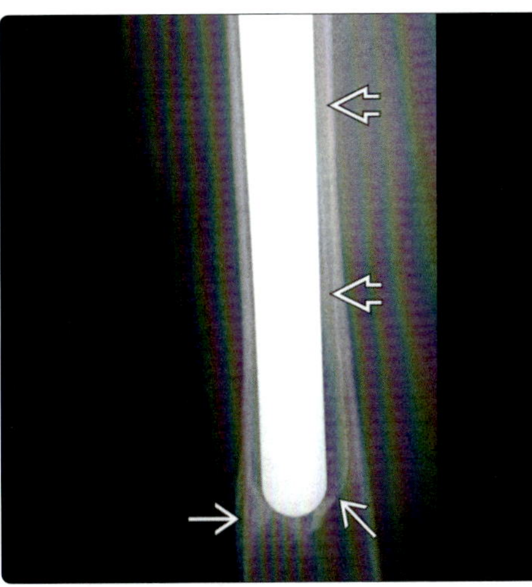

(Left) *AP radiograph shows moderate cortical and endosteal hypertrophy ➡ about the tip of the stem of a cementless femoral component. There is also a sclerotic line ➡ but no lucent bone-component interface. This appearance is normal for a cementless component.* **(Right)** *AP radiograph shows excessive cortical and endosteal hypertrophy ➡ bridging the medullary canal. Additionally, there is a lucency > 2 mm surrounding the component ➡. These findings are typical of loosening.*

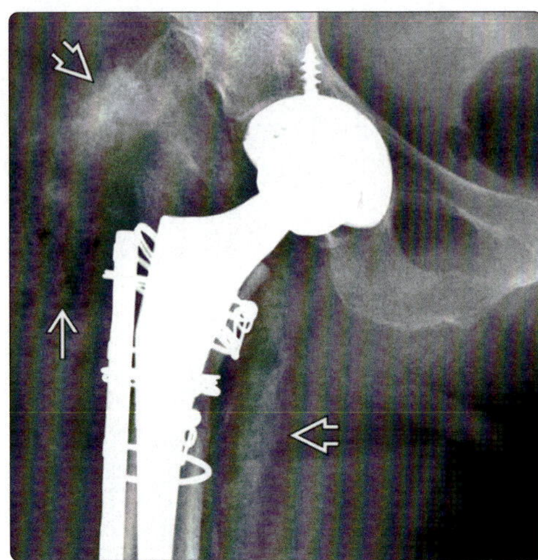

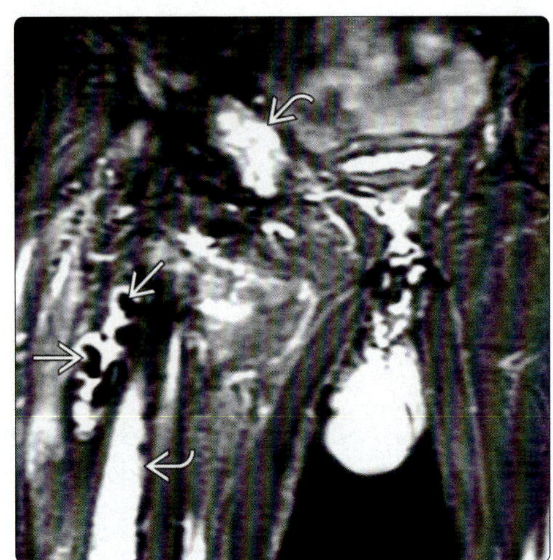

(Left) *AP radiograph shows a THA with uncommonly obvious findings of infection. There is air in the soft tissues* ➡ *as well as fluffy, immature heterotopic bone formation* ➡*. An infected arthroplasty usually appears normal; any clinical suspicion requires aspiration.* **(Right)** *Coronal T2WI MR shows ↓ signal intensity (SI) antibiotic beads* ➡ *placed in the defect following explant of an infected THA. Unfortunately, the treatment has not been effective, indicated by ↑ SI throughout the remaining acetabulum and shaft* ➡*.*

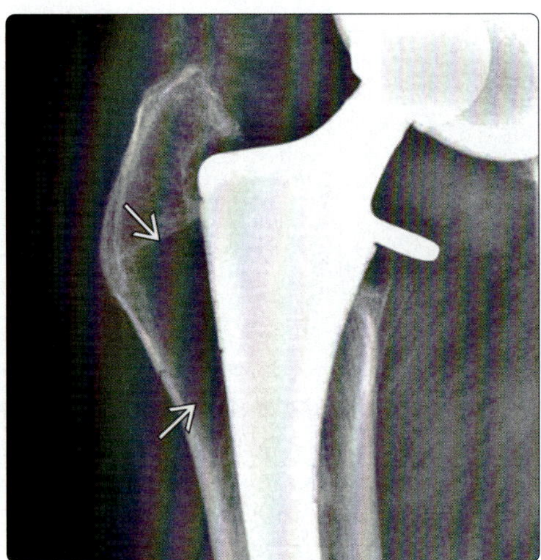

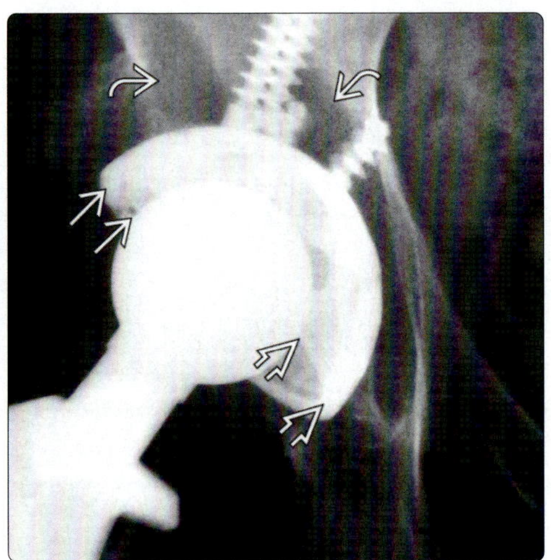

(Left) *AP radiograph shows metaphyseal lucency* ➡ *extending into the greater trochanter, noted several years following THA. This is the typical location of stress shielding and should not be misinterpreted as infection or a lytic lesion.* **(Right)** *AP radiograph shows polyethylene wear, demonstrated by thinning of the distance between the metal cup and head superiorly* ➡ *compared with the distance inferiorly* ➡*. This wear results in particle disease and lysis* ➡*.*

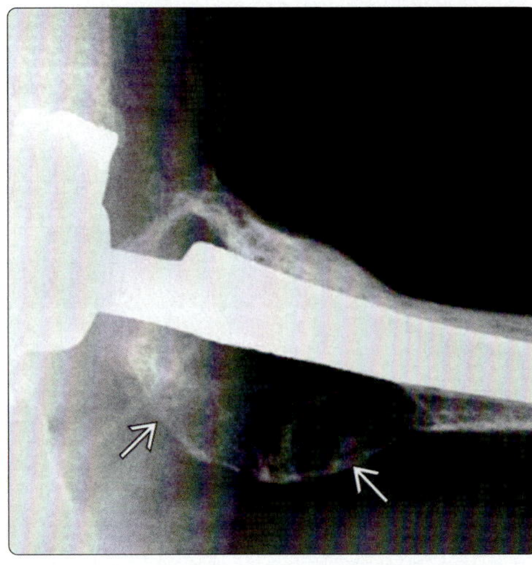

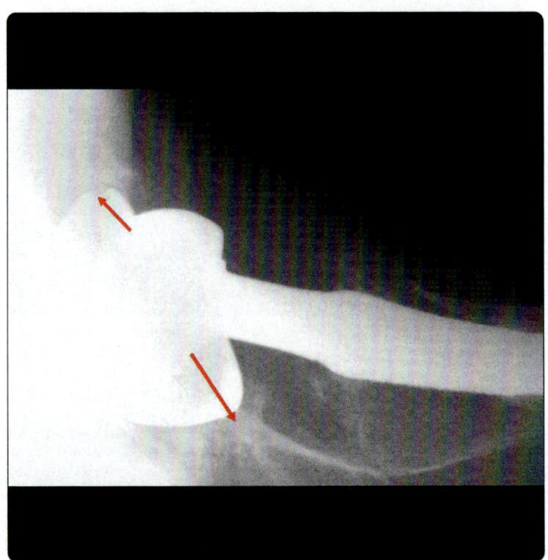

(Left) *Frog leg lateral radiograph shows an expanded lytic lesion involving the proximal metaphysis of the femur* ➡*. There is no other abnormality seen, and the AP radiograph was normal (not shown). This leaves a wide differential diagnosis, including tumor.* **(Right)** *Groin lateral in the same case does not show the lytic lesion as well, but polyethylene wear is readily seen, as outlined by the red arrows. With a source of particles demonstrated in this manner, the lytic lesion is highly likely to represent osteolysis.*

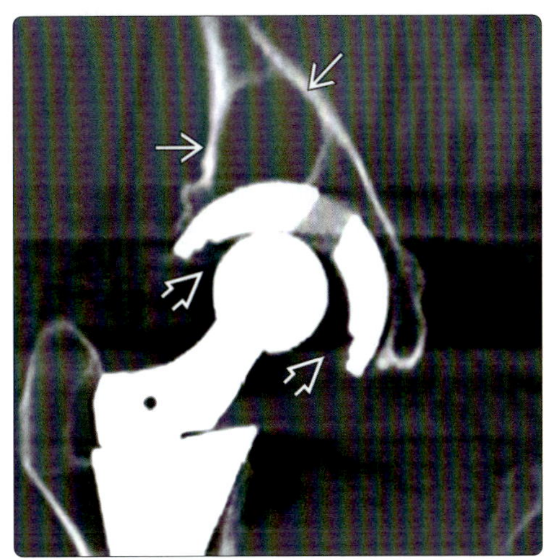

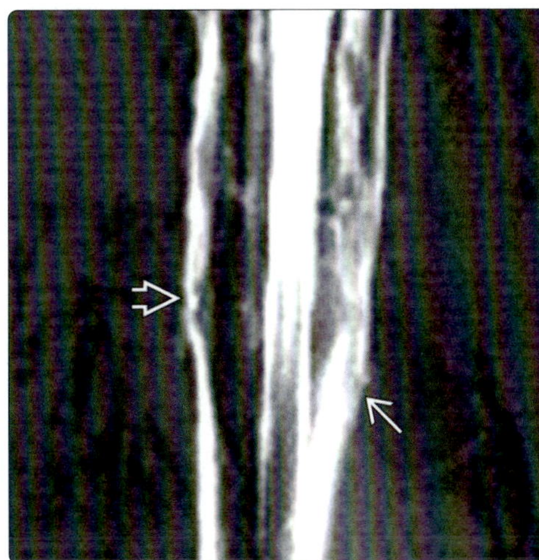

(Left) *Coronal reformat bone CT shows a large acetabular region of lysis* ➡ *as well as evidence of polyethylene wear (offset of head in cup* ➡*). The radiograph (not shown) was difficult to evaluate; CT adds important information regarding extent of osteolysis, which results in better planning of a substantial revision.* **(Right)** *Coronal bone CT shows extensive thinning of cortex* ➡ *with prosthetic loosening (note the wide bone-cement lucency), as well as fracture* ➡*. Neither subtlety was seen on radiograph.*

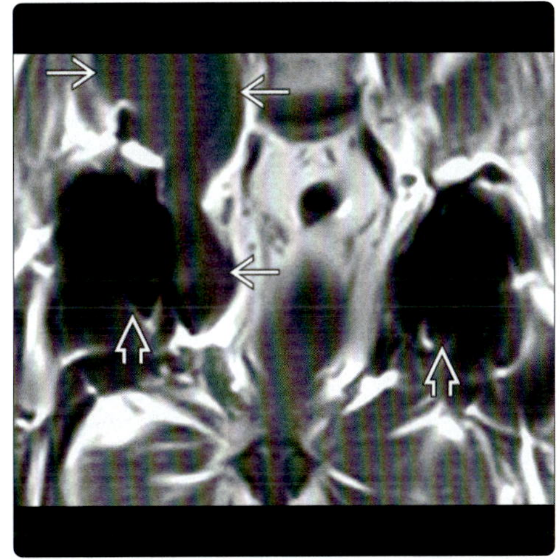

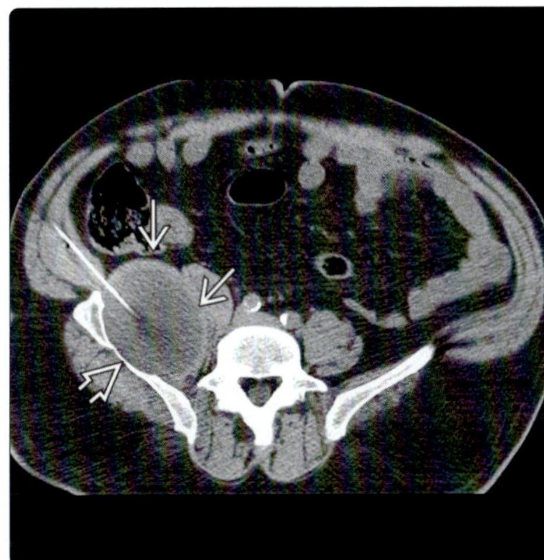

(Left) *Coronal T1WI MR shows bilateral THAs* ➡ *and an enormous fluid collection in the right iliopsoas bursa* ➡*. Concern was for infection vs. synovitis.* **(Right)** *Axial bone CT confirms a fluid collection in the iliacus bursa* ➡*. Aspiration yielded thick, gelatinous material and debris-laden macrophages. Debris formed from THA polyethylene wear and caused a synovitis, which decompressed into the iliopsoas bursa. Prominent thinning of the iliac wing* ➡ *may be due to pressure rather than particle lysis.*

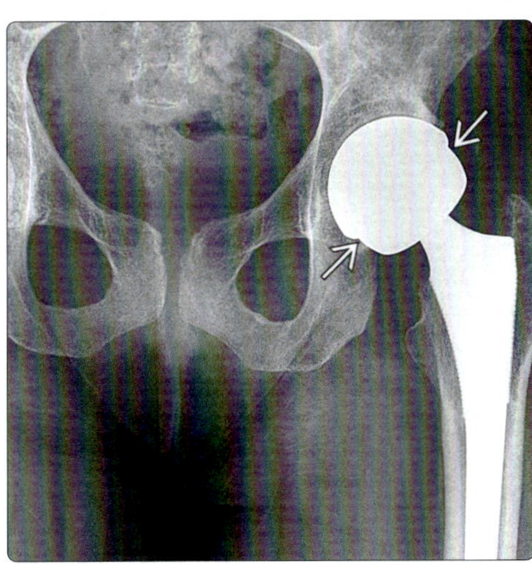

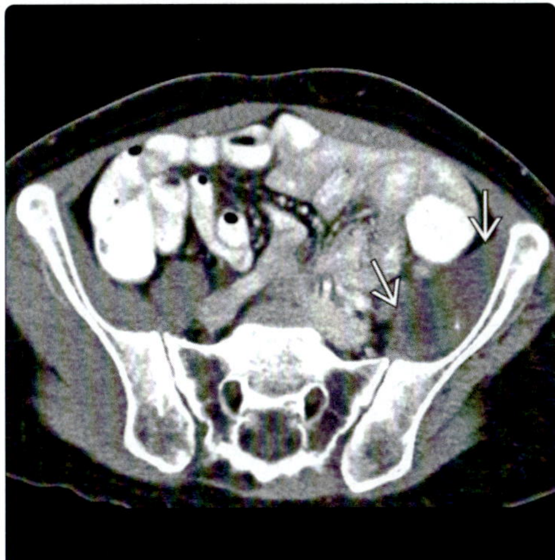

(Left) *AP radiograph shows a metal-on-metal prosthesis* ➡*; note the absence of polyethylene liner. This patient had pain, which is not explained by component positioning, which is normal.* **(Right)** *Axial CECT in the same case shows mild enhancement of an inhomogeneous iliacus mass* ➡*. Extensive biopsy showed only debris and necrotic tissue, typical of adverse local tissue reaction. Cross-sectional imaging should be suggested with this metal-on-metal arthroplasty and unexplained pain.*

KEY FACTS

TERMINOLOGY

- Revision arthroplasty: Placement of new component(s) following removal of failed implant
- Small revisions may not be obvious
  - Replacement of polyethylene component
  - Change of femoral head (modular; may be changed without extracting stem)
- Larger revisions of entire components

IMAGING

- Preop: Surgical planning
  - CT with reformats in coronal and sagittal planes to evaluate location and extent of lytic lesions
  - CT has greater sensitivity than radiograph for presence and amount of bone loss
  - Metal artifact-reduction techniques should be utilized
  - MR utilized only for problem solving
- Postop appearance depends on choice of material to anchor implant in deficient bone
  - Watch for periprosthetic fracture
    - Especially common with long-stem femoral shaft revisions
  - Expect graft (either structural or nonstructural) to compress and partially resorb as it matures and unites with host bone
  - Revision components should be expected to subside, sometimes > 1 cm for long stem
  - Evaluate for incorporation of onlay graft
  - Dislocation more likely following revision

DIAGNOSTIC CHECKLIST

- Revision arthroplasties cannot be evaluated with same stringency regarding loosening as original arthroplasties
  - Expect subsidence of components
  - Watch for stabilization over 6-12 months
- Do not be fooled by lucencies related to prior component failure
  - Compare with prerevision radiograph

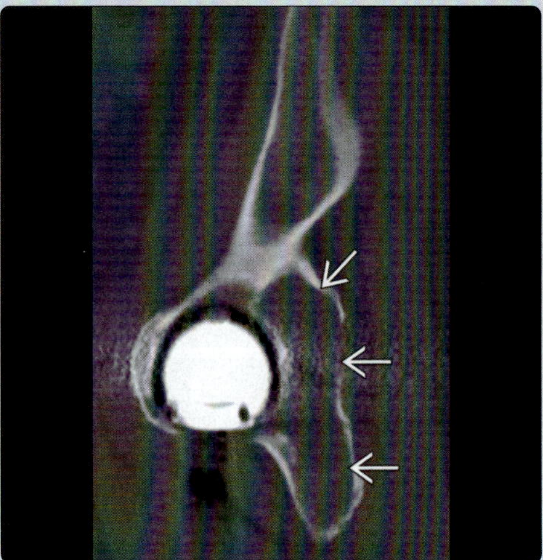

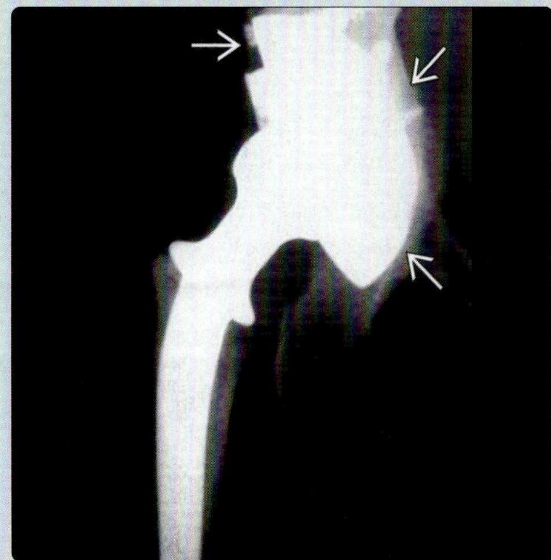

(Left) *Sagittal bone CT used for revision planning shows mild metal streak artifact. There is extensive posterior acetabular lysis ➡ extending well into the ischium. CT adds important information regarding extent of osteolysis, which suggests a highly substantial revision should be performed.* **(Right)** *AP radiograph shows an oversized acetabular component with augmentation ➡ used to fill a large superior acetabular defect. This type of component is one of several possible solutions for failed acetabular components.*

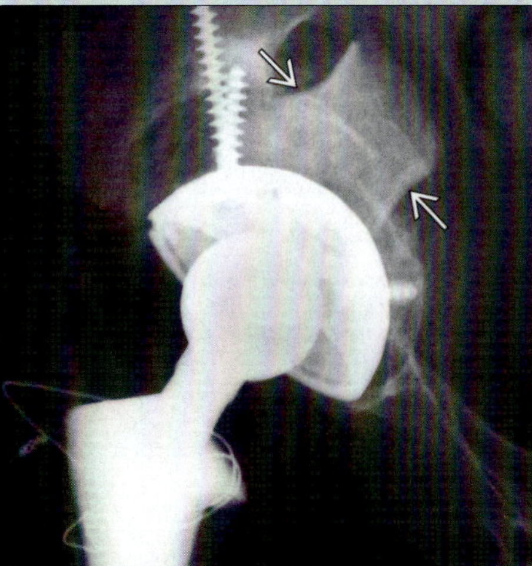

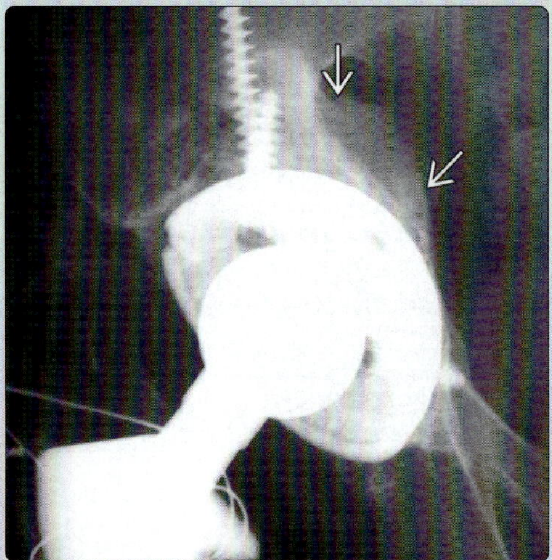

(Left) *AP x-ray shows a revision acetabular component that is normal in size. However, a large superior and superomedial acetabular defect is filled with a structural bone graft (note that it is a cadaver femoral neck ➡).* **(Right)** *AP x-ray of the same patient several months later shows that the structural graft has rounded, compressed ➡, and resorbed to some degree. The superior and medial acetabulum now gives solid osseous support to the acetabular component. There is slight associated component change in position.*

TERMINOLOGY

Definitions

- Revision arthroplasty: Placement of new component(s) following removal of failed implant
  - Some revisions have implications related to substantial bone loss: Large defects to fill, little bone to support arthroplasty
    - Loose components may fracture and lyse large regions of bone
    - Infection may destroy bone
    - Particle disease with massive osteolysis leaves osseous defects

IMAGING

Radiographic Findings

- Preop: Surgical planning must check for
  - Periprosthetic fracture
  - Cortical thinning or destruction
  - Lytic destructive bone sites
  - Amount and location of component migration
- Preop: Evaluation for residual infection
  - Evaluate for residual cement
    - If left in previously infected bone, may serve as nidus for ongoing infection
  - Aspiration and culture
- Postop appearance depends on choice of material to anchor implant in deficient bone
  - Acetabular defects, total hip arthroplasty (THA)
    - Widened, oversized cup augmentation
    - Cup with attached reconstructive plate and screw systems or reinforcement ring/cage
    - Defect filled with structural or nonstructural graft
  - Femoral defect, THA
    - SROM: Modular metaphyseal component
      - Wedge-shaped unit, which can be rotated around stem, used to fill proximal femoral metaphyseal defect
    - Clothespin femoral stem
      - Opens after insertion to help fill canal and stabilize stem
    - Long femoral stem
    - Onlay graft over femoral cortical defects with cerclage wiring
  - Total knee arthroplasty revisions
    - Generally long-stem components
    - May have wide polyethylene if soft tissue constraints are redundant
    - If knee is unstable, may place semiconstrained arthroplasty
      - Femoral and tibial components not hinged but connected by post
      - Post from femoral component can rotate slightly within tibial component, allowing normal rotation at end of full extension
      - Do not misinterpret lucency around this post as loosening
- Expected alterations in revision arthroplasty in follow-up examinations
  - Watch for periprosthetic fracture
    - More likely in revision
      - Disuse osteoporosis, cortical thinning
      - Long-stem components more likely to pierce cortex, especially anterior cortex in femur because there is normal anterior femoral bowing
    - 7.5% probability of fracture in revision THA
  - Lucency surrounding component
    - Do not misinterpret preexisting lucency from prior failed component as new loosening
      - Compare with radiograph of failed arthroplasty
  - Structural and nonstructural graft
    - Expect graft to compress and partially resorb as it matures and unites with host bone
      - Component placed in graft may change position, including new subsidence and tilt
      - Expect stabilization over 6-12 months
  - Subsidence of components
    - Revision components should be expected to subside, sometimes > 1 cm for long stem
      - Continue follow-up, watching for stabilization over 6-12 months
  - Evaluate for incorporation of onlay graft
    - Alternatively, watch for cerclage wire fracture and dissociation of graft from host bone
- Dislocation more likely following revision
  - Proper positioning of components may be compromised by bone stock loss
  - Stabilizing soft tissues may not be intact

CT Findings

- Preop: Surgical planning &/or follow-up
  - CT with reformats in coronal and sagittal planes to evaluate location and extent of lytic lesions
    - Greater sensitivity than radiograph for presence and amount of bone loss
  - Metal artifact-reduction techniques
    - Soft tissue image acquisition
    - ↑ kVp (140 kVp) and mAs (350-450 if 1 THA, 450-600 if bilateral)
    - Narrowed collimation
    - ↓ pitch (< 0.3)
    - Reconstruct with 1-mm section width with 0.5-mm reconstruction increment

DIFFERENTIAL DIAGNOSIS

Revision Failure vs. Expected Settling

- Revisions not judged by same strict criteria as 1st-time arthroplasty
- Stabilization takes longer to achieve; change in position of components expected

CLINICAL ISSUES

Natural History & Prognosis

- Prosthesis or liner dislocation in 12% of THA revisions
- Postoperative infections in 1-14%

SELECTED REFERENCES

1. Williams D et al: Revision arthroplasty: an update. Skeletal Radiol. 38(11):1031-6, 2009

(Left) *AP radiograph shows an acetabular revision component, normally sized and placed. There is a large defect within the superior acetabulum that has been filled with nonstructural bone graft* ➡. **(Right)** *AP radiograph of the same patient several months later shows that the nonstructural bone graft has matured and consolidated* ➡. *Although it would not be surprising to find that it had compressed, in this case it has not done so. There is no change in alignment of the cup over this time period; it is stable.*

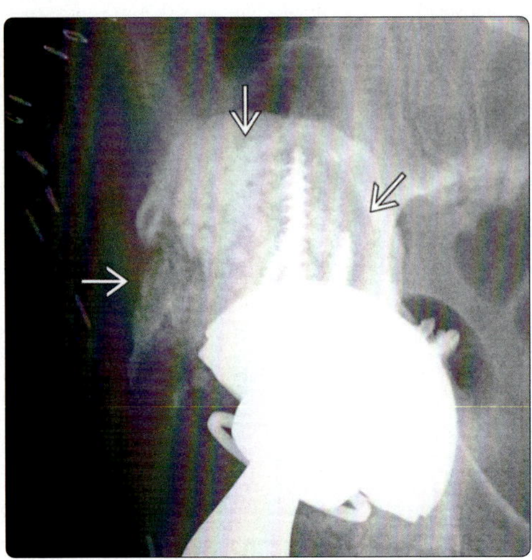

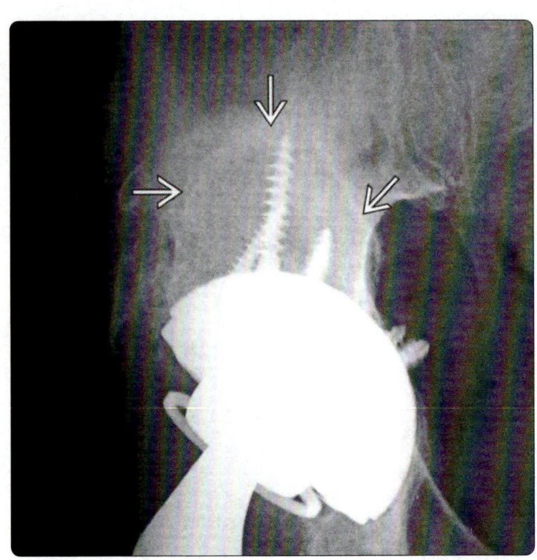

(Left) *Coronal bone CT shows a Girdlestone anatomy of the hip* ➡ *following explant of a loose prosthesis. The CT readily shows residual diaphyseal bone cement* ➡, *fractured and left during prosthesis removal. This will need to be removed prior to revision placement.* **(Right)** *AP radiograph shows a long-stem revision. There is a cortical lucency* ➡ *that is iatrogenic; a cortical window was cut in the diaphysis to extract a piece of fractured cement prior to revision placement. This should not be mistaken for fracture.*

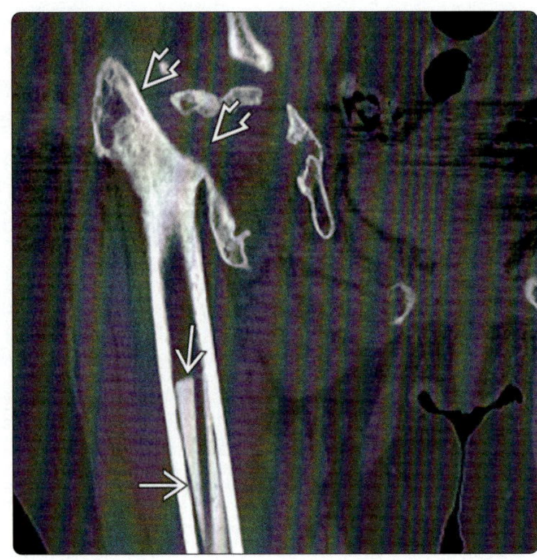

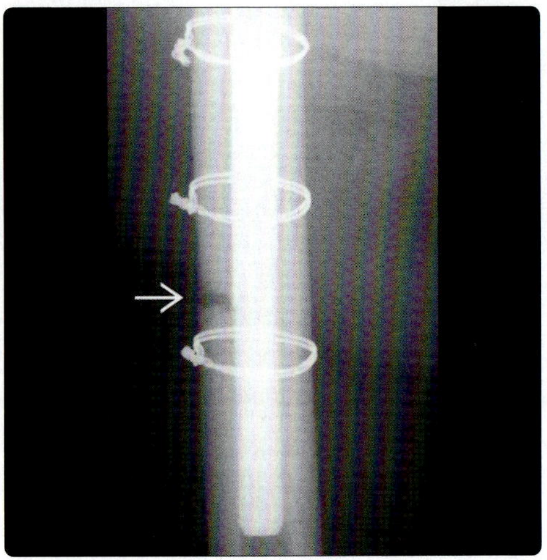

(Left) *Lateral radiograph shows the middiaphysis of the femur following revision arthroplasty surgery. The component has a clothespin design, commonly used in long stems. It has fractured through the anterior cortex* ➡ *of the anteriorly bowed femur. The fracture was heard intraoperatively; note cerclage wiring* ➡. **(Right)** *AP radiograph shows femoral onlay graft* ➡ *placed across a large lateral cortical defect. The graft is secured by cerclage wires and cables. It will be followed until it incorporates.*

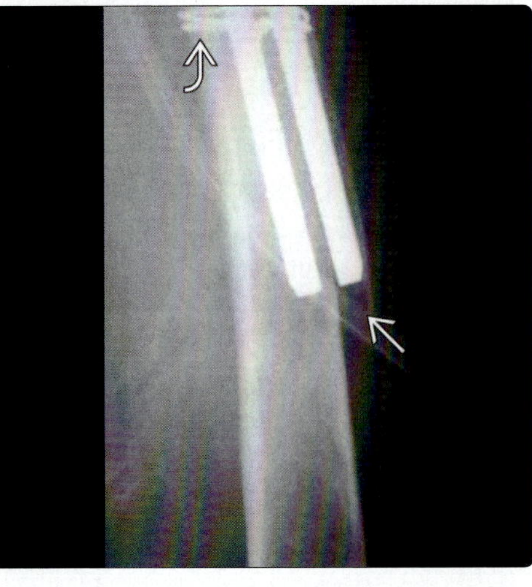

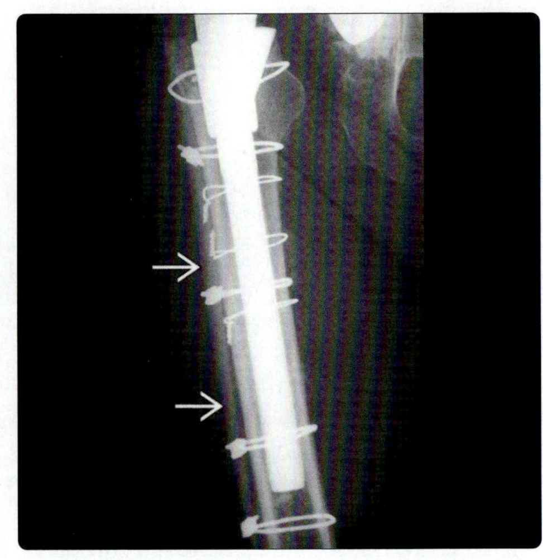

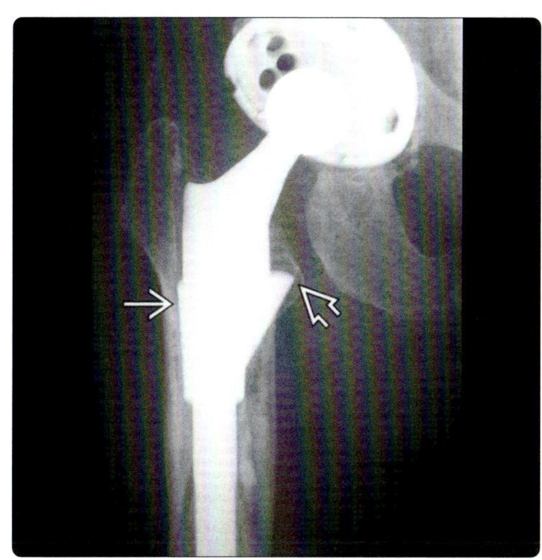

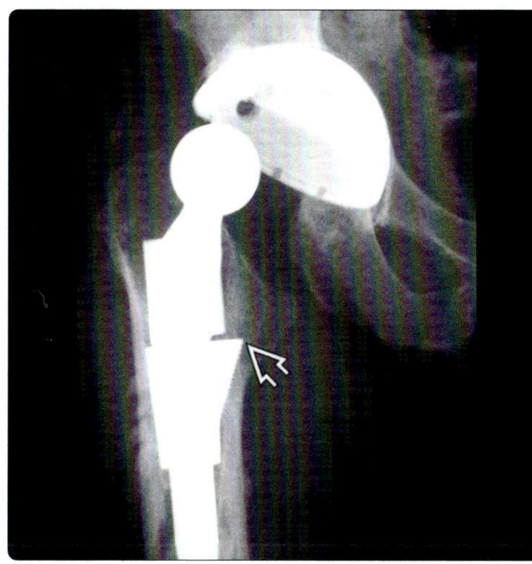

(Left) *AP radiograph shows a revision THA utilizing a SROM component ➡ to fill a large defect in the metaphysis. The component will be followed for stability. Use the relationship of the SROM to the lesser trochanter ➡ as a landmark.* **(Right)** *AP radiograph of the same patient 4 months later shows that the femoral component has subsided inferiorly substantially. Note the SROM ➡ relative to the lesser trochanter; the subsidence is so great that the femoral head is torqued out of the cup, resulting in dislocation.*

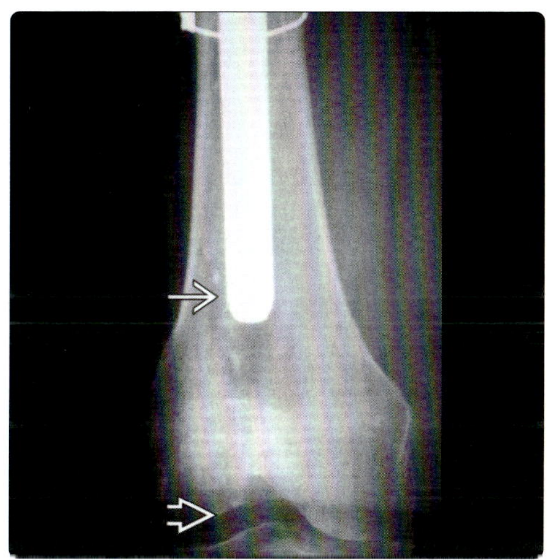

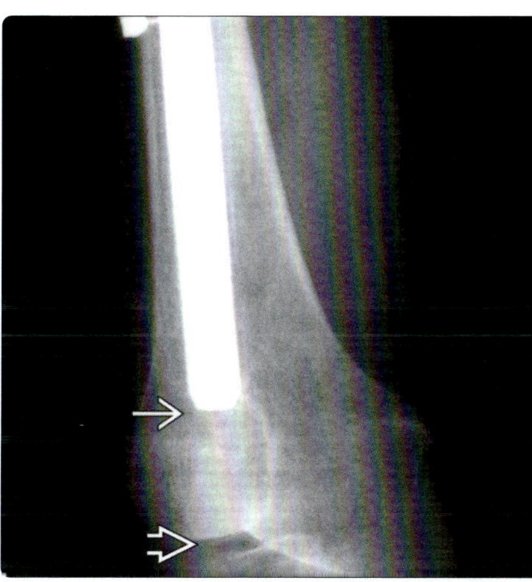

(Left) *AP radiograph shows a long-stem femoral component revision. Note the distance from the tip of the stem ➡ to the joint line ➡; this can be used as a landmark to follow any subsidence.* **(Right)** *AP radiograph of the same patient several months later shows the tip of the stem ➡ to be much closer to the joint line ➡. This shows substantial subsidence but may yet stabilize. If stabilization does not occur over 6-12 months, the revision will be considered loose.*

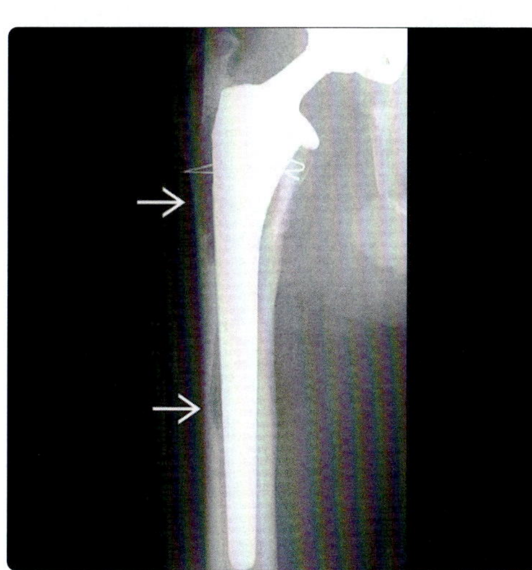

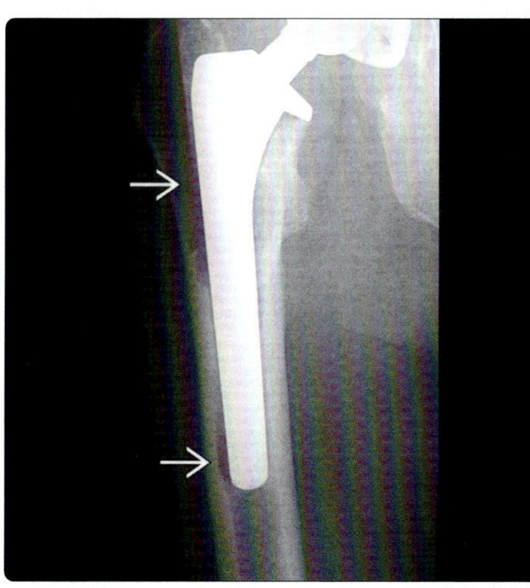

(Left) *AP radiograph of a slightly long-stem revision arthroplasty shows lucency along much of the bone-component interface ➡. This is concerning for either loosening, infection, or particle disease. However, comparison with preoperative radiograph should be made.* **(Right)** *AP radiograph of the same patient prior to revision shows the same lucencies ➡. This proves that they arose from the original failed prosthesis and are simply residua seen on the current exam. There is no evidence of revision failure.*

Knee Implant

KEY FACTS

TERMINOLOGY

- Total knee arthroplasty: Replacement of femoral, tibial, and patellar articular surfaces

IMAGING

- Component size matched to knee
- Initial placement of components
  - Femoral: 5° ± 5° to long axis of femoral axis on lateral
  - Femoral: 4-7° valgus on AP
  - Tibial: 90° ± 5° to long axis of tibial shaft on AP
  - Tibial: Component plus polyethylene → 10° posterior tilt
  - Rotational malalignment
    - Radiograph only shows significant malalignment; CT improves accuracy
- Complications, other than malalignment
  - Patellar button dislocation from cement or metal backing
  - Tibial polyethylene may dislocate from metal tray
  - Stress shielding: Occurs in anterior and mid femoral metaphysis, seen on lateral radiograph
    - Does not predict component failure
  - Loosening: Change in position (tilt or subsidence)
    - Patellar button usually subsides superiorly
    - Tibial component subsides inferiorly, usually with medial trabecular compression
  - Infection
    - Rare radiographic findings of serpiginous destruction
    - MR: Lamellated hyperintense synovitis differentiates infectious from noninfectious synovitis

DIAGNOSTIC CHECKLIST

- Keep in mind shape of polyethylene components; lucency of this shape in wrong location is hint of dislocation
- Periprosthetic fractures are easily missed; include them in your search pattern
  - Increased risk for periprosthetic fracture with osteoporosis &/or tibial tubercle transfer

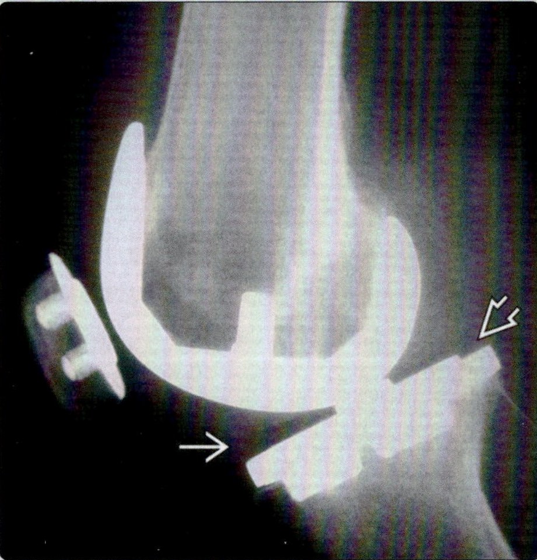

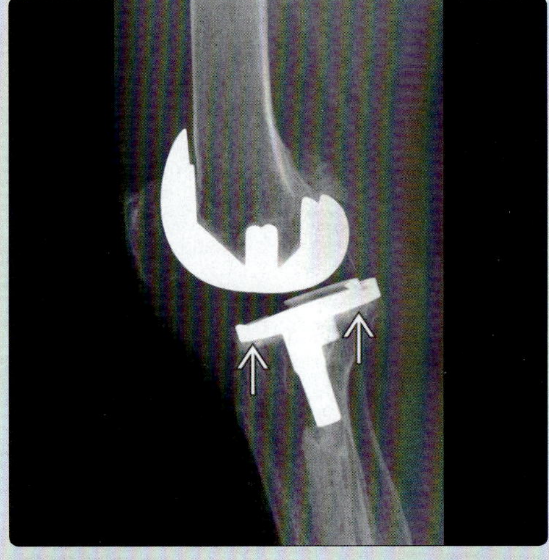

(Left) *Lateral radiograph shows a normal total knee arthroplasty (TKA). The sizing of the components is correct. Alignment is normal. Note the slight posterior tilt of the tibial component as well as the differential thickness of the anterior polyethylene ➡ compared with posterior ➡.* **(Right)** *Lateral radiograph shows anterior rather than posterior tilt of the tibial component ➡. The normal tibial plateau has a posterior tilt of approximately 7°, and the arthroplasty should approximate this angulation.*

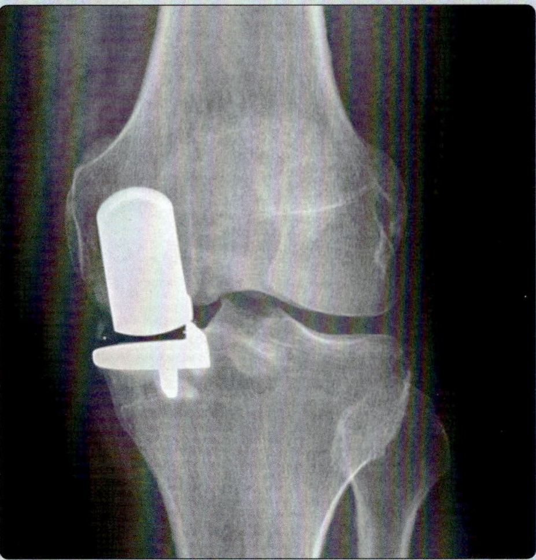

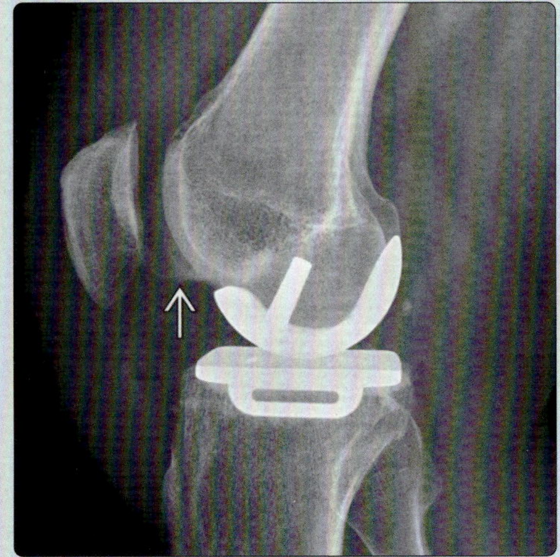

(Left) *AP radiograph shows a normal unicondylar knee arthroplasty. These components may be chosen when there is no significant arthritis in the remaining 2 compartments. Unicondylar arthroplasties are not used in patients with inflammatory arthritis.* **(Right)** *Lateral radiograph in the same patient shows the femoral implant is placed on the mid and posterior weight-bearing portions of the condyle; there is a notch formed in the anterior portion of the condyle ➡ to reduce the likelihood of patellar impingement.*

TERMINOLOGY

Definitions

- Total knee arthroplasty (TKA): Replacement of femoral, tibial, and patellar articular surfaces
  - Nonconstrained components
    - Generally, posterior cruciate ligament is retained
    - Other soft tissues, including collateral ligaments, provide stability
    - Concave polyethylene adds some constraint
  - Semiconstrained components
    - Usually long-stemmed
    - Peg extends from femoral side into central cylinder on tibial side; allows some rotation
      - Do not misinterpret lucency around peg as loosening of component
- Single compartment (unicompartmental) implant: Medial, lateral, or patellofemoral
  - Considered when only single compartment involved with significant osteoarthritis
  - Not used if underlying process is inflammatory

IMAGING

Radiographic Findings

- Component size matched to knee
  - Oversized femoral component seen as gap between anterior cortex and flange
    - Blocks full range of motion
  - Undersized femoral component → notching of anterior femoral cortex
    - At risk for fracture
  - Oversized tibial component → overhanging edge
    - Irritates adjacent tendons and ligaments
  - Undersized tibial component
    - Subsidence into tibia, eventual loosening
- Initial placement of components
  - Femoral component
    - 5° ± 5° to long axis of femoral axis on lateral
    - 4-7° valgus on AP
  - Tibial component
    - 90° ± 5° to long axis of tibial shaft on AP
    - Component plus polyethylene → 10° posterior tilt
      - Metal component may not appear tilted; made up by differential thickness of polyethylene
      - If no posterior tilt, blocks full flexion
  - Rotational malalignment
    - External rotation of tibial component → patellar dislocation, eccentric wear
- Implant fracture
  - Fracture of metallic backing ring, dissociates from patella
    - Indicates likely polyethylene fracture or dislocation
    - Fragments may line synovium or joint components: Metallosis
- Dislocation
  - Patellar button dislocated from cement or metal backing
    - Seen as convex lucency offset from patella
    - Patellar button may take ring or partial ring of metallic backing material with it
  - Tibial polyethylene may dislocate from metal tray
    - Displaces into joint, locking it
- Stress shielding
  - Occurs in anterior and mid femoral metaphysis, seen on lateral radiograph
    - Bone resorption and lucency at this site
    - Streaming ↑ bone density, extends from posterior femoral peg to posterior metaphyseal cortex
- Loosening
  - Change in position (tilt or subsidence)
    - Patellar button usually subsides superiorly
    - Tibial component subsides inferiorly, usually with medial compression
  - ≥ 2-mm lucency at bone-cement or bone-component interface
- Component wear
  - Asymmetric width of tibial polyethylene, medial compared with lateral (asymmetry normally expected anterior vs. posterior)
- Particle disease
  - Morphology
    - Focal lytic bone destruction; may mimic tumor
    - May extend along screw, with bone destruction appearing more elongated
    - Soft tissue mass or bursal collection
  - Search for particle source to establish diagnosis
    - Polyethylene dislocation or wear
    - Metallosis (bead shedding or other metal debris)
- Periprosthetic fracture
  - Most frequent fracture: Patella (usually transverse)
    - Thin bone, made even thinner and devascularized by osteotomy for patellar button
  - Proximal tibial metaphyseal fracture
    - Initial buckle, followed by linear sclerosis; fracture risk increased with prior tibial tubercle transfer

CT Findings

- Evaluation of rotational malalignment
- Evaluation of periprosthetic loosening, osteolysis, fracture
  - Presence and extent of osteolysis better evaluated by CT than radiograph
  - Used to evaluate location of lysis and adequacy of bone stock prior to revision

MR Findings

- Evaluation of soft tissue or bursal mass (particle disease)
  - T1WI: ↓ regions of synovitis and lysis in bone
  - STIR: ↑ SI synovitis, mass, bursal, bone lesions
- Differentiating infectious from noninfectious synovitis
  - Lamellated pattern of hyperintense synovitis has high sensitivity and specificity for infection

CLINICAL ISSUES

Natural History & Prognosis

- Revision-free survival of modern TKAs: 95%

SELECTED REFERENCES

1. Helito CP et al: Severe metallosis following total knee arthroplasty: a case report and review of radiographic signs. Skeletal Radiol. 43(8):1169-73, 2014
2. Plodkowski AJ et al: Lamellated hyperintense synovitis: potential MR imaging sign of an infected knee arthroplasty. Radiology. 266(1):256-60, 2013

(Left) *Lateral radiograph shows an unstable TKA. This prosthesis spares the posterior cruciate ligament (PCL), but PCL must be ruptured in this case.* **(Right)** *Lateral radiograph shows typical stress shielding, considered normal. There is resorption of bone in the anterior and mid femoral metaphysis ➡, while new bone is laid down posteriorly, extending from the peg to the posterior cortex ➡. There is no associated pain or risk of failure. The lucency must not be misinterpreted as osteolysis.*

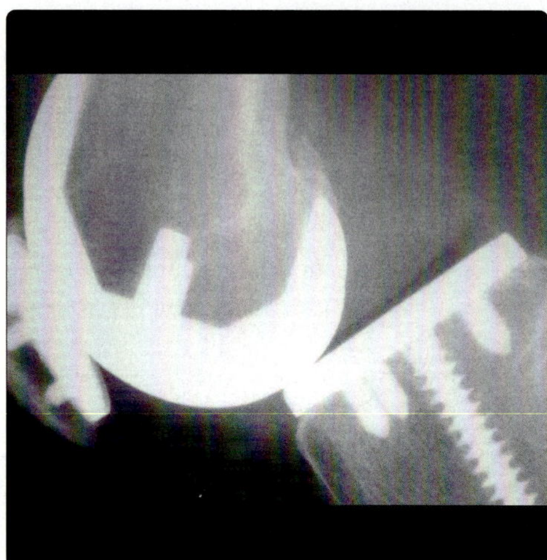

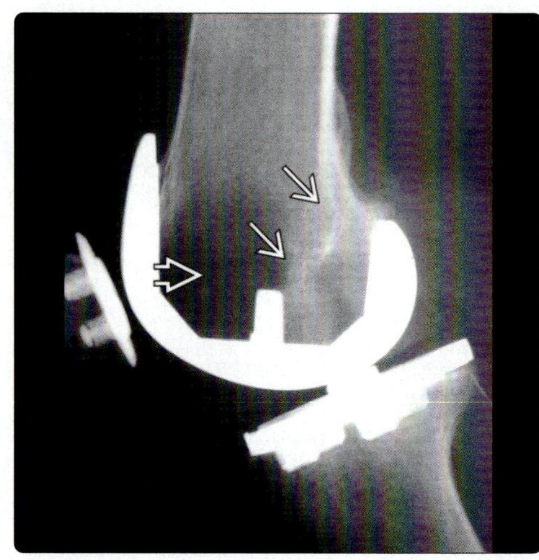

(Left) *AP radiograph shows a thin lucency at the bone-component interface ➡. This does not qualify as loosening but should be watched for progression.* **(Right)** *AP radiograph shows a cemented TKA that is grossly loose. There is abnormal tilt and a wide bone-cement lucency ➡. There is bead shedding ➡ as well. Note the wide polyethylene compared with that on the previous image; different widths are chosen based on stability requirements.*

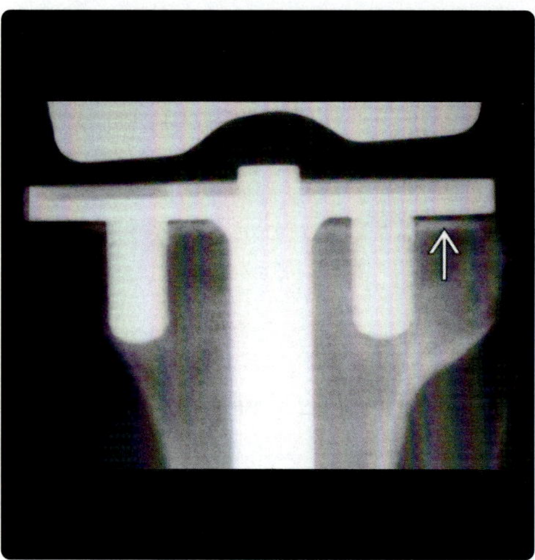

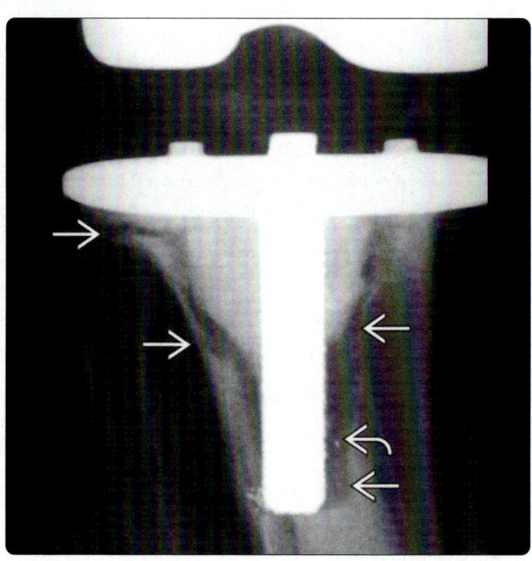

(Left) *Lateral radiograph shows a failed semiconstrained prosthesis. There is a loose screw ➡. More importantly, the constraining peg ➡ has dislocated, along with the plate ➡ by which it attaches to the tibial tray. This plate also attached to the tibial polyethylene, which has dislocated anteromedially into the soft tissues.* **(Right)** *AP radiograph obtained 4 months following TKA placement shows serpiginous osseous destruction ➡ not present on index postoperative exam. This represents infection.*

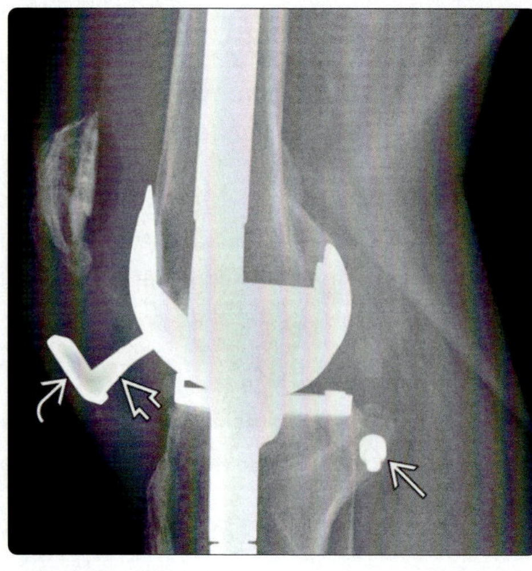

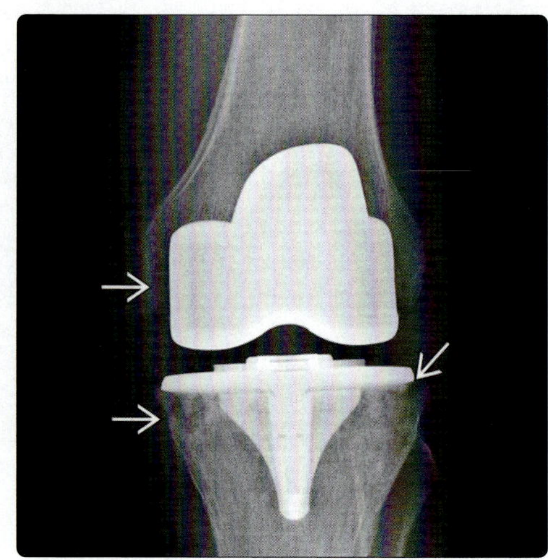

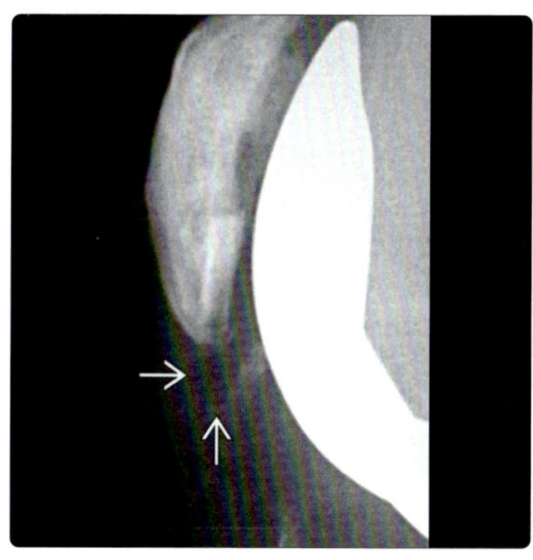

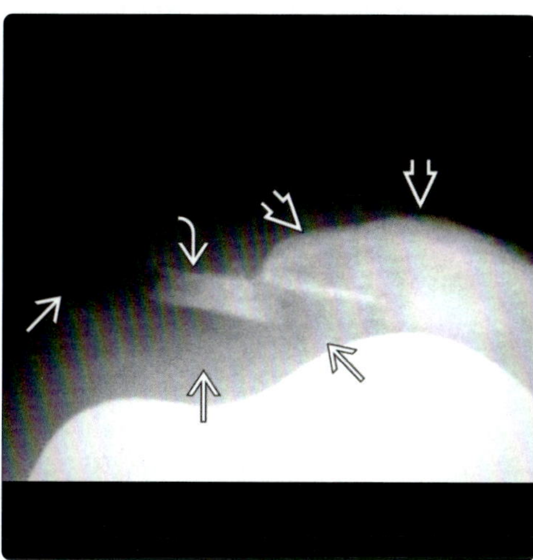

(Left) *Lateral radiograph shows the lucent patellar button to be dissociated from the patella and inferiorly displaced ➡. This abnormality is easily missed and depends on noting a subtle lucency in an abnormal location.* **(Right)** *Axial radiograph of the patellofemoral joint in the same patient shows that the entire patellar button is dislocated ➡ relative to the patella ➡. The cement ➡ has sheared off the bone, making visualization of the lucent patellar button easier.*

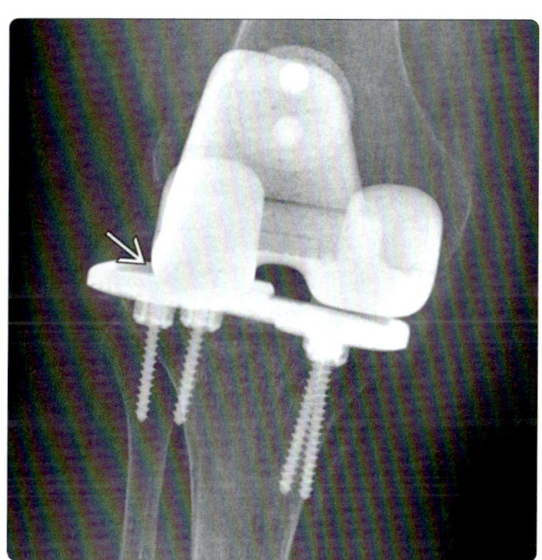

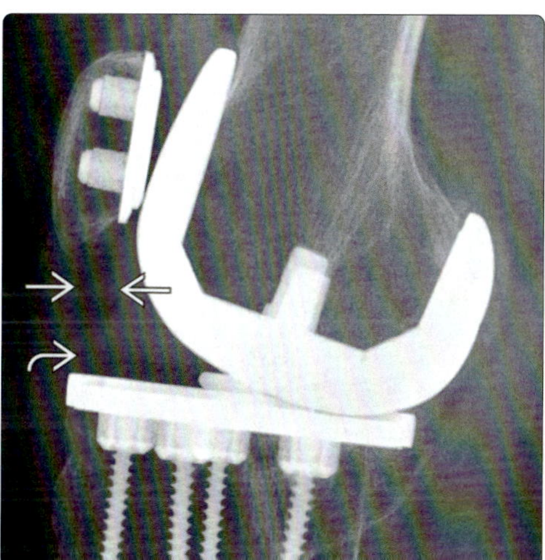

(Left) *AP radiograph shows significant offset and rotation of the tibia relative to the femur. This could represent soft tissue deficiency. However, there is no space for polyethylene on the tibial tray ➡. This should raise the question of polyethylene dislocation.* **(Right)** *Lateral radiograph in the same patient shows a fractured fragment of the lucent polyethylene ➡ with some residual polyethylene on the tibial tray ➡. The knee is locked in this abnormal position by the dislocated fragment.*

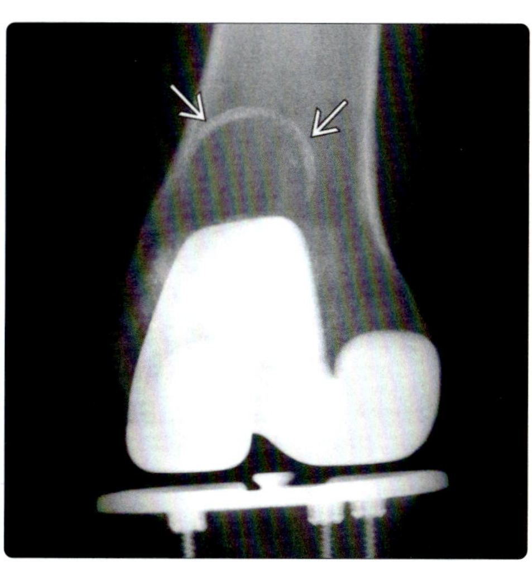

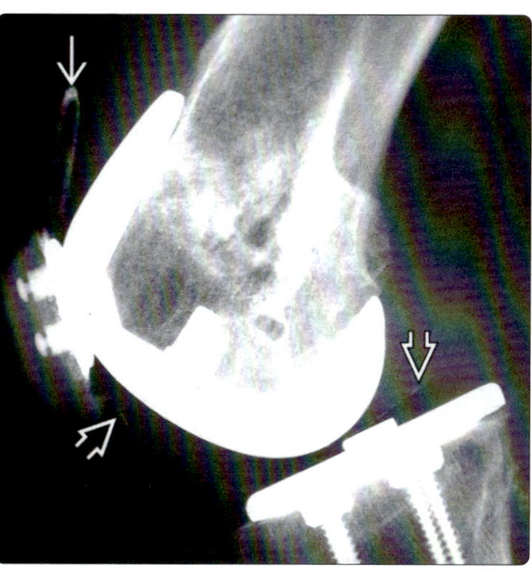

(Left) *AP radiograph shows a rounded metallic density ➡ located superior to the patella, representing dissociation of the metal backing from the patellar button.* **(Right)** *Lateral radiograph in the same patient confirms the superior displacement of the dissociated backing ➡. There are 2 areas of faint deposition of metal along the synovium anteriorly and along the tibial polyethylene ➡. The patellar button will go on to fail further; the metallosis will lead to a significant synovitis.*

(Left) *AP radiograph shows a lytic lesion in the subimplant bone ➡. Considerations include preexisting subchondral cyst or lytic lesion, such as metastasis, but in this case it is due to particle disease. The source of the particles are worn polyethylene; note the differential thickness ➡.* **(Right)** *AP radiograph shows massive osteolysis occurring around the medial tibial screw in this TKA ➡. Additionally, there is a subtle decrease in height of the polyethylene on the tibial tray ➡, indicating wear.*

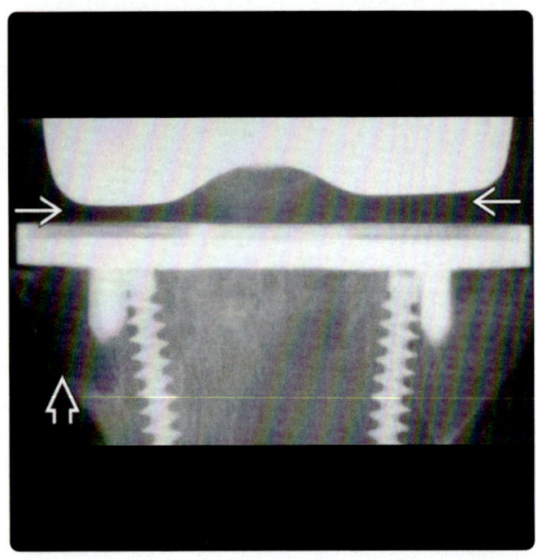

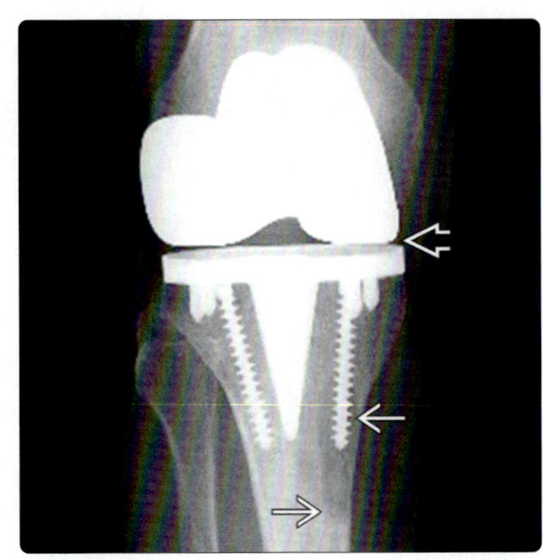

(Left) *Coronal CT in the same patient is obtained for further evaluation. It shows the degree of osteolysis surrounding the medial screw ➡. The lysis is much more extensive than would be expected based only on the radiograph. Note the relationship to the tibial screw; the particles are forced down along the screw track.* **(Right)** *Sagittal bone CT in the same patient shows a pathologic fracture at the posterior cortex along with a small amount of fracture callus ➡, indicating subacuity.*

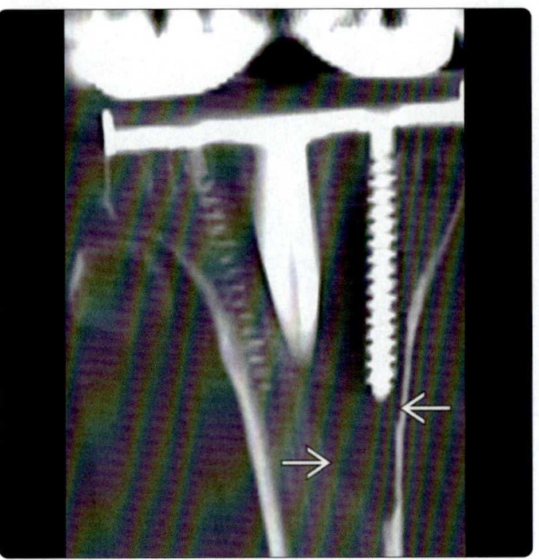

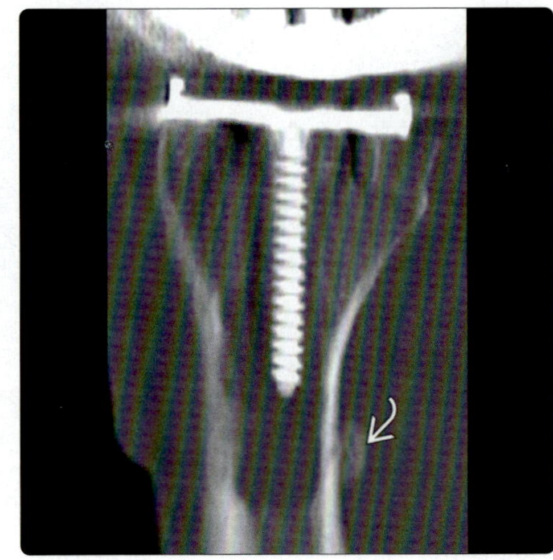

(Left) *AP radiograph demonstrates a TKA and large adjacent soft tissue mass ➡. The TKA shows mild thinning of the medial polyethylene ➡.* **(Right)** *Axial NECT in the same patient shows the mass ➡ along with a large lytic osseous lesion ➡. The femoral component is neutral relative to the surgical epicondyle axis, but the tibial component was externally rotated (not shown). Thus, particle sources may arise from either patellar or tibial polyethylene. The mass was necrotic granulomatous tissue, proven by biopsy.*

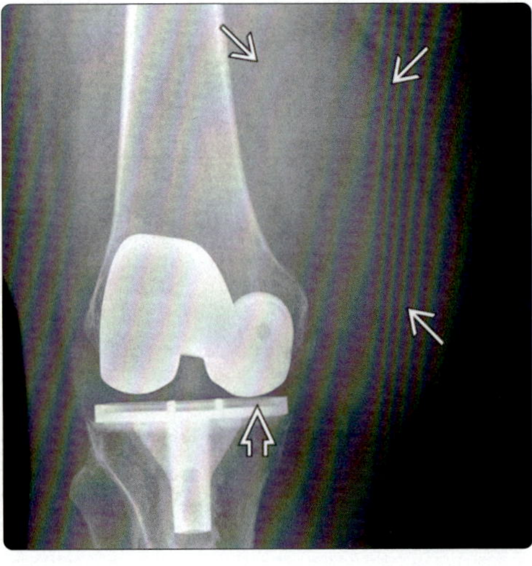

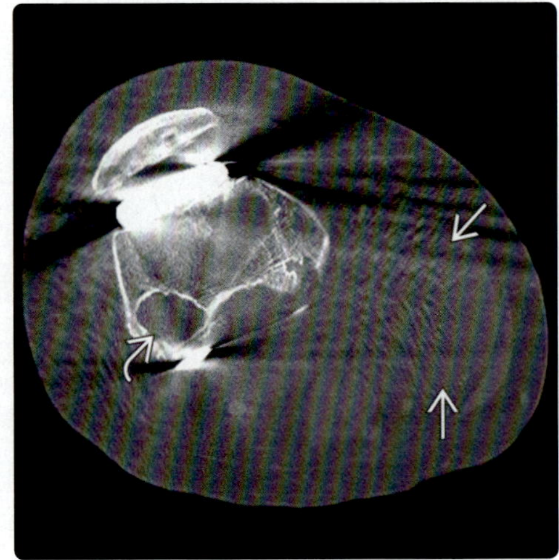

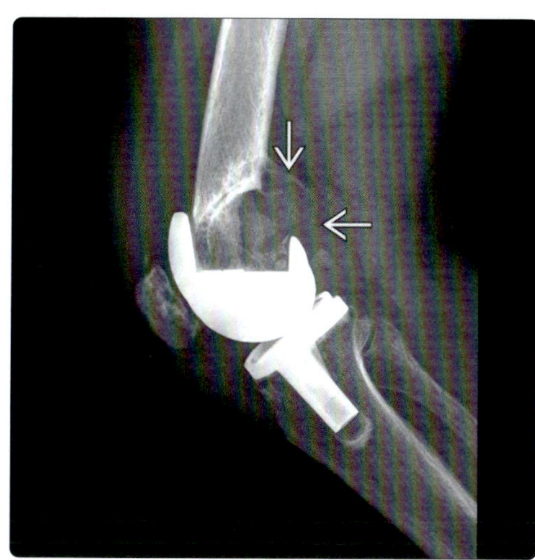

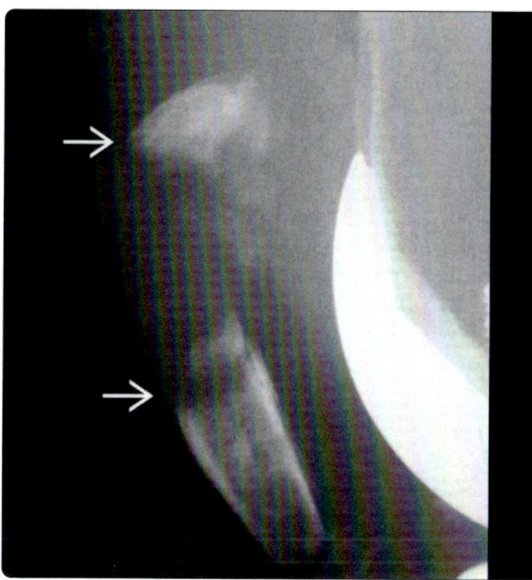

(Left) *Lateral radiograph shows a large, expansile mass that has destroyed the majority of the posterior distal left femur ➡. The smooth, sclerotic border and marginal heterotopic ossification suggest that this is a slowly progressive process. Biopsy confirmed particle disease.* **(Right)** *Lateral radiograph shows a displaced patellar fracture ➡ following placement of TKA. The patella is at risk due to the osteotomy for placement of the patellar button, which causes devascularization and thinning of the bone.*

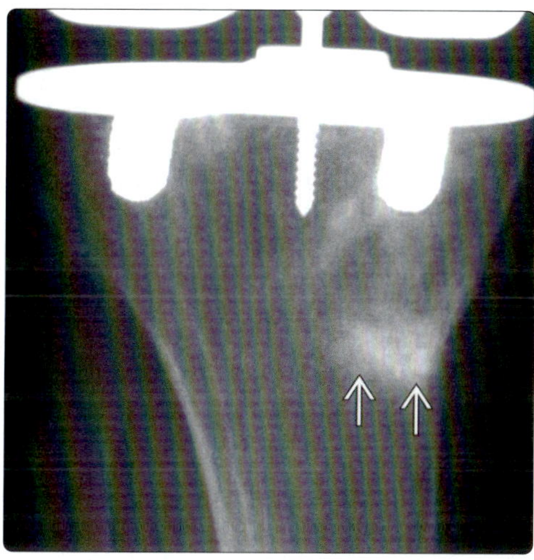

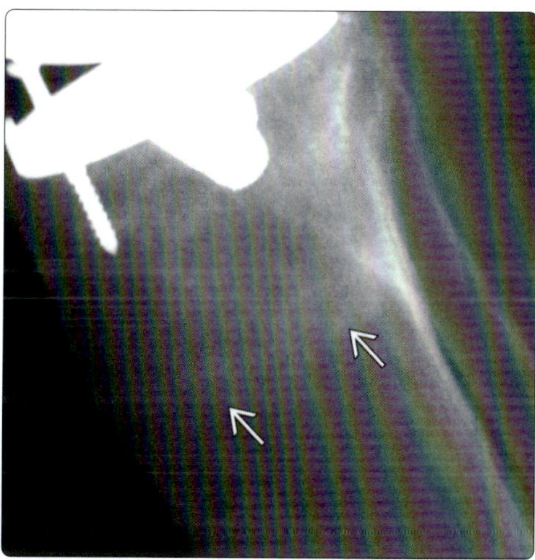

(Left) *AP radiograph shows TKA in osteoporotic bone. There is linear sclerosis ➡ in the tibial metaphysis, which is diagnostic of an insufficiency fracture.* **(Right)** *Lateral radiograph confirms the linear nature of the sclerosis ➡. Periprosthetic fractures are difficult to diagnose in the acute situation but should be sought and diagnosed once this impaction and healing sclerosis is demonstrated. Such fractures occur following TKA placement, particularly when the bone is osteoporotic and the patient increases activity.*

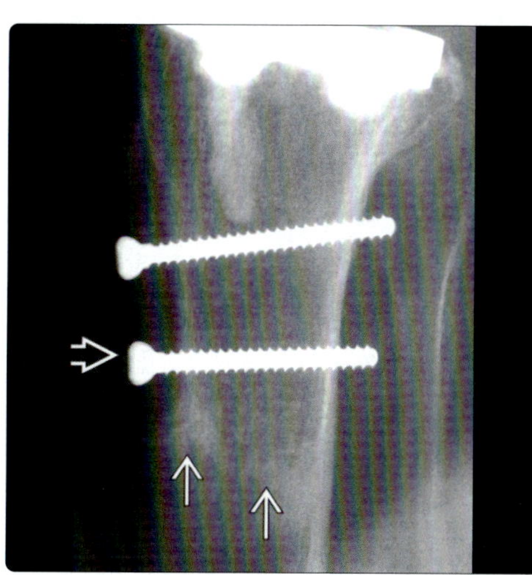

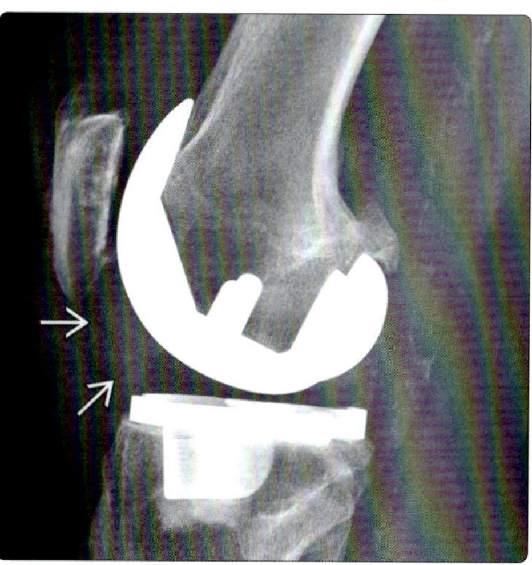

(Left) *Lateral radiograph shows a TKA but also shows a tibial tubercle transfer ➡. Additionally, there is linear sclerosis seen just distal to the transferred tubercle ➡. This represents a periprosthetic insufficiency fracture. There is added risk for development of a fracture when the patient has also had a tibial tubercle transfer, as in this case.* **(Right)** *Lateral radiograph of a patient with TKA shows intraarticular density ➡, which distorts the Hoffa fat pad. This proved to be arthrofibrosis.*

KEY FACTS

TERMINOLOGY

- Total shoulder arthroplasty (TSA): Implant replaces both glenoid and humeral head
- Shoulder hemiarthroplasty: Implant replaces only humeral head, native glenoid retained
- Reverse shoulder arthroplasty (RSA): Implant replaces both glenoid and humeral head but reverses normal ball-and-socket relationship
  - Used in patients with irreparable rotator cuff tear and secondary arthropathy, pain, and pseudoparalysis (inability to lift arm above 90°)
  - Reversing glenoid and head components changes center of rotation; allows greater control of shoulder motion by deltoid, especially anterior and posterior portions

IMAGING

- Initial placement and appearance in TSA
  - Glenoid component placed to replicate native glenoid, with slight anterior and inferior tilt
- Initial placement and appearance in RSA
  - Craniocaudad placement of metaglene and attached glenosphere is critical
  - Line starting at inferior edge of glenosphere must continue uninterrupted along line of axillary border of scapula
  - Neutral to inferior tilt of glenosphere is desirable
- Complications of shoulder arthroplasty
  - Glenoid component may dislocate from scapular neck in TSA; visualized by cement or lucent polyethylene in wrong location
  - Inferior glenoid &/or metaglene at risk for fracture or loosening, respectively, in RSA with substantial scapular notching on axillary border
  - Acromial stress fracture in RSA
    - Inferomedial displacement of center of rotation → ↑ stress on acromion by deltoid → stress fracture
  - Loosening: Lucency ≥ 2 mm at bone-component or bone-cement interface of either component

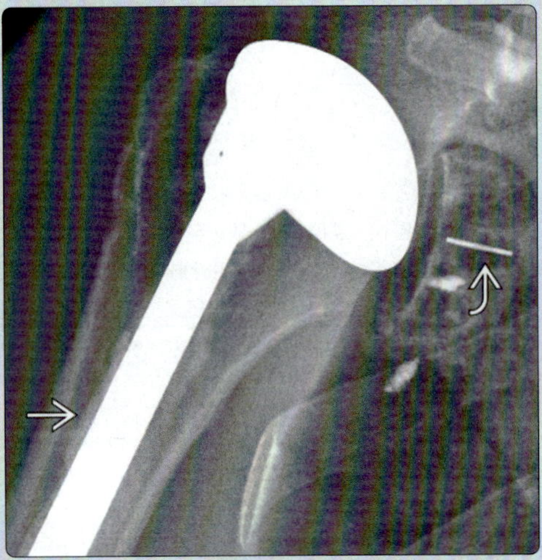

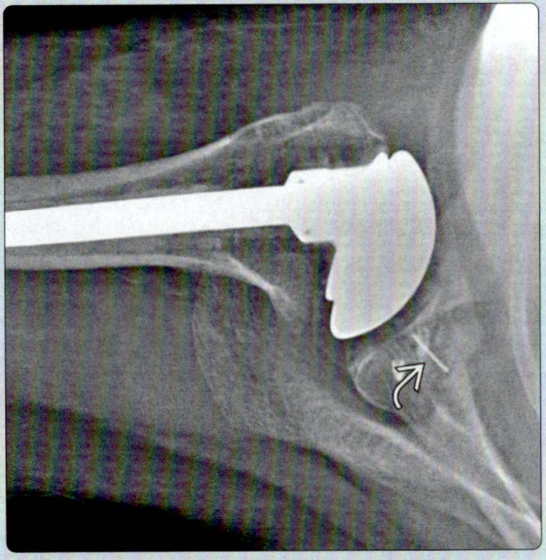

(Left) *AP radiograph shows a total shoulder arthroplasty (TSA) with components in appropriate position. There are 2 suture anchors (1 that has backed out of the bone) from prior Bankart repair. Polyethylene glenoid component is cemented; a marker wire is present within the peg ➲. Humeral component is cemented ➲; head is slightly elevated, but alignment is within acceptable limits.* **(Right)** *Axillary lateral, same patient, shows the wire marker in the central peg ➲ of the polyethylene glenoid. The head articulates normally.*

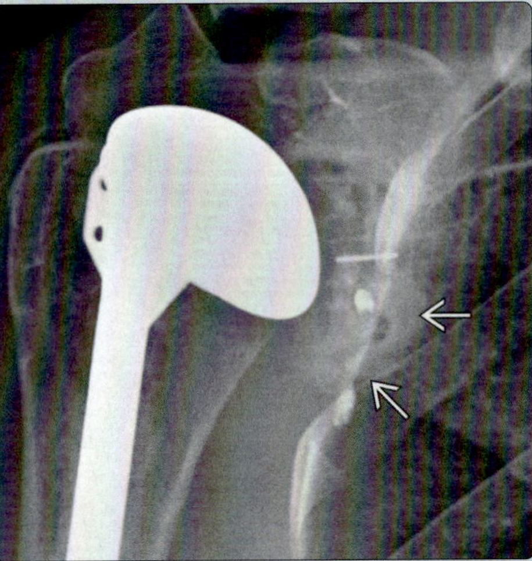

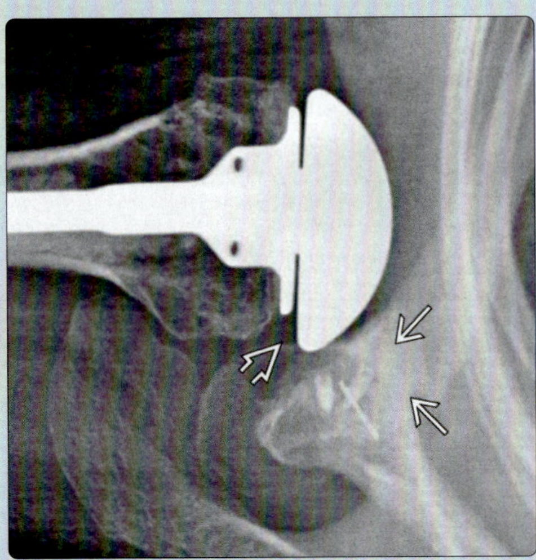

(Left) *AP radiograph 9 months later in the same patient shows sclerosis in the inferior glenoid ➲, which was not present postoperatively. The glenoid is oriented differently, with an inferior tilt, compared with the previous image.* **(Right)** *Axillary lateral in the same patient shows that the anterior glenoid was impacted ➲; the glenoid arthroplasty has displaced anteriorly and tilted compared to the prior image, indicating loosening. The humeral prosthesis is subluxated anteriorly ➲. Comparison images are crucial for diagnosis of failure.*

TERMINOLOGY

Definitions

- Total shoulder arthroplasty (TSA): Implant replaces both glenoid and humeral head
  - Used for several decades to replace arthritic shoulders
  - Humeral component is metal, with ball at end to act as humeral head
    - Either cemented or cementless
  - Glenoid component may be metal backed with polyethylene insert or may be entirely polyethylene (often containing metal markers)
    - Either cemented (cement surrounds flat backing and its pegs) or cementless (bone ingrowth, stabilized by pegs and cancellous screws)
- Shoulder hemiarthroplasty: Implant replaces only humeral head, native glenoid retained
  - Used for several decades, though infrequently
    - Primarily used for humeral head damage (osteonecrosis, severely comminuted fracture) without arthritic change
  - Stem and humeral head are metal
    - Either cemented or cementless
- Reverse shoulder arthroplasty (RSA): Implant replaces both glenoid and humeral head but reverses normal ball-and-socket relationship
  - Used in patients with irreparable rotator cuff tear and secondary arthropathy, pain, and pseudoparalysis (inability to lift arm above 90°)
  - Reversing glenoid and head components changes center of rotation
    - Arm lowered (lengthened) and medialized: Moves center of rotation distally and medially
      - Allows greater control of shoulder motion by anterior and posterior deltoid
  - 4 main components: Humeral stem, polyethylene cup, glenosphere (ball), and metaglene (base for glenoid)
    - Humeral stem: Metal, either cemented or cementless, with cup-shaped proximal portion
    - Polyethylene cup: Fits within proximal end of humeral component, deepening cup
    - Glenosphere: Metal ball, attached into metaglene
    - Metaglene: Metal base with flat attachment on glenoid surface, secured by cancellous screws

IMAGING

Radiographic Findings

- Initial placement and appearance
  - Humeral stem placement in all types of shoulder implants: Centered in proximal shaft
  - TSA
    - Glenoid component placed to replicate native glenoid, with slight anterior and inferior tilt
      - Screws/pegs well within scapular neck bone stock
  - RSA
    - Thickness of polyethylene insert may vary, depending on need to treat shoulder laxity
    - Correct craniocaudad placement of metaglene and attached glenosphere is critical
      - Line starting at inferior edge of glenosphere must continue uninterrupted along line of axillary border of scapula
      - Usually achieved by placing inferior edge of metaglene and glenosphere either neutral or slightly inferior to native glenoid inferior edge
      - Failure to achieve this placement → humeral component impinging on scapula → scapular notching → failure of glenosphere
    - Neutral to inferior tilt of glenosphere is desirable
      - Superior tilt of glenosphere results in humeral impingement on axillary border of scapula → scapular notching and failure
    - Anterior and superior glenoid often resorbed or deficient due to underlying arthritic process
      - May supplement by glenoid bone graft or more inferior placement of glenosphere
- Dislocation
  - Dislocation of humeral head from glenoid
    - May occur in TSA with malposition of glenoid or insufficient soft tissue stabilization
    - Early reports of dislocation in up to 20% of RSA, usually in immediate perioperative period
      - Improved surgical technique: Incidence ↓ to 2%
      - Late dislocations: Associated with soft tissue scarring or heterotopic ossification in axilla
  - Dislocation/separation of implant components (rare)
  - Dislocation or separation of components from bone
    - Glenoid component may dislocate from scapular neck in TSA; visualized by cement or lucent polyethylene in wrong location
- Periprosthetic fracture
  - Humeral shaft at risk for fracture with loose stem
    - Greatest risk at tip of stem
  - Inferior glenoid at risk for fracture in RSA with substantial scapular notching on axillary border (notching reported in 50-96% RSA)
  - Acromial stress fracture in RSA
    - Lengthening of arm results in deltoid lengthening
    - ↑ stress on acromion by deltoid → stress fracture
    - Usually occurs within first 2 weeks; patient feels distinct "pop"
    - May be surprisingly difficult to visualize on radiograph; CT may be required for diagnosis
- Loosening
  - Lucency ≥ 2 mm at bone-component or bone-cement interface of either component
  - Any change in alignment of component
    - Glenoid may show osseous impaction, especially anteriorly or inferiorly to component prior to gross loosening
  - In RSA, scapular notching (along axillary border) is often precursor to metaglene loosening and failure
    - Scapular notching should be evaluated for associated bone stock deficiency or screw loosening and cutout

SELECTED REFERENCES

1. Ha AS et al: Current concepts of shoulder arthroplasty for radiologists: Part 2–Anatomic and reverse total shoulder replacement and nonprosthetic resurfacing. AJR Am J Roentgenol. 199(4):768-76, 2012

(Left) *AP radiograph of a cemented total shoulder appears normal. Note the expected placement of the humeral component without evidence of loosening or other failure.* **(Right)** *Axillary lateral obtained from the same patient shows that the humeral component articulates with bare bone. The glenoid component is dislocated posteriorly from the scapular neck. The dislocated component is seen only as the lucent polyethylene ➔ with cement surrounding its base ➔ and pegs ➔.*

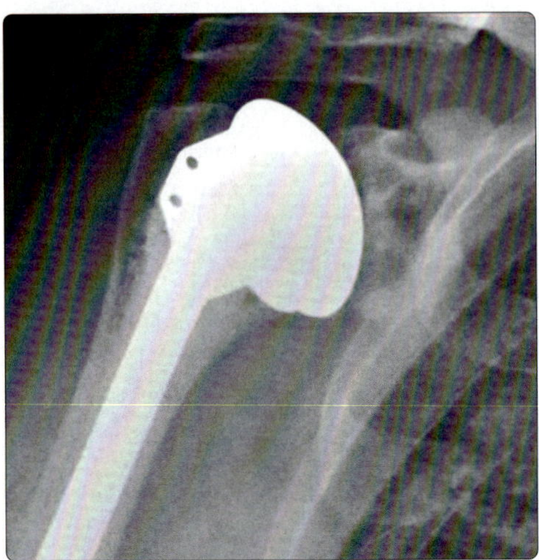

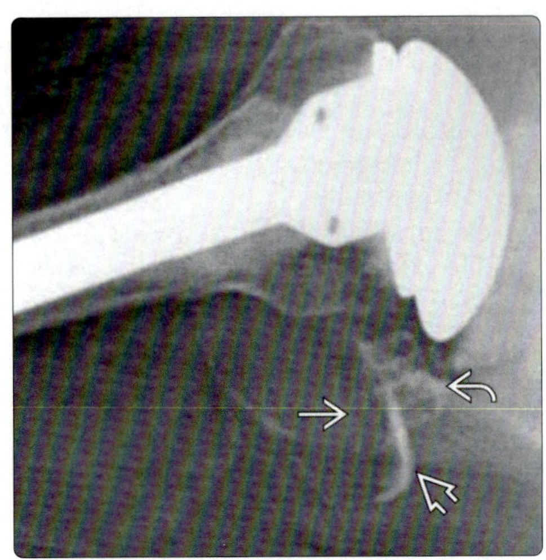

(Left) *Axillary x-ray shows failed glenoid component with lucency at the bone-cement interface ➔ around the glenoid with thinning of the scapular cortex. There is also a fractured piece of cement ➔ located posterior to the polyethylene.* **(Right)** *AP x-ray shows normal placement of an RSA. Metal glenoid base (metaglene) is placed such that a smooth line extends from it down the axillary scapular border ➔. The glenosphere ➔ attaches to the metaglene and articulates with the polyethylene ➔ of the cup.*

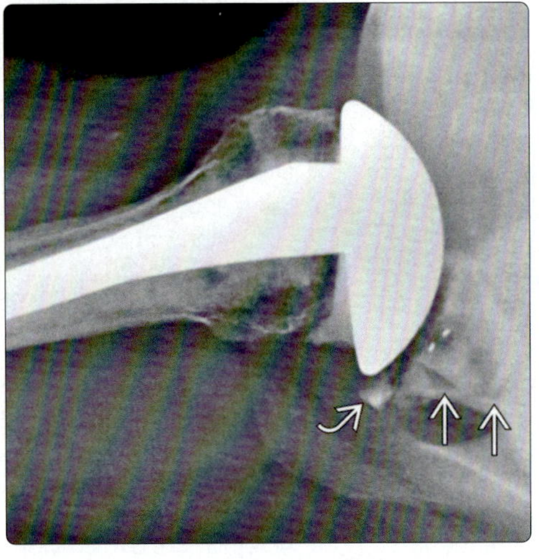

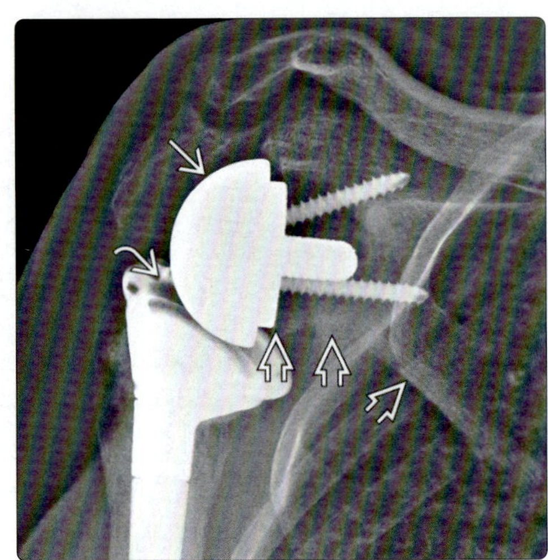

(Left) *Axillary lateral radiograph in the same patient shows the components are placed in appropriate position, with slight anterior tilt of the glenosphere and normal articulation of the ball and cup. There is no suggestion of complication.* **(Right)** *Bone CT 3D reformat of the same patient following arthrogram shows the reason for the patient's pain. There is a stress fracture of the acromion ➔. This patient remembers an audible "pop" and pain. The acromion is at risk for fracture due to arm lengthening with RSA.*

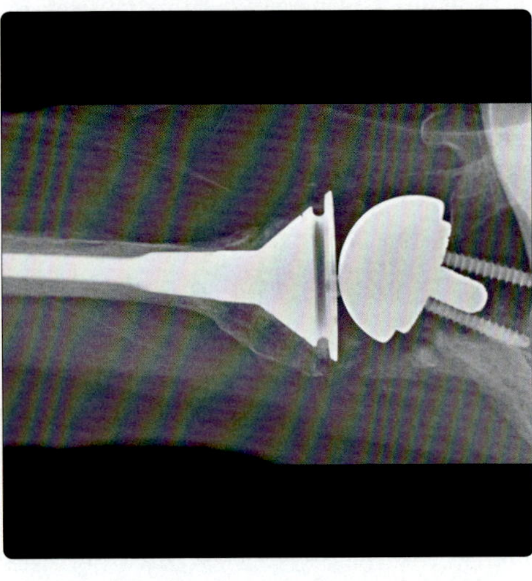

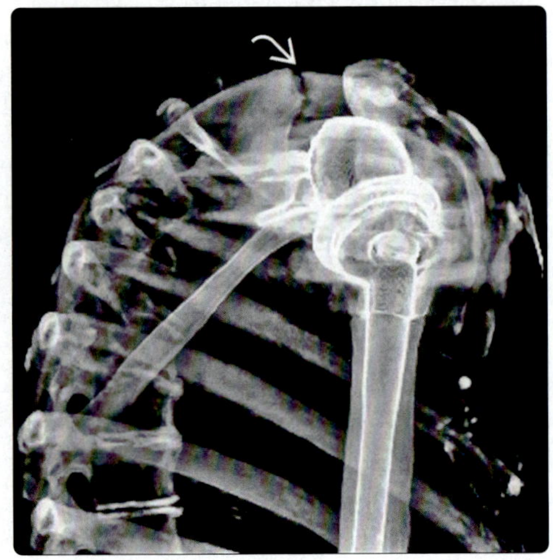

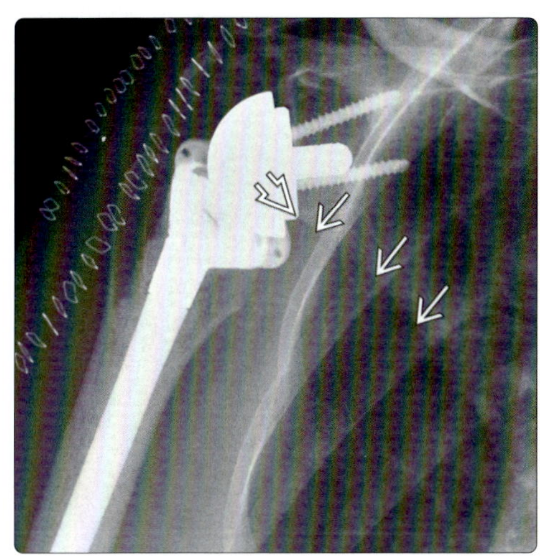

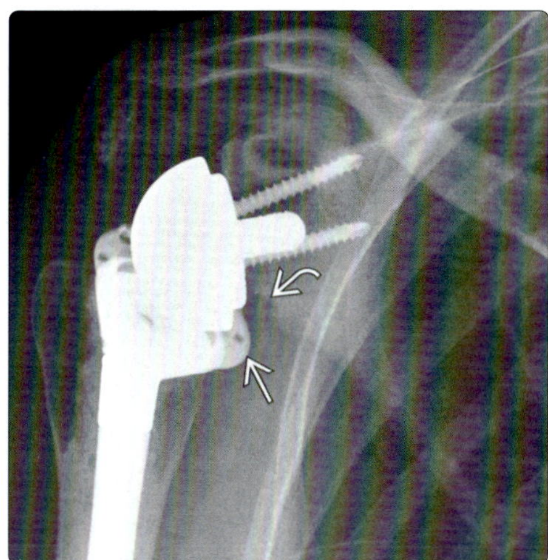

(Left) *AP radiograph shows normal placement of RSA. Note that the inferior edge of the metaglene* ⇨ *aligns with the axillary border of the scapula* ➡. **(Right)** *AP radiograph in the same patient 1 year later shows scapular notching* ↪ *due to impingement by the humeral component* ➡, *despite normal original placement of the arthroplasty. Notching is a common complication of RSA and is associated with metaglene failure (not yet seen in this case).*

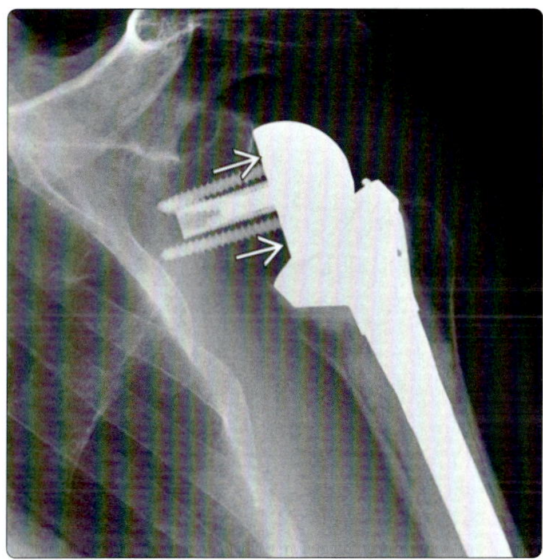

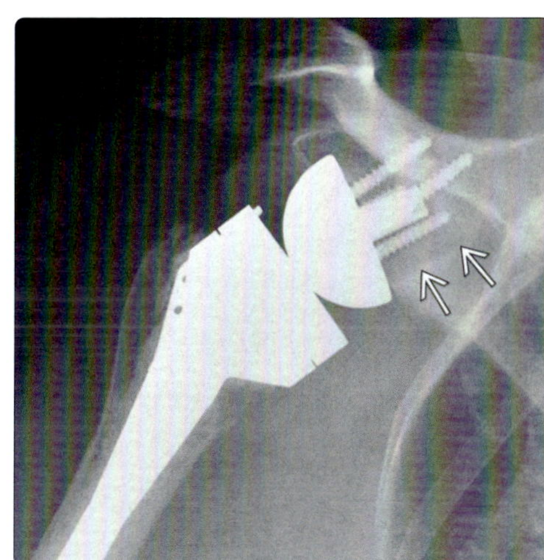

(Left) *AP radiograph shows initial malplacement of the metaglene and glenosphere* ➡. *There should normally be slight inferior and anterior tilt, not a superior tilt as is seen in this case.* **(Right)** *AP radiograph in a different patient shows wide lucency* ➡ *within the glenoid surrounding the peg and screws, indicating loosening.*

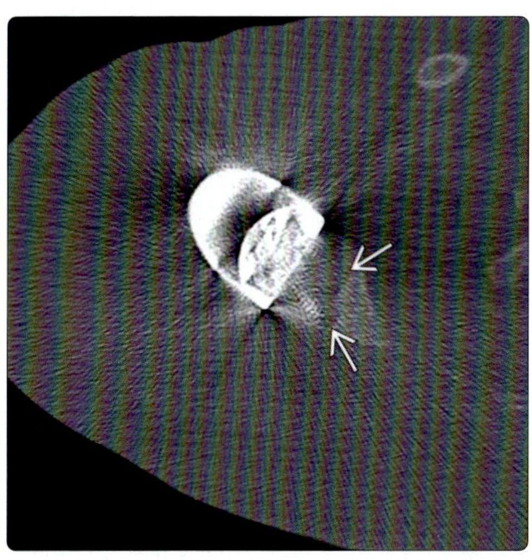

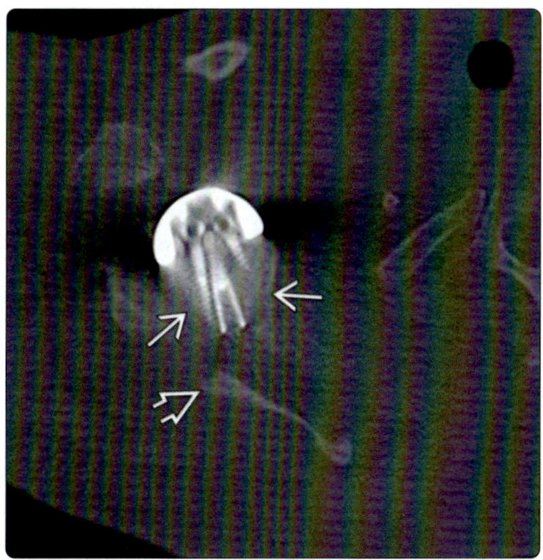

(Left) *Axial CT in the same patient obtained at the same time as the radiograph confirms the loosening and likely particle disease with osteolysis* ➡ *occupying the majority of the glenoid.* **(Right)** *Axial CT obtained 4 months later shows a new angulation of the glenoid* ➡, *fracture, and diastasis from the scapula* ⇨. *Note the difference in diagnostic quality between the 2 CT images; proper protocol for reducing metal artifact should be observed whenever possible.*

Elbow Implant

KEY FACTS

TERMINOLOGY

- Elbow arthroplasty: Replacement of distal humeral and proximal ulnar portions of elbow joint
  - Hinged implant (linked or coupled)
  - Semiconstrained linked implant
  - Unlinked or uncoupled implant
  - Hemiarthroplasty: Replacement of only 1 portion of elbow joint (radial implant is only 1 currently placed)

IMAGING

- Implant placement
  - Long stem must be centered in shaft without fracture
  - Normal mild valgus carrying angle of 154-178° should be maintained
  - Normal, congruent articulation of humeral and ulnar components
    - Radial head resection in total elbow arthroplasty
- Cementing technique
  - Thin mantle of cement surrounding entire stems
- Complications
  - Loosening
    - Change in position of component
    - Subsidence of component into shaft
  - Heterotopic ossification
  - Implant or periprosthetic fracture
  - Polyethylene (bushing) wear

CLINICAL ISSUES

- Elbow arthroplasty has higher rate of all types of complication and failure than hip or knee implants
- Loosening: Most frequent cause of long-term implant failure (18% in 1 study; likely more)
  - 47% for elbow implant in RA

DIAGNOSTIC CHECKLIST

- High rate of failure in implants placed for RA or young posttraumatic patients
  - Watch for early signs of loosening in these patients

(Left) *AP radiograph shows a typical hinged total elbow arthroplasty without evidence of complication. There has been resection of the radial head ➡, as is usually performed. The long stems extend within the humeral and ulnar shafts with a surrounding thin, regular cement mantle ➡. Note the normal valgus carrying angle.* **(Right)** *Lateral radiograph in the same patient shows the hinged arthroplasty. There is no evidence of loosening or other complications. The anterior humeral line ➡ confirms normal positioning.*

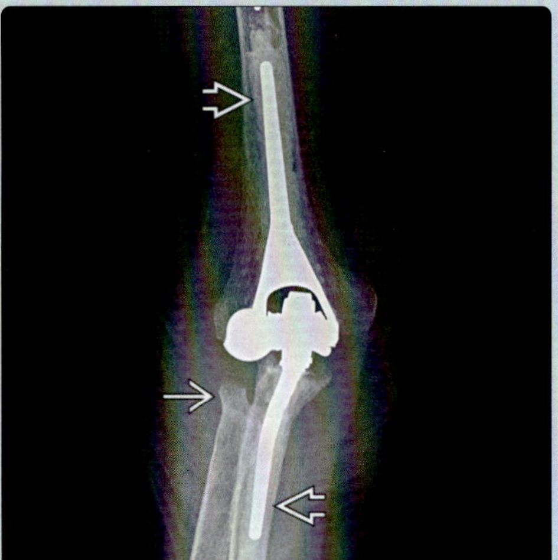

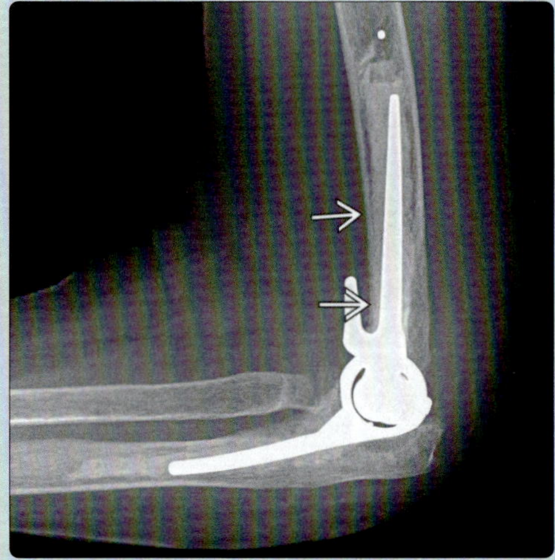

(Left) *Sagittal CT shows heterotopic ossification ➡ that is nonbridging. There is severe radiocapitellar osteoarthritis ➡, but there is no indication of loosening of the prosthesis.* **(Right)** *Sagittal T2WI FS MR shows a Silastic radial head prosthesis. The peg ➡ in the radial neck is intact and not loose, but there is a central fracture of the implant head ➡ with splaying of the fragments. Complete capitellar cartilage loss is seen, as well as significant synovitis ➡; massive osteolysis has not yet occurred.*

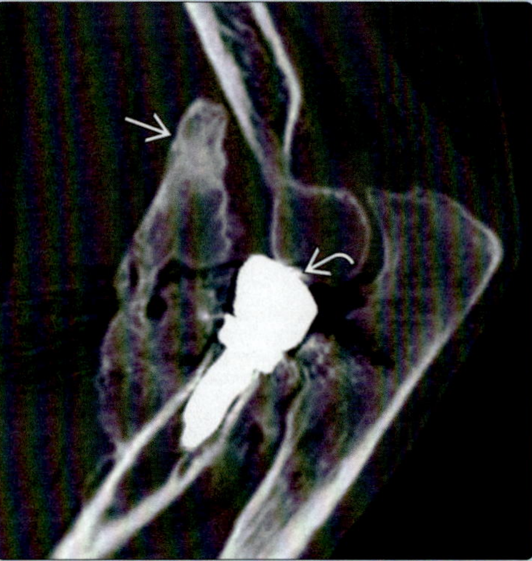

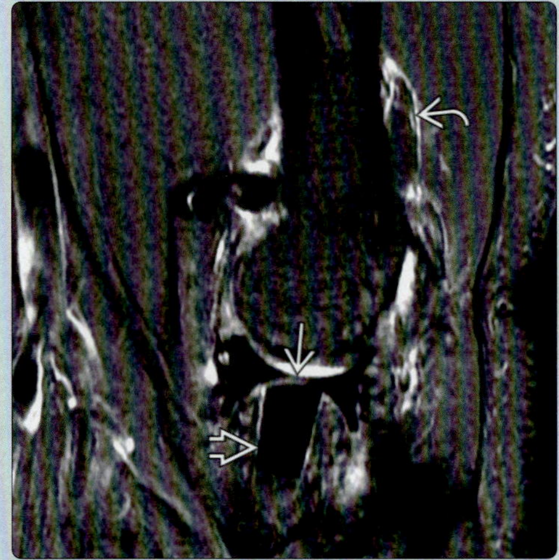

TERMINOLOGY

Definitions

- Elbow arthroplasty: Replacement of distal humeral and proximal ulnar portions of elbow joint
  - Hinged implant
    - Also termed linked or coupled
    - Implant is stable
    - Older components invariably loosened because hinge did not allow rotation
    - Newer design: Uses pin, which allows small amount of rotation and varus-valgus angulation (7-10°)
      - Termed semiconstrained linked implant
      - Most commonly used total elbow arthroplasty
  - Unlinked or uncoupled implant
    - Inherently less stable than hinged implant
      - Requires normal underlying bone stock
      - Stabilizing soft tissues must be intact (muscles, tendons, and radial and ulnar collateral ligaments)
    - Alignment is technically difficult
      - Requires excellent surgical technique
    - Increased rate of dislocation (13%) but decreased rate of loosening
- Hemiarthroplasty: Replacement of only 1 portion of joint
  - Humeral and ulnar hemiarthroplasties not used secondary to high failure rate
  - Radial head implant used but has high rate of failure
    - Unipolar or bipolar (allows rotation of head up to 15°)
- Cadaveric allograft
  - Salvage procedure
  - Prone to nonunion and instability

IMAGING

Radiographic Findings

- Implant placement
  - Long stem must be centered in shaft without fracture
    - On lateral view, line drawn along anterior humeral cortex should bisect distance between anterior humeral flange and posterior humeral cortex
  - Normal valgus carrying angle of 154-178° maintained
  - Normal, congruent articulation of components
    - Note: Radial head usually resected
- Cementing technique
  - Thin mantle of cement surrounding entire stems
    - Cementless techniques not used for arthroplasties but may be seen with radial head implant
- Loosening
  - Change in position of component
  - Subsidence of component into shaft
  - Bone-cement interface lucency ≥ 2 mm surrounding majority of stem
  - Cement fracture
- Infection
  - Lytic osseous destruction
  - Periosteal reaction
  - Soft tissue abscess
- Polyethylene (bushing) wear common, contributes to lysis
  - Suggested by change in varus or valgus (>10°) alignment
- Osteolysis
  - With frequent loosening and cement fracture, fragments arise from bone, cement, polyethylene, and metal, eliciting lytic reaction
- Heterotopic ossification (HO)
  - May occur anywhere, but antecubital fossa prone to HO formation; specify whether bridging or nonbridging

PATHOLOGY

Indications for Elbow Implant

- Intractable pain
- Progressive loss of extension beyond 60°
- Instability
- Comminuted intracondylar humeral fracture in elderly patients
- End-stage RA

Indications for Cadaveric Allograft

- Young patients with disabling disease
- Massive bone loss following trauma
- Elbow resection for tumor
- Revision arthroplasty

CLINICAL ISSUES

Natural History & Prognosis

- Elbow arthroplasty has higher rate of complications (all types) and failure than hip or knee implants
  - Loosening: Most frequent cause of long-term implant failure (18% in 1 study; likely more)
    - 47% for elbow implant in RA
  - Instability: 9%
  - Fracture: 6-22%
  - Infection: 2-5%; early mode of failure
  - Polyethylene (bushing) wear
- Semiconstrained elbow arthroplasty: 90% 10-year survival rate in all patient groups
  - Semiconstrained construct in young patients (< 40 years)
    - 22% require additional surgical procedure within 7.5 years
      - Most common reason: Loosening, wear
      - Posttraumatic arthroplasties more likely to require revision than postarthritis arthroplasties, perhaps due to higher mechanical demands
- Radial head arthroplasty complications
  - Nonbridging HO (38%)
  - Secondary osteoarthritis (27.9%)
  - Loosening (19.8%)
  - Bridging HO (8.9%)
  - Component dislocation (2.7%)
  - Fracture (2.3%)

DIAGNOSTIC CHECKLIST

Consider

- High rate of failure in implants placed for RA or young posttraumatic patients
  - Watch for early signs of loosening in these patients

SELECTED REFERENCES

1. Petscavage JM et al: Radiologic review of total elbow, radial head, and capitellar resurfacing arthroplasty. Radiographics. 32(1):129-49, 2012

KEY FACTS

TERMINOLOGY

- Tibial and talar implant for treatment of severe arthritis
- Two 2nd-generation design types, though many individual systems of each
  - 2-component (fixed-bearing): Tibial and talar metal implants; polyethylene spacer fixed to tibial implant
  - 3-component (mobile-bearing): Tibial and talar metal implants, separated by polyethylene spacer

IMAGING

- Generalizations
  - Bone ingrowth (porous) tibial and talar components
  - Implants anchored by stem, pegs, cylinders, or fins, depending on system chosen
  - Various conformable shapes of polyethylene, depending on system
  - Some systems incorporate fibula with syndesmotic screws and fusion to increase bone stock
- CT: Earlier and more accurate demonstration of loosening or lytic lesions than radiograph
- Most common complications
  - Periprosthetic fracture
  - Loosening
  - Syndesmotic fusion failure
  - Polyethylene wear, fracture, or dislocation
  - Particle disease with osteolysis
  - Infection

CLINICAL ISSUES

- Overall failure rate 10% over 5 years (includes all types of total ankle arthroplasties)
  - However, reoperation rate of 27%
    - Suggests failure may occur later than 5 years postop
  - Strong correlation of radiographic signs of failure to clinical failure
- Diabetes, especially if poorly controlled, adversely affects tibial and talar implant

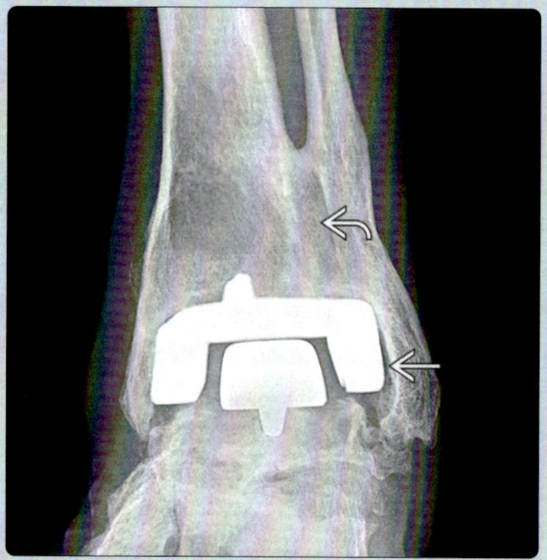

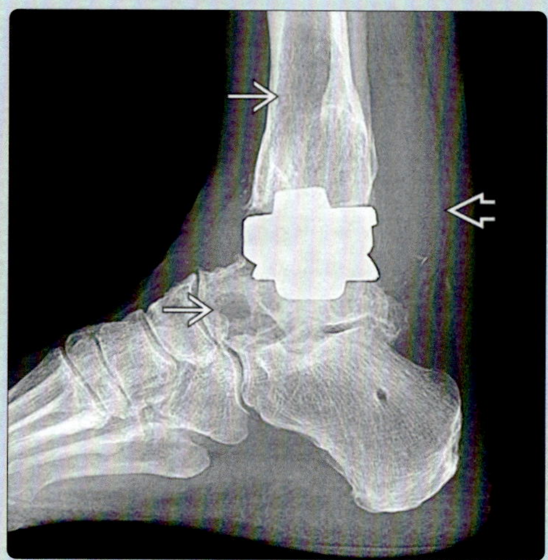

(Left) *AP radiograph shows the Agility Total Ankle, the most commonly placed 2-piece implant used in the USA. There is syndesmotic fusion ➡ increasing the osseous surface area for the tibial component, which decreases the likelihood of loosening and subsidence. The talar component is placed with 20° of external rotation. Minimal lucency is seen at the bone-component interface ➡, not indicating loosening.* **(Right)** *Lateral radiograph, same case, shows a complication with posterior soft tissue mass ➡ and lysis of the tibia/talus ➡.*

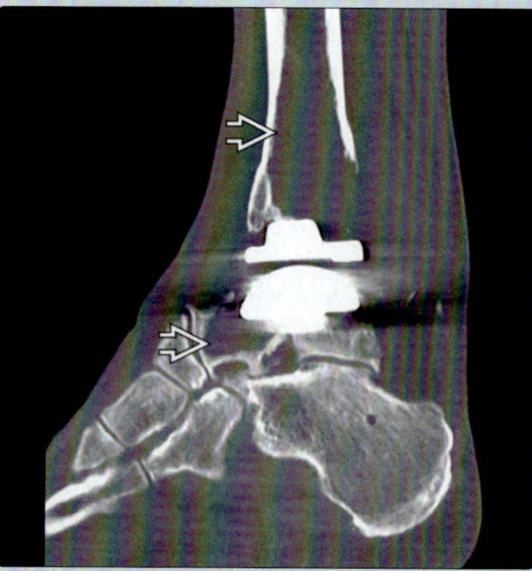

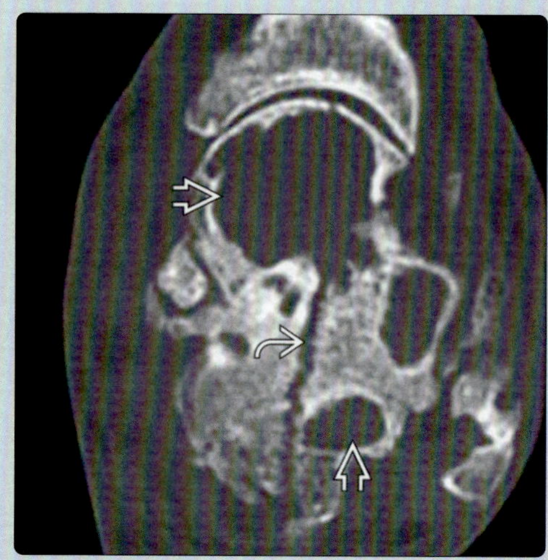

(Left) *Sagittal bone CT, same case, shows how much more sensitive CT is than radiograph in demonstrating the extent of the lytic lesions ➡. Note that the polyethylene appears symmetric, not indicating wear.* **(Right)** *Axial CT, same case, shows the source of the particles leading to the massive osteolysis ➡. The image is immediately below the fin that secures the talar prosthesis; a fracture ➡ extends from that stress riser. This chronic fracture is the source of osseous debris, which has resulted in massive osteolysis and failure.*

TERMINOLOGY

Definitions

- Tibial and talar implant for treatment of severe arthritis
  - 2nd-generation ankle arthroplasty
    - Cementless, requiring less bone resection
  - Two 2nd-generation design types, though many individual systems of each
    - 2-component (fixed-bearing): Tibial and talar metal implants, with polyethylene spacer fixed to tibial component
      - Polyethylene is partially conforming articulation
      - Most frequently used type of ankle implant in USA up to now
    - 3-component (mobile-bearing): Tibial and talar metal implants, separated by polyethylene spacer
      - Polyethylene is fully conforming and mobile
      - Has been used in Europe for many years; recently approved for use by FDA, so will be seen more frequently now in USA

IMAGING

Radiographic Findings

- Generalizations
  - Bone ingrowth (porous) tibial and talar components
  - Implants anchored by stem, pegs, cylinders, or fins, depending on system chosen
  - Various conformable shapes of polyethylene
  - Some systems incorporate fibula with syndesmotic screws and fusion to increase bone stock
- Initial placement
  - Tibial component perpendicular to long axis of tibia
- Incorrect sizing of component
  - Impingement if component overhangs
  - Larger component results in more bone loss
  - Puts malleolus at risk for fracture
- Periprosthetic fracture
  - Usually malleolar
  - Stress risers from pegs or fins may result in fracture of tibia or talus
- Loosening
  - Change in position of either component
    - Subsidence or tilt
    - May be subtle, requiring comparison with index postoperative radiograph
    - Choose landmarks to compare angles and position relative to subsidence
  - Lucency ≥ 2 mm at bone-component interface, substantially surrounding component
    - May have sclerotic line surrounding lucency
- Syndesmotic fusion failure
  - Lucency around screws indicating loosening
  - Screw fracture
  - Nonunion at syndesmosis
- Polyethylene wear
  - Asymmetry in lucent polyethylene
- Polyethylene fracture or dislocation
  - Watch for lucency in incorrect location; tibial and talar metal on metal
- Particle disease with osteolysis
  - Lytic lesions in tibia, talus, adjacent bones
  - Look for source of particles, including polyethylene, bone fragments, and bead shedding or metallosis
- Infection
  - Serpiginous lucency
  - Adjacent reactive sclerosis and periosteal reaction
  - Effusion
  - Differentiate from mechanical loosening/particle disease by clinical signs/symptoms; not always reliable
    - Aspiration may be required
- Heterotopic ossification
  - May irritate or limit range of motion
  - Talar component placed without varus or valgus, allowing normal alignment in line extending from bisecting tibia through to normal calcaneal alignment on weight-bearing AP view

CT Findings

- Earlier and more accurate demonstration of loosening or lytic lesions than radiograph

Imaging Recommendations

- Protocol advice
  - Minimize metal artifact on CT
    - Increased kVp, mAs
    - Decreased pitch
    - Narrow collimation, thin slice

CLINICAL ISSUES

Natural History & Prognosis

- Midterm (average: 44 months) analysis of Agility ankle arthroplasty (most frequently used 2-component device in USA)
  - Favorable clinical outcome (37/38 patients satisfied) despite radiographic abnormalities
    - 34/40 showed radiographic lucency or lysis (variable degree of involvement)
    - Migration or subsidence in 18/40
- One larger and longer-term study (n = 262) showed higher numbers of radiographic complications (62% overall)
  - Most common complications
    - Perihardware lucency (> 2 mm): 34%
    - Subsidence: 24%
    - Perihardware fracture: 11%
    - Syndesmotic screw loosening: 10%
    - Hardware fracture: 6.5%
    - Heterotopic ossification: 6%
    - ↑ varus or valgus: 5.4%
    - Ankle gutter narrowing: 5.4%
    - Syndesmotic nonunion or fracture: 2.7%
  - Strong positive association between radiographic findings and clinical outcome
    - Reoperations in 27%
- Diabetes, especially if poorly controlled, adversely affects total ankle arthroplasty
  - Higher rates of infection and osteolysis

SELECTED REFERENCES

1. Lee AY et al: Total ankle arthroplasty: a radiographic outcome study. AJR Am J Roentgenol. 200(6):1310-6, 2013

KEY FACTS

IMAGING

- **Normal findings after arthrodesis**
  - Early postoperative: Close apposition of articular surfaces
  - 2-6 months postoperative: Bridging trabeculae across joint
  - May initially involve only small portion of joint ("spot welding")
  - If 1 portion of joint fuses, remainder tends to fuse over time
  - Confluent bone graft material
- **Failure of arthrodesis**
  - Persistent visualization of joint space
  - CT more accurate than radiographs in assessing if joint space is still open
  - Lucency surrounding fixation screws or plates
    - Minimal lucency is okay and may stabilize
    - > 1-2-mm is concerning for motion
  - Fracture of hardware
  - Migration of hardware
  - Change in joint alignment
  - Periosteal reaction
    - May become exuberant with motion or infection

CLINICAL ISSUES

- Osteoarthritis of posterior subtalar joint is common sequela of ankle fusion
- Fusion of subtalar joint may be performed for persistent pain after isolated ankle joint fusion

DIAGNOSTIC CHECKLIST

- Radiographs not highly accurate in diagnosis of fusion vs. nonunion; CT scan more reliable
- Beware of partial volume artifact mimicking fusion where joint surfaces are tightly curving
  - Confirm diagnosis in 2 planes
- Watch for normal amount of dorsiflexion at tibiotalar joint

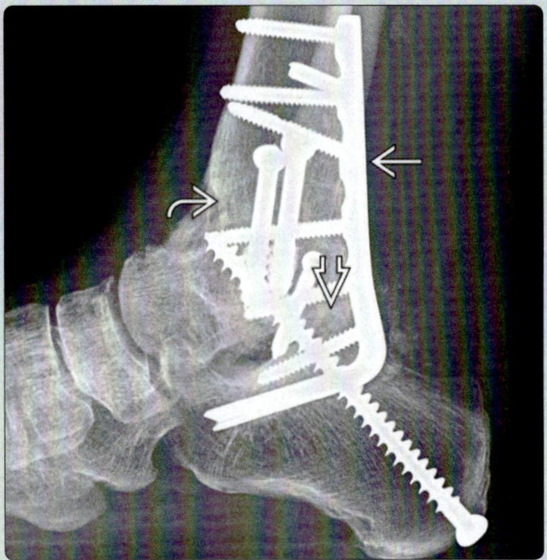

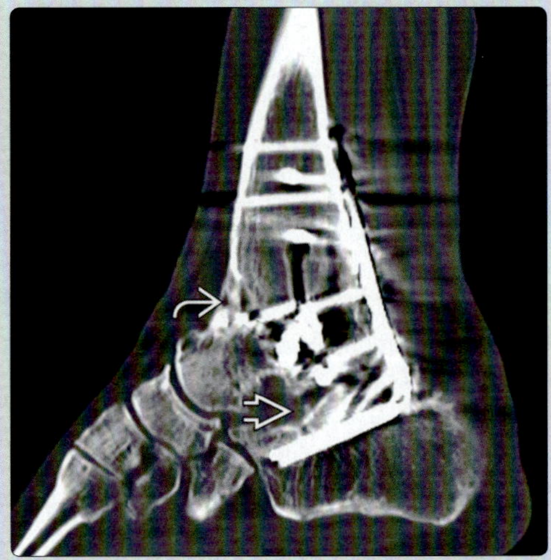

(Left) *Lateral radiograph 6 months after ankle and subtalar arthrodesis with a blade plate fixator ➡ shows the trabeculae appearing to bridge the tibiotalar ➡ and subtalar ➡ joints. However, radiographs may overestimate osseous fusion due to beam obliquity or superimposition of different portions of the joint.* **(Right)** *Sagittal reformatted bone CT in the same patient performed because of persistent pain shows bridging across the tibiotalar ➡ but not the subtalar ➡ joint.*

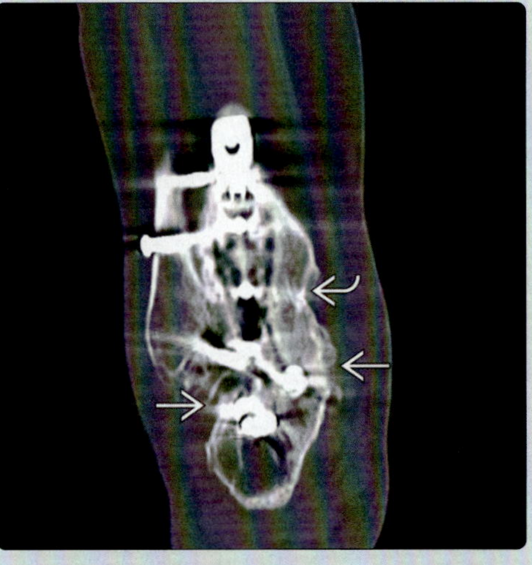

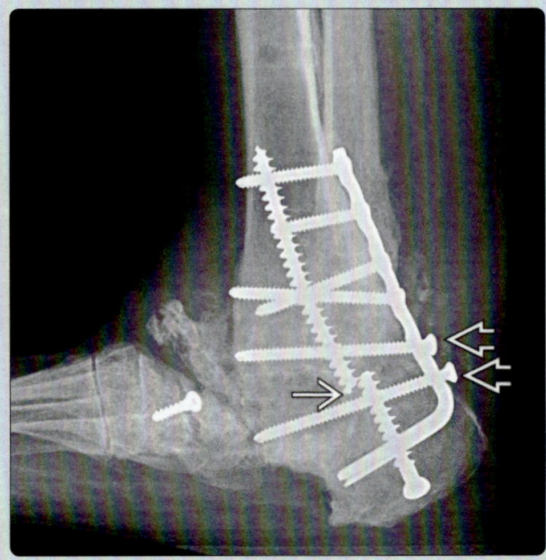

(Left) *Coronal reformatted bone CT from the same patient confirms the presence of tibiotalar fusion ➡ & the absence of subtalar fusion ➡. It is important to confirm findings on both coronal reformat & sagittal planes in order to avoid misdiagnosis because of partial volume artifact.* **(Right)** *Lateral radiograph after ankle & subtalar fusion shows fractured fixation screw ➡ indicating continued motion. Two fixation screws have backed out, & their heads are proud ➡. Charcot changes are seen in the midfoot.*

TERMINOLOGY

Synonyms

- Ankle fusion

Definitions

- Surgical bridging of tibiotalar joint with orthopedic hardware to establish osseous fusion of joint

IMAGING

General Features

- Best diagnostic clue
  - Trabecular bridging across joint

Radiographic Findings

- **Normal findings after arthrodesis**
  - Early postoperative
    - Some surgeons perform fibular osteotomy and fuse medial fibular cortex with tibia to act as strut across joint ("incorporation of fibula")
    - Close apposition of articular surfaces
    - Unincorporated bone graft material
  - 2-6 months postoperative
    - Bridging trabeculae across joint
      - May initially involve only small portion of joint ("spot welding")
      - If 1 portion of joint fuses, remainder tends to fuse over time
    - Confluent bone graft material; some resorption likely
  - Pitfalls in diagnosis
    - Obliquity of x-ray beam may result in nonvisualization of joint margins
    - Superimposition of nonarticular bone may also obscure joint margins
    - Either problem can lead to erroneous diagnosis of successful fusion
- **Failure of arthrodesis**
  - Persistent visualization of joint space
    - CT more accurate than radiographs in assessing if joint space is still open
  - Lucency surrounding fixation screws or plates
    - Minimal lucency is okay and may stabilize
    - > 1-2 mm is concerning for motion
  - Fracture of hardware
  - Migration of hardware
  - Change in joint alignment
  - Periosteal reaction
    - May become exuberant with motion or infection

CT Findings

- Same findings as for radiographs but far more clearly and unequivocally demonstrated
- If patient has pain after arthrodesis, CT may show fusion failure, which is not visible on radiographs
- Possible false-positive diagnosis of fusion if joint space curves in plane of scan
  - Carefully correlate sagittal and coronal reformations to accurately distinguish between partial volume artifact and true fusion

MR Findings

- Bone marrow and trabeculae across joint space
- Limited by metal artifact

Imaging Recommendations

- Best imaging tool
  - CT; ↑ kVp often useful
- Protocol advice
  - Coronal and sagittal reformations essential

DIFFERENTIAL DIAGNOSIS

Posttraumatic Fusion

- Usually fibrous, not osseous

Juvenile Idiopathic Arthritis

- Usually multiple hindfoot joints fused
- Ankle less commonly involved than subtalar joint
- Abnormal osseous growth (overgrowth or early fusion)

CLINICAL ISSUES

Presentation

- Most common signs/symptoms
  - Clinical failure of fusion presents with pain, which may be due to lack of osseous fusion, infection, degeneration of adjacent joint, impingement, or tendon abnormality

Natural History & Prognosis

- Subtalar and Chopart joints often develop increased mobility to compensate for loss of ankle motion
- Osteoarthritis of posterior subtalar joint is common sequela of ankle fusion
- High rate of fusion failure in neuropathic arthropathy

Treatment

- Fusion of subtalar joint may be performed for persistent pain after isolated ankle joint fusion

DIAGNOSTIC CHECKLIST

Image Interpretation Pearls

- Radiographs not highly accurate in diagnosis; CT scan more reliable
- Beware of partial volume artifact mimicking fusion where joint surfaces are tightly curving
  - Confirm diagnosis in 2 planes
  - Localizer lines on PACS very helpful to ensure both planes are through same region
- Assess for tibiotalar fusion in anatomic/functional alignment

SELECTED REFERENCES

1. Chalayon O et al: Factors affecting the outcomes of uncomplicated primary open ankle arthrodesis. Foot Ankle Int. 36(10):1170-9, 2015
2. Ling JS et al: Investigating the relationship between ankle arthrodesis and adjacent-joint arthritis in the hindfoot: a systematic review. J Bone Joint Surg Am. 97(6):513-20, 2015
3. Vulcano E et al: The spectrum of indications for subtalar joint arthrodesis. Foot Ankle Clin. 20(2):293-310, 2015
4. Dorsey ML et al: Correlation of arthrodesis stability with degree of joint fusion on MDCT. AJR Am J Roentgenol. 192(2):496-9, 2009
5. Coughlin MJ et al: Comparison of radiographs and CT scans in the prospective evaluation of the fusion of hindfoot arthrodesis. Foot Ankle Int. 27(10):780-7, 2006

KEY FACTS

TERMINOLOGY

- Small implants may be used to replace bone or joints in hands or feet
  - Variety of materials used; may have metal components but most are a variety of silicon

IMAGING

- Silastic implants are increased density on radiograph relative to adjacent osteoporotic bone
  - Smooth, homogeneous, in shape of bone but without trabeculae
- Fracture of hinge in Swanson arthroplasty difficult to visualize
  - Secondary sign: Discontinuity, especially between body and stem of implant
  - Abrupt change in alignment or displacement of phalanx, such that stem within phalanx can no longer be attached to body
  - High failure rate, particular in RA patients (26-34%)
- Periprosthetic fracture: Watch for sites at ↑ risk
  - Radiocarpal arthroplasty: Stem extends into thin 3rd metacarpal shaft, further weakening it
  - Swanson arthroplasty: Stem extending into phalanx &/or metacarpal/metatarsal shafts; subluxation also increases risk for fracture
- Prosthetic dislocation
  - Implants constrained only by shape (carpals, TMJ meniscus) may dislocate with any abnormal stress or motion
  - Stem of Swanson arthroplasty may pull out of phalanx without fracturing; elongated triangle noted in soft tissues
- Particle disease
  - Osteolysis, restricted to regions particles can access
  - MR: ↓ Silastic implant; synovitis, marrow edema/cysts

(Left) *PA radiograph shows a radiocarpal arthroplasty. The components are placed appropriately; the radial stem extends into the radius and carpal stem extends up the shaft of the 3rd MC ➡. The distal ulna is resected. Subluxation occurs because of the underlying ligamentous imbalance in patients with RA, often resulting in implant failure.* **(Right)** *PA x-ray shows the homogeneous density of scaphoid ➡ and lunate ➡ Silastic implants, both subluxated, and associated massive osteolysis involving multiple adjacent bones ➡.*

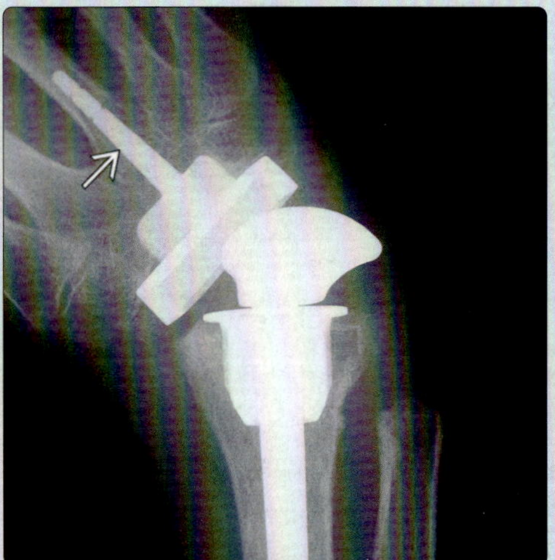

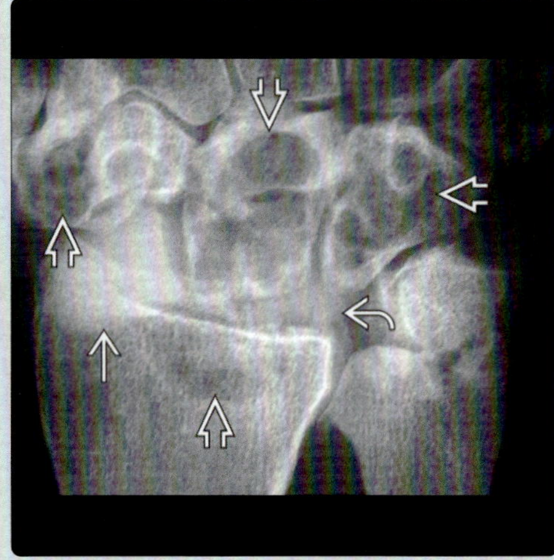

(Left) *PA radiograph shows fusion of the 1st MCP ➡ and a grossly loose ulnar Silastic implant ➡ in a patient with RA. Silastic stems from a radiocarpal implant can faintly be seen in the radius and 3rd MC ➡ from failed wrist arthroplasty.* **(Right)** *PA radiograph shows a radial column fusion ➡ including the scaphoid, trapezoid, and trapezium, performed for osteoarthritis (OA) following trauma. Since implants perform so poorly in the wrist, arthrodesis is preferred in some patients.*

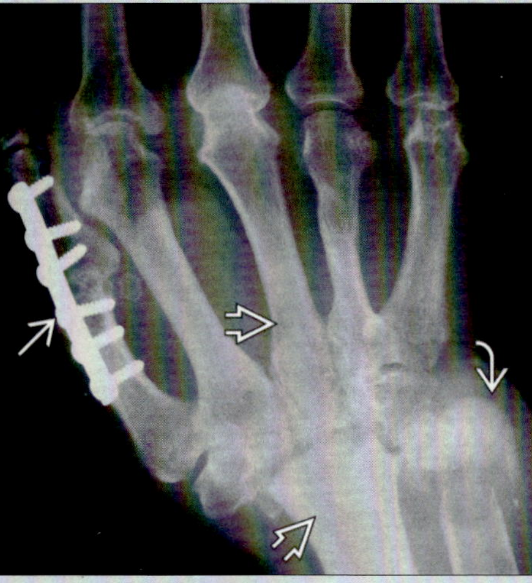

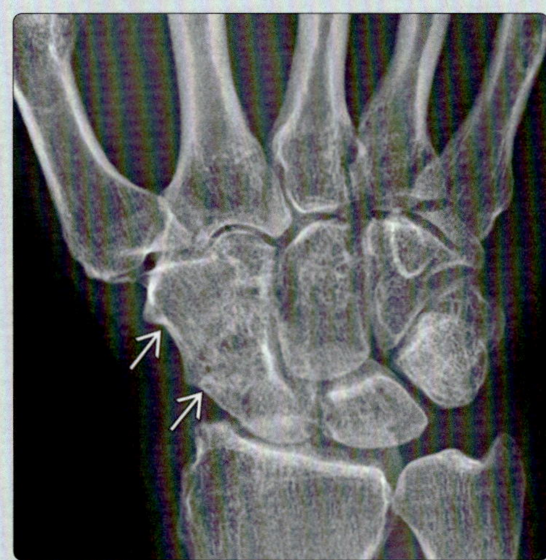

TERMINOLOGY

Definitions

- Small implants may be used to replace bone or joints in hands or feet
  - Variety of materials used; may have metal components but most are a variety of silicon
  - "Silastic" = silicon for purposes of this discussion
  - Carpal or other small implants are formed in shape of structure to be replaced [scaphoid, lunate, temporomandibular joint (TMJ) meniscus, base of 1st metacarpal (MC)/metatarsal (MT)]
  - Swanson arthroplasty: Silastic arthroplasty utilized for MCP, metatarsophalangeal (MTP), or interphalangeal (IP) joints of hand or feet
    - Other varieties (i.e., Sutter arthroplasty) are not distinguished here since appearance and complications are similar
    - Rectangular body with triangular flanges or stems extending into diaphyses of phalanges or MC/MT
    - Stems are usually not cemented within diaphyses, and there is no ingrowth potential
    - "Hinge" at site of joint is thinning of Silastic between body of prosthesis and its stem; at risk for fracture
    - May have metal grommets: Theoretical but not demonstrated protection against stem fracture

IMAGING

Radiographic Findings

- Silastic implants are increased in density relative to adjacent osteoporotic bone
  - Smooth, homogeneous, in shape of bone but without trabeculae
- Prosthetic fracture
  - Microfractures of bone implants may not be visible on radiograph
  - Implant fracture: Difficult to visualize
    - Look for interruption or irregularity of normally smooth shape of implant body
  - Fracture of hinge in Swanson arthroplasty
    - Fracture line in Silastic rarely directly seen
    - Secondary sign: Discontinuity, especially between body and stem of implant
      - ◻ Abrupt change in alignment or displacement of phalanx, such that stem within phalanx can no longer be attached to body
    - High failure rate, particular in RA patients (26-34%)
- Periprosthetic fracture: Watch for sites at particular risk
  - Radiocarpal arthroplasty: 1 stem extends into radius; other stem extends into 3rd metacarpal shaft; at particular risk for metacarpal fracture
  - Swanson arthroplasty: Stems extend into phalanx &/or MC/MT shafts; thin bone at significant risk for fracture
    - Fracture risk increased if there is associated
      - ◻ Subluxation of joint
      - ◻ Underlying osteoporosis with thin cortices (any abnormal motion of stem within shaft risks shaft fracture)
      - ◻ Osteolysis from particle disease
- Prosthetic dislocation
  - Implants constrained only by shape (carpals, TMJ meniscus) may dislocate with any abnormal stress or motion
  - Silastic implants at base of thumb (trapezium replacement) or at MT head of MTP arthroplasty may not have stem; dislocation in these seen as complete lack of articulation
  - Stem of Swanson arthroplasty may pull out of phalanx without fracturing implant or bone; elongated prosthesis triangle seen within soft tissues
- Particle disease
  - Osteolysis, restricted to regions particles can access
    - Swanson arthroplasties: Restricted to affected joint(s)
    - Carpal arthroplasties: Lysis affects all bones within joint
      - ◻ Implant at trapezium will affect base of 1st MC; if 1st carpometacarpal (CMC) joint capsule is disrupted, may affect any bone within middle wrist compartment (trapezoid, capitate, hamate, proximal portions of scaphoid, lunate, trapezium, and bases of metacarpals 2-5)
      - ◻ Scaphoid or lunate implant may affect all carpal bones, bases of MCs (except 1st), and radius/ulna, given disruption of scapholunate ligament
  - Lysis often seen as round lucencies, generally multiple
    - Sclerotic border often present
    - Underlying osteoporosis affects how distinctly lytic process is visualized
- Arthrodesis/resection in carpus
  - Complete arthrodesis of carpus generally not chosen since it is too limiting of motion
  - Partial arthrodesis/resection may accomplish 3 goals: ↓ pain, maintain some motion, avoid complications of Silastic implants
  - Various patterns of arthrodesis and resection chosen, depending on site of arthritis
    - 1st carpometacarpal (CMC) joint arthritis
      - ◻ Ligament reconstruction/tendon interposition: Resection of trapezium, lateral ligament reconstruction with flexor carpi radialis through tunnel at base of 1st MC, interposition of rolled-up tendon into trapezium defect (± small Silastic implant)
      - ◻ Fusion of CMC joint (fairly significant limitation of motion)
    - Radiocarpal arthritis, with various disruptions of scapholunate and lunatotriquetral ligaments and triangular fibrocartilage
      - ◻ Radial column fusion (scaphoid-trapezium-trapezoid)
      - ◻ Ulnar column fusion (4-corner: Capitate-hamate-lunate-triquetrum)
      - ◻ ± resection of all or part of proximal carpal row

MR Findings

- Silastic implants are low signal on all MR sequences
- Prosthetic fracture
  - Fractures more visible than on radiograph
  - Small fragments visible within fluid collections
- Particle disease
  - Synovitis
    - Low T1 SI, high T2 SI fluid

- Thickened synovium
- Remember extensive synovial sheaths in wrist and hand; distribution may be widespread
- Marrow edema, osteolysis
  - Low T1 SI, high T2 SI in marrow and cysts

Imaging Recommendations

- Best imaging tool
  - Implant and many complications should be identified on radiograph
  - MR demonstrates extent of synovitis and osseous destruction

DIFFERENTIAL DIAGNOSIS

Septic Arthritis

- Subchondral cysts, erosions mimic osteolysis of particle disease
- No implant (implants can be surprisingly easy to overlook)

Inflammatory Arthritis

- Subchondral cysts, erosions, cartilage damage of rheumatoid or pyrophosphate arthritis mimic particle disease osteolysis

PATHOLOGY

General Features

- Etiology
  - Flange of Swanson-type arthroplasty within small tubular bones is not cemented (no solid fixation)
    - Abnormal repetitive motion occurs at MCP, MTP, IP joints from soft tissue imbalance
      - Leads to fragmentation and failure of prosthesis or bone
    - Soft tissue imbalance or contractures (especially in RA patients) results in abnormal force occurring at hinge
      - Typical patterns: Volar subluxation at MCPs, ulnar deviation at MCPs
      - Increases risk of fracture at hinge or dislocation of stem from shaft
  - Carpal soft tissue imbalance (especially in RA) puts carpal prostheses at risk for dislocation
    - Ulnar translocation
    - Carpal instability patterns

Gross Pathologic & Surgical Features

- Retrieved implants show fracture, fragmentation
  - In vivo oxidation may play role
  - Mechanical factors (abnormal motion) also certain to play role

Microscopic Features

- Macrophages containing debris, either metal, Silastic, or bone

CLINICAL ISSUES

Presentation

- Most common signs/symptoms
  - Pain, malalignment
  - May be either sudden or slow in onset
  - Even with radiographic failure, patient may have functional result

Demographics

- Age
  - Older patients, related to likelihood of destructive arthritis and implant placement
- Gender
  - Male < female, related to incidence of RA (most common reason for small joint implants)

Natural History & Prognosis

- 17-year survivorship for Swanson-type implants: 63% (though 2/3 showed fractures on radiographs)
  - Improved survival with soft tissue balancing, crossed intrinsic transfer, and realignment of wrist
  - Use of metal grommets does not improve rate of implant fracture
- Failed arthroplasty generally progresses to worsening disruption
  - Fragmentation of polyethylene, metal, bone, cement
  - Osteolysis and fracture
- Unprotected periprosthetic fracture may complete and displace
- Pyrolytic carbon: New design
  - One study showed 30% required surgical revision or retrieval
  - Radiographic complications
    - Subsidence (32%)
    - Loosening (40%)
    - Periprosthetic fracture (8.5%)
    - Ulnar subluxation of joint (4.3%)
  - Clinical survival of implant significantly better than radiographic impression of survival

Treatment

- Failed, painful implant generally needs revision
  - Revision prior to disintegration of bone stock is advisable
  - Revision may require arthrodesis
- Failed small joint implant in RA patients may not require revision if not painful

DIAGNOSTIC CHECKLIST

Image Interpretation Pearls

- Watch for increased radiographic density (smooth, without trabeculation or differentiation of cortical surface) to identify Silastic implants
- Evaluate location of Silastic carpal implants, especially on lateral radiograph in order to detect dislocation
- Watch for joint malalignment (suggests Silastic failure)
- Watch for subtle buckle of implant or cortical change in alignment/buckle to suggest fracture of implant or bone
- Recognize where failures occur; search for subtle signs

SELECTED REFERENCES

1. Gaspar MP et al: Management of complications of wrist arthroplasty and wrist fusion. Hand Clin. 31(2):277-292, 2015
2. Satteson ES et al: The management of complications of small joint arthrodesis and arthroplasty. Hand Clin. 31(2):243-266, 2015

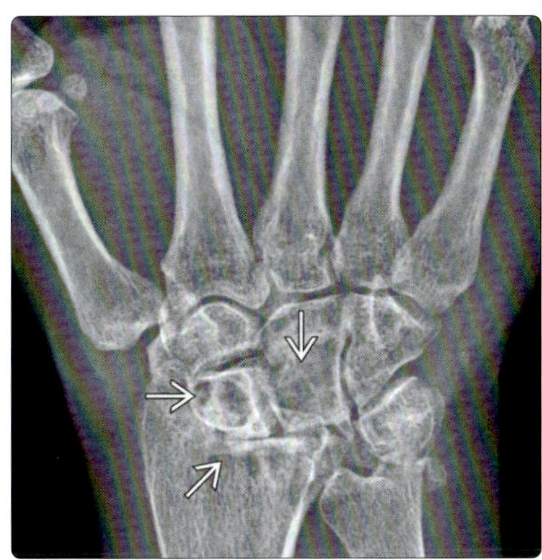

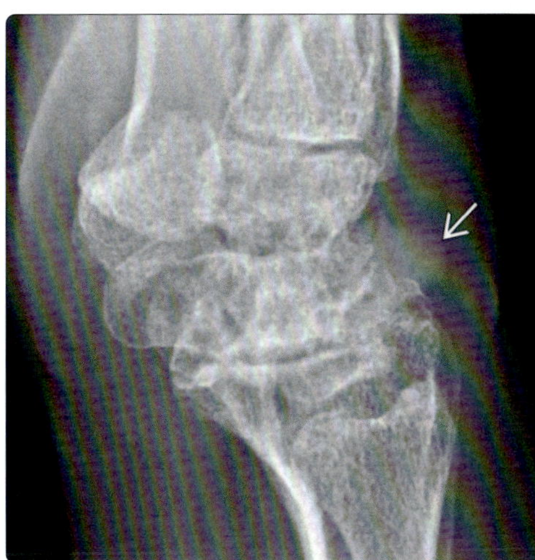

(Left) *PA radiograph shows an abnormal carpus with tremendous cyst formation within the scaphoid, capitate, and distal radius. There is complete cartilage loss at the radiocarpal joint and absent lunate. This appearance might be misinterpreted as RA or pyrophosphate arthropathy.* **(Right)** *Lateral radiograph, same case, shows a smooth, rounded density located posteriorly within the joint. This is a Silastic lunate implant, placed for lunate necrosis but now dislocated and the cause of massive osteolysis.*

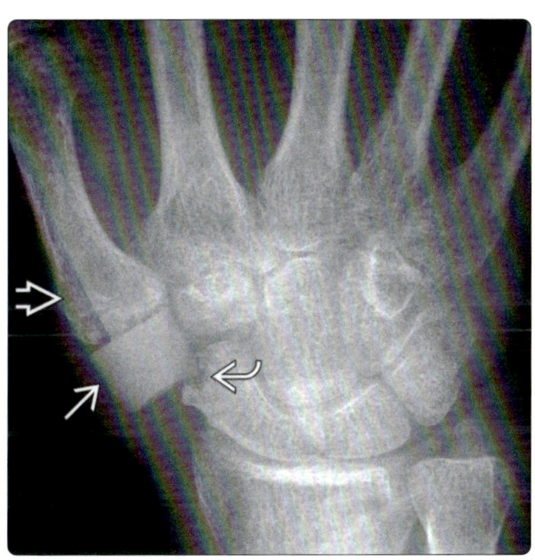

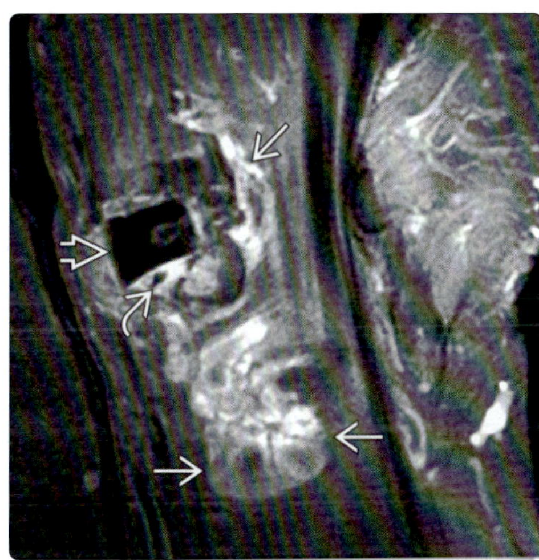

(Left) *PA radiograph shows resection of the trapezium and replacement by a Silastic implant with stem extending only into the 1st MC. This is already beginning to fail, as it is subluxated radially and has eroded the scaphoid. Note the resorption of bone about the stem of the implant as well.* **(Right)** *Coronal STIR MR near the palmar surface of the wrist shows extensive synovitis. This is in reaction to a Silastic trapezium implant. Note implant fragments, often seen adjacent to the implant.*

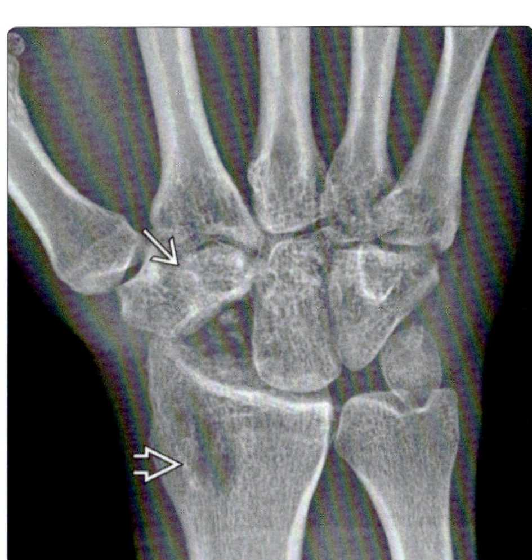

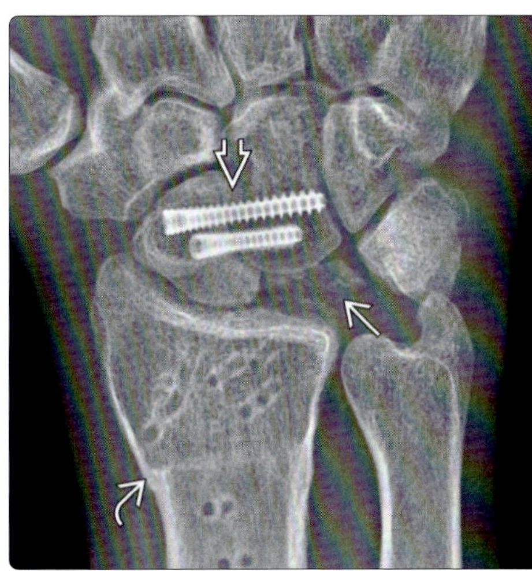

(Left) *PA radiograph shows proximal row carpectomy for osteonecrosis of the scaphoid and secondary OA. There is fusion of the trapezium and trapezoid. Note the lucency at the site of graft harvest in the distal radius.* **(Right)** *PA radiograph shows resection of the lunate for osteonecrosis. There is fusion of the scaphoid and capitate, performed in an effort to prevent proximal migration of the capitate. The osteotomy at the distal radius had previously been performed as a lengthening procedure.*

(Left) *PA radiograph shows a thin Silastic implant ➔ placed following resection of much of the trapezium for OA. There is also a radial ligament reconstruction, evidenced by the suture anchor ➔. Note the subluxation as well as fraying of the implant, which is beginning to fail secondary to insufficient support and abnormal motion.* **(Right)** *PA radiograph shows fusion of the trapezium, trapezoid, and base of 1st MC ➔ for OA. There is also a proximal row carpectomy (scaphoid, lunate, and triquetrum).*

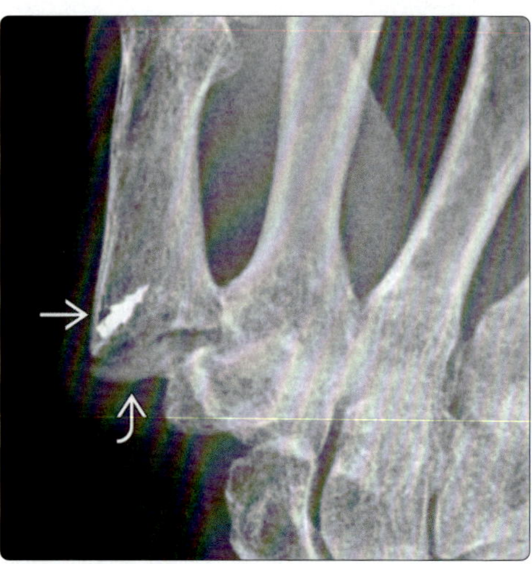

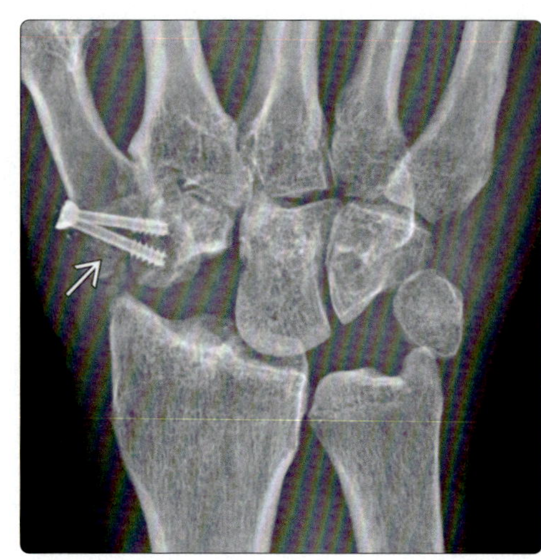

(Left) *PA radiograph shows gull wing erosive deformities of the DIP joints ➔, typical of erosive OA. Additionally, 2 of the PIP joints have been replaced with a Swanson arthroplasty; the bodies of the implants are seen as rectangular shapes ➔, and the stems extend into the shafts.* **(Right)** *PA radiograph shows the rectangular body ➔ and elongated triangular stems ➔ of a Swanson arthroplasty. There is ulnar deviation of the joint and some lysis and loosening around the phalangeal stem.*

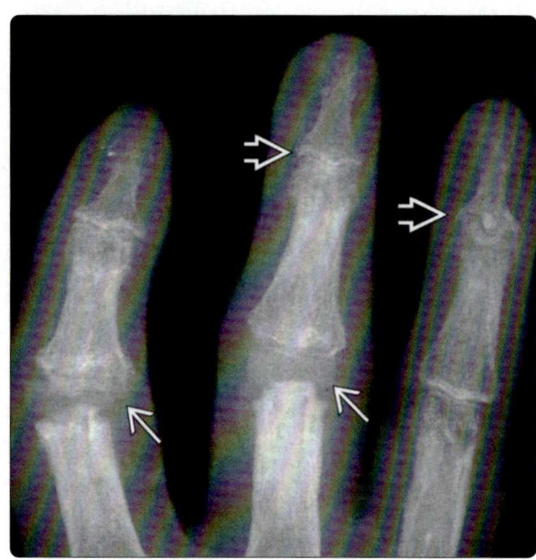

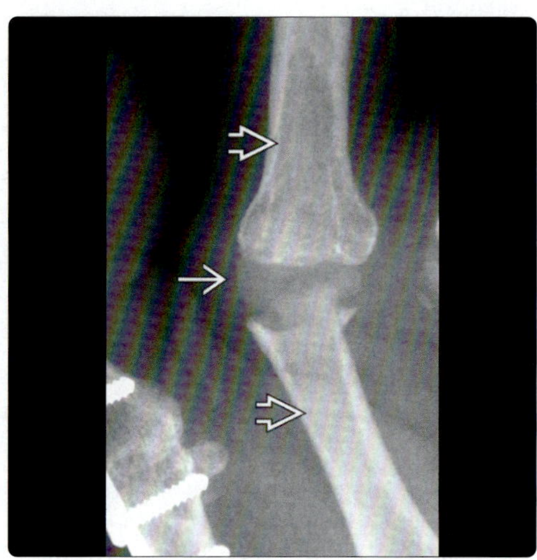

(Left) *PA radiograph shows a Swanson implant body ➔, which has fractured and been displaced from its stem ➔. Fractures at the hinge of the implant are common, as seen here. A 2nd implant shows fracture of the stem through the MC shaft ➔, another common form of failure of these implants.* **(Right)** *PA radiograph shows Swanson implants at MCP 2-5. At each, the distal flange (barely seen) has fractured from the body ➔ due to the stress from unopposed ulnar deviation at these joints. This is a common mode of failure.*

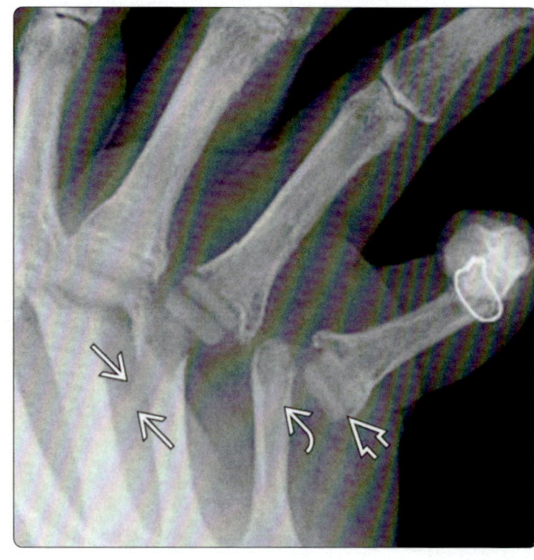

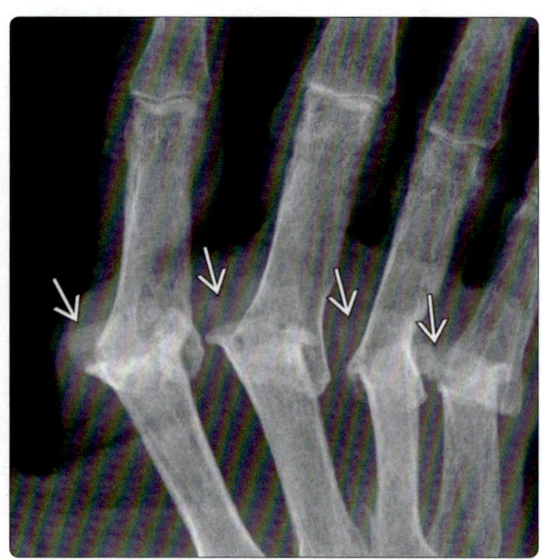

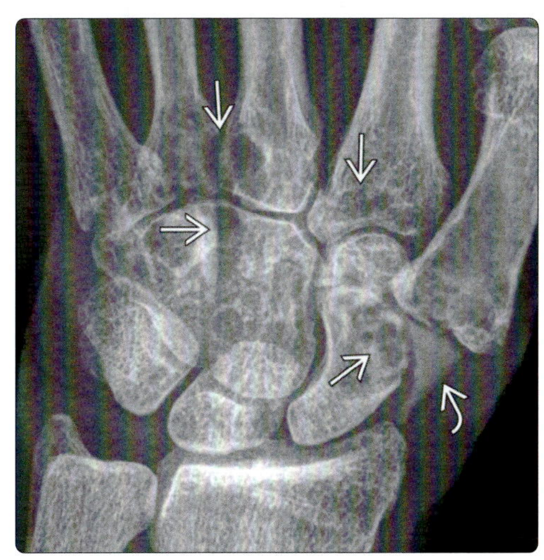

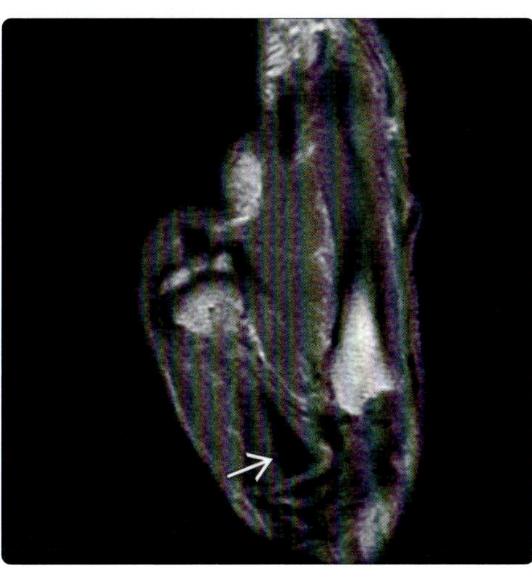

(Left) *PA radiograph shows a small residual fragment of a failed trapezium Silastic implant ➲, with the 1st MCP subluxed proximally. There are large cysts within virtually all of the nearby bones ➲ concerning for osteolysis.* **(Right)** *Coronal T1 MR of the thumb, same case, shows the fractured residual triangular-shaped flange ➲ of the trapezium implant, buried within the base of the 1st MC.*

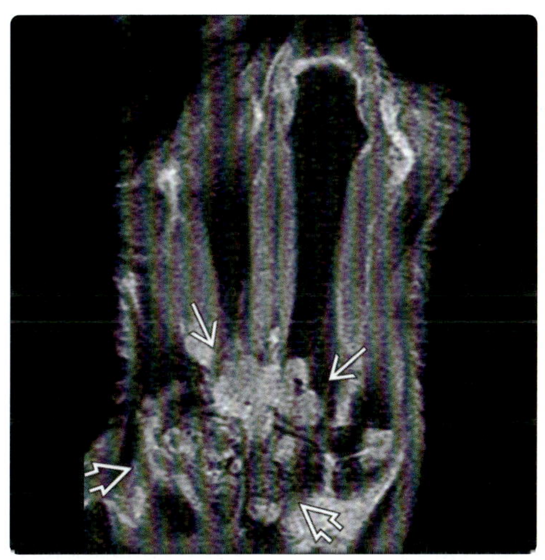

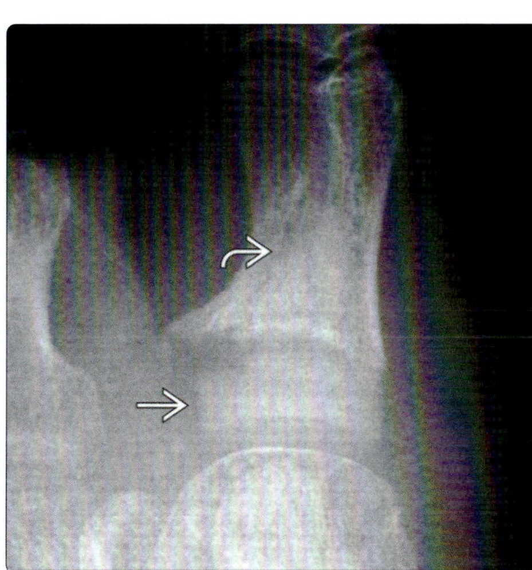

(Left) *Coronal T2FS MR, same case, shows the high signal rounded synovitis within osteolytic cysts of the 2nd and 3rd metacarpal bases ➲ as well as the trapezoid, capitate, and hamate ➲. This synovitis/osteolysis is massive.* **(Right)** *AP radiograph shows a Silastic implant at the 1st MTP. The body is at the joint ➲, and a single stem extends into the proximal phalanx of the great toe ➲. There is soft tissue swelling and a hint of lucency at the stem-bone interface. This early loosening is not surprising since the stem is not anchored in the bone.*

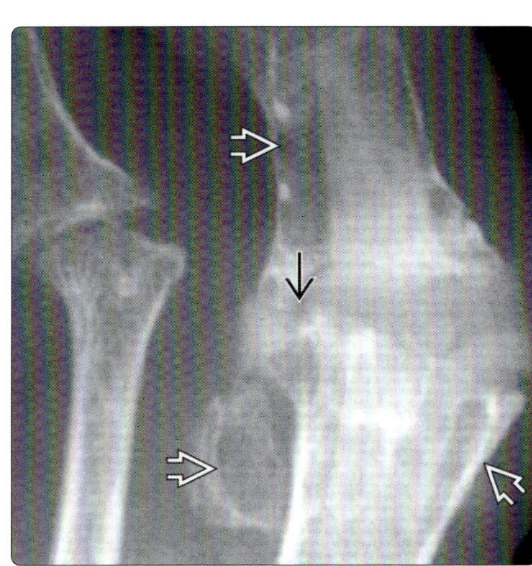

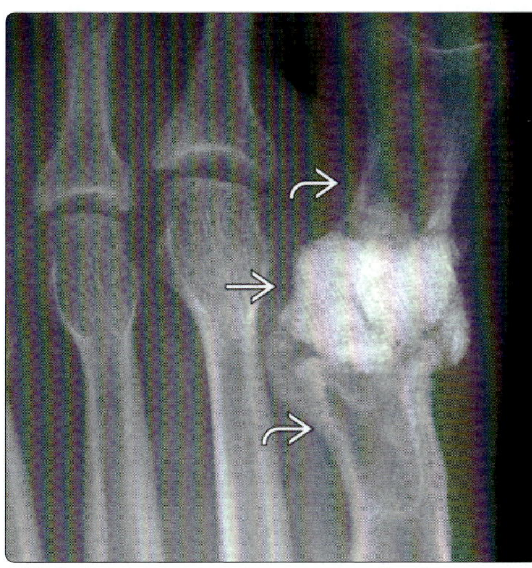

(Left) *AP radiograph of the great toe shows a Silastic MTP arthroplasty. The body of the arthroplasty has fractured ➲. The fractured piece produces particles, which in turn result in osteolysis ➲.* **(Right)** *AP radiograph shows defects from removal of a previously placed Silastic implant in the 1st MTP ➲. There is dense material placed for attempted arthrodesis ➲; this is coral, chosen as a strut material because of similar-sized cavities to haversian canals.*

Hallux Valgus Corrections

KEY FACTS

IMAGING

- Silver procedure (bunionectomy): Excision of medial bony prominence of 1st metatarsal (MT) head
  - Usually combined with some type of corrective osteotomy
- 1st MT osteotomies: Realignment of MT to improve orientation of metatarsophalangeal (MTP), tarsometatarsal (TMT) joints
  - Chevron osteotomy: V-shaped in sagittal plane
  - Scarf osteotomy: Z-shaped in sagittal plane
  - Wedge osteotomy of proximal MT
- Keller procedure: Bunionectomy + excision of proximal portion of 1st proximal phalanx
- Lapidus procedure: Bunionectomy + fusion of 1st TMT joint

PATHOLOGY

- Soft tissue components of procedures usually performed and are not directly seen on radiographs

CLINICAL ISSUES

- Surgical complications
  - Hallux varus: Due to release of lateral joint capsule &/or lateral sesamoidectomy
  - Recurrent hallux valgus: Due to incomplete correction of underlying deforming forces
  - Dorsiflexion of 1st MTP joint
  - Transfer metatarsalgia (significantly shortened 1st metatarsal)
  - Osteomyelitis
  - Osteonecrosis of 1st MT head
- Persistent sesamoid displacement

DIAGNOSTIC CHECKLIST

- Describe residual or new deformity, osteotomy healing
- Be alert for signs of stress transfer to 2nd MT
- Watch for malalignment of sesamoids

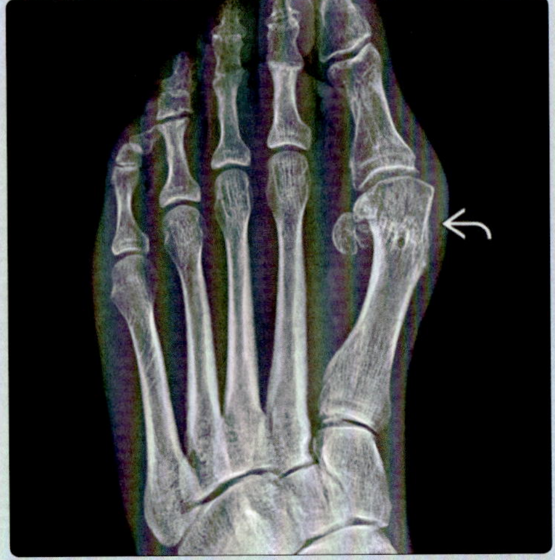

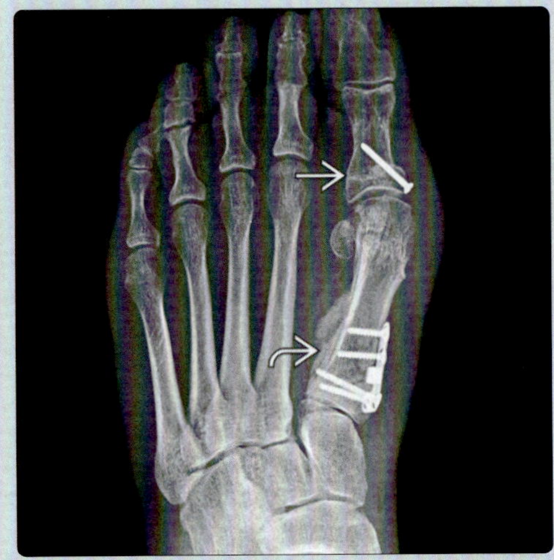

(Left) *AP radiograph shows Silver procedure ➡. This simple bunionectomy (resection of medial prominence of 1st MT head) did not address the deforming forces on the 1st toe. The patient has metatarsus primus varus (> 10° angle between 1st and 2nd metatarsals) and recurrent hallux valgus.* **(Right)** *AP radiograph in the same patient after osteotomies of the 1st proximal phalanx ➡ and 1st MT ➡ is shown. Iatrogenic shortening of the 1st toe is now seen and can lead to transfer metatarsalgia.*

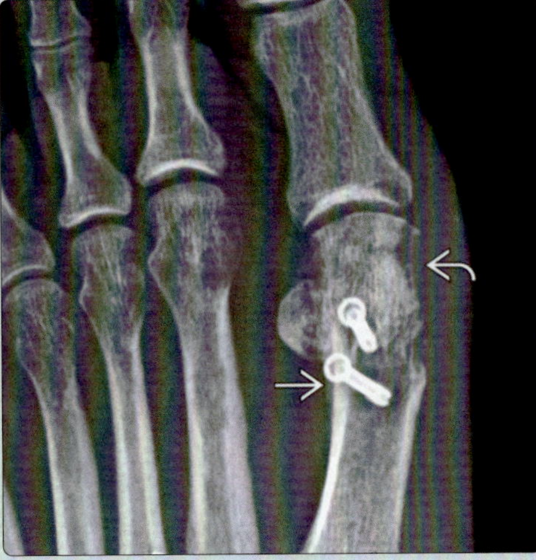

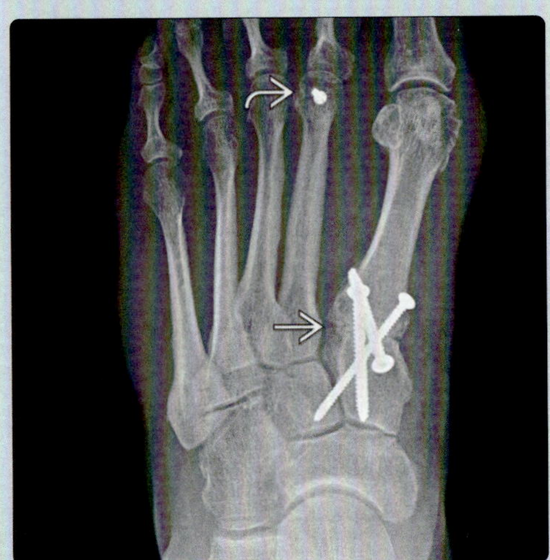

(Left) *AP radiograph shows bunionectomy ➡ and chevron osteotomy ➡ with lateral shifting of the 1st MT head across the osteotomy site. Chevron osteotomy is not well seen on AP radiograph, since it is V-shaped in the sagittal plane.* **(Right)** *AP radiograph shows osteotomy of 1st MT combined with fusion of 1st tarsometatarsal joint ➡ to correct for hypermobile 1st toe and metatarsus primus varus. A shortening osteotomy of the 2nd MT head ➡ was also performed to correct Morton foot alignment.*

TERMINOLOGY

Definitions

- Hallux valgus is well-entrenched misnomer
  - Valgus refers to deformity in vertical plane, apex medial
  - Hallux valgus is deformity of 1st metatarsophalangeal (MTP) joint in horizontal plane, apex medial
    - Correct term would be hallux abductus
  - Some sources use term hallux abductovalgus
- Metatarsus primus varus is also misnomer
  - Varus is deformity in vertical plane, apex lateral
  - Metatarsus primus varus is deformity of 1st tarsometatarsal (TMT) joint in horizontal plane, apex lateral
  - Some sources use term metatarsus primus adductus

IMAGING

General Features

- Location
  - Corrective osteotomies may be performed at multiple locations
    - Osteotomies of 1st metatarsal (MT): Proximal or distal
    - Osteotomies of 1st proximal phalanx

Radiographic Findings

- Silver procedure (bunionectomy): Excision of medial bony prominence of 1st MT head
  - Usually combined with some type of corrective osteotomy
- 1st MT osteotomies: Realignment of MT to improve orientation of MTP joint
  - Osteotomies may be fixed with K-wire or screws
  - Chevron osteotomy: V-shaped in sagittal plane
  - Scarf osteotomy: Z-shaped in sagittal plane
  - Wedge osteotomy of proximal MT
    - Lateral closing or medial opening wedge
  - Ludloff osteotomy: Oblique, oriented 30° from horizontal
    - Proximal margin is dorsal, distal margin is plantar
  - Mitchell osteotomy: L-shaped in axial plane
    - Lateral cortex "notched out"
    - Distal fragment repositioned laterally
  - Crescentic shelf osteotomy
    - In 2 planes, allows rotation of 1st MT
- Keller procedure: Bunionectomy + excision of proximal portion of 1st proximal phalanx
- Lapidus procedure: Bunionectomy + fusion of 1st TMT joint

Imaging Recommendations

- Best imaging tool
  - Radiographs
- Protocol advice
  - AP, lateral **weight-bearing** radiographs

Nuclear Medicine Findings

- Bone scan
  - May show decreased vascularity to 1st MT head, but symptomatic osteonecrosis is rare

PATHOLOGY

Gross Pathologic & Surgical Features

- Soft tissue components of procedures are not directly seen on radiographs and include
  - Modified McBride procedure: Release of adductor hallucis to improve sesamoid alignment
  - Medial capsular plication
  - Lateral capsule release

CLINICAL ISSUES

Surgical Complications

- Hallux varus: Due to release of lateral joint capsule &/or lateral sesamoidectomy
- Recurrent hallux valgus: Due to incomplete correction of underlying deforming forces
- Tendon injury
  - Injury to extensor hallucis longus rarely seen
- Persistent sesamoid displacement
- Dorsiflexion of 1st MTP joint
- Shortening of 1st MT
- Transfer metatarsalgia
  - Transfer of stress to 2nd MT from 1st MT
  - Seen when surgery shortens 1st MT or there is postoperative 1st MTP dorsiflexion
  - Results in Freiberg infraction, 2nd MTP instability, 2nd MT neck or head stress fracture
- Osteomyelitis
  - Fortunately rare
  - Look for erosions, focal osteopenia, cortical breakthrough, resorption around K-wires, screws
- Osteonecrosis of 1st MT head
- Pseudarthrosis or nonunion of attempted arthrodesis

Salvage Operations

- Additional osteotomies to improve alignment
- 1st MTP or 1st carpometacarpal arthrodesis

DIAGNOSTIC CHECKLIST

Reporting Tips

- Describe residual deformity, osteotomy healing
- Be alert for signs of stress transfer to 2nd MT
- Watch for malalignment of sesamoids

SELECTED REFERENCES

1. Chong A et al: Surgery for the correction of hallux valgus: minimum five-year results with a validated patient-reported outcome tool and regression analysis. Bone Joint J. 97-B(2):208-14, 2015
2. Harb Z et al: Adolescent hallux valgus: a systematic review of outcomes following surgery. J Child Orthop. 9(2):105-12, 2015
3. Kim YJ et al: A new measure of tibial sesamoid position in hallux valgus in relation to the coronal rotation of the first metatarsal in CT scans. Foot Ankle Int. 136(8): 944-52, 2015
4. Pentikainen I et al: Preoperative radiological factors correlated to long-term recurrence of hallux valgus following distal chevron osteotomy. Foot Ankle Int. 35(12):1262-7, 2014
5. Sorensen MD et al: Metatarsus primus varus correction: the osteotomies. Clin Podiatr Med Surg. 26(3):409-25, Table of Contents, 2009
6. Chhaya SA et al: Understanding hallux valgus deformity: what the surgeon wants to know from the conventional radiograph. Curr Probl Diagn Radiol. 37(3):127-37, 2008
7. Easley ME et al: Current concepts review: hallux valgus part II: operative treatment. Foot Ankle Int. 28(6):748-58, 2007

Intramedullary Rod/Nail

KEY FACTS

TERMINOLOGY

- Rods: Solid rigid structures
- Nails: Hollow rigid structures that can be locked
- Used to treat long bone fractures
  - Femur and tibia most common
- Share load, allowing for early weight-bearing
- Reaming: To remove intramedullary contents and widen canal by removing endosteal bone; reamed nails usually larger, provide greater stability
- Static locking: Locked at proximal and distal ends
  - Used for unstable fractures: Prevents collapse at fracture leading to leg-length discrepancy
- Dynamic locking: Locked 1 end only
  - Used for transverse or shallow oblique fractures with minimal comminution
- Antegrade placement: Placed from proximal end of bone to distal end of bone; most common direction of insertion
- Retrograde placement: Placed in distal aspect of bone and directed proximally

IMAGING

- Hardware integrity
  - Rod/nail rarely fracture
  - Locking screws may fracture, especially distal locking screws; may allow rod to migrate
- Hardware relationship to bone
  - Rod/nail migration; collapse at fracture site
  - Infection
- Healing: Occurs via periosteal callus

CLINICAL ISSUES

- Fat embolism: Greater risk with reamed nails
- Palpable lump if rods migrate out of bone
- Persistent pain, worsening pain: Nonunion, infection, bursa over protruding hardware
- Limited/painful motion if rod migrates into joint

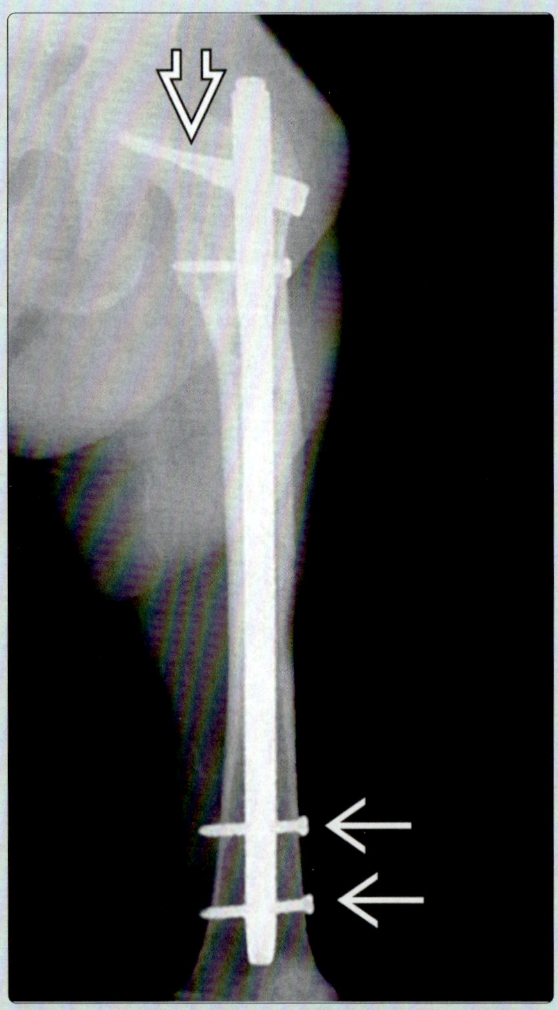

AP radiograph after fixation with a cephalomedullary nail locked distally ➡ is shown. By definition, the nail will have a proximal pin or screw extending into the femoral neck ➡.

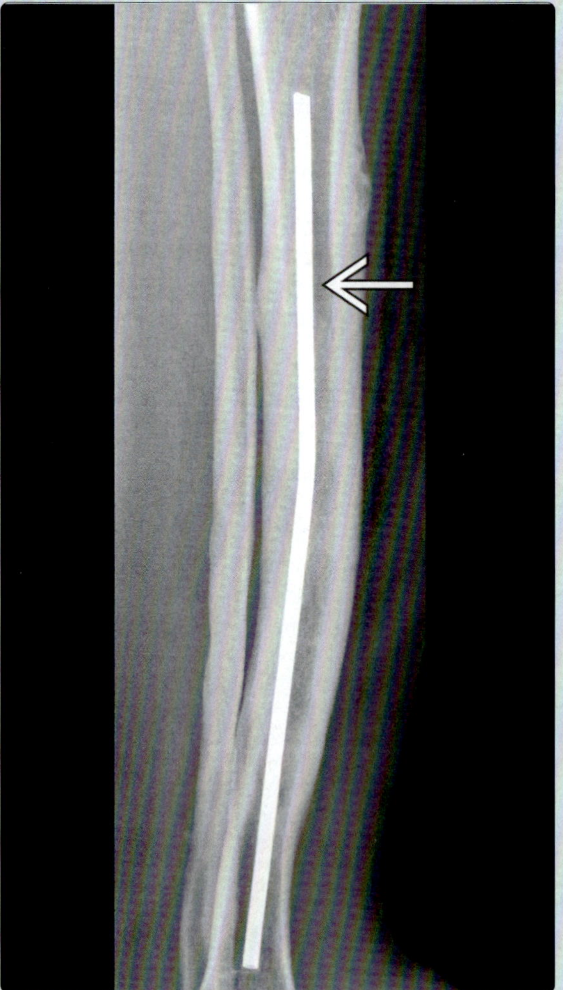

This is a case of recurrent adamantinoma. A flexible rod ➡ had been previously inserted for stabilization. Note the slight anterior bow in the rod. Flexible rods are thinner than rigid nails. Observe how this rod does not fill the entire medullary canal.

TERMINOLOGY

Definitions

- Orthopedic hardware is ever evolving field with constant introduction of new technology
  - Vendor-specific names are often erroneously used to describe hardware types
  - It is impossible to know all names and types
  - Best to understand concepts
- Rods: Solid, usually rigid structures
- Nails: Hollow rigid structures that can be locked
- Antegrade placement: Placed from proximal end of bone to distal end of bone; most common direction of insertion
- Retrograde placement
  - Placed in distal aspect of bone and directed proximally; for example, in femur placed through intercondylar notch and directed proximally
  - Indications for retrograde insertion in femur
    - Obese patients where entry point in proximal femur will be difficult to reach
    - Polytrauma patients to minimize surgical time
    - Distal femoral fractures to achieve better control/reduction

Concepts of Rod/Nail Placement and Use

- Used to treat long bone fractures
- Share load, allowing for early weight-bearing
  - Unlocked and dynamic locking allow micromotion, which stimulates healing
- Insertion with minimal soft tissue dissection
  - Antegrade vs. retrograde determined by site of fracture, ease of access to desired entry site
- Removed after healing achieved in children/young adults
- Dynamic locking
  - Interlocking screw, locked at 1 end only
  - To dynamize means to remove 1 set of screws of static (proximal and distal) locked rod
    - Dynamizing allows compression across fracture
    - Used for transverse or shallow oblique fractures with minimal comminution
- Static locking
  - Rod locked at proximal end and distal end
  - Provides axial and rotational stability
  - Allows immediate weight-bearing
  - Risk is overdistraction, which can lead to delayed healing
  - Used for unstable fractures
  - Prevents collapse at fracture, which could lead to leg-length discrepancy
- Reaming: To remove intramedullary contents and widen canal by removing endosteal bone
  - Disrupts internal blood supply, ↑ infection risk
  - Reamed nails usually larger, provide greater stability
  - May increase risk of fat embolism
- Flexible rods: Ender, Lottes, Rush
  - Less rigid, may require additional stabilization, such as splint/cast
  - Usually place multiple rods via multiple entry sites in metaphysis
  - Used in immature skeleton to avoid growth plate
- Cephalomedullary nails a.k.a. reconstruction or recon nails or proximal femoral nails
  - Placed antegrade in femur for treatment of proximal fractures; has proximal hole to allow insertion of pin/screw into femoral neck
- Gamma nails: Combination of intramedullary rod and sliding screw used for extracapsular proximal femoral fractures

IMAGING

General Features

- Location
  - Femur and tibia most common
- Morphology
  - Cross-sectional shape highly variable
    - Round, cloverleaf, trefoil

Radiographic Findings

- Assess fixation integrity: Hardware integrity, hardware relationship to bone, status of healing
- Healing: Occurs via periosteal callus
- Hardware integrity
  - Rods/nails rarely fracture
  - Locking screws may fracture, especially distal locking screws
    - May allow rod to migrate
    - Breakage during healing phase may produce dynamization where none is desired
- Hardware relationship to bone
  - Assess for collapse at fracture site, especially in comminuted fractures
  - Rod/nail migration
    - May be subtle, comparison with previous films essential
    - May migrate into joint space
    - May piston: Move back and forth within bone
  - Infection
    - Focal or diffuse lucency around rod
    - Cortical destruction, aggressive periostitis

CT Findings

- Useful if radiographs indeterminate for healing

CLINICAL ISSUES

Presentation

- Most common signs/symptoms
  - Palpable lump if rods migrate out of bone
  - Persistent pain, worsening pain: Nonunion, infection, bursa over protruding hardware
  - Limited/painful motion if migrates into joint
- Other signs/symptoms
  - Fat embolism: Clinical diagnosis
    - 2° to marrow displacement during rod placement
    - Greater risk with reamed nails

SELECTED REFERENCES

1. Georgiannos D et al: Subtrochanteric femoral fractures treated with the long Gamma3 nail: a historical control case study versus long trochanteric Gamma nail. Orthop Traumatol Surg Res. ePub, 2015
2. Queally JM et al: Intramedullary nails for extracapsular hip fractures in adults. Cochrane Database Syst Rev. 9:CD004961, 2014

(Left) *AP radiograph of the tibia following treatment of a diaphyseal fracture that had extensive segmental bone loss distally ➡ is shown. A locked ➡ intramedullary rod was placed to maintain length and alignment. In order to address the distal bone defect, a proximal osteotomy was performed ➡. As new bone grows at the osteotomy site, the external fixator ➡ moves the segmental fragment ➡ distally, leading to eventual healing of the fracture and normal length of the bone.* **(Right)** *Lateral radiograph following tibial osteotomy ➡ for treatment of bowing deformity secondary to fibrous dysplasia is shown. An antegrade nail was placed through the tibial tubercle, which is a common insertion site for tibial rods. The holes for insertion of locking screws ➡ are visible in this projection.*

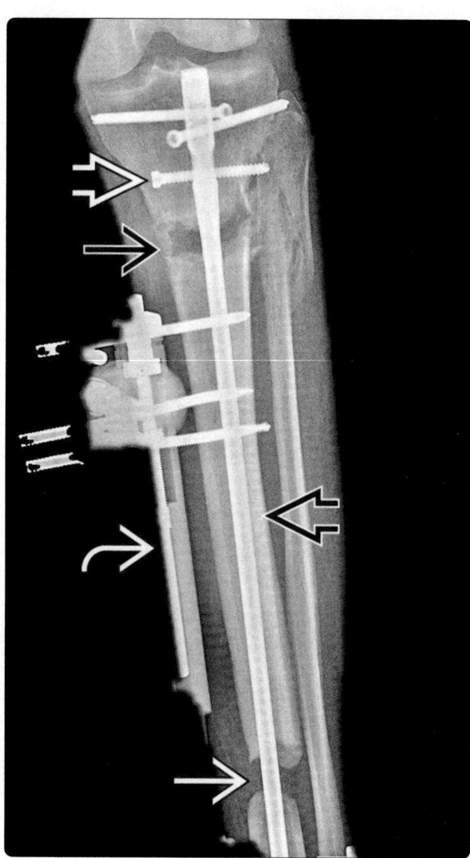

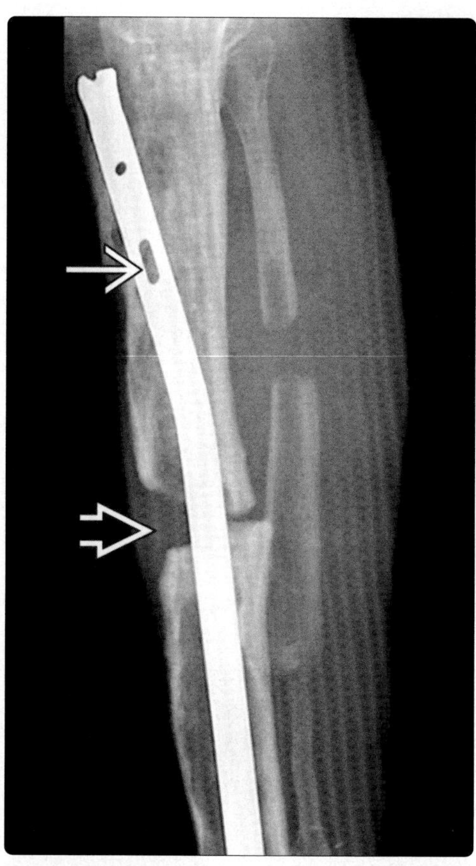

(Left) *AP radiograph of a humerus following placement of an intramedullary rod for fixation of a mildly comminuted midshaft fracture ➡ is shown. The rod is locked proximally and distally ➡. It is difficult to immobilize the humerus with a splint or a cast. The rod prevents displacement or angular deformity, and the locking prevents collapse with shortening across the fracture. Such shortening is especially likely with large butterfly fragments.* **(Right)** *AP radiograph shows an intramedullary nail with distal interlocking screw that has fractured ➡. The fractured screw allows too much motion and results in an ununited tibial fracture.*

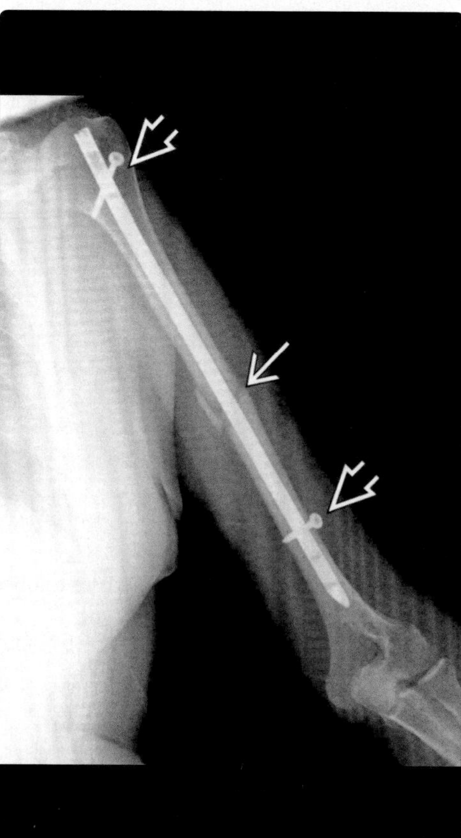

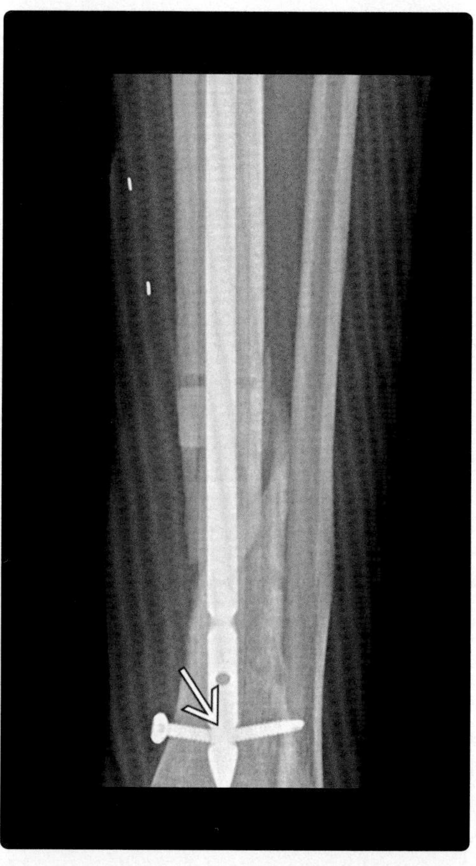

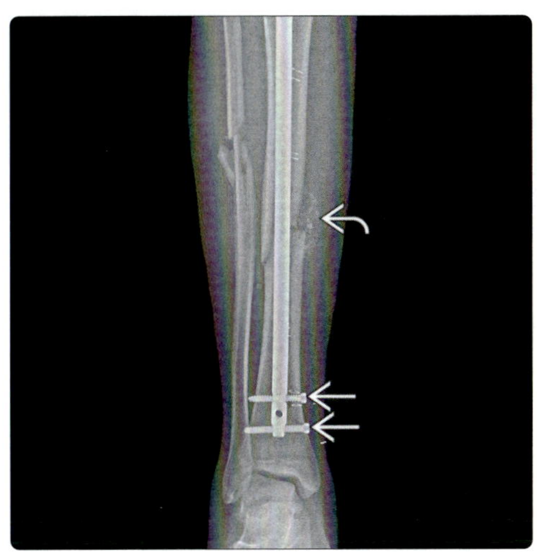

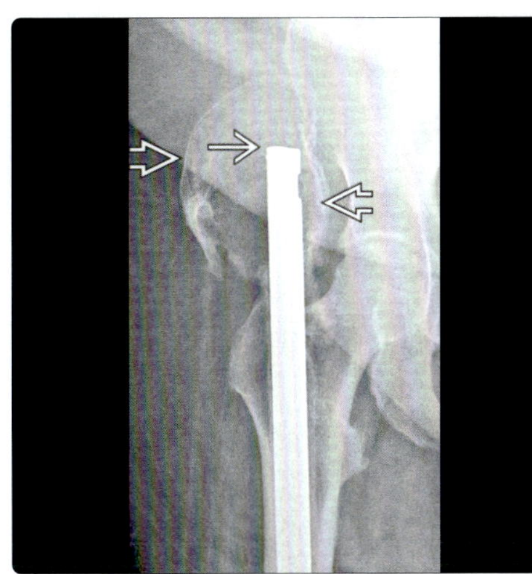

(Left) *AP x-ray shows an intramedullary nail placed antegrade with 2 locking screws ➡, commonly used to prevent migration into the joint. Bone graft is placed at the fracture site ↪. Tibial fractures are slow to heal relative to other long bones because of relatively poor soft tissue coverage.* **(Right)** *AP x-ray shows an intramedullary rod that protrudes several centimeters above the greater trochanter ➡. Heterotopic bone surrounds the tip of the rod ⇨. The rod may not be static and may piston with motion of the leg.*

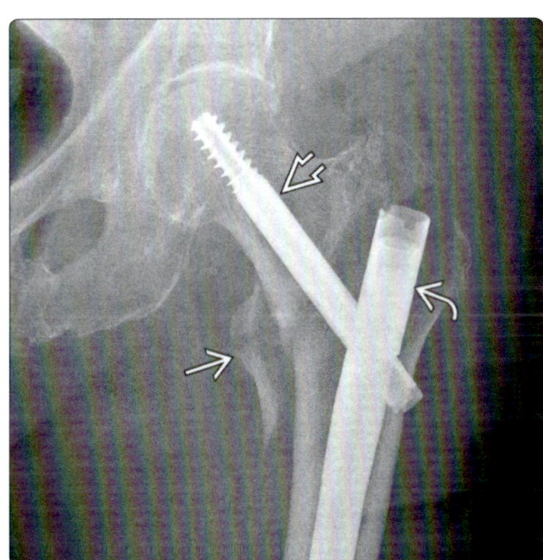

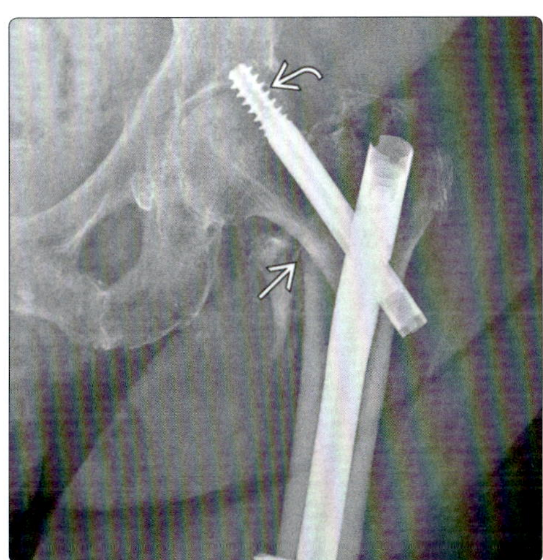

(Left) *AP radiograph shows a Gamma nail ↪ with sliding screw ⇨ securing an intertrochanteric fracture. Alignment at the calcar appears nearly anatomic, but the fragmented lesser trochanter and medial cortex ➡ affects stability.* **(Right)** *AP radiograph in the same patient obtained 4 weeks later shows that the intertrochanteric region has collapsed into varus ➡ and shortened. In addition, the screw has cut out of the femoral head and protrudes into the joint ↪.*

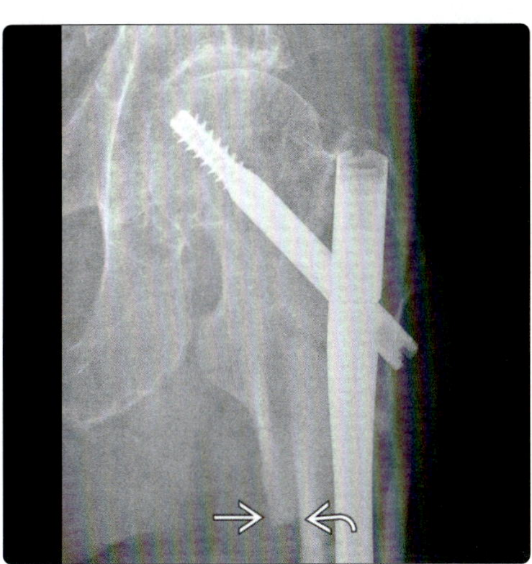

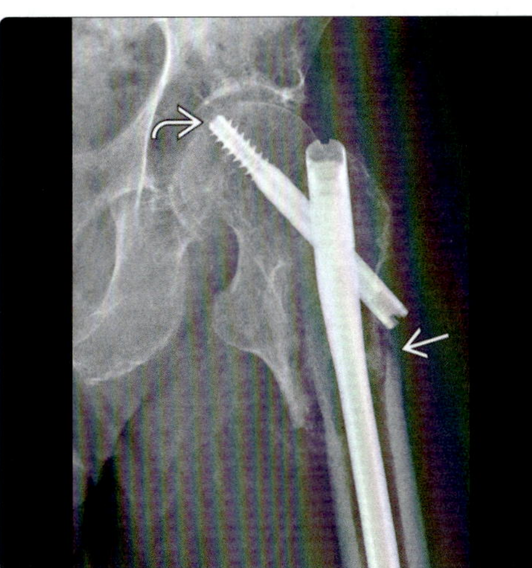

(Left) *AP radiograph shows a Gamma nail and sliding screw utilized for a subtrochanteric fracture. There is lateral displacement of the shaft fragment ↪ relative to the medial cortex ➡, resulting in potential instability. This construct must be followed closely for failure.* **(Right)** *AP radiograph, obtained 3 weeks later, shows collapse by ~ 1 cm; note the overlapping of the lateral cortices ➡. The screw has also migrated within the head ↪ and is close to extruding into the joint. There is minimal periosteal callus formation.*

KEY FACTS

TERMINOLOGY

- Metallic plates fixed to bone by screws; designed to immobilize bone during healing process; technology is ever evolving

IMAGING

- Must always include both ends of plate on follow-up films
- Every fracture evaluation requires at least 2 orthogonal views to assess alignment
- CT and MR imaging
  - Artifact varies from minimal to significant depending on type of metal; greater with stainless steel than titanium
  - Multiple strategies exist to reduce artifact
- Evaluate hardware placement, hardware integrity, fracture alignment, fracture healing
  - Plate should be flush with bone
  - Screws should be flush with plate
  - In healing phase (which will vary with bone quality and quantity, fracture type and location) must seek and report hardware fracture
  - Any change in alignment from immediate posthardware placement films must be reported
  - Healing occurs primarily through endosteal callus; minimal external callus seen

PATHOLOGY

- Compression across fracture stimulates bone healing
- Distraction across fracture creates gap, which new bone must span; may lead to delayed union, nonunion; may be created by misplaced plate
- Extensive soft tissue or periosteal dissection for placement may impair blood supply → impacts healing
- Some stress across fracture desirable to stimulate new bone formation
  - Excessive motion → nonunion
  - Fixation too rigid → inhibits healing

(Left) *AP radiograph shows a distal fibular fracture fixed with a lateral plate. The plate is closely applied to bone, and all of the screws are flush. There is bicortical fixation in the diaphysis ➡ and unicortical fixation ➡ in the metaphysis.* **(Right)** *AP radiograph shows blade plate fixation of the distal femur. The blade portion ➡ angles from the plate. This plate is a rigid form of fixation and can be used when bone contour prevents contact of the plate along the cortex ➡.*

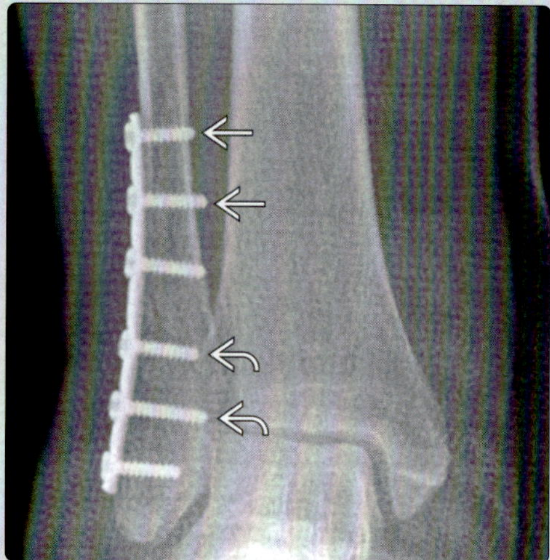

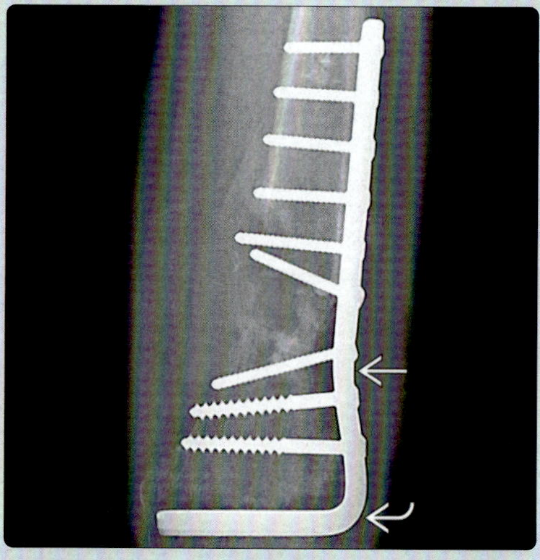

(Left) *AP radiograph following remote fixation of a proximal tibial osteotomy is shown. A buttress plate is commonly used for fixation in this region where weight-bearing produces axial loading forces. The widened ➡ end of the plate is used to support the proximal fragment.* **(Right)** *AP radiograph shows dynamic hip screw instrumentation. A lateral plate is used to secure the implant to the bone ➡. At this time no compression has occurred, as indicated by the lack of screw protruding proximally from the sleeve ➡.*

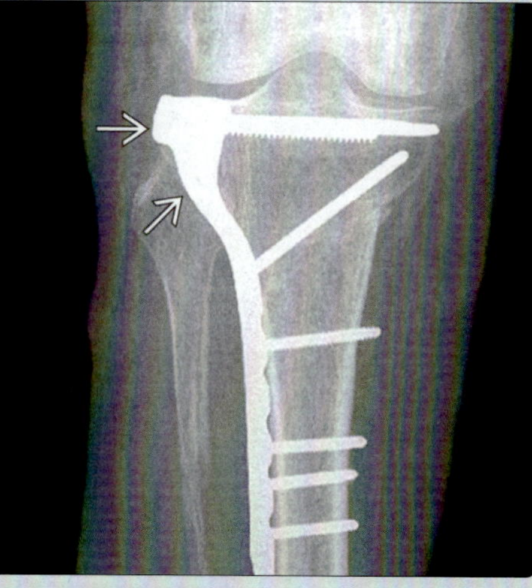

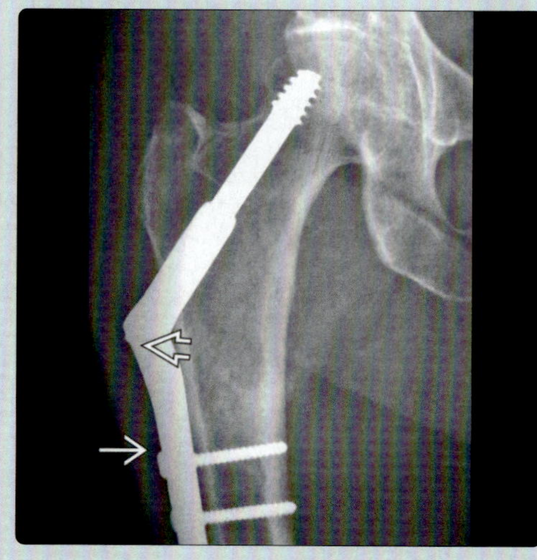

TERMINOLOGY

Definitions

- Metallic plates fixed to bone by screws; designed to immobilize bone during healing process; technology is ever evolving
- Blade plates
  - End of plate has angled extension that is inserted into bone
  - Provides rigid fixation when plate cannot contact entire cortex, such as condylar regions of long bones
- Bridging plates: Crosses comminuted segment
- Buttress plates and T plates
  - 1 end has increased width either through orthogonal bar (T) or some form of flare
  - Placed at sites of thin cortical bone, usually at metaphysis; often used for periarticular fractures
  - Used when deforming forces across fracture are axial/compression: Distal radius, proximal tibia
- Compression plating
  - Specific type of plate with ovoid screw holes
  - Dynamic compression plating: Ovoid holes are oriented so that as screw is tightened, both screw and attached bone are drawn to plate center, resulting in compression
  - Primarily for treatment of diaphyseal fractures
- Dynamic hip screw instrumentation
  - Cancellous lag screw within metal cannula attached to side plate; with weight-bearing screw slides within cannula, resulting in compression at fracture
  - Used for femoral neck and intertrochanteric fractures
- Locking plate: Screw heads threaded to lock with threaded screw hole; joins screws and plate to create single unit; prevents failure due to screws backing out
  - Does not require close application to bone surface
  - May only need unicortical screw fixation
  - ↓ soft tissue damage, ↓ disruption of blood supply
  - Concerns raised that construct is too rigid, inhibiting slight motion required to induce healing
- Neutralization plating
  - Refers to manner in which plate is applied to bone
  - Neutralizes external forces, such as rotation and bending so they are not transmitted to fracture
  - Used to treat comminuted fractures where compression not desirable and comminuted fragments are unable to resist those forces, resulting in collapse of reduction
- 1/3 tubular plates: 1/3 circumference of cylinder
  - Used for fixation of thin tubular bones, such as metatarsals, ulna, fibula
- Reconstruction (recon) plates
  - Low stiffness; notched to allow bending along 3 axes, up to 15° along each axis
  - Can be cut to size and bent to contour along desired shape
  - Fixation of osseous structures with complex anatomy, such as pelvic and acetabular fractures or osteotomies, also distal humerus, clavicle, calcaneus

IMAGING

Imaging Recommendations

- Best imaging tool
  - Radiographs are optimal imaging technique
- Protocol advice
  - Radiographs
    - Must always include entirety of plate on follow-up films
    - Every fracture evaluation requires at least 2 orthogonal views to assess alignment
  - CT and MR
    - Artifact varies from minimal to significant depending on type of metal
      - Greater with stainless steel than titanium
    - Multiple strategies exist to reduce artifact

Radiographic Findings

- Radiography
  - Evaluate hardware placement, hardware integrity, fracture alignment, fracture healing
  - Hardware placement
    - Fracture should be at center of plate
    - Plate should be along tension side of fracture
    - Plate should be flush with bone
    - Screws should be flush with plate
    - Screws may penetrate opposite cortical surface, should not penetrate articular surface
  - Hardware integrity
    - In healing phase (which will vary with bone quality and quantity, fracture type and location) must seek and report hardware fracture
    - Once healing has occurred plate and screws may break; despite efforts to match mechanical properties to bone, metal will eventually fatigue
  - Fracture alignment
    - Acceptable variation from true anatomic reduction depends on patient age and specific bone
    - Any change in alignment from immediate post-hardware placement films must be reported
      - Underlying reason for loss of reduction should be determined
  - Fracture healing
    - Minimal external callus will be seen with plating
    - Healing occurs primarily through endosteal callus

PATHOLOGY

Pertinent Factors Affecting Fracture Healing

- Compression across fracture stimulates bone healing
- Distraction across fracture creates gap, which new bone must span; may lead to delayed union, nonunion
  - Misplacement of plate may create distraction
- Extensive soft tissue or periosteal dissection for placement may impair blood supply, impairing healing
- Some stress across fracture desirable to stimulate new bone formation
  - Excessive motion → nonunion
  - Fixation too rigid → healing is inhibited

SELECTED REFERENCES

1. Zhang J et al: One-stage external fixation using a locking plate: experience in 116 tibial fractures. Orthopedics. 38(8):494-7, 2015
2. Lee MJ et al: Overcoming artifacts from metallic orthopedic implants at high-field-strength MR imaging and multi-detector CT. Radiographics. 27(3):791-803, 2007

(Left) *AP radiograph following internal fixation of a comminuted tibial diaphyseal fracture with a lateral plate and lag screw ➲ is shown.* **(Right)** *Lateral radiograph of the same patient shows that the screws are located in the outer aspect of each ovoid screw hole ➲. This screw position indicates that the compression function of the plate has not been employed. If compression mode had been used, the screws would be located on the side of the hole toward the center of the plate ➲.*

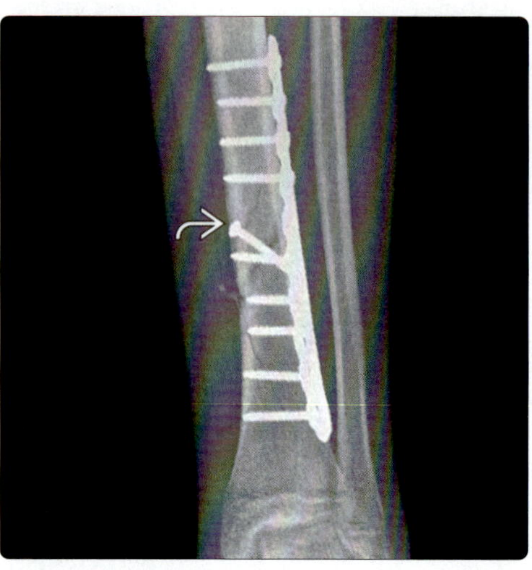

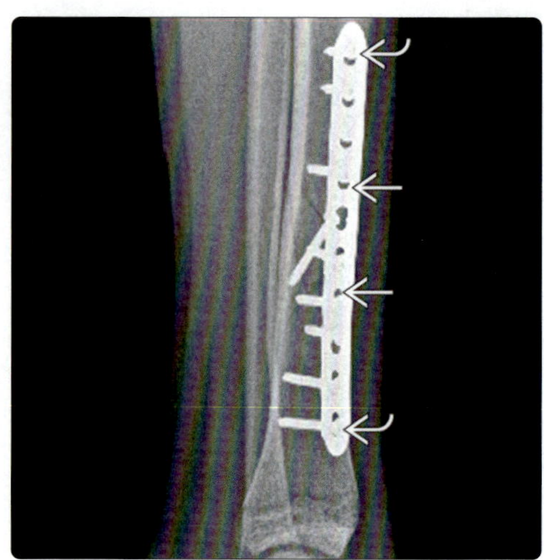

(Left) *AP radiograph shows an ulnar nonunion secondary to hardware failure. The plate has fractured ➲ and distal screws have backed out slightly ➲. The fracture line remains visible with nonbridging external callus ➲.* **(Right)** *Lateral radiograph from the same patient shows the changes are more difficult to appreciate. Several screws have backed out and the plate is discontinuous ➲. External callus is present ➲. External callus is rarely seen in a normal healing bone following plate fixation.*

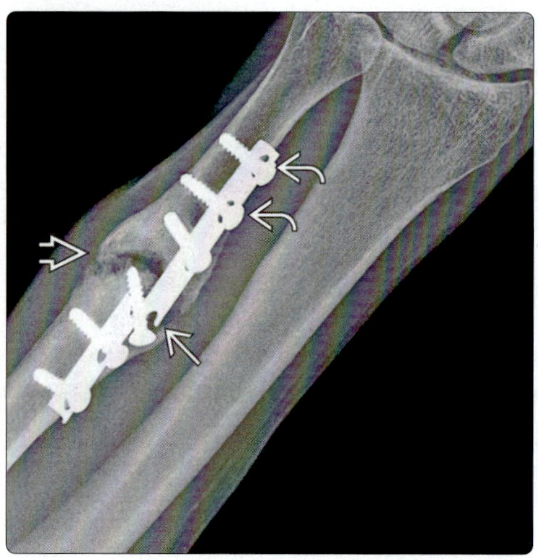

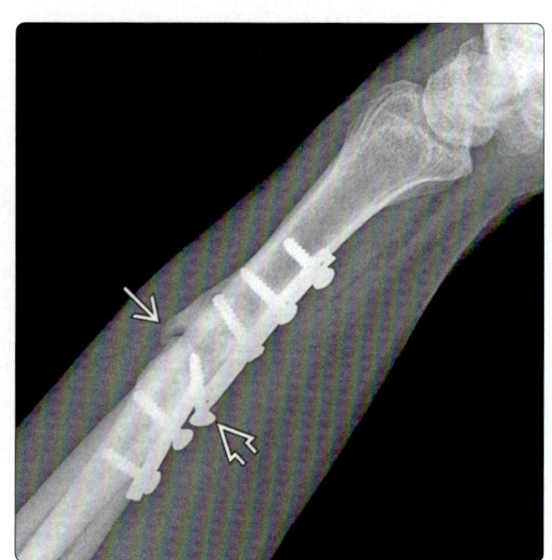

(Left) *AP x-ray of a femur following osteotomy. A blade plate has been used for fixation ➲. The plate is contoured to provide maximal contact with the cortex. Periacetabular osteotomy ➲ has also been performed.* **(Right)** *Lateral x-ray shows subtle fracture of the compression plate ➲. In addition, note that the head of the screw (visible in the hole ➲) is angled and discontinuous with its shaft ➲, indicating that the screw has fractured at the junction of the head and shaft (most typical site of screw fracture).*

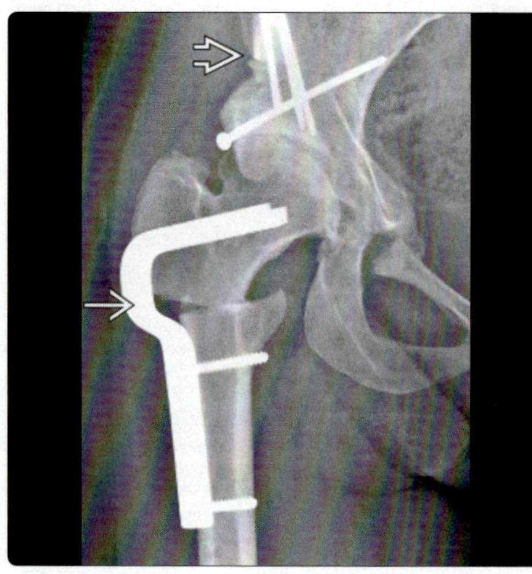

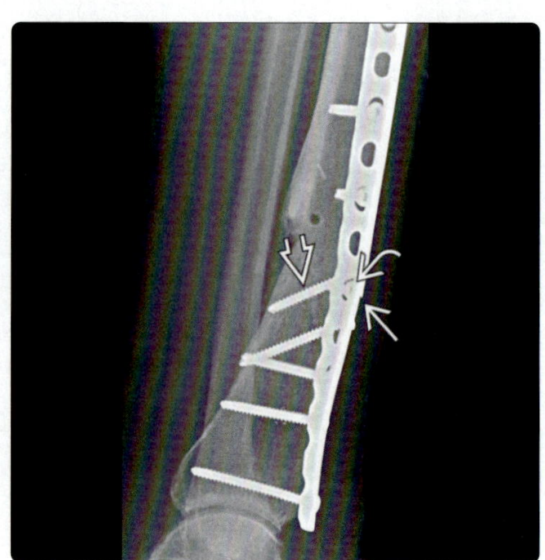

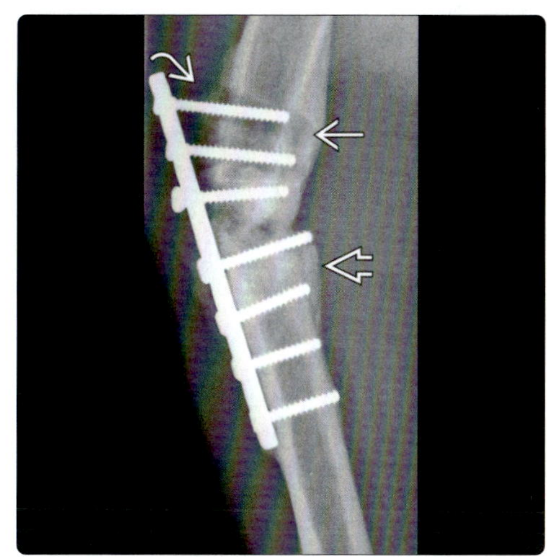

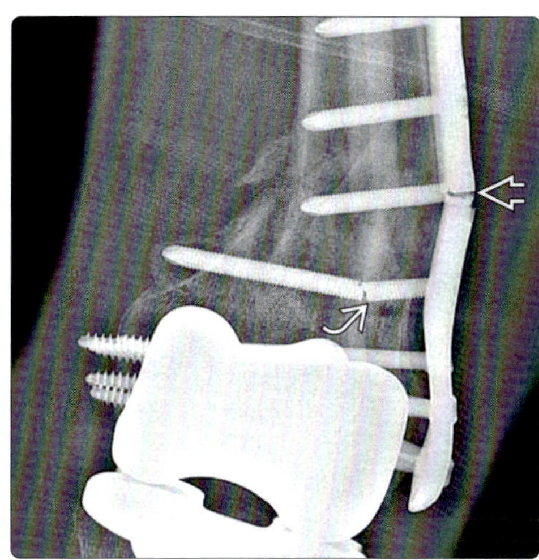

(Left) *AP radiograph shows femur with hypertrophic nonunion. Extensive lucency around the proximal screw is the result of motion →. The plate and screws have lifted off the bone →. Extensive periosteal callus is present without bridging the fracture →.* **(Right)** *AP radiograph shows the distal femur with hardware failure. The plate → and 1 screw → have fractured, allowing angulation between fracture fragments even though the plate has not lifted off the cortex.*

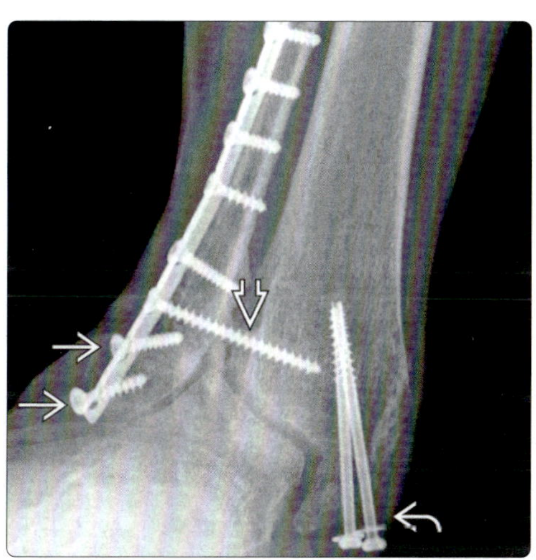

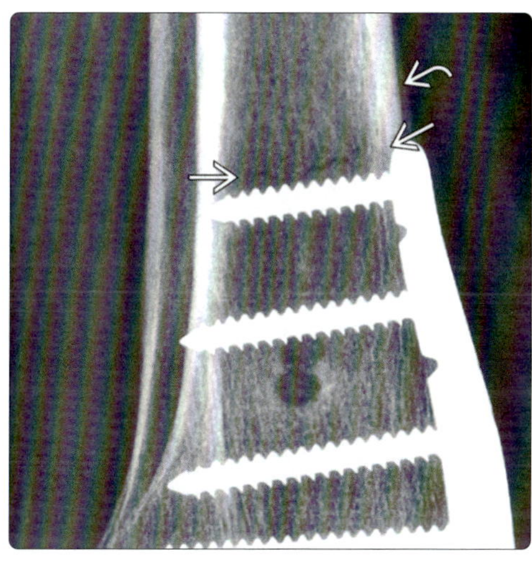

(Left) *AP radiograph shows failure of fixation. Medial malleolar screws → have backed out slightly. Fibular plate is intact with slight back out of distal screws →. The plate has not lifted off the cortex. The syndesmotic screw has backed out with widening of the distal tibiofibular articulation →.* **(Right)** *AP radiograph shows a stress fracture → at the proximal end of a plate. These fractures can be extremely subtle; in this case, a small amount of callus has formed →, which may lead one to the diagnosis.*

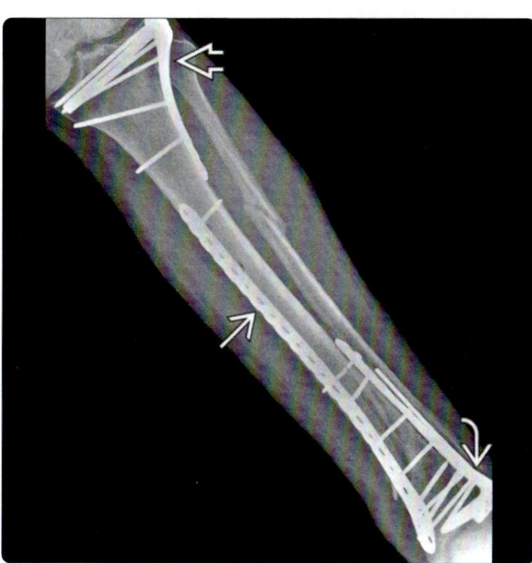

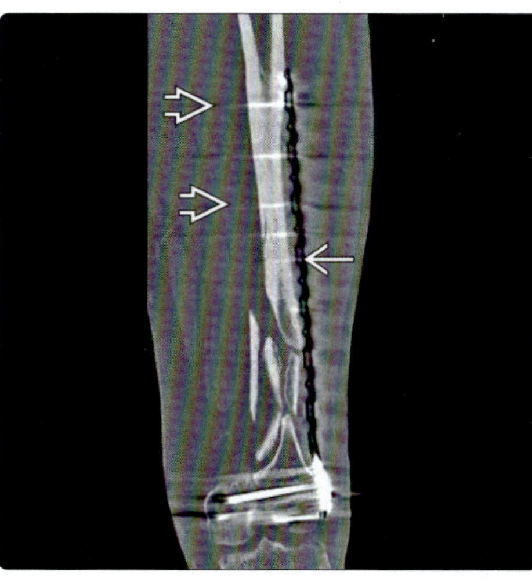

(Left) *AP radiograph shows extensive tibial instrumentation. Proximal lateral buttress plate →, long medial plate →, and distal lateral blade plate → have been used. Extensive instrumentation has a high likelihood of complication due to compromised blood supply.* **(Right)** *Coronal reformatted bone CT shows long lateral plate → and screws →. Artifact reduction techniques allow the bone around the hardware to be visualized. This technique allows assessment of healing status (atrophic nonunion in this case).*

Screw Fixation

KEY FACTS

TERMINOLOGY

- Cancellous screw
  - Deep, widely spaced threads; used in metaphyseal bone; weaker than cortical screw
- Cortical screw
  - Fully threaded with shallow, closely spaced threads
  - Used with plates and for fixation of diaphyseal bone
- Herbert screw/Acutrak screw
  - Produces compression as inserted into bone
  - Primarily used in scaphoid
- Interference screw
  - Fixation of tendon and bone grafts within osseous tunnel: Usually ACL repair
- Lag screw technique
  - Method of using screw, not specific screw type
  - Screw not engaged in proximal fragment; as screw is tightened in distal fragment it draws that fragment closer to proximal fragment

IMAGING

- Fixation integrity consists of hardware integrity, relationship with hardware, relationship between hardware and bone
  - Hardware integrity
    - Screw fracture during healing phase may lead to loss of stabilization
  - Hardware relationship to bone
    - Lucency around screws seen with motion &/or infection
    - Screw backing out may lead to loss of stabilization
- Pin tract sequestrum: Doughnut-shaped sclerotic focus at site of previous pin
- CT and MR: Difficulties arise because of metallic artifacts; stainless steel artifact > > titanium

CLINICAL ISSUES

- Indicators of fixation failure: Pain, palpable lump

(Left) *Oblique radiograph following fixation of a metatarsal fracture ➡ with a fully threaded screw is shown. The threads are deep and widely spaced, characteristic of a cancellous screw. These features make the threads easy to visualize.* **(Right)** *Sagittal cutaway graphic of distal radius with volar buttress plate is shown. The plate prevents the distal radius from collapsing into the shaft. Bicortical fixation with cortical screws ➡ is used in the diaphysis, while a cancellous screw ➡ is placed in the metaphysis.*

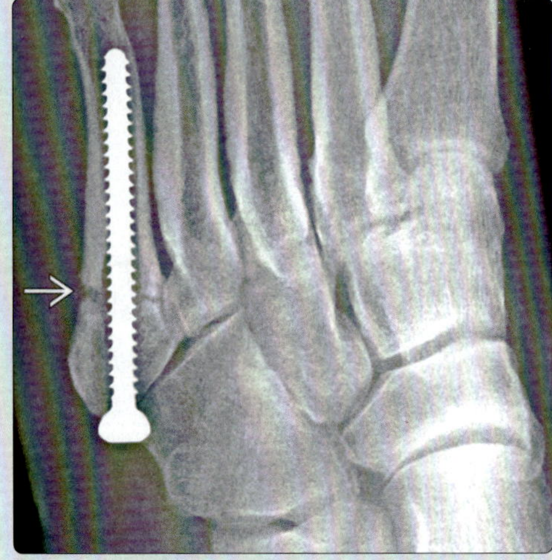

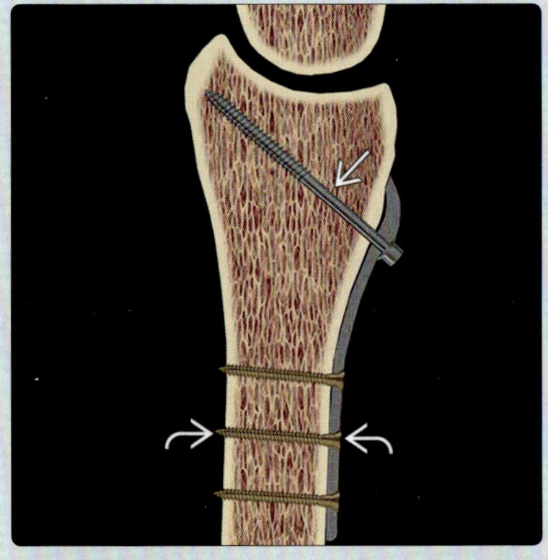

(Left) *AP radiograph shows a screw transfixing the medial epicondyle. This partially threaded screw ➡ was placed with lag screw technique, providing compression across the fracture. The absence of the threads proximally means that the screw is not engaged within the proximal fragment.* **(Right)** *AP radiograph of an ankle following internal fixation is shown. Lateral fibular plate ➡ and interfragmentary screw ➡ have been employed. A syndesmotic screw ➡ is present with tricortical (2 fibular and 1 tibial) fixation.*

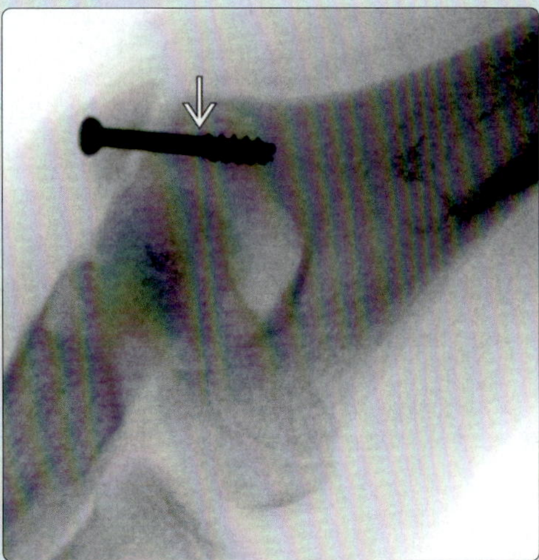

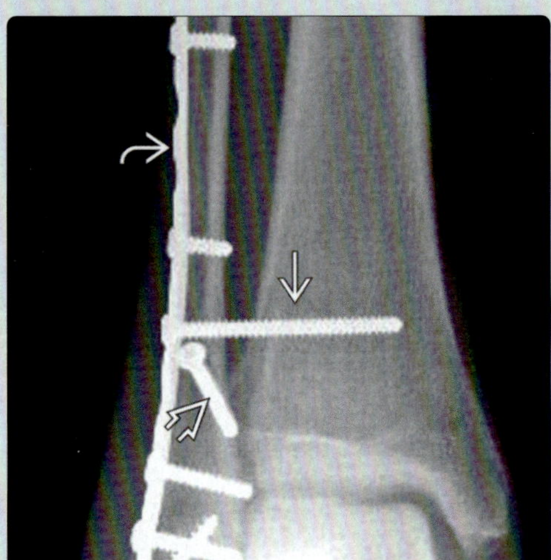

TERMINOLOGY

Definitions

- Cannulated screw: Hollow screw for placement over guidewire
- Core: Central tube around which threads are wound; may be hollow or solid
- Core diameter: Diameter of core portion of screw
- Head: Flat surface on screw opposite tip; helps prevent inserting screw too far
- Pitch: Distance between threads
- Pullout strength: Amount of energy required to pullout or disengage screw from bone
- Outer diameter (OD): Diameter of outer margin of threads measured from thread tip to thread tip
- Shaft: Nonthreaded portion of screw
- Shank: Threaded portion of screw
- Tap: Instrument inserted through predrilled hole to create threads (channel) for screw
  - Tapping: Process of inserting tap
- Thread: Inclined plane (semihorizontally oriented structure), which wraps around screw core
  - Converts rotational force of turning screw into linear force, driving screw forward into bone
  - Width of threads may vary (deep or shallow), depending on screw type
  - Screws may be **fully** or **partially** threaded depending on whether threads traverse part of or entire core
- Tip: Distal end of screw 1st inserted into bone
  - May be blunt
  - **Self-tapping**: Allows screw to be advanced without tapping
    - Screws cut their own path through bone
    - Require predrilling hole size of screw core into cortex
  - Nonself-tapping screws require tap to be advanced after drilling hole size of core diameter

Basic Screw Types

- Cancellous screw
  - Threads are deep, widely spaced
  - Relatively thin core
  - For same OD, weaker than cortical screws
  - Used for fixation of metaphyseal bone
  - Self-tapping or nonself-tapping
  - Fully or partially threaded
- Cortical screw
  - Threads are shallow, closely spaced
  - Fully threaded
  - For same OD, stronger than cancellous screw
  - For fixation of diaphyseal bone
  - For same OD, larger central core than cancellous screw
  - Blunt tip, nonself-tapping
  - Used for plate fixation
    - Fixation often described by number of cortices engaged
      - Unicortical fixation crosses 1 cortex; may be used with locking plate
      - Bicortical fixation engages both cortices, protrudes into soft tissues 1-2 mm
      - Tricortical and quadricortical fixation also used

Specialty Screws

- Arthroereisis screw
  - Bullet-shaped
  - Threads are blunted
  - Cannulated
  - Used to stabilize subtalar joint in flexible flat foot
- Dynamic hip screw
  - Cancellous lag screw within metal cannula attached to side plate
  - For fixation of femoral neck and intertrochanteric fractures
  - With weight bearing, screw slides within metal cannula resulting in compression across fracture
- Herbert screw/Acutrak screw
  - Cannulated screw
  - Distal end: Cancellous threads, smaller OD
  - Proximal end: Cortical threads greater OD
  - Produces compression as inserted into bone
  - With each screw turn, distal end travels further along longitudinal axis than proximal end due to greater thread pitch in distal portion of screw
- Interference screws
  - Fixation of tendon and bone grafts within osseous tunnel
  - Most commonly used in ACL repair
  - Bullet-shaped, cannulated, and fully threaded

Related Hardware

- Kirschner (K-) wires
  - Thin, sharp, smooth, stainless steel
  - Often used for temporary intraoperative fixation; allows control of fragments, aiding reduction and then maintaining reduction during placement of more definitive fixation
  - May be used as fracture fixation in small bones of hands and feet; often placed percutaneously for this application
- Steinman pins
  - Threaded or nonthreaded
  - Larger than K-wires
  - Previously known as traction pins
  - Rarely used today

Other

- Lag screw technique
  - Method of using screw, not specific screw type
  - Screw not engaged in proximal fragment; as screw is tightened in distal fragment, it draws that fragment closer to proximal fragment
  - Interfragmentary screws are placed as lag screws: Used to produce compression across fracture
  - Cortical or cancellous screws may be lag screws
    - With cortical screws, overdrilling proximal cortex so threads are not engaged converts to lag technique
  - Cannot identify lag screw by radiographic appearance
- Syndesmotic screw technique
  - Used to immobilize distal tibiofibular syndesmosis
  - Placed through fibula into tibia
  - Tricortical fixation most common
    - 2 fibular cortices, 1 tibial cortex

IMAGING

General Features

- Best diagnostic clue
  - Screws used for skeletal stabilization
    - Fracture fixation
      - Either in isolation or in conjunction with fixation plates, intramedullary rods
    - Postoperative stabilization
      - Pedicle screw instrumentation of spine
      - Plate fixation for spine fusion
      - Fixation of implants for joint replacement
      - Arthrodesis
      - Arthroereisis

Radiographic Findings

- Radiography
  - Assess
    - Fixation integrity, including screws, plates, nails, etc.
    - Healing
  - Fixation integrity: Hardware integrity, relationship among hardware, hardware relationship to bone
  - Hardware integrity: Screw fracture
    - Occurs in partially threaded screw at junction of threaded/nonthreaded segments
    - Often seen in distal interlocking screws of intramedullary rod
    - Screw fracture during healing phase indicates motion
      - Risk for nonunion
    - Once healing has occurred, screw fracture may occur
      - Bone is elastic structure, mechanical properties not matched by screw, metal fatigue may occur
  - Hardware relationship to bone
    - Screws backing out may lead to loss of stabilization
    - Rarely screws subside (sink further into bone)
    - Lucency around screws
      - Seen with motion: Usually mirrors shape of screw
      - Consider possibility of infection: Irregular shape, ill-defined margins
    - Pin tract sequestrum: Doughnut-shaped sclerotic focus at site of pin removal
    - Screws may serve as stress risers, resulting in stress fracture
  - Fracture healing
    - Screws not as rigid as plates or rods; may see periosteal callus
      - Periosteal callus more common in diaphyseal region; less common in metaphysis, condyles, tuberosities, carpal and tarsal bones

CT Findings

- CT may be desirable as sensitive method to assess fracture healing
  - Difficulties arise because of metallic artifacts
    - Artifact from stainless steel > > titanium
- Hardware artifact reduction techniques
  - Short axis of screw should be as parallel to imaging plane as possible
  - Use higher peak voltage, increase tube charge (higher photon flux)
    - Higher milliampere-seconds
    - Higher patient dose
  - Narrow collimation
  - Thin acquisition slices, thicker reconstructed slices
  - Use standard reconstruction algorithm; bone algorithm accentuates artifact
  - View with wide windows

MR Findings

- MR use to image directly around screw less frequent than CT
- May need to image structure around hardware, e.g., to evaluate status of reconstructed ACL
  - Difficulties arise because of metallic susceptibility artifacts
  - Artifact from stainless steel > > titanium
  - Artifacts create more image distortion with MR than CT
- Factors that decrease artifact
  - Orientation of screw along long axis parallel to main magnetic field
  - Fast spin-echo sequences better than spin-echo; gradient echo sequences have severe artifact
    - Use short echo spacing
  - STIR sequences better than fat-suppressed images
  - Lower field strength systems
  - Increased gradient strength
  - Smaller field of view, increased spatial resolution along frequency encoding axis
  - Increased matrix size
  - Increased echo train length

CLINICAL ISSUES

Presentation

- Most common signs/symptoms
  - Clinical indicators of failure of fixation
    - Pain
      - Motion at fixation site
      - Nonunion
      - Infection
      - Bursa may develop over screw heads
    - Palpable lump
      - Hardware backing out may be palpable under skin
      - Exuberant callus

DIAGNOSTIC CHECKLIST

Image Interpretation Pearls

- Comparison with immediate postoperative films provides most sensitive assessment for change in screw position

SELECTED REFERENCES

1. Downey MW et al: Fully threaded versus partially threaded screws: determining shear in cancellous bone fixation. J Foot Ankle Surg. 54(6):1021-4, 2015
2. Lee MJ et al: Overcoming artifacts from metallic orthopedic implants at high-field-strength MR imaging and multi-detector CT. Radiographics. 27(3):791-803, 2007
3. Douglas-Akinwande AC et al: Multichannel CT: evaluating the spine in postoperative patients with orthopedic hardware. Radiographics. 26 Suppl 1:S97-110, 2006

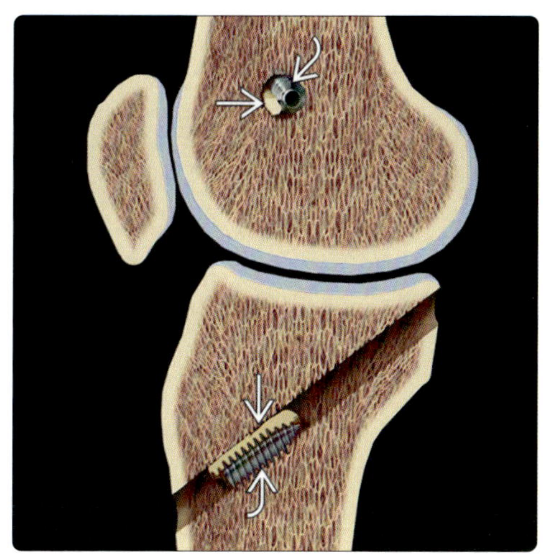

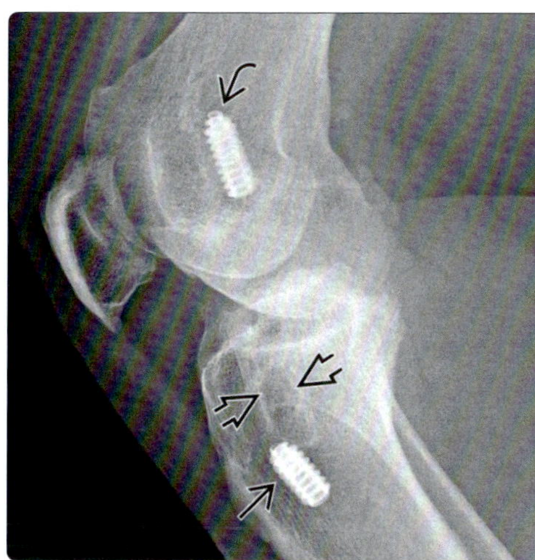

(Left) *Sagittal cutaway graphic following PCL reconstruction shows interference screws ➡ present in femoral and tibial tunnels. Each screw provides fixation for bone plug ➡ at each end of graft by pressing it against the tunnel wall (soft tissue portion not shown).* **(Right)** *Lateral x-ray following ACL reconstruction is shown. Interference screws have been used. The femoral screw is normally positioned ➡. The tibial screw ➡ is abnormally positioned relative to the tibial tunnel ➡ as a result of accidental graft pullout.*

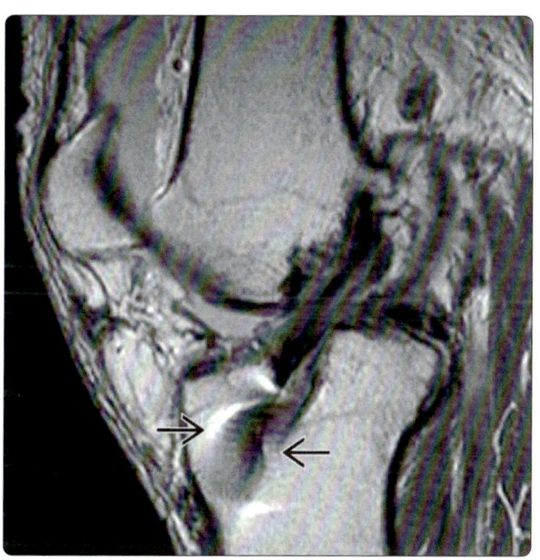

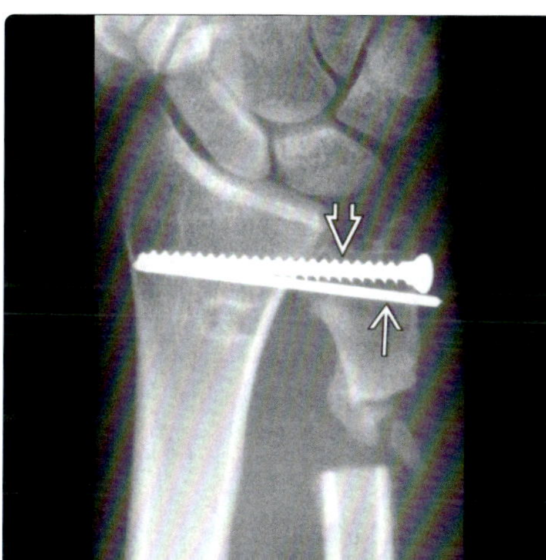

(Left) *Sagittal PD/intermediate MR of patient with prior ACL reconstruction and new onset pain is shown. Magnetic susceptibility artifact is confined to the region of the screw ➡ without distortion of the neo-ACL.* **(Right)** *PA radiograph demonstrates hardware for distal radioulnar joint arthrodesis. A smooth pin ➡ and a cancellous screw ➡ have been used to provide fixation. The relatively thin cortex of the distal ends of these bones favors use of cancellous screws over cortical screws.*

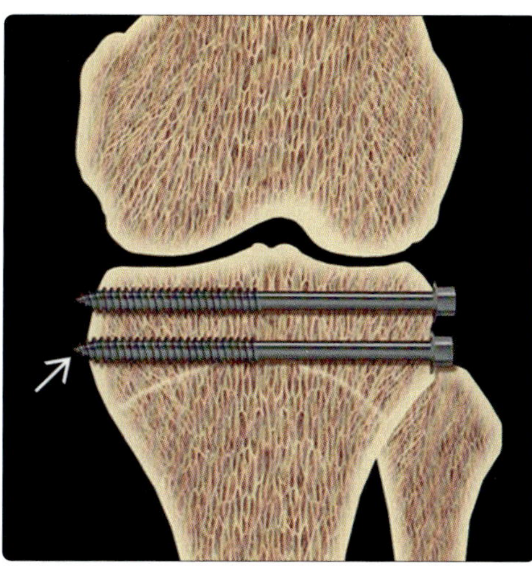

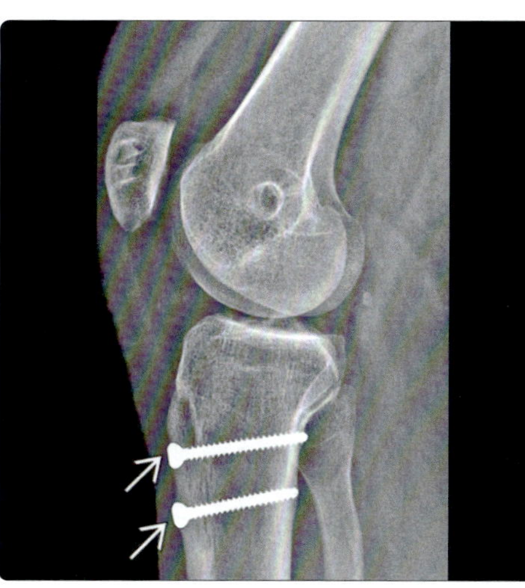

(Left) *Coronal cutaway graphic of tibia following fixation for a tibial plateau fracture is shown. Fractures without significant loss of bone stock or other indicators of instability do not require buttress plates. Lag screw technique is often employed. The screws may penetrate 1-2 mm beyond the opposite cortex ➡.* **(Right)** *Lateral radiograph following patellar realignment is shown. Cortical screws (small, closely spaced threads) ➡ have been used for fixation of the realigned tibial tubercle.*

(Left) *AP radiograph was obtained in the operating room during placement of cannulated screws. Guidepins ➡ have been placed & the screws are then inserted over the pins. Placement of thin guidepins allows for repositioning with minimal bone damage.* **(Right)** *AP radiograph shows the wrist with a Herbert screw. The proximal OD ➡ is > the distal OD ➡, allowing a channel to be drilled for passage of the distal end with subsequent placement & purchase of the larger proximal end of the screw.*

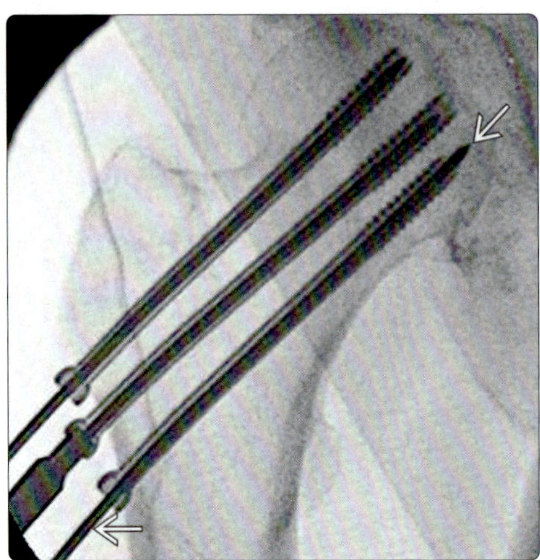

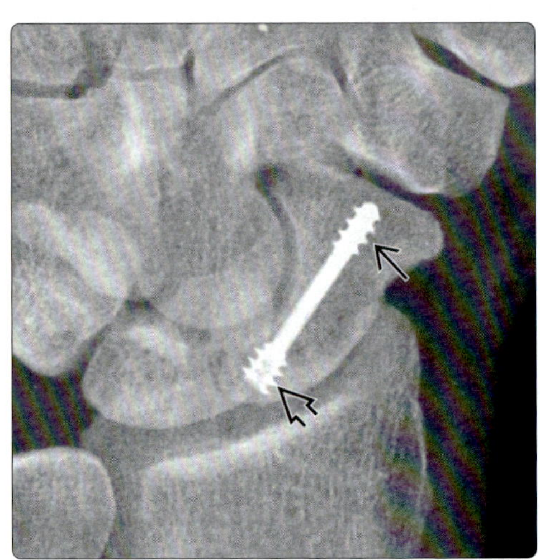

(Left) *Coronal T1WI MR following Herbert screw fixation of a scaphoid fracture ➡ shows minimal susceptibility artifact ➡. Spin-echo imaging helps reduce metallic artifact.* **(Right)** *PA radiograph after surgery for lunatomalacia shows buttress plate is present on the distal radius ➡. Capitoscaphoid fusion has been performed with screws that follow the same principle as a Herbert screw. The pitch between distal threads ➡ is greater than the proximal pitch ➡. As the screw is advanced, it compresses the bones.*

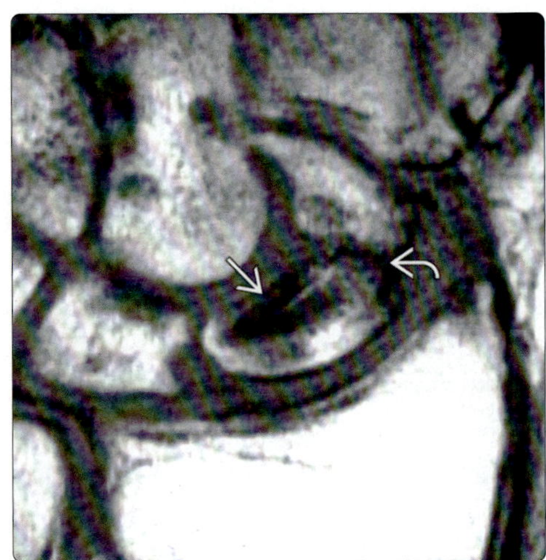

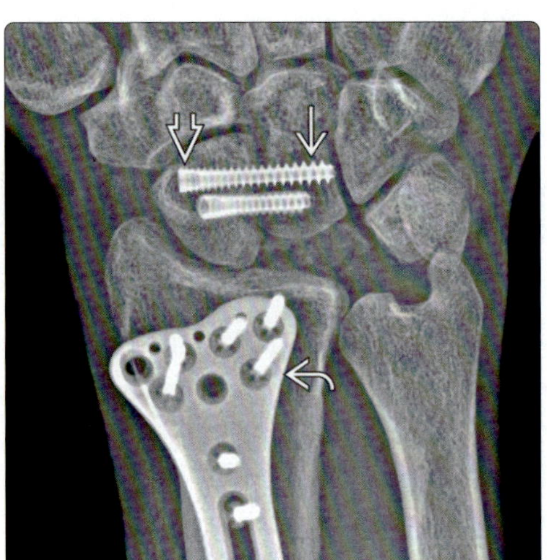

(Left) *Lateral x-ray following occipitocervical fusion. Several problems with fixation have developed, including backing out of occipital screw ➡ and complete loss of fixation of one of the transarticular screws ➡ (which now no longer crosses the C1-C2 articulation).* **(Right)** *Axial CT of vertebral body with pedicle screw instrumentation ➡ complicated by fracture ➡ of the pedicle as well as displacement of a cap ➡. The high trabecular content of vertebrae require deep threads to achieve satisfactory purchase.*

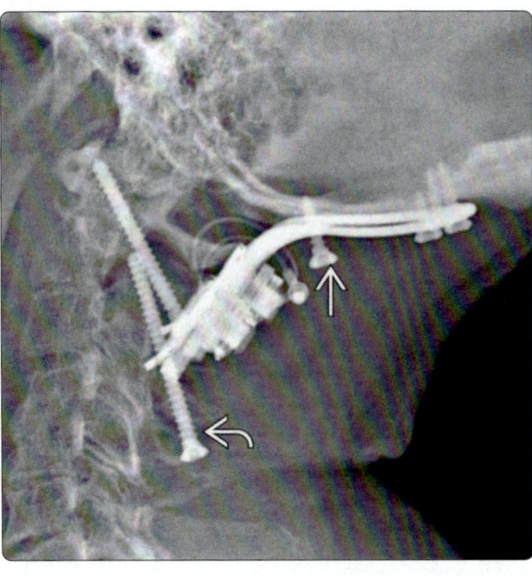

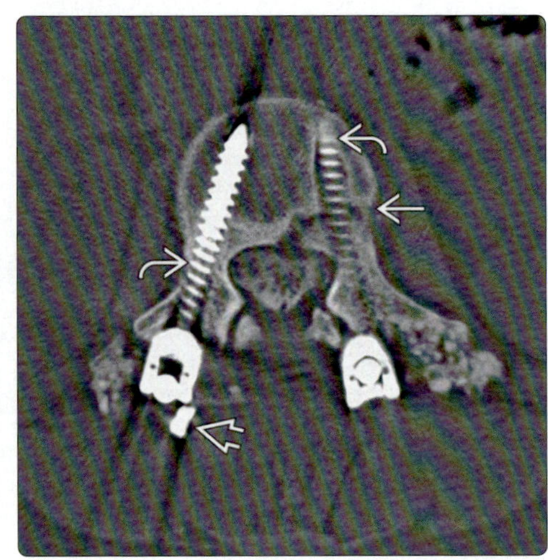

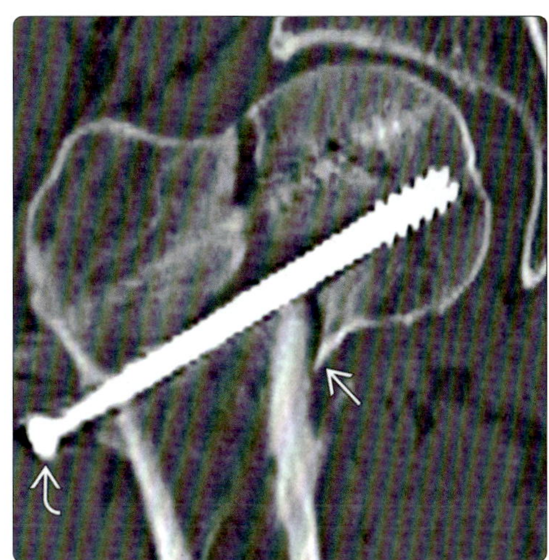

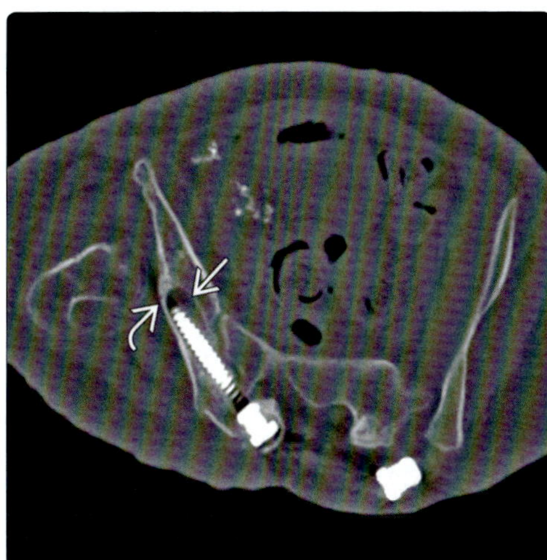

(Left) *Coronal reformat bone CT of a nonunion is shown. Significant resorption of the femoral neck has led to failure of healing. The head has collapsed onto the remnant of the neck ➡, driving the screw head away from the cortex ➡.* **(Right)** *Axial bone CT with SI joint screw fixation is shown. Extensive lucency ➡ is present around the right screw. Lucency is greatest at the screw tip. The finding indicates screw motion; nonunion is likely. Remodeling along the posterior iliac cortex ➡ indicates a longstanding process.*

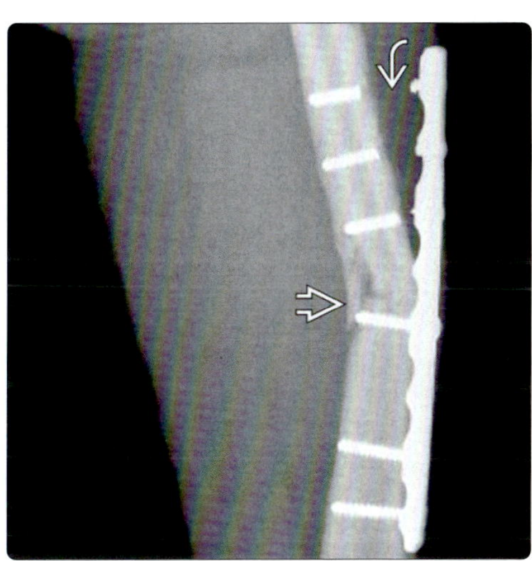

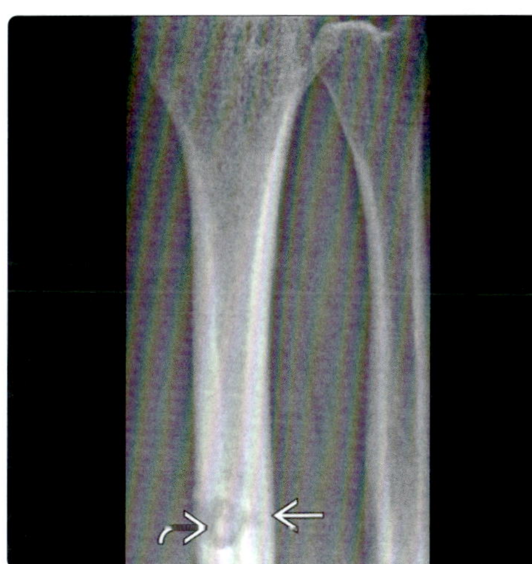

(Left) *AP radiograph of the femur following internal fixation is shown. The patient has been experiencing increasing pain. The proximal 3 screws of the plate have fractured ➡, allowing the plate to lift off bone and losing all fixation. The fracture has not healed and angulation has developed ➡.* **(Right)** *AP radiograph demonstrates an old thin pin tract ➡ that has widened into a round lytic lesion with central sclerosis ➡. The central sclerosis is a sequestrum in this pin tract infection.*

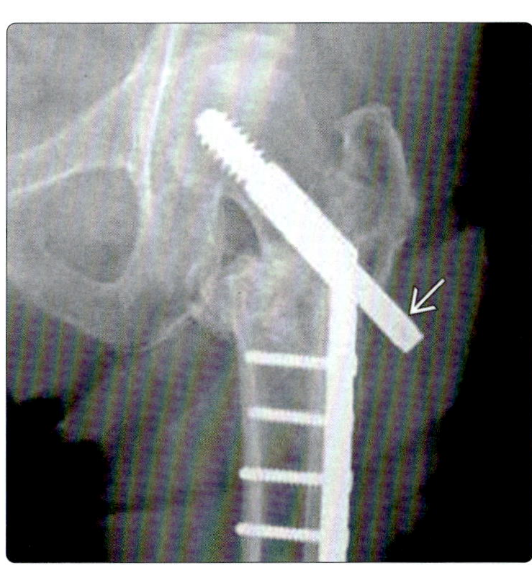

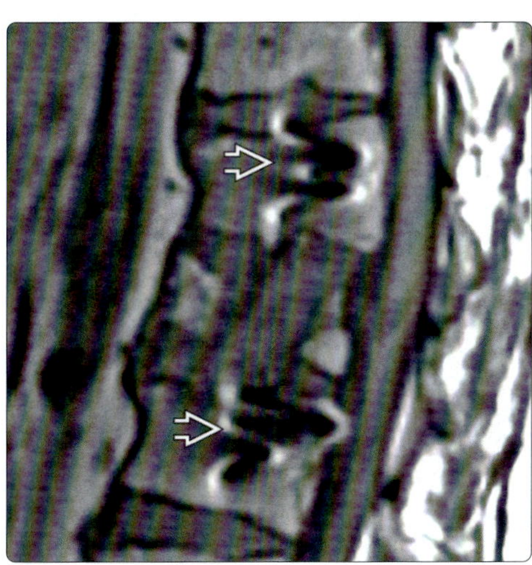

(Left) *AP radiograph with dynamic hip screw shows the screw is well positioned without penetration of the articular surface. Compression is evident with protrusion of screw from sleeve ➡, a satisfactory result since the fracture healed.* **(Right)** *Sagittal T1WI MR following screw fixation ➡ within the vertebral bodies shows typical arrow-shaped artifact visible along the short axis of the screw. The distortion occurs along the phase-encoding axis. Minimal artifact indicates that the screws are titanium.*

Cement and Bone Fillers

KEY FACTS

TERMINOLOGY

- Purpose: Different techniques used to fill defects, restore structure and strength, provide scaffold for bone ingrowth

IMAGING

- Radiographs are optimal for assessing position of graft and status of incorporation
- Requires serial films to assess incorporation or failure
- Techniques for filling defects
  - Bone cement
    - < 2-mm lucency with sclerotic rim at bone/cement or bone/component interface within normal limits
    - > 2-mm lucency following joint replacement concerning for loosening or particle disease
    - Irregular lucency following curettage and cementation of tumor concerning for recurrence
    - Cement shows signal void on all MR sequences
  - Cancellous graft
    - May initially mimic tumor matrix or mineralization
    - Over time resorbs as new bone incorporates graft
  - Cortical graft: Support for large defects
    - May be either structural or nonstructural
  - Bone autografts
    - Autograft: From self, contains marrow elements
    - Initially have same imaging characteristics as normal bone/marrow
    - Intermediate phase with granulation tissue
    - If successfully incorporated, over long term has appearance of normal marrow
  - Bone allografts
    - Allograft: Derived from different individual; lacks marrow elements; high rate of complications
    - Initially ↓ T1 and ↓ T2 signal due to lack of marrow elements
    - Persistent low signal indicates failure of incorporation

CLINICAL ISSUES

- Successful incorporation is asymptomatic

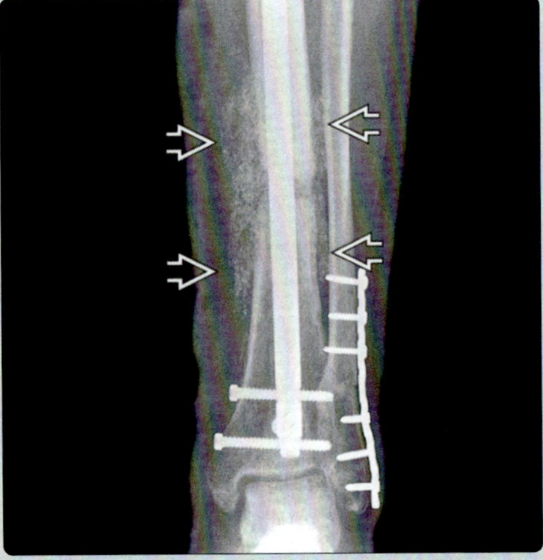

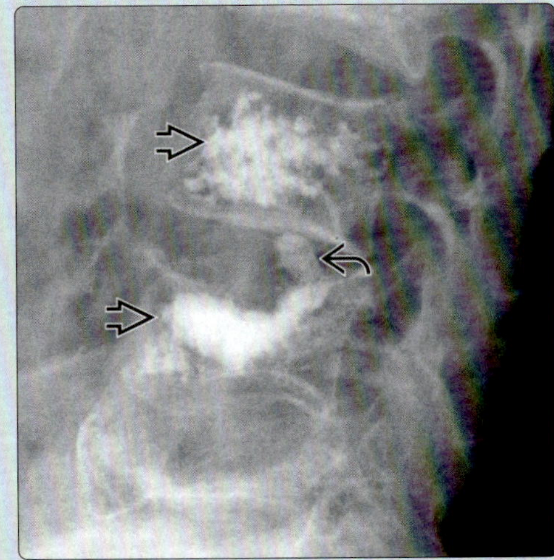

(Left) *AP radiograph following a tibial fracture fixation is shown. Morselized bone graft has been placed within and around the gap ➡. Graft fragments are relatively discrete, indicating they have been recently placed.* **(Right)** *Lateral radiograph following vertebral augmentation with cement is shown. The cement has a uniform density and is interspersed among the trabecula ➡ and into the disc space ➡. In this application, the cement is rarely confused with mineralization or ossification in a pathologic process.*

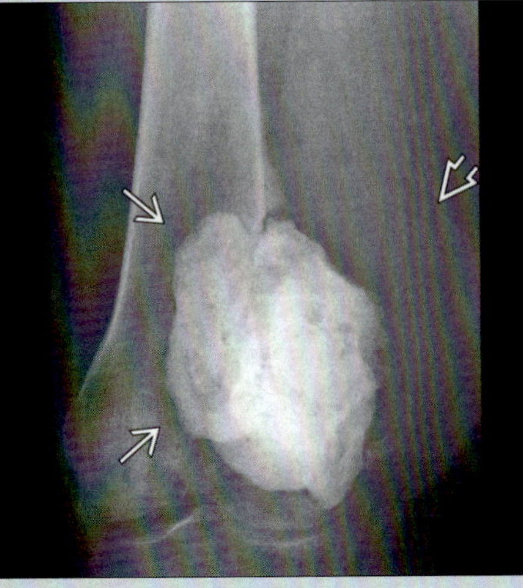

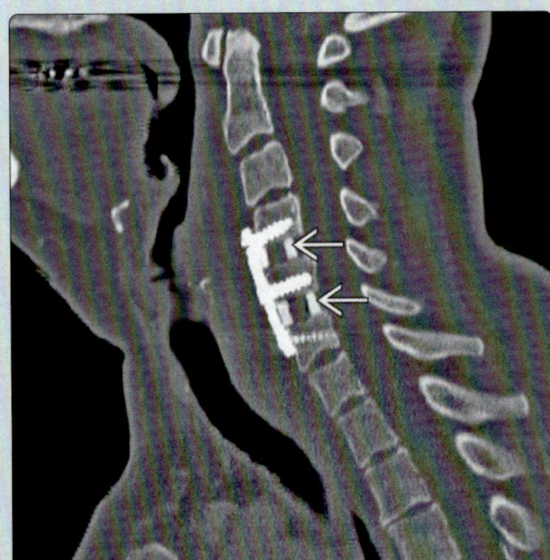

(Left) *AP radiograph following curettage and cement packing of distal femoral lesion is shown. There are regions of subtle irregular lucency at the interface ➡ suggesting tumor recurrence; the finding is substantiated by the presence of soft tissue mass ➡.* **(Right)** *Sagittal reformatted CT with 2-level interbody fusion with bicortical grafts ➡ is shown. The cortex of the graft provides structural support. The position of the graft provides contact between the debrided endplate and graft medullary bone, maximizing the opportunity for fusion.*

TERMINOLOGY

Abbreviations

- Bone morphogenic protein (BMP)
- Polymethylmethacrylate (PMMA) bone cement

Definitions

- Purpose: Various techniques used to fill defects, restore structure and strength, provide scaffold for bone ingrowth
- Ceramic: Inorganic material transformed during process of heating and cooling, often has crystalline structure
- Bone graft
  - Autograft: Taken from self, contains marrow elements leading to osteogenesis
  - Allograft: Derived from different individual
  - Xenograft: Derived from different species
  - Onlay graft: Placed along surface of bone
  - Strut graft: Spans defect in bone or segment of spine
  - Vascularized graft: Graft with blood supply, usually reestablished through microvascular techniques; fibula most common source, typically autograft
    - Sources: Iliac crest, fibula, rib, mandible
- Biologic activity of grafts
  - Osteoinductive: Recruits and then stimulates osteoprogenitor cells and undifferentiated stems cells to form osteoblasts
  - Osteoconductive: Scaffolding for bone ingrowth
  - Osteogenic: Stimulates new bone formation via implanted cells within graft, primarily autograft
    - Cancellous graft > potential than cortical graft

Bone Graft

- Autograft
  - Additional morbidity, especially pain, occurs at harvest site (especially iliac crest)
  - Cortical: Provides strength of cortical bone
    - Often used as onlay graft
    - Minimal marrow elements, so incorporation requires long period of time
  - Cancellous: Offers no structural support
    - Provides marrow elements stimulating bone ingrowth and more rapid incorporation
  - Corticocancellous
    - Provides structural support of cortical bone, combined with marrow elements with their osteogenic properties
  - Vascular grafts
    - Blood supply and marrow elements offer maximal opportunity by providing all elements needed for graft incorporation
- Allograft
  - Only contains mineralized component of bone; lacks marrow elements
  - Little risk of disease transmission
  - Frozen, freeze-dried; techniques reduce strength
  - Higher rate of complications
    - Nonunion, fracture, infection
    - Lacks ability to repair following damage
  - Incorporation requires balance between bone resorption and bone deposition

Bone Morphogenic Protein

- Group of 6 different proteins (BMP-2 through BMP-7) that stimulate formation of bone and cartilage
  - BMP-7, a.k.a. OP-1
- Derived from recombinant DNA techniques
- Requires carrier, usually mixed with bone graft or bone graft substitutes
- Provides osteoinductive influence
- Offers no structural support
- Use in spine may be associated with aggressive bone resorption mimicking infection

Ceramics

- Majority are calcium phosphate based
  - Hydroxyapatite forms most common
    - Mimics structure of calcium within bone
    - Available in pastes, powder, granular, block forms
    - Poor mechanical properties
    - Coralline hydroxyapatite derived from sea coral, others synthetic
  - Other less commonly used chemical forms: Tricalcium phosphate, calcium sulfate
- Density similar to or greater than bone
- Fills defects, provides scaffolding for new bone
  - Resorbs over long periods of time as new bone incorporated: Complete resorption indicates failure of incorporation or tumor recurrence
- Biologic activity
  - Osteointegrative (new bone binds to graft)
  - Osteoconductive
  - May be osteoinductive
  - Inert material, no toxicity

Demineralized Bone Matrix

- Type of allograft
- Useful because releases BMP
- No structural properties
- Often mixed with other bone fillers to introduce its osteoinductive properties
- Demineralized, therefore radiolucent; carrier usually has density

Injectable Cements

- Useful because of mechanical properties
  - Structural characteristics mimic bone
- Also provide 3D scaffold for bone ingrowth
- Polymer based; no biologic activity

Polymethylmethacrylate

- Same material used to make acrylic
- Supplied as liquid monomer and powder polymer
  - Monomer: Stabilizer, activator
  - Powder: Includes polymerization initiator
  - When mixed, creates exothermic reaction
- Uses
  - Fix joint implants to bone, sometimes pedicle screws
  - Fill defects in bone after curettage for tumor
  - May be mixed with slow-release antibiotics and placed in infected osseous defects
    - Most frequently following explant of infected implant
  - Treatment of painful vertebral and sacral fractures

- Low viscosity cements preferred for vertebral augmentation
- Function is to be load sharing
  - More flexible than cortical bone, less flexible than cancellous
  - Strength is in compression; fails along lines of shear
- No biologic activity
- Barium added to increase density
- Toxicity to user
  - Vapors permeate contact lenses
  - Mucous membrane irritation
  - Contact dermatitis, numbness, paresthesias
- Excess monomer may be toxic to patient
  - Small amounts always exist in tissues
  - Earlier vertebroplasties had different monomer:powder ratio resulting in increased amounts of free monomer; this caused damage to lungs and liver

IMAGING

Imaging Recommendations

- Best imaging tool
  - Radiographs are optimal for assessing position of graft, location of cement, status of incorporation, potential tumor recurrence

Radiographic and CT Findings

- Bone cement
  - Amorphous material with density greater than cortical bone
  - Usually appears as conglomerate mass
    - In vertebroplasty, may be interspersed among trabecular bone, creating lace-like appearance
    - Following curettage and packing of tumor or kyphoplasty has more solid ball-like appearance
  - May have < 2-mm lucency with sclerotic rim
    - Normal finding
    - Possibly secondary to rim of fibrosis created by exothermic reaction at time of placement
  - Increasing lucency at margin may indicate complication
    - Recurrence of underlying neoplasm
    - Loosening or particle disease following joint replacement
  - Fracture through cement
    - Indicates failure of joint replacement
    - Little significance when used to fill bone defect
- Cancellous graft
  - Cluster of irregularly shaped bodies with density similar to cortical bone
    - May mimic tumor matrix, mineralization, or ossification
      - Clinical history essential
    - Over time, resorbs as new bone incorporates graft
      - Requires serial films to assess incorporation
      - Following tumor resection, failure to see development of new bone suggests tumor recurrence
      - Development of cortical margins around graft at fracture site indicates nonunion
- Cortical graft
  - Onlay graft: Attached with cerclage wires or cables, less commonly by screws
  - May be seen spanning large defect
  - Graft incorporation requires long period of time, does not always occur
- Corticocancellous graft
  - Osseous incorporation assessed at edges of graft
    - Confirm incorporation when trabecula seen crossing from native bone to graft
  - Lucency at interface indicates nonunion
  - Femoral ring: Lumbar vertebral interbody fusion
  - Bicortical, tricortical, quadricortical grafts: Describes how many cortical surfaces on grafts; for example, bicortical grafts for cervical interbody fusion

MR Findings

- Autografts: Variable appearance depending on age
  - Initially have same imaging characteristics as normal bone/marrow
  - Intermediate phase with edematous-like changes
    - Result of granulation tissue ingrowth
    - ↓ T1 and ↑ T2 signal relative to normal marrow
  - If successfully incorporated, over long term resumes appearance of normal marrow
- Allografts
  - Initially ↓ T1 and ↓ T2 signal
    - Reflects lack of marrow elements
  - With successful incorporation of strut graft, marrow develops within medullary canal
    - Initially ↓ T1 and ↑ T2 signal of granulation tissue; begins at graft-native bone interfaces, progresses toward center of graft
  - Persistent low signal indicates failure of incorporation
- Bone cement
  - Signal void on all imaging sequences
  - No change over time
  - Surrounding marrow may have initial edematous changes

PATHOLOGY

Microscopic Features

- Incorporation of graft: Osteoblastic cells rim trabecula or crystal structure, which is resorbed as new bone is formed

CLINICAL ISSUES

Natural History & Prognosis

- Most common signs/symptoms
  - Successful incorporation is asymptomatic
  - Pain most common symptom of failure
    - Abnormal motion, occult fracture, infection, tumor recurrence
- BMP injected in vertebral bodies may result in aggressive resorption
  - Mimics infection

SELECTED REFERENCES

1. García-Gareta E et al: Osteoinduction of bone grafting materials for bone repair and regeneration. Bone. 81:112-121, 2015
2. Gupta A et al: Bone graft substitutes for spine fusion: a brief review. World J Orthop. 6(6):449-56, 2015

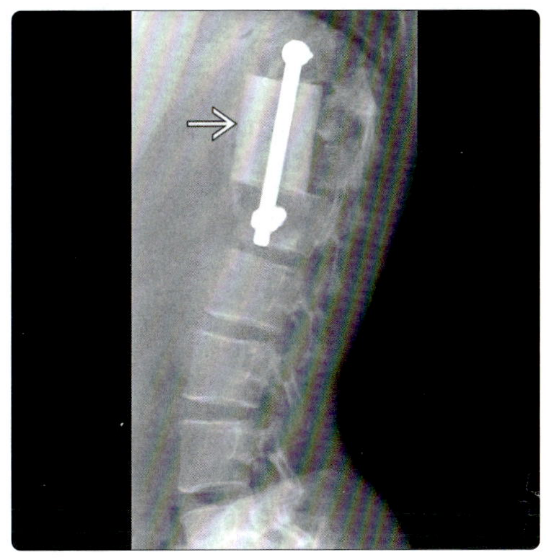

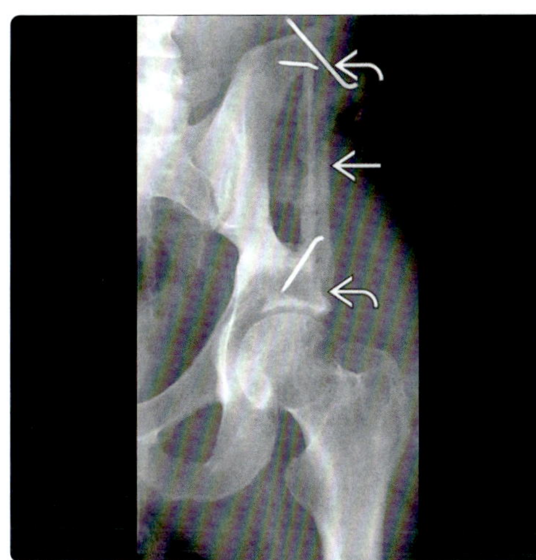

(Left) *Lateral radiograph with femoral strut graft ➡ fixation following corpectomy is shown. The strength of grafted bone is identical to native femur strength. Fusion occurs as granulation tissue migrates into the graft bone, blurring the margin between native bone and graft.* **(Right)** *AP radiograph after remote tumor resection is shown. A fibular strut graft ➡ was placed to provide structural support across the defect. The graft is well incorporated with trabecular continuity at its interface with the native bone ↪.*

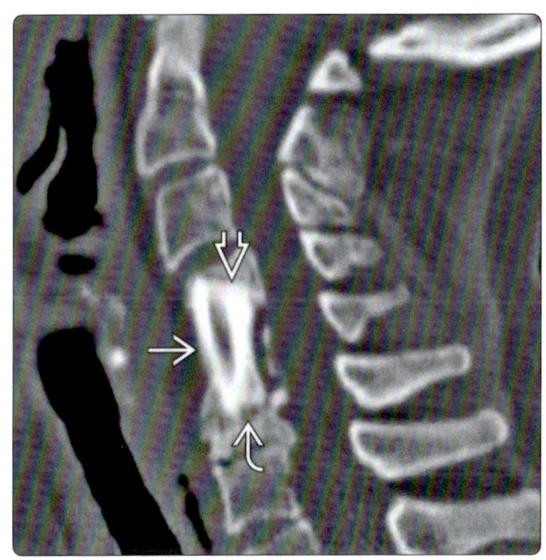

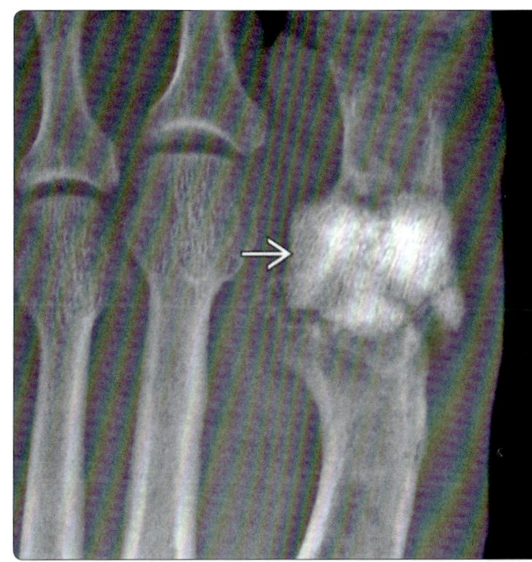

(Left) *Sagittal reformatted CT with pseudoarthrosis of a strut graft ➡ is shown. A lucent defect persists at the inferior bone-graft interface, indicating failure of bone formation across the site ↪. Superiorly the graft is well incorporated ⇨.* **(Right)** *AP radiograph with coral graft placement ➡ in an attempted arthrodesis is shown. Coral has a trabeculae-like structure. It is chosen as a graft because of its similar-sized cavities to haversian canals. It is inert; bone fusion is hoped for by means of creeping substitution.*

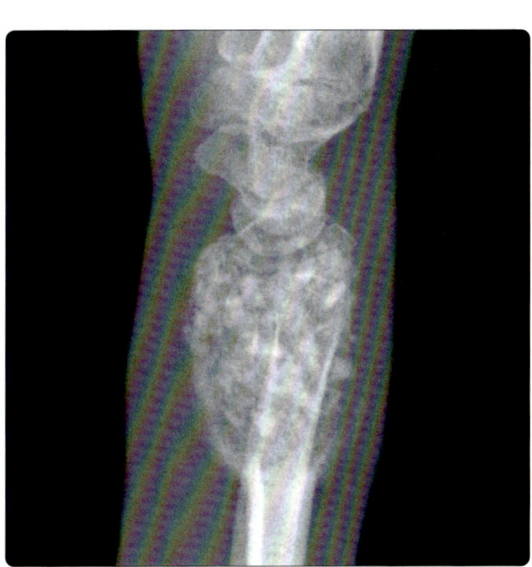

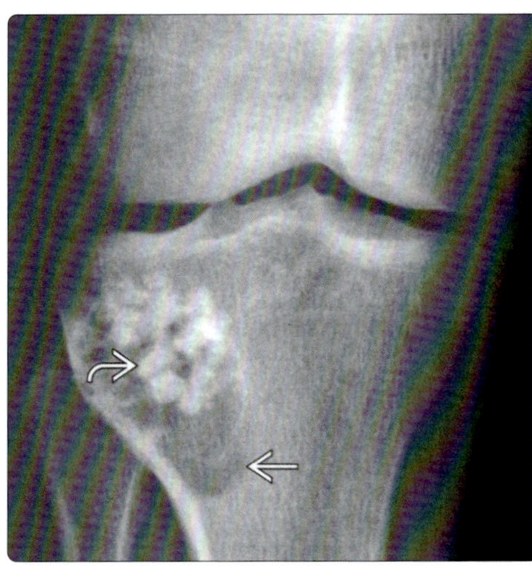

(Left) *Lateral radiograph shows curettage and packing of a distal radial giant cell tumor with cancellous graft. The graft could be confused with coarse calcification.* **(Right)** *AP radiograph shows multiple foci of mineralization ↪ eccentrically located within a lytic lesion ➡. The foci are relatively uniform in size with cuboidal shape, which is not a natural occurrence. Shape should be a clue. The margins are ill defined, indicating resorption that may be a part of the incorporation process or may indicate tumor recurrence.*

(Left) *AP radiograph shows changes following treatment of Langerhans cell histiocytosis. The lesion was curetted & packed with bone graft* ➡*. In the absence of old films, the solid amorphous nature of the density should indicate this is not something created by native bone.* **(Right)** *Sagittal reformatted CT after interesting use of cement to treat chronic osteomyelitis is shown. A chest tube was inserted into the medullary space & antibiotic impregnated cement* ➡ *injected as the tube was withdrawn.*

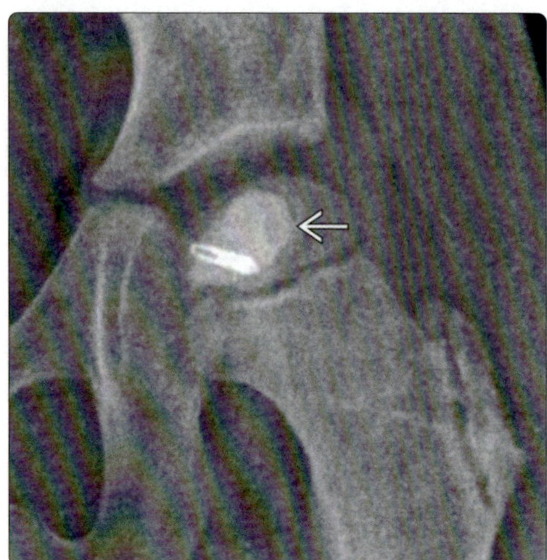

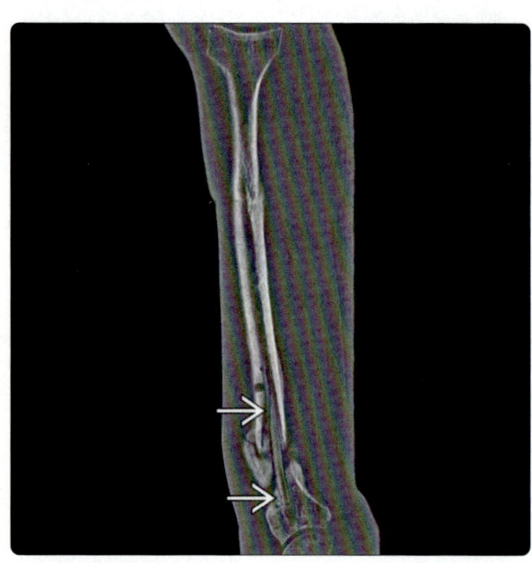

(Left) *AP radiograph was obtained for follow-up of a high tibial osteotomy & wedge graft. The graft is well healed, with trabecular continuity across the osteotomy* ➡*. Increased density is a result of new bone formation along the graft trabecula.* **(Right)** *Sagittal CT shows discectomy and placement of strut graft. There is lucency surrounding the graft* ➡*, concerning for infection or abnormal motion. It represents lysis, which can occur with overpacking of BMP. Clinical history helps confirm the diagnosis of BMP lysis.*

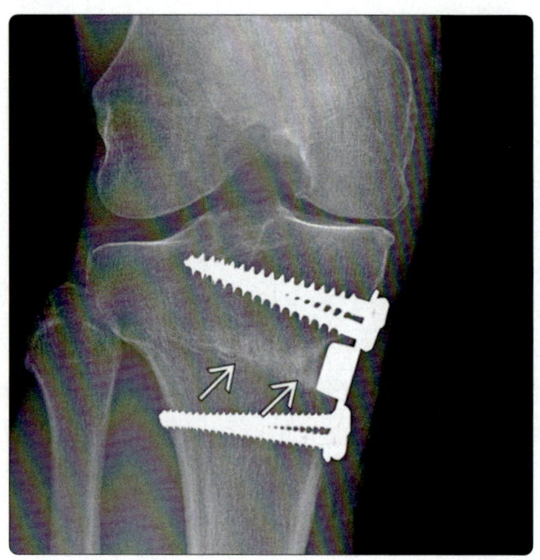

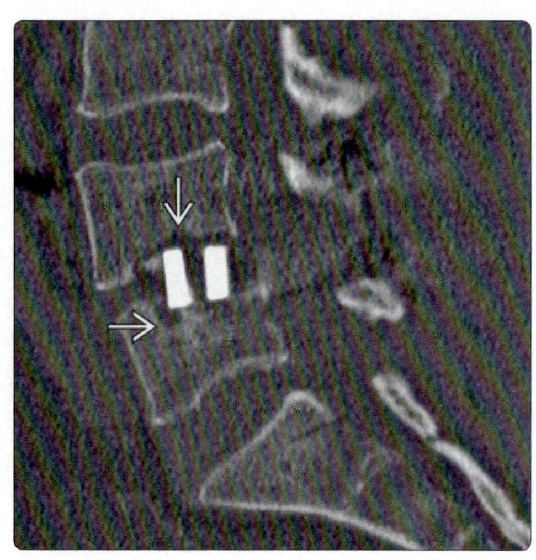

(Left) *AP radiograph following curettage of giant cell tumor is shown; the defect was filled with cement* ➡ *and a screw for additional support. The cement has an amorphous dense appearance.* **(Right)** *AP radiograph of the same patient was obtained in follow-up. A thin lucent border with a sclerotic line* ➡ *at the radial margin of the lesion is within normal limits and likely created by the exothermic curing process. However, the focal lytic lesion is an obvious tumor recurrence* ➡*.*

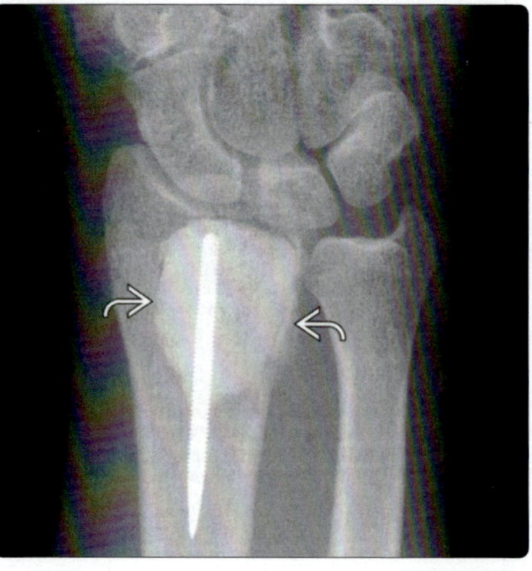

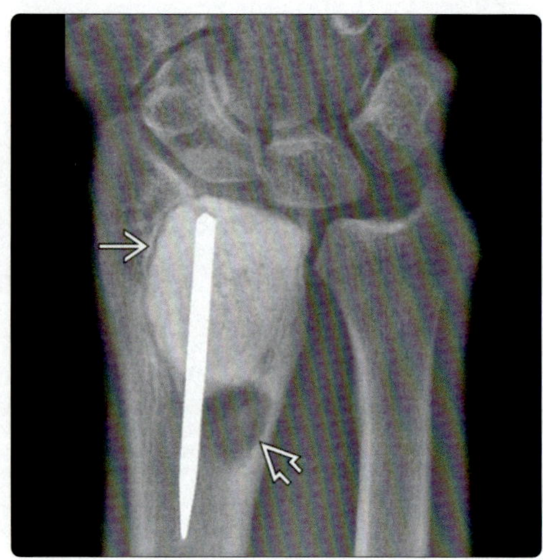

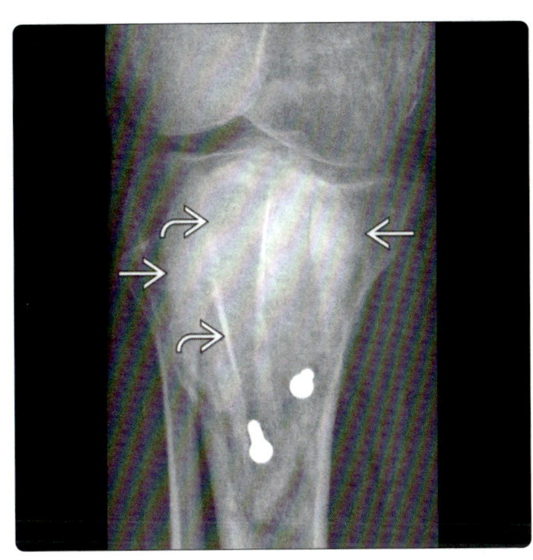

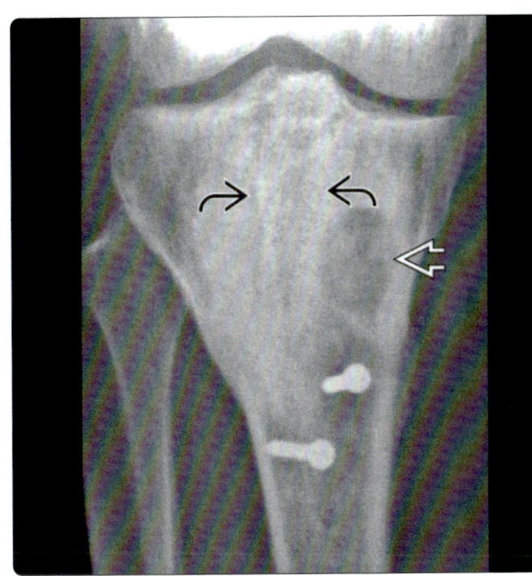

(Left) *AP radiograph following curettage and packing of giant cell tumor is shown. Mixed cortical* ➡ *and cancellous* ➡ *bone graft were used. Cortical graft provides structural support; cancellous graft provides lesion fill and surface area for osseous ingrowth.* **(Right)** *AP radiograph of the same patient shows incorporation of the graft material with hints of residual cortical graft* ➡*. Well-defined rounded lucency* ➡ *was not present on earlier radiographs. Development of such a finding indicates tumor recurrence.*

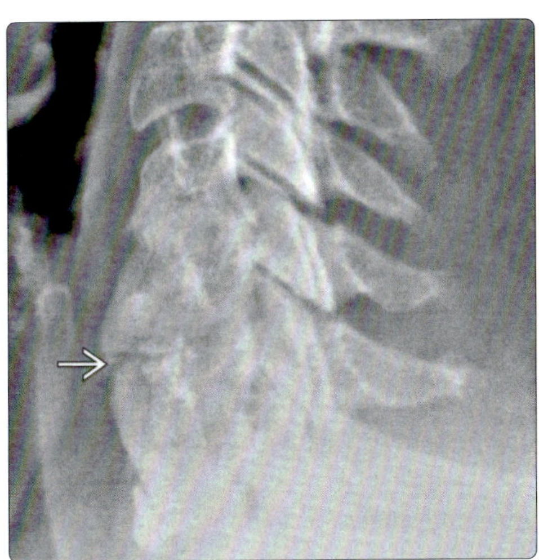

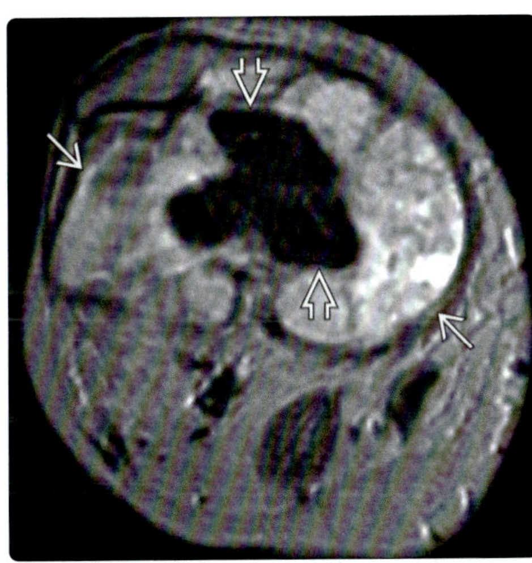

(Left) *Lateral radiograph shows a fibular strut graft used for a fusion attempt that has failed. The graft has fractured* ➡*. Proximal and distal pseudoarthroses are present. While the cortical graft is as strong as normal bone, it lacks the ability to repair itself.* **(Right)** *Axial T2WI MR shows recurrent chondrosarcoma* ➡*. Central signal void is present* ➡ *from cement inserted during previous curettage and packing of the lesion. The lack of field distortion helps differentiate this appearance from artifact due to hardware.*

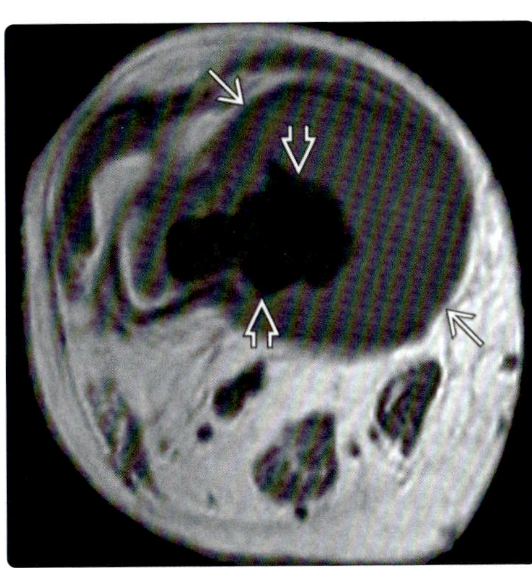

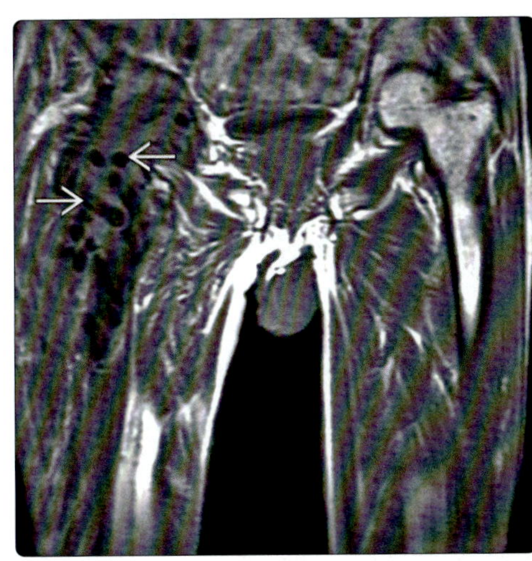

(Left) *Axial T1WI MR with a true signal void* ➡ *within a large tumor* ➡ *is shown. The signal void represents cement from a previous treatment. Once cured, cement has no mobile protons. Note the absence of any chemical shift artifact.* **(Right)** *Coronal T1WI MR following placement of antibiotic-impregnated cement beads* ➡ *after removal of an infected total hip is shown. Cement is commonly used as a vehicle for antibiotic delivery. Cement created a signal void on all imaging sequences.*

KEY FACTS

TERMINOLOGY

- Wire: Usually monofilament 18G stainless steel
  - Aids fracture fixation, not 1° means of stabilization
  - Tension provided by twisting ends; tension lost if ends untwist
  - Differs from K-wires (Kirschner wires), which are rigid and may be used for 1° fixation
- Cable: Multifilament structure
  - Fixed with locking device to maintain tension
  - Greater strength than wire
- FiberWire cerclage: Fiber is radiolucent; only lock is seen

IMAGING

- Tension band fixation (TBF) used for stabilization of fractures subject to tension forces: Patella, olecranon, greater trochanter, small avulsions
  - Placed along surface of greatest tension
  - Converts forces along tension side of fracture to compression along opposite side
  - Figure of 8 wire configuration placed around pins or screws placed perpendicular to fracture line
- Cerclage: Encircling bone with wire/cable
  - Common uses: Fracture fixation along femoral implant; cortical graft fixation to long bone, fixation of long oblique fractures
- Modes of failure
  - Metal fatigue: Loss of integrity
  - Dislodge from bone
  - TBF: Disengagement of wire from pins/screws
  - In early postoperative period, failure increases incidence of malunion, nonunion, delayed union
  - Late failure often inconsequential

CLINICAL ISSUES

- Discomfort / soft tissue irritation
- Infection
- Possible granulomatous reaction to FiberWire cerclage

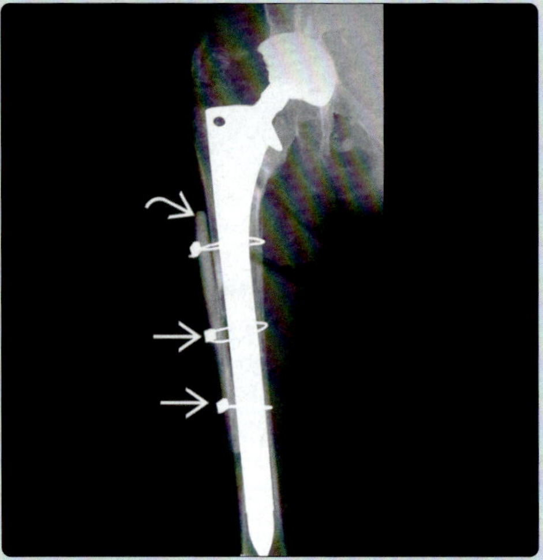

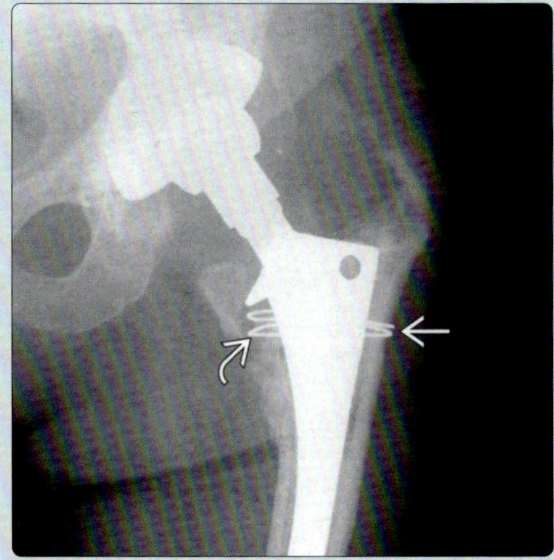

(Left) *AP radiograph following complex total hip revision is shown. Three cerclage cables were used for fixation of a long lateral cortical graft ➡ to the femoral shaft. Note the locks, which maintain tension within the cable ➡.* **(Right)** *AP radiograph for follow-up of a total hip replacement is shown. During surgery, 2 cerclage wires ➡ were placed for fixation of a minor crack. In the interim, the lesser trochanter has fractured and displaced. As a result, the wires no longer engage the proximal femur ➡.*

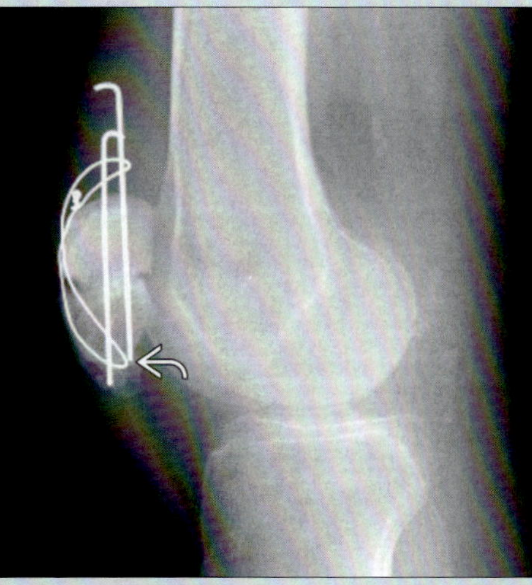

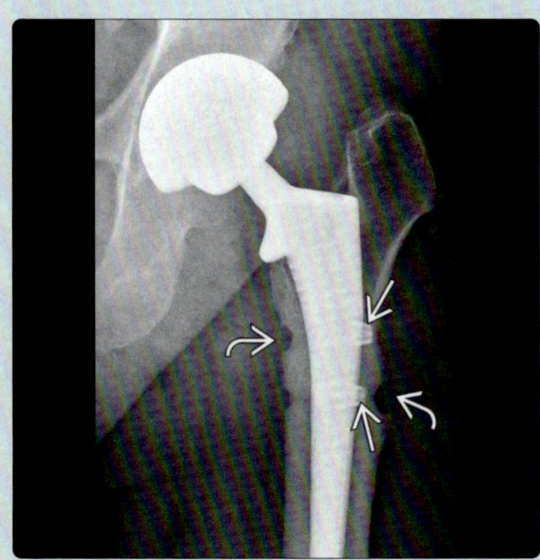

(Left) *Lateral radiograph following tension band fixation is shown. Figure of 8 wire has been placed along the external surface of the patella. When tension is applied to that surface, it results in compression along the articular surface. Fixation was lost when 1 of the pins backed out and no longer engaged the wire ➡.* **(Right)** *AP x-ray shows an implant. An incomplete femoral fracture was stabilized with FiberWire cerclage bands; only the locks ➡ are visualized. Over a year, bone has resorbed beneath the bands ➡.*

KEY FACTS

TERMINOLOGY

- Components
  - Anchor: Provides fixation to bone
  - Eyelet: Connects suture to anchor
  - Suture: Engages soft tissue
- Function: Provides method for attachment of soft tissues, primarily tendon and ligaments, to bone
  - Expected to maintain fixation until healing occurs
  - Not expected to provide permanent anchoring
  - Anchor may be screw-like or arrow-like

IMAGING

- Failure at bone interface
  - Pullout: More likely in osteoporotic bone
    - Cement augmentation techniques promising for osteoporotic bone
  - Migration to intraarticular location
  - Loosening: Lucency around screw, shift in screw position; uncommon
- Failure at soft tissue interface
  - Suture disengagement from tendon
  - Best detected on MR
- Radiography and CT
  - Titanium anchors visible as metallic object
  - Bioabsorbable anchors appear as bone defect
- MR
  - Used to assess integrity of soft tissue repair
  - Artifact from titanium screw may obscure soft tissue healing; requires use of magnetic susceptibility reduction techniques
  - Aids detection of bioabsorbable sutures that have pulled out; anchor appears as signal void

CLINICAL ISSUES

- Common uses: Rotator cuff repair, capsular fixation
- Low profile more commonly seen as apposed to previously used protruding screw and washer

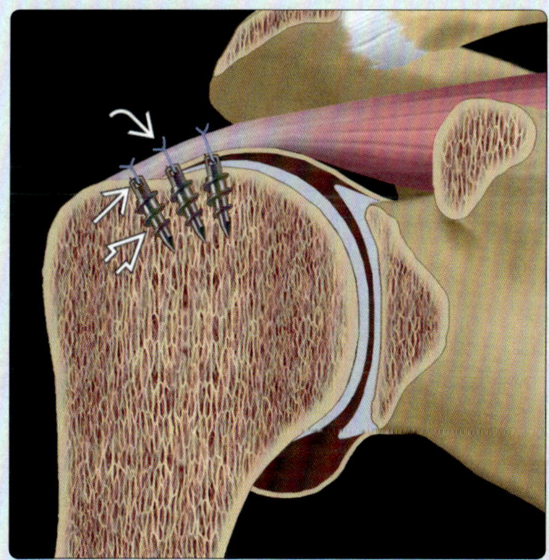

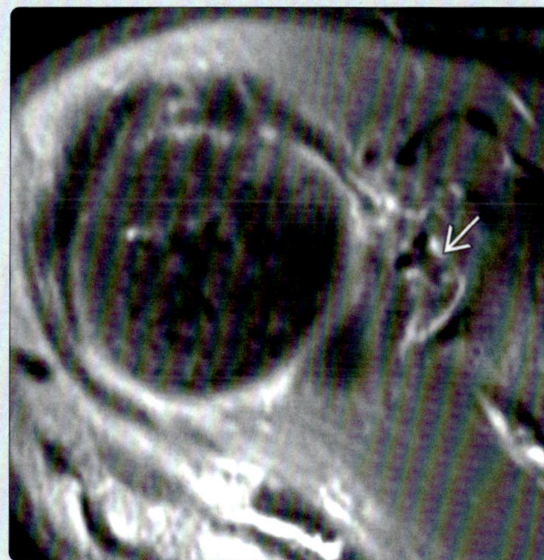

(Left) *Coronal section graphic shows a shoulder following rotator cuff repair. Threaded suture anchors were used ⇨. The sutures ⇨ have been passed through the eyelet ⇨ of the anchor, completing the connection between tendon and bone.* **(Right)** *Axial PD FSE FS MR shows shoulder with clinical findings of failure of a labral repair with bioabsorbable sutures. The MR examination was able to confirm pullout of the anchors. One of the dislodged anchors is located anterosuperiorly within the joint ⇨.*

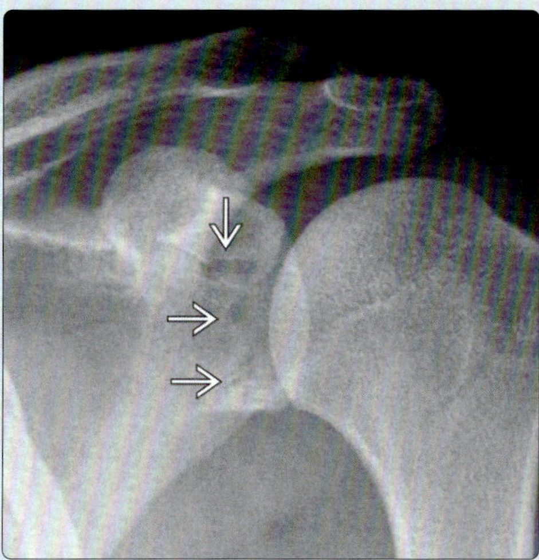

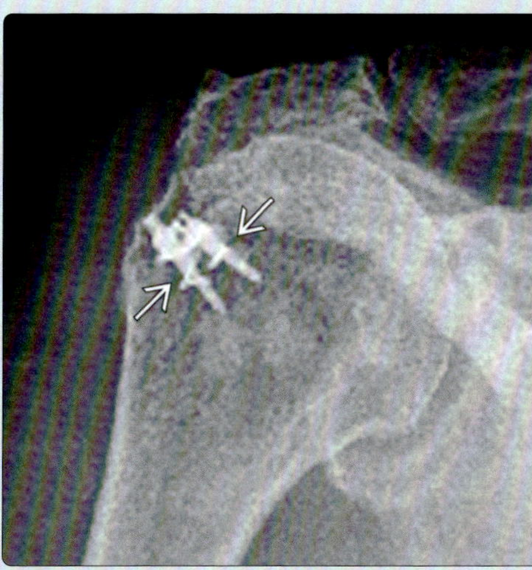

(Left) *AP radiograph shows multiple radiolucent tunnels ⇨ within the glenoid. These defects are the sites of bioabsorbable anchors, which have been used during a glenoid labral-capsular repair. MR would be required to detect dislodgement of such anchors.* **(Right)** *AP radiograph follows rotator cuff repair with 2 suture anchors ⇨ placed within the greater tuberosity. The anchors are "sunk" and do not protrude beyond the osseous margins. These particular screws are threaded.*

SECTION 8

Infection

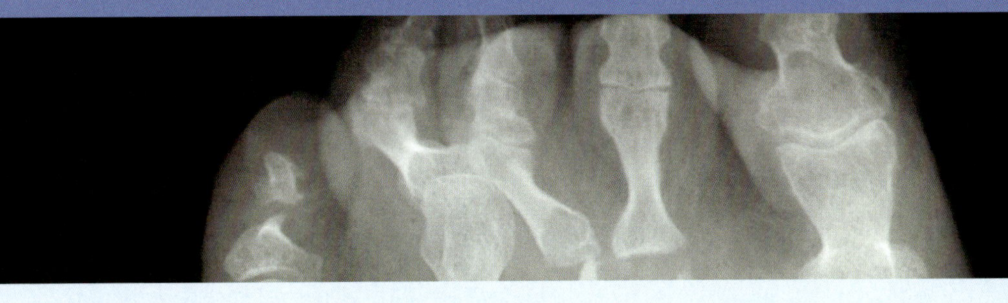

Osteomyelitis

Soft Tissue and Joints

Specific Pathogens

Conditions of Unknown Etiology

KEY FACTS

TERMINOLOGY

- Infection of bone, presenting within 1st 14 days

IMAGING

- Metaphysis of long bone most common
- Vertebral osteomyelitis accounts for 25% of cases
- Radiographs: Focal osteopenia, periostitis, ill-defined or permeative bone destruction
- MR: Edematous changes in marrow and soft tissues ± intraosseous, subperiosteal, soft tissue, epidural abscesses
- 3-phase bone scan sensitive & specific
    - ↑ activity on blood flow & blood pool
    - Focal uptake on delayed images
- Preferred imaging technique
    - MR or bone scan if focal symptoms
    - Bone scan preferred if nonlocalizing symptoms
    - Radiographs best to assess healing

TOP DIFFERENTIAL DIAGNOSES

- Ewing sarcoma
    - Less likely to have + bone scan, ↑ white cell count

PATHOLOGY

- Hematogenous seeding of metaphysis
- Bacterial infection most common, typically *Staphylococcus aureus*
- In 30% of cases, organism never identified

CLINICAL ISSUES

- Pain, fever, limited weight bearing, irritability
- Positive ESR in > 90%
- < 50% have elevated white cell count, left shift, or positive blood cultures
- Most common in children < 3 years old
- Untreated → extensive bone destruction, soft tissue abscess, draining sinuses, death

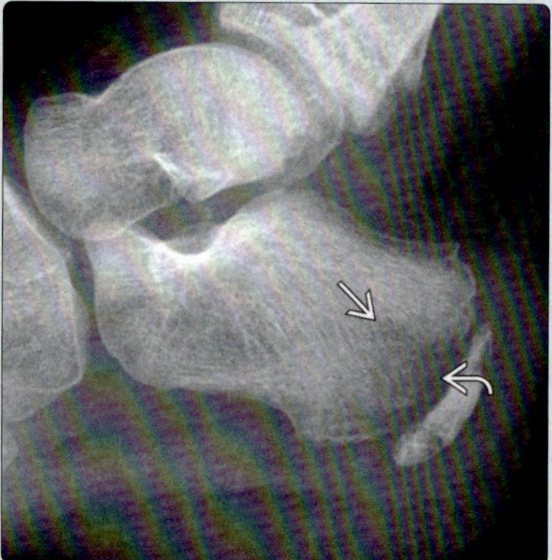
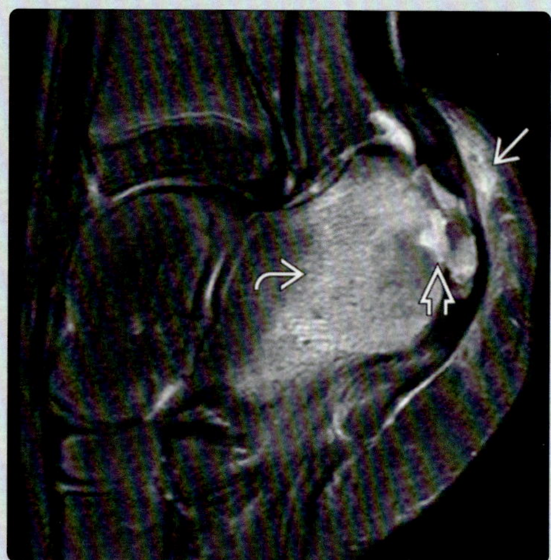

(Left) *Lateral radiograph shows how subtle the radiographic appearance of early osteomyelitis can be. Vague demineralization → is present in the metaphysis of the tuberosity with loss of the metaphyseal border of the growth plate →.* **(Right)** *Sagittal T2WI MR of the same patient reveals more extensive disease than one might expect. There is a focal lesion → that corresponds to the radiographic abnormality, diffuse marrow edema →, and soft tissue edema →, all typical findings of osteomyelitis.*

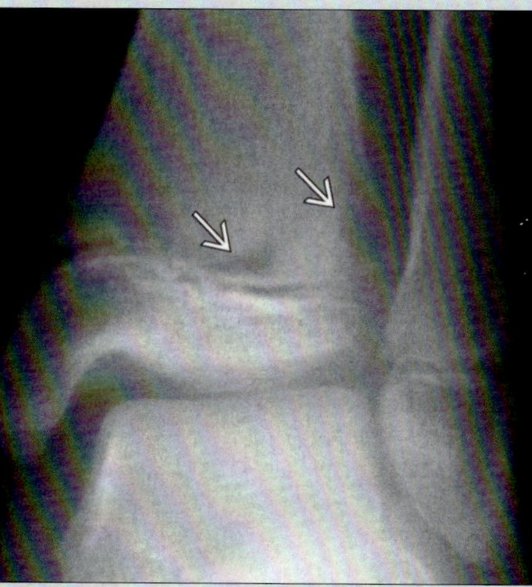
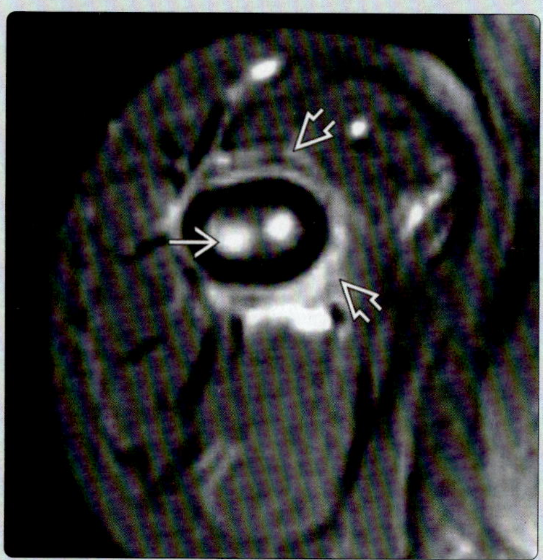

(Left) *AP radiograph was taken of a child who was limping. Close inspection reveals ill-defined areas of osteolysis in the metaphysis →. Hematogenous seeding is the most common mechanism and occurs primarily in the metaphysis where blood flow slows.* **(Right)** *Axial T1WI FS C+ MR shows classic findings of osteomyelitis. Enhancing foci are present within the marrow →, and there is diffuse enhancement of the periosteum →. This case is biopsy-proven Salmonella, a common pathogen in patients with sickle cell anemia.*

TERMINOLOGY

Definitions

- Infection of bone, presenting within 1st 14 days

IMAGING

General Features

- Best diagnostic clue
  - Ill-defined destruction, usually within metaphysis
- Location
  - Metaphysis of long bone most common
    - Femur, tibia, humerus
  - Vertebral osteomyelitis accounts for 25% of cases
  - Metaphyseal equivalent in pelvis in 10%
  - Multiple lesions in 5-10%

Radiographic Findings

- Radiography
  - Earliest finding: Deep soft tissue swelling
  - Advanced disease: Focal osteopenia, periostitis, ill-defined or permeative bone destruction
    - Seen at 10-14 days in approximately 20%

CT Findings

- ↑ sensitivity for bone destruction, periostitis
- Limited role in imaging algorithm, especially with concern for radiation use in children

MR Findings

- Edematous changes in marrow and soft tissues
  - T1WI: ↓ marrow signal, ill-defined fat planes
  - Fluid-sensitive: ↑ marrow & soft tissue signal
  - C+: Diffuse enhancement throughout edema
- Abscesses
  - ↓ T1 signal, ↑ signal on fluid-sensitive sequences
  - Peripheral enhancement
  - Intraosseous, subperiosteal, soft tissue, epidural
    - More with pelvic infection than long bone disease

Nuclear Medicine Findings

- Bone scan
  - 3-phase imaging sensitive & specific
    - ↑ activity on blood flow & blood pool
    - Focal uptake on delayed images
    - Positive in > 90% within 48 hours
    - Limitation is anatomic detail
    - Does not require sedation, relatively inexpensive
    - Useful for whole body screening
    - Cold (false-negative): ↑ in very young children
      - May initially have decreased uptake due to vascular occlusion, lasts < 3 days
    - Pinhole imaging to image adjacent to metaphysis
- Tc-99m sulfur colloid
  - Usually not positive during 1st week
  - Combined study with labeled white cell scans
    - Positive: Uptake on white cell scan without uptake on marrow scan
- Labeled leukocyte scintigraphy
  - Difficult to use alone 2° to variable marrow distribution

Image-Guided Biopsy

- Surgical biopsy often preferred 2° to patient age

Imaging Recommendations

- Best imaging tool
  - MR or bone scan if focal symptoms
  - Bone scan preferred if nonlocalizing symptoms
  - Radiographs best to assess healing

DIFFERENTIAL DIAGNOSIS

Ewing Sarcoma

- Less likely to have + bone scan, ↑ white cell count

PATHOLOGY

General Features

- Etiology
  - Hematogenous seeding of metaphysis where blood flow becomes sluggish
  - Bacterial infection most common
    - Most frequently *Staphylococcus aureus*
    - Tuberculous, fungal, parasitic infections rare
      - More commonly seen in immunocompromised patients and those from developing countries
    - *Haemophilus influenzae*, *Streptococcus pneumonia* in very young children
    - In 30% of cases, organism never identified

CLINICAL ISSUES

Presentation

- Most common signs/symptoms
  - Pain, fever, limited weight bearing, irritability
  - Young children: Irritability, refusal to bear weight
- Other signs/symptoms
  - Bacteremia, positive blood cultures
  - Positive ESR in > 90%
  - < 50% have elevated white cell count, left shift, or positive blood cultures

Demographics

- Age
  - Most common in children < 3 years of age
  - Pelvic osteomyelitis seen in slightly older group

Natural History & Prognosis

- Untreated → extensive bone destruction, soft tissue abscess, draining sinuses, death
- Complications: Growth arrest, deformity
- Undertreatment will lead to chronic osteomyelitis
- In young child, vessels cross physis; osteomyelitis may be associated with septic arthritis

Treatment

- Parenteral antibiotics followed by oral antibiotics
- If symptoms persist, consider MR to assess for abscess

SELECTED REFERENCES

1. Yoo WJ et al: Primary epiphyseal osteomyelitis caused by mycobacterium species in otherwise healthy toddlers. J Bone Joint Surg Am. 96(17):e145, 2014

(Left) *Frontal view from a delayed bone scan of a child with arm pain shows diffuse increased uptake throughout the right humerus involving the metaphysis and diaphysis →. Bone scans are often chosen as the 1st imaging modality due to their relative low cost and rapid acquisition that does not require sedation. They lack fine anatomic detail.* **(Right)** *Sagittal T1WI C+ FS MR from the same patient shows diffuse enhancement of the marrow → and periosteum →. Bone scans and MR are of equal sensitivity for the detection of osteomyelitis. Typically, both examinations are not required for initial evaluation. MR may be used for further evaluation to detect abscess if the patient does not improve. The use of contrast is essential for the characterization of abscesses, which are recognized by their peripheral enhancement.*

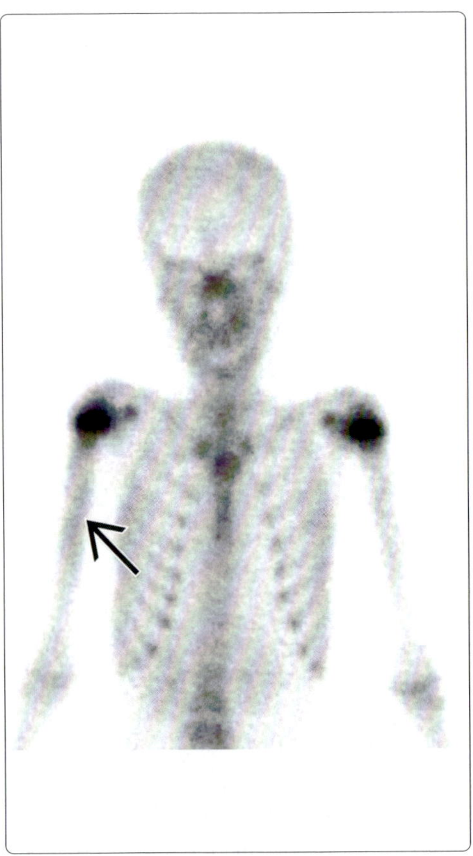

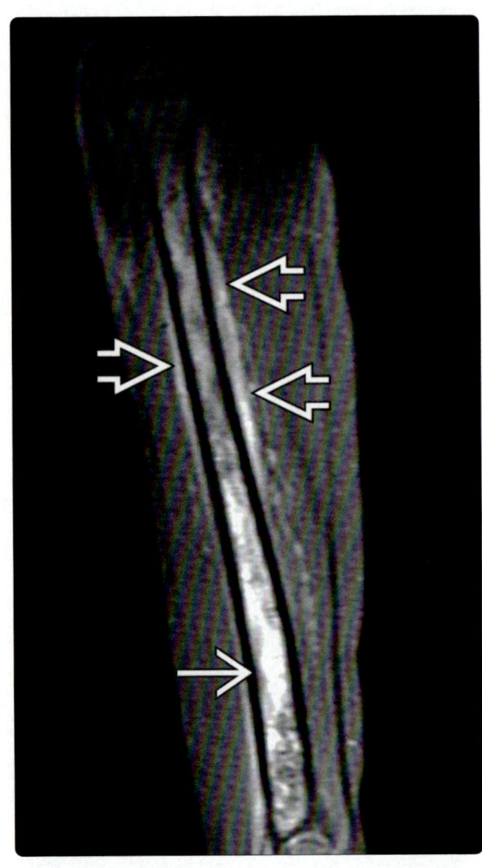

(Left) *Coronal T2WI FS MR shows ↑ signal intensity in the right sacral ala →, left posterior iliac wing →, right ischium →. Findings are nonspecific and consistent with osteomyelitis. Correlation with other studies aids diagnosis. The erythrocyte sedimentation rate will be elevated in almost all patients with osteomyelitis. Elevated white blood cell count, left shift are less reliable. Pelvic osteomyelitis often occurs in slightly older children and has a more nonspecific presentation and a greater incidence of abscesses.* **(Right)** *Lateral radiograph of the spine in a 15 year old shows disc space narrowing, endplate destruction, and vertebral sclerosis →. The spine is a common site of hematogenous osteomyelitis in children. Sluggish flow in the endplates mimics flow in the metaphyses. In younger children, the disc is vascular and may be directly seeded.*

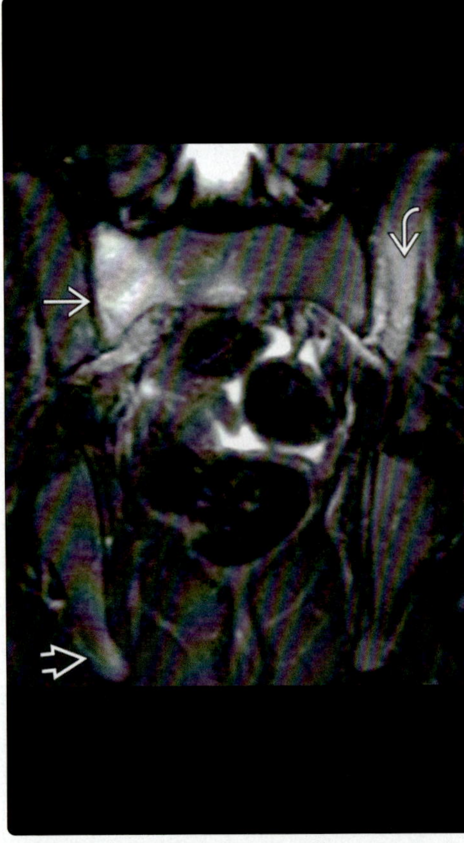

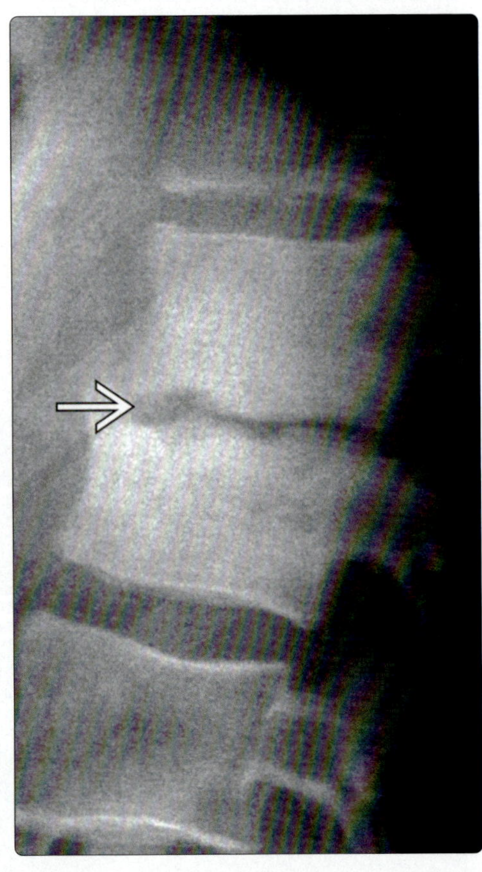

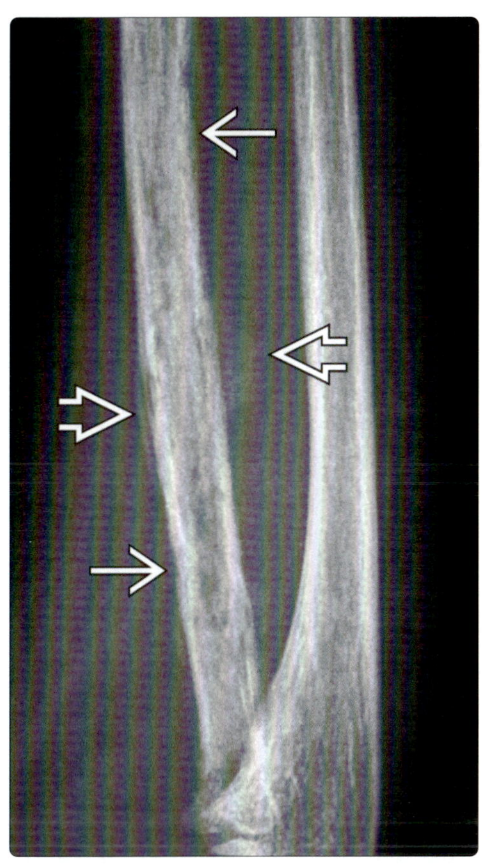

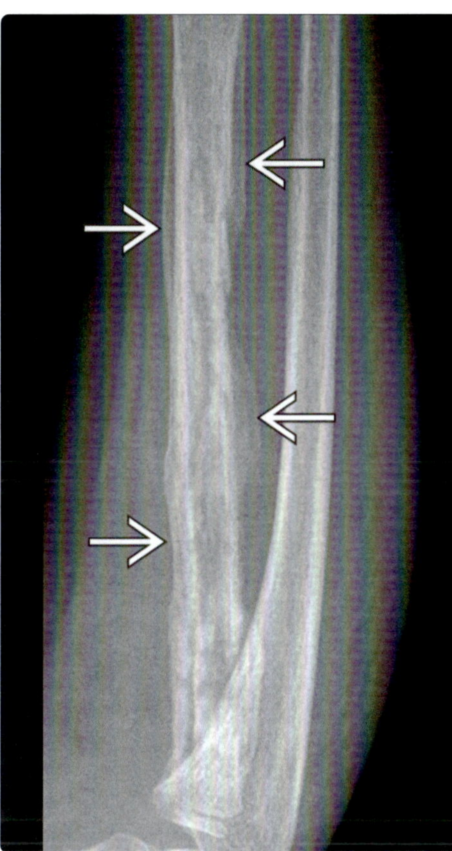

(Left) *AP radiograph shows extensive osteomyelitis. Permeative destruction of cortical and medullary bone is seen throughout the radius* ➡, *accompanied by immature periosteal new bone formation* ➡. **(Right)** *AP radiograph of the same patient was obtained in follow-up. The periostitis, while more extensive, is also more mature* ➡. *There is increasing sclerosis throughout the bone and better definition of the cortex. These osseous changes are the result of new reactive bone formation during the healing processes. In the 1st 7-10 days, radiographic changes are likely to progress, even in the face of appropriate therapy. It will take 2 weeks or more of appropriate therapy to see the changes depicted here.*

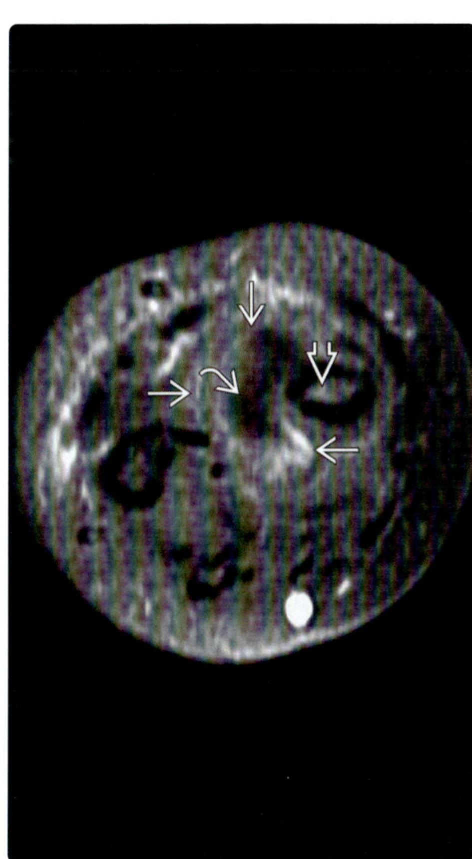

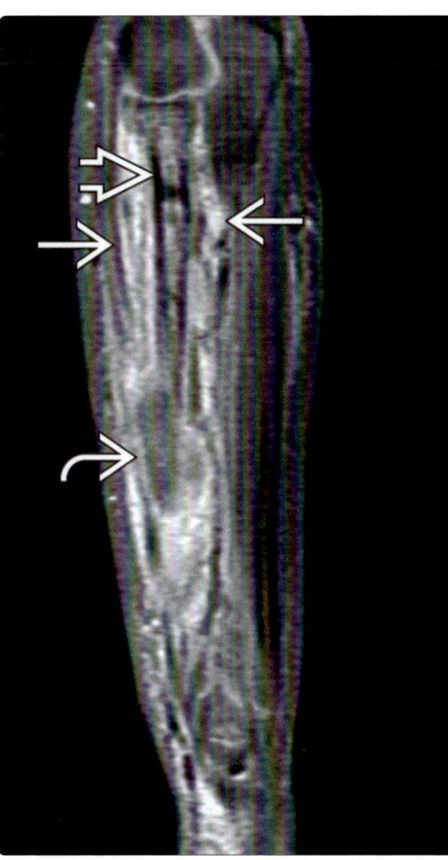

(Left) *Axial T1WI C+ MR in the same patient, obtained at the time of initial evaluation, shows mild marrow enhancement* ➡ *and diffuse soft tissue inflammation* ➡. *A nonenhancing relatively hypointense focus with peripheral enhancement is consistent with abscess* ➡. **(Right)** *Sagittal T1WI C+ FS MR of the same patient shows extensive enhancement along thickened periosteum* ➡, *which is better appreciated in this plane. Again seen is the irregular enhancement of the marrow of the radius* ➡ *and abscess in the adjacent soft tissues* ➡. *To confirm abscess, this focus should be bright on fluid-sensitive sequences. If this focus remains hypointense on a fluid-sensitive sequence, it more likely represents devitalized (devascularized) tissue, which occasionally accompanies extensive infection.*

KEY FACTS

IMAGING

- Long bones: With hematogenous spread, location of infection relates to vascular anatomy
- Destructive pattern of osteomyelitis has wide range
  - May appear as aggressive as round cell tumor
  - May be geographic with sclerotic margin
- Radiograph/CT
  - Obliteration of fat planes differentiates infectious mass from tumor, which cleanly distorts fat planes
  - Earliest osseous change is indistinctness of cortex
  - Permeative osseous destruction; may have serpiginous, branching pattern
  - Periosteal reaction usually dense, linear
  - Late osseous change: Sequestrum and involucrum
- MR of osteomyelitis
  - Air may be seen in soft tissue ulcer/sinus tract: Low signal on all sequences
  - T1: Confluent region of low signal intensity
    - Confluent low T1 SI differentiated from hazy reticulated pattern seen with bone reaction to adjacent soft tissue infection
    - Unequivocal confluence of decreased signal on T1 increases specificity of MR
  - Fluid-sensitive sequences: ↑ signal within bone and soft tissue abscess; overly sensitive for osteomyelitis when interpreted independently of corresponding T1 MR
  - Contrast shows enhancing rim around abscess and within bone
- Even with MR, differentiating osteomyelitis from abnormalities in Charcot foot is extremely difficult

DIAGNOSTIC CHECKLIST

- Consider: Time course of destructive changes in osteomyelitis is faster than tumor
  - Exception is Langerhans cell histiocytosis, which rarely may show extremely rapid destruction

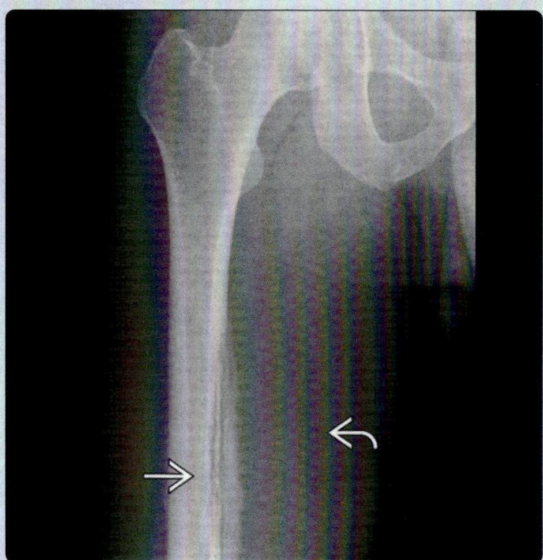

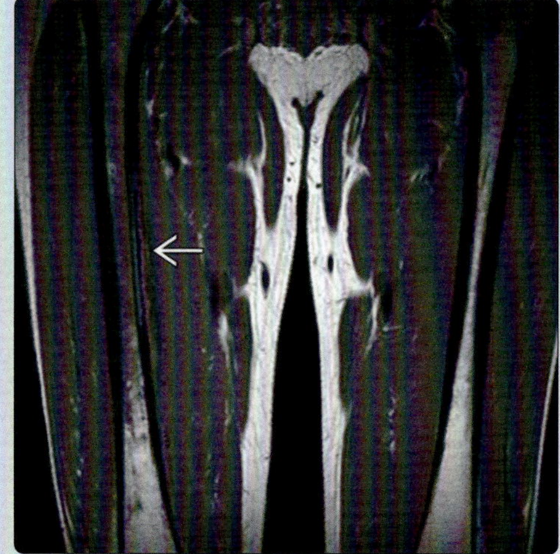

(Left) *AP radiograph shows intense, linear, somewhat disordered periosteal reaction ➡ and permeative change within the marrow. There is distortion of the soft tissue fat planes with partial obliteration ➡. The appearance of the soft tissues favors osteomyelitis.* **(Right)** *Coronal T1WI MR shows the extent of the marrow abnormality in the femur, as well as the linear character of much of the periosteal reaction ➡. Note that the majority of the T1 low signal is confluent, expected in osteomyelitis.*

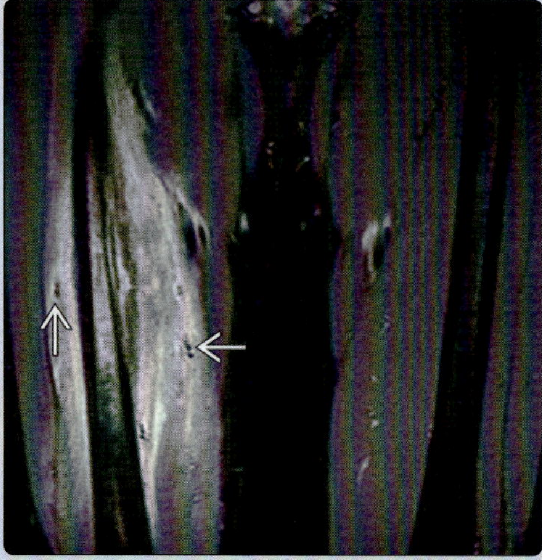

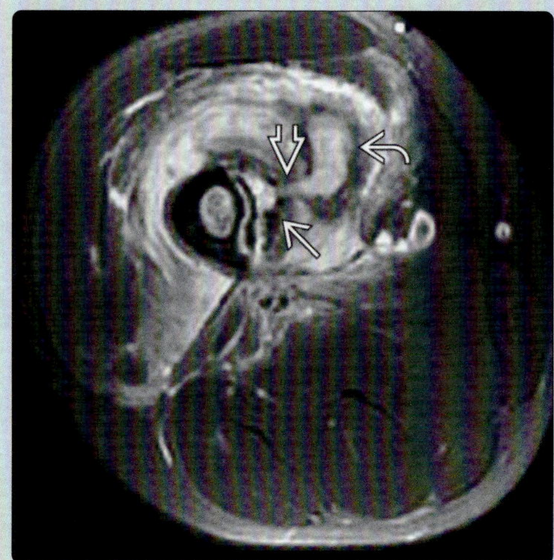

(Left) *Coronal T2WI FS MR in the same patient shows the extent of the high signal soft tissue abnormality, along with air bubbles ➡. The combination assures the diagnosis of osteomyelitis.* **(Right)** *Axial T2WI FS MR shows the thick periosteal reaction to be disrupted ➡. There is a sinus tract extending through the periosteal reaction ➡ into a complex high signal fluid collection ➡. The character of the periosteal reaction and presence of sinus tract, as well as presence of air, make the diagnosis of osteomyelitis.*

IMAGING

General Features

- Best diagnostic clue
  - Lytic destructive osseous change, often with osseous reaction (both periosteal and intramedullary)
- Location
  - Long bones: With hematogenous spread, location of infection relates to vascular anatomy
    - In infants up to 12 months of age, some metaphyseal vessels penetrate physis and anastomose with epiphyseal vessels
      - Infections in infants therefore involve metaphysis, epiphysis, and joint
      - Related to epiphyseal infection, infants may develop slipped epiphyses and growth deformities
    - In toddlers and older children, blood vessels terminate in loops within metaphysis
      - Blood flow is sluggish in these terminal loops; children develop osteomyelitis in metaphyses
    - In adults, terminal metaphyseal and epiphyseal vessels anastomose across physeal scar
      - Adult osteomyelitis therefore may involve joint more frequently than in children
  - Infection rarely may be located in cortex
  - With direct inoculation, may be diaphyseal
- Morphology
  - Destructive pattern of osteomyelitis has wide range
    - May appear aggressive, mimicking round cell tumor
    - May be geographic with sclerotic margin

Radiographic Findings

- Soft tissue abnormalities
  - ± cellulitis, soft tissue mass
    - Mass may blur or obliterate fat planes
    - Obliteration of fat planes differentiates infectious mass from tumor, which cleanly distorts fat planes
  - Rarely, air seen in sinus tract
- Osseous abnormalities
  - No osseous change for 1-2 weeks
  - Earliest osseous change is indistinctness of cortex
  - Subacute osseous change
    - Permeative osseous destruction; may have serpiginous, branching pattern
    - Endosteal scalloping or osseous reaction
    - Periosteal reaction
  - Late osseous change: Sequestrum and involucrum
    - Sequestrum: Necrotic bone, surrounded by purulent material or granulation tissue
    - Sequestrum is usually normal density (due to loss of blood supply), with surrounding osteopenia
    - Sequestrum may harbor bacteria, serving as source for chronic osteomyelitis
    - Involucrum: Bone shell surrounding purulent material and sequestrum
    - Cloaca: Cortical and periosteal defect through which pus drains from infected medullary cavity
  - Late osseous change: Brodie abscess
    - Lytic, generally oval lesion with sclerotic, well-marginated rim
    - Surrounding osseous sclerosis
    - Dense, regular periosteal reaction
    - Less aggressive appearance than acute osteomyelitis
    - Generally in child and located in metaphysis
    - May be found in epiphysis of very young child (differential of chondroblastoma and Langerhans cell histiocytosis)
    - May not have associated fever or laboratory abnormalities (↑ sedimentation rate or WBC)

CT Findings

- Osseous lytic destructive change, often with serpiginous tracking
- Reactive bone formation
  - Central, endosteal, or periosteal
- Obliteration of soft tissue planes
- Enhancing rim around bone or soft tissue abscess

MR Findings

- Highly sensitive and specific when contrast is utilized
- Air may be seen in soft tissue ulcer/sinus tract: Low signal on all sequences
- T1: Confluent region of low signal intensity
  - Unequivocal confluence of decreased signal increases specificity of MR
  - Differentiated from hazy reticulated pattern seen with bone reaction to adjacent soft tissue infection
- Fluid-sensitive sequences: ↑ signal within bone and soft tissue abscess; overly sensitive for osteomyelitis when interpreted independently of corresponding T1 MR
- Subcutaneous edema common
- Contrast shows enhancing rim around abscess and within bone
  - Remember that tumor necrosis may show central low signal with surrounding enhancement
- Even with MR, differentiating osteomyelitis from abnormalities in Charcot foot is extremely difficult

Nuclear Medicine Findings

- Multiphase Tc-99m bone scanning shows ↑ tracer uptake on all phases in acute osteomyelitis
- Osteomyelitis may be "cold" on delayed images of bone scan, especially in children in early acute phase
- Gallium-67 nearly 100% sensitive, but nonspecific
- Combined WBC imaging and complementary bone marrow imaging with Tc-99m sulfur colloid 90% accurate for diagnosing osteomyelitis
- Recent meta-analysis suggests high accuracy of FDG PET to diagnose chronic osteomyelitis

Imaging Recommendations

- Best imaging tool
  - Radiograph is appropriately 1st-line test; relatively insensitive; MR is gold standard
  - Even MR may be nonspecific for osteomyelitis in presence of Charcot joint changes
- Protocol advice
  - T1 imaging in at least 2 planes is useful to differentiate osseous changes due to osteomyelitis from those due to reactive bone change
  - Postcontrast imaging is mandatory

DIFFERENTIAL DIAGNOSIS

Round Cell Tumor

- Round cell tumor (Ewing sarcoma, lymphoma): Same degree of aggressiveness as osteomyelitis
- In children, metastatic neuroblastoma shows same degree of aggressiveness
- Langerhans cell histiocytosis: May occasionally be as aggressive as osteomyelitis

Cortical Osteomyelitis: Osteoid Osteoma or Stress Fracture With Reaction

- Osteoid osteoma may show rounded central lucency; however, this nidus may be masked by reactive bone
- Stress fracture may show linear pattern of sclerosis

Diabetic Foot: Charcot Changes vs. Osteomyelitis in Presence of Charcot

- Charcot foot may have large fluid collections with enhancing rim, even in absence of sepsis
- Charcot foot may have soft tissue ulceration
- Charcot foot may show reactive bone changes: Decreased T1 signal, increased signal on fluid-sensitive sequences, enhancement, even without sepsis
- Several factors help to differentiate Charcot from infection
  - Confluent T1 signal seen in bone with osteomyelitis; reticulated hazy signal in reactive bone
  - Osseous fragments more likely to be seen in Charcot fluid collections than abscess from infection
  - Sinus tracts and soft tissue fat replacement more common with infection
  - Diffuse joint fluid enhancement more common in infection; thin rim enhancement in Charcot

PATHOLOGY

General Features

- Etiology
  - Hematogenous spread is most frequent
    - Neonates: *Staphylococcus aureus*, group B *Streptococcus*, *Escherichia coli*
    - Normal child: *Staphylococcus aureus* most common
    - Children and adults with sickle cell disease: *Staphylococcus* predominates, but *Salmonella* has higher incidence than normal
    - Normal adults: *Staphylococcus* most frequent; enteric pathogens also seen
    - IV drug users: Often gram-negative species (*Pseudomonas*, *Klebsiella*)
  - Soft tissue ulceration and contiguous spread
  - Soft tissue infection of hand or foot spreads along fascial planes and tendon sheaths
    - Site of osteomyelitis may be distant from initial soft tissue injury
  - Hand bones at risk for infection from human bite (particularly if skin broken from punching mouth)
  - Stubbed toe with hematoma beneath nail bed at risk for infection (nail bed is adjacent to periosteum)
  - Direct blow with hematoma formation
  - Systemic diseases may increase risk of osteomyelitis
    - Diabetic patients
    - HIV/AIDS patients
    - Sickle cell anemia patients
  - Chronic recurrent multifocal osteomyelitis (plasma cell osteomyelitis)
    - Children and adolescents
    - Repeated episodes of pain and soft tissue swelling
    - Infectious organism identified only by biopsy (or may never be identified)
    - Radiographs often normal; diagnosed by MR

CLINICAL ISSUES

Presentation

- Most common signs/symptoms
  - Pain, fever, chills
  - Elevated sedimentation rate, WBC count
  - May present without systemic symptoms or abnormal laboratory values

Natural History & Prognosis

- Acute osteomyelitis
  - If untreated, may progress to aggressive destruction and abscess formation
  - If untreated, may be walled off by reactive bone and progress to chronic osteomyelitis
- Chronic osteomyelitis
  - May appear unchanged for years, then reactivate
  - Reactivation may be difficult to diagnose since changes of chronic osteomyelitis may mask it
  - Serial imaging may show new destruction
  - If no radiographic progression, bone scanning &/or tagged leukocyte nuclear medicine scanning may improve specificity
  - Chronic osteomyelitis with draining sinus tract may develop squamous cell carcinoma
    - Generally after several years of drainage
    - New pain and bone destruction in setting of chronic drainage should suggest diagnosis
    - Generally difficult to treat; high mortality rate

DIAGNOSTIC CHECKLIST

Consider

- Time course of destructive changes in osteomyelitis is faster than tumor
  - Exception is Langerhans cell histiocytosis, which rarely may show extremely rapid destruction

SELECTED REFERENCES

1. Prieto-Pérez L et al: Osteomyelitis: a descriptive study. Clin Orthop Surg. 6(1):20-5, 2014
2. van der Bruggen W et al: PET and SPECT in osteomyelitis and prosthetic bone and joint infections: a systematic review. Semin Nucl Med. 40(1):3-15, 2010
3. Sella EJ: Current concepts review: diagnostic imaging of the diabetic foot. Foot Ankle Int. 30(6):568-76, 2009
4. Fayad LM et al: Musculoskeletal infection: role of CT in the emergency department. Radiographics. 27(6):1723-36, 2007
5. Ahmadi ME et al: Neuropathic arthropathy of the foot with and without superimposed osteomyelitis: MR imaging characteristics. Radiology. 238(2):622-31, 2006
6. Collins MS et al: T1-weighted MRI characteristics of pedal osteomyelitis. AJR Am J Roentgenol. 185(2):386-93, 2005

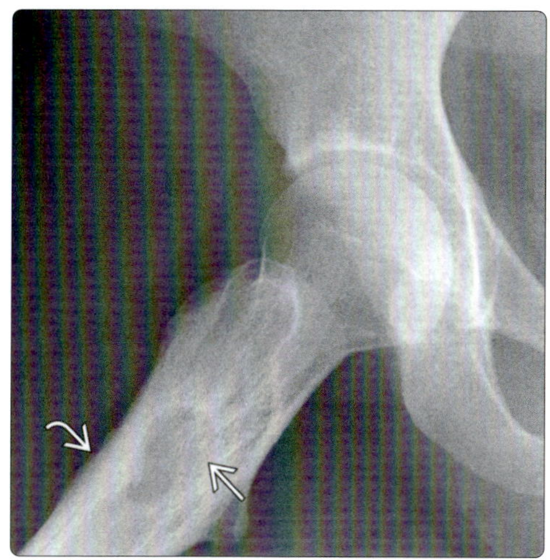

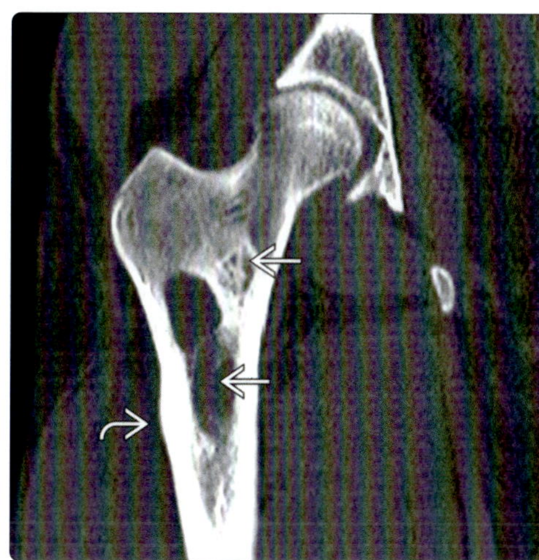

(Left) *Lateral radiograph shows a multiloculated lytic lesion ➡, which has adjacent prominent endosteal and periosteal cortical reactive bone formation ➡. The most cost-effective next step would be MR. However, in this case, CT was performed.* **(Right)** *Coronal bone CT confirms the radiographic findings, showing the multiple lytic lesions ➡ and reactive bone formation ➡. The pattern is highly typical of osteomyelitis, but confirmation is required.*

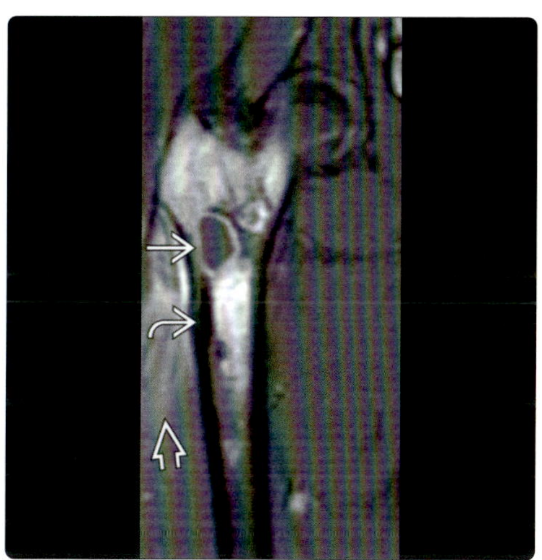

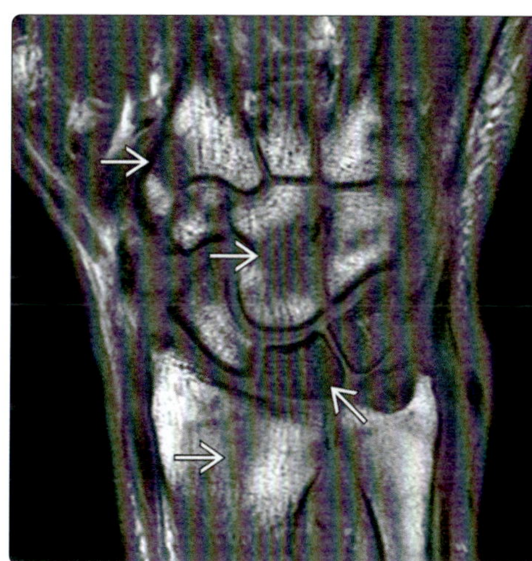

(Left) *Coronal T1WI C+ FS MR is confirmatory, with regions of marrow enhancement surrounding rim-enhancing fluid ➡ and cortical/endosteal reactive bone ➡. Adjacent soft tissue enhancement is without abscess ➡.* **(Right)** *Coronal T1 MR shows ↓ SI in multiple bones, including portions of radius, ulna, carpal bones, and base of 2nd metacarpal ➡. The T1 signal abnormality is confluent in many of these sites, more suggestive of marrow replacement (as by osteomyelitis) than reactive edema.*

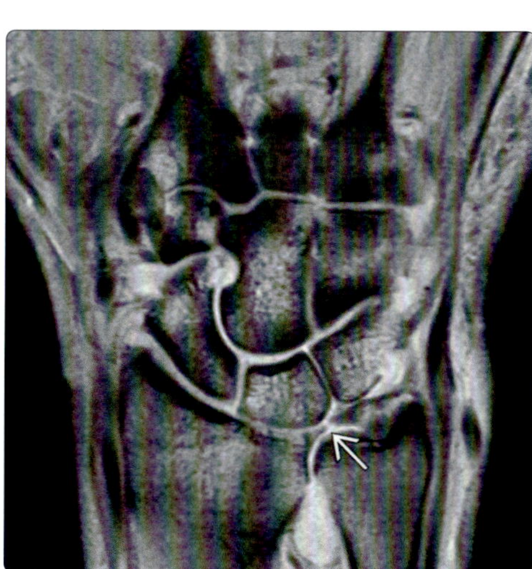

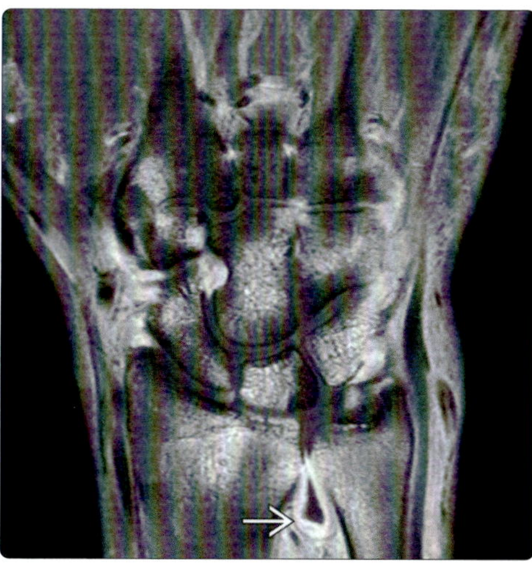

(Left) *Coronal PD FS MR shows corresponding high signal in the bones along with disruption of the triangular fibrocartilage complex ➡ and scapholunate ligaments. Fluid is seen in all 3 compartments.* **(Right)** *Coronal T1WI C+ FS MR shows enhancement of the synovium ➡ and osseous structures to be intense. The differential diagnosis is inflammatory arthritis vs. osteomyelitis with septic joints. At arthroscopy, purulent material was seen, along with destructive changes involving most of the osseous structures.*

(Left) *This patient recently arrived from Africa with shoulder pain and swelling. The radiograph shows air within the soft tissues ➡, as well as a lytic lesion in the scapula ➡. Note that soft tissue fat planes have been obliterated.* **(Right)** *Axial bone CT in the same patient shows lytic lesions within the body of the scapula ➡. It should be noted that CT is not the optimal study to demonstrate abscess formation, though the foci of osteomyelitis are confirmed. The more cost-effective study, MR, was then performed.*

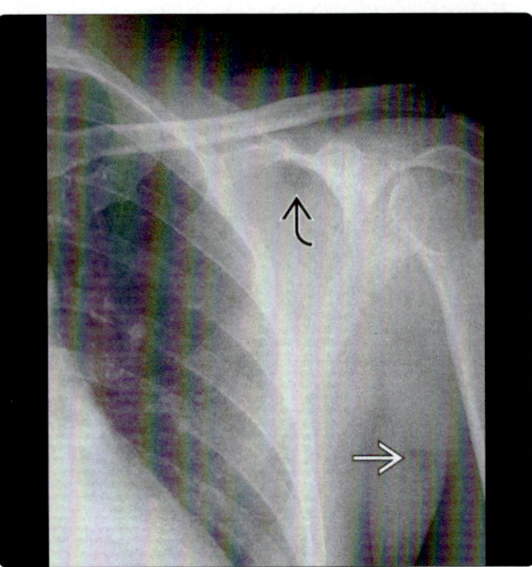

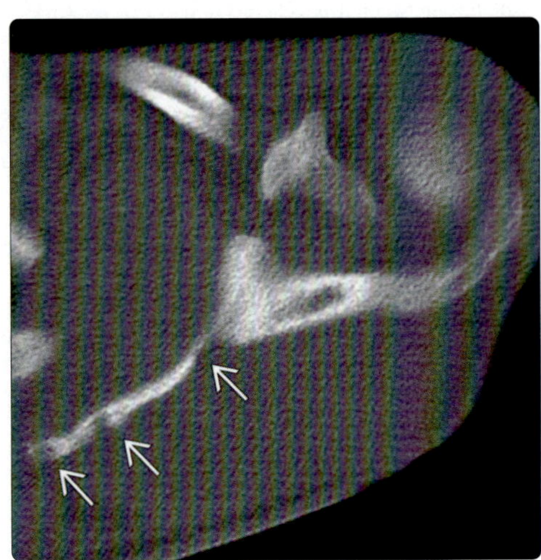

(Left) *Axial T1WI C+ FS MR shows abscess formation within the subscapularis ➡ and infraspinatus ➡ muscles as low signal fluid collections surrounded by high signal rim and muscle edema. The constellation of findings of osseous destruction with surrounding soft tissue abscess is diagnostic of osteomyelitis. Aspiration yielded Staphylococcus.* **(Right)** *AP radiograph shows a lytic lesion within the lateral portion of the patella ➡. There is a wide differential for this lesion; further work-up is required.*

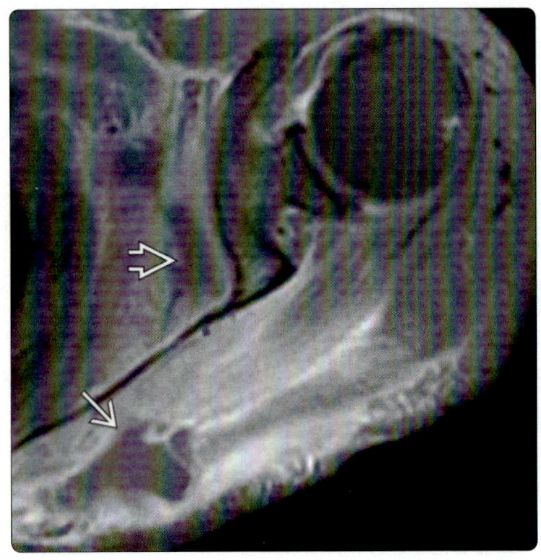

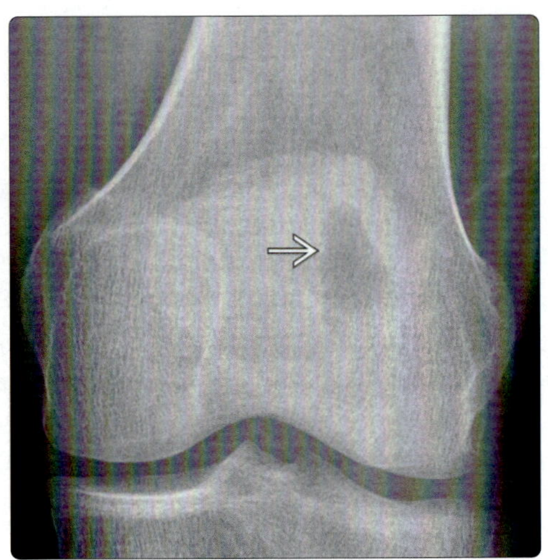

(Left) *Sagittal T2WI FS MR in the same patient shows the lesion to be fluid signal ➡ but also shows a low signal blooming metallic artifact within the superior patella ➡. This suggests penetrating injury with a metallic foreign body too small to be seen on a radiograph. There is edema within the adjacent Hoffa fat pad ➡, as well as a large effusion.* **(Right)** *Coronal T1WI C+ FS MR shows the patellar lesion to have an enhancing rim surrounding low signal fluid ➡; staphylococcal osteomyelitis was proven.*

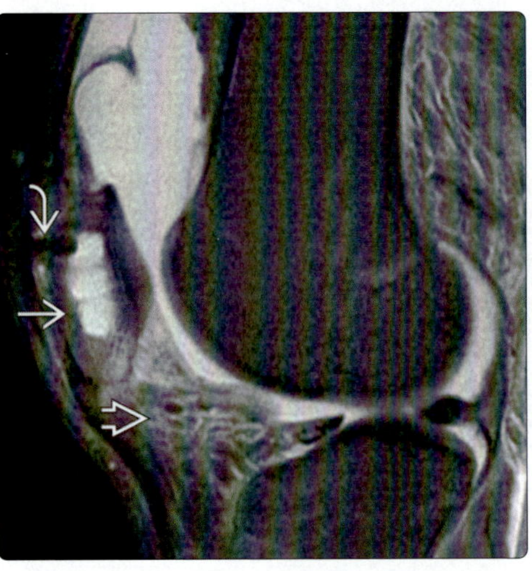

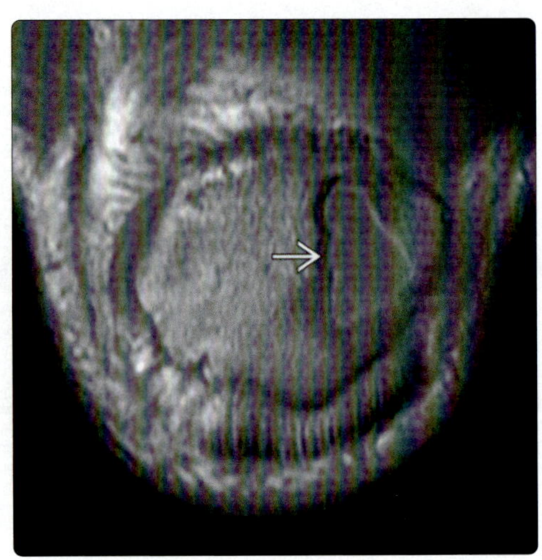

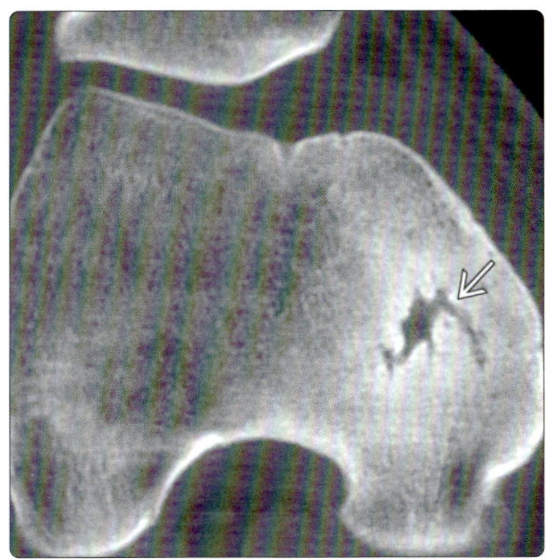

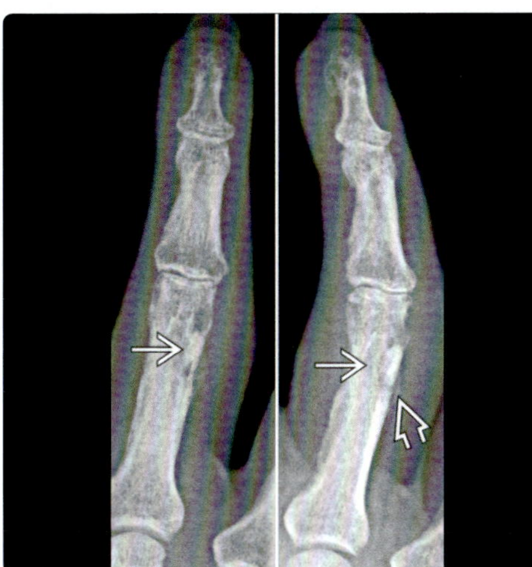

(Left) *Axial CT shows a permeative pattern of bone destruction and sclerotic reaction, which involves this entire cross section. There is a focal lytic region* ➡ *with serpiginous branching. This serpiginous pattern is almost pathognomonic for osteomyelitis.* **(Right)** *PA (left) & oblique (right) radiographs demonstrate soft tissue swelling about a proximal phalanx, as well as dense periosteal reaction* ➡*. There is a lytic focus containing an oval sclerotic piece of bone* ➡*, a sequestrum within an involucrum.*

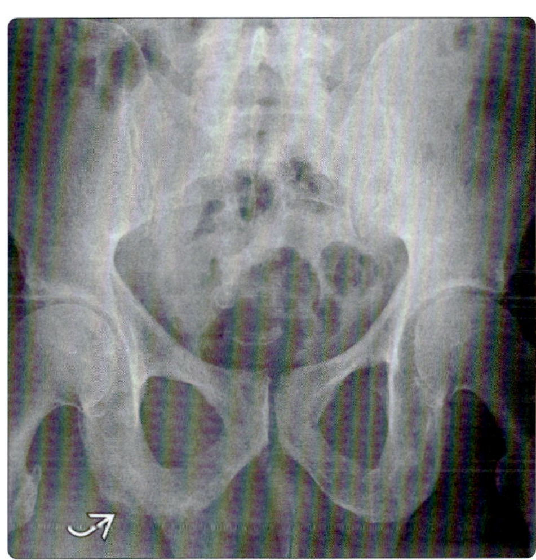

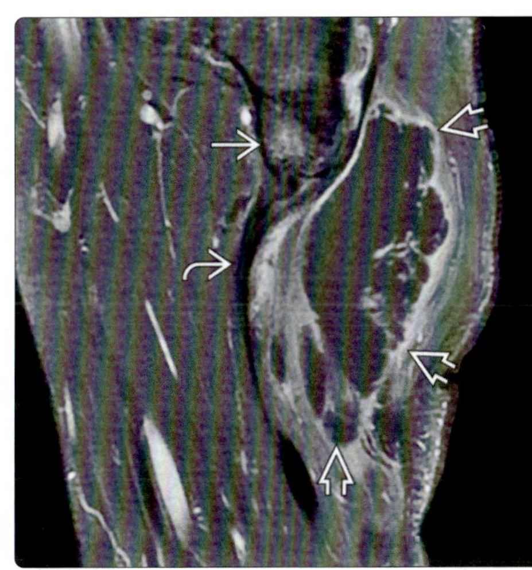

(Left) *AP radiograph demonstrates irregular lucency at the right ischial tuberosity* ➡*. This could represent trauma (tug lesion of the hamstrings), resorption from hyperparathyroidism, or osteomyelitis.* **(Right)** *Sagittal postcontrast T1FS MR in the same patient shows enhancement of the ischium* ➡*. The hamstrings* ➡ *are bowed forward but are intact. There is a large, multiloculated fluid collection with enhancing rim* ➡*, indicating soft tissue abscess and complicating this case of osteomyelitis.*

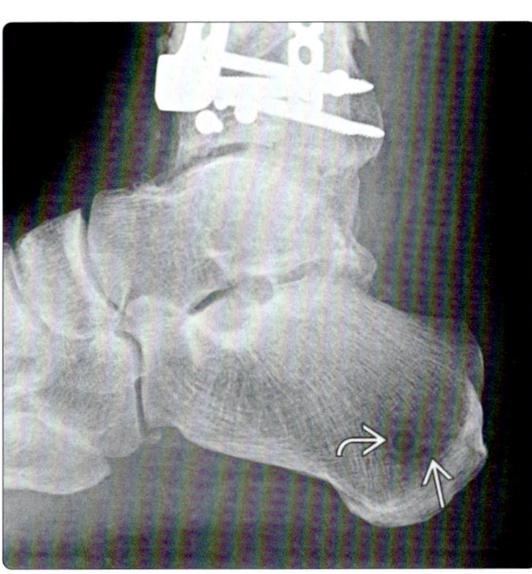

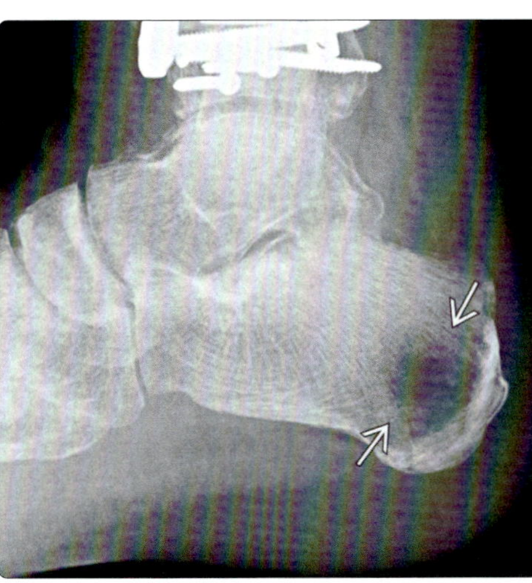

(Left) *Lateral radiograph shows a ring and button sequestrum* ➡ *at a pin tract (from traction for tibial fracture). While one might hope that there is healing at the pin tract, one should also note a slightly serpiginous track leading from it* ➡*. This is strongly suggestive of osteomyelitis.* **(Right)** *Lateral radiograph obtained in same patient 3 months later shows more extensive permeative change* ➡*, indicating progression of a relatively minor pin tract infection to a more extensive osteomyelitis.*

KEY FACTS

TERMINOLOGY

- Infectious spondylitis, discitis, vertebral body osteomyelitis

IMAGING

- Most common in lumbar spine
- Osteomyelitis
  - Focal destruction of endplate, progresses to extensive destruction, vertebral body collapse
  - Disc space narrowing
  - Malalignment, kyphosis → instability
  - MR: Bone marrow edema, changes begin at endplate, extend into vertebral body; paraspinal edema, phlegmon, abscess
- Septic arthritis
  - Subchondral edema, destruction
  - Periarticular soft tissue edema, joint effusion
- MR is most sensitive and specific
- Bone scan and labeled white cell scan: ↓ sensitivity compared to detection at other sites in body
- Percutaneous biopsy: Pathogen identified in < 50%
  - Sample endplate not disc, send for histology

TOP DIFFERENTIAL DIAGNOSES

- Amyloid deposition disease related to dialysis
  - Most common in cervical spine
- Inflammatory arthritis and crystal deposition
  - May require aspiration; send for crystal analysis

PATHOLOGY

- *Staphylococcus aureus* most common pathogen

CLINICAL ISSUES

- Severe pain, patient often unable to lie still
- 1st peak in children, 2nd peak in older adults
- If untreated → abscess, may progress to spinal instability with neurologic deficit, rarely death
- Treatment: Antimicrobial therapy is mainstay
  - Surgical debridement typically not indicated
  - Surgical stabilization if significant instability

(Left) *Lateral radiograph shows a classic case of vertebral osteomyelitis. The L4-5 disc space is narrowed ➔. Irregular destruction of both endplates is present with accompanying sclerosis.* **(Right)** *Sagittal T1WI MR in the same patient shows diffuse heterogeneous low signal present throughout the L4 and L5 vertebral bodies ➔. The normal low signal line of the endplate is absent, indicative of endplate destruction. The anterior paraspinal soft tissues are ill defined due to inflammation ➔.*

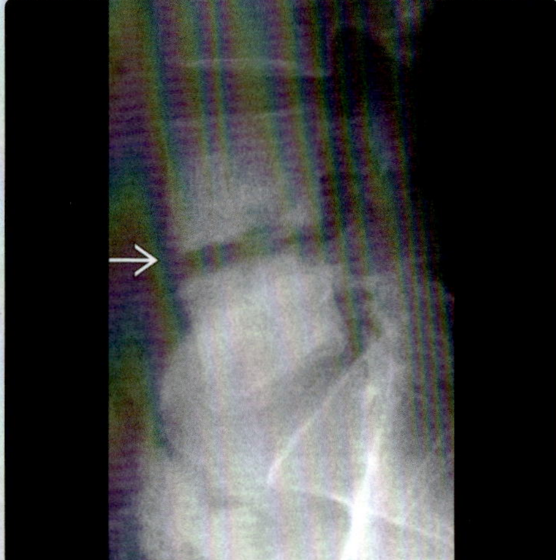

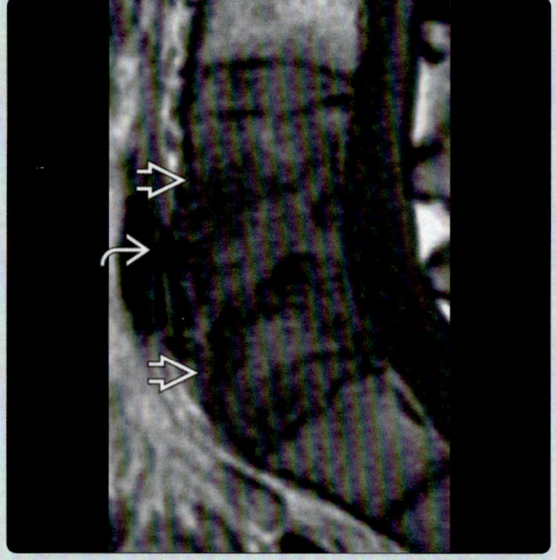

(Left) *Sagittal T2WI MR, same patient, shows ↑ SI throughout both vertebral bodies ➔ and bright intradiscal signal ➔. The low SI along the vertebral endplates ➔ is not an uncommon finding in vertebral osteomyelitis.* **(Right)** *Sagittal T1WI C+ MR in the same patient shows diffuse enhancement of vertebral bodies ➔ and disc enhancement, characteristic of vertebral body osteomyelitis. Irregular disc morphology with herniation into the vertebra ➔ results from endplate destruction.*

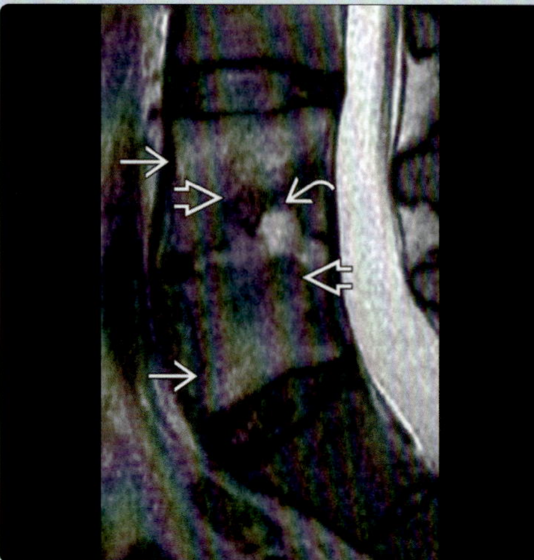

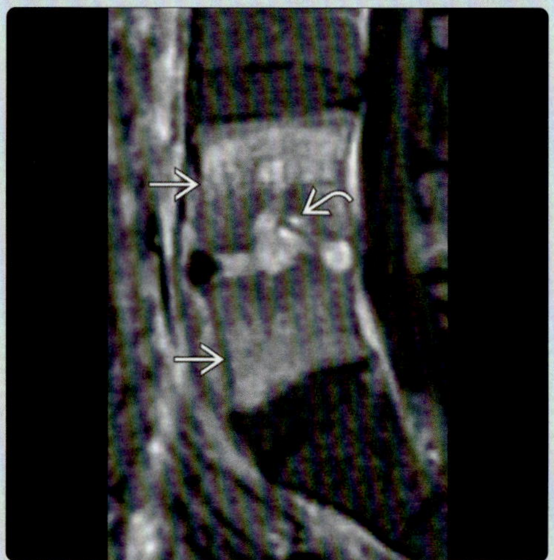

TERMINOLOGY

Synonyms

- Infectious spondylitis, discitis, vertebral body osteomyelitis, discitis osteomyelitis

Definitions

- Discitis: Infection of disc space, typically secondary phenomenon related to vertebral body osteomyelitis
  - Term vertebral osteomyelitis preferred to discitis
- Epidural abscess: Abscess in epidural space, may be isolated or related to osteomyelitis

IMAGING

General Features

- Best diagnostic clue
  - Vertebral osteomyelitis/discitis: Disc space narrowing, endplate destruction, bone marrow edema
  - Septic facet arthritis: Joint effusion, bone marrow edema, and surrounding soft tissue inflammation
- Location
  - Osteomyelitis: Most common in lumbar spine
    - 95% in vertebral body; spares posterior elements
  - Septic arthritis: Most common in facets of lumbar spine

Radiographic Findings

- Osteomyelitis/discitis
  - Osseous destruction: Begins with focal destruction of endplate, progresses to extensive destruction, vertebral body collapse
  - Disc space narrowing
  - Paraspinal new bone is immature during active infection, especially bacterial
  - Sclerosis not uncommon in bacterial disease
    - May be absent or more extensive in fungal disease
    - Limited with tuberculous disease
  - Healing
    - Increased vertebral body sclerosis
    - Maturing paraspinal new bone
    - May lead to ankylosis across disc space
  - Malalignment, kyphosis → instability
  - Intradisc vacuum phenomenon excludes infection
    - Use lateral extension view to evoke, may eliminate requirement for further evaluation
- Septic arthritis: Generally not visible on radiographs
- Epidural abscess: No radiographic findings

CT Findings

- Osteomyelitis/discitis
  - Endplate destructive changes
  - Immature paraspinal new bone formation
  - Paraspinal soft tissue inflammation with ill-defined fat planes
  - Paraspinal abscess: Peripheral enhancing rim
    - Pyogenic: Usually within psoas muscle
    - Tuberculous: Cold abscesses can be quite extensive
- Septic arthritis
  - Joint space widening early by effusion, narrowing late as articular cartilage destroyed
  - Cysts, foci of destruction articular surface
- Epidural infection
  - Epidural mass, diffuse enhancement with phlegmon, peripheral enhancement with abscess

MR Findings

- Osteomyelitis
  - Osseous changes
    - Bone marrow edema
      - ▫ T1WI: ↓ signal
      - ▫ Fluid-sensitive: ↑ signal
      - ▫ Changes on T2W images are least reliable: Low T2 signal may be seen
      - ▫ C+: Diffuse enhancement of involved bone
    - Early endplate destruction best seen on T1W images
    - Changes begin at endplate, extend into vertebral body
  - Paraspinal edema and phlegmon
    - T1WI: Ill-defined fat planes
    - Fluid-sensitive: Diffuse ↑ signal in fat and musculature
    - C+: Enhancement
      - ▫ Phlegmon: Mass-like, diffusely enhances
      - ▫ Abscess: Peripheral enhancement
  - Abscess
    - T1WI: Slightly hypointense to muscle; intramuscular abscess may not be visible
    - Fluid-sensitive: Focal fluid collection with ↑ signal
    - C+: Peripheral enhancement
    - May see in psoas muscle, paraspinal soft tissues, or epidural space
  - Disc space: Key to establishing diagnosis
    - Increased signal on fluid-sensitive sequences
    - Enhancement within disc space, may be subtle
  - Resolving soft tissue inflammation and ↓ epidural enhancement best indication of resolving disease
- Septic arthritis
  - Subchondral edema
    - T1WI: ↓ signal
    - Fluid-sensitive: ↑ signal
    - C+: Diffuse enhancement
      - ▫ ± synovial enhancement at joint periphery
  - Periarticular soft tissue edema
    - T1WI: Ill-defined fat planes
    - Fluid-sensitive: Diffuse ↑ signal in fat and musculature
    - C+: Diffuse enhancement
  - Joint effusion
    - T1WI: ↓ signal
    - Fluid-sensitive: ↑ signal
    - C+: Peripheral enhancement
    - May slightly widen joint space

Nuclear Medicine Findings

- Bone scan
  - Focal radioisotope uptake at site of infection
    - Diminished sensitivity compared to detection of osteomyelitis at other sites in body
    - Septic arthritis may be mistaken for arthrosis
- Ga-67 scintigraphy
  - Preferred nuclear medicine examination
- Labeled leukocyte scintigraphy
  - As with bone scan, has diminished sensitivity compared to other sites in body

Imaging Recommendations

- Best imaging tool
  - MR is most sensitive and specific
- Protocol advice
  - Osteomyelitis
    - MR imaging requires T1 and T2 images to detect bone marrow edema and soft tissue changes
    - Contrast use is essential to detect disc space enhancement, confirm abscesses
  - Septic arthritis
    - Often not suspected preimaging
    - Contrast enhancement may provide better delineation of abnormalities

Image-Guided Biopsy

- Pathogen identified in < 50%
- Diagnosis often rests on histologic identification of acute inflammatory changes
- Fine-needle aspiration less sensitive than core biopsy
- Sample vertebral endplate rather than disc
- Paraspinal approach: Easier to biopsy inferior endplate of superior vertebra to avoid nerve root
  - Transpedicular approach also avoids nerve root

Pathogen-Specific Comments

- Granulomatous disease
  - Subligamentous spread leads to noncontiguous vertebral infection
  - Coccidiomycosis may spare disc space
  - Blastomycosis may have associated rib destruction
  - Tuberculosis: Extensive paraspinal abscess formation
- Gram-negative organisms → gas formation: Multiple small bubbles in disc space and bone
  - Multiple bubbles have different appearance than linear disc vacuum sign

DIFFERENTIAL DIAGNOSIS

Amyloid Deposition Disease Related to Dialysis

- Most common in cervical spine
- Disc space narrowing, endplate destruction
- Lacks sclerosis, new bone formation, paraspinal inflammation/abscess, disc space enhancement

Bone Morphogenic Protein

- Postoperative disc space with interbody graft and surrounding endplate osteolysis
- Lacks extensive inflammatory changes of soft tissue and bone

Mechanical Disc Disease/Neuropathic Spine

- Lacks disc space enhancement, abscess formation

Neoplasms Crossing Disc Space

- Multiple myeloma, lymphoma, metastatic disease
- Lack surrounding inflammation, no abscess formation

Inflammatory Arthritis Crystal Deposition

- May require aspiration to differentiate from infection

PATHOLOGY

General Features

- Etiology
  - Most commonly result from hematogenous spread
  - Proposed spread via Batson plexus from genitourinary infection; common source in elderly individuals
  - *Staphylococcus aureus* most common pathogen
  - Pseudomonas seen in IV drug abusers
  - Fungal, tuberculous infections rare
    - Usually underlying compromised immune system
    - Seen in developing countries or immigrants and tourists from those countries
  - Increased risk in IV drug abusers
  - Other etiologies
    - Postoperative or postprocedure etiologies with direct implantation
    - Posttraumatic

CLINICAL ISSUES

Presentation

- Most common signs/symptoms
  - Severe pain, patient often unable to lie still
  - Children: Generalized symptoms of malaise, fever
- Other signs/symptoms
  - Fever
  - Neurologic deficit: Uncommon presentation

Demographics

- Age
  - 1st peak incidence in children
    - Separate mechanism: Disc is vascular, discitis results from direct seeding of disc
  - 2nd peak incidence in older adults
    - Increased incidence of immunocompromise, steroid use, malignancy, diabetes
- Gender
  - Male > female

Natural History & Prognosis

- Osteomyelitis
  - If untreated, extensive surrounding abscess develops, including epidural abscess
  - May progress to significant spinal instability with neurologic deficit, severe debility, and eventual death

Treatment

- Antimicrobial therapy is mainstay of treatment
  - Treatment failure relatively common and may occur early with *S. aureus*
- Surgical debridement typically not indicated
- Surgical stabilization if significant instability
- Rarely percutaneous drainage of psoas abscess

SELECTED REFERENCES

1. Gupta A et al: Long-term outcome of pyogenic vertebral osteomyelitis: a cohort study of 260 patients. Open Forum Infect Dis. 1(3):ofu107, 2014
2. Kowalski TJ et al: Follow-up MR imaging in patients with pyogenic spine infections: lack of correlation with clinical features. AJNR Am J Neuroradiol. 28(4):693-9, 2007

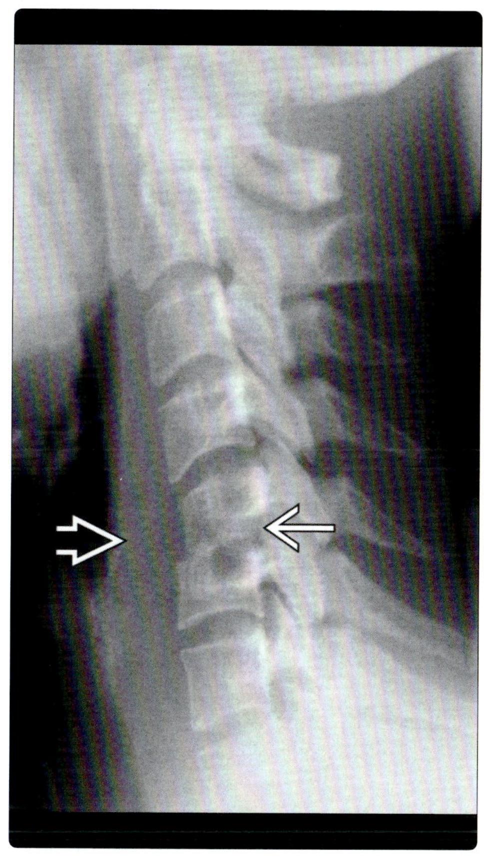

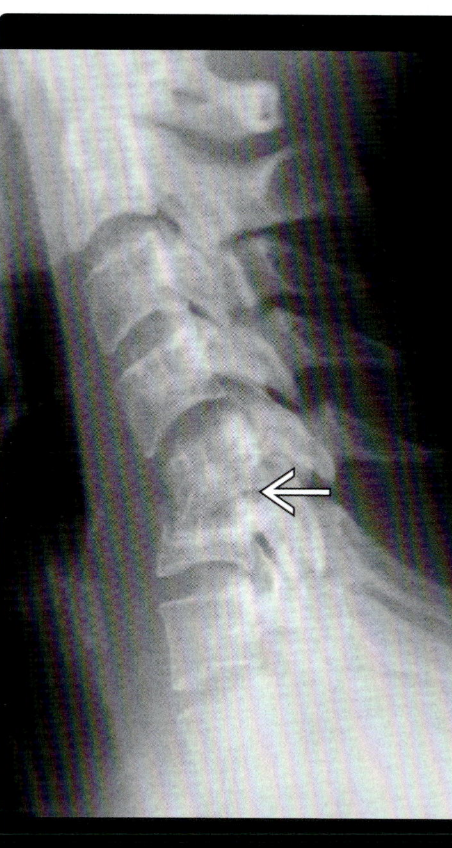

(Left) *Lateral radiograph of a patient with severe neck pain shows destruction of the C5-6 disc space and adjacent endplates ➡. At this time, there is no sclerosis or periosteal new bone. This appearance may be seen with either vertebral osteomyelitis or amyloid deposition disease. However, the patient had no supportive clinical history for amyloid. Soft tissue fullness is seen anteriorly ➡, either from diffuse soft tissue inflammation or, less likely, abscess. Soft tissue changes are uncommon with amyloid deposition disease.* **(Right)** *Lateral x-ray, same patient 2 weeks later, shows progression of the vertebral destruction & new kyphosis ➡. Even with appropriate therapy for infection, osseous changes will progress for a period of time. MR evidence of resolving soft tissue inflammatory changes is the best evidence of improving infection.*

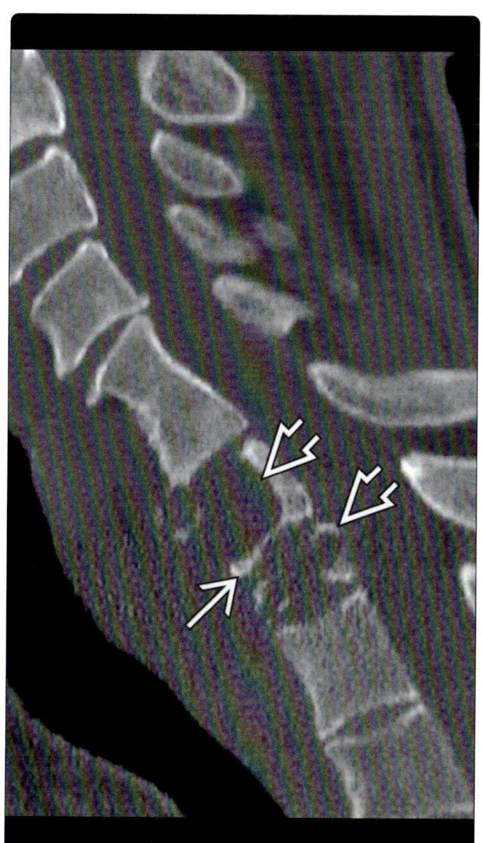

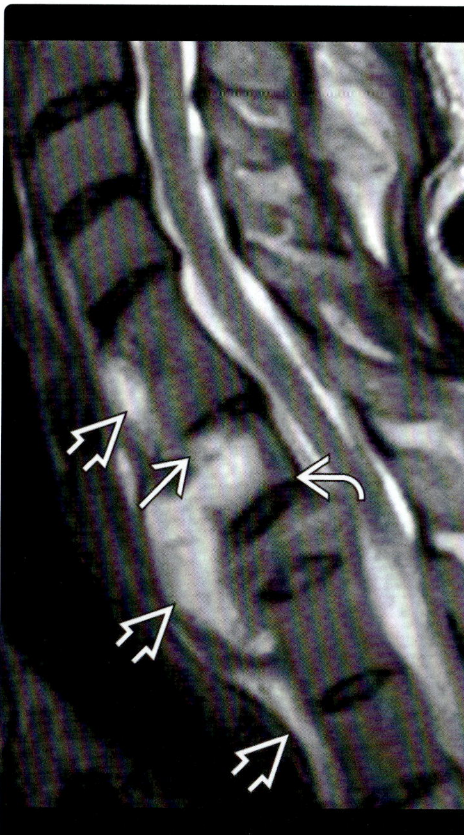

(Left) *Sagittal NECT of a patient with coccidiomycosis is shown. The osseous lesions ➡ have geographic, nonsclerotic margins that are typical of this pathogen. Extensive destruction at T1 has resulted in vertebral collapse. The C7-T1 disc space is preserved ➡ despite the extensive osseous disease, which is a characteristic feature of coccidiomycosis.* **(Right)** *Sagittal T2WI MR from the same patient confirms sparing of the C7-T1 disc space ➡. Bright T2 signal indicates early involvement of the C6-7 disc ➡. The osseous lesion has extended beyond the anterior vertebral cortex, resulting in extensive anterior soft tissue inflammation ➡. The inflammatory changes have spread across multiple levels, and it is easy to appreciate the subligamentous pattern of spread, which can lead to multilevel noncontiguous disease.*

(Left) *Axial NECT shows typical destruction and fragmentation of advanced osteomyelitis ➡. Paraspinal inflammatory changes are minimal; however, epidural disease is present ➡.* **(Right)** *Sagittal STIR MR shows typical increased signal throughout 2 contiguous thoracic vertebral bodies and the intervening disc, indicative of vertebral osteomyelitis. Somewhat unusual features in this case include involvement of posterior elements (facet joint ➡) and posteriorly located epidural phlegmon ➡.*

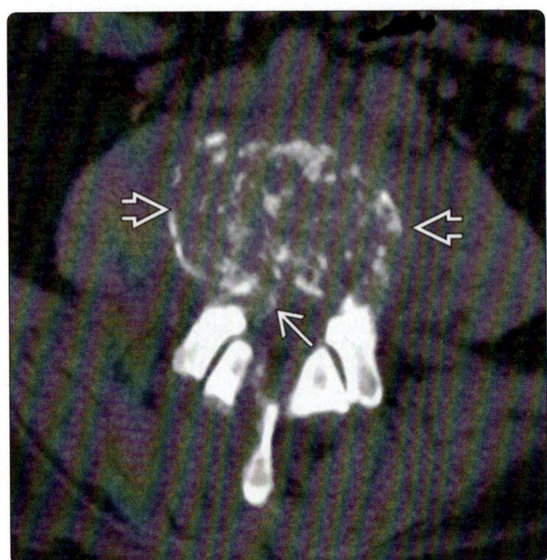

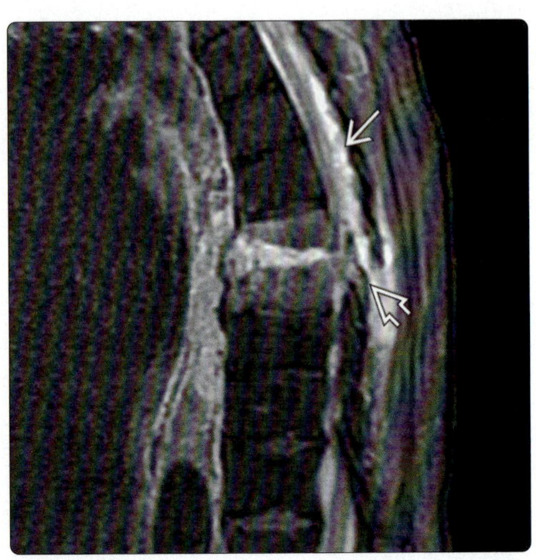

(Left) *Axial T1WI MR shows typical osteomyelitis. The marrow is diffusely hypointense ➡ and fat planes surrounding the vertebra and the epidural fat ➡ are ill defined as a result of the extensive inflammatory process.* **(Right)** *Axial T1WI C+ FS MR shows extensive inflammatory changes in the psoas ➡, posterior paraspinal muscles ➡, and epidural soft tissues ➡. This extensive inflammation is seen with pyogenic infections and is not expected in the cold abscesses of tuberculous disease.*

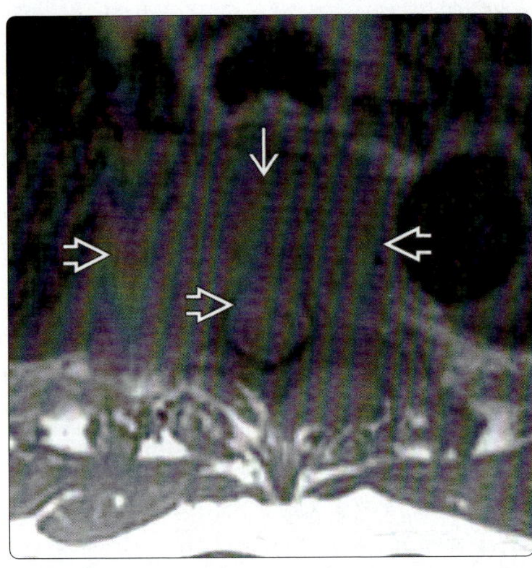

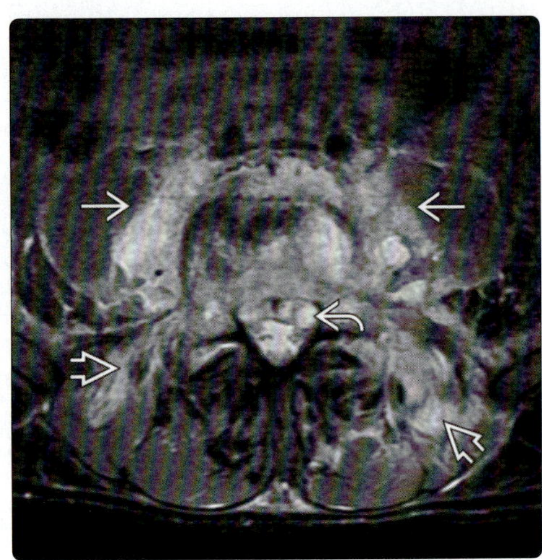

(Left) *Axial NECT shows destruction of the right C1-2 facet joint ➡ with malalignment and osseous fragmentation. This is a case where the location can turn a benign disease into a highly aggressive process because of the potential for neurologic compromise.* **(Right)** *Sagittal T1WI C+ MR of the same patient reveals the full extent of the disease. There is phlegmon throughout the upper spinal canal, extending cephalad ➡. The MR also shows the extent of osseous disease throughout the dens ➡.*

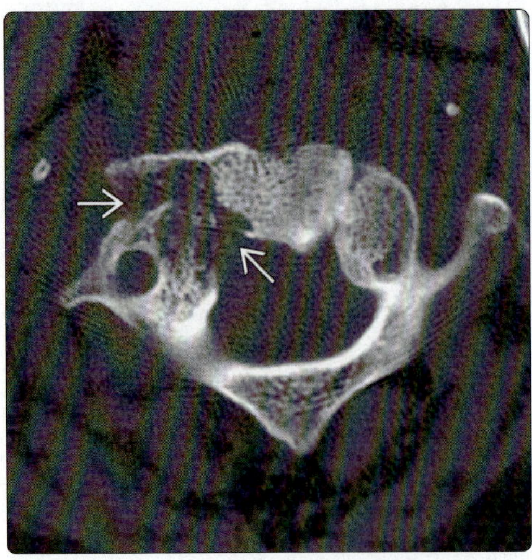

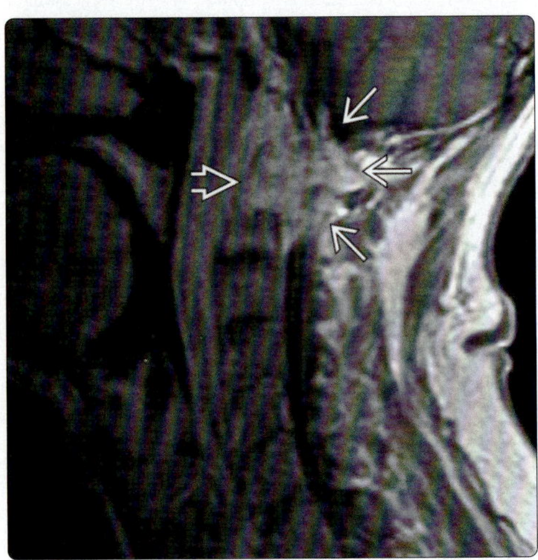

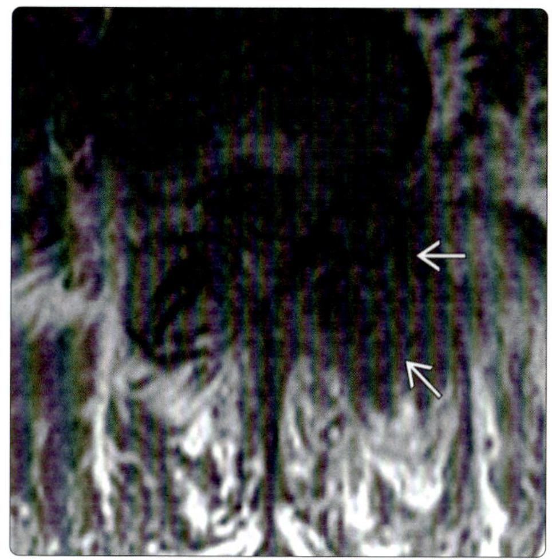

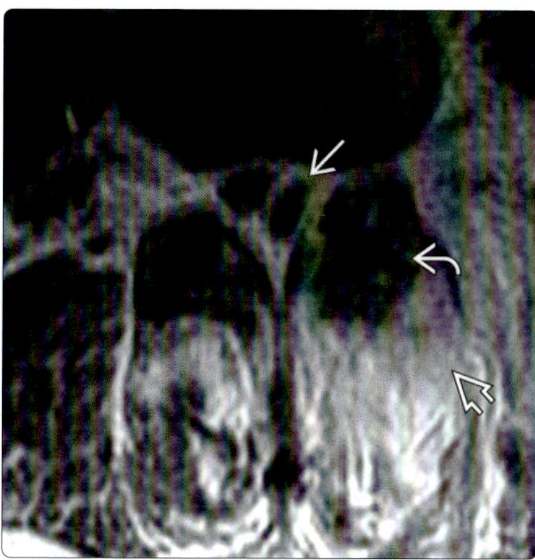

(Left) *Axial T1WI MR demonstrates ill definition of the articular surfaces of the left facet joint and the surrounding soft tissues. This appearance should raise concern for an inflammatory process, including the possibility of septic arthritis.* **(Right)** *Axial T1WI C+ MR in the same patient shows irregularity of the articular surfaces, indicative of early facet joint destruction as well as inflammatory change in the paraspinal muscles. Posterior epidural abscess is also present.*

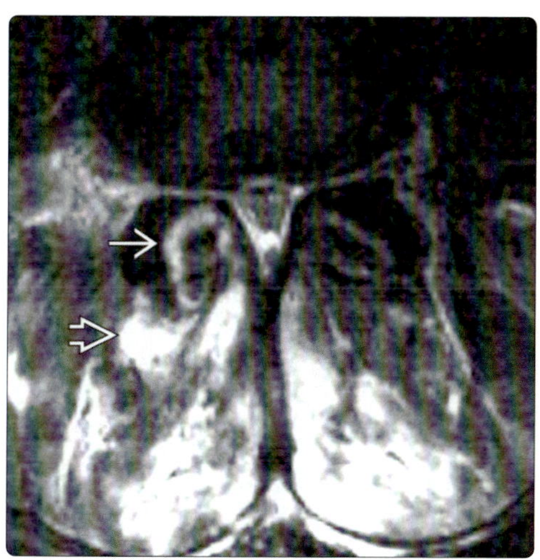

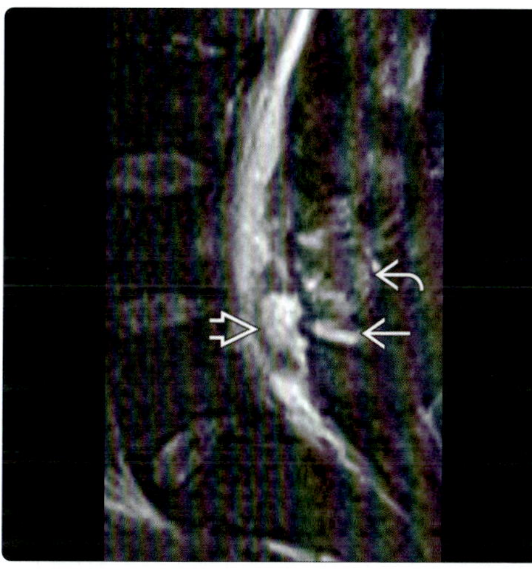

(Left) *Axial T2WI MR of the lumbar spine demonstrates asymmetric ↑ T2 signal in the right facet joint. While joint fluid is not uncommon with facet arthrosis, the edema/fluid in the surrounding musculature is a clue to the fact that a different process is at work.* **(Right)** *Sagittal T2WI demonstrates fluid within a facet joint, edema in the articular facet, and an epidural abscess. This constellation of findings should raise concern for septic arthritis of facet joint.*

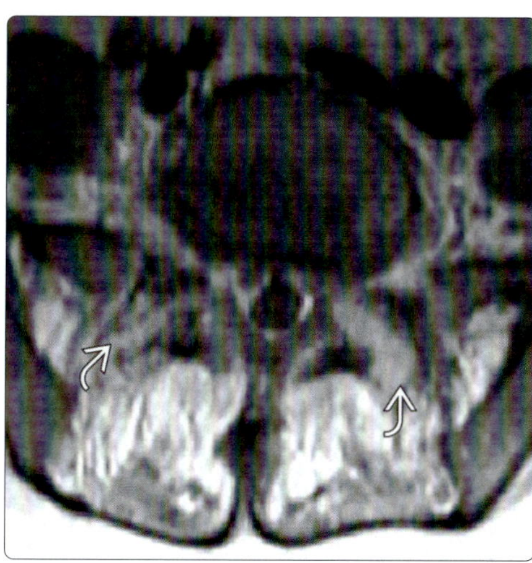

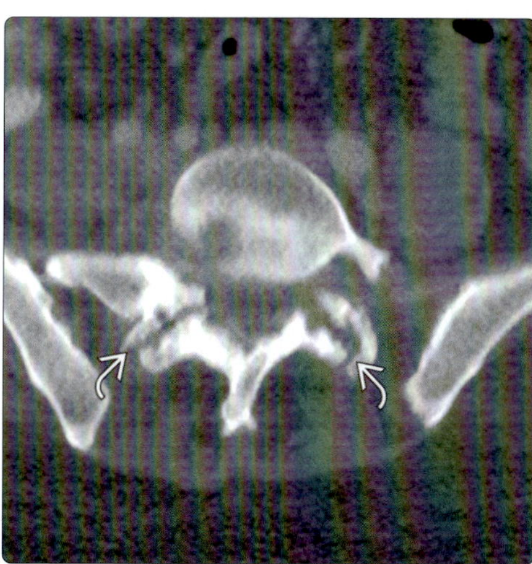

(Left) *Axial T1WI C+ MR shows diffuse enhancement in both facet joints, accompanied by destruction of the articular surfaces. While septic facet arthritis is uncommon, bilateral disease is even more rare.* **(Right)** *Axial NECT of the same patient shows the extent of joint space narrowing and destruction of the articular surfaces of both facet joints. Crystal deposition disease may have a similar appearance. In some instances, aspiration of the joint is required to confirm the diagnosis.*

KEY FACTS

TERMINOLOGY

- Brodie abscess: Subacute osteomyelitis with single focus of intraosseous abscess formation
- Chronic osteomyelitis: Persistent infection of bone despite treatment, evolves over months to years

IMAGING

- Long bones: Femur, tibia most common locations
- Brodie abscess
  - Radiographs: Lytic lesion with geographic nonsclerotic margins, metaphyseal location
  - MR: Well-defined intraosseous abscess with peripheral enhancement, typically metaphyseal
- Chronic active osteomyelitis
  - Radiographs: Thickened, irregular sclerotic bone
  - Periosteal bone formation, soft tissue swelling ± sequestrum
  - MR: Marrow and soft tissue edema, abscess, sinus tracts

TOP DIFFERENTIAL DIAGNOSES

- Brodie abscess: Langerhans cell histiocytosis, giant cell tumor
- Chronic active osteomyelitis: Neoplasm

PATHOLOGY

- Results from untreated or undertreated acute infection, leading to dead bone that continues to harbor bacteria

CLINICAL ISSUES

- Deep bone pain, draining sinus
- Risk factors: Diabetes, dialysis, IV drug abuse, poor nutrition, smoking, trauma
- Untreated: Abscess, sinuses, may require amputation
- Treatment: Surgical debridement and parenteral antibiotics
  - May use antibiotic impregnated cement within surgical defect
- Rarely develop squamous cell carcinoma 2° to metaplasia along sinus tract; occurs after 20-30 years

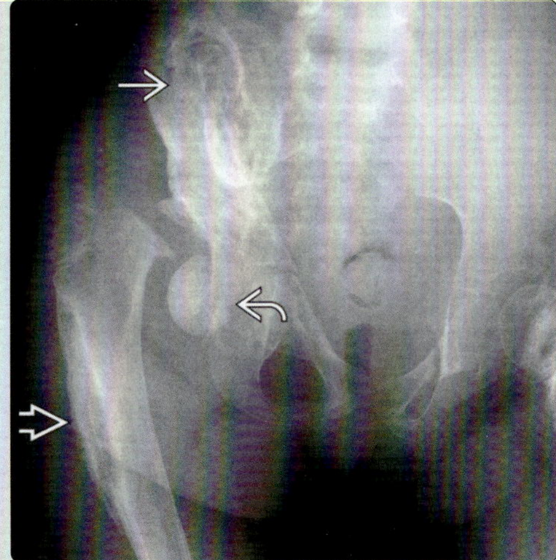

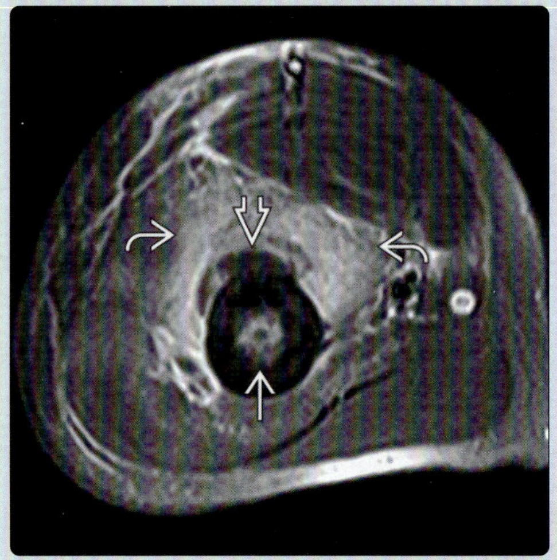

(Left) *AP radiograph of a pelvis shows multifocal chronic osteomyelitis. Irregular lucency and sclerosis are present throughout the right ilium ➡ and along the lateral right femur ➡. The femoral epiphysis has slipped and is sclerotic ➡, indicating ongoing infection.* **(Right)** *Axial T1WI C+ FS MR depicts typical changes of chronic osteomyelitis. There is marrow enhancement ➡, periosteal new bone formation ➡, cortical thickening, and extensive soft tissue inflammation ➡.*

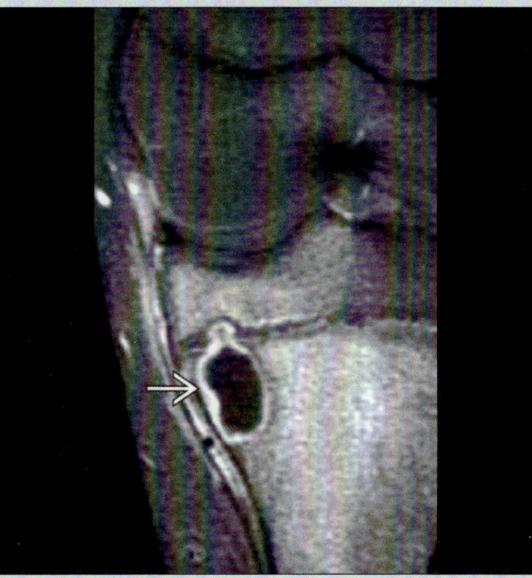

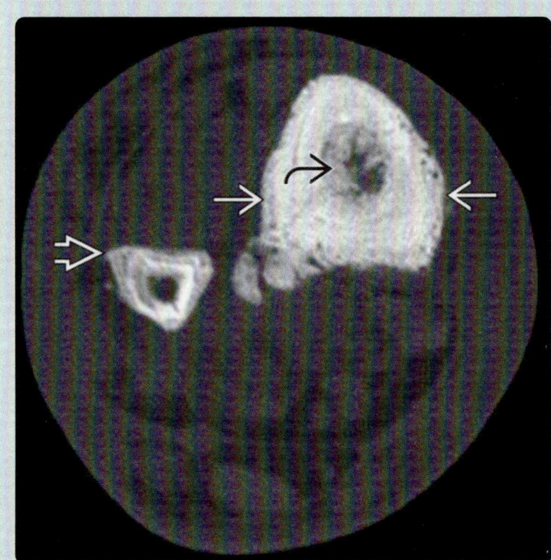

(Left) *Coronal T1 C+ MR shows a typical example of subacute osteomyelitis and Brodie abscess ➡. The abscess is located in the metaphysis and has crossed the growth plate. Peripheral enhancement confirms the diagnosis.* **(Right)** *Axial NECT reveals classic chronic osteomyelitis. Massive mature periosteal new bone formation is present around the tibial diaphysis ➡ and, to a lesser degree, along the fibula ➡. The cortical endosteum is markedly thickened as well ➡. This tremendous reaction is typical of chronic infection.*

TERMINOLOGY

Definitions

- Brodie abscess: Subacute osteomyelitis with intraosseous abscess formation
- Chronic osteomyelitis: Persistent infection of bone despite treatment, evolves over months to years
  - Chronic indolent osteomyelitis: Low-grade infection without episodes of activity/inflammation
  - Chronic relapsing course: Intermittent periods of active inflammation
- Cloaca: Defect in bone caused by spontaneous decompression of infection
- Involucrum: New bone formation by periosteum around infected bone, occurs in attempt to wall off infection; more common in children who have looser attachment of periosteum to cortex
- Sequestrum: Devascularized fragment of bone
  - Variable size from small fragment to entire bone

IMAGING

General Features

- Best diagnostic clue
  - Thickened, irregular sclerotic bone with periostitis
- Location
  - Long bones: Femur and tibia most common

Imaging Recommendations

- Best imaging tool
  - MR best for demonstrating inflammatory changes
  - CT useful for identifying sequestrum
- Protocol advice
  - MR and CT: Intravenous contrast material essential for detecting sinus tracts, abscesses

Radiographic Findings

- Comparison with old films may be useful
  - Interval changes often not radiographically evident, even with relapsing disease
- Chronic active osteomyelitis
  - Sclerotic bone with thickened cortex along endosteal and periosteal surfaces
  - Periosteal new bone formation, soft tissue swelling
  - Sequestrum may be evident
- Brodie abscess
  - Metaphyseal lytic lesion with geographic nonsclerotic margins

CT Findings

- ↓ sensitivity vs. MR for active inflammation

MR Findings

- Active inflammation in chronic active disease
  - Marrow and soft tissue edema: ↓ SI on T1WI, ↑ SI on fluid-sensitive sequences, diffuse enhancement
  - Abscess: ↓ SI on T1WI, ↑ SI on fluid-sensitive sequences, peripheral enhancement
  - Sinus tract: Thin tract of soft tissue enhancement that extends from site of inflammation to skin
- Brodie abscess
  - Well-defined intraosseous focus with peripheral enhancement, typically metaphyseal; minimal inflammation
- Sequestrum: May see marrow fat, lacks enhancement
- Reactive joint effusion may be present

Nuclear Medicine Findings

- Bone scan, labeled white cell scans lack sensitivity for detection of active disease: PET scans may offer greatest sensitivity

DIFFERENTIAL DIAGNOSIS

DDx of Brodie Abscess

- Langerhans cell histiocytosis, giant cell tumor
  - Lacks clinical evidence of infection

DDx of Chronic Active Osteomyelitis

- Neoplasm: Ewing sarcoma, fibroosseous lesions
  - Lacks inflammatory changes, sinus tracts, abscesses

PATHOLOGY

General Features

- Etiology
  - Results from untreated or undertreated acute infection, leading to dead bone → continues to harbor bacteria
    - Dead bone lacks blood supply → no delivery of antibiotics
  - Dead bone results from ↑ intramedullary pressure with vascular compression, thrombosis, and pus-stripping periosteum, disrupting blood supply
    - Associated bone sclerosis, inflammation and fibrosis in haversian canals and surrounding soft tissues further compromise blood supply

CLINICAL ISSUES

Presentation

- Most common signs/symptoms
  - Deep bone pain, draining sinus
- Other signs/symptoms
  - Fever and systemic manifestations uncommon

Demographics

- Epidemiology
  - Risk factors: Diabetes, dialysis, IV drug abuse, poor nutrition, smoking, trauma

Natural History & Prognosis

- Untreated: Abscess, sinuses, may require amputation
- Rarely develop squamous cell carcinoma 2° to metaplasia along sinus tract; occurs after 20-30 years
- Child: Leg length discrepancy

Treatment

- Surgical debridement and parenteral antibiotics

SELECTED REFERENCES

1. Panteli M et al: Malignant transformation in chronic osteomyelitis: recognition and principles of management. J Am Acad Orthop Surg. 22(9):586-594, 2014

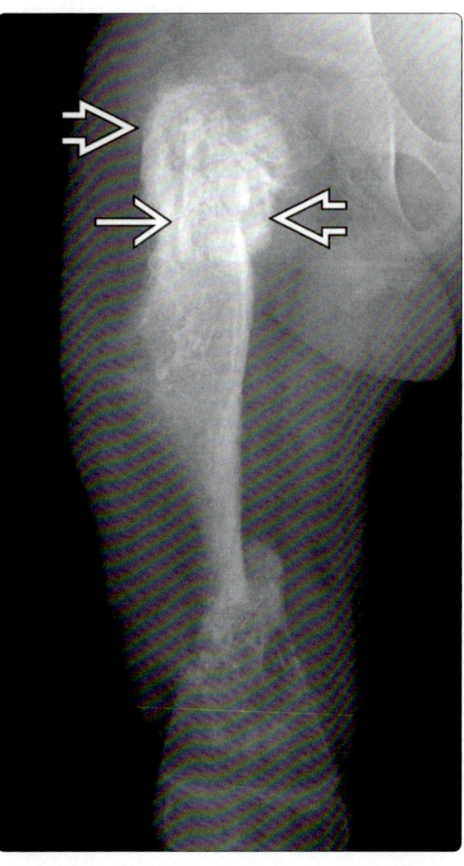

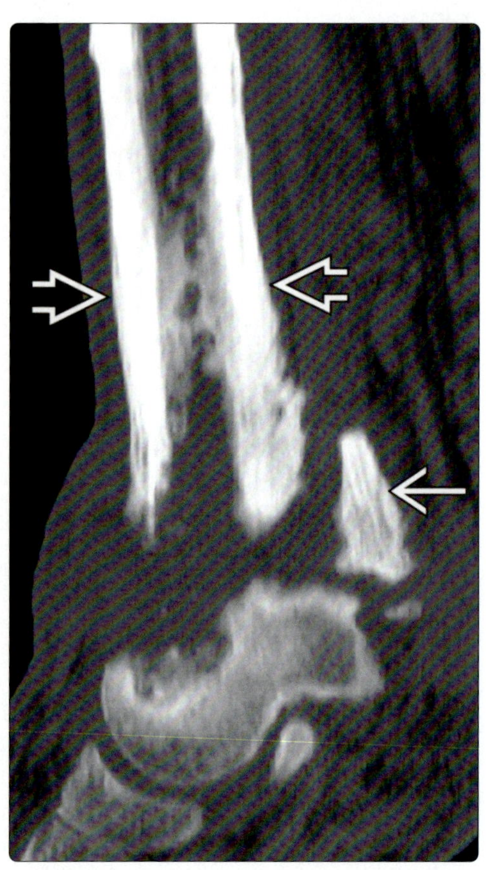

(Left) *AP radiograph shows a femur with extensive chronic osteomyelitis. Periosteal new bone is present, especially along the proximal aspect ➔ where the underlying original cortex remains visible ➔. The periosteal new bone formation is an involucrum, and it is attempting to wall off the infected femoral shaft. The femoral shaft appears to be a separate segment of bone, which is likely devascularized, representing sequestration.* **(Right)** *Sagittal reformatted NECT following explant of an infected total ankle arthroplasty is shown. Marked cortical thickening and periosteal new bone formation are present along the distal tibia ➔. These findings are rather nonaggressive in their appearance, reflecting the general low-grade nature of chronic osteomyelitis. The fibula is similarly involved ➔.*

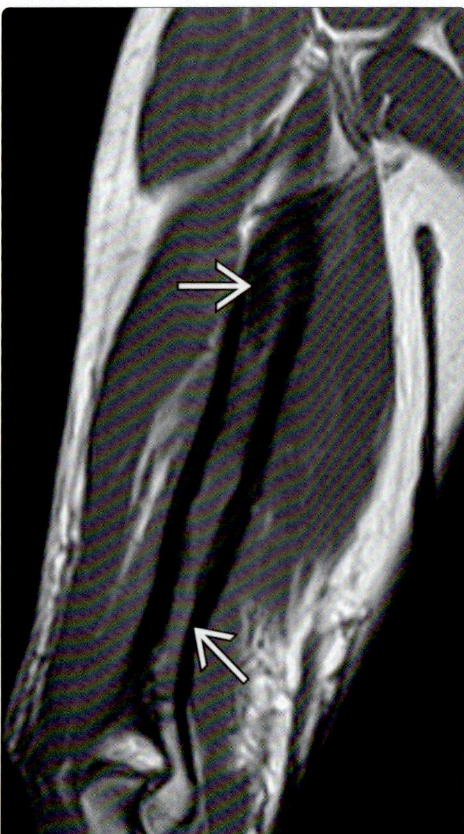

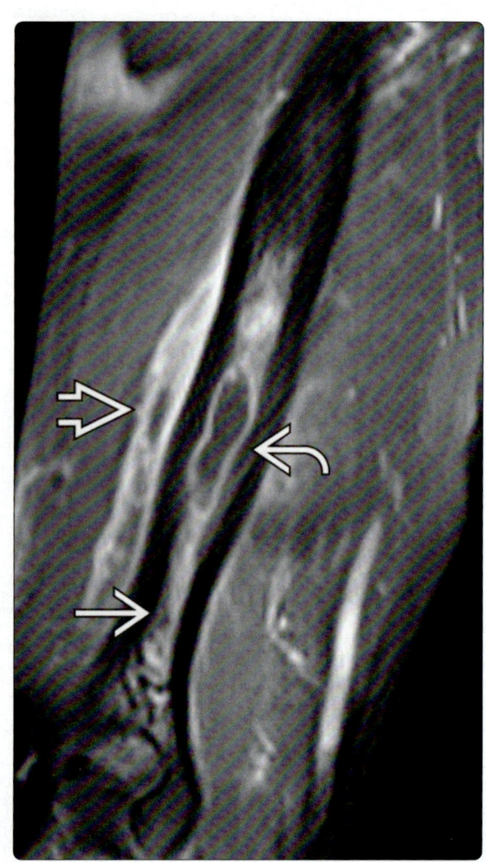

(Left) *Long axis T1WI MR shows abnormally low marrow signal throughout the entire humeral diaphysis ➔. The cortex is diffusely thickened along both the endosteal and periosteal surfaces.* **(Right)** *Long axis T1WI C+ FS MR of the same patient shows findings that indicate active inflammation include diffuse enhancement throughout the medullary canal ➔ and soft tissue inflammatory changes with a small abscess ➔. Central nonenhancing focus in the midshaft ➔ is most likely an intraosseous abscess; however, it could also represent a sequestrum. Correlation with radiographs or CT will help differentiate intraosseous abscess from sequestrum in this case. The MR findings of active inflammation establish the diagnosis of chronic active osteomyelitis.*

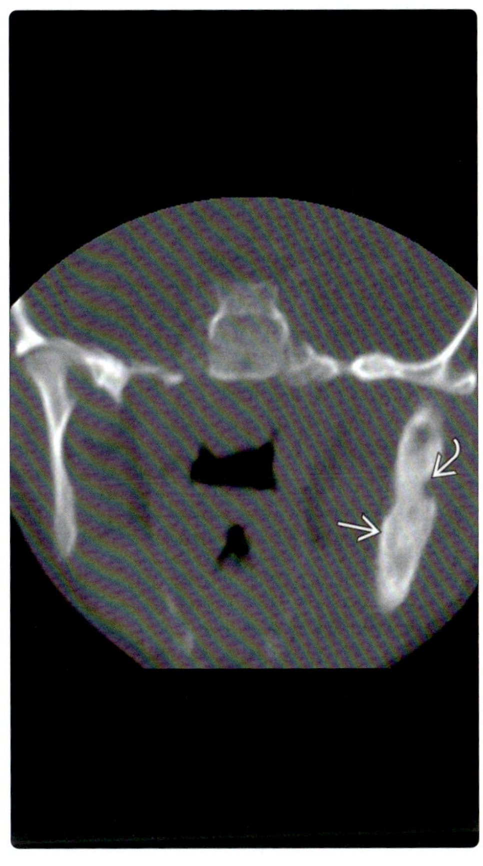

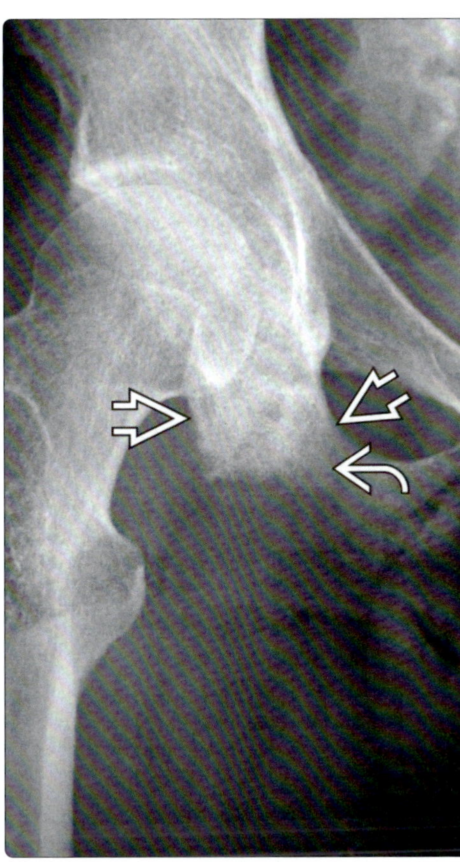

(Left) *Coronal CECT of the mandible shows enlargement and heterogeneous sclerosis throughout the left mandibular ramus ➡. A defect in the lateral cortex ➡ may represent a cloaca, a defect in bone through which infection/pus decompresses. This patient had actinomyces with multiple recurrence when he stopped taking antibiotics.* **(Right)** *AP x-ray shows a patient with longstanding chronic osteomyelitis of the ischial tuberosity, evidenced by patchy sclerosis ➡. The patient presented with a change in his symptoms, including a newly palpable lump. When compared to prior films, the margins of a preexisting defect in the tuberosity showed new ill-defined destruction ➡. Biopsy proved squamous cell carcinoma. These malignancies may occur after many years of draining sinus.*

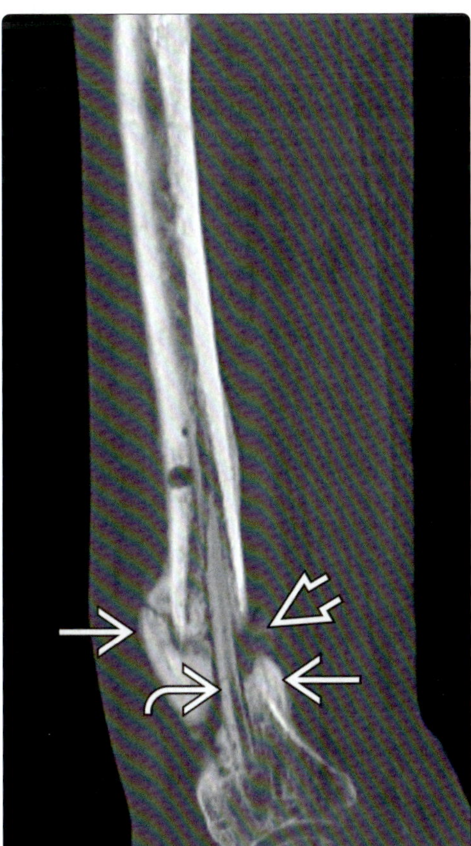

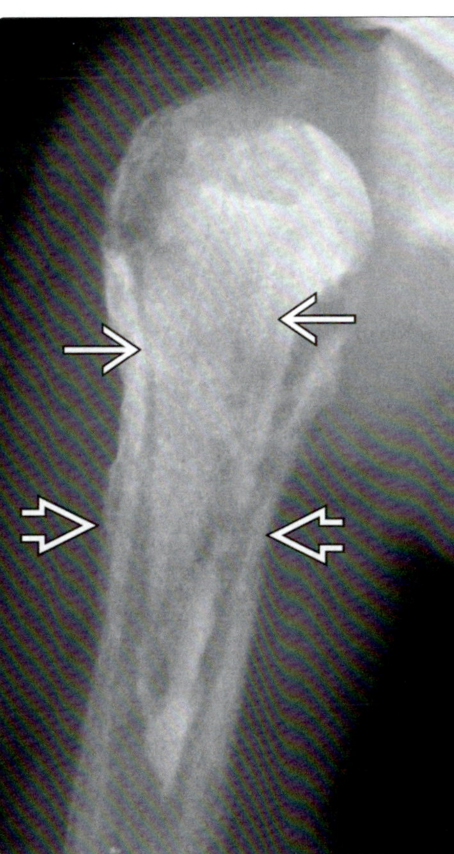

(Left) *Sagittal bone CT shows a patient with remote tibial fracture. The fracture remains nonunited ➡. Cortical thickening is seen along the tibial shaft, and periosteal new bone formation is seen around the fracture ➡. The hardware was removed. At the time of surgery, antibiotic-impregnated cement was injected through a chest tube into the defect ➡. Antibiotic-impregnated cement is often used to maximize delivery to relatively avascular areas of bone in patients with chronic osteomyelitis.* **(Right)** *AP radiograph shows a classic sequestrum of dead bone ➡ surrounded by an involucrum ➡. Prior to the widespread use of antibiotics, the only available treatment of chronic osteomyelitis was sequestrectomy. This appearance of osteomyelitis should no longer be seen, except perhaps in 3rd-world countries.*

KEY FACTS

IMAGING

- Location
  - Any joint is at risk; knee most common in adults
  - Hip especially at risk in children
  - Sacroiliac joint and sternoclavicular joint at particular risk in diabetics, HIV/AIDS patients, IV drug abusers
- Radiograph/CT
  - Early in process, radiographs are normal
  - 1st sign: Joint effusion
  - Hyperemia leads to periarticular osteoporosis
  - Cartilage destruction (joint space narrowing)
  - Cortical bone becomes indistinct
  - Marginal erosions
  - Sclerotic host reaction if septic joint is bacterial
  - Tuberculosis and fungal septic joints tend to elicit little or no osseous reaction
- MR imaging
  - MR abnormal within 24 hours of onset of septic joint
  - More sensitive (100%) and more specific (77%) than other imaging
  - T1-weighted sequence: Low signal within subchondral bone on both sides of joint
  - Fluid-sensitive sequences: Hyperintense effusion, hyperintense subchondral bone, perisynovial soft tissue enhancement
  - Postcontrast T1 fat-saturated imaging: Synovial thickening surrounding effusion, subchondral bone enhancement, occasional adjacent soft tissue abscess
- Ultrasound: Highly sensitive for joint fluid if joint is superficial enough to evaluate
  - US is diagnostic method of choice for hip effusion in children; also guides aspiration

CLINICAL ISSUES

- Patients who are symptomatic for > 7 days prior to diagnosis and treatment have more severe damage
- Septic hip is clinical emergency; immediate aspiration

(Left) *Frog leg lateral radiograph in a child with severe left hip pain shows only mild osteopenia in the left femoral neck and head. If there is clinical suspicion of septic hip in a child, US-guided aspiration should be performed emergently.* **(Right)** *Coronal T1 MR, same patient, shows a ↓ SI hip effusion. Even more importantly, there is confluent ↓ SI within the entire left femoral neck ➡ and head ⮌. This confluent pattern suggests marrow infiltration, as with osteomyelitis or tumor, rather than reactive change.*

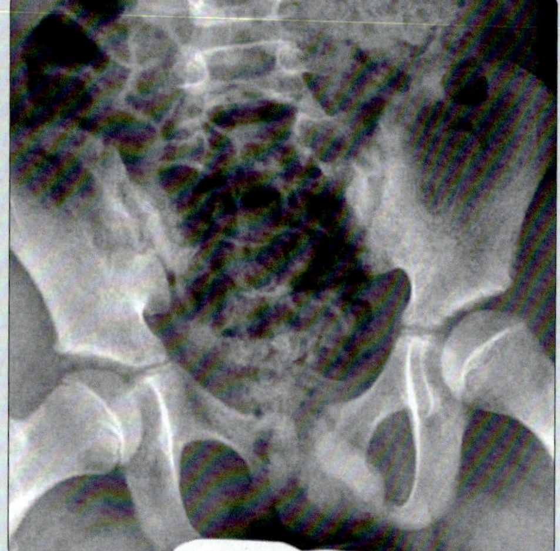

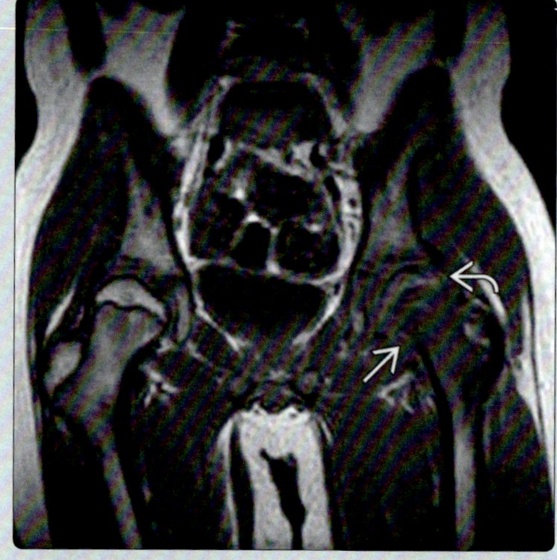

(Left) *Coronal STIR MR confirms the hip effusion ⇨ and high SI femoral head, neck ➡, and acetabulum. Additionally, there is high SI within surrounding muscles ⮌. The findings are typical of septic joint with superimposed osteomyelitis, proven at aspiration.* **(Right)** *AP radiograph was obtained 10 months after treatment for septic hip demonstrates osteopenia and overgrowth of the left proximal femur ➡, related to chronic hyperemia. There are erosions as well; this patient will develop early osteoarthritis.*

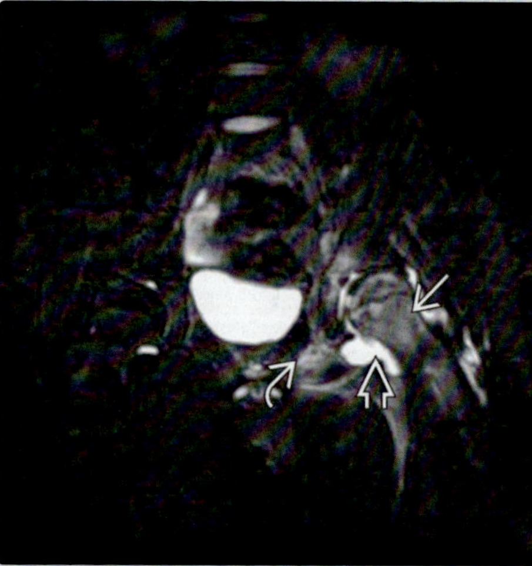

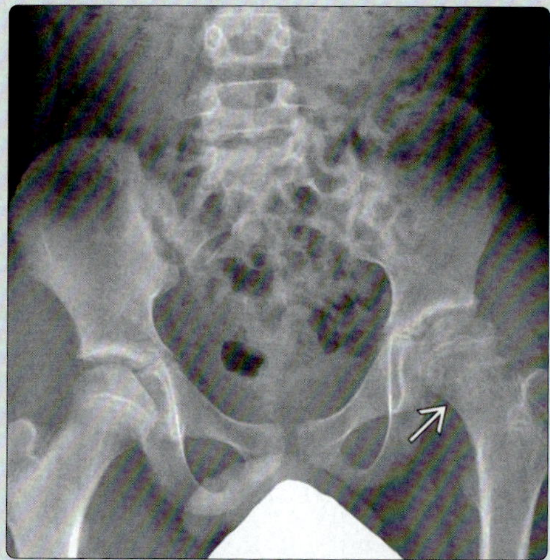

TERMINOLOGY

Synonyms

- Infectious arthritis, pyogenic arthritis, bacterial arthritis, nonpyogenic arthritis, nonbacterial arthritis

IMAGING

General Features

- Best diagnostic clue
  - Effusion seen by radiograph or ultrasound; may be associated with decreased joint space (cartilage destruction), osteopenia, and osseous destruction
- Location
  - Any joint is at risk; knee most common in adults
  - Hip especially at risk in children
  - Sacroiliac joint and sternoclavicular joint at particular risk in diabetics, HIV/AIDS patients, IV drug abusers

Radiographic Findings

- Early in process, radiographs are normal
- With progression, nonspecific findings
- 1st sign: Joint effusion
  - Bulging fat planes
  - Radiographic signs of hip effusion
    - Requires perfect AP pelvis with hips in internal rotation
    - Bulging fat planes: Obturator, gluteal, iliopsoas
    - Increased distance between radiographic teardrop and femoral metaphysis compared to contralateral hip
    - Air arthrogram with traction on hip rules out effusion
  - Radiographic signs of knee effusion
    - Suprapatellar effusion
    - Obliteration of Hoffa fat pad
  - Radiographic signs of ankle effusion
    - Bulging anterior fat pad at tibiotalar joint
    - False-positive if tibiotalar joint dorsiflexed
  - Radiographic signs of shoulder effusion
    - None; glenohumeral joint is large and can decompress into subscapularis bursa
  - Radiographic signs of elbow effusion
    - Bulging anterior fat pad (sail sign)
    - Presence of posterior fat pad
  - Radiographic signs of wrist effusion
    - Bulging pronator fat pad
- Hyperemia leads to periarticular osteoporosis
- Cartilage destruction (joint space narrowing)
- Cortical bone becomes indistinct
- Marginal erosions
- Osteomyelitis may develop in adjacent bone
- Sclerotic host reaction if infection is bacterial
  - Tuberculosis or fungal arthritis elicit little or no sclerotic host reaction
- Eventual ankylosis (rare; more frequent in tuberculous than pyogenic arthritis)
- Infected arthroplasties
  - Generally no abnormality seen
  - Rarely, serpiginous osseous destruction and periosteal reaction
  - Fluffy periarticular bone formation is suggestive

CT Findings

- Rarely used with suspicion of septic joint
- Findings similar to those of radiographs: Soft tissue swelling, joint effusion, joint space narrowing, bone and cartilage erosions
- May show erosions or sclerosis in joints which are difficult to evaluate (sacroiliac and sternoclavicular)
- Guides difficult aspirations (sternoclavicular, sacroiliac)

MR Findings

- MR sensitive (100%) and more specific (77%) than other imaging; abnormal within 24 hours of onset
- T1-weighted sequence: Low signal within subchondral bone on both sides of joint
- Fluid-sensitive sequences: Hyperintense effusion, hyperintense subchondral bone, perisynovial soft tissue enhancement
- Postcontrast T1 fat-saturated imaging: Synovial thickening surrounding effusion, subchondral bone enhancement, occasional adjacent soft tissue abscess
- Frequency of findings
  - Synovial enhancement (98%)
  - Marrow bare area changes (86%)
  - Abnormal T2 marrow signal (84%) and abnormal enhancement (81%)
  - Abnormal T1 marrow signal (66%)
  - Perisynovial edema (84%)
  - Joint effusion (70%) (almost 1/3 lack effusion; joints of hand or foot predominate)
- Following treatment, abscesses and joint effusions ↓ in size
  - Marrow edema, cellulitis, synovial thickening and enhancement persist even after resolution of infection

Ultrasonographic Findings

- Highly sensitive for joint fluid if joint is superficial enough to evaluate
- Not specific for type of effusion
- US is diagnostic method of choice for hip effusion in children; also guides aspiration

Nuclear Medicine Findings

- Bone scan
  - Sensitive (90-100%), nonspecific (75%) for septic joint
  - Blood flow and blood pool images show increased activity on both sides of joint
  - Delayed phase shows continued increase in activity if septic joint has progressed to osteomyelitis
- Arthroplasties are particularly problematic
  - Increased uptake with all nuclear medicine studies for variable amount of time following surgery

Image-Guided Aspiration

- Aspiration required with suspicion of septic joint
  - Sterile technique
  - Positioning may be difficult due to painful joint, often held in flexion
  - Large bore needle required since purulent material may be thick (18 gauge)
  - Local anesthetic; try to avoid injecting into joint (lidocaine is weakly bacteriostatic)

- If aspiration yields no fluid, inject nonbacteriostatic saline and then reaspirate (some orthopedic surgeons request this not be performed)
- If need to confirm intraarticular location, inject small amount of air or radiographic contrast (contrast is weakly bacteriostatic)
- Send fluid for Gram stain, culture (with appropriate sensitivities), glucose, leukocyte count/differential
  - Crystal analysis if pyrophosphate arthropathy is in differential
  - Leukocyte esterase ("dipstick") analysis shows high sensitivity (97%), positive predictive value (95%), and negative predictive value (100%) in periprosthetic aspirates

Imaging Recommendations

- Best imaging tool
  - With clinical suspicion, aspiration required
  - Radiograph may show signs of effusion and early destruction; insensitive early and nonspecific later
  - MR shows nonspecific abnormalities; useful in situations of clinical uncertainty
  - Suspicion of septic hip in child should be evaluated with ultrasound
- Protocol advice
  - MR evaluation must include postcontrast sequences

DIFFERENTIAL DIAGNOSIS

Inflammatory Arthritis

- Rheumatoid and other inflammatory arthritides may initially show only effusion/tenosynovitis
- MR likely to show marrow edema, possibly early erosions

PATHOLOGY

General Features

- Etiology
  - Hematogenous spread most common
    - From distant source, such as pneumonia, wound infection, endocarditis
  - Direct seeding through trauma or surgery
  - Spread from contiguous infection (osteomyelitis or cellulitis)
  - Pyogenic: *Staphylococcus aureus* most frequent (64%)
    - Other organisms include *Streptococcus pneumoniae* (20%), group B streptococci, *Gonococcus* (2%), *Escherichia coli* (10%), *Haemophilus*, *Klebsiella*, *Pseudomonas* (4%)
  - IV drug abusers often have unusual organisms: *Mycobacterium avium*, *Pseudomonas aeruginosa*, *Enterobacter* species
  - Septic hip in child: Common
    - Osteomyelitis develops in proximal femoral metaphysis
    - Metaphysis is within hip joint capsule
    - Extension from osteomyelitis to septic joint is common because of this anatomic arrangement
  - Nonpyogenic: Tuberculous or fungal septic arthritis
    - More chronic processes than bacterial
    - Elicit little or no host bone reaction
    - Phemister triad thought to be characteristic
      - Cartilage destruction is slower (joint width remains normal for some time)
      - Osteoporosis, especially juxtaarticular
      - Erosions develop late; once seen, well delineated
    - Most common sites: Hip > knee > wrist

CLINICAL ISSUES

Presentation

- Most common signs/symptoms
  - Traditionally clinical diagnosis, but findings are not specific; deep joint sepsis is particularly challenging
  - Warm, swollen joint, decreased range of motion
  - ± fever, chills
  - Monoarticular in 90%
  - Blood cultures positive in 50%
- Other signs/symptoms
  - Gonococcal arthritis: 66% have associated dermatitis, 25% have associated GU symptoms

Demographics

- Age
  - Septic hip in children generally < 3 years old
  - Septic joints increase in incidence in teenagers
  - Elderly most at risk due to prevalence of arthroplasties and chronic diseases
- Populations at increased risk
  - Chronic illness ± steroids
  - Rheumatoid arthritis
  - Diabetes, end-stage renal disease
  - IV drug use, HIV/AIDS
  - Joint surgery, ± prosthesis

Natural History & Prognosis

- With appropriate treatment, 60% recover completely
- Remainder have permanent damage to joint, resulting in deformity or mechanical arthritis
- Patients who are symptomatic for > 7 days prior to diagnosis and treatment have more severe damage
- *S. aureus* and gram-negative tend to be more destructive

Treatment

- Antibiotics, appropriate to infecting organism
- Drainage; needle aspiration or open drainage
- Arthroplasty is special case
  - Remove components plus all cement; anything remaining serves as nidus for continued infection
  - Antibiotic-impregnated cement often placed at defect for several weeks
  - Joint must be evaluated for continued infection prior to placement of revision prosthesis

SELECTED REFERENCES

1. Colvin OC et al: Leukocyte esterase analysis in the diagnosis of joint infection: Can we make a diagnosis using a simple urine dipstick? Skeletal Radiol. ePub, 2015
2. Bierry G et al: MRI findings of treated bacterial septic arthritis. Skeletal Radiol. 41(12):1509-16, 2012

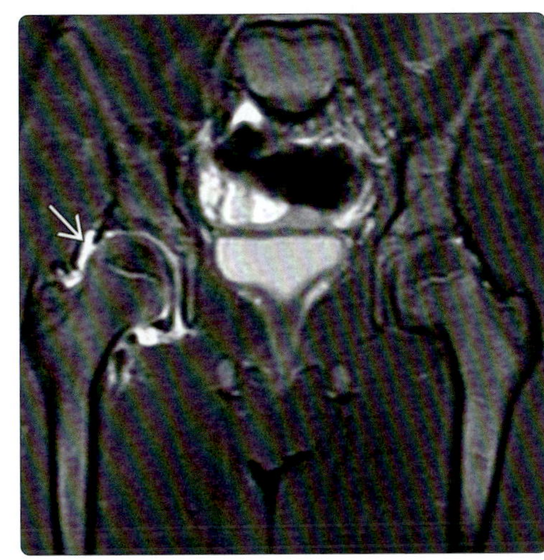

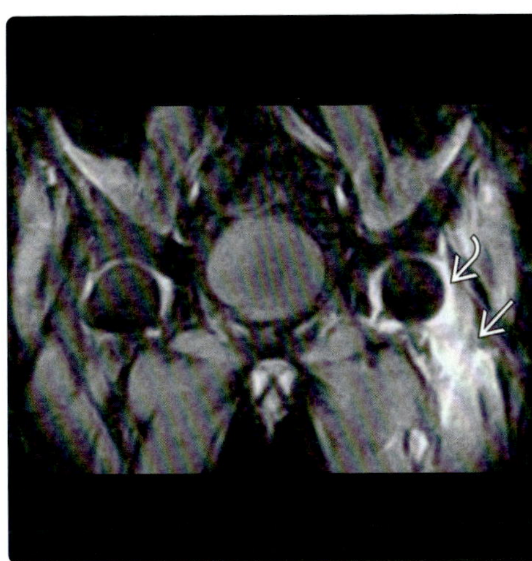

(Left) *Coronal PDWI FS MR shows right hip effusion ➡. There is no evidence of osteomyelitis or involvement of the femoral head physis. However, septic hip in a child should be considered an emergency since it is at high risk for developing osteomyelitis.* **(Right)** *Coronal STIR MR shows left hip effusion ➡. No defining arthritic features, such as joint space narrowing, subchondral signal change, cyst, or osteophyte formation, are present. However, there is soft tissue edema ➡; septic hip was proven by aspiration.*

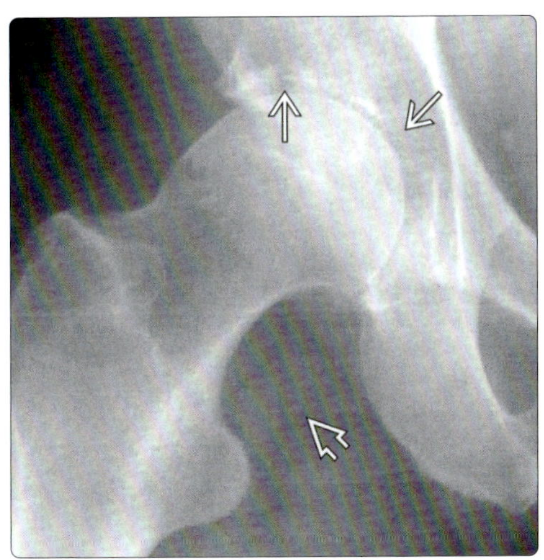

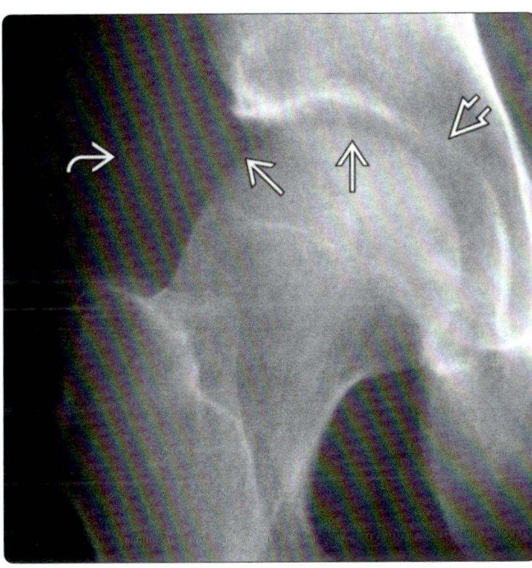

(Left) *AP radiograph of this hip shows classic radiographic signs of advanced septic joint. There is a distended iliopsoas fat pad ➡, indicating an effusion. Moreover, there is loss of the cortical distinctness of the superior and medial acetabulum ➡. There is cartilage loss as well.* **(Right)** *AP radiograph, in a different patient, should secure the diagnosis of septic joint. The gluteal fat pad of the right hip is distended ➡; this indicates a hip effusion. There is also deossification of the acetabular cortex ➡ as well as the femoral head ➡.*

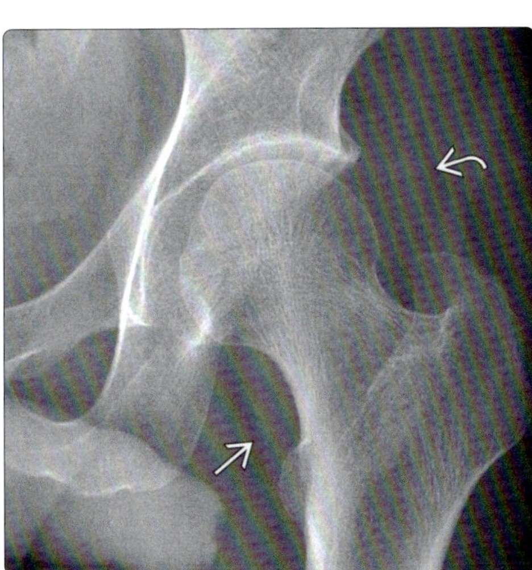

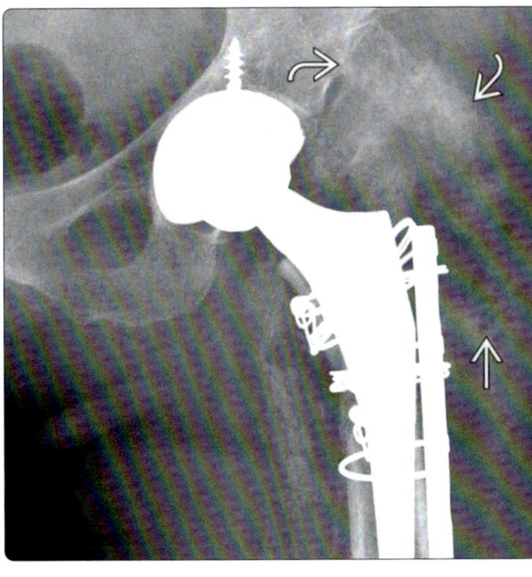

(Left) *AP radiograph in a young male patient shows distended gluteal ➡ and iliopsoas ➡ fat planes, indicating hip effusion. The patient had the hip injected with steroids 1 week earlier in the sports clinic and had worsening pain. Aspiration proved early septic hip, prior to radiographic evidence of osseous change.* **(Right)** *AP radiograph shows air in the soft tissues ➡ around a 5-year hip arthroplasty. There is fluffy heterotopic ossification present ➡. This combination of findings is typical for infection of an arthroplasty.*

(Left) *Axial T1WI C+ FS MR demonstrates thick enhancing synovium* ➔*, subcutaneous edema* ➔*, and vague patchy high signal in the femur* ➔*. These findings are nonspecific; they may represent an inflammatory arthritis with osseous reactive change or septic knee.* **(Right)** *Axial T1WI MR shows marginal ↓ SI around the subchondral bone of the femur* ➔*. This is nonspecific and may be seen either as osseous reaction to inflammatory or septic arthritis or as osteomyelitis related to septic joint.*

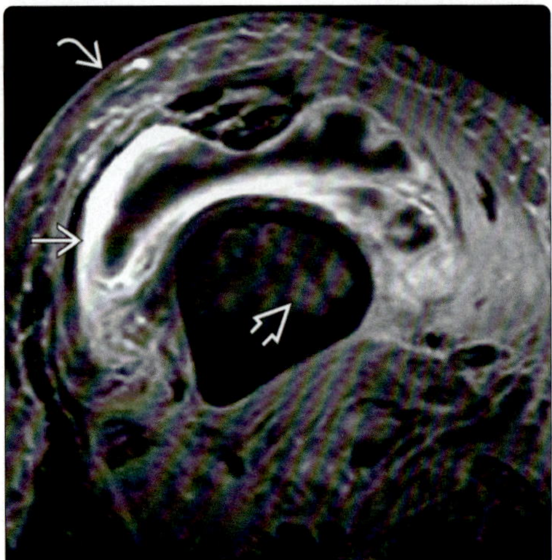

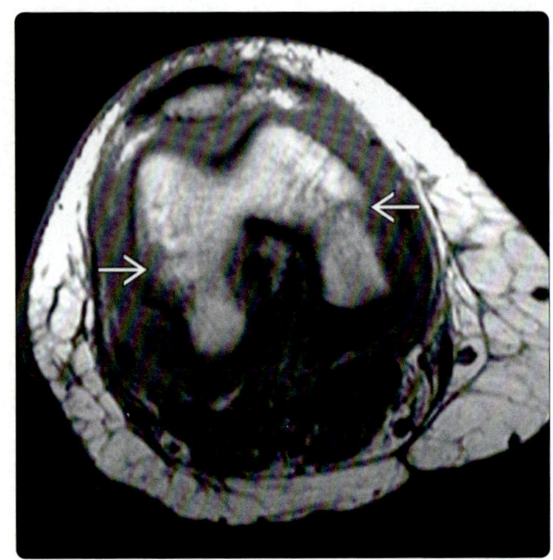

(Left) *Axial T1WI C+ FS MR at the same level shows the bone enhancement* ➔ *to be greater than expected for reactive marrow edema from a noninfective synovitis and is consistent with osteomyelitis related to the septic joint; gram-positive cocci were cultured from the joint aspirate.* **(Right)** *Axial T2WI MR shows fluid within the glenohumeral joint* ➔*, as well as complex fluid signal within the subdeltoid bursa* ➔*. This IV drug abuser shared needles and developed both septic joint and bursitis.*

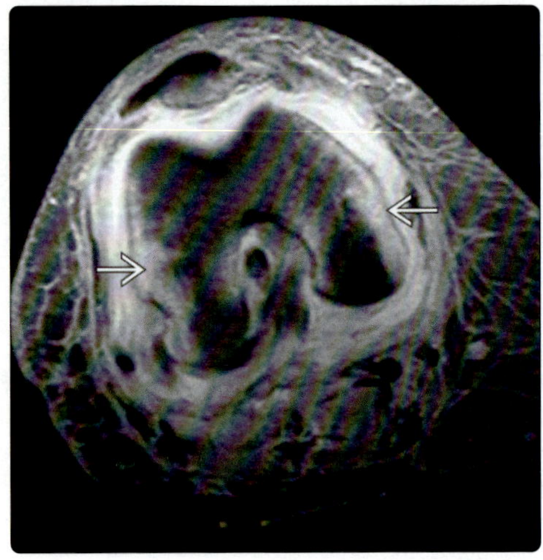

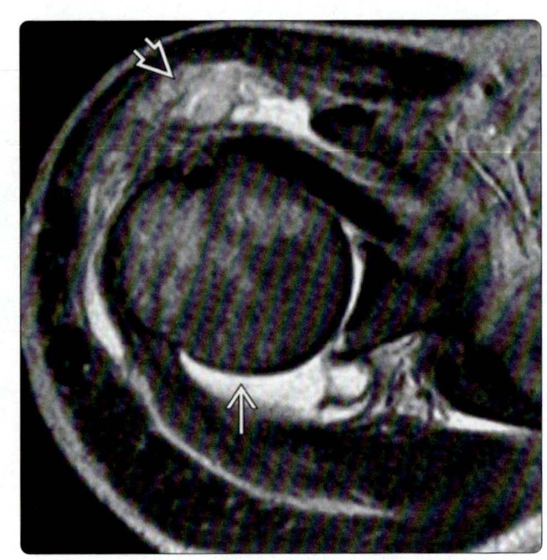

(Left) *Angled coronal T1WI MR shows decreased signal intensity in the clavicle* ➔ *and adjacent manubrium* ➔ *in a 65-year-old woman. The elderly are at particular risk for developing septic arthritis at the sternoclavicular joint.* **(Right)** *Angled coronal T2WI FS MR shows ↑ signal in the clavicle* ➔*, adjacent manubrium* ➔*, fluid within the joint, and normal disc in the joint* ➔*. Note how well the joint is depicted when angulated along the coronal plane of this joint. Aspiration proved septic arthritis.*

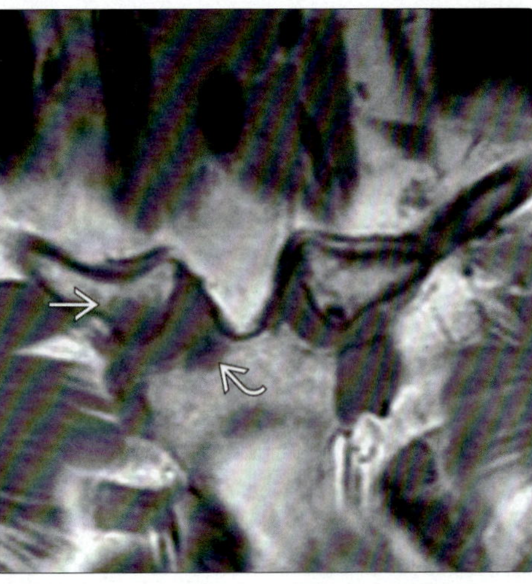

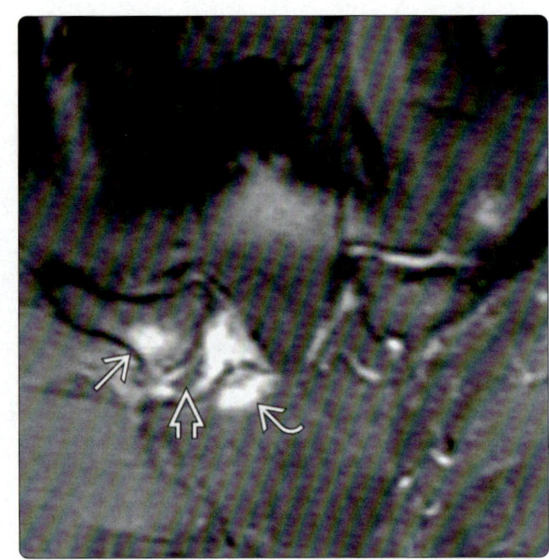

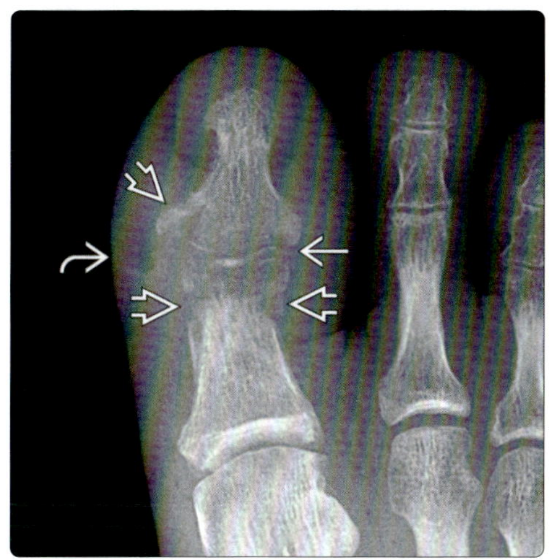

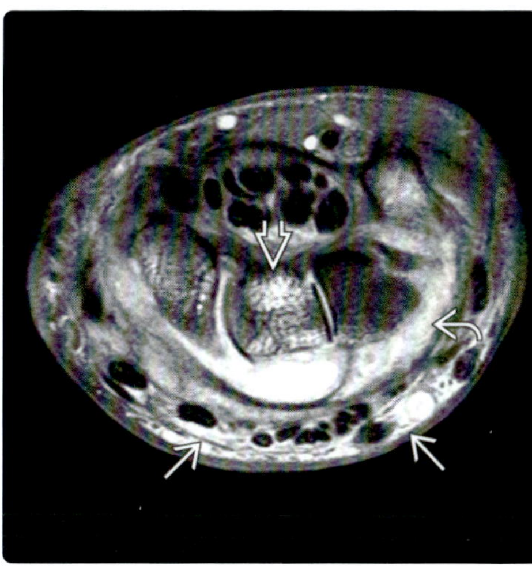

(Left) *AP radiograph shows severe osteopenia at the interphalangeal joint. There is osseous destruction involving both phalanges. There is periosteal reaction on the proximal phalanx and air in the soft tissues. The constellation of findings are classic for septic arthritis accompanied by osteomyelitis.* **(Right)** *Axial PDWI FS MR of the wrist shows extensive tenosynovitis as well as enhancement of the synovium. Osseous hyperintensity is seen as well in this patient with septic joint.*

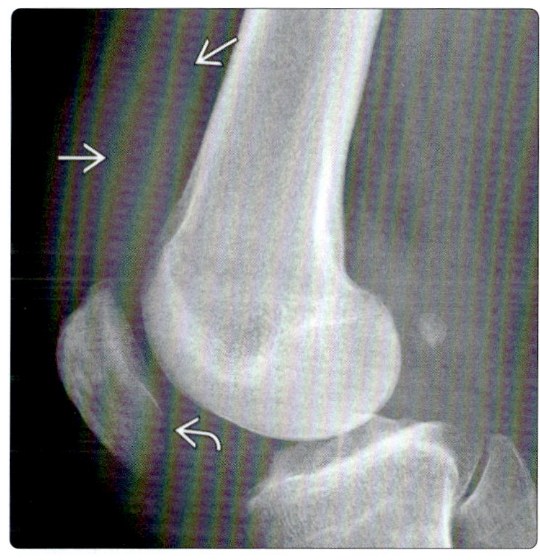

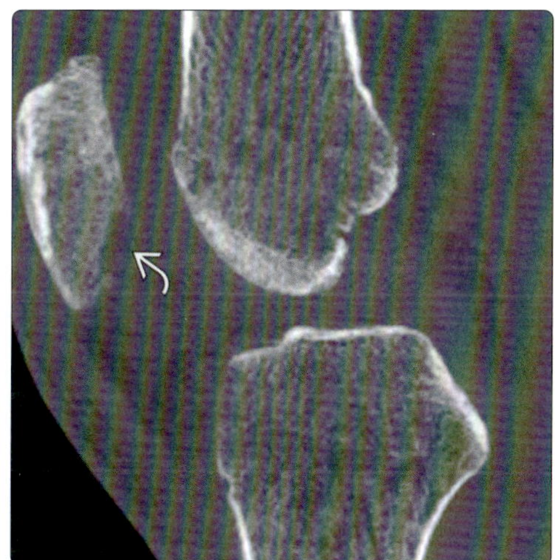

(Left) *Lateral radiograph of the knee in a 26-year-old man who complained of 2 months of worsening pain and swelling. He also had 4 episodes of fever and night sweats. The exam shows a large effusion and focal region of deossification in the patella. Septic joint must be presumed.* **(Right)** *Sagittal CT in the same patient shows diffuse osteopenia and a large erosion in the patella. There is no reactive change. History and imaging suggests either tuberculosis or a fungal septic joint. Aspiration showed coccidiomycosis.*

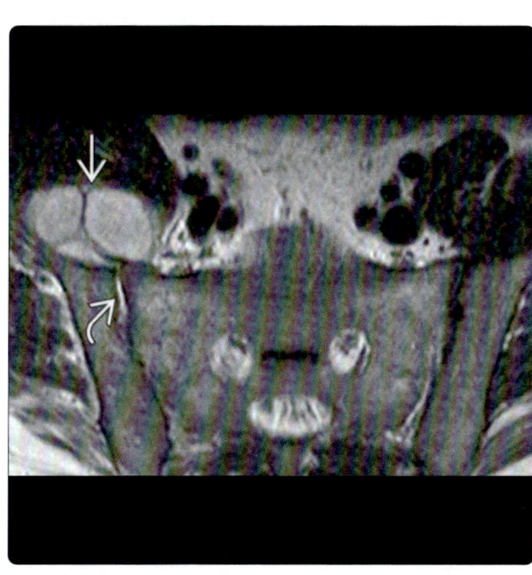

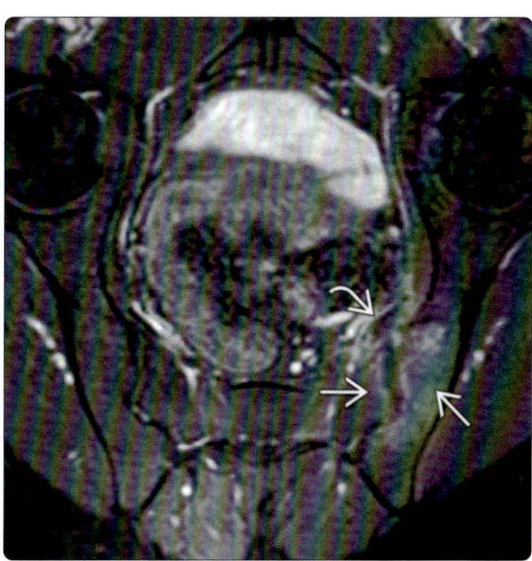

(Left) *Axial T2WI MR demonstrates fluid collections anterior to the right sacroiliac joint (SIJ) as well as fluid within the SIJ. This is a typical septic SIJ. Remember that SIJ pathology can present with hip pain (as did this patient), particularly when there is an iliopsoas abscess. This patient has HIV and is at added risk for infection.* **(Right)** *Axial oblique T1WI C+ FS MR shows enhancement of both sides of the left SIJ, along with a small abscess anterior to the joint, typical for a septic SIJ in this HIV-positive patient.*

KEY FACTS

IMAGING

- Radiograph: Swelling in tendon distribution
- MR: Thickened, enhancing synovium surrounding fluid within tendon sheath
  - Tendons may show high T2 signal damage
  - Tendon rupture if longstanding
  - Debris may be present within tendon sheaths
- US: Demonstrates fluid and integrity of tendon

TOP DIFFERENTIAL DIAGNOSES

- Inflammatory tenosynovitis
  - Thickened synovium surrounding fluid
  - May contain debris or rice bodies
  - Common manifestation of SLE, RA, and other inflammatory arthritic diseases
  - Infectious tenosynovitis not infrequently seen in patients with rheumatoid arthritis; aseptic inflammation should not be presumed
- Traumatic tenosynovitis
  - Injury; extensor carpi ulnaris is common
- HIV/AIDS-related tenosynovitis
  - If proven not to be infectious, may be related to immune reconstitution syndrome (IRS); IRS seen in 10-25% of patients starting HAART
- Sarcoidal tenosynovitis
  - Nonspecific MR appearance; clinical circumstance suggests diagnosis; proven by biopsy

PATHOLOGY

- Etiology: Usually trauma or needle puncture
- Work environment and underlying patient condition may suggest specific infectious agent
- Flexor tendon sheath: Location of aggressive closed space infection; early systemic antibiotics reduce morbidity
- Methicillin-resistant *Staphylococcus aureus* (MRSA) increasingly prevalent in hand infections
  - CDC: Empiric coverage for MRSA in hand infections if local rate of MRSA exceeds 10-15%

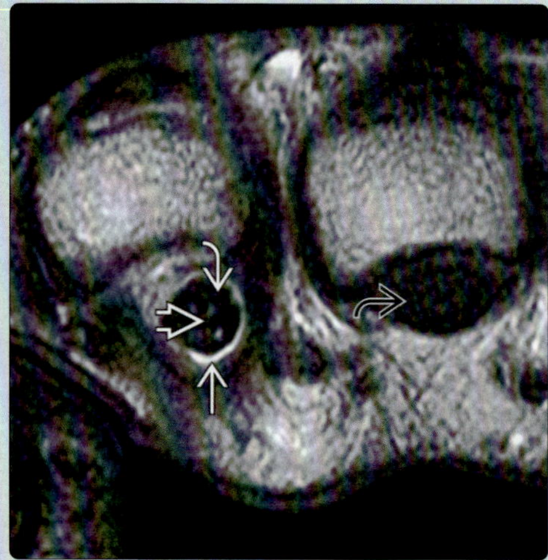

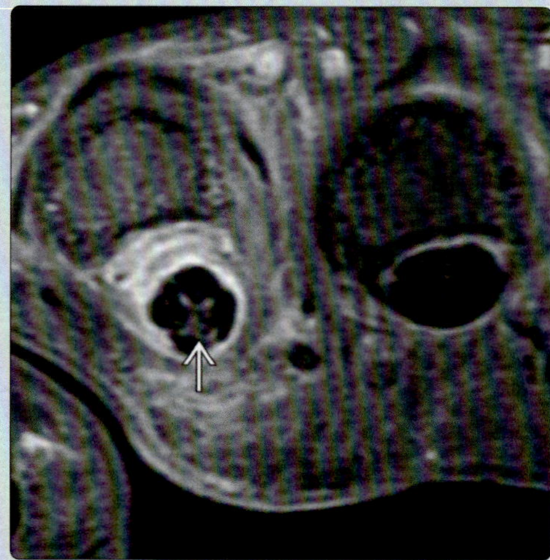

(Left) *Axial T2WI MR shows infectious tenosynovitis of the flexor units in the 2nd finger due to puncture wound, with high signal soft tissue ➡ around and particularly deep to the profunda ➡ and superficialis ➡ flexor tendons of the digit. Compare with the normal flexor unit of the 3rd digit ➡.* **(Right)** *Axial T1WI C+ FS MR, same case, confirms the tenosynovitis. There is also heterogeneity in the profunda unit ➡, indicating likely infection of the tendon (compare to the normal adjacent 3rd flexor units).*

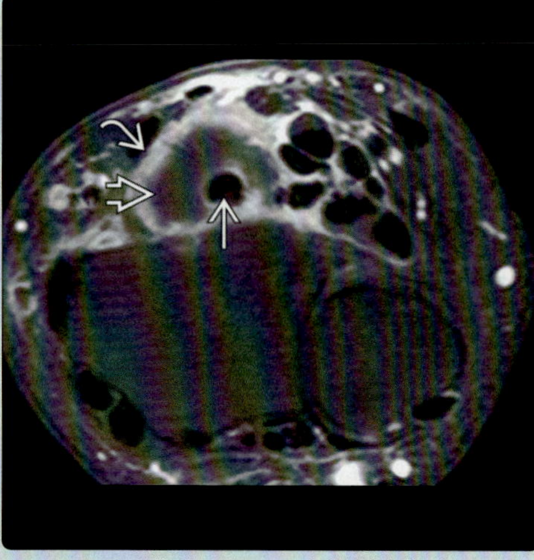

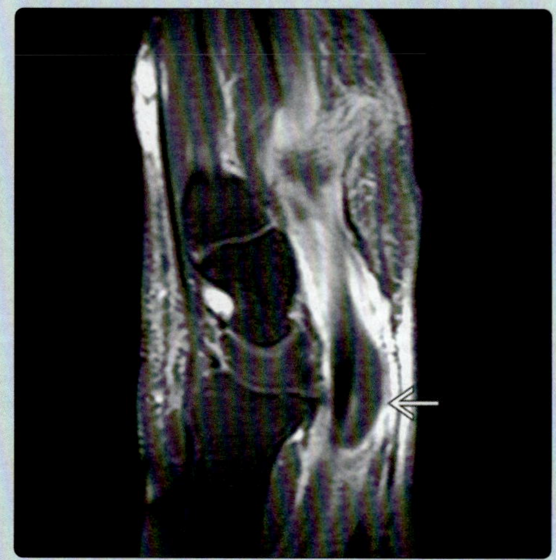

(Left) *Axial T1WI C+ FS MR demonstrates tremendous tenosynovitis of the flexor pollicis longus ➡. The contrast enhancement ➡ around the fluid-filled tendon sheath ➡ is thick, suggesting infection.* **(Right)** *Sagittal T1WI C+ FS MR, same case, again shows the thick enhancing rim ➡ surrounding fluid within the tendon sheath of flexor pollicis longus. There is edema in the surrounding soft tissues, but the adjacent bones are normal. Staphylococcus was cultured from the aspirate.*

KEY FACTS

IMAGING

- Location specific to bursa
  - Direct inoculation: Prepatellar, olecranon bursae
  - Extension from infected arthroplasty: Iliopsoas, subacromial/subdeltoid bursae
- Radiograph: Swelling, obliteration of adjacent fat planes
  - Adjacent subcutaneous edema
- MR: Distended bursa, ↓ SI on T1WI, ↑ SI on T2WI
  - Thick enhancing rim surrounding fluid, ± debris
- US: Detects bursal fluid, guides aspiration

TOP DIFFERENTIAL DIAGNOSES

- Inflammatory aseptic bursitis
  - Thick ↓ SI synovium surrounding bursal fluid
  - May contain rice bodies if patient has RA
  - Afebrile state may differentiate RA from infection
- Hematoma within bursa
  - Fluid levels and blood products shown on MR, depending on age of hematoma
- Synovial chondromatosis
  - May arise in bursa as well as joint
  - Bodies may be radiolucent; presents as bursal mass
  - Bodies demonstrated on T2WI MR
- Gouty tophus
  - May arise in bursa (especially olecranon)
  - Calcific density serves to differentiate, if present
- Rheumatoid nodule
  - May arise contiguous with a bursa
  - MR: Heterogeneous low to high SI, showing enhancement ± cystic regions

PATHOLOGY

- Etiology: Trauma, needle puncture, arthroplasty
  - Other predisposing factors: Diabetes, alcoholism, immunocompromised state, RA, or gout

CLINICAL ISSUES

- Treatment: Incision and drainage, appropriate antibiotics

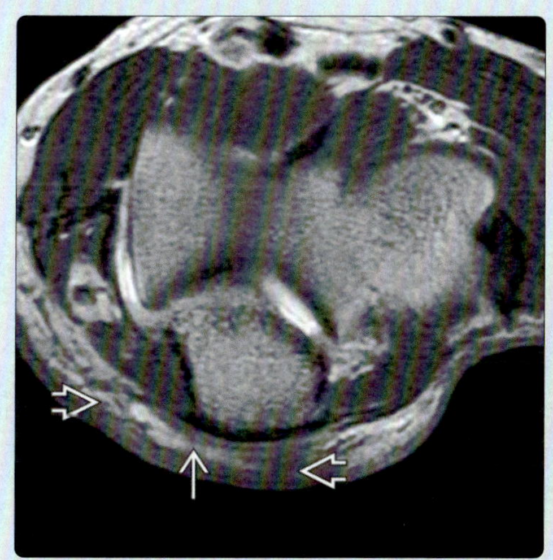

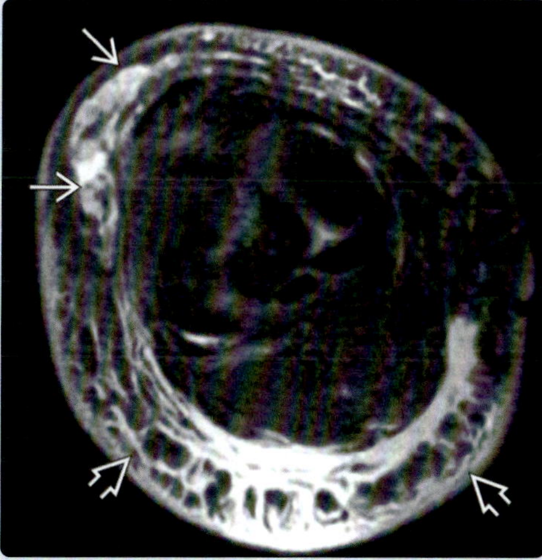

(Left) *Axial T2WI MR shows infectious olecranon bursitis. There is an irregular fluid collection ➡ in the subcutaneous tissues posterior to the olecranon with surrounding infiltrative changes in the fat ➡. Aspiration of the collection yielded Staphylococcus aureus. There was no evidence of osteomyelitis.* **(Right)** *Axial T2WI FS MR demonstrates heterogeneous debris within a fluid collection anterior to the patellar tendon ➡. There is no joint effusion; note subcutaneous edema ➡.*

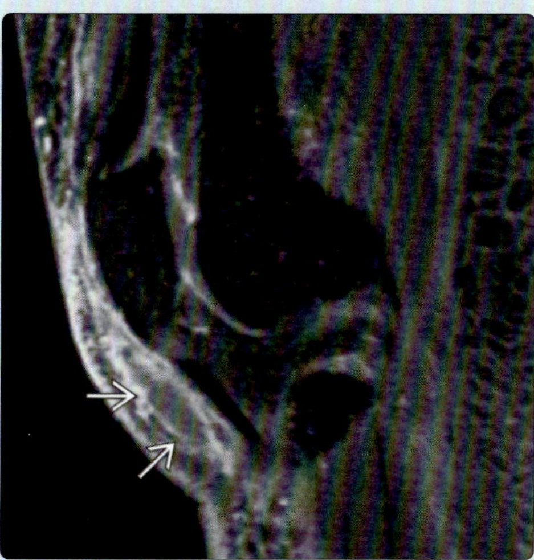

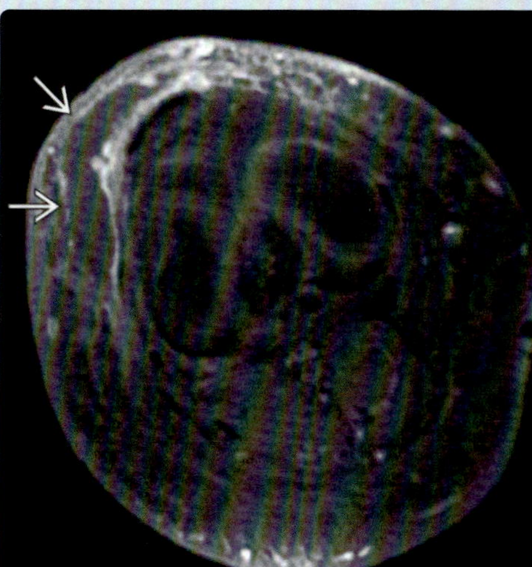

(Left) *Sagittal T1WI C+ FS MR, same case, shows a thickened enhancing rim around the low signal prepatellar bursal fluid collection ➡.* **(Right)** *Axial T1WI C+ FS MR again confirms the thickened enhancing rim around the prepatellar bursal fluid collection, consistent with synovitis ➡. There is no knee effusion nor abnormal signal in the adjacent tendon or bone. Subcutaneous cellulitis is prominent circumferentially about the knee. The fluid collection was aspirated and grew gram-positive bacteria.*

KEY FACTS

IMAGING

- Subtle radiographic findings, confirmed by CT, MR, or US
- Radiographic/CT findings
  - Soft tissue swelling
  - Obliteration of fat plane definition
  - Stranding in adjacent fat tissue
  - Adjacent reactive bone formation
  - Gas in soft tissues: Rare
- MR findings
  - Low SI T1, high SI T2 soft tissue mass + fluid
  - Thick enhancing rim and septa by MR
  - Associated cellulitis, fasciitis
  - ± saucerization of adjacent cortex and extension as osteomyelitis
- Ultrasound findings
  - Well-defined fluid collection
  - Hyperechoic rim, ± debris
- Aspirate/drain under US or CT guidance, depending on depth and accessibility

TOP DIFFERENTIAL DIAGNOSES

- Cellulitis
- Necrotizing fasciitis
- Distension, Charcot joint
- Infectious bursitis

CLINICAL ISSUES

- Etiology
  - Direct inoculation: Trauma, IV drug abusers
  - Additional risk factors: Diabetics, end-stage renal disease, steroid users

DIAGNOSTIC CHECKLIST

- Watch for adjacent involvement of bone
- Use character of fat plane displacement/obliteration to suggest tumor vs. abscess

(Left) *Lateral radiograph shows obliteration of fat planes ➡ in the popliteal fossa. Such obliteration suggests the soft tissue mass is due to abscess rather than tumor. There is also faint scalloping of the posterior cortex ➡ suggesting extrinsic bone destruction.* **(Right)** *Sagittal T2WI MR shows a large inhomogeneous mass in the popliteal fossa, which deviates the popliteal vessels ➡ and adjacent muscles. There is disruption of the posterior cortex of the femur ➡ by contiguity with the mass.*

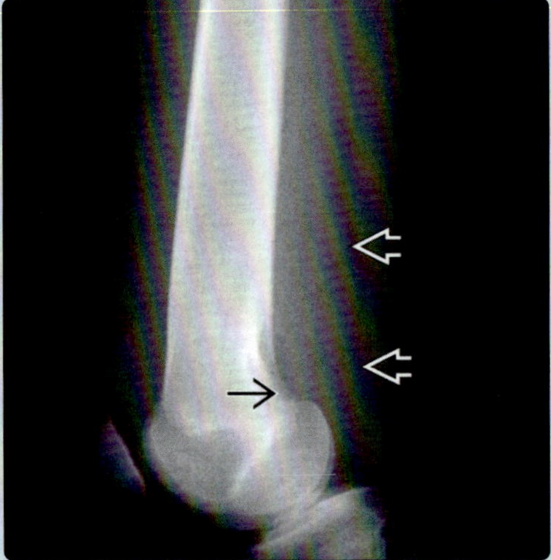

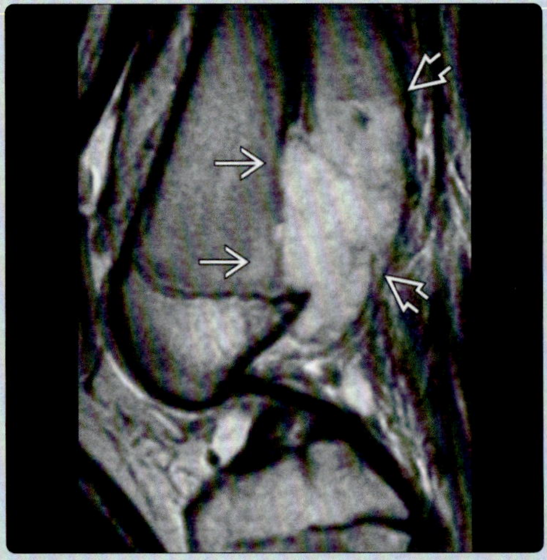

(Left) *Axial T1WI MR in same patient shows the inhomogeneous ↓ SI mass ➡ with adjacent confluent ↓ SI in the bone ➡ with peripheral patchy marrow. Considerations are infection vs. reactive osseous change.* **(Right)** *Sagittal T1WI C+ MR confirms a large abscess ➡ with thick rim enhancement surrounding a large fluid collection and adjacent invasion of cortex and focal osteomyelitis ➡. The patient had been camping near Reno, Nevada and had cervical and mediastinal adenopathy in this proven case of Yersinia pestis.*

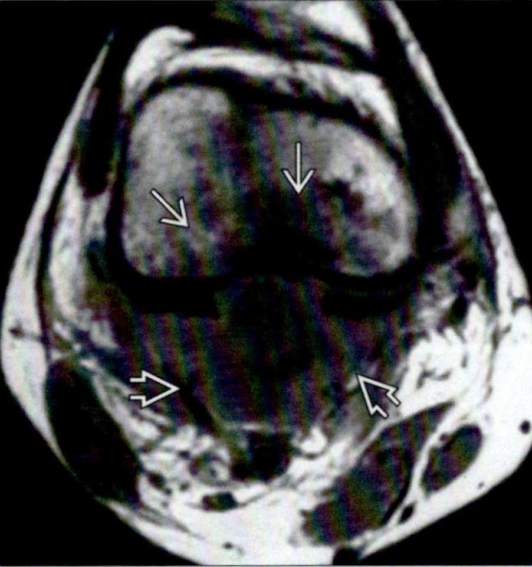

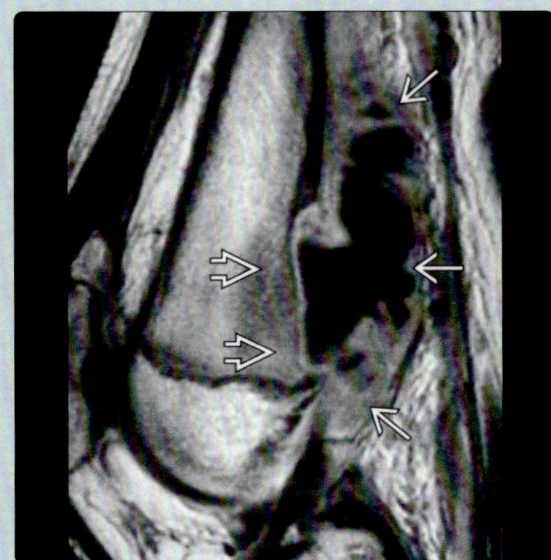

TERMINOLOGY

Definitions

- Infection in soft tissues: May be subcutaneous, inter- or intramuscular

IMAGING

General Features

- Best diagnostic clue
  - Subtle radiographic findings, confirmed by CT, MR, or US

Radiographic Findings

- Nonspecific and subtle radiographic findings
  - Soft tissue swelling, stranding in adjacent fat tissue
  - Obliteration of fat plane definition
    - Tumor displaces, but does not obliterate, fat planes, which may help differentiate from abscess
  - Adjacent reactive bone formation
    - Less frequently, scalloping/erosion
- Gas in soft tissues: Rare

CT Findings

- Fluid attenuation collection by CT
- Abscess walls and internal septa enhance with CT
- Associated cellulitis

MR Findings

- Low SI T1, high SI T2 soft tissue collection by MR
- Associated cellulitis, fasciitis
- Adjacent reactive bone formation
  - Periosteal/endosteal reaction
  - Patchy intermediate signal in bone; reactive vs. osteomyelitis (less patchy, more confluent)
- ± saucerization of adjacent cortex and extension as osteomyelitis
- Abscess: Thick enhancing rim and septa by MR
- Myositis: Intramuscular edema ± intermuscular edema, subcutaneous edema
- Pyomyositis: Intramuscular abscess with enhancing peripheral rim
  - Inflammation in adjacent tissue
  - ± periostitis/periosteal thickening

Ultrasonographic Findings

- Well-defined fluid collection, hyperechoic rim
- ± debris
- Elastography shows soft tissue induration

Imaging Recommendations

- Best imaging tool
  - MR most sensitive for deep abscess or pyomyositis; image to define disease extent and complications
  - Aspirate/drain under US or CT control, depending on depth and accessibility

DIFFERENTIAL DIAGNOSIS

Cellulitis

- Usually clinical diagnosis; image to rule out abscess or complications
- CT or MR: ↑ attenuation or signal (respectively) with enhancement in subcutaneous fat
- May have associated fascial thickening and fluid (usually only superficial)

Necrotizing Fasciitis

- Fluid extending along thickened fascial planes
- Superficial and deep involvement
- May have necrotic regions, simulating abscess

Distension, Charcot Joint

- Neuropathic joints develop tremendous joint distension
  - Fluid collections may dissect away from expected location, mimicking abscess formation

Infectious Bursitis

- Collection of fluid with enhancing rim
- Same MR characteristics as abscess
- Conforms to anatomic site of bursa

Inflammatory Myositis

- Generally multiple symmetric sites, not mass-like

CLINICAL ISSUES

Presentation

- Most common signs/symptoms
  - Pain, soft tissue swelling, redness

Demographics

- Epidemiology
  - Direct inoculation: Trauma, IV drug abusers
  - Tropical myositis: Not uncommon; usually seen in children and adolescents
  - Temperate myositis: Increasing incidence due to increase in immunocompromised individuals
    - Additional risk factors: Diabetics, end-stage renal disease, steroid users

Natural History & Prognosis

- Complications
  - May progress to severe systemic sepsis
  - Septic arthritis, tenosynovitis, osteomyelitis
  - Soft tissue ulceration, fistula formation

Treatment

- Drainage: Either incision or percutaneous
- Appropriate antibiotics

DIAGNOSTIC CHECKLIST

Image Interpretation Pearls

- Use character of fat plane displacement/obliteration to suggest tumor vs. abscess
- Adjacent bone may show patchy increased signal and enhancement as reaction and not be truly infected
- Confluent regions of low signal within marrow on T1 imaging makes osteomyelitis more likely than simple osseous reaction (patchy or reticulated pattern)

SELECTED REFERENCES

1. Turecki MB et al: Imaging of musculoskeletal soft tissue infections. Skeletal Radiol. 39(10):957-71, 2010

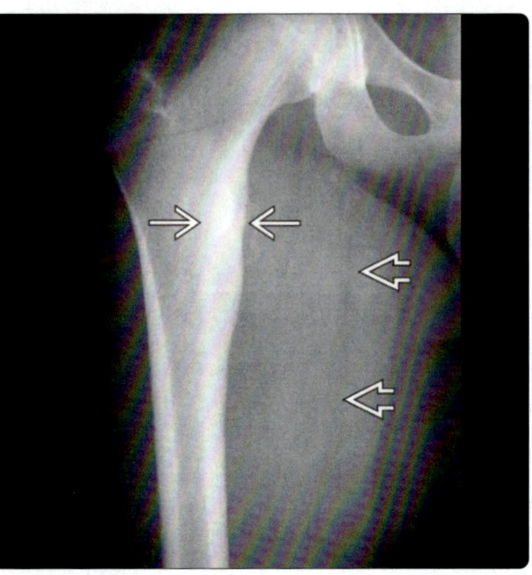

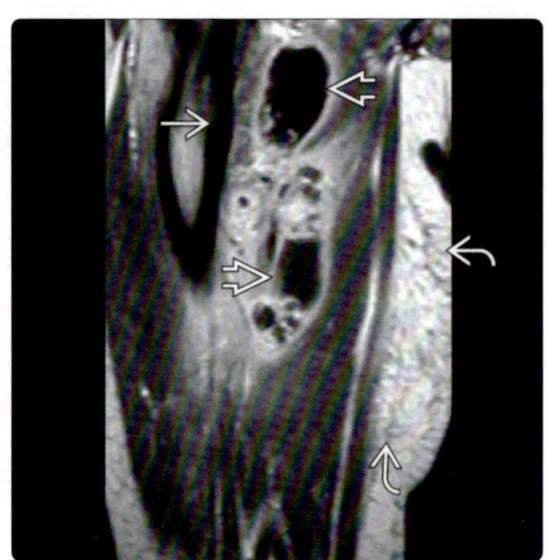

(Left) *AP radiograph shows near complete obliteration (rather than distortion) of fat planes ➡. There is thick periosteal reactive bone formation ➡. The appearance is typical of soft tissue abscess with adjacent osseous reaction.* **(Right)** *Coronal T1 C+ MR confirms multiloculated abscess ➡ with several fluid collections and rim enhancement. Note that the bone marrow is normal, but the cortex is thickened in reaction to the adjacent abscess ➡. There is subcutaneous swelling and stranding ➡.*

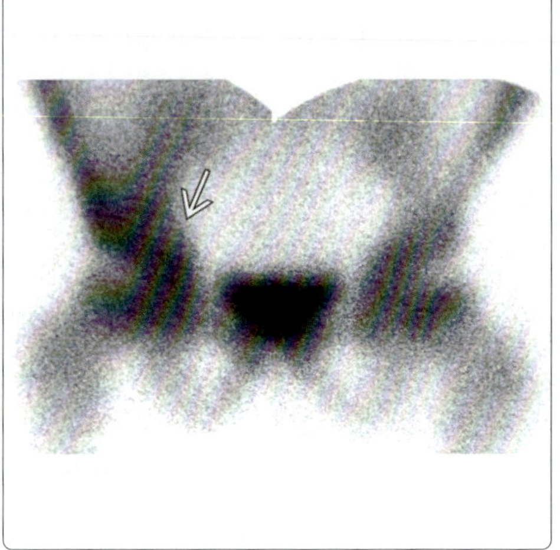

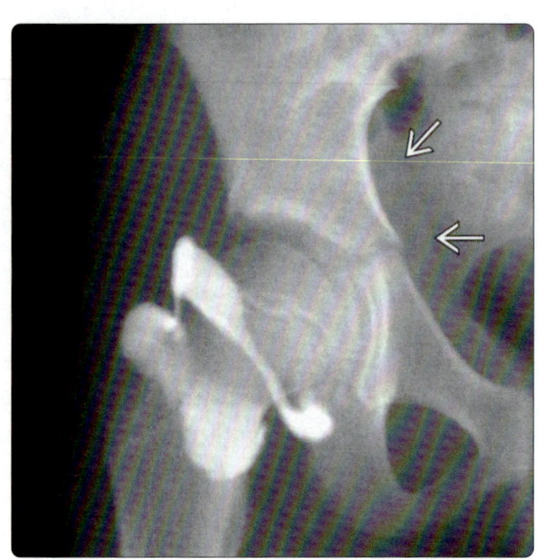

(Left) *Frontal bone scan shows abnormal uptake in the right acetabulum and femoral head ➡. In this child, the concern was for septic hip.* **(Right)** *AP radiograph in the same patient obtained during hip aspiration and arthrogram shows normal hip joint (culture and Gram stain negative). Note that there is a distorted, bulging obturator fat plane ➡. The underlying bone is normal. This proved to be an obturator muscle abscess with hyperemia and resulting bone scan uptake. Lesson: Not all cases of hip pain in a child are septic joints.*

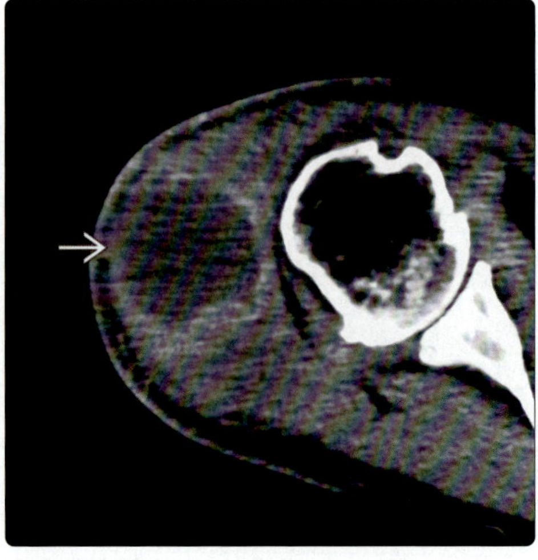

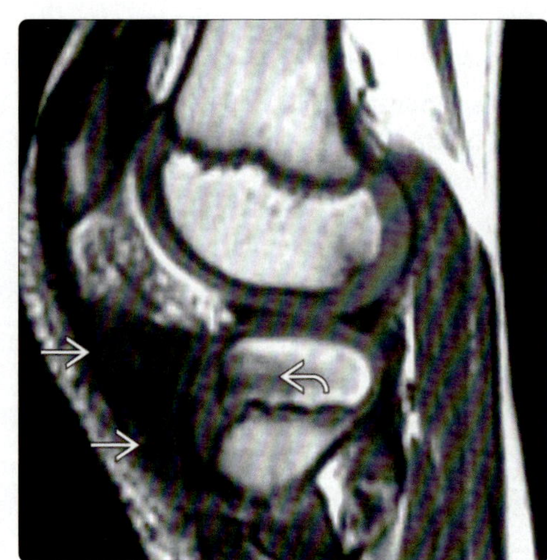

(Left) *Axial CECT demonstrates a low-density lesion with a thin enhancing rim ➡ located within the deltoid muscle. Etiology of this typical abscess was intramuscular injection.* **(Right)** *Lateral T1WI MR shows low signal replacing the fat signal of Hoffa fat pad ➡. This patient had fallen on his knee and had a direct inoculation, resulting in abscess formation. There is adjacent low signal in the tibial epiphysis ➡, which may be either osseous reaction or infection.*

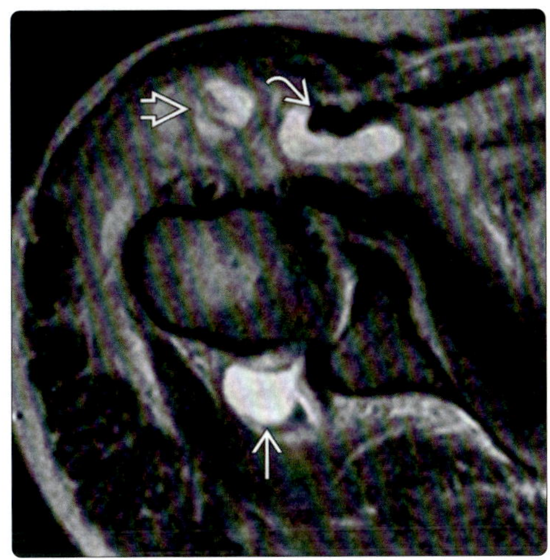

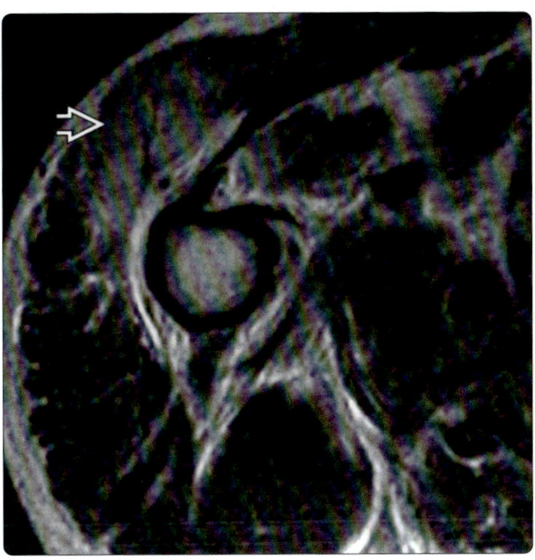

(Left) *Axial T2WI MR shows fluid within the glenohumeral joint ➡. Additionally, there is swelling and a complex fluid signal mass located within the anterior deltoid muscle ➡. Note that the pectoralis major tendon is ruptured and retracted ➡, and fluid is seen surrounding it.* **(Right)** *Axial T2WI MR located more distally shows heterogeneous high signal persisting within the more distal portion of the deltoid muscle. The muscle has lost its feathery texture ➡; the appearance is more typical of abscess than tumor.*

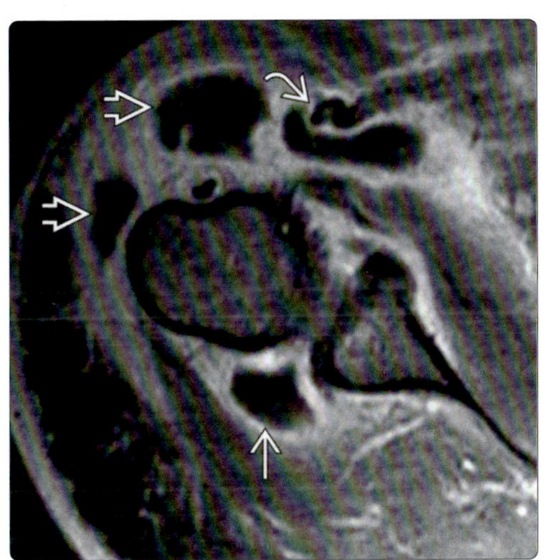

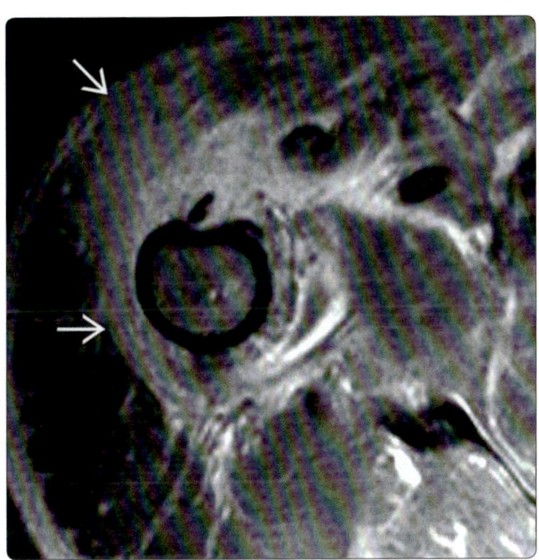

(Left) *Axial T1WI C+ FS MR in the same patient shows intramuscular abscesses within the anterior deltoid mass ➡ with thick rim enhancement. The ruptured, retracted pectoralis is seen in the same plane ➡. There is rim enhancement about the glenohumeral effusion as well ➡.* **(Right)** *Axial T1WI C+ FS MR located more distally shows diffuse enhancement of the soft tissues surrounding the humerus ➡. The intramuscular abscess and septic shoulder resulted from the patient sharing needles with her drug partner.*

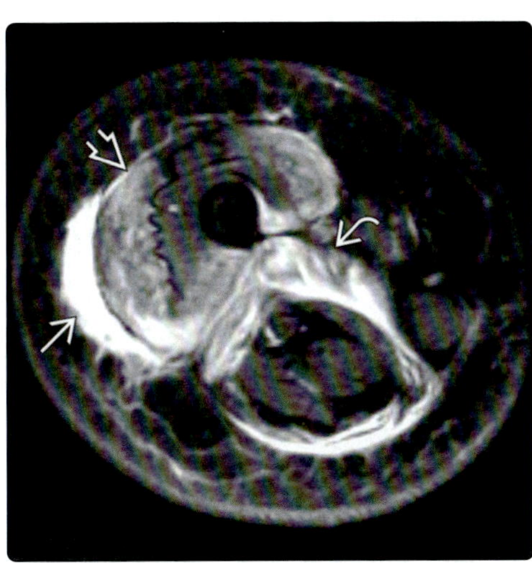

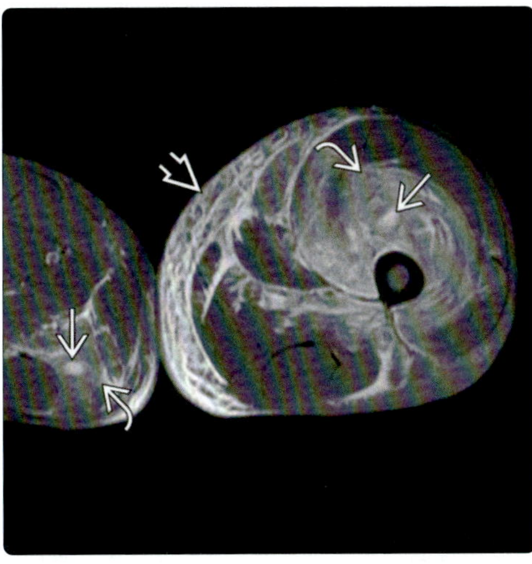

(Left) *Axial PDWI FS MR of a patient with HIV/AIDS shows diffuse intramuscular edema ➡ accompanied by extensive edema in the intermuscular fat planes ➡ and fluid in the superficial fascia ➡, indicating myositis in this immunocompromised patient.* **(Right)** *Axial T2WI FS MR in a patient with HIV/AIDS shows bilateral thigh intramuscular edema and enlargement ➡, as well as subcutaneous edema ➡ on the left. Small intramuscular abscesses ➡ indicate pyomyositis. Staphylococcus aureus was proven by culture.*

KEY FACTS

TERMINOLOGY

- Necrotizing fasciitis (NF): Aggressive, rapidly progressive soft tissue infection that tracks along both superficial (early) and deep fascial planes causing necrosis by microvascular occlusion

IMAGING

- Dissecting gas collections: Superficial &/or deep
  - In absence of penetrating trauma (including iatrogenic causes, such as surgery or chest tube), gas tracking along fascial planes is virtually pathognomonic (seen by radiograph, CT, or MR)
- Subcutaneous edema may be present
  - Less prominent in necrotizing fasciitis than in cellulitis
- Fascial thickening with increased T2 (fluid) signal is invariably present but not specific
  - In NF, fascial thickening almost always involves both superficial and deep fascia
- Nonenhancing islands within and surrounded by enhancing abnormal fascia suggest necrosis

TOP DIFFERENTIAL DIAGNOSES

- Nonnecrotizing fasciitis
- Deep venous thrombosis
- Cellulitis
- Compartment syndrome

PATHOLOGY

- Diabetics are at particular risk owing to both immunocompromise and vascular insufficiency

DIAGNOSTIC CHECKLIST

- Consider: If there is real clinical suspicion for NF, imaging should not delay surgical biopsy/treatment
- Reporting tip: With negative or nonspecific imaging findings, remind clinician that NF is clinical diagnosis
  - If there is real clinical suspicion of NF, surgical biopsy is necessary, regardless of imaging findings

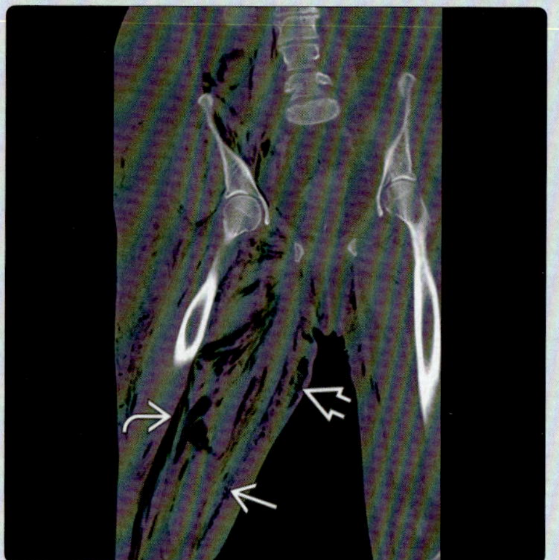

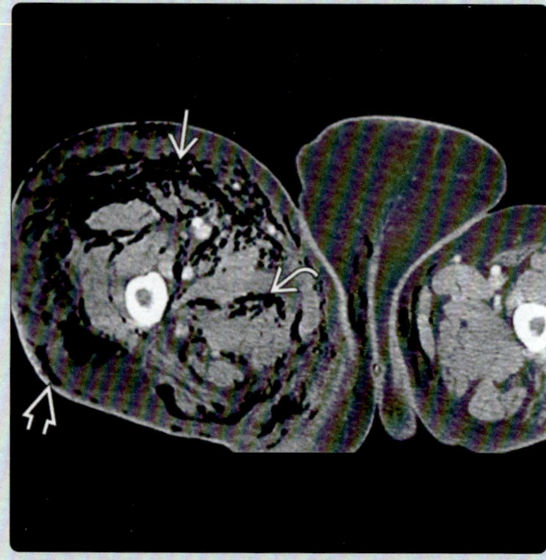

(Left) *Coronal CT in a 54-year-old diabetic who presented with vesico-enteric fistula but rapidly deteriorated shows air dissecting in subcutaneous ➡, superficial fascial ➡, and deep fascial ➡ tissues. It extends into the retroperitoneum along the iliopsoas planes.* **(Right)** *Axial CT, same patient, shows air dissecting along the subcutaneous ➡, superficial fascial ➡ and deep fascial ➡ tissue planes. The perineum and contralateral thigh are involved in this case of necrotizing fasciitis.*

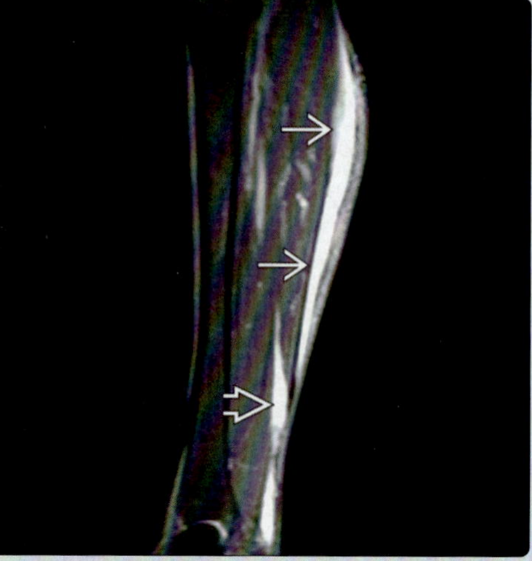

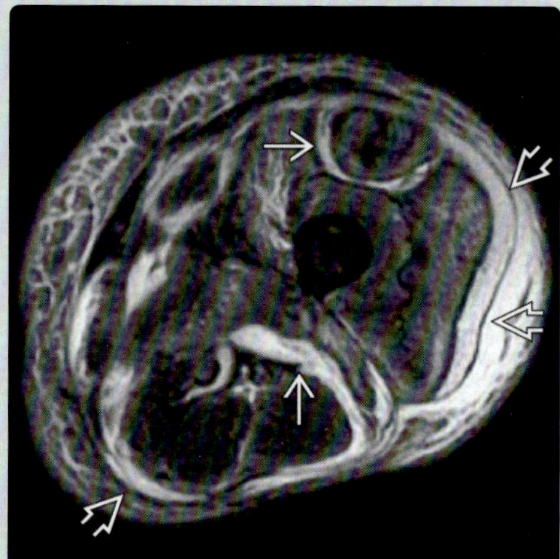

(Left) *Sagittal STIR MR shows high signal fluid extending between the medial gastrocnemius and subcutaneous tissue ➡. Deep fascial fluid collections are seen as well, between the deep flexors and Achilles tendon ➡. Findings are typical but nonspecific for NF.* **(Right)** *Axial T2WI FS MR shows extensive deep ➡ and superficial ➡ fascial fluid and thickening, as well as subcutaneous and muscle edema. This severe case of NF required amputation.*

TERMINOLOGY

Definitions

- Necrotizing fasciitis (NF): Aggressive, rapidly progressive soft tissue infection that tracks along both superficial (early) and deep fascial planes causing necrosis by microvascular occlusion
- Fournier gangrene: Necrotizing fasciitis of perineum

IMAGING

General Features

- Best diagnostic clue
  - In absence of penetrating trauma (including iatrogenic causes, such as surgery or chest tube), gas tracking along fascial planes is virtually pathognomonic
  - Thickened fascia with fluid plus regions of necrosis strongly suggestive of diagnosis

Radiograph and CT Findings

- Gas tracking in soft tissues, superficial &/or deep

MR Findings

- Subcutaneous tissue
  - Circumferential thickening and edema may be seen
  - Subcutaneous edema is less prominent feature in NF than in cellulitis
- Fascia
  - Dissecting gas collections: Superficial &/or deep
  - Fascial thickening with increased T2 (fluid) signal is invariably present but not specific
    - Generally smooth, fusiform, extending along length of muscle/compartment
  - In NF, fascial thickening almost always involves both superficial and deep fascia
    - NF begins in superficial fascia, so in very early NF, differentiation from cellulitis may be difficult
      - If only superficial fascia is abnormal, cellulitis is statistically more likely, but long segment involvement, smooth fusiform thickening, necrosis, fascial gas, and marked thickening should raise possibility of NF
  - Abnormal fascia generally enhances
    - May be uniform or patchy
    - Nonenhancing islands of tissue within and surrounded by enhancing abnormal fascia suggest necrosis
      - Most suggestive MR feature (besides fascial gas)
    - Rim-enhancing abscess may be present
- Muscle
  - Generally not swollen or enhancing
  - Uncommonly, intramuscular fluid is seen

Imaging Recommendations

- Best imaging tool
  - Clinical diagnosis; imaging may not be required
    - Imaging may be used for problem solving
      - **Entirely** normal fascia can rule out NF
    - CT used to search for gas
    - MR with contrast for evaluation of fascial fluid
  - Main utility of imaging in cases of suspected NF is to aid surgical planning

DIFFERENTIAL DIAGNOSIS

Nonnecrotizing Fasciitis

- Deep fascial thickening with enhancement
- No necrosis

Deep Venous Thrombosis

- Thrombus diagnosed on US; may be seen on MR
- May have deep fascial thickening with enhancement

Cellulitis

- Subcutaneous thickening and edema
- Deep fascial thickening not present; superficial fascial thickening/fluid may be seen
- Gas not present

Compartment Syndrome

- Follows length of muscle(s)
- Muscle swelling and edema; loss of normal striations
- May have intermuscular fascial fluid

PATHOLOGY

General Features

- Etiology
  - Predisposing factors: Immunocompromise, vascular insufficiency, and recent trauma or surgery
    - Diabetics are at particular risk owing to both immunocompromise and vascular insufficiency

CLINICAL ISSUES

Presentation

- Most common signs/symptoms
  - Sudden onset of pain, swelling, and often erythema
    - Early on, can be very difficult to differentiate from cellulitis, but pain is often much more severe
- Other signs/symptoms
  - As infection progresses, pain may disappear and area may become anesthetic
  - Skin may demonstrate patchy areas of bluish-purple discoloration &/or hemorrhagic bullae
  - Although patients may present in florid sepsis, many may appear remarkably well owing to blunted immune response

Natural History & Prognosis

- Extensive and rapid progression of soft tissue infection to sepsis and multiorgan system failure
  - Morbidity and mortality is as high as 70-80%

Treatment

- Broad spectrum antibiotics, general supportive measures, and early, extensive surgical debridement
  - 90% polymicrobial with aerobes and anaerobes
  - Only about 10% are due to isolated group A strep
- Hyperbaric oxygen therapy may reduce mortality

SELECTED REFERENCES

1. Paz Maya S et al: Necrotizing fasciitis: an urgent diagnosis. Skeletal Radiol. 43(5):577-89, 2014

KEY FACTS

IMAGING

- Location: 50% of musculoskeletal tuberculosis (TB) infections involve spine; next most common manifestation is septic arthritis; soft tissue involvement rare
  - Spondylitis: Lower thoracic and upper lumbar spine
  - Septic arthritis: Hip, knee most common
  - Pelvis, rib relatively common sites of osteomyelitis
- Septic arthritis: Phemister triad
  - Reactive hyperemia → juxtaarticular osteoporosis
  - Peripheral erosion
  - Late joint space narrowing
  - Septic arthritis often secondary to osteomyelitis
- Appendicular osteomyelitis
  - Hematogenous spread
  - May have multiple sites, especially in children
  - Osteoporosis
  - Osteolytic lesion with ill-defined margins
  - Periostitis and sclerosis are limited
- Tuberculous spondylitis
  - Infection originates in endplate, 1st site of destruction at superior or inferior anterior vertebral body corner
  - Secondary subligamentous spread
  - Children may primarily seed disc
  - May be isolated to 1 vertebral body or involve multiple vertebral bodies ± involvement of intervening disc space
  - Disc space narrowing is late finding
  - Extensive paraspinal abscess formation
  - Calcification within abscess is characteristic
  - May scallop anterior vertebral body
  - Vertebral destruction may lead to vertebra plana, kyphosis, gibbus deformity, ankylosis

CLINICAL ISSUES

- Concomitant pulmonary disease in 50%
- Often long diagnostic delays, which may be > 1 year

(Left) *Oblique radiograph shows an osteolytic lesion in the distal fibular metaphysis ➡. The lesion has crossed the growth plate ➡ to involve the epiphysis ➡. Transphyseal spread is seen with tuberculosis (TB) osteomyelitis and is not common with pyogenic osteomyelitis.* **(Right)** *AP radiograph shows typical findings of TB. Calcified masses are present in both upper lobes ➡ from previous pulmonary disease. Tuberculous septic arthritis has destroyed the right shoulder ➡.*

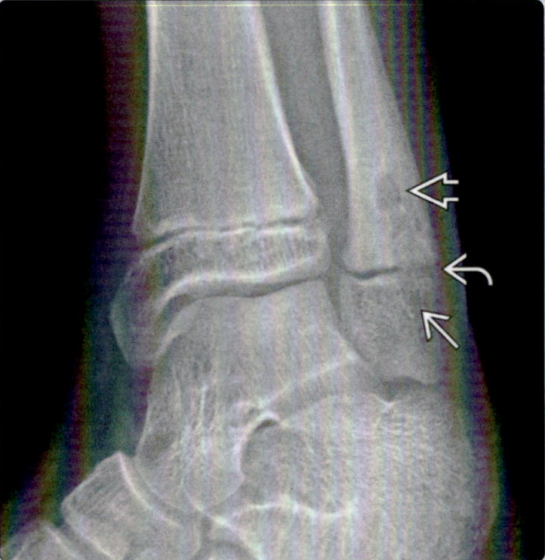

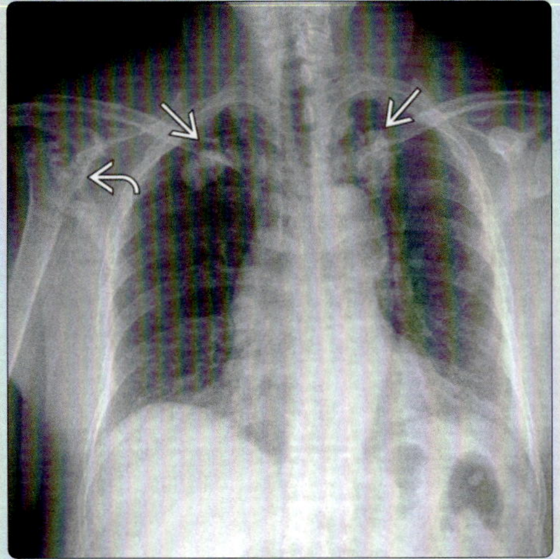

(Left) *Sagittal T1WI C+ MR shows destruction of the T4-T6 vertebra and intervening disc spaces ➡ with focal kyphosis. Large paraspinal abscesses ➡ are present with the posterior epidural mass causing significant canal compromise. Note the thick irregular peripheral enhancement of the abscesses.* **(Right)** *Axial NECT of the same patient shows extensive peripheral calcification at multiple sites ➡ throughout the paraspinal masses. The finding is virtually pathognomonic of tuberculous infection.*

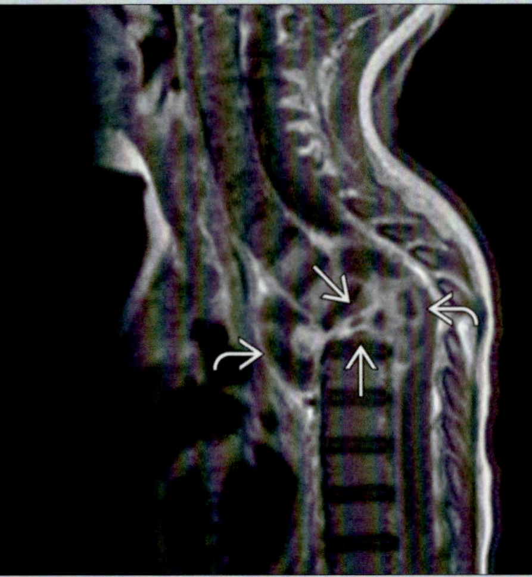

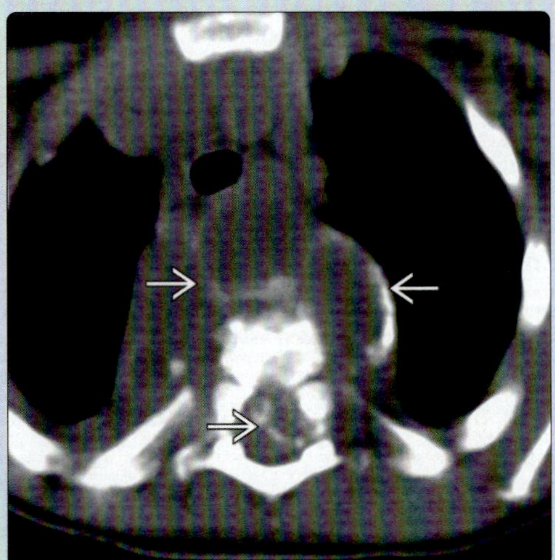

TERMINOLOGY

Definitions

- Cystic tuberculosis (TB): Well-defined intraosseous cystic lesions
- Cold abscess: Slowly developing abscesses, minimal surrounding inflammation, most common around spine
- Phemister triad: Findings seen in tuberculous arthritis
- Pott disease: Osteomyelitis of spine, tuberculous spondylitis
- Pott paraplegia: Paraplegia resulting from tuberculous spondylitis
- Pott puffy tumor: Osteomyelitis of frontal bone with anterior cortical destruction, overlying soft tissue swelling

IMAGING

General Features

- Best diagnostic clue
  - Arthritis: Phemister triad
    - Osteoporosis
    - Peripheral erosions
    - Late joint space narrowing
  - Spondylitis
    - Late disc space narrowing
    - Large paraspinal abscesses with calcification
  - Appendicular osteomyelitis
    - Transphyseal spread in child
- Location
  - 50% of musculoskeletal TB infections involve spine; next most common manifestation is septic arthritis; soft tissue involvement rare
    - Spondylitis: Lower thoracic and upper lumbar spine
    - Septic arthritis: Hip, knee most common
    - Pelvis, rib relatively common sites of osteomyelitis
- Morphology
  - Infection that incites little reaction in surrounding tissues
    - Late development of periostitis, sclerosis
    - Late destruction of articular cartilage and intervertebral disc
    - Cold abscesses, which may produce pressure erosions on adjacent bone

Imaging Recommendations

- Best imaging tool
  - Arthritis: Radiographs identify joint-based findings
    - Advanced imaging provides details of anatomic extent, does not aid differential diagnosis
  - Osteomyelitis: Radiographs to identify abnormality
    - CT and MR identify osseous and soft tissue extent of disease
  - Spondylitis
    - MR best depicts findings, extent of disease
  - Tissue/fluid sampling usually required to establish diagnosis

Radiographic Findings

- Septic arthritis
  - Phemister triad
    - Juxtaarticular osteoporosis 2° to reactive hyperemia
    - Peripheral erosion
    - Late joint space narrowing
  - Periostitis and sclerosis are limited
    - If present, seen late in disease
  - Often secondary to osteomyelitis
    - Adult: Epiphyseal osteomyelitis may seed joint
    - Child: Metaphyseal site of osteomyelitis with transphyseal spread into joint
  - Soft tissue masses and cold abscesses, sinus tract formation
  - Fibrous ankylosis common, osseous fusion less common than in pyogenic disease
- Appendicular osteomyelitis
  - Hematogenous spread
    - May have multiple sites, especially in children
  - Metaphyseal location most common
    - May spread to epiphysis
    - Diaphyseal disease rare
  - Usually associated with septic arthritis
    - Isolated osteomyelitis less common
  - Osteoporosis
  - Osteolytic lesion with ill-defined margins
    - Cystic TB: Lytic lesions with geographic well-defined margins, which may be sclerotic
  - Periostitis and sclerosis are limited
    - If present, seen late in disease
  - ± soft tissue mass
  - Sequestrum rare
  - Spina ventosa or tuberculous dactylitis
    - Begins with fusiform soft tissue swelling and periostitis
    - Progresses to balloon-like or fusiform enlargement of bone with internal septations
      - Diffuse cortical thickening without periosteal new bone
    - Hands more common than feet
    - Most are under 6 years of age
- Tuberculous spondylitis (vertebral body osteomyelitis)
  - Lower thoracic and upper lumbar spine
  - Hematogenous seeding of vertebral body
    - Infection originates in endplate, 1st site of destruction at superior or inferior anterior vertebral body corner
    - Secondary subligamentous spread
    - Children may primarily seed disc
  - May be isolated to 1 vertebral body or involve multiple vertebral bodies ± involvement of intervening disc space
    - Disc space narrowing is late finding
  - Extensive paraspinal abscess formation
    - Calcification within abscess is characteristic
    - May scallop anterior vertebral body
  - Vertebral destruction may lead to vertebra plana, kyphosis, gibbus deformity, ankylosis
  - Limited sclerosis, periosteal new bone formation
- Soft tissue infection rare
  - Tenosynovitis, bursitis, primary myositis

CT Findings

- Mirrors radiographic findings
- More sensitive than radiographs for identification of soft tissue and paraspinal abscesses
- Sensitive for detection of calcification in abscesses

- Contrast enhancement helps differentiate abscess from phlegmon and aids detection of sinus tracts

MR Findings

- Septic arthritis
  - Joint effusion and synovitis
    - ↓ T1W, ↑ T2W signal
    - C+: Enhancement within synovium
    - Synovial proliferation may be low SI on T2
  - Associated osteomyelitis will be seen
- Osteomyelitis
  - Bone marrow edema and inflammation
    - ↓ T1W, ↑ T2W signal
    - C+: Diffuse enhancement
      - May have intraosseous abscess with peripheral enhancement
  - Soft tissue masses
    - Heterogeneous ↓ T1W, ↑ T2W signal
    - Thick irregular peripheral enhancement in abscess is characteristic
    - Contrast enhancement along sinus tract
    - Abscesses may be invasive, extend to distant sites
      - With spondylitis, see large abscess within paraspinal muscles, may see epidural abscess

Nuclear Medicine Findings

- Bone scan
  - Useful to identify osteomyelitis
    - Nonspecific
    - High false-negative rate in TB due to relatively mild response of adjacent bone
- Ga-67 scintigraphy
  - Better than labeled white cells scans to identify paraspinal disease
    - High false-negative rate

Image-Guided Biopsy

- Core biopsy recommended to maximize yield
  - Diagnosis requires identification of *Mycobacterium* in sample
  - Should be sent for acid-fast stain

DIFFERENTIAL DIAGNOSIS

TB Spondylitis

- Bacterial infection: May have more sclerosis, new bone formation
- Brucellosis: May be indistinguishable from TB spondylitis
- Coccidiomycosis: Spares disc spaces
- Metastatic disease: Often involves posterior elements

TB Spina Ventosa

- Sickle cell disease: Laboratory confirmation
- Syphilis: Bilateral, symmetric

Tuberculous Osteomyelitis

- Metastatic disease and multiple myeloma: May require biopsy to differentiate
- Pyogenic infection: Does not cross growth plate

TB Septic Arthritis

- Inflammatory arthritides, pyogenic infection
  - More rapid joint destruction in inflammatory and pyogenic arthritis

PATHOLOGY

General Features

- Etiology
  - Organism: *Mycobacterium tuberculosis*
  - Hematogenous spread often from lung infection
  - Musculoskeletal (MSK) disease accounts for 1-3% of all TB infection
    - In developing countries, MSK disease in 10-15% of all TB infection

Microscopic Features

- Caseating granulomas
- Positive acid-fast bacilli stain

CLINICAL ISSUES

Presentation

- Most common signs/symptoms
  - Mild pain, low-grade fever
- Other signs/symptoms
  - Concomitant pulmonary disease (50%)
    - More extrapulmonary disease in immunocompromised patients
  - Often long diagnostic delays, which may be > 1 year

Demographics

- Age
  - Developed countries: TB more commonly in adults
  - Developing countries: TB often seen in children
- Gender
  - Males slightly greater
- Epidemiology
  - Increasing incidence due to increasing immunocompromised population

Natural History & Prognosis

- Spondylitis: Severe deformity, neurologic deficit, including paraplegia
- Osteomyelitis and septic arthritis progress to soft tissue abscess, draining sinuses

Treatment

- Surgical debridement, antituberculin medications
- Multidrug-resistant organisms are increasing
  - No difference in virulence
  - Greater morbidity due to inability to halt disease progression

SELECTED REFERENCES

1. Hirji H et al: Paediatric acquired pathological vertebral collapse. Skeletal Radiol. 43(4):423-36, 2014
2. De Backer AI et al: Imaging features of extraaxial musculoskeletal tuberculosis. Indian J Radiol Imaging. 19(3):176-86, 2009
3. Sanghvi DA et al: MRI features of tuberculosis of the knee. Skeletal Radiol. 38(3):267-73, 2009

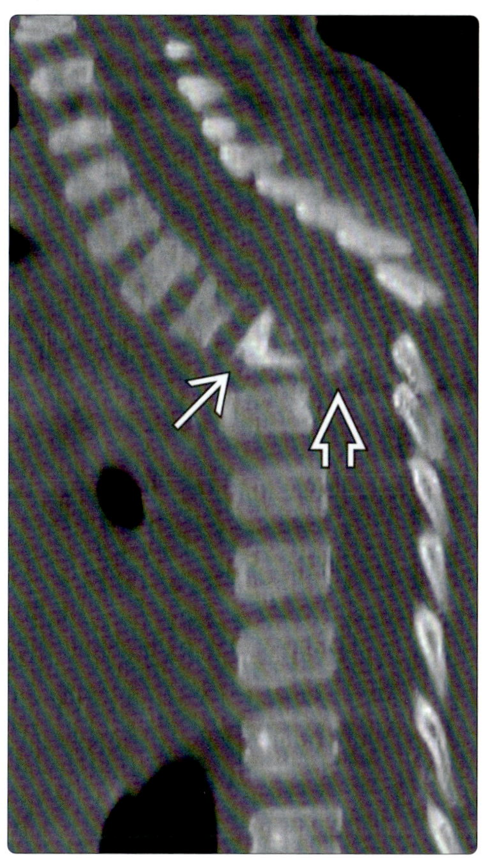

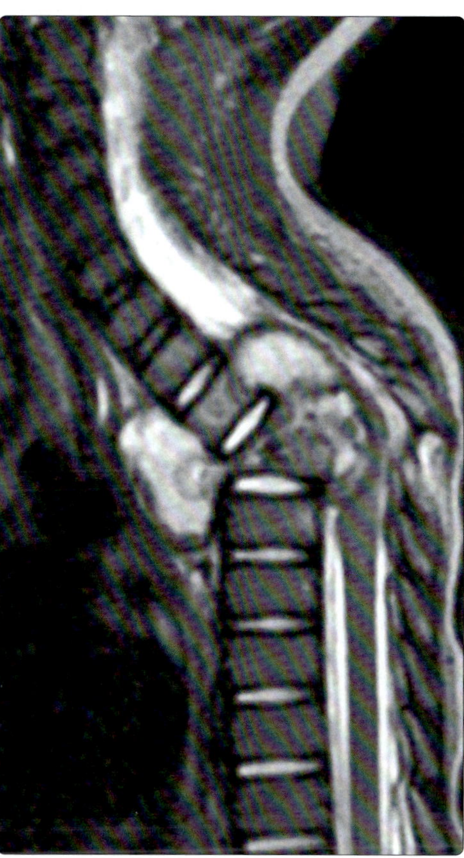

(Left) *Sagittal NECT shows a child with spinal TB. Slivers of endplates are all that remain of 3 contiguous vertebra* ➡. *Calcification within the spinal canal* ⇨ *is key to recognizing this as tuberculous infection.* **(Right)** *Sagittal T2WI MR of the same patient shows the heterogeneous appearance of the paraspinal masses. As seen here, these masses can be quite large. The masses may extend far from the original site of infection and may invade the mediastinum or pleural space. Neurologic complications are often associated. In this case, symptoms of cord compression are likely and may be the presenting symptom. The disease has a slowly progressive nature and is often quite advanced at the time of presentation for imaging.*

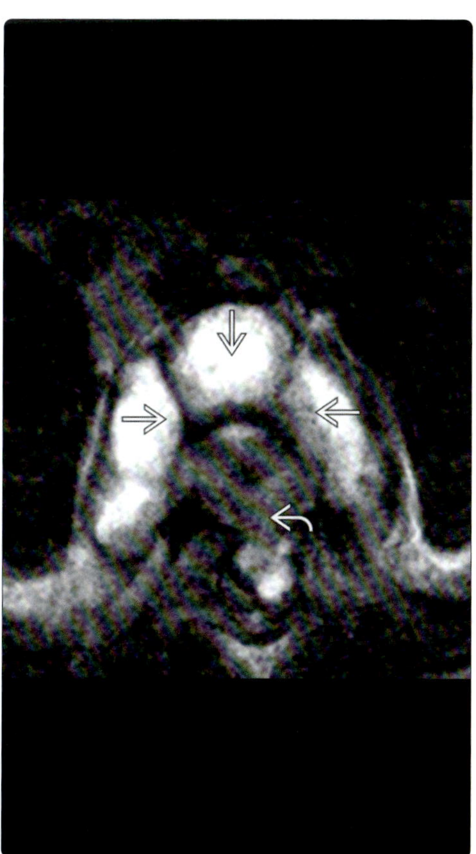

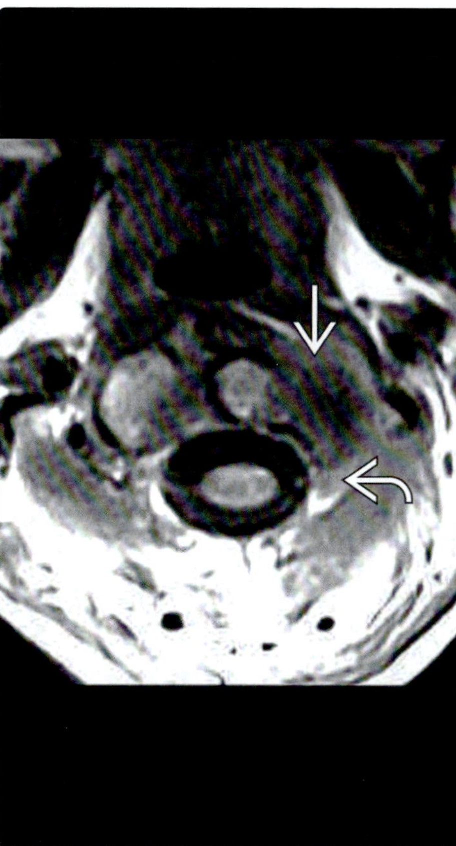

(Left) *Axial T2WI MR of large paraspinal* ➡ *and epidural* ↪ *abscesses accompanying tuberculous spondylitis shows signal characteristics that are nonspecific. However, their exuberance, both in size and extent, should suggest the possibility of tuberculous spondylitis. These abscesses are often known as cold abscesses, reflecting the findings of slow growth without inciting a significant inflammatory response. Often they cause pressure erosions on the adjacent anterior vertebral body.* **(Right)** *Axial T1WI MR shows abnormal low signal within the body of C2 on the left* ➡. *Adjacent inflammatory changes are present with ill-definition of the fat planes* ↪. *The appearance is nonspecific. TB involvement of the cervical spine is less common than thoracic or lumbar disease.*

(Left) *AP x-ray shows TB septic arthritis. The glenoid and humeral head are both destroyed ➡. Multiple osseous fragments are seen within the joint, including the axillary pouch ➡. The extent of destruction is not as aggressive as might be seen with pyogenic infection, and there is no sclerotic osseous reaction. Identification of the calcified lung mass ➡ provides a strong clue to the diagnosis of tuberculous septic arthritis.* **(Right)** *AP radiograph coned to lower ribs shows complete opacification of the left hemithorax and a lytic lesion in 1 of the lower ribs ➡. While the combination of lung disease and lytic lesions may be seen with metastatic disease, TB should be considered. The ribs are 1 of the more common sites for development of tuberculous osteomyelitis.*

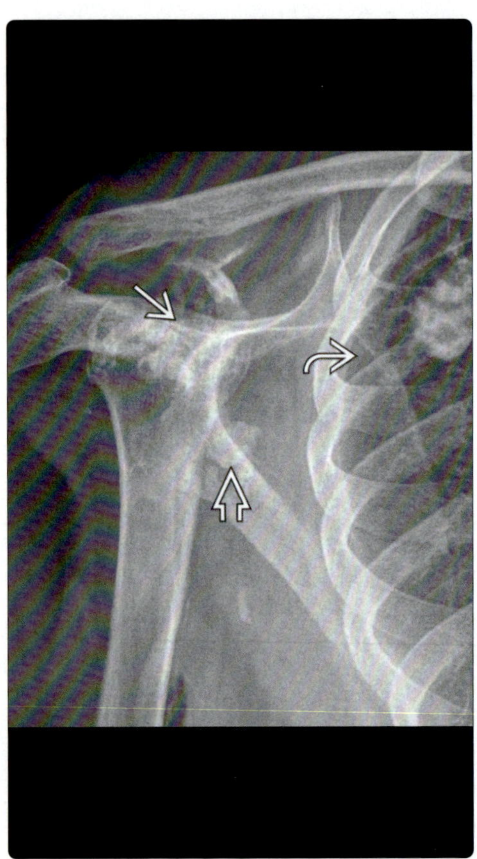

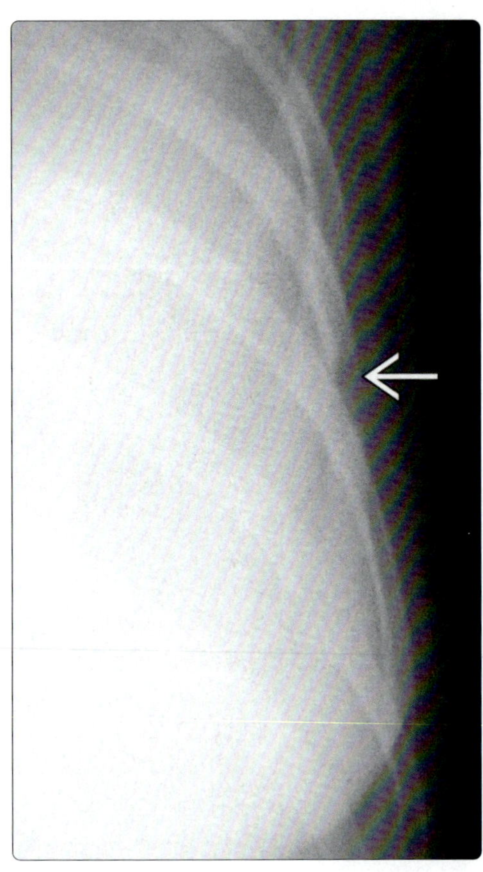

(Left) *Sagittal T1WI MR demonstrates multilevel TB vertebral osteomyelitis. In the lower thoracic spine, contiguous disease with involvement of the intervening disc is seen and is accompanied by subligamentous spread of infection ➡. Scattered vertebral involvement is present within the mid and upper thoracic spine. Epidural extension of disease is noted in the upper thoracic spine, mimicking neoplasm ➡.* **(Right)** *AP x-ray shows a well-defined lytic lesion in the femoral diaphysis with periostitis ➡. Imaging characteristics are slightly atypical for TB, which usually favors a metaphyseal location and has ill-defined borders without periostitis. Differential in a child would include eosinophilic granuloma, and, in an adult, one would consider metastatic disease. However, the lesion proved to be TB.*

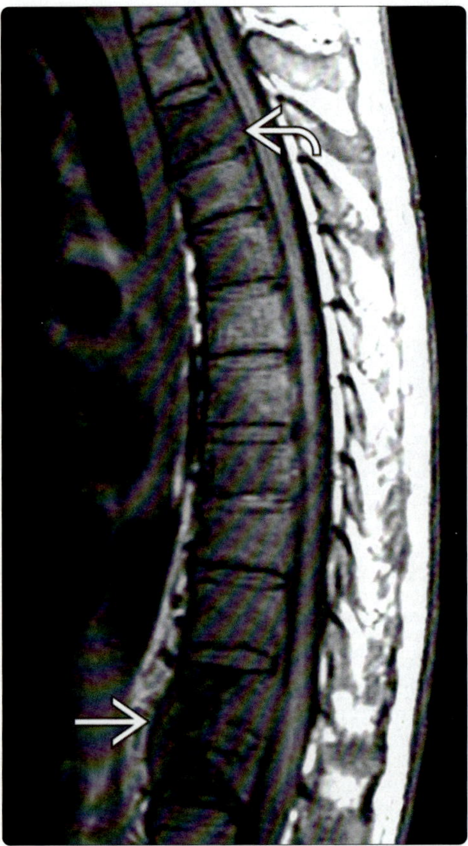

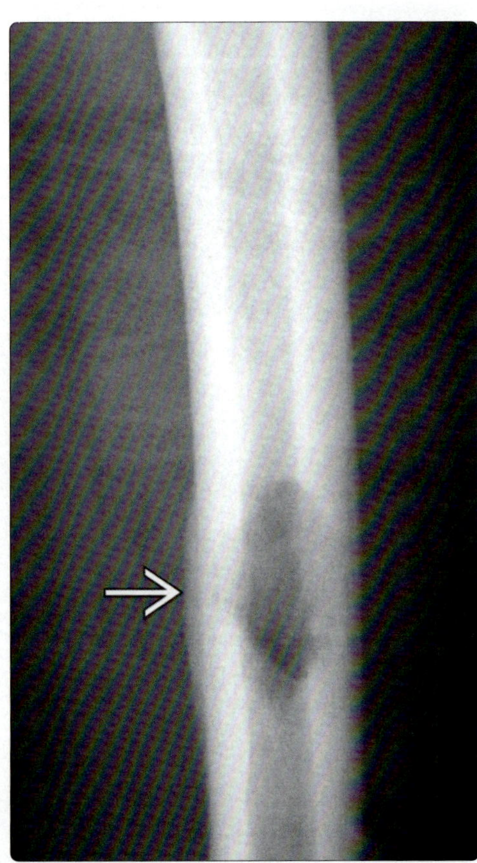

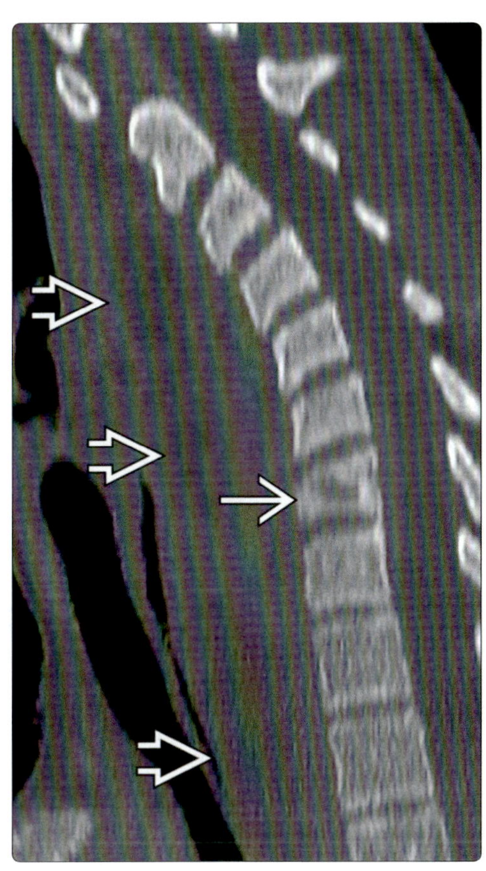

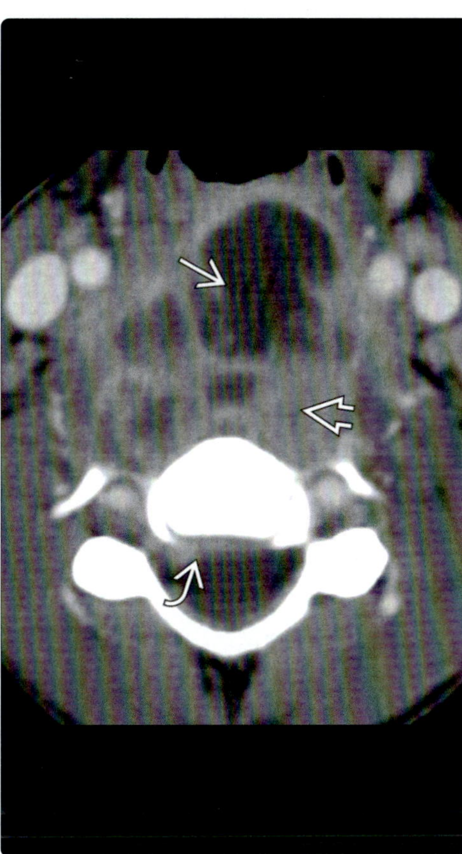

(Left) *Sagittal CT demonstrates limited C7 vertebral destruction ➡ with normal adjacent disc spaces. No other osseous lesions are seen. There is extensive anterior soft tissue abnormality with mass extending along the prevertebral space ➡.* **(Right)** *Axial CECT of the same patient shows extensive soft tissue changes accompanying the vertebral destruction resulting from tuberculous spondylitis. A small enhancing epidural phlegmon is present ➡. Large anterior soft tissue mass contains nonenhancing components ➡, indicative of abscess formation, as well as diffusely enhancing components ➡, which represent inflamed tissue of a phlegmon. The fact that a mass this large could develop in the neck without causing airway obstruction is a testament to the slowly progressive nature of this infection.*

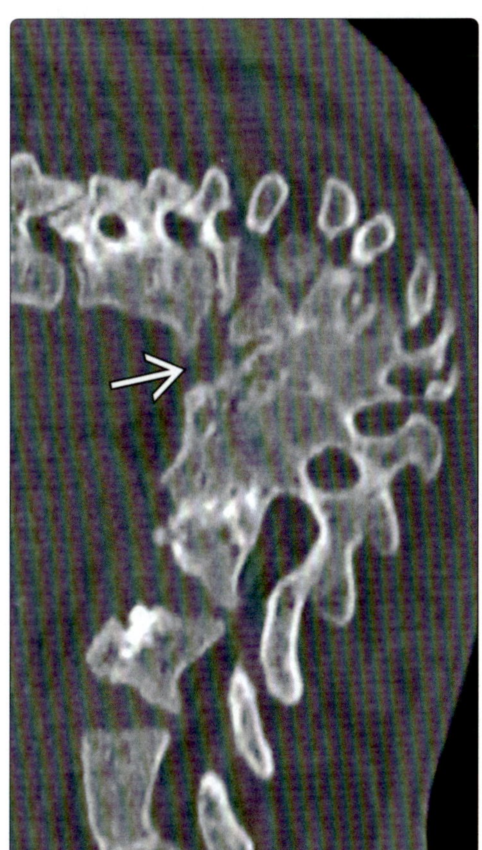

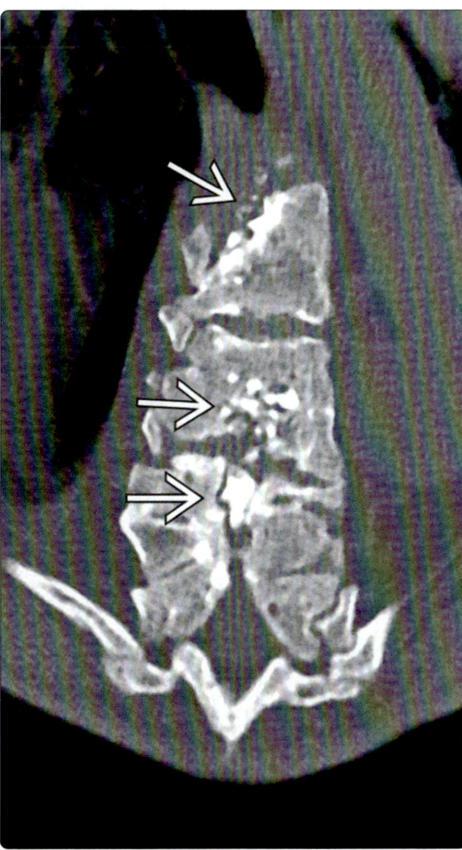

(Left) *Sagittal CT obtained in follow-up of TB spondylitis reveals a 90° kyphosis ➡. There is multilevel contiguous vertebral body destruction with involvement of the intervening disc spaces, leading to the angular deformity. Healing has resulted in fusion across the destroyed segments. While healing leads to fusion in the spine, it is less common following healing of septic discitis than TB.* **(Right)** *Axial CT in the same patient through the upper segment mimics a coronal view due to the deformity. Multiple chunky foci of mineralization are present within several vertebral bodies ➡. The intraosseous mineralization is a combination of vertebral body fragmentation, reactive bone formation from the healing process, and residual mineralization (which is commonly associated with the cold abscesses of TB).*

KEY FACTS

IMAGING

- Fungal osteomyelitis: Appendicular sites
  - 2 patterns: Permeative destruction **or** focal well-defined lytic lesions; ± sclerotic margins; ± periostitis, limited osteoporosis
  - Limited reactive change relative to pyogenic
  - May extend into joint if at end of long bone
- Fungal osteomyelitis: Axial sites
  - Extensive soft tissue phlegmon ± abscess
  - Spread along anterior longitudinal ligament leads to multiple noncontiguous levels of involvement
  - Coccidioidomycosis: Disc sparing is distinctive feature relative to any other spondylitis
  - Blastomycosis: Associated rib destruction
- Fungal septic arthritis
  - Joint space narrowing, well-defined foci of destruction, limited osteoporosis
  - Sporotrichosis: Septic arthritis > > osteomyelitis

TOP DIFFERENTIAL DIAGNOSES

- Tuberculosis: May be indistinguishable from fungal
  - May be more destructive, with ill-defined margins
  - Osteoporosis is significant feature
  - Disc space destruction more prominent than in coccidioidomycosis, less than in pyogenic

PATHOLOGY

- Soil inhabitants, often enter via lungs: *Actinomyces*, *Aspergillus*, *Blastomyces*, *Coccidioides*, *Cryptococcus*, *Sporothrix*

CLINICAL ISSUES

- Often underlying immune deficiency or diabetes
- Often misdiagnosed as malignancy
- High association with pulmonary disease
- Skin lesions, draining sinuses frequent
- Treatment: Surgical debridement, antifungal therapy

(Left) *AP radiograph of the elbow shows a well-defined lytic lesion in the medial epicondylar region ➡, biopsy proven to be blastomycosis. Lesion is well defined without sclerotic margins, periostitis, or sclerotic reactive bone.* **(Right)** *PA radiograph shows a patient with sporotrichosis septic arthritis. Marked narrowing of the radiocarpal compartment is present, along with several well-defined foci of destruction ➡. Unlike other fungal infection, sporotrichosis causes septic arthritis more frequently than osteomyelitis.*

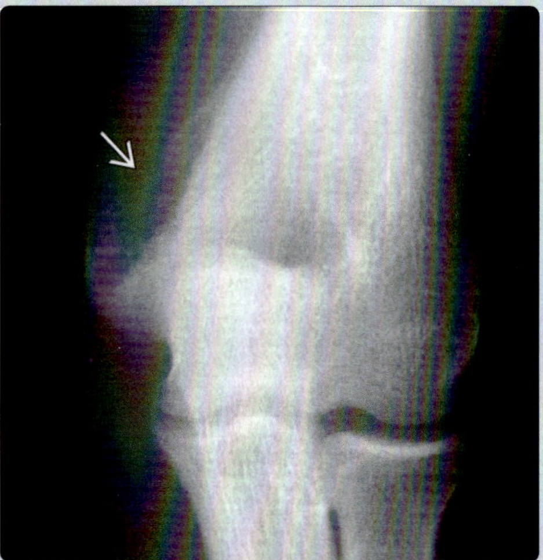

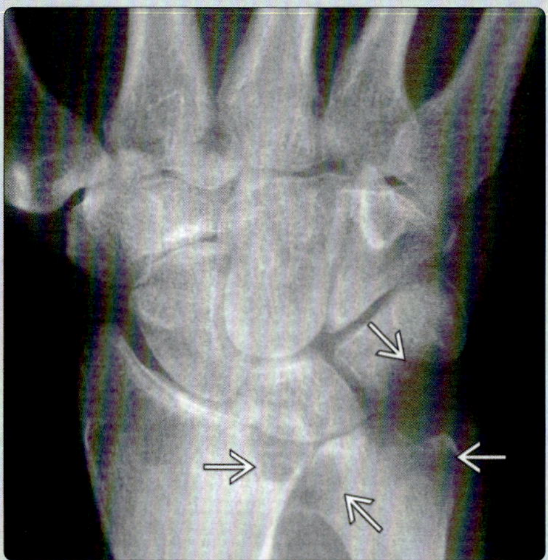

(Left) *Coronal T2WI MR with disseminated coccidioidomycosis shows multilevel vertebral involvement and extensive paraspinal phlegmon ➡. Note the paraspinal mode of spread and relative sparing of discs ➡.* **(Right)** *AP x-ray shows an adult who developed Candida septic arthritis after anterior cruciate ligament surgery 5 years earlier. Cartilage narrowing, marginal tibial erosion ➡, and deossification ➡ are seen. Aspiration proved active infection despite 2 years of therapy. Lack of reactive change is typical.*

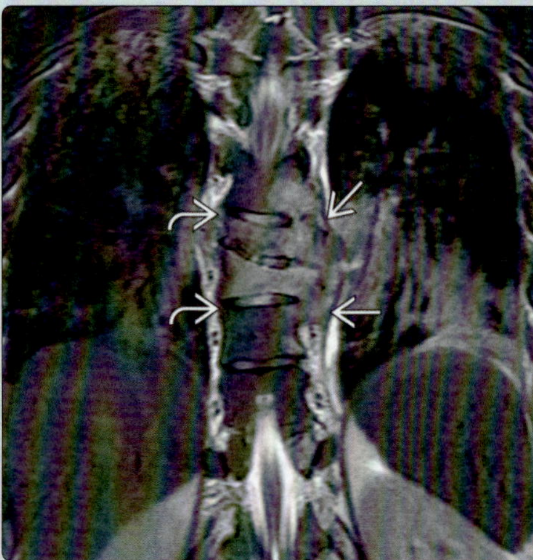

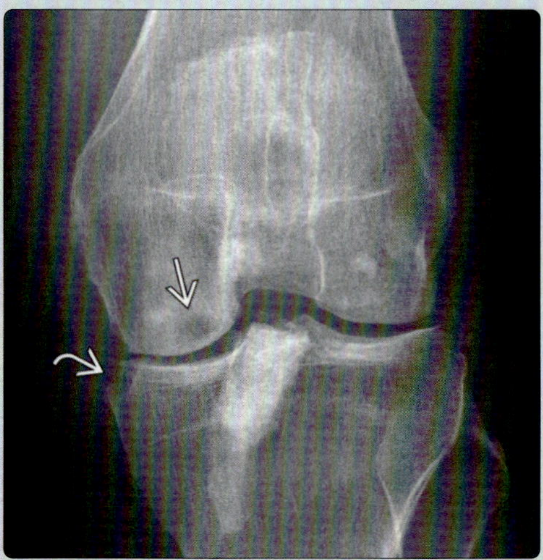

KEY FACTS

TERMINOLOGY

- Zoonotic disease caused by bacteria within *Brucella* genus
  - Systemic infection that can affect any organ
  - Musculoskeletal (MSK) abnormalities may be present in acute, subacute, or chronic stages

IMAGING

- Sacroiliac joints (SIJ) most common site of MSK involvement
  - 28% of those with brucellosis
  - 53% of patients with MSK abnormalities have sacroiliitis
  - 2/3 unilateral, 1/3 bilateral
  - Irregular erosions along synovial portion of SIJ
  - Mild sclerotic reaction
- Spondylodiscitis is common MSK manifestation
  - 10.5% of those with brucellosis
  - 19% of brucellosis patients with MSK abnormalities have spondylodiscitis
  - Lumbar spine most frequently involved
  - May have contiguous involvement > 1 disc space
  - May have noncontiguous multifocal involvement
  - Decreased disc height
  - Irregularity, destruction of adjacent endplates
  - Relatively slower disc height loss and sclerotic osseous response than seen in other more typical bacterial discitis
  - Gibbus deformity
  - Iliopsoas mass, ± dystrophic calcification
- Shoulders (16% of cases with MSK involvement)
- Osteomyelitis
  - Slow destructive change without significant reactive sclerosis
- Septic arthritis
  - Joint space narrowing, effusion
  - Deossification/outright destruction of subchondral bone
- CT: Bone destruction (including endplates if discitis)
  - Relatively mild sclerotic reactive bone formation
  - Abscess: ↓ attenuation collections/rim enhancement
- MR findings in brucellosis: Nonspecific
  - T1WI: Confluent low signal in affected regions
  - Fluid-sensitive sequences: Inhomogeneous ↑ SI
  - Postcontrast imaging: Inhomogeneous enhancement
  - Thick enhancing rim around abscess collections
  - Epidural and paravertebral extension
  - Septic arthritis: Same signal pattern plus effusion and articular cartilage/bone destruction

TOP DIFFERENTIAL DIAGNOSES

- Tuberculosis (TB)
  - Identical appearance of discitis preferentially centered at thoracolumbar junction
  - Disc space destruction, gibbus deformity
  - Iliopsoas abscesses, often containing calcification
  - May have multiple levels of vertebral involvement, with skip lesions
  - Clinical history and testing for TB serve to differentiate TB from brucellosis

PATHOLOGY

- Etiology: Direct or indirect exposure to animals
  - Transmission usually by milk or milk products
  - In USA, transmitted to workers in meat-packing plants
- Diagnosed by serologic analysis (*Brucella* agglutinin titer) or positive blood culture
  - Blood culture is frequently false-negative

CLINICAL ISSUES

- Clinical presentation
  - Fatigue, fever, sweating, headache
  - Arthralgias (84%), back pain (65%)
- Age: Wide range, 40-60 years most common
- Gender: Male < female
- Ethnicity: Mediterranean and Arabian regions > Indian subcontinent > Mexico, Central and South America
- Natural History: 40% of patients in large prospective study developed MSK abnormalities
  - Acute onset and rapid progression may occur
  - More frequently chronic and slowly progressive

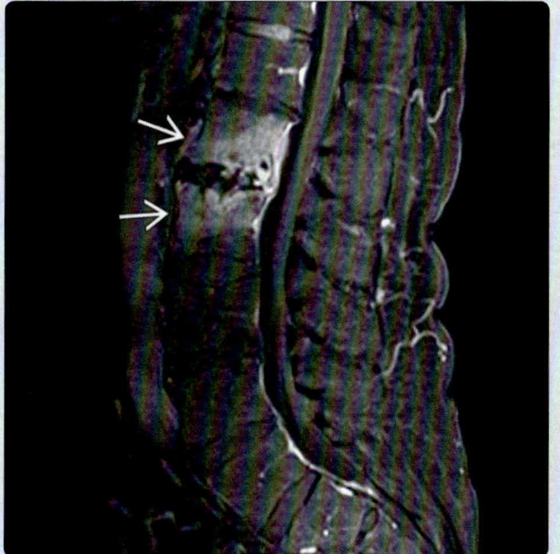

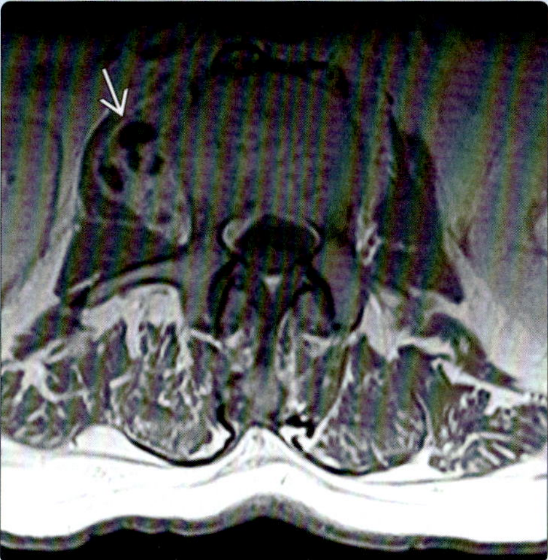

(Left) *Sagittal T2FS MR shows hyperintensity involving L1 and L2 adjacent endplates ➡, with partial destruction of the intervening disc. This indicates a disc space infection. Because of the location and slow disc destruction, tuberculosis should be considered.* **(Right)** *Axial postcontrast T1MR, same patient, shows abscess within the right psoas muscle ➡. The patient was a Mexican national who drank unpasteurized milk; serologic tests proved Brucellosis. The relatively slow destructive process is typical of this disease.*

KEY FACTS

TERMINOLOGY

- Mycetoma; eumycetoma (fungal infection); actinomycetoma (infection with *Actinomyces*)

IMAGING

- Multiple nodular soft tissue masses → pressure erosions and osseous distortion → periosteal new bone formation &/or sclerosis → bone destruction → osseous fusion
- Osseous invasion
  - May follow along single digit (vertical spread)
  - May spread from bone to adjacent bone (horizontal spread)
  - May have multidirectional spread
- Radiographs
  - Soft tissue mass(es)
  - Pressure erosions on bone, may become extensive and create appearance of melting snow
  - Bones become bowed, with interosseous widening
  - Late disease shows extensive osseous fusion
- MR
  - Soft tissue masses ± necrosis; sinus tracts
  - Periosteal inflammatory changes, marrow edema
  - Dot-in-circle sign described: High signal granuloma with central low signal fungal elements (grains)

PATHOLOGY

- Granulomatous infection 2° to *Actinomyces* (60%) or fungus (40%)
  - Soil-based organisms enter through breaks in skin, invade deep soft tissues, then bone

CLINICAL ISSUES

- M > F, ratio of 5:1; most common age 20-40
- Solitary/multiple hard tissue mass(es) with multiple draining sinuses may progress to extensive deformity
- Painless, slowly progressive disease
- Treatment: Antibiotics in early disease; advanced disease requires aggressive surgical resection, amputation necessary in large percentage

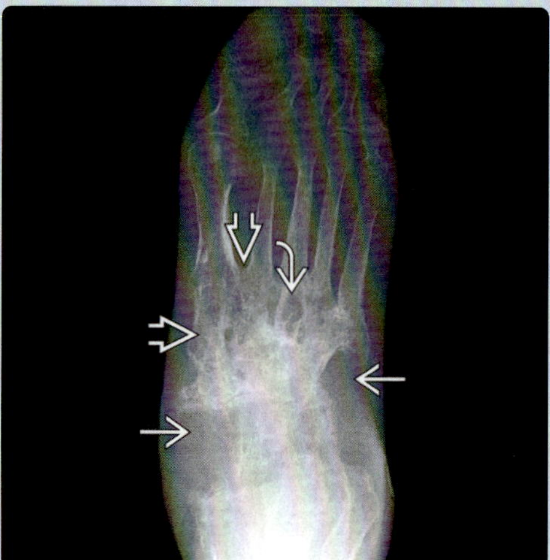

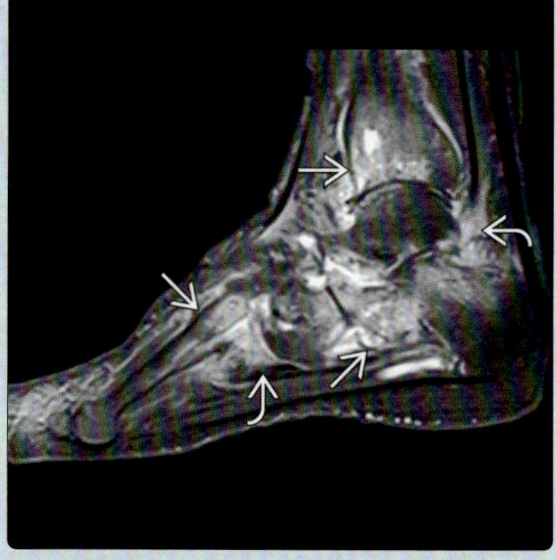

(Left) *AP radiograph shows large pressure erosions along the medial and lateral aspects of the midfoot* ➡. *Extensive osseous fusion is present in the intermetatarsal, tarsal-metatarsal, and intertarsal articulations* ➡. *Residual defects from pressure erosions are noted* ➡. **(Right)** *Sagittal T1WI C+ FS MR of the same patient shows extensive intraosseous enhancement* ➡ *and soft tissue inflammatory changes* ➡. *In this late stage, osseous changes dominate soft tissue changes.*

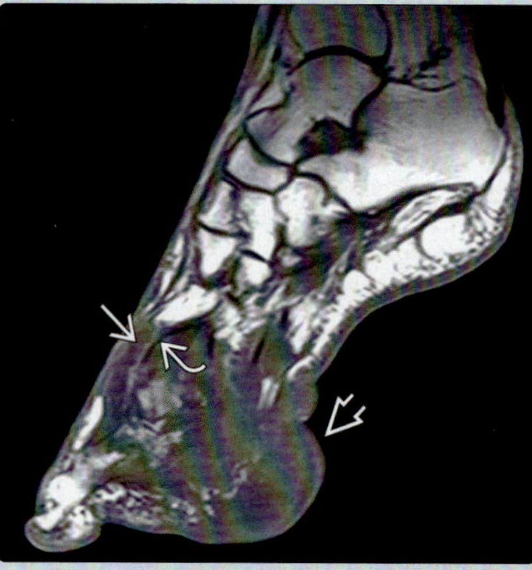

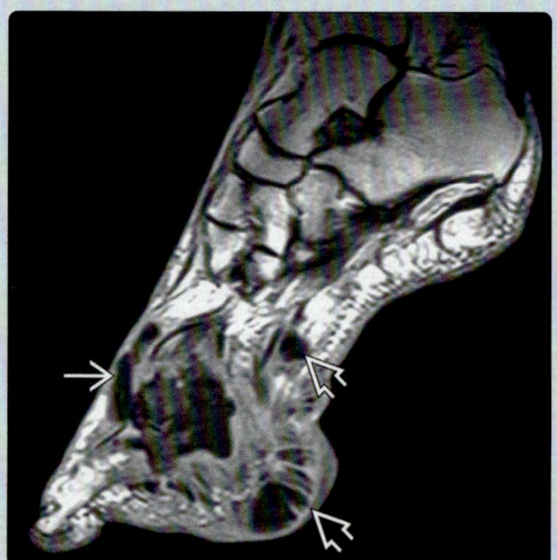

(Left) *Sagittal T1WI reveals a large soft tissue mass along the plantar surface of the foot* ➡. *The mass distorts the adjacent metatarsal, which is bowed* ➡. *Marrow changes within the metatarsal indicate osseous invasion* ➡. **(Right)** *Sagittal T1WI C+ MR of the same patient shows multiple soft tissue* ➡ *and intraosseous foci* ➡ *of necrosis. Clinically multiple draining sinuses were evident. The draining material had a granular appearance resulting from clumping of the organisms.*

KEY FACTS

TERMINOLOGY

- Rocky Mountain spotted fever: Disease caused by *Rickettsia rickettsii*

IMAGING

- Serpiginous pattern of bone infarction
  - Double line sign
- Neuro MR: Uncommon presence of abnormalities
  - Infarction, cerebral edema, enhancement of meninges, spinal cord, and cauda equina

PATHOLOGY

- Obligately intracellular bacterium spread to humans by ticks
- Causes ↑ permeability in vascular endothelial cells
  - Systemic ↑ in vascular permeability leads to edema, hypovolemia, and hypoalbuminemia
  - Necrotizing vasculitis → osseous infarction

CLINICAL ISSUES

- Fever (98%)
- Rash (97%): Begins on extremities, travels proximally to involve trunk
- Nausea and vomiting (73%)
- Headache (61%)
- Epidemiology
  - Endemic in southeastern USA (only 2% in Rocky Mountain states)
  - Seasonal outbreaks parallel tick activity
- Natural history
  - 1 of most virulent infections
  - Potentially fatal even in previously healthy young people (mortality rate: 1.4%)
  - Mortality greater in young children (5% if < 5 years old) and elderly
  - Treatment delay > 5 days leads to complications in 40-55% of cases

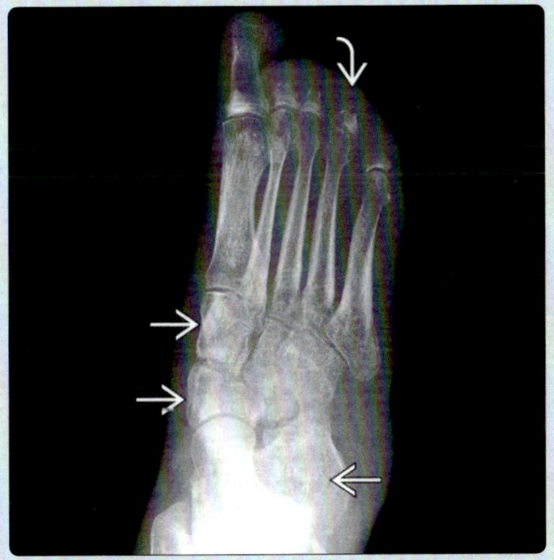

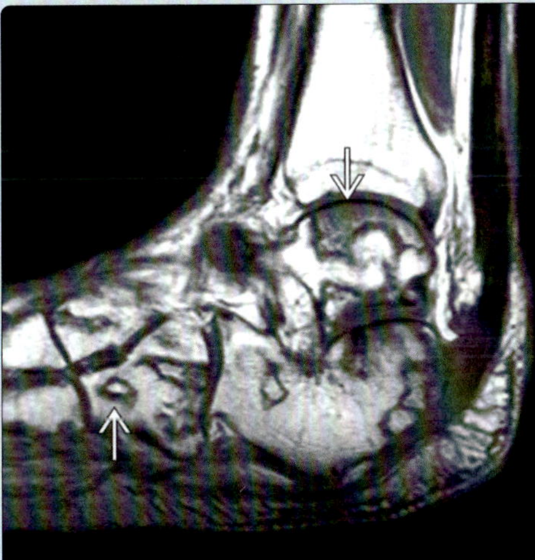

(Left) *This patient was hospitalized with encephalitis resulting from a tick bite; the diagnosis was Rocky Mountain spotted fever (RMSF). The radiograph shows most of the tarsales to have a mixed sclerotic and lytic appearance, typical of bone infarct ➡. The toes have been amputated ➡ due to vascular insufficiency.* **(Right)** *Sagittal T1WI MR in the same patient shows the irregular serpiginous pattern of bone infarcts ➡. The bone central to the low signal rim is variably low signal or normal marrow signal.*

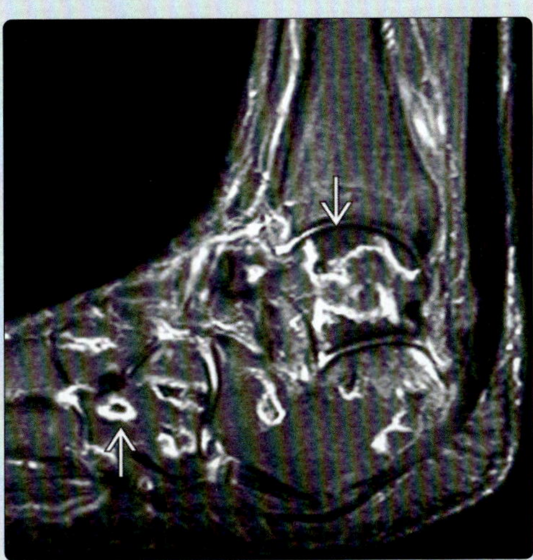

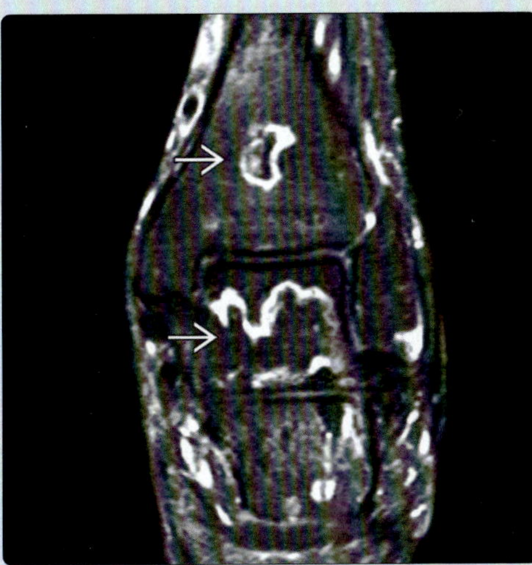

(Left) *Sagittal T2WI FS MR in the same patient shows the double line sign of high signal surrounding the low signal rim of multiple bone infarcts ➡.* **(Right)** *Coronal T2WI FS MR similarly shows a pattern typical of multiple infarcts ➡. RMSF, in which the vascular endothelial cells are targeted, may result in necrotizing vasculitis. This may in turn cause osseous infarction. Amputation may be required. In this case, several digits were amputated.*

Leprosy

KEY FACTS

TERMINOLOGY

- Synonym: Hansen disease
- Definition: Chronic infection caused by *Mycobacterium leprae*, which has 2 phases
  - Initial insult is infection, causing cellular immune response that results in neural injury
  - Second insult: Bony destruction 2° to peripheral neuropathy

IMAGING

- Most common nerves involved: Ulnar and peroneal
- Bony involvement: Digits (hands &/or feet), ankles, wrists
- Radiographic abnormalities
  - Neuropathic acroosteolysis, may be severe and involve much more than distal phalanx (20-70% of hospitalized cases)
  - Acral bone remnant may be sharply tapered or blunt
  - Neuropathic wrist or ankle joints
  - Periostitis, osteomyelitis (uncommon; 3-5% of hospitalized cases)
  - At risk for secondary infection as well due to decreased proprioception
  - Nerve calcification, considered pathognomonic (rare)
- MR findings of neural involvement
  - Nerve enlargement
  - Nerve bright on STIR, enhancing
- MR findings of other tissues
  - Nonspecific findings of reticulated abnormal signal in subcutaneous fat
  - Look for osteomyelitis and perineural abscess
- US shows nerve inflammation
  - Increased vascularity
  - Distorted echotexture, enlargement

TOP DIFFERENTIAL DIAGNOSES

- Thermal injury, burns
  - Contraction, acroosteolysis, ± calcifications
- Progressive systemic sclerosis
  - Acroosteolysis, ± calcifications
- Diabetes
  - Neuropathic joints, infection, vascular calcification
- Lesch-Nyhan
  - Delayed motor development, destruction of digits

PATHOLOGY

- Manifestation depends on individual's host response
- Vigorous cellular immune response: Tuberculoid form
  - Limited asymmetric number of skin and nerve lesions that contain small numbers of bacteria
- Minimal cellular immune response: Lepromatous form
  - Extensive symmetric skin involvement; large numbers of bacteria

CLINICAL ISSUES

- Clinical presentation
  - Painless skin patch accompanied by loss of sensation
  - Loss of sensory and motor function, resulting in trauma and amputation
  - Hand and foot ulcerations
  - Wasting and muscle weakness
  - Foot drop, claw hand
  - Nasal cartilage destruction
  - Ocular involvement
  - Thickening of skin
- Age: Peaks in children < 10 years old
- Gender: Male > female (1.5:1 ratio)
- Epidemiology: 500,000-700,000 new cases worldwide per year
  - 150 cases diagnosed in USA per year
- Natural history
  - Most individuals exposed to leprosy never develop disease
  - 33% of newly diagnosed cases display signs of nerve function impairment
  - Preservation of nerve function considered emergency in cases of early inflammation

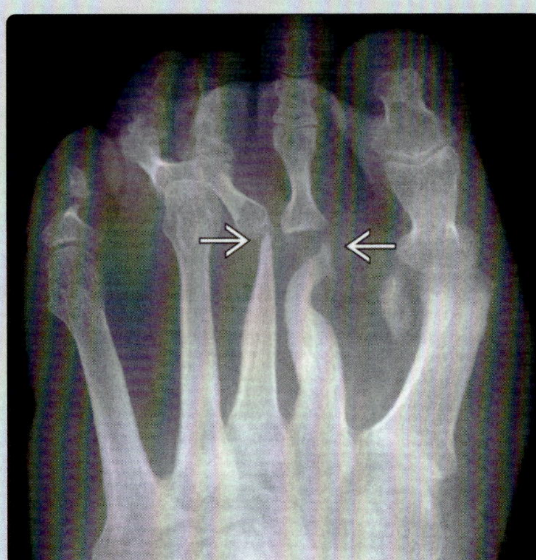

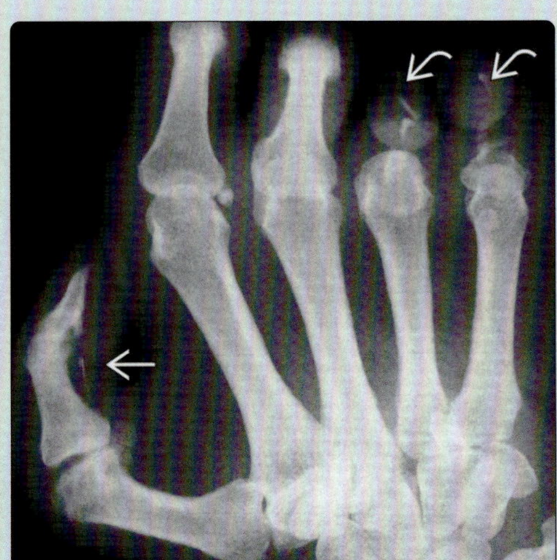

(Left) *AP radiograph in a patient with leprosy shows destruction of the metatarsals ➡ much more prominently than distal phalanges. This pattern does not fit that of other etiologies of acroosteolysis, making leprosy the most likely diagnosis, as was proven.* **(Right)** *PA radiograph shows this patient has tremendous acroosteolysis ➡, which has destroyed most of the phalanges. Additionally, there is linear calcification in the location of a digital nerve ➡. This combination of findings is pathognomonic for leprosy.*

Syphilis

KEY FACTS

IMAGING

- Congenital syphilis: Osteochondritis
  - Disturbance of endochondral ossification
  - Symmetric involvement of sites of endochondral ossification (epiphyseal-metaphyseal junction, costochondral junction, sites of ossification in sternum and spine)
  - Widening of zone of provisional calcification, metaphyseal irregularity
  - Horizontal lucent bands
  - Vertical ("celery stalk") alternating lucent and sclerotic lines
  - With progression, develop erosive-appearing lesions at metaphyses (histologically, granulomas): At medial proximal tibia, called Wimberger sign
- Congenital syphilis: Diaphyseal osteomyelitis (lytic destructive change with sclerotic reaction)
- Congenital syphilis: Periostitis
  - Painful; may be related to infiltration by syphilitic granulation tissue
  - Reactive periostitis related to osteochondritis or slipped epiphysis
- Acquired syphilis: Musculoskeletal findings usually in 3° stage
  - Proliferative periostitis: Dense, usually linear, often bilateral; tibia, skull, ribs, sternum most common
  - Osteomyelitis of skull characteristic of 2° syphilis (9%); uncommon elsewhere in 2°
  - Tertiary syphilis: Gummatous osseous lesions (mixed lytic and sclerotic lesions; may be large, with dense periosteal reactive change)
  - Tertiary syphilis: Nongummatous osseous lesions (periostitis, osteitis, osteomyelitis)
- Articular involvement
  - Septic or gummatous involvement uncommon at any stage; nonspecific
  - Charcot joints: Knee, hip, spine most common

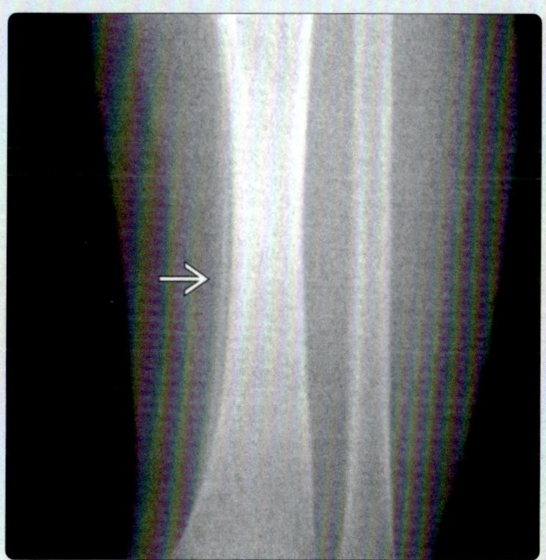

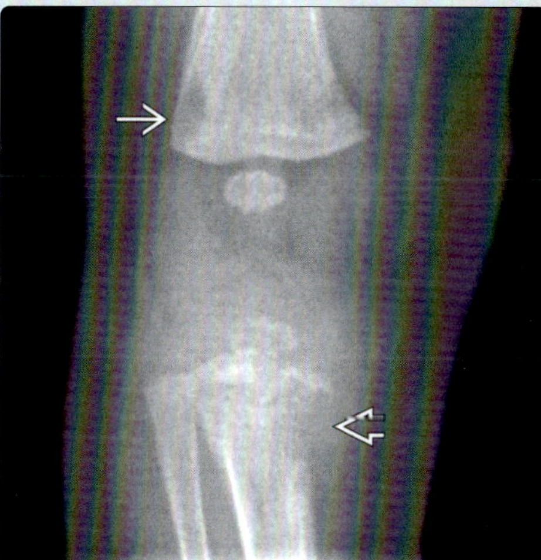

(Left) *AP x-ray shows periostitis ➡ in an infant with congenital syphilis. This periostitis is nonspecific since there are no metaphyseal or other findings more specific for syphilis; it could represent physiological or other causes of periostitis.* **(Right)** *AP x-ray shows generalized metaphyseal osteitis ➡, with lytic metaphyseal lesions. There is a particularly prominent site of osteitis at the proximal medial metaphysis ➡, which has been termed Wimberger sign and is highly suggestive of congenital syphilis.*

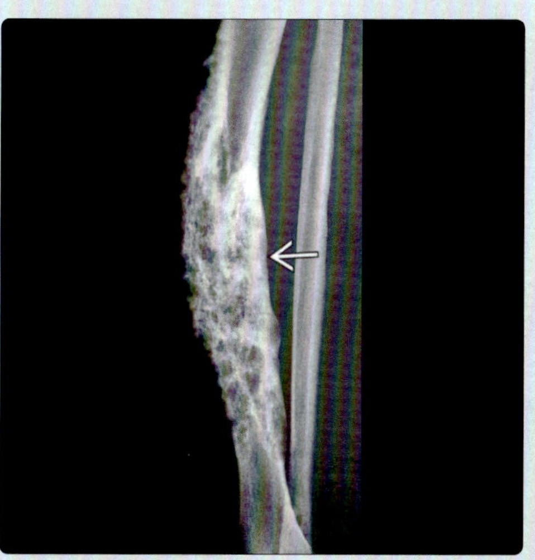

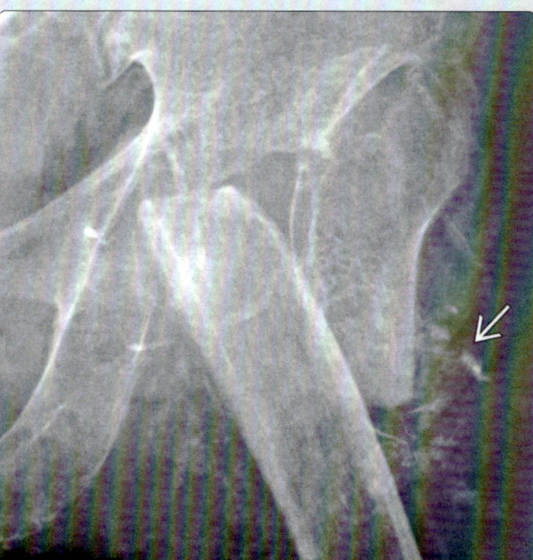

(Left) *Lateral radiograph shows a central diaphyseal tibial lesion ➡, which is overgrown, bowed anteriorly, with the appearance of chronicity. There is moderate destructive change with mixed lytic pattern and reactive sclerotic bone formation. This is typical of tertiary syphilis, so much that it has been termed the "saber shin" deformity.* **(Right)** *AP radiograph shows destruction of the hip joint, fracture, dislocation of the head, and debris scattered in and around the joint ➡, typical of a tabetic Charcot joint.*

Polio

KEY FACTS

TERMINOLOGY

- RNA virus that affects motor neurons in anterior horn/brainstem, resulting in flaccid paralysis
  - 5-10% of cases develop symptoms (majority silent)
  - Significant progress toward worldwide eradication by means of aggressive vaccine programs
  - Though no new cases, complications of old cases seen

IMAGING

- Osteoporosis of affected sites
  - Associated ↑ risk of fracture
- Soft tissue atrophy of affected sites
  - Muscle wasting, fatty infiltration
- Scoliosis
  - Usually single thoracolumbar curve
  - Degenerative spine disease associated with scoliosis and pelvic tilt
- Growth deformities on affected side
  - Hypoplasia of affected hemipelvis
  - Related to lack of muscle contraction &/or imbalance on growing skeleton
  - Valgus hip ± subluxation/dislocation
  - Gracile long tubular bones
- Premature physeal closure (9% in 1 series)
  - Restricted to feet (4th MT most common) or knees
  - Corresponds to sites involved in neurologic disease
  - May be coned; results in shortening
- Foot deformities
  - Pes cavus most common
- Heterotopic ossification: Rare
- Neuropathic (Charcot) joint: Rare
- Postpoliomyelitis syndrome
  - Usually 20-40 years after infection
  - Recurrences of weakness or fatigue
  - Usually same groups of initially involved muscles

CLINICAL ISSUES

- Mostly affects children; immunocompromised adults at risk

(Left) *AP radiograph shows pelvic asymmetry with hypoplastic right hemipelvis, valgus femoral neck, and gracile femoral shaft. Note the relatively increased soft tissues on the left compared with the right. This is a case of polio involving the right side. There is no hip subluxation, though such may be present in these cases.* **(Right)** *Lateral radiograph shows a foot with excessive plantar flexion of the talus but no equinus. There is a varus forefoot deformity. The overall appearance is of a cavus foot; this patient has polio.*

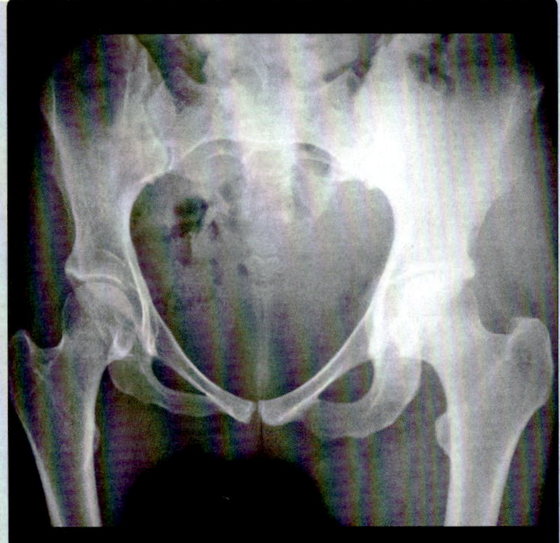

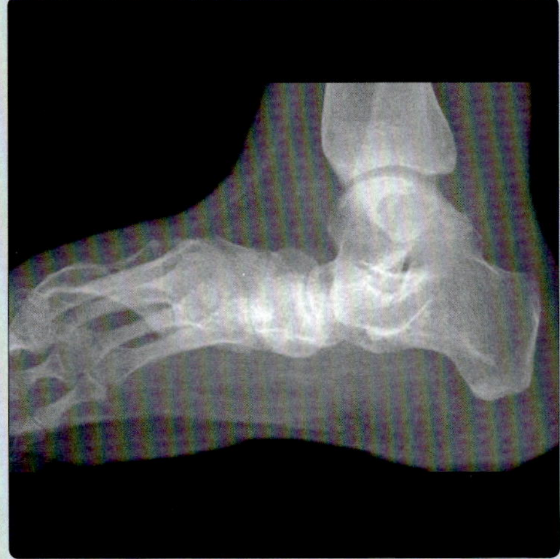

(Left) *Coronal T1WI MR in a patient with polio confirms nearly complete replacement of the right thigh musculature with hyperintense fat. The degree of muscular hemiatrophy is remarkable.* **(Right)** *Coronal STIR MR, same case, reveals some persistent high T2 signal in the remaining muscle. This may represent a small component of ongoing denervation even this late in the clinical course, although, clinically, an inflammatory process was suspected.*

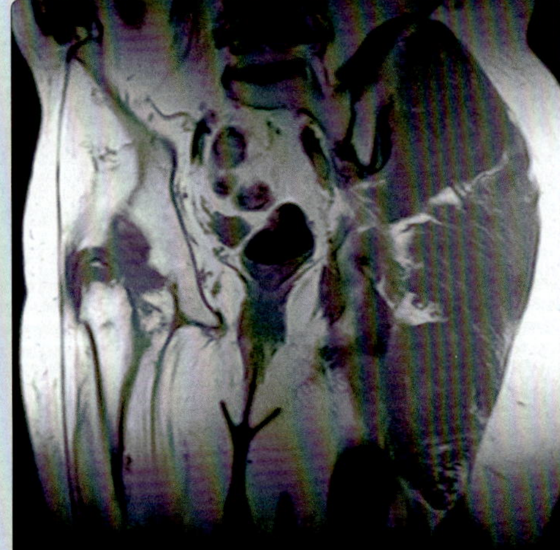

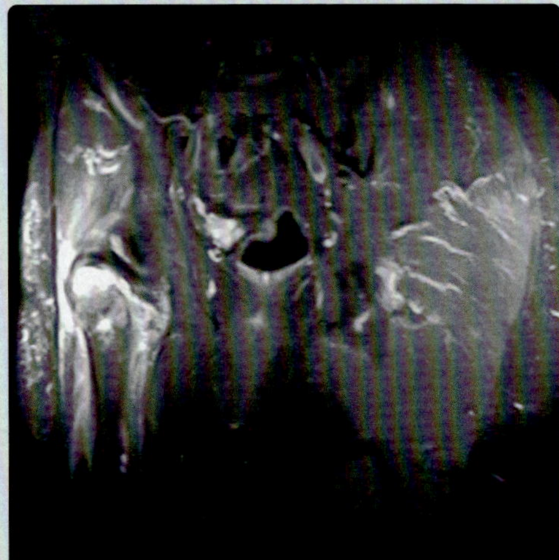

Parasitic Infection

KEY FACTS

IMAGING

- Characterized by soft tissue calcification 2° to calcification of dead worm
- Cysticercosis (pork tapeworm)
  - Numerous small linear/ovoid calcific foci oriented along long axis of muscle belly
  - Ingested worms exit small intestine and travel through subcutaneous tissues & muscle
  - Common sites of infection: Lungs, brain, eye, liver
  - ↑ incidence in American West, especially in Hispanic males
- Dracunculosis (guinea worm)
  - Calcified female worms: Linear, may be whorled or fragmented; favors lower extremity
  - Ingestion of contaminated water
  - Other: Sterile abscess, aseptic arthritis
- Echinococcal disease (hydatid disease)
  - Calcification is eggshell-like at cyst periphery
  - Organisms ingested; humans are accidental host
  - Most common sites: Lungs, liver
  - Musculoskeletal sites: Spine, pelvis, extremities
  - Classic appearance is multiple cysts (bundle of grapes appearance) with daughter cysts
  - Lesions may be soft tissue or osseous with lysis ± bone expansion
  - MR T1WI: Fluid has variable signal intensity from low to bright; depends on protein content
  - MR C+: Enhancement of cyst periphery & septa
- Filariasis
  - Sporadic calcification: Looks like granuloma
  - Organisms enter through mosquito bite
  - Lymphatic obstruction leads to elephantiasis
  - Other: Pulmonary eosinophilia, skin lesions

TOP DIFFERENTIAL DIAGNOSES

- Linear soft tissue calcification: Vascular, dermatomyositis
- Focal soft tissue calcification: Phleboliths, granulomas

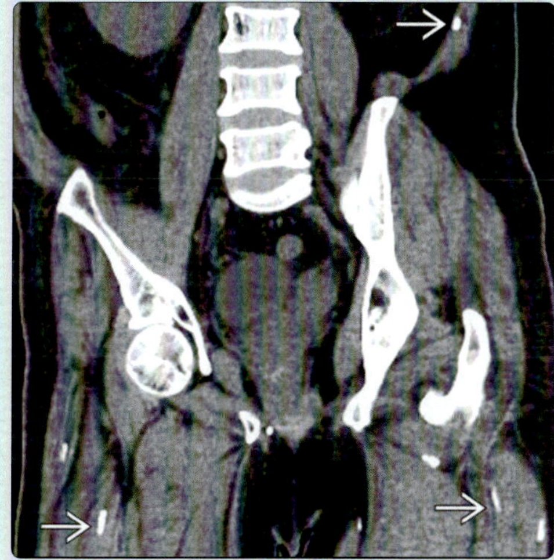

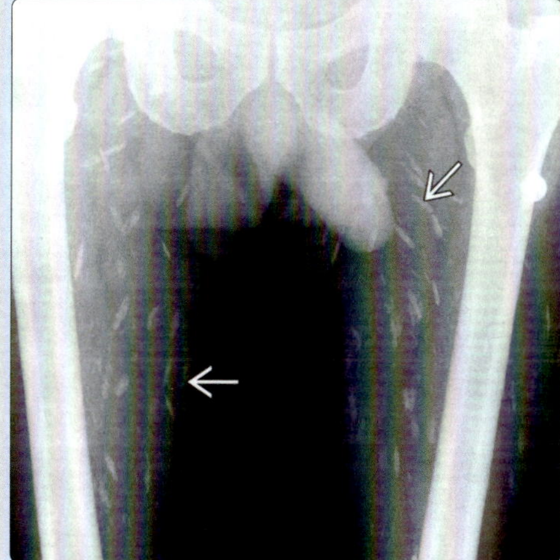

(Left) *Coronal CT shows multiple oval intramuscular calcifications → typical of cysticercosis. It should be noted that this parasitic infection is now seen more frequently in the western USA, particularly in Hispanic men. (Courtesy P. Tirman, MD.)* **(Right)** *AP radiograph reveals multiple ovoid rice-shaped calcifications oriented along the long axis of the muscle fibers of the thighs →. The appearance Is classic for cysticercosis.*

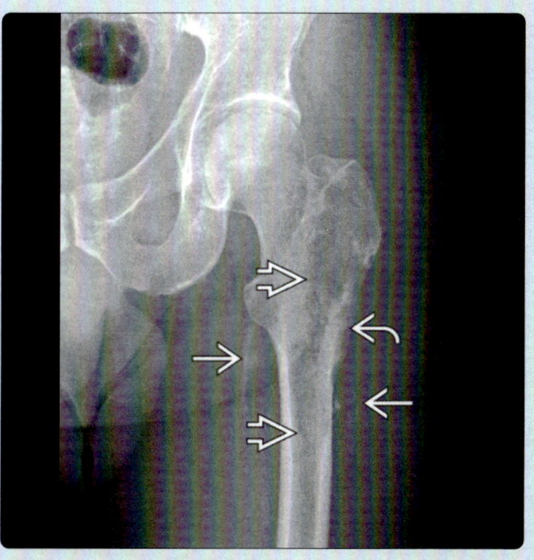

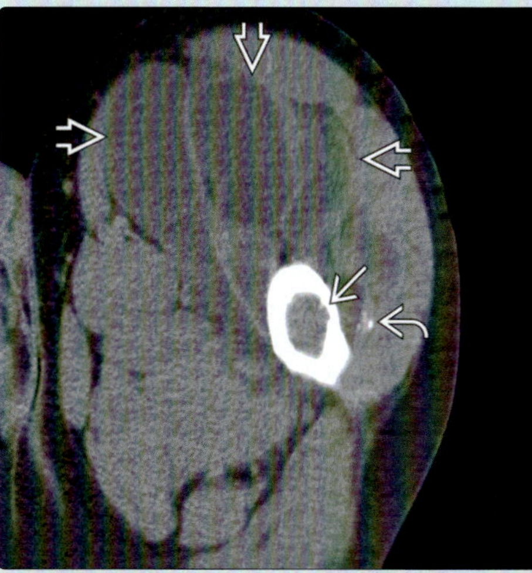

(Left) *AP radiograph shows an osteolytic process involving the proximal femur → with lateral cortical irregularity →. A soft tissue mass is present with peripheral mineralization →.* **(Right)** *Axial NECT of the same patient shows soft tissue within the marrow with endosteal destruction →. The soft tissue mass is a multilobulated cystic structure →. Mineralization in the wall of a cyst is noted →. The findings are typical for intraosseous and soft tissue echinococcal disease. (Courtesy M. Murphey, MD.)*

KEY FACTS

TERMINOLOGY

- Syndrome classically involving skin, bone, and joints, although skin changes may be absent

IMAGING

- Sternoclavicular joint involved in majority of cases ± 1st, 2nd costochondral articulations, sternomanubrial joint
  - Joint space narrowing, enthesopathy, sclerosis
  - Osteolysis and ankylosis less common
- Vertebral body sclerosis; disc space narrowing, endplate erosions, paravertebral ossification (syndesmophytes to extensive bridging bone)
- Long bones: Aggressive-appearing lucency and sclerosis
  - ± metaphyseal periostitis, especially around knee

PATHOLOGY

- May be exaggerated immune response in genetically susceptible individuals to *Propionibacterium acnes*
- Biopsy: Acute inflammation; culture often negative
- Often HLA-B27 positive; proposed association with seronegative spondyloarthropathies, especially psoriasis and chronic recurrent multifocal osteomyelitis

CLINICAL ISSUES

- Young to middle-aged adults most frequently; M=F
- Pain, tenderness, soft tissue swelling, warmth
- Limitation of motion, especially anterior chest wall
- Skin findings may occur prior to, during, or after bone manifestations
- Treatment usually symptomatic, may require steroids
- Chronic disease with exacerbations, no ↓ life expectancy

DIAGNOSTIC CHECKLIST

- **S**ynovitis: Anterior chest wall, unilateral sacroiliitis
- **A**cne: Hydradenitis suppurativa; acne conglobata
- **P**ustulosis: Palmoplantar pustulosis (50%)
- **H**yperostosis: Enthesopathy, sclerosis
- **O**steitis: Inflammatory changes, pain

(Left) *AP radiograph shows extensive sclerosis in the left clavicular head ➡. A single erosion is noted ➡. The changes are highly suggestive of sternoclavicular hyperostosis (another name for SAPHO syndrome). The term describes the most prominent features.* **(Right)** *Coronal reformatted CT shows extensive hyperostosis in the manubrium on the left ➡, which correlated with patient's pain. Sclerotic changes in the 1st and 2nd costochondral articulations (not shown) helped confirm the diagnosis.*

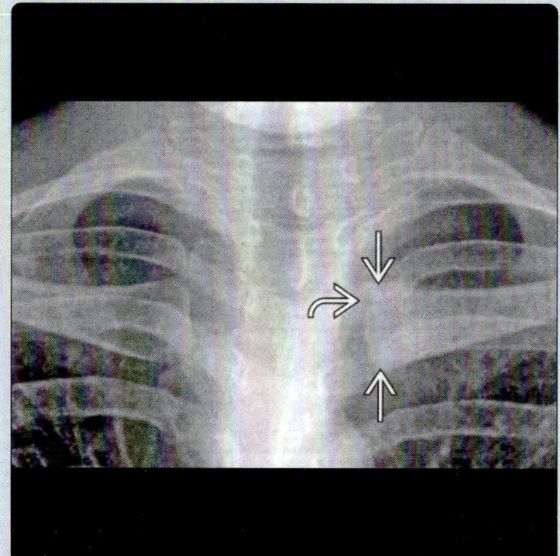

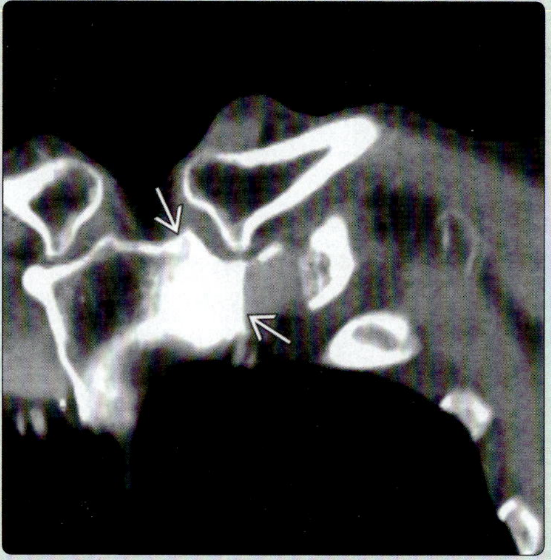

(Left) *Coronal T1WI shows marrow edema in the left clavicular head and shaft ➡. Both manubrial articular surfaces are also affected ➡. Osteitis (bone inflammation) is a common feature in SAPHO syndrome. Note the soft tissue thickening along the left sternoclavicular (SC) joint inferiorly ➡.* **(Right)** *Coronal T1WI C+ FS MR of the same patient demonstrates inflammatory changes in the soft tissues of the left SC joint ➡ and at the manubrial articular surfaces ➡. Acute inflammation is the hallmark of SAPHO.*

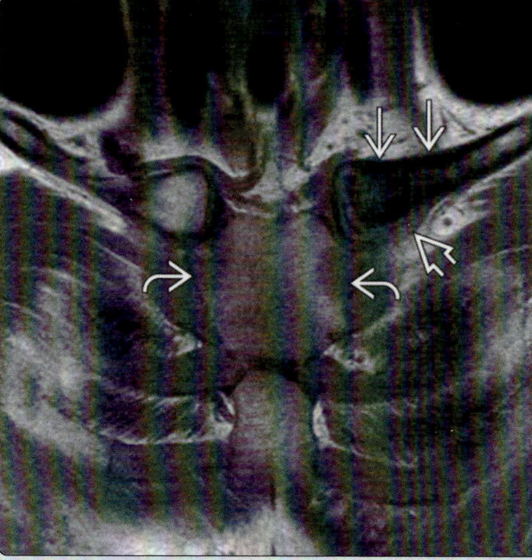

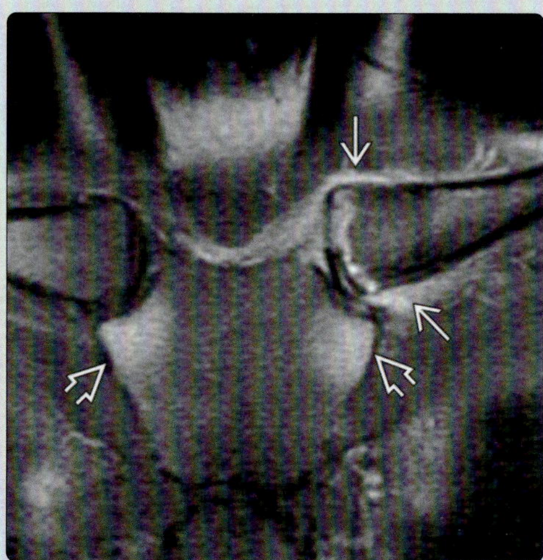

KEY FACTS

TERMINOLOGY

- Chronic recurrent multifocal osteomyelitis (CRMO)
- Multifocal aseptic osseous inflammatory lesions in children and adolescents

IMAGING

- Location: Metaphyseal sites of distal femur, proximal and distal tibia, distal fibula, clavicle most common
  - Often crosses into adjacent epiphysis
  - Spine, pelvis, epiphyseal equivalents in thorax
  - Upper extremity rarely involved; exception is clavicle (involved in 30%)
  - Clavicular involvement fairly unique for CRMO
- Radiographs: Lesions often not visible
  - Lytic, either ill- (27%) or well defined (73%)
  - Sclerotic reaction; tends to be associated with chronicity
    - Mixed, peripheral, or completely sclerotic
  - Periosteal reaction; occasionally large and dense
- MR: Patchy low SI on T1WI, high SI on fluid-sensitive sequences (marrow edema pattern)
  - Enhancement
  - Periostitis (50%); adjacent soft tissue edema
  - Sacroiliitis
  - Effusion, synovitis
  - No sequestrum or significant abscess
  - Whole body MR advocated to evaluate for multifocality
- Bone scan may show subtle abnormality but may be normal

TOP DIFFERENTIAL DIAGNOSES

- Ewing sarcoma
  - Same age group as CRMO
  - Lytic, highly aggressive, osseous lesion
  - Frequent osseous metastases, making lesion polyostotic
- Lymphoma of bone
  - 50% present as polyostotic lesions in children
  - Lytic, destructive osseous lesions
  - May not be visualized on radiograph
  - Positive on bone scan
- SAPHO
  - Some believe CRMO is in same spectrum of disease as SAPHO, the latter being the adult equivalent
  - Periostitis is important feature in SAPHO, along with inflammatory change
  - Greater incidence of palmoplantar pustulosis in SAPHO than CRMO

PATHOLOGY

- Etiology: Autoimmune cause, genetic susceptibility likely
- Histology: Chronic nonspecific inflammation
  - Histiocytes, lymphocytes, plasma cells

CLINICAL ISSUES

- Nonspecific musculoskeletal pain
- Many sites shown by MR are not clinically symptomatic
- Remission and exacerbation over many months
- Blood cultures usually negative for bacteria
- Bone biopsy usually shows no infectious agents
- Other signs/symptoms or associations
  - Fever, weight loss, lethargy all uncommon
  - Dermatologic disorders (palmoplantar pustulosis, psoriasis, acne fulminans)
  - Autoinflammatory disorders
  - Gastrointestinal disorders (Crohn, ulcerative colitis)
  - Spondyloarthropathies
- Age: Primarily disease of children (ages 9-14 most common); reported in adults as well
- Gender: Male < female (1:2)
- Natural history
  - Generally self limiting, but course can be prolonged and associated with significant morbidity
  - If uncontrolled, may be associated with growth disturbances, early physeal fusion, pathologic fracture (particularly in spine)
- Treatment: No current agreement
  - NSAIDs and other antiinflammatory drugs used
  - Bisphosphonates reported to dramatically relieve pain

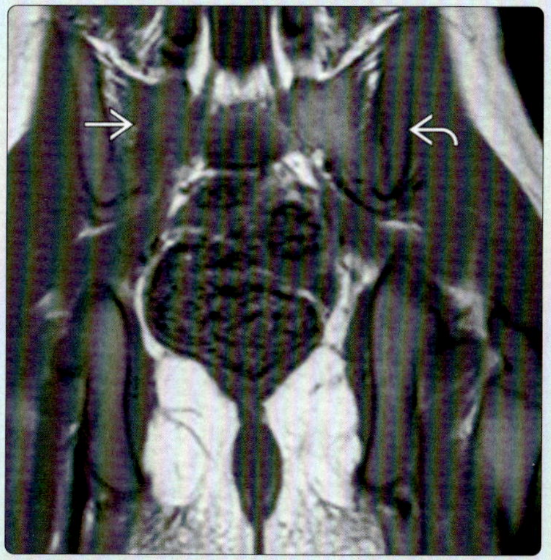

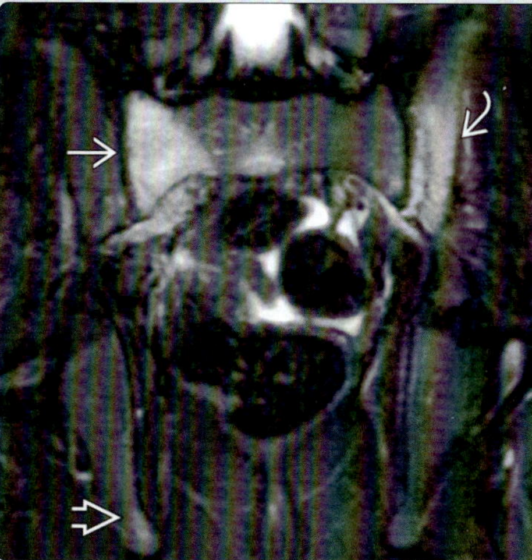

(Left) *Coronal T1WI MR in a 10 year old shows subtle changes of ↓ SI within the right sacral ala ➡ and left posterior iliac wing ↩. Note that T1 ↓ signal can be difficult to identify in children because much of their marrow has not yet converted to fat.* **(Right)** *Coronal T2WI FS MR, same case, shows ↑ SI within the marrow of the right sacral ala ➡, left posterior iliac wing ↩, and right ischial tuberosity ⇨. This patient had a normal radiograph, bone scan, and blood cultures; core biopsy proved chronic recurrent multifocal osteomyelitis.*

SECTION 9
Bone Marrow

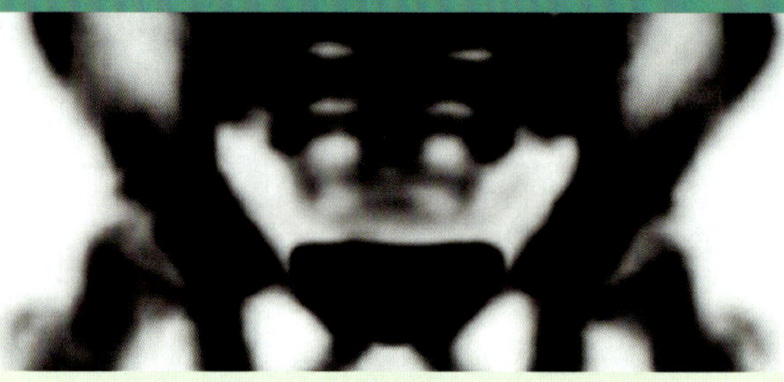

Distribution Pattern

KEY FACTS

TERMINOLOGY

- Hematopoietic (red) and fatty (yellow) marrow coexist within medullary space
- Dynamic relationship of red and yellow marrow
  - Changes throughout development in orderly fashion
  - Detectable as changes in SI on routine MR sequences

IMAGING

- T1 often is most useful sequence for evaluating marrow
  - T1WI depicts red marrow distribution against background of yellow marrow
    - Sensitive but not specific sequence
    - T1 signal intensity directly related to amount of marrow fat
  - Red marrow on T1WI before 10 years of age
    - Little (if any) fat admixed with red marrow
    - May be lower in SI than disc and muscle on T1WI sequence
  - Red marrow on T1WI in patients ≥ 10 years of age
    - Red marrow normally admixed with fat
      - **Internal standard of comparison**: Red marrow normally has greater SI than muscle/disc on T1WI
- T2 has **no internal standard** for comparison of marrow SI
- Gadolinium not useful for **routine** marrow assessment
  - Yellow marrow does not enhance
  - Red marrow enhances minimally in adults (< 10%)
  - Red marrow may enhance in hematopoietic islands in children

DIAGNOSTIC CHECKLIST

- Red/yellow marrow ratios vary between individuals
  - Ratio of fat to red marrow on MR varies based on
    - Patient age and anatomic location
    - Changes in normal physiologic stresses
- Distribution of red and yellow marrow should be fairly symmetric
- Use internal standard on T1WI where red marrow SI should be < disc or muscle SI

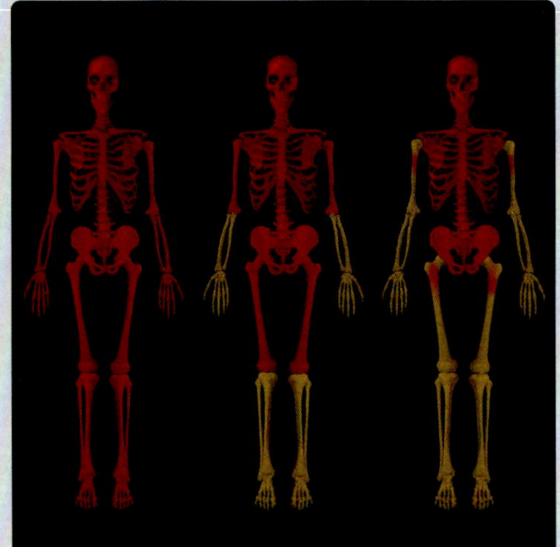

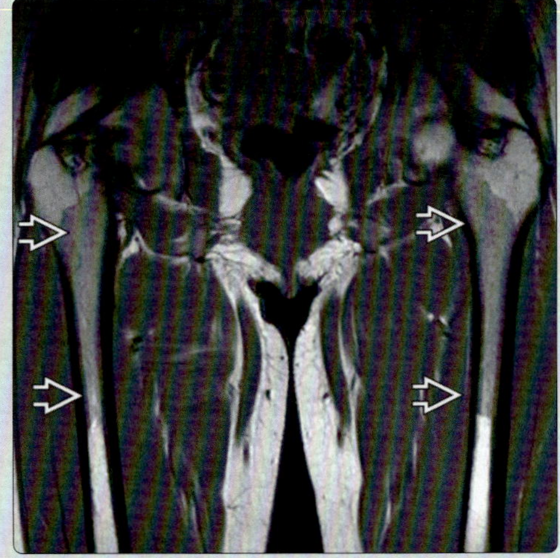

(Left) *Graphic shows normal developmental transformation of marrow in the skeleton. Left shows global red marrow (at birth), middle shows fatty conversion of distal extremities (in childhood), and right shows proximal fatty conversion (in adulthood). This process is completed by 25 years of age. Residual red marrow in the axial skeleton and humeral/femoral proximal metaphyses is normal in adults.* **(Right)** *Coronal T1WI MR shows normal red marrow residua ➲. The amount varies between individuals but should be symmetric.*

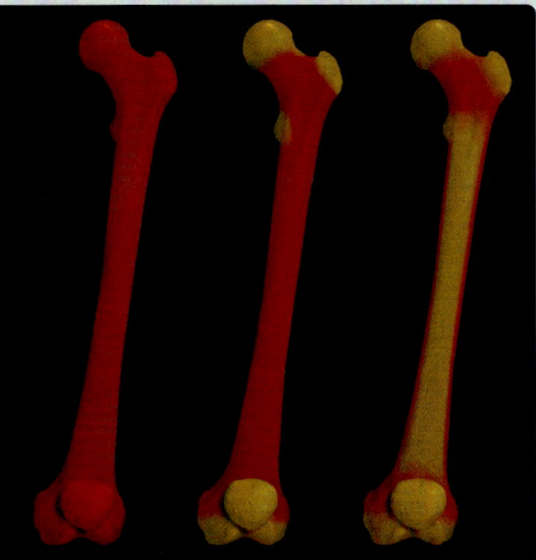

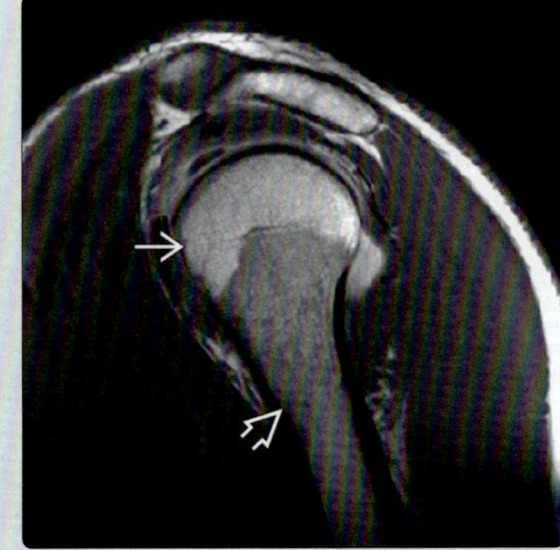

(Left) *Coronal graphic shows normal developmental transformation from complete red marrow in the long bones (left). Apophyses/epiphyses transform from red to fatty marrow shortly after ossification centers appear (middle). This is followed by the distal metaphysis and diaphysis, then proximal metaphysis, where residual red marrow may persist.* **(Right)** *Sagittal T1 MR shows yellow marrow in the epiphysis ➲ and red marrow admixed with fat in the metaphysis ➲, a normal distribution pattern in this young adult.*

TERMINOLOGY

Synonyms

- Marrow distribution: Normal developmental conversion of red to yellow marrow

Definitions

- Hematopoietic (red) and fatty (yellow) marrow coexist within medullary space
  - Relationship is dynamic
  - Changes throughout development in orderly fashion
  - Detectable as changes in SI on routine MR sequences

IMAGING

General Features

- Best diagnostic clue
  - Red and yellow marrow ratios vary significantly between individuals
  - Distribution of red and yellow marrow should be fairly symmetric
    - Red marrow before 10 years of age may be lower in SI than disc and muscle on T1WI sequence
    - Red marrow in patients ≥ 10 years of age should be slightly higher in SI than disc and muscle on T1WI
- Location
  - Birth: Almost all marrow is hematopoietic
  - Conversion to yellow marrow begins in distal extremities
    - Progresses proximally
    - Extremity conversion begins in epiphyses and apophyses within 6 months of ossification
    - Epiphyses/apophyses followed by diaphyseal conversion
    - Some red marrow retained at periphery of marrow space
      - Subcortical distribution of retained red marrow
      - Centripetal distribution of retained red marrow
    - Finally, metaphyses convert to yellow marrow
      - Distal metaphyses followed by proximal
  - By age 20-25, appendicular marrow mostly fatty
    - Red marrow retained in axial skeleton and proximal metaphyses of femora and humeri in adults
      - Diminishes with advancing age
  - By 60 years of age, axial marrow may be substantially yellow (fatty)
- Morphology
  - Hemopoietic marrow not usually geographic
    - May appear patchy
    - Vaguely demarcated

CT Findings

- CT of limited utility in assessment of normal marrow
  - Useful to assess trabecular bone
  - Useful to depict sclerosis

MR Findings

- T1WI
  - Depicts red marrow distribution against background of yellow marrow
    - Sensitive but not specific sequence
    - T1 SI directly related to amount of marrow fat
    - Red marrow is normally admixed with fat
      - **Internal standard of comparison**: Red marrow generally higher SI than muscle/disc in adults; if not, marrow infiltration should be suspected
      - Caveat: Normal T1 images do not exclude **early** marrow infiltration
      - Less admixture of fat in children < 10 years of age; same internal standard of comparison not as reliable in children as adults
- T2WI FS
  - Fat saturation increases conspicuity of fat-replacing lesions
    - May be masked on non-fat-saturated routine T2WI
  - Unlike T1, T2 imaging has **no internal standard** for comparison of SI of marrow
- PD/intermediate
  - Fatty and fluid-weighted constituents show similar signal intensity
    - PD therefore of limited utility to assess marrow
    - PD may mask lesions
- T1WI C+
  - Not useful for **routine** marrow assessment
    - Yellow marrow does not enhance
    - Red marrow enhances minimally in adults (< 10%)
    - Red marrow may enhance in hematopoietic islands in children, causing confusion
      - Number of foci and intensity of enhancement ↓ with maturation
- Inversion recovery FSE
  - Fat is suppressed uniformly
    - T1 and T2 contrast are additive
  - IR and fat-saturated intermediate intensity sequences demonstrate similar results in evaluation of marrow signal intensity changes
- Opposed phase (chemical shift) imaging
  - GRE sequences used
    - Minimal time penalty; available with all MR field strengths
  - Lesion opposed phase signal loss criteria: Generally < 20% accepted as suggestive of malignancy
    - One study showed yields of 100% sensitivity, 61% specificity, 75% PPV, 100% NPV, and 82% accuracy
      - Despite low specificity, need for biopsy obviated in 60% of benign lesions
  - Generally not routinely used, but good for problem solving

Imaging Recommendations

- Best imaging tool
  - MR: Provides noninvasive window for direct visualization of changes in ratio of fat and cellular constituents of marrow
    - Ratio of fat and red marrow varies based on
      - Patient age
      - Anatomic location
      - Location within specific bone
      - Physiologic stresses on patient
- Protocol advice
  - T1 conventional SE recommended
    - Marrow lesions may be obscured on T1 FSE sequences
  - T1 plus inversion recovery or T2 TSE fat-saturated sequences suffice for assessment of normal marrow

- Contrast imaging reserved for problem-solving
- Opposed-phase imaging used for problem-solving

DIFFERENTIAL DIAGNOSIS

Normal Dense Red Marrow

- May be difficult to differentiate from infiltrative pathology
- Diffusely present in early childhood
- Does not show abnormal uptake on bone scan
- Does not show abnormal uptake on FDG PET
- Red marrow islands seen in childhood
  - May enhance
  - Should drop in SI > 20% on opposed-phase imaging

Anemia

- Recovery involves conversion to red marrow
- May be patchy
- May follow reverse pattern of conversion to fatty marrow

Multiple Myeloma

- Distribution is similar to that of marrow reconversion
  - Vertebral bodies and posterior elements
  - Pelvis
  - Shoulder girdle
  - Proximal femora and humeri
- Radiographs may show diffuse osteopenia or focal lesions
- Low SI on T1WI, high SI on STIR
  - Lesions show enhancement

Leukemia

- Low SI on T1WI, high SI on STIR
  - Lesions show enhancement
- Radiographs may show diffuse osteopenia or focal lytic lesions

Multifocal Lymphoma of Bone

- Multifocal disease more frequently seen in childhood
- Low SI on T1WI, high SI on STIR
  - Lesions show enhancement

PATHOLOGY

Staging, Grading, & Classification

- Bone marrow consists of
  - Trabeculae
  - Hematopoietic cells
  - Adipocytes
  - Reticuloendothelial cells
  - Stroma
- Trabecular architecture composed of
  - Primary and secondary bridging trabeculae
  - Decrease in number with age
- Yellow marrow is composed of
  - 80% fat
  - 16% water
  - Poorly vascularized
    - Hence more at risk for osteonecrosis
- Red marrow is composed of
  - 40% water
  - 40% fat
  - Stroma
  - Richly vascularized

Gross Pathologic & Surgical Features

- Fatty marrow is predominantly yellow
- Hematopoietic marrow is pink to red

DIAGNOSTIC CHECKLIST

Consider

- If marrow darker than disc or muscle on T1WI MR, consider marrow infiltration or replacement

Image Interpretation Pearls

- Marrow signal is normally low on T1WI in children < 10 years of age
  - Pathology may be masked by low T1 signal in children
    - Conspicuity increased on fluid-sensitive sequences or with gadolinium administration

Reporting Tips

- Particularly in evaluating MR of young and elderly individuals, assess if marrow distribution is normal for age

SELECTED REFERENCES

1. Kohl CA et al: Accuracy of chemical shift MR imaging in diagnosing indeterminate bone marrow lesions in the pelvis: review of a single institution's experience. Skeletal Radiol. 43(8):1079-84, 2014
2. Chen BB et al: Dynamic contrast-enhanced MR imaging measurement of vertebral bone marrow perfusion may be indicator of outcome of acute myeloid leukemia patients in remission. Radiology. 258(3):821-31, 2011
3. Kung JW et al: Bone marrow signal alteration in the extremities. AJR Am J Roentgenol. 196(5):W492-510, 2011
4. Laor T et al: MR imaging insights into skeletal maturation: what is normal? Radiology. 250(1):28-38, 2009
5. Shabshin N et al: Age dependent T2 changes of bone marrow in pediatric wrist MRI. Skeletal Radiol. 38(12):1163-8, 2009
6. Van der Woude HJ et al: Contrast-enhanced magnetic resonance imaging of bone marrow. Semin Musculoskelet Radiol. 5(1):21-33, 2001
7. Ricci C et al: Normal age-related patterns of cellular and fatty bone marrow distribution in the axial skeleton: MR imaging study. Radiology. 177(1):83-8, 1990
8. Custer RP: An Atlas of the Blood and Bone Marrow. Philadelphia: Saunders, 1974
9. Ellis RE: The distribution of active bone marrow in the adult. Phys Med Biol. 5:255-8, 1961

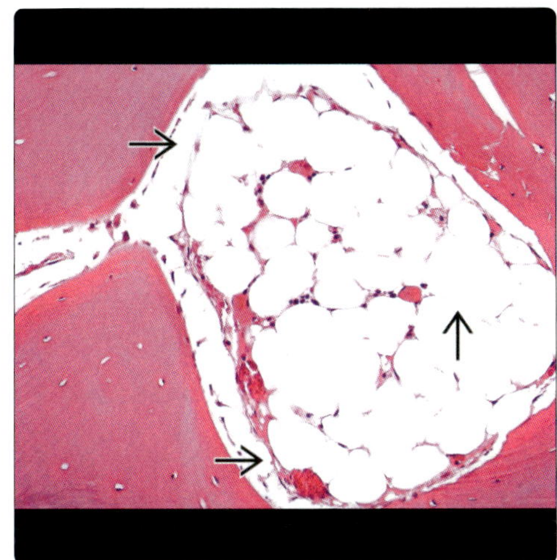

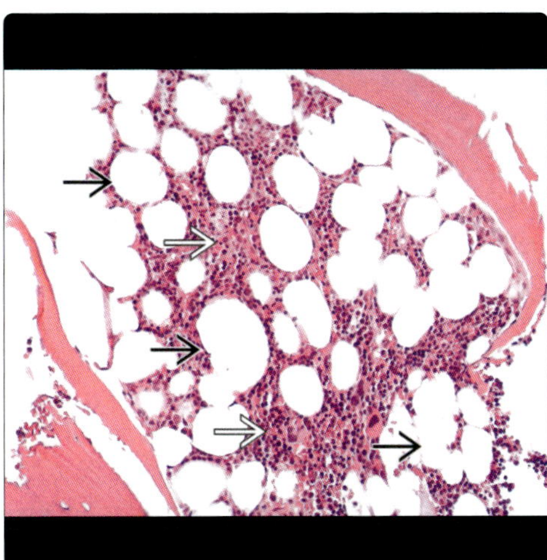

(Left) *Micrograph demonstrates normal fatty marrow. Adipocytes* ➡ *fill the space between trabeculae. Vascularity is sparse, and red cells are scant. (Courtesy P. Desai, MD.)* **(Right)** *Micrograph demonstrates normal red marrow. Red and white cells* ➡ *are admixed fairly equally with adipocytes* ➡*. (Courtesy P. Desai, MD.)*

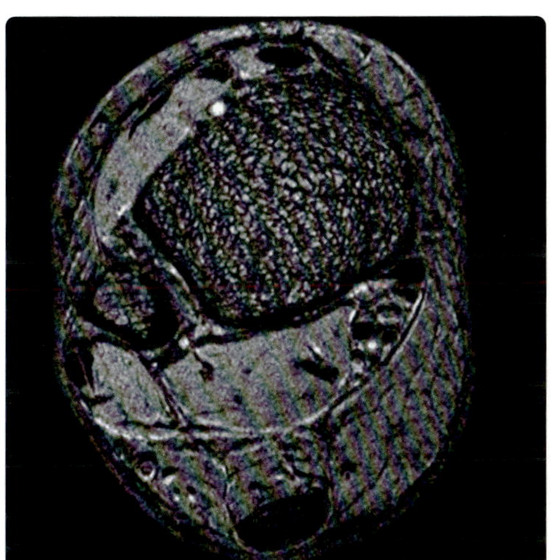

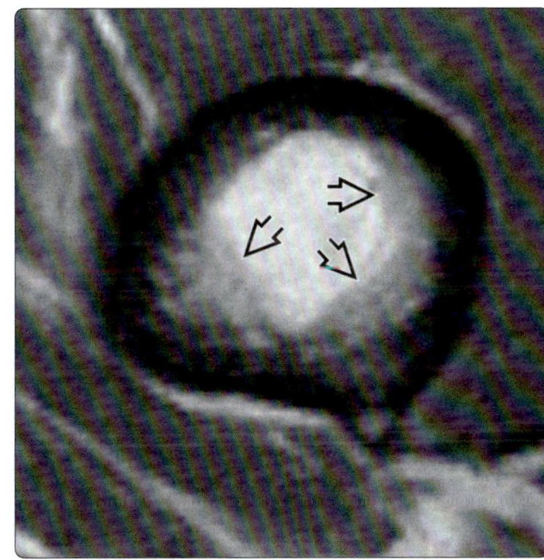

(Left) *7T axial gradient-echo high-resolution image of the distal tibia (matrix 156 μm x 156 μm x 1000 μm) depicts the individual trabeculae, revealed by susceptibility on this sequence. (Courtesy R. Regatte, PhD.)* **(Right)** *Axial T1WI MR demonstrates the normal centripetal distribution of red and yellow marrow in the diaphysis of a long bone. Yellow marrow is seen centrally; red marrow* ➡ *conforms to the marrow space periphery.*

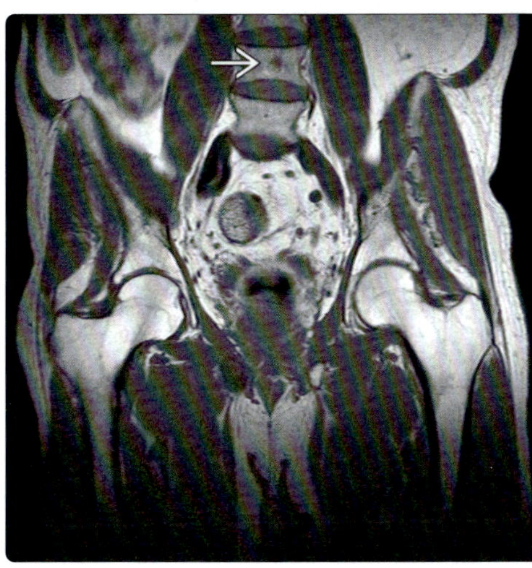

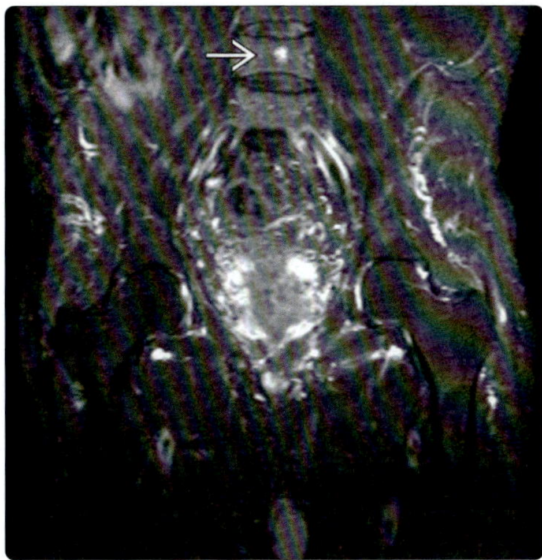

(Left) *Coronal T1WI MR shows normal adult marrow pattern. The marrow spaces of the proximal femora are nearly entirely filled with yellow marrow. Patchy but symmetric residual red marrow is seen in the vertebrae > pelvis. A focus of signal abnormality in L4* ➡ *is isointense with muscle, and therefore suspect for a lesion.* **(Right)** *Coronal STIR MR in the same patient shows uniform fat suppression. Additive T1 and T2 signal contrast make the L4 lesion* ➡ *conspicuous but are nonspecific for diagnosis.*

Increased or Decreased Marrow Cellularity

KEY FACTS

TERMINOLOGY

- Red and yellow marrow ratios fluctuate in response to multiple processes
- Increased red marrow seen with
  - Marrow reconversion: Otherwise normal patients confronting new stress
  - Marrow repopulation: Response to severe anemia
  - Marrow stimulation: Treatment with granulocyte &/or red cell stimulating factors
- Decreased red marrow seen with
  - Advanced age: Diffuse marrow depletion
  - Severe depletion: Aplastic anemia (global)
  - Radiation: Focal cellular marrow depletion
- Serous atrophy: Severe depletion 2° to starvation

IMAGING

- Best diagnostic clue: Red marrow amount and distribution
  - Related to patient age and clinical circumstances
- Red marrow reconversion, repopulation, stimulation follows specific pattern
  - Reverse order of physiologic marrow conversion
- Serous atrophy
  - Progresses from distal extremities to proximal extremities/axial skeleton

DIAGNOSTIC CHECKLIST

- Densely repopulated marrow may resemble diffuse marrow replacement by tumor
  - Treatment history may clarify diagnosis
- Marrow abnormalities are likely underdiagnosed
  - Be aware of normal patterns of red marrow and their relationship to patient age
- Watch for pattern of marrow abnormality
  - Axial vs. appendicular
  - Proximal to distal regions of involvement
  - Portions of long bones affected

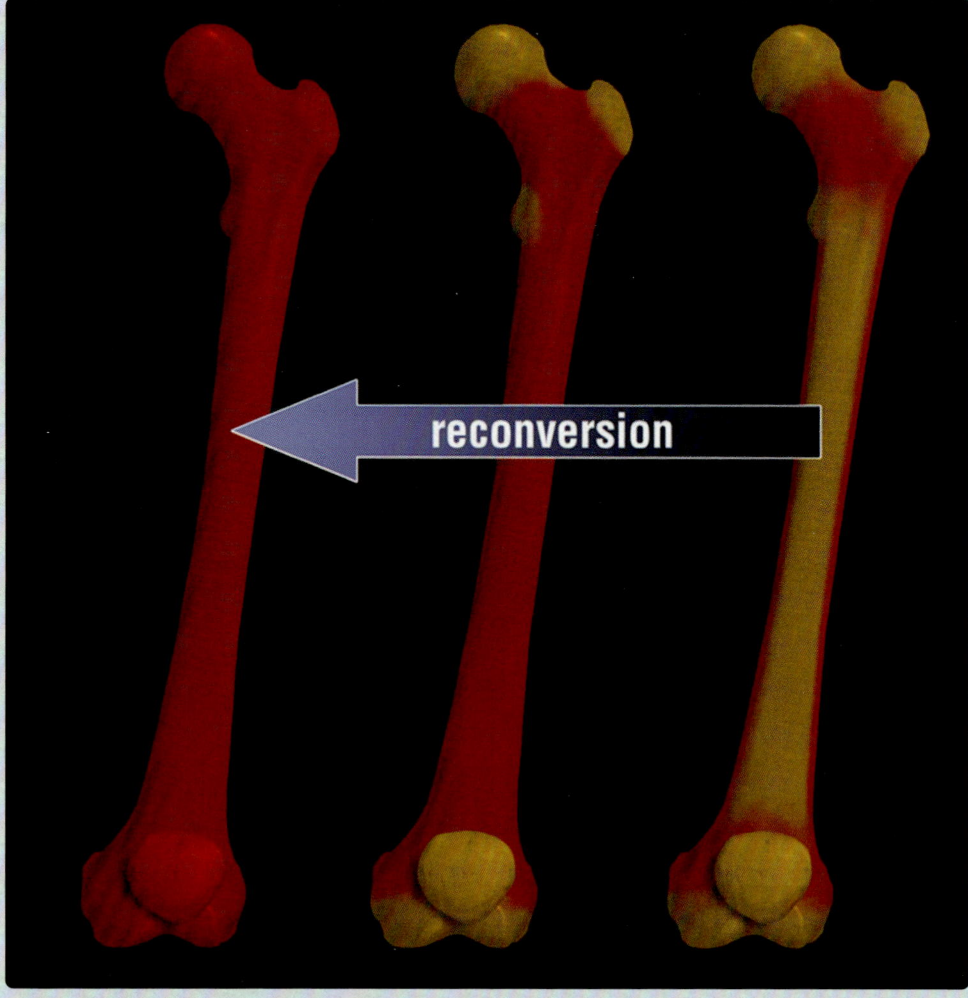

Graphic shows pattern of red marrow reconversion, repopulation, and stimulation in the long tubular bones. Red marrow reconversion occurs in the reverse order of developmental conversion. Thus, conversion 1st occurs in the axial skeleton, then distal appendicular bones. As shown in the diagram, red marrow conversion in the tubular bones commences in the proximal metaphyses, followed by distal metaphyses and diaphysis. Ultimately, in cases of extreme hematopoietic stress, the epiphyses show conversion to red marrow.

TERMINOLOGY

Definitions

- Red and yellow marrow ratios fluctuate in response to
  - Hematopoietic stress
  - Oxygen demand
  - Treatment/medications
  - Exposure to myelotoxins
- Increased red marrow seen with
  - Marrow reconversion
    - Otherwise normal patients confronting new stress
    - e.g., new athletic training, high altitude
  - Marrow repopulation
    - e.g., severe sickle cell anemia, thalassemia
  - Marrow stimulation
    - Treatment with granulocyte stimulating factor (GCSF) &/or red cell stimulating factors
- Decreased red marrow seen with
  - Advanced age: Diffuse marrow depletion
  - Severe depletion
    - Aplastic anemia: Global cellular marrow depletion
    - Radiation: Focal cellular marrow depletion
  - Serous atrophy
    - Related to starvation
      - ☐ Marrow fat usually sequestered from energy metabolism, except in starvation states
    - Depletion of **both** red and yellow marrow
    - Gelatinous transformation of marrow

IMAGING

General Features

- Best diagnostic clue
  - Red marrow amount and distribution, related to age and clinical circumstances
- Location
  - Red marrow reconversion, repopulation, stimulation
    - Reverse order of physiologic marrow conversion
      - ☐ Begins in vertebrae and flat bones
      - ☐ Progresses to long bones: Proximal metaphysis, followed by distal metaphysis, then diaphysis
      - ☐ Ultimately involves small bones (hands/feet)
      - ☐ Spares epiphyses except in severe stress
  - Red marrow depletion
    - May be diffuse in advanced age or aplastic anemia
    - Therapeutic radiation → focal (port-like) red marrow depletion with normal surrounding marrow
  - Serous atrophy
    - Progresses from distal extremities to proximal extremities/axial skeleton
- Morphology
  - Variable, depending on stage of marrow change
    - Reconverted red marrow may occur as focal islands, which then coalesce
    - Serous atrophy commences as small T2 bright foci, which coalesce over time

Imaging Recommendations

- Best imaging tool
  - MR: T1 and T2 (or STIR) used most frequently
    - Opposed-phase sequences can be performed rapidly (1-2 minutes) at any field strength
    - Contrast-enhanced imaging may be useful in differentiating infiltrative marrow disease from other marrow alteration
- Protocol advice
  - **Conventional** T1-weighted pulse sequences allow optimal evaluation of marrow
  - **High T2**-weighted (> 80 ms) pulse sequence is most sensitive for free water
    - Useful for evaluation of serous atrophy
  - Opposed-phase sequences highly recommended for problem solving
    - Chemical shift imaging exploits differences in resonant frequencies of lipid and water
      - ☐ Confirms small quantities of fat within tissue
    - Recognition of chemical shift may corroborate diagnosis of lesions with substantial fat elements
      - ☐ Repopulated or stimulated marrow
  - If using contrast imaging to differentiate marrow repopulation/stimulation from infiltration
    - Requires both pre- and postcontrast T1 FS to determine ratios

Radiographic Findings

- Generally increase or decrease in red marrow does not result in radiographic abnormality
- Rare exceptions: Aplastic anemia and serous atrophy
  - Insufficiency fractures may occur

MR Findings

- T1WI
  - Red marrow reconversion, repopulation, stimulation
    - Low SI, isointense to muscle or disc
  - Marrow depletion
    - High SI, increased fatty marrow
  - Serous atrophy
    - Intermediate marrow SI, appearing rather gray
      - ☐ Due to diminished red **and** yellow marrow
    - No high signal body fat (wasted)
- T2WI/STIR
  - Red marrow reconversion, repopulation, stimulation
    - Slightly hyperintense to muscle
  - Marrow depletion
    - Moderately high SI, isointense to fat
  - Serous atrophy
    - High SI (fluid signal)
- Gradient-echo imaging
  - Sites of marrow repopulation bloom with hemosiderin deposits from chronic transfusions
    - Patients treated for chronic severe anemia
- Opposed-phase imaging
  - Red marrow reconversion, repopulation, stimulation
    - Contain equal parts lipid and water
    - ↓ signal on out of phase imaging (distinguishes from tumor, which shows no drop in SI since fat is replaced by tumor)
      - ☐ ↓ SI by > 20% on out of phase sequence strongly suggests (but does not prove) benign process
- Contrast-enhanced T1 FS
  - Yellow marrow does not enhance

- Red marrow enhances by ~ 10%
  - Exception: Marrow islands in children can enhance significantly
- Stimulated marrow enhances no more than 35%

Nuclear Medicine Findings

- PET/CT
  - Rebound marrow following chemotherapy: Moderate ↑ uptake
  - Stimulated marrow from GCSF: Intense ↑ uptake
    - Duration uncertain, may be in range of 3-4 weeks

DIFFERENTIAL DIAGNOSIS

DDx of Increased Red Marrow

- Red marrow reconversion, repopulation, stimulation
- Rebound from chemotherapy
- Marrow deposition disease (including Gaucher)
- Myelofibrosis, myelodysplasia
- Tumor
  - Leukemia/lymphoma, multiple myeloma, carcinomatosis
  - Tend to show ↑ STIR, ↑ enhancement, ↑ SI on out of phase imaging compared to red marrow

DDx of Red Marrow Depletion

- Advanced age, aplastic anemia, focal radiation
- Cytoxic chemotherapy (transient marrow suppression)
  - Especially noted with methotrexate
- NSAIDs rarely may cause marrow suppression

PATHOLOGY

General Features

- Etiology
  - Marrow reconversion
    - Increased oxygen requirements
      - Rigorous athleticism, smoking, obesity, chronic obstructive pulmonary disease, high altitude
  - Marrow repopulation
    - Severe sickle cell disease, thalassemia
  - Marrow stimulation
    - GCSF
      - Augments high intensity chemotherapy and recovery from neutropenia after chemotherapy
      - Used in marrow donors to stimulate cellular precursors prior to leukapheresis
  - Aplastic anemia may develop from myelotoxins
    - Benzene, alkylating agents, chloramphenicol, some insecticides
    - Whole body irradiation
    - Hepatitis C
    - CMV, EBV, herpes zoster
    - 50% of cases idiopathic
  - Serous atrophy
    - Advanced cachexia, anorexia nervosa, HIV/AIDS
    - Following chemotherapy
    - Severe illness, such as chronic renal disease

Microscopic Features

- Normal adult red marrow
  - Approximately = ratio of cellular to fatty marrow
- Marrow repopulation
  - Normal red marrow with ↑ red:yellow ratio
- Aplastic anemia
  - Marrow hypocellular ("empty," < 30% red cells)
  - Populated by adipocytes, fibrous stroma, scattered lymphocytes, and plasma cells
  - May develop fibrosis or infarction
- Serous atrophy
  - Depletion of both hematopoietic and fat cells
  - Extracellular deposition of mucopolysaccharides

CLINICAL ISSUES

Presentation

- Most common signs/symptoms
  - Aplastic anemia usually gradual in onset
    - Weakness, pallor, dyspnea, petechiae, ecchymosis
    - Increased risk of infection
  - Serous atrophy
    - 80% present with anemia or weight loss

Demographics

- Age
  - Aplastic anemia seen in any age
  - Serous atrophy usually in adults
- Gender
  - Aplastic anemia: No gender preference
  - Serous atrophy: M:F = 1.5:1

Natural History & Prognosis

- Clinical course of aplastic anemia unpredictable
  - May be reversible if causative agent is treated
  - May be fatal
- Serous atrophy may reverse if etiologic condition (e.g., anorexia) eliminated

Treatment

- Aplastic anemia
  - Bone marrow transplant in younger patients
  - Immunosuppressive agents in older patients

DIAGNOSTIC CHECKLIST

Consider

- Densely repopulated marrow may resemble diffuse marrow replacement
  - Treatment history may clarify diagnosis
- Marrow abnormalities likely underdiagnosed
  - Be aware of normal patterns of red marrow and their relationship to patient age

Image Interpretation Pearls

- Diffuse marrow depletion involving large area (i.e., many vertebrae) most likely reflects aplastic anemia or pattern of advanced age
  - Radiated marrow has a port-like configuration, with normal marrow outside port
- Paucity of subcutaneous fat supports diagnosis of serous atrophy

SELECTED REFERENCES

1. Kohl CA et al: Accuracy of chemical shift MR imaging in diagnosing indeterminate bone marrow lesions in the pelvis: review of a single institution's experience. Skeletal Radiol. 43(8):1079-84, 2014

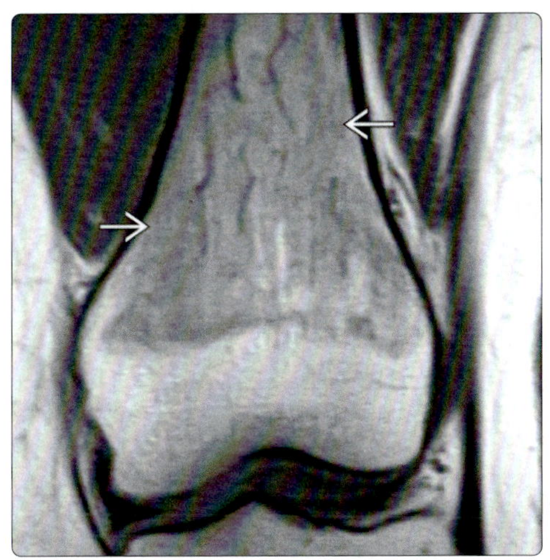

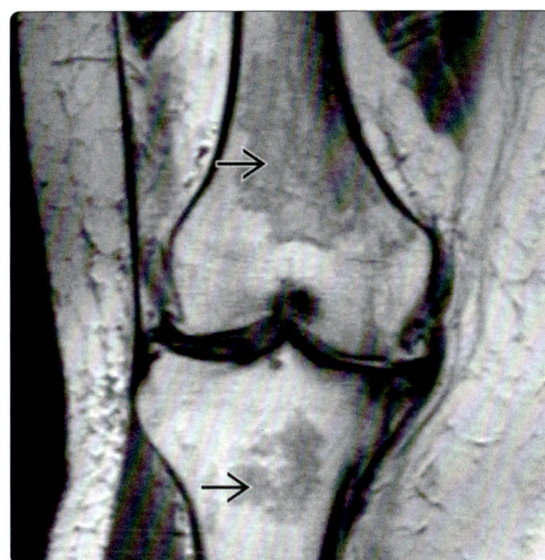

(Left) *Coronal T1WI MR in a normal young adult shows expected gray signal of red marrow residua occupying the metaphysis ➡, clearly admixed with fat. Fatty conversion is complete in the epiphysis.* **(Right)** *Coronal T1WI MR shows red marrow reconversion due to hypoxia in a middle-aged obese smoker. Patchy intermediate T1 signal is admixed with fat in the distal femoral and proximal tibial metaphyses ➡. A similar appearance can be seen in marathon runners and in individuals adjusting to high altitude.*

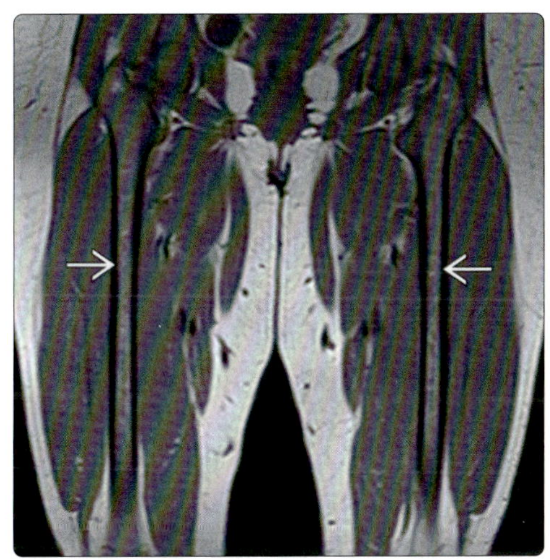

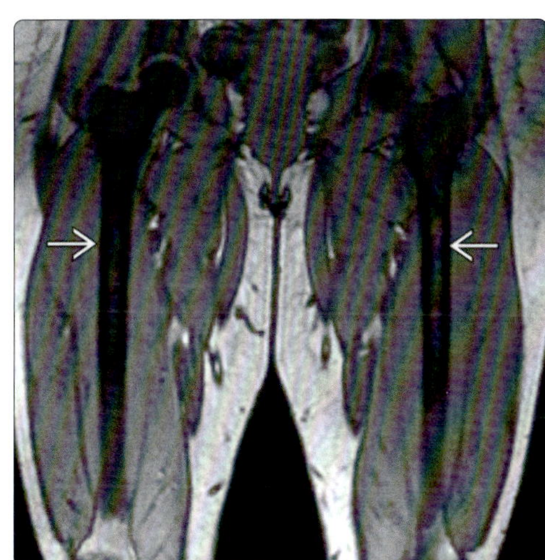

(Left) *Coronal T1WI MR shows marrow repopulation. The middle-aged woman has diffuse bilateral femoral T1 SI isointense to muscle ➡, except the distal femora and a portion of the proximal apophyses. Her clinician inquired as to whether this represented tumor infiltration.* **(Right)** *Out-of-phase chemical shift image demonstrates ↓ in femoral marrow SI of > 20% ➡, strongly suggesting red marrow repopulation. The patient was recovering from severe anemia.*

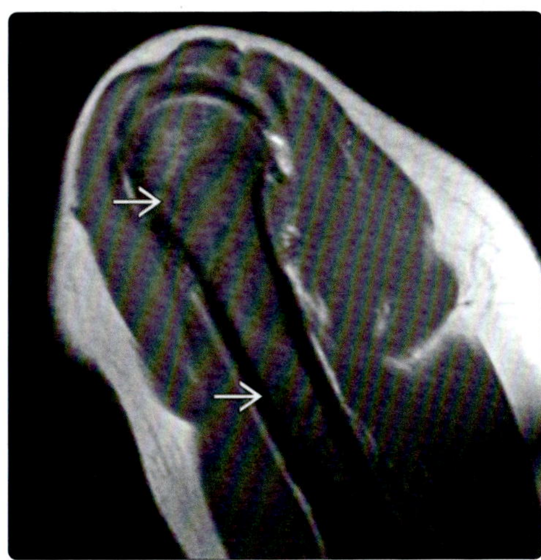

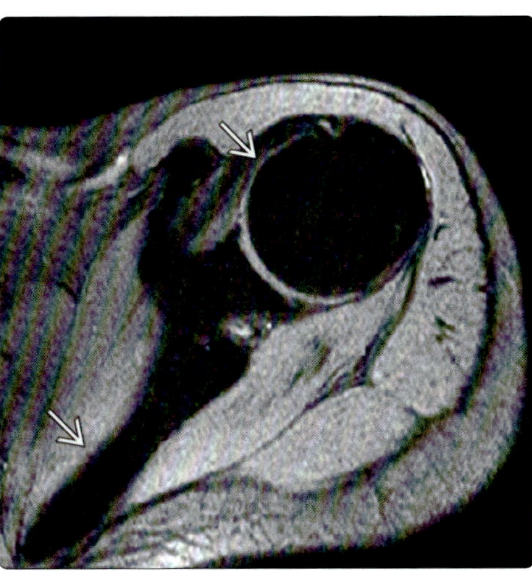

(Left) *Sagittal T1WI MR shows a patient in late adolescence with sickle cell anemia, status post multiple transfusions. There is diffuse low T1 signal throughout the marrow ➡, nearly isointense with muscle. Note that the abnormal signal involves even the epiphysis. This represents red marrow repopulation.* **(Right)** *Axial gradient echo MR in the same patient demonstrates blooming susceptibility artifact ➡. This reflects the iron content within the cellular marrow, secondary to multiple transfusions.*

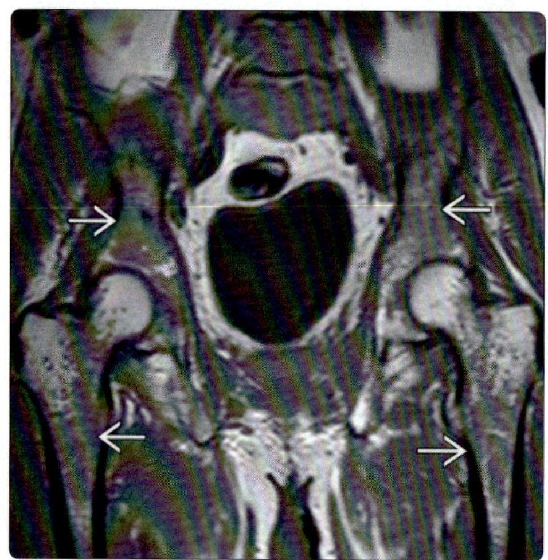

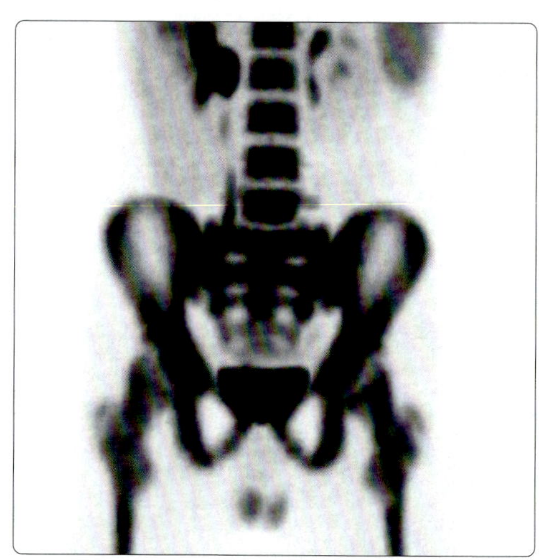

(Left) *Coronal T1WI MR of a middle-aged woman with bone metastases, treated with GCSF, shows confluent ↓ SI foci → isointense with muscle. Opposed-phase imaging (not shown) demonstrated > 20% ↓ in SI, indicating the abnormal foci are most likely due to marrow stimulation.* **(Right)** *PET shows avid axial and proximal appendicular activity in a patient treated with GCSF. The pattern is symmetric and conforms to the expected distribution of hematopoietic marrow. (Courtesy K. Friedman, MD.)*

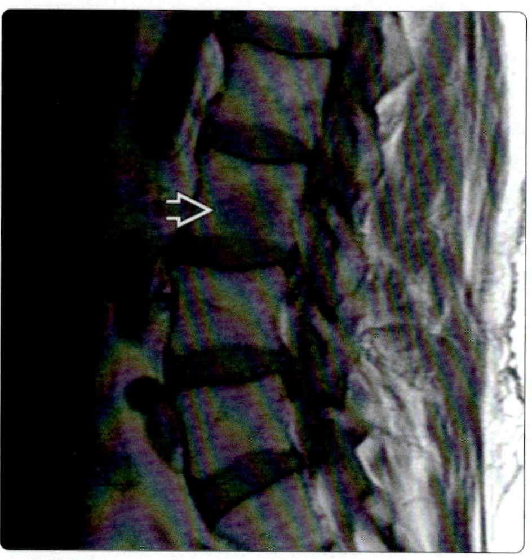

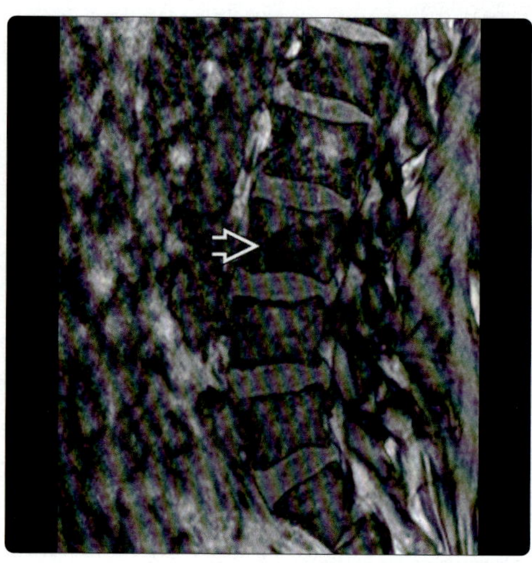

(Left) *Sagittal T1WI MR demonstrates a discretely marginated island of red marrow within a lumbar vertebral body →. This is not quite as dark as disc or muscle, but its morphology raised concern for a lesion. Opposed-phase imaging was obtained.* **(Right)** *Sagittal out-of-phase image in the same patient is shown. The region of interest measurement of the "lesion" in L3 → demonstrated > 20% ↓ in SI on out of phase compared to in-phase imaging, strongly suggesting a benign etiology, such as red marrow replacement.*

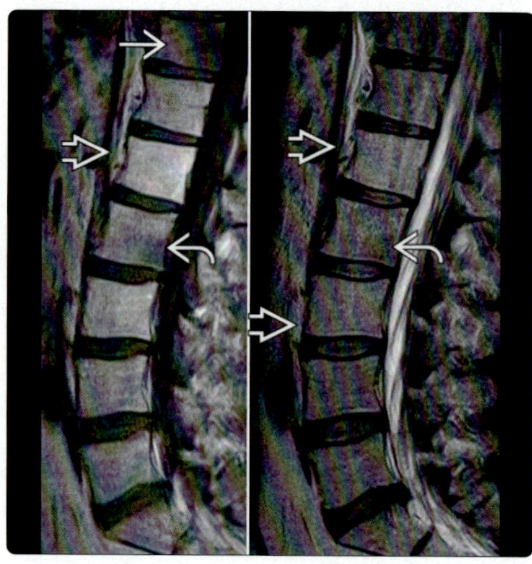

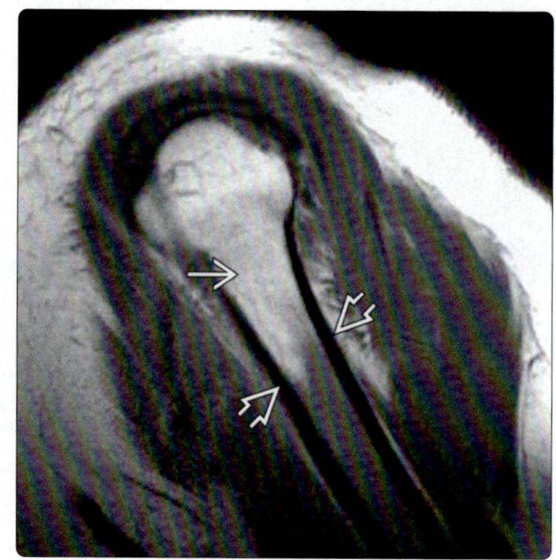

(Left) *Sagittal T1 (L) and T2 (R) MR images show a low signal treated tumor focus in L2 →. High T1/T2 signal at L1 and L3 → indicates fat replacement in the radiation port. Hypointense lesion is seen in T11 →, outside the radiation port, concerning for metastasis.* **(Right)** *Sagittal T1WI MR of a teenager post radiation of a scapular tumor shows focal ablation of red marrow in the proximal humerus →. Note the demarcation → between radiated fatty marrow and cellular marrow in the diaphysis.*

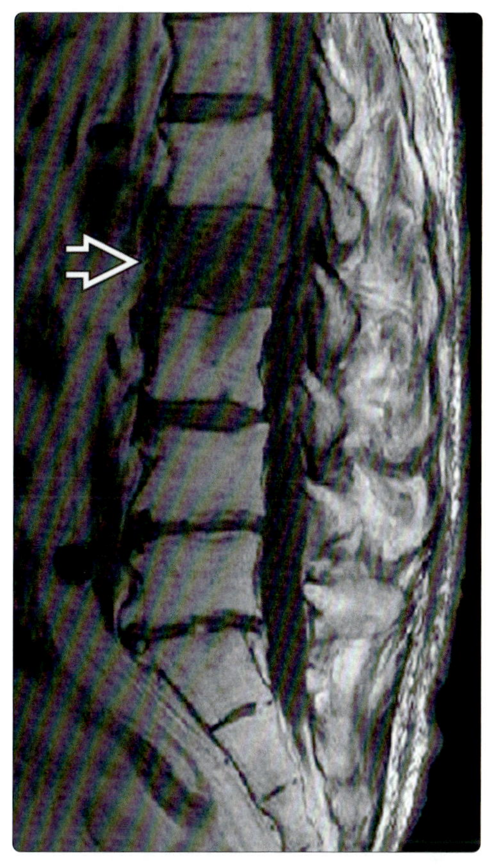

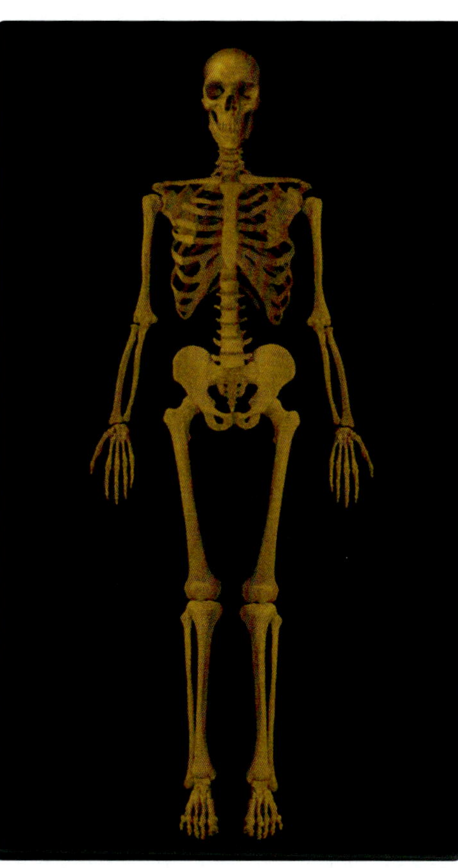

(Left) *Sagittal T1WI MR shows diffuse cellular marrow depletion. This middle-aged man has anemia and metastatic lung carcinoma. Pathologic fracture of L2* ➲ *shows diffuse low T1 signal. The spine otherwise demonstrates depletion of cellular marrow with diffuse fatty replacement. There was no history of radiation treatment; the depleted marrow conforms to a region larger than expected for a radiation port.* **(Right)** *Coronal graphic demonstrates the pattern of diffuse fatty marrow occupying the marrow space. This may be seen in advanced age &/or in aplastic anemia. Completely or mostly fat-replaced bones are at higher risk for fracture and ischemia.*

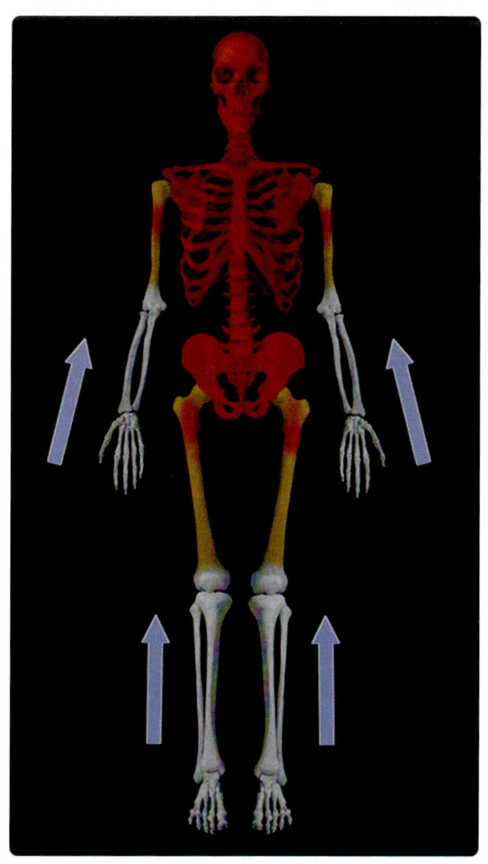

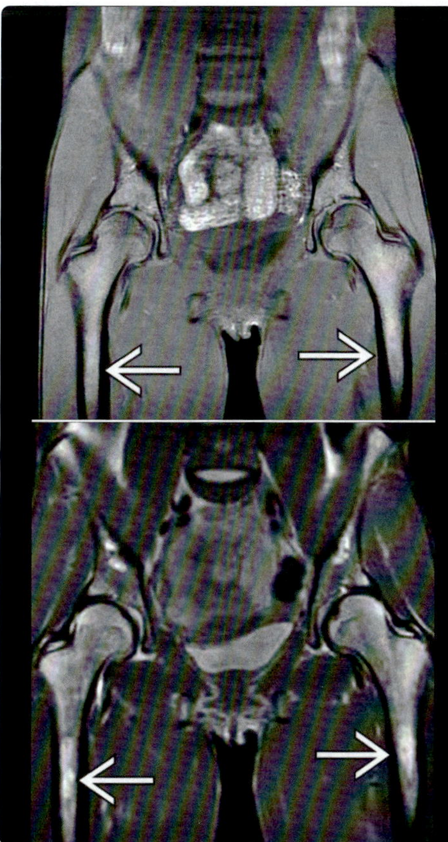

(Left) *Coronal graphic demonstrates the pattern of spread of serous atrophy. Gelatinous transformation of marrow progresses distal to proximal in the appendicular skeleton. The axial skeleton is involved last. Note that this pattern of marrow change allows differentiation from hematogenous distribution of osseous metastases. Gelatinous islands may initially be discrete and eventually coalesce.* **(Right)** *Serous atrophy of the marrow is shown in a 23-year-old female athlete with anorexia. T1 (top) shows gray rather than high signal regions in the femoral metadiaphysis* ➲. *Matched regions on STIR (bottom) shows high signal typical of serous atrophy. Note the diminished subcutaneous fat on the T1 image; this is an essential feature of serous atrophy. (Courtesy D. Blankenbaker, MD.)*

KEY FACTS

TERMINOLOGY

- "Marrow infiltration" and "replacement" refer to amount of cellular vs. adipocytes admixed in a lesion
- **Diffuse marrow infiltration**: Moderately cellular tissue admixed with fat, diffuse bone involvement
  - Regenerated/repopulated/stimulated red marrow
  - Chronic infection
  - HIV/AIDS
  - Marrow storage disorders
- **Diffuse marrow replacement**: Densely cellular lesions, with no significant adipocytes, distributed diffusely in skeleton
  - Osseous carcinomatosis
  - Multiple myeloma
  - Myelodysplasias: Diverse group of diseases 2° to ineffective production of myeloid elements
  - Myeloproliferative disorders: Overproduction of myeloid elements
- Diffuse marrow infiltration or replacement do not connote benignity or malignancy per se

IMAGING

- Conventional SE T1-weighted images are optimal: Infiltration or replacement of fatty marrow by low signal material
  - Diffuse marrow infiltration: Moderate ↓ in SI
  - Diffuse marrow replacement: Marked ↓ in SI
- Low T2 SI: Marrow fibrosis &/or collagen deposition
- PDWI: May underestimate or mask marrow signal abnormalities
- T1WI C+: Highly cellular lesions, such as myeloma, lymphoma, and metastases, usually enhance with SI increase > 35%
- Opposed phase/chemical shift imaging
  - Principle use is to differentiate red marrow regeneration/repopulation/stimulation from metastatic foci

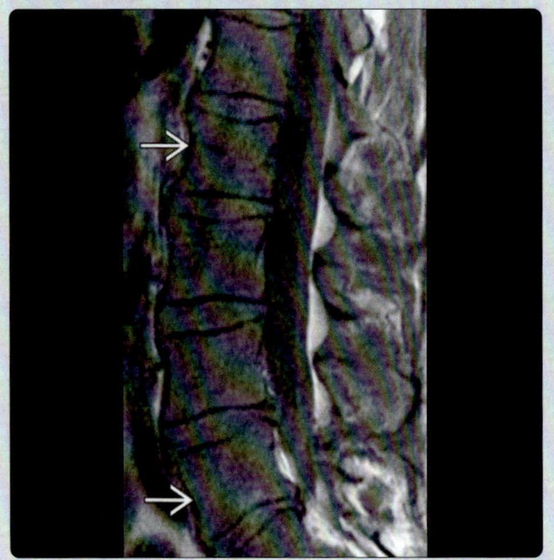

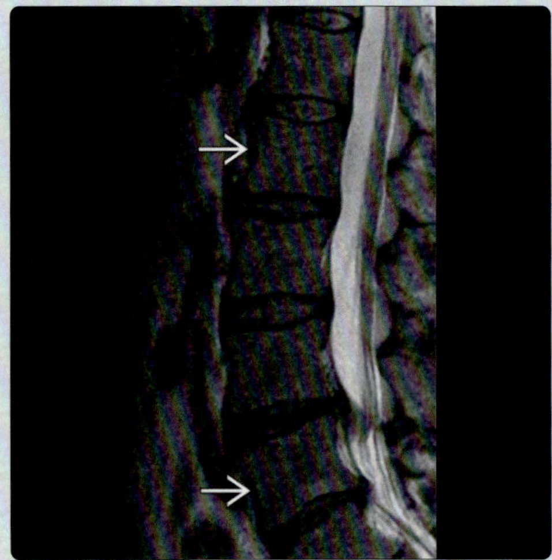

(Left) *Sagittal T1WI MR shows diffuse, fairly homogeneous low signal replacing the normal vertebral body marrow ➡. Note that the vertebral body signal is isointense with adjacent discs. This comparison is a useful internal standard of reference on T1WI.* **(Right)** *Sagittal T2WI MR, same case, shows persistence of diffusely homogeneous low marrow SI ➡. In this case, the marrow replacement is due to essential thrombocytosis; other myeloproliferative disorders may appear identical.*

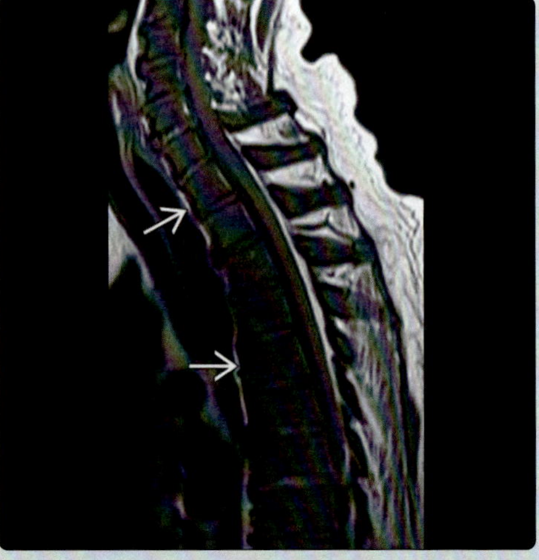

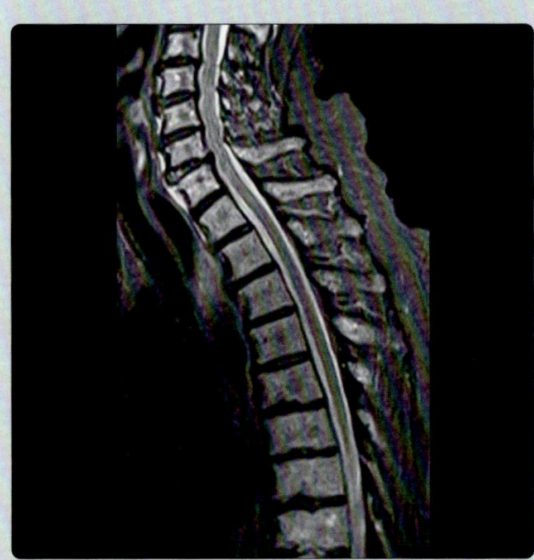

(Left) *Sagittal T1 MR in a 42-year-old man with nonspecific back pain and normal radiographs shows diffuse ↓ SI throughout the spine ➡. Note the internal comparison with disc material shows that the hypointensity is severe.* **(Right)** *Sagittal STIR MR, same case, shows hyperintensity at all levels. This diffuse marrow replacement proved to be due to multiple myeloma.*

TERMINOLOGY

Synonyms

- Myelodysplasia: Formerly known as preleukemia

Definitions

- "Marrow infiltration" and "replacement" refer to amount of cellular vs. adipocytes admixed in lesion
  - **Diffuse marrow infiltration**: Moderately cellular tissue admixed with fat, with diffuse bone involvement
    - Regenerated/repopulated/stimulated red marrow
    - Chronic infection
    - HIV/AIDS
    - Marrow storage disorders
    - Early (or treated) phase of myelodysplasia and myeloproliferative disorders
  - **Diffuse marrow replacement**: Densely cellular lesions, with no significant adipocytes, distributed diffusely in skeleton
    - Osseous carcinomatosis
    - Multiple myeloma
    - Myelodysplasias: Diverse group of hematologic conditions due to ineffective production of myeloid elements
      - Characterized by variety of refractory anemic conditions
    - Myeloproliferative disorders: Overproduction of myeloid elements
      - Platelets (essential thrombocytosis)
      - Reticulocytes (polycythemia vera)
      - Fibroblasts/collagen (myelofibrosis)
      - White cells (leukemia)
- Diffuse marrow infiltration or replacement do not connote benignity or malignancy per se

IMAGING

General Features

- Best diagnostic clue
  - Conventional SE T1-weighted images are optimal: Infiltration or replacement of fatty marrow by low signal material
- Location
  - Diffuse replacement
    - Dense in axial skeleton and proximal tubular bones
    - More infiltrative and sparse in distal extremities
- Size
  - Variable
    - Multiple discrete lesions throughout axial and proximal tubular bones
    - Coalescent/conglomerate large lesions
    - Complete marrow replacement
- Morphology
  - Variable, ranging from multifocal to diffuse marrow packing
    - Variability (and inconstant, sometimes confusing, appearance) often relates to
      - Severity of disease
      - Treatment regimen
      - Response to treatment
  - Multiple myeloma displays variety of MR patterns
    - Normal marrow
    - Dense cellular marrow
    - Variegated appearance
    - Salt and pepper pattern
    - Focal confluent lesions

Radiographic Findings

- Variable, depending on aggressiveness of marrow process relative to cortex and trabeculae
  - Not infrequently appears normal in any of these disease processes
  - Diffuse osteopenia
    - May be difficult to detect but may be only radiographic clue to extensive disease
      - Interpret bone density within context of patient age and gender
    - 40-50% of trabeculae must be destroyed to become radiographically apparent as osteopenia
  - Multifocal lytic or sclerotic lesions
  - Diffuse increased bone density
- Cortical disruption and pathologic fracture
- Periosteal reaction

CT Findings

- Varies by entity from nondetectable to intramedullary soft tissue deposition isoattenuated to muscle
- Abnormal bone density: Osteopenia or sclerosis
- Cortical disruption or fracture

MR Findings

- T1WI
  - Diffuse marrow infiltration: Moderate decrease in SI
    - Some residual and admixed fatty elements
  - Diffuse marrow replacement: Marked decrease in SI
    - Muscle/disc are useful as internal T1 signal standard: Diffuse replacement shows SI isointense or darker than these structures
- T2WI FS
  - Highly variable
    - Useful, but not definitive in differentiating etiologies of marrow infiltration/replacement
  - Low T2 SI: Marrow fibrosis &/or collagen deposition
    - Sclerotic and fibrotic lesions may not be discernible on IR and T2 fat-saturated images
  - High T2 SI: Edema/free fluid component
- PD/intermediate
  - May underestimate or mask marrow signal abnormalities
  - No role in detection or diagnosis of marrow pathology
- STIR
  - Variable, as T2WI FS
- T1WI C+
  - Highly cellular lesions, such as myeloma, lymphoma, and metastases, usually enhance with SI increase greater than 35%
    - Sclerotic lesions variably enhance
    - Without fat saturation, diffuse marrow replacement may be obscured
      - Comparison with precontrast images is required
- Opposed-phase/chemical shift imaging
  - GRE sequences used
    - Minimal time penalty; all MR field strengths

- Principle use is to differentiate red marrow regeneration/repopulation/stimulation from metastatic foci
  - Metastases and myeloproliferative disorders are highly cellular, and exclude marrow fat
    - SI does not decrease (and may increase) on out-of-phase sequence
  - Red marrow regeneration/repopulation/stimulation is mixed with adipocytes
    - SI decreases > 20% on out-of-phase sequence
- Highly suggestive, but not diagnostic, of benignancy vs. malignancy
  - False-negatives: Multiple myeloma and lymphoma (may entrap adipocytes and show ↓ SI on out-of-phase)

Imaging Recommendations

- Best imaging tool
  - MR is most reliable imaging tool to detect marrow infiltration/replacement
  - Current protocol for detecting osseous metastases
    - Usually bone scan, followed by radiographs of positive sites
  - This paradigm is currently shifting
    - For PET-avid lesions (such as multiple myeloma), PET may be performed with MR correlation of hypermetabolic sites
    - MR survey (usually combination of T1WI and STIR of osseous axial, and proximal appendicular skeleton) may be utilized
      - Often used to assess tumor burden &/or response to treatment
    - Whole body MR allows global assessment of marrow
      - Employed in some centers to survey for bone metastases, assess myeloma &/or bone lymphoma
      - Other findings (splenomegaly, primary tumor) may be revealed
    - No role for MR in diagnosis of leukemia and other myeloproliferative disorders
      - May be helpful in assessing treatment response and in surveying for biopsy sites if iliac crest biopsy does not yield diagnostic material
- Protocol advice
  - Conventional SE T1WI: Principle sequence for detection and evaluation of diffuse marrow infiltration/replacement
  - Opposed-phase and IV gadolinium contrast are useful for problem solving

DIFFERENTIAL DIAGNOSIS

DDx of Moderate Diffuse Low T1WI Signal

- Iron deposition following transfusion therapy
- Severe anemia: Sickle cell, thalassemia
- HIV/AIDS: Reticuloendothelial iron blockade
- Marrow stimulation [granulocyte cell stimulating factor (GCSF)]

DDx of Severe Diffuse Low T1WI Signal

- Mastocytosis
- Hemosiderosis
- Myelofibrosis
- Osteopetrosis/pycnodysostosis
- Myeloma, lymphoma

Multifocal ↑ SI on T2, Mimicking Metastases

- Sarcoidosis
- Brown tumors
- Postchemotherapy change
- Multiple infarcts
- Serous atrophy
- Disseminated fungal and hydatid infection

CLINICAL ISSUES

Presentation

- Most common signs/symptoms
  - Diffuse marrow replacement: Anemia, fatigue, shortness of breath

Natural History & Prognosis

- Varies by entity
  - ~ 1/3 of patients with myelodysplasia progress to acute myelogenous leukemia

DIAGNOSTIC CHECKLIST

Consider

- Diffuse marrow changes may be encountered on MR, related to cancer treatments
  - Marrow ablation, rebound, stimulation, widespread osteonecrosis, disseminated infection
  - Discuss treatment history with clinician prior to interpreting MR in these patients

Image Interpretation Pearls

- In children, diffuse red marrow may mask marrow infiltration and replacement on MR
  - Fluid-sensitive and contrast-enhanced sequences improve detection

Reporting Tips

- In many cases, diffuse marrow disorder has been diagnosed clinically prior to MR
  - Clinician may be seeking information regarding disease load &/or treatment response
  - MR may be useful for selection of biopsy sites if iliac biopsy is not diagnostic
    - Remember that replaced marrow offers better chance for diagnosis than infiltrated marrow

SELECTED REFERENCES

1. Kohl CA et al: Accuracy of chemical shift MR imaging in diagnosing indeterminate bone marrow lesions in the pelvis: review of a single institution's experience. Skeletal Radiol. 43(8):1079-84, 2014
2. Kung JW et al: Bone marrow signal alteration in the extremities. AJR Am J Roentgenol. 196(5):W492-510, 2011
3. Steinbach LS: "MRI in the detection of malignant infiltration of bone marrow"--a commentary. AJR Am J Roentgenol. 188(6):1443-5, 2007
4. Zajick DC Jr et al: Benign and malignant processes: normal values and differentiation with chemical shift MR imaging in vertebral marrow. Radiology. 237(2):590-6, 2005
5. Lecouvet FE et al: Magnetic resonance and computed tomography imaging in multiple myeloma. Semin Musculoskelet Radiol. 5(1):43-55, 2001
6. Walker RE et al: Whole-body magnetic resonance imaging: techniques, clinical indications, and future applications. Semin Musculoskelet Radiol. 5(1):5-20, 2001
7. Panicek DM et al: MR imaging of bone Marrow in patients with musculoskeletal tumors. Sarcoma. 3(1):37-41, 1999

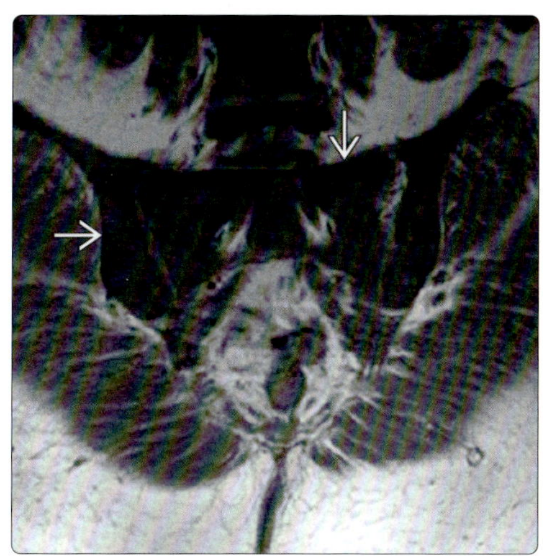

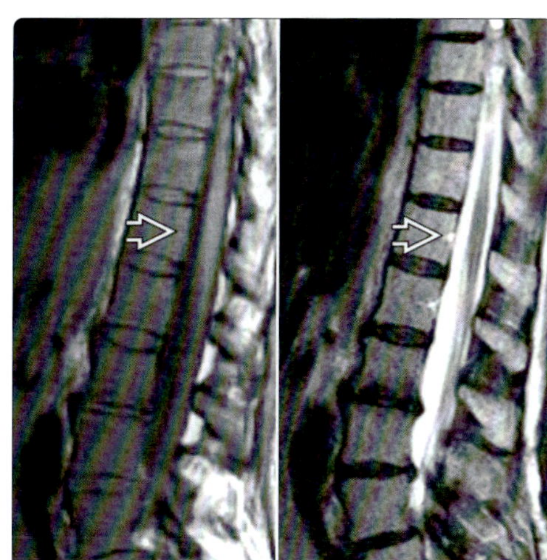

(Left) *Coronal oblique T1WI MR of the sacrum demonstrates diffuse marrow replacement ➡. The marrow SI is lower than muscle. This patient has polycythemia vera, but diffuse replacement by tumor cannot be ruled out without biopsy.* **(Right)** *Sagittal T1WI (left) and T2WI (right) of the lumbar spine in a patient with CML. T1 SI is isointense with the disc and effaces ➡ basivertebral vessels. This diffuse marrow replacement pattern may be easily missed since there are no focal lesions to draw one's attention.*

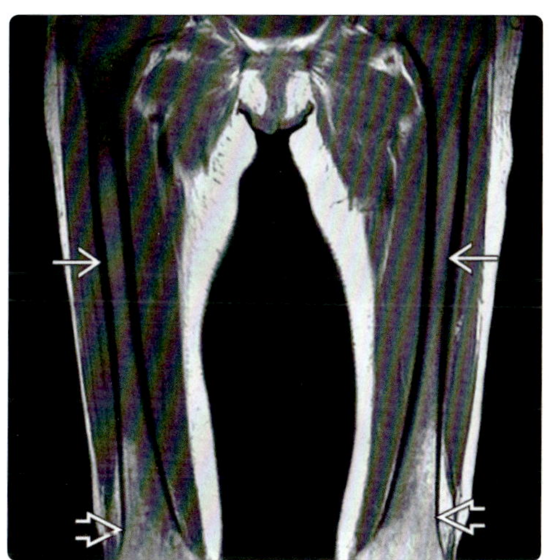

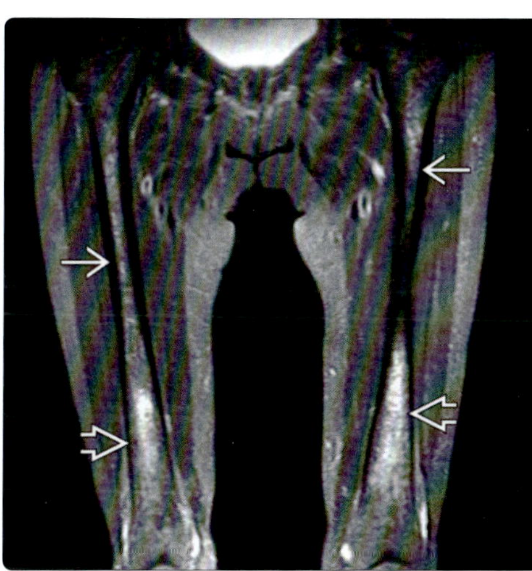

(Left) *Coronal T1WI MR in a patient with primary myelofibrosis shows T1 SI isointense with muscle in the bilateral femoral diaphyses ➡, with some residual fatty marrow in the distal femora ➡. The low T1 SI indicates fibrosis and collagen deposition within the medullary space.* **(Right)** *Coronal STIR MR in the same patient shows mixed SI in the proximal femora ➡, suggesting fibrosis. Vaguely demarcated high T2 SI in the distal femora ➡ may reflect marrow edema. Complaint was of lower thigh pain.*

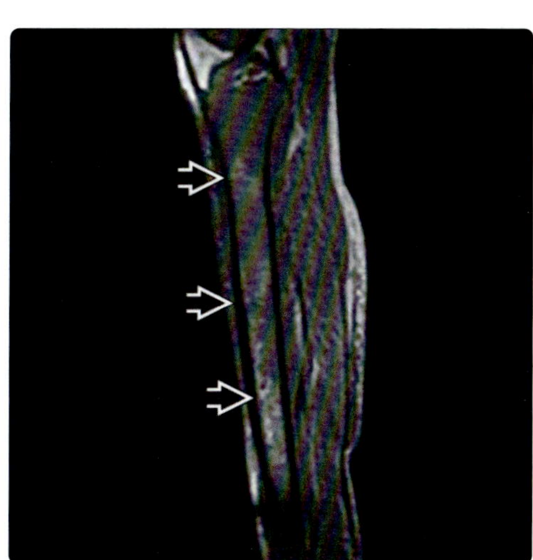

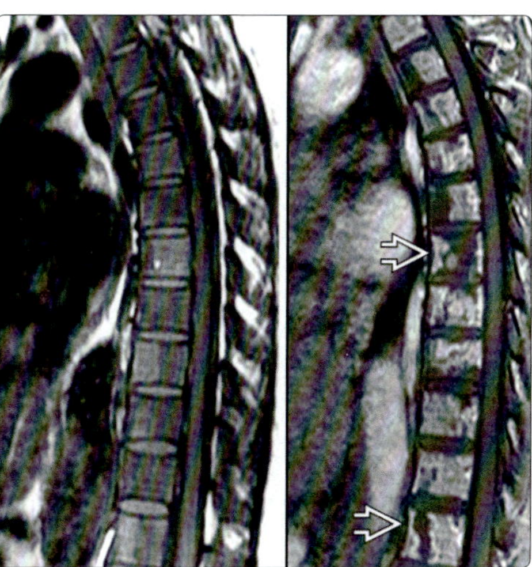

(Left) *Sagittal T1WI MR of the tibia in a patient with sickle cell disease shows diffuse low T1 SI, indicating iron deposition from transfusions, likely superimposed on marrow repopulation in this anemic patient. Against this background, geographically marginated infarcts ➡ are faintly seen.* **(Right)** *Graphic shows sagittal T1WI pre- (left) and postcontrast (right) images in a patient with bone lymphoma. Infarctions are seen on the contrast images ➡ that were concealed on T1. (Courtesy V. Sarkis-Oliveira, MD, and D. Amaral, MD.)*

(Left) *Coronal T1WI MR in a patient with biopsy-proven multiple myeloma shows the diffuse salt and pepper pattern of punctate low signal against marrow fat ➡, as well as larger focal sites of myeloma ➡.* **(Right)** *Coronal STIR MR in the same patient shows the salt and pepper pattern of multiple myeloma as innumerable diffuse minute bright foci ➡. The larger coalesced myeloma lesions ➡ are heterogeneously increased in SI on this sequence.*

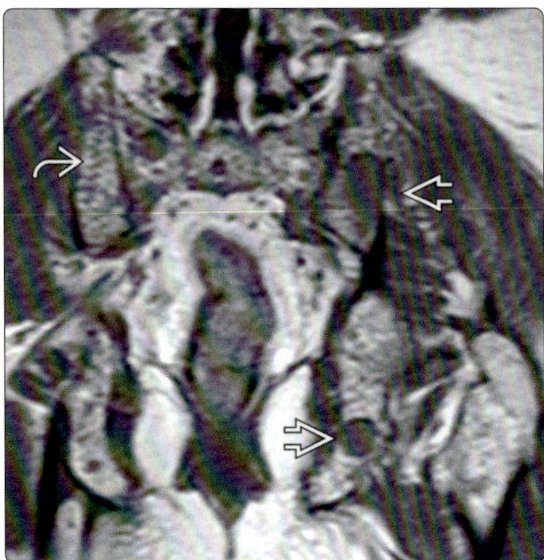

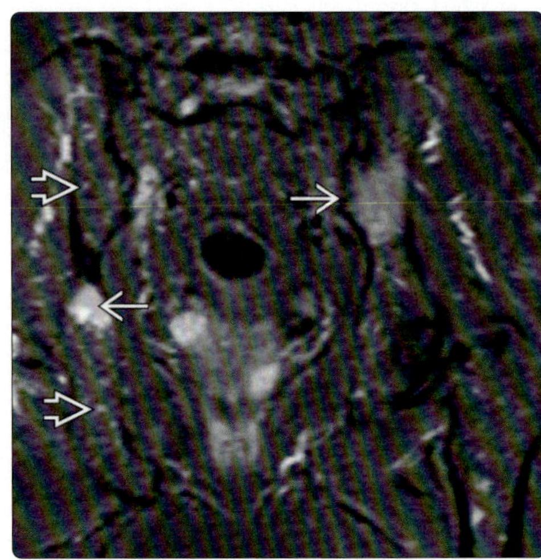

(Left) *Sagittal T1WI MR shows numerous metastatic deposits, all lower SI than disc ➡. Osseous carcinomatosis can range from multiple discrete foci to complete marrow replacement.* **(Right)** *Sagittal T1WI (left) and T2WI (right) show a variegated pattern of marrow replacement. Focal lesion in L5 ➡ is a biopsy-proven metastasis (note that metastases are not always hyperintense on T2). Patchy low T1 signal interspersed with fatty islands ➡ are indeterminate for metastases and may reflect red marrow.*

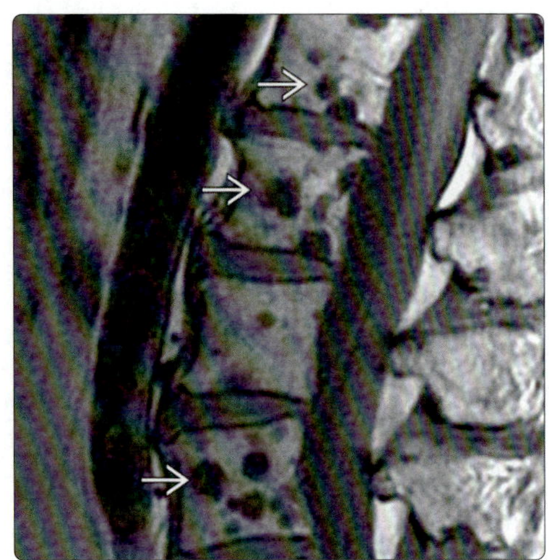

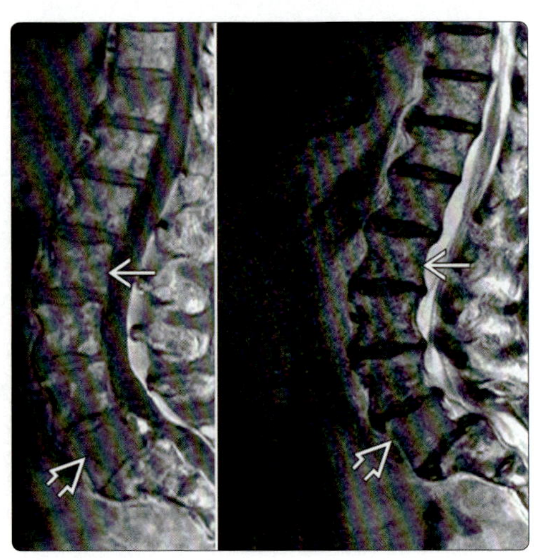

(Left) *Sagittal T1WI (left) and T2WI (right) demonstrate multiple scattered foci of low-signal marrow, isointense with disc on T1WI ➡, interspersed with fatty islands. This is a common pattern encountered in individuals of advancing age.* **(Right)** *Sagittal GRE in (left) and out-of-phase (right) sequence in the same patient shows the same patchy foci ➡ to demonstrate SI ↓ of > 20%, indicating fat admixed within the measured voxels. This militates for, but does not prove, that the regions of concern are red marrow.*

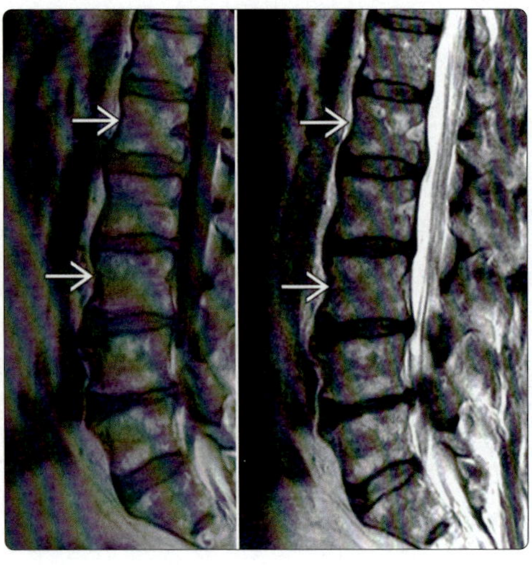

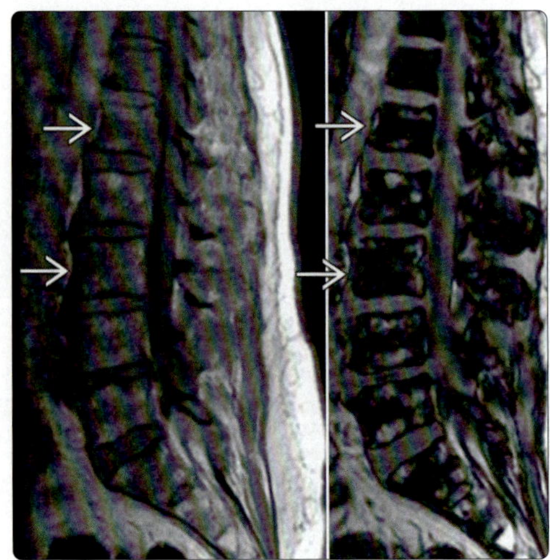

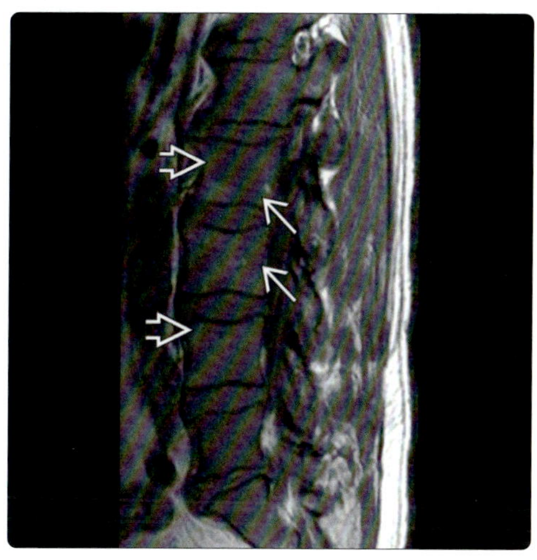

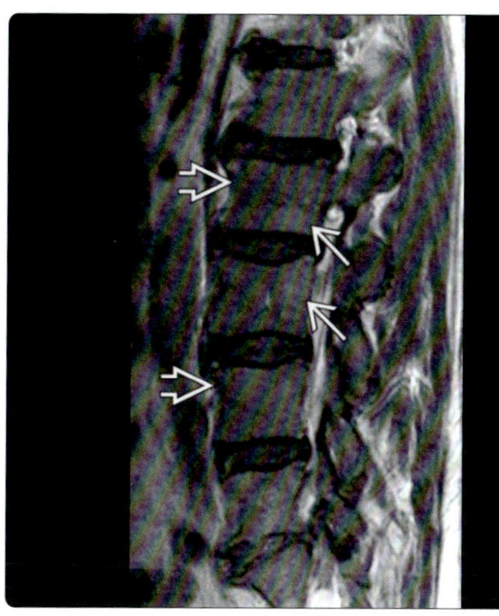

(Left) *Sagittal T1 MR in a middle-aged man shows coalescent regions of ↓ SI in the anterior ➡ and posterior bodies ➡. These regions are isointense with disc; they are concerning for metastatic deposits, though other etiologies must also be considered.* **(Right)** *Sagittal T2 MR, same case, suggests a faint ↑ in SI within the identified regions of the posterior bodies ➡, increasing concern for marrow replacement. The anterior lesions ➡ do not appear to have ↑ SI, making these sites less worrisome.*

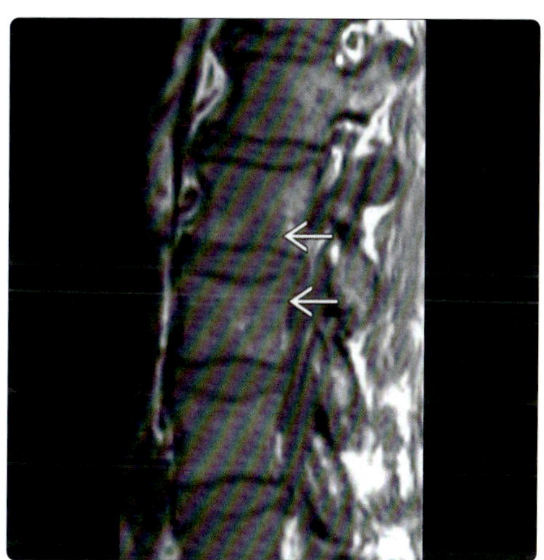

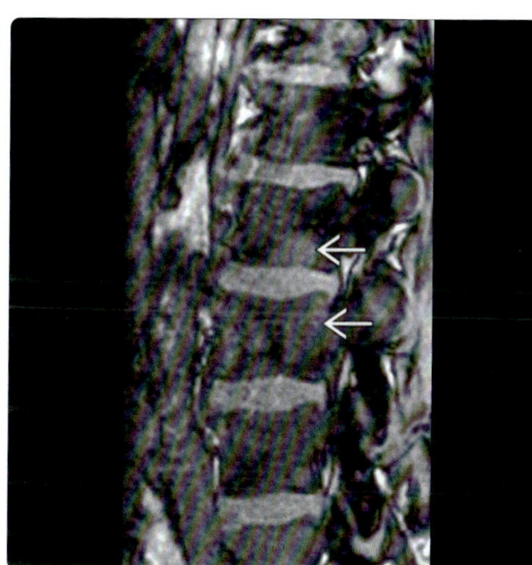

(Left) *Sagittal GRE opposed-phase sequence imaging, same case; this is the in-phase image. Note the signal in the regions of greatest concern ➡.* **(Right)** *Sagittal GRE opposed-phase imaging, out-of-phase matched image, shows ↑ SI in the 2 most concerning lesions ➡. This strongly suggests a marrow infiltrating lesion, such as metastases. Comparative region of interest measurements at the other sites varied but mostly showed > 20% decrease in SI, making the other sites less concerning for tumor.*

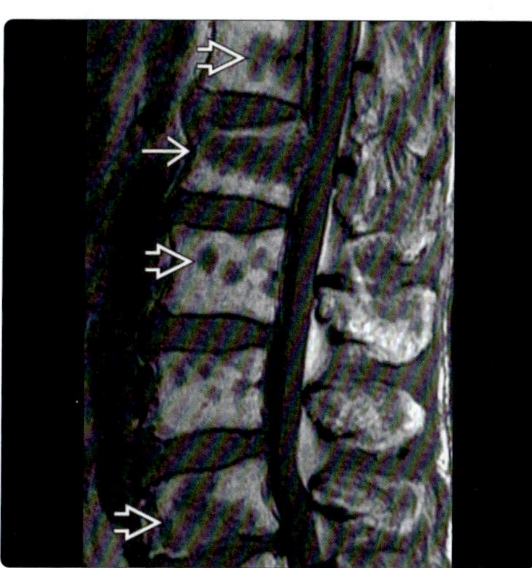

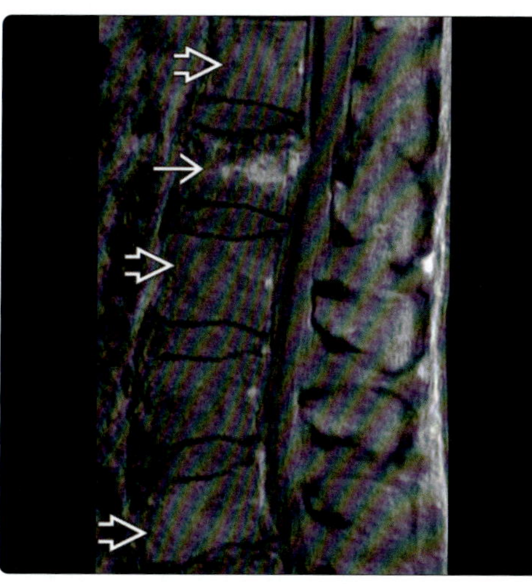

(Left) *Sagittal T1 MR in a 52-year-old man being evaluated for acute traumatic fracture ➡ also shows diffuse regions of marrow replacement ➡.* **(Right)** *Sagittal postcontrast T1FS MR shows edema at the fracture site ➡, but minimal significance at the other sites of concern ➡, making tumor less likely. By follow-up, this is determined to represent focal nodular marrow hyperplasia.*

KEY FACTS

TERMINOLOGY

- **Marrow infiltration** and **marrow replacement** refer to amount of cellularity vs. admixed fat in lesion
  - Focal marrow **infiltration** has residual and admixed fatty elements
  - Focal marrow **replacement** has no residual fat
- Terms do not imply benignity or malignancy per se
  - Focal infiltration seen at margins of fractures, tumors, infarctions, and sites of mechanical edema
  - Marrow replacement seen with highly cellular lesions, such as metastatic deposits, but can also be seen in nonmalignant processes, such as osteomyelitis

IMAGING

- Focal marrow **infiltration**: Moderate ↓ SI on T1WI, with residual and admixed fatty elements
- Focal marrow **replacement**: Marked ↓ SI on T1WI, isointense or darker than muscle/disc
- Biopsy more likely to yield diagnostic material of replaced than infiltrated marrow
- Contrast may be used for problem solving
  - Normal red marrow enhances by 10%
  - Stimulated marrow may enhance up to 30%
  - Increase in SI > 35% after IV gadolinium suspicious for infiltrating/replacing marrow lesion
- Chemical shift useful for differentiating red marrow island (which commingles with fatty marrow) from infiltrative tumor
  - Red marrow foci ↓ SI at least 20% on out-of-phase imaging
  - Hypercellular tumor with advancing front displaces adipocytes; should not drop significantly or should ↑ in SI on opposed-phase images
  - < 20% signal intensity decrease on out-of-phase imaging is threshold to suggest malignancy
    - Highly sensitive but specificity relatively poor

(Left) *Coronal T2WI FS MR shows the focal marrow infiltration pattern of edema. Note the indistinctly marginated ↑ T2 signal seen in the right femoral condyle ➡, admixed with suppressed fat. T1WI (not shown) would show a reticulated pattern of moderately low SI.* **(Right)** *Coronal T1WI MR shows focal marrow replacement in osteomyelitis of the great toe. Low SI replaces the fatty marrow of both phalanges ➡. High T2 SI and enhancement (not shown) were also noted but are nonspecific relative to this confluent T1 pattern.*

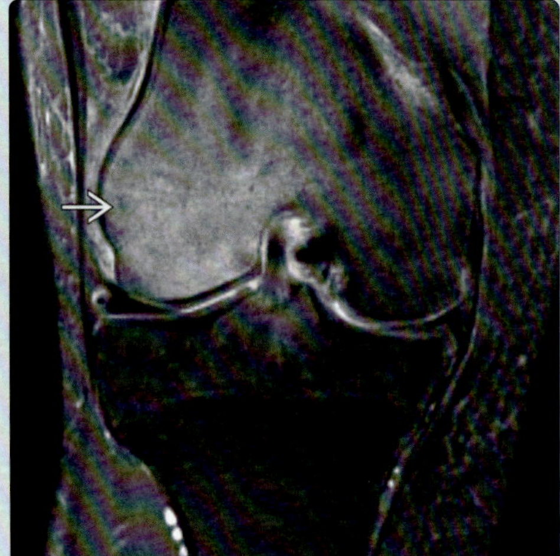

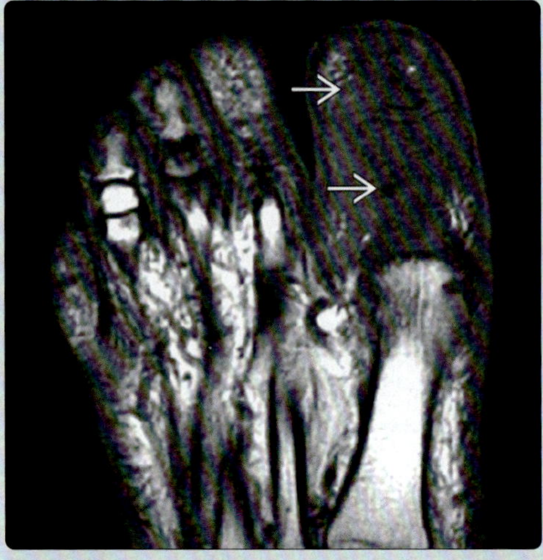

(Left) *Sagittal T1WI MR demonstrates marrow infiltration ➡ with indistinct margination and admixed fat. More proximally the marrow is replaced ➡, without perceivable fat; this latter site would be expected to have a better yield at biopsy.* **(Right)** *Sagittal pre- (left) and postcontrast (right) T1WI of the lumbar spine show marrow replacement in L4, which enhances ➡. A precontrast image is crucial, as enhancement may mask lesions on nonfat-saturated images.*

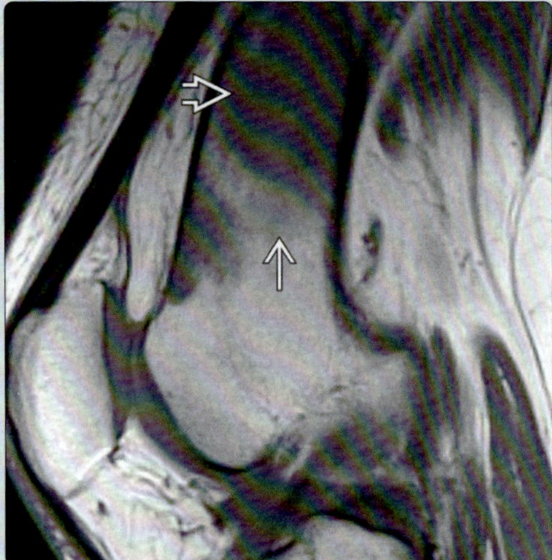

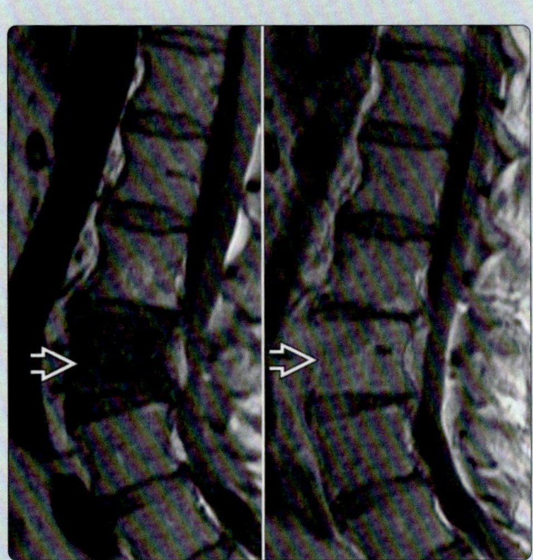

TERMINOLOGY

Definitions

- Focal lesions can **infiltrate** or **replace** normal marrow
  - Terms refer to amount of cellularity vs. admixed fat in lesion
  - Infiltration or replacement do not imply benignity or malignancy per se
- Focal infiltration can be seen
  - At margins of fractures, tumors, infarction
    - Represents marrow edema, reactive change
- Marrow replacement is seen with
  - Highly cellular lesions, such as tumor or osteomyelitis

IMAGING

General Features

- Best diagnostic clue
  - Focal marrow **infiltration** has residual and admixed fatty elements
    - Moderate decrease in SI on T1WI MR
    - Indistinct margin, with gradual zone of transition
    - Because of residual fat, infiltrated marrow may ↓ SI > 20% on out-of-phase chemical shift sequence
  - Focal marrow **replacement** has no residual fat
    - Marked ↓ SI on T1WI MR (isointense or darker than muscle/disc)
    - Margins may be sharp or indistinct (or marrow entirely replaced)
    - Because of fat replacement, SI on out-of-phase sequence may ↑ but at least will not ↓ > 20%
      - Margins of infiltrative lesions that have wide zone of transition may drop in SI > 20% on out-of-phase sequence
  - Marrow infiltration or replacement are variable in SI on fluid-sensitive sequences
- Location
  - Infiltrative lesions in adults that are spread hematogenously (metastases, multiple myeloma, infection)
    - Axial skeleton, proximal metadiaphyses
  - Infiltrative lesions of lymphoma and sarcoidosis may occur in distal extremities

Radiographic Findings

- When focus of marrow signal abnormality is encountered on MR, radiographs are recommended
  - If not occult, character of lesion may be diagnostic
    - Matrix, density, degree of aggressiveness
- Diffuse marrow replacement may present as diffuse osteopenia

CT Findings

- Range from occult lesion to soft tissue intramedullary lesion(s) isoattenuated to muscle
  - Characteristic matrix or features of lesion may be diagnostic

MR Findings

- T1WI
  - Conventional SE T1WI more sensitive to abnormal marrow foci than FSE
  - Focal marrow infiltration
    - Moderate ↓ SI, with interspersed fat signal
  - Marrow replacement
    - Marked ↓ SI, usually in confluent configuration
    - Lower SI or isointense to muscle or disc (standard reference tissue)
  - In setting of infection vs. reactive edema, character of T1 abnormality may differentiate
    - Osteomyelitis: Confluent geographic abnormality
    - Reactive edema: Hazy reticulated low signal interspersed with fat
- T2WI FS
  - Variable SI on T2WI or other fluid-sensitive sequences for both focal infiltration and marrow replacement processes
  - Low SI on T2WI does not necessarily connote sclerosis; clarify on radiograph or CT
  - Bone marrow edema: Common pattern of marrow infiltration, demonstrating ↑ SI on fluid-sensitive sequences
- PD/intermediate
  - Foci of cellular marrow demonstrate variable SI relative to marrow fat
    - Not helpful sequence for evaluating marrow lesions (may even be obscured)
- T2* GRE
  - Susceptibility artifact on GRE images can be exploited to detect and characterize lesions
    - Focal destruction of trabeculae detected on GRE images implies aggressive process
- DWI
  - Echo planar diffusion-weighted imaging being investigated to evaluate marrow pathology
    - Model: Benign vs. malignant vertebral body compression fracture
      - Utilizing DWI to differentiate benign (osteoporotic) from malignant marrow remains controversial
  - Based on concept that water molecules diffuse freely in normal tissue and have constricted motion in hypercellular tissue
    - Pathologic tissue is brighter in SI than normal tissue
    - Technical considerations
      - DWI requires strong gradients, and images are low resolution
      - Multishot DWI partially overcomes susceptibility artifact at interfaces in bone
      - DWI data presented as SI or as image map of apparent diffusion coefficient (ADC) from which quantitative measurements of SI can be obtained
      - ADC calculation requires at least 2 acquisitions with different diffusion weightings
      - Low ADC measurement corresponds to high SI (restricted diffusion) and is suspect for pathology
- T1WI C+
  - Extent of enhancement may differentiate processes
    - Normal red marrow enhances by 10%
      - Marrow foci in children may enhance significantly more
    - Stimulated marrow may enhance up to 30%
    - Enhancement > 35% suspicious for marrow infiltration or replacement

- Perceivable marrow enhancement raises concern for pathology but is nonspecific
  - Enhancement expected with marrow replacement by tumor or osteomyelitis
    - Radiographically sclerotic lesions do not invariably enhance (potential false-negative)
  - Reactive marrow edema and fractures enhance
- Other advantages of imaging with contrast
  - Differentiating cystic from solid lesions
  - Locating necrotic regions of lesion
  - Assessing soft tissue involvement
- Technical considerations for T1WI C+
  - Pre- and postcontrast images or fat-saturated images are required
    - Nonfat-saturated T1WI C+ may mask lesions
- Dynamic IV gadolinium to assess bone lesions not yet useful in clinical practice

- Chemical shift (opposed phase) imaging
  - Useful to help differentiate marrow replacement processes from repopulated/regenerated/stimulated red marrow
  - Basis of technique: Detects presence of lipid in lesion by exploiting differences in resonant frequencies of lipid and water
  - Chemical shift imaging of foci of red marrow repopulation/regeneration/stimulation
    - Red marrow foci commingle with fatty marrow
    - "Lesions" ↓ signal at least 20% on out-of-phase imaging
  - Chemical shift imaging of foci of tumor or infection
    - Hypercellular lesions have advancing front that displaces adipocytes
    - Because they lack fat, lesions do not show significant ↓ SI on opposed-phase imaging (often ↑ SI)
  - False-positive lesions on chemical shift imaging
    - Fracture
    - Schmorl node, endplate reactive change
    - Some inflammatory lesions
  - False-negative lesions on chemical shift imaging
    - Sclerotic lesions
    - Occasionally multiple myeloma or lymphoma (contain microscopic regions of fat)
    - Small lesions; volume averaging

Imaging Recommendations

- Best imaging tool
  - T1WI and T2WI fat-saturated or IR MR sequences exquisitely sensitive for foci of abnormal marrow
- Protocol advice
  - Conventional SE T1WI is most useful sequence for detecting hypercellular foci against background of fatty marrow
  - Problem solving: Pre- and postcontrast &/or opposed-phase imaging may allow confident differentiation of benign red marrow deposits from infiltrative foci
    - Use standard T1WI to localize focus to be measured on opposed-phase images
    - Make SI measurements from ROIs on matched in- and out-of-phase images; **eyeballing can be deceptive**

DIFFERENTIAL DIAGNOSIS

Red Marrow Islands

- Normal islands or due to reconversion (hypoxic demand)
- Same low SI on T1WI as marrow replacement
- Contrast imaging or opposed-phase imaging may differentiate from marrow replacement processes

Red Marrow Repopulation

- Rebound from red marrow ablation in chemotherapy
- Severe anemia (sickle cell, thalassemia)
  - Low signal repopulated cell appearance often complicated by infarction, fibrosis
  - Also show low signal hemosiderin deposition in marrow from transfusions

Red Marrow Stimulation

- Granulocyte cell stimulating factor
- May show intense uptake on PET imaging

Mastocytosis or Myelofibrosis

- Processes stimulate reticulin fibrosis
- Low signal on all sequences, usually diffuse

PATHOLOGY

Microscopic Features

- Marrow infiltration: Adipocytes usually admixed
- Marrow replacement: Few or no adipocytes

DIAGNOSTIC CHECKLIST

Consider

- Other imaging, which may solve problematic cases
  - Bone scan to assess for lesion multiplicity
  - PET to assess metabolic activity

Image Interpretation Pearls

- Biopsy more likely to yield diagnostic material of replaced rather than infiltrated marrow
- Soft tissue changes (reticulation of fat, phlegmon, abscess, tract) support diagnosis of osteomyelitis rather than reactive change

Reporting Tips

- ↓ in SI out-of-phase images > 20% **militates** for, but does not **prove**, benignity
  - Clinical context weighed with imaging findings
    - Early manifestation of, or healing response of, metastatic lesion may yield confounding findings

SELECTED REFERENCES

1. Lee EY et al: Bone marrow uptake of indolent non-Hodgkin lymphoma on PET/CT with histopathological correlation. Nucl Med Commun. 36(10):1035-41, 2015
2. Kohl CA et al: Accuracy of chemical shift MR imaging in diagnosing indeterminate bone marrow lesions in the pelvis: review of a single institution's experience. Skeletal Radiol. 43(8):1079-84, 2014
3. Kung JW et al: Bone marrow signal alteration in the extremities. AJR Am J Roentgenol. 196(5):W492-510, 2011
4. Collins MS et al: T1-weighted MRI characteristics of pedal osteomyelitis. AJR Am J Roentgenol. 185(2):386-93, 2005

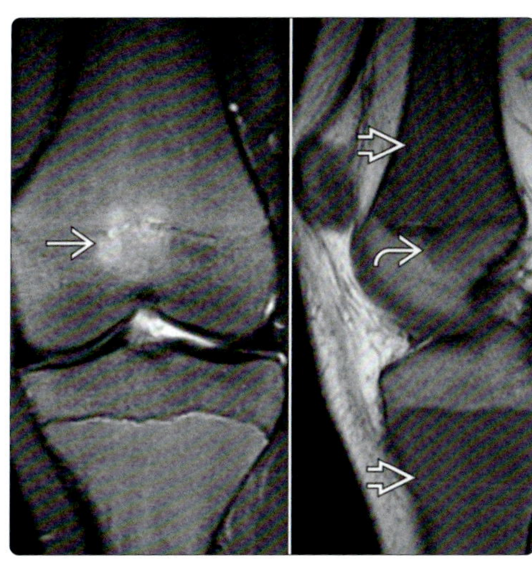

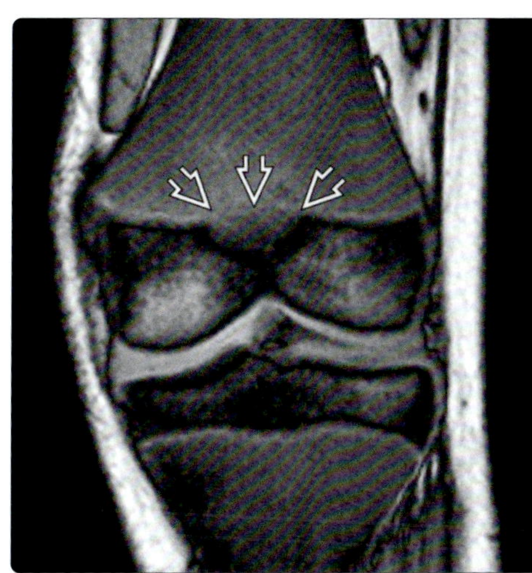

(Left) *Coronal T2WI FS MR (L) shows an indistinctly marginated focus of ↑ SI above the intercondylar notch ➔ in a teenager with treated Burkitt leukemia. Sagittal T1WI MR (R) shows stimulated dense red marrow ➔, as well as the same infiltrative lesion extending into the distal femoral epiphysis ➔.* **(Right)** *Coronal gradient echo image in the same patient demonstrates focal effacement of the trabeculae at the site of the lesion ➔. This finding is nonspecific but suggests an aggressive lesion.*

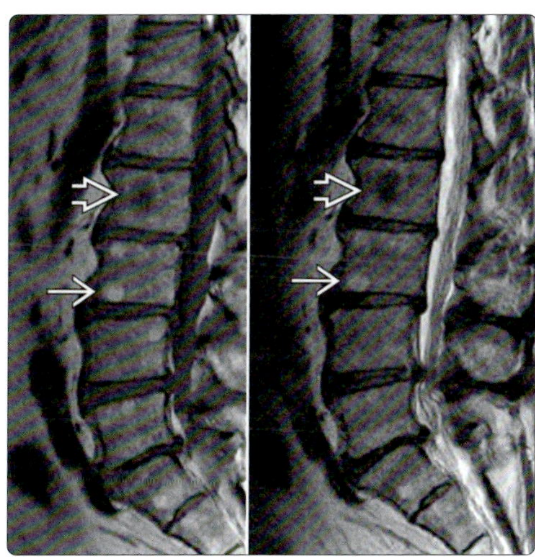

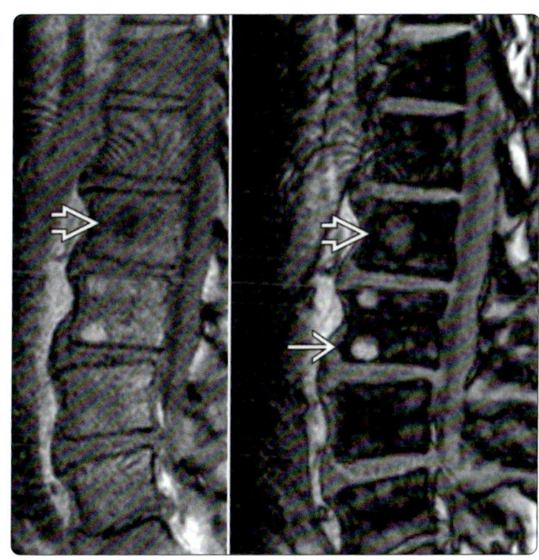

(Left) *Sagittal T1WI MR (L) and T2WI MR (R) show a rounded focus of low T1 and T2 SI in L2 ➔. The lesion was incidentally encountered on a study for low back pain. Note fatty island in L3 ➔.* **(Right)** *Sagittal opposed-phase GRE MR in the same patient shows the L2 focus ➔ has no ↓ in SI between in- (L) and out-of-phase (R) images by ROI measurement. Thus, this focus is unlikely to reflect a red marrow deposit and tumor must be considered. Bulk fatty island in L3 ➔ also does not ↓ SI on opposed phase.*

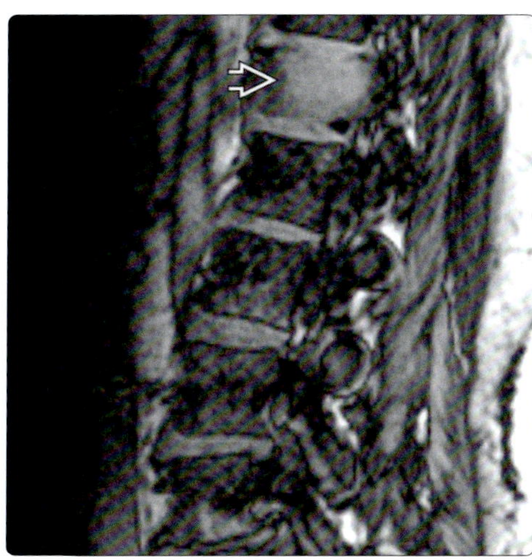

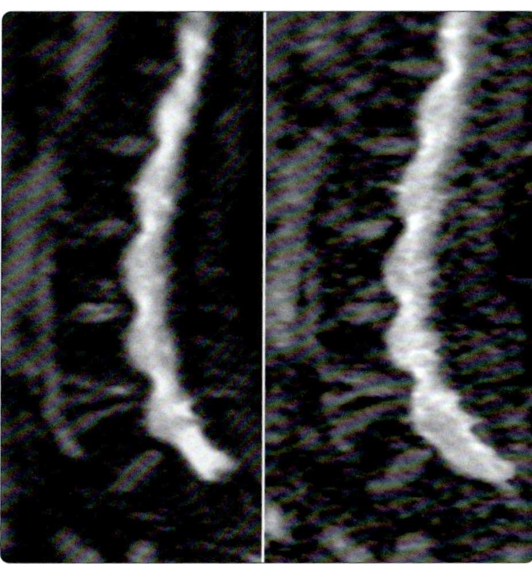

(Left) *Sagittal opposed-phase GRE MR in a patient with a focal myeloma lesion in L1 ➔ demonstrates a rise in SI (compared to in-phase image, not shown). This case shows a true positive, but note that myeloma lesions may be falsely negative on chemical shift sequences.* **(Right)** *Sagittal echoplanar multishot DWI MR shows the lumbar spine in a patient with lymphoma. No lesions were detected on routine MR, nor on the diffusion images (L) or the multiplanar ADC map (R). Diffusion-weighted images are low in resolution.*

SECTION 10

Bone Marrow Edema and Necrosis

Terminology

Osteonecrosis (ON) refers to the death of bone and marrow elements secondary to the loss of blood supply. A number of different terms are used to describe this condition, including **avascular necrosis**, **aseptic necrosis**, **ischemic necrosis**, and **bone infarct**. These terms are used relatively interchangeably since they all refer to necrosis of bone, but location is a factor that tends to differentiate "bone infarct." There are three different locations within bone where necrosis may be seen, including subchondral, within the metaphyseal or diaphyseal regions of long bones remote from the subchondral region, and within the small bones of the hands and feet. The term bone infarct is generally used to refer to the lesions that occur away from the subchondral region, and the other terms in general refer to foci of necrosis in the subchondral region or small bones of the hands and feet. ON of a vertebral body is also known by the name **Kümmel disease**.

Anatomy-Based Imaging Issues

The imaging appearance of ON and bone infarct varies depending on whether it occurs in the small bones of the hands and feet, subchondral region of long bones, or metaphysis and diaphysis of long bones. There are also differences in proposed etiologies at each of these sites.

The MR finding most characteristic of ON (**double line sign)** occurs in the subchondral region and in the metaphyses and diaphyses. The double line sign consists of an outer rim of low signal, usually serpiginous in shape. This line represents demarcation between living bone and necrotic bone. A bright line is located along the inner margin of the low signal line. This line represents the granulation tissue/inflammatory response of the healing process. Internal to the bright line most typically is fatty marrow. However, this marrow will undergo changes throughout the evolution of the infarct.

Initially, the infarcted marrow has a fat-like appearance with increased signal on T1W images, which decreases slightly on T2W images. The marrow then progresses through a hemorrhagic-like phase with bright signal on T1W and T2W images. This phase is not frequently seen with imaging. Next, the marrow has an edema-like appearance with decreased T1W signal and increased signal on T2W images. Lastly, the marrow becomes dark on both T1W and T2W images, indicative of fibrosis and sclerosis.

Infarcts within the metaphyses and diaphyses may come to clinical attention because of pain. More commonly, these are incidental findings either on radiographs or MR. On radiographs, these lesions may mimic other lesions, especially a chondroid lesion. MR may be used to differentiate these processes. The bone infarcts otherwise cause little morbidity, though they may rarely differentiate into malignant fibrous histiocytoma.

Unlike bone infarcts, ON in the subchondral bone can lead to significant morbidity. As healing occurs and bone is resorbed, the remaining bone becomes weakened. Continued stress via weight-bearing leads to characteristic findings of subchondral fracture, articular surface collapse, fragmentation, and secondary osteoarthritis.

Bone collapse and fragmentation are findings in advanced ON in small bones of the hands and feet. However, the MR imaging features leading to this point vary from those seen in subchondral bone. In these small bones, the characteristic double line sign is not typically observed. Rather the MR findings consist of bone marrow edema (↓ T1 and ↑ T2 signal), either focal or diffuse. In advanced stages, low signal is present on both T1W and T2W images. Radiographic findings in these bones may include patchy or diffuse sclerosis, which may progress to fracture, fragmentation, and collapse. One of the key clues to diagnosing subtle ON in these small bones is the location, for example, the lunate or tarsal navicular. Other predisposing factors, such as the correlation of an ulna negative variance with lunate ON, support the diagnosis.

Pathologic Issues

The microscopic appearance of ON does little to reveal the underlying etiology. The appearance is common to all forms of ON and includes empty lacunae, fibrovascular tissue surrounding necrotic bone, and amorphous debris in the marrow space. New bone formation is present at the periphery of the lesion.

A number of different mechanisms have been proposed to explain this condition. The end result of each mechanism is diminished blood flow within a region of bone. Disruption of blood flow may occur at many different levels from the macroscopic to microscopic.

True **vascular disruption** is the mechanism underlying posttraumatic etiologies, such as scaphoid waist fracture. The proximal pole is separated from the blood supply, which enters through the distal pole. A similar mechanism underlies posttraumatic ON of the femoral head. The femoral head and proximal pole of the scaphoid are the number 1 and 2 sites of posttraumatic ON, respectively. **Vasospasm** also contributes to posttraumatic ON. In cases of a dislocated femoral head, there is compression on the smaller vessels. If the compression is not resolved by prompt relocation of the hip, the vasospasm persists, leading to disrupted inflow of blood at the small vessel level.

Sickle cell disease is the typical example of **embolic phenomenon** limiting blood flow. The sickled cells clump within the microvasculature. Lipid emboli from the liver in alcoholism-associated ON and hyperlipidemia associated with corticosteroid use, as well as HIV/AIDS treatments, are additional examples of ON associated with emboli. Caisson disease or dysbaric ON is caused by nitrogen gas bubbles, which occlude blood flow.

Increased marrow pressure diminishes the pressure gradient across the vasculature leading to decreased or absence of blood flow. The conditions associated with this mechanism produce an increase in marrow fat. This is one mechanism for corticosteroid-associated ON (both endogenous and exogenous). Similarly, Gaucher disease with its lipid-laden cells increases marrow pressure. Gaucher disease is also accompanied by **vasospasm** 2° to vascular irritation, further limiting blood flow.

Vasculitis will disrupt blood flow by **diminishing vessel size**. Treatment of this condition with steroids may further increase the risk for ON.

In the small bones of the hands and feet, especially the lunate, tarsal navicular, and 2nd metatarsal head, the proposed mechanism is **chronic repetitive trauma**. While the changes in these bones are usually classified as ON, the etiology is likely multifactorial. Chronic trauma may produce microfractures, which weaken bone. The trauma itself, as well as associated fractures, likely lead to marrow edema, which then inhibits blood flow.

Pathology-Based Imaging Issues

The real pathology of ON is related to the healing process. Initially, dead bone is as strong as living bone. The process of healing includes "walling off" the dead bone by forming a fibrotic, and eventually sclerotic, margin at the interface between living and dead bone. From this interface there is an advancing front of granulation tissue. Osteoblasts rim the dead bone and their job is to produce new, healthy bone. Osteoclasts are responsible for resorbing the underlying dead bone. The problems arise as the body starts to remove the dead bone as part of this healing process. It is this activity that weakens bone, leading to the subchondral fractures and eventual articular surface collapse and fragmentation with subsequent secondary osteoarthritis.

The goal of imaging and treatment should be to identify ON before it undergoes the irreversible changes. Radiographic and MR classification systems have been developed to accurately describe the progression of ON. The lag is on the clinical side in terms of finding an appropriate treatment, which will either reverse the process of ischemia &/or support the bone through the healing process. While interventions, such as vascularized fibular grafts, for treatment of femoral head ON theoretically would fit the bill, they have had less than overwhelming success in the clinical arena.

Imaging Protocols

Radiographs

The number and type of views will vary with the anatomic site being imaged. The underlying radiographic principle of 2 orthogonal views remains relevant. Many findings, including articular surface collapse, may only be visible on a single view. For example, the crescentic fracture of the femoral head is often better seen on frog lateral view compared to the AP view.

MR

Imaging sequences should include, at minimum, T1W and fluid-sensitive images. T1W images provide excellent visualization of fat marrow within the infarct. T2W images are best for visualizing the pathognomonic double line sign. Contrast enhancement may be used to confirm devascularization. Avascular regions of bone will fail to enhance after contrast administration. Application of this principle, however, is not widely accepted. In general, if a bone does not enhance, it is avascular; however, the presence of enhancement does not preclude the development of complications of ON. The time frame for development of imaging-related changes is unknown and has been proposed to be as long as six months after the insult.

Identification of findings, especially articular surface collapse, is not equal for all imaging planes. In most sites, axial images will be least sensitive to articular surface collapse since this plane is along the short axis of the bone. Sagittal and coronal images oriented to the long axis of bone will best depict these abnormalities.

Bone scan

Delayed images can identify avascular bone in its early phases. Avascular bone will appear "cold" due to lack of radioisotope uptake. This finding is easiest to recognize in the large femoral head as compared to the small bones of the hand and feet. It really is not applicable to bone infarcts in the metaphyses or diaphyses. As healing progresses, uptake will occur in the ischemic bone, diminishing sensitivity after the earliest stages.

Clinical Implications

The greatest clinical implication of ON is the morbidity caused by the articular surface fracture, fragmentation, and collapse with secondary osteoarthritis. Up to 10% of all total hip replacements are performed for treatment of ON-associated ostearthritis. The pain and functional limitations associated with lunate or scaphoid ON can be significant.

Exogenous steroid use is a major contributor to the development of ON and bone infarcts. Approximately 2% of all patients using steroids will develop ON, and, interestingly, the risk is greater with short-term high doses as compared to chronic low-dose treatment. Renal transplant patients who receive steroids are at extremely high risk; over 40% of these patients will develop ON and bone infarcts. Another high-risk group is the bone marrow transplant population; 10% will develop ON and bone infarcts.

A number of different systemic conditions are associated with a high risk of ON and bone infarct. Such populations include patients with lupus. The underlying vasculitis and steroid treatment both increase risk. Patients with sickle cell disease are at risk and those with sickle cell thalassemia are at an even higher risk. Morphologic abnormalities, such as developmental dysplasia of the hip, and patients with previous slipped capital femoral epiphysis, have increased incidence of ON relative to the normal patient population.

Differential Diagnosis

Bone marrow edema is a nonspecific finding and may be the earliest manifestation of ON. In the femoral head, femoral condyles, and humeral head, there is an extensive differential diagnosis, which includes transient osteoporosis (especially in the lower extremity) as well as infection and neoplasm. Correlation with patient history, including patient age and gender, is crucial. The underlying etiology will usually declare itself over time.

Insufficiency fractures may also be confused with ON. This confusion is best described by reviewing the condition formerly known as SONK or spontaneous ON (of the knee). Previously thought to be a result of ischemia, this disease has several features that are atypical of ON of the knee. SONK is most commonly seen in elderly women with no risk factors for ON. These patients fall into the population at high risk for osteoporosis. Features that differentiate insufficiency fracture from ON include (1) the clinical profile: Patients with insufficiency fractures have no risk factors and are typically elderly women, (2) the lack of double line sign on T2W images, and (3) insufficiency fractures are directly seen with careful examination of the MR and are often concave to the articular surface, while subchondral crescent fractures of ON parallel the articular surface. Features common to both conditions include articular surface collapse, fragmentation, and 2° osteoarthritis.

Selected References

1. Lee GC et al: How do radiologists evaluate osteonecrosis? Skeletal Radiol. 43(5):607-14, 2014
2. Murphey MD et al: From the radiologic pathology archives imaging of osteonecrosis: radiologic-pathologic correlation. Radiographics. 34(4):1003-28, 2014

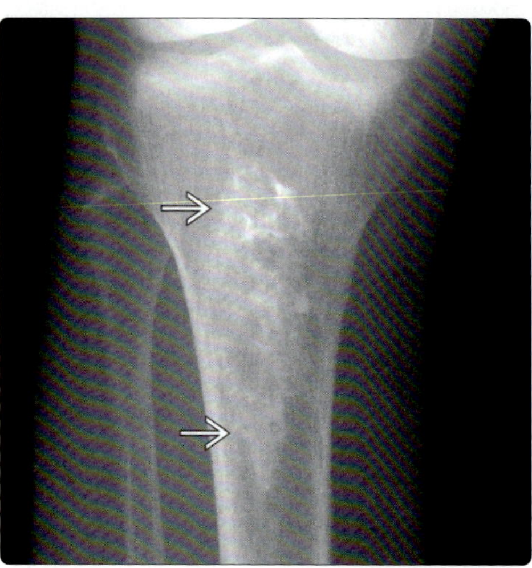

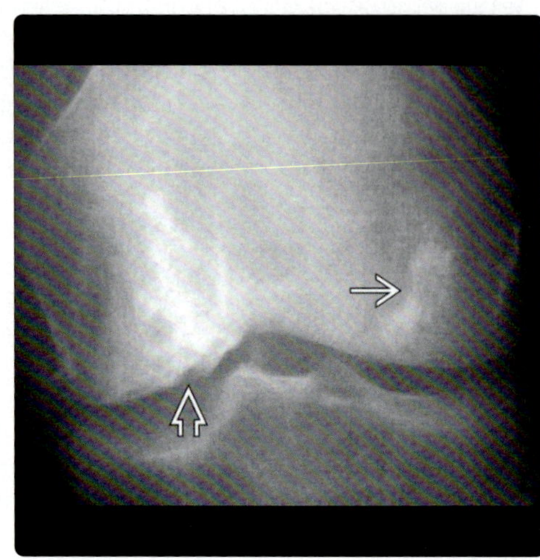

(Left) *AP radiograph shows a typical bone infarct, which appears as serpiginous sclerosis in the metadiaphyseal region of a long bone* ➡. **(Right)** *AP radiograph of a patient with osteonecrosis (ON) of the femoral condyles is shown. The lateral lesion shows the typical serpiginous sclerosis* ➡. *The medial lesion is more advanced with irregularity of the articular surface* ➡. *Once this stage has been reached, the lesion is irreversible; osteoarthritis is likely and may require eventual surgical intervention.*

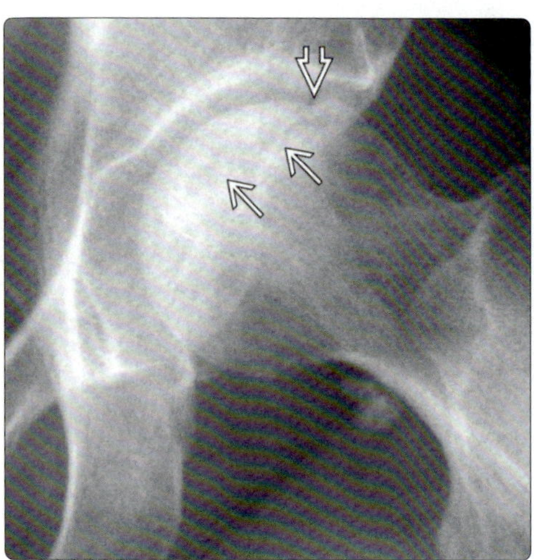

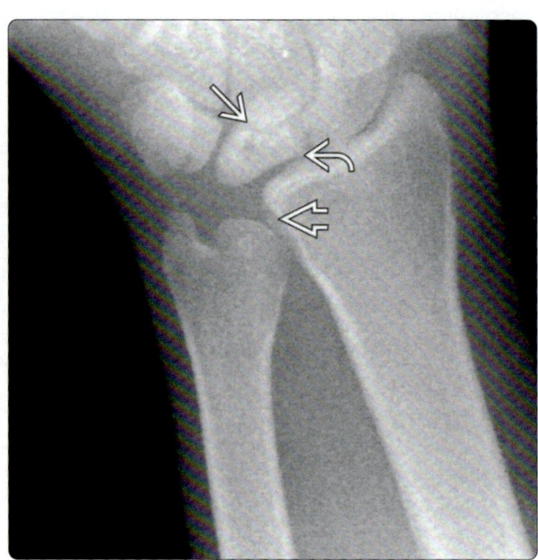

(Left) *AP radiograph shows a hip with stage IV ON. A subchondral crescentic fracture is present* ➡ *and is accompanied by articular surface collapse* ➡. **(Right)** *AP radiograph of a painful wrist shows a negative ulnar variance is present* ➡. *This alignment alters the mechanics through the wrist, placing increased stress on the lunate. In this case, there is advanced lunatomalacia. Changes include patchy sclerosis* ➡ *and collapse, especially along the proximal articular surface* ➡.

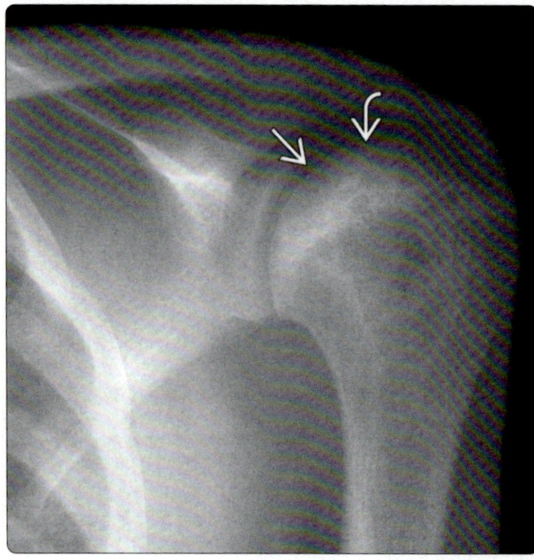

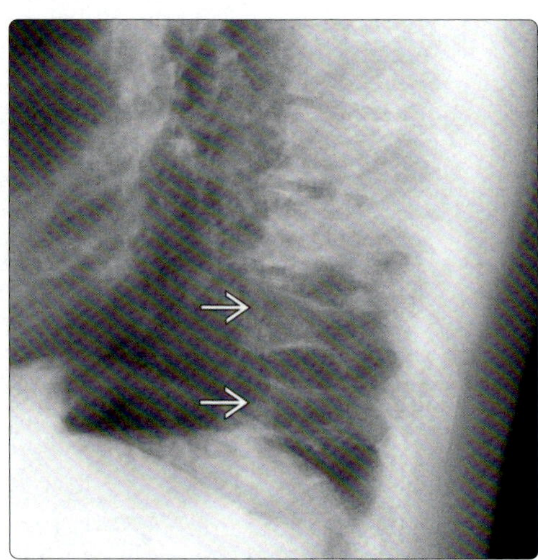

(Left) *AP radiograph shows the shoulder of a patient with sickle cell disease. Patchy sclerosis is present throughout the epiphysis of the proximal humerus* ➡ *with subtle collapse of the articular surface* ➡. *The findings are characteristic of ON.* **(Right)** *Lateral radiograph of the spine in the same patient shows the characteristic H-shaped vertebral bodies* ➡ *of ON in sickle cell disease. Central collapse of the endplate results from ON in the subchondral bone and is most commonly associated with the hemoglobinopathies.*

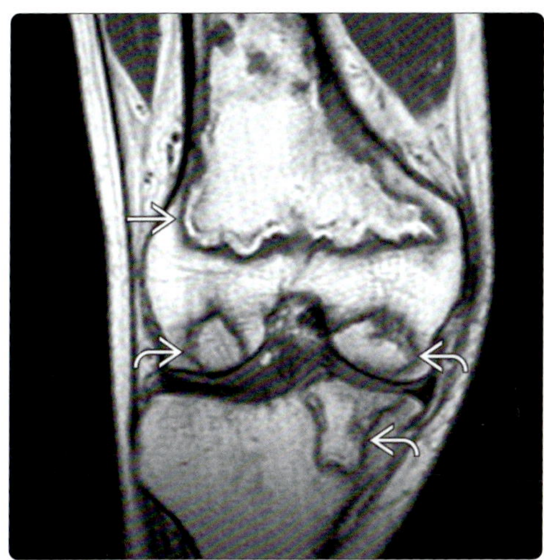

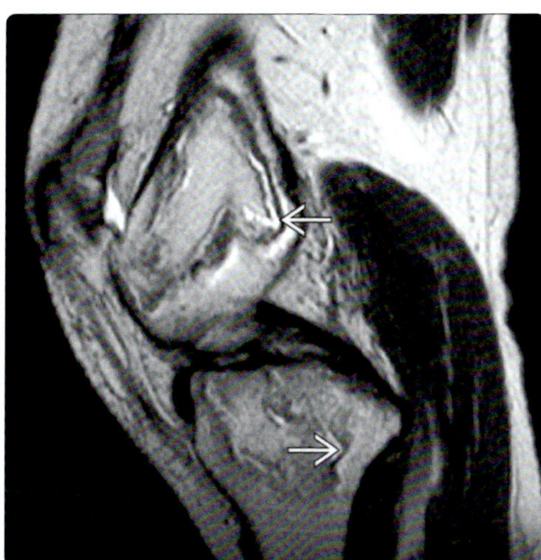

(Left) *Coronal T1WI MR shows classic ON and bone infarcts. Serpiginous low signal geographic abnormalities are present in the femoral metaphysis* → *and subchondral bone of both the femur and tibia* ↷. *The internal marrow signal on T1 is relatively maintained, differentiating this appearance of infarct from tumor.* **(Right)** *Sagittal T2WI MR of the same knee shows the classic double line sign* →, *which consists of a low signal peripheral line with an internal line of bright signal.*

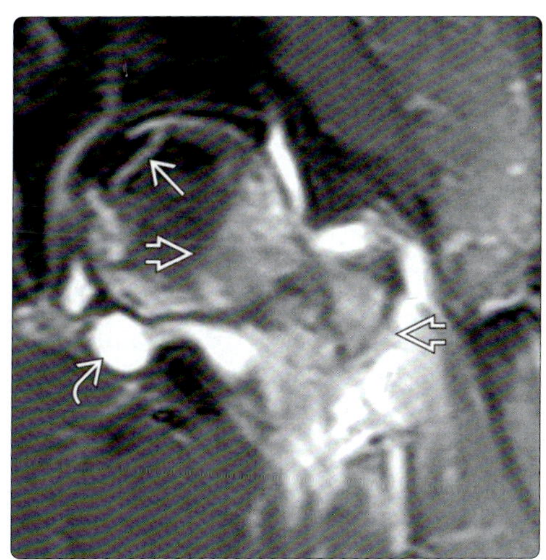

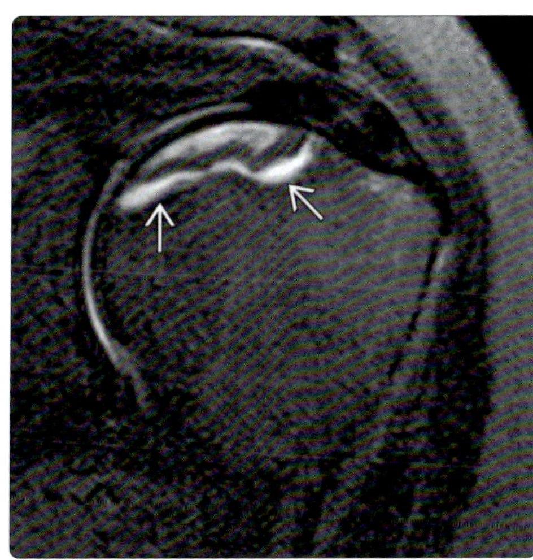

(Left) *Coronal STIR MR shows a subchondral crescentic fracture in a focus of avascular necrosis* →. *Extensive marrow edema* ⇨ *extends from the head into the neck and is accompanied by joint effusion* ↷. *This pattern of marrow edema has been correlated with pain. Joint effusion has not.* **(Right)** *Coronal MR arthrogram T1WI FS shows contrast material tracking within a subchondral fracture* →. *This fracture often marks the point of irreversible disease and usually continues to articular surface collapse.*

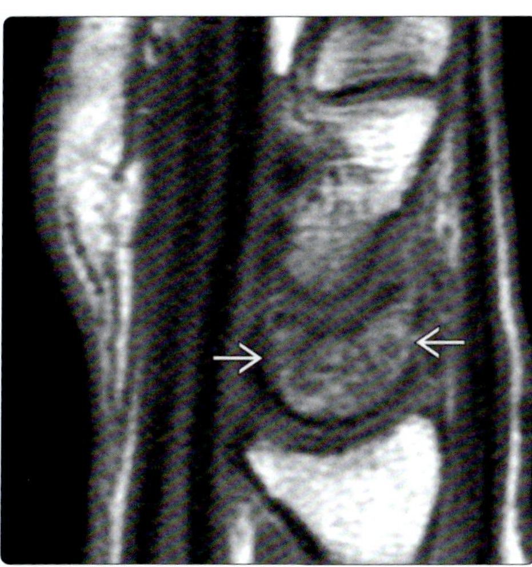

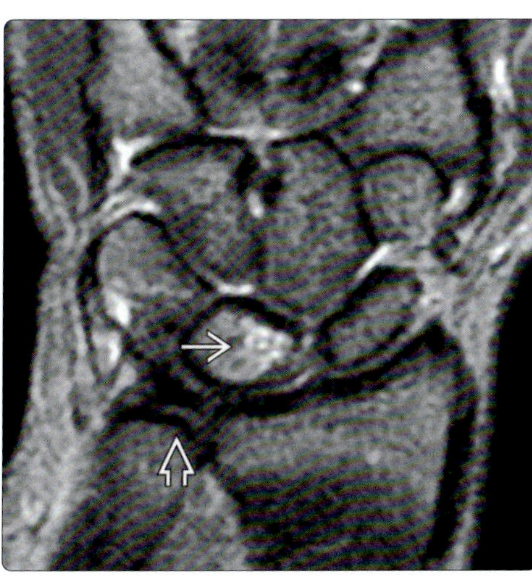

(Left) *Sagittal T1WI MR reveals marrow edema throughout the lunate* →. *While nonspecific, the possibility of ON should be considered.* **(Right)** *Coronal T2WI FS MR of the same patient shows an ulna negative variance* ⇨, *which predisposes to lunate ON. Marrow edema is again noted in the lunate* → *without fracture, articular surface collapse, or fragmentation. Correction of the ulna minus may lead to reversal of the lunate changes at this stage.*

Transient Bone Marrow Edema and Regional Migratory Osteoporosis

KEY FACTS

TERMINOLOGY

- Transient bone marrow edema syndrome: Painful bone marrow edema centered around joints; of unknown etiology and self-limited
  - Transient regional osteoporosis (TRO): Likely subset of transient bone marrow edema syndrome that shows bone marrow edema and osteoporosis
  - Regional migratory osteoporosis: TRO that shows migratory pattern
  - Transient osteoporosis of hip: TRO, specifically of hip (most common location)

IMAGING

- Lower extremity: Proximal femur > distal femur
- Diagnosis of TRO **requires** combined MR and radiographic findings: Marrow edema and osteoporosis, respectively
  - Femoral head marrow edema
    - ↓ T1W, ↑ T2W signal
    - Variable extension into femoral neck, ± involvement of acetabulum
  - Osteopenia within 8 weeks after onset of symptoms
- Changes of irreversible disease absent (subchondral curvilinear low T1 signal; articular surface irregularity)
- May have small joint effusion; adjacent soft tissue changes usually minimal or absent

TOP DIFFERENTIAL DIAGNOSES

- Bone marrow edema pattern
- Osteonecrosis
- Septic joint

PATHOLOGY

- Etiology unknown; self-limited

CLINICAL ISSUES

- Male > female
- Severe pain develops over days

(Left) *Coronal T1WI MR shows bone marrow edema through right femoral head extending into femoral neck ➔. Subchondral linear low signal and irregularity of articular surface are absent.* **(Right)** *AP radiograph from the same patient shows diffuse osteopenia of femoral head. There is poor definition of the cortical bone of the articular surface ➔. Acetabulum is unaffected, and the joint space is preserved. Diagnosis of transient osteoporosis of the hip requires both MR and radiographic findings, as in this case.*

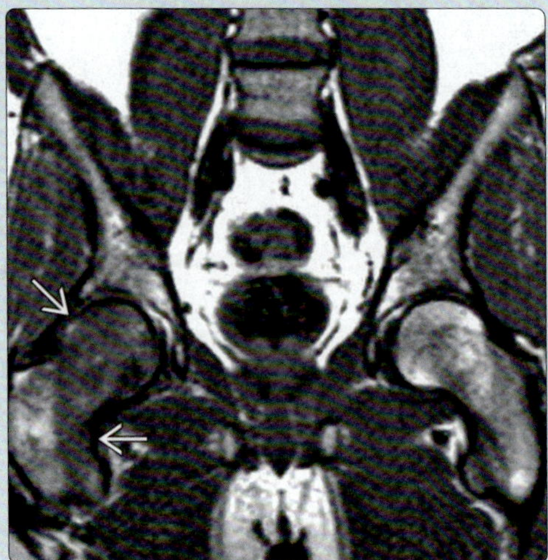

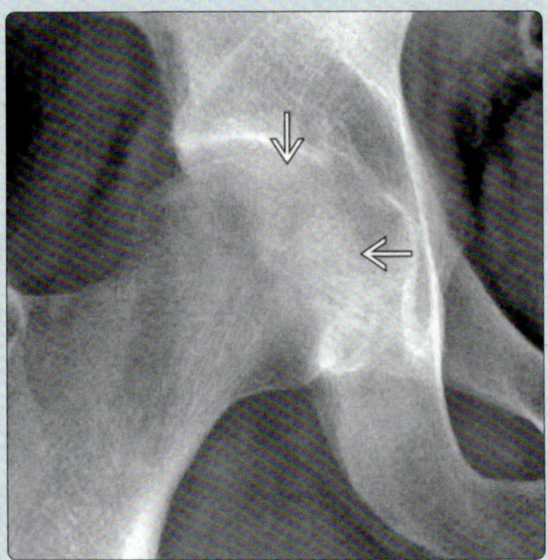

(Left) *Axial T2WI FS MR of a patient with regional migratory osteoporosis shows extensive marrow edema in lateral femoral condyle ➔, and mild soft tissues changes are seen ➔.* **(Right)** *Coronal T2W FS MR of the same patient several months later is shown. Pattern of edema has shifted, with less extensive changes laterally ➔ and new edema medially ➔ and in the proximal tibia ➔. Regional migratory osteoporosis may migrate from one joint to another, or as in this case, from one location to another in the same joint.*

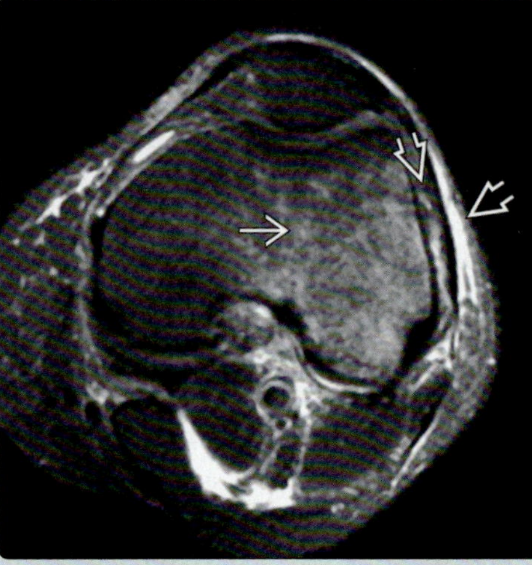

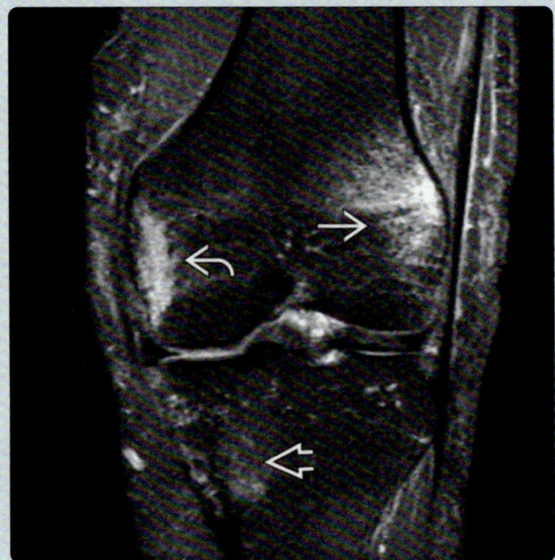

TERMINOLOGY

Definitions

- Transient bone marrow edema syndrome: Painful bone marrow edema centered around joints; of unknown etiology and self-limited
  - Transient regional osteoporosis (TRO): Likely subset of transient bone marrow edema syndrome that shows bone marrow edema and radiographic osteoporosis
    - Regional migratory osteoporosis: TRO that shows migratory pattern
    - Transient osteoporosis of hip (TOH): TRO, specifically of hip (most common location)

IMAGING

General Features

- Best diagnostic clue
  - Radiograph: Osteopenia of femoral head and neck within 8 weeks after onset of pain
  - MR: Edema pattern; highly sensitive but nonspecific
- Location
  - Lower extremity: Proximal femur > distal femur
  - Favors left hip in pregnant women
- Morphology
  - No morphologic changes: Presence of such indicates other etiology or complication by fracture

Imaging Recommendations

- Best imaging tool
  - Diagnosis of TRO **requires** combined MR and radiographic findings
- Protocol advice
  - Timing of imaging essential to making diagnosis
    - If too early, may not identify crucial osteopenia
    - ± follow-up MR to exclude osteonecrosis (ON), especially if osteopenia never develops

Radiographic Findings

- To confirm diagnosis of TOH, must have osteopenia within 8 weeks after onset of symptoms
- Osteopenia manifests as marked thinning or complete loss of femoral head cortex, trabecular thinning
  - No aggressive changes (bone destruction, ↓ joint space)
  - No arthritic changes (↓ joint space, erosions, cysts)

MR Findings

- Femoral head marrow edema
  - ↓ T1W, ↑ T2W signal; enhancement with contrast, peak enhancement may be delayed
  - Does not involve entire subchondral region
    - Portions of femoral head/neck/greater trochanter may exhibit completely normal signal
  - ± involvement of acetabulum
- No changes indicating irreversibility
  - Subchondral low signal; articular surface irregularity
- May have small joint effusion
- Adjacent soft tissue changes usually minimal or absent

Bone Scan Findings

- Increased uptake; nonspecific

DIFFERENTIAL DIAGNOSIS

Bone Marrow Edema Pattern

- Nonspecific descriptor applied to MR imaging pattern; extensive differential diagnosis includes TOH, early ON, infection, neoplasm

Osteonecrosis

- Marrow edema and effusion may be 1st manifestation
- Important to differentiate in follow-up, since ON may require early intervention to preserve joint integrity

Septic Joint

- Radiographically presents with osteoporosis and effusion
- MR more likely to have extensive soft tissue changes, limited osseous changes
- If advanced, cartilage is destroyed; bony erosions

PATHOLOGY

General Features

- Etiology
  - Unknown; self-limited

Gross Pathologic & Surgical Features

- Elevated pressure within bone marrow
- Normal articular cartilage and cortex
- Effusion and synovial inflammation

Microscopic Features

- Edema, reactive new bone formation

CLINICAL ISSUES

Presentation

- Most common signs/symptoms
  - Severe pain develops over days
  - Resolves over weeks to months

Demographics

- Age
  - 2nd, 3rd decades; may occur in children
- Gender
  - Initially described in pregnant females, yet more common in middle-aged men

Natural History & Prognosis

- Self-limited, usually reversing after several months; imaging returns to normal
- May be migratory, involving another joint (usually hip or knee) or another location within same joint
- May be complicated by insufficiency fracture

Treatment

- Conservative; protected weight-bearing
- For debilitating pain, core decompression has been suggested; shown to shorten course of disease

SELECTED REFERENCES

1. Joshi V et al: Painless transient bone marrow edema syndrome in a pediatric patient. Skeletal Radiol. 43(11):1615-9, 2014
2. Korompilias AV et al: Bone marrow edema syndrome. Skeletal Radiol. 38(5):425-36, 2009

Bone Infarct

KEY FACTS

TERMINOLOGY

- Bone infarct, osteonecrosis, avascular necrosis, aseptic necrosis (terms may be used interchangeably)
  - By convention, term bone infarct is used when lesion is not in subchondral location

IMAGING

- Classic uncomplicated infarct
  - Serpiginous or amorphous sclerosis on radiograph
  - Double line sign on MR
    - Outer rim of low signal, usually serpiginous (demarcation between living and necrotic bone)
    - Inner margin of bright line (granulation tissue/inflammatory response of healing)
    - Internal signal usually fat
- Wide range of other appearances, depending on stage of infarct or repair process or degeneration
  - Initially appears normal
  - Early infarct of digits may demonstrate periostitis
  - Over time may develop abnormal density with various patterns
- Cystic degeneration: Uncommon
- Rarely develop sarcomatous degeneration
  - Change in character from benign-appearing lesion to highly aggressive lytic lesion with cortical breakthrough and soft tissue mass
  - Usually transforms to malignant fibrous histiocytoma

PATHOLOGY

- Many patients have no predisposing factors, and infarcts considered idiopathic
- Sickle cell disease is strong predisposing factor
- Steroid use predisposes to bone infarct

DIAGNOSTIC CHECKLIST

- Although serpiginous pattern of calcification is classic finding, other radiographic appearances of infarct occur frequently and may mimic other diseases
  - MR usually definitive

(Left) *Lateral x-ray shows the typical serpiginous pattern of dystrophic calcification in bone infarcts of the calcaneus* ➡ *and distal tibia* ➡*. This is not the punctate calcification seen in enchondroma; the multiplicity of lesions also invokes the diagnosis of bone infarcts.* **(Right)** *Lateral x-ray shows a predominantly lytic lesion occupying the distal humeral diaphysis, causing mild cortical scalloping* ➡*. There is a focal region of punctate calcification* ➡*. This could represent either enchondroma or bone island; diagnosis was the latter.*

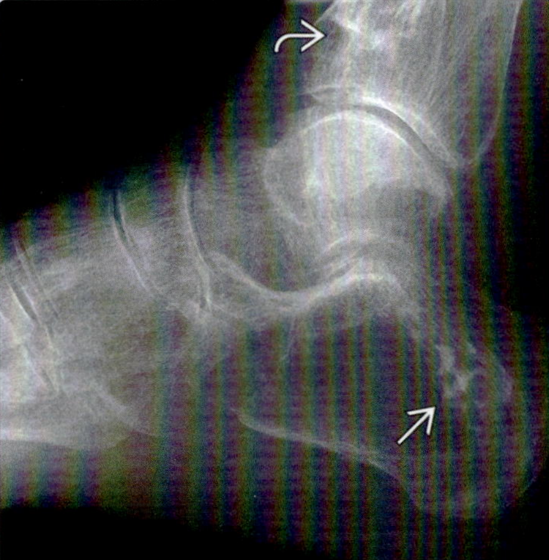

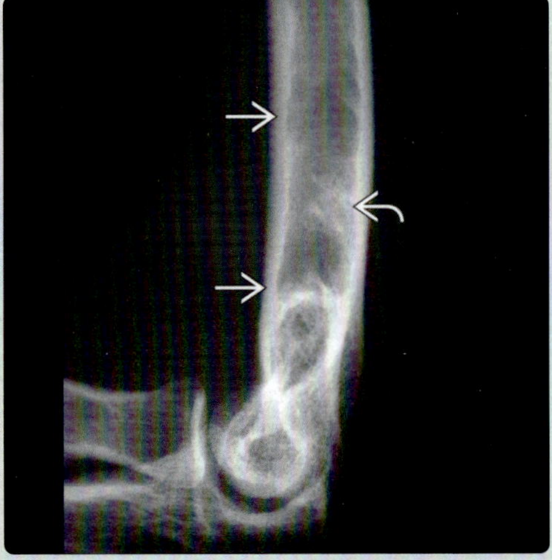

(Left) *Lateral radiograph shows subtle punctate calcification* ➡ *with adjacent region of disturbed trabeculae* ➡*. This lesion could represent either enchondroma or bone infarct.* **(Right)** *Lateral radiograph in the same patient, 2 years later, shows a more clear-cut serpiginous pattern typical of bone infarct* ➡*. Remember that the appearance of bone infarct may change as it evolves. There is also a subchondral infarct, more conventionally termed osteonecrosis, within the femoral condyle* ➡*.*

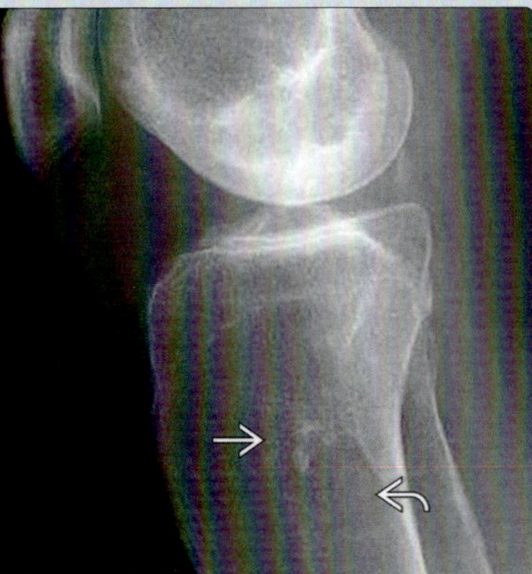

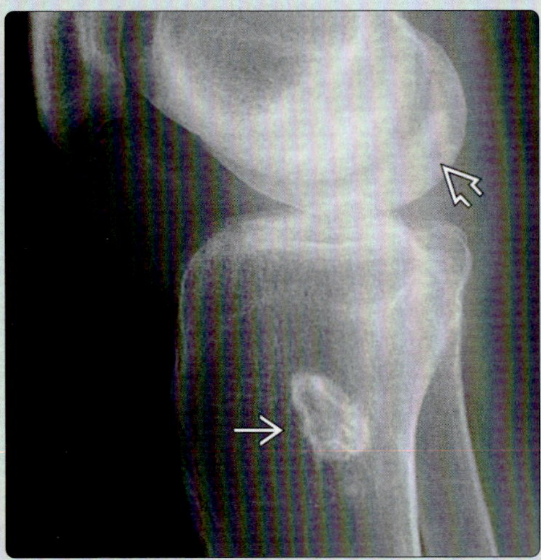

TERMINOLOGY

Synonyms

- Osteonecrosis, avascular necrosis, aseptic necrosis
  - Terms used interchangeably; all refer to necrosis of bone
  - By convention, term bone infarct used when lesion is not in subchondral location

Definitions

- Death of bone and marrow secondary to loss of blood supply

IMAGING

General Features

- Best diagnostic clue
  - Classic uncomplicated infarct
    - Serpiginous or amorphous sclerosis on radiograph
    - Double line sign on MR
  - Wide range of other appearances, depending on repair process or evolution of infarct
- Location
  - Long bones, metaphyseal or diaphyseal locations
  - Less frequently, flat bones

Radiographic Findings

- Wide range, depending on stage of infarct or repair process or degeneration
  - Initially appears normal
  - Early infarct of digits may demonstrate periostitis
  - May develop abnormal density with various patterns
    - Patchy or diffuse sclerosis
    - Serpiginous dystrophic calcification
  - Cystic degeneration: Uncommon
    - Mild expansion of involved region of bone
    - Cysts may develop thin, sclerotic rim
  - Rarely develop sarcomatous degeneration
    - Change in character from benign appearing lesion to highly aggressive lytic lesion with cortical breakthrough and soft tissue mass
    - Transformation usually to malignant fibrous histiocytoma

MR Findings

- Uncomplicated bone infarct
  - Double line sign on fluid-sensitive sequences
    - Outer rim of low signal, usually serpiginous (demarcation between living and necrotic bone)
    - Inner margin of bright line (granulation tissue/inflammatory response of healing)
  - Internal signal variable
    - Usually fat (high signal on T1WI, slightly low on T2WI, saturates out on fat-saturated sequences)
    - 2nd phase is hemorrhagic and infrequently seen (bright signal on both T1WI and T2WI sequences)
    - Next phase is edema-like signal (low signal on T1WI, high signal on T2WI)
    - With fibrosis and sclerosis of marrow, it is dark on both T1WI and T2WI sequences
- Dystrophic calcification → low signal on all sequences
  - May be serpiginous or focal, punctate
- Cystic degeneration: Uncommon
  - Decreased signal on T1WI
  - Heterogeneously bright on T2WI
  - Postcontrast imaging shows well-defined, enhancing rim surrounding low signal fluid
- Transformation to sarcoma
  - Change in character in portion of lesion
  - Cortical breakthrough with soft tissue mass
  - T2 hyperintense, heterogeneous
  - Postcontrast shows enhancement and regions of necrosis

Nuclear Medicine Findings

- Bone scan
  - "Cold" spot in bone early in process
  - As healing progresses, variably increased uptake

DIFFERENTIAL DIAGNOSIS

Bone Marrow Edema

- If early stage of infarct, without dystrophic calcification or double line sign

Marrow Replacement Processes, Diffuse or Focal

- If early stage of infarct, without dystrophic calcification or double line sign

PATHOLOGY

General Features

- Etiology
  - Diminished blood flow to bone with various etiologies
    - Embolic phenomenon: Sickle cell disease, lipid emboli
    - Increased marrow pressure: Steroids, Gaucher disease
    - Diminished vessel size: Vasculitis
  - Many patients have no predisposing factors, and infarcts considered idiopathic

CLINICAL ISSUES

Presentation

- Most common signs/symptoms
  - Usually incidental findings on radiograph or MR
  - May present with dull pain
  - Sickle cell patients may present with intense limb pain

Natural History & Prognosis

- Most metaphyseal or diaphyseal infarcts do not change and are inconsequential
- May develop cystic degeneration, also inconsequential
- Rare degeneration of bone infarct to osseous sarcoma
  - Usually malignant fibrous histiocytoma
  - 60% around knee
  - 1/3 have identifiable etiology for infarct
  - 2-year disease-free survival in range of 60%

Treatment

- No treatment of uncomplicated bone infarct

SELECTED REFERENCES

1. Inusa BP et al: Dilemma in differentiating between acute osteomyelitis and bone infarction in children with sickle cell disease: the role of ultrasound. PLoS One. 8(6):e65001, 2013

(Left) *Lateral radiograph shows a metadiaphyseal abnormality that includes dense sclerosis ➡, as well as areas of punctate calcification ➡. One might consider enchondroma vs. bone infarct for the diagnosis.* **(Right)** *Coronal T1 MR, same case, shows the serpiginous ➡ low-signal pattern of bone infarct, with fatty marrow in its center ➡, along with more punctate low-signal foci ➡ corresponding to that seen on the radiograph. The appearance is diagnostic of bone infarct.*

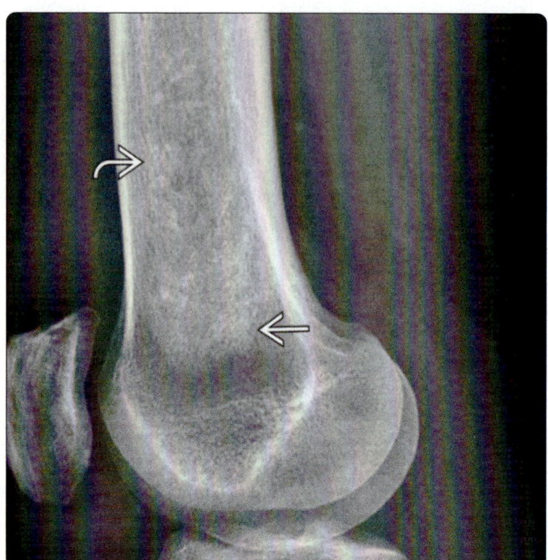

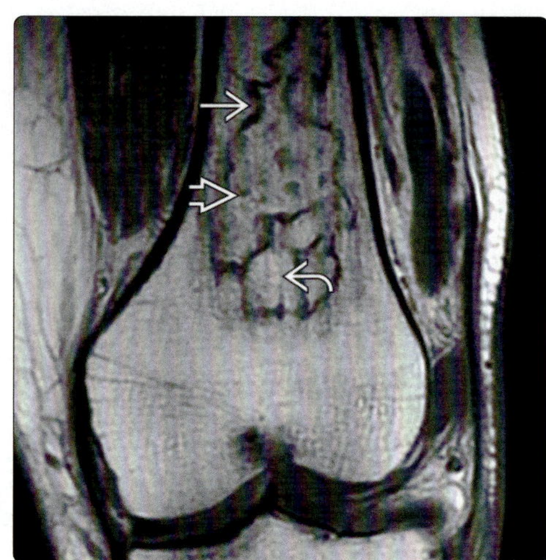

(Left) *Coronal T2FS MR, same case, shows the serpiginous high-signal rim ➡; the low signal surrounding the high signal is not well seen because of the fat saturation. However, it is present ➡, and this constitutes a double line sign of bone infarct.* **(Right)** *AP x-ray shows a lytic lesion within the femoral diaphysis ➡. There is no sclerotic margin and no dystrophic calcification. While this could represent intraosseous lipoma, biopsy proved bone infarct. A completely lytic lesion is an uncommon appearance of infarct.*

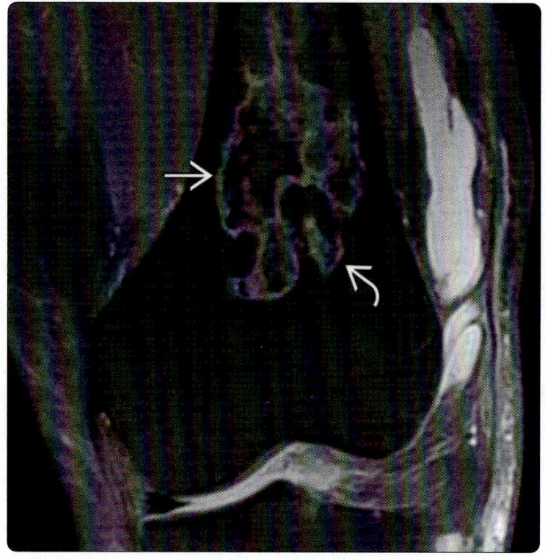

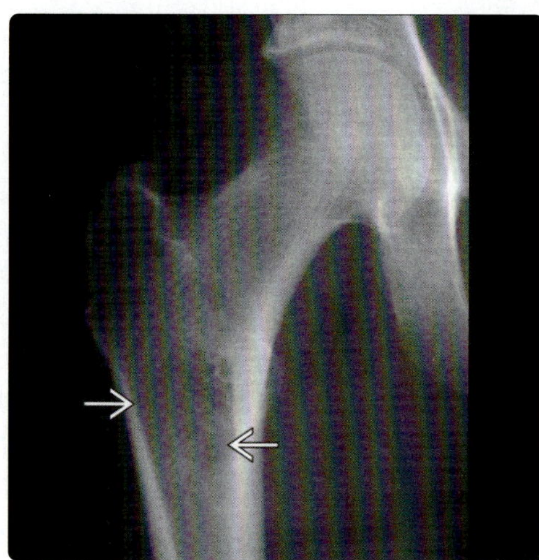

(Left) *AP x-ray in a patient with sickle cell anemia shows diffuse patchy areas of increased ➡ and decreased density. Although diagnosis of bone infarcts is often based on the presence of serpiginous calcification, frequently they present simply as diffuse patchy sclerosis.* **(Right)** *Sagittal T2WI FS MR shows typical pattern of multiple bone infarcts with a double line pattern ➡. This patient had Rocky Mountain spotted fever, which may result in necrotizing vasculitis, in turn resulting in osseous infarction.*

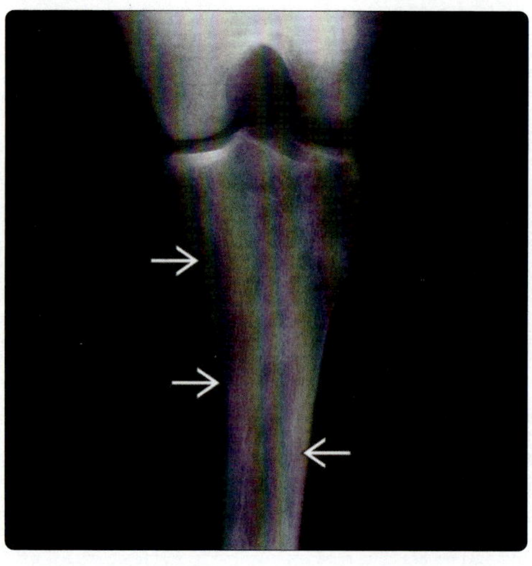

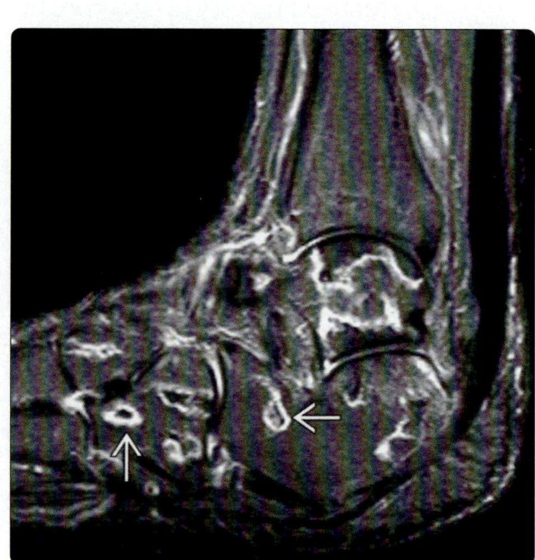

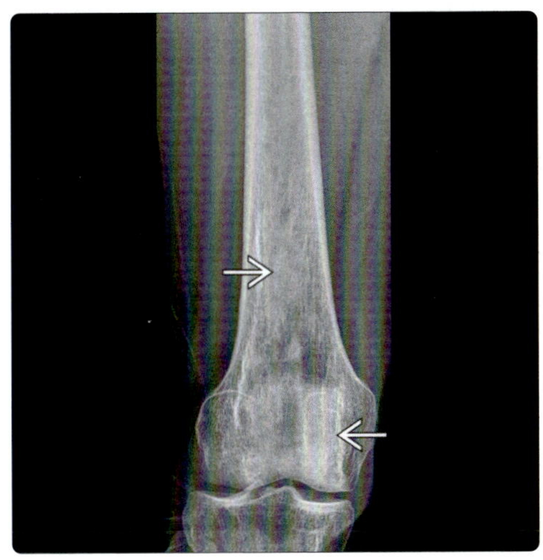

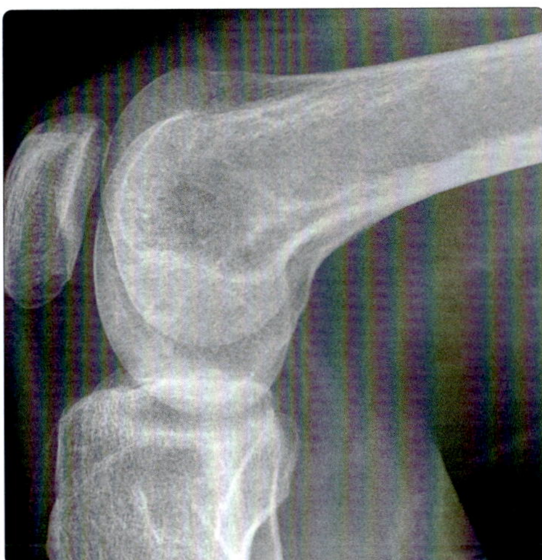

(Left) *AP radiograph shows diffuse inhomogeneous sclerosis ➡ in the metadiaphysis, extending into the subchondral region in a patient who is dependent on steroids. Although there is no serpiginous pattern seen on this radiograph, the distribution and density makes bone infarct the most likely diagnosis.* **(Right)** *Lateral radiograph, same patient, shows the diffuse abnormalities in density to be more subtle.*

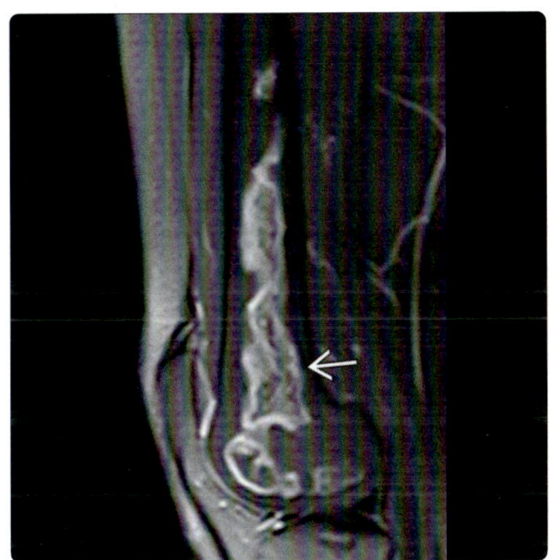

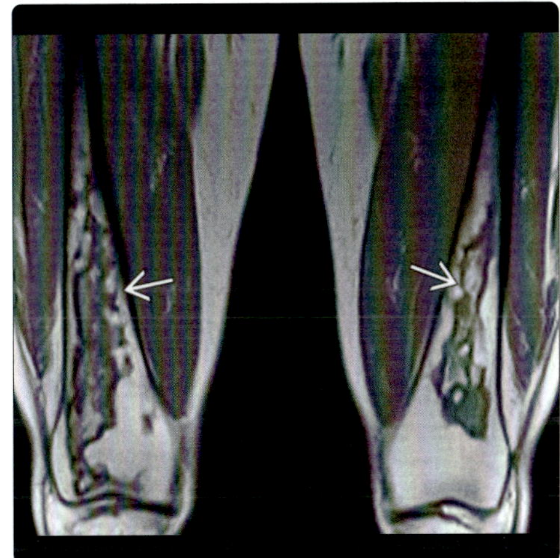

(Left) *Sagittal T2FS MR, same patient, shows the double line sign ➡ and serpiginous pattern typical of bone infarct. The infarcts involve the subchondral region as well as the metadiaphysis, although no articular collapse is seen at this time.* **(Right)** *Coronal T1 MR, same case, shows the bone infarcts to involve both femoral diaphyses extensively ➡. Of all bone infarcts, 1/3 have a diagnosable etiology; among these, chronic steroid use is common.*

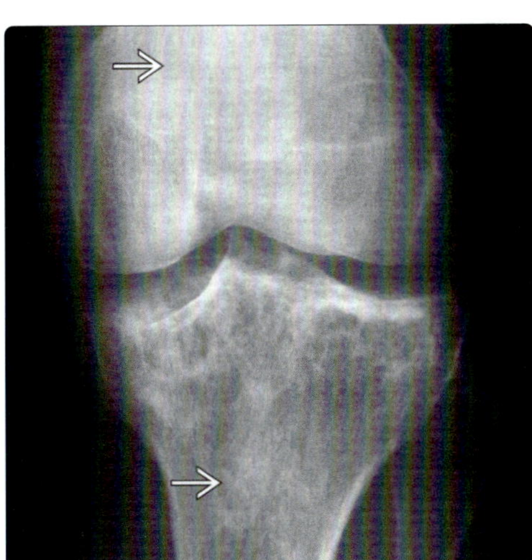

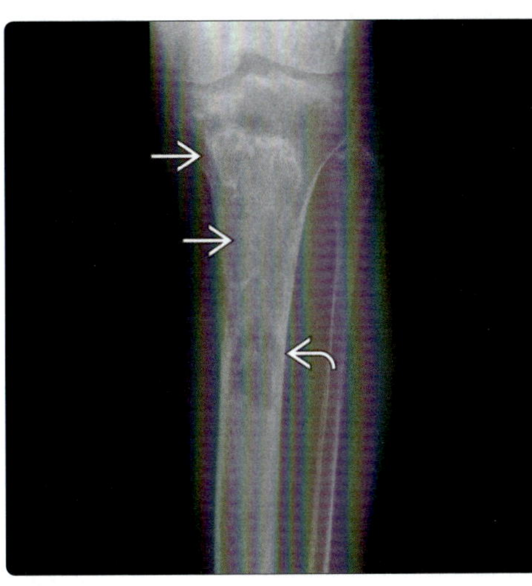

(Left) *AP x-ray shows patchy sclerosis within the metaphyses of the tibia and femur ➡. This is not serpiginous but is 1 pattern of abnormal density in bone infarct. This patient has polymyositis, treated with steroids.* **(Right)** *AP x-ray shows serpiginous calcification ➡ in the metadiaphysis, typical of bone infarct. More distally, there is a more aggressive lytic lesion ⮫ extending from the bone infarct; this proved to be malignant fibrous histiocytoma, a rare complication of bone infarct.*

KEY FACTS

TERMINOLOGY

- Necrosis of cellular elements of bone secondary to ischemia

IMAGING

- Early radiographs: Patchy sclerosis femoral head
- Late radiographs: Irregularity, fragmentation, collapse of femoral head articular surface; secondary osteoarthritis
  - Crescentic subchondral lucency indicative of fracture, may precede articular surface collapse
- MR is most sensitive and specific
  - Infarcted bone progresses from normal marrow → hemorrhage → edema → fibrosis
  - Double line sign: Low signal intensity line at periphery of infarct with bright inner line along interface with infarcted bone
- T1 C+: Decreased enhancement in early osteonecrosis (ON); later, absent enhancement of nonviable segments
- Adjacent edema correlates with pain, risk of collapse

TOP DIFFERENTIAL DIAGNOSES

- Bone marrow edema pattern
  - Extensive differential diagnosis; often requires time and evidence of progression before definitive diagnosis becomes apparent
- Insufficiency fracture of femoral head
  - Elderly, osteoporotic women; no double line sign

PATHOLOGY

- Posttraumatic: Disrupted blood supply
- Corticosteroid use: Enlargement of intramedullary fat cells and ↑ marrow pressure inhibits blood flow
- Major morbidity from ON is not from infarct, it is result of healing process and subsequent articular collapse

CLINICAL ISSUES

- Hip, groin pain; decreased range of motion
- 3rd-6th decades most common
- M:F = 4:1

(Left) *AP radiograph shows classic patchy sclerosis ➡ in the femoral head, indicative of osteonecrosis (ON). In this case, the articular surface is intact. Findings are indicative of stage II disease.* **(Right)** *AP radiograph shows stage IV ON. Patchy sclerosis ➡ is present in the femoral head, and there is subtle collapse of a large segment of the articular surface ➡. A subchondral fracture ➡ is present, paralleling the articular surface. The acetabulum and joint space are normal.*

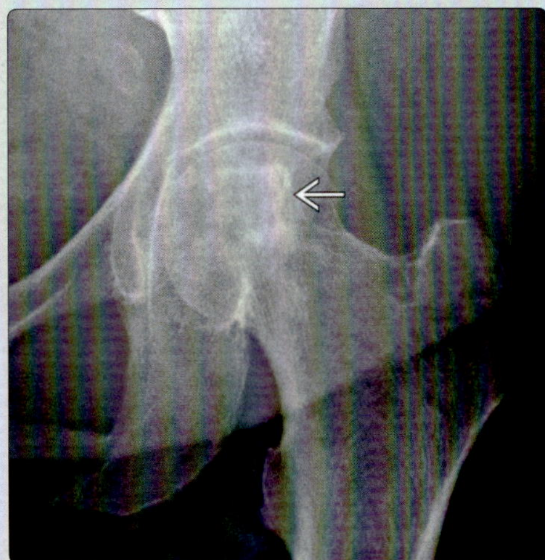

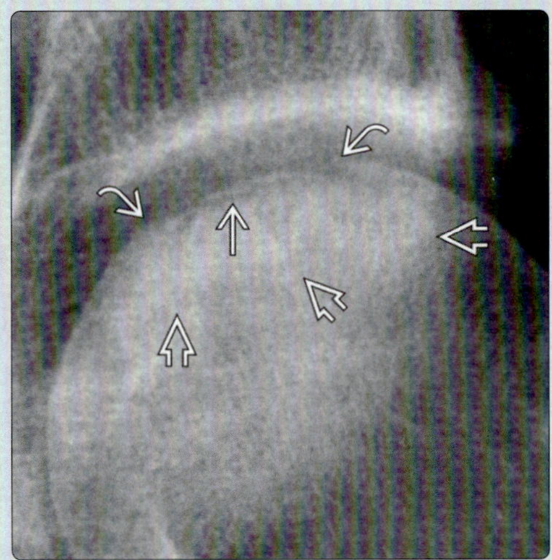

(Left) *AP radiograph shows advanced stage IV ON. Marked collapse of the entire articular surface of the femoral head ➡ is present. However, no radiographic changes of arthritis are seen within the acetabular articular surface.* **(Right)** *Coronal PD FS MR shows characteristic double line sign of ON. The hypointense outer dark line ➡ represents sclerosis at the border between the infarcted and normal bone. The bright line ➡ is created by the advancing granulation tissue/inflammatory response.*

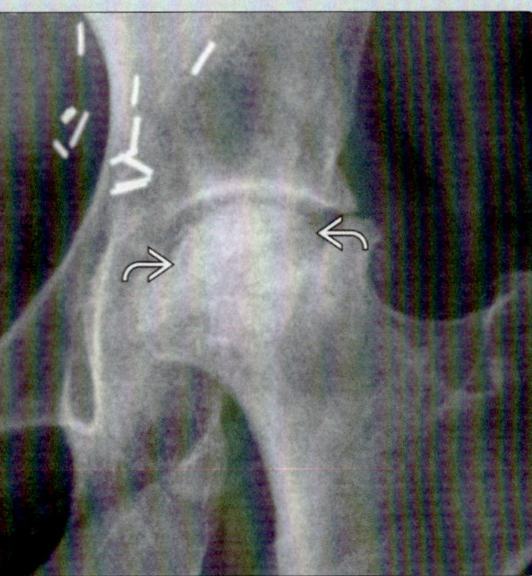

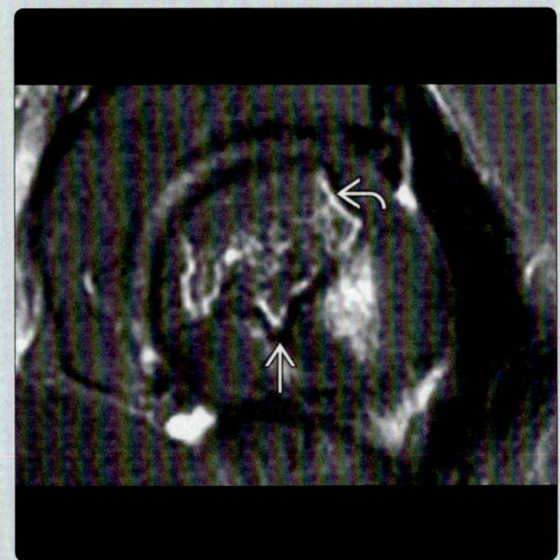

TERMINOLOGY

Synonyms

- Ischemic necrosis, osteonecrosis (ON), aseptic necrosis, avascular necrosis

Definitions

- Necrosis of cellular elements of bone 2° to ischemia

IMAGING

General Features

- Best diagnostic clue
  - Radiograph
    - Early: Patchy sclerosis in femoral head
    - Late: Irregularity, fragmentation, collapse of femoral head articular surface
  - MR: Double line sign
- Location
  - Early in disease: Anterior weight-bearing femoral head
- Size
  - Size of infarct quite variable, ranges from small focus to involvement of entire femoral head
    - Assess extent of disease using visual inspection
- Morphology
  - Factors associated with articular surface collapse: Size of infarct, lateral location within head

Imaging Recommendations

- Best imaging tool
  - MR is most sensitive and specific
- Protocol advice
  - Any MR protocol for hip pain should include at least 1 sequence that images opposite hip
    - Aids detection of asymptomatic disease
    - T1WI &/or STIR coronal ideal
  - MR imaging: Use coronal and sagittal planes to fully demonstrate extent; small FOV of each hip best

Radiographic Findings

- Early: Patchy sclerosis of femoral head due to new bone formation along necrotic trabecula
- Advanced findings
  - Crescentic subchondral lucency indicative of fracture, may precede articular surface collapse
    - Frog lateral or false profile lateral views show best
    - Orientation parallels articular surface
  - Articular surface collapse
    - May be subtle, requires close inspection, visible cortical break may not be evident
    - Often easier to appreciate on radiographs vs. MR
  - Articular surface fragmentation
  - 2° osteoarthritis (OA): Joint space narrowing, acetabular subchondral sclerosis, osteophytes

CT Findings

- Osteoporosis and distortion of bony asterisk of femoral head trabeculae on axial
- Most sensitive modality for subchondral fracture
  - Sagittal and coronal (to lesser degree 3D reformats) useful to visualize articular surface collapse
- Overall not as sensitive (55%) or accurate as MR

MR Findings

- MR is 97% sensitive, 98% specific for ON
- Initial MR findings: Nonspecific bone marrow edema
  - ↓ T1W signal, ↑ signal on fluid-sensitive sequences
  - Edema may extend from femoral head into femoral neck
- During 1st few months following infarct, infarcted bone will appear normal; other than edema, MR changes do not occur until healing has begun
  - Stages within infarcted bone progress from normal marrow → hemorrhage → edema → fibrosis
    - T1WI: Bright marrow → hypointense → dark
    - T2WI: Hypointense marrow → bright → dark
- Pathognomonic finding: Double line sign
  - Low signal intensity line at periphery of infarct with bright inner line forming reactive interface with infarcted bone
- MR ability to detect subtle articular surface collapse poorer than radiographs; often easier to appreciate on sagittal images, least apparent on axial images
  - Crescentic fracture may not be visible, does not always precede collapse
- Associated edema extending from infarct into head/neck correlates with pain, risk of collapse
  - Edema found in 48% of patients with ON
  - 72% of cases with edema occur in Steinberg stage III disease (ON with subchondral lucency)
  - May presage collapse of head and suggest latest point where core decompression may be efficacious
- Joint effusion: ↓ T1W signal, ↑ T2W signal (at any stage)
- T1 C+: Decreased enhancement in early ON; later, absent enhancement of nonviable segments

Nuclear Medicine Findings

- Bone scan
  - Very early: Photopenic femoral head
  - Later: ↑ radioisotope accumulation resulting from revascularization and repair
  - May be more sensitive than radiograph (85% sensitivity on SPECT), but significantly less than MR

DIFFERENTIAL DIAGNOSIS

Bone Marrow Edema Pattern

- Extensive differential diagnosis, including transient osteoporosis of hip, infection, neoplasm; may require time before definitive diagnosis becomes apparent

Insufficiency Fracture of Femoral Head

- Patient population: Elderly, osteoporotic women
- ± significant articular surface collapse, fragmentation
- Does not develop double line sign
- Usually absent risk factors for ON

PATHOLOGY

General Features

- Etiology
  - Posttraumatic: Disrupted blood supply
    - Hip dislocation: If not reduced within 12 hours, 50% develop ON
    - Subcapital fracture: 30% of displaced femoral fractures develop ON

- Corticosteroid use: Enlargement of intramedullary fat cells and ↑ marrow pressure inhibits blood flow
  - Of all patients on steroids, 2% develop ON
  - Risk greater with short duration (6 weeks) and high doses (> 20 mg); 5-25% of patients develop ON
  - Risk ↑ in renal transplant patients on steroids, with osteodystrophy (40% develop ON)
  - 10% of long-term survivors of bone marrow transplantation who received high doses of steroids develop ON
- Other etiologies
  - Sickle cell anemia: Sickled cells thrombose in microvasculature at low oxygen tension
  - Gaucher disease: Marrow packing → ↑ pressure
  - Systemic lupus erythematosus (SLE): Vasculitis + steroids; 5-40% develop ON
  - Caisson disease: Nitrogen air embolization from dysbaric phenomena
  - Radiation: Vasculitis results in ON
  - HIV/AIDS: May relate to antiretroviral therapy or hyperlipidemia
  - Alcohol abuse: Likely due to fat emboli from liver

- Associated abnormalities
  - Major morbidity from ON is not from infarct, but is result of healing process
    - Infarcted bone is as strong as normal bone
    - Healing weakens bone by resorbing dead bone

Staging, Grading, & Classification

- Steinberg classification: Based on radiographic appearance and location of lesion
  - Stage 0: Normal radiographs, MR, and bone scan of at-risk hip (often contralateral hip involved, or patient has risk factors and hip pain)
  - Stage I: Nl radiograph, abnormal bone scan/MR
  - Stage II: Cystic or sclerotic radiographic changes
  - Stage III: Subchondral lucency or crescent sign
  - Stage IV: Flattening of femoral head
  - Stage V: Joint space narrowing
  - Stage VI: Advanced degenerative disease

CLINICAL ISSUES

Presentation

- Most common signs/symptoms
  - Hip, groin, or referred pain to thigh
  - Decreased range of motion
  - Etiology of pain not well understood
    - Presence of marrow edema is very highly correlated with degree of pain
    - Relief of pressure by core decompression relieves pain promptly
    - Development of fracture may exacerbate pain
- Other signs/symptoms
  - Effusion especially with collapse contributes to pain
  - Atraumatic ON commonly bilateral (30-70% at time of presentation) but progresses asymmetrically
    - 1/3 of asymptomatic contralateral hips will go on to pain, collapse; with cystic changes, more likely to progress to collapse
    - Contralateral asymptomatic disease in 60%
  - Slipped capital femoral epiphysis and developmental dysplasia hip both at ↑ risk for ON
  - Average of 4 years between onset of symptoms between bilaterally involved hips

Demographics

- Age
  - 3rd-6th decades
- Gender
  - M:F = 4:1
- Epidemiology
  - 15,000 cases hip ON in USA per year
  - Steroids responsible for 30-40% of non-traumatic ON
  - Alcoholism responsible for 20-40%
  - 10% of hip arthroplasties performed for ON

Natural History & Prognosis

- Rarely may revascularize without progression
- Generally proceeds to flattening → collapse → 2° OA

Treatment

- Treatment of early disease not always straightforward
  - Pain occasionally lessens spontaneously with conservative management
  - Core decompression generally relieves pain promptly, likely from ↓ marrow edema and intraosseous hypertension; may elect to pack with graft
    - May be particularly useful in stage III patients (no significant collapse) with marrow edema
    - May continue with progression to collapse
  - Core decompression with vascularized fibular grafting is not proven to be more efficacious than core decompression alone
  - Small study suggests hyperbaric oxygen useful in stage I or II
- Treatment of later disease: Required in 50% of patients within 3 years of diagnosis
  - Collapse without OA: Hemiarthroplasty
  - Significant OA: Total hip arthroplasty

DIAGNOSTIC CHECKLIST

Consider

- Check history for trauma, steroid use, alcohol abuse, SLE, sickle cell disease
- Watch for clinically silent contralateral involvement

Reporting Tips

- Use face-of-clock terminology to describe location

SELECTED REFERENCES

1. Koren L et al: Hyperbaric oxygen for stage I and II femoral head osteonecrosis. Orthopedics. 38(3):e200-5, 2015
2. Lee GC et al: How do radiologists evaluate osteonecrosis? Skeletal Radiol. 43(5):607-14, 2014
3. Vahid Farahmandi M et al: Midterm results of treating femoral head osteonecrosis with autogenous corticocancellous bone grafting. Trauma Mon. 19(4):e17092, 2014

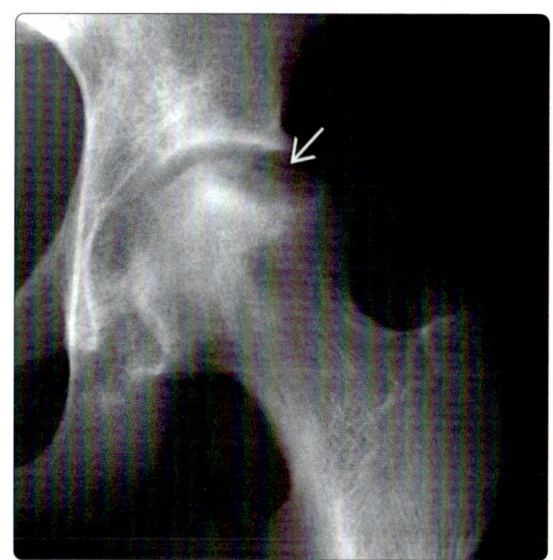

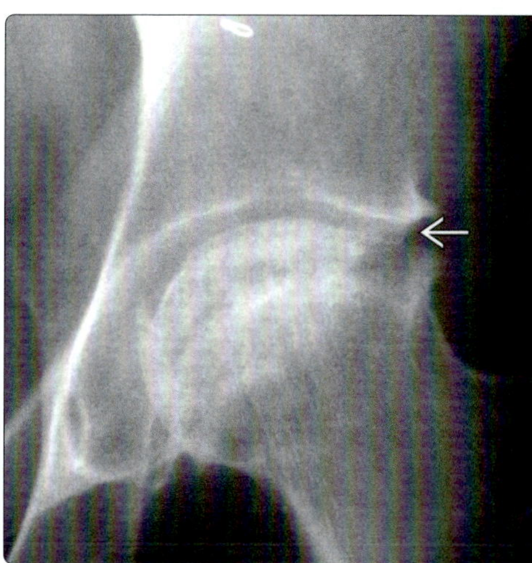

(Left) *AP radiograph with advanced ON is shown. Findings include patchy sclerosis and mild articular surface collapse* ➡*. The lateral location of the insult has a higher risk of collapse than a more medially positioned lesion.* **(Right)** *AP radiograph shows hip ON with severe articular surface collapse. Once collapse has occurred, surgical options are limited to hemiarthroplasty or total joint replacement. Mild superior joint space narrowing* ➡ *heralds onset of 2° osteoarthritis (OA).*

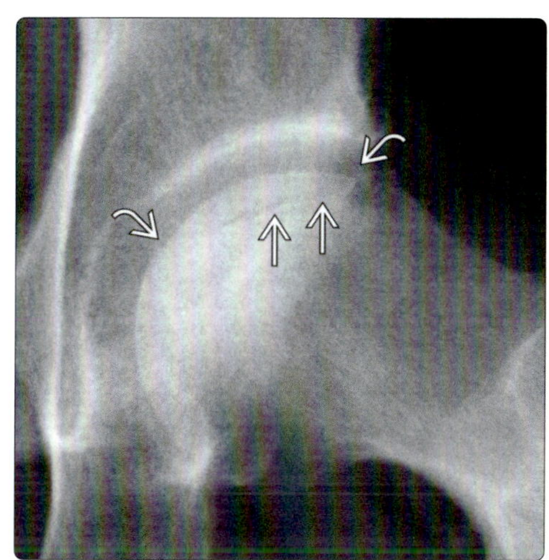

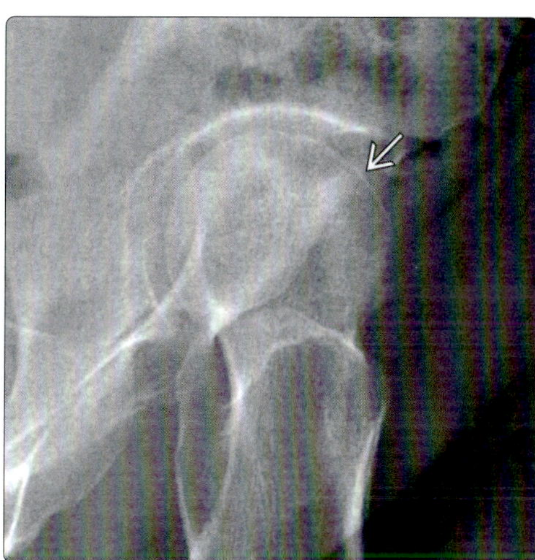

(Left) *Frog leg lateral radiograph nicely depicts an extensive subchondral fracture* ➡*. Such a finding should direct one's attention to the articular surface, which in this case is mildly collapsed* ➡*.* **(Right)** *False profile view of the hip of a different patient shows subtle sclerosis and collapse within the anterior superior weight-bearing portion of the femoral head* ➡*. An anterosuperior location is the most common site of ON, and subtle changes are best depicted on frog lateral or false profile views.*

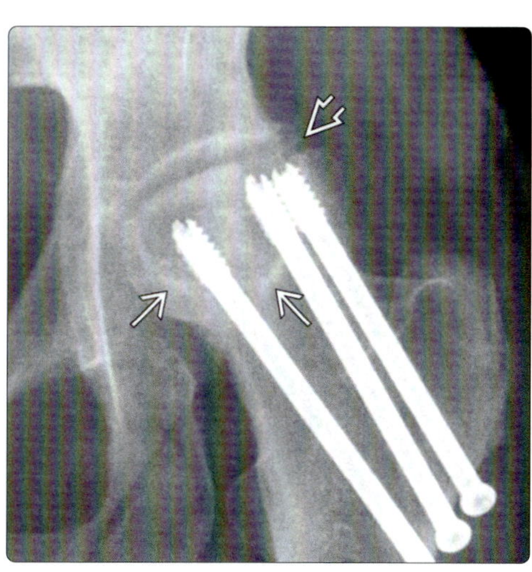

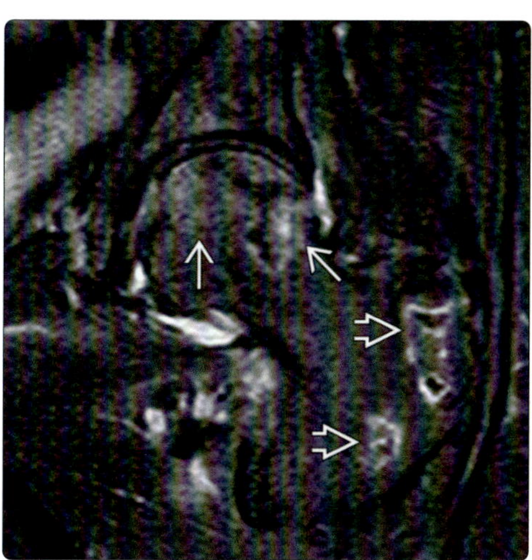

(Left) *AP radiograph with ON following subcapital femoral neck fracture and fixation is shown. Large infarct* ➡ *has led to marked flattening of the head. 2° OA is already present with joint space narrowing and osteophytes* ➡*.* **(Right)** *Coronal STIR MR with ON* ➡ *and bone infarcts* ➡ *2° to chemotherapy is shown. While the etiology is the same, terminology associated with these lesions is often confusing. ON and avascular necrosis refer to subchondral lesions, while bone infarct describes lesions distant to an articular surface.*

(Left) *Coronal T1WI MR of the earliest changes indicative of ON is shown. Band-like foci* ➡ *of low T1W signal are present in the anterior aspect of each femoral head.* **(Right)** *Sagittal T1WI MR with ON in a large segment of the anterior head is shown. A low signal line demarcates normal bone from infarcted bone* ➡*. The infarcted bone maintains normal fat signal* ⇨*. Edema* ↪ *is present in otherwise normal marrow adjacent to the infarct. Edematous marrow is associated with pain and may herald impending collapse.*

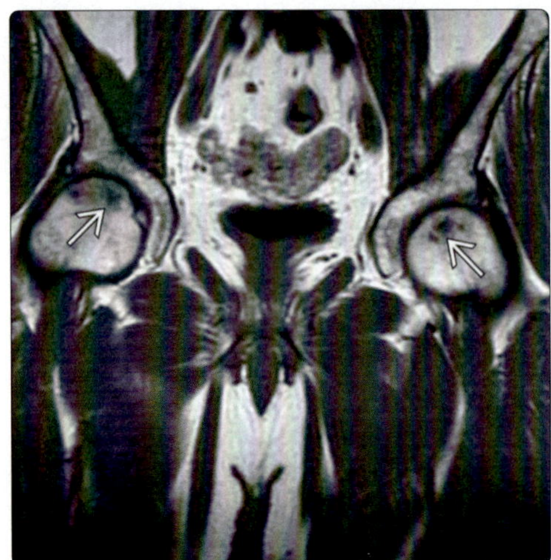

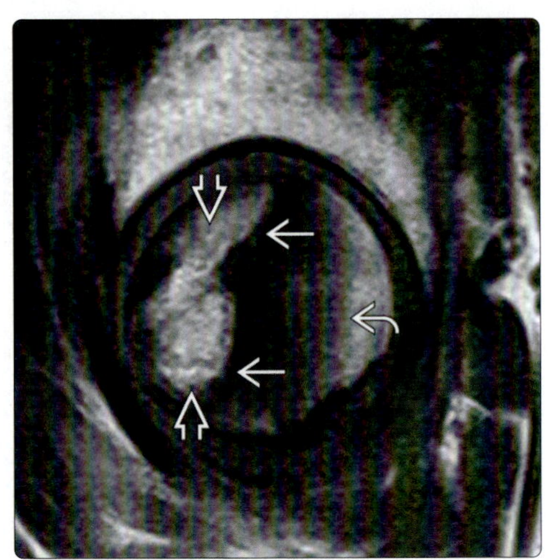

(Left) *Axial T2WI FS MR with double line sign, low signal band adjacent to normal bone* ➡*, and bright signal* ↪ *at the reparative zone is shown. Identification of this sign is necessary to confirm the diagnosis. Axial plane is least likely to reveal articular surface collapse, which usually involves the superior articular surface.* **(Right)** *Coronal MR arthrogram T2WI FS reveals a subchondral crescentic fracture* ➡ *involving 50% of the superior articular surface. The disease was clinically unsuspected and related to alcoholic use.*

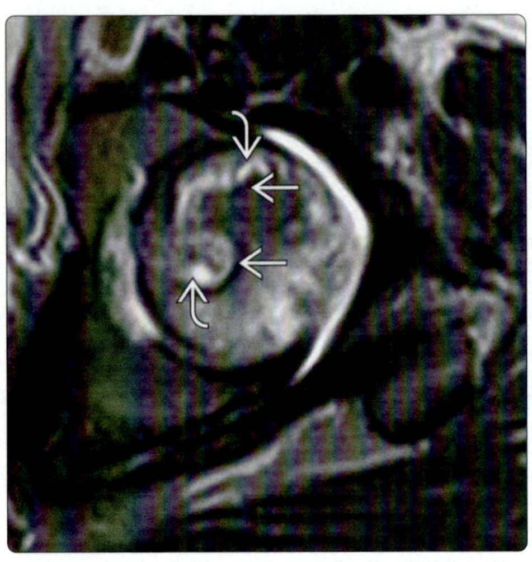

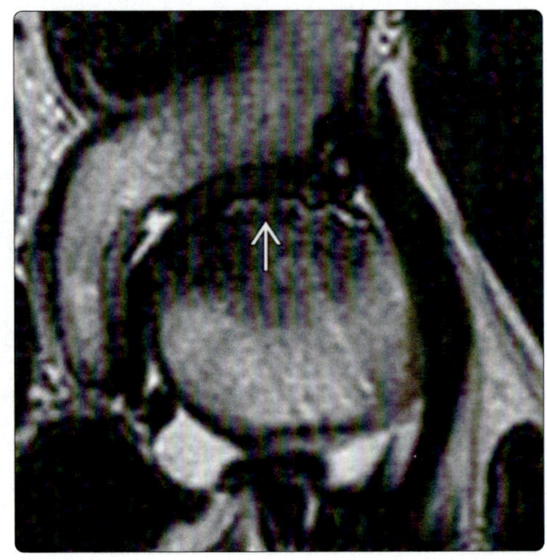

(Left) *Coronal PD FSE FS MR shows subtle subchondral fracture* ↪*, articular surface irregularity* ⇨*, and extended hyperintense bone marrow edema pattern* ➡ *in the femoral head and neck. This edema pattern is most common in stage III disease and is highly associated with pain.* **(Right)** *Coronal STIR MR shows bright lines of double line sign* ↪*, marrow edema* ➡*, and a large joint effusion* ⇨*. The significance of the joint effusion is unclear. Aspiration of the fluid may reduce the patient's pain.*

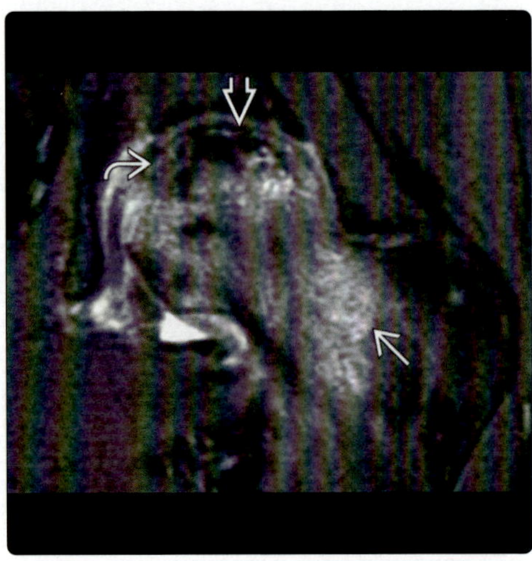

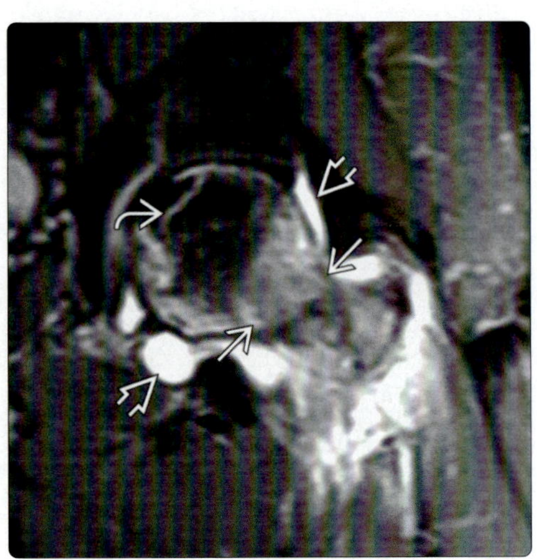

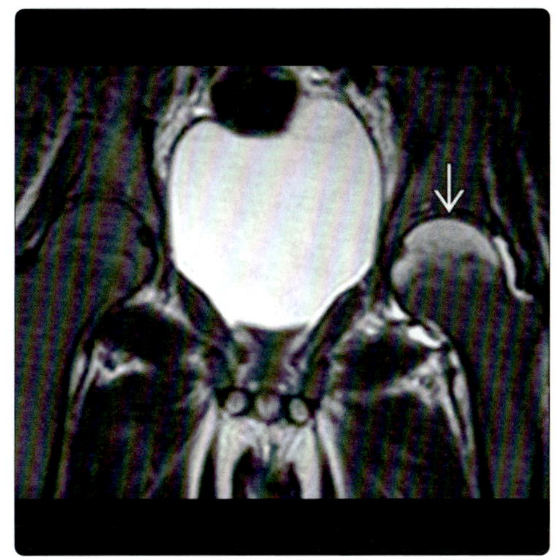

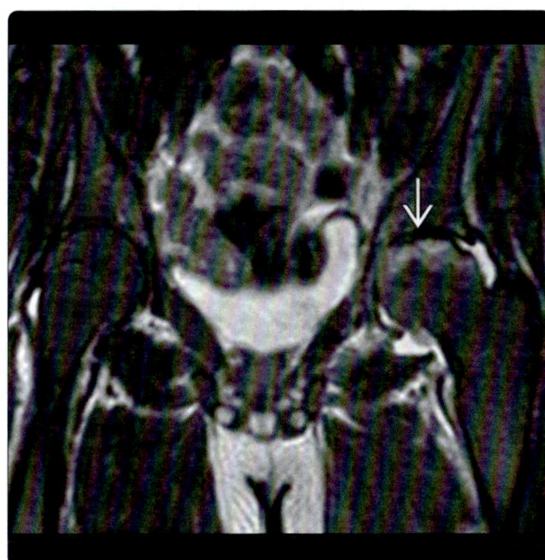

(Left) *Coronal T2 MR shows diffuse hematopoietic marrow 2° to sickle cell disease (SSD). SSD is a risk factor for ON. The hip is the most common site of involvement. Edema ➡ within the left femoral head is likely stage 1 ON.* **(Right)** *Coronal T2W1 MR of the same patient 7 months later shows progression with new collapse of the articular surface ➡; the diagnosis is now definitive and is stage IV. The right hip is stage 0 or "at risk." Statistically, disease in the right hip will develop in the next 3-4 years.*

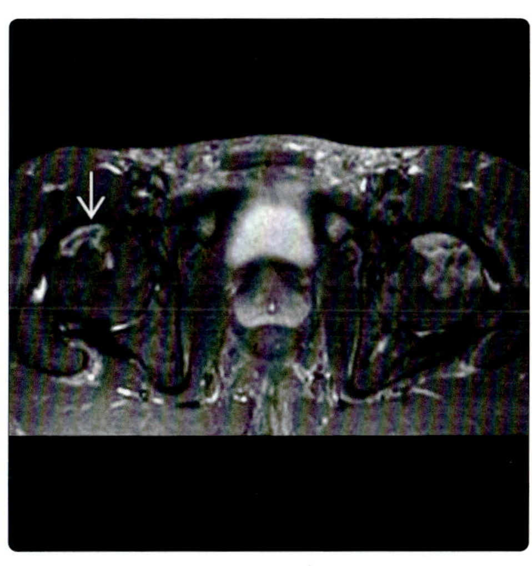

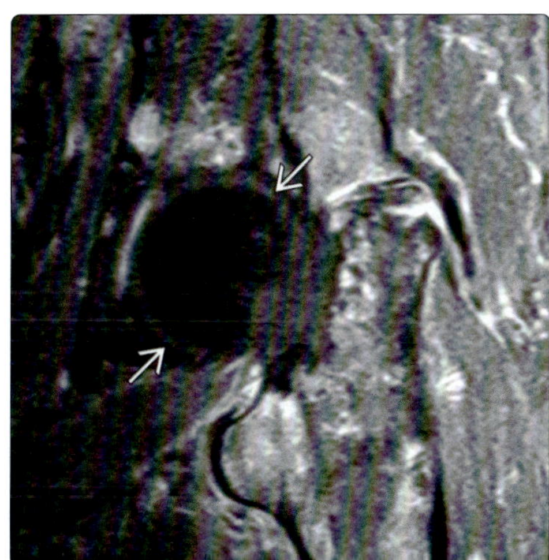

(Left) *Axial STIR MR in the same patient with SSD several months later shows that classic ON has now developed in the right femoral head ➡.* **(Right)** *Coronal T1WI C+ FS MR in a patient with femoral neck fracture is shown. Treatment options included percutaneous pinning vs. hemiarthroplasty. This study was done to evaluate blood flow to the femoral head. It demonstrates complete absence of enhancement within the head ➡, indicative of posttraumatic loss of blood supply and the need for replacement.*

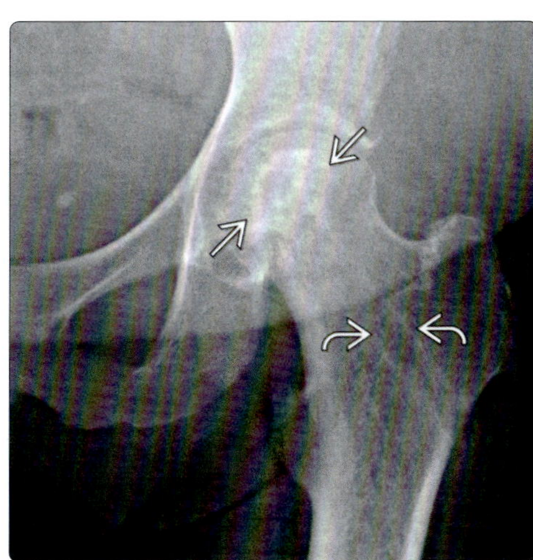

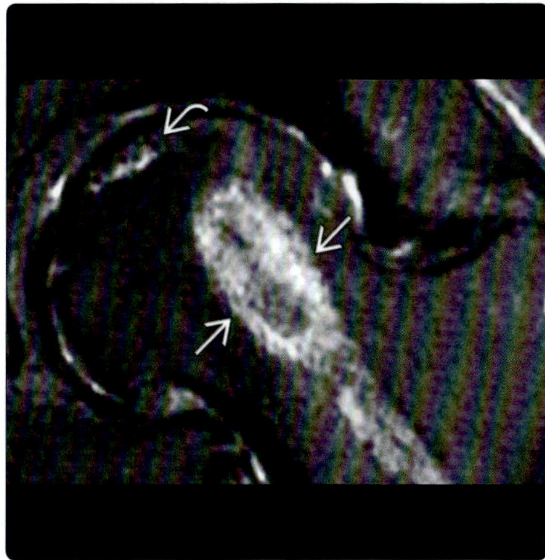

(Left) *AP radiograph of hip following core decompression ➡. Typical patchy sclerosis of ON is present ➡. Core decompression is designed to relieve intramedullary hypertension and improve blood flow. It also provides immediate relief of symptoms.* **(Right)** *Coronal PD FSE FS MR shows small focus of ON ➡. Core decompression track is present ➡. Core decompression is best used for stages I and II. Once fracture/collapse have occurred, the changes are irreversible.*

Osteonecrosis of Shoulder

KEY FACTS

TERMINOLOGY

- Osteonecrosis (ON), avascular necrosis, aseptic necrosis, bone infarct

IMAGING

- Cruess classification adapted from Ficat
  - Stage 1: Radiographs normal, MR positive
  - Stage 2: Sclerosis
  - Stage 3: Crescentic subchondral fracture (best seen in external rotation), ± minor collapse
  - Stage 4: More advanced collapse and fragmentation; glenoid normal
  - Stage 5: Secondary osteoarthritis
- Usually involves central, superior humeral head at site of greatest contact with glenoid
- Often large lesion; size correlates with risk of collapse
- MR: Characteristic double line on T2W images
- Bone scan: Donut sign

CLINICAL ISSUES

- Etiology: Steroid-induced most common in USA
  - Throughout world, sickle cell (SC) most common etiology, ON seen in 1/3-1/2 of SC patients
  - Posttraumatic: 15-30% of 4-part fracture develop ON; multivessel blood supply is protective
- Humeral head 2nd most common site for ON after femoral head; 75-90% humeral ON associated with disease at other sites, especially femoral head
- Presentation: Pain ± mechanical issues
  - Often present with advanced disease; shoulder movement involves multiple joints so limited ROM occurs late
- Treatment: Directed at symptoms, prevention of collapse; includes pain control, physical therapy, activity modification, debridement of cartilage and loose bodies, core decompression, eventual joint replacement

(Left) *AP radiograph demonstrates patchy sclerosis ➡ and minimal articular surface collapse ➡ of the humeral head in a patient with sickle cell (SC) disease. The osteonecrosis (ON) in patients with SC disease may follow a more benign course than that of other etiologies.* **(Right)** *AP radiograph shows an extensive subchondral fracture ➡ in the humeral head at the site of greatest contact with the glenoid. The finding is characteristic of ON even in the absence of other findings.*

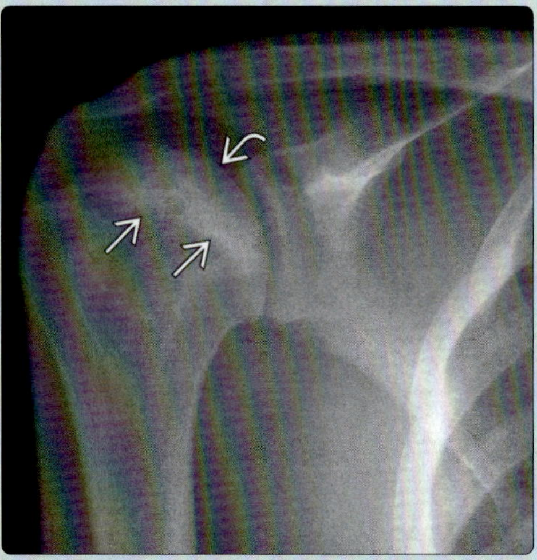

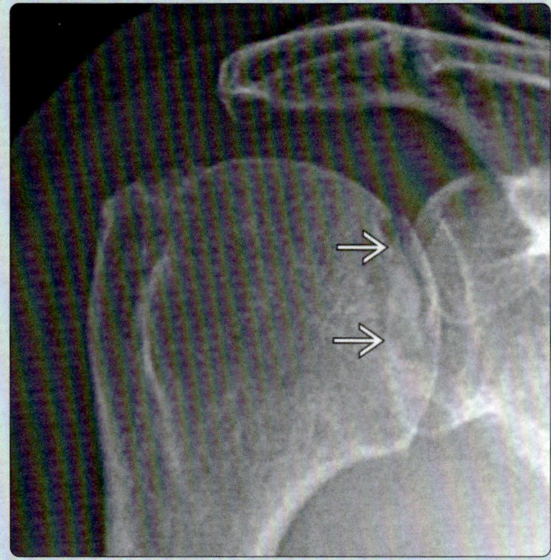

(Left) *AP radiograph reveals advanced changes of humeral ON. Note the typical superior and central location, subchondral lucency with characteristic serpentine sclerotic border ➡, and subchondral fracture with a large displaced flake of bone ➡.* **(Right)** *Coronal T2WI FS MR shows a bright line outlining the infarcted bone ➡. It is a result of healing at the interface between normal and infarcted bone. The typical central and superior location is at the site of maximal contact between the humerus and glenoid.*

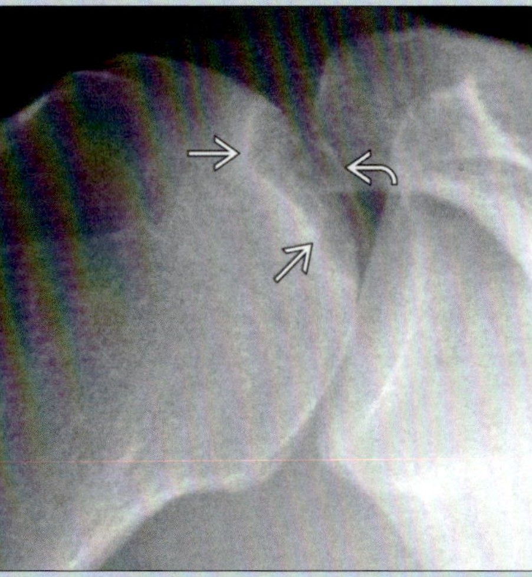

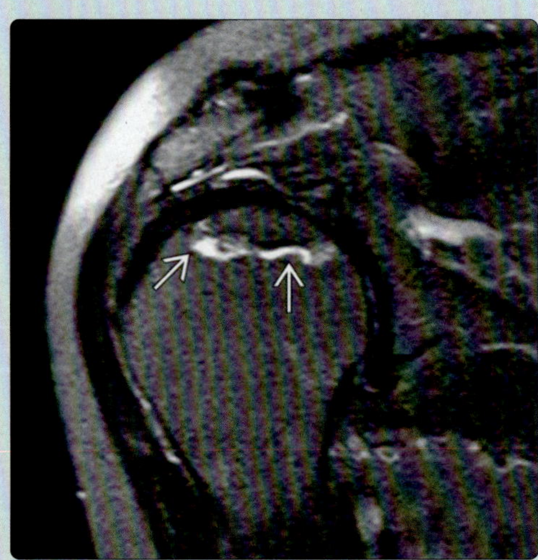

KEY FACTS

TERMINOLOGY

- Osteonecrosis (ON) located within osseous structures of knee; imaging appearance and clinical risks are not unique relative to other sites of ON

IMAGING

- Radiographs: Serpiginous or patchy sclerotic foci
  - Typically multifocal: May be seen in femoral condyles, tibial plateau, femoral and tibial diaphysis, patella (especially superior pole)
  - Involvement of articular surface may result in collapse, fragmentation
- MR
  - Initial presentation may be bone marrow edema: ↓ T1W and ↑ T2W signal
  - Double line sign on T2W images is diagnostic: Low signal rim at lesion periphery with bright inner signal at reactive interface

TOP DIFFERENTIAL DIAGNOSES

- Insufficiency fracture (formerly known as spontaneous ON of knee, SONK)
  - SONK originally considered 1° ON; now recognized as insufficiency fracture rather than ON
  - Male < female; over 60 years of age
  - Single site; femur > tibial; medial > lateral
  - More sudden onset than ON
- Regional migratory osteoporosis
  - Middle-aged males most frequently affected
  - Bone marrow edema; lacks subchondral curvilinear signal change, articular surface collapse
  - Develops radiographically evident osteopenia

CLINICAL ISSUES

- Gradual onset mild or vague pain
- Isolated patellar ON: Rare; may be idiopathic
  - Posttraumatic: Transverse patella fracture
  - Post arthroplasty: Associated with lateral release

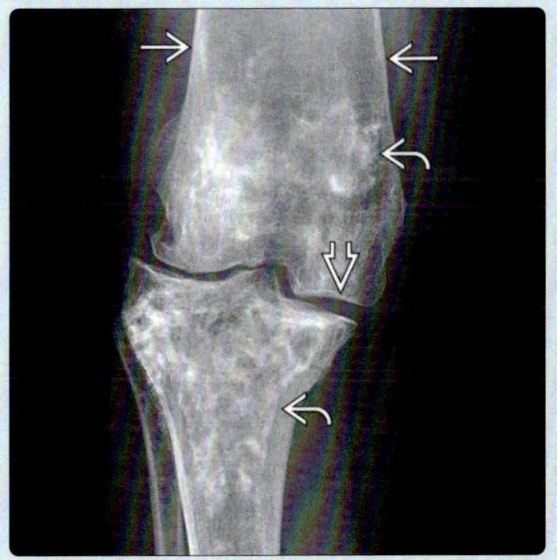

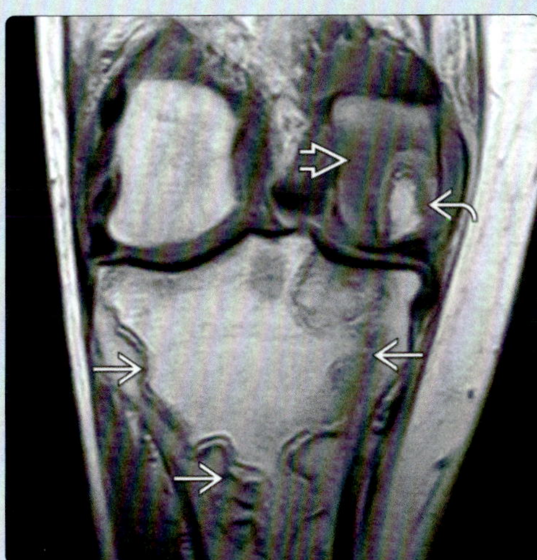

(Left) *AP radiograph shows Erlenmeyer flask deformity ➡ in this patient with Gaucher disease. Classic serpentine and patchy sclerosis ➡ is present in the distal femur and proximal tibia, indicative of extensive osteonecrosis (ON). The ON results in mild flattening of the medial femoral condylar articular surface ➡.* **(Right)** *Coronal T1WI shows extensive ON of the medial femoral condyle ➡ and proximal tibia ➡. Edema around the condylar lesion ➡ may indicate impending articular surface collapse.*

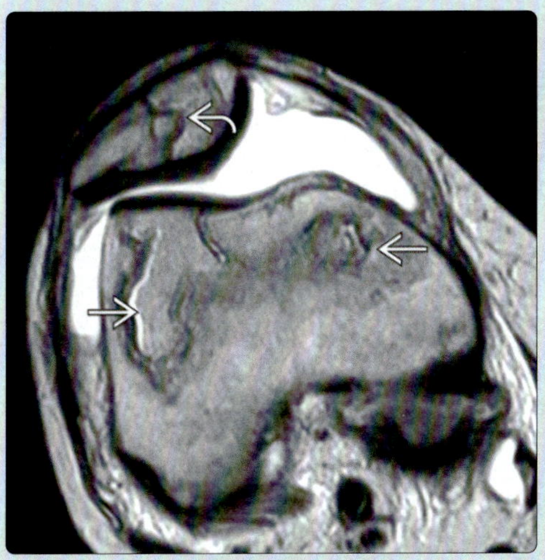

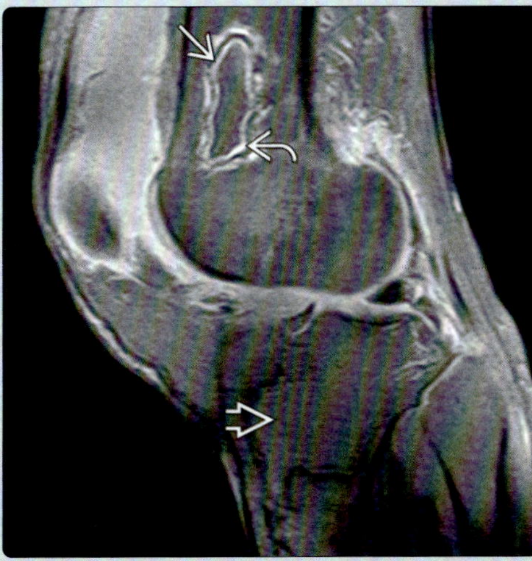

(Left) *Axial PDWI MR demonstrates multifocal ON. Lesions are present in both femoral condyles ➡ and within the patella ➡. Involvement of the patella is almost always associated with disease elsewhere in the knee.* **(Right)** *Lateral T2WI FS MR of ON shows variable imaging features. The distal femoral lesion has a characteristic double line sign with low signal outer line ➡ and an internal bright line ➡. The tibial lesion has only a low signal line. However, fat within the lesion ➡ is a strong diagnostic clue.*

Osteonecrosis of Wrist

KEY FACTS

IMAGING

- Radiographs: Normal bone density & morphology early → increased density → cysts, fragmentation, articular surface collapse → 2° osteoarthritis (OA)
- Associated findings/risk factors
  - Capitate: Transverse midbody fracture
  - Lunate: Ulnar minus, rarely ulnar positive
  - Scaphoid: Fracture proximal pole or waist ± nonunion with rounded, sclerotic fracture margins
- T1WI: ↓ signal intensity, may see low signal fracture line
- Fluid-sensitive sequences: Signal changes quite variable; typically early ↑ signal, late ↓ signal
- T1WI C+: Lack of enhancement suggests nonviable fragments
  - Revascularization may occur late in process
- MR: Distribution of signal changes quite variable

TOP DIFFERENTIAL DIAGNOSES

- Lunate: Ulnar impaction syndrome
  - Usually ulnar positive variance; chondromalacia, osteophyte & subchondral cysts
- Scaphoid: Fracture nonunion without osteonecrosis (ON)
  - Proximal pole or waist of scaphoid fracture may develop nonunion without necessarily having ON

PATHOLOGY

- Capitate: Rare; 2° severe trauma & midbody fracture
- Lunate: Chronic repetitive trauma
- Scaphoid: Posttraumatic etiology most common
  - Distribution of vascular supply → proximal pole at risk

CLINICAL ISSUES

- 20-40 yr old
- Pain, limited range of motion, grip weakness
- Chronic pain and arthrosis of radiocarpal & midcarpal joints
- May begin with conservative therapy; no accepted algorithm
- Vascularized bone grafting if fragment is nonviable

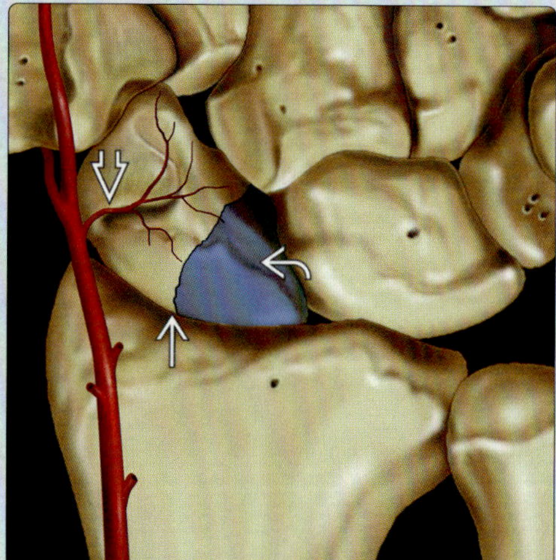

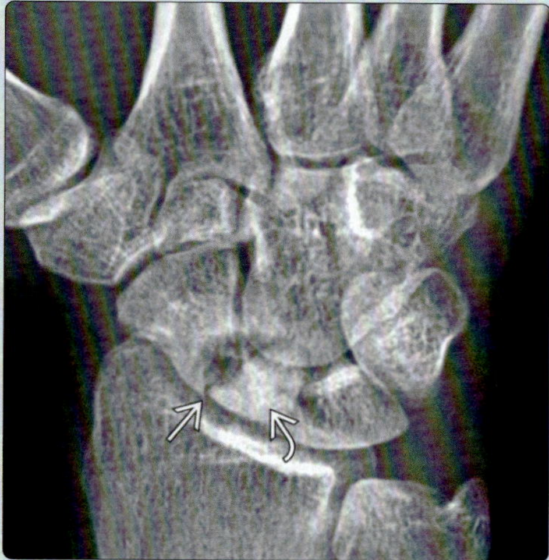

(Left) *Graphic of the carpus shows the blood supply to the scaphoid, which enters distally ⇨. Fracture of the scaphoid waist or proximal pole ➡ separates the proximal pole from its blood supply, leading to osteonecrosis (ON) ↪ of the proximal fragment.* **(Right)** *Oblique radiograph shows an ununited fracture through the proximal pole of scaphoid ➡. Note the increased density of the proximal pole ↪; this density, as well as the proximal location of the fracture, suggests that irreversible ON is highly probable.*

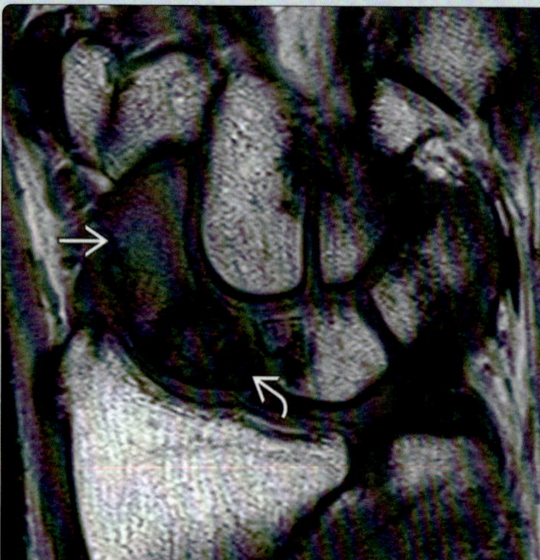

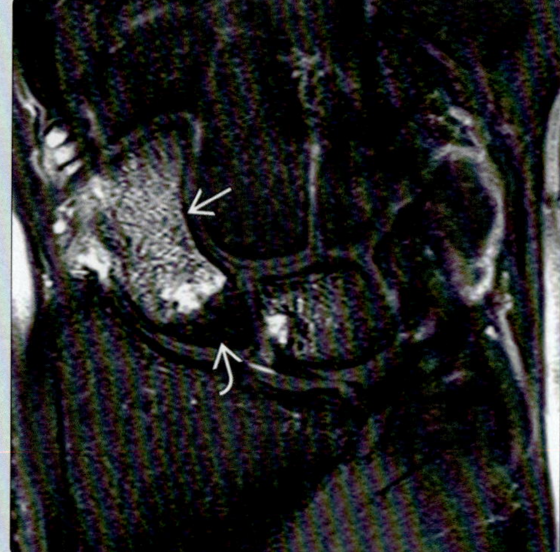

(Left) *Coronal T1 MR, same case, shows low signal edema in the distal pole ➡ and hypointense edema/sclerosis in proximal pole ↪ of scaphoid.* **(Right)** *Coronal postcontrast T1FS MR, same case, shows enhancement of the distal pole ➡ but distinct lack of enhancement of the proximal fragment ↪. Although late revascularization and healing of scaphoid fractures can be seen, it is extremely unlikely in this case; the proximal location of the fracture line has rendered the fragment nonviable.*

TERMINOLOGY

Synonyms

- Ischemic necrosis, aseptic necrosis, avascular necrosis

Definitions

- Preiser disease: Scaphoid osteonecrosis (ON) without known trauma
- Kienböck disease: ON of lunate; lunatomalacia

IMAGING

General Features

- Best diagnostic clue
  - Sclerosis ± fragmentation, collapse

Imaging Recommendations

- Best imaging tool
  - MR most sensitive & specific

Radiographic Findings

- General features
  - Normal bone density & morphology early → increased density → cysts, fragmentation, articular surface collapse → 2° osteoarthritis (OA)
- Associated findings
  - Capitate: Transverse midbody fracture
  - Lunate: Ulnar minus, rarely ulnar positive
    - As lunate collapses, capitate migrates proximally
  - Scaphoid: Fracture proximal pole or waist ± nonunion with rounded, sclerotic fracture margins

MR Findings

- T1WI: ↓ signal intensity, may see low signal fracture line
- Fluid-sensitive sequences: Signal changes quite variable; typically early ↑ signal, late ↓ signal
  - Fracture line low or bright, not always visible
- T1WI C+: Lack of enhancement suggests nonviable fragments
  - Not invariably specific; late revascularization may occur
- Distribution of signal changes quite variable
  - May involve small segment or entire bone, be patchy or diffuse, change between sequences
  - If 2° OA occurs, subchondral changes in adjacent bones
- Specific issues
  - Lunate: Earliest collapse along proximal radial border; if ulnar negative variance with lunatomalacia, triangular fibrocartilage complex may be thickened or torn
  - Scaphoid: Nonunion seen as discontinuity of trabecular bone, fluid signal within fracture line

Nuclear Medicine Findings

- Bone scan
  - Early: Absent uptake; late: Normal to ↑ uptake

DIFFERENTIAL DIAGNOSIS

Lunate: Ulnar Impaction Syndrome

- Usually ulnar positive variance
- Chondromalacia, osteophyte & subchondral cysts

Scaphoid: Fracture Nonunion Without Osteonecrosis

- Proximal pole or waist of scaphoid fracture may develop nonunion, without necessarily having ON

PATHOLOGY

General Features

- Etiology
  - Capitate: Rare; 2° to severe trauma & midbody fracture
  - Lunate: Chronic repetitive trauma
    - Risk factors: Ulnar negative variance, rarely ulnar positive; oblong or square lunate morphology; rarely associated with systemic lupus erythematosus, steroids
  - Scaphoid: Posttraumatic etiology most common
    - Nearly 100% proximal pole fractures develop ON
    - 30% scaphoid waist fractures develop ON
    - Fracture displacement increases risk of ON

Staging, Grading, & Classification

- Lunatomalacia: Lichtman classification
  - Stage I: Normal radiographs ± fracture
  - Stage II: Sclerosis without collapse
  - Stage III: Fragmentation + collapse (IIIA = no carpal instability, IIIB = carpal instability)
  - Stage IV: Sclerosis, collapse + perilunate OA

Gross Pathologic & Surgical Features

- Scaphoid blood supply enters midscaphoid; fracture of proximal pole/waist separates proximal pole from blood supply

CLINICAL ISSUES

Presentation

- Most common signs/symptoms
  - Pain, limited range of motion, grip weakness

Demographics

- Age: 20-40 yr old

Natural History & Prognosis

- Chronic pain, arthrosis radiocarpal & midcarpal joints

Treatment

- Lunate: Radial shortening in stage I & II to reduce mechanical stress & slow disease progression
- Scaphoid: Prior to surgical intervention for nonunion exclude ON in proximal fragment
- No generally accepted treatment algorithm
  - Multitude of different procedures speaks to limited success of any single procedure
  - Surgery usually for more advanced disease
    - Revascularization, bone graft, osteotomy
    - Resection of avascular bone, ± limited or extensive carpal resection; limited or extensive carpal fusion

SELECTED REFERENCES

1. Bervian MR et al: Scaphoid fracture nonunion: correlation of radiographic imaging, proximal fragment histologic viability evaluation, and estimation of viability at surgery: diagnosis of scaphoid pseudarthrosis. Int Orthop. 39(1):67-72, 2015

(Left) *AP radiograph of the left wrist reveals increased density within the lunate ➡. No height loss is present, and fragmentation is not seen. Findings correspond to stage II Kienböck disease.* **(Right)** *Coronal T1WI MR shows patchy hypointense ➡ to dark ➡ signal within the lunate. The dark signal corresponds to sclerosis/fibrosis in advanced disease. Morphologic changes were seen on other images and indicate that this is stage III Kienböck disease.*

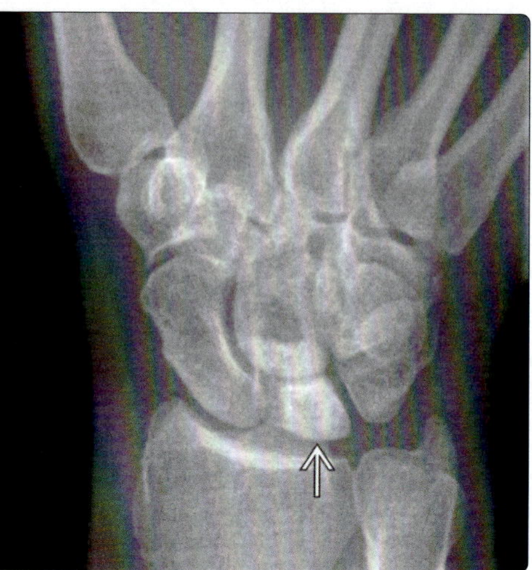

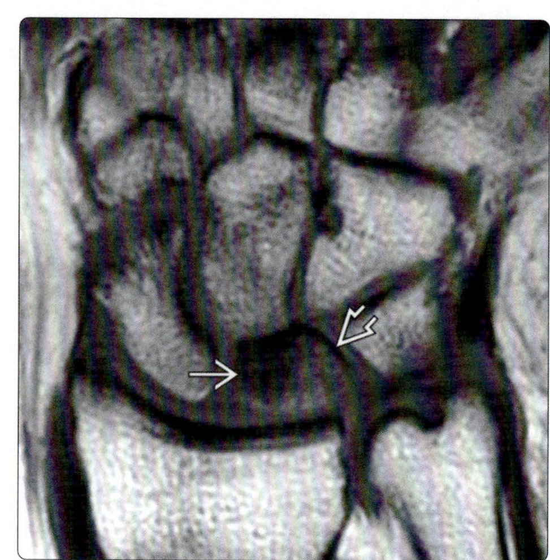

(Left) *PA radiograph shows patchy sclerosis throughout the lunate ➡ with significant collapse of the proximal articular surface ➡. Despite the advanced changes, radial shortening was performed. This surgery is used to correct negative ulnar variance in an attempt to reduce mechanical forces across the abnormal lunate.* **(Right)** *PA radiograph in the same patient after treatment for persistent pain is shown here. The lunate has been resected ➡ and a limited (capitohamate) carpal fusion performed ➡.*

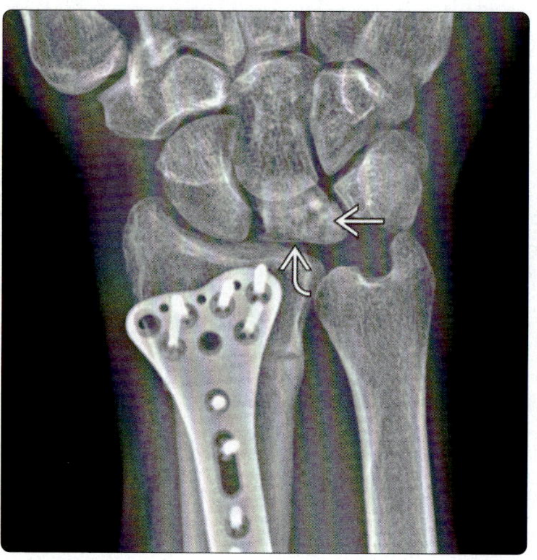

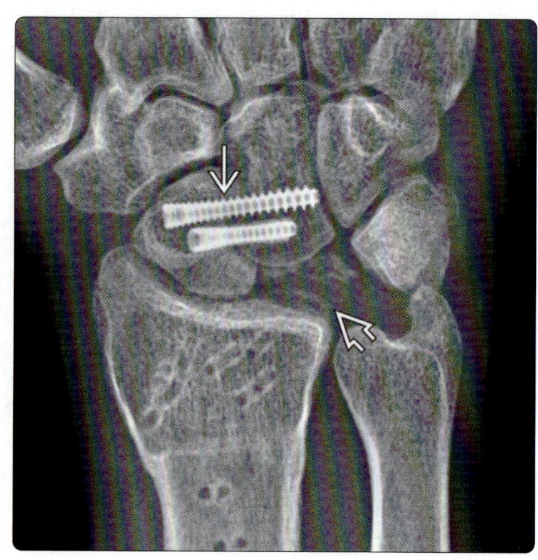

(Left) *Coronal T2WI FS MR shows stage I Kienböck disease. Ulnar minus deformity is present ➡. Marrow edema is seen in the lunate ➡ and capitate ➡. Capitate edema may be related to altered axial loading mechanics 2° to the short ulna.* **(Right)** *Coronal T1WI MR of the same patient shows the marrow edema within the lunate ➡. The main mechanical axis, radius to lunate to capitate to long finger ➡, is easy to appreciate. Normal radiographs make this stage I lunatomalacia.*

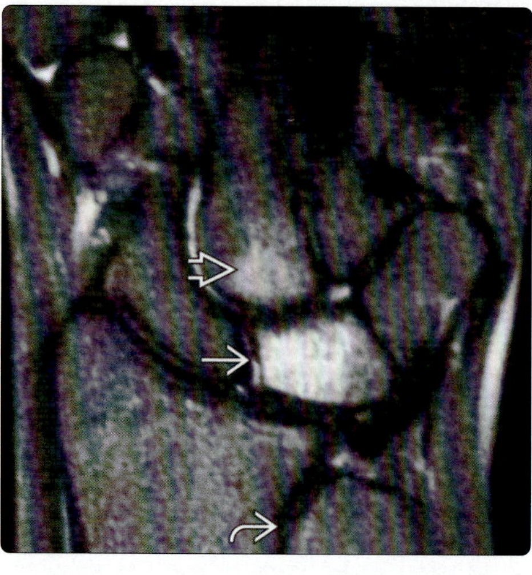

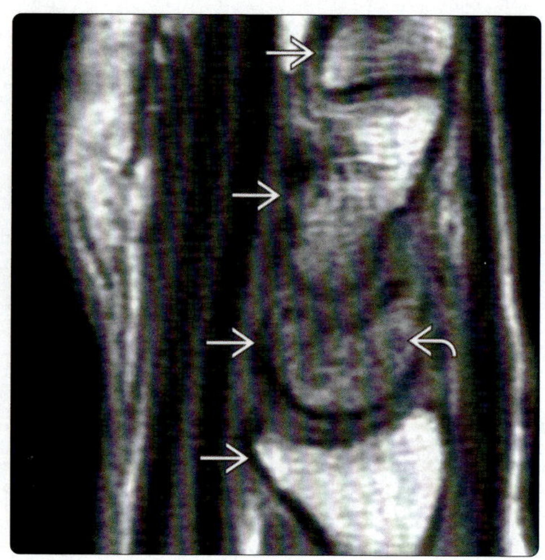

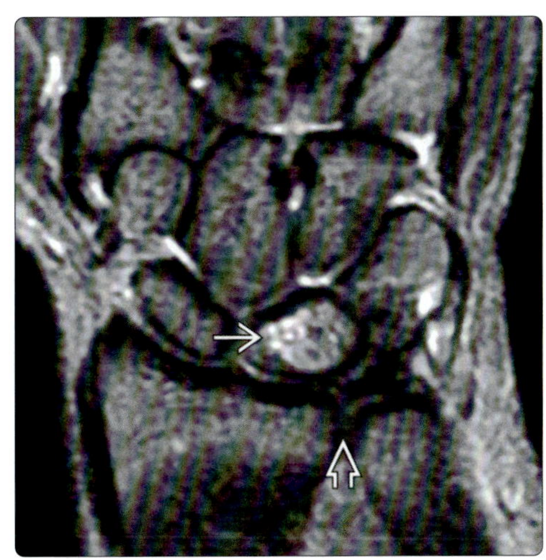

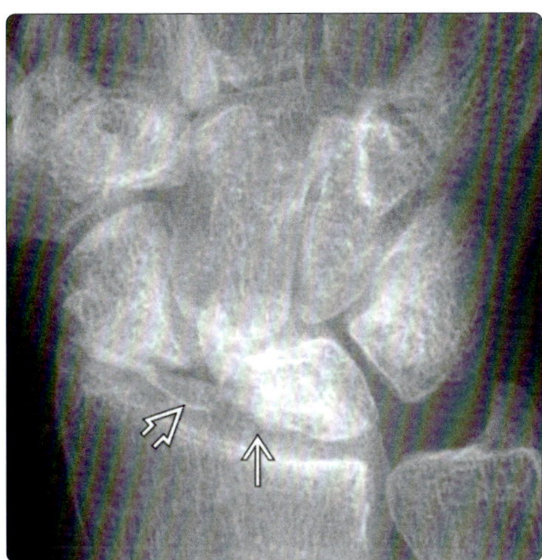

(Left) *Coronal fat-suppressed T2WI demonstrates irregular marrow edema in the lunate ➡ without morphologic change. An ulna minus deformity ➡ is present. The appearance is nonspecific and should raise concern for early ON.* **(Right)** *PA radiograph shows steroid-related ON at multiple sites. Lunate has patchy density & proximal articular surface collapse ➡. The proximal pole of the scaphoid is collapsed ➡. Although scaphoid ON is usually posttraumatic, steroid use is a risk factor.*

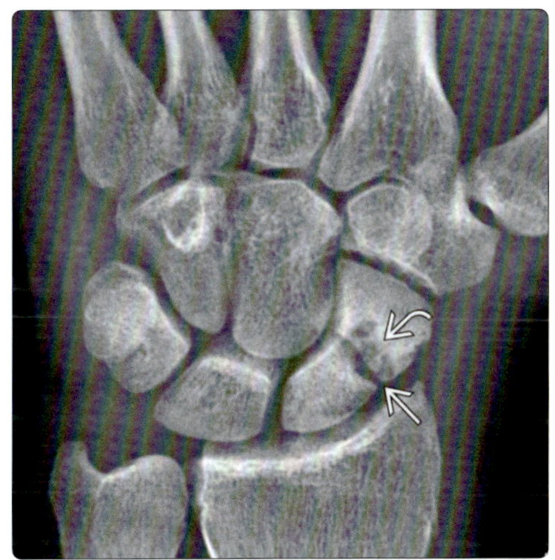

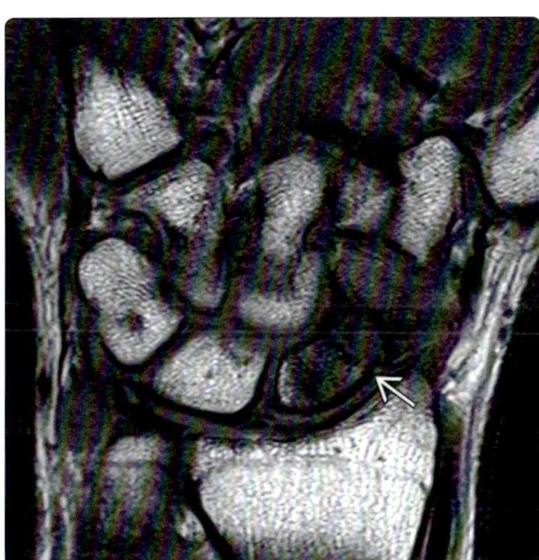

(Left) *PA radiograph shows an ununited waist of scaphoid fracture ➡. This is likely a true nonunion since the fracture lines are sclerotic and rounded, with subchondral cyst formation ➡. No definite sclerosis of the proximal pole is seen.* **(Right)** *Coronal T1 MR in the same case shows patchy low signal in both the proximal and distal poles of the scaphoid ➡. The fracture line is indistinctly seen.*

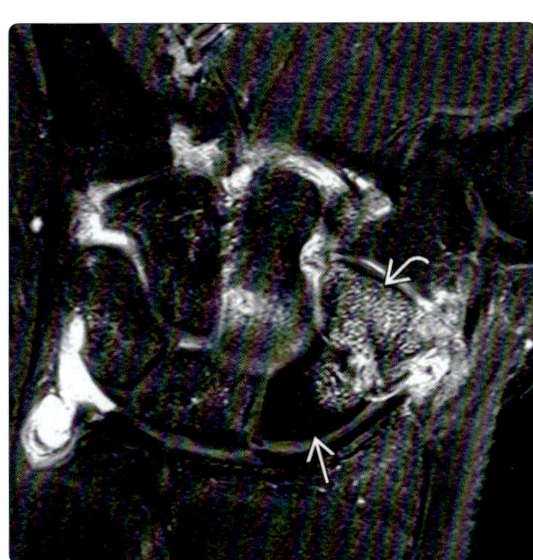

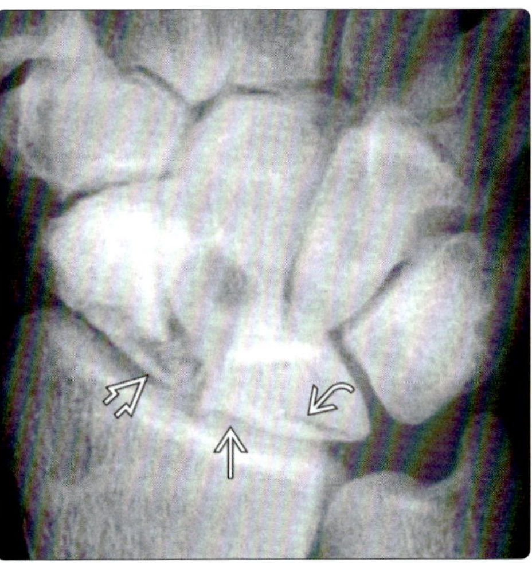

(Left) *Coronal postcontrast T1FS MR shows enhancement of distal pole ➡ but low signal in proximal pole ➡, indicating no blood supply. Though this is likely nonviable, it hasn't collapsed; surgery may be successful.* **(Right)** *PA radiograph of carpus from patient with systemic lupus erythematosus and ON shows collapsed proximal pole of scaphoid ➡. Irregularity along radial aspect of proximal lunate articular surface ➡ and subchondral fracture ➡ are seen. Radial-sided changes are more common than ulnar changes in Kienböck disease.*

KEY FACTS

IMAGING

- Radiographs: Sclerosis, articular surface irregularity ± collapse, fragmentation
- T1WI: Hypointense marrow signal
- Fluid-sensitive sequences
  - Acute/early: Bright marrow signal
  - Late: Low marrow signal
- Talar osteonecrosis (ON): Posttraumatic
  - Hawkins talar fracture classification used to estimate risk of ON
  - Hawkins sign: Relative ↑ lucency of talus indicates intact blood flow to talar body and predicts little risk of ON; occurs 6-8 weeks post injury
- Talar ON: Other causes
  - Ill-defined talar body sclerosis ± serpiginous margins on radiograph, less diffuse than posttraumatic causes
  - Classic MR appearance including serpiginous low signal periphery with central fat, double line sign
- Navicular ON: Mueller-Weiss (adult-onset) & Köhler (childhood-onset) disease
  - Changes initially occur laterally on navicular
  - Medial aspect subluxates medially and dorsally
- Metatarsals: 2nd metatarsal head most common, may involve 3rd metatarsal head in combination or isolation (Freiberg infraction)
- Sesamoids: Fibular sesamoid > tibial sesamoid

CLINICAL ISSUES

- Navicular & sesamoid ON, Freiberg infraction common in adolescent & young adult women
  - Chronic repetitive trauma may play role
- Initial stage of disease painful; may resolve or progress
- With progression at any of these sites, lesion develops fragmentation and sclerosis
  - ± articular surface collapse
  - May develop secondary osteoarthritis

(Left) *Oblique radiograph shows typical changes of advanced osteonecrosis (ON) of the talus. Irregular subchondral sclerosis is present ➡. Subtle collapse of the articular surface manifests as slight undulation in the articular surface ➡. Subchondral fracture appears as a lucent line ➡.* **(Right)** *Sagittal CT appearance of Freiberg infraction is shown. The metatarsal head is diffusely sclerotic ➡ and articular surface is flattened ➡. Secondary osteoarthritis is present with joint space narrowing & osteophytes ➡.*

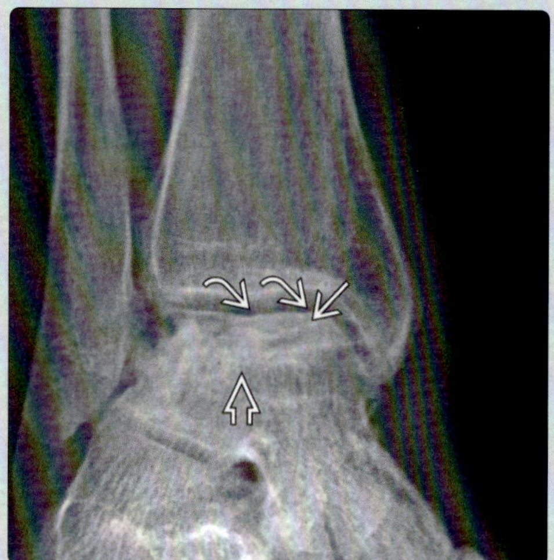

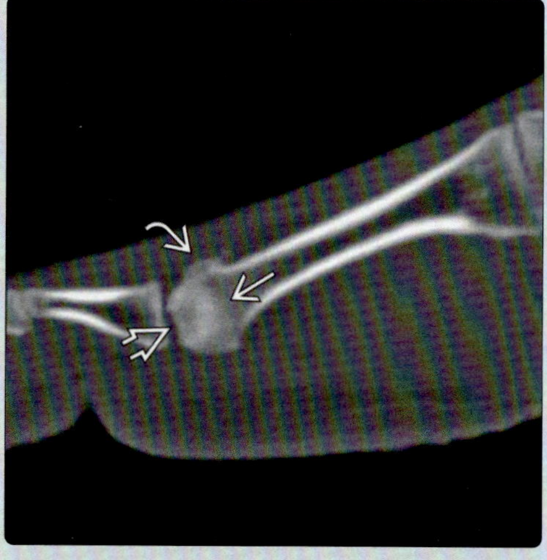

(Left) *Lateral radiograph in a young adult shows ON of the navicular, termed Mueller-Weiss. The navicular is highly fragmented, with some fragments being displaced superiorly ➡.* **(Right)** *AP radiograph, same case, shows the medial subluxation of the fragments ➡ that results in severe flattening of the navicular in its lateral aspect ➡. This morphology is typical of Mueller-Weiss.*

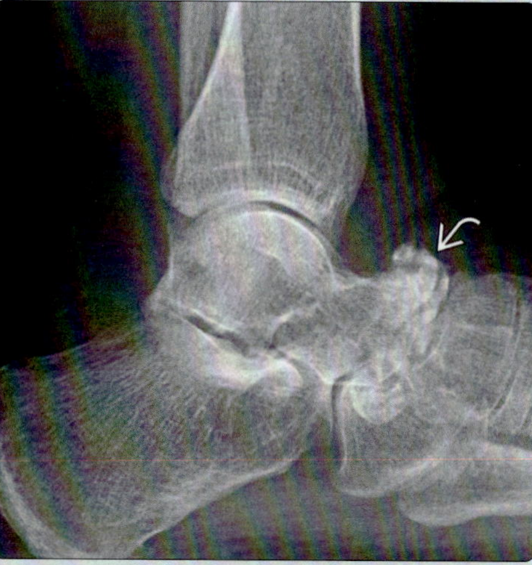

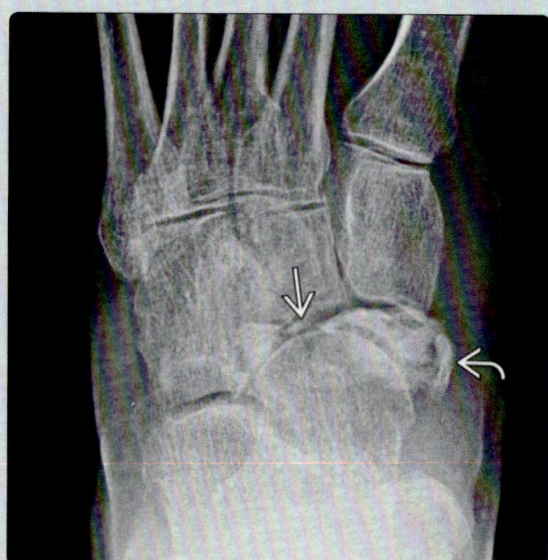

TERMINOLOGY

Definitions

- Hawkins sign: Subchondral ↑ lucency in talar dome
- Köhler disease: Childhood onset navicular disease
- Mueller-Weiss disease: Adult onset of navicular disease
- Freiberg infraction: Insult involving metatarsal head
- Sesamoiditis: Poorly defined term; may refer to any painful condition of sesamoid bones, including osteonecrosis (ON)

IMAGING

General Features

- Best diagnostic clue
  - Radiographs: Sclerosis, articular surface irregularity ± collapse, fragmentation
- Location
  - Freiberg infraction: 2nd metatarsal head most common, may involve 3rd metatarsal head in combination or isolation
  - Sesamoids: Fibular sesamoid > tibial sesamoid

Radiographic Findings

- Common constellation of findings
  - Sclerosis, fragmentation, articular surface collapse
- Talus: Posttraumatic etiology, most commonly talar neck fracture located distal to posterior facet
  - Vascularized bone becomes osteopenic; devascularized bone appears dense
  - As healing & new bone formation occur, devascularized fragment becomes even more dense
  - Hawkins sign: Indicates intact blood flow to talar body, predicts little risk of ON; occurs 6-8 weeks post injury
    - Partial Hawkins sign (subchondral lucency only present medially) indicative of necrosis isolated to lateral body
- Talus: ON due to other causes
  - Ill-defined talar body sclerosis ± serpiginous margins, less diffuse than posttraumatic causes
- Mueller-Weiss & Köhler disease: Commonly bilateral
  - Changes initially occur laterally
  - With disease progression lateral aspect collapses, may fragment or develop fracture
  - Medial aspect subluxes medially and dorsally

CT Findings

- Mirrors radiographs; more sensitive

MR Findings

- Common appearance for all described sites
  - T1WI: Hypointense marrow signal
  - Fluid-sensitive sequences
    - Acute/early: Bright marrow signal
    - Late: Low marrow signal
- Talus: Non-traumatic causes
  - Classic appearance including serpiginous low signal periphery with central fat, double line sign

Nuclear Medicine Findings

- Bone scan
  - Initially see focus of decreased uptake
    - May be difficult to appreciate in foot
  - Later disease shows increased uptake

PATHOLOGY

General Features

- Etiology
  - Köhler disease
    - Proposed etiologies other than ON: Abnormal enchondral ossification, normal variant
  - Sesamoid ON & Freiberg infraction
    - Unclear if idiopathic ON is etiology
    - Chronic repetitive trauma may play role
    - High-heeled shoes implicated as causative insult

Staging, Grading, & Classification

- Hawkins classification of talar neck fractures: Used to assess risk of ON
  - I: Nondisplaced talar neck fracture (0-15% risk)
  - II: Displaced fracture with subtalar subluxation/dislocation (20-50% risk)
  - III: Displaced fracture with tibiotalar and subtalar disruption (65-100% risk)
  - IV: III + talonavicular disruption (100% risk)

Gross Pathologic & Surgical Features

- Talus vascular supply: Branches of posterior tibial artery, dorsalis pedis artery, perforating peroneal artery
  - Blood supply to body is retrograde from neck
  - Fracture between body & neck separates body from its blood supply
  - Richer supply medially; lateral talus at greater risk

CLINICAL ISSUES

Presentation

- Most common signs/symptoms
  - Pain most common presenting symptom
  - Köhler disease: Asymptomatic or mild pain

Demographics

- Navicular & sesamoid ON, Freiberg infraction common in adolescent & young adult women

Natural History & Prognosis

- Initial stage of disease painful; may resolve or progress
- Köhler disease may resolve without treatment
- If progresses, → fragmentation, sclerosis ± articular surface collapse; may develop secondary osteoarthritis

Treatment

- Prior to onset of fragmentation & collapse nonweight-bearing may lead to resolution
- Once collapse & fragmentation occur, treatment if symptomatic, may require surgical intervention

SELECTED REFERENCES

1. Bartolotta RJ et al: Mueller-Weiss syndrome: imaging and implications. Clin Imaging. 38(6):895-8, 2014
2. Talusan PG et al: Freiberg's infraction: diagnosis and treatment. Foot Ankle Spec. 7(1):52-6, 2014
3. Buchan CA et al: Imaging of postoperative avascular necrosis of the ankle and foot. Semin Musculoskelet Radiol. 16(3):192-204, 2012

(Left) *Lateral radiograph of the talus taken 1 year after talar neck fracture is shown. The talar body is diffusely sclerotic, and the articular surface is irregular, indicative of osteonecrosis. While talar ON is more commonly seen in adults, it can occur at any age.* **(Right)** *AP radiograph shows a talus with avascular necrosis confined to the lateral body. The lateral articular surface is fragmented and collapsed. The medial body has a richer blood supply, which offers some protection against ON.*

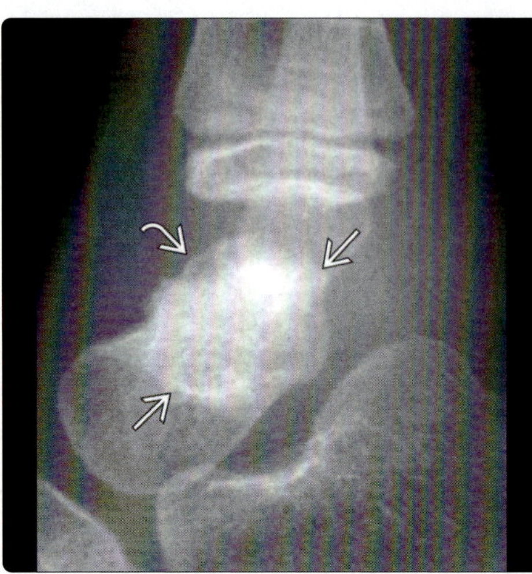

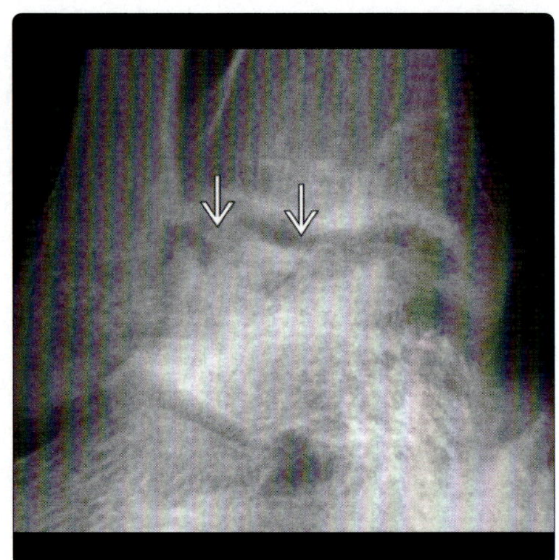

(Left) *Lateral radiograph shows a foot with ON of the navicular, also termed Mueller-Weiss. The typical superior subluxation of the medial aspect of the navicular is readily apparent.* **(Right)** *Axial CT, same case, shows the morphology of Mueller-Weiss syndrome. This condition may have associated fracture that is typically sagittally oriented, as in this case where the fracture is now healed. This fracture contributes to the medial subluxation of the navicular.*

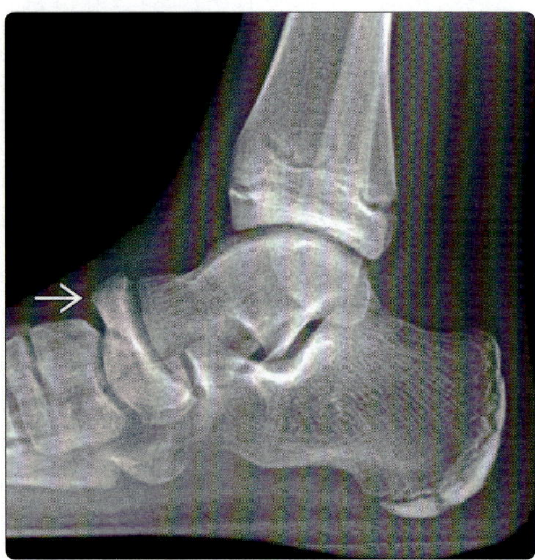

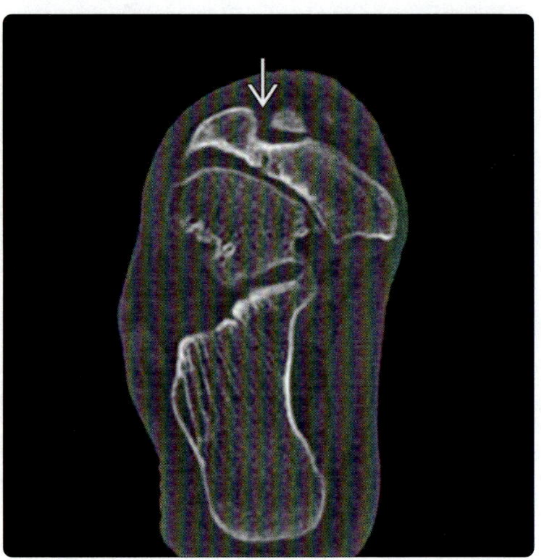

(Left) *Sagittal T1WI of the foot demonstrates the common appearance of navicular ON. There is low signal within the tarsal navicular and the bone is collapsed.* **(Right)** *Sagittal STIR MR of the foot shows the common appearance of acute or subacute ON with marrow edema. In addition, the typical fracture that accompanies Mueller-Weiss syndrome is evident.*

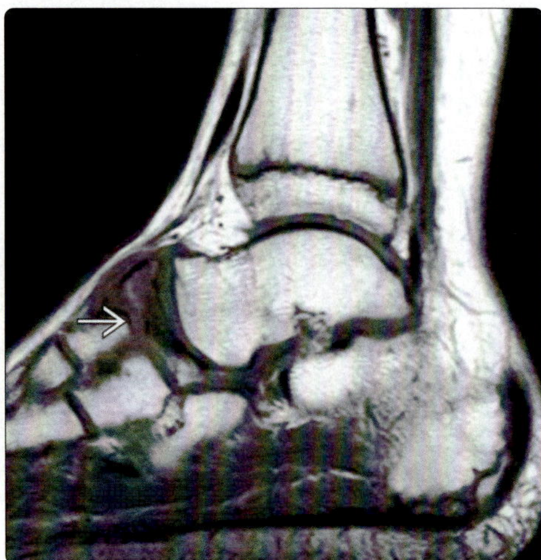

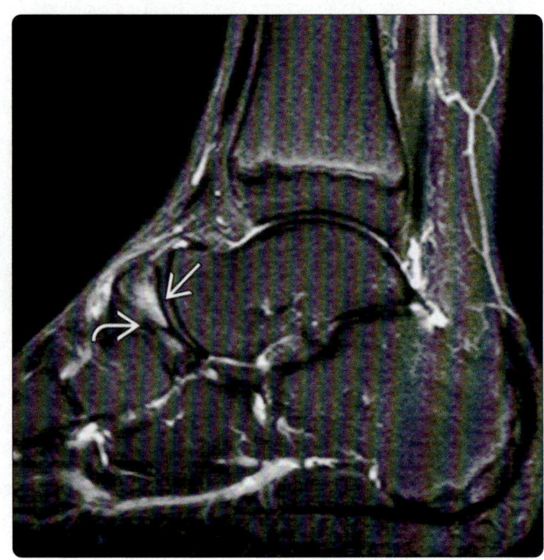

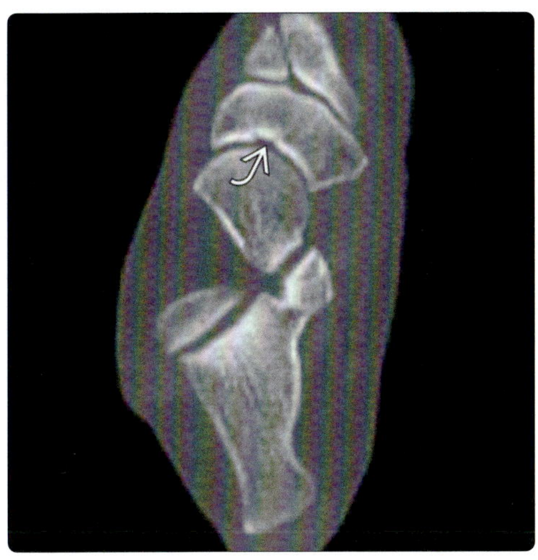

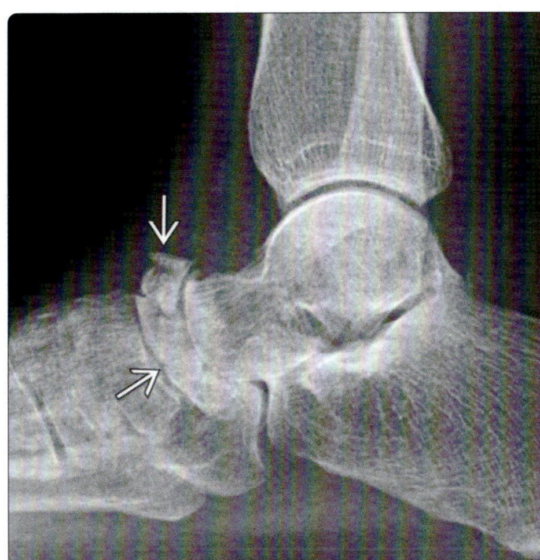

(Left) *Long axis CT of a young adult's foot that is newly painful shows a subtle depression ➩ in the proximal aspect of the navicular. This is the site where a fracture will subsequently develop, leading eventually to severe fragmentation and a more recognizable appearance of Mueller-Weiss.* **(Right)** *Lateral radiograph of the same patient obtained 2 years later shows the severe fragmentation of the navicular ➡ that has developed.*

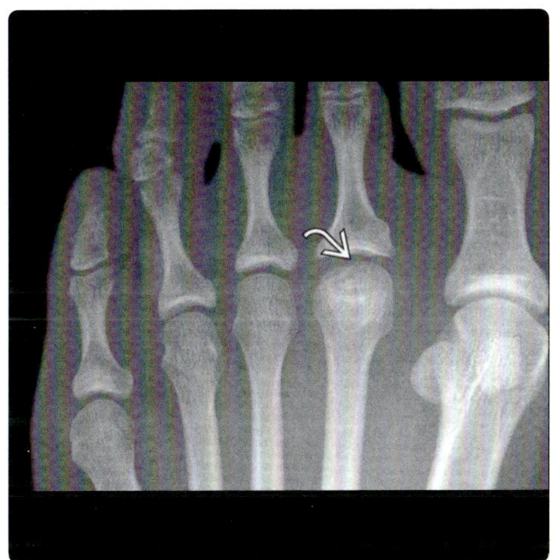

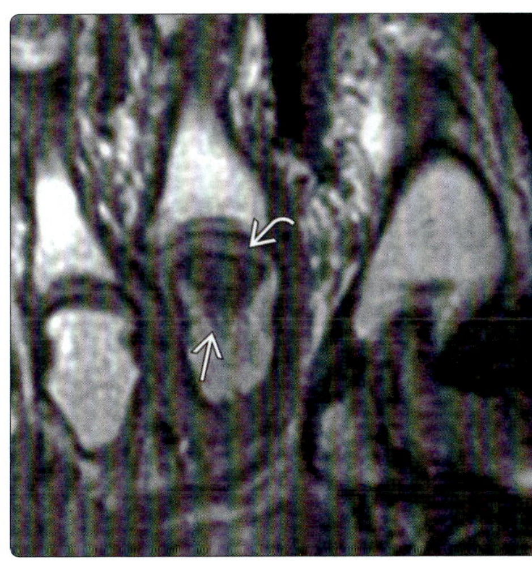

(Left) *AP radiograph of the toes shows that the 2nd metatarsal head has slightly increased density and the articular surface is flattened ➩. These findings are typical of Freiberg infraction.* **(Right)** *Axial T1WI MR shows typical Freiberg infraction. Low signal is present with the subchondral bone of the 2nd metatarsal head ➡. The articular surface is flattened ➩ without fracture or fragmentation.*

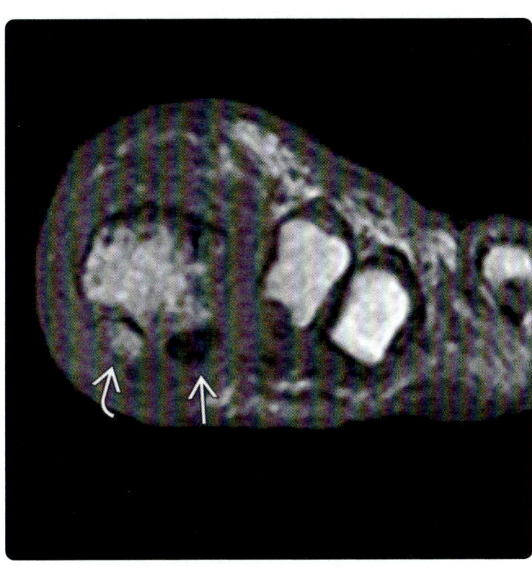

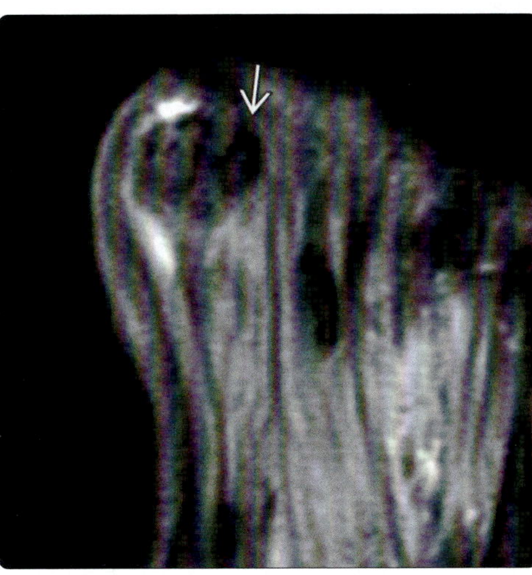

(Left) *Coronal T1WI MR through the 1st metatarsal shows expected changes of chronic ON of the lateral (fibular) hallux sesamoid with sclerosis and resultant low signal intensity of the marrow ➡. The medial (tibial) sesamoid is normal ➩.* **(Right)** *Axial T2WI FS MR shows the late phase of sesamoid ON. Diffuse low signal is present in the fibular sesamoid ➡. In the acute phase, edematous/bright signal will be seen.*

Legg-Calvé-Perthes Disease

KEY FACTS

TERMINOLOGY

- Legg-Calvé-Perthes: Osteonecrosis of femoral head epiphysis during childhood

IMAGING

- Early radiographic findings
  - Effusion and lateral subluxation of femoral head
  - Fragmentation of femoral capital epiphysis
  - Sclerosis and flattening of epiphysis
- Midterm radiographic findings, if progresses
  - Lateral extrusion of portion of femoral head
  - Metaphyseal irregularity, cystic changes
- Late radiographic findings with severe progression
  - Coxa plana deformity, ↓ acetabular congruence
  - Coxa magna deformity (short broad head/neck)
  - Growth disturbance (25% have premature physeal closure, 90% show decreased growth resulting in limb length discrepancy)
- MR: Early (avascular or necrotic) phase
  - Low or intermediate T1 signal epiphysis
  - Variable SI on T2WI/STIR: May see curvilinear low SI or high SI edema
  - Partial or complete nonenhancement (normal hip shows early and rapid enhancement)
- Revascularization and reparative phases
  - Heterogeneous epiphyseal signal on T1WI, T2WI/STIR
  - Revascularized areas of epiphysis show ↑ SI on T2WI/STIR and enhancement (even hyperenhancement)
  - Morphologic epiphyseal abnormalities
  - Abnormal; physeal enhancement 2° to presence of abnormal transphyseal blood vessels
  - Early bony bridging (physeal bar)
  - Metaphyseal abnormalities corresponding to "cysts" seen on radiograph (cartilage, fibrosis)

CLINICAL ISSUES

- Age: 3-12 years (median peak incidence: 6 years)
- Gender: M > F (4-5:1)

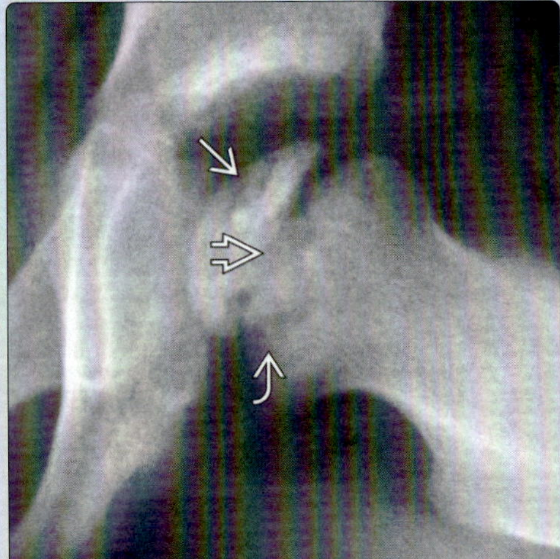

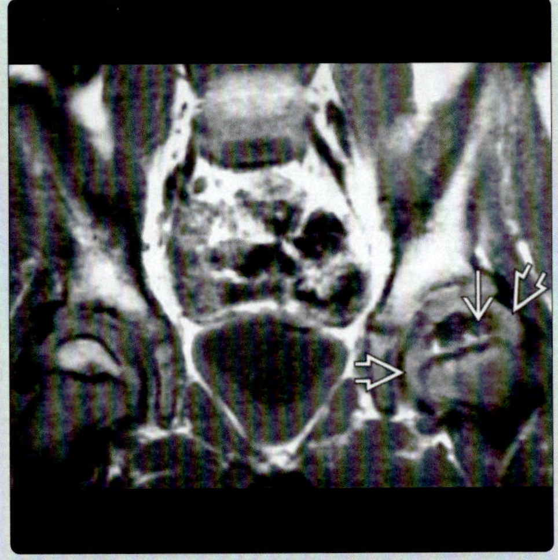

(Left) *Frog leg lateral radiograph shows classic Legg-Calvé-Perthes (LCP), with relative increase in density of the femoral capital epiphysis, flattening of the femoral head, & subchondral fracture in the weight-bearing portion of the head ➔. Metaphysis is widened, with "cystic" changes ➔. There is a physeal bar ➔, which will result in growth deformity.* **(Right)** *Coronal T1WI MR, same case, shows central low signal at the site of necrosis ➔. The cartilage is thicker, surrounding the necrotic epiphysis both medially and laterally ➔.*

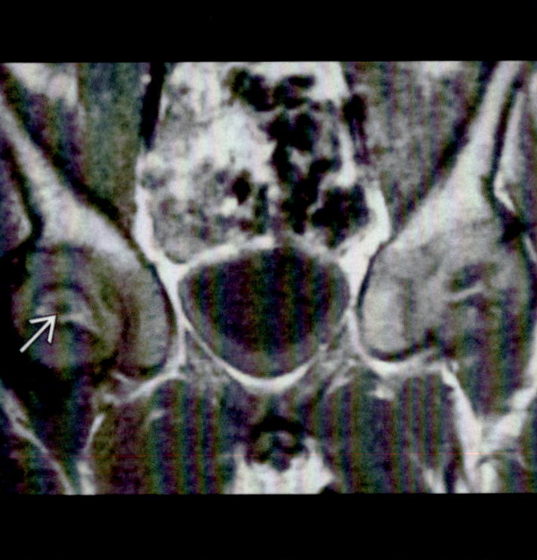

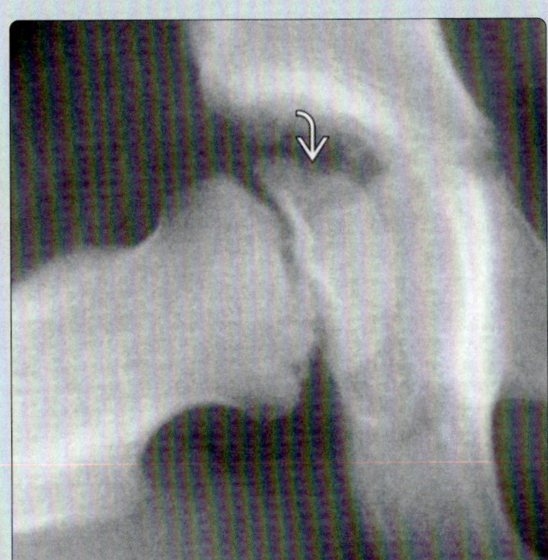

(Left) *Coronal T1WI MR more anteriorly in the same case shows the only focus of abnormality in the right epiphysis. This small, low signal focus ➔ indicates early LCP.* **(Right)** *Frog leg lateral radiograph, same case, shows a small focal region of lucency in the anterosuperior femoral head ➔, corresponding to the MR abnormality. There is no sclerosis or convincing flattening. AP of the right hip (not shown) was normal and only the left hip was symptomatic. LCP involves both hips in 15-20% of cases and is often asynchronous.*

TERMINOLOGY

Abbreviations

- Legg-Calvé-Perthes (LCP)

Definitions

- Osteonecrosis (ON) of femoral head epiphysis during childhood

IMAGING

Radiographic Findings

- Radiography
  - Early findings
    - Effusion and lateral subluxation of femoral head
    - Fragmentation of femoral capital epiphysis
    - Sclerosis and flattening of epiphysis
  - Midterm findings, if disease progresses
    - Lateral extrusion of portion of femoral head
    - Metaphyseal irregularity (rarefaction of lateral + medial metaphysis + cystic changes)
    - Catterall classification (group I-IV) estimates amount of femoral head involvement
  - Late findings with severe progression
    - Lateral subluxation
    - Coxa plana deformity (flattened head)
    - Loss of sphericity of head and congruence with acetabulum
    - Coxa magna deformity (short broad head and neck)
    - Growth disturbance (25% have premature physeal closure, 90% show decreased growth, resulting in limb length discrepancy)
    - Thigh atrophy
    - Eventual osteoarthritis (OA)

MR Findings

- Parameters to be evaluated on MR
  - Early disease
  - Percentage of femoral head involvement
  - Femoral head epiphyseal bone and cartilage height
  - Hypoperfusion of portions of head
- Early (avascular or necrotic) phase
  - Abnormality usually in subchondral and central epiphysis
    - Low or intermediate T1 signal
    - Variable signal intensity on T2WI/STIR: May see curvilinear low signal intensity or high signal intensity edema
    - Partial or complete nonenhancement (normal hip shows early and rapid enhancement)
    - If ossific surface is flattened, overlying cartilage may be thickened and abnormal in signal
    - If bone is low signal intensity on all sequences with no enhancement, advanced necrosis is likely
- Revascularization and reparative phases
  - Heterogeneous epiphyseal signal on T1WI, T2WI/STIR, enhanced MR
    - Combination of necrosis, revascularization, repair
    - Over time, necrotic bone replaced by granulation tissue, later replaced by fibrous tissue, and eventually replaced by mature bone with normal signal
  - Revascularized areas of epiphysis show increased signal intensity on T2WI/STIR and enhancement (even hyperenhancement)
    - Early reperfusion of lateral pillar (lateral 1/3 of head) correlates with improved prognosis
  - Morphologic epiphyseal abnormalities
    - Coxa plana, fragmentation
    - Lateral femoral head subluxation, ↓ containment by acetabulum
  - Physeal involvement
    - Irregularity of growth plate
    - Abnormal enhancement 2° to presence of abnormal transphyseal blood vessels
    - Early bony bridging (physeal bar)
    - Cystic change
  - Metaphyseal involvement
    - Abnormalities corresponding to "cysts" seen on radiograph
      - May consist of physeal cartilage extensions
      - Some contain granulation tissue, fibrosis, or fat necrosis
    - Coxa magna morphology (short, broad neck)
- Specialized MR techniques relating to prognosis
  - Dynamic gadolinium-enhanced subtracted T1 or SPGR
    - Lateral pillar enhancement correlates with vascularization and better prognosis
  - Diffusion-weighted MR imaging
    - Increased diffusivity shown in all affected hips
    - Increased diffusivity in metaphysis in those hips with absent lateral pillar enhancement
    - DWI appears to correlate with dynamic enhanced imaging for prognostic purposes
  - Delayed enhanced MR
    - Demonstrates complex cartilage damage pattern (glycosaminoglycan loss in medial cartilage)
- MR arthrography for adolescent/young adult patients with residual deformity
  - Labral tear
  - Cartilage thinning, defects

Nuclear Medicine Findings

- Bone scintigraphy
  - Early photopenia in epiphysis secondary to interruption of blood supply
  - Increased uptake late, following revascularization, repair, &/or degenerative arthritis

Imaging Recommendations

- Best imaging tool
  - MR for early detection/prognosis → early treatment
  - MR arthrogram for evaluation of associated femoral acetabular impingement and early OA
- Protocol advice
  - Coronal and sagittal planes emphasized on MR; 26% underestimated head flattening without sagittal

DIFFERENTIAL DIAGNOSIS

Immune-Mediated and Viral (Toxic) Synovitis

- Self-limiting acute synovitis (3-10 days)
- Boys < 4 years old (generally younger than LCP)
- Significant effusion; no epiphyseal abnormality

Septic Hip

- Acutely ill with fever
- Increased white blood cell count + sedimentation rate
- Hips held in flexion, abduction + external rotation vs. hip adduction in LCP
- Joint effusion ± joint debris ± reactive marrow edema

Juvenile Idiopathic Arthritis

- Epiphyseal crenulation or erosions may mimic LCP
- Chronic disease: Valgus hip, gracile femoral shaft, hypoplastic iliac wing
- Thigh muscle hypoplasia

Juvenile Osteonecrosis

- Distinction: Identifiable etiology of ON
  - Sickle cell, less likely thalassemia
  - Idiopathic thrombocytopenia purpura
  - Hip dislocation

Epiphyseal Dysplasias

- Not isolated to femoral capital epiphysis

Hypothyroidism and Cretinism

- Cretinoid hip: Fragmented, small femoral capital epiphysis
- Significant delay in skeletal maturation

DDx of Coxa Magna of Mature Legg-Calvé-Perthes

- Developmental dysplasia of hip
  - Acetabular dysplasia distinguishes this etiology
- Slipped capital femoral epiphysis
  - Posteromedial head prominence, even with coxa magna

PATHOLOGY

General Features

- Etiology
  - Insufficiency of capital epiphyseal blood supply with physis acting as barrier
    - Infarction → trabecular fracture with decreased epiphyseal height
    - Ischemia may be arterial or venous-based leading to intraepiphyseal infarction
    - Hypercoagulable disorders may play role
  - Overgrowth of articular cartilage medially and laterally
    - Contributes to flattening of head and coxa magna
  - Incongruity of head with acetabulum → femoral acetabular impingement → labral tear and cartilage defects → early OA

Staging, Grading, & Classification

- Catterall: Distribution of epiphyseal abnormalities based on AP + lateral radiographs
  - Group I: < 1/4 epiphysis involved
  - Group II: < 1/2 epiphysis involved
  - Group III: Most of epiphysis involved
  - Group IV: Total epiphysis involved
- Herring system: Based on lateral pillar involvement (lateral 30% of epiphysis = lateral pillar)
  - A = uninvolved lateral pillar
  - B = < 50% involvement of lateral pillar
  - C = > 50% involvement of lateral pillar

CLINICAL ISSUES

Presentation

- Most common signs/symptoms
  - Limp + groin, thigh, or knee pain (referred)

Demographics

- Age
  - 3-12 years (median peak incidence: 6 years)
- Gender
  - M > F (4-5:1)
- Ethnicity
  - Caucasians most frequently affected
- Epidemiology
  - 15-20% bilateral (usually asynchronous)
  - 5-15 per 100,000

Natural History & Prognosis

- 60-70% heal spontaneously without functional impairment at maturity
- Risk factors associated with poor outcome
  - Older skeletal age at time of presentation
  - Radiographic signs of worse prognosis
    - Lateral subluxation
    - Calcification lateral to epiphysis
    - Gage sign (radiolucent "V" in lateral epiphysis)
    - Metaphyseal "cyst" formation
    - > 20% epiphyseal extrusion
    - > 50% femoral head involvement
  - MR signs of worse prognosis
    - Extensive epiphyseal involvement, especially lateral pillar (lateral 1/3 head)
    - Transphyseal neovascularity (associated with growth disturbance)
    - Subchondral ossific nucleus fracture
    - Metaphyseal signal abnormalities and physeal bar
- Late adolescence/young adult developments
  - In young adults, deterioration of hip function correlates with residual hip deformity
    - Femoral acetabular impingement
    - Labral tear, cartilage damage, leading to early OA

Treatment

- Conservative for those judged at ↓ risk for progression
  - Bed rest + abduction stretching and bracing
- Surgical: Principle is containment and preservation of range of motion
  - Femoral/pelvic osteotomy to improve containment and head reduction osteotomy to improve sphericity

DIAGNOSTIC CHECKLIST

Consider

- MR useful for initial preradiography detection, determination of prognosis, and evaluation of complications at skeletal maturity

SELECTED REFERENCES

1. Accadbled F et al: "Femoroacetabular impingement". Legg-Calve-Perthes disease: from childhood to adulthood. Orthop Traumatol Surg Res. 100(6):647-9, 2014

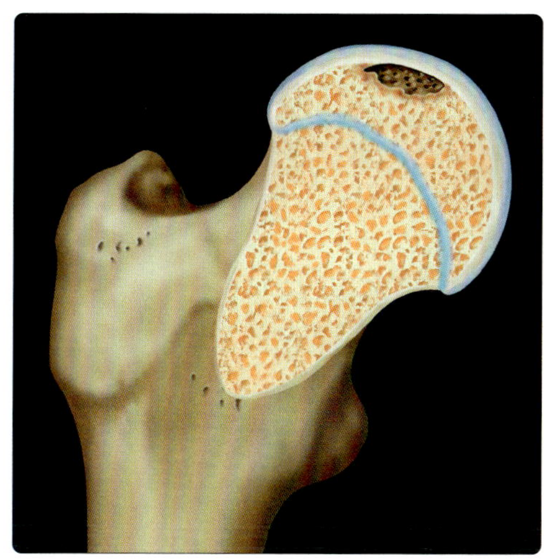

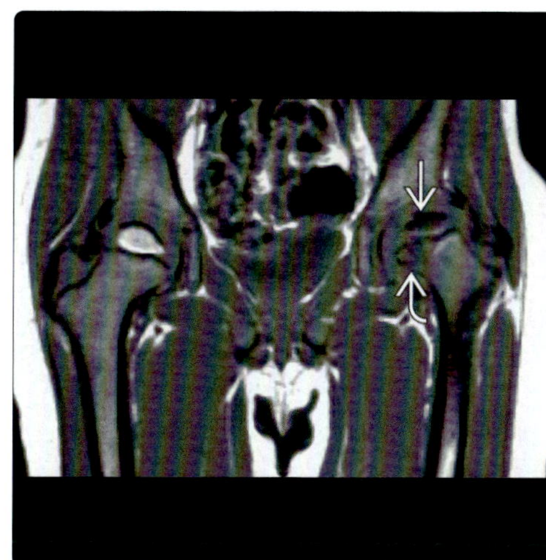

(Left) *Coronal graphic shows subchondral necrosis in the proximal femoral epiphysis in early LCP. This superolateral location is typical; earliest disease is often located farther anteriorly than depicted here.* **(Right)** *Coronal T1WI MR shows an ischemic left capital epiphysis ➡. Compare it to the normal fat density in the right. There is hypertrophy of the medial and lateral cartilage and medial metaphyseal sclerosis/cystic change ⮕.*

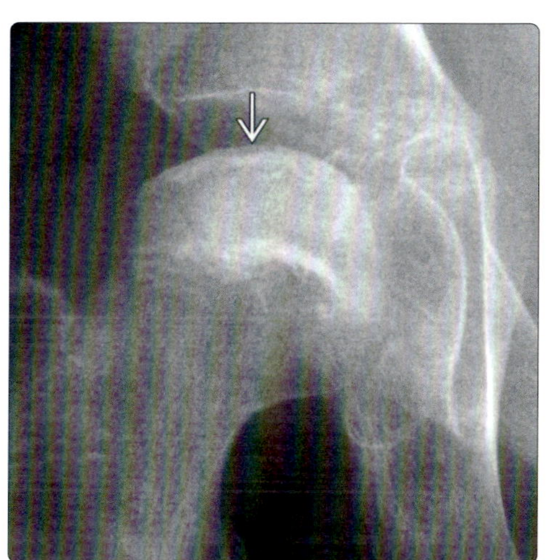

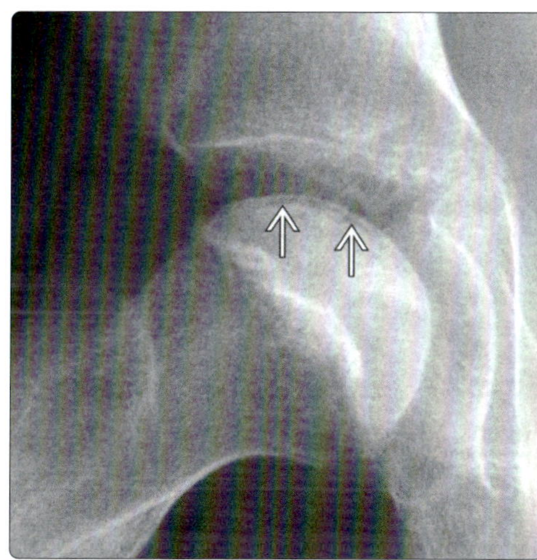

(Left) *AP radiograph shows a relative density of the right femoral capital epiphysis, seen prominently because of the osteoporosis of the surrounding bones. The hip shows mild flattening of the weight-bearing portion of the head, as well as a subchondral fracture ➡.* **(Right)** *Frog leg lateral radiograph, same case, shows the flattening and crescent sign of the subchondral fracture to better advantage ➡. LCP, as well as osteonecrosis in the adult patient, is a good indication for a frog lateral rather than a groin lateral.*

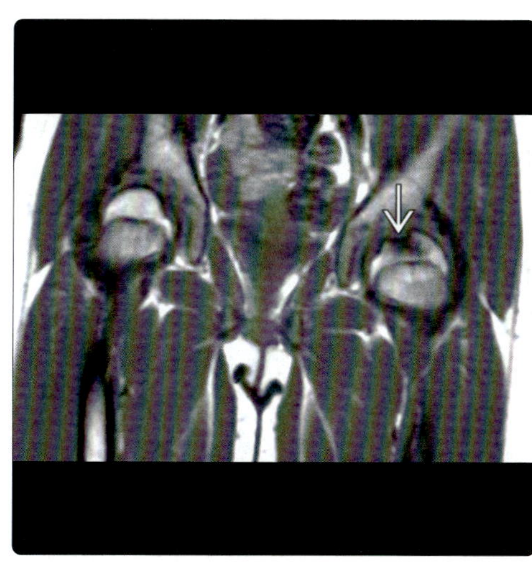

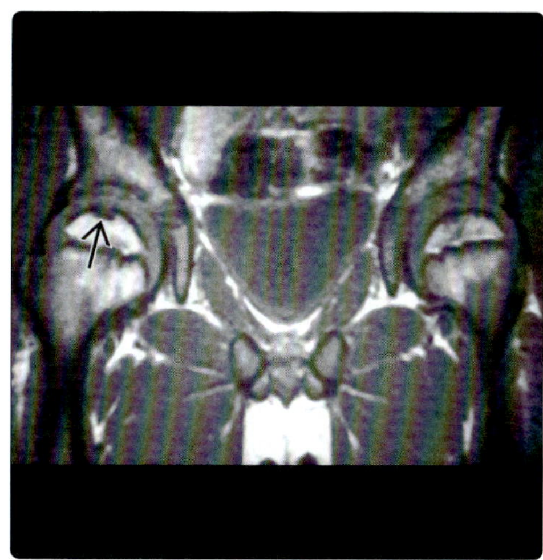

(Left) *Coronal T1WI MR shows left LCP with subchondral collapse ➡. This child is older than many that are imaged for LCP, as indicated by the greater proportion of femoral head ossification. A mild coxa plana has developed; the acetabulum has overgrown to contain the nonspherical femoral head.* **(Right)** *Coronal T1WI MR shows early LCP with hypointense ischemic change in the superior aspect of the right capital epiphysis ➡ and centrally in the left epiphysis. Bilateral physeal irregularity is present.*

(Left) *Frog leg lateral radiograph shows slight flattening ➡ and sclerosis ➡ of the left femoral capital epiphysis, typical of LCP. This child was 9.2 years of age, giving a poor prognosis for this hip.* **(Right)** *Coronal T2WI MR, same patient and obtained at the time of the radiograph, shows low signal necrosis within the epiphysis with associated flattening ➡. There is marrow edema in the femoral neck ➡ and a sizable joint effusion ➡. The physis is abnormal, with variable low and high signal.*

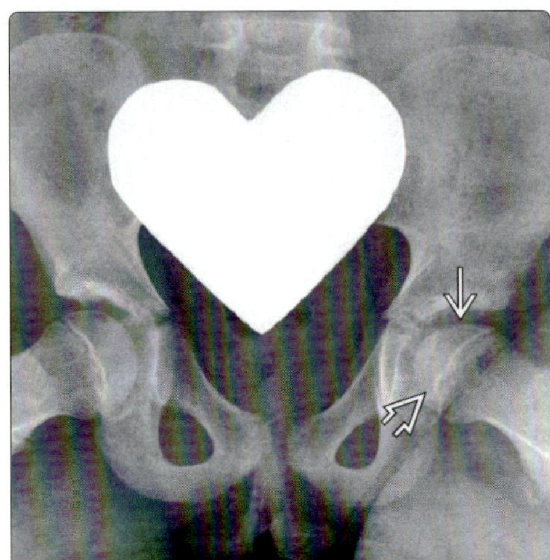

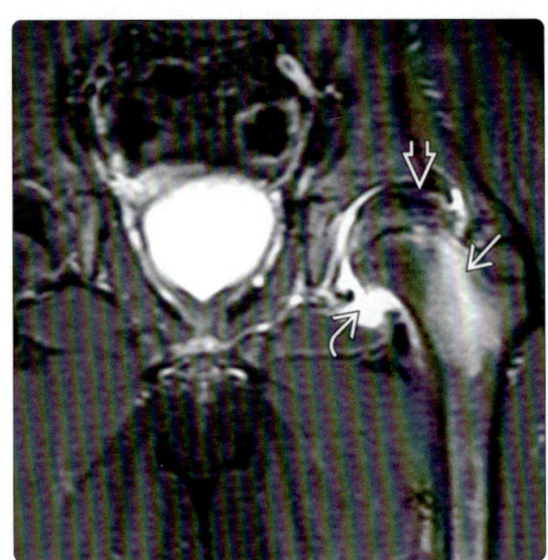

(Left) *Frog leg lateral radiograph in the same case 3 months later shows further collapse ➡ and sclerosis of the femoral ossification center and new development of pseudocystic changes in the femoral neck ➡. The concerns at the outset for poor prognosis were justified.* **(Right)** *Frog leg lateral shows left femoral flattening, coxa magna, and a small fragmented ossification center ➡. Though the head is likely to fully reossify at a later time, this deformity and extent of epiphyseal abnormality indicate a poor prognosis.*

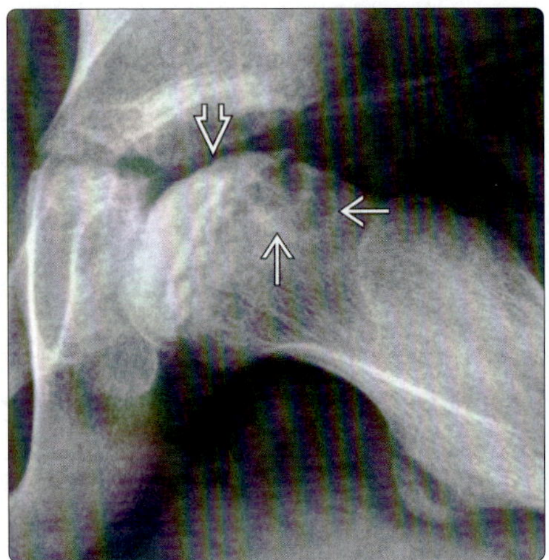

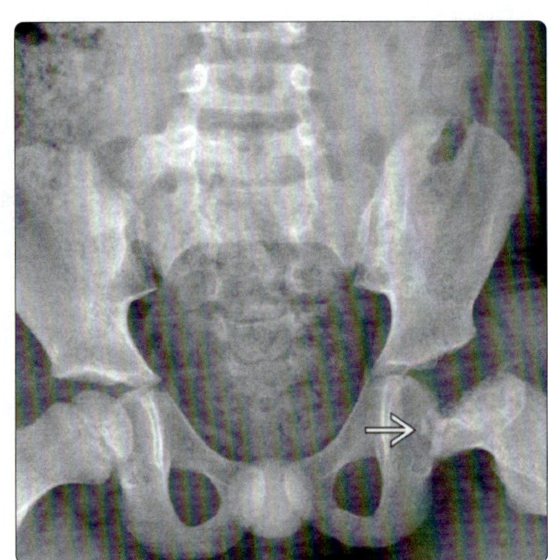

(Left) *Coronal STIR MR, same case, shows extrusion of the femoral head laterally with partial uncoverage ➡. There is increased signal at the physeal-metaphyseal junction ➡ due to revascularization and repair and a small joint effusion ➡.* **(Right)** *Axial T1WI C+ FS MR shows enhancement at the physeal-metaphyseal junction ➡, which may be granulation or fibrous tissue or transphyseal revascularization. These findings indicate a poor prognosis for a long-term functional outcome.*

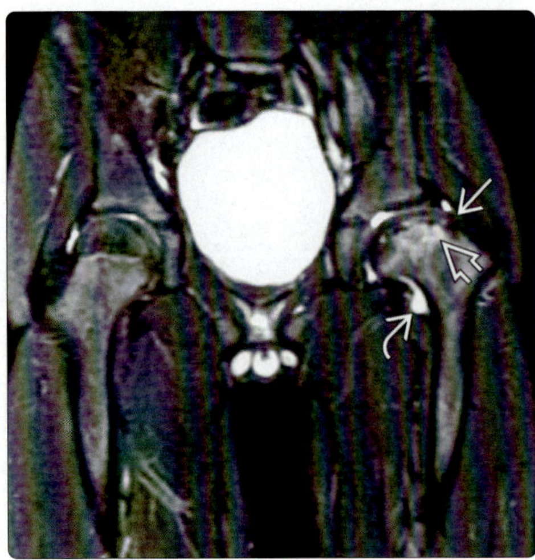

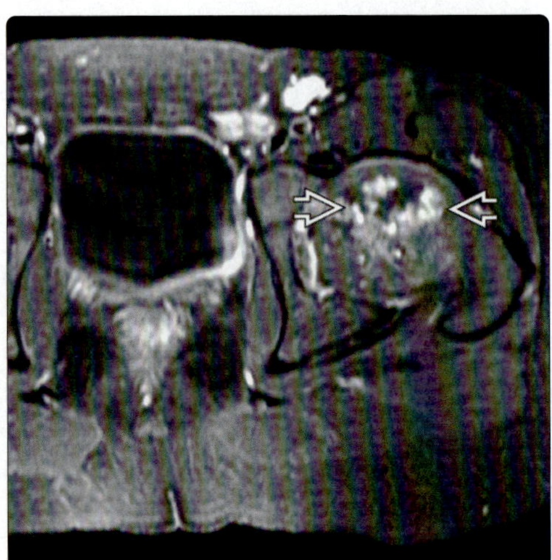

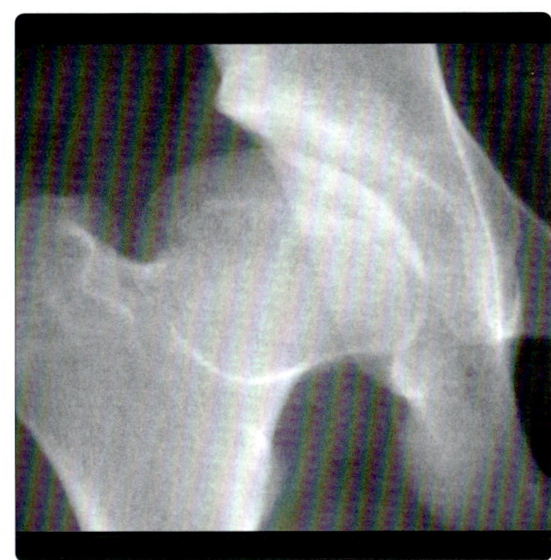

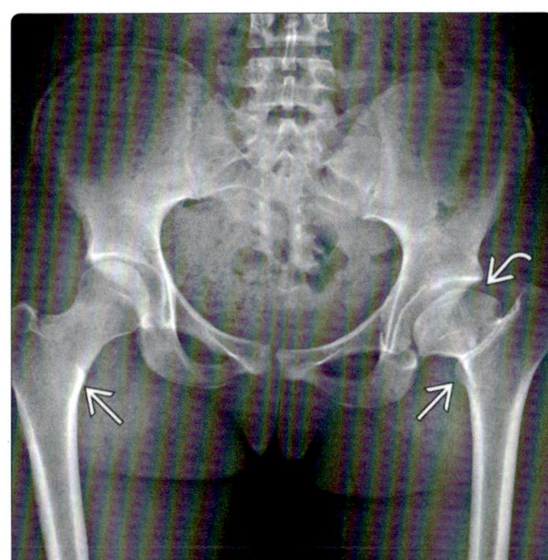

(Left) *AP radiograph obtained 8 years following diagnosis of LCP shows a typical coxa magna deformity with a large flattened femoral head and short wide femoral neck. The acetabulum is remodeled, resulting in a concentric but nonspherical joint.* **(Right)** *AP radiograph shows a coxa magna deformity ➡. There is relative shortening of the limb (compare levels of lesser trochanters ➡). This LCP is at risk for developing early osteoarthritis (OA) due to a morphology that predisposes to femoral acetabular impingement (FAI).*

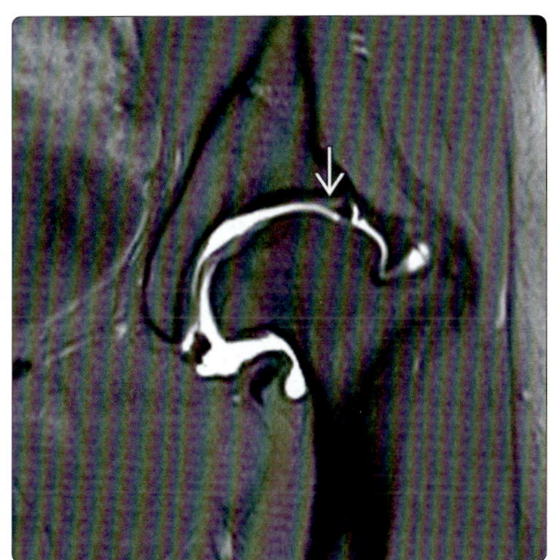

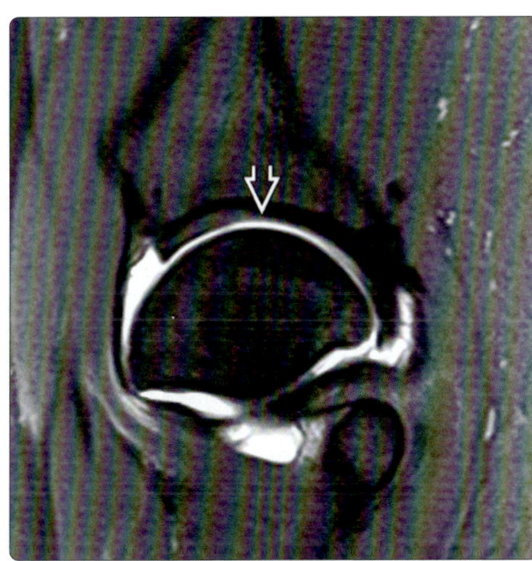

(Left) *Coronal MR arthrogram, same case, shows the coxa magna deformity with nonspherical head and a tear in the superior labrum ➡.* **(Right)** *Sagittal MR arthrogram, same case, shows a large region of cartilage damage in the weight-bearing portions of both the acetabulum and femoral head ➡. The cartilage and labral damage are already severe in this 15-year-old patient who developed LCP 8 years earlier and is now well on her way to developing debilitating OA.*

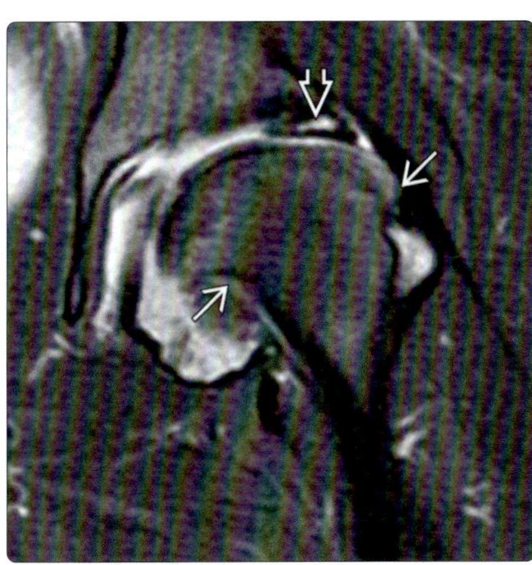

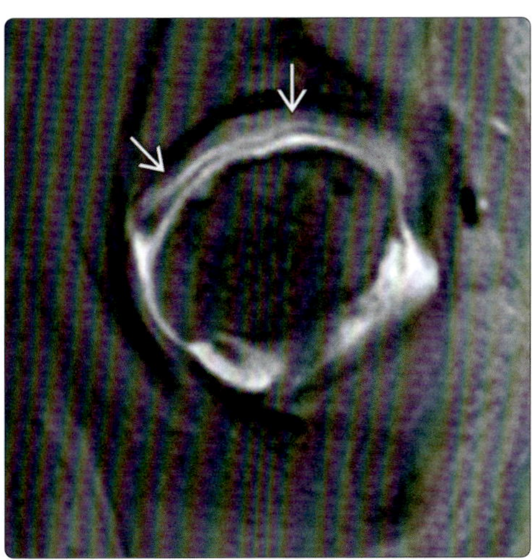

(Left) *Coronal T2WI FS MR following arthrogram demonstrates a coxa magna deformity ➡, which results in abnormal articulation and secondary hypertrophy of the labrum. The shape of the femoral head and neck results in a cam-type FAI, which often results in a labral tear and cartilage damage. Large labral tear is noted ➡.* **(Right)** *Sagittal T1WI FS MR arthrogram, same case, shows that the labral injury is a bucket handle tear ➡. Remember that coxa magna deformity contributes to FAI.*

SECTION 11

Metabolic Bone Disease

Introduction and Overview

Diseases of Calcium Homeostasis

Osteoporosis

Pituitary Disorders

Thyroid Disease

Miscellaneous Metabolic Conditions

General Comments

Metabolic bone disease is a topic which many find intimidating, others just plain boring. It does not require sexy MR imaging and often we are bystanders rather than active participants in the diagnostic process. However, when one takes the time to explore the topic, it can be as exciting as any other facet of musculoskeletal imaging.

The actual role of bone is often misunderstood. While certainly it serves a critical function in providing structure and protection to our soft tissues, bone also serves a crucial role as a reservoir for calcium and many other salts essential to life. Bone is a dynamic biologic system. Active bone remodeling involves a balance between bone formation and resorption that occurs throughout life.

Bone Metabolism: The Players

Salts

Calcium (Ca^{2+}) is essential to the function of skeletal muscle, cardiac muscle, nerve conduction, and the coagulation cascade. The body ensures that adequate Ca^{2+} is always available by storing Ca^{2+} within the mineralized component of bone. Over 99% of the body's Ca^{2+} is stored in bone as calcium hydroxyapatite.

Phosphorus is the chemical element required for almost all biological functions.

Phosphate ($PO4^{3-}$) is formed when phosphorus binds with oxygen to form phosphate, which is the most common form of phosphorus in the body.

Calcium hydroxyapatite [$Ca_{10}(PO4^{3-})_6(OH)_2$] is the primary form of calcium found within bones and teeth.

Hormones, prohormones, and enzymes

Parathyroid hormone (PTH) is produced in the parathyroid glands. Production is stimulated by low serum Ca^{2+}. PTH acts on the bone, kidney, and intestine to increase serum Ca^{2+} levels. Mechanisms of action include ↑ renal tubule reabsorption of Ca^{2+}, ↑ intestinal absorption of Ca^{2+}, and stimulation of renal formation of calcitriol. PTH also indirectly increases serum Ca^{2+} levels by diminishing renal reabsorption of $PO4^{3-}$, thus preventing its binding to Ca^{2+}, which would lead to decreased serum Ca^{2+} levels. The overall effects of PTH are to ↑ **serum Ca^{2+}**. Regarding its effect on $PO4^{3-}$, PTH blocks reabsorption of excreted $PO4^{3-}$ (resulting in $PO4^{3-}$ excretion) in the kidney and promotes absorption in the intestines and from the bones resulting in an **overall null effect on serum $PO4^{3-}$** levels.

Calcitonin is produced by parafollicular cells of the thyroid gland. An antagonist to PTH, its secretion results in **decreased serum Ca^{2+}**. Formation is stimulated by ↑ Ca^{2+} levels. Its importance in bone homeostasis is not clear.

Cholecalciferol or vitamin D_3 is the prohormone of active vitamin D. It is produced in the skin.

7- dehydrocholesterol is the supplemental and dietary precursor of vitamin D, converted in the skin to prohormone vitamin D_3. Conversion requires UV light.

Vitamin D_2 (ergosterol) is the artificial form of vitamin D that may be used for dietary supplementation. It follows the same conversion path as vitamin D_3.

25 hydroxycholecalciferol (25-OH-D_3, calcifediol, calcidiol) is formed by hydroxylation of vitamin D_3 in the liver; the responsible enzyme is **vitamin D-25 hydroxylase**.

1,25 dihydroxycholecalciferol [1,25$(OH)_2D_3$; calcitriol] is the active form of vitamin D, formed in the renal proximal tubule under control of the enzyme **1α hydroxylase.** Active vitamin D is actually a hormone. Its formation is stimulated by low serum Ca^{2+} and $PO4^{3-}$. Its primary target organs are the intestine and bone. In the intestines, it increases absorption of Ca^{2+} and $PO4^{3-}$. In bone, in conjunction with PTH, active vitamin D stimulates Ca^{2+} and $PO4^{3-}$ resorption. The kidney is a secondary target. In the kidney, it increases reabsorption of Ca^{2+} and stimulates 1α hydroxylase activity. The feedback loop is through its own levels and it is suppressed by PTH. The overall effect of active vitamin D is to **increase serum Ca^{2+} and $PO4^{3-}$**. It also promotes normal mineralization of bone.

Growth hormone (GH) is produced in the pituitary gland. It is necessary for normal **maturation** of bone and **maintenance** of normal bone remodeling.

Organs and Cells

The **skin** is the site of conversion of 7-dehydrocholesterol to 25-OH-D_3.

The **liver** is the site of conversion of 25-OH-D_3 to 1,25 $(OH)_2D_3$.

The **kidney** hydroxylates 25 hydroxycholecalciferol to 1,25 $(OH)_2D_3$ and excretes and resorbs Ca^{2+} and $PO4^{3-}$ in the proximal renal tubules. PTH and vitamin D regulate Ca^{2+} and $PO4^{3-}$ reabsorption.

Intestines absorb the dietary intake of Ca^{2+} and $PO4^{3-}$.

The **thyroid** is the source of calcitonin.

The **pituitary gland** forms GH.

Osteoblasts are the cells responsible for the *f***ormation** of new bone. They produce and mineralize osteoid and are stimulated by GH, thyroid hormone, estrogen, and androgens. Interestingly, vitamin D and PTH cause these cells to produce substances which induce progenitor cell conversion to osteoclasts and stimulate osteoclasts to resorb bone.

Osteocytes are the cells responsible for the **maintenance** of bone. They are mature osteoblasts, which have become entrapped in the bone they formed.

Osteoclasts are the cells responsible for the **resorption** of bone. They are stimulated by cytokines produced by osteoblasts. Calcitonin turns off their function.

Pathologic Issues

Metabolic bone disease results from any condition which interrupts the normal complex balance detailed above. Stress on the bones further helps to maintain the normal balance of bone formation and bone resorption. Disuse osteoporosis is an example of loss of this balance. The lack of stress on the bone results in rapid bone resorption with an aggressively lytic radiographic appearance. In addition, disease in other organs, such as the liver, intestines, and even skin disease can lead to disruption of the cycle by failing to provide the necessary building blocks. Resulting conditions affect bone quality, quantity, or both.

Osteoporosis is the condition of **decreased bone quantity**. It has both 1° and 2° forms and can result from **excessive bone resorption &/or decreased bone formation**. In 1° osteoporosis the bone is otherwise normal. With 2° osteoporosis diminished bone quantity may be accompanied by alterations in bone quality.

Hyperparathyroidism (HPTH) is the classic disease of bone resorption. With 1° HPTH, excessive levels of PTH result in unnecessary bone resorption. In 2° HPTH, the body tries to replenish serum Ca^{2+} by sacrificing bone Ca^{2+}. In addition to the focal sites of bone resorption associated with this disease, an overall decrease in the amount of bone will also be seen (2° osteoporosis).

Osteomalacia is a disease of **abnormal bone quality** due to the inability to form normal bone. The underlying condition is vitamin D deficiency resulting in an inability to adequately mineralize osteoid, resulting in bone softening. It is accompanied by an overall decrease in bone quantity (2° osteoporosis).

Conditions such as **renal osteodystrophy** affect both **bone resorption and bone formation**. Renal parenchymal disease leads to impaired formation of 1,25 hydroxycholecalciferol (active vitamin D_3). Further, hyperphosphatemia 2° to the inability to excrete excess $PO4^{3-}$ suppresses formation of active vitamin D, resulting in osteomalacia. Low levels of active vitamin D_3 lead to hypocalcemia, which is further worsened by Ca^{2+} binding with excess $PO4^{3-}$. The hypocalcemia, hyperphosphatemia, and low 1,25 dihydroxycholecalciferol levels result in increased PTH production, which creates the HPTH component of renal osteodystrophy. The underlying cause of the neoostosis in this condition is not clear. Proposed mechanisms include osteoblast stimulation and increased calcitonin, which inhibits bone resorption.

GH is necessary for normal bone development. The absence of GH in a child results in **delayed skeletal maturation** as well as **slow bone growth**. Too much of the hormone leads to the *excess* **bone formation**, which occurs with acromegaly.

Imaging Protocols

Radiographs and CT are the imaging modalities of choice when the goal is to evaluate integrity and structure of bone. DEXA and quantitative CT are the tools for assessing the overall amount of bone. Bone scans are not used as a primary modality for assessing metabolic bone disease; however, metabolic bone disease can create some rather dramatic changes. MR also is not a primary imaging modality. It may be useful when assessing secondary changes, such as brown tumors of HPTH. MR is also useful for evaluating complications of poor bone quality, such as insufficiency fracture.

DEXA scanning

DEXA scans are the most widely accepted and widely employed imaging modality for measuring bone mineral density (BMD) and thus the amount of bone. DEXA scans do not evaluate bone quality. Standards for DEXA scanning and certification for interpretation have been established by the International Society for Clinical Densitometry and are available on their website.

Appropriate scanning **technique** requires attention to detail. Proper positioning is critical and is manufacturer specific. Individual error measurements for each technologist, for each body site, need to be determined to know the measurement error. This information is necessary when comparing follow-up studies, enabling one to determine if BMD changes are beyond the error of measurement. At least 2 sites should be measured, typically AP spine and the dominant hip. Nondominant hip measurements add additional information. The forearm is an additional measurement site. The nondominant forearm measurement should be employed when the hips cannot be measured, in morbidly obese patients, and in those with suspected HPTH.

Optimal **interpretation** requires more than just reporting T scores and Z scores. Images must be evaluated for appropriate positioning and lack of confounding factors and artifacts. Ideally each lumbar vertebra measurement should be within 1 standard deviation of the other vertebra. The appropriate region of interest must be employed and should follow current recommendations. Current recommended measurements are AP lumbar spine L1-L4 and total femur and femoral neck. If the forearm is measured, the distal 1/3 radius measurement should be reported. The patient's age and sex need to be considered to ensure that appropriate reference standards are employed. In the pediatric population, only the Z score should be reported, and the terms osteoporosis and osteopenia should not be used. In the male population, osteoporosis should not be determined solely by BMD measurement. When performing follow-up scans, only measurements from the same machine should be compared.

Pathology-Based Imaging Issues

Bone is a highly organized organ. It consists of a dense outer shell, the **cortex** or compact bone, and a porous internal **trabecular** network. Bones with a higher ratio of cortical bone to trabecular bone are stronger than bones with relatively more trabecular bone. Different conditions will affect cortical and trabecular bone differently, and thus have different implications for bone strength. Since the main musculoskeletal morbidity in many metabolic diseases results from fracture, there will be variable morbidity. Bones that have high cortical to trabecular ratios include the femur, radius, and ulna. Vertebra have a lower cortical to trabecular bone ratio and are therefore more likely to fracture than femora.

The **growth plate** is a site of highly active new bone formation and is extremely vulnerable to factors which alter normal bone formation. Enchondral ossification within the epiphyses and apophyses is less susceptible. Different underlying mechanisms result in the common radiologic appearance of widening, irregular margins, cupping, and fraying. In osteomalacia, the normal highly organized structure of the hypertrophic zone is disrupted by the inability to mineralize the cartilage. This unmineralized cartilage then accumulates. In HPTH, bone resorption occurs at the metaphyseal margin of the growth plate and around the periphery of the epiphysis and apophyses, creating irregularity at that interface.

Selected References

1. International Society for Clinical Densitometry. www.ISCD.org. Updated 2015
2. Binkovitz LA et al: Pediatric DXA: technique, interpretation and clinical applications. Pediatr Radiol. 38 Suppl 2:S227-39, 2008
3. Christiansen P: The skeleton in primary hyperparathyroidism: a review focusing on bone remodeling, structure, mass, and fracture. APMIS Suppl. (102):1-52, 2001

(Left) *The major responder to a low-serum calcium is the parathyroid gland with production of parathyroid hormone (PTH). Target organs of PTH are the kidneys, intestines, and bone.* **(Right)** *In the intestines, PTH stimulates resorption of calcium and phosphate. $PO4^{3-}$ absorption is shown in red on the graphic because this action works against the goal of increasing serum calcium. Any serum phosphate will lower serum calcium because the two bind together, effectively making calcium unavailable for other functions.*

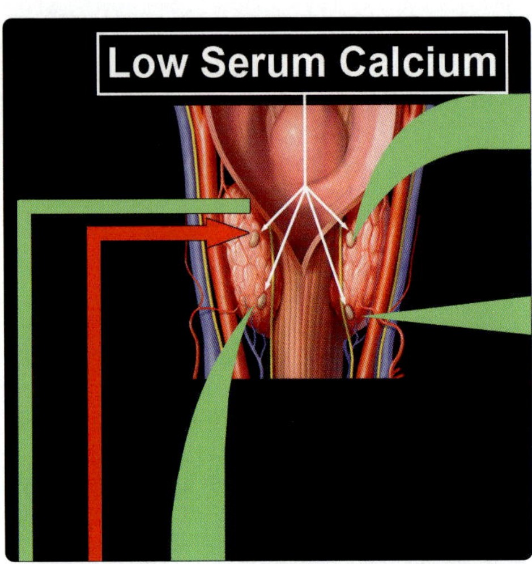

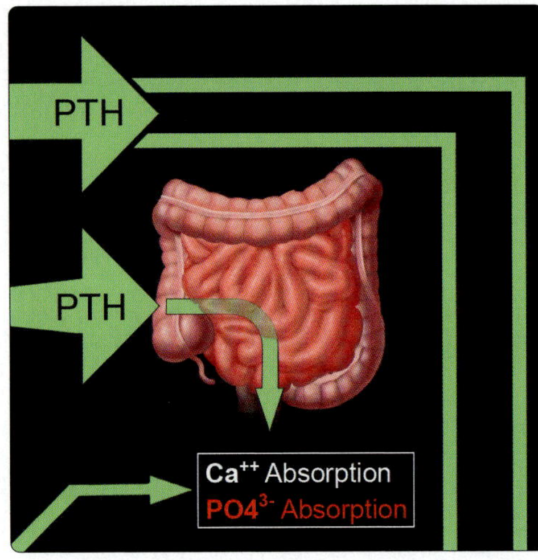

(Left) *The kidney is a 1° target organ of PTH, serving 2 functions: (1) PTH stimulates Ca^{2+} reabsorption and $PO4^{3-}$ excretion in renal tubules, and (2) $1,25(OH)_2D_3$ is formed within the renal parenchyma. This active form of vitamin D targets the bone and intestines. It has a negative feedback on its own production and PTH production (red arrows).* **(Right)** *PTH has both long- and short-term affects on bone. Short term, it works in conjunction with vitamin D to stimulate bone resorption, → ↑ Ca^{2+} and $PO4^{3-}$.*

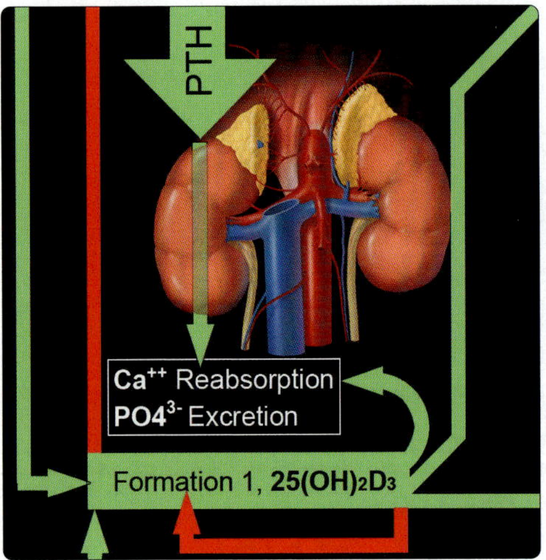

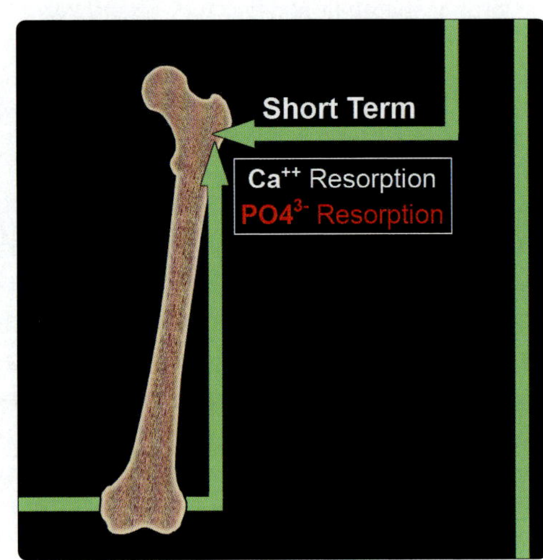

(Left) *Skin and liver play critical roles in Ca^{2+} metabolism through formation of cholecalciferol from its precursor 7-dehydroxycholesterol (obtained through dietary intake). This function requires UV light. In the liver, cholecalciferol is converted to prohormone $25(OH)D_3$.* **(Right)** *Long term, PTH inhibits osteoblasts, preventing bone formation (which requires consumption of serum Ca^{2+}). It stimulates progenitor cell conversion to osteoclasts, which then resorb bone, releasing calcium.*

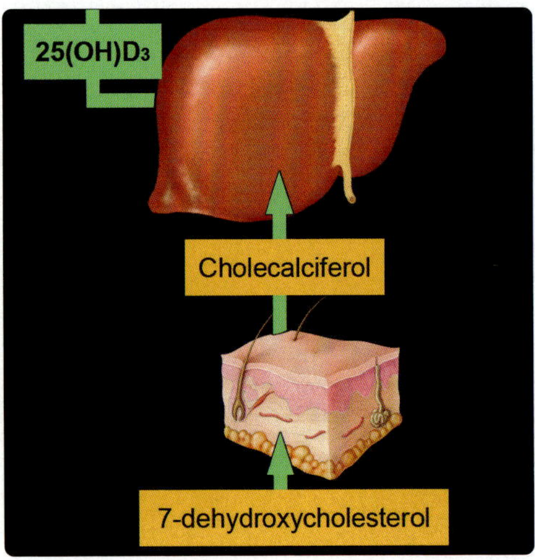

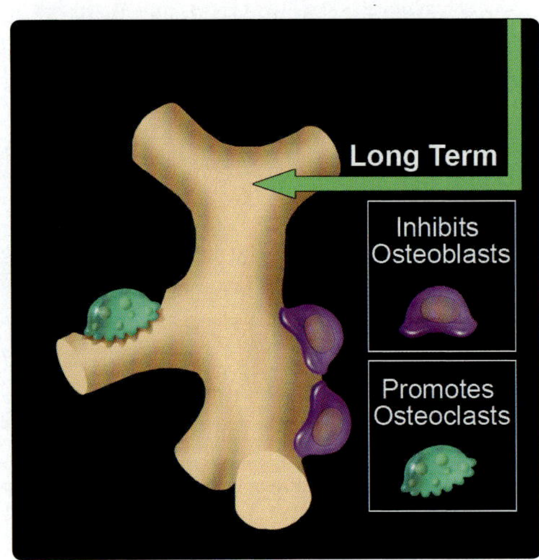

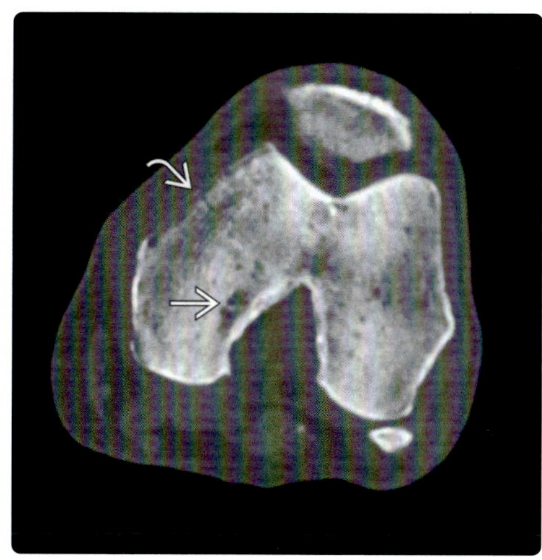

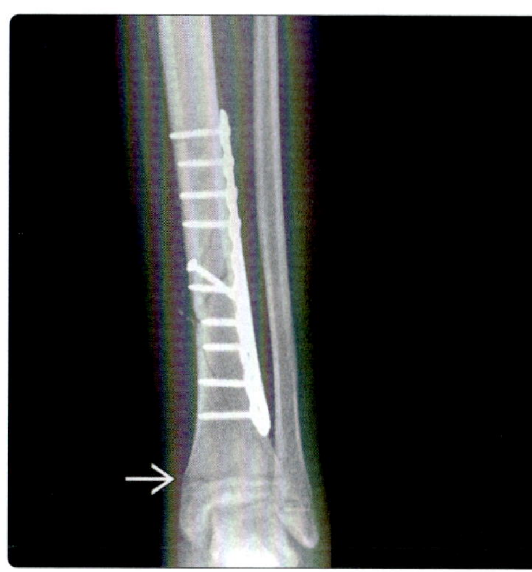

(Left) *Axial bone CT reveals changes of disuse osteoporosis. This is a true osteoporosis brought on by the lack of weight-bearing stress. In this case, it manifests as small, patchy lucencies in the medullary bone ➡ and extensive intracortical bone resorption ➡.* **(Right)** *AP radiograph shows a patient with disuse osteoporosis following limited weight-bearing after fracture fixation. In this instance, the osteoporosis takes on the appearance of a linear metaphyseal lucency ➡.*

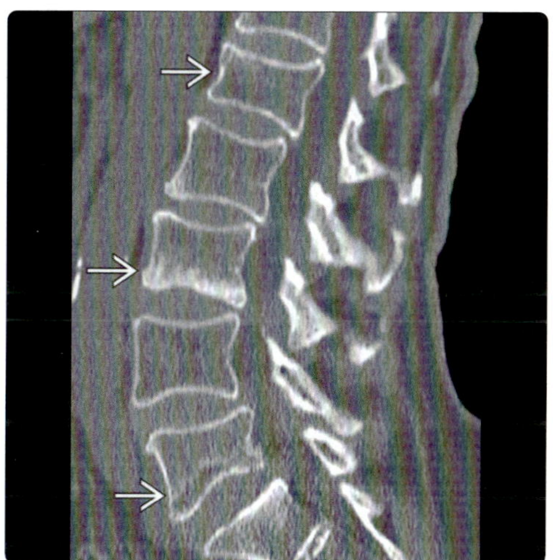

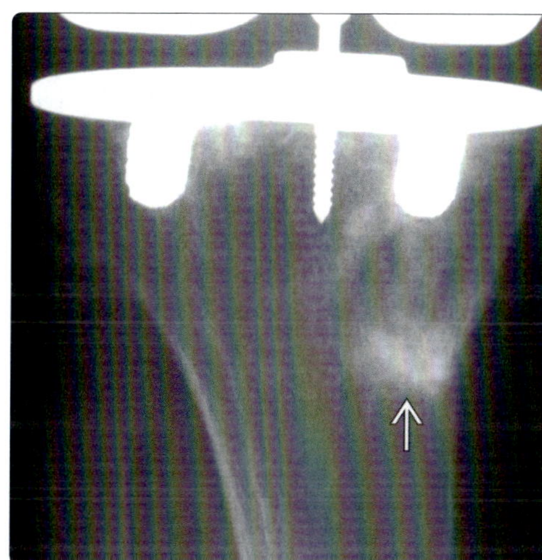

(Left) *Sagittal reformatted CT shows varied appearance of vertebral compression fractures ➡. Such fractures are a significant cause of morbidity in patients with osteoporosis.* **(Right)** *AP radiograph of a patient with osteoporosis and new onset of pain shows arthroplasty has redistributed forces through the knee, placing greater stress medially than was previously experienced. The bone is unable to respond to these stresses, and insufficiency fracture ➡ results.*

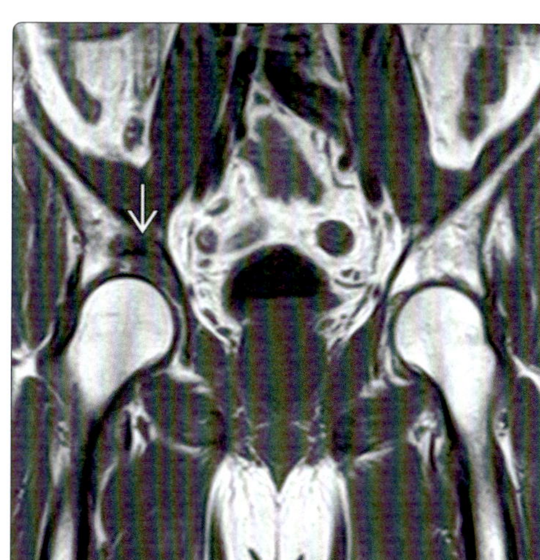

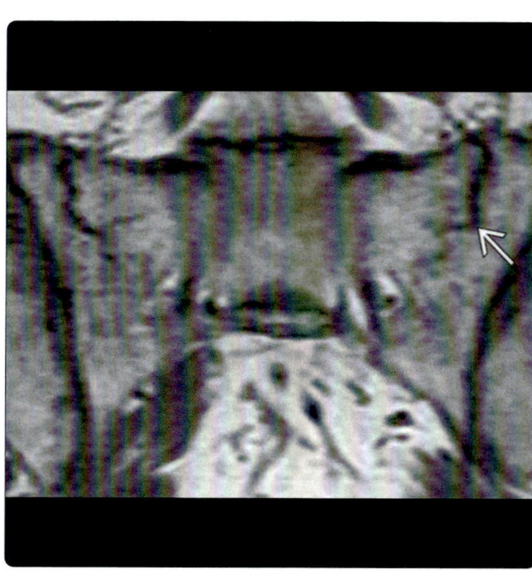

(Left) *Coronal T1WI MR shows a patient with new hip pain and osteoporosis. Differential included arthritis, but radiographs were unremarkable. Pain is a result of acetabular insufficiency fracture ➡, a complication of osteoporosis.* **(Right)** *Coronal T1WI MR shows classic vertically oriented sacral insufficiency fractures ➡. Pain from such fractures is a major cause of osteoporosis-associated morbidity. Associated limited mobility causes further complications, such as muscle loss and deep vein thrombosis.*

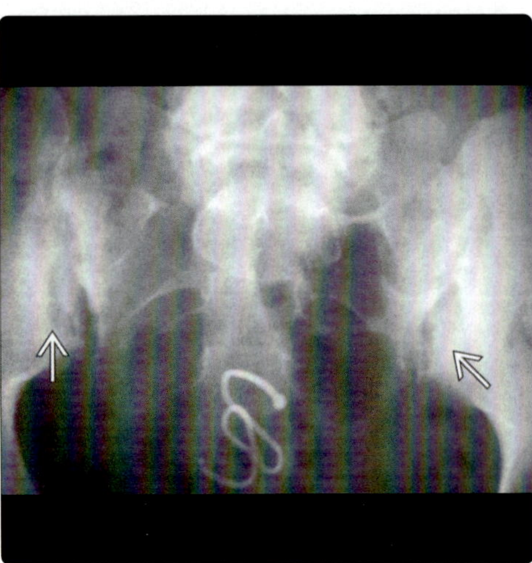

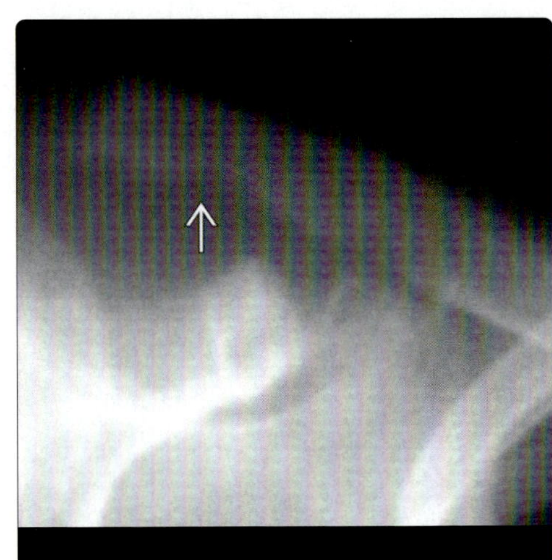

(Left) *AP radiograph shows typical subchondral bone resorptive changes of hyperparathyroidism (HPTH), seen predominantly on the ilial side of the SI joint ➡. This could be confused with a spondyloarthropathy, such as ankylosing spondylitis.* **(Right)** *AP radiograph of the distal clavicle demonstrates characteristic bone resorptive changes of HPTH ➡. In cases of renal osteodystrophy (the most common cause of HPTH), the body is trying to reclaim calcium from the skeleton in response to hypocalcemia.*

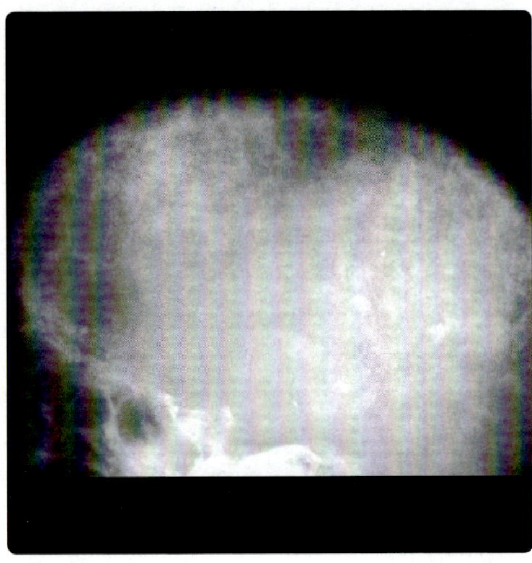

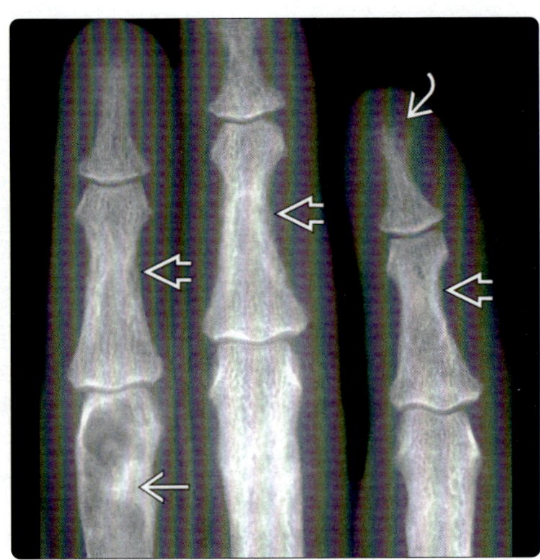

(Left) *Lateral radiograph shows a typical salt and pepper skull. The appearance is created by foci of bone resorption and bone formation in renal osteodystrophy. It is usually not seen until the disease is relatively advanced.* **(Right)** *PA radiograph shows multiple findings of 2° HPTH. Subperiosteal resorption along the radial aspect of the middle phalanges is a characteristic finding ➡. More advanced findings in this hand include subcortical resorption ➡ of the distal phalanges and brown tumors ➡.*

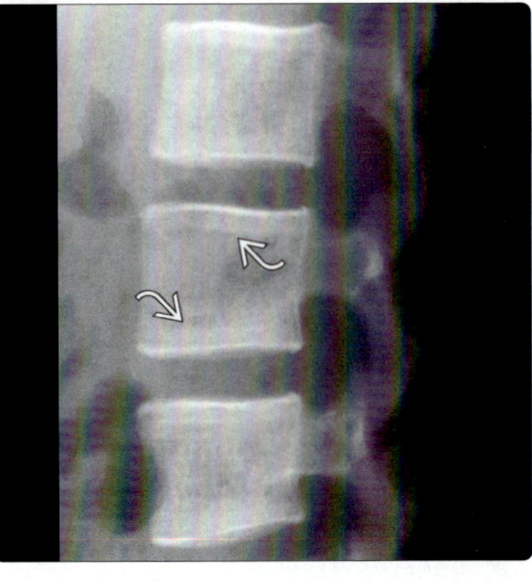

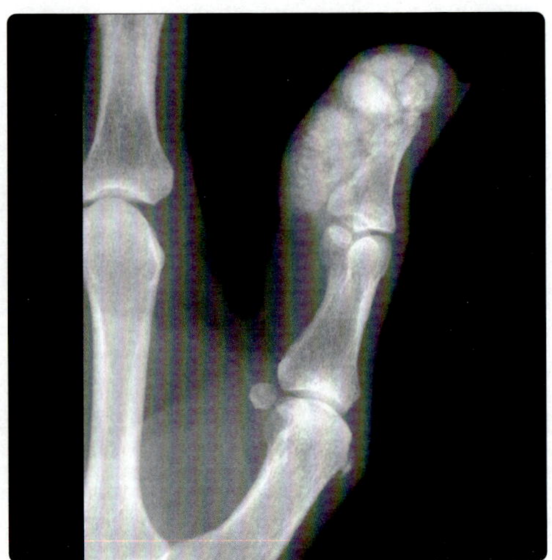

(Left) *Lateral radiograph of the spine demonstrates dense lines at the endplates of the vertebral bodies ➡. This results from osteoblastic activity, which occurs in addition to the osteoclastic activity in renal osteodystrophy. The appearance is of horizontal stripes, as are seen on the shirts of rugby players.* **(Right)** *Lateral x-ray of the thumb shows intense dystrophic calcification in a patient with renal osteodystrophy. Soft tissue deposits are particularly commonly seen in patients on dialysis.*

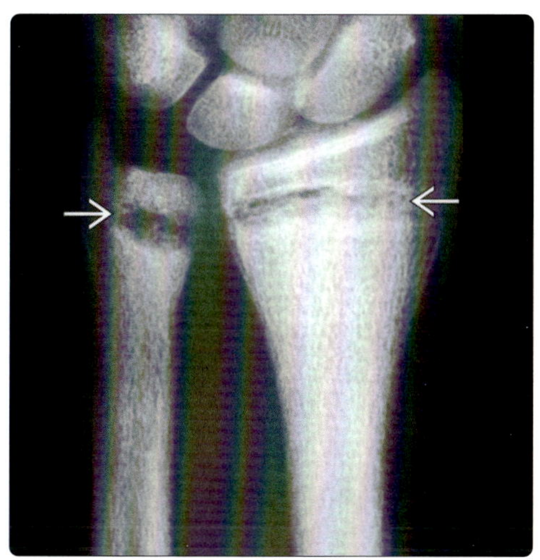

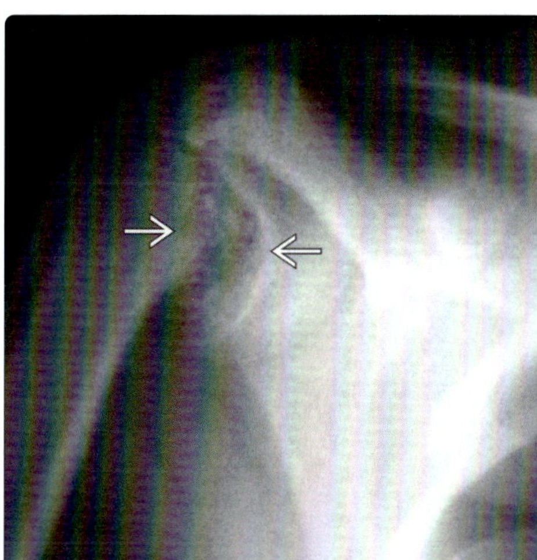

(Left) *PA radiograph shows findings of renal osteodystrophy. Typical physeal changes of bone resorption include widening and irregularity* ➨*. Additionally, in this patient the bones are diffusely dense, a manifestation of the neoostosis of this condition.* **(Right)** *AP radiograph shows marked widening of the growth plate with slipped epiphysis* ➨*. The growth plate is a site of ↑ metabolic activity related to bone formation. As such, it is sensitive to any metabolic bone disease.*

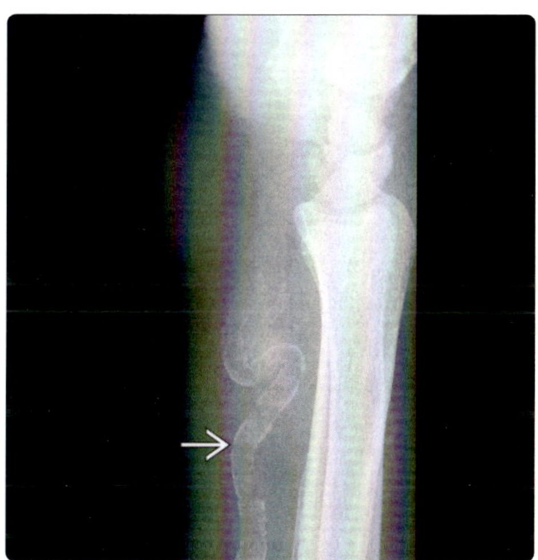

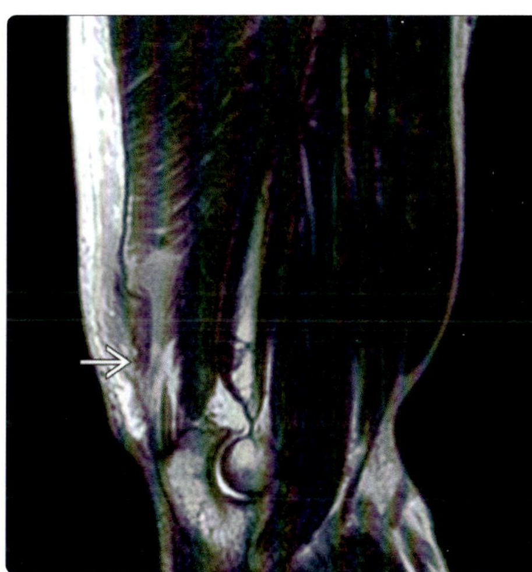

(Left) *Lateral radiograph shows extensive calcification of medium-sized vessels in the wrist* ➨*. Metabolic bone disease affects not only the bones, but also various soft tissues. Metastatic calcification within vessel walls is a common finding in HPTH.* **(Right)** *Sagittal T2WI MR shows disruption of the triceps tendon* ➨*. Poor integrity of tendons and other soft tissues is another nonosseous feature that accompanies renal osteodystrophy.*

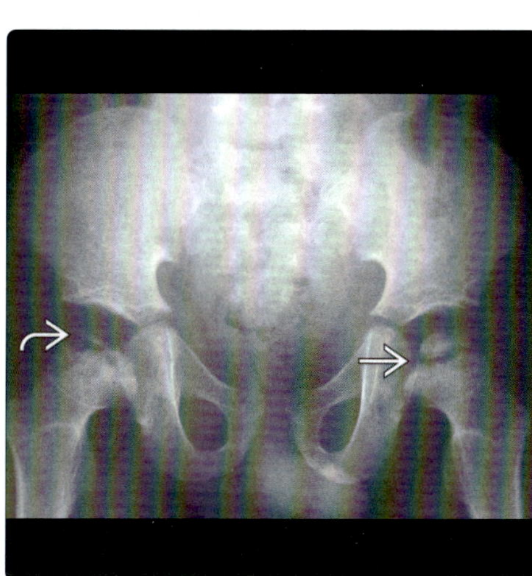

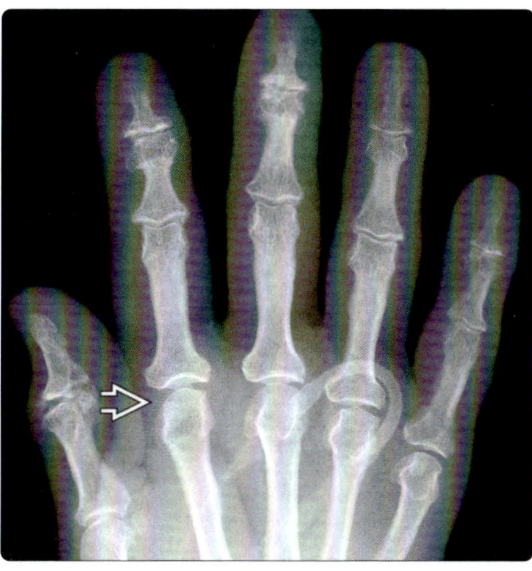

(Left) *AP radiograph shows changes which accompany hypothyroidism. There is severely delayed bone age. Growth plates are abnormal with slight widening* ➨*. The right femoral capital epiphysis is fragmented (termed cretinoid hip)* ➨*.* **(Right)** *PA radiograph shows changes of acromegaly. This condition results in overgrowth of bone and cartilage, which is not uniformly distributed throughout the skeleton. This hand demonstrates widened MCP joint spaces, indicating cartilage overgrowth* ➨*.*

KEY FACTS

IMAGING

- Resorption is essential radiograph feature
  - Subperiosteal, endosteal, subchondral, intracortical, subtendinous, subligamentous, along trabecula
- Physeal resorption, especially along metaphyseal aspect, creates widening & irregularity
- Generalized osteopenia due to osteoporosis
- Metastatic soft tissue calcification, chondrocalcinosis
- Brown tumor: Expansile, lytic lesion with geographic nonsclerotic margins
- Salt and pepper or pepper pot skull
- Weakened tendons & ligaments, may rupture or cause joint laxity
- Bowing deformities resulting from bone softening
- Fragility fractures
- Erosive arthritis-like appearance
- Bone scan has Superscan appearance
- Mixed signal intensities: Variable depending on degree of fibrous tissue, cyst formation, & hemorrhage

TOP DIFFERENTIAL DIAGNOSES

- Brown tumor may mimic giant cell tumor, fibrous dysplasia, metastatic disease, multiple myeloma
- Sacroiliac joint & symphyseal changes mimic ankylosing spondylitis
- Subchondral resorption & collapse of hand, feet, knees mimic rheumatoid arthritis

PATHOLOGY

- 1° HPTH: Parathyroid adenoma (75-85%)
- 2° HPTH: Chronic renal disease most common

DIAGNOSTIC CHECKLIST

- Resorption along radial aspect of middle phalanx of index finger considered pathognomonic

(Left) *PA radiograph shows resorptive changes of hyperparathyroidism (HPTH). The cortex along the radial and ulnar aspects of the middle phalanges has a lace-like appearance resulting from subperiosteal resorption and intracortical tunneling ➡. Tuft resorption of the 2nd and 5th distal phalanges ➦.* **(Right)** *PA radiograph shows subchondral resorption at the margins of the DIP joints ➡. The adjacent articular surface has collapsed, mimicking erosions. Prior imaging showed subperiosteal resorption, now resolved.*

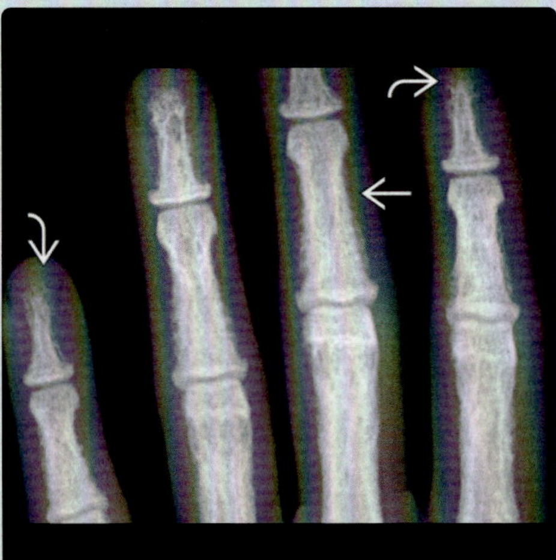

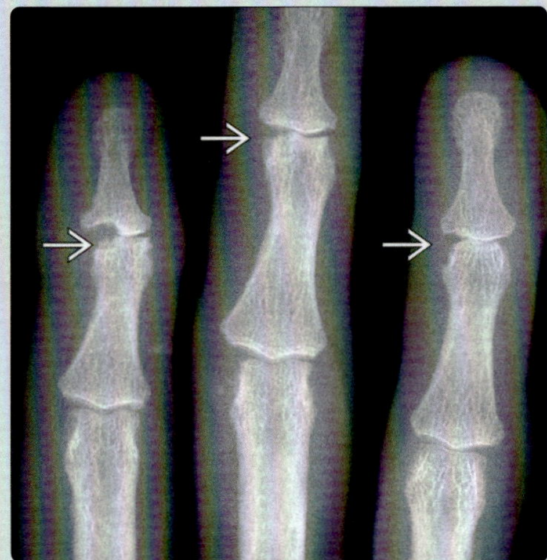

(Left) *Lateral radiograph shows a skull with salt and pepper changes resulting from generalized but irregular bone resorption accompanied by ill-defined foci of sclerosis. Note the loss of definition of the inner and outer tables.* **(Right)** *Axial bone CT shows dramatic changes, including ill definition of the inner and outer tables, as well as multiple ill-defined sclerotic foci within the medullary space. This appearance is the CT equivalent of the salt and pepper skull.*

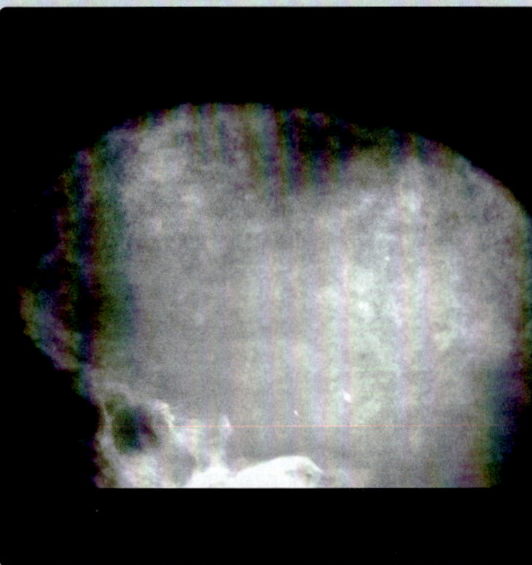

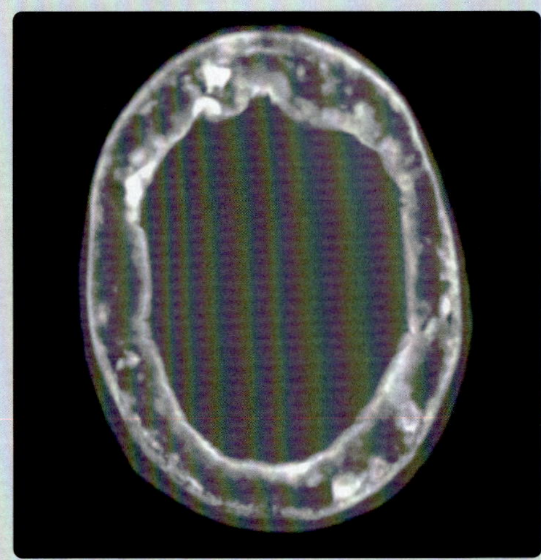

TERMINOLOGY

Abbreviations

- Hyperparathyroidism (HPTH)

Synonyms

- Advanced osseous changes
  - (von) Recklinghausen disease of bone
  - Osteitis fibrosis cystica
- Brown tumor: Osteoclastoma

Definitions

- Disease resulting from ↑ parathyroid hormone

IMAGING

General Features

- Best diagnostic clue
  - Bone resorption is diagnostic feature
    - Subperiosteal resorption along radial aspect of middle phalanges of index & middle fingers pathognomonic
- Location
  - Resorption may be subperiosteal, endosteal, subchondral, subtendinous, subligamentous, intracortical, along trabecula

Imaging Recommendations

- Best imaging tool
  - Radiographs best for demonstrating osseous changes
- Protocol advice
  - High-resolution radiographs of hands most sensitive for bone involvement

Radiographic Findings

- General findings
  - Osteoporosis
  - Bone resorption: Typically bilateral & symmetric
    - Subperiosteal resorption
      - Radial cortices of middle phalanges of hand, especially index & middle fingers
      - Medial cortices of proximal humerus, femur, tibia
    - Subchondral resorption (often with associated collapse, mimicking erosion)
      - Acromioclavicular (AC) joints, especially distal clavicle
      - Sternoclavicular (SC) joints
      - Subchondral ends of carpals, metacarpals, phalanges
      - Discovertebral junctions
      - Sacroiliac (SI) joints, especially iliac side
      - Symphysis pubis
    - Subtendinous/subligamentous resorption
      - Clavicular attachments of coracoclavicular ligaments
      - Humeral tuberosities at rotator cuff insertion
      - Triceps tendon insertion onto olecranon
      - Ischial tuberosities
      - Greater trochanter
      - Calcaneal attachment plantar fascia
    - Physeal resorption, especially along metaphyseal aspect, creates widening & irregularity (mimics rickets)
    - Endosteal/intracortical/trabecular resorption
      - Metacarpal intracortical tunneling (lace-like)
      - Acroosteolysis (especially band-like pattern)
    - Lamina dura of teeth
  - Brown tumor
    - Greater incidence in 1° HPTH than 2°
    - Overall, more commonly seen with 2° HPTH due to greater prevalence of 2° HPTH relative to 1°
    - Mandible, clavicle, ribs, pelvis, femur
    - Solitary or multiple
    - Nonaggressive imaging features: Expansile lytic lesion, geographic nonsclerotic margins; no cortical destruction, periostitis, soft tissue mass or matrix
    - Most commonly metaphyseal; may extend into epiphysis or originate in diaphysis
  - Soft tissue abnormalities
    - Metastatic soft tissue calcification
      - More common in 2° HPTH
      - Favors periarticular sites: Hip, shoulder
      - Medium-sized arteries, lungs, heart, liver
    - Weakened tendons & ligaments, may rupture or cause joint laxity
  - Osteosclerosis
    - More often seen following treatment (hyperossifying)
    - Mechanism unknown
    - Most commonly seen in axial skeleton; also seen in skull, metaphyses
    - 1° HPTH: Most often patchy, unusual to be generalized, seen with healing brown tumors
    - 2° HPTH: May be generalized; not necessarily manifestation of HPTH
  - Periostitis
    - More common with 2° HPTH; especially during healing phase
- Additional findings
  - Chondrocalcinosis
    - Menisci, triangular fibrocartilage, symphysis pubis More common with 1° HPTH
  - Renal stones & nephrocalcinosis
  - Salt and pepper or pepper pot skull due to generalized bone resorption and more focal cystic areas of resorption ± patchy sclerosis
  - Spine: Schmorl nodes, widened disc spaces, & endplate compressions
  - Bowing deformities resulting from bone softening
  - Fragility fractures
  - Erosive arthritis-like appearance
    - Subchondral erosion & collapse at articular margins mimics erosions: SI, AC, SC joints, symphysis pubic, discovertebral margins
      - Especially 2° HPTH
    - Subperiosteal resorption at joint margins creates appearance of erosive arthritis, involves hands, wrist, feet; AC, SC & SI joints; symphysis pubis
  - Osteitis fibrosa cystica
    - Marrow replacement by fibrous & vascular tissue
    - Structurally weakened bone becomes deformed

MR Findings

- Sensitive for identification of parathyroid adenoma
- No significant role in identification of bone disease

- Nonspecific changes: Hematopoietic marrow, widened medullary cavity, thinned cortices
- Brown tumor
  - Mixed signal intensities: Variable depending on degree of fibrous tissue, cyst formation, & hemorrhage

Nuclear Medicine Findings

- Bone scan
  - Superscan: Intense skeletal uptake, visualization of fingers & toes, no renal uptake
  - May have soft tissue uptake at sites of calcium deposition, especially in lungs, liver, heart
  - Brown tumors: Intense focal uptake
- Parathyroid imaging (Tc-99m sestamibi)
  - Increased uptake in parathyroid adenoma

Other Modality Findings

- DEXA & quantitative CT diagnose osteoporosis

DIFFERENTIAL DIAGNOSIS

Brown Tumor

- Giant cell tumor, fibrous dysplasia, metastatic disease, multiple myeloma
- Differentiate on basis of serum calcium, other radiographic findings of HPTH

Ankylosing Spondylitis

- SI joint & symphysis changes of HPTH may mimic ankylosing spondylitis

Rheumatoid Arthritis

- Arthritis-like changes of HPTH, especially in hand, may mimic RA

PATHOLOGY

General Features

- Etiology
  - 1° HPTH
    - Parathyroid adenoma: 75-85%
      - Multiple endocrine neoplasia rare
    - Parathyroid hyperplasia: 10-20%
    - Parathyroid carcinoma: 1-5%
  - 2° HPTH
    - Chronic renal disease most common
    - Calcium deficiency, vitamin D disorders, disrupted phosphate metabolism
  - Tertiary HPTH
    - Parathyroid hyperplasia with lack of response to calcium levels (autonomously functioning glands)
    - Result of longstanding HPTH
  - Brown tumor: Reactive process, not neoplastic
    - Results from osteoclastic bone resorption, subsequent fibrous replacement, hemorrhage & necrosis leading to cyst formation
- Associated abnormalities
  - 1° HPTH serum chemistries
    - Serum calcium: Elevated
    - Serum phosphorus: Normal or decreased
  - 2° HPTH serum chemistries
    - Serum calcium: Normal or low
    - Serum phosphorus: Increased
    - Calcium-phosphate product: Elevated
    - Vitamin D: Low (from renal parenchymal disease)

Microscopic Features

- Generalized
  - Medullary bone: Decrease bone trabecula, increased vascular spaces, increased fibrovascular tissue
  - Cortical bone: Increased vascular channels
  - Increased number of osteoclasts
  - Osteoblasts along trabecula

CLINICAL ISSUES

Presentation

- Most common signs/symptoms
  - Usually asymptomatic: When symptomatic, most common presentation is related to nephrolithiasis
- Other signs/symptoms
  - "Stones, bones, abdominal groans, psychiatric moans"
  - Nonspecific bone, joint, muscle pain & weakness
  - Pancreatitis, peptic ulcer disease
  - Nausea, constipation, vomiting, anorexia

Demographics

- Age
  - 1° HPTH: Most common in middle-aged to older adults, rare in children
  - 2° HPTH: Most patients over 40 years old
- Epidemiology
  - 1° HPTH: 42 per 100,000 individuals
  - 2° HPTH: Present in majority of dialysis patients

Natural History & Prognosis

- 1° & 2° HPTH are reversible
  - If left untreated, progresses to 3° disease, which does not respond to treatment

Treatment

- 1° HPTH
  - Normal/slightly ↑ serum calcium: Close observation
  - Elevated serum calcium: Removal of adenoma
- 2° HPTH
  - Aim to increase serum calcium levels
  - Renal transplant

DIAGNOSTIC CHECKLIST

Image Interpretation Pearls

- Resorption along radial aspect of middle phalanx of index finger considered pathognomonic

SELECTED REFERENCES

1. Bandeira F et al: Bone disease in primary hyperparathyroidism. Arq Bras Endocrinol Metabol. 58(5):553-61, 2014
2. Hoang JK et al: How to perform parathyroid 4D CT: tips and traps for technique and interpretation. Radiology. 270(1):15-24, 2014
3. Genant HK et al: Primary hyperparathyroidism. A comprehensive study of clinical, biochemical and radiographic manifestations. Radiology. 109(3):513-24, 1973

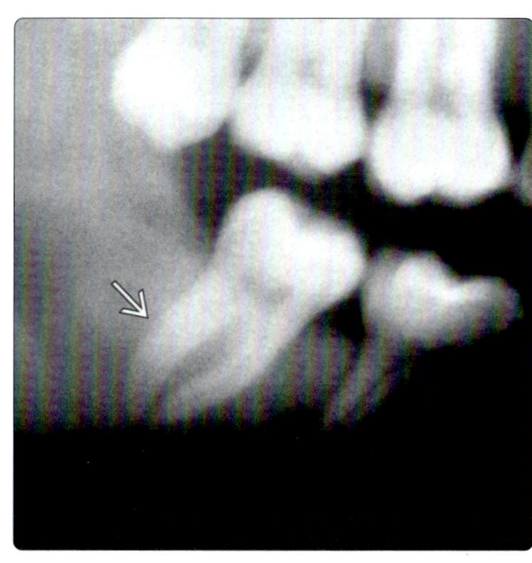

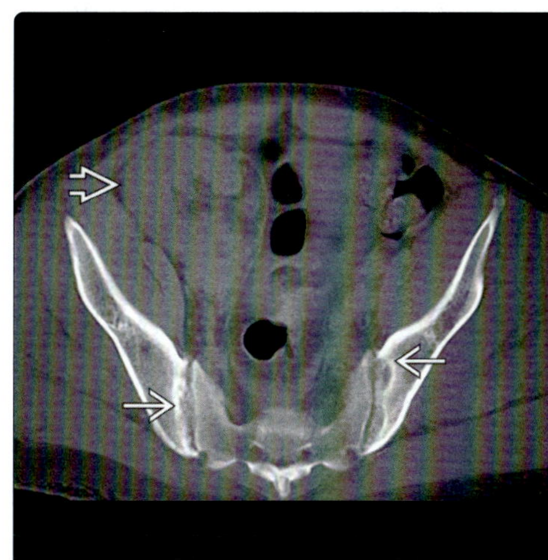

(Left) *Frontal radiograph coned down to provide tooth detail shows subperiosteal resorption of the lamina dura ➡, which normally appears as a white line surrounding the root of the tooth.* **(Right)** *Axial bone NECT depicts the sacroiliac joint changes of HPTH ➡, with subchondral resorption primarily of the iliac side of the joints. The transplanted kidney in the right lower quadrant is a strong clue to the etiology of these changes ➡ (HPTH 2° to renal osteodystrophy).*

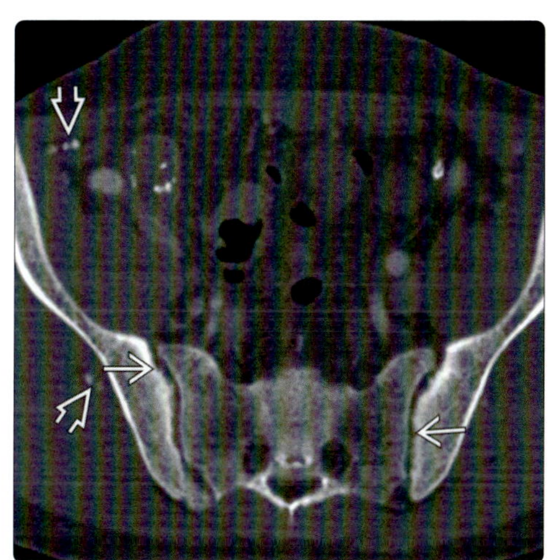

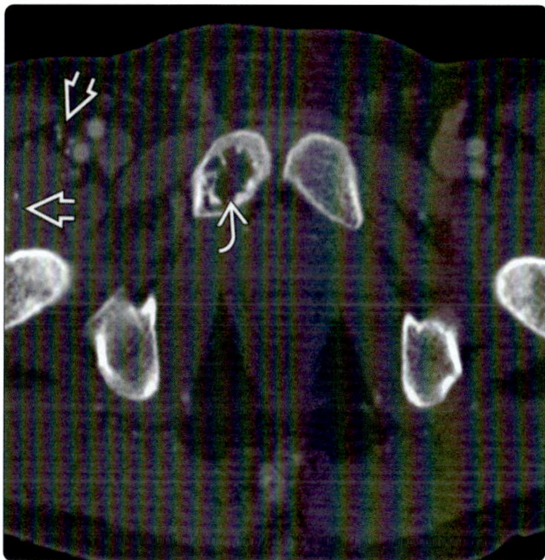

(Left) *Axial bone CT shows smudgy trabeculae typical of HPTH, along with resorption of the iliac side of the sacroiliac joints ➡. In addition, there is soft tissue calcification ➡. All findings point to HPTH.* **(Right)** *Axial bone CT in the same patient shows more abnormal soft tissue calcification ➡ as well as a lytic slightly bubbly lesion ➡ in the pubic ramus that is typical of brown tumor of HPTH. While occasionally there is only a single finding to suggest the diagnosis of HPTH, more commonly there are many.*

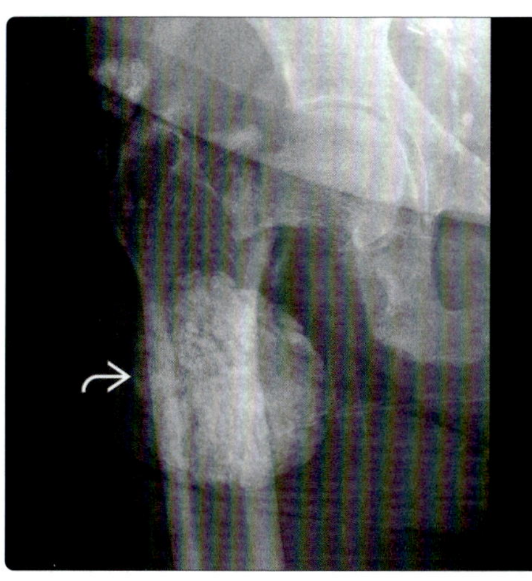

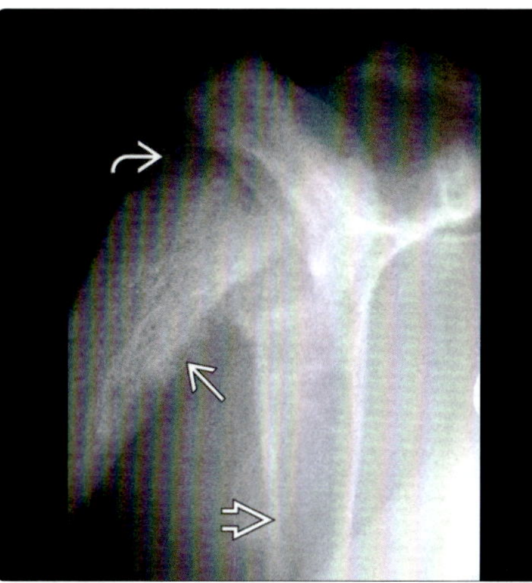

(Left) *AP radiograph in a patient with primary HPTH shows vascular calcification, abundant soft tissue calcification ➡, and a combination of osteopenia and thickened trabeculae. The fragile femur has fractured.* **(Right)** *AP radiograph shows dramatic changes of HPTH. Typical physeal changes are present ➡. Characteristic subperiosteal resorption of the medial cortex of the proximal humerus is evident ➡, and a large brown tumor is present in the scapula ➡.*

(Left) *PA radiograph in a young adult shows diffuse osteopenia and coarsening of trabeculae. Subchondral resorption is seen at the lunate and there is dense amorphous calcification in a periarticular distribution. All are findings expected in HPTH.* **(Right)** *AP radiograph reveals prominent nephrocalcinosis. While nonspecific in its appearance, identification of associated osseous changes helps narrow the differential diagnosis to HPTH.*

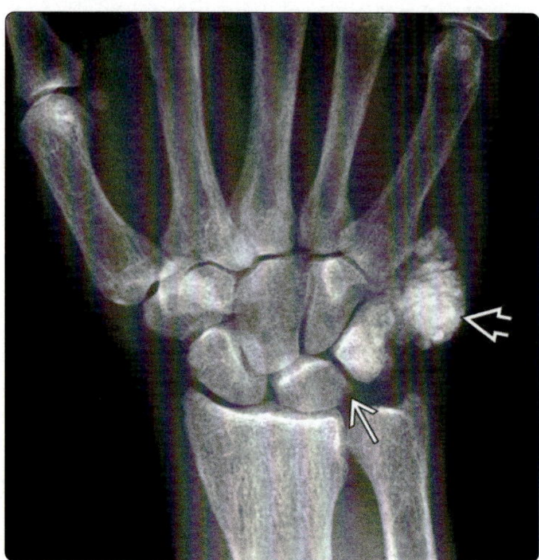

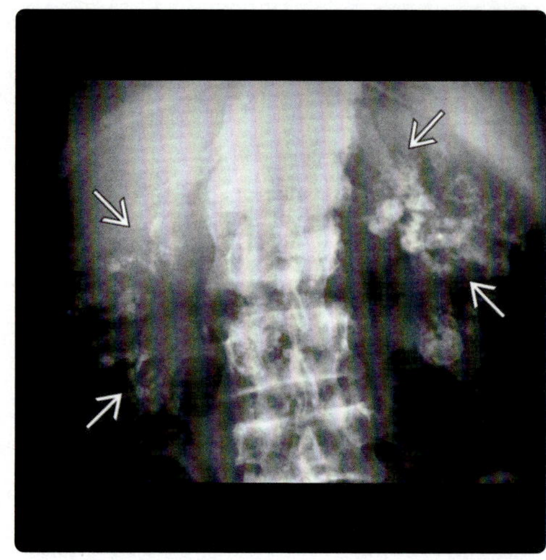

(Left) *Lateral radiograph demonstrates the extensive vascular calcification that accompanies HPTH. Medium-sized vessels are typically involved, as opposed to the larger vessels affected by atherosclerosis and smaller vessels, which are calcified in diabetics. Note the abnormal bone density and ill-defined trabeculae.* **(Right)** *AP radiograph of the lower leg shows nonspecific changes of HPTH, including severe osteopenia, not explained by age and gender, and diffuse soft tissue calcification.*

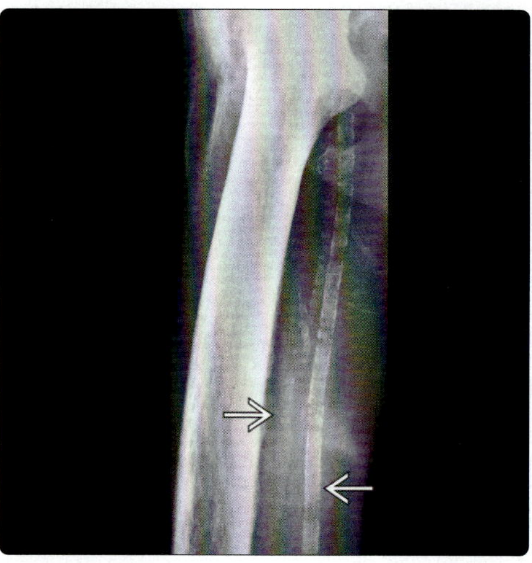

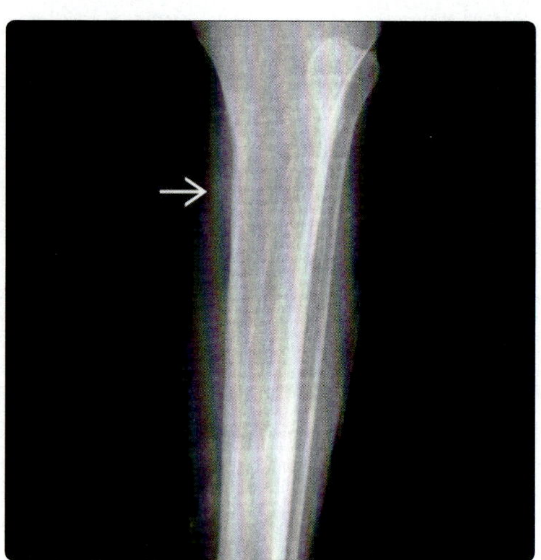

(Left) *PA radiograph shows physeal changes. Both growth plates are widened, and the margins are irregular (especially at the metaphyseal border), mimicking rickets. Intracortical tunneling is present. The trabecula are coarsened.* **(Right)** *AP radiograph shows a typical brown tumor, lytic with geographic margins and no aggressive features. This resembles other fibroosseous lesions. The bone density is highly abnormal; if the patient is a young adult, HPTH with brown tumor must be considered.*

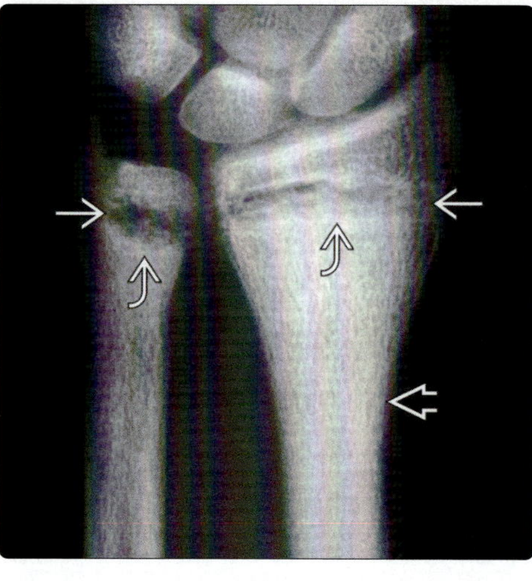

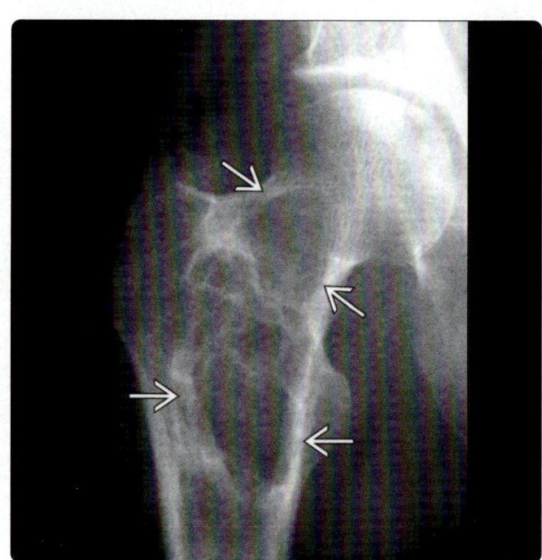

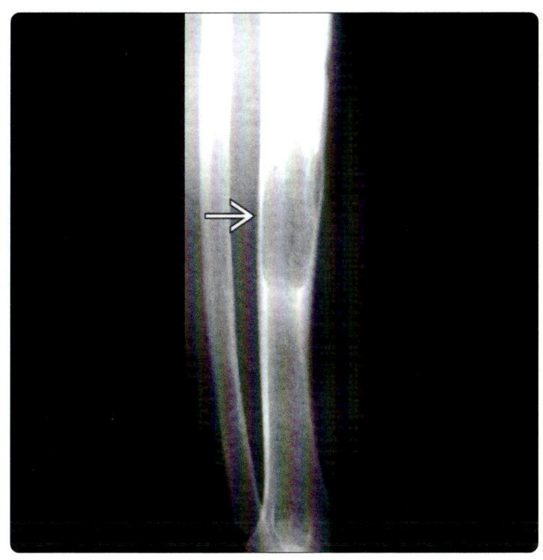

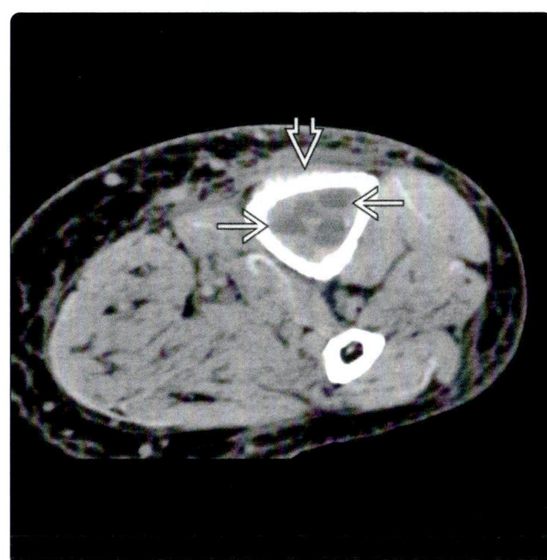

(Left) *AP radiograph shows a typical brown tumor. The tumor is lytic and mildly expansile with nonsclerotic geographic margins ➡. No aggressive features are evident. The lesions can occur anywhere in bone, including the diaphysis as seen here.* **(Right)** *Axial NECT through a mid tibial, mildly expansile lytic lesion reveals multiple fluid-fluid levels ➡ resulting from hemorrhage and necrosis leading to cyst formation. Ill-defined changes along the cortical surface are a reflection of subperiosteal resorption ➡.*

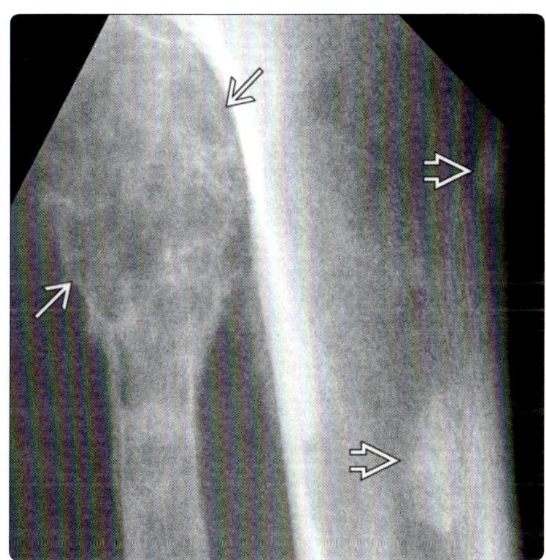

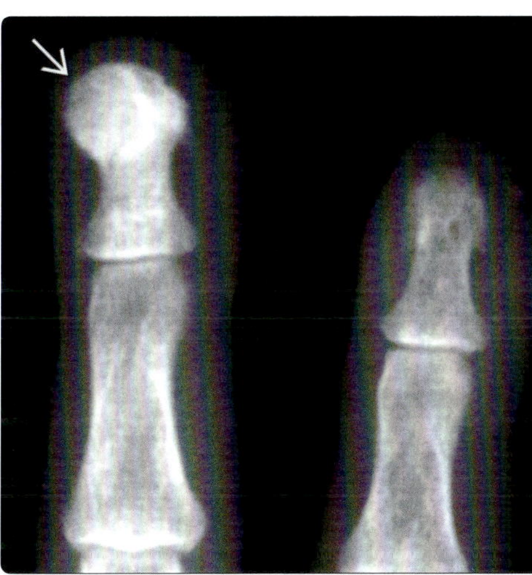

(Left) *AP radiograph reveals a mix of expansile lytic lesions ➡ and patchy sclerotic lesions ➡. Few processes have this mixed radiographic appearance. While well-defined mildly expansile lytic lesions are typical for brown tumors, this case reveals the wide variability of these lesions.* **(Right)** *PA radiograph shows a brown tumor within the distal phalanx ➡. The expansile nature is still evident. Following treatment, this previously lytic lesion became sclerotic, indicating healing.*

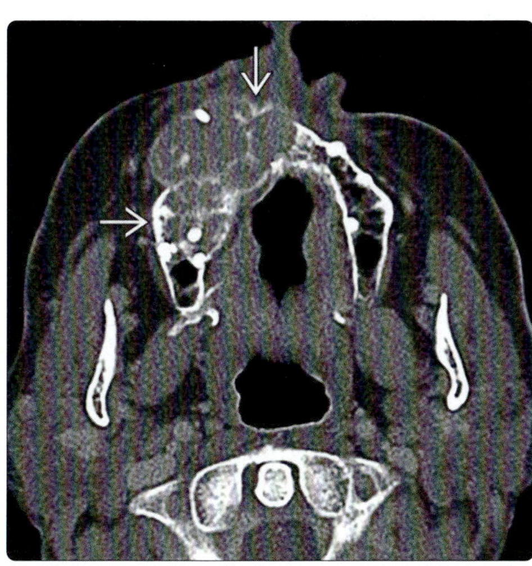

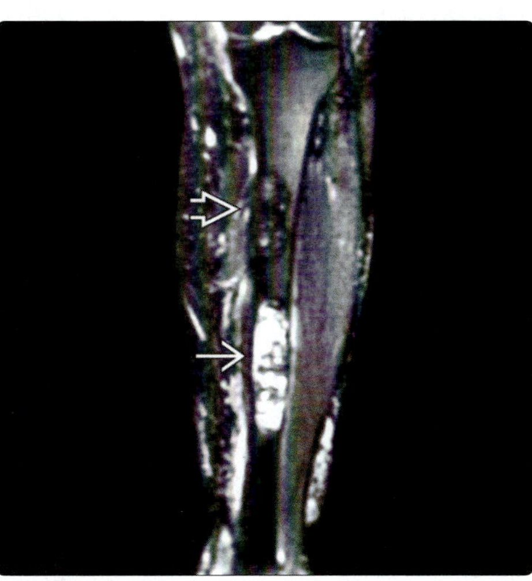

(Left) *Axial bone CT reveals a multiloculated lesion arising from the mandible ➡. The mandible and maxilla are common sites of brown tumor, in addition to the ribs, clavicle, pelvis, and femur.* **(Right)** *Coronal STIR MR of the tibia reveals 2 lesions with different imaging characteristics. The proximal lesion is heavily mineralized ➡, and the more distal lesion has nonspecific ↑ signal intensity ➡. Brown tumors have variable signal intensities depending on the mix of mineralization, hemorrhage, cyst formation, and fibrosis.*

Osteomalacia and Rickets

KEY FACTS

TERMINOLOGY

- Osteomalacia: Abnormal mineralization in trabecular and cortical bone
- Rickets: Abnormal mineralization of growth plates, concomitant osteomalacia

IMAGING

- Adult with osteomalacia
  - Looser zones, Milkman fractures, pseudofractures
  - Common sites: Lateral border scapula, medial femur, ribs, pubic rami, ischii
  - Bilateral, symmetric, ill-defined, horizontal, linear lucencies ± focal periostitis ± sclerotic margins
- Child with rickets
  - Widening, fraying, cupping of growth plate
  - Common sites: Ribs, distal femur, proximal and distal tibia, proximal humerus, distal radius and ulna
- Findings in both adults and children
  - Generalized osteopenia; coarse, ill-defined trabecula
  - Deformities 2° to bone softening
- Hypophosphatemic osteomalacia, adult onset
  - Enthesopathy, especially pelvis and proximal femur
  - Spinal hyperostotic changes

TOP DIFFERENTIAL DIAGNOSES

- Insufficiency fractures mimic Looser zones
- Physeal injuries and infection mimic rickets

PATHOLOGY

- Most common cause: Renal osteodystrophy
- Other causes: Malabsorption, liver disease, nutritional, abnormal vitamin D or phosphate metabolism, anticonvulsants, tumor induced

CLINICAL ISSUES

- Nonspecific bone pain and muscle weakness
- Progressive bone deformities and fractures
- Treatment: Vitamin D replacement

(Left) *Graphic depicting transection through a child's knee affected by rickets shows widening of the epiphyseal growth plate region. Physeal tongues of cartilage are seen penetrating into the metaphyseal bone. Note the thickened, sparse, and irregular trabeculae.* **(Right)** *AP radiograph shows typical physeal changes of rickets, including widening of the growth plate, widening at the end of the metaphysis, cupping at the margins, and irregularity along the metaphyseal margin.*

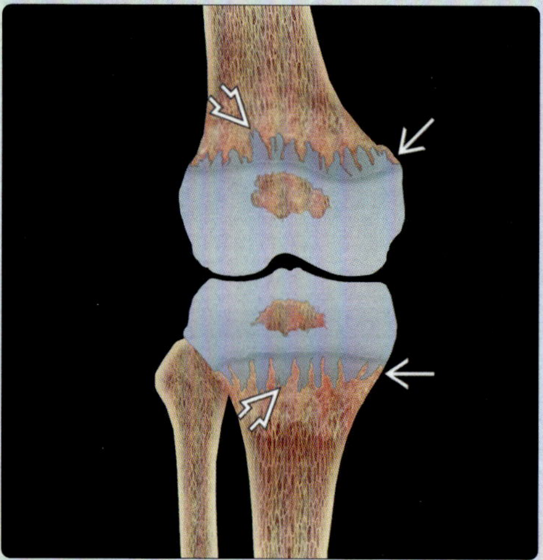

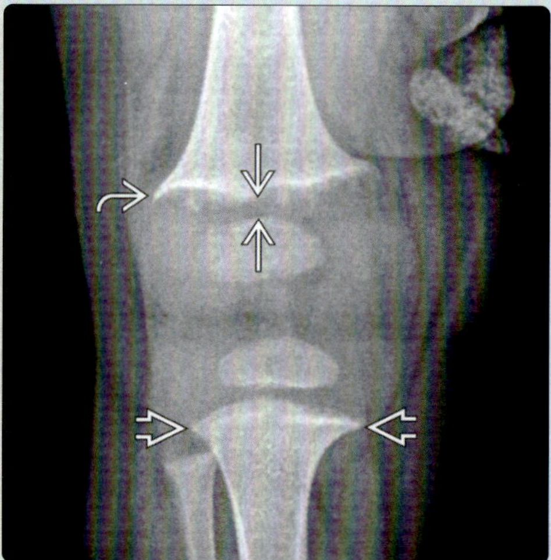

(Left) *AP radiograph shows a typical Milkman fracture. It is located at the site of compressive forces as opposed to the pseudofractures of Paget disease, which occur along the tensile side of the femur. The pseudofracture is perpendicular to the cortex, ill-defined, and with faint periostitis.* **(Right)** *Lateral radiograph of the elbow shows a Looser zone of the ulna. This pseudofracture happens to be fairly well defined. Note the background of ill-defined trabecula typical of osteomalacia.*

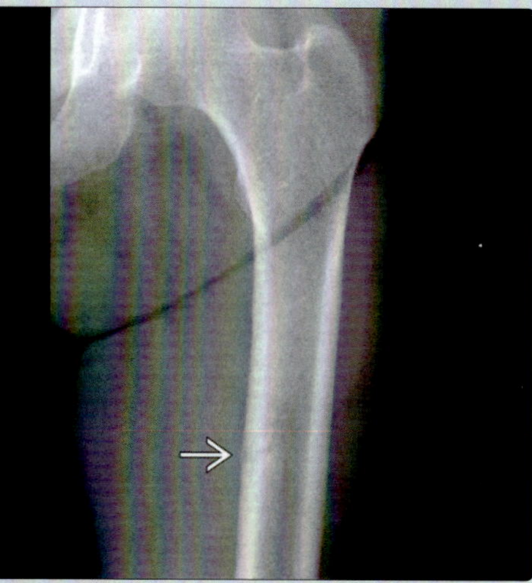

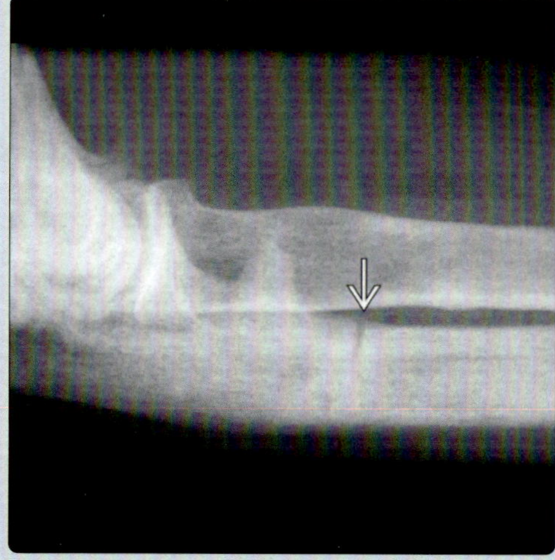

TERMINOLOGY

Definitions

- Osteomalacia: Abnormal mineralization in trabecular and cortical bone
- Rickets: Abnormal mineralization of growth plates
  - Only seen in skeletally immature individuals
  - Concomitant osteomalacia

IMAGING

General Features

- Best diagnostic clue
  - Adult: Looser zones
  - Child: Widening, fraying, cupping of growth plate
- Location
  - Common sites of physeal involvement: Ribs, distal femur, proximal and distal tibia, proximal humerus, distal radius and ulna
  - Common sites of Looser zones: Lateral border scapula, medial femur, ribs, pubic rami, ischii

Radiographic Findings

- Looser zones (Milkman fractures, pseudofractures)
  - Bilateral, symmetric, ill-defined, horizontal, linear lucencies ± focal periostitis ± sclerotic margins
  - Result from local accumulations of unmineralized osteoid
  - May progress to true and complete fracture
- Generalized osteopenia
- Coarse ill-defined (smudgy) trabecula
- Deformities 2° to bone softening
  - Craniotabes: Flattening of posterior skull in infants
  - Basilar invagination, vertebral endplate compressions, scoliosis
  - Triradiate pelvis and acetabular protrusio
  - Shepherd crook deformity: Laterally bowed proximal femur
  - Saber shin tibia: Anterior bowing
- Physis
  - Widening along long axis and short axis
  - Fraying, cupping, increased lucency
  - Slipped capital femoral epiphysis and disruption of other physes, including proximal humerus
  - Rachitic rosary due to accumulation of osteoid at costochondral junction
  - Delayed ossification and skeletal maturation
- X-linked hypophosphatemic (vitamin D-resistant) rickets/osteomalacia
  - Early onset: Presents in 1st few months of life
  - Adult onset: Enthesopathy, especially pelvis and proximal femur, spinal hyperostotic changes

Nuclear Medicine Findings

- Bone scan
  - Superscan: Intense diffuse skeletal uptake

DIFFERENTIAL DIAGNOSIS

Insufficiency Fractures

- Mimic Looser zones but lack bilateral symmetry

Physeal Injuries/Infection

- Mimic rickets: Typically isolated to single growth plate

PATHOLOGY

General Features

- Etiology
  - Most common cause: Renal osteodystrophy
  - Vitamin D deficiency or abnormal metabolism
    - Nutritional: ↓ intake, especially during pregnancy
    - Malabsorption states (short gut, celiac disease)
    - Lack of sunlight exposure
    - Chronic renal parenchymal disease
    - Liver disease
  - Abnormal phosphate metabolism
    - Renal tubular acidosis
  - Hypophosphatemic rickets
    - ↑ urinary excretion of phosphorus
  - Oncogenic (tumor-induced) osteomalacia
    - Paraneoplastic syndrome, may be reversible
    - Most common with mesenchymal tumors
  - Anticonvulsant therapy: Phenytoin, phenobarbital
  - Rickets of prematurity: Nutritional, metabolic causes
  - Hereditary vitamin D-resistant (pseudovitamin D deficient) rickets: Malabsorption of calcium
- Genetics
  - Hypophosphatemic rickets (X-linked dominant)
    - *PHEX* or *FGF23* gene abnormalities
  - Oncogenic osteomalacia: ↑ production *FGF23* gene

Microscopic Features

- Unmineralized osteoid rimming trabecula
- Abnormal hypertrophic zone of physeal plate and periphery epiphyses and apophyses
  - Loss of columnar organization; accumulation of chondrocytes; poorly mineralized cartilaginous bars

CLINICAL ISSUES

Presentation

- Most common signs/symptoms
  - Nonspecific bone pain and muscle weakness
- Other signs/symptoms
  - Growth retardation and joint swelling (actually enlarged growth plates)

Natural History & Prognosis

- Progressive bone deformities and fractures

Treatment

- Vitamin D replacement

DIAGNOSTIC CHECKLIST

Image Interpretation Pearls

- Osteomalacia difficult to appreciate radiographically

SELECTED REFERENCES

1. Hautmann AH et al: Tumor-induced osteomalacia: an up-to-date review. Curr Rheumatol Rep. 17(6):512, 2015

(Left) *Axial bone CT nicely reveals the ill-defined and coarsened trabecula of osteomalacia. The poor definition results from unmineralized osteoid rimming the trabecular margins.* **(Right)** *AP radiograph reveals markedly abnormal physis of the proximal humerus. The growth plate is extremely thick with extensive fragmentation ➡ and ill definition of the metaphyseal margin. The epiphysis is displaced similar to a slipped capital femoral epiphysis.*

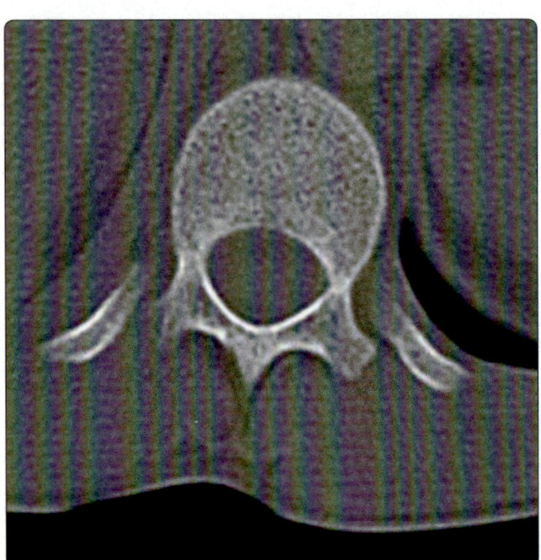

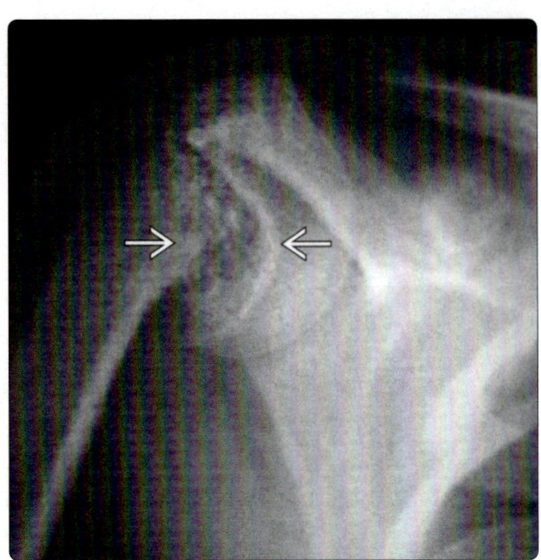

(Left) *PA radiograph of the hand with abnormal physes of the 3rd-5th metacarpal growth plates ➡ demonstrates that any physis can be affected by rickets. The coarsened trabecula in the proximal phalanges is a manifestation of concomitant osteomalacia ➡.* **(Right)** *AP radiograph shows marked distortion of the pelvic contour on the right ➡ resulting from the bone softening of osteomalacia. When distortion involves both sides of the pelvis, it creates the triradiate pelvis appearance.*

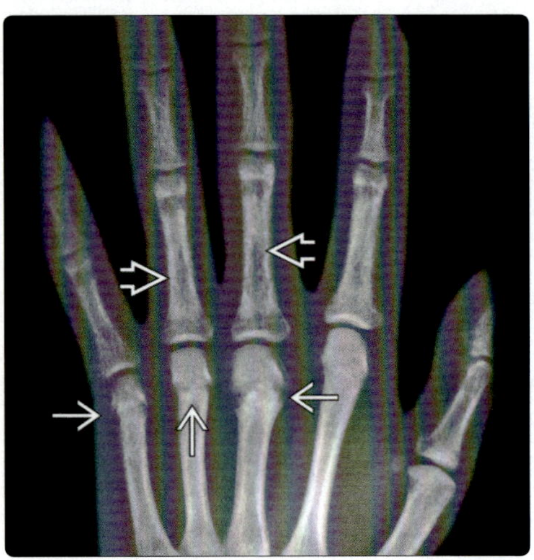

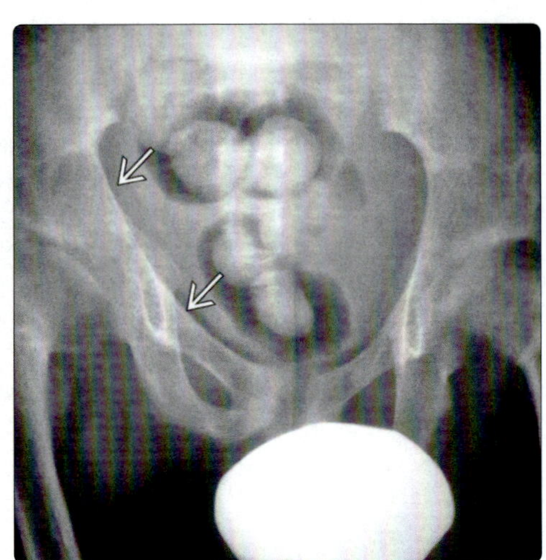

(Left) *AP radiograph of an infant with renal rickets is shown. The proximal femoral epiphyses ➡ are much smaller than anticipated for this 5 year old, and the growth plates are abnormal ➡.* **(Right)** *AP radiograph of the chest coned down to the anterior costochondral junctions shows the radiographic appearance of a rachitic rosary. The ends of the ribs are widened, cupped, and frayed ➡, identical to the changes seen at the growth plates. The term refers to the clinically evident prominent beads along the chest wall.*

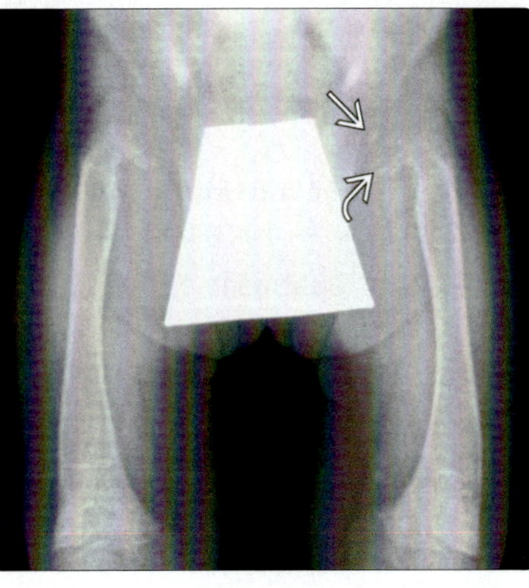

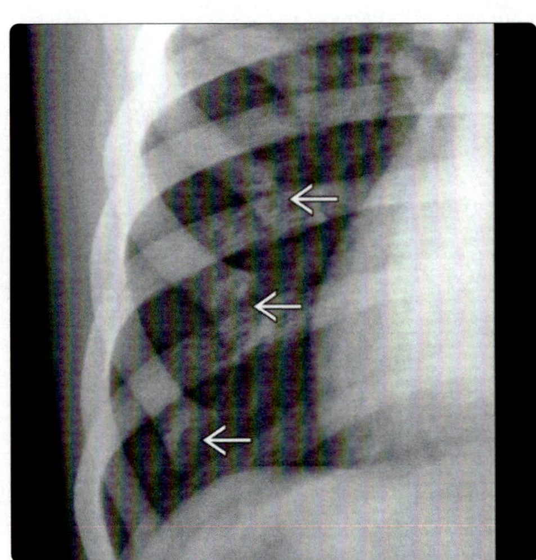

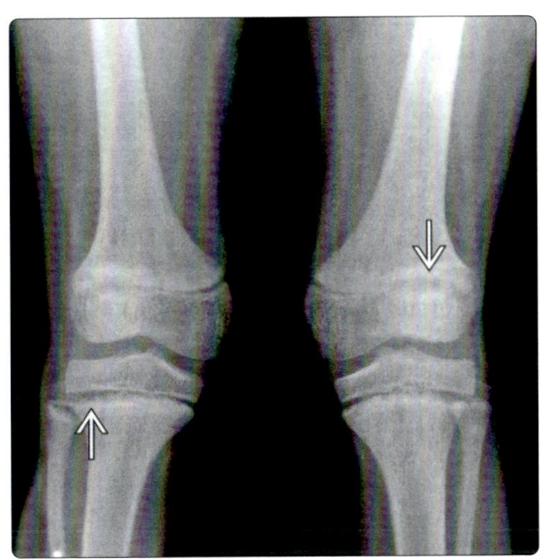

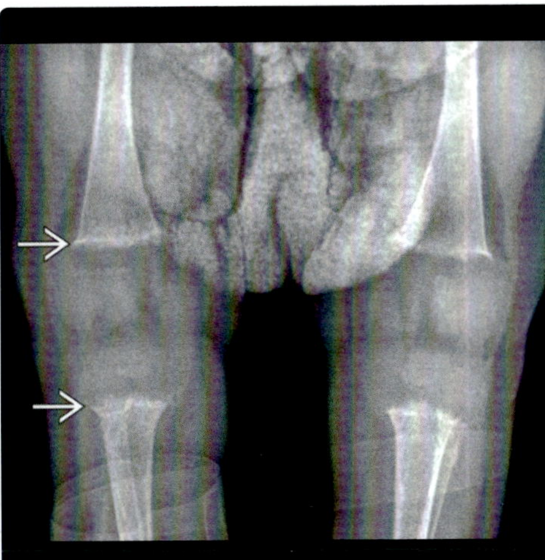

(Left) *This child has developed nutritional rickets, an extremely uncommon disease in the USA. However, the appearance is classic, with a widened zone of provisional calcification at all the physes of the knee ➡. The weakened physes have allowed a valgus deformity to develop.* **(Right)** *AP radiograph of the knees reveals poorly mineralized epiphyses and irregular mildly widened physes ➡ in this child with rickets secondary to biliary atresia.*

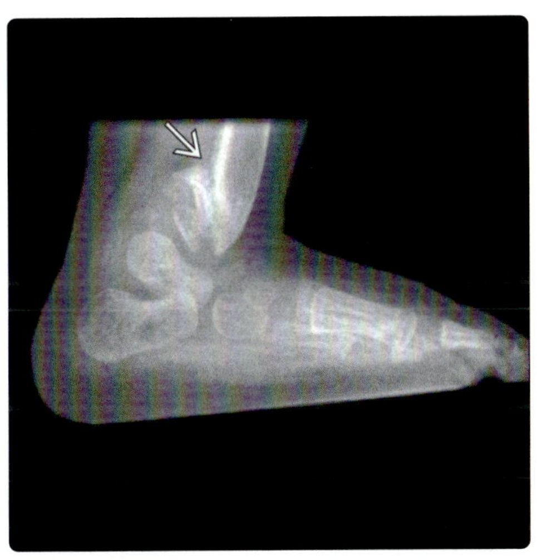

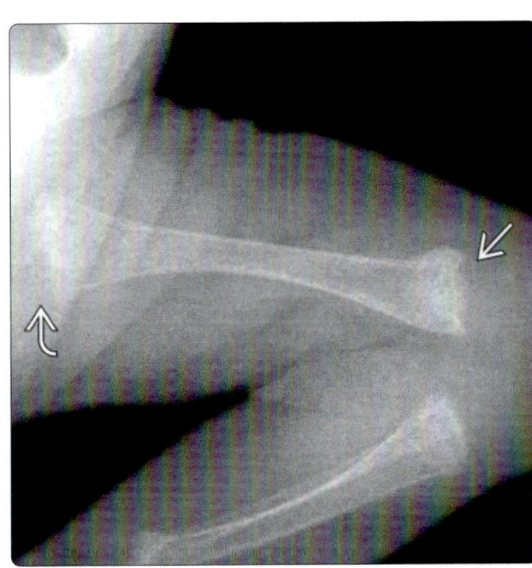

(Left) *Lateral radiograph shows angular deformity of the tibial metaphysis ➡. An underlying Salter II fracture through osteomalacic bone results in this malalignment.* **(Right)** *AP radiograph in a 3 month old shows delayed skeletal age, osteopenia, and widened frayed metaphyses at the knee ➡ and proximal femur ⮫. Generally one would not expect to see rickets at this age. However, a premature child spending a long time in the NBICU is at risk for rickets, with nutritional, liver, and renal deficiencies all contributing.*

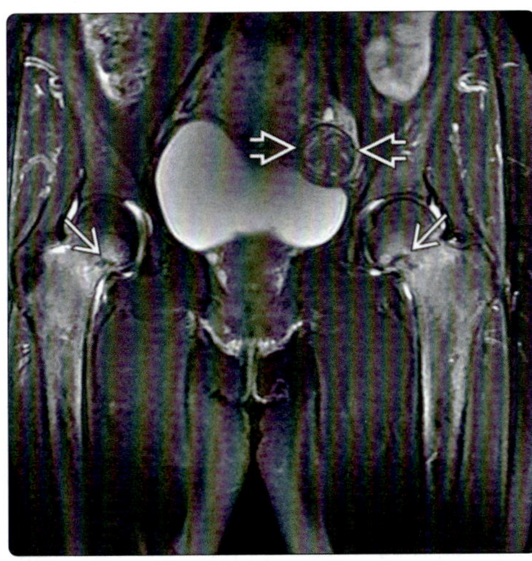

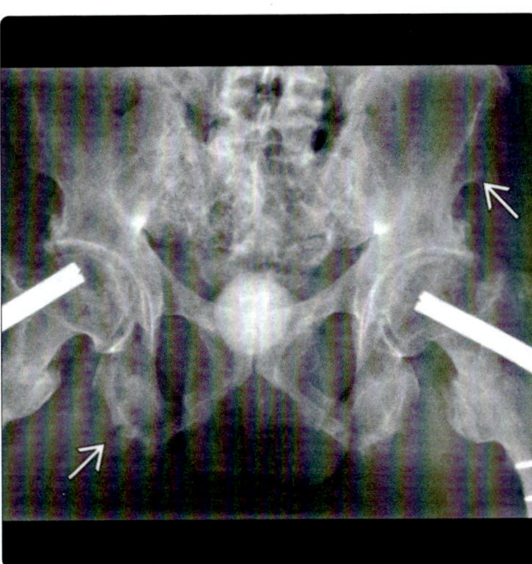

(Left) *Coronal PD FS MR shows incomplete insufficiency fractures of the subcapital region ➡ with adjacent edema. There is also an ovarian mass ➡ that is inhomogeneous and contains fat. This is a dermoid, and the patient has associated oncogenic osteomalacia.* **(Right)** *AP radiograph shows vitamin D-resistant rickets due to a renal tubular disorder. The patient must take massive doses of vitamin D, resulting in enthesopathy ➡ and osteopenic fragile bone.*

KEY FACTS

TERMINOLOGY

- Combination of 2° hyperparathyroidism (HPTH), osteomalacia, osteoporosis, neoostosis

IMAGING

- 2° HPTH manifests as bone resorption; brown tumors; metastatic soft tissue, arterial & visceral mineralization
- Osteomalacia: Looser zones (pseudofractures, Milkman fractures)
- Rickets: Physeal cupping, fraying, irregularity, growth plate disruption
- Neoostosis: Pelvis, ribs, clavicles
- Amyloid deposition in bursa, tendons, tenosynovium, bones, joints, vertebral disc, articular cartilage, muscle
  - Considered almost epidemic in dialysis patients
- Crystal deposition disease: Gout, chondrocalcinosis, oxalosis, hydroxyapatite
- Osteonecrosis: Usually from steroids (usually relates to transplant)
- Tendon & ligament laxity, disruption
- Olecranon bursitis, osteomyelitis, septic arthritis
- Aluminum toxicity, presenting as worsening of osteomalacia

TOP DIFFERENTIAL DIAGNOSES

- Soft tissue calcification: Collagen vascular disease (scleroderma, systemic lupus erythematosus)
- Destructive spondyloarthropathy radiographically similar to vertebral osteomyelitis
- Subchondral resorption & collapse mimic erosions of rheumatoid arthritis, ankylosing spondylitis
- Trauma & infection may mimic rickets

PATHOLOGY

- Acquired forms: Glomerulonephritis most common
  - Diabetes, hypertension most common etiologies of glomerulonephritis
- Congenital forms: Inborn errors of metabolism affecting renal tubules

(Left) *Lateral radiograph shows typical salt & pepper skull. The bone has ill-defined appearance. Note the absence of well-defined inner & outer tables. Superimposed foci of sclerosis & more focal areas of bone resorption contribute to overall mottled appearance.* **(Right)** *AP radiograph shows apparent widening of the acromioclavicular joint, which is in fact the result of subchondral resorption & collapse of the distal end of the clavicle ➡, resulting from the hyperparathyroidism (HPTH) component of renal osteodystrophy.*

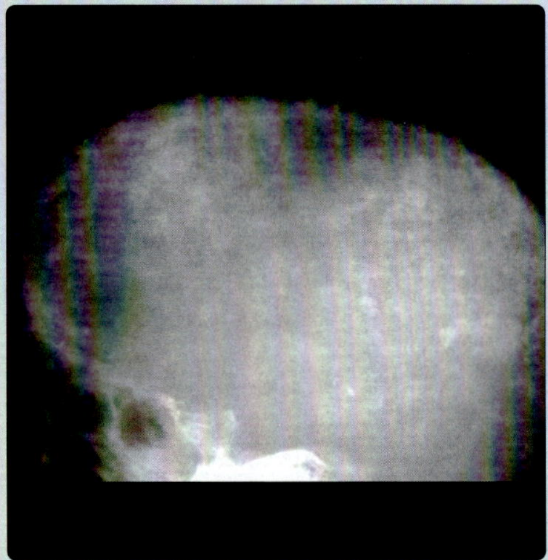

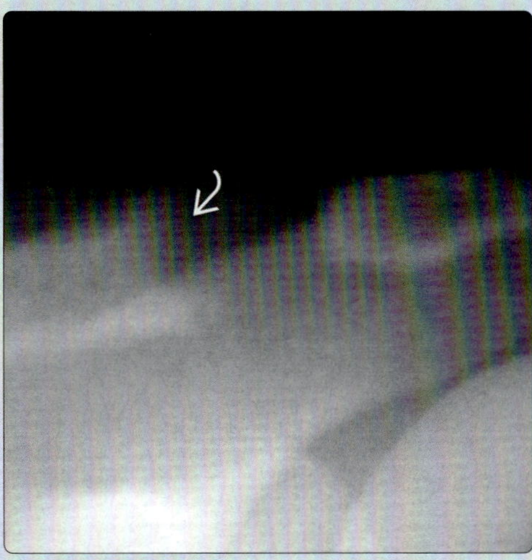

(Left) *Lateral radiograph shows dramatic appearance of rugger jersey spine with thick, ill-defined sclerosis along the superior & inferior endplates ➡. Lumbar & thoracic vertebrae are uniformly involved.* **(Right)** *PA radiograph shows a hand with classic changes of renal osteodystrophy. Osteomalacia causes the coarsened appearance of the trabecula, while 2° HPTH leads to resorption at the tufts of the distal phalanges ➡ & pathognomonic subperiosteal resorption along the middle phalanges ➡.*

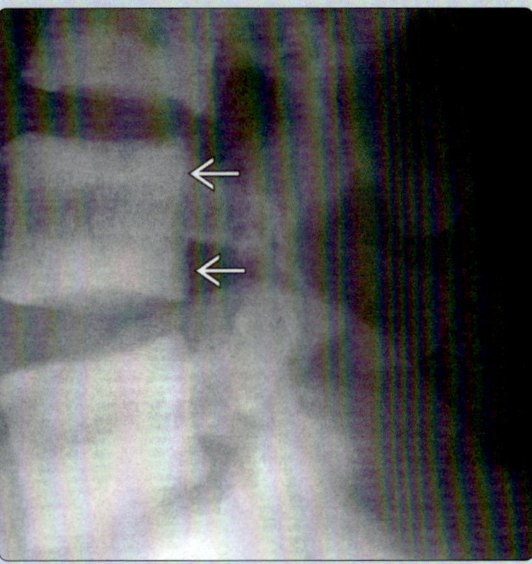

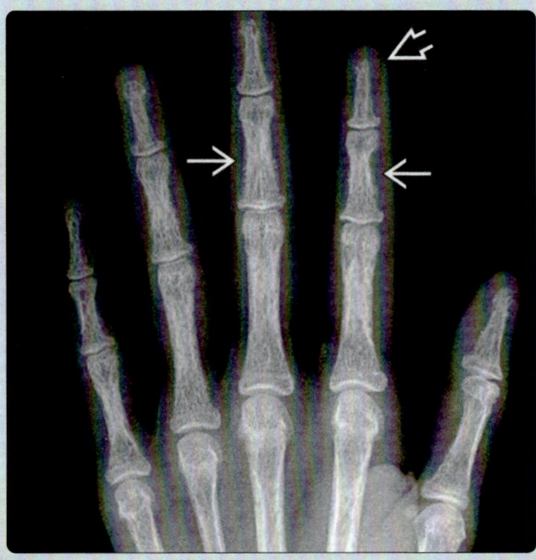

TERMINOLOGY

Definitions

- Bone & soft tissue disease resulting from end-stage renal disease (ESRD)
  - Combination of 2° hyperparathyroidism (HPTH), osteomalacia, osteoporosis, neoostosis

IMAGING

General Features

- Best diagnostic clue
  - Bone resorption patterns of 2° HPTH & osteosclerosis of rugger jersey spine

Imaging Recommendations

- Best imaging tool
  - Radiographs are best for characterizing osseous changes & associated soft tissue abnormalities

Radiographic Findings

- 2° HPTH manifests as bone resorption
  - Subperiosteal, subchondral, subligamentous, subtendinous, intracortical tunneling, trabecular, physeal (in child)
  - Result of osteoclastic activity; reversible
  - Characteristic findings
    - Subperiosteal resorption radial cortex 2nd & 3rd middle phalanges considered pathognomonic
    - Bilateral distal clavicular subchondral osteolysis & collapse; subligamentous resorption at coracoclavicular ligament attachments
    - Bilateral subchondral bone resorption at sacroiliac joints, especially along ilial surface
    - Subchondral collapse, especially metacarpal heads, may mimic erosive arthritis
    - Salt & pepper or pepper pot skull
      - Generalized osteopenia with cystic areas of bone resorption & patchy foci of sclerosis
    - Brown tumors
      - Expanded lytic lesions with geographic nonsclerotic margins; no matrix, soft tissue mass, cortical destruction, periostitis
      - Multiple or solitary: Metaphyseal ± epiphyseal extension; may originate in diaphysis
      - Mandible, clavicle, ribs, pelvis, femur, patella
  - Metastatic soft tissue, arterial, visceral calcification
    - Soft tissue calcification: Favors periarticular locations, especially shoulders & hips
      - Severity & extent increases on dialysis therapy
      - Can cause pressure erosions on adjacent bone
      - May have fluid-fluid levels
      - Calcium hydroxyapatite crystals
    - Vascular calcification: Medium-sized vessels, such as common femoral artery, as well as small vessels
    - Visceral calcification
      - Heart, lungs, kidneys, stomach
    - Other sites: Tendons, bursa, tenosynovium
  - Chondrocalcinosis
    - Calcium pyrophosphate crystals
    - Knees, symphysis pubis, triangular fibrocartilage
    - Associated arthritic findings uncommon
  - Periostitis
    - Lamellar in appearance
    - Incorporation may produce cortical thickening
- Osteomalacia & rickets
  - Coarse, ill-defined trabecula
  - Rickets: Physeal cupping, fraying, irregularity, growth plate disruption, such as slipped capital femoral epiphysis
  - Osteomalacia: Looser zones, pseudofractures, Milkman fractures
  - Bowing deformities 2° to bone softening
- Osteoporosis
  - Generalized osteopenia
  - Vertebral compression deformities
  - Insufficiency fractures
    - Increased incidence on dialysis therapy
  - May be superimposed on reparative ↑ density
    - Mixed pattern of ↑ and ↓ density possible
- Neoostosis
  - Focal areas of bone sclerosis
  - Pelvis, ribs, clavicles
  - Metaphysis, epiphysis
  - Characteristic appearance: Rugger jersey spine
    - Wide bands of ill-defined sclerosis along vertebral endplates throughout thoracic & lumbar spine
- Other findings
  - Osteonecrosis: Usually from steroids, especially following renal transplantation
  - Ligament & tendon abnormalities
    - Laxity; may cause joint instability
    - Disruption, especially quadriceps & patellar tendons, may be within tendon substance due to poor tissue quality
    - Result of HPTH, chronic acidosis, steroid use, intratendinous crystal & amyloid deposits
  - Dialysis-related conditions
    - Olecranon bursitis, osteomyelitis, septic arthritis
  - Crystal deposition disease: Gout, chondrocalcinosis, oxalosis, hydroxyapatite
  - Amyloid deposition
    - Most common sites of deposition different from other causes of amyloid
      - Bursa, tendons, tenosynovium, bones, joints, vertebral disc, articular cartilage, muscle
    - Shoulder especially common site; creates "shoulder pad" sign
    - Contributes to carpal tunnel syndrome
    - Subchondral cystic changes (hemodialysis cysts): Carpus, especially scaphoid, lunate, capitate; metacarpophalangeal joints, hip, elbow
    - Sites of deposition in bone prone to fractures
    - Destructive spondyloarthropathy
      - Disc space narrowing, minimal endplate sclerosis & fragmentation, malalignment, hyperostosis
  - Aluminum toxicity
    - Radiographic changes identical to osteomalacia
    - Presents as worsening of osteomalacia

CT Findings

- Mirrors radiographic findings, provides greater detail
- Musculoskeletal findings usually incidental

MR Findings

- Brown tumor
  - Variable signal intensity related to variable degrees of fibrosis, hemorrhage, cyst formation
- Tendon rupture: MR helps identify site of disruption, site of gap, degree of retraction
  - Unable to determine underlying etiology of rupture
- Amyloid deposition: Low signal intensity on all imaging sequences; enhances post contrast

Nuclear Medicine Findings

- Bone scan
  - Superscan: Diffuse intense skeletal uptake in context of no renal uptake
  - Focal uptake in pseudofracture, brown tumor
  - Focal uptake at sites of soft tissue calcification

Other Modality Findings

- DEXA & quantitative CT diagnose osteoporosis

DIFFERENTIAL DIAGNOSIS

Soft Tissue Calcification

- Includes collagen vascular disease, such as progressive systemic sclerosis, systemic lupus erythematosus
  - These conditions may also lead to ESRD
  - Calcific deposits in these conditions, usually small, favor hands

Osteoporosis

- Complex series of etiologies, many of which overlap in patient with renal osteodystrophy

Destructive Spondyloarthropathy

- Radiographically similar to vertebral osteomyelitis; lacks disc enhancement on MR
  - Vacuum phenomenon if present excludes infection
- Identical appearance to neuropathic spine

Subchondral Resorption & Collapse

- Rheumatoid arthritis (RA) type changes
  - "Erosions" in HPTH appear better defined than true erosions in RA
  - HPTH favors DIP, MCPs, shoulder
- Resorption on calcaneus, SI, symphysis mimics ankylosing spondylitis

Physeal Abnormalities

- Trauma & infection may have similar appearance; usually isolated to single growth plate

PATHOLOGY

General Features

- Etiology
  - Disease is combination of HPTH, osteomalacia and rickets, & neoostosis
  - HPTH
    - Damaged kidneys fail to excrete phosphate
    - Excess phosphate binds with calcium, leading to hypocalcemia
    - Hypocalcemia stimulates parathyroid hormone production
    - Parathyroid hormone (PTH) stimulates bone resorption to increase serum calcium levels
  - Osteomalacia
    - Damaged kidneys fail to convert vitamin D_3 to calcitriol
  - Neoostosis poorly understood
    - Proposed etiologies
      - PTH stimulation of osteoclasts
      - Calcium phosphate deposition in bone
  - ESRD
    - Acquired forms: Glomerulonephritis most common etiology; diabetes, hypertension most common causes of glomerulonephritis
    - Congenital forms: Inborn errors of metabolism affecting renal tubules
      - Vitamin D-resistant rickets
      - Fanconi syndrome
      - Renal tubular acidosis
  - Aluminum toxicity
    - Due to excess aluminum in oral phosphate binders; previously dialysate was also source
    - Aluminum replaces calcium in osteoid mineralization

Microscopic Features

- Osteoporosis: Thinning cortical & trabecular bone
- Osteomalacia: Osteoid rimming trabecula
- 2° HPTH: Fibrovascular tissue, ↑ number osteoclasts
- Brown tumors: Aborted new bone formation, hemorrhage of varying age, fibrovascular tissue
- Amyloid: β_2 microglobulin, stains positive with Congo red; apple-green birefringence in polarized light

Laboratory Analysis

- Decreased serum calcium, calcitriol
- Elevated serum phosphate, parathyroid hormone

CLINICAL ISSUES

Presentation

- Most common signs/symptoms
  - Bone & joint pain: ↑ incidence when on dialysis
- Other signs/symptoms
  - Weakness; skeletal deformity

Demographics

- Age
  - Majority of patients will be over 40 years old
- Gender
  - ESRD slightly more common in men
- Ethnicity
  - ↑ incidence of ESRD in African Americans, Native Americans
- Epidemiology
  - 0.01% of population
  - Nearly 1,000,000 individuals currently undergoing renal dialysis

SELECTED REFERENCES

1. Babayev R et al: Bone disorders in chronic kidney disease: an update in diagnosis and management. Semin Dial. 28(6):645-53, 2015
2. Degrassi F et al: Imaging of haemodialysis: renal and extrarenal findings. Insights Imaging. 6(3):309-21, 2015

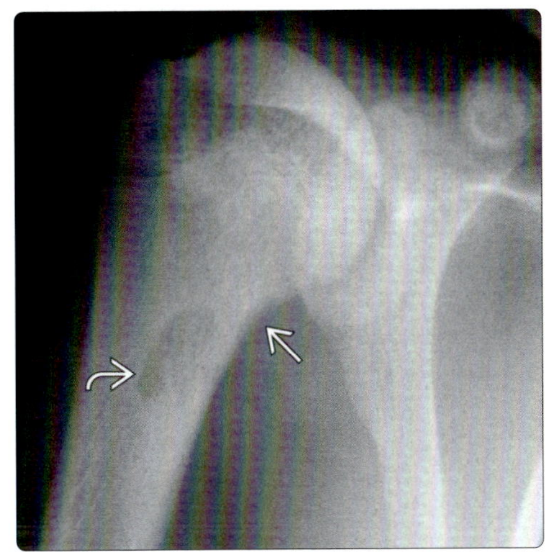

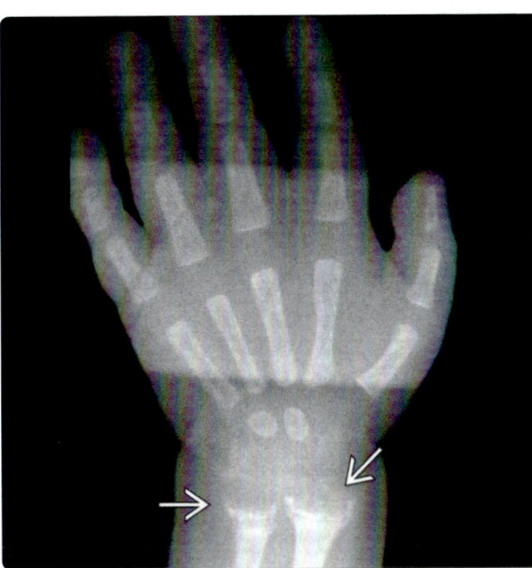

(Left) *AP radiograph shows proximal humerus with generalized increased density & smudgy trabeculae. There is subtle subperiosteal resorption at the medial humeral metaphysis ➡. A small lytic lesion within the humeral metaphysis ➡, in the context of known renal osteodystrophy, can reliably be considered a brown tumor.* **(Right)** *PA radiograph shows a skeletally immature hand in a patient with renal rickets. The growth plates are abnormal, with widening, cupping, and fraying ➡.*

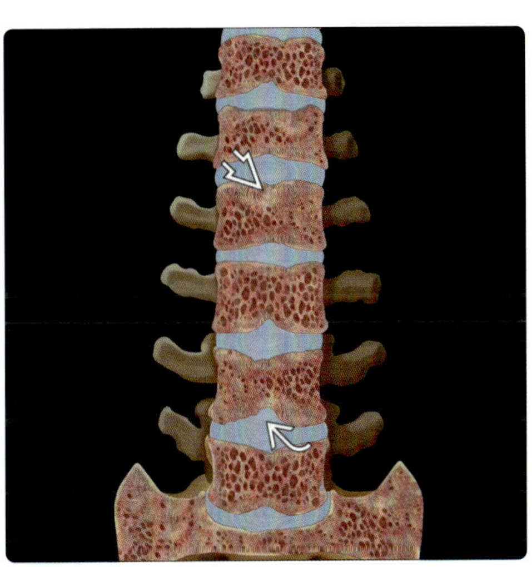

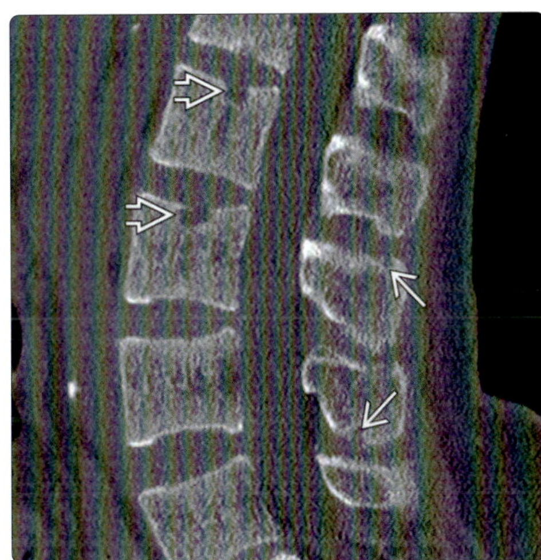

(Left) *Graphic depicts the transected spine in a patient with renal osteodystrophy. Note the loss of normal trabecular organization. There is also an increase in sclerosis, particularly at the endplates ➡, & otherwise nonfocal, as well as some collapse ➡.* **(Right)** *Sagittal bone CT shows coarsened and ill-defined trabecula and multiple Schmorl nodes ➡, all the result of osteomalacia. Several small foci of bone resorption ➡ are the result of HPTH.*

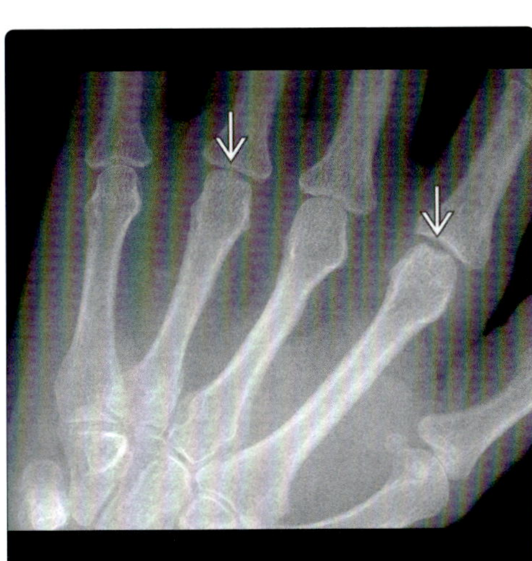

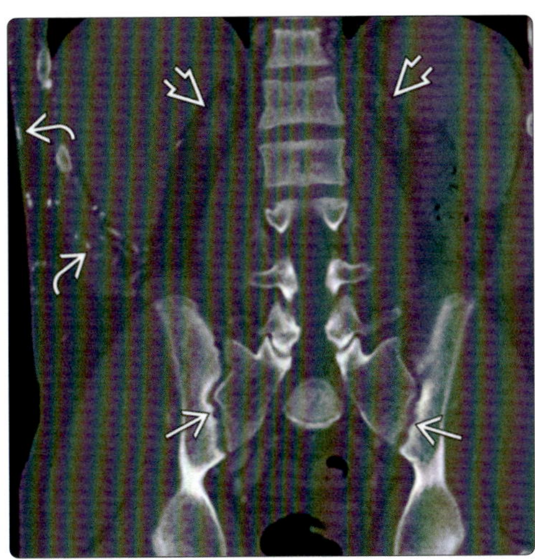

(Left) *PA radiograph shows erosive-like deformities on heads of 2nd & 4th metacarpals ➡ resulting from subchondral resorption and collapse in patient with end-stage renal disease (ESRD). Appearance may be mistaken for rheumatoid arthritis.* **(Right)** *Coronal CT in 33-year-old man shows many findings of renal osteodystrophy, including atrophic kidneys ➡, SI joint subchondral resorption ➡, and metastatic soft tissue calcification ➡. Note in addition the ill-defined trabeculae, indicating osteomalacia.*

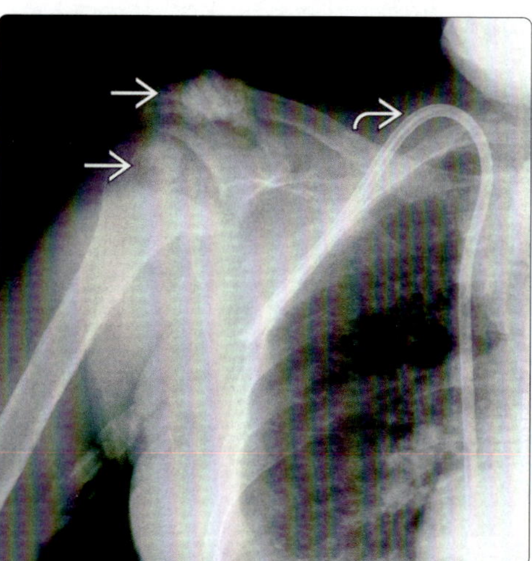

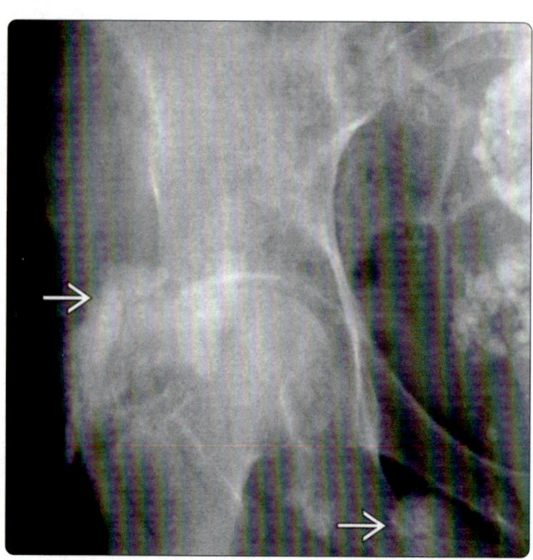

(Left) *AP radiograph shows amorphus calcific deposits surrounding the shoulder . The shoulder and hip are common sites for such calcium deposits. The dialysis catheter provides a clue to the underlying etiology.* **(Right)** *AP radiograph shows a hip with amorphous calcium deposits . Such periarticular calcifications are common in renal osteodystrophy. They are in part attributable to 2° HPTH and increase in size once the patient is placed on dialysis.*

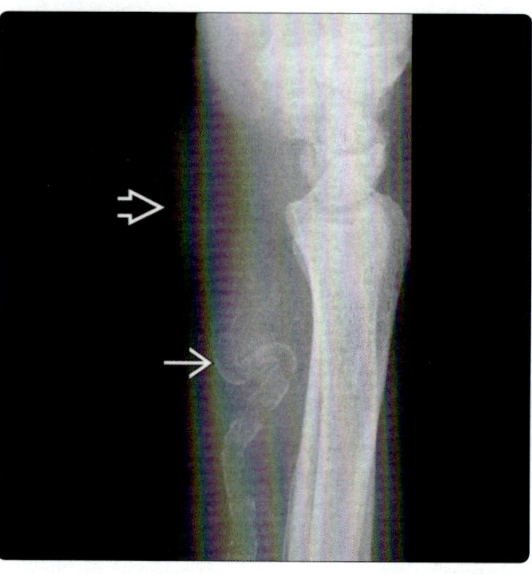

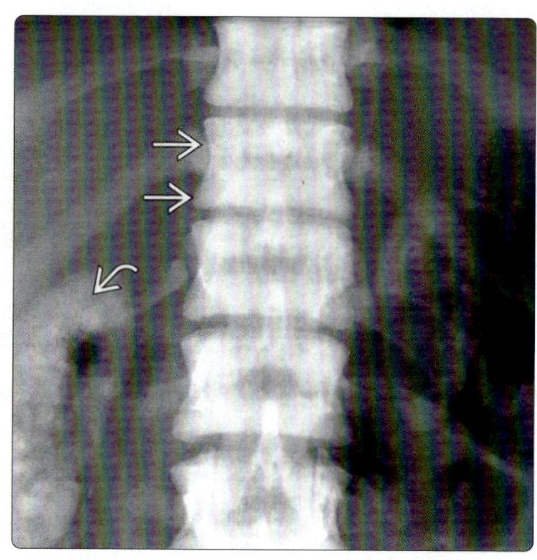

(Left) *Lateral radiograph demonstrates extensive vascular calcification , which is often seen as part of the HPTH component of renal osteodystrophy. A prominent soft tissue mass on the volar surface of the wrist may be due to either gout or amyloid deposition (proven in this case).* **(Right)** *AP radiograph has all the findings needed to make a diagnosis. The left kidney is small, and extensive nephrocalcinosis is present in the right kidney . Dramatic changes of rugger jersey spine are evident .*

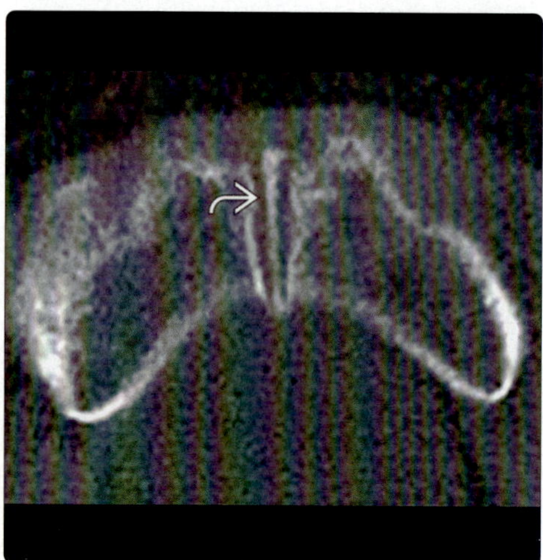

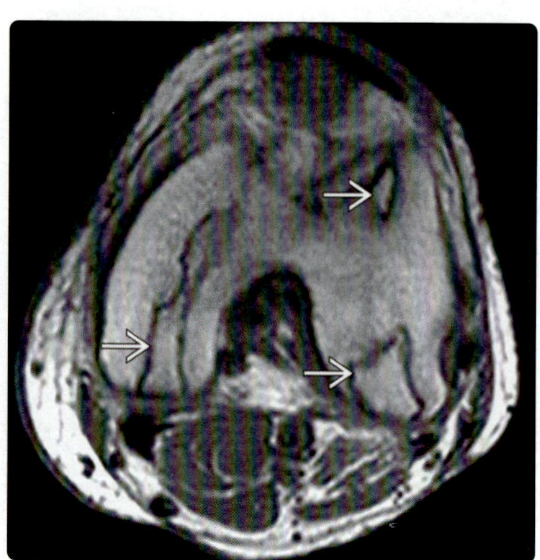

(Left) *Axial NECT shows a symphysis pubis with extensive chondrocalcinosis . Arthritic changes are absent, which is typical of calcium pyrophosphate deposition in renal osteodystrophy.* **(Right)** *Axial T1WI MR with multiple bone infarcts is classic in appearance. The multiplicity should trigger a search for an underlying condition. In patients with ESRD, multiple infarcts often occur after transplantation when steroids are used to prevent rejection.*

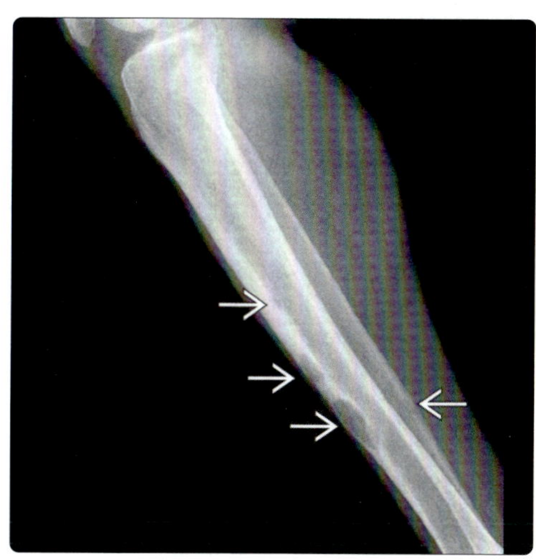

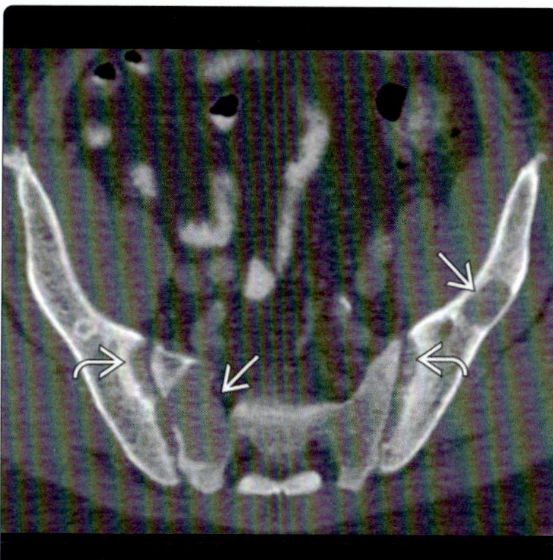

(Left) *Lateral radiograph shows a tibia with multiple brown tumors ➡. In this case, the lesions are cortically based, which is somewhat unusual although these tumors have an extremely variable presentation.* **(Right)** *Axial bone CT reveals 2 lytic lesions with geographic nonsclerotic margins ➡. Similar lesions were seen elsewhere, and the possibility of multiple myeloma was considered. Subchondral resorption at the SI joint ➡ is a clue to the underlying diagnosis of brown tumors in ESRD.*

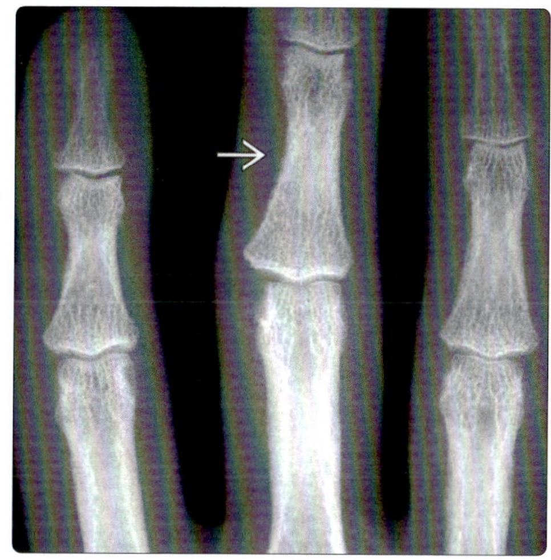

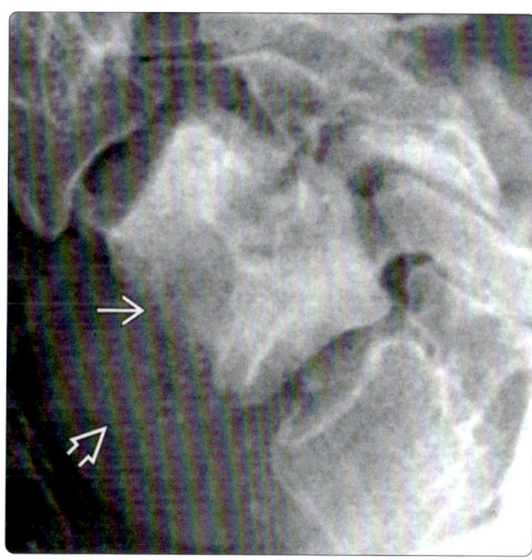

(Left) *PA x-ray shows subtle subperiosteal resorption along the radial cortex of the 3rd middle phalanx ➡; this is one of the earliest findings of HPTH, as may be seen with renal osteodystrophy.* **(Right)** *Lateral radiograph shows endplate destruction and vertebral body erosions at the C4/5 level ➡. Vertebral bodies are sclerotic due to longstanding reparative process. Punctate calcifications anteriorly ➡ are due to crystal deposition. This is hemodialysis-related spondyloarthropathy.*

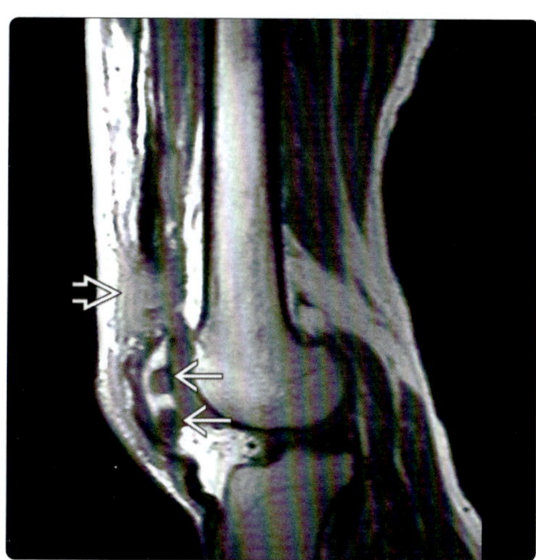

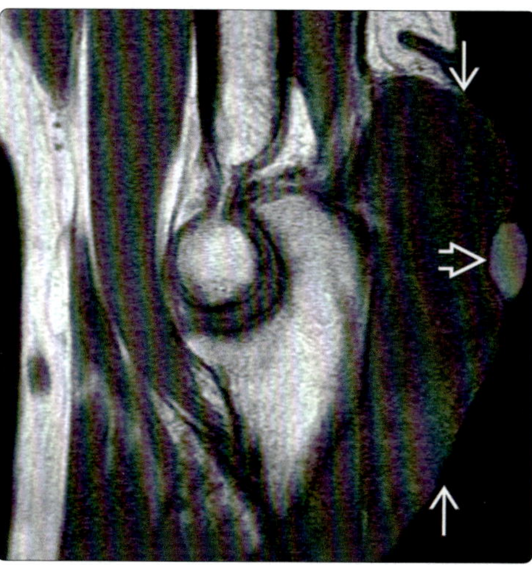

(Left) *Sagittal T1WI MR shows a full thickness quadriceps tendon tear ➡. Such tears almost always occur in the face of systemic disease, which weakens the tendon. The associated lesions in the patella ➡ are likely brown tumors.* **(Right)** *Sagittal T1WI MR reveals a large fluid collection in the olecranon bursa ➡. In a dialysis patient, diagnostic possibilities include gout and "dialysis elbow," which is bursitis resulting from prolonged pressure on an immobilized elbow (marker is present ➡).*

KEY FACTS

TERMINOLOGY

- Metastatic calcification: Transport of calcium from 1 part of body to another

IMAGING

- Common sites
  - Soft tissues: Especially periarticular deposits
  - Vascular: Medium size arteries
  - Viscera: Lung, liver, stomach, kidneys, heart
- Periarticular deposits: Muscles, tenosynovium, joint capsule, usually bilateral ± symmetric
  - May occur anywhere; hips & shoulders common
  - May erode adjacent bone
- Radiographs: Amorphous, cloud-like densities of variable size, often quite large
- CT: Variably dense masses
- Bone scan: ↑ uptake at sites of soft tissue calcification
- T1WI MR: Heterogeneous hypointense to low signal
- Fluid-sensitive MR sequences: Low signal
- US: Diffuse echogenicity throughout mass
- ± adjacent soft tissue inflammation

TOP DIFFERENTIAL DIAGNOSES

- Collagen vascular disease: Small foci, often in hands, may have associated renal failure
- Hydroxyapatite deposition disease: Small deposits, usually solitary

PATHOLOGY

- Dialysis alters calcium phosphate product (> 70)

CLINICAL ISSUES

- Hard, mobile, ± tender mass(es)
- Control of phosphate levels may reduce size
- Vascular calcifications contribute to ↑ morbidity
- Conjunctival & corneal calcifications reportedly are common
- Rare reports of associated spinal cord compression
- No correlation to onset/duration of dialysis

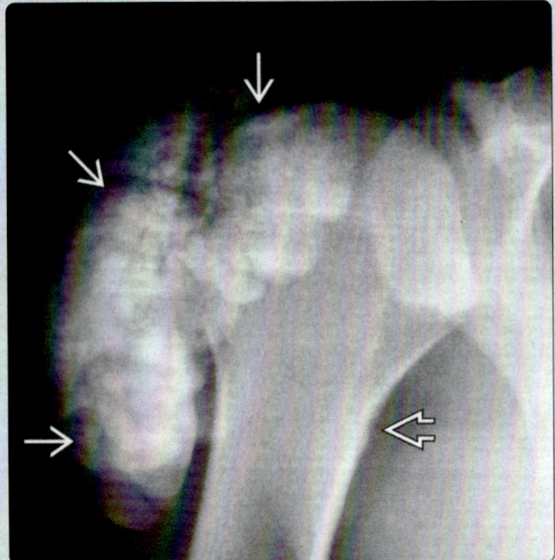

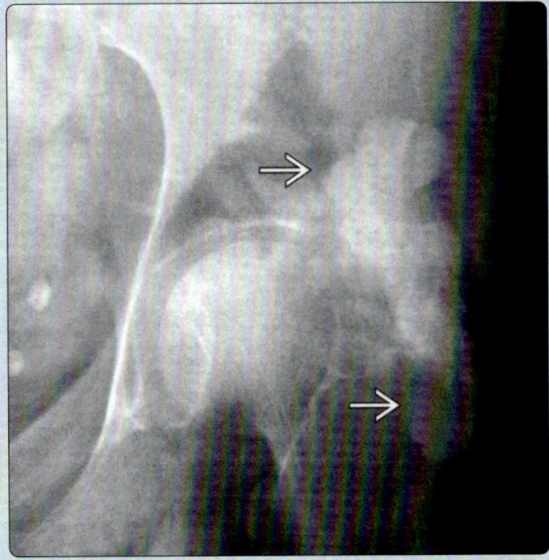

(Left) *AP radiograph shows large cloud-like collection of calcification adjacent to the shoulder ➡. Subperiosteal resorption at the proximal medial humeral metaphysis ➡ is a clue to the underlying renal osteodystrophy. The patient was undergoing dialysis.* **(Right)** *AP radiograph reveals typical periarticular amorphous mineralization ➡. The hip is a common site of involvement for dialysis-related metastatic calcification. The deposits are often bilateral and present as hard, mobile, asymptomatic masses.*

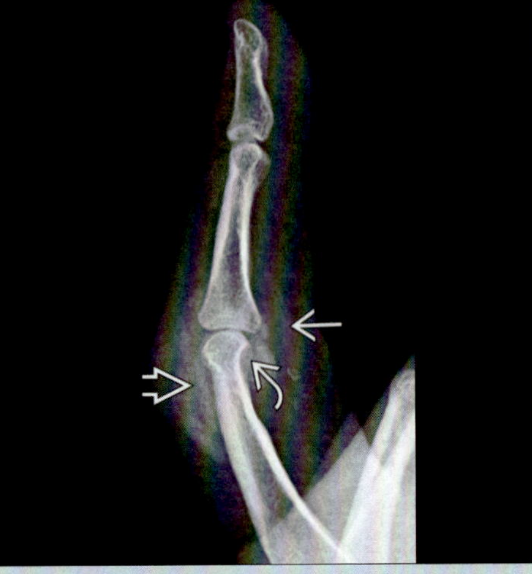

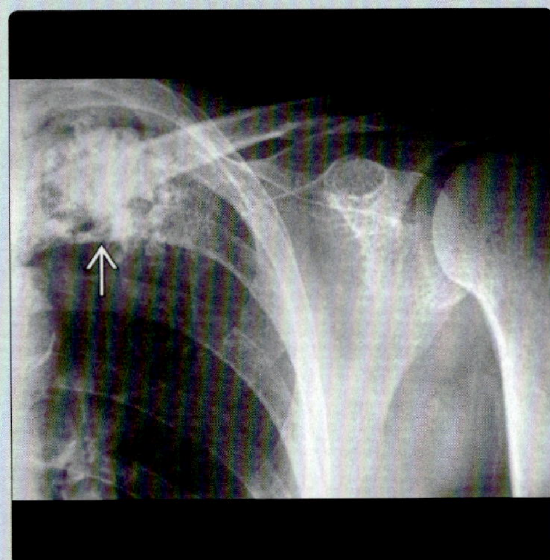

(Left) *Lateral x-ray in a 50-year-old man on dialysis shows fluffy metastatic calcification ➡ in a periarticular distribution. Note a related mechanical erosion of the phalangeal head ➡. Vascular calcifications ➡ complete image.* **(Right)** *AP x-ray reveals a large focus of mineralization in the upper left lung ➡. The lung is a less frequent location than are the soft tissues of the musculoskeletal system, but when it occurs, there is a preferential upper lobe distribution of the calcification, thought to be due to pH differences.*

KEY FACTS

TERMINOLOGY

- Destructive discovertebral changes in dialysis patients 2° to amyloid & crystal deposition

IMAGING

- Radiograph & CT: Disc space narrowing, endplate erosions & cysts, malalignment, minimal sclerosis/hyperostosis
- MR: Amyloid deposits in bone & soft tissue have ↓ T1W & variable T2W (low to slight ↑) signal
  - MR examination may differentiate from infection & obviate need for biopsy
    - Lack of soft tissue mass in spondyloarthropathy
    - Different signal characteristics from infection, particularly if MR contrast used
- Rapid progression (weeks to months)
- Multiple levels; favors cervical & lumbar segments
- Other changes of renal osteodystrophy seen as well
  - Schmorl nodes, rugger jersey spine, small foci of bone resorption, periarticular soft tissue crystal deposition

TOP DIFFERENTIAL DIAGNOSES

- Vertebral body osteomyelitis (discitis)
  - ↑ signal & enhancement in disc space on MR
  - Inflammatory soft tissue changes/mass
- Neuropathic spine: More sclerosis, hyperostosis, fragmentation, significant malalignment
- Rheumatoid arthritis with erosions, ligamentous laxity

PATHOLOGY

- Amyloid deposits in intervertebral disc, facet joint synovium, ligamentum flavum
  - β_2 microglobulin fibrils stain with Congo red; apple-green birefringence with polarized light
- Crystal deposition & ligamentous laxity may contribute
- Previously incorrectly attributed to aluminum toxicity

CLINICAL ISSUES

- Increased incidence with longer duration dialysis (either hemodialysis or peritoneal dialysis)

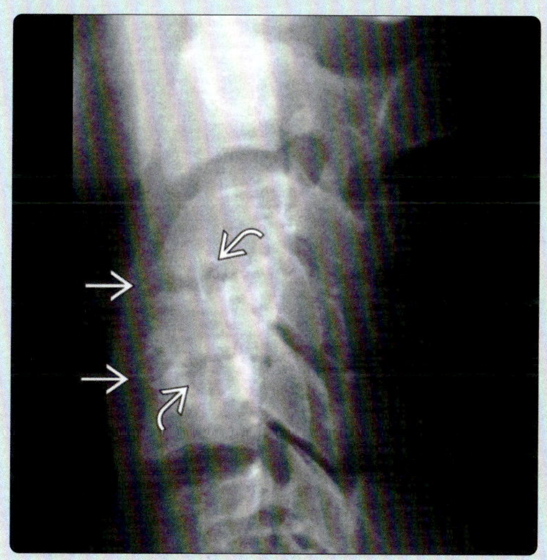

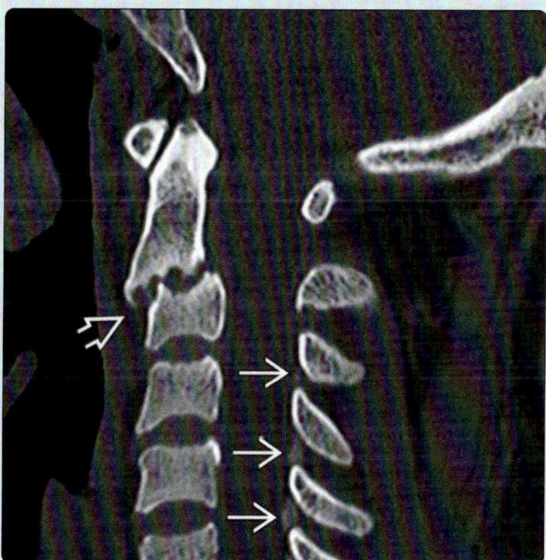

(Left) *Lateral x-ray depicts spondyloarthropathy of dialysis. The involved disc spaces are narrowed ➡, & the endplates are destroyed with multiple erosions of varying size ➡. Note the absence of sclerosis or new bone formation.* **(Right)** *Sagittal CT in a 33-year-old man with renal disease on dialysis, shows disc space narrowing, offset, & erosions ➡, but no evidence of soft tissue mass. There are also calcific deposits at multiple levels of the ligamentum flavum ➡, typical of dialysis-related spondyloarthropathy.*

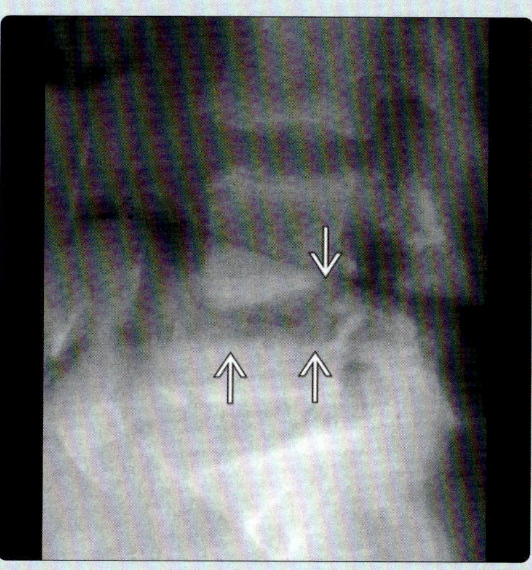

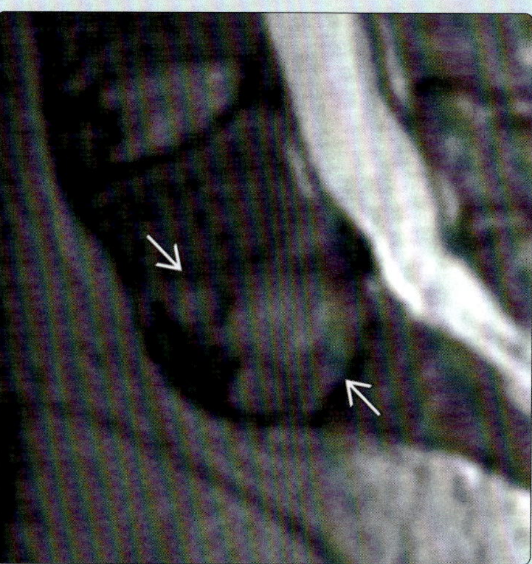

(Left) *Lateral radiograph shows endplate destruction ➡, disc-space narrowing with mild sclerosis, & minimal hyperostosis. There are no findings to reliably differentiate dialysis spondyloarthropathy from infection.* **(Right)** *Sagittal T2WI MR, same case, shows the slight hyperintensity of amyloid that has invaded the disc space & adjacent vertebral bodies ➡. Note the absence of marrow edema in the destroyed vertebra. This is a pertinent negative, helping differentiate amyloid deposition from infection.*

Hypoparathyroidism, Pseudo- and Pseudopseudohypoparathyroidism

KEY FACTS

TERMINOLOGY

- Hypoparathyroidism (HP)
- Pseudohypoparathyroidism (PHP)
- Pseudopseudohypoparathyroidism (PPHP)

IMAGING

- Common features in HP, PHP, PPHP
  - Subcutaneous calcification, basal ganglia calcification, thick skull, abnormal dentition
- HP: Childhood
  - Osteosclerosis, spinal calcification/ossification enthesopathy (especially around pelvis)
- PHP and PPHP
  - Short stature and premature physeal fusion
  - Brachydactyly
    - Especially 1st, 4th, and 5th metacarpal, but others also affected
    - Short distal phalanges ± short middle phalanges
    - 3rd and 4th metatarsal shortening and widening common
  - Coned epiphyses, exostoses, bowing deformities

TOP DIFFERENTIAL DIAGNOSES

- Soft tissue calcification: Scleroderma, hydroxyapatite deposition, hyperparathyroidism/renal osteodystrophy
- Spinal ossification/calcification: Diffuse idiopathic skeletal hyperostosis

PATHOLOGY

- HP: ↓ hormone production
- PHP: End organ insensitivity
- PPHP: Incomplete expression of PHP

CLINICAL ISSUES

- HP and PHP: Hypocalcemia and hyperphosphatemia
- PHP: Elevated levels of parathyroid hormone
- PHP: Obesity, round face, intellectual disability

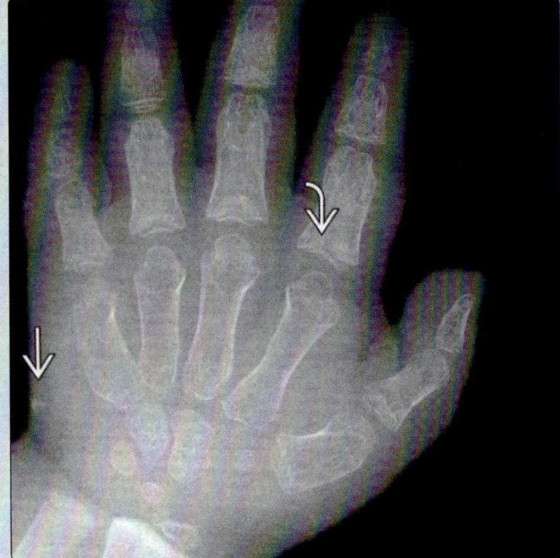

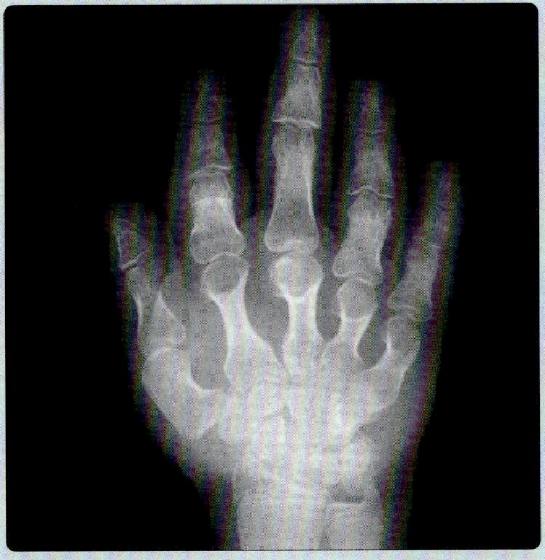

(Left) *PA radiograph shows a hand with findings typical of pseudohypoparathyroidism (PHP) or pseudopseudohypoparathyroidism (PPHP). Small round foci of soft tissue calcification are present ➡. There is diffuse shortening and widening of all bones of the hand, and coned epiphyses are evident ➡.* **(Right)** *PA radiograph shows a hand with varying degrees of shortening and widening in the metacarpals and phalanges. The 1st, 4th, and 5th metacarpals are most significantly involved, common in patients with PHP or PPHP.*

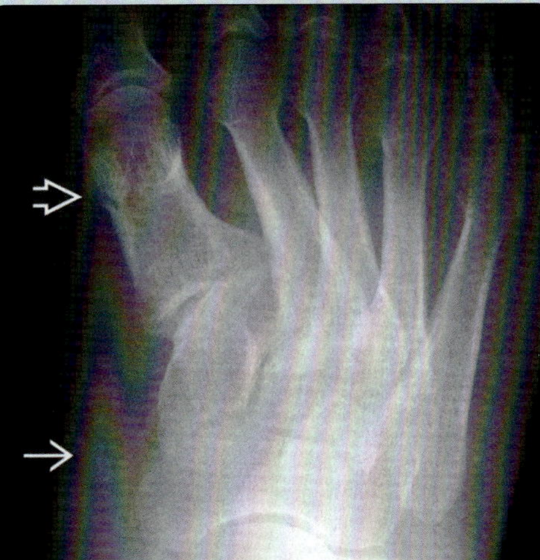

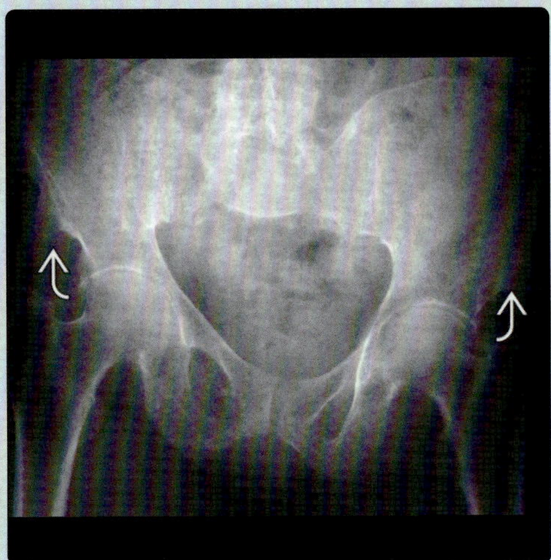

(Left) *AP radiograph of the foot shows multiple foci of soft tissue calcification ➡. Marked shortening and widening of the 1st metatarsal ➡ is present while the remaining metatarsals are relatively normal.* **(Right)** *AP radiograph shows the pelvis with typical exostoses ➡ of PHP or PPHP. The osseous outgrowths are short, broad-based, and oriented perpendicular to the cortex.*

Hypoparathyroidism, Pseudo- and Pseudopseudohypoparathyroidism

TERMINOLOGY

Abbreviations

- Hypoparathyroidism (HP)
- Pseudohypoparathyroidism (PHP)
- Pseudopseudohypoparathyroidism (PPHP)

Definitions

- Albright hereditary osteodystrophy: Phenotype, including short 4th and 5th metacarpals, round face, short stature seen in autosomal dominant PHP

IMAGING

General Features

- Best diagnostic clue
  - HP: Osteosclerosis, soft tissue calcification
  - PHP and PPHP: Short metacarpals/metatarsals and phalanges, coned epiphyses

Imaging Recommendations

- Best imaging tool
  - Radiographs reveal characteristic findings

Radiographic Findings

- Common features of HP, PHP, and PPHP
  - Subcutaneous calcification
  - Basal ganglia calcification
    - PHP > PPHP
  - Dense metaphyseal bands and growth arrest lines
  - Thickened skull, abnormal dentition
- HP: Adult (postoperative)
  - Limited radiographic findings
- HP: Childhood (autoimmune)
  - Osteosclerosis prominent feature
  - Spinal calcification/ossification
    - Anterior longitudinal ligament, paraspinal ligaments, osteophyte formation
  - Enthesopathy, especially around pelvis
- PHP and PPHP
  - Short stature and premature physeal fusion
  - Brachydactyly, usually symmetric
    - Disproportionately short even for short stature
    - Metacarpal shortening, 1st, 4th, and 5th most common
    - Metatarsal shortening, 3rd and 4th most common
    - Short distal phalanges ± short middle phalanges
    - Coned epiphyses of phalanges and metacarpals
    - Widening of metacarpals/metatarsals
  - Exostoses: Short and broad-based, metaphyseal or more central, perpendicular to long axis of bone
  - Bowing deformities
  - Osteosclerosis or osteoporosis
  - May have hyperparathyroidism with subperiosteal resorption of radial aspect middle phalanges
- General comments on soft tissue calcification and ossification
  - Skin, subcutaneous tissues, connective tissue
    - Independent of serum calcium and phosphate levels
    - Not within muscle or viscera
    - Small rounded foci, especially around joints
    - Plaque-like in skin, subcutaneous tissues
  - Other sites of calcification are dependent on calcium and phosphate levels

CT Findings

- NECT: Basal ganglia calcification

DIFFERENTIAL DIAGNOSIS

Soft Tissue Calcification

- Scleroderma: Acroosteolysis, tuft soft tissue resorption
- Hydroxyapatite deposition disease: Often solitary, globular, intratendinous/bursal
- Hyperparathyroidism/renal osteodystrophy: Evidence of bone resorption

Spinal Ossification/Calcification

- Diffuse idiopathic skeletal hyperostosis: Usually older individuals, often symptomatic

PATHOLOGY

General Features

- Etiology
  - HP
    - Child: Decreased hormone production, possible autoimmune etiology
    - Adult: Inadvertent removal of parathyroid glands during thyroidectomy
    - Adult: Hypomagnesemia 2° to long-term use of proton-pump inhibitors
  - PHP: End organ insensitivity
  - PPHP: Incomplete expression of PHP
- Genetics
  - PHP: X-linked dominant, autosomal recessive or dominant
  - PHP & PPHP: Likely genetically related

CLINICAL ISSUES

Presentation

- Most common signs/symptoms
  - Often asymptomatic
  - Symptomatic hypocalcemia (PH and PHP)
    - Typically present around age 5
    - Delayed cases present during times of high calcium demand: Pregnancy, growth spurt
- Other signs/symptoms
  - HP and PHP: Hypocalcemia and hyperphosphatemia
    - PHP: Elevated levels of parathyroid hormone
  - PPHP: Normal calcium and phosphate levels
  - PHP: Obesity, round face, intellectual disability

Demographics

- Gender
  - PH, PHP, PPHP: M < F

Treatment

- Oral calcium replacement and vitamin D supplements

SELECTED REFERENCES

1. Janett S et al: Hypomagnesemia induced by long-term treatment with proton-pump inhibitors. Gastroenterol Res Pract. 2015:951768, 2015

KEY FACTS

TERMINOLOGY

- Osteoporosis: ↓ amount of histologically normal bone
- Primary osteoporosis encompasses postmenopausal (type I) & senile (type II) osteoporosis
- Fragility fracture: Results from minor trauma, such as fall from standing height
- Insufficiency fracture: Results from normal stress on abnormal bone

IMAGING

- Decreased thickness of cortical bone; decreased number of trabecula, which are thinner than normal
- Complications: Insufficiency fractures, fragility fractures, vertebral compressions
- Dual energy x-ray absorptiometry (DEXA): Preferred modality to determine bone mineral density
- MR: Extremely useful for detection of incomplete fragility or insufficiency fractures

TOP DIFFERENTIAL DIAGNOSES

- Secondary osteoporosis
- False DEXA

PATHOLOGY

- Abnormality of bone formation &/or bone resorption
- Postmenopausal: Decreased estrogen levels resulting in increased bone resorption
- Senile osteoporosis: Age-related changes in bone formation/resorption balance leading to bone loss

CLINICAL ISSUES

- Increasing incidence with increasing age
- M < < F
- Symptoms arise from complications (fractures)
- Fractures lead to ↑ morbidity & mortality
  - Disuse osteoporosis may be superimposed

(Left) *Graphic depicting transected spine shows senile osteoporosis on the left ➡ compared with normal appearance on the right. Note that with osteoporosis there is less bone, but the bone that is present is normal both grossly and histologically.* **(Right)** *CT study shows marked osteoporosis involving all vertebral bodies and posterior elements with maintained vertebral body shape and height. Findings include diffuse cortical thinning ➡ and decrease in the number of trabecula ↪.*

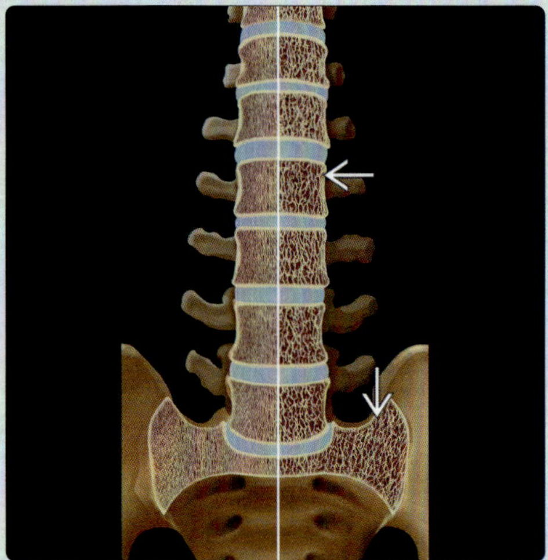

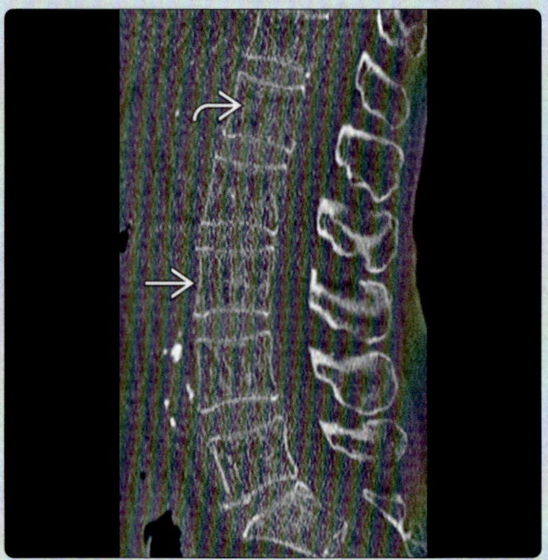

(Left) *Coronal T1 MR in a 61-year-old woman with hip pain shows a linear hypointensity in the subchondral acetabulum ➡. This represents an insufficiency fracture.* **(Right)** *Sagittal T2FS MR, same patient, shows the linear fracture ➡ of the acetabulum with surrounding edema ↪. It is easy to neglect evaluation of the acetabulum in a patient with hip pain and also to dismiss this appearance as osteoarthritis. Insufficiency fractures of the acetabulum in osteoporotic patients are now recognized as not uncommon.*

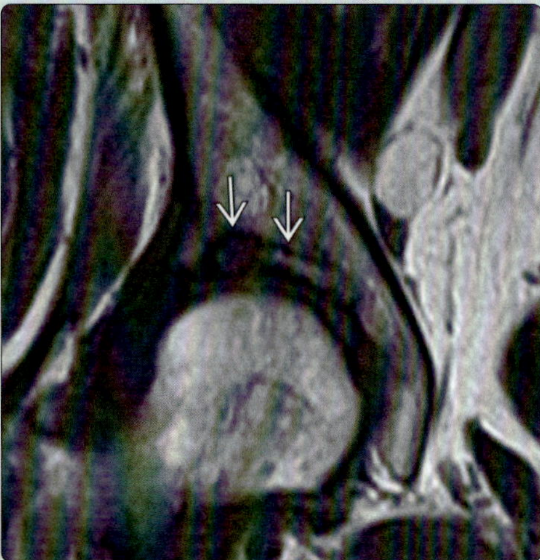

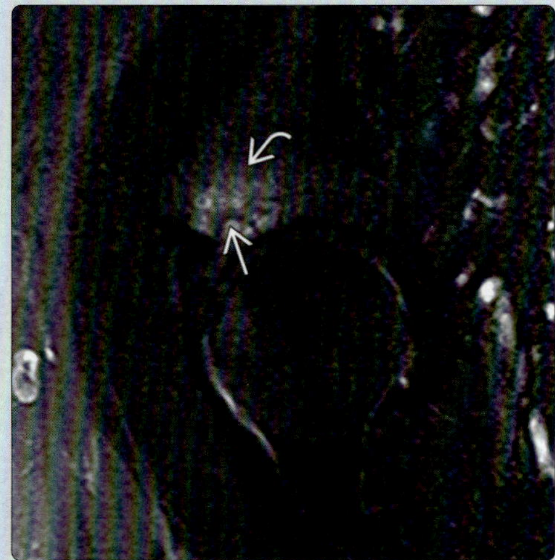

TERMINOLOGY

Abbreviations

- Dual-energy x-ray absorptiometry (DEXA)
- Bone mineral density (BMD)

Synonyms

- Primary osteoporosis encompasses postmenopausal (type I) & senile (type II) osteoporosis
  - Other terms: Age related or involutional

Definitions

- Osteoporosis: ↓ amount of histologically normal bone
  - For clinical purposes, defined by BMD relative to standard population
- Senile osteoporosis: Osteoporosis occurring in individuals > 75 years old
- Osteopenia: Different meanings depending on context
  - **Radiographic appearance** of decreased bone density
    - Osteoporosis is one of many causes
  - **DEXA** interpretation applies to BMD between normal & osteoporosis; T score between -1 and -2.5
- Fragility fracture: Results from minor trauma, such as fall from standing height
  - Typically occurs in vertebral body, femoral neck, or distal radius (Colles fracture)
- Insufficiency fracture: Results from normal stress on abnormal bone
- Severe or established osteoporosis
  - T score ≤ -2.5 **and** fragility fracture

IMAGING

General Features

- Best diagnostic clue
  - Abnormal DEXA
- Location
  - Generalized process involving axial & appendicular skeleton
  - Hip, vertebra, & distal radius have highest trabecular to cortical bone ratios, most prone to fractures
- Morphology
  - Decreased thickness of cortical bone; decreased number of trabecula, which are thinner than normal

Imaging Recommendations

- Best imaging tool
  - DEXA
- Protocol advice
  - AP lumbar spine
    - Report total spine BMD
    - Use L1 to L4; exclude vertebra with anomalies & focal abnormalities, such as discogenic sclerosis
    - Must use at least 2 vertebra
  - Hip
    - Bilateral if > 65 years old
    - Nondominant hip if < 65 years old
    - Report total hip and proximal femur measurements
  - Forearm, nondominant: Use 1/3 radius measurement
    - As replacement for spine, hip when unavailable
    - If patient has hyperparathyroidism or is obese

Radiographic Findings

- Diffuse osteopenia
  - Unreliable finding
  - Can be mimicked by poor technique, absent overlying soft tissues
- Complications
  - Insufficiency fractures: Sacrum, pubic rami, supraacetabular ilium, superolateral femoral neck, proximal medial tibia
  - Vertebral compressions: Thoracic & lumbar
    - Wedge: Anterior > posterior height loss
    - Biconcave: Central height loss
    - Crush: Generalized height loss
  - Fragility fractures: Vertebral bodies, femoral neck, distal radius (Colles fracture)

CT Findings

- Quantitative CT
  - Advantage of separate measurements for cortical & trabecular bone
  - Not as widespread as DEXA

MR Findings

- No clinically accepted role in diagnosis of osteoporosis
  - Research focusing on use of different techniques to evaluate bone architecture
- Extremely useful for identification of fractures
  - Long bones
    - Bone marrow edema (↓ T1W, ↑ fluid-sensitive sequences) in common location
    - Fracture line not always evident; when visible may be seen on any sequence & will not be visible on every sequence
  - Vertebral body
    - Acute: Variable degree/extent of marrow edema ± height loss
    - Subacute: Decrease in edema from previous scan, otherwise difficult to confirm as subacute
    - Chronic or remote: Decreased vertebral body height, no marrow edema
    - Cleft or pseudoarthrosis may develop in subacute to chronic phase
      - Fluid-filled cavity paralleling endplate, usually superior or central vertebral body
      - May widen with spinal extension

Ultrasonographic Findings

- Quantitative US; calcaneus
  - Low cost, no ionizing radiation
  - Well accepted, not as widespread as DEXA

Dual-Energy X-Ray Absorptiometry

- T score: BMD relative to young adult at peak bone mass, gender specific
  - ≥ -1: Normal
  - Between -1 and -2.5: Osteopenia
  - ≤ -2.5: Osteoporosis
- Z score: BMD relative to individuals of same age, gender, body weight
- Pediatric patients & men require comparison to appropriate population

- In men < 50 years old, cannot diagnosis osteoporosis on basis of BMD alone
- Follow-up studies must be done on same machine; otherwise comparison unreliable

DIFFERENTIAL DIAGNOSIS

Secondary Osteoporosis

- Steroid-induced, alcoholism, multiple myeloma

False Dual-Energy X-Ray Absorptiometry

- Incorrect technique
- Lytic lesion or focal osteoporosis

PATHOLOGY

General Features

- Etiology
  - Abnormality of bone formation &/or bone resorption
    - Postmenopausal: Decreased estrogen levels resulting in increased bone resorption
    - Senile osteoporosis: Age-related changes in bone formation/resorption balance leading to bone loss
  - Contributing factors
    - Diminished exercise: Development & maintenance of normal BMD requires bones to be stressed
    - Poor nutrition leads to diminished bone formation
      - Poor calcium intake
      - Vitamin D deficiency
      - Excess caffeine or alcohol intake
      - Smoking
    - Low-peak bone mass: Requires less bone loss to reach osteoporotic range

Staging, Grading, & Classification

- WHO classifies osteoporosis as primary or secondary
  - Primary osteoporosis includes those conditions that are result of normal aging process
- Grading vertebral compression deformities: Genant visual semiquantitative method

Microscopic Features

- Thinned cortex
- Decreased number & thickness of trabecula
- Disruption of normal trabecular architecture
  - Microfractures through individual trabecula

CLINICAL ISSUES

Presentation

- Most common signs/symptoms
  - Osteoporosis itself asymptomatic
  - Symptoms arise from complications
    - Typically pain following fracture
- Other signs/symptoms
  - Vertebral compression
    - Breathing difficulties due to ↓ thoracic volume
    - Early satiety secondary to ↓ intraabdominal volume
    - Increased risk of additional fractures
  - Femoral neck fractures
    - High incidence of mortality within 1 year

Demographics

- Age
  - Increasing incidence with increasing age
- Gender
  - M < < F
- Epidemiology
  - Risk factors
    - Family history of osteoporosis, hip fracture, or insufficiency fracture after 40 years old in 1st-degree female relative
    - Race: Highest incidence of osteoporosis in Caucasian > Asian > Hispanic > African American
    - Low body weight
    - Menstrual history: Late onset (after 15 years old), periods of amenorrhea, premature menopause

Natural History & Prognosis

- Progressive disease
  - Continual loss of BMD
  - Increasing fracture risk with decreasing BMD
  - Fractures result in significant morbidity & increased mortality

Treatment

- Medications
  - Treatment directed at reducing rate of bone resorption: Bisphosphonates, selective estrogen receptor modulators
    - Some studies suggest that though bisphosphonates ↑ bone density, they may not prevent fractures
  - Treatment directed at increasing rate of bone formation: None in routine use
- Vertebral augmentation for treatment of painful vertebral compression
  - Vertebroplasty, kyphoplasty, sacroplasty

Future Directions

- Bone architecture is determinant of bone strength irrespective of BMD (bone quality more important than bone quantity)
  - This may be more appropriate parameter to evaluate

DIAGNOSTIC CHECKLIST

Image Interpretation Pearls

- Important to comment on vertebral compression deformities whenever seen, including on chest x-rays

Reporting Tips

- DEXA: Do not qualify osteopenia or osteoporosis as mild, moderate, or severe

SELECTED REFERENCES

1. Marques A et al: The accuracy of osteoporotic fracture risk prediction tools: a systematic review and meta-analysis. Ann Rheum Dis. 74(11):1958-67, 2015
2. Krappinger D et al: Preoperative assessment of the cancellous bone mineral density of the proximal humerus using CT data. Skeletal Radiol. 41(3):299-304, 2012
3. Adams JE: Quantitative computed tomography. Eur J Radiol. 71(3):415-24, 2009
4. Bauer JS et al: Advances in osteoporosis imaging. Eur J Radiol. 71(3):440-9, 2009
5. Krestan C et al: Imaging of insufficiency fractures. Eur J Radiol. 71(3):398-405, 2009

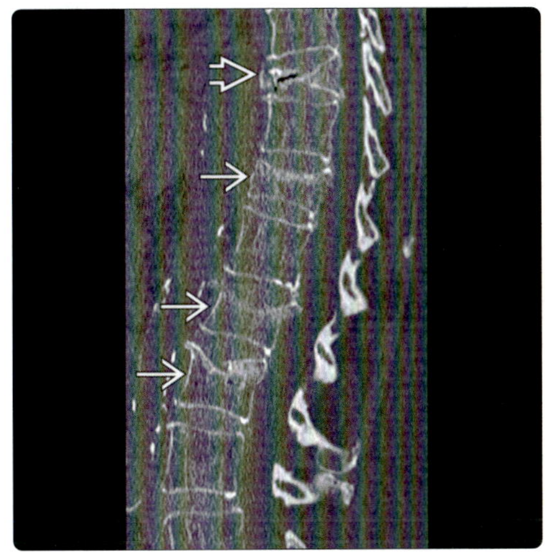

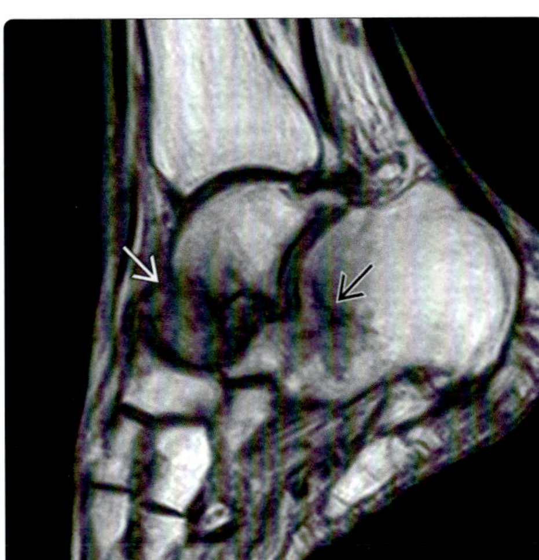

(Left) *Sagittal NECT shows the lumbar spine in a patient with severe osteoporosis complicated by multiple compression deformities. In this case, the fractures are wedge type ➡ and crush type ➡. In patients with osteoporosis, fractures are a significant source of morbidity.* **(Right)** *Sagittal T1WI shows typical insufficiency fractures. The talar neck ➡ is a common site. The posterior calcaneal tuberosity is more commonly involved than the body ⇨. Fracture lines are apparent at both sites.*

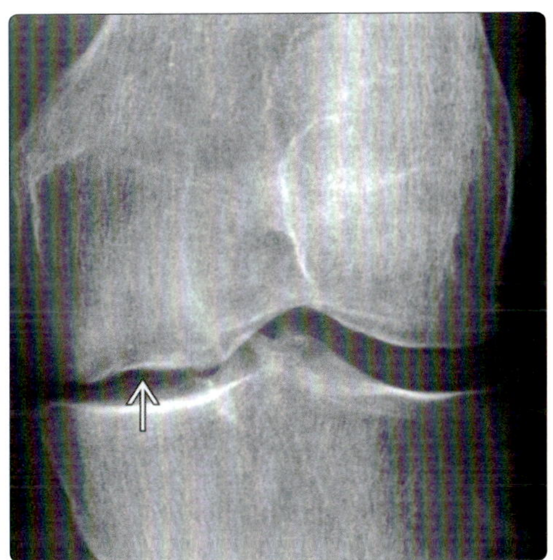

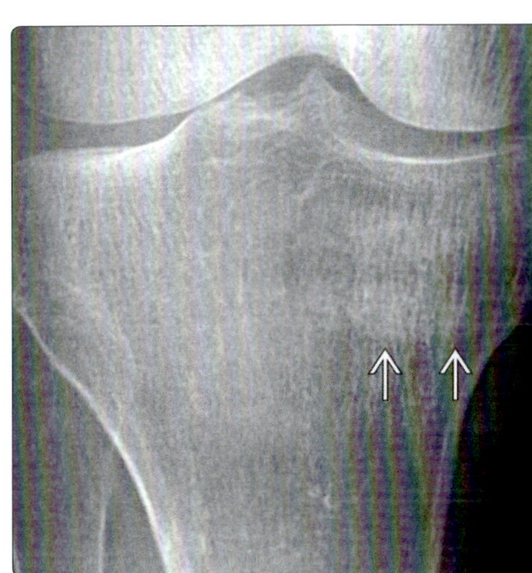

(Left) *AP radiograph shows a knee with osteopenia resulting from osteoporosis. Insufficiency fracture of the medial femoral condyle has resulted in articular surface collapse ➡.* **(Right)** *AP radiograph shows insufficiency fracture of the proximal medial tibia ➡. The fracture presents as a horizontally oriented ill-defined smudgy line of sclerosis in a typical location for insufficiency fracture.*

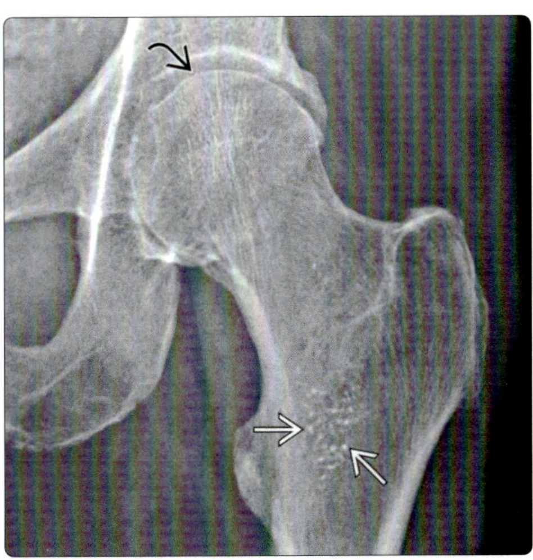

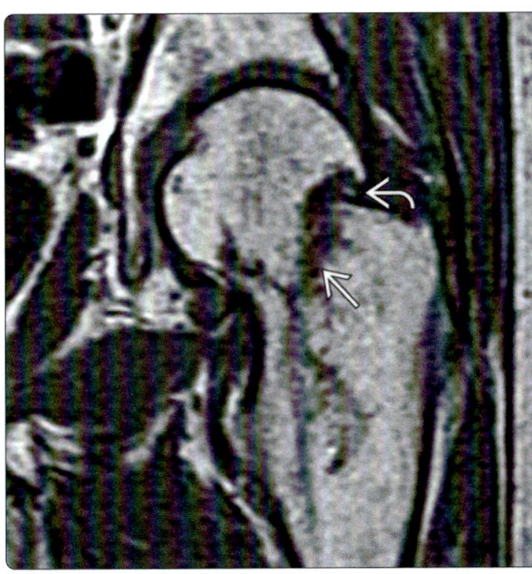

(Left) *AP radiograph shows typical osteopenia. Note the thin cortex of the femoral head ⇨. While generally trabecula are thin, in certain areas of stress they may remain normal and stand out against the osteoporotic bone, as seen here with coarse primary trabeculae ➡.* **(Right)** *Coronal T1WI shows subcapital femoral fracture ➡. One theory states that insufficiency fractures of the hip, which begin superolaterally ➡, go on to completion leading to a fall, rather than the fall leading to the fracture.*

KEY FACTS

IMAGING

- Regional distribution of osteopenia, most commonly centered around joint
  - Radiographs and CT will be abnormal
  - MR, bone scan expected to be normal at site of disuse osteoporosis
- Different patterns of osteopenia
  - Linear: Metaphyseal or subchondral
  - Spotty, speckled, permeative
  - Intracortical tunneling (double cortical sign)
  - Generalized decrease in density

TOP DIFFERENTIAL DIAGNOSES

- Identification of recent nonweight-bearing status is key to differentiation from other etiologies of osteoporosis
- Linear pattern mimics fracture
  - Fracture thinner, more sharply marginated
  - Fracture may have associated callus
- Permeative and generalized patterns mimic infiltrative process; tumor or infection distinguished by
  - Usually confined to single bone, rarely cross joint
  - May have soft tissue mass
  - MR abnormality with infiltration

PATHOLOGY

- Nonweight-bearing status decreases stress on bone
  - → ↑ bone turnover: ↑ resorption &/or ↓ bone formation
- If nonweight-bearing due to fracture, healing → ↑ blood flow, → bone resorption

CLINICAL ISSUES

- Reversible
- Associated with recent onset nonweight-bearing: Fracture ± immobilization/ORIF, stroke, paralysis
- More common in lower extremity (knee, ankle)
- More common in elderly (except postop fracture)
- May be complicated by insufficiency fracture

(Left) *AP radiograph in a young adult, 2 weeks postop for ankle fracture, shows disuse osteoporosis as a linear metaphyseal lucency ➡ in the tibia, and as a distinct subchondral lucency in both the talus ➡ and medial malleolus ➡. These patterns of osteoporosis can appear aggressive.* **(Right)** *AP radiograph reveals aggressive osteopenia of the proximal tibia ➡ and distal femur. Recognizing the regional pattern and identifying a femur fracture (not shown) aid in establishing the correct diagnosis.*

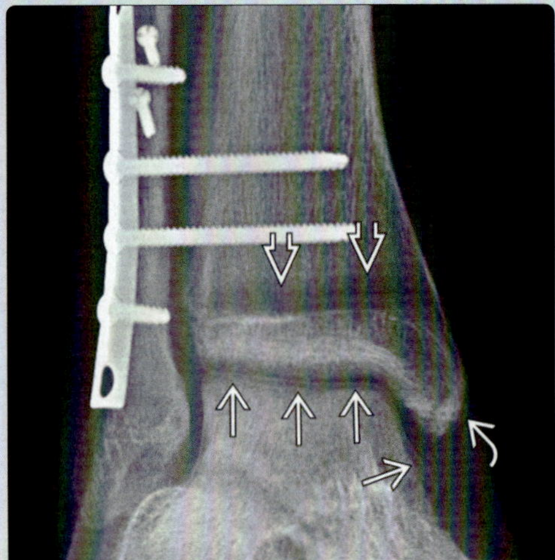

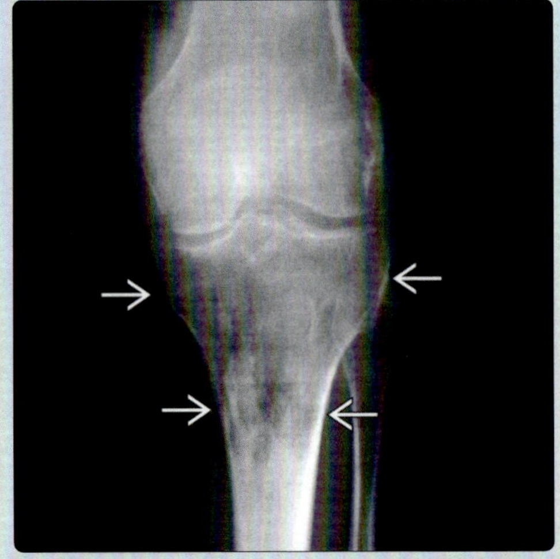

(Left) *Axial NECT shows several patterns of disuse osteoporosis. Multiple small, subchondral, rounded lucent foci in the distal femur ➡, scattered lucencies within the medullary bone ➡, and intracortical bone loss ➡ are typical but not specific for disuse osteoporosis.* **(Right)** *Axial images of the distal tibia and fibula reveal multiple small lucencies throughout the medullary canal. In addition, several small lucent foci are present within cortical bone ➡. Intracortical tunneling is seen in, but not unique to, disuse osteoporosis.*

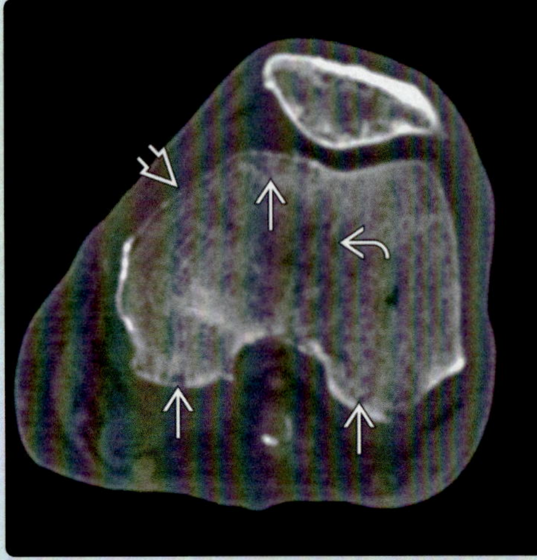

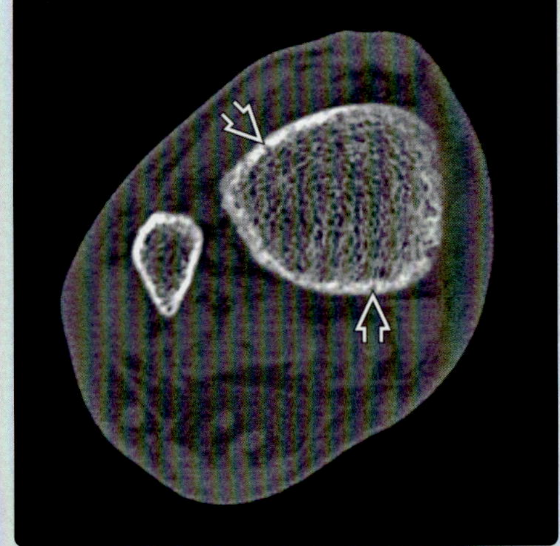

KEY FACTS

TERMINOLOGY

- Idiopathic osteoporosis of young

IMAGING

- Radiographs may show diffuse osteopenia of axial and appendicular skeleton
- Complications include vertebral compressions and various long bone fractures
- Neoosseous osteoporosis: Formation of osteoporotic new bone; appears as wide zone of rarefaction adjacent to physis at metaphysis; leads to collapse, especially of ankles, knees
- If treated with bisphosphonates, may acquire bone-in-bone appearance
- Dual energy x-ray absorptiometry
  - Interpret in conjunction with clinical factors, including height, weight, Tanner stage, bone age
  - Term low bone density advocated over terms osteopenia and osteoporosis
  - Only use Z score in juvenile evaluation

TOP DIFFERENTIAL DIAGNOSES

- Osteogenesis imperfecta
  - Does not show resolution over time
- Secondary osteoporosis: Rickets, chronic renal disease, malabsorption syndromes

PATHOLOGY

- Likely heterogeneous bone disorder
- Poor bone remodeling: Trabecular compartment severely involved with ↓ bone formation and ↑ bone resorption

CLINICAL ISSUES

- Rare condition
- Diagnosis of exclusion; laboratory tests normal
- Prepubertal onset with spontaneous remission as puberty progresses: May start at any age, some differentiate types based on age of onset
- M = F; starts earlier in girls

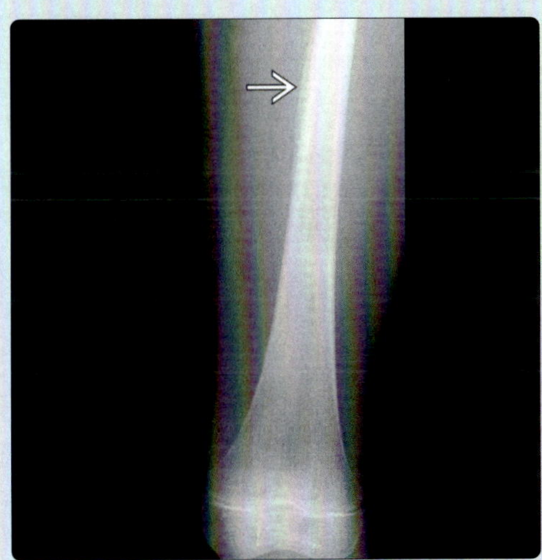

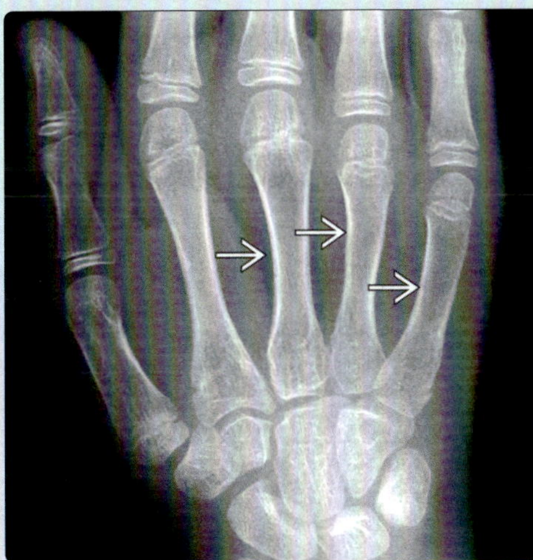

(Left) *AP radiograph shows the femur of a 7 year old with leg pain. There is periosteal new bone formation* ➡, *which proved to be a fatigue fracture. Dual energy x-ray absorptiometry scan revealed low bone mineral density. Fractures range in severity in this population.* **(Right)** *AP radiograph shows the hand of a child with a significant lower extremity fracture in the absence of trauma. This film, 1 year after initial presentation, shows marked thinning in the cortices of the metacarpals* ➡, *indicative of osteoporosis.*

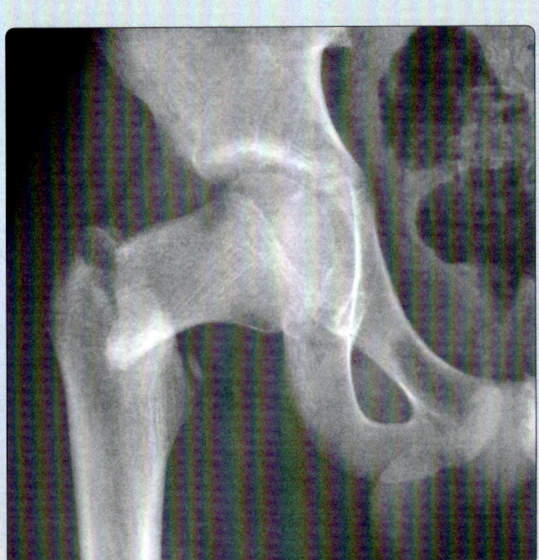

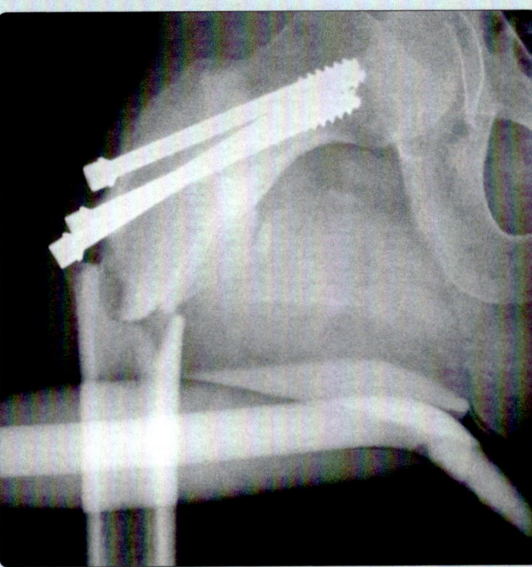

(Left) *AP radiograph shows a proximal femur in a child without any history of significant trauma. Such a fracture indicates severely weakened bone. After extensive evaluation, idiopathic juvenile osteoporosis (a diagnosis of exclusion) was established.* **(Right)** *AP radiograph in the same patient obtained several months after fixation of the basicervical fracture shows a new subtrochanteric fracture. Again there was no significant trauma. Fractures are a major cause of morbidity in patients with juvenile osteoporosis.*

KEY FACTS

TERMINOLOGY

- Eating disorder that involves limiting intake of food
  - Effects on musculoskeletal system depend on severity and length of process
    - Osteoporosis, muscle wasting, delayed skeletal maturation, bone marrow depletion

IMAGING

- Delayed skeletal maturation in teenager
  - Open physes beyond expected age of closure
  - Delayed pattern of fatty marrow replacement on MR: Epiphyses may not show complete fatty replacement in young adult; metaphyses may retain red marrow
- Osteoporosis not appropriate for age
  - Thin metacarpal cortices
  - Abnormal DEXA values
  - Flat-panel volume CT shows trabecular structural abnormality even when bone mineral density is normal on DEXA
- Insufficiency fractures in young patients
  - MR of insufficiency fractures: Linear low SI on T1WI, high SI with edema on fluid-sensitive sequences
- Serous atrophy of marrow (rare)
  - Severe reduction in subcutaneous fat
  - Focal gray signal on T1; not as low SI as seen in marrow-replacement processes
  - Very high fluid signal on fluid-sensitive sequences
  - Usually coalescent, although may initially show several small foci

CLINICAL ISSUES

- Effect on bone: Osteoporosis and its consequent bone fragility
  - 7x ↑ in fracture risk; may persist despite recovery
  - Greater deficit in bone mineral density if onset of anorexia is during adolescence
- Reduced muscle mass
- Serous atrophy associated with true starvation

(Left) *T1WI MR shows delayed physeal fusion in a 19-year-old elite female gymnast. There is also delayed replacement of red marrow, with only partial replacement by fat (note the subchondral rim of low signal red marrow ➡). There is no replacement of red marrow in the metaphysis ➡, indicating a significant delay in marrow maturation.* **(Right)** *PA x-ray, same patient, shows osteoporosis ➡ and open physes ➡, indicating a delay in skeletal maturation. This athlete was anorexic, given the degree of exercise required for her training.*

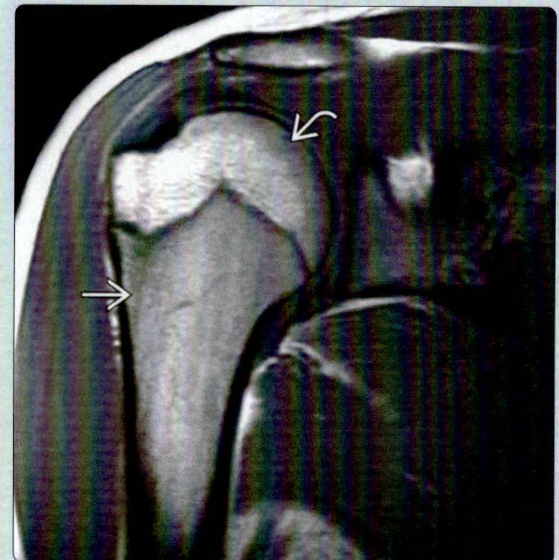

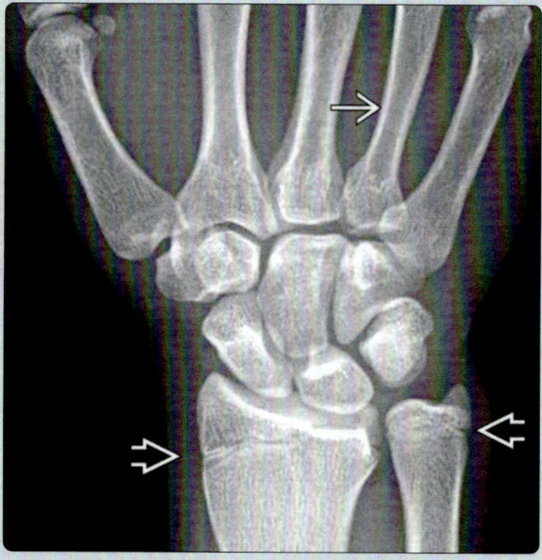

(Left) *AP radiograph in a 44-year-old woman addicted to running shows a basicervical left hip fracture ➡. The bones are not obviously osteoporotic, but the woman measured 5' 6" in height and weighed only 105 pounds; she admitted to "not eating well." MR (not shown) also showed insufficiency fracture in the right hip.* **(Right)** *Coronal CT, same patient 9 months after pinning of insufficiency fracture, shows no evidence of healing ➡. Contralateral hip showed the same abnormality, an inability to heal due to anorexia-related osteoporosis.*

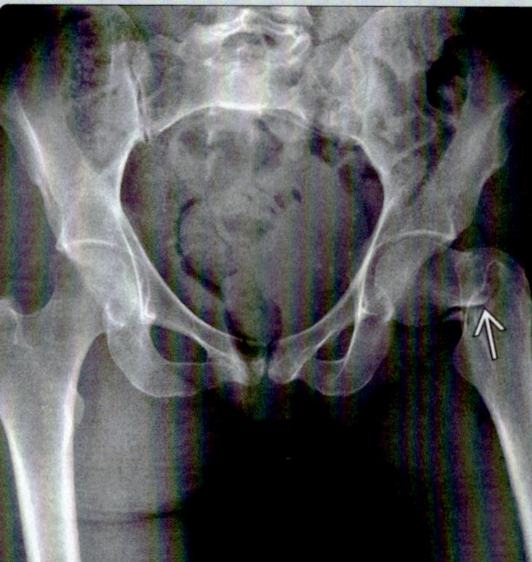

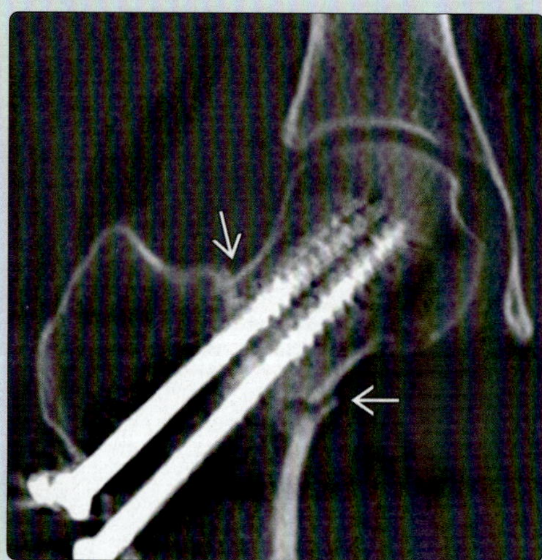

KEY FACTS

TERMINOLOGY

- Osteoporosis unrelated to postmenopausal state or process of aging

IMAGING

- Diffuse process involving axial and appendicular skeleton: Thinning of cortex with decreased number of thinned trabeculae
- Abnormal DEXA to establish diagnosis
- Appears as decreased bone density on radiographs
- Radiographs useful to identify characteristic findings of underlying condition
  - Hyperparathyroidism (HPTH): Bone resorption
  - Osteomalacia: Coarse, ill-defined trabeculae
  - Rickets: Physeal widening, fraying, cupping
  - Renal osteodystrophy: Osteomalacia and HPTH
  - Rheumatoid arthritis: Bilateral, symmetric erosive arthropathy

TOP DIFFERENTIAL DIAGNOSES

- Incorrect DEXA: Poor technique, bone destruction at sites of measurement
- Primary osteoporosis: May coexist

PATHOLOGY

- Other underlying conditions to consider: Chronic liver failure, tumor infiltration (myeloma, leukemia, lymphoma), ankylosing spondylitis, juvenile idiopathic arthropathy, anorexia, malabsorption syndromes, hyperthyroidism, diabetes, steroids, chronic lung disease, alcohol abuse

CLINICAL ISSUES

- Treatment directed at underlying condition

DIAGNOSTIC CHECKLIST

- Use of screening form for DEXA essential to help identify risk factors for both 1° and 2° osteoporosis

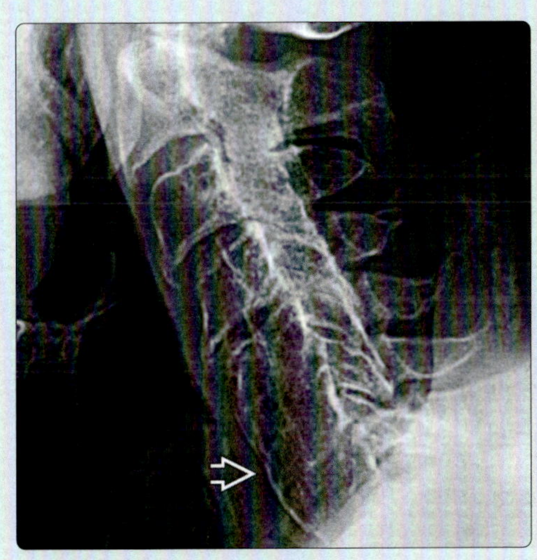

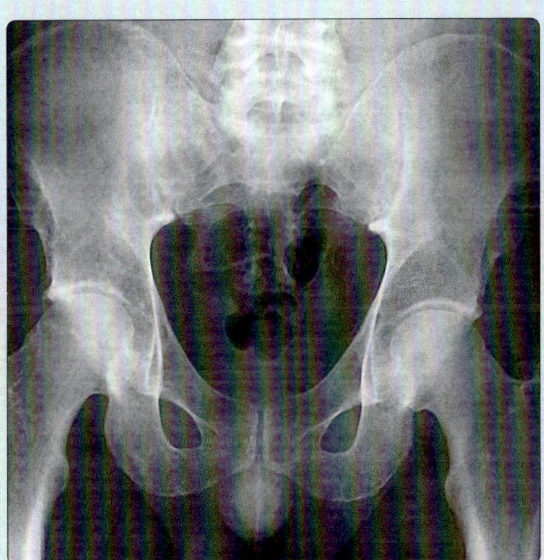

(Left) *Lateral radiograph of a middle-aged man reveals osteopenia atypical for his age. Fusion through the lower disc spaces ➡ is a clue to the underlying ankylosing spondylitis (AS). AS and rheumatoid arthritis are commonly associated with osteoporosis.* **(Right)** *AP x-ray shows diffuse osteopenia in a 32-year-old man. Thoracic spine had a similar appearance. Osteopenia is uncommon in young men; its presence should prompt a search for an underlying condition such as multiple myeloma, found in this case.*

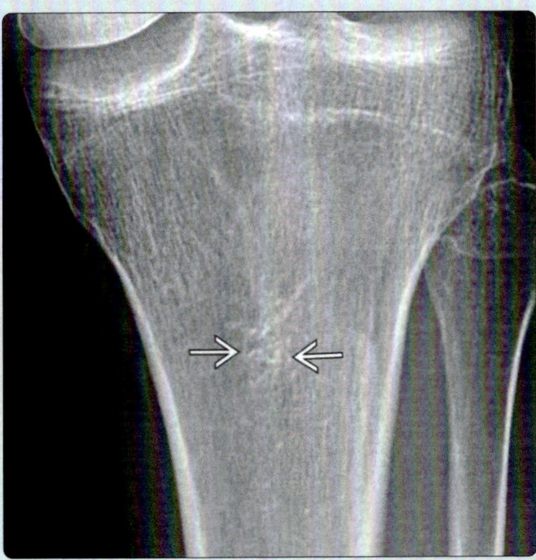

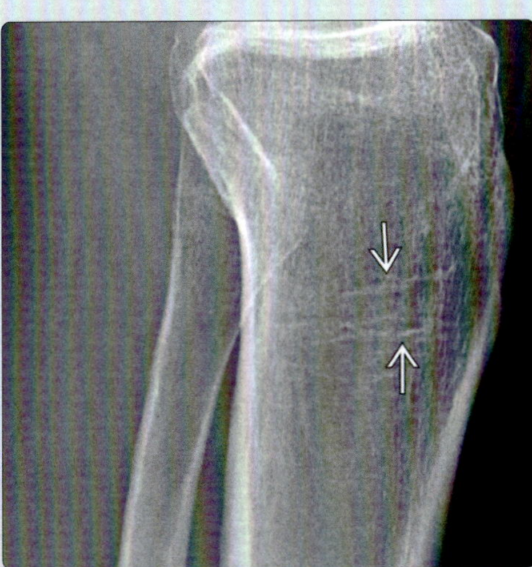

(Left) *AP radiograph in a 33-year-old Polynesian man shows "stippling" ➡ in the metaphysis of the tibia. Lateral view is required to prove the etiology.* **(Right)** *Lateral radiograph, same patient, shows the stippling seen on the AP, which is in fact due to linear 1° trabeculae ➡. While always present, these trabeculae appear more prominent in osteopenic bone once secondary trabeculae are resorbed. The cause in this 33-year-old was alcoholism and associated malnutrition.*

Pituitary Disorders: Acromegaly and Growth Hormone Deficiency

KEY FACTS

TERMINOLOGY

- Acromegaly: Onset of disease after physeal closure
- Gigantism: Onset of disease prior to physeal closure

IMAGING

- Acromegaly
  - Joint space widening: Interphalangeal, metacarpophalangeal, metatarsophalangeal, knee
  - Widened disc spaces, posterior vertebral scalloping
  - Cranial thickening, enlarged protuberances
  - Osteophytosis hips, knee, spine
  - Thickened diaphyses of long bones
  - Spade-like terminal tufts
  - Soft tissue enlargement: Especially hands and feet
  - Degenerative arthropathy
- Hypopituitarism (child)
  - Delayed skeletal maturation: Late appearance epiphyses, late fusion physes, slow rate of growth

TOP DIFFERENTIAL DIAGNOSES

- Hypopituitarism: Other causes of short stature
- Acromegaly: Diffuse idiopathic skeletal hyperostosis

PATHOLOGY

- Acromegaly and gigantism: ↑ GH
- Hypopituitarism: ↓ pituitary hormones including GH

CLINICAL ISSUES

- Acromegaly: Headaches, abnormal facial features, back pain, painful swelling of knees and hands
- Hypopituitarism (child): Poor physical and mental development
- Acromegaly: Diagnosed around age 40, often delayed due to insidious onset
- Gigantism: Childhood; ↑ longitudinal growth = ↑ height
- Hypopituitarism: Variable relative to etiology

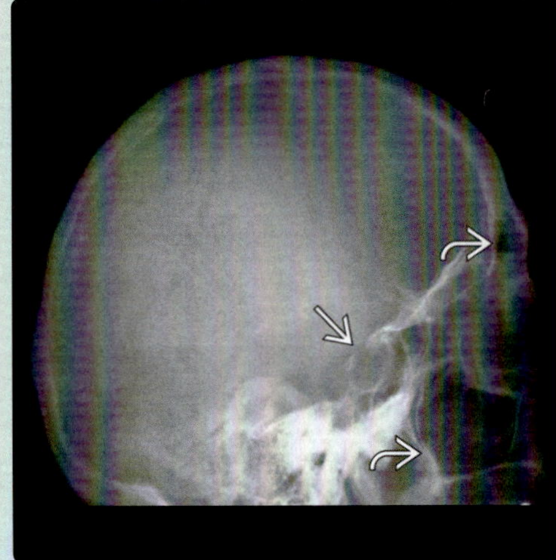

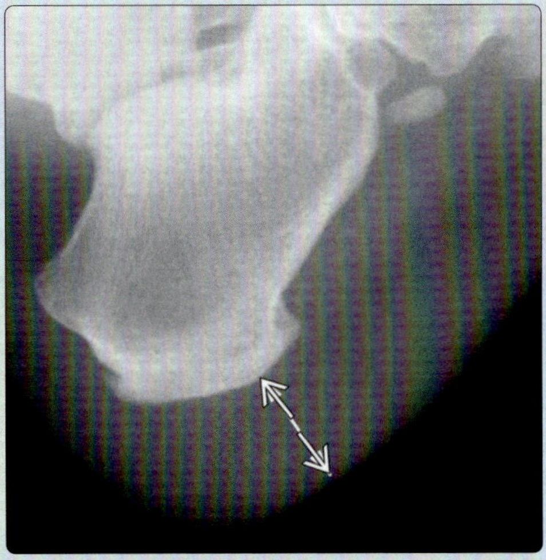

(Left) *Lateral radiograph of the skull reveals an enlarged sella ➡ due to the longstanding pituitary adenoma, which has caused remodeling. The paranasal sinuses, especially the maxillary sinuses, are enlarged ➡. In this patient, the skull has not thickened significantly.* **(Right)** *Lateral radiograph of the foot demonstrates overgrowth of soft tissues, with a thickened heel pad ➡. Thickening > 2.30 cm and 2.15 cm in male and female patients, respectively, is considered abnormal.*

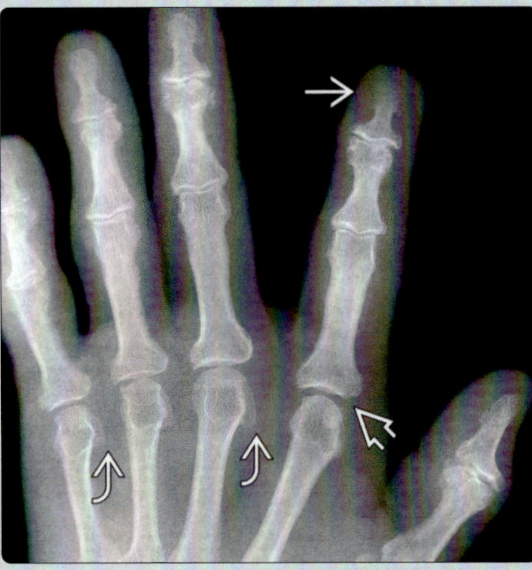

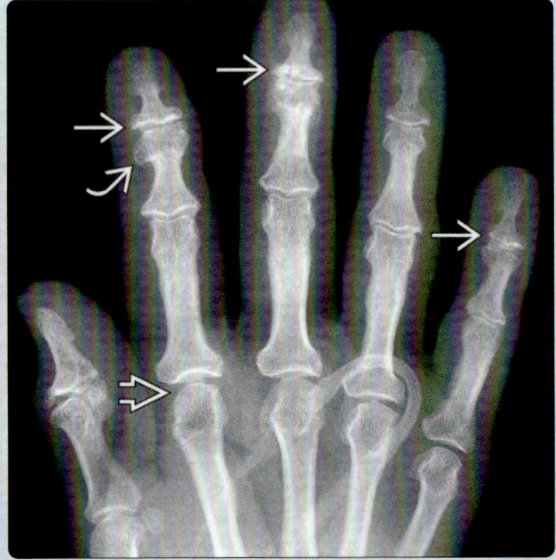

(Left) *PA radiograph of the hand shows enlarged, spade-like tufts ➡ and widened joint space at the 2nd metacarpophalangeal (MCP) ➡. Beaked osteophytes are present on the metacarpal heads ➡. These findings result from stimulation of new bone and cartilage formation.* **(Right)** *PA radiograph of the hand demonstrates MCP joint space widening ➡ and osteophyte-like growths at articular margins ➡, which are typical findings associated with acromegaly. There are degenerative changes at the DIP joints ➡.*

TERMINOLOGY

Definitions

- Acromegaly: Onset of disease after physeal closure
- Gigantism: Onset of disease prior to physeal closure

IMAGING

General Features

- Best diagnostic clue
  - Acromegaly: Soft tissue and osseous enlargement, widened cartilage spaces
  - Gigantism: ↑ bone length and width
  - Hypopituitarism: Delayed skeletal maturation

Imaging Recommendations

- Best imaging tool
  - Radiograph best for musculoskeletal changes
  - Bone age: Method of Greulich and Pyle
  - MR crucial for pituitary assessment

Radiography: Acromegaly

- Enlargement of cartilage spaces
  - Joint space widening: Interphalangeal, metacarpophalangeal, metatarsophalangeal, knee
  - Widened intervertebral disc spaces
  - Prominent costochondral articulations
- Bone formation: Periosteal surfaces, tendon and ligament attachments (enthesopathy), articular margins (osteophytes), capsular calcification/ossification
  - Cranial thickening, enlarged protuberances
  - Hypertrophy of paranasal sinuses
  - Ossification of anterior vertebral body and disc space
  - Osteophytosis of hips, knee, spine
  - Thickened diaphyses of long bones
  - Squaring metacarpal heads
  - Phalangeal widening, outgrowths at base
  - Spade-like terminal tufts
- Soft tissue enlargement: Especially hands and feet
  - Thickened heel pad is classic finding
- Bone resorption: Less common finding
  - May see generalized osteopenia
  - May sporadically present as undertubulation
  - Posterior vertebral scalloping: Common finding
- Other musculoskeletal findings
  - Mild chondrocalcinosis, no arthropathy
  - Degenerative arthropathy: Hips, knees, shoulders, hands; end result of increased cartilage thickness

Radiography: Hypopituitarism

- Delayed skeletal maturation: Late appearance of epiphyses, late fusion of physes, slow rate of growth
- Osteopenia (childhood and adult disease)

DIFFERENTIAL DIAGNOSIS

Hypopituitarism: Other Causes of Short Stature

- Correlate radiographic, clinical, laboratory findings

Acromegaly: Diffuse Idiopathic Skeletal Hyperostosis

- Diffuse idiopathic skeletal hyperostosis lacks joint space and disc space widening
- Clinically has associated stiffness, whereas acromegaly has hypermobility of extremities and spine

PATHOLOGY

General Features

- Etiology
  - Acromegaly and gigantism: Excess production GH and IGF-1 by pituitary adenoma
    - GH stimulates bone and cartilage production, collagen formation in soft tissue and solid organs
  - Hypopituitarism: Deficiency of pituitary hormones; GH deficiency most common
    - Usually from pituitary tumor, most commonly craniopharyngioma; 10% idiopathic, familial

CLINICAL ISSUES

Presentation

- Most common signs/symptoms
  - Acromegaly: Headaches and abnormal features
    - Thick, widened nose, bulging forehead, thick lips, mandibular overgrowth, enlarged maxilla, separation of teeth, malocclusion
    - Back pain, painful swelling of knees, hands
  - Hypopituitarism (child): Poor physical and mental development
- Other signs/symptoms
  - Acromegaly
    - Carpal tunnel syndrome: Median nerve edema
    - Sweaty, oily skin; deepening voice
    - Hypertension, cardiac disease, valve disease
    - ↑ risk of colonic polyps and colorectal cancer
    - Diabetes, renal failure, goiter
    - ↑ lean muscle mass, enlarged solid organs
  - Gigantism: ↑ longitudinal growth = ↑ height
  - Hypopituitarism: GH deficiency
    - Children: Proportional short stature, slow rate of growth; child-like face and body fat distribution
    - Adult: GH deficiency syndrome: ↓ skeletal muscle, ↑ central/truncal body fat; impaired cardiac function, insulin resistance

Demographics

- Age
  - Acromegaly: Diagnosed around age 40, often delayed 10+ years secondary to insidious onset of changes
  - Gigantism: Childhood
  - Hypopituitarism: Variable relative to etiology
- Gender
  - All conditions: M = F
- Epidemiology
  - Acromegaly: 60/1,000,000 people
  - GH deficiency: Estimated 1/3,500 children

Treatment

- Acromegaly and gigantism: Treat pituitary tumor
- Hypopituitarism: Growth hormone replacement

SELECTED REFERENCES

1. Colao A et al: The effects of somatostatin analogue therapy on pituitary tumor volume in patients with acromegaly. Pituitary. ePub, 2015

Hypothyroidism and Cretinism

KEY FACTS

IMAGING

- Congenital hypothyroidism: Delayed skeletal maturation, absent or small epiphyses, stippled epiphyses, short thick bones
- Juvenile & adolescent onset disease: Bone age delay of 1-2 years, slipped capital femoral epiphysis

TOP DIFFERENTIAL DIAGNOSES

- Delayed skeletal maturation: Extensive differential; measurement of thyroid hormones helpful

PATHOLOGY

- Congenital hypothyroidism: Maternal iodine deficiency most common, major public health concern in underdeveloped countries
- Juvenile, adolescent, adult onset hypothyroidism: Autoimmune (Hashimoto) thyroiditis most common; other causes include pituitary disorders, subacute (viral) thyroiditis, idiopathic

CLINICAL ISSUES

- Greater morbidity with neonatal/childhood onset or long duration of hypothyroid state
- Congenital: Mental retardation & growth retardation, which may be severe
  - Dull face, thick protruding tongue, swelling of face, umbilical hernia, cardiac failure
  - Jaundice, poor appetite, hoarse cry, constipation
  - Prevent morbidity if treated before 6 weeks of age
  - Leading cause of preventable mental retardation
- Juvenile onset: Delayed skeletal maturation, late puberty, delayed eruption of teeth
- Juvenile & adult onset
  - Puffy face, slowed speech, droopy eyelids
- All conditions: M < F
- Autoimmune disease: Variable course depending on severity of disease; initially hyperthyroid → euthyroid → hypothyroid (usually over years)

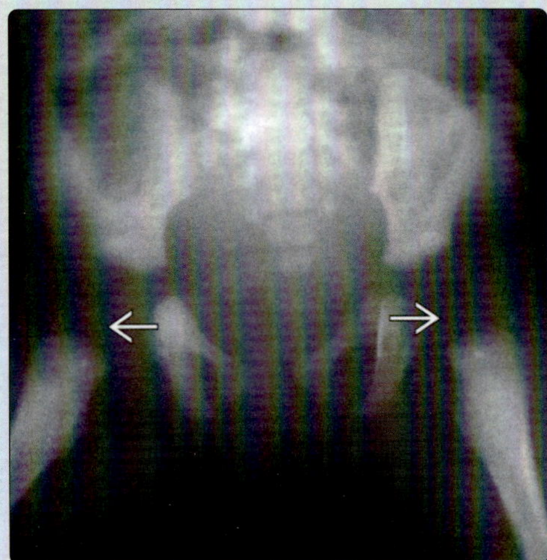

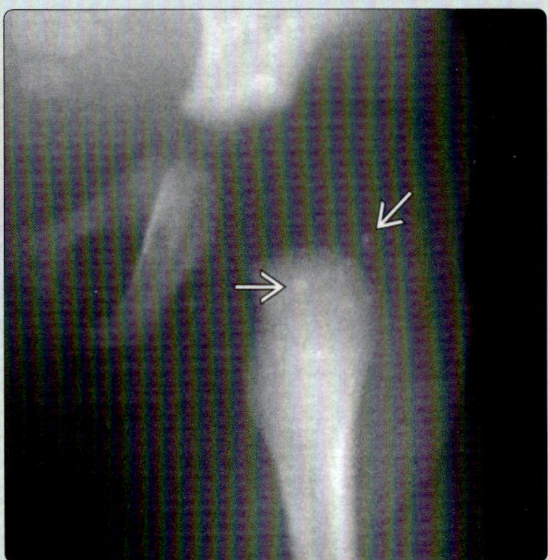

***(Left)** AP radiograph shows the pelvis in a newborn. The femoral capital epiphysis is not ossified ➡, indicative of delayed skeletal development. Recognition of this finding and its association with hypothyroidism is crucial to preventing the devastating sequelae of this condition. **(Right)** AP radiograph of the left hip in the same patient shows stippling of the greater trochanteric apophysis ➡, a subtle finding in this case. Stippled epiphyses are characteristic of hypothyroidism.*

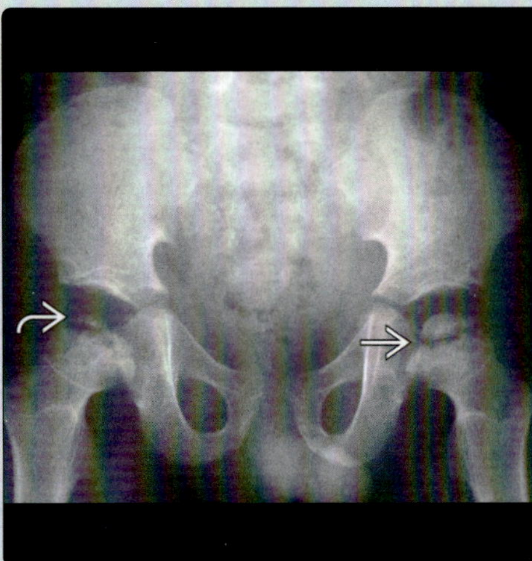

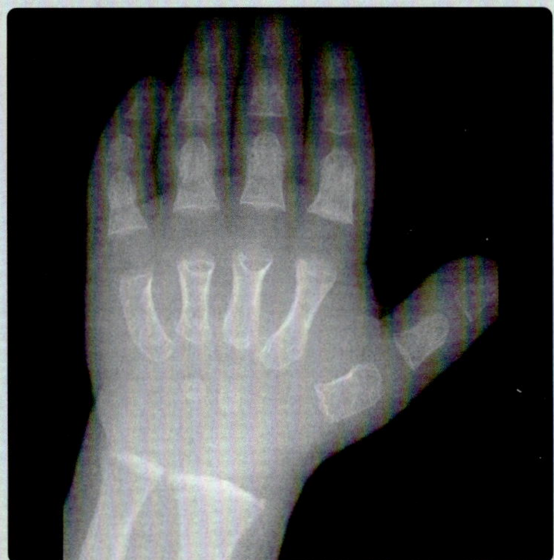

***(Left)** AP radiograph of the pelvis of a 4 year old reveals fragmentation of the femoral capital epiphysis (termed cretinoid hip) ➡. Both hips show widening of growth plate ➡. Findings indicate delayed skeletal maturation. **(Right)** AP radiograph of the same patient's hand is remarkable for what is missing. Multiple carpal bones are not yet visible, and phalangeal epiphyses are absent. The hands show the skeletal maturity of an infant rather than a 4 year old. The findings are all typical of hypothyroidism.*

TERMINOLOGY

Synonyms

- Cretinism: Neonatal hypothyroidism; congenital hypothyroidism
- Hashimoto thyroiditis: Autoimmune/chronic lymphocytic thyroiditis

IMAGING

General Features

- Best diagnostic clue
  - Congenital: Delayed bone age
  - Juvenile, adolescent, adult: Abnormal thyroid scan

Imaging Recommendations

- Best imaging tool
  - Radiographs (bone age) to assess skeletal maturation
  - Thyroid scan to evaluate thyroid gland

Radiographic Findings

- Radiography
  - Congenital hypothyroidism
    - Delayed skeletal maturation
    - Absent or small epiphyses; stippled epiphyses
    - Short thick bones, delayed closure of fontanelles
  - Juvenile & adolescent onset disease
    - Bone age delay of 1-2 years
    - Slipped capital femoral epiphysis
    - Enlarged sella turcica

Nuclear Medicine Findings

- Labeled iodine scans
  - Athyroid states: No uptake
  - Inborn errors of thyroid metabolism: Normal
  - Hashimoto thyroiditis: Increased uptake early → irregular patchy uptake midcourse → diminished uptake; ± hot or cold nodules in late disease

DIFFERENTIAL DIAGNOSIS

Delayed Skeletal Maturation

- Extensive differential diagnosis
- Measurement of thyroid hormones aids differentiation

PATHOLOGY

General Features

- Etiology
  - Congenital hypothyroidism: Maternal iodine deficiency most common, major public health concern in underdeveloped countries
    - Absent thyroid gland, inborn errors of thyroid metabolism, pituitary-related process less common
  - Juvenile, adolescent, adult onset hypothyroidism
    - Autoimmune (Hashimoto) thyroiditis most common; other causes include pituitary disorders, subacute (viral) thyroiditis, idiopathic
- Genetics
  - Autoimmune disease has familial pattern
  - Inborn errors of thyroid metabolism: Autosomal recessive & dominant patterns

CLINICAL ISSUES

Presentation

- Most common signs/symptoms
  - Congenital: Mental retardation & growth retardation, which may be severe
  - Other etiologies: Itchy & dry skin, thin hair, myxedema, cold intolerance, weight gain, fatigue
- Other signs/symptoms
  - Greater morbidity with neonatal/childhood onset or long duration of hypothyroid state
  - Palpable goiter with iodine deficiency, early autoimmune disease
  - Congenital hypothyroidism
    - Dull face, thick protruding tongue, swelling of face, umbilical hernia, cardiac failure
    - Jaundice, poor appetite, hoarse cry, constipation
  - Juvenile onset
    - Delayed growth & short stature; with treatment, accelerated skeletal growth allowing catch-up
    - Delayed appearance of deciduous & permanent teeth
    - Delayed onset of puberty or precocious puberty if condition leads to hyperpituitarism
  - Juvenile & adult onset
    - Puffy face, slowed speech, droopy eyelids
    - Reversible dementia, depression

Demographics

- Age
  - Congenital disease presents during infancy; otherwise quite variable
- Gender
  - All conditions: M < F
- Ethnicity
  - Hispanic > Caucasian > African American
- Epidemiology
  - Congenital hypothyroidism: 1:6,000 live births
  - Autoimmune thyroiditis: 1-5% of population

Natural History & Prognosis

- Congenital hypothyroidism
  - Prevent morbidity if treated before 6 weeks of age
  - Neonatal screening programs have been developed because condition is asymptomatic until changes are irreversible; despite treatment, intelligence at lower limits of normal
  - Leading cause of preventable mental retardation
- Autoimmune disease: Variable course depending on severity of disease; typical pattern has initial hyperthyroid state followed by euthyroid period with progression to hypothyroid state, usually over years

Treatment

- Hormone replacement

SELECTED REFERENCES

1. Wassner AJ et al: Congenital hypothyroidism: recent advances. Curr Opin Endocrinol Diabetes Obes. 22(5):407-12, 2015
2. Rajatanavin R et al: Endemic cretinism in Thailand: a multidisciplinary survey. Eur J Endocrinol. 137(4):349-55, 1997
3. Newland CJ et al: Congenital hypothyroidism–correlation between radiographic appearances of the knee epiphyses and biochemical data. Postgrad Med J. 67(788):553-6, 1991

KEY FACTS

IMAGING

- Radiographs
  - ↓ bone density resulting from osteoporosis
  - Intracortical tunneling
  - Insufficiency fractures & fragility fractures; common sites include vertebral bodies, femoral neck, distal radius
  - Changes more conspicuous in men & older patients
  - Children: Accelerated skeletal maturation, craniosynostosis
  - Thyroid acropachy: Occurs during healing phase
- Dual energy x-ray absorptiometry (DEXA): Bone mineral density indicative of osteopenia or osteoporosis

TOP DIFFERENTIAL DIAGNOSES

- Osteoporosis has extensive differential diagnosis
- No specific distinguishing features of hyperthyroidism

PATHOLOGY

- Complex pathology
  - Thyroid hormone stimulates osteoclasts
  - Osteoblast-mediated bone resorption
- Cortical bone loss > trabecular bone loss
- One of most common causes of 2° osteoporosis
- Suppressive hyperthyroid states for treatment of thyroid cancer
  - TSH levels normal: No osteoporosis
  - Low TSH levels: Controversial as to whether or not at risk for osteoporosis

CLINICAL ISSUES

- Hyperthyroid states
  - Graves disease
  - Toxic nodular goiter
- Symptoms: Fatigue, weight loss, heat intolerance, tachycardia, palpitations, ocular abnormalities
- Myopathy
  - Weakness
  - Muscle wasting

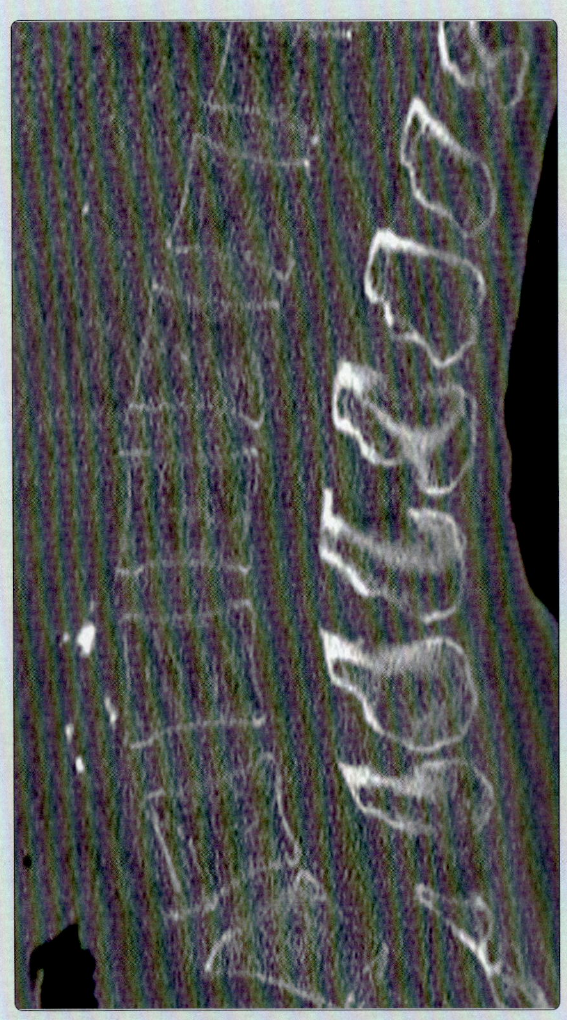

Sagittal NECT demonstrates severely decreased bone density due to osteoporosis. Excess thyroid hormone results in an imbalance between bone formation and bone resorption that favors osteoclast activity and bone resorption.

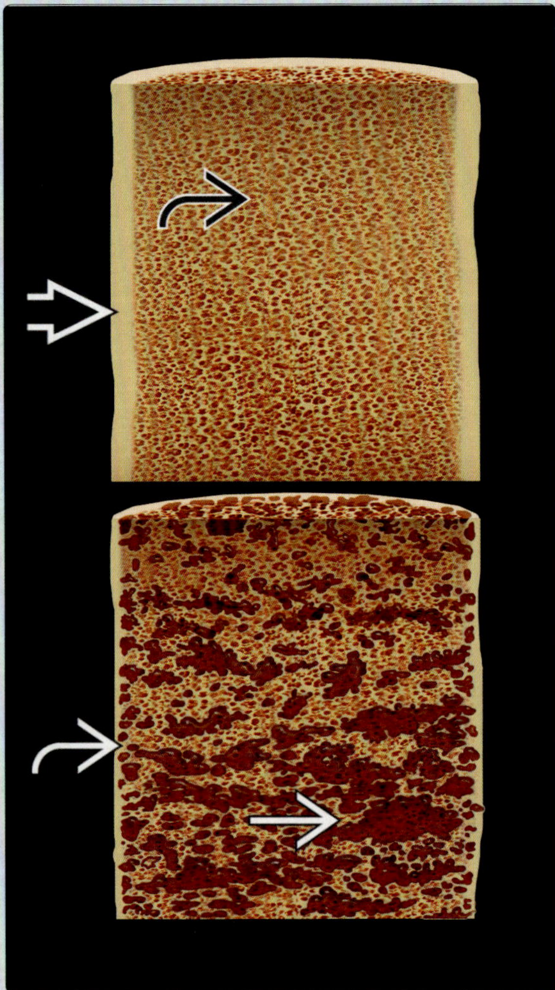

Graphic representation shows normal trabecular ⮫ and cortical bone ➡ (above), compared with osteoporosis of hyperthyroidism (below), which affects both trabecular ➡ and cortical bone ⮫ (greatest impact on cortical bone).

KEY FACTS

IMAGING

- Radiographs: Periosteal new bone formation
  - Spiculated, lacy appearance
  - Metacarpals, metatarsals most common
  - Radial aspect metacarpals 1st through 4th
  - Ulnar aspect 5th metacarpal
  - Middle & distal phalanges less common
  - Favors upper extremity
  - Asymmetric distribution

TOP DIFFERENTIAL DIAGNOSES

- Hypertrophic osteoarthropathy
  - Involves tibia & fibula, radius & ulna
  - Diaphyseal
  - Linear periosteal reaction
  - Symmetric distribution
- Pachydermoperiostitis
  - Involves tibia & fibula, radius & ulna
  - Predominates in diaphysis, may extend into metaphysis
  - Symmetric distribution
  - Characteristic facies

CLINICAL ISSUES

- Occurs following initiation of treatment of Graves
  - Patient euthyroid or hypothyroid
  - Often years after diagnosis
- Acropachy typically asymptomatic
- Acropachy relatively uncommon (0.3% Graves patients)
- Male < female
- Associated findings
  - Ophthalmopathy (25% Graves patients)
  - Soft tissue swelling of fingers & toes
  - Dermopathy: Pretibial myxedema (1.5% Graves patients)
  - Clubbing most common finding
  - Acropachy almost always associated with ophthalmopathy & dermopathy; reverse not true

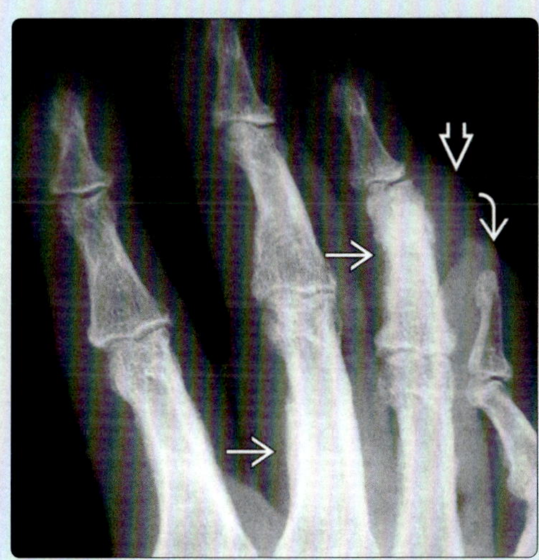

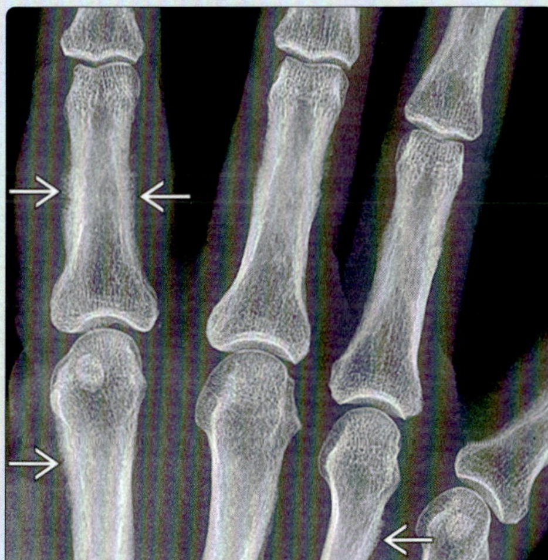

(Left) *PA radiograph shows characteristic changes of thyroid acropachy. Clubbing is best seen in the 5th finger ➩. Fluffy periosteal new bone formation is present along the 3rd proximal phalanx & 4th middle phalanx ➡. Soft tissue swelling is most prominent about the 4th finger ➪.* **(Right)** *PA radiograph of a 74-year-old woman with Graves disease shows the lacey periostitis ➡ along metacarpals and proximal phalangeals that is typical of thyroid acropachy.*

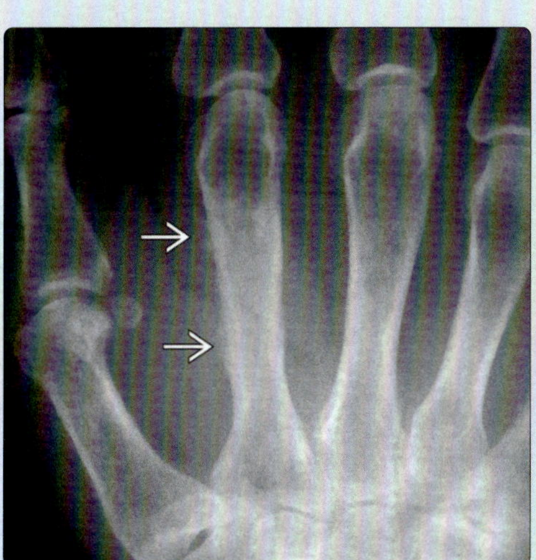

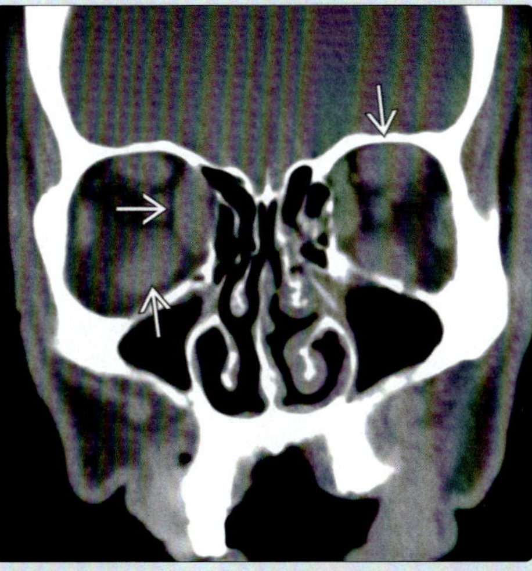

(Left) *PA radiograph shows characteristic periostitis along the radial aspect of the 2nd metacarpal ➡. The appearance in thyroid acropachy has been described as fluffy, spiculated, or lace-like, as opposed to the lamellar periostitis of other conditions like hypertrophic osteoarthropathy.* **(Right)** *Coronal NECT shows benign appearing enlargement of the extraocular muscles bilaterally ➡. This ophthalmopathy almost always accompanies thyroid acropachy. Involvement is inferior > medial > superior.*

Hypophosphatasia

KEY FACTS

IMAGING

- Perinatal form: Lethal type
  - Micromelia; markedly diminished bone density, skeleton may appear completely unmineralized
- Perinatal form: Benign type
  - Skeletal changes show spontaneous resolution
- Infantile form: Severe rachitic-like changes
- Childhood form
  - Short stature, rickets-like changes, falsely widened-appearing sutures, & functional craniosynostosis
- Adult form: Osteopenia, osteomalacia-like changes
  - Pseudofracture in lateral cortex proximal femur
- Odontohypophosphatasia: Affects teeth only
- Prenatal ultrasound: 3rd trimester
  - Excellent brain detail: ↓ mineralization of skull allows ↑ through transmission
  - Micromelia

TOP DIFFERENTIAL DIAGNOSES

- Osteogenesis imperfecta
- Rickets
- Achondrogenesis

PATHOLOGY

- Mutation in *ALPL* gene → deficient production TNSALP (tissue nonspecific alkaline phosphatase)

CLINICAL ISSUES

- Perinatal lethal: Stillborn or death within days/weeks
- Infantile: Appears in first 6 months of life, symptoms related to hypercalcemia
- Childhood: Delayed walking, waddling gait, bone pain, respiratory difficulties 2° to rib deformities
- Adult: Bone pain, skeletal deformities, fractures
- Treatment is symptomatic only: Cannot adequately address underlying metabolic abnormality

(Left) *AP radiograph shows a stillborn infant with the most severe & lethal form of hypophosphatasia. Note the near complete absence of mineralization of the skeleton* ➡ *and severe micromelia* ➡*.* **(Right)** *AP radiograph of the humerus with typical findings of the childhood form of hypophosphatasia. The humeral diaphysis is slightly bowed* ➡ *and an exostosis is present* ➡*. While classically described arising from the tibia or ulna, these excrescences can arise on any bone. The physis is minimally widened* ➡*.*

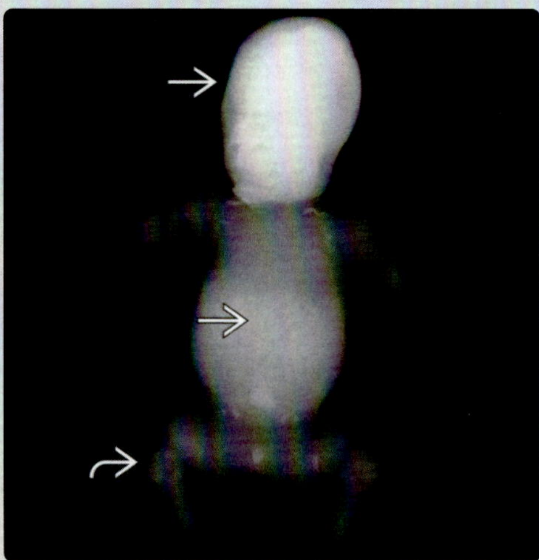

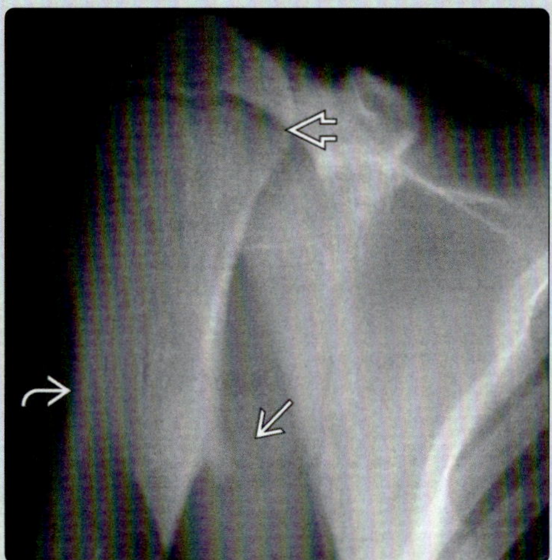

(Left) *AP radiograph shows both femora in a child with significant hypophosphatasia. The physes are grossly abnormal, showing widening and irregularity* ➡*. Bone softening has resulted in bowing of both femora proximally as well as the diaphysis of the left femur* ➡*. Bilateral protrusio deformities of the hips are seen* ➡*, indicating softening of the bone.* **(Right)** *Coronal graphic depicts hypophosphatasia, with marked irregularity of the growth plates and tongues of cartilage extending into the metaphyseal region* ➡*.*

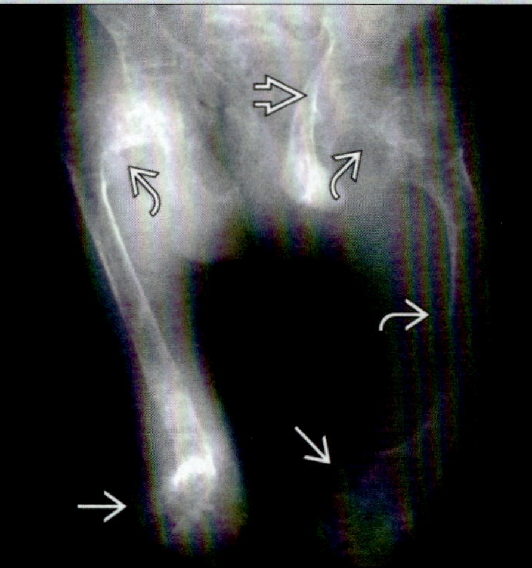

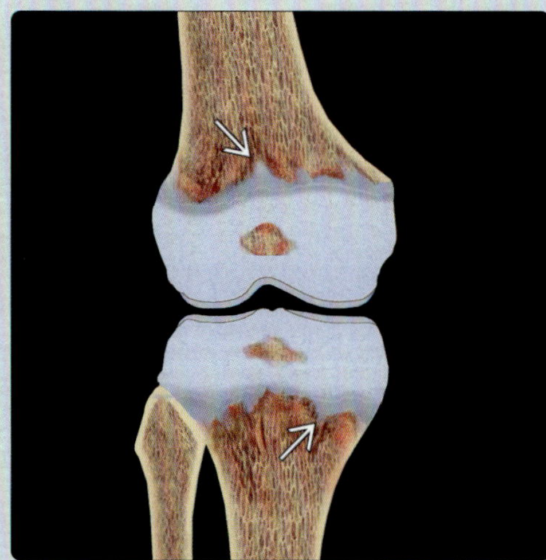

IMAGING

General Features

- Best diagnostic clue
  - Perinatal: Severe hypomineralization of skeleton
  - Infantile: Severe rachitic-like changes
  - Childhood: Rachitic-like changes of varying severity
  - Adult: Osteomalacia-like changes

Radiographic Findings

- Perinatal form: Lethal type
  - Markedly diminished bone density
    - Skeleton may appear completely unmineralized
  - Micromelia
  - Soft bones that become deformed
    - Chest deformity → respiratory difficulties → death
  - Bowdler (bone) spurs midshaft ulna & fibulae
  - False appearance of widened sutures with functional craniosynostosis
- Perinatal form: Benign type
  - Same skeletal manifestations as lethal type
  - Skeletal changes show spontaneous resolution
- Infantile form
  - Severe rachitic-like changes
  - Radiolucent tongues protrude into metaphyses from growth plate
  - Falsely widened sutures, functional craniosynostosis
  - Abnormal vertebral body formation
  - Short stature
- Childhood form
  - Short stature
  - Rickets-like changes
  - Bowdler spurs
  - Falsely widened sutures, functional craniosynostosis
- Adult form
  - Osteopenia, osteomalacia-like changes
  - Pseudofracture in lateral cortex of proximal femur
    - Osteomalacia pseudofractures in medial cortex
  - ± calcium pyrophosphate deposition disease
  - Multiple insufficiency fractures, especially in feet
  - Bowdler spurs, particularly on ulna, fibula
  - Functional craniosynostosis
- Odontohypophosphatasia: Affects teeth only
  - Early loss of deciduous teeth
  - Abnormal development of permanent teeth
  - Loose permanent teeth

Ultrasonographic Findings

- Prenatal ultrasound: 3rd trimester
  - Excellent brain detail: ↓ mineralization of skull allows ↑ through transmission
  - Micromelia

DIFFERENTIAL DIAGNOSIS

Osteogenesis Imperfecta

- Multiple fractures produce asymmetric limb shortening; small amount of skull ossification

Osteomalacia and Rickets

- Hypomineralization and deformities not as profound

Achondrogenesis

- Absent mineralization mainly vertebra, more normal mineralization in appendicular skeleton and skull

PATHOLOGY

General Features

- Etiology
  - Mutation in *ALPL* gene → deficient production TNSALP (tissue nonspecific alkaline phosphatase)
    - Poor hydrolyzation of inorganic phosphate, which accumulates and prevents formation of hydroxyapatite (mineralized bone)
- Genetics
  - Infantile, perinatal forms: Autosomal recessive
  - Less severe forms: Autosomal recessive or dominant
- Associated abnormalities
  - Infantile form: Hypercalcemia resulting from failure to incorporate calcium into bone

Microscopic Features

- Increased osteoid and unmineralized cartilage
- Physis: Disrupted hypertrophic zone as seen in rickets, calcified zone may be completely absent

CLINICAL ISSUES

Presentation

- Most common signs/symptoms
  - Variable presentation depending on form
  - All forms have early loss of deciduous teeth
  - Perinatal lethal: Stillborn or death within days/weeks 2° to respiratory difficulties
  - Infantile: Appears in 1st 6 months of life, symptoms related to hypercalcemia
    - Irritability, poor feeding, vomiting, renal stones & renal damage, seizures
  - Childhood: Delayed walking, waddling gait, bone pain, respiratory difficulties 2° to rib deformities
  - Adult: Bone pain, skeletal deformities, fractures

Demographics

- Gender
  - Severe forms: Male = female
- Epidemiology
  - Severe forms: 1/100,000 births

Natural History & Prognosis

- Perinatal lethal: Stillbirth or death in days/weeks
- Infantile: Limited life span
- Childhood: May resolve spontaneously, reappear in adulthood
- Childhood & adult: Varying deformities & fractures

Treatment

- Symptomatic only: Cannot adequately address underlying metabolic abnormality
  - Enzyme replacement therapy experimental

SELECTED REFERENCES

1. Bianchi ML: Hypophosphatasia: an overview of the disease and its treatment. Osteoporos Int. 26(12):2743-57, 2015

Cushing Syndrome

KEY FACTS

TERMINOLOGY

- Cushing syndrome (CS): Hypercortisolism from exogenous or endogenous causes
  - Adrenocorticotrophic hormone (ACTH) independent: 1° adrenal disease, usually adenoma
  - Ectopic ACTH syndrome: Paraneoplastic syndrome, #1 cause is lung cancer; male > female
  - Cushing disease: ACTH dependent, usually from pituitary microadenoma; male < < female
  - Exogenous = iatrogenic: Treatment for asthma, suppression following renal transplantation
- Cushing disease: 65-80% of endogenous CS
  - Adults: Male < < female
  - Pediatric disease: Male > female

IMAGING

- Radiographs: Osteopenia worse in appendicular skeleton, more severe in men; osteonecrosis; insufficiency fractures; hypertrophic callus
- DEXA: Osteopenia or osteoporosis
- MR: Detects pituitary adenomas, useful to diagnose insufficiency fractures
- Ga88 somatostatin receptor analogs & FDG PET for identification of ectopic Cushing etiologies

TOP DIFFERENTIAL DIAGNOSES

- Osteoporosis of other etiologies
  - Children: Idiopathic juvenile osteoporosis
  - Adults: Extensive differential diagnosis

PATHOLOGY

- Bone resorption: Trabecular bone > cortical bone

CLINICAL ISSUES

- Truncal obesity, rounded (moon) face, irregular menses, weight gain, lethargy, hirsutism, acne, striae, myopathy, thin skin, easy bruising
- Delayed skeletal maturation; resultant short stature

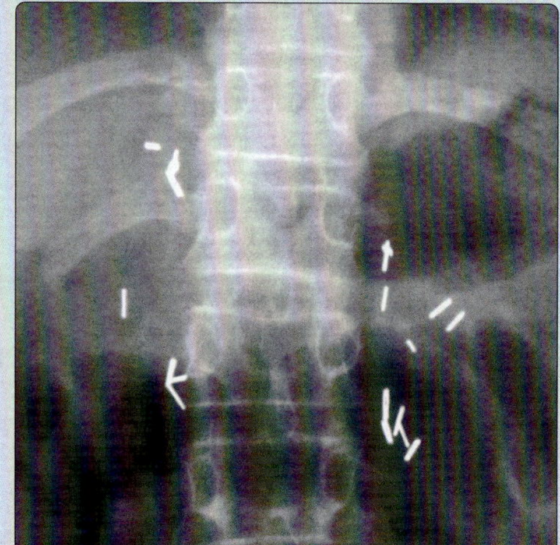

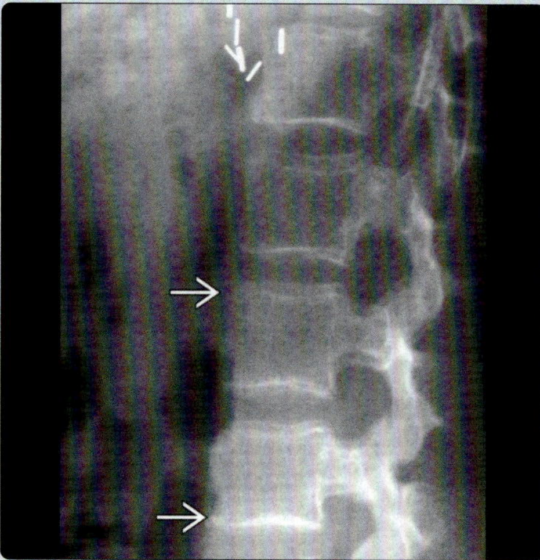

(Left) *AP radiograph of the lumbar spine from a 19-year-old woman who underwent bilateral adrenalectomy for ACTH independent Cushing syndrome (CS) shows diffuse osteopenia.* **(Right)** *Lateral radiograph of the same patient shows radiographic findings of osteoporosis. Note the very thin cortical bone of the endplates ➡. Due to the higher percentage of trabecular bone, vertebra are more severely affected by the osteoporosis of CS than appendicular bones, such as the femur, that have a greater percentage of cortical bone.*

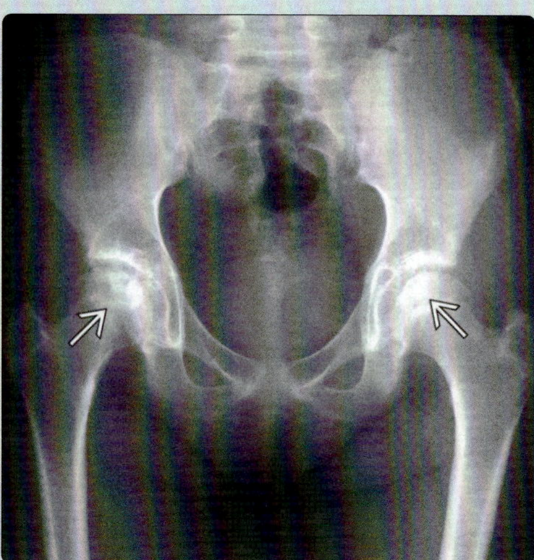

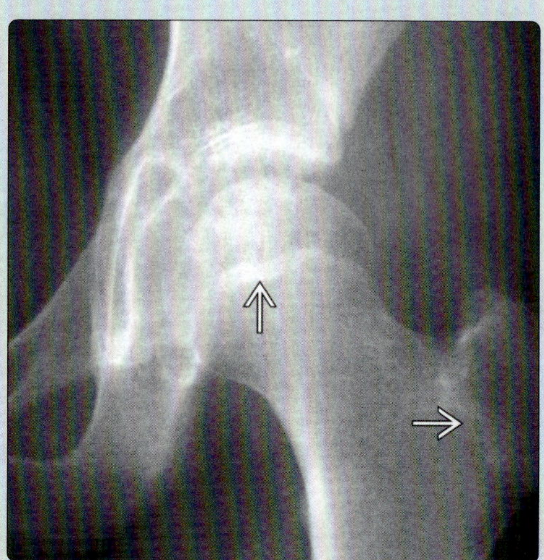

(Left) *AP radiograph of the pelvis shows diffuse osteopenia & focal sclerosis in the femoral heads ➡. Patchy sclerosis is an early radiographic finding of osteonecrosis (ON). The incidence of ON is less in endogenous CS than in exogenous CS. While osteoporosis may reverse following treatment, the sequelae of ON will be lifelong.* **(Right)** *AP radiograph of the hip reveals that the physes of the patient are not yet fused ➡, indicating delayed skeletal maturation, another feature of CS.*

KEY FACTS

IMAGING

- Radiographs: Cloud-like densities; may be quite large and enlarge over time, rarely regress
  - Periarticular: Within bursa, along extensor tendons; hips, shoulders, elbows, feet
  - Marrow deposits: Uncommon, ± periostitis
  - Other sites: Skin, retina, pulp stones in teeth
- CT, active phase: Multiple small cystic areas with peripheral mineralization, sedimentation phenomenon (fluid-calcium levels)
- CT, inactive phase: Solid lobules of calcification
- Bone scan: Uptake at sites of calcium deposition
- MR T1WI: Heterogeneous hypointense/low SI
- MR fluid-sensitive sequence
  - Active phase: Cystic areas bright; bright periphery 2° to foreign body reaction, edema in adjacent tissues, sedimentation with low signal
  - Inactive phase: Low signal foci with little edema

TOP DIFFERENTIAL DIAGNOSES

- Hyperparathyroidism/renal osteodystrophy
  - Dialysis-related deposits have similar appearance
  - Radiographic evidence of bone resorption

PATHOLOGY

- Calcium hydroxyapatite crystal deposition, rim of chronic foreign body reaction, fibrosis
- Hyperphosphatemia; ↑ 1,25 dihydroxy vitamin D

CLINICAL ISSUES

- Appears in childhood/adolescence although onset may occur at any age from infants to elderly
- Predominately African American
- Symptoms arise from compression of adjacent structures including nerves and skin
- Rare, autosomal dominant
- Abnormal fibroblast growth factor 23
- Bisphosphonate therapy may be useful

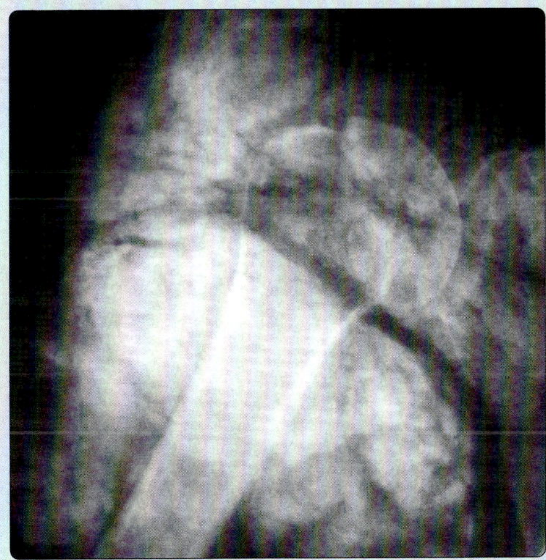

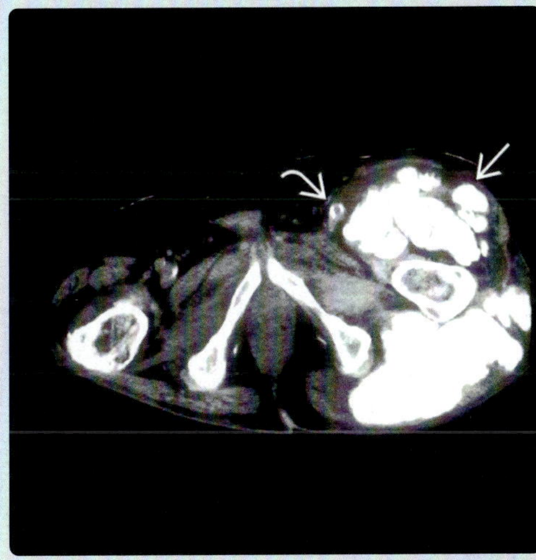

(Left) *AP radiograph shows dense cloud-like calcification surrounding an otherwise normal-appearing shoulder. While the more common etiologies of this include renal osteodystrophy in a patient on dialysis or collagen vascular diseases, one should also consider tumoral calcinosis.* **(Right)** *Axial NECT of a thigh shows dense mineralization in the musculature surrounding the left hip ➡. In this older individual (note vascular calcification ➡), the mineralization is solid rather than cystic, indicating inactive deposition.*

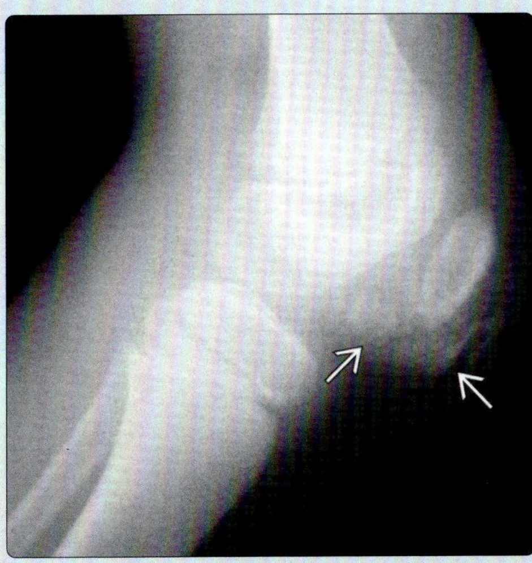

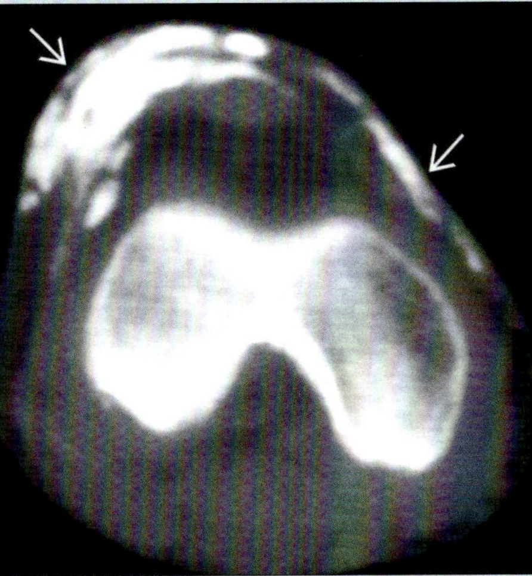

(Left) *Lateral radiograph demonstrates amorphous dense calcifications, which appear to be entirely extraarticular ➡. As in this case, the deposits often occur along the extensor surface. In this younger patient, the depositions are likely to continue to enlarge. The knee is a common site of tumoral calcinosis.* **(Right)** *Axial bone CT shows that, in this patient, the mineralization has deposited in the skin and subcutaneous tissues ➡. Deposits may be seen in a number of different periarticular tissues.*

SECTION 12

Drug-Induced and Nutritional MSK Conditions

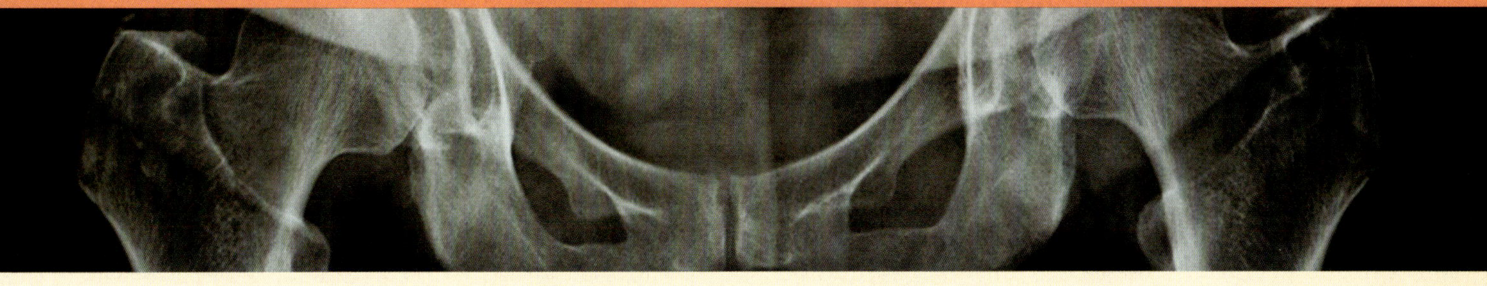

Drug-Induced Conditions

Nutritional Deficiency

KEY FACTS

IMAGING

- Osteoporosis
  - Likely direct inhibition of bone formation and indirect stimulation of bone resorption (↓ intestinal absorption of calcium → ↑ PTH)
  - Results in insufficiency fractures, particularly in spine, sacrum, pubic rami, hips
- Osteonecrosis (ON) and bone infarcts
  - Of all patients on steroids, 2% develop ON
  - High risk with short duration (6 weeks) and high doses (> 20 mg): 5-25% develop ON
  - ↑ risk of ON in renal transplant patients on steroids who also have renal osteodystrophy (40% develop ON)
  - Mechanism may be vascular compression 2° to enlarged marrow fat cells
  - Steroids responsible for 30-40% of non-traumatic ON of hip
  - ON in vertebral bodies: Several patterns of collapse, but may develop lucent cleft in body
- Soft tissue fat accumulation
  - Mediastinal, paraspinal, subcutaneous
  - Epidural: May lead to cord compression
- Tendinopathy
  - May be induced by steroids; delayed healing
- Myopathy
  - Glucocorticoid rhabdomyolysis: Rare complication
- Steroid arthropathy
  - Related to intraarticular injection of steroids
  - Neuropathic-like arthropathy, with bony debris and collapse that may be rapid
  - Hip and knee most frequently involved
- Intraarticular calcification: Infrapatellar fat pad, synovium, joint capsule
  - Periarticular calcification may also occur
  - Both intra- and periarticular related to steroid injection
- Osteomyelitis, septic arthritis
  - Rare complication

(Left) *Sagittal T1WI MR in a patient with chronic steroid use shows multiple insufficiency fractures, seen as low signal intensity lines crossing thoracic vertebral bodies ⇒. Epidural fat deposition ⇒ may eventually put the spinal cord at risk. Increased fat deposition in the dorsal subcutaneous tissue ⇒ results in the buffalo hump appearance.* **(Right)** *AP radiograph in a 30-year-old man shows an incomplete but subacute basicervical fracture ⇒, as well as severe osteoporosis. The etiology was steroid use for asthma.*

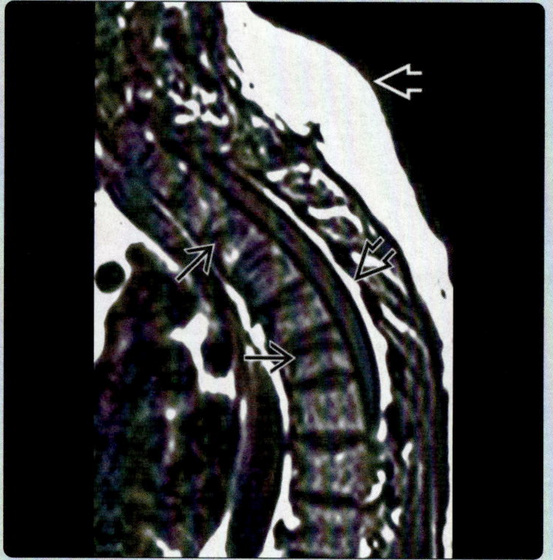

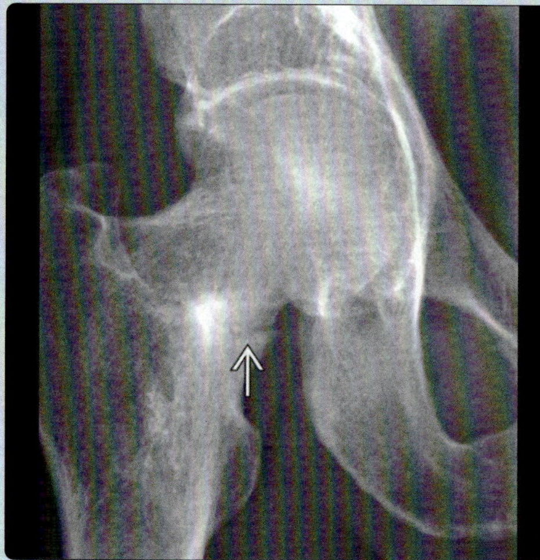

(Left) *Lateral radiograph shows severe osteoporosis, fragmentation, and collapse of both femoral condyles ⇒. Additionally, there is calcification lining the suprapatellar recess ⇒. Both of these findings may result from intraarticular injection of steroids over an extended period of time, as occurred in this patient with severe RA.* **(Right)** *Coronal T1 MR demonstrates serpiginous ↓ SI geographic abnormalities in the metaphyses and subchondral bone ⇒, diagnostic of bone infarcts in a patient dependent on steroids.*

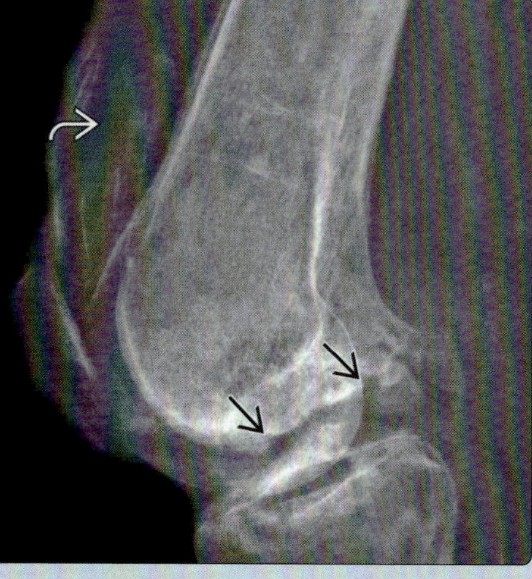

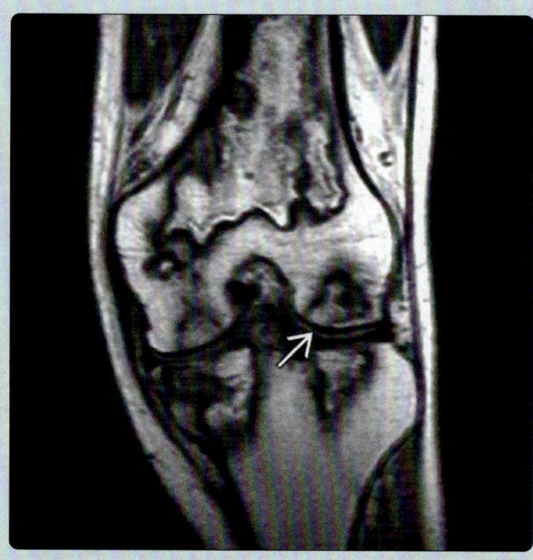

KEY FACTS

TERMINOLOGY

- Osteoporosis
  - Difficult to quantify as to how much an individual's osteoporosis is related to alcohol
  - Osteoporosis also related to generally poor nutritional status in alcoholics
- Osteonecrosis (ON)
  - Hip or shoulder most frequently involved
  - Alcohol accounts for 20-40% of ON of hip in USA
  - Extent of alcohol use may not be obvious; must ask appropriate questions to elicit history
  - Likely due to fat emboli from liver
  - Patchy sclerosis within femoral head
  - Curvilinear subchondral lucency, often followed by collapse
  - Double line sign on MR
- Neuropathic joint
  - Neuropathic hip is rare
  - May be associated with alcohol abuse
- Fetal alcohol syndrome
  - Ethanol metabolism → production of free radicals → apoptosis, DNA damage, and lipid peroxidation
  - No lower threshold of safety for alcohol use during pregnancy
  - 1-3 per 1,000 live births in USA
  - Growth retardation
  - Microcephaly, behavioral and cognitive disorders
  - Cardiac: Atrial and ventricular septal defects, aberrant great vessels, conotruncal heart defects
  - Skeletal: Radioulnar synostosis, contractures, vertebral segmentation abnormalities, scoliosis
  - Renal: Aplastic/hypoplastic/dysplastic kidneys, horseshoe kidneys, hydronephrosis
  - Ophthalmologic: Strabismus, retinal vascular abnormalities, ptosis, optic nerve hypoplasia
  - Hearing loss: Neurosensory and conductive

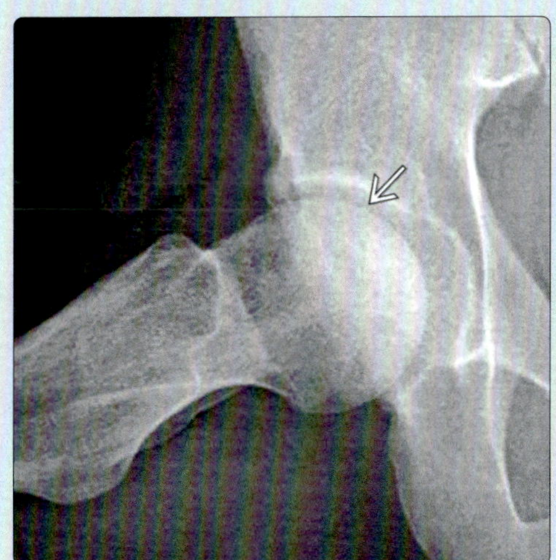

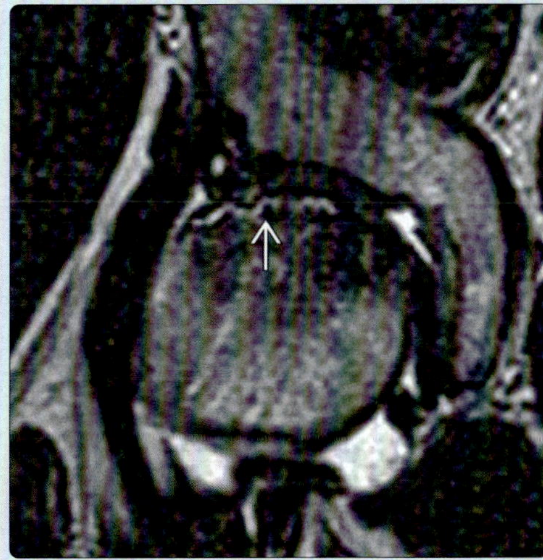

(Left) *Frog lateral x-ray demonstrates subtle flattening of the femoral head in the weight-bearing portion ➡. Though there is no lucent crescent sign, this is typical of osteonecrosis.* **(Right)** *Coronal MR arthrogram T2WI FS, same case, shows osteonecrosis ➡. This is easily demonstrated on MR and is the cause of the patient's hip pain. Though there were no overt signs of alcoholism, on careful questioning the patient admitted to "probably drinking too much with clients" several nights per week.*

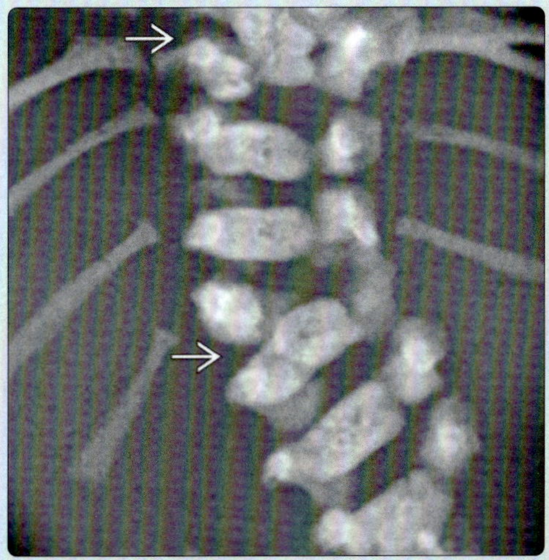

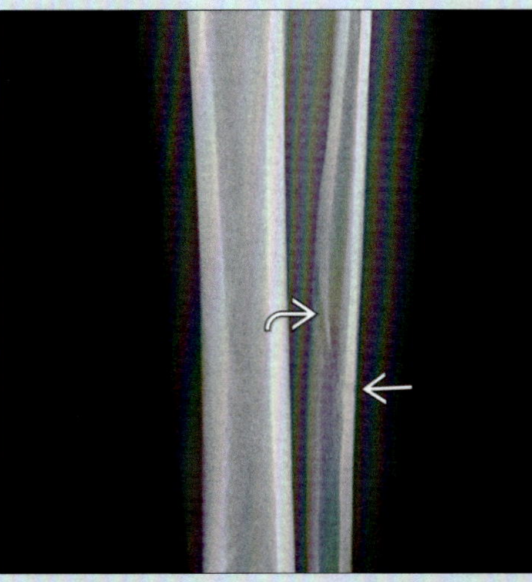

(Left) *AP radiograph shows vertebral segmentation defects ➡, which are nonspecific but typical of those found in fetal alcohol syndrome. Other osseous abnormalities include forearm synostosis, contractures, scoliosis, and delayed maturation.* **(Right)** *AP x-ray of a 35-year-old alcoholic Polynesian man with a painful leg shows a subtle insufficiency fracture of the fibula ➡ (proximal lucency is nutrient vessel ↪). This man proved to be severely osteopenic related to his alcoholism/malnutrition.*

Vitamin A: Complications

KEY FACTS

TERMINOLOGY

- Musculoskeletal abnormalities associated with hypervitaminosis A

IMAGING

- Subacute toxicity in child (appears after 6 months of ingestion)
  - Periosteal reaction (cortical hyperostosis): Regular or wavy, dense, along long bones
  - May have skin nodules associated
  - Most common locations: Ulna, tibia, metacarpals, metatarsals, clavicles
- Chronic toxicity in child
  - Coned epiphyses with possible early fusion across physes
- Chronic toxicity related to dermatologic retinoid use
  - Hyperostosis along spinal ligaments
  - Enthesopathy
- Chronic subtoxicity in adult
  - May occur with intake of just twice recommended daily allowance of vitamin A
  - Osteoporosis (nonspecific), ↑ risk fracture

TOP DIFFERENTIAL DIAGNOSES

- Periosteal reaction in child
  - Child abuse: May present with periosteal reaction
  - Caffey disease: Present at birth; self-limited
  - Neonatal diffuse infection: Usually infant in intensive care unit or TORCH infections
- Coned epiphyses
  - Vascular or thermal insult, multiple syndromes
- Retinoid hyperostosis: DISH

PATHOLOGY

- Excessive oral intake or as retinoid skin application
- Vitamin A is fat soluble, so is stored in body, making it more likely to cause toxicity with excessive intake

(Left) *PA radiograph shows cortical hyperostosis of the ulnar diaphysis ➡, which is typical of hypervitaminosis A. The periosteal change is generally not seen prior to 6 months of age, as it takes several months of overdosing to develop the osseous changes.* **(Right)** *AP radiograph in the same child shows bilateral tibial and fibular diaphysis cortical hyperostosis ➡. Note this cortical thickening does not involve the metaphyses or epiphyses. However, if it is longstanding, physeal changes will occur.*

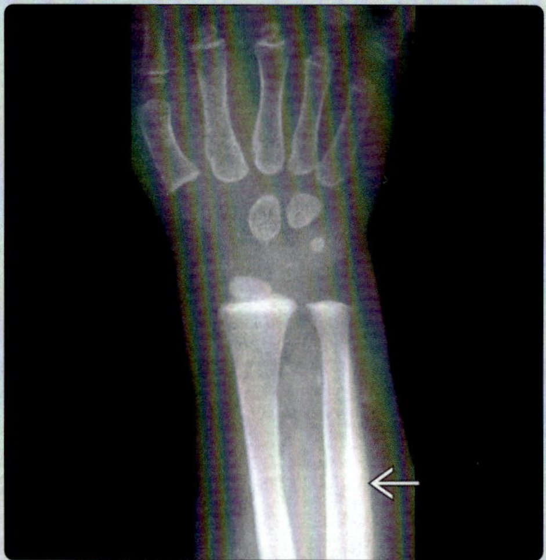

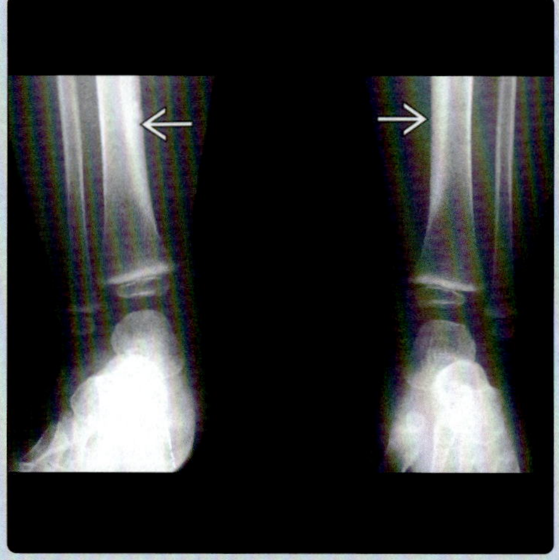

(Left) *AP radiograph of the foot shows early fusion of the proximal phalanges ➡. There is a coned epiphysis of the great toe showing early fusion ⇨. Multiple coned epiphyses are associated with a number of syndromes. They are also seen with thermal injury. Hypervitaminosis A can also result in coned epiphyses, as in this case.* **(Right)** *PA radiograph in the same case shows early fusion of epiphyses of middle phalanges ➡ and coning of epiphysis of phalanges of the thumb ⇨. The contralateral hand had similar findings.*

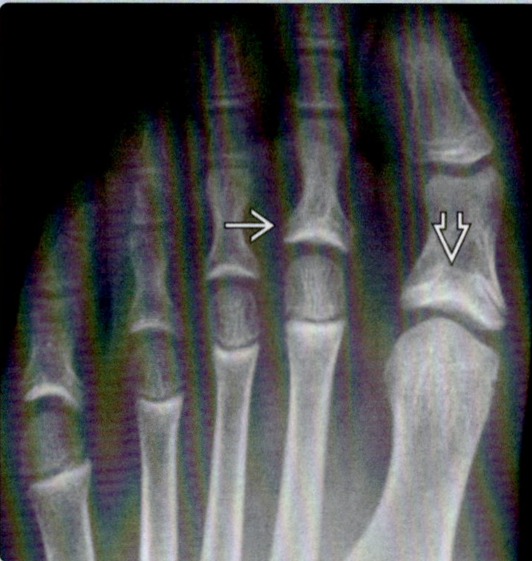

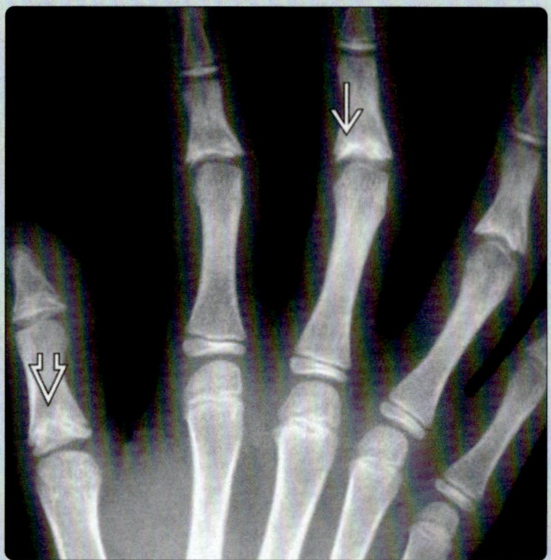

KEY FACTS

TERMINOLOGY

- Hypervitaminosis D
  - Excessive intake of vitamin D
    - May occur in patients with vitamin D-resistant rickets
    - Overzealous dosage of cholecalciferol or other forms of vitamin D (infants especially vulnerable)
    - High variability in vitamin D content on over-the-counter supplements
  - Manifest as enthesopathy (occasionally severe)
  - Although bone density may appear increased, fragility is still present if there is resistance to vitamin D; Looser zones seen in typical locations
  - Vascular & soft tissue calcifications
- Hypovitaminosis D in general population
  - Nutritional deficiency (rare in USA except in elderly, common in 3rd-world countries)
  - Renal deficiency, liver damage, intestinal malabsorption, inadequate sun exposure; end-stage renal disease is most common cause in USA
  - Manifest in children as rickets: Widened zone of provisional calcification, metaphyseal fraying and cupping, ↓ bone density with coarsened trabeculae
  - Manifest in adults as osteomalacia: Wide transverse fractures in ribs, lateral border scapula, pubic rami, medial femur (Looser zones)
- Hypovitaminosis D in the elderly
  - High prevalence: May be in up to 87% of adults > 65 yr
  - Etiologies include poor dietary intake, intestinal malabsorption of precursors, disease-related or drug-induced alterations in vitamin D metabolism, reduced cutaneous production (age-dependent ↓ in synthesis by skin, plus inadequate exposure)
  - Affects bone primarily: May even result in osteomalacia
  - Associated with decline in physical performance and loss of muscle strength with ↓ muscle mass; may result in ↑ number and severity of falls
  - Thigh muscle atrophy with fatty substitution correlates strongly with ↓ in 25-OHD serum levels

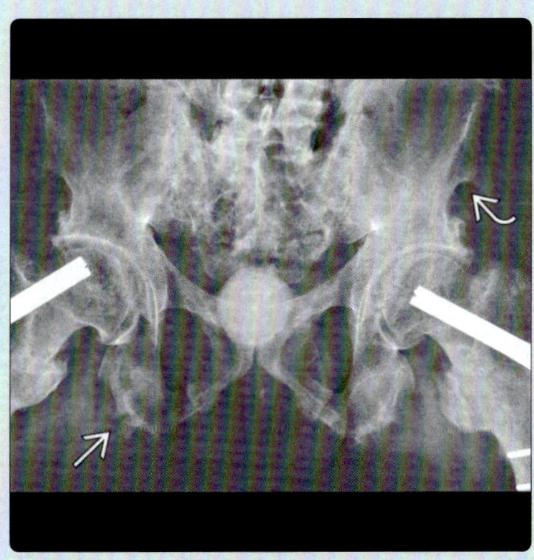

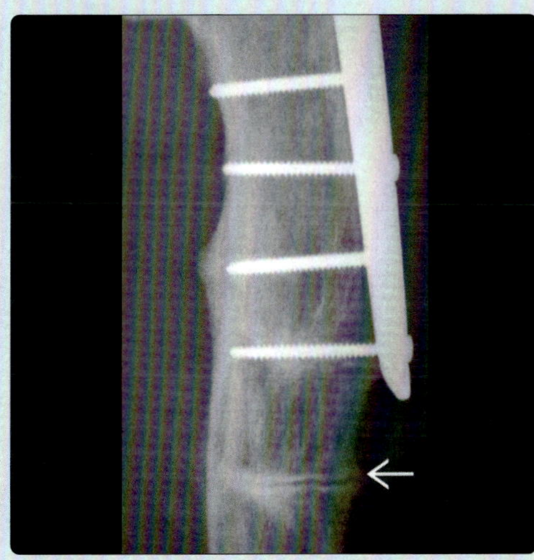

(Left) *AP radiograph of a patient who has vitamin D-resistant rickets due to a renal tubular disorder is shown. He must take massive doses of vitamin D. This results in prominent enthesopathy, seen at the ischial tuberosity ➡ and ASIS ⮫.* **(Right)** *AP radiograph in the same patient shows a transverse fracture that is chronic, with sclerosis at the edges and lucency remaining ➡. This represents a Looser zone, a region of osteoid that is not mineralized at a fracture site and the typical radiographic sign of osteomalacia in adults.*

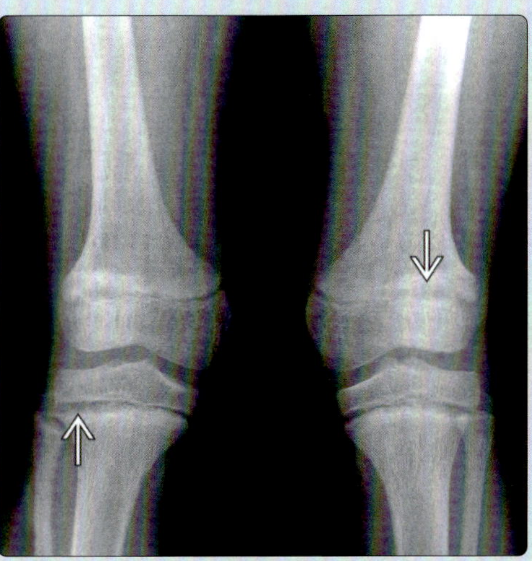

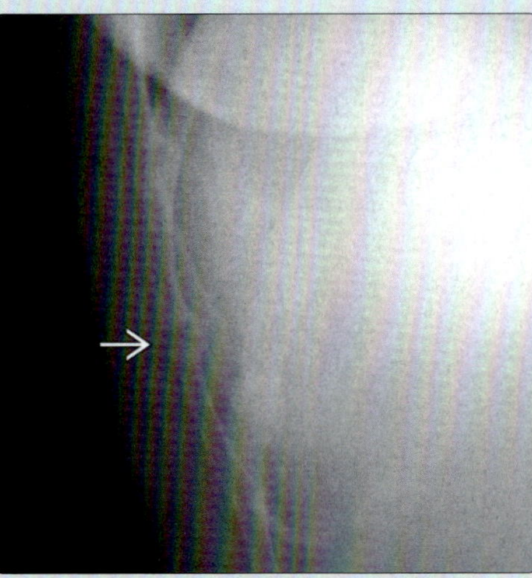

(Left) *AP radiograph of the knees in a child who has developed nutritional rickets, an extremely uncommon disease in the USA. However, the appearance is classic, with a widened zone of provisional calcification at all the physes of the knee ➡.* **(Right)** *AP radiograph shows typical Looser zones of osteomalacia. This produces wide lucencies at the fracture sites ➡ and is the radiographic manifestation of osteomalacia. The scapula, pubic rami, as well as long weight-bearing bones are also typical locations.*

KEY FACTS

TERMINOLOGY

- Chronic fluorine intoxication resulting in skeletal abnormalities
  - 99% of fluoride retained in body is deposited in bone
  - Half life: 8 years; slow improvement after cessation

IMAGING

- Combination of triad of findings is diagnostic: Osteosclerosis, osteophytosis, ligamentous Ca++
  - Usually evident on pelvis and spine imaging
- Osteosclerosis
  - Dense, with condensation along trabeculae obscures osseous architecture
  - Osseous fragility remains, despite sclerosis
  - Many years after cessation of intake, sclerosis improves but coarsened trabecular pattern remains
  - Location of osteosclerosis
    - Spine, pelvis, thorax
    - Spares skull & tubular bones
- Vertebral osteophytosis and enthesopathy
  - Excrescences at iliac crests, ischial tuberosities & other sites of tendinous & ligamentous attachment
- Ligamentous calcification of axial skeleton
  - Sacrotuberous, sacrospinous, iliolumbar, paraspinal, intraspinal, posterior longitudinal
- Other extraaxial findings: Periostitis
- Dental root irregularities and resorption

TOP DIFFERENTIAL DIAGNOSES

- Osteosclerosis
  - Myelofibrosis
  - Mastocytosis
- Ligamentous proliferative changes
  - DISH
  - Spondyloarthropathies
- Periostitis
  - Hypertrophic osteoarthropathy, 1° or 2°

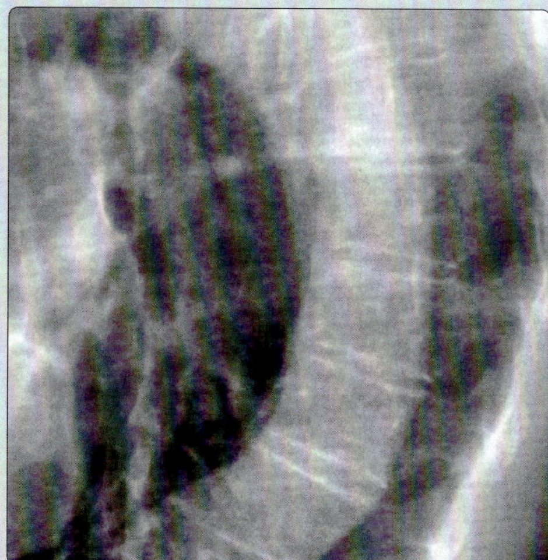

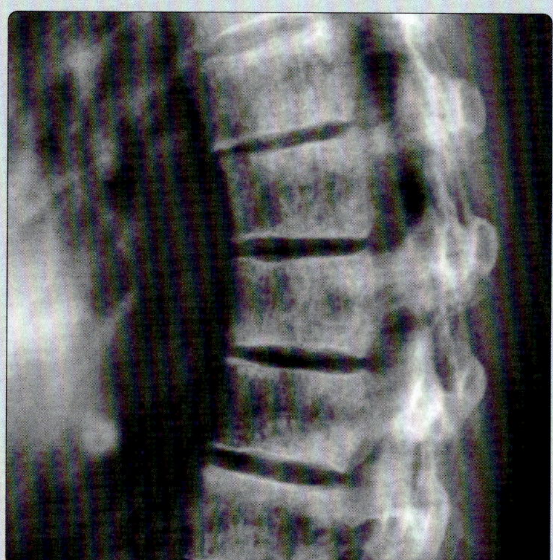

(Left) *Lateral radiograph, coned to the thoracic spine, shows ectatic aorta overlying severe osteoporosis; the severe degree of bone mineral loss was consistent with the age and gender. The patient started a regimen to treat the osteoporosis, including regular doses of fluoride.* **(Right)** *Lateral radiograph, same patient, coned to the same region and obtained 2 years following institution of fluoride treatment shows osteosclerosis, with thickening and indistinctness of the trabeculae. The findings are typical of fluorosis.*

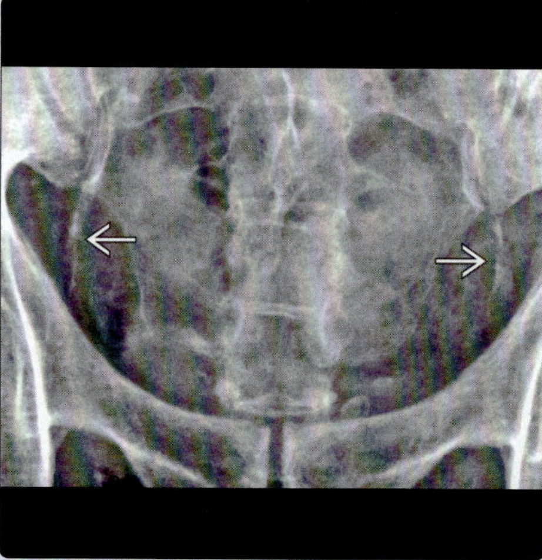

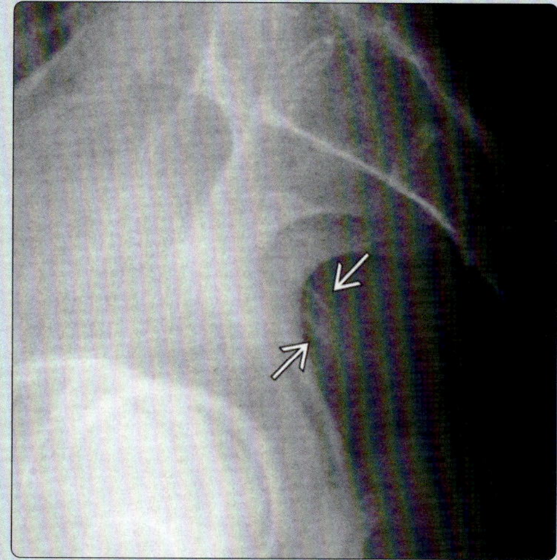

(Left) *AP radiograph shows 1 hallmark of fluorosis: Calcification of the sacrospinous and sacrotuberous ligaments. This image shows the calcified sacrospinous ligaments ➡ extending toward the ischial spines. Note that the character as well as the location of the calcification is slightly different than more frequently seen pelvic arterial calcification.* **(Right)** *Lateral radiograph, same case, shows linear calcifications extending posteriorly toward the ischial spines ➡, confirming this as sacrospinous ligament Ca++.*

KEY FACTS

TERMINOLOGY

- Hyperostosis related to chronic use of retinoids
  - Retinoids: Synthetic derivatives of vitamin A

IMAGING

- Axial hyperostosis
  - Entire axial skeleton, most notably cervical spine
  - Early appearance: Osteophytes extending from vertebral body adjacent to disc, giving appearance of spondylosis
  - Continued bone formation results in bridging across disc space
  - Long term may appear undulating and flowing, bulky enough to mimic anterior longitudinal ligament ossification of diffuse idiopathic skeletal hyperostosis (DISH)
- Ossification of atlantoaxial, stylohyoid, atlantooccipital, and coracoclavicular ligaments
- Enthesopathy, especially around pelvis and hip

TOP DIFFERENTIAL DIAGNOSES

- Spondylosis deformans
  - Osteophytes extending from anterior vertebral bodies indistinguishable from those of osteoarthritis
- DISH: Long-term retinoid use results in such prominent ossification that it mimics this
- Normal discs and facet joints as well as young patient age helps to avoid misdiagnosis

CLINICAL ISSUES

- Retinoids used in standard medical practice to treat
  - Acne, psoriasis, and other rare skin diseases
  - Rarely, certain skin and squamous cancers
- Etiology uncertain
  - Appears to accelerate bone maturation and formation
- Changes appear to be irreversible

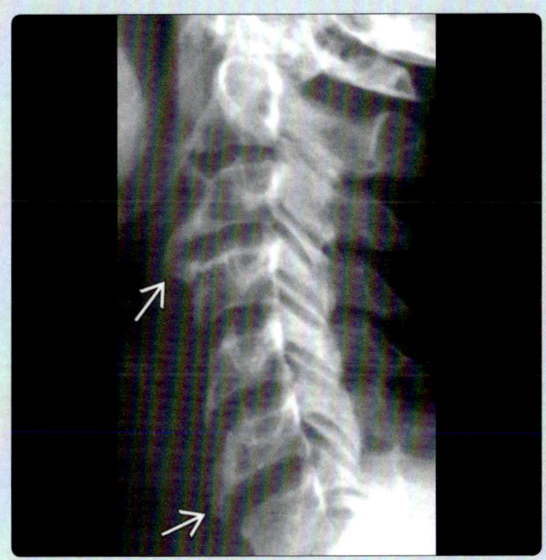

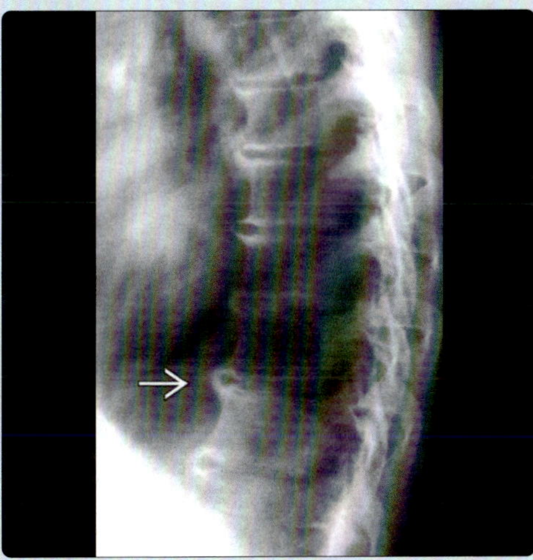

(Left) *Lateral radiograph of the cervical spine shows diffuse prominent spondylosis ➡ so prominent that it nears the appearance of the anterior flowing osteophytes seen with diffuse idiopathic skeletal hyperostosis (DISH). This patient was a young man, not at risk for DISH. He had been using retinoids for a skin condition.* **(Right)** *Lateral radiograph of the thoracic spine in the same patient shows similar findings ➡ involving the entire thoracic spine. Use of retinoids puts patients at risk for this bone formation.*

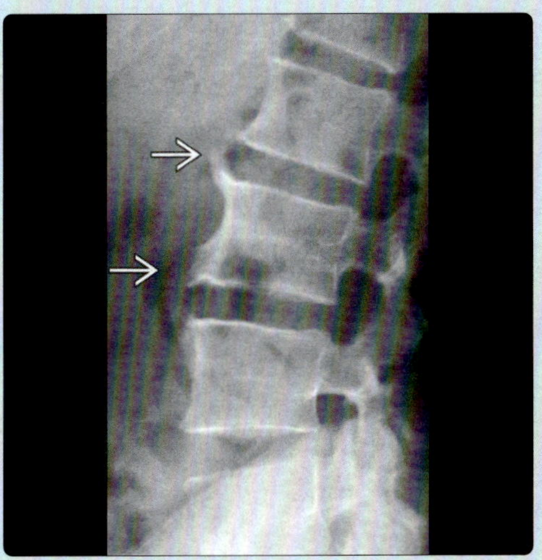

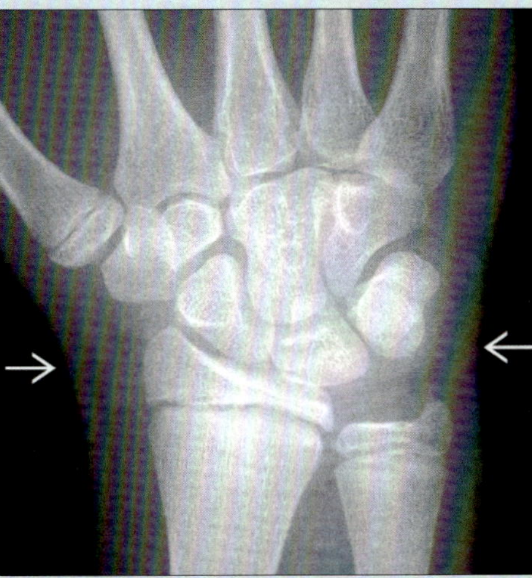

(Left) *Lateral radiograph of the lumbar spine in the same patient emphasizes the bone production ➡.* **(Right)** *PA radiograph of the hand in the same patient taken several years earlier shows diffuse irregularity of the soft tissues ➡. This patient has ichthyosis, which has been aggressively treated with retinoids. The drug treatment carries the risk of bone formation, particularly in the axial skeleton, and relative risk is related to length of time of treatment.*

Lead Poisoning

KEY FACTS

IMAGING

- Dense lead lines in metaphysis of child
- Lead chips within bowel
- Intraarticular shrapnel
  - Degree of intraarticular fragmentation correlates with symptoms of lead intoxication (increased surface area of exposure)
- Neuroimaging: Cerebral edema, microhemorrhages

TOP DIFFERENTIAL DIAGNOSES

- Normal variant metaphyses
  - Normal growing skeleton may have dense horizontal metaphyseal lines
  - Normal fibula in normal variant; differentiates from lead lines
- Growth arrest lines
  - Variable distance from metaphysis depending on age of insult
  - Sharply defined, thin dense lines

PATHOLOGY

- Source of lead intake
  - Oral ingestion: Lead paint chips, toys, food or liquid stored in lead containers or pipes
  - Gunshot wounds; Retained lead shrapnel within joints
  - Inhalation; workplace exposure
  - Environmental maternal exposure transfers through placenta and nursing
- Adults may absorb 20% of ingested lead; children and pregnant women may absorb as much as 70%
  - Once in body, rapidly excreted by kidneys/liver
  - That portion not excreted accumulates in bones (not considered harmful) and soft tissues (particularly liver, kidney, lungs, brain)
- Mechanism of activity
  - Promotes axonal degeneration in spinal cord
  - Lead replaces calcium in bone; highest concentration in growing bone (metaphyses around knee, distal radius)

(Left) *AP radiograph shows dense metaphyseal lines ➡ from lead poisoning. This is especially well seen in the knee, the fastest site of bony growth, with corresponding deposition of radiodense lead. While children may have physiologic dense metaphyseal lines, these generally are not seen in the fibula, serving to distinguish normal from abnormal.* **(Right)** *AP radiograph, same case, shows metallic flakes throughout the bowel ➡. These proved to be paint chips, the most common source of lead in children.*

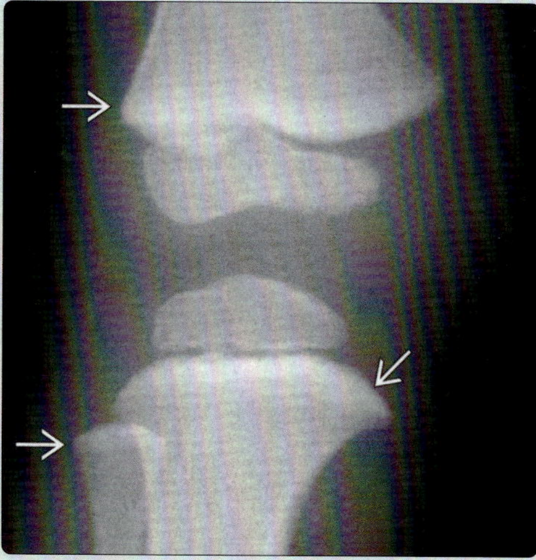

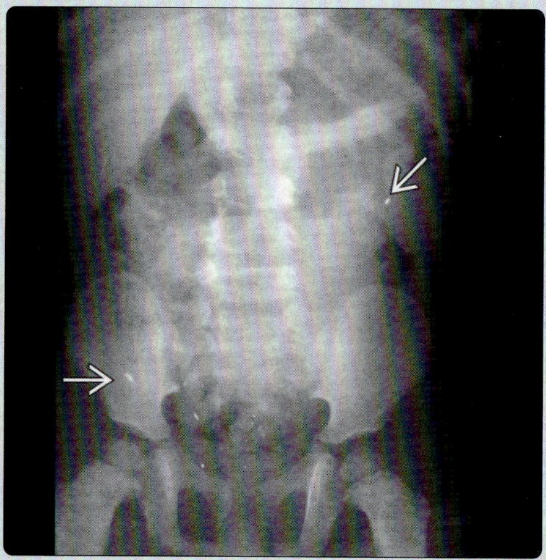

(Left) *AP radiograph shows intraarticular shrapnel ➡. Generally, if the shrapnel is remote from important structures, the metal is inert & is not removed. However, if shrapnel is in an intraarticular position, it causes a reactive synovitis, resulting in systemic resorption of lead. High enough levels of lead can result in systemic symptoms.* **(Right)** *AP radiograph shows multiple bullet fragments ➡. This intraarticular lead creates a synovial inflammatory process, resulting in osteoarthritis. Cystic lesions ➡ are reactive.*

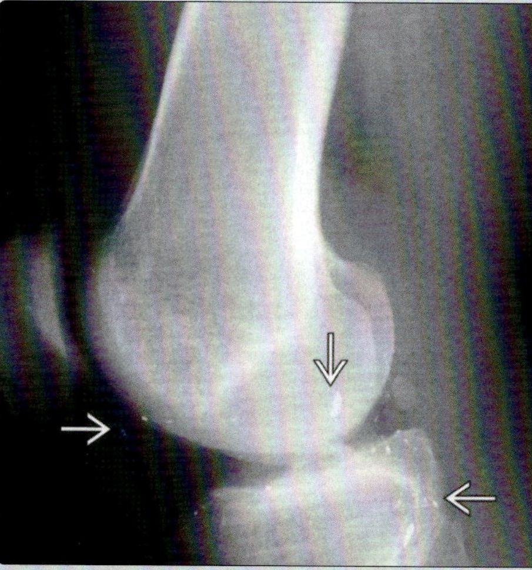

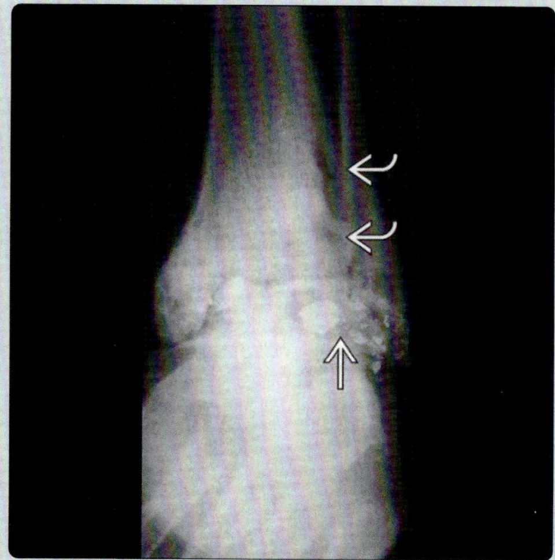

KEY FACTS

TERMINOLOGY

- Warfarin embryopathy: Fetal abnormalities resulting from maternal use of warfarin during pregnancy

IMAGING

- Skeletal location: Epiphyses and apophyses
- Radiographic abnormalities
  - Stippled epiphyses and apophyses
  - Nasal hypoplasia
  - Early ossification of hyoid

TOP DIFFERENTIAL DIAGNOSES

- Chondrodysplasia punctata
  - Nonrhizomelic type: Conradi-Hünermann (nonlethal and autosomal dominant)
  - Rhizomelic type: Lethal autosomal recessive; multiple other abnormalities
- Hypothyroidism and cretinism
  - Infantile stippled epiphyses (nonspecific)
  - Child: Severe delay in skeletal maturation and fragmentation of femoral capital epiphysis

PATHOLOGY

- Low molecular weight drug that readily crosses the placenta → clinically significant levels in fetus
- Greatest vulnerability for midfacial and epiphyseal abnormalities: 6-12 weeks gestation
- Neurological effects seem related to 2nd or 3rd trimester exposure
  - At least partially related to hemorrhagic episodes
  - Hemorrhage, hydrocephalus

CLINICAL ISSUES

- Incidence of 5.7-7.4% of exposed pregnancies
- Stippled epiphyses usually disappear within 1st few months of life
- ± residual epiphyseal and vertebral deformities
- Respiratory, dental, nasal, and speech complications

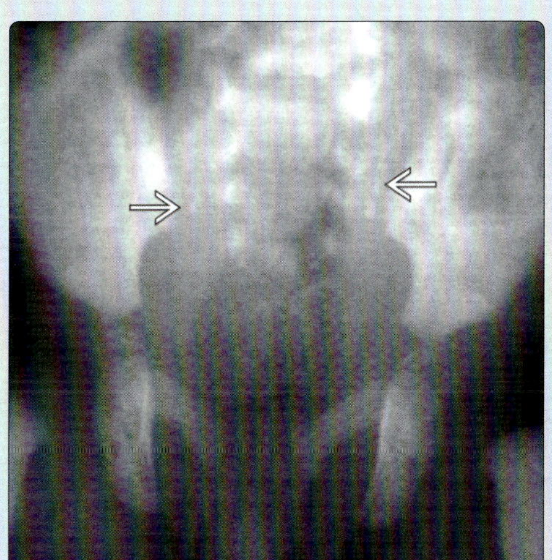

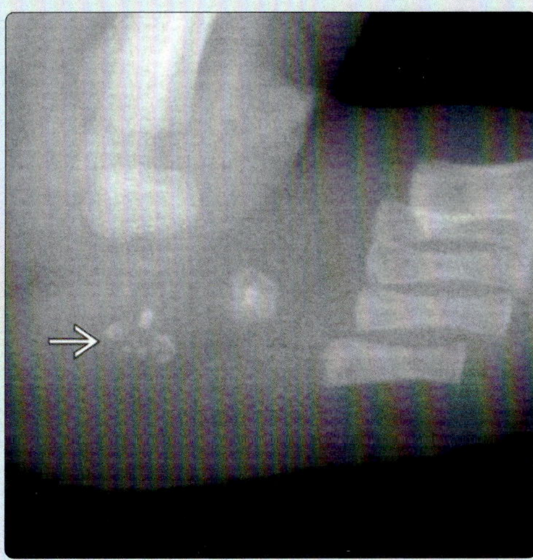

(Left) *Anteroposterior radiograph shows subtle findings in the pelvis. Small stippled epiphyses are seen along the sacral ala ➡. This infant's mother had been treated with warfarin (Coumadin) for deep venous thrombosis during her pregnancy. Osseous manifestations are stippled epiphyses.* **(Right)** *Lateral radiograph of the foot shows stippled epiphysis of the calcaneus ➡. The foot otherwise appears normal.*

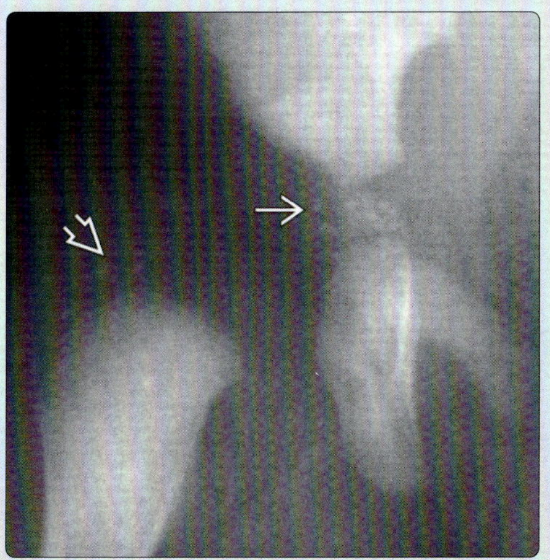

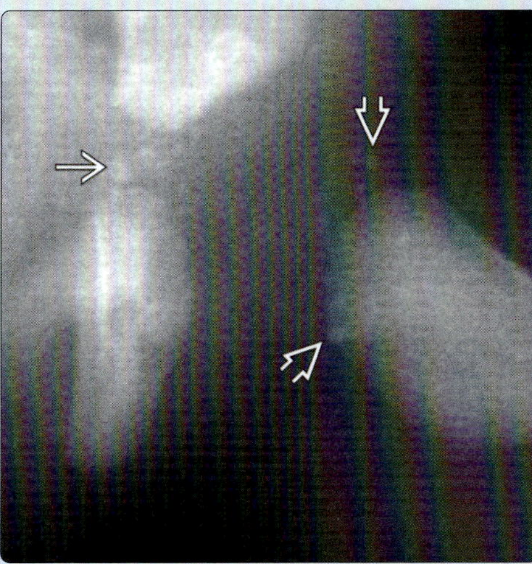

(Left) *AP radiograph shows stippled epiphyses in both the triradiate cartilage of the acetabulum ➡ and the greater trochanter ➡.* **(Right)** *AP radiograph, contralateral hip, also shows triradiate cartilage ➡ and greater trochanteric stippled epiphyses ➡. Stippled epiphyses are seen in several disease processes, one of which is warfarin (Coumadin) embryopathy. Other considerations in the differential include hypothyroidism and chondrodysplasia punctata (Conradi-Hünermann disease).*

KEY FACTS

TERMINOLOGY

- Periostitis related to therapeutic ingestion of Voriconazole
  - Used as treatment or prophylaxis for aspergillosis
    - Aspergillus infection following lung transplantation ranges from 6-17%
  - Commonly used in immunosuppressed patients following organ transplant
    - Lung, cardiac, liver transplants

IMAGING

- Dense periostitis
  - May be linear, but often heaped up, irregular & focal
  - Though diffuse, often asymmetric
- Capsular & entheseal ossification described as well
- Location: Multiple sites, including ribs, shoulder & hip girdles, digits
  - Often no associated digital clubbing
- Absent in pretransplant images

TOP DIFFERENTIAL DIAGNOSES

- Secondary hypertrophic osteoarthritis
  - Similar-appearing dense periostitis; usually linear but may be focal
  - Involves predominantly tibia & fibula, radius & ulna
  - Diaphyseal, symmetric distribution
  - Associated with pulmonary malignancies, congenital cyanotic heart disease
- Periostitis deformans
  - Subacute fluoride poisoning

CLINICAL ISSUES

- May present with diffuse bone pain
- Palpable lump
- Symptoms develop 6 months-3 years following chronic treatment with Voriconazole
- Treatment: Symptoms resolve when Voriconazole treatment stopped

(Left) *AP radiograph in a 68-year-old man who obtained a liver transplant 14 months earlier shows dense solid-appearing periostitis along the upper ribs ➡. This is the typical appearance of voriconazole-related periostitis, given the clinical history of recent transplant.* **(Right)** *AP radiograph was obtained in a 64-year-old woman who complained of a lump on her finger. The lump corresponds to the dense periostitis ➡ seen on the radiograph. Clinical history of recent lung transplant leads to the correct diagnosis.*

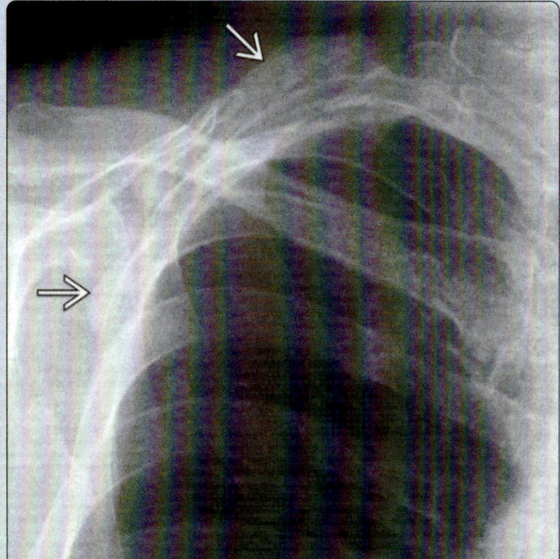

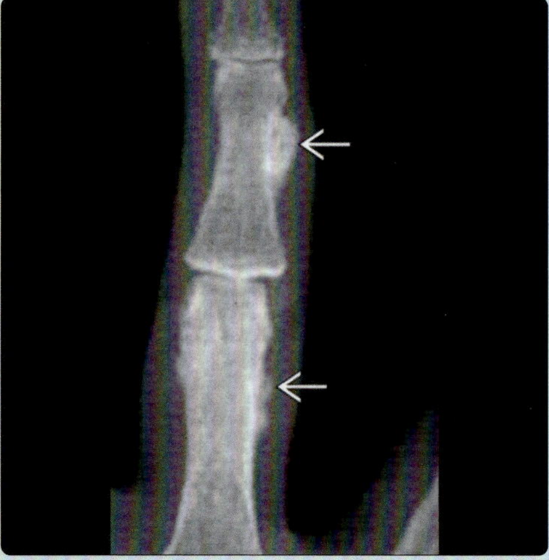

(Left) *Axial CT shows fibrotic left lung with reduced volume and right lung transplant. The ribs show subtle periosteal reaction ➡ in this patient who takes voriconazole prophylactically against an aspergillus infection.* **(Right)** *AP radiograph in a patient following cardiac transplant shows a small focus of periostitis ➡ along the lateral femoral neck. The contralateral hip showed a similar but less dense deposit. Clinical history of organ transplant leads to the correct diagnosis.*

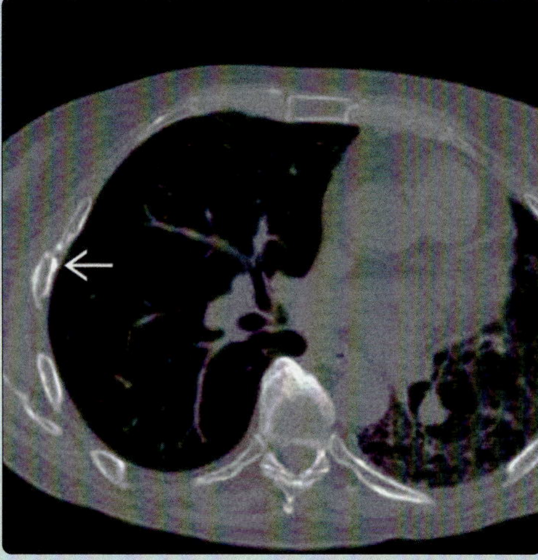

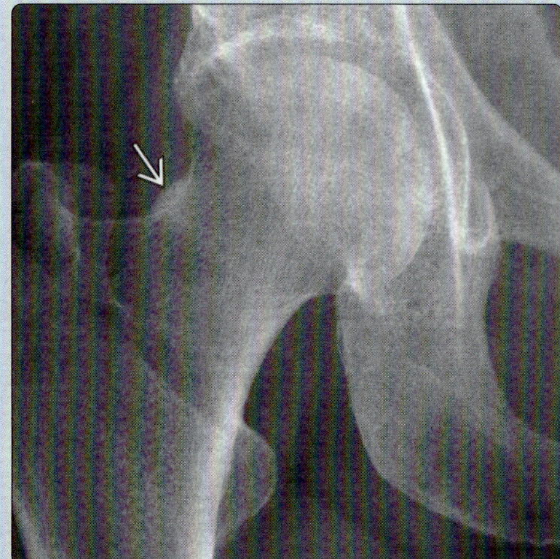

KEY FACTS

IMAGING

- Subtrochanteric femoral structural abnormalities
  - Focal lateral cortical hypertrophy precedes fracture
  - Fractures: Transverse orientation, cortical beak; occur with low velocity trauma
  - May have poor or delayed bone healing
- Long bone osteonecrosis (ON): Rare, tibia and femur
- ON of jaw: Focal or diffuse bone loss

PATHOLOGY

- Femoral lesions
  - Occur at sites of stress; 2° to inhibited bone turnover due to osteoclast inactivity
- ON of jaw: Histologic bone necrosis and infection

CLINICAL ISSUES

- Bisphosphonates used for treatment of osteoporosis, Paget disease, metastatic disease, multiple myeloma to reduce bone turnover
  - Mechanism of action: Inhibit osteoclast activity
- Assess risk/benefit ratio: Whether morbidity/mortality associated with osteoporotic fractures outweighs risk of bisphosphonate-induced fracture
- ON of jaw: Bisphosphonate association unclear
  - Doubtful in doses used to treat osteoporosis
  - Possible association in cancer patients who receive high-dose therapy: Related to duration of treatment, presence of periodontal disease
  - Clinical diagnosis: Exposed bone of mandible or maxilla that does not heal within 8 weeks after identification by healthcare worker
- Bisphosphonate-related femur fractures
  - Pain may precede onset of fractures by months
  - Condition often bilateral (63%), screen opposite femur even if asymptomatic
    - Prophylactic rodding may be considered
  - Risk may be as great as 1/1,000
  - Usually bisphosphonate treatment > 4 years in duration

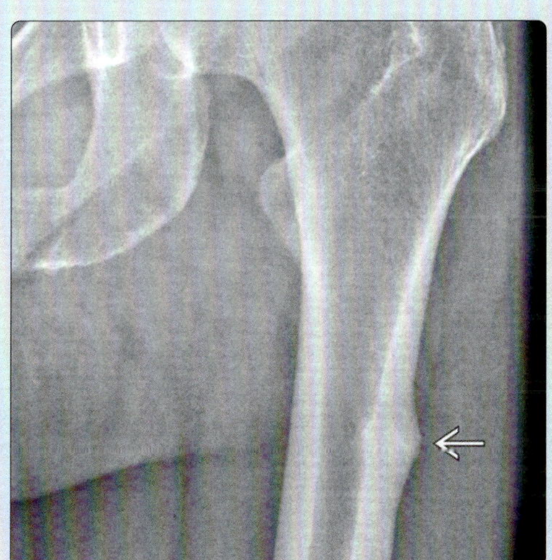

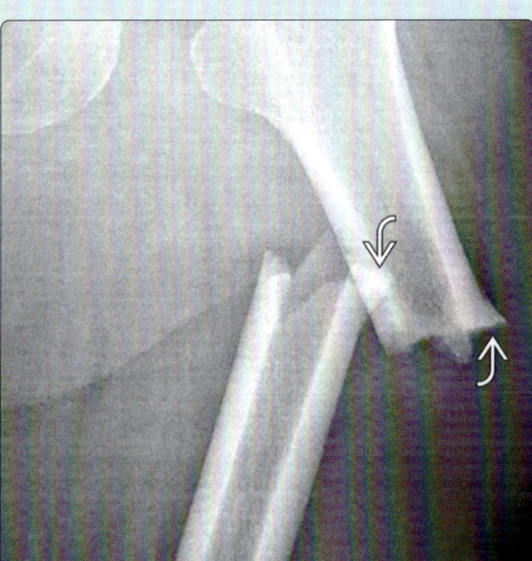

(Left) *AP x-ray shows focal cortical thickening of the lateral femoral cortex ➡. This thickening results from inability to adequately respond to normal stress due to impaired osteoclast activity, 2° to use of bisphosphonates.* **(Right)** *AP x-ray, same patient, shows a fracture that occurred with no significant trauma. Femoral fractures typically require significant energy; fracture without such history should raise concerns for an underlying process. In this case, cortical beak ➡ at the fracture is a clue to the underlying condition.*

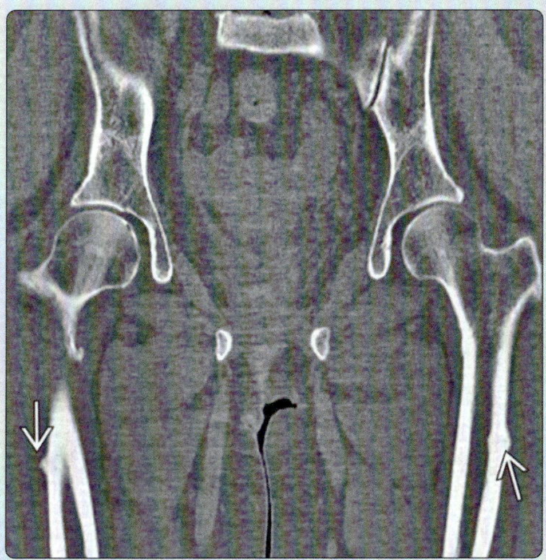

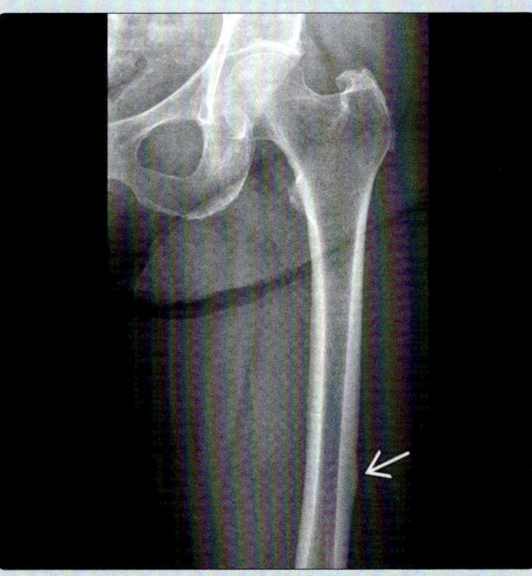

(Left) *Coronal CT shows a patient with faint bone scan uptake in the subtrochanteric femora who was experiencing aching left thigh pain. CT shows focal lateral cortical thickening ➡; faint fracture lines are already evident. Due to high bilaterality of this condition, the opposite femur should be screened even if asymptomatic.* **(Right)** *For a painful thigh in an elderly woman, an AP x-ray shows subtle cortical abnormality ➡ initially thought to be osteoid osteoma (unusual lesion in older patient). Clinical history showed bisphosphonate use.*

Fluoroquinolone Tendinopathy

KEY FACTS

TERMINOLOGY

- Fluoroquinolone: Antibiotic commonly used for treatment of bacterial infections
  - Most commonly used: Ciprofloxacin, levofloxacin, and moxifloxacin
  - Broad-spectrum coverage against common pathogens
  - Good tissue penetration
  - High bioavailability

IMAGING

- Tendinopathy nonspecific in appearance compared with sports-related tendinopathy
  - In Achilles, abnormality generally occurs at musculotendinous junction
    - Tendon thickens, with axial morphology changing from anterior concavity to rounded appearance
  - T1: ↑ signal intensity in normally low signal tendon
  - Fluid-sensitive sequences: ↑ signal intensity
    - If complete rupture, ↑ signal fluid within tendon gap

CLINICAL ISSUES

- Associated risk of tendinopathy
  - Full tendon rupture less frequent than tendinopathy
  - Risk appears greater in
    - Elderly patients
    - Nonobese patients
    - Concurrent use of glucocorticoids
    - Concurrent chronic renal disease
  - Contraindicated in children except for life-threatening circumstances
    - Animal studies show destruction of immature joint cartilage
    - Arthralgia, arthritis, tendinitis, gait abnormality reported in 1 nonblinded comparison study in children
  - Achilles most commonly involved tendon
    - Shoulder and hip tendons and plantar fasciitis also reported

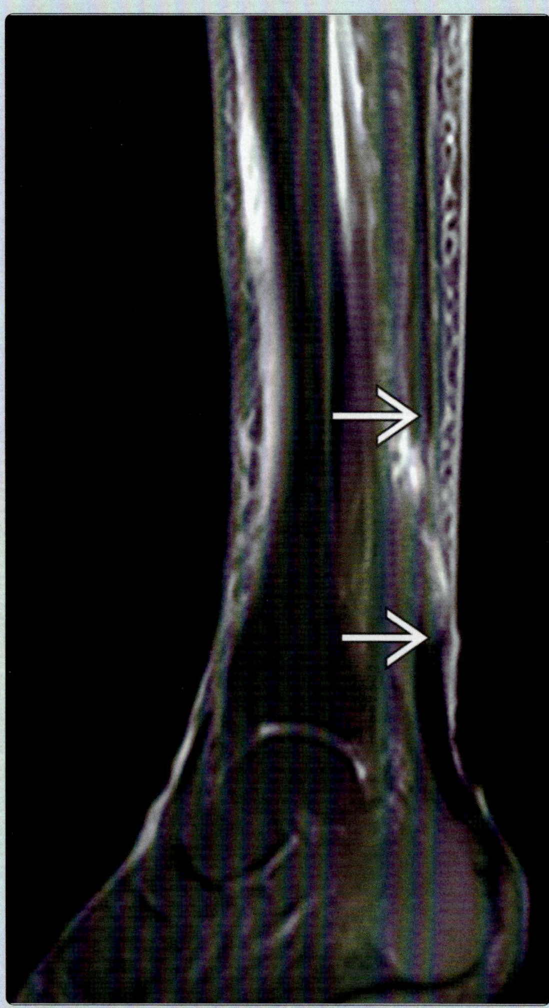

Sagittal T2FS MR of the ankle in a 72-year-old woman known to be taking antibiotics, but otherwise healthy, shows a complete tear of the Achilles tendon ➡, with significant gap between the tendon fragments.

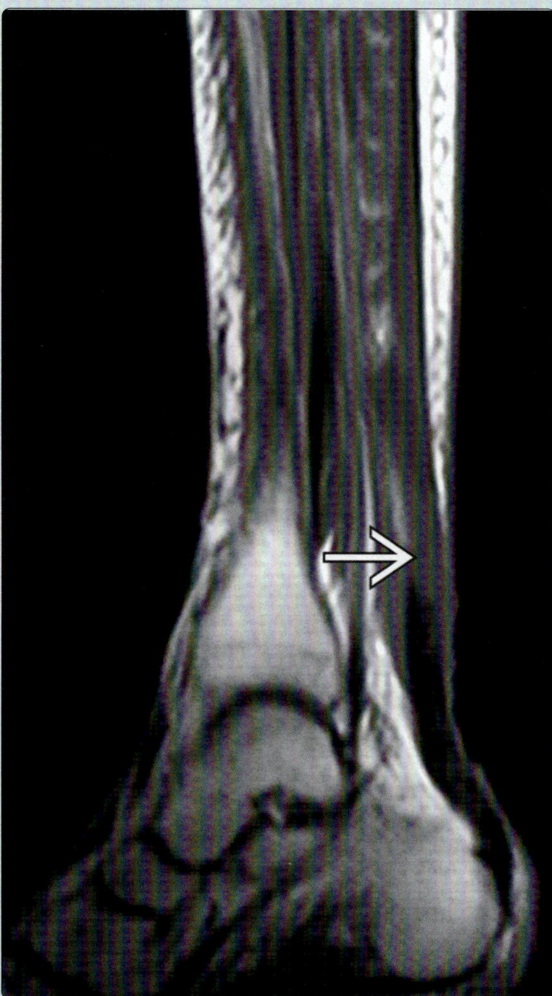

Sagittal T1 MR, same patient, shows the disrupted tendon ➡. There is nothing specific in the appearance to suggest Fluoroquinolone-related tendinopathy; however the patient age and gender would be unusual for a sports-related Achilles tear, and she was ingesting Levaquin.

KEY FACTS

TERMINOLOGY

- Disease resulting from insufficient vitamin C, manifesting as defective collagen

IMAGING

- Dense epiphyseal ring with central lucency: Wimberger sign
- Dense metaphyseal line with adjacent lucent scurvy line
- Metaphyseal excrescences ± corner fracture
- Slipped epiphysis (uncommon)
- Later metaphyseal cupping, growth disturbance (uncommon)
- Elevation of periosteum, subperiosteal hemorrhage
    - Results in extremely wide periosteal reaction ("shell")
- Diffuse osteopenia
- Hemarthrosis
- Teeth: Cyst formation, interruption of lamina dura

TOP DIFFERENTIAL DIAGNOSES

- Leukemia
    - Diffuse osteoporosis, metaphyseal lines
- Neuroblastoma metastases
    - Lytic destruction of metaphyses

PATHOLOGY

- Vitamin C has positive effect on trabecular bone formation by influencing expression of bone matrix genes in osteoblasts

CLINICAL ISSUES

- Mental status alteration
- Gum disease and tooth loss
- Heart and skeletal muscle damage
- Gastrointestinal blood loss
- Other concomitant vitamin deficiencies and alcoholism may be seen in adults
- Usually children 6-18 months old; however, may occur at any age
- Male = female

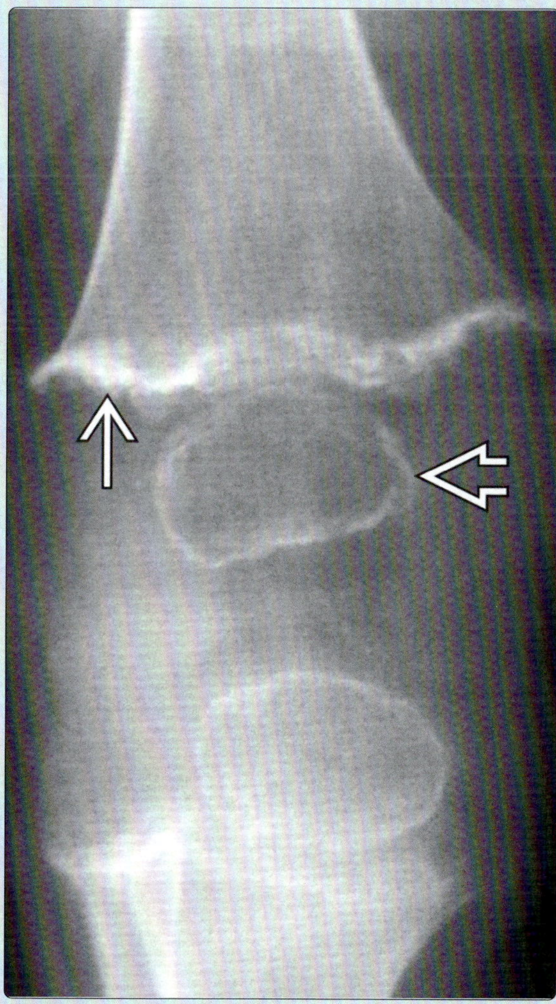

AP radiograph shows classic signs of scurvy. The bones are diffusely osteopenic. There are dense lines at the metaphyses ➡ and epiphyses ⇨; the underlying osteopenia makes the dense lines even more prominent.

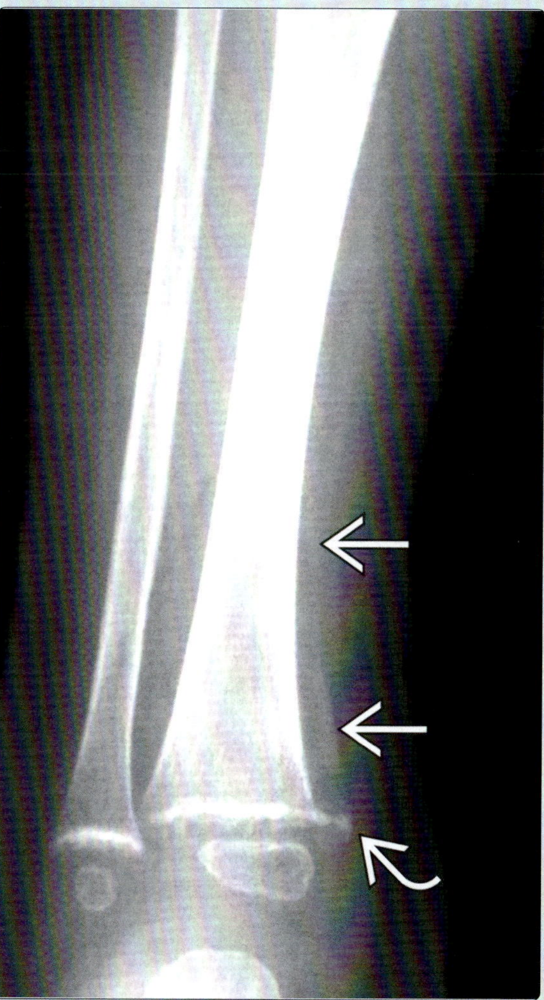

AP radiograph shows a metaphyseal excrescence that has developed a corner fracture ↪. With these fractures, the patients may develop an extensive subperiosteal bleed, raising the periosteum ➡, which can result in a wide periosteal shell.

INDEX

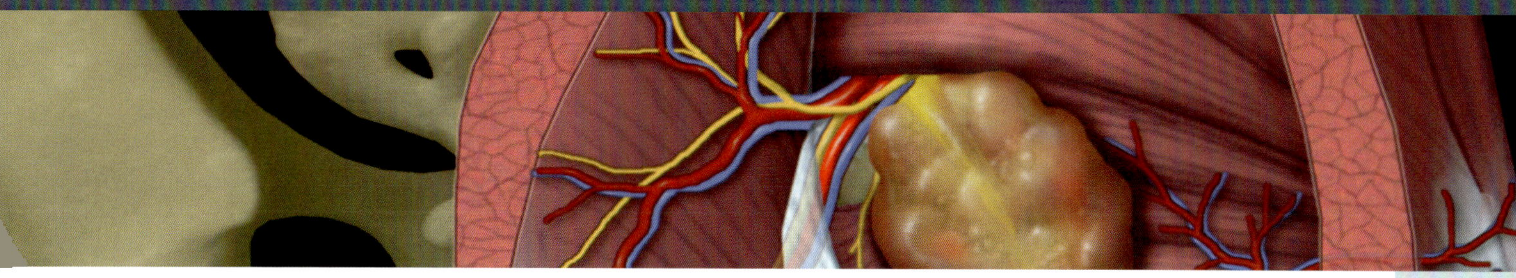

A

INDEX

INDEX

INDEX

B

INDEX

INDEX

INDEX

INDEX

INDEX

D

INDEX

INDEX

INDEX

INDEX

INDEX

G

H

INDEX

I

INDEX

INDEX

J

INDEX

K

L

INDEX

INDEX

M

INDEX

INDEX

INDEX

N

INDEX

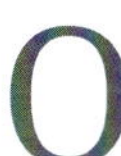

INDEX

P

INDEX

INDEX

R

INDEX

S

INDEX

INDEX

INDEX

T

INDEX

U

V

INDEX

W

X

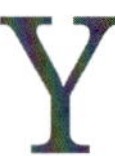

Z